AF675593

Hazel Henderson
John Kilner Diabetic Unit
Epsom General Hospital
Epsom, Surrey
KT18 7EG

International Textbook of Diabetes Mellitus

THIRD EDITION

Editorial Board

International Textbook of Diabetes Mellitus

THIRD EDITION

Editors-in-Chief

Ralph A. DeFronzo

The University of Texas Health Science Centre, San Antonio, TX, USA

Ele Ferrannini

Department of Internal Medicine, University of Pisa School of Medicine, Pisa, Italy

Harry Keen

Department of Diabetes Endocrinology and Metabolism, Guy's Hospital, London, UK

Paul Zimmet

International Diabetes Institute, Melbourne, Australia

VOLUME ONE

John Wiley & Sons, Ltd

Telephone (+44) 1243 779777

Email (for orders and customer service enquiries): cs-books@wiley.co.uk
Visit our Home Page on www.wileyeurope.com or www.wiley.com

Other Wiley Editorial Offices

John Wiley & Sons Inc., 111 River Street,
Hoboken, NJ 07030, USA

Jossey-Bass, 989 Market Street,
San Francisco, CA 94103-1741, USA

Wiley-VCH Verlag GmbH, Boschstr. 12,
D-69469 Weinheim, Germany

John Wiley & Sons Australia Ltd, 33 Park Road,
Milton, Queensland 4064, Australia

John Wiley & Sons (Asia) Pte Ltd, 2 Clementi Loop #02-01,
Jin Xing Distripark, Singapore 129809

John Wiley & Sons Canada Ltd, 22 Worcester Road,
Etobicoke, Ontario, Canada M9W 1L1

Wiley also publishes its books in a variety of electronic formats. Some content that appears in print may not be available in electronic books.

Library of Congress Cataloging- in-Publication Data

International textbook of diabetes mellitus / editors, Ralph A. DeFronzo
. . . [et al.]. – 3rd ed.
p. ; cm.
Includes bibliographical references and index.
ISBN 0-471-48655-8 (cloth : alk. paper)
1. Diabetes
[DNLM: 1. Diabetes Mellitus. WK 810 I60359 2004] I. DeFronzo, Ralph
A. II. Series.
RC660.I585 2004
616.4'62–dc21 2003009069

British Library Cataloguing in Publication Data

A catalogue record for this book is available from the British Library

ISBN 0-471-48655-8

Typeset in 10/12 pt Times by Techbooks, Delhi, India.
Printed and bound by Rotolito Lombarda, Milan, Italy.
This book is printed on acid-free paper responsibly manufactured from sustainable forestry in which at least two trees are planted for each one used for paper production.

About the Editors-in-Chief

Professor Ralph A. DeFronzo, MD, is a Professor of Medicine and Chief of the Diabetes Division at the University of Texas Health Science Center and the Audie L. Murphy Memorial VA Hospital in San Antonio, Texas. He also functions as the Deputy Director of the Texas Diabetes Institute. Dr DeFronzo is a graduate of Harvard Medical School and did his training in internal medicine at the Johns Hopkins Hospital. Later, he completed fellowships in endocrinology at the National Institutes of Health (NIH) and Baltimore City Hospitals and in nephrology at the Hospital of the University of Pennsylvania.

His major interests focus on the pathogenesis and treatment of type 2 diabetes mellitus, the central role of insulin resistance in the metabolic-cardiovascular cluster of disorders known collectively as the *insulin resistance syndrome*, and the etiology and treatment of diabetic nephropathy. Using the euglycemic insulin clamp technique in combination with radioisotope turnover methodology, limb catheterization, indirect calorimetry, and muscle biopsy, he has helped to define the biochemical and cellular disturbances responsible for insulin resistance in type 2 diabetes mellitus.

For his work in this area, Dr DeFronzo has received the prestigious Lilly Award from the American Diabetes Association (ADA), the Banting Lectureship from the Canadian Diabetes Association as well as many other national and international awards. He is also the recipient of the ADA's Albert Renold Award for lifetime commitment to the training of young diabetes investigators. Previously, he served on the ADA Board of Directors and as Chairman of the ADA's Medical and Scientific Oversight Committee, Research Policy Committee, Research Review Committee, and Professional Education Committee.

He is the past-editor of *Diabetes Reviews*, a co-editor of the ADA's *Physicians' Guide to Type 1 Diabetes* and the ADA's *Physicians' Guide to Type 2 Diabetes,* a co-editor of the *International Textbook of Diabetes*, and a past member of the editorial board of *Diabetologia*. With more than 400 articles published in peer-reviewed medical journals, Dr DeFronzo is a distinguished clinician, teacher, and investigator who has been an invited speaker at major national and international conferences on diabetes mellitus.

Professor Ele Ferrannini is the Professor of Internal Medicine, University of Pisa School of Medicine; Chief of the Metabolism Unit of the CNR (National Research Council) Institute of Clinical Physiology, Pisa; and Clinical Professor of Medicine, Diabetes Division, University of Texas Health Science Center at San Antonio.

From 1977 to 1978, Professor Ferrannini was a Visiting Investigator at the Karolinska Institute in Stockholm, Sweden. In 1979 he became a Post-doctoral Fellow of the Fogarty International Centre of the National Institutes of Health, Yale University School of Medicine, Connecticut, USA, in 1988 he was appointed Clinical Professor of Medicine, Diabetes Division at the University of Texas Health Science Center at San Antonio, and in 1994 he assumed his current position in Italy.

Professor Ferrannini has been involved in over 250 publications in the field of diabetes, metabolism, hypertension, obesity, and cardiovascular risk factors. He was formerly the Editor-in-Chief of *Diabetologia*, the official journal of the European Association for the Study of Diabetes (EASD) and is currently the Chairman of the European Group for the Study of Insulin Resistance.

Professor Harry Keen, CBE, MD, FRCP, qualified in 1948 at St Mary's Hospital Medical School, London, where he worked, after service in the Royal Army Medical Corps, with Sir George Pickering and Sir Stanley Peart in the Professorial Medical Unit. From 1953 to 1960 Professor Keen was Senior Clinical Assistant to Dr R.D. Lawrence and Dr W.G. Oakley in the Diabetic Department, King's College Hospital. After an International Post-doctoral Research Fellowship at NIH, Bethesda, MD, USA (1960–1961), he joined Lord Butterfield at Guy's Hospital, London, as Senior Lecturer, Reader, and from 1971, as Professor of Human Metabolism, heading the Academic Unit for Metabolic Medicine and as Consultant Physician till his retirement in 1990. He continues to work in the Department, School, and University as Professor and Consultant Physician Emeritus.

His main research and clinical interests have been in diabetes and its complications and have included basic laboratory studies, clinical research, and clinical epidemiology.

Professor Keen has published many papers, reviews, and book chapters and is editor and co-editor of various books and international peer-reviewed journals. He has received numerous honors including the Banting Memorial Lecturer of the British Diabetic Association (1984), Claude Bernard Lecturer of the European Association for the Study of Diabetes (EASD) (1987), Harold Rifkin

Distinguished Fellow of the American Diabetes Association (1979, 1987, and 1989), James Watt Lecturer of the Royal College of Physicians of Edinburgh (1988), and the Juhling Award for Diabetes Research (1995). Professor Keen was the first recipient of the United Nations/ UNESCO Hellmut Mehnert Award for the Prevention of Diabetes and its Complications (1998) and was presented with the Novartis Distinguished Service Award UK (1999). Professor Keen was awarded a CBE in 1998.

Professor Keen was appointed Director of the Diabetes and Metabolism Unit and Honorary Consultant Physician, Guy's Group of Hospitals in 1967 and was involved in research, clinical care, and undergraduate and postgraduate teaching. Following this, he was appointed Director of Medicine (1985–1990), Chairman of the British Diabetic Association (1990–1996) and has been Honorary President of the International Diabetes Federation (IDF) since 1991. Appointed Emeritus Professor of the University of London Faculty of Medicine in 1990, he continues clinical research and teaching activities at the Guy's Hospital Campus of the (now) King's College London School of Medicine, London.

Professor Paul Zimmet is currently Foundation Director of the International Diabetes Institute, a position he has held since 1985, and Professor of Diabetes at Monash University. He is also a Professor at Deakin University and is Adjunct Professor in the Graduate School of Public Health, the University of Pittsburgh. He also serves on the Australian Government's Strategic Taskforce on Diabetes. His current research interests include epidemiological, environmental, and molecular biological components in the causation of type 2 diabetes, and he has published over 500 scientific papers, chapters, and reviews in peer-reviewed journals and books.

Professor Zimmet is a member of the Editorial Board of a number of international peer-reviewed journals, and has received many awards, including the Kelly West Medal from the American Diabetes Associated, Eli Lilly Award from the IDF, and the AM Cohen Award Lecture from the EASD. In 1997, at the *16th IDF Congress* in Finland, he received the first Peter Bennett Diabetes Epidemiology Award for outstanding contributions to research on the epidemiology of diabetes. In 2002, he received the Harold Rifkin Award of the American Diabetes Association for contributions to diabetes internationally. In 1993, he was awarded the Order of Australia for distinguished services to medicine and education, particularly in the field of diabetes. In 2001, he was further honored with the Order of Australia (AO) for services to medical research of national and international significance, particularly in the field of diabetes, as a leader of investigations into social, nutritional, and lifestyle diseases, and to biotechnology development in Australia.

Contents

VOLUME ONE

Contributors

Carl-David Agardh	Malmö University Hospital, Malmö, Sweden
Elisabet Agardh	Malmö University Hospital, Malmö, Sweden
Intekhab Ahmed	Jefferson Medical College, Thomas Jefferson University, Philadelphia, PA, USA
Bo Ahrén	Lund University, Lund, Sweden
Lloyd M. Aiello	Joslin Diabetes Center, Boston, MA, USA, and Harvard Medical School, Boston, MA, USA
J. Akwe	University of Perugia, Perugia, Italy
Abdulaziz R. Al-Harthi	University of Michigan, Ann Arbor, MI, USA
K.G.M.M. Alberti	University of Newcastle upon Tyne, Newcastle upon Tyne, UK
Marie-Christine Alessi	University Hospital Timone, Marseille, France
Stephanie A. Amiel	King's College, London, UK
James H. Anderson, Jr.	Eli Lilly and Company, Indianapolis, IN, USA
Morsi Arab	University of Alexandria, Alexandria, Egypt
Pablo Arias	University of Buenos Aires Medical School, Buenos Aires, Argentina
Arne Astrup	The Royal Veterinary and Agricultural University, Frederiksberg, Denmark
Shigeaki Baba	International Institute for Diabetes Education and Study, Kobe, Japan
Laurie L. Baggio	Banting and Best Diabetes Centre, Toronto General Hospital, University of Toronto, Toronto, Canada
Clifford J. Bailey	Aston University, Birmingham, UK
Stephen C. Bain	University of Birmingham, Birmingham, UK and Birmingham Heartlands Hospital, Birmingham, UK
Mandeep Bajaj	University of Texas Health Science Center at San Antonio, San Antonio, TX, USA
George L. Bakris	Rush Presbyterian/St. Luke's Medical Centre, Chicago, IL, USA
Alberto Barcelo	Pan American Health Organization, Washington, DC, USA
Anthony H. Barnett	University of Birmingham, Birmingham, UK, and Birmingham Heartlands Hospital, Birmingham, UK

Eugene J. Barrett	University of Virginia Health System, Charlottesville, VA, USA
M. Massi Benedetti	University of Perugia, Perugia, Italy
Richard M. Bergenstal	International Diabetes Center, Park Nicollet Institute, Minneapolis, MN, USA
Richard N. Bergman	University of Southern California, Los Angeles, CA, USA
Rudy W. Bilous	James Cook University Hospital, Middlesbrough, UK
Per Björntorp (deceased)	University of Göteborg, Göteborg, Sweden
Henry R. Black	Rush Presbyterian/St. Luke's Medical Centre, Chicago, IL, USA
Geremia B. Bolli	University of Perugia, Perugia, Italy
Riccardo C. Bonadonna	University of Verona School of Medicine, Verona, Italy
Claude Bouchard	Louisiana State University, Baton Rouge, LA, USA
Michael Brownlee	Albert Einstein College of Medicine, Bronx, NY, USA
G. Calabrese	University of Perugia, Perugia, Italy
Jerry D. Cavallerano	Joslin Diabetes Center, Boston, MA, USA
A. Cesarini	"Pretura Circondariale" of Perugia, Italy
Juliana C.N. Chan	The Chinese University of Hong Kong, Shatin, Hong Kong, China
Sudesna Chatterjee	Leicester Royal Infirmary, University Hospitals of Leicester NHS Trust, Leicester, UK
Chee W. Chia	The Johns Hopkins University School of Medicine, Baltimore, MD, USA
Jean-Louis Chiasson	Research Centre, Centre Hospitalier de l'Université de Montréal, Montréal, Canada, and Université de Montréal, Montréal, Canada
Theodore P. Ciaraldi	University of California San Diego, San Diego, CA, USA
A. Clark	Oxford Centre for Diabetes, Endocrinology and Metabolism, Oxford, UK
Deborah J. Clegg	University of Cincinnati, Cincinnati, OH, USA
Clive S. Cockram	The Chinese University of Hong Kong, Shatin, Hong Kong, China
Peter G. Colman	The Walter and Eliza Hall Institute of Medical Research, Parkville, Australia
Alberto Coppelli	University of Pisa, Pisa, Italy
Catherine Cowie	National Institutes of Health, Bethesda, MD, USA
Philip E. Cryer	Washington University School of Medicine, St. Louis, MO, USA

Michael H. Cummings	Queen Alexandra Hospital, Portsmouth, UK
M.J. Davies	Leicester Royal Infirmary, University Hospitals of Leicester NHS Trust, Leicester, UK
J.L. Day	Ipswich Hospital, Ipswich, Suffolk, UK
Ralph A. DeFronzo	University of Texas Health Science Center, San Antonio, TX, USA
Thanh L. Dinh	Harvard Medical School, Boston, MA, USA
Gary Dowse	Department of Health, Perth, Australia
Daniel J. Drucker	Banting and Best Diabetes Centre, Toronto General Hospital, University of Toronto, Toronto, Canada
Jean-Luc Dulong	Technological University of Compiègne, Compiègne, France
Michael Edmonds	Kings College Hospital, London, UK
George S. Eisenbarth	Barbara Davis Center for Childhood Diabetes, University of Colorado Health Sciences Center, Denver, CO, USA
Karin Ekberg	Karolinska Institute, Stockholm, Sweden
Jean-Marie Ekoe	Centre de Reserche CHUM, Montreal, Canada
Alison L. Every	The Walter and Eliza Hall Institute of Medical Research, Parkville, Australia
Stephen R. Farmer	Boston University School of Medicine, Boston, MA, USA
M. Orsini Federici	University of Perugia, Perugia, Italy
Ele Ferrannini	Department of Internal Medicine, University of Pisa School of Medicine, Pisa, Italy
Samuel Edwin Fineberg	Indiana University School of Medicine, Indianapolis, IN, USA
Spiros Fourlanos	The Walter and Eliza Hall Institute of Medical Research, Parkville, Australia
Brian M. Frier	Royal Infirmary, Edinburgh, Scotland
David P. Funda	The Walter and Eliza Hall Institute of Medical Research, Parkville, Australia
Henrik Galbo	University of Copenhagen, Copenhagen, Denmark
Alan J. Garber	Baylor College of Medicine, Houston, TX, USA
Abhimanyu Garg	The University of Texas Southwestern Medical Center at Dallas, Dallas, TX, USA
W. Timothy Garvey	University of Alabama at Birmingham, and the Birmingham Veterans Affairs Medical Center, Birmingham, AL, USA
Robert J. Genco	State University of New York at Buffalo, Buffalo, NY, USA
G.V. Gill	University of Liverpool, Liverpool, UK
Barry J. Goldstein	Jefferson Medical College, Thomas Jefferson University, Philadelphia, PA, USA

Christopher S. Gray University of Newcastle upon Tyne, Newcastle upon Tyne, UK

Rosaire P. Gray Whittington Hospital, London, UK

Leif Groop Lund University, Malmö, Sweden

Leonard C. Harrison The Walter and Eliza Hall Institute of Medical Research, Parkville, Australia

Andrew T. Hattersley Peninsula Medical School, Exeter, UK

Zhiheng He Joslin Diabetes Center, Harvard Medical School, Boston, MA, USA

Robert R. Henry VA San Diego Healthcare System, and University of California San Diego, San Diego, CA, USA

William H. Herman University of Michigan, Ann Arbor, MI, USA

Rury Holman Diabetes Trials Unit, Radcliffe Infirmary, Oxford, UK

Margo C. Honeyman The Walter and Eliza Hall Institute of Medical Research, Parkville, Australia

Barbara V. Howard MedStar Research Institute, Washington, DC, USA

Katrin Hücking University of Southern California, Los Angeles, CA, USA

Giuseppina Imperatore Centers for Disease Control and Prevention, National Center for Chronic Disease Prevention and Health Promotion, Atlanta, GA, USA

Serge Jabbour Jefferson Medical College, Thomas Jefferson University, Philadelphia, PA, USA

Alan M. Jacobson Joslin Diabetes Center, Harvard Medical School, Boston, MA, USA

Dimitrije Jakovljevic National Public Health Institute, Helsinki, Finland

Kent P. Jensen The Walter and Eliza Hall Institute of Medical Research, Parkville, Australia

Bo-Lennart Johansson Karolinska Institute, Stockholm, Sweden

Jan Johansson Karolinska Institute, Stockholm, Sweden

Stephen C. Jones James Cook University Hospital, Middlesbrough, UK

Hans Jörnvall Karolinska Institute, Stockholm, Sweden

Lois Jovanovic Sansum Medical Research Foundation, Santa Barbara, CA, USA

Irène Juhan-Vague University Hospital Timone, Marseille, France

Steven E. Kahn VA Puget Sound Health Care System and University of Washington, Seattle, WA, USA

M. Ann Kelly University of Birmingham, Birmingham, UK

George L. King Joslin Diabetes Center, Harvard Medical School, Boston, MA, USA

Abbas E. Kitabchi University of Tennessee Health Science Center, Memphis, TN, USA

Peter J.E.M Kitslaar University Hospital Maastricht, Maastricht, The Netherlands, and Cardiovascular Research Institute Maastricht (CARIM), Maastricht, The Netherlands

Leslie P. Kozak Pennington Biomedical Research Center, Baton Rouge, LA, USA

M.F. Laker University of Newcastle upon Tyne, Newcastle upon Tyne, UK

Jonathan R.T. Lakey University of Alberta, Edmonton, Canada

Karen S.L. Lam The University of Hong Kong, Queen Mary Hospital, Hong Kong, China

H.E. Lebovitz State University of New York, Brooklyn, NY, USA

Warren Lee KK Women's and Children's Hospital, Singapore

Pierre J. Lefèbvre University of Liège, Liège, Belgium

Cécile Legallais Technological University of Compiègne, Compiègne, France

Eldon D. Lehmann St Bartholomew's Hospital, London, UK, and Imperial College, London, UK

R.D.G. Leslie St Bartholomew's Hospital, London, UK

Naomi S. Levitt University of Cape Town, Cape Town, South Africa

N.J. Lewis-Barned University of Newcastle Medical School, Newcastle upon Tyne, UK and North Tyneside General Hospital, Tyne and Wear, UK

Astrid M. Libman University of Rosario Medical School, Rosario, Argentina

Julio Libman University of Rosario Medical School, Rosario, Argentina

Robert S. Lindsay MedStar Research Institute, Washington, DC, USA

Jaana Lindstrom National Public Health Institute, Helsinki, Finland

Zhenqi Liu University of Virginia Health System, Charlottesville, VA, USA

Pierre Maechler University Medical Centre, Geneva, Switzerland

Lawrence Mandarino University of Texas Health Science Center, San Antonio, TX, USA

J.I. Mann University of Otago, Dunedin, New Zealand and Diabetes Service, Dunedin Hospital, Dunedin, New Zealand

Stuart I. Mannering The Walter and Eliza Hall Institute of Medical Research, Parkville, Australia

Sally M. Marshall The Medical School, University of Newcastle upon Tyne, Newcastle upon Tyne, UK

Nathan R. Martinez The Walter and Eliza Hall Institute of Medical Research, Parkville, Australia

Jean Claude Mbanya University of Yaoundé I, Yaoundé, Cameroon

Arne Melander The NEPI Foundation, Medical Research Centre, University Hospital, Malmö, Sweden

Anoop Misra The University of Texas Southwestern Medical Center at Dallas, Dallas, TX, USA

Braxton D. Mitchell University of Maryland School of Medicine, Baltimore, MD, USA

Pierre Emmanuel Morange University Hospital Timone, Marseille, France

Sunder Mudaliar	VA San Diego Healthcare System, San Diego, CA, USA and University of California at San Diego, CA, USA
Dara Murphy	Centers for Disease Control, Division of Diabetes, Atlanta, GA, USA
Mary Beth Murphy	University of Tennessee Health Science Center, Memphis, TN, USA
Seiki Nambu	Mukogawa Women's University, Nishinomiya, Japan
K.M.Venkat Narayan	Centers for Disease Control and Prevention, National Center for Chronic Disease Prevention and Health Promotion, Atlanta, GA, USA
Parth Narendran	The Walter and Eliza Hall Institute of Medical Research, Parkville, Australia
R.D.G. Neely	Newcastle upon Tyne Hospitals NHS Trust, Newcastle upon Tyne, UK
Christopher B. Newgard	Duke University Medical Center, Durham, NC, USA
Jens Høiriis Nielsen	University of Copenhagen, Copenhagen, Denmark
Jane Overland	Royal Prince Alfred Hospital, Camperdown, Australia, and The University of Sydney, Sydney, Australia
David R. Owens	University of Wales College of Medicine, Cardiff, Wales, UK
Johanna Paronen	Barbara Davis Center for Childhood Diabetes, University of Colorado Health Sciences Center, Denver, CO, USA, and University of Helsinki, Helsinki, Finland
Breay W. Paty	University of Alberta, Edmonton, Canada
Ewan R. Pearson	Peninsula Medical School, Exeter, UK
Louis Pérusse	Laval University, Québec, Canada
John C. Pickup	Guy's Hospital, London, UK
Vincent Poitout	Pacific Northwest Research Institute, Seattle, WA, USA
Daniel Porte, Jr.	VA Puget Sound Health Care System and University of Washington, Seattle, WA, USA
Paolo Pozzilli	University Campus Bio Medico, Rome, Italy, and St Bartholomew's Hospital, London, UK
Stefano Del Prato	University of Pisa, Pisa, Italy
Deepanwita Prusty	Boston University School of Medicine, Boston, MA, USA
Qing Qiao	University of Helsinki, Helsinki, Finland and National Public Health Institute, Helsinki, Finland
Rémi Rabasa-Lhoret	Research Centre, Centre Hospitalier de l'Université de Montréal, Montréal, Canada and Université de Montréal, Montréal, Canada
Ambady Ramachandran	Diabetes Research Centre, M.V. Hospital for Diabetes and WHO Collaborating Centre for Research Education and Training in Diabetes, Chennai, India
Lawrence I. Rand	Joslin Diabetes Center, Boston, MA, USA, and Harvard Medical School, Boston, MA, USA

Christian Rask-Madsen	Joslin Diabetes Center, Harvard Medical School, Boston, MA, USA
Daiva Rastenyte	Kaunas Institute of Cardiology, Kaunas, Lithuania
Eric Ravussin	Pennington Biomedical Research Center, Baton Rouge, LA, USA
Gérard Reach	Hôpital Avicenne, Assistance Publique-Hôpitaux de Paris, Bobigny, France
Jane E.-B. Reusch	University of Colorado School of Medicine, Denver, CO, USA
Marian J. Rewers	University of Colorado Health Sciences Center, Denver, CO, USA
Christopher J. Rhodes	Pacific Northwest Research Institute, Seattle, WA, USA
Erik A. Richter	University of Copenhagen, Copenhagen, Denmark
Martin Ridderstråle	Lund University, Malmö, Sweden
R. Paul Robertson	Pacific Northwest Research Institute, Seattle, WA, USA
Arlan L. Rosenbloom	University of Florida College of Medicine, Gainesville, FL, USA
Kathy Rufo	Centers for Disease Control, Division of Diabetes, Atlanta, GA, USA
Giacomo Ruotolo	MedStar Research Institute, Washington, DC, USA
Sue Rutherford	University of Maryland School of Medicine, Baltimore, MD, USA
Edmond A. Ryan	University of Alberta, Edmonton, Canada
Christopher D. Saudek	The Johns Hopkins University School of Medicine, Baltimore, MD, USA
Simon A. Saunders	University Hospital Aintree, Liverpool, UK
Casper G. Schalkwijk	VU University Medical Centre, Amsterdam, The Netherlands
Nicolaas C. Schaper	University Hospital Maastricht, Maastricht, The Netherlands, and Cardiovascular Research Institute Maastricht (CARIM), Maastricht, The Netherlands
Michael W. Schwartz	Harborview Medical Center and University of Washington, Seattle, WA, USA
Randy J. Seeley	University of Cincinnati, Cincinnati, OH, USA
Palle Serup	Hagedorn Research Institute Gentofte, Denmark
Jawed Shafqat	Karolinska Institute, Stockholm, Sweden
A.M. James Shapiro	University of Alberta, Edmonton, Canada
Jonathan E. Shaw	International Diabetes Institute, Melbourne, Australia
A. Samad Shera	Diabetes Association of Pakistan and WHO Collaborating Centre, Karachi, Pakistan
Alan R. Shuldiner	University of Maryland School of Medicine, Baltimore, MD, USA
Kamran Siddiqi	University of Leeds, Leeds, UK
Richard W. Simpson	Monash University, Box Hill Hospital, Victoria, Australia

Alan J. Sinclair	University of Warwick, Coventry, UK
Jay S. Skyler	University of Miami, FL, USA
Chamukuttan Snehalatha	Diabetes Research Centre, M.V. Hospital for Diabetes and WHO Collaborating Centre for Research Education and Training in Diabetes, Chennai, India
Thomas J. Songer	University of Pittsburgh, Pittsburgh, PA, USA
Andrea K. Steck	University of Colorado Health Sciences Center, Denver, CO, USA
Coen D.A. Stehouwer	VU University Medical Centre, Amsterdam, The Netherlands
Roland Stein	Vanderbilt University Medical Center, Nashville, TN, USA
Raymond J. Steptoe	The Walter and Eliza Hall Institute of Medical Research, Parkville, Australia
Nelia P. Steyn	South African Medical Research Council, Tygerberg, Cape Town, South Africa
William V. Tamborlane	Yale University School of Medicine, New Haven, CT, USA
Kathryn C.B. Tan	The University of Hong Kong, Queen Mary Hospital, Hong Kong, China
Nauman Tarif	King Fiassel University, Riyadh, Saudi Arabia
Marja-Riitta Taskinen	University of Helsinki, Helsinki, Finland
P.K. Thomas	Institute of Neurology, London, UK
Antonio Tiengo	University of Padova, Padova, Italy
P. Tong	The Chinese University of Hong Kong, Hong Kong, China
John E. Tooke	Peninsula Medical School, Plymouth, UK
Russell P. Tracy	College of Medicine, The University of Vermont, Burlington, VT, USA
Jaakko Tuomilehto	University of Helsinki, Helsinki, Finland and National Public Health Institute, Helsinki, Finland
Guillermo E. Umpierrez	University of Tennessee Health Science Center, Memphis, TN, USA
Kristina M. Utzschneider	VA Puget Sound Health Care System and University of Washington, Seattle, WA, USA
Aristidis Veves	Harvard Medical School, Boston, MA, USA
Frank Vinicor	Centers for Disease Control, Division of Diabetes, Atlanta, GA, USA
Vijay Viswanathan	Diabetes Research Centre, MV Hospital for Diabetes and WHO Collaborating Centre for Research Education and Training in Diabetes, Chennai, India
John Wahren	Karolinska Institute, Stockholm, Sweden
Richard M. Watanabe	University of Southern California, Los Angeles, CA, USA
Stuart A. Weinzimer	Yale University School of Medicine, New Haven, CT, USA

Desmond E. Williams	Centers for Disease Control and Prevention, National Center for Chronic Disease Prevention and Health Promotion, Atlanta, GA, USA
Gareth Williams	University of Bristol, Bristol, UK
Rhys Williams	University of Leeds, Leeds, UK
Claes B. Wollheim	University Medical Centre, Geneva, Switzerland
Stephen C. Woods	University of Cincinnati, Cincinnati, OH, USA
Hannele Yki-Järvinen	Helsinki University, Helsinki, Finland
David A. York	Louisiana State University, Baton Rouge, LA, USA
John S. Yudkin	Royal Free and University College Medical School, London, UK
Paul Zimmet	International Diabetes Institute, Melbourne, Australia
Bernard Zinman	Mount Sinai Hospital, Toronto, Canada

Preface

The late and lamented David Pyke used to say that two notable things happened in 1921. First, he was born. Second, insulin was isolated. Although little has happened in diabetes since to match either event, especially the latter, our knowledge of the disease, its surrounding pathophysiology, and its roots in the basic sciences has grown stupendously. Those working with diabetes, whether in the clinics, in the laboratories, or, increasingly, in government or international health agencies, are overwhelmed by the sheer torrent of new diabetes-related information that flows daily from professional journals, from the media, and from cyberspace. In many parts of the world, the prospects for the person with diabetes have never been better. The threat of diabetic blindness has receded, kidney failure can be anticipated and its progression greatly attenuated, the spectre of gangrene and limb amputation has retreated, we have almost come to expect a successful outcome of pregnancy, and even the great atherosclerotic behemoth begins to shrink.

Nonetheless, although the devastating complications of the disease have been mollified, they are still with us and still of uncertain mechanisms. To many people with diabetes, the benefits of these advances are not available. Despite the explosion in understanding, the breathtaking technological bravura, and our well-furnished therapeutic armoury, we are actually losing the battle against diabetes and, at best, engaged in a fighting retreat. Paradoxically, this "failure" is an almost direct consequence of "success" elsewhere. The global population continues to expand, with the biggest contribution from peoples seemingly most susceptible to diabetes. A growing abundance of foods coincides with falling physical energy requirements as machines take on the hard labor. Adaptation falls far short of perfect, and obesity inexorably engulfs a growing portion of the population at an earlier age. Our much sought-after increasing longevity comes at a price, of which greater risk of diabetes is only part. In many industrialized countries, these threats to health have been recognized, often by the better educated and financially more privileged members of society, who have successfully adapted their lifestyle to maintain higher levels of physical activity and to reduce the risk of obesity and the complications which follow in its wake.

Diabetes is often represented as a prime exemplar of a maladaptive response of a genetic constitution fashioned to fit a human environment subject to intermittent famine, exotic infections, and frequent recourse to "fight and flight." This entirely plausible (but untestable) hypothesis, memorably given literary immortality by J. V. Neel with his "thrifty genotype," carried the implication that in type 2 diabetes the genetic component(s) would be likely to be found among the genomic elements concerned with adapting insulin production or insulin effects (or both) to the prevailing "nutritional climate." The clear evidence of bimodality in the distribution of glucose tolerance/intolerance in, first, the Pima Indian and then the Nauruan, Mexican American, and other high diabetes prevalence societies raised the expectation that a single gene, or at most a very small number of genes, of substantial effect would distinguish between the upper and lower modes of the distribution. To date, despite the wide application of the powerful methods of genetic analysis now available, such offending genes have not been identified and bimodality remains unexplained.

We have always been conscious of the wide front on which diabetes knowledge advances and have tried to reflect this in the breadth of subject and versatility of authorship of the *International Textbook of Diabetes Mellitus* (ITDM). At the same time, we have always tried to highlight the growing points of knowledge and, more difficult, to anticipate growth areas and to set some authoritative pointers to the future. Backing the whole enterprise, we have also attempted to present, as far as we are able to in two volumes, the firm foundation of validated knowledge on which our day-to-day clinical decisions and our broad strategies and directions of research are based. Even these laudable activities and objectives are in flux. The very process of information storage, organization, and transfer has been revolutionized by the Internet and this has affected us all. Not least, ITDM has responded to the challenge and is bringing its content to the diabetes community both in familiar hard copy and, hot from the keyboard, through the Internet (http://www.mrw.interscience.wiley.com/itdm). This will allow existing chapters to be updated as new information becomes available, and new chapters to be added, without the necessarily longer turnaround time, which has been the case with print publication. In due course it is possible that a more interactive element may also be added, allowing readers and authors a forum to comment on and discuss points of interest. We certainly welcome feedback on this latest edition of ITDM and will seriously consider readers' suggestions for future inclusions and improvements.

Harry Keen

April 2004

Introduction

INTRODUCTION TO THE THIRD EDITION

The *International Textbook of Diabetes Mellitus* (ITDM), now in its third edition, has become the most widely referenced textbook of diabetes worldwide. It is the only textbook that truly engages the expertise of clinicians, educators, and investigators from widely diverse regions of the world. It provides a comprehensive overview of the treatment of diabetes and its associated microvascular and macrovascular complications. However, it is unique in that it also addresses the specific pathogenic mechanisms, the diverse epidemiological features of diabetes and its complications, clinical presentations, diagnostic evaluation, and therapeutic approaches, that are unique to different ethnic groups and countries throughout the world.

The current edition of the *International Textbook of Diabetes Mellitus* has been extensively reorganized, with 11 major subdivisions (Epidemiology; Normal Physiology of Pancreatic Function; Normal Physiology of Insulin Action; Pathogenesis; Obesity; Management of Diabetes: Diet, Exercise, and Drugs; Management of Diabetes: Monitoring and Other Interventions; Complications: General and Microvascular; Complications: Macrovascular Disease; Management of Diabetes: Glucose and Lipid Monitoring, Specific Subgroups; and Diabetes and Public Health), each headed by a Section Editor who is an internationally recognized authority in his/her area. A number of new chapters have been added, among them:

- Development and Life Cycle of a β-Cell
- Mechanisms of Insulin Signal Transduction
- Monogenic Disorders of the β-Cell
- Is Type 2 Diabetes the Result of a "Thrifty Genotype" or a "Thrifty Phenotype"?
- The Genetics of Human Obesity
- Role of the Adipocyte in Type 2 Diabetes
- Treatment of Obesity
- The Role of the Hypothalamus in the Maintenance of Energy Balance and Peripheral Glucose Control
- Thiazolidinediones as PPAR Agonists
- Combination Therapy in Type 2 Diabetes
- Periodontal Disease and Diabetes Mellitus
- Erectile Dysfunction in Diabetes Mellitus
- The Syndrome of Insulin Resistance and Its Links to Atherosclerosis
- Endothelial Function and Dysfunction
- Cerebrovascular Disease in Diabetes Mellitus
- Prevention of Type 1 Diabetes
- Prevention of Type 2 Diabetes

In addition, several previous chapters have been combined, and all chapters (including those combined) have been revised extensively since the last edition of the Textbook seven years ago. In an attempt to introduce fresh looks and perspectives to keep the *International Textbook of Diabetes Mellitus* current, approximately one third of the authors have been replaced since the previous edition. An innovative feature of the current edition is the availability of all chapters online (http://www.mrw.interscience.wiley.com/itdm), with regular updates scheduled depending upon scientific advances and growth of knowledge in specific areas.

Ralph A. DeFronzo
Ele Ferrannini
Harry Keen
Paul Zimmet

April 2004

INTRODUCTION TO THE SECOND EDITION

It has been four years since the first edition of *International Textbook of Diabetes Mellitus* appeared. At that time we attempted to give a broader sweep to our coverage of diabetes than was customary in the available "Northern" textbooks. This was due in part to the pandemic of diabetes that was, and still is, sweeping the globe, and in part to the lack of texts dealing with diabetes in non-Europids. We felt that much could be learned by considering diabetes in relation to different ethnic groups, cultures, and geographical settings. We also attempted to cover the whole of diabetes, from the gene and cell biology to the social and economic aspects. Further background to the rationale of ITDM is given in the original introduction, which is reprinted below.

We have been encouraged by the response to the first edition: hence the present volumes. This second edition does not, however, just represent a reworking of the previous volumes. Several new chapters have been added, others replaced, and many new authors introduced. We hope that we have been able to enhance the previous edition and also remain current and relevant.

K.G.M.M. Alberti
P.Z. Zimmet
R.A. DeFronzo

INTRODUCTION TO THE FIRST EDITION

A modern textbook of diabetes should be international in scope. Not only does it draw on the knowledge and expertise of people from all over the world, but it also reminds us that no race of mankind is immune from the diabetic state. Ethnic susceptibility to diabetes varies tremendously, a variation in liability that must depend both upon the widely differing conditions in which the human species exists and upon the diversity of the genetic endowment. It is important to our understanding of the nature of diabetes mellitus and our attempts to prevent and treat it that we view the diabetic state as the outcome of the interplay of a multiplicity of causal factors, potentially varying in both the genetic and the environmental components of the mix. Although the diabetic state can itself be clearly defined—we, after all, are responsible for creating the definition—it is, nevertheless, heterogeneous in its causation and in its consequences. In investigating its mechanisms we should be prepared to find differences between, and even within, populations in the nature of the underlying susceptibility and in the factors that provoke its emergence and its pathological sequelae.

Before attempting to explain the diabetic state, we should agree upon its definition. Those who coined the term *diabetes mellitus* had little doubt: originally, it described a grave sickness characterized by dramatic symptoms—intense thirst, profuse urination, rapid wasting, inexorably proceeding through the stages of vomiting and drowsiness to coma and death. The term *diabetes* was no more than a description of these characteristic symptoms; *mellitus* was added when the sweetness of the urine indicated its high sugar content and distinguished it from the insipid, sugar-free variety.

Identification of the urinary sugar as glucose can be said to have ushered in the era of clinical chemistry. However, it was not until laboratory methods were sufficiently refined that the central importance of hyperglycemia in the diabetic state and its primacy in diabetes diagnosis were recognized. This transition from clinical to chemical diagnosis had a profound effect on the diagnostic concept of diabetes: it resulted in the addition to the same diagnostic rubric of ever-larger numbers of cases with ever-lessening degrees of symptomatology. This conceptual inflation reached its limits with the application of preemptive screening tests for diabetes to large sections of the general population. Now, the diagnosis was called upon to accommodate cases without symptoms or signs, sometimes even without glucose in the urine. The existence of a state of "pathological hyperglycemia" had become the main justification for including in the same diagnostic category a spectrum of abnormality which ranged from a totally asymptomatic transgression of an arbitrary blood glucose norm at the one extreme, to a potentially lethal metabolic catastrophe at the other. A further justification for retaining the single diagnostic term was the common liability to the ultimate development of a characteristic set of organ and tissue abnormalities—the complications of diabetes.

Population surveys for diabetes, with the new diagnostic perspectives that they generated, stemmed from the recognition of the high prevalence of unsuspected diabetes and the hope that early detection and treatment might avert its complications. Large population samples were tested, many being submitted to measurements of blood glucose concentration in response to a glucose challenge. It was difficulty with interpretation of the results of such surveys that brought the diagnostic definition of diabetes to critical review. Unexpectedly large numbers of apparently healthy people had blood glucose levels at the suspiciously high end of the range, their frequency increasing with age. At no age could a "natural" dividing line be found separating normal from diabetic glycemic responses. Depending on which set of diagnostic criteria were adopted, the estimates of diabetes frequency in a given population could vary as much as 10-fold. As a consequence, an individual diagnosed as unquestionably diabetic by one doctor could be equally emphatically reassured of normality by another. Add to this the substantial variation introduced by differences in the methods of diagnostic testing, and the reasons for the moves toward national and international standardization of the 1970s and early 1980s become clear. A measure of order was introduced in consensus meetings of a number of national diabetes organizations, principally the US National Diabetes Data Group, and soon after by the World Health Organization (WHO). They agreed upon a set of glycemic criteria for diabetes diagnosis and interposed a new category of "impaired glucose tolerance" (IGT) between clearly normal and clearly diabetic glycemic responses. Although these proposals are by no means above criticism, they have been increasingly widely applied in both clinical practice and epidemiological investigation, and provide a degree of comparability and uniformity that was previously lacking.

The international perspective is also appropriate to the classification of the diabetic state, which also has been the subject of concern and revision over the past decade. The two major types of diabetes mellitus, insulin dependent (IDDM or type 1) and non-insulin dependent

(NIDDM or type 2), are essentially defined by their clinical characteristics, although these largely correspond (in people of European origin) to underlying etiological mechanisms and, perhaps, to genetic liabilities. The frequency of IDDM or type 1 diabetes—the severe disease of classic description—is notably higher in peoples of European origin, although it has been reported almost universally in others. NIDDM also has rather different characteristics in Europeans, compared with most other ethnic groups: its prevalence is lower, it appears later in life, and it is, perhaps, less liable to lead to renal failure, possibly because of its later appearance. Malnutrition-related diabetes mellitus (MRDM) appeared in the most recent WHO classification as an independent type. Its existence as a tropical variant of diabetes, secondary to pancreatic damage and etiologically related to dietary protein deficiency or to toxic food contaminants, has been the subject of debate and investigation in recent years. More systematic investigation is needed before the size and nature of this problem can be confidently documented.

NIDDM is by far the largest problem numerically on a global scale. In the most susceptible populations, up to one person in two may expect to develop the disease. The Pima tribe of American Indians, currently topping the league tables for diabetes prevalence, has shown what appears to be an explosive increase in incidence over the course of this century. The tribe was visited in the early 1930s by Dr E.P. Joslin, the doyen of diabetes in the United States, who was interested in the reputed rarity of diabetes among its members. This dramatic transformation must have been the response to some widespread environmental change affecting a relatively inbred population carrying some underlying genetic susceptibility to the disease: a steeply rising prevalence of obesity is widely held to have been the environmental determinant; the genetic susceptibility factor has as yet eluded definition. At the present pace of genetic research and discovery, its detection can only be a matter of time. When it is found, however, will it prove to be the same as that determining susceptibility to NIDDM in other populations? On the face of it, it seems unlikely that NIDDM is a single homogeneous entity *within* populations, let alone *between* them. Its associations with age, adiposity, and clinical progression appear so diverse that a multiplicity of underlying mechanisms appears probable.

In recent years some part of this broad spectrum of NIDDM and IGT have been linked with a number of other common disorders and conditions, such as hypertension, hyperlipidemia, and hyperinsulinemia. From this has emerged the view that this form of glucose intolerance may only be part—and not an obligatory part at that—of some much more general disturbance of adaptation to the conditions of modern life. Characterized by diminished tissue sensitivity to the effects of insulin and associated with a centripetal distribution of body fat and increased liability to atherosclerosis, this so-called syndrome X currently attracts the attention of many investigators. In a continuum of interacting mechanisms that may contribute to a number of important human disorders, glucose intolerance or diabetes may have a small or even nonexistent role. Other broad classes of NIDDM may be described, without obesity, with early age of onset, and with evidence of islet autoimmunity, which highlight its probable heterogeneity.

It is the so-called complications of diabetes that today constitute the main burden for patients, their families, and the societies in which they live. Blindness due to retinopathy, such a dreaded hazard a generation ago, is now in large part a preventable disaster, provided that facilities for eye screening and timely photocoagulation are available. The long period of ill health as diabetic renal disease neared its termination in end-stage renal failure can now be reversed with modern renal substitution methods of dialysis and transplantation; there is reason to suppose that the stage of renal failure may be postponed and the number of patients entering renal failure greatly diminished, again depending upon facilities for the early recognition of those at risk and their appropriately monitored treatment. There is some evidence that people with the increased arterial disease risk of diabetes are sharing in the general diminution in coronary heart disease morbidity and mortality documented in some societies over the past 20 years. This strongly suggests that much of the aggravated risk of atherosclerotic disease in diabetes could be reduced. Even the morbid effects of that most intransigent of diabetic complications—neuropathy—can be ameliorated by the application of quite simple preventative measures. The scope of diabetes care has expanded dramatically in recent years, with the promise of longer and healthier years of life for many and (that prize so beloved of health politicians) a reduction in the enormous costs of health-care provision for diabetic complications. The remarkable advances of knowledge have firmly placed on the agenda even the prevention of diabetes itself.

It is our hope that we have been able, in this book, to cover most of this broad panorama of diabetes, from the molecular structures responsible for susceptibility, through the hormonal and biochemical mechanisms responsible for the clinical manifestations and complications of the disease, to the therapeutic agencies and their availability to ameliorate, arrest, reverse, or even prevent its damaging impact. Much remains to be discovered; we are still far short of a full understanding of the disease. Much that is known remains to be applied; it is important to translate what we know into what we do. We hope that this book will enhance the understanding of diabetes mellitus and help in applying that understanding to the better care of people with diabetes.

Harry Keen
George Alberti
Ralph DeFronzo
Paul Zimmet

Epidemiology

1

Classification of Diabetes Mellitus and Other Categories of Glucose Intolerance

Paul Zimmet*, Catherine Cowie†, Jean-Marie Ekoe‡, and Jonathan E. Shaw*

**International Diabetes Institute, Melbourne, Australia, †National Institutes of Health, Bethesda, MD, USA, and ‡Centre de Reserche CHUM, Montreal, Canada*

INTRODUCTION

The major requirement for orderly epidemiologic, genetic, and clinical research on diabetes mellitus and glucose intolerance, and indeed for its clinical management, is an appropriate classification. Furthermore, a hallmark in the process of understanding the etiology of a disease and studying its natural history is the ability to identify and differentiate its various forms and place them into a rational etiopathologic framework. While there have been a number of sets of nomenclature and diagnostic criteria proposed for diabetes, no systematic categorization existed until just over 20 years ago [1]. Now diabetes mellitus is recognized as being a syndrome, a collection of disorders that have hyperglycemia and glucose intolerance as their hallmark, because of insulin deficiency or impaired effectiveness of insulin action, or because of a combination of these.

HISTORICAL PERSPECTIVE AND PREVIOUS CLASSIFICATIONS

Credit for the initial recognition that diabetes mellitus was not a single disorder rests with two Indian physicians, Chakrata and Susruta (600 BC). They differentiated two forms of the disease, although most of the descriptions in the classic literature probably relate to what we know today as type 1 diabetes. During the eighteenth and nineteenth centuries, a less clinically symptomatic variety of the disorder, identified by marked glycosuria, often detected in later life and commonly associated with overweight rather than wasting, was noted. This form today is recognized as type 2 diabetes. In the twenieth century, when screening programs for diabetes commenced, it became apparent that there were many people who could be classified as having diabetes but who were generally "asymptomatic." It has become apparent subsequently that the term diabetes mellitus covers a wide spectrum of disease, from the acute and sometimes explosive onset of type 1 diabetes to asymptomatic individuals whose type 2 diabetes is discovered by accident.

In the mid-1930s, Himsworth [2] proposed that there were at least two clinical types of diabetes, insulin-sensitive and insulin-insensitive, the former being due to insulin deficiency. Confirmation of his clinical observations came with Bornstein's development of a bioassay for insulin [3]. The Nobel Prize winning discovery of a radioimmunoassay for insulin by Berson and Yalow a decade later saw the confirmation of Bornstein's observations [4]. The widespread acceptance of the terms *juvenile-onset* and *maturity-onset diabetes* at this time was affirmation of the concept that there were at least two major forms of the disease.

Previous Classifications

In 1965, a World Health Organization (WHO) Expert Committee on Diabetes Mellitus published the first WHO report containing a classification of patients according to age of recognized onset [5]. The report of this committee includes one of the first attempts at international consensus on a classification. They decided to "...make the

International Textbook of Diabetes Mellitus, Third Edition. Edited by R. A. DeFronzo, E. Ferrannini, H. Keen, and P. Zimmet.
 ISBN: 0-471-48655-8.

following strong recommendations, based on the age of recognized onset, which seemed to be the only reliable means of classification for universal use."

They also recognized, in addition to the age classification, other characteristics to define diabetes including juvenile-type, brittle, insulin-resistant, gestational, pancreatic, endocrine, and iatrogenic diabetes. Their suggested classification was really the first attempt to bring some international consensus on criteria for diagnosis and classification of the diabetes syndrome. Since that time, other pathogenic mechanisms have been described and long-term studies have shown different courses and outcomes of different types of diabetes. Some of the new classifications proposed tried to incorporate various aspects of diabetes, which, in fact, sometimes reflected the specific research interests of particular investigators on the committees. For example, a new major class of malnutrition-related diabetes mellitus (MRDM) was introduced in the 1985 WHO classification and removed in the most recent one. Considerable confusion arose from this and it became quite difficult to construct a simple classification that met all interests.

In order to overcome these setbacks and establish a new classification that included all possible forms of diabetes mellitus and glucose intolerance, a revised classification of diabetes was formulated by the National Diabetes Data Group (NDDG) [6]. This was reviewed, amended, and adopted in the second report of the WHO Expert Committee in 1980 [7] and in a modified form in 1985. The 1980 [7] and 1985 [8] classifications of diabetes and allied categories of glucose intolerance included clinical classes and two statistical risk classes. The 1980 Expert Committee proposed two major classes of diabetes mellitus and named them insulin-dependent diabetes mellitus (IDDM) or type 1, and non-insulin-dependent diabetes mellitus (NIDDM) or type 2 [7]. In the 1985 Study Group Report the terms type 1 and type 2 were omitted, but the classes IDDM and NIDDM were retained and a new class of MRDM was introduced [8]. The 1985 WHO classification was essentially based on clinical descriptions (e.g., insulin-dependent, non-insulin-dependent) and did not include terms that might indicate etiological mechanisms (such as type 1or type 2). The question whether certain clinical forms of diabetes (such as the so-called tropical diabetes) were given adequate priority to correct hierarchic order that was raised many years before probably led to the introduction of MRDM although more precise epidemiological data and a better assessment were needed, and called for. The statistical risk classes included individuals having a previous abnormality of glucose tolerance (PrevAGT) and those with a potential abnormality of glucose tolerance (PotAGT) e.g., those of higher risk ethnic groups and those exhibiting a genetic predisposition.

Both the 1980 and 1985 reports included other types of diabetes, e.g. pancreatic and drug-induced, and impaired glucose tolerance (IGT) as well as gestational diabetes mellitus (GDM). The 1985 classification was widely accepted, was used internationally, and represented a compromise between clinical and etiological classifications. Furthermore, it permitted classification of individual subjects and patients in a clinically useful manner even when the specific cause of etiology is unknown. Based on emerging research that drew attention to the need to refine the classification of diabetes to reflect clinical characteristics, etiology, and the stages in the natural history of the disease(s), the 1999 WHO [9] as well as the 1997 ADA (American Diabetes Association) [10] classifications have been developed. They include clinical descriptive criteria with a complementary classification according to etiology recommended by both organizations.

The 1999 WHO Classification of Diabetes Mellitus and Other Categories of Glucose Tolerance

The etiological classification of diabetes mellitus is summarized in Table 1. The etiological and clinical stages are presented in Figure 1. The concepts for this new staging/etiological classification were reported by Kuzuya and Matsuda [11]. The proposal sought to separate clearly the criteria related to etiology and those related to degree of deficiency of insulin or insulin action and to define each patient on the basis of these two criteria.

Working on a similar basis, the new WHO [9] and indeed ADA [10] classifications encompass both the clinical stages and etiological types of diabetes and other categories of glucose intolerance (Table 1 and Figure 1). It is now well established that diabetes may progress through several clinical stages during its natural history, quite independent of its etiology. The clinical staging reflects this and, indeed, individuals may move from one stage to another stage in both directions (Figure 1). Even if there is no information concerning the underlying etiology, persons with diabetes or those who are developing the disease can be categorized by stage according to clinical characteristics. The classification by etiological type results from improved understanding of the causes of diabetes, although this is still far from complete.

The new classification also takes into account the various degrees of hyperglycemia in individual subjects with any of the disease processes that could lead to diabetes. These are glycemic stages ranging from normal glucose tolerance to the hyperglycemia in established diabetes where insulin is required for survival. All individuals with the disorder can be categorized according to clinical stage (9). The stage of glycemia may change over time, depending on the extent of the underlying disease processes. As shown in Figure 1, the disease process may be present but may not have progressed far enough to cause hyperglycemia. The etiological classification is useful as the defect or process that may lead to diabetes may be

Table 1 Etiological classification of disorders of glycemia*†

Type 1 (β-cell destruction, usually leading to absolute insulin deficiency)
Autoimmune
Idiopathic
Type 2 (may range from predominantly insulin resistance with relative insulin deficiency to a predominantly secretory defect with or without insulin resistance)
Other specific types (see Table 3)
Genetic defects of β-cell function
Genetic defects in insulin action
Diseases of the exocrine pancreas
Endocrinopathies
Drug- or chemical-induced
Infections
Uncommon forms of immune-mediated diabetes
Other genetic syndromes sometimes associated with diabetes
Gestational diabetes‡

* Reproduced by permission of WTO [9].
† As additional sub types are discovered it is anticipated hat they will be reclassified within their own specific category.
‡ Includes the former categories of gestational impaired glucose tolerance and gestational diabetes.

identifiable at any stage in the development of diabetes, even at the stage of normoglycemia. As an example, the presence of islet cell antibodies (ICA) or antibodies to glutamic acid decarboxylase (anti-GAD) in a normoglycemic individual makes it likely that the individual has the type 1 autoimmune process [9, 12]. For type 2 diabetes, there are few useful highly specific indicators. It is hoped that future research will reveal them.

The same disease process can cause various degrees of impaired glucose metabolism, such as IFG (impaired fasting glycemia) and/or IGT, without fulfilling the criteria for the diagnosis of diabetes [9]. In some persons with type 2 diabetes, weight reduction, exercise, and/or oral hypoglycaemic therapy can achieve satisfactory glycemic control [13]. These persons, therefore, do not require insulin. Other persons with type 2 diabetes require insulin for adequate glycemic control but can survive without it. By definition these persons have some residual insulin secretion. Patients with extensive β-cell destruction (no residual insulin secretion) do require insulin

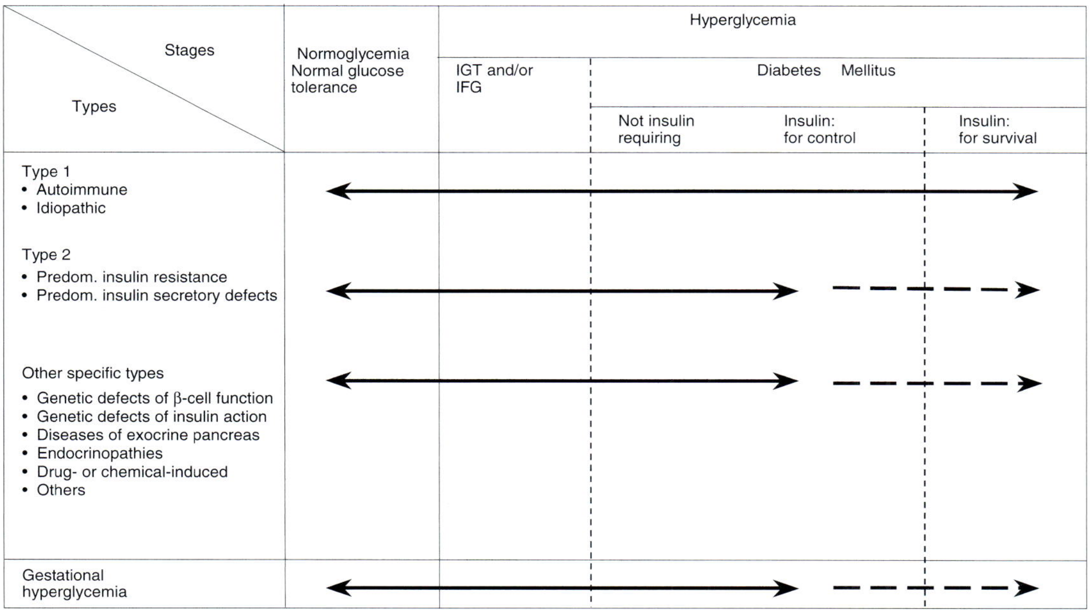

Figure 1 Disorders of glycemia: etiological types and clinical stages. (Reproduced by permission of WTO [9])

Table 2 Values for diagnosis* of diabetes and other categories of hyperglycemia†

	Glucose concentration (mmol/l)			
	Plasma		Whole blood	
	Venous	Capillary	Venous	Capillary
Diabetes mellitus				
Fasting	≥7.0	≥7.0	≥6.1	≥6.1
or				
2-h post-glucose load	≥11.1	≥12.2	≥10.0	≥11.1
Impaired glucose tolerance				
Fasting concentration	<7.0	<7.0	<6.1	<6.1
and				
2-h post-glucose load	7.8–11.0	8.9–12.1	6.7–9.9	7.8–11.0
Impaired fasting glucose				
Fasting	6.1–6.9	6.1–6.9	5.6–6.0	5.6–6.0
and (if measured)				
2-h post-glucose load	<7.8	<8.9	<6.7	<7.8

* Note that diabetes can only be diagnosed in an individual when these diagnostic values are confirmed on another day. Ranges of values are inclusive, i.e. 6.1–6.9 means ≥6.1 and <7.0.
* Reproduced by permission of WTO [9].

for survival and this is the hallmark of type 1 diabetes [9, 12].

Terminology Changes Resulting from New Classification

Both the most recent WHO [9] and ADA [10] classifications have dropped the terms *insulin-dependent diabetes mellitus, non-insulin-dependent diabetes mellitus*, and their acronyms IDDM and NIDDM. These terms were very confusing and frequently resulted in misclassification and so the patients were classified on the basis of their treatment rather than on pathogenesis. In the new classification, the terms *type 1* and *type* 2 are retained (using arabic rather than roman numerals) [9]. People with any form of diabetes may require insulin treatment at some stage of their disease [13].

The etiological form of diabetes called type 1 encompasses the majority of cases that are primarily due to pancreatic islet β-cell destruction and are prone to ketoacidosis. Type 1 includes those cases attributable to an autoimmune process, as well as those with β-cell destruction and those who are prone to ketoacidosis for which neither an etiology nor a pathogenesis is known (idiopathic). Those forms of β-cell destruction that are unrelated to an autoimmune process but to which other specific causes can be assigned are not included in type 1 diabetes (e.g., cystic fibrosis, mitochondrial defects). These issues are discussed in greater detail below.

The form named type 2 includes the common major form of diabetes that results almost always from insulin resistance and often from defect(s) in insulin secretion. MRDM has been deleted in the latest WHO classification (9). Of its two subtypes, protein-deficient pancreatic diabetes (PDPD or PDDM) needs more studies for a better definition. The other former subtype of MRDM, fibrocalculous pancreatic diabetes (FCPD), is now classified as a disease of the exocrine pancreas, called fibrocalculous pancreatopathy, which may lead to diabetes (see Chapter 29).

The class called IGT is reclassified as a stage of impaired glucose regulation, since it can be observed in any hyperglycemic disorder, and in itself, is not a state of diabetes.

Gestational diabetes is retained but now encompasses the groups formerly classified as GIGT (gestational impaired glucose tolerance) and GDM according to the new WHO criteria [9] (Table 2).

THE NEW WHO CLASSIFICATION BASED ON ETIOLOGY

The new classification proposes that hyperglycemia, irrespective of the underlying cause, can be subcategorized into the following clinical stages:

Diabetes Mellitus

Diabetes mellitus, regardless of underyling cause, is subdivided into three stages:

(1) *Insulin requiring for survival* (corresponding to the former clinical class of IDDM), e.g. C-peptide deficient
(2) *Insulin requiring for control*, i.e. for metabolic control, rather than for survival, e.g. some endogenous insulin secretion but insufficient to achieve normoglycemia without added exogenous insulin, and *not insulin requiring*, i.e. those who may be treated

and controlled satisfactorily by nonpharmacological methods or drugs other than insulin. These two categories correspond to the former NIDDM.

(3) *Not insulin requiring*

Impaired Glucose Regulation (Impaired Glucose Tolerance and Impaired Fasting Glycemia)

IGT was considered a class in the previous WHO classification [8]. It is now categorized as a stage in the natural history of disordered carbohydrate metabolism. A stage called *impaired fasting hyperglycemia* or *impaired fasting glycemia* (IFG) or *nondiabetic fasting hyperglycemia* is now included, as subjects with this disorder also appear to be at greater risk for progression to diabetes and macrovascular disease (9). IFG refers to fasting glucose concentrations that are lower than those required to diagnose diabetes but higher than the "normal" reference range (Table 2).

IGT and IFG are not proposed as clinical entities in their own right but rather as risk categories for future diabetes and/or cardiovascular disease (CVD) [9,10]. They represent impaired glucose regulation, which refers to a metabolic state intermediate between normal glucose homeostasis and diabetes. Individuals who meet criteria for IGT or IFG are euglycemic in the circumstances of their day-to-day life as confirmed by normal or near-normal glycosylated hemoglobin levels [9]. IGT is often associated with the metabolic or insulin resistance syndrome [9, 10, 14].

An individual with a fasting plasma glucose (FPG) concentration of 6.1 mmol/l (110 mg/dl) or greater (whole blood 5.6 mmol/l; 100 mg/dl) but less than 7.0 mmol/l (126 mg/dl) (whole blood 6.1 mmol/l; 110 mg/dl) is considered to have IFG (Table 2). If an oral glucose tolerance test (OGTT) is performed, some individuals with IFG will have IGT (2-h post-glucose load plasma concentration 7.8–11.0 mmol/l, whole blood 6.7–9.9 mmol/l). Some may have diabetes (2-h post-glucose load plasma concentration >11.1 mmol/l; whole blood concentration >10.0 mmol/l) but this cannot be determined without an OGTT. If sufficient resources are available, then it is recommended that subjects with IFG should have an OGTT to exclude diabetes [9].

A major question to be addressed is whether IGT and IFG are the same conditions in disguise? A large body of data is now available on the epidemiology, natural history, and consequences of IGT. However, it is only recently that data have become available on IFG as it was only first defined in 1997 [10]. There is a need to establish whether IGT and IFG should only be considered risk factors for type 2 diabetes, with IGT also being a risk determinant of CVD, or are they diseases in their own right. This issue has been considered in depth by the recent International Diabetes Federation (IDF) IGT/IFG Consensus Workshop [15].

The IDF workshop sought to address three questions:

(1) Are the current definitions of IGT and IFG appropriate?
(2) Are IFG and IGT risk factors, risk markers or diseases?
(3) What interventions (if any) should be recommended for people with IFG and IGT?

As a result of epidemiological data, both the ADA [10] and WHO [9] had recommended that the latest classification of glucose intolerance be based on stages of glucose tolerance with complementary subclassifications based on etiology. As a result, in the new WHO and ADA classifications and criteria, first the FPG threshold for the diagnosis of diabetes was lowered from 7.8 to 7.0 mol/l, and second, IFG (FPG 6.1–6.9 mol/l) was introduced as a new category for abnormal glucose metabolism, being above "normal" but not diagnostic of diabetes. The ADA [10], but not the WHO [10], recommended that the FPG rather than the OGTT should be the diagnostic test of choice both for clinical and epidemiological purposes. The ADA recommendation was mainly made on the basis of inconvenience of performing the OGTT in clinical practice.

If the purpose of diagnosing intermediate categories of glucose metabolism is to initiate treatment (lifestyle modification or drug therapy) that will reduce the risk of progressing to diabetes, then it is important that IFG identifies either the same subjects as does IGT, or at least a group with a similar risk for progression [15, 16]. From the population perspective, the considerably lower sensitivity of IFG indicates that far fewer cases of diabetes could be prevented by targeting preventive measures on subjects with IFG than could be by targeting IGT subjects [15].

The published data [15, 16] show that IGT has a much higher sensitivity for predicting progression to diabetes than does IFG. This occurs at the cost of only a small reduction in specificity and positive predictive value. Thus, while the new category of IFG may broaden and improve our description of states of intermediate glucose metabolism, it should be seen as complementary to rather than a replacement for IGT [15]. If data from other populations confirm these findings, then screening programs aimed at identifying people at risk of diabetes would lose a considerable amount of information by relying on fasting values alone rather than the OGTT.

This is consistent with the recommendations of the IDF Consensus group [16] who concluded that IGT and IFG differ in their prevalence, population distribution, phenotype, gender distribution, and risk of total mortality and CVD. The workshop findings can be summarized as follows:

(1) The diagnostic thresholds for all categories of impaired glucose regulation should be revisited in light of the latest evidence. There was no clear consensus

(with current evidence) on whether IFG and IGT should be classified as diseases but they clearly represent risk factors and risk markers for diabetes and CVD.

(2) Both IGT and IFG are similarly associated with an increased risk of diabetes but IGT is more strongly associated with CVD outcomes.
(3) Risks are higher when IGT and IFG coexist.
(4) Life style interventions are highly effective in delaying or preventing the onset of diabetes in people with IGT, as are pharmacological agents such as metformin and acarbose. Lifestyle interventions may reduce cardiovascular and total mortality but this requires further studies addressing this issue directly.

Normoglycemia

A fasting venous plasma glucose concentration of less than 6.1 mmol/l (110 mg/dl) has been chosen as "normal" (Table 2). Values above this are associated with progressively greater risks of developing micro- and macrovascular complications [9, 10, 16]. The etiological processes that often lead to diabetes begin and may be recognizable in some subjects who have normal glucose tolerance [9]. Recognition of the pathological process at an early stage may be useful if progression to more advanced stages can be prevented. The new classification includes a stage of normoglycemia in which persons who have evidence of the pathological processes that may lead to diabetes mellitus, or in whom a reversal of the hyperglycemia has occurred, are classified (Figure 1).

THE NEWLY PROPOSED ETIOLOGICAL CLASSIFICATION BASED ON TYPES OF DIABETES

The etiological types listed represent processes or disorders that may result in diabetes mellitus.

Type 1 Process

Type 1 indicates the processes of β-cell destruction that may ultimately lead to diabetes in which "insulin is required for survival" in order to prevent the development of ketoacidosis, coma, and death. This category is composed of the following:

(1) *Immune-mediated diabetes mellitus*: This form of diabetes, previously encompassed by the terms IDDM, type 1 diabetes, or juvenile-onset diabetes, appear to result from a cell-mediated autoimmune destruction of the pancreatic β-cells. The type 1 process is characterized by the presence of ICA, anti-GAD, IA-2, or insulin autoantibodies that identify the autoimmune process associated with β-cell destruction [12]. Other autoimmune disorders such as Grave's disease, Hashimoto's thyroiditis, and Addison's disease may be associated with type 1 diabetes mellitus [12, 17].

The rate of β-cell destruction is quite variable. It can be rapid in children but a slowly progressive form, latent autoimmune diabetes in adults (LADA), is well described in adults [18, 19]. It is recognized that the type 1 process can occur at any age and type 1 diabetes in an adult may masquerade as type 2 diabetes at presentation with a slow deterioration in metabolic control, and subsequent progression to insulin-dependency. We named this phenomenon as LADA [18] and in the new classification, LADA falls within type 1 autoimmune diabetes but in a slowly progressive form.

In some cases of the Type 1 process, there is no evidence of the presence of antibodies and these are classified as type 1 idiopathic (see below).

(2) *Idiopathic*: There are some forms of type 1 diabetes that have no known etiology. Some of these patients have permanent insulinopenia and are prone to ketoacidosis, but have no evidence of autoimmunity [20]. This form is more common among individuals of African and Asian origin [21]. In another form found in Africans, an absolute requirement for insulin replacement therapy in affected patients may fluctuate with time, wax and wane, and patients periodically develop ketoacidosis [21].

Type 2 Process

Type 2 diabetes is the commonest form of diabetes and is characterized by disorders of insulin resistance and insulin secretion, either of which may be the predominant feature. Both are usually present at the time that the diabetes is clinically manifest. The specific reasons for the development of these is not yet known. This form of diabetes mellitus, previously referred to as NIDDM or adult-onset diabetes, is a term used for individuals who have relative (rather than absolute) insulin deficiency. People with type 2 diabetes frequently are resistant to the action of insulin [22].

At least initially, and often throughout their lifetime, these individuals do not need insulin treatment to survive. type 2 diabetes is frequently undiagnosed for many years because the hyperglycemia is often not severe enough to provoke noticeable symptoms of diabetes [23]. Nevertheless, such patients are at increased risk of developing macro- and microvascular complications. This form of diabetes is very heterogeneous with many different causes [24], and it is likely that the number of patients in this category will decrease in the future as identification of specific pathogenic processes and genetic defects permit better differentiation and a more definitive classification. Although the specific etiologies of this form of diabetes are not known, autoimmune destruction of the pancreas

Table 3 Other specific types of diabetes*

Genetic defects of β-cell function
Chromosome 20, HNF-4α (MODY1)
Chromosome 7, glucokinase (MODY2)
Chromosome 12, HNF-1α (MODY3)
Chromosome 13, IPF-1 (MODY4)
Mitochondrial DNA 3243 mutation
Others
Genetic defects in insulin action
Type A insulin resistance
Leprechaunism
Rabson–Mendenhall syndrome
Lipoatrophic diabetes
Others
Diseases of the exocrine pancreas
Fibrocalculous pancreatopathy
Pancreatitis
Trauma/pancreatectomy
Neoplasia
Cystic fibrosis
Hemochromatosis
Others
Endocrinopathies
Cushing's syndrome
Acromegaly
Pheochromocytoma
Glucagonoma
Hyperthyroidism
Somatostatinoma
Others
Drug- or chemical-induced (see Table 4)
Infections
Congenital rubella
Cytomegalovirus
Others
Uncommon forms of immune-mediated diabetes
Insulin autoimmune syndrome (antibodies to insulin)
Anti-insulin receptor antibodies
"Stiff Man" syndrome
Others
Other genetic syndromes (see Table 5)

* Reproduced by permission of WTO [9].

does not occur and patients do not have any other known causes of diabetes as listed in Table 3.

Most patients with the type 2 process of diabetes are obese, and obesity itself causes insulin resistance [25]. Many of those not obese by traditional criteria, e.g. body mass index (BMI), may have an increased percentage of body fat distributed predominantly in the abdominal region [26]. Ketoacidosis seldom occurs in type 2 diabetes and when seen, it usually arises in association with the stress of another illness such as infection. This was described by us as "Flatbush diabetes" [27].

Often, insulin secretion is defective in patients with the type 2 process and insufficient to compensate for the insulin resistance. On the other hand, insulin action is essentially normal in some individuals, but insulin secretion is markedly impaired. Insulin resistance may improve with weight reduction, increased physical activity, and/or pharmacologic treatment of hyperglycemia, but it is not restored to normal [28, 29].

The risk of developing type 2 diabetes increases with age, obesity, and lack of physical activity [30]. It occurs more frequently in women with prior GDM, in those with hypertension or dyslipidemia, and its frequency varies in different ethnic subgroups [9, 30, 31]. type 2 diabetes is often associated with strong familial, likely genetic, predisposition but the genetics of type 2 diabetes are quite complex and not clearly defined [24]. Some patients who present a clinical picture consistent of type 2 diabetes have been shown to have antibodies similar to those found in type 1 diabetes [19]. As described above, this form known as LADA, may masquerade as type 2 diabetes if antibody determinations are not made.

Although diagnosis in most patients with type 2 diabetes is made in adult years, the disease also occurs in young persons who do not require insulin and are not ketotic, and hence could not be considered to have the type 1 process [32]. In addition, the age at diagnosis of type 2 diabetes now tends to occur much earlier in high prevalence groups such as North American Indians and Pacific Islanders. Consequently, age at onset is not recommended as a criterion by which to determine whether a patient should be classified as having type 2 diabetes, and the previously used terms *adult-onset* and *maturity-onset diabetes* have been abandoned [9].

Other Specific Types

The other specific types are less common, but are those in which the underlying defect or disease process can be identified, in a relatively specific manner, particularly those where a monogenic defect has been identified, e.g., in maturity-onset diabetes of the young (MODY) [33, 34]. These include identified genetic, exocrine pancreatic, endocrine, and drug-induced causes [9]. A more comprehensive breakdown is provided in Table 3.

Genetic Defects of β-Cell Function

The diabetic state may be associated with monogenetic defects in β-cell function. These forms are characterized by onset of mild hyperglycemia at an early age (generally <25 years). They are inherited in an autosomal dominant pattern. Patients with these forms of diabetes, formerly referred to as MODY, have impaired insulin secretion with minimal or no defect in insulin action [34]. Abnormalities at a number of gene loci on different chromosomes have been identified to date. The most common form is associated with mutations on chromosome 12 in a hepatic transcription factor referred to as hepatocyte nuclear factor 1α (HNF-1α) [35]. A second form is associated with mutations in the glucokinase gene on chromosome 7p [33, 36] and results in a reduction in glucokinase. Glucokinase converts glucose to glucose-6-phosphate, the metabolism of which in turn stimulates insulin secretion by the β-cell. Thus, glucokinase serves as the "glucose sensor" for the β-cell. Because of defects in the glucokinase gene, increased levels of glucose are necessary to elicit normal levels of insulin secretion. A mutation in the HNF-4α gene on chromosome 20q characterizes the third form [37]. HNF-4α is a transcription factor that is involved in the regulation of the expression of HNF-12. A fourth variant has recently been described to mutations in another transcription factor gene, IPF-1, which in its homozygous form leads to total pancreatic agenesis [38]. Specific genetic defects in other individuals who have a similar clinical presentation are currently being investigated.

In addition, point mutations in mitochondrial DNA have been found to be associated with deafness [34, 39]. The most common mutation occurs at position 3243 in the tRNA leucine gene, leading to an A → G substitution. An identical lesion occurs in the MELAS syndrome (mitochondrial myopathy, encephalopathy, lactic acidosis, and stroke-like syndrome). Diabetes is not part of this syndrome and this suggests that there is different phenotypic expressions of this genetic lesion [40].

Genetic abnormalities that result in the inability to convert proinsulin to insulin have been identified in a few families. Usually such traits are inherited in an autosomal dominant pattern [41, 42] and the resultant carbohydrate intolerance is mild. Mutant insulin molecules with impaired receptor binding have been identified in a few families. These are also associated with autosomal dominant inheritance and either normal or only mildly impaired carbohydrate metabolism [42].

Genetic Defects in Insulin Action

These causes of diabetes are unusual and result from genetically determined abnormalities of insulin action. The metabolic abnormalities associated with mutations of the insulin receptor may range from hyperinsulinemia and modest hyperglycemia to severe symptomatic diabetes [43, 44]. Acanthosis nigricans may be present in some of these individuals. Women may have virilization and have enlarged cystic ovaries. This syndrome was termed *type A insulin resistance* in the past [45]. Two pediatric syndromes that have mutations in the insulin receptor gene with subsequent alterations in insulin receptor function and extreme insulin resistance are called leprechaunism and the Rabson–Mendenhall syndrome [46]. Leprechaunism has characteristic facial features while the Rabson–Mendenhall syndrome is associated with abnormalities of teeth, nails, and pineal gland hyperplasia. In patients with insulin-resistant lipoatrophic diabetes, alterations in the structure and function of the insulin receptor cannot be demonstrated. Therefore it is assumed that the lesion(s) must reside in the postreceptor signal transduction pathways.

Diseases of the Exocrine Pancreas

Pancreatitis, trauma, infection, pancreatic carcinoma, and pancreatectomy are some of the acquired processes of the pancreas that can cause diabetes. Any process that diffusely injures the pancreas may cause diabetes [47, 48]. With the exception of cancer, damage to the pancreas must be extensive for diabetes to occur. However, adenocarcinomas that involve only a small portion of the pancreas have been associated with diabetes. This implies a mechanism other than solely reduction in β-cell mass [49]. Depending on their extension, cystic fibrosis and hemochromatosis will also damage β-cells and impair insulin secretion [50, 51]. Fibrocalculous pancreatopathy may be accompanied by abdominal pain radiating to the back, pancreatic calcification on X-ray, and ductal dilatation (see Chapter 29). Pancreatic fibrosis and calcified stones in the exocrine ducts are found at autopsy [52].

Endocrinopathies

Insulin action can be antagonized by several hormones (e.g. growth hormone, cortisol, glucagon, and epinephrine). Diseases associated with excess secretion of these hormones can cause diabetes (e.g. acromegaly, Cushing's syndrome, glucagonoma, and phaechromocytoma) [9, 53]. These forms of hyperglycemia resolve when the hormone excess is removed. Somatostinoma and aldosteronoma-induced hypokalemia can cause diabetes at least in part by inhibiting insulin secretion [54, 55]. Hyperglycemia generally resolves following successful removal of the tumor.

Drug- or Chemical-induced Diabetes

Insulin secretion may be impaired by many drugs. They may not, by themselves, cause diabetes but may precipitate diabetes in persons with insulin resistance [56, 57]. Classification is ambiguous in such cases as the primacy of β-cell destruction or insulin resistance is unknown. Pancreatic β-cell destruction may occur with the use of certain toxins such as Vacor (a rat poison) [58] and pentamidine [59]. There are also many drugs and hormones that can impair insulin action. The list shown in Table 4 is not all-inclusive, but reflects the more commonly recognized drug-, hormone-, or toxin-induced forms of diabetes and hyperglycemia.

Table 4 Drug- or chemical-induced diabetes*

Nicotinic acid
Glucocorticoids
Thyroid hormone
α-Adrenergic agonists
β-Adrenergic agonists
Thiazides
Dilantin
Pentamidine
Vacor
Interferon α therapy
Others

* Reproduced by permission of WTO [9].

Infections

Certain viruses have been associated with β-cell destruction. Diabetes occurs in some patients with congenital rubella [60]. Coxsackie B, cytomegalovirus, and other viruses (e.g. adenovirus and mumps) have been implicated in inducing diabetes [61–63].

Uncommon but Specific Forms of Immune-mediated Diabetes Mellitus

Diabetes may be associated with several immunological diseases with a pathogenesis or etiology different from that which leads to the type 1 diabetes process. Postprandial hyperglycemia of a severity sufficient to fulfill the criteria for diabetes has been reported in rare individuals who spontaneously develop insulin autoantibodies. However, these individuals generally present with symptoms of hypoglycemia rather than hyperglycemia [64]. The *stiff man syndrome* is an autoimmune disorder of the central nervous system, characterized by stiffness of the axial muscles with painful spasms. Affected people usually have high titers of anti-GAD and approximately one-third to half will develop type 1 diabetes [65]. Patients receiving interferon alpha have been reported to develop diabetes associated with islet cell autoantibodies and, in certain instances, severe insulin deficiency [66].

Anti-insulin receptor antibodies can cause diabetes by binding to the insulin receptor, thereby reducing the binding of insulin to target tissues [67]. However, these antibodies can also act as an insulin agonist after binding to the receptor and can thereby cause hypoglycemia [68]. Anti-insulin receptor antibodies are occasionally found in patients with systemic lupus erythematosus and other autoimmune diseases [69]. As in other states of extreme insulin resistance, patients with anti-insulin receptor antibodies often have acanthosis nigricans. In the past, this syndrome was termed *type B insulin resistance*.

Other Genetic Syndromes Associated with Diabetes

Many genetic syndromes are accompanied by an increased incidence of diabetes mellitus. These include the chromosomal abnormalities of Down syndrome, Klinefelter's syndrome, and Turner's syndrome. Wolfram's syndrome is an autosomal recessive disorder characterized by insulin-deficient diabetes and the absence of β-cells at autopsy [70]. Additional manifestations include diabetes insipidus, hypogonadism, optic atrophy, and neural deafness. These and other similar disorders are listed in Table 5.

Gestational Diabetes Mellitus

Gestational diabetes is carbohydrate intolerance resulting in hyperglycemia of variable severity with onset or first recognition during pregnancy. The definition applies irrespective of whether or not insulin is used for treatment or the condition persists after pregnancy. It does not exclude the possibility that the glucose intolerance may antedate pregnancy but has been previously unrecognized [9, 10].

Women who become pregnant and who are known to have diabetes that antedates pregnancy do not have gestational diabetes but have "diabetes mellitus and pregnancy" and should be treated accordingly before, during, and after the pregnancy [9, 10].

Fasting and postprandial glucose concentrations are normally lower in the early part of pregnancy (e.g. first trimester and first half of second trimester) than in normal, nonpregnant women. Elevated fasting or postprandial plasma glucose levels at this time in pregnancy may well reflect the presence of diabetes that has antedated pregnancy, but criteria for designating abnormally high glucose concentrations at this time have not yet been established. The occurrence of higher than normal plasma glucose levels at this time in pregnancy mandates careful management and may be an indication for carrying out an OGTT. Nevertheless, normal glucose tolerance in the early part of pregnancy does not itself establish that gestational diabetes may not develop later.

Individuals at high risk for gestational diabetes include older women, those with previous history of glucose intolerance, those with a history of large for gestational age babies, women from ethnic groups with a high risk of

Table 5 Other genetic syndromes sometimes associated with diabetes

Down syndrome
Friedreich's ataxia
Huntington's chorea
Klinefelter's syndrome
Lawrence–Moon–Biedel syndrome
Myotonic dystrophy
Porphyria
Prader–Willi syndrome
Turner's syndrome
Wolfram's syndrome
Others

diabetes (e.g. Hispanic American, Native American, Asian American, African American, Pacific islander) [30], and any pregnant woman who has elevated fasting, or casual, blood glucose levels [9, 10] that are not in the diabetic range. It may be appropriate to screen pregnant women belonging to high-risk populations during the first trimester of pregnancy in order to detect previously undiagnosed diabetes. Formal systematic testing for gestational diabetes is usually done between 24 and 28 weeks of gestation [9].

If a woman has been determined to have gestational diabetes, she should be reclassified 6 weeks or more after pregnancy as having diabetes, IFG, IGT, or normal glucose tolerance. Although the majority of patients will have glucose levels that return to normal, the lifetime risk for glycemic disorders is substantially increased in women who have had gestational diabetes.

The final word with respect to the classification of diabetes may still be coming, and neither the ADA nor the WHO Expert groups have discounted this possibility. As the research into diabetes is a continuing and dynamic process, and epidemiological and clinical studies are in progress, there undoubtedly will be revision and refinement of the classification system, especially as more knowledge emerges about the etiology of type 2 diabetes process.

REFERENCES

1. Harris M, Zimmet P. Classification of diabetes mellitus and other categories of glucose intolerance. In Alberti KGMM, Zimmet P, DeFronzo RA, Keen H (eds) *International Textbook of Diabetes Mellitus*, 2nd edn. Chichester: Wiley, 1985; pp 9–23.
2. Himsworth HP. Diabetes mellitus: its differentiation into insulin-sensitive and insulin-insensitive types. *Lancet* 1936; i: 117–9.
3. Bornstein J, Lawrence RD. Plasma insulin in human diabetes mellitus. *Br Med J* 1951; 2: 1541–4.
4. Berson SA, Yalow RS. Antigens in insulin determinants of specificity of porcine insulin in man. *Science* 1963; 139: 844–5.
5. WHO Expert Committee. *Diabetes Mellitus First Report*. Technical Report Series 310. Geneva: WHO, 1965.
6. National Diabetes Data Group. Classification and diagnosis of diabetes mellitus and other categories of glucose intolerance. *Diabetes* 1979; 28: 1039–57.
7. World Health Organization. *Second Report of the WHO Expert Committee on Diabetes Mellitus*. Technical Report Series 646. Geneva: WHO, 1980.
8. World Health Organization. *Diabetes Mellitus, Report of a WHO Study Group*. Technical Report Series 727. Geneva: WHO, 1985.
9. World Health Organization. *Definition, Diagnosis and Classification of Diabetes Mellitus and its Complications Report of a WHO Consultation, Part 1: Diagnosis and Classification of Diabetes Mellitus*. Geneva. WHO, 1999.
10. American Diabetes Association. Report of the expert committee on the diagnosis and classification of diabetes mellitus. *Diabetes Care* 1997; 20: 1183–97.
11. Kuzuya T, Matsuda A Classification of diabetes on the basis of etiologies versus degree of insulin deficiency. *Diabetes Care* 1997; 20: 1185–97.
12. Atkinson MA, Maclaren NK. The pathogenesis of insulin-dependent diabetes mellitus. *New Engl J Med* 1994; 331: 1428–36.
13. Nathan DM. Initial management of glycemia in type 2 diabetes mellitus *New Engl J Med* 2002; 347: 1342–9.
14. Zimmet P. Diabetes epidemiology as a trigger to diabetes research. *Diabetologia* 1999; 42: 499–518.
15. Shaw JE, Zimmet PZ, de Courten M, Dowse GK, Chitson P, Gareeboo H, Hemraj F, Fareed D, Tuomilehto J, Alberti KGMM. Impaired fasting glucose or impaired glucose tolerance: what best predicts future diabetes in Mauritius? *Diabetes Care* 1999; 22: 399–402.
16. Unwin N, Shaw J, Zimmet P, Alberti G. International Diabetes Federation IGT/IFG Consensus Statement. Report of an Expert Consensus Workshop 1–4 August 2001, Stoke Poges, UK. *Diabet Med* 2002; 19: 708–23.
17. Betterle C, Zanette F, Pedini B, Presotto F, Rap LB, Monsciotti CM, Rigon F. Clinical and subclinical organ-specific autoimmune manifestations in type 1 (insulin-dependent) diabetic patients and their first-degree relatives. *Diabetologia* 1983; 26: 431–36.
18. Tuomi T, Groop LC, Zimmet PZ, Rowley MJ, Knowles W, Mackay IR. Antibodies to glutamic acid decarboxylase reveal latent autoimmune diabetes mellitus in adults with a non-insulin-dependent onset of disease. *Diabetes* 1993; 42: 358–62.
19. Zimmet P, Turner R, McCarty D, Rowley M, Mackay IR. Crucial points at diagnosis—NIDDM or slow IDDM. *Diabetes Care* 1999; 22 (suppl 2): B59-64.
20. McLarty DG, Athaide I, Bottazzo GF, Swai ABM, Alberti KGMM. Islet cell antibodies are not specifically associated with insulin-dependent diabetes in rural Tanzanian Africans. *Diabetes Res Clin Pract* 1990; 9: 219–24.
21. Ahrén B, Corrigan CB. Intermittent need for insulin in a subgroup of diabetic patients in Tanzania. *Diabet Med* 1984; 2: 262–64.
22. DeFronzo RA, Bonadonna RC, Ferrannini E. Pathogenesis of NIDDM. In Alberti KGMM, Zimmet P, DeFronzo RA (eds) *International Textbook of Diabetes Mellitus*, 2nd edn. Chichester: Wiley, 1997; pp 635–712.
23. Harris MI, Klein R, Welborn TA, Knuiman MW. Onset of NIDDM occurs at least 4–7 yr before clinical diagnosis. *Diabetes Care* 1992; 15: 815–19.
24. Groop L. The molecular genetics of non-insulin dependent diabetes mellitus. *J Intern Med* 1997; 241: 95–110.
25. Bogardus C, Lillioja S, Mott DM, Hollenbeck C, Reaven G. Relationship between degree of obesity and in vivo insulin action in man. *Am J Physiol* 1985; 248: E286–91.
26. Kissebah AH, Vydelingum N, Murray R, Evans DF, Hartz AJ, Kalkhoff RK, Adams PW. Relationship of body fat distribution to metabolic complications of obesity. *J Clin Endocrinol Metab* 1982; 54: 254–60.
27. Banerji MA, Chaiken RI, Huey H, Tuomi T, Norin AJ, MacKay IR, Rowley MJ, Zimmet PZ, Lebovitz HE. GAD antibody negative NIDDM in adult black subjects with diabetic ketoacidosis and increased frequency of human leukocyte antigen DR3 and DR4: Flatbush diabetes. *Diabetes* 1994; 43: 741–45.
28. Simonson DC, Ferrannini E, Bevilacqua S, Smith D, Barrett E, Carlson R, Defronzo RA. Mechanism of improvement in glucose metabolism after chronic glyburide therapy. *Diabetes* 1984; 33: 838–45.
29. Wing RR, Blair EH, Bononi P, Marcus MD, Watanabe R, Bergman RN. Caloric restriction per

se is a significant factor in improvements in glycemic control and insulin sensitivity during weight loss in obese NIDDM patients. *Diabetes Care* 1994; 17: 30–6.

30. de Courten M, Bennett PH, Tuomilehto J, Zimmet P. Epidemiology of NIDDM in non-Europids. In Alberti KGMM, Zimmet P, DeFronzo RA (eds) *International Textbook of Diabetes Mellitus*, 2nd edn. Chichester: Wiley, 1997; pp 143–70.
31. Valle T, Tuomilehto J, Eriksson J. Epidemiology of NIDDM in Europids. In Alberti KGMM, Zimmet P, DeFronzo RA (eds) *International Textbook of Diabetes Mellitus*, 2nd edn. Chichester: Wiley, 1997; pp 125–42.
32. Zimmet P, Alberti KGMM, Shaw J. Global and societal implications of the diabetes epidemic. *Nature* 2001; 414: 782–7.
33. Froguel P, Vaxillaire M, Sun F, Velho G, Zouali H, Butel MO, Lesage S, Vionnet N, Clement K, Fougerousse F, et al. Close linkage of glucokinase locus on chromosome 7p to early-onset non-insulin-dependent diabetes. *Nature* 1992; 356: 162–4.
34. Hattersley AT. Maturity-onset diabetes of the young: clinical heterogeneity explained by genetic heterogeneity. *Diabet Med* 1998; 15: 15–24.
35. Yamagata K, Oda N, Kaisaki PJ, Menzel S, Furuta H, Vaxillaire M, Southam L, Cox RD, Lathrop GM, Boriraj VV, Chen X, Cox NJ, Oda Y, Yano H, Le Beau MM, Yamada S, Nighigori H, Takeda J, Fajans SS, Hattersley AT, Iwasaki N, Hansen T, Pedersen O, Polonsky KS, Bell GI, et al. Mutations in the hepatocyte nuclear factor-1α gene in maturity-onset diabetes of the young (MODY 3). *Nature* 1996; 384: 455–8.
36. Vionnet N, Stoffel M, Takeda J, Yasuda K, Bell GI, Zouali H, Lesage S, Velho G, Iris S, Passa PH, Froguel PH, Cohen D. Nonsense mutation in the glucokinase gene causes early-onset non-insulin-dependent diabetes. *Nature* 1992; 356: 721–2.
37. Yamagata K, Furuta H, Oda N, Kaisaki PJ, Menzel S, Cox NJ, Fajans SS, Signorini S, Stoffel M, Bell GI. Mutations in the hepatocyte nuclear factor-4α gene in maturity-onset diabetes of the young (MODY 1). *Nature* 1996; 384: 458–60.
38. Stoffers DA, Ferrer J, Clarke WL, Habener JF. Early-onset type-II diabetes mellitus (MODY 4) linked to IPF1. *Nat Genet* 1997; 117: 138–9.
39. Walker M, Turnbull DM. Mitochondrial related diabetes: a clinical perspective. *Diabet Med* 1997; 14: 1007–9.
40. Johns DR. Mitochondrial DNA and disease. *N Engl J Med* 1995; 333: 638–44.
41. Gruppuso PA, Gorden P, Kahn CR, Cornblath M, Zeller WP, Schwartz R. Familial hyperproinsulinemia due to a proposed defect in conversion of proinsulin to insulin. *N Engl J Med* 1984; 311: 629–34.
42. Robbins DC, Shoelson SE, Rubenstein AH, Tager HS. Familial hyperproinsulinemia: two cohorts secreting indistinguishable type II intermediates of proinsulin conversion. *J Clin Invest* 1984; 73: 714–9.
43. Haneda M, Polonsky KS, Bergenstal RM, Jaspan JB, Shoelson SE, Blix PM, Chan SJ, Kwok SC, Wishner WB, Zeidler A, Olefsky JM, Freidenberg G, Tager HS, Steiner DF, Rubinstein AH. Familial hyperinsulinemia due to a structurally abnormal insulin. Definition of an emerging new clinical syndrome. *N Engl J Med* 1984; 310: 1288–94.
44. Sanz N, Karam JH, Horita S, Bell GI. Prevalence of insulin-gene mutations in non-insulin-dependent diabetes mellitus. *N Engl J Med* 1986; 314: 1322–3.
45. Kahn CR, Flier JS, Bar RS, Archer JA, Gorden P, Martin MM, Roth J. The syndromes of insulin resistance and acanthosis nigricans. *N Engl J Med* 1976; 294: 739–45.
46. Taylor SI. Lilly Lecture. Molecular mechanisms of insulin resistance: lessons from patients with mutations in the insulin-receptor gene. *Diabetes* 1992; 41: 1473–90.
47. Gullo L, Pezzilli, R, Morselli-Labate AM, and the Italian Pancreatic Cancer Study Group. Diabetes and the risk of pancreatic cancer. *N Engl J Med* 1994; 331: 81–4.
48. Larsen S, Hilsted J, Tronier B, Worning H. Metabolic control and β-cell function in patients with insulin-dependent diabetes mellitus secondary to chronic pancreatitis. *Metabolism* 1987; 36: 964–7.
49. Permert J, Larsson J. Westermark GT, Herrington MK, Christmanson L, Pour PM, Westermark P, Adrian TE. Islet amyloid polypeptide in patients with pancreatic cancer and diabetes. *N Engl J Med* 1994; 330: 313–8.
50. Moran A, Pyzdrowski KL, Weinreb J, Khan BB, Smith SA, Adams KS, Seaquist ER. Insulin sensitivity in cystic fibrosis. *Diabetes* 1994; 43: 1020–6.
51. Phelps G, Chapman I, Hall P, Braund W, Mackinnon M. Prevalence of genetic haemochromatosis among diabetic patients. *Lancet* 1989; ii: 233–4.
52. Yajnik CS, Shelgikar KM, Naik SS, Kanitkar SV, Orskov H, Alberti KGMM, Hockaday TDR. The ketoacidosis-resistance in fibro-calculous-pancreatic-diabetes. *Diabetes Res Clin Pract* 1992; 15: 149–56.
53. MacFarlane IA. Endocrine diseases and diabetes mellitus. In Pickup JC, Williams G (eds) *Textbook of Diabetes,* 2nd edn. Oxford: Blackwell, 1997; pp 1–64.
54. Krejs GJ, Orci L, Conlon JM, Ravazzola M, Davis GR, Raskin P, Collins SM, McCarthy DM, Baetens D, Rubinstein A, Aldor TA, Unger RH. Somatostatinoma syndrome. *N Engl J Med* 1979; 301: 285–92.
55. Conn JW. Hypertension, the potassium ion and impaired carbohydrate tolerance. *N Engl J Med* 1965; 273: 1135–43.
56. Pandit MK, Burke J, Gustafson AB, Minocha A, Peiris AN. Drug-induced disorders of glucose tolerance. *Ann Intern Med* 1993; 118: 529–40.
57. O' Byrne S, Feely J. Effects of drugs on glucose tolerance in non-insulin-dependent diabetes (parts 1 and II). *Drugs* 1990; 40: 203–19.
58. Karam JH, Lewitt PA, Young CW, Nowlain RE, Frankel BJ, Fujiya H, Freedman ZR, Grodsky GM. Insulinopenic diabetes after rodenticide (Vacor) ingestion: a unique model of acquired diabetes in man. *Diabetes* 1980; 29: 971–8.
59. Assan R, Perronne C, Assan D, Chotard L, Mayaud C, Matheron S, Zucman D. Pentamidine-induced derangements of glucose homeostasis. *Diabetes Care* 1995; 18: 47–55.
60. Forrest JA, Menser MA, Burgess JA. High frequency of diabetes mellitus in young patients with congenital rubella. *Lancet* 1971; ii: 332–4.
61. King ML, Bidwell D, Shaikh A, Voller A, Banatvala JE. Coxsackie-B-virus-specific IgM responses in children with insulin-dependent (juvenile-onset; type 1) diabetes mellitus. *Lancet* 1983; i: 1397–9.
62. Karjalainen J, Knip M, Hyoty H, Linikki P, Ilonen J, Kaar M-L, Akerblom HK. Relationship between serum insulin antibodies, islet cell antibodies and Coxsackie-B4

and mumps virus-specific antibodies at the clinical manifestation of type 1 (insulin-dependent) diabetes. *Diabetologia* 1988; 31: 146–52.

63. Pak CY, Eun H, McArthur RG, Yoon J. Association of cytomegalovirus infection with autoimmune type 1 diabetes. *Lancet* 1988; ii: 1–4.
64. Hirata Y, Ishizu H, Ouchi N, et al. Insulin autoimmunity in a case of spontaneous hypoglycaemia. *J Jpn Diabet Soc* 1970; 13: 312–20.
65. Solimena M, De Camilli P. Autoimmunity to glutamic acid decarboxylase (GAD) in Stiff-Man syndrome and insulin-dependent diabetes mellitus. *Trends Neurosci* 1991; 14: 452–7.
66. Fabris P, Betterle C, Floreani A, Greggio NA, de Lazzari F, Naccarato R, Chiaramonte M. Development of type 1 diabetes mellitus during interferon alfa therapy for chronic HCV hepatitis [letter]. *Lancet* 1992; 340: 548.
67. Flier JS. Lilly Lecture. Syndromes of insulin resistance: from patient to gene and back again. *Diabetes* 1992; 41: 1207–19.
68. Khan CR, Baird KL, Flier JS, Jarrett DB. Effects of autoantibodies to the insulin receptor on isolated adipocytes. *J Clin Invest* 1977; 60: 1094–106.
69. Tsokos GC, Gorden P, Antonovych T, Wilson CB, Balow JE. Lupus nephritis and other autoimmune features in patients with diabetes mellitus due to autoantibody to insulin receptors. *Ann Intern Med* 1985; 102: 176–81.
70. Barrett TG, Bundey SE, Macleod AF. Neurodegeneration and diabetes: UK nationwide study of Wolfram (DIDMOAD) syndrome. *Lancet* 1995; 346; 1458–63.

This chapter is based in part on a chapter of the same title which was published in an earlier edition of the *International Textbook of Diabetes Mellitus*, by Maureen I. Harris and Paul Zimmet.

2

Epidemiology and Geography of Type 1 Diabetes Mellitus

Andrea K. Steck and Marian J. Rewers

University of Colorado Health Sciences Center, Denver, CO, USA

INTRODUCTION

Type 1 diabetes is one of the most prevalent severe chronic disease of childhood, affecting approximately 1.4 million people in the United States and 10–20 million people globally [1–3]. In the United States, where 30 000 new cases occur each year, 1:300 children and 1:100 adults are diagnosed with type 1 diabetes during the life span [4]. Type 1 diabetes is the leading cause of end-stage renal disease, blindness, and amputation, and a major cause of cardiovascular disease and premature death in the general population [5]. The economic impact of diabetes is large, with an annual average total direct cost of medical care in the United States in 1997 of $10 071 per person with diabetes compared to $2669 per person without diabetes [6]. These expenditures include all types of diabetes and are likely to underestimate type 1 diabetes related costs. The incidence of type 1 diabetes appears to be increasing by 3–5% per year [7, 8]. The high incidence, associated severe morbidity, mortality, and associated health care expenditures [9, 10] make type 1 diabetes a prime target for prevention. Population-based epidemiological studies as well as family studies and clinical trials have provided new insights into the pathogenesis and natural history of type 1 diabetes. Such studies are essential for appropriate diagnosis and for evidence-based programs of prevention and treatment.

Classification of Diabetes

The new classification of diabetes, revised by the American Diabetes Association and the World Health Organization [11, 12], is now primarily based on pathogenesis rather than on the requirement for insulin therapy (for details see Chapter 1). The current classification of diabetes mellitus distinguishes four types; however the vast majority of cases belong to type 1A or type 2 categories.

Type 1 diabetes is caused by β-cell destruction, usually leading to absolute insulin deficiency. Type 1A, previously defined as insulin-dependent or juvenile-onset diabetes, results from a cellular-mediated autoimmune destruction of the β-cells of the pancreas. Type 1B diabetes, also called idiopathic type 1 diabetes, includes cases that are not immune mediated, but also characterized by absolute insulin deficiency (insulinopenia). Type 2 diabetes, previously referred to as non-insulin-dependent diabetes or adult-onset diabetes, includes cases characterized by insulin resistance and insulin deficiency (often relative rather than absolute).

Type 1A is the most common form of diabetes among children and adolescents of European origin, usually characterized by acute onset and dependence on exogenous insulin for survival. In adults, the disease is nearly as frequent as in children, but often less dramatic onset may lead to misclassification as type 2 and a delayed insulin treatment. About 60% of persons with type 1 diabetes are diagnosed as adults.

Type 1B Diabetes

According to the recent American Diabetes Association classification, type 1 diabetic patients who do not show evidence of humoral islet autoimmunity at disease onset are referred to as idiopathic (type 1B) diabetic subjects. This heterogeneous group is responsible for 3–40% of type 1

International Textbook of Diabetes Mellitus, Third Edition. Edited by R. A. DeFronzo, E. Ferrannini, H. Keen, and P. Zimmet.
 ISBN: 0-471-48655-8.

diabetes [13, 14], depending on classification and countries: in Caucasians, only a small number of patients seem to have type 1B diabetes [15], whereas the incidence is much higher in Japan, which interestingly is one of the countries with the lowest incidence of childhood type 1 diabetes in the world [16, 17]. Idiopathic type 1 diabetes has been further divided into at least two subgroups, both of which are characterized by absence of insulitis and absence of diabetes-related autoantibodies [16]. The nonautoimmune nonfulminant type 1 diabetes has a relatively slow progression of β-cell loss after the onset of diabetes. The nonautoimmune fulminant type 1 diabetes is characterized by lymphocytic infiltration in the exocrine pancreatic tissue, elevated serum pancreatic enzyme levels, and a remarkably aggressive course of disease [17, 18]. A study in Japan also showed that patients with type 1B diabetes were significantly younger at diagnosis, displayed more severe metabolic decompensation, and had a higher frequency of preceding viral infection before onset compared to those with type 1A diabetes [14].

NATURAL HISTORY OF TYPE 1A DIABETES

The natural history of type 1A diabetes (Figure 1) includes four distinct stages:

(1) preclinical β-cell autoimmunity with progressive defect of insulin secretion;
(2) onset of clinical diabetes;
(3) transient remission; and
(4) established diabetes associated with acute and chronic complications and premature death.

β-Cell Autoimmunity

Type 1A diabetes results from a chronic autoimmune destruction of the pancreatic β-cells, probably initiated by exposure of a genetically susceptible individual to environmental agent(s). This preclinical period is marked by the presence of autoantibodies to pancreatic β-cell antigens such as insulin, GAD65 (glutamic acid decarboxylase), or ICA512 (called also IA-2), and precedes the onset of hyperglycemia by a few years. Several prospective studies have reported that these autoantibodies can appear early in childhood and the presence of two or more of these antibodies is highly predictive for the development of diabetes [20, 21]. However, the etiology of the autoimmune process and β-cell destruction is not known. The islet cell antibody (ICA) assay using immunofluorescence and pancreatic tissue has been notoriously difficult to standardize and has been replaced by a combination of radioassays for autoantobodies to insulin [22–24], GAD [25, 26], and IA-2 [27]. These tests have been shown to be quite sensitive and predictive in relatives of type 1 diabetic patients [20] and in the general population [21]. Several prospective cohort studies investigate early genetic and environmental factors contributing to risk of β-cell autoimmunity and progression to diabetes in relatives of patients with type 1A diabetes and in a general newborn population [28–31].

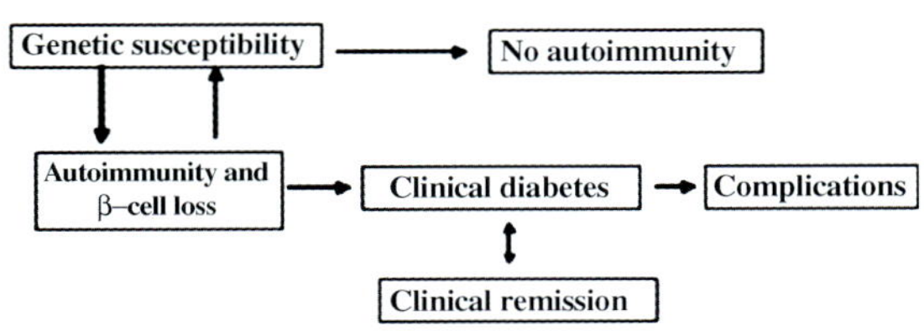

Figure 1 Natural history of type 1A diabetes (reproduced with permission from reference 19)

Progression from β-Cell Autoimmunity to Clinical Diabetes

The duration of preclinical β-cell autoimmunity is variable and precedes the diagnosis of diabetes by up to 13 years [32, 33]. In persons with persistent autoantibodies, there is an early loss of spontaneous pulsatile insulin secretion, progressive reduction in the acute insulin response to intravenous glucose load, followed by decreased response to other β-cell secretagogues, impaired oral glucose tolerance, and fasting hyperglycemia [34].

Studies in first-degree relatives of type 1 diabetic patients [33, 35, 36] and in school children with no family history of type 1 diabetes [37–39] have reported ICA "remission" rates between 10 and 78%. Newer data suggest that while individual islet-specific autoantibodies may fluctuate in titers, it is very unusual to observe remission after two or more of such autoantibodies were present for even a few months. Age also plays a role, because children younger than 10 years have a threefold increased risk of progressing from autoimmunity to type 1 diabetes compared to older relatives [40].

Markers of autoimmunity can be detected in 14–33% of diabetic patients classified on clinical grounds as "type 2" [41, 42] and are associated with early failure of oral hypoglycemic drug therapy and insulin dependence in these patients. A term "latent autoimmune diabetes of adults" (LADA) [43] has been coined for this slowly progressive form of type 1 diabetes.

CLINICAL ONSET OF TYPE 1 DIABETES

In industrialized countries, 20–40% of type 1 diabetic patients younger than 20 years present with diabetic ketoacidosis [44–47]. Younger age, female gender, HLA-DR4 allele [48], lower socioeconomical status, and lack of family history of diabetes have been associated with more severe presentation. Younger children present with more severe symptoms at diagnosis, because children younger than 7 years old have lost on average 80% of the islets compared to 60% in those 7–14 years old and 40% in those older than 14 years old [49]. Case fatality in industrialized countries ranges between 0.4 and 0.9% [50]. Both diabetic ketoacidosis and onset death are largely preventable, because most of the patients have typical symptoms of polyuria, polydipsia, and weight loss 2–4 weeks prior to diagnosis. The diagnosis is straightforward in almost all cases, based on the symptoms, random blood glucose over 200 mg/dl, and/or $HbA_{1c} > 7\%$.

Traditionally, nearly all children with newly diagnosed type 1 diabetes were hospitalized. More recently, increasing proportion of children with new-onset diabetes have been managed on an outpatient basis, especially in urban centers with specialized diabetes education and treatment facilities. In Colorado, USA, the proportion of children receiving only outpatient care at diabetes diagnosis increased from 6% in 1978 to 35% in 1988 [51]. Hospitalization at onset does not improve short-term outcomes such as readmission for diabetic ketoacidosis or severe hypoglycemia [44, 47] if adequate family education and follow-up is available on outpatient basis.

The SEARCH for Diabetes in Youth Study is a project sponsored by the Centers for Disease Control to understand the occurrence, classification, progression of diabetes and care patterns in childhood. Six centers in the United States are establishing registries of youth who develop diabetes, by identifying all children who develop diabetes before the age of 20 years.

Prevalence of Type 1 Diabetes

The prevalence of type 1 diabetes, that is the proportion of people in the population who have the disease at a given point in time, is determined not only by disease incidence but also by case survival, which may vary markedly in populations.

The prevalence of β-cell autoimmunity appears to be roughly proportional to the incidence of type 1 diabetes in different population. In contrast, the prevalence of β-cell autoimmunity in first-degree relatives of type 1 diabetic persons does not differ a lot between high- and low-risk countries for type 1 diabetes. The prevalence of type 1 diabetes in children aged less than 15 years ranges from 0.05 to 0.3% in most European and North American populations (1). Selected estimates of type 1 diabetes prevalence in different populations with at least 90% ascertainment of cases are shown in Table 1.

Incidence of Type 1 Diabetes

Incidence is the rate at which new cases of disease appear in the population and is usually expressed as the annual number of new cases per 100 000 persons. Incidence of type 1 diabetes varies by geographic location, ethnicity, age, gender, and time. The incidence of type 1 diabetes is increasing worldwide both in low- and high-incidence populations. By the year 2010 the incidence will be 50/100 000 a year in Finland and will exceed 30/100 000 a year in many other populations [8].

Table 1 Prevalence of childhood type 1 diabetes, 1977–1993

Location	Year of study	Age (years)	Prevalence (per 100 000)
Europe			
Estonia	1988	0–14	60
Finland	1979	0–14	191
Iceland	1979	0–14	45
	1989	0–14	57
Leicester, UK	1984–1985	0–14	99
Scotland	1993	0–14	150
Sweden	1977	0–14	300
United States			
Colorado	1981	0–14	170
Kentucky	1978–1979	0–17	208
North Dakota	1983	0–18	130
Oceania			
Canterbury, New Zealand	1986	0–19	105
Tasmania, Australia	1984	0–14	57

Geographic Location

One of the most striking characteristics of type 1 diabetes is the large geographic variability in the incidence [52–54] (Figure 2). The incidence rates of type 1 diabetes vary from 0.1/100 000 per year in China and Venezuela to 36.8 and 36.5/100 000 per year in Sardinia and Finland respectively. A child in Finland is 400 times more likely to develop diabetes than a child in China. A clear difference appears between Northern and Southern hemispheres, with no countries below the equator having an incidence greater than 15/100 000; in contrast, above the equator the disease is common [55]. The largest intracontinental variation in incidence appears to be in Europe, varying from the highest in Finland to the lowest in Greece. There are also noticeable within-country variations in incidence rates (Figure 2), which can only be partially explained by racial composition of the population.

The geographic and ethnic variation in type 1 diabetes risk may reflect different pools of susceptibility genes or different prevalence of causative environmental factors, or a combination of both.

Race and Ethnicity

There are also striking racial differences in type 1 diabetes risk within the same population, although they are not as important as the geographic differences (Table 2). In the United States, non-Hispanic Whites are about 1.5 times as likely to develop type 1 diabetes as African Americans or Hispanics [52, 56]. There are similar differences

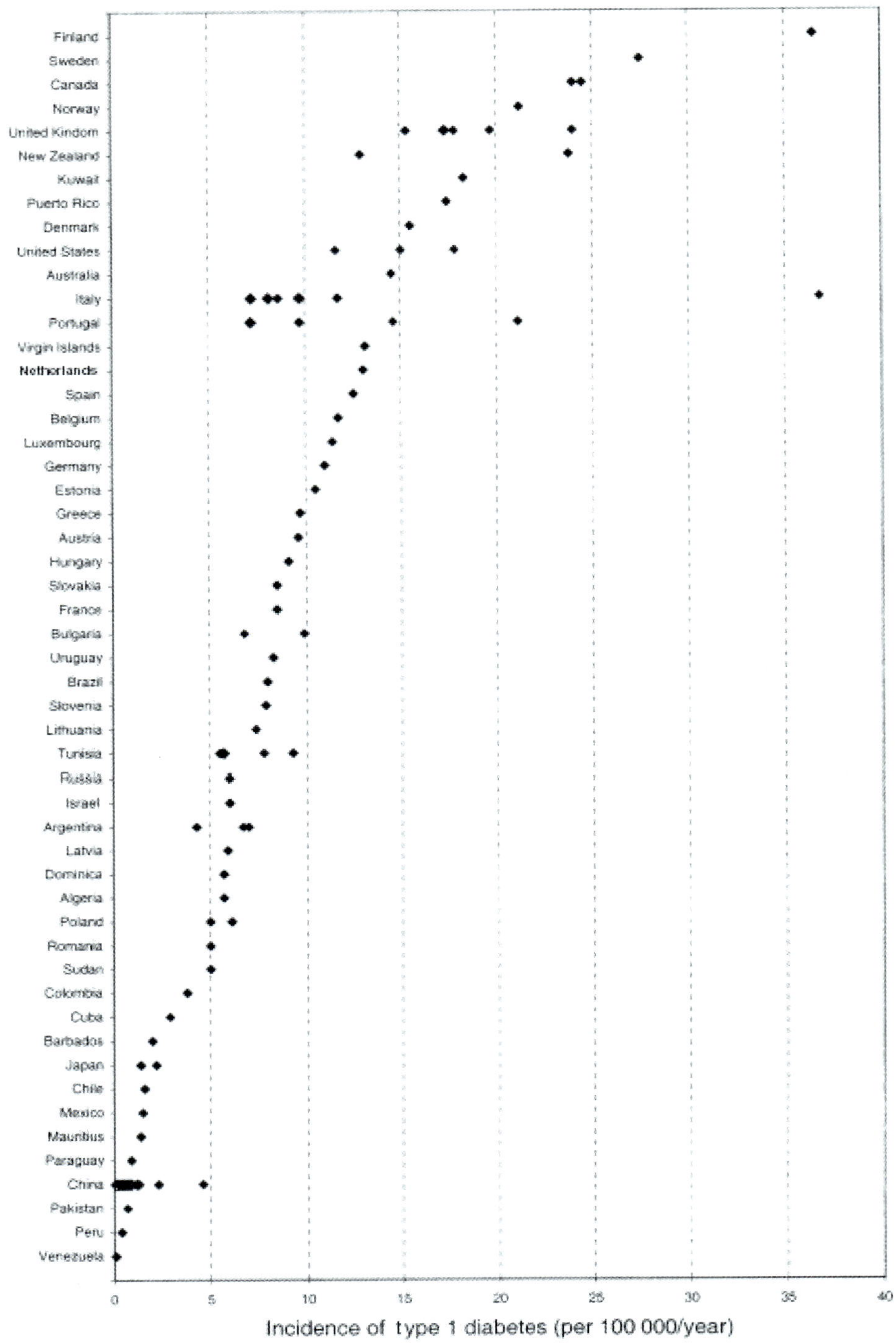

Figure 2 Geographic variation in childhood type 1 diabetes incidence. (Copyright © 2000 American Diabetes Association. From Diabetes, Vol 23, 2000; 1516–1526. Reprinted with permission from *The American Diabetes Association* [54])

reported from Montreal, where children of French descent have about two-thirds the risk of type 1 diabetes compared to children of other origins, mainly British and other Europeans [57]. This mimics the patterns of risk in Europe, where France is reported to have lower rates than does Britain and Scandinavia.

Interestingly, there is also evidence that migrants from a country with low incidence of type 1 diabetes soon have the higher rate incidence of the country where they live; for example, South Asian children living in the United Kingdom have similar overall rates of type 1 diabetes compared to indigenous White children [58]. Genetic factors

Table 2 Childhood incidence of type 1 diabetes, by ethnic group

Location	Years of study	Incidence 100 000 per year	95% Confidence interval
Colorado	1978–1983		
White		16.4	15.0–17.8
Hispanic		9.7	7.4–12.4
Montreal, Canada	1971–1985		
French		8.2	7.5–8.9
British		15.3	12.8–17.8
Italian		10.7	7.5–13.9
Jewish		17.2	10.4–24.0
Philadelphia, PA, USA	1985–1989		
White		13.3	11.0–16.1
African American		11.0	8.8–13.6
Hispanic		15.2	8.8–24.3
San Diego, CA, USA	1978–1980		
White		13.8	9.8–18.9
African American		3.3	0.4–11.9
Oriental		6.4	1.3–18.7
Hispanic		4.1	1.3–9.6

are unlikely to explain such a rapid change, implying an influence of environmental factors in disease etiology.

Age

Type 1 diabetes incidence peaks at the ages of 2, 4–6, and 10–14 years, perhaps because of alterations in the pattern of infections or increases in insulin resistance (Figure 3). The main incidence peak occurs at puberty, with females having a pubertal peak about 1 year earlier. Few cases of type 1 diabetes develop in the first year of life. There is little information concerning the incidence of type 1 diabetes in adults, but the incidence seems to decrease in the third decade of life [59] and increase again in the fifth to seventh decades of life [60, 61]. The prevalence of ICA decreases with age in first-degree relatives participating in the Diabetes Prevention Trial (DPT-1 screening). It is not known whether there are etiologic differences between

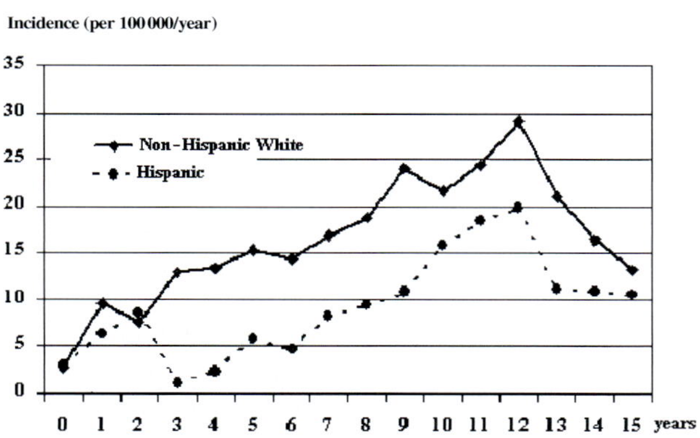

Figure 3 Incidence of type 1 diabetes in Colorado, by age (reproduced with permission from reference 51)

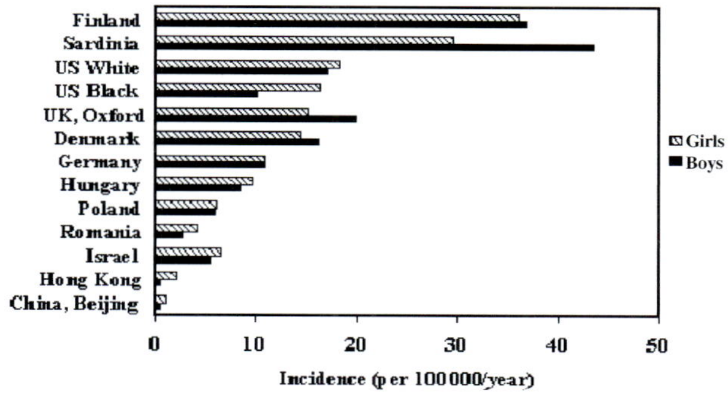

Figure 4 Incidence of childhood type 1 diabetes, by gender. (Copyright © 2000 American Diabetes Association. From Diabetes, Vol 23, 2000; 1516–1526. Reprinted with permission from *The American Diabetes Association* [54])

child- and adult-onset type 1 diabetes, but it was not apparent among adult participants in the United Kingdom Prospective Diabetes Study (UKPDS).

Gender

In general, males and females have similar risk of type 1 diabetes [62] (Figure 4). In lower risk populations, such as Japan or African Americans, there is a female preponderance, while in high-risk groups, there is a slight male excess [52, 63]. DPT-1 screening data have suggested higher prevalence of ICA in male first-degree relatives (4.3%) than in females (3.3%). Interestingly, even within Europe, all populations with an incidence higher than 20/100 000 (Sardinia, United Kingdom, Italy, Finland, Norway, etc.) had male excess, whereas those with a rate below 4.5/100 000 (the Baltic countries, Macedonia, Yugoslavia, Romania, etc.) had female excess [1, 64].

Increasing Incidence and Seasonality

There is evidence for marked variations in the incidence of type 1 diabetes over time, both seasonally and annually. In the Northern Hemisphere, the incidence declines during the warm summer months; similarly in the Southern Hemisphere, the seasonal pattern exhibits a decline during the warm months of December and January, implicating a climatic factor [65] (Figure 5). This seasonal pattern appears to occur predominantly in older children [56, 66, 67], suggesting that factors triggering diabetes may be related to school attendance.

Most population-based registries have shown increasing type 1 diabetes incidence over time [68–73] (Figure 6). Several studies have observed periodic outbreaks superimposed on a steady secular increase in incidence.

While the increase in type 1 diabetes incidence has affected all age groups, several studies have reported a particular increase among the youngest children [74–76]. In the youngest age group (0–4 years) an increase of 11%

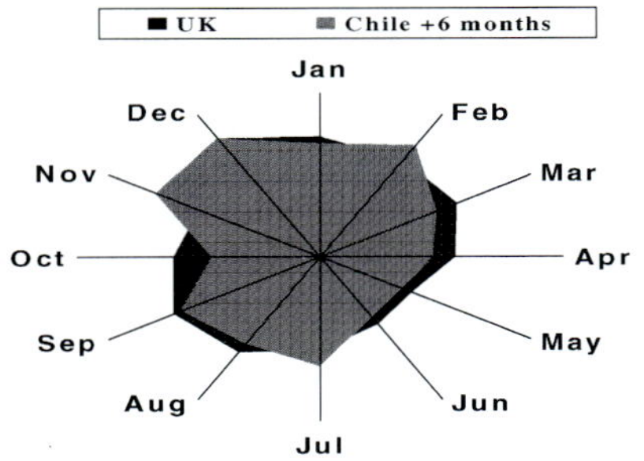

Figure 5 Seasonality of type 1 diabetes. (Reproduced by permission from Oxford University Press [65])

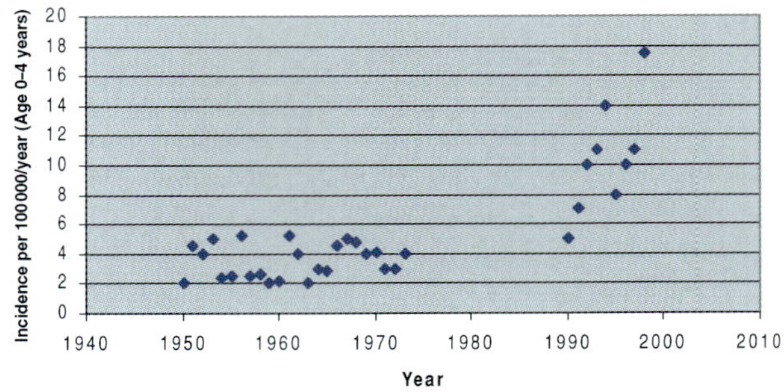

Figure 7 Incidence of type 1 diabetes in Swiss boys. (Reproduced by permission of Springer-Verlag [7])

and 24% per year was reported in, respectively, the United Kingdom [77] and Switzerland [7] (Figure 7). On the contrary, some studies show the highest increase in incidence in children 10–14 years old [54, 78].

The EURODIAB ACE Study Group, representing most European countries and Israel, found an average annual incidence rate during the period 1989–1994 ranging from 3.2 cases/100 000 per year in the former Yugoslav Republic of Macedonia to 40.2 cases/100 000 per year in two regions of Finland. Pooled over centers and sexes, the rates of increase were 6.3% [4.1–8.5%] for children aged 0–4 years, 3.1% [1.5–4.8%] for 5–9 years, and 2.4% [1.0–3.8%] for 10–14 years [73].

Genetic Factors

Family History of Type 1 Diabetes

In moderate type 1 diabetes risk areas, such as the United States, the risk of type 1 diabetes by the age of 20 years is approximately 1:300 (Table 3). The risk is increased to about 1:50 in offspring of type 1 diabetic mothers and 1:15 in offspring of type 1 diabetic fathers (the reason for this parental gender difference is not known). The risk to siblings of type 1 diabetic probands ranges from 1:12 to 1:35 [79, 80] and is further increased in HLA-identical siblings. It is estimated that by the age of 60 years approximately 10% of the first-degree relatives develop type 1 diabetes [81]. Family history of type 1 diabetes is a surrogate measure of the combination of type 1 diabetes genes and environmental exposures shared by family members. The risk of β-cell autoimmunity is higher, because not all autoantibody positive children develop diabetes by the age of 20 or even during the life span.

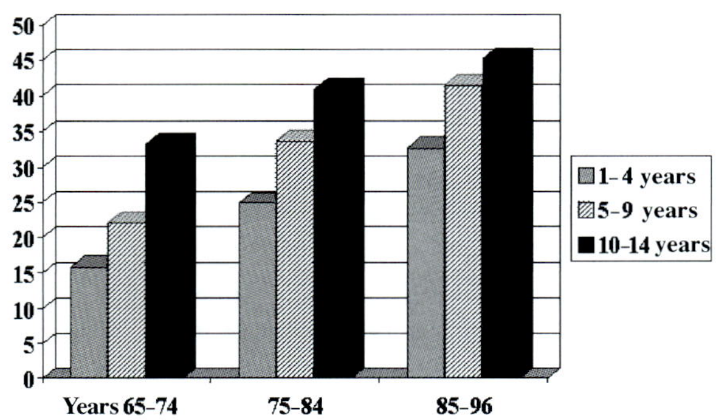

Figure 6 Increase in incidence of type 1 diabetes in Finland, 1965–1996. (Copyright © 2000 American Diabetes Association. From Diabetes, Vol 23, 2000; 1516–1526. Reprinted with permission from *The American Diabetes Association* [74])

"Familial" cases represent about 10% of type 1 diabetes and do not appear to be etiologically different from "sporadic" cases in terms of the HLA-DR,DQ genotype frequencies, seasonality of onset, and prevalence of islet autoantibodies [82]. Familial cases tend to have lower HbA_{1c} and higher C-peptide levels than do sporadic cases, because relatives recognize diabetic symptoms earlier; however, these differences disappear soon after diagnosis.

Candidate Genes

Type 1 diabetes is associated with susceptibility genes in the HLA region on chromosome 6p21 that accounts for 40–50% of the familial clustering of type 1 diabetes in Caucasians [83–85]. While 50% of non-Hispanic Whites in the United States have HLA-DR3 or -DR4 allele, at

Table 3 Risk, by the age of 20 years, of type 1 diabetes and β-cell autoimmunity in the general population and family members of type 1 diabetic patients*

Risk group	Type 1 diabetes	Prediabetic autoimmunity
General population		
All HLA genotypes	1:300	1:30–1:100
HLA-DR3/4,DQB1*0302	1:15	1:10 (?)
Family members		
Maternal offspring	1:50	1:15
Paternal offspring	1:15	1:5
Siblings (all)	1:12–1:35	1:5
Monozygotic twins	1:3	1:1 (?)
HLA-identical siblings	1:4	1:2 (?)

Note. "?" indicates that these numbers are based on very limited published data.
* From reference 19.

least one of these alleles is present in 95% of patients with type 1 diabetes. The estimated risk of developing type 1 diabetes for the general population children who have the HLA-DR3/4,DQB1*0302 genotype is approximately 1:15–1:25 [28]. Only 2.4% of the general population carries this genotype compared to 30–40% of type 1 diabetic patients. In siblings, HLA-DR3/4 heterozygosity identifies higher risk of type 1 diabetes than HLA-identity [86].

Candidate genes outside the HLA region are being identified. The insulin gene on chromosome 11p15, which regulates transcription of insulin, confers about 10% of genetic susceptibility to type 1 diabetes and at least 10 additional susceptibility genes are under investigation [87–93] (for more detail see Chapter 30).

Environmental Factors

Twin [94] and family studies indicate that genetic factors alone cannot explain the etiology of type 1 diabetes. Seasonality, increasing incidence, and epidemics of type 1 diabetes as well as numerous ecological, cross-sectional, and retrospective studies suggest a critical role of environmental factors, such as infections with certain viruses (especially enteric infections in early life) and effects of early childhood diet. Natural history studies that follow children at increased risk of type 1 diabetes provide the best opportunity to study environmental triggers.

Viruses

Herpesviruses [95, 96], mumps [97, 98], rubella [99, 100], and retroviruses [101, 102] have been implicated. Viral infections appear to initiate autoimmunity and perhaps also precipitate diabetes in subjects with autoimmunity. ICA or IAA have been detected after mumps [97], rubella, measles, chickenpox [103], coxsackie [104], ECHO-4, and rotavirus [105] infections. Newborns and infants are particularly likely to develop a persistent infection, and among patients with congenital rubella syndrome, 70% have ICA [99] as well as an increased incidence of type 1 diabetes.

Enteroviruses have been most strongly linked to human type 1 diabetes. Enteroviral infections are seen more frequently in prediabetic children and prior to the onset of islet autoimmunity in Finnish cohorts, implying a temporal relationship between enterovirus infections and the induction of β-cell autoimmunity [106–108]. Although multiple studies support an association between enteroviruses and the onset of type 1 diabetes [109–112], convincing proof of causality remains elusive [113, 114]. Enteroviral infection could initiate β-cell autoimmunity through molecular mimicry between CBV P2-C protein and GAD [113, 115], or limited capacity of β-cells to neutralize free radicals released in the infectious process could initiate β-cell autoimmunity. Interestingly, studies from Finland [108] and Sweden [116, 117] have even suggested that *in utero* enteroviral infections can lead to type 1 diabetes in a significant proportion of cases.

Rotavirus contains peptide sequences highly similar to T-cell epitopes in the islet autoantigens GAD and tyrosine phosphatase IA-2, suggesting that T-cells to rotavirus could trigger islet autoimmunity by molecular mimicry [105]. The Australian BabyDiab Study, which has followed approximately 500 babies from birth who have a first-degree relative with type 1 diabetes, demonstrated a relationship between rotavirus infection and the first appearance or an increase in islet autoantibodies [118].

Effect of Childhood Infections and Day Care Exposure

Early infectious exposure may play a role in the development of immunoregulatory mechanisms that protect against diabetes. Social mixing through attendance at day care in early infancy appears to confer protection against the development of childhood diabetes [119]. Although several other well-designed case-control studies show a statistically significant protective effect of day care exposure on type 1 diabetes [57, 120, 121], meta-analysis reveals too much heterogeneity to accept overall synthesis [122]. However, day care exposure does seem to have a protective effect in the two studies that included children diagnosed with type 1 diabetes before age 5 years [119, 123].

Improvement in Hygiene

Genetic models are unable to explain the apparent temporal changes in the incidence of type 1 diabetes [124, 125]. Alternative explanations look at environmental factors and some invoke the congenital rubella model. Briefly, increased hygiene in Western World has led to a decline in immunity to common infections among women of childbearing age. These women are more likely to develop viremia during pregnancy, resulting in congenital persistent infection of β-cells and early-onset type 1 diabetes in the offspring. This model could explain both the increasing incidence of diabetes and the decreasing age of disease onset.

Routine Childhood Immunization

Neither type nor quantity or timing of vaccinations, including BCG vaccine, HIB vaccine, diphtheria, tetanus and pertussis vaccine, measles, mumps, and rubella vaccine, hepatitis B vaccine, varicella vaccine, or tick-borne encephalitis vaccine, have been associated with the development of islet antibodies and diabetes [121, 126–132]. At least two studies even showed a possible protective effect of the measles–mumps–rubella vaccine [98, 128].

Perinatal Factors

Environmental risk factors may play a role early in life, possibly *in utero* [133]. Several studies have investigated perinatal determinants for developing type 1 diabetes. Offsprings of a type 1 diabetic parent have an increased risk of developing diabetes, the risk being higher if the father has diabetes. Although the relation of maternal age and birth order to risk of type 1 diabetes is complex, several studies found that maternal age over 35–40 years [123, 134–136] and/or increasing birth order [137–139] were associated with an increase in type 1 diabetes. There also seems to be a relatively weak but significant association between increasing birth weight and increasing risk of type 1 diabetes [140–143], although several other case-control studies have not found any association [123, 144–147].

Interestingly, others studies suggest that early weight gain and/or rapid linear growth are risk factors for development of not only type 2 but also type 1 diabetes in children [148, 149].

Dietary factors

Cow's milk or wheat introduced at weaning triggers insulitis and diabetes in animal models [150] perhaps through a molecular mimicry [151]. Breastfeeding may be viewed as a surrogate for the delay in the introduction of diabetogenic substances present in formula or early childhood diet. Several human studies have suggested an association between short duration of breastfeeding and increase in type 1 diabetes [152–157]. More recent cohort studies failed to find an association between cow's milk and β-cell autoimmunity [132, 158–163]. Interestingly, a study from Finland suggested that children's current consumption of cow's milk was more closely linked to prediabetic autoimmunity and diabetes than was infant exposure to the same [159]. To resolve this controversy, a dietary intervention trial to prevent type 1 diabetes by a short-term elimination of cow's milk from infant diet (TRIGR) is underway.

Concerning the introduction of cereals, the DAISY (J.M. Norris, unpublished data, 2002) and the German BabyDiab (A.G. Ziegler, unpublished data, 2002) studies recently found that early introduction of gluten before the age of 3 months increases the risk of development of β-cell autoimmunity.

Vitamins and Dietary Supplements

Studies *in vitro* have shown that vitamin D_3 is immunosuppressive or immunomodulating and studies in experimental models of autoimmunity have shown vitamin D to be protective [164]. Several recent European studies showed a protective effect of vitamin D supplementation in infancy against type 1 diabetes [165–168]. These findings indicate that activated vitamin D might contribute to immune modulation and thereby protect or arrest an ongoing immune process initiated in susceptible people by early environmental exposures. A study in Norway [168] found that cod liver oil taken during pregnancy was associated with reduced risk of type 1 diabetes, suggesting that vitamin D and/or the omega-3 fatty acids in the cod liver oil have a protective effect.

Exposures to Toxins

Circumstantial evidence suggest a connection between type 1 diabetes and consumption of foods and water containing nitrates, nitrites, or nitrosamines [169–172]. A recent study in the Netherlands [173] shows no convincing evidence that nitrate in drinking water at current exposures levels is a risk factor for type 1 diabetes, although a threshold value > 25 mg/l for the occurrence of the disease cannot be excluded.

Gene–Environment Interaction in Clinical Type 1 Diabetes

Type 1 diabetes is likely caused by an interactive effect of genetic and environmental factors within a limited age-window. While both the susceptibility genes and the candidate environmental exposures appear to be quite common, the likelihood of these causal components meeting within the susceptibility age-window is low [174]. To investigate the environmental causes of type 1 diabetes, the study subjects have to be screened for known susceptibility gene markers so that gene–environment interactions can be accounted for.

Interaction Between HLA Class II Alleles and Viral Infection

Susceptibility to diabetogenic enteroviruses in humans appears to be genetically restricted by HLA-DR and -DQ alleles [113]. However, the allelic specificity is controversial [48, 175–177] and may depend on the viral type and epidemicity. In general, the HLA-DR3 allele, present in most patients with type 1 diabetes, is associated with viral persistence.

Interaction Between HLA Class II Alleles and Infant Diet

Few studies to date have examined a possibility of an interaction between the HLA genes and dietary exposures [178, 179]. The epidemiological data are limited, but suggest that an early exposure to cow's milk in relatives with HLA-DR3/4,DQB1*0302, -DR3/3, or -DRx/4,DQB1*0302 is not associated with development of β-cell autoantibodies [158].

Primary Prevention

Early primary prevention includes all strategies aimed at decreasing the risk of developing type 1 diabetic in individuals without any signs of β-cell damage. Primary prevention trials include either relatives of type 1 diabetic patients or individuals at high genetic risk for developing type 1 diabetes. For instance, if early exposure to cow's milk triggers β-cell autoimmunity, primary prevention could include avoidance of cow's milk, especially in those with type 1 diabetes associated HLA alleles. Such an intervention has been piloted in newborn relatives of type 1 diabetic patients [180] and a large multicenter trial (TRIGR = Trial to Reduce IDD in the Genetically at Risk) is underway.

Late primary prevention trials target nondiabetic individuals who already have developed β-cell autoimmunity [181–183]. For instance, the DENIS Group (Deutsche Nicotinamide Intervention Study) [184] and the ENDIT study (European Nicotinamide Diabetes Intervention Trial) [185] (ENDIT, unpublished data, 2002) evaluated the clinical efficacy of oral nicotinamide in children at high risk of developing type 1 diabetes. However, both trials showed no efficacy of nicotinamide in preventing diabetes.

Promising results of a pilot trial with parenteral insulin [186] gave impetus to a large randomized unmasked trial of low-dose SC/IV isulin in relatives with confirmed ICA positivity and low acute insulin response to IV glucose (DPT-1) [187]. The results of this trial unfortunately showed no efficacy of insulin injections in preventing or delaying diabetes onset. The oral insulin arm of the DPT-1 is in progress, but results of smaller studies in newly diagnosed patients have not been encouraging [188, 189].

Secondary Prevention

Secondary prevention aims to reduce the incidence of type 1 diabetes by stopping β-cell destruction in individuals with new-onset diabetes. A number of the placebo-controlled randomized trials using azathioprine, cyclosporin A, nicotinamide, prednisone, and other immunosupressive agents attempted to increase the rate and the duration of type 1 diabetes remission. Only cyclosporin A treatment has been shown to be partially effective, inducing total remission in 25–40% and sustaining it for 1 year in 18–24% of newly diagnosed patients compared to 0–10% in the placebo group [190, 191]. However, the drug is nephrotoxic, of little value in children, and effective for only as long as it is administered [192], rendering this approach to secondary prevention of type 1 diabetes unacceptable. Several new studies are underway or in the planning phases through the United States type 1 diabetes prevention TrialNet, using immunosupression with mycophenolate mofetil [193], antigen-based therapies with GAD65 or B9–23 fragment of insulin [194], or immunomodulation with humanized anti-CD3 antibodies [195].

REMISSION (HONEYMOON PERIOD)

Shortly after clinical onset, most type 1 diabetic patients experience a transient fall in insulin requirement due to improved β-cell function. Total and partial remissions have been reported in, respectively, 2–12% and 18–62% of young type 1 diabetic patients [47, 196, 197]. Older age and less severe initial presentation of type 1 diabetes [196–199] and low or absent ICA [199–201] or IA-2 [202] have been consistently associated with deeper and longer remission. Evidence relating GAD autoantibodies [199, 202, 203], non-Caucasian origin, HLA-DR3 allele, female gender, and family history of type 1 diabetes to a less severe presentation, greater frequency of remission, and slower deterioration of insulin secretion is inconclusive. Most studies agree that preserved β-cell function is associated with better glycemic control (lower HbA_{1c}) and preserved α-cell glucagon response to hypoglycemia [204]. The prevalence of ICA (but not GAA) decreases from 87% at the time of type 1 diabetes diagnosis to 38–62% 2–3 years later [200, 205], faster in young boys and in subjects lacking HLA-DR3 and -DR4.

The natural remission is always temporary, ending with a gradual or abrupt increase in exogenous insulin requirements. Destruction of β-cells is complete within 3 years of diagnosis in most young children, especially those with the HLA-DR3/4 genotype [206]. It is much slower and often only partial in older patients [207], 15% of whom have still some β-cell function preserved 10 years after diagnosis [208].

ESTABLISHED TYPE 1 DIABETES

Acute Complications

Acute complications of type 1 diabetes (diabetic ketoacidosis, hypoglycemia, and infections) are described in detail in other chapters. The risk of hospital admission for acute complication is 30/100 patient-years in the first year of the disease and 20/100 patient-years in the subsequent 3 years [47]. An estimated 26% of the patients have at least one episode of severe hypoglycemia within the initial 4 years of diagnosis. The incidence of severe hypoglycemic episodes varies between 6 and 20/100 person-years, and increases with younger age, longer duration of diabetes, intensity of insulin treatment, lower levels of HbA_{1c}, and in older children with presence of underinsurance and psychiatric disorders [47, 209]. The incidence of ketoacidosis is about 8/100 person-years and increases with age in girls; the risk of ketoacidosis also increases with higher HbA_{1c}, higher reported insulin dose, and in older children limited access to care due to underinsurance and presence of psychiatric disorders [209]. Interestingly, most of ketoacidosis and/or hypoglycemic episodes occur among 20% of children who have recurrent events.

Morbidity and Mortality

Insulin treatment dramatically prolongs survival but it does not cure diabetes. Although the absolute mortality at onset and within the first 20 years of type 1 diabetes is low (3–6%), it is 5 times higher for diabetic males and 12 times higher for diabetic females compared to the general population [210]. This excess mortality is lowest in Scandinavia, intermediate in the United States, and highest in countries where type 1 diabetes is rare, e.g. Japan [211, 212], probably because of a combination of the quality of care and access. Even in Finland, at least half of the deaths are due to currently preventable causes such as acute complications, infections, and suicide [213]. On the other hand, 40% of the patients survive over 40 years and half of these have no major complications. Survival and avoidance of complications has been related to better metabolic control [214]. However, genetic factors also appear to be involved; inconsistent associations have been reported between diabetic nephropathy and HLA-DR4 [215] and several genes involved in blood pressure regulation [216–222].

Tertiary Prevention

The objective of tertiary prevention is to restore β-cell function or prevent complications in patients with overt type 1 diabetes. The Diabetes Control and Complication Trial [223] and a number of smaller studies have demonstrated that intensive insulin therapy that maintains blood glucose concentrations close to the normal range can delay the onset and slow the progression of diabetic retinopathy, nephropathy, and neuropathy. Additional research is needed to determine the basis for genetic susceptibility to micro- and macrovascular complications [224] and to develop successful tertiary prevention of hypertension and accelerated atherosclerosis in persons with type 1 diabetes.

REFERENCES

1. Rewers M, LaPorte RE, King H, Tuomilehto J. Trends in the prevalence and incidence of diabetes: insulin-dependent diabetes mellitus in childhood. *World Health Stat Q* 1988; 41: 179–89.
2. Rewers M. The changing face of the epidemiology of insulin-dependent diabetes mellitus (IDDM): research designs and models of disease causation. *Ann Med* 1991; 23: 419–26.
3. Libman I, Songer T, LaPorte R. How many people in the U.S. have IDDM? *Diabetes Care* 1993; 16 (5): 841–2.
4. Patrick SL, Moy CS, LaPorte RE. The world of IDDM: what international epidemiologic studies reveal about the etiology and natural history of IDDM. *Diabetes Metab Rev* 1989; 5: 571–8.
5. *Diabetes in America*, 2nd edn. Bethesda, MD: NIH, NIDDK, 1995.
6. American Diabetes Association. Economic consequences of diabetes mellitus in the U.S. in 1997. *Diabetes Care* 1998; 21 (2): 296–309.
7. Schoenle EJ, Lang-Muritano M, Gschwend S, Laimbacher J, Mullis PE, Torresani T, Biason-Lauber A, Molinari L. Epidemiology of type I diabetes mellitus in Switzerland: steep rise in incidence in under 5 year old children in the past decade. *Diabetologia* 2001; 44 (3): 286–9.
8. Onkamo P, Vaananen S, Karvonen M, Tuomilehto J. Worldwide increase in incidence of type I diabetes—the analysis of the data on published incidence trends. *Diabetologia* 1999; 42 (12): 1395–403.
9. Songer TJ. Health services and costing in diabetes. *Med J Aust* 1990; 152: 115–7.
10. Songer TJ, LaPorte R, Lave JR, Dorman JS, Becker DJ. Health insurance and the financial impact of IDDM in families with a child with IDDM. *Diabetes Care* 1997; 20 (4): 577–84.
11. Report of the Expert Committee on the Diagnosis and Classification of Diabetes Mellitus. *Diabetes Care* 1997; 20 (7): 1183–97.
12. Alberti KG, Zimmet PZ. Definition, diagnosis and classification of diabetes mellitus and its complications. Part 1: diagnosis and classification of diabetes mellitus provisional report of a WHO consultation [see comments]. *Diabet Med* 1998; 15 (7): 539–53.
13. Fajardo C, Pinon F, Carmona E, Sanchez-Cuenca JM, Merino JF, Carles C. Influence of age on clinical and immunological characteristics of newly diagnosed type 1 diabetic patients. *Acta Diabetol* 2001; 38 (1): 31–6.
14. Urakami T, Inami I, Morimoto S, Kubota S, Owada M. Clinical characteristics of non-immune-mediated, idiopathic type 1 (type 1B) diabetes mellitus in Japanese children and adolescents. *J Pediatr Endocrinol Metab* 2002; 15 (3): 283–8.
15. Tiberti C, Buzzetti R, Anastasi E, Dotta F, Vasta M, Petrone A, Cervoni M, Torresi P, Vecci E, Multari G, Di Mario U. Autoantibody negative new onset type 1 diabetic patients lacking high risk HLA alleles in a caucasian population: are these type 1b diabetes cases? *Diabetes Metab Res Rev* 2000; 16 (1): 8–14.
16. Imagawa A, Hanafusa T, Miyagawa J, Matsuzawa Y. A proposal of three distinct subtypes of type 1 diabetes mellitus based on clinical and pathological evidence. *Ann Med* 2000; 32 (8): 539–43.
17. Abiru N, Kawasaki E, Eguch K. Current knowledge of Japanese type 1 diabetic syndrome. *Diabetes Metab Res Rev* 2002; 18 (5): 357–66.
18. Imagawa A, Hanafusa T, Miyagawa J, Matsuzawa Y, for the Osaka IDDM Study Group. A novel subtype of type 1 diabetes mellitus characterized by a rapid onset and an absence of diabetes-related antibodies. *N Engl J Med* 2000; 342 (5): 301–7.
19. Eisenbarth GS, Lafferty K. *Type 1 Diabetes: Cellular, Molecular and Clinical Immunology* [on line book]. Available at: www.uchsc.edu/misc/diabetes/books.html.
20. Verge CF, Gianani R, Kawasaki E, Yu L, Pietropaolo M, Jackson RA, Chase HP, Eisenbarth GS. Prediction of type I diabetes in first-degree relatives using a combination of insulin, GAD, and ICA512bdc/IA-2 autoantibodies. *Diabetes* 1996; 45 (7): 926–33.

21. Bingley PJ, Bonifacio E, Williams AJ, Genovese S, Bottazzo GF, Gale EA. Prediction of IDDM in the general population: strategies based on combinations of autoantibody markers. *Diabetes* 1997; 46 (11): 1701–10.
22. Palmer JP, Asplin CM, Clemons P, Lyen K, Tatpati O, Raghu PK, Paquette TL. Insulin antibodies in insulin-dependent diabetics before insulin treatment. *Science* 1983; 222 (4630): 1337–9.
23. Vardi P, Dib SA, Tuttleman M, Connelly JE, Grinbergs M, Radizabeh A, Riley WJ, Maclaren NK, Eisenbarth GS, Soeldner JS. Competitive insulin autoantibody assay. Prospective evaluation of subjects at high risk for development of type I diabetes mellitus. *Diabetes* 1987; 36 (11): 1286–91.
24. Williams AJ, Bingley PJ, Bonifacio E, Palmer JP, Gale EA. A novel micro-assay for insulin autoantibodies. *J Autoimmun* 1997; 10 (5): 473–8.
25. Baekkeskov S, Nielsen JH, Marner B, Bilde T, Ludvigsson J, Lernmark Å. Autoantibodies in newly diagnosed diabetic children immunoprecipitate specific human pancreatic islet cell proteins. *Nature* 1982; 298 (5870): 167–9.
26. Baekkeskov S, Aanstoot HJ, Christgau S, Reetz A, Solimena M, Cascalho M, Folli F, Richter-Olesen H, DeCamilli P. Identification of the 64K autoantigen in insulin-dependent diabetes as the GABA-synthesizing enzyme glutamic acid decarboxylase. *Nature* 1990; 347 (6289): 151–6.
27. Rabin DU, Pleasic SM, Shapiro JA, Yoo-Warren H, Oles J, Hicks JM, Goldstein DE, Rae PM. Islet cell antigen 512 is a diabetes-specific islet autoantigen related to protein tyrosine phosphatases. *J Immunol* 1994; 152 (6): 3183–8.
28. Rewers M, Bugawan TL, Norris JM, Blair A, Beaty B, Hoffman M, McDuffie RS, Hamman RF, Klingensmith G, Eisenbarth GS, Erlich HA. Newborn screening for HLA markers associated with IDDM: diabetes autoimmunity study in the young (DAISY). *Diabetologia* 1996; 39 (7): 807–12.
29. Robles DT, Eisenbarth GS, Wang T, Erlich HA, Bugawan TL, Babu SR, Barriga K, Norris JM, Hoffman M, Klingensmith G, Yu L, Rewers M. Identification of children with early onset and high incidence of anti-islet autoantibodies. *Clin Immunol* 2002; 102 (3): 217–24.
30. Roll U, Christie MR, Fuchtenbusch M, Payton MA, Hawkes CJ, Ziegler AG. Perinatal autoimmunity in offspring of diabetic parents. The German Multicenter BABY-DIAB Study: detection of humoral immune responses to islet antigens in early childhood. *Diabetes* 1996; 45 (7): 967–73.
31. Kupila A, Keskinen P, Simell T, Erkkila S, Arvilommi P, Korhonen S, Kimpimaki T, Sjoroos M, Ronkainen M, Ilonen J, Knip M, Simell O. Genetic risk determines the emergence of diabetes-associated autoantibodies in young children. *Diabetes* 2002; 51 (3): 646–51.
32. Bonifacio E, Bingley PJ, Shattock M, Dean BM, Dunger D, Gale EAM, Bottazzo GF. Quantification of islet-cell antibodies and prediction of insulin-dependent diabetes. *Lancet* 1990; 335: 147–9.
33. Johnston C, Millward BA, Hoskins P, Leslie RD, Bottazzo GF, Pyke DA. Islet-cell antibodies as predictors of the later development of type 1 (insulin-dependent) diabetes. A study in identical twins. *Diabetologia* 1989; 32 (6): 382–6.
34. McCulloch DK, Palmer JP. The appropriate use of B-cell function testing in the preclinical period of type 1 diabetes. *Diabet Med* 1991; 8: 800–4.
35. Spinas GA, Matter L, Wilkin T, Staffelbach O, Berger W. Islet-cell and insulin autoantibodies in first-degree relatives of type I diabetics: a 5-year follow-up study in a Swiss population. *Adv Exp Med Biol* 1988; 246: 209–14.
36. Thivolet C, Beaufrere B, Betuel H, Gebuhrer L, Chatelain P, Durand A, Tourniaire J, Francois R. Islet cell and insulin autoantibodies in subjects at high risk for development of type 1 (insulin-dependent) diabetes mellitus: the Lyon family study. *Diabetologia* 1988; 31 (10): 741–6.
37. Landin-Olsson M, Palmer JP, Lernmark A, Blom L, Sundkvist G, Nystrom L, Dahlquist G. Predictive value of islet cell and insulin autoantibodies for type 1 (insulin-dependent) diabetes mellitus in a population-based study of newly-diagnosed diabetic and matched control children. *Diabetologia* 1992; 35 (11): 1068–73.
38. Karjalainen JK. Islet cell antibodies as predictive markers for IDDM in children with high background incidence of disease. *Diabetes* 1990; 39 (9): 1144–50.
39. Lindberg BA, Ericsson UB, Kockum I, Lernmark A, Landin-Olsson M, Sundkvist G, Ivarsson SA. Prevalence of β-cell and thyroid autoantibody positivity in schoolchildren during three-year follow-up. *Autoimmunity* 1999; 31 (3): 175–85.
40. Riley WJ, Maclaren NK, Krischer J, Spillar RP, Silverstein JH, Schatz DA, Schwartz S, Malone J, Shah S, Vadheim C, Rotter JI. A prospective study of the development of diabetes in relatives of patients with insulin-dependent diabetes. *N Engl J Med* 1990; 323: 1167–72.
41. Groop LC, Bottazzo GF, Doniach D. Islet cell antibodies identify latent type I diabetes in patients aged 35–75 years at diagnosis. *Diabetes* 1986; 35 (2): 237–41.
42. Tuomi T, Groop LC, Zimmet PZ, Rowley MJ, Knowles W, Mackay IR. Antibodies to glutamic acid decarboxylase reveal latent autoimmune diabetes mellitus in adults with a non-insulin-dependent onset of disease. *Diabetes* 1993; 42 (2): 359–62.
43. Zimmet PZ, Tuomi T, Mackay IR, Rowley MJ, Knowles W, Cohen M, Lang DA. Latent autoimmune diabetes mellitus in adults (LADA): the role of antibodies to glutamic acid decarboxylase in diagnosis and prediction of insulin dependency. *Diabet Med* 1994; 11: 299–303.
44. Hamman RF, Cook M, Keefer S, Young WF, Finch JL, Lezotte D, McLaren B, Orleans M, Klingensmith G, Chase HP. Medical care patterns at the onset of insulin-dependent diabetes mellitus: association with severity and subsequent complications. *Diabetes Care* 1985; 8 (suppl 1): 94–100.
45. Karjalainen J, Salmela P, Ilonen J, Surcel HM, Knip M. A comparison of childhood and adult type I diabetes mellitus. *N Engl J Med* 1989; 320: 881–6.
46. Levy-Marchal C, Papoz L, de Beaufort C, Doutreix J, Froment V, Voirin J, Czernichow P. Clinical and laboratory features of type I diabetic children at time of diagnosis. *Diabet Med* 1992; 9 (3): 279–84.
47. Pinkey JH, Bingley PJ, Sawtell PA, Dunger DB, Gale EA, for the Bart's-Oxford Study Group. Presentation and progress of childhood diabetes mellitus: a prospective population-based study. *Diabetologia* 1994; 37 (1): 70–4.
48. Eberhardt MS, Wagener DK, Orchard TJ, LaPorte RE, Cavender DE, Rabin BS, Atchison RW, Kuller LH, Drash AL, Becker DJ. HLA heterogeneity of insulin-dependent diabetes mellitus at diagnosis. The Pittsburgh IDDM Study. *Diabetes* 1985; 34 (12): 1247–52.
49. Foulis AK, Liddle CN, Farquharson MA, Richmond JA, Weir RS. The histopathology of the pancreas in type 1

(insulin-dependent) diabetes mellitus: a 25-year review of deaths in patients under 20 years of age in the United Kingdom. *Diabetologia* 1986; 29 (5): 267–74.

50. Childhood Diabetes Research Committee, Ministry of Health and Welfare, Japan; Polish Diabetes Research Group, Poznan; The Netherlands Institute for Preventive Health Care, Leiden; Diabetes Research Center of Pittsburgh, Pennsylvania. How frequently do children die at the onset of insulin-dependent diabetes? Analyses of registry data from Japan, Poland, the Netherlands, and Allegheny County, Pennsylvania. *Diab Nutr Metab* 1990; 3: 57–62.
51. Kostraba JN, Gay EC, Rewers M, Chase HP, Klingensmith GJ, Hamman RF. Increasing trend of outpatient management of children with newly diagnosed IDDM. Colorado IDDM Registry, 1978–1988. *Diabetes Care* 1992; 15 (1): 95–100.
52. Diabetes Epidemiology Research International Group. Geographic patterns of childhood insulin-dependent diabetes mellitus. *Diabetes* 1988; 37(8):1113–9.
53. Green A, Gale EAM, Patterson CC. Incidence of childhood-onset insulin-dependent diabetes mellitus: the EURODIAB ACE Study. *Lancet* 1992; 339 (8798): 905–9.
54. Karvonen M, Viik-Kajander M, Moltchanova E, Libman I, LaPorte R, Tuomilehto J, for the Diabetes Mondiale (DiaMond) Project Group. Incidence of childhood type 1 diabetes worldwide. *Diabetes Care* 2000; 23 (10): 1516–26.
55. Karvonen M, Tuomilehto J, Libman I, LaPorte R, for the World Health Organization DIAMOND Project Group. A review of the recent epidemiological data on the worldwide incidence of type 1 (insulin-dependent) diabetes mellitus. *Diabetologia* 1993; 36 (10): 883–92.
56. Kostraba JN, Gay EC, Cai Y, Cruickshanks KJ, Rewers MJ, Klingensmith GJ, Chase HP, Hamman RF. Incidence of insulin-dependent diabetes mellitus in Colorado. *Epidemiology* 1992; 3: 232–8.
57. Siemiatycki J, Colle E, Campbell S, Dewar RA, Belmonte MM. Case-control study of IDDM. *Diabetes Care* 1989; 12 (3): 209–16.
58. Gujral JS, McNally PG, Botha JL, Burden AC. Childhood-onset diabetes in the white and South Asian population in Leicestershire, UK. *Diabet Med* 1994; 11 (6): 570–2.
59. Joner G, Sovik O. The incidence of type 1 (insulin-dependent) diabetes mellitus 15–29 years in Norway 1978–1982. *Diabetologia* 1991; 34 (4): 271–4.
60. Christau B, Kromann H, Andersen OO, Christy M, Buschard K, Arnung K, Kristensen IH, Peitersen B, Steinrud J, Nerup J. Incidence, seasonal and geographical patterns of juvenile-onset insulin-dependent diabetes mellitus in Denmark. *Diabetologia* 1977; 13 (4): 281–4.
61. Melton LJ III, Palumbo PJ, Chu CP. Incidence of diabetes mellitus by clinical type. *Diabetes Care* 1983; 6 (1): 75–86.
62. Gale EA, Gillespie KM. Diabetes and gender. *Diabetologia* 2001; 44 (1): 3–15.
63. Karvonen M, Pitkaniemi M, Pitkaniemi J, Kohtamaki K, Tajima N, Tuomilehto J, for the World Health Organization DIAMOND Project Group. Sex difference in the incidence of insulin-dependent diabetes mellitus: an analysis of the recent epidemiological data. *Diabetes Metab Rev* 1997; 13 (4): 275–91.
64. ONROCAD Study Group (National Romanian Organisation for the Care of Diabetic Children and Adolescents). Serban V, Timar R, Dabelea D, Green A, McKinney P, Law G. The epidemiology of childhood-onset type 1 diabetes mellitus in Romania. *J Pediatr Endocrinol Metab* 2001; 14 (5): 535–41.
65. Gamble DR. The epidemiology of insulin-dependent diabetes, with particular reference to the relationship of virus infection to its etiology. *Epidemiol Rev* 1980; 2: 49–70.
66. Dahlquist G, Gustavsson KH, Holmgren G, Hagglof B, Larsson Y, Nilsson KO, Samuelsson G, Sterky G, Thalme B, Wall S. The incidence of diabetes mellitus in Swedish children 0–14 years of age. A prospective study 1977–1980. *Acta Paediatr Scand* 1982; 71 (1): 7–14.
67. Dahlquist G, Blom L, Holmgren G, Hagglof B, Larsson Y, Sterky G, Wall S. The epidemiology of diabetes in Swedish children 0–14 years—a six-year prospective study. *Diabetologia* 1985; 28 (11): 802–8.
68. Rewers M, LaPorte RE, Walczak M, Dmochowski K, Bogaczynska E. Apparent epidemic of insulin-dependent diabetes mellitus in Midwestern Poland. *Diabetes* 1987; 36 (1): 106–13.
69. Diabetes Epidemiology Research International Group. Secular trends in incidence of childhood IDDM in 10 countries. *Diabetes* 1990; 39 (7): 858–64.
70. Nystrom L, Dahlquist G, Rewers M, Wall S. The Swedish childhood diabetes study. An analysis of the temporal variation in diabetes incidence 1978–1987. *Int J Epidemiol* 1990; 19 (1): 141–6.
71. Tuomilehto J, Rewers M, Reunanen A, Lounamaa P, Lounamaa R, Tuomilehto-Wolf E, Akerblom HK. Increasing trend in type 1 (insulin-dependent) diabetes mellitus in childhood in Finland. Analysis of age, calendar time and birth cohort effects during 1965 to 1984. *Diabetologia* 1991; 34 (4): 282–7.
72. Dokheel TM, for the Pittsburgh Diabetes Epidemiology Research Group. An epidemic of childhood diabetes in the United States? Evidence from Allegheny County, Pennsylvania. *Diabetes Care* 1993; 16 (12): 1606–11.
73. EURODIAB ACE Study Group. Variation and trends in incidence of childhood diabetes in Europe. *Lancet* 2000; 355 (9207): 873– 6.
74. Karvonen M, Pitkaniemi J, Tuomilehto J, for the Finnish Childhood Diabetes Registry Group. The onset age of type 1 diabetes in Finnish children has become younger. *Diabetes Care* 1999; 22 (7): 1066–70.
75. Rosenbauer J, Herzig P, von Kries R, Neu A, Giani G. Temporal, seasonal, and geographical incidence patterns of type I diabetes mellitus in children under 5 years of age in Germany. *Diabetologia* 1999; 42 (9): 1055–9.
76. Cinek O, Lanska V, Kolouskova S, Sumnik Z, Snajderova M, Ronningen KS, Vavrinec J. for the Collaborators of the Czech Childhood Diabetes Registry. Type 1 diabetes mellitus in Czech children diagnosed in 1990–1997: a significant increase in incidence and male predominance in the age group 0–4 years. *Diabetic Med* 2000; 17 (1): 64–9.
77. Gardner SG, Bingley PJ, Sawtell PA, Weeks S, Gale EA, for the Bart's-Oxford Study Group. Rising incidence of insulin dependent diabetes in children aged under 5 years in the Oxford region: time trend analysis [see comments]. *BMJ* 1997; 315 (7110): 713–7.
78. Rangasami JJ, Greenwood DC, McSporran B, Smail PJ, Patterson CC, Waugh NR, for the Scottish Study Group

for the Care of Young Diabetics. Rising incidence of type 1 diabetes in Scottish children, 1984–93. *Arch Dis Child* 1997; 77 (3): 210–3.

79. Wagener DK, Sacks JM, LaPorte RE, Macgregor JM. The Pittsburgh study of insulin-dependent diabetes mellitus. Risk for diabetes among relatives of IDDM. *Diabetes* 1982; 31 (2): 136–44.
80. Allen C, Palta M, D'Alessio DJ. Risk of diabetes in siblings and other relatives of IDDM subjects. *Diabetes* 1991; 40 (7): 831–6.
81. Lorenzen T, Pociot F, Hougaard P, Nerup J. Long-term risk of IDDM in first-degree relatives of patients with IDDM. *Diabetologia* 1994; 37 (3): 321–7.
82. O'Leary LA, Dorman JS, LaPorte RE, Orchard TJ, Becker DJ, Kuller LH, Eberhardt MS, Cavender DE, Rabin BS, Drash AL. Familial and sporadic insulin-dependent diabetes: Evidence for heterogeneous etiologies? *Diab Res Clin Pract* 1991; 14: 183–90.
83. Erlich HA, Griffith RL, Bugawan TL, Ziegler R, Alper C, Eisenbarth G. Implication of specific DQB1 alleles in genetic susceptibility and resistance by identification of IDDM siblings with novel HLA-DQB1 allele and unusual DR2 and DR1 haplotypes. *Diabetes* 1991; 40 (4): 478–81.
84. Bertrams J. The HLA association of insulin-dependent (type I) diabetes mellitus. *Behring Inst Mitt* 1984; (75): 89–99.
85. Todd JA. The role of MHC class II genes in susceptibility to insulin-dependent diabetes mellitus. *Curr Top Microbiol Immunol* 1990; 164: 17–40.
86. Deschamps I, Boitard C, Hors J, Busson M, Marcelli-Barge A, Mogenet A, Robert JJ. Life table analysis of the risk of type 1 (insulin-dependent) diabetes mellitus in siblings according to islet cell antibodies and HLA markers. An 8-year prospective study. *Diabetologia* 1992; 35 (10): 951–7.
87. Owerbach D, Gabbay KH. Localization of a type I diabetes susceptibility locus to the variable tandem repeat region flanking the insulin gene. *Diabetes* 1993; 42 (12): 1708–14.
88. Davies JL, Kawaguchi Y, Bennett ST, Copeman JB, Cordell HJ, Pritchard LE, Reed PW, Gough SCL, Jenkins SC, Palmer SM, Balfour KM, Rowe BR, Farrall M, Barnett AH, Bain SC, Todd JA. A genome-wide search for human type 1 diabetes susceptibility genes. *Nature* 1994; 371 (6493): 130–6.
89. Delepine M, Pociot F, Habita C, Hashimoto L, Frougel P, Rotter J, Cambon-Thomsen A, Deschamps I, Djoulah S, Weissenbach J, Nerup J, Lathrop M, Julier C. Evidence of a non-MHC susceptiblity locus in type I diabetes linked to HLA on chromosome 6. *Am J Hum Genet* 1997; 60: 174–87.
90. Owerbach D, Gabbay KH. The HOXD8 locus (2q31) is linked to type I diabetes. Interaction with chromosome 6 and 11 disease susceptibility genes. *Diabetes* 1995; 44 (1): 132–6.
91. Field LL, Tobias R, Magnus T. A locus on chromosome 15q26 (*IDDM3*) produces susceptibility to insulin- dependent diabetes mellitus. *Nat Genet* 1994; 8 (2): 189–94.
92. Copeman JB, Cucca F, Hearne CM, Cornall RJ, Reed PW, Ronningen KS, Undlien DE, Nistico L, Buzzetti R, Tosi R, et al. Linkage disequilibrium mapping of a type 1 diabetes susceptibility gene (*IDDM7*) to chromosome 2q31–q33. *Nat Genet* 1995; 9 (1): 80–5.
93. Cox NJ, Wapelhorst B, Morrison VA, Johnson L, Pinchuk L, Spielman RS, Todd JA, Concannon P. Seven regions of the genome show evidence of linkage to type 1 diabetes in a consensus analysis of 767 multiplex families. *Am J Hum Genet* 2001; 69 (4): 820–30.
94. Kaprio J, Tuomilehto J, Koskenvuo M, Romanov K, Reunanen A, Eriksson J, Stengard J, Kesaniemi YA. Concordance for type 1 (insulin-dependent) and type 2 (non-insulin-dependent) diabetes mellitus in a population-based cohort of twins in Finland. *Diabetologia* 1992; 35 (11): 1060–7.
95. Pak CY, Hyone-Myong E, McArthur RG, Yoon JW. Association of cytomegalovirus infection with autoimmune type 1 diabetes. *Lancet* 1988; 2: 1–3.
96. Sairenji T, Daibata M, Sorli CH, Qvistback H, Humphreys RE, Ludvigsson J, Palmer J, Landin-Olsson M, Sundkvist G, Michelsen B. Relating homology between the Epstein–Barr virus BOLF1 molecule and HLA-DQw8 beta chain to recent onset type 1 (insulin-dependent) diabetes mellitus. *Diabetologia* 1991; 34 (1): 33–9.
97. Helmke K, Otten A, Willems WR, Brockhaus R, Mueller-Eckhardt G, Stief T, Bertrams J, Wolf H, Federlin K. Islet cell antibodies and the development of diabetes mellitus in relation to mumps infection and mumps vaccination. *Diabetologia* 1986; 29 (1): 30–3.
98. Hyoty H, Hiltunen M, Reunanen A, Leinikki P, Vesikari T, Lounamaa R, Tuomilehto J, Akerblom HK. for the Childhood Diabetes in Finland Study Group. Decline of mumps antibodies in type 1 (insulin-dependent) diabetic children and a plateau in the rising incidence of type 1 diabetes after introduction of the mumps-measles-rubella vaccine in Finland. *Diabetologia* 1993; 36 (12): 1303–8.
99. Ginsberg-Fellner F, Witt ME, Yagihashi S, Dobersen MJ, Taub F, Fedun B, Mcevoy RC, Roman SH, Davies RG, Cooper LZ, et al. Congenital rubella syndrome as a model for type 1 (insulin-dependent) diabetes mellitus: increased prevalence of islet cell surface antibodies. *Diabetologia* 1984; 27 (suppl): 87–9.
100. Menser MA, Forrest JM, Bransby RD. Rubella infection and diabetes mellitus. *Lancet* 1978; 1: 57–60.
101. Suenaga K, Yoon JW. Association of β-cell-specific expression of endogenous retrovirus with development of insulitis and diabetes in NOD mouse. *Diabetes* 1988; 37 (12): 1722–6.
102. Conrad B, Weidmann E, Trucco G, Rudert WA, Behboo R, Ricordi C, Rodriquez-Rilo H, Finegold D, Trucco M. Evidence for superantigen involvement in insulin-dependent diabetes mellitus aetiology. *Nature* 1994; 371 (6495): 351–5.
103. Bodansky HJ, Dean BM, Bottazzo GF, Grant PJ, McNally J, Hambling MH. Islet-cell antibodies and insulin autoantibodies in association with common viral infections. *Lancet* December 1986; 13: 1351–3.
104. Champsaur H, Bottazzo GF, Bertrams J, Assan R, Bach C. Virologic, immunologic and genetic factors in insulin-dependent diabetes mellitus. *J Pediatr* 1982; 100 (1): 15–20.
105. Honeyman MC, Coulson BS, Stone NL, Gellert SA, Goldwater PN, Steele CE, Couper JJ, Tait BD, Colman PG, Harrison LC. Association between rotavirus infection and pancreatic islet autoimmunity in children at risk of developing type 1 diabetes. *Diabetes* 2000; 49 (8): 1319–24.

106. Lonnrot M, Korpela K, Knip M, Ilonen J, Simell O, Korhonen S, Savola K, Muona P, Simell T, Koskela P, Hyoty H. Enterovirus infection as a risk factor for β-cell autoimmunity in a prospectively observed birth cohort: the Finnish Diabetes Prediction and Prevention Study. *Diabetes* 2000; 49 (8): 1314–8.
107. Lonnrot M, Salminen K, Knip M, Savola K, Kulmala P, Leinikki P, Hyypia T, Akerblom HK, Hyoty H. for the Childhood Diabetes in Finland (DiMe) Study Group. Enterovirus RNA in serum is a risk factor for β-cell autoimmunity and clinical type 1 diabetes: a prospective study. *J Med Virol* 2000; 61 (2): 214–20.
108. Hyoty H, Hiltunen M, Knip M, Laakkonen M, Vahasalo P, Karjalainen J, Koskela P, Roivainen M, Leinikki P, Hovi T. for the Childhood Diabetes in Finland (DiMe) Study Group. A prospective study of the role of coxsackie B and other enterovirus infections in the pathogenesis of IDDM. *Diabetes* 1995; 44 (6): 652–7.
109. Helfand RF, Gary HE Jr, Freeman CY, Anderson LJ, Pallansch MA, for the Pittsburgh Diabetes Research Group. Serologic evidence of an association between enteroviruses and the onset of type 1 diabetes mellitus. *J Infect Dis* 1995; 172 (5): 1206–11.
110. Jenson AB, Rosenberg HS, Notkins AL. Pancreatic islet-cell damage in children with fatal viral infections. *Lancet* August 1980; 16: 354–8.
111. Yoon JW, Austin M, Onodera T, Notkins AL. Virus-induced diabetes mellitus: isolation of a virus from the pancreas of a child with diabetic ketoacidosis. *N Engl J Med* 1979; 300: 1173–9.
112. Wagenknecht LE, Roseman JM, Herman WH. Increased incidence of insulin-dependent diabetes mellitus following an epidemic of coxsackievirus B5. *Am J Epidemiol* 1991; 133: 1024–31.
113. Rewers M, Atkinson M. The possible role of enteroviruses in diabetes mellitus. In Rotbart HA, (ed) *Human Enterovirus Infections*. Washington: *ASM*, 1996; 353–85.
114. Graves PM, Norris JM, Pallansch MA, Gerling IC, Rewers M. The role of enteroviral infections in the development of IDDM: limitations of current approaches. *Diabetes* 1997; 46 (2): 161–8.
115. Kaufman DL, Clare-Salzler M, Tian J, Forsthuber T, Ting GS, Robinson P, Atkinson MA, Sercarz EE, Tobin AJ, Lehmann PV. Spontaneous loss of T-cell tolerance to glutamic acid decarboxylase in murine insulin-dependent diabetes [see comments]. *Nature* 1993; 366: 69–72.
116. Dahlquist G, Frisk G, Ivarsson SA, Svanberg L, Forsgren M, Diderholm H. Indications that maternal coxsackie B virus infection during pregnancy is a risk factor for childhood-onset IDDM. *Diabetologia* 1995; 38 (11): 1371–3.
117. Dahlquist GG. Viruses and other perinatal exposures as initiating events for β-cell destruction. *Ann Med* 1997; 29 (5): 413–7.
118. Couper JJ. Environmental triggers of type 1 diabetes. *J Paediatr Child Health* 2001; 37 (3): 218–20.
119. McKinney PA, Okasha M, Parslow RC, Law GR, Gurney KA, Williams R, Bodansky HJ. Early social mixing and childhood type 1 diabetes mellitus: a case-control study in Yorkshire, UK. *Diabet Med* 2000; 17 (3): 236–42.
120. Verge CF, Howard NJ, Irwig L, Simpson JM, Mackerras D, Silink M. Environmental factors in childhood IDDM. A population-based, case-control study. *Diabetes Care* 1994; 17 (12): 1381–9.
121. The EURODIAB Substudy 2 Study Group. Infections and vaccinations as risk factors for childhood type I (insulin-dependent) diabetes mellitus: a multicentre case-control investigation. *Diabetologia* 2000; 43 (1): 47–53.
122. Kaila B, Taback SP. The effect of day care exposure on the risk of developing type 1 diabetes: a meta-analysis of case-control studies. *Diabetes Care* 2001; 24 (8): 1353–8.
123. Blom L, Dahlquist G, Nystrom L, Sandstrom A, Wall S. The Swedish childhood diabetes study—social and perinatal determinants for diabetes in childhood. *Diabetologia* 1989; 32 (1): 7–13.
124. Cordell HJ, Todd JA. Multifactorial inheritance in type 1 diabetes [review]. *Trends Genet* 1995; 11 (12): 499–504.
125. Zinkernagel RM. Maternal antibodies, childhood infections, and autoimmune diseases. *N Engl J Med* 2001; 345 (18): 1331–5.
126. Dahlquist G, Gothefors L. The cumulative incidence of childhood diabetes mellitus in Sweden unaffected by BCG-vaccination. *Diabetologia* 1995; 38 (7): 873–4.
127. Heijbel H, Chen RT, Dahlquist G. Cumulative incidence of childhood-onset IDDM is unaffected by pertussis immunization. *Diabetes Care* 1997; 20 (2): 173–5.
128. Blom L, Nystrom L, Dahlquist G. The Swedish childhood diabetes study. Vaccinations and infections as risk determinants for diabetes in childhood. *Diabetologia* 1991; 34 (3): 176–81.
129. Karvonen M, Cepaitis Z, Tuomilehto J. Association between type 1 diabetes and *Haemophilus influenzae* type b vaccination: birth cohort study. *BMJ* 1999; 318 (7192): 1169–72.
130. Lindberg B, Ahlfors K, Carlsson A, Ericsson UB, Landin-Olsson M, Lernmark A, Ludvigsson J, Sundkvist G, Ivarsson SA. Previous exposure to measles, mumps, and rubella—but not vaccination during adolescence—correlates to the prevalence of pancreatic and thyroid autoantibodies. *Pediatrics* 1999; 104 (1): e12.
131. Graves PM, Barriga KJ, Norris JM, Hoffman MR, Yu L, Eisenbarth GS, Rewers M. Lack of association between early childhood immunizations and β-cell autoimmunity. *Diabetes Care* 1999; 22 (10): 1694–7.
132. Hummel M, Fuchtenbusch M, Schenker M, Ziegler AG. No major association of breast-feeding, vaccinations, and childhood viral diseases with early islet autoimmunity in the German BABYDIAB Study. *Diabetes Care* 2000; 23 (7): 969–74.
133. Leslie RD, Elliott RB. Early environmental events as a cause of IDDM. Evidence and implications. *Diabetes* 1994; 43 (7): 843–50.
134. Soltesz G, Jeges S, Dahlquist G, Hungarian Childhood Diabetes Epidemiology Study Group. Non-genetic risk determinants for type 1 (insulin-dependent) diabetes. *Acta Paediatr* 1994; 83: 730–5.
135. Patterson CC, Carson DJ, Hadden DR, Waugh NR, Cole SK. A case-control investigation of perinatal risk factors for childhood IDDM in Northern Ireland and Scotland. *Diabetes Care* 1994; 17 (5): 376–81.
136. Bingley PJ, Douek IF, Rogers CA, Gale EA, for the Bart's-Oxford Family Study Group. Influence of maternal age at delivery and birth order on risk of type 1 diabetes in childhood: prospective population based family study. *BMJ* 2000; 321 (7258): 420–4.
137. Stene LC, Magnus P, Lie RT, Sovik O, Joner G. Maternal and paternal age at delivery, birth order, and risk of childhood onset type 1 diabetes: population based cohort study. *BMJ* 2001; 323 (7309): 1–4.

138. Rami B, Schneider U, Imhof A, Waldhor T, Schober E. Risk factors for type I diabetes mellitus in children in Austria. *Eur J Pediatr* 1999; 158 (5): 362–6.
139. Tai TY, Wang CY, Lin LL, Lee LT, Tsai ST, Chen CJ. A case-control study on risk factors for type 1 diabetes in Taipei City. *Diabetes Res Clin Pract* 1998; 42 (3): 197–203.
140. Stene LC, Magnus P, Lie RT, Sovik O, Joner G. Birth weight and childhood onset type 1 diabetes: population based cohort study. *BMJ* 2001; 322A (7291): 889–92.
141. Dahlquist G, Bennich SS, Kallen B. Intrauterine growth pattern and risk of childhood onset insulin dependent (type I) diabetes: population based case-control study. *BMJ* 1996; 313 (7066): 1174–7.
142. Dahlquist GG, Patterson C, Soltesz G, for the EURODIAB Substudy 2 Study Group. Perinatal risk factors for childhood type 1 diabetes in Europe. *Diabetes Care* 1999; 22 (10): 1698–702.
143. Podar T, Onkamo P, Forsen T, Karvonen M, Tuomilehto-Wolf E, Tuomilehto J, for the DiMe Study Group. Neonatal anthropometric measurements and risk of childhood-onset type 1 diabetes. *Diabetes Care* 1999; 22 (12): 2092–4.
144. Lawler-Heavner J, Cruickshanks KJ, Hay WH Jr, Gay EC, Hamman RF. Birth size and risk of insulin-dependent diabetes mellitus (IDDM). *Diab Res Clin Pract* 1994; 24: 153–9.
145. Bock T, Pedersen CR, Volund A, Pallesen CS, Buschard K. Perinatal determinants among children who later develop IDDM. *Diabetes Care* 1994; 17 (10): 1154–7.
146. McKinney PA, Parslow R, Gurney KA, Law GR, Bodansky HJ, Williams R. Perinatal and neonatal determinants of childhood type 1 diabetes. A case-control study in Yorkshire, U.K. *Diabetes Care* 1999; 22 (6): 928–32.
147. Kyvik KO, Bache I, Green A, Beck-NielsenH, Buschard K. No association between birth weight and type 1 diabetes mellitus—a twin-control study. *Diabet Med* 2000; 17 (2): 158–62.
148. Johansson C, Samuelsson U, Ludvigsson J. A high weight gain early in life is associated with an increased risk of type 1 (insulin-dependent) diabetes mellitus. *Diabetologia* 1994; 37 (1): 91–4.
149. Hypponen E, Virtanen SM, Kenward MG, Knip M, Akerblom HK. Obesity, increased linear growth, and risk of type 1 diabetes in children. *Diabetes Care* 2000; 23 (12): 1755–60.
150. Atkinson MA, Winter WE, Skordis N, Beppu H, Riley WM, Maclaren NK. Dietary protein restriction reduces the frequency and delays the onset of insulin dependent diabetes in BB rats. *Autoimmunity* 1988; 2: 11–20.
151. Martin JM, Trink B, Daneman D, Dosch H-M, Robinson B. Milk proteins in the etiology of insulin-dependent diabetes mellitus (IDDM). *Ann Med* 1991; 23: 447–52.
152. Borch-Johnsen K, Joner G, Mandrup-Poulsen T, Christy M, Zachau-Christiansen B, Kastrup K, Nerup J. Relation between breast-feeding and incidence rates of insulin-dependent diabetes mellitus. A hypothesis. *Lancet* 1984; 2 (8411): 1083–6.
153. Nigro G, Campea L, De Novellis A, Orsini M. Breast-feeding and insulin-dependent diabetes mellitus [letter]. *Lancet* 1985; 1 (8426): 467.
154. Mayer EJ, Hamman RF, Gay EC, Lezotte DC, Savitz DA, Klingensmith GJ, for the Colorado IDDM Registry. Reduced risk of IDDM among breast-fed children. *Diabetes* 1988; 37 (12): 1625–32.
155. Virtanen SM, Rasanen L, Aro A, Ylonen K, Lounamaa R, Tuomilehto J, Akerblom HK, for the Childhood Diabetes in Finland Study Group. Feeding in infancy and the risk of type 1 diabetes mellitus in Finnish children. *Diabet Med* 1992; 9: 815–9.
156. Gerstein HC. Cow's milk exposure and type I diabetes mellitus. A critical overview of the clinical literature. *Diabetes Care* 1994; 17 (1): 13–9.
157. Norris JM, Scott FW. A meta-analysis of infant diet and insulin-dependent diabetes mellitus: do biases play a role? *Epidemiology* 1996; 7: 87–92.
158. Norris JM, Beaty B, Klingensmith G, Yu L, Hoffman M, Chase HP, Erlich HA, Hamman RF, Eisenbarth GS, Rewers M. Lack of association between early exposure to cow's milk protein and β-cell autoimmunity. Diabetes Autoimmunity Study in the Young (DAISY). *JAMA* 1996; 276 (8): 609–14.
159. Virtanen SM, Hypponen E, Laara E, Vahasalo P, Kulmala P, Savola K, Rasanen L, Aro A, Knip M, Akerblom HK. for the Childhood Diabetes in Finland Study Group. Cow's milk consumption, disease-associated autoantibodies and type 1 diabetes mellitus: a follow-up study in siblings of diabetic children. *Diabet Med* 1998; 15 (9): 730–8.
160. Couper JJ, Steele C, Beresford S, Powell T, McCaul K, Pollard A, Gellert S, Tait B, Harrison LC, Colman PG. Lack of association between duration of breast-feeding or introduction of cow's milk and development of islet autoimmunity. *Diabetes* 1999; 48 (11): 2145–9.
161. Kyvik KO, Green A, Svendsen A, Mortensen K. Breast feeding and the development of type 1 diabetes mellitus. *Diabet Med* 1992; 9: 233–5.
162. Samuelsson U, Johansson C, Ludvigsson J. Breast-feeding seems to play a marginal role in the prevention of insulin-dependent diabetes mellitus. *Diabetes Res Clin Pract* 1993; 19: 203–10.
163. Bodington MJ, McNally PG, Burden AC. Cow's milk and type 1 childhood diabetes: no increase in risk. *Diabet Med* 1994; 11: 663–5.
164. Mathieu C, Laureys J, Sobis H, Vandeputte M, Waer M, Bouillon R. 1,25-Dihydroxyvitamin D3 prevents insulitis in NOD mice. *Diabetes* 1992; 41 (11): 1491–5.
165. Harris S. Can vitamin D supplementation in infancy prevent type 1 diabetes? *Nutr Rev* 2002; 60 (4): 118–21.
166. The EURODIAB Substudy 2 Study Group. Vitamin D supplement in early childhood and risk for type I (insulin-dependent) diabetes mellitus. *Diabetologia* 1999; 42 (1): 51–4.
167. Hypponen E, Laara E, Reunanen A, Jarvelin MR, Virtanen SM. Intake of vitamin D and risk of type 1 diabetes: a birth-cohort study. *Lancet* 2001; 358 (9292): 1500–3.
168. Stene LC, Ulriksen J, Magnus P, Joner G. Use of cod liver oil during pregnancy associated with lower risk of type I diabetes in the offspring. *Diabetologia* 2000; 43 (9): 1093–8.
169. Helgason T, Jonasson MR. Evidence for a food additive as a cause of ketosis-prone diabetes. *Lancet* 1981; 2: 716–20.
170. Dahlquist GG, Blom LG, Persson LA, Sandstrom AI, Wall SG. Dietary factors and the risk of developing insulin dependent diabetes in childhood. *BMJ* 1990; 300: 1302–6.

171. Kostraba JN, Gay EC, Rewers M, Hamman RF. Nitrate levels in community drinking waters and risk of IDDM. An ecological analysis. *Diabetes Care* 1992; 15 (11): 1505–8.
172. Virtanen SM, Jaakkola L, Rasanen L, Ylonen K, Aro A, Lounamaa R, Akerblom HK, for the Childhood Diabetes in Finland Study Group. Nitrate and nitrite intake and the risk for type I diabetes in Finnish children. *Diabet Med* 1994; 11: 656–62.
173. van Maanen JM, Albering HJ, de Kok TM, van Breda SG, Curfs DM, Vermeer IT, Ambergen AW, Wolffenbuttel BH, Kleinjans JC, Reeser HM. Does the risk of childhood diabetes mellitus require revision of the guideline values for nitrate in drinking water? *Environ Health Perspect* 2000; 108 (5): 457–61.
174. Khoury MJ, Flanders WD, Greenland S, Adams MJ. On the measurement of susceptibility in epidemiologic studies. *Am J Epidemiol* 1989; 129: 183–90.
175. Fohlman J, Bohme J, Rask L, Frisk G, Diderholm H, Friman G, Tuvemo T. Matching of host genotype and serotypes of Coxsackie B virus in the development of juvenile diabetes. *Scand J Immunol* 1987; 26: 105–10.
176. D'Alessio DJ. A case-control study of group B Coxsackievirus immunoglobulin M antibody prevalence and HLA-DR antigens in newly diagnosed cases of insulin-dependent diabetes mellitus. *Am J Epidemiol* 1992; 135: 1331–8.
177. Schernthaner G, Banatvala JE, Scherbaum W, Bryant J, Borkenstein M, Schober E, Mayr WR. Coxsackie-B-virus-specific IgM responses, complement-fixing islet-cell antibodies, HLA DR antigens, and C-peptide secretion in insulin-dependent diabetes mellitus. *Lancet* 1985; 2: 630–2.
178. Kostraba JN, Cruickshanks KJ, Lawler-Heavner J, Jobim LF, Rewers MJ, Gay EC, Chase HP, Klingensmith G, Hamman RF. Early exposure to cow's milk and solid foods in infancy, genetic predisposition, and risk of IDDM. *Diabetes* 1993; 42 (2): 288–95.
179. Virtanen SM, Laara E, Hypponen E, Reijonen H, Rasanen L, Aro A, Knip M, Ilonen J, Akerblom HK. for the Childhood diabetes in Finland Study Group. Cow's milk consumption, HLA-DQB1 genotype, and type 1 diabetes: a nested case-control study of siblings of children with diabetes. *Diabetes* 2000; 49 (6): 912–7.
180. Paronen J, Knip M, Savilahti E, Virtanen SM, Ilonen J, Akerblom HK, Vaarala O. Effect of cow's milk exposure and maternal type 1 diabetes on cellular and humoral immunization to dietary insulin in infants at genetic risk for type 1 diabetes Finnish Trial to Reduce IDDM in the Genetically at Risk Study Group. Finnish Trial to Reduce IDDM in the Genetically at Risk Study Group. *Diabetes* 2000; 49 (10): 1657–65.
181. Eisenbarth GS, Verge CF, Allen H, Rewers MJ. The design of trials for prevention of IDDM. *Diabetes* 1993; 42 (7): 941–7.
182. Bingley PJ, Bonifacio E, Ziegler AG, Schatz DA, Atkinson MA, Eisenbarth GS. Proposed guidelines on screening for risk of type 1 diabetes. *Diabetes Care* 2001; 24 (2): 398.
183. Schatz DA, Bingley PJ. Update on major trials for the prevention of type 1 diabetes mellitus: the American Diabetes Prevention Trial (DPT-1) and the European Nicotinamide Diabetes Intervention Trial (ENDIT). *J Pediatr Endocrinol Metab* 2001; 14 (suppl 1): 619–22.
184. Lampeter EF, Klinghammer A, Scherbaum WA, Heinze E, Haastert B, Giani G, Kolb H. for the DENIS Group. The Deutsche Nicotinamide Intervention Study: an attempt to prevent type 1 diabetes. *Diabetes* 1998; 47 (6): 980–4.
185. Knip M, Douek IF, Moore WP, Gillmor HA, McLean AE, Bingley PJ, Gale EA. Safety of high-dose nicotinamide: a review. *Diabetologia* 2000; 43 (11): 1337–45.
186. Keller RJ, Eisenbarth GS, Jackson RA. Insulin prophylaxis in individuals at high risk of type I diabetes. *Lancet* 1993; 341 (8850): 927–8.
187. DPT-1 Study Group. The Diabetes Prevention Trial-type 1 diabetes (DPT-1): implementation of screening and staging of relatives. *Transplant Proc* 1995; 27 (6): 3377.
188. Pozzilli P, Pitocco D, Visalli N, Cavallo MG, Buzzetti R, Crino A, Spera S, Suraci C, Multari G, Cervoni M, Manca BM, Matteoli MC, Marietti G, Ferrazzoli F, Cassone FM, Giordano C, Sbriglia M, Sarugeri E, Ghirlanda G. for the IMDIAB Group. No effect of oral insulin on residual β-cell function in recent-onset type I diabetes (the IMDIAB VII). *Diabetologia* 2000; 43 (8): 1000–4.
189. Chaillous L, Lefevre H, Thivolet C, Boitard C, Lahlou N, Atlan-Gepner C, Bouhanick B, Mogenet A, Nicolino M, Carel JC, Lecomte P, Marechaud R, Bougneres P, Charbonnel B Sai P. Oral insulin administration and residual β-cell function in recent-onset type 1 diabetes: a multicentre randomised controlled trial. *Lancet* 2000; 356 (9229): 545–9.
190. Feutren G, Assan G, Karsenty G, DuRostu H, Sirmai J, Papoz L, Vialettes B, Vexiau P, Rodier M, Lallemand A, Bach JF. Cyclosporin increases the rate and length of remissions in insulin dependent diabetes of recent onset. Results of a multicentre double-blind trial. *Lancet* 1986; 2 (8499): 119–24.
191. The Canadian-European Randomized Control Trial Group. Cyclosporin-induced remission of IDDM after early intervention. Association of 1 yr of cyclosporin treatment with enhanced insulin secretion. *Diabetes* 1988; 37 (11): 1574–82.
192. Martin S, Schernthaner G, Nerup J, Gries FA, Koivisto VA, Dupre J, Standl E, Hamet P, McArthur R, Tan MH. Follow-up of cyclosporin A treatment in type 1 (insulin-dependent) diabetes mellitus: lack of long-term effects. *Diabetologia* 1991; 34 (6): 429–34.
193. Hao L, Chan S-M, Lafferty KJ. Mycophenolate mofetil can prevent the development of diabetes in BB rats. *Ann NY Acad Sci* 1994; 696: 328–32.
194. Alleva DG, Gaur A, Jin L, Wegmann D, Gottlieb PA, Pahuja A, Johnson EB, Motheral T, Putnam A, Crowe PD, Ling N, Boehme SA, Conlon PJ. Immunological characterization and therapeutic activity of an altered- peptide ligand, NBI-6024, based on the immunodominant type 1 diabetes autoantigen insulin B-chain (9–23) peptide. *Diabetes* 2002; 51 (7): 2126–34.
195. Herold KC, Bluestone JA, Montag AG, Parihar A, Wiegner A, Gress RE, Hirsch R. Prevention of autoimmune diabetes with nonactivating anti-CD3 monoclonal antibody. *Diabetes* 1992; 41 (3): 385–91.
196. Knip M, Sakkinen A, Huttunen NP, Kaar ML, Lankela S, Mustonen A, Akerblom HK. Postinitial remission in diabetic children—an analysis of 178 cases. *Acta Paediatr Scand* 1982; 71 (6): 901–8.
197. Agner T, Damm P, Binder C. Remission in IDDM: prospective study of basal C-peptide and insulin dose in

268 consecutive patients. *Diabetes Care* 1987; 10 (2): 164–9.

198. Sochett EB, Daneman D, Clarson C, Ehrlich RM. Factors affecting and patterns of residual insulin secretion during the first year of type 1 (insulin-dependent) diabetes mellitus in children. *Diabetologia* 1987; 30 (7): 453–9.
199. Ortqvist E, Falorni A, Scheynius A, Persson B, Lernmark A. Age governs gender-dependent islet cell autoreactivity and predicts the clinical course in childhood IDDM. *Acta Paediatr* 1997; 86 (11): 1166–71.
200. Schiffrin A, Suissa S, Poussier P, Guttmann R, Weitzner G. Prospective study of predictors of β-cell survival in type I diabetes. *Diabetes* 1988; 37 (7): 920–5.
201. Wallensteen M, Dahlquist G, Persson B, Landin-Olsson M, Lernmark A, Sundkvist G, Thalme B. Factors influencing the magnitude, duration, and rate of fall of B-cell function in type 1 (insulin-dependent) diabetic children followed for two years from their clinical diagnosis. *Diabetologia* 1988; 31 (9): 664–9.
202. Sabbah E, Savola K, Kulmala P, Veijola R, Vahasalo P, Karjalainen J, Akerblom HK, Knip M, for the Childhood Diabetes in Finland Study Group. Diabetes-associated autoantibodies in relation to clinical characteristics and natural course in children with newly diagnosed type 1 diabetes. *J Clin Endocrinol Metab* 1999; 84 (5): 1534–9.
203. Petersen JS, Dyrberg T, Karlsen AE, Molvig J, Michelsen B, Nerup J, Mandrup-Poulsen T, for the Canadian-European Randomized Control Trial Group. Glutamic acid decarboxylase (GAD65) autoantibodies in prediction of β-cell function and remission in recent-onset IDDM after cyclosporin treatment. *Diabetes* 1994; 43 (11): 1291–6.
204. Fukuda M, Tanaka A, Tahara Y, Ikegami H, Yamamoto Y, Kumahara Y, Shima K. Correlation between minimal secretory capacity of pancreatic β-cells and stability of diabetic control. *Diabetes* 1988; 37 (1): 81–8.
205. Kolb H, Dannehl K, Gruneklee D, Zielasek J, Bertrams J, Hubinger A, Gries FA. Prospective analysis of islet cell antibodies in children with type 1 (insulin-dependent) diabetes. *Diabetologia* 1988; 31 (4): 189–94.
206. Knip M, Ilonen J, Mustonen A, Akerblom HK. Evidence of an accelerated B-cell destruction in HLA-Dw3/Dw4 heterozygous children with type 1 (insulin-dependent) diabetes. *Diabetologia* 1986; 29 (6): 347–51.
207. Pipeleers D, Ling Z. Pancreatic β-cells in insulin-dependent diabetes. *Diabetes Metab Rev* 1992; 8 (3): 209–27.
208. Madsbad S, Faber OK, Binder C, McNair P, Christiansen C, Transbol I. Prevalence of residual β-cell function in insulin-dependent diabetics in relation to age at onset and duration of diabetes. *Diabetes* 1978; 27 (suppl 1): 262–4.
209. Rewers A, Chase HP, Mackenzie T, Walravens P, Roback M, Rewers M, Hamman RF, Klingensmith G. Predictors of acute complications in children with type 1 diabetes. *JAMA* 2002; 287 (19): 2511–8.
210. Dorman JS, LaPorte RE, Kuller LH, Cruickshanks KJ, Orchard TJ, Wagener DK, Becker DJ, Cavender DE, Drash AL. The Pittsburgh insulin-dependent diabetes mellitus (IDDM) morbidity and mortality study. Mortality results. *Diabetes* 1984; 33 (3): 271–6.
211. Diabetes Epidemiology Research International Mortality Study Group. Major cross-country differences in risk of dying for people with IDDM. *Diabetes Care* 1991; 14 (1): 49–54.
212. Matsushima M, LaPorte RE, Maruyama M, Shimizu K, Nishimura R, Tajima N, for the DERI Mortality Study Group. Diabetes Epidemiology Research International. Geographic variation in mortality among individuals with youth-onset diabetes mellitus across the world. *Diabetologia* 1997; 40 (2): 212–6.
213. Diabetes Epidemiology Research International Mortality Study Group. International evaluation of cause-specific mortality and IDDM. *Diabetes Care* 1991; 14 (1): 55–60.
214. Borch-Johnsen K, Nissen H, Henriksen E, Kreiner S, Salling N, Deckert T, Nerup J. The natural history of insulin-dependent diabetes mellitus in Denmark, 1: long-term survival with and without late diabetic complications. *Diabet Med* 1987; 4: 201–10.
215. Chowdhury TA, Dyer PH, Mijovic CH, Dunger DB, Barnett AH, Bain SC. Human leucocyte antigen and insulin gene regions and nephropathy in type I diabetes. *Diabetologia* 1999; 42 (8): 1017–20.
216. Doria A, Onuma T, Gearin G, Freire MB, Warram JH, Krolewski AS. Angiotensinogen polymorphism M235T, hypertension, and nephropathy in insulin-dependent diabetes. *Hypertension* 1996; 27 (5): 1134–9.
217. Doria A, Warram JH, Krolewski AS. Genetic predisposition to diabetic nephropathy. Evidence for a role of the angiotensin I-converting enzyme gene. *Diabetes* 1994; 43 (5): 690–5.
218. Fogarty DG, Harron JC, Hughes AE, Nevin NC, Doherty CC, Maxwell AP. A molecular variant of angiotensinogen is associated with diabetic nephropathy in IDDM. *Diabetes* 1996; 45 (9): 1204–8.
219. Nagi DK, Mansfield MW, Stickland MH, Grant PJ. Angiotensin converting enzyme (ACE) insertion/deletion (I/D) polymorphism, and diabetic retinopathy in subjects with IDDM and NIDDM. *Diabet Med* 1995; 12 (11): 997–1001.
220. Parving HH, Jacobsen P, Tarnow L, Rossing P, Lecerf L, Poirier O, Cambien F. Effect of deletion polymorphism of angiotensin converting enzyme gene on progression of diabetic nephropathy during inhibition of angiotensin converting enzyme: observational follow up study. *BMJ* 1996; 313 (7057): 591–4.
221. Tarnow L, Cambien F, Rossing P, Nielsen FS, Hansen BV, Lecerf L, Poirier O, Danilov S, Parving HH. Lack of relationship between an insertion/deletion polymorphism in the angiotensin I-converting enzyme gene and diabetic nephropathy and proliferative retinopathy in IDDM patients. *Diabetes* 1995; 44 (5): 489–94.
222. Tarnow L, Cambien F, Rossing P, Nielsen FS, Hansen BV, Ricard S, Poirier O, Parving HH. Angiotensinogen gene polymorphisms in IDDM patients with diabetic nephropathy. *Diabetes* 1996; 45 (3): 367–9.
223. The Diabetes Control and Complications Trial Research Group. The effect of intensive treatment of diabetes on the development and progression of long-term complications in insulin-dependent diabetes mellitus. *New Engl J Med* 1993; 329: 977–86.
224. The Diabetes Control and Complications Trial Research Group. Clustering of long-term complications in families with diabetes in the diabetes control and complications trial. *Diabetes* 1997; 46 (11): 1829–39.

3

Epidemiology and Geography of Type 2 Diabetes Mellitus

Qing Qiao*†, Desmond E. Williams‡, Giuseppina Imperatore‡, K.M. Venkat Narayan‡, and Jaakko Tuomilehto*†

**University of Helsinki, Helsinki, Finland, †National Public Health Institute, Helsinki, Finland, and ‡Centers for Disease Control and Prevention, National Center for Chronic Disease Prevention and Health Promotion, Atlanta, GA, USA*

AGE- AND SEX-SPECIFIC PREVALENCE OF TYPE 2 DIABETES IN DIFFERENT ETHNIC GROUPS

Type 2 diabetes mellitus is now taking its place as one of the main threats to human health in the twenty-first century [1]. In 1921, Dr Elliot Joslin was already concerned that according to his count there had been a doubling of diabetes in three decades [2]. The impact of type 2 diabetes is increasingly felt around the world, with its prevalence rising dramatically over the recent decades. The World Health Organization (WHO) estimated that there were 150 million people 20 years and older living with diabetes in 2000, and by 2025, this will be 300 million (Figure 1). There will be a 42% increase, from 51 to 72 million, in developed countries and a 170% increase, from 84 to 228 million, in developing countries [3]. The top 10 countries with the highest estimated number of people with diabetes in 2025 are listed in Table 1.

Diagnostic Criteria for Diabetes

In the past two decades there have been several important developments, which have had significant impact on the definition of diabetes and thereby on the assessment of its magnitude. In 1979, the 2-h 75-g oral glucose tolerance test (OGTT) was proposed as a standard test for diagnosis of diabetes by the National Diabetes Data Group (NDDG) [4], and endorsed by WHO in 1980 [5]. In 1985, WHO made a minor modification on the diagnostic criteria [6]. This has created order out of the confusion in the diagnostic criteria for diabetes. Before that enormous variations existed in diagnostic cutoff values for both fasting as well as after glucose loading. The glucose load varied between 50 and 100 g or was body weight related. The differences in glucose assay methods, glucose load, and the time after loading made the comparison between different studies difficult. Near-universal adoption of the WHO criteria has had a significant influence on epidemiological studies of diabetes.

In 1997, a revision of the diagnostic criteria was approved by American Diabetes Association (ADA) [7] and adopted by WHO Consultation in 1999 [8]. The major changes were lowering the positive cutoff value of fasting venous plasma glucose from 7.8 mmol/l (140 mg/dl) to 7.0 mmol/l (126 mg/dl). The positive cutoff value for 2-h plasma glucose remained unchanged, i.e. 11.1 mmol/l (200 mg/dl) and over. For epidemiological studies and for routine clinical practice, the ADA did not recommend the primary use of OGTT, but WHO Consultation still retained the OGTT as the standard test procedure. The prevalence data assembled in this chapter are estimated mainly according to the WHO 1999 criteria [8], except for those noted otherwise.

Conversion Factors for Glucose Concentrations

Glucose concentration can be measured using different blood specimens such as venous plasma glucose, capillary

International Textbook of Diabetes Mellitus, Third Edition. Edited by R. A. DeFronzo, E. Ferrannini, H. Keen, and P. Zimmet.
 ISBN: 0-471-48655-8.

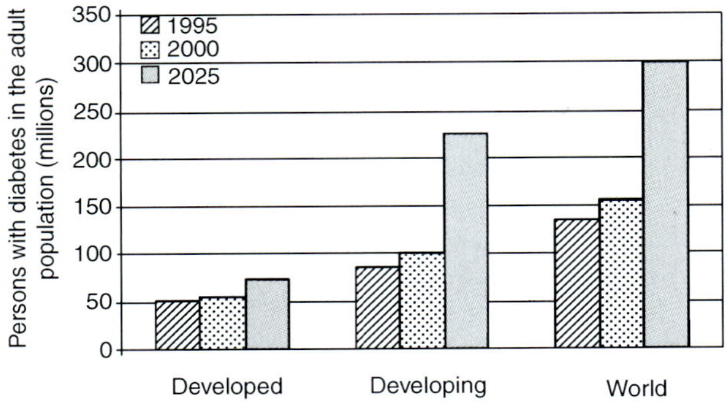

Figure 1 Number of people with diabetes mellitus, 1995–2025. (Adapted from reference 3)

whole blood glucose, and venous whole blood glucose. The cutoff points for the classification of stages of glucose abnormalities from different specimens are different. Currently, there are no internationally accepted conversion factors for glucose concentrations in the literature. Recently, Tuomilehto et al. (J. Tuomilehto and B. Carstensen, personal communication, 2003) developed conversion factors for changing glucose concentrations between different blood samples on the basis of data from a Finnish study and applied them in the DECODE study (Diabetes Epidemiology: Collaborative Analysis of Diagnostic Criteria in Europe) [9–11]. The equations were derived based on 294 matched samples of whole blood (capillary and serum) glucose and plasma glucose concentrations drawn from a standard 75-g OGTT in 74 individuals at 0, 30, 60, and 120 min at the Diabetes and Genetic Epidemiology Unit, National Public Health Institute in Finland. The relationships between glucose concentrations as measured by the different methods used were

Table 1 Top 10 countries for estimated number of adults with diabetes, 1995 and 2025*

Rank	Country	1995 (millions)	Country	2025 (millions)
1	India	19.4	India	57.2
2	China	16.0	China	37.6
3	United States	13.9	U.S.	21.9
4	Russian Federation	8.9	Pakistan	14.5
5	Japan	6.3	Indonesia	12.4
6	Brazil	4.9	Russian Federation	12.2
7	Indonesia	4.5	Mexico	11.7
8	Pakistan	4.3	Brazil	11.6
9	Mexico	3.8	Egypt	8.8
10	Ukraine	3.6	Japan	8.5
	All other countries	49.7		103.6
	Total	*135.3*		*300.0*

* From reference 3.

estimated. The formulas derived are as follows:

Venous plasma glucose (mmol/l)

$= 0.558 + 1.119 \times$ whole blood glucose (mmol/l)

Venous plasma glucose (mmol/l)

$= 0.102 + 1.066 \times$ capillary blood glucose (mmol/l)

Venous plasma glucose (mmol/l)

$= -0.137 + 1.047 \times$ serum glucose (mmol/l)

Age- and Sex-specific Plasma Glucose Concentration

The age- and sex-specific mean fasting and 2-h plasma glucose after 75-g glucose load were estimated in general Caucasian populations in Europe, and in Chinese, Japanese, and Indians in Asia, who did not have prior history of diabetes. The participants are included in the DECODE and the DECODA studies (Diabetes Epidemiology: Collaborative Analysis of Diagnostic Criteria in Asia), the two largest epidemiological studies for diabetes in Europe and Asia, with a total of 15 606 subjects from Europe [10] and 19 845 subjects from Asia [12]. The data presented here are based on the pooled data from 13 DECODE and the 11 DECODA participating cohorts. A standard OGTT was carried out in all populations, and subjects with prior history of diabetes were not included in the analysis. The plasma glucose concentrations rose with age and reached a peak at 60–69 years of age and then started to decline in Indians but continued to increase after 70 years of age in Europeans (Figure 2). At each age group, the mean 2-h plasma glucose was significantly higher for Indians than for Chinese and Japanese, and the same was also true for fasting plasma glucose in most of the age groups (Figure 2). The mean fasting and 2-h glucose concentrations did not differ between Chinese and Japanese except at 40–49 years of age where the glucose values were higher in the Japanese. The mean glucose levels were lower in Europeans than in Asians younger than 70 years, whereas they were higher in Europeans than in Asians 70 years or older. The mean glucose levels were similar in Asian men and women. In Europe, the mean fasting glucose concentration was higher in men than in women at 30–69 years of age but after 70 years of age, it was higher in women. The 2-h glucose was higher in women than in men throughout the age range. Two-hour glucose increased more with age than did fasting glucose.

Age- and Sex-specific Prevalence of Diabetes

Europe

The prevalence of diabetes has been estimated by applying the WHO 1999 criteria [8] for 13 European and 11 Asian cohorts participating in the DECODE and the DECODA

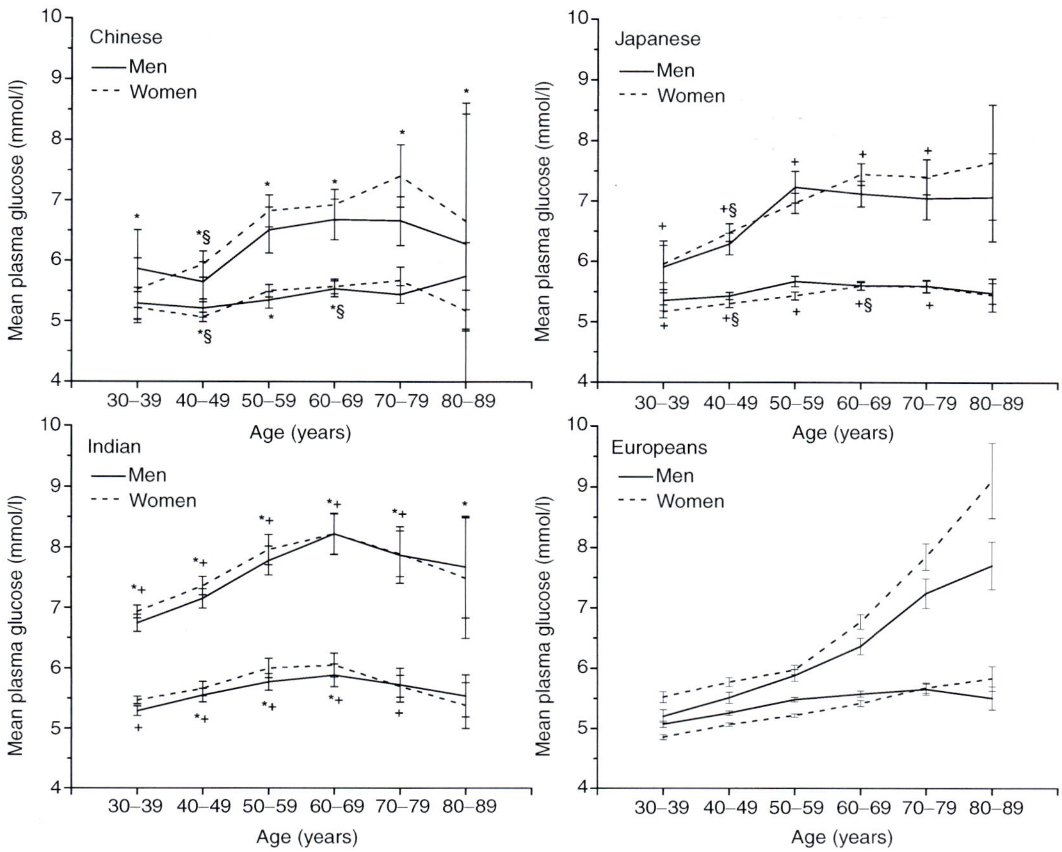

Figure 2 Mean fasting (the two lower lines) and 2-h (the two upper lines) plasma glucose concentrations and their 95% confidence intervals (vertical bars) for the DECODE and the DECODA study populations. *Indians vs. Chinese, +Indians vs. Japanese, §Japanese vs. Chinese, all for $p < 0.05$ for both genders combined. [Adapted from the DECODE [10] and the DECODA [12] Study Groups]

studies. In Europe, the age-specific prevalence of diabetes rose with age up to 70s and 80s in both men and women [10] (Figure 3). In most of the studies, the prevalence was less than 10% in subjects younger than 60 years and between 10 and 20% at 60–79 years of age. They were higher in Malta than in other populations. The prevalence of isolated postload hyperglycemia (2-h glucose ≥11.1 mmol/l and fasting glucose <7.0 mmol/l) increased more with age than did isolated fasting hyperglycemia (fasting glucose ≥7.0 mmol/l and 2-h glucose <11.1 mmol/l), particularly in women.

A recent German study using WHO 1999 criteria [8] showed that the prevalence of diabetes in Germany in 2000 was 16.7% in men and 8.6% in women at 55–59 years of age and 23.1% in men and 17.0% in women at 70–74 years of age [13]; i.e., rates are within the variation reported for the DECODE study. In the Turkish Diabetes Epidemiology Study (TURDEP) made in 1997–1998, where a single 2-h postload glucose test was applied, the prevalence of diabetes increased with age, reaching the peak of 19.4% in men and 25.7% in women at 60–69 years of age in the urban population and of 19.1% in men and 18.2% in women at 70 years or older in the rural population [14]. These rates are higher than those reported by another earlier Turkish study in 1994 [15].

Compared with most of the other racial and ethnic groups worldwide, where age- and sex-specific prevalence of diabetes has been reported, Europeans have a moderate to low prevalence of diabetes [10].

United States

In the United States, the prevalence of diabetes varies considerably among different ethnic groups. The prevalence was 1.9 times greater in Latino Americans and 1.6 times in African Americans than in White of the same age in the Third National Health and Nutrition Examination Survey (NHANES III) [16]. In NHANES III, where a single fasting plasma glucose ≥7.0 mmol/l was applied for the diagnosis of diabetes, the prevalence of diabetes in US Whites in 1988–1994 was 5.9% in men and 4.8% in women at 40–49 years of age and reached peak of 19.2% in men and 16.6% in women at 75 years or older [16]. The prevalence of undiagnosed diabetes according to the same fasting

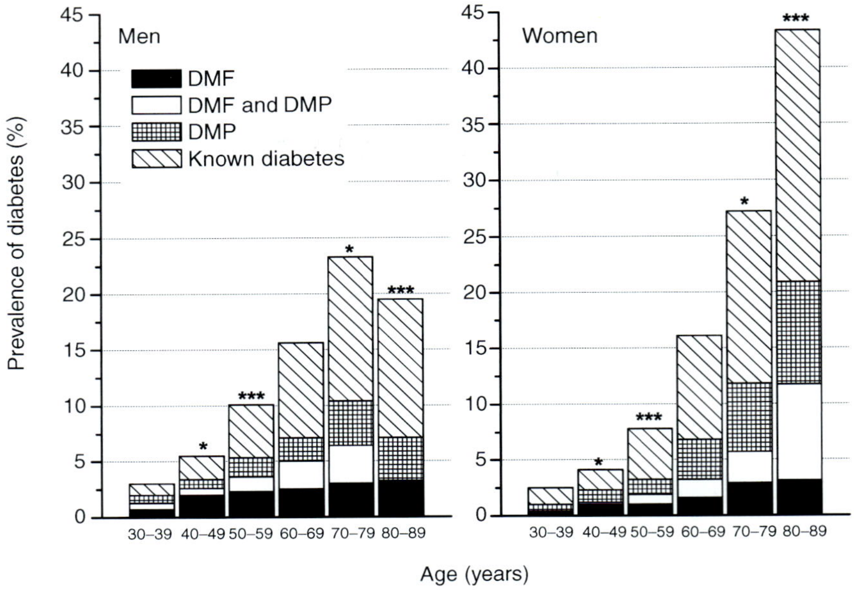

Figure 3 Age- and sex-specific prevalence of diabetes in the DECODE study population. DMF: diabetes by FPG $\geq$7.0 mmol/l and 2hPG $<$11.1 mmol/l; DMP: diabetes by 2hPG $\geq$11.1 mmol/l and FPG $<$7.0 mmol/l; DMF&DMP: Diabetes by FPG $\geq$7.0 mmol/l and 2hPG $\geq$11.1 mmol/l. $^{*}p<0.05$, $^{**}p<0.01$, $^{***}p<0.001$, for the difference between men and women. (Adapted from the DECODE Study Group [10])

glucose criteria at a comparable age range of 40–59 years was higher in US Whites than in most of the female and in half of the male European populations participating in the DECODE study [10]. The rates were higher in Mexican Americans than in the US Whites, and were higher than seen in any of the populations included in the DECODE study.

The Pima Indians have the highest prevalence of diabetes in the world, being 50% at 30–64 years of age, estimated using 2-h postload glucose test alone [17]. The prevalence of diabetes in Native Hawaiians (Polynesian population of Hawaii) in two rural communities was estimated using WHO 1985 criteria [18]. At 30–39 years of age, the prevalence was 6.5% in women and 10.7% in men, reaching the peak of 34.6% in women and 40.0% in men at 70 years or older. Other Native American tribes also have higher prevalence of diabetes than do Caucasoids.

Central and South America

The age-standardized prevalence of diabetes using 2-h glucose criteria alone was investigated in Brazilian population in Sao Paulo in 1987 and in Colombian population in Bogota in 1988–1989 [17]. The prevalences in both populations were similar, around 7% for men and 9% for women. The age-specific prevalence of diabetes in Mexican population in Mexico City was 4.2% in men and 3.2% in women at 35–39 years of age and reached 23.1% in men and 41.7% in women at 60–64 years of age [17].

Australia

The Australia Diabetes, Obesity and Lifestyle Study (AusDiab) took place in 1999–2000 applying WHO 1999 criteria mainly in Caucasoids. The prevalence of diabetes increased with age, from 2.7% in men and 2.2% in women at 35–44 years of age to 23.5% and 22.7% at 75 years or older [19]. These rates were higher than those in most of the DECODE populations [10].

Asia and Pacific Islands

Asia The prevalence of diabetes varies markedly among Asian populations. In those participating in the DECODA study, it rises with age up to 70s and 80s in Chinese and Japanese, and in Indian men and women with age up to 60s and then declines [12] (Figure 4a and b). The age- and sex-specific prevalence and the peak prevalence of diabetes were higher in cohorts from India and Singapore than in most of the Chinese and Japanese cohorts. In Chinese and Japanese, the prevalence was less than 10% at 30–49 years of age; the peak prevalence was less than 20% in most of the cohorts and none exceeded 30%. In contrast, in India and Singapore the prevalence was over 10% among people aged 40–49 years, and over 30% among those aged 50–69 years for most of the cohorts. The urban Chinese and Japanese had significantly higher prevalences of diabetes than their rural counterparts at 40–69 years of age in men and at 50–79 years of age in women (Figure 4). The prevalence of diabetes in Korea was within the range observed in China and Japan [20].

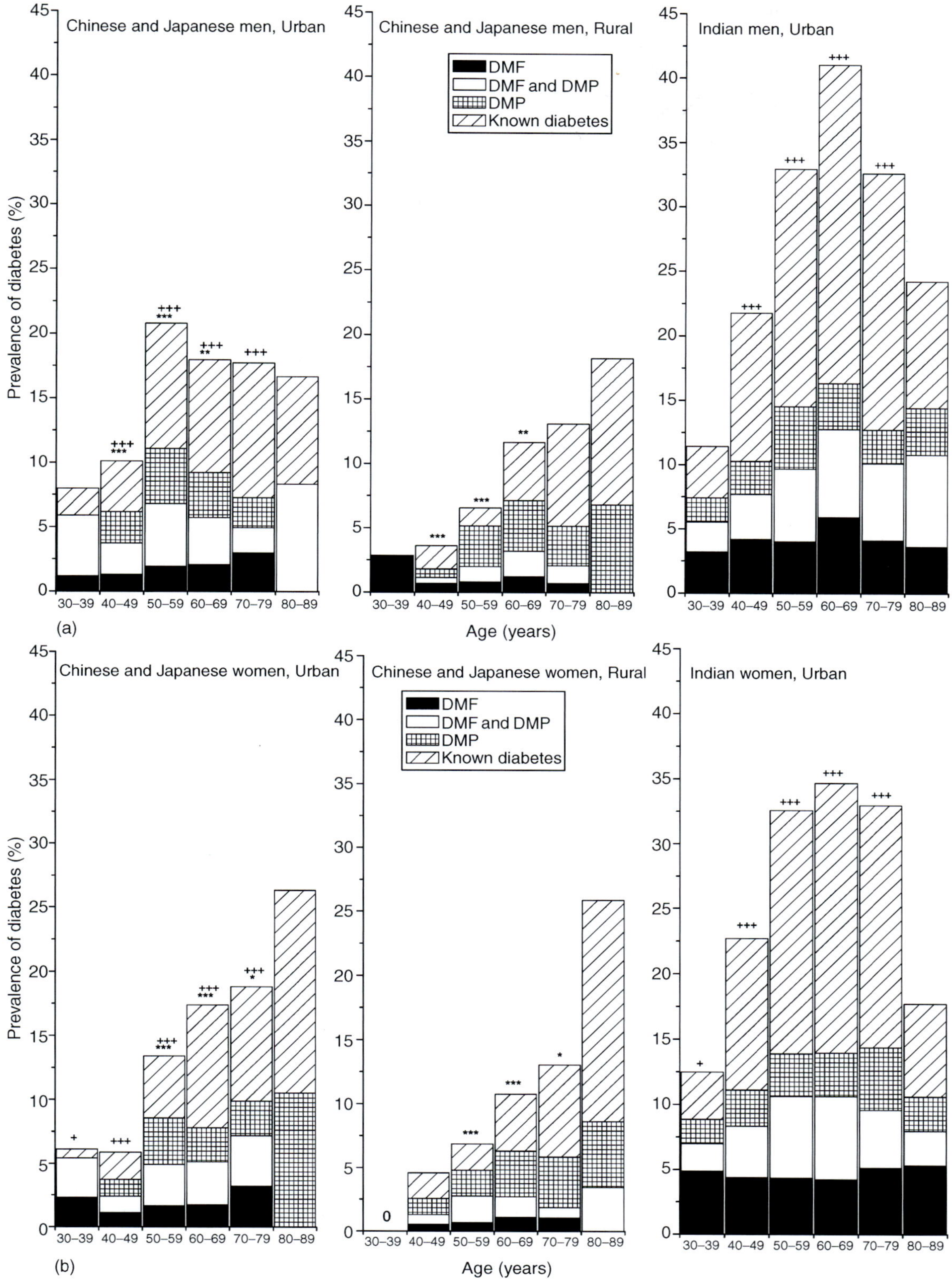

Figure 4 Age- and sex-specific prevalence of diabetes in Asia men (a) and women (b) in the DECODA study. DMF: diabetes determined by FPG $\geq$7.0 mmol/l and 2hPG $<$11.1 mmol/l; DMP: diabetes determined by 2hPG $\geq$11.1 mmol/l and FPG $<$7.0 mmol/l; DMF&DMP: diabetes determined by FPG $\geq$7.0 mmol/l and 2hPG $\geq$11.1 mmol/l. $^{*}p < 0.05$, $^{**}p < 0.01$, $^{***}p < 0.001$, for the difference between urban and rural Chinese and Japanese; $+p < 0.05$, $+++p < 0.001$, for the difference between Chinese and Japanese combined and Indians. (Adapted from the DECODA Study Group [12])

Type 2 diabetes was found at a relatively younger age in Pakistan and the prevalence reached the peak in the age group 55–64 years [21–23]; the prevalence pattern was similar to that in India. In a rural community the prevalence was over 13% at 35–44 years of age, with the highest prevalence of 30% in men at 65–74 years of age [22], indicating diabetes has already become a major health threat in Pakistan as in India.

In the late 1990s, King et al. carried out a series of surveys on diabetes in Uzbekistan and Mongolia using WHO 1985 criteria [6]. In Uzbekistan, the prevalence did not differ markedly between rural and urban communities [24, 25]. It was relatively rare in people younger than 45 years, around 1%, and 10–15% at 65 years or older. The prevalence in Mongolia [26] was relatively low with a peak of less than 5% at the age of 65 years or older, comparable to the prevalence reported from China in 1994 [27]. Taking into account the high positive cutoff value of 7.8 mmol/l for fasting glucose for diabetes in the WHO 1985 criteria, the prevalence reported in these studies would be somewhat higher if the current cutoff value of 7.0 mmol/l were used. Because different diagnostic criteria have been applied, the results from some of these studies cannot be compared directly with those from the DECODA study [12].

Compared with the European populations included in the DECODE study [10], the age-specific prevalence of diabetes in urban Chinese and Japanese was slightly higher than that in Europeans at 30–69 years of age, but was lower than that in Indians. In the elderly population, however, the peak prevalence was higher in a few European populations than in Indians, such as in Maltese, in Finnish women in Oulu, and in women living in the Canary Island, Spain. The age at which the peak prevalence of diabetes was reached was similar for Europeans, Chinese, and Japanese (over 70 years), while Indians had their highest prevalence at the age up to 60s and then started to decline. These differences in prevalence in the elderly (women, in particular) are probably due to selective mortality associated with diabetes.

In all Asian populations included in the DECODA study, the prevalence of isolated fasting hyperglycemia (fasting plasma glucose $\geq$7.0 mmol/l and 2-h plasma glucose $<$11.1 mmol/l) did not increase with age (Figure 4). The prevalence of isolated 2-h hyperglycemia (2-h plasma glucose $\geq$11.1 mmol/l and fasting plasma glucose $<$7.0 mmol/l) tended to increase with age in Chinese and Japanese but not in Asian Indians [12].

Pacific Islands There are remarkable differences in the prevalence of diabetes among the Melanesia, Micronesian, and Polynesian populations of the Pacific Islands. According to the 2-h postload glucose criteria alone [6], an age-standardized diabetes prevalence of more than 40% was revealed in the Micronesia population of Nauru in 1980s [28, 29]. The prevalence of diabetes in the Melanesia population of Papua New Guinea had been reported close to 0% in highland populations [30], whereas in the urbanized Koki people the age-standardized rate exceeds 40%, approaching that of Nauru [29], exhibiting an extreme urban–rural gradient. Intermediate rates are seen in other Pacific Island populations. In the Polynesia population of the Western Samoa, the crude prevalence rates were 3.4 and 8.7% in rural and urban populations, respectively. By 1991, these rates had risen to 6.5 and 9.0% in two rural communities and to 16% in the urban settings of Apia [31]. A recent study in the Polynesia population of Tonga in 1998–2000 using 2-h OGTT showed that the peak prevalence of diabetes reached 20% in men and 40% in women aged 60 years or older [32].

Middle East

The prevalences of diabetes in Arabian countries, calculated according to the WHO 1985 criteria [6], have been reported to be high [33–35]. It is relatively low before the age of 30 years and starts to increase at 40s, with the highest in the oldest age group (Figure 5). In a rural Palestinian village, in 1996 the prevalence of diabetes was less than 4.0% in people younger than 40 years but increased to 11.0% at 40–49 years of age, with a peak of 21.7% in men and 31.6% in women at 60–65 years of age [35]. The prevalence in Palestine was similar to that in rural Saudi Arabia, but both were lower than that in urban Saudi Arabia [33]. The prevalence of type 2 diabetes in 1995–1996 in Kuwait was recalculated using ADA 1997 criteria [7]. It was lower than 3% at age of 20–29 years, around 9% at age of 30–39 years and higher than 15% at age of 40–49 [36]. Diabetes is prevalent in all Arab countries despite the differences in the economic status among these countries, indicating that genetic susceptibility and cultural factors may play an important role in the development of the disease.

The age-specific rate ranged from 8% at 40–44 years of age to 25% at 60–64 years of age in Israeli Jews [17].

Africa

In subjects aged 30–64 years, the age-standardized prevalence of diabetes using 2-h glucose alone has been reported to be higher in Hindu and Muslim Indians living in Mauritius [37] and Tanzania [38], around 10% in Tanzania and 13–18% in Mauritius. The age-standardized rate was very low in Bantu in Tanzania, less than 1% in women and 0.9–3.3% in men [39]. The prevalence was 8% in Tunisia [17]. It is interesting to notice that the age-standardized prevalence was much high in Chinese living in Mauritius than that in Da Qing in China in the middle of the 1980s [17, 37], indicating the importance of the impact of the environmental factors.

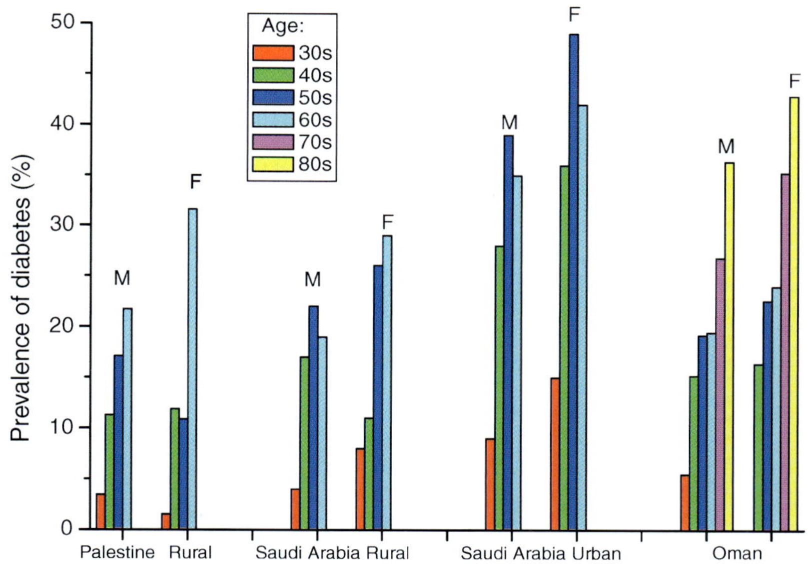

Figure 5 Prevalence of diabetes in men and women in three Arabian countries

In Native People: Mapuche and Aymara in Chile and in Siberia in Russian Federation

The native people who still practice their traditional lifestyle and have considerable physical activity have extremely low prevalences of diabetes despite their high prevalence of obesity [40, 41]. Among Aymara the prevalence of diabetes in 1997 was almost undetectable despite the fact that 13% of the men and 24% of the women had body mass index (BMI) higher than 30 kg/m^2 [40]. Similar findings have been reported among native Mapuche [41, 42]. The indigenous groups in northern Siberia also showed a very low prevalence, being less than 1% in 1994 [43]. This suggests that a healthy lifestyle with much physical activity provides protection from the development of diabetes. A recent report from Mapuche [41] showed that the prevalence in 1998 was higher than that reported 15 years ago, as was the prevalence of obesity [42], suggesting a possible impact of lifestyle changes on the trends in prevalence of diabetes.

Previously Undiagnosed Diabetes

The proportion with previously undiagnosed diabetes varies with age. It seems to be highest at 30–39 years of age (70–80%), and the lowest in the elderly (around 40%) [10, 12]. The only exception was seen in European women where the proportion of undiagnosed diabetic cases was around 40–45% in all age groups. The proportion of undiagnosed diabetes was higher in European men than in European women. In Asians, it was slightly higher in women than in men at youngest age groups.

PREVALENCE OF IMPAIRED GLUCOSE TOLERANCE AND IMPAIRED FASTING GLYCAEMIA IN DIFFERENT ETHNIC GROUPS

A category of nondiabetic fasting hyperglycemia was defined only recently, by ADA in 1997 [7] and adopted also by WHO in 1999 [8], and named impaired fasting glycemia (IFG). It was introduced by consensus to define impaired glucose homeostasis intermediate between diabetes and normal glucose homeostasis and to be analogous to impaired glucose tolerance (IGT), but without any epidemiological evidence of possible risks associated with it. Since the introduction of the category of IFG, prospective studies have examined the relationship between IFG and future morbidity and mortality with a comparison to IGT, and shown that the risk of cardiovascular disease (CVD) morbidity and mortality is higher for IGT than for IFG [44–47]. Thus far the data are scanty on the risk of progression to diabetes in subjects with IFG as compared with those with normal fasting glucose or those with IGT. A few studies, which have examined the issue, agree that the risk of developing diabetes is high in subjects with either IFG or IGT and highest in those with both IFG and IGT, as compared with subjects with normal fasting and normal 2-h glucose [48–52]. At present neither IFG nor IGT is considered a clinical entity, but as a risk category for the future development of diabetes [53]. Each represents metabolic state intermediate between normal glucose homeostasis and diabetic hyperglycemia, and are combined and defined formally as impaired glucose regulation (IGR) by WHO Consultation in 1999 [8]. All studies agree that only IGT but not IFG is a risk factor for CVD.

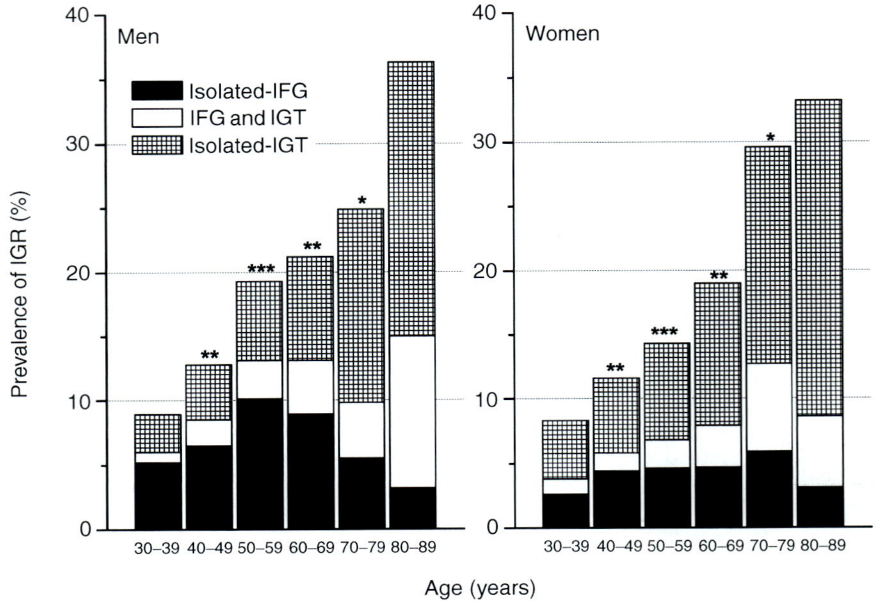

Figure 6 Age- and sex-specific prevalence of impaired glucose regulation (IGR) in the DECODE study populations. Isolated-IFG: FPG 6.1–6.9 mmol/l and 2hPG <7.8 mmol/l; Isolated-IGT: 2hPG 7.8–11.0 mmol/l and FPG < 6.1 mmol/l; IFG&IGT: FPG 6.1–6.9 mmol/l and 2hPG 7.8–11.0 mmol/l. $^{*}p < 0.05$, $^{**}p < 0.01$, $^{***}p < 0.001$, for the difference in the total prevalence between men and women. (Adapted from the DECODE Study Group [10])

The prevalences of IGT and IFG in Europe and Asia were reported recently by the DECODE and the DECODA Study Groups [8, 12].

Europe

The prevalence of IGR rose with age in each study [10] (Figure 6). In most of the study populations, the prevalence of IGR was less than 15% at 30–59 years of age and between 15 and 30% after 60 years of age. The prevalence of IGT increased linearly with age, but the prevalence of IFG did not (Figure 6). The increase in the prevalence of undiagnosed diabetes and IGR in the elderly population resulted mainly from the proportionately larger increase in postload hyperglycemia than in fasting hyperglycemia.

Asia

The prevalence of IGR rose with age up to 70s and 80s in most of the study cohorts [12] (Figure 7a and b). The increase was graded with aging in Chinese, Japanese, and Singaporean populations, as observed in Europeans, but not in Indians where the prevalence of IGR started to increase by the age of 30–39 years and did not change much with increasing age. The peak prevalences of IGR were not different among different populations, but the age-specific prevalence of IGR was higher in Indians than in Chinese and Japanese at 30–49 years of age for both men and women. In the urban populations the prevalence was higher than in the rural populations aged 40–69 years in men and 50–59 years in women in Chinese and Japanese (Figure 7). The difference in the prevalence pattern in different ethnic groups may not be completely explained by living environments and geographic locations, suggesting that genetic differences play a role, too.

IGT was more prevalent than IFG in almost all age groups in Asian subjects (Figure 7). The prevalence of IGT increases with age whereas IFG does not. This pattern is consistent with that among the European populations [10]. The concordance for IFG and IGT was very poor in all populations, particularly in Asians [10, 12, 54–56]. The finding that postload hyperglycemia was more prevalent in the elderly in Europe and Asia is consistent with the report from NHANES III [57]. Thus, the prevalence of undiagnosed diabetes and IGR would be underestimated to a large extent, especially in female and elderly population, if only fasting glucose determination were used. The primary purpose of population-based testing for blood glucose is to detect previously undiagnosed diabetes and IGR in order to apply early intervention to reduce the serious diabetic complications and to prevent worsening from IGT to diabetes as demonstrated by the recent diabetes prevention trials [58–62].

SEX DIFFERENCES IN PREVALENCE OF DIABETES, IGT, AND IFG

The ratio of prevalences of glucose abnormality between men and women has been estimated in many studies, but

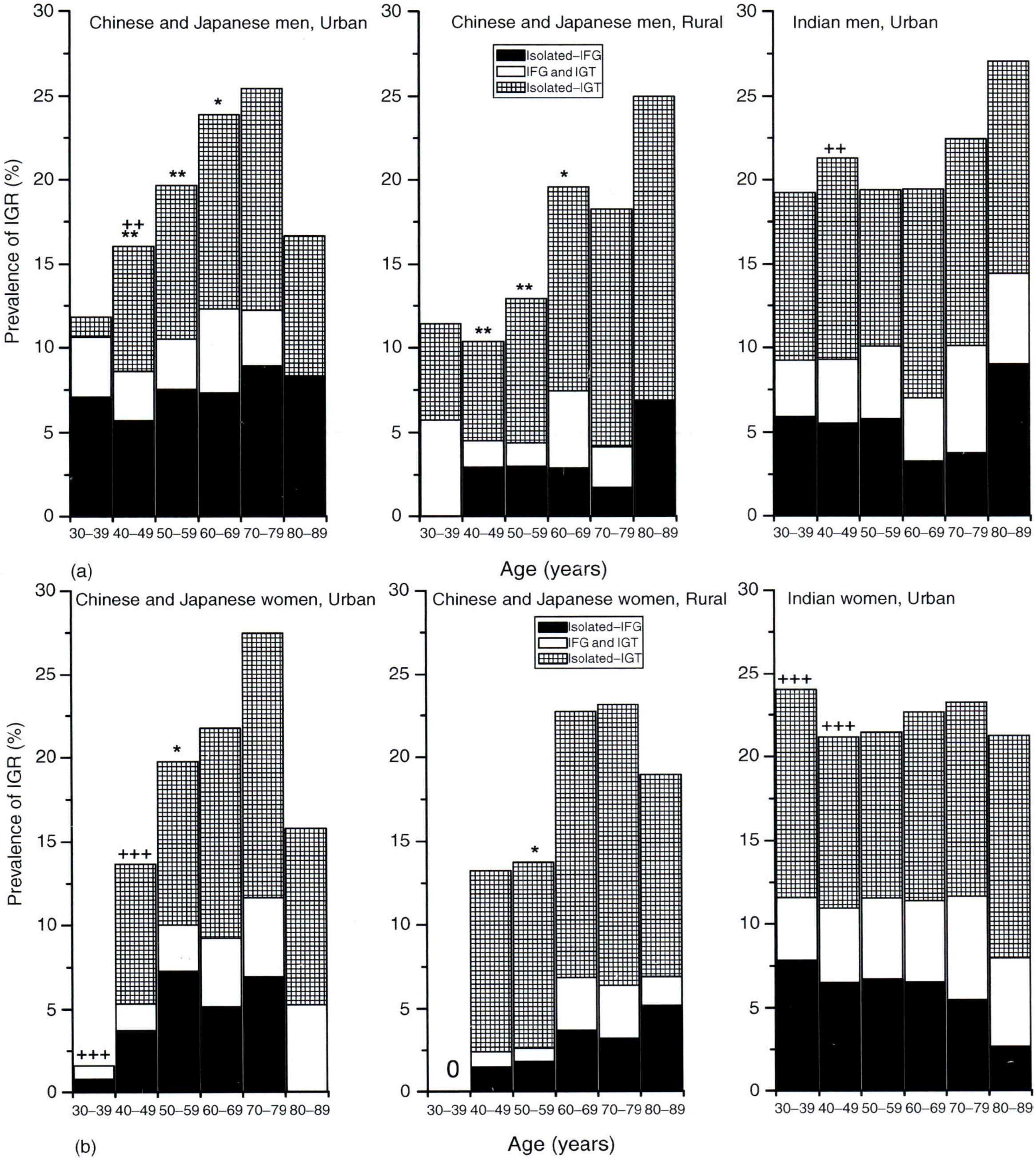

Figure 7 Age- and sex-specific prevalence of impaired glucose regulation in the DECODA study populations in men (a) and women (b). Isolated-IFG: FPG 6.1–6.9 mmol/l and 2hPG <7.8 mmol/l; Isolated-IGT: 2hPG 7.8–11.0 mmol/l and FPG <6.1 mmol/l; IFG&IGT: FPG 6.1–6.9 mmol/l and 2hPG 7.8–11.0 mmol/l. $^{*}p < 0.05$, $^{**}p < 0.01$, $^{***}p < 0.001$, for the difference between urban and rural Chinese and Japanese; $+p < 0.05$, $+{+}+p < 0.001$, for the difference between Chinese and Japanese combined and Asian Indian populations combined. (Adapted from the DECODA Study Group [12])

so far there has been no consistent trend [16, 17]. In the DECODE study, we found there is a clear gender pattern in the prevalence of postload hyperglycemia and the prevalence of fasting hyperglycemia [10]. Undiagnosed diabetes and IFG defined by isolated fasting hyperglycemia was more common in men than in women at 30–69 years of age, whereas the prevalence of isolated postload hyperglycemia was higher in women than in men and was particularly high in the elderly population [10]. In the DECODA study, gender difference was not as clear as

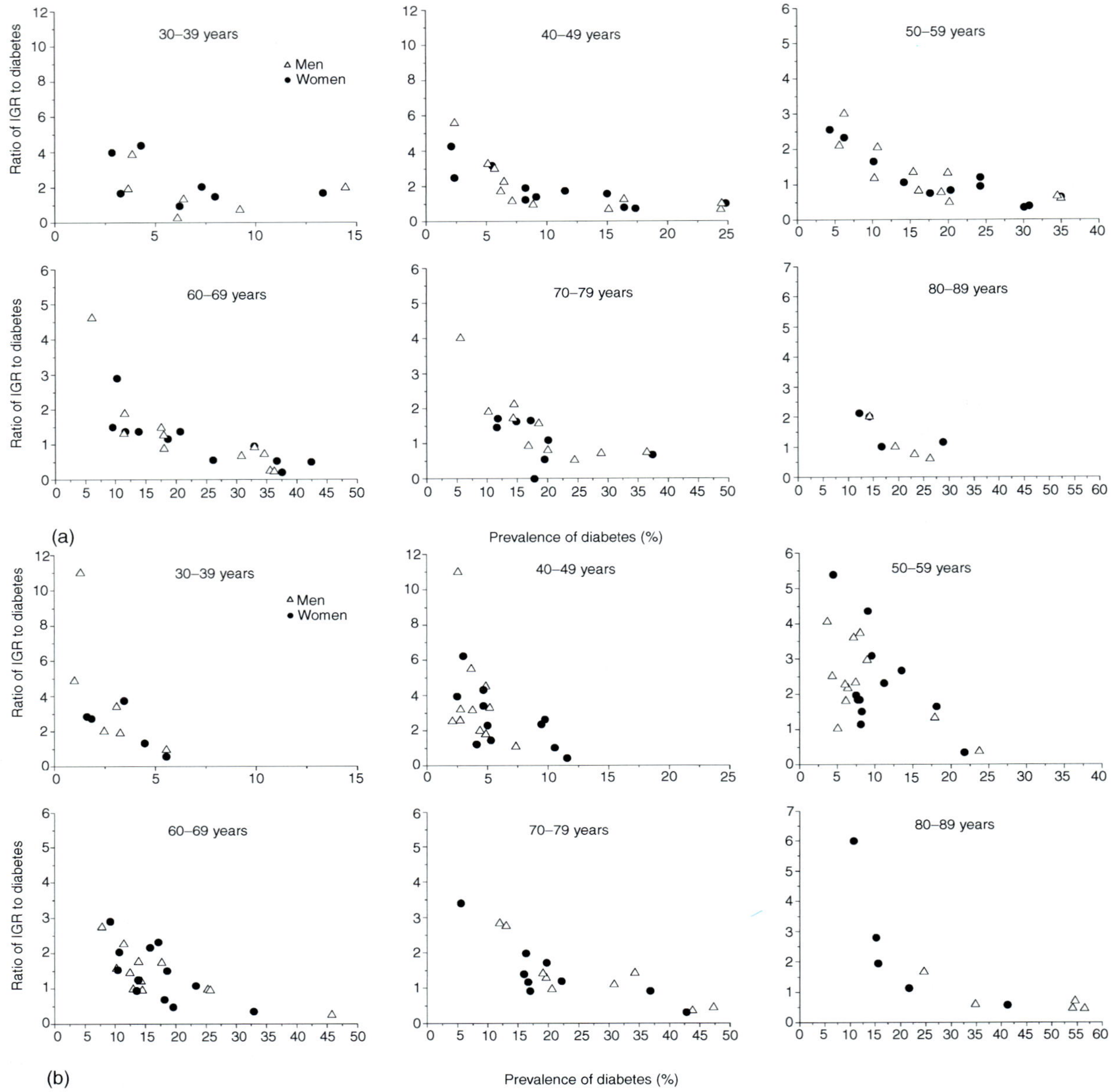

Figure 8 Age- and sex-specific scatter plot of ratios of IGR to diabetes against the prevalence of diabetes (diagnosed and undiagnosed) separately for 11 Asian (a) and 13 European studies (b). (Adapted from the DECODE [10] and the DECODA [12] Study Groups)

in Europe. The prevalence of IFG also seems higher in Chinese and Japanese men than in women, whereas it was higher in women than in men in Indians. IGT was more prevalent in Chinese and Japanese women than in men, but such a difference was not observed in Indians [12]. Gender differences in the prevalence of diabetes and IGR depend on how the prevalence was estimated, by fasting or by postload hyperglycemia, on the age distributions, and on the ethnic groups. Asian Indians, who have a very high risk of diabetes, show abnormalities in fasting glucose values at an earlier age than other populations.

THE RATIO OF IGT TO DIABETES

The ratio of IGT to diabetes has been reported to decrease as prevalence of diabetes rises [17] and may have some predictive value in determining the stage of a glucose intolerance epidemic within a population [63]. When the ratio is high, but the prevalence of diabetes is low, the early stage of a diabetes epidemic may be occurring [17]. The age- and sex-specific ratios of IGR to diabetes according to the newly revised diagnostic criteria for diabetes [8] are shown in Figure 8a for Asian and Figure 8b for European populations [10, 12]. The ratio of IGR to diabetes declines when the prevalence of diabetes increased in both Asian and European populations. It has been estimated that there will be a 57% increase in the prevalence of diabetes in Asia and 24% in Europe from 2000 to 2010 [1]. According to this, a higher ratio of IGR to diabetes might be expected in Asia than in Europe, given the same age and same prevalence of diabetes, but this was not observed.

SECULAR TRENDS IN PREVALENCE OF TYPE 2 DIABETES

Accumulating evidence shows that the prevalence of diabetes is increasing with time during the last decades. This upward trend was seen primarily in developing countries [3, 64] (Figure 1). A series of studies in the southern Indian city of Chennai showed a steady increase in the prevalence of diabetes in the Indian population. The age-standardized prevalence increased from 8.2% in 1988–1989 [65] to 11.6% in 1994–1995 [66] and reached 13.5% in 2000 [67], a 65% increase within the two decades. During the last two decades a considerable amount of information has been obtained from China. Studies conducted in China between 1980 and 1990 consistently show low diabetes prevalence rates of approximately 1.5% or less, even in urban populations such as in Shanghai in 1980 [68–71]. The prevalence of diabetes in Shanghai in 1980 was close to 1%. In rural Guangdong province it was 0.33% [69]. Studies made in the later 1990s, however, indicate a sharply rising prevalence rates in China [72–74] and the prevalence estimated at the beginning of the current century shows that diabetes in an urban Chinese population in mainland China [75] is already as prevalent as in Hong Kong and Taiwan in the middle of the 1990s (Figure 9) [76–78]. The prevalence of both diabetes and

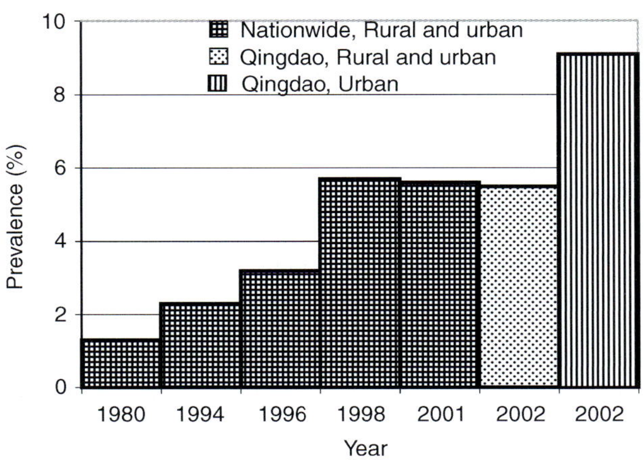

Figure 9 Age-standardized prevalence of type 2 diabetes mellitus in a series nationwide surveys in China and a recent study in Qingdao city (personal communication with Weiguo Gao)

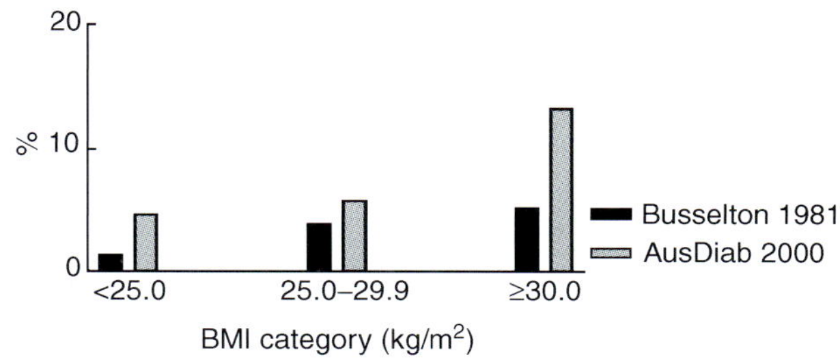

Mean BMI			
Busselton	22.5	27.1	33.0
AusDiab	22.4	27.3	34.1

Figure 10 Diabetes prevalence (diagnosed and undiagnosed) in Australia according to survey and BMI. Mean values for each BMI category are provided for both surveys. Prevalence data on BMI were adjusted for each population to the 1998 Australia resident population. (Adapted from reference 19)

its microvascular complications in Pacific Island population (20 years or older) of Western Samoa has been examined by Zimmet's group in 1978 and 1991 [31]. In 1978, the crude prevalence rates were 3.4 and 8.7% in rural and urban populations, respectively. By 1991, these rates had risen to 6.5 and 9.0% in two rural communities and to 16.0% in the urban setting of Apia.

Recent studies indicate that diabetes prevalence continues to increase even in developed countries. According to the data from the US NHANES II and NHANES III surveys, using ADA criteria, the prevalence of type 2 diabetes in the US adult population aged 40–74 years of age increased from 8.9% in the period 1976–1980 to 12.3% by 1988–1994. A similar increase was found when WHO criteria were applied (11.4 and 14.3%) [16]. In Australia, the total prevalence of diabetes had increased from 3.4 to 7.2% from 1981 to 1999–2000 and the difference persisted after adjustment for BMI [19] (Figure 10). In adult Norwegian population [79], the crude prevalence of known diabetes in men increased from 2.6% in 1984–1986 to 3.3% in 1995–1997, an increase of 24%, but the increase was not found in women. At the same time period, an increase of 86% in the prevalence of obesity defined by BMI ≥ 30 kg/m^2 was observed in men, which was much higher than the increase of 38% in women. In a Denmark study of a 60-year-old cohort, during a 22-year period an increase of 58% in men and of 21% in women in the prevalence of diabetes was observed, which was fully explained by a concurrent increase in BMI [80]. Rising trends in the prevalence of diabetes and obesity have also been reported in other European countries [81, 82]. In addition to the increase in obesity, reduced physical activity resulting from changes in work-related activity and sedentary lifestyle has contributed to the rising trend in type 2 diabetes.

Prevalence, which reflects the accumulation of the patients at any given time, can be influenced by many factors such as the increase in the number of new cases and the reduction in the mortality attributed to the disease. There is evidence that mortality in diabetes has declined in men in the United States [83]. Thus, a rise in prevalence could be a result of an improved survival of diabetic subjects. However, studies also show increasing trend in diabetes incidence due to the increase in the obesity and decrease in exercise. Knowler et al. [84] compared the incidence rates over two 10-year time periods, 1965–1975 and 1975–1985 in Arizona Pima Indians, and found that over the 10-year period the incidence rates increased by 50% in most age and sex groups. The San Antonio Heart Study revealed an increasing secular trend in the 7- to 8-year incidence of type 2 diabetes occurring from 1987 to 1996 in Mexican American and non-Hispanic Whites [85]. Therefore, both increased incidence and decreased mortality among diabetic subjects have contributed to the increased trend in the prevalence of diabetes.

TYPE 2 DIABETES IN CHILDREN

Prevalence and Incidence

Type 2 diabetes was historically a rare occurrence in children but recent studies have reported marked increases in the prevalence of type 2 diabetes in children. Type 2 diabetes was first reported in a population-based study in children in 1979 in American Indians in Arizona [86]. This American Indian community has one of the highest rates of type 2 diabetes in adults and obesity in both adults and children [87]. After 30 years of follow-up in this population, the youngest age of onset of type 2 diabetes was 4 years and the prevalence of type 2 diabetes in 15–19-year-old children increased from 2.4 to 3.8% in boys and from 2.7 to 5.3% in girls in this community [88]. Data from the Indian Health Service (IHS) in the United States confirmed an increase in the prevalence of diabetes in American Indian populations in the United States, with a 68% increase in the prevalence of diagnosed diabetes in American Indian and Alaska Natives adolescents between the age of 15 and 19 years between 1990 and 1998. Although these IHS estimates were for all diabetes and not type 2 diabetes, type 1 diabetes is very rare in some of these American Indian populations [89, 90].

The increase in type 2 diabetes is not limited to the American Indians. Very few population-based studies have been conducted in other racial and ethnic groups but results from diabetes registries, case reports, and cross-sectional studies from Canada [91], Cincinnati [92], Japan [93–95], Libya [96], Thailand [97], United Kingdom [98–100], India [101], Taiwan [102] and numerous case reports from the United States [103–107] have all indicated a significant increase in the prevalence of type 2 diabetes in children, although all these studies did not use a standard method to differentiate between type 1 and type 2 diabetes (see Table 2). The incidence of type 2 diabetes in African American adolescents in Cincinnati increased 10-fold from 0.7 to 7.2 per 100 000 in a 12-year period [92]. The proportion of type 2 diabetes in children diagnosed with diabetes has increased from 2–4% in 1992 to 8–45% in the last decade [108]. The proportion of type 1 to type 2 diabetic children is highly variable according to their different age and racial and ethnic groups (see Table 2).

Characteristics and Diagnosis

The majority of children with type 2 diabetes are non-Caucasian and in one review about 94% of cases were from minority groups [109]. The cause of this increased risk in non-Caucasian groups is unclear but will involve genetic predisposition and cultural and environmental risk factors. African American [110, 111] and Hispanic [112] children, for example, have been shown to have higher insulin resistance than do non-Hispanic White children.

The majority of type 2 diabetes cases occur in overweight and obese children and they may have clinical signs of insulin resistance, such as acanthosis nigricans. The prevalence of type 2 diabetes in these children is higher in girls who may be two to six times more likely to have type 2 diabetes. The mean age of onset is around puberty in most population.

Cases may present with classical signs and symptoms of diabetes but the disease may have an insidious onset and only detected by opportunistic screening. In a series from a referral center in Cincinnati, 32% of children with type 2 diabetes were discovered by opportunistic screening [92]. Therefore, underreporting of cases of type 2 diabetes in children may be as common as in adults.

The differentiation of type 2 diabetes from type 1 diabetes may be difficult in some cases (see Table 3). Currently, the mainstay of differentiating diabetes in children is inadequate and includes the use of clinical characteristics like obesity, severity of onset, use of insulin, age of onset, diabetic ketoacidosis, and family history of diabetes. With the rising prevalence of obesity in children, more type 1 diabetes cases are presenting with obesity [113]. In addition, some cases of type 2 diabeties may present with diabetic ketoacidosis [114, 115]. Diabetes-related autoantibodies that include the glutamic acid decarboxylase (GAD), tyrosine phosphatase-like molecule (IA2), islet cell antibody (ICA), and C-peptide (which is co-secreted with insulin) concentrations are currently being investigated as a means of improving the differentiation of diabetes type in children. The use of diabetes autoantibodies is limited by problems with assay methodology and the transient nature of some of these autoantibodies in cases of type 1 diabetes

Table 2 Selected studies of type 2 diabetes in children and adolescents

Study and reference*	Years	Race/ethnicity	Age (years)	Sample size	No. of cases	Estimates
Population-based studies†						
New Mexico, USA [136]	1991–1992	Navajo Indians	12–19	142	2‡	14.1 *[0–33.5]*‡
Arizona, USA [88]	1992–1996	Pima Indians	10–14	672	15	22.3 *[11.1–33.5]*
			15–19	530	27	50.9 *[32.2–69.6]*
Manitoba, Canada [137]	1996–1997	Cree and Ojibway Indians	4–19	717	8	11.1 *[3.4–18.8]*
			10–19	U	7	0 for boys and 36.0 for girls
NHANES III, USA [138]	1988–1994	Whites, and African and Mexican Americans, all Americans	12–19	2 867	13‡	4.1 [0–8.6]‡
Taiwan [102]	1993–1999	Thai	School age children	2 932 855	2 066‡	0.08 in boys and 0.12 in girls‡
Clinic-based studies†						
Indian Health Services, USA [89]	1996	American Indians, all Americans	0–14	402 580	518‡	1.3‡
			15–19	111 239	498‡	4.5‡
United Kingdom [100]	1993–2000	British	0–18	261 811	21	0.038
Clinic-based study§						
Libya [96]	1981–1990	Libyan	0–14	11 846	12	0.5 (0.26–0.87)
			15–34	75 836	1 027	70.9 (66.6–75.5)
Cincinnati, OH, USA [92]	1994	Whites and African Americans	0–19	U	U	3.5
			10–19	U	U	7.2
Case series‖				¶		
Cincinnati, OH, USA [92]	1982–1994	Whites and African Americans	0–19	1 027#	54#	16# (in 1994)
			10–19	U	U	33# (in 1994)
Charleston, SC, USA [104]	1997	African Americans	10–19	97	45	46
Little Rock, AR, USA [139]	1988–1995	Whites, Hispanics, and African Americans	0–19	U	50	U
San Diego, CA, USA [105]	1993–1994	Whites, Hispanics, and African and Asian Americans	0–16	160#	13#	8#
San Antonio, TX, USA [106]	1990–1997	Whites, Hispanics	U	560#	101#	18#
Ventura, CA, USA [103]	1990–1994	Hispanics	0–17	31#	14#	45#
Thailand [97]	1986–1995	Thai	0–14	59	3	5
	1996–1999	Thai	0–14	39	7	17.9

Note. Numbers in italics are estimates. NHANES III = National Health and Nutrition Examination Survey III; U = unknown data.
* Table updated from Fagot-Campagna et al., *J Pediatr* 2000 [112].
† Estimates are given as prevalence per 1000 and 95% CI.
‡ Estimates include cases of type 1 diabetes.
§ Estimates are given as incidence per 100 000/year.
‖ Estimates are given as percentage of type 2 diabetes among new cases of diabetes.
¶ In case series, the sample size refers to the total number of cases of diabetes (types 1 and 2).
\# Incident cases.

[116, 117]. The use of C-peptide to differentiate the type of diabetes in children is made especially difficult by varying levels of residual β-cell function in type 1 diabetic cases. Current efforts are underway in a CDC (Centers for Disease Control) and NIDDK (National Institute of Diabetes and Digestive and Kidney Diseases) sponsored study, the SEARCH for Diabetes in Youth Study, to develop cutoff points and algorithms that include diabetes autoantibodies and C-peptide concentration that may be used to diagnose and differentiate diabetes in children.

Risk Factors

Very few studies have examined the risk factors for type 2 diabetes in children. Some of the established risk factors for adult type 2 diabetes, discussed in other sections of this chapter, may play a role in the development of type 2 diabetes in children. Overweight and obesity are some of the strongest risk factors for insulin resistance and type 2 diabetes in adults. The rising prevalence of overweight in children may thus play a role in the

Table 3 Challenges in the classification of diabetes in children

Type 1 diabetes	Type 2 diabetes	Comments
Not overweight	Overweight or obese	Rising obesity means >30% of type 1 are obese
Severe onset	Insidious	Presentations may vary
Weight loss	Some	Presentation may vary
Polyuria	Polyuria	Common to both
Polydipsia	Polydipsia	Common to both
Insulinopenia	No insulinopenia	Not present in all type 1 diabetes in honeymoon phase
Autoantibodies	No Autoantibodies	Usually occur in type 1, absence does not exclude type 1
No insulin resistance	Insulin resistance	Usually occur in type 2

risk of type 2 diabetes in children. In the United States, the prevalence of overweight in children has increased sharply over the last three decades to 15% in a 1999–2000 survey [118]. Over 20% of Hispanic and African American children are overweight compared to 12% in non-Hispanic White children [119]. This difference in prevalence of obesity may in part explain the higher prevalence of type 2 diabetes in ethnic minority children like American Indians, African Americans, and Hispanics in the United States [88, 92, 103] and Asian Indians in the United Kingdom [100].

Most cases of type 2 diabetes occur around puberty. The reason for this increased risk around puberty is unclear but may be related to the physiological 30% increase in insulin resistance observed in children as they go through Tanner stages II to IV [120–124]. This physiological increase in insulin resistance is thought to be related to increased growth hormone production during puberty [121, 122] but not related to the increase of sex hormones [121]. In the presence of increased insulin resistance produced by overweight and physical inactivity the reduction in insulin resistance around puberty may precipitate type 2 diabetes in these children especially if they have inadequate compensatory insulin secretion (see Figure 11).

Prenatal and early childhood events may also increase the risk of developing type 2 diabetes in children. Among siblings from the same nuclear family, the child of a mother who had diabetes during pregnancy has a threefold risk of developing early onset diabetes as their sibling who was born before the mother became diabetic [125]. This increased risk is mainly due to exposure to diabetes *in utero* since these siblings share the same environment and a similar probability of inheriting the same genetic composition.

Low birth weight and disproportionate growth *in utero* has also been shown to be associated with both type 2 diabetes and insulin resistance [126, 127]. Breast-feeding is also protective against obesity and type 2 diabetes [128, 129, 130] especially when sustained for long durations.

Complications and Comorbid Conditions

The development of type 2 diabetes in children is alarming. In adults, type 2 diabetes is associated with the development of complications like retinopathy, renal disease, and CVD. Recent reports of type 2 diabetes in children suggest that diabetes carries the similar risk for the development of complications in early adulthood. In a study on the development of complications in Pima Indian children with type 2 diabetes, the rate of development of nephropathy was as severe in children as in adults over 30 years of follow-up [131]. The rate of development of retinopathy was however lower in cases that developed diabetes in childhood. A small series of young adults from the First Nation in Canada who had been diagnosed with type 2 diabetes before their 17th birthday were traced and followed up for the prevalence of diabetic complications and adverse outcomes by their 36th birthday. In this small series 9% had died, and 6.3% were already on dialysis and their blood glucose control was poor [132].

At diagnosis, a number of children have comorbid conditions like dyslipidemia and hypertension both of which are risk factors for CVD [133]. Cardiovascular risk is strongly related to duration of diabetes [134] and type 2 diabetes in children will increase their risk to develop CVD later on in life.

The apparent rise in the prevalence of type 2 diabetes in children is presenting new challenges in the management and classification of diabetes in children. Adolescents are more likely to be noncompliant and may find it more difficult to follow the lifestyle modifications and treatment regimen that would be necessary to control blood glucose [108, 135]. Furthermore, very few medications have been approved for use in treating type 2 diabetic children. Insulin and metformin are the only medications currently licensed for treatment of type 2 diabetes in children in the United States.

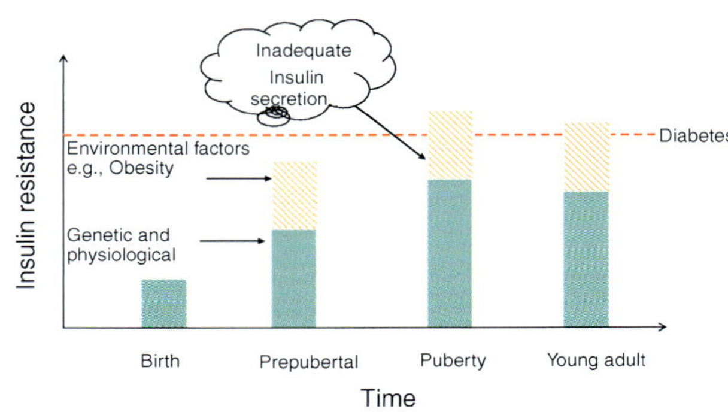

Figure 11 Type 2 diabetes, insulin resistance, and puberty in children

MODIFIABLE RISK FACTORS FOR TYPE 2 DIABETES

Obesity

Obesity and weight gain have consistently been shown to be the one of the strongest modifiable risk factors for diabetes [140–142]. The ratio of a persons weight in kilograms divided by the square of their height in meters called the body mass index (BMI) has been used in numerous studies as a surrogate for obesity. In a representative sample of the US population, each unit increase in BMI was associated with a 12% increased risk of type 2 diabetes [143]. Compared to people with BMI < 22 kg/m^2 those with BMI of 25–27 kg/m^2 had 2.75 times the risk of diabetes, and each kilogram increase in body weight over 10 years was associated with a 4.5% increase in diabetes risk. Numerous studies have found similar results in different populations [144, 145], but the magnitude of risk associated with a given BMI may differ across populations. The distribution of weight and weight gain are also important risk factors for diabetes. Central obesity, i.e. deposition of fat in the trunk and abdominal areas, has been shown to be strong risk factors for diabetes. The surrogate measures of central obesity include circumference of waist, waist-to-hip ratio, and waist-to-thigh ratio. More recent technological advances like dual-energy X-ray absorptiometry (DEXA) and magnetic resonance imaging (MRI), and computer tomography have made it possible to measure subcutaneous and intra-abdominal fat. Intra-abdominal fat has been shown to increase the risk of insulin resistance and diabetes in a number of studies in different populations [145–148] and this effect may be independent of the effects of total body obesity [149, 150]. Obesity always occurs when energy intake exceeds energy expenditure.

Physical Activity

Physical activity has been consistently reported to be inversely related to future risk of diabetes in most populations. Higher levels of physical activity are associated with a lower risk of diabetes in observational studies [151]. Increased physical activity reduces the risk of obesity but its effect on diabetes risk has been shown to be independent of its effect on body weight. Numerous studies have shown that exercise is related to acute and long-term improvements in insulin sensitivity and reduction in insulin concentrations [152, 153]. Several epidemiologic studies in diverse populations [154–161] confirm a dose–response relationship between levels of physical activity and diabetes incidence. One study among Finnish men [160] found a strong gradient of diabetes risk associated with intensity of physical activity regardless of duration, but most evidence indicates that the total amount (i.e., number of days or minutes) of physical activity per week is a more important determinant.

Sedentary Lifestyle

Sedentary lifestyle has also been shown to be a risk factor for both diabetes and obesity. Prolonged television (TV) watching as a surrogate of a sedentary lifestyle has also been reported to be a risk factor for diabetes [162, 163]. Compared to men spending 0–1 h/week watching TV, those spending 2–10 h had 66% higher risk of diabetes, and the risk increased progressively to 187% higher incidence among those spending >40 h/week [162]. In women, every 2 h/day increment in TV watching was associated with a 23% increase in risk of obesity and 14% increase in risk of diabetes [163]. Furthermore, each 2-h increment in sitting at work was associated with a 5% increase in diabetes risk. It is estimated that a relatively active lifestyle (<10 h/week of TV watching and ≥ 30 min/day of brisk walking) can prevent 43% of new cases of diabetes [163].

Evidence from Intervention Studies

Results from a number of intervention studies have clarified the role of physical activity as a risk factor for diabetes. Results from Malmö trial in Sweden [164], Da Qing trial in China [58], Diabetes Prevention Study (DPS) in Finland [59], and the Diabetes Prevention Program in the Unites States [60] have all shown that moderate physical activity reduces the progression of IGT to diabetes by 30–58%. In these studies moderate physical activity was included in a lifestyle intervention arm of the trials with dietary changes that include reduction in caloric intake and in the percentage of dietary fat and increase in fiber intake (Table 4). In most of these studies it is difficult to discern the individual effect of the dietary intervention as it was combined with modifications in physical activity.

Dietary Factors

Diet is a phenomenon that is made up of complex interactions between numerous foods and nutrients that are highly correlated and are determined by personal preference, cultural heritage, and socioeconomic factors. Diet is traditionally measured using questionnaires and food diaries. A number of studies have examined the relationship between diabetes and different aspects of diet including absolute intake of nutrients, nutrient intake as a percentage of total energy, dietary patterns, and bioavailability characteristics of foods like glycemic index.

Nutrients and Diabetes Risk

Dietary fat Animal studies and clinical human studies suggest several plausible mechanisms relating diet to the etiology of type 2 diabetes. High-fat diet have been

Table 4 Lifestyle changes in the primary prevention of type 2 diabetes mellitus*

Study	Population	Age (years)	Interventions	Results	Comments
Mälmö [164]	181 Swedish men with IGT	47–49	Diet, physical activity, and training	50% with IGT reverted to normal; blood sugars normalized in 50% with diabetes	6-year follow-up; participants were not randomized
Da Qing [58]	577 Chinese men and women with IGT	>25 (mean age 44.9)	Diet only, exercise only, and diet + exercise	Diet only: 31% ↓ in diabetes risk; exercise only: 46% ↓; diet + exercise 42% ↓	6-year follow-up; randomization by clinic
Diabetes Prevention Study (DPS) [59]	522 overweight Finnish men and women with IGT	Middle age (mean age 55)	Increased physical activity, increased fiber intake, and reduced fat intake	58% decrease in diabetes risk	3.2-year follow-up
DPP [60]	3324 overweight US men and women with IGT	Mean age 50.6	Lifestyle (increased physical activity, weight loss, reduced fat intake), and drug (metformin)	Lifestyle 58% ↓ in diabetes risk; metformin 31% ↓	2.8-year follow-up; subjects from several different race/ethnic groups. Lifestyle interventions were effective in all race/ethnic and age groups

Note: IGT = impaired glucose tolerance.
* Modified from Bowman et al. *J Public Health Manage Pract* 2003; 9 (suppl): S8–14.

associated with obesity [165], increased body fat for a given weight [166], and altered fat distribution [166]. Furthermore, alterations in cell membrane composition induced by the composition of dietary fat could alter membrane fluidity and/or insulin-mediated signal transduction as well as subsequent insulin action [167].

The results from epidemiological studies on the relationship of total fat and type 2 diabetes have been controversial. In general, most of the migrant [168, 169] and retrospective [170, 171] studies show a positive relationship between high-fat, low-carbohydrate diets and type 2 diabetes, whereas results from prospective studies from different populations have been mixed [172–174] and not as consistent.

The effect of different subtypes of fat like saturated, polyunsaturated, monounsaturated fat [175, 176] and ω-3 fatty acids [177–179] on diabetes risk has also been investigated. An extensive review [180] concluded that while neither total fat nor total carbohydrate as proportions of total energy play a major part in the development of type 2 diabetes, specific types of fat and carbohydrate are important. For example, they concluded that (1) higher intake of polyunsaturated fat and long-chain n-3 fatty acids (fish oil) may be beneficial, and (2) higher intake of saturated fat and trans-fatty acids may be deleterious.

Dietary Carbohydrate

The possibility of the risk of diabetes being related to carbohydrate consumption has been frequently raised. This hypothesis was generated because of the stronger, more direct, and more immediate challenge that ingestion of carbohydrate presents to the β-cells, compared with ingestion of proteins or fats. Results from studies on carbohydrate and diabetes risk have however been inconclusive [169, 181, 182]. Other aspects of carbohydrate composition and metabolism including glycemic index and fiber content have also been examined.

Glycemic index The glycemic index [183] of food is a measure of the postprandial excursion of glucose as a result of the ingestion of a fixed amount of food. Foods with high glycemic index cause greater excursions of glucose. The postprandial excursions are dependent on the rate of absorption of glucose, which in turn is dependent on a number of factors including the type of carbohydrate (simple or complex) and the amount of fiber. Food with lower glycemic index has been associated with a lower risk of developing diabetes in some studies [182, 184], but others have failed to show any association between the glycemic index of foods and the risk of developing diabetes [185, 186].

Fiber intake High-fiber intakes have been related to a reduction in the risk of diabetes in some populations [182, 184, 187–190]. The mechanism by which high fiber reduces the risk of diabetes is unknown. High-fiber diets usually have a lower glycemic index but some studies that have shown a relationship between fiber intake and diabetes have failed to demonstrate a beneficial effect of the glycemic index of the diet [185]. Thiamine and vegetable protein are found in high concentrations in foods that are rich in fiber and have also been shown to reduce 2-h glucose concentration in women and may explain some of the association between fiber intake and diabetes [191, 192].

Vegetable and Fruit Intake

Higher intakes of vegetables have been shown to be associated with a reduction in the risk of diabetes [172, 173, 193]. The component of vegetables that confers lower risk has not been clearly identified but may include antioxidants such as carotenoids and tocopherols [194], higher fiber intake, and vitamins [172, 195, 196]. The effect of fruit consumption on diabetes risk has been inconclusive [173, 193].

Dietary Patterns and Scores

Studies have examined the effect of the whole composition and quality of diet on diabetes risk using various scores and dietary patterns identified by principal component and factor analyses [197, 198] on diabetes risk. The results from these studies have shown that diet that has relatively higher intakes of vegetables and fruits and lower intakes of fat-rich foods has been associated with a reduction in diabetes risk [197, 198].

Self-rated dietary patterns can be used to discriminate differences in the nutrient composition in diet. Pima Indians who self-reported a diet more similar to their traditional Pima diet had a lower risk of developing diabetes over a 12-year period [199] when compared to a more Westernized dietary preference. The traditional Pima diet had a higher fiber and lower fat intake when compared to the more Westernized diet. The traditional diets of most ingenious populations have a higher intake of fiber and lower glycemic index [200, 201] than the more recent Westernized diets that most of these populations have adopted.

NONTRADITIONAL MODIFIABLE RISK FACTORS FOR TYPE 2 DIABETES

Inflammation

Although insulin resistance and relative insulin deficiency represent the main characteristics of type 2 diabetes, the underlying mechanism responsible for these abnormalities remains largely unknown. On the basis of hypothesis that both type 2 diabetes and atherosclerosis may generate from a "common soil" [202, 203], more recently a growing body of evidence points out that inflammation may constitute the common factor that leads to the development of both type 2 diabetes and atherosclerotic vascular disease. One of the most used markers of subclinical inflammation is the C-reactive protein (CRP). A number of cross-sectional studies have shown that increased concentrations of CRP are associated with abnormalities characterizing the metabolic syndrome, including obesity, insulin resistance, low HDL cholesterol, and hypertriglyceridemia [204–206]. In addition, prospective studies have demonstrated that high levels of CRP increase the risk of developing type 2 diabetes [207–212]. These findings have opened new avenues for understanding the pathogenesis of type 2 diabetes and, eventually, for preventing the disease. Indeed, if, as these data have indicated, subclinical inflammation is an important determinant of type 2 diabetes, then the use of anti-inflammatory drugs may prevent diabetes. In this regard, it is noteworthy that in patient with type 2 diabetes high-dose aspirin reduces insulin resistance and improves glucose tolerance [213].

Smoking

Numerous prospective studies have indicated that smoking is associated with the development of diabetes. In the US Nurses' Health Study, women who smoked at least 25 cigarettes per day compared to those who never smoked had a relative risk of developing diabetes of 1.42, even after controlling for known risk factors [214]. Similar results were shown in men [215]. These findings were confirmed by Will et al. in a prospective study involving over 275 000 men and 434 000 women from the US Cancer Prevention Study [216]. Among those who smoked at least 2 packs per day at baseline, men had a 45% higher diabetes rate than do men who had never smoked; in women the comparable increase was 74%. More important, quitting smoking reduced the rate of diabetes to that of nonsmokers after 5 years in women and after 10 years in men. In support of these findings are cross-sectional data on the association between cigarettes smoking and hemoglobin A_{1c} (HbA_{1c}) from the East Anglian component of the European Prospective Investigation into Cancer (EPIC-Norfolk) [196]. In this study, current smokers had highest mean HbA_{1c} concentrations, lowest levels were observed in never smokers, and intermediate in former smokers. HbA_{1c} levels also correlated in a dose–response manner both with the number of cigarettess smoked per day and with total amount of smoking as measured by pack-years.This association persisted even after adjusting for potential confounders including BMI, waist-to-hip ratio, physical activity, and dietary variables. However, to better assess the role of smoking as determinant of type 2 diabetes we need cohort studies to further confirm that this association exists in different populations.

There is evidence that smoking is associated with insulin resistance [217, 218]. In a study by Facchini et al. [217] chronic smokers compared to nonsmokers had significantly higher plasma triglycerides and lower HDL-cholesterol levels and higher insulin concentrations after a 75-g oral glucose challenge. Well-designed clinical studies of the effects of acute and chronic smoking on insulin resistance are needed to elucidate the mechanism by which smoking induces insulin resistance. It is plausible that oxidative stress caused by smoking may induce endothelial dysfunction, resulting in insulin resistance into muscle and liver.

The possibility that smoking may play a causal role in the development of type 2 diabetes has important implication for prevention. Both diabetes and smoking are conditions common enough that even a small increase in the risk of diabetes associated with smoking may have important public health impact.

REFERENCES

1. Zimmet P, Alberti KG, Shaw J. Global and societal implications of the diabetes epidemic. *Nature* 2001; 414 (6865): 782–7.
2. Joslin EP. The prevention of diabetes mellitus. *JAMA* 1921; 76: 79–84.
3. King H, Aubert RE, Herman WH. Global burden of diabetes, 1995–2025: prevalence, numerical estimates, and projections. *Diabetes Care* 1998; 21: 1414–31.
4. National Diabetes Data Group. Classification and diagnosis of diabetes mellitus and other categories of glucose intolerance. *Diabetes* 1979; 28 (12): 1039–57.
5. World Health Organization. WHO Expert Committee on Diabetes Mellitus: Second Report. Technical Report Series No. 646. Geneva: WHO, 1980.
6. World Health Organisation. Diabetes Mellitus: Report of a Study Group. Technical Report Series No. 727. Geneva: WHO, 1985.
7. Expert Committee on the Diagnosis and Classification of Diabetes Mellitus. Report of the Expert Committee on the Diagnosis and Classification of Diabetes Mellitus. *Diabetes Care* 1997; 20 (7): 1183–97.
8. WHO Consultation. Definition, Diagnosis and Classification of Diabetes Mellitus and Its Complications. Part 1: Diagnosis and Classification of Diabetes Mellitus. Report No. 99.2. Geneva: WHO, 1999.
9. The DECODE Study Group. Is the current definition for diabetes relevant to mortality risk from all-cause, cardiovascular and non-cardiovascular disease? *Diabetes Care* 2003; 26 (3): 688–96.
10. The DECODE Study Group. Age- and sex-specific prevalences of diabetes and impaired glucose regulation in 13 European cohorts. *Diabetes Care* 2003; 26 (1): 61–9.
11. The DECODE Study Group. Gender difference in all-cause and cardiovascular mortality related to hyperglyaemia and newly-diagnosed diabetes. *Diabetologia* 2003; 46: 608–17.
12. The DECODA Study Group. Age- and sex-specific prevalences of diabetes and impaired glucose regulation in 11 Asian cohorts. *Diabetes Care* 2003; 26 (6): 1770–80.
13. Rathmann W, Haastert B, Icks A, Lowel H, Meisinger C, Holle R, Giani G. High prevalence of undiagnosed diabetes mellitus in Southern Germany: target populations for efficient screening. The KORA Survey 2000. *Diabetologia* 2003; 46 (2): 182–9.
14. Satman I, Yilmaz T, Sengul A, Salman S, Salman F, Uygur S, Bastar I, Tutuncu Y, Sargin M, Dinccag N, Karsidag K, Kalaca S, Ozcan C, King H. Population-based study of diabetes and risk characteristics in Turkey: results of the Turkish Diabetes Epidemiology Study (TURDEP). *Diabetes Care* 2002; 25 (9): 1551–6.
15. Kelestimur F, Cetin M, Pasaoglu H, Coksevim B, Cetinkaya F, Unluhizarci K, Unal S, Koker AH. The prevalence and identification of risk factors for type 2 diabetes mellitus and impaired glucose tolerance in Kayseri, central Anatolia, Turkey. *Acta Diabetol* 1999; 36 (1–2): 85–91.
16. Harris MI, Flegal KM, Cowie CC, Eberhardt MS, Goldsten DE, Little RR, Wiedmeyer H-M, Byrd-Holt DD. Prevalence of diabetes, impaired fasting glucose, and impaired glucose tolerance in U.S. adults. *Diabetes Care* 1998; 21: 518–24.
17. King H, Rewers M, WHO Ad Hoc Diabetes Reporting Group. Global estimates for prevalence of diabetes mellitus and impaired glucose tolerance in adults. *Diabetes Care* 1993; 16: 157–77.
18. Grandinetti A, Chang HK, Mau MK, Curb JD, Kinney EK, Sagum R, Arakaki RF. Prevalence of glucose intolerance among Native Hawaiians in two rural communities. Native Hawaiian Health Research (NHHR) Project. *Diabetes Care* 1998; 21 (4): 549–54.
19. Dunstan DW, Zimmet PZ, Welborn TA, de Courten MP, Cameron AJ, Sicree RA, Dwyer T, Colagiuri S, Jolley D, Knuiman M, Atkins R, Shaw JE. The rising prevalence of diabetes and impaired glucose tolerance: the Australian Diabetes, Obesity and Lifestyle Study. *Diabetes Care* 2002; 25 (5): 829–34.
20. Park Y, Lee H, Koh CS, Min H, Yoo K, Kim Y, Shin Y. Prevalence of diabetes and IGT in Yonchon County, South Korea. *Diabetes Care* 1995; 18 (4): 545–8.
21. Shera AS, Rafique G, Khawaja IA, Baqai S, King H. Pakistan National Diabetes Survey: prevalence of glucose intolerance and associated factors in Baluchistan province. *Diabetes Res Clin Pract* 1999; 44 (1): 49–58.
22. Shera AS, Rafique G, Khwaja IA, Ara J, Baqai S, King H. Pakistan National Diabetes Survey: prevalence of glucose intolerance and associated factors in Shikarpur, Sindh Province. *Diabet Med* 1995; 12 (12): 1116–21.
23. Shera AS, Rafique G, Khwaja IA, Baqai S, Khan IA, King H, Ahmed KI. Pakistan National Diabetes Survey: prevalence of glucose intolerance and associated factors in North West at Frontier Province (NWFP) of Pakistan. *J Pak Med Assoc* 1999; 49 (9): 206–11.
24. King H, Djumaeva S, Abdullaev B, Gacic Dobo M. Epidemiology of glucose intolerance and associated factors in Uzbekistan: a survey in Sirdaria province. *Diabetes Res Clin Pract* 2002; 55 (1): 19–27.
25. King H, Abdullaev B, Djumaeva S, Nikitin V, Ashworth L, Dobo MG. Glucose intolerance and associated factors in the Fergana Valley, Uzbekistan. *Diabet Med* 1998; 15 (12): 1052–62.
26. Suvd J, Gerel B, Otgooloi H, Purevsuren D, Zolzaya H, Roglic G, King H. Glucose intolerance and associated factors in Mongolia: results of a national survey. *Diabet Med* 2002; 19 (6): 502–8.
27. Pan XR, Yang WY, Li GW, Liu J. Prevalence of diabetes and its risk factors in China, 1994. *Diabetes Care* 1997; 20: 1664–9.
28. Zimmet P, King H, Taylor R, Raper LR, Balkau B, Borger J, et al. The high prevalence of diabetes mellitus, impaired glucose tolerance and diabetic retinopathy in Nauru—the 1982 survey. *Diabetes Res* 1984; 1 (1): 13–8.
29. Dowse GK, Zimmet PZ, Finch CF, Collins VR. Decline in incidence of epidemic glucose intolerance in Nauruans: implications for the "thrifty genotype." *Am J Epidemiol* 1991; 133 (11): 1093–104.
30. King H, Finch C, Collins A, Koki G, King LF, Heywood P, et al. Glucose tolerance in Papua New Guinea: ethnic differences, association with environmental and

behavioural factors and the possible emergence of glucose intolerance in a highland community. *Med J Aust* 1989; 151 (4): 204–10.
31. Collins VR, Dowse GK, Toelupe PM, Imo TT, Aloaina FL, Spark RA, et al. Increasing prevalence of NIDDM in the Pacific island population of Western Samoa over a 13-year period. *Diabetes Care* 1994; 17 (4): 288–96.
32. Colagiuri S, Colagiuri R, Na'ati S, Muimuiheata S, Hussain Z, Palu T. The prevalence of diabetes in the kingdom of Tonga. *Diabetes Care* 2002; 25 (8): 1378–83.
33. Al-Nuaim AR. Prevalence of glucose intolerance in urban and rural communities in Saudi Arabia. *Diabet Med* 1997; 14 (7): 595–602.
34. Asfour MG, Lambourne A, Soliman A, Al-Behlani S, Al-Asfoor D, Bold A, Mahtab H, King H. High prevalence of diabetes mellitus and impaired glucose tolerance in the Sultanate of Oman: results of the 1991 National Survey. *Diabet Med* 1995; 12 (12): 1122–5.
35. Husseini A, Abdul-Rahim H, Awartani F, Jervell J, Bjertness E. Prevalence of diabetes mellitus and impaired glucose tolerance in a rural Palestinian population. *East Mediterr Health J* 2000; 6 (5–6): 1039–45.
36. Abdella N, Al Nakhi A, Al Arouj M, Assoussi A, Moussa M. Impact of the 1997 American Diabetes Association criteria on classification of glucose intolerance among Kuwaitis below 50 years of age. *Acta Diabetol* 1999; 36 (3): 133–40.
37. Dowse GK, Gareeboo H, Zimmet PZ, Alberti KG, Tuomilehto J, Fareed D, Brissonnette LG, Finch CF, for the Mauritius Noncommunicable Disease Study Group. High prevalence of NIDDM and impaired glucose tolerance in Indian, Creole, and Chinese Mauritians. *Diabetes* 1990; 39 (3): 390–6.
38. Swai AB, McLarty DG, Sherrif F, Chuwa LM, Maro E, Lukmanji Z, Kermali W, Makene W, Alberti KG. Diabetes and impaired glucose tolerance in an Asian community in Tanzania. *Diabetes Res Clin Pract* 1990; 8 (3): 227–34.
39. McLarty DG, Swai AB, Kitange HM, Masuki G, Mtinangi BL, Kilima PM, Makene WJ, Chuwa LM, Alberti KG. Prevalence of diabetes and impaired glucose tolerance in rural Tanzania. *Lancet* 1989; 1 (8643): 871–5.
40. Santos JL, Perez-Bravo F, Carrasco E, Calvillan M, Albala C. Low prevalence of type 2 diabetes despite a high average body mass index in the Aymara natives from Chile. *Nutrition* 2001; 17 (4): 305–9.
41. Perez-Bravo F, Carrasco E, Santos JL, Calvillan M, Larenas G, Albala C. Prevalence of type 2 diabetes and obesity in rural Mapuche population from Chile. *Nutrition* 2001; 17 (3): 236–8.
42. Larenas G, Arias G, Espinoza O. Prevalence of diabetes mellitus in an indigenous (Mapuche) community of the IX region in Chile. *Rev Med Chile* 1985; 113: 1121–5.
43. Dogadin SA, Mashtakov BP, Taranushenko TE. Prevalence of type 2 diabetes in northern populations of Siberia. *Int J Circumpolar Health* 2001; 60 (2): 205–10.
44. The DECODE Study Group. Glucose tolerance and mortality: comparison of WHO and American Diabetes Association diagnostic criteria. *Lancet* 1999; 354 (9179): 617–21.
45. The DECODE Study Group. Glucose tolerance and cardiovascular mortality: comparison of fasting and 2-hour diagnostic criteria. *Arch Intern Med* 2001; 161 (3): 397–405.
46. Qiao Q, Pyorala K, Pyorala M, Nissinen A, Lindstrom J, Tilvis R, Tuomilehto J. Two-hour glucose is a better risk predictor for incident coronary heart disease and cardiovascular mortality than fasting glucose. *Eur Heart J* 2002; 23 (16): 1267–75.
47. Tominaga M, Eguchi H, Manaka H, Igarashi K, Kato T, Sekikawa A. Impaired glucose tolerance is a risk factor for cardiovascular disease, but not impaired fasting glucose: the Funagata Diabetes Study. *Diabetes Care* 1999; 22 (6): 920–4.
48. Shaw JE, Zimmet PZ, de Courten M, Dowse GK, Chitson P, Gareeboo H, Hemraj F, Fareed D, Tuomilehto J, Alberti KG. Impaired fasting glucose or impaired glucose tolerance. What best predicts future diabetes in Mauritius? *Diabetes Care* 1999; 22 (3): 399–402.
49. Vaccaro O, Ruffa G, Imperatore G, Iovino V, Rivellese A, Riccardi G. Risk of diabetes in the new diagnostic category of impaired fasting glucose: a prospective analysis. *Diabetes Care* 1999; 22 (9): 1490–3.
50. Gabir MM, Hanson RL, Dabelea D, Imperatore G, Roumain J, Bennett PH, Knowler WC. The 1997 American Diabetes Association and 1999 World Health Organization criteria for hyperglycemia in the diagnosis and prediction of diabetes. *Diabetes Care* 2000; 23 (8): 1108–12.
51. de Vegt F, Dekker JM, Jager A, Hienkens E, Kostense PJ, Stehouwer CD, Nijpels G, Bouter LM, Heine RJ. Relation of impaired fasting and postload glucose with incident type 2 diabetes in a Dutch population: the Hoorn Study. *JAMA* 2001; 285 (16): 2109–13.
52. Qiao Q, Lindström J, Valle TT, Tuomilehto J. Progression to clinically diagnosed and treated diabetes from impaired glucose tolerance and impaired fasting glycaemia. *Diabet Med* 2003; 20: 1027–33.
53. Unwin N, Shaw J, Zimmet P, Alberti KG. Impaired glucose tolerance and impaired fasting glycaemia: the current status on definition and intervention. *Diabet Med* 2002; 19 (9): 708–23.
54. The DECODE Study Group on behalf of the European Diabetes Epidemiology Study Group. Will new diagnostic criteria for diabetes mellitus change phenotype of patients with diabetes? Reanalysis of European epidemiological data. *BMJ* 1998; 317 (7155): 371–5.
55. The DECODE Study Group. Is fasting glucose sufficient to define diabetes? Epidemiological data from 20 European studies. *Diabetologia* 1999; 42 (6): 647–54.
56. Qiao Q, Nakagami T, Tuomilehto J, Borch-Johnsen K, Balkau B, Iwamoto Y, Tajima N. Comparison of the fasting and the 2-hour glucose criteria for diabetes in different Asian cohorts. *Diabetologia* 2000; 43: 1470–5.
57. Resnick HE, Harris MI, Brock DB, Harris TB. American Diabetes Association diabetes diagnostic criteria, advancing age, and cardiovascular disease risk profiles. Results from the Third National Health and Nutrition Examination Survey. *Diabetes Care* 2000; 23 (2): 176–80.
58. Pan X, Li G, Hu Y, Wang J, Yang W, An Z, Hu Z, Lin J, Xiao J, Cao H, Liu P, Jiang X, Jiang Y, Wang J, Zheng H, Zhang H, Bennett P, Howard B. Effects of diet and exercise in preventing NIDDM in people with impaired glucose tolerance: the Da Qing IGT and Diabetes Study. *Diabetes Care* 1997; 20 (4): 537–44.
59. Tuomilehto J, Lindstrom J, Eriksson JG, Valle TT, Hamalainen H, Ilanne-Parikka P, Keinanen-Kiukaanniemi S, Laakso M, Louheranta A, Rastas M,

Salminen V, Uusitupa M. Prevention of type 2 diabetes mellitus by changes in lifestyle among subjects with impaired glucose tolerance. *N Engl J Med* 2001; 344 (18): 1343–50.

60. Knowler WC, Barrett-Connor E, Fowler SE, Hamman RF, Lachin JM, Walker EA, Nathan DM. Reduction in the incidence of type 2 diabetes with lifestyle intervention or metformin. *N Engl J Med* 2002; 346 (6): 393–403.
61. Chiasson JL, Josse RG, Gomis R, Hanefeld M, Karasik A, Laakso M. Acarbose for prevention of type 2 diabetes mellitus: the STOP-NIDDM randomised trial. *Lancet* 2002; 359 (9323): 2072–7.
62. Yang W, Lin L, Qi J, Yu Z, Pei H, He G, Yang Z, Wang F, Li G, Pan X. The preventive effect of acarbose and metformin on the progression to diabetes mellitus in the IGT population: a 3-year multicenter prospective study. *Clin J Endocrinol Metab* 2001; 17 (3): 131–5.
63. Dowse GK, Zimmet PZ, King H. Relationship between prevalence of impaired glucose tolerance and NIDDM in a population. *Diabetes Care* 1991; 14 (11): 968–74.
64. Coughlan A, McCarty DJ, Jorgensen LN, Zimmet P. The epidemic of NIDDM in Asian and Pacific Island populations: prevalence and risk factors. *Horm Metab Res* 1997; 29 (7): 323–31.
65. Ramachandran A, Snehalatha C, Dharmaraj D, Viswanathan M. Prevalence of glucose intolerance in Asian Indians. Urban–rural difference and significance of upper body adiposity. *Diabetes Care* 1992; 15 (10): 1348–55.
66. Ramachandran A, Snehalatha C, Latha E, Vijay V, Viswanathan M. Rising prevalence of NIDDM in an urban population in India. *Diabetologia* 1997; 40 (2): 232–7.
67. Ramachandran A, Snehalatha C, Kapur A, Vijay V, Mohan V, Das AK, Rao PV, Yajnik CS, Kumar KMP, Nair JD. High prevalence of diabetes and impaired glucose tolerance in India: National Urban Diabetes Survey. *Diabetologia* 2001; 44: 1094–101.
68. National Diabetes Co-operative Study Group. A mass survey of diabetes mellitus in a population of 300 000 in 14 provinces and municipalities in China. *Clin J Intern Med* 1981; 20 (11): 678–83.
69. Shanghai Diabetes Research Cooperative Group. A survey of diabetes mellitus among the population in Shanghai. *Natl Med J Chin* 1980; 60: 323–9.
70. Pan XR, Hu YH, Li GW, Liu PA, Bennett PH, Howard BV. Impaired glucose tolerance and its relationship to ECG-indicated coronary heart disease and risk factors among Chinese: Da Qing IGT and Diabetes Study. *Diabetes Care* 1993; 16 (1): 150–6.
71. Hu YH, Li GW, Pan XR. Incidence of NIDDM in Daqing and forecasting of NIDDM in China in 21st century. *Zhonghua Nei Ke Za Zhi* 1993; 32 (3): 173–5.
72. Xiang HD, Wu W, Liu CQ, Li K, Feng JG, Zhang YT, Wang FQ, Yan SL, Wang CJ, Xu YC, Xu DR, Fu ZZ, Liu ZY, Li TL, Bai J, Fu ZY, Wang KA. An epidemiological study on diabetes mellitus 1995–1996, in China. *Chin J Diabetes* 1998; 6 (3): 131–3.
73. Yang Z, Zheng H, Tong Z. Prevalence of diabetes and IGT in elderly population of Beijing in 1997. *Chin J Geriatr* 2001; 20: 290–3.
74. Jia WP, Xiang KS, Chen L, Lu JX, Wu YM. Epidemiological study on obesity and its comorbidities in urban Chinese older than 20 years of age in Shanghai, China. *Obes Rev* 2002; 3 (3): 157–65.
75. Dong YH, Gao WG, Nan H, for the Qingdao Epidemiology Study Group. The prevalence of diabetes and the risk factor in Chinese population in Qingdao city (abstract). In *18th International Diabetes Federation Congress*, August 24–29, 2003, Paris, France, 2003.
76. Cockram CS, Woo J, Lau E, Chan JC, Chan AY, Lau J, Swaminathan R, Donnan SP. The prevalence of diabetes mellitus and impaired glucose tolerance among Hong Kong Chinese adults of working age. *Diabetes Res Clin Pract* 1993; 21 (1): 67–73.
77. Janus ED, Watt NM, Lam KS, Cockram CS, Siu ST, Liu LJ, Lam TH. The prevalence of diabetes, association with cardiovascular risk factors and implications of diagnostic criteria (ADA 1997 and WHO 1998) in a 1996 community-based population study in Hong Kong Chinese. *Diabet Med* 2000; 17 (10): 741–5.
78. Chen HD, Shaw CK, Tseng WP, Chen HI, Lee ML. Prevalence of diabetes mellitus and impaired glucose tolerance in Aborigines and Chinese in eastern Taiwan. *Diabetes Res Clin Pract* 1997; 38 (3): 199–205.
79. Midthjell K, Kruger O, Holmen J, Tverdal A, Claudi T, Bjorndal A, et al. Rapid changes in the prevalence of obesity and known diabetes in an adult Norwegian population. The Nord-Trondelag Health Surveys: 1984–1986 and 1995–1997. *Diabetes Care* 1999; 22 (11): 1813–20.
80. Drivsholm T, Ibsen H, Schroll M, Davidsen M, Borch-Johnsen K. Increasing prevalence of diabetes mellitus and impaired glucose tolerance among 60-year-old Danes. *Diabet Med* 2001; 18: 126–32.
81. Andersson DK, Svardsudd K, Tibblin G. Prevalence and incidence of diabetes in a Swedish community 1972–1987. *Diabet Med* 1991; 8 (5): 428–34.
82. Laakso M, Reunanen A, Klaukka T, Aromaa A, Maatela J, Pyorala K. Changes in the prevalence and incidence of diabetes mellitus in Finnish adults, 1970–1987. *Am J Epidemiol* 1991; 133 (9): 850–7.
83. Gu K, Cowie CC, Harris MI. Diabetes and decline in heart disease mortality in US adults. *JAMA* 1999; 281 (14): 1291–7.
84. Knowler WC, Pettitt DJ, Saad MF, Bennett PH. Diabetes mellitus in the Pima Indians: incidence, risk factors and pathogenesis. *Diabetes Metab Rev* 1990; 6 (1): 1–27.
85. Burke JP, Williams K, Gaskill SP, Hazuda HP, Haffner SM, Stern MP. Rapid rise in the incidence of type 2 diabetes from 1987 to 1996: results from the San Antonio Heart Study. *Arch Intern Med* 1999; 159 (13): 1450–6.
86. Savage PJ, Bennett PH, Senter RG, Miller M. High prevalence of diabetes in young Pima Indians: evidence of phenotypic variation in a genetically isolated population. *Diabetes* 1979; 28 (10): 937–42.
87. Knowler WC, Pettitt DJ, Savage PJ, Bennett PH. Diabetes incidence in Pima Indians: contributions of obesity and parental diabetes. *Am J Epidemiol* 1981; 113 (2): 144–56.
88. Dabelea D, Hanson RL, Bennett PH, Roumain J, Knowler WC, Pettitt DJ. Increasing prevalence of Type II diabetes in American Indian children. *Diabetologia* 1998; 41 (8): 904–10.
89. Acton KJ, Burrows NR, Moore K, Querec L, Geiss LS, Engelgau MM. Trends in diabetes prevalence among American Indian and Alaska native children, adolescents, and young adults. *Am J Public Health* 2002; 92 (9): 1485–90.
90. Burrows NR, Geiss LS, Engelgau MM, Acton KJ. Prevalence of diabetes among Native Americans and Alaska

Natives, 1990–1997: an increasing burden. *Diabetes Care* 2000; 23 (12): 1786–90.
91. Harris SB, Perkins BA, Whalen-Brough E. Non-insulin-dependent diabetes mellitus among First Nations children. New entity among First Nations people of northwestern Ontario. *Can Fam Physician* 1996; 42: 869–76.
92. Pinhas-Hamiel O, Dolan LM, Daniels SR, Standiford D, Khoury PR, Zeitler P. Increased incidence of non-insulin-dependent diabetes mellitus among adolescents. *J Pediatr* 1996; 128 (5, pt 1): 608–15.
93. Kitagawa T, Owada M, Urakami T, Tajima N. Epidemiology of type 1 (insulin-dependent) and type 2 (non-insulin-dependent) diabetes mellitus in Japanese children. *Diabetes Res Clin Pract* 1994; 24 (suppl): S7–13.
94. Kitagawa T, Owada M, Urakami T, Yamauchi K. Increased incidence of non-insulin dependent diabetes mellitus among Japanese schoolchildren correlates with an increased intake of animal protein and fat. *Clin Pediatr (Phila)* 1998; 37 (2): 111–5.
95. Owada M, Hanaoka Y, Tanimoto Y, Kitagawa T. Descriptive epidemiology of non-insulin dependent diabetes mellitus detected by urine glucose screening in school children in Japan. *Acta Paediatr Jpn* 1990; 32 (6): 716–24.
96. Kadiki OA, Reddy MR, Marzouk AA. Incidence of insulin-dependent diabetes (IDDM) and non-insulin-dependent diabetes (NIDDM) (0–34 years at onset) in Benghazi, Libya. *Diabetes Res Clin Pract* 1996; 32 (3): 165–73.
97. Likitmaskul S, Kiattisathavee P, Chaichanwatanakul K, Punnakanta L, Angsusingha K, Tuchinda C. Increasing prevalence of type 2 diabetes mellitus in Thai children and adolescents associated with increasing prevalence of obesity. *J Pediatr Endocrinol Metab* 2003; 16 (1): 71–7.
98. Drake AJ, Smith A, Betts PR, Crowne EC, Shield JP. Type 2 diabetes in obese white children. *Arch Dis Child* 2002; 86 (3): 207–8.
99. Ehtisham S, Barrett TG, Shaw NJ. Type 2 diabetes mellitus in UK children—an emerging problem. *Diabet Med* 2000; 17 (12): 867–71.
100. Ehtisham S, Kirk J, McEvilly A, Shaw N, Jones S, Rose S, et al. Prevalence of type 2 diabetes in children in Birmingham. *BMJ* 2001; 322 (7299): 1428.
101. Ramachandran A, Snehalatha C, Satyavani K, Sivasankari S, Vijay V. Type 2 diabetes in Asian-Indian urban children. *Diabetes Care* 2003; 26 (4): 1022–5.
102. Wei JN, Chuang LM, Lin CC, Chiang CC, Lin RS, Sung FC. Childhood diabetes identified in mass urine screening program in Taiwan, 1993–1999. *Diabetes Res Clin Pract* 2003; 59 (3): 201–6.
103. Neufeld ND, Raffel LJ, Landon C, Chen YD, Vadheim CM. Early presentation of type 2 diabetes in Mexican-American youth. *Diabetes Care* 1998; 21 (1): 80–6.
104. Willi SM, Kennedy A, Wojciechowski B, Garvey W. Insulin resistance and defective glucose-insulin coupling in ketosis-prone type 2 diabetes of African-American youth. *Diabetes* 1998; 47 (suppl 1): A306.
105. Glaser NS, Jones KL. Non-insulin dependent diabetes mellitus in Mexican-American children. *West J Med* 1998; 168 (1): 11–6.
106. Hale DE, Dabbey MM. Non-insulin dependent diabetes in Hispanic youth (type 2Y). *Diabetes* 1998; 47 (suppl 1): A82.
107. Macaluso CJ, Bauer UE, Deeb LC, Malone JI, Chaudhari M, Silverstein J, Eidson M, Goldberg R, Gaughan-Bailey B, Brooks RG, Rosenbloom AL. Type 2 diabetes mellitus among Florida children and adolescents, 1994 through 1998. *Public Health Rep* 2002; 117: 373–9.
108. Rosenbloom AL, Joe JR, Young RS, Winter WE. Emerging epidemic of type 2 diabetes in youth. *Diabetes Care* 1999; 22 (2): 345–54.
109. Fagot-Campagna A, Pettitt DJ, Engelgau MM, Burrows NR, Geiss LS, Valdez R, et al. Type 2 diabetes among North American children and adolescents: an epidemiologic review and a public health perspective. *J Pediatr* 2000; 136 (5): 664–72.
110. Freedman DS, Srinivasan SR, Burke GL, Shear CL, Smoak CG, Harsha DW, Webber LS, Berenson GS. Relation of body fat distribution to hyperinsulinemia in children and adolescents: the Bogalusa Heart Study. *Am J Clin Nutr* 1987; 46 (3): 403–10.
111. Arslanian S, Suprasongsin C. Insulin sensitivity, lipids, and body composition in childhood: is "syndrome X" present? *J Clin Endocrinol Metab* 1996; 81 (3): 1058–62.
112. Haffner SM, Stern MP, Mitchell BD, Hazuda HP, Patterson JK. Incidence of type II diabetes in Mexican Americans predicted by fasting insulin and glucose levels, obesity, and body-fat distribution. *Diabetes* 1990; 39 (3): 283–8.
113. Thomas-Dobersen DA, Butler-Simon N, Fleshner M. Evaluation of a weight management intervention program in adolescents with insulin-dependent diabetes mellitus. *J Am Diet Assoc* 1993; 93 (5): 535–40.
114. Pinhas-Hamiel O, Dolan LM, Zeitler PS. Diabetic ketoacidosis among obese African-American adolescents with NIDDM. *Diabetes Care* 1997; 20 (4): 484–6.
115. Pihoker C, Scott CR, Lensing SY, Cradock MM, Smith J. Non-insulin dependent diabetes mellitus in African-American youths of Arkansas. *Clin Pediatr (Phila)* 1998; 37 (2): 97–102.
116. Savola K, Laara E, Vahasalo P, Kulmala P, Akerblom HK, Knip M. Dynamic pattern of disease-associated autoantibodies in siblings of children with type 1 diabetes: a population-based study. *Diabetes* 2001; 50 (11): 2625–32.
117. Kimpimaki T, Kulmala P, Savola K, Kupila A, Korhonen S, Simell T, Ilonen J, Simell O, Knip M. Natural history of beta-cell autoimmunity in young children with increased genetic susceptibility to type 1 diabetes recruited from the general population. *J Clin Endocrinol Metab* 2002; 87 (10): 4572–9.
118. Ogden CL, Flegal KM, Carroll MD, Johnson CL. Prevalence and trends in overweight among US children and adolescents, 1999–2000. *JAMA* 2002; 288 (14): 1728–32.
119. Strauss RS, Pollack HA. Epidemic increase in childhood overweight, 1986–1998. *JAMA* 2001; 286 (22): 2845–8.
120. Amiel SA, Sherwin RS, Simonson DC, Lauritano AA, Tamborlane WV. Impaired insulin action in puberty. A contributing factor to poor glycemic control in adolescents with diabetes. *N Engl J Med* 1986; 315 (4): 215–9.
121. Arslanian S, Suprasongsin C. Testosterone treatment in adolescents with delayed puberty: changes in body composition, protein, fat, and glucose metabolism. *J Clin Endocrinol Metab* 1997; 82 (10): 3213–20.
122. Caprio S, Plewe G, Diamond MP, Simonson DC, Boulware SD, Sherwin RS, Tamborlane WV. Increased insulin secretion in puberty: a compensatory response to reductions in insulin sensitivity. *J Pediatr* 1989; 114 (6): 963–7.

123. Goran MI, Gower BA. Longitudinal study on pubertal insulin resistance. *Diabetes* 2001; 50 (11): 2444–50.
124. Bloch CA, Clemons P, Sperling MA. Puberty decreases insulin sensitivity. *J Pediatr* 1987; 110 (3): 481–7.
125. Dabelea D, Hanson RL, Lindsay RS, Pettitt DJ, Imperatore G, Gabir MM, Roumain J, Bennett PH, Knowler WC. Intrauterine exposure to diabetes conveys risks for type 2 diabetes and obesity: a study of discordant sibships. *Diabetes* 2000; 49 (12): 2208–11.
126. Barker DJ, Martyn CN. The maternal and fetal origins of cardiovascular disease. *J Epidemiol Community Health* 1992; 46 (1): 8–11.
127. Hales CN, Barker DJ, Clark PM, Cox LJ, Fall C, Osmond C, Winter PD. Fetal and infant growth and impaired glucose tolerance at age 64. *BMJ* 1991; 303 (6809): 1019–22.
128. Young TK, Martens PJ, Taback SP, Sellers EA, Dean HJ, Cheang M, Flett B. Type 2 diabetes mellitus in children: prenatal and early infancy risk factors among native Canadians. *Arch Pediatr Adolesc Med* 2002; 156 (7): 651–5.
129. Pettitt D, Knowler WC. Long-term effects of the intrauterine environment, birth weight, and breast-feeding in Pima Indians. *Diabetes Care* 1998; 21 (suppl 2): B138–41.
130. Pettitt DJ, Forman MR, Hanson RL, Knowler WC, Bennett PH. Breastfeeding and incidence of non-insulin-dependent diabetes mellitus in Pima Indians. *Lancet* 1997; 350 (9072): 166–8.
131. Krakoff J, Lindsay RS, Looker HC, Nelson RG, Hanson RL, Knowler WC. Incidence of retinopathy and nephropathy in youth-onset compared with adult-onset type 2 diabetes. *Diabetes Care* 2003; 26 (1): 76–81.
132. Dean HJ, Flett B. Natural history of type 2 diabetes diagnosed in childhood: long term follow-up in young adult years. *Diabetes* 2002; 51: A24–5.
133. Ferrara A, Imperatore G, Quesenberry CP, Karter AJ, Fagot-Campagna A, Ergas IJ, Selby V. Characteristics and quality of health care of type 1 (T1DM) and type 2 (T2DM) diabetic youths: the Northern California Kaiser Permanente (NCKP) Diabetes Registry. *Diabetes* 2002; 51 (suppl 2): 105.
134. Nelson RG, Sievers ML, Knowler WC, Swinburn BA, Pettitt DJ, Saad MF, Liebow IM, Howard BV, Bennett PH. Low incidence of fatal coronary heart disease in Pima Indians despite high prevalence of non-insulin-dependent diabetes. *Circulation* 1990; 81 (3): 987–95.
135. American Diabetes Association. Type 2 diabetes in children and adolescents. *Diabetes Care* 2000; 23: 381–9.
136. Freedman DS, Serdula MK, Percy CA, Ballew C, White L. Obesity, levels of lipids and glucose, and smoking among Navajo adolescents. *J Nutr* 1997; 127: 2120S–7S.
137. Dean HJ, Young TK, Flett B, Wood-Steiman P. Screening for type 2 diabetes in aboriginal children in northern Canada. *Lancet* 1998; 352: 1523–4.
138. Fagot-Campagna A, Saadine JB, Fiegal KM, Beckles GL. Diabetes, impaired fasting glucose, and elevated HbA_{1c} in US adolescents; the Third National Health and Nutrition Examination Survey. *Diabetes Care* 2001; 24: 834–7.
139. Scott CR, Smith JM, Creddock MM, Pihoker C. Characteristics of youth-onset noninsulin-dependent diabetes mellitus and insulin-dependent diabetes mellitus at diagnosis. *Pediatrics* 1997; 100: 84–91.
140. O'Dea K. Obesity and diabetes in "the land of milk and honey." *Diabetes Metab Rev* 1992; 8 (4): 373–88.
141. Knowler WC, Saad MF, Pettitt DJ, Nelson RG, Bennett PH. Determinants of diabetes mellitus in the Pima Indians. *Diabetes Care* 1993; 16 (1): 216–27.
142. Haffner SM. Epidemiology of type 2 diabetes: risk factors. *Diabetes Care* 1998; 21 (suppl 3): C3–6.
143. Ford ES, Williamson DF, Liu S. Weight change and diabetes incidence: findings from a national cohort of US adults. *Am J Epidemiol* 1997; 146 (3): 214–22.
144. Colditz GA, Willett WC, Rotnitzky A, Manson JE. Weight gain as a risk factor for clinical diabetes mellitus in women. *Ann Intern Med* 1995; 122 (7): 481–6.
145. Chang CJ, Wu CH, Lu FH, Wu JS, Chiu NT, Yao WJ. Discriminating glucose tolerance status by regions of interest of dual-energy X-ray absorptiometry. Clinical implications of body fat distribution. *Diabetes Care* 1999; 22 (12): 1938–43.
146. Goodpaster BH, Krishnaswami S, Resnick H, Kelley DE, Haggerty C, Harris TB, Schwartz AV, Kritchevsky S, Newman AB. Association between regional adipose tissue distribution and both type 2 diabetes and impaired glucose tolerance in elderly men and women. *Diabetes Care* 2003; 26 (2): 372–9.
147. Despres JP. Abdominal obesity as important component of insulin-resistance syndrome. *Nutrition* 1993; 9 (5): 452–9.
148. Rush EC, Plank LD, Mitchelson E, Laulu MS. Central obesity and risk for type 2 diabetes in Maori, Pacific, and European young men in New Zealand. *Food Nutr Bull* 2002; 23 (3, suppl): 82–6.
149. Hayashi T, Boyko EJ, Leonetti DL, McNeely MJ, Newell-Morris L, Kahn SE, Fujimoto WY. Visceral adiposity and the risk of impaired glucose tolerance: a prospective study among Japanese Americans. *Diabetes Care* 2003; 26 (3): 650–5.
150. Cruz ML, Bergman RN, Goran MI. Unique effect of visceral fat on insulin sensitivity in obese Hispanic children with a family history of type 2 diabetes. *Diabetes Care* 2002; 25 (9): 1631–6.
151. Hu FB, Sigal RJ, Rich-Edwards JW, Colditz GA, Solomon CG, Willett WC, Speizer FE, Manson JE. Walking compared with vigorous physical activity and risk of type 2 diabetes in women: a prospective study. *JAMA* 1999; 282 (15): 1433–9.
152. Mayer-Davis EJ, D'Agostino R Jr, Karter AJ, Haffner SM, Rewers MJ, Saad M, Bergman RN. Intensity and amount of physical activity in relation to insulin sensitivity: the Insulin Resistance Atherosclerosis Study. *JAMA* 1998; 279 (9): 669–74.
153. Kriska AM, Pereira MA, Hanson RL, Court D, Zimmet PZ, Alberti KG, Chitson P, Bennett PH, Narayan KM, Knowler WC. Association of physical activity and serum insulin concentrations in two populations at high risk for type 2 diabetes but differing by *BMI* 2001; 24 (7): 1175–80.
154. Manson JE, Nathan DM, Krolewski AS, Stampfer MJ, Willett WC, Hennekens CH. A prospective study of exercise and incidence of diabetes among US male physicians. *JAMA* 1992; 268 (1): 63–7.
155. Helmrich SP, Ragland DR, Leung RW, Paffenbarger RS Jr. Physical activity and reduced occurrence of non-insulin-dependent diabetes mellitus. *N Engl J Med* 1991; 325 (3): 147–52.
156. Manson JE, Rimm EB, Stampfer MJ, Colditz GA, Willett WC, Krolewski AS, Rosner B, Hennekens CH, Speizer FE. Physical activity and incidence of non-insulin-dependent diabetes mellitus in women. *Lancet* 1991; 338 (8770): 774–8.

157. Schranz A, Tuomilehto J, Marti B, Jarrett RJ, Grabauskas V, Vassallo A. Low physical activity and worsening of glucose tolerance: results from a 2-year follow-up of a population sample in Malta. *Diabetes Res Clin Pract* 1991; 11: 127–36.
158. Burchfiel CM, Sharp DS, Curb JD, Rodriguez BL, Hwang LJ, Marcus EB, Yano K. Physical activity and incidence of diabetes: the Honolulu Heart Program. *Am J Epidemiol* 1995; 141 (4): 360–8.
159. Lynch J, Helmrich SP, Lakka TA, Kaplan GA, Cohen RD, Salonen R, Salonen JT. Moderately intense physical activities and high levels of cardiorespiratory fitness reduce the risk of non-insulin-dependent diabetes mellitus in middle-aged men. *Arch Intern Med* 1996; 156 (12): 1307–14.
160. Haapanen N, Miilunpalo S, Vuori I, Oja P, Pasanen M. Association of leisure time physical activity with the risk of coronary heart disease, hypertension and diabetes in middle-aged men and women. *Int J Epidemiol* 1997; 26 (4): 739–47.
161. Folsom AR, Kushi LH, Hong CP. Physical activity and incident diabetes mellitus in postmenopausal women. *Am J Public Health* 2000; 90 (1): 134–8.
162. Hu FB, Leitzmann MF, Stampfer MJ, Colditz GA, Willett WC, Rimm EB. Physical activity and television watching in relation to risk for type 2 diabetes mellitus in men. *Arch Intern Med* 2001; 161 (12): 1542–8.
163. Hu FB, Li TY, Colditz GA, Willett WC, Manson JE. Television watching and other sedentary behaviors in relation to risk of obesity and type 2 diabetes mellitus in women. *JAMA* 2003; 289 (14): 1785–91.
164. Eriksson KF, Lindgarde F. Prevention of type 2 (non-insulin-dependent) diabetes mellitus by diet and physical exercise. The 6-year Malmö feasibility study. *Diabetologia* 1991; 34 (12): 891–8.
165. Danforth E Jr. Diet and obesity. *Am J Clin Nutr* 1985; 41 (5, suppl): 1132–45.
166. Storlien LH, James DE, Burleigh KM, Chisholm DJ, Kraegen EW. Fat feeding causes widespread in vivo insulin resistance, decreased energy expenditure, and obesity in rats. *Am J Physiol* 1986; 251 (5, pt 1): E576–83.
167. Storlien LH, Pan DA, Kriketos AD, Baur LA. High fat diet-induced insulin resistance. Lessons and implications from animal studies. *Ann N Y Acad Sci* 1993; 683: 82–90.
168. Kawate R, Yamakido M, Nishimoto Y, Bennett PH, Hamman RF, Knowler WC. Diabetes mellitus and its vascular complications in Japanese migrants on the Island of Hawaii. *Diabetes Care* 1979; 2 (2): 161–70.
169. Stern MP, Gonzalez C, Mitchell BD, Villalpando E, Haffner SM, Hazuda HP. Genetic and environmental determinants of type II diabetes in Mexico City and San Antonio. *Diabetes* 1992; 41 (4): 484–92.
170. Tsunehara CH, Leonetti DL, Fujimoto WY. Diet of second-generation Japanese-American men with and without non-insulin-dependent diabetes. *Am J Clin Nutr* 1990; 52 (4): 731–8.
171. Marshall JA, Hamman RF, Baxter J. High-fat, low-carbohydrate diet and the etiology of non-insulin-dependent diabetes mellitus: the San Luis Valley Diabetes Study. *Am J Epidemiol* 1991; 134 (6): 590–603.
172. Feskens EJ, Virtanen SM, Rasanen L, Tuomilehto J, Stengard J, Pekkanen J, Nissinen A, Kromhout D. Dietary factors determining diabetes and impaired glucose tolerance. A 20-year follow-up of the Finnish and Dutch cohorts of the seven countries study. *Diabetes Care* 1995; 18 (8): 1104–12.
173. Colditz GA, Manson JE, Stampfer MJ, Rosner B, Willett WC, Speizer FE. Diet and risk of clinical diabetes in women. *Am J Clin Nutr* 1992; 55 (5): 1018–23.
174. Lundgren H, Bengtsson C, Blohme G, Isaksson B, Lapidus L, Lenner RA, et al. Dietary habits and incidence of noninsulin-dependent diabetes mellitus in a population study of women in Gotnenburg, Sweden. *Am J Clin Nutr* 1989; 49: 708–12.
175. Virtanen SM, Rasanen L, Maenpaa J, Akerblom HK. Dietary survey of Finnish adolescent diabetics and non-diabetic controls. *Acta Paediatr Scand* 1987; 76 (5): 801–8.
176. Marshall JA, Bessesen DH, Hamman RF. High saturated fat and low starch and fibre are associated with hyperinsulinaemia in a non-diabetic population: the San Luis Valley Diabetes Study. *Diabetologia* 1997; 40 (4): 430–8.
177. Adler AI, Boyko EJ, Schraer CD, Murphy NJ. Lower prevalence of impaired glucose tolerance and diabetes associated with daily seal oil or salmon consumption among Alaska Natives. *Diabetes Care* 1994; 17 (12): 1498–501.
178. Vessby B. Effects of omega 3 fatty acids on glucose and lipid metabolism in non-insulin-dependent diabetes mellitus. *World Rev Nutr Diet* 1991; 66: 407–16.
179. Storlien LH, Kraegen EW, Chisholm DJ, Ford GL, Bruce DG, Pascoe WS. Fish oil prevents insulin resistance induced by high-fat feeding in rats. *Science* 1987; 237 (4817): 885–8.
180. Hu FB, van Dam RM, Liu S. Diet and risk of Type II diabetes: the role of types of fat and carbohydrate. *Diabetologia* 2001; 44 (7): 805–17.
181. Feskens EJ, Bowles CH, Kromhout D. Carbohydrate intake and body mass index in relation to the risk of glucose intolerance in an elderly population. *Am J Clin Nutr* 1991; 54 (1): 136–40.
182. Wolever TM, Hamad S, Gittelsohn J, Gao J, Hanley AJ, Harris SB, Zinman B. Low dietary fiber and high protein intakes associated with newly diagnosed diabetes in a remote aboriginal community. *Am J Clin Nutr* 1997; 66 (6): 1470–4.
183. Jenkins DJ, Wolever TM, Taylor RH, Barker H, Fielden H, Baldwin JM, Bowling AC, Newman HC, Jenkins AL, Goff DV. Glycemic index of foods: a physiological basis for carbohydrate exchange. *Am J Clin Nutr* 1981; 34 (3): 362–6.
184. Salmeron J, Ascherio A, Rimm EB, Colditz GA, Spiegelman D, Jenkins DJ, Stampfer MJ, Wing AL, Willett WC. Dietary fiber, glycemic load, and risk of NIDDM in men. *Diabetes Care* 1997; 20 (4): 545–50.
185. Meyer KA, Kushi LH, Jacobs DR Jr, Slavin J, Sellers TA, Folsom AR. Carbohydrates, dietary fiber, and incident type 2 diabetes in older women. *Am J Clin Nutr* 2000; 71 (4): 921–30.
186. van Dam RM, Visscher AW, Feskens EJ, Verhoef P, Kromhout D. Dietary glycemic index in relation to metabolic risk factors and incidence of coronary heart disease: the Zutphen Elderly Study. *Eur J Clin Nutr* 2000; 54 (9): 726–31.
187. Trowell HC. Dietary-fiber hypothesis of the etiology of diabetes mellitus. *Diabetes* 1975; 24 (8): 762–5.
188. Burkitt DP, Trowell HC. Dietary fibre and western diseases. *Ir Med J* 1977; 70 (9): 272–7.

189. Salmeron J, Manson JE, Stampfer MJ, Colditz GA, Wing AL, Willett WC. Dietary fiber, glycemic load, and risk of non-insulin-dependent diabetes mellitus in women. *JAMA* 1997; 277 (6): 472–7.
190. Fung TT, Hu FB, Pereira MA, Liu S, Stampfer MJ, Colditz GA, Willett WC. Whole-grain intake and the risk of type 2 diabetes: a prospective study in men. *Am J Clin Nutr* 2002; 76 (3): 535–40.
191. Bakker SJ, Hoogeveen EK, Nijpels G, Kostense PJ, Dekker JM, Gans RO, Heine RJ. The association of dietary fibres with glucose tolerance is partly explained by concomitant intake of thiamine: the Hoorn Study. *Diabetologia* 1998; 41 (10): 1168–75.
192. Jenkins DJ, Axelsen M, Kendall CW, Augustin LS, Vuksan V, Smith U. Dietary fibre, lente carbohydrates and the insulin-resistant diseases. *Br J Nutr* 2000; 83 (suppl 1): S157–63.
193. Williams DE, Wareham NJ, Cox BD, Byrne CD, Hales CN, Day NE. Frequent salad vegetable consumption is associated with a reduction in the risk of diabetes mellitus. *J Clin Epidemiol* 1999; 52 (4): 329–35.
194. Ylonen K, Alfthan G, Groop L, Saloranta C, Aro A, Virtanen SM. Dietary intakes and plasma concentrations of carotenoids and tocopherols in relation to glucose metabolism in subjects at high risk of type 2 diabetes: the Botnia Dietary Study. *Am J Clin Nutr* 2003; 77 (6): 1434–41.
195. Ford ES, Mokdad AH, Giles WH, Brown DW. The metabolic syndrome and antioxidant concentrations: findings from the Third National Health and Nutrition Examination Survey. *Diabetes* 2003; 52 (9): 2346–52.
196. Sargeant LA, Khaw KT, Bingham S, Day NE, Luben RN, Oakes S, Welch A, Wareham NJ. Cigarette smoking and glycaemia: the EPIC-Norfolk Study. *Int J Epidemiol* 2001; 30 (3): 547–54.
197. Williams DE, Prevost AT, Whichelow MJ, Cox BD, Day NE, Wareham NJ. A cross-sectional study of dietary patterns with glucose intolerance and other features of the metabolic syndrome. *Br J Nutr* 2000; 83 (3): 257–66.
198. van Dam RM, Rimm EB, Willett WC, Stampfer MJ, Hu FB. Dietary patterns and risk for type 2 diabetes mellitus in U.S. men. *Ann Intern Med* 2002; 136 (3): 201–9.
199. Williams DE, Knowler WC, Smith CJ, Hanson RL, Roumain J, Saremi A, Kriska AM, Bennett PH, Nelson RG. The effect of Indian or Anglo dietary preference on the incidence of diabetes in Pima Indians. *Diabetes Care* 2001; 24 (5): 811–6.
200. Brand JC, Snow BJ, Nabhan GP, Truswell AS. Plasma glucose and insulin responses to traditional Pima Indian meals. *Am J Clin Nutr* 1990; 51 (3): 416–20.
201. Thorburn AW, Brand JC, O'Dea K, Spargo RM, Truswell AS. Plasma glucose and insulin responses to starchy foods in Australian aborigines: a population now at high risk of diabetes. *Am J Clin Nutr* 1987; 46 (2): 282–5.
202. Jarrett RJ, Shipley MJ. Type 2 (non-insulin-dependent) diabetes mellitus and cardiovascular disease—putative association via common antecedents; further evidence from the Whitehall Study. *Diabetologia* 1988; 31 (10): 737–40.
203. Stern MP. Diabetes and cardiovascular disease. The "common soil" hypothesis. *Diabetes* 1995; 44 (4): 369–74.
204. Yudkin JS, Stehouwer CD, Emeis JJ, Coppack SW. C-reactive protein in healthy subjects: associations with obesity, insulin resistance, and endothelial dysfunction: a potential role for cytokines originating from adipose tissue? *Arterioscler Thromb Vasc Biol* 1999; 19 (4): 972–8.
205. Festa A, D'Agostino R Jr, Howard G, Mykkanen L, Tracy RP, Haffner SM. Chronic subclinical inflammation as part of the insulin resistance syndrome: the Insulin Resistance Atherosclerosis Study (IRAS). *Circulation* 2000; 102 (1): 42–7.
206. Forouhi NG, Sattar N, McKeigue PM. Relation of C-reactive protein to body fat distribution and features of the metabolic syndrome in Europeans and South Asians. *Int J Obes Relat Metab Disord* 2001; 25 (9): 1327–31.
207. Pradhan AD, Manson JE, Rifai N, Buring JE, Ridker PM. C-reactive protein, interleukin 6, and risk of developing type 2 diabetes mellitus. *JAMA* 2001; 286 (3): 327–34.
208. Barzilay JI, Abraham L, Heckbert SR, Cushman M, Kuller LH, Resnick HE, Tracy RP. The relation of markers of inflammation to the development of glucose disorders in the elderly: the Cardiovascular Health Study. *Diabetes* 2001; 50 (10): 2384–9.
209. Freeman DJ, Norrie J, Caslake MJ, Gaw A, Ford I, Lowe GD, et al. C-reactive protein is an independent predictor of risk for the development of diabetes in the West of Scotland Coronary Prevention Study. *Diabetes* 2002; 51 (5): 1596–600.
210. Festa A, D'Agostino R Jr, Tracy RP, Haffner SM. Elevated levels of acute-phase proteins and plasminogen activator inhibitor-1 predict the development of type 2 diabetes: the insulin resistance atherosclerosis study. *Diabetes* 2002; 51 (4): 1131–7.
211. Han TS, Sattar N, Williams K, Gonzalez-Villalpando C, Lean ME, Haffner SM. Prospective study of C-reactive protein in relation to the development of diabetes and metabolic syndrome in the Mexico City Diabetes Study. *Diabetes Care* 2002; 25 (11): 2016–21.
212. Thorand B, Lowel H, Schneider A, Kolb H, Meisinger C, Frohlich M, Koenig W. C-reactive protein as a predictor for incident diabetes mellitus among middle-aged men: results from the MONICA Augsburg Cohort Study, 1984–1998. *Arch Intern Med* 2003; 163 (1): 93–9.
213. Hundal RS, Petersen KF, Mayerson AB, Randhawa PS, Inzucchi S, Shoelson SE, Shulman GI. Mechanism by which high-dose aspirin improves glucose metabolism in type 2 diabetes. *J Clin Invest* 2002; 109 (10): 1321–6.
214. Rimm EB, Manson JE, Stampfer MJ, Colditz GA, Willett WC, Rosner B, Hennekens CH, Speizer FE. Cigarette smoking and the risk of diabetes in women. *Am J Public Health* 1993; 83 (2): 211–4.
215. Rimm EB, Chan J, Stampfer MJ, Colditz GA, Willett WC. Prospective study of cigarette smoking, alcohol use, and the risk of diabetes in men. *BMJ* 1995; 310 (6979): 555–9.
216. Will JC, Galuska DA, Ford ES, Mokdad A, Calle EE. Cigarette smoking and diabetes mellitus: evidence of a positive association from a large prospective cohort study. *Int J Epidemiol* 2001; 30 (3): 540–6.
217. Facchini FS, Hollenbeck CB, Jeppesen J, Chen YD, Reaven GM. Insulin resistance and cigarette smoking. *Lancet* 1992; 339 (8802): 1128–30.
218. Attvall S, Fowelin J, Lager I, Von Schenck H, Smith U. Smoking induces insulin resistance—a potential link with the insulin resistance syndrome. *J Intern Med* 1993; 233 (4): 327–32.

Normal Physiology of Pancreatic Function

4

Development and Life Cycle of a β-Cell

Palle Serup* and Jens Høiriis Nielsen†

*Hagedorn Research Institute Gentofte, Denmark, and †University of Copenhagen, Copenhagen, Denmark

INTRODUCTION

The understanding of the molecular biology of the pancreas β-cell began 25 years ago with the cloning of the insulin cDNA, followed by the determination of the genomic organization and the identification of multiple *cis-* and *trans*-acting elements in the 5′-flanking region. The developmental biology of the pancreas started earlier but was put on hold until the molecular biological technology allowed approaching the questions raised some 30 years ago. A major breakthrough happened 8 years ago when disruption of the gene for an insulin gene transcription factor was found to ablate the development of the pancreas. This has greatly stimulated the search for new transcription factors and their regulation by growth and differentiation factors in order to understand the basal molecular mechanisms involved in the formation of the pancreas β-cell and the perspectives for prevention, treatment, and cure of diabetes. The maintenance of an appropriate β-cell mass depends on neogenesis from progenitor cells, proliferation of existing β-cells, and β-cell death. The balance between these processes is regulated by a complex interaction of metabolites, hormones, and growth factors. Under normal conditions there appears to be a close correspondence between insulin demand and the functional β-cell mass. The function of the β-cell is not only under acute regulation by nutrients following a meal but is also subject to regulation by chronic changes in the insulin demand as in pregnancy or obesity, which result in adjustment of the β-cell number. The hypothetical changes in the β-cell mass during normal and diabetic conditions are outlined in Figure 1.

PATTERNING OF PANCREAS ENDODERM: "THE TOUCH OF MESODERM"

The first morphological signs of pancreas development in vertebrates are a dorsal and one or two ventral evaginations of the primitive gut epithelium. The pancreas epithelium subsequently grows, branches, and fuses to form a single organ. The earliest molecular signs of pancreas development in the gut epithelium occur well before morphological signs are evident [1–3]. The gut tube forms from the endoderm when a crescent-shaped fold, the so-called anterior intestinal portal (AIP), which appears at the anterior tip of the endoderm, moves in a caudal direction and meets a similar, rostrally moving fold, called the caudal intestinal portal (CIP), which appears slightly later at the posterior end of the embryo. Domains in the forming gut tube that contribute to various digestive and other gut-tube-associated organs overlap, although regions of different fates can be distinguished. This rough regional differentiation is progressively refined, likely through interactions with the surrounding tissues [2]. By the 15-somite stage, expression of distinct sets of transcription factors marks presumptive organ territories such as the esophagus, stomach, liver, pancreas, duodenum, and small and large intestines [3]. Thus, the pancreas region is recognizable in the anterior endoderm before gut tube closure by expression of the transcription factor Pdx-1 (pancreatic and duodenal homeobox 1) [1]. Pdx1 is expressed in precursors of all pancreas cells (i.e., endocrine, acinar, and duct cells) [4] before eventually being confined to β-cells and some δ-cells at late stages of development [1, 5]. Initiation of Pdx1 expression in the

International Textbook of Diabetes Mellitus, Third Edition. Edited by R. A. DeFronzo, E. Ferrannini, H. Keen, and P. Zimmet.
 ISBN: 0-471-48655-8.

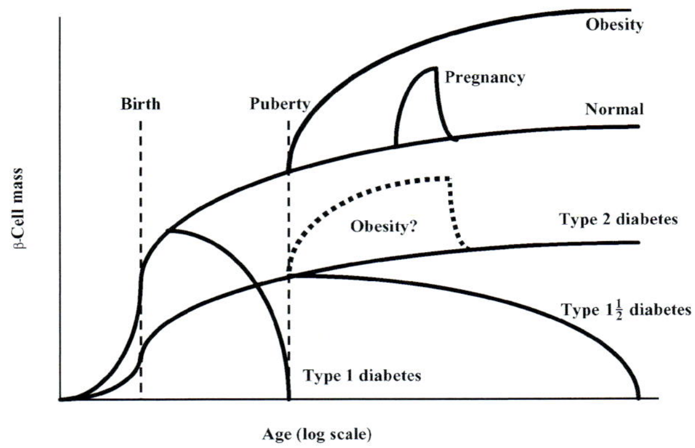

Figure 1 Hypothetical changes in the β-cell mass with age. See text for explanations

endoderm depends on signals received from the surrounding mesodermal tissues. In chicken, early studies demonstrated that axial mesoderm (the notochord) is required for the initiation of pancreas-specific gene expression [6]. Support for the requirement of notochord–endoderm signaling (Figure 2a) for proper pancreas formation comes from studies in zebrafish, as *floating head (flh)* mutants lacking a notochord display spectacularly reduced expression of the pancreas markers Pdx1 and insulin in the presumptive pancreas area. Later studies in chicken revealed that notochord-derived signals function to exclude sonic hedgehog (Shh) expression from part of the dorsal endoderm, including the pancreas primordium. This pattern suggests that Shh might function to restrict pancreas development and that ectopic expression within pancreas tissue may interfere with normal development [7]. These ideas have been tested by a combination of gain-of-function and loss-of-function experiments in chicken, mice, and fish. Analysis of *in vitro* cultured pancreas epithelium isolated from 15-somite chicken embryos revealed loss of Pdx1 and insulin expression concurrent with increased Shh expression. Expression of both genes could be rescued by co-culturing the epithelium with either notochord or function-blocking anti-Shh antibodies [7]. These results suggest that inhibition of Shh signaling is required to initiate or maintain pancreas gene expression. Furthermore, Edlund and coworkers [8] directly demonstrated that presence of Shh in pancreas endoderm is incompatible with pancreas organogenesis. In contrast to amniotes and Xenopus, hedgehog signaling in zebrafish is required for early pancreas development [7]. However, this apparent contradiction might be explained by the fact that zebrafish carrying mutations in the hedgehog pathway show defects in the development of the vascular system. Vascular defects do not normally prevent the development of zebrafish embryos since their small size allows sufficient oxygen to reach even deeply located tissues by diffusion, but vascular endothelial cells might be a source of inductive

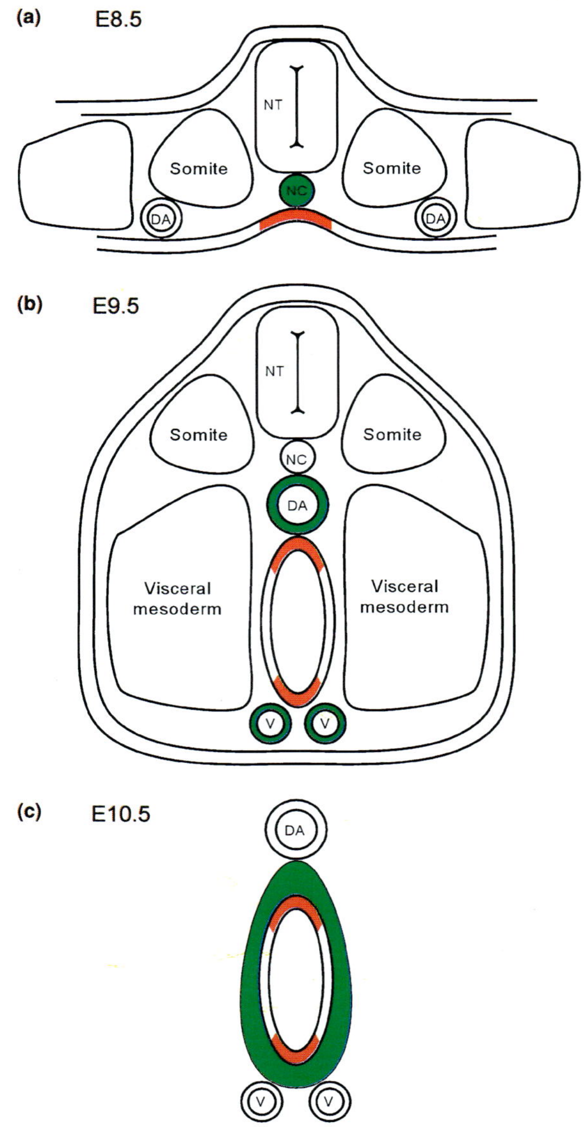

Figure 2 Signaling from mesoderm to endoderm. (a) At embryonic day 8.5 (E8.5) the future dorsal pancreas is in contact with the notochord. Activin B and FGF-2 secreted by the notochord act on the endoderm that responds by repressing Shh expression and initiation of *pdx1* expression (shown in red). At this stage lateral endoderm is in contact with splanchnic mesoderm and the paired dorsal aortas and these tissues may act as signaling centers that instruct lateral endoderm to acquire a ventral pancreas fate. (b) At E9.5, fusion of the paired dorsal aortas displace the notochord from contact with the endoderm. Endothelial cells from the dorsal aorta and the vitelline veins secrete an unknown signal that initiates endocrine differentiation in the pancreas endoderm. (c) At E10.5, visceral mesoderm migrates between the pancreas endoderm and the dorsal aorta and separates contact between these tissues. FGF-10 produced by the mesoderm is critical for normal proliferation of the pancreas endoderm. Other secreted factors from the mesoderm also acts to control pancreas development. Despite the displacement of the larger vessels endothelial cells from smaller vessels are still in contact with the pancreas endoderm. NT = neural tube; DA = dorsal aorta; V = vitelline veins

signals (Figure 2b) required for early pancreas gene expression [9].

Proper development of the posterior foregut also depends on signaling by activins, members of the TGF-β (transforming growth factor β) superfamily of signaling molecules. Phenotypes similar to those observed with ectopic hedgehog expression are observed in mice carrying mutations in type II activin receptors, ActRIIA and ActRIIB [10]. Activins have been shown to inhibit Shh expression in developing gut endoderm [7], suggesting that activin signaling can block Shh expression within the forming pancreas. Evidence that TGF-β signaling is important for organ formation comes from studies of ActRIIB$^{-/-}$ and ActRIIA$^{+/-}$; ActRIIB$^{-/-}$ double mutant mice had revealed anteriorization of the stomach, reduction in pancreas and islet mass, and significantly decreased expression of endocrine marker proteins [11]. An expansion of the Shh expression domain from its normal boundary within the anterior region of the stomach toward the posterior part was detected in ActRIIA$^{+/-}$, with ActRIIB$^{-/-}$ embryos further support the hypothesis that the observed defects are caused by ectopic hedgehog signaling. A summary of the various mesoderm to endoderm signaling events are shown in Figure 2.

MORPHOGENESIS OF THE PANCREAS: "THE MASTER SWITCH, Pdx1"

The outcome of these signaling events is that part of the endoderm is set aside to a pancreas fate. This fate can be monitored by the expression of a distinct set of transcription factors. Among these the best known factor is Pdx1. *pdx1* expression is initiated at the 8–10-somite stage, i.e., before hormone gene expression, in the ventral part of the foregut at the position where ventral pancreas will later form, followed slightly later by dorsal expression [1, 12]. The pattern of *pdx1* expression and the ability of Pdx-1 to stimulate transcription of many β-cell-specific genes suggest that *pdx1* functions both in the regionalization of the primitive gut endoderm and in the function of the mature β-cell. Homozygous mutations in the *pdx1* gene, in mice and humans, result in pancreas agenesis [13–15]. *pdx1* does not seem to be required for the initial bud formation, but rather it appears to permit the early pancreas epithelium to proliferate and subsequently differentiate. However, introduction of PDX-1 in the prospective intestinal endoderm of chicken embryos is sufficient to induce formation of bud-like structures [16], suggesting that PDX-1 may be sufficient (but with redundancy) for some aspects of bud formation. Thus, the initial stages of pancreas development involving the early events leading to the formation of the pancreas buds and the appearance of the early insulin and glucagon cells, still occur in the *pdx1*-deficient embryos [12]. These results suggest that additional transcriptional factors exist that act upstream of *pdx1* in the initial specification of the pancreas endoderm. However, the subsequent morphogenesis of the pancreas epithelium and the progression of differentiation of the endocrine cells are arrested in the *pdx1*$^{-/-}$ embryos. In contrast, the pancreas mesenchyme grows and develops both morphologically and functionally independent of the epithelium. The pancreas epithelium in the *pdx1* mutants is, however, unable to respond to the mesenchymal-derived signal(s) that normally promotes pancreas morphogenesis [12]. Together, these data provide evidence that *pdx1* acts cell-autonomously and that the lack of a pancreas in the *pdx1*$^{-/-}$ mice is due to a defect in the pancreas epithelium. Later in development strong *pdx1* expression becomes restricted to mature β-cells, where it is required also for normal GLUT-2 and Nkx-6-1 expression [17]. Numerous other transcription factors are also required for normal pancreas endocrine development (Table 1). A detailed description of the function of these can be found in reference 18.

FORMATION OF THE EXOCRINE PANCREAS: "THE ROLE OF p48"

The above transcription factors are or become endocrine-specific, and mutations in these genes generally affect various aspects of pancreas endocrine differentiation. In contrast, p48, which is a basic helix–loop–helix (bHLH) transcription factor, becomes restricted to acinar cells in the adult pancreas [19]. However, during development p48 expression can be detected as early as E10 in both pancreas buds [20], and lineage tracing has revealed that all pancreas cells derive from p48-expressing progenitors [20]. The pancreas agenesis observed in *p48*$^{-/-}$ mice points toward a crucial role for p48 in pancreas development. Acinar development is completely impaired in these mice, whereas some duct and endocrine cell differentiation still occurs. However, most of the prospective pancreas cells switch fate and become incorporated into the duodenal epithelium in the absence of p48 [20]. p48 is thus the first exocrine-specific transcription factor that has been isolated and whose function has been genetically tested. Further analysis of p48 function will be of vital importance for our understanding of pancreas ontogeny.

EXPANSION OF THE PANCREAS EPITHELIUM: "THE PLEIOTROPIC FIBROBLAST GROWTH FACTOR FAMILY"

The proliferation of early pancreas epithelium, marked by the expression of these transcription factors, is dependent on fibroblast growth factor (FGF) signaling [21]. The FGF family consists of at least 22 structurally related polypeptides that play key roles in morphogenesis, development,

Table 1 Transcription factors involved in pancreas development

Factor	Family	Expression*	Mouse mutations†	Human mutations
Neurogenin3	bHLH	All endocrine progenitors	Diabetes, no islet cells	
NeuroD1/BETA2	bHLH	Islet cells	Diabetes, decreased islet cells	Het. late-onset diabetes
P48/PTF	bHLH	Pancreatic progenitors Acinar cells	Pancreatic agenesis, few islet cells in spleen	
Mist-1	bHLH	Acinar cells	Exocrine pancreas disorganized	
Pdx-1/IPF-1	Homeobox	Pancreatic progenitors Acinar cells	Pancreatic agenesis	Het. MODY4 Hom. pancreatic agenesis
HB-9	Homeobox	Pancreatic progenitors β-Cells	Dorsal pancreas agenesis, β-cells abnormal	
Pax-4	Paired-homeobox	Some endocrine precursors β-Cells	Diabetes, no β- and δ-cells, more α-cells	
Pax-6	Paired-homeobox	Islet cells	Reduced islet cells	Aniridia, glucose intolerance
Nkx-2.2	NK-homeobox	Pancreatic progenitors α-, β-, and PP-Cells	Diabetes, no insulin-producing cells	
Nkx-6.1	NK-homeobox	Pancreatic progenitors β-Cells	Very few β-cells	
Nkx-6.2	NK-homeobox	Pancreatic progenitors		
Cdx-2	Caudal-homeobox	Islet cells	Het. intestinal tumors	
Isl-1	LIM-homeobox	Islet cells	No islet cells	
Brn-4	POU-homeobox	α-Cells		
HNF-1α	POU-homeobox	Islet cells	Diabetes, impaired glucose sensing	Het. MODY3
HNF-1β	POU-homeobox	Islet and duct cells	Embryonic lethal	Het. MODY5
HNF-6	Cut-homeobox	Pancreatic progenitors Duct cells	Small islets, improved glucose tolerance	
Foxa-1/HNF-3α	Forkhead/winged helix	Islet cells	Hypoglycemia	
Foxa-2/HNF-3β	Forkhead/winged helix	All pancreas cells	Embryonic lethal	
Foxa-3/HNF-3γ	Forkhead/winged helix	Islet cells	No pancreas phenotype	
HNF-4α	Nuclear receptor		Embryonic lethal	Het. MODY1
MafA	bZIP	β-Cells		
c-Maf	bZIP	α-Cells		
Arx	Homeobox	Some endocrine precursors α-Cells		
Irx-1/2	Homeobox	Some endocrine precursors α-Cells		

*Only pancreas expression is included.
†All mouse phenotypes are for homozygous mutants unless stated otherwise. Only pancreas defects are included.

angiogenesis, and wound healing [22]. FGF-stimulated processes are mediated by four FGF RTKs (FGFR-1–4). A large number of the FGFs are expressed in the developing pancreas. Others and we have detected FGF-1, -2, -7, and -10 [23], but additionally we have found FGF-4, -9, and -18 to be expressed [24]. Expression of all four known FGF receptors is also detected in the developing pancreas, indicating a complex role for FGF signaling in pancreas organogenesis [24]. However, the precise splice forms present in the pancreas are not known, with the exception of FGFR-2(IIIb) through which FGF-7 and FGF-10 act. Several types of experiments that implicate FGF1, -7, and -10 in pancreas epithelial cell proliferation have been done *in vitro*. First, when the embryonic epithelium depleted of its mesenchyme is grown in culture in the presence of FGF-1, -7, or -10, epithelial cell proliferation is activated [25, 26]. Second, when the epithelium surrounded by its mesenchyme is grown in culture in the presence of inhibitory FGFR-2b-Fc recombinant protein, a small reduction in proliferation is observed [25, 26]. These results confirmed earlier ones in various animal models in which FGF-7 caused proliferation of pancreas ductal epithelium in adult rats after 1–2 weeks of treatment [27] and transgenic mice overexpressing FGF-7 in either liver [28] or pancreas β-cells [29] showed ductal hyperplasia. Additionally, transgenic mice expressing a soluble dominant-negative FGFR-2(IIIb) under control of the metallothionein promoter display greatly reduced acinar differentiation [30]. Finally, mice lacking FGF-10 show severely reduced proliferation of early PDX-1^+ pancreas epithelial cells [21]. Our knowledge of the role of FGF signaling in pancreas development is still rudimentary, but in general, proper growth of the embryonic epithelium and acinar differentiation are dependent on FGF signaling (Figure 2c).

DEVELOPMENT OF ENDOCRINE CELLS: "THE NOTCH RECIPROCITY"

Close to appearance of pancreas evaginations, endocrine precursor cells can be distinguished by expression of the transcription factor gene *neurogenin3 (ngn3)* [31, 32]. Pancreatic cells that express *ngn3* seem to be irreversibly committed to adopt an endocrine fate [4]. *ngn3* encodes a member of the bHLH family of transcription factors (NGN-3), and acts upstream of *neuroD* in a bHLH cascade [31, 32]. Detailed analysis of *ngn3*/PAX-6 and *neuroD*/PAX-6 co-expression shows that the two bHLH factors are expressed in a largely nonoverlapping set of cells, but such analysis also suggests that the *neuroD*$^+$ cells arise from cells transiently expressing *ngn3*. Analyses of *ngn3* mutant mice support this idea, as no endocrine cells are formed in these animals [31]. However, direct evidence for the notion that NGN-3^+ cells are endocrine precursors comes from elegant genetic lineage tracing studies by Melton and coworkers. Using an *ngn3* promoter to drive expression of Cre recombinase, they demonstrated that NGN-3^+ progenitor cells give rise to all four types of endocrine cells [4]. When NGN-3^+ cells were labeled and their descendents followed at different developmental stages, it was found that they were always differentiated endocrine cells and never maintained *ngn3* expression. This result suggests that NGN-3^+ cells do not self-renew even though a small number do apparently divide [4, 32]. Therefore, NGN-3^+ cells are likely to be transient progenitors. Since NGN-3^+ cells are detected throughout pancreas development they must therefore be generated from NGN-3^- cells, which presumably are mitotically active. Their identification is of supreme importance for the attempts to generate β-cells *in vitro*.

Formation and/or differentiation of NGN-3^+ endocrine progenitor cells appear to be regulated by Notch signaling. There are four vertebrate *NOTCH* genes (*NOTCH-1, -2, -3*, and *-4*) andthese are highly related to each other and to the *Drosophila notch* and *Candida elegans lin-12* and *glp-1* genes [33]. There also are multiple Notch ligands in vertebrates and these are homologous to the *Drosophila* ligands Delta and Serrate and the *C. elegans* ligand Lag-2 [34]. In mammals, Delta homologues are called "Delta-like" (Dll) and the Serrate homologues "Jagged." Notch receptors and ligands contain multiple epidermal growth factor (EGF)-like repeats in their extracellular domains. There are three Dll genes (*Dll-1, -3*, and *-4*) and two Jagged genes (*Jagged-1* and *-2*) in the mouse. Upon ligand stimulation Notch receptors are cleaved in the transmembrane region and the intracellular part translocates to the nucleus where it interacts with RBP-jκ, which provides a DNA-binding domain and activates a set of target genes (Figure 3). Among these are bHLH transcriptional

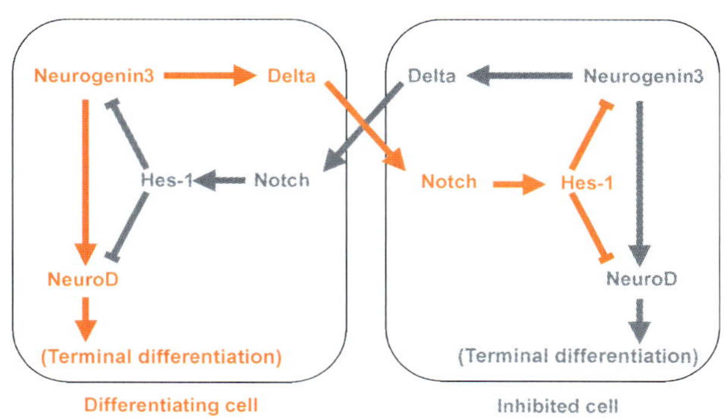

Figure 3 Lateral inhibition mediated by the Notch signaling pathway controls endocrine differentiation. Two adjacent cells of developing pancreas tissue are shown interacting. One cell, the winner in the lateral-inhibition competition, differentiates as an endocrine cell, whereas the other as a result is inhibited. Activated components of the regulatory system are shown in red, whereas inactive components are grey

repressors of the hairy and enhancer of split homologue (HES) family [35, 36].

Notch signaling was recently shown to be important for proper pancreas development. Mice lacking the Notch pathway genes *Dll-1, RBP-j*κ, or *hes-1* showed accelerated differentiation of endocrine cells in the pancreas [37, 38]. This signaling pathway most likely inhibits *ngn3* function (Figure 3). However, the presence of Notch-1 and Notch-2 as well as another ligand Jagged-1 in the epithelium and several Notch modifying glycosyltransferases suggests a complex role in pancreas development [32, 38, 39]. Furthermore, Notch-3 is expressed in the mesenchyme. Forced expression of a constitutive active form of Notch-1 in embryonic mouse pancreas epithelium thus leads to a block in acinar development and completely inhibits branching morphogenesis (J. Hald, personal communication). Not surprisingly, *ngn3* expression is reduced but some endocrine development, albeit at reduced level, still occurs in these animals. The remaining epithelium appears to be retained in an immature embryonic-like state. Targeted mutation of Notch genes leads to embryonic death at the time when pancreas development begins, but none have been analyzed for defects in pancreas development. Together, these findings suggest that Notch agonists and antagonists could be used to control the proliferation and differentiation of endocrine precursor cells *in vitro*.

OTHER SIGNALING PATHWAYS IN ENDOCRINE DEVELOPMENT: "A NETWORK OF GROWTH FACTORS"

Proper development of the pancreas also requires signaling through the EGF receptor (ErbB) family. ErbB proteins belong to the RTK superfamily. There are four members of ErbB, and all four are expressed in embryonic pancreas epithelium [40, 41]. However, there are conflicting reports as to the cellular distribution of ErbB-3 in either mesenchyme [42] or epithelium [41]. A family of ligands, the EGF-related peptide growth factors, binds the extracellular domain of ErbB receptors, leading to the formation of both homo- and heterodimers. Consequently, numerous ErbB homo- and heterodimer combinations are possible, which can provide a high degree of signaling diversity. There are four categories of ligands that bind ErbB family receptors. EGF, amphiregulin and TGF-α bind ErbB-1; betacellulin, heparin binding EGF (HB-EGF), and epiregulin bind ErbB-1 and ErbB-4; neuregulin (NRG) 1 and NRG-2 bind ErbB-3 and ErbB-4; and NRG-3 and NRG-4 bind Erb-B-4. Betacellulin [43, 44], TGF-α [45], HB-EGF [46], NRG-4 [47], and the NRG-1 isoforms HRG-α and HRG-β3 [41] have been reported to be expressed in the developing pancreas. Genetic evidence for the importance of ErbB signaling in pancreas development comes from mice lacking the ErbB-1 and ErbB-3 receptors. ErbB-1 (EGF receptor) mutant mice display a generalized proliferation defect with reduced branching of the pancreas epithelia associated with a delay in β-cell development [40]. However, on other genetic backgrounds pancreas development appears normal [41]. ErbB-3 mutant embryos have retarded pancreas development with variable penetrance; islet development occurs but at very reduced levels [42]. The precise role of the individual ligands and receptors is thus still unclear, but proper growth of the embryonic epithelium and endocrine differentiation seem to require some form of ErbB signaling.

Another RTK family important for normal endocrine development is the insulin-IGF (insulin growth factor) receptor family. Islets are reduced in size in *igf1r*$^{+/-}$ mice, and develop poorly in *igf1r*$^{-/-}$ mice as reduced numbers of α- and β-cells fail to form typical islet structures. *igf1r*$^{-/-}$ mice die at birth, whereas *igf1r*$^{+/-}$ mice survive with reduced β-cell mass, but never develop diabetes; however, combined with an insulin receptor substrate 2 (IRS-2) disruption, *igf1r*$^{+/-}$/*irs2*$^{-/-}$ mice die at 30 days of age with severe hyperglycemia, owing to small islets containing a reduced number of α-cells and nearly no β-cells. IRS-2 plays a special role in carbohydrate metabolism as it regulates both peripheral insulin action and pancreas β-cell function. This relation is revealed in *irs1*$^{-/-}$/*irs2*$^{+/-}$ mice. Although very small at birth, these lean mice are insulin resistant and become glucose intolerant with age, but β-cell compensation is robust and diabetes never develops. By contrast, the larger *irs1*$^{+/-}$/*irs2*$^{-/-}$ littermates fail to compensate for peripheral insulin resistance and die by 30 days of age with few β-cells and extreme hyperglycemia. Apparently the presence of a single allele of *irs2* promotes sufficient β-cell expansion and survival to compensate for severe peripheral insulin resistance, whereas IRS-1 fails to do so [48]. These results suggest that the IGF-1R–IRS-2 signaling pathway is critical for both the embryonic development and postnatal growth of β-cells, and reveals an important interface between the insulin and IGF signaling pathways as will be discussed later.

Additional growth factors and their receptors are expressed during pancreas development but little is known about their function. Hepatocyte growth factor (HGF) is expressed in the mesenchyme and its RTK-receptor c-Met in the epithelium [49]. HGF could thus be an important component of the mesenchymal signals that govern epithelial growth and differentiation. HGF stimulates growth of adult human duct cells in culture, but not of β-cells [50]. Several members of the nerve growth factor (NGF)/neurotrophin family and its cognate receptors (TrkA–C) are expressed in the developing pancreas, but their role is unknown, although they may serve as survival factors analogous to their function in the nervous system. NGF is expressed in the mesenchyme and TrkA in the embryonic epithelium and in mature β-cells [51].

Additionally, the NT-3 (neurotrophin 3) receptor TrkC is expressed in INS-1 (rat insulinoma cell line 1) cells [52]. The Wnt morphogen family and its receptors, the Frizzled proteins, have several members expressed during pancreas development [53]. However, little is known about the cellular distribution and the function of these factors. Finally, several Eph (ephrin receptor) RTKs and their ligands, the ephrins, are expressed, but again the cellular expression pattern and function of these molecules are not known [54].

SPECIFICATION OF ENDOCRINE SUBTYPES: "HOW TO BECOME A β-CELL"

How the four different endocrine cell types are specified is still to a large degree unknown. It seems that β- and δ-cells both depend on the function of the *pax4* gene. *pax4* expression is evident as early as E9.5 in both pancreas buds, but later in development *pax4* expression becomes restricted to the emerging β-cells. It is still not entirely clear whether *pax4* is co-expressed with *ngn3* or whether *pax4* is found only in differentiated β-cells, albeit transiently. However, ectopic expression of NGN-3 in adult human duct cells induces expression of the *pax4* gene [55], consistent with the idea that *pax4* is expressed in NGN-3$^+$ progenitor cells. Mice lacking a functional *pax4* gene lack differentiated insulin and somatostatin cells; in addition, there is an associated increase in the number of glucagon-producing cells [56]. This could possibly suggest that *pax4* is responsible for an insulin$^+$ cell fate choice and that in the absence of *pax4*, the default fate would be to become a glucagon$^+$ cell. The increase in glucagon$^+$ cells is, however, similar to the islet phenotype of the β-cell-specific *pdx1* mutants, and it is thus possible that *pax4* is directly or indirectly involved in repressing glucagon expression [57, 58].

The POU-homeodomain protein POU-3F4 (also know as Brn-4) is the earliest marker of the developing α-cells [32]. However, analysis of *pou3f4* mutant mice shows that this gene is not required for α-cell formation (R. S. Heller, personal communication). However, whether the *pou3f4*-deficient α-cells express their normal repertoire of genes is not known. Additional transcription factors with expression restricted to particular endocrine cell types are currently being investigated and will undoubtedly bring novel insights into this topic.

ADHESION MOLECULES: "HOW TO ORGANIZE THE ISLET"

Classical cell dissociation/reaggregation experiments with embryonic tissue and cultured cells have demonstrated that cellular cohesiveness, mediated by cell adhesion molecules (CAMs), is important for the organization of cells within tissues and organs; this includes the pancreas islets [59, 60]. Islet cells express a number of CAMs, including the immunoglobulin superfamily members N-CAM and I-CAM, the cadherin superfamily members E-, N-, and R-cadherin, as well as Ep-CAM [61–64]. A study of N-CAM-deficient mice showed that N-CAM plays a functional role in the proper segregation of cells during the development of islets. In N-CAM-deficient mice the normal localization of α-cells in the periphery of pancreas islets is lost, resulting in a more randomized cell distribution. However, increased clustering of cadherins, F-actin, and cell–cell junctions suggests enhanced cadherin-mediated adhesion in the absence of N-CAM. Furthermore, islet cell polarity is affected and the β-cells appear degranulated, suggesting that N-CAM is required for normal turnover of β-cell secretory granules. Cadherin function is also required for normal β-cell adhesiveness. Overexpression of a dominant-negative version of mouse E-cadherin lacking nearly all extracellular amino acids in transgenic mice displaces both E- and N-cadherin from pancreas β-cells. As a result, the aggregation of β-cells, which normally begins at E13.5–14.5, is perturbed. As a result, the clustering of endocrine cells into islets, which normally begins at E17.5–18, is abrogated. Instead, transgenic β-cells were found dispersed in the tissue as individual cells, while α-cells selectively aggregated into islet-like clusters devoid of β-cells [65]. Cell–matrix interactions play a critical role also in tissue morphogenesis and homeostasis of adult tissues. The integrin family of adhesion receptors regulates cellular interactions with the extracellular matrix. Cirulli and coworkers have demonstrated that pancreas expression and function of alpha(v)beta(3) and alpha(v)beta(5) integrins are developmentally regulated, and mediate adhesion and migration of putative endocrine progenitor cells both *in vitro* and *in vivo* in a model of pancreas islet development [66].

β-CELL GROWTH IN LATE FETAL AND NEONATAL LIFE: "THE THRIFTY PHENOTYPE"

Following the embryonic determination, differentiation, and morphogenesis of the islet organ described in the preceding section, there is a marked increase in the number of β-cells at the time around birth in the rat [67], which is partly due to proliferation of differentiated β-cells and partly to neogenesis from progenitor cells [67, 68]. The growth of the fetal β-cells depends on nutritional and hormonal factors. Thus restriction of nutrients, in particular amino acids, during pregnancy results in reduced β-cell mass in the offspring [69, 70] that may be due to reduced neogenesis and proliferation, or excessive apoptosis. This is in agreement with *in vitro* studies where it has been shown that glucose and amino acids stimulate the mitotic activity in fetal but not in adult islets [67]. In the rat a remarkable remodeling of the endocrine pancreas takes place at 2–3 weeks of age, characterized by an increase in apoptotic activity [71]. This is reflected in a plateau in the age-dependent growth curve for the β-cells, as shown for rats [67] and mice [72]. In agreement with the earlier appearance of insulin-producing cells in the human fetus [69, 73], this remodeling probably occurs already in the third trimester [69]. As it has been shown that IGF-1 and -2 can stimulate proliferation of fetal islets and prevent apoptosis in adult islets, it is conceivable that in particular IGF-2, which is expressed in fetal and neonatal islets up to 2 weeks of age coinciding with the apoptotic burst, contributes to the β-cell growth in the fetal and neonatal period [69]. However β-cell-specific knockout of either the insulin receptor or the IGF-1 receptor did not change β-cell mass but resulted in hyperinsulinemia and glucose intolerance [74]. A role of fetal insulin as growth factor for the β-cell also seems to be ruled out by the knockout of both insulin genes in mice that resulted in increased proliferation of fetal β-cells [75]. The significance of this remodeling is not known, but an intriguing hypothesis proposes that the apoptotic event under certain circumstances may trigger the autoimmune reaction to β-cell antigens, leading to type 1 diabetes [76–78]. Interestingly, the finding of a negative correlation between birth weight and type 2 diabetes has resulted in the *thrifty phenotype hypothesis* [79] where intrauterine malnutrition will lead to impaired β-cell development, thus making the offspring unable to compensate for the increased insulin demand if exposed to hypercaloric diet and sedentary life style. The reduction of the β-cell mass in neonatal rats by streptozotocin treatment results in recovery from acute diabetes but increased susceptibility to develop glucose intolerance as an adult [80]. The Goto-Kakisaki rat, which serves as genetic model for type 2 diabetes, has a reduced β-cell mass at birth, which was found to be due to impaired development of the pancreas [81]. Although this hypothesis has ample support from animal experiments, it is difficult to prove it in humans and thus remains controversial. In conclusion, neither insulin nor IGFs seem to be indispensable for the fetal and neonatal growth of the β-cell, suggesting that other factors are involved and may compensate for their lack during this period.

POSTNATAL β-CELL GROWTH: "ADAPTATION TO DEMAND"

Although islets are formed late in fetal life, a considerable growth in the islet cell mass occurs postpartum. This was studied in detail in rodents 30 years ago [82] when it was observed that after a temporary reduction in the growth rate in the young rat, corresponding to the apoptotic episode mentioned above, the islets like most other organs follow the body weight in a linear pattern in a double-logarithmic plot. It was also found that the postnatal growth of the endocrine pancreas was associated with an increase in average islet size in humans also [82], suggesting that proliferation of existing β-cells is responsible for the major part of the growth. The β-cell mass continues to grow with age, although analysis in greater detail indicates that in the aged animal hypertrophy of the β-cell may contribute to the observed growth [83]. Mitotic activity, measured either *in vivo* or *in vitro*, decreases markedly with age [67]. Although clinical onset of type 1 diabetes seems to occur only after destruction of more than 80% of the β-cells, the apparent surplus of β-cells may be important in protecting the organism under extreme conditions of metabolic stress. Thus, it has been reported that individuals who were hemipancreatectomized so as to transplant part of their pancreas to their identical twin subsequently developed glucose intolerance [84]. That the proper β-cell mass is strictly regulated is supported by transplantation of islets to streptozotocin diabetic rats concurrently treated with insulin, resulting in downsizing of the transplant by apoptosis [85]. Also in the case of β-cell hyperplasia in pregnancy it has been observed that the "surplus" β-cells are deleted by apoptosis after delivery [86]. As shown in animals transplanted with insulinomas, the apoptotic atrophy of the endogenous β-cells [87] can be prevented by simultaneous glucose infusion (K. Lindberg and J.H.N., unpublished data), suggesting that hypoglycemia rather than insulin is responsible for "downsizing". The stimulus for compensatory growth of the β-cell mass is the insulin "demand," an ill-defined term that integrates genetic background, body mass, adiposity, physical activity, and the insulin sensitivity of various tissues. An extensive number of substances have been shown to influence β-cell growth, as listed in [67, 88] Table 2.

β-CELL GROWTH IN OBESITY AND TYPE 2 DIABETES: "COMPENSATION AND DECOMPENSATION"

Glucose is not only the most important regulator of insulin secretion in mammals, but also an essential regulator of β-cell growth. It is most probably the main indicator of insulin "demand." Thus, glucose infusion for only 48 h results in both hypertrophy and hyperplasia of β-cells [71]. This effect was even more pronounced in mildly diabetic rats where the β-cells were more than doubled after 24 h of glucose infusion [89]. The increase was not only due to replication of the existing β-cells but also due to neogenesis from ductal cells [89]. *In vitro*, glucose has been shown to recruit β-cells to undergo mitosis, without changing cell cycle velocity [67]. Several animal models of obesity and diabetes exhibit hyperplasia of the β-cells. Most pronounced are *ob/ob* mice with combined hyperglycemia

Table 2 List of factors that inhibit or stimulate β-cell growth and/or function

	Inhibitors	Stimulators
Metabolites	Glucose,	Glucose, FFA, amino acids
Cytokines	Interleukin-1, leptin	GH, PRL, PL
IGF family	IGF -1	IGF-1, IGF-2, insulin
EGF family		TGF-α, betacellulin, HB-EGF
FGF family		FGF
VEGF/PDGF family		VEGF, PDGF
HGF	HGF	HGF
Glucagon family		GLP-1, GIP, glucagon
Somatostatin	Somatostatin	
CGRP family	IAPP/amylin	
Gastrin family		Gastrin, CCK
TGF-β family	TGF-β	ActivinA
Neurotrophins		NGF, NT-3
Neurotransmitters	(Nor)epinephrine	Acetycholine
Delta-like		Pref-1/FA-1
Lectins		Reg/INGA
Drugs	Diazoxide	Nicotinamide, sulfonylurea
Toxins	Streptazotocin, alloxan	

and hyperinsulinemia [67]. Also diet-induced obesity is associated with β-cell hyperplasia [67]. In humans, obese nondiabetic subjects have previously been reported to have an increased islet mass, but this could not be confirmed in a more recent study [73]. Neither could the previous data on reduced β-cell mass in type 2 diabetic patients be reproduced, except for the insulin-treated group [73, 90]. This discrepancy could be due to the recruitment of more severe cases of type 2 diabetes, or inclusion of late-onset type 1 diabetes in earlier studies. Most recently, however, data from a larger material showed increased β-cell volume in obese nondiabetic individuals compared to lean subjects, and furthermore both lean and obese type 2 diabetic subjects showed reduced β-cell volume when compared with weight-matched control subjects, as shown in Figure 4 [91]. Similar results were found in nonobese patients with type 2 diabetes in Korea [92]. Several animal models of diabetes show a transient compensatory hyperplasia of β-

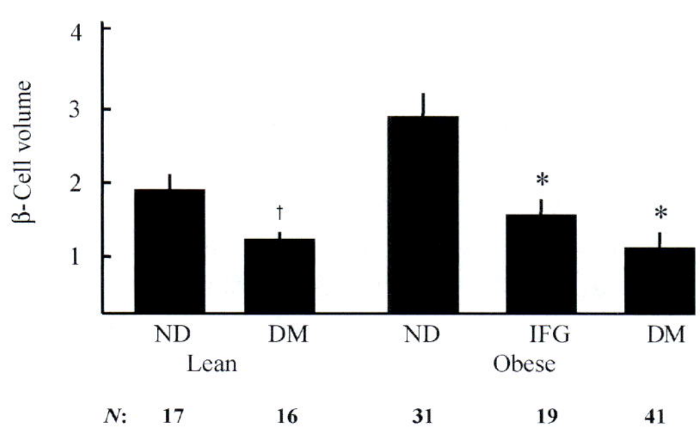

Figure 4 β-cell volume in percent in lean and obese nondiabetic (ND) patients, patients with type 2 diabetes (DM), and patients with increased fasting blood glucose (IFG).*$p < 0.01$; †$p < 0.05$. (Copyright © 2003 American Diabetes Association. From Diabetes, Vol 52, 2003; 102–110. Reprinted with permission from The American Diabetes Association. [91])

cells followed by reduction, as in the *db/db* mouse [67], the diabetes-prone sand rat *Psammomys obesus* [93], and the Zucker diabetic *fa/fa* rat [94]. The phenotype of the *db/db* and *ob/ob* mice depends on the genetic background and, interestingly, the capacity of the β-cells to replicate was found to be significantly higher in the C57Bl/6J strain than in the C57Bl/KsJ, emphasizing the genetic control of the proliferative capacity [67]. The hyperplasia of the β-cells is supposed to be secondary to insulin resistance and hyperglycemia, but it has also been suggested that hyperinsulinemia *per se* is the driving force in the "vicious cycle." Thus, transgenic mice expressing IGF-2 in the β-cells have marked hyperplasia of the β-cells but develop hyperglycemia [95]. This finding indicates that β-cell hyperplasia may be a double-edged sword: on one hand it may compensate for increased demand, but on the other hand it may aggravate the insulin resistance. The recent use of targeted gene disruption techniques may elucidate the molecular mechanisms involved. While mice with homozygous double knockout of the insulin receptor and the IRS-1 died from diabetic ketoacidosis, the heterozygous mice developed normally but showed marked hyperinsulinemia and β-cell hyperplasia; at age 4–6 months some of these animals became diabetic [96]. Also combined heterozygous double knockout for IRS-1 and glucokinase resulted in β-cell hyperplasia and type 2 diabetes [96]. The finding that transplantation of islets to normoglycemic IRS-1/IR heterozygous double knockout mice or to hyperglycemic *ob/ob* mice resulted in hyperplasia of the transplanted β-cells suggests that a circulating growth factor is present in insulin-resistant states [97]. These results support the view that moderate insulin resistance can be compensated for by concomitant β-cell growth, at least for a period of time, but may eventually lead to β-cell failure and overt diabetes. Whether the failure is due to the persistent hyperglycemia, known as *glucose toxicity*, or lack of proliferative capacity or both, is not clear. Lack of first-phase insulin release in type 2 diabetes was described more than 30 years ago [98]. A similar loss of glucose responsiveness is found in rats after removal of 90% of the pancreas, supporting the "overworking β-cell" hypothesis [99]. Persistent hyperglycemia may result in loss of β-cell-specific transcription factors like Pdx-1, but an increase in c-myc expression may also be implicated, since it was shown that in transgenic mice overexpressing c-myc in the β-cells either proliferation or apoptosis of β-cells was observed depending on the concomitant expression of antiapoptotic genes [100–102]. When an insufficient number of islets are transplanted to streptozotocin-treated diabetic rats a marked loss of β-cells by apoptosis and necrosis occurs because of the persistent hyperglycemia [85]. Increased apoptosis has been observed in isolated rat islets and purified β-cells at either high or low glucose [103, 104], and in human islets exposed to high glucose in culture [105, 106]. The glucose-induced apoptosis seems to involve increased Fas expression and could be prevented by upregulation of the caspase-8 inhibitory protein FLIP that resulted in a switch from apoptosis to replication [107]. It is known from islet transplantation experiments in diabetic mice that the genetic background plays an important role in the fate of the transplanted β-cells [108]. The nature of the difference in susceptibility to hyperglycemia is not known but could be related to variations in expression of pro- and antiapoptotic genes that may be reflected in differences in the proliferative capacity, as mentioned above.

The other major metabolite that affects the function and viability of the β-cell is fatty acids. Studies in the Zucker diabetic rat, which like the *db/db* mouse carries a mutation in the leptin receptor, have shown that accumulation of fat hampers the function and viability of the β-cells; this motivated the lipotoxicity hypothesis [94]. Interestingly, it has also been reported that low concentrations of free fatty acid (FFA) can stimulate proliferation of rat β-cells *in vitro* [94], in agreement with the stimulatory effects of low concentrations of FFA in glucose-induced insulin secretion. The initial hyperplasia is however followed by lipid accumulation in the β-cells, which may then deteriorate the function and viability and lead to β-cell apoptosis, probably involving ceramide and NO formation [94]. Studies *in vitro* have confirmed the toxic effects of palmitate in cultured human islets [109]. The apoptotic effect has been shown to involve ceramide formation and reduced Bcl-2 expression [110]. Interestingly peroxisome proliferator-activated receptor agonists like thiazolidinediones protect against the toxic effects of lipids [94, 110].

A new aspect of β-cell function in obesity comes from the discovery of leptin and its receptor, the Ob or leptin receptor. Interestingly, the functional receptor is expressed in the β-cells and leptin has been shown to inhibit insulin release and gene expression, although contradictory results have been published [111]. Leptin treatment of *ob/ob* mice reversed the diabetic phenotype, and in the Zucker rat reconstitution of the leptin receptor prevented diabetes [94]. Leptin has been reported to stimulate fetal islet cell proliferation [112], which may offer an explanation for the adaptive β-cell proliferation in obesity under normoglycemic conditions. In another study leptin was found to suppress apoptosis but not to stimulate proliferation in serum-deprived rat islets [113]. In contrast to the β-cell compensation mechanism discussed above, the β-cell hyperplasia in the *ob/ob*, *db/db*, and *fa/fa* animals may support yet another hypothesis: the absence of a negative feed back loop between β-cells and adipocytes results in excessive β-cell growth due to insulin-induced insulin resistance and the ensuing hyperglycemia [111]. The leptin receptor belongs to the cytokine receptor superfamily including the receptors for growth hormone and prolactin that will be dealt with below. While the latter activates both STAT-3 and STAT-5 in the β-cells, leptin only activates STAT-3, which may explain their common inhibitory effect on lipid accumulation but divergent effects on insulin expression. The role of lipids, leptin, and other adipocyte factors like resistin, adiponectin, and TNF-α in compensation and decompensation of the β-cell in obesity and type 2 diabetes needs further investigations.

In summary, both glucose and fatty acids may exert a dual effect on the β-cells, i.e. stimulation of function and growth at moderate concentrations, and adverse suppressive or toxic effects on function and viability at excessive concentrations or prolonged exposure. Both genetic and environmental factors determine the transition from trophic to atrophic fate.

THE ROLE OF GROWTH HORMONE AND PREGNANCY HORMONES IN β-CELL GROWTH: "CONCERTED ACTIONS"

Although the proliferative capacity of the mature, terminally differentiated β-cells is considered to be limited in the adult, there are conditions like pregnancy where β-cells can undergo mitosis. In the rat a marked increase in the islet cell proliferation has been observed during pregnancy as shown in Figure 5 [114]. During pregnancy the placental lactogen(s) (PL), prolactin (PRL), and (placental) growth hormone (GH) appear to be the main growth factors for the β-cells [114, 115]. Expression of receptors for both GH and PRL has been demonstrated in islet cells, and both have been shown to be upregulated during pregnancy. Interestingly, PRL receptor expression is stimulated by GH and PRL, which is not the case for the GH receptor [115]. The signaling pathway for GH and PRL includes activation of the tyrosine kinase JAK-2 and members of the STAT (signal transducers and activators of

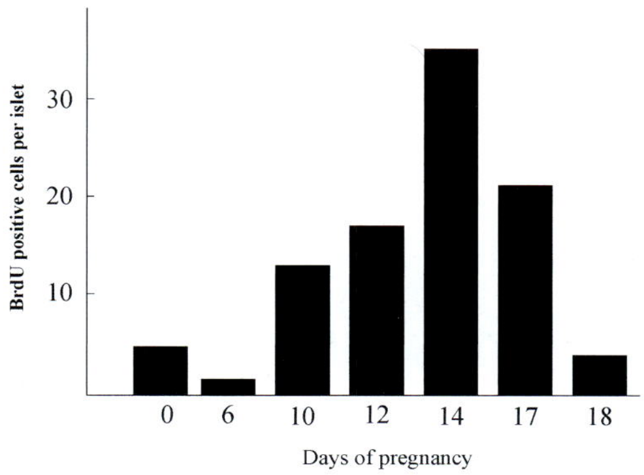

Figure 5 Islet cell proliferation in rats during pregnancy shown as number of BrdU (5-bromo-2′-deoxyuridine) positive cells per islet. (Reprinted with permission from S. Karger AG, Basel (Pancreatic Growth and Regeneration 1997: pp. 1–30) [114])

transcription) family, in particular STAT5. The increased insulin gene expression is at least in part due to a STAT5 binding element that was identified in the rat insulin-1 promoter [115]. STAT5 activation was shown to be essential for GH- and PRL-induced β-cell proliferation that also involves upregulation of cyclin D2 [116]. Studies are ongoing in transgenic mice expressing dominant-negative and constitutive active mutants of STAT5 in the β-cells, and are expected to clarify the role of STAT5 in compensatory β-cell growth in pregnancy (J.H.N., unpublished data). Recently GH and PRL were found to induce the expression of SOCS (suppressors of cytokine action) proteins that may act as negative modulators of the STAT signaling pathway in β-cells. Thus, overexpression of SOCS-3 abolished the mitogenic effect of GH in β-cells [117] and prevented the cytotoxic action of the cytokines IL-1, TNF-α, and IFN-γ [118]. β-Cell hyperplasia during pregnancy seems to depend on elevated blood glucose levels, since insulin treatment prevents the growth in spite of elevated PLs [119]; this was also reported *in vitro* [120]. Also in pregnant women islet cell hyperplasia has been reported [84], although the *in vitro* effect of PRL on human islets is modest [114]. Lack of compensatory β-cell hyperplasia in pregnancy may give rise to gestational diabetes, which occurs in 1–2% of pregnant women. It may be speculated that reduced expression of PRL receptors in β-cells may be involved. The paradoxical role of GH as both a diabetogenic hormone resulting in insulin resistance and hyperglycemia, as well as a trophic factor for the β-cell resulting in proliferation and increased insulin production, may be explained by age and species variation in the β-cell responsiveness to GH. Thus, GH is not diabetogenic in normal rats because they can compensate by increasing the β-cell mass. In contrast, GH is diabetogenic in adult dogs but not in puppies or pregnant dogs [121]. A similar situation may occur in humans where GH is diabetogenic in the adult but not in children treated with GH. In the absence of GH, as in Snell dwarf mice and Ames dwarf mice, the β-cell mass is reduced, which is in accordance with a decreased demand due to increased insulin sensitivity [122]. Conversely, transgenic mice expressing hGH under the metallothionein or phosphoenolpyruvate carboxykinase promoters have increased β-cell mass comparable to pregnant mice [122]. Also expression of mouse PL-1 under the insulin promoter results in β-cell hyperplasia [123]. As adult human islets express very low levels of GH and PRL receptor mRNA (J.H.N., unpublished data), the factors that regulate the expression of these receptors in human β-cells remain to be identified.

GH and PRL do not seem to induce IGF-1 expression in postnatal rat islets [115], but have been shown to upregulate a novel islet protein, Pref-1, which was recently cloned from the 3T3-L1 preadipocyte-like cell line [124]. Pref-1 is a transmembrane protein containing six EGF-like motifs and can be converted to a soluble form by proteolytic cleavage, which was recently isolated from human amniotic fluid as FA-1 (fetal antigen 1). It was shown to be expressed in most epithelial cells in the early embryonic pancreas but became confined to the β-cells close to term both in humans and in rats. The level of expression is low in adult β-cells but is markedly upregulated in pregnancy [124]. The function of Pref-1/FA-1 remains to be elucidated, but as it shares some homology with the Notch ligands Delta and Jagged (see above) it may be speculated to play a role in maintaining β-cells in a proliferative state without being a growth factor *per se* [125].

THE ROLE OF STEROID HORMONES IN β-CELL GROWTH: "INDIRECT ACTIONS"

Although glucocorticoid hormones have been reported to stimulate β-cell proliferation *in vivo*, their effect *in vitro* is inhibitory [121]. Therefore the increased β-cell proliferation found *in vivo* is probably secondary to the hyperglycemia that results from the peripheral insulin resistance and augmented gluconeogenesis induced by glucocorticoids. As hydrocortisone increases the expression of GH receptors in neonatal rat islets in culture, this effect may also contribute to the β-cell hyperplasia observed *in vivo*. Similarly, estradiol has been reported to stimulate β-cell proliferation *in vivo* but not *in vitro*, suggesting that the effect is secondary to, e.g., stimulation of GH or PRL release or increase in the expression of PRL receptors, as reported in neonatal rat islets in culture [115]. Progesterone and glucocorticoids inhibit β-cell proliferation *in vitro* and may contribute to the cessation of the β-cell proliferation in close-to-term pregnancy [121, 126]. As receptors for the steroid hormones have been identified in β-cells, these hormones can influence other functions, such as glucose-induced insulin release [121]. Glucocorticoid hormones have been shown to influence pancreas development without affecting the β-cells [67].

THE ROLE OF GASTROINTESTINAL HORMONES IN β-CELL GROWTH: "THE MAGIC BULLET"

Interestingly, members of the "incretin" family of intestinal hormones, glucagon-like peptide 1 (GLP-1) and glucose-dependent insulinotropic polypeptide (GIP), well-known for their augmentation of glucose-stimulated insulin secretion, recently have been found to stimulate both β-cell proliferation and β-cell differentiation, *in vivo* as well as *in vitro* [127] (see also Chapter 12). The signaling pathway for the mitogenic effect depends on adenylate cyclase activation and PKA activity [128] as well as PKC-ζ [129]. Also other agents that increase the level of cAMP like IBMX and forskolin stimulate β-cell proliferation [130]. In insulin-resistant aged rats the GLP-1 analogue exendin-4 was found to increase the number of Pdx-1-expressing cells in the pancreas, suggesting promotion of β-cell neogenesis [127]. In patients with type 2 diabetes GLP-1 and exendin-4 have been shown to normalize blood glucose levels [127]. Whether the β-cell mass is increased remains to be studied but the treatment certainly holds great promise with regard to reversal of the disease.

Other gastrointestinal hormones like secretin, cholecystokinin (CCK), and gastrin have been reported to stimulate insulin secretion *in vivo* and have been implicated in β-cell growth, but their effects are rather on neogenesis than proliferation of differentiated β-cells, as discussed below.

THE ROLE OF INSULIN AND INSULIN-LIKE GROWTH FACTORS IN β-CELL GROWTH: "AUTOCRINE REGULATION"

Although the role of IGF-2 in β-cell growth is mainly confined to early life, as mentioned above, IGF-1 and insulin may be important for the postnatal growth of the β-cells. Although no direct mitogenic effect of IGF-1 was detected in rat islets *in vitro* [115], the recent mutations in IRS-2 and the β-cell-specific deletion of the insulin and IGF-1 receptors have demonstrated that the insulin and/or IGF-1 signaling pathways may be of importance for normal β-cell function and growth. Thus, IRS-2-deficient mice were unable to respond to increased insulin demand by compensatory β-cell growth [131]. The studies suggest that increased apoptosis rather than decreased proliferation is responsible for this defect [131]. Recently overexpression of a constitutive active form of Akt-1/PKB-α, which is part of the insulin signaling cascade, was shown to result in marked β-cell hyperplasia and hypertrophy [132, 133]. Evidence for a direct stimulatory effect of insulin on insulin secretion and gene transcription has been published [134]. These results have recently found support in a study where activation of mTOR (mammalian target of rapamycin) by insulin is augmented by amino acids like leucine and glutamine that increase ATP production. Activation of mTOR results in increased protein biosynthesis that may stimulate the growth and function of β-cells [135]. To what extent insulin contributes to the regulation of β-cell growth and function *in vivo* is uncertain as the high local concentration of insulin in the islets probably results in occupation and maximal activation of the insulin receptors on the β-cells. The different signal pathways that may lead to β-cell proliferation are outlined in Figure 6.

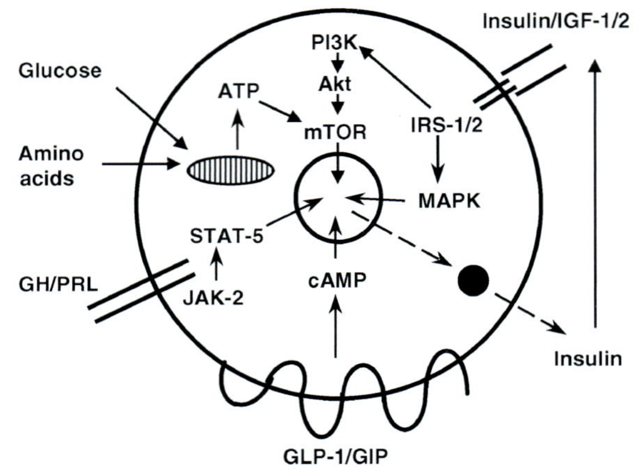

Figure 6 Signaling pathways involved in β-cell proliferation. For explanation, see text

REGENERATION OF β-CELLS IN DIABETES: "PLEIOTROPIC CYTOKINES"

According to the idea of compensatory β-cell growth in response to increased demand for insulin it is to be expected that β-cell destruction in type 1 diabetes will result in at least a temporary growth response. As the proinflammatory cytokines IL-1, IFN-γ, and TNF-α are supposed to contribute to β-cell destruction in type 1 diabetes and indeed are cytotoxic to β-cells *in vitro*, it is of considerable interest to study the effects of these cytokines on β-cell growth. IL-1 has been shown to exert a bimodal effect on insulin secretion and insulin gene transcription in rat islets *in vitro*, and transient stimulation of β-cell proliferation has been reported [136]. Surprisingly, evidence has recently been presented for induction of IL-1 expression in human β-cells exposed to 33 mM glucose for prolonged time *in vitro* [137]. IL-1 immunoreactivity was also seen in islets on sections of pancreas from type 2 diabetic patients, suggesting that IL-1 may be involved in the pathogenesis of both types of diabetes. When IL-1-induced β-cell gene or protein expression is analyzed, it is striking that several factors involved in β-cell survival and growth are upregulated, at least temporarily [138, 139]. If compensatory β-cell regeneration does take place in type 1 diabetes, this phenomenon may escape detection because of recurrent autoimmune destruction. In the diabetic NOD mouse islets Pdx-1/somatostatin positive cells appeared whereas insulin co-expressing cells were absent probably because of autoimmune destruction [88]. An exception is the transgenic mouse expressing IFN-γ driven by the insulin promoter. Massive inflammation and destruction of the β-cells occur but new β-cells appear in the lumen of the ducts where they are inaccessible for lymphocytes.

Although regenerated β-cells are destroyed by the immune system in the NOD mouse, evidence for islet regeneration has been found in the observation of duct cell proliferation and expression of tyrosine hydroxylase, neuropeptide Y, and glucagon [88]. These findings indicate that β-cell regeneration and proliferation do take place in type 1 diabetes, but will only be apparent if the autoimmune process is ablated.

In addition to the increased proliferation of β-cells in animal models of type 2 diabetes, there are indications for neogenesis of β-cells from ducts. Thus, in patients with type 2 diabetes an increased number of insulin-positive cells were found in the ducts [140]. These cells are obviously insufficient to correct the hyperglycemia, but their presence indicates that means that augment their number could lead to increased β-cell mass in patients with type 2 diabetes, possibly with a clinical benefit.

NEOGENESIS OF β-CELLS FROM DUCT CELLS *IN VIVO*: "RESPONSE TO INJURY"

Several models have been employed in order to study regeneration of the endocrine pancreas after damage [141]. They include partial pancreatectomy, duct ligation, and treatment with streptozotocin or alloxan. Common for these models is that the main pathway of regeneration is neogenesis from duct cells either by differentiation of putative stem cells or by dedifferentiation of other cells to stem cells that are reprogrammed to follow the β-cell lineage ("transdifferentiation") [142]. Several growth factors and receptors have been implicated in the regeneration process, including EGF, betacellulin, TGF-α, HGF, PDGF, VEGF, NGF, activin A, and TGF-β [88, 143]. Some of these have been shown to be involved in the embryonic development of the pancreas (see above), suggesting that the same pathways are involved in regeneration and neogenesis. Gastrin and CCK are normally expressed in the developing pancreas but not in the adult. Recently gastrin was found to stimulate proliferation of duct-like cells in the pancreas that express CCK_B receptors [144]. CCK was expressed in the islet-regenerating areas of the duct in IFN-γ transgenic mice [145], and in duct-ligated regenerating pancreas CCK can stimulate β-cell neogenesis [146]. Betacellulin, a member of the EGF family, originally isolated as an angiogenic factor from SV40 T-antigen-induced insulinoma, was reported to promote β-cell regeneration in both partial pancreatectomized rats [147] and alloxan-treated mice [148]. GLP-1 and exendin-4 were found to stimulate β-cell neogenesis in streptozotocin-treated neonatal rats with persistent improvement, but not normalization, of glucose homeostasis [80]. Regeneration of β-cells from intraislet progenitor cells in streptozotocin-treated diabetic rats has been shown to be favored under normoglycemic conditions induced by insulin treatment [149].

After several years of attempts to isolate the putative growth factor(s) involved in the neogenesis of islets in the hamster, where the pancreas was wrapped in cellophane, INGAP (islet neogenesis associated peptide) was identified in the regenerating tissue [150]. This was shown to be a peptide of 15 amino acids, able to stimulate duct cell proliferation. INGAP is expressed in acinar cells and shares homology with the reg (Regeneration gene) or pancreas stone protein family. Reg was identified in regenerating islets from rats after 90% pancreatectomy and treatment with nicotinamide [151]. This family of proteins belongs to the mammalian lectins. The function of reg is thought to be stimulation of β-cell neogenesis from ductal cells. Upregulation of reg expression has also been observed in diabetic NOD mice and BB rats where it has been proposed to play a role in β-cell regeneration [151]. Recently a member of the multiple exostoses (EXT) family (EXTL-3/EXTR-1) was found to be expressed in islets and suggested to function as a reg receptor [152]. The mechanism of action of reg remains to be elucidated.

In conclusion, surgical or chemical injury of the pancreas can elicit neogenesis of β-cells. Although exposure to β-cytotoxic agents or partial pancreatectomy leads to β-cell depletion and therefore to an increased demand for insulin, it is not obvious why duct ligation results in β-cell hyperplasia. Interestingly, it has been reported that duct ligation did not result in acinar cell apoptosis and duct cell proliferation in p53 knockout mice, suggesting that signals from the apoptotic acinar cells trigger the proliferation [153]. The stimulus could be cytokines released from inflammatory cells that may invade the site of injury.

GENERATION OF β-CELLS FROM DUCT CELLS *IN VITRO*: "DOES TRANSDIFFERENTIATION OCCUR?"

A number of intriguing observations of islet cell neogenesis in cultured islet and duct cell preparations have been published during recent years. Thus, long-term culture of islets from prediabetic NOD mice was reported to give rise to the outgrowth of a non-endocrine population of rapidly proliferating cells that can form islet-like structures with low level of hormone expression, which upon transplantation into diabetic NOD mice can reduce the blood sugar level and cure the disease [154]. Culture of adult human islets in collagen resulted in formation of large cysts consisting of duct cells, some of which eventually differentiate to single endocrine cells [155]. Expansion of ductal cells from human pancreas was obtained in cultures on Matrigel, with formation of cysts from which insulin-containing cells were budding [156]. In a similar setup, human or canine islets cultured on an extracellular matrix and exposed to cAMP-stimulating agents transdifferentiated to duct-like cells [157]. Similar transdifferentiation of human islet cells to exocrine and undifferentiated cells after long-term culture has been reported [158]. Transdifferentiation of adult hepatic oval cells to endocrine-like cells when cultured for a very long time in a medium with high glucose was recently reported [159]. In attempts to promote differentiation of human pancreas duct cells to insulin-producing cells, GLP-1 was claimed to stimulate expression of Pdx-1 and insulin in nestin-positive progenitor cells derived from human islets [160]. It is certainly pertinent to dissect the molecular mechanism involved in this hitherto unrecognized plasticity of "terminally" differentiated cells, and to investigate the significance of this plasticity for the regulation of the β-cell mass *in vivo* [89].

β-CELLS FROM EMBRYONIC STEM CELLS: "A BIOLOGICAL AND ETHICAL CHALLENGE"

Although all cells in the body originate from the fertilized egg it came as a surprise that a highly specialized and low abundant cell type like the pancreas β-cells can differentiate directly from embryonic stem (ES) cells. Within the last 2 years a number of publications have reported that ES cells indeed can differentiate to insulin-producing cells. Thus, mouse ES cells were transfected with a DNA construct consisting of a neomycin selection system under the control of the insulin promoter and cultured under standard conditions except for a last step where they were allowed to aggregate at low glucose concentration [161]. The resulting insulin-producing cells were able to normalize hyperglycemia when transplanted to streptozotocin-treated diabetic mice. Using another strategy, mouse ES cells were allowed to form embryoid bodies, which were then plated in serum-free medium that favors the survival of cells that express the intermediary filament protein nestin, which is a marker for neural progenitor cells [162]. These cells were expanded by addition of basic FGF (bFGF), and after withdrawal of the growth factor the cells were allowed to differentiate in the presence of nicotinamide, resulting in cells containing insulin, but not Pdx-1. In an attempt to differentiate human ES cells, a cell line cloned from human ES cells was cultured in the presence of eight growth factors, bFGF, TGF-β1, activin-A, BMP-4, HGF, EGF, NGF, and retinoic acid, known to be involved in embryonic development of various tissues including the pancreas, as discussed above. It was found that each growth factor had specific effects on the differentiation to various cell types. Although insulin and Pdx-1 were already expressed in the embryoid bodies, only NGF favored Pdx-1 expression in the differentiated ES cells [163]. Spontaneous differentiation of human ES cells to insulin-producing cells expressing glucokinase, GLUT-2, Pdx-1, and Ngn3 has been reported [164]. It has however been questioned whether the insulin-producing cells derived from ES cells are true β-cells, or rather neuronal cells expressing low levels of insulin as has been observed in transgenic mice expressing the SV40 T-antigen under the insulin promoter [165]. It is obvious that much more work is needed in the stem cell field before definite conclusions can be made. As employment of human ES cells has raised considerable ethical concerns, the possibility of using adult stem cells that may have a broader differentiation potential than hitherto recognized is being considered, although the potential pitfalls that some of the promising results may be due to fusion of the stem cell with an already differentiated cell in the host cannot as yet be excluded [166].

An overview of the possible sources of β-cells is outlined in Figure 7.

FUTURE ASPECTS

The β-cell mass exhibits a marked degree of plasticity to adapt to variations in insulin demand under physiological and pathological conditions. Identification of the molecular mechanisms involved in the embryonic development of the pancreas is at present under intensive research. Defective development due to either fetal malnutrition or mutations in certain transcription factors may result in later development of type 2 diabetes. β-Cell regeneration in response to various types of damage has been documented. The course of regeneration resembles a recapitulation of the embryonic development with respect to growth and transcription factors. The question that

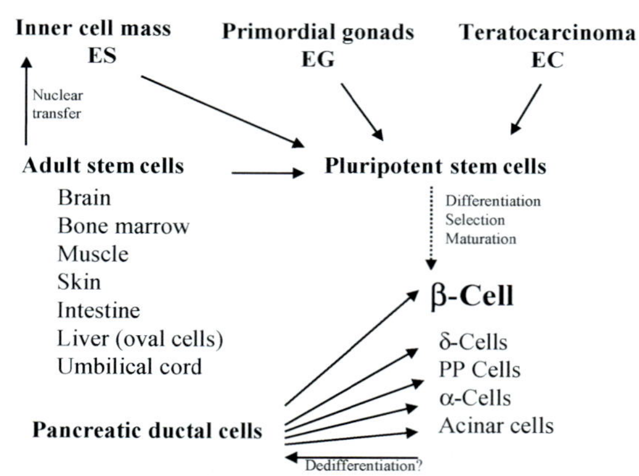

Figure 7 Potential sources of stem cells for β-cells

remains open is to what extent these events take place *in vivo* in the diabetic patient. Compensatory increase in the β-cell mass occurs under conditions of increased insulin demand, such as pregnancy and obesity. However, both genetic and environmental factors may determine at which point the compensation fails and turns into decompensation. It may be expected that identification of growth and survival factors can lead to extension of the compensatory capacity. In type 1 diabetes regeneration of β-cells implies abrogation of the autoimmune reaction. The fact that some individuals even after many years with type 1 diabetes retain some C-peptide production indicates that spontaneous abrogation of the autoimmune state can occur. As complete remission from diabetes does not seem to occur, either β-cells are unable to regenerate in the adult human, or the regenerative capacity is exhausted during the long period of autoimmune destruction. Another possibility is that dormant progenitor or stem cells persist but that proper stimulus for their activation is missing, since already differentiated cells can dedifferentiate to stem cells if given the proper conditions. Therefore the hope is that embryonic or adult stem cells can be propagated and programmed to acquire the β-cell lineage and become normally glucose-responsive β-cells; these could then be transplanted into diabetic patients.

Acknowledgments

The authors want to acknowledge the support from the Juvenile Diabetes Research Foundation (P.S., J.H.N.), National Institutes of Health (P.S.), Danish Research Council for Health Sciences (J.H.N.), the Danish Diabetes Association (J.H.N.), and the Novo Nordisk Foundation (J.H.N.).

REFERENCES

1. Li H, Arber S, Jessell TM, Edlund H. Selective agenesis of the dorsal pancreas in mice lacking homeobox gene Hlxb9. *Nat Genet* 1999; 23: 67–70.
2. Wells JM, Melton DA. Vertebrate endoderm development. *Annu Rev Cell Dev Biol* 1999; 15: 393–410.
3. Grapin-Botton A, Melton DA. Endoderm development: from patterning to organogenesis. *Trends Genet* 2000; 16: 124–30.
4. Gu G, Brown JR, Melton DA. Direct lineage tracing reveals the ontogeny of pancreatic cell fates during mouse embryogenesis. *Mech Dev* 2003; 120: 35–43.
5. Jensen J, Serup P, Karlsen C, Nielsen TF, Madsen OD. mRNA profiling of rat islet tumors reveals Nkx6.1 as a beta-cell-specific homeodomain transcription factor. *J Biol Chem* 1996; 271: 18749–58.
6. Kim SK, Hebrok M, Melton DA. Notochord to endoderm signaling is required for pancreas development. *Development* 1997; 124: 4243–52.
7. Hebrok M. Hedgehog signaling in pancreas development. *Mech Dev* 2003; 120: 45–57.
8. Apelqvist A, Ahlgren U, Edlund H. Sonic hedgehog directs specialised mesoderm differentiation in the intestine and pancreas. *Curr Biol* 1997; 7: 801–4.
9. Lammert E, Cleaver O, Melton D. Role of endothelial cells in early pancreas and liver development. *Mech Dev* 2003; 120: 59–64.
10. Massague J, Wotton D. Transcriptional control by the TGF-beta/Smad signaling system. *EMBO J* 2000; 19: 1745–54.
11. Kim SK, Hebrok M, Li E, Oh SP, Schrewe H, Harmon EB, Lee JS, Melton DA. Activin receptor patterning of foregut organogenesis. *Genes Dev* 2000; 14: 1866–71.
12. Ahlgren U, Jonsson J, Edlund H. The morphogenesis of the pancreatic mesenchyme is uncoupled from that of the pancreatic epithelium in IPF1/PDX-1-deficient mice. *Development* 1996; 122: 1409–16.
13. Jonsson J, Carlsson L, Edlund T, Edlund H. Insulin-promoter-factor 1 is required for pancreas development in mice. *Nature* 1994; 371: 606–9.
14. Offield M, Jetton T, Labosky P, Ray M, Stein R, Magnuson M, Hogan B, Wright C. PDX-1 is required for pancreatic outgrowth and differentiation of the rostral duodenum. *Development* 1996; 122: 983–95.
15. Stoffers D, Zinkin N, Stanojevic V, Clarke W, Habener J. Pancreatic agenesis attributable to a single nucleotide deletion in the human IPF1 gene coding sequence. *Nat Genet* 1997; 15: 106–10.
16. Grapin-Botton A, Majithia AR, Melton DA. Key events of pancreas formation are triggered in gut endoderm by ectopic expression of pancreatic regulatory genes. *Genes Dev* 2001; 15: 444–54.
17. Ahlgren U, Jonsson J, Jonsson L, Simu K, Edlund H. Beta-cell-specific inactivation of the mouse Ipf1/Pdx1 gene results in loss of the beta-cell phenotype and maturity onset diabetes. *Genes Dev* 1998; 12: 1763–8.
18. Wilson ME, Scheel D, German MS. Gene expression cascades in pancreatic development. *Mech Dev* 2003; 120: 65–80.
19. Krapp A, Knofler M, Ledermann B, Burki K, Berney C, Zoerkler N, Hagenbuchle O, Wellauer PK. The bHLH protein PTF1-p48 is essential for the formation of the exocrine and the correct spatial organization of the endocrine pancreas. *Genes Dev* 1998; 12: 3752–63.
20. Kawaguchi Y, Cooper B, Gannon M, Ray M, MacDonald RJ, Wright CV. The role of the transcriptional regulator Ptf1a in converting intestinal to pancreatic progenitors. *Nat Genet* 2002; 32: 128–34.
21. Bhushan A, Itoh N, Kato S, Thiery JP, Czernchow P, Bellusci S, Scharfmann R. Fgf10 is essential for maintaining the proliferative capacity of epithelial progenitor cells during early pancreatic organogenesis. *Development* 2001; 128: 5109–17.
22. Yamashita T, Yoshioka M, Itoh N. Identification of a novel fibroblast growth factor, FGF-23, preferentially expressed in the ventrolateral thalamic nucleus of the brain. *Biochem Biophys Res Commun* 2000; 277: 494–8.
23. Scharfmann R. Control of early development of the pancreas in rodents and humans: implications of signals from the mesenchyme. *Diabetologia* 2000; 43: 1083–92.
24. Dichmann D, Miller C, Jensen J, Heller R, Serup P. Expression and misexpression of members of the FGF and TGFb families of growth factors in the developing mouse pancreas. *Dev Dyn* 2000; 226: 663–74.
25. Le Bras S, Miralles F, Basmaciogullari A, Czernichow P, Scharfmann R. Fibroblast growth factor 2 promotes pancreatic epithelial cell proliferation via functional fibroblast growth factor receptors during embryonic life. *Diabetes* 1998; 47: 1236–42.

26. Miralles F, Czernichow P, Ozaki K, Itoh N, Scharfmann R. Signaling through fibroblast growth factor receptor 2b plays a key role in the development of the exocrine pancreas. *Proc Natl Acad Sci USA* 1999; 96: 6267–72.
27. Yi ES, Yin S, Harclerode DL, Bedoya A, Bikhazi NB, Housley RM, Aukerman SL, Morris CF, Pierce GF, Ulich TR. Keratinocyte growth factor induces pancreatic ductal epithelial proliferation. *Am J Pathol* 1994; 145: 80–5.
28. Nguyen HQ, Danilenko DM, Bucay N, DeRose ML, Van GY, Thomason A, Simonet WS. Expression of keratinocyte growth factor in embryonic liver of transgenic mice causes changes in epithelial growth and differentiation resulting in polycystic kidneys and other organ malformations. *Oncogene* 1996; 12: 2109–19.
29. Krakowski ML, Kritzik MR, Jones EM, Krahl T, Lee J, Arnush M, Gu D, Sarvetnick N. Pancreatic expression of keratinocyte growth factor leads to differentiation of islet hepatocytes and proliferation of duct cells. *Am J Pathol* 1999; 154: 683–91.
30. Celli G, LaRochelle WJ, Mackem S, Sharp R, Merlino G. Soluble dominant-negative receptor uncovers essential roles for fibroblast growth factors in multi-organ induction and patterning. *EMBO J* 1998; 17: 1642–55.
31. Gradwohl G, Dierich A, LeMeur M, Guillemot F. Neurogenin3 is required for the development of the four endocrine cell lineages of the pancreas. *Proc Natl Acad Sci USA* 2000; 97: 1607–11.
32. Jensen J, Heller RS, Nielsen TF, Pedersen EE, Lindsell C, Weinmaster G, Madsen OD, Serup P. Independent development of pancreatic a- and β-cells from neurogenin3 expressing presursors. A role for the Notch pathway in repression of premature differentiation. *Diabetes* 2000; 49: 163–76.
33. Lardelli M, Williams R, Lendahl U. Notch-related genes in animal development *Int J Dev Biol* 1995; 39: 769–80.
34. Weinmaster G. The ins and outs of notch signaling. *Mol Cell Neurosci* 1997; 9: 91–102.
35. Kageyama R, Ohtsuka T. The Notch–Hes pathway in mammalian neural development. *Cell Res* 1999; 9: 179–88.
36. Weinmaster G. Notch signal transduction: a real rip and more. *Curr Opin Genet Dev* 2000; 10: 363–9.
37. Apelqvist A, Li H, Sommer L, Beatus P, Anderson DJ, Honjo T, Hrabe de Angelis M, Lendahl U, Edlund H. Notch signaling controls pancreatic cell differentiation. *Nature* 1999; 400: 877–81.
38. Jensen J, Pedersen EE, Galante P, Hald J, Heller RS, Ishibashi M, Kageyama R, Guillemot F, Serup P, Madsen OD. Control of endodermal endocrine development by Hes-1. *Nat Genet* 2000; 24: 36–44.
39. Lammert E, Brown J, Melton DA. Notch gene expression during pancreatic organogenesis. *Mech Dev* 2000; 94: 199–203.
40. Miettinen PJ, Huotari M, Koivisto T, Ustinov J, Palgi J, Rasilainen S, Lehtonen E, Keski-Oja J, Otonkoski T. Impaired migration and delayed differentiation of pancreatic islet cells in mice lacking EGF-receptors. *Development* 2000; 127: 2617–27.
41. Kritzik MR, Krahl T, Good A, Gu D, Lai C, Fox H, Sarvetnick N. Expression of ErbB receptors during pancreatic islet development and regrowth. *J Endocrinol* 2000; 165: 67–77.
42. Erickson SL, O'Shea KS, Ghaboosi N, Loverro L, Frantz G, Bauer M, Lu LH, Moore MW. ErbB3 is required for normal cerebellar and cardiac development: a comparison with ErbB2- and heregulin-deficient mice. *Development* 1997; 124: 4999–5011.
43. Seno M, Tada H, Kosaka M, Sasada R, Igarashi K, Shing Y, Folkman J, Ueda M, Yamada H. Human betacellulin, a member of the EGF family dominantly expressed in pancreas and small intestine, is fully active in a monomeric form. *Growth Factors* 1996; 13: 181–91.
44. Miyagawa J, Hanafusa O, Sasada R, Yamamoto K, Igarashi K, Yamamori K, Seno M, Tada H, Nammo T, Li M, Yamagata K, Nakajima H, Namba M, Kuwajima M, Matsuzawa Y. Immunohistochemical localization of betacellulin, a new member of the EGF family, in normal human pancreas and islet tumor cells. *Endocr J* 1999; 46: 755–64.
45. Wang RN, Rehfeld JF, Nielsen FC, Kloppel G. Expression of gastrin and transforming growth factor-alpha during duct to islet cell differentiation in the pancreas of duct-ligated adult rats. *Diabetologia* 1997; 40: 887–93.
46. Kaneto H, Miyagawa J, Kajimoto Y, Yamamoto K, Watada H, Umayahara Y, Hanafusa T, Matsuzawa Y, Yamasaki Y, Higashiyama S, Taniguchi N. Expression of heparin-binding epidermal growth factor-like growth factor during pancreas development. A potential role of PDX-1 in transcriptional activation. *J Biol Chem* 1997; 272: 29137–43.
47. Harari D, Tzahar E, Romano J, Shelly M, Pierce JH, Andrews GC, Yarden Y. Neuregulin-4: a novel growth factor that acts through the ErbB-4 receptor tyrosine kinase. *Oncogene* 1999; 18: 2681–9.
48. Withers DJ, Burks DJ, Towery HH, Altamuro SL, Flint CL, White MF. Irs-2 coordinates Igf-1 receptor-mediated beta-cell development and peripheral insulin signaling. *Nat Genet* 1999; 23: 32–40.
49. Otonkoski T, Cirulli V, Beattie M, Mally MI, Soto G, Rubin JS, Hayek A. A role for hepatocyte growth factor/scatter factor in fetal mesenchyme-induced pancreatic beta-cell growth. *Endocrinology* 1996; 137: 3131–9.
50. Beattie GM, Rubin JS, Mally MI, Otonkoski T, Hayek A. Regulation of proliferation and differentiation of human fetal pancreatic islet cells by extracellular matrix, hepatocyte growth factor, and cell-cell contact. *Diabetes* 1996; 45: 1223–8.
51. Kanaka-Gantenbein C, Tazi A, Czernichow P, Scharfmann R. In vivo presence of the high affinity nerve growth factor receptor Trk-A in the rat pancreas: differential localization during pancreatic development. *Endocrinology* 1995; 136: 761–9.
52. Tazi A, Le Bras S, Lamghitnia HO, Vincent JD, Czernichow P, Scharfmann R. Neurotrophin-3 increases intracellular calcium in a rat insulin-secreting cell line through its action on a functional TrkC receptor. *J Biol Chem* 1996; 271: 10154–60.
53. Heller RS, Dichmann DS, Jensen J, Miller C, Wong G, Madsen OD, Serup P. Expression patterns of Wnts, Frizzleds, sFRPs, and misexpression in transgenic mice suggesting a role for Wnts in pancreas and foregut pattern formation. *Dev Dyn* 2002; 225: 260–70.
54. LeBras S, Czernichow P, Scharfmann R. A search for tyrosine kinase receptors expressed in the rat embryonic pancreas. *Diabetologia* 1998; 41: 1474–81.
55. Heremans Y, Van De Casteele M, in't Veld P, Gradwohl G, Serup P, Madsen O, Pipeleers D, Heimberg H. Recapitulation of embryonic neuroendocrine differentiation in adult human pancreatic duct cells expressing neurogenin 3. *J Cell Biol* 2002; 159: 303–12.

56. Sosa-Pineda B, Chowdhury K, Torres M, Oliver G, Gruss P. The Pax4 gene is essential for differentiation of insulin-producing beta cells in the mammalian pancreas. *Nature* 1997; 386: 399–402.
57. Petersen HV, Jorgensen MC, Andersen FG, Jensen J, T FN, Jorgensen R, Madsen OD, Serup P. Pax4 represses pancreatic glucagon gene expression. *Mol Cell Biol Res* 2000; 3: 249–54.
58. Smith SB, Ee HC, Conners JR, German MS. Paired-homeodomain transcription factor PAX4 acts as a transcriptional repressor in early pancreatic development. *Mol Cell Biol* 1999; 19: 8272–80.
59. Rouiller DG, Cirulli V, Halban PA. Uvomorulin mediates calcium-dependent aggregation of islet cells, whereas calcium-independent cell adhesion molecules distinguish between islet cell types. *Dev Biol* 1991; 148: 233–42.
60. Rouiller DG, Cirulli V, Halban PA. Differences in aggregation properties and levels of the neural cell adhesion molecule (NCAM) between islet cell types. *Exp Cell Res* 1990; 191: 305–12.
61. Sjodin A, Dahl U, Semb H. Mouse R-cadherin: expression during the organogenesis of pancreas and gastrointestinal tract. *Exp Cell Res* 1995; 221: 413–25.
62. Cirulli V, Baetens D, Rutishauser U, Halban PA, Orci L, Rouiller DG. Expression of neural cell adhesion molecule (N-CAM) in rat islets and its role in islet cell type segregation. *J Cell Sci* 1994; 107: 1429–36.
63. Cirulli V, Ricordi C, Hayek A. E-cadherin, NCAM, and EpCAM expression in human fetal pancreata. *Transplant Proc* 1995; 27: 3335.
64. Moller CJ, Christgau S, Williamson MR, Madsen OD, Niu ZP, Bock E, Baekkeskov S. Differential expression of neural cell adhesion molecule and cadherins in pancreatic islets, glucagonomas, and insulinomas. *Mol Endocrinol* 1992; 6: 1332–42.
65. Dahl U, Sjodin A, Semb H. Cadherins regulate aggregation of pancreatic beta-cells *in vivo*. *Development* 1996; 122: 2895–902.
66. Cirulli V, Beattie GM, Klier G, Ellisman M, Ricordi C, Quaranta V, Frasier F, Ishii JK, Hayek A, Salomon DR. Expression and function of alpha(v)beta(3) and alpha(v)beta(5) integrins in the developing pancreas: roles in the adhesion and migration of putative endocrine progenitor cells. *J Cell Biol* 2000; 150: 1445–60.
67. Hellerström C, Swenne I. Growth pattern of pancreatic islets in animals. In Volk B, Arquilla E (eds) *The Diabetic Pancreas*. New York: Plenum, 1985; pp 53–79.
68. Rosselin G, Emami S. Growth and differentiation of the islet cells in neonates. In Sarvetnick N (ed) *Pancreatic Growth and Rregeneration*. Basel: Karger, 1997; pp 44–95.
69. Fowden AL, Hill DJ. Intra-uterine programming of the endocrine pancreas. *Br Med Bull* 2001; 60: 123–42.
70. Bertin E, Gangnerau MN, Bellon G, Bailbe D, Arbelot De, Vacqueur A, Portha B. Development of beta-cell mass in fetuses of rats deprived of protein and/or energy in last trimester of pregnancy. *Am J Physiol Regul Integr Comp Physiol* 2002; 283: R623–30.
71. Bonner-Weir S, Weir G. Mechanisms of postnatal β-cell mass regulation. In Habener J, Hussain M (eds) *Molecular Basis of Pancreas Development*. Norwell: Kluwer, 2001; pp 289–97.
72. Bonner-Weir S. Islet growth and development in the adult. *J Mol Endocrinol* 2000; 24: 297–302.
73. Klöppel G-W, in't Veld P. Morphology of the pancreas in normal and diabetic states. In Alberti K, Zimmet P, DeFronzo R, Keen H (eds) *International Textbook of Diabetes Mellitus*. Chichester: Wiley, 1997; pp 287–313.
74. Kulkarni RN, Holzenberger M, Shih DQ, Ozcan U, Stoffel M, Magnuson MA, Kahn CR. Beta-cell-specific deletion of the Igf1 receptor leads to hyperinsulinemia and glucose intolerance but does not alter beta-cell mass. *Nat Genet* 2002; 31: 111–5.
75. Duvillie B, Currie C, Chrones T, Bucchini D, Jami J, Joshi RL, Hill DJ. Increased islet cell proliferation, decreased apoptosis, and greater vascularization leading to beta-cell hyperplasia in mutant mice lacking insulin. *Endocrinology* 2002; 143: 1530–7.
76. Homo-Delarche F. Is pancreas development abnormal in the non-obese diabetic mouse, a spontaneous model of type 1 diabetes? *Braz J Med Biol Res* 2001; 34: 437–47.
77. O'Brien BA, Huang Y, Geng X, Dutz JP, Finegood DT. Phagocytosis of apoptotic cells by macrophages from NOD mice is reduced. *Diabetes* 2002; 51: 2481–8.
78. Trudeau JD, Dutz JP, Arany E, Hill DJ, Fieldus WE, Finegood DT. Neonatal beta-cell apoptosis: a trigger for autoimmune diabetes? *Diabetes* 2000; 49: 1–7.
79. Hales CN, Barker DJ. The thrifty phenotype hypothesis. *Br Med Bull* 2001; 60: 5–20.
80. Tourrel C, Bailbe D, Meile MJ, Kergoat M, Portha B. Glucagon-like peptide-1 and exendin-4 stimulate beta-cell neogenesis in streptozotocin-treated newborn rats resulting in persistently improved glucose homeostasis at adult age. *Diabetes* 2001; 50: 1562–70.
81. Miralles F, Portha B. Early development of beta-cells is impaired in the GK rat model of type 2 diabetes. *Diabetes* 2001; 50: S84–8.
82. Hellerström C. Growth pattern of pancreatic islets in animals. In Volk B, Wellmann K (eds) *The Diabetic Pancreas*. London: Bailliere Tindall, 1977; pp 61–97.
83. Bonner-Weir S. Perspective: postnatal pancreatic beta cell growth. *Endocrinology* 2000; 141: 1926–9.
84. Nielsen J, Møldrup A, Billestrup N, Petersen E, Allevato G, Stahl M. The role of growth hormone and prolactin in beta cell growth and regeneration. In Vinik A (ed) *Pancreatic Islet Regeneration and Growth* New York: Plenum, 1992; pp 9–17.
85. Biarnes M, Montolio M, Nacher V, Raurell M, Soler J, Montanya E. Beta-cell death and mass in syngeneically transplanted islets exposed to short- and long-term hyperglycemia. *Diabetes* 2002; 51: 66–72.
86. Scaglia L, Smith FE, Bonner-Weir S. Apoptosis contributes to the involution of beta cell mass in the post partum rat pancreas. *Endocrinology* 1995; 136: 5461–8.
87. Blume N, Skouv J, Larsson L-I, Holst JJ, Madsen OD. Potent inhibitory effects of transplantable rat glucagonomas and insulinomas on the respective endogenous islet cells are associated with pancreatic apoptosis. *J Clin Invest* 1995; 96: 2227–35.
88. Nielsen JH, Serup P. Molecular basis for islet development, growth, and regeneration. *Curr Opin Endocrinol Diabet* 1998; 5: 97–107.
89. Bernard-Kargar C, Ktorza A. Endocrine pancreas plasticity under physiological and pathological conditions. *Diabetes* 2001; 50 (suppl 1): S30–5.
90. Guiot Y, Sempoux C, Moulin P, Rahier J. No decrease of the beta-cell mass in type 2 diabetic patients. *Diabetes* 2001; 50 (suppl 1): S188.
91. Butler A, Janson J, Bonner-Weir S, Ritzel R, Rizza R, Butler P. Beta-cell deficit and increased beta-cell

apoptosis in humans with type 2-diabetes mellitus. *Diabetes* 2003; 52: 102–10.

92. Yoon K, Ko S, Cho J, Lee J, Ahn Y, Song K, Yoo S, Kang M, Cha B, Lee K, Don H, Kang S, Kim D, Lee I, Bonner-Weir S. Selective β-cell loss and α-cell expansion in patients with type 2 diabetes mellitus in Korea. *J Clin Endocrinol Metab* 2003; 88: 2300–8.
93. Shafrir E, Ben-Sasson R, Ziv E, Bar-On H. Insulin resistance, β-cell survival, and apoptosis in type 2 diabetes: animal models and human implications. *Diabetes Rev* 1999; 7: 114–23.
94. Unger RH. Lipotoxic diseases. *Annu Rev Med* 2002; 53: 319–36.
95. Devedjian JC, George M, Casellas A, Pujol A, Visa J, Pelegrin M, Gros L, Bosch F. Transgenic mice overexpressing insulin-like growth factor-II in beta cells develop type 2 diabetes. *J Clin Invest* 2000; 105: 731–40.
96. Kulkarni R, Kahn C. Genetic models of insulin resistance: alterations in β-cell biology. In Habener J, Hussain M (eds) *Molecular Basis of Pancreas Development*. Norwell: Kluwer, 2001; pp 299–323.
97. Flier SN, Kulkarni RN, Kahn CR. Evidence for a circulating islet cell growth factor in insulin-resistant states. *Proc Natl Acad Sci USA* 2001; 98: 7475–80.
98. Cerasi E. Insulin deficiency and insulin resistance in the pathogenesis of NIDDM: is a divorce possible? *Diabetologia* 1995; 38: 992–7.
99. Leahy J. Impaired β-cell function with chronic hyperglycemia: "overworked β-cell" hypothesis *Diabetes Rev* 1996; 4: 298–319.
100. Laybutt DR, Weir GC, Kaneto H, Lebet J, Palmiter RD, Sharma A, Bonner-Weir S. Overexpression of c-Myc in beta-cells of transgenic mice causes proliferation and apoptosis, downregulation of insulin gene expression, and diabetes. *Diabetes* 2002; 51: 1793–804.
101. Pelengaris S, Khan M, Evan GI. Suppression of Myc-induced apoptosis in beta cells exposes multiple oncogenic properties of Myc and triggers carcinogenic progression. *Cell* 2002; 109: 321–34.
102. Laybutt DR, Kaneto H, Hasenkamp W, Grey S, Jonas JC, Sgroi DC, Groff A, Ferran C, Bonner-Weir S, Sharma A, Weir GC. Increased expression of antioxidant and anti-apoptotic genes in islets that may contribute to beta-cell survival during chronic hyperglycemia. *Diabetes* 2002; 51: 413–23.
103. Efanova IB, Zaitsev SV, Zhivotovsky B, Kohler M, Efendic S, Orrenius S, Berggren PO. Glucose and tolbutamide induce apoptosis in pancreatic beta-cells. A process dependent on intracellular Ca^{2+} concentration. *J Biol Chem* 1998; 273: 33501–7.
104. Hoorens A, Van de Casteele M, Kloppel G, Pipeleers D. Glucose promotes survival of rat pancreatic beta cells by activating synthesis of proteins which suppress a constitutive apoptotic program. *J Clin Invest* 1996; 98: 1568–74.
105. Federici M, Hribal M, Perego L, Ranalli M, Caradonna Z, Perego C, Usellini L, Nano R, Bonini P, Bertuzzi F, Marlier LN, Davalli AM, Carandente O, Pontiroli AE, Melino G, Marchetti P, Lauro R, Sesti G, Folli F. High glucose causes apoptosis in cultured human pancreatic islets of Langerhans: a potential role for regulation of specific Bcl family genes toward an apoptotic cell death program. *Diabetes* 2001; 50: 1290–301.
106. Maedler K, Spinas GA, Lehmann R, Sergeev P, Weber M, Fontana A, Kaiser N, Donath MY. Glucose induces beta-cell apoptosis via upregulation of the Fas receptor in human islets. *Diabetes* 2001; 50: 1683–90.
107. Maedler K, Fontana A, Ris F, Sergeev P, Toso C, Oberholzer J, Lehmann R, Bachmann F, Tasinato A, Spinas GA, Halban PA, Donath MY. FLIP switches Fas-mediated glucose signaling in human pancreatic beta cells from apoptosis to cell replication. *Proc Natl Acad Sci USA* 2002; 99: 8236–41.
108. Korsgren O, Jansson L, Sandler S, Andersson A. Hyperglycemia-induced B cell toxicity. The fate of pancreatic islets transplanted into diabetic mice is dependent on their genetic background. *J Clin Invest* 1990; 86: 2161–8.
109. Maedler K, Spinas GA, Dyntar D, Moritz W, Kaiser N, Donath MY. Distinct effects of saturated and monounsaturated fatty acids on beta-cell turnover and function. *Diabetes* 2001; 50: 69–76.
110. Lupi R, Dotta F, Marselli L, Del Guerra S, Masini M, Santangelo C, Patane G, Boggi U, Piro S, Anello M, Bergamini E, Mosca F, Di Mario U, Del Prato S, Marchetti P. Prolonged exposure to free fatty acids has cytostatic and proapoptotic effects on human pancreatic islets: evidence that beta-cell death is caspase mediated, partially dependent on ceramide pathway, and Bcl-2 regulated. *Diabetes* 2002; 51: 1437–42.
111. Ceddia RB, Koistinen HA, Zierath JR, Sweeney G. Analysis of paradoxical observations on the association between leptin and insulin resistance. *FASEB J* 2002; 16: 1163–76.
112. Islam MS, Sjoholm A, Emilsson V. Fetal pancreatic islets express functional leptin receptors and leptin stimulates proliferation of fetal islet cells. *Int J Obes Relat Metab Disord* 2000; 24: 1246–53.
113. Okuya S, Tanabe K, Tanizawa Y, Oka Y. Leptin increases the viability of isolated rat pancreatic islets by suppressing apoptosis. *Endocrinology* 2001; 142: 4827–30.
114. Brelje T, Sorenson R. The physiological roles of prolactin, growth hormone and placental lactogen in the regulation of islet cell proliferation. In Sarvetnick N (ed) *Pancreatic Growth and Rregeneration*. Basel: Karger, 1997; pp 1–30.
115. Nielsen JH, Galsgaard ED, Moldrup A, Friedrichsen BN, Billestrup N, Hansen JA, Lee YC, Carlsson C. Regulation of β-cell mass by hormones and growth factors. *Diabetes* 2001; 50: S25–9.
116. Friedrichsen BN, Galsgaard ED, Nielsen JH, Moldrup A. Growth hormone- and prolactin-induced proliferation of insulinoma cells, INS-1, depends on activation of STAT5 (signal transducer and activator of transcription 5). *Mol Endocrinol* 2001; 15: 136–48.
117. Rønn SG, Hansen JA, Lindberg K, Karlsen AE, Billestrup N. The effect of suppressor of cytokine signaling 3 on GH signaling in β-cells. *Mol Endocrinol* 2002; 16: 2124–34.
118. Karlsen AE, Ronn SG, Lindberg K, Johannesen J, Galsgaard ED, Pociot F, Nielsen JH, Mandrup-Poulsen T, Nerup J, Billestrup N. Suppressor of cytokine signaling 3 (SOCS-3) protects β-cells against interleukin-1beta- and interferon-gamma-mediated toxicity. *Proc Natl Acad Sci USA* 2001; 98: 12191–6.
119. Nieuwenhuizen AG, Schuiling GA, Moes H, Koiter TR. Role of increased insulin demand in the adaptation of the endocrine pancreas to pregnancy. *Acta Physiol Scand* 1997; 159: 303–12.

120. Rhodes CJ. IGF-I and GH post-receptor signaling mechanisms for pancreatic β-cell replication. *J Mol Endocrinol* 2000; 24: 303–11.
121. Nielsen JH. Growth and function of the pancreatic beta cell *in vitro*: effects of glucose, hormones and serum factors on mouse, rat and human pancreatic islets in organ culture. *Acta Endocrinol Suppl (Copenh)* 1985; 266: 1–39.
122. Parsons JA, Bartke A, Sorenson RL. Number and size of islets of Langerhans in pregnant, human growth hormone-expressing transgenic, and pituitary dwarf mice: effect of lactogenic hormones. *Endocrinology* 1995; 136: 2013–21.
123. Garcia-Ocana A, Vasavada RC, Takane KK, Cebrian A, Lopez-Talavera JC, Stewart AF. Using beta-cell growth factors to enhance human pancreatic Islet transplantation. *J Clin Endocrinol Metab* 2001; 86: 984–8.
124. Carlsson C, Tornehave D, Lindberg K, Galante P, Billestrup N, Michelsen B, Larsson LI, Nielsen JH. Growth hormone and prolactin stimulate the expression of rat preadipocyte factor-1/delta-like protein in pancreatic islets: molecular cloning and expression pattern during development and growth of the endocrine pancreas. *Endocrinology* 1997; 138: 3940–8.
125. Friedrichsen B, Carlsson C, Møldrup A, Michelsen B, Jensen C, Teisner B, Nielsen J. Expression, biosynthesis and release of Pref-1/dlk/FA1 in pancreatic β-cells: possible physiological implications. *J Endocrinol* 2003; 176: 257–66.
126. Weinhaus AJ, Bhagroo NV, Brelje TC, Sorenson RL. Dexamethasone counteracts the effect of prolactin on islet function: implications for islet regulation in late pregnancy. *Endocrinology* 2000; 141: 1384–93.
127. Habener J. Glucagonlike peptide-1 agonits stimulation of β-cell growth and differentiation. *Curr Opin Endocrinol Metab* 2001; 8: 74–81.
128. Trümper A, Trümper K, Trusheim H, Arnold R, Goke B, Horsch D. Glucose-dependent insulinotropic polypeptide is a growth factor for beta (INS-1) cells by pleiotropic signaling. *Mol Endocrinol* 2001; 15: 1559–70.
129. Buteau J, Foisy S, Rhodes CJ, Carpenter L, Biden TJ, Prentki M. Protein kinase Czeta activation mediates glucagon-like peptide-1-induced pancreatic beta-cell proliferation. *Diabetes* 2001; 50: 2237–43.
130. Swenne I. Pancreatic β-cell growth and diabetes mellitus. *Diabetologia* 1992; 35: 193–201.
131. White MF. IRS proteins and the common path to diabetes. *Am J Physiol Endocrinol Metab* 2002; 283: E413–22.
132. Bernal-Mizrachi E, Wen W, Stahlhut S, Welling CM, Permutt MA. Islet β cell expression of constitutively active Akt1/PKB alpha induces striking hypertrophy, hyperplasia, and hyperinsulinemia. *J Clin Invest* 2001; 108: 1631–8.
133. Tuttle RL, Gill NS, Pugh W, Lee JP, Koeberlein B, Furth EE, Polonsky KS, Naji A, Birnbaum MJ. Regulation of pancreatic β-cell growth and survival by the serine/threonine protein kinase Akt1/PKBalpha. *Nat Med* 2001; 7: 1133–7.
134. Leibiger IB, Leibiger B, Moede T, Berggren PO. Exocytosis of insulin promotes insulin gene transcription via the insulin receptor/PI-3 kinase/p70 s6 kinase and CaM kinase pathways. *Mol Cell* 1998; 1: 933–8.
135. McDaniel ML, Marshall CA, Pappan KL, Kwon G. Metabolic and autocrine regulation of the mammalian target of rapamycin by pancreatic β-cells. *Diabetes* 2002; 51: 2877–85.
136. Nielsen J, Billestrup N. The role of cytokine receptor signaling in β-cell growth and function. In Sarvetnick N (ed) *Pancreatic Growth and Regeneration*. Basel: Karger, 1997; pp 31–43.
137. Maedler K, Sergeev P, Ris F, Oberholzer J, Joller-Jemelka HI, Spinas GA, Kaiser N, Halban PA, Donath MY. Glucose-induced beta cell production of IL-1beta contributes to glucotoxicity in human pancreatic islets. *J Clin Invest* 2002; 110: 851–60.
138. Cardozo AK, Kruhoffer M, Leeman R, Orntoft T, Eizirik DL. Identification of novel cytokine-induced genes in pancreatic β-cells by high-density oligonucleotide arrays. *Diabetes* 2001; 50: 909–20.
139. Larsen PM, Fey SJ, Larsen MR, Nawrocki A, Andersen HU, Kahler H, Heilmann C, Voss MC, Roepstorff P, Pociot F, Karlsen AE, Nerup J. Proteome analysis of interleukin-1beta-induced changes in protein expression in rat islets of Langerhans. *Diabetes* 2001; 50: 1056–63.
140. Jones LC, Clark A. Beta-cell neogenesis in type 2 diabetes. *Diabetes* 2001; 50 (suppl 1): S186–7.
141. Risbud MV, Bhonde RR. Models of pancreatic regeneration in diabetes. *Diabetes Res Clin Pract* 2002; 58: 155–65.
142. Bouwens L. Transdifferentiation versus stem cell hypothesis for the regeneration of islet β-cells in the pancreas. *Microsc Res Tech* 1998; 43: 332–6.
143. Yamaoka T, Itakura M. Development of pancreatic islets (review). *Int J Mol Med* 1999; 3: 247–61.
144. Rooman I, Lardon J, Flamez D, Schuit F, Bouwens L. Mitogenic effect of gastrin and expression of gastrin receptors in duct-like cells of rat pancreas. *Gastroenterology* 2001; 121: 940–9.
145. Liu G, Pakala SV, Gu D, Krahl T, Mocnik L, Sarvetnick N. Cholecystokinin expression in the developing and regenerating pancreas and intestine. *J Endocrinol* 2001; 169: 233–40.
146. Rooman I, Lardon J, Bouwens L. Gastrin stimulates β-cell neogenesis and increases islet mass from transdifferentiated but not from normal exocrine pancreas tissue. *Diabetes* 2002; 51: 686–90.
147. Li L, Seno M, Yamada H, Kojima I. Promotion of β-cell regeneration by betacellulin in ninety percent-pancreatectomized rats. *Endocrinology* 2001; 142: 5379–85.
148. Yamamoto K, Miyagawa J, Waguri M, Sasada R, Igarashi K, Li M, Nammo T, Moriwaki M, Imagawa A, Yamagata K, Nakajima H, Namba M, Tochino Y, Hanafusa T, Matsuzawa Y. Recombinant human betacellulin promotes the neogenesis of β-cells and ameliorates glucose intolerance in mice with diabetes induced by selective alloxan perfusion. *Diabetes* 2000; 49: 2021–7.
149. Guz Y, Nasir I, Teitelman G. Regeneration of pancreatic beta cells from intra-islet precursor cells in an experimental model of diabetes. *Endocrinology* 2001; 142: 4956–68.
150. Rafaeloff R, Pittenger GL, Barlow SW, Qin XF, Yan B, Rosenberg L, Duguid WP, Vinik AI. Cloning and sequencing of the pancreatic islet neogenesis associated protein (INGAP) gene and its expression in islet neogenesis in hamsters. *J Clin Invest* 1997; 99: 2100–9.
151. Okamoto H. The Reg gene family and Reg proteins: with special attention to the regeneration of pancreatic β-cells. *J Hepatobiliary Pancreat Surg* 1999; 6: 254–62.

152. Kobayashi S, Akiyama T, Nata K, Abe M, Tajima M, Shervani NJ, Unno M, Matsuno S, Sasaki H, Takasawa S, Okamoto H. Identification of a receptor for reg (regenerating gene) protein, a pancreatic β-cell regeneration factor. *J Biol Chem* 2000; 275: 10723–6.
153. Scoggins CR, Meszoely IM, Wada M, Means AL, Yang L, Leach SD. p53-dependent acinar cell apoptosis triggers epithelial proliferation in duct-ligated murine pancreas. *Am J Physiol Gastrointest Liver Physiol* 2000; 279: G827–36.
154. Ramiya VK, Maraist M, Arfors KE, Schatz DA, Peck AB, Cornelius JG. Reversal of insulin-dependent diabetes using islets generated *in vitro* from pancreatic stem cells. *Nat Med* 2000; 6: 278–82.
155. Kerr-Conte J, Pattou F, Lecomte-Houcke M, Xia Y, Boilly B, Proye C, Lefebvre J. Ductal cyst formation in collagen-embedded adult human islet preparations. A means to the reproduction of nesidioblastosis in vitro. *Diabetes* 1996; 45: 1108–14.
156. Bonner-Weir S, Taneja M, Weir GC, Tatarkiewicz K, Song KH, Sharma A, O'Neil JJ. In vitro cultivation of human islets from expanded ductal tissue. *Proc Natl Acad Sci USA* 2000; 97: 7999–8004.
157. Wang R, Li J, Rosenberg L. Factors mediating the transdifferentiation of islets of Langerhans to duct epithelial-like structures. *J Endocrinol* 2001; 171: 309–18.
158. Schmied BM, Ulrich A, Matsuzaki H, Ding X, Ricordi C, Weide L, Moyer MP, Batra SK, Adrian TE, Pour PM. Transdifferentiation of human islet cells in a long-term culture. *Pancreas* 2001; 23: 157–71.
159. Yang L, Li S, Hatch H, Ahrens K, Cornelius JG, Petersen BE, Peck AB. In vitro trans-differentiation of adult hepatic stem cells into pancreatic endocrine hormone-producing cells. *Proc Natl Acad Sci USA* 2002; 99: 8078–83.
160. Abraham EJ, Leech CA, Lin JC, Zulewski H, Habener JF. Insulinotropic hormone glucagon-like peptide-1 differentiation of human pancreatic islet-derived progenitor cells into insulin-producing cells. *Endocrinology* 2002; 143: 3152–61.
161. Soria B, Roche E, Berna G, Leon-Quinto T, Reig JA, Martin F. Insulin-secreting cells derived from embryonic stem cells normalize glycemia in streptozotocin-induced diabetic mice. *Diabetes* 2000; 49: 157–62.
162. Lumelsky N, Blondel O, Laeng P, Velasco I, Ravin R, McKay R. Differentiation of embryonic stem cells to insulin-secreting structures similar to pancreatic islets. *Science* 2001; 292: 1389–94.
163. Schuldiner M, Yanuka O, Itskovitz-Eldor J, Melton DA, Benvenisty N. Effects of eight growth factors on the differentiation of cells derived from human embryonic stem cells. *Proc Natl Acad Sci USA* 2000; 97: 11307–12.
164. Assady S, Maor G, Amit M, Itskovitz-Eldor J, Skorecki KL, Tzukerman M. Insulin production by human embryonic stem cells. *Diabetes* 2001; 50: 1691–7.
165. Edlund H. Pancreatic organogenesis–developmental mechanisms and implications for therapy. *Nat Rev Genet* 2002; 3: 524–32.
166. Wurmser AE, Gage FH. Stem cells: cell fusion causes confusion. *Nature* 2002; 416: 485–7.

5

Morphology of the Pancreas in Normal and Diabetic States

A. Clark

Oxford Centre for Diabetes, Endocrinology and Metabolism, Oxford, UK

THE NORMAL PANCREAS

Macroscopy

The pancreas lies adjacent to the larger curvature of the stomach and is so called since it appears to permeate the supporting membranes of the gut, particularly in rodents—hence *pan creas* from the Greek, which means "tissue throughout." It has two separate functions: the larger exocrine component produces digestive enzymes, which drain into the duodenum via the pancreatic duct, and the much smaller and more diffuse endocrine pancreas, which secretes hormones into the circulation. An adult human pancreas typically weighs 40–150 g and the dispersed islets of Langerhans comprise the endocrine pancreas, which is 2–5% of the total pancreatic mass [1, 2]. For descriptive purposes it is anatomically divided into three regions: the head, which lies adjacent to the duodenum and consists of tissue derived from both the ventral and dorsal embryonic primordium [3]; the body, which is the central part lying under the greater curvature of the stomach; and the tail, the portion adjacent to the spleen. However, the pancreas is a homogeneous structure with continuous drainage of all of the lobules of the exocrine tissue via branches of the pancreatic duct that empty into the duodenum.

Islets of Langerhans

The endocrine cell clusters (islets), which are visible only with the microscope, were first identified by Paul Langerhans in his thesis of 1869 [4], and were named after Langerhans 24 years later by Laguess [5]. This generated considerable interest in the world of pathology and careful observations were made of the tinctorial properties of the different cells in the islets. The significance of these small cellular masses in the control of glucose metabolism was identified in 1889 when removal of the pancreas by von Mering and Minkowski was shown to induce hyperglycemia [6].

The islets of Langerhans are surrounded by a "sea" of exocrine tissue. The number of islets in humans has been estimated to be between 1 000 000 and 10 000; these numbers have been determined in different ways and the classification of what constitutes an islet also differs [2, 7]. While the islet shape is roughly spherical in rodents, in humans, islets are less regular and vary in size from less than 50 μm to more than 500 μm in diameter [8]. Islets appear to be randomly distributed throughout the exocrine tissue when viewed in a histological section. However, as a result of their embryological origin from the pancreatic ducts, islets can be seen in rodents (particularly in the mouse where islets are relatively large) to remain relatively close to the ducts and the islet vascular stalk is in close proximity to the ductal structures [9]. Islet density is considered to be higher in the tail of the pancreas compared to the body region, but it is highest in the portion of the head derived from the ventral primordium where islets consist largely of cells containing pancreatic polypeptide [10, 11].

Structure of the Islet

The endocrine cells have many features in common with neuroendocrine cells. Both types have a large central

International Textbook of Diabetes Mellitus, Third Edition. Edited by R. A. DeFronzo, E. Ferrannini, H. Keen, and P. Zimmet.
 ISBN: 0-471-48655-8.

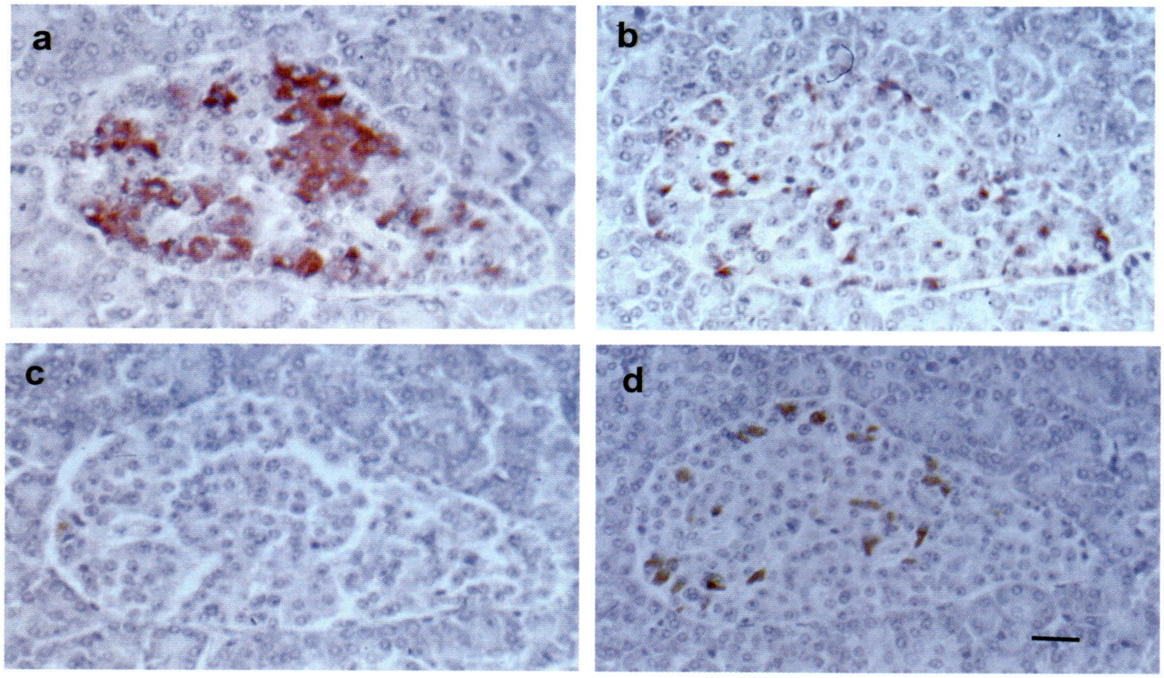

Figure 1 Distribution of different types of endocrine cells in islets. Serial sections of a normal human islet from the body region of the pancreas immunolabeled for different hormones: (a) insulin-containing β-cells (brown) are mostly in clusters and are situated toward the central region of the islet. (b) Cells immunoreactive for glucagon (α-cells) are distributed throughout the islet section. These cells border capillaries that surround the islet and penetrate into the central region. (c) Pancreatic-polypeptide-containing cells are infrequent in islets from this part of the pancreas. (d) Somatostatin-containing δ-cells are elongated and also line islet capillaries. Scale bar = 50 μm

nucleus and relatively clear cytoplasm containing the machinery for production and storage of secretory granules. Islets consist of four main cell types. Islet β-cells secreting insulin are the most numerous, forming 60–80% of the islet mass. α-Cells form up to 25% of the islet and produce glucagon. These cell types were first identified by Lane [12]. δ-Cells secreting somatostatin form 2–8% of the islet mass [13] and cells containing pancreatic polypeptide (PP-cells) [14] are very infrequent (1–2%) in islets in the major part of the pancreas (Figure 1a–d). More than 90% of the endocrine cell mass is present in islets; some isolated endocrine cells are found in or adjacent to the ductal epithelium in an adult human and some small single cells and cell clusters (defined as consisting of less than five cells) are found adjacent to ducts or scattered within the exocrine tissue [15, 16]. It is unclear if these are functional units with intact machinery to enable hormone release in response to a stimulus such as glucose. In the portion of the head that lies adjacent to the duodenum and is derived during organogenesis from the ventral primordium, the islets consist largely of PP-cells [17]. The islets in this region are not ovoid but irregular in shape, spreading between the exocrine lobules. In the remainder of the pancreas, derived from the dorsal primordium, the islets have the characteristic cellular composition and semiovoid shape.

Insulin-secreting β-Cells

This was the second cell type to be identified by silver staining in 1907, the first being the A-cells (named due to fixation by Alcohol) [12]. The hormone within β-cells was later identified as being isletin, or insulin [18]. The cells containing insulin are located in clusters (Figure 1a) within the islet and are connected by tight junctions to form a functional syncytium [19]. This allows coordinated secretion from β-cells within an islet. In rodents, β-cells are located toward the center of the islet and surrounded by a mantle of non-β-cells. However, in humans, this cellular architecture is less clear; in cross sections of islets, non-β-cells are also found within the central portion of the islet. This is due to differences in the capillary network of the islet. Non-β-cells line the islet capillaries, which, in humans, penetrate the central region of the islet. Islet architecture is significantly different in cats, guinea pigs [20], and horses [21], where non-β-cells still line the capillaries but are located largely toward the central region of the islet.

Insulin is stored in β-cells in secretory granules that have an electron dense core and an electron lucent halo (Figure 2). Immature granules containing the precursor peptide proinsulin are less electron dense and lack a halo;

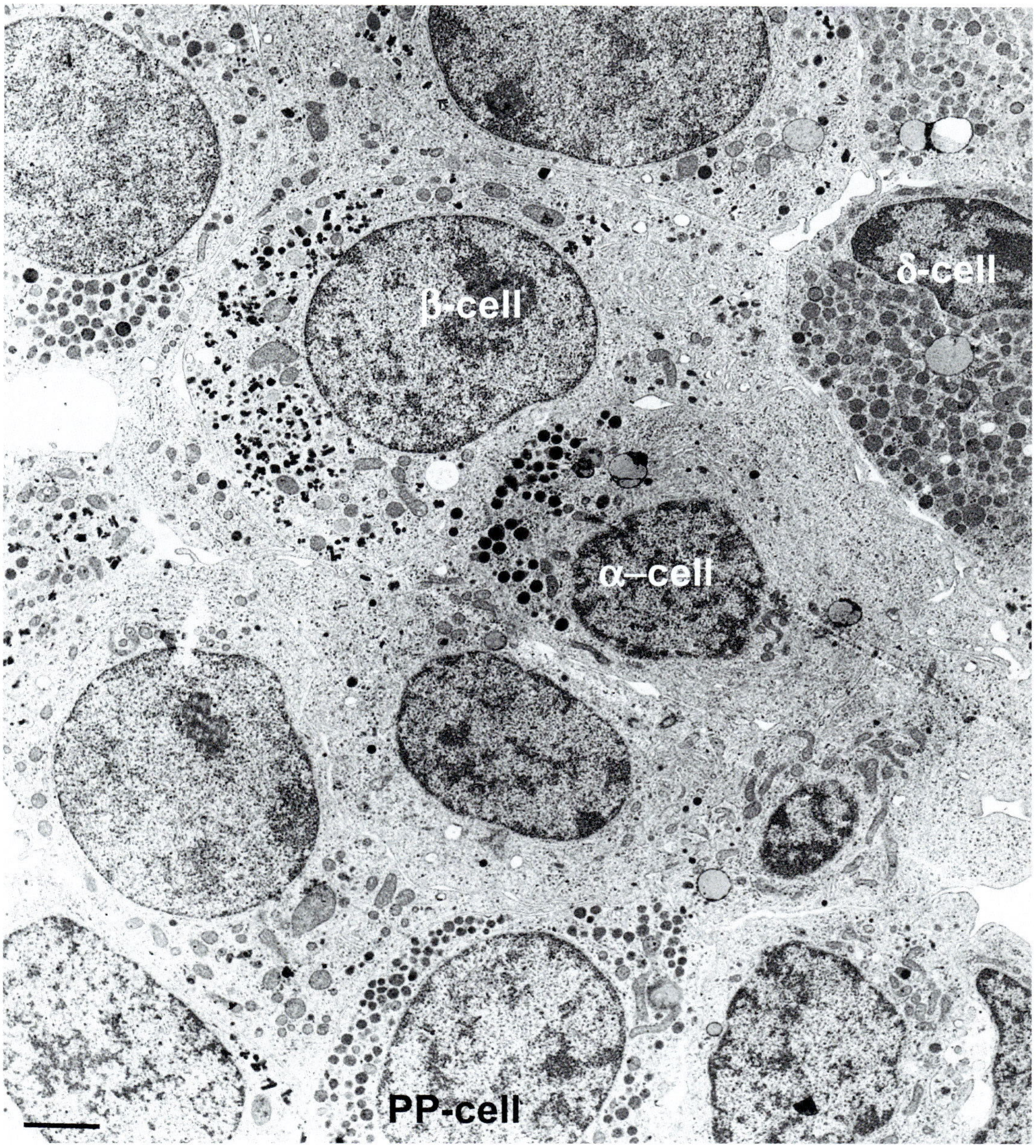

Figure 2 Electron micrograph of a cross section of a human islet. Cells are in close apposition with each other with connections through tight junctions. β-Cells contain granules that have a characteristic electron dense core and an electron lucent halo. The dense core is often crystalline in appearance in mature granules, indicating hexameric assemblies of insulin with zinc. Granules in α-cells are electron dense and relatively uniform in size whereas granules in PP-cells are electron dense but heterogeneous in size. Somatostatin-containing cells are usually packed with granules that are relatively pale and large. Scale bar = 1 μm

as the granule matures, proteolytic cleavage results in separation of insulin, which assembles into an insoluble hexameric complex with zinc, which forms the dense core [22–24]. The secretory granule contains many other compounds including high concentrations of calcium, the proteolytic enzymes (prohormone convertase 1/3 and 2 and carboxypeptidase), chromogranin, and the connecting peptide of proinsulin, C-peptide. In addition, islet amyloid polypeptide is co-stored in β-cell granules and co-released with insulin [25]; this peptide is the component peptide of islet amyloid deposits that form in type 2 diabetes [26]. Granule content of β-cells is variable and has been estimated as 10 000 granules per cell. As a result of stimulus–secretion coupling, granules docked at the plasma membrane are released by exocytosis into the extracellular space [27] where the hexamer dissociates and insulin diffuses to the islet capillaries. It has been estimated that the granule concentration of insulin is 40 mM;

this high concentration necessitates strategies such as hexamer formation to prevent precipitation and inactivation of this relatively insoluble peptide within the cell.

Glucagon-secreting α-Cells

Glucagon-containing cells line the islet capillaries and are adjacent to other cell types including β-cells (Figure 1b). This situation permits receipt of signaling from the blood supply and communication within the islet by locally released hormone, known as paracrine signaling; in addition, glucagon acts at distant sites by hormone released into the capillaries. Glucagon granules are electron dense, with a slightly paler peripheral region (Figure 2). Like proinsulin, proglucagon is processed into pancreatic glucagon by proteolysis in the secretory granules [28]. Glucagon release is stimulated by insulin and by low concentrations of glucose.

Somatostatin-containing δ-Cells

Somatostatin regulates cellular secretion in all cells by hypopolarizing the cell membrane [29]. These cells are filled with large granules and possess long processes that allow contact with many cells within the islet (Figure 2). In this way they are similar to neuroendocrine δ-cells found in the hypothalamus where secretion of somatostatin also inhibits hormone secretion [30]. Unlike other hormones secreted from the islet, the half-life of somatostatin is very short, and therefore its action is largely paracrine, inhibiting secretion from adjacent cells and acting via tight junctions.

Pancreatic-Polypeptide-containing PP-Cells

The function of this hormone and control of its secretion are largely unknown. Cells are infrequent in islets of the body and tail. Cells can be identified by the granule population, which is electron dense but very heterogeneous in size (Figure 2), and the relatively infrequent distribution in islets. Pancreatic polypeptide is also found in endocrine cells of the duodenum and has been shown to modulate gastric secretion and motility. It is closely related to other gastrointestinal peptides such as peptide YY and NPY that have important roles in control of appetite. The highest concentration of PP-cells is in islets of the pancreatic head, where the islet density of PP-cells is up to 75% and the density of α-cells and β-cells is lower than that found in the major part of the pancreas [1, 10, 11, 31].

TYPE 1 (INSULIN-DEPENDENT) DIABETES

Macroscopy and Pathophysiology

The age of onset of type 1 diabetes is typically in the first and second decades but the age of diagnosis is getting lower, with many children being diagnosed under the age of 3 years. The pancreas in patients with recent-onset type 1 diabetes is macroscopically normal compared with age-matched specimens from nondiabetic subjects. After many years of disease, pancreatic size is reduced [32–36]. Erosion of exocrine tissue occurs specifically adjacent to islets with insulitis [37], suggesting that both exocrine and endocrine functions are compromised during the early acute stages of the disease. This has been attributed to the lack of local high concentrations of insulin, which are required for normal functioning of the exocrine cells [38, 39]. The degree of pancreatic reduction is very variable and is also dependent upon the age and obesity of the subject.

The sequence of events that leads to autoimmune destruction of β-cells remains largely unknown [40]. As with other autoimmune diseases, a characteristic feature is the presence in the circulation of autoantibodies directed against components of the affected organ. These autoantibodies are markers of an incipient or active autoimmune process and can be used for diagnosis of the disease. In type 1 diabetes, patients can possess several autoantibodies that can indicate either the stages or the severity of the disease process; these are antibodies to nonspecified islet proteins (ICA), to insulin (IAA), to glutamic acid decarboxylase (GAD; either GAD65 or the related but different molecule GAD67), to insulin granule proteins phogrin (IA12), or to islet antigen 2 (IA-2). These specific, antigenic proteins are all found at intracellular sites in islet β-cells.

The causative factors for and the associated islet pathology in type 1 diabetes still remain unclear [41, 42]. There is a genetic predisposition for autoimmune diabetes [43] but environmental factors are also important. The MHC locus (*IDDM1*) is the most important gene region for type 1 diabetes susceptibility [44]. This has led to hypotheses suggesting that class II MHC molecules become aberrantly expressed on β-cells and autoantigens are presented either by β-cells or indirectly by antigen-presenting cells such as macrophages or dendritic cells within the islets. This process leads to cell death.

Islet Changes

In the acute phase of onset of type 1 diabetes the islets demonstrate insulitis, and mononuclear cells including macrophages and dendritic cells accumulate within the islets [37, 45]; β-cells show decreased immunoreactivity for insulin and are progressively destroyed (Figure 3a and b). The affected islets at the initiation of the disease are distributed in a lobular fashion such that all islets in one pancreatic lobule can have insulitis but islets appear normal in adjacent lobules [37]. As the disease progresses, all islets can become affected, β-cells are destroyed, and the insulitis disappears [46]. At the very early stages in

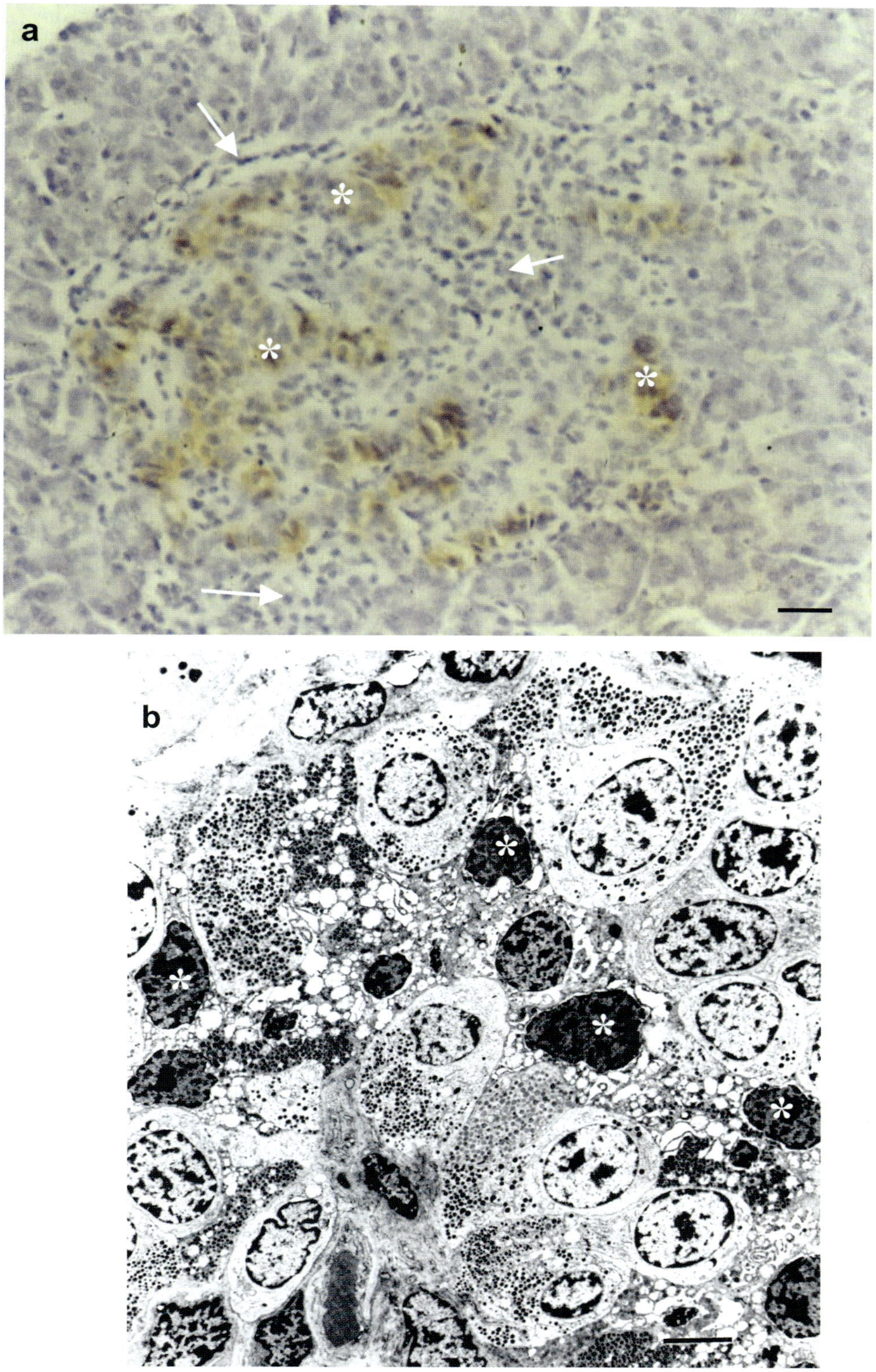

Figure 3 Islets from a type 1 diabetic subject in the acute phase of the disease. (a) Light microscopy with cells labeled for insulin (brown) demonstrating diffuse insulin staining (∗) in the remaining β-cells. Lymphocytic infiltration (⟹) is extensive. Scale bar = 50 μm. (b) Electron micrograph of islet from the same patient. Apoptotic β-cells (∗) are present, which have degenerating, vacuolated cytoplasm. Other endocrine cell types are also present, which contain many granules and are not affected by the autoimmune attack. Scale bar = 2 μm

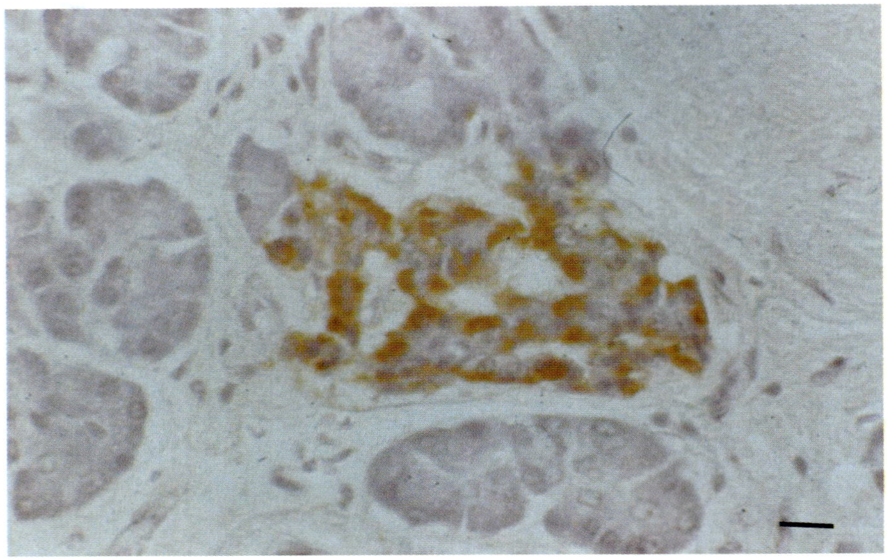

Figure 4 Islet morphology after many years of type 1 diabetes. Cells immunolabeled for glucagon fill most of the islet, which is irregular in shape. The islet appears to have imploded following loss of the centrally clustered β-cells. Scale bar = 14 μm

unaffected islets, immunoreactivity for HLA-DR can be found in islets that are apparently not yet affected [47, 48]. This supports the theory that there is increased expression of HLA preceding the immune attack. Since the pathological factors, the genetics, the age of onset, and severity of the acute autoimmune reaction are quite variable, it is likely that more than one process is involved in the destruction of the islet cells in type 1 diabetes. The outcome of the destructive process, which can last from 1 week to several months or even years, is loss of β-cells but other cell types remain. The islets become irregular in shape as if the islet became imploded as a result of the loss of the core of β-cells and consist of cells containing, glucagon, somatostatin, and PP (Figure 4).

Autoimmune diabetes can develop in older patients, e.g. over the age of 35 years. It is then described as latent autoimmune diabetes in adults (LADA). The onset of the disease is generally less severe and often mistakenly diagnosed as type 2 diabetes. However, these patients are autoantibody positive and require insulin-replacement therapy at an earlier stage than subjects with classical type 2 diabetes [49]. There are no data on pancreatic pathology in well-characterized subjects with LADA but insulin-positive cells have been identified in islets after more than 20 years of autoimmune, insulin-requiring diabetes [34], suggesting that, at least in these subjects, some islets/cells can be protected against the total autoimmune destruction of β-cells seen in classical type 1 diabetes. This may be one condition when β-cell mass, rather than cellular function, is an important contributor to the severity of the disease. However, whether LADA is a separate disease entity or a slowly developing form of type 1 diabetes remains to be elucidated.

TYPE 2 (NON-INSULIN-DEPENDENT) DIABETES

Macroscopy and Pathophysiology

The macroscopic appearance of the pancreas from patients with type 2 (non-insulin-dependent) diabetes is largely unchanged; many patients are, however, obese and this is apparent in the pancreas in the form of enlarged adipocytes within the exocrine lobules and connective tissue matrix (Figure 5). The degree of lipid deposition, with or without diabetes, is related to the extent of adiposity with more and larger adipocytes in very obese subjects [50]. The overall weight of the pancreas is therefore proportionally increased in these obese subjects. However, when the degree of lipid deposition is subtracted, the pancreatic tissue mass is either unchanged or reduced. Deposition of fat in the pancreas is reversible, often with increased pancreatic function if obese subjects lose weight [51]. In type 2 diabetes there is also evidence for fibrotic changes in the exocrine tissue, suggesting a degree of subclinical pancreatitis. Decreased exocrine function as assessed by exocrine secretion studies has been described in patients with type 2 diabetes [52].

The pathophysiology of type 2 diabetes includes insulin resistance of peripheral tissues but also islet dysfunction resulting in an inappropriate insulin secretion in relation to glucose concentrations [53, 54]. Thus, most type 2 diabetic patients at diagnosis have the capacity to secrete insulin but lack the usual sensitive control of insulin production. The factors that modify insulin secretion in type 2 diabetes are poorly understood. The pancreatic islets of type 2 diabetic subjects in postmortem tissue always contain insulin-immunoreactive cells and there

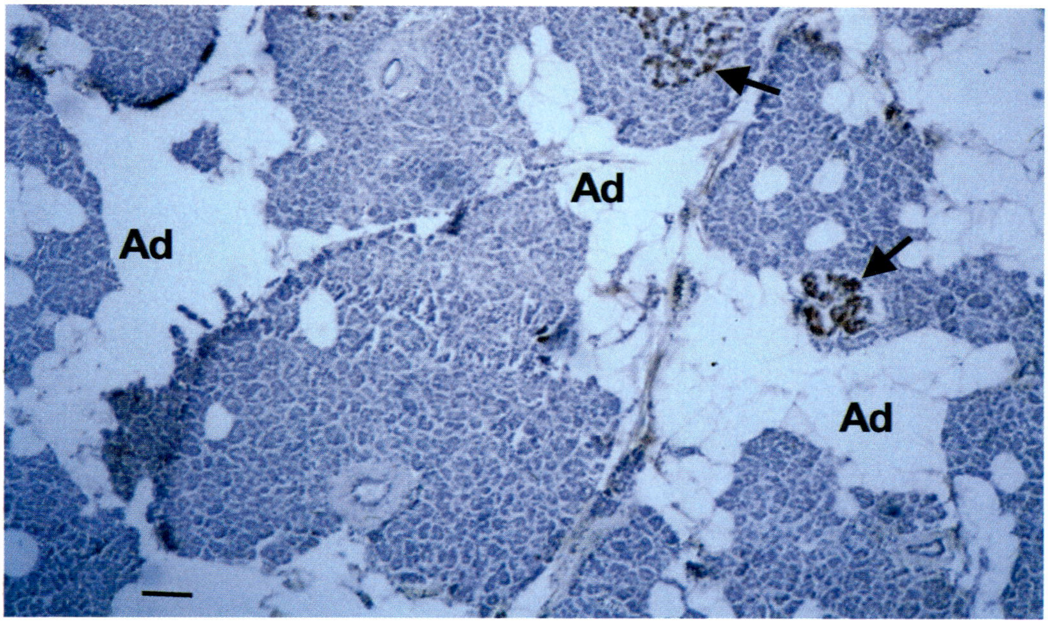

Figure 5 Pancreatic lipid deposition in an obese patient with type 2 diabetes. Swollen adipocytes (Ad) are present both between and within the exocrine lobules. There are some lipid accumulations within the islets that are immunolabeled for insulin (⇨). Scale bar = 200 μm

appears to be no evidence for decreased immunoreactivity for insulin which would be consistent with cellular degranulation. This has been proposed as an explanation for the lack of first-phase insulin secretion associated with β-cell dysfunction in type 2 diabetes. There is an increase in the proportion of unprocessed proinsulin secreted in these patients and it has been reported that increased labeling for proinsulin is found in islets of type 2 diabetic subjects [55], suggesting that there are more granules containing unprocessed propeptide than would normally occur. However, expression of the (pro)insulin gene is not affected in islets of diabetic subjects [11].

Islets in patients with type 2 diabetes contain β-cells and many islets are identical in appearance to those found in similarly aged nondiabetic subjects; the only abnormal feature of some islets in type 2 diabetes is deposition of islet amyloid [56]. While the reduction in insulin secretion in type 1 diabetes is related to a severe decline in the population of β-cells, this is not the situation in most patients with type 2 diabetes. It is therefore unclear if the important etiological factors for the onset of this form of diabetes are functional or result from modest changes in endocrine cellular proportion [57].

Changes in Mass of Endocrine Cells in Diabetes

The proportions of endocrine cells in type 2 diabetes have been reported to be unchanged; data vary from no-change in β-cells to a 30–50% reduction [1, 7, 10, 11, 31, 58, 59]. The variability of these data reflects not only the heterogeneous nature of the disease but also other problems inherent in such studies, such as the necessity of using postmortem material and selection of appropriate controls for this elderly population of type 2 diabetic subjects for additional features of pancreatic pathology, such as obesity, pancreatitis, duration of disease [59]. Quantitative changes are expressed in different ways by different authors, e.g. β-cell volume or mass, and β-cells as a proportion to exocrine or islet area. All features of the exocrine tissue will influence the outcome. Also, changes in pancreatic pathology can be induced by the immediate premortem period when poor circulation and glucose intolerance may have occurred.

The relationship between functional and quantitative changes of islet cells has been more clearly identified in rodent models than in humans [60]. While a 95% partial pancreatectomy is required to induce hyperglycemia in rodents [61], removal of 30% of the pancreas in monkeys results in diabetes [62]. Hemipancreatectomy in a normal adult human was reported to not induce diabetes [63]. This suggests that, under normal conditions, the β-cell population exceeds that required to maintain normoglycemia in most species. Conditions of severe insulin resistance, if β-cell secretion can be more than doubled, do not automatically result in hyperglycemia; therefore there must be considerable reserve capacity for insulin production in the human pancreas. It is unlikely that any moderate reduction in β-cell mass would

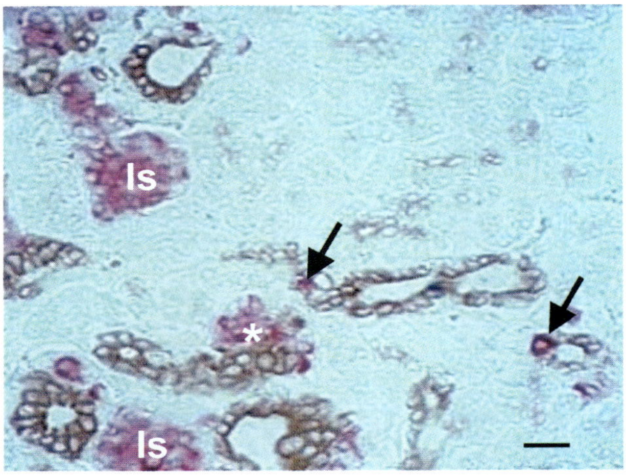

Figure 6 Neogenesis of β-cells from ductal stem cells in adult human pancreas. Specimen from a type 2 diabetic subject immunolabeled for insulin (red – ⇒) and cytokeratin 19 (brown-marker for ductal epithelial cells). Islets (Is) and small islet cell clusters (∗) are present close to ducts. Insulin-positive cells are situated within the ductal epithelial layer (⇒), suggesting neoformation from a ductal stem cell. Ductal endocrine cells containing all pancreatic hormone types and β-cell clusters have been identified in human nondiabetic and diabetic pancreas. Scale bar = 20 μm

be important unless function was also compromised [57].

It has been suggested from studies in rodents that diabetes results from an imbalance of a normal cycle of turnover of islet cells [64]: an increase in apoptosis or a decreased neogenesis of β-cells [65, 66]. At present there is little evidence for extensive regeneration of β-cells by division of differentiated islet cells or death by apoptosis in normal human islets [16]. However, single β-cells associated with ducts and clusters of β-cells have been identified in specimens of pancreas from both nondiabetic and type 2 diabetic subjects (Figure 6) [15, 16], suggesting that there is potential for neogenesis of islet cells in adults. It is unclear if these cells, which form less than 1% of pancreatic β-cell mass, contribute to the functional mass of endocrine cells or any active turnover process.

Islet Amyloid and Type 2 Diabetes

Deposits of amyloid within the islets is a characteristic feature of type 2 diabetes (Figure 7a and b): at postmortem, more than 90% of type 2 diabetic subjects have amyloid deposits in islets [67–69]; the deposits are less frequently (up to 12%) found in nondiabetic subjects of similar age [70]. Islet amyloid is not associated with systemic amyloidosis and deposits are restricted to pancreatic islets. Hyaline deposits in pancreatic islets in diabetes were first described by Opie [71] and subsequently shown to be amyloid [72]. Islet amyloidosis has been identified in diabetic patients in every ethnic group examined including Pima Indians [73], Asian Indians [73, 74], and Japanese [11, 58]. The deposition of islet amyloid within a pancreas is heterogeneous; not all islets have amyloid in type 2 diabetic subjects [75] and affected islets are often clustered in a

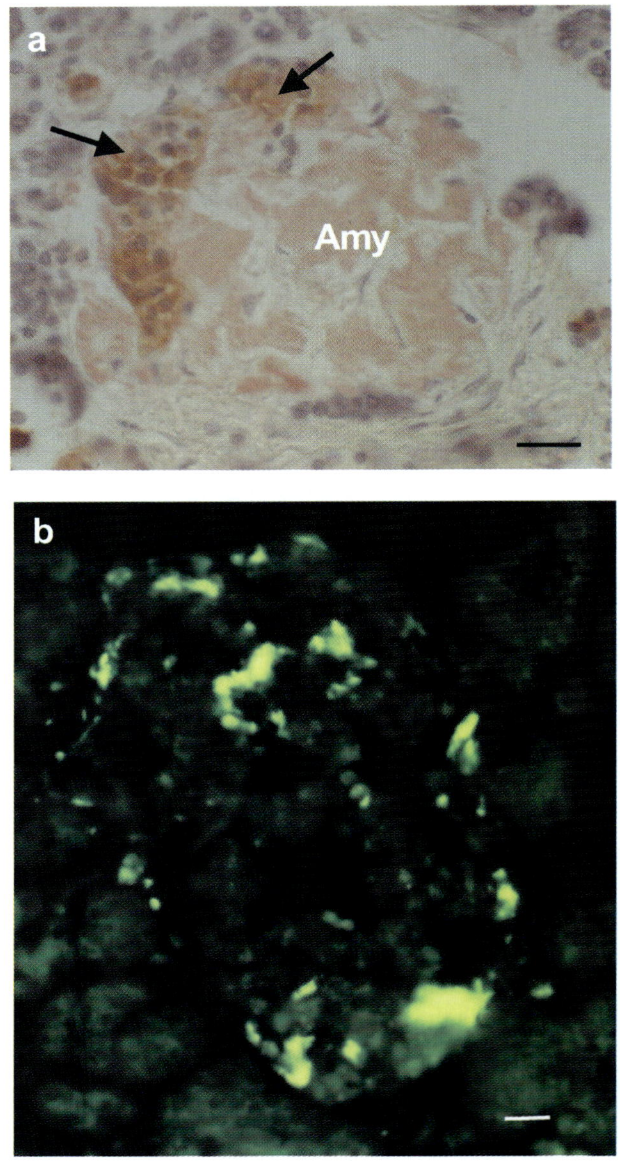

Figure 7 Islet amyloid deposition in type 2 diabetes. (a) Insulin-containing β-cells (brown – ⇒) have been replaced by amyloid (Amy) (pink – labeled with congo-red) that occupies more than 50% of the islet space. This patient had been diabetic for 12 years and was on oral diabetic therapy, and more than 80% islets examined throughout the pancreas were affected. (b) Islet demonstrating less amyloid deposition. Amyloid is labeled fluorescent green with thioflavine S and fibril accumulations are mostly adjacent to capillaries at the periphery of the islet (⇒). This patient had been diabetic for 10 years and was on oral diabetic therapy, and less than 1% of the islets examined were affected. Scale bars = 20 μm

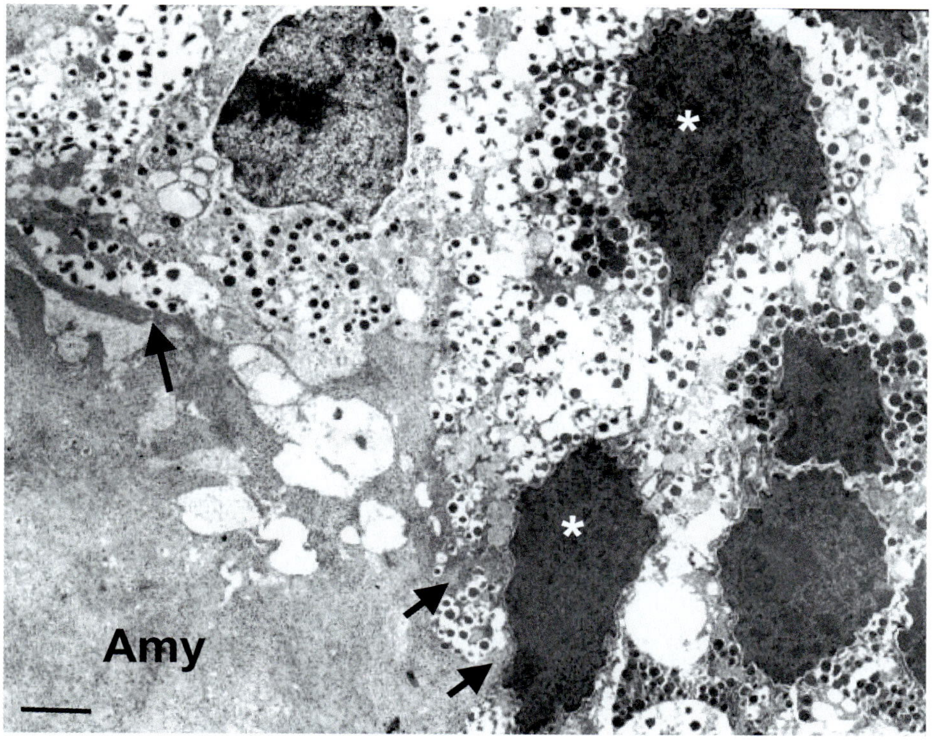

Figure 8 Amyloid accumulates in islets adjacent to endocrine cells in type 2 diabetes. Amorphous amyloid deposits lie in invaginations of the β-cells (⟹) and cause apoptosis of adjacent cells (black nuclei – ∗) in a human type 2 diabetic islet. Cells contain the usual population of insulin granules in diabetes. Scale bar = 2.5 μm

lobular distribution in the body and tail of the pancreas. Amyloid is not found in the islets derived from the ventral primordium in the head of the pancreas where few β-cells are present [76].

Islet amyloid fibrils are formed from islet amyloid polypeptide (IAPP), also known as amylin. This 37-amino acid peptide was identified in 1987 as the component peptide of islet amyloid deposits [77, 78] and found to be a normally occurring peptide of the β-cell, co-stored with insulin in secretory granules and co-released in response to β-cell secretagogues [25, 79–81]. The causal factors for refolding of IAPP into a β-sheet conformation and molecular oligomerization to form amyloid fibrils are largely unknown, but variations in the region IAPP 20–29 contribute to the absence of islet amyloid in rodent models of diabetes [82, 83]. Unlike some other types of amyloidosis, there is no evidence for production of a genetically determined abnormal IAPP molecule in type 2 diabetes [84, 85]. Proposed causal factors for islet amyloidosis include overproduction of IAPP or abnormal cleavage of proIAPP, and decreased clearance of secreted peptide or its association with basement membrane components in the extracellular space [57, 82]. However, there is no evidence that amyloid is a major factor for the onset of the disease in humans; some patients with diabetes of many years' duration have less than 1% of their islets affected, suggesting that amyloid deposition is a complication rather than an etiological factor for the pathogenesis of the disease [82].

Initially IAPP fibrils accumulate in the perivascular space between islet cells and the islet capillary basement membrane: fibrils are found in close apposition to the membrane of β-cells and in invagination of the membrane (Figure 8). This localization could compromise glucose signaling, insulin secretion, and mobility of membrane components. Progressively, the fibril accumulations increase in size and occupy more of the islet interior (Figure 7a). Amyloid deposits gradually replace endocrine cells and, in some patients, more than 80% of the islet endocrine cell mass is replaced with fibrils [10]. Increased degree of amyloidosis (more islets affected and more amyloid mass per islet) is related to the requirement for insulin replacement therapy in type 2 diabetic subjects [69, 86], suggesting that amyloidosis is a causal factor for the severe decline of islet function that occurs later in the diabetic syndrome. This hypothesis is supported by studies *in vitro* showing that synthetic human IAPP fibrils are toxic to cells by induction of apoptosis [87], and islet amyloidosis progressively replaces islet β-cells in diabetic monkeys [88] and transgenic mice expressing the gene for human IAPP (hIAPP TM) [90].

In experimental models such as hIAPP TM, fibrils form only against a background of overexpression of the transgene, obesity (high-fat diet or expression of obesity genes), or increased insulin resistance [89–92]. This suggests that overproduction and decreased clearance of hIAPP in the islet are important factors for amyloid formation. However, current data indicate that IAPP production in humans parallels changes in insulin secretion that accompany increased insulin resistance in normal subjects or those with IGT or with diabetes [93], and there is no evidence for a disproportionate increased secretion of IAPP in type 2 diabetes. The factors that initiate fibrillogenesis in type 2 diabetes are therefore still obscure.

IAPP amyloid also forms in human insulinomas [94]. These tumors secrete high concentrations of β-cell products including IAPP, insulin, and proinsulin. Increased production of abnormally processed proIAPP could be a factor in amyloidosis. ProIAPP fragments have been identified in IAPP amyloid deposits [95], and proIAPP binds to heparan sulfate, which is a basement membrane proteoglycan and has been shown to accelerate IAPP fibril formation [96]. Increased production of incompletely processed proinsulin is a characteristic feature of type 2 diabetes [97] and could be accompanied by increased proIAPP, which could initiate fibrillogenesis.

THE PANCREAS IN DEFINED SUBGROUPS OF TYPE 2 DIABETES

There are now several well-defined, genetic or environmental conditions that result in diabetes and some of which result in pancreatic changes.

Maturity-Onset Diabetes of the Young (MODY)

Maturity-onset diabetes of the young (MODY) describes a group of conditions of genetically determined type 2 diabetes developing at a younger age [98–100]. The genes involved are expressed in the pancreatic β-cell and mutations are likely to result in changes in islet development and morphology [101, 102]. However, little is known of the pancreatic pathology in these conditions. In one subject diagnosed with MODY2 (mutation in the gene for glucokinase), the islet proportion in postmortem pancreas was unchanged and no islet amyloid was present [103]. This lack of islet amyloid was confirmed in a transgenic mouse model expressing the human IAPP gene and a mutation in glucokinase [104]. Since MODY2 is associated with reduced β-cell secretion of both IAPP and insulin, it could be expected that amyloid would not be formed. MODY types 1, 3, 4, 5, and 6 are all associated with heterozygous mutations in transcription factors [102] and affect not only transcriptional control of insulin and other β-cell genes but the development of the pancreatic β-cell [105]. The pancreas from subjects with these forms of MODY have not been examined. However, deletions in *PDX-1* gene (MODY5) result in pancreatic agenesis in humans [106] and mutations in the hepatic nuclear factor (HNF) genes are associated with abnormal pancreatic development in rodents [105]. It is likely therefore that the pancreatic islets in patients with other forms of MODY involving transcription factors would demonstrate some changes in endocrine cell populations.

Mitochondrial Gene Mutations

Mutations in genes for mitochondrial proteins are associated with type 2 diabetes [107–110] and patients with mtDNA mutations have reduced insulin secretion [108] and decreased β-cell population [111]. In a patient with a severe mitochondrial myopathy, Kearns-Sayre syndrome, who developed diabetes at age 8 years and died aged 20, islets were substantially smaller, suggesting that adequate cellular energy requirements are essential for islet growth *in utero* and development and function in the early years [112]. The frequency of mitochondrial gene mutations is less than 1.0% in classical type 2 diabetes [109] and can be considered to be a genetically distinct subtype of type 2 diabetes.

Wolfram Syndrome

Wolfram syndrome or DIDMOAD (diabetes insipidus, diabetes mellitus, optical atrophy, and deafness) is a rare congenital and complex neurological and endocrinological condition [113]. These subjects possess mutations in the Wolfram gene *WFS1* on chromosome 4p16.3 and develop diabetes mellitus in the course of the disease, often at puberty [114]. In these patients, pancreatic islets are small as in mitochondrial disease, suggesting that β-cell growth and development is inadequate to sustain normoglycemia.

DIABETES SECONDARY TO OTHER CONDITIONS

Pancreatitis

The relationship of pancreatitis to the pathophysiology of diabetes is unclear; acute pancreatitis can result in temporary impaired glucose tolerance or overt diabetes. Chronic pancreatitis is associated with diabetes in up to 50% of patients whose principal diagnosis is exocrine disease but it is also relatively common in type 2 diabetic subjects. Chronic pancreatitis is associated with recurrent attacks of pancreatic inflammation, which can be asymptomatic or cause severe pain. In extreme conditions ductal calcification occurs owing to impaired drainage of calcium-rich secretions; pancreatic stones formed from calcium carbonate accretions are formed in ducts and further reduce drainage (Figure 9). Pancreatitis is apparent in surgical or postmortem specimens as a mononuclear cell infiltrate into acinar tissue and periductular spaces. Later, the process

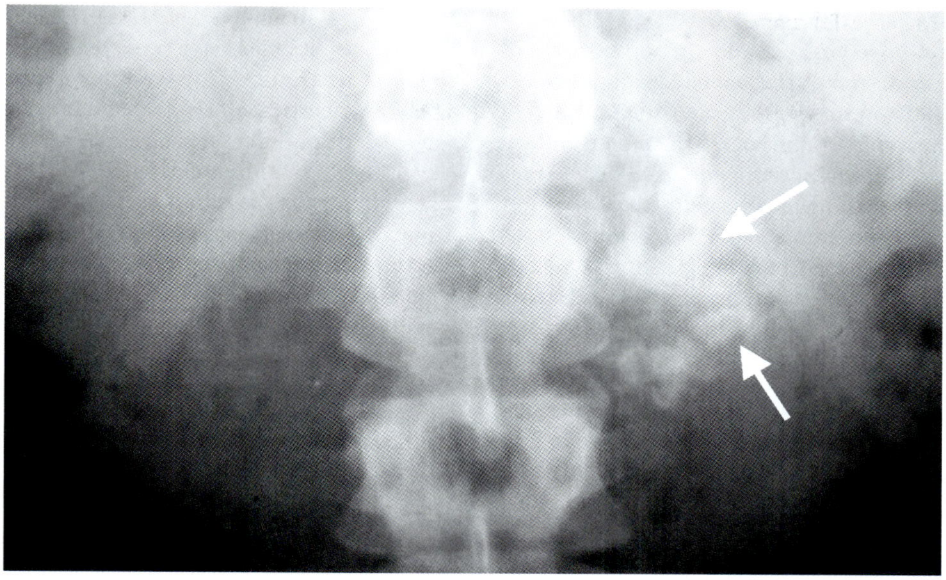

Figure 9 X-ray of a patient with calcific pancreatic nodules (⟹) associated with chronic pancreatitis

is apparent as replacement of exocrine tissue with fibrotic material. This is present as interlobular and intralobular fibrosis. Quantitation indicates an increase of this material in postmortem pancreas in type 2 diabetes [10]. Reduced exocrine function has been described in type 2 diabetes [52]. However, islet tissue remains relatively unaffected; the islets become embedded in the fibrotic tissue and may cluster together, apparently isolated from the remaining exocrine tissue; this gives the appearance of a small adenoma or a neogenic structure. Quantitative immunocytochemistry has demonstrated a reduction in the proportion of β-cells to α-cells in these islets [115]. Pancreatitis is associated with proliferation of larger ductular structures as the disease progresses; neogenesis of both ductular epithelium and endocrine cells occurs with "new" islet cell clusters appearing adjacent to ducts (Figure 10).

Although the role of the exocrine pancreas in endocrine pancreas function is not at all clear, the association of

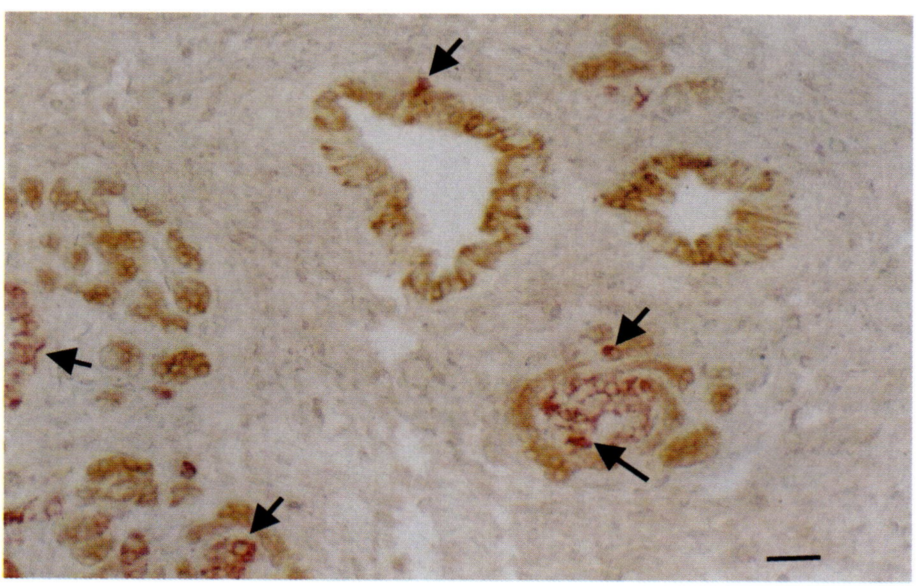

Figure 10 Pancreatic ductal proliferation and endocrine neogenesis in pancreatitis. Ductal epithelial cells (brown – labeled for cytokeratin19) form new branching ductules in fibrotic regions of the pancreas. There is an increase in the neogenesis of insulin-positive cells (red – ⟹) in the dividing ducts. Scale bar = 25 μm

diseases of the exocrine tissue with diabetes, e.g. pancreatitis and cystic fibrosis, indicates the importance of the proximity of the two organs. Islets embedded in sclerosed or fibrotic material appear normal with a similar proportion of β-cells; impaired insulin secretion could therefore result from abnormal vascular supply/drainage or aberrant stimulus–secretion coupling as a result of their isolation from the exocrine tissue. In diabetes, where the origin of the pathology is in the islets, exocrine function could become impaired, resulting in decreased exocrine mass. This suggests that the symbiotic relationship of the two organs is essential to normal function.

Cystic Fibrosis and Diabetes

Patients with cystic fibrosis as a result of mutations in the chloride channel gene *CFTR* [116, 117] develop diabetes in the course of the disease; this has become more apparent with improved treatment and increased longevity of the patients, and at the age of 30 years, more than 50% of patients have diabetes. Insulin replacement therapy is the common form of treatment [118]. Many of the clinical features and the pancreatic morphological changes are similar to those of chronic pancreatitis. Abnormal exocrine and ductal secretions result in poor ductal drainage, exocrine atrophy, and replacement by sclerosed and lipid-containing tissues. Pancreatic islets become embedded in the fibrotic or lipid-containing material (Figure 11). The mechanics of insulin secretion are not affected by the mutation in *CFTR* gene but islet function is reduced; patients progress through glucose intolerance to frank diabetes [119]. Initially the islets have the normal population of endocrine cells [120, 121] but as the exocrine disease progresses, amyloid is deposited and β-cell population is reduced [122, 123]. Although the treatment of choice is insulin in cystic fibrosis, the pathophysiological progression of the diabetes and the presence of amyloid deposits suggest that abnormal islet function is related to type 2 diabetes rather than autoimmune type 1 diabetes. This further supports the hypothesis for an interrelationship of the exocrine and endocrine tissues; impaired vascular supply to the islets embedded in the connective tissue could be a major factor in the reduced insulin secretion.

Hemochromatosis

There is an association of diabetes with diseases that promote iron accumulation [124]. Iron is deposited in the exocrine tissue, giving the pancreas a typical brown color. There is less iron in the islets than in the exocrine tissue and islet size has been reported to be unchanged [125]; there was no evidence for death of β-cells in these patients but there was a significant reduction in insulin secretory granules. This suggests that iron overload could affect insulin gene expression and/or stimulus–secretion coupling.

Fibrocalculous Pancreatic Diabetes

This form of pancreatic pathology—FCPD (fibrocalculous pancreatic diabetes)—is widespread in countries within the tropics in Asia, India, and South America [126]. This condition was also known as tropical calcific pancreatic diabetes and/or malnutrition-related diabetes mellitus [127]. This form of the disease was originally considered

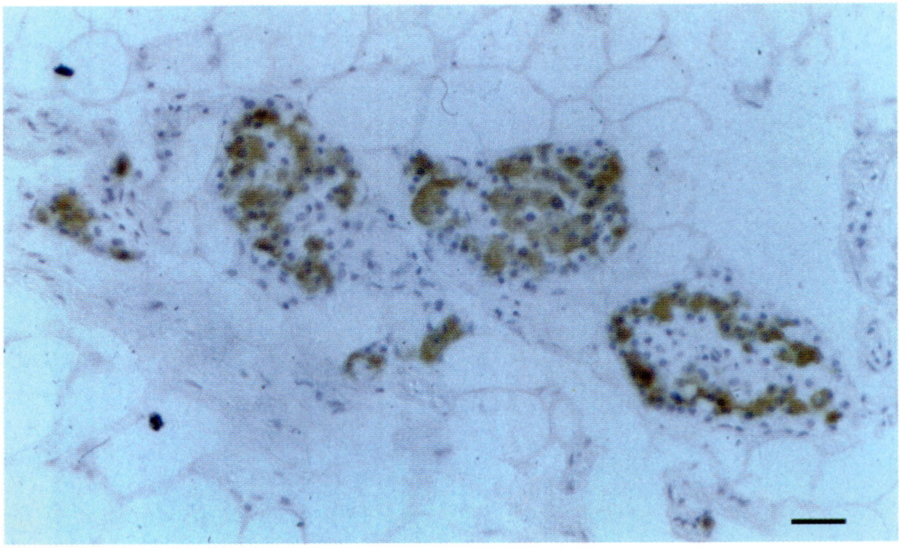

Figure 11 Pancreas from a diabetic patient with cystic fibrosis. The exocrine tissue has been replaced by a matrix of fibrotic and lipid-containing material in which the islets are suspended. In diabetic subjects, the islets contain the normal population of β-cells (brown) and islet amyloid is present in older patients. Scale bar = 38 μm

to be related to low protein diets and/or ingestion of some food toxins, in particular cassava [128, 129]. Diagnosis is made between the ages of 10–40 and is frequently associated with severe chronic pancreatitis [126]. The severity of the diabetes is variable, which is reflected in the heterogeneity of the pancreatic changes. In severe cases, the pancreas is small, fibrotic, and contains calcific nodules in the ducts, that are visible in abdominal X-rays [130]. These are similar to those found in other forms of chronic pancreatitis, which are composed largely of calcium carbonate in the form of calcite and include other metals laid down in layers. As the disease progresses, the exocrine tissue becomes atrophic and the islets, which contain the normal distribution of cells without amyloid deposition, become embedded in fibrous tissue [131]. Recent studies have demonstrated genetic susceptibility for FCPD at the MHC locus [132] and an association with a mutation in the serine protease inhibitor, Kazal type 1 gene *SPINK1* [133, 135].

Pancreatic Carcinoma

Adenocarcinomas of the pancreas can result in transient or persistent glucose intolerance or diabetes [135]. Commonly, these tumors develop in the head of the pancreas and result in impaired ductal drainage and features similar to those of pancreatitis in adjacent areas of the pancreas. In tissue adjacent to the tumor, ductal proliferation occurs and there is considerable increase in neogenesis of endocrine cells, resulting in the presence of single β-cells and islet clusters. These cells have been shown to contain high concentrations of other β-cell peptides, including IAPP, which has been associated with some of the symptoms of pancreatic carcinoma [136, 137].

Insulinoma

Small β-cell adenomas occur within the pancreas [138]. These are rarely malignant and are identified only by persistent hypoglycemia and hyperinsulinemia when surgery is required [139], which is an effective treatment. The adenomas are usually small, less than 2 cm in diameter and, by themselves, they have no relationship to diabetes. There is a persistent secretion of insulin and proinsulin, which can be ameliorated by inhibitors such as diazoxide or somatostatin. In older patients, insulinoma is occasionally associated with, and masks, the clinical features of type 2 diabetes [140]; an underlying susceptibility for impaired insulin secretion and hyperglycemia is masked by hypersecretion of insulin by the tumor and hypoglycemia. In these patients, postoperatively, when the source of the increased insulin secretion has been removed, the diabetes will become apparent [141]. Such a combination of pathologies can be identified by detection of amyloid deposits within islets adjacent to the tumor in the surgical specimen, indicating an established pathology for type 2 diabetes.

Insulin-Receptor Mutations: Rabson–Mendenhall Syndrome

Mutations in the insulin-receptor gene result in severe insulin-resistant syndromes which are characterized by fasting hyperglycemia, acute diabetic ketoacidosis, postprandial hyperglycemia, and extremely elevated insulin concentrations and growth retardation. Children with leprechaunism usually die before 1 year of age [142]. These conditions in the different syndromes have been shown to be associated with different mutations in the insulin-receptor gene [143]. Insulin concentrations progressively decline with time in patients with Rabson–Mendenhall syndrome [144]. This decline in insulin secretion is consistent with pancreatic pathology showing enlarged islets with extensive islet amyloidosis. Such features have also been demonstrated in a patient with congenital lipodystrophy [145] and insulin resistance due to insulin-receptor antibodies [146].

Acknowledgments

I am grateful to our local surgeons, physicians, and our research team for contributions and to Dr Fredrik Karpe for helpful advice on the manuscript, and to The Wellcome Trust for financial support.

REFERENCES

1. Rahier J, Goebbels RM, Henquin JC. Cellular composition of the human diabetic pancreas. *Diabetologia* 1983; 24: 355–71.
2. Olgivie RF. A quantitative study of the pancreatic islet tissue. *Q J Med* 1937; 6: 278–91.
3. Stefan Y, Grasso S, Perrelet A, Orci L. The pancreatic polypeptide-rich lobe of the human pancreas: definitive identification of its derivation from the ventral pancreatic primordium. *Diabetologia* 1982; 23: 141–2.
4. Langerhans P. *Beiträge zur mikroskopischen Anatomie der Bauchspeicheldrüse* [Inaugural dissertation]. Berlin, 1869.
5. Laguess EL. Sur la formation des ilôts de Langerhans das le pancréas. *C R Soc Biol (Paris)* 1893; 45: 819–920.
6. von Mering J, Minkowski O. Diabetes mellitus nach pankreas-extirpation. *Arch Exp Pathol Pharmacol* 1889; 26: 371–87.
7. MacLean N, Ogilvie RF. Quantitative estimation of pancreatic islet tissue in diabetic subjects. *Diabetes* 1955; 4: 367–76.
8. Hellman B. A method for rapid estimation of islet volume in the rat pancreas based on counting instead of measuring the islet sections. *Acta Pathol Microbiol Scand* 1959; 47: 21.
9. Bertelli E, Regoli M, Orazioli D, Bendayan M. Association between islets of Langerhans and pancreatic ductal

system in adult rat. Where endocrine and exocrine meet together? *Diabetologia* 2001; 44: 575–84.
10. Clark A, Wells CA, Buley ID, Cruickshank JK, Vanhegan RI, Matthews DR, Cooper GJ, Holman RR, Turner RC. Islet amyloid, increased A-cells, reduced B-cells and exocrine fibrosis: quantitative changes in the pancreas in type 2 diabetes. *Diabetes Res* 1988; 9: 151–9.
11. Sakuraba H, Mizukami H, Yagihashi N, Wada R, Hanyu C, Yagihashi S. Reduced beta-cell mass and expression of oxidative stress-related DNA damage in the islet of Japanese type II diabetic patients. *Diabetologia* 2002; 45: 85–96.
12. Lane MA. The cytological characteritics of the areas of Langerhans. *Am J Anat* 1907; 7: 409–22.
13. Bloom W. A new type of granular cell in the pancreatic islets of Langerhans of man. *Anat Rec* 1931; 49: 363–71.
14. Larsson LS, Sundler F, Håkansson R, Pollock HG, Kimmel JR. Localisation of APP, a postulated new hormone to a pancreatic endocrine cell type. *Histochemistry* 1974; 42: 377–82.
15. Jones LC, Clark A. Beta-cell neogenesis in type 2 diabetes. *Diabetes* 2001; 50 (suppl 1): S186–7.
16. Bouwens L, Pipeleers DG. Extra-insular beta cells associated with ductules are frequent in adult human pancreas. *Diabetologia* 1998; 41: 629–33.
17. Malaisse-Lagae F, Stefan Y, Cox J, Perrelet A, Orci L. Identification of a lobe in the adult human pancreas rich in pancreatic polypeptide. *Diabetologia* 1979; 17: 361–5.
18. Banting FG, Best CH. The internal secretion of the pancreas. *J Lab Clin Med* 1922; 7: 465–80.
19. Nadal A, Quesada I, Soria B. Homologous and heterologous asynchronicity between identified alpha-, beta- and delta-cells within intact islets of Langerhans in the mouse. *J Physiol* 1999; 517 (pt 1): 85–93.
20. Baskin DG, Gorray KC, Fujimoto WY. Immunocytochemical identification of cells containing insulin, glucagon, somatostatin and pancreatic polypeptide in the islets of Langerhans of the guinea pig pancreas with light and electron microscopy. *Anat Rec* 1984; 208: 567–78.
21. Helmstaedter V, Feurle GE, Forssmann WG. Insulin, glucagon and somatostatin-immunoreactive endocrine cells in the equine pancreas. *Cell Tissue Res* 1976; 172: 447–54.
22. Orci L. Macro and micro-domains in the endocrine pancreas. *Diabetes* 1982; 31: 538–65.
23. Orci L. The insulin factory: a tour of the plant and a visit to the assembly line. *Diabetologia* 1985; 28: 528–46.
24. Hutton JC. Insulin secretory granule biogenesis and the proinsulin-processing endopeptidases. *Diabetologia* 1994; 37 (suppl 2): S48–56.
25. Clark A, Edwards CA, Ostle LR, Sutton R, Rothbard JB, Morris JF, Turner RC. Localisation of islet amyloid peptide in lipofuscin bodies and secretory granules of human beta-cells and in islets of type-2 diabetic subjects. *Cell Tissue Res* 1989; 257: 179–85.
26. Westermark P, Wernstedt C, Wilander E, Hayden DW, O'Brien TD, Johnson KH. Amyloid fibrils in human insulinoma and islets of Langerhans of the diabetic cat are derived from a neuropeptide-like protein also present in normal islet cells. *Proc Natl Acad Sci USA* 1987; 84: 3881–5.
27. Barg S, Eliasson L, Renström E, Rorsman P. A subset of 50 secretory granules in close contact with L-type calcium channels accounts for first-phase insulin secretion in mouse beta-cells. *Diabetes* 2002; 51 (suppl 1): S74–82.
28. Holst JJ (ed). *Post-translational Processing of Proglucagon and Post-secretory fate of Proglucagon Peptides*. Basle: Kärger, 1987.
29. Pace CS, Tarvin JT. Somatostatin: mechanism of action in pancreatic islet beta-cells. *Diabetes* 1981; 30: 836–42.
30. Koerker DJ, Ruch W, Chideckel EJP, Goodner CJ, Ensinck J, Gale CC. Somatostatin: hypothalamic inhibitor of the endocrine pancreas. *Science* 1974; 184: 482–84.
31. Stephan Y, Orci L, Malaisse-Lagae F, Perrelet A, Patel Y, Unger RH. Quantitation of endocrine cell content in the pancreas of nondiabetic and diabetic humans. *Diabetes* 1982; 31: 694–700.
32. MacLean N, Ogilvie RF. Observations on the pancreatic islet tissue of young diabetic subjects. *Diabetes* 1959; 8: 83–91.
33. Gepts W. Pathologic anatomy of the pancreas in juvenile diabetes mellitus. *Diabetes* 1965; 14: 619–33.
34. Löhr M, Klöppel G. Residual insulin positivity and pancreatic atrophy in relation to duration of chronic, type 1 (insulin-dependent) diabetes mellitus and microangiopathy. *Diabetologia* 1987; 30: 757–62.
35. Fonseca V, Berger LA, Beckett AG, Dandona P. Size of pancreas in diabetes mellitus: a study based on ultra sound. *BMJ* 1985; 291: 1240–1.
36. Chiarelli F, Verrotti A, Altobelli E, Blasetti A, Morgese G. Size of the pancreas in type I diabetic children and adolescents. *Diabetes Care* 1995; 18: 1505–6.
37. Foulis AK, Stewart JA. The pancreas in recent onset type 1 (insulin-depdendent) diabetes mellitus: insulin content of islets, insulitis and associated changes in the exocrine and acinar tissue. *Diabetologia* 1984; 26: 456–61.
38. Williams JA, Goldfine ID. The insulin-pancreatic acinar axis. *Diabetes* 1985; 34: 980–6.
39. Owerbach D, Quinto C, Rutter WJ. Pancreatic-acinar cell interaction: amylase messenger RNA levels are determined by insulin. *Science* 1981; 213: 351–3.
40. Gale EA. The discovery of type 1 diabetes. *Diabetes* 2001; 50: 217–26.
41. Rosmalen JG, Leenen PJ, Pelegri C, Drexhage HA, Homo-Delarche F. Islet abnormalities in the pathogenesis of autoimmune diabetes. *Trends Endocrinol Metab* 2002; 13: 209–14.
42. Klöppel G, Clemens A. Insulin-dependent diabetes mellitus: islet changes in relation to etiology and pathogenesis. *Endocr Pathol* 1997; 8: 273–82.
43. Pociot F, McDermott MF. Genetics of type 1 diabetes. *Genes Immunol* 2002; 3: 235–49.
44. Nerup J, Platz P, Andersen OO, Christy M, Lyngsoe J, Poulsen JE, Ryder LP, Nielsen LS, Thomsen M, Svejgaard A. HLA antigens and diabetes mellitus. *Lancet* 1974; ii: 864–6.
45. Rosmalen JG, Martin T, Dobbs C, Voerman JS, Drexhage HA, Haskins K, Leenen PJ. Subsets of macrophages and dendritic cells in nonobese diabetic mouse pancreatic inflammatory infiltrates: correlation with the development of diabetes. *Lab Invest* 2000; 80: 23–30.
46. Foulis AK, Liddle CN, Farquharson MA, Richmond JA, Wier RS. The histopathology of the pancreas in type 1 (insulin dependent) diabetes mellitus: a 25-year review of deaths in patients under 20 years of age in the United Kingdom. *Diabetologia* 1986; 29: 267–74.
47. Foulis AK, Farquharson MA, Hardman R. Aberrant expression of Class II major histocompatibility complex

molecules by B-cells and hyperexpression of Class I major histocompatibility complex molecules by insulin containing islets in type 1 (insulin-dependent) diabetes mellitus. *Diabetologia* 1987; 30: 333–43.

48. Foulis AK, Farquharson MA. Aberrant expression of HLA-DR antigens by insulin-containing cells in recent-onset type 1 diabetes mellitus. *Diabetes* 1986; 35: 1215–24.
49. Turner RC, Stratton I, Horton V, Manley S, Zimmett P, MacKay IR, Shattock M, Bottazzo GF, Holman RR. UKPDS 25: autoantibodies to islet cell cytoplasm and glutamic acid decarboxylase for prediction of insulin requirement in type 2 diabetes. *Lancet* 1997; 350: 1288–93.
50. Olsen TS. Lipomatosis of the pancreas in autopsy material and its relation to age and overweight. *Acta Path Microbiol Scand [A]* 1978; 86: 367–73.
51. Dreiling DA, Elsbach P, Schaffner F, Schwartz IL. The effects of restriction of protein and total calories on pancreatic function in obese patients. *Gastroenterology* 1961; 42: 686–90.
52. Dandona P, Freedman DB, Foo Y, Perkins J, Katrak A, Mikhailidis DP, Rosalki SB, Beckett AG. Exocrine pancreatic functions in diabetes mellitus. *J Clin Pathol* 1984; 37: 302–6.
53. Ahmed SA, Clark A, Matthews DR. Progressive decline of beta cell function in non-insulin dependent diabetes. *Curr Opin Endocrinol Diabetes* 1997; 4: 300–7.
54. Kahn SE. Clinical review 135: the importance of beta-cell failure in the development and progression of type 2 diabetes. *J Clin Endocrinol Metab* 2001; 86: 4047–58.
55. Sempoux C, Guiot Y, Dubois D, Moulin P, Rahier J. Human type 2 diabetes: morphological evidence for abnormal beta-cell function. *Diabetes* 2001; 50 (suppl 1): S172–7.
56. Westermark P. Quantitative studies on amyloid in the islets of Langerhans. *Ups J Med Sci* 1972; 77: 91–4.
57. Porte D Jr, Kahn SE. Beta-cell dysfunction and failure in type 2 diabetes: potential mechanisms. *Diabetes* 2001; 50 (suppl 1): S160–3.
58. Saito K, Yaginuma N, Takahashi T. Differential volumetry of A, B and D cells in the pancreatic islets of diabetic and nondiabetic subjects. *Tohoku J Exp Med* 1979; 129: 273–83.
59. Guiot Y, Sempoux C, Moulin P, Rahier J. No decrease of the β-cell mass in type 2 diabetic patients. *Diabetes* 2001; 50 (suppl 1): S188.
60. Topp B, Promislow K, de Vries G, Miura RM, Finegood DT. A model of beta-cell mass, insulin, and glucose kinetics: pathways to diabetes. *J Theor Biol* 2000; 206: 605–19.
61. Bonner-Weir S, Trent DF, Weir G. Partial pancreatectomy in the rat and subsequent defect in glucose-induced insulin release. *J Clin Invest* 1981; 71: 1544–54.
62. McCulloch DK, Koerker DJ, Kahn SE, Bonner-Weir S, Palmer JP. Correlations of in vivo beta-cell function tests with beta-cell mass and pancreatic insulin content in streptozotocin-administered baboons. *Diabetes* 1991; 40: 673–9.
63. Kendall DM, Sutherland DE, Najarian JS, Goetz FC, Robertson RP. Effects of hemipancreatectomy on insulin secretion and glucose tolerance in healthy humans. *N Engl J Med* 1990; 322: 898–903.
64. Bonner-Weir S. Islet growth and development in the adult. *J Mol Endocrinol* 2000; 24: 297–302.
65. Bonner-Weir S, Sharma A. Pancreatic stem cells. *J Pathol* 2002; 197: 519–26.
66. Finegood DT, Scaglia L, Bonner-Weir S. Dynamics of beta-cell mass in the growing rat pancreas. Estimation with a simple mathematical model. *Diabetes* 1995; 44: 249–56.
67. Westermark P. Amyloid and polypeptide hormones: what is their interrelationship? *Int J Exp Clin Invest* 1994; 1: 47–60.
68. Cecil RL. A study of the pathological anatomy of the pancreas in ninety cases of diabetes mellitus. *J Exp Med* 1909; 11: 266–90.
69. Schneider HM, Störkel S, Will W. Das amyloid der Langerhansschen inseln und seine beziehung zum diabetes mellitus. [Amyloid of islets of Langerhans and its relation to diabetes mellitus (author's transl)]. *Dtsch Med Wochenschr* 1980; 105: 1143–7.
70. Wright A. Hyaline degeneration of the islets of Langerhans in nondiabetics. *Am J Pathol* 1927; 3: 461–81.
71. Opie EL. The relation of diabetes mellitus to lesions of the pancreas. Hyaline degeneration of the islands of Langerhans. *J Exp Med* 1901; 5: 527–40.
72. Ehrlich J, Ratner M. Amyloidosis of the islets of Langerhans. A study of islet hyaline in diabetic and nondiabetic individuals. *Am J Pathol* 1961; 38: 49–59.
73. Clark A, Saad MF, Nezzer T, Uren C, Knowler WC, Bennett PH, Turner RC. Islet amyloid polypeptide in diabetic and nondiabetic Pima Indians. *Diabetologia* 1990; 33: 285–9.
74. Vishwanathan KA, Bazaz-Malik G, Dandekar J, Vaishnava O. A qualitative and quantitative histological study of the islets of Langerhans in diabetes mellitus. *Indian J Med Sci* 1972; 26: 807–12.
75. Maloy AL, Longnecker DS, Greenberg ER. The relation of islet amyloid to the clinical type of diabetes. *Hum Pathol* 1981; 12: 917–22.
76. Clark A, Holman R, Matthews D, Hockaday T, Turner R. Non-uniform distribution of islet amyloid in the pancreas of "maturity-onset" diabetic patients. *Diabetologia* 1984; 27: 527–28.
77. Westermark P, Wernstedt C, O'Brien TD, Hayden DW, Johnson KH. Islet amyloid in type 2 human diabetes mellitus and adult diabetic cats contains a novel putative polypeptide hormone. *Am J Pathol* 1987; 127: 414–7.
78. Clark A, Cooper GJ, Lewis CE, Morris JF, Willis AC, Reid KB, Turner RC. Islet amyloid formed from diabetes-associated peptide may be pathogenic in type-2 diabetes. *Lancet* 1987; 2: 231–4.
79. Lukinius A, Wilander E, Westermark GT, Engström U, Westermark P. Co-localization of islet amyloid polypeptide and insulin in the B cell secretory granules of the human pancreatic islets. *Diabetologia* 1989; 32: 240–4.
80. Sanke T, Hanabusa T, Nakano Y, Oki C, Okai K, Nishimura S, Kondo M, Nanjo K. Plasma islet amyloid polypeptide (amylin) levels and their responses to oral glucose in type 2 (non-insulin-dependent) diabetic patients. *Diabetologia* 1991; 34: 129–32.
81. Butler PC, Chou J, Carter WB, Wang YN, Bu BH, Chang D, Chang JK, Rizza RA. Effects of meal ingestion on plasma amylin concentration in NIDDM and nondiabetic humans. *Diabetes* 1990; 39: 752–6.
82. Jaikaran ETAS, Clark A. Islet amyloid and type 2 diabetes: from molecular misfolding to islet pathophysiology. *Biochim Biophys Acta* 2001; 1537: 179–203.

83. Betsholtz C, Christmansson L, Engström U, Rorsman F, Svensson V, Johnson KH, Westermark P. Sequence divergence in a specific region of islet amyloid polypeptide (IAPP) explains differences in islet amyloid formation between species. *FEBS Lett* 1989; 251: 261–4.
84. Cook JT, Patel PP, Clark A, Höppener JW, Lips CJ, Mosselman S, O'Rahilly S, Page RC, Wainscoat JS, Turner RC. Non-linkage of the islet amyloid polypeptide gene with type 2 (non-insulin-dependent) diabetes mellitus. *Diabetologia* 1991; 34: 103–8.
85. Nishi M, Bell GI, Steiner DF. Islet amyloid polypeptide (amylin): no evidence of an abnormal precursor sequence in 25 type 2 (non-insulin-dependent) diabetic patients. *Diabetologia* 1990; 33: 628–30.
86. Röcken C, Linke RP, Saeger W. Immunohistology of islet amyloid polypeptide in diabetes mellitus: semi-quantitative studies in a postmortem series. *Virchows Arch A Pathol Anat Histopathol* 1992; 421: 339–44.
87. Lorenzo A, Razzaboni B, Weir G, Yankner B. Pancreatic islet cell toxicity of amylin associated with type-2 diabetes mellitus. *Nature* 1994; 368: 756–60.
88. de Koning EJ, Bodkin NL, Hansen BC, Clark A. Diabetes mellitus in *Macaca mulatta* monkeys is characterised by islet amyloidosis and reduction in beta-cell population. *Diabetologia* 1993; 36: 378–84.
89. Janson J, Soeller WC, Roche PC, Nelson RT, Torchia AJ, Kreutter DK, Butler PC. Spontaneous diabetes mellitus in transgenic mice expressing human islet amyloid polypeptide. *Proc Natl Acad Sci USA* 1996; 93: 7283–8.
90. Höppener JW, Verbeek JS, de Koning EJP, Oösterwijk C, van Hulst KL, Visser Vernooy HJ, Hofhuis FM, van Gaalen S, Berends MJ, Hackeng WH, et al. Chronic overproduction of islet amyloid polypeptide/amylin in transgenic mice: lysosomal localization of human islet amyloid polypeptide and lack of marked hyperglycemia or hyperinsulinemia. *Diabetologia* 1993; 36: 1258–65.
91. Verchere CB, D'Alessio DA, Palmiter RD, Weir GC, Bonner Weir S, Baskin DG, Kahn SE. Islet amyloid formation associated with hyperglycemia in transgenic mice with pancreatic beta cell expression of human islet amyloid polypeptide. *Proc Natl Acad Sci USA* 1996; 93: 3492–6.
92. Höppener JWM, Oösterwijk C, Nieuwenhuis MG, Posthuma G, Thijssen JHH, Vroom TM, Ahren B, Lips CJM. Extensive islet amyloid formation is induced by development of type II diabetes mellitus and contributes to its progression: pathogenesis of diabetes in a mouse model. *Diabetologia* 1999; 42: 427–34.
93. MacNamara CM, Barrow BA, Manley SE, Levy JC, Clark A, Turner RC. Parallel changes of proinsulin and islet amyloid polypeptide in glucose intolerance. *Diabetes Res Clin Pract* 2000; 50: 117–26.
94. O'Brien TD, Butler AE, Roche PC, Johnson KH, Butler PC. Islet amyloid polypeptide in human insulinomas. Evidence for intracellular amyloidogenesis. *Diabetes* 1994; 43: 329–36.
95. Clark A, de Koning EJP, Baker CA, Charge S, Morris JF. Localisation of N-terminal pro-islet amyloid polypeptide in beta cells of man and transgenic mice. *Diabetologia* 1993; 36: A136.
96. Park K, Verchere CB. Identification of a heparin-binding domain in the N-terminal cleavage site of pro-islet amyloid polypeptide: implications for islet amyloid formation. *J Biol Chem* 2001; 276: 16611–6.
97. Porte D, Kahn SE. Hyperproinsulinaemia and amyloid in NIDDM: clues to etiology of islet β-cell dysfunction. *Diabetes* 1989; 38: 1333–6.
98. Tattersall RB. Maturity-onset diabetes of the young: a clinical history. *Diabet Med* 1998; 15: 11–4.
99. Hattersley AT. Maturity-onset diabetes of the young: clinical heterogeneity explained by genetic heterogeneity. *Diabet Med* 1998; 15: 15–24.
100. Frayling T, Evans JC, Bulman MP, Pearson E, Allen L, Owen K, Bingham C, Hannemann M, Shepherd M, Ellard S, Hattersley AT. Beta-cell genes and diabetes: molecular and clinical characterisation of mutations in transcription factors. *Diabetes* 2001; 50 (suppl 1): S94–100.
101. Johansson KA, Grapin-Botton A. Development and diseases of the pancreas. *Clin Genet* 2002; 62: 14–23.
102. Velho G, Robert J-J. Maturity-onset diabetes of the young (MODY): genetic and clinical characteristics. *Horm Res* 2002; 57: 29–33.
103. Clark A, de Koning EJP, Hattersley AT, Hansen BC, Yajnik CS, Poulton J. Pancreatic pathology in non-insulin depdendent diabetes (NIDDM). *Diabetes Res Clin Pract* 1995; 28 (suppl): S39–47.
104. Andrikopoulos S, Verchere CB, Terauchi Y, Kadowaki T, Kahn SE. Beta cell glucokinase deficiency and hyperglycemia are associated with reduced islet amyloid deposition in a mouse model of type 2 diabetes. *Diabetes* 2000; 49: 2056–62.
105. Edlund H. Pancreatic organogenesis—developmental mechanisms and implications for therapy. *Nat Rev Genet* 2002; 3: 524–32.
106. Stoffers DA, Zinkin NT, Stanojevek V, Clarke WL, Habener JF. Pancreatic agenesis attributable to a single nucleotide deletion in the human IPF1 gene coding sequence. *Nat Genet* 1997; 15: 106–10.
107. van den Ouweland JM, Lemkes HHPJ, Ruitenbeek W, Sandkuijl LA, de Vijlder MF, Struyvenberg PAA, van de Kamp JJP, Maasen JA. Mutation in mitochondrial $sRNA^{Leu(UUR)}$ gene in a large pedigree with maternally transmitted type II diabetes mellitus and deafness. *Nat Genet* 1992; 1: 368–71.
108. Otobe S, Sakura H, Shimokawa K, Mori Y, Kadowaki K, Yasuda K, Nonaka K, Hagura R, Akanuma Y, Tazaki Y, Kadowaki T. The high prevalence of diabetic patients with a mutation in the mitochondrial gene in Japan. *J Clin Endocrinol Metab* 1994; 79: 768–71.
109. Saker PJ, Hattersley AT, Barrow B, Hammersley MS, Horton V, Gilmer MD, Turner RC. UKPDS 21: low prevalence of the mitochondrial transfer RNA gene ($tRNA^{Leu(UUR)}$) mutation at position 3243bp in UK caucasian type 2 diabetic patients. *Diabet Med* 1997; 14: 42–5.
110. Kadowaki T, Kadowaki H, Mori Yl, Tobe K, Sakuta R, Suzuki Y. A subtype of diabetes mellitus associated with a mutation of mitochondrial DNA. *N Engl J Med* 1994; 330: 962–68.
111. Kobayashi T, Nakanishi K, Nakase H, Kajio H, Okubo M, Murase T, Kosaka K. In situ characterization of islets in diabetes with a mitochondrial DNA mutation at nucleotide position 3243. *Diabetes* 1997; 46: 1567–71.
112. Poulton J, O'Rahilly S, Morten KJ, Clark A. Mitochondrial DNA, diabetes and pancreatic pathology in Kearns-Sayre syndrome. *Diabetologia* 1995; 38: 868–71.
113. Barrett TG, Bundey SE, MacLeod AF. Neurodegeneration and diabetes: UK nationwide study of

Wolfram (DIDMOAD) syndrome. *Lancet* 1995; 346: 1458–63.

114. Collier DA, Barrett TG, Curtis D, MacLeod A, Arranz MJ, Maassen JA, Bundey S. Linkage of Wolfram syndrome to chromosome 4p16.1 and evidence for heterogeneity. *Am J Hum Genet* 1996; 59: 855–63.
115. Klöppel G, Bommer G, Heitz PH. Immunocytochemistry of the endocrine pancreas in chronic pancreatitis and pancreatic carcinoma. In Podolsky SVM (ed) *Secondary Diabetes: The Spectrum of the Diabetic Syndromes*. New York: Raven Press, 1980.
116. Riordan JR, Rommens JM, Kerem B-S, Alon N, Rozmahel R, Grzelczak Z, Zielenski J, Lok S, Plavsic N, Chou J-L, Drumm ML, Iannuzzi MC, Collins FS, Tsui L-C. Identification of the cystic fibrosis gene: cloning and characterisation of complementary DNA. *Science* 1989; 245: 1066–73.
117. Rommens JM, Iannuzzi MC, Kerem B-S, Drumm ML, Melmer G, Dean M, Rozmahel R, Cole JL, Kennedy D, Hidaka N, Zsiga M, Buchwald M, Riordan JR, Tsui L-C, Collins FS. Identification of the cystic fibrosis gene: chromosome walking and jumping. *Science* 1989; 245: 1059–65.
118. Lanng S. Glucose intolerance in cystic fibrosis patients. *Paediatr Respir Rev* 2001; 2: 253–9.
119. Lippe BM, Sperling MA, Dooley RR. Pancreatic alpha and beta cell functions in cystic fibrosis. *J Pediatr* 1977; 90: 751–55.
120. Löhr M, Goertchen H, Nizze H, Gould VE, Gould M, Oberholzer M, Heitz UPh, Klöppel G. Cystic fibrosis associated islet changes may provide a basis for diabetes. *Virchows Arch A Pathol Anat* 1989; 414: 179–85.
121. Iannucci A, Mukai K, Johnson D, Burke B. Endocrine pancreas in cystic fibrosis: an immunohistochemical study. *Hum Pathol* 1984; 15: 278–84.
122. Kopito LE, Shwachman H, Vawter GF, Edlow J. The pancreas in cystic fibrosis: chemical composition and comparative morphology. *Pediatr Res* 1976; 10: 742–9.
123. Clark A, Stead RJ, Hodson ME, Batten JC, Turner RC. Quantitative morphometry of pancreatic islet cells in cystic fibrosis. *Diabet Med* 1985; 2: 514A.
124. Balcerzak SP, Mitz DH, Westerman MP. Diabetes mellitus and idiopathic haemochromotosis. *Am J Med Sci* 1968; 255: 53–62.
125. Rahier J, Loozen S, Goebbels RM, Abrahem M. The haemochromatotic pancreas: a quantitative immunohistochemical and ultrastructural study. *Diabetologia* 1987; 30: 5–12.
126. Mohan V, Nagalotimath SJ, Yajnik CS, Tripathy BB. Fibrocalculous pancreatic disease. *Diabetes Metab Rev* 1998; 14: 153–70.
127. WHO. Report of the Expert Committee on the Diagnosis and Classification of Diabetes Mellitus. *Diabetes Care* 2000; 23 (suppl 1): S4–19.
128. Petersen JM. Tropical pancreatitis. *J Clin Gastroenterol* 2002; 35: 61–6.
129. McLarty DG, Pollitt C, Swai ABM. Diabetes in Africa. *Diabet Med* 1990; 7: 670–84.
130. Chari S, Jayanthi V, Mohan V, Malathi S, Madanagopalan N, Viswanathan M. Radiological appearance of pancreatic calculi in tropical versus alcoholic chronic pancreatitis. *J Gastroenterol Hepatol* 1992; 7: 42–4.
131. Clark A, de Koning EJ, Hattersley AT, Hansen BC, Yajnik CS, Poulton J. Pancreatic pathology in non-insulin dependent diabetes (NIDDM). *Diabetes Res Clin Pract* 1995; 28 (suppl): S39–47.
132. Chowdhury ZM, McDermott MF, Davey S, Hassan Z, Sinnott PJ, Hemmatpour SK, Sherwin S, Ali L, Aganna E, Allotey RA, North BV, Cassell PG, Azad Khan AK, Hitman GA. Genetic susceptibility to fibrocalculous pancreatic diabetes in Bangladeshi subjects: a family study. *Genes Immun* 2002; 3: 5–8.
133. Hassan Z, Mohan V, Ali L, Allotey R, Barakat K, Faruque MO, Deepa R, McDermott MF, Jackson AE, Cassell P, Curtis D, Gelding SV, Vijayaravaghan S, Gyr N, Whitcomb DC, Khan AK, Hitman GA. *SPINK1* is a susceptibility gene for fibrocalculous pancreatic diabetes in subjects from the indian subcontinent. *Am J Hum Genet* 2002; 71: 964–8.
134. Bhatia E, Choudhuri G, Sikora SS, Landt O, Kage A, Becker M, Witt H. Tropical calcific pancreatitis: strong association with SPINK trypsin inhibitor mutations. *Gastroenterology* 2002; 123: 1020–5.
135. Pour PM, Permert J, Mogaki M, Fuji H, Kazakoff K. Endocrine aspects of exocrine cancer of the pancreas–their patterns and suggested biologic significance. *Am J Clin Pathol* 1993; 100: 223–30.
136. Permert J, Larsson J, Westermark GT, Herrington MK, Christmansson L, Pour PM. Islet amyloid polypeptide in patients with pancreatic cancer. *N Engl J Med* 1994; 330: 313–8.
137. Permert J, Larsson J, Fruin AB, Tatemoto K, Herrington MK, Von Schenk H, Adrian TE. Islet hormone secretion in pancreatic cancer patients with diabetes. *Pancreas* 1997; 15: 60–8.
138. Stabile BE. Islet cell tumors. *Gastroenterologist* 1997; 5: 213–32.
139. Azzoni C, D'Adda T, Tamburrano G, Coscelli C, Madsen OD, Scopsi L, Bordi C. Functioning human insulinomas. An immunohistochemical analysis of intracellular insulin processing. *Virchows Arch* 1998; 433: 495–504.
140. Arioglu E, Gottlieb NA, Koch CA, Doppman JL, Grey NJ, Gorden P. Natural history of a proinsulin-secreting insulinoma: from symptomatic hypoglycemia to clinical diabetes. *J Clin Endocrinol Metab* 2000; 85: 3628–30.
141. Gittler RD, Zucker R, Eisinger R, Stoller N. Amelioration of diabetes mellitus by an insulinoma. *N Engl J Med* 1958; 258: 932–5.
142. Kadowaki T, Bevins CL, Cama A, Ojamaa K, Marcus-Samuels B, Kadowaki H, Beitz L, McKeon C, Taylor SI. Two mutant alleles of the insulin receptor gene in a patient with extreme insulin resistance. *Science* 1988; 240: 787–90.
143. Krook A, Kumar S, Laing I, Boulton AJM, Wass AH, O'Rahilly S. Molecular scanning of the insulin receptor gene in syndromes of insulin resistance. *Diabetes* 1994; 43: 357–68.
144. Longo N, Wang Y, Pasquali M. Progressive decline in insulin levels in Rabson–Mendenhall syndrome. *J Clin Endocrinol Metab* 1999; 84: 2623–9.
145. Garg A, Chandalia M, Vuitch F. Severe islet amyloidosis in congenital generalised lipodystrophy. *Diabetes Care* 1996; 19: 28–31.
146. O'Brien TD, Rizza RA, Carney JA, Butler PC. Islet amyloidosis in a patient with chronic massive insulin resistance due to antiinsulin receptor antibodies. *J Clin Endocrinol Metab* 1994; 79: 290–2.

6

Insulin Gene Expression and Biosynthesis

Vincent Poitout*, Roland Stein†, and Christopher J. Rhodes*

**Pacific Northwest Research Institute, Seattle, WA, USA, and †Vanderbilt University Medical Center, Nashville, TN, USA*

INTRODUCTION

The unique property of the pancreatic β-cell is the ability to secrete insulin to allow circulating glucose levels to be maintained within a narrow physiological range, despite wide fluctuations in energy supply. Indeed, the β-cell is able to sense the glucose concentration in the extracellular milieu, and adapt its insulin secretion rate via a complex interplay between nutrients, hormones, and neuronal signals [1]. As the minute-to-minute regulation of insulin secretion probably occurs at the level of exocytosis of preformed insulin, adaptation to longer term changes in the environment also involves regulated changes in the transcription rate of the insulin gene, translation of the mRNA, and processing of the proinsulin molecule into fully mature insulin [2–4]. The first section of this chapter focuses on the regulation of insulin gene transcription, of which much has been uncovered in recent years, and a number of *trans*-activating factors regulating insulin gene 5′-flanking control region driven expression have been identified. In the second section, the successive steps leading from translation of the insulin mRNA molecule to the storage of mature insulin into readily releasable secretory granules are presented, as well as the metabolic regulation of these processes.

INSULIN GENE EXPRESSION

Structure of the Insulin Gene

The insulin gene is specifically expressed in pancreatic β-cells, although low levels of expression have been detected in the brain [5–7], the thymus [8, 9], and in the yolk sac during fetal development [10]. Insulin is expressed at very high levels in primary β-cells, on the order of approximately 100 000 molecules of insulin mRNA under stimulatory glucose conditions, which represents about 2 orders of magnitude greater level than β-actin mRNA [11].

The sequence of the insulin gene is remarkably conserved throughout evolution [12], and is present as a single copy in most species, including humans, where it is located on chromosome 11 between the genes for tyrosine hydroxylase and insulin-like growth factor 2 [13, 14]. In rodents, there are two nonallelic insulin genes (I and II), probably resulting from duplication of the original insulin II gene [15]. The human insulin gene contains three exons and two introns. The first intron is within the 5′-untranslated region (UTR), whereas the second intron interrupts the C-peptide coding sequence [12]. The mature preproinsulin mRNA is 446 bp long.

Most of the tissue-specific expression and metabolic regulation of the insulin gene is conferred by a highly conserved region lying approximately 340 bp immediately upstream of the transcription initiation start, composing the insulin gene enhancer/promoter control region [2–4]. A hybrid construct spanning these insulin 5′-flanking sequences linked to an unrelated reporter gene is expressed specifically in β-cells both *in vitro* [16–20] and *in vivo* [21–24]. In the last 15 years, considerable progress has been made in identifying the *cis*-acting regulatory sequences and corresponding *trans*-activating factors that influence transcription. The organization of the human and rat insulin transcription control region sequences have been reviewed in detail recently [2–4], and only the control factors pertinent to the metabolic regulation of insulin gene expression are presented here. The many control factors that act upon this region form a highly sophisticated transcriptional network that ensures precise transcriptional regulation. Among these, those most critical for activation

International Textbook of Diabetes Mellitus, Third Edition. Edited by R. A. DeFronzo, E. Ferrannini, H. Keen, and P. Zimmet.
 ISBN: 0-471-48655-8.

of transcription in cell transfection experiments were highly conserved and termed the C2 (−317/−311 bp) [18, 25, 26], A3 (−201/−196 bp) [25, 27, 28], C1 (−115/−107 bp) [20, 29], and E1 (−100/−91 bp) [18, 30, 31] sites (labeled in accordance with the adopted consensus nomenclature [32]). Although these elements are also likely to be of importance for expression of the insulin gene *in vivo*, this hypothesis has not been tested directly.

Pancreatic and duodenal homeobox-1 (PDX-1; also called IPF-1 [33], STF-1 [34], IUF-1 [35], or IDX-1 [36]), is a homeodomain protein orthologous to the *Xenopus laevis* XIHbox 8 [37], which plays a major role in pancreatic β-cell development and function [38, 39]. PDX-1 binds to the AT-rich A3 box and activates transcription [28, 33, 40–43]. PDX-1 is essential in the normal development of the pancreas [44], although inactivation in the adult animal does not lead to complete absence of insulin production [45]. Both homozygous [46] and heterozygous [47] mutations in the PDX-1 gene have been identified in humans, which lead, respectively, to complete agenesis of the pancreas and a form of maturity-onset diabetes of the young (MODY4).

PDX-1 functionally interacts with the proteins of the basic helix–loop–helix (bHLH) family that bind to the E1 box [42, 48]. The E1 bHLH activator is a heterodimer composed of ubiquitous class A (E12/E47 and E2/5) and cell-restricted class B (BETA2/NeuroD) members of the bHLH family [20, 49–54]. The cooperation between PDX-1 and bHLH proteins also involves interactions with other DNA-binding proteins [55] and coactivators [56], thus forming a unique network of protein–protein and protein–DNA interactions. In mice lacking BETA2, severe defects in islet cell formation (i.e., β-, α-, and δ-cells) [53] were found, although insulin was still produced. Heterozygous mutations in this gene can also contribute to diabetes [57, 58].

The rat insulin promoter element 3b (RIPE3b) motif is juxtaposed between the A2 and C1 sites [20]. The activator of the C1 site, previously referred to as RIPE3b1 [19, 59–62], has recently been identified as the mammalian homologue of MafA/L-Maf (mMafA) [29] (T. Matsuoka and R.S., unpublished data). Although mMafA appears to be the principal C1 activator, two other large Maf proteins (c-Maf, MafB) are also enriched in β-cells and capable of binding and activating (T. Matsuoka and R.S., unpublished data). Because of their apparent importance in myeloid [63, 64] and lens [65–68] development, it is likely that the large Maf proteins (especially mMafA) will also be important in islet β-cell differentiation.

The C2 element binds the paired homeodomain proteins PAX6 and PAX4, respectively acting as either activator [26] or repressor [69–71]. These factors also act at specific stages of islet development, affecting α- (PAX6 [72]) or β- and δ-cell (PAX4 [73]) development. Collectively, these results have established a central role for at least PAX6, PDX-1, and BETA2 in islet cell development and function, although it is interesting that insulin gene expression is still observed in mice lacking any one of these genes. Because recent chromatin immunoprecipitation assays have established that PAX6, PDX-1, BETA2, and the MAF proteins bind within insulin control region sequences *in vivo* (R.S., unpublished observation), it is likely that insulin expression in PAX6, PDX-1, or BETA2 *null* mice results from compensation by the remaining factors.

In contrast, the role of hepatic nuclear factors (HNFs) in insulin gene transcription is still unclear. The interest in a potential involvement of HNFs comes from the observation that three forms of MODY are due to mutations in HNF genes: MODY1 (HNF-4α [74]), MODY3 (HNF-1α [75]), and MODY5 (HNF-1β [76]). The homeodomain transcription factor HNF-1α is expressed in an insulinoma cell line and *trans*-activates the rat insulin I gene through binding to an A-like box [77]. Furthermore, dominant-negative suppression of HNF-1α [78] or mutations of the HNF-1α gene [79] inhibit insulin gene transcription in transformed cells, although insulin gene expression is unaffected in HNF-1α *null* mice [80]. On the other hand, dominant-negative suppression of HNF-4α reduces HNF-1α gene transcription and insulin gene expression [81], suggesting that HNF-4α regulates HNF-1α, which in turn binds to and *trans*-activates the insulin gene, similar to the hierarchy of HNFs in the liver [82]. Recent observations, however, suggest that the relationship between HNF-1α and HNF-4α in the pancreatic β-cell is more complex. Thus, HNF-1α *trans*-activates the HNF-4α promoter in β-cells [83, 84], and HNF-4α can directly bind to the insulin gene promoter [85]. In addition, both HNF-1α and HNF-3β (*Foxa2*) regulate PDX-1 gene transcription [86, 87].

In conclusion, a highly sophisticated network of transcription factors provide the infrastructure for precise cell-type specific transcription of the insulin gene, which relies on the cooperative and synergistic interactions between DNA-binding factors and coactivators. In the following section, the most physiologically relevant metabolic regulators of insulin gene expression are presented.

Physiological Regulation of Insulin Gene Expression

Glucose Regulation of Insulin Promoter Activity

Glucose is the major physiological regulator of β-cell function, and, as such, plays a major role in the metabolic control of insulin gene expression. Since the early studies demonstrating the effects of glucose on preproinsulin mRNA levels in rat [88] and human [89] islets *in vitro* and in rats *in vivo* [10], it has been appreciated that glucose regulates all levels of insulin gene expression, including transcription [90], preRNA splicing [91], and mRNA stability [92] (Figure 1). Transient transfection experiments using

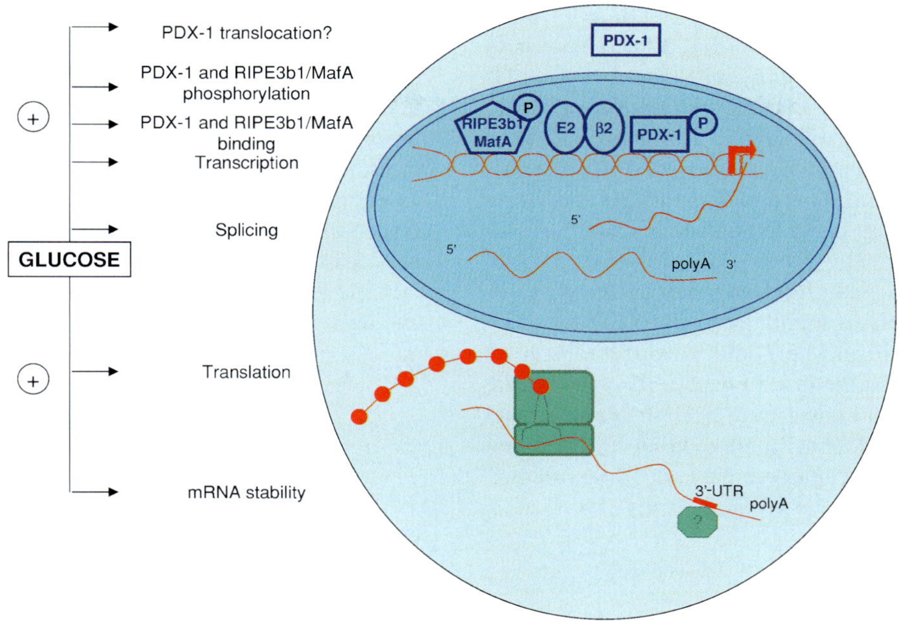

Figure 1 Various levels of glucose regulation of insulin gene expression. Glucose was proposed to stimulate nuclear translocation of PDX-1 [93], although the significance of PDX-1 translocation has been questioned [94]. Glucose promotes PDX-1 [35] and RIPE3b1/MafA [61, 62] phosphorylation, PDX-1 [40, 41, 95] and RIPE3b1/MafA [19, 60] binding to the insulin promoter, transcription [90], pre-mRNA splicing [91], translation [96], and mRNA stability [92]. *Note*: the question mark indicates that the effects of glucose on PDX-1 translocation are uncertain

insulin gene 5′-flanking region driven chimeric reporter constructs have demonstrated that the tissue-specific control region confers responsiveness to glucose, and that this also requires a rise in cytosolic calcium [95, 97]. The main glucose-responsive elements are the A3, E1, and C1 sites. In addition, a more distal glucose-responsive element at −292/−243 bp in the human gene seems to bind a glucose-sensitive complex specifically present in primary islets [98].

Activation of both RIPE3b1/mMafA and BETA2/E47 is stimulated in response to glucose [19, 60]. Although it is unclear how BETA2/E47 activation is regulated, RIPE3b1/mMafA binding is directly activated by glucose, possibly via tyrosine phosphorylation [61, 62].

Much more is known about the activation of PDX-1 activity by glucose. Initially, a rat insulin I mini-enhancer consisting of the E2 motif juxtaposed to the A3/A4 box (the FF mini-enhancer) was shown to be responsive to glucose [95]. The glucose-responsive element was further mapped to the A3 site [41], and was shown to bind PDX-1 [40]. Furthermore, mutation of PDX-1 binding sites abolishes the response to glucose [28, 40]. The signal transduction mechanisms involved in glucose-dependent PDX-1 binding are not fully understood. However, the decrease in PDX-1 binding activity in the presence of low glucose concentrations likely involves protein dephosphorylation [35]. PDX-1 phosphorylation does not appear to be mediated by protein kinase A (PKA) or protein kinase C [35]; rather, glucose-induced PDX-1 binding appears to require p38 mitogen-activated protein kinase (MAPK) activity, since inhibition of p38 MAPK prevents glucose-induced PDX-1 activation, whereas its overexpression activates it [93, 99]. Furthermore, glucose may promote translocation of a cytoplasmic, 31-kDa inactive PDX-1 form to a nuclear, 46-kDa active form, via activation of p38 MAPK [93], an event that appears essential for PDX-1-dependent transcription [100]. However, these results were in conflict with a more recent study in which PDX-1 nuclear translocation was unaffected by inhibition of p38 MAPK (although it was blocked by inhibitors of phosphatidylinositol 3 (PI3) kinase), and was not associated with the 31–46 kDa change in molecular mass [94]. These data also questioned the relevance of massive translocation of PDX-1 to the nucleus under physiological circumstances [94]. On the other hand, inhibition of the extracellular-signal-regulated kinases (ERK) was found to independently prevent insulin transcription [101]. The fact that insulin gene expression is stimulated by non-glucose secretagogues such as leucine (or its metabolite α-ketoisocaproic acid) [102, 103] or glyceraldehyde [104] and that glucose stimulation is blocked by inhibitors of glucose metabolism [104, 105] indicates that activation of the insulin gene is regulated by intracellular signals emanating from glucose metabolism. Furthermore, early observations demonstrating that calcium channel blockers impede the transcriptional response to glucose

[95, 97] have led to the concept that calcium influx is required. However, this was challenged in studies in both insulin-secreting cells [105, 106] and isolated islets [107] that showed that calcium blockers fail to affect glucose-induced insulin gene transcription. If glucose-regulated insulin gene expression is indeed independent from calcium influx, the signal transduction pathways mediating this glucose effect are likely to be distinct from those involved in secretion.

In conclusion, the nature of the signal transduction pathways mediating glucose-stimulated insulin gene transcription by PDX-1 is still unclear. Although glucose increases binding of PDX-1 to the insulin gene, it is questionable if glucose stimulates PDX-1 translocation from an inactive cytoplasmic pool. Finally, in addition to increasing PDX-1 binding activity, glucose also potentiates PDX-1 *trans*-activation potency [28, 108].

Glucose Regulation of Insulin mRNA Stability

In addition to its major effects on transcription of the insulin promoter, glucose markedly stabilizes the preproinsulin mRNA. Indeed, the half-life of the message has been estimated to increase from 29 to 77 h when switched from low to high glucose [92]. Two elements located in the 3′-UTR of the mRNA molecule have been proposed as mediators of the glucose-stabilizing effect—the conserved UUGAA sequence [109] and the pyrimidine-rich sequence (insPRS) [11]. Stabilization appears to involve binding of a polypyrimidine-tract-binding (PTB) protein to the insPRS, as binding was induced by glucose and prevented upon mutating the core PTB site [11].

Glucose Regulation of the Insulin Gene In Vivo

Variations in the amount of insulin mRNA at any given time represent the net effect of metabolic, hormonal, and neuronal stimuli on insulin gene transcription and mRNA stability. From the *in vitro* effects described in the previous sections, it is predicted that an increase in blood glucose should rapidly elevate preproinsulin mRNA levels in the endocrine pancreas (due to rapid stimulation of transcription), whereas a decrease in blood glucose would be followed by a slow decline in preproinsulin mRNA levels (due to reduced transcription and the long half-life of the message). Indeed, early studies in rats showed that 4 days of starvation are necessary to detect significant decreases in preproinsulin mRNA, which returned to basal values only 6 h after re-feeding [110] or 12 h after glucose injection [111]. The delay in the disappearance of the message upon fasting appears to be directly due to the stability of the mRNA, as insulin-induced hypoglycemia is followed by a rapid (2 h) decrease in the level of precursors for insulin mRNA [112].

An additional level of complexity in the regulation of insulin gene expression *in vivo* is the potential interaction between β-cells and non-β- (i.e. α-, δ-, and PP-) cells within the intact islet. Indeed, it is known that isolated β-cells behave differently in terms of insulin secretion than in the context of the islet [113], a phenomenon which has also been demonstrated at the level of insulin gene transcription [107]. Thus, the global response measured in an entire islet represents the integration of the individual responses. This fact should be kept in mind when interpreting experiments performed in clonal cell lines, which lack the level of regulation provided by islet architecture and the neighboring non-β-cells.

Regulation of Insulin Gene Expression by Glucagon-like Peptide-1, Growth Hormone, and Lactogenic Hormones

Glucagon-like peptide 1 (GLP-1) is an incretin hormone that strongly potentiates glucose-induced insulin secretion (reviewed in reference 114). The GLP-1 receptor is expressed on the β-cell surface and transduces GLP-1 signaling mostly through the heterotrimeric Gs protein and by activation of adenylyl cyclase [115, 116], although GLP-1 can also activate a number of second messengers in β-cells, including MAPK [117, 118], phospholipase C [119], PI3 kinase [120], and intracellular calcium [121, 122] (see also Chapter 12). GLP-1 stimulates insulin gene expression [115, 123, 124] by various mechanisms. First, it directly activates the cyclic AMP (cAMP) response element (CRE) within the 5′-proximal control sequences of the insulin gene, by a mechanism that seems at least partly independent from PKA activation [125]. Second, GLP-1 can augment the glucose-stimulated binding activity of PDX-1 [126]. Third, GLP-1 can stimulate transcription of the PDX-1 gene (the promoter of which also contains a CRE) [127]. Fourth, GLP-1 potentiates glucose-induced insulin gene transcription by activating the nuclear factor of activated T-cells, of which there are three binding sites on the rat insulin I promoter, via calcium/calmodulin-dependent protein phosphatase 2B (calcineurin) activation in response to a rise in intracellular calcium [128, 129]. This signaling pathway is thought to be the mechanism by which FK506, an inhibitor of calcineurin used clinically as an immunosuppressant, inhibits insulin gene transcription [128, 130].

In addition to being major stimulators of β-cell proliferation, growth hormone (GH) and the lactogenic hormones prolactin (PRL) and placental lactogen stimulate insulin gene transcription [131]. GH and PRL induce nuclear translocation [132] and activate DNA binding [131, 133] of the STAT5 transcription factor in insulin-secreting cells. The STAT5 binding sequence in the rat insulin I gene is at −330/−322 bp [131], although it has recently been suggested that PRL can induce transcription in a STAT5-independent manner [134].

Physiological Inhibitors of Insulin Gene Expression

Several physiological inhibitors of insulin secretion also impair insulin gene expression. Epinephrine and somatostatin, two hormones acting through G-protein-coupled receptors and known inhibitors of insulin release (reviewed in reference 135), also inhibit the rate of insulin gene transcription [136, 137]. In addition, somatostatin decreases the stability of insulin mRNA [138]. Glucagon, a key hormone in the counterregulatory response to hypoglycemia *in vivo*, stimulates expression of the inducible cAMP early repressor, which inhibits insulin gene transcription [139]. Finally, the adipocyte-secreted hormone leptin, which reduces the levels of cAMP by activation of phosphodiesterase 3B [140], decreases stimulated insulin secretion [141–143] and gene expression [144], possibly via activation of STAT3 [145]. Thus, physiological modulators of insulin secretion coordinately inhibit insulin gene expression, thereby ensuring that the long-term biosynthetic rate of insulin matches the secretory demand.

Short-term Regulation of Insulin Gene Expression by Insulin

The above description of the regulatory mechanisms by which insulin gene expression is controlled is based on the premise, confirmed by a large number of studies, that several hours are needed between the time the stimulus is applied and the time one can detect significant differences in the levels of insulin mRNA. This implies that the short-term signals regulating insulin secretion are distinct from the long-term signals regulating insulin gene transcription and that these two processes, although regulated in a coordinated fashion by most of the physiological modulators, are independent from each other. Recently, this view has been challenged by the observation that a 15-min glucose stimulation is sufficient to trigger a transcriptional response, which can be detected 60–100 min after glucose stimulation in HIT-T15 β-cells [146]. It was proposed that insulin acts in an autocrine manner to stimulate insulin gene transcription by binding to the insulin receptor and activating the PI3 kinase and CaM kinase pathways [147]. The role of insulin and PI3 kinase activation in glucose stimulation of insulin gene transcription was also supported by da Silva Xavier et al. [148] in insulin-secreting MIN6 β-cells, and by the observation that insulin promotes PDX-1 binding activity [149]. The fact that mice lacking insulin receptor function specifically in pancreatic β-cells *in vivo* exhibit defective insulin secretion is also consistent with a role for insulin signaling in β-cell function, although insulin gene expression has yet to be examined in this model [150]. However, the majority of studies have failed to detect significant changes in preproinsulin mRNA levels upon 1 h of glucose [11, 109] or insulin [11] stimulation, and it has been shown that glucose can activate insulin gene expression independently from insulin secretion [105–107]. Thus, the relevance of a putative short-term, insulin-mediated regulation of insulin gene transcription is still unclear.

Dysregulation of Insulin Gene Expression

There is convincing evidence that abnormalities in insulin gene sequence or function plays a role in pancreatic β-cell dysfunction in pathologic states, primarily in diabetes mellitus. Abnormalities in the insulin gene structure consist of rare control region mutations, while insulin gene expression appears to be reduced by metabolic conditions associated with the diabetic state.

Polymorphisms of the Insulin Gene

A highly polymorphic region located 360 bp upstream of the transcription initiation site in the human insulin gene consists of a variable number of tandem repeats (VNTR) of a G-rich consensus sequence [151, 152]. The diabetes susceptibility gene *IDDM2* has been mapped to the insulin VNTR [153]. VNTRs are classified as class I, II, or III, depending on the number of tandem repeats. While the short class I VNTR gene predisposes to type 1 diabetes, the long class III allele is thought to confer a protective effect against type 1 diabetes, but predispose to type 2 diabetes (reviewed in reference 154). Moreover, variations in VNTR number are associated with changes in transcriptional activity *in vivo* [155]. The zinc-finger Pur-1 transcription factor can bind to the VNTR and activate transcription [156], although how VNTR confers susceptibility to diabetes remains unexplained [154].

Glucose Toxicity and the Insulin Gene

The glucose toxicity hypothesis proposes that chronic hyperglycemia is deleterious to β-cell function by contributing to the deterioration of insulin secretion (reviewed in reference 157). These adverse effects of chronically elevated glucose levels in type 2 diabetic patients include impairment of insulin gene expression [158]. A decrease in preproinsulin mRNA levels has also been observed in several animal models of diabetes [159–164]; however, the specific mechanisms involved in glucose-mediated inhibition have principally been studied in insulin-secreting cell lines [165–173] and isolated rat [174] and human [175, 176] islets.

In the insulin-secreting HIT-T15 and INS-1 cells, impairment of insulin gene expression is associated with diminished activity of PDX-1 [166, 167, 170, 172] and RIPE3b1/Maf [168, 170, 177]. In HIT-T15 cells, decreased binding activity of PDX-1 is due to diminished expression, which cannot be accounted for by decreased PDX-1 gene transcription, therefore suggesting a post-transcriptional mechanism [167]. Overexpression of exogenous PDX-1 in glucotoxic HIT-T15 cells partially restores insulin gene activity [172]. In the mouse βTC-6 cell line, binding of RIPE3b1/mMaf is strongly reduced upon prolonged exposure to high glucose, but PDX-1 is unaffected [168], suggesting regulatory differences between cell lines. Importantly, PDX-1 protein levels are reduced *in vivo* in partially pancreatectomized, hyperglycemic rats [162] and in the diabetic gerbil *Psammomys obesus* [164], and binding activity is decreased in Zucker diabetic fatty (ZDF) rats [178]. Insulin gene expression may also be decreased by the CCAAT/enhancer-binding protein beta (C/EBPβ) [179, 180]. C/EBPβ directly binds the bHLH protein E47, thereby preventing formation of the BETA2/E47 activator complex required for insulin E1 stimulation [179].

The biochemical mechanisms whereby chronically elevated glucose impairs insulin gene expression have received considerable attention in the past few years. The prevailing hypothesis is that high glucose induces the excessive production of reactive oxygen species (ROS) and the formation of advanced glycation end products (AGE) [171, 181–185]. The β-cell is particularly sensitive to ROS because of low expression of antioxidant enzymes [186]. Induction of glycation reactions in the presence of a reducing sugar [171] or chronic exposure to elevated glucose [184] leads, in HIT-T15 cells, to decreased transcription of the insulin gene, an effect that is prevented by the antioxidants aminoguanidine and *N*-acetyl-cysteine (NAC). Chronic exposure of isolated islets to elevated glucose levels *in vitro* leads to accumulation of AGE, impaired β-cell function, and increased apoptosis, all of which can be prevented by aminoguanidine and NAC [181, 187]. Importantly, treatment of ZDF rats with aminoguanidine or NAC normalizes plasma glucose levels and restores insulin secretion, insulin content, and preproinsulin mRNA levels, whereas administration of the inhibitor of nitric oxide synthase SMT is ineffective, thus excluding the involvement of nitric oxide production as a mediator of glucose toxicity in this animal model [184].

These findings support the hypothesis that glucose toxicity is mediated in part by chronic oxidative stress, a phenomenon known to play a role in secondary complications of diabetes in other tissues [188]. Interestingly, activation of the hexosamine pathway, a mediator of glucose toxicity in peripheral tissues [189], decreases insulin gene expression and insulin secretion in isolated islets via generation of oxidative stress but not via O-linked glycosylation [190]. Oxidative stress-mediated impairment in PDX-1 binding activity is prevented by overexpression of a dominant-negative c-*jun* N-terminal kinase (JNK), and is mimicked by overexpression of wild-type JNK, without apparent changes in c-*jun* expression [191]. Since c-*jun* can also inhibit insulin gene transcription by interfering with bHLH-mediated transcriptional activity [192, 193], it is conceivable that several distinct pathways might be involved in the negative regulation of insulin gene transcription by oxidative stress (Figure 2). For example, chronic exposure to elevated glucose levels may lead to dedifferentiation and loss of genes associated with β-cell function. In addition, this state may result in expression of genes normally repressed in differentiated β-cells [200, 201]. For instance, the c-*myc* transcription factor is upregulated in diabetic islets [194] and is induced by high glucose in normal islets [195]. In turn, c-*myc* can inhibit insulin gene transcription [202] by competing for BETA2 binding at the E-box [203] (Figure 2).

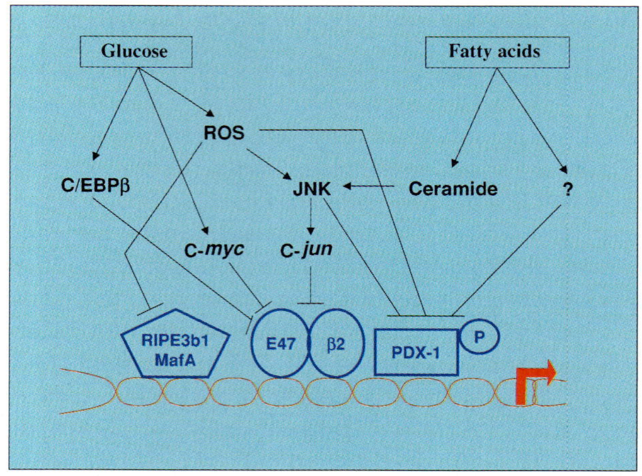

Figure 2 Proposed mechanisms whereby chronically elevated glucose and fatty acid levels impair insulin gene transcription. Prolonged exposure to high glucose decreases binding activity of MafA [168, 170, 177] and PDX-1 [162, 164, 166, 167, 170, 172, 177, 178] to the insulin promoter. The adverse effects of high glucose on the insulin gene are at least in part mediated by generation of ROS [171, 181–185], which can activate JNK [191], and impair insulin gene transcription both via c-*jun*-dependent [192, 193] and -independent [191] pathways. In addition, chronically elevated glucose induces C/EBPβ [179, 180] and c-*myc* [194, 195], which both interfere with bHLH-protein-mediated transcription. Prolonged exposure to elevated fatty acids impair insulin gene expression [196–199] and PDX-1 binding [196]. We propose that activation of JNK might be a common mechanism whereby chronically elevated glucose (via ROS generation) and fatty acids (via ceramide synthesis) inhibit insulin gene transcription. *Note*: the question mark indicates that fatty acids might interfere with PDX-1 via ceramide-independent, as yet unknown mechanisms

Lipotoxicity and the Insulin Gene

Like chronic hyperglycemia, hyperlipidemia has been proposed to contribute to β-cell dysfunction in type 2 diabetes [204–206]. Among other effects, chronically elevated fatty acid levels decrease insulin gene expression [196–199]. Initially, Gremlich et al. reported that a 48-h exposure of islets to 0.6 mM palmitate decreases insulin gene transcription in the presence of 30 mM glucose through negative regulation of PDX-1 [196]. In contrast, Bollheimer et al. found that a 24-h exposure of islets to 0.125 mM oleate at 5.6 mM glucose modestly increased preproinsulin mRNA levels [207]. In view of this apparent discrepancy, we hypothesized that fatty acids inhibit insulin gene expression only in the presence of elevated glucose levels, and tested this hypothesis in isolated rat islets and HIT-T15 cells [198]. We found that prolonged exposure of isolated islets to elevated levels of palmitic acid does not reduce preproinsulin mRNA levels in the presence of low glucose levels, but does so in the presence of high glucose [198]. This is associated with a decrease in human insulin promoter activity in transfected HIT cells [198] and isolated islets (C. L. Kelpe and V.P., unpublished data). Deleterious effects of fatty acids on insulin gene expression in isolated islets are associated with increased accumulation of intracellular triglycerides (TG), suggesting a role for neutral lipid synthesis [199]. However, increasing TG synthesis by overexpression of the TG-synthesizing enzyme diacylglycerol-acyltranferase inhibits glucose-induced insulin secretion but not preproinsulin mRNA levels [208], suggesting that TG accumulation is associated with, but not causally related to, decreased insulin gene expression. We have recently observed that culturing islets in the presence of palmitate is associated with generation of ceramide, and that blockade of ceramide synthesis prevents palmitate inhibition of insulin gene expression (C.L. Kelpe, P. Moore, C. Sutton, and V.P., unpublished observation). On the basis of these preliminary results, we propose that intracellular ceramide generation might mediate, at least in part, the deleterious effects of chronic fatty acids on insulin gene expression (Figure 2), in addition to its established role as a mediator of fatty acid induced apoptosis (reviewed in reference 209). Since ceramide is known to activate JNK in a variety of cells (reviewed in reference 210), it is tempting to speculate that ceramide-induced JNK activation might inhibit insulin gene transcription both via c-*jun*-dependent [192, 193] and -independent pathways [191].

INSULIN BIOSYNTHESIS

Introduction

From the previous section, one has ascertained that transcription of the insulin gene is a highly controlled process. Moreover, and somewhat unusually, preproinsulin mRNA is highly stable in pancreatic β-cells, with its half-life measured in excess of 36 h compared to 4–6 h for most eukaryotic mRNAs [211], and the preproinsulin mRNA stability is even extended further as glucose concentrations increase [92, 211] (see under Glucose Regulation of Insulin mRNA Stability). As such, there is normally an abundant source of preproinsulin mRNA in the β-cell cytosol available for translation. In this section we shall find that, under most circumstances, the production of insulin is also highly regulated at the translational level. Indeed, this is the predominant control mechanism in the β-cell whereby intracellular insulin stores are efficiently maintained. This enables the β-cell to rapidly replenished insulin stores back to optimal levels after they have been depleted by stimulated insulin secretion, and is more economic energy-wise to the β-cell, as translational control of insulin production bypasses the need for insulin gene transcription and preproinsulin mRNA maturation.

Structure of the Insulin Molecule

The primary structure of the A- and B-chains and of insulin itself has been known for close to 50 years [212, 213]. However, it was not until at least 10 years after this discovery that it was realized insulin is actually synthesized as a precursor molecule, preproinsulin (Figure 3) [214, 215].

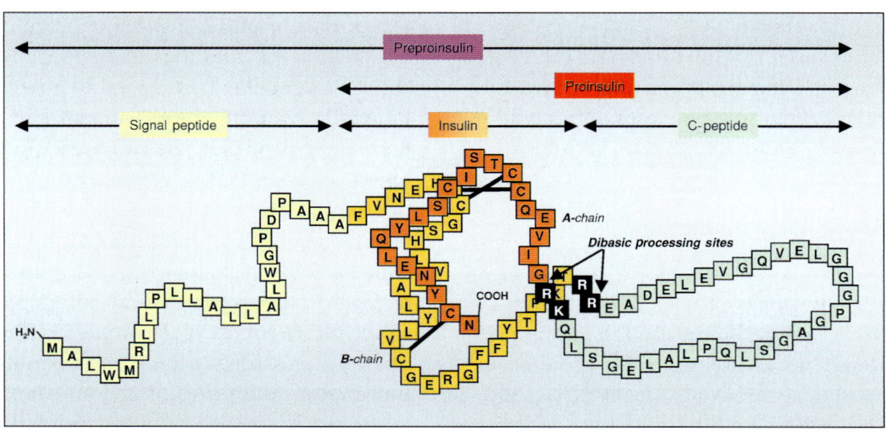

Figure 3 The primary structure of human preproinsulin. The figure indicates the N-terminal signal peptide, followed by the insulin B-chain, the C-peptide, and the C-terminal insulin A-chain. The two dibasic proteolytic conversion sites and the endoproteases that cleave these are also indicated (PC3 at Arg^{31}—Arg^{32} and PC2 at Lys^{64}—Arg^{65}). The signal peptide + insulin + C-peptide moieties comprise the preproinsulin, and the insulin + C-peptide moieties comprise proinsulin

Human preproinsulin is a single polypeptide chain consisting of the sequence of the proinsulin preceded by an N-terminal signal peptide (24 amino acids) that is relatively short-lived since this single peptide is removed co-translationally to yield proinsulin as the final product of preproinsulin mRNA translation [216, 217]. The proinsulin molecule is a 12-kDa single-chain polypeptide that encompasses the B-chain (30 amino acids) and the A-chain (21 amino acids) of insulin joined by the connecting peptide, C-peptide (Figure 3). It contains two interchain disulfide bonds between the A- and B-chains, and one A-chain intrachain disulfide bridge. Proinsulin to insulin conversion occurs by cleavage at two dibasic amino acid sequences in the B-chain/C-peptide and C-peptide/A-chain junctions to release the C-peptide moiety, yielding the insulin molecule with the two independent disulfide-linked A- and B-chains correctly aligned [218, 219]. Generally, the proinsulin primary amino acid sequence is highly conserved in higher vertebrates, mainly within the insulin A- and B-chains. The C-peptide sequence shows greater species variation, including in length, varying between 26 and 38 residues. However, the position of the disulfide bonds and dibasic conversion sites are very highly conserved among species [220]. The C-peptide moiety of proinsulin, which essentially promotes the correct structural alignment and disulfide linkage of the insulin A- and B-chains, has little secondary structure itself [221, 222]. In contrast, the insulin moiety within the proinsulin molecule has a close resemblance to that of insulin itself [221, 223]. Initially, proinsulin dimerizes and then three proinsulin dimers in the presence of Zn^{2+} form a hexameric structure similar to that of insulin [224, 225], yet proinsulin has only <5% of insulin's biological activity [226, 227]. As such, it is thought that the flexibility of the structureless C-peptide moiety leads to interaction with the insulin A- and B-chains, accounting for reduced biological activity of proinsulin. Nonetheless, the two dibasic conversion sites on proinsulin are very close to each other and located on the outer surface of the proinsulin molecule [221], thus facilitating an efficient proinsulin conversion process (see later under Proteolytic Enzymes of Proinsulin Conversion).

Proinsulin Biosynthesis: Translation and Translocation

The first step in proinsulin biosynthesis is translation of preproinsulin mRNA. Essentially, translation of the preproinsulin mRNA template to preproinsulin protein occurs in a fashion typical of most eukaryotic mRNAs [228]. First, binding of the free 40S and 60S ribosomal subunits and methionyl-tRNA to the AUG start codon on preproinsulin mRNA occurs in the β-cell cytosol, to form an 80S translation initiation complex. The construction of such a translational initiation complex is specifically catalyzed and coordinately controlled by a group of cytosolic proteins known as eukaryotic initiation factors (eIFs) in the intiation phase of protein synthesis translation [229–233]. Translation of preproinsulin mRNA then proceeds to the elongation phase of protein synthesis [229, 230]. Elongation involves the sequential recruitment of codon-directed aminoacyl-tRNAs to the ribosomal/preproinsulin mRNA translation complex, catalyzed and controlled by cytosolic proteins known as elongation factors (EFs) [229, 230]. The codon sequence on preproinsulin mRNA directs the order of aminoacyl-tRNAs brought into the ribosomal cleft of the ribosomal/preproinsulin mRNA complex, and peptide bonds form between amino acids successively and the correct amino acid sequence of preproinsulin begins to emerge. As the ribosome scans along the preproinsulin mRNA vacating the AUG start codon, another translation initiation step can occur so that several ribosomal complexes can form on the preproinsulin mRNA template to form a polysome. Ribosomal complexes can follow each other along the template to yield several preproinsulin polypeptides from a single preproinsulin mRNA. As elongation proceeds, the emerging signal sequence of preproinsulin binds the signal recognition particle (SRP), a cytosolic ribonucleoprotein complex, and translation is momentarily arrested. The signal-sequence-bound SRP then docks to the SRP receptor, which is an integral membrane protein of the rough endoplasmic reticulum (RER), thereby locating the preproinsulin mRNA/ribosomal complex to the RER, the major site of proinsulin biosynthesis in the β-cell [234]. As SRP binds to the SRP receptor, the nascent signal peptide of the newly forming preproinsulin dissociates from SRP and is transferred to another RER integral membrane protein called the signal sequence receptor (SSR). SSR is part of a "translocation pore" that facilitates transport of the newly forming preproinsulin polypeptide across the RER membrane into the RER lumen, marking the entrance of the newly synthesized preproinsulin into the β-cell's secretory pathway. Elongation then resumes increasing the length of the preproinsulin polypeptide. The signal peptide is cleaved cotranslationally by another RER-membrane-associated protein, the signal peptidase, before preproinsulin mRNA translation is complete. Eventually, preproinsulin polypeptide elongation is halted at the UAG stop codon on preproinsulin mRNA, catalyzed by a GTP-binding protein called releasing factor (RF). RF promotes release of the newly formed preproinsulin polypeptide from preproinsulin mRNA/ribosomal complex, allowing the recycling of ribosomes for another round of preproinsulin mRNA translation initiation/elongation. The C-terminal portion of the newly formed preproinsulin polypeptide then completes translocation across the RER, resulting in a soluble nascent proinsulin molecule in the RER lumen. Once in the RER lumen, the proinsulin molecule undergoes appropriate folding so that the intrachain disulfide bond of the insulin A-chain, and the two A/B interchain disulfide bridges within the proinsulin molecule can be correctly aligned. The folding process is likely catalyzed by the molecular chaperons, such as BiP, and disulfide bonds catalyzed by disulfide isomerase activity found in the RER lumen of β-cells [235].

Proinsulin Biosynthesis: Effectors and Stimulus–Response Coupling Mechanisms

Proinsulin biosynthesis is controlled by certain nutrients, neurotransmitters, and hormones at the translational level [236, 237], but of these glucose is probably physiologically the most relevant. In general, nutrients that stimulate insulin secretion also stimulate proinsulin biosynthesis at the translational level. This provides a means whereby insulin stores lost via nutrient-regulated secretion can be rapidly replenished by a parallel upregulation of proinsulin translation/biosynthesis. Glucose metabolism is required for glucose-induced proinsulin biosynthesis [96, 238–241]. The threshold concentration of glucose required to stimulate insulin secretion is 4–6 mM, but that required to stimulate proinsulin biosynthesis is only 2–4 mM [241–244]. A maximum rate of proinsulin biosynthesis is reached at a glucose concentration of 10–12 mM, which is lower than that for maximal glucose-induced insulin secretion at >15 mM [238, 240, 241]. The short-term stimulation (<2 h) appears to be entirely mediated at the translational level [245, 247]. Significant glucose-induced proinsulin biosynthesis can be observed after a 20-min lag period, and reaches a maximum rate (~20–30-fold increase above basal) by 60 min [240, 241, 247]. Once the glucose stimulus is removed, the "off-rate" of proinsulin biosynthesis is relatively slow, taking more than 1 h to return to basal rate [247]. Put together, these characteristics of glucose-induced proinsulin biosynthesis ensure that intracellular stores of insulin are maintained at optimal levels, so as not to compromise efficient insulin secretion.

Of the peptide hormones that stimulate proinsulin biosynthesis, perhaps the incretins, GLP-1 and GIP (glucose-dependent insulin-releasing polypeptide), are the most physiologically relevant [248]. GLP-1/GIP do not increase proinsulin biosynthesis in their own right, but potentiate glucose-induced proinsulin biosynthesis as they do glucose-induced insulin secretion [249]. The means by which GLP-1/GIP upregulate proinsulin biosynthesis is thought to be via the Gαs-linked GLP-1/GIP receptors, to increase adenylate cyclase activity and consequently intracellular cAMP concentration, leading to PKA activation [248]. As to how PKA increases the proinsulin biosynthesis is unknown. Epinepherine is also worthy of mention for specifically inhibiting glucose-induced proinsulin biosynthesis as it does glucose-induced insulin secretion [250].

Unlike glucose-induced insulin secretion [1, 251–253], the secondary signals that lead to an increase in proinsulin biosynthesis are less well defined. Glucose metabolism is required for glucose induction of both proinsulin biosynthesis and insulin secretion [238], but several lines of evidence indicate that the stimulus–response coupling mechanism for these β-cell functions are quite distinct. As previously mentioned, the threshold glucose concentration to stimulate proinsulin biosynthesis is lower than that to evoke insulin secretion [238]. In marked contrast to glucose-induced insulin secretion, glucose-induced proinsulin biosynthesis requires Mg^{2+} but is independent of extracellular Ca^{2+} [254–256]. Although sulfonylureas stimulate and diazoxide inhibit glucose-induced insulin secretion, these compounds have no effect on glucose-induced proinsulin biosynthesis, indicating that the signal transduction mechanism for regulating proinsulin biosynthesis is independent of the K_{ATP} channel, unlike that for glucose-stimulated insulin secretion [256–260]. Somatostatin is a potent inhibitor of insulin secretion, but has no effect on proinsulin biosynthesis [261, 262]. Long-chain fatty acids, when applied acutely, are marked potentiators of glucose-induced insulin secretion [263–265], but only if anything modestly inhibit glucose-induced proinsulin biosynthesis [207, 266]. Analogous to general protein synthesis, proinsulin biosynthesis has a dependence for GTP, which likely resides in the GTP requirement for the action of the 54-kDa subunit of SRP [267] or eIF2. [229, 230, 232, 233, 268]. In addition, general protein biosynthesis in the β-cell requires ATP [229, 232, 233], but it has been shown that ATP does not act as a *specific* stimulus–response coupling factor for glucose-induced proinsulin biosynthesis as it does for glucose-induced insulin secretion [262]. Recently, it has been indicated that a secondary signal for glucose-induced proinsulin biosynthesis does not emanate from β-cell glycolysis or electron transport chain/oxidative phosphorylation but from anaplerosis in the Krebs cycle [262, 266, 269]. In this regard, it has been suggested that mitochondrial export of succinate and cytosolic accumulation of succinyl-CoA are key "signals" specific for glucose-induced proinsulin biosynthesis [262], but the effectors downstream of succinate/succinyl-CoA to specifically upregulate the preproinsulin mRNA translational machinery require further investigation.

Proinsulin Biosynthesis: Translational Control Mechanism

In general, glucose modestly increases total protein synthesis in the β-cell (1.5–2-fold). This likely occurs via phosphorylation-regulation of certain eIFs, in particular, eIF2α, eIF-2B, and eIF-4E-BP. In addition, the signal peptide region can facilitate a modest 1.5–2-fold increase in the synthesis of secretory pathway proteins [246, 270].

However, the effect of glucose on proinsulin synthesis is much greater, reaching >15-fold stimulation above basal. This indicates a *specific* effect of glucose on translational control of proinsulin biosynthesis. Recently, it has been shown that such *specific* control of glucose-induced proinsulin biosynthesis in the β-cell resides in *cis*-elements in the 5′- and 3′-UTRs of preproinsulin mRNA itself [109]. Indeed, in the 5′-UTR there is a "stem-loop" secondary structure (not necessarily primary sequence) that is highly conserved across mammalian preproinsulin mRNAs [271, 272]. In addition in the 3′-UTR of preproinsulin mRNA, downstream of and close to the polyadenylation signal, there is a highly conserved primary sequence containing a UUGAA *cis*-element core [109]. The 5′-UTR stem-loop element of the preproinsulin mRNA is required for glucose-induced proinsulin biosynthesis, since the translation of a preproinsulin mRNA variant that lacks this 5′-UTR does not undergo glucose-induced translational regulation [109]. The 3′-UTR *cis*-element does not in itself upregulate glucose-induced proinsulin biosynthesis, but may be involved in maintaining preproinsulin mRNA stability specifically in β-cells [11, 109] (see under Glucose Regulation of Insulin mRNA Stability). However, when the 5′-UTR stem-loop is present, the 3′-UTR *cis*-element appears to mediate glucose-induced alleviation of a translational block [109]. Thus, it appears that there is cooperativity between the preproinsulin mRNA 5′- and 3′-UTRs for the *specific* translational control of proinsulin biosynthesis influenced by extracellular glucose concentrations [109]. Recently, it has been shown that flanking a luciferase-coding mRNA with the 5′- and 3′-UTRs of preproinsulin mRNA can confer *specific* glucose-induced luciferase biosynthesis in islet β-cells [273], emphasizing the important role of these 5′- and 3′-UTRs in the translational control of proinsulin biosynthesis. Intriguingly, some preliminary RNA-gel shift evidence has indicated that different *trans*-acting proteins specifically bind to the 5′- and 3′-UTR *cis*-elements of preproinsulin mRNA in a glucose-regulated manner [273]. However, the identity of such *trans*-acting factors has not been revealed. Characterization of such factors will improve our understanding of the control mechanisms behind proinsulin production in the β-cell.

It should be noted that proinsulin is only one of a small subset of β-cell proteins (~50 in all) [257, 274] whose biosynthesis is regulated by glucose at the translational level. Other glucose-regulated proteins include a common β-granule matrix protein, chromogranin A [240]; a β-granule membrane glycoprotein, SGM-110 [275]; and the proinsulin processing endopeptidases, proprotein convertase 2 (PC2) and proprotein convertase 3 (PC3) [241, 276, 277] (see later). Glucose-induced biosynthesis of these β-cell proteins appear to be coupled to that of proinsulin [240, 241, 275, 276]. Thus, the translational control mechanism for chromogranin-A, SGM-110, PC2, and PC3 biosyntheses are likely common to that of proinsulin [272] and important for the biogenesis of β-granules. Indeed, a stem-loop structure similar to that of the preproinsulin mRNA 5′-UTR is predicted in the 5′-UTR of the mRNA encoding these β-granule proteins [272]. However, glucose does not regulate the biosynthesis of a number of other β-granule proteins in rat islets, including the proinsulin converting exopeptidase, carboxypeptidase-H (CP-H) [240, 276]. Interestingly, however, the preproCP-H mRNA does not encode a predicted stem-loop in its 5′-UTR [272]. Notwithstanding, it should be noted that CP-H is a relatively abundant β-granule protein, and the lack of glucose-induced translational control of its biosynthesis does not appear to adversely affect proinsulin conversion [240] (see under Proteolytic Enzymes of Proinsulin Conversion). In contrast, glucose-induced translational control of the proinsulin processing endopeptidases, proPC2 and proPC3, provides a means whereby proinsulin conversion is not compromised upon increased proinsulin biosynthesis [241, 278] (see under Regulation of Proinsulin Conversion).

Transport of Proinsulin from the RER to the Golgi Apparatus

After proinsulin is translocated into the lumen of the RER, correctly folded proinsulin can then be delivered in transport vesicles to the *cis*-Golgi apparatus in an ATP-dependent process [279] (Figure 4). The RER to *cis*-Golgi transport mechanism also requires the integrity of the β-cell's microfilament/microtubular network [280], and other cofactors including [Ca^{2+}], GTP hydrolysis, and some cytosolic proteins [281–284]. The newly synthesized proinsulin is then transported from the *cis*-stack, via the *medial*- to the *trans*-stack of the Golgi apparatus in COP-coated vesicles [285–287] (Figure 4). The COP coat consists of a protein complex of cytosolic coatmer proteins (α-, β-, δ-, and γ-COPs) [285]. Fusion of a COP-coated vesicle with a target Golgi stack membrane requires loss of the coat in a GTP-dependent process just prior to fusion, and the GTP-binding protein, ARF, interacting with phospholipase-D [285]. In addition, intercisternal transport between Golgi stacks also requires cytosolic factors and various Golgi-membrane proteins [282, 285, 288]. The newly synthesized proinsulin eventually accumulates in clathrin-coated regions of the *trans*-Golgi network (TGN) [234], which are the sites of secretory granule biogenesis (Figure 4). Recently, a 3D-morphometric analysis of the Golgi apparatus in pancreatic β-cells has revealed that newly forming immature β-granules seem to emerge from a particular compartment of the TGN, distinct from other regions of the TGN where other secretory vesicles emerge (including unregulated constitutive vesicles) [289] (Figure 4). Pulse-chase radiolabeling experiments have revealed that the transit time from the initiation

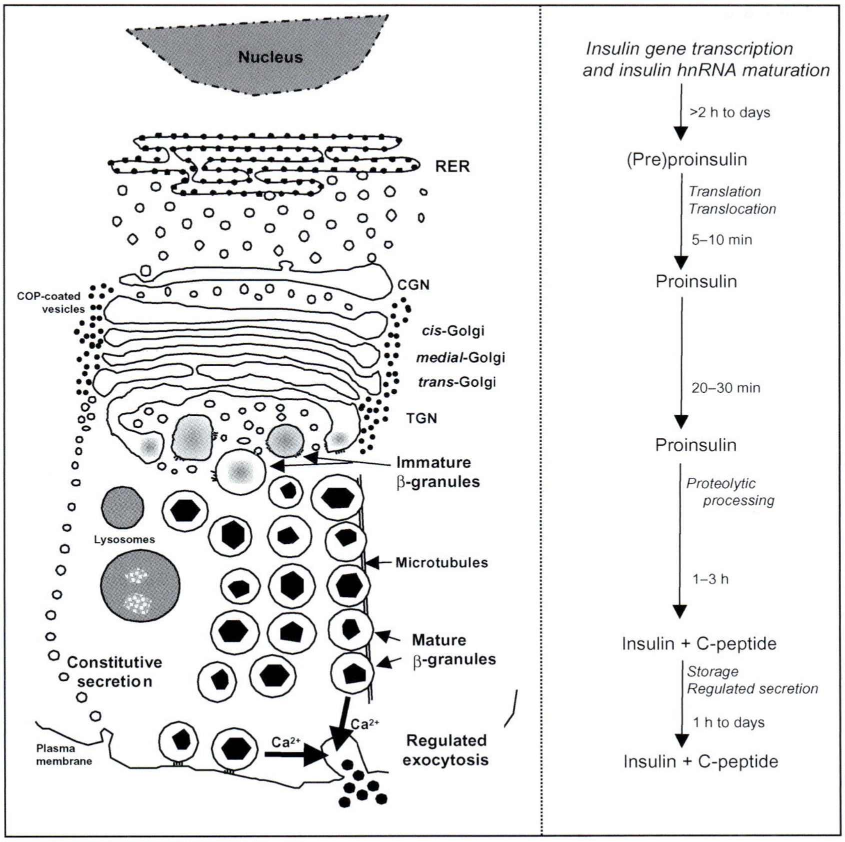

Figure 4 The cell biology of proinsulin trafficking and processing. The site of preproinsulin biosynthesis is on the ribosomes of the RER. The signal peptide is cleaved cotranslationally, enabling proinsulin translocation into the RER lumen. The newly synthesized proinsulin is then transported to the *cis*-Golgi and transferred through the stacks of the *medial*- and *trans*-Golgi to clathrin-coated regions of the TGN. Immature β-granules bud off from the TGN, which is the major site of proinsulin conversion (~30-min posttranslation). Proinsulin conversion proceeds as a β-granule matures. Mature β-granules form the intracellular insulin storage compartment of the β-cells and do not undergo Ca^{2+}-dependent exocytosis unless triggered by an appropriate stimulus. The left panel shows the intracellular compartments through which proinsulin is sequentially transported, and the right panel indicates the kinetics of the preproinsulin biosynthetic/processing/secretory process in these compartments

of preproinsulin biosynthesis to the TGN is around 20–30 min [234] (Figure 2).

The means by which newly synthesized proinsulin (and other specific proteins destined to the β-granule) is specifically targeted to sites of β-granule biogenesis in clathrin-coated regions of the TGN remains a matter of debate [290, 291]. However, it is known to be a highly efficient process, with >99% efficiency for newly synthesized proinsulin to be sorted to the β-granule and the regulated secretory pathway under normal conditions [292]. Essentially, there are two schools of thought for the process of sorting proinsulin to β-granules: either by an active process, perhaps via a receptor-mediated sorting mechanism (as for lysosomal proteins that are also sorted in the TGN [293] or RER proteins in the *cis*-Golgi network, CGN [294]), or a more passive process resulting from selective aggregation/condensation of proinsulin (in the presence of Zn^{2+}) and other β-granule proteins [291, 295]. Several candidate "receptors" for sorting mechanisms in the TGN have been proposed, including CP-H [296, 297] and chromogranin-A [298]. However, CP-H is an unlikely sorting receptor in β-cells, since proinsulin is efficiently and conventionally sorted in CP-H deficient mice [299, 300]. It has also been proposed that a so-called amphipathic hairpin loop structure in prohormones could act as a positive sorting signal to the regulated secretory pathway [301], but this is also not relevant to β-cells as this structure is not present in the proinsulin molecule [295, 302]. Currently, sorting to the β-granule by aggregation is the favored hypothesis [291, 295]. This model proposes that common physicochemical properties of β-granule proteins make them prone to a possible Zn^{2+}/Ca^{2+}-dependent aggregation in the mildly acidic internal environment of the TGN [291, 295]. However, sorting by aggregation is likely to be a complex mechanism requiring other yet to be defined nuances, considering that >50 β-granule proteins must be coordinately delivered to the site of β-granule biogenesis in the TGN. Nonetheless, this model appears to be quite pertinent to the β-cell, since a mutation in human proinsulin (B-chain His-10 to Asp-10) [303], which removes the Zn^{2+}-binding motif and prevents proinsulin hexamer formation, disrupted proinsulin sorting to β-granules and consequently proinsulin processing, and increased constitutive proinsulin/insulin secretion [304, 305].

Generally, analogous to other neuroendocrine cells, the process of β-granule biogenesis should also require other factors including intraluminal acidic milieu (pH 6.5) [306], Ca^{2+} [306], ATP [307], GTP-hydrolysis [308], cytosolic proteins [309–311], and protein tyrosine phosphorylation [312]. Although β-granule biogenesis occurs in limited clathrin-coated regions of the TGN [234], the role that clathrin itself plays is unclear. Clathrin is not an essential component of vesicular traffic along the biosynthetic secretory pathway [313], but may be involved in a post-Golgi editing mechanism that retrieves TGN-membrane proteins and "minor missorted protein contaminants" after a newly formed immature β-granule has budded off from the TGN [313, 314]. In β-cells, the minor degree of "constitutive-like" proinsulin secretion observed could be symptomatic of such a post-TGN editing mechanism [315, 316]. Once an immature, partly clathrin-coated β-granule has budded off from the TGN, it undergoes a maturation process [234]. The immature β-granule is the intracellular compartment where the vast majority of proinsulin-to-insulin conversion takes place (see the next subsection; Figure 4) [234, 317–319]. Maturation of β-granules involves proinsulin conversion, progressive intragranular acidification, loss of the clathrin-coated regions, and formation of hexameric insulin crystals [234, 257, 316]. Acidification provides the correct intragranular pH (pH 5.0–5.5) for proinsulin processing to proceed [234, 317–319], and optimal insulin crystal formation around insulin's isoelectric point (pK_i 5.3) [226, 257]. Delivery of newly synthesized proinsulin to an immature β-granule occurs around 30–40-min posttranslation where proinsulin processing begins and is >90% completed ~3 h later [234, 292] (Figure 4).

Proteolytic Enzymes of Proinsulin Conversion

The major site for processing of proinsulin to biologically active insulin is the immature granule compartment of the β-cell [234] (Figure 4). Production of insulin (and C-peptide) occurs via limited proteolysis of the proinsulin precursor molecule, which is catalyzed by two Ca^{2+}-dependent endopeptidases, PC2 and PC3 (also known as PC-1) [320–323], and a Ni^{2+}-dependent exopeptidase, CP-H [324, 325]. There are two dibasic sites on the human proinsulin molecule, Arg^{31}—Arg^{32} and Lys^{64}—Arg^{65} (Figure 3), that signal limited endoproteolytic cleavage of proinsulin to excise the C-peptide moiety and to generate insulin with its disulfide-linked A- and B-chains correctly aligned [226, 257, 278]. Endoproteolytic peptide bond cleavage of proinsulin occurs on the carboxylic side of the Arg^{31}—Arg^{32} or Lys^{64}—Arg^{65}, followed by rapid and specific exopeptidic removal of the newly exposed basic amino acids by CP-H [324, 325]. The two distinct β-granule proinsulin-processing endopeptidase activities were originally discovered as Ca^{2+}-dependent with an acidic pH optimum [318]. One (type I) cleaved specifically at the Arg^{31}—Arg^{32} site of proinsulin, whereas the other (type II) had a strong preference for the Lys^{64}—Arg^{65} site [318]. These activities were later found to be the cloned PC3 [326–328] and PC2 [328–330] endopeptidases, respectively.

A scheme of proinsulin conversion is illustrated in Figure 5. Proinsulin conversion could occur by two possible routes. Either PC2 first cleaves on the carboxylic side of Lys^{64}—Arg^{65} to yield a split-65,66-proinsulin intermediate, followed by CP-H trimming of the newly exposed lysine and arginine residues to yield des-64,65-proinsulin. Then PC3 can cleave des-64,65-proinsulin at Arg^{31}—Arg^{32}, which together with CP-H trimming of the exposed arginine residues, yields insulin and C-peptide (Figure 5). Alternatively, PC3 first could cleave at the carboxylic side of Arg^{31}—Arg^{32} to yield a split-32,33-proinsulin intermediate, followed by CP-H trimming of the revealed arginine residues to yield des-31,32-proinsulin. PC2 can then cleave des-32,33- proinsulin at Lys^{64}—Arg^{65}, which together with CP-H trimming of the lysine and arginine residues, yields insulin and C-peptide (Figure 5). However, although both of these routes can occur in the β-cell *in vivo*, several lines of evidence indicate that the latter route (via the des-31,32-proinsulin intermediate) is predominant [221, 223, 278, 327, 331–333]. Most pronounced is that PC2 has a much stronger preference for the des-31,32-proinsulin substrate than for proinsulin [221, 223]. In contrast, PC3 has an equivalent preference for proinsulin or des-64,65-proinsulin substrates [223]. As such, in humans, the sequential processing of proinsulin via des-31,32-proinsulin is the predominant route, where PC3 cleaves intact proinsulin first, followed by PC2 cleavage of des-31,32-proinsulin (Figure 5). This is consistent with the presence of the des-31,32-proinsulin conversion intermediate in the human circulation, but of negligible levels of des-64,65-proinsulin [332, 333]. As example, HPLC analysis of proinsulin conversion intermediates is illustrated in Figure 6, where purified rat [^{3}H]leucine-proinsulin 1 has been incubated *in vitro* with a purified β-granule preparation containing the PC2, PC3, and CP-H enzymes at 30°C for 1 h. Even in this *in vitro* analysis, des-31,32-proinsulin (and split-32,33-proinsulin) is more abundant than des-64,65-proinsulin (and split-65,66-proinsulin) (Figure 6), emphasizing the preferred des-31,32-proinsulin processing route (Figure 5).

PC2, PC3, and CP-H are generally expressed in most neuroendocrine cells where they are involved in

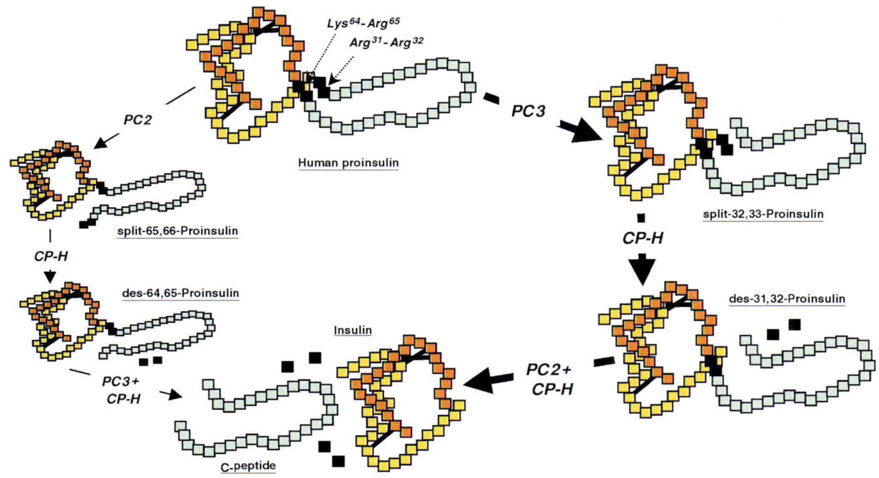

Figure 5 Proteolytic conversion of proinsulin. There are two potential pathways of proteolytic conversion of proinsulin to insulin. Either PC2 first cleaves proinsulin at Lys^{64}—$Arg^{65}$to yield split-65,66-proinsulin, followed by CP-H trimming of the newly exposed lysine and arginine residues to yield des-64,65-proinsulin. PC3 can then cleave des-64,65-proinsulin at Arg^{31}—Arg^{32}, which together with trimming of the exposed arginine residues by CP-H, yields insulin and C-peptide. Alternatively, PC3 cleaves at Arg^{31}—Arg^{32} to yield split-32,33-proinsulin, followed by CP-H trimming of the revealed arginine residues, producing des-31,32-proinsulin. PC2 can then cleave des-32,33-proinsulin at Lys^{64}—Arg^{65}, which together with trimming of the lysine and arginine residues by CP-H, generates insulin and C-peptide. In human β-cells, the route via des-31,32-proinsulin predominates as illustrated by the larger size of this pathway

posttranslational processing of other prohormone precursors [337]. The role of these proteolytic enzymes in proinsulin conversion has been substantiated in various gene-deletion studies. However, PC2, PC3, or CP-H deficiencies also generate multiple endocrine deficiencies, which is not too surprising, given the wider role these enzymes have in general prohormone processing. PC2 knockout mice have defective proinsulin processing with increased levels of the split proinsulin conversion intermediate des-31,32-proinsulin, consistent with PC2 preferentially cleaving at the Lys^{64}—Arg^{65} site on proinsulin, and the preferred sequential proinsulin processing route [338, 339] (Figure 5). PC2 *null* mice have a polyendocrine phenotype, the most obvious being fasting hypoglycemia and glucose intolerance due to a deficiency of circulating glucagon levels rather than increased insulin levels [338, 339]. In contrast, PC3 *null* mice are embryonic lethal. However, a human mutation of both PC3 alleles exists that results in negligible PC3 activity [340]. This generates a complicated phenotype of multiple endocrine

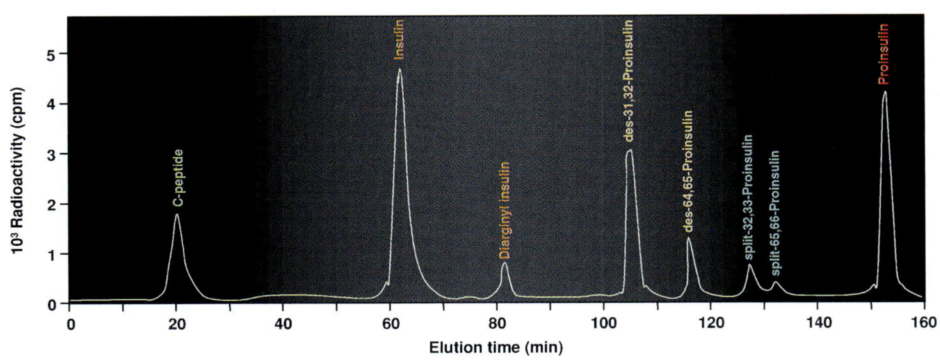

Figure 6 HPLC analysis of proinsulin processing: intermediates and products. Isolated rat islets were pulse-radiolabeled with [^{3}H]leucine at a stimulatory glucose concentration (17 mM) for 30 min, and then the [^{3}H]proinsulin was extracted from the islet lysates in 100 mM HCl as previously described [334]. The rat-1 [^{3}H]proinsulin was then purified using HPLC and lyophilization [335]. The purified rat [^{3}H]proinsulin 1 was then incubated with a purified β-granule preparation, which contains the PC2, PC3, and CP-H proinsulin processing enzymes, for 60 min at 30°C *in vitro* as described [223, 336], and analyzed for proinsulin processing intermediates and products as described, using acetontrile elution gradients [223, 334, 336]. An example HPLC rat [^{3}H]proinsulin 1 processing profile analysis (after a 30-min incubation) is shown with the elution positions of unprocessed proinsulin, split proinsulin conversion intermediates, diarginyl insulin, insulin, and C-peptide indicated

disorders due to general abnormal prohormone processing, one of which is very low insulin concentrations and high proinsulin levels, together with abnormal glucose homeostasis, consistent with defective proinsulin processing [340]. Finally, the obese *Fat/Fat* mice have been found to have a mutation in the CP-H gene, resulting in negligible CP-H activity [341]. These CP-H *null* animals are hyperproinsulinemic [341], suggesting that CP-H trimming of basic amino acids after PC2/PC3 endopeptidic cleavage accelerates proinsulin proteolytic maturation to insulin [278, 300]. Moreover diarginyl insulin (that has >50% reduced biological activity) rather than insulin is produced, indicating the role that CP-H plays in trimming basic amino acids during the proinsulin conversion process [341].

Regulation of Proinsulin Conversion

PC2 and PC3 are Ca^{2+}-dependent enzyme activities with an acidic pH 5–5.5 optimum [223, 318, 326, 327]. Fortunately, the β-granule contains an intraorganellar environment of 1–10 mM free [Ca^{2+}] [342] and acidic pH 5.5 [343], which ideally suits the requirements for optimal PC2/PC3 and CP-H activities within this organelle [318, 325]. This also ensures that insulin is produced mainly in the intracellular β-granule compartment in which it is stored [278, 318]. To render PC2 and PC3 fully active for proinsulin processing in a newly formed β-granule, it follows that activation of the proton-pumping ATPase [319, 343, 344] and Ca^{2+}-translocation proteins [345] are key regulatory events that control proinsulin conversion.

Both PC2 and PC3 are initially synthesized as preproPC2/PC3 precursor molecules, with the "pre" signal peptide region enabling translocation into the RER lumen during translation as with the signal peptide region of proinsulin (see under Proinsulin Biosynthesis: Translation and Translocation). proPC2 and proPC3 are transported to β-granules along with their proinsulin substrate in the β-cell's secretory pathway and undergo maturation beginning in the TGN [241, 346]. However, unlike proinsulin, proPC2 and proPC3 are accompanied by individual chaperon molecules, 7B2 and proSAAS respectively, that specifically inhibit these endopeptidase's activity [347–350]. Proteolytic cleavage of 7B2 by PC2, and proSAAS by PC3, in the TGN/immature β-granule compartment alleviates the inhibition on proPC2 and proPC3, promoting their maturation and activation to mature PC2 and PC3. This then provides an additional degree of proPC2 and proPC3 regulation, by restricting their activation and proinsulin conversion to the β-granule compartment. It appears that 7B2 has an important role in controlling PC2 activity *in vivo*. The 7B2 knockout mouse has multiple neuroendocrine disorders, similar yet more severe than the PC2 *null* mouse [338, 339], including hypoglycemia, hyperproinsulinemia, defective glucagon production, and also Cushing's syndrome due to defective ACTH production in the pituitary [351].

As previously indicated, the short-term (<4 h) biosynthesis of proPC2 and proPC3 is stimulated predominately at a translational level coordinately with that of proinsulin [241, 276, 277]. However, in the long term (>12 h), glucose regulates PC2 and PC3 gene transcription in parallel with the preproinsulin gene [211]. Thus, it seems that proinsulin conversion is adaptable to changes in glucose by coordinate regulation of the endopeptidases that catalyze processing [352].

The Mature β-Granule Storage Pool

A mature β-granule is retained from anywhere between a few hours to several days, awaiting transport to the β-cell's plasma membrane and exocytosis under stimulatory conditions, characteristic of a regulated secretory pathway [290, 291] (Figure 4). It should be noted that under normal conditions, the storage compartment of insulin in mature β-granules far exceeds the compartment undergoing transport/exocytosis, so that during a 1-h stimulation by glucose only ~1–2% of the insulin content of a primary islet β-cell is secreted [262, 292]. The insulin content of a β-cell is kept at a relatively constant level under normal physiological conditions where secreted insulin is rapidly replaced by regulation at the biosynthetic level (see under Proinsulin Biosynthesis: Effectors and Stimulus–Response Coupling Mechanisms). However, in the long term there is also an additional regulatory component that maintains insulin stores at optimal levels, via insulin degradation [353–355]. The half-life of a β-granule is several days, but if it is not used for exocytosis it is eventually degraded by fusion with lysosomes, a process known as *crinophagy* [234, 353, 354].

Dysfunctional Proinsulin Processing in Diabetes

In type 1 diabetes, where there is autoimmune destruction of β-cells, proinsulin production is distinctly decreased in line with the marked reduction in β-cell mass. In type 2 diabetes, where there is apparent hyperinsulinemia to compensate for peripheral insulin resistance, an increased proportion of the secreted insulin is actually proinsulin or split proinsulin conversion intermediates (mostly des-31,32-proinsulin) so that it is in fact a hyperproinsulinemic state [278, 332, 333, 356–364]. Some have gone as far as to suggest hyperproinsulinemia as a predictive marker of non-insulin-dependent diabetes mellitus (NIDDM) [357]. How might hyperproinsulinemia occur? It is possible that genetic defects in the proinsulin conversion enzyme genes or the insulin gene itself hamper proinsulin conversion, resulting in an increased proportion of secreted proinsulin [303, 304, 338–341, 351, 365]. However, these genetic mutations are relatively rare occurrences, yet hyperproinsulinemia is a common trait of NIDDM [278]. As such, an increased proportion of secreted proinsulin likely occurs as a consequence of β-cell dysfunction in NIDDM [356, 366–368]. In type 2 diabetes there is chronic hyperglycemia and hyperlipidemia [206, 366, 367, 369]), both of which could have long-term detrimental effects on proinsulin processing and insulin production in the β-cell. As a consequence of chronically elevated glucose levels, the β-cell works very hard with both proinsulin synthesis and insulin secretion being upregulated [278, 362]. Yet one should consider that there is preferential release of newly synthesized (pro)insulin [292, 370], so that newly formed β-granules are preferentially targeted for exocytosis before they are fully matured (<90 min). Thus, newly synthesized proinsulin is not retained long enough to be fully converted to insulin and C-peptide, and a greater proportion of proinsulin (as well as des-31,32-proinsulin) is secreted [278]. It should also be recognized that newly synthesized proPC2 and proPC3 also undergo a zymogen-like maturation/activation process guided by their specific chaperons, 7B2 and proSAAS [347–350], that might be adversely affected by chronically elevated glucose. As for proinsulin processing in hyperglycemia, an immature β-granule may not be held long enough for full autocatalytic proteolytic activation of PC2 and PC3, which in turn compromises proinsulin processing, and contributes to the hyperproinsulinemia in NIDDM. In addition, while proPC2 and proPC3 synthesis is translationally regulated by glucose in parallel to proinsulin [241, 276–278], it is currently unclear whether synthesis of the 7B2 and proSAAS chaperons are regulated in parallel. If not, activation of proPC2 and proPC3 may be impaired, causing increased proinsulin accumulation and consequently an increased proportion of proinsulin secreted. It should also be noted that proPC2 passage along the β-cell's secretory pathway is significantly slower than that of proPC3 and proinsulin [346], and during chronic hyperglycemia the availability of PC2 delivered to an immature β-granule could be reduced, adversely affecting proinsulin processing, again contributing to the hyperproinsulinemia. Unlike proinsulin, PC2, and PC3 biosyntheses, CP-H biosynthesis is not translationally regulated [240, 241]. Although CP-H is relatively abundant in β-granules [371], during chronic hyperglycemia the availability of CP-H delivered to β-granules may become limited in type 2 diabetes. If so, then hyperproinsulinemia should ensue as observed in the CP-H *null* mouse [341].

Chronic hyperlipidemia found in type 2 diabetes might also affect proinsulin production. Chronically elevated fatty acid levels can increase the amount of insulin secreted from the β-cell [207], but in contrast, fatty acids modestly inhibit glucose-induced proinsulin biosynthesis [266], which can markedly decrease the insulin content of β-cells *in vivo* [207]. As such, insulin secretory capacity (the availability of β-granules for exocytosis) can be reduced by chronic hyperlipidemia in type 2 diabetes. This in turn places a greater demand for increased β-granule biogenesis, perhaps driven by the concurrent hyperglycemia in type 2 diabetes, and a greater proportion of immature β-granules are targeted for secretion. A similar situation might also be envisaged with the prolonged use of sulfonylureas, which though potent inducers of insulin secretion, do not stimulate proinsulin synthesis, and therefore decrease the insulin content [256, 258, 259, 372], thus reducing the insulin secretory capacity of the β-cell. As a result, hyperproinsulinemia can also ensue with long-term use of sulfonylureas, and ultimately alternative therapies, including insulin replacement therapy, are used to treat type 2 diabetes [373]. In general, the chronic hyperlgycemia and hyperlipidemia of type 2 diabetes make the β-cell constantly work harder to produce sufficient insulin to compensate for peripheral insulin resistance [373, 374]. This, in turn, leads to β-cell dysfunction of which the hyperproinsulinemia is a symptom [278]. Interestingly, if the β-cell in type 2 diabetic patients is allowed to rest, the secretory dysfunction *in vivo* is very much reduced [375]. This emphasizes the importance of protecting the β-cell mass and function in the treatment of type 2 diabetes [373–375].

Acknowledgment

Work from our laboratories cited in this chapter was supported by the following grants: R01 DK 47919, R01 DK 50610, and R01 DK 55267 (C.J. Rhodes); R01 DK 58096, Grant-in-Aid from the American Heart Association and a Career Development Award from the ADA (V. Poitout); and R01 DK 50203, R01 DK55091, and R01 DK 42502 (R. Stein).

REFERENCES

1. Newgard CB, McGarry JD. Metabolic coupling factors in pancreatic β-cell signal transduction. *Annu Rev Biochem* 1995; 64: 689–719.
2. Stein R. Insulin gene transcription: the factors involved in cell-type specific and glucose-regulated expression in islet β-cells are also essential during pancreatic development. In Cherrington A, Jefferson J (eds) *Handbook of Physiology. Section 7: The Endocrine System.* Washington, DC: American Physiology Society, 2001; pp 25–78.
3. Ohneda K, Ee H, German M. Regulation of insulin gene transcription. *Semin Cell Dev Biol* 2000; 11: 227–33.
4. Melloul D, Marshak S, Cerasi E. Regulation of insulin gene transcription. *Diabetologia* 2002; 45: 309–326.
5. Havrankova J, Brownstein M, Roth J. Insulin and insulin receptors in rodent brain. *Diabetologia* 1981; 20 (suppl): 268–73.
6. Le Roith D, Hendricks SA, Lesniak MA, Rishi S, Becker KL, Havrankova J, Rosenzweig JL, Brownstein MJ, Roth J. Insulin in brain and other extrapancreatic tissues of

vertebrates and nonvertebrates. *Adv Metab Disord* 1983; 10: 303–40.

7. Gannon M, Shiota C, Postic C, Wright CV, Magnuson M. Analysis of the Cre-mediated recombination driven by rat insulin promoter in embryonic and adult mouse pancreas. *Genesis* 2000; 26: 139–42.
8. Jolicoeur C, Hanahan D, Smith KM. T-cell tolerance toward a transgenic β-cell antigen and transcription of endogenous pancreatic genes in thymus. *Proc Natl Acad Sci USA* 1994; 91: 6707–11.
9. Smith KM, Olson DC, Hirose R, Hanahan D. Pancreatic gene expression in rare cells of thymic medulla: evidence for functional contribution to T cell tolerance. *Int Immunol* 1997; 9: 1355–65.
10. Giddings SJ, Carnaghi L. Rat insulin II gene expression by extraplacental membranes. A non-pancreatic source for fetal insulin. *J Biol Chem* 1989; 264: 9462–9.
11. Tillmar L, Carlsson C, Welsh N. Control of insulin mRNA stability in rat pancreatic islets. Regulatory role of a 3′-untranslated region pyrimidine-rich sequence. *J Biol Chem* 2002; 277: 1099–106.
12. Steiner DF, Chan SJ, Welsh JM, Kwok SC. Structure and evolution of the insulin gene. *Annu Rev Genet* 1985; 19: 463–84.
13. Owerbach D, Bell GI, Rutter WJ, Shows TB. The insulin gene is located on chromosome 11 in humans. *Nature* 1980; 286: 82–4.
14. Harper ME, Ullrich A, Saunders GF. Localization of the human insulin gene to the distal end of the short arm of chromosome 11. *Proc Natl Acad Sci USA* 1981; 78: 4458–60.
15. Soares MB, Schon E, Henderson A, Karathanasis SK, Cate R, Zeitlin S, Chirgwin J, Efstratiadis A. RNA-mediated gene duplication: the rat preproinsulin I gene is a functional retroposon. *Mol Cell Biol* 1985; 5: 2090–103.
16. Walker MD, Edlund T, Boulet AM, Rutter WJ. Cell-specific expression controlled by the 5′-flanking region of insulin and chymotrypsin genes. *Nature* 1983; 306: 557–61.
17. German MS, Wang J. The insulin gene contains multiple transcriptional elements that respond to glucose. *Mol Cell Biol* 1994; 14: 4067–75.
18. Karlsson O, Edlund T, Moss JB, Rutter WJ, Walker MD. A mutational analysis of the insulin gene transcription control region: expression in beta cells is dependent on two related sequences within the enhancer. *Proc Natl Acad Sci USA* 1987; 84: 8819–23.
19. Sharma A, Stein R. Glucose-induced transcription of the insulin gene is mediated by factors required for β-cell-type-specific expression. *Mol Cell Biol* 1994; 14: 871–9.
20. Shieh S-Y, Tsai M-J. Cell-specific and ubiquitous factors are responsible for the enhancer activity of the rat insulin II gene. *J Biol Chem* 1991; 266: 16708–14.
21. Hanahan D. Heritable formation of pancreatic β-cell tumors in transgenic mice expressing recombinant insulin/SV40 oncogenes. *Nature* 1985; 315: 115–22.
22. Aronheim A, Shiran R, Rosen A, Walker MD. The E2A gene product contains two separable and functionally distinct transcription activation domains. *Proc Natl Acad Sci USA* 1993; 90: 8063–7.
23. Bucchini D, Ripoche MA, Stinnakre MG, Desbois P, Lores P, Monthioux E, Absil J, Lepesant JA, Pictet R, Jami J. Pancreatic expression of human insulin gene in transgenic mice. *Proc Natl Acad Sci USA* 1986; 83: 2511–5.
24. Stellrecht CM, DeMayo FJ, Finegold MJ, Tsai MJ. Tissue-specific and developmental regulation of the rat insulin II gene enhancer, RIPE3, in transgenic mice. *J Biol Chem* 1997; 272: 3567–72.
25. German MS, Moss LG, Wang J, Rutter WJ. The insulin and islet amyloid polypeptide genes contain similar cell-specific promoter elements that bind identical β-cell nuclear complexes. *Mol Cell Biol* 1992; 12: 1777–8.
26. Sander M, Neubuser A, Kalamaras J, Ee HC, Martin GR, German MS. Genetic analysis reveals that PAX6 is required for normal transcription of pancreatic hormone genes and islet development. *Genes Dev* 1997; 11: 1662–73.
27. Peshavaria M, Gamer L, Henderson E, Teitelman G, Wright CV, Stein R. XIHbox 8, an endoderm-specific Xenopus homeodomain protein, is closely related to a mammalian insulin gene transcription factor. *Mol Endocrinol* 1994; 8: 806–16.
28. Petersen HV, Serup P, Leonard J, Michelsen BK, Madsen OD. Transcriptional regulation of the human insulin gene is dependent on the homeodomain protein STF1/IPF1 acting through the CT boxes. *Proc Natl Acad Sci USA* 1994; 91: 10465–9.
29. Olbrot M, Rud J, Moss LG, Sharma A. Identification of β-cell-specific insulin gene transcription factor RIPE3b1 as mammalian MafA. *Proc Natl Acad Sci USA* 2002; 99: 6737–42.
30. Crowe DT, Tsai M-J. Mutagenesis of the rat insulin II 5′-flanking region defines sequences important for expression in HIT cells. *Mol Cell Biol* 1989; 9: 1784–9.
31. Whelan J, Cordle SR, Henderson E, Weil PA, Stein R. Identification of a pancreatic β-cell insulin gene transcription factor that binds to and appears to activate cell-type-specific expression: its possible relationship to other cellular factors that bind to a common insulin gene sequence. *Mol Cell Biol* 1990; 10: 1564–72.
32. German M, Ashcroft S, Docherty K, Edlund E, Edlund T, Goodion S, Imura H, Kennedy G, Madsen O, Melloul D, Moss L, Olson K, Permutt MA, Philippe J, Robertson RP, Rutter WJ, Serup P, Stein R, Steiner D, Tsai M-J, Walker MD. The Insulin gene promoter. A simplified nomenclature. *Diabetes* 1995; 44: 1002–4.
33. Ohlsson H, Karlsson K, Edlund T. IPF-1, a homeodomain-containing transactivator of the insulin gene. *EMBO J* 1993; 12: 4251–9.
34. Leonard J, Peers B, Johnson T, Ferreri K, Lee S, Montminy MR. Characterization of somatostatin transactivating factor-1, a novel homeobox factor that stimulates somatostatin expression in pancreatic islet cells. *Mol Endocrinol* 1993; 7: 1275–83.
35. Macfarlane WM, Read ML, Gilligan M, Bujalska I, Docherty K. Glucose modulates the binding activity of the β-cell transcription factor IUF1 in a phosphorylation-dependent manner. *Biochem J* 1994; 303 (pt 2): 625–31.
36. Miller CP, McGehee RE Jr, Habener JF. IDX-1: a new homeodomain transcription factor expressed in rat pancreatic islets and duodenum that transactivates the somatostatin gene. *EMBO J* 1994; 13: 1145–56.
37. Wright CV, Schnegelsberg P, De Robertis EM. XlHbox 8: a novel Xenopus homeo protein restricted to a narrow band of endoderm. *Development* 1989; 105: 787–94.
38. Stoffers DA, Thomas MK, Habener JF. Homeodomain protein IDX-1. A master regulator of pancreas

development and insulin gene expression. *Trends Endocrinol Metab* 1997; 8: 145–51.
39. Jonsson J, Ahlgren U, Edlund T, Edlund H. IPF-1, a homeodomain protein with dual function in pancreas development. *Int J Dev Biol* 1995; 39: 789–98.
40. Marshak S, Totary H, Cerasi E, Melloul D. Purification of the β-cell glucose-sensitive factor that transactivates the insulin gene differentially in normal and transformed islet cells. *Proc Natl Acad Sci USA* 1996; 93: 15057–62.
41. Melloul D, Ben-Neriah Y, Cerasi E. Glucose modulates the binding of an islet-specific factor to a conserved sequence within the rat I and the human insulin promoters. *Proc Natl Acad Sci USA* 1993; 90: 3865–9.
42. Peers B, Leonard J, Sharma S, Teitelman G, Montminy MR. Insulin expression in pancreatic islet cells relies on cooperative interactions between the helix loop helix factor E47 and the homeobox factor STF-1. *Mol Endocrinol* 1994; 8: 1798–806.
43. Serup P, Petersen HV, Pedersen EE, Edlund H, Leonard J, Petersen JS, Larsson LI, Madsen OD. The homeodomain protein IPF-1/STF-1 is expressed in a subset of islet cells and promotes rat insulin 1 gene expression dependent on an intact E1 helix–loop–helix factor binding site. *Biochem J* 1995; 310 (pt 3): 997–1003.
44. Jonsson J, Carlsson L, Edlund T, Edlund H. Insulin-promoter factor 1 is required for pancreatic development in mice. *Nature* 1994; 371: 606–9.
45. Ahima RS, Prabakaran D, Mantzoros C, Qu D, Lowell B, Maratos-Flier E, Flier JS. Role of leptin in the neuroendocrine response to fasting. *Nature* 1996; 382: 250–2.
46. Stoffers DA, Zinkin NT, Stanojevic V, Clarke WL, Habener JF. Pancreatic agenesis attributable to a single nucleotide deletion in the human IPF1 gene coding sequence. *Nat Genet* 1997; 15: 106–10.
47. Stoffers DA, Ferrer J, Clarke WL, Habener JF. Early-onset type-II diabetes mellitus (MODY4) linked to IPF1. *Nat Genet* 1997; 17: 138–9.
48. Peshavaria M, Henderson E, Sharma A, Wright CVE, Stein R. Functional characterization of the transactivation properties of the PDX-1 homeodomain protein. *Mol Cell Biol* 1997; 17: 3987–96.
49. Aronheim A, Ohlsson H, Park CW, Edlund T, Walker MD. Distribution and characterization of helix–loop–helix enhancer-binding proteins from pancreatic beta cells and lymphocytes. *Nucleic Acids Res* 1991; 19: 3893–9.
50. German MS, Blanar MA, Nelson C, Moss LG, Rutter WJ. Two related helix–loop–helix proteins participate in separate cell-specific complexes that bind the insulin enhancer. *Mol Endocrinol* 1991; 5: 292–9.
51. Cordle SR, Henderson E, Masuoka H, Weil PA, Stein R. Pancreatic β-cell-type-specific transcription of the insulin gene is mediated by basic helix–loop–helix DNA-binding proteins. *Mol Cell Biol* 1991; 11: 1734–8.
52. Peyton M, Moss LG, Tsai MJ. Two distinct class A helix–loop–helix transcription factors, E2A and BETA1, form separate DNA binding complexes on the insulin gene E box. *J Biol Chem* 1994; 269: 25936–41.
53. Naya FJ, Huang H-P, Qiu Y, Mutoh H, DeMayo FJ, Leiter AB, Tsai M-J. Diabetes, defective pancreatic morphogenesis, and abnormal enteroendocrine differentiation in BETA2/NeuroD-deficient mice. *Genes Dev* 1997; 11: 2323–34.
54. Lee JE, Hollenberg SM, Snider L, Turner DL, Lipnick N, Weintraub H. Conversion of *Xenopus ectoderm* into neurons by NeuroD, a basic helix–loop–helix protein. *Science* 1995; 268: 836–44.
55. Ohneda K, Mirmira RG, Wang J, Johnson JD, German MS. The homeodomain of PDX-1 mediates multiple protein–protein interactions in the formation of a transcriptional activation complex on the insulin promoter. *Mol Cell Biol* 2000; 20: 900–11.
56. Qiu Y, Guo M, Huang S, Stein R. Insulin gene transcription is mediated by interactions between the p300 coactivator and PDX-1, BETA2, and E47. *Mol Cell Biol* 2002; 22: 412–20.
57. Kristinsson SY, Thorolfsdottir ET, Talseth B, Steingrimsson E, Thorsson AV, Helgason T, Hreidarsson AB, Arngrimsson R. MODY in Iceland is associated with mutations in HNF-1alpha and a novel mutation in NeuroD1. *Diabetologia* 2001; 44: 2098–103.
58. Malecki MT, Jhala US, Antonellis A, Fields L, Doria A, Orban T, Saad M, Warram JH, Montminy M, Krolewski AS. Mutations in NEUROD1 are associated with the development of type 2 diabetes mellitus. *Nat Genet* 1999; 23: 323–328.
59. Read ML, Masson MR, Docherty K. A RIPE3b1-like factor binds to a novel site in the human insulin promoter in a redox-dependent manner. *FEBS Lett* 1997; 418: 68–72.
60. Sharma A, Fusco-DeMane D, Henderson E, Efrat S, Stein R. The role of the insulin control element and RIPE3b1 activators in glucose-stimulated transcription of the insulin gene. *Mol Endocrinol* 1995; 9: 1468–76.
61. Zhao L, Cissell MA, Henderson E, Colbran R, Stein R. The RIPE3b1 activator of the insulin gene is composed of a protein(s) of approximately 43 kDa, whose DNA binding activity is inhibited by protein phosphatase treatment. *J Biol Chem* 2000; 275: 10532–7.
62. Matsuoka T, Zhao L, Stein R. The DNA binding activity of the RIPE3b1 transcription factor of insulin appears to be influenced by tyrosine phosphorylation. *J Biol Chem* 2001; 276: 22071–6.
63. Friedman AD. Transcriptional regulation of granulocyte and monocyte development. *Oncogene* 2002; 21: 3377–90.
64. Sieweke MH, Tekotte H, Frampton J, Graf T. MafB is an interaction partner and repressor of Ets-1 that inhibits erythroid differentiation. *Cell* 1996; 85: 49–60.
65. Kawauchi S, Takahashi S, Nakajima O, Ogino H, Morita M, Nishizawa M, Yasuda K, Yamamoto M. Regulation of lens fiber cell differentiation by transcription factor c-Maf. *J Biol Chem* 1999; 274: 19254–60.
66. Kim JI, Li T, Ho IC, Grusby MJ, Glimcher LH. Requirement for the c-Maf transcription factor in crystallin gene regulation and lens development. *Proc Natl Acad Sci USA* 1999; 96: 3781–5.
67. Ogino H, Yasuda K. Induction of lens differentiation by activation of a bZIP transcription factor, L-Maf. *Science* 1998; 280: 115–8.
68. Ring BZ, Cordes SP, Overbeek PA, Barsh GS. Regulation of mouse lens fiber cell development and differentiation by the *Maf* gene. *Development* 2000; 127: 307–17.
69. Smith SB, Ee HC, Conners JR, German MS. Paired-homeodomain transcription factor PAX4 acts as a transcriptional repressor in early pancreatic development. *Mol Cell Biol* 1999; 19: 8272–80.
70. Campbell SC, Cragg H, Elrick LJ, Macfarlane WM, Shennan KI, Docherty K. Inhibitory effect of pax4 on

the human insulin and islet amyloid polypeptide (IAPP) promoters. *FEBS Lett* 1999; 463: 53–7.

71. Fujitani Y, Kajimoto Y, Yasuda T, Matsuoka TA, Kaneto H, Umayahara Y, Fujita N, Watada H, Miyazaki JI, Yamasaki Y, Hori M. Identification of a portable repression domain and an E1A-responsive activation domain in Pax4: a possible role of Pax4 as a transcriptional repressor in the pancreas. *Mol Cell Biol* 1999; 19: 8281–91.
72. St-Onge L, Sosa-Pineda B, Chowdhury K, Mansouri A, Gruss P. Pax6 is required for differentiation of glucagon-producing alpha-cells in mouse pancreas. *Nature* 1997; 387: 406–9.
73. Sosa-Pineda B, Chowdhury K, Torres M, Oliver G, Gruss P. The *Pax4* gene is essential for differentiation of insulin-producing β-cells in the mammalian pancreas. *Nature* 1997; 386: 399–402.
74. Yajima H, Komatsu M, Yamada S, Straub SG, Kaneko T, Sato Y, Yamauchi K, Hashizume K, Sharp GW, Aizawa T. Cerulenin, an inhibitor of protein acylation, selectively attenuates nutrient stimulation of insulin release: a study in rat pancreatic islets. *Diabetes* 2000; 49: 712–7.
75. Yamagata K, Oda N, Kaisaki PJ, Menzel S, Furuta H, Vaxillaire M, Southam LRDC, Lathrop GM, Boriraj VV, et al. Mutations in the hepatocyte nuclear factor-1alpha gene in maturity-onset diabetes of the young (MODY3). *Nature* 1996; 384: 455–8.
76. Horikawa Y, Iwasaki N, Hara M, Furuta H, Hinokio Y, Cockburn BN, Lindner T, Yamagata K, Ogata M, Tomonaga O, Kuroki H, Kasahara T, Iwamoto Y, Bell GI. Mutation in hepatocyte nuclear factor-1 beta gene (*TCF2*) associated with MODY [letter]. *Nat Genet* 1997; 17: 384–5.
77. Emens LA, Landers DW, Moss LG. Hepatocyte nuclear factor 1 is expressed in a hamster insulinoma line and transactivated the rat insulin I gene. *Proc Natl Acad Sci USA* 1992; 89: 7300–4.
78. Wang H, Maechler P, Hagenfeldt KA, Wollheim CB. Dominant-negative suppression of HNF-1alpha function results in defective insulin gene transcription and impaired metabolism–secretion coupling in a pancreatic β-cell line. *EMBO J* 1998; 17: 6701–13.
79. Okita K, Yang Q, Yamagata K, Hangenfeldt KA, Miyagawa J, Kajimoto Y, Nakajima H, Namba M, Wollheim CB, Hanafusa T, Matsuzawa Y. Human insulin gene is a target gene of hepatocyte nuclear factor-1alpha (HNF-1alpha) and HNF-1beta. *Biochem Biophys Res Commun* 1999; 263: 566–9.
80. Pontoglio M, Sreenan S, Roe M, Pugh W, Ostrega D, Doyen A, Pick AJ, Bladwin A, Velho G, Froguel P, Levisetti M, Bonner-Weir S, Bell GI, Yaniv M, Polonsky KS. Defective insulin secretion in hepatocyte nuclear factor 1α-deficient mice. *J Clin Invest* 1998; 101: 2215–22.
81. Wang H, Maechler P, Antinozzi PA, Hagenfeldt KA, Wollheim CB. Hepatocyte nuclear factor 4alpha regulates the expression of pancreatic beta-cell genes implicated in glucose metabolism and nutrient-induced insulin secretion. *J Biol Chem* 2000; 275: 35953–9.
82. Kuo CJ, Conley PB, Chen L, Sladek FM, Darnell JE Jr, Crabtree GR. A transcriptional hierarchy involved in mammalian cell-type specification. *Nature* 1992; 355: 457–61.
83. Boj SF, Parrizas M, Maestro MA, Ferrer J. A transcription factor regulatory circuit in differentiated pancreatic cells. *Proc Natl Acad Sci USA* 2001; 98: 14481–6.
84. Thomas H, Jaschkowitz K, Bulman M, Frayling TM, Mitchell SM, Roosen S, Lingott-Frieg A,Tack CJ, Ellard S, Ryffel GU, Hattersley AT. A distant upstream promoter of the HNF-4alpha gene connects the transcription factors involved in maturity-onset diabetes of the young. *Hum Mol Genet* 2001; 10: 2089–97.
85. Bartoov-Shifman R, Hertz R, Wang H, Wollheim CB, Bar-Tana J, Walker MD. Activation of the insulin gene promoter through a direct effect of hepatocyte nuclear factor 4 alpha. *J Biol Chem* 2002; 277: 25914–9.
86. Gerrish K, Cissell MA, Stein R. The role of hepatic nuclear factor 1 alpha and PDX-1 in transcriptional regulation of the *pdx-1* gene. *J Biol Chem* 2001; 276: 47775–84.
87. Ben-Shushan E, Marshak S, Shoshkes M, Cerasi E, Melloul D. A pancreatic beta-cell-specific enhancer in the human *PDX-1* gene is regulated by hepatocyte nuclear factor 3beta (HNF-3beta), HNF-1alpha, and SPs transcription factors. *J Biol Chem* 2001; 276: 17533–40.
88. Brunstedt J, Chan SJ. Direct effect of glucose on the preproinsulin mRNA level in isolated pancreatic islets. *Biochem Biophys Res Commun* 1982; 106: 1383–9.
89. Hammonds P, Schofield PN, Ashcroft SHJ, Sutton R, Gray DWR. Regulation and specificity of glucose-stimulated insulin gene expression in human islets of Langerhans. *FEBS Lett* 1987; 223: 131–7.
90. Nielsen DA, Welsh M, Casadaban MJ, Steiner DF. Control of insulin gene expression in pancreatic β-cells and in an insulin producing cell line, RIN-5F cells, 1: effects of glucose and cyclic AMP on the transcription of insulin mRNA. *J Biol Chem* 1985; 260: 13585–9.
91. Wang J, Shen L, Najafi H, Kolberg J, Matchinsky FM, Urdea M, German M. Regulation of insulin pre-RNA splicing by glucose. *Proc Natl Acad Sci USA* 1997; 94: 4360–5.
92. Welsh M, Nielsen DA, MacKrell AJ, Steiner DF. Control of insulin gene expression in pancreatic β-cells and in an insulin producing cell line, RIN-5F cells, 2: regulation of insulin mRNA stability. *J Biol Chem* 1985; 260: 13590–94.
93. Macfarlane WM, McKinnon CM, Felton-Edkins ZA, Cragg H, James RF, Docherty K. Glucose stimulates translocation of the homeodomain transcription factor PDX1 from the cytoplasm to the nucleus in pancreatic β-cells. *J Biol Chem* 1999; 274: 1011–6.
94. Rafiq I, da Silva Xavier G, Hooper S, Rutter GA. Glucose-stimulated preproinsulin gene expression and nuclear trans-location of pancreatic duodenum homeobox-1 require activation of phosphatidylinositol 3-kinase but not p38 MAPK/SAPK2. *J Biol Chem* 2000; 275: 15977–84.
95. German MS, Moss LG, Rutter WJ. Regulation of insulin gene expression by glucose and calcium in transfected primary islet culture. *J Biol Chem* 1990; 265: 22063–6.
96. Ashcroft S, Bunce J, Lowry M, Hansen S, Hedeskov C. The effect of sugars on (pro)insulin biosynthesis. *Biochem J* 1978; 174: 517–26.
97. Efrat S, Surana M, Fleischer N. Glucose induces insulin gene transcription in a murine pancreatic β-cell line. *J Biol Chem* 1991; 266: 11141–3.
98. Sander M, Griffen SC, Huang J, German MS. A novel glucose-responsive element in the human insulin gene functions uniquely in primary cultured islets. *Proc Natl Acad Sci USA* 1998; 95: 11572–7.
99. Macfarlane WM, Smith SB, James RFL, Clifton AD, Doza YN, Cohen P, Docherty K. The p38/reactivating kinase mlitogen-activated protein kinase cascade mediates

the activation of the transcription factor insulin upstream factor 1 and insulin gene transcription by high glucose in pancreatic β-cells. *J Biol Chem* 1997; 272: 20936–44.

100. Rafiq I, Kennedy HJ, Rutter GA. Glucose-dependent translocation of insulin promoter factor-1 (IPF-1) between the nuclear periphery and the nucleoplasm of single MIN6 β-cells. *J Biol Chem* 1998; 273: 23241–7.
101. Benes C, Poitout V, Marie JC, Martin-Perez J, Roisin MP, Fagard R. Mode of regulation of the extracellular signal-regulated kinases in the pancreatic β-cell line MIN6 and their implication in the regulation of insulin gene transcription. *Biochem J* 1999; 340: 219–25.
102. Welsh N, Welsh M, Steiner DF, Hellerstrom C. Mechanisms of leucine- and theophylline-stimulated insulin biosynthesis in isolated rat pancreatic islets. *Biochem J* 1987; 246: 245–8.
103. Welsh M, Brunstedt J, Hellerstrom C. Effects of D-glucose, L-leucine, and 2-ketoisocaproate on insulin mRNA levels in mouse pancreatic islets. *Diabetes* 1986; 35: 228–31.
104. Ferrer J, Gomis R, Fernandez Alvarez J, Casamitjana R, Vilardell E. Signals derived from glucose metabolism are required for glucose regulation of pancreatic islet GLUT2 mRNA and protein. *Diabetes* 1993; 42: 1273–80.
105. Goodison S, Kenna S, Ashcroft SJ. Control of insulin gene expression by glucose. *Biochem J* 1992; 285 (pt 2): 563–8.
106. Kennedy H, Rafiq I, Pouli A, Rutter G. Glucose enhances insulin promoter activity in MIN6 β-cells independently of changes in intracellular Ca^{2+} concentration and insulin secretion. *Biochem J* 1999; 342: 275–80.
107. Moitoso de Vargas L, Sobolewski J, Siegel R, Moss LG. Individual β-cells whithin the intact islet differentially respond to glucose. *J Biol Chem* 1997; 272: 26573–7.
108. Shushan EB, Cerasi E, Melloul D. Regulation of the insulin gene by glucose: stimulation of trans-activation potency of human PDX-1 N-terminal domain. *DNA Cell Biol* 1999; 18: 471–9.
109. Wicksteed B, Herbert TP, Alarcon C, Lingohr MK, Moss LG, Rhodes CJ. Cooperativity between the preproinsulin mRNA untranslated regions is necessary for glucose-stimulated translation. *J Biol Chem* 2001; 276: 22553–8.
110. Giddings SJ, Chirgwin J, Permutt MA. The effects of fasting and feeding on preproinsulin messenger RNA in rats. *J Clin Invest* 1981; 67: 952–60.
111. Giddings SJ, Chirgwin J, Permutt MA. Effects of glucose on proinsulin messenger RNA in rats *in vivo*. *Diabetes* 1982; 31: 624–9.
112. Shalwitz RA, Herbst T, Carnaghi LR, Giddings SJ. Time course for effects of hypoglycemia on insulin gene transcription *in vivo*. *Diabetes* 1994; 43: 929–34.
113. Pipeleers DG. Heterogeneity in pancreatic β-cell population. *Diabetes* 1992; 41: 777–81.
114. Habener JF. Insulinotropic glucagon-like peptides. In LeRoith D, Taylor SI, Olefsky JM (eds) *Diabetes Mellitus: A Fundamental and Clinical Text*. Second edition. Philadelphia: Lippincott Williams & Wilkins, 2000: pp 94–105.
115. Drucker DJ, Philippe J, Mojsov S, Chick WL, Habener JF. Glucagon–like peptide I stimulates insulin gene expression and increases cyclic AMP levels in a rat islet cell line. *Proc Natl Acad Sci USA* 1987; 84: 3434–8.
116. Widmann C, Burki E, Dolci W, Thorens B. Signal transduction by the cloned glucagon-like peptide-1 receptor: comparison with signaling by the endogenous receptors of beta cell lines. *Mol Pharmacol* 1994; 45: 1029–35.
117. Frodin M, Sekine N, Roche E, Filloux C, Prentki M, Wollheim CB, Van Obberghen E. Glucose, other secretagogues, and nerve growth factor stimulate mitogen-activated protein kinase in the insulin-secreting β-cell line, INS-1. *J Biol Chem* 1995; 270: 7882–9.
118. Kemp DM, Habener JF. Insulinotropic hormone glucagon-like peptide 1 (GLP-1) activation of insulin gene promoter inhibited by p38 mitogen-activated protein kinase. *Endocrinology* 2001; 142: 1179–87.
119. Wheeler MB, Lu M, Dillon JS, Leng XH, Chen C, Boyd AE III. Functional expression of the rat glucagon-like peptide-I receptor, evidence for coupling to both adenylyl cyclase and phospholipase-C. *Endocrinology* 1993; 133: 57–62.
120. Buteau J, Roduit R, Susini S, Prentki M. Glucagon-like peptide-1 promotes DNA synthesis, activates phosphatidylinositol 3-kinase and increases transcription factor pancreatic and duodenal homeobox gene 1 (PDX-1) DNA binding activity in beta (INS-1)-cells. *Diabetologia* 1999; 42: 856–64.
121. Holz GG, Leech CA, Habener JF. Activation of a cAMP-regulated Ca(2+)-signaling pathway in pancreatic β-cells by the insulinotropic hormone glucagon-like peptide-1. *J Biol Chem* 1995; 270: 17749–57.
122. Holz GG, Leech CA, Heller RS, Castonguay M, Habener JF. cAMP-dependent mobilization of intracellular Ca^{2+} stores by activation of ryanodine receptors in pancreatic β-cells. A Ca^{2+} signaling system stimulated by the insulinotropic hormone glucagon-like peptide-1-(7-37). *J Biol Chem* 1999; 274: 14147–56.
123. Fehmann HC, Habener JF. Galanin inhibits proinsulin gene expression stimulated by the insulinotropic hormone glucagon-like peptide-I(7-37) in mouse insulinoma beta TC-1 cells. *Endocrinology* 1992; 130: 2890–6.
124. Wang Y, Egan JM, Raygada M, Nadiv O, Roth J, Montrose-Rafizadeh C. Glucagon-like peptide-1 affects gene transcription and messenger ribonucleic acid stability of components of the insulin secretory system in RIN 1046-38 cells. *Endocrinology* 1995; 136: 4910–7.
125. Smith PA, Sakura H, Coles B, Gummerson N, Proks P, Ashcroft FM. Electrogenic arginine transport mediates stimulus–secretion coupling in mouse pancreatic β-cells. *J Physiol* 1997; 499: 625–35.
126. Hussain MA, Habener JF. Glucagon-like peptide 1 increases glucose-dependent activity of the homeoprotein IDX-1 transactivating domain in pancreatic β-cells. *Biochem Biophys Res Commun* 2000; 274: 616–9.
127. Wang X, Cahill CM, Pineyro MA, Zhou J, Doyle ME, Egan JM. Glucagon-like peptide-1 regulates the beta cell transcription factor, PDX-1, in insulinoma cells. *Endocrinology* 1999; 140: 4904–7.
128. Lawrence MC, Bhatt HS, Watterson JM, Easom RA. Regulation of insulin gene transcription by a Ca(2+)-responsive pathway involving calcineurin and nuclear factor of activated T cells. *Mol Endocrinol* 2001; 15: 1758–67.
129. Lawrence MC, Bhatt HS, Easom RA. NFAT regulates insulin gene promoter activity in response to synergistic pathways induced by glucose and glucagon-like peptide-1. *Diabetes* 2002; 51: 691–8.
130. Redmon JB, Olson LK, Armstrong MB, Greene MJ, Robertson RP. Effects of tacrolimus (FK506) on human insulin gene expression, insulin mRNA levels, and insulin

secretion in HIT-T15 cells. *J Clin Invest* 1996; 98: 2786–93.

131. Galsgaard ED, Gouilleux F, Groner B, Serup P, Nielsen JH, Billestrup N. Identification of a growth hormone-responsive STAT5-binding element in the rat insulin 1 gene. *Mol Endocrinol* 1996; 10: 652–60.
132. Straub SG, James RF, Dunne MJ, Sharp GW. Glucose activates both K(ATP) channel-dependent and K(ATP) channel-independent signaling pathways in human islets. *Diabetes* 1998; 47: 758–63.
133. Galsgaard ED, Nielsen JH, Moldrup A. Regulation of prolactin receptor (PRLR) gene expression in insulin-producing cells. Prolactin and growth hormone activate one of the rat *prlr* gene promoters via STAT5a and STAT5b. *J Biol Chem* 1999; 274: 18686–92.
134. Fleenor DE, Freemark M. Prolactin induction of insulin gene transcription: roles of glucose and signal transducer and activator of transcription 5. *Endocrinology* 2001; 142: 2805–10.
135. Sharp GW. Mechanisms of inhibition of insulin release. *Am J Physiol* 1996; 271: C1781–99.
136. Zhang HJ, Redmond JB, Andresen JM, Robertson RP. Somatostatin and epinephrin decrease insulin messenger ribonucleic acid in HIT cells through a pertussis toxin-sensitive mechanism. *Endocrinology* 1991; 129: 2409–14.
137. Redmon JB, Towle HC, Robertson RP. Regulation of human insulin gene transcription by glucose, epinephrine, and somatostatin. *Diabetes* 1994; 43: 546–51.
138. Philippe J. Somatostatin inhibits insulin-gene expression through a posttranscriptional mechanism in a hamster islet cell line. *Diabetes* 1993; 42: 244–9.
139. Hussain MA, Daniel PB, Habener JF. Glucagon stimulates expression of the inducible cAMP early repressor and suppresses insulin gene expression in pancreatic β-cells. *Diabetes* 2000; 49: 1681–90.
140. Zhao AZ, Bornfeldt KE, Beavo JA. Leptin inhibits insulin secretion by activation of phosphodiesterase 3B. *J Clin Invest* 1998; 102: 869–73.
141. Kieffer T, Scott-Heller R, Leech CA, Holz GG, Habener JF. Leptin suppression of insulin secretion by the activation of ATP-sensitive K^+ channels in pancreatic β-cells. *Diabetes* 1997; 46: 1087–93.
142. Emilsson V, Liu Y-L, Cawthorne MA, Morton NM, Davenport M. Expression of the functional leptin receptor mRNA in pancreatic islets and direct inhibitory action of leptin on insulin secretion. *Diabetes* 1997; 46: 313–6.
143. Poitout V, Rouault C, Guerre-Millo M, Briaud I, Reach G. Inhibition of insulin secretion by leptin in normal rodent islets of Langerhans. *Endocrinology* 1998; 139: 822–6.
144. Seufert J, Kieffer TJ, Habener JF. Leptin inhibits insulin gene transcription and reverses hyperinsulinemia in leptin-deficient *ob/ob* mice. *Proc Natl Acad Sci USA* 1999; 96: 674–9.
145. Morton NM, Emilsson V, de Groot P, Pallett AL, Cawthorne MA. Leptin signalling in pancreatic islets and clonal insulin-secreting cells. *J Mol Endocrinol* 1999; 22: 173–84.
146. Leibiger B, Moede T, Schwarz T, Brown G, Kohler M, Leibiger I, Berggren P. Short-term regulation of insulin gene transcription by glucose. *Proc Natl Acad Sci USA* 1998; 95: 9307–12.
147. Leibiger IB, Leibiger B, Moede T, Berggren PO. Exocytosis of insulin promotes insulin gene transcription via the insulin receptor/PI-3 kinase/p70 s6 kinase and CaM kinase. *Mol Cell* 1998; 1: 933–8.
148. da Silva Xavier G, Varadi A, Ainscow EK, Rutter GA. Regulation of gene expression by glucose in pancreatic beta-cells (MIN6) via insulin secretion and activation of phosphatidylinositol 3′-kinase. *J Biol Chem* 2000; 275: 36269–77.
149. Wu H, MacFarlane WM, Tadayyon M, Arch JR, James RF, Docherty K. Insulin stimulates pancreatic-duodenal homoeobox factor-1 (PDX1) DNA-binding activity and insulin promoter activity in pancreatic beta cells. *Biochem J* 1999; 344 (pt 3): 813–8.
150. Kulkarni RN, Bruning JC, Winnay JN, Postic C, Magnuson MA, Kahn CR. Tissue-specific knockout of the insulin receptor in pancreatic beta cells creates an insulin secretory defect similar to that in type 2 diabetes. *Cell* 1999; 96: 329–39.
151. Bell GI, Karam JH, Rutter WJ. Polymorphic DNA region adjacent to the 5′ end of the human insulin gene. *Proc Natl Acad Sci USA* 1981; 78: 5759–63.
152. Bell GI, Selby MJ, Rutter WJ. The highly polymorphic region near the human insulin gene is composed of simple tandemly repeating sequences. *Nature* 1982; 295: 31–5.
153. Bennett ST, Lucassen AM, Gough SC, Powell EE, Undlien DE, Pritchard LE, Merriman ME, Kawaguchi Y, Dronsfield MJ, Pociot F, et al.: Susceptibility to human type 1 diabetes at IDDM2 is determined by tandem repeat variation at the insulin gene minisatellite locus. *Nat Genet* 1995; 9: 284–92.
154. Pugliese A, Miceli D. The insulin gene in diabetes. *Diabetes Metab Res Rev* 2002; 18: 13–25.
155. Lucassen AM, Screaton GR, Julier C, Elliott TJ, Lathrop M, Bell JI. Regulation of insulin gene expression by the IDDM associated, insulin locus haplotype. *Hum Mol Genet* 1995; 4: 501–6.
156. Kennedy GC, German MS, Rutter WJ. The minisatellite in the diabetes susceptibility locus *IDDM2* regulates insulin transcription. *Nat Genet* 1995; 9: 293–8.
157. Robertson RP, Harmon JS, Tanaka Y, Sacchi G, Tran POT, Gleason CE, Poitout V. Glucose toxicity of the β-cell: cellular and molecular mechanisms. In Le Roith D, Taylor SI, Olefsky JM (eds) *Diabetes Mellitus. A Fundamental and Clinical Text*. 2nd edition. Philadelphia, Lippincott Williams & Wilkins, 2000; pp 125–32.
158. Robertson RP, Olson LK, Zhang HJ. Differentiating glucose toxicity from glucose desensitization: a new message from the insulin gene. *Diabetes* 1994; 43: 1085–9.
159. Permutt MA, Kakita K, Malinas P, Karl I, Bonner-Weir S, Weir G, Giddings SJ. An *in vivo* analysis of pancreatic protein and insulin biosynthesis in a rat model for non-insulin-dependent diabetes. *J Clin Invest* 1984; 73: 1344–50.
160. Orland MJ, Permutt MA. Quantitative analysis of pancreatic proinsulin mRNA in genetically diabetic (*db/db*) mice. *Diabetes* 1987; 37: 341–7.
161. Tokuyama Y, Sturis J, DePaoli AM, Takeda J, Stoffel M, Tang J, Sun X, Polonsky KS, Bell GI. Evolution of β-cell dysfunction in the male Zucker diabetic fatty rat. *Diabetes* 1995; 44: 1447–57.
162. Zangen DH, Bonner-Weir S, Lee CH, Latimer JB, Miller CP, Habener JF. Reduced insulin, GLUT2, and IDX-1 in β-cells after partial pancreatectomy. *Diabetes* 1997; 46: 258–64.
163. Briaud I, Rouault C, Bailbe D, Portha B, Reach G, Poitout V. Glucose-induced insulin mRNA accumulation is

impaired in islets from neonatal streptozotocin-treated rats. *Horm Metab Res* 2000; 32: 103–6.

164. Leibowitz G, Ferber S, Apelqvist A, Edlund H, Gross DJ, Cerasi E, Melloul D, Kaiser N. IPF1/PDX1 deficiency and β-cell dysfunction in *Psammomys obesus*, an animal with type 2 diabetes. *Diabetes* 2001; 50: 1799–806.
165. Robertson RP, Zhang HJ, Pyzdrowski KL, Walseth TF. Preservation of insulin mRNA levels and insulin secretion in HIT cells by avoidance of chronic exposure to high glucose concentrations. *J Clin Invest* 1992; 90: 320–5.
166. Olson LK, Redmon JB, Towle HC, Robertson RP. Chronic exposure of HIT cells to high glucose concentrations paradoxically decreases insulin gene transcription and alters binding of insulin gene regulatory protein. *J Clin Invest* 1993; 92: 514–9.
167. Olson LK, Sharma A, Peshavaria M, Wright CVE, Towle HC, Robertson RP, Stein R. Reduction of insulin gene transcription in HIT-T15 cells chronically exposed to a supraphysiologic glucose concentration is associated with loss of STF-1 transcription factor expression. *Proc Natl Acad Sci USA* 1995; 92: 9127–31.
168. Poitout V, Olson LK, Robertson RP. Chronic exposure of βTC-6 cells to supraphysiologic concentrations of glucose decreases binding of the RIPE-3b1 insulin gene transcription activator. *J Clin Invest* 1996; 97: 1041–6.
169. Moran A, Zhang H-J, Olson LK, Harmon JS, Poitout V, Robertson RP. Differentiation of glucose toxicity from β-cell exhaustion during the evolution of defective insulin gene expression in the pancreatic islet cell line, HIT-T15. *J Clin Invest* 1997; 99: 534–9.
170. Olson LK, Qian J, Poitout V. Glucose rapidly and reversibly decreases insulin gene transcription in INS-1 cells via decrements in binding activity of STF-1 and C1 activator. *Mol Endocrinaol* 1998; 12: 207–19.
171. Matsuoka TA, Kajimoto Y, Watada H, Kaneto H, Kishimoto M, Umayahara Y, Fujitani Y, Kamada T, Kawamori R, Yamakasi Y. Glycation-dependent, reactive oxygen species mediated suppression of the insulin gene promoter activity in HIT cells. *J Clin Invest* 1997; 99: 144–50.
172. Harmon JS, Tanaka Y, Olson LK, Robertson RP. Reconstitution of glucotoxic HIT-T15 cells with somatostatin transcritpion factor-1 partially restores insulin promoter activity. *Diabetes* 1998; 47: 900–4.
173. Gleason CE, Gonzalez M, Harmon JS, Robertson RP. Determinants of glucose toxicity and its reversibility in the pancreatic islet β-cell line, HIT-T15. *Am J Physiol Endocrinol Metab* 2000; 279: E997–1002.
174. Briaud I, Rouault C, Reach G, Poitout V. Long-term exposure of isolated rat islets of Langerhans to supraphysiologic glucose concentrations decreases insulin mRNA levels. *Metabolism* 1999; 48: 319–23.
175. Eizirik DL, Korbutt GS, Hellerstrom C. Prolonged exposure of human pancreatic islets to high glucose concentrations in vitro impairs the β-cell function. *J Clin Invest* 1992; 90: 1263–8.
176. Marshak S, Leibowitz G, Bertuzzi F, Socci C, Kaiser N, Gross DJ, Cerasi E, Melloul D. Impaired β-cell functions induced by chronic exposure of cultured human pancreatic islets to high glucose. *Diabetes* 1999; 48: 1230–6.
177. Sharma A, Olson LK, Robertson RP, Stein R. The reduction of insulin gene transcription in HIT-T15 β cells chronically exposed to high glucose concentration is associated with the loss of RIPE3b1 and STF-1 transcription factor expression. *Mol Endocrinol* 1995; 9: 1127–34.
178. Harmon JS, Gleason CE, Tanaka Y, Oseid EA, Hunter-Berger KK, Robertson RP. *In vivo* prevention of hyperglycemia also prevents glucotoxic effects on PDX-1 and insulin gene expression. *Diabetes* 1999; 48: 1995–2000.
179. Lu M, Seufert J, Habener JF. Pancreatic β-cell-specific repression of insulin gene transcription by CCAAT/enhancer-binding protein β. Inhibitory interactions with basic helix–loop–helix transcription factor E47. *J Biol Chem* 1997; 272: 28349–59.
180. Seufert J, Weir GC, Habener JF. Differential expression of the insulin gene transcriptional repressor CCAAT/enhancer-binding protein beta and transactivator iselt duodenum homeobox-1 in rat pancreatic beta cells during the development of diabetes mellitus. *J Clin Invest* 1998; 101: 2528–39.
181. Tajiri Y, Moller C, Grill V. Long term effects of aminoguanidine on insulin release and biosynthesis: evidence that the formation of advanced glycosylation end products inhibits β-cell function. *Endocrinology* 1997; 138: 273–80.
182. Abdel-Wahab YHA, O'Harte FPM, Ratcliff H, McClenaghan NH, Barnett CR, Flatt PR. Glycation of insulin in the islets of Langerhans of normal and diabetic animals. *Diabetes* 1996; 45: 1489–96.
183. Kaneto H, Kajimoto Y, Fujitani Y, Matsuoka T, Sakamoto K, Matsuhisa M, Yamasaki Y, Hori M. Oxidative stress induces p21 expression in pancreatic islet cells: possible implication in β-cell dysfunction. *Diabetologia* 1999; 42: 1093–7.
184. Tanaka Y, Gleason CE, Tran POT, Harmon JS, Robertson RP. Prevention of glucose toxicity in HIT-T15 cells and Zucker diabetic fatty rats by antioxidants. *Proc Natl Acad Sci USA* 1999; 96: 10857–62.
185. Ihara Y, Toyokuni S, Uchida K, Odaka H, Tanaka T, Ikeda H, Hiai H, Seino Y, Yamada Y. Hyperglycemia causes oxidative stress in pancreatic β-cells of GK rats, a model of type 2 diabetes. *Diabetes* 1999; 48: 927–32.
186. Tiedge M, Lortz S, Drinkgern J, Lenzen S. Relation between antioxidant enzyme gene expression and antioxidative defense status of insulin-producing cells. *Diabetes* 1997; 46: 1733–42.
187. Kaneto H, Fujii J, Myint T, Miyazawa N, Islam KN, Kawasaki Y, Suzuki K, Makamura M, Tatsumi H, Yamasaki Y, Taniguchi N. Reducing sugars trigger oxidative modification and apoptosis in pancreatic β-cells by provoking oxidative stress through the glycation reaction. *Biochem J* 1996; 320 (pt 3): 855–63.
188. Baynes JW, Thorpe SR. Role of oxidative stress in diabetic complications: a new perspective on an old paradigm. *Diabetes* 1999; 48: 1–9.
189. Hawkins M, Barzilai N, Liu R, Hu M, Chen W, Rossetti L. Role of the glucosamine pathway in fat-induced insulin resistance. *J Clin Invest* 1997; 99: 2173–82.
190. Kaneto H, Xu G, Song KH, Suzuma K, Bonner-Weir S, Sharma A, Weir GC. Activation of the hexosamine pathway leads to deterioration of pancreatic β-cell function through the induction of oxidative stress. *J Biol Chem* 2001; 276: 31099–104.
191. Kaneto H, Xu G, Fujii N, Kim S, Bonner-Weir S, Weir GC. Involvement of c-*Jun* N-terminal kinase in oxidative stress-mediated suppression of insulin gene expression. *J Biol Chem* 2002; 277: 30010–8.
192. Henderson E, Stein R. c-*jun* inhibits transcriptional activation by the insulin enhancer, and the insulin control

element is the target of control. *Mol Cell Biol* 1994; 14: 655–62.

193. Robinson GL, Henderson E, Massari ME, Murre C, Stein R. c-*jun* inhibits insulin control element-mediated transcription by affecting the transactivation potential of the E2A gene products. *Mol Cell Biol* 1995; 15: 1398–404.
194. Jonas JC, Sharma A, Hasenkamp W, Ilkova H, Patane G, Laybutt R, Bonner-Weir S, Weir GC. Chronic hyperglycemia triggers loss of pancreatic beta cell differentiation in an animal model of diabetes. *J Biol Chem* 1999; 274: 14112–21.
195. Jonas JC, Laybutt DR, Steil GM, Trivedi N, Pertusa JG, Van de Casteele M, Weir GC, Henquin JC. High glucose stimulates early response gene c-*Myc* expression in rat pancreatic beta cells. *J Biol Chem* 2001; 276: 35375–81.
196. Gremlich S, Bonny C, Waeber G, Thorens B. Fatty acids decrease IDX-1 expression in rat pancreatic islets and reduce GLUT2, glucokinase, insulin, and somatostatin levels. *J Biol Chem* 1997; 272: 30261–9.
197. Ritz-Laser B, Meda P, Constant I, Klages N, Charollais A, Morales A, Magnan C, Ktorza A, Philippe J. Glucose-induced preproinsulin gene expression is inhibited by the free-fatty acid palmitate. *Endocrinology* 1999; 140: 4005–14.
198. Jacqueminet S, Briaud I, Rouault C, Reach G, Poitout V. Inhibition of insulin gene expression by long-term exposure of pancreatic β-cells to palmitate is dependent upon the presence of a stimulatory glucose concentration. *Metabolism* 2000; 49: 532–6.
199. Briaud I, Harmon JS, Kelpe CL, Segu VB, Poitout V. Lipotoxicity of the pancreatic β-cell is associated with glucose-dependent esterification of fatty acids into neutral lipids. *Diabetes* 2001; 50: 315–21.
200. Weir GC, Sharma A, Zangen DH, Bonner-Weir S. Transcription factor abnormalities as a cause of beta cell dysfunction in diabetes: a hypothesis. *Acta Diabetol* 1997; 34: 177–84.
201. Laybutt DR, Sharma A, Sgroi DC, Gaudet J, Bonner-Weir S, Weir GC. Genetic regulation of metabolic pathways in β-cells disrupted by hyperglycemia. *J Biol Chem* 2002; 277: 10912–21.
202. Laybutt DR, Weir GC, Kaneto H, Lebet J, Palmiter RD, Sharma A, Bonner-Weir S. Overexpression of c-*Myc* in β-cells of transgenic mice causes proliferation and apoptosis, downregulation of insulin gene expression, and diabetes. *Diabetes* 2002; 51: 1793–804.
203. Kaneto H, Sharma A, Suzuma K, Laybutt DR, Xu G, Bonner-Weir S, Weir GC. Induction of c-*Myc* expression suppresses insulin gene transcription by inhibiting NeuroD/BETA2-mediated transcriptional activation. *J Biol Chem* 2002; 277: 12998–3006.
204. Unger RH. Lipotoxicity in the pathogenesis of obesity-dependent NIDDM. Genetic and clinical implications. *Diabetes* 1995; 44: 863–70.
205. McGarry JD, Dobbins RL. Fatty acids, lipotoxicity and insulin secretion. *Diabetologia* 1999; 42: 128–38.
206. Poitout V, Robertson RP. Secondary β-cell failure in type 2 diabetes: a convergence of glucotoxicity and lipotoxicity. *Endocrinology* 2002; 143: 339–42.
207. Bollheimer LC, Skelly RH, Chester MW, McGarry JD, Rhodes CJ. Chronic exposure to free fatty acid reduces pancreatic beta cell insulin content by increasing basal insulin secretion that is not compensated for by a corresponding increase in proinsulin biosynthesis translation. *J Clin Invest* 1998; 101: 1094–101.
208. Kelpe CL, Johnson LM, Poitout V. Increasing triglyceride synthesis inhibits glucose-induced insulin secretion in isolated rat islets of Langerhans. A study using adenoviral expression of diacylglycerol acyltransferase. *Endocrinology* 2002; 143: 3326–32.
209. Unger RH, Zhou YT, Orci L. Lipotoxicity. In LeRoith D, Taylor SI, Olefsky JM (eds) *Diabetes Mellitus: A Fundamental and Clinical Text. Second edition.* Philadelphia: Lippincott Williams & Wilkins, 2000; pp. 132–141.
210. Mathias S, Pena LA, Kolesnick RN. Signal transduction of stress via ceramide. *Biochem J* 1998; 335 (pt 3): 465–80.
211. Schuppin GT, Rhodes CJ. Specific co-ordinated regulation of *PC3* and *PC2* gene expression with that of preproinsulin in insulin-producing beta TC3 cells. *Biochem J* 1996; 313 (pt 1): 259–68.
212. Brown H, Sanger F, Kitai R. The structure of pig and sheep insulins. *Biochem J* 1955; 60: 556–65.
213. Sanger F. Chemistry of insulin: determination of the structure of insulin opens the way to greater understanding of life processes. *Science* 1959; 129: 1340–4.
214. Steiner DF, Oyer PE. The biosynthesis of insulin and a probable precursor of insulin by a human islet cell adenoma. *Proce Nat Acad Sci USA* 1967; 57: 473–80.
215. Steiner DF, Cunningham D, Spigelman L, Aten B. Insulin biosynthesis: evidence for a precursor. *Science* 1967; 157: 697–700.
216. Steiner DF, Clark JL, Nolan C, Rubenstein AH, Margoliash E, Melani F, Oyer PE. The biosynthesis of insulin and some speculations regarding the pathogenesis of human diabetes. In Cerasi E, Luft T (eds) *The Biosynthesis of Insulin and Some Speculations Regarding the Pathogenesis of Human Diabetes*. Stockholm: Almqvist & Wiksells, 1970; pp 123–32.
217. Steiner DF, Kemmler W, Clark JL, Oyer PE, Rubenstein AH. The biosynthesis of insulin. In Greep RO, Astwood EB (eds) *The Biosynthesis of Insulin.* Washington, DC: American Physiological Society, 1972; pp. 175–98.
218. Steiner DF. On the role of the proinsulin C-peptide. *Diabetes* 1978; 27 (suppl 1): 145–8.
219. Snell CR, Smyth DG. Proinsulin: a proposed three-dimensional structure. *J Biol Chem* 1975; 250: 6291–5.
220. Gross DJ, Villa-Komaroff L, Kahn CR, Weir GC, Halban PA. Deletion of a highly conserved tetrapeptide sequence of the proinsulin connecting peptide (C-peptide) inhibits proinsulin to insulin conversion by transfected pituitary corticotroph (AtT20) cells. *J Biol Chem* 1989; 264: 21486–90.
221. Weiss MA, Frank BH, Khait I, Pekar A, Heiney R, Shoelson SE, Neuringer LJ. NMR and photo-CIDNP studies of human proinsulin and prohormone processing intermediates with application to endopeptidase recognition. *Biochemistry* 1990; 29: 8389–401.
222. Derewenda U, Derewenda Z, Dodson GG, Hubbard RE, Korber F. Molecular structure of insulin: the insulin monomer and its assembly. *Br Med Bull* 1989; 45: 4–18.
223. Rhodes CJ, Lincoln B, Shoelson SE. Preferential cleavage of des-31,32-proinsulin over intact proinsulin by the insulin secretory granule type II endopeptidase. Implication of a favored route for prohormone processing. *J Biol Chem* 1992; 267: 22719–27.
224. Steiner DF. Cocrystallization of proinsulin and insulin. *Nature* 1973; 243: 528–30.

225. Frank BH, Veros AJ. Interaction of zinc with proinsulin. *Biochem Biophys Res Commun* 1970; 38: 284–9.
226. Steiner DF, Bell GI, Tager HS. Chemistry and biosynthesis of pancreatic protein hormones. In de Groot P (ed) *Chemistry and Biosynthesis of Pancreatic Protein Hormones* Philadelphia: Saunders, 1990; pp 1263–89.
227. Galloway JA, Hooper SA, Spradlin CT, Howey DC, Frank BH, Bowsher RR, Anderson JH. Biosynthetic human proinsulin. Review of chemistry, in vitro and *in vivo* receptor binding, animal and human pharmacology studies, and clinical trial experience. *Diabetes Care* 1992; 15: 666–92.
228. Blobel G, Dobberstein B. Transfer of proteins across membranes, I: Presence of proteolytically processed and unprocessed nascent immunoglobulin light chains on membrane-bound ribosomes of murine myeloma. *J Cell Biol* 1975; 67: 835–51.
229. Merrick WC. Mechanism and regulation of eukaryotic protein synthesis. *Microbiol Rev* 1992; 56: 291–315.
230. Clemens MJ. Regulatory mechanisms in translational control. *Curr Opin Cell Biol* 1989; 1: 1160–7.
231. Hershey JW. Translational control in mammalian cells. *Annu Rev Biochem* 1991; 60: 717–55.
232. Redpath NT, Proud CG. Molecular mechanisms in the control of translation by hormones and growth factors. *Biochim Biophys Acta* 1994; 1220: 147–62.
233. Pain VM. Initiation of protein synthesis in eukaryotic cells. *Eur J Biochem* 1996; 236: 747–71.
234. Orci L. The insulin factory: a tour of the plant surroundings and a visit to the assembly line. The Minkowski lecture 1973 revisited. *Diabetologia* 1985; 28: 528–46.
235. Tang JG, Wang CC, Tsou CL. Formation of native insulin from the scrambled molecule by protein disulphide-isomerase. *Biochem J* 1988; 255: 451–5.
236. Campbell IL, Hellquist LN, Taylor KW. Insulin biosynthesis and its regulation. *Clin Sci (Lond)* 1982; 62: 449–55.
237. Shoelson SE, Halban PA. Insulin biosynthesis and chemistry. In Malvern PA, Weir GC (eds) *Insulin Biosynthesis and Chemistry*. 13 edn. Malvern: Lea & Febiger, 1994; pp 29–55.
238. Ashcroft SJ. Glucoreceptor mechanisms and the control of insulin release and biosynthesis. *Diabetologia* 1980; 18: 5–15.
239. Lin BJ, Haist RE. Insulin biosynthesis: effects of carbohydrates and related compounds. *Can J Physiol Pharmacol* 1969; 47: 791–801.
240. Guest P, Rhodes C, Hutton J. Regulation of the biosynthesis of insulin secretory granule proteins: coordinate translational control is exerted on some but not all granule matrix constituents. *Biochem. J.* 1989; 257: 431.
241. Alarcon C, Lincoln B, Rhodes CJ. The biosynthesis of the subtilisin-related proprotein convertase PC3, but no that of the PC2 convertase, is regulated by glucose in parallel to proinsulin biosynthesis in rat pancreatic islets. *J Biol Chem* 1993; 268: 4276–80.
242. Guest PC, Rhodes CJ, Hutton JC. Regulation of the biosynthesis of insulin-secretory-granule proteins. Coordinate translational control is exerted on some, but not all, granule matrix constituents. *Biochem J* 1989; 257: 431–7.
243. Pipeleers DG, Marichal M, Malaisse WJ. The stimulus-secretion coupling of glucose-induced insulin release, XIV; glucose regulation of insular biosynthetic activity. *Endocrinology* 1973; 93: 1001–11.
244. Maldonato A, Renold AE, Sharp GW, Cerasi E. Glucose-induced proinsulin biosynthesis. Role of islet cyclic AMP. *Diabetes* 1977; 26: 538–45.
245. Itoh N, Okamoto H. Translational control of proinsulin synthesis by glucose. *Nature* 1980; 283: 100–2.
246. Welsh M, Scherberg N, Gilmore R, Steiner DF. Translational control of insulin biosynthesis. Evidence for regulation of elongation, initiation and signal-recognition-particle-mediated translational arrest by glucose. *Biochem J* 1986; 235: 459–67.
247. Kaelin D, Renold AE, Sharp GW. Glucose stimulated proinsulin biosynthesis rates of turn off after cessation of the stimulus. *Diabetologia* 1978; 14: 329–35.
248. Fehmann HC, Goke R, Goke B. Cell and molecular biology of the incretin hormones glucagon-like peptide-I and glucose-dependent insulin releasing polypeptide. *Endocr Rev* 1995; 16: 390–410.
249. Fehmann HC, Habener JF. Insulinotropic hormone glucagon-like peptide-I(7-37) stimulation of proinsulin gene expression and proinsulin biosynthesis in insulinoma beta TC-1 cells. *Endocrinology* 1992; 130: 159–66.
250. Malaisse WJ, Pipeleers DG, Levy J. The stimulus-secretion coupling of glucose-induced insulin release, XVI: a glucose-like and calcium-independent effect of cyclic AMP. *Biochim Biophys Acta* 1974; 362: 121–8.
251. Prentki M. New insights into pancreatic β-cell metabolic signaling in insulin secretion. *Eur J Endocrinol* 1996; 134: 272–86.
252. Prentki M, Tornheim K, Corkey BE. Signal transduction mechanisms in nutrient-induced insulin secretion. *Diabetologia* 1997; 40: S32–41.
253. Ashcroft FM, Proks P, Smith PA, Ammala C, Bokvist K, Rorsman P. Stimulus-secretion coupling in pancreatic beta cells. *J Cell Biochem* 1994; 55 (suppl): 54–65.
254. Pipeleers DG, Marichal M, Malaisse WJ. The stimulus–secretion coupling of glucose-induced insulin release, XV: participation of cations in the recognition of glucose by the β-cell. *Endocrinology* 1973; 93: 1012–8.
255. Prentki M, Matschinsky FM. $Ca2^{+}$, cAMP, and phospholipid-derived messengers in coupling mechanisms of insulin secretion. *Physiol Rev* 1987; 67: 1185–248.
256. Lin B, Haist R. Effects of some modifiers of insulin secretion and insulin biosynthesis. *Endocrinology* 1973; 92: 735–42.
257. Bailyes EM, Guest PC, Hutton JC. Insulin synthesis. In Ashcroft FM, Ashcroft SJ (eds) *Insulin Synthesis*, 1st edn. Oxford, UK: Oxford University Press, 1992; pp 64–92.
258. Levy J, Malaisse WJ. The stimulus–secretion coupling of glucose-induced insulin release, XVII: effects of sulfonylureas and diazoxide on insular biosynthetic activity. *Biochem Pharmacol* 1975; 24: 235–9.
259. Morris GE, Korner A. The effect of glucose on insulin biosynthesis by isolated islets of Langerhans of the rat. *Biochim Biophys Acta* 1970; 208: 404–13.
260. Ashcroft FM, Ashcroft SJ. Mechanism of insulin secretion. In Ashcroft FM, Ashcroft SJ (eds) *Mechanism of Insulin Secretion*, 1st edn. Oxford, UK: Oxford University Press, 1992; pp 97–150.
261. Olsson SE, Anderson A, Petersson B, Hellerstrom C. Effects of somatostatin on the biosynthesis and release of insulin from isolated pancreatic islets. *Diabete Metab* 1976; 2: 199–202.
262. Alarcon C, Wicksteed B, Prentki M, Corkey BE, Rhodes CJ. Succinate is a preferential metabolic

stimulus-coupling signal for glucose-induced proinsulin biosynthesis translation. *Diabetes* 2002; 51: 2496–504.

263. Stein DT, Stevenson BE, Chester MW, Basit M, Daniels MB, Turley SD, McGarry JD. The insulinotropic potency of fatty acids is influenced profoundly by their chain length and degree of saturation. *J Clin Invest* 1997; 100: 398–403.
264. Stein DT, Esser V, Stevenson BE, Lane KE, Whiteside JH, Daniels MB, Chen S, McGarry JD. Essentiality of circulating fatty acids for glucose-stimulated insulin secretion in the fasted rat. *J Clin Invest* 1996; 97: 2728–35.
265. Prentki M, Vischer S, Glennon MC, Regazzi R, Deeney JT, Corkey BE. Malonyl-CoA and long chain acyl-CoA esters as metabolic coupling factors in nutrient-induced insulin secretion. *J Biol Chem* 1992; 267: 5802–10.
266. Skelly RH, Bollheimer C, Wicksteeed BL, Corkey BE, Rhodes CJ. A distinct difference in the metabolic stimulus–response coupling pathways for regulating proinsulin biosynthesis and insulin secretion that lies at the level of a requirement for fatty acyl moieties. *Biochem J* 1998; 331: 553–61.
267. Welsh N, Oberg C, Welsh M. GTP-binding proteins may stimulate insulin biosynthesis in rat pancreatic islets by enhancing the signal-recognition-particle-dependent translocation of the insulin mRNA poly-/mono-some complex to the endoplasmic reticulum. *Biochem J* 1991; 275 (pt 1): 23–8.
268. Gilligan M, Welsh GI, Flynn A, Bujalska I, Diggle TA, Denton RM, Proud CG, Docherty K. Glucose stimulates the activity of the guanine nucleotide-exchange factor eIF-2B in isolated rat islets of Langerhans. *J Biol Chem* 1996; 271: 2121–5.
269. Skelly RH, Wicksteed B, Antinozzi PA, Rhodes CJ. Glycerol-stimulated proinsulin biosynthesis in isolated pancreatic rat islets via adenoviral-induced expression of glycerol kinase is mediated via mitochondrial metabolism. *Diabetes* 2001; 50: 1791–8.
270. Rusnak F, Mertz P. Calcineurin: form and function. *Physiol Rev* 2000; 80: 1483–521.
271. Knight S, Docherty K. RNA–protein interactions in the 5′-untranslated region of preproinsulin mRNA. *J Mol Endocrinol* 1992; 8: 225–34.
272. Herbert TP, Alarcon C, Skelly RH, Bollheimer LC, Schuppin GT, Rhodes CJ. Regulation of prohormone conversion by coordinated control of processing endopeptidase biosynthesis with that of the prohormone substrate. In Hook Y (ed) *Regulation of Prohormone Conversion by Coordinated Control of Processing Endopeptidase Biosynthesis with that of the Prohormone Substrate*. Austin, TX: RG Landes Co., 1998; pp 105–20.
273. Wicksteed B, Alarcon C, Rhodes CJ. RNA-protein interactions regulate proinsulin biosynthesis. *Diabetes* 2002; 51: A385.
274. Guest PC, Bailyes EM, Rutherford NG, Hutton JC. Insulin secretory granule biogenesis. Co-ordinate regulation of the biosynthesis of the majority of constituent proteins. *Biochem J* 1991; 274 (pt 1): 73–8.
275. Grimaldi KA, Siddle K, Hutton JC. Biosynthesis of insulin secretory granule membrane proteins. Control by glucose. *Biochem J* 1987; 245: 567–73.
276. Skelly RH, Schuppin GT, Ishihara H, Oka Y, Rhodes CJ. Glucose-regulated translational control of proinsulin biosynthesis with that of the proinsulin endopeptidases PC2 and PC3 in the insulin-producing MIN6 cell line. *Diabetes* 1996; 45: 37–43.
277. Martin SK, Carroll R, Benig M, Steiner DF. Regulation by glucose of the biosynthesis of PC2, PC3 and proinsulin in (*ob/ob*) mouse islets of Langerhans. *FEBS Lett* 1994; 356: 279–82.
278. Rhodes CJ, Alarcon C. What β-cell defect could lead to hyperproinsulinemia in NIDDM? Some clues from recent advances made in understanding the proinsulin-processing mechanism. *Diabetes* 1994; 43: 511–7.
279. Howell SL. Role of ATP in the intracellular translocation of proinsulin and insulin in the rat pancreatic B cell. *Nat New Biol* 1972; 235: 85–6.
280. Howell SL. The mechanism of insulin secretion. *Diabetologia* 1984; 26: 319–27.
281. Schwaninger R, Plutner H, Bokoch GM, Balch WE. Multiple GTP-binding proteins regulate vesicular transport from the ER to Golgi membranes. *J Cell Biol* 1992; 119: 1077–96.
282. Balch WE. Small GTP-binding proteins in vesicular transport. *Trends Biochem Sci* 1990; 15: 473–7.
283. Rothman JE, Wieland FT. Protein sorting by transport vesicles. *Science* 1996; 272: 227–34.
284. Zerial M, Stenmark H. Rab GTPases in vesicular transport. *Curr Opin Cell Biol* 1993; 5: 613–20.
285. Rothman JE, Orci L. Molecular dissection of the secretory pathway. *Nature* 1992; 355: 409–15.
286. Rothman JE. The compartmental organization of the Golgi apparatus. *Sci Am* 1985; 253: 74–89.
287. Rothman JE. The golgi apparatus: two organelles in tandem. *Science* 1981; 213: 1212–9.
288. Sollner T. SNAREs and targeted membrane fusion. *FEBS Lett* 1995; 369: 80–3.
289. Marsh BJ, Mastronarde DN, Buttle KF, Howell KE, McIntosh JR. Organellar relationships in the Golgi region of the pancreatic beta cell line, HIT-T15, visualized by high resolution electron tomography. *Proc Natl Acad Sci USA* 2001; 98: 2399–406.
290. Burgess TL, Kelly RB. Constitutive and regulated secretion of proteins. *Annu Rev Cell Biol* 1987; 3: 243–93.
291. Molinete M, Irminger JC, Tooze SA, Halban PA. Trafficking/sorting and granule biogenesis in the β-cell. *Semin Cell Dev Biol* 2000; 11: 243–51.
292. Rhodes CJ, Halban PA. Newly synthesized proinsulin/insulin and stored insulin are released from pancreatic B cells predominantly via a regulated, rather than a constitutive, pathway. *J Cell Biol* 1987; 105: 145–53.
293. Kornfeld S, Mellman I. The biogenesis of lysosomes. *Annu Rev Cell Biol* 1989; 5: 483–525.
294. Pelham HR. Control of protein exit from the endoplasmic reticulum. *Annu Rev Cell Biol* 1989; 5: 1–23.
295. Arvan P, Castle D. Sorting and storage during secretory granule biogenesis: looking backward and looking forward. *Biochem J* 1998; 332 (pt 3): 593–610.
296. Cool DR, Normant E, Shen F, Chen HC, Pannell L, Zhang Y, Loh YP. Carboxypeptidase E is a regulated secretory pathway sorting receptor: genetic obliteration leads to endocrine disorders in Cpe(fat) mice. *Cell* 1997; 88: 73–83.
297. Cool DR, Loh YP. Carboxypeptidase E is a sorting receptor for prohormones: binding and kinetic studies. *Mol Cell Endocrinol* 1998; 139: 7–13.
298. Kim T, Tao-Cheng JH, Eiden LE, Loh YP. Chromogranin A, an "on/off" switch controlling dense-core secretory granule biogenesis. *Cell* 2001; 106: 499–509.

299. Irminger JC, Verchere CB, Meyer K, Halban PA. Proinsulin targeting to the regulated pathway is not impaired in carboxypeptidase E-deficient Cpefat/Cpefat mice. *J Biol Chem* 1997; 272: 27532–4.
300. Varlamov O, Fricker LD, Furukawa H, Steiner DF, Langley SH, Leiter EH. β-cell lines derived from transgenic Cpe(fat)/Cpe(fat) mice are defective in carboxypeptidase E and proinsulin processing. *Endocrinology* 1997; 138: 4883–92.
301. Cool DR, Fenger M, Snell CR, Loh YP. Identification of the sorting signal motif within pro-opiomelanocortin for the regulated secretory pathway. *J Biol Chem* 1995; 270: 8723–9.
302. Tooze SA. Biogenesis of secretory granules in the *trans*-Golgi network of neuroendocrine and endocrine cells. *Biochim Biophys Acta* 1998; 1404: 231–44.
303. Chan SJ, Seino S, Gruppuso PA, Schwartz R, Steiner DF. A mutation in the B chain coding region is associated with impaired proinsulin conversion in a family with hyperproinsulinemia. *Proc Natl Acad Sci USA* 1987; 84: 2194–7.
304. Carroll RJ, Hammer RE, Chan SJ, Swift HH, Rubenstein AH, Steiner DF. A mutant human proinsulin is secreted from islets of Langerhans in increased amounts via an unregulated pathway. *Proc Natl Acad Sci USA* 1988; 85: 8943–7.
305. Gross DJ, Halban PA, Kahn CR, Weir GC, Villa-Komaroff L. Partial diversion of a mutant proinsulin (B10 aspartic acid) from the regulated to the constitutive secretory pathway in transfected AtT-20 cells. *Proc Natl Acad Sci USA* 1989; 86: 4107–11.
306. Gerdes HH, Rosa P, Phillips E, Baeuerle PA, Frank R, Argos P, Huttner WB. The primary structure of human secretogranin II, a widespread tyrosine-sulfated secretory granule protein that exhibits low pH- and calcium-induced aggregation. *J Biol Chem* 1989; 264: 12009–15.
307. Tooze SA, Huttner WB. Cell-free protein sorting to the regulated and constitutive secretory pathways. *Cell* 1990; 60: 837–47.
308. Tooze SA, Weiss U, Huttner WB. Requirement for GTP hydrolysis in the formation of secretory vesicles. *Nature* 1990; 347: 207–8.
309. Nuoffer C, Balch WE. GTPases: multifunctional molecular switches regulating vesicular traffic. *Annu Rev Biochem* 1994; 63: 949–90.
310. Barr FA, Leyte A, Mollner S, Pfeuffer T, Tooze SA, Huttner WB. Trimeric G-proteins of the *trans*-Golgi network are involved in the formation of constitutive secretory vesicles and immature secretory granules. *FEBS Lett* 1991; 294: 239–43.
311. Tooze SA, Martens GJ, Huttner WB. Secretory granule biogenesis: rafting to the SNARE. *Trends Cell Biol* 2001; 11: 116–22.
312. Austin CD, Shields D. Formation of nascent secretory vesicles from the *trans*-Golgi network of endocrine cells is inhibited by tyrosine kinase and phosphatase inhibitors. *J Cell Biol* 1996; 135: 1471–83.
313. Payne GS, Schekman R. Clathrin: a role in the intracellular retention of a Golgi membrane protein. *Science* 1989; 245: 1358–65.
314. Bauerfeind R, Huttner WB. Biogenesis of constitutive secretory vesicles, secretory granules and synaptic vesicles. *Curr Opin Cell Biol* 1993; 5: 628–35.
315. Kuliawat R, Arvan P. Protein targeting via the "constitutive-like" secretory pathway in isolated pancreatic islets: passive sorting in the immature granule compartment. *J Cell Biol* 1992; 118: 521–9.
316. Halban PA, Irminger JC. Sorting and processing of secretory proteins. *Biochem J* 1994; 299 (pt 1): 1–18.
317. Kemmler W, Steiner DF. Conversion of proinsulin to insulin in a subcellular fraction from rat islets. *Biochem Biophys Res Commun* 1970; 41: 1223–30.
318. Davidson HW, Rhodes CJ, Hutton JC. Intraorganellar calcium and pH control proinsulin cleavage in the pancreatic beta cell via two distinct site-specific endopeptidases. *Nature* 1988; 333: 93–6.
319. Rhodes CJ, Lucas CA, Mutkoski RL, Orci L, Halban PA. Stimulation by ATP of proinsulin to insulin conversion in isolated rat pancreatic islet secretory granules. Association with the ATP-dependent proton pump. *J Biol Chem* 1987; 262: 10712–7.
320. Smeekens SP, Steiner DF. Identification of a human insulinoma cDNA encoding a novel mammalian protein structurally related to the yeast dibasic processing protease Kex2. *J Biol Chem* 1990; 265: 2997–3000.
321. Seidah NG, Gaspar L, Mion P, Marcinkiewicz M, Mbikay M, Chretien M. cDNA sequence of two distinct pituitary proteins homologous to Kex2 and furin gene products: tissue-specific mRNAs encoding candidates for prohormone processing proteinases. *DNA Cell Biol* 1990; 9: 415–24.
322. Smeekens SP, Avruch AS, LaMendola J, Chan SJ, Steiner DF. Identification of a cDNA encoding a second putative prohormone convertase related to PC2 in AtT20 cells and islets of Langerhans. *Proc Natl Acad Sci USA* 1991; 88: 340–4.
323. Seidah NG, Marcinkiewicz M, Benjannet S, Gaspar L, Beaubien G, Mattei MG, Lazure C, Mbikay M, Chretien M. Cloning and primary sequence of a mouse candidate prohormone convertase PC1 homologous to PC2, Furin, and Kex2: distinct chromosomal localization and messenger RNA distribution in brain and pituitary compared to PC2. *Mol Endocrinol* 1991; 5: 111–22.
324. Docherty K, Hutton JC. Carboxypeptidase activity in the insulin secretory granule. *FEBS Lett* 1983; 162: 137–41.
325. Davidson HW, Hutton JC. The insulin-secretory-granule carboxypeptidase H. Purification and demonstration of involvement in proinsulin processing. *Biochem J* 1987; 245: 575–82.
326. Bailyes EM, Shennan KI, Seal AJ, Smeekens SP, Steiner DF, Hutton JC, Docherty K. A member of the eukaryotic subtilisin family (PC3) has the enzymic properties of the type 1 proinsulin-converting endopeptidase. *Biochem J* 1992; 285 (pt 2): 391–4.
327. Bailyes EM, Bennett DL, Hutton JC. Proprotein-processing endopeptidases of the insulin secretory granule. *Enzyme* 1991; 45: 301–13.
328. Smeekens SP, Montag AG, Thomas G, Albiges-Rizo C, Carroll R, Benig M, Phillips LA, Martin S, Ohagi S, Gardner P, et al. Proinsulin processing by the subtilisin-related proprotein convertases furin, PC2, and PC3. *Proc Natl Acad Sci USA* 1992; 89: 8822–6.
329. Bennett DL, Bailyes EM, Nielsen E, Guest PC, Rutherford NG, Arden SD, Hutton JC. Identification of the type 2 proinsulin processing endopeptidase as PC2, a member of the eukaryote subtilisin family. *J Biol Chem* 1992; 267: 15229–36.
330. Hutton JC. Insulin secretory granule biogenesis and the proinsulin-processing endopeptidases. *Diabetologia* 1994; 37 (suppl 2): S48–56.

331. Sizonenko S, Irminger JC, Buhler L, Deng S, Morel P, Halban PA. Kinetics of proinsulin conversion in human islets. *Diabetes* 1993; 42: 933–6.
332. Sobey WJ, Beer SF, Carrington CA, Clark PM, Frank BH, Gray IP, Luzio SD, Owens DR, Schneider AE, Siddle K, et al. Sensitive and specific two-site immunoradiometric assays for human insulin, proinsulin, 65-66 split and 32-33 split proinsulins. *Biochem J* 1989; 260: 535–41.
333. Temple RC, Carrington CA, Luzio SD, Owens DR, Schneider AE, Sobey WJ, Hales CN. Insulin deficiency in non-insulin-dependent diabetes. *Lancet* 1989; 1: 293–5.
334. Rhodes CJ, Halban PA. The intracellular handling of insulin-related peptides in isolated pancreatic islets. Evidence for differential rates of degradation of insulin and C-peptide. *Biochem J* 1988; 251: 23–30.
335. Rhodes CJ, Lucas CA, Halban PA. Glucose stimulates the biosynthesis of rat I and II insulin to an equal extent in isolated pancreatic islets. *FEBS Lett* 1987; 215: 179–82.
336. Docherty K, Rhodes CJ, Taylor NA, Shennan KI, Hutton JC. Proinsulin endopeptidase substrate specificities defined by site-directed mutagenesis of proinsulin. *J Biol Chem* 1989; 264: 18335–9.
337. Steiner DF, Smeekens SP, Ohagi S, Chan SJ. The new enzymology of precursor processing endoproteases. *J Biol Chem* 1992; 267: 23435–8.
338. Furuta M, Yano H, Zhou A, Rouille Y, Holst JJ, Carroll R, Ravazzola M, Orci L, Furuta H, Steiner DF. Defective prohormone processing and altered pancreatic islet morphology in mice lacking active SPC2. *Proc Natl Acad Sci USA* 1997; 94: 6646–51.
339. Furuta M, Carroll R, Martin S, Swift HH, Ravazzola M, Orci L, Steiner DF. Incomplete processing of proinsulin to insulin accompanied by elevation of des-31,32 proinsulin intermediates in islets of mice lacking active PC2. *J Biol Chem* 1998; 273: 3431–7.
340. Jackson RS, Creemers JW, Ohagi S, Raffin-Sanson ML, Sanders L, Montague CT, Hutton JC, O'Rahilly S. Obesity and impaired prohormone processing associated with mutations in the human prohormone convertase 1 gene. *Nat Genet* 1997; 16: 303–6.
341. Naggert JK, Fricker LD, Varlamov O, Nishina PM, Rouille Y, Steiner DF, Carroll RJ, Paigen BJ, Leiter EH. Hyperproinsulinaemia in obese fat/fat mice associated with a carboxypeptidase E mutation which reduces enzyme activity. *Nat Genet* 1995; 10: 135–42.
342. Hutton JC, Penn EJ, Peshavaria M. Low-molecular-weight constituents of isolated insulin-secretory granules. Bivalent cations, adenine nucleotides and inorganic phosphate. *Biochem J* 1983; 210: 297–305.
343. Hutton JC. The internal pH and membrane potential of the insulin-secretory granule. *Biochem J* 1982; 204: 171–8.
344. Orci L, Ravazzola M, Amherdt M, Madsen O, Perrelet A, Vassalli JD, Anderson RG. Conversion of proinsulin to insulin occurs coordinately with acidification of maturing secretory vesicles. *J Cell Biol* 1986; 103: 2273–81.
345. Formby B, Capito K, Egeberg J, Hedeskov CJ. Ca-activated ATPase activity in subcellular fractions of mouse pancreatic islets. *Am J Physiol* 1976; 230: 441–8.
346. Guest PC, Arden SD, Bennett DL, Clark A, Rutherford NG, Hutton JC. The post-translational processing and intracellular sorting of PC2 in the islets of Langerhans. *J Biol Chem* 1992; 267: 22401–6.
347. Martens GJ, Braks JA, Eib DW, Zhou Y, Lindberg I. The neuroendocrine polypeptide 7B2 is an endogenous inhibitor of prohormone convertase PC2. *Proc Natl Acad Sci USA* 1994; 91: 5784–7.
348. Muller L, Zhu X, Lindberg I. Mechanism of the facilitation of PC2 maturation by 7B2: involvement in ProPC2 transport and activation but not folding. *J Cell Biol* 1997; 139: 625–38.
349. Qian Y, Devi LA, Mzhavia N, Munzer S, Seidah NG, Fricker LD. The C-terminal region of proSAAS is a potent inhibitor of prohormone convertase 1. *J Biol Chem* 2000; 275: 23596–601.
350. Fortenberry Y, Hwang JR, Apletalina EV, Lindberg I. Functional characterization of ProSAAS: similarities and differences with 7B2. *J Biol Chem* 2002; 277: 5175–86.
351. Westphal CH, Muller L, Zhou A, Zhu X, Bonner-Weir S, Schambelan M, Steiner DF, Lindberg I, Leder P. The neuroendocrine protein 7B2 is required for peptide hormone processing *in vivo* and provides a novel mechanism for pituitary Cushing's disease. *Cell* 1999; 96: 689–700.
352. Nagamatsu S, Bolaffi JL, Grodsky GM. Direct effects of glucose on proinsulin synthesis and processing during desensitization. *Endocrinology* 1987; 120: 1225–31.
353. Halban PA, Wollheim CB. Intracellular degradation of insulin stores by rat pancreatic islets in vitro. An alternative pathway for homeostasis of pancreatic insulin content. *J Biol Chem* 1980; 255: 6003–6.
354. Halban PA, Renold AE. Influence of glucose on insulin handling by rat islets in culture. A reflection of integrated changes in insulin biosynthesis, release, and intracellular degradation. *Diabetes* 1983; 32: 254–61.
355. Schnell AH, Swenne I, Borg LA. Lysosomes and pancreatic islet function. A quantitative estimation of crinophagy in the mouse pancreatic B-cell. *Cell Tissue Res* 1988; 252: 9–15.
356. Porte D Jr, Kahn SE. Hyperproinsulinemia and amyloid in NIDDM. Clues to etiology of islet β-cell dysfunction? *Diabetes* 1989; 38: 1333–6.
357. Kahn SE, Leonetti DL, Prigeon RL, Boyko EJ, Bergstrom RW, Fujimoto WY. Proinsulin as a marker for the development of NIDDM in Japanese-American men. *Diabetes* 1995; 44: 173–9.
358. Nagi DK, Hendra TJ, Ryle AJ, Cooper TM, Temple RC, Clark PM, Schneider AE, Hales CN, Yudkin JS. The relationships of concentrations of insulin, intact proinsulin and 32-33 split proinsulin with cardiovascular risk factors in type 2 (non-insulin-dependent) diabetic subjects. *Diabetologia* 1990; 33: 532–7.
359. Levy JC, Clark PM, Hales CN, Turner RC. Normal proinsulin responses to glucose in mild type II subjects with subnormal insulin response. *Diabetes* 1993; 42: 162–9.
360. Heaton DA, Millward BA, Gray IP, Tun Y, Hales CN, Pyke DA, Leslie RD. Increased proinsulin levels as an early indicator of B-cell dysfunction in non-diabetic twins of type 1 (insulin-dependent) diabetic patients. *Diabetologia* 1988; 31: 182–4.
361. Roder ME, Porte D Jr, Schwartz RS, Kahn SE. Disproportionately elevated proinsulin levels reflect the degree of impaired B cell secretory capacity in patients with noninsulin-dependent diabetes mellitus. *J Clin Endocrinol Metab* 1998; 83: 604–8.
362. Alarcon C, Leahy JL, Schuppin GT, Rhodes CJ. Increased secretory demand rather than a defect in the proinsulin conversion mechanism causes hyperproinsulinemia in a glucose-infusion rat model of non-insulin-dependent diabetes mellitus. *J Clin Invest* 1995; 95: 1032–9.

363. Leahy JL, Halban PA, Weir GC. Relative hypersecretion of proinsulin in rat model of NIDDM. *Diabetes* 1991; 40: 985–9.
364. Haffner SM. Risk factors for non-insulin-dependent diabetes mellitus. *J Hypertens Suppl* 1995; 13: S73–6.
365. Oohashi H, Ohgawara H, Nanjo K, Tasaka Y, Cao QP, Chan SJ, Rubenstein AH, Steiner DF, Omori Y. Familial hyperproinsulinemia associated with NIDDM. A case study. *Diabetes Care* 1993; 16: 1340–6.
366. Polonsky KS. Evolution of β-cell dysfunction in impaired glucose tolerance and diabetes. *Exp Clin Endocrinol Diabetes* 1999; 107 (suppl 4): S124–7.
367. Leahy JL. Natural history of β-cell dysfunction in NIDDM. *Diabetes Care* 1990; 13: 992–1010.
368. Leahy JL, Bonner-Weir S, Weir G. β-cell dysfunction induced by chronic hyperglycemia. Current ideas on mechanism of impaired glucose-induced insulin secretion. *Diabetes Care* 1992; 15: 442–55.
369. Kahn SE. Regulation of B-cell function *in vivo*. *Diabetes Rev* 1996; 4: 372–89.
370. Halban PA. Differential rates of release of newly synthesized and of stored insulin from pancreatic islets. *Endocrinology* 1982; 110: 1183–8.
371. Guest PC, Pipeleers D, Rossier J, Rhodes CJ, Hutton JC. Co-secretion of carboxypeptidase H and insulin from isolated rat islets of Langerhans. *Biochem J* 1989; 264: 503–8.
372. Hosokawa YA, Leahy JL. Parallel reduction of pancreatic insulin content and insulin secretion in 48-h tolbutamide-infused normoglycemic rats. *Diabetes* 1997; 46: 808–13.
373. Gerich JE. Redefining the clinical management of type 2 diabetes: matching therapy to pathophysiology. *Eur J Clin Invest* 2002; 32 (suppl 3): 46–53.
374. Porte D Jr. Clinical importance of insulin secretion and its interaction with insulin resistance in the treatment of type 2 diabetes mellitus and its complications. *Diabetes Metab Res Rev* 2001; 17: 181–8.
375. Laedtke T, Kjems L, Porksen N, Schmitz O, Veldhuis J, Kao PC, Butler PC. Overnight inhibition of insulin secretion restores pulsatility and proinsulin/insulin ratio in type 2 diabetes. *Am J Physiol Endocrinol Metab* 2000; 279: E520–8.

7

β-Cell Biology of Insulin Secretion

Claes B. Wollheim and Pierre Maechler

University Medical Centre, Geneva, Switzerland

INTRODUCTION

Role of β-Cell in Glucose Homeostasis

Blood glucose control depends on the normal regulation of insulin secretion from the pancreatic β-cells and the action of insulin on its target tissues. The initial stages of type 1 diabetes, before β-cell destruction, are characterized by impaired glucose-stimulated insulin secretion. The large majority of diabetic patients are classified as type 2 diabetes, or non-insulin-dependent diabetes mellitus. The patients display dysregulation of insulin secretion, often but not always combined with insulin resistance of liver, muscle, and fat. The etiology of type 2 diabetes is still poorly understood and has been elucidated in only a limited number of subtypes. Among these, maturity-onset diabetes of the young (MODY) and mitochondrial diabetes have been linked to specific gene mutations and primary β-cell dysfunction. The impact of such mutations on the β-cell highlights the importance of the mitochondria in the control of insulin secretion.

The human β-cells constitute about 70% of the islets of Langerhans, which are spread throughout the pancreas and represent only 1–2% of this organ [1]. The cytoplasm of each β-cell is filled with insulin secretory granules, estimated to amount to 13 000 in the mouse [2]. In the granule, insulin forms crystals with Zn^{2+} and each granule stores about 200 000 insulin molecules. During glucose stimulation only a small proportion of the granules undergo exocytosis. The exocytotic process is tightly controlled by signals generated by nutrient metabolism, as well as by neurotransmitters and circulating hormones. Through its particular gene expression profile, the β-cell is poised to rapidly adapt the rate of insulin secretion to fluctuations in the blood glucose concentration (Figure 1). This chapter describes the molecular basis of metabolism–secretion coupling of glucose-stimulated insulin release.

The reader is referred to other sections of this book for information on the mode of action of receptor agonists known to potentiate or inhibit insulin secretion.

FROM GLUCOSE ENTRY TO THE MITOCHONDRIA

Glucose Transport

In several insulin target tissues, notably muscle and fat, stimulated glucose entry into the cell depends on insulin-induced glucose transporter (Glut-4) translocation. This contrasts with the rapid equilibration of glucose across the plasma membrane of hepatocytes and β-cells [3]. In rodent β-cells the principal glucose transporter is Glut-2, as demonstrated by the hyperglycemia and impaired insulin secretion of mice lacking this transporter [4]. In human β-cells the role of Glut-2 has been debated [5, 6], and the major glucose transporter is probably Glut-1, as genetic defects in Glut-2 do not cause diabetes [7]. Nonetheless, glucose equilibrates across the β-cell plasma membrane and is trapped by phosphorylation ensuring efficient glycolysis.

Glucose Phosphorylation

The facilitated glucose entry into hepatocytes and β-cells necessitates a specific glucose-phosphorylating enzyme with a much higher K_m than that of hexokinase expressed in muscle, fat, and other tissues. Therefore, a high K_m hexokinase IV, or glucokinase, catalyzes the formation of glucose-6-phosphate and determines the rate of glycolysis in β-cells [8, 9]. As glucokinase acts as a pacemaker of

International Textbook of Diabetes Mellitus, Third Edition. Edited by R. A. DeFronzo, E. Ferrannini, H. Keen, and P. Zimmet.
 ISBN: 0-471-48655-8.

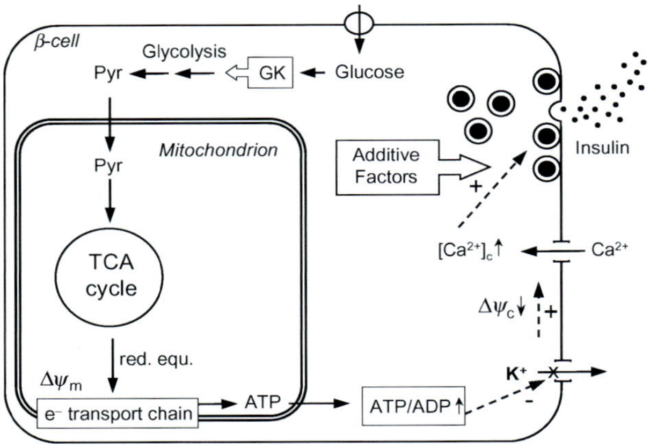

Figure 1 Model for coupling of glucose metabolism to insulin secretion in the β-cell. Glucose equilibrates across the plasma membrane and is phosphorylated by glucokinase (GK). Further glycolysis produces pyruvate (Pyr). Pyr preferentially enters the mitochondria and fuels the TCA cycle, resulting in the transfer of reducing equivalents (red. equ.) to the respiratory chain, leading to hyperpolarization of the mitochondrial membrane potential ($\Delta\psi_m$) and generation of ATP. ATP is then transferred to the cytosol, raising the ATP/ADP ratio. Subsequently, closure of K_{ATP} channels depolarizes the cell membrane potential ($\Delta\psi_c$). This opens voltage-dependent Ca^{2+} channels, increasing cytosolic Ca^{2+} concentration ($[Ca^{2+}]_c$), which triggers insulin exocytosis

glycolysis, it is generally considered as a glucose sensor in the β-cells.

Glycolysis

Attesting to the importance of glucokinase, its overexpression leads to accumulation of glucose-6-phosphate since

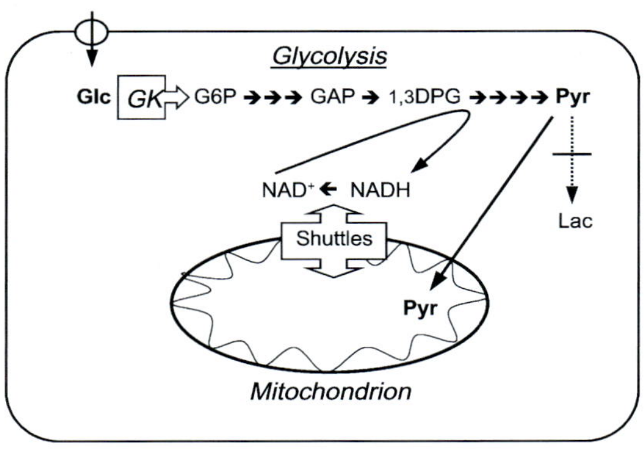

Figure 2 Glucose entry to the mitochondria. Glucose is phosphorylated by glucokinase (GK), initiating glycolysis. Following isomerization and further phosphorylation, the resulting six-carbon fructose 1,6-diphosphate is split into the three-carbon molecules dihydroxyacetone phosphate plus glyceraldehyde 3-phosphate (GAP). The next step generates 1,3-diphosphoglycerate (1,3DPG) plus NADH. The latter requires mitochondrial shuttles in order to ensure NAD^+ regeneration, compensating for low lactate (Lac) formation. As a consequence, pyruvate (Pyr) is the major end product of glycolysis in the β-cell

phosphofructokinase is the next flux-determining enzyme of glycolysis [10]. In contrast to other tissues, neither the pentose phosphate shunt nor glucose-6-phosphatase activity significantly influences the fate of glucose in normal β-cells [3, 9]. The subsequent steps of glycolysis following glucose phosphorylation are not flux-determining through the pathway, which rather depends on the mass action of glucose metabolites (Figure 2).

Pyruvate Handling

Pyruvate kinase catalyzes the formation of pyruvate, which is the essential end product of glycolysis as only little lactate is produced in β-cells. Accordingly, both lactate dehydrogenase and the plasma membrane monocarboxylic transporter levels are low in this cell type [11–13]. This particular feature confers glucose selectivity and may avoid undesired pyruvate- and lactate-induced insulin secretion during exercise. The β-cells are uniquely poised to metabolize pyruvate inside the mitochondria since as much as 90% of glucose-derived carbons end up in the organelle [14].

Mitochondrial Proton Shuttles

In most tissues, lactate dehydrogenase ensures NADH oxidation so as to avoid inhibition of glycolysis by NADH. However, in β-cells high rates of glycolysis are maintained through the activity of mitochondrial proton shuttles. These are mainly the glycerophosphate and malate/aspartate shuttles [15, 16]. Simultaneous blockade of the two shuttles inhibits glucose-stimulated insulin secretion [16]. Reoxidation to dihydroxyacetonephosphate permits the transfer of electrons from cytosolic glycerophosphate to mitochondrial $FADH_2$. In the second shuttle, electrons from cytosolic NADH are transferred to malate, which is reoxidized to oxaloacetate in the mitochondrial matrix. The shuttle is completed by transamination of oxaloacetate, forming aspartate, which returns to the cytosol. Other shuttles generating cytosolic NADPH have also been described [17, 18]. The dependence on these proton shuttles explains the tight coupling between glycolysis and mitochondrial metabolism: any attenuation of the latter will inhibit the former [3, 11, 19].

JOURNEY THROUGH THE MITOCHONDRION

Fate of Pyruvate

After its entry into the mitochondria, pyruvate is converted to acetyl-CoA by pyruvate dehydrogenase [20] or to oxaloacetate by pyruvate carboxylase [21]. Different methodological approaches concur in emphasizing the importance of pyruvate carboxylase in β-cell mitochondria

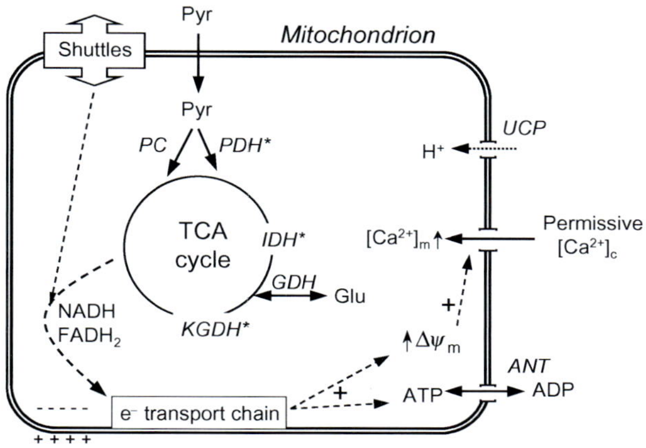

Figure 3 Journey through the mitochondrion. In the mitochondria, pyruvate (Pyr) is a substrate both for pyruvate dehydrogenase (PDH) and pyruvate carboxylase (PC). The TCA cycle generates reducing equivalents in the form of NADH and $FADH_2$, which are transferred to the electron transport chain. The elevation of $[Ca^{2+}]_c$ following cell activation is relayed to the mitochondria via a Ca^{2+} uniporter. At permissive $[Ca^{2+}]_c$ (about 300 nM), Ca^{2+} entry is favored by hyperpolarization of $\Delta\psi_m$ secondary to respiratory chain activation. The rise in $[Ca^{2+}]_m$ further activates (*) (PDH) pyruvate dehydrogenase (PDH), isocitrate dehydrogenase (IDH), and α-ketoglutarate dehydrogenase (KGDH). In certain conditions, glutamate is produced from α-ketoglutarate by glutamate dehydrogenase (GDH). The uncoupling protein (UCP) diminishes the proton gradient

[14, 18, 22–24]. The enzyme provides anaplerotic input (carbon skeleton) to the tricarboxylic acid (TCA) cycle (Figure 3). The high anaplerotic activity suggests that the loss of TCA-cycle-derived coupling factors, such as citrate [18] or glutamate [25], is compensated for by oxaloacetate. Approximately 50% of pyruvate is oxidized to acetyl-CoA by pyruvate dehydrogenase. The activity of this multienzyme complex is regulated by specific kinases and a dedicated phosphatase [20]. This phosphatase is activated by Ca^{2+}, which results in stimulation of the pyruvate dehydrogenase activity.

The TCA Cycle

The TCA cycle is an important crossroad of metabolism, enabling fuel oxidation as well as provision of building blocks for lipids and proteins. Oxaloacetate is condensed with acetyl-CoA, both originating from glucose metabolism, to form citrate, which undergoes stepwise oxidation and decarboxylation, yielding α-ketoglutarate. The fate of α-ketoglutarate is either a further oxidative decarboxylation to succinyl-CoA or a reductive transamination forming glutamate, a main spin-off product of the TCA cycle [26]. Succinyl-CoA is converted to succinate, the substrate of succinate dehydrogenase. This enzyme is unique in the TCA cycle as it is also a constituent of the electron transport chain. The cycle is completed via fumarate and malate, in turn producing oxaloacetate. It should be noted that the TCA cycle also oxidizes fatty acids and amino acids, although in the β-cell, carbohydrates are the most important fuel under physiological conditions.

Transfer of Reducing Equivalents

Through activation of the TCA cycle, electrons are transferred to the respiratory chain, resulting in hyperpolarization of the mitochondrial membrane and generation of ATP. The electrons are transferred by the pyridine nucleotide NAD^+ and the flavin adenine nucleotide FAD. In the mitochondrial matrix, NADH is formed by several dehydrogenases: pyruvate, isocitrate, α-ketoglutarate, and malate dehydrogenases. The former three are activated by Ca^{2+} [27, 28], thereby reinforcing the production of reducing equivalents during cell activation. $FADH_2$, on the other hand, is generated in the succinate dehydrogenase reaction.

The Electron Transport Chain and ATP Generation

The electron transport chain activity results in proton export from the mitochondrial matrix across the inner membrane, thereby establishing a strong mitochondrial membrane potential ($\Delta\psi_m$), inside negative (−180 mV). The respiratory chain comprises five complexes, the subunits of which are encoded both by the nuclear and mitochondrial genomes [29]. Complex I is the only acceptor of electrons from NADH in the inner mitochondrial membrane and its blockade abolishes glucose-induced insulin secretion [3, 30]. Complex II (succinate dehydrogenase) receives electrons from $FADH_2$, which is generated both by the oxidative activity of the TCA cycle and the glycerophosphate shuttle. Together with complex I, complexes III and IV accomplish proton pumping. Complex IV also ensures respiration, i.e. oxygen reduction to water. Through complex V (ATP synthase) protons leak back into the mitochondrial matrix, thereby driving ATP formation from ADP and inorganic phosphate. Fuel oxidation accelerates proton extrusion from the mitochondria, causing hyperpolarization of $\Delta\psi_m$. The synthesized ATP is translocated to the cytosol in exchange for ADP by the adenine nucleotide translocator (ANT). Thus, the work of the separate complexes of the electron transport chain and the ANT is consorted to ensure the coupling between respiration and ATP supply.

Ca^{2+} and Mitochondrial Metabolism

At the inner mitochondrial membrane, hyperpolarization of $\Delta\psi_m$ increases the driving force for Ca^{2+} entry through the Ca^{2+} uniporter [28]. Hereby, relatively modest increases in cytosolic Ca^{2+} result in larger Ca^{2+} elevations in the mitochondrial matrix [31]. The Ca^{2+} concentrations reached are sufficient for the activation of the NADH-generating dehydrogenases, in particular pyruvate dehydrogenase and α-ketoglutarate dehydrogenase [27, 32]. In this manner, increases in cytosolic Ca^{2+} occurring during glucose activation are relayed to the mitochondria to enhance the production of NADH and other coupling factors participating in the stimulation of insulin secretion [33–35].

FROM THE MITOCHONDRIA TO THE PLASMA MEMBRANE

Changes in Cytosolic ATP/ADP

The ATP formed in the mitochondria by oxidative phosphorylation is transferred to the cytosol. A major part of cytosolic ATP serves to maintain the ionic homeostasis of the cell. The transmembrane ionic gradients are established by the activity of ion-selective pumps consuming ATP, or ATPases. The plasma membrane Na^+/K^+-ATPase controls the sodium gradient (∼10-fold lower inside) and the potassium gradient (∼20-fold higher inside). The cytosolic concentration of the second messenger calcium is maintained at ∼100 nM under resting conditions essentially by two pumps, the plasma membrane Ca^+-ATPase and the sarcoplasmic/endoplasmic reticulum Ca^+-ATPase (SERCA). These pumps achieve the impressive Ca^+ gradients of ∼10 000 relative to the extracellular space and ∼3000 with respect to the reticulum [36, 37]. The paramount importance of continued ATP provision for Ca^{2+} homeostasis is illustrated on the one hand by the lowering of intrareticular Ca^{2+} when mitochondrial ATP synthesis is inhibited [38], and on the other hand by the elevation of cytosolic ATP upon blockade of the SERCA activity [39]. In the β-cell, as in other neuroendocrine cells, ATP (and ADP) is sequestered by the secretory granules, accounting for approximately half of the total cellular adenine nucleotide pool [40]. The nucleotide uptake may be mediated by a vesicular transporter [41]. The compartmentalization of ATP could explain the relatively modest glucose-evoked elevation of cytosolic ATP [34, 42]. Consequently, for the messenger function of ATP, the ATP/ADP ratio is considered most relevant, in particular since glucose stimulation is accompanied by a decrease in ADP [9]. Accordingly, such effector systems as ion channels and the exocytotic machinery are regulated in opposite directions by ATP and ADP.

The ATP-sensitive K^+-Channel Controls Membrane Potential

Like neurones and muscle cells, β-cells are excitable. The plasma membrane is kept polarized (−70 mV, inside negative) at basal glucose concentrations <5 mM, corresponding to the fasting condition. The polarized state is maintained by the efflux of the cation K^+ through ATP-sensitive K^+ channels (K_{ATP} channels). It is known since 1984 that stimulatory glucose concentrations close K_{ATP} channels, thus explaining the coinciding depolarization of the plasma membrane [43]. The K_{ATP} channel is a hetero-octamer composed of four pore-forming units, Kir6.2, surrounded by four sulfonylurea receptors, SUR1 [44]. The antidiabetic sulfonylurea drugs are ligands for the SUR, thereby closing the K_{ATP} channels independent of metabolic activity (Figure 4). This is the initiating mechanism by which sulfonylureas stimulate insulin secretion and lower blood glucose in type 2 diabetic patients. On the other hand, the metabolism of glucose increases the ATP/ADP ratio, which in turn closes the K_{ATP} channel. As a consequence, the plasma membrane is depolarized and displays bursting electrical activity at suboptimal glucose concentrations [45]. Direct stimulation of mitochondrial ATP synthase (complex V) has been shown to promote K_{ATP}-channel closure [46], emphasizing the link between the mitochondria and the plasma membrane. The effects of glucose and sulfonylureas are counteracted by K_{ATP}-channel openers such as diazoxide [44].

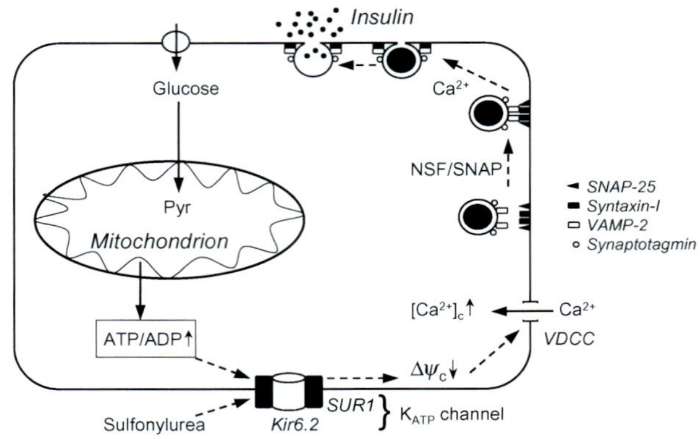

Figure 4 Exocytosis. Elevation of the ATP/ADP ratio closes the K_{ATP} channels (an action mimicked by sulfonylureas), leading to depolarization of the plasma membrane potential ($\Delta\psi_c$) and subsequent opening of voltage-dependent Ca^{2+} channels (VDCC). VAMP-2 (vesicle-associated membrane protein 2), located in the vesicle membrane, associates with syntaxin-I and SNAP-25 (synaptosome-associated protein of 25 kDa), which are found on the plasma membrane. Such association is facilitated by NSF (*N*-ethyl-maleimide-sensitive factor) and SNAP (soluble NSF attachment proteins), leading to vesicle fusion with the target membrane and insulin exocytosis

The Voltage-sensitive Ca^{2+} Channels

Closure of the K_{ATP} channels is the key step by which glucose raises cytosolic Ca^{2+}. The β-cells express voltage- and dihydropyridine-sensitive L-type Ca^{2+} channels similar to those of other excitable cells [47]. These channels are active in the membrane potential range −40 mV to 0 mV.

Other voltage-sensitive Ca^{2+} channels are expressed in β-cells but are much less abundant [48]. Ca^{2+} enters the cell during the Ca^{2+} action potentials, which are superimposed on the oscillatory changes of the membrane potential evoked by glucose [45]. The bursts have been shown to coincide with oscillations in insulin secretion [49, 50]. Upon glucose stimulation, the global patterns of membrane potential, cytosolic Ca^{2+}, and insulin secretion are biphasic with a transient first phase, lasting a few minutes, followed by a second sustained phase [49]. Blockade of L-type Ca^{2+} channels abolishes both phases of insulin secretion, whereas activators of the channels stimulate secretion [51]. This illustrates the absolute requirement for the elevation of cytosolic Ca^{2+} in the insulin release process.

Elevation of Cytosolic Ca^{2+}

Although the importance of Ca^{2+} in β-cell stimulus–secretion coupling was already emphasized in the 1960s, the detailed characterization only became possible by introduction of fluorescent Ca^{2+} indicators in 1982 (for review, see reference 51). Nutrients (such as glucose and L-leucine) and depolarizing agents (such as potassium, arginine, and sulfonylureas) raise cytosolic Ca^{2+} primarily through the opening of L-type Ca^{2+} channels. The neurotransmitter acetylcholine and the gastrointestinal hormone cholecystokinin generate the second messenger molecules inositol 1,4,5-trisphopsphate (IP_3) and diacylglycerol (DAG) through the activation of phospholipase C [51]. IP_3 binds its specific receptors on the membrane of the endoplasmic reticulum, thereby promoting Ca^{2+} efflux through the channel pore of the receptors. This permits the rapid increase of cytosolic Ca^{2+} [36, 52]. The lowering of the reticular Ca^{2+} stimulates Ca^{2+} entry through voltage-independent Ca^{2+} channels, which is detected as Ca^{2+}-release-activated Ca^{2+} current (ICRAC) [53]. The β-cells also express low levels of ryanodine receptors, another class of ligand-operated endoplasmic reticulum Ca^{2+} channels [54]. The physiological role of ryanodine receptors in glucose-stimulated insulin secretion is debated. The receptors mediate Ca^{2+}-induced Ca^{2+} release (CICR) in other cell types. Direct measurements of endoplasmic reticulum Ca^{2+} in insulin-secreting cells did not show CICR during either glucose or potassium stimulation, but on the contrary these secretagogues increased reticular Ca^{2+} [36, 55]. It is peculiar that cyclic ADP ribose, a ryanodine receptor ligand, mobilizes Ca^{2+} from secretory granules [56]. The gastrointestinal hormones glucagon-like peptide 1 (GLP-1) and gastric inhibitory polypeptide (GIP) potentiate glucose-induced insulin secretion by raising cellular cAMP levels [57]. cAMP-dependent protein kinase may increase cytosolic Ca^{2+} by phosphorylation of both L-type Ca^{2+} channels [58] and ryanodine receptors [54]. Hereby, the two universal second messengers Ca^{2+} and cAMP are able to cross talk during β-cell activation. Taken together, the endoplasmic reticulum in β-cells serves more as a Ca^{2+} sink than a source for trigger Ca^{2+} (in contrast to IP_3-generating-agonists) in glucose-stimulated insulin secretion. Accordingly, compounds that empty the reticular Ca^{2+} store do not alter glucose-evoked biphasic insulin release, while oscillations in cytosolic Ca^{2+} are abolished [59].

Movement of Secretory Granules to the Plasma Membrane

The β-cell cytosol contains approximately 10 000 insulin secretory granules [2], also called large dense-core vesicles [60]. Only a small fraction of the granule pool is located at the plasma membrane, part of which is competent for exocytosis. This docked pool contains the readily releasable granule pool (<5%), while the majority, referred to as the reserve pool (>95%), requires further translocation and priming. Sustained insulin release, as evoked by glucose or other nutrients, necessitates movement of the granules along microtubules [61]. The directed movement is accomplished by ATP-dependent kinesins and possibly other motor proteins [62, 63]. Protein phopshorylation mediated by cAMP-dependent protein kinase (PKA), protein kinase C (PKC), and myosin light chain kinase increase granule translocation [64]. On the other hand, kinesin dephosphorylation by calcineurin (phosphoprotein phosphatase 2B, Ca^{2+}/calmodulin activated) is thought to favor granule movement during stimulation of secretion [65]. This is an attractive proposal, as an increase in cytosolic Ca^{2+} also promotes the liberation of granules tethered to the cytoskeleton composed of an actin microfilamentous network [66]. At the same time, cortical actin situated beneath the plasma membrane limits the access of the granules to their docking sites [67]. The further characterization of proteins participating in granule tethering and transport as well as the shaping of the cortical actin remains to be accomplished.

In Preparation for Exocytosis

Insulin, like neurotransmitters and other peptide hormones, exits from the cells by regulated exocytosis. In addition to the regulated pathway, β-cells share constitutive exocytosis with all other cell types. It is possible that a very minor proportion of secreted insulin employs the constitutive pathway [68], which occurs in the absence of external signals. Regulated exocytosis is a specialized pathway in particular present in cells whose secretory products require tightly controlled release. Vesicles in this pathway undergo exocytosis only in response to particular stimuli such as an increase in cytosolic Ca^{2+}. Several sequential steps during regulated exocytosis constitute the prelude to the final release of vesicular contents into the extracellular space. These steps are (1) recruitment of vesicles to the membrane (see above), (2) vesicle docking to the plasma membrane, (3) priming to achieve release competence, and (4) fusion with the plasma membrane. Docking of recruited vesicles to the plasma membrane was initially characterized by electron microscopy but little is known of the biochemical dynamics of this process [60]. Patch clamp capacitance studies have shown that the subsequent priming reaction requires ATP and Ca^{2+} (in the submicromolar range) while membrane fusion is triggered by micromolar amounts of Ca^{2+} [69–71]. Electrophysiological studies have distinguished a small readily releasable pool (RRP) of vesicles or granules from a larger, more slowly released pool, suggesting that the former represents primed vesicles [45, 72]. In fact, at least three functional pools of secretory vesicles can be distinguished: the large reserve pool not associated with the plasma membrane, a docked pool not release-competent, and the docked readily releasable vesicles, or RRP [73]. Fusion of the vesicle to the plasma membrane results in the formation of a pore, initially similar to a small ion channel, which subsequently widens to allow release of the granule contents [73]. However, scarce information is available on the relative contributions of proteins and lipids in this process [74, 75]. The most extensively studied and best-understood form of regulated exocytosis is synaptic neurotransmitter release. Interestingly, analysis of exocytosis in endocrine cells revealed strong similarities between the two systems. Indeed, proteins important in synaptic vesicle exocytosis were shown to be present and functional also in pancreatic β-cells [76].

Machinery of Exocytosis

A unifying hypothesis has been proposed to account in molecular terms for membrane docking and fusion of vesicles throughout the secretory pathway from the endoplasmic reticulum to the plasma membrane [77]. The SNARE hypothesis suggests that this process is induced by the specific pairing of the v-SNARE protein VAMP-2 (vesicle-associated membrane protein 2/synaptobrevin), located in the vesicle membrane, with the cognate t-SNARE proteins syntaxin-I and SNAP-25 (synaptosome-associated protein of 25 kDa), which are found on the target (plasma) membrane. These proteins interact mainly via coiled–coiled regions present in distinct helices and are capable of forming extremely stable complexes arranged in ring-like structures. They form stable heterotrimeric complexes consisting of a four-helix bundle of one α-helix each contributed by VAMP and by syntaxin and two helices provided by SNAP-25 [70, 78]. Association of v-SNAREs with t-SNAREs to form SNARE complexes is facilitated by the recruitment of several cytosolic proteins including NSF (*N*-ethylmaleimide-sensitive factor) and SNAPs (soluble NSF attachment proteins). These soluble proteins assemble with the SNARE complex, ultimately leading to vesicle fusion with the target membrane. Botulinum and tetanus neurotoxins, which compromise neurotransmission by cleaving specifically v- or t-SNARE proteins, have been instrumental in placing the action of SNAREs downstream of vesicle docking [79]. The identification of multiple SNAREs within a single eukaryotic cell, with each isoform having a distinct subcellular distribution, suggests that these proteins may confer spatial specificity to vesicle trafficking [77]. Although the SNARE complex is important for exocytosis, several assumptions of the initial SNARE hypothesis remain a matter of debate. Among these, the spatial organization, the temporal sequence of events and the precise function of docking, priming, and fusion of vesicles are still unresolved. Each step of this complex pathway involves the action of additional proteins (for review see reference 80). An additional mechanism completing the cycle is the disassembly of the SNARE complex through the ATP-hydrolizing action of NSF [70, 80].

GETTING OUT OF THE CELL (INSULIN EXOCYTOSIS)

Regulation of Exocytosis

The SNARE proteins VAMP-2 [81], syntaxin-I [82, 83], and SNAP-25 [84] are expressed in β-cells and their function in Ca^{2+}-induced insulin exocytosis has been demonstrated by the use of tetanus and botulinum neurotoxins [76]. These toxins are proteases that specifically cleave these SNARE proteins. Other proteins have been implicated in the regulation of exocytosis by Ca^{2+} and GTP. The Ca^{2+}-binding protein synaptotagmin is expressed both on synaptic vesicles and on insulin secretory granules, whereas some of its 13 isoforms are also expressed on the plasma membrane [85–88]. Specific synaptotagmin isoforms are functional in neurotransmitter release, but their role in insulin exocytosis remains to be clarified. The results obtained in β-cell lines are not unequivocal as important differences exist between primary β-cells and β-cell lines. Exocytosis is also controlled by G-proteins, which are active in their GTP-bound form. The monomeric G-proteins Rab3A, B, C, and D are all associated with insulin granules [89]. A current model for their action suggests that the plasma-membrane-associated Rab3-interacting molecule (RIM) binds Rab3 to allow exocytosis to proceed [90, 91]. Using recombinant proteins, Ca^{2+} affects the binding of RIM to the membrane, to SNAREs and to Ca^{2+}-channel subunits [91]. It has been suggested that SNARE proteins can modulate L-type Ca^{2+}-channel function and that there is tight spatial coupling between the channels and the exocytotic event [92].

The universal second messenger cAMP, generated at the plasma membrane from ATP, potentiates glucose-stimulated insulin secretion. Many neurotransmitters and hormones, including glucagon as well as the intestinal hormones GLP-1 and GIP, increase cAMP levels in the β-cell by activating adenyl cyclase [93]. Although glucose itself is inefficient in producing cAMP, permissive levels of cAMP are necessary for normal responsiveness of secretion [94]. The most important target of cAMP is the exocytotic machinery, where the messenger acts both in a PKA-dependent and -independent manner [95–99]. Among other putative nucleotide messengers, NADH and NADPH are generated by glucose metabolism [3]. The rise in pyridine nucleotides precedes the increase in cytosolic Ca^{2+} [100] and the elevation in the cytosol is reached more rapidly than the elevation in the mitochondria [101]. It remains to be determined whether pyridine nucleotides participate in β-cell activation through effects on ion fluxes or on the process of exocytosis.

Insulin Secretion Profiles

A square wave increase of the glucose concentration reaching the β-cells results in biphasic insulin secretion. It is characterized by a transient first phase lasting a few minutes, followed by a nadir and a second sustained phase lasting for the entire glucose stimulation period [102–104]. The square wave glucose challenge tests the β-cell performance in terms of secretory capacity. Under conditions of meal ingestion, blood glucose levels increase gradually, which is mimicked experimentally by ramp-like elevation of glucose concentration. Such a protocol leads to a graded increase in plasma insulin levels [105]. Both the square wave and ramp protocols have yielded consistent secretory profiles when applied *in vivo* and in several *in vitro* preparations, including the perfused rat pancreas and perifused isolated islets.

Insulin secretion is oscillatory under steady state conditions (basal and stimulated). The oscillations display different periodicity ranging from one every 5–10 min *in vivo* [106] to 2–7 per min in isolated islet preparations [107]. In the latter preparation, the rapid oscillations are correlated with the bursting activity of oxygen consumption, membrane potential, and cytosolic Ca^{2+} transients [108]. These results as well as measurements of additional metabolic parameters [33, 109] suggest that the pattern of insulin release is shaped by the oscillations in β-cell metabolism. For further details on this vast research topic, we refer the reader to the cited reviews and the references therein [106–108].

Biphasic Insulin Secretion

Several hypotheses have attempted to account for the transient nature of the first phase of glucose-induced insulin secretion [110]. Clues come from the use of potassium concentrations that depolarize the membrane potential and promote Ca^{2+} influx [111]. The ensuing rise in cytosolic Ca^{2+} results in a monophasic insulin secretory response, not reproducing the sustained release evoked by glucose. It is noteworthy that the amplitudes of potassium-induced insulin release and of the first phase of glucose-stimulated secretion are similar [111]. This strongly suggests that the glucose-induced rise in cytosolic Ca^{2+} is sufficient to explain the first phase of the biphasic insulin secretion. The monophasic response to potassium is generally believed to result from the uncompensated exhaustion of the readily releasable pool of secretory granules and/or of the entire pool docked to the plasma membrane [72, 110, 112]. The latter may be further compartmentalized according to measurements of exocytosis by electrophysiological techniques [112]. Interestingly, pretreatment with glucose can replenish the readily releasable pool and reestablish a second response to the sole increase in cytosolic Ca^{2+} concentration [72]. Nutrient secretagogues, in particular glucose, evoke a long-lasting second phase of insulin secretion. In contrast to the transient secretion induced by potassium and Ca^{2+}-mobilizing receptor agonists, the sustained insulin release depends on the generation of metabolic factors including ATP. The elevation of cytosolic Ca^{2+} is also a prerequisite for this phase of secretion, as demonstrated, among others, by the inhibitory action of voltage-sensitive Ca^{2+}-channel blockers.

The K_{ATP}-Channel-independent Pathway

The Ca^{2+} signal in the cytosol is necessary but not sufficient for the full development of biphasic insulin secretion. It was proposed around 1900 that glucose evokes K_{ATP}-channel-independent stimulation of insulin secretion [113–115]. This K_{ATP}-channel-independent pathway, or amplifying pathway [116], was unmasked by clamping cytosolic Ca^{2+} at permissive levels using sulfonylureas or the combination of high potassium and the K_{ATP}-channel-opener diazoxide during glucose stimulation [113–115]. In addition, knockout mouse models lacking either of the two functional subunits of the K_{ATP} channel show marked reduction, albeit not abolished, glucose-stimulated insulin secretion [117, 118]. The β-cells in these mice exhibit a partial secretory response to glucose, not accompanied by changes in their constitutively elevated cytosolic Ca^{2+}. Taken together, these studies suggest the existence of metabolic coupling factors generated by glucose.

Metabolic Factors Implicated in Secretion

ATP is a primary metabolic factor implicated in K_{ATP}-channel regulation [44], secretory granule movement [63, 64], as well as the process of insulin exocytosis [96, 112]. Glucose also promotes the elevation of GTP [119], which could trigger insulin exocytosis via GTPases [76, 95, 96]. GTP is formed in the mitochondria by the

TCA cycle but it is trapped in the organelle. In the cytosol, GTP is mainly formed through the action of nucleoside diphosphate kinase from GDP and ATP. In contrast to ATP, GTP is a *bona fide* messenger molecule, since it is capable of initiating insulin exocytosis in a Ca^{2+}-independent manner [95, 96, 120]. It is not known whether GTP acts via a monomeric or heterotrimeric G-protein directly controlling exocytosis [76, 90].

In glucose-stimulated β-cells, citrate exported from the mitochondria to the cytosol reacts with coenzyme-A (CoA) to form malonyl-CoA, which is a lipid precursor. This favors the accumulation of long-chain acyl-CoAs such as palmitoyl-CoA in the cytosol [121, 122], suggested to couple glucose metabolism to insulin secretion [123]. The long-chain acyl-CoA hypothesis was substantiated by the observation that palmitoyl-CoA enhances Ca^{2+}-evoked insulin exocytosis [124]. Since abrogation of malonyl-CoA accumulation during glucose stimulation did not attenuate the secretory response [125], the role of long-chain acyl-CoA derivatives remains a matter of debate [116, 126].

The amino acid glutamate is another metabolic factor proposed to participate in the amplifying pathway [25, 127]. Glutamate can be produced from the TCA cycle intermediate α-ketoglutarate or by transamination reactions [26]. During glucose stimulation total cellular glutamate levels are increased in human, mouse, and rat islets as well as in clonal β-cells [23, 25, 128, 129], whereas there was no change in other islet studies [130, 131]. The model for the effect of glutamate was based on the finding that mitochondrial activation in permeabilized β-cells directly stimulates insulin exocytosis [132] and that glutamate is the putative mediator [25, 133]. At present, the mechanism of glutamate action on exocytosis is unknown.

GENETIC β-CELL DEFECTS AND PATHOPHYSIOLGY OF INSULIN SECRETION

Glucokinase Mutations

Mutations in the glucokinase gene that result in decreased glucose sensitivity affect blood glucose regulation and are associated with maturity-onset diabetes of the young, type 2 (MODY2) [134]. Conversely, glucokinase mutations resulting in a gain of function of the enzyme cause one form of a syndrome of persistent hyperinsulinemic hypoglycemia of infancy (PHHI) [135]. These phenotypes illustrate the role of the glucokinase enzyme as a gatekeeper determining the flux of intermediates undergoing glycolysis.

Glucose Metabolism and MODY Disease

Five of the six forms of MODY described to date have been associated with mutations in nuclear transcription factors: hepatocyte nuclear factor 4α (HNF-4α) (MODY1), HNF-1α (MODY3), human insulin promoter factor-1 corresponding to rodent PDX-1 (MODY4), HNF-1β (MODY5), and NeuroD or Beta2 (MODY6) [136, 137]. These syndromes are characterized by β-cell dysfunction with impaired glucose-stimulated insulin secretion [138, 139]. Transgenic mouse models have demonstrated that the β-cell defects are the primary cause of MODY3 and MODY4 [140–143]. In cellular model systems, the molecular basis of the MODY1 and MODY3 genes has been attributed to deranged mitochondrial metabolism [144, 145]. In both models, the defective respiratory chain activation correlated with downregulation of the TCA cycle enzyme α-ketoglutarate dehydrogenase accompanied by an upregulation of the uncoupling protein 2 (UCP2) [144, 145]. UCP2 is an inner mitochondrial membrane protein that tends to diminish the proton gradient generated by the respiratory chain. Its overexpression in β-cells attenuates ATP synthesis and insulin secretion in response to glucose [146]. Whether changes in glucose metabolism underlie β-cell dysfunction in other forms of MODY remains to be established.

MITOCHONDRIAL DNA MUTATIONS

In view of the importance of mitochondrial activation in metabolism–secretion coupling, it is not surprising that mutations in the mitochondrial genome have been associated with diabetes [147, 148]. The phenotype has been characterized in transgenic mice lacking expression of the mitochondrial genome specifically in the β-cells [149]. These mice are diabetic and their islets are unable to release insulin in response to glucose. Mitochondrial DNA-deficient cellular models are also glucose unresponsive and are defective in mitochondrial function, but retain depolarization-mediated (potassium and sulfonylurea) insulin secretion [150–152]. These models of various forms of diabetes demonstrate the fragility of nutrient-stimulated insulin secretion, caused primarily by defective mitochondrial ATP generation.

Mutations in the ATP-sensitive K^+-Channel and Metabolic Enzymes

Mutations in both subunits of the K_{ATP}-channel SUR1 and Kir6.2 cause neonatal hyperinsulinism, referred to as PHHI [153]. On the other hand, a polymorphism in the Kir6.2 subunit is more frequent in type 2 diabetic patients than in the general population. The variant decreases the sensitivity to ATP, thereby increasing channel open state probability [154]. Surprisingly, deletion of each of the two K_{ATP}-channel subunits in mice does not lead to the PHHI syndrome. The animals exhibit impaired glucose-stimulated insulin secretion, which is counterbalanced by increased peripheral insulin sensitivity [117, 118, 155]. As expected by the absence of K_{ATP}-channel function, β-cell resting cytosolic Ca^{2+} levels are increased, but the islets still retain some responsiveness to insulin secretagogues [117, 118, 155]. A cell line has been derived from the pancreas of a PHHI patient. The secretory defect of these cells was restored for a while by triple transfection with PDX1, SUR1, and Kir6.2 [156]. The PHHI syndrome is not restricted to mutations in K_{ATP}-channel subunits and glucokinase, but has also been linked to activating mutations of the mitochondrial enzyme glutamate dehydrogenase [157], as well as impaired β-oxidation due to mutated short-chain L-3-hydroxyacyl-CoA dehydrogenase [158].

CONCLUSIONS

The expression profile of the carbohydrate-metabolizing enzymes is optimized to accomplish the key role of the β-cell, i.e. the coupling of blood glucose increases to enhanced insulin exocytosis. To this end, most of the glucose carbons are funneled to the mitochondria where they are converted to various molecules implicated in the triggering of the exocytotic process. These signals include ATP, which promotes the elevation of cytosolic Ca^{2+} levels, constituting the main and obligatory step in secretion. In addition, citrate-derived long-chain acyl-CoAs as well as glutamate have been proposed to participate in the final steps of insulin release. There are close similarities between neurotransmitter and insulin exocytosis, explained by the related expression profile of SNARE proteins and other molecules controlling exocytosis in neurons and β-cells. Impaired insulin secretion has already been linked to mutations in metabolic enzymes. Polymorphisms of ion channels may also be implicated and alterations in exocytotic proteins could well underlie defects in metabolism–secretion coupling in the β-cell.

REFERENCES

1. Rahier J, Goebbels RM, Henquin JC. Cellular composition of the human diabetic pancreas. *Diabetologia* 1983; 24: 366–71.
2. Dean PM. Ultrastructural morphometry of the pancreatic β-cell. *Diabetologia* 1973; 9: 115–9.
3. Newgard CB, McGarry JD. Metabolic coupling factors in pancreatic beta-cell signal transduction. *Annu Rev Biochem* 1995; 64: 689–719.
4. Guillam MT, Hummler E, Schaerer E, Yeh JI, Birnbaum MJ, Beermann F, Schmidt A, Deriaz N, Thorens B, Wu JY. Early diabetes and abnormal postnatal pancreatic islet development in mice lacking Glut-2. *Nat Genet* 1997; 17: 327–30.
5. Ferrer J, Benito C, Gomis R. Pancreatic islet GLUT2 glucose transporter mRNA and protein expression in humans with and without NIDDM. *Diabetes* 1995; 44: 1369–74.
6. De Vos A, Heimberg H, Quartier E, Huypens P, Bouwens L, Pipeleers D, Schuit F. Human and rat beta cells differ in glucose transporter but not in glucokinase gene expression. *J Clin Invest* 1995; 96: 2489–95.
7. Santer R, Schneppenheim R, Dombrowski A, Gotze H, Steinmann B, Schaub J. Mutations in *GLUT2*, the gene for the liver-type glucose transporter, in patients with Fanconi–Bickel syndrome. *Nat Genet* 1997; 17: 324–6.
8. Iynedjian PB. Mammalian glucokinase and its gene. *Biochem J* 1993; 293 (pt 1): 1–13.
9. Matschinsky FM. Banting Lecture 1995. A lesson in metabolic regulation inspired by the glucokinase glucose sensor paradigm. *Diabetes* 1996; 45: 223–41.
10. Wang H, Iynedjian PB. Acute glucose intolerance in insulinoma cells with unbalanced overexpression of glucokinase. *J Biol Chem* 1997; 272: 25731–6.
11. Sekine N, Cirulli V, Regazzi R, Brown LJ, Gine E, Tamarit-Rodriguez J, Girotti M, Marie S, MacDonald MJ, Wollheim CB. Low lactate dehydrogenase and high mitochondrial glycerol phosphate dehydrogenase in pancreatic beta-cells. Potential role in nutrient sensing. *J Biol Chem* 1994; 269: 4895–902.
12. Zhao C, Wilson MC, Schuit F, Halestrap AP, Rutter GA. Expression and distribution of lactate/monocarboxylate transporter isoforms in pancreatic islets and the exocrine pancreas. *Diabetes* 2001; 50: 361–6.
13. Ishihara H, Wang H, Drewes LR, Wollheim CB. Overexpression of monocarboxylate transporter and lactate dehydrogenase alters insulin secretory responses to pyruvate and lactate in beta cells. *J Clin Invest* 1999; 104: 1621–9.
14. Schuit F, De Vos A, Farfari S, Moens K, Pipeleers D, Brun T, Prentki M. Metabolic fate of glucose in purified islet cells. Glucose-regulated anaplerosis in beta cells. *J Biol Chem* 1997; 272: 18572–9.
15. MacDonald MJ. High content of mitochondrial glycerol-3-phosphate dehydrogenase in pancreatic islets and its inhibition by diazoxide. *J Biol Chem* 1981; 256: 8287–90.
16. Eto K, Tsubamoto Y, Terauchi Y, Sugiyama T, Kishimoto T, Takahashi N, Yamauchi N, Kubota N, Murayama S, Aizawa T, Akanuma Y, Aizawa S, Kasai H, Yazaki Y, Kadowaki T. Role of NADH shuttle system in glucose-induced activation of mitochondrial metabolism and insulin secretion. *Science* 1999; 283: 981–5.
17. MacDonald MJ. Feasibility of a mitochondrial pyruvate malate shuttle in pancreatic islets. Further implication of cytosolic NADPH in insulin secretion. *J Biol Chem* 1995; 270: 20051–8.
18. Farfari S, Schulz V, Corkey B, Prentki M. Glucose-regulated anaplerosis and cataplerosis in pancreatic beta-cells: possible implication of a pyruvate/citrate shuttle in insulin secretion. *Diabetes* 2000; 49: 718–26.
19. Ishihara H, Wollheim CB. What couples glycolysis to mitochondrial signal generation in glucose-stimulated insulin secretion? *IUBMB Life* 2000; 49: 391–5.
20. Behal RH, Buxton DB, Robertson JG, Olson MS. Regulation of the pyruvate dehydrogenase multienzyme complex. *Annu Rev Nutr* 1993; 13: 497–520.
21. Jitrapakdee S, Wallace JC. Structure, function and regulation of pyruvate carboxylase. *Biochem J* 1999; 340 (pt 1): 1–16.
22. MacDonald MJ. Influence of glucose on pyruvate carboxylase expression in pancreatic islets. *Arch Biochem Biophys* 1995; 319: 128–32.
23. Brennan L, Shine A, Hewage C, Malthouse JP, Brindle KM, McClenaghan N, Flatt PR, Newsholme P. A nuclear magnetic resonance-based demonstration of substantial oxidative L-alanine metabolism and L-alanine-enhanced

glucose metabolism in a clonal pancreatic beta-cell line: metabolism of L-alanine is important to the regulation of insulin secretion. *Diabetes* 2002; 51: 1714–21.
24. Lu D, Mulder H, Zhao P, Burgess SC, Jensen MV, Kamzolova S, Newgard CB, Sherry AD. ^{13}C NMR isotopomer analysis reveals a connection between pyruvate 23 cycling and glucose-stimulated insulin secretion (GSIS). *Proc Natl Acad Sci USA* 2002; 99: 2708–13.
25. Maechler P, Wollheim CB. Mitochondrial glutamate acts as a messenger in glucoseinduced insulin exocytosis. *Nature* 1999; 402: 685–9.
26. Nissim I. Newer aspects of glutamine/glutamate metabolism: the role of acute pH changes. *Am J Physiol* 1999; 277: F493–7.
27. McCormack JG, Halestrap AP, Denton RM. Role of calcium ions in regulation of mammalian intramitochondrial metabolism. *Physiol Rev* 1990; 70: 391–425.
28. Duchen MR. Contributions of mitochondria to animal physiology: from homeostatic sensor to calcium signalling and cell death. *J Physiol* 1999; 516: 1–17.
29. Wallace DC. Mitochondrial diseases in man and mouse. *Science* 1999; 283: 1482–88.
30. Antinozzi PA, Ishihara H, Newgard CB, Wollheim CB. Mitochondrial metabolism sets the maximal limit of fuel-stimulated insulin secretion in a model pancreatic beta cell: a survey of four fuel secretagogues. *J Biol Chem* 2002; 277: 11746–55.
31. Kennedy ED, Rizzuto R, Theler JM, Pralong WF, Bastianutto C, Pozzan T, Wollheim CB. Glucose-stimulated insulin secretion correlates with changes in mitochondrial and cytosolic Ca^{2+} in aequorin-expressing INS-1 cells. *J Clin Invest* 1996; 98: 2524–38.
32. Rutter GA, Burnett P, Rizzuto R, Brini M, Murgia M, Pozzan T, Tavare JM, Denton RM. Subcellular imaging of intramitochondrial Ca^{2+} with recombinant targeted aequorin: significance for the regulation of pyruvate dehydrogenase activity. *Proc Natl Acad Sci USA* 1996; 93: 5489–94.
33. Pralong WF, Spat A, Wollheim CB. Dynamic pacing of cell metabolism by intracellular Ca^{2+} transients. *J Biol Chem* 1994; 269: 27310–4.
34. Kennedy HJ, Pouli AE, Ainscow EK, Jouaville LS, Rizzuto R, Rutter GA. Glucose generates sub-plasma membrane ATP microdomains in single islet beta-cells. Potential role for strategically located mitochondria. *J Biol Chem* 1999; 274: 13281–91.
35. Wollheim CB, Maechler P. Beta-cell mitochondria and insulin secretion: messenger role of nucleotides and metabolites. *Diabetes* 2002; 51 (suppl 1): S37–42.
36. Maechler P, Kennedy ED, Sebo E, Valeva A, Pozzan T, Wollheim CB. Secretagogues modulate the calcium concentration in the endoplasmic reticulum of insulin-secreting cells. Studies in aequorin-expressing intact and permeabilized ins-1 cells. *J Biol Chem* 1999; 274: 12583–92.
37. Carafoli E. Calcium signaling: a tale for all seasons. *Proc Natl Acad Sci USA* 2002; 99: 1115–22.
38. Maechler P, Jornot L, Wollheim CB. Hydrogen peroxide alters mitochondrial activation and insulin secretion in pancreatic beta cells. *J Biol Chem* 1999; 274: 27905–13.
39. Ainscow EK, Rutter GA. Glucose-stimulated oscillations in free cytosolic ATP concentration imaged in single islet beta-cells: evidence for a Ca(2+)-dependent mechanism. *Diabetes* 2002; 51 (suppl 1): S162–70.
40. Detimary P, Jonas JC, Henquin JC. Possible links between glucose-induced changes in the energy state of pancreatic B cells and insulin release. Unmasking by decreasing a stable pool of adenine nucleotides in mouse islets. *J Clin Invest* 1995; 96: 1738–45.
41. Gualix J, Abal M, Pintor J, Garcia-Carmona F, Miras-Portugal MT. Nucleotide vesicular transporter of bovine chromaffin granules. Evidence for a mnemonic regulation. *J Biol Chem* 1996; 271: 1957–65.
42. Maechler P, Wang H, Wollheim CB. Continuous monitoring of ATP levels in living insulin secreting cells expressing cytosolic firefly luciferase. *FEBS Lett* 1998; 422: 328–32.
43. Ashcroft FM, Harrison DE, Ashcroft SJ. Glucose induces closure of single potassium channels in isolated rat pancreatic beta-cells. *Nature* 1984; 312: 446–8.
44. Miki T, Nagashima K, Seino S. The structure and function of the ATP-sensitive K^+ channel in insulin-secreting pancreatic beta-cells. *J Mol Endocrinol* 1999; 22: 113–23.
45. Rorsman P. The pancreatic beta-cell as a fuel sensor: an electrophysiologist's viewpoint. *Diabetologia* 1997; 40: 487–95.
46. Duchen MR, Smith PA, Ashcroft FM. Substrate-dependent changes in mitochondrial function, intracellular free calcium concentration and membrane channels in pancreatic beta-cells. *Biochem J* 1993; 294 (pt 1): 35–42.
47. Ligon B, Boyd AE III, Dunlap K. Class A calcium channel variants in pancreatic islets and their role in insulin secretion. *J Biol Chem* 1998; 273: 13905–11.
48. Horvath A, Szabadkai G, Varnai P, Aranyi T, Wollheim CB, Spat A, Enyedi P. Voltage dependent calcium channels in adrenal glomerulosa cells and in insulin producing cells. *Cell Calcium* 1998; 23: 33–42.
49. Bergsten P. Slow and fast oscillations of cytoplasmic Ca^{2+} in pancreatic islets correspond to pulsatile insulin release. *Am J Physiol* 1995; 268: E282–87.
50. Barbosa RM, Silva AM, Tome AR, Stamford JA, Santos RM, Rosario LM. Control of pulsatile 5-HT/insulin secretion from single mouse pancreatic islets by intracellular calcium dynamics. *J Physiol* 1998; 510 (pt 1): 135–43.
51. Wollheim CB, Lang J, Regazzi R. The exocytotic process of insulin secretion and its regulation by Ca^{2+} and G-proteins. *Diabetes Rev* 1996; 4: 276–97.
52. Parekh AB, Penner R: Store depletion and calcium influx. *Physiol Rev* 1997; 77: 901–30.
53. Bertram R, Smolen P, Sherman A, Mears D, Atwater I, Martin F, Soria B. A role for calcium release-activated current (CRAC) in cholinergic modulation of electrical activity in pancreatic beta-cells. *Biophys J* 1995; 68: 2323–32.
54. Islam MS. The ryanodine receptor calcium channel of beta-cells: molecular regulation and physiological significance. *Diabetes* 2002; 51: 1299–309.
55. Tengholm A, Hellman B, Gylfe E. Glucose regulation of free Ca(2+) in the endoplasmic reticulum of mouse pancreatic beta cells. *J Biol Chem* 1999; 274: 36883–90.
56. Mitchell KJ, Pinton P, Varadi A, Tacchetti C, Ainscow EK, Pozzan T, Rizzuto R, Rutter GA. Dense core secretory vesicles revealed as a dynamic Ca(2+) store in neuroendocrine cells with a vesicle-associated membrane protein aequorin chimaera. *J Cell Biol* 2001; 155: 41–51.

57. Ahren B. Autonomic regulation of islet hormone secretion–implications for health and disease. *Diabetologia* 2000; 43: 393–410.
58. Kanno T, Suga S, Wu J, Kimura M, Wakui M. Intracellular cAMP potentiates voltage-dependent activation of L-type Ca^{2+} channels in rat islet beta-cells. *Pflugers Arch* 1998; 435: 578–80.
59. Roe MW, Philipson LH, Frangakis CJ, Kuznetsov A, Mertz RJ, Lancaster ME, Spencer B, Worley JF III, Dukes ID. Defective glucose-dependent endoplasmic reticulum Ca^{2+} sequestration in diabetic mouse islets of Langerhans. *J Biol Chem* 1994; 269: 18279–82.
60. Orci L. A portrait of the pancreatic B-cell. The Minkowski Award Lecture delivered on July 19, 1973, during the 8th Congress of the International Diabetes Federation, held in Brussels, Belgium. *Diabetologia* 1974; 10: 163–87.
61. Boyd AE III, Bolton WE, Brinkley BR. Microtubules and beta cell function: effect of colchicine on microtubules and insulin secretion in vitro by mouse beta cells. *J Cell Biol* 1982; 92: 425–34.
62. Meng YX, Wilson GW, Avery MC, Varden CH, Balczon R. Suppression of the expression of a pancreatic beta-cell form of the kinesin heavy chain by antisense oligonucleotides inhibits insulin secretion from primary cultures of mouse beta-cells. *Endocrinology* 1997; 138: 1979–87.
63. Varadi A, Ainscow EK, Allan VJ, Rutter GA. Involvement of conventional kinesin in glucose-stimulated secretory granule movements and exocytosis in clonal pancreatic beta-cells. *J Cell Sci* 2002; 115: 4177–89.
64. Yu W, Niwa T, Fukasawa T, Hidaka H, Senda T, Sasaki Y, Niki I. Synergism of protein kinase A, protein kinase C, and myosin light-chain kinase in the secretory cascade of the pancreatic beta-cell. *Diabetes* 2000; 49: 945–52.
65. Donelan MJ, Morfini G, Julyan R, Sommers S, Hays L, Briaud I, Kajio H, Easom RA, Molkentin JD, Brady ST, Rhodes CJ. Ca^{2+}-dependent dephosphorylation of kinesin heavy chain on {beta}-granules in pancreatic {beta}-cells: implications for regulated {beta}-granule transport and insulin exocytosis. *J Biol Chem* 2002; 277: 24232–42.
66. Ort T, Voronov S, Guo J, Zawalich K, Froehner SC, Zawalich W, Solimena M. Dephosphorylation of beta2-syntrophin and Ca^{2+}/mu-calpain-mediated cleavage of ICA512 upon stimulation of insulin secretion. *EMBO J* 2001; 20: 4013–23.
67. Li G, Rungger-Brandle E, Just I, Jonas JC, Aktories K, Wollheim CB. Effect of disruption of actin filaments by *Clostridium botulinum* C2 toxin on insulin secretion in HIT-T15 cells and pancreatic islets. *Mol Biol Cell* 1994; 5: 1199–213.
68. Kuliawat R, Arvan P. Protein targeting via the "constitutive-like" secretory pathway in isolated pancreatic islets: passive sorting in the immature granule compartment. *J Cell Biol* 1992; 118: 521–9.
69. Bokvist K, Eliasson L, Ammala C, Renstrom E, Rorsman P. Co-localization of L-type Ca^{2+} channels and insulin-containing secretory granules and its significance for the initiation of exocytosis in mouse pancreatic β-cells. *EMBO J* 1995; 14: 50–7.
70. Klenchin VA, Martin TF. Priming in exocytosis: attaining fusion-competence after vesicle docking. *Biochimie* 2000; 82: 399–407.
71. Barg S, Huang P, Eliasson L, Nelson DJ, Obermuller S, Rorsman P, Thevenod F, Renstrom E. Priming of insulin granules for exocytosis by granular Cl(−) uptake and acidification. *J Cell Sci* 2001; 114: 2145–54.
72. Olofsson CS, Gopel SO, Barg S, Galvanovskis J, Ma X, Salehi A, Rorsman P, Eliasson L. Fast insulin secretion reflects exocytosis of docked granules in mouse pancreatic β-cells. *Pflugers Arch* 2002; 444: 43–51.
73. Barg S, Olofsson CS, Schriever-Abeln J, Wendt A, Gebre-Medhin S, Renstrom E, Rorsman P. Delay between fusion pore opening and peptide release from large densecore vesicles in neuroendocrine cells. *Neuron* 2002; 33: 287–99.
74. Lollike K, Borregaard N, Lindau M. The exocytotic fusion pore of small granules has a conductance similar to an ion channel. *J Cell Biol* 1995; 129: 99–104.
75. Chanturiya A, Chernomordik LV, Zimmerberg J. Flickering fusion pores comparable with initial exocytotic pores occur in protein-free phospholipid bilayers. *Proc Natl Acad Sci USA* 1997; 94: 14423–8.
76. Lang J. Molecular mechanisms and regulation of insulin exocytosis as a paradigm of endocrine secretion. *Eur J Biochem* 1999; 259: 3–17.
77. Rothman JE, Warren G. Implications of the SNARE hypothesis for intracellular membrane topology and dynamics. *Curr Biol* 1994; 4: 220–33.
78. Sutton RB, Fasshauer D, Jahn R, Brunger AT. Crystal structure of a SNARE complex involved in synaptic exocytosis at 2.4 Å resolution. *Nature* 1998; 395: 347–53.
79. Schiavo G, Matteoli M, Montecucco C. Neurotoxins affecting neuroexocytosis. *Physiol Rev* 2000; 80: 717–66.
80. Lin RC, Scheller RH. Mechanisms of synaptic vesicle exocytosis. *Annu Rev Cell Dev Biol* 2000; 16: 19–49.
81. Regazzi R, Sadoul K, Meda P, Kelly RB, Halban PA, Wollheim CB. Mutational analysis of VAMP domains implicated in Ca^{2+}-induced insulin exocytosis. *EMBO J* 1996; 15: 6951–9.
82. Martin F, Moya F, Gutierrez LM, Reig JA, Soria B. Role of syntaxin in mouse pancreatic beta cells. *Diabetologia* 1995; 38: 860–3.
83. Lang J, Zhang H, Vaidyanathan VV, Sadoul K, Niemann H, Wollheim CB. Transient expression of botulinum neurotoxin C1 light chain differentially inhibits calcium and glucose induced insulin secretion in clonal beta–cells. *FEBS Lett* 1997; 419: 13–7.
84. Sadoul K, Lang J, Montecucco C, Weller U, Regazzi R, Catsicas S, Wollheim CB, Halban PA. SNAP-25 is expressed in islets of Langerhans and is involved in insulin release. *J Cell Biol* 1995; 128: 1019–28.
85. Lang J, Fukuda M, Zhang H, Mikoshiba K, Wollheim CB. The first C2 domain of synaptotagmin is required for exocytosis of insulin from pancreatic beta-cells: action of synaptotagmin at low micromolar calcium. *EMBO J* 1997; 16: 5837–46.
86. Brown H, Meister B, Deeney J, Corkey BE, Yang SN, Larsson O, Rhodes CJ, Seino S, Berggren PO, Fried G. Synaptotagmin III isoform is compartmentalized in pancreatic beta-cells and has a functional role in exocytosis. *Diabetes* 2000; 49: 383–91.
87. Gao Z, Reavey-Cantwell J, Young RA, Jegier P, Wolf BA. Synaptotagmin III/VII isoforms mediate Ca^{2+}-induced insulin secretion in pancreatic islet beta -cells. *J Biol Chem* 2000; 275: 36079–85.
88. Gut A, Kiraly CE, Fukuda M, Mikoshiba K, Wollheim CB, Lang J. Expression and localisation of synaptotagmin isoforms in endocrine beta-cells: their function in insulin exocytosis. *J Cell Sci* 2001; 114: 1709–16.

89. Iezzi M, Escher G, Meda P, Charollais A, Baldini G, Darchen F, Wollheim CB, Regazzi R. Subcellular distribution and function of Rab3A, B, C, and D isoforms in insulin-secreting cells. *Mol Endocrinol* 1999; 13: 202–12.
90. Iezzi M, Regazzi R, Wollheim CB. The Rab3-interacting molecule RIM is expressed in pancreatic beta-cells and is implicated in insulin exocytosis. *FEBS Lett* 2000; 474: 66–70.
91. Coppola T, Magnin-Luthi S, Perret-Menoud V, Gattesco S, Schiavo G, Regazzi R. Direct interaction of the Rab3 effector RIM with Ca^{2+} channels, SNAP-25, and synaptotagmin. *J Biol Chem* 2001; 276: 32756–62.
92. Wiser O, Trus M, Hernandez A, Renstrom E, Barg S, Rorsman P, Atlas D. The voltage sensitive Lc-type Ca^{2+} channel is functionally coupled to the exocytotic machinery. *Proc Natl Acad Sci USA* 1999; 96: 248–53.
93. Schuit FC, Huypens P, Heimberg H, Pipeleers DG. Glucose sensing in pancreatic beta-cells: a model for the study of other glucose-regulated cells in gut, pancreas, and hypothalamus. *Diabetes* 2001; 50: 1–11.
94. Huypens P, Ling Z, Pipeleers D, Schuit F. Glucagon receptors on human islet cells contribute to glucose competence of insulin release. *Diabetologia* 2000; 43: 1012–9.
95. Wollheim CB, Ullrich S, Meda P, Vallar L. Regulation of exocytosis in electrically permeabilized insulin-secreting cells. Evidence for Ca^{2+} dependent and independent secretion. *Biosci Rep* 1987; 7: 443–54.
96. Vallar L, Biden TJ, Wollheim CB. Guanine nucleotides induce Ca^{2+}-independent insulin secretion from permeabilized RINm5F cells. *J Biol Chem* 1987; 262: 5049–56.
97. Jones PM, Fyles JM, Howell SL. Regulation of insulin secretion by cAMP in rat islets of Langerhans permeabilised by high-voltage discharge. *FEBS Lett* 1986; 205: 205–9.
98. Ammala C, Eliasson L, Bokvist K, Berggren PO, Honkanen RE, Sjoholm A, Rorsman P. Activation of protein kinases and inhibition of protein phosphatases play a central role in the regulation of exocytosis in mouse pancreatic beta cells. *Proc Natl Acad Sci USA* 1994; 91: 4343–7.
99. Ozaki N, Shibasaki T, Kashima Y, Miki T, Takahashi K, Ueno H, Sunaga Y, Yano H, Matsuura Y, Iwanaga T, Takai Y, Seino S. cAMP-GEFII is a direct target of cAMP in regulated exocytosis. *Nat Cell Biol* 2000; 2: 805–11.
100. Pralong WF, Bartley C, Wollheim CB. Single islet beta-cell stimulation by nutrients: relationship between pyridine nucleotides, cytosolic Ca^{2+} and secretion. *EMBO J* 1990; 9: 53–60.
101. Patterson GH, Knobel SM, Arkhammar P, Thastrup O, Piston DW. Separation of the glucose-stimulated cytoplasmic and mitochondrial NAD(P)H responses in pancreatic islet beta cells. *Proc Natl Acad Sci USA* 2000; 97: 5203–7.
102. Blackard WG, Nelson NC. Portal vein insulin concentrations in diabetic subjects. *Diabetes* 1971; 20: 286–8.
103. Grodsky GM. A threshold distribution hypothesis for packet storage of insulin and its mathematical modeling. *J Clin Invest* 1972; 51: 2047–59.
104. Hosker JP, Rudenski AS, Burnett MA, Matthews DR, Turner RC. Similar reduction of first- and second-phase B-cell responses at three different glucose levels in type II diabetes and the effect of gliclazide therapy. *Metabolism* 1989; 38: 767–72.
105. Cavaghan MK, Ehrmann DA, Polonsky KS. Interactions between insulin resistance and insulin secretion in the development of glucose intolerance. *J Clin Invest* 2000; 106: 329–33.
106. Porksen N. The in vivo regulation of pulsatile insulin secretion. *Diabetologia* 2002; 45: 3–20.
107. Gilon P, Ravier MA, Jonas JC, Henquin JC. Control mechanisms of the oscillations of insulin secretion in vitro and in vivo. *Diabetes* 2002; 51 (suppl 1): S144–51.
108. Bergsten P. Role of oscillations in membrane potential, cytoplasmic Ca(2+), and metabolism for plasma insulin oscillations. *Diabetes* 2002; 51 (suppl 1): S171–6.
109. Nilsson T, Schultz V, Berggren PO, Corkey BE, Tornheim K. Temporal patterns of changes in ATP/ADP ratio, glucose 6-phosphate and cytoplasmic free Ca^{2+} in glucose-stimulated pancreatic beta-cells. *Biochem J* 1996; 314 (pt 1): 91–4.
110. Wollheim CB, Sharp GW. Regulation of insulin release by calcium. *Physiol Rev* 1981; 61: 914–73.
111. Ravier MA, Gilon P, Henquin JC. Oscillations of insulin secretion can be triggered by imposed oscillations of cytoplasmic Ca^{2+} or metabolism in normal mouse islets. *Diabetes* 1999; 48: 2374–82.
112. Rorsman P, Eliasson L, Renstrom E, Gromada J, Barg S, Gopel S. The cell physiology of biphasic insulin secretion. *News Physiol Sci* 2000; 15: 72–7.
113. Panten U, Schwanstecher M, Wallasch A, Lenzen S. Glucose both inhibits and stimulates insulin secretion from isolated pancreatic islets exposed to maximally effective concentrations of sulfonylureas. *Naunyn Schmiedebergs Arch Pharmacol* 1988; 338: 459–62.
114. Gembal M, Gilon P, Henquin JC. Evidence that glucose can control insulin release independently from its action on ATP-sensitive K^+ channels in mouse B cells. *J Clin Invest* 1992; 89: 1288–95.
115. Sato Y, Aizawa T, Komatsu M, Okada N, Yamada T. Dual functional role of membrane depolarization/Ca^{2+} influx in rat pancreatic B-cell. *Diabetes* 1992; 41: 438–43.
116. Henquin JC. Triggering and amplifying pathways of regulation of insulin secretion by glucose. *Diabetes* 2000; 49: 1751–60.
117. Miki T, Nagashima K, Tashiro F, Kotake K, Yoshitomi H, Tamamoto A, Gonoi T, Iwanaga T, Miyazaki J, Seino S. Defective insulin secretion and enhanced insulin action in KATP channel-deficient mice. *Proc Natl Acad Sci USA* 1998; 95: 10402–6.
118. Seghers V, Nakazaki M, DeMayo F, Aguilar-Bryan L, Bryan J. *Sur1* knockout mice. A model for K(ATP) channel-independent regulation of insulin secretion. *J Biol Chem* 2000; 275: 9270–7.
119. Detimary P, Van den Berghe G, Henquin JC. Concentration dependence and time course of the effects of glucose on adenine and guanine nucleotides in mouse pancreatic islets. *J Biol Chem* 1996; 271: 20559–65.
120. Proks P, Eliasson L, Ammala C, Rorsman P, Ashcroft FM. Ca(2+)- and GTP-dependent exocytosis in mouse pancreatic beta-cells involves both common and distinct steps. *J Physiol* 1996; 496: 255–64.
121. Liang Y, Matschinsky FM. Content of CoA-esters in perifused rat islets stimulated by glucose and other fuels. *Diabetes* 1991; 40: 327–33.
122. Prentki M, Vischer S, Glennon MC, Regazzi R, Deeney JT, Corkey BE. Malonyl-CoA and long chain acyl-CoA esters as metabolic coupling factors in nutrientinduced insulin secretion. *J Biol Chem* 1992; 267: 5802–10.

123. Prentki M, Corkey BE. Are the beta-cell signaling molecules malonyl-CoA and cystolic long-chain acyl-CoA implicated in multiple tissue defects of obesity and NIDDM? *Diabetes* 1996; 45: 273–83.
124. Deeney JT, Gromada J, Hoy M, Olsen HL, Rhodes CJ, Prentki M, Berggren PO, Corkey BE. Acute stimulation with long chain acyl-CoA enhances exocytosis in insulin-secreting cells (HIT T-15 and NMRI beta-cells). *J Biol Chem* 2000; 275: 9363–8.
125. Antinozzi PA, Segall L, Prentki M, McGarry JD, Newgard CB. Molecular or pharmacologic perturbation of the link between glucose and lipid metabolism is without effect on glucose-stimulated insulin secretion. A re-evaluation of the longchain acyl-CoA hypothesis. *J Biol Chem* 1998; 273: 16146–54.
126. Newgard CB. While tinkering with the beta-cell. Metabolic regulatory mechanisms and new therapeutic strategies: American Diabetes Association Lilly Lecture, 2001. *Diabetes* 2002; 51: 3141–50.
127. Maechler P, Wollheim CB. Mitochondrial signals in glucose-stimulated insulin secretion in the beta cell. *J Physiol* 2000; 529: 49–56.
128. Rubi B, Ishihara H, Hegardt FG, Wollheim CB, Maechler P. GAD65-mediated glutamate decarboxylation reduces glucose-stimulated insulin secretion in pancreatic beta cells. *J Biol Chem* 2001; 276: 36391–6.
129. Bertrand G, Ishiyama N, Nenquin M, Ravier MA, Henquin JC. The elevation of glutamate content and the amplification of insulin secretion in glucose-stimulated pancreatic islets are not causally related. *J Biol Chem* 2002; 277: 32883–91.
130. Danielsson A, Hellman B, Idahl LA. Levels of alpha-ketoglutarate and glutamate in stimulated pancreatic β-cells. *Horm Metab Res* 1970; 2: 28–31.
131. MacDonald MJ, Fahien LA. Glutamate is not a messenger in insulin secretion. *J Biol Chem* 2000; 275: 34025–7.
132. Maechler P, Kennedy ED, Pozzan T, Wollheim CB. Mitochondrial act ivation directly triggers the exocytosis of insulin in permeabilized pancreatic beta-cells. *EMBO J* 1997; 16: 3833–41.
133. Hoy M, Maechler P, Efanov AM, Wollheim CB, Berggren PO, Gromada J. Increase in cellular glutamate levels stimulates exocytosis in pancreatic beta-cells. *FEBS Lett* 2002; 531: 199–203.
134. Froguel P, Zouali H, Vionnet N, Velho G, Vaxillaire M, Sun F, Lesage S, Stoffel M, Takeda J, Passa P. Familial hyperglycemia due to mutations in glucokinase. Definition of a subtype of diabetes mellitus. *N Engl J Med* 1993; 328: 697–702.
135. Glaser B, Kesavan P, Heyman M, Davis E, Cuesta A, Buchs A, Stanley CA, Thornton PS, Permutt MA, Matschinsky FM, Herold KC. Familial hyperinsulinism caused by an activating glucokinase mutation. *N Engl J Med* 1998; 338: 226–30.
136. Fajans SS, Bell GI, Polonsky KS. Molecular mechanisms and clinical pathophysiology of maturity-onset diabetes of the young. *N Engl J Med* 2001; 345: 971–80.
137. Ryffel GU. Mutations in the human genes encoding the transcription factors of the hepatocyte nuclear factor (HNF)1 and HNF4 families: functional and pathological consequences. *J Mol Endocrinol* 2001; 27: 11–29.
138. Byrne MM, Sturis J, Menzel S, Yamagata K, Fajans SS, Dronsfield MJ, Bain SC, Hattersley AT, Velho G, Froguel P, Bell GI, Polonsky KS. Altered insulin secretory responses to glucose in diabetic and nondiabetic subjects with mutations in the diabetes susceptibility gene MODY3 on chromosome 12. *Diabetes* 1996; 45: 1503–10.
139. Clocquet AR, Egan JM, Stoffers DA, Muller DC, Wideman L, Chin GA, Clarke WL, Hanks JB, Habener JF, Elahi D. Impaired insulin secretion and increased insulin sensitivity in familial maturity-onset diabetes of the young 4 (insulin promoter factor 1 gene). *Diabetes* 2000; 49: 1856–64.
140. Pontoglio M, Sreenan S, Roe M, Pugh W, Ostrega D, Doyen A, Pick AJ, Baldwin A, Velho G, Froguel P, Levisetti M, Bonner-Weir S, Bell GI, Yaniv M, Polonsky KS. Defective insulin secretion in hepatocyte nuclear factor 1 alpha-deficient mice. *J Clin Invest* 1998; 101: 2215–22.
141. Hagenfeldt-Johansson KA, Herrera PL, Wang H, Gjinovci A, Ishihara H, Wollheim CB. Beta-cell-targeted expression of a dominant-negative hepatocyte nuclear factor-1 alpha induces a maturity-onset diabetes of the young (MODY)3-like phenotype in transgenic mice. *Endocrinology* 2001; 142: 5311–20.
142. Yamagata K, Nammo T, Moriwaki M, Ihara A, Iizuka K, Yang Q, Satoh T, Li M, Uenaka R, Okita K, Iwahashi H, Zhu Q, Cao Y, Imagawa A, Tochino Y, Hanafusa T, Miyagawa J, Matsuzawa Y. Overexpression of dominant-negative mutant hepatocyte nuclear fctor-1 alpha in pancreatic beta-cells causes abnormal islet architecture with decreased expression of E-cadherin, reduced beta-cell proliferation, and diabetes. *Diabetes* 2002; 51: 114–23.
143. Brissova M, Shiota M, Nicholson WE, Gannon M, Knobel SM, Piston DW, Wright CV, Powers AC. Reduction in pancreatic transcription factor PDX-1 impairs glucose-stimulated insulin secretion. *J Biol Chem* 2002; 277: 11225–32.
144. Wang H, Maechler P, Antinozzi PA, Hagenfeldt KA, Wollheim CB. Hepatocyte nuclear factor 4alpha regulates the expression of pancreatic beta-cell genes implicated in glucose metabolism and nutrient-induced insulin secretion. *J Biol Chem* 2000; 275: 35953–9.
145. Wang H, Antinozzi PA, Hagenfeldt KA, Maechler P, Wollheim CB. Molecular targets of a human HNF1 alpha mutation responsible for pancreatic beta-cell dysfunction. *EMBO J* 2000; 19: 4257–64.
146. Chan CB, De Leo D, Joseph JW, McQuaid TS, Ha XF, Xu F, Tsushima RG, Pennefather PS, Salapatek AM, Wheeler MB. Increased uncoupling protein-2 levels in beta-cells are associated with impaired glucose-stimulated insulin secretion: mechanism of action. *Diabetes* 2001; 50: 1302–10.
147. Maassen JA, van Essen E, van den Ouweland JM, Lemkes HH. Molecular and clinical aspects of mitochondrial diabetes mellitus. *Exp Clin Endocrinol Diabetes* 2001; 109: 127–34.
148. Maechler P, Wollheim CB. Mitochondrial function in normal and diabetic beta-cells. *Nature* 2001; 414: 807–12.
149. Silva JP, Kohler M, Graff C, Oldfors A, Magnuson MA, Berggren PO, Larsson NG. Impaired insulin secretion and beta-cell loss in tissue-specific knockout mice with mitochondrial diabetes. *Nat Genet* 2000; 26: 336–40.
150. Soejima A, Inoue K, Takai D, Kaneko M, Ishihara H, Oka Y, Hayashi JI. Mitochondrial DNA is required for regulation of glucose-stimulated insulin secretion in a

mouse pancreatic beta cell line, MIN6. *J Biol Chem* 1996; 271: 26194–9.

151. Kennedy ED, Maechler P, Wollheim CB. Effects of depletion of mitochondrial DNA in metabolism secretion coupling in INS-1 cells. *Diabetes* 1998; 47: 374–80.
152. Tsuruzoe K, Araki E, Furukawa N, Shirotani T, Matsumoto K, Kaneko K, Motoshima H, Yoshizato K, Shirakami A, Kishikawa H, Miyazaki J, Shichiri M. Creation and characterization of a mitochondrial DNA-depleted pancreatic beta-cell line: impaired insulin secretion induced by glucose, leucine, and sulfonylureas. *Diabetes* 1998; 47: 621–31.
153. Aguilar-Bryan L, Bryan J. Molecular biology of adenosine triphosphate-sensitive potassium channels. *Endocr Rev* 1999; 20: 101–35.
154. Schwanstecher C, Meyer U, Schwanstecher M. K(IR)6.2 polymorphism predisposes to type 2 diabetes by inducing overactivity of pancreatic beta-cell ATP-sensitive K(+) channels. *Diabetes* 2002; 51: 875–9.
155. Shiota C, Larsson O, Shelton KD, Shiota M, Efanov AM, Hoy M, Lindner J, Kooptiwut S, Juntti-Berggren L, Gromada J, Berggren PO, Magnuson MA. Sulfonylurea receptor type 1 knock-out mice have intact feeding-stimulated insulin secretion despite marked impairment in their response to glucose. *J Biol Chem* 2002; 277: 37176–83.
156. MacFarlane WM, Chapman JC, Shepherd RM, Hashmi MN, Kamimura N, Cosgrove KE, O'Brien RE, Barnes PD, Hart AW, Docherty HM, Lindley KJ, Aynsley-Green A, James RF, Docherty K, Dunne MJ. Engineering a glucose-responsive human insulin-secreting cell line from islets of Langerhans isolated from a patient with persistent hyperinsulinemic hypoglycemia of infancy. *J Biol Chem* 1999; 274: 34059–66.
157. Stanley CA, Lieu YK, Hsu BY, Burlina AB, Greenberg CR, Hopwood NJ, Perlman K, Rich BH, Zammarchi E, Poncz M. Hyperinsulinism and hyperammonemia in infants with regulatory mutations of the glutamate dehydrogenase gene. *N Engl J Med* 1998; 338: 1352–7.
158. Clayton PT, Eaton S, Aynsley-Green A, Edginton M, Hussain K, Krywawych S, Datta V, Malingre HE, Berger R, van den Berg IE. Hyperinsulinism in short-chain L-3-hydroxyacyl-CoA dehydrogenase deficiency reveals the importance of betaoxidation in insulin secretion. *J Clin Invest* 2001; 108: 457–65.

8

Normal Insulin Secretion in Humans

Kristina M. Utzschneider, Daniel Porte, Jr., and Steven E. Kahn

VA Puget Sound Health Care System and University of Washington, Seattle, WA, USA

INTRODUCTION

Normal insulin secretion is highly regulated by glucose and involves feedback between the liver, peripheral tissues, and the pancreas, with moment-to-moment changes in insulin secretion resulting in relatively stable glucose levels. While a change in the glucose level is the main regulator of insulin secretion, other nutrients, hormones, and neural inputs modulate the insulin response so that efficient glucose absorption and disposal occurs after meals while hypoglycemia is avoided in times of fasting or stress. In addition, another important aspect involves the ability of the islet to adapt over time to changes in insulin sensitivity, thereby ensuring appropriate insulin output in the basal state and in response to stimulation.

Advances in the techniques for measuring human β-cell function have improved our understanding of the importance of the insulin secretion in health and disease. This chapter reviews our current understanding of normal insulin secretion *in vivo*. Understanding the normal mechanisms responsible for maintaining euglycemia will provide the basis for understanding β-cell dysfunction that ultimately leads to hyperglycemia and type 2 diabetes, which are discussed in greater detail in the chapter on type 2 diabetes (see Chapter 25).

REGULATION OF BASAL AND POSTPRANDIAL GLUCOSE LEVELS

In the fasting state most of the glucose is produced by the liver via gluconeogenesis and glycogenolysis, but up to 25% is produced in the kidney via gluconeogenesis [1]. About 80% of glucose utilization in the basal state occurs by insulin-independent mechanisms [2]. Of this, the central nervous system accounts for approximately 80% with about 20% occurring in other tissues such as red blood cells, peripheral nerves, and a small amount in muscle [2, 3]. On the other hand, muscle accounts for most of insulin-dependent glucose uptake both at euglycemia and under conditions of hyperglycemia [2].

In the basal state, a classic feedback loop maintains glucose concentrations at a relatively constant level (Figure 1). Insulin release is regulated by glucose, although other nutrients, hormones, and neural factors play an important role. Insulin and glucagon, which have divergent actions, act in concert to maintain glucose levels while avoiding hyperglycemia and hypoglycemia. Their release is determined in part by the sensitivity of the liver and peripheral tissues to insulin as well as the sensitivity of the islet to glucose, with small changes in the glucose level leading to alterations in insulin and glucagon release to ensure maintenance of the steady state. Thus, with a small increase in glucose, insulin levels increase and glucagon levels decline, resulting in a reduction in glucose production and an increase in glucose utilization. Conversely, with a small decline in glucose, in order to achieve an increase in glucose release and a decrease in glucose uptake, insulin levels fall and glucagon levels rise.

During the anabolic state that typically occurs after a meal, when glucose is in excess and amino acids and fatty acids are being absorbed, insulin levels increase and glucagon levels increase or remain relatively stable depending on the composition of the meal [4]. The greater increase in insulin relative to glucagon results in a change from a state of glucose production to one of glucose storage [5]. Thus, the increase in insulin acts in the liver to inhibit hepatic glucose production while promoting glucose uptake and glycogen formation in the liver and peripheral tissues.

International Textbook of Diabetes Mellitus, Third Edition. Edited by R. A. DeFronzo, E. Ferrannini, H. Keen, and P. Zimmet, 2004.
 ISBN: 0-471-48655-8.

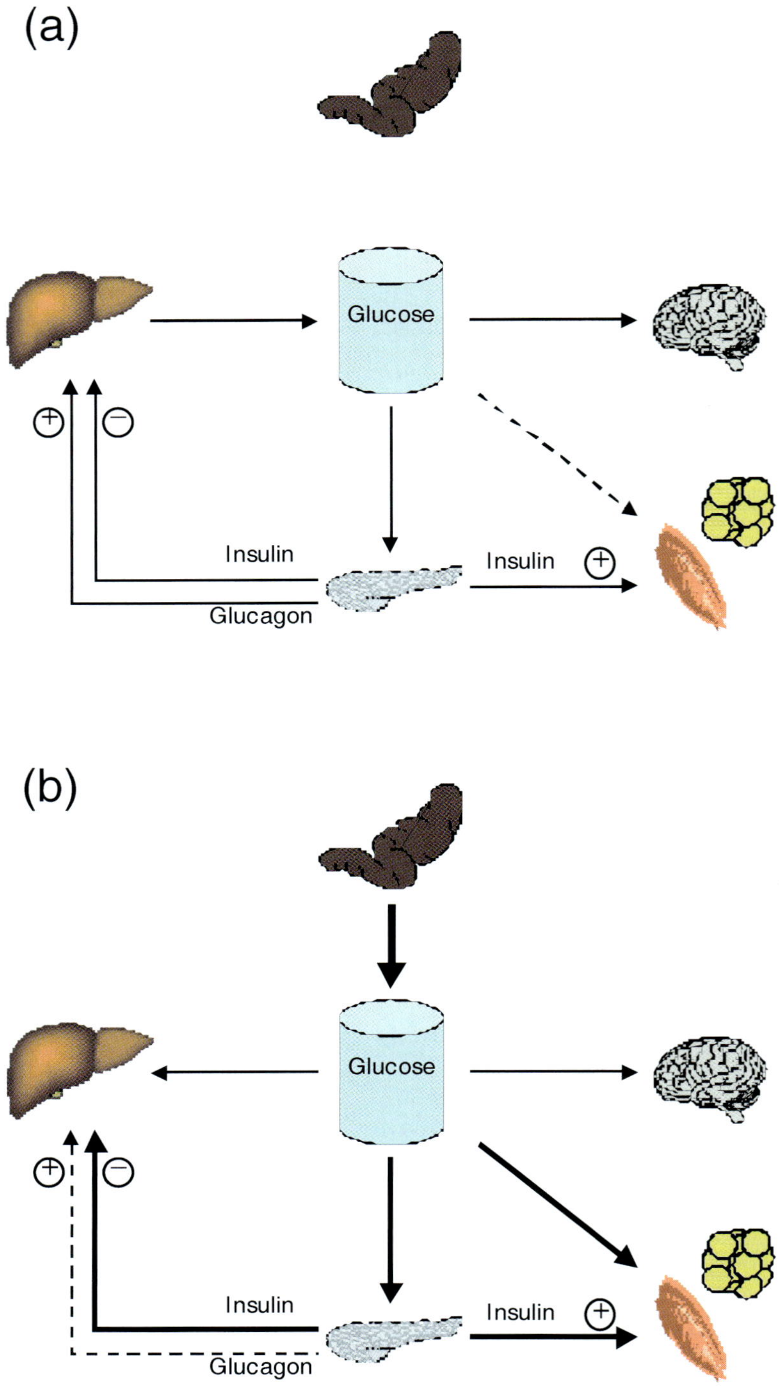

Figure 1 A model for regulation of plasma glucose. Plasma glucose has direct effects on the pancreatic islet to increase insulin release from the β-cell and decrease glucagon release from the α-cell during hyperglycemia and to increase glucagon release and reduce insulin secretion during hypoglycemia. Glucagon acts to stimulate glucose production by the liver while insulin suppresses glucagon production and increases glucose uptake in the insulin-sensitive tissues such as muscle and fat. Glucose uptake in the brain is insulin independent. (a) In the fasting state, glucose production by the liver maintains the plasma glucose in the normal range. Any change in hormone release will be modulated by this feedback loop to ensure fuel availability for the tissues. (b) Following nutrient ingestion, the increase in plasma glucose results in increased insulin secretion and reduced glucagon release from the islet. Thus, the liver changes from a state of glucose production to one of glucose storage. The increase in insulin release also results in increased glucose uptake and storage by the insulin-dependent tissues such as muscle and fat while glucose uptake by the insulin-independent tissues such as the brain remains fairly constant

PHYSIOLOGY OF NORMAL BASAL INSULIN SECRETION

General Considerations

The β-cell converts proinsulin to insulin and C-peptide, resulting in the equimolar release of these two peptides [6] (see also Chapter 6). Of this secreted insulin, not all appears in the peripheral circulation as about 60% of it is removed during its initial passage through the liver [7–9]. Thus, the insulin concentration in the portal vein is two- to threefold greater than in the peripheral circulation [10]. Insulin clearance also occurs in the kidney, with the normal kidney removing about 40% of the insulin that is presented to it [11]. The resultant basal plasma insulin concentrations in normal lean individuals are typically 18–90 pmol/l (3–15 μU/ml). To maintain ongoing basal insulin levels, insulin secretion varies from 0.25 to 1.5 units/h in normal subjects, and accounts for 50% or more of 24-h integrated insulin release [12]. The half-life of insulin in plasma is about 5–8 min [13], which is shorter than that of C-peptide, which is about 35 min [14]. This difference in half-life is due to the fact that the liver does not clear C-peptide [7].

Pulsatile Insulin Secretion

Insulin is secreted in a rapid pulsatile pattern that is intrinsic to the β-cell, occurring at a frequency of 6–10 min [15–17]. *In vitro* studies have shown that these discrete pulses [18] are most likely linked to cyclic glycolysis [19] and apparently not dependent on intact neural input from the brain. Rather, the coordinated pulsatile response of the thousands of β-cells within an islet is thought to occur as the result of an electrophysiological coupling of cells or an intraislet neuronal network [20]. Increases in pulse amplitude have been demonstrated under exposure to high glucose concentrations *in vitro* [21, 22]. An increased pulse amplitude and frequency have also been observed under conditions of increased secretory demand as occurs in insulin resistance states such as obesity in humans [23, 24]. As with a number of other hormones, pulsatile release appears to be critical to ensure an adequate insulin effect. Pulsatile delivery of insulin has been shown to have a greater hypoglycemic effect than continuous delivery, primarily through greater suppression of hepatic glucose production [25, 26].

Ultradian Oscillatory Insulin Secretion

While the rapid pulsatile pattern of insulin release was recognized first, it is now also clear that insulin is secreted in an oscillatory pattern of 11–15 insulin oscillations per 24 h, having a periodicity of every 80–150 min [12]. These ultradian oscillations closely follow oscillations in the glucose level, but they are not associated with changes in either glucagon or cortisol levels [27]. Ultradian β-cell oscillations can be entrained by glucose, so that administration of a variable rate glucose infusion that produces oscillations in the plasma glucose level in healthy adults is associated with the release of insulin in concert with these exogenously induced glucose cycles [28].

GLUCOSE REGULATION OF INSULIN SECRETION

General Considerations

Insulin release following stimulation of the β-cell is a complex event that is modulated by a number of variables. The response of the β-cell to the oral ingestion of calories integrates these variables. Our understanding of parameters that determine insulin release in humans has come in part from studies that have revolved around the intravenous administration of secretagogues. The information gleaned from these studies has provided insight into the regulation of insulin secretion in response to oral intake. The discussion that follows first addresses factors that regulate secretion based on assessments of the β-cell's response to intravenous stimulation and is then followed by a discussion of the integration of the response to oral ingestion.

Glucose Stimulation of Insulin Secretion

Examining the response to an intravenous glucose stimulus is one of the most common methods of assessing the kinetics of insulin secretion. While this does not replicate the physiologic slow absorption of glucose in response to glucose ingestion, it has allowed for closer study of the components of the insulin response. This approach has demonstrated two distinct phases of insulin secretion [29] (Figure 2).

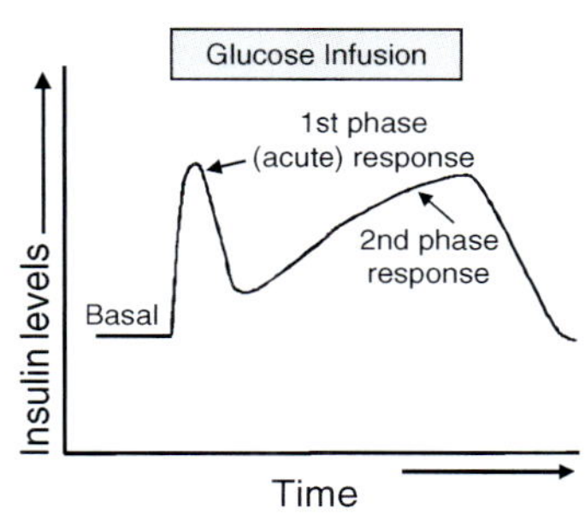

Figure 2 The biphasic insulin response to a constant glucose stimulus. The response to a constant (square-wave) glucose infusion comprises two phases. The first phase in humans develops rapidly, peaking between 3 and 5 min and lasting for 10 min. The second phase begins at the time of commencement of glucose administration but does not become apparent until after 10 min. This phase continues to increase slowly as long as the glucose level remains elevated

The first phase of the response consists of the rapid release of insulin that appears in the portal vein within 60–120 s and in the peripheral circulation within 3–5 min following intravenous glucose administration [30, 31]. This response lasts up to 10 min and represents the rapid release of insulin that has already been synthesized and is stored in secretory granules that reside near the cell membrane [29, 32, 33] (see also Chapter 7). The magnitude of the first phase response is dependent on two important factors. The first is the rate and amount of glucose that is administered, with a 20-g intravenous bolus administered rapidly over 2–3 min providing a maximal stimulus in human subjects [34, 35]. The second factor is the prevailing degree of insulin sensitivity that results in greater responses in healthy insulin-resistant individuals compared to those observed in insulin-sensitive subjects [36, 37].

The second phase response begins immediately after the glucose bolus is administered but is masked during the first 10 min after glucose administration by first phase insulin secretion. From 10 min on it comprises the entire insulin response and continues as long as the glucose level remains elevated. The insulin released during this phase depends primarily on insulin stores, but also comprises the release of newly synthesized insulin [29, 32, 33]. The magnitude of the response is related to the prevailing glucose level at the time the intravenous glucose is administered, increasing linearly to a plasma glucose concentration of 13.9 mmol/l (250 mg/dl) and being maximal at a glucose concentration of above 25.0 mmol/l (450 mg/dl) [38, 39]. The nature of the relationship between the prestimulus glucose level and the second phase response makes it very important that the prestimulus conditions be matched in groups of subjects that are being compared.

Glucose Priming of Insulin Secretion

Elevated concentrations of glucose have the ability to modulate the β-cell's response to a subsequent glucose challenge administered shortly after the glucose level has returned to its basal concentration [40]. This ability of glucose to increase the responsiveness of the β-cell to subsequent stimulation is often referred to as priming. The effect of priming is observed when sequential glucose infusions are administered with a 40–70-min rest interval between them, during which the glucose levels are allowed to return to normal. The insulin response to the second challenge is enhanced with amplification of both the first and second phases [40]. The magnitude and duration of the original glucose stimulus determines the amount of subsequent priming, and the priming effect is decreased by lengthening the time between exposures [41]. *In vitro* studies suggest that this enhancement of β-cell responsiveness to glucose may be mediated by an upregulation of the enzyme glucokinase [42, 43].

Glucose Potentiation of Insulin Secretion

The ability of the prestimulus glucose level to modulate the magnitude of the acute insulin response following administration of a non-glucose secretagogue such as the amino acid arginine [39], the β-adrenergic agent isoproterenol [44], and peptides such as secretin [44] is known as potentiation. Thus, the non-glucose secretagogue stimulated insulin response is proportionate to the steady-state glucose concentration immediately preceding the challenge. The magnitude of the acute insulin response (AIR) is a curvilinear function of the plasma glucose level, but between 3.3 mmol/l (60 mg/dl) and 13.9 mmol/l (250 mg/dl) it is essentially linear [39]. If one determines two or more AIRs to a non-glucose secretagogue at plasma glucose levels between 3.3 and 13.9 mmol/l, one can calculate the slope of the least-squares regression line relating these insulin responses to the glucose level (Figure 3). This measurement has been termed the glucose potentiation slope and is an index of the ability of hyperglycemia to potentiate the AIR to the non-glucose secretagogue. It thus provides a measure of β-cell modulation by glucose. Maximal potentiation of the AIR to the non-glucose secretagogue (AIR_{max}) occurs at a plasma glucose level of 25 mmol/l (450 mg/dl) and above, and is a measure of the maximal responsiveness of the system to glucose [39]. From this value and the slope of potentiation, the glucose level at half-maximal response can be calculated. This measure is termed PG_{50} and is a measure of the β-cell's sensitivity to glucose. These are useful indices, which permit functional characterization of the β-cell.

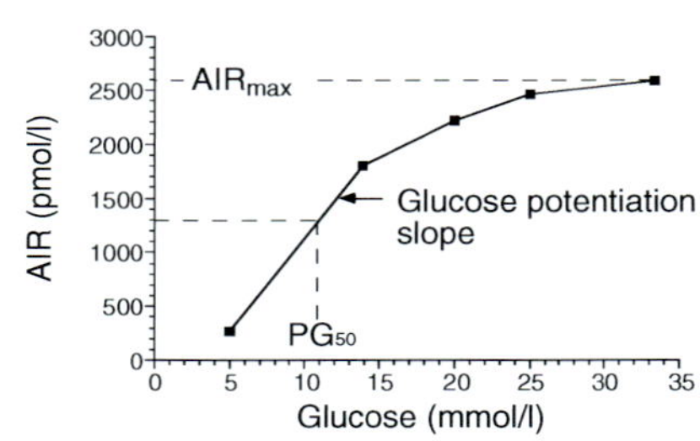

Figure 3 The acute insulin response (AIR) to intravenous arginine at different glucose levels in a normal individual. The magnitude of the AIR is a linear function of the plasma glucose level between 3.3 and 13.9 mmol/l. The least-squares regression line relating these two measures, termed the glucose potentiation slope, is a measure of β-cell modulation by glucose. Maximal potentiation of the AIR by glucose (AIR_{max}) occurs at a glucose level above 25 mmol/l and is a measure of β-cell secretory capacity. The glucose level at half-maximal response can be calculated from AIR_{max} and the glucose potentiation slope and this level, termed the PG_{50}, provides an assessment of β-cell sensitivity to glucose

NON-GLUCOSE REGULATION OF INSULIN SECRETION

General Considerations

A number of non-glucose regulators affect insulin release and include amino acids, fatty acids, hormones, and neural mechanisms. While these factors are critical in determining the β-cell's response, studies examining the effects of these regulators have frequently been performed under conditions that obviate the gastrointestinal tract in order to gain a better understanding of their role.

Amino Acids

Amino acids are important stimulators of insulin secretion. Arginine has been the primary amino acid used in research as it is safely administered to humans and is a powerful β-cell stimulant [45]. The insulin response to arginine occurs rapidly, peaking within 3 min following injection, with the acute response typically lasting for about 10 min. As is the case for the second phase response to glucose, the magnitude of the insulin response is dependent on the glucose level that prevails at the time of arginine injection [39]. Thus, the response increases as the plasma glucose level at which the arginine is administered increases.

Fatty Acids

Free fatty acids (FFAs) acutely stimulate insulin secretion both *in vivo* and *in vitro*, but this effect is moderate [46–48]. In humans, plasma FFA levels have been elevated by intravenous infusion of a lipid emulsion along with heparin under hyperglycemic clamp conditions. Under this experimental scenario, insulin secretion initially increases but later decreases in keeping with a reduction in β-cell function with longer term exposure to FFAs [49, 50]. Under fasting conditions, FFAs appear to be important in maintaining basal insulin secretion, as acute depletion of FFAs results in a significant fall in insulin secretion [51].

Medications

Administration of the β-adrenergic agent isoproterenol [44] and the sulfonylurea drugs such as tolbutamide [52] is also followed by an acute insulin response. Thus, these agents have commonly been employed in studies to evaluate insulin secretion and β-cell function. In addition to these medications, salicylates also increase insulin release and can induce hypoglycemia in people with or without diabetes [53, 54]. Other medications shown to induce hypoglycemia by increasing insulin release include quinine [55], disopyramide [56], and monoamine oxidase inhibitors [57].

A number of agents are capable of impairing insulin release. These include commonly used medications such as glucocorticoids [58, 59], potassium depleting diuretics [60], β-blockers [61], phenytoin [62], centrally acting α-blockers [63], and phenothiazines [64].

Cytotoxic agents such as streptozotocin and alloxan reduce insulin release by virtue of their effect to destroy β-cells [65]. Pentamidine, a biguanide derivative used to treat *Pneumocystis carinii* pneumonia, can cause initial hypoglycemia followed by insulin-dependent diabetes [66, 67]. This loss of β-cells is due to cytotoxic damage, which is initially associated with insulin release [68].

OTHER REGULATORY INFLUENCES ON INSULIN SECRETION

Neural Regulation

The nervous system plays an important role in regulating islet secretory function. The autonomic nervous system innervates and regulates the function of many endocrine organs in the body including the islet, which is innervated by both sympathetic and parasympathetic nerve fibers.

Activation of α-adrenergic receptors inhibits insulin secretion [69] while β-adrenergic receptor activation stimulates insulin release [44]. Normally α-adrenergic activation is the predominant component, resulting in a net inhibition of stimulus-induced insulin secretion when the sympathetic nervous system is activated. During stress the combination of systemic epinephrine release from the adrenal and/or local norepinephrine release from the nerves innervating the pancreas leads to a suppression of insulin responses to glucose, contributing to an increase in plasma glucose.

On the other hand, parasympathetic cholinergic activation mediated by the vagal nerve results in an increase in insulin secretion that is glucose dependent [70]. Activation of the parasympathetic nerves is thought to mediate the cephalic phase of insulin secretion that occurs even before the absorption of glucose or other nutrients [71, 72]. This component of the neural regulation of the islet also appears to play an important role in insulin secretion during the absorptive phase of meal ingestion [73, 74].

A host of neuropeptides are found in pancreatic neurons and appear to have a role in regulating islet function. Their important role has been demonstrated by the infusion of peptides such as vasoactive intestinal peptide, calcitonin gene-related peptide, neuropeptide Y, galanin, substance P, and enkephalins [75]. These studies have provided evidence of the importance of the peptidergic system as a determinant of insulin secretion. Vasoactive intestinal peptide has been shown to have dose-dependent stimulatory effects on the β-cell when administered to healthy human subjects [76], while calcitonin has been demonstrated to suppress insulin in humans, the rapidity of the response suggesting a direct effect [77]. Galanin, a peptide that is present in humans, has been shown to inhibit glucose-stimulated insulin release in animal models, but human studies have not shown any effects on insulin secretion [78–81].

The neural regulation of insulin release by the brain appears to be mediated through hypothalamic control centers. The ventral medial hypothalamus is the sympathetic center, while the lateral hypothalamus is the parasympathetic center; these two centers regulate glucose and fat metabolism in a reciprocal manner [82]. The role of the hypothalamus in these aspects of insulin secretion appears to be only a portion of the critical role played by this brain region, which is also strategically involved in the regulation of satiety and body weight [83]. (The reader is also referred to Chapter 9.)

Hormonal Influences

Many hormones have effects on the β-cell, either by stimulating or inhibiting insulin release or by modulating the insulin response to glucose. A number of gastrointestinal tract derived hormones have important effects on insulin release. Two of these, glucagon-like peptide 1 (GLP-1) and glucose-dependent insulinotropic polypeptide (GIP), also known as gastric inhibitory peptide, enhance the insulin response during a meal. GLP-1 is a potent insulin secretagogue and after just a short period of administration it is capable of enhancing glucose-induced insulin secretion [84]. This effect appears to occur in part by amplification of secretory burst mass and not pulse frequency [85]. Both GLP-1 and GIP as well as gastrin [86, 87], and secretin [44, 87, 88] have stimulatory effects on the β-cell, resulting in a glucose-dependent increase in insulin release. Cholecystokinin has been shown to potentiate the insulin response to arginine or mixed amino acids in humans, but does not change basal insulin release or glucose-stimulated insulin release [89]. (For greater detail, see Chapter 12.)

Intraislet paracrine effects may also occur, although the general consensus is that these are minimal based in large part on the fact that islet blood flow is in the direction of β-cell to α-cell to δ-cell [90]. Infusions of somatostatin and glucagon have clearly demonstrated their ability to modulate insulin release. Somatostatin has broad inhibitory properties that can affect both basal and postprandial release of insulin [91]. It may also affect insulin secretion through changes in other hormones, e.g. by reducing GIP and to a lesser extent gastrin [92] and CCK release [91]. On the other hand, glucagon, secreted by the islet α-cell, is capable of stimulating insulin secretion [93].

The stress hormones play a role in the body's response to a variety of conditions such as hypoglycemia, exercise, illness, trauma, and emotional responses such as anxiety and fear. Catecholamines released by the adrenal as well as those released by sympathetic nerves in the pancreas can serve to modulate insulin release. This effect is in large part due to the effect of epinephrine to suppress glucose-stimulated insulin secretion and inhibit insulin-stimulated glucose utilization [94]. Corticosteroids also inhibit β-cell function in humans but this effect is not always apparent as they also produce insulin resistance [95]. Thus, while absolute insulin release is increased in response to the augmentation in secretory demand, the response is not adequate, given the change in insulin sensitivity. Growth hormone is also known to affect glucose metabolism. Its effects are largely mediated by insulin-like growth factor-1, which has been shown to suppress insulin secretion both *in vivo* [96, 97] and *in vitro* [98] (see Chapter 4).

Insulin Sensitivity

The most common cause of insulin resistance in humans is obesity. The islets in obese individuals are larger and it has long been recognized that obesity is associated with enhanced insulin release [99–101]. The enhancement of insulin release in obesity can be demonstrated in the basal state [102] and following administration of glucose [100, 102] and non-glucose secretagogues [103]. With the application of measures of insulin sensitivity and resistance, it appears that obesity *per se* may not be responsible for the greater insulin responses, but that variations in insulin sensitivity modulate β-cell function, leading to compensatory hyperinsulinemia. The nature of this interaction between tissue insulin sensitivity and β-cell function has been measured in a large cohort of young, apparently healthy subjects, and has been demonstrated to be nonlinear in nature as best described by a hyperbolic function [36] (Figure 4a). The product of the insulin sensitivity index and $AIR_{glucose}$ provides an index of β-cell compensation to insulin sensitivity and has been called the disposition index [37]. This hyperbolic relationship exists regardless of whether β-cell function is assessed in response to glucose or non-glucose stimulation. The variations in insulin release in response to insulin sensitivity reflect changes in β-cell secretory capacity (AIR_{max}) [36] (Figure 4b). This increase in β-cell function that occurs with insulin resistance is an adaptive response and minimizes the development of hyperglycemia in insulin-resistant individuals. If this compensatory response does not occur, hyperglycemia will ensue.

Delineation of this relationship has also allowed for assessments of the ability of the β-cell to adapt to experimental changes in insulin sensitivity. An adaptive increase in insulin secretion can occur relatively quickly. In young healthy human subjects given nicotinic acid to induce insulin resistance, enhanced insulin release was seen after 2 weeks [104]. Although insulin secretion increased within 2 weeks, this compensatory increase was incomplete so that a mild deterioration of glucose tolerance was observed. With alterations in insulin sensitivity that are produced for longer periods of time, such as with

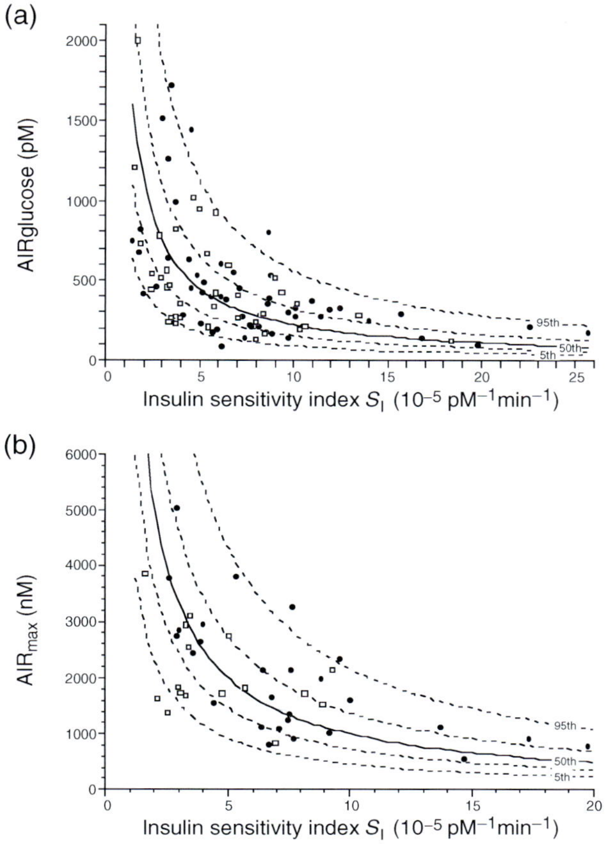

Figure 4 The hyperbolic relationship between insulin sensitivity (S_I) and the first phase (acute) insulin response to glucose ($AIR_{glucose}$; $n = 93$) (a) and the maximal acute insulin response to arginine (AIR_{max}; $n = 43$) (b) in a cohort of healthy individuals. The solid line depicts the best-fit relationship (50th percentile), while the broken lines represent the 5th, 25th, 75th, and 95th percentiles. A reduction in insulin sensitivity, as measured by a decrease in S_I, results in a compensatory reciprocal and proportionate increase in glucose-stimulated insulin secretion and an increase in maximal acute insulin response to arginine, the latter a measure of β-cell secretory capacity. These compensatory changes in β-cell function contribute to maintenance of euglycemia in healthy individuals. (Copyright © 1993 American Diabetes Association. From Diabetes, Vol 42, 1993; 1663–1672. Reprinted with permission from *The American Diabetes Association* [36])

6 months of exercise training in older subjects, insulin sensitivity improves with a concomitant reciprocal and proportionate decrease in insulin secretion, resulting in no net change in overall glucose tolerance assessed both by intravenous and oral glucose tolerance tests [105]. Weight loss also produces an improvement in insulin sensitivity with a corresponding decrease in insulin secretion. However, what distinguishes weight loss from exercise training is that after a 3-month period of weight loss in obese, older individuals, the relationship between insulin sensitivity and insulin release does not change proportionately. Thus, while insulin sensitivity improves with weight loss and insulin release decreases, the change in insulin levels is not proportionate to that of insulin sensitivity so that the net effect is an overall improvement in β-cell function (unpublished observations). This finding of an overall improvement in β-cell function provides a potential explanation for the effect of weight loss to improve glucose tolerance in obese individuals.

The nature of the relationship describing the interaction between insulin sensitivity and insulin levels has important implications for the estimation of β-cell function in humans. Although insulin responses may be identical in two groups of individuals, if insulin sensitivity is not the same, then glucose tolerance also has to differ between the two groups. On the basis of the concept that insulin responses should be assessed relative to insulin sensitivity, subjects at risk for developing diabetes have been shown to have poorer β-cell function than controls [106–109]. This aspect is discussed in further detail in the chapter on type 2 diabetes (see Chapter 25).

The mechanism that regulates this adaptation of the β-cell to changes in insulin sensitivity is not known. A variety of humoral factors have been suggested to be important including glucose, FFAs, and GLP-1. However, none of these have been clearly demonstrated to be critically important, although glucose is able to enhance insulin output when administered for periods of 20–42 h [110, 111]. This adaptation involves a variety of different parameters of β-cell function that are all associated with increased insulin release. It has also been demonstrated to involve the α-cell, resulting in a diminution of glucagon release [111], thus limiting the development of hyperglycemia.

INTEGRATED INSULIN SECRETION DURING NUTRIENT INGESTION

During meals a complex interplay of the aforementioned hormonal and neural elements is triggered to help coordinate the efficient absorption and tissue uptake of nutrients and to minimize the postprandial rise in glucose levels. This interplay results in the conversion from a state of glucose production to one of glucose storage, as the calories absorbed following meal ingestion are stored for subsequent breakdown and utilization.

Insulin secretion following oral ingestion can be evaluated following either a glucose load or a standardized mixed meal. In healthy individuals following oral glucose administration, the glucose level peaks within 30–60 min of ingestion and has largely returned to baseline by 2–3 h [112]. Plasma insulin levels follow a similar pattern although they tend to be a little delayed, peaking at around 60 min and then returning to baseline within about 3 h [112] (Figure 5). The ratio of the 30-min increment in insulin to the 30-min increment in glucose concentration during the oral glucose tolerance test (OGTT) correlates

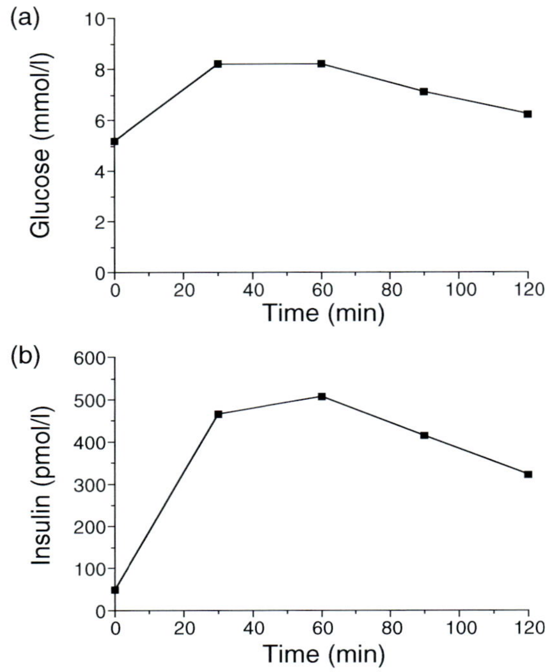

Figure 5 Plasma glucose (a) and insulin (b) levels after an oral glucose tolerance test in healthy individuals. Plasma glucose levels peak at 30 min and subsequently return slowly toward baseline. Plasma insulin levels also increase rapidly, peaking after the glucose peak at 60 min and then declining slowly

well in healthy subjects with the first phase insulin secretion following intravenous glucose administration [113]. However, the insulin response following oral glucose administration is more variable than that following intravenous stimulation for a number of reasons. First, the rate of appearance of oral glucose in the bloodstream is dependent on the rate of gastric emptying and gut motility. Second, the contribution of the neural and incretin components invoked during oral ingestion is variable while it is bypassed by intravenous administration of glucose. Nevertheless, the response to oral glucose has been commonly used and has proven to be valuable, especially in large studies where the variability of the response poses less of a challenge.

Since the β-cell responds to other nutrients besides glucose, insulin secretion can also be assessed using a standardized meal. The necessity to standardize the meal is based on the fact that the magnitude of the insulin response is dependent on which amino acid is present and if it is a mixed carbohydrate/protein meal or a pure protein meal. The greater the carbohydrate content of a meal, the greater the rise in insulin and the smaller the rise in glucagon [114]. A meal lacking carbohydrate will still result in stimulation of insulin release, but a larger rise in glucagon secretion will occur, as protein is a strong stimulus of glucagon release. Thus, glucagon released in response to protein ingestion enhances hepatic glucose production and prevents insulin-induced hypoglycemia [115, 116].

The magnitude of the insulin response to oral nutrient ingestion is greater than that observed when a similar stimulus is administered intravenously. This observation has been termed the incretin effect. The concept of an incretin effect was postulated in the 1960s when it was observed that even with matched plasma glucose concentrations, there was a greater insulin response to oral glucose than there was following intravenous glucose administration [117, 118]. It was suggested that this effect was due to the release of gastrointestinal tract derived hormones that enhanced glucose-stimulated insulin secretion [99, 118]. The major incretins currently recognized are GLP-1 and GIP.

GLP-1 is secreted within minutes of nutrient ingestion [119, 120] from the intestinal L-cells of the ileum and colon [121]. Nutrients such as fat and carbohydrate stimulate endocrine and neural mediators, which then signal the release of GLP-1 from the distal gut [122]. GLP-1 has potent effects on glucose-mediated insulin secretion. Studies in healthy humans given exogenous GLP-1 have demonstrated improved glucose tolerance and increases in the acute insulin response to intravenous glucose [84, 123]. GLP-1 has a short half-life as it is rapidly degraded by the enzyme DDP-IV as well as being cleared by the kidneys [124, 125]. It is this rapid degradation of GLP-1 that tends to limit its ability to enhance insulin release.

The islet effects of GLP-1 are not limited to enhancing exocytosis of secretory granules by the β-cell. The peptide affects the α-cell, resulting in a reduction in glucagon release that also acts to limit the postprandial rise in glucose [126]. Finally, there is currently a great deal of interest in the potential effect of GLP-1 to increase islet regeneration by virtue of its action on transcription factors such as PDX-1 [127, 128]. This growth effect of GLP-1 may play a role in the adaptation of islets under conditions associated with increased β-cell secretory demand such as the insulin resistance occurring with obesity. In addition to its effects on the islet, GLP-1 has extra-pancreatic effects that include the inhibition of gastric motility [129, 130], insulin-independent glucose disposal [131], and improving insulin sensitivity [84, 131–133].

The second incretin, GIP, is released from enteroendocrine K-cells located predominantly in the duodenum and proximal jejunum [134]. GIP reaches peak concentrations 15–30 min after oral ingestion of glucose or lipids [135–137]. Stimulation of insulin secretion by GIP has been shown in humans [138–140], but this effect has only been observed in the presence of elevated glucose concentrations [141]. Thus this peptide enhances insulin release by enhancing glucose-dependent insulin secretion [142, 143]. Like GLP-1, GIP is rapidly degraded by the enzyme dipeptidyl peptidase IV [124, 144, 145], resulting in a short biologic half-life.

Similar to GLP-1, GIP has been shown to stimulate cellular proliferation of β-cells [146]. However, unlike GLP-1, infusion of GIP does not influence glucagon secretion in healthy humans [147, 148]. GIP has also been demonstrated to have extra-pancreatic effects. Animal studies have shown a potential role for GIP in triglyceride uptake in fat [149, 150] but no clear effect on lipid metabolism has been demonstrated in humans [151]. While GLP-1 has been shown to inhibit gastric emptying, GIP appears to have the opposite effect in that it accelerates emptying of the stomach [152] (see Chapter 12).

CONCLUSIONS

Insulin secretion is a highly complex process, and its regulation *in vivo* involves the integrated influences of the ambient glucose level, hormones, neural activation, and other nutrients. Our improved understanding of normal β-cell physiology and function has helped better understand the abnormalities in β-cell function that are critical in the pathogenesis of type 2 diabetes. These are discussed in greater detail in the chapter on type 2 diabetes.

REFERENCES

1. Stumvoll M, Meyer C, Mitrakou A, Nadkarni V, Gerich JE. Renal glucose production and utilization: new aspects in humans. *Diabetologia* 1997; 40: 749–57.
2. Baron AD, Brechtel G, Wallace P, Edelman SV. Rates and tissue sites of non-insulin- and insulin-mediated glucose uptake in humans. *Am J Physiol* 1988; 255: E769–74.
3. Huang SC, Phelps ME, Hoffman EJ, Sideris K, Selin CJ, Kuhl DE. Noninvasive determination of local cerebral metabolic rate of glucose in man. *Am J Physiol* 1980; 238: E69–82.
4. Gutniak M, Grill V, Efendic S. Effect of composition of mixed meals—low-versus high-carbohydrate content—on insulin, glucagon, and somatostatin release in healthy humans and in patients with NIDDM. *Diabetes Care* 1986; 9: 244–9.
5. Taylor R, Magnusson I, Rothman DL, Cline GW, Caumo A, Cobelli C, Shulman GI. Direct assessment of liver glycogen storage by ^{13}C nuclear magnetic resonance spectroscopy and regulation of glucose homeostasis after a mixed meal in normal subjects. *J Clin Invest* 1996; 97: 126–32.
6. Horwitz DL, Starr JI, Mako ME, Blackard WG, Rubenstein AH. Proinsulin, insulin, and C-peptide concentrations in human portal and peripheral blood. *J Clin Invest* 1975; 55: 1278–83.
7. Polonsky K, Jaspan J, Pugh W, Cohen D, Schneider M, Schwartz T, Moossa AR, Tager H, Rubenstein AH. Metabolism of C-peptide in the dog. In vivo demonstration of the absence of hepatic extraction. *J Clin Invest* 1983; 72: 1114–23.
8. Eaton RP, Allen RC, Schade DS. Hepatic removal of insulin in normal man: dose response to endogenous insulin secretion. *J Clin Endocrinol Metab* 1983; 56: 1294–300.
9. Eaton RP, Friedman N, Allen RC, Schade DS. Insulin removal in man: in vivo evidence for a receptor-mediated process. *J Clin Endocrinol Metab* 1984; 58: 555–9.
10. Ferrannini E, Cobelli C. The kinetics of insulin in man, II: role of the liver. *Diabetes Metab Rev* 1987; 3: 365–97.
11. Rabkin R, Simon NM, Steiner S, Colwell JA. Effect of renal disease on renal uptake and excretion of insulin in man. *N Engl J Med* 1970; 282: 182–7.
12. Polonsky KS, Given BD, Van Cauter E. Twenty-four-hour profiles and pulsatile patterns of insulin secretion in normal and obese subjects. *J Clin Invest* 1988; 81: 442–8.
13. Porksen N, Nyholm B, Veldhuis JD, Butler PC, Schmitz O. In humans at least 75% of insulin secretion arises from punctuated insulin secretory bursts. *Am J Physiol* 1997; 273: E908–14.
14. Van Cauter E, Mestrez F, Sturis J, Polonsky KS. Estimation of insulin secretion rates from C-peptide levels. Comparison of individual and standard kinetic parameters for C-peptide clearance. *Diabetes* 1992; 41: 368–77.
15. Stagner JI, Samols E, Weir GC. Sustained oscillations of insulin, glucagon, and somatostatin from the isolated canine pancreas during exposure to a constant glucose concentration. *J Clin Invest* 1980; 65: 939–42.
16. Matthews DR, Hermansen K, Connolly AA, Gray D, Schmitz O, Clark A, Orskov H, Turner RC. Greater *in vivo* than *in vitro* pulsatility of insulin secretion with synchronized insulin and somatostatin secretory pulses. *Endocrinology* 1987; 120: 2272–8.
17. Goodner CJ, Walike BC, Koerker DJ, Ensinck JW, Brown AC, Chideckel EW, Palmer J, Kalnasy L. Insulin, glucagon, and glucose exhibit synchronous, sustained oscillations in fasting monkeys. *Science* 1977; 195: 177–9.
18. Hellman B, Gylfe E, Bergsten P, Grapengiesser E, Lund PE, Berts A, Tengholm A, Pipeleers DG, Ling Z. Glucose induces oscillatory Ca^{2+} signalling and insulin release in human pancreatic beta cells. *Diabetologia* 1994; 37 (suppl 2): S11–20.
19. Chou HF, Berman N, Ipp E. Oscillations of lactate released from islets of Langerhans: evidence for oscillatory glycolysis in beta-cells. *Am J Physiol* 1992; 262: E800–5.
20. Bergstrom RW, Fujimoto WY, Teller DC, de Haen C. Oscillatory insulin secretion in perifused isolated rat islets. *Am J Physiol* 1989; 257: E479–85.
21. Cunningham BA, Deeney JT, Bliss CR, Corkey BE, Tornheim K. Glucose-induced oscillatory insulin secretion in perifused rat pancreatic islets and clonal beta-cells (HIT). *Am J Physiol* 1996; 271: E702–10.
22. Bergsten P, Hellman B. Glucose-induced amplitude regulation of pulsatile insulin secretion from individual pancreatic islets. *Diabetes* 1993; 42: 670–4.
23. Radetti G, Ghizzoni L, Paganini C, Iughetti L, Caselli G, Bernasconi S. Insulin pulsatility in obese and normal prepubertal children. *Horm Res* 1998; 50: 78–82.
24. Zarkovic M, Ciric J, Stojanovic M, Penezic Z, Trbojevic B, Dresgic M, Nesovic M. Effect of insulin sensitivity on pulsatile insulin secretion. *Eur J Endocrinol* 1999; 141: 494–501.
25. Bratusch-Marrain PR, Komjati M, Waldhausl WK. Efficacy of pulsatile versus continuous insulin administration on hepatic glucose production and glucose utilization in type I diabetic humans. *Diabetes* 1986; 35: 922–6.
26. Paolisso G, Scheen AJ, Giugliano D, Sgambato S, Albert A, Varricchio M, D'Onofrio F. Lefebvre PJ. Pulsatile insulin delivery has greater metabolic effects than continuous hormone administration in man: importance of pulse frequency. *J Clin Endocrinol Metab* 1991; 72: 607–15.
27. Shapiro ET, Tillil H, Polonsky KS, Fang VS, Rubenstein AH, Van Cauter E. Oscillations in insulin secretion

during constant glucose infusion in normal man: relationship to changes in plasma glucose. *J Clin Endocrinol Metab* 1988; 67: 307–14.
28. O'Meara NM, Sturis J, Van Cauter E, Polonsky KS. Lack of control by glucose of ultradian insulin secretory oscillations in impaired glucose tolerance and in non-insulin-dependent diabetes mellitus. *J Clin Invest* 1993; 92: 262–71.
29. Porte D Jr, Pupo AA. Insulin responses to glucose: evidence for a two pool system in man. *J Clin Invest* 1969; 48: 2309–19.
30. Blackard WG, Nelson NC. Portal and peripheral vein immunoreactive insulin concentrations before and after glucose infusion. *Diabetes* 1970; 19: 302–6.
31. Cerasi E, Hallberg D, Luft R. Simultaneous determination of insulin in brachial and portal veins during glucose infusion in normal and prediabetic subjects. *Horm Metab Res* 1970; 2: 302–3.
32. Grodsky GM. A threshold distribution hypothesis for packet storage of insulin and its mathematical modeling. *J Clin Invest* 1972; 51: 2047–59.
33. Daniel S, Noda M, Straub SG, Sharp GW. Identification of the docked granule pool responsible for the first phase of glucose-stimulated insulin secretion. *Diabetes* 1999; 48: 1686–90.
34. Chen M, Porte D Jr. The effect of rate and dose of glucose infusion on the acute insulin response in man. *J Clin Endocrinol Metab* 1976; 42: 1168–75.
35. Lerner RL, Porte D Jr. Relationship between intravenous glucose loads, insulin responses and glucose disappearance rate. *J Clin Endocrinol Metab* 1971; 33: 409–17.
36. Kahn SE, Prigeon RL, McCulloch DK, Boyko EJ, Bergman RN, Schwartz MW, Neifing JL, Ward WK, Beard JC, Palmer JP, et al. Quantification of the relationship between insulin sensitivity and beta-cell function in human subjects. Evidence for a hyperbolic function. *Diabetes* 1993; 42: 1663–72.
37. Bergman RN, Phillips LS, Cobelli C. Physiologic evaluation of factors controlling glucose tolerance in man: measurement of insulin sensitivity and beta-cell glucose sensitivity from the response to intravenous glucose. *J Clin Invest* 1981; 68: 1456–67.
38. Halter JB, Graf RJ, Porte D Jr. Potentiation of insulin secretory responses by plasma glucose levels in man: evidence that hyperglycemia in diabetes compensates for impaired glucose potentiation. *J Clin Endocrinol Metab* 1979; 48: 946–54.
39. Ward WK, Bolgiano DC, McKnight B, Halter JB, Porte D Jr. Diminished B cell secretory capacity in patients with noninsulin-dependent diabetes mellitus. *J Clin Invest* 1984; 74: 1318–28.
40. Cerasi E. Potentiation of insulin release by glucose in man, I: quantitative analysis of the enhancement of glucose-induced insulin secretion by pretreatment with glucose in normal subjects. *Acta Endocrinol (Copenh)* 1975; 79: 483–501.
41. Grill V. Time and dose dependencies for priming effect of glucose on insulin secretion. *Am J Physiol* 1981; 240: E24–31.
42. Liang Y, Najafi H, Smith RM, Zimmerman EC, Magnuson MA, Tal M, Matschinsky FM. Concordant glucose induction of glucokinase, glucose usage, and glucose-stimulated insulin release in pancreatic islets maintained in organ culture. *Diabetes* 1992; 41: 792–806.
43. Matschinsky FM. Glucokinase as glucose sensor and metabolic signal generator in pancreatic beta-cells and hepatocytes. *Diabetes* 1990; 39: 647–52.
44. Halter JB, Porte D Jr. Mechanisms of impaired acute insulin release in adult onset diabetes: studies with isoproterenol and secretin. *J Clin Endocrinol Metab* 1978; 46: 952–60.
45. Floyd JC Jr, Fajans SS, Conn JW, Knopf RF, Rull J. Stimulation of insulin secretion by amino acids. *J Clin Invest* 1966; 45: 1487–502.
46. Crespin SR, Greenough WB III, Steinberg D. Stimulation of insulin secretion by long-chain free fatty acids. A direct pancreatic effect. *J Clin Invest* 1973; 52: 1979–84.
47. Pelkonen R, Miettinen TA, Taskinen MR, Nikkila EA. Effect of acute elevation of plasma glycerol, triglyceride and FFA levels on glucose utilization and plasma insulin. *Diabetes* 1968; 17: 76–82.
48. Malaisse WJ, Malaisse-Lagae F. Stimulation of insulin secretion by noncarbohydrate metabolites. *J Lab Clin Med* 1968; 72: 438–48.
49. Paolisso G, Gambardella A, Amato L, Tortoriello R, D'Amore A, Varricchio M, D'Onofrio F. Opposite effects of short- and long-term fatty acid infusion on insulin secretion in healthy subjects. *Diabetologia* 1995; 38: 1295–9.
50. Carpentier A, Mittelman SD, Lamarche B, Bergman RN, Giacca A, Lewis GF. Acute enhancement of insulin secretion by FFA in humans is lost with prolonged FFA elevation. *Am J Physiol* 1999; 276: E1055–66.
51. Dobbins RL, Chester MW, Daniels MB, McGarry JD, Stein DT. Circulating fatty acids are essential for efficient glucose-stimulated insulin secretion after prolonged fasting in humans. *Diabetes* 1998; 47: 1613–8.
52. Varsano-Aharon N, Echemendia E, Yalow RS, Berson SA. Early insulin responses to glucose and to tolbutamide in maturity-onset diabetes. *Metabolism* 1970; 19: 409–17.
53. Gilgore S. The influence of salicylate on hyperglycemia. *Diabetes* 1960; 9: 392–3.
54. Hecht A, Goldner M. Reappraisal of the hypoglycemic action of acetylsalicylate. *Metabolism* 1959; 8: 418–28.
55. White NJ, Warrell DA, Chanthavanich P, Looareesuwan S, Warrell MJ, Krishna S, Williamson DH, Turner RC. Severe hypoglycemia and hyperinsulinemia in falciparum malaria. *N Engl J Med* 1983; 309: 61–6.
56. Croxson MS, Shaw DW, Henley PG, Gabriel HD. Disopyramide-induced hypoglycaemia and increased serum insulin. *N Z Med J* 1987; 100: 407–8.
57. Cooper AJ, Ashcroft G. Potentiation of insulin hypoglycaemia by M.A.O.I. antidepressant drugs. *Lancet* 1966; 1: 407–9.
58. Kalhan SC, Adam PA. Inhibitory effect of prednisone on insulin secretion in man: model for duplication of blood glucose concentration. *J Clin Endocrinol Metab* 1975; 41: 600–10.
59. Barseghian G, Levine R. Effect of corticosterone on insulin and glucagon secretion by the isolated perfused rat pancreas. *Endocrinology* 1980; 106: 547–52.
60. Helderman JH, Elahi D, Andersen DK, Raizes GS, Tobin JD, Shocken D, Andres R. Prevention of the glucose intolerance of thiazide diuretics by maintenance of body potassium. *Diabetes* 1983; 32: 106–11.
61. Cerasi E, Luft R, Efendic S. Effect of adrenergic blocking agents on insulin response to glucose infusion in man. *Acta Endocrinol (Copenh)* 1972; 69: 335–46.

62. Cudworth AG, Cunningham JL. The effect of diphenylhydantoin on insulin response. *Clin Sci Mol Med* 1974; 46: 131–6.
63. Metz SA, Halter JB, Robertson RP. Induction of defective insulin secretion and impaired glucose tolerance by clonidine. Selective stimulation of metabolic alpha-adrenergic pathways. *Diabetes* 1978; 27: 554–62.
64. Erle G, Basso M, Federspil G, Sicolo N, Scandellari C. Effect of chlorpromazine on blood glucose and plasma insulin in man. *Eur J Clin Pharmacol* 1977; 11: 15–8.
65. Rerup CC. Drugs producing diabetes through damage of the insulin secreting cells. *Pharmacol Rev* 1970; 22: 485–518.
66. Bouchard P, Sai P, Reach G, Caubarrere I, Ganeval D, Assan R. Diabetes mellitus following pentamidine-induced hypoglycemia in humans. *Diabetes* 1982; 31: 40–5.
67. Shen M, Orwoll ES, Conte JE Jr, Prince MJ. Pentamidine-induced pancreatic beta-cell dysfunction. *Am J Med* 1989; 86: 726–8.
68. Sai P, Boillot D, Boitard C, Debray-Sachs M, Reach G, Assan R. Pentamidine, a new diabetogenic drug in laboratory rodents. *Diabetologia* 1983; 25: 418–23.
69. Robertson RP, Halter JB, Porte D Jr. A role for alpha-adrenergic receptors in abnormal insulin secretion in diabetes mellitus. *J Clin Invest* 1976; 57: 791–5.
70. Bergman RN, Miller RE. Direct enhancement of insulin secretion by vagal stimulation of the isolated pancreas. *Am J Physiol* 1973; 225: 481–6.
71. Ahren B. Autonomic regulation of islet hormone secretion—implications for health and disease. *Diabetologia* 2000; 43: 393–410.
72. Teff KL, Engelman K. Oral sensory stimulation improves glucose tolerance in humans: effects on insulin, C-peptide, and glucagon. *Am J Physiol* 1996; 270: R1371–9.
73. D'Alessio DA, Kieffer TJ, Taborsky GJ Jr, Havel PJ. Activation of the parasympathetic nervous system is necessary for normal meal-induced insulin secretion in rhesus macaques. *J Clin Endocrinol Metab* 2001; 86: 1253–9.
74. Benthem L, Mundinger TO, Taborsky GJ Jr. Meal-induced insulin secretion in dogs is mediated by both branches of the autonomic nervous system. *Am J Physiol Endocrinol Metab* 2000; 278: E603–10.
75. Ahren B, Taborsky GJ Jr, Porte D Jr. Neuropeptidergic versus cholinergic and adrenergic regulation of islet hormone secretion. *Diabetologia* 1986; 29: 827–36.
76. Fahrenkrug J, Pedersen JH, Yamashita Y, Ottesen B, Hokfelt T, Lundberg JM. Occurrence of VIP and peptide HM in human pancreas and their influence on pancreatic endocrine secretion in man. *Regul Pept* 1987; 18: 51–61.
77. Stevenson JC, Adrian TE, Christofides ND, Bloom SR. Effect of calcitonin on gastrointestinal regulatory peptides in man. *Clin Endocrinol (Oxf)* 1985; 22: 655–60.
78. Dunning BE, Ahren B, Veith RC, Bottcher G, Sundler F, Taborsky GJ Jr. Galanin: a novel pancreatic neuropeptide. *Am J Physiol* 1986; 251: E127–33.
79. Holst JJ, Bersani M, Hvidberg A, Knigge U, Christiansen E, Madsbad S, Harling H, Kofod H. On the effects of human galanin in man. *Diabetologia* 1993; 36: 653–7.
80. Carey DG, Iismaa TP, Ho KY, Rajkovic IA, Kelly J, Kraegen EW, Ferguson J, Inglis AS, Shine J, Chisholm DJ. Potent effects of human galanin in man: growth hormone secretion and vagal blockade. *J Clin Endocrinol Metab* 1993; 77: 90–3.
81. Gilbey SG, Stephenson J, O'Halloran DJ, Burrin JM, Bloom SR. High-dose porcine galanin infusion and effect on intravenous glucose tolerance in humans. *Diabetes* 1989; 38: 1114–6.
82. Shimazu T. Innervation of the liver and glucoregulation: roles of the hypothalamus and autonomic nerves. *Nutrition* 1996; 12: 65–6.
83. Schwartz MW, Woods SC, Porte D Jr, Seeley RJ, Baskin DG. Central nervous system control of food intake. *Nature* 2000; 404: 661–71.
84. D'Alessio DA, Kahn SE, Leusner CR, Ensinck JW. Glucagon-like peptide 1 enhances glucose tolerance both by stimulation of insulin release and by increasing insulin-independent glucose disposal. *J Clin Invest* 1994; 93: 2263–6.
85. Porksen N, Grofte B, Nyholm B, Holst JJ, Pincus SM, Veldhuis JD, Schmitz O, Butler PC. Glucagon-like peptide 1 increases mass but not frequency or orderliness of pulsatile insulin secretion. *Diabetes* 1998; 47: 45–9.
86. Rehfeld JF, Stadil F. The effect of gastrin on basal- and glucose-stimulated insulin secretion in man. *J Clin Invest* 1973; 52: 1415–26.
87. Dupre J, Curtis JD, Unger RH, Waddell RW, Beck JC. Effects of secretin, pancreozymin, or gastrin on the response of the endocrine pancreas to administration of glucose or arginine in man. *J Clin Invest* 1969; 48: 745–57.
88. Lerner RL, Porte D Jr. Studies of secretin-stimulated insulin responses in man. *J Clin Invest* 1972; 51: 2205–10.
89. Rushakoff RJ, Goldfine ID, Carter JD, Liddle RA. Physiological concentrations of cholecystokinin stimulate amino acid-induced insulin release in humans. *J Clin Endocrinol Metab* 1987; 65: 395–401.
90. Stagner JI, Samols E, Bonner-Weir S. Beta–alpha–delta pancreatic islet cellular perfusion in dogs. *Diabetes* 1988; 37: 1715–21.
91. Emoto T, Miyata M, Izukura M, Yumiba T, Mizutani S, Sakamoto T, Matsuda H. Simultaneous observation of endocrine and exocrine functions of the pancreas responding to somatostatin in man. *Regul Pept* 1997; 68: 1–8.
92. Creutzfeldt W, Lembcke B, Folsch UR, Schleser S, Koop I. Effect of somatostatin analogue (SMS 201-995, Sandostatin) on pancreatic secretion in humans. *Am J Med* 1987; 82: 49–54.
93. Samols E MG, Marks V. Promotion of insulin secretion by glucagon. *Lancet* 1965; 2: 415–6.
94. Havel PJ, Taborsky GJ Jr. Stress-induced activation of the neuroendocrine system and its effects on carbohydrate metabolism. In Porte D Jr, Sherwin RS, Baron AD (eds) *Ellenberg and Rifkin's Diabetes Mellitus*. New York: McGraw-Hill, 2003; pp 127–49.
95. Beard JC, Halter JB, Best JD, Pfeifer MA, Porte D Jr. Dexamethasone-induced insulin resistance enhances B cell responsiveness to glucose level in normal men. *Am J Physiol* 1984; 247: E592–6.
96. Rennert NJ, Caprio S, Sherwin RS. Insulin-like growth factor I inhibits glucose-stimulated insulin secretion but does not impair glucose metabolism in normal humans. *J Clin Endocrinol Metab* 1993; 76: 804–6.
97. Zenobi PD, Graf S, Ursprung H, Froesch ER. Effects of insulin-like growth factor-I on glucose tolerance, insulin levels, and insulin secretion. *J Clin Invest* 1992; 89: 1908–13.
98. Leahy JL, Vandekerkhove KM. Insulin-like growth factor-I at physiological concentrations is a potent

inhibitor of insulin secretion. *Endocrinology* 1990; 126: 1593–8.
99. Perley MJ, Kipnis DM. Plasma insulin responses to oral and intravenous glucose: studies in normal and diabetic sujbjects. *J Clin Invest* 1967; 46: 1954–62.
100. Karam JH GG, Forsham PH. Excessive insulin response to glucose in obese subjects as measured by immunochemical assay. *Diabetes* 1963; 12: 197–204.
101. Bagdade JD, Bierman EL, Porte D Jr. The significance of basal insulin levels in the evaluation of the insulin response to glucose in diabetic and nondiabetic subjects. *J Clin Invest* 1967; 46: 1549–57.
102. Bagdade JD, Porte D Jr, Brunzell JD, Bierman EL. Basal and stimulated hyperinsulinism: reversible metabolic sequelae of obesity. *J Lab Clin Med* 1974; 83: 563–9.
103. Beard JC, Ward WK, Halter JB, Wallum BJ, Porte D Jr. Relationship of islet function to insulin action in human obesity. *J Clin Endocrinol Metab* 1987; 65: 59–64.
104. Kahn SE, Beard JC, Schwartz MW, Ward WK, Ding HL, Bergman RN, Taborsky GJ Jr, Porte D Jr. Increased beta-cell secretory capacity as mechanism for islet adaptation to nicotinic acid-induced insulin resistance. *Diabetes* 1989; 38: 562–8.
105. Kahn SE, Larson VG, Beard JC, Cain KC, Fellingham GW, Schwartz RS, Veith RC, Stratton JR, Cerqueira MD, Abrass IB. Effect of exercise on insulin action, glucose tolerance, and insulin secretion in aging. *Am J Physiol* 1990; 258: E937–43.
106. Ehrmann DA, Sturis J, Byrne MM, Karrison T, Rosenfield RL, Polonsky KS. Insulin secretory defects in polycystic ovary syndrome. Relationship to insulin sensitivity and family history of non-insulin-dependent diabetes mellitus. *J Clin Invest* 1995; 96: 520–7.
107. Ryan EA, Imes S, Liu D, McManus R, Finegood DT, Polonsky KS, Sturis J. Defects in insulin secretion and action in women with a history of gestational diabetes. *Diabetes* 1995; 44: 506–12.
108. Ward WK, Johnston CL, Beard JC, Benedetti TJ, Halter JB, Porte D Jr. Insulin resistance and impaired insulin secretion in subjects with histories of gestational diabetes mellitus. *Diabetes* 1985; 34: 861–9.
109. Johnston C, Ward WK, Beard JC, McKnight B, Porte D Jr. Islet function and insulin sensitivity in the non-diabetic offspring of conjugal type 2 diabetic patients. *Diabet Med* 1990; 7: 119–25.
110. Byrne MM, Sturis J, Polonsky KS. Insulin secretion and clearance during low-dose graded glucose infusion. *Am J Physiol* 1995; 268: E21–7.
111. Ward WK, Halter JB, Beard JC, Porte D Jr. Adaptation of B and A cell function during prolonged glucose infusion in human subjects. *Am J Physiol* 1984; 246: E405–11.
112. Ganda OP, Day JL, Soeldner JS, Connon JJ, Gleason RE. Reproducibility and comparative analysis of repeated intravenous and oral glucose tolerance tests. *Diabetes* 1978; 27: 715–25.
113. Phillips DI, Clark PM, Hales CN, Osmond C. Understanding oral glucose tolerance: comparison of glucose or insulin measurements during the oral glucose tolerance test with specific measurements of insulin resistance and insulin secretion. *Diabet Med* 1994; 11: 286–92.
114. Shulman GI, Liljenquist JE, Williams PE, Lacy WW. Glucose disposal during insulinopenia in somatostatin-treated dogs. The roles of glucose and glucagon. *J Clin Invest* 1978; 62: 487–91.
115. Unger RH, Ohneda A, Aguilar-Parada E, Eisentraut AM. The role of aminogenic glucagon secretion in blood glucose homeostasis. *J Clin Invest* 1969; 48: 810–22.
116. Felig P, Wahren J, Hendler R. Influence of physiologic hyperglucagonemia on basal and insulin-inhibited splanchnic glucose output in normal man. *J Clin Invest* 1976; 58: 761–5.
117. Creutzfeldt W. The incretin concept today. *Diabetologia* 1979; 16: 75–85.
118. Elrick H, Stimmler L, Hlad CJ Jr, Plasma insulin response to oral and intravenous glucose administration. *J Clin Endocrin* 1964; 24: 1076–82.
119. Orskov C, Holst JJ, Knuhtsen S, Baldissera FG, Poulsen SS, Nielsen OV. Glucagon-like peptides GLP-1 and GLP-2, predicted products of the glucagon gene, are secreted separately from pig small intestine but not pancreas. *Endocrinology* 1986; 119: 1467–75.
120. Roberge JN, Brubaker PL. Secretion of proglucagon-derived peptides in response to intestinal luminal nutrients. *Endocrinology* 1991; 128: 3169–74.
121. Eissele R, Goke R, Willemer S, Harthus HP, Vermeer H, Arnold R, Goke B. Glucagon-like peptide-1 cells in the gastrointestinal tract and pancreas of rat, pig and man. *Eur J Clin Invest* 1992; 22: 283–91.
122. Roberge JN, Brubaker PL. Regulation of intestinal proglucagon-derived peptide secretion by glucose-dependent insulinotropic peptide in a novel enteroendocrine loop. *Endocrinology* 1993; 133: 233–40.
123. Ritzel R, Orskov C, Holst JJ, Nauck MA. Pharmacokinetic, insulinotropic, and glucagonostatic properties of GLP-1 [7-36 amide] after subcutaneous injection in healthy volunteers. Dose–response-relationships. *Diabetologia* 1995; 38: 720–5.
124. Kieffer TJ, McIntosh CH, Pederson RA. Degradation of glucose-dependent insulinotropic polypeptide and truncated glucagon-like peptide 1 *in vitro* and *in vivo* by dipeptidyl peptidase IV. *Endocrinology* 1995; 136: 3585–96.
125. Deacon CF, Johnsen AH, Holst JJ. Degradation of glucagon-like peptide-1 by human plasma *in vitro* yields an N-terminally truncated peptide that is a major endogenous metabolite *in vivo*. *J Clin Endocrinol Metab* 1995; 80: 952–7.
126. Komatsu R, Matsuyama T, Namba M, Watanabe N, Ioth H, Kono N, Tarui S. Glucagonostatic and insulinotropic action of glucagonlike peptide I-(7-36)-amide. *Diabetes* 1989; 38: 902–5.
127. Perfetti R, Zhou J, Doyle ME, Egan JM. Glucagon-like peptide-1 induces cell proliferation and pancreatic-duodenum homeobox-1 expression and increases endocrine cell mass in the pancreas of old, glucose-intolerant rats. *Endocrinology* 2000; 141: 4600–5.
128. Doyle ME, Egan JM. Glucagon-like peptide-1. *Recent Prog Horm Res* 2001; 56: 377–99.
129. Wettergren A, Schjoldager B, Mortensen PE, Myhre J, Christiansen J, Holst JJ. Truncated GLP-1 (proglucagon 78-107-amide) inhibits gastric and pancreatic functions in man. *Dig Dis Sci* 1993; 38: 665–73.
130. Nauck MA, Niedereichholz U, Ettler R, Holst JJ, Orskov C, Ritzel R, Schmiegel WH. Glucagon-like peptide 1 inhibition of gastric emptying outweighs its insulinotropic effects in healthy humans. *Am J Physiol* 1997; 273: E981–8.
131. D'Alessio DA, Prigeon RL, Ensinck JW. Enteral enhancement of glucose disposition by both insulin-dependent and insulin-independent processes. A

physiological role of glucagon-like peptide I. *Diabetes* 1995; 44: 1433–7.
132. Gutniak M, Orskov C, Holst JJ, Ahren B, Efendic S. Antidiabetogenic effect of glucagon-like peptide-1 (7-36)amide in normal subjects and patients with diabetes mellitus. *N Engl J Med* 1992; 326: 1316–22.
133. Villanueva-Penacarrillo ML, Alcantara AI, Clemente F, Delgado E, Valverde I. Potent glycogenic effect of GLP-1(7-36)amide in rat skeletal muscle. *Diabetologia* 1994; 37: 1163–6.
134. Buffa R, Polak JM, Pearse AG, Solcia E, Grimelius L, Capella C. Identification of the intestinal cell storing gastric inhibitory peptide. *Histochemistry* 1975; 43: 249–55.
135. Ross SA, Dupre J. Effects of ingestion of triglyceride or galactose on secretion of gastric inhibitory polypeptide and on responses to intravenous glucose in normal and diabetic subjects. *Diabetes* 1978; 27: 327–33.
136. Cataland S, Crockett SE, Brown JC, Mazzaferri EL. Gastric inhibitory polypeptide (GIP) stimulation by oral glucose in man. *J Clin Endocrinol Metab* 1974; 39: 223–8.
137. Falko JM, Crockett SE, Cataland S, Mazzaferri EL. Gastric inhibitory polypeptide (GIP) stimulated by fat ingestion in man. *J Clin Endocrinol Metab* 1975; 41: 260–5.
138. Dupre J, Ross SA, Watson D, Brown JC. Stimulation of insulin secretion by gastric inhibitory polypeptide in man. *J Clin Endocrinol Metab* 1973; 37: 826–8.
139. Andersen DK, Elahi D, Brown JC, Tobin JD, Andres R. Oral glucose augmentation of insulin secretion. Interactions of gastric inhibitory polypeptide with ambient glucose and insulin levels. *J Clin Invest* 1978; 62: 152–61.
140. Elahi D, Andersen DK, Brown JC, Debas HT, Hershcopf RJ, Raizes GS, Tobin JD, Andres R. Pancreatic alpha- and beta-cell responses to GIP infusion in normal man. *Am J Physiol* 1979; 237: E185–91.
141. Nauck MA, Homberger E, Siegel EG, Allen RC, Eaton RP, Ebert R, Creutzfeldt W. Incretin effects of increasing glucose loads in man calculated from venous insulin and C-peptide responses. *J Clin Endocrinol Metab* 1986; 63: 492–8.
142. Creutzfeldt W, Ebert R. New developments in the incretin concept. *Diabetologia* 1985; 28: 565–73.
143. Fehmann HC, Goke R, Goke B. Cell and molecular biology of the incretin hormones glucagon-like peptide-I and glucose-dependent insulin releasing polypeptide. *Endocr Rev* 1995; 16: 390–410.
144. Mentlein R, Gallwitz B, Schmidt WE. Dipeptidyl-peptidase IV hydrolyses gastric inhibitory polypeptide, glucagon-like peptide-1(7-36)amide, peptide histidine methionine and is responsible for their degradation in human serum. *Eur J Biochem* 1993; 214: 829–35.
145. Mentlein R. Dipeptidyl-peptidase IV (CD26)—role in the inactivation of regulatory peptides. *Regul Pept* 1999; 85: 9–24.
146. Trumper A, Trumper K, Trusheim H, Arnold R, Goke B, Horsch D. Glucose-dependent insulinotropic polypeptide is a growth factor for beta (INS-1) cells by pleiotropic signaling. *Mol Endocrinol* 2001; 15: 1559–70.
147. Meier JJ, Hucking K, Holst JJ, Deacon CF, Schmiegel WH, Nauck MA. Reduced insulinotropic effect of gastric inhibitory polypeptide in first-degree relatives of patients with type 2 diabetes. *Diabetes* 2001; 50: 2497–504.
148. Nauck MA, Heimesaat MM, Orskov C, Holst JJ, Ebert R, Creutzfeldt W. Preserved incretin activity of glucagon-like peptide 1 [7-36 amide] but not of synthetic human gastric inhibitory polypeptide in patients with type-2 diabetes mellitus. *J Clin Invest* 1993; 91: 301–7.
149. Wasada T, McCorkle K, Harris V, Kawai K, Howard B, Unger RH. Effect of gastric inhibitory polypeptide on plasma levels of chylomicron triglycerides in dogs. *J Clin Invest* 1981; 68: 1106–7.
150. Ebert R, Nauck M, Creutzfeldt W. Effect of exogenous or endogenous gastric inhibitory polypeptide (GIP) on plasma triglyceride responses in rats. *Horm Metab Res* 1991; 23: 517–21.
151. Jorde R, Pettersen JE, Burhol PG. Lack of effect of exogenous or endogenous gastric inhibitory polypeptide on the elimination rate of Intralipid in man. *Acta Med Scand* 1984; 216: 19–23.
152. Creutzfeldt W, Nauck M. Gut hormones and diabetes mellitus. *Diabetes Metab Rev* 1992; 8: 149–77.

9

Neuropeptides and Insulin Secretion

Bo Ahrén

Lund University, Lund, Sweden

INTRODUCTION

Circulating nutrients, such as glucose, amino acids, and free fatty acids, and the gut hormones, which function as incretins, mainly glucagon-like peptide 1 (GLP-1) and gastric inhibitory polypeptide (GIP), are all important for a normal insulin secretion. However, for an optimal minute-to-minute regulation of insulin secretion, the autonomic nerves, which innervate the islets, are also important [1]. These nerves belong to the parasympathetic, sympathetic, or sensory branches of the autonomic nervous system, and their nerve terminals end in close apposition to the islet endocrine cells. The islet nerves harbor both the classical neurotransmitters, acetylcholine and noradrenaline, as well as a number of neuropeptides [1] (Figure 1). Through activation of these nerves, the neurotransmitters are liberated to affect the β-cells, thereby optimizing insulin secretion to meet the demand of insulin under various conditions. Therefore, for a complete understanding of the complex regulation of insulin secretion, knowledge of these neuropeptides and their involvement in islet function is necessary. It is also possible that the neuro-islet interaction is involved in the pathogenesis of type 2 diabetes, in view of the vital importance of islet failure for the development of this disease [2].

ISLET PARASYMPATHETIC NERVES

The islet parasympathetic nerve fibers originate in the pancreatic ganglia, which in turn are controlled by preganglionic nerves, originating in the dorsal motor nucleus of the vagus [1]. Activation of the parasympathetic nerves stimulates insulin secretion. This is of main physiological importance during the cephalic phase of meal-induced insulin secretion, i.e., the rapid and early increase in insulin secretion during the first few minutes after food intake initiated by anticipation or ingestion of food before nutrients have reached the islets. This importance of the nerves is evident by findings that insulin secretion during the cephalic phase is abolished by ganglionic blockade [3]. The cephalic phase of meal-induced insulin secretion is of major physiological relevance in spite that it is short-lived and in magnitude corresponding to only 1–3% of the total insulin secretion after intake of a meal. Thus, inhibition of the cephalic phase of insulin secretion results in glucose intolerance [3].

An important mechanism explaining the stimulated insulin secretion during vagal nerve activation is the release of the classical neurotransmitter acetylcholine, which stimulates β-cell secretion through a direct action on the cells. An important mechanism underlying the insulinotropic action of acetylcholine is activation of phospholipase C (PLC), which increases the formation of inositol-1,4,5-trisphosphate (IP_3) and liberation of calcium from intracellular stores in conjunction with formation of diacyl glycerol (DAG) and subsequent activation of protein kinase C (PKC), although other mechanisms may also contribute [4]. Besides acetylcholine, neuropeptides confined to islet parasympathetic nerve terminals also contribute to vagally induced insulin secretion. Evidence for such a noncholinergic mechanism is that vagally induced insulin secretion is not abolished by atropine but abolished by ganglionic blockade by hexamethonium [1]. This shows that the postganglionic nerves are regulated by nicotinic receptors but use noncholinergic neurotransmitters in addition to acetylcholine for eliciting effects. The neuropeptides localized to islet parasympathetic nerve terminals and therefore potential mediators of the

International Textbook of Diabetes Mellitus, Third Edition. Edited by R. A. DeFronzo, E. Ferrannini, H. Keen, and P. Zimmet.
 ISBN: 0-471-48655-8.

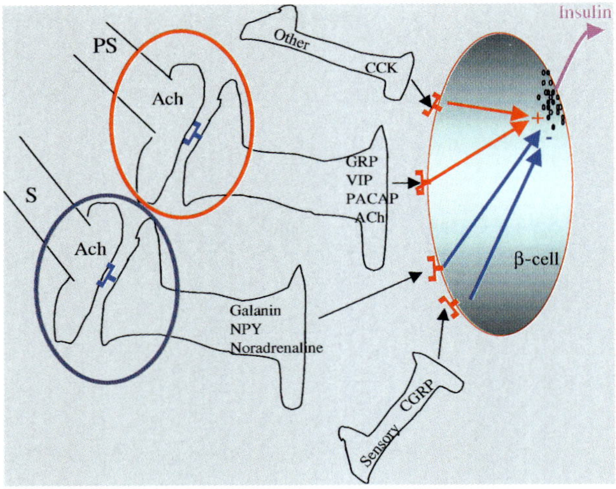

Figure 1 Schematic view of the innervation of the pancreatic islets with the main branches of the autonomic nerves (PS = parasympathetic nerve, S = sympathetic nerve, sensory nerves, and other nerves) with the neurotransmitters localized to these nerves and their net effect on insulin secretion (Ach = acetylcholine, NPY = neuropeptide Y, CCK = cholecystokinin, GRP = gastrin releasing peptide, VIP = vasoactive intestinal polypeptide, PACAP = pituitary adenylate cyclase activating polypeptide, CGRP = calcitonin gene related polypeptide). + and − indicate positive and negative influences on exocytosis of insulin, respectively

noncholinergic effects are gastrin releasing polypeptide (GRP), vasoactive intestinal polypeptide (VIP), and pituitary adenylate cyclase activating polypeptide (PACAP).

GASTRIN RELEASING POLYPEPTIDE

GRP is one of the neuropeptides in islet cholinergic nerves. This neuropeptide is the mammalian homologue of the amphibian peptide bombesin. In mammals, GRP was isolated from the porcine gastrointestinal tract in 1979, and since the peptide was found to stimulate gastrin release from the stomach, it was called GRP [5]. GRP consists of a 27-amino acid residue, which is α-amidated in its C-terminal methionine (Figure 2). The peptide is highly conserved during evolution, having identical N-terminal end as bombesin, and the human and porcine forms of the peptide differ in only two residues. The gene for GRP is located on chromosome 18q21 and GRP is formed after processing of a 125-amino acid proform [6]. GRP is widely distributed in mammalian tissues, with particular abundancy in the lung, the central nervous system, and the gut. In the pancreas, GRP has been shown to be a neuropeptide in islet nerves in several different species including humans [1, 7]. GRP is also localized to nerves in the pancreatic ganglia, is released from the isolated pig pancreas during vagal nerve activation, and stimulates insulin secretion, as shown in several species [1, 8–11]. This suggests that GRP is a neuropeptide in cholinergic nerves involved in the regulation of insulin secretion. Its stimulatory effect on insulin secretion is executed through a direct action on the islets [12], which is supported by the demonstration of specific GRP binding sites in the islets [13] and the expression of mRNA of the GRP receptor (GRPR) in isolated mouse islets [14]. *In vivo* studies have, however, also demonstrated that the ganglionic antagonist hexamethonium and the muscarinic antagonist atropine both partially inhibit GRP-stimulated insulin secretion, suggesting that a portion of GRP-stimulated insulin secretion is executed through a ganglionic action of GRP [1, 9]. Therefore, GRP stimulates insulin secretion both through a direct action on the islet and indirectly through stimulating postganglionic nerves.

The insulinotropic action of GRP is accompanied by increased cytoplasmic concentration of calcium due to stimulation of both calcium uptake from extracellular space and release from intracellular stores [12, 15, 16]. This latter process has been studied in detail in clonal HIT-cells, in which GRP induces a rapid and transient increase in cytoplasmic calcium also in the absence of extracellular calcium and through a mechanism that is prevented by thapsigargin, i.e., a compound inhibiting microsomal calcium-ATPase activity, thereby preventing intracellular calcium stores from being refilled [15, 16]. It should be emphasized, however, that an increase in cytoplasmic calcium may not be the only mechanism for GRP

```
            1   5    10   15   20   25   30   35   40
hGRP        VPLPAGGGTVLTKMYPRGNHWAVGHLM*
pGRP        APVSVGGGTVLAKMYPRGNHWAVGHLM*
bombesin               EQRLGNQWAVGHLM*
VIP         HSDAVFTDNYTRLRKQMAVKKYLNSILN*
Glucagon    HSQGTFTSDYSKYLDSRRAQDFVQWLMNT
hPHM        HADGVFTSDFSKLLGQLSAKKYLESLM*
Secretin    HSDGTFTSELSRLREGARLQRLLQGLV*
hGIP        YAEGTFISDYSIAMDKIHQQDFVNWLLAQKGKKNDWKHNITQ
PACAP       HSDGIFTDSYSRYRKQMAVKKYLAAVLGKRYKQRVKNK*
hNPY        YPSKPDNPGEDAPAEDMARYYSALRHYINLITRQRY*
hPP         APLEPVYPGDNATPEQMAQYAADLRRYINMLTRPRY*
hPYY        YPIKPEAPGEDASPEELNRYYASLRHYLNLVTRQRY*
hgalanin    GWTLNSAGYLLGPHAVGNHRSFSDKNGLTS
pgalanin    GWTLNSAGYLLGPHAIDNHRSFHDKYGLA*
rgalanin    GWTLNSAGYLLGPHAIDNHRSFSDKHGLT*
hαCGRP      ACDTATCVTHRLAGLLSRSGGVVKNNFVPTNVGSKAF*
hßCGRP      ACNTATCVTHRLAGLLSRSGGMVKSNFVPTNVGSKAF*
hIAPP       KCNTATCATQRLANFLVHSSNNFGAILSSTNVGSNTY*
hcalcitonin CGNLSTCMLGTYTQDFNKFHTFPQTAIGVGAP*
CCK33       KAPSGRMSIVKNLQNLDPSHRISDRDYMGWMDF*
CCK8                                  DYMGWMDF*
CCK4                                      WMDF*
```

Figure 2 The amino acid sequences of the islet neuropeptides and biologically active peptides showing resemblances to these. The amino acids are abbreviated according to the one-letter system: A ala, C cys, D asp, E glu, F phe, G gly, H his, I ile, K lys, L leu, M met, N asn, P pro, Q gln, R arg, S ser, T thr, V val, W trp, and Y tyr. * indicates amidation. GRP = gastrin releasing polypeptide, VIP = vasoactive intestinal polypeptide, PHM = peptide histidine methionine, GIP = gastric inhibitory polypeptide, PACAP = pituitary adenylate cyclase-activating polypeptide, NPY = neuropeptide Y, PP = pancreatic polypeptide, PYY = peptide YY, CGRP = calcitonin gene-related polypeptide, IAPP = islet amyloid polypeptide, CCK = cholecystokinin, h = human, p = porcine, r = rat

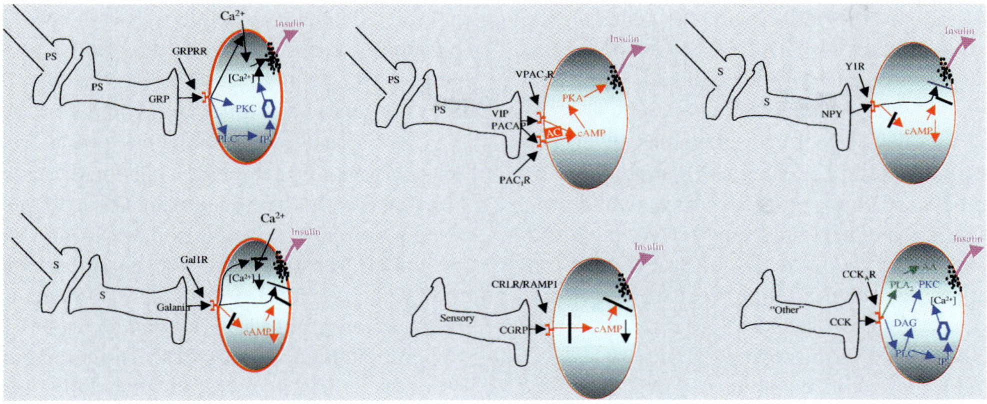

Figure 3 Schematic view of nerves innervating islet β-cells, with focus on neuropeptides released from islet nerve terminals affecting β-cell receptors, leading to perturbations of β-cell signaling pathways and altered insulin secretion. PS = parasympathetic nerve, S = sympathetic nerve. For more detailed information of β-cell signaling, see Figure 4

in stimulating insulin secretion. Thus, it has also been shown that GRP-induced insulin secretion is inhibited by downregulation of PKC [15] and that PKC is activated by GRP, in particular the subspecies of PKC—PKCα, PKCβ, and PKCζ [17]. It is also possible, although not yet convincingly demonstrated, that activation of phospholipase D (PLD) with formation of DAG contributes to GRP-induced insulin secretion [1]. Hence, activation of several different signaling mechanisms may together contribute to the insulinotropic action of GRP (Figure 3).

Four different receptor subtypes with affinity for bombesin-like peptides have been cloned in mammals: the GRP receptor, the neuromedin B receptor, and the bombesin receptor subtypes 3 and 4 [1, 14, 18]. Recent studies have shown that it is the GRPR that is the receptor subtype responsible for GRP-stimulated insulin secretion, because mRNA for the GRPR has been demonstrated in isolated islets and GRP does not stimulate insulin from islets isolated from mice genetically deleted of the GRPR [14]. The gene for the GRPR is localized to the chromosome Xp21.2-p21.3, and the receptor, which consists of 384 amino acids, shows a high degree of conservation during evolution, with homology of approximately 90% between species [6]. To study the physiology of GRP for islet function, mice genetically deleted of the GRPR have been studied. These mice exhibit impaired insulin secretion in response to autonomic nerve activation by neuroglycopenia induced by 2-deoxyglucose (2-DG) [14]. 2-DG is known to activate the autonomic nerves, thereby increasing insulin secretion in mice by an effect that is counteracted by ganglionic blockade by hexamethonium [1]. The involvement of GRP in the neural activation of insulin secretion is also supported by the finding that vagal nerve activation releases GRP from the pig pancreas [8]. Also insulin secretion in response to oral glucose is impaired in the GRPR-deleted mice [19]. In contrast, insulin secretion in response to intravenous glucose is augmented in GRPR-deleted mice. This suggests that neurally activated insulin secretion is dependent on GRP and that a compensatory increase in glucose-stimulated insulin secretion from the β-cells develops in GRPR-deleted mice. Thus, augmented response to glucose compensates for impaired neural response. This compensatory increased insulin secretion is sensitive to ganglionic blockade by hexamethonium and parallelled by increased insulin secretion to cholinergic activation by carbachol and may therefore be instituted by a cholinergic mechanism [14]. Hence, results so far suggest that GRP is involved in neural regulation of insulin secretion and that long-term prevention of this effect leads to compensatory cholinergic hyperresponsiveness.

VASOACTIVE INTESTINAL POLYPEPTIDE

VIP was originally isolated from the porcine small intestine in the early 1970s and found to consist of a 28-amino acid residue, with a C-terminal α-amidation showing structural similarities to other members of the glucagon superfamily of peptides [20] (Figure 2). VIP is formed by processing of a 149-amino acid proVIP and is highly conserved as illustrated by human, porcine, and rat VIP being identical, differing from guinea pig VIP in only two amino acids. The human gene coding for VIP is located on chromosome 6q24 and encodes also for peptide histidine methionine (PHM), the function of which remains to be established [6].

VIP nerves are localized both to the central nervous system and to the respiratory, gastrointestinal, and genitourinary systems, and the neuropeptide exerts a variety of actions, like relaxation of smooth muscle cells and stimulation of exocrine and endocrine secretions. In the pancreas, a neural VIP network surrounding the islets has been demonstrated both in humans and experimental animals and it has also been demonstrated that islet VIP nerves show particular association with the centrally located insulin-producing cells [6, 21–23]. VIP has also been demonstrated in ganglionic nerve cell bodies, showing that VIP is a neuropeptide of postganglionic nerves [23]. Like GRP, also VIP is released from the pancreas when the vagal nerves are activated [22], suggesting that also VIP is a parasympathetic, noncholinergic neurotransmitter involved in the regulation of islet function. VIP is a powerful stimulator of insulin secretion as demonstrated after exogenous administration *in vivo* and *in vitro* [1]. Similarly, transgenic mice overexpressing the VIP gene in the islet β-cells show increased insulin secretion [24].

Two VIP binding receptors exist and because they also show affinity for PACAP they are called the $VPAC_1$ and $VPAC_2$ receptors ($VPAC_1R$ and $VPAC_2R$) [25]. They are both G-protein-coupled receptors of the seven transmembraneous domain type. *In situ* hybridization using probes for the messages of $VPAC_1R$ and $VPAC_2R$ has demonstrated that $VPAC_2R$ but not the $VPAC_1R$ are expressed in the rat and mouse islets as well as in insulin-producing clonal cells [26]. This suggests that it is the $VPAC_2R$ that transmits the signal of VIP in islet endocrine cells. Through activation of $VPAC_2R$, VIP activates adenylate cyclase, which increases the formation of cyclic AMP (cAMP), as has been demonstrated in islet cells [27]. cAMP in turn activates PKA, which enhances exocytosis in both direct and indirect manners [28] (Figure 3). It has also been demonstrated that wortmannin inhibits VIP-stimulated insulin secretion [27], suggesting that pathways independent from cAMP formation may also be involved, like for example a direct action on the exocytosis or an action through augmented activity of phosphatidylinositol 3 kinase. Nevertheless, the stimulation by insulin secretion of VIP seems largely to be a classical cAMP–PKA-mediated process. Hence, VIP is localized to parasympathetic islet nerves, is released from the pancreas when these nerves are activated, and stimulates insulin secretion. The functional role of VIP in islet function, however, remains to be established.

PITUITARY ADENYLATE CYCLASE ACTIVATING POLYPEPTIDE

PACAP was originally extracted from the pituitary in 1989 [29]. It exists in two forms, consisting of 27 and 38 amino acids and, like VIP, belongs to the glucagon peptide family. The two neuropeptides, VIP and PACAP, show 68% identity (Figure 2). The gene for PACAP is located on the chromosome 18p11. proPACAP consists of 152 amino acids and PACAP27 is cleaved from PACAP38 being its 27 N-terminal amino acids ($PACAP38_{1-27}$). The main form of the peptide is PACAP38 [6, 29].

PACAP is a neuropeptide mainly in nerves in the central nervous system, in the lungs, and in the gastrointestinal tract. The neuropeptide is also localized to islet nerve terminals and in pancreatic ganglia, as has been demonstrated in mice and rats [23, 29]. The islet PACAP nerves are thought to be mainly parasympathetic nerves, because PACAP is costored with VIP in some islets nerves, is released from the pancreas during electrical activation of the vagal nerves, and the pancreatic PACAP content is reduced by vagotomy [29]. In addition, however, PACAP may also be a neurotransmitter in islet sensory nerves [23].

PACAP potently stimulates insulin secretion as demonstrated both *in vivo* and *in vitro* in a number of experimental conditions [29]. It also augments glucose-stimulated insulin secretion in healthy volunteers upon exogenous administration, showing that PACAP is an insulinotropic neuropeptide in humans also [30]. The neuropeptide stimulates insulin secretion in a glucose-dependent manner accompanied by increased action of adenylate cyclase with increased formation of cAMP and activation of PKA [29]. PACAP also increases the cytoplasmic concentration of calcium and sodium through opening of membraneous calcium and sodium channels [29], and stimulates a distal effect on the exocytosis machinery [27]. The potency of PACAP to stimulate insulin secretion, which exceeds that of VIP, is therefore most likely due to the diversity of signaling actions induced by PACAP in islet β-cells (Figure 3).

There is a close relation between PACAP and VIP, which is evident by the structural similarity of the peptides and by the affinity of both peptides to $VPAC_1R$ and $VPAC_2R$. However, PACAP also stimulates a third subtype of the PACAP receptors, which is specific for PACAP. This receptor is called the PAC_1 receptor (PAC_1R), and this receptor is, like the two VPAC receptors, G-protein-coupled receptors of the seven transmembraneous domain type [25, 29]. Gene expression and *in situ* hybridization studies have shown that PAC_1 receptors and $VPAC_2$ receptors are expressed in the islets [26, 29].

To study the physiology of PACAP, PAC_1R-deficient mice ($PAC_1R^{-/-}$) have been developed by homologous recombination in embryonic stem cells [31]. In this model, the 18-exon-containing PAC_1R gene was disrupted by deletion of a fragment containing exons 8–11. This resulted in expression of a truncated PAC_1R, which does not bind PACAP. The PAC_1R-deleted mice were viable and developed normally, and baseline glucose and insulin levels were normal as was the pancreatic insulin content. The insulin response to PACAP was markedly reduced in these mice (by 50%), showing that a main mediator of the PACAP-induced insulin secretion is the PAC_1 receptors. The most interesting phenotype in the PAC_1R-deleted mice, however, is that they exhibit impaired insulin response to glucose, both *in vivo* and *in vitro*. Thus, the insulin response to an increase in the glucose concentration from 4.2 to 16.7 mmol/l in the perfused pancreas is impaired by approximately 50% in the $PAC_1R^{-/-}$ mice, and, furthermore, the insulin response to exogenously added glucose *in vivo* to these mice is accompanied by impaired glucose-stimulated insulin secretion. This suggests that PAC_1R contributes both to PACAP- and glucose-induced insulin secretion, i.e., PACAP is of physiological importance for glucose-stimulated insulin secretion. In regard to these PAC_1R-deleted mice, it is important to remember that expression of $VPAC_1R$ and $VPAC_2R$ are still intact, which enables PACAP to affect islet function through activating these receptors. This explains why PACAP-induced insulin secretion is not abolished, but reduced only by approximately 50% in the mice. Future studies on $VPAC_1R$- and $VPAC_2R$-deleted mice are now of importance for a more complete understanding of the insulinotropic action of PACAP. Recently mice deleted of the PACAP gene have also been developed [32]. These mice exhibit high mortality and also marked changes in psychomotor phenotype; their phenotype in relation to islet function has not been described.

Because of its localization to parasympathetic nerves in the pancreas and release from the pancreas after vagal nerve activation, and its potent stimulation of insulin secretion, PACAP might be of physiological relevance for neural regulation of islet function after a meal intake. Results showing that the insulin response to oral glucose is inhibited by a PACAP receptor antagonist and impaired in PAC_1R-deleted mice support this [29, 31]. However, the exact involvement of PACAP in islet physiology remains to be established.

ISLET SYMPATHETIC NERVES

The pancreatic islets are also densely innervated by the sympathetic nerves, as demonstrated by fluorescence microscopy, electron microscopy, and immunocytochemistry [1]. The sympathetic nerves are postganglionic with most nerve cell bodies located in the celiac ganglion or in the paravertebral sympathetic ganglia, and the peripheral nerve endings are localized in close connection to the β-cells. Electrical activation of these sympathetic nerves inhibits insulin secretion, which is physiologically of importance during various forms of stresses or physical exercise to achieve or maintain hyperglycemia [1]. The inhibitory effect of sympathetic nerves on insulin secretion is partially mediated by the classical neurotransmitter noradrenaline. This is executed through inhibition of adenyl cylcase, with reduced formation of cAMP, through hyperpolarization with closure of the voltage-sensitive calcium channels, and through a direct exocytotic action. However, in addition to noradrenaline, neuropeptides may also contribute to sympathetically induced inhibition of insulin secretion. The evidence for this is that combined α_2- and β-adrenoceptor blockade by yohimbine and propranolol does not prevent the effect of sympathetic activation, and that exogenous administration of noradrenaline does, as sympathetic activation, inhibit basal insulin secretion [1]. Two neuropeptides may be of relevance in this context—galanin and neuropeptide Y (NPY)—because these two neuropeptides are localized to the islet sympathetic nerve terminals and to nerve cell bodies in the celiac ganglion, are released from the pancreas in response to electrical activation of the sympathetic nerves, and inhibit insulin secretion as demonstrated both *in vivo* and *in vitro* [1].

GALANIN

Galanin was isolated from the porcine gastrointestinal tract in 1983 and named galanin because of its glycine C-terminus and alanin N-terminus [33]. It consists of 29 amino acids in most species, being C-terminally amidated, although the human form consists of a 30-amino acid residue, which is not C-terminally amidated (Figure 2). The human galanin gene is located on chromosome 11q13.3-q13.5 and progalanin is a 123 residue peptide [6].

Galanin is a widely distributed neuropeptide both in the central and peripheral nervous systems. In the islets, a dense galanin innervation of the islets was first demonstrated in dogs, where galanin nerve fibers have been visualized in close association with the islets [33]. In other species also, a dense islet galanin innervation has been demonstrated, including humans [33]. However, species differences exist; for example, islet galanin innervation is more abundant in dogs and cats than in other species [33]. The islet galanin nerves stain immunocytochemically for tyrosine hydroxylase, and nerve cell bodies in the celiac ganglion have been shown to costore galanin and tyrosine hydroxylase, as shown in dogs [33]. This suggests that islet galanin nerves are sympathetic, which is also supported by results that a substantial, although not total, reduction of pancreatic galanin nerves develops after chemical sympathectomy by means of 6-hydroxydopamine treatment of the rodent pancreas [33]. Furthermore, in the dog, galanin is released from the pancreas after sympathetic nerve activation, and in the mouse, pancreatic galanin content is reduced by exercise stress, which is known to activate sympathetic nerves [33]. Therefore, although galanin may also be localized to nonsympathetic nerves, most results suggest that islet galanin is mainly a sympathetic neuropeptide.

Galanin has been demonstrated to potently inhibit basal and stimulated insulin secretion in a number of experimental systems both *in vivo* as demonstrated in dogs, rats, and mice and *in vitro* from isolated islets of several species including humans, and in perfused rat pancreas [33]. The mechanism underlying this inhibitory action has been shown to involve several signaling pathways including inhibition of the cellular uptake of calcium by closure of voltage-sensitive calcium channels through hyperpolarization, inhibition of the formation of cAMP through involvement of a pertussis toxin sensitive G-protein, and through a direct action, inhibiting the exocytosis of secretory granules [33–35] (Figure 3). The actions of galanin have been shown to be transmitted by signals induced by activation of three different galanin receptor subtypes, which are called GalR1, GalR2, and GalR3, respectively. These receptor subtypes are encoded by different genes and are G-protein-coupled receptors [6]. The receptor subtype form GalR1 is the form that is expressed in insulin-producing cells and therefore most likely mediating the inhibitory influence of galanin on insulin secretion [36].

Functional studies have demonstrated that galanin is released from the dog pancreas during sympathetic nerve activation in a quantity that is sufficient to mimic the inhibition of insulin secretion induced by sympathetic nerve stimulation [37]. This would suggest that galanin contributes to sympathetically induced inhibition of insulin secretion, which is also supported by a study in an experimental model in mice, in which swimming for 2 min is accompanied by a 50% inhibition of glucose-stimulated insulin secretion as a sign of the stress associated with the physical exercise. When galanin was immunoneutralized in these mice by pretreatment with a high-titer galanin antiserum, no inhibition of glucose-stimulated insulin secretion during the swimming was seen [38]. Therefore, immunoneutralization of galanin prevents exercise stress from inhibiting insulin secretion in mice, supporting that galanin is a contributor of this response. Studies to conclusively establish this remain to be performed, however. Such studies could take use of specific galanin receptor antagonists, such as galantide [39] or mice lacking galanin through gene deletion [40].

NEUROPEPTIDE Y

NPY was isolated from the porcine brain in 1982 and since it was demonstrated to consist of tyrosine both in its N- and C-terminal ends, it was named NPY [41]. It consists of a 36-amino acid residue and shows structural homology to peptide YY (PYY) and pancreatic polypeptide (PP). The human NPY gene is located on chromosome 7p15.11 and the 68 residue proNPY is processed to NPY at its N-terminal end [6].

NPY is widely distributed in the central and peripheral tissues and in most locations, the peptide is localized to perivascular adrenergic nerve fibers [41]. In the pancreas, NPY-containing neurons have been demonstrated around vessels, in the exocrine portion of the islets as well as in the islets as demonstrated in dogs, pigs, and mice [1, 42, 43]. NPY is in some of these nerve terminals colocalized with tyrosine hydroxylase, showing that in the islets too, NPY is an adrenergic neuropeptide, which is supported by the localization of NPY to nerve cell bodies in the celiac ganglion (also staining for tyrosine hydroxylase and galanin), and that electrical activation of the pancreatic nerves releases NPY [1, 43]. However, islet nerve terminals expressing NPY but not tyrosine hydroxylase have also been described [43]. This suggests a possible dual function of islet NPY as both a sympathetic and a nonsympathetic neuropeptide.

NPY is released from the pancreas during nerve activation [43] and most studies on the islet effects of NPY have shown that the peptide inhibits glucose-stimulated insulin secretion, i.e., it exerts sympathetic-like effect, both *in vivo* and *in vitro* [1, 42, 44, 45]. However, also only marginal effects have been reported [1], which has questioned the physiological role of NPY in the regulation of insulin secretion. Instead, the marked vasoconstrictor action of NPY has suggested that a main physiological role of NPY in the islets is regulation of islet blood flow [1]. Nevertheless, an inhibitory effect is evident from most studies. Six different NPY receptors have been cloned, which are called the Y1, Y2, Y3, Y4, Y5, and Y6 receptors [46]. These receptor subtypes are all of the G-protein-coupled seven transmembraneous domain type. In insulin-producing cells, it is the Y1 receptor subtype (Y1R) that mediates islet actions of NPY [45]. The gene for human Y1R is located at chromosome 4q31.3-32 and the human and mouse forms of the receptor show 93% identity, suggesting a high degree of conservation of the Y1R during evolution. The Y1R consists of two subtypes, called Y1α and Y1β receptors, showing a high degree of identity [6].

The mechanism underlying the inhibition by NPY of glucose-stimulated insulin secretion seems to involve inhibition of adenylate cyclase with reduced formation of cAMP [44] (Figure 3). However, NPY also seems to inhibit insulin secretion through a distal mechanism in relation to formation of cAMP because insulin secretion stimulated by a cAMP analogue is also inhibited by NPY [1]. The physiological importance of NPY for islet function remains to be established. One study has demonstrated that immunoneutralization of NPY in isolated islets leads to increased insulin secretion [44], which would suggest a physiological inhibitory effect of islet NPY on insulin secretion. Such a hypothesis might be further tested in NPY- or Y1R-deficient animals [47, 48].

SENSORY NEUROPEPTIDES

Besides by the sympathetic and parasympathetic nerves, the islets are also innervated by sensory nerves that harbor sensory neuropeptides, mainly calcitonin-gene-related peptide (CGRP) [1]. These sensory islet nerves innervate mainly the peripheral portions of the islets although nerve fibers are occasionally also found in the central portion of the islets [1, 49]. The fibers leave the pancreas along the sympathetic fibers within the splanchnic nerves to reach the spinal cord. A tool for examining the role of the islet sensory nerves is capsaicin, which causes deafferentation of small unmyelinated C-fibers, leading to sensory denervation in conjunction with a substantial reduction of the number of islet CGRP nerves [50]. Such studies have shown that following capsaicin, insulin secretion and glucose elimination are increased both in mice [51] and in Zucker diabetic fatty rats [52], suggesting that the sensory nerves inhibit insulin secretion.

CALCITONIN-GENE-RELATED POLYPEPTIDE

CGRP was originally described in a medullary thyroid carcinoma cell line, where CGRP was found to be encoded in the same gene as calcitonin [49, 53]. This gene is currently called the calcitonin complex gene A (*CALCA*), is located on chromosome 11p15.2-p15.1, and encodes for two different mRNAs, one being translated to preprocalcitonin and the other to the 128-amino acid preproCGRP, which is processed to α-CGRP. Later, another gene was described, named calcitonin complex gene B (*CALCB*), which is located at chromosome 11p12-14.2 and encodes for β-CGRP. The two CGRPs are both 37-amino acid peptides and show a high degree of similarity and they resemble islet amyloid polypeptide (IAPP) and adrenomedullin [53] (Figure 3). CGRP is localized both to the central and peripheral nervous systems and mainly seems to be localized to sensory nerves. In the pancreas, CGRP nerves are scattered throughout the parenchyma, with particular density along small blood vessels and within the islets where nerve endings are in close apposition to the endocrine cells [49]. This shows that CGRP is an islet neuropeptide.

Exogenous administration of CGRP inhibits insulin secretion [49]. In isolated islets, this inhibition is accompanied by reduction of the formation of cAMP by an effect which is prevented by pertussis toxin and therefore most likely mediated by an inhibitory G_i-protein [49] (Figure 3). Recent studies have, furthermore, disclosed an interesting mode of regulation of the islet CGRP influences, because CGRP, as well as IAPP, calcitonin, and adrenomedullin, acts through the calcitonin-receptor-like receptor (CRLR) and the calcitonin receptor (CTR) and that the affinity of these receptors for the different ligands is under active regulation. Thus, three different receptor-activity-modifying proteins (RAMPs) govern the specificity of the receptors for the different ligands: RAMP1-transported CRLR is a CGRP receptor, whereas RAMP2- or RAMP3-transported CRLR is an adrenomedullin receptor, and IAPP binding is more related to RAMP-transported CTR [54]. Of particular interest for islet physiology is the demonstration that CRLR and RAMP are both expressed in β-cells [54], suggesting that the regulation of RAMP1 expression and function governs the islet influence of CGRP. The detailed involvement of this regulation for an islet function, however, remains to be established. In conclusion, CGRP is a neuropeptide in islet sensory nerves and inhibits insulin secretion.

CHOLECYSTOKININ

Besides the sympathetic, parasympathetic, or sensory nervous system, nerves not related to these main branches of the autonomic nervous system also seem to innervate the endocrine pancreas. These nerve fibers have been shown to harbor other neurotransmitters than the other types of autonomic nerve terminals. One such neurotransmitter is cholecystokinin (CCK), which is located in islet nerves and exerts marked stimulatory influence on insulin secretion [55]. CCK was initially demonstrated as a gut hormone released into the circulation, stimulating gallbladder contraction. During the 1970s and 1980s it was demonstrated that CCK is a neuropeptide with localization both to central and peripheral neurons, and in 1980, it was reported that CCK is a neuropeptide in pancreatic islets [56]. The human gene for CCK is located on chromosome 3q12-3pter and encodes for a proCCK with a 115-amino acid residue, the initial translational product of which is CCK83, which is further processed to CCK variants with 58, 39, 33, 25, 22, 18, 12, 8, 7, 5, and 4 residues, respectively. The mechanisms of the CCK processing and the function of all these intermediates or CCK forms are still not established. In neurons, most evidence favors that it is the smaller CCK forms, mainly CCK4, that are the main products and therefore probably function as neurotransmitter [56].

In the pancreatic islets, CCK has been shown to potently stimulate insulin secretion and since this action is executed at levels of CCK above those circulating after meal intake, it is most likely that the stimulation by CCK of insulin secretion does not reflect an incretin action but rather a neural action [55]. Of the two different types of CCK receptor subtypes that have been described, it seems as it is the CCK_A receptor subtype, which consists of 428 amino acids, that mediates the insulinotropic action of CCK. This is based on findings that specific CCK_A receptor antagonists inhibit CCK-induced insulin secretion [55]. This receptor type shows almost a 1000-fold higher affinity for CCK than for gastrin. In contrast, the CCK_B receptor type does not seem to be involved in CCK-induced insulin secretion.

The insulinotropic activation of CCK is mainly mediated by PLC that stimulates the hydrolysis of phosphoinositides. The phosphoinositide hydrolysis in turn yields

IP_3, releasing calcium from intracellular calcium stores to raise the cytosolic concentration of calcium. Consequently, CCK increases the cytosolic concentration of calcium independently from uptake of extracellular calcium, which is accompanied by a rapid stimulation of exocytosis and insulin secretion [55]. CCK has also been shown to stimulate the generation of arachidonic acid (AA) through activation of phospholipase A_2 (PLA_2), which has emerged as an important mechanism underlying insulin secretion and is affected not only by CCK but also by, for example, the cholinergic agonist carbachol [57]. Finally, downregulation of PKC inhibits CCK-induced insulin secretion [55]. The combined action by CCK to release calcium from intracellular stores to raise the cytosolic concentration of calcium, to stimulate the formation of AA, and to activate PKC seems to contribute to the insulinotropic action after activation of the CCK_A receptors (Figure 3). The physiological role of the islet CCK nerves for the regulation of insulin secretion, however, remains to be established.

CONCLUSION

The pancreatic islets are innervated by the autonomic nerves and these nerves harbor neuropeptides besides the classical neurotransmitters, noradrenaline and acetylcholine [1]. Today we know that several neuropeptides are localized to islet nerve terminals and that they are released from the pancreas upon nerve activation. These neuropeptides therefore contribute to the regulation of insulin secretion. Table 1 summarizes the islet neuropeptides and the action of these neuropeptides. Thus galanin and NPY, localized to sympathetic nerve endings, inhibit insulin secretion, whereas PACAP, VIP, and GRP, localized to parasympathetic nerve endings, stimulate insulin secretion. Since, furthermore, the actions of the neuroeptides are in general glucose-dependent, it may be suggested that the function of the neuropeptides is to transmit neural effects in adjusting the fine regulation of insulin secretion by being permissive factors for glucose. To do so, the neuropeptides affect different signaling pathways in the islet

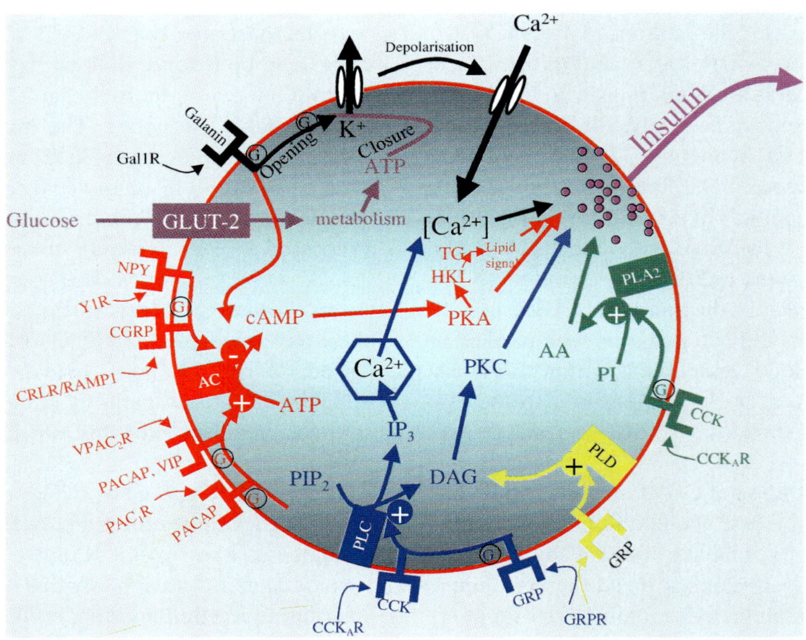

Figure 4 Schematic view of integrated β-cell signaling highlighting four pathways perturbed by islet neuropeptides. (1) Glucose is transported into the cells by means of GLUT-2 and is metabolized, which increases the cytosolic ratio of ATP/ADP, which in turn depolarizes the plasma membrane through closure of ATP-regulated K^+ channels, ensuing opening of voltage-sensitive calcium channels and uptake of extracellular calcium to raise the cytosolic concentration of calcium. (2) Phosphoinositide hydrolysis achieved by phospholipase C (PLC), which yields diacyl glycerol (DAG), activating protein kinase C (PKC), as well as inositol-1,4,5-trisphophate (IP_3), stimulating the liberation of Ca^{2+} from intracellular storage sites. (3) Activation of adenylate cyclase, which induces formation of cAMP and activation of protein kinase A (PKA). PKA phosphorylates proteins of importance for exocytosis as well as hormone-sensitive lipase (HSL), which generates lipid-derived signal(s) from lipolysis of stored triglycerides, activating exocytosis. (4) Activation of phospholipase A_2 (PLA_2), which generates arachidonic acid (AA), which in turn through several mechanisms stimulate insulin secretion. These second messengers (cytosolic calcium, PKC, PKA, lipid signals, and AA) activate the exocytotic machinery that releases insulin. The neurotransmitters affecting insulin secretion execute their actions either by affecting any of these signaling mechanisms or by directly affecting the final exocytosis of insulin-storing granules. It should be emphasized first that the figure is simplified and does not take into account extensive cross talk between pathways, and second that for most actions of neuropeptides a primary initiating effect of glucose is required

Table 1 Islet neuropeptides, islet neuropeptide receptors, their main signaling pathways, and their effects on insulin secretion

Neuropeptide	Localization	Islet receptor	Release after nerve activation	Effect on insulin secretion	Main signaling pathway	Mouse model as tool
GRP	Islet PS nerves	GRPR	Yes (vagal)	Stimulation	Ca^{2+}, PLC, PKC	Yes (GRPR deletion)
VIP	Islet PS nerves	$VPAC_2$	Yes (vagal	Stimulation	cAMP/PKA	Yes ($VPAC_2R$ deletion)
PACAP	Mainly islet PS nerves	PAC_1, $VPAC_2$	Yes (vagal)	Stimulation	cAMP/PKA	Yes (PAC_1R and $VPAC_2R$ deletion)
Galanin	Islet S nerves	Gal1R	Yes (sympathetic)	Inhibition	K^+/Ca^{2+}, cAMP/PKA	Yes (galanin deletion)
NPY	Islet S nerves	Y1	Yes	Inhibition	K^+/Ca^{2+}, cAMP/PKA	Yes (NPY and Y1 deletion)
CGRP	Islet sensory nerves	CRLR/ RAMP	Not established	Inhibition	K^+/Ca^{2+}, cAMP/PKA	Yes (capsaicin)
CCK	"Other islet nerves"	CCK_A	Not established	Stimulation	PLC/PLA_2	No

Note. PS = parasympathetic, S = sympathetic.

β-cells, which are summarized in Figure 4. Therefore, numerous studies in this productive field during the last three decades have fairly well established the localisation of islet neuropeptides, their actions on insulin secretion, and their signaling mechanisms in the β-cells. In contrast, the detailed involvement of the neuropeptides in islet physiology and their possible involvement in the pathophysiology of glucose intolerance, type 2 diabetes, and obesity, is less known and, therefore, now remains to be established in more detail. In such studies, besides classical pharmacological techniques, genetically modified mice will also be valuable tools.

Acknowledgments

The work by the author has been supported by grants from the Swedish Research Council (Grant No. 6834); Albert PÅhlsson, Crafoord and Novo Nordic Foundations; Swedish Diabetes Association; and the Faculty of Medicine, Lund University. For this study, the author is grateful to Lilian Bengtsson, Kerstin Knutsson, and Lena Kvist for expert technical assistance.

REFERENCES

1. Ahrén B. Autonomic regulation of islet hormone secretion—implications for health and disease. *Diabetologia* 2000; 43: 393–410.
2. Kahn SE. The importance of beta-cell failure in the development and progression of type 2 diabetes. *J Clin Endocrinol Metab* 2001; 86: 4047–58.
3. Ahrén B, Holst JJ. The cephalic insulin response to meal ingestion in humans is dependent both on cholinergic and noncholinergic mechanisms and is important for postprandial glycemia. *Diabetes* 2001; 50: 1030–8.
4. Gilon P, Henquin JC. Mechanisms and physiological significance of cholinergic control of pancreatic beta-cell function. *Endocr Rev* 2001; 22: 565–604.
5. McDonald TJ, Jörnvall H, Nilsson G, Vagne M, Ghatei M, Bloom SR. Characterization of a gastrin-releasing peptide from porcine non-antral gastric tissue. *Biochem Biophys Res Commun* 1979; 90: 277–33.
6. Ahrén B. Neuropeptides in the control of islet function. In Ramachandran VS (ed) *Encyclopedia of the Human Brain*. San Diego: Academic Press, 2002, pp 525–40.
7. Shimosegawa T, Asakura T, Kashimura J, Yoshida K, Meguro T, Koizumi M, Mochizuki T, Yanaihara N, Toyota T. Neurons containing gastrin releasing peptide-like immunoreactivity in the human pancreas. *Pancreas* 1993; 8: 403–12.
8. Knuthsen S, Holst JJ, Baldissera FG, Skak-Nielsen T, Poulsen SS, Jensen SL, Nielsen OV. Gastrin-releasing peptide in the porcine pancreas. *Gastroenterology* 1987; 92: 1153–8.
9. Karlsson S, Sundler F, Ahrén B. Insulin secretion by gastrin-releasing peptide in mice: ganglionic versus direct islet effect. *Am J Physiol* 1998; 274: E124–9.
10. Wood SM, Jung RT, Webster JD, Ghatei MA, Adrian TE, Yanaihara N, Yanaihara C, Bloom SR. The effect of the mammalian neuropeptide, gastrin releasing peptide (GRP), on gastrointestinal and pancreatic hormone secretion in man. *Clin Sci* 1983; 65: 365–71.
11. Hermansen K, Ahrén B. Gastrin releasing peptide stimulates the secretion of insulin, but not that of glucagon or somatostatin, from the isolated perfused dog pancreas. *Acta Physiol Scand* 1990; 138: 175–9.
12. Gregersen S, Ahrén B. Studies on the mechanisms by which gastrin releasing peptide potentiates glucose-induced insulin secretion from mouse islets. *Pancreas* 1996; 12: 48–57.
13. Wahl MA, Landsbeck EA, Ammon HPT, Verspohl EJ. Gastrin-releasing peptide: binding and functional studies in mouse pancreatic islets. *Pancreas* 1992; 7: 345–51.
14. Persson K, Pacini G, Ahrén B. Islet function phenotype in gastrin releasing peptide receptor gene deficient mice. *Eudocrinology* 2002; 143: 3717–26.
15. Karlsson S, Ahrén B. Gastrin-releasing peptide mobilizes calcium from intracellular stores in HIT-T15 cells. *Peptides* 1996; 17: 909–16.
16. Karlsson S, Ahrén B. Cytosolic Ca^{2+} oscillations by gastrin releasing peptide in single HIT-T15 cells. *Peptides* 1999; 230: 579–87.
17. Bihlmayer A, Ammon HPT, Wahl MA. Distribution and stimulation by gastrin-releasing peptide of protein kinase C subfamilies in insulin-secreting cells. *Neuroendocrinology* 2001; 73: 352–7.
18. Wada E, Watase K, Yamada K, Ogura H, Yamano M, Imomata Y, Eguchi J, Yamamoto K, Sunday ME, Maeno H, Mikoshiba K, Ohk-Hamazaki H, Wada K. Generation and characterization of mice lacking gastrin-releasing peptide receptor. *Biochem Biophys Res Commun* 1997; 239: 28–33.
19. Persson K, Gingerich RL, Nayak S, Wada K, Wada E, Ahrén B. Reduced GLP-1 and insulin responses and glucose intolerance after gastric glucose in GRP receptor deleted mice. *Am J Physiol* 2000; 279: E956–62.
20. Mutt V. Vasoactive intestinal polypeptide and related peptides. Isolation and chemistry. *Ann N Y Acad Sci* 1988; 527: 1–19.
21. Bishop AE, Polak JM, Gren IC, Bryant MG, Bloom SR. The location of VIP in the pancreas of man and rat. *Diabetologia* 1980; 18: 73–8.
22. Havel PJ, Dunning BE, Verchere CB, Baskin DG, O'Dorisio T, Taborsky GJ Jr. Evidence that vasoactive intestinal polypeptide is a parasympathetic neurotransmitter in the endocrine pancreas in the dog. *Regul Pept* 71; 163–70.
23. Hannibal J, Fahrenkrug J. Pituitary adenylate cyclase-activating polypeptide in intrinsic and extrinsic nerves of the rat pancreas. *Cell Tissue Res* 2000; 299: 59–70.
24. Kato I, Suzuki Y, Kabane A, Yonekura H, Tanaka O, Kondo H, Takasawa S, Yoshimoto T, Okamoto H. Transgenic mice overexpressing human vasoactive intestinal peptide (VIP) gene in pancreatic beta cells. Evidence for improved glucose tolerance and enhanced insulin secretion by VIP and PHM-27 *in vivo*. *J Biol Chem* 1994; 269: 1223–8.
25. Vaudry D, Gonzales BJ, Basille M, Yon L, Fournier A, Vaudry H. Pituitary adenylate cyclase-activating polypeptide and its receptors: from structure to functions. *Pharmacol Rev* 2000; 52: 269–324.
26. Filipsson K, Sundler F, Hannibal J, Ahrén B. PACAP and PACAP receptors in insulin producing tissues: localization and effects. *Regul Pept* 1998; 74: 167–75.
27. Straub SG, Sharp GW. A wortmannin-sensitive signal transduction pathway is involved in the stimulation of

insulin release by vasoactive intestinal polypeptide and pituitary adenylate cyclase-activating polypeptide. *J Biol Chem* 1996; 271: 1660–8.
28. Howell SL, Jones PM, Persaud SJ. Regulation of insulin secretion: the role of second messengers. *Diabetologia* 1994; 37: (suppl 2): S30–5.
29. Filipsson K, Kvist Reimer M, Ahrén B. The neuropeptide pituitary adenylate cyclase-activating polypeptide and islet function. *Diabetes* 2001; 50: 1959–69.
30. Filipsson K, Tornoe K, Holst JJ, Ahrén B: Pituitary adenylate cyclase-activating polypeptide stimulates insulin and glucagon secretion in humans. *J Clin Endocrinol Metab* 1997; 82: 3093–8.
31. Jamen F, Persson K, Bertrand G, Rodriguez-Henche N, Puech R, Bockaert J, Ahrén B, Brabet P: PAC1 receptor-deficient mice display impaired insulinotropic response to glucose and reduced glucose tolerance. *J Clin Invest* 2000; 105: 1307–15.
32. Hashimoto H, Shintani N, Tanaka K, Mori W, Hirose M, Matsuda T, Sakaue M, Miyazaki J, Niwa H, Tashiro F, Yamamoto K, Koga K, Tomimoto S, Kunugi A, Suetake S, Baba A. Altered psychomotor behaviors in mice lacking pituitary adenylate cycloase-activating polypeptide (PACAP). *Proc Natl Acad Sci USA* 2001; 98: 13355–60.
33. Ahrén B, Lindskog S. Galanin and the regulation of islet hormone secretion. *Int J Pancreatol* 1992; 11: 147–60.
34. Ahrén B, Berggren PO, Bokvist K, Rorsman P. Does galanin inhibit insulin secretion by opening of the ATP-regulated K^+-channel in the β-cell? *Peptides* 1989; 10: 453–7.
35. Lindskog S, Ahrén B. Studies on the mechanism by which galanin inhibits insulin secretion in islets. *Eur J Pharmacol* 1991; 205: 21–7.
36. Parker EM, Izzarelli DG, Nowak MP, Mahle CD, Iben LD, Wang J, Goldstein ME. Cloning and characterization of the rat GALR1 galanin receptor from RIN 14B insulinoma cells. *Mol Brain Res* 1995; 34: 179–89.
37. Dunning BE, Taborsky GJ Jr. Galanin release during pancreatic nerve stimulation is sufficient to influence islet function. *Am J Physiol* 1989; 256: E191–8.
38. Dunning BE, Karlsson S, Ahrén B. Contribution of galanin to stress-induced impairment of insulin secretion in swimming mice. Acta Physiol Scand 1991; 143: 145–52.
39. Lindskog S, Ahrén B, Land T, Langel Ü, Bartfai T. The novel high-affinity antagonist, galantide, blocks the galanin-mediated inhibition of glucose-induced insulin secretion. *Eur J Pharmacol* 1992; 210: 183–8.
40. Wynick D, Small CJ, Bloom SR, Pachnis V. Targeted disruption of the murine galanin gene. *Ann N Y Acad Sci* 1998; 863: 22–47.
41. Colmers WF, Wahlestedt C. *The Biology of Neuropeptide Y and Related Peptides*. Totowa, NJ: Humana Press, 1993.
42. Pettersson M, Ahrén B, Lundquist I, Böttcher G, Sundler F. Neuropeptide Y: Intrapancreatic neuronal localization and effects on insulin secretion in the mouse. *Cell Tissue Res* 1987; 248: 43–8.
43. Sheikh SP, Holst JJ, Skak-Nielsen T, Knigge U, Warberg J, Theodorsson-Norheim E, Hökfelt T, Lundberg JM, Schwartz TW. Release of NPY in pig pancreas: dual parasympathetic and sympathetic regulation. *Am J Physiol* 1988; 255: G46–54.
44. Wang ZL, Bennet WM, Wang RM, Ghatei MA, Bloom SR. Evidence of a paracrine role of neuropeptide Y in the regulation of insulin release from pancreatic islets of normal and dexamethasone treated rats. *Endocrinology* 1994; 135: 200–6.
45. Morgan DG, Kulkarni RN, Hurley JD, Wang ZL, Wang RM, Ghatei MA, Karlsen AE, Bloom SR, Smith DM. Inhibition of glucose-stimulated insulin secretion by neuropeptide Y is mediated via the Y1 receptor and inhibition of adenylyl cyclase in RIN 5AH insulinoma cells. *Diabetologia* 1998; 41: 1482–91.
46. Balasubramaniam A. Neuropeptide Y family of hormones: receptor subtypes and anatgonists. *Peptides* 1997; 18: 445–57.
47. Erickson JC, Clegg KE, Palmiter RD. Sensitivity to leptin and susceptibility to seizures on mice lacking neuropeptide Y. *Nature* 1996; 381: 415–8.
48. Burcelin R, Brunner HR, Seydoux J, Thorens B, Pedrazzini T. Increased insulin concentrations and glucose storage in neuropeptide Y Y1 receptor-deficient mice. *Peptides* 2001; 22: 421–7.
49. Ahrén B, Pettersson M. Calcitonin gene-related peptide (CGRP) and amylin and the endocrine pancreas. *Int J Pancreatol* 1990; 6: 1–15.
50. Karlsson S, Sundler F, Ahrén B. Neonatal capsaicin-treatment in mice: effects on pancreatic peptidergic nerves and 2-deoxy-D-glucose-induced insulin and glucagon secretion. *J Autonom Nerv Syst* 1992; 39: 51–60.
51. Karlsson S, Scheurink AJW, Steffens AB, Ahrén B. Involvement of capsaicin-sensitive nerves in regulation of insulin secretion and glucose tolerance in conscious mice. *Am J Physiol* 1994; 267: R1071–7.
52. Gram DX, B Ahrén, F Sundler, UB Olsen, AJ Hansen, RD Carr, CL Brand: Sensory nerve desentisation in Zucker diabetic fatty rats preserves *in vitro* insulin secretion. *Diabetologia* 2000; 43 (suppl 1): A130.
53. Wimalawansa SJ. Amylin, calcitonin gene-related peptide, calcitonin and adrenomedullin: a peptide superfamily. *Crit Rev Neurobiol* 1997; 11: 167–239.
54. Martinez A, Kapas S, Miller MJ, Ward Y, Cuttitta F. Coexpression of receptors for adrenomedullin, calcitonin gene-related peptide, and amylin in pancreatic β-cells. *Endocrinology* 2000; 141: 406–11.
55. Karlsson S, Ahrén B. Cholecystokinin and the regulation of insulin secretion. *Scand J Gastroenterol* 1992; 27: 161–5.
56. Rehfeld JF, Larsson LI, Goltermann NR, Schwartz TW, Holst JJ, Jensen SL, Morley JS. Neural regulation of pancreatic hormone secretion by the C-terminal tetrapeptide of CCK. *Nature* 1980; 284: 33–8.
57. Simonsson E, Ahrén B. Phospholipase A_2 and its potential regulation of islet function. *Int J Pancreatol* 2000; 27: 1–11.

10

Biological Effects of C-peptide and Proinsulin

John Wahren, Karin Ekberg, Jawed Shafqat, Jan Johansson, Bo-Lennart Johansson, and Hans Jörnvall

Karolinska Institute, Stockholm, Sweden

C-PEPTIDE

Introduction

C-peptide or connecting peptide is cleaved off from proinsulin in the course of insulin biosynthesis [1, 2] (see Chapter 6 for details). It is stored in the secretory granules of β-cells and eventually released to the portal circulation, essentially stoichiometrically with insulin [3]. C-peptide plays an important role in the synthesis of insulin by serving as a flexible linker between the A- and B-chains, thus facilitating proper folding and the formation of the disulfide bridges. Following the discovery of C-peptide and the development of radioimmunoassays for measuring its plasma concentration [4], several early studies attempted, without success, to define a physiological role for C-peptide. Insulin-like effects on glucose metabolism were searched for but not found [5, 6]. It was also recognized that C-peptide shows considerable interspecies variability [7] in contrast to the well-conserved structure of insulin. Gradually, the view prevailed that C-peptide does not possess physiological effects, and has no other role than to participate in insulin biosynthesis. Interest in C-peptide shifted to its pharmacokinetic properties and to the use of plasma C-peptide concentrations as a marker of β-cell function in healthy subjects and patients with diabetes [8].

Since then, a series of studies has provided direct evidence that C-peptide is after all a biologically active, endogenous peptide hormone. C-peptide binds specifically to cell membranes, with resultant activation of intracellular signaling pathways [9]. Direct studies in C-peptide-deficient type 1 diabetic patients have demonstrated that replacement of the peptide has important physiological effects. Blood circulation in several tissues is improved, and renal and nerve dysfunctions ameliorated [10]. On the basis of these new biochemical, biophysical, and clinical findings it has been suggested that C-peptide administration, together with insulin therapy, may be beneficial in the treatment and prevention of long-term complications in type 1 diabetes [9–11]. In this chapter, we review the currently available information on the cellular and *in vivo* effects of C-peptide.

Indirect evidence implying biological effects of C-peptide has been available earlier. Thus, type 1 diabetic patients with low but sustained plasma C-peptide levels are less prone to develop long-term complications involving the kidneys [12, 13], eyes [14], or nerves [13] than patients who have become totally C-peptide- and insulin-deficient. Moreover, pancreas transplantation, resulting in restoration of endogenous insulin and C-peptide levels, significantly reverses the structural lesions of diabetic nephropathy, albeit after considerable time [15]. Pancreas or islet transplantation is also accompanied by significant amelioration of diabetic neuropathy [16, 17]. These beneficial effects have partly been ascribed to restored endogenous insulin secretion, improved glycemic control, or immunosuppressive therapy, but the possibility of a positive C-peptide effect has also been recognized [18].

Structural Properties of C-peptide

C-peptide is a 31-residue peptide with a primary structure that varies considerably between species. Thus, the human and pig sequences differ at no less than 11 positions and comparison of all known mammalian C-peptides shows that most, but not all, residues are susceptible to variation.

International Textbook of Diabetes Mellitus, Third Edition. Edited by R. A. DeFronzo, E. Ferrannini, H. Keen, and P. Zimmet.
 ISBN: 0-471-48655-8.

Table 1 C-peptide structural variability in mammalian species

E	**A**	**E**	**D**	**L**	**Q**	**V**	**G**	**Q**	**V**	**E**	**L**	**G**	**G**	**G**	**P**	**G**	**A**	**G**	**S**	**L**	**Q**	**P**	**L**	**A**	**L**	**E**	**G**	**S**	**L**	**Q**
G	V	D	N	P		A	R	A	L			A	A	A	L	E	S	I	T	G	S	L	P	P		A	L	P	M	
	L		G			M	P	E	A				M	S			L	D	D	E	R	A	G	G			V	A	P	
			E				A	D	T				L	E			E		G			T	S				M	I	Q	
							E																						R	

The top sequence (in bold) shows the primary structure of human C-peptide. Residues indicated below are alternatives found at the same positions in C-peptides of other mammalian species. Data from reference 19.

Among 20 mammalian forms, however, five residues—at positions 6 (Gln), 11 (Glu), 12 (Leu), 26 (Leu), and 31 (Gln)—are conserved (Table 1). Similarly, residues at positions 1, 3, and 27 (all Glu) vary in only one species each. Regarding the 3-D structure, C-peptide does not assume a stable conformation in solution, as judged by circular dichroism measurements [20]. Random structure in solution is compatible with the overall interspecies variability of C-peptide. Like many other small peptides, C-peptide appears to have a "random coil" structure. Elements of defined secondary structure may be induced by special solvents (trifluoroethanol) and have also been suggested as explanation for C-peptide–membrane interactions [21] and other functions, but evidence for defined structures under physiological conditions has not been reported.

The species variability and the lack of defined conformational properties made it difficult to understand the molecular mechanisms of C-peptide action. Hormones often exhibit structural conservation of their binding segments. Insulin is an example, with all but one of its residues conserved between human and pig (Table 2), explaining why pig insulin is active in humans. In contrast, many residues differ between human and pig C-peptide. Hence, the structural properties of C-peptide differ markedly from those of insulin. Nevertheless, C-peptide is not unique in its variability. Other peptide hormones, including relaxin of the same peptide family as insulin and C-peptide, are even more variable than C-peptide [19] (Table 2). Thus, the structural variability of C-peptide is large but not exceptional compared to other biopeptides, and does not exclude hormonal action and specific binding of C-peptide to cell membranes [22].

Table 2 Structural variability among peptide hormones originating from or acting on the pancreas

Hormone	Variability between human and pig biopeptides/ Variable residues out of total residues
Somatostatin	0 of 14
Glucagon	0 of 29
VIP	0 of 28
IGF-1	0 of 70
IGF-2	1 of 67
Insulin	1 of 51
GIP	2 of 42
Pancreatic polypeptide	2 of 36
Secretin	2 of 27
CCK	4 of 33
GRP	5 of 27
C-peptide	11 of 31
Relaxin	31 of 54

Data from reference 19.

The overall structural variability of C-peptide suggests that its receptor interactions are exceptional. C-peptide binding may depend on a single or few residues, conserved in mammals. Thus, free Glu is able to partially displace membrane-bound C-peptide [23]. Nevertheless, there is no strong support for only single-residue interactions as an explanation for C-peptide variability. A second alternative is that receptors may co-vary with the ligand structure in different species. However, experimental support in the case of C-peptide is not available. A third, and perhaps more likely, alternative is for the C-peptide binding interactions to be of recent origin, with only higher mammals needing C-peptide function, which would explain the great variability in the earlier forms. Four internal residues are conserved in mammalian C-peptide (Gln6, Glu11, Leu12, and Leu26; Table 1). An additional residue, Glu27, is conserved in all but one of the mammals and has been ascribed special importance for C-peptide–membrane interactions [23]. A similar situation may exist in the case of relaxin, whose effect on the symphysis [24] is not needed before mammals.

In conclusion, the structural and evolutionary features of C-peptide demonstrate that it lacks a defined tertiary structure and a strictly conserved primary structure. Nevertheless, its structural properties are compatible with specific receptor binding, and the hypothesis is offered that in the course of evolution, C-peptide has assumed a hormonal role by affecting specific cellular processes in higher mammals.

Membrane Interactions and Cellular Effects

Binding of C-peptide to Cell Membranes

With a radioligand binding technique, an early study found specific binding of tyrosylated ^{125}I-labeled homologous C-peptide to cultured rat islet cells [25]. However, subsequent attempts to document specific binding of human radiolabeled C-peptide to crude cell membranes from human skeletal muscle [26] and renal tubular cells [22] were not successful. Neither could binding to human lymphoblasts be demonstrated [27], but bound labeled proinsulin could be displaced by C-peptide [27, 28]. The relative paucity of binding sites per cell surface area [22, 25] may have contributed to the difficulty in demonstrating binding of C-peptide using radioligand techniques.

Other ligand binding assays have been more successful, in particular fluorescence correlation spectroscopy (FCS), and more recently the surface plasmon resonance technique. In FCS, the spontaneous molecular movements of a fluorophore-marked ligand (rhodamine-labeled C-peptide) are observed after excitation by a focused laser beam. Measurements are performed in a small volume element ($<10^{-15}$ l), which can be shifted from the incubation medium above a cell growing in culture to the cell membrane. Compared to the radioligand binding method, the FCS technique offers higher detection sensitivity and improved signal-to-noise ratio [29, 30]. The method can also be used for studies of C-peptide binding to solubilized membrane components [31].

Specific binding of human C-peptide in the nanomolar range to human renal tubular cells, skin fibroblasts, and endothelial cells in primary culture has been demonstrated using the FCS technique [22]. The specificity of the binding was evidenced by the consistent displacement of bound C-peptide following the addition of a molar excess of unlabeled C-peptide. Addition of a peptide with residues arranged in random order ("scrambled C-peptide"), or of an all D-amino acid C-peptide, failed to displace bound, native C-peptide, demonstrating the stereospecific nature of the binding. Likewise, incubation with insulin, proinsulin, IGF-I, IGF-II, or neuropeptide Y did not displace bound C-peptide, indicating absence of cross-reactivity with these hormones and their receptors. Moreover, labeled insulin bound to cell membranes was not displaced by addition of C-peptide, suggesting that C-peptide does not interact with the insulin receptor. Pretreatment of cells with pertussis toxin abolishes the binding of C-peptide to the cell membrane at physiological concentrations, suggesting involvement of G-proteins [22]. The estimated association constant for C-peptide binding is 3×10^{9} M^{-1}; the binding curve is illustrated in Figure 1. Half-saturation of C-peptide binding to renal tubular cells occurs already at approximately 0.3 nM. Consequently, it is likely that in healthy humans near-saturation of the receptor is reached at physiological plasma C-peptide concentrations (0.5–1 nM). This finding helps explain the consistent observation that effects of C-peptide cannot be demonstrated in nondiabetic animals or healthy subjects [6, 32–34]; it is only in diabetic animals or patients with C-peptide deficiency that specific effects of C-peptide have been observed. Species specificity with regard to C-peptide binding has not been studied, but human C-peptide is reported to elicit effects in the diabetic rat, although only at supraphysiological concentrations [21]. Likewise, a bioassay based on Ca^{2+} release (see below) shows cross-reactivity and effects of both rat C-peptide and the rat C-terminal pentapeptide in human cells [35].

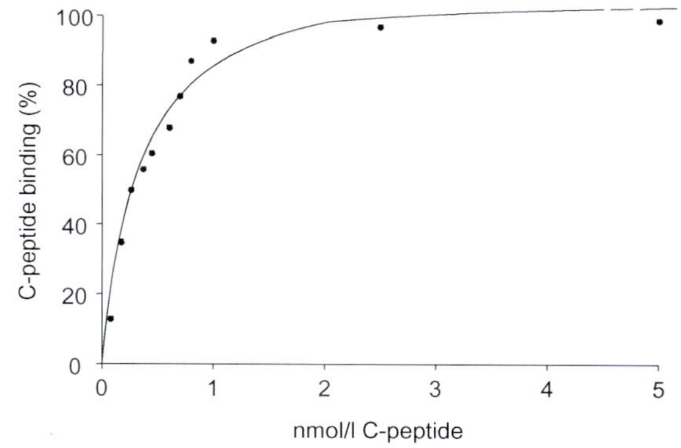

Figure 1 Binding of rhodamine-labeled C-peptide to cell membranes of renal tubular cells. Fractional saturation of the membrane-bound-labeled ligand is presented as a function of the C-peptide concentration in the binding medium. The binding curve corresponds to $K_{\text{ass}} = 3.3 \times 10^{9}$ M^{-1} (data from reference 22)

C-peptide binding has also been studied using surface plasmon resonance spectroscopy [36]. With this method interactions with a chip-bound ligand are studied during exposure to solubilized cell or tissue extracts, and binding is evaluated via changes in the refractive index. Higher binding of cell lysate components to C-peptide than to scrambled C-peptide is observed when presented to the immobilized peptides (Figure 2). Preincubation of the detergent-solubilized cellular extracts with free C-peptide selectively decreases the binding to the immobilized C-peptide [36]. These observations confirm the finding from FCS studies that molecules capable of binding C-peptide are present in cell lysates [31].

Usually, bioactive peptides exert their effects via specific binding of a limited region of the ligand molecule to the receptor. The C-terminal pentapeptide of human C-peptide (EGSLQ) is able to competitively displace the bound, full-length peptide, indicating the involvement of the C-terminal segment as an "active site" in the binding process. With the help of sequential alanine substitution of the pentapeptide, it could be determined that the pentapeptide N-terminal glutamic acid residue (Glu27) is of particular importance for the binding process [23].

In summary, direct-binding studies with C-peptide demonstrate specific binding to cell surfaces and to solubilized cell components, thus far most clearly documented with the FCS and the surface plasmon resonance techniques. Association constants, binding curves, and displacement characteristics have been established at physiologically relevant concentrations. The C-terminal pentapeptide is able to competitively displace the bound, full-length peptide, indicating the involvement of this

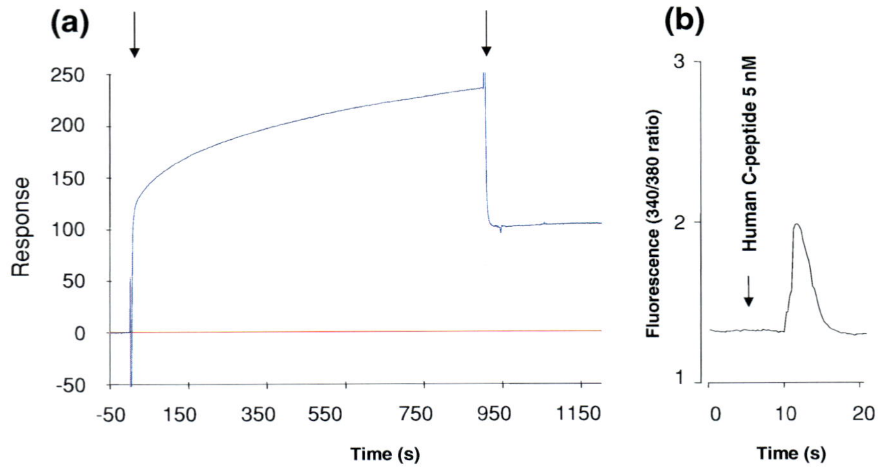

Figure 2 C-peptide–membrane interaction and cellular effects. In part (a) binding of cell lysate components to C-peptide is demonstrated by the difference plasmon resonance signal. Crude cell lysate from HEK-293 cells in 0.4% deoxycholate was presented to C-peptide and scrambled C-peptide, respectively, immobilized on a streptavidine-coated chip (data from reference 36). The top curve shows binding to C-peptide relative to scrambled C-peptide. The first arrow marks the start of the injection and the curve shows the progress in differential binding during sample injection. The second arrow indicates the end of injection and the subsequent stable difference line represents actual binding to C-peptide, i.e. about 100 RU higher than for scrambled C-peptide. Part (b) shows a transient increase in the intracellular Ca^{2+} concentration in human renal tubular cells exposed to 5 nM C-peptide. Changes in intracellular Ca^{2+} were measured by fluorescence from the indicator fura-2/AM (data from reference 35)

segment as an active site in the binding process. Although identification of a functional receptor remains to be reported, the available data on C-peptide's binding to cell membranes provide a molecular basis for its cellular effects, discussed below.

Cellular Effects of C-peptide

Intracellular calcium concentrations C-peptide has been shown to activate Ca^{2+}-dependent intracellular signaling pathways. Exposure of rat renal tubular cells in primary culture to homologous C-peptide in the physiological range results in prompt elevation of intracellular Ca^{2+} [37]. Both the human full-length C-peptide (Figure 2) and its C-terminal pentapeptide, but not scrambled C-peptide, increase intracellular Ca^{2+} in human renal cells, confirming the specificity of the signal [35]. A pentapeptide analogue with Glu replaced by Ala had no effect, emphasizing the importance of this residue for the binding process [23]. Addition of a calcium chelator abolishes the effect of C-peptide, suggesting that it is elicited via influx of extracellular Ca^{2+} [37]. Addition of pertussis toxin also prevents the effect of both C-peptide and the pentapeptide segment on intracellular Ca^{2+}, again indicating G-protein involvement [35].

Mitogen-activated protein kinase phosphorylation C-peptide has been shown to induce phosphorylation of the mitogen-activated protein kinase (MAP-kinase) extracellular signal-regulated kinases (ERK 1/2) in Swiss 3T3 fibroblasts [38]. Moreover, ERK 1/2 phosphorylation is observed in human renal tubular cells upon incubation with homologous C-peptide [39]. Preincubation of the cells with pertussis toxin or with PD98059, a MAP-kinase kinase 1 inhibitor, abolishes this effect. Interestingly, C-peptide stimulated both p38 stress-activated protein kinase (p38 MAP-kinase) and ERK 1/2 activity and phosphorylation in mouse lung capillary endothelial cells [40]. C-peptide stimulation also induces phosphorylation and DNA binding of transcription factors, and these effects are blocked by a p38 MAP-kinase inhibitor, but not by an ERK 1/2 inhibitor. Altogether, these data provide evidence that MAP-kinase phosphorylation is involved in C-peptide signal transduction.

Na^+,K^+-ATPase In experimental and human diabetes, Na^+,K^+-ATPase activity is reduced in several tissues [21, 41]. C-peptide is reported to stimulate Na^+,K^+-ATPase activity under both *in vitro* and *in vivo* conditions. Exposure of rat renal tubular segments to homologous C-peptide results in a concentration-dependent increase in Na^+,K^+-ATPase activity [37, 42, 43] (Figure 3). In rat medullary thick ascending limb cells the effect is mediated via protein kinase Cα (PKCα) [43]. Similarly, studies using human tubular cells in primary culture and ouabain-sensitive uptake of $^{86}Rb^+$ as a marker of Na^+,K^+-ATPase activity have confirmed a concentration-dependent effect of human C-peptide on Na^+,K^+-ATPase activity at physiological concentrations [39]. Interestingly, the C-peptide ability to stimulate Na^+,K^+-ATPase is augmented by more than 2 orders of magnitude in the presence of subthreshold concentrations of neuropeptide Y [37],

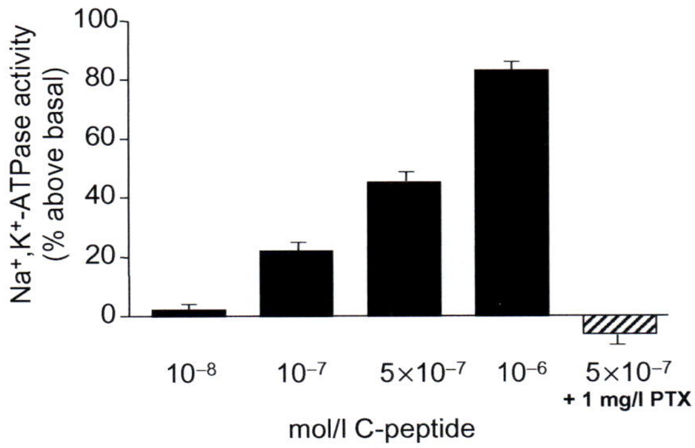

Figure 3 Effect of C-peptide on Na^+,K^+-ATPase activity in rat proximal convoluted tubular segments. The segments were incubated with rising concentrations of rat C-peptide and with pertussis toxin (PTX; 1 μg/ml, 37°C, 4 h) (data from reference 37)

suggesting a possible interaction between the two peptides at sympathetic nerve endings, the primary site of neuropeptide Y release. Pretreatment of tubular segments or cells with pertussis toxin or incubation of the cells in a Ca^{2+}-free medium block the C-peptide effect [37, 39]. Likewise, pretreatment with FK 506, a specific inhibitor of the Ca^{2+}-calmodulin-dependent protein phosphatase 2B, abolishes C-peptide-elicited stimulation of Na^+,K^+-ATPase [37]. The C-terminal pentapeptide is as potent as the full-length C-peptide in stimulating Na^+,K^+-ATPase [39, 42].

Administration of C-peptide to diabetic rats for 2–8 weeks results in partial restoration of nerve Na^+,K^+-ATPase activity [20, 33]. Red blood cell Na^+,K^+-ATPase activity is reduced in type 1 diabetic patients [44, 45] proportionately to the decrease in plasma C-peptide concentration [41], and can be corrected by C-peptide administration [46]. Thus, the available evidence strongly supports the existence of a direct relationship between C-peptide levels and Na^+,K^+-ATPase activity under both *in vitro* and *in vivo* conditions.

Endothelial nitric oxide synthase stimulation Administration of C-peptide to type 1 diabetic patients and to animals with experimental diabetes is accompanied by increased blood flow in several tissues [32, 47–51], reduced vascular resistance, and increased capillary recruitment [52]. Coadministration of a NO-synthase inhibitor completely abolishes the blood flow effects of C-peptide, suggesting that the vasodilatory effect is mediated by stimulation of NO formation in the endothelium [48, 53]. Support for this notion is found in the increased expression of endothelial nitric oxide synthase (eNOS) mRNA levels in lung tissue of rats injected with C-peptide [54]. A stimulatory effect of C-peptide on NO production has also been demonstrated *in vitro*; using a reporter cell assay and bovine aortic endothelial cells, C-peptide increased the release of NO in a concentration- and time-dependent manner [55]. In keeping with the *in vivo* findings, there was no stimulation of NO production in the presence of a NO-synthase inhibitor or when a calcium-binding agent was added to the incubation medium [55]. Likewise, C-peptide, in the presence of small amounts of insulin, is reported to elicit NO-mediated dilatation of rat skeletal muscle arterioles [56]. Taken together, these data demonstrate that C-peptide is capable of eliciting vasodilatation in several tissues and that its effect is mediated via Ca^{2+}-dependent endothelial NO-release.

Besides eliciting vasodilatation, C-peptide-induced stimulation of endothelial NO-release may exert several other effects, e.g. reduction of the adhesion of blood cells to the vascular wall. It has been suggested that C-peptide may exert a cardioprotective effect against leukocyte-mediated reperfusion injury in the isolated rat heart [57]. It has also been shown that C-peptide is a potent inhibitor of leukocyte–endothelium interactions and that this effect is specifically related to inhibition of endothelial cell adhesion molecules via stimulation of NO release from the vascular endothelium [54]. Further studies in this area may improve our understanding of the physiological role and therapeutic potential of C-peptide in disorders of the microcirculation in the diabetic state.

Insulinomimetic effects of C-peptide Additional receptor systems, not involving G-proteins, have also been implicated for C-peptide. Interactions between C-peptide and receptors with catalytic activity are indicated by results showing that C-peptide may attenuate protein tyrosine phosphatase activity [58]. Protein tyrosine phosphatases inactivate the insulin signaling pathway by dephosphorylation of the insulin receptor, insulin receptor substrates, and MAP-kinases. C-peptide at physiological concentrations is reported to mimic insulin effects in myoblasts; it activates insulin receptor tyrosine kinase, insulin receptor substrate-1 tyrosine phosphorylation, PI3-kinase activity, and MAP-kinase phosphorylation [59]. Thus, C-peptide and insulin may exert a synergistic effect on the insulin signaling pathway. It has been suggested that low C-peptide levels may enhance insulin effects, while at supraphysiological concentrations they blunt insulin action [59]. However, C-peptide, unlike insulin, does not activate protein kinase B (Akt), suggesting that C-peptide also works via mechanisms distinct from those of insulin. C-peptide-induced stimulation of glycogen synthesis in myoblasts is blocked by Wortmannin, an inhibitor of PI3-kinase, but not by pertussis toxin [59]. However, another study indicates that C-peptide stimulates glucose transport in human muscle strips without affecting the insulin receptor or tyrosine kinase activation [26]. C-peptide interactions with ligand-gated ion channels coupled to glutamate receptors have also been considered in view of the capacity of free glutamic acid to partly displace C-peptide from cell membranes, and the importance of N-terminal Glu in intact C-peptide and its C-terminal pentapeptide in binding and biological activity [23, 60].

Nonreceptor interactions It has been suggested that the effects of C-peptide may be mediated by a direct membranotropic action, rather than by binding to a stereospecific receptor [21]. Human C-peptide, an all D-amino acid C-peptide, and a retro-sequence C-peptide were all found to partially correct diabetes-induced vascular dysfunction in a rat model of type 1 diabetes [21]. The findings were taken to indicate that the C-peptide effects may have been mediated in a manner similar to that for amphipathic antimicrobial peptides involving pore or ion channel formation [61]. However, direct measurements indicate that C-peptide fails to associate in a stable manner with lipid membranes or micelles [20]. Moreover, C-peptide does not possess the characteristics of a channel-forming peptide; it does not show tendency to self-associate, is overall hydrophilic and negatively charged, and lacks a specific structure in solution [20]. Consequently, it is unlikely that the effects of C-peptide are mediated via conformation-dependent, nonchiral membrane interactions.

In summary, the available information provides a general outline of the intracellular signal transduction pattern for C-peptide (Figure 4). It involves binding to a G-protein coupled membrane receptor, activation of Ca^{2+}-dependent intracellular signaling pathways, and phosphorylation of the MAP-kinase system, eliciting increased activities of both Na^+,K^+-ATPase and eNOS. In addition, some studies indicate that C-peptide and insulin may interact synergistically on the insulin signaling pathway.

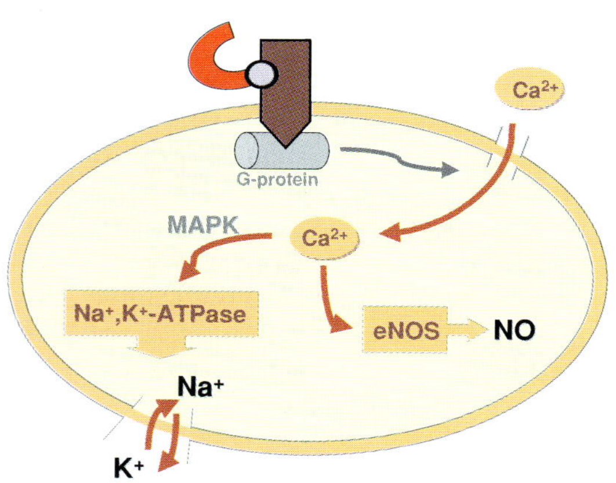

Figure 4 Schematic representation of C-peptide's molecular effects. The available evidence is compatible with the hypothesis that C-peptide binds specifically to a cell membrane receptor coupled to a pertussis toxin sensitive G-protein. The G-protein signal opens Ca^{2+}-channels, resulting in rise of intracellular Ca^{2+} and stimulation of eNOS activity, NO formation, and vasodilatation. There is also stimulation of the MAP-kinase signaling pathway, resulting in augmented Na^+,K^+-ATPase activity. In addition, C-peptide and insulin may interact synergistically on the insulin signaling pathway

Metabolism and Pharmacokinetics of C-peptide

Insulin and C-peptide are secreted from the pancreas in equimolar amounts [8, 62]. Unlike insulin, C-peptide escapes hepatic extraction [63–65]. Approximately 30–50% of the C-peptide secreted in the basal state is removed and catabolized by the kidneys [65, 66], about 20% by skeletal muscle [32], and the remainder elsewhere, possibly as membrane bound to the vascular endothelium. Release of C-peptide in skeletal muscle venous effluent has been observed during physical exercise, suggesting that C-peptide may be reversibly retained by the endothelium [32]. Following an intravenous bolus injection of C-peptide the concentration decay curves can be described as the sum of two exponentials with half disappearance times of approximately 5 and 35 min, respectively [67, 68]. The metabolic clearance rate is independent of the plasma concentration over a wide range and is similar in healthy subjects and in patients with type 1 diabetes [67]. Some studies indicate that when C-peptide is infused intravenously, the plasma concentration fails to change in direct proportion to infusion rate [32, 69]; the observed kinetics require the assumption of a two-compartment model for C-peptide distribution [70].

C-peptide has been used extensively as a peripheral marker of β-cell secretory activity. The validity of this approach depends on several assumptions, the most important being (1) absence of hepatic C-peptide extraction, (2) constant metabolic clearance rate within the physiological concentration range, and (3) distribution kinetics of C-peptide that allow plasma concentrations to accurately reflect secretion rates. Available evidence indicates that assumptions (1) and (2) are fulfilled under most circumstances but (3) may not be valid, at least not under non-steady-state conditions [71]. Despite these limitations, peripheral C-peptide concentrations are very useful for clinical assessments of endogenous insulin secretion under steady-state conditions or when the rate of insulin secretion changes slowly. Likewise, plasma C-peptide measurements are helpful in the evaluation of patients with hypoglycemia, as in the diagnosis of insulinoma.

C-peptide and Nerve Function in Type 1 Diabetes

Peripheral Nerve Effects

A variety of disturbances affecting the peripheral and autonomic nervous system may be encountered in patients with diabetes [72]. The commonest type of neuropathy in diabetes is distal symmetric sensory polyneuropathy, with underlying structural changes consisting of distal axonal degeneration of "dying back" type [73, 74]. There is currently no established causal therapy for diabetic

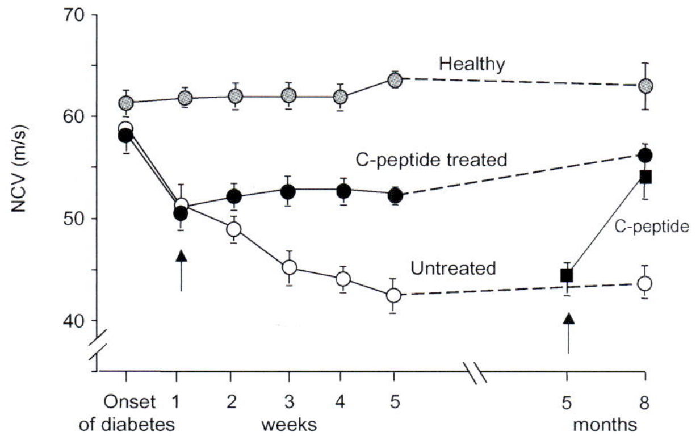

Figure 5 Sciatic-tibial nerve conduction velocity (NCV) in BB/Wor and healthy rats before and after onset of diabetes. Arrows indicate start of C-peptide administration at 1 week or 5 months after onset of diabetes. Data from reference 33

neuropathy; several compounds have been tested, but none has been proven successful so far, because of both limited efficacy and the occurrence of adverse reactions [75, 76].

Studies in animal models of type 1 diabetes and in patients demonstrate that C-peptide replacement has the ability to improve peripheral nerve function and prevent or reverse the development of nerve structural changes. Thus, replacement of C-peptide for 2 months in diabetic BB/Wor rats reduces the development of the acute nerve conduction velocity (NCV; sciatic-tibial nerve) defect by 60% [33]. Administration of C-peptide for 8 months reduces the NCV defect by 70% (Figure 5) and has a beneficial effect on the structural changes that otherwise occur. The latter effect includes prevention of diabetes-induced paranodal swelling, axoglial dysjunction and paranodal demyelination of sural nerve fibers [33]. The introduction of C-peptide treatment after 5 months of diabetes, when neuropathy had become established, led not only to a significant improvement in NCV (+13%) but also to marked repair of diabetes-induced axonal degeneration and increase in nerve fiber regeneration (sural nerve) [33]. The above effects on nerve function and structure in the diabetic rat can be elicited also by human C-peptide, albeit at higher concentrations [21]; increasing doses of human C-peptide result in less marked early structural abnormalities and a rising frequency of regenerating sural nerve fibers, demonstrating not only cross-species activity of human C-peptide but also dose dependency of the C-peptide effect [77]. Neurovascular function in streptozotocin-diabetic rats has been further evaluated in a study involving infusion of rat C-peptide in replacement doses for 2 weeks, starting at 6 weeks after induction of diabetes [48]. Diabetes caused significant reductions in both motor (sciatic) and sensory (saphenous) nerve conduction velocities. C-peptide administration to physiological concentrations prevented 60% of the motor conduction deficit and 80% of the sensory deficit. Coadministration of C-peptide and a NO-synthase inhibitor completely abolished the C-peptide effects on nerve conduction velocity, indicating the involvement of a neurovascular mechanism [48].

Beneficial effects of C-peptide on nerve function have been demonstrated also in type 1 diabetic patients. In a randomized double-blind placebo-controlled study, 46 patients without overt symptoms of diabetic neuropathy and with an average diabetes duration of 10 years were given C-peptide or placebo, together with their regular insulin regimen for 3 months [78]. At the onset of the study, both sensory (sural) and motor (peroneal) nerve conduction velocities were reduced. A significant increase in sensory nerve conduction velocity was recorded after 3 months in the C-peptide group, representing 80% correction of the initial defect. Vibration perception thresholds improved but the motor nerve conduction velocity remained unchanged [78]. Similar findings are reported for a smaller group of patients, in whom lowered thermal perception thresholds were observed after 3 months of C-peptide replacement, suggesting ameliorated sensory nerve function [79]. These data provide evidence of therapeutic improvement of diabetes-induced peripheral nerve dysfunction following C-peptide administration in patients with type 1 diabetes.

Autonomic Nervous System

C-peptide effects have been evaluated in type 1 diabetic patients with early signs of autonomic dysfunction [80]. Patients were studied under normoglycemic conditions and during a 3-h intravenous infusion of either human C-peptide or saline in a double-blind study. Plasma concentrations of C-peptide during the infusion reached levels within the physiological range. Heart rate variability during deep breathing (an index of autonomic, primarily vagal, nerve activity) decreased before the study and rose by 50% during C-peptide infusion [80] (Figure 6). A significant improvement was also seen in the brake index during tilting in those patients who showed a reduced index before the study. Autonomic nerve function has also been evaluated in type 1 diabetic patients receiving C-peptide replacement for 3 months in a double-blind cross-over study [79]. A 20% improvement in heart rate variability was recorded during C-peptide administration, while no change or a slight deterioration was observed in the same patients during the control period.

C-peptide and the Pathogenesis of Neuropathy

The mechanisms involved in the development of distal symmetric sensory polyneuropathy and related forms of diabetic neuropathy are incompletely understood. The discussion of pathogenic mechanisms has focused primarily on two possible causes, metabolic effects mediated

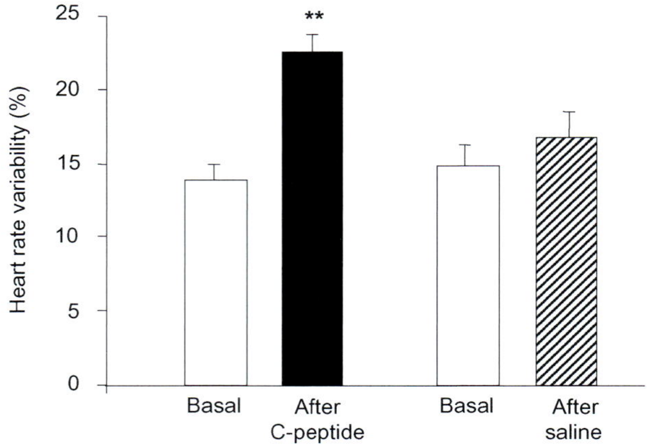

Figure 6 Heart rate variability in type 1 diabetic patients before and during 3 h administration of C-peptide or saline. The infusions were given on different study days 1–2 weeks apart. Asterisks denote a significant difference between data obtained after C-peptide and in the basal state, $P < 0.01$ (data from reference 80)

directly or indirectly by hyperglycemia, and hypoxia caused by microvascular disease, or a combination of the two [73]. The Diabetes Control and Complications Trial documented that strict metabolic control will retard but not prevent the development of diabetic neuropathy, indicating that factors in addition to hyperglycemia and its sequel are of importance [81]. In the context of C-peptide and its influence on nerve function, it is noteworthy that blood glucose levels, HbA_{1c} levels, and insulin requirements remained unchanged in all of the above studies describing positive effects on nerve function and structure. Consequently, it is unlikely that improved metabolic control contributed to the C-peptide effects. Impaired nerve blood flow secondary to perturbed nitric oxide metabolism [82, 83] and reduced levels of nerve Na^+,K^+-ATPase activity [21, 82] are both factors that have been implicated in the pathogenesis of the distal symmetric sensory polyneuropathy [73]. Consequently, it is possible that C-peptide's ability to partially correct the reduced Na^+,K^+-ATPase activity in experimental diabetes [21, 33] contributes to the positive effects of the peptide. In addition, direct measurements of sciatic nerve blood flow in streptozotocin-diabetic rats show that C-peptide administration results in significant amelioration of the diabetes-induced reduction; this effect is elicited via NO release in the endoneural vasculature [48]. Consequently, while the mechanism underlying the beneficial influence of C-peptide on peripheral nerve function and structure and on the autonomic nervous system is not known in detail, it appears likely that improvements elicited by C-peptide in Na^+,K^+-ATPase activity and nerve blood flow are contributory factors. It is recognized that many of the observations were made under *in vitro* conditions or in animal models of diabetes and that the extent to which these findings translate to the human disorder remains to be examined.

C-peptide and Renal Function in Type 1 Diabetes

The early signs of diabetic nephropathy [84, 85] are followed by structural changes [86] and microalbuminuria [87], continuing to overt nephropathy with decreasing glomerular filtration, and clinical albuminuria. The influence of C-peptide administration on renal function and structure in diabetic nephropathy has been examined both in animal models of diabetes and in type 1 diabetic patients, with focus on early stages of the disorder.

In a short-term study of 60-min human C-peptide infusion in streptozotocin-diabetic rats, glomerular hyperfiltration decreased (Figure 7), albumin excretion fell, and renal functional reserve rose [88]. Homologous C-peptide replacement for 14 days was subsequently studied in diabetic rats [89]; glomerular hyperfiltration and reduction of functional reserve were almost completely prevented, and urinary albumin excretion was significantly reduced. Moreover, morphological studies showed that C-peptide replacement partially normalized the diabetes-induced augmentation of glomerular volume [89]. When increasing doses of the human peptide was used in diabetic rats, C-peptide dose-dependently lowered the increased glomerular filtration rate and albumin excretion [90]. Renal function in healthy animals was unresponsive to C-peptide administration [90].

The possible effect of C-peptide on renal function has also been examined in type 1 diabetic patients with varying renal involvement. Short-term C-peptide administration in young, otherwise healthy type 1 diabetic patients reduced the characteristic glomerular hyperfiltration and elicited a small increase in renal blood flow [47]. These observations have been extended to more prolonged administration. In type 1 diabetic patients with hyperfiltration and

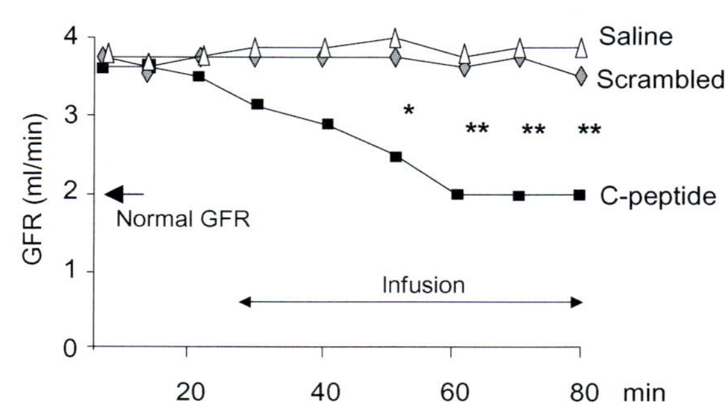

Figure 7 Glomerular filtration rate (GFR) before and during infusion of C-peptide (filled squares), scrambled C-peptide (diamonds), and saline (open triangles) in streptozotocin-diabetic rats. Asterisks denote a significant difference between the C-peptide and saline treated group, $^{*}P < 0.05$ and $^{**}P < 0.01$ (data from reference 88)

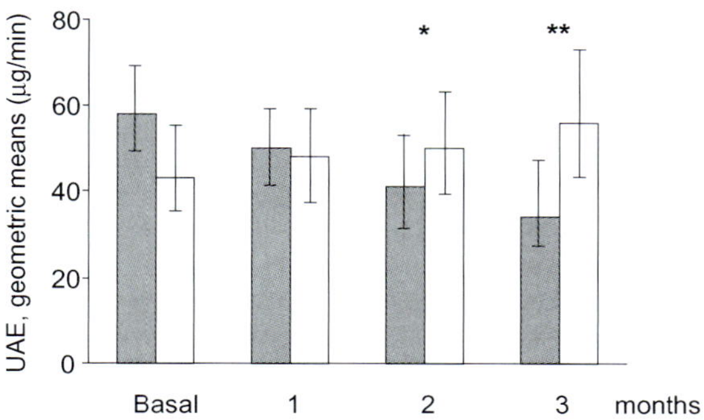

Figure 8 Urinary albumin excretion rate (UAE) in type 1 diabetic given C-peptide plus insulin (filled columns) and placebo plus insulin (open columns) for 3 months. Asterisks denote a significant difference from baseline during the C-peptide treatment period, $^{*}P < 0.05$ and $^{**}P < 0.01$. (data from reference 79)

a low level urinary albumin excretion, C-peptide plus insulin, administered by subcutaneous pump infusion for 4 weeks in a double-blind randomized study [91], elicited reduction of the glomerular hyperfiltration, together with significantly diminished albumin excretion. In a further study, C-peptide was given for 3 months in a double-blind randomized crossover design, together with insulin [79]; urinary albumin decreased progressively during C-peptide treatment but not during the control period (Figure 8). A significant fall in albumin excretion was seen after 2 months, the reduction at the end of the 3-month study amounting to 40%. No change in blood pressure or blood glucose was observed and are therefore unlikely to have contributed to the improvement of renal function. Taken together, the present evidence from studies in diabetic animals and in type 1 diabetic patient supports the view that C-peptide has the ability to limit glomerular hyperfiltration and reduce urinary albumin excretion in the early stages of diabetes-induced renal dysfunction.

C-peptide and the Pathogenesis of Diabetic Nephropathy

The pathogenesis of the characteristic structural and functional abnormalities of the kidneys that frequently accompany diabetes includes both metabolic and hemodynamic factors [92]. Hyperglycemia and glucose-related metabolic processes are likely to contribute to the genesis of renal diabetic complications both directly [93] and by cytokine activation involving, e.g., transforming growth factor (TGF_{β}) [94]. Intraglomerular pressure distribution may be altered in diabetes, leading to increased glomerular pressure even in the absence of systemic hypertension [95]. In addition, decreased erythrocyte deformability in diabetes has been proposed to interfere with glomerular function [96].

The mechanism underlying the beneficial effects of C-peptide on renal function and structure in diabetes is incompletely understood. However, Na^{+},K^{+}-ATPase activity is reduced in kidney cells of diabetic animals [97], and several studies demonstrate that C-peptide effectively stimulates Na^{+},K^{+}-ATPase in glomerular cells [98] and renal tubular segments in a concentration-dependent manner [37, 43]. In addition, stimulation of eNOS activity [55] may increase renal blood flow [47] and possibly modify intraglomerular pressure distribution. Finally, C-peptide has been shown to correct the deficit in red blood cell deformability in type 1 diabetes via stimulation of erythrocyte Na^{+},K^{+}-ATPase activity [99, 100], thereby contributing to improved intraglomerular rheological conditions. Consequently, it can be hypothesized that C-peptide may influence glomerular membrane permeability and transport, as well as the regional circulation of the kidney, possibly accounting for the observed improvement in renal function associated with C-peptide administration.

Other C-peptide Effects

Blood Flow

It has been demonstrated in aortic endothelial cells that C-peptide has the capacity to stimulate eNOS activity via a calcium-dependent mechanism [55]. This effect has also been confirmed *in vivo*; infusion of C-peptide into the brachial artery of type 1 diabetic patients results in an immediate blood flow increase of approximately 35% [53]. The stimulatory effect of C-peptide is abolished when an eNOS inhibitor is coinfused with the peptide, confirming that the effect is mediated via NO release.

Forearm blood flow in type 1 diabetic patients increases in response to intravenous infusion of C-peptide in a concentration-dependent manner in the range 0–1 nM; no additional circulatory effect of C-peptide could be seen when the concentration was raised above 1 nM [49]. This observation is in keeping with the demonstration that the C-peptide binding curve reaches saturation at approximately 1 nM [22]. Forearm vascular dynamics and influence of C-peptide have also been studied during rhythmic forearm exercise in type 1 diabetic patients [32]. Both forearm blood flow and capillary diffusion capacity increased, while vascular resistance decreased in response to C-peptide administration, to levels similar to those observed in healthy subjects. These results and those of a subsequent study using the perfused rat hindquarter model [52] indicate that the circulatory effect of C-peptide is achieved primarily by capillary recruitment. The effect of C-peptide on the endothelial function of the large arteries has been examined in type 1 diabetes, using ultrasound measurements of brachial artery blood flow and vascular diameter during reactive hyperemia [101]. Shear-stress-induced arterial dilatation was reduced in diabetic patients. C-peptide administration resulted in augmented basal blood flow but the response to reactive hyperemia was unchanged, indicating that C-peptide exerts its effect primarily on the distal resistance vessels. A C-peptide-induced improvement in blood flow has been reported not only for forearm tissue, which is mostly muscle [32, 49, 53, 102], but also for skin [103], kidney [47], and nerve [48]. In addition, studies of C-peptide's effect on myocardial blood flow in patients with type 1 diabetes without signs of heart disease, using tissue contrast echocardiography and PET techniques, respectively, have demonstrated marked increases in myocardial blood flow in the basal state [50] and during adenosine-induced myocardial hyperemia [51]. Both studies also showed C-peptide-induced improvements in left ventricular performance as reflected by augmented rates of ventricular contraction and relaxation [50] and increased left ventricular ejection fraction and stroke volume [51]. C-peptide's circulatory effects also involve rheological factors. Erythrocyte deformability is impaired in diabetes [44, 104], with potentially negative effects on the microcirculation. It now emerges that C-peptide is able to ameliorate the altered erythrocyte deformability; this effect is blocked by ouabain, indicating that it is mediated by restoration of Na^+,K^+-ATPase activity [100].

The available evidence thus indicates that in animal models of diabetes and in type 1 diabetic patients, C-peptide stimulates eNOS and local release of NO primarily at the level of the resistance vessels, resulting in capillary recruitment and augmented blood flow in several tissues. Improved rheological conditions secondary to increased erythrocyte deformability may also contribute to the flow augmentation.

Glucose Utilization

C-peptide effects on blood glucose concentration and disposal of an oral glucose load were examined in early studies, but with negative results [5, 6]. However, more recent *in vitro* measurements of glucose transport in skeletal muscle indicate that C-peptide is able to stimulate 3-*O*-methylglucose transport in incubated muscle strips from both healthy subjects and type 1 diabetic patients [105]. The maximal C-peptide effect, seen at 1 nM, was approximately two thirds of the corresponding insulin effect. The mechanism by which this stimulation occurs is not apparent; it does not seem to involve either the insulin receptor or tyrosine kinase activation [26]. C-peptide is reported to stimulate glycogen synthesis in isolated human muscle strips [105] and in L6 myoblasts [59] but the effect could not be confirmed in mouse soleus muscles [106].

In vivo, human C-peptide at supraphysiological concentrations stimulated whole body glucose utilization in streptozotocin-diabetic rats, as determined by euglycemic insulin clamp technique [107]. The two forms of C-peptide in the rat, which differ at two positions (8 and 17), were equipotent in the physiological concentration range in stimulating glucose utilization [108]; raising the C-peptide concentration two- to threefold caused doubling of the basal glucose utilization in diabetic but not in nondiabetic rats. Coinfusion of a NO-synthase inhibitor completely inhibited the C-peptide effect, suggesting a NO-mediated pathway [108].

The stimulatory influence of C-peptide on whole body glucose appears to be less prominent in humans. Type 1 diabetic patients have been studied under euglycemic conditions with infusion of C-peptide at two dose levels in short-term studies. Whole body glucose turnover rose by 20–25% when C-peptide levels were increased to approximately 0.8 nM. No further increase in glucose utilization was observed when C-peptide was raised to 1.9–2.6 nM [47]. Likewise, when C-peptide is infused together with insulin in type 1 diabetic patients, the resultant fall in blood glucose is more marked than when insulin only is administered [109]. The question arises whether the short-term effects of C-peptide on glucose utilization in type 1 diabetic patients, observed in some but not all studies [110], will result in lower blood glucose levels and/or diminished insulin requirements during long-term C-peptide administration. Although not studied directly, this does not seem to be the case because average blood glucose concentrations, levels of HbA_{1c}, and insulin doses were unchanged in patients receiving C-peptide plus insulin for 3 months [78, 79]. In summary, C-peptide's ability to augment glucose utilization under *in vitro* conditions and in animal studies may be NO mediated, and appears to be less pronounced in humans than in rats.

C-peptide and Type 2 Diabetes

In type 2 diabetes both insulin and C-peptide are often elevated initially. Nevertheless, patients frequently develop long-term complications as in type 1 diabetes. It is debated whether the long-term complications of type 1 and type 2 diabetes differ in nature and pathogenesis. It has been suggested that while hyperglycemia is an important factor in both conditions, other contributory factors may also be involved [111–113]. Specifically, C-peptide deficiency has been suggested to be of importance in type 1 diabetes. Limited information is available regarding C-peptide effects in type 2 diabetes. However, physiological concentrations of C-peptide, known to stimulate glucose uptake in muscle strips from healthy subjects or type 1 diabetic patients [26, 105], are reported not to do so in skeletal muscle strips from type 2 diabetic patients [114]. Taken together these findings and previous reports [26, 105] establish in the same experimental model a stimulatory effect of C-peptide on glucose transport in insulin-sensitive, but not insulin-resistant human skeletal muscle [114]. It may be hypothesized that in type 2 diabetes tissue resistance extends to both insulin and C-peptide; the possibility that muscle from type 2 diabetic patients may respond to higher concentrations of C-peptide should be studied.

PROINSULIN

Introduction

Proinsulin is converted into insulin, C-peptide, and conversion intermediates in the β-cells; for a detailed description of proinsulin processing, see references 1 and 115 and Chapter 6 here. The plasma concentration of proinsulin in fasting humans is in the low picomolar range (about 10 pM) and its half-life in the circulation is approximately 90 min. Uptake and degradation by the kidneys appear to be the major route of proinsulin elimination [66, 116]; urinary excretion makes only a minimal contribution [117]. Patients with chronic renal failure show marked elevations of plasma proinsulin concentrations and a prolonged half-life of the peptide [118], in keeping with the findings that renal mechanisms dominate in proinsulin removal. Hepatic extraction of proinsulin is reported to be less than 5% [119]. *In vitro* studies suggest that proinsulin catabolism may also occur via receptor-mediated cellular degradation in muscle, liver, kidney, and other tissues [120, 121], but the extent to which this occurs *in vivo* is not known.

Two major proinsulin conversion intermediates, des-31,32-proinsulin and des-64,65-proinsulin, may be released from the β-cells and are present in plasma [122] in low but approximately equal proportions [122]. Type 2 diabetic patients show consistently increased plasma proinsulin and elevated proinsulin/insulin ratios; with marked hyperglycemia, proinsulin may contribute as much as 50% of the total insulin immunoreactivity [123]. Likewise, the concentrations of proinsulin conversion intermediates are increased in patients with type 2 diabetes [124]. The measurement of proinsulin in plasma is complicated by the presence of the conversion intermediates, but specific immunoradiometric techniques based on monoclonal antibodies are available, making individual analyses possible [125–127]. No extra-pancreatic conversion of proinsulin to insulin has been reported [128].

Proinsulin Binding to Cell Membranes

Proinsulin can bind directly to the insulin receptor in various cell types, albeit with significantly lower affinity [129–131]. This is due to restriction of proinsulin's access to the receptor imposed by the C-peptide segment [132]. Certain biological effects of proinsulin, relating to growth stimulation, may differ from those of insulin [133]. Although there are structural similarities between proinsulin and IGF-I, these effects are unlikely to be mediated via proinsulin binding to the IGF-I receptor, which is minimal [134]. The existence of a specific proinsulin receptor has been suggested [135], and is supported by recent reports of high affinity binding of proinsulin to human umbilical vein endothelial cells [136] and to transformed human lymphoblasts [27]; the role of such receptors is as yet unclear and further study is required to determine whether proinsulin influences growth in some tissues [28]. In this context it is noteworthy that the expression of plasminogen activator inhibitor type 1 in endothelial cells and in visceral adipose tissue *in vitro* is stimulated by both proinsulin and its conversion intermediates [137, 138], with potential clinical effects on the fibrinolytic system [139].

Biological Effects of Proinsulin and Clinical Implications

In vivo studies in humans using the glucose clamp technique indicated that proinsulin's inhibitory effect on hepatic glucose production may be more pronounced than that of insulin [140]. It was therefore suggested that a hepatospecific effect of proinsulin could be advantageous in the treatment of excessive glucose production by the liver in type 2 diabetes. However, extensive clinical testing revealed that the effect of proinsulin on the liver did not differ from that of insulin either in healthy subjects or in patients with diabetes [117]. On account of its longer elimination half-life and lower metabolic clearance rate, proinsulin has been considered for use as an intermediate-acting insulin agonist. However, clinical trials in type 2 diabetic patients failed to document superior effects on glycemic control [117]. Plasma triglyceride and HDL-cholesterol concentrations were improved in 3-month proinsulin-treated patients [141, 142]. It was suggested that in type 2 diabetic patients with hypertriglyceridemia, proinsulin may exert a selective beneficial influence on lipid profiles. Studies of the possible therapeutic use of proinsulin were, however, discontinued following the detection of an unexpected increase in the incidence of myocardial infarction in a clinical study on type 2 diabetic patients, although there was no definite proof of a causal effect of proinsulin [143].

Measurements of plasma proinsulin concentrations are appropriate in the evaluation of patients with hypoglycemia. Proinsulin has been found in human insulinomas [2] and several studies have documented elevated plasma levels of proinsulin in patients with islet cell tumors [144, 145]. Inappropriately increased insulin levels together with elevated proinsulin and C-peptide concentrations in the face of hypoglycemia are diagnostic of islet cell tumors. The elevated proinsulin levels of islet tumors do not appear to be secondary to lack of proconvertases [146] but may be a consequence of defective granule formation, maturation, or secretion [147, 148]. Elevated plasma levels of proinsulin may also be found in multiple endocrine neoplasia type 1 [144].

It is possible that plasma levels of proinsulin may have a role in predicting the risk of developing diabetes or coronary heart disease. In a large, population-based study of type 2 diabetic patients, glucose levels and insulin resistance parameters were directly related to levels of proinsulin or proinsulin/insulin ratios. However, there was no evidence of a relationship between family history of diabetes and proinsulin-related variables, suggesting that elevated proinsulin concentrations and increased proinsulin/insulin ratios primarily reflect increased demands on β-cell secretion caused by hyperglycemia [149]. Proinsulin has also been used in the prediction of coronary heart disease. Thus, in a population-based cohort of 50-year-old men with a follow-up period of 27 years, elevated proinsulin concentrations predicted coronary heart disease related morbidity and death independently of other major risk factors [150].

SUMMARY AND CONCLUSIONS

C-peptide, previously regarded as biologically inert, has now been found to be biologically active. Although the structural variability of C-peptide is considerable, five amino acid residues in the N- and C-terminal regions are conserved in mammals. Available data indicate that C-peptide in nanomolar concentrations binds specifically to cell membranes, probably to a G-protein coupled receptor, resulting in subsequent activation of Ca^{2+}- and MAP-kinase-dependent signaling pathways. C-peptide's binding to cell membranes is stereospecific and the C-terminal pentapeptide segment participates in the process. There is no binding competition with insulin, proinsulin, IGF-I, IGF-II, or neuropeptide Y, but some studies indicate that C-peptide and insulin may exert a synergistic effect on the insulin signaling pathway. C-peptide stimulates Na^+,K^+-ATPase and eNOS activities. C-peptide administration in replacement dosage in animal models of diabetes or in type 1 diabetic patients results in increased blood flow in skeletal muscle, myocardium, kidney, nerve, and skin. C-peptide replacement decreases glomerular hyperfiltration, reduces urinary albumin excretion, and corrects glomerular expansion. It also increases nerve conduction velocity, improves sensory nerve function, and reduces or reverses the characteristic diabetes-induced nodal and paranodal nerve structural changes. It is concluded that C-peptide shows the characteristics of an endogenous peptide hormone. The evidence suggests that replacement of C-peptide together with insulin may be beneficial in patients with type 1 diabetes and serve to retard or prevent the development of long-term complications.

Only a very small proportion of proinsulin is released in its intact form to the circulation in healthy subjects. In contrast, in type 2 diabetes, plasma proinsulin and its conversion intermediates may be higher than in healthy individuals. Proinsulin binds to the insulin receptor with approximately 10% of insulin's affinity. The suggestion of a specific effect of proinsulin in lowering hepatic glucose output has not been verified in direct studies. Clinical trials designed to evaluate the usefulness of proinsulin as an insulin analogue in type 2 diabetic patients were discontinued because of increased incidence of myocardial infarction. Recent reports of specific high affinity proinsulin receptors in several tissues are intriguing and warrant further investigation.

REFERENCES

1. Steiner DF, Bell GI, Rubenstein AH, Chan SJ. Chemistry and biosynthesis of the islet hormones: insulin, islet amyloid polypeptide (amylin), glucagon, somatostatin and pancreatic polypeptide. In DeGroot LJ, Jameson JL (eds) *Endocrinology*. Philadelphia: WB Saunders, 2001; pp 667–96.
2. Steiner DF, Oyer PE. Biosynthesis of insulin and a probable precursor of insulin by a human islet cell adenoma. *Proc Natl Acad Sci USA* 1967; 57: 473–81.
3. Rubenstein AH, Clark JL, Melani F, Steiner DF. Secretion of proinsulin C-peptide by pancreatic beta cells and its circulation in blood. *Nature (Lond)* 1969; 224: 697–9.
4. Heding LG. Radioimmunological determination of human C-peptide in serum. *Diabetologia* 1975; 11: 541–8.
5. Hagen C, Faber OK, Binder C, Alberti KGMM. Lack of metabolic effect of C-peptide in normal subjects and juvenile diabetic patients. *Acta Endocrinol* 1977; 85: 29.
6. Hoogwerf BJ, Bantle JP, Gaenslen HE, Greenberg BZ, Senske BJ, Francis R, Goetz FC. Infusion of synthetic human C-peptide does not affect plasma glucose, serum insulin, or plasma glucagon in healthy subjects. *Metabolism* 1986; 35: 122–5.
7. Steiner DF. The biosynthesis of insulin: generic, evolutionary and pathophysiologic aspects. In Gotshlich EC (ed) *The Harvey Lectures, Series 78*. New York: Academic Press, 1984; pp 191–8.
8. Polonsky KS, Rubenstein AH. C-peptide as a measure of the secretion and hepatic extraction of insulin. Pitfalls and limitations. *Diabetes* 1984; 33: 486–94.
9. Johansson J, Ekberg K, Shafqat J, Henriksson M, Chibalin A, Wahren J, Jörnvall H. Molecular effects of proinsulin C-peptide. *Biochem Biophys Res Commun* 2002; 295: 1035–40.
10. Wahren J, Ekberg K, Johansson J, Henriksson M, Pramanik A, Johansson B-L, Rigler R, Jörnvall H. Role of C-peptide in human physiology. *Am J Physiol Endocrinol Metab* 2000; 278: E759–68.
11. Steiner DF, Rubenstein AH. Proinsulin C-peptide—biological activity? *Science* 1997; 277: 531–2.
12. Zerbini G, Mangili R, Luzi L. Higher post-absorptive C-peptide levels in type 1 diabetic patients without renal complications. *Diabet Med* 1999; 16: 1048–9.
13. Sjöberg S, Gunnarsson R, Gjötterberg M, Lefvert AK, Persson A, Östman J. Residual insulin production, glycemic control and prevalence of microvascular lesions and polyneuropathy in long-term type 1 (insulin-dependent) diabetes mellitus. *Diabetologia* 1987; 30: 208–13.
14. Sjöberg S, Gjötterberg M, Berglund L, Möller E, Östman J. Residual C-peptide excretion is associated with better long-term glycemic control and slower progress of

retinopathy in type 1 (insulin-dependent) diabetes mellitus. *J Diabetes Complications* 1991; 5: 18–22.
15. Fioretto P, Steffes MW, Sutherland DER, Goetz FC, Mauer M. Reversal of lesions of diabetic nephropathy after pancreas transplantation. *N Engl J Med* 1998; 339: 69–75.
16. Navarro X, Sutherland DE, Kennedy WR. Long-term effects of pancreatic transplantation on diabetic neuropathy. *Ann Neurol* 1997; 42: 727–36.
17. Maffi P, Furiani S, Castelnuovo A, DiCarlo V, Galardi G, Pozza G. Relationship between C-peptide levels and diabetic neuropathy in type 1 diabetic patients after islet transplantation. *Diabetes* 1999; 48: A55.
18. Luzi L. Pancreas transplantation and diabetic complications. *N Engl J Med* 1998; 339: 115–7.
19. Jörnvall H, Nordling E, Persson B, Shafqat J, Ekberg K, Wahren J, Johansson J. A structural basis for proinsulin C-peptide activity. *Cell Mol Life Sci* (in press).
20. Henriksson M, Shafqat J, Liepinsh E, Tally M, Wahren J, Jörnvall H, Johansson J. Unordered structure of proinsulin C-peptide in aqueous solution and in the presence of lipid vesicles. *Cell Mol Life Sci* 2000; 57: 337–42.
21. Ido Y, Vindigni A, Chang K, Stramm L, Chance R, Heath WF, DiMarchi RD, DiCera E, Williamson JR. Prevention of vascular and neural dysfunction in diabetic rats by C-peptide. *Science* 1997; 277: 563–6.
22. Rigler R, Pramanik A, Jonasson P, Kratz G, Jansson O, Nygren P-Å, Ståhl S, Ekberg K, Johansson B-L, Uhlén S, Uhlén M, Jörnvall H, Wahren J. Specific binding of proinsulin C-peptide to human cell membranes. *Proc Natl Acad Sci USA* 1999; 96: 13318–23.
23. Pramanik A, Ekberg K, Zhong Z, Shafqat T, Henriksson M, Tally M, Tibell A, Jansson OT, Wahren J, Jörnvall H, Rigler R, Johansson J. C-peptide binding to human cell membranes: importance of Glu^{27}. *Biochem Biophys Res Commun* 2001; 284: 94–8.
24. Hsu SY, Nakabayashi K, Nishi S, Kumagai J, Kudo M, Sherwood OD, Hsueh AJ. Activation of orphan receptors by the hormone relaxin. *Science* 2002; 295: 671–4.
25. Flatt PR, Swanston-Flatt SK, Hampton SM, Bailey CJ, Marks V. Specific binding of the C-peptide of proinsulin to cultured B-cells from a transplantable rat islet cell tumor. *Biosci Rep* 1986; 6: 193–9.
26. Zierath J, Handberg A, Tally M, Wallberg-Henriksson Harriet. C-peptide stimulates glucose transport in isolated human skeletal muscle independent of insulin receptor and tyrosine kinase activation. *Diabetologia* 1996; 39: 306–13.
27. Jehle PM, Lutz MP, Fussgänger RD. High affinity binding sites for proinsulin in human IM-9 lymphoblasts. *Diabetologia* 1996; 39: 421–32.
28. Jehle PM, Fussgänger RD, Angelus NK, Jungwirth RJ, Saile B, Lutz MP. Proinsulin stimulates growth of small intestinal crypt-like cells acting via specific receptors. *Am J Physiol* 1999; 276: E262–8.
29. Eigen M, Rigler R. Sorting single molecules: application to diagnostics and evolutionary biotechnology. *Proc Natl Acad Sci USA* 1994; 91: 5740–7.
30. Maiti S, Haupts U, Webb WW. Fluorescence correlation spectroscopy: diagnostics for sparse molecuales. *Proc Natl Acad Sci USA* 1997; 94: 11753–7.
31. Henriksson M, Pramanik A, Shafqat J, Zhong Z, Tally M, Ekberg K, Wahren J, Rigler R, Johansson J, Jörnvall H. Specific binding of proinsulin C-peptide to detergent-solubilised human skin fibroblasts. *Biochem Biophys Res Commun* 2001; 280: 423–7.
32. Johansson B-L, Linde B, Wahren J. Effects of C-peptide on blood flow, capillary diffusion capacity and glucose utilization in the exercising forearm of Type I (insulin-dependent) diabetic patients. *Diabetologia* 1992; 35: 1151–8.
33. Sima AF, Zhang W, Sugimoto K, Henry D, Li Z, Wahren J, Grunberger G. C-peptide prevents and improves chronic type 1 diabetic neuropathy in the BB/Wor rat. *Diabetologia* 2001; 44: 889–97.
34. Wójcikowski Cz, Maier V, Dominiak K, Fussgänger R, Pfeiffer EF. Effects of synthetic rat C-peptide in normal and diabetic rats. *Diabetologia* 1983; 25: 288–90.
35. Shafqat J, Juntti-Berggren L, Zhong Z, Ekberg K, Köhler M, Berggren P-O, Johansson J, Wahren J, Jörnvall H. Proinsulin C-peptide and its analogues induce intracellular Ca^{2+} increases in human renal tubular cells. *Cell Mol Life Sci* 2002; 59: 1185–9.
36. Shafqat J, Wiberg D, Sigmundson K, Ekberg K, Johansson J, Wahren J, Öberg B, Jörnvall H. Binding to C-peptide of proteins in tissue extracts. *Cell Mol Life Sci* (in press).
37. Ohtomo Y, Aperia A, Sahlgren B, Johansson B-L, Wahren J. C-peptide stimulates rat renal tubular Na^+,K^+ATPase activity in synergism with neuropeptide Y. *Diabetologia* 1996; 39: 199–205.
38. Kitamura T, Kimura K, Okamoto S, Canas X, Sakane N, Yoshida T, Saito M. Proinsulin C-peptide rapidly stimulates mitogen-activated protein kinases in Swiss 3T3 fibroblasts: requirement of protein kinase C, phosphoinositide 3-kinase and pertussis toxin-sensitive G-protein. *Biochem J* 2001; 355: 123–9.
39. Chibalin A, Dumitresco A, Ehrén I, Ekberg K, Wahren J. C-peptide stimulates Na, K-ATPase activity via MAP-kinase dependent pathway in human renal tubular cells. *Diabetologia* 2002; 45 (suppl 2): A350.
40. Kitamura T, Kimura K, Jung BD, Makondo K, Sakane N, Yoshida T, Saito M. Proinsulin C-peptide activates cAMP response element-binding proteins through the p38 mitogen-activated protein kinase pathway in mouse lung capillary endothelial cells. *Biochem J* 2002; 366: 737–44.
41. Dufayet De La Tour D, Raccah D, Jannot MF, Coste T, Rougerie C, Vague P. Erythrocyte Na/K ATPase activity and diabetes: relationship with C-peptide level. *Diabetologia* 1998; 41: 1080–4.
42. Ohtomo Y, Bergman T, Johansson B-L, Jörnvall H, Wahren J. Differential effects of proinsulin C-peptide fragments on Na^+,K^+-ATPase activity of renal tubule segments. *Diabetologia* 1998; 41: 287–91.
43. Tsimaratos MT, Roger F, Chabardès D, Mordasini D, Hasler U, Doucet A, Martin P-Y, Féraille E. C-peptide stimulates Na, K-ATPase via PKC alpha in rat medullary thick ascending limb. *Diabetologia* 2003; 46: 124–31.
44. McMillan DE, Utterback NG, La Puma J. Reduced erythrocyte deformability in diabetes. *Diabetes* 1978; 27: 895–901.
45. Finotti P, Palatini P. Reduction of erythrocyte (Na^+-K^+)ATPase activity in type 1 (insulin-dependent) diabetic subjects and its activation by homologous plasma. *Diabetologia* 1986; 26: 623–8.
46. Forst T, Dufayet De La Tour D, Kunt T, Pfützner A, Goitom K, Pohlmann T, Schneider S, Johansson B-L, Wahren J, Löbig M, Engelbach M, Beyer J, Vague P. Effects of proinsulin C-peptide on nitric oxide, microvascular blood flow and erythrocyte Na^+K^+ATPase

activity in diabetes mellitus type 1. *Clin Sci* 2000; 98: 283–90.
47. Johansson B-L, Sjöberg S, Wahren J. The influence of human C-peptide on renal function and glucose utilization in Type I (insulin-dependent) diabetic patients. *Diabetologia* 1992; 35: 121–8.
48. Cotter M, Cameron N. C-peptide effects on nerve conduction and blood flow in streptozotocin-induced diabetic rats: modulation by nitric oxide synthase inhibition. *Diabetes* 2001; 50: A184.
49. Ekberg K, Johansson B-L, Wahren J. Stimulation of blood flow by C-peptide in patients with type 1 diabetes. *Diabetologia* 2001; 44 (suppl 1): A323.
50. Hansen A, Johansson B-L, Wahren J, von H Bibra. C-peptide exerts beneficial effects on myocardial blood flow and function in patients with type 1 diabetes. *Diabetes* 2002; 51: 3077–82.
51. Johansson B-L, Sundell J, Ekberg K, Jonsson C, Wahren J, Nuutila P, Knuuti J, Raitakari O, Seppänen M, Luotolahti M. Adenosine-induced myocardial vasodilatation is improved by C-peptide in type 1 diabetes. *Diabetologia* 2002; 45 (suppl 2): A197.
52. Lindström K, Johansson C, Johnsson E, Haraldsson B. Acute effects of C-peptide on the microvasculature of isolated perfused skeletal muscle and kidneys in rat. *Acta Physiol Scand* 1996; 156: 19–25.
53. Johansson B-L, Pernow J, Wahren J. Muscle vasodilatation by C-peptide is NO-mediated. *Diabetologia* 1999; 42 (suppl 1): A324.
54. Scalia R, Coyle KM, Levine BJ, Booth G, Lefer AM. C-peptide inhibits leukocyte–endothelium interaction in the microcirculation during endothelial dysfunction. *FASEB J* 2000; 14: 2357–64.
55. Kunt T, Forst T, Closs E, Wallerath U, Förstermann R, Lehamnn R, Pfützner A, Harzer O, Engelback M, Beyer J. Activation of endothelial nitric oxide synthase (eNOS) by C-peptide. *Diabetologia* 1998; 41: A176.
56. Jensen JM, Messina EJ. C-peptide induces a concentration-dependent dilation of skeletal muscle arterioles only in presence of insulin. *Am J Physiol Heart Circ* 1999; 276: H1223–8.
57. Young L, Ikeda Y, Scalia R, Lefer AM. C-peptide exerts cardioprotective effects in myocardial ischemia-reperfusion. *Am J Physiol Heart Circ* 2000; 279: H1453–9.
58. Li Z-G, Qiang X, Sima AAF, Grunberger G. C-peptide attenuates protein tyrosine phosphatase activity and enhances glycogen synthesis in L6 myoblasts. *Biochem Biophys Res Commun* 2001; 280: 615–9.
59. Grunberger G, Qiang X, Li Z, Mathews ST, Sbrissa D, Shisheva A, Sima AAF. Molecular basis for the insulinomimetic effects of C-peptide. *Diabetologia* 2001; 44: 1247–57.
60. Bourguignon JP, Alvarez Gonzalez ML, Gerard A, Franchimont P. Gonadotropin relasing hormone inhibitory autofeed back by subproducts antagonist at *N*-methyl-D-aspartate receptors: a model of autocrine regulation of peptide secretion. *Endocrinology* 1994; 134: 1589–92.
61. Bessalle R, Kapitkovsky A, Gorea A, Shalit I, Fridkin M. All-D-magainin: chirality, antimicrobial activity and proteolytic resistance. *FEBS Lett* 1990; 274: 151–5.
62. Polonsky KS, Rubenstein AH. Current approaches to measurements of insulin secretion. *Diab Metab Rev* 1986; 2: 315–29.
63. Polonsky KS, Jaspan JB, Pugh W, Cohen D, Schneider M, Schwartz T, Moossa AR, Tager HS, Rubenstein AH. The metabolism of C-peptide in the dog: in vivo demonstration of the absence of hepatic extraction. *J Clin Invest* 1983; 72: 1114–23.
64. Bratusch-Marrain P, Waldhäusl WK, Gasic S, Hofer A. Hepatic disposal of biosynthetic human insulin and porcine proinsulin in humans. *Metabolism* 1984; 33: 151–7.
65. Sjöberg S, Johansson B-L, Östman J, Wahren J. Renal and splanchnic exchange of human biosynthetic C-peptide in Type I (insulin-dependent) diabetes mellitus. *Diabetologia* 1991; 34: 423–8.
66. Henriksen JH, Tronier B, Bülow JB. Kinetics of circulating endogenous insulin, C-peptide, and proinsulin in fasting nondiabetic man. *Metabolism* 1987; 36: 463–8.
67. Faber OK, Hagen C, Binder C, Markussen J, Naithani VK, Blix PM, Kuzuya H, Horwitz DL, Rubenstein AH, Rossing N. Kinetics of human connecting peptide in normal and diabetic subjects. *J Clin Invest* 1978; 62: 197–203.
68. Licinia-Paixao J, Polonsky K, Given BD, Pugh W, Ostrega D, Frank BH, Rubenstein A. Ingestion of a mixed meal does not affect the metabolic clearance rate of biosynthetic human C-peptide. *J Clin Endocrinol Metab* 1986; 63: 401–3.
69. Polonsky K, Licinia-Paixao J, Given BD, Pugh W, Rue P, Galloway J, Karrison T, Frank B. Use of biosynthetic human C-peptide in the measurement of insulin secretion rates in nirmal volunteers and Type 1 diabetic patients. *J Clin Invest* 1986; 77: 98–105.
70. Eaton RP, Allen RC, Schade DS, Erickson KM, Standefer J. Prehepatic insulin production in man: kinetic analysis using peripheal connecting peptide behaviour. *J Clin Endocrinol Metab* 1980; 51: 520–8.
71. Van Cauter E, Mestrez F, Sturis J, Polonsky K. Estimation of insulin secretion rates from C-peptide levels: comparison of individual and standard kinetic parameters for C-peptide clearance. *Diabetes* 1992; 41: 368–77.
72. Watkins PJ, Thomas PK. Diabetes mellitus and the nervous system. *J Neurol Neurosurg Psychiatry* 1998; 65: 620–32.
73. Thomas PK. Diabetic neuropathy: mechanisms and future treatment options. *J Neurol Neurosurg Psychiatry* 1999; 67: 277–9.
74. Said G, Slama G, Selva J. Progressive centripetal degeneration of axons in small fibre diabetic polyneuropathy. *Brain* 1983; 106: 791–807.
75. Jaspan JB, Towle VL, Maselli R, Herold K. Clinical studies with an aldose reductase inhibitor in the autonomic and somatic neuropathies of diabetes. *Metabolism* 1986; 35: 83–92.
76. Foppiano M, Lombardo G. Worldwide pharmacovigilance systems and tolrestat withdrawal. *Lancet* 1997; 349: 399–400.
77. Zhang W, Yorek M, Pierson CR, Murakawa Y, Breidenbach A, Sima AAF. Human C-peptide dose dependently prevents early neuropathy in the BB/Wor rat. *Int J Experimental Diab Res* 2001; 2: 187–93.
78. Ekberg K, Brismar T, Johansson B-L, Jonsson B, Lindström P, Wahren J. Amelioration of sensory nerve dysfunction by C-peptide in patients with type 1 diabetes. *Diabetes* 2003; 52: 536–41.

79. Johansson B-L, Borg K, Fernqvist-Forbes E, Kernell A, Odergren T, Wahren J. Beneficial effects of C-peptide on incipient nephropathy and neuropathy in patients with type I diabetes—a three-month study. *Diabe Medi* 2000; 17: 181–9.
80. Johansson B-L, Borg K, Fernqvist-Forbes E, Odergren T, Remahl S, Wahren J. C-peptide improves autonomic nerve function IDDM patients. *Diabetologia* 1996; 39: 687–95.
81. DCCT Group. The effect of intensive diabetes therapy on the development and progression of neuropathy. *Ann Intern Med* 1995; 122: 561–8.
82. Stevens MJ, Dananberg J, Feldman EL, Lattimer SA, Kamijo M, Thomas TP, Shindo H, Sima AA, Greene DA. The linked roles of nitric oxide, aldose reductase and (Na^+/K^+)-ATPase in the slowing of nerve conduction in the streptozotocin diabetic rat. *J Clin Invest* 1994; 94: 853–9.
83. Cameron NE, Cotter MA, Basso M, Hohman TC. Comparison of the effects of inhibitors of aldose reductase and sorbitol dehydrogenase on neurovascular function, nerve conduction and tissue polyol pathway metabolites in streptozotocin-diabetic rats. *Diabetologia* 1997; 40: 271–81.
84. Krolewski AS, Warram JH, Christlieb AR, Busick EJ, Kahn CR. The changing natural history of nephropathy in type I diabetes. *Am J Med* 1985; 78: 785–94.
85. Bosch JP, Saccaggi A, Lauer A, Ronco C, Belledonne M, Glabman S. Renal functional reserve in humans. Effect of protein intake on glomerular filtration rate. *Am J Med* 1983; 75: 943–50.
86. Fioretto P, Steffes MW, Brown DM, Mauer SM. An overview of renal pathology in insulin-dependent diabetes mellitus in relationship to altered glomerular hemodynamics. *Am J Kidney Dis* 1992; 20: 549–58.
87. Mogensen CE. Prediction of clinical diabetic nephropathy in IDDM patients. Alternatives to microalbuminuria? *Diabetes* 1990; 39: 761–7.
88. Sjöquist M, Huang W, Johansson B-L. Effects of C-peptide on renal function at the early stage of experimental diabetes. *Kidney Int* 1998; 54: 758–64.
89. Samnegård B, Jacobson S, Jaremko G, Johansson B-L, Sjöquist M. Effects of C-peptide on glomerular and renal size and renal function in diabetic rats. *Kidney Int* 2001; 60: 1258–65.
90. Huang D-Y, Richter K, Breidenbach A, Vallon V. Human C-peptide acutely lowers glomerular hyperfiltration and proteinuria in diabetic rats: a dose–response study. *Naunyn Schmiedebergs Arch Pharmacol* 2002; 365: 67–73.
91. Johansson B-L, Kernell A, Sjöberg S, Wahren J. Influence of combined C-peptide and insulin administration on renal function and metabolic control in diabetes type 1. *J Clin Endocrinol Metab* 1993; 77: 976–81.
92. Cooper ME. Pathogenesis, prevention and treatment of diabetic nephropathy. *Lancet* 1998; 352: 213–9.
93. Vlassara H. Protein glycation in the kidney: role in diabetes and aging. *Kidney Int* 1996; 49: 1795–804.
94. Gilbert RE, Cox A, Dziadek M, Cooper ME, Jerums G. Extracellular matrix and its interactions in the diabetic kidney: a molecular biological approach. *J Diabetes Complications* 1995; 9: 252–4.
95. Zatz R, Dunn BR, Meyer TW, Brenner B. Prevention of diabetic glomerulopathy by pharmacological amelioration of glomerular capillary hypertension. *J Clin Invest* 1986; 77: 1925–30.
96. Simpson LO. Intrinsic stiffening of red blood cells as the fundamental cause of diabetic nephropathy and microangiopathy: a new hypothesis. *Nephron* 1985; 39: 344–51.
97. Wald HP, Scherzer P, Rasch R, Popovtzer MM. Renal tubular Na^+-K^+-ATPase in diabetes mellitus: relationship to metabolic abnormality. *Am J Physiol* 1993; 265: F96–101.
98. Körner A, Wahren J, Johansson B-L, Aperia A. Effect of C-peptide on glomerular Na^+,K^+-ATPase activity in streptozotocin diabetic rats. *Diabetologia* 2000; 43 (suppl 1): A258.
99. Djemli-Shipkolye A, Gallice P, Coste T, Jannot MF, Tsimaratos M, Raccah D, Vague P. The effects ex vivo and in vitro of insulin and C-peptide in Na/K adenosine triphosphatase activity red blood cell membranes of type 1 diabetic patient. *Metbolism* 2000; 49: 868–72.
100. Kunt T, Schneider S, Pfützner A, Goitum K, Engelbach M, Schauf B, Beyer J, Forst T. The effect of human proinsulin C-peptide on erythrocyte deformability in patients with type 1 diabetes mellitus. *Diabetologia* 1999; 42: 465–71.
101. Fernqvist-Forbes E, Johansson B-L, Eriksson MJ. Effects of C-peptide on forearm blood flow and brachial artery dilatation in patients with type 1 diabetes. *Acta Physiol Scand* 2001; 172: 159–65.
102. Johansson B-L, Pernow J. C-peptide potentiates the vasoconstrictor effect of neuropeptide Y in insulin dependent diabetic patients. *Acta Physiol Scand* 1999; 165: 39–44.
103. Forst T, Kunt T, Pohlmann T, Goitom K, Engelbach M, Beyer J, Pfützner A. Biological activity of C-peptide on the skin microcirculation in patients with insulin dependent diabetes mellitus. *J Clin Invest* 1998; 101: 2036–41.
104. Ernst E, Matrai A. Altered red and white blood cell rheology in type II diabetes. *Diabetes* 1986; 35: 1412–5.
105. Zierath J, Galuska D, Johansson B-L, Wallberg-Henriksson H. Effect of human C-peptide on glucose transport in in vitro incubated human skeletal muscle. *Diabetologia* 1991; 34: 899–901.
106. Shashkin PN, Jiao Y, Westerblad H, Katz A. C-peptide does not alter carbohydrate metabolism in isolated mouse muscle. *Am J Physiol* 1997; 272: E245–7.
107. Wu W, Oshida Y, Yang W-P, Ohsawa I, Sato J, Iwao S, Johansson B-L, Wahren J, Sato Y. Effect of C-peptide administration on whole body glucose utlilization in STZ-induced diabetic rats. *Acta Physiol Scand* 1996; 157: 253–8.
108. Ling L, Oshida Y, Kusunoki M, Yamanouchi K, Johansson B-L, Wahren J, Sato Y. Rat C-peptide I and II stimulate glucose utilization in STZ-induced diabetic rats. *Diabetologia* 1999; 42: 958–64.
109. Oskarsson P, Johansson B-L, Adamson U, Lins P-E. Effects of C-peptide on insulin-induced hypoglyaemia and its counterregulatory responses in IDDM patients. *Diabet Med.* 1997; 14: 655–9.
110. Forst T, Rave K, Pfüetzner A, Buchholz R, Pohlmann T, Heinemann L. Effect of C-peptide on glucose metabolism in patients with type 1 diabetes. *Diabetes Care* 2002; 25: 1096–7.
111. Dalla Vestra M, Saller A, Bortoloso E, Mauer M, Fioretto P. Structural involvement in type 1 and type 2 diabetic nephropathy. *Diabetes Metab* 2000; 26 (suppl 4): 8–14.

112. Schmitz A, Gundersen HJ, Österby R. Glomerular morphology by light microscopy in non-insulin-dependent diabetes mellitus. Lack of glomerular hypertrophy. *Diabetes* 1988; 37: 38–43.
113. Sima AFF, Sugimoto K. Experimental diabetic neuropathy: an update. *Diabetologia* 1999; 42: 773–88.
114. Zierath J. In vitro studies of human skeletal muscle: hormonal and metabolic regulation of glucose transport. *Acta Physiol Scand* 1995; 155 (suppl 626): 1–96.
115. Steiner DF. New aspects of proinsulin and pathophysiology. *J Pediatr Endocrinol Metab* 2000; 13: 229–39.
116. Katz AI, Rubenstein AH. Metabolism of proinsulin, insulin and C-peptide in the rat. *J Clin Invest* 1973; 52: 1113–21.
117. Galloway JA, Hooper SA, Spradlin CT, Howey DC, Frank BH, Bowsher RR, Anderson JH. Review of chemistry, in vitro and in vivo receptor binding, animal and human pharmacology studies and clinical trial experience. *Diabetes Care* 1992; 15: 666–92.
118. Jaspan JB, Mako ME, Kuzuya H, Blix PM, Horowitz DL, Rubenstein A. Abnormalities in circulating beta cell peptides in chronic renal failure: comparison of C-peptide, proinsulin and insulin. *J Clin Endocrinol Metab* 1977; 45: 441–6.
119. Waldhaüsl WK, Bratusch-Marrain P, Gasic S, Komjati M, Heding L. Inhibition by proinsulin of endogenous C-peptide release in healthy man. *Am J Physiol* 1986; 251: E139–45.
120. Podlecki DA, Frank BH, Olefsky JM. In vitro characterization of biosynthetic human proinsulin. *Diabetes* 1984; 33: 111–8.
121. Ciaraldi TP, Brady D, Olefsky JM. Kinetics of biosynthetic human proinsulin action in isolated rat adipocytes. *Diabetes* 1986; 35: 318–23.
122. De Haen C, Little SA, May JM, William RH. Characterization of proinsulin–inslin intermediates in human plasma. *J Clin Invest* 1978; 62: 727–37.
123. Saad M, Kahn SE, Nelson R, Pettitt DJ, Knowler WC, Schwartz MW, Kowalyk S, Bennett PH, Porte D Jr. Disproportionately elevated proinsulin in Pima Indians with noninsulin-dependent diabetes mellitus. *J Clin Endocrinol Metab* 1990; 70: 1247–53.
124. Kahn SE, Halban PA. Release of incompletely processed proinsulin is the cause of the disproportionate proinuslinemia of NIDDM. *Diabetes* 1997; 46: 1725–32.
125. Temple RC, Carrington CA, Luzio SD, Owens DR, Schneider AE, Sobey WJ, Hales CN. Insulin deficiency in non-insulin-dependent diabetes. *Lancet* 1989; 1: 293–5.
126. Temple RC, Clark PM, Nagi DK, Schneider AE, Yudkin JS, Hales CN. Radioimmunoassay may overestimate insulin in non-insulin-dependent diabetics. *Clin Endocrinol (Oxf)* 1990; 32: 689–93.
127. Zilker TR, Rainbow SJ, Hales CN, Saldern S, Gray IP. Determination of proinsulin intermediates by means of an immunoradiometric method using polyclonal antibodies. *Horm Metab Res* 1988; 18 (suppl): 48–55.
128. Root MA, Ellis RM, Chance RE, Galloway JA. Preparation and use of purified porcine proinsulin antiserum. *Diabetes* 1970; 19: 359–65.
129. Freychet P. The interaction of proinsulin with insulin receptors on the plasma membrane in the liver. *J Clin Invest* 1974; 54: 1020–31.
130. Peavy DE, Abram JD, Frank BH, Duckworth WC. In vitro activity of biosynthetic human proinsulin: receptor binding and biological potency of proinsulin and insulin in isolated rat adipocytes. *Diabetes* 1984; 33: 1062–7.
131. Yu SS, Kitabchi AE. Biological activity of proinsulin and related polypeptides in the fat tissue. *J Biol Chem* 1973; 248: 3753–61.
132. Gliemann J, Sorenson HH. Assay of insulin-like activity by the isolated fat cell method, IV: the biological activity of proinsulin. *Diabetologia* 1970; 6: 499–504.
133. Nissley SP, Rechler MM, Moses AC, Short PA, Podskalny JM. Proinsulin binds to a growth peptide receptor and stimulates DNA synthesis in chick embryo fibroblasts. *Endocrinology* 1977; 101: 708–16.
134. Gruppuso PA, Frank BH, Schwartz R. Binding of proinsulin and proinsulin conversion intermediates to human placental insulin-like growth factor I receptors. *J Clin Endocrinol Metab* 1988; 67: 194–7.
135. Rausch UW, Fussgänger RD. Qualitative dissimilarities of insulin and proinsulin binding and action in vitro at IM-9-lymphocytes. *Horm Metab Res* 1988; 18: 89–92.
136. Faehling M, Fussgänger RD, Jehle PM. High affinity binding sites for proinsulin on human umbilical vein endothelial cells (HUVEC). *Diabetologia* 1999; 42: 259–60.
137. Schneider DJ, Nordt TK, Sobel BE. Stimulation by proinsulin of expression of plasminogen activator inhibitor type-1 in endothelial cells. *Diabetes* 1992; 41: 890–5.
138. Nordt TK, Bode C, Sobel BE. Stimulation in vivo of expression of intra-abdominal adipose tissue plasminogen activator inhibitor Type 1 by proinsulin. *Diabetologia* 2001; 44: 1121–4.
139. Lindahl B, Dinesen B, Eliasson M, Roder M, Jansson JH, Huhtasaari F, Hallmans G. High proinsulin concentration preceedes acute myocardial infarction in a nondiabetic population. *Metabolism* 1999; 48: 1197–202.
140. Revers RR, Henry R, Schmeiser L, Kolterman O, Cohen R, Bergenstal R, Polonsky K, Jaspan J, Rubenstein A, Frank B, Galloway JA, Olefsky JM. The effects of biosynthetic human proinsulin on carbohydrate metabolism. *Diabetes* 1984; 33: 762–70.
141. Drexel H, Hopferwieser T, Braunsteiner H, Patsch JR. Effects of biosynthetic human proinsulin on plasma lipids in type 2 diabetes mellitus. *Klin Wochenschr* 1988; 66: 1171–4.
142. Winocour PH, Mallik TH, Ishola M, Baker RD, Bhatnagar D, Durrington PN, Anderson DC. A randomized cross-over study of the effects on proinsulin on lipid metabolism in type 2 diabetes. *Diabet Med* 1991; 8: 22–7.
143. Spradlin CT, Galloway JA, Anderson JH. Apparent increase in coronary heart disease with human proinsulin (HPI)—randomization failure or HPI effect? *Diabetologia* 1990; 33 (suppl): A60.
144. Gordon P, Sjarulis MC, Roach P, Comi RJ, Fraker DL, Norton JA, Alexander HR, Doppman JL. Plasma proinsulin-like component in insulinoma: a 25-year experience. *J Clin Endocrinol Metab* 1995; 80: 2884–7.
145. Nakamori S, Ishikawa O, Ohigashi H, Sasakuma F, Shimizu T, Nakaizumi A, Furukawa H, Sasaki Y, Imaoka S. Increased blood proinsulin and decreased C-peptide levels in patients with pancreatic cancer. *Hepatogastroenerology* 1999; 46: 16–24.
146. Azzoni C, D'Adda T, Tamburrano G, Coscelli C, Madsen OD, Scopsi L, Bordi C. Functioning human insulinomas. An immunohistochemical analysis of intracellular insulin processing. *Virchows Arch* 1998; 433: 495–504.

147. Roth J, Komminoth P, Heitz P. Topograpical abnormalities of proinsulin to insulin conversion in functioning human insulinomas. Comparison of immunoelectron microscopic and clinical data. *Am J Pathol* 1995; 147: 489–502.
148. Hiura A, Kim E-C, Ikahara T, Mishima K, Shindo K, Ohta T, Satake K. Insulinoma with hyperproinsulinemia during hypoglycemia and loss of expression of vascular-type H^+-ATPase (V-ATPase) in the tumor tissue. *Int J Pancreatol* 1999; 25: 11–6.
149. Grill V, Dinesen B, Crlsson S, Efendic S, Pedersen O, Östenson C-G. Hyperproinsulinemia and proinsulin-to-insulin ratios in Swedish middle-aged men: association with glycemia and insulin resistance but not with family history of diabetes. *Acta Endocrinol* 2002; 155: 834–41.
150. Zethelius B, Byberg L, Hales N, Lithell H, Berne C. Proinsulin is an independent predictor of coronary heart disease. *Circulation* 2002; 105: 2153–8.

11

Biosynthesis, Secretion, and Action of Glucagon

Pierre J. Lefèbvre

University of Liège, Liège, Belgium

Glucagon, discovered in 1923 as a contaminant of early insulin preparations, has long been a neglected hormone. Our knowledge of the physiology of glucagon is based on the work of Stahl, Foà, Sutherland, and de Duve and on the work performed since the late 1950s in Dallas by Unger and his coworkers, joined in the 1970s by Orci and his team in Geneva. Glucagon was among the very first polypeptide hormones to be isolated, purified, sequenced, and synthesized. Thanks to the pioneer work of Unger, it was the second polypeptide hormone to become measurable by radioimmunoassay, only a few months after insulin. It has served two Nobel Prize winners as a unique tool, which permitted Sutherland and his associates to discover cyclic AMP (cAMP), and Rodbell and his coworkers to discover the role of G-proteins in cell-membrane receptors. Subsequently, the nucleotide sequence of the glucagon gene has been determined and the structure of the human glucagon precursor (preproglucagon) has been deduced. This discovery has been fundamental for clarifying the relationships of glucagon itself with various other peptides derived from the same common precursor, and originating from both the pancreas and the gut. A comprehensive bibliography on glucagon, up to 1983, has been edited by Lefèbvre [1] and subsequently updated [2, 3]. Dr D. Drucker in Toronto maintains a Web site (http://www.glucagon.com) where information on glucagon and its related peptides is permanently updated.

AMINO ACID COMPOSITION, EXTRACTION, SYNTHESIS, AND BIOSYNTHESIS

The amino acid sequence is identical for glucagon isolated from the pancreas of pigs, cattle, and humans. Guinea-pig glucagon is different from all other glucagons that have been isolated, while avian glucagons differ from the predominant mammalian glucagon only by a few conservative replacements. This extreme conservation of primary structure exhibited by glucagon has been considered "at least unusual and at most extraordinary" [4]. In fact, it has now been recognized that glucagon belongs to what has been called the pituitary adenylate cyclase activating polypeptide (PACAP)/glucagon superfamily that includes nine hormones that are related by structure, distribution (especially the brain and the gut), function (often by activation of cAMP), and receptors (a subset of seven *trans*-membrane receptors) [5]. The nine hormones include glucagon, GLP-1 (glucagon-like peptide 1), GLP-2 (glucagon-like peptide 2), GIP (gastric inhibitory polypeptide), GRF (growth-hormone-releasing factor), PHM (peptide histidine methionine), PACAP, secretin, and VIP (vasoactive intestinal peptide). The origin of the ancestral superfamily members is at least as old as the invertebrates. The most ancient and tightly conserved members are PACAP and glucagon. As reviewed by Sherwood et al. [5] evidence to date suggests that the superfamily began with a gene or exon duplication and then continued to diverge with some gene duplications in vertebrates. Mammalian glucagon contains 29 amino acid residues and has a molecular mass of 3485 Da (Figure 1). Glucagon can be synthesized *in vitro* by either classic solution synthesis or solid-phase synthesis; in both cases, two substrategies can be used—either fragment assembly or stepwise assembly [6]. All procedures have given highly purified materials that are homogeneous and indistinguishable from natural glucagon by a range of sensitive analytic methods. The *glucagon gene* has been extensively

International Textbook of Diabetes Mellitus, Third Edition. Edited by R. A. DeFronzo, E. Ferrannini, H. Keen, and P. Zimmet.
 ISBN: 0-471-48655-8.

H-His-Ser-Gln-Gly-Thr-Phe-Thr-Ser-Asp-Tyr-Ser-Lys-Tyr-Leu-Asp-
1 2 3 4 5 6 7 8 9 10 11 12 13 14 15

Ser-Arg-Arg-Ala-Gln-Asp-Phe-Val-Gln-Trp-Leu-Met-Asn-Thr-OH
16 17 18 19 20 21 22 23 24 25 26 27 28 29

Figure 1 The primary structure of human–porcine glucagon

investigated by Habener and his coworkers (see review in reference 7). Consisting of six exons and five introns spanning 10 kb, the human glucagon gene is located on chromosome 2. It encodes for a preprohormone of 180 amino acids that contains not only glucagon but several other peptides including two glucagon-like peptides whose amino acid structures are distinct from, but closely resemble, that of glucagon and other members of the glucagon superfamily of peptides. The glucagon gene is expressed in the A-cells of the islets of Langerhans, the intestinal L-cells, and in some parts of the brain. While the functional relevance of glucagon gene expression in the brain is still poorly understood, a better image has recently emerged regarding the processing of proglucagon into several bioactive peptides in the pancreas and in the gut [8] (Figure 2).

In the pancreas glucagon is the predominant peptide produced, together with glucagon-related polypeptide (GRPP), while the glucagon-like peptides remain in an incompletely processed prohormone fragment. *In the gut* two glucagon-like peptides (GLP-1 and GLP-2) are produced, while glucagon remains, in part, as a prohormone fragment, glicentin. However, glicentin can be further processed to oxyntomodulin and GRPP. Of these peptides of the glucagon superfamily, oxyntomodulin and

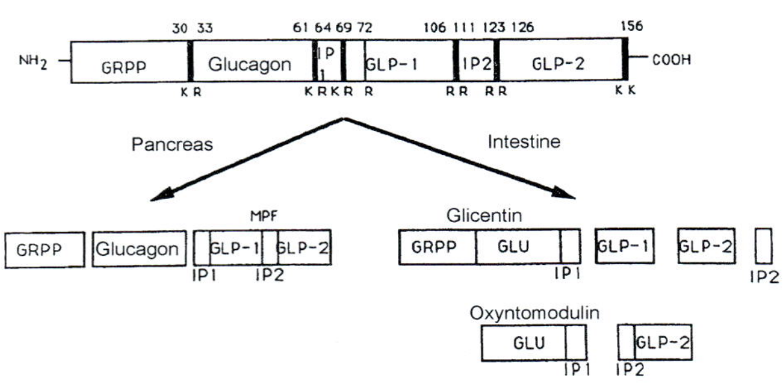

Figure 2 Differential processing of proglucagon in the pancreas and large intestine. Peptides released from the pancreas are glucagon, and the amino- and carboxy-terminal ends of the precursor, respectively. Very small amounts of GLP-1 are also liberated. Glicentin (GRPP + glucagon + IP1), GLP-1, GLP-2, IP2, and oxyntomodulin (glucagon + IP1) are secreted from the intestinal L-cells. The amino- and carboxy-terminal ends of proglucagon are indicated by NH_2 and COOH, respectively. Numbers refer to the first and last amino acids of processed peptides, starting from the first amino acid of proglucagon. K (lysine) and R (arginine) indicate basic amino acids where processing sites have been localized. IP: intervening peptide (from reference 7, with permission, ©1991, The Endocrine Society)

possibly glicentin are implicated in the physiological negative control of gastric acid secretion. On the other hand, the glucagon-like peptide GLP-1-(7-37), a peptide of 31 amino acids, or the equally potent isopeptide GLP-1-(7-36), an amide of 30 amino acids, has major insulinotropic action on pancreatic B-cells (see reviews in references 9 and 10). This peptide binds to specific receptors on islet B-cells, stimulating cAMP formation, insulin release, proinsulin gene transcription, and proinsulin biosynthesis, all in a glucose-dependent manner [11]. It has recently been suggested that GLP-1-(7-36) amide has an antidiabetogenic effect and that it may therefore be useful in the treatment of patients with non-insulin-dependent diabetes mellitus. This topic is reviewed in detail in Chapter 12.

GLP-2 has emerged recently as a most intriguing regulator of intestinal growth and function [12]. Its secretion is stimulated by nutrient intake. It has specific trophic effects on the gut, which appear mediated by stimulation of cell proliferation and inhibition of apoptosis and proteolysis. Preliminary studies suggest a great therapeutic potential in total parenteral nutrition, massive small bowel resections, nonsteroidal drug-induced enteritis, inflammatory bowel diseases, ischemic bowel, and so forth.

Studies by Bataille and his coworkers [13, 14] have shown that both glucagon and oxyntomodulin are further processed into N-terminal and C-terminal fragments by cleavage at a dibasic site (Arg^{17}-Arg^{18}). The C-terminal fragments are of particular interest: glucagon-(19-29) modulates the plasma membrane calcium flow in the nanomolar range, whereas oxyntomodulin-(19-37) inhibits gastric acid secretion, as does oxyntomodulin itself. Finally, studies performed by Pavoine et al. [15] have shown that glucagon processing to glucagon-(19-29) (mini-glucagon) is probably essential for the positive inotropic effect of glucagon on heart contraction. Thus, the concept has emerged that glucagon and oxyntomodulin are first released into the blood and then processed at the level of their respective targets into the corresponding biologically active C-terminal fragments. Recent studies have indicated that mini-glucagon inhibits insulin secretion at picomolar concentrations [16]. It has been proposed that mini-glucagon acts as a local inhibitory regulator of insulin release by turning off the main external calcium source for islet B-cells via a specific receptor linked to ion channels that control cell polarity [17].

The tissue-specific liberation of proglucagon is controlled by cell-specific expression of enzymes known as prohormone convertases (PC). A major defect in the processing of proglucagon to mature pancreatic glucagon is seen in the PC-2 knockout mouse. These animals exhibit mild hypoglycemia and hyperplasia of the A-cells in the islets of Langerhans [18, 19]. These abnormalities are corrected by glucagon replacement via a microosmotic pump [20]. Numerous studies have recently investigated the mechanisms regulating the transcription of the proglucagon gene. Most of these studies concerned the rat proglucagon gene. The transcription factors identified until now include isl-1, cdx-2/3, pax-6, HNF-3α, NHF-3β, and brn 4 [21–25]. Studies about the regulation of the human proglucagon gene are still scarce [26].

PHYSIOLOGICAL EFFECTS OF GLUCAGON

Glucagon acts through binding to specific receptors located at the target cell plasma membrane. The major common effect of glucagon is to activate adenylate cyclase and to increase the intracellular production of cAMP. There is considerable evidence that binding of glucagon to its receptor activates an intermediate transduction process that involves the participation of guanosine triphosphate (GTP), divalent cations, and adenosine (or other similar natural substances). The glucagon receptor has been characterized; it is a 62-kDa glycoprotein that contains at least four N-linked oligosaccharide chains and intramolecular disulfide bonds. The use of various mutated glucagon receptors has permitted Buggy et al. [27] to demonstrate that a five-amino acid domain within the membrane proximal portion of the COOH-terminal tail is required for cell surface expression; that most of the COOH-terminal tail is not required for glucagon binding, cAMP accumulation, or Ca^{2+} mobilization; and that phosphorylation of the COOH-terminal tail is required for glucagon-stimulated receptor internalization. Studies of Unson et al. [28] have shown that positively charged residues at positions 12, 17, and 18 of the glucagon molecule contribute strongly to the stabilization of the binding interaction with the glucagon receptor that leads to maximal biological potency.

Elimination of signaling through the glucagon receptor in the mouse has now been reported. Glucagon receptor knockout mice are viable; they exhibit high circulating levels of glucagon, mild hypoglycemia, and improved glucose tolerance [29]. The expression of the glucagon receptor gene is markedly increased by glucose (see review in reference 30).

The hepatocyte is a major target cell of glucagon. The main effect of glucagon on the liver is to increase glucose output, an effect that results from inhibition of glycogen synthesis and stimulation of liver glycogenolysis and gluconeogenesis. The studies of Cherrington and his colleagues [31, 32] have established the importance of basal glucagon in maintaining hepatic glucose production during a prolonged fast and have shown that gluconeogenesis and glycogenolysis are equally sensitive to stimulation by glucagon *in vivo*. However, subsequent studies of Chhibber et al. [33] using mass isotopomers suggest that low doses of glucagon stimulate only nongluconeogenic glucose release while higher doses stimulate both the gluconeogenic and nongluconeogenic pathways. Interestingly, hyperglucagonemia stimulated endogenous glucose production during fructose infusion, but this effect was not secondary to stimulation of gluconeogenesis but rather to channeling of glucose-6-phosphate toward systemic release [34, 35]. There is ample evidence that most of these effects are mediated by cAMP, but the possibility has been raised that part of the glycogenolytic effect of glucagon may occur by a cAMP-independent mechanism. *In vitro* studies have shown that pulsatile delivery of glucagon is more efficient than continuous exposure to stimulate hepatic glucose production. Similarly, pulsatile delivery of glucagon in humans has greater effects in stimulating endogenous glucose production than continuous infusion [36]. Furthermore, when both insulin and glucagon are delivered intermittently and out of phase, the greater effect of glucagon in stimulating glucose production prevails over the greater effect of insulin in inhibiting this parameter [36]. Another major effect of glucagon on the liver is to stimulate ketogenesis. The elegant studies of McGarry and Foster [37] have convincingly shown that liver ketogenesis depends upon both the flux of free fatty acids (FFA) into the liver and the pathway status of this organ, which is influenced in a crucial manner by the glucagon/insulin ratio in the blood perfusing the liver. The studies of these authors have shown that a high glucagon/insulin ratio increases the intracellular level of cAMP, reduces glycolysis and acetyl-CoA carboxylase activity, and reduces the intracellular concentration of malonyl-CoA. This fall in malonyl-CoA brings fatty acid synthesis to a halt and causes derepression of the enzyme carnitine acyltransferase such that incoming fatty acids (made abundant through stimulation of lipolysis) are efficiently converted into the ketone bodies acetoacetate and 3-hydroxybutyrate.

The effects of glucagon on the adipocyte markedly depend upon the species considered. Although glucagon is a potent lipolytic hormone in birds and in rodents, its effects on the human adipose cell have long been disputed. Recent investigations have shown that glucagon is indeed strongly lipolytic in the human adipocyte *in vitro*, but that this effect is difficult to demonstrate using incubation of adipocytes or adipose tissue pieces because glucagon is rapidly destroyed by a proteolytic activity associated with those cells. When perfusion techniques are used, the lipolytic effect of glucagon on human adipocytes can easily be demonstrated, an effect confirmed using an advanced *in vitro* system, pH stat titration [38]. A study performed by Paolisso et al. [39] in humans has shown that in the presence of somatostatin-induced insulin deficiency, pulsatile glucagon exerts greater effects than its continuous delivery not only on blood glucose (see above) but also on plasma FFA, glycerol, and 3-hydroxybutyrate levels. Interestingly, in the older population the lipolytic and ketogenic, but not the hyperglycemic, responses to pulsatile glucagon are significantly reduced [39]. Observations of Carlson et al. [40] in healthy volunteers have shown that

Table 1 Stimulators of glucagon release

Substrates	Hypoglycemia or cytoglycopenia (2-deoxyglucose), low circulating levels of FFA, most amino acids, fumarate and glutamate
Neural factors	Stimulation of adrenergic and cholinergic nervous systems, stimulation of ventromedial (and ventrolateral?) hypothalamus
Local transmitters or factors	Epinephrine, norepinephrine, acetylcholine, dopamine, VIP, neurotensin, bombesin, substance P, prostaglandins, cAMP, β-endorphin
Hormones	Gastrin, cholecystokinin-pancreozymin (CCK-PZ), GIP, growth hormone
Ions	Total absence of calcium; lack of phosphate, lack of magnesium, presence of potassium (?)
Pharmacological	Furosemide, scorpion venom, phospholipase A_2, L-dopa, clonidine, oxymetazoline, clonbuterol
Environmental factors	Starvation, exercise, stress, balanced meal

Note: In this table, "?" indicates uncertain or conflicting data.

moderate hyperglucagonemia undoubtedly stimulates the rate of appearance in the plasma of both glycerol and FFA, while more recent microdialysis studies performed by others failed to demonstrate a lipolytic effect of glucagon [41, 42].

OTHER EFFECTS OF GLUCAGON

Other metabolic effects of glucagon include modification of the circulatory pattern of plasma amino acids (partly due to the stimulation of gluconeogenesis), a reduction in circulating levels of cholesterol and triglycerides, and a stimulation of fibrinogen formation. Glucagon also stimulates insulin release but the physiological character of this effect is questionable [43]. It has a major role, together with insulin, in liver regeneration [44]. Under certain circumstances, glucagon increases renal blood flow and glomerular filtration rate, and promotes renal loss of sodium and other ions [45]. At pharmacological doses, glucagon stimulates adrenal catecholamine release, an effect that has been used for the diagnosis of pheochromocytoma. Combining glucagon stimulation and clonidine suppression testing has given a sensitivity of 100% and a specificity of 79% for the diagnosis of pheochromocytoma [46]. Glucagon also exerts positive inotropic and chronotropic effects on the heart [47], effects that might be useful, for instance, in treating the cardiodepressive manifestations of poisoning by β-receptor blocking agents. Glucagon and several of its analogues (like glucagon-(1-21), which is devoid of metabolic effects) exert a potent smooth-muscle spasmolytic action, largely used for various diagnostic procedures or for therapeutic applications like bronchospasm [48].

CONTROL OF GLUCAGON RELEASE

Table 1 lists the factors and conditions demonstrated as stimulators of glucagon secretion. The main physiological or pathophysiological stimulators of glucagon release are hypoglycemia (insulin-induced, associated with starvation or intense muscular exercise), hyperaminoacidemia (the rise in plasma glucagon levels after a balanced meal is probably due mainly to amino acid induced glucagon release), stimulation of the adrenergic system (stress, exercise, and possibly hypoglycemia [49]), and stimulation of the vagal system (which together with hormones like GIP and CCK-PZ probably participate in the mixed meal induced glucagon rise).

The factors and conditions associated with inhibition of glucagon release are listed in Table 2. The main physiological inhibitors of glucagon release are probably hyperglycemia and hyperinsulinemia (in a glucose-rich or carbohydrate-rich meal) and high circulating levels of FFA. It has been suggested that glucokinase may serve as a metabolic glucose sensor in pancreatic A-cells, and hence constitute a mechanism for direct regulation of glucagon

Table 2 Inhibitors of glucagon release

Substrates	Hyperglycemia (also fructose and xylitol), high circulating levels of FFA (and ketone bodies)
Local transmitters or factors	Serotonin, somatostatin
Hormones	Insulin, secretin, GLP-1, estrogens, amylin
Ions	Calcium, magnesium
Pharmacological	Atropine, β-receptor blocking agents, α_2-receptor blocking agents, indomethacin, meclofenemate, ibuprofen, diphenylhydantoin, procaine, diazepam, phenformin, various somatostatin analogues, diazoxide (?), sulfonylureas (?), pramlintide, exendin-4
Environmental factors	Carbohydrate meal, pregnancy

Note: In this table, "?" indicates uncertain or conflicting data.

release by extracellular glucose [50]. Pharmacological inhibition of glucagon release may participate in various drug-induced hypoglycemic syndromes. Samols and his coworkers [51] have emphasized the delicate mechanisms by which intraislet insulin, glucagon, and somatostatin release may be interrelated. In such paracrine mechanisms, further data have suggested that the oscillatory pattern of islet hormone release may be particularly important [52]. Recent studies have shown that intraislet hyperinsulinemia prevents the glucagon response to hypoglycemia despite an intact autonomic response and a low A-cell glucose concentration [53].

SOME ASPECTS OF GLUCAGON PHYSIOLOGY AND PATHOPHYSIOLOGY

Glucagon as a Counterregulatory Hormone

Numerous studies have shown that the liver is the main site at which moment-to-moment control of glucose homeostasis takes place and that in normal humans glucagon is the major glucose counterregulatory hormone; by antagonizing the suppressive effects of insulin on glucose production and by stimulating glucose production when appropriate, glucagon not only defends the organism against hypoglycemia, but also restores normoglycemia if hypoglycemia occurs. Perturbation of the mechanisms controlling hypoglycemia-induced glucagon release in some diabetic patients markedly increases the risk of severe hypoglycemia in these subjects. Other hormones, such as epinephrine (acutely) and growth hormone and cortisol (more slowly), participate in the counterregulation of the effects of insulin, but careful clinical observations suggest that indeed glucagon is the first line of defense against hypoglycemia [54].

Glucagon in Exercise

Glucagon levels increase progressively during prolonged exercise [55], during which blood glucose remains relatively constant thanks to a fine balance between muscle glucose uptake and liver glucose production. Although a rise in plasma glucagon does not appear to be essential for increased glucose production during exercise, the presence of glucagon does appear to be necessary [56].

Glucagon in Stress

Hyperglucagonemia is a classic feature of stress [57]. It occurs mainly as a result of the β-adrenergic stimulation associated with stress and undoubtedly contributes to the hyperglycemia, which is a classical finding in this condition.

Glucagon in Starvation

Starvation is accompanied by a decline in circulating insulin and a moderate rise in plasma glucagon. The main effects of glucagon during starvation are at the liver, where it contributes to the maintenance of continuous liver glucose output (initially by stimulating glycogenolysis, and later by promoting gluconeogenesis) and the induction of ketogenesis [58]. Whether glucagon contributes to the stimulation of adipose tissue lipolysis during starvation is still disputed.

Glucagon and Adaptation to Extrauterine Life

A significant rise in plasma glucagon occurs soon after birth in all the species investigated so far, which suggests that glucagon has a crucial role in neonatal glucose homeostasis. Furthermore, an important role of glucagon in thermogenic regulation has been suggested.

Glucagon and Diabetes

Plasma levels of glucagon have been found increased in all experimental and clinical forms of diabetes mellitus. This disturbance undoubtedly contributes to the hyperglycemia of the disease and to the excessive ketogenesis of diabetic coma. More recent studies have shown that failure of glucagon suppression contributes to postprandial hyperglycemia in type 1 [59] and type 2 [60, 61] diabetes. Impaired glucagon suppression contributed with impaired insulin release to the excessive blood glucose levels in early type 1 diabetes [62] and in subjects with impaired glucose tolerance [63, 64]. Studies are in progress to identify inhibitors of glucagon secretion or action to decrease hepatic glucose production in patients with diabetes. Compounds like amylin [65, 66], pramlintide [66, 67], or GLP-1 [68, 69] reduce glucagon release and this is considered as an important component of their antidiabetic action. Numerous glucagon antagonists, either peptidic or nonpeptidic, have been identified and several have been entered in clinical trials [70–77].

The Glucagonoma Syndrome

The glucagonoma syndrome is a rare disorder associating necrolytic migratory erythema, cheilosis, usually mild diabetes mellitus, anemia, weight loss, venous thrombosis, and, frequently, neuropsychiatric symptoms. The clinical and pathologic features in 21 patients from a single institution has been reported by Wermers et al. [78] and guidelines for management can be found in Scheen and Lefèbvre [79].

CONCLUSIONS

Glucagon is a very ancient and tightly conserved molecule and is an important hormone exerting numerous metabolic effects, including stimulation of hepatic glycogenolysis, gluconeogenesis, and ketogenesis; inhibition of liver glycogen synthesis; and, at least in some species, stimulation of adipose tissue lipolysis. All these effects of glucagon are strongly antagonized by insulin. Glucagon originates in the A-cells of the islets of Langerhans of the pancreas, where it is synthesized in the form of a large precursor, preproglucagon. Several peptides derived from the preproglucagon molecule are also expressed in the gut and the brain; they include glicentin, oxyntomodulin, glucagon, and GLP-1 and GLP-2, while a smaller molecule, mini-glucagon, is generated at the hormone target cells. Glucagon release is increased in various physiological situations including hypoglycemia, low circulating levels of FFAs, high levels of numerous amino acids, and stimulation of both vagal and adrenergic nervous systems. Prolonged starvation, long-lasting exercise, stress, and adaptation to the extrauterine life are also associated with high circulating levels of glucagon. All these effects of glucagon make it above all a "hormone of energy need." Diabetes is characterized by excessive circulating levels of glucagon, which are now considered to stem largely from the absolute or relative insulin deficiency that is observed in this syndrome. Studies are in progress to identify inhibitors or glucagon secretion or action as new tools in the pharmacological treatment of diabetes.

Acknowledgment

I acknowledge the expert secretarial help of E. Vaessen-Petit.

REFERENCES

1. Lefèbvre PJ (ed). *Glucagon* (Handbook of Experimental Pharmacology 66, vols I and II). Berlin: Springer, 1983.
2. Lefèbvre PJ (ed). *Glucagon III* (Handbook of Experimental Pharmacology 123). Berlin: Springer, 1996.
3. Lefèbvre PJ. Glucagon and its family revisited. *Diabetes Care* 1995; 18: 715–30.
4. Bromer WW. Chemical characteristics of glucagon. In Lefèbvre PJ (ed). *Glucagon, Vol I*. Berlin: Springer, 1983; pp 1–22.
5. Sherwood NM, Krueckl SL, McRory JE. The origin and function of the pituitary adenylate cyclase-acivating polypeptide (PACAP)/glucagon superfamily. *Endocr Rev* 2000; 21: 619–70.
6. Merrifield RB, Mojsov S. The chemical synthesis of glucagon. In Lefèbvre PJ (ed). *Glucagon, Vol I*. Berlin: Springer, 1983; pp 23–5.
7. Philippe J. Structure and pancreatic expression of the insulin and glucagon genes. *Endocr Rev* 1991; 12: 252–71.
8. Lefèbvre PJ. The intriguing diversity of the glucagon gene products. *Curr Diabetes Rep* 2002; 2: 201–2.
9. Kieffer TJ, Habener JF. The glucagon-like peptides. *Endocr Rev* 1999; 20: 876–913.
10. Drucker DJ. Biological actions and therapeutic potential of the glucagon-like peptides. Gastroenterology 2002; 122: 531–44.
11. Ørskov C. Glucagon-like peptide-1, a new hormone of the entero-insular axis. Diabetologia 1992; 35: 701–11.
12. Drucker DJ. Glucagon-like peptide 2. *J Clin Endocrinol Metab* 2001; 86: 1759–64.
13. Blache P, Kervran A, Dufour M, et al. Glucagon-(19-29), a Ca^{2+} pump inhibitory peptide, is processed from glucagon in the rat liver plasma membrane by a thiol endopeptidase. *J Biol Chem* 1990; 265: 21514–9.
14. Bataille D, Jarrousse C, Blache P, et al. Oxyntomodulin and glucagon: are the whole molecules and their C-terminal fragments different biological entities? *Biomed Res* 1988; 9 (suppl 3): 169–79.
15. Pavoine C, Brechler V, Kervran A, et al. Mini-glucagon glucagon-(19-29) is a component of the positive inotropic effect of glucagon. *Am J Physiol Cell Physiol* 1991; 260 (29): C993–9.
16. Dalle S, Fontés G, Lajoix AD, et al. Mini-glucagon (glucagon 19-29). A novel regulator of the pancreatic islet physiology. *Diabetes* 2002; 51: 406–12.
17. Dalle S, Smith P, Blache P, et al. Mini-glucagon (glucagon 19-29), a potent and efficient inhibitor of secretagogue-induced insulin release through a Ca^{2+} pathway. *J Biol Chem* 1999; 274: 10869–76.
18. Furuta M, Yano H, Zhou A, et al. Defective prohormone processing and altered pancreatic islet morphology in mice lacking active SPC2. *Proc Natl Acad Sci USA* 1997; 94: 6646–51.
19. Furuta M, Zhou A, Webb G, et al. Severe defect in proglucagon processing in islet A-cells of prohormone convertase 2 null mice. *J Biol Chem* 2001; 276: 27197–202.
20. Webb GC, Akbar MS, Zhao C, et al. Glucagon replacement via micro-osmotic pump corrects hypoglycemia and α-cell hyperplasia in prohormone convertase 2 knockout mice. *Diabetes* 2002; 51: 398–405.
21. Kaestner KH, Katz K, Liu Y, et al. Inactivation of the winged helix transcription factor HNF3α affects glucose homeostasis and islet glucagon gene expression *in vivo*. *Gene Dev* 1999; 13: 495–504.
22. Trinh KY, Jin T, Drucker DJ. Identification of domains mediating transcriptional activation and cytoplasmic export in the *caudal* homeobox protein Cdx-3. *J Biol Chem* 1999; 274: 6011–9.
23. Hill FM, Asa SL, Drucker DJ. Essential requirement for Pax6 in control of enteroendocrine proglucagon gene transcription. *Mol Endocrinol* 1999; 13: 1474–86.
24. Fürstenau U, Schwaninger M, Blume R, et al. Characterization of a novel protein kinase C response element in the glucagon gene. *Mol Cell Biol* 1997; 17: 1805–16.
25. Laser B, Meda P, Constant I, Philippe J. The *caudal*-related homeodomain protein Cdx-2/3 regulated glucagon gene expression in islet cells. *Biol Chem* 1996; 46: 28984–94.
26. Nian M, Gu J, Irwin D, Drucker DJ. Human glucagon gene promoter sequences regulating tissue-specific versus nutrient-regulated gene expression. *Am J Physiol* 2002; 282: R173–83.
27. Buggy JJ, Heurich RO, MacDougall M, et al. Role of the glucagon receptor COOH-terminal domain in glucagon-mediated signaling and receptor internalization. *Diabetes* 1997; 46: 1400–5.
28. Unson CG, Wu CR, Cheung CP, Merrifield RB. Positively charged residues at positions 12, 17, and 18 of glucagon ensure maximum biological potency. *J Biol Chem* 1998; 273: 10308–12.
29. Parker JC, Andrews KM, Allen MR, et al. Glycemic control in mice with targeted disruption of the glucagon

receptor gene. *Biochem Biophys Res Commun* 2002; 290: 839–43.
30. Svoboda M, Portois L, Malaisse WJ. Glucose regulation of the expression of the glucagon receptor gene. *Mol Genet Metab* 1999; 68: 258–67.
31. Hendrick GT, Wasserman DH, Tyler Frizzel R, et al. Importance of basal glucagon in maintaining hepatic glucose production during a prolonged fast in conscious dogs. *Am J Physiol Endocrinol Metab* 1992; 263 (26): E541–9.
32. Steiner KE, Williams PE, Lacy WW, Cherrington AD. Effects of insulin on glucagon-stimulated glucose production in the conscious dog. *Metabolism* 1990; 39: 1325–33.
33. Chhibber VL, Soriano C, Tayek JA. Effects of low-dose and high-dose glucagon on glucose production and gluconeogenesis in humans. *Metabolism* 2000; 49: 39–46.
34. Paquot N, Schneiter Ph, Jéquier E, et al. Effects of ingested fructose and infused glucagon on endogenous glucose production in obese NIDDM patients, obese non-diabetic subjects, and healthy subjects. *Diabetologia* 1996; 39: 580–6.
35. Surmely JF, Schneiter Ph, Henry S, et al. Effects of glucagon in the control of endogenous glucose production in man. *Nutrition* 1999; 15: 267–73.
36. Paolisso G, Scheen AJ, Albert A, Lefèbvre PJ. Effects of pulsatile delivery of insulin and glucagon in humans. *Am J Physiol Endocrinol Metab* 1989; 257 (20): E686–96.
37. McGarry JD, Foster DW. Glucagon and ketogenesis. In Lefèbvre PJ (ed) *Glucagon, Vol I*. Berlin: Springer, 1983; pp 383–98.
38. Richter WO, Robl W, Schwandt P. Human glucagon and vasoactive intestinal polypeptide (VIP) stimulate free fatty acid release from human adipose tissue *in vitro*. *Peptides, Vol. 10*. Oxford: Pergamon Press, 1989; pp 333–5.
39. Paolisso G, Buonocore S, Gentile S, et al. Pulsatile glucagon has greater hyperglycaemic, lipolytic and ketogenic effects than continuous hormone delivery in man: effect of age. *Diabetologia* 1990; 33: 272–7.
40. Carlson MG, Snead WL, Campbell PJ. Regulation of free fatty acid metabolism by glucagon. *J Clin Endocrinol Metab* 1993; 77: 11–5.
41. Højberg Gravholt C, Møller N, Jensen MD, et al. Physiological levels of glucagon do not influence lipolysis in abdominal adipose tissue as assessed by microdialysis. *J Clin Endocrinol Metab* 2001; 86: 2085–9.
42. Bertin E, Arner P, Bolinder J, Hagström-Toft E. Action of glucagon and glucagon-like peptide-1-(7-36) amide on lipolysis in human subcutaneous adipose tissue and skeletal muscle *in vivo*. *J Clin Endocrinol Metab* 2001; 86: 1229–34.
43. Moens K, Berger V, Ahn JM, et al. Assessment of the role of interstitial glucagon in the acute glucose secretory responsiveness of in situ pancreatic β-cells. *Diabetes* 2002; 51: 669–75.
44. Leffert HL, Koch KS, Lad PJ, De Hemptinne B, Skelly H. Glucagon and liver regeneration. In Lefèbvre PJ (ed) *Glucagon, Vol I*. Berlin: Springer, 1983; pp 453–84.
45. Ahloulay M, Bouby N, Machet F, Kubrusly M, Coutaud C, Bankir L. Effects of glucagon on glomerular filtration rate and urea and water excretion. *Am J Physiol Renal Fluid Electrolyte Physiol* 1992; 263 (32): F24–36.
46. Grossman E, Goldstein DS, Hoffman A, Keiser HR. Glucagon and clonidine testing in the diagnosis of pheochromocytoma. *Hypertension* 1991; 17: 733–41.
47. Farah AH, Glucagon and the heart. In Lefèbvre PJ (ed) *Glucagon, Vol II*. Berlin: Springer, 1983; pp 553–609.
48. Melanson SW, Bonfante G, Heller MB. Nebulized glucagon in the treatment of bronchospasm in asthmatic patients. *Am J Emerg Med* 1998; 16: 272–5.
49. Taborsky GJ Jr, Ahrén B, Havel J. Autonomic mediation of glucagon secretion during hypoglycemia. Implications for impaired α-cell responses in Type 1 diabetes. *Diabetes* 1998; 47: 995–1005.
50. Heimberg H, De Vos A, Moens K, et al. The glucose sensor protein glucokinase is expressed in glucagon-producing α-cells. *Cell Biol* 1996; 93: 7036–41.
51. Samols E, Weir GC, Bonner-Weir S. Intra-islet insulin–glucagon–somatostatin relationships. In Lefèbvre PJ (ed) *Glucagon, Vol II*. Berlin: Springer, 1983; pp 133–73.
52. Paolisso G, Sgambato S, Passariello N, Varrichio M, Scheen A, D'Onofrio F, Lefèbvre PJ. Pulsatile insulin delivery is more efficient than continuous infusion in modulating islet-cell function in normal subjects and in patients with type-1 diabetes. *J Clin Endocrinol Metab* 1988; 66: 1220–6.
53. Banarer S, McGregor VP, Cryer PE. Intraislet hyperinsulinemia prevents the glucagon response to hypoglycemia despite an intact autonomic response. *Diabetes* 2002; 51: 958–65.
54. Cryer PE. Hypoglycaemia: the limiting factor in the glycaemic management of Type I and Type II diabetes. *Diabetologia* 2002; 45: 937–48.
55. Luyckx AS, Pirnay F, Lefèbvre PJ. Effect of glucose on plasma glucagon and free fatty acids during prolonged exercise. *Eur J Appl Physiol* 1978; 39: 53–61.
56. Lickley HLA, Kemmer FW, Wasserman DH, Vranic M. Glucagon and its relationship to other glucoregulatory hormones in exercise and stress in normal and diabetic subjects. In Lefèbvre PJ (ed) *Glucagon, Vol II*. Berlin: Springer, 1983; pp 297–350.
57. Lindsey CA, Faloona GR, Unger RH. Plasma glucagon levels during rapid exsanguination with and without adrenergic blockade. *Diabetes* 1975; 24: 313–9.
58. Gelfand RA, Sherwin RS. Glucagon and starvation. In Lefèbvre PJ (ed) *Glucagon, Vol II*. Berlin: Springer, 1983; pp 223–37.
59. Dinneen S, Alzaid A, Turk D, Rizza R. Failure of glucagon suppression contributes to postprandial hyperglycaemia in IDDM. *Diabetologia* 1995; 38: 337–43.
60. Shah P, Basu A, Basu R, Rizza R. Impact of lack of suppression of glucagon on glucose tolerance in humans. *Am J Physiol* 1999; 277: E283–90.
61. Shah P, Vella A, Basu A, Schwenk WF, Rizza RA. Lack of suppression of glucagon contributes to postprandial hyperglycemia in subjects with Type 2 diabetes mellitus. *J Clin Endocrinol Metab* 2000; 85: 4053–9.
62. Greenbaum CJ, Prigeon RL, D'Alessio DA. Impaired β-cell function, incretin effect, and glucagon suppression in patients with Type 1 diabetes who have normal fasting glucose. *Diabetes* 2002; 51: 951–7.
63. Ipp E. Impaired glucose tolerance. The irrepressible α-cell? *Diabetes Care* 2000; 23: 569–70.
64. Larsson H, Ahrén B. Islet dysfunction in insulin resistance involves impaired insulin secretion and increased glucagon secretion in postmenopausal women with impaired glucose tolerance. *Diabetes Care* 2000; 23: 650–7.
65. Young A, Moore C, Herich J, et al. Neuroendocrine actions of amylin. In Poyner D, Marshall I, Brain S (eds) *Calcitonin Gene-related Peptide (CGRP)*. Austin, TX: Landes, 1999; pp 91–102.
66. Weyer C, Maggs DG, Young AA, et al. Amylin replacement with pramlintide as an adjunct to insulin therapy in type 1 and type 2 diabetes mellitus: a physiological

approach toward improved metabolic control. *Curr Pharm Des* 2001; 7: 1353–73.
67. Fineman MS, Koda JE, Shen LZ, et al. The human amylin analog, pramlintide, corrects postprandial hyperglucagonemia in patients with type 1 diabetes. *Metabolism* 2002; 51: 636–41.
68. Drucker DJ. The glucagon-like peptides. *Endocrinology* 2001; 142: 521–7.
69. Drucker DJ. Development of glucagon-like peptide-1-based pharmaceuticals as therapeutic agents for the treatment of diabetes. *Curr Pharm Des* 2001; 7: 1399–442.
70. Azizeh BY, Van Tine BA, Trivedi D, Hruby VJ. Pure glucagon antagonists: biological activities and cAMP accumulation using phosphodiesterase inhibitors. *Peptides* 1997; 18: 633–41.
71. Madsen P, Knudsen LB, Wiberg FC, Carr RD. Discovery and structure–activity relationship of the first non-peptide competitive human glucagon receptor antagonists. *J Med Chem* 1998; 41: 5150–7.
72. de Laszlo SE, Hacker C, Li B, et al. Potent, orally absorbed glucagon receptor antagonists. *Bioorg Med Chem Lett* 1999; 9: 641–6.
73. Cascieri MA, Koch GE, Ber E. Characterization of a novel, non-peptidyl antagonist of the human glucagon receptor. *J Biol Chem* 1999; 274: 8694–7.
74. Madsen P, Brand CL, Holst JJ, Knudsen LB. Advances in non-peptide glucagon receptor antagonists. *Curr Pharm Des* 1999; 5: 683–91.
75. Connell RD. Glucagon antagonists for the treatment of type 2 diabetes. *Exp Opin Ther Patents* 1999; 9: 701–9.
76. Parker JC, MdPherson RK, Andrews KM, et al. Effects of skyrin, a receptor-selective glucagon antagonists, in rat and human hepatocytes. *Diabetes* 2000; 49: 2079–86.
77. Petersen KF, Sullivan JT. Effects of a novel glucagon receptor antagonist (Bay 27-9955) on glucagon-stimulated glucose production in humans. *Diabetologia* 2001; 44: 2018–24.
78. Wermers RA, Fatourechi V, Wynne AG, et al. The Glucagonoma Syndrome. Clinical and pathologic features in 21 patients. *Medicine* 1996; 75: 53–63.
79. Scheen AJ, Lefèbvre PJ. Glucagonoma and its management. In Lefèbvre PJ (ed) *Glucagon III* (Handbook of Experimental Pharmacology, Vol 123). Berlin: Springer, 1996; pp 239–54.

12

Islet Amyloid Polypeptide/GLP-1/Exendin

Laurie L. Baggio and Daniel J. Drucker

Banting and Best Diabetes Centre, Toronto General Hospital, University of Toronto, Toronto, Canada

INTRODUCTION

The maintenance of glucose homeostasis is tightly regulated by integration of hepatic glucose production, glucose uptake and utilization by peripheral tissues, and islet hormone secretion. Insulin is secreted in response to elevated blood glucose levels, controls hepatic glucose flux, and promotes glucose uptake from the blood into adipocytes and muscle cells. Defects in insulin secretion or action lead to impaired glucose tolerance and the development of diabetes mellitus.

The primary regulator of insulin synthesis and secretion is the level of ambient plasma glucose concentration. Insulin secretion is also modulated by peptide hormones secreted from endocrine cells in the gastrointestinal tract. The concept that factors released from the gut in response to nutrient ingestion can stimulate secretion from the endocrine pancreas was first proposed in the early 1900s [1–4], and in 1929, the term *incretin* was introduced to describe these putative gut factors [5]. This connection between the gastrointestinal tract and the endocrine pancreas was dubbed the *enteroinsular axis* [6]. The subsequent observation that oral glucose administration stimulates a greater increase in insulin secretion from pancreatic β-cells than an isoglycemic intravenous infusion [7–11] was attributed to the action of incretins [3, 4]. Thus, the term incretin refers to an agent released from the gut in response to nutrient ingestion that acts to potentiate glucose-stimulated insulin secretion [12].

The first incretin hormone to be identified was glucose-dependent insulinotropic polypeptide (GIP) [13–17]. Consistent with its role as an incretin, GIP is synthesized in and released from intestinal K-cells, primarily in response to ingestion of glucose or fat, and enhances glucose-stimulated insulin secretion. However, GIP alone cannot account fully for the incretin effect *in vivo*, based on the following findings: (1) A portion of the incretin activity is preserved in rat gut extracts, despite immunoneutralization of endogenous GIP activity [18, 19]; (2) Anti-GIP antiserum depresses but does not eliminate insulin secretion in response to an oral glucose load in rats [20]; (3) The incretin effect is reduced in patients following surgical resection of the ileum [21].

The cloning and sequencing of mammalian genes and cDNAs encoding proglucagon [22–24] led to the discovery of a second candidate incretin hormone, glucagon-like peptide 1 (GLP-1). GLP-1, a posttranslational product of the proglucagon gene, is released from intestinal L-cells in response to ingestion of glucose or a mixed meal and potentiates glucose-stimulated insulin secretion [25]. GLP-1 also lowers blood glucose via non-incretin effects, including inhibition of gastric emptying and glucagon secretion.

To date, only GIP and GLP-1 have been identified as incretin hormones. These two peptides augment glucose-stimulated insulin secretion in an additive manner and are thought to account fully for the incretin effect [26, 27]. Exendin-4, a naturally occurring, long-acting GLP-1R (GLP-1R) agonist, was originally purified from the venom of the *Heloderma suspectum* lizard [28] and subsequently found to elicit biological effects that mimic the physiological actions of GLP-1.

Islet amyloid polypeptide (IAPP) or amylin is co-localized with insulin in β-cells and co-secreted with insulin in response to nutrient intake and may play a role in the regulation of glucose metabolism. IAPP is also a major component of amyloid deposits found in the islets of Langerhans in subjects with type 2 (noninsulin-dependent) diabetes [29, 30]. Whether IAPP is responsible

International Textbook of Diabetes Mellitus, Third Edition. Edited by R. A. DeFronzo, E. Ferrannini, H. Keen, and P. Zimmet.
 ISBN: 0-471-48655-8.

for the formation of amyloid deposits in the pancreas of diabetic patients, and thus contributes to the pathogenesis of type 2 diabetes, remains under active investigation [31–33].

The following sections summarize our current knowledge regarding the synthesis, secretion, and biological activities of IAPP, GLP-1, GIP, and exendin-4.

IAPP Gene and Coding Sequence

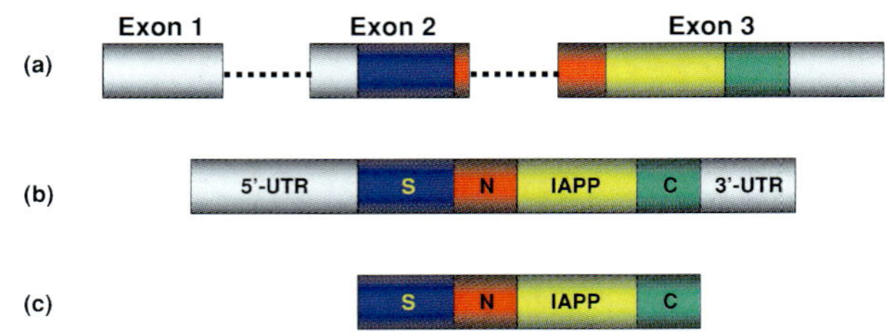

Figure 1 IAPP gene (a), mRNA (b) and protein (c) structures. The IAPP gene is composed of three exons and two introns, with the coding region for IAPP located within exon 3. In addition to IAPP, preproIAPP mRNA encodes N- and C-terminal propeptides of unknown function. IAPP is liberated from proIAPP by PC-mediated cleavage of the flanking N- and C-terminal propeptides. UTR: untranslated region; S: signal peptide; N: N-terminal propeptide; C: C-terminal propeptide

ISLET AMYLOID POLYPEPTIDE

Discovery of IAPP

IAPP was originally identified in 1987 as a major constituent of amyloid deposits in the islets of Langerhans of type 2 diabetic patients and in insulinomas [29, 30, 34, 35]. Subsequent purification and characterization of IAPP, originally termed diabetes-associated peptide, revealed that this 37-amino acid peptide is a normal component of pancreatic β-cells that is stored and released, along with insulin, from β-cell secretory granules in response to nutritional stimuli. IAPP shares approximately 45% amino acid sequence identity with calcitonin gene-related peptide (CGRP) and belongs to the CGRP family of peptides that also includes adrenomedullin and calcitonin [36].

Islet amyloid deposits are found only in humans, nonhuman primates, and cats; however, amyloidogenesis never occurs naturally in rodents. This species-dependent susceptibility to amyloid formation is likely due to amino acid sequence differences at positions 20–29 of IAPP. However, because humans synthesize and secrete IAPP, but not all humans develop islet amyloid deposits, the presence of amyloidogenic sequences between residues 20 and 29 alone is not sufficient to promote amyloid formation [33, 37].

IAPP Gene Structure and Expression

IAPP is derived from an 89-amino acid preproIAPP precursor protein that also contains N- and C-terminal propeptide sequences. The human IAPP gene is located on the short arm of chromosome 12 and consists of three exons and two introns [38] (Figure 1). Exon 1 encodes most of the 5′-untranslated region (UTR) of the IAPP mRNA; exon 2 encodes the remainder of the 5′-UTR, a putative 22-amino acid signal peptide and five amino acids of the N-terminal propeptide; exon 3 encodes the remainder of the N-terminal propeptide, IAPP, the C-terminal propeptide, and the 3′-UTR [38].

Although IAPP is predominantly expressed in and released from pancreatic β-cells, IAPP immunoreactivity and mRNA are also present in islet δ-cells, lung, stomach, duodenum, jejunum, ileum, colon, rectum, and throughout the central nervous system [39].

Systematic analyses of the 5′-flanking sequences of the human IAPP gene identified regulatory regions similar to sequences within the rat and human insulin gene 5′-flanking region, including A/T-rich elements and binding of a basic helix–loop–helix (B-HLH) transcription factor [40]. Transgenic mouse studies reveal that the sequences regulating tissue-specific expression of the human IAPP gene are located between nucleotides −2798 and +450 [41]. Mutagenesis experiments indicate that β-cell-specific expression of the human IAPP gene is mediated by a proximal promoter region spanning nucleotides −222 and −91 that modulates islet-specific transcription, and an intronic region between nucleotides +104 and +434 that modifies expression at a posttranscriptional level [41]. Linker scanning mutagenesis analysis of sequences located within −211 and −32 of the 5′-flanking region of the human IAPP gene identified a negative-acting element at −111 to −21 and positive-acting elements that include a B-HLH binding site at −138 to −131 and three A/T-rich regions at −172 to −163, −154 to −142, and −91 to −84 [41]. The transcription factor PDX-1 (pancreatic and duodenal homeobox 1) which is required for insulin gene transcription in β-cells, has been identified as the factor that binds to the −154 to −142 and −91 to −84 positive-acting A/T-rich elements in the human IAPP gene 5′-flanking sequences [41]. The B-HLH binding site in the IAPP promoter cannot substitute for the analogous B-HLH site in the insulin gene promoter. Thus, differences in IAPP and insulin gene expression are likely mediated, at least in part, by the A/T-rich element located between −172 and −163 and the B-HLH binding site at −138 to −131 [41].

Although co-expressed in pancreatic β-cells, IAPP and insulin mRNA levels are regulated independently [42]. Studies in rats indicate that, at the level of the β-cell, IAPP mRNA levels are upregulated in response to glucose and dexamethasone [43], whereas prolonged fasting, chronic hypoglycemia, and high-dose streptozotocin are associated with reductions in IAPP mRNA [44, 45]. The PDX-1 transcription factor, which plays an important role in the regulation of insulin gene transcription by glucose, is also essential for glucose-stimulated activation of IAPP gene expression [42]. However, in contrast to regulation of the insulin promoter, glucose regulation of the IAPP promoter is also calcium-dependent [42].

Both glucose and forskolin increase IAPP gene expression but only the effect of forskolin is abolished by inhibition of protein kinase A (PKA) activity in the INS-1 β-cell line [46]. Thus, glucose-dependent transcription of the IAPP gene is regulated by a PKA-independent pathway. Glucose and forskolin appear to have a synergistic effect on IAPP gene expression, and electrophoretic mobility shift assays (EMSAs) indicate that glucose and forskolin regulate IAPP gene transcription via distinct promoter elements [46].

IAPP Posttranslational Processing, Secretion, and Clearance

IAPP is synthesized as a larger 89-amino acid precursor propeptide that contains an N-terminal propeptide, followed by the sequence for IAPP and then a C-terminal propeptide [47, 48]. IAPP is generated from proIAPP by removal of the adjacent N- and C-terminal flanking propeptides (Figure 1). The cleavage sites that flank the IAPP sequence consist of pairs of basic amino acids that constitute the recognition motif for the prohormone convertase (PC) enzymes [49]. Transcription/translation studies in *Xenopus* oocytes [50] and reconstitution experiments [51] indicate that proIAPP is processed to IAPP largely by the action of PC2, and PC2 null mice exhibit major defects in the formation of mature processed IAPP [52]. Since PC2 is active under conditions of low pH and high calcium, proIAPP processing likely occurs within secretory granules where the pH and calcium levels are optimal for PC2 activity [50].

IAPP undergoes two posttranslational modifications to generate mature IAPP, including the formation of an intramolecular disulfide bond and C-terminal amidation [39]. Both posttranslational modifications appear to be essential for IAPP bioactivity [39].

Circulating levels of IAPP are increased in response to nutritional stimuli; however, the molecular mechanisms whereby nutrients stimulate IAPP secretion are largely unknown. Studies in diabetic animals and humans implicate the pancreas as the predominant origin of circulating IAPP [39]. Experiments utilizing cultured β-cells or perfused rat pancreas preparations indicate that IAPP secretion is stimulated by glucagon and GLP-1 and inhibited by somatostatin and insulin [53–56]. Cholinergic agonists also stimulate IAPP release from isolated rat islets [57].

Plasma levels of circulating IAPP in healthy fasting humans are approximately 4–8 pM and reach concentrations up to 15–25 pM following a meal [58, 59]. IAPP levels are elevated in type 2 diabetic and insulin-resistant obese patients, as well as in individuals with impaired glucose tolerance [60]. In contrast, because of an absolute loss of functional β-cell mass, individuals with type 1 diabetes are IAPP deficient [58].

IAPP is cleared in part via the kidney; hence, plasma levels of IAPP are elevated in patients with chronic renal failure, and hemodialysis reduces plasma IAPP concentrations [61]. IAPP-like immunoreactivity is also detectable in urine from healthy humans [61]. IAPP may be partly metabolized by the liver, as portal but not peripheral infusion of IAPP in dogs is associated with reduced biological activity of IAPP [62].

The IAPP Receptor

High-affinity IAPP binding sites have been detected in skeletal muscle, kidney, lung, brain, and pancreatic β-cells [63, 64]. Attempts to isolate a single IAPP-specific receptor had been unsuccessful until the discovery that functional IAPP receptors are generated by co-expression of the G-protein-coupled calcitonin receptor (CTR) gene and receptor-activity-modifying proteins (RAMPs) [65]. The RAMP family of proteins, which consists of RAMP1, RAMP2, and RAMP3, are integral membrane proteins that have a large extracellular N-terminus, a single transmembrane domain, and a short intracellular C-terminal tail [65]. RAMP expression modifies the pharmacological phenotype of receptors, with high-affinity IAPP receptors consisting of the CTR and either RAMP1 or RAMP3 [65]. RAMP1 and RAMP3 mRNAs are colocalized with CTR mRNA in mouse pancreatic β-cells and brain [64, 66]. Studies with chimeric RAMP proteins indicate that receptor-binding properties are determined by the N-terminal domain of RAMP proteins, whereas the C-terminal and/or the transmembrane domains of these proteins interact with the CTR and regulate receptor expression [67].

Biological Actions of IAPP

To date, few effects have been ascribed to either proamylin or the N- and C-terminal propeptides. In contrast, as described below, IAPP exerts a diverse array of physiological actions (Table 1) that, together, modulate the rate of glucose influx into the bloodstream.

Pancreas

A role for IAPP as a negative regulator of insulin secretion has been controversial. While some studies indicate that IAPP has no effect on insulin secretion [68, 69] IAPP inhibits insulin secretion in isolated rat β-cells or islets, in the perfused rat pancreas [70, 71] as well as in rats and humans *in vivo* [71, 72]. Blockade of IAPP activity using IAPP antiserum dose-dependently increases

Table 1 Biological actions of IAPP

Pancreas
Negatively regulates insulin secretion
Inhibits glucagon secretion
Gastrointestinal system
Inhibits gastric emptying
Inhibits gastric acid secretion
CNS
Inhibits food intake
Stimulates prandial-drinking behavior
Muscle
Inhibits insulin-stimulated glucose uptake
Reduces glycogen content
Kidney
Activates renin activity
Stimulates sodium and water reabsorption in proximal tubule
Bone
Inhibits bone resorption
Reduces plasma calcium levels
Stimulates osteoblast proliferation
Vasculature
Induces vasodilatation

arginine-stimulated insulin, glucagon, and somatostatin secretion from isolated rat islets, indicating that endogenous IAPP has a tonic inhibitory effect on pancreatic β-, α-, and δ-cells [73]. Suppression of IAPP action with specific peptide antagonists increases insulin secretion from perfused rat islets *in vitro* and from anesthetized rats *in vivo* [74, 75]. Inhibition of IAPP expression with antisense oligodeoxynucleotides increases insulin mRNA and protein in the HIT-T15 hamster insulinoma cell line [76]. In human studies, antagonism of IAPP activity has no effect on insulin levels under basal conditions, but significantly augments glucose-stimulated insulin secretion [77].

Transgenic mice overexpressing human IAPP (hIAPP) [78] and IAPP null mice [79] have provided additional evidence implicating IAPP as a negative regulator of insulin secretion. hIAPP transgenic mice exhibit a diminished insulin response and are glucose intolerant following enteral glucose challenge. Conversely, male mice with a targeted deletion of the IAPP gene have elevated insulin levels and improved glucose tolerance in response to glucose challenge. Expression of an insulin-promoter-hIAPP fusion gene in β-cells reverses the enhanced insulin response and abnormal blood glucose profiles in IAPP null males [80]. In contrast, female IAPP-deficient mice have improved glucose tolerance but normal plasma insulin responses to a glucose challenge, suggesting that extra-pancreatic effects of IAPP may also contribute to the regulation of glucose homeostasis.

IAPP stimulates proliferation of neonatal rat islet cells, but does not significantly modulate β-cell apoptosis [81]. IAPP is expressed early in mouse development (embryonic day 12); however, whether IAPP regulates fetal pancreatic growth and development remains unclear [81]. IAPP also inhibits glucagon secretion as physiological levels of IAPP inhibit arginine-stimulated glucagon secretion during a hyperinsulinemic euglycemic clamp in rats [82], and in type 1 diabetic patients administration of an IAPP analogue decreases levels of postprandial glucagon [82]. IAPP selectively inhibits arginine-induced, but not hypoglycemia-induced glucagon secretion in anesthetized rats *in vivo* [83].

Gastrointestinal System

IAPP is produced in the gastrointestinal tract and studies in both animals and humans demonstrate that IAPP, whether infused peripherally [84, 85] or centrally [86], is a potent inhibitor of gastric emptying and gastric acid secretion. The effect of IAPP on inhibition of gastric emptying delays nutrient transit in the gastrointestinal tract, thereby reducing the rate of glucose appearance in the circulation. A direct effect of IAPP on the gastrointestinal tract is unlikely as binding sites for this peptide have not been detected in the stomach. However, the peripheral and central nervous systems likely mediate the inhibitory effects of IAPP in the gut. Subdiaphragmatic vagotomy abolishes the gastric inhibitory effects of IAPP, and insulin-induced hypoglycemia overcomes the IAPP-mediated inhibition of gastric emptying in rats [85]. IAPP binding sites are present in the area postrema, a blood–brain-barrier-free region of the central nervous system (CNS) through which circulating peptides can gain access to the brain [87]. The area postrema and the dorsal motor nucleus of the vagus nerve constitute a neural loop implicated in the regulation of gastric motility.

Central Nervous System

IAPP is a potent satiety factor in rodents, with both central and peripheral administration of IAPP associated with significant reductions in short-term food intake [88–90]. Furthermore, chronic subcutaneous or intracerebroventricular infusion of IAPP promotes anorexia, weight loss, and a decrease in total body adiposity in rats [91–93]. Moreover, IAPP null mice exhibit increased body weight relative to control mice, and in rats, chronic inhibition of central IAPP signaling using a specific IAPP peptide antagonist leads to increases in food intake and total fat mass [94], suggesting that endogenous IAPP produced in the CNS contributes to the long-term maintenance of energy homeostasis [79]. The effects of either central or peripheral IAPP do not elicit a conditioned taste aversion, indicating that the anorectic effects of IAPP do not involve activation of interoceptive stress pathways [95].

As gastric distention can reduce food intake, IAPP may induce anorexia in part via inhibition of gastric emptying

[96]. However, the mechanism whereby IAPP regulates food intake most likely involves the CNS. Total subdiaphragmatic vagotomy does not impair the anorectic effect of peripherally administered IAPP, nor does capsaicin-mediated destruction of vagal and splanchnic afferent nerve fibers [97, 98], suggesting that IAPP receptors located within the CNS are responsible for modulating its anorectic effect. In support of this notion, destruction of the area postrema in rats significantly impairs the anorectic effect of IAPP [99]. The area postrema contains a high density of IAPP binding sites [87]. Furthermore molecular components of functional IAPP receptors (RAMP1, RAMP3, and CTR) are expressed in the area postrema [66]. Experiments using slice preparations of the rat area postrema demonstrate that IAPP activates neuronal activity in this region via a mechanism involving cyclic guanosine monophosphate (cGMP) [100].

IAPP is also implicated in the stimulation of prandial-drinking behavior. High levels of IAPP receptors are located in the subfornical organ (SFO), a second blood–brain-barrier-free CNS site [87]. Activation of SFO neurons by circulating angiotensin II potently stimulates water intake [101]. Similarly, studies using slice preparations of rat brain indicate that IAPP stimulates SFO neurons, an effect that can be prevented by co-perfusion with an IAPP receptor antagonist, and subcutaneous administration of IAPP increases short-term water intake in rats [102]. Thus, IAPP released in response to meal ingestion may play a role in meal-associated drinking.

Muscle and Kidney

High-affinity IAPP binding sites are present in skeletal muscle, consistent with the observation that IAPP inhibits insulin-stimulated glucose uptake in isolated rat soleus muscle [63, 103, 104]. IAPP also decreases muscle glycogen content and enhances glycogenolysis and lactate production via inhibition of glycogen synthase and stimulation of glycogen phosphorylase [105–107]. Studies using isolated rat soleus muscle strips suggest that IAPP mediates its effects in muscle by activating adenylyl cyclase and increasing intracellular cyclic adenosine monophosphate (cAMP) [108]. Whether IAPP also plays a physiological role as a mediator of insulin sensitivity remains uncertain. Although IAPP inhibits insulin-stimulated glucose disposal in rats [104], neither exogenous infusion of IAPP nor inhibition of endogenous IAPP activity using a specific antagonist has any effect on insulin action in human studies [77, 109].

In the kidney, high-affinity IAPP binding sites are localized to the proximal tubules of the renal cortex [110]. IAPP activates plasma renin activity in rats and humans and selectively stimulates sodium and water reabsorption from the external, rather than the luminal, side of the proximal tubule [110–112]. As intravenous administration of an IAPP receptor antagonist decreases proximal tubular sodium and water reabsorption, endogenous IAPP likely plays a role in sodium homeostasis [110–112]. The exact mechanism whereby IAPP mediates these effects in the kidney is not known, but likely involves activation of adenylyl cyclase and generation of cAMP [110, 112]. IAPP may also influence renal growth and development as it stimulates cellular proliferation in primary cultures of proximal-tubule-derived epithelial cells, an effect that is inhibited by IAPP receptor antagonism [112]. Consistent with these findings, IAPP mRNA is transiently expressed in the proximal tubules of the developing nephron, where it may act as a growth factor for brush border epithelial cells in both the developing and adult kidney [113].

Other Tissues

IAPP also exerts effects on calcium and bone metabolism. In cultured cells from the neonatal mouse cranium, IAPP inhibits both basal and parathyroid-hormone-stimulated bone resorption via inhibition of osteoclast activity and prevention of osteoblast retraction [114]. IAPP also reduces circulating calcium levels in both rats and rabbits, and stimulates osteoblast proliferation and increases the amounts of mineralized bone in mice [115, 116]. IAPP also stimulates cell proliferation and osteocalcin production in a dose-dependent manner in human osteoblast-like primary cell cultures [117].

In the vasculature, IAPP has vasodilatory effects in the rabbit, in the kidney and mesenteric vascular bed of the rat, and in the pulmonary vascular bed of the cat [118]. IAPP also induces vasorelaxation in rat pulmonary artery rings [119]. However, the vasodilatory response to IAPP appears to be dependent on the species and type of vascular bed under examination. Studies using isolated mesenteric arteries from the rat indicate that IAPP mediates its effects on the mesenteric vascular bed by a mechanism that is independent of nitric oxide release and elevation in cGMP levels [118]. In contrast, the effects of IAPP on pulmonary artery rings seem to be nitric oxide dependent [119].

IAPP, Diabetes Pathophysiology, and Treatment

IAPP was originally discovered as a major component of amyloid fibrils found in human insulinomas and in pancreatic islets of patients with type 2 diabetes [34, 35, 120]. Although rodent amylin does not form islet amyloid deposits, transgenic mice that overexpress hIAPP develop amyloid formation following high-fat feeding [121]. This ability to initiate amyloidogenesis, associated with impaired β-cell function and decreased β-cell mass, suggests that IAPP may be involved in the development of diabetes [122, 123]. However, the role of local islet versus circulating IAPP in the pathogenesis of diabetes remains unclear, as this peptide elicits several physiological responses that lower meal-related glucose excursions, including an ability to inhibit food intake, gastric emptying, and postprandial glucagon levels.

A potential therapeutic role for amylin agonists in the treatment of diabetes derives in part from observations that individuals with diabetes fail to suppress postprandial glucagon secretion and hepatic glucose production [124–126] and exhibit accelerated gastric emptying [127–129]. Although exogenous insulin administration lowers fasting and postprandial glucose in diabetic subjects, HbA_{1c} values are still significantly elevated because of persistent postprandial hyperglycemia, indicating that insulin therapy alone is unable to completely correct the glucoregulatory defects in these patients [130]. Therefore, IAPP therapy has been proposed as an adjunctive approach for the restoration of normal glucose control in subsets of diabetic patients [131–133]. To this end, pramlintide, a synthetic human IAPP analogue, has been developed as a potential clinical agent for the treatment of diabetes. In patients with type 1 diabetes, acute intravenous or 14-day subcutaneous administration of pramlintide significantly lowers postprandial hyperglycemia [134, 135]. In 4-week studies, subcutaneous pramlintide reduced 24-h plasma glucose profiles, levels of serum fructosamine, and HbA_{1c} in patients with either type 1 or late-stage (insulin-requiring) type 2 diabetes [136, 137]. Subcutaneous administration of pramlintide three times a day for 52 weeks significantly decreases HbA_{1c} and body weight in insulin-treated patients with type 2 diabetes [138]. Thus, pramlintide therapy may offset the undesirable weight gain often associated with intensive insulin treatment. Pramlintide also reduces the levels of postprandial glucagon and delays gastric emptying in type 1 diabetic patients, thereby improving postprandial glucose control [84, 139, 140]. Finally, IAPP administration did not blunt the counterregulatory response to hypoglycemia in subjects with type 1 diabetes [135], and pramlintide therapy may be associated with modest but significant weight loss [141] in insulin-treated subjects.

GLP-1

Discovery of GLP-1

GLP-1, a posttranslational product of the proglucagon gene, is a member of the glucagon superfamily of peptide hormones, which includes glucagon, glucagon-like peptide 2 (GLP-2), GIP, and exendin-4. The existence of GLP-1 was first predicted following the discovery that the anglerfish pancreatic proglucagon cDNA encodes an additional C-terminal glucagon-like sequence [142]. The subsequent cloning and sequencing of proglucagon cDNAs from several species confirmed the presence of GLP-1 encoded within mammalian proglucagon genes [22–24].

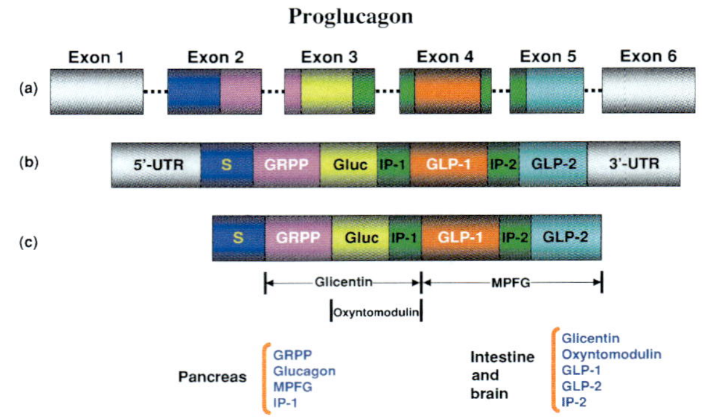

Figure 2 Proglucagon gene (a), mRNA (b) and protein (c). The proglucagon gene contains six exons that encode functional peptide domains within the proglucagon precursor protein. The gene gives rise to a single, identical mRNA transcript in the pancreas, brain, and intestine. Proglucagon undergoes tissue-specific posttranslational processing in the pancreas, intestine, and brain to liberate the indicated proglucagon-derived peptides. UTR: untranslated region; S: signal peptide; GRPP: glicentin-related pancreatic polypeptide; Gluc: glucagon; IP-1 and IP-2: intervening peptide 1 and 2; GLP-1 and GLP-2: glucagon-like peptide 1 and 2; MPGF: major proglucagon fragment

Proglucagon Gene Structure and Regulation of Expression

The human proglucagon gene is located on the long arm of chromosome 2 [143] and consists of six exons, with the sequence encoding GLP-1 contained within exon 4 [3] (Figure 2). In mammals, the proglucagon gene gives rise to a single, identical mRNA transcript in the α-cells of the endocrine pancreas, the enteroendocrine L-cells of the intestine, and in hypothalamic nuclei and brainstem neuronal cell bodies in the CNS [3, 144, 145].

Pancreatic proglucagon gene expression is stimulated by fasting and hypoglycemia and inhibited by insulin [146, 147], whereas in the intestine, proglucagon gene expression is upregulated by nutrients [148] and possibly by peptides such as gastrin-releasing peptide (GRP) and GIP [149, 150]. Agents that activate the cAMP and PKA signaling pathway also increase proglucagon gene expression in both the pancreas and the intestine [151–153], whereas activation of the protein kinase C (PKC) pathway is associated with increased levels of proglucagon mRNA in an islet cell line [154].

Tissue-specific control of proglucagon gene expression has been studied using islet and intestinal endocrine cell lines and transgenic mice [4, 155]. Several *cis*-acting sequences within the rat proglucagon gene promoter have been identified as important control regions for pancreas-specific gene expression (Figure 3). G1, a proximal promoter element, restricts proglucagon gene expression to the α-cells of the endocrine pancreas, and binds the transcription factors Brn4, Pax-6, Cdx-2/3, Isl-1, and members of the hepatocyte nuclear factor 3 (HNF-3 or Foxa)

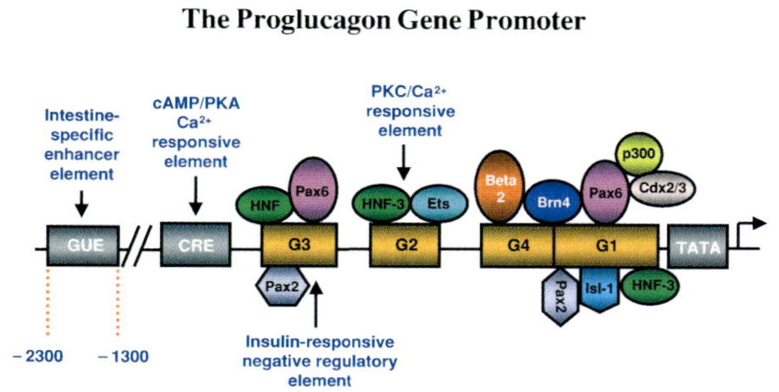

Figure 3 DNA regulatory elements and their associated transcription factors within the 5′-flanking region of the rat proglucagon gene. G1 confers α-cell specific expression to the proglucagon gene. G2, G3, and G4 are islet-specific enhancer elements that promote pancreas-specific expression of the proglucagon gene. GUE: glucagon upstream enhancer; CRE: cAMP response element; TATA: TATA box. The right-angled arrow marks the site of transcription initiation

family [156–163]. Pax6 and Cdx2/3, in association with a coactivator protein, p300, interact synergistically to regulate proglucagon gene expression in islet cells [164]. G2, G3, and G4 represent proglucagon gene islet cell-specific enhancer-like elements [156]. The G2 element binds members of the HNF-3 family of transcription factors to either enhance or repress proglucagon gene expression [163, 165, 166]. G2 also interacts with members of the Ets family of transcription factors [167], and mediates PKC-stimulated glucagon gene transcription in islet cell lines [154, 168]. The G3 element interacts with transcription factors belonging to the HNF family [169], as well as Pax-6 [170]. The transcription factor Pax-2 has been shown to bind to the G1 and G3 elements of the proglucagon gene [171], but whether Pax-2 plays a role in the control of proglucagon gene expression remains uncertain. G3 also contains an insulin response element believed to modulate insulin-mediated negative regulation of proglucagon expression in α-cells [172]. Insulin responsiveness is also conferred to the proglucagon gene promoter via synergistic interactions between proximal promoter elements and more distal enhancer-like elements [173]. G4 is a subelement of G1 that binds the transcription factor Beta2/NeuroD [4, 174]. The proglucagon gene 5′-flanking sequences also contain a cAMP response element (CRE), which binds to a cAMP response element binding protein (CREB), conferring cAMP responsivity to proglucagon gene transcription in pancreas and intestine [151–153, 175]. CAP-binding sites (CBS) are located adjacent to the CRE, on either side, and are binding sites for CREB-associated proteins (CAPs), which inhibit CREB-mediated cAMP stimulation of proglucagon gene expression [176]. The rat proglucagon CRE is also activated by membrane depolarization or influx of calcium [177]. A second calcium response element has been identified in G2, and calcium responsiveness is mediated through an interaction between HNF-3β and the calcium/calcineurin-regulated transcription factor NFATp at the G2 element [178].

In contrast to proglucagon expression in the endocrine pancreas, very little is known about the factors that specify proglucagon gene expression in the intestine and brain. Studies in transgenic mice indicate that approximately 1.3 kb of the rat proglucagon gene 5′-flanking region are sufficient to direct gene expression to the pancreatic α-cells and brain [179], whereas a larger (2.3 kb) region of 5′-flanking sequences directs proglucagon gene expression to the pancreas, brain, and intestine [180], suggesting that sequences between −1252 and −2292 in the rat proglucagon promoter are essential for specifying intestinal proglucagon expression. The sequences between −1252 and −2292 in the rat proglucagon gene have been designated the proglucagon upstream enhancer (GUE) element [181]. Transfection and EMSA experiments in enteroendocrine cell lines indicate that the proglucagon gene GUE is functionally composed of multiple positive and negative *cis*-acting DNA regulatory subdomains that contribute to the integrated transcriptional control of proglucagon gene expression in both islet and intestinal cells [181].

For some transcription factors, loss-of-function experiments provide direct evidence implicating transcription factor action with proglucagon gene expression. Genetic inactivation of the murine Foxa1 (HNF-3α) gene results in mice with hypoglycemia, inappropriately low levels of pancreatic proglucagon mRNA transcripts, and reduced levels of circulating glucagon, implicating Foxa1 as an essential factor for α-cell proglucagon gene transcription [163, 182]. Inactivation of the murine Pax-6 gene results in major defects in formation of islet cell lineages [170] whereas mice homozygous for a dominant negative form of Pax-6 (SEY^{Neu}) have significantly reduced levels of proglucagon mRNA transcripts in the pancreas [183] and both the small and large bowel, indicating that this transcription factor is essential for proglucagon gene expression in both islet and enteroendocrine cells [184].

Although the rat proglucagon promoter has been extensively studied, there is little information available regarding regulation of human proglucagon gene expression. The rat and human proglucagon genes share a similar structural organization [185] and display significant nucleotide sequence identity encompassing the G1–G4 promoter and enhancer elements [186]. Analysis of human proglucagon promoter activity in transgenic mice indicates that the human proglucagon gene appears to utilize transcription factors and DNA sequences that are distinct from those used by the rat to specify tissue-specific gene transcription [186]. Approximately 1.6 kb of human proglucagon gene 5′-flanking sequences direct proglucagon gene transcription to the brain and intestine, but not to the pancreas in transgenic mice [186]. Cell transfection studies examining human proglucagon promoter reporter plasmids in rodent islet cell lines suggest that sequences within the first 6 kb of the human proglucagon gene 5′-flanking sequences are required for pancreatic expression [186].

Proglucagon Posttranslational Processing

In the pancreas, intestine, and brain, proglucagon mRNA is translated into a single 160-amino acid precursor protein, which undergoes tissue-specific posttranslational processing [144, 187] to liberate the proglucagon-derived peptides (PGDPs) (Figure 2).

In pancreatic α-cells, the predominant posttranslational processing products of proglucagon are glicentin-related pancreatic polypeptide (GRPP), glucagon, intervening peptide 1 (IP-1), and the major proglucagon fragment (MPGF) [3, 4] (Figure 2). Glucagon increases blood glucose primarily by stimulating hepatic glycogenolysis and gluconeogenesis [188] and is essential for maintaining glucose homeostasis in the fasting state. Mice with an inactivating mutation in the glucagon receptor exhibit mild hypoglycemia, consistent with the central importance of glucagon for glucoregulation [189]. The functions, if any, of GRPP, IP-1, and MPGF are currently not known.

In gut L-cells and brain, posttranslational processing of proglucagon gives rise to glicentin, oxyntomodulin, GLP-1, intervening peptide-2 (IP-2), and GLP-2 [3, 4] (Figure 2). Glicentin exerts trophic effects in the rodent small intestine [190, 191] and oxyntomodulin inhibits gastric acid secretion and food intake [192–194]. Specific receptors that transduce the actions of glicentin or oxyntomodulin have not been identified.

The amino acid sequence of GLP-1 is completely conserved in mammals [3] and GLP-1 displays several biological actions that are discussed below. A biological function for IP-2 has not yet been identified. The major biological action of GLP-2 appears to be that of an intestinal trophic factor [191, 195, 196]. GLP-2 mediates its trophic effects by induction of intestinal crypt cell proliferation and inhibition of apoptosis in both the crypt and villus compartments [195, 197]. GLP-2 also upregulates intestinal glucose transport [198, 199], inhibits gastric emptying [200] and gastric acid secretion [201], and improves intestinal barrier function by reducing intestinal epithelial permeability [155, 202, 203]. GLP-2 has also been shown to inhibit food intake following intracerebroventricular administration in rodents [204, 205].

The posttranslational processing of proglucagon is mediated by PC enzymes. The PGDPs are flanked by pairs of basic amino acid residues, the recognition sites for PC cleavage. The C-terminal basic residues exposed following cleavage by the PCs are removed by the actions of carboxypeptidase E [206]. PC1/3 and PC2 have been detected in proglucagon-expressing cells [207, 208]. PC1/3 has been localized to intestinal L-cells and is both necessary and sufficient for the posttranslational processing of proglucagon to intestinal PGDPs, including GLP-1 and GLP-2 [209–214]. In contrast, PC2, but not PC1/3, has been localized to adult pancreatic α-cells [215] and is believed to be responsible, at least in part, for the posttranslational processing of proglucagon to glucagon in these cells [216–219]. Intriguingly, PC1/3 has been localized to α-cells in the embryonic pancreas, raising the possibility that GLP-1 may be liberated during development of the endocrine pancreas [220]. The PC enzymes responsible for liberation of PGDPs in the brain have not been conclusively identified; however, high levels of PC1/3 and PC2 mRNA are present in numerous regions of the CNS, including the hypothalamus [49] where proglucagon-expressing neurons have also been detected. PC1/3 expression has also been localized in α-cells in the setting of experimental diabetes; however, the biological implications of this finding remains uncertain [220, 221].

Multiple forms of GLP-1 are released *in vivo*, including GLP-1(1-37) and GLP-1(1-36)NH_2, which thus far appear to be biologically inactive [222–224], and GLP-1(7-37) and GLP-1(7-36)NH_2, which are biologically active. A major proportion of GLP-1 is amidated at the C-terminal glycine residue [GLP-1(1-36)NH_2 and GLP-1(7-36)NH_2], likely via the activity of peptidylglycine α-amidating monooxygenase (PAM) [225]. C-terminal amidation may enhance the survival of GLP-1 in plasma [226]. GLP-1(7-37) and GLP-1(7-36)NH_2 are generated by the action of PC1/3 [211], and both forms of peptide appear equipotent [226–228]. In humans, the majority of circulating GLP-1 is in the form GLP-1(7-36)NH_2 [229]. In pigs and rats approximately half of the GLP-1 is glycine-extended, while in dogs the glycine-extended forms of GLP-1 predominate.

Regulation of GLP-1 Secretion

GLP-1 is produced in enteroendocrine L-cells, the majority of which are found in the distal ileum and colon [230–233]. GLP-1 secretion from gut endocrine cells is regulated by several intracellular signals, including PKA, PKC, and calcium [150, 234–236]. Studies with fetal rat intestinal cultures and isolated perfused rat ileum and experiments in humans, rodents, and dogs have demonstrated that GLP-1 secretion is controlled by nutrients, and neural and endocrine factors [3, 4, 25]. In humans, basal plasma levels of intact GLP-1 are typically within the 5–10 pM range, and increase to approximately 50 pM postprandially [229, 237].

GLP-1 is secreted in response to mixed meals, or individual nutrients such as glucose, fatty acids, and dietary fiber [4, 25, 238–242]. Oral administration of glucose in humans produces a biphasic increase in plasma GLP-1, whereas intravenous infusion of glucose has minimal effects [241]. As the majority of GLP-1-producing L-cells are located in the distal portion of the small intestine the rapid increase in plasma GLP-1 levels observed following nutrient ingestion are likely mediated by indirect stimulatory effects. Thus, the existence of a proximal–distal loop that transmits nutrient-induced stimulatory signals from the proximal gut, via neural or endocrine effectors, to distal L-cells has been proposed [243]. Candidate mediators of this indirect response in rats include the more proximally located duodenal hormone GIP and the neurotransmitter acetylcholine [243–245]. However, in humans GIP does not stimulate GLP-1 secretion [246, 247]. The neuropeptide GRP stimulates GLP-1 secretion in both humans [248] and rodents [249], and mice with targeted inactivation of the GRP receptor exhibit a reduced plasma GLP-1 response to gastric glucose [250]. Furthermore, the stimulatory effects of GIP on GLP-1 secretion in rodents may be mediated indirectly, via GRP [249]. A role for the neuropeptide CGRP in the regulation of GLP-1 release has also been proposed [251]. The vagus nerve plays a major role in mediating the rapid release of GLP-1 from the distal L-cells in response to ingested nutrients [252]. Thus, the biphasic nature of GLP-1 release appears to be mediated through integration of hormonal and neural factors, which stimulate early (within 10–15 min) GLP-1 release, and direct nutrient contact with L-cells to promote the second phase (30–60 min) of GLP-1 secretion [4]. Although less well studied, inhibition of gut GLP-1 release has been attributed to insulin and somatostatin-28 [213, 253], as well as the neuropeptide galanin [254].

GLP-1 Metabolism and Clearance

The half-life of circulating, biologically active GLP-1 is less than 2 min [255, 256]. This short plasma half-life has been attributed to the protease activity of dipeptidyl peptidase IV (DPP-IV), a ubiquitously expressed serine protease that can be found anchored to the surface of cells or as a circulating soluble form in plasma [257, 258]. DPP-IV specifically cleaves dipeptides from the amino terminus of oligopeptides or proteins that contain alanine or proline in the penultimate position. DPP-IV is widely expressed in many tissues including the pancreas, CNS, and the vascular endothelium of the small intestine, adjacent to the sites of GLP-1 release [255, 257, 258]. DPP-IV catalyzes the cleavage of GLP-1 at the position 2 Ala residue to yield GLP-1-(9-37) or GLP-1-(9-36)NH_2. In rats, greater than 50% of an intravenous bolus of GLP-1 is metabolized to its N-terminal truncated form by DPP-IV within 2 min of peptide administration [259]. In contrast, N-terminal truncation is absent when GLP-1 is infused into a strain of rats that is DPP-IV deficient, and inhibition of DPP-IV activity prolongs the half-life of the bioactive form of GLP-1 [259–261]. GLP-1 is rapidly degraded to GLP-1-(9-37) or GLP-1-(9-36)NH_2 as it enters the DPP-IV-containing blood vessels, which drain the intestinal mucosa [255]. In human studies intravenous or subcutaneous GLP-1 is similarly rapidly degraded (within 30 min) to GLP-1- (9-36)NH_2, which accounts for more than 75% of the immunodetectable circulating GLP-1 [256].

A search for potential biological actions of GLP-1 metabolites has revealed that GLP-1-(9-36)NH_2 can function as a competitive pharmacological antagonist of the GLP-1R in the gastrointestinal system [262]. However, experiments in anesthetized pigs treated with DPP-IV inhibitors revealed that GLP-1-(9-36)NH_2 could paradoxically elicit modest insulin-independent antihyperglycemic effects [263]. Thus, the biological importance of N-terminally cleaved GLP-1 peptides remains uncertain. Neutral endopeptidase (NEP-24.11) has endoproteolytic activity on GLP-1 and may also contribute to the metabolism of GLP-1 [264, 265].

The primary route of GLP-1 clearance appears to be through the kidney via mechanisms that include glomerular filtration and tubular catabolism [266, 267]. Uremic patients have elevated levels of circulating, immunoreactive GLP-1 [268], and bilateral nephrectomy or ureteral ligation in rats is associated with increases in the circulating half-life of GLP-1 [266]. A role for tissues other than the kidney, such as the liver and lung, in GLP-1 clearance has not been clearly established [266].

The GLP-1 Receptor

The GLP-1R belongs to the seven-transmembrane-spanning, heterotrimeric G-protein-coupled family of receptors, and was originally cloned from a rat pancreatic islet cDNA library [269]. The human GLP-1R gene has been mapped to chromosome 6, band p21.1 [270]. In humans and rodents, GLP-1R is expressed in lung, stomach, heart, intestine, α-, β-, and δ-cells of the pancreatic islets, kidney, and regions of the CNS, including the brainstem, hypothalamus, and pituitary [271–275]. Only a single GLP-1R has been identified, which is structurally identical in all tissues examined [272]. Nevertheless, the potential presence of GLP-1Rs in human peripheral tissues such as muscle, liver, and fat remains controversial [276, 277] and has prompted the suggestion that structural GLP-1R variants or a second, closely related receptor may exist in these tissues [4, 278].

The GLP-1R can couple to multiple G-proteins, including $G\alpha_s$, $G\alpha_{q/11}$, and $G\alpha_{i1,2}$, and interaction of GLP-1 with its receptor activates multiple intracellular signaling pathways [279, 280]. GLP-1 binding stimulates adenylate cyclase and phospholipase C and activation of PKA and PKC, respectively [269, 277, 281], as well as increases in intracellular calcium [282–286] and activation of the phosphatidylinositol 3 kinase (PI3K) and mitogen-activated protein kinase (MAPK) signaling pathways [279, 287].

Table 2 Biological actions of GLP-1

Pancreas
Enhances glucose-stimulated insulin secretion
Stimulates insulin gene transcription, mRNA stability, and biosynthesis
Inhibits glucagon secretion
Stimulates somatostatin secretion
Regulates β-cell K_{ATP}-channel expression and activity
Enhances β-cell responsivity and glucose competence
Induces β-cell neogenesis and proliferation
Gastrointestinal system
Inhibits gastric emptying
Inhibits gastric acid secretion
Cardiovascular system
Increases heart rate and blood pressure
CNS
Inhibits food and water intake
Stimulates LHRH secretion from hypothalamic neuronal cell lines
Stimulates TSH, LH, and corticosterone secretion *in vivo*
Muscle, Adipose tissue, and liver
Enhances insulin-stimulated glucose metabolism in adipocytes
Stimulates glucose incorporation into glycogen in hepatocytes and skeletal muscle
Mediates hepatoportal glucose sensing
Thyroid, lung, and kidney
Stimulates release of calcitonin from thyroid gland
Enhances mucous secretion, pulmonary muscle relaxation, and surfactant secretion in lung
Promotes diuresis and natriuresis in kidney

Structure–function studies reveal that the N-terminal histidine residue and the C-terminal residues 34–37 of GLP-1 are essential for GLP-1R activation and binding, respectively [288]. The N-terminal extracellular domain of the GLP-1R is required for GLP-1 binding [289, 290], whereas the third intracellular loop is necessary for efficient coupling of the GLP-1R to adenylyl cyclase and subsequent activation of PKA [291, 292].

Little is known about the factors that regulate GLP-1R gene expression. GLP-1R expression is downregulated in response to GLP-1, activation of PKC, high glucose, or dexamethasone [293–296], whereas treatment of diabetic rodents with DPP-IV inhibitors is associated with upregulation of pancreatic GLP-1R expression [297]. GLP-1R promoter activity is positively regulated by Sp1 and Sp3 transcription factors [298], whereas cell- and tissue-specific GLP-1R expression is negatively regulated by more distal elements [299]. A distal cell-specific silencer element has been identified in the 5′-flanking sequences of the GLP-1R gene that represses human GLP-1R promoter activity in fibroblast and pancreatic α-cells, but not in β- or δ-cells [300].

The GLP-1R undergoes homologous and heterologous desensitization [301–304] and internalization [304, 305] in islet cell lines, which are both correlated with receptor phosphorylation [302–304]. However, desensitization of the GLP-1R has not been observed *in vivo* [4]. Exendin-(9-39), an N-terminally truncated fragment of the lizard GLP-1R agonist exendin-4, binds to the GLP-1R and functions as a specific GLP-1R antagonist [306–309]. Exendin-(9-39) is commonly used as a tool to examine the physiological consequences of loss of GLP-1R signaling.

Biological Actions of GLP-1

GLP-1 exerts multiple physiological actions in different tissues, which are listed in Table 2 and described in greater detail below.

Pancreas

The original physiological role described for GLP-1 was that of an incretin hormone: GLP-1, released from the gut in response to nutrient ingestion, is secreted into the circulation, and augments glucose-stimulated insulin secretion [246]. GLP-1 stimulates insulin secretion through mechanisms that involve (1) inhibition of ATP-sensitive K^+ channels (K_{ATP}), resulting in membrane depolarization; (2) increases in intracellular Ca^{2+} levels through voltage-dependent Ca^{2+} channels, activation of nonselective cation channels, and release of Ca^{2+} from intracellular stores; and (3) potentiation of Ca^{2+}-induced secretion via direct effects on the β-cell exocytotic machinery [310]. The molecular signaling pathways that mediate the insulinotropic effects of GLP-1 include elevations in intracellular cAMP and activation of PKA, as well as cAMP-dependent, PKA-independent mechanisms involving activation of guanine nucleotide exchange factors (GEFs) [311, 312]. GLP-1 also increases insulin gene transcription, mRNA stability, and biosynthesis by mechanisms that involve both cAMP/PKA-dependent and -independent pathways, as well as increases in the levels of intracellular Ca^{2+} [280, 313, 314]. Thus, GLP-1 replenishes β-cell insulin stores and prevents exhaustion of β-cell reserves. GLP-1 also regulates the expression and function of the β-cell K_{ATP} channel, a key molecular component of glucose-dependent insulin secretion. GLP-1 increases expression of the sulfonylurea receptor (SUR1) and inwardly rectifying potassium channel (Kir 6.2) in the INS-1 β-cell line, and prevents glucose-dependent inhibition of K_{ATP} channel activity [315].

The physiological importance of GLP-1 has been demonstrated using GLP-1R antagonists, immunoneutralizing antisera, and GLP-1R knockout mice. Elimination of GLP-1 activity with GLP-1 immunoneutralizing antisera or the GLP-1R antagonist exendin-(9-39) results in impaired glucose tolerance and diminished glucose-stimulated insulin levels in both animals and humans [316–319]. Similarly, mice with a targeted inactivation of the GLP-1R gene (GLP-1R$^{-/-}$) are glucose intolerant and exhibit defective glucose-stimulated insulin secretion [320]. GLP-1 confers glucose sensitivity to β-cells, thereby improving the ability of the endocrine pancreas to sense and respond to glucose [321, 322]. The demonstration that GLP-1 upregulates the expression of components of the β-cell glucose sensing system (i.e. glucose transporters and glucokinase) may provide a partial mechanism for the effects of GLP-1 on β-cell glucose responsivity [323, 324].

GLP-1 also inhibits glucagon and stimulates somatostatin secretion. The increase in somatostatin secretion appears to be direct, via GLP-1Rs on somatostatin-secreting pancreatic δ-cells [325], whereas the inhibitory effect of GLP-1 on glucagon secretion may be indirect, through stimulation of insulin and somatostatin, both of which inhibit glucagon secretion [326]. However, GLP-1 may also inhibit glucagon secretion directly, via interaction with GLP-1Rs on α-cells [273]. Basal GLP-1 signaling in the fasting state is important for glucoregulation as administration of exendin-(9-39) to humans produces significant elevations in fasting glucose and glucagon, suggesting that even the very low basal levels of GLP-1 exert a tonic inhibitory effect on glucagon-secreting α-cells [327]. The insulinotropic and glucagonostatic effects of GLP-1 are glucose-dependent [328, 329]. Thus, when blood glucose levels fall, GLP-1 no longer stimulates insulin secretion or inhibits glucagon secretion, thereby reducing the possibility of hypoglycemia [329].

GLP-1 administration is also associated with induction of proliferation and neogenesis of pancreatic β-cells. GLP-1 activates the expression of immediate early genes whose products encode for transcription factors that regulate islet cell proliferation and differentiation, increases DNA synthesis in β-cell lines, and induces differentiation of pancreatic exocrine cells into insulin-secreting cells with endocrine properties [330–332]. GLP-1 agonists also stimulate β-cell neogenesis and proliferation, and increase β-cell mass in both normal and diabetic rodents [333–336]. Additionally, disruption of GLP-1R signaling pathways in the mouse is associated with reduced numbers of large β-cell clusters and alterations in islet α-cell topography [337]. The intracellular signal transduction pathways whereby GLP-1 mediates its proliferative effects have not been clearly defined, but likely involve the induction of PI3K and activation of p38 MAPK and PKCζ [331].

Gastrointestinal System

GLP-1 inhibits pentagastrin- and meal-induced gastric acid secretion, and gastric emptying in both humans and animals [192, 338]. Inhibition of gastric emptying promotes attenuation of meal-associated increases in blood glucose by slowing the transit of nutrients from the stomach to the small intestine. The inhibitory effects of GLP-1 on the gut are dependent on the vagus nerve and likely involve both central and peripheral GLP-1 actions [339]. Vagal afferent denervation or GLP-1R antagonism with exendin-(9-39) eliminates the effects of central and peripheral GLP-1 on the rate of gastric emptying.

Cardiovascular System

GLP-1Rs are expressed in the heart and in the nucleus of the solitary tract in the CNS, a region important for the central control of cardiovascular function [340]. Consistent with these observations, GLP-1 increases systolic, diastolic, and mean arterial blood pressures and heart rate in rats [341] and increases heart rate in conscious calves [342]. These effects of GLP-1 are not mediated by catecholamines and are blocked by exendin-(9-39). The stimulatory effects of GLP-1 on the cardiovascular system appear to be mediated through both central and peripheral mechanisms [341, 343, 344]. Thus GLP-1, released in the brain or from the intestinal L-cell, can activate CNS pathways that transmit signals to the cardiovascular system via the vagus nerve. Alternatively, GLP-1 may exert a direct effect on cardiovascular parameters through interaction with GLP-1Rs in the heart [345].

Central Nervous System

GLP-1Rs and GLP-1-immunoreactive nerve fibers are detected in brain regions that regulate diverse homeostatic functions, including ingestive behavior [274, 346, 347]. Central administration of GLP-1 inhibits short-term food and water intake in rodents [348, 349], and peripheral administration promotes satiety and suppresses energy intake in normal, diabetic, and obese humans [350–354].

The inhibitory effects of GLP-1 on food intake may be mediated by a direct interaction of GLP-1 with hypothalamic centers in the CNS, which modulate feeding behavior, or indirectly via the inhibitory effects of GLP-1 on gastric emptying. Alternatively, GLP-1 may modify feeding behavior through mechanisms involving induction of modest interoceptive stress, a term that includes endocrine, autonomic, and behavioral responses to visceral illness [355, 356]. GLP-1 and noxious substances such as lithium chloride induce a similar pattern of neuronal activity in the rodent CNS and elicit comparable aversive behavioral responses that are indicative of visceral illness [356–359]. Importantly, many of the responses produced by GLP-1 and noxious stimuli are blocked by pharmacological antagonism of the GLP-1R. Moreover, GLP-1 activates neurons in the central nucleus of the amygdala, a CNS region that modulates fear and anxiety [360]. Thus, GLP-1-mediated effects on feeding behavior may also reflect physiological responses to activation of central aversive signaling pathways.

Muscle, Fat, and Liver

GLP-1 may enhance glucose disposal indirectly through peripheral effects on liver, skeletal muscle, and adipose tissue. GLP-1 enhanced insulin-stimulated glucose metabolism in adipocyte cell cultures and isolated rat adipocytes and increased glucose incorporation into glycogen in isolated rat hepatocytes and skeletal muscle [361]. However, not all experimental analyses substantiate these conclusions [362, 363] and the existence of GLP-1Rs within these peripheral tissues remains controversial [271, 276, 277, 364, 365]. Although GLP-1 enhances insulin sensitivity in pancreatectomized dogs [366] and following chronic infusion in diabetic subjects [367], mechanistic studies in normal and diabetic humans do not support a direct role for GLP-1 in the modulation of insulin sensitivity [368, 369].

Activation of GLP-1R signaling pathways also appears to be essential for the glucose-sensing mechanism in the murine hepatoportal system. Infusion of glucose into the portal vein increases glucose clearance in mice and rats [370, 371] and the effects of intraportal glucose are suppressed by coadministration of the GLP-1R antagonist exendin-(9-39) into the portal vein. Similarly, enhanced glucose clearance following portal glucose infusion is abrogated in GLP-1R$^{-/-}$ mice [371].

Hypothalamus, Pituitary, Thyroid, Lung, and Kidney

GLP-1 may also modulate the hypothalamic–pituitary axis. GLP-1Rs are present on rat pituitary cells [347, 372] and GLP-1 stimulates cAMP formation and thyroid-stimulating hormone (TSH) release from cultured mouse pituitary thyrotrophs and isolated rat anterior pituitary cells [373]. GLP-1 also stimulates luteinizing hormone-releasing hormone (LHRH) secretion from rodent hypothalamic neuronal cell lines, and central GLP-1 administration stimulates TSH, LH, corticosterone, and vasopressin secretion in rats [374, 375]. Nevertheless, complete disruption of GLP-1R signaling in the mouse is not associated with major impairment of hypothalamic–pituitary function [376]. GLP-1 can promote the release of calcitonin from normal rat thyroid and rat medullary thyroid carcinoma cell lines that express the GLP-1R [377]; however, thyroid hormone levels are normal in GLP-1R$^{-/-}$ mice [376].

High levels of GLP-1Rs are expressed in the lung in the submucosal glands of the trachea, pulmonary artery smooth muscle cells, and in rat and human type II pneumocytes, where GLP-1 increases mucous secretion, pulmonary muscle relaxation, and surfactant secretion, respectively [378, 379]. Despite the comparatively abundant levels of GLP-1Rs in the lung, whether GLP-1 actions are essential for normal pulmonary physiology remains uncertain.

GLP-1Rs are expressed in the kidney and infusion of GLP-1 has diuretic and natriuretic effects in rats that are associated with inhibition of proximal tubule reabsorption and increase in glomerular filtration rate. The precise mechanisms whereby GLP-1 exerts these actions are not known, but may involve activation of sympathetic outflow as well as direct effects on renal GLP-1Rs [380].

GIP

Biosynthesis and Secretion of GIP

The second major incretin hormone is GIP, a 42-amino acid peptide that is released into the circulation in response to ingestion of nutrients. GIP was originally isolated from crude extracts of porcine small intestine and named gastric inhibitory polypeptide on the basis of its ability to inhibit gastric acid secretion in dogs [381, 382]. However, subsequent analyses revealed that GIP is an incretin hormone that potentiates glucose-stimulated insulin secretion [13, 383, 384]. Accordingly, the peptide was renamed glucose-dependent insulinotropic peptide [3, 385].

The human GIP gene is located on the long arm of chromosome 17, and like the proglucagon gene, consists of six exons, with the majority of sequences encoding GIP contained within exon 3 [386] (Figure 4). The predicted amino acid sequences encoded by human and rat GIP cDNA clones indicate that GIP is derived from a larger proGIP prohormone precursor that sequentially encodes a signal peptide, an N-terminal peptide, GIP, and a C-terminal peptide [387–389] (Figure 4). The mature 42-amino acid bioactive form of GIP is released from proGIP via posttranslational cleavage at single arginine residues that flank the hormone. The sequence of GIP is highly conserved across species, with over 90% identity at the amino acid level in human, rat, mouse, porcine, and bovine GIP.

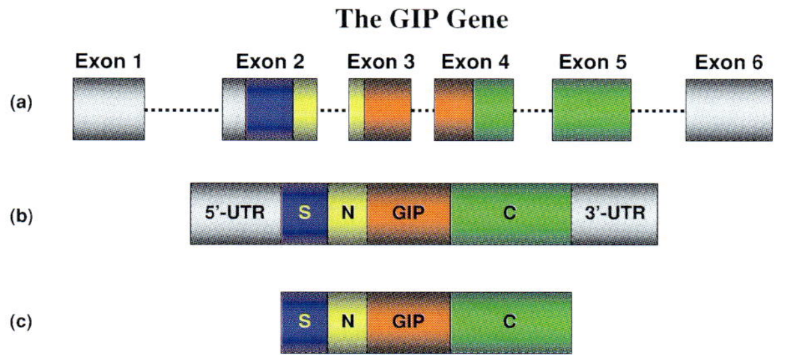

Figure 4 GIP gene (a), mRNA (b) and protein (c) structures. The GIP gene consists of six exons and five introns, with the majority of GIP encoded within exon 3. In addition to GIP, preproGIP mRNA also encodes N- and C-terminal propeptides of unknown function. Bioactive GIP is liberated from its proGIP protein precursor by posttranslational cleavage at single arginine residues that flank the hormone. UTR: untranslated region; S: signal peptide; N: N-terminal propeptide; C: C-terminal propeptide

The peptides encoded within the N- and C-terminal segments of proGIP have no known biological function.

In rodents and humans the GIP gene is expressed in the stomach and in the K-cells of the small intestine. GIP mRNA is also present in the submandibular salivary gland of the rat [3]. However, there is very little information regarding the factors that regulate GIP gene expression. The promoter region of the human GIP gene contains putative binding sites for Sp1, AP-1, and AP-2, and transient expression assays using insulinoma cells indicate that basal promoter activity of the GIP gene is regulated by two cAMP responsive elements [390]. In the rat, GIP gene promoter sequences between −193 and −182 contain a functional GATA element and are responsible for regulating cell-specific promoter activity [391]. Administration of a glucose- or fat-rich meal upregulates GIP mRNA levels in the rat duodenum and submandibular salivary gland, whereas prolonged fasting is associated with significant reductions in the levels of GIP mRNA [392, 393].

Basal circulating levels of GIP range from 0.06 to 0.1 nM, depending on the assay used to measure total versus intact GIP immunoreactivity, and increase to levels that vary between 0.2 and 0.5 nM following a meal [237, 394]. GIP is synthesized in and released from K-cells of the duodenum and proximal jejunum primarily in response to the ingestion of glucose or fat [3, 385], although peptones can also potently increase GIP secretion in rats [394]. Moreover, GIP secretion is dependent on the rate of nutrient absorption, rather than the simple presence of nutrients in the small intestine [395]. The nutritional regulation of GIP secretion appears to be species-specific, with fat a more potent secretory stimulus than carbohydrates in humans, whereas in rodents and pigs carbohydrates are more effective [385]. GIP is secreted from canine gut cells in response to the activation of adenylyl cyclase, elevations in intracellular Ca^{2+}, K^+ mediated depolarization, and glucose, GRP, and β-adrenergic stimulation [396].

GIP Metabolism and Clearance

The half-life of total immunoreactive GIP was initially determined to be approximately 20 min. However, this determination did not reflect the half-life of biologically active intact GIP, which is estimated to be less than 2 min in rats [259] and approximately 7 and 5 min in normal subjects and patients with type 2 diabetes, respectively [397].

A role for DPP-IV in the degradation of GIP-(1-42) to the biologically inactive fragment GIP-(3-42) has been established [398]. Experiments in rats and both normal and diabetic human subjects implicate DPP-IV as the primary GIP-inactivating enzyme *in vivo* [259, 397]. However, a direct comparison of the levels of intact GIP and GLP-1 following intravenous infusion in humans indicates that intact bioactive GIP accounts for approximately 40% of the total detectable amount of immunoreactive GIP, whereas only about 20% of total immunoreactive GLP-1 remained intact in the same studies [397]. Thus, GIP appears to be less susceptible to DPP-IV-mediated degradation *in vivo* and this is reflected in its slightly longer plasma half-life relative to GLP-1. The main route of GIP clearance is likely through the kidney as levels of GIP are elevated in patients with uremia or chronic renal failure and GIP clearance is decreased in nephrectomized rats [399–401]. Measurement of arteriovenous concentration differences of GIP across various organ beds in anesthetized pigs indicates that the kidney is the major site of GIP degradation, but the liver and extremities also contribute to GIP extraction [402].

The GIP Receptor

The GIP receptor (GIPR) was originally cloned from a rat cerebral cortex cDNA library in 1993 and the hamster and human GIPRs were cloned shortly thereafter [385, 403–405]. Genetic mapping and linkage studies have localized the human GIPR gene to chromosome 19, band q13.3 [406]. GIPR is expressed in the pancreas, stomach, small intestine, adipose tissue, adrenal cortex, lung, pituitary, heart, testis, vascular endothelium, bone, and several regions of the brain [407–409]. It belongs to the seven-transmembrane domain, heterotrimeric G-protein-coupled glucagon receptor superfamily [407].

Very little is known about regulation of GIPR expression. Cloning and analysis of the 5′-flanking region of the rat GIPR gene identified a number of potential regulatory elements, including a cAMP response element, an octamer binding site, three Spl sites, as well as a transcription initiator element consensus sequence [410]. However, there are no TATA or CAAT box motifs upstream of the

Table 3 Biological actions of GIP

Pancreas
Enhances glucose-stimulated insulin secretion
Stimulates insulin gene transcription
Adipose tissue
Stimulates insulin-dependent glucose uptake
Increases insulin receptor affinity and sensitivity of insulin-stimulated glucose transport
Enhances fatty acid synthesis and incorporation into triglyceride
Augments lipoprotein lipase synthesis and activity
Decreases glucagon-stimulated lipolysis
Modifies fat accumulation in setting of nutritional excess
Bone
Augments alkaline phosphatase activity and collagen type I mRNA levels
Increases bone mineral density in a rodent model of postmenopausal osteoporosis
Other tissues
Upregulates intestinal hexose transport
Stimulates glucocorticoid secretion
Induces vascular bed type dependent vasoconstriction or vasodilatation

transcription initiation site [410]. *Cis*-acting negative regulatory elements that influence cell-specific GIPR promoter activity have been localized to more distal 5′-flanking sequences [410].

GIPR signaling is coupled to cAMP activation and increase in intracellular calcium [411]. Activation of the GIPR increases intracellular cAMP in pancreatic islet cells, adipocytes, osteoblast cells, endothelial cells, and heterologous cell lines transfected with GIPR [408, 409, 411, 412]. GIPR-mediated elevation in intracellular Ca^{2+} involves mobilization of Ca^{2+} from intracellular stores and activation of cell surface cation channels [411]. The GIPR also signals via activation of PI3K, MAPK, and phospholipase A2 pathways [413–415]. The N-terminus of GIP is essential for biological activity, as GIP-(3-42) is biologically inactive [416]. The N-terminal domain and the first extracellular loop of the GIPR are necessary for high-affinity GIP binding, whereas the distal part of the N-terminal domain and the first transmembrane domain are essential for receptor activation and coupling to cAMP [417]. Most of the C-terminal tail of GIPR is not required for intracellular signaling, but a minimum receptor length of approximately 405 amino acids is required for efficient receptor transport and plasma membrane insertion [418].

The GIPR undergoes rapid and reversible homologous desensitization [3]. A combination of site-directed mutagenesis and C-terminal deletion experiments indicate that specific serine residues in the C-terminal tail of the GIPR, especially serines 426 and 427, are necessary for regulating the rate of receptor internalization, whereas serine residues 406 and 411 contribute to receptor desensitization [418]. Moreover, studies using the βTC3 islet cell line implicate a role for regulator of G-protein signaling 2, G-protein receptor kinase 2, and β-arrestin 1 in GIP-induced receptor desensitization [419].

Biological Actions of GIP

GIP exerts actions in different tissues, which are listed in Table 3 and summarized below.

Pancreas

GIP is released from intestinal K-cells following nutrient ingestion and functions as an incretin to augment glucose-stimulated insulin secretion. The molecular mechanisms by which GIP potentiates glucose-dependent insulin secretion are similar to those identified for GLP-1 and include elevation of intracellular cAMP, inhibition of ATP-sensitive K^+ channels, increase in intracellular Ca^{2+}, and direct interactions with the β-cell secretory machinery [310]. GIP may also enhance insulin gene transcription and upregulate the expression of glucose transporters and glucokinase, components of cellular glucose sensors [420]. The signaling pathways that mediate the insulin secretory action of GIP include activation of PKA, as well as PKA-independent mechanisms involving cAMP-GEFs and specific protein kinase signaling pathways [311, 421]. The importance of GIP as an incretin hormone is illustrated by disruption of GIP action *in vivo*. Elimination of GIPR activation with GIPR peptide antagonists or GIPR immunoneutralizing antisera leads to impaired oral glucose tolerance and reduced insulin secretion in rodents [422, 423]. Similarly, mice with a targeted deletion of the GIPR gene ($GIPR^{-/-}$) exhibit impaired glucose tolerance with a significant reduction in insulin secretion [424]. GIP, like GLP-1, may also function as a β-cell growth factor. The molecular signaling pathways that transmit the proliferative and antiapoptotic effects of GIP on β-cells include activation of cAMP/PKA, MAPK, and PI3K [425, 426].

Adipose Tissue

GIP acts as an anabolic hormone for adipocyte lipid metabolism [385, 427]. GIP stimulates glucose uptake and increases both the affinity of insulin for its receptor and the sensitivity of insulin-stimulated glucose transport in isolated adipocytes. GIP also enhances fatty acid production and insulin-stimulated incorporation of fatty acids into triglyceride, augments lipoprotein lipase synthesis and activity, and reduces glucagon-stimulated lipolysis in adipose tissue.

GIP may also have lipolytic effects [428]: it increases intracellular cAMP levels and stimulates glycerol release in the 3T3-L1 adipocyte cell line. GIP-induced lipolysis is inhibited by insulin in 3T3-L1 cells, suggesting that the lipolytic effects of GIP would likely occur in the fasting or postabsorptive state, when insulin levels are low. The signaling mechanism(s) activated by GIP in adipocytes has not been elucidated [385]. However, functional GIPRs are expressed on adipocytes [407, 408, 428], and GIP binding promotes increase in intracellular cAMP in adipocyte cultures [408, 428].

Bone

GIPR mRNA and protein are also found in normal bone and osteoblast-like cell lines [409]. GIP elevates cAMP and intracellular calcium in osteoblast cells and these effects are coupled to increases in both alkaline phosphatase activity and levels of collagen type I mRNA, events associated with bone formation [409]. In the ovariectomized rat, an animal model for postmenopausal osteoporosis, GIP treatment increases bone mineral density [429].

Other Tissues

In the stomach, GIP was originally shown to inhibit gastric acid secretion, but only at supraphysiological doses [430]. GIP upregulates hexose transport in the intestine [198] and attenuates glucagon-stimulated hepatic glucose production [431, 432], likely through an indirect mechanism, as GIPRs have not been detected in the liver [407]. GIP can enhance insulin-dependent glucose disposal in animals, although this effect is not seen in humans [433]. GIP also stimulates glucocorticoid secretion in rats via a cAMP/PKA-dependent signaling pathway [434], and aberrant expression of the GIPR in adrenocortical adenomas is associated with meal-induced Cushing's syndrome [435, 436]. The GIPR is present in the vascular endothelium, and infusion of GIP into dogs induces either vasoconstriction or vasodilatation, depending on the vascular bed involved [412]. The opposing effects of GIP in different vascular beds are attributed to variation in the degree of activation of signal transduction pathways in different endothelial cell types. GIP receptor mRNA is also detected in the heart, testis, lung, and several regions of the brain, including the telencephalon, diencephalon, cerebellum, and brain stem [385, 407]. The effects of GIP receptor activation in these tissues are not known.

EXENDIN

The majority of glucagon superfamily peptides have a highly conserved histidine residue at their amino terminus (His^1) [437]. To identify novel bioactive peptides in lizard venom, amino-terminal sequencing was used as a strategy to screen for novel His^1 peptides [438]. Using this technique, a 39-amino acid carboxy-terminal amidated peptide, designated exendin-4, was identified and purified from the venom of a *H. suspectum* lizard. The designation *exen*din-4 is derived from the observation that this peptide is found in an *ex*ocrine secretion and has *en*docrine activity, as described below.

Exendin-4 shares 53% amino acid sequence identity with mammalian GLP-1 (Figure 5) and functions as a GLP-1R agonist [307–309, 439]. Exendin-4 binds to the GLP-1R and conveys biological actions similar to those of GLP-1, including regulation of glucose-stimulated insulin secretion and insulin gene transcription, feeding behavior, gastric emptying, heart rate and blood pressure, and β-cell neogenesis and proliferation [28, 307, 308, 438]. Moreover, the actions of exendin-4 are blocked by the specific GLP-1R antagonist exendin-(9-39) [438].

As GLP-1 and exendin-4 exhibit 53% amino acid identity, and exendin-4 functions as a GLP-1R agonist, it was originally thought that exendin-4 may represent the reptilian GLP-1 homologue. However, the cloning and sequencing of cDNAs for both lizard proglucagon and exendin-4 demonstrated that exendin-4 was not the reptilian equivalent of GLP-1 [439]. In the lizard two different proglucagon cDNAs, lizard proglucagon I and II (LPI and LPII), with unique 3′-untranslated regions have been identified. LPI encodes glucagon and GLP-1 and its expression is restricted to the lizard pancreas. In contrast, LPII encodes glucagon, GLP-1, and GLP-2 and is expressed in both the lizard pancreas and intestine. Lizard exendin-4 is encoded by a single RNA transcript of approximately 500 nucleotides that also encodes a 45-amino acid peptide of unknown biological function N-terminal to the exendin-4 sequence. This peptide, designated exendin

GLP-1-(7-36)NH_2 ····HAEGTFTSDVSSYLEGQAAKEFIAWLVKGR-NH_2

Exendin-4 ···············HGEGTFTSDLSKQMEEEAVRLFIEWLKNGGPSSGAPPPS-NH_2

Figure 5 Comparison of the amino acid sequences of N-terminally truncated bioactive GLP-1 and exendin-4. The lizard-derived exendin-4 shares 53% amino acid sequence identity with mammalian GLP-1. Amino acid residues that are identical between the two sequences are in red

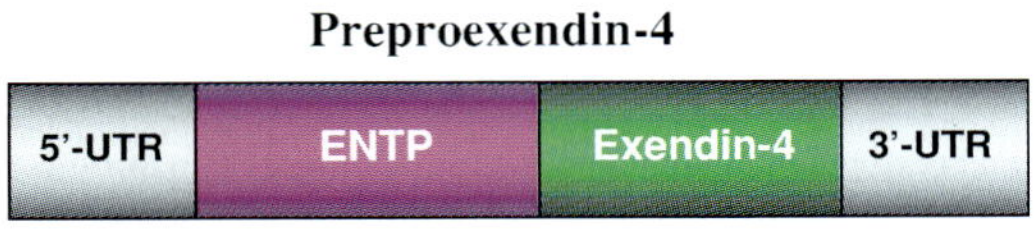

Figure 6 Lizard proexendin-4 mRNA structure. In addition to exendin-4, proexendin-4 also encodes ENTP, a 45-amino acid sequence, which likely encodes a signal peptide and a smaller peptide of unknown function. UTR: untranslated region; ENTP: exendin N-terminal peptide

N-terminal peptide, is followed by a pair of basic amino acids (characteristic of PC cleavage sites) and the 40-amino acid exendin sequence [439] (Figure 6). Lizard exendin-4 mRNA transcripts were detected in the lizard salivary gland, but not in the pancreas or intestine. The discovery that proglucagon and exendin-4 are encoded by unique genes in the lizard suggests that other species, including mammals, may possess an exendin-4 gene. However, attempts to clone a mammalian exendin-4 homologue have been unsuccessful [440].

Exendin-4 exhibits greater potency and more protracted physiological effects relative to GLP-1 [441, 442]. This is likely due, in part, to the longer plasma half-life of exendin-4 (18–41 min following intravenous bolus in rats) [443] compared to that of GLP-1 (less than 2 min) [259]. GLP-1 contains an alanine residue in position 2 and thus is rapidly catabolized by DPP-IV and is also a potential target for the endoproteolytic activity of NEP-24.11. In contrast, exendin-4 contains a glycine residue in position 2 and is not a substrate for DPP-IV-mediated catabolism. Furthermore, exendin-4 is a very poor substrate for NEP-24.11 [264]. This greater potency and extended plasma half-life, relative to GLP-1, renders exendin-4 a potential long-acting therapeutic agent for the treatment of diabetes.

GLP-1 and GLP-1 Analogues as a Therapy for Type 2 Diabetes

The actions of GLP-1 and GIP are essential for maintaining normal glucose homeostasis as disruption of their biological activity leads to impaired glucose tolerance. Several studies indicate that the incretin effect is lost or significantly reduced in type 2 diabetic patients [444, 445]. However, population studies and linkage analysis suggest that inherited mutations within or near the GLP-1R gene are unlikely to contribute to a predisposition to type 2 diabetes [270, 446]. Similarly, mutations in the gene encoding the GIPR have not been linked to the reduced incretin effect observed in type 2 diabetic patients and no mutations have been reported in the coding region of the GIP gene in diabetic patients [447].

Although enhancement of GIP action would appear to represent a useful strategy for the treatment of diabetes, circulating levels of GIP are normal or elevated in diabetic patients [448, 449], with the inactive truncated catabolite (GIP-(3-42)) representing the predominant molecular form [397]. Moreover, native GIP has little insulinotropic or glucagon-lowering activity in diabetic subjects [247, 450]. These observations are consistent with reports that elevated levels of plasma GIP promote chronic homologous desensitization of the GIP receptor [451]. It has been suggested that such a mechanism could contribute to the impaired insulin secretion seen in subjects with type 2 diabetes [451]. The diminished incretin effect in type 2 diabetes might result from defects in the GIPR, at the level of either GIPR mRNA expression or postreceptor signal transduction pathways. Indeed, levels of GIPR mRNA and protein are reduced in the pancreatic β-cells of Zucker diabetic fatty rats, a rodent model of type 2 diabetes [452]. As a consequence of the defective insulinotropic activity of human GIP, current therapeutic interventions are more focused on the use of GLP-1 and its analogues for the treatment of type 2 diabetes.

In healthy human subjects, GLP-1 augments glucose-stimulated insulin secretion, inhibits glucagon secretion and gastric emptying, and lowers both fasting and postprandial glucose levels [25]. Moreover, stimulatory and inhibitory effects of GLP-1 on insulin and glucagon levels, respectively, are glucose-dependent. Thus, under conditions of hypoglycemia, GLP-1 does not stimulate insulin secretion or suppress glucagon secretion [329]. The insulinotropic, glucagonostatic, and gastric inhibitory effects of GLP-1 are also preserved in the setting of type 2 diabetes. GLP-1 normalizes both fasting and postprandial glycemia by enhancing β-cell function and inhibiting glucagon secretion and gastric emptying in diabetic subjects [367, 453, 454]. GLP-1 also improves glycemic control in diabetic patients unresponsive to sulfonylureas [455], suggesting that GLP-1 restores β-cell function in patients with more advanced stages of the disease. In type 1 diabetic patients, GLP-1 reduces fasting and postprandial glucose levels and lowers meal-related insulin requirements, likely via inhibition of glucagon secretion and/or gastric emptying [456, 457]. In longer term studies, 3 weeks of subcutaneous administration of GLP-1, three times a day prior to a standard test meal, lowered postprandial glycemic excursions and plasma glucagon levels in patients with type 2 diabetes [458]. Continuous subcutaneous infusion of GLP-1 for 6 weeks in patients with type 2 diabetes decreased fasting and mean plasma glucose and free fatty acid levels, reduced hemoglobin A_{1c} (HbA_{1c}) values, inhibited gastric emptying, decreased appetite and body weight, and improved insulin sensitivity and β-cell function [367]. Thus, GLP-1 seems to retain its glucose-lowering effects in diabetic subjects even with extended treatment. In short-term studies, GLP-1 and its more potent analogue exendin-4 decreased food intake and promoted satiety in both healthy humans and patients with type 2 diabetes [352, 353, 459]. More prolonged and sustained GLP-1 infusion leads to a reduction in body weight in type 2 diabetic individuals [367]. Since there is a strong correlation between obesity and the development of insulin resistance and type 2 diabetes, the ability of GLP-1 and its analogs to suppress energy intake and reduce body weight imparts an additional beneficial mechanism for improving glucose tolerance in these patients.

The capacity of GLP-1 to (1) lower elevated blood glucose levels through multiple mechanisms including stimulation of insulin secretion and inhibition of glucagon secretion and gastric emptying, (2) reduce food intake and body weight, (3) function in a highly glucose-dependent manner, and (4) induce β-cell neogenesis and proliferation implicates a potential therapeutic role for GLP-1 in type 2 diabetes. Moreover, defects in GLP-1 secretion have been observed in type 2 diabetic and obese individuals, as well as in subjects with insulin resistance [448, 460]. However, native GLP-1 has a very short plasma half-life (less than 2 min) and thus would require continuous infusion or multiple injections to achieve adequate glycemic control. Consequently, alternative strategies for maintaining sustained GLP-1 action have been developed and include elimination of DPP-IV activity with specific inhibitors [260] and the development of GLP-1 analogs or formulations that prolong GLP-1 action *in vivo* [461–463].

DPP-IV and Incretin Action

The use of agents that inhibit DPP-IV activity has been proposed as an alternative to GLP-1 therapy for the treatment of type 2 diabetes [256, 260, 464]. The DPP-IV inhibitor valine pyrrolidide increases the plasma levels of intact biologically active GLP-1, both in the basal (endogenous) state and following GLP-1 infusion, and is associated with enhanced insulinotropic and glucagonostatic GLP-1 actions [465]. In rats, pharmacological inhibition of DPP-IV activity with isoleucine thiazolide increases the plasma half-life of intact, endogenous GLP-1 released in response to intraduodenal glucose, which reduces the time required to reach peak insulin levels and thus results in a more rapid clearance of blood glucose [466]. In lean and obese Zucker rats, oral administration of the DPP-IV inhibitors isoleucine thiazolide or 1-[[[2-[(5-cyanopyridin-2-yl)amino]ethyl]amino]acetyl]-2-cyano-(*S*)-pyrrolidine (NVP-DPP728) enhances insulin secretion and improves glucose tolerance [467, 468]. In control and high-fat fed glucose intolerant mice, inhibition of DPP-IV activity raises the levels of endogenous GLP-1 and improves glucose tolerance and insulin secretion [469]. In more long-term studies, inhibition of DPP-IV activity leads to sustained improvements in β-cell function and insulin action [470, 471]. Mice with a targeted inactivation of their DPP-IV gene clear an oral glucose load more rapidly than their wild-type littermates and exhibit significant increases in the glucose-stimulated insulin levels, in association with elevated plasma levels of intact biologically active GLP-1 [472]. Inhibition of DPP-IV activity for up to 4 months is associated with sustained improvements in glucose tolerance, peripheral insulin sensitivity, and β-cell glucose responsiveness in diabetic rats [470], and 8 weeks of DPP-IV inhibition improves glucose tolerance, enhances insulin secretion and GLUT-2 expression, and preserves islet function in insulin-resistant diabetic mice [473]. Preliminary analysis of the use of DPP-IV inhibitors in human subjects with type 2 diabetes demonstrated improvements in both fasting and postprandial glucose and HbA_{1c} in a 4-week placebo controlled randomized study with NVP-DPP728, a selective, orally active inhibitor of DPP-IV [474].

The available data suggest that DPP-IV inhibition represents a potential therapeutic approach for treatment of patients with type 2 diabetes. However, DPP-IV can also degrade cytokines and regulatory peptides that contain an alanine or proline in the penultimate N-terminal position, including neuropeptide Y, growth-hormone-releasing factor, and peptide YY [257]. Furthermore, DPP-IV has been implicated in the co-stimulation and activation of T-cells [475, 476]. Thus, the long-term use of DPP-IV inhibitors as a therapeutic treatment for diabetes may be associated with unanticipated side effects, and monitoring of immune function in treated patients appears warranted.

An alternative approach to circumvent DPP-IV-mediated incretin degradation is through the use of DPP-IV-resistant GLP-1 analogues. Substitution of the N-terminal penultimate alanine residue of GLP-1 with a glycine or serine residue, α-aminoisobutyric acid, or the D-amino acid form generates DPP-IV-resistant molecules with increased plasma stability and similar or greater insulin-releasing activity compared to the native peptide [477–480]. Removal of the α-amino group or insertion of a glucitol adduct at the N-terminal histidine residue of GLP-1 produces stable analogues with comparable or more potent glucose-lowering effects than wild-type GLP-1 [481, 482]. Studies in normal and diabetic rodents indicate that linkage of acyl chains to the α-amino group of the N-terminal histidine residue or insertion of 6-aminohexanoic acid between the N-terminal histidine and alanine residues yields more potent GLP-1 derivatives with sustained biological activity [480, 483]. Fatty acid derivitization of amino acids located in the C-terminal region of GLP-1 promotes albumin binding and produces GLP-1 analogs with plasma half-lives of up to approximately 10 h in humans [484, 485]. Subchronic treatment with these long-acting acylated GLP-1 derivatives decreases food intake and reduces body weight and adiposity in both normal and diabetic rats [485]. In type 2 diabetic patients, a single subcutaneous injection of an acylated GLP-1 analogue increased insulin release, suppressed both glucagon secretion and gastric emptying, and significantly reduced fasting and postprandial glucose excursions [462].

SUMMARY

(1) IAPP secreted from β-cells exerts diverse actions on gastrointestinal motility and islet hormone secretion.
(2) Exogenous IAPP analogue administration lowers blood glucose in subjects with type 1 and type 2 diabetes.
(3) IAPP action is mediated through a unique receptor dependent on RAMP activity.
(4) GLP-1 is secreted from gut endocrine cells in a nutrient-dependent manner and regulates both postprandial and fasting glycemia.
(5) Exogenous GLP-1 administration reduces food intake and inhibits gastric emptying.
(6) Native GLP-1 is rapidly degraded by DPP-IV.
(7) DPP-IV-resistant GLP-1 analogues appear effective in clinical trials for the treatment of type 2 diabetes.
(8) The lizard salivary gland peptide exendin-4 is a potent DPP-IV-resistant GLP-1R agonist that exerts similar glucose-lowering actions compared to native GLP-1.

REFERENCES

1. Bayliss WM, Starling EH. On the causation of the so-called "peripheral reflex secretion" of the pancreas. *Proc R Soc Lond* [Biol] 1902; 69: 352–3.
2. Moore B, Edie ES, Abram JH. On the treatment of diabetes mellitus by acid extract of duodenal mucous membrane. *Biochem J* 1906; 1: 28–38.
3. Fehmann H-C, Goke R, Goke B. Cell and molecular biology of the incretin hormones glucagon-like peptide 1 and glucose-dependent releasing polypeptide. *Endocrine Rev* 1995; 16: 390–410.
4. Kieffer TJ, Habener JF. The glucagon-like peptides. *Endocr Rev* 1999; 20: 876–913.
5. Zunz E, LaBarre J. Contributions a l'etude des variations physiologiques de la secretion interne du pancreas: realations entre les secretions extern et interne du pancreas. *Arch Int Phsiol Biochim* 1929; 31: 20–44.
6. Unger RH, Eisentraut AM. Entero-insular axis. *Arch Int Med* 1969; 123: 261–6.
7. Elrick H, Stimmler L, Hlad CJ Jr, Arai Y. Plasma insulin response to oral and intravenous glucose administration. *J Clin Invest* 1964; 24: 1076–82.
8. Perley MJ, Kipnis DM. Plasma insulin responses to oral and intravenous glucose: studies in normal and diabetic subjects. *J Clin Invest* 1967; 46: 1954–62.
9. McIntyre N, Holsworth DC, Turner DS. New interpretation of oral glucose tolerance. *Lancet* 1964; 2: 20–1.
10. Arnould Y, Bellens R, Franckson JRM, Conard V. Insulin response and glucose-C14 disappearance rate during the glucose tolerance test in the unanesthetized dog. *Metabolism* 1963; 12: 1122–31.
11. Dupre J, Beck JC. Stimulation of release of insulin by an extract of intestinal mucosa. *Diabetes* 1966; 15: 555–9.
12. Creutzfeld WO. The incretin concept today. *Diabetologia* 1979; 16: 75–85.
13. Dupre J, Ross SA, Watson D, Brown JC. Stimulation of insulin secretion by gastric inhibitory polypeptide in man. *J Clin Endocrinol Metab* 1973; 37: 826–8.
14. Pederson RA, Schubert HE, Brown JC. Gastric inhibitory polypeptide. Its physiological release and insulinotropic action in the dog. *Diabetes* 1975; 24: 1050–6.
15. Elahi D, Andersen DK, Brown JC, Debas HT, Hershcopf RJ, Raizes GS, Tobin JD, Andres R. Pancreatic alpha- and beta-cell responses to GIP infusion in normal man. *Am J Physiol* 1979; 237: E185–91.
16. Cleator IG, Gourlay RH. Release of immunoreactive gastric inhibitory polypeptide (IR-GIP) by oral ingestion of food substances. *Am J Surg* 1975; 130: 128–35.
17. Ross SA, Dupre J. Effects of ingestion of triglyceride or galactose on secretion of gastric inhibitory polypeptide and on responses to intravenous glucose in normal and diabetic subjects. *Diabetes* 1978; 27: 327–33.
18. Ebert R, Creutzfeldt W. Influence of gastric inhibitory polypeptide antiserum on glucose-induced insulin secretion in rats. *Endocrinology* 1982; 111: 1601–6.
19. Ebert R, Unger H, Creutzfeld W. Preservation of incretin activity after removal of gastric inhibitory polypeptide (GIP) from rat gut extracts by immunoadsorption. *Diabetologia* 1983; 24: 449–54.
20. Lauritsen KB, Holst JJ, Moody AJ. Depression of insulin release by anti-GIP serum after oral glucose tolerance in rats. *Scand J Gastroenterol* 1981; 16: 417–21.
21. Lauritsen KB, Moody AJ, Christensen KC, Lindkaer Jensen S. Gastric inhibitory polypeptide (GIP) and insulin release after small-bowel resection in man. *Scand J Gastroenterol* 1980; 15: 833–40.
22. Heinrich G, Gros P, Lund PK, Bentley RC, Habener JF. Pre-proglucagon messenger ribonucleic acid: nucleotide and encoded amino acid sequences of the rat pancreatic complementary deoxyribonucleic acid. *Endocrinology* 1984; 115: 2176–81.
23. Bell GI, Santerre RF, Mullenbach GT. Hamster preproglucagon contains the sequence of glucagon and two related peptides. *Nature* 1983; 302: 716–8.
24. Lopez LC, Frazier ML, Su CJ, Kumar A, Saunders GF. Mammalian pancreatic preproglucagon contains three glucagon-related peptides. *Proc Natl Acad Sci USA* 1983; 80: 5485–9.
25. Drucker DJ. The glucagon-like peptides. *Diabetes* 1998; 47: 159–69.
26. Nauck MA, Bartels E, Orskov C, Ebert R, Creutzfeld W. Additive insulinotropic effects of exogenous synthetic human gastric inhibitory polypeptide and glucagon-like peptide-1-(7-36) amide infused at near-physiological insulinotropic hormone and glucose concentrations. *J Clin Endocrinol Metab* 1993; 76: 912–7.
27. Fehmann HC, Goke B, Goke R, Trautmann ME, Arnold R. Synergistic stimulatory effect of glucagon-like peptide-1 (7-36) amide and glucose-dependent insulin-releasing polypeptide on the endocrine pancreas. *FEBS Lett* 1989; 252: 109–12.
28. Eng J, Kleinman WA, Singh L, Singh G, Raufman JP. Isolation and characterization of exendin 4, an exendin 3 analogue from Heloderma suspectum venom. *J Biol Chem* 1992; 267: 7402–5.
29. Cooper GJ, Willis AC, Clark A, Turner RC, Sim RB, Reid KB. Purification and characterization of a peptide from amyloid-rich pancreases of type 2 diabetic patients. *Proc Natl Acad Sci USA* 1987; 84: 8628–32.
30. Westermark P, Wernstedt C, Wilander E, Sletten K. A novel peptide in the calcitonin gene related peptide family as an amyloid fibril protein in the endocrine pancreas. *Biochem Biophys Res Commun* 1986; 140: 827–31.

31. Porte D Jr, Kahn SE. Beta-cell dysfunction and failure in type 2 diabetes: potential mechanisms. *Diabetes* 2001; 50 (suppl 1): S160–3.
32. Hoppener JW, Ahren B, Lips CJ. Islet amyloid and type 2 diabetes mellitus. *N Engl J Med* 2000; 343: 411–9.
33. Kahn SE, Andrikopoulos S, Verchere CB. Islet amyloid: a long-recognized but underappreciated pathological feature of type 2 diabetes. *Diabetes* 1999; 48: 241–53.
34. Westermark P, Wilander E, Westermark GT, Johnson KH. Islet amyloid polypeptide-like immunoreactivity in the islet B cells of type 2 (non-insulin-dependent) diabetic and non-diabetic individuals. *Diabetologia* 1987; 30: 887–92.
35. Westermark P, Wernstedt C, Wilander E, Hayden DW, O'Brien TD, Johnson KH. Amyloid fibrils in human insulinoma and islets of Langerhans of the diabetic cat are derived from a neuropeptide-like protein also present in normal islet cells. *Proc Natl Acad Sci USA* 1987; 84: 3881–5.
36. Wimalawansa SJ. Amylin, calcitonin gene-related peptide, calcitonin, and adrenomedullin: a peptide superfamily. *Crit Rev Neurobiol* 1997; 11: 167–239.
37. Jaikaran ET, Clark A. Islet amyloid and type 2 diabetes: from molecular misfolding to islet pathophysiology. *Biochim Biophys Acta* 2001; 1537: 179–203.
38. Nishi M, Sanke T, Seino S, Eddy RL, Fan Y-S, Byers MG, Shows TB, Bell GI, Steiner DF. Human islet amyloid polypeptide gene: complete nucleotide sequence, chromosomal localization, and evolutionary history. *Mol Endocrinol* 1989; 3: 1775–81.
39. Cooper GJS. Amylin compared with calcitonin gene-related peptide: structure, biology and relevance to metabolic disease. *Endocrine Rev* 1994; 15: 163–201.
40. Bretherton-Watt D, Gore N, Boam DS. Insulin upstream factor 1 and a novel ubiquitous factor bind to the human islet amyloid polypeptide/amylin gene promoter. *Biochem J* 1996; 313 (pt 2): 495–502.
41. Carty MD, Lillquist JS, Peshavaria M, Stein R, Soeller WC. Identification of *cis*- and *trans*-active factors regulating human islet amyloid polypeptide gene expression in pancreatic beta-cells. *J Biol Chem* 1997; 272: 11986–93.
42. Macfarlane WM, Campbell SC, Elrick LJ, Oates V, Bermano G, Lindley KJ, Aynsley-Green A, Dunne MJ, James RF, Docherty K. Glucose regulates islet amyloid polypeptide gene transcription in a PDX1- and calcium-dependent manner. *J Biol Chem* 2000; 275: 15330–5.
43. O'Brien TD, Westermark P, Johnson KH. Islet amyloid polypeptide and insulin secretion from isolated perfused pancreas of fed, fasted, glucose-treated, and dexamethasone-treated rats. *Diabetes* 1991; 40: 1701–6.
44. Bretherton-Watt D, Ghatei MA, Bloom SR, Jamal H, Ferrier GJ, Girgis SI, Legon S. Altered islet amyloid polypeptide (amylin) gene expression in rat models of diabetes. *Diabetologia* 1989; 32: 881–3.
45. Alam T, Chen L, Ogawa A, Leffert JD, Unger RH, Luskey KL. Coordinate regulation of amylin and insulin expression in response to hypoglycemia and fasting. *Diabetes* 1992; 41: 508–14.
46. Ding WQ, Holicky E, Miller LJ. Glucose and forskolin regulate IAPP gene expression through different signal transduction pathways. *Am J Physiol Endocrinol Metab* 2001; 281: E938–45.
47. Sanke T, Bell GI, Sample C, Rubenstein AH, Steiner DF. An islet amyloid peptide is derived from an 89-amino acid precursor by proteolytic processing. *J Biol Chem* 1988; 263: 17243–6.
48. Leffert JD, Newgard CB, Okamoto H, Milburn JL, Luskey KL. Rat amylin: cloning and tissue-specific expression in pancreatic islets. *Proc Natl Acad Sci USA* 1989; 86: 3127–30.
49. Seidah NG, Chretien M. Proprotein and prohormone convertases: a family of subtilases generating diverse bioactive polypeptides. *Brain Res* 1999; 848: 45–62.
50. Badman MK, Shennan KI, Jermany JL, Docherty K, Clark A. Processing of pro-islet amyloid polypeptide (proIAPP) by the prohormone convertase PC2. *FEBS Lett* 1996; 378: 227–31.
51. Higham CE, Hull RL, Lawrie L, Shennan KI, Morris JF, Birch NP, Docherty K, Clark A. Processing of synthetic pro-islet amyloid polypeptide (proIAPP) "amylin" by recombinant prohormone convertase enzymes, PC2 and PC3, *in vitro*. *Eur J Biochem* 2000; 267: 4998–5004.
52. Wang J, Xu J, Finnerty J, Furuta M, Steiner DF, Verchere CB. The prohormone convertase enzyme 2 (PC2) is essential for processing pro-islet amyloid polypeptide at the NH_2-terminal cleavage site. *Diabetes* 2001; 50: 534–9.
53. Inoue K, Hisatomi A, Umeda F, Nawata H. Release of amylin from perfused rat pancreas in response to glucose and glucagon. *Diabetes Res Clin Pract* 1992; 15: 85–8.
54. Inoue K, Hisatomi A, Umeda F, Nawata H. Effects of exogenous somatostatin and insulin on islet amyloid polypeptide (amylin) release from perfused rat pancreas. *Horm Metab Res* 1992; 24: 251–3.
55. Moore CX, Cooper GJ. Co-secretion of amylin and insulin from cultured islet beta-cells: modulation by nutrient secretagogues, islet hormones and hypoglycemic agents. *Biochem Biophys Res Commun* 1991; 179: 1–9.
56. Inoue K, Hisatomi A, Umeda F, Nawata H. Effects of glucagon-like peptide 1 (7-36) amide and glucagon on amylin release from perfused rat pancreas. *Horm Metab Res* 1991; 23: 407–9.
57. Jamal H, Suda K, Bretherton-Watt D, Ghatei MA, Bloom SR. Molecular form of islet amyloid polypeptide (amylin) released from isolated rat islets of Langerhans. *Pancreas* 1993; 8: 261–6.
58. Koda JE, Fineman M, Rink TJ, Dailey GE, Muchmore DB, Linarelli LG. Amylin concentrations and glucose control. *Lancet* 1992; 339: 1179–80.
59. Pittner RA, Albrandt K, Beaumont K, Gaeta LS, Koda JE, Moore CX, Rittenhouse J, Rink TJ. Molecular physiology of amylin. *J Cell Biochem* 1994; 55 (suppl): 19–28.
60. Hayden MR, Tyagi SC. "A" is for amylin and amyloid in type 2 diabetes mellitus. *JOP* 2001; 2: 124–39.
61. Leckstrom A, Bjorklund K, Permert J, Larsson R, Westermark P. Renal elimination of islet amyloid polypeptide. *Biochem Biophys Res Commun* 1997; 239: 265–8.
62. Sowa R, Sanke T, Hirayama J, Tabata H, Furuta H, Nishimura S, Nanjo K. Islet amyloid polypeptide amide causes peripheral insulin resistance *in vivo* in dogs. *Diabetologia* 1990; 33: 118–20.
63. Muff R, Born W, Fischer JA. Adrenomedullin and related peptides: receptors and accessory proteins. *Peptides* 2001; 22: 1765–72.
64. Martinez A, Kapas S, Miller MJ, Ward Y, Cuttitta F. Coexpression of receptors for adrenomedullin, calcitonin gene-related peptide, and amylin in pancreatic beta-cells. *Endocrinology* 2000; 141: 406–11.

65. Christopoulos G, Perry KJ, Morfis M, Tilakaratne N, Gao Y, Fraser NJ, Main MJ, Foord SM, Sexton PM. Multiple amylin receptors arise from receptor activity-modifying protein interaction with the calcitonin receptor gene product. *Mol Pharmacol* 1999; 56: 235–42.
66. Ueda T, Ugawa S, Saishin Y, Shimada S. Expression of receptor-activity modifying protein (RAMP) mRNAs in the mouse brain. *Brain Res Mol Brain Res* 2001; 93: 36–45.
67. Zumpe ET, Tilakaratne N, Fraser NJ, Christopoulos G, Foord SM, Sexton PM. Multiple ramp domains are required for generation of amylin receptor phenotype from the calcitonin receptor gene product. *Biochem Biophys Res Commun* 2000; 267: 368–72.
68. Tedstone AE, Nezzer T, Hughes SJ, Clark A, Matthews DR. The effect of islet amyloid polypeptide (amylin) and calcitonin gene-related peptide on glucose removal in the anaesthetized rat and on insulin secretion from rat pancreatic islets *in vitro*. *Biosci Rep* 1990; 10: 339–45.
69. Nagamatsu S, Carroll RJ, Grodsky GM, Steiner DF. Lack of islet amyloid polypeptide regulation of insulin biosynthesis or secretion in normal rat islets. *Diabetes* 1990; 39: 871–4.
70. Ohsawa H, Kanatsuka A, Yamaguchi T, Makino H, Yoshida S. Islet amyloid polypeptide inhibits glucose-stimulated insulin secretion from isolated rat pancreatic islets. *Biochem Biophys Res Commun* 1989; 160: 961–7.
71. Degano P, Silvestre RA, Salas M, Peiro E, Marco J. Amylin inhibits glucose-induced insulin secretion in a dose-dependent manner. Study in the perfused rat pancreas. *Regul Pept* 1993; 43: 91–6.
72. Bretherton-Watt D, Gilbey SG, Ghatei MA, Beacham J, Macrae AD, Bloom SR. Very high concentrations of islet amyloid polypeptide are necessary to alter the insulin response to intravenous glucose in man. *J Clin Endocrinol Metab* 1992; 74: 1032–5.
73. Wang F, Adrian TE, Westermark GT, Ding X, Gasslander T, Permert J. Islet amyloid polypeptide tonally inhibits beta-, alpha-, and delta-cell secretion in isolated rat pancreatic islets. *Am J Physiol* 1999; 276: E19–24.
74. Wang ZL, Bennet WM, Ghatei MA, Byfield PG, Smith DM, Bloom SR. Influence of islet amyloid polypeptide and the 8-37 fragment of islet amyloid polypeptide on insulin release from perifused rat islets. *Diabetes* 1993; 42: 330–5.
75. Young AA, Carlo P, Rink TJ, Wang MW. 8-37hCGRP, an amylin receptor antagonist, enhances the insulin response and perturbs the glucose response to infused arginine in anesthetized rats. *Mol Cell Endocrinol* 1992; 84: R1–5.
76. Kulkarni RN, Smith DM, Ghatei MA, Jones PM, Bloom SR. Investigation of the effects of antisense oligodeoxynucleotides to islet amyloid polypeptide mRNA on insulin release, content and expression. *J Endocrinol* 1996; 151: 341–8.
77. Mather KJ, Paradisi G, Leaming R, Hook G, Steinberg HO, Fineberg N, Hanley R, Baron AD. Role of amylin in insulin secretion and action in humans: antagonist studies across the spectrum of insulin sensitivity. *Diabetes Metab Res Rev* 2002; 18: 118–26.
78. Ahren B, Oosterwijk C, Lips CJ, Hoppener JW. Transgenic overexpression of human islet amyloid polypeptide inhibits insulin secretion and glucose elimination after gastric glucose gavage in mice. *Diabetologia* 1998; 41: 1374–80.
79. Gebre-Medhin S, Mulder H, Pekny M, Westermark G, Tornell J, Westermark P, Sundler F, Ahren B, Betsholtz C. Increased insulin secretion and glucose tolerance in mice lacking islet amyloid polypeptide (amylin). *Biochem Biophys Res Commun* 1998; 250: 271–7.
80. Gebre-Medhin S, Olofsson C, Mulder H. Islet amyloid polypeptide in the islets of Langerhans: friend or foe? *Diabetologia* 2000; 43: 687–95.
81. Karlsson E, Sandler S. Islet amyloid polypeptide promotes beta-cell proliferation in neonatal rat pancreatic islets. *Diabetologia* 2001; 44: 1015–8.
82. Gedulin BR, Rink TJ, Young AA. Dose-response for glucagonostatic effect of amylin in rats. *Metabolism* 1997; 46: 67–70.
83. Silvestre RA, Rodriguez-Gallardo J, Jodka C, Parkes DG, Pittner RA, Young AA, Marco J. Selective amylin inhibition of the glucagon response to arginine is extrinsic to the pancreas. *Am J Physiol Endocrinol Metab* 2001; 280: E443–9.
84. Kong MF, King P, Macdonald IA, Stubbs TA, Perkins AC, Blackshaw PE, Moyses C, Tattersall RB. Infusion of pramlintide, a human amylin analogue, delays gastric emptying in men with IDDM. *Diabetologia* 1997; 40: 82–8.
85. Young A, Denaro M. Roles of amylin in diabetes and in regulation of nutrient load. *Nutrition* 1998; 14: 524–7.
86. Clementi G, Caruso A, Cutuli VM, de Bernardis E, Prato A, Amico-Roxas M. Amylin given by central or peripheral routes decreases gastric emptying and intestinal transit in the rat. *Experientia* 1996; 52: 677–9.
87. Sexton PM, Paxinos G, Kenney MA, Wookey PJ, Beaumont K. *In vitro* autoradiographic localization of amylin binding sites in rat brain. *Neuroscience* 1994; 62: 553–67.
88. Bouali SM, Wimalawansa SJ, Jolicoeur FB. *In vivo* central actions of rat amylin. *Regul Pept* 1995; 56: 167–74.
89. Lutz TA, Del Prete E, Scharrer E. Reduction of food intake in rats by intraperitoneal injection of low doses of amylin. *Physiol Behav* 1994; 55: 891–5.
90. Morley JE, Flood JF. Amylin decreases food intake in mice. *Peptides* 1991; 12: 865–9.
91. Arnelo U, Permert J, Adrian TE, Larsson J, Westermark P, Reidelberger RD. Chronic infusion of islet amyloid polypeptide causes anorexia in rats. *Am J Physiol* 1996; 271: R1654–9.
92. Rushing PA, Hagan MM, Seeley RJ, Lutz TA, Woods SC. Amylin: a novel action in the brain to reduce body weight. *Endocrinology* 2000; 141: 850–3.
93. Rushing PA, Lutz TA, Seeley RJ, Woods SC. Amylin and insulin interact to reduce food intake in rats. *Horm Metab Res* 2000; 32: 62–5.
94. Rushing PA, Hagan MM, Seeley RJ, Lutz TA, D'Alessio DA, Air EL, Woods SC. Inhibition of central amylin signaling increases food intake and body adiposity in rats. *Endocrinology* 2001; 142: 5035–8.
95. Chance WT, Balasubramaniam A, Chen X, Fischer JE. Tests of adipsia and conditioned taste aversion following the intrahypothalamic injection of amylin. *Peptides* 1992; 13: 961–4.
96. Reidelberger RD, Arnelo U, Granqvist L, Permert J. Comparative effects of amylin and cholecystokinin on food intake and gastric emptying in rats. *Am J Physiol Regul Integr Comp Physiol* 2001; 280: R605–11.
97. Lutz TA, Althaus J, Rossi R, Scharrer E. Anorectic effect of amylin is not transmitted by capsaicin-sensitive

nerve fibers. *Am J Physiol* 1998; 274: R1777–82.
98. Lutz TA, Del Prete E, Scharrer E. Subdiaphragmatic vagotomy does not influence the anorectic effect of amylin. *Peptides* 1995; 16: 457–62.
99. Lutz TA, Senn M, Althaus J, Del Prete E, Ehrensperger F, Scharrer E. Lesion of the area postrema/nucleus of the solitary tract (AP/NTS) attenuates the anorectic effects of amylin and calcitonin gene-related peptide (CGRP) in rats. *Peptides* 1998; 19: 309–17.
100. Riediger T, Schmid HA, Lutz T, Simon E. Amylin potently activates AP neurons possibly via formation of the excitatory second messenger cGMP. *Am J Physiol Regul Integr Comp Physiol* 2001; 281: R1833–43.
101. Johnson AK, Thunhorst RL. The neuroendocrinology of thirst and salt appetite: visceral sensory signals and mechanisms of central integration. *Front Neuroendocrinol* 1997; 18: 292–353.
102. Riediger T, Rauch M, Schmid HA. Actions of amylin on subfornical organ neurons and on drinking behavior in rats. *Am J Physiol* 1999; 276: R514–21.
103. Leighton B, Cooper GJ. Pancreatic amylin and calcitonin gene-related peptide cause resistance to insulin in skeletal muscle *in vitro*. *Nature* 1988; 335: 632–5.
104. Koopmans SJ, van Mansfeld AD, Jansz HS, Krans HM, Radder JK, Frolich M, de Boer SF, Kreutter DK, Andrews GC, Maassen JA. Amylin-induced *in vivo* insulin resistance in conscious rats: the liver is more sensitive to amylin than peripheral tissues. *Diabetologia* 1991; 34: 218–24.
105. Deems RO, Deacon RW, Young DA. Amylin activates glycogen phosphorylase and inactivates glycogen synthase via a cAMP-independent mechanism. *Biochem Biophys Res Commun* 1991; 174: 716–20.
106. Young AA, Crocker LB, Wolfe-Lopez D, Cooper GJ. Daily amylin replacement reverses hepatic glycogen depletion in insulin-treated streptozotocin diabetic rats. *FEBS Lett* 1991; 287: 203–5.
107. Young AA, Mott DM, Stone K, Cooper GJ. Amylin activates glycogen phosphorylase in the isolated soleus muscle of the rat. *FEBS Lett* 1991; 281: 149–51.
108. Pittner R, Beaumont K, Young A, Rink T. Dose-dependent elevation of cyclic AMP, activation of glycogen phosphorylase, and release of lactate by amylin in rat skeletal muscle. *Biochim Biophys Acta* 1995; 1267: 75–82.
109. Wilding JP, Khandan-Nia N, Bennet WM, Gilbey SG, Beacham J, Ghatei MA, Bloom SR. Lack of acute effect of amylin (islet associated polypeptide) on insulin sensitivity during hyperinsulinaemic euglycaemic clamp in humans. *Diabetologia* 1994; 37: 166–9.
110. Wookey PJ, Tikellis C, Du HC, Qin HF, Sexton PM, Cooper ME. Amylin binding in rat renal cortex, stimulation of adenylyl cyclase, and activation of plasma renin. *Am J Physiol* 1996; 270: F289–94.
111. Cooper ME, McNally PG, Phillips PA, Johnston CI. Amylin stimulates plasma renin concentration in humans. *Hypertension* 1995; 26: 460–4.
112. Harris PJ, Cooper ME, Hiranyachattada S, Berka JL, Kelly DJ, Nobes M, Wookey PJ. Amylin stimulates proximal tubular sodium transport and cell proliferation in the rat kidney. *Am J Physiol* 1997; 272: F13–21.
113. Wookey PJ, Tikellis C, Nobes M, Casley D, Cooper ME, Darby IA. Amylin as a growth factor during fetal and postnatal development of the rat kidney. *Kidney Int* 1998; 53: 25–30.
114. Pietschmann P, Farsoudi KH, Hoffmann O, Klaushofer K, Horandner H, Peterlik M. Inhibitory effect of amylin on basal and parathyroid hormone-stimulated bone resorption in cultured neonatal mouse calvaria. *Bone* 1993; 14: 167–72.
115. Datta HK, Zaidi M, Wimalawansa SJ, Ghatei MA, Beacham JL, Bloom SR, MacIntyre I. *In vivo* and *in vitro* effects of amylin and amylin-amide on calcium metabolism in the rat and rabbit. *Biochem Biophys Res Commun* 1989; 162: 876–81.
116. Cornish J, Callon KE, Cooper GJ, Reid IR. Amylin stimulates osteoblast proliferation and increases mineralized bone volume in adult mice. *Biochem Biophys Res Commun* 1995; 207: 133–9.
117. Villa I, Rubinacci A, Ravasi F, Ferrara AF, Guidobono F. Effects of amylin on human osteoblast-like cells. *Peptides* 1997; 18: 537–40.
118. Champion HC, Pierce RL, Bivalacqua TJ, Murphy WA, Coy DH, Kadowitz PJ. Analysis of responses to hAmylin, hCGRP, and hADM in isolated resistance arteries from the mesenteric vascular bed of the rat. *Peptides* 2001; 22: 1427–34.
119. Golpon HA, Puechner A, Welte T, Wichert PV, Feddersen CO. Vasorelaxant effect of glucagon-like peptide-(7-36)amide and amylin on the pulmonary circulation of the rat. *Regul Pept* 2001; 102: 81–6.
120. Westermark P, Wernstedt C, O'Brien TD, Hayden DW, Johnson KH. Islet amyloid in type 2 human diabetes mellitus and adult diabetic cats contains a novel putative polypeptide hormone. *Am J Pathol* 1987; 127: 414–7.
121. Verchere CB, D'Alessio DA, Palmiter RD, Weir GC, Bonner-Weir S, Baskin DG, Kahn SE. Islet amyloid formation associated with hyperglycemia in transgenic mice with pancreatic beta cell expression of human islet amyloid polypeptide. *Proc Natl Acad Sci USA* 1996; 93: 3492–6.
122. Johnson KH, O'Brien TD, Betsholtz C, Westermark P. Islet amyloid, islet-amyloid polypeptide, and diabetes mellitus. *N Engl J Med* 1989; 321: 513–8.
123. Johnson KH, O'Brien TD, Jordan K, Westermark P. Impaired glucose tolerance is associated with increased islet amyloid polypeptide (IAPP) immunoreactivity in pancreatic beta cells. *Am J Pathol* 1989; 135: 245–50.
124. Pehling G, Tessari P, Gerich JE, Haymond MW, Service FJ, Rizza RA. Abnormal meal carbohydrate disposition in insulin-dependent diabetes. Relative contributions of endogenous glucose production and initial splanchnic uptake and effect of intensive insulin therapy. *J Clin Invest* 1984; 74: 985–91.
125. Dinneen S, Alzaid A, Turk D, Rizza R. Failure of glucagon suppression contributes to postprandial hyperglycaemia in IDDM. *Diabetologia* 1995; 38: 337–43.
126. Cline GW, Rothman DL, Magnusson I, Katz LD, Shulman GI. 13C-nuclear magnetic resonance spectroscopy studies of hepatic glucose metabolism in normal subjects and subjects with insulin-dependent diabetes mellitus. *J Clin Invest* 1994; 94: 2369–76.
127. Frank JW, Saslow SB, Camilleri M, Thomforde GM, Dinneen S, Rizza RA. Mechanism of accelerated gastric emptying of liquids and hyperglycemia in patients with type II diabetes mellitus. *Gastroenterology* 1995; 109: 755–65.

128. Schwartz JG, Green GM, Guan D, McMahan CA, Phillips WT. Rapid gastric emptying of a solid pancake meal in type II diabetic patients. *Diabetes Care* 1996; 19: 468–71.
129. Nowak TV, Johnson CP, Kalbfleisch JH, Roza AM, Wood CM, Weisbruch JP, Soergel KH. Highly variable gastric emptying in patients with insulin dependent diabetes mellitus. *Gut* 1995; 37: 23–9.
130. DeFronzo RA. Pharmacologic therapy for type 2 diabetes mellitus. *Ann Intern Med* 1999; 131: 281–303.
131. Barlocco D. Pramlintide (amylin). *Curr Opin Investig Drugs* 2001; 2: 1575–81.
132. Nyholm B, Brock B, Orskov L, Schmitz O. Amylin receptor agonists: a novel pharmacological approach in the management of insulin-treated diabetes mellitus. *Expert Opin Investig Drugs* 2001; 10: 1641–52.
133. Weyer C, Maggs DG, Young AA, Kolterman OG. Amylin replacement with pramlintide as an adjunct to insulin therapy in type 1 and type 2 diabetes mellitus: a physiological approach toward improved metabolic control. *Curr Pharm Des* 2001; 7: 1353–73.
134. Kolterman OG, Gottlieb A, Moyses C, Colburn W. Reduction of postprandial hyperglycemia in subjects with IDDM by intravenous infusion of AC137, a human amylin analogue. *Diabetes Care* 1995; 18: 1179–82.
135. Kolterman OG, Schwartz S, Corder C, Levy B, Klaff L, Peterson J, Gottlieb A. Effect of 14 days' subcutaneous administration of the human amylin analogue, pramlintide (AC137), on an intravenous insulin challenge and response to a standard liquid meal in patients with IDDM. *Diabetologia* 1996; 39: 492–9.
136. Thompson RG, Pearson L, Kolterman OG. Effects of 4 weeks' administration of pramlintide, a human amylin analogue, on glycaemia control in patients with IDDM: effects on plasma glucose profiles and serum fructosamine concentrations. *Diabetologia* 1997; 40: 1278–85.
137. Thompson RG, Pearson L, Schoenfeld SL, Kolterman OG. Pramlintide, a synthetic analogue of human amylin, improves the metabolic profile of patients with type 2 diabetes using insulin. The pramlintide in Type 2 Diabetes Group. *Diabetes Care* 1998; 21: 987–93.
138. Ratner RE, Want LL, Fineman MS, Velte MJ, Ruggles JA, Gottlieb A, Weyer C, Kolterman O, Schmitz O. Adjunctive therapy with the amylin analogue pramlintide leads to a combined improvement in glycemic and weight control in insulin-treated subjects with type 2 diabetes. *Diabetes Technol Ther* 2002; 4: 51–61.
139. Nyholm B, Orskov L, Hove KY, Gravholt CH, Moller N, Alberti KG, Moyses C, Kolterman O, Schmitz O. The amylin analogue pramlintide improves glycemic control and reduces postprandial glucagon concentrations in patients with type 1 diabetes mellitus. *Metabolism* 1999; 48: 935–41.
140. Fineman MS, Koda JE, Shen LZ, Strobel SA, Maggs DG, Weyer C, Kolterman OG. The human amylin analogue, pramlintide, corrects postprandial hyperglucagonemia in patients with type 1 diabetes. *Metabolism* 2002; 51: 636–41.
141. Whitehouse F, Kruger DF, Fineman M, Shen L, Ruggles JA, Maggs DG, Weyer C, Kolterman OG. A randomized study and open-label extension evaluating the long-term efficacy of pramlintide as an adjunct to insulin therapy in type 1 diabetes. *Diabetes Care* 2002; 25: 724–30.
142. Lund PK, Goodman RH, Dee PC, Habener JF. Pancreatic preproglucagon cDNA contains two glucagon-related coding sequences arranged in tandem. *Proc Natl Acad Sci USA* 1982; 79: 345–9.
143. White JW, Saunders GF. Structure of the human glucagon gene. *Nucl Acids Res* 1986; 14: 4719–30.
144. Mojsov S, Heinrich G, Wilson IB, Ravazzola M, Orci L, Habener JF. Preproglucagon gene expression in pancreas and intestine diversifies at the level of posttranslational processing. *J Biol Chem* 1986; 261: 11880–9.
145. Drucker DJ, Asa S. Glucagon gene expression in vertebrate brain. *J Biol Chem* 1988; 263: 13475–8.
146. Chen L, Komiya I, Inman L, McCorkle K, Alam T, Unger RH. Molecular and cellular responses of islets during perturbations of glucose homeostasis determined by *in situ* hybridization histochemistry. *Proc Natl Acad Sci USA* 1989; 86: 1367–71.
147. Chen L, Komiyo I, Inman L, O'Neill J, Appel M, Alam T, Unger RH. Effects of hypoglycemia and prolonged fasting on insulin and glucagon gene expression. *J Clin Invest* 1989; 84: 711–4.
148. Rountree DB, Ulshen MH, Selub S, Fuller CR, Bloom SR, Ghatei MA, Lund PK. Nutrient-independent increases in proglucagon and ornithine decarboxylase messenger RNAs after jejunoileal resection. *Gastroenterology* 1992; 103: 462–8.
149. Lu F, Jin T, Drucker DJ. Activation of proglucagon gene expression by gastrin-releasing peptide in a mouse enteroendocrine cell line. *Endocrinology* 1996; 137: 3710–6.
150. Huang THJ, Brubaker PL. Synthesis and secretion of glucagon-like peptide-1 by fetal rat intestinal cells in culture. *endocrine* 1995; 3: 499–503.
151. Drucker DJ, Brubaker PL. Proglucagon gene expression is regulated by a cyclic AMP-dependent pathway in rat intestine. *Proc Natl Acad Sci* 1989; 86: 3953–7.
152. Drucker DJ, Campos R, Reynolds R, Stobie K, Brubaker PL. The rat glucagon gene is regulated by a cyclic AMP-dependent pathway in pancreatic islet cells. *Endocrinology* 1991; 128: 394–400.
153. Drucker DJ, Jin T, Asa SL, Young TA, Brubaker PL. Activation of proglucagon gene transcription by protein kinase A in a novel mouse enteroendocrine cell line. *Mol Endocrinol* 1994; 8: 1646–55.
154. Philippe J, Drucker DJ, Habener JF. Glucagon gene transcription in an islet cell line is regulated via a protein kinase C-activated pathway. *J Biol Chem* 1987; 262: 1823–8.
155. Lovshin J, Drucker DJ. Synthesis, secretion and biological actions of the glucagon-like peptides. *Pediatric Diabetes* 2000; 1: 49–57.
156. Philippe J, Drucker DJ, Knepel W, Jepeal L, Misulovin Z, Habener JF. Alpha-cell-specific expression of the glucagon gene is conferred to the glucagon promoter element by the interactions of DNA-binding proteins. *Mol Cell Biol* 1988; 8: 4877–88.
157. Hussain MA, Lee J, Miller CP, Habener JF. POU domain transcription factor brain 4 confers pancreatic a-cell-specific expression of the proglucagon gene through interaction with a novel proximal promoter G1 element. *Mol Cell Biol* 1997; 17: 7186–94.
158. Ritz-Laser B, Estreicher A, Klages N, Saule S, Philippe J. Pax-6 and Cdx-2/3 interact to activate glucagon gene expression on the G1 control element. *J Biol Chem* 1999; 274: 4124–32.
159. Jin T, Drucker DJ. Activation of proglucagon gene transcription through a novel promoter element by the

caudal-related homeodomain protein cdx-2/3. *Mol Cell Biol* 1996; 16: 19–28.
160. Wang M, Drucker DJ. The LIM domain homeobox gene isl-1 is a positive regulator of islet cell-specific proglucagon gene transcription. *J Biol Chem* 1995; 270: 12646–52.
161. Morel C, Cordier-Bussat M, Philippe J. The upstream promoter element of the glucagon gene, G1, confers pancreatic alpha cell-specific expression. *J Biol Chem* 1995; 270: 3046–55.
162. Gauthier BR, Schwitzgebel VM, Zaiko M, Mamin A, Ritz-Laser B, Philippe J. Hepatic nuclear factor-3 (HNF-3 or Foxa2) regulates glucagon gene transcription by binding to the G1 and G2 promoter elements. *Mol Endocrinol* 2002; 16: 170–83.
163. Kaestner KH, Katz J, Liu Y, Drucker DJ, Schutz G. Inactivation of the winged helix transcription factor HNF3α affects glucose homeostasis and islet glucagon gene expression *in vivo*. *Genes Dev* 1999; 13: 495–504.
164. Hussain MA, Habener JF. Glucagon gene transcription activation mediated by synergistic interactions of pax-6 and cdx-2 with the p300 co-activator. *J Biol Chem* 1999; 274: 28950–7.
165. Philippe J. Hepatocyte-nuclear factor 3β gene transcripts generate protein isoforms with different transactivation properties on the glucagon gene. *Mol Endocrinol* 1995; 9: 368–74.
166. Philippe J, Morel C, Prezioso VR. Glucagon gene expression is negatively regulated by hepatocyte nuclear factor 3β. *Mol Cell Biol* 1994; 14: 3514–23.
167. Philippe J, Morel C, Cordier-Bussat M. Islet-specific proteins interact with the insulin-response element of the glucagon gene. *J Biol Chem* 1995; 270: 3039–45.
168. Furstenau U, Schwaninger M, Blume R, Kennerknecht I, Knepel W. Characterization of a novel protein kinase C response element in the glucagon gene. *Mol Cell Biol* 1997; 17: 1805–16.
169. Diedrich T, Furstenau U, Knepel W. Glucagon gene G3 enhancer: Evidence that activity depends on combination of an islet-specific factor and a winged helix protein. *Biol Chem* 1997; 378: 89–98.
170. St-Onge L, Sosa-Pineda B, Chowdhury K, Mansouri A, Gruss P. Pax6 is required for differentiation of glucagon-producing a-cells in mouse pancreas. *Nature* 1997; 387: 406–9.
171. Ritz-Laser B, Estreicher A, Gauthier B, Philippe J. The paired homeodomain transcription factor pax-2 is expressed in the endocrine pancreas and transactivates the glucagon gene promoter. *J Biol Chem* 2000; 275: 32708–15.
172. Philippe J. Insulin regulation of the glucagon gene is mediated by an insulin-responsive DNA element. *Proc Natl Acad Sci USA* 1991; 88: 7224–7.
173. Grzeskowiak R, Amin J, Oetjen E, Knepel W. Insulin responsiveness of the glucagon gene conferred by interactions between proximal promoter and more distal enhancer-like elements involving the paired-domain transcription factor pax6. *J Biol Chem* 2000; 275: 30037–45.
174. Cordier-Bussat M, Morel C, Philippe J. Homologous DNA sequences and cellular factors are implicated in the control of glucagon and insulin gene expression. *Mol Cell Biol* 1995; 15: 3904–16.
175. Knepel W, Chafitz J, Habener JF. Transcriptional activation of the rat glucagon gene by the cyclic AMP-responsive element in pancreatic islet cells. *Mol Cell Biol* 1990; 10: 6799–804.
176. Miller CP, Lin JC, Habener JF. Transcription of the rat glucagon gene by the cyclic AMP response element-binding protein CREB is modulated by adjacent CREB-associated proteins. *Mol Cell Biol* 1993; 13: 7080–90.
177. Schwaninger M, Lux G, Blume R, Oetjen E, Hidaka H, Knepel W. Membrane depolarization and calcium influx induce glucagon gene transcription in pancreatic islet cells through the cyclic AMP-responsive element. *J Biol Chem* 1993; 268: 5168–77.
178. Furstenau U, Schwaninger M, Blumes R, Jendrusch E-M, Knepel W. Characterization of a novel calcium response element in the glucagon gene. *J Biol Chem* 1999; 274: 5851–60.
179. Efrat S, Teitelman G, Anwar M, Ruggiero D, Hanahan D. Glucagon gene regulatory region directs oncoprotein expression to neurons and pancreatic alpha cells. *Neuron* 1988; 1: 605–13.
180. Lee YC, Asa SL, Drucker DJ. Glucagon gene 5′-flanking sequences direct expression of SV40 large T antigen to the intestine producing carcinoma of the large bowel in transgenic mice. *J Biol Chem* 1992; 267: 10705–8.
181. Jin T, Drucker DJ. The proglucagon gene upstream enhancer contains positive and negative domains important for tissue-specific proglucagon gene transcription. *Mol Endocrinol* 1995; 9: 1306–20.
182. Shih DQ, Navas MA, Kuwajima S, Duncan SA, Stoffel M. Impaired glucose homeostasis and neonatal mortality in hepatocyte nuclear factor 3alpha-deficient mice. *Proc Natl Acad Sci USA* 1999; 96: 10152–7.
183. Sander M, Neubuser A, Kalamaras J, Ee HC, Martin GR, German MS. Genetic analysis reveals that PAX6 is required for normal transcription of pancreatic hormone genes and islet development. *Genes Dev* 1997; 11: 1662–73.
184. Hill MF, Asa SL, Drucker DJ. Essential requirement for Pax6 in control of enteroendocrine proglucagon gene transcription. *Mol Endocrinol* 1999; 13: 1474–86.
185. Irwin DM. Molecular evolution of proglucagon. *Regul Pept* 2001; 98: 1–12.
186. Nian M, Drucker DJ, Irwin D. Divergent regulation of human and rat proglucagon gene promoters *in vivo*. *Am J Physiol* 1999; 277: G829–37.
187. Drucker DJ, Mojsov S, Habener JF. Cell-specific post-translational processing of preproglucagon expressed from a metallothionein-glucagon fusion gene. *J Biol Chem* 1986; 261: 9637–43.
188. Lefebvre PJ. Glucagon and its family revisited. *Diabetes Care* 1995; 18: 715–30.
189. Parker JC, Andrews KM, Allen MR, Stock JL, McNeish JD. Glycemic control *in mice* with targeted disruption of the glucagon receptor gene. *Biochem Biophys Res Commun* 2002; 290: 839–43.
190. Myojo S, Tsujikawa T, Sasaki M, Fujiyama Y, Bamba T. Trophic effects of glicentin on rat small-intestinal mucosa *in vivo* and *in vitro*. *J Gastroenterol* 1997; 32: 300–5.
191. Drucker DJ, Ehrlich P, Asa SL, Brubaker PL. Induction of intestinal epithelial proliferation by glucagon-like peptide 2. *Proc Natl Acad Sci USA* 1996; 93: 7911–6.
192. Schjoldager BTG, Mortensen PE, Christiansen J, Orskov C, Holst JJ. GLP-1 (glucagon-like peptide 1) and truncated GLP-1, fragments of human proglucagon, inhibit gastric acid secretion in humans. *Dig Dis Sci* 1989; 34: 703–8.

193. Veyrac M, Ribard D, Daures JP, Mion H, Lequellec A, Martinez J, Bataille D, Michel H. Inhibitory effect of the C-terminal octapeptide of oxyntomodulin on pentagastrin-stimulated gastric acid secretion in man. *Scand J Gastroenterol* 1989; 24: 1238–42.
194. Dakin CL, Gunn I, Small CJ, Edwards CM, Hay DL, Smith DM, Ghatei MA, Bloom SR. Oxyntomodulin inhibits food intake in the rat. *Endocrinology* 2001; 142: 4244–50.
195. Tsai C-H, Hill M, Asa SL, Brubaker PL, Drucker DJ. Intestinal growth-promoting properties of glucagon-like peptide 2 in mice. *Am J Physiol* 1997; 273: E77–84.
196. Drucker DJ. Intestinal growth factors. *Am J Physiol* 1997; 273: G3–6.
197. Tsai C-H, Hill M, Drucker DJ. Biological determinants of intestinotrophic properties of GLP-2 *in vivo*. *Am J Physiol* 1997; 272: G662–8.
198. Cheeseman CI, Tsang R. The effect of gastric inhibitory polypeptide and glucagon like peptides on intestinal hexose transport. *Am J Physiol Gastrointest Liver Physiol* 1996; 271: G477–82.
199. Cheeseman CI. Upregulation of SGLT-1 transport activity in rat jejunum induced by GLP-2 infusion *in vivo*. *Am J Physiol* 1997; 273: R1965–71.
200. Wojdemann M, Wettergren A, Hartmann B, Holst JJ. Glucagon-like peptide-2 inhibits centrally induced antral motility in pigs. *Scand J Gastroenterol* 1998; 33: 828–32.
201. Wojdemann M, Wettergren A, Hartmann B, Hilsted L, Holst JJ. Inhibition of sham feeding-stimulated human gastric acid secretion by glucagon-like peptide-2. *J Clin Endocrinol Metab* 1999; 84: 2513–7.
202. Benjamin MA, McKay DM, Yang P-C, Perdue MH. Glucagon-like peptide-2 enhances epithelial barrier function of both transcellular and paracellular pathways in the mouse. *Gut* 2000; 47: 112–9.
203. Boushey RP, Yusta B, Drucker DJ. Glucagon-like peptide 2 decreases mortality and reduces the severity of indomethacin-induced murine enteritis. *Am J Physiol* 1999; 277: E937–47.
204. Tang-Christensen M, Larsen PJ, Thulesen J, Romer J, Vrang N. The proglucagon-derived peptide, glucagon-like peptide-2, is a neurotransmitter involved in the regulation of food intake. *Nat Med* 2000; 6: 802–7.
205. Lovshin J, Estall J, Yusta B, Brown TJ, Drucker DJ. Glucagon-like peptide (GLP)-2 action in the murine central nervous system is enhanced by elimination of GLP-1R signaling. *J Biol Chem* 2001; 276: 21489–99.
206. Bergeron F, Leduc R, Day R. Subtilase-like pro-protein convertases: from molecular specificity to therapeutic applications. *J Mol Endocrinol* 2000; 24: 1–22.
207. Tanaka S, Kurabuchi S, Mochida H, Kato T, Takahashi S, Watanabe T, Nakayama K. Immunocytochemical localization of prohormone convertases PC1/PC2 in rat pancreatic islets. *Arch Histol Cytol* 1996; 59: 261–71.
208. Scopsi L, Gullo M, Rilke F, Martin S, Steiner DF. Proprotein convertases (PC1/PC3 and PC2) in normal and neoplastic human tissues: their use as markers of neuroendocrine differentiation. *J Clin Endocrinol Metab* 1995; 80: 294–301.
209. Rothenberg ME, Eilertson CD, Klein K, Zhou Y, Lindberg I, McDonald JK, Mackin RB, Noe BD. Processing of mouse proglucagon by recombinant prohormone convertase 1 and immunopurified prohormone convertase 2 *in vitro*. *J Biol Chem* 1995; 270: 10136–46.
210. Rothenberg ME, Eilertson CD, Klein K, Mackin RB, Noe BD. Evidence for redundancy in propeptide/prohormone convertase activities in processing proglucagon: an antisense study. *Mol Endocrinol* 1996; 10: 331–41.
211. Dhanvantari S, Seidah NG, Brubaker PL. Role of prohormone convertases in the tissue-specific processing of proglucagon. *Mol Endocrinol* 1996; 10: 342–55.
212. Rouille Y, Kantengwa S, Irminger JC, Halban PA. Role of the prohormone convertase PC3 in the processing of proglucagon to glucagon-like peptide-1. *J Biol Chem* 1997; 272: 32810–6.
213. Brubaker PL, Drucker DJ. Intestinal proglucagon-derived peptides. In Greeley GH, Jr (ed) *Gastrointestinal Endocrinology*. Totowa, NJ: Humana Press, 1998: pp 493–514.
214. Zhu X, Zhou A, Dey A, Norrbom C, Carroll R, Zhang C, Laurent V, Lindberg I, Ugleholdt R, Holst JJ, Steiner DF. Disruption of PC1/3 expression in mice causes dwarfism and multiple neuroendocrine peptide processing defects. *Proc Natl Acad Sci USA* 2002; 99: 10293–8.
215. Marcinkiewicz M, Ramla D, Seidah NG, Cretien M. Developmental expression of the prohormone convertases PC1 and PC2 in mouse pancreatic islets. *Endocrinology* 1994; 135: 1651–60.
216. Rouille Y, Westermark G, Martin SK, Steiner DF. Proglucagon is processed to glucagon by prohormone convertase PC2 in aTC1-6 cells. *Proc Natl Acad Sci USA* 1994; 91: 3242–6.
217. Rouille Y, Martin S, Steiner DF. Differential processing of proglucagon by the subtilisin-like prohormone convertases PC2 and PC3 to generate either glucagon or glucagon-like peptide. *J Biol Chem* 1995; 270: 26488–96.
218. Furuta M, Yano H, Zhou A, Rouille Y, Holst JJ, Carroll R, Ravazzola M, Orci L, Furuta H, Steiner DF. Defective prohormone processing and altered pancreatic islet morphology in mice lacking active SPC2. *Proc Natl Acad Sci USA* 1997; 94: 6646–51.
219. Dhanvantari S, Brubaker PL. Proglucagon processing in an islet cell line: effects of PC1 overexpression and PC2 depletion. *Endocrinology* 1998; 139: 1630–7.
220. Wilson ME, Kalamaras JA, German MS. Expression pattern of IAPP and prohormone convertase 1/3 reveals a distinctive set of endocrine cells in the embryonic pancreas. *Mech Dev* 2002; 115: 171–6.
221. Nie Y, Nakashima M, Brubaker PL, Li QL, Perfetti R, Jansen E, Zambre Y, Pipeleers D, Friedman TC. Regulation of pancreatic PC1 and PC2 associated with increased glucagon-like peptide 1 in diabetic rats. *J Clin Invest* 2000; 105: 955–65.
222. Ghiglione M, Uttenthal LO, George SK, Bloom SR. How glucagon-like is glucagon-like peptide-1? *Diabetologia* 1984; 27: 599–600.
223. Schmidt WE, Siegel EG, Creutzfeldt W. Glucagon-like peptide-1 but not glucagon-like peptide-2 stimulates insulin release from isolated rat pancreatic islets. *Diabetologia* 1985; 28: 704–7.
224. Kawai K, Suzuki S, Ohashi S, Mukai H, Ohmori H, Murayama Y, Yamashita K. Comparison of the effects of glucagon-like peptide-1-(1-37) and -(7-37) and glucagon on islet hormone release from isolated perfused canine and rat pancreases. *Endocrinology* 1989; 124: 1768–73.
225. Martinez A, Burrell MA, Kuijk M, Montuenga LM, Treston A, Cuttitta F, Polak JM. Localization of

amidating enzymes (PAM) in rat gastrointestinal tract. *J Histochem Cytochem* 1993; 41: 1617–22.

226. Wettergren A, Pridal L, Wojdemann M, Holst JJ. Amidated and non-amidated glucagon-like peptide-1 (GLP-1): non-pancreatic effects (cephalic phase acid secretion) and stability in plasma in humans. *Regul Pept* 1998; 77: 83–7.
227. Mojsov S, Kopczynski MG, Habener JF. Both amidated and nonamidated forms of glucagon-like peptide I are synthesized in the rat intestine and the pancreas. *J Biol Chem* 1990; 265: 8001–8.
228. Orskov C, Wettergren A, Holst JJ. Biological effects and metabolic rates of glucagonlike peptide-1 7-36 amide and glucagonlike peptide-1 7-37 in healthy subjects are indistinguishable. *Diabetes* 1993; 42: 658–61.
229. Orskov C, Rabenhoj L, Wettergren A, Kofod H, Holst JJ. Tissue and plasma concentrations of amidated and glycine-extended glucagon-like peptide I in humans. *Diabetes* 1994; 43: 535–9.
230. Moody AJ. Gut glucagon-like immunoreactivity. *Clin Gastroenterol* 1980; 9: 699–709.
231. Bryant MG, Bloom SR, Polak JM. Measurement of gut hormonal peptides in biopsies from human stomach and proximal intestine. *Gut* 1983; 24: 114–9.
232. Sjolund K, Sanden G, Hakanson R, Sundler F. Endocrine cells in human intestine: an immunocytochemical study. *Gastroenterology* 1983; 85: 1120–30.
233. Eissele R, Goke R, Willemer S, Harthus H-P, Vermeer H, Arnold R, Goke B. Glucagon-like peptide 1 cells in the gastrointestinal tract and pancreas of rat, pig, and man. *Eur J Clin Invest* 1992; 22: 283–91.
234. Buchan AMJ, Barber DL, Gregor M, Soll AH. Morphologic and physiologic studies of canine ileal enteroglucagon-containing cells in short-term culture. *Gastroenterology* 1987; 93: 791–800.
235. Brubaker P. Control of glucagon-like immunoreactive peptide secretion from fetal rat intestinal cultures. *Endocrinology* 1988; 123: 220–6.
236. Brubaker PL, Schloos J, Drucker DJ. Regulation of glucagon-like peptide-1 synthesis and secretion in the GLUTag enteroendocrine cell line. *Endocrinology* 1998; 139: 4108–14.
237. Vilsboll T, Krarup T, Deacon CF, Madsbad S, Holst JJ. Reduced postprandial concentrations of intact biologically active glucagon-like peptide 1 in type 2 diabetic patients. *Diabetes* 2001; 50: 609–13.
238. Roberge JN, Brubaker PL. Secretion of proglucagon-derived peptides in response to intestinal luminal nutrients. *Endocrinology* 1991; 128: 3169–74.
239. Elliott RM, Morgan LM, Tredger JA, Deacon S, Wright J, Marks V. Glucagon-like peptide-1(7-36)amide and glucose-dependent insulinotropic polypeptide secretion in response to nutrient ingestion in man: Acute postprandial and 24-h secretion patterns. *J Endocrinol* 1993; 138: 159–66.
240. D'Alessio D, Thirlby R, Laschansky E, Zebroski H, Ensinck J. Response of tGLP-1 to nutrients in humans. *Digestion* 1993; 54: 377–9.
241. Hermann C, Goke R, Richter G, Fehmann HC, Arnold R, Goke B. Glucagon-like peptide-1 and glucose-dependent insulin-releasing polypeptide plasma levels in response to nutrients. *Digestion* 1995; 56: 117–26.
242. Massimino SP, McBurney MI, Field CJ, Thomson AB, Keelan M, Hayek MG, Sunvold GD. Fermentable dietary fiber increases GLP-1 secretion and improves glucose homeostasis despite increased intestinal glucose transport capacity in healthy dogs. *J Nutr* 1998; 128: 1786–93.
243. Roberge JN, Brubaker PL. Regulation of intestinal proglucagon-derived peptide secretion by glucose-dependent insulinotropic peptide in a novel enteroendocrine loop. *Endocrinology* 1993; 133: 233–40.
244. Brubaker PL. Regulation of intestinal proglucagon-derived peptide secretion by intestinal regulatory peptides. *Endocrinology* 1991; 128: 3175–82.
245. Herrmann-Rinke C, Voge A, Hess M, Goke B. Regulation of glucagon-like peptide-1 secretion from rat ileum by neurotransmitters and peptides. *J Endocrinol* 1995; 147: 25–31.
246. Kreymann B, Ghatei MA, Williams G, Bloom SR. Glucagon-like peptide-1 7-36: a physiological incretin in man. *Lancet* 1987; ii: 1300–4.
247. Nauck MA, Heimesaat MM, Orskov C, Holst JJ, Ebert R, Creutzfeldt W. Preserved incretin activity of glucagon-like peptide 1 [7-36 amide] but not of synthetic human gastric inhibitory polypeptide in patients with type-2 diabetes mellitus. *J Clin Invest* 1993; 91: 301–7.
248. Bruzzone R, Tamburrano G, Lala A, Mauceri M, Annibale B, Severi C, DeMagistris L, Leonetti F, DelleFave G. Effect of bombesin on plasma insulin, pancreatic glucagon, and gut glucagon in man. *J Clin Endocrinol Metab* 1983; 56: 643–47.
249. Roberge JN, Gronau KA, Brubaker PL. Gastrin-releasing peptide is a novel mediator of proximal nutrient-induced proglucagon-derived peptide secretion from the distal gut. *Endocrinology* 1996; 137: 2383–8.
250. Persson K, Gingerich RL, Nayak S, Wada K, Wada E, Ahren B. Reduced GLP-1 and insulin responses and glucose intolerance after gastric glucose in GRP receptor-deleted mice [In Process Citation]. *Am J Physiol Endocrinol Metab* 2000; 279: E956–62.
251. Herrmann-Rinke C, McGregor GP, Goke B. Calcitonin gene-related peptide potently stimulates glucagon-like peptide-1 release in the isolated perfused rat ileum. *Peptides* 2000; 21: 431–7.
252. Rocca AS, Brubaker PL. Role of the vagus nerve in mediating proximal nutrient-induced glucagon- like peptide-1 secretion. *Endocrinology* 1999; 140: 1687–94.
253. Hansen L, Hartmann B, Bisgaard T, Mineo H, Jorgensen PN, Holst JJ. Somatostatin restrains the secretion of glucagon-like peptide-1 and -2 from isolated perfused porcine ileum. *Am J Physiol Endocrinol Metab* 2000; 278: E1010–8.
254. Herrmann-Rinke C, Horsch D, McGregor GP, Goke B. Galanin is a potent inhibitor of glucagon-like peptide-1 secretion from rat ileum. *Peptides* 1996; 17: 571–6.
255. Hansen L, Deacon CF, Orskov C, Holst JJ. Glucagon-like peptide-1-(7-36)amide is transformed to glucagon-like peptide-1-(9-36)amide by dipeptidyl peptidase IV in the capillaries supplying the L cells of the porcine intestine. *Endocrinology* 1999; 140: 5356–63.
256. Deacon CF, Nauck MA, Toft-Nielsen M, Pridal L, Willms B, Holst JJ. Both subcutaneously and intra- venously administered glucagon-like peptide 1 are rapidly degraded from the NH2-terminus in type II diabetic patients and in healthy subjects. *Diabetes* 1995; 44: 1126–31.
257. Mentlein R. Dipeptidyl-peptidase IV (CD26)—role in the inactivation of regulatory peptides. *Regul Pept* 1999; 85: 9–24.
258. De Meester I, Korom S, Van Damme J, Scharpe S. CD26, let it cut or cut it down. *Immunol Today* 1999; 20: 367–75.

259. Kieffer TJ, McIntosh CHS, Pederson RA. Degradation of glucose-dependent insulinotropic polypeptide and truncated glucagon-like peptide 1 *in vitro* and *in vivo* by dipeptidyl peptidase IV. *Endocrinology* 1995; 136: 3585–96.
260. Holst JJ, Deacon CF. Inhibition of the activity of dipeptidyl-peptidase IV as a treatment for type 2 diabetes. *Diabetes* 1998; 47: 1663–70.
261. Mitani H, Takimoto M, Hughes TE, Kimura M. Dipeptidyl peptidase IV inhibition improves impaired glucose tolerance in high-fat diet-fed rats: study using a Fischer 344 rat substrain deficient in its enzyme activity. *Jpn J Pharmacol* 2002; 88: 442–50.
262. Wettergren A, Wojdemann M, Holst JJ. The inhibitory effect of glucagon-like peptide-1 (7-36)amide on antral motility is antagonized by its N-terminally truncated primary metabolite GLP-1 (9-36)amide. *Peptides* 1998; 19: 877–82.
263. Deacon CF, Plamboeck A, Moller S, Holst JJ. GLP-1-(9-36) amide reduces blood glucose in anesthetized pigs by a mechanism that does not involve insulin secretion. *Am J Physiol Endocrinol Metab* 2002; 282: E873–9.
264. Hupe-Sodmann K, McGregor GP, Bridenbaugh R, Rudiger G, Burkhard G, Thole H, Zimmermann B, Voigt K. Characterisation of the processing by human neutral endopeptidase 24.11 of GLP-1(7-36) amide and comparison of the substrate specificity of the enzyme for other glucagon-like peptides. *Regul Pept* 1995; 58: 149–56.
265. Hupe-Sodmann K, Goke R, Goke B, Thole HH, Zimmermann B, Voigt K, McGregor GP. Endoproteolysis of glucagon-like peptide (GLP)-1 (7-36) amide by ectopeptidases in RINm5F cells. *Peptides* 1997; 18: 625–32.
266. Ruiz-Grande C, Alarcon C, Alcantara A, Castilla C, Lopez Novoa JM, Villanueva-Penacarrillo ML, Valverde I. Renal catabolism of truncated glucagon-like peptide 1. *Horm Metab Res* 1993; 25: 612–6.
267. Deacon CF, Pridal L, Klarskov L, Olesen M, Holst JJ. Glucagon-like peptide 1 undergoes differential tissue-specific metabolism in the anesthetized pig. *Am J Physiol* 1996; 271: E458–64.
268. Orskov C, Andreasen J, Holst JJ. All products of proglucagon are elevated in plasma from uremic patients. *J Clin Endocrinol Metab* 1992; 74: 379–84.
269. Thorens B. Expression cloning of the pancreatic β cell receptor for the gluco-incretin hormone glucagon-like peptide 1. *Proc Natl Acad Sci USA* 1992; 89: 8641–5.
270. Stoffel M, Espinosa III R, Le Beau MM, Bell GI. Human glucagon-like peptide-1 receptor gene. *Diabetes* 1993; 42: 1215–8.
271. Campos RV, Lee YC, Drucker DJ. Divergent tissue-specific and developmental expression of receptors for glucagon and glucagon-like peptide-1 in the mouse. *Endocrinology* 1994; 134: 2156–64.
272. Wei Y, Mojsov S. Tissue-specific expression of the human receptor for glucagon-like peptide 1: brain, heart and pancreatic forms have the same deduced amino acid sequences. *FEBS Lett* 1995; 358: 219–24.
273. Heller RS, Kieffer TJ, Habener JF. Insulinotropic glucagon-like peptide I receptor expression in glucagon-producing alpha-cells of the rat endocrine pancreas. *Diabetes* 1997; 46: 785–91.
274. Merchenthaler I, Lane M, Shughrue P. Distribution of pre-pro-glucagon and glucagon-like peptide-1 receptor messenger RNAs in the rat central nervous system. *J Comp Neurol* 1999; 403: 261–80.
275. Satoh F, Beak SA, Small CJ, Falzon M, Ghatei MA, Bloom SR, Smith DM. Characterization of human and rat glucagon-like peptide-1 receptors in the neurointermediate lobe: lack of coupling to either stimulation or inhibition of adenylyl cyclase. *Endocrinology* 2000; 141: 1301–9.
276. Bullock BP, Heller RS, Habener JF. Tissue distribution of messenger ribonucleic acid encoding the rat glucagon-like peptide 1 receptor. *Endocrinology* 1996; 137: 2968–78.
277. Wheeler MB, Lu M, Dillon JS, Leng X-H, Chen C, Boyd AE, III. Functional expression of the rat glucagon-like peptide-I receptor, evidence for coupling to both adenylyl cyclase and phospholipase-C. *Endocrinology* 1993; 133: 57–62.
278. Yang H, Egan JM, Wang Y, Moyes CD, Roth J, Montrose MH, Montrose-Rafizadesh C. GLP-1 action in L6 myotubes is via a receptor different from the pancreatic GLP-1R. *Am J Physiol* 1998; 275: C675–83.
279. Montrose-Rafizadeh C, Avdonin P, Garant MJ, Rodgers BD, Kole S, Yang H, Levine MA, Schwindinger W, Bernier M. Pancreatic glucagon-like peptide-1 receptor couples to multiple G proteins and activates mitogen-activated protein kinase pathways in Chinese hamster ovary cells. *Endocrinology* 1999; 140: 1132–40.
280. Chepurny OG, Hussain MA, Holz GG. Exendin-4 as a stimulator of rat insulin I gene promoter activity via bZIP/CRE interactions sensitive to serine/threonine protein kinase inhibitor Ro 31-8220. *Endocrinology* 2002; 143: 2303–13.
281. Drucker DJ, Philippe J, Mojsov S, Chick WL, Habener JF. Glucagon-like peptide I stimulates insulin gene expression and increases cyclic AMP levels in a rat islet cell line. *Proc Natl Acad Sci USA* 1987; 84: 3434–8.
282. Lu M, Wheeler MB, Leng X-H, Boyd AE III. The role of the free cytoplasmic calcium level in β-cell signal transduction by gastric inhibitory polypeptide and glucagon-like peptide I(7-37). *Endocrinology* 1993; 132: 94–100.
283. Gromada J, Dissing S, Bokvist K, Renstrom E, Frokjaer-Jensen J, Wulff BS, Rorsman P. Glucagon-like peptide I increases cytoplasmic calcium in insulin-secreting bTC3-cells by enhancement of intracellular calcium mobilization. *Diabetes* 1995; 44: 767–74.
284. Holz GG, Leech CA, Habener JF. Activation of a cAMP-regulated Ca^{2+}-signaling pathway in pancreatic b-cells by the insulinotropic hormone glucagon-like peptide-1. *J Biol Chem* 1995; 270: 17749–57.
285. Goke R, Trautmann ME, Haus E, Richter G, Fehmann HC, Arnold R, Goke B. Signal transmission after GLP-1(7-36)amide binding in RINm5F cells. *Am J Physiol* 1989; 257: G397–401.
286. Holz GG, Leech CA, Heller RS, Castonguay M, Habener JF. cAMP-dependent mobilization of intracellular Ca^{2+}stores by activation of ryanodine receptors in pancreatic beta-cells. A Ca^{2+}signaling system stimulated by the insulinotropic hormone glucagon-like peptide-1-(7-37). *J Biol Chem* 1999; 274: 14147–56.
287. Buteau J, Roduit R, Susini S, Prentki M. Glucagon-like peptide-1 promotes DNA synthesis, activates phosphatidylinositol 3-kinase and increases transcription factor pancreatic and duodenal homeobox gene 1 (PDX-1) DNA binding activity in beta (INS-1)-cells. *Diabetologia* 1999; 42: 856–64.
288. Gefel D, Hendrick GK, Mojsov S, Habener J, Weir GC. Glucagon-like peptide-I analogs: effects on insulin

secretion and adenosine 3′,5′-monophosphate formation. *Endocrinology* 1990; 126: 2164–8.
289. Wilmen A, Goke B, Goke R. The isolated N-terminal extracellular domain of the glucagon-like peptide-1 (GLP)-1 receptor has intrinsic binding activity. *FEBS Lett* 1996; 398: 43–7.
290. Van Eyll B, Goke B, Wilmen A, Goke R. Exchange of W39 by A within the N-terminal extracellular domain of the GLP-1R results in a loss of receptor function. *Peptides* 1996; 17: 565–70.
291. Takhar S, Gyomorey S, Su RC, Mathi SK, Li X, Wheeler MB. The third cytoplasmic domain of the GLP-1[7-36 amide] receptor is required for coupling to the adenylyl cyclase system. *Endocrinology* 1996; 137: 2175–8.
292. Mathi SK, Chan Y, Li X, Wheeler MB. Scanning of the glucagon-like peptide-1 receptor localizes G protein-activating determinants primarily to the N terminus of the third intracellular loop. *Mol Endocrinol* 1997; 11: 424–32.
293. Jiang J, Fehmann HC, Loth H, Goke R, Goke B. Regulation of GLP-1R mRNA levels and GLP-1 binding sites by forskolin, PMA and dexamethasone in RINm5F cells. *Exp Clin Endrocrinol* 1994; 102 (suppl 1): 117.
294. Abrahamsen N, Nishimura E. Regulation of glucagon and glucagon-like peptide-1 receptor messenger ribonucleic acid expression in cultured rat pancreatic islets by glucose, cyclic adenosine 3′,5′-monophosphate, and glucocorticoids. *Endocrinology* 1995; 136: 1572–8.
295. Fehmann HC, Jiang J, Pitt D, Schweinfurth J, Goke B. Ligand-induced regulation of glucagon-like peptide-I receptor function and expression in insulin-secreting beta cells. *Pancreas* 1996; 13: 273–82.
296. Fehmann HC, Schweinfurth J, Jiang J, Goke B. Regulation of glucagon-like peptide-1 receptor expression and transcription by the protein kinase C pathway. *Res Exp Med* 1996; 196: 219–25.
297. Sudre B, Broqua P, White RB, Ashworth D, Evans DM, Haigh R, Junien JL, Aubert ML. Chronic inhibition of circulating dipeptidyl peptidase IV by FE 999011 delays the occurrence of diabetes in male zucker diabetic fatty rats. *Diabetes* 2002; 51: 1461–9.
298. Wildhage I, Trusheim H, Goke B, Lankat-Buttgereit B. Gene expression of the human glucagon-like peptide-1 receptor is regulated by Sp1 and Sp3. *Endocrinology* 1999; 140: 624–31.
299. Galehshahi FS, Goke B, Lankat-Buttgereit B. Contribution of a PS1-like element to the tissue- and cell-specific expression of the human GLP-1R gene. *FEBS Lett* 1998; 436: 163–8.
300. Galehshahi FS, Goke B, Lankat-Buttgereit B. A novel silencer element repressing expression of the GLP-1R gene in fibroblasts and pancreatic A-cells, but not in pancreatic B- and D-cells. *Peptides* 2000; 21: 1169–76.
301. Fehmann HC, Habener JF. Homologous desensitization of the insulinotropic glucagon-like peptide-I(7-37) receptor on insulinoma (HIT-T15) cells. *Endocrinology* 1991; 128: 2880–8.
302. Widmann C, Dolci W, Thorens B. Heterologous desensitization of the glucagon-like peptide-1 receptor by phorbol esters requires phosphorylation of the cytoplasmic tail at four different sites. *J Biol Chem* 1996; 271: 19957–63.
303. Widmann C, Dolci W, Thorens B. Desensitization and phosphorylation of the glucagon-like peptide-1 (GLP-1) receptor by GLP-1 and 4-phorbol 12-myristate 13-acetate. *Mol Endocrinol* 1996; 10: 62–75.
304. Widmann C, Dolci W, Thorens B. Internalization and homologous desensitization of the GLP-1R depend on phosphorylation of the receptor carboxyl tail at the same three sites. *Mol Endocrinol* 1997; 11: 1094–102.
305. Widmann C, Dolci W, Thorens B. Agonist-induced internalization and recycling of the glucagon-like peptide-1 receptor in transfected fibroblasts and in insulinomas. *Biochem J* 1995; 310: 203–14.
306. Thorens B, Porret A, Buhler L, Deng S-P, Morel P, Widmann C. Cloning and functional expression of the human islet GLP-1R: Demonstration that exendin-4 is an agonist and exendin-(9-39) an antagonist of the receptor. *Diabetes* 1993; 42: 1678–82.
307. Goke R, Fehmann H-C, Linn T, Schmidt H, Krause M, Eng J, Gške B. Exendin-4 is a high potency agonist and truncated exendin-(9-39)-amide an antagonist at the glucagon-like peptide 1-(7-36)-amide receptor of insulin-secreting β-cells. *J Biol Chem* 1993; 268: 19650–5.
308. Schepp W, Schmidtler J, Riedel T, Dehne K, Schusdziarra V, Holst JJ, Eng J, Raufman J-P, Classen M. Exendin-4 and exendin-(9-39)NH2: agonist and antagonist, respectively, at the rat parietal cell receptor for glucagon-like peptide-1-(7-36)NH_2. *Eur J Pharmacol Mol Pharmacol* 1994; 269: 183–91.
309. Fehmann HC, Jiang J, Schweinfurth J, Wheeler MB, Boyd AE III, Göke B. Stable expression of the rat GLP-I receptor in CHO cells: activation and binding characteristics utilizing GLP-I(7-36)-amide, oxyntomodulin, exendin-4, and exendin(9-39). *Peptides* 1994; 15: 453–6.
310. Gromada J, Bokvist K, Ding WG, Holst JJ, Nielsen JH, Rorsman P. Glucagon-like peptide 1 (7-36) amide stimulates exocytosis in human pancreatic beta-cells by both proximal and distal regulatory steps in stimulus-secretion coupling. *Diabetes* 1998; 47: 57–65.
311. Kashima Y, Miki T, Shibasaki T, Ozaki N, Miyazaki M, Yano H, Seino S. Critical role of cAMP-GEFII–Rim2 complex in incretin-potentiated insulin secretion. *J Biol Chem* 2001; 276: 46046–53.
312. Kang G, Chepurny OG, Holz GG. cAMP-regulated guanine nucleotide exchange factor II (Epac2) mediates Ca^{2+}-induced Ca^{2+} release in INS-1 pancreatic beta-cells. *J Physiol* 2001; 536: 375–85.
313. Skoglund G, Hussain MA, Holz GG. Glucagon-like peptide 1 stimulates insulin gene promoter activity by protein kinase A-independent activation of the rat insulin I gene cAMP response element. *Diabetes* 2000; 49: 1156–64.
314. Lawrence MC, Bhatt HS, Easom RA. NFAT regulates insulin gene promoter activity in response to synergistic pathways induced by glucose and glucagon-like peptide-1. *Diabetes* 2002; 51: 691–8.
315. Moritz W, Leech CA, Ferrer J, Habener JF. Regulated expression of adenosine triphosphate-sensitive potassium channel subunits in pancreatic beta-cells. *Endocrinology* 2001; 142: 129–38.
316. D'alessio DA, Vogel R, Prigeon R, Laschansky E, Koerker D, Eng J, Ensinck JW. Elimination of the action of glucagon-like peptide 1 causes an impairment of glucose tolerance after nutrient ingestion by healthy baboons. *J Clin Invest* 1996; 97: 133–8.
317. Edwards CM, Todd JF, Mahmoudi M, Wang Z, Wang RM, Ghatei MA, Bloom SR. Glucagon-like peptide 1 has a physiological role in the control of postprandial glucose in humans: studies with the antagonist exendin 9-39. *Diabetes* 1999; 48: 86–93.

318. Wang Z, Wang RM, Owji AA, Smith DM, Ghatei MA, Bloom SR. Glucagon-like peptide 1 is a physiological incretin in rat. *J Clin Invest* 1995; 95: 417–21.
319. Baggio L, Kieffer TJ, Drucker DJ. GLP-1 but not GIP regulates fasting and non-enteral glucose clearance in mice. *Endocrinology* 2000; 141: 3703–9.
320. Scrocchi LA, Brown TJ, MacLusky N, Brubaker PL, Auerbach AB, Joyner AL, Drucker DJ. Glucose intolerance but normal satiety *in mice* with a null mutation in the glucagon-like peptide receptor gene. *Nature Med* 1996; 2: 1254–8.
321. Dachicourt N, Serradas P, Bailbe D, Kergoat M, Doare L, Portha B. Glucagon-like peptide-1(7-36)-amide confers glucose sensitivity to previously glucose-incompetent beta-cells in diabetic rats: *in vivo* and *in vitro* studies. *J Endocrinol* 1997; 155: 369–76.
322. Byrne MM, Gliem K, Wank U, Arnold R, Katschinski M, Polonsky KS, Goke B. Glucagon-like peptide-1 improves the ability of the beta-cell to sense and respond to glucose in subjects with impaired glucose tolerance. *Diabetes* 1998; 47: 1259–65.
323. Wang YH, Egan JM, Raygada M, Nadiv O, Roth J, Montrose-Rafizadeh C. Glucagon-like peptide-1 affects gene transcription and messenger ribonucleic acid stability of components of the insulin secretory system in RIN 1046-38 cells. *Endocrinology* 1995; 136: 4910–17.
324. Wang Y, Perfetti R, Greig NH, Holloway HW, DeOre KA, Montrose-Rafizadeh C, Elahi D, Egan JM. Glucagon-like peptide-1 can reverse the age-related decline in glucose tolerance in rats. *J Clin Invest* 1997; 99: 2883–9.
325. Fehmann HC, Habener JF. Functional receptors for the insulinotropic hormone glucagon-like peptide-I(7-37) on a somatostatin secreting cell line. *FEBS Lett* 1991; 279: 335–40.
326. Samols E, Bonner-Weir S, Weir GC. Intra-islet insulin-glucagon-somatostatin relationships. *Clin Endocrinol Metab* 1986; 15: 33–58.
327. Schirra J, Sturm K, Leicht P, Arnold R, Goke B, Katschinski M. Exendin-(9-39)amide is an antagonist of glucagon-like peptide-1(7- 36)amide in humans. *J Clin Invest* 1998; 101: 1421–30.
328. Goke R, Wagner B, Fehmann HC, Goke B. Glucose-dependency of the insulin stimulatory effect of glucagon-like peptide-1 (7-36) amide on the rat pancreas. *Res Exp Med (Berl)* 1993; 193: 97–103.
329. Nauck MA, Heimesaat MM, Behle K, Holst JJ, Nauck MS, Ritzel R, Hufner M, Schmiegel WH. Effects of glucagon-like peptide 1 on counterregulatory hormone responses, cognitive functions, and insulin secretion during hyperinsulinemic, stepped hypoglycemic clamp experiments in healthy volunteers. *J Clin Endocrinol Metab* 2002; 87: 1239–46.
330. Susini S, Roche E, Prentki M, Schlegel W. Glucose and glucoincretin peptides synergize to induce c-*fos*, c-*jun*, *jun*B, *zif*-268, and *nur*-77 gene expression in pancreatic beta(INS-1) cells. *FASEB J* 1998; 12: 1173–82.
331. Buteau J, Foisy S, Rhodes CJ, Carpenter L, Binden TJ, Prentki M. Protein kinase C activation mediates glucagon-like peptide-1-induced pancreatic B-cell proliferation. *Diabetes* 2001; 50: 1–7.
332. Zhou J, Wang X, Pineyro MA, Egan JM. Glucagon-like peptide 1 and exendin-4 convert pancreatic AR42J cells into glucagon- and insulin-producing cells. *Diabetes* 1999; 48: 2358–66.
333. Xu G, Stoffers DA, Habener JF, Bonner-Weir S. Exendin-4 stimulates both beta-cell replication and neogenesis, resulting in increased beta-cell mass and improved glucose tolerance in diabetic rats. *Diabetes* 1999; 48: 2270–6.
334. Edvell A, Lindstrom P. Initiation of increased pancreatic islet growth in young normoglycemic mice (Umea +/?). *Endocrinology* 1999; 140: 778–83.
335. Stoffers DA, Kieffer TJ, Hussain MA, Drucker DJ, Egan JM, Bonner-Weir S, Habener JF. Insulinotropic glucagon-like peptide-1 agonists stimulate expression of homeodomain protein IDX-1 and increase β-cell mass in mouse pancreas. *Diabetes* 2000; 49: 741–8.
336. Perfetti R, Zhou J, Doyle ME, Egan JM. Glucagon-like peptide-1 induces cell proliferation and pancreatic-duodenum homeobox-1 expression and increases endocrine cell mass in the pancreas of old, glucose-intolerant rats. *Endocrinology* 2000; 141: 4600–5.
337. Ling Z, Wu D, Zambre Y, Flamez D, Drucker DJ, Pipeleers DG, Schuit FC. Glucagon-like peptide 1 receptor signaling influences topography of islet cells in mice. *Virchows Arch* 2001; 438: 382–7.
338. Wettergren A, Schjoldager B, Mortensen PE, Petersen H, Orskov C, Holst JJ. Effect of GLP-1 on gastric motility and gastric and pancreatic secretion in man. *Digestion* 1993; 54: 384–5.
339. Imeryuz N, Yegen BC, Bozkurt A, Coskun T, Villanueva-Pennacarrillo ML, Ulusoy NB. Glucagon-like peptide-1 inhibits gastric emptying via vagal afferent-mediated central mechanisms. *Am J Physiol* 1997; 273: G920–7.
340. Cechetto DF. Central representation of visceral function. *Federation Proc* 1987; 46: 17–23.
341. Barragan JM, Eng J, Rodriuez R, Blazquez E. Neural contribution to the effect of glucagon-like peptide-1-(7-36) amide on arterial blood pressure in rats. *Am J Physiol* 1999; 277: E784–91.
342. Edwards CM, Edwards AV, Bloom SR. Cardiovascular and pancreatic endocrine responses to glucagon-like peptide-1(7-36) amide in the conscious calf. *Exp Physiol* 1997; 82: 709–16.
343. Barragan JM, Rodriguez RE, Blazquez E. Changes in arterial blood pressure and heart rate induced by glucagon-like peptide-1-(7-36 amide) in rats. *Am J Physiol* 1994; 266: E459–66.
344. Barragan JM, Rodriguez RE, Eng J, Blazquez E, Defize LHK. Interactions of exendin-(9-39) with the effects of glucagon-like peptide-1-(7-36) amide and of exendin-4 on arterial blood pressure and heart rate in rats. *Regul Pept* 1996; 67: 63–8.
345. Vila Petroff MG, Egan JM, Wang X, Sollott SJ. Glucagon-like peptide-1 increases cAMP but fails to augment contraction in adult rat cardiac myocytes. *Circ Res* 2001; 89: 445–52.
346. Larsen PJ, Tang-Christensen M, Holst JJ, Orskov C. Distribution of glucagon-like peptide-1 and other preproglucagon-derived peptides in the rat hypothalamus and brainstem. *Neuroscience* 1997; 77: 257–70.
347. Alvarez E, Roncero I, Chowen JA, Thorens B, Blazquez E. Expression of the glucagon-like peptide-1 receptor gene in rat brain. *J Neurochem* 1996; 66: 920–7.
348. Turton MD, O'Shea D, Gunn I, Beak SA, Edwards CMB, Meeran K, Choi SJ, Taylor GM, Heath MM, Lambert PD, Wilding JPH, Smith DM, Ghatei MA, Herbert J, Bloom SR. A role for glucagon-like peptide-1 in the central regulation of feeding. *Nature* 1996; 379: 69–72.

349. Tang-Christensen M, Larsen PJ, Goke R, Fink-Jensen A, Jessop DS, Moller M, Sheikh SP. Central administration of GLP-1(7-36) amide inhibits food and water intake in rats. *Am J Physiol* 1996; 271: R848–56.
350. Toft-Nielsen MB, Madsbad S, Holst JJ. Continuous subcutaneous infusion of glucagon-like peptide-1 lowers plasma glucose and reduces appetite in type 2 diabetic patients. *Diabetes Care* 1998; 22: 1137–43.
351. Flint A, Raben A, Astrup A, Holst JJ. Glucagon-like peptide 1 promotes satiety and suppresses energy intake in humans. *J Clin Invest* 1998; 101: 515–20.
352. Gutzwiller JP, Drewe J, Goke B, Schmidt H, Rohrer B, Lareida J, Beglinger C. Glucagon-like peptide-1 promotes satiety and reduces food intake in patients with diabetes mellitus type 2. *Am J Physiol* 1999; 276: R1541–4.
353. Gutzwiller J-P, Goke B, Drewe J, Hildebrand P, Ketterer S, Handschin D, Winterhalder R, Conen D, Beglinger C. Glucagon-like peptide-1: a potent regulator of food intake in humans. *Gut* 1999; 44: 81–6.
354. Naslund E, Barkeling B, King N, Gutniak M, Blundell JE, Holst JJ, Rossner S, Hellstrom PM. Energy intake and appetite are suppressed by glucagon-like peptide-1 (GLP-1) in obese men. *Int J Obes Relat Metab Disord* 1999; 23: 304–11.
355. Seeley RJ, Blake K, Rushing PA, Benoit S, Eng J, Woods SC, D'Alessio D. The role of CNS glucagon-like peptide-1 (7-36) amide receptors in mediating the visceral illness effects of lithium chloride. *J Neurosci* 2000; 20: 1616–21.
356. Rinaman L. Interoceptive stress activates glucagon-like peptide-1 neurons that project to the hypothalamus. *Am J Physiol* 1999; 277: R582–90.
357. Thiele TE, Van Dijk G, Campfield LA, Smith FJ, Burn P, Woods SC, Bernstein H, Seeley RJ. Central infusion of GLP-1, but not leptin, produces conditioned taste aversion in rats. *Am J Physiol* 1997; 272: R726–30.
358. Thiele TE, Seeley RJ, D'Alessio D, Eng J, Bernstein IL, Woods SC, van Dijk G. Central infusion of glucagon-like peptide-1-(7-36) amide (GLP-1) receptor antagonist attenuates lithium chloride-induced c-Fos induction in rat brainstem. *Brain Res* 1998; 801: 164–70.
359. Rinaman L. A functional role for central glucagon-like peptide-1 receptors in lithium chloride-induced anorexia. *Am J Physiol* 1999; 277: R1537–R1540.
360. Moller C, Sommer W, Thorsell A, Rimondini R, Heilig M. Anxiogenic-like action of centrally administered glucagon-like peptide-1 in a punished drinking test. *Prog Neuropsychopharmacol Biol Psychiatry* 2002; 26: 119–22.
361. Valverde I, Villanueva-Penacarrillo ML. *In vitro* insulinomemetric effects of GLP-1 in liver, muscle and fat. *Acta Physiol Scand* 1996; 157: 359–60.
362. Nakagawa Y, Kawai K, Suzuki H, Ohashi S, Yamashita K. Glucagon-like peptide-1(7-36)amide and glycogen synthesis in the liver. *Diabetologia* 1996; 39: 1241–2.
363. Furnsinn C, Ebner K, Waldhausl W. Failure of GLP-1 (7-36) amide to affect glycogenesis in rat skeletal muscle. *Diabetologia* 1995; 38: 864–7.
364. Blackmore PF, Mojsov S, Exton JH, Habener JF. Absence of insulinotropic glucagon-like peptide-I(7-37) receptors on isolated rat liver hepatocytes. *FEBS Lett* 1991; 283: 7–10.
365. Valverde I, Merida E, Delgado E, Trapote MA, Villanueva-Penacarillo ML. Presence and characterization of glucagon-like peptide-1(7-36) amide receptors in solubilized membranes of rat adipose tissue. *Endocrinology* 1993; 132: 75–9.
366. Sandhu H, Wiesenthal SR, MacDonald PE, McCall RH, Tchipashvili V, Rashid S, Satkunarajah M, Irwin DM, Shi ZQ, Brubaker PL, Wheeler MB, Vranic M, Efendic S, Giacca A. Glucagon-like peptide 1 increases insulin sensitivity in depancreatized dogs. *Diabetes* 1999; 48: 1045–53.
367. Zander M, Madsbad S, Madsen JL, Holst JJ. Effect of 6-week course of glucagon-like peptide 1 on glycaemic control, insulin sensitivity, and beta-cell function in type 2 diabetes: a parallel-group study. *Lancet* 2002; 359: 824–30.
368. Orskov L, Holst JJ, Moller J, Orskov C, Moller N, Alberti KG, Schmitz O. GLP-1 does not acutely affect insulin sensitivity in healthy man. *Diabetologia* 1996; 39: 1227–32.
369. Vella A, Shah P, Basu R, Basu A, Holst JJ, Rizza RA. Effect of glucagon-like peptide 1(7-36) amide on glucose effectiveness and insulin action in people with type 2 diabetes. *Diabetes* 2000; 49: 611–7.
370. Balkan B, Li X. Portal GLP-1 administration in rats augments the insulin response to glucose via neuronal mechanisms. *Am J Physiol Regul Integr Comp Physiol* 2000; 279: R1449–54.
371. Burcelin R, Da Costa A, Drucker D, Thorens B. Glucose competence of the hepatoportal vein sensor requires the presence of an activated glucagon-like peptide-1 receptor. *Diabetes* 2001; 50: 1720–8.
372. Goke R, Larsen PJ, Mikkelsen JD, Sheikh SP. Distribution of GLP-1 binding sites in the rat brain: evidence that exendin-4 is a ligand of brain GLP-1 binding sites. *Eur J Neurosci* 1995; 7: 2294–300.
373. Beak SA, Small CJ, Ilovaiskaia I, Hurley JD, Ghatei MA, Bloom SR, Smith DM. Glucagon-like peptide-1 (GLP-1) releases thyrotropin (TSH): characterization of binding sites for GLP-1 on alpha-TSH cells. *Endocrinology* 1996; 137: 4130–8.
374. Larsen PJ, Tang-Christensen M, Jessop DS. Central administration of glucagon-like peptide-1 activates hypothalamic neuroendocrine neurons in the rat. *Endocrinology* 1997; 138: 4445–55.
375. Beak SA, Heath MM, Small CJ, Morgan DGA, Ghatei MA, Taylor AD, Buckingham JC, Bloom SR, Smith DM. Glucagon-like peptide-1 stimulates luteinizing hormone releasing hormone secretion in a rodent hypothalamic neuronal cell line (GT1-7). *J Clin Invest* 1998; 101: 1334–41.
376. MacLusky N, Cook S, Scrocchi L, Shin J, Kim J, Vaccarino F, Asa SL, Drucker DJ. Neuroendocrine function in mice with complete disruption of GLP-1R signaling. *Endocrinology* 2000; 141: 752–62.
377. Crespel A, De Boisvilliers F, Gros L, Kervran A. Effects of glucagon and glucagon-like peptide-1-(7-36) amide on C cells from rat thyroid and medullary thyroid carcinoma CA-77 cell line. *Endocrinology* 1996; 137: 3674–80.
378. Richter G, Feddersen O, Wagner U, Barth P, Göke R, Gške B. GLP-1 stimulates secretion of macromolecules from airways and relaxes pulmonary artery. *Am J Physiol Lung Cell Mol Physiol* 1993; 265: L374–81.
379. Vara E, Arias-Diaz J, Garcia C, Balibrea JL, Blazquez E. Glucagon-like peptide-1(7-36) amide stimulates surfactant secretion in human type II pneumocytes. *Am J Respir Crit Care Med* 2001; 163: 840–6.

380. Moreno C, Mistry M, Roman RJ. Renal effects of glucagon-like peptide in rats. *Eur J Pharmacol* 2002; 434: 163–7.
381. Brown JC. A gastric inhibitory polypeptide, I: the amino acid composition and the tryptic peptides. *Can J Biochem* 1971; 49: 255–61.
382. Brown JC, Dryburgh JR. A gastric inhibitory polypeptide, II: the complete amino acid sequence. *Can J Biochem* 1971; 49: 867–72.
383. Pederson RA, Schubert HE, Brown JC. Gastric inhibitory polypeptide. Its physiologic release and insulinotropic action in the dog. *Diabetes* 1975; 24: 1050–6.
384. Pederson RA, Schubert HE, Brown JC. The insulinotropic action of gastric inhibitory polypeptide. *Can J Physiol Pharmacol* 1975; 53: 217–23.
385. Yip RGC, Wolfe MM. GIP biology and fat metabolism. *Life Sci.* 2000; 66: 91–103.
386. Inagaki N, Seino Y, Takeda J, Yano H, Yamada Y, Bell GI, Eddy RL, Fukushima Y, Byers MG, Shows TB, Gastric inhibitory polypeptide: structure and chromosomal localization of the human gene. *Mol Endocrinol* 1989; 3: 1014–21.
387. Takeda J, Seino Y, Tanaka K, Fukumoto H, Kayano T, Takahashi H, Mitani T, Kurono M, Suzuki T, Tobe T, Sequence of an intestinal cDNA encoding human gastric inhibitory polypeptide precursor. *Proc Natl Acad Sci USA* 1987; 84: 7005–8.
388. Higashimoto Y, Simchock J, Liddle RA. Molecular cloning of rat glucose-dependent insulinotropic peptide (GIP). *Biochim Biophys Acta* 1992; 1132: 72–4.
389. Sharma SK, Austin C, Howard A, Lo G, Nicholl CG, Legon S. Characterization of rat gastric inhibitory peptide cDNA. *J Mol Endocrinol* 1992; 9: 265–72.
390. Someya Y, Inagaki N, Maekawa T, Seino Y, Ishii S. Two 3′,5′-cyclic-adenosine monophosphate response elements in the promoter region of the human gastric inhibitory polypeptide gene. *FEBS Lett* 1993; 317: 67–73.
391. Boylan MO, Jepeal LI, Jarboe LA, Wolfe MM. Cell-specific expression of the glucose-dependent insulinotropic polypeptide gene in a mouse neuroendocrine tumor cell line. *J Biol Chem* 1997; 272: 17438–43.
392. Higashimoto Y, Opara EC, Liddle RA. Dietary regulation of glucose-dependent insulinotropic peptide (GIP) gene expression in rat small intestine. *Comp Biochem Physiol C Pharmacol Toxicol Endocrinol* 1995; 110: 207–14.
393. Tseng CC, Jarboe LA, Landau SB, Williams EK, Wolfe MM. Glucose-dependent insulinotropic peptide: structure of the precursor and tissue-specific expression in rat. *Proc Natl Acad Sci USA* 1993; 90: 1992–6.
394. Wolfe MM, Zhao KB, Glazier KD, Jarboe LA, Tseng CC. Regulation of glucose-dependent insulinotropic polypeptide release by protein in the rat. *Am J Physiol Gastrointest Liver Physiol* 2000; 279: G561–6.
395. Sykes S, Morgan LM, English J, Marks V. Evidence for preferential stimulation of gastric inhibitory polypeptide secretion in the rat by actively transported carbohydrates and their analogues. *J Endocrinol* 1980; 85: 201–7.
396. Kieffer TJ, Buchan AMJ, Barker H, Brown JC, Pederson RA. Release of gastric inhibitory polypeptide from cultured canine endocrine cells. *Am J Physiol* 1994; 267: E489–96.
397. Deacon CF, Nauck MA, Meier J, Hucking K, Holst JJ. Degradation of endogenous and exogenous gastric inhibitory polypeptide in healthy and in type 2 diabetic subjects as revealed using a new assay for the intact peptide. *J Clin Endocrinol Metab* 2000; 85: 3575–81.
398. Mentlein R, Gallwitz B, Schmidt WE. Dipeptidyl-peptidase IV hydrolyses gastric inhibitory polypeptide, glucagon-like peptide-1(7-36)amide, peptide histidine methionine and is responsible for their degradation in human serum. *Eur J Biochem* 1993; 214: 829–35.
399. O'Doriso TM, Sirinek KR, Mazzaferri EL, Cataland S. Renal effects on serum gastric inhibitory polypeptide (GIP). *Metabolism* 1977; 26: 651–6.
400. Jorde R, Burhol PG, Gunnes P, Schulz TB. Removal of IR-GIP by the kidneys in man, and the effect of acute nephrectomy on plasma GIP in rats. *Scand J Gastroenterol* 1981; 16: 469–71.
401. Sirinek KR, O'Dorisio TM, Gaskill HV, Levine BA. Chronic renal failure: effect of hemodialysis on gastrointestinal hormones. *Am J Surg* 1984; 148: 732–5.
402. Deacon CF, Nauck MA, Meier J, Hucking K, Holst JJ. Degradation of endogenous and exogenous gastric inhibitory polypeptide in healthy and in type 2 diabetic subjects as revealed using a new assay for the intact peptide. *J Clin Endocrinol Metab* 2000; 85: 3575–81.
403. Yamada Y, Hayami T, Nakamura K, Kaisaki PJ, Someya Y, Wang CZ, Seino S, Seino Y. Human gastric inhibitory polypeptide receptor: cloning of the gene (GIPR) and cDNA. *Genomics* 1995; 29: 773–6.
404. Volz A, Goke R, Lankat-Buttgereit B, Fehmann HC, Bode HP, Goke B. Molecular cloning, functional expression, and signal transduction of the GIP-receptor cloned from a human insulinoma. *FEBS Lett* 1995; 373: 23–9.
405. Yasuda K, Inagaki N, Yamada Y, Kubota A, Seino S, Seino Y. Hamster gastric inhibitory polypeptide receptor expressed in pancreatic islets and clonal insulin-secreting cells: its structure and functional properties. *Biochem Biophys Res Commun* 1994; 205: 1556–62.
406. Gremlich S, Porret A, Hani EH, Cherif D, Vionnet D, Froguel P, Thorens B. Cloning, functional expression, and chromosomal localization of the human pancreatic islet glucose-dependent insulinotropic polypeptide receptor. *Diabetes* 1995; 44: 1202–8.
407. Usdin TB, Mezey E, Button DC, Brownstein MJ, Bonner TI. Gastric inhibitory polypeptide receptor, a member of the secretin- vasoactive intestinal peptide receptor family, is widely distributed in peripheral organs and the brain. *Endocrinology* 1993; 133: 2861–70.
408. Yip RGC, Boylan MO, Kieffer TJ, Wolfe MM. Functional GIP receptors are present on adipocytes. *Endocrinology* 1998; 139: 4004–7.
409. Bollag RJ, Zhong Q, Phillips P, Min L, Zhong L, Cameron R, Mulloy AL, Rasmussen H, Qin F, Ding KH, Isales CM. Osteoblast-derived cells express functional glucose-dependent insulinotropic peptide receptors. *Endocrinology* 2000; 141: 1228–35.
410. Boylan MO, Jepeal LI, Wolfe MM. Stucture of the rat glucose-dependent insulinotropic polypeptide receptor gene. *Peptides* 1999; 20: 219–28.
411. McIntosh CHS, Wheeler MB, Gelling RW, Brown JC, Pederson RA. GIP receptors and signal-transduction mechanisms. *Acta Physiol Scand* 1996; 157: 361–5.
412. Zhong Q, Bollag RJ, Dransfield DT, Gasalla-Herraiz J, Ding KH, Min L, Isales CM. Glucose-dependent insulinotropic peptide signaling pathways in endothelial cells. *Peptides* 2000; 21: 1427–32.

413. Straub SG, Sharp GWG. Glucose-dependent insulinotropic polypeptide stimulates insulin secretion via increased cyclic AMP and $[Ca^{2+}]_i$ and a wortmannin-sensitive signalling pathway. *Biochem Biophys Res Commun* 1996; 224: 369–74.
414. Kubota A, Yamada Y, Yasuda K, Someya Y, Ihara Y, Kagimoto S, Watanabe R, Kuroe A, Ishida H, Seino Y. Gastric inhibitory polypeptide activates MAP kinase through the wortmannin-sensitive and -insensitive pathways. *Biochem Biophys Res Commun* 1997; 235: 171–5.
415. Ehses JA, Lee SS, Pederson RA, McIntosh CH. A new pathway for glucose-dependent insulinotropic polypeptide (GIP) receptor signaling: evidence for the involvement of phospholipase A2 in GIP-stimulated insulin secretion. *J Biol Chem* 2001; 276: 23667–73.
416. Schmidt WE, Siegel EG, Kummel H, Gallwitz B, Creutzfeldt W. Commercially available preparations of porcine glucose-dependent insulinotropic polypeptide (GIP) contain a biologically inactive GIP-fragment and cholecystokinin-33/-39. *Endocrinology* 1987; 120: 835–7.
417. Gelling RW, Wheeler MB, Xue J, Gyomorey S, Nian C, Pederson RA, McIntosh CH. Localization of the domains involved in ligand binding and activation of the glucose-dependent insulinotropic polypeptide receptor. *Endocrinology* 1997; 138: 2640–3.
418. Wheeler MB, Gelling RW, Hinke SA, Tu B, Pederson RA, Lynn F, Ehses J, McIntosh CH. Characterization of the carboxyl-terminal domain of the rat glucose-dependent insulinotropic polypeptide (GIP) receptor. A role for serines 426 and 427 in regulating the rate of internalization. *J Biol Chem* 1999; 274: 24593–601.
419. Tseng CC, Zhang XY. Role of G protein-coupled receptor kinases in glucose-dependent insulinotropic polypeptide receptor signaling. *Endocrinology* 2000; 141: 947–52.
420. Wang Y, Montrose-Rafizadeh C, Adams L, Raygada M, Nadiv O, Egan JM. GIP regulates glucose transporters, hexokinases, and glucose-induced insulin secretion in RIN 1046-38 cells. *Mol Cell Endocrinol* 1996; 116: 81–7.
421. Ehses JA, Pelech SL, Pederson RA, McIntosh CH. Glucose-dependent insulinotropic polypeptide (GIP) activates the Raf-Mek 1/2-ERK 1/2 module via a cyclic AMP/PKA/Rap1-mediated pathway. *J Biol Chem* 2002; 277: 37088–97.
422. Tseng CC, Kieffer TJ, Jarboe LA, Usdin TB, Wolfe MM. Postprandial stimulation of insulin release by glucose-dependent insulinotropic polypeptide (GIP). Effect of a specific glucose-dependent insulinotropic polypeptide receptor antagonist in the rat. *J Clin Invest* 1996; 98: 2440–5.
423. Lewis JT, Dayanadan B, Habener JF, Kieffer TJ. Glucose-dependent insulinotropic polypeptide confers early phase insulin release to oral glucose in rats: demonstration by a receptor antagonist. *Endocrinology* 2000; 141: 3710–6.
424. Miyawaki K, Yamada Y, Yano H, Niwa H, Ban N, Ihara Y, Kubota A, Fujimoto S, Kajikawa M, Kuroe A, Tsuda K, Hashimoto H, Yamashita T, Jomori T, Tashiro F, Miyazaki J, Seino Y. Glucose intolerance caused by a defect in the entero-insular axis: a study in gastric inhibitory polypeptide receptor knockout mice. *Proc Natl Acad Sci USA* 1999; 96: 14843–7.
425. Trumper A, Trumper K, Trusheim H, Arnold R, Goke B, Horsch D. Glucose-dependent insulinotropic polypeptide is a growth factor for beta (INS-1) cells by pleiotropic signaling. *Mol Endocrinol* 2001; 15: 1559–70.
426. Trumper A, Trumper K, Horsch D. Mechanisms of mitogenic and anti-apoptotic signaling by glucose-dependent insulinotropic polypeptide in beta(INS-1)-cells. *J Endocrinol* 2002; 174: 233–46.
427. Morgan LM. The metabolic role of GIP: physiology and pathology. *Biochem Soc Trans* 1996; 24: 585–91.
428. McIntosh CH, Bremsak I, Lynn FC, Gill R, Hinke SA, Gelling R, Nian C, McKniht G, Jaspers S, Pederson RA. Glucose-dependent insulinotropic polypeptide stimulation of lipolysis in differentiated 3T3-L1 cells: wortmannin-sensitive inhibition by insulin. *Endocrinology* 1999; 140: 398–404.
429. Bollag RJ, Zhong Q, Ding KH, Phillips P, Zhong L, Qin F, Cranford J, Mulloy AL, Cameron R, Isales CM. Glucose-dependent insulinotropic peptide is an integrative hormone with osteotropic effects. *Mol Cell Endocrinol* 2001; 177: 35–41.
430. Nauck MA, Bartels E, Orskov C, Ebert R, Creutzfeldt W. Lack of effect of synthetic human gastric inhibitory polypeptide and glucagon-like peptide 1 [7-36 amide] infused at near-physiological concentrations on pentagastrin-stimulated gastric acid secretion in normal human subjects. *Digestion* 1992; 52: 214–21.
431. Andersen DK, Putnam WS, Hanks JB, Wise JE, Lebovitz HE, Jones RS. Gastric inhibitory polypeptide (GIP) suppression of hepatic glucose production. *Regul Pept* 1980; 1: 4–9.
432. Hartmann H, Ebert R, Creutzfeld WO. Insulin-dependent inhibition of hepatic glycogenolysis by gastric inhibitory polypeptide (GIP) in perfused rat liver. *Diabetologia* 1986; 29: 112–4.
433. Deacon CF, Danielsen P, Klarskov L, Olesen M, Holst JJ. Dipeptidyl peptidase IV inhibition reduces the degradation and clearance of GIP and potentiates its insulinotropic and antihyperglycemic effects in anesthetized pigs. *Diabetes* 2001; 50: 1588–97.
434. Mazzocchi G, Rebuffat P, Meneghelli V, Malendowicz LK, Tortorella C, Gottardo G, Nussdorfer GG. Gastric inhibitory polypeptide stimulates glucocorticoid secretion in rats, acting through specific receptors coupled with the adenylate cyclase-dependent signaling pathway. *Peptides* 1999; 20: 589–94.
435. Lacroix A, Bolte E, Tremblay J, Dupre J, Poitras P, Fournier H, Garon J, Garrel D, Bayard F, Taillefer R. Gastric inhibitory polypeptide-dependent cortisol hypersecretion—a new cause of Cushing's syndrome. *N Engl J Med* 1992; 327: 974–80.
436. de Herder WW, Hofland LJ, Usdin TB, de Jong FH, Uitterlinden P, van Koetsveld P, Mezey E, Bonner TI, Bonjer HJ, Lamberts SW. Food-dependent Cushing's Syndrome resulting from abundant expression of gastric inhibitory polypeptide receptors in adrenal adenoma cells. *J Clin Endocrinol Metabol* 1996; 81: 3168–72.
437. Bell GI. The glucagon superfamily: precursor structure and gene organization. *Peptides* 1986; 7: 27–36.
438. Raufman J-P. Bioactive peptides from lizard venoms. *Regul Pept* 1996; 61: 1–18.
439. Chen YE, Drucker DJ. Tissue-specific expression of unique mRNAs that encode proglucagon-derived peptides or exendin 4 in the lizard. *J Biol Chem* 1997; 272: 4108–15.
440. Pohl M, Wank SA. Molecular cloning of the helodermin and exendin-4 cDNAs in the lizard. Relationship to

vasoactive intestinal polypeptide/pituitary adenylate cyclase activating polypeptide and glucagon-like peptide 1 and evidence against the existence of mammalian homologues. *J Biol Chem* 1998; 273: 9778–84.

441. Greig NH, Holloway HW, De Ore KA, Jani D, Wang Y, Zhou J, Garant MJ, Egan JM. Once daily injection of exendin-4 to diabetic mice achieves long-term beneficial effects on blood glucose concentrations. *Diabetologia* 1999; 42: 45–50.
442. Young AA, Gedulin BR, Bhavsar S, Bodkin N, Jodka C, Hansen B, Denaro M. Glucose-lowering and insulin-sensitizing actions of exendin-4: studies in obese diabetic (ob/ob, db/db) mice, diabetic fatty Zucker rats, and diabetic rhesus monkeys (*Macaca mulatta*). *Diabetes* 1999; 48: 1026–34.
443. Parkes DG, Young AA, Petrella E, Hiles R. Pharmacokinetics of exendin-4 in the rat following intravenous, subcutaneous and intraperitoneal administration [Abstract]. In *Program and Abstracts: 81st Annual Meeting of the Endocrine Society*. Bethesda, MD, 1999.
444. Nauck M, Stockmann F, Ebert R, Creutzfeldt W. Reduced incretin effect in type 2 (non-insulin-dependent) diabetes. *Diabetologia* 1986; 29: 46–52.
445. Tronier B, Dejgaard A, Andersen T, Madsbad S. Absence of incretin effect in obese type 2 and diminished effect in lean type 2 and obese subjects. *Diab Res Clin Pract* 1985; 48 (suppl): S568.
446. Zhang Y, Cook JTE, Hattersley AT, Firth R, Saker PJ, Warren-Perry M, Stoffel M, Turner RC. Non-linkage of the glucagon-like peptide-1 receptor gene with maturity onset diabetes of the young. *Diabetologia* 1994; 37: 721–4.
447. Kubota A, Yamada Y, Hayami T, Yasuda K, Someya Y, Ihara Y, Kagimoto S, Watanabe R, Taminato T, Tsuda K, Seino Y. Identification of two missense mutations in the GIP receptor gene: a functional study and association analysis with NIDDM: no evidence of association with Japanese NIDDM subjects. *Diabetes* 1996; 45: 1701–5.
448. Toft-Nielsen MB, Damholt MB, Madsbad S, Hilsted LM, Hughes TE, Michelsen BK, Holst JJ. Determinants of the impaired secretion of glucagon-like peptide-1 in type 2 diabetic patients. *J Clin Endocrinol Metab* 2001; 86: 3717–23.
449. Vaag AA, Holst JJ, Volund A, Beck-Nielsen HB. Gut incretin hormones in identical twins discordant for non-insulin- dependent diabetes mellitus (NIDDM)—evidence for decreased glucagon-like peptide 1 secretion during oral glucose ingestion in NIDDM twins. *Eur J Endocrinol* 1996; 135: 425–32.
450. Elahi D, McAloon-Dyke M, Fukagawa NK, Meneilly GS, Sclater AL, Minaker KL, Habener JF, Andersen DK. The insulinotropic actions of glucose-dependent insulinotropic polypeptide (GIP) and glucagon-like peptide-1 (7-37) in normal and diabetic subjects. *Regul Pept* 1994; 51: 63–74.
451. Tseng CC, Boylan MO, Jarboe LA, Usdin TB, Wolfe MM. Chronic desensitization of the glucose-dependent insulinotropic polypeptide receptor in diabetic rats. *Am J Physiol* 1996; 270: E661–6.
452. Lynn FC, Pamir N, Ng EH, McIntosh CH, Kieffer TJ, Pederson RA. Defective glucose-dependent insulinotropic polypeptide receptor expression in diabetic fatty Zucker rats. *Diabetes* 2001; 50: 1004–11.
453. Nauck MA, Sauerwald A, Ritzel R, Holst JJ, Schmiegel W. Influence of glucagon-like peptide 1 on fasting glycemia in type 2 diabetic patients treated with insulin after sulfonylurea secondary failure. *Diabetes Care* 1998; 21: 1925–31.
454. Toft-Nielsen MB, Madsbad S, Holst JJ. Continuous subcutaneous infusion of glucagon-like peptide 1 lowers plasma glucose and reduces appetite in type 2 diabetic patients. *Diabetes Care* 1999; 22: 1137–43.
455. Gutniak MK, Juntti -BL, Hellstrom PM, Guenifi A, Holst JJ, Efendic S. Glucagon-like peptide I enhances the insulinotropic effect of glibenclamide in NIDDM patients and in the perfused rat pancreas. *Diabetes Care* 1996; 19: 857–63.
456. Gutniak M, Orskov C, Holst JJ, Ahren B, Efendic S. Antidiabetogenic effect of glucagon-like peptide-1 (7-36)amide in normal subjects and patients with diabetes mellitus. *N Engl J Med* 1992; 326: 1316–22.
457. Dupre J, Behme MT, Hramiak IM, McFarlane P, Williamson MP, Zabel P, McDonald TJ. Glucagon-like peptide I reduces postprandial glycemic excursions in IDDM. *Diabetes* 1995; 44: 626–30.
458. Todd JF, Edwards CM, Ghatei MA, Mather HM, Bloom SR. Subcutaneous glucagon-like peptide-1 improves postprandial glycaemic control over a 3-week period in patients with early type 2 diabetes. *Clin Sci (Colch)* 1998; 95: 325–9.
459. Edwards CM, Stanley SA, Davis R, Brynes AE, Frost GS, Seal LJ, Ghatei MA, Bloom SR. Exendin-4 reduces fasting and postprandial glucose and decreases energy intake in healthy volunteers. *Am J Physiol Endocrinol Metab* 2001; 281: E155–61.
460. Rask E, Olsson T, Soderberg S, Johnson O, Seckl J, Holst JJ, Ahren B. Impaired incretin response after a mixed meal is associated with insulin resistance in nondiabetic men. *Diabetes Care* 2001; 24: 1640–5.
461. Agerso H, Jensen LB, Elbrond B, Rolan P, Zdravkovic M. The pharmacokinetics, pharmacodynamics, safety and tolerability of NN2211, a new long-acting GLP-1 derivative, in healthy men. *Diabetologia* 2002; 45: 195–202.
462. Juhl CB, Hollingdal M, Sturis J, Jakobsen G, Agerso H, Veldhuis J, Porksen N, Schmitz O. Bedtime administration of NN2211, a long-acting GLP-1 derivative, substantially reduces fasting and postprandial glycemia in type 2 diabetes. *Diabetes* 2002; 51: 424–9.
463. Drucker DJ. Development of glucagon-like peptide-1-based pharmaceuticals as therapeutic agents for the treatment of diabetes. *Curr Pharm Des* 2001; 7: 1399–412.
464. Deacon CF, Holst JJ. Dipeptidyl peptidase IV inhibition as an approach to the treatment and prevention of type 2 diabetes: a historical perspective. *Biochem Biophys Res Commun* 2002; 294: 1–4.
465. Deacon CF, Hughes TE, Holst JJ. Dipeptidyl peptidase IV inhibition potentiates the insulinotropic effect of glucagon-like peptide 1 in the anesthetized pig. *Diabetes* 1998; 47: 764–9.
466. Pauly RP, Demuth HU, Rosche F, Schmidt J, White HA, Lynn F, McIntosh CH, Pederson RA. Improved glucose tolerance in rats treated with the dipeptidyl peptidase IV (CD26) inhibitor Ile-thiazolidide. *Metabolism* 1999; 48: 385–9.
467. Pederson RA, White HA, Schlenzig D, Pauly RP, McIntosh CH, Demuth HU. Improved glucose tolerance in Zucker fatty rats by oral administration of the dipeptidyl peptidase IV inhibitor isoleucine thiazolidide. *Diabetes* 1998; 47: 1253–8.

468. Balkan B, Kwasnik L, Miserendino R, Holst JJ, Li X. Inhibition of dipeptidyl peptidase IV with NVP-DPP728 increases plasma GLP-1 (7-36 amide) concentrations and improves oral glucose tolerance in obese Zucker rats. *Diabetologia* 1999; 42: 1324–31.

469. Ahren B, Holst JJ, Martensson H, Balkan B. Improved glucose tolerance and insulin secretion by inhibition of dipeptidyl peptidase IV in mice [In Process Citation]. *Eur J Pharmacol* 2000; 404: 239–45.

470. Pospisilik JA, Stafford SG, Demuth HU, Brownsey R, Parkhouse W, Finegood DT, McIntosh CH, Pederson RA. Long-term treatment with the dipeptidyl peptidase IV inhibitor P32/98 causes sustained improvements in glucose tolerance, insulin sensitivity, hyperinsulinemia, and beta-cell glucose responsiveness in VDF (*fa/fa*) Zucker rats. *Diabetes* 2002; 51: 943–50.

471. Pospisilik JA, Stafford SG, Demuth HU, McIntosh CH, Pederson RA. Long-term treatment with dipeptidyl peptidase IV inhibitor improves hepatic and peripheral insulin sensitivity in the VDF Zucker rat: a Euglycemic-Hyperinsulinemic Clamp Study. *Diabetes* 2002; 51: 2677–83.

472. Marguet D, Baggio L, Kobayashi T, Bernard AM, Pierres M, Nielsen PF, Ribel U, Watanabe T, Drucker DJ, Wagtmann N. Enhanced insulin secretion and improved glucose tolerance in mice lacking CD26. *Proc Natl Acad Sci USA* 2000; 97: 6874–9.

473. Reimer MK, Holst JJ, Ahren B. Long-term inhibition of dipeptidyl peptidase IV improves glucose tolerance and preserves islet function in mice. *Eur J Endocrinol* 2002; 146: 717–27.

474. Ahren B, Simonsson E, Larsson H, Landin-Olsson M, Torgeirsson H, Jansson PA, Sandqvist M, Bavenholm P, Efendic S, Eriksson JW, Dickinson S, Holmes D. Inhibition of dipeptidyl peptidase IV improves metabolic control over a 4-week study period in type 2 diabetes. *Diabetes Care* 2002; 25: 869–75.

475. Morimoto C, Schlossman SF. The structure and function of CD26 in the T-cell immune response. *Immunol Rev* 1998; 161: 55–70.

476. Fleischer B. CD26: A surface protease involved in T-cell activation. *Immunol Today* 1994; 15: 180–4.

477. Ritzel U, Leonhardt U, Ottleben M, Ruhmann A, Eckart K, Spiess J, Ramadori G. A synthetic glucagon-like peptide-1 analogue with improved plasma stability. *J Endocrinol* 1998; 159: 93–102.

478. Deacon CF, Knudsen LB, Madsen K, Wiberg FC, Jacobsen O, Holst JJ. Dipeptidyl peptidase IV resistant analogues of glucagon-like peptide-1 which have extended metabolic stability and improved biological activity. *Diabetologia* 1998; 41: 271–8.

479. Burcelin R, Dolci W, Thorens B. Long-lasting antidiabetic effect of a dipeptidyl peptidase IV-resistant analogue of glucagon-like peptide-1. *Metabolism* 1999; 48: 252–8.

480. Xiao Q, Giguere J, Parisien M, Jeng W, St-Pierre SA, Brubaker PL, Wheeler MB. Biological activities of glucagon-like peptide-1 analogues *in vitro* and *in vivo*. *Biochemistry* 2001; 40: 2860–9.

481. Siegel EG, Gallwitz B, Scharf G, Mentlein R, Morys-Wortmann C, Folsch UR, Schrezenmeir J, Dresher K, Schmidt WE. Biological activity of GLP-1-analogues with N-terminal modifications. *Regul Pept* 1999; 79: 93–102.

482. O'Harte FPM, Mooney MH, Lawlor A, Flatt PR. N-terminally modified glucagon-like peptide-1(7-36)amide exhibits resistance to enzymatic degradation while maintaining its antihyperglycaemic activity *in vivo*. *Biochim Biophys Acta* 2000; 1474: 13–22.

483. Doyle ME, Greig NH, Holloway HW, Betkey JA, Bernier M, Egan JM. Insertion of an N-terminal 6-aminohexanoic acid after the 7 amino acid position of glucagon-like peptide-1 produces a long-acting hypoglycemic agent. *Endocrinology* 2001; 142: 4462–8.

484. Knudsen LB, Nielsen PF, Huusfeldt PO, Johansen NL, Madsen K, Pedersen FZ, Thogersen H, Wilken M, Agerso H. Potent derivatives of glucagon-like peptide-1 with pharmacokinetic properties suitable for once daily administration [In Process Citation]. *J Med Chem* 2000; 43: 1664–9.

485. Larsen PJ, Fledelius C, Knudsen L-B, Tang-Christensen M. Systemic Administration of the long-acting GLP-1 derivative NN2211 induces lasting and reversible weight loss in both normal and obese rats. *Diabetes* 2001; 50: 2530–9.

Normal Physiology of Insulin Action

13

Mechanisms of Insulin Signal Transduction

W. Timothy Garvey

University of Alabama at Birmingham, and the Birmingham Veterans Affairs Medical Center, Birmingham, AL, USA

INTRODUCTION

Fuel Homeostasis

The peptide hormone insulin is secreted from pancreatic β-cells, and exerts a broad spectrum of anabolic effects in multiple tissues. In response to a meal, insulin stimulates uptake and storage of carbohydrate, fat, and amino acids, while at the same time, antagonizing the catabolism of these fuel reserves. During periods of fasting, a fall in circulating insulin combined with increased secretion of counterregulatory hormones leads to breakdown of stored fuels and increased availability of metabolic substrates for cellular energy. In particular, insulin plays a key role in maintaining blood glucose level within a narrowly defined range despite large fluctuations in food intake. After a meal, insulin returns the organism to postabsorptive homeostasis by promoting uptake and storage of glucose as glycogen in skeletal muscle and liver, and by inhibiting hepatic glucose production via decrements in glycogenolysis and gluconeogenesis. Insulin also promotes triglyceride storage by suppressing fatty acid oxidation, increasing lipid synthesis in liver and adipose tissues, and via an antilipolytic effect in fat cells. Insulin's actions extend to protein accretion through a diminution in protein catabolism and an increase in translation to cell growth and differentiation and to cell survival as a consequence of mitogenicity and antiapoptosis.

Changing Perspectives of Insulin Action

In mediating its pleiotrophic actions, insulin engages multiple networks of signal transduction molecules and a wide array of effector systems. Insulin alters activity of enzymatic pathways, subcellular localization of enzymes, and activation state of membrane transport systems by regulating the posttranslational modification, translation, and degradation of proteins in cells, and by affecting gene transcription and expression. The classical approach to the review of insulin action is to describe a linear cascade of sequentially interacting signal transduction molecules, which then engage specific effector systems, such as membrane transport proteins or the activities of rate-limiting enzymes (e.g., glycogen synthase). This narrow perspective is myopic for three reasons. First, signal transduction and effector functions are not clearly distinct. For example, phosphatidylinositide 3 kinase (PI-3 kinase), which is a component of linear signal transduction from insulin receptor to activation of Akt/protein kinase B (Akt/PKB) and protein kinase C (PKC) isoforms, is integrally involved in glucose transport system effector functions such as vesicle trafficking and the actin cytoskeleton [1].

Secondly, it has become clear, partly through the study of genetic disruption and hyperexpression in mice, that insulin activates numerous systems of signal transduction. These systems are at least partially redundant and are able to interact in modulating signal transduction and ultimate biological effects. One example is the ability of Akt/PKB, activated through the PI-3 kinase "metabolic" signaling pathway, to impact mitogenic responses through regulation of gene transcription factors. Furthermore, signal transduction systems and effector systems must work in concert to mediate a given biological effect. For example, stimulation of glucose transport requires parallel activation of PI-3 kinase and CAP/Cbl/TC10 signal pathways, as well as interaction between two effector systems, the glucose transport system (i.e., trafficking of GLUT-4-containing vesicles) and effects on the cellular cytoskeleton. Thus, promulgation of the insulin action is most accurately viewed as a changing pattern of network interactions involving a web of signal molecule cascades and effector

International Textbook of Diabetes Mellitus, Third Edition. Edited by R. A. DeFronzo, E. Ferrannini, H. Keen, and P. Zimmet.
 ISBN: 0-471-48655-8.

systems. The final biological action represents the net synergism of the combined facilitative, inhibitory, and complementary signaling pathways that interact with more terminal functional systems in cell biology. Certain aspects of linear insulin signal transduction are evolutionarily conserved and are quite similar in mammals and invertebrates. However, complex patterns of interactions between signal and effector systems are more pronounced in mammals and allow for greater plasticity in adaptive responses.

Thirdly, the classic descriptions of insulin signaling pathways emphasize insulin action mechanisms within certain target cells, especially fat cells. However, these actions at the level of cells and tissues affect substrate flux and release of hormones and tissue factors, resulting in the coordinated function of multiple organs as whole organisms adapt to the nutritional environment. The reader is encouraged to think about insulin action in the context of systems biology and integrative physiology. This chapter will emphasize insulin action involving stimulation of glucose transport and glucose metabolism, for reasons outlined below. However, this information will complement other chapters depicting insulin's ability to regulate protein metabolism (Chapter 18), fat metabolism (Chapters 19 and 34), and intermediary metabolism (Chapter 15).

Insulin Resistance

Interest in defining molecular mechanisms mediating insulin action has accelerated with the recognition that insulin resistance is both a primary abnormality in the evolution of type 2 Diabetes and is also associated with a cluster of risk factors predisposing to cardiovascular disease (the insulin resistance syndrome) [2]. The cardinal clinical manifestations of insulin resistance include hyperinsulinemia in conjunction with normoglycemia or hyperglycemia. Investigators have used various *in vivo* metabolic techniques that assess glucose uptake during insulin infusions to demonstrate that insulin resistance was due to impaired insulin action in peripheral tissues. These conclusions were subsequently confirmed with the demonstration that insulin-stimulated glucose transport was diminished in fat and muscle tissues removed from insulin resistant subjects and studied *ex vivo*. Therefore, while insulin resistance could apply to any of insulin's pleiotrophic effects, the term generally applies to insulin's ability to stimulate tissue glucose uptake and suppress hepatic glucose production, since these actions are most directly relevant to its clinical manifestations (hyperinsulinemia and impaired glucose tolerance). This chapter will primarily focus on mechanisms of insulin action related to the regulation of glucose transport and metabolism. While many key aspects remain to be elucidated, this field is rapidly advancing. Over the past decade, the application of new and improved methodologies in molecular biology have facilitated the study of insulin action, resulting in new knowledge and new way to conceptualize the effects of this powerful and interesting hormone.

INSULIN RECEPTORS

Ligand Binding

The insulin action sequence is initiated with specific binding to high-affinity receptors on the plasma membrane of target cells. The insulin receptor is a large transmembrane glycoprotein consisting of two α and two β subunits that form a heterotetramer as depicted in Figure 1. The insulin receptor is synthesized from a single gene as a polypeptide proreceptor composed of α and β subunit sequences in tandem. The proreceptor is processed into separate α and β subunits that then assemble as a disulfide-linked holoenzyme of stoichiometry $(\alpha\beta)_2$ [3]. The 135 kDa α subunits, derived from the amino-terminal portion of the proreceptor, reside entirely on the outside of the cell, tethered to the membrane via the 95 kDa β subunits that span the membrane. Insulin binds to the extracellular α subunit. Studies using chimeric receptors containing structural domains from the homologous insulin-like growth factor 1 (IGF-1) receptor have established that multiple extracellular regions including glycine-centered repeats in the α-subunit establish the specificity for insulin binding [4]; however, a cysteine-rich domain has been shown to directly interact with the ligand. Insulin binding results in conformational changes that bring the α subunits closer together, and enables ATP to bind to the intracellular domain of the β subunit.

Tyrosine Kinase Activity

The β subunits possess tyrosine kinase activity [5, 6]. The initial event following insulin binding appears to be phosphorylation of one β subunit catalyzed by a specific domain in the other β subunit within the same heterotetramer, a reaction that has been termed transphosphorylation or autophosphorylation [7]. Autophosphorylation of the kinase renders it considerably more active, allowing the accelerated transfer of phosphate to other tyrosine sites within the same receptor, as well as exogenous substrates [8]. Ligand-dependent stimulation of the β subunit tyrosine kinase activity is critical for promulgation of the insulin signal. There is an ATP-binding domain in the β subunit, and at least six tyrosine residues undergoing phosphorylation that have been shown in mutagenesis experiments to subserve different roles in insulin signaling, as shown in Figure 1. These phosphotyrosines lie within three functional groups. Tyrosine phosphorylation sites at positions Y^{1158}, Y^{1162}, and Y^{1163} are essential for mediating an increase in subunit tyrosine kinase activity and signal transduction, and lie in the active loop of the kinase catalytic domain. When phosphorylated, a juxtamembrane

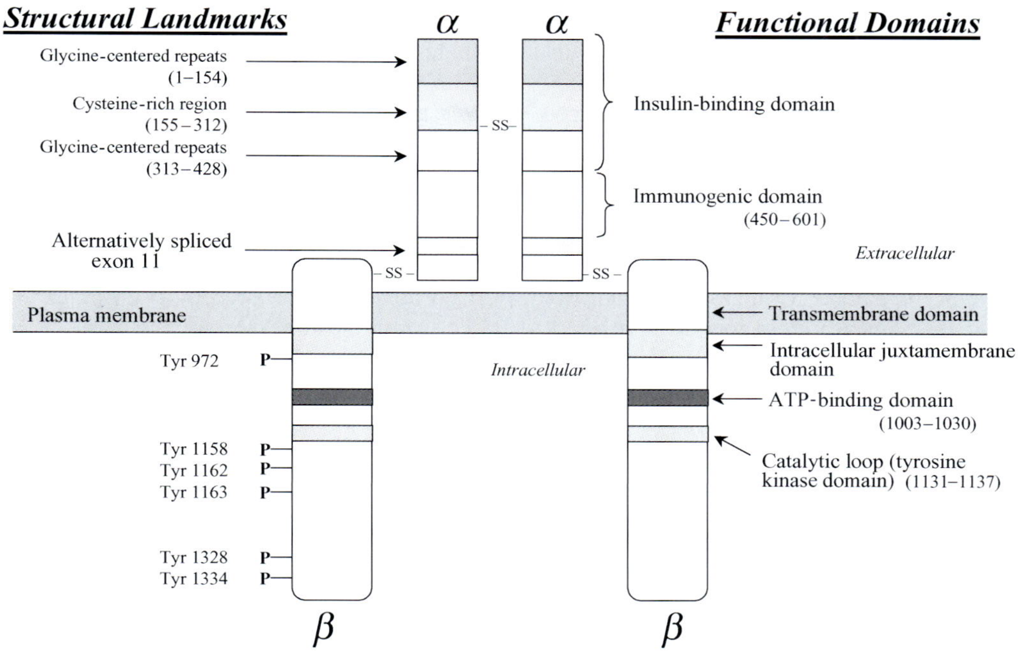

Figure 1 Structural and functional domains of the insulin receptor. Schematic diagram of the insulin receptor showing structural landmarks (left side) and functional domains (right side). (Numbering of amino acids based on translation of the alternatively spliced exon 11)

tyrosine at position Y^{972} becomes part of a recognition motif and provides a docking site for several intracellular substrates. Y^{972} is required to assure sufficient stability of the receptor/substrate complex for substrate phosphorylation. Y^{972} also lies within a domain that mediates endocytosis of ligand-bound insulin receptors. Phosphorylation sites Y^{1328} and Y^{1334} near the COOH terminus are not essential for stimulation of glucose transport but may affect the sensitivity of Ras/MAP kinase pathway activation, and so are involved in the receptor's mitogenic responses [9]. Phosphorylation of serine and threonine residues within the insulin receptor also occurs following insulin binding, and, as described below, phosphorylation of these residues by intracellular serine kinases can diminish receptor tyrosine kinase activity and represents a regulatory feedback mechanism [10].

Insulin-Like Growth Factors

The insulin receptor is similar in structure to IGF-1 and other growth factor and cytokine receptors [all $(\alpha\beta)_2$ stoichiometry], and IGF-2 receptors [$(\alpha\beta)$ stoichiometry], in having an extracellular ligand-binding domain that activates an intracellular tyrosine kinase domain [11]. In fact, both IGF-1 and IGF-2 can bind to cell surface insulin receptors. The affinity of IGF-1 for the insulin receptor is 100- to 1000-fold less than that for insulin. Nevertheless, circulating IGF-1 concentrations can be 100-fold higher than insulin such that there is some potential for IGF-1 binding and action through the insulin receptor. IGF-2 binds insulin receptors during embryogenesis in rodents, and promotes fetal growth. This capability may be associated with expression of an alternatively spliced form of the insulin receptor with high affinity for IGF-2 [12]. Alternative splicing in exon 11 determines the insertion or deletion of 12 amino acids near the COOH terminus of the α subunit. Isoform A lacking the 12 amino acids has high affinity for IGF-2, predominates during fetal development, and promotes growth as a consequence of IGF-2 binding. Isoform B containing the 12 amino acids predominates postnatally and is activated mainly by insulin. Some evidence supports the contention that dysregulated expression toward the fetal pattern could occur in adult tissues and result in insulin resistance [12, 13].

Insulin Receptor Mutations

Identification of functional domains within the insulin receptor has been accomplished by studying site-directed mutations, knockout and transgenic mice, and rare native mutations of the insulin receptor in patients with severe forms of insulin resistance. Native insulin receptor gene mutations have been detected in all major structural and functional domains, and generally either diminish ligand binding and/or impair β subunit tyrosine kinase activity [14]. Five major categories of insulin receptor mutations have been delineated that cause severe defects in insulin binding. These include (i) nonsense or frame-shift mutations that lead to premature termination of translation and decreased receptor synthesis; (ii) mutations that impair intracellular transport and posttranslational processing of receptors such that fewer receptors reach the cell surface; (iii) mutations in the insulin-binding domain that affect ligand affinity; (iv) mutations that enhance ligand-mediated endocytosis and degradation of insulin receptors; and (v) mutations that cause defects in receptor kinase activity. These latter mutations usually consist of point mutations in one of three areas within the β subunit: the ATP-binding site, the tyrosine kinase domain, or other areas in the intracellular domain. Phenotypically, patients with syndromes of severe insulin resistance can exhibit mild diabetes or glucose intolerance with marked hyperinsulinemia, acanthosis nigricans, hyperandrogenism, and abnormalities of growth and development with precocious pseudopuberty and cardiac enlargement. Related disease categories include type a severe insulin resistance, lipoatrophic diabetes, leprechaunism, and Rabson–Mendenhall syndrome [15, 16].

INSULIN RECEPTOR SUBSTRATE MOLECULES

Receptor Substrate/Docking Proteins

Following insulin binding and receptor autophosphorylation, the next committed step in signal transduction is tyrosine phosphorylation of intracellular proteins. To accomplish this, autophosphorylation of the β subunit mediates noncovalent but stable interactions between the receptor and intracellular substrate proteins, and this positions these molecules for tyrosine phosphorylation by the activated insulin receptor kinase [17–19]. Several proteins are rapidly phosphorylated on tyrosine residues by ligand-bound insulin receptors, including four insulin receptor substrate proteins (IRS-1, IRS-2, IRS-3, IRS-4) [20–23], Src-homology-collagen proteins (SHC) [24] and, growth factor receptor bound 2 (Grb-2) associated binder 1 (Gab-1) [25], signal-regulatory protein (SIRP) family members [26, 27], the CAP/c–Cbl complex [28, 29], an adapter protein with a pleckstrin homology (PH) and Src homology 2 (SH-2) domain (APS) [30], signal transducer and activator of transcription 5B (STAT-5B) [31], and five proteins referred to as downstream of kinase (DOK 1–5) [32, 33].

Although no enzymatic activity has been found associated with IRS molecules, their primary structure is noteworthy for multiple sites capable of interaction with other proteins. The receptor substrates are characterized by a representative architecture, particularly with respect to three functional domains. These include an N-terminal PH domain, an intermediate phosphotyrosine-binding (PTB) domain, and a carboxy-terminal region of variable length that contains the multiple tyrosine and serine phosphorylation sites [17–19]. The PH domain helps position the insulin receptor for coupling with IRS, possibly by binding to charged headgroups of certain phosphatidylinositides in adjacent membrane structures. PTB domains recognize the phosphotyrosine in an amino acid sequence asparagine–proline–any amino acid–phosphotyrosine (NPXpY), and this motif is present in the insulin receptor and other receptors with tyrosine kinase activity, such as the IGF-1 receptor. In this manner, the PTB domain enables receptor substrates to directly bind Y^{972} of the insulin receptor β subunit. All of the receptor substrate molecules have PH domains except SHC, and all have a PTB domain except Gab-1. These domains facilitate binding of the receptor substrates to the phosphorylated insulin receptor, allowing for phosphorylation of tyrosine residues in their COOH-terminal domain.

In the carboxy end of IRS molecules, the phosphotyrosines provide binding sites (pYMXM) for other proteins containing SH-2 domains. This term relates to homology with $pp60^{v\text{-}src}$, the sarc oncogene product and first protein kinase demonstrated to possess activity toward tyrosine residues [34]. Noncovalent attachment of SH-2-containing signaling molecules allows receptor substrates to function as docking proteins that appose proteins in the transduction cascade. Receptor substrates thus propagate the insulin signal via the docking, apposition, interaction, and activation of downstream signal molecules, rather than as a consequence of any intrinsic enzymatic activity *per se*. This system provides for extensive plasticity and regulation. For example, the multiple receptor substrate molecules exhibit differences in tissue specific expression and in their capacity to activate various downstream signal pathways. In addition, the receptor substrates can be acted upon by multiple receptor tyrosine kinases, such as IGF-1, interleukin, and integrin receptors, as well as serine kinases (see below), in a manner that allows for modulation of insulin signal and integration of responses to extracellular factors. Thus, these docking molecules provide for divergence, heterogeneity, and regulation of insulin signal transduction processes.

Insulin Receptor Substrate Family of Docking Proteins

IRS-1 and IRS-2 exhibit a wide range of tissue expression, including muscle, fat, liver, and pancreatic islets, although their relative levels can vary in different tissues [18–21]. IRS-3 is expressed in adipose tissue, fibroblasts, and liver cells, while IRS-4 has been detected in brain, thymus, and embryonic kidney [22, 23]. Knockout mouse models have highlighted functional differences among the IRS protein family. Genetic ablation of IRS-1 leads to severe growth retardation reflecting a decrease in growth-promoting effects of insulin and other factors that signal through IRS-1 [35, 36]. These mice were also insulin resistant but did not develop overt diabetes. On the other hand, ablation of IRS-2 produced insulin resistance, impaired insulin secretion, and overt diabetes in mice that were normal in size [37]. The IRS-2 knockout mice were observed to have decreased β-cell mass and insulin content, indicative of a trophic role for insulin signaling through IRS-2 in β-cell development. Genetic ablation of IRS-2 recapitulates the pathogenesis of type 2 diabetes in that diabetes arises only when insulin resistance and insulin secretion are both impaired in these knockout mouse models. IRS-3 knockout mice do not have an obvious phenotype, and IRS-3 has not been detected in the human genome. IRS-4 null mice also appear normal with the exception of reduced fertility. Therefore, IRS-1 and IRS-2 are the IRS isoforms critically important in glucose homeostasis. The consensus that has arisen from these studies is that, while the IRS family members to some extent represent duplicative pathways for insulin signal transduction, IRS-1 functions as the principal IRS in skeletal muscle, and that IRS-2 predominates in liver and β-cells where insulin action is required for normal β-cell growth and development.

In addition to PH and PTB domains assuring close apposition to the insulin receptor, IRS-2 (but not other IRSs) contains another region that interacts with the phosphorylated regulatory loop of the insulin receptor kinase, and this region has been designated the kinase regulatory loop-binding domain (KRLB) [31, 38, 39]. While the KRLB domain could confer some measure of signal specificity, it is unclear whether the presence of the KRLB explains the differences in phenotype between IRS-1 and IRS-2 knockout mice.

Other receptor substrates

Like IRSs, SHC proteins are phosphorylated in response to insulin, lack any known catalytic activity, and interact with SH-2 domain-containing proteins through their tyrosine phosphorylation sites [24]. A phosphorylation site on SHC can bind Grb-2, which can lead to the activation of the Ras/MAP kinase mitogenic signaling pathway. Therefore, SHC constitutes an additional substrate for the insulin receptor kinase and transduces the insulin signal via its protein-docking properties. There are at least three known SHC isoforms (46, 52, and 66 kDa), and all contain an amino-terminal PTB domain, a central region that is homologous to the α1 chain of collagen, and a carboxy terminal SH-2 domain.

Gab-1 contains only a PH domain at the amino terminus and a domain containing several tyrosine phosphorylation sites, but lacks a PTB domain [25]. In this case, the PH is sufficient for positioning Gab-1 adjacent to the insulin receptor and enabling phosphorylation, although a tight anchor is not possible due to the lack of a PTB domain. Gab-1 is most heavily phosphorylated by the ligand-activated epidermal growth factor receptors, another receptor containing tyrosine kinase activity, and less well by activated insulin receptors.

The DOK proteins 1 through 5 can all be phosphorylated by the insulin receptor and are similar to IRS family members in domain architecture [32, 33]. DOK proteins appear to have functional effects in lymphocytes and myeloid cells, and can be phosphorylated by both membrane-associated and cytoplasmic tyrosine kinases. DOKs are docking proteins that have been observed to associate with Ras GTPase-activating protein (RasGAP), Nck, and c-Abl, and in cultured cells can be involved in cytoskeletal reorganization. Their role in mediating the biological effects of insulin has not been elucidated.

Proteins that Dock with Receptor Substrate Molecules

SH-2-containing proteins, which bind to phosphotyrosine motifs and dock with IRS proteins, include proteins with enzymatic activity, such as PI-3 kinase, Fyn (tyrosine kinase), Csk (tyrosine kinase), and SHIP-2 (phosphotyrosine phosphatase), and other adapter proteins such as Grb-2, Crk, APS, and Nck [18, 19]. In addition to SH-2 domains, the adapter proteins also contain SH-3 domains, which bind to proline-rich sequences in other proteins with consensus sequence PXXP. In this way, the adapter proteins associate with receptor substrates via their SH-2 domains and bring with them other proteins bound to their SH-3 domains. The SH-3-bound proteins represent downstream signaling molecules and catalytic subunits, which participate in transduction of the insulin signal. The proteins that dock with receptor substrates, whether binding directly or via adapters, have different enzymatic activities that activate specific downstream molecules as a result of their juxtaposition on receptor substrate docking molecules. In this way, IRSs provide the first major point of divergence of insulin signal transduction pathways, leading to activation of mitogenic (Ras/MAP kinase) and metabolic (PI-3 kinase) pathways. This is illustrated in Figure 2.

RAS/MAP KINASE PATHWAY: MITOGENIC SIGNALING

One component of signal divergence emanating from IRS docking proteins is the engagement of the Ras/MAP kinase mitogenic signaling pathway (Figure 2). One of the SH-2 domain-containing proteins that docks with IRS is Grb-2, a small cytosolic adapter protein. Grb-2 also contains an SH-3-binding domain that binds proteins via interaction with proline-rich sequences, and one of these proteins is SOS (mammalian homologue of the *Drosophila* son-of-sevenless protein), a GDP/GTP exchange factor. Following insulin stimulation, Grb-2 is able to bind IRS via its SH-2 domain, and position SOS

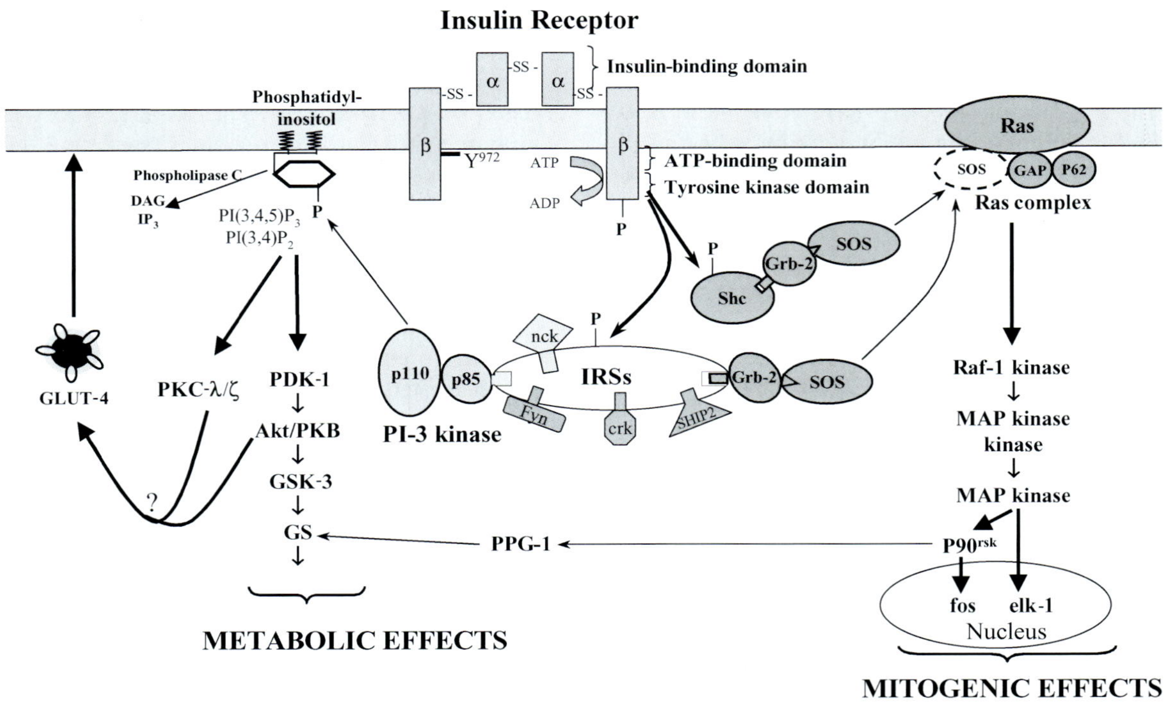

Figure 2 Metabolic and mitogenic signaling pathways in insulin action. Abbreviations: DAG – diacylglycerol; IP3 – inositol-3-phosphates; $PI(3,4)P_2$ – phosphatidylinositide 3,4-diphosphate; $PI(3,4,5)P_3$ – phosphatidylinositide 3,4,5-triphosphate; PI-3 kinase – phosphatidylinositide-3 kinase; PDK-1 – phosphoinositide-dependent kinase 1; GSK-3 – glycogen synthase kinase 3; GS – glycogen synthase; GLUT-4 – glucose transport protein 4; IRSs – family of insulin receptor substrate proteins; SHIP-2 – SH-2-containing inositol phosphatase 2; Grb-2 – growth factor receptor bound 2; SOS – mammalian homologue of *Drosophila* son-of-sevenless protein; Akt/PKB – protein kinase B; Shc – adapter protein with homology with Src and collagen; Ras – rat sarcoma protein; Gap – GTPase-activating protein; MAP kinase kinase – mitogen-activated protein kinase kinase; MAP kinase – mitogen-activating protein kinase; PPG-1 – glycogen-associated protein phosphatase 1

for activation of the Ras signaling pathway. SOS facilitates GTP activation of membrane-bound Ras, the 21 kDa small molecular weight GTPase, which has been demonstrated to play a major role in cell growth and oncogenesis. The GTP-bound form of Ras complexes with and activates Raf-1 kinase, and initiates a cascade, leading to sequential phosphorylation and activation of MAP kinase kinase, (MAPKK), MAP kinase, and $p90^{RSK}$. Insulin receptors can also mediate activation of the Ras/MAP kinase pathway through another substrate-docking molecule, SHC [40]. Similar to IRSs, SHC activates Ras and the MAP kinase pathway by forming a complex with Grb-2/SOS in response to insulin. Whether activated through IRS or SHC, MAP kinase translocates into the nucleus where it phosphorylates transcription factors mediating the mitogenic and growth promoting effects of insulin [41]. Phosphorylation of nuclear transcription factors modulates their DNA-binding properties and ability to regulate gene transcription. For example, $p90^{RSK}$ phosphorylates c-fos, and MAP kinase phosphorylates Elk-1, increasing transcriptional factor activity in both instances. The MAP kinase cascade is also one of the pathways with the potential to stimulate glycogen synthase, since p90 S6 kinase is able to activate the glycogen-associated protein phosphatase 1 (PPG-1), which in turn dephosphorylates and activates glycogen synthase. In this way, the MAP kinase pathway has the potential to interact with metabolic signaling pathways (see below). However, the MAP kinase pathway is not necessary for stimulation of glucose transport, and is not viewed as being critically related to the metabolic effects of insulin. For example, inhibition of the pathway in adipocytes using dominant negative forms of Ras [42] or inhibitors of MAPKK [43] will block transcriptional effects associated with the MAP kinase pathway, but will not interfere with insulin stimulation of either glucose transport or glycogen synthesis.

PI-3 KINASE PATHWAYS: REGULATION OF METABOLISM AND GENE EXPRESSION

Phosphatidylinositide-3 Kinase

Signal transduction for insulin's metabolic effects also diverges from IRS proteins and proceeds via the PI-3 kinase pathway (Figure 2). The first committed step involves type 1A PI-3 kinase, a heterodimer consisting of a p85 regulatory subunit and a p110 catalytic subunit [44]. In quiescent cells, the regulatory subunit maintains a state of low activity for the catalytic subunit. Upon insulin-mediated tyrosine phosphorylation, IRS-1 and IRS-2 (and other docking proteins) bind PI-3 kinase via interaction with the SH-2 domain on the p85 regulatory subunit [45]. Insulin stimulation increases the amount of PI-3 kinase associated with IRS, and the binding process increases the specific activity of the p110 catalytic subunit. Activation of PI-3 kinase is critical for transducing the metabolic actions of insulin, including stimulation of GLUT-4 translocation to the plasma membrane, with subsequent stimulation of glucose transport activity. This has been demonstrated in several lines of investigation. Treatment of adipocytes with (i) inhibitors of PI-3 kinase, including wortmannin or LY-294002, (ii) hyperexpression of dominant negative mutants of PI-3 kinase that interfere with endogenous wild-type enzyme function, and (iii) microinjection of neutralizing antibodies to the p110 catalytic subunits all result in abrogation of insulin's biological effect [46]. Conversely, hyperexpression of wild-type PI-3 kinase, or a constitutively active mutant leads to stimulation of both glucose transport activity and GLUT-4 translocation from 50 to 100% of insulin's maximal effect, depending on the study [47].

Several proteins can serve as the regulatory subunit of PI-3 kinase [19]. Six isoforms arise through alternative splicing of the p85α gene (p85α, p55α/AS53, and p50α each occurring with and without a spliced insert), and two other isoforms represent products of different genes (p85β, $p55^{PIK}$). All regulatory subunit isoforms associate with IRS phosphotyrosines and mediate activation of the associated p110 catalytic subunit. While p85α is ubiquitously expressed and is the dominant form in many tissues, the other isoforms exhibit differential tissue-specific expression. It remains possible that the various isoforms could serve to modulate or direct signal transduction via different affinities for IRS proteins or differences in subcellular compartmentalization, although there do not yet exist substantial data to support this hypothesis.

The function of the activated PI-3 kinase is to phosphorylate the inositol ring in plasma membrane glycolipids at the D-3 position, thereby converting phosphatidylinositol 4,5-bisphosphate to phosphatidylinositol 3,4,5-trisphosphate [PI(3,4,5)P_3], and to a lesser extent phosphatidylinositol 4-phosphate to phosphatidylinositol 3,4-bisphosphate [PI(3,4)P_2] [48, 49]. In skeletal muscle, the PI-3 kinase inhibitor, wortmannin, has been shown to prevent both the formation of 3′ phospholipids and the increase in glucose uptake in response to insulin. While the proximal physiological targets for the D-3 phosphoinositides have not been fully elucidated, phosphorylation of the inositol ring at the 3′ position in membrane glycolipids recruits certain signaling proteins with PH domains to the plasma membrane. Binding to membrane-associated phosphoinositides both activates these proteins and positions them for downstream signal transduction. In addition, phospholipase C may participate in the release of the 3′ inositol phosphate moieties and may be activated by insulin through an IRS-independent mechanism [50]. More research is necessary to determine the importance of phospholipase action in mediating or modulating insulin signaling.

While the role of PI-3 kinase in stimulation of glucose transport has been widely recognized, it has also become clear that PI-3 kinase activation is necessary for mediating multiple other metabolic effects of insulin as well as regulation of gene transcription. Thus, PI-3 kinase is the second major step, following IRSs, providing for broad divergence of insulin signal transduction, as illustrated in Figure 3. This is well demonstrated by experiments wherein suppression of PI-3 kinase has been shown to impact a host of insulin bioeffects including stimulation of glucose transport, glycogen synthesis, and glycolysis; promotion of lipogenesis via effects on fatty acid synthase and acetyl-CoA carboxylase; suppression of gluconeogenesis; stimulation of protein synthesis; stimulation of DNA synthesis; attenuation [phosphoenolpyruvate carboxykinase (PEPCK) and glucose-6-phosphatase] and induction [glucose-6-phosphate dehydrogenase and hexokinase II] of gene transcription; cell survival; and cell cycle progression. In order to propagate many of these effects, PI-3 kinase activates three serine–threonine kinases and their downstream pathways, namely, Akt or protein kinase B (Akt/PKB), atypical PKC isoforms (ζ, λ), and phosphoinositide-dependent kinases (PDK-1 and PDK-2).

Akt/Protein Kinase B

There are 3 isoforms of Akt/PKB; Akt-1 is expressed in a variety of tissues, while Akt-2 is most highly expressed in adipocytes and Akt-3 in certain cultured cell models [51–54]. Phosphorylation and activation of Akt/PKB isoforms involve 3′ phosphoinositides and the action of PDK. 3′ phosphoinositides in membrane glycolipids bind directly to the PH domain of Akt/PKB, and this process results in the uncovering of phosphorylation sites. At the same time, 3′ phosphoinositides activate PDK-1, which in turn phosphorylates threonine 308 of Akt/PKB. Full activation of Akt/PKB also requires phosphorylation of serine 473, and this could be accomplished in either of three ways. This could arise through the action of another putative phosphoinositide-dependent protein kinase, PDK-2, or could be accomplished by PDK-1, following a change in substrate recognition that results from threonine 308 phosphorylation, or may be the consequence of autophosphorylation.

Regardless of the mechanism of phosphorylation, there are several lines of evidence that implicate a role for

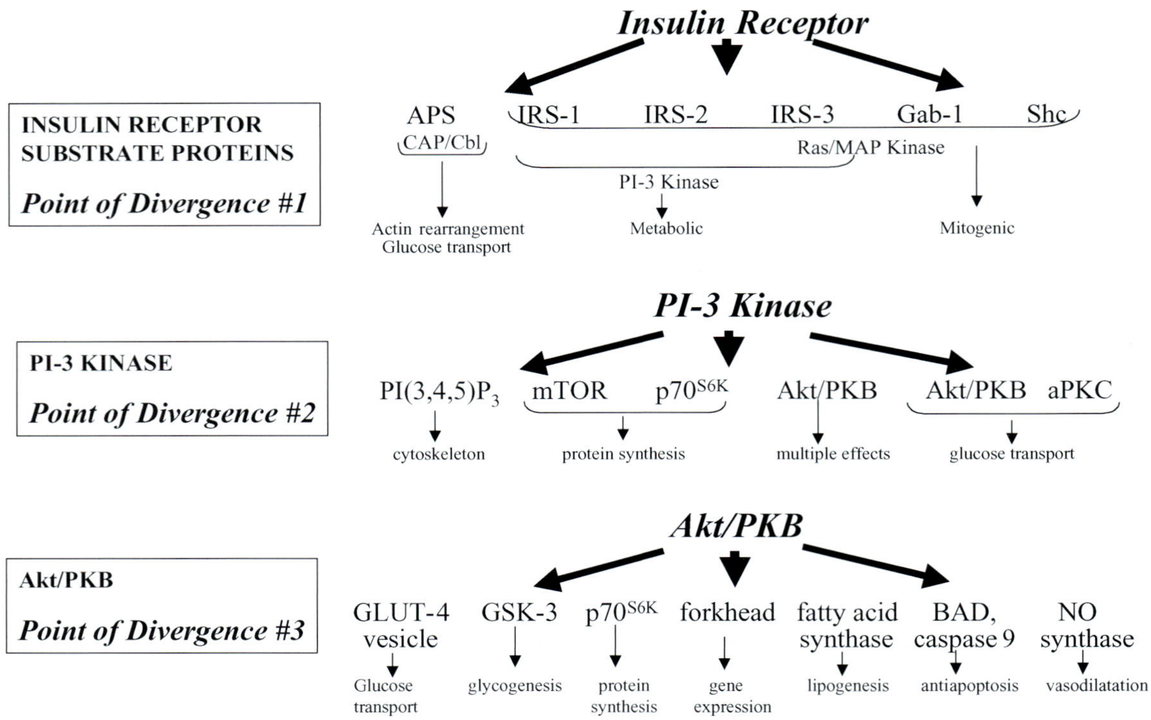

Figure 3 Three major steps providing for functional divergence of insulin signal transduction. The insulin receptor substrate docking proteins PI-3 kinase and Akt/PKB are sequentially activated by insulin, but then each factor engages multiple downstream signal molecules and pathways resulting in divergence, capacity for interaction, and complementarity of insulin signaling pathways. Abbreviations: APS – adaptor protein containing PH and SH-2 domains; IRS – insulin receptor substrate protein; Gab-1 – Grb-2-associated binding protein 1; Shc – adapter protein with homology with Src and collagen; $PI(3,4,5)P_3$ – phosphatidylinositide 3,4,5-triphosphate; mTOR – mammalian target of rapamycin; $p70^{S6K}$ – p70 S6 kinase; Akt/PKB – protein kinase B; aPKC – atypical protein kinase C isoforms; GSK-3 – glycogen synthase kinase 3; BAD – Bcl2 antagonist of cell death; NO – nitric oxide

Akt/PKB activation in the stimulation of glucose transport. Expression of constitutively active membrane-bound forms of Akt results in persistent translocation of GLUT-4 to the plasma membrane in muscle, fat, and cultured cell systems [55]. Interestingly, insulin stimulation is accompanied by association of Akt-2 with GLUT-4-containing vesicles in rat adipocytes, resulting in phosphorylation of constituent proteins [56]. Conversely, cellular introduction of neutralizing antibodies, substrate peptides, and dominant negative mutant blocked insulin-stimulated GLUT-4 translocation in adipocytes, albeit by only ~50%. These experiments constitute strong evidence for a role of Akt/PKB in insulin stimulation of glucose transport. However, these results are somewhat controversial because other investigators demonstrated that a dominant-interfering mutant, while blocking insulin-stimulated protein synthesis, did not inhibit GLUT-4 translocation [57]. Furthermore, in muscle from insulin-resistant diabetic humans, insulin-stimulated Akt phosphorylation was intact despite gross impairment in glucose uptake [58]. These discrepant results regarding a role for Akt/PKB do not exclude a role in the stimulation of glucose transport, perhaps working in concert with parallel activating pathways (e.g., PKC-λ/ζ, CAP/Cbl/TC10). Mice deficient in Akt2 exhibit mild insulin resistance in muscle, glucose intolerance, and an inability to suppress hepatic glucose production, whereas Akt-1 gene disruption produces growth reduction but has little effect on glucose tolerance [59, 60]. These results are indicative of an important role for Akt/PKB in insulin regulation of glucose homeostasis and also suggest that Akt-1 and Akt-2 may compensate for each other's absence to varying degrees. Nevertheless, the downstream targets of Akt/PKB connecting this signaling pathway to stimulation of the glucose transport effector system have not been identified.

Akt/PKB activation is involved in multiple other insulin responses [60]. One of the first substrates identified for Akt/PKB was a serine 9 residue in glycogen synthase kinase 3β (GSK-3β) [61, 62]. Thus, one pathway that could contribute to insulin-stimulated glycogen synthesis involves Akt/PKB-mediated phosphorylation and inactivation of GSK-3β resulted in activation of glycogen synthase activity (see Chapter 15). Akt/PKB also is capable of phosphorylating and activating mammalian target of rapamycin (mTOR), which in turn phosphorylates 4E-BP1/PHAS-1, leading to release of translation initiation factor eIF-4E, and recruitment of mRNA to the 40S ribosomal subunit [63]. The ribosomal S6 protein ($p70^{S6K}$) is phosphorylated and activated either through PDK-1, Akt/PKB, or mTOR, and similarly enhances translation of select populations of mRNA by increasing their interaction with the 40S ribosome [64]. In this way, Akt/PKB helps mediate insulin's effect to stimulate protein synthesis (see Chapter 18). Another apparent action is the phosphorylation and activation of endothelial NO synthase, leading to increased NO generation and vasodilatation [65]. Additional substrates for Akt/PKB include BAD and caspase 9, which are involved in antiapoptotic effects and alteration of cell survival pathways [66]. Finally, Akt/PKB phosphorylates forkhead transcription factors [67, 68] altering expression patterns of genes involved in carbohydrate and lipid metabolism. In fact, the gene regulatory effects of MAP kinase and Akt/PKB-activated forkhead transcription factors generally oppose each other. In this way, Akt/PKB represents an important mechanism for "cross-talk" between the PI-3 kinase pathway and other pathways regulating gene transcription and mitogenic effects, in the web of insulin signal transduction (Figure 3).

Protein Kinase C

The IRS/PI-3 kinase pathway also activates PKC-ζ and PKC-λ, two serine–threonine PKC isoforms in the "atypical" class that is not activated by calcium binding, diacylglycerol, or, phorbol esters [69, 70]. PI-3-kinase-dependent activation of PKC-ζ/λ has been observed in multiple target tissues and cultured cell models in response to insulin [71]. The activation of PKC-ζ/λ occurs proximal to Akt/PKB as a result of direct interaction with 3′ phosphoinositides and/or through phosphorylation and activation by PDK-1. Overexpression of constitutively active forms of PKC ζ or PKC λ increases glucose transport activity and GLUT-4 translocation by 50–100% of the extent observed in response to maximal insulin [71]. Also, expression of dominant-interfering PKC mutants, lacking a critical lysine in the kinase domain or at the site phosphorylated by PDK-1, inhibits insulin's ability to promote glucose transport and GLUT-4 translocation by ~50%. As is common in the insulin action field, discrepant results have also been reported where overexpression of wild-type or dominant negative mutant forms in adipocytes did not affect basal or insulin-stimulated glucose transport [72]. This type of recurring controversy indicates that hyperexpression and gene knockout experiments should be interpreted cautiously, especially when expression levels are altered well above or below the physiological range, and also reflects overlapping and complementary pathways that comprise the web of insulin signal transduction. Nevertheless, the available data indicate the PKC-ζ/λ participate in insulin's metabolic signaling pathways [71]. As is the case for Akt/PKB, the downstream targets of PKC-ζ/λ have not been identified, and this will be necessary for understanding of the relative participation of these two signaling proteins in the stimulation of glucose transport and other metabolic effects. Atypical PKCs can also mediate insulin simulation of general protein synthesis in a rapamycin-insensitive manner [73].

Degradation of the PI-3 Kinase Signal

At least two different types of phosphatases can degrade phosphoinositides, leading to deactivation of the PI-3 kinase signal [49]. Overactivity of these enzymes have the potential for inhibiting insulin signal transduction distal to the generation of 3′ phosphoinositides and causing insulin resistance. SH-2-containing inositol phosphatases (SHIP-1 and SHIP-2) dephosphorylate the 5′ position of $PI(3,4,5)P_3$ to form $PI(3,4)P_2$. Genetic disruption and loss of SHIP-2 results in a marked increase in insulin sensitivity, implying that PI-3-kinase-mediated formation of $PI(3,4,5)P_3$, rather than $PI(3,4)P_2$, is the critical 3′ phosphoinositide in insulin signaling. Another phosphatase, phosphatase and tensin homolog (PTEN), dephosphorylates the 3′ position converting $PI(3,4,5)P_3$ to $PI(4,5)P_2$. Some human cancers are associated with loss of PTEN expression, suggesting that unrestrained production of 3′ phosphoinositides could result in oncogenesis.

PI-3 KINASE-INDEPENDENT PATHWAYS FOR STIMULATION OF GLUCOSE TRANSPORT

The CAP/Cbl/TC10 Pathway

Substantial evidence confirms the presence of PI-3 kinase independent pathways for stimulation of glucose transport. It had long been clear that other growth factor receptors [i.e., the platelet-derived growth factor (PDGF) receptor, cytokine receptors such as interleukin 4 (IL-4), and certain integrins] activate PI-3 kinase to the same extent as the insulin receptor with generation of $PI(3,4,5)P_3$, yet still do not stimulate glucose transport [74, 75]. Since stimulation of transport was blocked by PI-3 kinase inhibitors (e.g., wortmannin), investigators concluded that PI-3 kinase is necessary but not sufficient for this key metabolic effect of insulin [76]. The additional factor that endows the insulin receptor with the specific capacity to stimulate glucose transport could include another parallel signaling pathway, compartmentalization of the PI-3 kinase response, or the utilization of specific signal protein isoforms in insulin target cells.

Multiple observations support a second parallel complementary pathway for insulin-stimulated glucose transport [76, 77]. For example, adenovirus-mediated hyperexpression of dominantly interfering PH and PTB domains block insulin receptor/IRS interaction and inhibit some responses involving PI-3 kinase, such as membrane ruffling and DNA synthesis, without any effect on GLUT-4 translocation. Similarly, blockade of PI-3 kinase activation, via prolonged pretreatment with PDGF or overexpression of GSK-3β, inhibits association of PI-3 kinase with IRS proteins without affecting stimulation of glucose transport or GLUT-4 translocation. In addition, specific mutations in the insulin receptor have been identified that exhibit a near normal ability to activate PI-3 kinase but completely fail to induce GLUT-4 translocation [78]. Finally, introduction of a cell permeable analogue of $PI(3,4,5)P_3$ does not have any effect to stimulate basal glucose transport, but in the presence of wortmannin plus insulin does elicit a maximal glucose transport response [79]. These data indicate that insulin signaling requires a separate wortmannin-insensitive pathway, which must operate in parallel with the PI-3 kinase pathway, for stimulation of glucose transport.

Evidence has accumulated strongly supporting the CAP/Cbl/TC10 pathway as the complementary pathway for insulin-stimulated glucose transport [76, 77], as illustrated in Figure 4. This pathway was elucidated as a linear sequence of interacting factors, using technologies such as the yeast two-hybrid system and co-immunoprecipitation of interacting factors. The pathway diverges from the PI-3-kinase pathway at the level of the insulin receptor kinase, which mediates tyrosine phosphorylation of Cbl protooncogene through a process that does not involve IRSs. c-Cbl phosphorylation does require another adapter protein, APS, which binds the insulin receptor via SH-2 domain–phosphotyrosine interaction and couples the receptor to Cbl [80]. c-Cbl is also complexed with another adapter protein, the c-Cbl associating protein (CAP), which helps facilitate recruitment of CAP/Cbl to the microdomain of the insulin receptor [81]. Tyrosine phosphorylation of Cbl results in disengagement of the CAP/Cbl complex from the insulin receptor.

CAP contains three tandem SH-3 domains in the COOH-terminus that binds to a proline-rich domain of Cbl, and, in the NH2-terminal region, also contains a sorbin homology (SoHo) domain. After disengagement of CAP/Cbl from the insulin receptor, the CAP SoHo domain binds to flotillin in caveolin-containing lipid raft domains of the plasma membrane [82]. Lipid rafts are plasma membrane domains, enriched in cholesterol, glycolipids, and sphingolipids, which coordinate signaling events by accumulating specific protein constituents. One class of lipid rafts contains caveolin proteins in invaginated

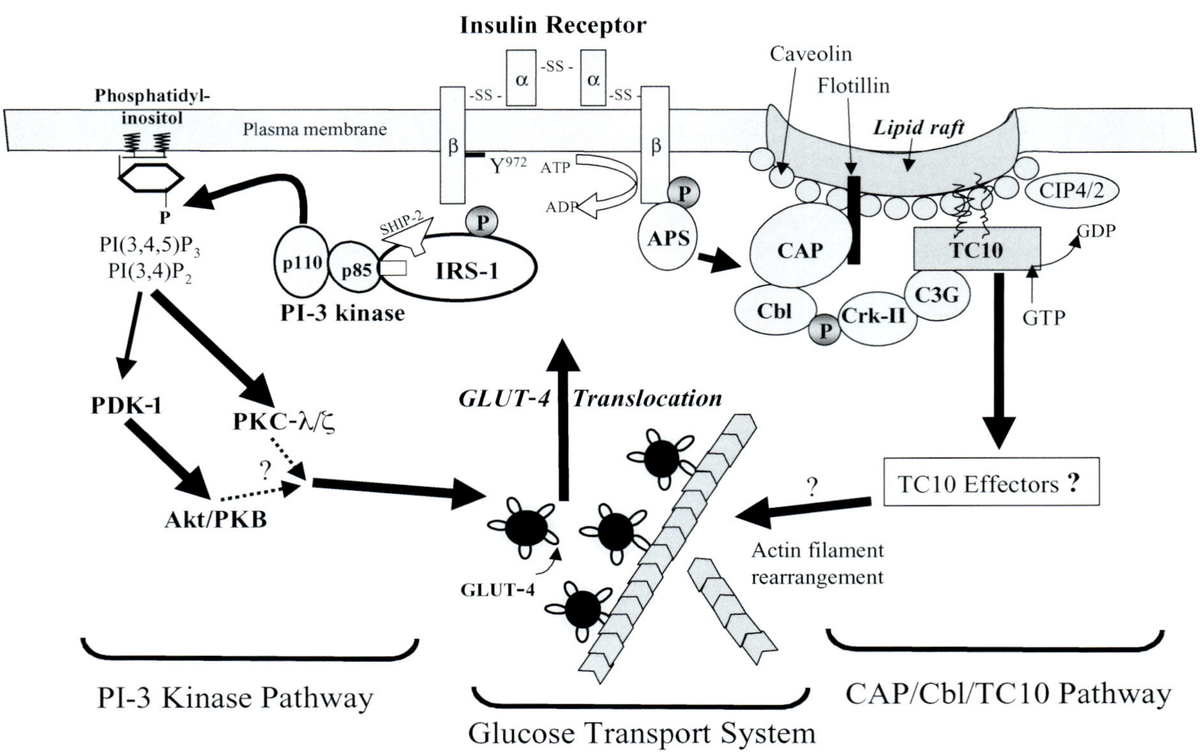

Figure 4 Two complementary pathways for stimulation of GLUT-4 translocation. IRS-1 – insulin receptor substrate 1; SHIP-2 – SH-2-containing inositol phosphatase 2; PI-3 kinase – phosphatidylinositide-3 kinase; PKC – protein kinase C; Akt/PKB – protein kinase B; PDK-1 – phosphoinositide-dependent kinase 1; APS – adaptor protein containing PH and SH-2 domains; CAP – c-Cbl associating protein; Cbl – Cbl proto-oncogene; Crk-II – Crk oncogene; C3G – guanine nucleotide-releasing protein C3G; TC10 – ras-like protein TC10; CIP4/2 – Cdc42-interacting protein; GTP – guanosine triphosphate; GDP – guanosine diphosphate

structures referred to as caveolae ("little caves"). Flotillin is anchored in lipid raft domains via its interaction with caveolin proteins. Thus, CAP is responsible for relocation of the CAP/Cbl complex to lipid raft domains. Once bound to flotillin, tyrosine phosphorylated Cbl presents a recognition site for recruitment of the Crk-II/C3G complex to the lipid raft. Crk-II is a small adapter protein that contains an SH-2 domain that binds phosphorylated Cbl, and SH-3 domains that interact with a proline-rich region of C3G. C3G is a guanyl nucleotide exchange factor for TC10 and other small molecular weight GTP-binding proteins [83]. TC10 is a member of the Rho family of GTPases, and is also targeted to lipid raft domains as a result of its capacity to undergo posttranslational modification by farnesylation and palmitoylation [84]. Insulin-mediated recruitment of C3G to the lipid raft results in the activation of TC10 via GTP exchange for GDCIP4/2P. TC10 in turn interacts with and recruits Cdc42-interacting protein 4/2 (CIP4/2) to the lipid raft [85]. The signaling events between TC10-CIP4/2 and translocation of GLUT-4-containing vesicles have not yet been elucidated. It is tempting to hypothesize that TC10, as a Rho family member, participates in the regulation of the actin cytoskeleton, given that investigators have demonstrated a functional requirement for filamentous actin in GLUT-4 translocation [86].

Experiments involving transgene expression in adipocytes have provided strong support for the contribution of the CAP/Cbl/TC10 pathway. Deletion of CAP SH-3 domains creates a dominant-interfering mutant that blocks binding to Cbl and recruitment of Cbl to lipid rafts, and prevents GLUT-4 translocation and stimulation of glucose transport without loss PI-3 kinase or MAP kinase activation [87]. SoHo deletion mutations in CAP, which prevent binding of the CAP/Cbl complex to flotillin in lipid rafts, also block GLUT-4 translocation and glucose transport stimulation [88]. Hyperexpression of C3G potentiates insulin action and shifts the insulin dose response curve to the left [89]. Overexpression of TC10 (but not other Rho family members) results in miss-targeting to nonlipid raft regions of the plasma membrane, and inhibits recruitment of GLUT-4 translocation associated with disruption of cortical actin in adipocytes [84]. Mutant forms of CIP4/2 also inhibit GLUT-4 translocation. To illustrate the dependence on caveolin-containing lipid rafts, disruption of rafts by cholesterol-extracting drugs (β-cyclodextrin) or by expression of mutant caveolins blocks insulin stimulation of TC10 and glucose transport [90, 91]. These experiments demonstrate that the CAP/Cbl/TC10 pathway is necessary for insulin stimulation of glucose transport.

In future research, it will be important to elucidate the mechanisms by which activation of Akt/PKB, PKC-ζ/λ, and TC10 interact with insulin's metabolic effector systems and, in particular, with the trafficking and translocation of GLUT-4 vesicles (see below). Detailed study of these processes will be necessary to better define defects causing insulin resistance in human disease.

Muscle Contraction

Acute exercise or muscle contraction results in GLUT-4 translocation and stimulates muscle glucose transport activity [92]. This effect occurs without any change in serum insulin concentrations and does not involve activation of PI-3 kinase or Akt/PKB. The mobilization of GLUT-4 to the cell surface by acute exercise involves a different intracellular pool of GLUT-4 than that recruited by insulin, and the effects of acute exercise and insulin are partially additive [92]. These observations indicate that signaling systems mediating glucose transport stimulation are different in response to acute exercise versus insulin [93]. This is underscored by the finding that, in muscle from insulin resistant humans and rodents, GLUT-4 translocation is impaired in response to insulin but normal in response to acute exercise.

While signal transduction mechanisms are not fully understood, this response to acute exercise appears to be at least partially dependent on increments in intracellular 5′AMP induced by acute exercise, and subsequent activation of 5′ AMP-activated protein kinase (AMPK) [93–95]. Hypoxia and mitochondrial uncoupling agents also increase 5′ AMP levels and increase cellular glucose transport rates. Investigators in this field have made frequent use of 5-aminoimidazole-4-carboxamide-1-β-D-riboside (AICAR), which acts as a 5′AMP analog by being phosphorylated after cellular uptake and then activating AMPK. AICAR administration mimics acute exercise by stimulating both GLUT-4 translocation and glucose transport in a PI-3 kinase independent manner [94, 95]. AMPK is an enzyme consisting of one catalytic subunit (α) and two regulatory subunits (β and γ), and exhibits a complex mechanism of regulation that "senses" fuel status in the cell. When ATP levels are low and 5′AMP is elevated, AMPK activates pathways for ATP regeneration and limits further ATP utilization by modifying activity of multiple metabolic enzymes, including acetyl-CoA carboxylase, hydroxymethylglutaryl-CoA reductase, creatine kinase, and hormone-sensitive lipase [96]. However, the downstream mechanisms leading to translocation of a distinct intracellular GLUT-4 pool have not been identified. It is also important to keep in mind that AICAR is a nonspecific stimulus, and that calcium, nitric oxide, bradykinin, atypical PKCs, and other factors may be involved in glucose transport stimulation by acute exercise. While the responsible signaling pathway operates independent of the insulin receptor and PI-3 kinase, additional research is needed to elucidate this important mechanism.

THE GLUCOSE TRANSPORT EFFECTOR SYSTEM

GLUT-4 Vesicle Translocation and Trafficking

Glucose transport proteins are the key functional units of the glucose transport effector system. Multiple glucose transporter genes have been identified [47, 97] that encode a family of homologous proteins exhibiting different functional properties and marked differences in tissue-specific expression. Members of the *GLUT* gene family are delineated in Table 1. On the basis of hydrophobicity plots, GLUT proteins contain 12 α-helical transmembrane-spanning domains with both the NH_2 and COOH terminals extending into the cytoplasm. This model forms six exofacial loops and five endofacial loops. Regarding GLUT-1 to 4 isoforms (class I in Table 1), the first exofacial loop is the largest and contains an asparagine-linked glycosylation site, and the five endofacial loops include a large hydrophilic central loop. Thus, GLUT proteins are intimately embedded in membranes, and the most highly conserved regions are the putative membrane-spanning domains that subserve a common function, the creation of a pore for facilitative diffusion of monosaccharides.

The major mechanism by which insulin activates glucose transport activity is by recruiting intracellular glucose transport proteins to the plasma membrane. Increased numbers of cell surface transporters augment facilitative diffusion of glucose into the cell where glucose is rapidly phosphorylated by hexokinase, and metabolized. Importantly, the glucose transport step is rate-limiting for insulin-stimulated glucose uptake and metabolism in peripheral target tissues under physiological conditions [97]. Upon dissipation of the insulin signal, deactivation of glucose transport activity is the result of a net reverse translocation of transporters back into the cell interior. The major insulin-responsive glucose transporter isoform is GLUT-4, which is predominately expressed in target tissues such as skeletal and cardiac muscle and adipose tissue.

Based on subcellular membrane fractionation experiments, insulin-mediated translocation was initially conceptualized as a two-compartment process with recruitment of GLUT-4 from Golgi-enriched microsomal membranes to the plasma membrane. However, these studies consistently indicated that only ~50–60% of microsomal GLUT-4 translocated to the plasma membrane fraction, suggesting that there were both insulin responsive and nonresponsive intracellular pools. It is now clear that GLUT-4 trafficking involves multiple intracellular membrane compartments [47, 76, 99, 100]. In basal cells, morphological studies employing immunohistochemistry and electron microscopy have detected GLUT-4 in perinuclear trans-Golgi membranes, in cytosolic tubulovesicular elements, and in subplasma membrane vesicles. Insulin results in a dramatic increase in plasma membrane GLUT-4 concomitant with a decrement in intracellular GLUT-4, although the intracellular translocating pool still has not been precisely defined. In one study, disruption of Golgi and trans-Golgi using the antibiotic brefeldin A did not impair insulin-stimulated glucose transport activity or surface appearance of GLUT-4, which were largely recruited from small vesicles located near the endofacial surface of the plasma membrane [100]. Other morphological data have implicated tubulovesicular structures as the source of the translocating GLUT-4 pool [99]. In addition to the intracellular translocating pool, GLUT-4 also cycles through an early endosomal

Table 1 The GLUT gene family

Isoform designation*	Class*	HUGO gene nomenclature	Major tissue distribution	Characteristics
GLUT-1	I	*SLC2A1*	Brain microvessels, erythrocytes, placenta, kidney	Ubiquitous, functions as basal transporter, predominates in cultured cell systems
GLUT-2	I	*SLC2A2*	Liver, kidney, β-cell, small intestine	High K_m transporter
GLUT-3	I	*SLC2A3*	Brain, placenta, fetal muscle	Low K_m transporter, found in tissues metabolically dependent on glucose
GLUT-4	I	*SLC2A4*	Skeletal muscle, adipocytes, heart	Sequestered intracellularly and translocates to cell surface in response to insulin
GLUT-5	II	*SLC2A5*	Testes, small intestine	High affinity for fructose
GLUT-6	III	*SLC2A6*	Spleen, leukocytes, brain	Transports glucose
GLUT-7	II	*SLC2A7*	Unknown	
GLUT-8	III	*SLC2A8*	Testes, blastocyst, brain	Transports glucose, mediates insulin-stimulable glucose transport in blastocyst
GLUT-9	II	*SLC2A9*	Liver, kidney	
GLUT-10	III	*SLC2A10*	Liver, pancreas	
GLUT-11	II	*SLC2A11*	Heart, muscle	Fructose-inhibitable glucose transport
GLUT-12	III	*SLC2A12*	Heart, prostate	
HMIT	III	*SLC2A13*	Brain	H^+-myoinositol transporter

Note: Four untranslated pseudogenes have been reported, including a pseudogene previously designated as GLUT-6.
* Isoform designation and class conforms to nomenclature proposed in reference 98.

compartment in an endocytotic/exocytotic pathway (distinct from fluid-phase endocytosis) analogous to that described for other insulin-responsive proteins, such as the mannose-6-phosphate/IGF-2 receptor and the transferrin receptor. GLUT-4 in the endosomal recycling system is clearly distinct from the intracellular inducible GLUT-4 storage compartment [102–106]. For example, ablation of the recycling compartment, accomplished via internalization of a transferrin–horseradish peroxidase conjugate, eliminates vesicles containing transferrin receptors and VAMP-3/cellubrevin (endosomal markers) but leaves intact a large fraction of GLUT-4-containing vesicles. This intracellular GLUT-4 storage compartment is purported to sequester GLUT-4 under basal conditions, and to be the major source for insulin-mediated exocytosis and translocation of GLUT-4 to the plasma membrane. This unique GLUT-4 storage compartment can explain why insulin's effect to augment cell surface proteins is much greater for GLUT-4 (10–40 fold over basal) compared with IGF-1 and transferrin receptors that traffic only in the endosomal recycling pathway.

A model for GLUT-4 traffic and translocation is shown in Figure 5, based on a consensus of current data. Following early endocytosis, GLUT-4 is sorted from other receptor and channel proteins in the recycling pathway and sequestered in a unique storage compartment composed of vesicles and tubulovesicular elements. Insulin recruits GLUT-4 primarily by stimulating exocytotic fusion of storage vesicles with the plasma membrane, resulting in exofacial exposure of functional glucose channels. In basal cells, constitutive cycling of GLUT-4 between intracellular and cell surface compartments has been demonstrated which may reflect a proportion of GLUT-4 remaining in the endosomal recycling pathway. Insulin increases numbers of plasma membrane GLUT-4 primarily by augmenting net exocytosis and also exerts a smaller effect to retard endocytosis. Stimulation of exocytosis proceeds primarily from the inducible storage compartment with a smaller contribution from the constitutive recycling pathway.

The proposed pathways for GLUT-4 vesicle traffic are determined by two general mechanisms, targeting motifs intrinsic to GLUT-4 and multiple proteins known to regulate the vectorial flow of cellular vesicles and their cargo proteins. In terms of intrinsic signals, a di-leucine motif at positions 489 and 490 in the cytosolic C-terminal of GLUT-4, and an aromatic-based motif (FQQI) in the NH_2 terminus, function as internalization signals for endocytosis [99, 107]. The COOH-terminus di-leucine motif is adjacent to a phosphorylation site (serine at 488) that, when mutated, can impair internalization when expressed in host cells. While these intrinsic motifs help direct internalization, the signal for intracellular retention in the inducible storage compartment have still not been identified with certainty. Some evidence has been obtained suggesting that an acidic cluster of amino acids (TELEYLGP) downstream from the di-leucine motif is important for

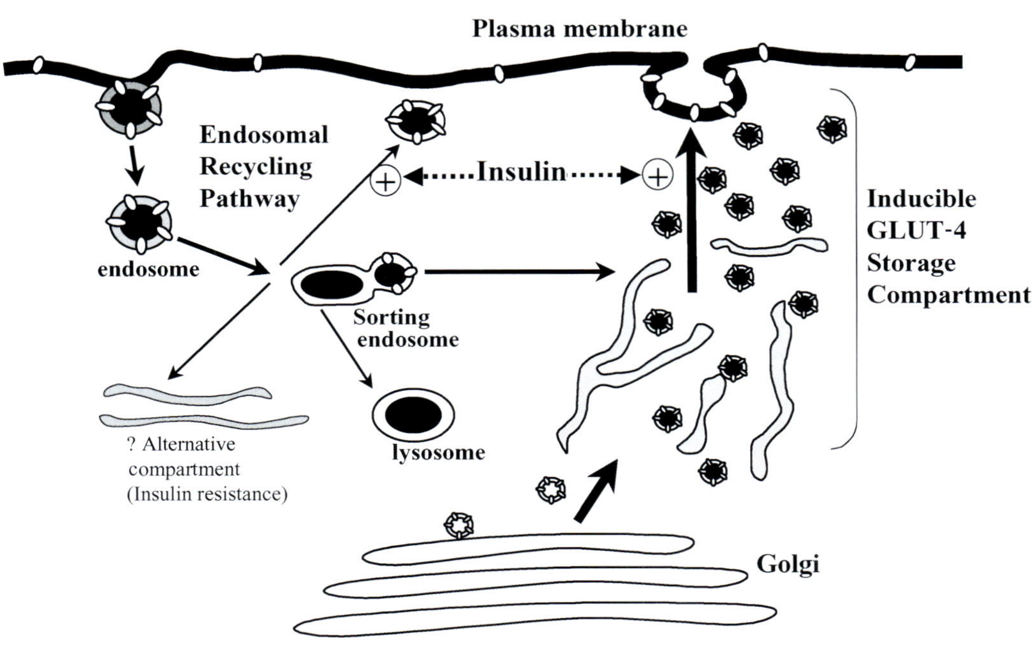

Figure 5 Cellular trafficking and itinerary of GLUT-4 glucose transporter proteins. The model is based on a consensus of current data, and includes an endosomal recycling pathway, a separate intracellular inducible GLUT-4 storage compartment that supplies the majority of GLUT-4 recruited by insulin to the cell surface, and an alternative compartment where accumulated GLUT-4 does not respond to insulin in insulin resistant states (see text)

targeting GLUT-4 to the inducible storage compartment [108]. In other experiments, overproduction of the GLUT-4 C-terminus, or the homologous cytoplasmic domain of IRAP, resulted in partial GLUT-4 translocation and activation of glucose transport, suggesting that these peptides are interacting with an intracellular retention protein [109]. The identity of such a protein remains elusive.

In addition, GLUT-4 vesicular traffic is controlled by multiple protein subclasses, also known to be involved in the regulated endocytosis/exocytosis of synaptic and neurosecretory vesicles [97, 99, 100, 102–107]. Multiple trafficking proteins are actual constituents of the GLUT-4 vesicle; GLUT-4 vesicle cargo proteins include vesicle-associated membrane protein 2 (VAMP-2) or synaptobrevin, VAMP-3/cellulobrevin, syntaxin 4, 35–39 kDa secretory carrier-associated membrane proteins (SCAMPs), sortilin, cellugyrin, acyl-CoA synthetase 1, and small molecular weight GTP-binding proteins in the Rab and Arf subclasses. Of these proteins, VAMP-2, VAMP-3/cellubrevin, SCAMPs, and cellulgyrin are known to be constituents of GLUT-4-containing vesicles in the endosomal recycling pathway where they co-localize with IGF-1 and transferrin receptors. Of these, only VAMP-2 is present together with GLUT-4 in the intracellular storage compartment. Another constituent of GLUT-4 vesicles is an aminopeptidase with as yet unknown function, referred to as the insulin-regulated aminopeptidase (IRAP) [110]. IRAP translocates with GLUT-4 and has been used to track the cellular itinerary of GLUT-4 vesicles. Given that there is a marked degree of insulin-stimulated recruitment of IRAP from intracellular to plasma membranes, GLUT-4 vesicles in the inducible storage compartment may be particularly enriched in IRAP.

The above-described trafficking proteins operate according to the v-SNARE/t-SNARE model developed by Rothman and others that explains how vesicles traffic to specific membrane compartments [111]. In this model, shown in Figure 6, a docking and fusion reaction is initiated via the high affinity interaction between a ligand on the transport vesicle (v-SNARE) and a receptor in the target membrane (t-SNARE). In the case of GLUT-4 vesicle translocation from the inducible storage compartment to the cell surface, evidence suggests that VAMP-2 functions as the v-SNARE and syntaxin 4 as the plasma membrane t-SNARE [97, 99, 100, 102–107]. Other proteins facilitate and regulate this interaction. The *N*-ethylmaleimide

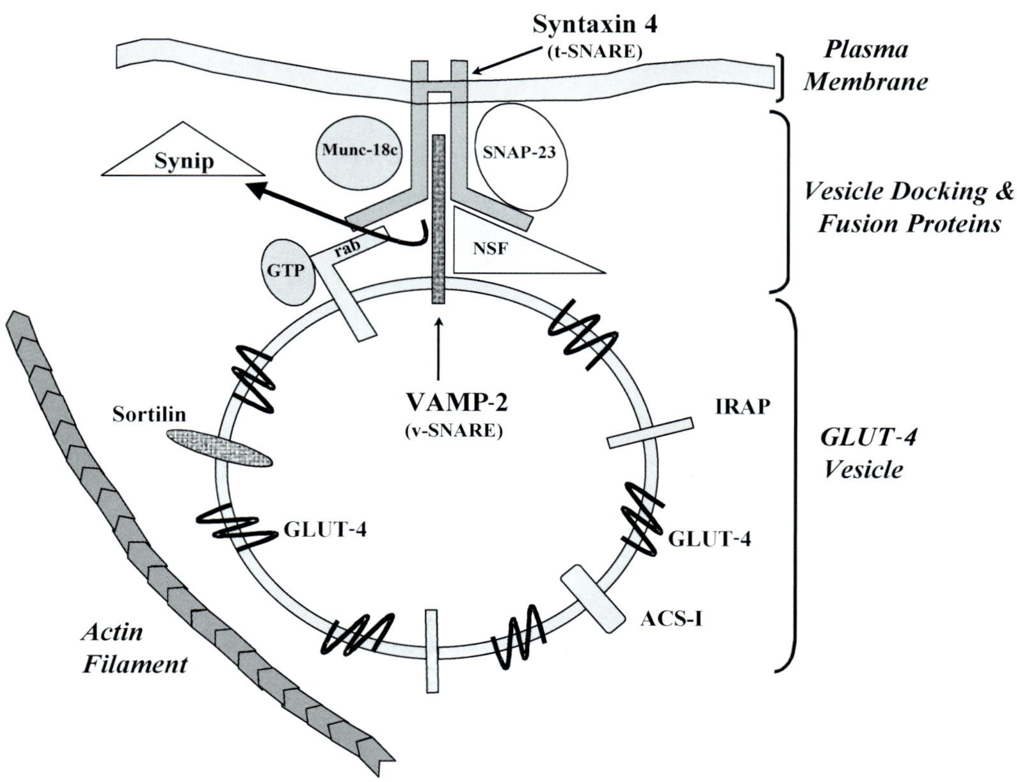

Figure 6 Proteins regulating the docking of exocytotic GLUT-4 vesicles at the plasma membrane. Abbreviations: IRAP – insulin-regulated aminopeptidase; ACS-1 – acyl-CoA synthetase 1; VAMP-2 – vesicle-associated membrane protein 2; NSF – *N*-ethylmaleimide-sensitive factor; SNAP-23 – soluble NSF attachment 23 kDa protein; Munc-18c – mouse Unc homologue 18c; synip – syntaxin 4 interacting protein; rab – monomeric GTPase in the rab subclass; t-SNARE and v-SNARE refer to target membrane and vesicle-associated soluble *N*-ethylmaleimide-sensitive attachment protein receptors, respectively

sensitive factor (NSF) activates the v-SNARE for docking competency, and three proteins, the soluble NSF attachment 23 kDa protein (SNAP-23), the mouse Unc homologue 18c (Munc-18c), and the syntaxin 4 interacting protein (Synip), regulate docking efficiency at the level of the t-SNARE by facilitating or blocking access to syntaxin4 [112]. While SNAP-23, Munc-18c, and Synip form a complex with syntaxin 4 at the endofacial plasma membrane, their precise roles in modulating interaction between VAMP-2 and syntaxin 4 are not fully understood. Synip appears to block access of VAMP-2 to syntaxin 4 under basal conditions and is released from the complex, following insulin stimulation allowing docking of v-SNARE (VAMP-2) to the t-SNARE (syntaxain 4). The function of Munc18c appears to be more complex with evidence that it can both inhibit (basal conditions) and facilitate (insulin-stimulated condition) VAMP-2-syntaxin 4 interaction. The Rab family of monomeric GTPases also play an important role in vesicle traffic; different isoforms are targeted to specific organelle membranes and direct the vectorial flow of vesicle proteins from one compartment to another [113, 114]. Rab GTPases also appear to catalyze the union of v- and t-SNARES in the docking process. Rab-4 has been demonstrated to be associated with GLUT-4 vesicles in basal cells, but is redistributed to cytosol in response to insulin where it associates with its GDP-association inhibitor [115]. Furthermore, Rab-4 has been shown to interact with syntaxin 4 *in vitro*, and overexpression of Rab-4 or a COOH-terminal domain peptide, prevented insulin-stimulated GLUT-4 translocation in adipocytes [116]. Undoubtedly, there are additional factors participating in GLUT-4 vesicle targeting, docking, and fusion in insulin target tissues that remain undiscovered.

The Cellular Cytoskeleton

There is increasing recognition that GLUT-4 translocation involves the actin cytoskeleton [47, 117–119]. One line of evidence supporting this hypothesis is that disruption of the actin cytoskeleton by cytochalasin D or latrunculin also inhibits insulin-mediated GLUT-4 translocation [117, 118]. In addition, insulin stimulates cytoskeletal rearrangement, in particular the cortical actin fibers subtending the plasma membrane, and regulates molecules that control actin polymerization, such as the Rho family of small molecular weight GTPases. The dependence of the glucose transport system on actin filaments may revolve around Rho GTPases, since inhibition of Rho function, either by *Clostridium difficile* toxin B or expression of a dominant-interfering TC10 mutant, blocks GLUT-4 translocation and disrupts the actin cytoskeleton in adipocytes [47, 86]. It is attractive to hypothesize that activation of TC10 via the CAP/Cbl/TC10 pathway could mediate regulation of the actin cytoskeleton in response to insulin, since TC10 and other Rho GTPases are generally known to affect biochemical modulators of cytoskeletal function [120]. However, PI-3 kinase can also affect cortical actin polymerization and events such as membrane ruffling and filopodia formation; therefore, other insulin signaling pathways could also contribute to this biological effect. The exact role of the actin cytoskeleton has not yet been delineated; however, one proposal is that actin filaments serve as a scaffold to direct GLUT-4 vesicle trafficking, using actin-based motility as a motor for vesicle movement.

The microtubule cytoskeleton is also involved in GLUT-4 vesicle trafficking [100, 121, 122]. Microtubules are believed to contain the intracellular depot of GLUT-4 that translocates to the plasma membrane in response to insulin, and it is not surprising that microtubule proteins such as dynein and kinesin have been co-purified with GLUT-4. Disruption of microtubules, using depolymerizing agents inhibits GLUT-4 translocation and glucose transport stimulation, and expression of a dominant-interfering dynein mutant was shown to inhibit GLUT-4 endocytosis in a process that might require Rab5 [123]. An emerging hypothesis is that GLUT-4 begins exocytosis in a microtubular compartment, and then transfers to actin scaffolds that connect the microtubule cytoskeleton with the plasma membrane, which then positions GLUT-4 vesicles for docking and membrane fusion. Upon endocytosis, GLUT-4 traffics in an endosomal compartment regulated by actin filaments and eventually is sorted back to the microtubular inducible storage compartment. While this model is compelling, additional research is necessary to define the role of cytoskeletal elements in GLUT-4 translocation. In any case, these considerations emphasize the complex nature of the glucose transport effector system, which functionally incorporates both vesicle traffic and cytoskeletal systems.

Insulin Resistance and the Glucose Transport Effector System

Given the rate-limiting role of plasma membrane transport in cellular glucose metabolism, GLUT-4 defects could readily result in insulin resistance at the level of the glucose transport effector system. These defects could involve either a decrease in cellular expression, diminished functional activity, or impaired translocation of GLUT-4 to the cell surface [124]. The multicompartmental nature of GLUT-4 cellular trafficking, requiring a multiplicity of regulatory proteins, indicates that there are many potential sites for defects that could impair GLUT-4 translocation. Indeed, defects intrinsic to glucose transport system are an important cause of insulin resistance in muscle and fat tissues from insulinresistant and diabetic patients. In adipocytes, cellular depletion of GLUT-4 transporters is a major mechanism of insulin resistance in obesity and type 2 diabetes [125], while GLUT-4 expression is relatively normal in skeletal muscle [126]. However, in both muscle and fat, GLUT-4 accumulates or is redistributed to a dense membrane compartment under basal conditions, and this abnormality is linked to impaired GLUT-4 translocation to the plasma membrane in response to insulin [127–129] (see Figure 6). These data are indicative of a trafficking or targeting abnormality impairing GLUT-4 translocation and causing human insulin resistance. Additional study of pathways and factors involved in abnormal GLUT-4 traffic may elucidate mechanisms causing human insulin resistance and establish targets for drug development.

MODULATION OF INSULIN ACTION

Important recent advances in the study of insulin signaling include the elucidation of multiple mechanisms for dampening or inhibiting insulin signal transduction. The studies have provided insight into the extensive regulation of insulin action, and have also identified potential therapeutic targets, since blocking these inhibitory mechanisms could enhance insulin sensitivity. These mechanisms are summarized in Figure 7.

Serine-Threonine Phosphorylation of the Insulin Receptor and IRS Proteins

Serine-threonine phosphorylation of insulin receptors and insulin substrate docking proteins has emerged as a major mechanism for modulation of insulin signal transduction. Serine phosphorylation of the insulin receptor diminishes its tyrosine kinase activity [10]. Serine phosphorylation of IRS-1 (and other IRSs) decreases receptor–IRS coupling by inhibiting insulin-mediated receptor phosphorylation, tyrosine phosphorylation of IRS-1, binding and activation of PI-3 kinase, and stimulation of glucose transport [130–132]. There are consensus sequences in IRS-1 that make it susceptible to a wide variety of serine–threonine kinases including PKC, PKA, Akt/PKB, MAP kinase, GSK-3, casein kinase II, Cdc-2 kinase, and c-Jun NH_2-terminal Kinase (JNK). Several of these kinases have been shown to function as physiological modulators causing desensitization of insulin signaling pathways.

Protein Kinase C

Protein kinase C isoforms are categorized as classic (α, β, γ), novel (δ, θ, ε, η, μ), and atypical (ζ, λ, β) depending

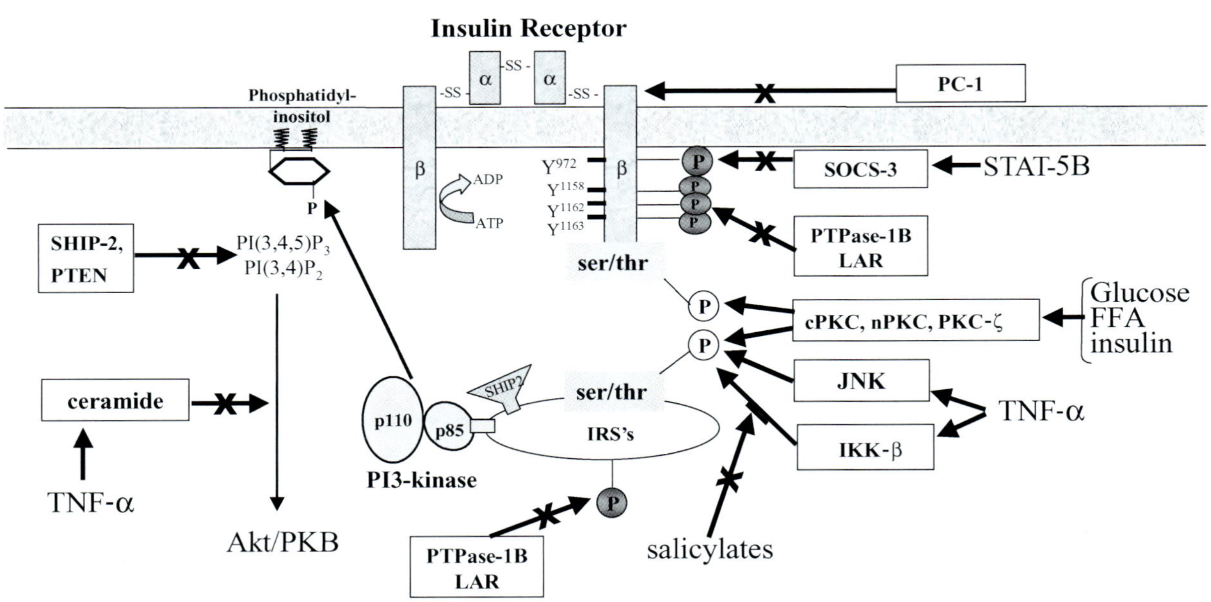

Figure 7 Mechanisms for modulation of insulin signal transduction. The figure illustrates pathways resulting in the desensitization of insulin signal transduction, including serine–threonine phosphorylation of the insulin receptor or IRS by PKC, IKK-β, or JNK; inhibition of the insulin receptor tyrosine kinase by PC-1; tyrosine phosphatase action of PTPase-1B and LAR; catabolism of 3′ phosphoinositide moieties by SHIP-2 or PTEN; inhibition of Akt/PKB activation by ceramide; and interference with substrate binding (STAT-5B) to the insulin receptor β subunit by SOCS-3. Abbreviations: PC-1 – plasma cell membrane glycoprotein PC-1; SOCS-3 – suppressor of cytokine signaling 3; STAT-5B – signal transducer and activator of transcription 5B; PTPase-1B – protein tyrosine phosphatase 1B; LAR – leukocyte antigen-related tyrosine phosphatase; cPKC – classic protein kinase C isoforms; nPKC – novel protein kinase C isoforms; PKC-ζ – protein kinase Cζ; JNK – c-Jun N-terminal kinase; IKK-β – kinase of inhibitor of kappa light chain gene enhancer in B cells β; TNF-α – tumor necrosis factor α; IRS – insulin receptor substrate protein; ser/thr – a serine or threonine residue; Y – tyrosine residue; PI-3 kinase – phosphatidylinositide-3 kinase; SHIP-2 – SH-2-containing inositol phosphatase 2; PTEN – phosphatase and tensin homolog; Akt/PKB – protein kinase B

on their ability to be activated by calcium and diacylglycerol. There are serine–threonine kinases with multiple substrates, including IRS docking proteins and the insulin receptor [10, 130, 131]. Serine-threonine phosphorylation of IRS impairs its ability to associate with the insulin receptor and with PI-3 kinase, resulting in desensitization of the PI-3 kinase pathway. Hyperinsulinemia, hyperglycemia, and elevated circulating free fatty acids increase intracellular DAG, which in turn activates conventional and novel PKC isoforms principally via recruitment to the plasma membrane. These conditions are associated with increased serine–threonine phosphorylation and diminished function of insulin receptors and IRS proteins. In addition, insulin activates atypical PKCs, such as PKC-ζ, via the PI-3 kinase pathway, which are also capable of phosphorylating and desensitizing IRS [133, 134]. Thus, PKC-ζ could be involved both in direct promulgation (Figure 2) and in feedback inhibition (Figure 7) of insulin signal transduction.

Tumor Necrosis Factor α

Tumor necrosis factor α TNF-α is a cytokine produced by immune cells and also by adipocytes and muscle tissue. While having little impact on systemic circulating concentrations, TNF-α expression is increased in adipose and muscle tissues as a function of insulin resistance [135, 136], raising the possibility that the cytokine could be inducing cellular insulin resistance via autocrine/paracrine effects. Consistent with this idea, TNF-α has been shown to cause insulin resistance in cultured cell models. While the mechanisms underlying desensitization have not been fully elucidated, TNF-α induces serine phosphorylation of IRS-1, thereby decreasing both insulin receptor tyrosine kinase activity and downstream insulin signal transduction [137–139]. One possible branch of the TNF-α signaling pathway that could mediate IRS phosphorylation results in the activation of the stress-induced kinase, JNK. JNK is a serine kinase with many interacellular substrates including IRS-docking proteins, IRS-1, IRS-2, Shc, and Gab-1. These docking molecules contain JNK-binding motifs that facilitate JNK-mediated phosphorylation of serine residues. In the case of IRS-1, JNK action results in the phosphorylation of a serine residue (ser^{307} in mice or ser^{312} in humans) that lies within the PTB domain; phosphorylation at this site interferes with PTB function reducing interaction between insulin receptor and IRS-1 [140]. Another potential mechanism involves insulin stimulation of sphingomyelinase activity, causing release of ceramide from sphingomyelin in lipid raft domains [54, 141]. Exogenous ceramide induces insulin resistance in cultured adipocytes associated with decreased Akt/PKB phosphorylation and GLUT-4 translocation. Regardless of underlying mechanisms, abrogation of TNF-α action by targeted disruption of TNF-α receptor isoforms (p55 and p75) results in enhanced insulin sensitivity in mice [141].

IκB Kinase β

Treatment with high doses of salicylates improves glucose tolerance and enhances insulin sensitivity in humans and rodents [142]. An important biological effect of salicylates is the inhibition of the IκB kinase β (IKK-β). Because IKK-β is a serine kinase, these observations implicate this serine kinase cascade in desensitization of the insulin signal, perhaps through serine phosphorylation of IRS or the insulin receptor. Predictably, salicylates would then enhance insulin sensitivity by causing a subsequent decrease in IKK-β-mediated serine phosphorylation of IRS. Consistent with this hypothesis, heterozygous ablation of the IKK-β gene in mice prevents insulin resistance induced by high fat feeding or lipid-infusion, and in obese leptin-deficient *ob/ob* mice [143, 144]. Interestingly, TNF-α also activates IKK-β, suggesting that the desensitizing effects of TNF-α, as a consequence of IRS serine phosphorylation, may in part be mediated through IKK-β.

Protein Phosphotyrosine Phosphatases

Endogenous phosphotyrosine phosphatases (PTPase) are able to dephosphorylate tyrosine residues on the insulin receptor β subunit and IRS-docking molecules, resulting in a dampening of insulin signal transduction [145]. Membrane-associated PTPase activity is increased in skeletal muscle from patients with type 2 diabetes [146], principally because of increments in cytosolic PTPase-1B and membrane-associated leukocyte antigen-related phosphatase (LAR) [147, 148]. The ability of PTPases to modulate insulin signaling has been demonstrated in mice with genetic ablation of PTPase-1B, which exhibit enhanced insulin sensitivity, increased insulin-mediated tyrosine phosphorylation of the receptor and IRS, and a failure to develop insulin resistance when fed a high fat diet [149]. The data demonstrate that PTPase-1B is able to negatively modulate insulin signaling through dephosphorylation of tyrosine residues in the insulin receptor and IRSs. Inhibition of PTPase action represents a clinically-attractive therapeutic target for increasing insulin sensitivity.

Other Mechanisms

Suppressor of Cytokine Signaling 3

Observations pertaining to suppressor of cytokine signaling 3 (SOCS-3) point to a new mechanism for insulin signal modulation [31]. The SOCS family of proteins (CIS and SOCS-1 to -7) were originally described as a negative feedback loop for cytokine receptor signaling through Janus kinase (JaK). JaK phosphorylates and activates signal transducer and activator of transcription (STAT), which is a transcription factor that augments SOCS gene expression. SOCS proteins then feedback to inhibit tyrosine-phosphorylated cytokine receptors, via either competitive binding through their SH-2 domain preventing phosphorylation of cytokine receptor substrates or by binding and inhibiting Jak tyrosine kinases. Evidence suggests that a similar mechanism may be operative for the insulin receptor [150]. Insulin stimulates STAT-5B activation by direct tyrosine phosphorylation after STAT-5B binds to insulin receptor phosphotyrosine 972 via its SH-2 domain (i.e., this interaction does not involve a PTB as is the case with IRS). STAT-5B induces expression of SOCS-3, which then competes with STAT-5B binding to the insulin receptor, inhibiting further STAT-5B activation. Thus, SOCS-3 could function as a new negative regulator for insulin signaling, not only with respect to STAT-5B activation, but also for other signaling pathways to the extent that SOCS-3 could prevent the interaction between the PTB domain of IRS and the insulin receptor. It is intriguing that several factors that induce cellular insulin resistance also induce SOCS-3 expression, including TNF-α [151], growth hormone [152], and leptin [153].

Plasma Differentiation Factor 1

Plasma differentiation factor 1 (PC-1) is a membrane glycoprotein with pyrophosphatase activity that appears to act as an intrinsic inhibitor of the insulin receptor tyrosine kinase through an undefined mechanism [154–156]. Muscle expression of PC-1 is elevated in diabetes and in obesity, and correlates with diminished insulin receptor tyrosine phosphorylation and muscle glucose uptake [157].

REGULATION OF GENE TRANSCRIPTION

Insulin Response Elements

Insulin regulates the expression of many individual proteins through effects on translation, mRNA stability, and gene transcription. The stimulatory effect on translation generally results from increases in the initial phase of translation of mRNA by ribosomes, and is discussed in Chapter 18. Regulation of gene transcription can be due to effects on transcription factors that are directly modified via insulin signaling mechanisms, or that are indirect as the result of stimulation of glucose metabolism. For example, genes encoding pyruvate kinase, fatty acid synthase, acetyl-CoA carboxylase, and stearoyl-CoA desaturase require increases in both insulin and glucose for induction, and PEPCK expression can be suppressed independently by insulin or glucose. The promoter elements (*cis*-acting sequences) that mediate changes in gene transcription are referred to as insulin response sequences or insulin response elements (IRE). There clearly exist multiple distinct classes of IREs that participate in the regulation of different gene promoters, rather than a single consensus nucleotide sequence [158]. These IREs can mediate either positive effects (GAPDH, pyruvate kinase, fatty acid synthase, somatostatin, c-fos, glucokinase, apoA1) or negative effects (e.g., PEPCK, glucose-6-phosphatase, tyrosine aminotransferase, apoCIII, glucagon) on gene transcription. It is also important to consider the identity of the transcription factors (*trans*-acting factors) activated by insulin that bind to the IREs and alter gene transcription rates. While the identification of transcription factors has progressed more slowly than with IREs, there has recently been exciting progress in identifying new transcription factors and signaling mechanisms involved in insulin regulation of specific genes.

Insulin regulation of gene expression has been most readily attributed to the mitogenic MAP kinase pathway. However, insulin inhibition of PEPCK, IGFBP-1, and glucose-6-phosphatase genes employs the PEPCK-like IRE with consensus sequence T(G/A)TTT(T/G)(G/T) in the core motif, and this occurs through a PI-3-kinase-dependent pathway [158]. The downstream targets of PI-3 kinase are somewhat controversial with studies arguing for and against the involvement of Akt/PKB and a recent study supporting a role for GSK-3 in the inhibition of PEPCK and glucose-6-phosphatase genes [159]. Nevertheless, PI-3 kinase pathways can also regulate gene transcription, and this calls into question notions of distinct and separate metabolic and mitogenic insulin action pathways in the web of insulin signal transduction.

TPA and Serum Response Elements

The ability of insulin to alter gene expression via the mitogenic MAP kinase pathway has long been recognized [160]. This classic mechanism involves phosphorylation of transcription factors in the activating protein 1 (AP-1) family such as c-Jun and c-fos that interact with the 12-O-tetradecanoylphorbol-13-acetate response element (TRE); and ternary complex factors such as Elk-1, SAP-1, and SAP-2 that interact with the serum response element (SRE). Both elements can be found in single gene promoters, for example, in the *c-fos* gene that is induced by insulin through activation of both c-jun and Elk-1.

Forkhead Transcription Factors

Genetic studies in the nematode, *Caenorhabtidis elegans*, have led to the discovery of a new pathway for insulin-regulated gene expression [161]. One of the developmental stages in *C. elegans* is the *dauer* stage characterized by increased longevity, reduced metabolic activity, and increased body fat. A series of specific gene mutations, termed Daf alleles, has defined a signal transduction pathway leading to a constitutive *dauer* phenoptype. Daf genes include the homologs of the insulin/IGF-1 receptor, PI-3 kinase, PDK-1, and Akt/PKB isoform genes in mammals, as well as Daf-16 that encodes a transcription factor with homology to the mammalian forkhead family of transcription factors. Forkhead transcription factors were first identified as being involved in the forkhead mutation in *Drosophila*, and the subclass of mammalian forkhead proteins with greatest homology to Daf-16 was first identified in alveolar rhabdomyosarcoma; this latter subclass is referred to as forkhead in human rhabdomyosarcoma (FKHR). The FKHR family is composed of three expressed genes, *FKHR* or *Foxo1*, *FKHRL1* or *Foxo3*, and *AFX* or *Foxo4* [162]. *Foxo1* is the most highly expressed FKHR isoform in insulin-responsive tissues such as liver, adipose tissue, and pancreatic β-cells.

In nematodes and in mammals, the FKHR proteins represent an important signal transduction pathway by which insulin receptors modulate gene expression. Insulin stimulation results in PI-3-kinase-dependent phosphorylation of FKHR transcription factors by Akt/PKB at three different phosphorylation sites (Thr 24, Ser 253, and Ser 316 in Foxo1) [163]. Under basal conditions, FKHR proteins reside within the nucleus, but, upon phosphorylation, dissociate from their DNA-binding site, and are then excluded from the nucleus and retained in the cytosol. Replacement of Thr 24 or Ser 253 by alanine results in loss of phosphorylation by Akt/PKB, lack of *Foxo1* nuclear export, and failure of insulin-mediated promoter suppression [164]. The relocation of FKHR out of the nucleus represents an effective mechanism for insulin in the suppression of transcriptional activity. For example, FKHR proteins bind to *cis* elements in the promoters of the PEPCK, glucose-6-phosphatase, and IGFBP-1 genes and augment transcriptional activity. Transactivation by FKHR is prevented when cells are stimulated by insulin [164–166]. The effects on PEPCK and glucose-6-phosphatase genes have led some investigators to the conclusion that FKRH could help coordinate the overall suppression of gluconeogenesis and hepatic glucose production by insulin. However, FKHR proteins are not involved in the regulation of all genes that are suppressed by insulin. Furthermore, even in the case of PEPCK and glucose-6-phosphatase, FKHR cannot by itself account for all of transcriptional inhibition under physiological conditions. FKHR can clearly mediate transactivation and insulin suppression of glucose-6-phosphatase and PEPCK when FKHR is overexpressed in cells; however, at physiological levels, FKHR may not be essential for gene regulation, suggesting that other transcription factors predominate in the regulation of these two genes [166, 167].

Another transcription factor, peroxisome proliferative activated receptor γ coactivator 1 (PGC-1), was first identified as a factor involved in brown fat adipogenesis [168]. PGC-1 also plays a important role in the regulated expression of gluconeogenic enzymes, even at physiological concentrations within hepatocytes [169, 170]. In addition, PGC-1 is induced in the liver by glucagon and glucocorticoids in the context of fasting, insulin deficiency, and diabetes, and then participates in the induction of the gluconeogenic program. However, in regulating hepatic gluconeogensis, PGC-1 may physically interact with *Foxo1* and function as its coactivator [171]. In this role, *Foxo1* function appears to be necessary for full induction of gluconeogenic genes by PGC-1 in hepatic cells and mouse liver. Several observations indicate that insulin may suppress gluconeogenic genes by interfering with the interaction between PGC-1 and *Foxo1*. For example, Akt/PKB is able to phosphorylate Foxo1, and this prevents the binding and coactivation by PGC-1. Also, insulin is able to suppress the induction of gluconeogenic genes by PGC-1 but not in the presence of a constitutively active Foxo1 mutant that is insensitive to insulin [171]. These studies indicate that a physiological role for Foxo1 in regulating gluconeogenic gene expression may only become evident when this is examined in the context of coactivation by PGC-1.

FKHR may also play other import roles in the biology of insulin-responsive cells. Foxo1 is involved in the stimulation of pancreatic β-cell proliferation and regulation of Pdx-1 expression by insulin [172]. *Foxo*1 also appears to contribute to the complex coordination of transcriptional events involved in adipocyte differentiation. Expression of a constitutively active Foxo1 mutant prevents differentiation of pre-adipocytes, and *Foxo1* haploinsufficiency in mice protects from diet-induced glucose intolerance and hyperinsulinemia [173].

Sterol Response Element Binding Protein-1c

Another exciting development pertains to the role of Sterol response element binding protein 1c (SREBP-1c) in insulin-regulated gene expression. The sterol response element binding protein (SREBP) family of transcription factors is classically viewed as being involved in the regulation of genes in response to the cellular availability of cholesterol [174]. This family includes SREBP-1a and SREBP-1c, which are encoded by a single gene and differ only in their first exon through use of alternative transcription start sites, and the homologous SREBP-2 encoded by a second gene [175]. Evidence has accumulated that SREBP-1c is regulated primarily by insulin rather than cholesterol availability, and is also involved in adipocyte differentiation, which explains the factor's alternative designation as adipocyte determination and differentiation factor 1 (ADD-1) [176]. SREBP-1c/ADD-1 is most highly expressed in liver, white adipose tissue, muscle, adrenal gland, and brain.

SREBPs contain an NH2-terminal domain consisting of a basic helix-loop-helix leucine zipper transcription factor, a central domain comprised of two transmembrane-spanning regions, and a COOH-terminal regulatory domain. In this form, SREBPs are associated with membranes in the endoplasmic reticulum. When membrane cholesterol concentrations are decreased, SREBP-1a and SREBP-2 undergo two sequential proteolytic cleavages, releasing the transcriptional domain, and allowing for its translocation into the nucleus [177]. These transcription factors then bind sterol responsive elements (SREs) in specific gene promoters and induce genes involved in cholesterol biosynthesis (i.e., HMG-CoA reductase, HMG-CoA synthase) and the LDL receptor, resulting in the cellular replenishment of cholesterol. Primarily regulation of SREBP-1c by insulin was first manifested in livers of fasted rodents re-fed with a high carbohydrate diet [178–180]. Subsequently, insulin was demonstrated to stimulate the expression and transcription of SREBP-1c in cell lines and in adipose, liver, and muscle tissues. This insulin effect is mediated through IRS-1 and PI-3 kinase, and possibly Akt/PKB [181], although downstream targets and transcription factors mediating induction of SREBP-1c gene transcription have not been elucidated. Regardless, SREBP-1c appears to play an important role in the regulation of specific genes in response to insulin. In experiments involving overexpression of wild type, constitutively active, and dominant interfering mutants, SREBP-1c has been shown to be involved in the induction of fatty acid synthase and leptin in adipose cells, and glucokinase, pyruvate kinase, fatty acid synthase, and acetyl-CoA carboxylase in the liver [182]. Thus, SREBP-1c mediates a positive transcriptional effect on genes promoting glycolysis and lipogenesis, and seems to prepare the liver for carbohydrate availability following a meal. While containing SREs in their promoter regions, the above-mentioned genes are regulated by multiple hormones as well as metabolic substrates, and the relative contribution of SREBP-1c in overall transactivation by insulin has not been defined. It is also not clear how insulin causes proteolytic cleavage of the transcriptional domain so that it can be free to translocate to the nucleus, although evidence suggest that, in the case of SREBP-1c, this could be a constitutive nonregulated process.

Signal Transducer and Activator of Transcription 5B

As discussed above in relationship to SOCS-3, the insulin receptor directly activates the STAT-5B transcription factor via tyrosine phosphorylation [31]. STAT-5B binds phosphotyrosine 972 of the insulin receptor, which is the same juxtamembrane phosphotyrosine involved in IRS binding via their PTB domains. Binding of STAT-5B is the result of a SH-2 domain interaction as opposed to the NPXpY-consensus sequence characterizing PTB domain interactions. Direct tyrosine phosphorylation of STAT-5B by the insulin receptor kinase allows for dimerization through SH-2 domain interactions and translocation into the nucleus [183, 184]. This is in contrast to the general mechanism of Stat factor activation by cytokine receptors, which employs JaK kinase as the activating kinase. Insulin activation of STAT-5B has only recently been described, and the complement of genes regulated through this mechanism has not been extensively studied. However, both glucokinase and SOCS-3 genes have STAT-5 binding sites in their promoter regions, and transcriptional activity is stimulated by insulin via STAT-5B [31, 184].

Acknowledgments

The work was supported by research grants from the National Institutes of Health (DK-38765, P01 HL-55782), the American Diabetes Association, and the Merit Review program of the Department of Veterans Affairs.

REFERENCES

1. Avruch J. Insulin signal transduction through protein kinase cascades. *Mol Cell Biochem* 1998; 182: 31–48.
2. Reaven GM. Pathophysiology of insulin resistance in human disease. *Physiol Rev* 1995; 75: 473–86.
3. Jacobs S, Cuatrecasas P. Insulin receptor. Structure and function. *Endocrinol Rev* 1981; 2: 251–63.
4. Zhang B, Roth RA. Binding properties of chimeric insulin receptors containing the cysteine-rich domain of either the insulin-like growth factor 1 receptor or the insulin receptor related receptor. *Biochemistry* 1991; 30: 5113–7.
5. Kasuga M, Karlsson FA, Kahn CR. Insulin stimulates the phosphorylation of the 95,000-dalton subunit of its own receptor. *Science* 1982; 215: 185–7.
6. Roth RA, Cassell MP. Insulin receptor. Evidence that it is a protein kinase. *Science* 1983; 219: 299–301.
7. Frattali AL, Treadway JL, Pessin JE. Transmembrane signaling by the human insulin receptor kinase. Relationship between intramolecular beta subunit trans- and cis autophosphorylation and substrate kinase activation. *J Biol Chem* 1992; 267: 19521–8.
8. Rosen OM. Structure and function of insulin receptors. *Diabetes* 1989; 38: 1508–11.
9. Cheatham B, Kahn CR. Insulin action and the insulin signaling network. *Endocrinol Rev* 1995; 16: 117–42.
10. Danielson AG, Liu F, Hosomi Y, Shii K, Roth RA. Activation of protein kinase C alpha inhibits signaling by members of the insulin receptor family. *J Biol Chem* 1995; 270: 21600–5.
11. Ullrich A, Bell JR, Chen EY, Herrera R, Petruzzelli LM, Dull TJ, Gray A, Coussens L, Liao YC, Tsubokawa M, Mason A, Seeburg PH, Grunfeld C, Rosen OM, Ramachandran J. Human insulin receptor and its relationship to the tyrosine kinase family of oncogenes. *Nature* 1985; 313: 756–61.
12. Frasca F, Pandini G, Scalia P, Sciacca L, Mineo R, Constantino A, Goldfine ID, Belfiore A, Vigneri R. Insulin receptor isoform A, a newly recognized, high-affinity insulin-like growth factor receptor II receptor in fetal and cancer cells. *Mol Cell Biol* 1999; 19: 3278–88.

13. Savkur RS, Philips AV, Cooper TA. Aberrant regulation of insulin receptor alternative splicing is associated with insulin resistance in myotonic dystrophy. *Nature Genet* 2001; 29: 40–7.
14. Taylor SI, Wertheimer E, Hone J, Levy-Toledano R, Quon MJ, Barbetti F, Suzuki Y, Roach P, Koller E, Haft CR, de la Luz M, Cama A, Accili D. Mutations in the insulin receptor gene in patients with genetic syndromes of extreme insulin resistance. In Draznin B, LeRoith D (eds), *Molecular Biology of Diabetes Vol* 2. Philadelphia: Humana Press; 1994: 1–23.
15. Kahn CR, Flier JS, Bar RS, Archer JA, Gorden P, Martin MM, Roth J. The syndromes of insulin resistance and acanthosis nigricans: insulin receptor disorders in man. *N Engl J Med* 1976; 294: 739–45.
16. O'Rahilly S, Moller DE. Mutant insulin receptors in syndromes of insulin resistance. *Clin Endocrinol* 1992; 36: 121–32.
17. Pawson T, Scott JD. Signaling through scaffold, anchoring, and adaptor proteins. *Science* 1997; 278: 2975–80.
18. White MF. IRS proteins and the common path to diabetes. *Am J Physiol* 2002; 283: E413–22.
19. Virkamaki A, Ueki K, Kahn CR. Protein-protein interaction in insulin signaling and the molecular mechanism of insulin resistance. *J Clin Invest* 1999; 103: 931–43.
20. Sun XJ, Rothenberg P, Kahn CR, Backer JM, Araki E, Wilden PA, Cahill DA, Goldstein BJ, White MF. The structure of the insulin receptor substrate IRS-1 defines a unique signal transduction protein. *Nature* 1991; 352: 73–7.
21. Sun XJ, Wang LM, Zhang Y, Yenush L, Myers MG, Glasheen E, Lane WS, Pierce JH, White MF. Role of IRS-2 in insulin and cytokine signaling. *Nature* 1995; 377: 173–7.
22. Lavan BE, Lane WS, Lienhard GE. The 60-kDa phosphotyrosine protein in insulin-treated adipocytes is a new member of the insulin receptor substrate family. *J Biol Chem* 1997; 272: 11439–43.
23. Lavan BE, Fantin VR, Chang ET, Lane WS, Keller SR, Lienhard GE. A novel 160-kDa phosphotyrosine protein in insulin-treated embyronic kidney cells is a new member of the insulin receptor substrate family. *J Biol Chem* 1997; 272: 21403–7.
24. Pelicci G, Lanfrancone L, Grignani F, McGlade J, Cavallo F, Forni G, Nicoletti I, Grignani F, Pawson T, Pelicci PG. A novel transforming protein (SHC) with an SH2 domain is implicated in mitogenic signal transduction. *Cell* 1992; 70: 93–104.
25. Holgado-Madruga M, Emlet DR, Moscatello DK, Goodwin AK, Wong AJ. AGrb-2 associated docking protein in EGF- and insulin-receptor signaling. *Nature* 1996; 379: 560–3.
26. Fujioka Y, Matozaki T, Noguchi T, Iwamatsu A, Yamao T, Takahashi N, Tsuda M, Takada T, Kasuga M. A novel membrane glycoprotein, SHPS-1, that binds the SH2-domain-containing protein tyrosine phosphatase SHP-2 in response to mitogens and cell adhesion. *Mol Cell Biol* 1996; 16: 6887–99.
27. Kharitonenkov A, Chen Z, Sures I, Wang H, Schilling J, Ullrich A. A family of proteins that inhibit signaling through tyrosine kinase receptors. *Nature* 1997; 386: 181–6.
28. Ribon V, Saltiel AR. Insulin stimulates tyrosine phosphorylation of the proto-oncogene product of c-Cbl in 3T3-L1 adipocytes. *Biochem J* 1997; 324: 839–45.
29. Baumann CA, Ribon V, Kanzaki M, Thurmond DC, Mora S, Shigematsu S, Bickel PE, Pessin JE, Saltiel AR. CAP defines a second signaling pathway required for insulin-stimulated glucose transport. *Nature* 2000; 407: 202–7.
30. Moodie SA, Alleman-Sposeto J, Gustafson TA. Identification of the APS protein as a novel insulin receptor substrate. *J Biol Chem* 1999; 274: 11186–93.
31. Van Obberghen E, Baron V, Delahaye L, Emanuelli B, Filippa N, Giogetti-Peraldi S, Lebrun P, Mothe-Satney I, Peraldi P, Rocchi S, Sawka-Verhelle D, Tartare-Deckert S, Giudicelli J. Surfing the insulin signaling web. *Eur J Clin Invest* 2001; 31: 966–77.
32. Carpino N, Wisniewski D, Strife A, Marshak D, Kobayashi R, Stillman B, Clarkson B. p62dok: a constitutively tyrosine-phosphorylated, GAP-associated protein in chronic myelogenous leukemia progenitor cells. *Cell* 1997; 88: 197–204.
33. Cai D, Dhe-Paganon S, Melendez PA, Lee J, Shoelson SE. Two new substrates in insulin signaling, IRS5/DOK4 and IRS6/DOK5 *J Biol Chem* 2003; 278: 25323–30.
34. Collett MS, Erikson RL. Protein kinase activity associated with the avian sarcoma virus src gene product. *Proc Natl Acad Sci USA* 1978; 75: 2021–4.
35. Tamemoto H, Kadowaki T, Tobe K, Yagi T, Sakura H, Hayakawa T, Terauchi Y, Ueki K, Kaburagi Y, Satoh S, Sekihara H, Yoshioka S, Horikoshi H, Furuta Y, Ikawa Y, Kasuga M, Yazaki Y, Aizawa S. Insulin resistance and growth retardation in mice lacking insulin receptor substrate-1. *Nature* 1994; 372: 182–6.
36. Araki E, Lipes MA, Patti ME, Bruning JC, Haag B, Johnson RS, Kahn CR. Alternative pathway of insulin signaling in mice with targeted disruption of the IRS-1 gene. *Nature* 1994; 372: 186–90.
37. Withers DJ, Gutierrez JS, Towery H, Burks DJ, Ren JM, Pervis S, Zhang Y, Bernal D, Pons S, Shulman GI, Bonner-Weir S, White MF. Disruption of IRS-2 causes type 2 diabetes in mice. *Nature* 1998; 391: 900–4.
38. Sawka-Verhelle D, Tartare-Deckert S, White MF, Van Obberghen E. Insulin receptor substrate-2 binds to the insulin receptor through its phosphotyrosine-binding domain and through a newly identified domain comprising amino acids 591-786. *J Biol Chem* 1996; 271: 5980–3.
39. Sawka-Verhelle D, Baron V, Mothe I, Filloux C, White MF, Van Obberghen E. Tyr624 and Tyr628 in insulin receptor substrate-2 mediate its association with the insulin receptor. *J Biol Chem* 1997; 272: 16414–20.
40. Egan SE, Weinberg RA. The pathway to signal achievement. *Nature* 1993; 365: 781–3.
41. Boulton TG, Hye SH, Robbins DJ, Ip NY, Radziejewska E, Morgenbesser SD, DePinho RA, Panayotatos N, Cobb MH, Yancopoulos GD. ERKs: a family of protein-serine/threonine kinases that are activated and tyrosine phosphorylated in response to insulin and NGF. *Cell* 1991; 65: 663–75.
42. Hausdorff SF, Frangioni JV, Birnbaum MJ. Role of p21ras in insulin-stimulated glucose transport in 3T3-L1 adipocytes. *J Biol Chem* 1994; 269: 21391–4.
43. Lazar DF, Wiese RJ, Brady MJ, Mastick CC, Waters SB, Yamauchi K, Pessin JE, Cuatracasas P, Saltiel AR. Mitogen-activated protein kinase kinase inhibition does not block the stimulation of glucose utilization by insulin. *J Biol Chem* 1995; 270: 20801–7.
44. Fruman DA, Meyers RE, Cantley LC. Phosphoinositide kinases. *Annu Rev Biochem* 1998; 67: 481–507.
45. Backer JM, Myers MG, Shoelson SE, Chin DJ, Sun XJ, Miralpeix M, Hu P, Margolis B, Skolnik EY,

Schlessinger J, White MF. Phosphatidylinositol 3′-kinase is activated by association with IRS during insulin stimulation. *EMBO J* 1992; 11: 3469–79.
46. Cheatham B, Kahn CR. Insulin action and the insulin signaling network. *Endocrinol Rev* 1995; 16: 117–42.
47. Khan AH, Pessin JE. Insulin regulation of glucose uptake: a complex interplay of intracellular signaling pathways. *Diabetologia* 2002; 45: 1475–83.
48. Rameh LE, Cantley LC. The role of phosphoinositide 3 kinase lipid products in cell function. *J Biol Chem* 1999; 274: 8347–50.
49. Cantley LC. The phosphoinositide 3-kinase pathway. *Science* 2002; 296: 1655–7.
50. Stralfors P. Insulin second messengers. *Bioessays* 1997; 19: 327–35.
51. Bellacosa A, Testa JR, Staal SP, Tsichlis P. A retroviral oncogene, akt, encoding a serine-threonine kinase containing an SH2-like region. *Science* 1991; 254: 274–7.
52. Bellacosa A, Chan TO, Ahmed NN, Datta K, Malstrom S, Stokoe D, McCormick F, Feng J, Tsichlis P. Akt activation by growth factors is a multiple-step process: the role of the PH domain. *Oncogene* 1998; 17: 313–25.
53. Kohn AD, Takeuchi F, Roth RA. Akt, a pleckstrin homology containing kinase, is activated primarily by phosphorylation. *J Biol Chem* 1996; 271: 21920–6.
54. Summers SA, Yin VP, Whiteman EL, Garza LA, Cho H, Tuttle RL, Birnbaum MJ. Signaling pathways mediating insulin-stimulated glucose transport. *Ann NY Acad Sci* 1999; 892: 169–86.
55. Kohn AD, Summers SA, Birnbaum MJ, Roth RA. Expression of a constitutively active akt ser/thr kinase in 3T3-L1 adipocytes stimulates glucose uptake and glucose transporter 4 translocation. *J Biol Chem* 1996; 271: 31372–8.
56. Calera MR, Martinez C, Liu H, Jack AK, Birnbaum MJ, Pilch PF. Insulin increases the association of akt-2 with Glut4-containing vesicles. *J Biol Chem* 1998; 273: 7201–4.
57. Kitamura T, Ogawa W, Sakaue H, Hino Y, Kuroda S, Takata M, Matsumoto M, Maeda T, Konishi H, KIKKawa U, Kasuga M. Requirement for activation of the serine–threonine kinase Akt (protein kinase B) in insulin stimulation of protein synthesis but not of glucose transport. *Mol Cell Biol* 1998; 18: 3708–17.
58. Kim YB, Nikoulina SE, Ciaraldi TP, Henry RR, Kahn BB. Normal insulin-dependent activation of Akt/protein kinase B, with diminished activity of phosphoinositide 3-kinase, in muscle in type 2 diabetes. *J Clin Invest* 1999; 104: 733–41.
59. Cho H, Mu J, Kim JK, Thorvaldsen JL, Chu Q, Crenshaw EB III, Kaestner KH, Bartolomei MS, Shulman GI, Birnbaum MJ. Insulin resistance and a diabetes mellitus-like syndrome in mice lacking the protein kinase Akt2 (PKBβ). *Science* 2001; 292: 1728–31.
60. Whiteman EL, Cho H, Birnbaum MJ. Role of Akt/protein kinase B in metabolism. *Trends Endocrinol Metab* 2002; 13: 444–51.
61. Cross DA, Alessi DR, Cohen P, Andjelkovitch M, Hemmings BA. Inhibition of glycogen synthase 3 by insulin mediated by protein kinase B. *Nature* 1995; 378: 785–9.
62. Summers SA, Kao AW, Kohn AD, Backus GS, Roth RA, Pessin JE, Birnbaum MJ. The role of glycogen synthase 3β in insulin-stimulated glucose metabolism. *J Biol Chem* 1999; 274: 17934–40.
63. Scott PH, Brunn GJ, Kohn AD, Roth RA, Lawrence JC. Evidence of insulin-stimulated phosphorylation and activation of the mammalian target of rapamycin mediated by a protein kinase B signaling pathway. *Proc Natl Acad Sci USA* 1998; 95: 7772–7.
64. Gingras AC, Raught B, Sonenberg N. Regulation of translation initiation by FRAP/mTOR. *Genes Dev* 2001; 15: 807–26.
65. Fulton D, Gratton JP, McCabe TJ, Fontana J, Fujio Y, Walsh K, Franke TF, Papapetropoulos A, Sessa WC. Regulation of endothelium-derived nitric oxide production by the protein kinase Akt. *Nature* 1999; 399: 597–601. [Erratum in. *Nature* 1999; 400: 792]
66. Datta SR, Brunet A, Greenberg ME. Cellular survival: a play in three Akts. *Genes Dev* 1999; 13: 2905–27.
67. Nakae J, Park B-C, Accili D. Insulin stimulates phosphorylation of the forkhead transcription factor FKHR on serine 253 through a wortmannin-sensitive pathway. *J Biol Chem* 1999; 274: 15982–5.
68. Biggs WH, Meisenhelder J, Hunter T, Cavenee WK, Arden KC. Protein kinase B/Akt-mediated phosphorylation promotes nuclear exclusion of the winged helix transcription factor FKHR1 *Proc Natl Acad Sci USA* 1999; 96: 7421–6.
69. Standaert ML, Galloway L, Karnam P, Bandyopadhyay G, Moscat J, Farese RV. Protein kinase C-zeta as a downstream effector of phosphatidylinositol 3-kinase during insulin stimulation in rat adipocytes: potential role in glucose transport. *J Biol Chem* 1997; 272: 30075–82.
70. Kotani K, Ogawa W, Matsumoto M, Kitamura T, Sakaue H, Hino Y, Miyake K, Sano W, Akimoto K, Ohno S, Kasuga M. Requirement of atypical protein kinase C lambda for insulin stimulation of glucose uptake but not for akt activation in 3T3-L1 adipocytes. *Mol Cell Biol* 1998; 18: 6971–82.
71. Farese RV. Function and dysfunction of aPKC isoforms for glucose transport in insulin-sensitive and insulin-resistant states. *Am J Physiol* 2002; 283: E1–11
72. Tsuru M, Katagiri H, Asano T, Yamada T, Ohno S, Ogihara T, Oka Y. Role of PKC isoforms in glucose transport in 3T3-L1 adipocytes: insignificance of atypical PKC. *Am J Physiol* 2002; 283: E338–45.
73. Mendez R, Kollmorgen G, White MF, Rhoads RE. Requirement of protein kinase C zeta for stimulation of protein synthesis by insulin. *Mol Cell Biol* 1997; 17: 5184–92.
74. Isakoff SJ, Taha C, Rose E, Marcusohn J, Klip A, Skolnik EY. The inability of phosphatidylinositol 3-kinase activation to stimulate GLUT-4 translocation indicates additional signaling pathways are required for insulin-stimulated glucose uptake. *Proc Natl Acad Sci USA* 1995; 92: 10247–51.
75. Guilherme A, Czech MP. Stimulation of IRS-1-associated phosphatidylinositol 3-kinase and Akt/protein kinase B but not glucose transport by beta1-integrin signaling in rat adipocytes. *J Biol Chem* 1998; 273: 33119–22.
76. Watson RT, Pessin JE. Intracellular organization of insulin signaling and GLUT-4 translocation. *Recent Prog Horm Res* 2001; 56: 175–93.
77. Saltiel AR, Pessin JE. Insulin signaling pathways in time and space. *Trends Cell Biol* 2002; 12: 65–71.
78. Krook A, Whitehead JP, Dobson SP, Griffiths MR, Ouwens M, Baker C, Hayward AC, Sen SK, Maassen JA,

Siddle K, Tavare JM, O'Rahilly S. Two naturally occurring insulin receptor tyrosine kinase domain mutants provide evidence that phosphoinositide 3-kinase activation alone is not sufficient for the mediation of insulin's metabolic and mitogenic effects. *J Biol Chem* 1997; 272: 30208–14.
79. Jiang T, Sweeney G, Rudolf MT, Klip A, Traynor-Kaplan A, Tsien RY. Membrane-permeant esters of phosphatidylinositol 3,4,5-trisphosphate. *J Biol Chem* 1998; 273: 11017–24.
80. Liu J, Kimura A, Baumann C, Saltiel A. APS facilitates c-Cbl tyrosine phosphorylation and GLUT-4 translocation in response to insulin in 3T3-L1 adipocytes. *Mol Cell Biol* 2002; 11: 3599–609.
81. Ribon V, Saltiel A. A novel, multifunctional c-Cbl binding protein in insulin receptor signaling in 3T3-L1 adipocytes. *Mol Cell Biol* 1998; 18: 872–9.
82. Bickel PE. Lipid rafts and insulin signaling. *Am J Physiol* 2002; 282: E1–10.
83. Chiang SH, Baumann CA, Kanzaki M, Thurmond DC, Watson RT, Neudauer CL, Macara IG, Pessin JE, Saltiel AR. Insulin-stimulated GLUT-4 translocation requires the CAP-dependent activation of TC10. *Nature* 2001; 410: 944–8.
84. Chiang S, Hou J, Hwang J, Pessin J, Saltiel A. Cloning and functional characterization of related TC10 isoforms, a subfamily of Rho proteins involved in insulin-stimulated glucose transport. *J Biol Chem* 2002; 277: 13067–73.
85. Chang L, Adams RD, Saltiel AR. The TC10-interacting protein CIP4/2 is required for insulin-stimulated Glut4 translocation in 3T3L1 adipocytes. *Proc Natl Acad Sci USA* 2002; 99: 12835–40.
86. Kanzaki M, Watson RT, Hou JC, Stamnes M, Saltiel AR, Pessin JE. Small GTP-binding protein TC10 differentially regulates two distinct populations of filamentous actin in 3T3L1 adipocytes. *Mol Biol Cell* 2002; 13: 2334–46.
87. Baumann CA, Ribon V, Kanzaki M, Thurmond DC, Mora S, Shigematsu S, Bickel PE, Pessin JE, Saltiel AR. CAP defines a second signalling pathway required for insulin-stimulated glucose transport. *Nature* 2000; 407: 202–7.
88. Kimura A, Baumann C, Chiang S, Saltiel A. The sorbin homology domain: a motif for the targeting of proteins to lipid rafts. *Proc Natl Acad Sci USA* 2001; 98: 9098–103.
89. Chiang SH, Baumann CA, Kanzaki M, Thurmond DC, Watson RT, Neudauer CL, Macara IG, Pessin JE, Saltiel AR. Insulin-stimulated GLUT-4 translocation requires the CAP-dependent activation of TC10. *Nature* 2001; 410: 944–8.
90. Gustavsson J, Parpal S, Stralfors P, Insulin-stimulated glucose uptake involves the transition of glucose transporters to a caveolin-rich fraction within the plasma membrane: implications for type II diabetes. *Mol Med* 1996; 2: 367–72.
91. Watson RT, Shigematsu S, Chiang SH, Mora S, Kanzaki M, Macara IG, Saltiel AR, Pessin JE. Lipid raft microdomain compartmentalization of TC10 is required for insulin signaling and GLUT-4 translocation. *J Cell Biol* 2001; 154: 829–40.
92. Hayashi T, Wojtaszewski JF, Goodyear LJ. Exercise regulation of glucose transport in skeletal muscle. *Am J Physiol* 1997; 273: E1039–51.
93. Goodyear LJ, AMP-activated protein kinase: a critical signaling intermediary for exercise-stimulated glucose transport. *Exerc Sport Sci Rev* 2000; 28: 113–6.
94. Merrill GF, Kurth EJ, Hardie DG, Winder WW. AICA riboside increases AMP-activated protein kinase, fatty acid oxidation, and glucose uptake in rat muscle. *Am J Physiol* 1997; 273: E1107–12.
95. Mu J, Brozinick JT Jr, Valladares O, Bucan M, Birnbaum MJ. A role for AMP-activated protein kinase in contraction- and hypoxia-regulated glucose transport in skeletal muscle. *Mol Cell* 2001; 7: 1085–94.
96. Hardie DG, Carling D, Carlson M. The AMP-activated/SNF1 protein kinase subfamily: metabolic sensors of the eukaryotic cell. *Annu Rev Biochem* 1998; 67: 821–55.
97. Garvey WT, Birnbaum MJ. Cellular insulin action and insulin resistance. *Baillieres Clin Endocrinol Metab* 1993; 7: 785–873.
98. Joost HG, Bell GI, Best JD, Birnbaum MJ, Charron MJ, Chen YT, Doege H, James DE, Lodish HF, Moley KH, Moley JF, Mueckler M, Rogers S, Schurmann A, Seino S, Thorens B. Nomenclature of GLUT/SLC2A family of sugar/polyol transport facilitators. *Am J Physiol* 2002; 282: E974–6.
99. Rea S, James DE. Moving GLUT4: the biogenesis and trafficking of GLUT4 storage vesicles. *Diabetes* 1997; 46: 1667–77.
100. Mora S, Pessin JE. An adipocentric view of signaling and intracellular trafficking. *Diabetes/Metab Res Rev* 2002; 18: 345–56.
101. Bao S, Smith RM, Jarett L, Garvey WT. The effects of brefeldin A on the glucose transport system in rat adipocytes: implications regarding the intracellular locus on insulin sensitive GLUT4. *J Biol Chem* 1995; 270: 30199–204.
102. Kandror KV, Pilch PF. Compartmentalization of protein traffic in insulin-sensitive cells. *Am J Physiol* 1996; 271: E1–14.
103. Rice JE, Livingstone C, Gould GW. Trafficking, targeting and translocation of the insulin-responsive glucose transporter, GLUT4, in adipocytes. *Biochem Soc Trans* 1996; 24: 540–6.
104. Holman GD, Kasuga M. From receptor to transporter: insulin signalling to glucose transport. *Diabetologia* 1997; 40: 910–1003.
105. Malide D, Dwer NK, Blanchette-Mackie EJ, Cushman SW. Immunocytochemical evidence that GLUT4 resides in a specialized translocation post-endosomal VAMP-2 positive compartment in rat adipose cells in the absence of insulin. *J Histochem Cytochem* 1997; 45: 1083–96.
106. Aledo JC, Lavoie L, Volchuk A, Keller SR, Klip A, Hundal HS. Identification and characterization of two distinct intracellular GLUT4 pools in rat skeletal muscle. Evidence for an endosomal and an insulin-sensitive GLUT4 compartment. *Biochem J* 1997; 325: 727–32.
107. Watson RT, Pessin JE. Subcellular compartmentalization and trafficking of the insulin-responsive glucose transporter, GLUT4. *Exp Cell Res* 2001; 271: 75–83.
108. Shewan AM, Marsh BJ, Melvin DR, Martin S, Gould GW, James DE. The cytosolic C-terminus of the glucose transporter GLUT4 contains an acidic cluster endosomal targeting motif distal to the dileucine signal. *Biochem J* 2000; 350: 99–107.
109. Lee W, Jung CY. A synthetic peptide corresponding to the GLUT4 C-terminal cytoplasmic domain causes insulin-like glucose transport stimulation and GLUT4 recruitment in rat adipocytes. *J Biol Chem* 1997; 272: 21572–31.

110. Kandror KV, Pilch PF. gp160, a tissue specific marker for insulin-activated glucose transport. *Proc Natl Acad Sci USA* 1994; 91: 8017–21.
111. Sollner TH, Rothman JE. Molecular machinery mediating vesicle budding, docking, and fusion. *Cell Struct Funct* 1996; 21: 407–12.
112. Pevsner J, Hsu S-C, Braun JE, Calakos N, Ting AE, Bennett MK, Scheller RH. Specificity and regulation of a synaptic vesicle docking complex. *Neuron* 1994; 13: 353–61.
113. Novick P, Zerial M. The diversity of rab proteins in vesicle transport. *Curr Opin Cell Biol* 1997; 9: 496–504.
114. Seabra M, Mules E, Hume A. Rab GTPases, intracellular traffic and disease. *Trends Mol Med* 2002; 8: 23–30.
115. Cormont M, Bortoluzzi MN, Gautier N, Mari M, Van Obberghen E, Le Marchand-Brustel Y. Potential role of Rab4 in the regulation of subcellular localization of Glut4 in adipocytes. *Mol Cell Biol* 1996; 16: 6879–86.
116. Shibata H, Omata W, Suzuki Y, Tanaka S, Kojima I. A synthetic peptide corresponding to the Rab4 hypervariable carboxyl-terminal domain inhibits insulin action on glucose transport in rat adipocytes. *J Biol Chem* 1996; 271: 9704–9.
117. Wang Q, Bilan PJ, Tsakiridis T, Hinek A, Klip A. Actin filaments participate in the relocation of phosphatidylinositol 3-kinase to glucose transporter-containing compartments and in the stimulation of glucose uptake in 3T3-L1 adipocytes. *Biochem J* 1998; 331: 917–28.
118. Kanzaki M, Pessin JE. Insulin-stimulated GLUT4 translocation in adipocytes is dependent upon cortical actin remodeling. *J Biol Chem* 2001; 276: 42436–44.
119. Jiang ZY, Chawla A, Bose A, Way M, Czech MP. A phosphatidylinositol 3-kinase-independent insulin signaling pathway to N-WASP/Arp2/3/F-actin required for GLUT4 glucose transporter recycling. *J Biol Chem* 2002; 277: 509–15.
120. Murphy GA, Solski PA, Jillian SA, Perez de la Ossa P, D'Eustachio P, Der CJ, Rush MG. Cellular functions of TC10, a Rho-family GTPase: regulation of morphology, signal transduction, and cell growth. *Oncogene* 1999; 18: 3831–45.
121. Semiz S, Park JG, Nicoloro SM, Furcinitti P, Zhang C, Chawla A, Leszyk J, Czech MP. Conventional kinesin KIF5B mediates insulin-stimulated GLUT4 movements on microtubules. *EMBO J* 2003; 22: 2387–99.
122. Olson A, Trumbly A, Gibson G. Insulin-mediated GLUT4 translocation is dependent on the microtubular network. *J Biol Chem* 2001; 276: 10706–14.
123. Huang J, Imamura T, Olefsky J. Insulin can regulate GLUT4 internalization by signaling to Rab5 and the motor protein dynein. *Proc Natl Acad Sci USA* 2001; 98: 1 3084–9.
124. Hunter S, Garvey WT. Insulin action and insulin resistance: diseases involving defects in insulin receptors, signal transduction, and the glucose transport effector system. *Am J Med* 1998; 105: 331–45.
125. Garvey WT, Maianu L, Huecksteadt TP, Birnbaum MJ, Molina JM, Ciaraldi TP. Pretranslational suppression of a glucose transporter protein causes cellular insulin resistance in non-insulin-dependent diabetes mellitus and obesity. *J Clin Invest* 1991; 87: 1072–81.
126. Garvey WT, Maianu L, Hancock JA, Golichowski AM, Baron A. Gene expression of GLUT4 glucose transporters in skeletal muscle from insulin-resistant patients with obesity, impaired glucose tolerance, gestational diabetes, and non-insulin-dependent diabetes mellitus. *Diabetes* 1992; 41: 465–75.
127. Garvey WT, Maianu L, Zhu J-H, Hancock JA, Golichowski AM. Multiple defects in the adipocyte glucose transport system cause cellular insulin resistance in gestational diabetes: heterogeneity in the number and a novel abnormality in subcellular localization of GLUT4 glucose transporters. *Diabetes* 1993; 42: 1773–85.
128. Garvey WT, Maianu L, Zhu J-H, Brechtel-Hook G, Wallace P, Baron AD. Evidence for defects in the trafficking and translocation of GLUT4 glucose transporters in skeletal muscle as a cause of human insulin resistance. *J Clin Invest* 1998; 101: 2377–86.
129. Maianu L, Keller SR, Garvey WT. Adipocytes express abnormalities in translocation and trafficking of vesicles containing GLUT4 and insulin-regulated aminopeptidase in type 2 diabetes. *J Clin Endocrinol Metab* 2001; 86: 5450–6.
130. Tanti JF, Gremeaux T, Van Obberghen E, Le Marchand-Brustel Y. Serine-threonine phosphorylation of insulin receptor substrate-1 modulates insulin receptor signaling. *J Biol Chem* 1994; 269: 6051–7.
131. Mothe I, Van Obberghen E. Phosphorylation of insulin receptor substrate-1 on multiple serine residues, 612, 632, 662, and 731, modulates insulin action. *J Biol Chem* 1996; 271: 11222–7.
132. Paz K, Hemi R, LeRoith D, Karasik A, Elhanany E, Kanety H, Zick Y. A molecular basis for insulin resistance. Elevated serine/threonine phosphorylation of IRS-1 and IRS-2 inhibits their binding to the juxtamembrane region of the insulin receptor and impairs their ability to undergo insulin-induced tyrosine phosphorylation. *J Biol Chem* 1997; 272: 29911–8.
133. Liu YF, Paz K, Herschkovitz A, Alt A, Tennenbaum T, Sampson SR, Ohba M, Kuroki T, LeRoith D, Zick Y. Insulin stimulates PKC zeta-mediated phosphorylation of insulin receptor substrate-1: a self-attenuated mechanism to negatively regulate the function of IRS proteins. *J Biol Chem* 2001; 276: 14459–65.
134. Ravichandran LV, Esposito DL, Chen J, Quon MJ. Protein kinase C zeta phosphorylates insulin receptor substrate-1 and impairs its ability to activate phosphatidylinositol 3-kinase in response to insulin. *J Biol Chem* 2001; 276: 3543–9.
135. Hotamisligil GS, Spiegelman BM. Adipose expression of TNFα direct role in obesity-linked insulin resistance. *Science* 1993; 259: 87–91.
136. Saghizadeh M, Ong JM, Garvey WT, Henry RR, Kern PA. The expression of TNFα by human muscle: relationship to insulin resistance. *J Clin Invest* 1996; 97: 1111–6.
137. Hotamisligil GS, Peraldi P, Budvari A, Ellis RW, White MF, Spiegelman BM. IRS-1 mediated inhibition of insulin receptor tyrosine kinase activity in TNF-α-induced and obesity-induced insulin resistance. *Science* 1996; 271: 665–8.
138. Kanety H, Feinstein R, Papa MZ, Hemi R, Karasik A. Tumor necrosis factor alpha-induced phosphorylation of of insulin receptor substrate-1 (IRS-1): possible mechanism for suppression of insulin-stimulated tyrosine phosphorylation of IRS-1. *J Biol Chem* 1995; 270: 23780–4.
139. Peraldi P, Xu M, Spiegelman BM. Thiazolidinediones block tumor necrosis factor-alpha-induced inhibition of insulin signaling. *J Clin Invest* 1997; 100: 1863–9.
140. Aguirre V, Werner ED, Giraud J, Lee YH, Shoelson SE, White MF. Phosphorylation of ser307 in insulin receptor

substrate-1 blocks interactions with the insulin receptor and inhibits insulin action. *J Biol Chem* 2002; 277: 1531–7.

141. Peraldi P, Hotamisligil GS, Buurman WA, White MF, Spiegelman BM. Tumor necrosis factor (TNF)-α inhibits insulin signaling through stimulation of the p55 TNF receptor and activation of sphingomyelinase. *J Biol Chem* 1996; 271: 13018–22.
142. Hundal RS, Petersen KF, Mayerson AB, Randhawa PS, Inzucchi S, Shoelson SE, Shulman GI. Mechanism by which high-dose aspirin improves glucose metabolism in type 2 diabetes. *J Clin Invest* 2002; 109: 1321–6.
143. Yuan M, Konstantopoulos N, Lee J, Hansen L, Li Z-W, Karin M, Shoelson SE. Reversal of obesity- and diet-induced insulin resistance with salicylates or targeted disruption of IKKβ. *Science* 2001; 293: 1673–7.
144. Kim JK, Kim YJ, Fillmore JJ, Chen Y, Moore I, Lee J, Yuan M, Li ZW, Karin M, Perret P, Shoelson SE, Shulman GI. Prevention of fat-induced insulin resistance by salicylate. *J Clin Invest* 2001; 108: 437–46.
145. Asante-Appiah E, Kennedy BP. Protein tyrosine phosphatases: the quest for negative regulators of insulin action. *Am J Physiol* 2003; 284: E663–70.
146. Ahmad F, Azevedo J, Cortright R, Dohm GL, Goldstein BJ. Alterations in skeletal muscle protein-tyrosine phosphatase activity and expression in insulin-resistant human obesity and diabetes. *J Clin Invest* 1997; 100: 449–58.
147. Goldstein BJ, Ahmad F, Ding W, Li PM, Zhang WR. Regulation of the insulin signaling pathways by cellular protein-tyrosine phosphatases. *Mol Cell Biochem* 1998; 182: 91–9.
148. Drake PJ, Posner BI. Insulin receptor-associated protein tyrosine phosphatases: role in insulin action. *Mol Cell Biochem* 1998; 182: 79–89.
149. Elchebly M, Payette P, Michaliszyn E, Cromlish W, Collins S, Loy AL, Normandin D, Cheng A, Himms-Hagen J, Chan CC, Ramachandran C, Gresser MJ, Tremblay ML, Kennedy BP. Increased insulin sensitivity and obesity resistance in mice lacking the protein tyrosine phosphatase-1B gene. *Science* 1999; 283: 1544–8.
150. Emanuelli B, Peraldi P, Filloux C, Sawka-Verhelle D, Hilton D, Van Obberghen E, SOCS-3 is an insulin-induced negative regulator of insulin signaling. *J Biol Chem* 2000; 275: 15985–91.
151. Starr R, Willson TA, Viney EM, Murray LJ, Rayner JR, Jenkins BJ, Gonda TJ, Alexander WS, Metcalf D, Nicola NA, Hilton DJ. A family of cytokine-inducible inhibitors of signalling. *Nature* 1997; 387: 917–21.
152. Luger A, Prager R, Gaube S, Graf H, Klauser R, Schernthaner G. Decreased peripheral insulin sensitivity in acromegalic patients. *Exp Clin Endocrinol* 1990; 95: 339–43.
153. Cohen B, Novick D, Rubinstein M. Modulation of insulin activities by leptin. *Science* 1996; 274: 1185–8.
154. Goldfine ID, Maddux BA, Youngren JF, Frittitta L, Trischitta V, Dohm GL. Membrane glycoprotein PC-1 and insulin resistance. *Mol Cell Biochem* 1998; 182: 177–84.
155. Frittitta L, Spampinato D, Solini A, Nosadini R, Goldfine ID, Vigneri R, Trischitta V. Elevated PC-1 content in cultured skin fibroblasts correlates with decreased in vivo and in vitro insulin action in non-diabetic subjects: evidence that PC-1 may be an intrinsic factor in impaired insulin receptor signaling. *Diabetes* 1998; 47: 1095–100.
156. Kumakura S, Maddux BA, Sung CK. Overexpression of membrane glycoprotein PC-1 can influence insulin action at a post-receptor site. *J Cell Biochem* 1998; 3: 366–77.
157. Youngren JF, Maddux BA, Sasson S, Sbraccia P, Tapscott EB, Swanson MS, Dohm GL, Goldfine ID. Skeletal muscle content of membrane glycoprotein PC-1 in obesity: relationship to muscle glucose transport. *Diabetes* 1996; 10: 1324–8.
158. O'Brien RM, Streeper RS, Ayala JE, Stadelmaier BT, Hornbuckle LA. Insulin-regulated gene expression. *Biochem Soc Trans* 2001; 29: 552–8.
159. Lochhead PA, Coghlan M, Rice SQ, Sutherland C. Inhibition of GSK-3 selectively reduces glucose-6-phosphatase and phosphoenolpyruvate carboxykinase gene expression. *Diabetes* 2001; 50: 937–46.
160. Pearson G, Robinson F, Beers Gibson T, Xu BE, Karandikar M, Berman K, Cobb MH. Mitogen-activated protein (MAP) kinase pathways: regulation and physiological functions. *Endocrinol Rev* 2001; 22: 153–83.
161. Paradis S, Ruvkun G. *Caenorhabditis elegans*: Akt/PKB transduces insulin receptor-like signals from AGE-1 PI3 kinase to the DAF-16 transcription factor. *Genes Dev* 1998; 12: 2488–98.
162. Anderson MJ, Viars CS, Czekay S, Cavenee WK, Arden KC. Cloning and characterization of three human forkhead genes that comprise an FKHR-like gene subfamily. *Genomics* 1998; 47: 187–99.
163. Tang ED, Nunez G, Barr FG, Guan KL. Negative regulation of the forkhead transcription factor FKHR by Akt. *J Biol Chem* 1999; 274: 16741–6.
164. Nakae J, Park B-C, Accili D. Insulin stimulates phosphorylation of the forkhead transcription factor FKHR on serine 253 through a wortmannin-sensitive pathway. *J Biol Chem* 1999; 274: 15982–5.
165. Guo S, Rena G, Cichy S, He X, Cohen P, Unterman T. Phosphorylation of serine 256 by protein kinase B disrupts transactivation by FKHR and mediates effects of insulin on insulin-like growth factor-binding protein-1 promoter activity through a conserved insulin response sequence. *J Biol Chem* 1999; 274: 17184–92.
166. Hall RK, Yamasaki T, Kucera T, Waltner-Law M, O'Brien R, Granner DK. Regulation of phosphoenolpyruvate carboxykinase and insulin-like growth factor-binding protein-1 gene expression by insulin: the role of winged helix/forkhead proteins. *J Biol Chem* 2000; 275: 30169–75.
167. Yeagley D, Guo S, Unterman T, Quinn PG. Gene- and activation-specific mechanisms for insulin inhibition of basal and glucocorticoid-induced insulin-like growth factor binding protein-1 and phosphoenolpyruvate carboxykinase transcription: roles of forkhead and insulin response sequences. *J Biol Chem* 2001; 276: 33705–10.
168. Puigserver P, Wu Z, Park CW, Graves R, Wright M, Spiegelman BM. A cold-inducible coactivator of nuclear receptors linked to adaptive thermogenesis. *Cell* 1998; 92: 829–39.
169. Yoon JC, Puigserver P, Chen G, Donovan J, Wu Z, Rhee J, Adelmant G, Stafford J, Kahn CR, Granner DK, Newgard CB, Spiegelman BM. Control of hepatic gluconeogenesis through the transcriptional coactivator PGC-1 *Nature* 2001; 413: 131–8.
170. Herzig S, Long F, Jhala US, Hedrick S, Quinn R, Bauer A, Rudolph D, Schutz G, Yoon C, Puigserver P, Spiegelman B, Montminy M. CREB regulates hepatic

gluconeogenesis through the coactivator PGC-1 *Nature* 2001; 413: 179–83. [Erratum in *Nature* 2001; 413: 652]

171. Puigserver P, Rhee J, Donovan J, Walkey CJ, Yoon JC, Oriente F, Kitamura Y, Altomonte J, Dong H, Accili D, Spiegelman BM. Insulin-regulated hepatic gluconeogenesis through FOXO1-PGC-1α interaction. *Nature* 2003; 423: 550–5.
172. Kitamura T, Nakae J, Kitamura Y, Kido Y, Biggs W, Wright C, White M, Arden K, Accili D. The transcription factor Foxo1 links insulin signaling to Pdx1 regulation of pancreatic β-cell growth. *J Clin Invest* 2002; 110: 1839–47.
173. Nakae J, Kitamura T, Kitamura Y, Biggs WH, Arden KC, Accili D. The forkhead transcription factor Foxo1 regulates adipocyte differentiation. *Dev Cell* 2003; 4: 119–29.
174. Wang X, Sato R, Brown MS, Hua X, Goldstein JL. SREBP-1, a membrane-bound transcription factor released by sterol-regulated proteolysis. *Cell* 1994; 77: 53–62.
175. Hua X, Wu J, Goldstein JL, Brown MS, Hobbs HH. Structure of the human gene encoding sterol regulatory element binding protein-1 (SREBF1) and localization of SREBF1 and SREBF2 to chromosomes 17p11.2 and 22q13. *Genomics* 1995; 25: 667–73.
176. Tontonoz P, Kim JB, Graves RA, Spiegelman BM. ADD1: a novel helix-loop-helix transcription factor associated with adipocytes determination and differentiation. *Mol Cell Biol* 1993; 13: 4753–9.
177. Brown MS, Goldstein JL. A proteolytic pathway that controls the cholesterol content of membranes, cells, and blood. *Proc Natl Acad Sci USA* 1999; 96: 11041–8.
178. Horton JD, Bashmakov Y, Shimomura Y, Shimano H. Regulation of sterol regulatory element binding proteins in livers of fasted and refed mice. *Proc Natl Acad Sci USA* 1998; 95: 5987–92.
179. Kim JB, Sarraf P, Wright M, Yao K, Mueller M, Solanes G, Lowell BB, Spiegelman B. Nutritional and insulin regulation of fatty acid synthetase and leptin gene expression through ADD1/SREBP1. *J Clin Invest* 1998; 101: 1–9.
180. Foretz M, Pacot C, Dugail I, Lemarchand P, Guichard C, Le Liepvre X, Berthelier-Lubrano C, Spiegelman B, Kim JB, Ferre P, Foufelle F. ADD1/SREBP-1c is required in the activation of hepatic lipogenic gene expression by glucose. *Mol Cell Biol* 1999; 19: 3760–8.
181. Matsumoto M, Ogawa W, Teshigawara K, Inoue H, Miyake K, Sakaue H, Kasuga M. Role of the insulin receptor 1 and phosphatidylinositol 3-kinase signaling pathway in insulin-induced expression of sterol regulatory element binding protein 1c and glucokinase genes in rat hepatocytes. *Diabetes* 2002: 51: 1672–80.
182. Foufelle F, Ferre P. New perspectives in the regulation of hepatic glycolytic and lipogenic genes by insulin and glucose: a role for the transcription factor sterol regulatory element binding protein-1c. *Biochem J* 2002; 366: 377–91.
183. Sawka-Verhelle D, Filloux C, Tartare-Deckert S, Mothe I, Van Obberghen E. Identification of Stat 5B as a substrate of the insulin receptor. *Eur J Biochem* 1997; 250: 411–7.
184. Sawka-Verhelle D, Tartare-Deckert S, Decaux JF, Girard J, Van Obberghen E. Stat 5B, activated by insulin in a JaK-independent fashion, plays a role in glucokinase gene transcription. *Endocrinology* 2000; 141: 1977–88.

14

Regulation of Glucose Metabolism in the Liver

Christopher B. Newgard

Duke University Medical Center, Durham, NC, USA

INTRODUCTION AND OVERVIEW

A hallmark of type 2 diabetes is the disruption of the normal balance between glucose disposal and glucose production in liver, such that net hepatic glucose output is increased. This chapter is devoted to a discussion of fundamental mechanisms by which carbohydrate metabolism is controlled in liver. This has been the subject of intense investigation for more than a century, with key ideas advanced by pioneers such as Claude Bernard remaining central to our understanding of events. For some readers, this probably suggests that little remains to be learned in the field. However, the past decade has seen a startling emergence of new transcription factors, new regulatory proteins and allosteric factors, and new ideas about the role of spatial organization and compartmentalization in regulation of glucose metabolism in liver. Much of this new knowledge has been gained via a surge in the application of the tools of molecular biology and genetics to the field. Importantly, these fresh insights into mechanisms of control of hepatic glucose balance are beginning to suggest new targets for diabetes therapy. A review of recent developments therefore seems timely. The chapter focuses almost exclusively on regulation of carbohydrate metabolism in liver, but attempts to compare and contrast regulatory paradigms in this tissue with those in muscle or pancreatic islet β-cells where appropriate and illustrative.

In normal animals, hepatic glucose production occurs at a high rate in the fasted state. This high rate of glucose production from the liver is curtailed in the fasted to fed transition in response to the rise in blood glucose and the consequent stimulation of insulin secretion from islet β-cells. The net rate of hepatic glucose production represents the balance between pathways that contribute to formation of glucose (gluconeogenesis and glycogenolysis), and pathways that consume or store glucose (glycogen synthesis, glycolysis, and the pentose monophosphate shunt). Tight control of these opposing pathways allows remarkable maintenance of glucose homeostasis in the fed and fasted states in normal subjects. The relative activities of these opposing pathways are controlled in large measure by the ratio of the pancreatic hormones insulin and glucagon. A low insulin/glucagon ratio in the fasted state favors glycogenolysis and gluconeogenesis, while a high insulin/glucagon ratio in the fed state favors glycogen synthesis, glycolysis, and other pathways of glucose disposal.

In diabetes, insulin insufficiency and/or insulin resistance are the prevalent conditions. Under these circumstances, the liver functions in a manner analogous to the fasted state, with a preferential activation of gluconeogeneis and glycogenolysis. The severity of dysfunction in terms of hepatic glucose balance is largely determined by the extent to which insulin concentration or action is impaired. Thus, subjects with poorly controlled, insulin-deficient type 1 diabetes exhibit a gross defect in suppression of hepatic glucose production following glucose ingestion, in concert with a failure to take up glucose and a severe defect in liver glycogen storage. These patients also have increased rates of gluconeogenesis, ascribable both to increased levels of expression of key gluconeogenic genes in response to unopposed glucagon action, and to increased delivery of gluconeogenic substrates from the periphery to the liver, including glycerol generated from

International Textbook of Diabetes Mellitus, Third Edition. Edited by R. A. DeFronzo, E. Ferrannini, H. Keen, and P. Zimmet.
 ISBN: 0-471-48655-8.

activation of lipolysis [1, 2]. In type 2 diabetes, where insulin levels and action are partially retained, defects in suppression of hepatic glucose production and liver glycogen storage are also observed, but to a lesser extent than in poorly controlled type 1 diabetes. Nevertheless, the defect in suppression of hepatic glucose production in type 2 diabetes is thought to account for approximately one third of the defect in total body glucose homeostasis [1]. Thus, in both major forms of diabetes, an imbalance in hepatic glucose production and disposal makes a major contribution to development of hyperglycemia and other perturbations in fuel homeostasis.

The important role played by impaired control of hepatic glucose balance in development of diabetes has motivated research into fundamental regulatory mechanisms involved in control of liver glucose metabolism for more than a century. Some of the most important insights in the entire history of biochemistry and medicine have arisen from studies in this area, including Claude Bernard's discovery of glucose storage in the form of liver glycogen [3], and the discovery of the "glycogenolytic cascade" of kinase reactions leading to activation of glycogen phosphorylase in liver cells by Sutherland and coworkers [4]. With the advent of the tools of molecular biology and genetics, coupled with continued application of more traditional tools of biochemistry and physiology, a surprising amount of new information about mechanisms controlling hepatic glucose metabolism has emerged in the past decade. The remainder of the chapter is devoted to integrating this new information with the bedrock of prior knowledge so as to synthesize new regulatory paradigms for control of glycolysis, gluconeogenesis, and glycogen metabolism in liver.

GLYCOLYSIS

General Considerations

Glycolysis is a series of 10 enzymatic reactions resulting in the conversion of glucose, an aldose with six carbons, to pyruvate, a three-carbon carboxylic acid. A balanced equation for this pathway is as follows:

$$\text{Glucose} + 2\,\text{Pi} + 2\,\text{NAD}^+ + 2\,\text{ADP} \rightleftharpoons 2\,\text{Pyruvate} + 2\,\text{ATP} + 2\,\text{NADH} + 2\,\text{H}^+ + 2\,\text{H}_2\text{O}$$

Among the 10 steps in the pathway, 7 are catalyzed by enzymes with equilibrium constants that allow the reaction to proceed in either the "forward" (glycolytic) or the "reverse" (gluconeogenic) direction, depending upon physiological changes in the relative concentrations of substrates and products of the reactions. Three other enzymatic steps, glucose phosphorylation by members of the hexokinase family (mainly hexokinase IV or glucokinase in liver), the conversion of fructose-6-phosphate to fructose-1,6-bisphosphate by phosphofructokinase (PFK), and the conversion of phosphoenolpyruvate to pyruvate by pyruvate kinase are considered to be essentially irreversible because of a large release of free energy associated with these reactions. Free energy is provided by the hydrolysis of ATP in the case of the glucokinase and PFK reactions, and via the favorable thermodynamics inherent in the conversion of an enol phosphate to a ketone in the pyruvate kinase reaction. In tissues that are capable of gluconeogenesis, such as kidney and liver, distinct enzymes have evolved to circumvent the otherwise irreversible glycolytic steps (see following section for further discussion).

Regulation of glycolysis occurs primarily through modulation of the concentration and activity of the three enzymes that catalyze irreversible steps in glycolysis—glucokinase, PFK, and pyruvate kinase. Until recently, most of the control strength (the relative contribution of a single enzyme to the overall flux through a metabolic pathway) for control of glycolysis in liver cells was thought to reside with PFK, a well-studied and highly regulated enzyme. However, a new modality of regulation has recently been discovered for glucokinase, involving its binding to a glucokinase regulatory protein (GKRP) in the nucleus, and its translocation from the nucleus to the cytosol in the transition from fasted to fed states. This has led to a more holistic model of regulation of glycolysis in liver, and our discussion summarizes the contributions made by each of the three key irreversible steps.

Regulation of Glucose Phosphorylation

Glucose phosphorylation in liver is primarily catalyzed by glucokinase (hexokinase IV). This enzyme has a lower affinity for glucose and a higher catalytic capacity than do the other members of its gene family, hexokinases I, II, and III [5, 6]. Glucokinase is limited in terms of its tissue distribution to liver, the islets of Langerhans, and certain specialized neuroendocrine cells in the pituitary and gastrointestinal tract [6–8], whereas hexokinase I is found in brain, red blood cells, and many other tissues, and hexokinase II is predominantly expressed in muscle and adipose tissue [5]. Glucokinase has an $S_{0.5}$ of about 8 mM for glucose, sigmoidal substrate dependency (indicated by a Hill coefficient of 1.7), and unlike hexokinases I and II, is not allosterically inhibited by the product of its reaction, G6P [5, 6]. The K_m for its other substrate Mg ATP^{2-} is about 0.4 mM, meaning that the enzyme operates at near-saturation in mammalian cells where ATP levels average approximately 2–4 mM. Liver cells are also equipped with the high capacity, high K_m facilitated glucose transporter, GLUT-2 (see later sections for more discussion). The glucose concentration in blood of normal subjects ranges from approximately 4 mM in the fasted state to a maximum of 8–9 mM in the fed state, a range very similar to the K_m of GLUT-2 and glucokinase. Thus, liver cells contain proteins that mediate glucose transport and phosphorylation with kinetic features that allow glucose metabolism to be regulated in response to changes in the external glucose concentration. Pancreatic islet β-cells and other "glucose sensing" cells in the gastrointestinal tract and central nervous system also co-express GLUT-2 and glucokinase [7–9]. In contrast, muscle and adipose cells contain mainly GLUT-4 and hexokinase II, making glucose transport and phosphorylation dependent upon insulin signaling in these tissues, while brain contains predominantly GLUT-1 and hexokinase I, both of which have a high affinity (low K_m) for glucose, ensuring that glucose transport and phosphorylation are near-maximal at all physiological glucose concentrations.

Until recently, transcriptional control was thought to be the predominant mechanism affecting glucokinase activity in liver. Indeed, levels of glucokinase mRNA are tightly controlled by insulin, such that levels fall in fasting or insulinopenic diabetes, and are increased dramatically (20–30-fold) by feeding or insulin injection [10–12]. These large changes in glucokinase mRNA are accompanied by significant, but more modest changes in glucokinase enzyme activity [12]. The time frame for changes in glucokinase enzyme activity due to activation of transcription and new protein synthesis is on the order of 30–60 min. However, a new mechanism for regulation of glucokinase activity has recently been described that appears more relevant for mediating acute changes in hepatic glucose phosphorylation (Figure 1). This regulatory paradigm emerged with the discovery of an activity in cellular extracts that could inhibit glucokinase enzyme activity in a fashion antagonized by fructose-1-phosphate [13]. This led to the identification of a GKRP, and the cloning of its cDNA [14]. Shortly thereafter, GKRP was shown to reside in the nucleus [15, 16]. Subsequent studies demonstrated that the protein has a nuclear import signal that allows it to carry glucokinase from the cytosol to the nucleus [17]. This transport of glucokinase to the nucleus occurs actively under fasting conditions *in vivo*, and when isolated hepatocytes are incubated at low glucose concentrations. Exposure of isolated hepatocytes to high concentrations of glucose, fructose or sorbitol, or ingestion of a carbohydrate-containing meal in animals, stimulates dissociation of glucokinase from the regulatory protein and translocation of the enzyme from the nucleus to the cytosol [15, 16, 18]. In this fashion, glucose phosphorylation is suppressed under fasting conditions, allowing hydrolysis of glucose-6-phosphate (G6P) via the glucose-6-phosphatase (G6Pase) enzyme complex to occur in an unimpeded fashion. Conversely, translocation of glucokinase from the nucleus to the cytoplasm in response to meal ingestion is a rapid means of increasing glucose phosphorylation, which is supplemented at later stages of absorption of the meal by an insulin-mediated increase in glucokinase gene expression.

In light of this, one might predict that genetic ablation of GKRP expression would remove the principle for

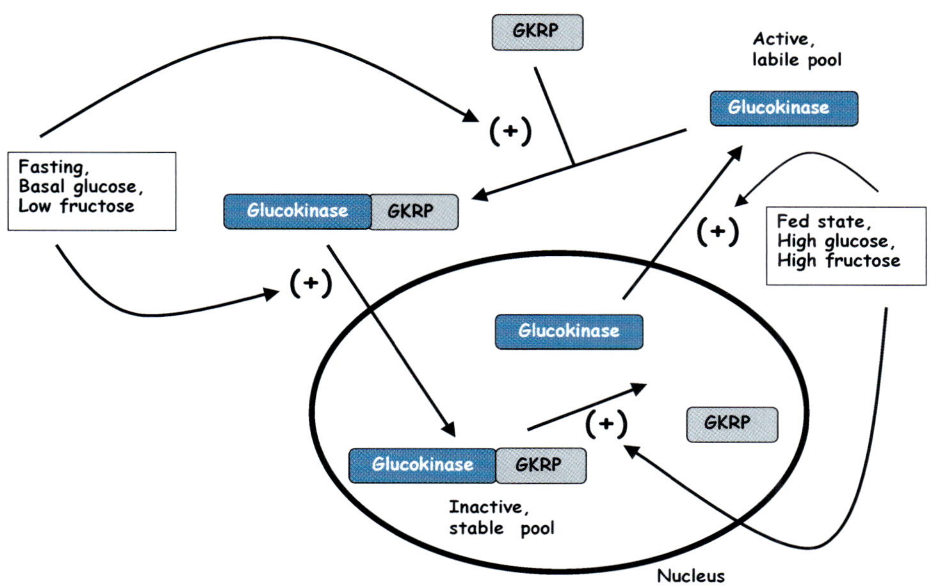

Figure 1 Interaction of glucokinase with the glucokinase regulatory protein (GKRP) in liver. In the fasted state, binding of glucokinase to GKRP is promoted. GKRP contains a nuclear import signal that facilitates transport of the glucokinase/GKRP complex into the nucleus. When bound to GKRP in the nucleus, glucokinase is catalytically inactive but protected against proteolytic degradation. In the transition from the fasted to the fed state, glucokinase dissociates from GKRP and is translocated from the nucleus to the cytosol, via a nuclear export sequence residing in the glucokinase protein. When present in the cytosol and dissociated from GKRP, glucokinase is fully active but more accessible to proteolytic enzymes.

nuclear sequestration and inhibition of glucokinase activity. However, this is not the case, as evidenced by two studies in which GKRP was knocked out in transgenic mice [19, 20]. Both heterozygous and homozygous knockout mice had decreased rather than increased glucokinase enzyme activity in liver. The knockout animals had normal blood glucose levels in the fasted state, but displayed an abnormal excursion of blood glucose concentrations during a glucose tolerance test. It is proposed that in addition to its inhibitory function, binding of GKRP to glucokinase protects the enzyme from degradation, thus maintaining a large stable pool of the protein in the fasted state that can be rapidly recruited in response to influx of metabolic fuels. Conversely, as the period of meal absorption comes to a close, glucokinase can be either degraded or rebound to GKRP for return to the nucleus, thus preventing inappropriate glucose disposal during the transition from the fed to the fasted state. This is the first of several examples reviewed in this chapter of important elements of spatial organization and compartmentalization that contribute to regulation of hepatic carbohydrate metabolism. The regulation of glucokinase by GKRP is summarized schematically in Figure 1.

Regulation of Phosphofructokinase

Another highly regulated reaction of glycolysis in liver is catalyzed by PFK. PFK catalyzes the conversion of fructose-6-phosphate to fructose-1,6-bisphosphate, with ATP serving as the phosphate donor. The enzyme displays sigmoidal kinetics, typical of enzymes that are regulated by allosteric ligands. PFK activity is regulated by the energy charge of the cell, such that increases in the ratio of ATP/ADP + AMP inhibit enzyme activity. Citrate, the product of the first committed step of the TCA cycle, is also a potent inhibitor of PFK activity, allowing glycolysis to slow when TCA cycle intermediates are replete and energy production is high. However, the most important allosteric regulator of PFK activity in liver is fructose-2,6-bisphosphate (F-2,6-P_2), discovered by three laboratories as a highly potent activator of PFK activity in the early 1980s [21–23]. F-2,6-P_2 activates PFK at low micromolar concentrations via two main actions. First, it converts the kinetic profile of PFK from sigmoidal to hyperbolic with respect to the concentration of the PFK substrate fructose-6-phosphate. This change in activity increases the affinity (lowers the K_m) of PFK for fructose-6-phosphate. Second, F-2,6-P_2 relieves inhibition of PFK by ATP, such that higher concentrations of the nucleotide are required to suppress enzyme activity.

Subsequent biochemical and molecular studies revealed that the synthesis and degradation of F-2,6-P_2 is catalyzed by a single protein with two distinct catalytic sites [24, 25]. This protein was named 6-phosphofructose-2-kinase/fructose-2,6-bisphosphatase but is also known more simply as *the bifunctional enzyme*. The bifunctional enzyme found in liver is regulated by cAMP-dependent protein kinase (PKA) mediated phosphorylation of a serine residue near its N-terminus (serine 32) [26]. Phosphorylation at this site inhibits the 2-kinase activity of the enzyme, and increases its bisphosphatase activity, resulting in a net decrease in F-2,6-P_2 concentration within cells. The discovery of F-2,6-P_2 and the bifunctional enzyme was a major contribution to our understanding of hormone-mediated regulation of liver glycolysis. In the fasted state, insulin levels decline and glucagon levels increase. Glucagon effects predominate under these conditions, and in liver, this is manifest by a rise in cAMP levels elicited by the binding of glucagon to its receptor, via activation of adenylate cyclase. The increase in cAMP activates PKA, which in turn phosphorylates the bifunctional enzyme at serine 32, resulting in a net decrease in cellular F-2,6-P_2 levels. This in turn leads to a decrease in the affinity of PFK for its substrate fructose-6-phosphate and an increase in sensitivity of the enzyme to the inhibitory effects of ATP, leading to a net decrease in enzyme activity.

In the transition from the fasted to the fed state, this regulation is reversed. Following a mixed meal, insulin and glucose levels rise in the blood while glucagon levels are decreased. Under these conditions, dephosphorylation of the bifunctional enzyme is stimulated, restoring its 2-kinase activity and causing a rapid increase in F-2,6-P_2 levels. The dephosphorylation of the bifunctional enzyme appears to be mediated by a xylulose-5-phosphate (Xu5P) activated protein phosphatase 2A [27]. Xu5P is formed in the pentose monophosphate shunt, and its levels rise in liver in response to an increase in glucose concentration. Thus, the Xu5P-regulated protein phosphatase provides a direct link between the postprandial change in glucose concentration and the reactivation of the 2-kinase activity of the bifunctional enzyme. In addition to the effect of glucose to activate the Xu5P-regulated phosphatase, the increase in insulin levels in the postprandial state serves to stimulate degradation of cAMP to AMP via phosphodiesterases, thus decreasing the activity of PKA and contributing to maintenance of the bifunctional enzyme in a nonphosphorylated state. Regulation of PFK via changes in bifunctional enzyme activity and F-2,6-P_2 levels is summarized schematically in Figure 2.

Pyruvate kinase catalyzes the last of the irreversible steps of glycolysis in liver, and is subject to both allosteric and transcriptional regulation. For example, the liver isoform of pyruvate kinase (L-PK) is activated by the product of the PFK reaction, fructose-1,6-bisphosphate [28]. This represents a "feed-forward" mechanism by which flux through an early step in glycolysis activates a later step. Similar to PFK, L-PK is sensitive to the energy charge of the cell, and its activity is decreased in the presence of a high ATP/ADP + AMP ratio. Similar to the bifunctional enzyme, L-PK is inhibited by PKA-mediated serine

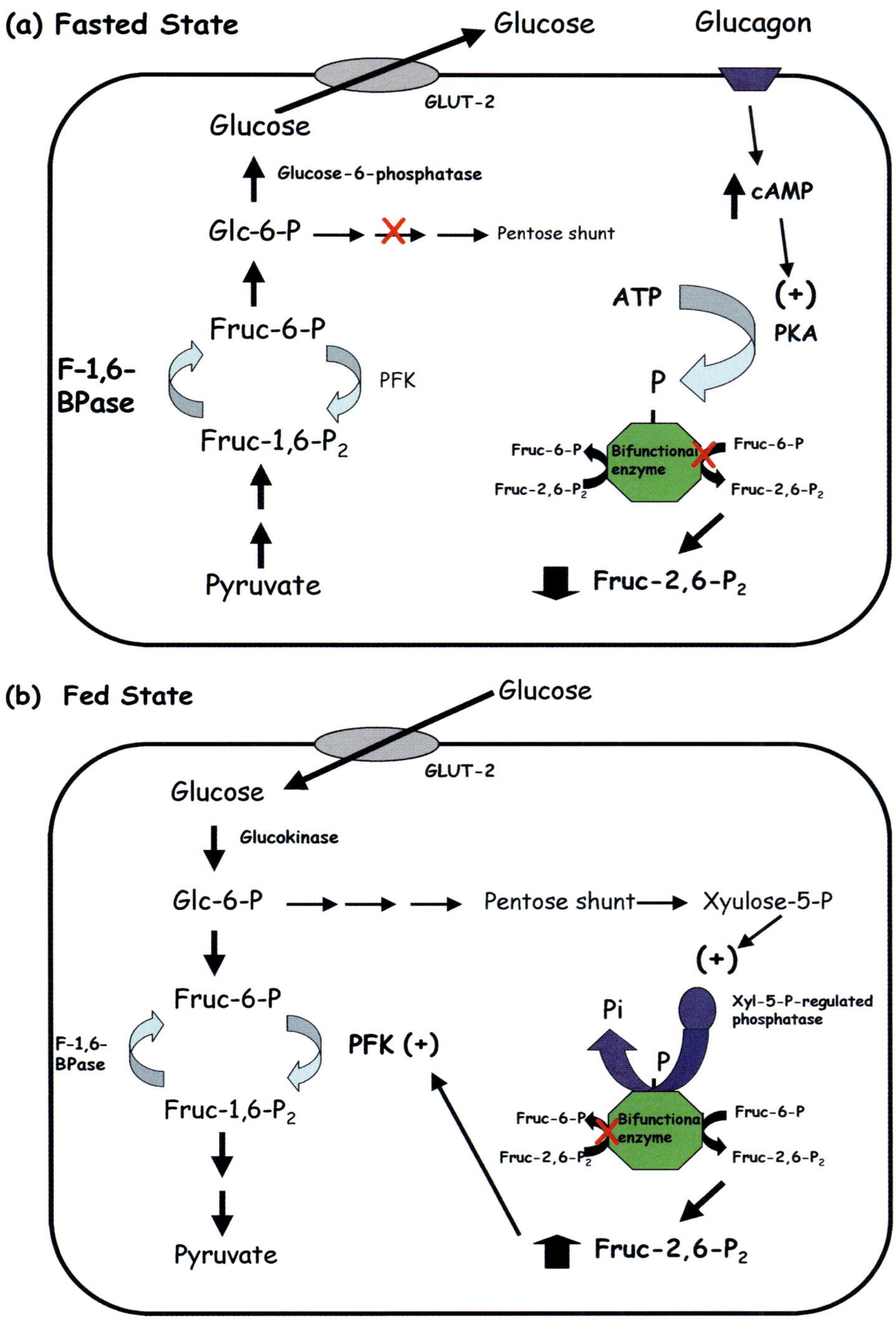

Figure 2 Regulation of glycolysis and gluconeogenesis by fructose-2,6-bisphosphate. (a) In the fasted state, glucagon levels are elevated, resulting in increased levels of cAMP in liver cells. cAMP activates cAMP-dependent protein kinase (PKA), which phosphorylates 6-phosphofructo-2-kinase/fructose-2,6-bisphosphatase (bifunctional enzyme), resulting in inhibition of 2-kinase activity, but retention of fructose-2,6-bisphosphatase activity. The resultant fall in fructose-2,6-bisphosphate concentrations removes a key allosteric activator of phosphofructokinase, favoring gluconeogenic flux through fructose-1,6-bisphosphatase. (b) In the fed state, cAMP levels fall, and glucose uptake and phosphorylation are increased. This leads to an increase in xyulose-5-phosphate synthesis in the pentose monophosphate shunt pathway, which in turn leads to activation of a xylulos-5-phosphate-regulated protein phosphatase 2A. This phosphatase dephosphorylates the bifunctional enzyme, thereby activating its kinase function and inhibiting its phosphatase activity. The resultant rise in fructose-2,6-bisphosphate concentration stimulates phosphofructokinase and glycolysis

phosphorylation [29]. Phosphorylation increases the apparent K_m of the enzyme for its substrate PEP, and renders the enzyme more sensitive to inhibition by a high-energy charge (elevated ATP/ADP + AMP ratio).

Like the other key glycolytic enzymes, glucokinase, PFK, and the bifunctional enzyme, transcription of the L-PK gene is decreased by fasting or insulinopenic diabetes, and is increased in the fed state or by insulin injection. Glucose appears to be a more direct and potent regulator of L-PK transcription than does insulin, which may be acting mostly to antagonize the effects of glucagon by activating phosphodiesterases and lowering cellular cAMP levels. Interestingly, the same Xu5P-regulated protein phosphatase that dephosphorylates the bifunctional enzyme under anabolic conditions also dephosphorylates and activates a recently discovered transcription factor termed carbohydrate responsive element binding protein or ChREBP [30, 31]. This factor has been shown to stimulate transcription of L-PK, as well as lipogenic genes such as acetyl-CoA carboxylase and fatty acid synthase. Thus, a rise in circulating glucose concentration and a proportional increase in the rate of hepatic glycolysis and pentose monophosphate shunt activity in the fasted to fed transition is translated into an increase in 2-kinase activity of the bifunctional enzyme via activation of the Xu5P-regulated protein phosphatase, resulting in an increase in F-2,6-P_2 levels and increased flux through PFK to generate fructose-1,6-bisphosphate. This intermediate, pyruvate kinase, then serves as a feed-forward activator of a later step in glycolysis. Finally, this allosteric activation of pyruvate kinase is supplemented by another action of the Xu5P-regulated protein phosphatase, the dephosphorylation and activation of the ChREBP transcription factor, which stimulates L-PK gene transcription.

Insights from Metabolic Engineering Studies Targeting Glucokinase or PFK Activity in Liver

The foregoing discussion suggests that glucokinase and PFK are enzymes with significant control strength for modulation of glycolysis in liver. The implication of this is that these enzymes might be important targets for overcoming the impairment in hepatic glucose disposal that exists in type 2 diabetes. The validity of this idea is supported by genetic studies and other work involving alterations in expression of glucokinase or the bifunctional enzyme in isolated hepatocytes or liver; these are summarized below.

A key illustration of the importance of glucokinase in controlling human fuel homeostasis comes from the discovery that a form of non-insulin-dependent diabetes mellitus known as maturity-onset diabetes of the young (MODY) type 2 is caused by mutations in the glucokinase gene [32]. Subsequent studies have identified a large number of mutations, mostly point mutations occurring in the protein-coding region of the gene, in French, English, and Japanese MODY2 pedigrees [33, 34]. All MODY2 patients are heterozygous, with one normal and one mutated glucokinase allele. Structural modeling studies based on the X-ray structure of yeast hexokinase suggest that mutations in glucokinase that cause severe reduction in enzyme activity are mostly found within the postulated glucose-binding cleft [35]. The effect of the mutations on glucokinase enzymatic activity has been evaluated by expression of the mutant genes in bacteria and kinetic analyses of the purified, expressed proteins [34, 36]. Most of the mutant enzymes exhibit large decreases in enzymatic activity due to changes in k_{cat}, $S_{0.5}$ for glucose, or both. Alterations in the K_m for ATP have also been reported. However, amino acid substitution mutations such as E300K are also associated with MODY2, despite the fact that the expressed enzymes exhibit little alteration in their kinetic properties. Mutants of this class are less effectively expressed in heterologous systems and exhibit reduced stability at elevated temperatures in *in vitro* studies [36]. Patients with MODY2 have a defect in glucose-stimulated insulin secretion, due to the important role that glucokinase plays in regulating the rate of glycolysis and thereby the production of key stimulus/secretion coupling factors in islet β-cells [37–39]. In addition, MODY2 patients have impaired hepatic glucose disposal, leading to an increase in net hepatic glucose production [33]. Patients with glucokinase mutations also store significantly less glycogen in liver than do normal subjects [40].

Two groups have independently produced transgenic mice heterozygous for disruption of a segment of the glucokinase gene, which affects gene expression in both the liver and the islets of Langherhans [41, 42]. This maneuver resulted in an approximate 30–40% decrease in glucokinase activity in both tissues, significant reduction in glucose-stimulated insulin secretion, and mild hyperglycemia. Interestingly, animals homozygous for knockout of the glucokinase gene die at an embryonic stage or shortly after birth [41–43].

The foregoing studies of glucokinase-deficient states imply that modulation of liver glucokinase activity may be an effective means of lowering blood glucose in diabetes. *In vitro* studies of hepatic glucose phosphorylation using recombinant adenoviruses encoding glucokinase or hexokinase I demonstrated that glucokinase overexpression causes marked increases in glycolytic rate and glycogen deposition in hepatocytes, while hexokinase I did not [44, 45]. This difference in efficacy is most likely explained by the fact that the product of the reaction, G6P, strongly inhibits hexokinase I but not glucokinase [45].

The impact of glucokinase overexpression in liver has also been studied in normal and diabetic animals. Infusion of a recombinant adenovirus containing the glucokinase cDNA into normal rats at rates designed to cause moderate (3-fold) or large (7-fold) increases in hepatic glucokinase enzymatic activity, resulted in a significant lowering of blood glucose levels only in the latter group, accompanied by a 67% decline in circulating insulin levels, and a large increase in liver glycogen stores [46]. Similar findings were reported in transgenic mice containing multiple copies of the glucokinase gene [47]. At first glance this result appears promising; however, closer examination reveals that this result came at the expense of a 190% increase in circulating triglycerides (TGs) and a 310% increase in circulating free fatty acids (FFAs) in normal rats with adenovirus-mediated glucokinase overexpression [46]. The lipid profile of animals with overexpression of hepatic glucokinase puts into question the manipulation of glucokinase activity as part of a viable therapy for diabetes.

However, studies in rodent models of diabetes have been more promising. In streptozotocin- (STZ)- diabetic mice transgenic for glucokinase expression under control of the phosphoenolpyruvate carboxykinase (PEPCK) promoter, near-normalization of blood glucose levels was achieved [48]. In addition, the high levels of fatty acids, TGs, and ketone bodies found in the diabetic mice were lowered, albeit not fully normalized. An explanation for the improved lipid profile in this animal model could be that the glucose-lowering effect of glucokinase resulted in a greater dependence on lipid oxidation for energy production throughout the body. It must also be pointed out that these animals are completely insulin deficient, making it difficult to extrapolate these findings to patients with type 1 diabetes or type 2 diabetes, who will have either residual endogenous or exogenously administered insulin available in the blood.

The effects of glucokinase overexpression in mouse models of high-fat-diet-induced type 2 diabetes have been reported by two groups of investigators [49, 50]. The first group reported a fall in circulating glucose and insulin levels, with an increase in liver TG content in response to high-fat feeding, but with a similar increase in hepatic TGs found in both glucokinase transgenic and nontransgenic mice. The second group reported that circulating FFA and TG levels were not raised by the high-fat diet, and subsequently not affected by adenovirus-mediated overexpression of glucokinase in the liver. Again, insulin and glucose levels were substantially reduced [21]. In these two studies the animals exhibited a 40% [20] or a 2.2-fold [21] increase in hepatic glucokinase activity, which is clearly less than the 6-fold increase achieved in adenovirus studies in normal rats [18].

Another interesting approach for manipulation of glucose phosphorylation in liver is to alter the expression of the GKRP. Remarkably, adenovirus-mediated overexpression of GKRP in liver of mice fed on a high-fat diet caused a dramatic lowering of their elevated blood glucose levels and restored insulin levels to near-normal, suggesting that insulin resistance was ameliorated [51]. Curiously, glucokinase enzymatic activity in liver was actually reduced in the GKRP-expressing mice, but this is probably explained by the fall in insulin levels and the consequent decrease in glucokinase gene transcription. Also, the measurement of enzyme activity was performed 3 weeks after the administration of the GKRP adenovirus; it is likely that glucokinase activity was increased at earlier time points. In support of this idea, adenovirus-mediated co-expression of glucokinase and GKRP in isolated hepatocytes resulted in higher levels of glucokinase protein and enzyme activity when GKRP and glucokinase were co-expressed compared with overexpression of glucokinase alone, consistent with our earlier discussion of a potential role for GKRP in stabilization of the glucokinase protein and maintenance of a pool of recruitable enzyme. Administration of GKRP virus to mice fed on the high-fat diet did not affect their circulating TG or FFA levels, but curiously, lipid levels did not rise in mice fed the high-fat diet relative to controls fed on a low-fat diet. Thus, while this initial study seems promising, further evaluation of the metabolic impact of hepatic overexpression of GKRP is warranted.

Further evidence for the potential utility of glucokinase as a target in diabetes therapy comes from a recent study with a newly developed small molecule activator of the enzyme [52]. Administration of this drug, which stimulates glucokinase activity in both the liver and the pancreatic islets, was shown to improve glucose homeostasis in an animal model of type 2 diabetes [52]. While no information about circulating lipids was provided, hyperlipidemia is actually not anticipated, given that the agent stimulates islet glucokinase activity and insulin secretion, which should result in suppression of lipolysis and increased lipid storage. In contrast, adenovirus-mediated overexpression of glucokinase in normal rats leads to reduced rather than increased insulin levels, secondary to the fall in blood glucose [46].

A summary of knowledge gained from glucokinase overexpression studies is as follows. At carefully regulated doses, an increase in glucokinase activity in liver can lead to improved glucose homeostasis in normal rodents, and in models of type 1 and type 2 diabetes. However, higher levels of glucokinase overexpression result in increases in circulating lipids, because of lowering of insulin levels and consequent impairment of lipid storage and increased hepatic lipogenesis. While studies with the new glucokinase activator clearly demonstrate a capacity of this approach for lowering of blood glucose, with no anticipated acute hyperlipidemia, the long-term effects of chronic elevations in insulin levels due to activation of islet glucokinase activity is a potential concern. Chronic hyperinsulinemia represents a sustained anabolic state, possibly leading to overstorage of lipids in tissues such as muscle and liver. Tissue lipid overstorage has been linked to the development of insulin resistance [1, 2]. A small molecule activator of glucokinase may also have the potential for causing hypoglycemia, as both hepatic glucose clearance and insulin secretion are stimulated by these molecules. Indeed, there was some evidence of hypoglycemia in animals that received the small molecule glucokinase activator [52]. Further investigation of these issues is required.

Glucokinase overexpression has also been applied to skeletal muscle [53–58]. An important finding that stimulated work in this area was the demonstration that adenovirus-mediated overexpression of glucokinase in isolated human myocytes enhanced glucose uptake and glycogen synthesis in an insulin-independent manner [53, 57]. Moreover, glucokinase overexpression altered the glucose dose–response relationship for glucose uptake to reflect the kinetic features of glucokinase, such that engineered cells responded to glucose in a range of 1–30 mM, as opposed to control cells that express endogenous hexokinase II, that exhibited maximal glucose uptake at <5 mM glucose [53]. Myoblasts engineered for glucokinase overexpression were able to lower blood glucose levels when transplanted into mice with STZ-induced diabetes [57]. Also, adenovirus-mediated expression of glucokinase in hind limb skeletal muscle of normal [54] or Zucker diabetic fatty (ZDF) [56] rats enhanced glucose tolerance and improved insulin sensitivity, respectively. Finally, expression of glucokinase in transgenic mice under control of a muscle-specific promoter protected against diet-induced insulin resistance and hyperglycemia [58]. The transgenic mice also exhibited increased expression of uncoupling protein 3 in skeletal muscle, possibly contributing to an increase in energy expenditure in these animals. While studies in this area have clearly been of interest, obstacles such as long-term safety and appropriate methods for introducing the glucokinase gene into human muscle remain to be considered.

On the basis of earlier discussion, one might also presume that glycolytic flux and hepatic glucose disposal could be modulated at steps distal to glucose phosphorylation. Accordingly, recombinant adenoviruses containing native and mutant forms of 6-phosphofructo-2-kinase/fructose-2,6-bisphosphate (the bifunctional enzyme) have been prepared and tested. A doubly mutated form of the bifunctional enzyme (Ser32Ala, His258Ala) has diminished fructose-2,6-bisphosphatase activity and cannot be phosphorylated by PKA; phosphorylation by PKA normally suppresses bifunctional enzyme 2-kinase function. Thus the mutated enzyme has a very high kinase/phosphatase ratio, and this favors formation of F-2,6-P_2. Overexpression of the wild-type or doubly mutated form of the bifunctional enzyme increases F-2,6-P_2 levels in isolated cells [59] and in the liver of whole animals [60, 61], with larger increases seen when the mutant form is expressed.

The metabolic impact of bifunctional enzyme overexpression is similar to that described for glucokinase. Thus, overexpression of the bifunctional enzyme lowers blood glucose levels in normal mice, but also causes a significant increase in circulating FFA and TG levels [60]. Blood glucose levels are also lowered in mice with STZ-induced type 1 diabetes, more effectively by the doubly mutated bifunctional enzyme than the wild-type enzyme [60]. The doubly mutated bifunctional enzyme also partially normalized circulating FFA and TG levels in these animals. Finally, the doubly mutated form of bifunctional enzyme has been overexpressed in liver of two mouse strains that develop syndromes resembling type 2 diabetes (KK/HIJ and KK.Cg-A^y/J strains), resulting again in partial normalization of blood glucose levels, lowering of circulating insulin levels, and a modest reduction in the elevated circulating FFA and TG levels [61]. Liver TG level were not changed by expression of bifunctional enzyme, similar to what was noted in glucokinase transgenic mice. As proposed for the case of glucokinase, the modest decrease in circulating lipids caused by overexpression of the bifunctional enzyme in both type 1 and type 2 diabetes models may have occurred in response to the fall in circulating glucose, making the animals more dependent upon lipid oxidation for energy production. However, as was also the case for glucokinase, more detailed analysis of metabolic consequences of long-term expression of the bifunctional enzyme is required, including better understanding of changes in lipid metabolism and the potential for hypoglycemia.

GLUCONEOGENESIS

General Considerations

Gluconeogenesis is the process by which certain mammalian tissues, primarily liver and kidney, are able to synthesize glucose from three carbon precursors such as alanine, pyruvate, lactate, and glycerol. Alanine and lactate are converted to pyruvate via transaminase and lactate dehydrogenase, respectively, whereas glycerol is phosphorylated to glycerol phosphate and then converted to the glycolytic intermediate dihydroxyacetone phosphate by cytosolic glycerol phosphate dehydrogenase. In considering the pathway for gluconeogenesis from pyruvate, a total of 13 enzymatic steps are required. Seven of these involve enzymes that catalyze the reversible steps of glycolysis such as aldolase and triose phosphate isomerase. The other six reactions are catalyzed by enzymes that are not used in glycolysis. These six unique reactions are required in order to circumvent the irreversible steps of glycolysis. Several of the unique reactions are deployed to facilitate conversion of pyruvate to phosphoenolpyruvate (Figure 3). Beginning with pyruvate, the first step in gluconeogenesis is carboxylation to yield oxaloacetate, catalyzed by the mitochondrial enzyme pyruvate carboxylase. Oxaloacetate is then converted to malate by mitochondrial malate dehydrogenase. Malate is transported out of the mitochondria

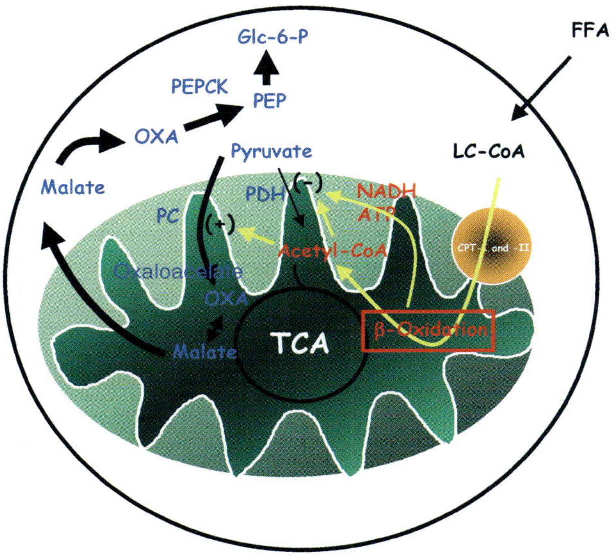

Figure 3 Regulation of pyruvate dehydrogenase and pyruvate carboxylase by products of lipid metabolism in the fasted state. In the fasted state, the elevated glucagon/insulin ratio promotes lipolysis in adipose tissue, leading to an increase in circulating free fatty acids (FFAs). FFAs are transported to liver through the bloodstream and converted to long-chain acyl-CoA (LC-CoA) by long-chain acyl-CoA synthetase. In the fasted state, malonyl-CoA levels are low, promoting transport of LC-CoA into mitochondria for β-oxidation via the carnitine palmitoyltransferase I and II enzymes (CPT-I and -II). The products of fatty acid oxidation—NADH, ATP, and acetyl-CoA—inhibit pyruvate dehydrogenase (PDH) activity directly and via activation of PDH kinases. Acetyl-CoA is also a potent allosteric activator of pyruvate carboxylase (PC) activity. Thus, the increase in hepatic fatty acid oxidation in the fasted state stimulates gluconeogenesis by diverting pyruvate away from entry into the TCA cycle toward conversion to phosphoenolpyruvate (PEP) via PC and phosphoenolpyruvate carboxykinase (PEPCK)

and then reconverted to oxaloacetate by cytosolic malate dehydrogenase. Finally, oxaloacetate is decarboxylated to yield the glycolytic intermediate phosphoenolpyruvate by PEPCK. These initial steps of gluconeogenesis are energetically expensive, with consumption of a mole of ATP in the pyruvate carboxylase reaction, and a mole of GTP in the PEPCK reaction for every mole of pyruvate converted to PEP. The energy is supplied in large part by the oxidation of fatty acids, which is promoted in the fasted state via a fall in the concentration of malonyl-CoA, an important allosteric inhibitior of carnitine palmitoyltransferase I (CPT-I), the enzyme that gates the entry of long-chain fatty acyl-CoAs into the mitochondria for oxidation [62].

Phosphoenolpyruvate is converted to fructose-1,6-bisphosphate via six enzymatic steps common to glycolysis. However, conversion of fructose-1,6-bisphosphate to fructose-6-phosphate requires a new enzyme, fructose-1,6-bisphosphatase, as the ATP-consuming PFK reaction is not reversible. Fructose-6-phosphate is then converted to G6P by reversal of the hexose phosphate isomerase reaction of glycolysis. The terminal step of gluconeogenesis is the hydrolysis of G6P to free glucose, catalyzed by the G6Pase enzyme complex. The complex comprises a catalytic subunit sequestered within the endoplasmic reticulum (ER), a G6P translocase known as T1 that delivers G6P to the catalytic subunit, and putative ER glucose and inorganic phosphate transporters (T2, T3) that move the reaction products back into the cytosol [63, 64]. Thus, gluconeogenesis from pyruvate serves as another example of compartmentalization and spatial organization in hepatic carbohydrate metabolism, in that it involves enzymatic reactions occurring in the mitochondrial lumen, the cytosol, and the lumen of the ER. The sequestration of G6Pase in the ER may be explained by the fact that the catalytic subunit of the complex is a nonspecific phosphohydrolase that will remove phosphate groups from several different phosphorylated sugars. Specificity of the system is conferred by the T1 translocase component, which transports G6P, but not its closely related epimer mannose-6-phosphate [65]. This prevents uncontrolled hydrolysis of phosphorylated sugars and spares energy.

Acute Regulation of Gluconeogenesis

Mirroring our discussion of regulation of glycolysis, regulation of gluconeogenesis in response to nutritional and physiologic changes occurs primarily via regulation of the amount and activity of those enzymes that counter the nonreversible steps in glycolysis. Gluconeogenesis is most active in the fasted condition or in insulinopenic states. Under these conditions, glucagon acts to enhance the rate of fatty acid oxidation in the liver, which results in diversion of pyruvate away from the pyruvate dehydrogenase reaction and oxidation in the TCA cycle toward the pyruvate carboxylase reaction and gluconeogenesis. The mechanism by which this occurs is both logical and elegant (Figure 3). A rise in the glucagon/insulin ratio in the fasted state or in insulinopenic diabetes results in binding of glucagon to its receptor in adipose tissue. This leads to activation of hormone-sensitive lipase, which catalyzes the hydrolysis of TGs to yield FFAs and glycerol, causing an increase in the concentrations of these metabolites in the blood. The FFAs are transported to the liver and imported for oxidation. Oxidation is favored in this condition because the decreased glycolytic flux mediated by changes in glucokinase, PFK, and pyruvate kinase activity described earlier results in a decreased rate of synthesis of malonyl-CoA. A fall in malonyl-CoA relieves inhibition of CPT-I, which, in combination with the increase in substrate supply, increases the rate of fatty acid oxidation [62]. Fatty acid oxidation occurs in the mitochondrial lumen. The products of fatty acid oxidation include acetyl-CoA, NADH, and ATP. The ATP produced from fatty acid oxidation provides energy for the early steps of gluconeogenesis. Acetyl-CoA, NADH, and ATP are all allosteric inhibitors of the mitochondrial enzyme pyruvate dehydrogenase [66, 67]. In addition, pyruvate dehydrogenase activity is regulated by a family of pyruvate dehydrogenase kinases [68]. Phosphorylation of pyruvate dehydrogenase is favored under fasting or catabolic conditions, and results in inactivation of the enzyme. Pyruvate dehydrogenase kinase activity is stimulated by the same set of allosteric effectors, acetyl-CoA, NADH, and ATP, that inhibit pyruvate dehydrogenase activity directly [68, 69]. Thus, these by-products of fatty acid oxidation cause highly efficient suppression of pyruvate dehydrogenase activity by a two-tiered mechanism. Furthermore, acetyl-CoA is a potent activator of pyruvate carboxylase [70, 71]. As summarized in Figure 3, fatty acid oxidation in the mitochondrial lumen generates by-products that interact with two mitochondrial enzymes that determine the metabolic fate of pyruvate. This regulatory mechanism preserves pyruvate for gluconeogenesis in fasting or insulinopenic diabetes.

Allosteric regulatory mechanisms have not been uncovered for other key gluconeogenic enzymes such as PEPCK or the G6Pase complex, although these enzymes are tightly regulated at the transcriptional level, as discussed below. The activity of fructose-1,6-bisphosphatase has long been thought to be regulated by F-2,6-P_2, the product of the bifunctional enzyme, based on findings from several laboratories that F-2,6-P_2 inhibits the activity of fructose-1,6-bisphosphatase *in vitro* [72, 73]. However, a recent study provides evidence that this regulatory mechanism is not operative in liver of intact animals [74]. The study involved the use of [U-^{13}C]glucose and D_2O infusion, followed by NMR analysis of the labeling pattern of glucose purified from plasma, to assess the relative contributions of gastric emptying, glycogenolysis, and gluconeogenesis to plasma glucose in 24-h fasted rats that received an oral bolus of glucose. The authors found that whereas the oral glucose load caused F-2,6-P_2 levels to rise by more than 10-fold, the fractional contribution of gluconeogenesis to plasma glucose was unchanged over the 150-min study period. These data strongly suggest that F-2,6-P_2 has little acute effect on fructose-1,6-bisphosphatase in the *in vivo* setting. They also suggest that allosteric regulation generally plays a small role in suppressing gluconeogenesis in the transition from the fasted to the fed state.

It is of interest to briefly compare the acute regulation of the bifunctional enzyme in liver and muscle. In muscle, glycolysis can remain active even under circumstances in which cellular cAMP levels are elevated such as in response to catecholamines in "fight or flight" situations. Based on events just described for liver, the expectation would be that the bifunctional enzyme would be phosphorylated and inactivated under these conditions. Instead, this mode of regulation is obviated by the expression of an isoform of bifunctional enzyme in muscle that lacks serine 32, eliminating the enzyme as a target for cAMP-dependent protein kinase [75].

Regulation of Gluconeogenesis at the Level of Gene Transcription

The transition from the fed to the fasted state occurs gradually, as opposed to the transition from the fasted to the fed state, in which fuels enter the system rapidly, requiring equally rapid activation of fuel disposal pathways. It is therefore not surprising that much of the regulation of gluconeogenesis occurs at the level of transcription of genes encoding key gluconeogenic enzymes. Accordingly, as the glucagon/insulin ratio rises, transcription of the PEPCK, fructose-1,6-bisphosphatase, and glucose-6-phosphtase catalytic subunit genes is increased in a gradual and coordinated fashion.

cAMP and glucocorticoids increase PEPCK activity by stimulating transcription of the PEPCK gene [76]. The increase in transcription results in increased levels of PEPCK mRNA, an effect supplemented by mRNA stabilization [77, 78]. cAMP enhances PEPCK gene transcription by PKA-mediated phosphorylation of the cAMP response element binding (CREB) protein, which binds to the cAMP response element (CRE) in the PEPCK gene promoter [79, 80]. Binding of phosphorylated CREB to its CRE site nucleates the assembly of a larger protein complex that causes transcription to be initiated from the PEPCK gene promoter [81]. Employing a similar paradigm, glucocorticoids bind to the cytosolic glucocorticoid receptor (GR), causing its dissociation from a chaperone protein and its translocation to the nucleus where it binds to a glucocorticoid response element (GRE) in the PEPCK promoter. Formation of the GR/GRE complex leads to recruitment of other proteins (albeit different ones than those bound to the CREB/CRE complex), again leading to stimulation of PEPCK gene transcription [82, 83]. Insulin antagonizes these actions of glucagon or glucocorticoids, by incompletely understood mechanisms [82, 84].

Similar to the case with PEPCK, fructose-1,6-bisphosphatase and G6Pase activity are increased several-fold in response to fasting or insulinopenic diabetes, and return to baseline in response to feeding or insulin injection. The molecular mechanism by which fructose-1,6-bisphosphatase is regulated in this fashion is not well understood, but regulation of G6Pase expression has been better studied. In addition to the stimulatory effect of agents that raise hepatic cAMP, variables associated with the diabetic state such as hyperglycemia and hyperlipidemia cause increased expression of the G6Pase catalytic subunit both *in vitro* and in whole-animal studies [85–89]. Insulin inhibits transcription of this gene when studied alone, and exerts a dominant inhibitory effect over the actions of cAMP and glucose [87, 90]. In the ZDF rat, the concentration of the G6Pase catalytic subunit and the overall enzymatic activity of the G6Pase complex are increased by approximately 2.5-fold relative to lean ZDF Wistar controls [91]. As ZDF rats are severely insulin resistant, these data are consistent with the idea that the normal dominant effect of insulin to suppress G6Pase expression is weakened in insulin-resistant states, and further challenged by increases in circulating glucose and lipid levels, leading to an increase in hepatic G6Pase expression. Data proving that an increase in G6Pase catalytic subunit expression is sufficient to cause several metabolic abnormalities associated with early stage diabetes are summarized below.

Recently, new information has appeared about the mechanism of coordinate control of key gluconeogenic genes in the fasted and fed states, based on the discovery of new functions of the PGC-1α transcriptional coactivator (PGC-1α is an acronym for peroxisome proliferator-activated receptor γ coactivator 1α). PGC-1α was originally discovered as a factor mediating mitochondrial biogenesis and thermogenesis in response to cold stress [92], and was not thought to be expressed in liver at significant levels. Subsequent studies, however, indicated that PGC-1α levels rise dramatically in liver in fasting and in several models of type 1 and type 2 diabetes, conditions under which gluconeogenic enzymes are coordinately induced [93]. Modest adenovirus-mediated overexpression of PGC-1α in isolated hepatocytes and liver of normal rats was subsequently shown to be sufficient to activate expression of the three key gluconeogenic enzymes, PEPCK, fructose-1,6-bisphosphatase, and the catalytic subunit of the G6Pase complex [93]. PGC-1α is able to mediate its effects on transcription of these genes by coactivating hepatocyte nuclear factor 4α (HNF-4α) or a member of the forkhead transcription factor gene family, FOXO-1 [93, 94]. The interaction of PGC-1 with FOXO-1 may be particularly relevant, as this protein is known to be phosphorylated by Akt-1, a component of the insulin signaling cascade. Phosphorylation of FOXO-1 by Akt-1 impairs its capacity to stimulate the expression of gluconeogenic genes. Thus, a unifying model for coordinate regulation of gluconeogenic gene expression is that the rise in cAMP levels engendered by glucagon action in the fasted state increases PGC-1 expression, which via FOXO-1 and HNF-4α stimulates expression of the gluconeogenic genes. These effects are antagonized by insulin in the fed state via Akt-1-mediated phosphorylation of FOXO-1, resulting in suppression of gluconeogenesis. How these regulatory elements may interact with other players such as CREB and the GR remains to be defined.

Insights from Metabolic Engineering Studies Targeting PEPCK or G6Pase Activity in Liver

As was the case for glycolysis, the metabolic impact of individual gluconeogenic enzymes has been investigated via genetic engineering experiments. For example, PEPCK has been overexpressed and knocked out in transgenic mice. Overexpression of PEPCK results in a condition resembling type 2 diabetes, with an increase in fasting blood glucose and a clear impairment in glucose disposal in response to a glucose challenge [95]. Surprisingly, tissue-specific knockout of PEPCK in liver causes little to no change in fasting blood glucose levels, but does result in hepatic steatosis despite an increase in expression of enzymes of fatty acid oxidation in the absence of any change in glucagon or insulin levels [96]. Further investigation of the mechanism by which blood glucose levels are maintained in the absence of hepatic PEPCK reveals that gluconeogenesis from lactate or pyruvate is almost completely suppressed, whereas total hepatic gluconeogenesis is only mildly diminished, because of normal gluconeogenesis from glycerol [97]. Extrahepatic gluconeogenesis may also be increased in these animals.

Another mechanism for impairing normal hepatic glucose disposal might be to increase the activity of the G6Pase enzyme complex. Whereas several studies have demonstrated a strong correlation between the level of expression of the G6Pase catalytic subunit and syndromes of dysregulated fuel homeostasis, they do not prove that G6Pase catalytic subunit overexpression directly contributes to impaired metabolic regulation. Moreover, the potential contribution of the T1 translocase component of the complex is not addressed by these studies. Overexpression of the G6Pase catalytic subunit in rat hepatocytes caused a large increase in G6P hydrolysis and an attendant reduction in intracellular G6P levels [98]. This led to substantial decreases in glycolytic flux and glycogen deposition, and a parallel increase in gluconeogenesis. Overexpression of the T1 translocase in rat hepatocytes caused a smaller but still significant increase in G6P hydrolysis [99]. This resulted in a similar inhibition of glycogen formation as observed with overexpression of the catalytic subunit, but a much smaller impairment of glycolytic flux [99]. The more pronounced effect of T1 on glycogen deposition may be explained by activation of glucose-1-phosphate by T1 translocase overexpression, whereas this maneuver had no effect on fructose-6-phosphate hydrolysis; note that the former is an intermediate in glycogen synthesis but not glycolysis [99]. Thus, overexpression of either the T1 translocase or the G6Pase catalytic subunit is sufficient to alter the overall rate of G6P hydrolysis by the G6Pase enzyme complex, but with a more pronounced metabolic impact achieved by expression of the catalytic subunit.

Normal rats infused with an adenovirus encoding the G6Pase catalytic subunit exhibited a 2–3-fold increase in enzyme activity in liver, with no change in other tissues surveyed, and showed several of the abnormalities associated with early-stage type 2 diabetes, including glucose intolerance, hyperinsulinemia, a marked decrease in hepatic glycogen content, and increased peripheral (muscle) TG stores [91]. These findings are consistent with the idea that increased activity of the G6Pase complex in liver can make a significant contribution to the development of type 2 diabetes, and clearly establish the importance of tight control of the balance between glucose phosphorylation and G6P hydrolysis in regulation of hepatic glucose balance.

GLYCOGEN METABOLISM

General Considerations

Mammalian cells are able to store glucose in the form of large polymers known as glycogen. Fully formed glycogen particles can contain thousands of glucose molecules, and can easily have a molecular mass in excess of 1×10^6 Da. In liver, glycogen can be synthesized via a "direct" pathway, involving transport of glucose from the blood, phosphorylation of glucose by glucokinase to yield G6P, conversion of G6P to glucose-1-phosphate by phosphoglucomutase, "activation" of glucose-1-phosphate by conversion to UDP-glucose by UDP-glucose pyrophosphorylase, and finally, addition of glucose molecules one at a time to a growing glycogen particle by glycogen synthase. The mature glycogen particle has a highly branched structure, which is created by a branching enzyme that moves blocks of glucose residues and links them in α-1,6-glycosidic linkages. Glycogen can also be synthesized by an "indirect" pathway involving synthesis of G6P from gluconeogenic precursors, after which G6P enters the same sequence of glycogenic reactions as utilized in the direct pathway [100]. This is made possible by continued gluconeogenesis in the early phases of the fasted to fed transition, as discussed earlier. Early studies revealed that the indirect pathway can account for as much as 80% of the glycogen synthesized in response to oral glucose infusion in overnight fasted rats [101, 102]. Subsequent studies have shown that approximately 30–60% of liver glycogen synthesis occurs via the indirect pathway in humans, with the exact percentage contribution determined by the time elapsed between meals [103, 104]. The difference in relative contributions of this pathway in the two species may relate to the fact that rats in an overnight fasted condition degrade nearly all of their liver glycogen, making them reliant on high rates of gluconeogenesis to protect against hypoglycemia, whereas humans degrade a much smaller fraction of their liver glycogen stores in an overnight fast. A schematic summary of the direct and indirect pathways of glycogen synthesis is provided in Figure 4.

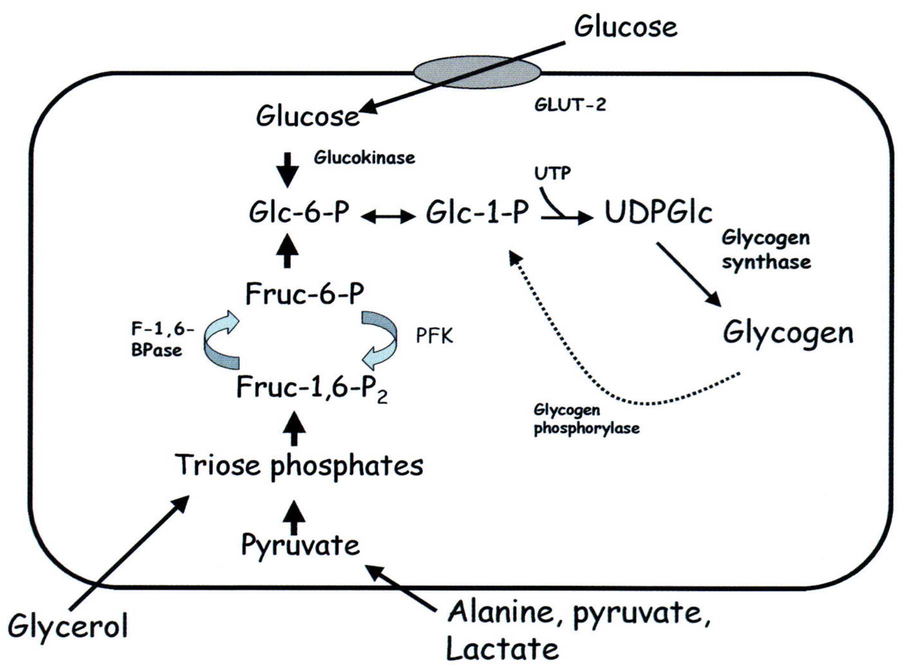

Figure 4 Direct and indirect pathways of glycogen synthesis in liver. In the transition from the fasted to the fed state, glycogen can be synthesized via a direct pathway, involving transport of glucose into liver cells, phosphorylation by glucokinase, conversion of glucose-6-phosphate (Glc-6-P) to glucose-1-phosphate (Glc-1-P) by phosphoglucomutase, "activation" of Glc-1-P by conversion to UDP-glucose (UDPGlc) by UDP-Glc pyrophosphorylase, and addition of glucose residues one by one to a growing glycogen particle in the glycogen synthase reaction. The indirect pathway of glycogen synthesis involves the synthesis of Glc-6-P from alanine, pyruvate, lactate, and glycerol via gluconeogenesis. Whereas in the fasted state the Glc-6-P derived from gluconeogenesis is hydrolyzed to free glucose, in the transition from the fasted to the fed state, gluconeogenically derived Glc-6-P is diverted into glycogen synthesis. The enzymatic reactions that convert Glc-6-P to glycogen in the indirect pathway are the same as those used in the direct pathway

Glycogen degradation, or glycogenolysis, is initiated by removal of glucose residues one at a time from the outer, nonreducing termini of the glycogen particle, catalyzed by the active form of glycogen phosphorylase (phosphorylase a). The enzyme catalyzes phosphorolytic cleavage of the α-1,4-glycosidic bonds of the glucose polymer to yield glucose-1-phosphate. Glucose-1-phosphate is then converted to G6P by the same phosphoglucomutase employed for glycogenesis. Glycogen degradation in liver is most active in fasting or insulinopenic states, and the physiological goal is to deliver glucose to the circulation to support the needs of the brain and the central nervous system. Thus, most of the G6P that is formed from glycogenolysis in the fasted state is hydrolyzed to free glucose via the G6Pase complex, and then transported into the circulation by GLUT-2 and other emergent mechanisms discussed below.

Regulation of Glycogen Metabolism

Glycogen metabolism is regulated in large part via reciprocal changes in the activities of the rate-limiting enzyme of glycogenesis, glycogen synthase, and the rate-limiting enzyme of glycogenolysis, glycogen phosphorylase. Activation of glycogen phosphorylase in fasted or insulinopenic conditions occurs as the culmination of a "glycogenolytic cascade" that is initiated by the binding of glucagon or β-adrenergic agonists to their receptors in liver cells [4]. Activation of adenylate cyclase by the Gαs heterotrimeric GTP-binding protein results in accumulation of cAMP and activation of cAMP-dependent protein kinase (PKA). This is turn leads to phosphorylation and activation of phosphorylase kinase. Finally, phosphorylase kinase phosphorylates glycogen phosphorylase on serine 14, thereby converting the enzyme from its inactive (phosphorylase b) to its active (phosphorylase a) form [105].

Similar to glycogen phosphorylase, glycogen synthase is phosphorylated under fasting conditions, albeit at a cluster of serine residues rather than a single one [106]. However, unlike phosphorylase, phosphorylation of glycogen synthase *inactivates* rather than activates the enzyme. Phosphorylation of glycogen synthase is catalyzed primarily by PKA and glycogen synthase kinase 3. In sum, a net activation of glycogenolysis is promoted under fasted or insulinopenic conditions via phosphorylation of glycogen phosphorylase and glycogen synthase, leading to activation of the former and decreased activity of the latter. It should be noted, however, that this reciprocal regulation of phosphorylase and synthase may not always be complete. Thus, in controlled experimental circumstances, such as during hyperinsulinemic, euglycemic clamp protocols in humans, a decrease in net hepatic glycogenolysis can be demonstrated, which is due to a large activation of glycogen synthase flux, but without a decrease in phosphorylase flux [107]. This and related studies [108] demonstrate that glycogenolysis can continue during periods of net glycogen synthesis, suggesting that a significant portion of the phosphorylated glucose derived from glycogenolysis in liver can be recycled back into glycogen. Thus, control of liver glycogen metabolism should not be viewed simply as regulation of perfectly reciprocal "on" and "off" switches, but more as control of net flux via a predominance of activity of one pathway relative to the other.

Whereas glycogenolysis is promoted by phosphorylation of glycogen synthase and glycogen phosphorylase, it follows that a central regulatory event for stimulating glycogen synthesis in the transition from the fasted to the fed state is to dephosphorylate these key regulatory enzymes. A common protein phosphatase, protein phosphatase 1 (PP-1), is used to dephosphorylate both glycogen synthase and glycogen phosphorylase. The dephosphorylation mechanism is complemented by several other regulatory events. G6P binds to glycogen synthase, causing a conformational change that renders it a better substrate for PP-1 [106, 109]. Similarly, glucose binds to glycogen phosphorylase a, again causing a conformational change that enhances its rate of PP-1-mediated dephosphorylation and decreases enzyme activity [105]. The expression of the glucose transporter GLUT-2 and the glucose phosphorylating enzyme glucokinase in liver allows the levels of free glucose and G6P to rise in proportion to changes in circulating glucose concentrations, contributing to effective regulation of glycogen phosphorylase and glycogen synthase activities. In addition, the rise in insulin levels in the postprandial state stimulates phosphorylation and inhibition of glycogen synthase kinase 3 (GSK-3), via a branch of the insulin signaling pathway that includes PI-3 kinase and Akt-1 (protein kinase B) [106, 110]. This results in less GSK-3-mediated phosphorylation of glycogen synthase, leaving the enzyme in a less phosphorylated, and therefore more active condition.

Spatial Organization of Glycogen Metabolism: Emergent Role of Glycogen-targeting Subunits of PP-1

The common use of PP-1 for dephosphorylation of both glycogen synthase and glycogen phosphorylase is not accidental, and brings us to yet another example of the importance of spatial organization in regulation of hepatic carbohydrate metabolism. It is now appreciated that enzymes of glycogen metabolism, including the regulatory enzyme PP-1, are assembled in a multi-protein complex that is also associated with the glycogen particle. Moreover, this spatial association contributes to appropriate activation or suppression of glycogen synthesis in response to changes in nutritional conditions. The scaffolding proteins that organize glycogen metabolism are known collectively as glycogen-targeting subunits of PP-1 (hereafter referred to generally as glycogen-targeting subunits) [111]. These proteins are part of a much larger family of more than 50 PP-1-binding proteins that deliver the enzyme to a wide array of substrates and cellular addresses, allowing PP-1 to participate in diverse cellular processes such as glycogen metabolism, cell division, vesicle fusion, and ion channel function [112, 113]. PP-1-binding proteins target the enzyme to the nucleus, plasma membrane, neuronal dendrites, myosin filaments, or glycogen particles [112, 113]. These interactions allow for compartmentalized activation of the phosphatase by a variety of extracellular signals, resulting in the specific dephosphorylation of discrete pools of proteins within the cell.

Four members of the glycogen-targeting subunit gene family have been well described [111]. The targeting subunit that is preferentially expressed in striated skeletal muscle, termed G_M/R_{Gl}, was the first to be cloned [114, 115]. G_L is a 35-kDa protein that is preferentially expressed in liver [116]. Protein targeting to glycogen (PTG) [117], also known as PPP1R5 [118], and a fourth form, PPP1R6 [119], are similar in size to G_L but differ from G_L and G_M/R_{Gl} in that they are expressed in a wide variety of tissues based on Northern blot analysis. All of the targeting subunits are able to bind glycogen and PP-1, and exhibit varying capacities for binding of glycogen synthase, glycogen phosphorylase, and phosphorylase kinase [111]. The sequence homology among family members is centered around the PP-1- and putative-glycogen-binding regions. All four family members contain the consensus PP-1-binding motif (R/K) (V/I) XF. An obvious distinguishing feature of G_M/R_{Gl} is that it is approximately three times as large as the other family members. The NH_2-terminal domain of G_M/R_{Gl} is homologous to the other family members and contains its PP-1- and glycogen-binding regions. The large COOH-terminal domain of G_M/R_{Gl} shares no homology with other family members, and contains a hydrophobic sarcoplasmic-reticulum binding domain [114]. G_M/R_{Gl} also contains two potential phosphorylation site, a unique site 1 with RRGS (serine 46 in the human G_M/R_{Gl} sequence) and a PKA-mediated phosphorylation site 2 (serine 65 in the human G_M/R_{Gl} sequence). A schematic rendering of these various targeting subunits is provided in Figure 5.

Some important insights into the biological function of the various targeting subunits as well as their potential utility for improving control of hepatic glucose disposal have been gleaned from overexpression studies in hepatocytes and liver of normal and diabetic animals [111]. In early studies of this type, overexpression of PTG in adipocytes or hepatocytes resulted in potent activation of glycogen synthesis, with a concomitant increase in

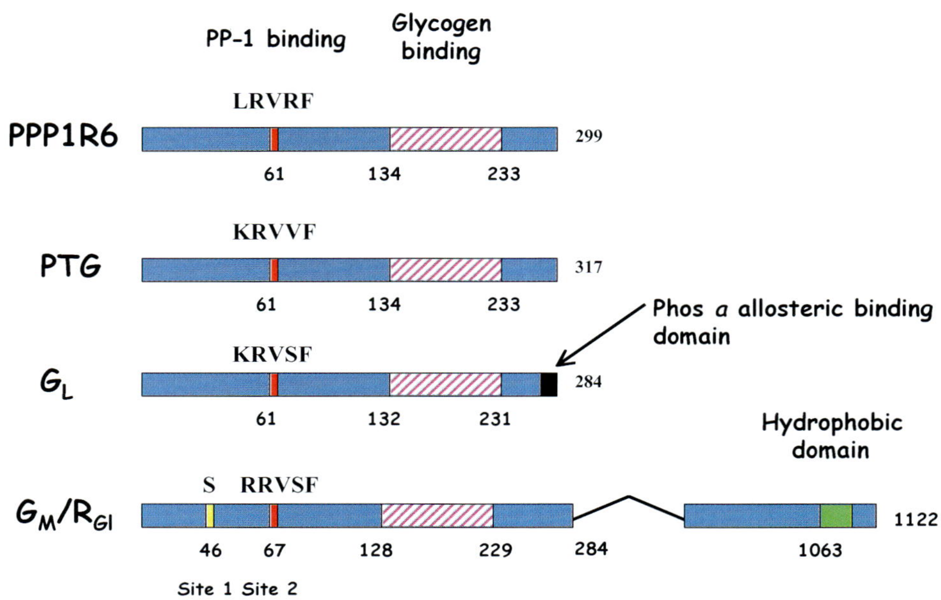

Figure 5 Schematic alignment of the mammalian glycogen-targeting subunits of protein phosphatase-1. Four members of the family are shown. G_M/R_{Gl} is expressed primarily in striated muscle, G_L is expressed primarily in liver, and protein targeting to glycogen (PTG) and PPP1R6 are expressed in many tissues. G_M/R_{Gl} is approximately three times larger than the other forms, and its C-terminal extension has no homology to the other family members. The C-terminal domain of G_M/R_{Gl} contains a patch of hydrophobic amino acids that are thought to mediate its binding to sarcoplasmic reticulum. G_M/R_{Gl} also contains two serines (designated site 1 and site 2) that are phosphorylated in response to glycogenolytic agents. None of the other forms contain serine at site 1, and contain varying sequences at site 2, as shown for each form. A conserved glycogen-binding motif is also indicated. Finally, G_L is the only targeting subunit that exhibits allosteric regulation by phosphorylase a, via binding of the enzyme to the C-terminal tail of the G_L molecule. Numbers under each targeting subunit refer to the amino acid sequence of each protein

G6P-independent glycogen synthase activity, which was likely due to activation of the enzyme by PP-1-mediated dephosphorylation [117, 120]. In hepatocytes with PTG overexpression, a large increase in glycogen synthesis was observed even in the complete absence of carbohydrates or insulin in the culture medium [120]. These data suggest that PTG overexpression activates the conversion of gluconeogenic precursors into glycogen. PTG overexpression also prevented the normal glycogenolytic action of agents such as forskolin and glucagon [120]. Overexpression of PTG in liver of normal rats improved whole-body glucose tolerance [121], but in contrast to studies involving overexpression of glucokinase or the bifunctional enzyme summarized earlier, this was achieved without perturbation of lipid homeostasis. ^{13}C-glucose NMR was used to study the pathways of glycogen synthesis in these animals, with the finding that PTG overexpression activated both direct and indirect pathways of glycogen synthesis [121]. Finally, overexpression of PTG in liver of normal rats prevented the normal activation of glycogenolysis in response to fasting, consistent with the finding of impaired glycogenolysis in response to forskolin and glucagon in PTG-overexpressing hepatocytes. Thus PTG expression resulted in improved glucose tolerance, but also appeared to cause a form of glycogen storage disease when overexpressed in liver of normal animals.

These findings led to investigation of the possibility that other members of the family of glycogen-targeting subunits, such as G_M/R_{Gl} or G_L, might have regulatory features that would allow them to stimulate glucose disposal while still allowing substrate- and hormone-mediated regulation of glycogen turnover. To this end, recombinant adenoviruses containing G_L, G_M/R_{Gl}, and a truncated version of G_M/R_{Gl} that lacked its C-terminal 700 amino acids, termed $G_M\Delta C$, were prepared. When controlled for extent of overexpression, the targeting subunits were found to exhibit a rank order of glycogenic potency in hepatocytes of $G_L > PTG > G_M\Delta C > G_M/R_{Gl}$ [122, 123]. Furthermore, cells with overexpressed $G_M\Delta C$ were unique in that only in these cells was glycogen efficiently degraded in response to lowering of media glucose concentrations, stimulation with forskolin, or the combination of both maneuvers [123].

The effects of two types of genes that stimulate glucose disposal, glucokinase, and glycogen-targeting subunits were compared in more detail in isolated hepatocytes [123]. Overexpression of either glycogen-targeting subunits or glucokinase stimulated glycogen synthesis in response to glucose and insulin. Glycogen synthesis in glucokinase-overexpressing cells was more dependent on the extracellular glucose concentration than in cells with overexpressed glycogen-targeting subunits. Overexpression of glucokinase also caused a much larger stimulation of radiolabeled glucose uptake than did overexpression of glycogen-targeting subunits. Glucokinase overexpression, but not glycogen-targeting subunit overexpression, significantly increased lactate production. Interestingly, co-overexpression of a single glycogen-targeting subunit and glucokinase resulted in an additive effect on glycogen synthesis, while co-overexpression of two different glycogen-targeting subunits did not. This suggests that targeting subunits and glucokinase activate glycogen synthesis through different pathways. To investigate this further, NMR was used to measure the labeling pattern of carbons in glycogen-glucose in hepatocytes incubated with ^2H_2O [123]. This allowed an estimate of the relative contributions of carbon emanating from the level of TCA cycle intermediates, triose phosphates, or hexose phosphates to glycogen synthesis, as reflected by the relative deuterium labeling of carbons 6, 5, and 2 [124, 125]. This analysis demonstrated that cells with overexpressed glycogen-targeting subunits synthesize a larger portion of their glycogen from the level of TCA cycle intermediates than do cells with overexpressed glucokinase. Therefore, overexpression of glucokinase may increase the pool of G6P, consequently activating glycolysis, glucose uptake, and glycogen synthesis through a "push" mechanism. Overexpression of glycogen-targeting subunits has little effect on G6P levels [120], and therefore seems to activate glycogen synthesis more through a "pull" mechanism that increases the contribution made by gluconeogenesis to glycogen synthesis. The increased glycogen synthesis from gluconeogenic precursors in cells with glycogen-targeting-subunit overexpression suggests that the effect of these molecules to enhance glucose tolerance may occur in part via diversion of gluconeogenic flux away from hepatic glucose production and into glycogen deposition.

Metabolic Engineering Studies with Glycogen-targeting Subunits *In Vivo*

These *in vitro* findings led to a comparison of the metabolic effects of hepatic overexpression of $G_M\Delta C$ and the most glycogenic of all the isoforms, G_L, *in vivo*. At similar levels of overexpression in liver, $G_M\Delta C$ but not G_L lowered blood glucose levels toward normal during an oral glucose tolerance test (OGTT) in rats made insulin resistant by feeding on a high-fat diet [126]. Liver glycogen levels after OGTT were increased by more than 100% in both G_L and $G_M\Delta C$ overexpressing rats compared with control animals. However, rats with overexpression of G_L had significantly increased liver glycogen content in the fed state and failed to efficiently remove the accumulated glycogen in the fasted state compared with control animals. In contrast, rats with overexpression of $G_M\Delta C$ had normal liver glycogen content in the fed state and efficiently degraded liver glycogen in the fasted state to near-normal fasting levels. Thus, overexpression of the highly glycogenic targeting subunit G_L caused glycogen stores to be replete in the fasted state, allowing little further synthesis of glycogen to occur during glucose challenge. In contrast, animals with overexpressed $G_M\Delta C$ were able to respond to glycogenolytic signals, thereby allowing them to maintain low fasting glycogen levels, in turn providing storage capacity during the glucose challenge.

In light of these encouraging findings in a model of diet-induced glucose intolerance, the capacity of $G_M\Delta C$ to reverse frank hyperglycemia associated with STZ-induced diabetes in rats was investigated [127]. Three new findings emerged from these studies. First, $G_M\Delta C$ expression in liver was found to be sufficient to fully normalize blood glucose levels and glycogen storage in this model of insulin-deficient diabetes. Second, this normalization occurred despite very low levels of liver glucokinase expression. Finally, $G_M\Delta C$ expression in liver curtailed food intake in STZ-injected rats, which were otherwise hyperphagic. This reduction in food intake occurred despite dramatic lowering of circulating insulin and leptin levels in the STZ-injected animals.

These findings concerning hepatic expression of $G_M\Delta C$ in liver of STZ-induced diabetic rats deserve some additional comment. The normalization of blood glucose and liver glycogen by hepatic $G_M\Delta C$ expression is remarkable in that it occurred in the face of a 68% reduction in circulating insulin levels. This is consistent with the observation that glycogen synthesis in hepatocytes with overexpressed glycogen-targeting subunits is glucose-dependent, but largely insulin-independent [122, 123]. Thus, the data in sum argue that *appropriately regulated* augmentation of hepatic glycogen storage is sufficient to reverse perturbations in glucose homeostasis caused by either impaired insulin action or impaired insulin secretion. In support of this idea, overexpression of another targeting subunit, G_L, in liver of insulin-resistant [126] or STZ-injected diabetic rats [127] resulted in unregulated glycogen overstorage in liver, and a consequent failure to stably reverse glucose intolerance or hyperglycemia, respectively.

Glucokinase is generally thought of as a key regulatory step in hepatic glucose metabolism, as described in detail earlier. It was therefore quite surprising that $G_M\Delta C$ expression in liver was able to lower blood glucose levels and normalize liver glycogen content in STZ-injected rats in the face of a dramatic reduction in glucokinase expression. The mechanism by which $G_M\Delta C$ overcomes the decrease in glucokinase expression in insulin-deficient animals remains to be defined. One possibility is that $G_M\Delta C$, by activating glycogen synthesis, exerts a "pull" on the G6P pool, preventing a rise in G6P levels that would normally cause product inhibition of hexokinase I. Alternatively, $G_M\Delta C$ expression may divert gluconeogenic precursors away from the G6Pase reaction and into the glycogen storage pathway, thereby contributing to lowering of glucose levels via a decrease in hepatic glucose production as suggested earlier and in agreement with ^2H_2O NMR studies [123]. While these ideas will require further investigation, it has become clear that normalization of blood glucose can be achieved by manipulation of steps distal to glucokinase, even when this important enzyme is present at very low levels.

Another possible mechanism contributing to lowering of blood glucose in animals with hepatic $G_M\Delta C$ expression is their decrease in food intake relative to controls. This is clearly not the only mechanism at work, however, based on a study of the effects of leptin infusion in STZ-induced diabetic rats [128]. In these studies, infusion of leptin at a rate that allowed circulating levels of the hormone to be restored to those found in non-STZ-injected controls resulted in complete normalization of food intake. Hyperglycemia was partially ameliorated in these animals, but clearly not normalized. Pair-fed studies were also performed and failed to normalize blood glucose levels in STZ-treated animals [129, 130]. In contrast, expression of $G_M\Delta C$ in STZ-injected animals not only normalized food intake but also completely normalized blood glucose levels.

There are several possible mechanisms by which $G_M\Delta C$ expression in liver could lead to normalization of food intake in STZ-injected animals, including alteration of leptin levels, amelioration of caloric spilling in the urine secondary to control of hyperglycemia, and a direct effect of liver glycogen repletion on food intake. STZ injection caused a large decrease in circulating leptin levels in both control and AdCMV-$G_M\Delta C$-treated rats, making it unlikely that leptin is playing an important role in $G_M\Delta C$-mediated change in food intake [127]. However, $G_M\Delta C$ expression caused a clear reduction in excretion of glucose in the urine. This amelioration of caloric "spilling" was proportional to the reduction in food intake [127]. This finding is consistent with the idea that $G_M\Delta C$ expression lowered food intake secondary to its effect on blood glucose. However, the factors that allowed $G_M\Delta C$-expressing rats to sense the reduction in caloric spilling and translate this into a reduction in food intake remain to be defined, especially since these changes occurred at a time when hormones known to regulate food intake such as insulin and leptin [131] were present at low levels. It remains possible that levels of peptides that influence feeding behaviors and metabolic homeostasis such as adiopnectin, glucagon-like peptide 1, ghrelin, or members of the pancreatic polypeptide gene family could be altered by $G_M\Delta C$ expression, and this will require further investigation.

Finally, it is possible that food intake in STZ-injected, $G_M\Delta C$-expressing rats is related to changes in glucose disposal and storage in the liver. Fifty years ago, Mayer [132] developed a "glucostatic theory" of feeding behavior in which changes in glucose utilization rates were proposed to regulate hunger and satiety. Russek [133] first proposed that hepatic glucosensors respond to the difference in arterial–portal glucose levels to control food intake. Later, a "glycogenostatic" model in which hepatic

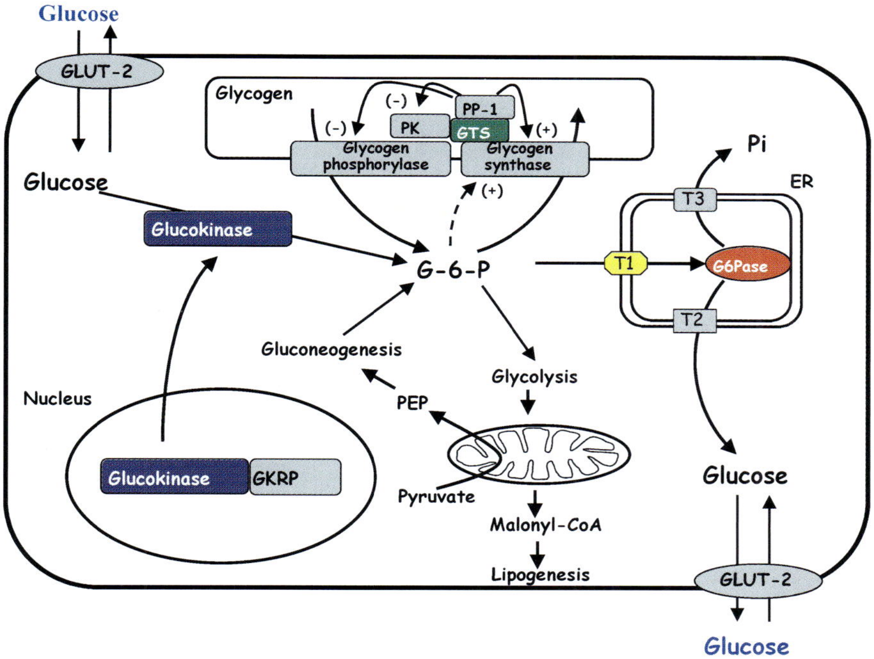

Figure 6 Spatial organization of glucose and glycogen metabolism in liver cells. The figure shows some of the key regulatory steps controlling hepatic glucose disposal and production, and emphasizes how these steps are compartmentalized. Examples of this include translocation of glucokinase from the nucleus to the cytoplasm in response to nutritional stimulation, conversion of pyruvate to phosphoenolpyruvate (PEP) via a series of enzymatic reactions occurring in the mitochondria and cytosol, localization and regulation of enzymes of glycogen metabolism via the glycogen-targeting subunits (GTS) of protein phosphatase 1 (pp-1), and sequestration of the glucose-6-phosphatase (G6Pase) catalytic subunit in the endoplasmic reticulum (ER). Other abbreviations used: PK = phosphorylase kinase; T1, T2, T3 = components of the glucose-6-phosphatase enzyme complex serving as translocases for glucose-6-phosphate, glucose, and inorganic phosphate, respectively; GKRP = glucokinase regulatory protein; G-6-P = glucose-6-phosphate

glycogen stores play a central role in regulating food intake and energy balance was proposed [134–136], but direct and consistent experimental support for this idea has not emerged. Interestingly, expression of the targeting subunit G_L in STZ-injected animals caused sharp but transient decreases in food intake and circulating glucose levels, with a return to high rates of food consumption in parallel with the return of hyperglycemia. Because the G_L-expressing animals had much higher liver glycogen content than did the $G_M\Delta C$-expressing animals at sacrifice, these data argue against a primary role for liver glycogen stores as a regulator of food intake. However, it remains possible that a sudden increment in hepatic glycogen storage, such as induced upon initial overexpression of G_L, could generate satiety signals.

It is remarkable that expression of $G_M\Delta C$ in liver not only reverses glucose intolerance in insulin-resistant rats but also normalizes blood glucose in STZ-induced diabetic animals. However, we recognize that while $G_M\Delta C$ is an effective reagent for treatment of diabetes in rodents, its application to human diabetes is hampered by the lack of safe and efficacious vectors for delivery of foreign genes to liver of diabetic patients. Small molecules that affect glycogen-targeting subunit in useful ways in liver may be difficult to design, as liver expresses a mixture of G_L and PTG, which are targeting subunit isoforms that when overexpressed seem to confer a lack of response to normal glycogenolytic signals. Nevertheless, the surprising demonstration of a glucose lowering effect of $G_M\Delta C$ in the background of depressed hepatic glucokinase expression and insulin insufficiency may place new focus on drugs that activate liver glycogen storage as a means of controlling blood glucose.

Glycogen-targeting subunits represent another example of agents that provide spatial organization to pathways of hepatic glucose metabolism. In light of the several examples that have been provided in this chapter, an overall schematic rendering is provided in Figure 6.

Potential Drug Targets Related to Glycogen Metabolism

Other groups have focused on proteins other than glycogen-targeting subunits as potential drug targets for altering hepatic glucose disposal via changes in glycogen metabolism, including glycogen phosphorylase and GSK-3. Several compounds have been described that directly inhibit glycogen phosphorylase and glycogenolysis in primary cell cultures [137, 138]. Interestingly, some of these inhibitors [e.g., compound 13 (CP-91,149) and compound 14 (CP-320,626)] also inhibit gluconeogenesis *in vitro* [137]. Moreover, chronic administration of compound 14 caused sustained improvement in glucose tolerance and fed glucose levels in diabetic *ob/ob* mice.

GSK3 inhibitors mimic the effect of insulin to activate glycogen synthesis *in vitro* [139]. Interestingly, some of the compounds also repress the expression of gluconeogenic genes *in vitro* [140]. Further studies show that GSK3 inhibitors (CHIR98023, CHIR99021) improve oral glucose tolerance in ZDF rats, mostly by enhancing liver glycogen synthesis [141]. However, since GSK3 plays a key role in the regulation of many cellular functions [110], the potential side effects of this class of compounds must be carefully evaluated.

Finally, a recent study suggests a strategy for enhancing hepatic glucose disposal that simultaneously activates glycolysis and glycogen synthesis. As discussed earlier, exposure of isolated hepatocytes to fructose leads to potent activation of glucokinase, probably via stimulation of dissociation of the glucokinase/GKRP complex. One predicted consequence of this maneuver will be to raise G6P levels via increased flux through the glucokinase step. To evaluate the impact of fructose administration *in vivo*, ^{13}C NMR was used to study liver glycogen metabolism noninvasively in normal human subjects under euglycemic, hyperinsulinemic conditions [142]. These studies revealed a clear increase in net hepatic glycogen synthesis in subjects that received a low-dose infusion of fructose relative to control subjects. The findings are consistent with a model of an effect of fructose to increase glucokinase activity and G6P content in liver, leading in turn to activation of glycogen synthase by a G6P allosteric mechanism. This relatively nontoxic approach for enhancing hepatic glucose disposal deserves further investigation.

GLUCOSE TRANSPORT IN LIVER—MULTIPLE MECHANISMS?

Having discussed several of the major metabolic pathways for catabolism, storage, and synthesis of glucose in liver, the chapter concludes with a discussion of glucose transport into and out of liver cells. Again, this topic is relevant because of very recent insights. A family of facilitated glucose transporters with analogy to the family of hexokinase genes in terms of tissue distribution and kinetic properties emerged from the work of several laboratories in the late 1980s and the early 1990s [143, 144]. The major glucose transporter isoform of liver and pancreatic islets, GLUT-2, was the second member of the family identified [145, 146]. Like glucokinase, GLUT-2 has a low affinity (high K_m) for glucose and a high capacity of glucose transport relative to other members of its gene family. All of the facilitated glucose transporters are equilibrium-based transporters that are capable of bidirectional glucose transport across cellular membranes, with the directionality of activity determined by the relative glucose concentrations on the outside versus the inside of the cell. Based on these findings, it was assumed that GLUT-2-mediated transport represented the only mechanism for import and export of glucose in liver cells. Indeed, mice with homozygous knockout of the GLUT-2 gene were found to be hyperglycemic and hypoinsulinemic, with elevated levels of FFAs and ketones [147]. However, further analysis of hepatic function in these animals revealed normal hepatic glucose production in terms of the hyperglycemic response to glucagon injection and the rate of release of glucose from isolated hepatocytes [148]. The non-GLUT-2-dependent pathway of glucose transport was found to be inhibited by exposure of cells to reduced temperatures, and by progesterone, leading the authors to suggest the possible involvement of a membrane-traffic-based mechanism for glucose transport in liver cells that complements the facilitated transport mechanism. Further study revealed that GLUT-2-deficient hepatocytes are defective in activation of glycogenolysis in response to a lowering of blood glucose [149]. This may be ascribable to their failure to appropriately lower G6P levels during fasting, leading in turn to sustained allosteric activation of glycogen synthase, and possible increases in glucokinase activity via effects on GKRP. The authors ascribe the elevation in G6P to an impairment in glucose export during fasting, resulting in rephosphorylation of a cytosolic glucose pool. Further study will be required to fully understand the physiological significance of this alternative mechanism for glucose export in liver.

SUMMARY AND PERSPECTIVE

Regulation of hepatic carbohydrate metabolism has been a field of intensive study for more than 100 years. This undoubtably leads many scientists and clinicians to assume that a complete understanding of all of the biochemical and molecular machinery required for achieving regulation of glycolysis, gluconeogensis, and glycogen metabolism in liver has long been in hand. It is hoped that this chapter will give pause to those who have made such assumptions, and reinvigorate others who continue to investigate unresolved issues in the field. The explosion in recent knowledge gained by investigation of transcriptional networks, the role of protein/protein interactions, and novel small molecule regulators of key enzymes, while impressive, still represents an unfinished canvas. Further investigation is likely to guide the development of novel pharmaceutical agents that can ameliorate the imbalance in glucose disposal and glucose production that afflicts patients with diabetes.

REFERENCES

1. Cusi K, DeFronzo RA. Pathogenesis of type 2 diabetes. In Jefferson LS, Cherrington AD (eds), *Handbook of Physiology—The Endocrine Pancreas and Regulation of Metabolism.* Oxford: Oxford University Press, 2001; pp 1115–68.
2. Shulman GI, Barrett EJ, Sherwin RS. Integrated fuel metabolism. In Porte D, Sherwin RS, Baron A (eds), *Ellenberg and Rifkin's Diabetes mellitus*, 6th edn. New York: McGraw-Hill, 2003; pp 1–14.
3. Young FC. Claude Bernard and the theory of the glycogenic function of the liver. *Ann Sci* 1937; 2: 47–83.
4. Sutherland EW, Robinson GA. The role of cyclic AMP in the control of carbohydrate metabolism. *Diabetes* 1969; 18: 797–819.
5. Wilson JE. Regulation of mammalian hexokinase activity. In Beitner R (ed), *Regulation of Carbohydrate Metabolism.* Boca Raton, FL: CRC Press, 1984; pp 45–85.
6. Matschinsky FM. Regulation of pancreatic beta-cell glucokinase: from basics to therapeutics. *Diabetes* 2002; 51 (suppl 3): S394–404.
7. Hughes SD, Quaade C, Milburn JL, Cassidy L, Newgard CB. Expression of normal and novel glucokinase mRNAs in anterior pituitary and islet cells. *J Biol Chem* 1991; 266: 4521–30.
8. Jetton TL, Liang Y, Pettepher CC, Zimmerman EC, Cox FG, Horvath K, Matschinsky FM, Magnuson MA. Analysis of upstream glucokinase promoter activity in transgenic mice and identification of glucokinase in rare neuroendocrine cells in the brain and gut. *J Biol Chem* 1994; 269: 3641–54.
9. Newgard CB. Regulatory role of glucose transport and phosphorylation in pancreatic islet β-cells. *Diabetes Rev* 1996; 4: 191–205.
10. Iynedjian PB, Ucla C, Mach B. Molecular cloning of glucokinase cDNA: developmental and dietary regulation of glucokinase mRNA in rat liver. *J Biol Chem* 1987; 262: 6032–8.
11. Andreone TL, Printz RL, Pilkis SJ, Magnuson MA, Granner DK. The amino acid sequence of rat liver glucokinase deduced from cloned cDNA. *J Biol Chem* 1989; 264: 363–9.
12. Iynedjian PB, Pilot P-R, Nouspikel T, Milburn JL, Quaade C, Hughes S, Newgard CB. Differential expression and regulation of the glucokinase gene in liver and islets: implications for control of glucose homeostasis. *Proc Natl Acad Sci USA* 1989; 86: 7838–42.
13. Malaisse WJ, Malaisse-Lagae F, Davies DR, Vandercammne A, VanSchaftingen E. Regulation of glucokinase by a fructose-1-phosphate-sensitive protein in pancreatic islets. *Eur J Biochem* 1990; 190: 539–45.
14. Dethuex M, Vandekerckhove J, Van Schaftingen E. Cloning and sequencing of rat liver cDNAs encoding the regulatory protein of glucokinase. *FEBS Lett* 1994; 321: 111–5.
15. Toyoda Y, Miwa I, Satake S, Anai M, Oka Y. Nuclear location of the regulatory protein of glucokinase in rat liver and translocation of the regulator to the cytoplasm in response to high glucose. *Biochem Biophys Res Commun* 1995; 215: 467–73.
16. Brown KS, Kalinowski SS, Megill JR, Durham SK, Mookhtiar KA. Glucokinase regulatory protein may interact with glucokinase in the hepatocyte nucleus. *Diabetes* 1997; 46: 179–86.
17. Shiota C, Coffey J, Grimsby J, Grippo JF, Magnuson MA. Nuclear import of hepatic glucokinase depends upon glucokinase regulatory protein, whereas export is due to a nuclear export signal sequence in glucokinase. *J Biol Chem* 1999; 274: 37125–30.
18. Niculescu L, Veiga-da-Cunha M, Van Schaftingen E. Investigation of the mechanism by which fructose, hexitols, and other compounds regulate the translocation of glucokinase in rat hepatocytes. *Biochem J* 1997; 321: 239–46.
19. Farrelly D, Brown KS, Tieman A, Ren J, Lira SA, Hagan D, Gregg R, Mookhtiar KA, Hariharan N. Mice mutant for glucokinase regulatory protein exhibit decreased liver glucokinase: a sequestration mechanism in metabolic regulation. *Proc Natl Acad Sci USA* 1999; 96: 14511–6.
20. Grimsby J, Coffey JW, Dvorozniak MT, Magram K, Li G, Matschinsky FM, Shiota C, Kaur S, Magnuson MA, Grippo JF. Characterization of glucokinase regulatory protein-deficient mice. *J Biol Chem* 2000; 275: 7826–31.
21. Van Schaftingen E, Hue L, Hers HG. Fructose-2,6-bisphosphate, the probable structure of the glucose and glucagon-sensitive stimulator of phosphofructokinase. *Biochem J* 1980; 192: 897–901.
22. Pilkis SJ, El-Maghrabi MR, Pilkis J, Claus TH, Cumming DA. Fructose-2,6-bisphosphate: a new activator of phosphofructokinase. *J Biol Chem* 1981; 256: 3171–4.
23. Uyeda K, Furuya E, Sherry AD. The structure of "activation factor" for phosphofructokinase. *J Biol Chem* 1981; 256: 8679–84.
24. El-Maghrabi MR, Claus TH, Pilkis J, Fox E, Pilkis SJ. Regulation of rat liver fructose-2,6-bisphosphatase. *J Biol Chem* 1982; 257: 7603–7.
25. Pilkis SJ, Chrisman T, Burgress B, McGrane M, Colosia A, Pilkis J, Claus TH, El-Maghrabi MR. Rat hepatic 6-phosphofructo 2-kinase/fructose-2,6-bisphosphatase: a unique bifunctional enzyme. *Adv Enzyme Regul* 1983; 21: 147–73.
26. Murray KJ, El-Maghrabi MR, Kountz PD, Lukas TJ, Soderling TR, Pilkis SJ. Amino acid sequence of the phosphorylation site of rat liver 6-phosphofructo-2-kinase/fructose-2,6-bisphosphatase. *J Biol Chem* 1984; 259: 7673–81.
27. Nishimura M, Uyeda K. Purification and characterization of a novel xyulose 5-phosphate-activated protein phosphatase catalyzing dephosphorylation of fructose-6-phosphate, 2 kinase:fructose-2,6-bisphosphatase. *J Biol Chem* 1995; 270: 26341–6.
28. Florey W, Peczon BD, Koeppe RE, Spivey HO. Kinetic properties of rat liver pyruvate kinase at cellular concentrations of enzyme, subtrates and modifiers. *Biochem J* 1974; 141: 127–31.
29. Engstrom D, Ekman P, Humble E, Zellergvist O. Pyruvate kinase. *Enzymes* 1987; 18: 47–75.
30. Yamashita H, Takenoshita M, Sakurai M, Bruick RK, Henzel WJ, Shillinglaw W, Arnot D, Uyeda K. A glucose-responsive transcription factor that regulates carbohydrate metabolism in the liver. *Proc Natl Acad Sci USA* 2001; 98: 9116–21.
31. Kabashima T, Kawaguchi T, Wadzinski BE, Uyeda K. Xyulose-5-phosphate mediates glucose-induced lipogenesis by xylulose 5-phosphate-activated protein phosphatase in rat liver. *Proc Natl Acad Sci USA* 2003; 100: 5107–12.

32. Frougel P, Vaxillaire M, Sun F, Vehlo G, Zouali H. Close linkage of glucokinase locus on chromosome 7p to early-onset noninsulin-dependent diabetes mellitus. *Nature* 1992; 356: 162–4.
33. Frougel P, Zouali H, Vionnet N, Velho G, Vaxillaire M, Sun F, Lesage S, Stoffel M, Takeda J, Passa P, Permutt A, Beckmann JS, Bell GI, Cohen D. Familial hyperglycemia due to mutations in glucokinase. *N Engl J Med* 1993; 328: 697–702.
34. Gidh-Jain M, Takeda J, Xu LZ, Lange AJ, Vionnet N, Stoffel M, Froguel P, Velho G, Sun F, Cohen D, Patel P, Lo Y-M, Hattersley AT, Luthman H, Wedell A, St Charles R, Harrison RW, Weber IT, Bell GI, Pilkis SJ. Glucokinase mutations associated with noninsulin-dependent (type 2) diabetes mellitus have decreased enzymatic activity: implications for structure/function relationships. *Proc Natl Acad Sci USA* 1993; 90: 1932–6.
35. Pilkis SJ, Weber IT, Harrison RW, Bell GI. Glucokinase: structural analysis of a protein involved in susceptibility to diabetes. *J Biol Chem* 1994; 269: 21925–8.
36. Liang Y, Kesavan P, Wang L, Niswender K, Tanizawa Y, Permutt MA, Magnuson MA, Matschinsky FM. Variable effects of maturity-onset-diabetes of youth (MODY)-associated glucokinase mutations on substrate interactions and stability of the enzyme. *Biochem J* 1995; 309: 167–73.
37. Vehlo G, Frougel P, Clement K, Pueyo ME, Rakotoambininia B, Zouali H, Passa P, Cohen D, Robert JJ. Primary pancreatic beta-cell secretory defect caused by mutations in glucokinase gene in kindreds of maturity onset diabetes of the young. *Lancet* 1992; 340: 444–8.
38. Byrne MM, Sturis J, Clement K, Vionnet N, Pueyo ME, Stoffel M, Takeda J, Passa P, Cohen D, Bell GI, Velho G, Froguel P, Polonsky KS. Insulin secretory abnormalities in subjects with hyperglycemia due to glucokinase mutations. *J Clin Invest* 1994; 93: 1122–30.
39. Newgard CB, Matschinsky FM. Substrate control of insulin release. In Jefferson J, Cherrington A (eds), *Handbook of Physiology, Vol II*. Oxford: Oxford University Press, 2001; pp 125–52.
40. Velho G, Petersen KF, Perseghin G, Hwang JH, Rothman DL, Pueyo ME, Cline GW, Froguel P, Shulman GI. Impaired hepatic glycogen synthesis in glucokinase-deficient (MODY-2) subjects. *J Clin Invest* 1996; 98: 1755–61.
41. Grupe A, Hultgren B, Ryan A, Ma YH, Bauer M, Stewart TA. Transgenic knockouts reveal a critical requirement for pancreatic β-cell glucokinase in maintaining glucose homeostasis. *Cell* 1995; 83: 69–78.
42. Bali D, Svetlanov A, Lee H-W, Fusco-Demane D, Leiser M, Li B, Barzilai N, Surana M, Hou H, Fleischer N, DePinho R, Rossetti L, Efrat S. Animal model for maturity-onset diabetes of the young generated by disruption of the mouse glucokinase gene. *J Biol Chem* 1995; 270: 21464–7.
43. Terauchi Y, Sakura H, Yasuda K, Iwamoto K, Takahashi N, Ito K, Kasai H, Suzuki H, Ueda O, Kamada N, Jishage K, Komeda K, Noda M, Kanazawa Y, Taniguchi S, Miwa I, Akanuma Y, Kodama T, Yazaki Y, Kadowaki T. Pancreatic β-cell-specific targeted disruption of glucokinase gene. *J Biol Chem* 1995; 270: 30253–6.
44. O'Doherty RM, Lehman DL, Seoane J, Gomez-Foix AM, Guinovart JJ, Newgard CB. Differential metabolic effects of adenovirus-mediated glucokinase and hexokinase I overexpression in rat primary hepatocytes. *J Biol Chem* 1996; 271: 20524–30.
45. Seoane J, Gomez-Foix AM, O'Doherty RM, Gomez-Ara C, Newgard CB, Guinovart JJ. Glucose-6-phosphate produced by glucokinase, but not hexokinase is the signal for the activation of hepatic glycogen synthase. *J Biol Chem* 1996; 271: 23756–60.
46. O'Doherty RM, Lehman DL, Telemaque-Potts S, Newgard CB. Metabolic impact of glucokinase overexpression in liver: lowering of blood glucose in fed rats is accompanied by hyperlipidemia. *Diabetes* 1999; 48: 2022–7.
47. Niswender KD, Shiota M, Postic C, Cherrington AD, Magnuson MA. Effects of increased glucokinase gene copy number on glucose homeostasis and hepatic glucose metabolism. *J Biol Chem* 1997; 272: 22570–5.
48. Ferre T, Pujol A, Riu E, Bosch F, Valera A. Correction of diabetic alterations by glucokinase. *Proc Natl Acad Sci USA* 1996; 93: 7225–30.
49. Shiota M, Postic C, Fujimoto Y, Jetton TL, Dixon K, Pan D, Grimsby J, Grippo JF, Magnuson MA, Cherrington AD. Glucokinase gene locus transgenic mice are resistant to the development of obesity-induced type 2 diabetes. *Diabetes* 2001; 50: 622–9.
50. Desai UJ, Slosberg ED, Boettcher BR, Caplan SL, Fanelli B, Spephan Z, Gunther VJ, Kaleko M, Connelly S. Phenotypic correction of diabetic mice by adenovirus-mediated glucokinase expression. *Diabetes* 2001; 50: 2287–95.
51. Slosberg ED, Desai UJ, Fanelli B, St Denny I, Connelly S, Kaleko M, Boettcher BR, Caplan SL. Treatment of type 2 diabetes by adenoviral-mediated overexpression of the glucokinase regulatory protein. *Diabetes* 2001; 50: 1813–20.
52. Grimsby J, Sarabu R, Corbett WL, Haynes NE, Bizzarro FT, Coffey JW, Guertin KR, Hilliard DW, Kester RF, Mahaney PE, Marcus L, Qi L, Spence CL, Tengi J, Magnuson MA, Chu CA, Dvorozniak MT, Matschinsky FM, Grippo JF. Allosteric activators of glucokinase: potential role in diabetes therapy. *Science* 2003; 301: 370–3.
53. Baque S, Montell E, Guinovart JJ, Newgard CB, Gomez-Foix AM. Expression of glucokinase in cultured human muscle cells confers insulin-independent and glucose concentration-dependent increases in glucose disposal and storage. *Diabetes* 1998; 47: 1392–8.
54. Jimenez-Chillaron JC, Newgard CB, Gomez-Foix AM. Increased glucose disposal induced by adenovirus-mediated transfer of glucokinase to skeletal muscle in vivo. *FASEB J* 1999; 13: 2153–60.
55. Otaegui PJ, Ferre T, Pujol A, Riu E, Jimenez R, Bosch F. Expression of glucokinase in skeletal muscle: a new approach to counteract diabetic hyperglycemia. *Hum Gene Ther* 2000; 11: 1543–52.
56. Jimenez-Chillaron JC, Telemaque-Potts S, Gomez-Valades AG, Anderson P, Newgard CB, Gomez-Foix AM. Glucokinase gene transfer to skeletal muscle of diabetic Zucker fatty rats improves insulin-sensitive glucose uptake. *Metabolism* 2002; 51: 121–6.
57. Otaegui PJ, Ontiveros M, Ferre T, Riu E, Jimenez R, Bosch F. Glucose-regulated glucose uptake by transplanted muscle cells expressing glucokinase counteracts diabetic hyperglycemia. *Hum Gene Ther* 2002; 13: 2125–33.
58. Otaegui PJ, Ferre T, Riu E, Bosch F. Prevention of obesity and insulin resistance by glucokinase expression in skeletal muscle of transgenic mice. *FASEB J* 2003; 17: 2097–9.
59. Argaud D, Lange AJ, Becker TC, Okar DA, El-Maghrabi MR, Newgard CB, Pilkis SJ. Adenovirus-mediated

overexpression of liver 6-phosphofructo-2-kinase/fructose-2,6-bisphosphatase in gluconeogenic rat hepatoma cells. Paradoxical effect on Fru-2,6-P2 levels. *J Biol Chem* 1995; 270: 24229–36.
60. Wu C, Okar DA, Newgard CB, Lange AJ. Overexpression of 6-phosphofructo-2-kinase/fructose-2,6-bisphosphatase in mouse liver lowers blood glucose by suppressing hepatic glucose production. *J Clin Invest* 2001; 107: 91–8.
61. Wu C, Okar DA, Newgard CB, Lange AJ. Increasing fructose 2,6-bisphosphate overcomes hepatic insulin resistance of type 2 diabetes. *Am J Physiol Endocrinol Metab* 2002; 282: E38–45.
62. McGarry JD. Banting lecture 2001: dysregulation of fatty acid metabolism in the etiology of type 2 diabetes. *Diabetes* 2002; 51: 7–18.
63. Nordlie RC. Metabolic regulation by multifunctional glucose-6-phosphatase. *Curr Top Cell Regul* 1974; 8: 33–117.
64. Arion WJ, Lange AJ, Walls EH, Ballas IM. Evidence for the participation of independent translocation for phosphate and glucose 6-phosphate in the microsomal glucose-6-phosphatase system. Interactions of the system with orthophosphate, inorganic pyrophosphate, and carbamyl phosphate. *J Biol Chem* 1980; 255: 10396–406.
65. Lange AJ, Arion WJ, Beaudet AL. Type 1b glycogen storage disease is caused by a defect in the glucose-6-phosphate translocase of the glucose-6-phosphatase system. *J Biol Chem* 1980; 255: 8381–4.
66. Tsai CS, Burgett MW, Reed LJ. α-Keto acid dehydrogenase complexes XX: a kinetic study of the pyruvate dehydrogenase complex from bovine kidney. *J Biol Chem* 1973; 248: 8348–52.
67. Denton RM, Randle PJ, Bridges BJ, Cooper RH, Kerbey AL, Pask HT, Severson DL, Stansbie D, Whitehouse S. Regulation of mammalian pyruvate dehydrogenase. *Mol Cell Biochem* 1975; 9: 27–53.
68. Sugden MC, Holness MJ. Recent advances in mechanisms regulating glucose oxidation at the level of the pyruvate dehydrogenase complex by PDKs. *Am J Physiol* 2003; 284: E855–62.
69. Pettit FH, Pelley JW, Reed LJ. Regulation of pyruvate dehydrogenase kinase and phosphatase by acetyl CoA/CoA and NADH/NAD ratios. *Biochem Biophys Res Commun* 1975; 65: 575–82.
70. Ashman LK, Wallace JC, Keech DB. Desensitization of pyruvate carboxylase against acetyl CoA stimulation by chemical modification. *Biochem Biophys Res Commun* 1975; 51: 924–31.
71. Warren GB, Tipton KF. The role of acetyl CoA in the reaction pathway of pig-liver pyruvate carboxylase. *Eur J Biochem* 1974; 47: 549–54.
72. Pilkis SJ, El-Maghrabi MR, Pilkis J, Claus T. The role of fructose-2,6-bisphosphate in regulation of fructose-1,6-bisphosphatase. *J Biol Chem* 1981; 256: 11489–95.
73. Van Schaftingen E, Hers HG. Inhibition of fructose-1,6-bisphosphatase by fructose-2,6-bisphosphate. *Proc Natl Acad Sci USA* 1981; 78: 2861–3.
74. Jin ES, Uyeda K, Kawaguchi T, Burgess SC, Malloy CR, Sherry AD. Increased hepatic fructose-2,6-bisphosphate after an oral glucose load does not affect gluconeogenesis. *J Biol Chem* 2003; 278: 28427–33.
75. Kitamura K, Uyeda K, Kangawa K, Matsuo H. Purification and characterization of rat skeletal muscle fructose-6-phosphate, 2 kinase:fructose-2,6-bisphosphatase. *J Biol Chem* 1989; 264: 9799–806.
76. Pilkis SJ, Granner DK. Molecular physiology of the regulation of hepatic gluconeogenesis and glycolysis. *Ann Rev Physiol* 1992; 54: 885–909.
77. Petersen DD, Koch SR, Granner DK. 3′ non-coding region of phosphoenolpyruvate carboxykinase mRNA contains a glucocorticoid-responsive mRNA-stabilizing element. *Proc Natl Acad Sci USA* 1989; 86: 7800–4.
78. Hod Y, Hanson RW. Cyclic AMP stabilizes the mRNA for phosphoenolpyruvate carboxykinase (GTP) against degradation. *J Biol Chem* 1988; 263: 7747–52.
79. Quinn PG, Wong TW, Magnuson MA, Shabb JB, Granner DK. Identification of the basal and cAMP regulatory elements in the promoter of the phosphoenolpyruvate carboxykinase gene. *Mol Cell Biol* 1988; 8: 3467–75.
80. Park EA, Roesler WJ, Liu J, Klemm DJ, Gurney AG, Thatcher JD, Shuman J, Friedman A, Hanson RW. The role of the CCAAT/enhancer-binding protein in the transcriptional regulation of the gene for phosphoenolpyruvate carboxykinase (GTP). *Mol Cell Biol* 1990; 10: 6264–72.
81. Waltner-Law M, Duong D, Daniels MC, Herzog B, Wang XL, Prasad R, Granner DK. Elements of the glucocorticoid and retinoic acid response units are involved in cAMP-mediated expression of the PEPCK gene. *J Biol Chem* 2003; 278 (12): 10427–35.
82. Sasaki K, Cripe TP, Koch SR, Andreone T, Petersen DD, Beale EG, Guanner DK. Multihormonal regulation of phosphoenolpyruvate carboxykinase gene transcription: dominant role of insulin. *J Biol Chem* 1984; 259: 15242–51.
83. Duong DT, Waltner-Law M, Sears R, Sealy L, Granner DK. Insulin inhibits hepatocellular glucose production by disrupting the association of CBP and RNA polymerase II with the PEPCK gene promoter. *J Biol Chem* 2002; 277: 32234–42.
84. Sasaki K, Granner DK. Regulation of phosphoenolpyruvate carboxykinase gene transcription by insulin and cAMP: reciprocal actions on initiation and elongation. *Proc Natl Acad Sci USA* 1988; 85: 2954–8.
85. Liu Z, Barrett EJ, Dalkin AC, Zwart AD, Chou JY. Effect of acute diabetes on rat hepatic glucose-6-phosphatase activity and its messenger RNA level. *Biochem Biophys Res Commun* 1994; 205: 680–6.
86. Massillon D, Barzilai N, Chen W, Hu M, Rossetti L. Glucose regulates in vivo glucose-6-phosphatase gene expression in the liver of diabetic rats. *J Biol Chem* 1996; 271: 9871–4.
87. Argaud D, Zhang Q, Pan W, Maitra S, Pilkis SJ, Lange AJ. Regulation of rat liver glucose-6-phosphatase gene expression in different nutritional and hormonal states: gene structure and 5′-flanking sequence. *Diabetes* 1996; 45: 1563–71.
88. Mithieux G, Vidal H, Zitoun C, Bruni N, Daniele N, Minassian C. Glucose-6-phosphatase mRNA and activity are increased to the same extent in kidney and liver of diabetic rats. *Diabetes* 1996; 45: 891–6.
89. Argaud D, Kirby TL, Newgard CB, Lange AJ. Glucose stimulation of glucose-6-phosphatase gene expression in primary hepatocytes and Fao hepatoma cells: requirement for glucokinase expression. *J Biol Chem* 1997; 272: 12854–61.
90. O'Brien RM, Streeper RS, Ayala JE, Stadelmaier BT, Hornbuckle LA. Insulin-regulated gene expression. *Biochem Soc Trans* 2001; 29: 552–8.
91. Trinh KY, O'Doherty RM, Anderson P, Lange AJ, Newgard CB. Perturbation of fuel homeostasis caused

by overexpression of the glucose-6-phosphatase catalytic subunit in liver of normal rats. *J Biol Chem* 1998; 273: 31615–20.

92. Wu Z, Puigserver P, Andersson U, Zhang C, Adelmant G, Mootha V, Troy A, Cinti S, Lowell B, Scarpulla RC, Spiegelman BM. Mechanisms controlling mitochondrial biogenesis and respiration through the thermogenic coactivator PGC-1. *Cell* 1999; 98: 115–24.
93. Yoon JC, Puigserver P, Chen G, Donovan J, Wu Z, Rhee J, Adelmant G, Stafford J, Kahn CR, Granner DK, Newgard CB, Spiegelman BM. Control of hepatic gluconeogenesis through the transcriptional activator PGC-1. *Nature* 2001; 413: 131–8.
94. Puigserver P, Rhee J, Donovan J, Walkey CJ, Yoon JC, Oriente F, Kitamura Y, Altomonte J, Dong H, Accili D, Spiegelman BM. Insulin-regulated hepatic gluconeogenesis through FOXO1–PGC-1alpha interaction. *Nature* 2003; 423: 550–5.
95. Valera A, Pujol A, Pelegrin M, Bosch F. Transgenic mice overexpressing phosphoenolpyruvate carboxykinase develop non-insulin-dependent diabetes mellitus. *Proc Natl Acad Sci USA* 1994; 91: 9151–4.
96. She P, Shiota M, Shelton KD, Chalkley R, Postic C, Magnuson MA. Phosphoenolpyruvate carboxykinase is necessary for integration of hepatic energy metabolism. *Mol Cell Biol* 2000; 20: 6508–17.
97. She P, Burgess SC, Shiota M, Flakoll P, Donahue EP, Malloy CR, Sherry AD, Magnuson MA. Mechanisms by which liver-specific PEPCK knockout mice preserve euglycemia during starvation. *Diabetes* 2003; 52: 1649–54.
98. Seoane J, Trinh K, O'Doherty RM, Gomez-Foix AM, Lange AJ, Newgard CB, Guinovart JJ. Metabolic impact of adenovirus-mediated overexpression of the glucose-6-phosphatase catalytic subunit in primary hepatocytes. *J Biol Chem* 1997; 272: 26972–7.
99. An J, Li Y, van De Werve G, Newgard CB. Overexpression of the P46 (T1) translocase component of the glucose-6-phosphatase complex in hepatocytes impairs glycogen accumulation via hydrolysis of glucose 1-phosphate. *J Biol Chem* 2001; 276: 10722–79.
100. McGarry JD, Kuwajima M, Newgard CB, Foster DW, Katz J. From dietary glucose to liver glycogen—the full circle round. *Annu Rev Nutr* 1986; 7: 51–73.
101. Newgard CB, Hirsch L, Foster DW, McGarry JD. Studies on the mechanism by which exogenous glucose is converted into liver glycogen in the rat—a direct or an indirect pathway? *J Biol Chem* 1983; 258: 8046–52.
102. Newgard CB, Moore SV, Foster DW, McGarry JD. Efficient hepatic glycogen synthesis in refeeding rats requires continued carbon flow through the gluconeogenic pathway. *J Biol Chem* 1984; 259: 6958–63.
103. Shulman GI, Cline G, Schumann WC, Chandramouli V, Kumaran K, Landau BR. Quantitative comparison of pathways of hepatic glycogen repletion in fed and fasted humans. *Am J Physiol* 1990; 259: E335–41.
104. Petersen KF, Cline GW, Gerard DP, Magnusson I, Rothman DL, Shulman GI. Contribution of net hepatic glycogen synthesis to disposal of an oral glucose load in humans. *Metabolism* 2001; 50: 598–601.
105. Newgard CB, Hwang PK, Fletterick RJ. The family of glycogen phosphorylases: structure and function. *CRC Crit Rev Biochem Mol Biol* 1989; 24: 69–99.
106. Lawrence JC Jr, Roach PJ. New insights into the role and mechanism of glycogen synthase activation by insulin. *Diabetes* 1997; 46: 541–7.
107. Petersen KF, Laurent D, Rothman DL, Cline GW, Shulman GI. Mechanism by which glucose and insulin inhibit net hepatic glycogenolyis in humans. *J Clin Invest* 1998; 101: 1203–9.
108. Magnusson I, Rothman DL, Jucker B, Cline GW, Shulman RG, Shulman GI. Liver glycogen turnover in fed and fasted humans. *Am J Physiol* 1994; 266: E796–803.
109. Ferrer JC, Favre C, Gomis RR, Fernandez-Novell JM, Garcia-Roach M, de la Iglesia N, Cid E, Guinovart JJ. Control of glycogen deposition. *FEBS Lett* 2003; 546: 127–32.
110. Frame S, Cohen P. GSK3 takes centre stage more than 20 years after its discovery. *Biochem J* 2001; 359: 1–16.
111. Newgard CB, Brady MJ, O'Doherty RM, Saltiel AR. Organizing glucose disposal: emerging roles of the glycogen targeting subunits of protein phosphatase-1. *Diabetes* 2000; 49: 1967–77.
112. Hubbard MJ, Cohen P. On target with a new mechanism for the regulation of protein phosphorylation. *Trends Biochem Sci* 1993; 18: 172–7.
113. Watanabe T, Huang HB, Horiuchi A, da Cruze Silva EF, Hsieh-Wilson L, Allen PB, Shenolikar S, Greengard P, Nairn AC. Protein phosphatase 1 regulation by inhibitors and targeting subunits. *Proc Natl Acad Sci USA* 2001; 98: 3080–5.
114. Tang PM, Bondor JA, Swiderek KM, DePaoli-Roach AA. Molecular cloning and expression of the regulatory (RG1) subunit of the glycogen-associated protein phosphatase. *J Biol Chem* 1991; 266: 15782–9.
115. Chen YH, Hansen L, Chen MX, Bjorbaek C, Vestergaard H, Hansen T, Cohen PT, Pedersen O. Sequence of the human glycogen-associated regulatory subunit of type 1 protein phosphatase and analysis of its coding region and mRNA level in muscle from patients with NIDDM. *Diabetes* 1994; 43: 1234–41.
116. Doherty MJ, Moorhead G, Morrice N, Cohen P, Cohen PT. Amino acid sequence and expression of the hepatic glycogen-binding (GL)-subunit of protein phosphatase-1. *FEBS Lett* 1995; 375: 294–8.
117. Printen JA, Brady MJ, Saltiel AR. PTG, a protein phosphatase 1-binding protein with a role in glycogen metabolism. *Science* 1997; 275: 1475–8.
118. Doherty MJ, Young PR, Cohen PT. Amino acid sequence of a novel protein phosphatase 1 binding protein (R5) which is related to the liver- and muscle-specific glycogen binding subunits of protein phosphatase 1. *FEBS Lett* 1996; 399: 339–43.
119. Armstrong CG, Browne GJ, Cohen P, Cohen PT. PPP1R6, a novel member of the family of glycogen-targetting subunits of protein phosphatase 1. *FEBS Lett* 1997; 418: 210–4.
120. Berman HK, O'Doherty RM, Anderson P, Newgard CB. Overexpression of protein targeting to glycogen (PTG) in rat hepatocytes causes profound activation of glycogen synthesis independent of normal hormone- and substrate-mediated regulatory mechanisms. *J Biol Chem* 1998; 273: 26421–5.
121. O'Doherty RM, Jensen PB, Anderson P, Jones JG, Berman HK, Kearney D, Newgard CB. Activation of direct and indirect pathways of glycogen synthesis by hepatic overexpression of protein targeting to glycogen. *J Clin Invest* 2000; 105: 479–88.
122. Gasa R, Jensen P-B, Berman H, Brady MJ, Roach AD, Newgard CB. Differential regulatory and metabolic

properties of glycogen targeting subunits (PTG, G_L, G_M) expressed in hepatocytes. *J Biol Chem* 2000; 275: 26396–403.

123. Yang R, Cao L, Gasa R, Brady MJ, Sherry AD, Newgard CB. Glycogen-targeting subunits and glucokinase differentially affect pathways of glycogen metabolism and their regulation in hepatocytes. *J Biol Chem* 2002; 277: 1514–23.
124. Landau BR, Wahren J, Chandramouli V, Schumann WC, Ekberg K, Kalhan SC. Contributions of gluconeogenesis to glucose production in the fasted state. *J Clin Invest* 1996; 98: 378–85.
125. Jones JG, Solomon MA, Cole SM, Sherry AD, Malloy CR. An integrated ^{2}H and ^{13}C NMR study of gluconeogenesis and TCA cycle flux in humans. *Am J Physiol* 2001; 281: E848–56.
126. Gasa R, Clark C, Yang R, DePaoli-Roach AA, Newgard CB. Reversal of diet-induced glucose intolerance by hepatic expression of a variant glycogen-targeting subunit of protein phosphatase-1. *J Biol Chem* 2002; 277: 1524–30.
127. Yang R, Newgard CB. Hepatic expression of a targeting subunit of protein phosphatase-1 in streptozotocin-diabetic rats reverses hyperglycemia and hyperphagia despite depressed glucokinase expression. *J Biol Chem* 2003; 278: 23418–25.
128. Sindelar DK, Havel PJ, Seeley RJ, Wilkinson CW, Woods SC, Schwartz MW. *Diabetes* 1999; 48: 1275–80.
129. Chinookoswong N, Wang JL, Shi ZQ. Leptin restores euglycemia and normalizes glucose turnover in insulin-deficient diabetes in the rat. *Diabetes* 1999; 48: 1487–92.
130. Cam MC, Rodrigues B, McNeill JH. Distinct glucose lowering and beta cell protective effects of vanadium and food restriction in streptozotocin-diabetes. *Eur J Endocrinol* 1999; 141: 546–54.
131. Schwartz MW, Woods SC, Porte D Jr, Seeley RJ, Baskin DG. Central nervous system control of food intake. *Nature* 2000; 404: 661–71.
132. Mayer J. Glucostatic mechanism of regulation of food intake. *N Engl J Med* 1953; 249: 13–6.
133. Russek M. Participation of hepatic glucoreceptors in the control of intake of food. *Nature* 1963; 197: 79–80.
134. Russek M. Current status of the hepatostatic theory of food intake control. *Appetite* 1981; 2: 137–43.
135. Flatt JP. Dietary fat, carbohydrate balance, and weight maintenance: effects of exercise. *Am J Clin Nutr* 1987; 45: 296–306.
136. Flatt JP. The difference in the storage capacities for carbohydrate and for fat, and its implications in the regulation of body weight. *Ann N Y Acad Sci* 1987; 499: 104–23.
137. Martin WH, Hoover DJ, Armento SJ, Stock IA, McPherson RK, Danley DE, Stevenson RW, Barrett EJ, Treadway JL. Discovery of a human liver glycogen phosphorylase inhibitor that lowers blood glucose in vivo. *Proc Natl Acad Sci USA* 1998; 95: 1776–81.
138. Treadway JL, Mendys P, Hoover DJ. Glycogen phosphorylase inhibitors for treatment of type 2 diabetes mellitus. *Expert Opin Investig Drugs* 2001; 10: 439–54.
139. Coghlan MP, Culbert AA, Cross DA, Corcoran SL, Yates JW, Pearce NJ, Rausch OL, Murphy GJ, Carter PS, Roxbee Cox L, Mills D, Brown MJ, Haigh D, Ward RW, Smith DG, Murray KJ, Reith AD, Holder JC. Selective small molecule inhibitors of glycogen synthase kinase-3 modulate glycogen metabolism and gene transcription. *Chem Biol* 2000; 7: 793–803.
140. Lochhead PA, Coghlan M, Rice SQ, Sutherland C. Inhibition of GSK-3 selectively reduces glucose-6-phosphatase and phosphatase and phosphoenolypyruvate carboxykinase gene expression. *Diabetes* 2001; 50: 937–46.
141. Cline GW, Johnson K, Regittnig W, Perret P, Tozzo E, Xiao L, Damico C, Shulman GI. Effects of a novel glycogen synthase kinase-3 inhibitor on insulin-stimulated glucose metabolism in Zucker diabetic fatty (*fa/fa*) rats. *Diabetes* 2002; 51: 2903–10.
142. Petersen KF, Laurent D, Yu C, Cline GW, Shulman GI. Stimulating effects of low-dose fructose on insulin-stimulated hepatic glycogen synthesis in humans. *Diabetes* 2001; 50: 1263–8.
143. Bell GI, Kayano T, Buse JB, Burant CF, Takeda J, Lin D, Fukumoto H, Seino S. Molecular biology of mammalian glucose transporters. *Diabetes Care* 1990; 13: 198–208.
144. Thorens B, Charron MJ, Lodish HF. Molecular physiology of glucose transporters. *Diabetes Care* 1990; 13: 209–18.
145. Thorens B, Sarkar HK, Kaback HR, Lodish HF. Cloning and functional expression in bacteria of a novel glucose transpoter in liver, intestine, kidney, and beta-pancreatic islet cells. *Cell* 1988; 55: 281–90.
146. Johnson JH, Newgard CB, Milburn JL, Lodish HF, Thorens B. The high K_m glucose transporter of islets of Langerhans is functionally similar to the low affinity transporter of liver and has an identical primary sequence. *J Biol Chem* 1990; 265: 6548–51.
147. Guillam MT, Hummler E, Schaerer E, Yeh JI, Birnbaum MJ, Beermann F, Schmidt A, Deriaz N, Thorens B, Wu JY. Early diabetes and abnormal postnatal pancreatic islet development in mice lacking GLUT-2. *Nat Genet* 1997; 17: 327–30.
148. Guillam MT, Burcelin R, Thorens B. Normal hepatic glucose production in the absence of GLUT2 reveals an alternative pathway for glucose release from hepatocytes. *Proc Natl Acad Sci USA* 1998; 95: 12317–21.
149. Burcelin R, del Carmen Munoz M, Guillan MT, Thorens B. Liver hyperplasia and paradoxical regulation of glycogen metabolism and glucose-sensitive gene expression in GLUT2-null hepatocytes. Further evidence for the existence of a membrane-based glucose release pathway. *J Biol Chem* 2000; 275: 10930–6.

15

Insulin Actions *In Vivo*: Glucose Metabolism

Ele Ferrannini* and Ralph A. DeFronzo†

**Department of Internal Medicine, University of Pisa School of Medicine, Pisa, Italy, and* †*University of Texas Health Science Center, San Antonio, TX, USA*

INTRODUCTION

Glucose

Glucose is widespread in living organisms, in which, with protein and fat, it completes the triad of the major metabolic fuels. To a much lesser extent than in plants, glucose also constitutes a building block for structural and enzymatic components of cells as well as the extracellular matrix. As a metabolic substrate, glucose is present in organisms essentially in its simple, monomeric form (α-D-glucopyranose), and as a branched polymer of α-glucose, namely glycogen. Disaccharides of glucose (lactose, maltose, and sucrose) are quantitatively less important.

Glucose is present in plasma water at a concentration that—in a healthy adult who has fasted overnight—ranges between 3.6 and 5.6 mmol/l (65–100 mg/dl). A family of proteins residing in the plasma membrane (and in microsomal membranes) can specifically and reversibly bind glucose molecules, and transfer them across cell membranes in both directions. Of such proteins, known as glucose transporters (or, more generally, solute carriers 2A or SLC2A), there are 13 different species that have so far been identified and at least partially characterized [1]. They differ from one another in both tissue distribution and physiologic regulation, particularly in respect to sensitivity to insulin stimulation. More than one species of glucose transporter is usually expressed in a tissue. Present knowledge in this rapidly evolving field indicates that only one type of glucose transporter (termed GLUT-4) shows clear sensitivity to acute insulin stimulation *in vivo*, and it is this transporter that is abundantly expressed in the classic insulin-sensitive tissues (adipocyte, brown fat, skeletal, heart, and smooth muscle). Variable dominance of the other types of glucose transporters is found in tissues in which glucose metabolism does not respond to insulin acutely (erythrocyte, liver, kidney, brain, pancreatic B cells). Some basic features of glucose distribution and metabolism can be suitably interpreted on the basis of current information on glucose transport.

A non-insulin-regulatable transporter (GT1) effects facilitated glucose diffusion in red blood cells (RBCs). The abundance of this transporter in RBCs has the following physiological consequences. First, glucose diffuses very rapidly across RBC membranes, with an estimated equilibration time of only 4 s (a total RBC mass of 25×10^9 cells with a mean diameter of 7 μm and a spherical shape occupies a surface area of approximately 4 m^2) [2]. The rate of glycolytic utilization of transported glucose by the erythrocyte mass is estimated to be 25 μmol/min, or about 6 μmol/min/m^2 of diffusion surface. As such a rate is about 17 000 times less than the rate of glucose transport in these cells, glucose concentration will, in general, be the same in plasma and erythrocyte water. Plasma proteins make up some 8% of plasma volume, while RBC proteins and ghost occupy about 38% of packed red cell volume (which, in turn, averages 40% of blood volume). Thus, 20% (i.e. $0.38 \times 0.4 + 0.08 \times 0.6 = 0.2$) of total blood volume is inaccessible to glucose. It follows that glucose concentration should be identical in plasma and RBC water under most circumstances, and that a *blood water* glucose concentration of 5.0 mmol/l translates into a *plasma* glucose concentration of 4.6 mmol/l and a whole-blood glucose concentration of 4.0 mmol/l, i.e. a 15% systematic difference between plasma and *whole-blood* glucose level under typical conditions of hematocrit, proteinemia, and erythrocyte volume.

Second, as both RBC and plasma convey glucose, the total amount of the sugar reaching any given organ is

International Textbook of Diabetes Mellitus, Third Edition. Edited by R. A. DeFronzo, E. Ferrannini, H. Keen, and P. Zimmet.

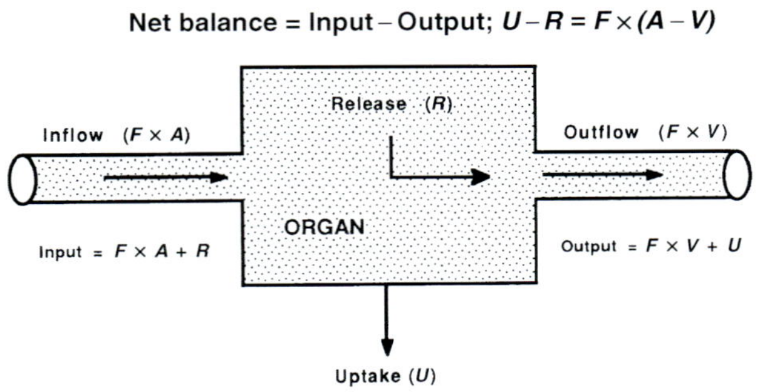

Figure 1 Scheme of an organ perfused by a blood flow (F) carrying a substrate that is both removed by irreversible metabolism and produced *de novo* by intraorgan synthesis. All equations shown are valid when blood flow, arterial substrate concentration, and rates of intraorgan substrate metabolism are constant (Fick principle)

the product of arterial whole-blood glucose concentration times the total blood flow to that organ. Similarly, the total amount of glucose leaving a body region is the product of whole-blood glucose level in the venous effluent times the blood flow rate. Thus, under steady-state conditions of blood flow (F), arterial glycemia (A), and organ metabolism, the net balance of glucose movements across a body region is given by the product of blood flow and the arterio-venous ($A - V$) whole-blood glucose concentration difference [$(A - V) \times F$, or Fick principle] (Figure 1) [3]. It is evident that the use of *plasma* flow rates and glucose concentrations systematically underestimates the net organ balance of glucose (and, for that matter, of any substance that travels in plasma as well as in erythrocytes, e.g. lactate and some amino acids). In fact, plasma flow is less than blood flow by an amount equal to the hematocrit (~40%), while plasma glucose is higher than whole-blood glucose by only 15% ($0.6 \times 1.15 = 0.69$, i.e. a 31% underestimation).

At least two non-insulin-regulatable glucose transporters (GLUT-1 and GLUT-3) have been identified in the blood–brain barrier and placenta [1], where transendothelial glucose passage occurs via facilitated diffusion. This is the structural basis for the long-held notion that brain and placental glucose utilization are subtracted from insulin control, so that vital functions for the adult and fetal organism can be maintained in the face of variable metabolic conditions. In other tissues, the mechanism of extravascular glucose transfer is still undefined.

In general, diffusion of glucose from the intravascular compartment into the interstitial fluid space is known to be very rapid. Whether this is accomplished by facilitated diffusion mediated by specific cell transporters (as in the brain) or by simple diffusion through intercellular clefts of endothelial cells is still uncertain. A lower limit of glucose diffusion through endothelial membranes is represented by cellular glucose uptake (which does not include glucose back-diffusion into the intravascular compartment), and can be estimated by carrying out the following calculation. In healthy subjects under conditions of maximal stimulation (i.e. combined hyperinsulinemia and hyperglycemia), whole-body glucose uptake can reach 12 mmol/min, which, for a total capillary surface of 700 m^2 available for diffusion (and considering a mean surface of 19 000 μ^2 per capillary [4]), corresponds to 0.3 pmol/min per capillary. Thus, about 200 billion glucose molecules must pass through each capillary surface each minute to travel cell-bound through the interstitial space. What kind of radial gradient (from the center of the capillary to the cell surface) is generated by the irreversible removal of glucose by cell metabolism *in vivo* is not known exactly, but theoretically this gradient is a function of the rate of diffusion through the endothelium, the distance between the capillary and the cell, and the rate of net glucose transport through the cell membrane. Furthermore, the presence of active glucose uptake also creates a longitudinal glucose concentration gradient along the axis of the capillary, as the glucose supplied at the arterial end of the capillary tree is progressively lost to cells and subtracted from the venous return. The two gradients are obviously dependent on one another, and together determine, at any given rate of cellular glucose uptake, the concentration of glucose at the cell surface (Figure 2). Further complexity is added by the three-dimensional structure of

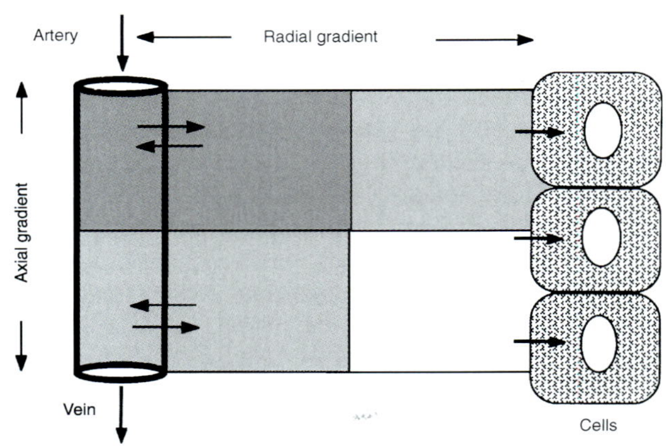

Figure 2 Schematic representation of substrate gradients in an idealized tissue. A capillary (human mean capillary length is 0.75–1.00 mm) receives the substrate from the arterial end (with a flow of 0.5×10^{-6} µl/min at a linear velocity of 17 mm/min) and delivers it back to the circulation at the venous end. During its transit time along the capillary (3.5 s), the substrate permeates the capillary endothelial membrane by facilitated diffusion (through a surface that averages 19 000 µm^2 per capillary), distributes radially into the tissue interstitium (in about 0.1 s), and is actively removed by cell metabolism. Because of the latter, there exists a dynamic steady state whereby a radial substrate gradient is compounded by an axial gradient along the capillary. Four degrees of shading represent in the scheme what must be a continuous distribution of interstitial gradients

tissues. Direct measurement of interstitial glucose concentrations has proven to be difficult, and has yielded conflicting results. Collection of subcutaneous filtrate, equilibration of perfusates through ultrafiltration membranes, and microdialysis-based methods have been employed. In one study in which these techniques were used simultaneously in the abdominal subcutaneous tissue of healthy volunteers, interstitial fluid glucose concentrations were found to be ~50% lower than venous blood glucose levels both under fasting circumstances and in response to IV glucose-induced hyperglycemia [4]. Difficult as it may be to measure or calculate this "bathing" concentration of glucose, it is this concentration that dictates the activity of cellular glucose transport together with the state of specific activation of the transporter.

In addition to hormonal stimulation and substrate mass action, cellular glucose uptake is influenced by changes in blood flow in at least two ways.

(1) An increase in blood supply to a given tissue unit will dissipate—at least in part—the longitudinal glucose gradient (along the axis of the capillary tree), thereby also flattening the radial gradient (capillary to cell surface) and raising the glucose concentration bathing the cell. Intuitively, this increase in the operating glucose level should by itself enhance glucose transport; the converse will happen if blood flow slows down. To quantitate this phenomenon, it is pertinent to recall the laws that govern cellular uptake of permeable solutes. According to the Renkin–Crone model of capillary exchange and tissue metabolism [5, 6], the following general equation applies:

$$J_s = [\mathrm{S}]_a \times F \times \left(1 - e^{-PS/F}\right)$$

where J_s is the net flux of solute from blood into tissue, $[\mathrm{S}]_a$ is the arterial blood solute concentration, F is the blood flow rate, and PS is the product of permeability of exchange surface to solute (P) and exchange surface area (S). Although such model is only valid for uniformly perfused capillary networks, it can be applied to real (heterogeneous) systems to dissect out the relative role of blood flow and the PS product in regulating glucose uptake. Note that the PS product for glucose refers to the slower one of the two exchange surfaces (namely, the capillary exchange surface and the cell membrane surface) that are interposed between the bloodstream and intracellular glucose disposition. Thus, as alluded to above, the glucose PS underestimates the actual unidirectional transfer of glucose across the capillary walls. For a given capillary surface, P is equivalent to net transmembrane glucose transport, and therefore is the target of hormonal influences. By combining the above equation (with $[\mathrm{S}]_a = A$) with the Fick equation [$J_s = F(A - V)$], one can estimate PS from perfused forearm experiments,

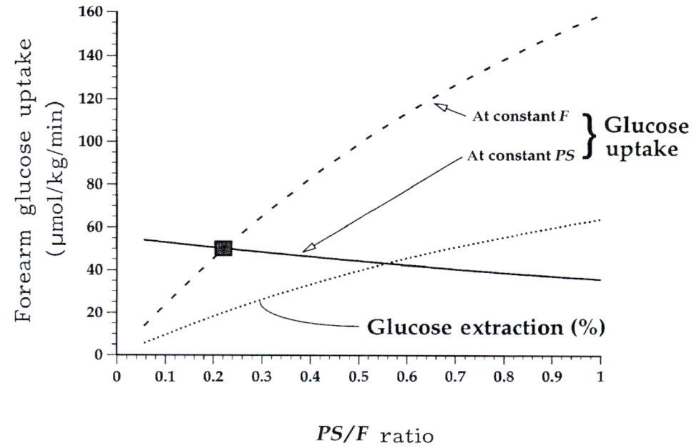

Figure 3 Forearm glucose uptake as a function of the PS/F ratio. The hatched square indicates the actual values of PS/F ratio (0.223) and forearm glucose uptake (50 μmol/min/kg) as measured in healthy volunteers during a euglycemic (5 mM) hyperinsulinemic (~80 mU/l) clamp experiment. Forearm glucose uptake is then calculated over a 20-fold range of PS/F values once by varying blood flow (at constant PS) and again by varying PS (at constant F). In the face of the same extraction ratio, glucose uptake changes little at constant PS and markedly at constant flow

in which forearm blood flow and the $A - V$ glucose gradient are directly measured, by using the following equation:

$$PS = -F \times \log_e(V/A)$$

As exemplified in Figure 3, in healthy subjects under conditions of physiological hyperinsulinemia at an arterial glycemia of 5 mM, one measures a deep forearm venous glucose level of 4 mM combined with a total forearm blood flow of 50 ml/min/kg of deep forearm tissues. The corresponding value (0.223) of the glucose PS/F ratio (corresponding to a PS of 11 ml/min/kg of tissue) is indicated by the hatched box in the figure. If the value of PS/F is allowed to vary over a 20-fold range of forearm blood flow (200 to 11 ml/min/kg) while holding PS constant, forearm glucose uptake declines sluggishly, by some 30% at most. Thus, blood flow has little effect on glucose uptake, provided that the permeability–surface product is maintained.

(2) Additional metabolic units may be recruited by vasodilation, i.e. through the opening-up of previously unperfused or hypoperfused capillary sectors. Capillaries display vasomotion under the control of feeding arterioles and precapillary sphincters. In response to exercise or hypoxia, the number of capillaries open at any moment and the integrated time that capillaries remain open increase. As a consequence, PS increases because of a larger capillary exchange surface. To the extent that a corresponding surface of cell membranes is exposed to perfusion (i.e. metabolic recruitment),

glucose uptake will be stimulated. As shown in Figure 3, when the forearm PS/F is allowed to vary over the same range by changing PS while holding flow constant, forearm glucose uptake increases sharply with PS. In other words, changes in the PS product are much more important than blood flow changes in regulating glucose uptake. Of note is that the glucose extraction ratio [i.e. $\mathrm{ER} = (A - V)/A)$] across forearm tissues, which in Crone–Renkin terms is equal to

$$\mathrm{ER} = 1 - e^{-PS/F}$$

is the same regardless of whether the PS/F ratio changes as a result of changes in PS or F. Thus, although the extraction ratio is a measure of the specific ability of cells to extract glucose from the arterial influx, it does not discriminate between simple acceleration of blood flow through already perfused areas and true metabolic recruitment. If both the extraction ratio and the blood flow rate through metabolically active tissue are known, glucose (and other substrates) metabolism can be determined with good accuracy. The key condition is that the measured changes in blood flow do occur in the tissue that drains into the sampling vein.

With regard to flow-dependent metabolic recruitment, several investigators have fostered the concept that insulin itself is a vasodilator in humans, and that this hemodynamic effect contributes to the metabolic actions of the hormone [7]. In these investigators' hands the response to systemic insulin administration—either with maintenance of euglycemia or with graded changes in plasma glucose from basal to high levels—consists in an increase in glucose uptake by leg tissues paralleled by a major (two- to threefold) increase in leg blood flow. The simultaneous infusion of somatostatin—to paralyze endogenous insulin release—abolishes the vasodilatory effect of hyperglycemia. In obese or diabetic subjects with insulin resistance, insulin fails to cause leg vasodilation. In healthy, insulin-sensitive volunteers, insulin-mediated increments in leg blood flow correlate with both glucose utilization and blood pressure levels. These findings have been interpreted to indicate that insulin-induced vasodilation recruits metabolically responsive muscle tissue and, in this capacity, it is a mechanism, or prerequisite, of insulin-mediated glucose uptake (or insulin sensitivity): resistance to insulin action on blood vessels contributes to metabolic insulin resistance.

This interpretation presents with some difficulties. In other laboratories and with a different experimental model (e.g. the forearm), insulin-induced vasodilation has generally been modest (25–40%), particularly at physiological insulin levels [8]. Differences in patient selection, experimental conditions, and techniques to measure blood flow (thermodilution, strain-gauge plethysmography, indicator dilution) possibly account for this discrepancy. More importantly, no direct evidence has been provided in humans that the observed increase in limb blood flow involves recruitment of muscle tissue rather than increased blood velocity through already well-perfused regions. Finally, if the increase in blood flow was rate limiting for insulin action on glucose metabolism, forcing vasodilation should overcome insulin resistance. However, in lean patients with essential hypertension, doubling forearm blood flow by a local intraarterial adenosine infusion does not increase oxygen uptake (which should follow recruitment of metabolically active tissue) and fails to modify insulin-stimulated glucose uptake [9]. Thus, impaired insulin-induced vasodilation appears to be another manifestation (possibly, even a consequence) of insulin resistance rather than a causally related phenomenon.

Another form of non-insulin-regulatable glucose transporter (GLUT-2) is amply expressed in the plasma membrane of liver, kidney, intestinal cells, and pancreatic B-cells. In liver and kidney, net glucose release occurs *in vivo*. Thus, in the only organs in the body in which the presence of glucose-6-phosphatase (G6Pase)—the enzyme catalyzing the formation of free intracellular glucose from glucose-6-phosphate (G6P)—makes glucose available to the circulation, the transporter is of a type that only responds to the concentration gradient between the internal and external side of the plasma membrane. This ensures that, when insulin is around to stimulate inward glucose transport in tissues with sensitive transporters, the liver can release glucose into the blood stream as long as sufficient G6P is derived from glycogenolysis or gluconeogenesis (or both) and sufficient G6Pase activity is there to accumulate free glucose on the inside of the plasma membrane. Under these conditions of reversed gradient, the presence of insulin-responsive glucose transport activity on hepatocyte cell membranes would enhance glucose *outflow*, thereby opposing the plasma glucose-lowering action of insulin. In contrast, the physiologic control of the direction and rate of glucose flux through the hepatocyte membrane is not on the transport step but on intracellular processes.

In summary, the differential distribution and acute insulin sensitivity of the various classes of glucose transporters appear to provide the backbone for the functional characteristics of glucose diffusion and exchange in the body. On the whole, free glucose is present in blood water, interstitial fluid, and the intracellular water compartment of insulin-independent tissues (liver, brain, kidney, intestine, placenta) in total amounts which, in the overnight-fasted healthy adult, average 80 mmol (14 g or 1.2 mmol/kg of body weight), of which one-fifth is in the blood volume. Free glucose is found at concentrations that (a) are uniform in the intravascular water compartment;

(b) decline across the interstitial space toward the cell; (c) fall precipitously within cells that consume glucose avidly (e.g. brain) or in which glucose transport is relatively slow in the basal state (e.g. muscle, adipose tissue); (d) are increased in the cytoplasm of cells that produce free glucose (mostly liver); and (e) gradually and continuously decrease in the vascular bed as arterial blood turns into capillary blood and then runs back toward the right heart as venous blood. The regional characteristics of tissue composition, blood flow rate, capillary density (i.e., the average distance between the capillary axis and the cell surface), and cellular glucose uptake concur to determine the $A - V$ glucose gradient in any region of the body (Figure 2).

Glycogen

Glycogen is present in most cells in cytoplasmic granules that encase the enzymes that regulate its metabolism. In normal humans, the largest part of glycogen stores is in liver and skeletal muscle. In the former, 3–4 g of glycogen are packed in each 100 g of parenchyma; in striated muscle, the concentration is much lower (0.7–1.0% weight by weight). As a consequence, a normal human liver (1.5 kg) contains some 60 g of glycogen, whereas muscle (28 kg) depots keep 250 g. Thus, approximately 25 times more glycosyl units are stored in intracellular depots as glycogen than are dissolved in body water as free glucose.

Glycogen metabolism is controlled by irreversible cascades of enzymatic reactions ultimately acting upon the proximal enzymes that catalyze glycogen synthesis (glycogen synthase) and degradation (glycogen phosphorylase). For the two symmetric pathways, reverse phosphorylation/dephosphorylation cycles convert inactive enzymes into their active counterparts [10]. Both synthesis and breakdown of glycogen are regulated by multiple, complex mechanisms involving substrates as well as hormones [11]. In this chapter, we recall only those established notions of glycogen metabolism that are the key to understanding some aspects of *in vivo* glucose metabolism.

Points of Clinical Interest

(1) Glucose concentration is an average 15% higher in the plasma than the whole-blood glucose under ordinary circumstances.
(2) Arterial glucose levels are higher than capillary glucose concentrations, which in turn are higher than venous levels. The extent of these differences depends on the circulatory region and on its rate of glucose utilization.
(3) Both plasma and erythrocytes carry glucose to and from consuming tissues.
(4) In brain, liver, kidney, intestine, and placenta, glucose uptake is insulin independent; in adipose tissue, skeletal and heart muscle, glucose uptake depends on insulin.
(5) The whole-body reserves of carbohydrate are quite small.

GLUCOSE METABOLISM

Introduction

Any given concentration of glucose in plasma (and in the space in equilibrium with plasma) is the result of simultaneous release of glucose into the circulation and uptake of glucose from the blood stream into cells. Whenever plasma glucose concentration is stable, the concurrent rates of its release and overall uptake must be equal. Glucose turnover (TR) is this rate of constant flux through its system. Accepted terminology refers to stationary conditions of glucose concentrations and flux rate as the "steady state," with the understanding that any physiological steady state is only an approximation of the true, ideal steady state. Furthermore, the "glucose system" refers to the whole space or volume into which glucose is present as free glucose, regardless of how many compartments this system consists of, where they are physically located in the body, and how they are interconnected. Finally, the reference pool for glucose kinetics customarily is the plasma (or whole blood), for in most clinical or experimental circumstances the plasma is the only site accessible for sampling.

When the plasma glucose concentration changes over time, one rate of glucose flux (entry or removal) is being exceeded by the other. Under these non-steady-state conditions, the glucose rates of entry and removal are conventionally termed rate of appearance (R_a) and disappearance (R_d), respectively. The glucose system is strongly homeostatic with respect to glucose levels, in that the normal variations in human plasma glucose concentration throughout a day of life are confined within a surprisingly narrow range. This in itself implies that multiple mechanisms must contribute to controlling glycemia in a highly integrated fashion. It should also be recalled that glycosuria is called upon whenever glycemia exceeds the renal threshold, as if a safety measure had been set to cope with emergency when metabolic control fails. These considerations alone suggest that the body does not tolerate either hypoglycemia or hyperglycemia. For the former, the obligate dependence of brain function on the use of glucose as fuel has classically offered a rational explanation. For hyperglycemia, the evidence—and hence the concept—that high glucose levels, if not immediately life-threatening, are nonetheless intolerable to bodily functions, is more recent but no less compelling, and currently goes under the name of "glucose toxicity" (see Chapter 26).

Methods

Under the conditions of an overnight fast the liver is the only organ that makes free glucose and pours it into the systemic circulation. In theory, therefore, placing catheters across the splanchnic bed (one in a hepatic vein and another one in any artery) and measuring splanchnic blood flow (e.g. by infusing a dye, such as indocyanine green, that is only cleared by the hepatocyte) would allow the measurement of glucose turnover as the product of $A - V$ difference and blood flow (Figure 1). However, the liver and extrahepatic splanchnic tissues (gut, pancreas, spleen, etc.) also take up glucose; the application of the Fick principle will therefore estimate the net balance between glucose uptake and release in the splanchnic area, not the total rate of glucose turnover (Figure 1). One must therefore resort to glucose tracers, such as radioactive (e.g. ^{3}H-glucose or ^{14}C-glucose) or stable (e.g. ^{2}H-glucose or ^{13}C-glucose) isotopes of glucose. The use of the isotope dilution method to measure glucose turnover has become popular among clinical investigators because of its good feasibility, and has generated large amounts of information; it therefore warrants description here. The details of the tracer technique as applied to glucose turnover measurement can be found in several reviews and treatises [12–14]. In brief, the choice of a tracer is dictated essentially by cost (of the isotope and the experimental apparatus to measure it) and safety (in terms of radiation burden to the patient in the case of radioactive isotopes). The format of tracer administration (pulse injection or constant intravenous infusion or combinations thereof) can also be chosen on the basis of practical ease. Problems arise in the calculation and interpretation of the data, however. Under steady-state conditions applying to both tracee (i.e. glucose) and tracer, glucose turnover rate is simply given by the ratio of the tracer infusion rate (IR) to the equilibrium plasma glucose specific activity (SA = tracer/tracee concentration). Equilibrium is the time (usually 2 h after starting the tracer infusion) when unchanging plasma tracer concentrations indicate that glucose specific activity has become uniform throughout its distribution space. This formula, IR/SA, is not based on any assumptions other than the attainment of equilibrium. On the other hand, in the nonsteady state this approach cannot be used because either the tracer or the tracee concentration (or both) change over the period of measurement. Unfortunately, in the patient with diabetes the glucose system is unsteady for most of the time, precisely because homeostasis has been lost. Using a steady state means to probe an ever-changing state sounds like a violation of Heisenberg's principle of indetermination (one cannot precisely measure position and speed of a subatomic particle at the same time). Practicable ways around the problem do, however, exist. Their common rationale is provided by the theory [15] which proves that the degree and rate of change in glucose specific activity are the principal factors affecting non-steady-state analysis of isotope data. The larger the swings in glucose specific activity the more uncertain is the estimation of actual rates of appearance and disappearance from plasma data. Intuitively, when a change occurs at the cellular level, the interposition of an undetermined number of compartments, each with its own kinetics of distribution and metabolism, blurs the image of that change that is reconstructed from a narrow window such as plasma. All the formal models that have been proposed to represent the glucose system become progressively weaker as plasma specific activity is allowed to fluctuate freely. Therefore, one of two strategies can be followed: either the tracer administration is repeated when the glucose system has reached a new, reasonably steady state, or the format of tracer infusion is adjusted empirically to follow plasma cold glucose changes. In both cases, the aim is to minimize the changes in specific activity, thereby meeting the conditions under which steady-state equations can be used reliably. In reporting results of glucose turnover obtaining under non-steady-state conditions, we shall have to make some selection of available data, and the reader will have to use some caution in accepting them at face value.

Glucose tracers are also useful in the study of regional metabolism in two respects. First, for organs in which glucose uptake and release occur simultaneously (typically, the liver) the $A - V$ difference for the tracer offers a measure of absolute uptake (for the tracer is not produced by the organ), while absolute release can be calculated as the difference between net balance (as measured by the Fick principle) and uptake. In formula, if A^* and V^* and A and V are the arterial and venous tracer and tracee concentrations respectively, and F is the blood flow, then

$$\begin{aligned}\text{Absolute uptake rate (GU)} &= (A^* - V^*)/A^* \times A \times F \\ \text{Net balance (NB)} &= (A - V) \times F \\ \text{Absolute release rate (GP)} &= \text{NB} - \text{GU} \\ &= F \times A \times (V^*/A^* - V/A)\end{aligned}$$

Second, as tracer glucose is metabolized its label will appear in one or more degradation products (P^*). For any degradation product, the ratio of its labeled moiety to the specific activity of glucose (i.e., $P^* \times [A^*/A]^{-1}$) is the amount of that product generated from glucose (in units of concentration). For example, measuring ^{14}C-lactate and ^{14}C-carbon dioxide during the infusion of ^{14}C-glucose makes it possible to estimate the amounts of glucose that were glycolyzed and completely oxidized, respectively. If, then, the kinetics of precursor and product are separately determined, all of these precursor–product relationships can be converted into fluxes of interconversion, regionally as well as at the whole-body level.

An important concept in kinetics and physiology is that of glucose clearance. When referred to the plasma volume, glucose clearance is the volume of plasma that is completely cleared of glucose per unit time. Glucose clearance (CR) is related to glucose turnover rate as follows: $TR = CR \times G$ (where G is the glucose concentration in the same pool, plasma or blood, arterial or venous, in which the tracer concentration was determined). At the level of an organ that only consumes glucose—i.e. in which $U = F \times (A - V)$ (Figure 1)—glucose clearance is also given by U/A or $[F \times (A - V)/A]$. The latter formula calculates *net* glucose clearance in organs in which there is simultaneous glucose uptake and release. As the ratio $(A - V)/A$ is the extraction ratio (or fractional extraction) of glucose, the product $[F \times (A - V)/A]$ is the fraction of the flow to an organ that is totally cleared of glucose at any glucose concentration. Thus, the clearance rate is a measure of the efficiency of glucose removal regardless of glycemia; as such, it "feels" the impact of specific stimuli (e.g. insulin) independently of the mass action of glucose. It is important in this context to bear in mind that the tracer method actually measures glucose clearance (as the ratio of the tracer infusion rate to the equilibrium plasma tracer concentration), and derives glucose turnover rate as the product of clearance and glycemia. For a detailed discussion of the merits and pitfalls of the various protocols of tracer administration and data analysis, the reader is referred to the excellent review by Radziuk [16].

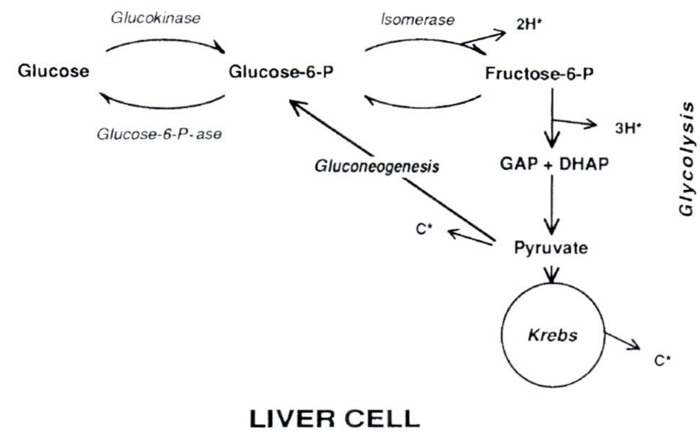

Figure 4 In liver cells, hydrogen labels in position 3 of the glucose molecule are almost exclusively lost at the triosephosphate step: they can therefore travel backwards through the phosphoglucoisomerase reaction to glucose-6-phosphate, and on to free glucose via glucose-6-phosphatase. In contrast, hydrogen labels in position 2 are largely lost in the isomerase reaction (by 75% for each complete cycle), and are therefore prevented from recycling to the free glucose pool. Carbon labels of glucose are lost to carbon dioxide following complete oxidation of glucose in the Krebs cycle, but can also recycle to glucose *de novo* through three-carbon precursors via gluconeogenesis

THE BASAL STATE

Glucose Production

By convention, the basal state is the metabolic condition prevailing in the morning after an overnight (10–14 h) fast. This time marks the end of the longest period of fasting in ordinary life (for the rest of the day humans are in a more or less fed state); this time is also the most common point of clinical observation and physiological measurements.

The true value of basal endogenous glucose production is the one that would be reproducibly measured with the use of an irreversible glucose tracer, which loses its label at the earliest possible intracellular step without ever getting it reincorporated into a circulating tracer molecule [14]. Carbon isotopes systematically underestimate glucose turnover because of the efficient reincorporation of carbons (via three-carbon fragments such as lactate) into new glucose in the liver (via gluconeogenesis) (Figure 4). Obviously, gluconeogenesis can occur in other tissues (e.g. skeletal muscle [17]), but the absence of significant G6Pase activity in tissues other than the liver prevents labeled breakdown products from re-entering the circulation as glucose, where they would alter the estimation of glucose turnover. As for tritiated or deuterated isotopes, labels in positions 3, 4, 5, and 6 are lost at the triosephosphate step or further downstream in anaerobic glycolysis, while a label in position 2 is largely lost at the (phosphogluco)isomerase step (a near-equilibrium reaction) soon after phosphorylation [18] (Figure 4). In neither case does the detached label (essentially in equilibrium with the hydrogen of the body water pool) recycle back into a new glucose molecule to any detectable extent. Therefore, everywhere in the body the clearance of any species of tritiated or deuterated glucose reflects the first, irreversible step in intracellular glucose metabolism, i.e. phosphorylation (=hexokinase activity). In the liver, in contrast, hydrogen isotopes can retrace their way back to free glucose because phosphorylation is reversed by G6Pase. ^{2}H isotopes are an exception because they lose most of their label (75%) in one turn of the isomerase cycle; the latter being faster than the phosphorylation/dephosphorylation cycle, very little labeled hexose regurgitates back to the free glucose pool. For this reason, the closest estimate of "true" glucose clearance is that provided by ^{3}H-2-glucose or ^{2}H-2-glucose, which reflects the activity of glucokinase for the forward reaction, and that of G6Pase for the reverse reaction (Figure 4).

It should be recalled that any free glucose molecule produced via the G6Pase reaction but reutilized before secretion into the central hepatic vein will not be detected by any tracer method precisely because it does not contribute to diluting the circulating tracer. Glucose production and reuptake can occur in the same cell; alternatively, since pericentral and periportal liver cells appear to be specialized metabolically (i.e. metabolic zonation [19]), intrahepatic exchange of free glucose may exist. Thus, for free glucose *biochemical production* may be in excess of *physiologic secretion*.

In the basal state, glucose output in healthy adults averages 840 μmol/min (or 12 μmol/min/kg of body weight). The dispersion around this mean estimate is significant (20–30%), with an unknown contribution of genetic and environmental factors. Whether, and how much, fasting glucose output varies as a consequence of changes in dietary habits, caloric intake, physical fitness, etc., has not been investigated. Recent studies measuring fasting glucose output in a large number of nondiabetic subjects [20] have established that total body endogenous glucose output variability is wide and is largely explained by the amount of lean mass; this, in turn, explains differences in total endogenous glucose output due to sex, obesity, and age. Intrafamilial covariance of this physiological variable is undetermined. Under standard nutritional conditions, the fasting liver depletes its glycogen stores at a rate of about 0.6 mmol/min or 11% per hour, such that glycogen depots would empty after about 10 h. Since fasting can be prolonged well beyond 10 h, obviously gluconeogenesis must progressively replace glycogenolysis as fast continues. Note that in animal species in which the basal rate of glucose turnover is higher than in humans (e.g. dogs, 20 μmol/min/kg; rats, 40 μmol/min/kg), the limited capacity of the liver to store glycogen confers an increasing role to gluconeogenesis for the maintenance of basal glycemia. This limitation on glycogen accumulation has an anatomical basis: overcrowding of cytoplasm with glycogen granules impairs cellular functions, leading to infiltration of nuclei, and, eventually, to cell death. Such is in fact the sequence of events in several glycogen storage diseases associated with damage of liver function [21].

In normal healthy adults in the overnight fasted state, gluconeogenesis is classically reputed to contribute to hepatic glucose release. The size of this contribution has been, however, somewhat controversial [22]. Studies in humans employing a multiple tracer method estimated that gluconeogenesis is responsible for ~30% of basal hepatic glucose release, the remaining 64% being, by default, a result of glycogenolysis [23]. Estimates of gluconeogenesis made from the incorporation of ^{14}C from ^{14}C-2-acetate into glucose and hydroxybutyrate are inaccurate because of extensive metabolism of acetate in tissues other than liver, and dilution of the specific activity of hydroxybutyrate formed in the liver by unlabeled hydroxybutyrate formed in muscle. Rothman and coworkers [24], by measuring ^{13}C-glycogen in human liver *in situ* with the use of ^{13}C nuclear magnetic resonance spectroscopy, reversed these estimates, and concluded that only 36% of fasting liver glucose output is supplied by glycogenolysis. Recent studies [25, 26] have used deuterated water to measure gluconeogenesis in humans. The technique, developed and validated by Landau and coworkers [27], is based on the differential incorporation of deuterium from labeled water at carbon 2 versus carbon 5 in the glucose molecule. With reference to Figure 4, the precursor of the hydrogen bound to C5 of glucose is the hydrogen bound to carbon 2 of glyceraldehyde-3-phosphate (GAP). That hydrogen equilibrates with the hydrogen of body water in the isomerization of GAP with dihydroxyacetone phosphate (DHAP), an intermediate in the conversion of glycerol to glucose, and binds in the hydration of phosphoenolpyruvate (PEP) (formed in the conversion of pyruvate to glucose). Since during glycogen breakdown there is no binding of hydrogen from body water to C5 of the glucose formed, enrichment at C5 in blood glucose versus water reflects the fractional contribution of total gluconeogenesis, i.e. from both PEP precursors and glycerol. In healthy subjects who have fasted for 15 h, gluconeogenesis contributes ~50% of endogenous glucose output. This contribution clearly increases as fasting is prolonged. By studying subjects with variable degrees of overweight and hyperglycemia, it has been established that the percent contribution of gluconeogenesis to fasting glucose release rises with increasing body mass index (by ~1% per body mass index unit) and increasing fasting hyperglycemia (by ~3% per mmol/l) [25]. In healthy subjects, physiological hyperinsulinemia suppresses percent gluconeogenesis by ~20% while completely blocking glycogenolysis [26]. As long as hyperinsulinemia restrains glycogenolysis—as is the case of obese nondiabetic subjects—endogenous glucose release will be normal in absolute terms. As glycogenolysis also becomes resistant to the inhibitory effect of insulin—as in the case of type 2 diabetic patients—fasting glucose output will increase.

The source of the substrates for *de novo* glucose synthesis has not identified with certainty. Circulating lactate, pyruvate, glycerol, alanine, and other gluconeogenic amino acids are natural candidate precursors, and undoubtedly transfer their carbons to newly synthesized glucose molecules (as proven, for example, by the incorporation of labeled lactate into glucose, or the Cori cycle). However, transsplanchnic catheterization in humans has shown that net uptake of circulating precursors is rather scanty in the basal state, accounting for only about 15–20% of endogenous glucose production [28]. The discrepancy (amounting to 1–2 μmol/min/kg) between radioisotopic estimates of basal gluconeogenic rate [25] and accountable circulating precursors [28] suggests that the blood may not be the only route of gluconeogenic supply. Within the splanchnic area, the intestine returns 10–20% of its glucose uptake to the liver as alanine (0.5 μmol/min/kg) [29], thereby filling part of the gap. Intrahepatic lipolysis (i.e. glycerol), proteolysis, and glycolysis theoretically could guarantee ample provision of precursors as an alternative or in addition to those in the circulation. However, the liver can supply gluconeogenic amino acids only at the cost of breaking down liver tissue. It has been calculated that to produce glucose at a rate of 5.6 μmol/min/kg (i.e. ~50% of fasting hepatic output) would require the consumption of all the protein in 40 g of liver tissue every hour [22]. Thus, both the amount and source of the gluconeogenic flux in fasting humans remain elusive.

In general, and with reference to the schemes in Figures 1 and 4, a complete description of a precursor–product pathway in any organ requires (1) measuring the rate of intraorgan conversion of the precursor into the product, for which the specific activity and flux rate of both are needed; and (2) measuring the net exchange of the precursor across the organ. For Cori cycle activity, for example, one must determine whole-body glucose and lactate kinetics with tracers, then measure the lactate label appearing in glucose, next determine the intrahepatic specific activity of the *immediate* precursor of new glucose (i.e. fructose 1,6-bisphosphate, triosephosphates, or phosphoenolpyruvate), and finally the net hepatic balance of lactate. This painstaking sequence is imposed by the facts that (a) lactate carbons can be found in new glucose without there being net lactate incorporation into glucose (as the liver simultaneously produces and takes up lactate), and (b) lactate specific activity is progressively diluted as other gluconeogenic precursors enter the oxaloacetate pool (e.g. alanine) or the triosephosphate pool (e.g. glycerol). This discussion is also meant to exemplify the intricacies and experimental difficulties that are involved in furnishing answers even to basic physiologic questions in glucose metabolism.

The main control of basal hepatic glucose production is exerted by the sum of several neurohormonal and metabolic influences, some stimulatory, others inhibitory. Figure 5 sketches the control system as a simple balance between inhibition and stimulation. Both parasympathetic and sympathetic fibers reach the liver via the splanchnic nerves, thereby supplying autonomic nervous modulation of both glucose production and uptake. An increase in parasympathetic impulses restrains glycogenesis and enhances glycogen synthesis (at least in animals), while an increase in sympathetic outflow to the liver stimulates

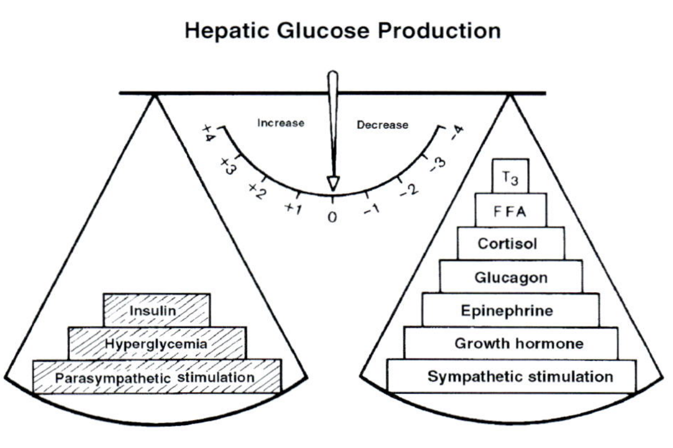

Figure 5 Inhibitory (on the left) and stimulatory (on the right) factors controlling hepatic glucose production

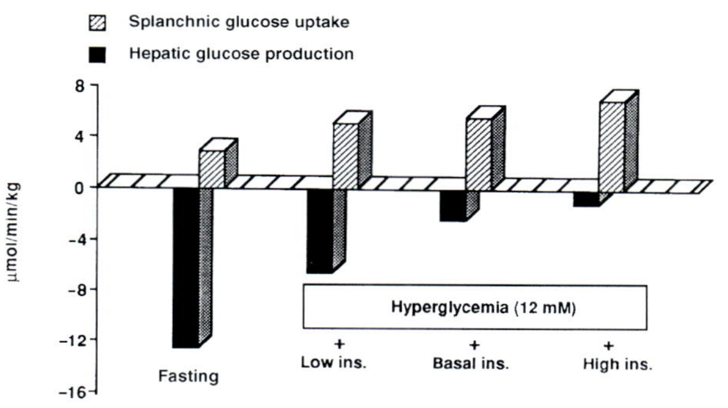

Figure 6 Splanchnic glucose uptake (cross-hatched bars) and hepatic glucose production (solid bars) in healthy adults under four experimental conditions: (1) overnight fast; (2) hyperglycemia with somatostatin block of endogenous insulin release (low ins.) (3) hyperglycemia with somatostatin block but replacement of fasting insulin concentrations (basal ins.); and (4) hyperglycemia and unopposed endogenous insulin release (high ins.). Note that hyperglycemia *per se* inhibits glucose production, and that hyperglycemia synergizes insulin in suppressing liver glucose output. In contrast, hyperglycemia stimulates splanchnic glucose uptake to approximately the same extent whether an insulin response is present or not, i.e. mostly by mass action

glucose output via potentiation of both glycogenolysis and gluconeogenesis [30]. In the human, the influence of the sympathetic nervous system on hepatic glucose metabolism can be demonstrated under conditions of acute stimulation, but the contribution of the autonomic nervous system to the maintenance of basal glucose production remains undetermined.

As for metabolic signals, hyperglycemia *per se* can effectively inhibit liver glucose output in normal humans. As shown in Figure 6, during constant hyperglycemia (maintained by a hyperglycemic clamp) hepatic glucose production is significantly reduced in comparison with euglycemia, even when the endogenous insulin response to hyperglycemia is blocked by somatostatin. It is evident from Figure 6 that normally the two inhibitory signals, hyperglycemia and endogenous hyperinsulinemia, concur to shut off glucose production [31]. That hypoglycemia by itself may trigger an increase in hepatic glucose release is suggested by the fact that during insulin-induced hypoglycemia the rise in tracer-determined R_a of glucose occurs even when one or more counterregulatory influences are paralyzed [32] and seems to precede in time any measurable increment in circulating anti-insulin hormones. Within the limits of reliability of current tracer methods, the evidence does suggest that glucose *per se* is a signal for liver cell glucose metabolism. This concept is, on the other hand, fully compatible with the idea that the net movement of glucose across the hepatocyte membrane is ultimately determined by the transmembrane gradient, which is the result of intracellular events (i.e. the balance between free glucose generation and disposition) and the extracellular glucose level. Recent studies in the dog have established a role for a portosystemic glucose concentration gradient in controlling hepatic glucose handling [33–35]. Thus, intraportal glucose infusion specifically alters partitioning of a glucose load among tissues, by stimulating net hepatic glucose uptake and reducing peripheral glucose uptake.

Of other metabolic signals not very much is known, except that it is very difficult to demonstrate in humans a detectable augmentation of hepatic glucose production by infusing large quantities of glycerol, lactate, or a mixture of amino acids, at least as long as there is physiological hyperinsulinemia to balance out such gluconeogenic push. Note that an increased provision of precursors may well lead to increased intrahepatic formation of G6P, but the eventual fate of this intermediate may be glycogen rather than free glucose if control of the rate-limiting step for free glucose production, namely G6Pase activity, is not simultaneously loosened. However, free fatty acids (FFAs) stand out as one substrate that may play an important part in setting the level of hepatic glucose production. Only odd-chain FFAs (i.e. propionate) can donate their carbon to oxaloacetate in the tricarboxylic acid cycle; most physiological FFAs, being even-chain, exchange their carbon moieties with tricarboxylic acid cycle intermediates but do not contribute to *de novo* glucose synthesis. Nevertheless, enriching the perfusion medium of isolated rat liver with oleate or palmitate induces an increase in new glucose formation from lactate or pyruvate [36–38]. Moreover, FFAs (or, rather, products of their oxidation such as citrate and acetyl-CoA) activate key enzymes of gluconeogenesis such as pyruvate carboxylase, phophoenol-pyruvate carboxykinase, and G6Pase [38]. In addition, raised FFA concentrations *in vivo* are accompanied by raised glycerol levels, both resulting from hydrolysis of triglycerides; therefore, accelerated lipolysis normally supplies both the stimulus (FFA) and the substrate (glycerol) for gluconeogenesis. Finally, the liver takes up FFAs avidly (with an extraction ratio of ~30%), and oxidizes them efficiently (as indicated by the low respiratory quotient of the organ) [39–41]. Thus, there are all the requisites to consider FFA oxidation in the liver as the energy-providing process that is coupled to energy-requiring gluconeogenesis. In isolated hepatocytes, FFAs in micromolar amounts have also been shown to inhibit glycogen synthase [42], which suggests that an additional interaction of this substrate with hepatic glucose metabolism may be at the level of glycogen metabolism. In healthy volunteers, short-term infusion of triglycerides (with heparin, to activate lipoprotein lipase) results in an increase in hepatic glucose output under conditions (hyperglycemia and somatostatin block of endogenous insulin response) mimicking the key features of diabetes [43]. A large part of this effect can be reproduced by infusing, under the same experimental circumstances, glycerol alone. On the other hand, when endogenous insulin is allowed to rise, or when exogenous insulin is administered, the stimulatory effect of triglyceride infusion or hepatic glucose release is easily overcome [43]. In summary, long-chain FFAs may regulate glucose production both by acting upon key enzymes of gluconeogenesis (through products of FFA oxidation) and by virtue of the substrate push of glycerol. In the normal subject, this regulatory loop would appear to be operative particularly when insulin secretion is not stimulated, i.e. in the basal state.

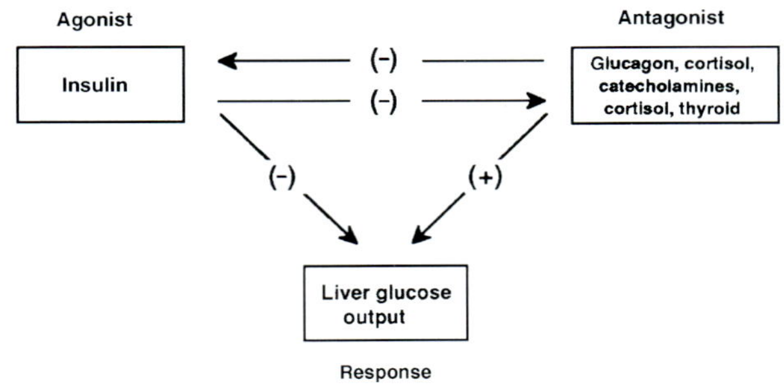

Figure 7 Insulin and the counterinsulin hormones make a complete regulatory system for hepatic glucose production

Insulin and the classic counterregulatory hormones—glucagon, cortisol, growth hormone (GH), catecholamines and triiodothyronine (T_3)—form one of the best-described agonist–antagonist regulatory systems (Figure 7). Insulin is a potent, specific, and rapid-acting inhibitor of hepatic glucose production. It restricts both glycogenolysis and gluconeogenesis, although with different dose–response characteristics (gluconeogenesis being less sensitive [26, 44]). Moreover, by restraining lipolysis and proteolysis, insulin also reduces the delivery of potential glucose precursors (glycerol, amino acids) to the liver. In its capacity as the inhibitory signal for glucose release, insulin is greatly favored by the anatomical connection between the pancreas and the liver. In fact, the pancreatic venous effluent being a tributary of the portal vein, secreted insulin reaches the liver at a concentration that in fasting humans is three to four times higher than the peripheral (arterial) concentration [45]. Such portosystemic gradient is maintained by a high rate of insulin degradation by hepatic tissues (with a fractional extraction of about 50%). Thus, a small secretory stimulus to the B-cell will raise mostly portal insulin levels, thereby selectively acting upon glucose production rather than also enhancing peripheral glucose utilization. In addition to short-circuiting the systemic circulation, pancreatic insulin release is potentiated by several gastrointestinal hormones (e.g. cholecystokinin–pancreozymin, gastric inhibitory polypeptide, glucagon-like peptide 1). Therefore, anatomical and physiologic connections in the gut–liver–pancreas circle ensure that the primary station for the handling of foodstuff, the liver, is under close control by a nearby, well-informed unit, the B-cell.

The role of insulin in regulating basal glucose production is best exemplified by the situation observed in type 1 diabetes: selective B-cell failure is associated with a marked increase in fasting glucose production despite the inhibitory influence of hyperglycemia. Furthermore, in the natural history of type 1 diabetes, progressive exhaustion of B-cell function is marked by a gradual rise in hepatic glucose output, and insulin treatment of even extreme diabetic hyperglycemia essentially aims at cutting down glucose release.

The anti-insulin hormones all counter insulin action on the liver by facilitating both glycogenolysis and gluconeogenesis. They do so, however, with different dose–response kinetics and time courses. Thus, glucagon and catecholamines act rapidly, while cortisol, GH, and thyroid hormones (in that order) are involved in the long-term control of glucose release. Glucagon has been shown to play a major part in the tonic support of hepatic glucose release: in the dog, suppression of glucagon release with preservation of basal insulin secretion causes a fall of glucose production of over one-third [46]. The precise quantitative contribution of the other hormones of the counterregulatory system to the maintenance of basal glucose output has not been assessed. What has become established, however, is the strongly synergistic pattern of interaction between the anti-insulin hormones, such that their cumulative effect is larger than the sum of the individual effects [47, 48]. This interaction may also be expressed at the level of the components of glucose production, glycogenolysis and gluconeogenesis, as well as at the level of peripheral tissues (as discussed later in this chapter). An added feature of this homeostatic complex is the dual negative feedback between agonists and antagonists (Figure 7). A-cells and B-cells "talk" to each other in the islets of Langerhans via paracrine influences (some of which may possibly be mediated by somatostatin). For example, insulin infusion *in vivo* reduces circulating glucagon levels by 20–30% even when changes in glycemia are prevented. Another example is the direct modulation of B-cell secretion by catecholamines, α-adrenergic stimulation (mostly, α-2) depressing, and β-adrenergic stimulation exciting, B-cell secretory activity. Of note in this control system is that a host of hormones is required to balance the action of only one agonist, insulin; such redundance of the antagonistic setup is typical of any system involved in a vital function. This fact must arise from the inhibitory nature of insulin's effect on the production of a fuel on which brain cell viability depends in an obligatory manner.

Points of Clinical Interest

(1) After a subject has fasted overnight, all the glucose entering the circulation (at a mean rate of 12 μmol/min/kg, or about 220 g/day) derives from liver glycogenolysis and gluconeogenesis, in approximately equal proportions.

(2) As fasting continues, glucose production becomes progressively more dependent on gluconeogenesis, and the kidneys may contribute to it. Consequently, substances interfering with gluconeogenesis (e.g. ethanol) may cause dangerous hypoglycemia in the fasting individual.

(3) Any given rate of glucose output is the net result of the inhibitory actions of insulin, hyperglycemia, parasympathetic nervous activity, and substrate shortage on the one hand, and the stimulatory actions of counterregulatory hormones, hypoglycemia, sympathetic nervous activity, and gluconeogenic substrate load on the other. Among substrates, lipids may have an added regulatory value for glucose output.

(4) Inappropriate insulin can be life-threatening in the fasting state by shutting off endogenous glucose supply to the brain. Insulin counterregulation therefore is entrusted to several hormones, providing both short-term and long-term control. The entire hormonal system is the best known in metabolism, and one of the best known in the whole of human physiology.

Glucose Disposal

In the basal state, whole-body glucose disposal equals endogenous (mostly hepatic) glucose production (by definition). Data on the individual contribution of organs and tissues to total glucose uptake have been obtained in regional catheterization studies. In the case of the splanchnic area, in which glucose uptake and production both occur, such data have been derived from the combined use of glucose tracers and indwelling catheters, as diagrammatically shown in Figure 1. By collating the available information, the organ-circulation model of Figure 8 can be drawn, in which steady-state interorgan exchanges of blood and glucose, and regional glucose gradients, are calibrated at a rate of endogenous glucose release of 840 μmol/min (or 12 μmol/min/kg or 1.2 mol/day). In this model, it is seen that roughly 70% of basal glucose disposal takes place in insulin-independent tissues (brain, liver, kidney, intestine, erythrocytes). It can also be appreciated that the fractional extraction of glucose (as defined earlier) is quite low everywhere in the body (ranging from 1.7 to 2.8%) except in the brain (9%). In particular, if it is assumed that skeletal muscle (40% of body weight) receives 16% of cardiac output and is responsible for one quarter of overall glucose disposal (~245 μmol/min; Figure 8), then muscle glucose clearance averages 1.3 ml/min/kg of tissue. This value can be compared with those of other organs and tissues (Table 1) similarly obtained by dividing the organ glucose clearance by the estimated organ weight. In the rank of efficiency of glucose utilization in the basal state, resting muscle is last, being 10 times less active than the liver,

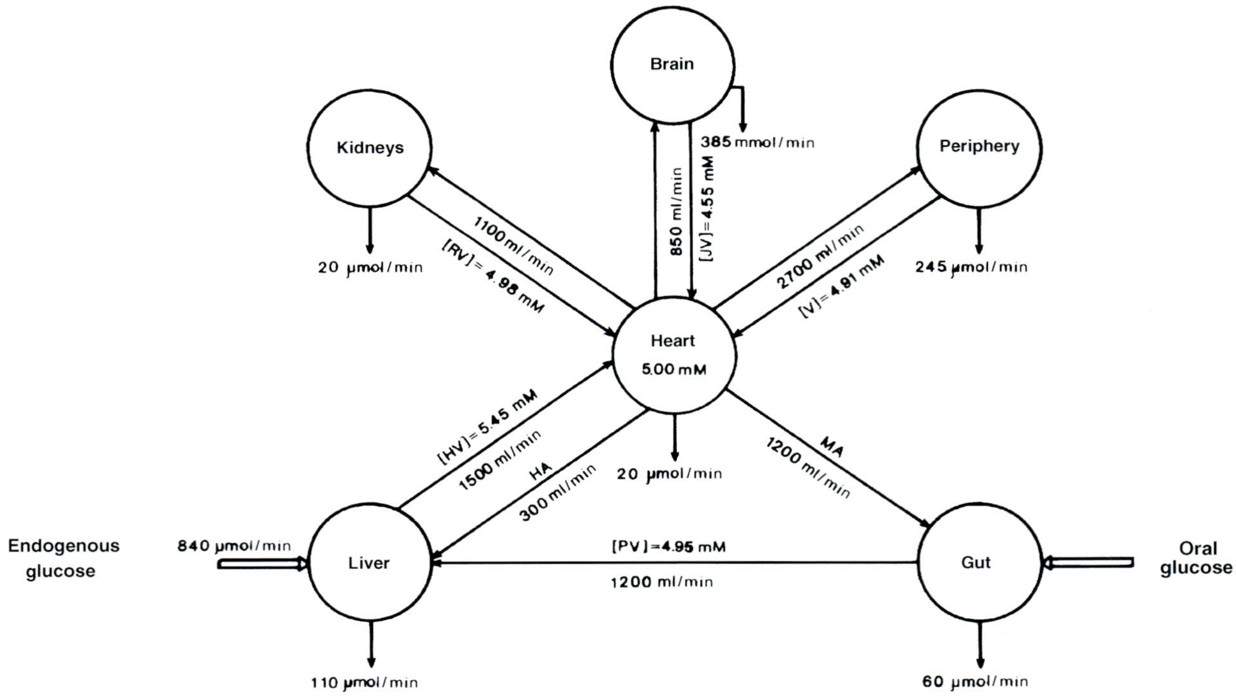

Figure 8 Organ circulation model for glucose metabolism in the basal state. Average data for healthy adults (from various literature sources) are indicated. The arrow labeled "oral glucose" indicates the site of dietary glucose entry in the postprandial state. "Periphery" encompasses all tissues other than liver, gut, kidneys, brain, and heart; "gut" includes organs (spleen, pancreas, etc.) draining their blood supply into the portal circulation. Abbrevations: PV, portal vein; MA, mesenteric arteries, HA, hepatic artery; HV, hepatic veins; RV, renal veins; JV, jugular veins; V, peripheral veins. Numbers are blood flow rates (ml/min) or glucose flux rates (μmol/min); blood glucose concentrations are given as mM

and 50 times less avid than the brain. In tissues in which specific glucose clearance is already high (brain, liver, kidneys), the effect on glucose uptake of acutely raising plasma insulin levels above fasting values is small or absent, while in muscle glucose clearance can increase by a factor of 10 over the physiological range of insulin concentrations. The intermediate position of heart muscle in the list is likely accounted for by its working state. As mentioned earlier, these characteristics can now be seen as the physiologic equivalent of the type and abundance of specific glucose transporters with which the various tissues are endowed. They also narrow the concept of insulin-independent tissue: in the latter, if raising insulin does not accelerate glucose clearance, lowering insulin may reduce the efficiency of glucose removal. In fact, even non-insulin-regulatable glucose transporters are subject to chronic regulation, as proven by the fact that animal models of insulin-deficient diabetes are associated with a depletion of all types of glucose transporters. This prediction has recently been verified in humans for at least two insulin-independent tissues: the liver and the brain. For the former, selective hypoinsulinemia (induced with somatostatin and glucagon replacement) lowers splanchnic glucose uptake below the basal value in healthy volunteers [31] (Figure 6). For the latter, indirect calculations indicate that brain glucose clearance is reduced in type 2 diabetic patients with moderate fasting hyperglycemia [49].

The intracellular disposition of transported glucose can be studied by using glucose tracers, and then tracking down the appearance of the label in specific metabolic

Table 1 Regional glucose disposal in the basal state

Organ	Weight (kg)	Blood flow (l/min)	Uptake (μmol/min)	Extraction (%)	Clearance* (ml/min/kg)
Brain	1.2	0.85	385	9.1	64
Liver	1.5	1.50	110	2.3	15
Kidneys	0.28	1.10	20	1.9	15
Heart	0.30	0.25	20	1.7	13
Gut	5.00	1.20	60	1.0	2.4
Muscle	28.00	1.05	245	3.5	1.3

* Organ clearance rate divided by organ weight.

products, such as lactate (i.e. anaerobic glycolysis) or carbon dioxide (i.e. complete oxidation) (see earlier). It is self-evident that these techniques, even when correctly applied, provide estimates of the metabolic fate of *plasma* glucose, which is the labeled pool. If, for example, there should be direct oxidation of glycogen in muscle, the plasma glucose specific activity would miss it (because of the lack of G6Pase in muscle tissue). Total carbon dioxide production, however, would include the oxidized glycogen together with all the other oxidized substrates. In general, measuring the exchange of oxygen and carbon dioxide makes it possible to obtain estimates of net rates of substrate oxidation. The method, which goes under the name of indirect calorimetry, does depend on a number of assumptions and, consequently, suffers from limitations. Theoretical analysis has, however, at least set the boundaries of validity of indirect calorimetry [50], which has the formidable advantage over tracer methods of being easy to apply and fully noninvasive. Furthermore, indirect calorimetry also supplies a close estimate of the rate of energy expenditure, can be done at the bedside, and complements information obtained by tracer methods.

In the basal state and under ordinary nutritional circumstances, oxygen consumption averages 250 ml/min, while carbon dioxide production is 200 ml/min, i.e. a whole-body respiratory quotient of 0.8 (RQ = carbon dioxide production/oxygen consumption). Simple calculations (Table 2) thus estimate whole-body net carbohydrate oxidation at about 60% of total glucose uptake. As the brain uses 46% of glucose turnover (Table 1) and readily oxidizes the transported sugar, it follows that three quarters (i.e. 46/60 = 77%) of basal glucose oxidation occurs in the brain. Little is left for other tissues, which preferentially derive their metabolic energy from the oxidation of fatty substrates and return most of the glucose to the liver after conversion into lactate (Cori cycle). Skeletal muscle, for example, has a respiratory quotient of 0.75 and relies on fat oxidation for the production of 80% of the energy it needs in the resting state [51]. Thus, the basal state is characterized by parsimonious usage of glucose as fuel, which is selectively channeled to organs that cannot rely on alternative energy sources. Altogether over one half of total energy production (5 kJ/min) is generated via oxidation of fat, of which there are plentiful (~500 MJ) and almost unlimited stores (e.g. morbid obesity). The role of insulin in maintaining this metabolic setup is permissive rather than determinant. Through a loose brake on lipolysis, insulin lets FFA override glucose in the competition between the two chief substrates, keeps glucose transport and metabolism in its own target tissues at a minimum, and restrains protein breakdown (which contributes only about 15% to energy metabolism). The part that counterregulation plays in basal glucose uptake is less well defined, but probably is centered upon maintenance of lipolysis, since all the anti-insulin hormones are more or less potent lipolytic stimuli.

Table 2 Formulae of indirect calorimetry

Net carbohydrate oxidation (μmol/min)	$= 25.3\dot{V}CO_2 - 17.8\dot{V}O_2 - 16.0N$
Net lipid oxidation (μmol/min)	$= 6.5(\dot{V}O_2 - \dot{V}CO_2) - 7.5N$
Energy expenditure (kJ/min)	$= 0.0164\dot{V}O_2 + 0.0046\dot{V}CO_2 - 0.014N$

Note. $\dot{V}O_2$ = oxygen consumption (in ml/min); $\dot{V}CO_2$ = carbon dioxide production (in ml/min); N = urinary non-protein nitrogen excretion (in mg/min).

Glucose Cycles

After transport through the plasma membrane, glucose does not necessarily follow a straight path to its eventual fate—be it glycogen, pyruvate, or pentoses—but may go around in what are known as *futile cycles*. A metabolic futile cycle is one in which a precursor is converted into a product by a forward reaction, which is then reversed to resynthesize the precursor. In this way, no net product accumulates, but energy (ATP) is used. One example of a futile cycle, G6P to fructose 6-phosphate and back through the phosphoglucoisomerase reaction, has been previously discussed in relation to the possibility of measuring it (as the difference between the turnover rate as estimated by ^2H and ^3H isotopes of glucose). Another example is glucose to G6P via glucokinase and back via G6Pase. In general terms, whenever bidirectional flux through a metabolic pathway is simultaneously operative, there exists a cycle, regardless of the number of intermediate reactions and of whether one or more tissues are involved. In this sense, lipolysis in adipose tissue, followed by partial reesterification of FFA in the liver, is a complete cycle. Another one is protein breakdown in skeletal muscle with reincorporation of amino acids into proteins in the liver. The negative connotation of futility has traditionally been reserved for those cycles that go on in the same cell. They are, however, anything but futile. As elegantly discussed by Newsholme [10], a metabolic cycle with an internal loop is the best kinetic stratagem to keep the enzymes of a dormant pathway at a minimum of activity, and to ensure a sensitivity gain for ready amplification of incoming signals. The ATP cost of these cycles is itself a means of increasing the efficiency of energy dissipation. The fact that the activity of these cycles is under hormonal control (e.g. catecholamines and thyroid hormones enhance the cycling rate) makes room for modulation; in this way, these cycles become components of facultative thermogenesis (see below).

Points of Clinical Interest

(1) Of fasting glucose uptake, 70% occurs in insulin-independent tissues, and two thirds of the glucose is

completely oxidized. Much of this distribution is due to the obligatory use of glucose as fuel by the brain.

(2) In insulin-independent tissues, raising insulin does not stimulate glucose metabolism, but insulin lack may decrease the efficiency of glucose utilization (glucose clearance).

(3) Fat is the preferred substrate of insulin-dependent tissues in the basal state.

(4) Over 50% of basal energy production relies on fat oxidation.

THE FED STATE

Introduction

The fed state is the absorptive period between meals. Carbohydrates are normally mixed with lipids and protein in the diet, of which they make up 40–60% of the caloric contents. Absorption of dietary carbohydrates is influenced by their chemical form (refined sugars or complex carbohydrates) and by other components of food. Furthermore, disposition of dietary carbohydrate is indirectly affected by fats and protein to the extent that these latter (a) compete with glucose as substrates, and (b) interfere with glucoregulatory hormones (both FFA and some amino acids are insulin secretagogues).

To circumvent the difficulties of study of glucose ingestion, the regulation of glucose homeostasis during the fed state has classically been investigated with the use of intravenous glucose, which can be administered in formats more suitable for formal analysis.

Methods

Glucose can be injected intravenously as a single bolus—0.33 or 0.5 g (1.8 or 2.8 mmol) per kg of body weight—and the decline in plasma glucose concentration after the initial peak followed for 60–90 min (intravenous glucose tolerance test or IVGTT). As, between 10 and 60 min, glycemia decreases approximately as a single exponential function of time, a decay constant (k value) can be easily calculated, and taken to estimate tolerance to intravenous glucose (Figure 10). The IVGTT has several drawbacks. First, the time course of glucose fall in reality is a multiexponential function of time, so that the decay constant takes on different values according to which segment of the curve is used for analysis. Second, over the same time interval, different curves can have similar k values (as exemplified in Figure 9); for this reason, the area under the glycemic excursion is sometimes used instead of the k value. The area under the curve, on the other hand, is also influenced by the volume into which the injected glucose is distributed. Third, and most important, the shape of the glucose curve is heavily affected by the endogenous insulin response to the acute hyperglycemia caused by

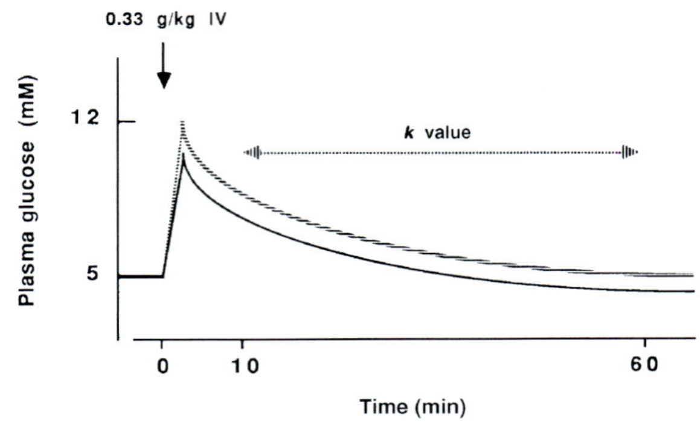

Figure 9 Schematic representation of the time course of plasma glucose concentrations following the bolus injection of 0.33 g/kg of glucose in a healthy individual. The k value is the rate constant of glucose removal from the plasma between 10 and 60 min after injection (calculated after logarithmic transformation of plasma glucose values). The two curves shown have similar k values but different areas under the time–concentration curve

the intravenous bolus. Such response is highly irregular, and after an initial peak proceeds in two or three smaller spikes tightly synchronized with similar glycemic spikes [52]. In general, in the presence of an intact feedback loop between glucose and insulin, glucose tolerance is the integrated outcome of multiple changes in the glucose as well as the insulin system: distribution of the exogenous glucose, stimulation of peripheral glucose uptake by insulin and hyperglycemia, suppression of hepatic glucose output, and secretion, distribution, and degradation of insulin. It is therefore not surprising that the information provided by an IVGTT is somewhat ambiguous, and that the test itself is neither very sensitive nor very well reproducible.

A modern version of the IVGTT is that which interprets the changes in glucose and peripheral insulin concentrations (measured at frequent intervals following the bolus) on the basis of a 'minimal' mathematical model of the glucose and insulin systems and their interactions [53]. The model generates a parameter reflecting the ability of hyperglycemia to stimulate insulin secretion, another parameter estimating the ability of insulin to stimulate glucose metabolism, and an index of the ability of glucose to promote its own disposal. Although attractive for its simplicity, the minimal model approach generally falls short of its ambitious goal, i.e. to describe all aspects of glucose tolerance with a minimum of data. In particular, the minimal model does not work when the endogenous insulin response is scarce, e.g. in diabetic patients. Not minimal is the problem that the data analysis requires a computer program that, like all package deals, deprives users of critical evaluation. Several updates of the technique have been devised. Labeled (tritiated or deuterated) glucose can be coinjected with cold glucose; appropriate model analysis of the tracer data makes it possible to dissect out the effects of insulin on the liver and on peripheral tissues [54]. For complexity of use and interpretation, the latter remains a purely investigative tool. A secondary injection of exogenous insulin or tolbutamide has been used to circumvent the failure of the minimal model in case of insufficient endogenous insulin response [55]. Other formats of intravenous glucose infusion (e.g. a constant 30-min infusion, with monitoring of the initial rise and subsequent fall in plasma glucose concentrations) must be considered investigative tools to the extent that the interpretation of their results relies on more or less complex mathematical models.

A simple way to estimate whole-body sensitivity to insulin is to paralyze endogenous insulin release with a constant infusion of somatostatin (at a rate of 0.3–0.5 mg/h) while simultaneously infusing glucose (at a rate of 1.35 mmol/min/m^2 of body surface area) and regular insulin (at a rate of 50 mU/min/m^2). With this technique (also known as the pancreatic suppression test) [55], steady hyperinsulinemia (of about 80 mU/l) is associated with a level of hyperglycemia that is inversely proportional to the ability of whole-body tissues to increment their glucose utilization in response to insulin. This test suffers from the fact that somatostatin inhibits the release of other glycoactive hormones (e.g. glucagon). With this limitation, however, it is simple and reliable enough for clinical use. Before synthetic somatostatin became commercially available, pancreatic suppression was achieved by an infusion of epinephrine (to inhibit endogenous insulin secretion via α-adrenergic stimulation) and propranolol (to block the pancreatic effects of β-adrenergic stimulation).

The glucose clamp technique has made a major breakthrough and has become the reference method in the study of glucose metabolism [56]. Figure 10 exemplifies the euglycemic, or insulin, version of the clamp technique. An exogenous infusion of regular insulin is started at time zero in a format comprising a prime followed by a constant infusion (usually at a rate of 1 mU/min/kg); such infusion quickly establishes a hyperinsulinemic plateau of about 60–70 mU/l. A few minutes after starting the insulin infusion, an infusion of glucose is begun, at a

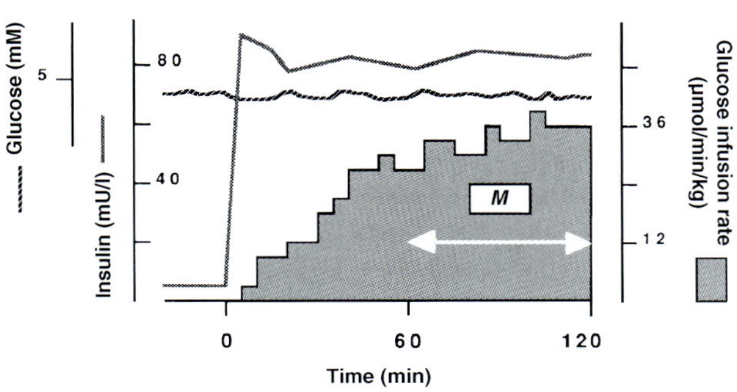

Figure 10 The euglycemic insulin clamp (see text for explanation)

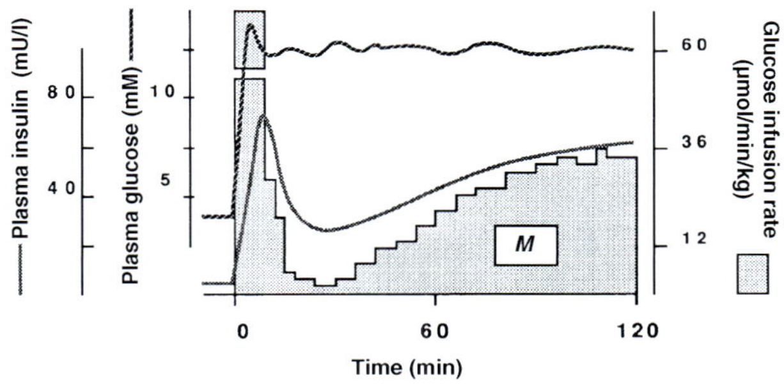

Figure 11 The hyperglycemic glucose clamp (see text for explanation)

rate which is adjusted every 5–10 min on the basis of on-line plasma glucose measurements obtained with the same frequency. Over the second hour of a 2-h experiment, euglycemia in the face of constant hyperinsulinemia is maintained by an approximately constant glucose infusion, which in a healthy adult ranges between 20 and 50 μmol/min/kg (a mean value is shown in the figure). Such a rate equals the overall rate of glucose uptake (also called *M* for metabolism) in a subject in whom endogenous glucose production is nil. Relative insulin insensitivity or insulin resistance is a low *M* value at comparable levels of glycemia and insulinemia. The technique has the following advantages: (a) any preset combination of plasma glucose and insulin levels can be easily achieved; (b) the time course of insulin action can be determined with a time resolution of about 10 min; (c) controlled hypoglycemia can be realized for study purposes; (d) other techniques, such as tracer glucose infusion and indirect calorimetry, can be readily combined with a clamp protocol; (e) the interference of other hormones or substances with insulin action can be quantitated by coinfusing them during a clamp study; and (f) although computerized algorithms are available to run a clamp, manual operation with a minimum of experience does just as well. The drawbacks of the euglycemic clamp are the need to draw frequent blood samples from an arterialized vein (e.g. a heated wrist or hand vein), and the cost of the equipment (glucose analyzer and infusion pumps). Expert hands usually elicit excellent patient compliance in the clinical use of the technique.

The hyperglycemic version of the glucose clamp (schematized in Figure 11) consists of acutely raising plasma glucose to any desired level, and then clamping it at that level, by means of a primed glucose infusion followed by an adjustable infusion (as in the euglycemic version). The hyperglycemic step evokes an endogenous insulin response that typically is biphasic: an early output (presumably of preformed hormone) lasts 10–15 min, and is followed by a gradual, continuous rise in insulin levels, reflecting glucose-induced triggering and potentiation of B-cell secretory activity. By analogy with the

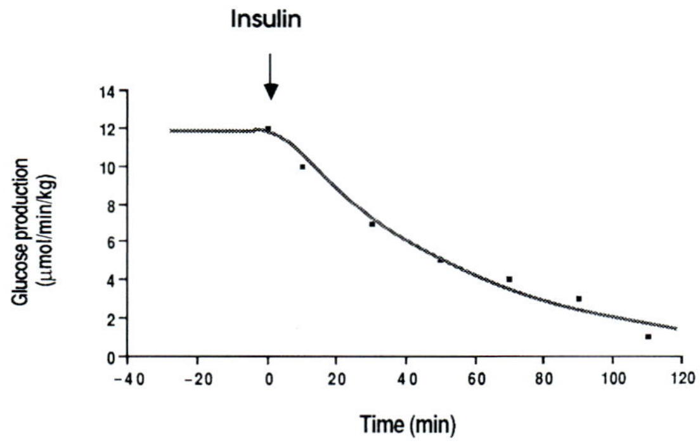

Figure 12 The time course of hepatic glucose production at euglycemia in response to insulin infusion (plasma levels of ~80 mU/l) in a healthy adult as reconstructed by using a tritium-labeled glucose isotope and non-steady-state analysis of the data. (Reproduced by permission of the American Physiological Society [31])

euglycemic counterpart, the hyperglycemic clamp provides an M value, which represents the combined effect of endogenous hyperinsulinemia and hyperglycemia on whole-body glucose disposal.

Intravenous Glucose

Even when euglycemia is maintained—thereby avoiding the inhibitory effect of raised plasma glucose levels—insulin displays a potent suppressive action on hepatic glucose production, such that portal insulin concentrations of less than 100 mU/l abolish glucose entry into the circulation. Figure 12 shows a typical time course for endogenous glucose production following an acute increase in plasma insulin to levels of 60–70 mU/l in a healthy subject. Dose–response curves relating calculated portal plasma insulin concentrations to suppression of glucose production (such as that in Figure 13) indicate a half-maximal effect at levels of about 30 mU/l, corresponding to increments in portal insulin in the range of only 5–10 mU/l. Note that in its capacity of a glucose-producing organ the liver is very sensitive to insulin; physiological hyperinsulinemia, on the other hand, does activate glucokinase, but the resulting increment in hepatic glucose uptake is very small [57]. Hyperglycemia induced by intravenous glucose administration strongly synergizes this inhibitory action of insulin on hepatic glucose release (see Figure 6): in normal adults, a rise in arterial plasma glucose levels of only about 2 mmol/l is sufficient to reduce glucose output promptly by over 80% [31].

Figure 13 also shows the dose–response of insulin-stimulated whole-body glucose disposal. The apparent maximum at euglycemia is in the order of 60 μmol/min/kg in healthy adult subjects, whereas the half-maximum lies around 70–110 mU/l of peripheral (systemic) plasma insulin concentrations. A dose–response curve of similar shape is derived when progressively higher insulin doses are applied locally in forearm tissues, about 70%

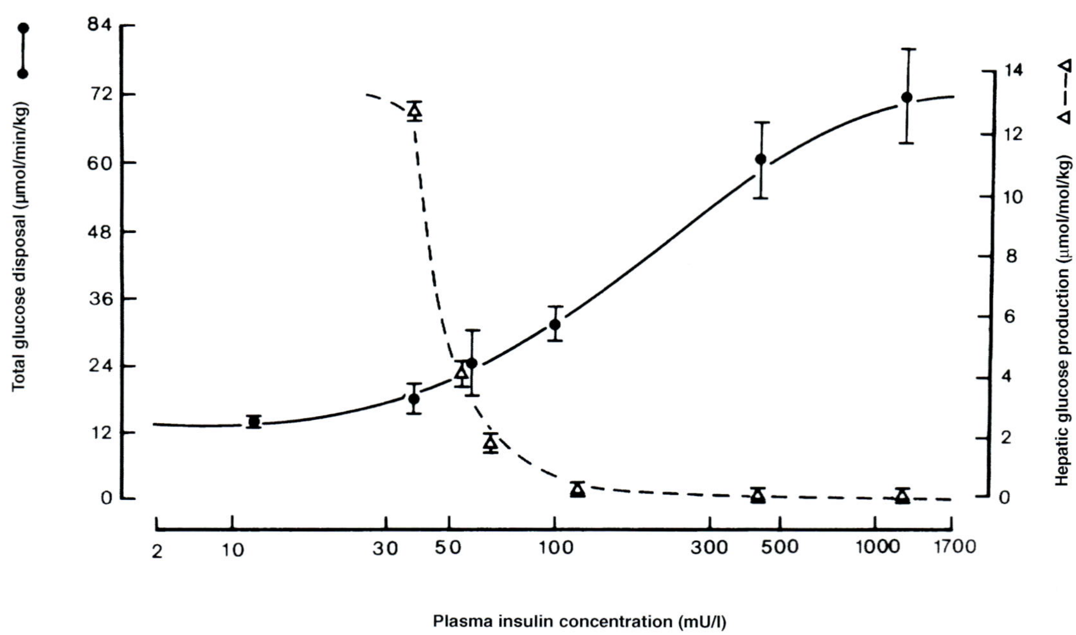

Figure 13 Dose–response curves for hepatic glucose production and whole-body glucose disposal in healthy subjects studied at five steady plasma insulin concentrations with euglycemia by the insulin clamp technique. The insulin concentrations shown are peripheral levels in the case of total glucose disposal, and portal levels in the case of hepatic glucose production. Note the logarithmic scale for insulin. (Copyright © 1983 American Diabetes Association. From Diabetes, Vol 32, 1983; 35–45. Reprinted with permission from the American Diabetes Association [31])

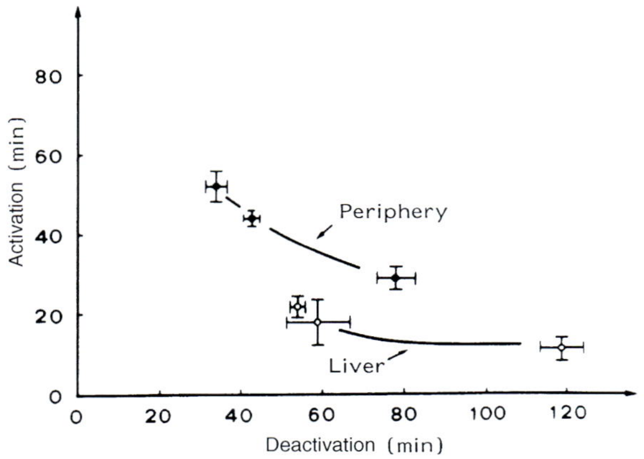

Figure 14 Relationship between activation and deactivation times for insulin stimulation of peripheral glucose uptake and inhibition of hepatic glucose production at three insulin infusion rates (15, 40, and 120 mU/min/m^2 of body surface area). (Reproduced by permission of the Journal of Clinical Investigation [59])

of which consists of skeletal muscle [58]. Extrapolating the latter data to total body muscle mass makes it possible to estimate that, with prevailing peripheral plasma insulin concentrations in the high physiological range (60–90 mU/l), 50–70% of a total glucose flux of 30–40 μmol/min/kg is disposed of in muscle tissue. Obviously, this percentage increases further at still higher insulin levels as the contribution of insulin-independent tissues declines.

The control of glucose production and utilization by insulin is dependent on both concentration and time. At any given hormone concentration, there is a finite time before the effect sets in and reaches its maximum. Such onset time is the sum of a circulatory delay (from arterial blood to cell surface, see Figure 1) and a cellular lag (intracellular diffusion and effector activation). Similarly, insulin's effect is present for some time (offset) after the circulating concentrations have returned to prestimulatory levels. Figure 14 shows the activation and deactivation times of insulin calculated at euglycemia over a wide range of plasma hormone levels (up to 1000 mU/l) [59]. With the reservations inherent in the analysis of non-steady-state tracer data, these results provide evidence that activation and deactivation are inversely related to one another; thus, at higher insulin doses the effect is more rapid and takes longer to wane. Also of physiological interest is that the relationship between onset and offset time is different for the liver (in terms of suppression of glucose release) and for peripheral tissue (as stimulation of glucose uptake): at any insulin dose, the liver is activated more rapidly and more persistently. The latter phenomenon may have to do with the shorter diffusion time of blood-borne substances into highly perfused organs (1 ml/min/g of tissue in the liver versus a corresponding value of 0.04 ml/min/g in resting skeletal muscle; Table 1).

The interindividual variation of insulin-stimulated glucose disposal is large, covering a severalfold span even in relatively homogeneous groups of healthy subjects. Adipose mass and degree of physical fitness are powerful determinants of insulin sensitivity, in that weight loss and regular aerobic training are associated with demonstrable gains in insulin sensitivity. On the other hand, age, gender, distribution of body fat, diet, and menstrual phase are general physiological covariates of insulin sensitivity. Evidence obtained in Pima Indians [60] has indicated that genetic factors are at work in the distribution of insulin sensitivity (estimated as the glucose disposal occurring at euglycemia with submaximal doses of insulin) in the population.

By combining indirect calorimetry with dose–response studies using the clamp technique, it has been possible to quantitate the two major components of whole-body glucose disposal, i.e. glucose oxidation and nonoxidative glucose disposal—the latter consisting of glycogen synthesis for the most part (>90%), the remainder being net lactate production. Figure 15 shows that the two daughter curves retain the sigmoidal shape of the mother curve but with distinctly different dose kinetics. Thus, glucose oxidation is more sensitive (lower apparent half-maximum) but saturates earlier (lower maximum) than glycogen synthesis; the latter behaves as a pathway with low sensitivity and high capacity. Whereas skeletal muscle has been identified as the predominant site of insulin-mediated net glycogen synthesis, the increment in carbohydrate oxidation that follows systemic insulin administration occurs in muscle as well as other tissues (possibly the liver) in an approximate ratio of 1 to 2. Insulin inhibits lipolysis and lipid utilization very effectively. As shown in Figure 16, plasma FFA concentrations decline steeply in response to small increments in circulating insulin levels at euglycemia; this is the result of a drastic reduction of the rate of FFA appearance into the circulation. The consequence of the reduced availability of FFA is a parallel reduction in both FFA oxidation and nonoxidative FFA disposal, i.e. reesterification (Figure 17).

The reciprocal pattern of changes of glucose disposal and oxidation on the one hand, and lipid utilization on the other, introduces the issue of substrate competition. Glucose and long-chain FFA are the first and best-known example of substrates in mutual competition for use by insulin-dependent tissues as fuels. Physiologically, a rise in plasma glucose concentration increases the rate of glucose uptake into cells by mass action; the resulting increase in the generation of α-glycerolphosphate during anaerobic glycolysis supplies the substrate for augmented reesterification of tissue FFA, thereby limiting their release into the blood stream. This effect is reinforced by the glucose-induced rise in insulin, which further reduces the supply of lipid substrates by directly inhibiting lipolysis. This glucose-on-FFA feedback is balanced by an

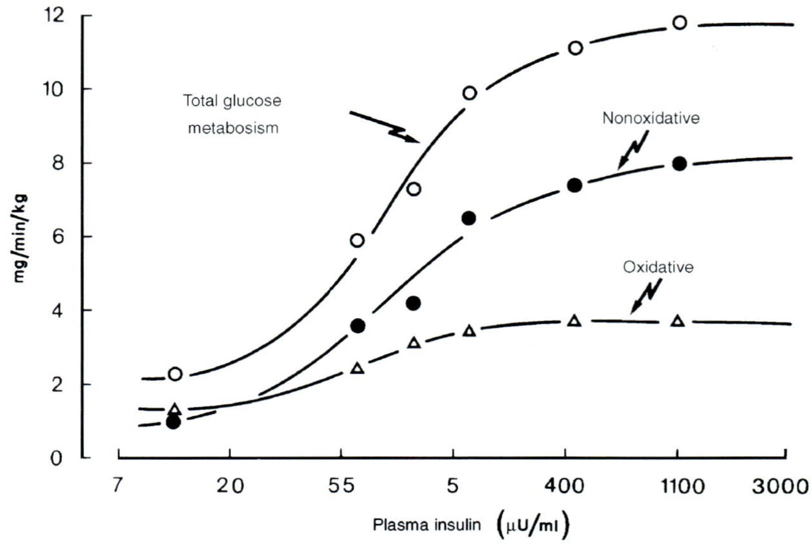

Figure 15 Dose–response curves for total glucose disposal and its components, oxidation, and nonoxidative glucose uptake, in healthy subjects during euglycemic insulin clamps

FFA-on-glucose negative feedback. A rise in FFA availability enhances lipid oxidation, and restrains pyruvate oxidation (at the pyruvate dehydrogenase step) and glycolysis (at the phosphofructokinase step), causing a backward accumulation of glycolytic intermediates, of which G6P in particular has the potential of slowing down glucose transport by allosterically inhibiting phosphorylation (at the hexokinase step). This sequence of biochemical events and the intracellular signals that trigger it (citrate, ATP and a high acetyl-CoA/CoA ratio) were elucidated by Randle and coworkers in an elegant series of experiments in rat hearts and diaphragms [61]. In the human, experimental elevations in FFA concentrations inhibit insulin-mediated glucose disposal [62] in a fashion that is both dose dependent and time dependent [63]. The insulin dose–response curves for glucose oxidation and glycogen synthesis are both shifted downwards during concomitant administration of an intravenous lipid load (Figure 18), supporting the idea that an excess of lipid supply may have inhibitory effects not only on glucose oxidation but also on glycogen synthase [42] and on glucose transport.

The extent to which insulin action in target tissues is direct rather than mediated by shifts in substrate supply can be appreciated by comparing systemic with local insulin administration. When infused intra-arterially into the forearm, insulin does not alter the circulating substrate supply, in that neither FFA nor glucose levels change in the arterial blood recirculating to the forearm tissues. Under these conditions, insulin stimulates forearm glucose uptake and lactate release (Figure 19), but induces only minimal changes in the local respiratory quotient (0.76). This indicates that the forearm tissues continue to rely mostly on lipid oxidation for energy production, and that the vast majority of insulin-stimulated glucose uptake is channeled to glycogen [51]. In contrast, when comparable hyperinsulinemia is created by systemic insulin administration (with maintenance of euglycemia), the leg respiratory quotient increases from 0.74 to almost 1.00, i.e. glucose oxidation increases while lipid oxidation is markedly depressed [64]. Thus, the direct effects of insulin are to promote glucose transport, glycolysis, and glycogen synthesis; the effect of the hormone on glucose oxidation is largely mediated by a fall in lipid availability. The insulin–glucose system therefore offers a paradigm of coordinate actions at multiple levels within the cell (transport, enzymes of glycolysis, glycogen synthesis, and pyruvate oxidation) as well at the whole-body level (suppression of glucose release, stimulation of glucose uptake, inhibition of lipolysis).

Amino acids, too, can enter a competition cycle with glucose, although somewhat less effectively than FFAs. Increased amino acid provision enhances glucose production under conditions of insulin deficiency or resistance, and limits glucose utilization in the insulinized state [65]. Furthermore, raising FFAs has a hypoaminoacidemic effect in humans [66]. In summary, each of the three major substrates, if present in excessive amounts (whether by endogenous production or exogenous administration), can lower the level of the other two by stimulating insulin release. In this capacity, glucose is obviously favored, being a much more potent secretagogue than fat or amino acids. In addition, multiple substrate effects (not mediated by changes in insulin release) participate in the regulation of the substrates themselves: high FFAs and amino acids raise glucose, high FFAs lower amino acids (Figure 20).

Intravenous glucose administration is thermogenic. Thus, during a standard euglycemic insulin clamp (such

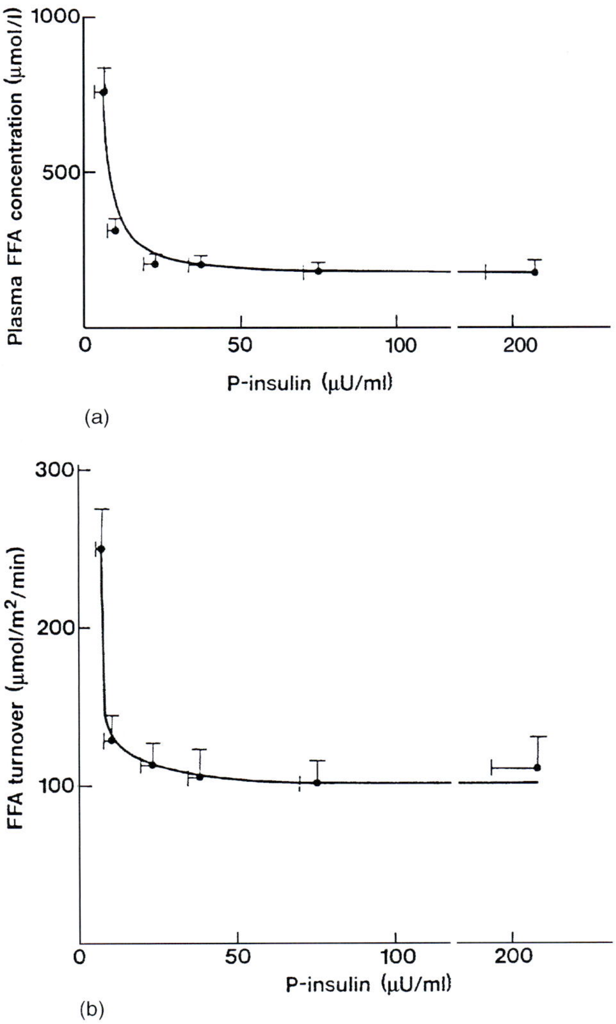

Figure 16 Dose–response curves for plasma FFA concentrations (a) and rates of FFA turnover (b), as estimated by ^{14}C-palmitate turnover, in healthy subjects during euglycemic insulin clamps

as that schematized in Figure 10), basal resting energy expenditure consistently increases by 6–10%. This effect, termed diet-induced thermogenesis (DIT), is also observed with fat and protein [67]. Part of the increase in energy production is evidently directed at meeting the cost of transporting and storing the excess nutrient. This obligatory component of DIT is even larger when the nutrients are ingested rather than infused, because of the added expense of absorbing foodstuffs. The remaining component of DIT is called facultative; substrate cycling, in the form of interconversion or futile cycles, is believed to make up this component. The adrenergic system and thyroid hormones effect short-term and long-term adjustments, respectively, of facultative DIT; dysregulation of these adjustments is reputed to have pathogenetic relevance for the development of obesity. With regard to this, it is important to note that obesity and type 2 diabetes, both states of insulin resistance, are characterized by a defective DIT, and that in both cases normalization of glucose utilization with extra insulin brings about a recovery of DIT [67]. It is therefore logical to suppose that an intact insulin action on carbohydrate oxidation is required for DIT. In support of this are the following observations in healthy volunteers: (a) if the same total glucose flux is realized by a combination of high insulin (80 mU/l) and euglycemia (5 mM) or low insulin (20 mU/l) plus hyperglycemia (15 mM), the intracellular routing of the transported glucose is different; with less insulin, glucose oxidation is significantly lower and the thermogenic effect of glucose is abolished [68]; (b) when insulin is infused locally into the forearm, muscle glucose oxidation is not stimulated and no thermogenic effect is evident [51]. In contrast, systemic hyperinsulinemia

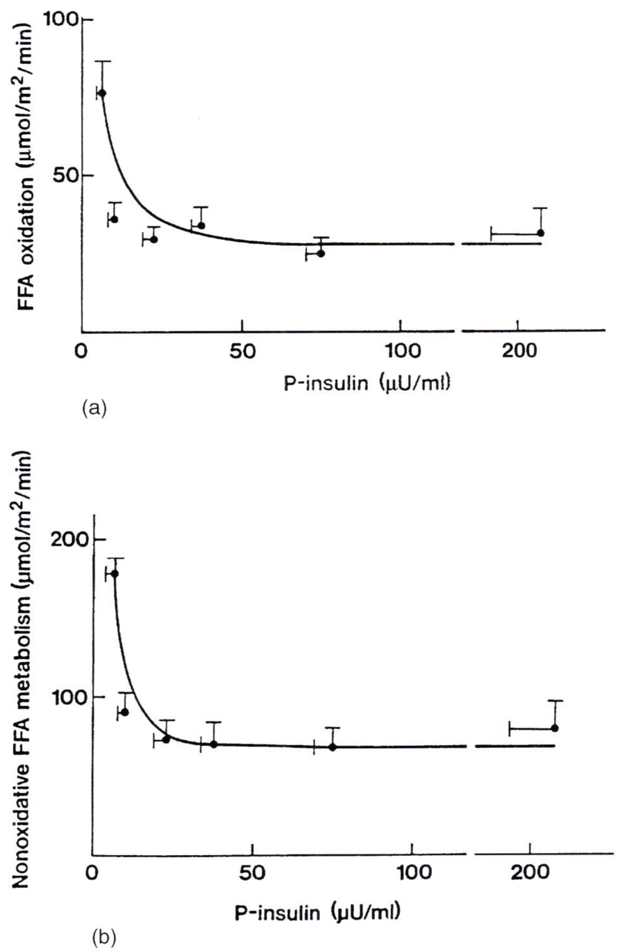

Figure 17 Dose–response curves for whole-body rates of FFA oxidation (a) and nonoxidative disposal (i.e. reesterification) (b) estimated from ^{14}C-carbon dioxide production during ^{14}C-palmitate infusion in healthy subjects during euglycemic insulin clamps

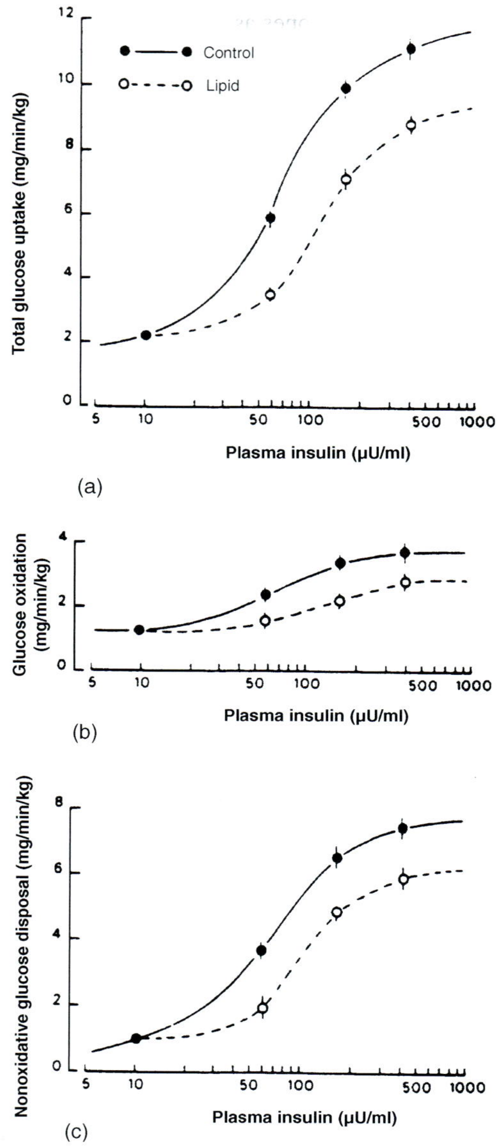

Figure 18 Dose–response curves for total glucose metabolism (a), glucose oxidation (b), and nonoxidative glucose disposal (i.e. glycogen synthesis) (c) in healthy subjects during euglycemic insulin clamps with (lipid) or without (control) a concomitant infusion of a triglyceride emulsion

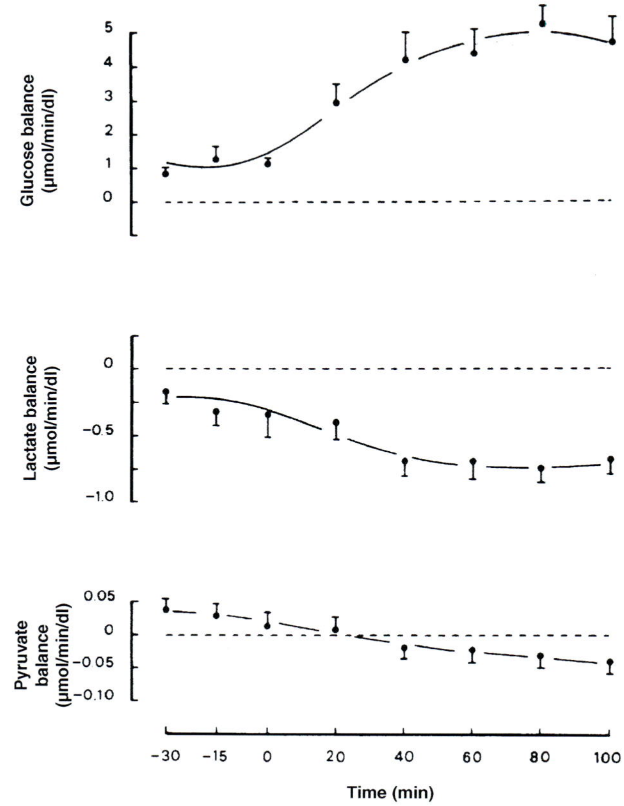

Figure 19 Net glucose, lactate, and pyruvate balances across the human forearm of healthy volunteers in the fasting state (time –30 min to 0) and during 100 min of intra-arterial insulin infusion, raising local insulin concentrations to ~120 mU/l. (Copyright © 1990 American Diabetes Association. From Diabetes, Vol 39, 1990; 490–500. Reprinted with permission from the American Diabetes Association [51])

increases both glucose oxidation and energy expenditure in leg tissues [64].

As discussed at the start of this chapter, whole-body glucose disposal may be influenced by hemodynamic responses. In particular, vasodilation can potentiate the effect of insulin on glucose uptake by exposing more sensitive tissue to hormone action; the converse can happen with vasoconstriction. Current evidence suggests that high rates of glucose uptake, whether maintained by hyperinsulinemia or a combination of hyperinsulinemia and hyperglycemia, are associated with reduced peripheral vascular

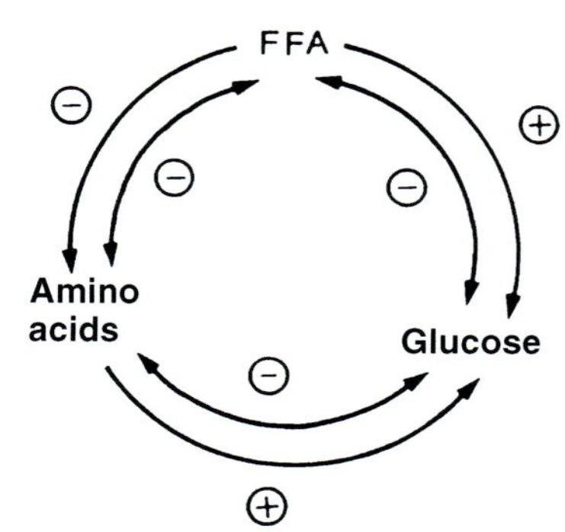

Figure 20 The glucose–FFA–amino acid cycle. Because glucose, FFA, and amino acids are all insulin secretagogues, isolated increases of each of them will lower the circulating levels of the other two via hyperinsulinemia (inner ring of the scheme). By substrate competition (outer ring), an increased supply of either FFA or amino acids will spare glucose; in addition, FFAs have a hypoaminoacidemic effect of their own (see text for further explanation)

resistance; the attending vasodilatation may contribute to overall glucose disposition by recruiting metabolically responsive tissue [69, 70].

Prolonged intravenous administration of insulin at a constant rate impairs insulin action *in vivo*, possibly through downregulation of insulin binding to its receptors [71]. Such an effect might be prevented by pulsatile, rather than constant, insulin infusion [72], the rationale being that basal endogenous insulin secretion oscillates cyclically [73].

Counterregulatory hormones in general impede insulin-stimulated glucose metabolism. Both direct effects on glucose transport (or some intracellular step of glucose utilization) and indirect effects are implicated. The latter comprise an increased supply of competitive substrates (notably, FFA) via stimulation of lipolysis. The mechanisms and time courses of action of the various member hormones of the counterregulatory system are different. For example, the inhibition of insulin-mediated glucose disposal by epinephrine or cortisol is acute, whereas it takes prolonged hyperglucagonemia or a chronic, large excess of thyroid hormones to impair glucose metabolism (see references 74 and 75 for reviews). Once again, the anti-insulin system operates in a synergistic, coordinated fashion to oppose insulin action on glucose uptake.

Oral Glucose

At any point in time, the glycemic response to exogenous glucose is the balance between the rate at which glucose appears in the systemic circulation (from oral as well as endogenous sources) and the rate at which glucose is disposed of. Oral glucose appearance in the peripheral circulation depends on (a) the rate at which the gastric contents are passed on to the small intestine; (b) the rate of intestinal glucose absorption; (c) the extent of gut glucose utilization; (d) the degree of hepatic glucose trapping; and (e) the dynamics of glucose transfer through gut, liver, and posthepatic circulation on to the right heart. The contribution of endogenous glucose to the glycemic response to feeding depends on the extent and rate of change of hepatic glucose release. Finally, glucose disposition depends on changes in the pattern of hormonal stimuli and substrate availability. Being a summation phenomenon, the response to oral glucose explores the whole of glucose tolerance, not the individual contribution of the various components.

The rate-limiting step in the transfer of ingested glucose from the stomach to the liver is the rate of gastric emptying. This depends on the volume, temperature, and osmolarity of the glucose solution in the case in which glucose alone is ingested. Glucose absorption through the intestinal lining cells is rapid and efficient, the capacity of the whole small intestine being far in excess of ordinary needs. The presence of sodium chloride in the glucose drink enhances glucose absorption, and potentiates the release of such gut hormones as gastric inhibitory polypeptide [76]. Glucose utilization by intestinal tissues is small when glucose is presented on the vascular side, i.e. when there is no oral glucose (Table 1); whether the presence of glucose at relatively high concentrations on the luminal side increases gut glucose metabolism is likely (in view of the increased energy needs for absorption) but undetermined in the human. The possibility also exists that systemic hyperglycemia and/or hyperinsulinemia may interfere with intestinal glucose absorption. Experimentally induced hyperglycemia impairs gastric motility and slows down gastric emptying, thereby delaying the absorption of sulfonylurea drugs [77].

Glucose uptake by the liver is stimulated by portal hyperglycemia (see below), but traversing the hepatic space is unlikely to significantly delay in the systemic appearance of oral glucose. On the whole, the dynamics of oral glucose appearance are essentially driven by gastric emptying, while intestinal transit, crossing of the mucosa to enter portal blood, and transhepatic passage together introduce only a small time delay. In other words, if neither gut nor liver tissues used glucose, the time course of oral glucose appearance would only follow gastric emptying, with a time shift of a few minutes. For this reason, the absorption step is a major component of the shape of the glycemic response to glucose.

Figure 21 shows the pattern of appearance of ingested glucose in the systemic circulation in healthy individuals,

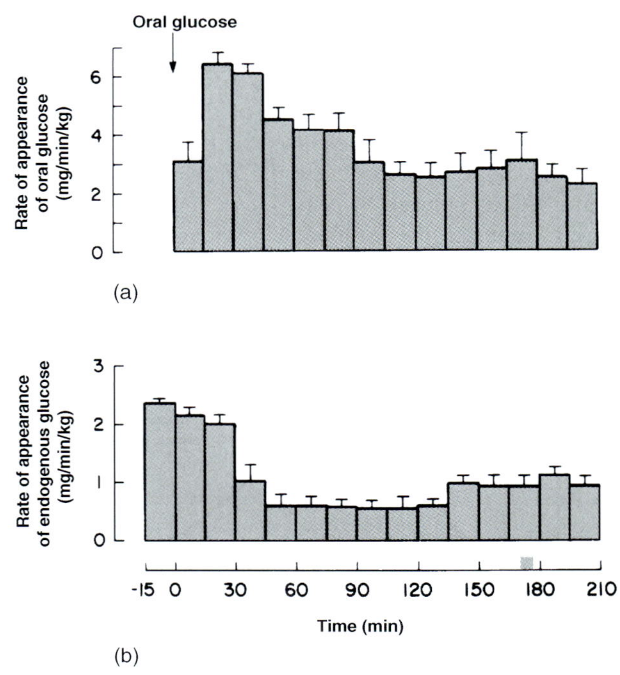

Figure 21 Rates of appearance of oral (a) and endogenous (b) glucose following the ingestion of 1 g/kg of glucose in healthy subjects. (Reproduced by permission of John Wiley & Sons, Ltd [78])

as reconstructed by a double tracer technique [78]. Glucose arrival peaks within 30–45 min, declines slowly thereafter, and is still significantly above zero 210 min after glucose ingestion. A secondary rise in oral glucose appearance is sometimes seen between 2 and 3 h after ingestion. Figure 21 also shows the time course of suppression of endogenous glucose release by oral glucose. A sustained nadir between 45 and 135 min is followed by a slow return toward fasting rates; hepatic glucose production is still significantly inhibited 210 min after the glucose challenge. Overall suppression of endogenous glucose production during 3–4 h after ingestion averages 50%, surprisingly less than what would be expected on the basis of the combined portal hyperglycemia and hyperinsulinemia (see Figure 6). Relative to intravenous glucose/insulin administration, glucose ingestion evidently reinforces counterregulatory influences (circulating catecholamines? adrenergic discharge?) which keep liver glucose outflow open.

In Figure 22 the observed arterial plasma glucose concentration is broken down into the component contributed by oral glucose appearance and that provided by hepatic glucose production. While the resemblance of oral *R*a to the plasma glucose curve is evident (especially during the first 60–90 min), less appreciated is the fact that absorption is still incomplete 3–4 h after ingestion. Figure 23 depicts the time course of total glucose disposal (R_d) following oral glucose: with a lag of some 30 min, glucose uptake is stimulated by 50–110% throughout the period of observation. Hyperglycemia contributes more to whole-body glucose disposal during the first half of the test; thereafter, hyperinsulinemia predominates. Oral glucose elicits vasodilation of the splanchnic vascular bed; this, too, is a change that persists for at least 4 h [79]. Thus, both the metabolic and the hemodynamic perturbations induced by oral glucose extend beyond the time of return of plasma glucose to preingestion levels.

The tissue destination of absorbed glucose has been the subject of intense investigation. While the liver was classically reputed to be responsible for the eventual disposal of the majority of oral glucose [79], the weight of more recent evidence [80, 81] favors the view that peripheral tissues collect between one half and two thirds of glucose uptake, while the splanchnic tissues account for the remainder. Naturally, these approximate proportions vary according to the time period over which they are observed, as well as the nature of individual responses to glucose ingestion. A robust insulin secretory response directs more posthepatic glucose to the periphery, while a large increase in splanchnic blood flow increases the delivery of incoming sugar to the liver. In humans, for example, a glucose drink sipped over 3.5 h rather than swallowed in one bolus generates the same overall glucose curve but a 50% smaller endogenous insulin response [82].

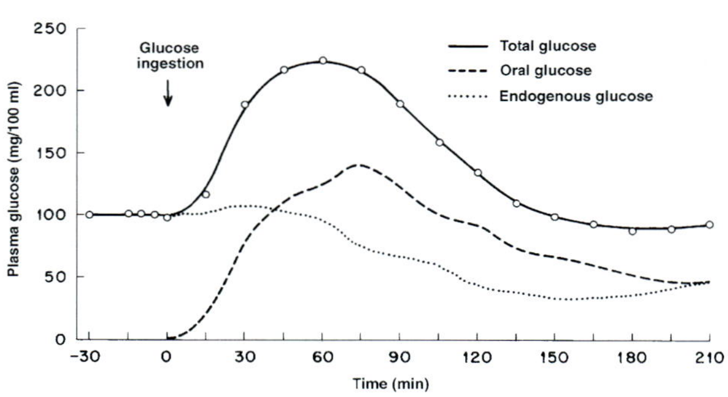

Figure 22 Separation of actual arterial plasma glucose concentration into its components contributed by endogenous and oral glucose (reconstructed by tracer analysis)

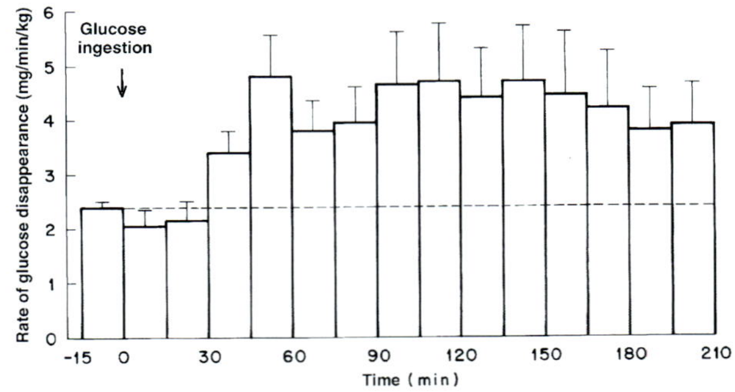

Figure 23 Total whole-body rates of glucose disappearance in healthy subjects following the ingestion of a glucose load of 1 g/kg. (Reproduced by permission of John Wiley & Sons, Ltd [78])

In animals, the route of administration seems to influence the metabolic fate of glucose [83, 84], in that the portosystemic glucose gradient *per se* enhances liver glucose uptake independently of portal glycemia and total glucose delivery to the organ (as previously discussed). In humans, however, good evidence for such a phenomenon is lacking. In fact, the available data (together with inevitable assumptions and approximations) rather suggest that the human liver takes up glucose in simple proportion to delivery (i.e. with a fixed efficiency) regardless of the route of administration [85].

Limited information is available on the intracellular fate of ingested glucose. While glucose oxidation in the brain continues unabated during the absorptive period, some 50% of the glucose taken up by peripheral tissues (muscle) is oxidized, the remainder being stored as muscle glycogen or as lactate in the lactate pool [80]. During absorption, there is an increase in lactate release by both the splanchnic area as a whole and the intestine [28, 29]. In the latter, it has been estimated that some 5% of the ingested load is converted into three-carbon precursors of glucose (lactate, pyruvate, and alanine) and passed on to the liver [29, 86]. The net release of lactate by the splanchnic area therefore suggests that the sum of hepatic lactate production and gut lactate formation exceeds hepatic lactate extraction. Liver glycogen formation during absorption of oral glucose certainly occurs both directly from glucose and indirectly via gluconeogenesis. The relative contribution of the direct versus indirect pathway to hepatic glycogen synthesis is somewhat uncertain owing to methodological difficulties [87]. Current data [88] suggest that gluconeogenesis participates in liver glycogen repletion to a lesser extent in humans than in rats [89, 90].

Points of Clinical Interest

(1) The liver (hepatic glucose production) is more sensitive to the inhibitory action of insulin than are peripheral tissues (glucose uptake) to the stimulatory action of the hormone.
(2) Insulin action on glucose metabolism is both direct (enhancement of glucose transport, glycolytic breakdown, and incorporation into glycogen) and indirect (inhibition of lipolysis, lipid oxidation, and protein degradation).
(3) In insulin-sensitive tissues, the three major substrates (glucose, FFAs, amino acids) are in competition with one another.
(4) The counterregulatory hormones oppose both the direct and the indirect actions of insulin on glucose disposal.
(5) Stimulation of glucose uptake by insulin increases energy production (diet-induced thermogenesis).
(6) The shape of the oral glucose tolerance curve is dominated by absorption processes, especially early after ingestion. Later on, insulin action prevails.
(7) Insulin controls oral glucose tolerance by suppressing endogenous glucose production and promoting glucose uptake into muscle. Hyperglycemia enhances splanchnic glucose uptake.

REFERENCES

1. Joost H-G, Thorens B. The extended GLUT-family of sugar/polyol transport facilitators: nomenclature, sequence characteristics, and potential function of its novel members [review]. *Mol Membr Biol* 2001; 18: 247–56.
2. Jacquez JA. Red blood cell as glucose carrier: significance for placental and cerebral glucose transfer. *Am J Physiol* 1984; 246: R289–98.
3. Zierler KL. Theory of the use of arteriovenous concentration differences for measuring metabolism in steady and non-steady states. *J Clin Invest* 1961; 40: 2111–25.
4. Schmidt FJ, Sluiter WJ, Schoonen AJM. Glucose concentration in subcutaneous extracellular space. *Diabetes Care* 1993; 16: 695–700.
5. Crone C, Levitt DG. Capillary permeability to small solutes. *Handbook of Physiology. The Cardiovascular System*, Vol 4. Bethesda, MD: American Physiological Society, 1984; pp 411–66 (sect 2: Microcirculation).
6. Renkin E. Control of microcirculation and blood tissue exchange. *Handbook of Physiology. The Cardiovascular System*, Vol 4. Bethesda, MD: American Physiological Society, 1984; pp 627–87 (sect 4: Microcirculation).
7. Baron AD. Cardiovascular actions of insulin in humans. Implications for insulin sensitivity and vascular tone. In Ferrannini E (ed) *Insulin Resistance and Disease. Bailliere's Clinical Endocrinology and Metabolism*, Vol 7, No 4. London: WB Saunders, 1993; pp 961–88.
8. Ferrannini E. Effects of insulin on the kidney and the cardiovascular system. In Mogensen CE (ed) *The Kidney and Hypertension in Diabetes Mellitus*, 5th edn. Boston: Kluwer Academic Publishers, 2000; pp 139–51.
9. Natali A, Bonadonna R, Santoro D, Quiñones Galvan A, Baldi S, Frascerra S, Palombo C, Ghione S, Ferrannini E. Insulin resistance and vasodilatation in essential hypertension: studies with adenosine. *J Clin Invest* 1994; 94: 1570–6.
10. Newsholme EA, Leech AR. *Biochemistry for the Medical Sciences*. Chichester: Wiley, 1983; pp 308–10.
11. Hers HG. The control of glycogen metabolism in the liver. *Ann Rev Biochem* 1976; 45: 167–89.
12. Shipley RA, Clark RE. *Tracer Methods for In Vivo Kinetics*. New York: Academic Press, 1972.
13. Wolfe RR. *Tracers in Metabolic Research. Radioisotope and Stable Isotope/Mass Spectrometry Methods*. New York: Alan R. Liss, 1984.
14. Ferrannini E, Del Prato S, DeFronzo RA. Glucose kinetics: tracer methods. In Clarke WL, Larner J, Pohl SL (eds) *Methods in Diabetes Research, Vol 11: Clinical Methods*. New York: Wiley, 1986; pp 107–42.
15. Cobelli C, Mari A, Ferrannini E. The non-steady state problem: error analysis of Steele's model and developments for glucose kinetics. *Am J Physiol* 1987; 252: E679–87.
16. Radziuk J, Pye S. Quantitation of basal endogenous glucose production in Type II diabetes: importance of the volume of distribution [review]. *Diabetologia* 2002; 45: 1053–84.
17. Bonen A, McDermott JC, Tan MH. Glycogenesis and glyconeogenesis in skeletal muscle: effects of pH and hormones. *Am J Physiol* 1990; 258: E693–700.
18. Katz J, Golden S, Dunn A, Chenoweth M. Estimation of glucose turnover in rats in vivo with tritium labeled glucoses. *Hoppe-Seyler's Z Physiol Chem* 1976; 357: 1387–94.
19. Jungerman K. Metabolic zonation of liver parenchyma: significance for the regulation of glycogen metabolism, gluconeogenesis and glycolysis. *Diabetes Metab Rev* 1987; 3: 260–93.
20. Natali A, Toschi E, Camastra S, Gastaldelli A, Groop L, Ferrannini E, for the European Group for the Study of Insulin Resistance (EGIR). Determinants of postabsorptive endogenous glucose output in non-diabetic subjects. *Diabetologia* 2000; 43: 1266–72.
21. Hers H-G, Van Hoof F, de Barsy T. Glycogen storage diseases. In Scriver CR, Beaudet AL, Sly NS, Valle D (eds) *The Metabolic Basis of Inherited Disease*. New York: McGraw-Hill, 1989; pp 425–52.
22. Barrett EJ, Liu Z. Hepatic glucose metabolism and insulin resistance in NIDDM. In Ferrannini E (ed) *Insulin Resistance and Disease. Bailliere's Clinical Endocrinology and Metabolism*, Vol 7, No 4. London: WB Saunders, 1993; pp 875–902.
23. Consoli A, Kennedy FP, Miles J, Gerich JE. Determination of Krebs cycle metabolic carbon exchange in vivo and its use to estimate individual contributions of gluconeogenesis and glycogenolysis to overall glucose output in man. *J Clin Invest* 1987; 80: 1303–10.

24. Rothman DL, Magnusson I, Katz LD, Shulman RG, Shulman GI. Quantitation of hepatic glycogenolysis and gluconeogenesis in fasting human with ^{13}C NMR. *Science* 1991; 254: 573–6.
25. Gastaldelli A, Baldi S, Pettiti M, Toschi E, Camastra S, Natali A, Landau BR, Ferrannini E. Influence of obesity and type 2 diabetes on gluconeogenesis and glucose output in humans: a quantitative study. *Diabetes* 2000; 49: 1367–73.
26. Gastaldelli A, Toschi E, Pettiti M, Frascerra S, Quiñones-Galvan A, Sironi AM, Natali A, Ferrannini E. Effect of physiological hyperinsulinemia on gluconeogenesis in nondiabetic subjects and in type 2 diabetic patients. *Diabetes* 2001; 50: 1807–12.
27. Landau BR, Wahren J, Chandramouli V, Schumann WC, Ekberg K, Kalhan SC. Contribution of gluconeogenesis to glucose production in the fasted state. *J Clin Invest* 1996; 98: 378–85.
28. Felig P, Sherwin RS. Carbohydrate homeostasis, liver and diabetes. *Prog Liver Dis* 1976; 5: 169–71.
29. Bjorkman O, Eriksson LS, Nyberg B, Wahren J. Gut exchange of glucose and lactate in basal state and after oral glucose ingestion in postoperative patients. *Diabetes* 1990; 39: 747–51.
30. Shimazu T. Neuronal regulation of hepatic glucose metabolism in mammals. *Diabetes Metab Rev* 1987; 3: 185–206.
31. DeFronzo RA, Ferrannini E, Hendler R, Felig P, Wahren J. Regulation of splanchnic and peripheral glucose uptake by insulin and hyperglycemia in man. *Diabetes* 1983; 32: 35–45.
32. Gerich JE, Campbell PJ. Overview of counter-regulation and its abnormalities in diabetes mellitus and other conditions. *Diabetes Metab Rev* 1988; 4: 93–112.
33. Galassetti P, Chu CA, Neal DW, Reed GW, Wasserman DH, Cherrington AD. A negative arterial–portal venous glucose gradient increases net hepatic glucose uptake in euglycemic dogs. *Am J Physiol* 1999; 277: E126–34.
34. Hsieh PS, Moore MC, Marshall B, Pagliassotti MJ, Shay B, Szurkus D, Neal DW, Cherrington AD. The head arterial glucose level is not the reference site for generation of the portal signal in conscious dogs. *Am J Physiol* 1999; 277: E678–84.
35. Hsieh PS, Moore MC, Neal DW, Cherrington AD. Importance of the hepatic arterial glucose level in generation of the portal signal in conscious dogs. *Am J Physiol* 2000; 279: E284–92.
36. Struck E, Ashmore J, Wieland O. Effects of glucagon and long-chain fatty acids on glucose production by isolated perfused rat liver. *Adv Enzyme Regul* 1966; 4: 219–24.
37. Williamson JR, Kreisberg RA, Felts PW. Mechanism for the stimulation of gluconeogenesis by fatty acids in perfused rat liver. *Proc Natl Acad Sci USA* 1966; 56: 247–54.
38. Friedman B, Goodman EH Jr, Weinhouse S. Effects of insulin and fatty acids on gluconeogenesis in the rat. *J Biol Chem* 1967; 242: 3620–7.
39. Havel RJ, Kane JP, Balasse EO, Segel N, Basso LV. Splanchnic metabolism of free fatty acids and production of triglycerides of very low density lipoproteins in normotriglyceridemic and hypertriglyceridemic humans. *J Clin Invest* 1970; 49: 2017–35.
40. Basso LV, Havel RJ. Hepatic metabolism of free fatty acids in normal and diabetic dogs. *J Clin Invest* 1970; 49: 537–47.
41. Wahren J, Hagenfeldt L, Felig P. Splanchnic and leg exchange of glucose, amino acids, and free fatty acids during exercise in diabetes mellitus. *J Clin Invest* 1975; 55: 1303–14.
42. Wititsuwannakul D, Kim K. Mechanism of palmityl coenzyme A inhibition of liver glycogen synthase. *J Biol Chem* 1977; 252: 7812–7.
43. Ferrannini E, Barrett EJ, Bevilacqua S, DeFronzo RA. Effect of fatty acids on glucose production and utilization in man. *J Clin Invest* 1983; 72: 1737–47.
44. Chiasson JL, Liljenquist JE, Finger FE, Lacy WW. Differential sensitivity of glycogenolysis and gluconeogenesis to insulin infusion in the dog. *Diabetes* 1976; 25: 283–91.
45. Ferrannini E, Cobelli C. The kinetics of insulin in man, II: Role of the liver. *Diabetes Metab Rev* 1987; 3: 365–97.
46. DeFronzo RA, Ferrannini E. Regulation of hepatic glucose metabolism in humans. *Diabetes Metab Rev* 1987; 3: 415–59.
47. Eigler NL, Sacca L, Sherwin RS. Synergistic interactions of physiologic increments of glucagon, epinephrine, and cortisol in the dog. A model for stress-induced hyperglycemia. *J Clin Invest* 1979; 63: 114–23.
48. Gerich J, Cryer P, Rizza R. Hormonal mechanisms in acute glucose counterregulation: the relative roles of glucagon, epinephrine, norepinephrine, growth hormone and cortisol. *Metabolism* 1980; 29: 1164–75.
49. Gerich JE, Mitrakou A, Kelley D, Mandarino L, Nurjhan N, Reilly J, Jenssen T, Veneman T, Consoli A. Contribution of impaired muscle glucose clearance to reduced postabsorptive systemic glucose clearance in NIDDM. *Diabetes* 1990; 39: 211–6.
50. Ferrannini E. The theoretical bases of indirect calorimetry: a review. *Metabolism* 1988; 37: 287–301.
51. Natali A, Buzzigoli G, Taddei S, Santoro D, Cerri M, Pedrinelli R, Ferrannini E. Effects of insulin on hemodynamics and metabolism in human forearm. *Diabetes* 1990; 39: 490–500.
52. Ferrannini E, Pilo A. Pattern of insulin delivery after intravenous glucose injection, and its relation to plasma glucose disappearance. *J Clin Invest* 1979; 64: 243–54.
53. Bergman RN, Ider YZ, Bowden CR, Cobelli C. Quantitative estimation of insulin sensitivity. *Am J Physiol* 1979; 236: E667–77.
54. Cobelli C, Pacini G, Toffolo G, Sacca L. Estimation of insulin sensitivity and glucose clearance from minimal model: new insights from labeled IVGTT. *Am J Physiol* 1986; 253: E551–64.
55. Bergman RN, Finegood DT, Ader M. Assessment of insulin sensitivity in vivo. *Endocr Rev* 1985; 6: 45–86.
56. DeFronzo RA, Tobin J, Andres R. Glucose clamp technique: a method for quantifying insulin secretion and insulin resistance. *Am J Physiol* 1979; 237: E214–23.
57. Iozzo P, Geisler F, Oikonen V, Maki M, Takala T, Solin O, Ferrannini E, Knuuti J, Nuutila P. Insulin stimulates liver glucose uptake in humans: an 18F-FDG PET Study. *J Nucl Med* 2003; 44: 682–9.
58. Yki-Järvinen H, Young AA, Lamkin C, Foley J. Kinetics of glucose disposal in whole body and across the forearm in man. *J Clin Invest* 1987; 79: 1713–9.
59. Prager R, Wallace P, Olefsky JM. In vivo kinetics of insulin action on peripheral glucose disposal and hepatic output in normal and obese subjects. *J Clin Invest* 1986; 78: 472–81.
60. Lillioja S, Mott DM, Zawadzki JK, et al. In vivo insulin action is familial characteristic in non-diabetic Pima Indians. *Diabetes* 1987; 36: 1329–35.

61. Randle PJ, Newsholme EA, Garland PB. Regulation of glucose uptake by muscle. Effects of fatty acids, ketone bodies, and pyruvate, and of alloxan diabetes and starvation, on the uptake and metabolic fate of glucose in rat heart and diaphragm muscles. *Biochem J* 1964; 93: 652–65.
62. Thiebaud D, Jacot E, DeFronzo RA, Maeder E, Jequier E, Felber JP. The effect of graded doses of insulin on total glucose uptake, glucose oxidation, and glucose storage in man. *Diabetes* 1982; 31: 957–63.
63. Bonadonna RC, Zych K, Boni C, Ferrannini E, DeFronzo RA. Time dependence of the interaction between glucose and lipid in man. *Am J Physiol* 1989; 257: E49–57.
64. Kelley DE, Reilly JP, Veneman T, Mandarino LJ. Effects of insulin on skeletal muscle glucose storage, oxidation, and glycolysis in humans. *Am J Physiol* 1990; 258: E923–9.
65. Ferrannini E, Bevilacqua S, Lanzone L, Bonadonna R, Brandi L, Oleggini M, Boni C, Buzzigoli G, Ciociaro D, Luzi L, DeFronzo RA. Metabolic interactions of amino acids and glucose in healthy humans. *Diab Nutr Metab* 1988; 3: 175–86.
66. Ferrannini E, Barrett EJ, Bevilacqua S, Jacob R, Walesky M, Sherwin RS, DeFronzo RA. Effect of free fatty acids on blood amino acid levels in humans. *Am J Physiol* 1986; 250: E686–94.
67. Jequier E, Schutz Y. Energy expenditure in obesity and diabetes. *Diabetes Metab Rev* 1988; 4: 583–94.
68. Ferrannini E, Locatelli L, Jequier E, Felber JP. Differential effects of insulin and hyperglycemia on intracellular glucose disposition in man. *Metabolism* 1989; 38: 459–67.
69. Edelman SV, Laakso M, Wallace P, Brechtel G, Olefsky JM, Baron AD. Kinetics of insulin-mediated and non-insulin-mediated glucose uptake in humans. *Diabetes* 1990; 39: 955–64.
70. Laakso M, Edelman SV, Brechtel G, Baron AD. Decreased effect of insulin to stimulate skeletal muscle blood flow in obese man. A novel mechanism for insulin resistance. *J Clin Invest* 1990; 85: 1844–52.
71. Rizza RA, Mandarino LJ, Genest J, Baker BA, Gerich JE. Production of insulin resistance by hyperinsulinaemia in man. *Diabetologia* 1985; 28: 70–5.
72. Ward GM, Walters J, Aitken PM, Best JD, Alford FP. Effects of prolonged pulsatile hyperinsulinemia in humans: enhancement of insulin sensitivity. *Diabetes* 1990; 39: 501–7.
73. Lang DA, Matthews DR, Peto J, Turner RC. Cyclic oscillations of basal plasma glucose and insulin concentrations in human beings. *N Engl J Med* 1979; 301: 1023–7.
74. Gerich JE, Rizza R, Haymond M, Cryer P. Hormonal mechanisms in acute glucose counter-regulation: the relative roles of glucagon, epinephrine, norepinephrine, growth hormone and cortisol. *Metabolism* 1981; 29 (suppl 2): 1164–75.
75. Bratusch-Marrain PR. Insulin-counteracting hormones: their impact on glucose metabolism. *Diabetologia* 1983; 24: 74–9.
76. Ferrannini E, Barrett E, Bevilacqua S, Dupre J, DeFronzo RA. Sodium elevates the plasma glucose response to glucose ingestion in man. *J Clin Endocrinol Metab* 1982; 54: 455–8.
77. Groop LC, Luzi L, DeFronzo RA, Melander A. Hyperglycaemia and absorption of sulphonylurea drugs. *Lancet* 1989; 2 (8655): 129–30.
78. Pilo A, Ferrannini E, Biorkman O, Wahren J, Reichard GA, Felig P, DeFronzo RA. Analysis of subjects: a double tracer approach. In Cobelli C, Bergman RN (eds) *Carbohydrate Metabolism*. New York: Wiley, 1981; pp 221–38.
79. Felig P, Wahren J, Hendler R. Influence of maturity-onset diabetes on splanchnic balance after oral glucose ingestion. *Diabetes* 1978; 27: 121–6.
80. Ferrannini E, Bjorkman O, Reichard GA, Pilo A, Olsson M, Wahren J, DeFronzo RA. The disposal of an oral glucose load in healthy subjects. A quantitative study. *Diabetes* 1985; 34: 580–8.
81. Kelley D, Mitrakou A, Marsh H, et al. Skeletal muscle glycolysis, oxidation, and storage of an oral glucose load. *J Clin Invest* 1988; 81: 1563–71.
82. Jenkins DJA, Wolever TMS, Ocana AM, et al. Metabolic effects of reducing rate of glucose ingestion by single bolus versus continuous sipping. *Diabetes* 1990; 39: 775–81.
83. Ishida T, Chap Z, Chen J, Lewis R, Hartley C, Entman M, Field J. Differential effects of oral, peripheral intravenous, and intraportal glucose on hepatic glucose uptake and insulin and glucagon extraction in conscious dogs. *J Clin Invest* 1983; 72: 590–601.
84. Adkins BA, Myers SR, Hendrick GK, Williams PE, Stevenson RW, Cherrington AD. Importance of route of intravenous glucose delivery on hepatic glucose balance in the conscious dog. *J Clin Invest* 1987; 79: 557–65.
85. Ferrannini E, Katz LD, Glickman MG, DeFronzo RA. Influence of combined intravenous and oral glucose administration on splanchnic glucose uptake in man. *Clin Physiol* 1990; 10: 527–38.
86. Abumrad NN, Cherrington AD, Williams PE, Lacy WW, Rabin D. Absorption and disposition of a glucose load in the conscious dog. *Am J Physiol* 1982; 242: E398–406.
87. Radziuk J. Mathematical basis for the measurement of the rates of glucose appearance and synthesis in vivo. In Clarke WL, Larner J, Pohl SL (eds) *Methods in Diabetes Research, Vol II: Clinical Methods*. New York: Wiley, 1986; pp 143–64.
88. Radziuk J. Carbon transfer in the measurement of glycogen synthesis from precursors during absorption of an ingested glucose load. *Fed Proc* 1982; 41: 88–90.
89. Newgard CB, Hirsch LJ, Foster DW, McGarry JD. Studies on the mechanism by which exogenous glucose is converted into liver glycogen in the rat. *J Biol Chem* 1983; 258: 8046–52.
90. Shulman GI, Rothman DL, Smith D, Johnson CM, Blair JB, Shulman RG, DeFronzo RA. Mechanism of liver glycogen repletion in vivo by nuclear magnetic resonance spectroscopy. *J Clin Invest* 1985; 76: 1229–36.

16

Measuring Insulin Action *In Vivo*

Richard N. Bergman, Katrin Hücking, and Richard M. Watanabe

University of Southern California, Los Angeles, CA, USA

HISTORICAL PERSPECTIVE

The heralded isolation of insulin in Toronto in 1921 was followed immediately by treatment of diabetes. It soon became clear that while insulin was effective in regulating the blood glucose levels in most patients, there were some subjects in whom insulin appeared to be ineffective [1, 2]. This lack of insulin effect was termed "insulin resistance" as early as 1925 [3]. In a remarkable but unfortunately forgotten study, Bainbridge observed that rats and mice, fed a carbohydrate-free, excess-fat diet, developed a high degree of resistance to insulin. In 1936, Himsworth noted that the effect of insulin injection was less pronounced in obese subjects and subjects with "mild" diabetes [4]. He suggested that obesity and diabetes are related to insulin resistance [5] and that insulin sensitivity could be increased by high-carbohydrate, low-fat diets [6]. However, lack of ability to measure the hormone directly made difficult the interpretation of Himsworth's elegant studies.

Introduction of the radioimmunoassay by Berson and Yalow provided compeling evidence for the existence of insulin resistance. These authors were aware that higher insulin after oral glucose implied insulin resistance, and suggested insulin resistance in obese patients, and patients with "maturity-onset" (type 2) diabetes [7, 8]. However, absent a direct assessment of insulin resistance, the putative role of this presumed defect in type 2 diabetes remained controversial. Adding to the controversy was Kipnis' elegant demonstration of a β-cell defect in type 2 diabetic patients. Kipnis reported a diminished plasma insulin response to a matched plasma glucose pattern in type 2 diabetic patients compared to nondiabetic patients [9]. Thus as of 1970 supportive evidence existed suggesting a defect in β-cell function was responsible for "maturity onset" diabetes; *au contraire*, insulin resistance could likewise be implicated.

Opening the Loop: The Pancreatic Suppression Test

Controversy regarding insulin resistance in type 2 diabetes was due to the "closed-loop" feedback system, which regulates the blood glucose concentration (Figure 1). In normal individuals ingestion of a meal increases glucose and other secretagogues, including glucagon-like peptide 1 (GLP-1), which act in concert to stimulate insulin secretion. Hyperinsulinemia in turn acts to renormalize the plasma glucose level by suppressing glucose production and increasing glucose utilization. In the presence of insulin resistance *per se*, the elevated insulin will be less able to normalize glucose, therefore resulting in a secondary stimulus to the β-cells and hyperinsulinemia. In fact, postprandial hyperinsulinemia was considered by Berson and Yalow to be the signature for insulin resistance [7, 8]. However, β-cell oversecretion could also account for postprandial hyperinsulinism. Because of the closed-loop relationship between insulin secretion and insulin action it is problematic to infer the existence of insulin resistance directly from a "closed-loop" procedure such as the oral glucose tolerance test (OGTT). Equally important, it appeared impossible to assign a quantitative value to insulin resistance based solely on the closed-loop response to oral glucose.

Shen and Reaven made the breakthrough that showed definitively the existence of insulin resistance in patients with type 2 diabetes [10–12]. These investigators intervened experimentally to interrupt the closed-loop; they made the β-cells unresponsive to ambient blood glucose. Initially this was done with epinephrine [11, 12] and later with somatostatin [13, 14]. Infusing a compound that renders the β-cells unresponsive and concomitantly infusing glucose, they argued persuasively that the resultant steady-state glucose concentration is proportional to insulin resistance. They reported that the steady-state plasma

International Textbook of Diabetes Mellitus, Third Edition. Edited by R. A. DeFronzo, E. Ferrannini, H. Keen, and P. Zimmet.
 ISBN: 0-471-48655-8.

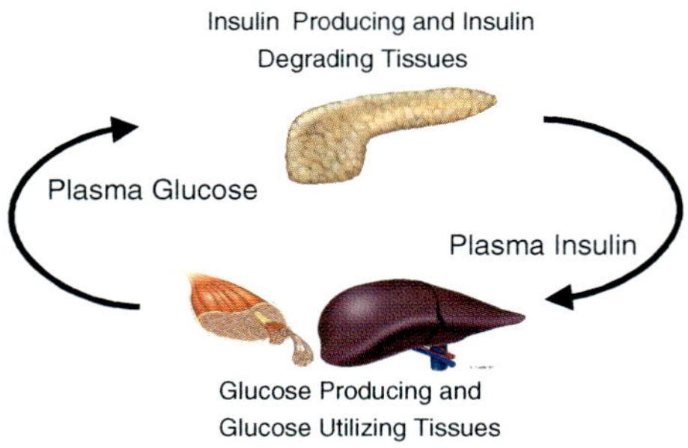

Figure 1 Closed-loop relationship between insulin and glucose

glucose (SSPG) concentration is a measure of insulin resistance, and that SSPG concentration was higher in obesity, but highest in type 2 diabetes [15, 16]. Thus, there was persuasive evidence that insulin resistance existed concomitant with type 2 diabetes. However, the existence of insulin resistance did not rule out the possibility that β-cell deficiency could play a role in the pathogenesis of type 2 diabetes. Also, the degree of hyperglycemia, while indicative of apparent insulin resistance, does not represent a quantitative *in vivo* index of the reduction of insulin sensitivity of the tissues. In fact, the debate regarding the relative importance of resistance versus insulin secretory defects in type 2 diabetes raged for several decades beyond the introduction of the pancreatic suppression test, which confirmed the insulin-resistant state [17–21].

Qualitative Versus Quantitative

Often it is not sufficient to establish whether insulin resistance exists, relative to a normative population. Much more common is the need to measure insulin resistance, i.e., to attach a number to it. A drawback of the qualitative resistance concept is that (as discussed above) virtually complete insensitivity to insulin can exist. It is much more practical to think in terms of "insulin sensitivity," where the latter concept is the inverse of resistance. Thus, insulin sensitivity determined by whatever method may have a minimum value near zero (total resistance), and values may extend to a finite number representing great sensitivity to the hormone. The first quantitative method to measure insulin sensitivity was originated by Dr Ruben Andres, and it is still called the glucose clamp [22].

THE GLUCOSE CLAMP

Rather than using agents that suppress β-cell insulin secretion, the glucose clamp uses an external feedback control to "open the loop" between insulin secretion and sensitivity (Figure 2). The glucose clamp is a powerful and widely used method to attain a quantitative measure of insulin sensitivity, and has been applied in literally thousands of experimental studies.

Performing the Clamp

DeFronzo and colleagues published the most widely applied clamp methodology [22, 23]. In the simplest manifestation, catheters are inserted in the right and left arms and basal samples are collected after which insulin is infused intravenously at a constant rate. The dose of insulin has varied widely [22–30]; however, the usual dose is 40 mU/min/m^2. Infusing insulin would normally lower the blood glucose; however, the lowering is prevented by infusing glucose concomitant with the insulin infusion. It is not possible *a priori* to know the rate of glucose infusion to prevent insulin from changing; therefore, a separate *external* feedback loop is established wherein glucose is measured frequently (usually every 5 min) and infusion rate is chosen to attempt to keep the plasma glucose concentration from changing.

In normal subjects plasma glucose concentration is usually "clamped" at or near 5 mM. Clearly, if a subject is totally insulin *resistant* (sensitivity = 0) no exogenous glucose would be needed; if a subject is very sensitive to insulin, the needed exogenous glucose infusion rate can be substantial. The rate of glucose infusion is considered a reflection of insulin sensitivity. Insulin sensitivity is normalized to body size in some manner: either per kg body weight [31], per surface area [32, 33], or per unit fat free mass [34, 35].

It is not a simple matter to determine in real time the exact glucose infusion rate needed to keep glucose at a predetermined "target" value. There have been numerous attempts to automate the external feedback loop, which includes the glucose measuring device as well as the glucose infusion pump. The "Biostator" device was used for some

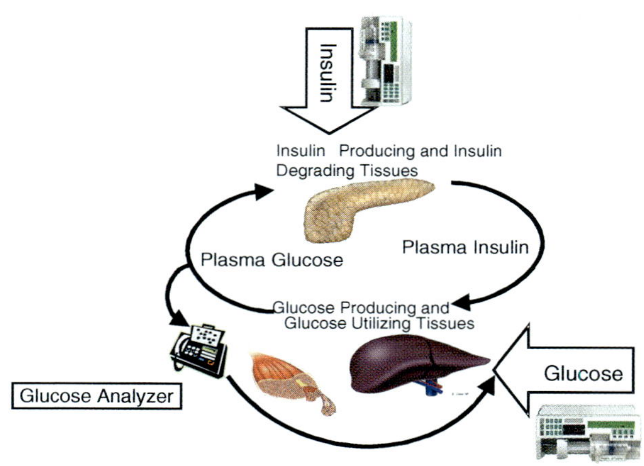

Figure 2 The glucose clamp as an open-loop method for measuring insulin sensitivity *in vivo*. Details in the text

years to do this [36, 37], although it is no longer available. Also, various algorithms have been made available to calculate glucose infusion rate independently [22, 38–40]. These algorithms have the advantage of objectivity; however, in most laboratories even today exogenous glucose infusion rate is determined at the bedside by a trained individual. The need for frequent monitoring of the blood glucose, and the need for a practiced individual to control the glucose infusion rate as a function of time, renders the glucose clamp method labor-intensive and costly. Although providing an accurate measure of insulin sensitivity, under most circumstances three trained individuals are needed to carry on a safe and effective glucose clamp experiment on a human subject.

Components of Insulin Action Calculated from the Euglycemic Clamp

Under fasting conditions in normal individuals the blood glucose is determined by a balance between endogenous glucose production by the liver (and kidneys) and glucose uptake by insulin-independent (brain, red blood cells, gut) and insulin-dependent tissues (skeletal muscle, heart, adipose). Infusing insulin lowers the blood glucose both by inhibiting endogenous glucose production (EGP) and by stimulating glucose uptake. One of the great assets of the glucose clamp is the potential for teasing apart these two effects of insulin on glucose handling. Over three decades accurate methods were established to measure rates of endogenous glucose production—even under conditions of substantial glucose turnover that is observed during clamps [22, 41–44]. These methods involve the infusion of glucose either labeled with radioactive tracer (usually ^{3}H-3-glucose) or stable isotopes such as 6,6-dideuterated glucose. Glucose output is calculated based upon the dilution by unlabeled endogenously produced glucose of the labeled glucose pool in extracellular fluid (Figure 3).

Great care is necessary to make accurate calculations of endogenous glucose production and glucose uptake during glucose clamps [42–48]. The large potential error is due to the considerable glucose turnover stimulated by hyperinsulinemia. Endogenous production is the difference between two large numbers: total rate of glucose disposal minus the rate of exogenous glucose infusion. Small errors in estimating either of these rates will cause a very large error in calculation of glucose output. Finegood and colleagues proved that to make an accurate calculation, exogenous glucose must be labeled at a specific activity or enrichment similar to that attained when labeled moiety is infused into the fasting patient [42]. Under such conditions plasma-specific activity remains near steady state and accurate EGP is calculated. Rizza et al. discovered that impurities in commercial labeled glucose preparations can lead to spurious results [47]. Also, even being unaware that so-called 50% D/W dextrose solution is only 45.4% glucose can lead to large errors. Thus, it is important to be vigilant in these calculations and to be familiar with the literature on these subjects.

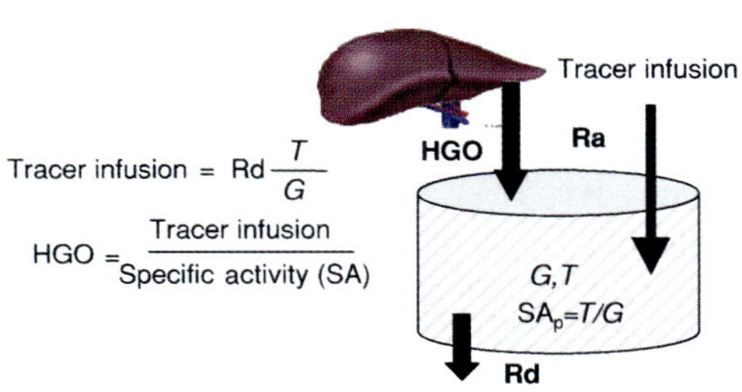

Figure 3 One-compartment model of glucose kinetics for estimation of endogenous glucose output (HGO equal to Ra) and glucose uptake (Rd). G: plasma glucose concentration (mg/dl), *T*: plasma tracer concentration (μCI/dl)

Based upon accurate methods applied to normal individuals, suppression of glucose output by liver is much more sensitive to insulin ($ED_{50} \sim 25$ mU/l) than stimulation of glucose uptake ($ED_{50} \sim 60$ mU/l) [46, 48]. Reduced insulin sensitivity as assessed by the clamp method has been demonstrated in a great many physiological and pathophysiological situations including fasting, impaired glucose tolerance (IGT), pregnancy, children of low birth weight, sedentary lifestyle, obesity, and acromegaly.

A Quantitative Index from the Glucose Clamp

As stated, glucose infusion rate during the clamp is an index of insulin sensitivity. Because insulin suppresses endogenous glucose output and increase glucose disposal the infusion rate is the sum of these two effects under euglycemic conditions:

$$\begin{aligned}&\text{Glucose infusion rate}\\&\quad = \text{Increase in glucose disposal}\\&\qquad + \text{Suppression of endogenous glucose production}\end{aligned}$$

Either of these components on the right-hand side may be regarded as reflecting insulin sensitivity; percent suppression of EGP is often considered hepatic insulin sensitivity whereas increase in glucose disposal (Rd: expressed as mass per unit time per unit body size) is reflective of "peripheral" insulin sensitivity. In populations of normal subjects these indices are often sufficient; however, in pathological conditions they may be misleading. Glucose uptake is a nonlinear function of glucose and insulin [41, 49, 50]. It is therefore not correct to compare Rd values in individuals assessed at different glucose levels [41, 49]. Generally subjects with fasting hyperglycemia may have their fasting glucose values normalized by infusing exogenous insulin acutely, or overnight [51–53]. However, insulin itself can affect insulin sensitivity [54–57]; therefore infusing the hormone can alter the measured variable. A better approach is to represent glucose disposal terms of metabolic clearance rate—dividing glucose uptake by the ambient glucose level [41]. This correction is appropriate at or near the normal fasting glucose value, but may result in underestimation of insulin action under severe hyperglycemic conditions where the relationship between glucose uptake and glucose concentration "flattens" and incremental changes in plasma glucose have a reduced effect on Rd.

An additional problem may occur due to alterations in metabolic clearance rate of insulin. Generally insulin clearance is reduced in insulin-resistant situations, resulting in proportionately greater plasma insulin levels during insulin infusion during the clamp [58–60]. This has resulted in some investigators dividing Rd by the increment in insulin under steady-state conditions. We have proposed a single variable, the "insulin sensitivity index," which attempts to correct or normalize for differences in plasma glucose and insulin concentration at which clamps may be performed [61–64].

The clamp-based index is defined as the following:

$$S_{IP(Clamp)} = \frac{\Delta Rd}{G \times \Delta I}$$

which relates the increase in glucose uptake to the ambient (clamp) glucose value and the increase in plasma insulin due to the exogenous infusion. The concept underlying the $S_{IP(Clamp)}$ is depicted in Figure 4. The relationship between glucose concentration and whole-body glucose uptake is practically linear at levels of glucose near the physiological range. Of course, it is necessary to demonstrate this using a complex protocol in which endogenous insulin does not respond to the increment in glucose. It is important to realize that what is being assessed is the increase in total glucose uptake—uptake not only by skeletal muscle, but also by liver itself, and hepatic glucose uptake is very sensitive to the glucose level [65–68]. The effect of increasing insulin is to enhance the rate of glucose uptake at each glucose level. Thus, with insulin increased, the slope of the relationship between glucose and glucose uptake is increased. Therefore, the effect of insulin on glucose uptake—that is, insulin sensitivity—is to increase the slope of the relationship between glucose and glucose uptake estimated under quasi-steady-state conditions. As shown in Figure 4, the $S_{IP(Clamp)}$ value shown above is equal to this definition of insulin sensitivity.

It remains problematic to compare insulin sensitivity among individuals with different glucose levels. One approach—to normalize glycemia acutely or chronically—is fraught with the problem that insulin itself alters sensitivity to the hormone. Use of the $S_{IP(Clamp)}$ has within it implicit assumptions regarding approximate linear relationships between glucose and glucose uptake, as well as effects of insulin on whole-body glucose utilization. Thus, this too must be considered an approximation,

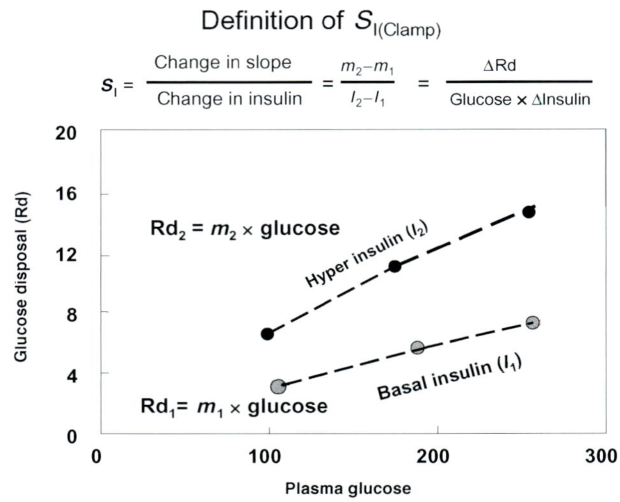

Figure 4 Relationship between plasma glucose concentration and whole-body glucose uptake at two levels of insulinemia

because we are aware that such linearity is only true in a limited range of glucose or insulin. However, we have calculated $S_{IP(Clamp)}$ at different levels of glucose and insulin in the same subjects, and have found similar values [41]. Therefore, given the widespread use of $S_{IP(Clamp)}$ as an index of insulin sensitivity, further study of the limits of its applicability seems appropriate.

While this index corrects for differences in target glucose from the clamp and differences in insulin clearance, it is more appropriate to prenormalize glucose overnight in subjects with fasting hyperglycemia.

Insulin Action Dynamics

Insulin sensitivity from the clamp is expressed in terms of the steady-state value reached after a period of hyperinsulinemia. A dose–response can be constructed and sensitivity can be expressed as the ED_{50}, i.e. the concentration for half-maximal stimulation of Rd as a function of dose. Alternatively, sensitivity can be expressed (as it usually is) as the Rd at a specific dose of insulin, which may be low, intermediate, or a maximum dose. It is often assumed that steady-state rate of glucose uptake is reached by 180 min after onset of the insulin infusion. In fact, Chen and Reaven reported that steady-state glucose uptake is nowhere nearly reached at 3 h [69], and we have recently confirmed this for normal individuals [70]. Glucose uptake rate at 3 h is only 2/3 the "true" steady state, which is not achieved until 6 h (Figure 5). Certainly, shorter periods (e.g., 120 min) are inadequate to reflect steady-state rates of uptake [41, 64, 71].

Rd at "steady-state" does not incorporate the events that account for the slow time course of activation of glucose uptake [41, 64, 72]. Events that may determine the time course of glucose uptake in the face of hyperinsulinemia

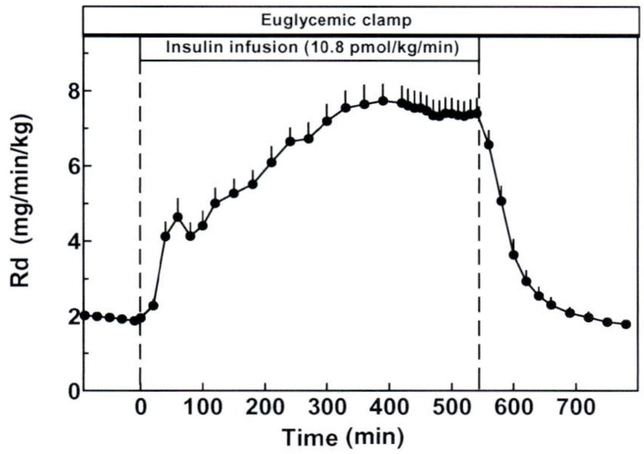

Figure 5 Time course of glucose uptake (Rd) during infusion of regular insulin (Novolin-R) does not reach steady state at 3 h after the start of the insulin infusion [70]

include dynamics of plasma insulin itself [71], access of insulin to the insulin-sensitive tissues (primarily skeletal muscle, liver, and adipose tissue) [73, 74], binding of insulin to receptors, and the downstream signaling pathways and mobilization of glucose transporters (primarily glucose transporter 4 [75–82]). It is of interest to examine the *in vivo* pathway of insulin action during clamps to identify the rate-limiting step, which determines insulin dynamics *in vivo*. It is possible that changes in *access* to insulin-sensitive cells could contribute to a "dynamic" insulin resistance, because insulin action does not generally reach the hyperinsulinemic steady-state value assessed during euglycemic clamp studies.

Access to sensitive cells includes the actual process of movement of insulin across the endothelial cells as well as any effect of insulin to access so-called "nutritive" capillaries (i.e., those that perfuse insulin-sensitive and glucose-utilizing or glucose-storing tissues). By measuring insulin in plasma and lymph simultaneously we were able to determine that it was the movement of insulin between the plasma and the interstitial fluid compartment that was the determinant of insulin action dynamics [73, 83].

Our conclusions were elegantly confirmed in human volunteers by Lonnroth and colleagues [84–86]. In fact, while the insulin concentration in interstitial fluid lagged in time behind plasma dynamics, indicating slow transport across the capillary endothelium, there was a dynamic equilibrium between interstitial insulin and glucose storage, suggesting little temporal delay at the level of insulin action on cells, confirming rapid insulin action *in vitro* [84].

That "dynamic resistance" exists was provided by Olefsky and colleagues who demonstrated that activation of the tyrosine kinase activity of the insulin receptor was slower in obese subjects [87–90]. Additionally, Baron has elegantly demonstrated the role of the nitric oxide system as a mediator of insulin's effect to increase blood flow in sensitive tissues [91–94]. Blood flow *per se* may be less important in that insulin's putative effect alters blood flow from so-called nonnutritive to nutritive skeletal muscle tissues. Thus, Clark and his colleagues have emphasized that insulin may act to increase the availability of insulin to so-called "nutritive" capillaries; i.e., those that perfuse insulin-sensitive cells [95]. We have recently found a profound increase in distribution volume of *inulin,* an inert molecule of molecular weight similar to insulin when insulin is incremented within the physiological range [96]. Thus, even in normal individuals it appears that insulin does enhance access to insulin-sensitive tissues, and that this ability of insulin is impaired, for example, in visceral adiposity [96]. Therefore, insulin sensitivity may well reflect a reduced capacity of insulin to enhance contact of glucose with insulin-sensitive cells via nutritive capillaries, resulting in a flow-dependent component of insulin resistance.

It is clear that cellular sensitivity to the hormone is not the only action of insulin on carbohydrate metabolism, which results in insulin resistance. The ability of the hormone to *access* sensitive tissues is reduced because of reduced transendothelial transport as well as failure to increase flow through nutritive capillaries. The relative importance of these "dynamic" components of insulin action under different conditions remains to be established. Given the various dynamic features that contribute to overall insulin action, it is reasonable to utilize the *dynamics* of insulin action, rather than quasi-steady-state alone to represent *in vivo* insulin sensitivity. One approach that utilizes insulin action dynamics is the "minimal model" approach.

Dynamic Insulin Action: The Minimal Model

In the normal 24-h day the insulin-sensitive tissues are never exposed to steady-state conditions. After a meal, glucose and insulin are changing, and the rate of glucose uptake lags in time behind the time courses of glucose and insulin. It may be preferable to measure insulin action from a dynamic relationship between glucose, the primary nutritive carbohydrate, insulin, the primary anabolic hormone, and the rate of glucose disposition. One approach to such a measurement is the frequently sampled intravenous glucose tolerance test (FSIGT) coupled with the "minimal model." The underlying concept behind the minimal model approach will be outlined herein, but the reader should refer to more extensive presentations for added information and detail [41, 61, 97–101].

Concept

As discussed, intervening to "open the loop" to perform a glucose clamp requires resources in dollars and labor.

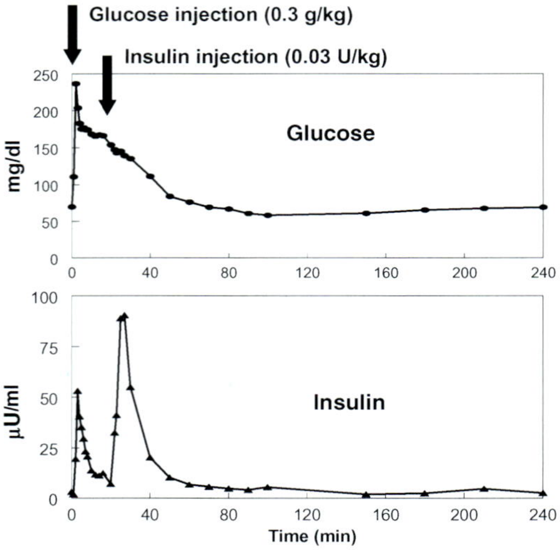

Figure 6 Plasma glucose and insulin dynamics during a frequently sampled intravenous glucose tolerance test (FSIGT). Unpublished data courtesy of Anne E. Sumner, MD

Using the power of the digital computer and modeling obviates the necessary to maintain constant plasma glucose and insulin to obtain a sensitivity measure.

To measure dynamic sensitivity the insulin/glucose regulating system must be perturbed. While the administration of oral glucose might be considered the simplest approach given the acceptance of the OGTT as a diagnostic procedure, oral glucose has substantial limitations due to lack of control over the rate of glucose appearance in the extracellular fluid [102, 103] (see below). Therefore intravenous administration was the protocol of choice. The explicit detailed dynamic relationship between glucose and insulin following intravenous glucose is measured by collecting frequent blood samples (Figure 6).

While many hormonal and neural signals can impact plasma dynamics, it has been shown that in the main a few factors dominate the time course of glucose and insulin following glucose injection. These are (1) endogenous glucose production (by liver predominantly and also kidney), (2) insulin secretion and insulin clearance, (3) effect of insulin to alter the rate of glucose uptake by insulin-dependent tissues (mostly skeletal muscle) by a variety of mechanisms including transporter mobilization, enzyme activation, changes in perfusion of nutritive tissues, endothelial transport, and (4) glucose uptake by tissues independent of insulin (brain, gut, red blood cells).

The Model

It was a challenge to develop a computer model that could account for plasma dynamics in a compact but accurate package. The model was the simplest representation we could devise, which was based upon known physiology, and which could accurately describe moment-by-moment plasma dynamics. The model continues to thrive in that it continues to be the basis for a large number of clinical investigations (~50/year) as well as a robust literature related to its mathematical and computer characteristics [41, 61, 62, 97–100, 104–114].

Practical Application of the Minimal Model

In contrast to the glucose clamp procedure neither on-line measurements nor external control of infusions are necessary to perform the minimal model procedure. Temporary intravenous lines are placed in antecubital veins in a relaxing subject. After basal sampling, glucose is injected and frequent sampling is begun. To facilitate the computer's ability to estimate metabolic parameters (cf. Table 1) insulin is injected at 20 min and sampling continued until 3 h [110, 111]. Samples are spun and plasma is stored frozen for later analysis of glucose and insulin. It is straightforward for two experimenters to perform the FSIGT on one subject.

Yields from the Minimal Model

By computer analysis using the program MINMOD Millennium, a set of values is calculated for each individual subjected to the FSIGT test (Table 1).

Insulin sensitivity from the model is expressed as parameter S_I. The latter parameter from the minimal model is analogous to the previously mentioned $S_{IP(Clamp)}$ estimated from the euglycemic clamp. In fact, the parameters are strongly correlated [61–63, 115–117]. The correlation is not perfect however. This may be due to inherent errors in measurement of each (errors in plasma measurements, sampling times, etc). Or, it may be due to the fact that the minimal model S_I is estimated from a dynamic test, whereas the analogous clamp parameter is from a steady-state test [100]. It is apparent that these very different tests—the FSIGT versus the clamp—may well be measuring somewhat different things. The clamp emphasizes

Table 1 Metabolic parameters estimated from a FSIGT by computer analysis using the MINMOD program

$AIR_{glucose}$	*First-phase insulin release*: Reflects β-cell functionality.
S_I	*Insulin sensitivity index*: Reflects ability of insulin to enhance effect of glucose to normalize its own concentration after injection.
S_G	*Glucose effectiveness*: Effect of glucose to enhance glucose disappearance, at basal insulin in absence of dynamic insulin response.
k_I	*Fractional metabolic clearance rate of insulin*: Reflects rate of clearance of injected insulin from the circulation. Related to first-pass hepatic insulin clearance.
DI	*Disposition index*: Equals S_I times $AIR_{glucose}$. Reflects insulin sensitivity *normalized to the degree of insulin resistance*.

steady-state effects of insulin on glucose uptake and production often at a single insulin level. The minimal model also measures the factors that determine the rates of distribution of insulin as well as glucose among different compartments of the organism, and factors that determine how rapidly insulin can stimulate glucose metabolism by accessing tissues (whether by changing blood flow distribution or endothelial transport) and by mobilizing transporters, activating enzymes, changing expression, and so on. The relative importance of insulin resistance to pathogenesis disease, whether measured by a steady-state or a dynamic approach, is of great interest.

Hyperbolic Relationship Between Insulin Sensitivity and Insulin Secretion: The Disposition Index

Diabetes, characterized by elevated blood glucose concentration, is reflective of an inability of the patient to regulate the plasma glucose concentration within normal limits. How is this regulation maintained in the normal individual?

Insulin resistance is common in Westernized societies. Yet, most insulin-resistant individuals do not have diabetes. Diabetes is prevented by the compensatory characteristics of the pancreatic β-cells. Insulin sensitivity is reduced in many normal as well as pathophysiological states. Among the normal states are pregnancy and puberty; pathologies include obesity and infection. Pathologies include not only type 2 diabetes, but hypertension, colon cancer, and polycystic ovarian syndrome.

Diabetes is prevented in many states of severe insulin resistance by the robust compensatory function of the β-cells of the pancreas. In fact, there is a predictable β-cell response to insulin resistance (Figure 7) [118]:

$$S_{\mathrm{I}} \times \mathrm{AIR}_{\mathrm{glucose}} = \mathrm{DI}$$

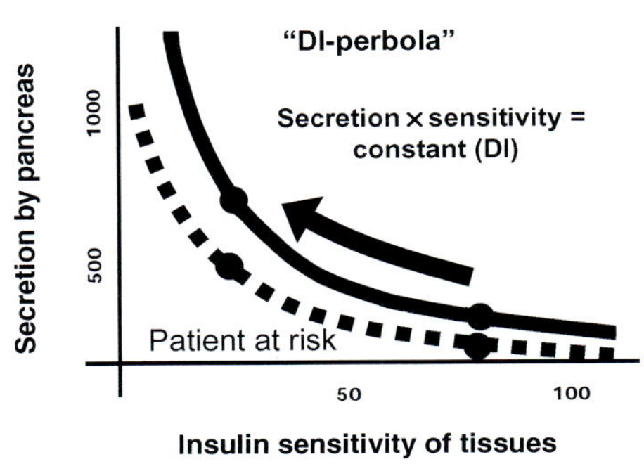

Figure 7 The hyperbolic insulin sensitivity/secretion curve. It is hypothesized that in the course of environmentally induced reduction in insulin sensitivity, "normal" pancreatic islets will respond by upregulation of insulin response (solid hyperbolic curve). The failure to upregulate would result in a curve nearer the origin, with a lesser value of DI (dashed hyperbolic curve)

where the three variables are defined as in Table 1. This equation is an *hyperbola*, which predicts that for a given decrease in insulin sensitivity, there will be a proportionately equal and opposite increase in β-cell sensitivity to glucose stimulation. The disposition index defines the position of the hyperbolic curve on the sensitivity/secretion plot. IF the DI is *high*, then the β-cells mount a robust response to a decrease in S_{I}; if the DI is *low*, such a value is reflective of unresponsive β-cells. Subjects at risk for type 2 diabetes have a low disposition index [107, 118–121]. There is strong evidence that the DI value is determined by genetics as well as environment [100, 122, 123].

The minimal model, therefore, provides a method for assessing insulin sensitivity in the intact organism by combining a relatively straightforward experimental protocol with the power of the digital computer to model real data. Software to calculate parameters has been available for some years making the methodology available to all clinical investigators. The method continues to be used in laboratories throughout the world.

Surrogate Measures of Insulin Sensitivity

Laboratory methods for measuring insulin action have been shown to be accurate. However under some conditions application of these methods is difficult if not impractical. Some studies call for assessment of insulin action in thousands of subjects. The minimal model has been used in studies of populations in excess of 1000 [112, 122, 124]. This latter study was expensive in time and money. Are there simpler but accurate methods for use in large populations? We shall focus on two classes of "surrogate" measures of insulin sensitivity: indices based upon fasting measures, and indices based upon the OGTT.

FASTING INSULIN

Kahn and his colleagues have reported a curvilinear relationship between *fasting insulin* and insulin sensitivity [125], one that is similar to stimulated insulin release. In an individual with healthy β-cells, because there is a defined relationship between secretion and insulin sensitivity, it could be argued that measuring one is as good as measuring the other. Thus, if insulin sensitivity is low, fasting insulin will be elevated, and vice versa. Therefore in a group of subjects with *identical β-cell function* we may expect elevated insulin to reflect insulin resistance. Similarly, with healthy β-cells, insulin resistance will be reflected in elevated β-cell secretory response to stimuli such as glucose, arginine, GLP-1, or other secretagogues. It is arguably appropriate to utilize fasting insulin or a provocative index of β-cell function as a surrogate with the following caveat: fasting insulin or other indices of insulin secretion may be considered accurate surrogates

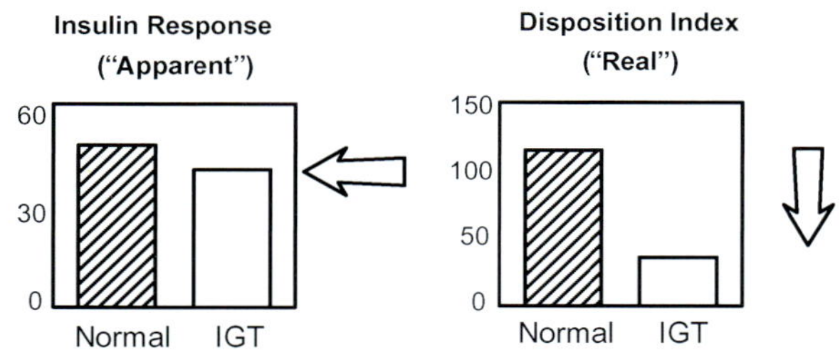

Figure 8 Reduced insulin secretory response in patients with IGT. A relative small reduction in insulin response (left panel) in subjects with IGT underestimates the severe β-cell defect, which is masked by upregulation secondary to insulin resistance (right panel)

for insulin sensitivity *only when comparing between or among individuals with equivalent functional activity of the pancreatic β-cells.*

The downside associated with using fasting insulin (or other related indices of insulin secretion) becomes clear if we consider comparing among groups or individuals with differing islet secretory function. Let us consider as an example comparison of fasting insulin between normal individuals and individuals with IGT. The latter group is not only insulin resistant, but is characterized by a β-cell defect of at least 50% [126–128].

As Figure 8 demonstrates, comparing the normal subjects with insulin-resistant subjects with IGI, plasma insulin concentration, or insulin response to glucose could be identical (Figure 8). Thus, the fasting insulin concentration will not represent an accurate reflection of insulin sensitivity comparing individuals or groups for whom β-cell function is not identical. In practice, individuals with similar β-cell function are not often compared; it is more usual to compare normal subjects with those at risk for disease (e.g., IGT [126–128], gestational diabetes after term [105, 119], first-degree relatives of type 2 diabetic patients [129, 130]).

The previous discussion demonstrates that *fasting insulin per se cannot be considered an accurate surrogate for insulin sensitivity (or resistance) under most conditions*. Nevertheless, there is a substantial literature using the fasting insulin value for just this purpose [131–133]. At the very least the careful observer must consider with care reports of fasting insulin as a surrogate for insulin resistance. If there is even a subtle β-cell defect in a group of subjects, any reported value of fasting insulin will likely underestimate the degree of insulin resistance.

Other Surrogate Measures

Besides fasting insulin itself, there are various other surrogate measures based upon fasting values alone, which have been exploited in population studies. The first to appear in the literature was the index proposed by Dr Peter Bennett. Others include the homeostasis model assessment index (HOMA) insulin resistance measure, and the "Quicki" [134–147]. Note that these indices are indeed similar; they represent insulin resistance as proportional to either the product or the inverse of the product of fasting insulin and fasting glucose. In fact, in nondiabetic subjects plasma glucose differs little compared to fasting plasma insulin. Therefore in nondiabetic subjects both HOMA index and Bennett's index are approximately proportional to the fasting insulin concentration. As discussed, similar to fasting insulin these indices will not reflect insulin sensitivity accurately in nondiabetic subjects with differing β-cell function.

Quon and colleagues have recently introduced the "Quicki" index [136]. Quon et al. equates insulin resistance to the inverse of the sum of the logarithms of fasting plasma glucose and fasting plasma insulin. The value of insulin resistance emerging from this index will depend upon the units of glucose and insulin, and the relative importance of these components will depend upon whether they are expressed in European (SI) units (mM glucose and pmol insulin) or in units used in the United States (mg/dl glucose and μU/ml). Also, despite the logarithmic transformation, Quicki values exhibit nonlinear proportionality to fasting plasma insulin and will, like fasting insulin, underestimate insulin resistance in a population with a latent decrease in β-cell function.

Thus, indices based upon fasting measurements of insulin alone or fasting insulin plus fasting glucose should not be considered accurate indices of insulin-resistance comparing groups with possible inequalities in β-cell health. Because we are often comparing between individuals or groups with differing islet function, it must be concluded that fasting insulin, as well as other surrogate measures based upon fasting values alone, may not be accurate. Certainly they are less accurate than measures available from laboratory procedures such as the euglycemic clamp or the minimal model.

Insulin Sensitivity Based upon the OGTT

The previous discussion suggests that "quick and dirty" indices from fasting values may not be accurate, and it is often true that laboratory procedures are impractical. Recently, it has been suggested that indices calculated from the OGTT may be useful for population studies.

For decades the OGTT has been used as a screening test and a diagnostic tool for diabetes and IGT [148, 149]. It might be ideal if one could classify the state of carbohydrate tolerance and simultaneously measure insulin sensitivity and β-cell function. As long ago as 1980, Voors et al. suggested the mathematical product of the 1-h glucose and the 1-h insulin concentration as "peripheral insulin resistance" [150]. Ten years later Cederholm and Wibell expressed sensitivity as the ratio of the glucose

Table 2 OGTT-derived and fasting indices of insulin sensitivity are correlated with clamp-derived estimations of insulin sensitivity

Insulin sensitivity indices	Equation	n^*	r	Reference
$ISI_{0,120}$ index	$\frac{75000\,mg - (Gk_0 - Gk_{120})^*0.19^*BW}{120^*Glc_{mean}{}^*\log[Ins_{mean}]}$	135	0.63	[152]
Stumvoll index	$0.226 - (0.0032^*BMI) - (0.0000645^*Ins_{120}) - (0.0037^*Glc_{90})$	104	0.79	[154]
Matzuda index	$\frac{10000}{SQRT[(Ins_0{}^*GLC_0)^*(Ins_{mean}{}^*Glc_{mean})]}$	153	0.73	[153]
HOMA-IR	$\frac{(Ins^*Glc)}{22.5}$	115	−0.82	[147]
Quickie	$\frac{1}{(\log[Ins] + \log[Glc])}$	56	0.78	[146]

$^*n$ = number of subjects in respective study.

metabolic clearance rate to the logarithmic transformed mean serum insulin concentration [151]. This latter index was later modified by Gutt et al. and shown to correlate with insulin sensitivity values derived from the euglycemic clamp [152]. In a recently proposed composite, Matsuda and DeFronzo applied a square-root conversion of the products of fasting OGTT glucose and insulin to correct for the nonlinearity of the values [153]. Stumvoll et al. performed multiple regression of several demographic parameters (body mass index, sex, waist-to-hip ratio, OGTT glucose and insulin) upon sensitivity from the euglycemic hyperinsulinemic clamp test [154]. Thus, their approach included as independent variables metabolic characteristics which themselves can alter insulin action [155–158].

The OGTT-derived estimates of insulin sensitivity mentioned above correlated with insulin sensitivity values obtained by the euglycemic clamp technique (Table 2). Several of the indices were additionally tested in different ethnic groups [159–161]. Kanauchi et al. showed that Matsuda's ($r = 0.45$), Gutt's ($r = 0.64$), and Stumvoll's ($r = 0.53$) formulas correlated modestly in the Japanese population with insulin sensitivity data from euglycemic clamps [161]. Kuo et al. reported the Matsuda index and the homeostatic model assessment equally applicable for estimation of insulin sensitivity in Chinese diabetic patients and their offspring [160]. In contrast, Chiu et al. [159] found that the estimated indices (Matsuda and Stumvoll) correlate with clamp-derived insulin sensitivity in a wide spectrum of glucose-tolerant healthy subjects, but that they are less likely to detect differences in insulin sensitivity among different ethnic groups (Asian Americans, African Americans, Caucasian Americans, and Mexico-Americans). Additionally a recently published study reported that the estimations of insulin sensitivity and β-cell function by OGTT-derived methods failed to reproduce the hyperbolic relation [162], which is well established for the relation between β-cell function and insulin sensitivity when measured by more established methods [118]. Therefore, as of this writing it remains a matter of debate whether the above-mentioned indices are in fact a suitable tool to measure insulin sensitivity.

It is clear that a correlation between proposed OGTT-derived indices and clamp-derived insulin sensitivity may exist. However, the OGTT-derived indices contain endogenous insulin response as an important term in their calculation and it cannot be excluded that reported correlations reflect islet-cell response rather than insulin sensitivity *per se*. If it is true that OGTT-based methods reflect secretion rather than sensitivity, application of the OGTT methods to subjects with impaired β-cell secretory capacity (e.g., those with impaired glucose tolerance, gestational diabetes, type 2 diabetes) would incorrectly underestimate insulin resistance as postload hyperinsulinemia would be reduced and they may not be accurate for diabetic patients. Confirming this latter weakness, correlations between OGTT-based indices and clamp-based sensitivity [153, 163] were lower when the indices are employed in subjects with type 2 diabetes.

Poor reproducibility of the 75-g OGTT also limits the value of the OGTT [164]. The overall test-to-test reproducibility (coefficient of variation) of the OGTT is no more than 65% [165]. The inherent variability is likely due, at least in part, to high day-to-day variability in gastrointestinal function (gastric emptying, absorption, incretin effect). It is well established that a delay in gastric emptying or reduced glucose absorption will result in lower glucose excursions as well as lower insulin levels [102, 166, 167]. In fact it has been demonstrated that gastric emptying alone accounts for 35% of the variance in peak plasma glucose after a 75-g OGTT in both healthy volunteers and patients with type 2 diabetes [102].

We have investigated the possible effects of variability in islet-cell function as well as variability in intestinal glucose absorption on glucose and insulin patterns and OGTT-based indices using a computer model [168]. The glucose and insulin time series simulated for a normal healthy subject closely match published data

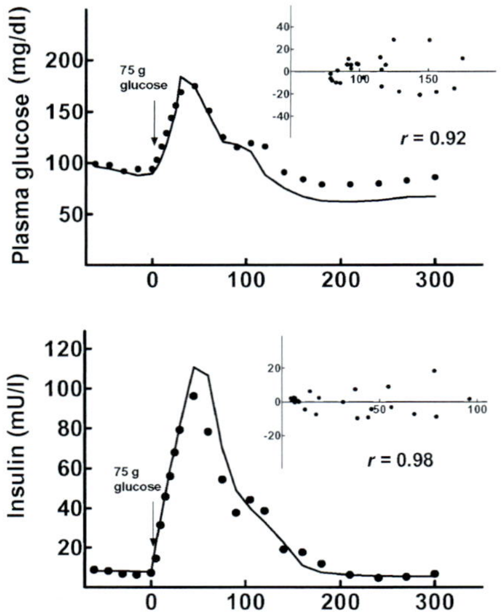

Figure 9 Plasma glucose and insulin excursions in response to an OGTT as predicted by our model (solid line) closely matches the "real" glucose and insulin data [169]

[169] (Figure 9). The OGTT data simulated under these conditions indicate that ±50% changes in β-cell sensitivity or glucose absorption have a far greater impact on the pattern of glucose and insulin than alterations of insulin sensitivity itself (Figure 10). A simulated 50% reduction of insulin sensitivity caused only very minor changes in sensitivity calculated by those indices (Table 3). In contrast isolated alterations of β-cell sensitivity and glucose absorption resulted in considerably higher or lower *apparent* values of insulin sensitivity from almost all indices. While these results are from a simulation study, they suggest strongly that one must be very careful in interpreting differences in OGTT values in terms of insulin sensitivity *per se* because differences in metabolic parameters *other than insulin sensitivity* may have greater effects on OGTT. Therefore alterations in OGTT cannot be readily interpreted to reflect changes in insulin sensitivity but rather changes in gastric emptying, insulin secretion, glucose effectiveness, etc. It may not be possible to support the use of the OGTT for assessing insulin resistance at this juncture.

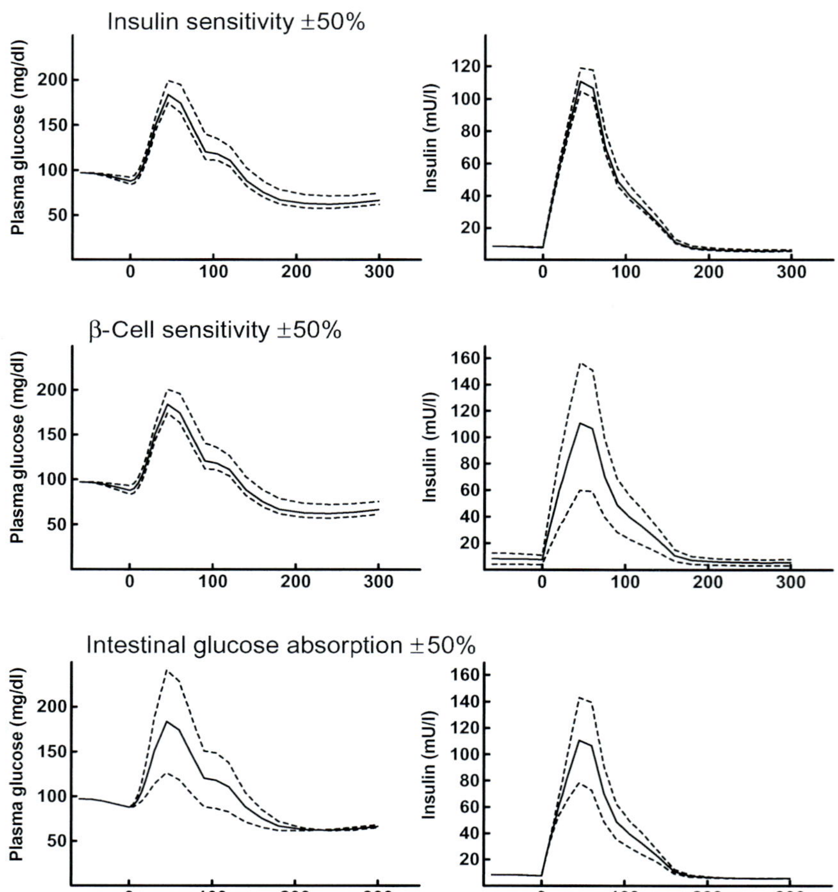

Figure 10 Model simulation of plasma glucose and insulin concentrations in response to an oral glucose load (75 g) under the assumption of a 50% increase or reduction (dashed line) in insulin sensitivity (upper panel), β-cell sensitivity (middle panel), or glucose absorption from the intestine (lower panel)

Table 3 OGTT-derived and fasting indices were calculated from the model-predicted glucose and insulin concentrations

		Imposed changes in metabolic variables					
		ΔInsulin sensitivity		Δβ-cell sensitivity		ΔGlucose absorption	
	Normal value	+50%	−50%	+50%	−50%	+50%	−50%
		Relative change in Insulin sensitivity values					
$ISI_{0,120}$ index	83.2	8	−14	−5	10	−21	34
Stumvoll index	0.11	2	−6	−3	1	−9	9
Matzuda index	4.0	10	−14	−26	69	−21	37
HOMA-IR	1.64	−8	10	36	−44	0	0
Quickie	0.36	2	−2	−5	10	0	0

Note: Relative changes of the individual sensitivity values under assumption of isolated 50% changes of insulin sensitivity, insulin secretion, and glucose absorption are shown in this table.

CONCLUSIONS

The goal to accurately measure insulin sensitivity (i.e., "insulin resistance") in patients remains an important goal. Insulin resistance is a risk factor for a plethora of chronic diseases (diabetes, cardiovascular disease, hypertension, colon cancer). To study these diseases, and to intervene early in their, pathogenesis, requires that we quantify risk factors and insulin resistance is one important candidate. *To accurately measure sensitivity it is important to use a method that observes in some fashion the metabolic effect of insulin given intravenously*. Thus, the glucose clamp and the minimal model are accurate and reproducible methods. One must remain vigilant regarding limitations of these methods. However, they may be applied with confidence under a wide variety of conditions.

Unfortunately it is not possible to recommend simpler (i.e. surrogate) methods, which can be applied with confidence. While it might be appropriate to use fasting insulin to reflect insulin resistance in patients without any degree of β-cell failure, it is usually not possible to determine *a priori* whether any such defect exists. Thus, one can report fasting insulin simply as a *qualitative reflection* of insulin resistance. Indices, which also include glucose appear to add little to the fasting insulin itself. If β-cell failure progresses, the interpretation of fasting insulin *per se* becomes impossible.

Finally, as of this writing it is not possible to recommend insulin sensitivity measures calculated from the OGTT due to confounds related to differences in gastric emptying, β-cell function, and glucose effectiveness. Clearly, studies to identify and validate simpler methods to assess insulin action accurately in the intact subject should be continued.

Acknowledgments

RNB was supported by the National Institutes of Health (DK27619 and DK29867). We are grateful to Anne E. Sumner, MD, for the data in Figure 6.

REFERENCES

1. Falta W. Diabetes refractory to insulin. *Klin Wchnschr* 1924; 3: 1315–7.
2. Meythaler F, Kotlorz H. Insulinresistenz. Formen der Insulinresistenz, Haeufigkeit und immunologische Mechanismen. *Aerztl Forsch* 1965; 19: 325–38.
3. Bainbridge HW. The reduced sensitivity to insulin of rats and mice fed on a carbohydrate-free excess-fat diet. *J Physiol* 1925; 60: 293–300.
4. Himsworth HP. Diabetes mellitus: its differentiation into insulin-sensitive and insulin insensitive types. *Lancet* 1936; 1: 127–30.
5. Himsworth HP. The syndrome of diabetes mellitus and its causes. *Lancet* 1949; 2: 465–72.
6. Himsworth HP. The diabetic factor determining the glucose tolerance and sensitivity to insulin of healthy men. *Clin Sci* 1935; 2: 67–71.
7. Yalow RS, Berson SA. Assay of plasma insulin in human subjects by immunological methods. *Nature* 1959; 184: 1648–9.
8. Yalow RS, Berson SA. Immunoassay of endogenous insulin in man. *J Clin Invest* 1960; 39: 1157–75.
9. Kipnis DM. Insulin secretion in diabetes mellitus. *Ann Intern Med* 1968; 69: 891–901.
10. Shen SW, Reaven GM, Farquhar JW. Comparison of impedance to insulin-mediated glucose uptake in normal subjects and in subjects with latent diabetes. *J Clin Invest* 1970; 49: 2151–60.
11. Reaven GM, Sageman WS, Swenson RS. Development of insulin resistance in normal dogs following alloxan-induced insulin deficiency. *Diabetologia* 1977; 13: 459–62.
12. Davis BM, Bernstein R, Kolterman O, Olefsky JM, Reaven GM. Defect in glucose removal in nonketotic diabetic patients with fasting hyperglycemia. *Diabetes* 1979; 28: 32–4.
13. Ratzmann KP, Besch W, Witt S, Schulz B. Evaluation of insulin resistance during inhibition of endogenous insulin and glucagon secretion by somatostatin in non-obese subjects with impaired glucose tolerance. *Diabetologia* 1981; 21: 192–7.
14. Harano Y, Ohgaku S, Hidaka H, Haneda K, Kikkawa R, Shigeta Y, Abe H. Glucose, insulin and somatostatin infusion for the determination of insulin sensitivity. *J Clin Endocrinol Metab* 1977; 45: 1124–7.
15. Harano Y, Ohgaku S, Kosugi K, Yasuda H, Nakano T, Kobayashi M, Hidaka H, Izumi K, Kashiwagi A, Shigeta Y. Clinical significance of altered insulin sensitivity

in diabetes mellitus assessed by glucose, insulin, and somatostatin infusion. *J Clin Endocrinol Metab* 1981; 52: 982–7.
16. Nagulesparan M, Savage PJ, Unger RH, Bennett PH. A simplified method using somatostatin to assess in vivo insulin resistance over a range of obesity. *Diabetes* 1979; 28: 980–3.
17. Porte D Jr. Banting Lecture 1990. Beta-cells in type II diabetes mellitus. *Diabetes* 1991; 40: 166–80.
18. Gerich JE. Is insulin resistance the principal cause of type 2 diabetes? *Diabetes Obes Metab* 1999; 1: 257–63.
19. Ferrannini E. Insulin resistance versus insulin deficiency in non-insulin-dependent diabetes mellitus: problems and prospects. *Endocr Rev* 1998; 19: 477–90.
20. Poitout V, Robertson RP. An integrated view of beta-cell dysfunction in type-II diabetes. *Annu Rev Med* 1996; 47: 69–83.
21. O'Rahilly SP, Nugent Z, Rudenski AS, Hosker JP, Burnett MA, Darling P, Turner RC, Beta-cell dysfunction, rather than insulin insensitivity, is the primary defect in familial type 2 diabetes. *Lancet* 1986; 2: 360–4.
22. DeFronzo RA, Tobin JD, Andres R. Glucose clamp technique: a method for quantifying insulin secretion and resistance. *Am J Physiol* 1979; 237: E214–23.
23. Bonadonna RC, Groop L, Kraemer N, Ferrannini E, Del Prato S, DeFronzo RA. Obesity and insulin resistance in humans: a dose–response study. *Metabolism* 1990; 39: 452–9.
24. Abate N, Garg A, Peshock RM, Stray-Gundersen J, Grundy SM. Relationships of generalized and regional adiposity to insulin sensitivity in men. *J Clin Invest* 1995; 96: 88–98.
25. Danadian K, Balasekaran G, Lewy V, Meza MP, Robertson R, Arslanian SA. Insulin sensitivity in African-American children with and without family history of type 2 diabetes. *Diabetes Care* 1999; 22: 1325–9.
26. Torlone E, Britta M, Rambotti AM, Perriello G, Santeusanio F, Brunetti P, Bolli GB. Improved insulin action and glycemic control after long-term angiotensin-converting enzyme inhibition in subjects with arterial hypertension and type II diabetes. *Diabetes Care* 1993; 16: 1347–55.
27. Schmitz O, Klebe J, Moller J, Arnfred J, Hermansen K, Orskov H, Beck-Nielsen H. In vivo insulin action in type 1 (insulin-dependent) diabetic pregnant women as assessed by the insulin clamp technique. *J Clin Endocrinol Metab* 1985; 61: 877–81.
28. McGuinness OP, Myers SR, Neal D, Cherrington AD. Chronic hyperinsulinemia decreases insulin action but not insulin sensitivity. *Metabolism* 1990; 39: 931–7.
29. Pratley RE, Coon PJ, Muller DC, Rogus EM, Goldberg AP. The effects of single and sequential insulin infusions on glucose disposal in older men. *Exp Gerontol* 1993; 28: 381–91.
30. Kraegen EW, Lazarus L, Campbell LV. Failure of insulin infusion during euglycemia to influence endogenous basal insulin secretion. *Metabolism* 1983; 32: 622–7.
31. Yu JG, Javorschi S, Hevener AL, Kruszynska YT, Norman RA, Sinha M, Olefsky JM. The effect of thiazolidinediones on plasma adiponectin levels in normal, obese, and type 2 diabetic subjects. *Diabetes* 2002; 51: 2968–74.
32. Merkel PA, Simonson DC, Amiel SA, Plewe G, Sherwin RS, Pearson HA, Tamborlane WV. Insulin resistance and hyperinsulinemia in patients with thalassemia major treated by hypertransfusion. *N Engl J Med* 1988; 318: 809–14.
33. Amiel SA, Sherwin RS, Simonson DC, Lauritano AA, Tamborlane WV. Impaired insulin action in puberty. A contributing factor to poor glycemic control in adolescents with diabetes. *N Engl J Med* 1986; 315: 215–9.
34. Bonora E, Gulli G, Bonadonna R, Del Prato S, Solini A, DeFronzo RA. Insulin sensitivity is not impaired in Mexican-American women without a family history of diabetes. *Diabetes Care* 1995; 18: 825–33.
35. Zuniga-Guajardo S, Jimenez J, Angel A, Zinman B. Effects of massive obesity on insulin sensitivity and insulin clearance and the metabolic response to insulin as assessed by the euglycemic clamp technique. *Metabolism* 1986; 35: 278–82.
36. Verdonk CA, Rizza RA, Westland RE, Nelson RL, Gerich JE, Service FJ. Glucose clamping using the Biostator GCIIS. *Horm Metab Res* 1980; 12: 133–5.
37. Heinemann L, Ampudia-Blasco FJ. Glucose clamps with the Biostator: a critical reappraisal. *Horm Metab Res* 1994; 26: 579–83.
38. Campostano A, Altomonte F, Bessarione D, Casu M, Triolo A, Lamedica G. A new glucose clamp algorithm: clinical validation. *Int J Artif Organs* 1991; 14: 441–7.
39. Matthews DR, Edge JA, Dunger DB. An unbiased glucose clamp method using a variable insulin infusion: its application in diabetic adolescents. *Diabet Med* 1990; 7: 246–51.
40. Furler SM, Zelenka GS, Kraegen EW. Development and testing of a simple algorithm for a glucose clamp. *Med Biol Eng Comput* 1986; 24: 365–70.
41. Bergman RN, Finegood DT, Ader M. Assessment of insulin sensitivity in vivo. *Endocr Rev* 1985; 6: 45–86.
42. Finegood DT, Bergman RN, Vranic M. Estimation of endogenous glucose production during hyperinsulinemic-euglycemic glucose clamps. Comparison of unlabeled and labeled exogenous glucose infusates. *Diabetes* 1987; 36: 914–24.
43. Radziuk J, Pye S. Quantitation of basal endogenous glucose production in Type II diabetes: importance of the volume of distribution. *Diabetologia* 2002; 45: 1053–84.
44. Neely RD, Harper R, Rooney DP, Ennis CN, Bell PM, Trimble ER. Failure of complete suppression of endogenous glucose production by euglycaemic hyperinsulinaemia in normal humans. *Eur J Clin Invest* 1995; 25: 447–53.
45. Bergman RN. Pathogenesis and prediction of diabetes mellitus: lessons from integrative physiology. *Mt Sinai J Med* 2002; 69: 280–90.
46. Rizza RA, Mandarino LJ, Gerich JE, Dose-response characteristics for effects of insulin on production and utilization of glucose in man. *Am J Physiol* 1981; 240: E630–9.
47. McMahon MM, Schwenk WF, Haymond MW, Rizza RA. Underestimation of glucose turnover measured with [6-^{3}H]- and [6,6-^{2}H]- but not [6-^{14}C]glucose during hyperinsulinemia in humans. *Diabetes* 1989; 38: 97–107.
48. Campbell PJ, Mandarino LJ, Gerich JE. Quantification of the relative impairment in actions of insulin on hepatic glucose production and peripheral glucose uptake in non-insulin-dependent diabetes mellitus. *Metabolism* 1988; 37: 15–21.
49. Verdonk CA, Rizza RA, Gerich JE. Effects of plasma glucose concentration on glucose utilization and glucose clearance in normal man. *Diabetes* 1981; 30: 535–7.

50. Gottesman I, Mandarino L, Gerich J. Use of glucose uptake and glucose clearance for the evaluation of insulin action in vivo. *Diabetes* 1984; 33: 184–91.
51. Mokan M, Gerich JE. A simple insulin infusion algorithm for establishing and maintaining overnight near-normoglycemia in type I and type II diabetes. *J Clin Endocrinol Metab* 1992; 74: 943–5.
52. Mevorach M, Giacca A, Aharon Y, Hawkins M, Shamoon H, Rossetti L. Regulation of endogenous glucose production by glucose per se is impaired in type 2 diabetes mellitus. *J Clin Invest* 1998; 102: 744–53.
53. Miyazaki Y, Glass L, Triplitt C, Wajcberg E, Mandarino LJ, DeFronzo RA. Abdominal fat distribution and peripheral and hepatic insulin resistance in type 2 diabetes mellitus. *Am J Physiol Endocrinol Metab* 2002; 283: E1135–43.
54. Pirola L, Bonnafous S, Johnston AM, Chaussade C, Portis F, Van Obberghen E. Phosphoinositide 3-kinase-mediated reduction of insulin receptor substrate-1/2 protein expression via different mechanisms contributes to the insulin-induced desensitization of its signaling pathways in L6 muscle cells. *J Biol Chem* 2003; 278: 15641–51.
55. Gavin JR III, Roth J, Neville DM Jr, de Meyts P, Buell DN. Insulin-dependent regulation of insulin receptor concentrations: a direct demonstration in cell culture. *Proc Natl Acad Sci USA* 1974; 71: 84–8.
56. Tong P, Khayat ZA, Huang C, Patel N, Ueyama A, Klip A. Insulin-induced cortical actin remodeling promotes GLUT4 insertion at muscle cell membrane ruffles. *J Clin Invest* 2001; 108: 371–81.
57. Buren J, Liu HX, Lauritz J, Eriksson JW. High glucose and insulin in combination cause insulin receptor substrate-1 and -2 depletion and protein kinase B desensitisation in primary cultured rat adipocytes: possible implications for insulin resistance in type 2 diabetes. *Eur J Endocrinol* 2003; 148: 157–67.
58. Mittelman SD, Van Citters GW, Kim SP, Davis DA, Dea MK, Hamilton-Wessler M, Bergman RN. Longitudinal compensation for fat-induced insulin resistance includes reduced insulin clearance and enhanced beta-cell response. *Diabetes* 2000; 49: 2116–25.
59. Flier JS, Minaker KL, Landsberg L, Young JB, Pallotta J, Rowe JW. Impaired in vivo insulin clearance in patients with severe target-cell resistance to insulin. *Diabetes* 1982; 31: 132–5.
60. Arslanian SA, Saad R, Lewy V, Danadian K, Janosky J. Hyperinsulinemia in African-American children: decreased insulin clearance and increased insulin secretion and its relationship to insulin sensitivity. *Diabetes* 2002; 51: 3014–9.
61. Bergman RN, Prager R, Volund A, Olefsky JM. Equivalence of the insulin sensitivity index in man derived by the minimal model method and the euglycemic glucose clamp. *J Clin Invest* 1987; 79: 790–800.
62. Beard JC, Bergman RN, Ward WK, Porte D Jr. The insulin sensitivity index in nondiabetic man. Correlation between clamp-derived and IVGTT-derived values. *Diabetes* 1986; 35: 362–9.
63. Finegood DT, Pacini G, Bergman RN. The insulin sensitivity index. Correlation in dogs between values determined from the intravenous glucose tolerance test and the euglycemic glucose clamp. *Diabetes* 1984; 33: 362–8.
64. Ader M, Bergman RN. Insulin sensitivity in the intact organism. *Baillieres Clin Endocrinol Metab* 1987; 1: 879–910.
65. Basu A, Basu R, Shah P, Vella A, Johnson CM, Nair KS, Jensen MD, Schwenk WF, Rizza RA. Effects of type 2 diabetes on the ability of insulin and glucose to regulate splanchnic and muscle glucose metabolism: evidence for a defect in hepatic glucokinase activity. *Diabetes* 2000; 49: 272–83.
66. DeFronzo RA, Ferrannini E, Hendler R, Felig P, Wahren J. Regulation of splanchnic and peripheral glucose uptake by insulin and hyperglycemia in man. *Diabetes* 1983; 32: 35–45.
67. DeFronzo RA, Ferrannini E, Hendler R, Wahren J, Felig P. Influence of hyperinsulinemia, hyperglycemia, and the route of glucose administration on splanchnic glucose exchange. *Proc Natl Acad Sci USA* 1978; 75: 5173–7.
68. Davidson MB. Autoregulation by glucose of hepatic glucose balance: permissive effect of insulin. *Metabolism* 1981; 30: 279–84.
69. Liu G, Chen YD, Hollenbeck CB, Lardinois CK, Reaven GM. Insulin-stimulated glucose disposal increases with time in patients with non-insulin-dependent diabetes mellitus. *Diabetes* 1984; 33: 643–7.
70. Hamilton-Wessler M, Buchanan TA, Buchanan BS, Hanks S, Bajwa R, Berrios F, Nakao S, Bergman RN. Lesser equimolar effect in humans of fatty acid acylated insulin is not due to increased liver extraction. *Diabetes* 2000; 49 (suppl 1:) 443–P.
71. Sherwin RS, Kramer KJ, Tobin JD, Insel PA, Liljenquist JE, Berman M, Andres R. A model of the kinetics of insulin in man. *J Clin Invest* 1974; 53: 1481–92.
72. Doberne L, Greenfield MS, Schulz B, Reaven GM. Enhanced glucose utilization during prolonged glucose clamp studies. *Diabetes* 1981; 30: 829–35.
73. Poulin RA, Steil GM, Moore DM, Ader M, Bergman RN. Dynamics of glucose production and uptake are more closely related to insulin in hind limb lymph than in thoracic duct lymph. *Diabetes* 1994; 43: 180–90.
74. Yang YJ, Hope ID, Ader M, Bergman RN. Insulin transport across capillaries is rate limiting for insulin action in dogs. *J Clin Invest* 1989; 84: 1620–8.
75. Livingstone C, Collison M. Sex steroids and insulin resistance. *Clin Sci (Lond)* 2002; 102: 151–66.
76. Grunberger G, Taylor SI, Dons RF, Gorden P. Insulin receptors in normal and disease states. *Clin Endocrinol Metab* 1983; 12: 191–219.
77. Comi RJ, Grunberger G, Gorden P. Relationship of insulin binding and insulin-stimulated tyrosine kinase activity is altered in type II diabetes. *J Clin Invest* 1987; 79: 453–62.
78. Brillon DJ, Freidenberg GR, Henry RR, Olefsky JM. Mechanism of defective insulin-receptor kinase activity in NIDDM. Evidence for two receptor populations. *Diabetes* 1989; 38: 397–403.
79. Olefsky JM, Garvey WT, Henry RR, Brillon D, Matthaei S, Freidenberg GR. Cellular mechanisms of insulin resistance in non-insulin-dependent (type II) diabetes. *Am J Med* 1988; 85: 86–105.
80. Kadowaki T. Insights into insulin resistance and type 2 diabetes from knockout mouse models. *J Clin Invest* 2000; 106: 459–65.
81. Pessin JE, Saltiel AR. Signaling pathways in insulin action: molecular targets of insulin resistance. *J Clin Invest* 2000; 106: 165–9.

82. Shepherd PR, Kahn BB. Glucose transporters and insulin action—implications for insulin resistance and diabetes mellitus. *N Engl J Med* 1999; 341: 248–57.
83. Yang YJ, Hope ID, Ader M, Bergman RN. Importance of transcapillary insulin transport to dynamics of insulin action after intravenous glucose. *Am J Physiol* 1994; 266: E17–25.
84. Sjostrand M, Gudbjornsdottir S, Holmang A, Lonn L, Strindberg L, Lonnroth P. Delayed transcapillary transport of insulin to muscle interstitial fluid in obese subjects. *Diabetes* 2002; 51: 2742–8.
85. Sjostrand M, Holmang A, Strindberg L, Lonnroth P. Estimations of muscle interstitial insulin, glucose, and lactate in type 2 diabetic subjects. *Am J Physiol Endocrinol Metab* 2000; 279: E1097–103.
86. Sjostrand M, Holmang A, Lonnroth P. Measurement of interstitial insulin in human muscle. *Am J Physiol* 1999; 276: E151–4.
87. Kolterman OG, Reaven GM, Olefsky JM. Relationship between in vivo insulin resistance and decreased insulin receptors in obese man. *J Clin Endocrinol Metab* 1979; 48: 487–94.
88. Kolterman OG, Gray RS, Griffin J, Burstein P, Insel J, Scarlett JA, Olefsky JM. Receptor and postreceptor defects contribute to the insulin resistance in non-insulin-dependent diabetes mellitus. *J Clin Invest* 1981; 68: 957–69.
89. Ciaraldi TP, Kolterman OG, Olefsky JM. Mechanism of the postreceptor defect in insulin action in human obesity. Decrease in glucose transport system activity. *J Clin Invest* 1981; 68: 875–80.
90. Olefsky JM. Lilly lecture 1980. Insulin resistance and insulin action. An in vitro and in vivo perspective. *Diabetes* 1981; 30: 148–62.
91. Baron AD, Zhu JS, Marshall S, Irsula O, Brechtel G, Keech C. Insulin resistance after hypertension induced by the nitric oxide synthesis inhibitor L-NMMA in rats. *Am J Physiol* 1995; 269: E709–15.
92. Baron AD, Brechtel-Hook G, Johnson A, Cronin J, Leaming R, Steinberg HO. Effect of perfusion rate on the time course of insulin-mediated skeletal muscle glucose uptake. *Am J Physiol* 1996; 271: E1067–72.
93. Baron AD. The coupling of glucose metabolism and perfusion in human skeletal muscle. The potential role of endothelium-derived nitric oxide. *Diabetes* 1996; 45 (suppl 1): S105–9.
94. Shankar R, Zhu JS, Ladd B, Henry D, Shen HQ, Baron AD. Central nervous system nitric oxide synthase activity regulates insulin secretion and insulin action. *J Clin Invest* 1998; 102: 1403–12.
95. Clark MG, Wallis MG, Barrett EJ, Vincent MA, Richards SM, Clerk LH, Rattigan S. Blood flow and muscle metabolism: a focus on insulin action. *Am J Physiol Endocrinol Metab* 2003; 284: E241–58.
96. Ellmerer M, Kim SP, Bergman RN. Diminished effect of physiological hyperinsulinemia to stimulate tissue recruitment after fat feeding in dogs. *Diabetes* 2003; 52 (suppl 1): 1418–P.
97. Bergman RN, Ider YZ, Bowden CR, Cobelli C. Quantitative estimation of insulin sensitivity. *Am J Physiol* 1979; 236: E667–77.
98. Bergman RN, Cobelli C. Minimal modeling, partition analysis, and the estimation of insulin sensitivity. *Fed Proc* 1980; 39: 110–5.
99. Bergman RN, Phillips LS, Cobelli C. Physiologic evaluation of factors controlling glucose tolerance in man: measurement of insulin sensitivity and beta-cell glucose sensitivity from the response to intravenous glucose. *J Clin Invest* 1981; 68: 1456–67.
100. Bergman RN. Lilly Lecture 1989. Toward physiological understanding of glucose tolerance: Minimal-model approach. *Diabetes* 1989; 38: 1512–27.
101. Cobelli C, Bier DM, Ferrannini E. Modeling glucose metabolism in man: theory and practice. *Horm Metab Res Suppl* 1990; 24: 1–10.
102. Horowitz M, Edelbroek MA, Wishart JM, Straathof JW. Relationship between oral glucose tolerance and gastric emptying in normal healthy subjects. *Diabetologia* 1993; 36: 857–62.
103. Abumrad NN, Cherrington AD, Williams PE, Lacy WW, Rabin D. Absorption and disposition of a glucose load in the conscious dog. *Am J Physiol* 1982; 242: E398–406.
104. Amoah AG, Owusu SK, Schuster DP, Osei K. Pathogenic mechanism of type 2 diabetes in Ghanaians—the importance of beta cell secretion, insulin sensitivity and glucose effectiveness. *S Afr Med J* 2002; 92: 377–84.
105. Buchanan TA, Metzger BE, Freinkel N, Bergman RN. Insulin sensitivity and B-cell responsiveness to glucose during late pregnancy in lean and moderately obese women with normal glucose tolerance or mild gestational diabetes. *Am J Obstet Gynecol* 1990; 162: 1008–14.
106. Cutfield WS, Bergman RN, Menon RK, Sperling MA. The modified minimal model: application to measurement of insulin sensitivity in children. *J Clin Endocrinol Metab* 1990; 70: 1644–50.
107. Elbein SC, Wegner K, Kahn SE. Reduced beta-cell compensation to the insulin resistance associated with obesity in members of Caucasian familial type 2 diabetic kindreds. *Diabetes Care* 2000; 23: 221–7.
108. Pacini G, Bergman RN. MINMOD: a computer program to calculate insulin sensitivity and pancreatic responsivity from the frequently sampled intravenous glucose tolerance test. *Comput Methods Programs Biomed* 1986; 23: 113–22.
109. Petrus DJ, Jackson MW, Kemnitz JW, Finegood DT, Panciera D. Assessing insulin sensitivity in the cat: evaluation of the hyperinsulinemic euglycemic clamp and the minimal model analysis. *Res Vet Sci* 1998; 65: 179–81.
110. Saad MF, Steil GM, Kades WW, Ayad MF, Elsewafy WA, Boyadjian R, Jinagouda SD, Bergman RN. Differences between the tolbutamide-boosted and the insulin-modified minimal model protocols. *Diabetes* 1997; 46: 1167–71.
111. Saad MF, Steil GM, Riad-Gabriel M, Khan A, Sharma A, Boyadjian R, Jinagouda SD, Bergman RN. Method of insulin administration has no effect on insulin sensitivity estimates from the insulin-modified minimal model protocol. *Diabetes* 1997; 46: 2044–8.
112. Valle T, Tuomilehto J, Bergman RN, Ghosh S, Hauser ER, Eriksson J, Nylund SJ, Kohtamaki K, Toivanen L, Vidgren G, Tuomilehto-Wolf E, Ehnholm C, Blaschak J, Langefeld CD, Watanabe RM, Magnuson V, Ally DS, Hagopian WA, Ross E, Buchanan TA, Collins F, Boehnke M. Mapping genes for NIDDM. Design of the Finland–United States Investigation of NIDDM Genetics (FUSION) Study. *Diabetes Care* 1998; 21: 949–58.
113. Welch S, Gebhart SS, Bergman RN, Phillips LS. Minimal model analysis of intravenous glucose tolerance

test-derived insulin sensitivity in diabetic subjects. *J Clin Endocrinol Metab* 1990; 71: 1508–18.

114. Yang YJ, Youn JH, Bergman RN. Modified protocols improve insulin sensitivity estimation using the minimal model. *Am J Physiol* 1987; 253: E595–602.
115. Swan JW, Walton C, Godsland IF. Assessment of insulin sensitivity in man: a comparison of minimal model- and euglycaemic clamp-derived measures in health and heart failure. *Clin Sci (Lond)* 1994; 86: 317–22.
116. Saad MF, Anderson RL, Laws A, Watanabe RM, Kades WW, Chen YD, Sands RE, Pei D, Savage PJ, Bergman RN. A comparison between the minimal model and the glucose clamp in the assessment of insulin sensitivity across the spectrum of glucose tolerance. Insulin Resistance Atherosclerosis Study. *Diabetes* 1994; 43: 1114–21.
117. Korytkowski MT, Berga SL, Horwitz MJ. Comparison of the minimal model and the hyperglycemic clamp for measuring insulin sensitivity and acute insulin response to glucose. *Metabolism* 1995; 44: 1121–5.
118. Bergman RN, Ader M, Huecking K, Van Citters G. Accurate assessment of beta-cell function: the hyperbolic correction. *Diabetes* 2002; 51 (suppl 1): S212–20.
119. Buchanan TA, Xiang AH, Peters RK, Kjos SL, Berkowitz K, Marroquin A, Goico J, Ochoa C, Azen SP. Response of pancreatic beta-cells to improved insulin sensitivity in women at high risk for type 2 diabetes. *Diabetes* 2000; 49: 782–8.
120. McManus RM, Cunningham I, Watson A, Harker L, Finegood DT, Beta-cell function and visceral fat in lactating women with a history of gestational diabetes. *Metabolism* 2001; 50: 715–9.
121. Bergman RN, Finegood DT, Kahn SE. The evolution of beta-cell dysfunction and insulin resistance in type 2 diabetes. *Eur J Clin Invest* 2002; 32 (suppl 3): 35–45.
122. Watanabe RM, Valle T, Hauser ER, Ghosh S, Eriksson J, Kohtamaki K, Ehnholm C, Tuomilehto J, Collins FS, Bergman RN, Boehnke M, for the Finland–United States Investigation of NIDDM Genetics (FUSION) Study Investigators. Familiality of quantitative metabolic traits in Finnish families with non-insulin-dependent diabetes mellitus. *Hum Hered* 1999; 49: 159–68.
123. Bergman RN, Zaccaro DJ, Watanabe RM, Haffner SM, Saad MF, Norris JM, Wagenknecht LE, Hokanson JE, Rotter JI, Rich SS. Minimal model-based insulin sensitivity has greater heritability and a different genetic basis than homeostasis model assessment or fasting insulin. *Diabetes* 2003; 52: 2168–74.
124. Haffner SM, Howard G, Mayer E, Bergman RN, Savage PJ, Rewers M, Mykkanen L, Karter AJ, Hamman R, Saad MF. Insulin sensitivity and acute insulin response in African-Americans, non-Hispanic whites, and Hispanics with NIDDM: the Insulin Resistance Atherosclerosis Study. *Diabetes* 1997; 46: 63–9.
125. Kahn SE, Prigeon RL, McCulloch DK, Boyko EJ, Bergman RN, Schwartz MW, Neifing JL, Ward WK, Beard JC, Palmer JP. Quantification of the relationship between insulin sensitivity and beta-cell function in human subjects. Evidence for a hyperbolic function. *Diabetes* 1993; 42: 1663–72.
126. Yoneda H, Ikegami H, Yamamoto Y, Yamato E, Cha T, Kawaguchi Y, Tahara Y, Ogihara T. Analysis of early-phase insulin responses in nonobese subjects with mild glucose intolerance. *Diabetes Care* 1992; 15: 1517–21.
127. Weyer C, Bogardus C, Pratley RE. Metabolic characteristics of individuals with impaired fasting glucose and/or impaired glucose tolerance. *Diabetes* 1999; 48: 2197–203.
128. Breda E, Toffolo G, Polonsky KS, Cobelli C. Insulin release in impaired glucose tolerance: oral minimal model predicts normal sensitivity to glucose but defective response times. *Diabetes* 2002; 51 (suppl 1): S227–33.
129. Guerrer-Romer F, Rodriguez-Moran M, Gonzalez-Ortiz M, Martinez-Abundis E. Insulin action and secretion in healthy Hispanic-Mexican first-degree relatives of subjects with type 2 diabetes. *J Endocrinol Invest* 2001; 24: 580–6.
130. Jansson PA, Eliasson B, Lindmark S, Eriksson JW. Endocrine abnormalities in healthy first-degree relatives of type 2 diabetes patients—potential role of steroid hormones and leptin in the development of insulin resistance. *Eur J Clin Invest* 2002; 32: 172–8.
131. Laakso M. How good a marker is insulin level for insulin resistance? *Am J Epidemiol* 1993; 137: 959–65.
132. Perseghin G, Caumo A, Sereni LP, Battezzati A, Luzi L. Fasting blood sample-based assessment of insulin sensitivity in kidney–pancreas-transplanted patients. *Diabetes Care* 2002; 25: 2207–11.
133. Paolisso G, Tagliamonte MR, De Lucia D, Palmieri F, Manzella D, Rinaldi C, Bossone A, Colaizzo D, Margaglione M, Varricchio M. ACE gene polymorphism and insulin action in older subjects and healthy centenarians. *J Am Geriatr Soc* 2001; 49: 610–4.
134. Hrebicek J, Janout V, Malincikova J, Horakova D, Cizek L. Detection of insulin resistance by simple quantitative insulin sensitivity check index QUICKI for epidemiological assessment and prevention. *J Clin Endocrinol Metab* 2002; 87: 144–7.
135. Abbasi F, Reaven GM. Evaluation of the quantitative insulin sensitivity check index as an estimate of insulin sensitivity in humans. *Metabolism* 2002; 51: 235–7.
136. Quon MJ. QUICKI is a useful and accurate index of insulin sensitivity. *J Clin Endocrinol Metab* 2002; 87: 949–51.
137. Duncan GE, Hutson AD, Stacpoole PW. QUICKI is not a useful and accurate index of insulin sensitivity following exercise training. *J Clin Endocrinol Metab* 2002; 87: 950–1.
138. Katsuki A, Sumida Y, Gabazza EC, Murashima S, Urakawa H, Morioka K, Kitagawa N, Tanaka T, Araki-Sasaki R, Hori Y, Nakatani K, Yano Y, Adachi Y. QUICKI is useful for following improvements in insulin sensitivity after therapy in patients with type 2 diabetes mellitus. *J Clin Endocrinol Metab* 2002; 87: 2906–8.
139. Uwaifo GI, Fallon EM, Chin J, Elberg J, Parikh SJ, Yanovski JA. Indices of insulin action, disposal, and secretion derived from fasting samples and clamps in normal glucose-tolerant black and white children. *Diabetes Care* 2002; 25: 2081–7.
140. Rajala U, Laakso M, Paivansalo M, Pelkonen O, Suramo I, Keinanen-Kiukaanniemi S. Low insulin sensitivity measured by both quantitative insulin sensitivity check index and homeostasis model assessment method as a risk factor of increased intima-media thickness of the carotid artery. *J Clin Endocrinol Metab* 2002; 87: 5092–7.
141. Katsuki A, Sumida Y, Urakawa H, Gabazza EC, Murashima S, Morioka K, Kitagawa N, Tanaka T, Araki-Sasaki R, Hori Y, Nakatani K, Yano Y, Adachi Y. Neither homeostasis model assessment nor quantitative insulin

sensitivity check index can predict insulin resistance in elderly patients with poorly controlled type 2 diabetes mellitus. *J Clin Endocrinol Metab* 2002; 87: 5332–5.

142. Vanhala P, Vanhala M, Kumpusalo E, Keinanen-Kiukaanniemi S. The quantitative insulin sensitivity check index QUICKI predicts the onset of type 2 diabetes better than fasting plasma insulin in obese subjects: a 5-year follow-up study. *J Clin Endocrinol Metab* 2002; 87: 5834–7.
143. Hanson RL, Pratley RE, Bogardus C, Narayan KM, Roumain JM, Imperatore G, Fagot-Campagna A, Pettitt DJ, Bennett PH, Knowler WC. Evaluation of simple indices of insulin sensitivity and insulin secretion for use in epidemiologic studies. *Am J Epidemiol* 2000; 151: 190–8.
144. Haffner SM, Kennedy E, Gonzalez C, Stern MP, Miettinen H. A prospective analysis of the HOMA model. The Mexico City Diabetes Study. *Diabetes Care* 1996; 19: 1138–41.
145. Emoto M, Nishizawa Y, Maekawa K, Hiura Y, Kanda H, Kawagishi T, Shoji T, Okuno Y, Morii H. Homeostasis model assessment as a clinical index of insulin resistance in type 2 diabetic patients treated with sulfonylureas. *Diabetes Care* 1999; 22: 818–22.
146. Katz A, Nambi SS, Mather K, Baron AD, Follmann DA, Sullivan G, Quon MJ. Quantitative insulin sensitivity check index: a simple, accurate method for assessing insulin sensitivity in humans. *J Clin Endocrinol Metab* 2000; 85: 2402–10.
147. Bonora E, Targher G, Alberiche M, Bonadonna RC, Saggiani F, Zenere MB, Monauni T, Muggeo M. Homeostasis model assessment closely mirrors the glucose clamp technique in the assessment of insulin sensitivity: studies in subjects with various degrees of glucose tolerance and insulin sensitivity. *Diabetes Care* 2000; 23: 57–63.
148. Baron AD. Impaired glucose tolerance as a disease. *Am J Cardiol* 2001; 88: 16H–9H.
149. Berger H, Crane J, Farine D, Armson A, De La RS, Keenan-Lindsay L, Leduc L, Reid G, Van Aerde J. Screening for gestational diabetes mellitus. *J Obstet Gynaecol Can* 2002; 24: 894–912.
150. Voors AW, Radhakrishnamurthy B, Srinivasan SR, Webber LS, Berenson GS. Plasma glucose level related to blood pressure in 272 children, ages 7–15 years sampled from a total biracial population. *Am J Epidemiol* 1981; 113: 347–56.
151. Cederholm J, Wibell L. Evaluation of insulin release and relative peripheral resistance with use of the oral glucose tolerance test: a study in subjects with normoglycaemia, glucose intolerance and non-insulin-dependent diabetes mellitus. *Scand J Clin Lab Invest* 1985; 45: 741–51.
152. Gutt M, Davis CL, Spitzer SB, Llabre MM, Kumar M, Czarnecki EM, Schneiderman N, Skyler JS, Marks JB. Validation of the insulin sensitivity index (ISI(0, 120)): comparison with other measures. *Diabetes Res Clin Pract* 2000; 47: 177–84.
153. Matsuda M, DeFronzo RA. Insulin sensitivity indices obtained from oral glucose tolerance testing: comparison with the euglycemic insulin clamp. *Diabetes Care* 1999; 22: 1462–70.
154. Stumvoll M, Mitrakou A, Pimenta W, Jenssen T, Yki-Jarvinen H, Van Haeften T, Renn W, Gerich J. Use of the oral glucose tolerance test to assess insulin release and insulin sensitivity. *Diabetes Care* 2000; 23: 295–301.
155. Souissi S, Rakotoambinina B, Foussier V, Lienhardt A, Laborde K, Jos J, Robert JJ. Insulin resistance and excess weight in adolescent insulin-dependent diabetic girls. *Diabete Metab* 1993; 19: 52–7.
156. Campbell PJ, Carlson MG. Impact of obesity on insulin action in NIDDM. *Diabetes* 1993; 42: 405–10.
157. Misra A, Garg A, Abate N, Peshock RM, Stray-Gundersen J, Grundy SM. Relationship of anterior and posterior subcutaneous abdominal fat to insulin sensitivity in nondiabetic men. *Obes Res* 1997; 5: 93–9.
158. Goodpaster BH, Thaete FL, Simoneau JA, Kelley DE. Subcutaneous abdominal fat and thigh muscle composition predict insulin sensitivity independently of visceral fat. *Diabetes* 1997; 46: 1579–85.
159. Chiu KC, Martinez DS, Yoon C, Chuang LM. Relative contribution of insulin sensitivity and beta-cell function to plasma glucose and insulin concentrations during the oral glucose tolerance test. *Metabolism* 2002; 51: 115–20.
160. Kuo CS, Hwu CM, Kwok CF, Hsiao LC, Weih MJ, Lee SH, Lee YS, Ho LT. Surrogate estimates of insulin sensitivity in Chinese diabetic patients and their offspring. *Diabet Med* 2002; 19: 735–40.
161. Kanauchi M, Tsujimoto N, Hashimoto T. Validation of simple indices to assess insulin sensitivity based on the oral glucose tolerance test in the Japanese population. *Diabetes Res Clin Pract* 2002; 55: 229–35.
162. Albareda M, Rodriguez-Espinosa J, Murugo M, de Leiva A, Corcoy R. Assessment of insulin sensitivity and beta-cell function from measurements in the fasting state and during an oral glucose tolerance test. *Diabetologia* 2000; 43: 1507–11.
163. Mari A, Pacini G, Murphy E, Ludvik B, Nolan JJ. A model-based method for assessing insulin sensitivity from the oral glucose tolerance test. *Diabetes Care* 2001; 24: 539–48.
164. Sievenpiper JL, Jenkins DJ, Josse RG, Vuksan V. Dilution of the 75-g oral glucose tolerance test improves overall tolerability but not reproducibility in subjects with different body compositions. *Diabetes Res Clin Pract* 2001; 51: 87–95.
165. Ko GT, Chan JC, Woo J, Lau E, Yeung VT, Chow CC, Cockram CS. The reproducibility and usefulness of the oral glucose tolerance test in screening for diabetes and other cardiovascular risk factors. *Ann Clin Biochem* 1998; 35 (pt 1): 62–7.
166. Moyses C, Young A, Kolterman O. Modulation of gastric emptying as a therapeutic approach to glycaemic control. *Diabet Med* 1996; 13: S34–8.
167. Phillips WT, Schwartz JG, McMahan CA. Reduced postprandial blood glucose levels in recently diagnosed non-insulin-dependent diabetics secondary to pharmacologically induced delayed gastric emptying. *Dig Dis Sci* 1993; 38: 51–8.
168. Hucking K, Bergman RN, Watanabe R, OGTT-derived measures of insulin sensitivity may be confounded by other factors. *Diabetes 3*; 52 (suppl 1): 1242–P.
169. Shapiro ET, Tillil H, Miller MA, Frank BH, Galloway JA, Rubenstein AH, Polonsky KS. Insulin secretion and clearance. Comparison after oral and intravenous glucose. *Diabetes* 1987; 36: 1365–71.

17

Protein Metabolism in Health and Diabetes

Zhenqi Liu and Eugene J. Barrett

University of Virginia Health System, Charlottesville, VA, USA

INTRODUCTION

Hamish Munro provided a scholarly description of the historical roots of protein metabolic studies in the introduction to his three-volume book *Mammalian Protein Metabolism* in 1964 [1]. Particularly noteworthy were the contributions by the French scientist Francois Magendie who wrote in 1817 that the

> life of man, and that of other organized bodies, is founded upon this, that they eventually assimilate to themselves certain quantitative matter which we named aliment. The privation of that matter during even a very limited period brings with it necessarily the cessation of life. On the other side, daily observation teaches that the organs of man, as well as those of all living beings, lose, at each instant a certain quantity of that matter which composes them; Nay, it is on the necessity of repairing those habitual losses that the want of aliment is founded. From these two data and from others which we will make known afterwards we justly conclude that living bodies are by no means always composed of the same matter at every period of its existence ... it is extremely probable of all parts of the body of man experience an intestinal movement, which has a double effect of expelling the molecules that can or ought no longer to compose the organs, and replacing them by new molecules. This internal, intimate motion, constitutes nutrition. [2]

Subsequently, he wrote,

> nutrition is more or less rapid according to the tissues. The glands, the muscles, skin, etc. change their volume, color, consistence, with great quickness; the tendons, fibrous membranes, the bones, the cartilages, appear to have a much slower nutrition, for physical properties changed slowly by the effect of aging and disease.

With brilliant deductive reasoning, Magendie had articulated three important principles: the first that the body's protein pool is in a state of constant turnover, the second that some essential dietary components are required to maintain the balance between factors that build and dissipate body protein, and finally that tissues vary in the rates at which its protein mass turns over. Full articulation of these principles would only come more than a century later when Schoenheimer [3] initiated the use of isotopic labeling techniques to quantify the turnover of body proteins and with the painstaking studies of Rose and colleagues characterizing the dietary essential amino acids. Magendie's conclusion to his experiments is rendered even more remarkable in that it preceded by 20 years the description by the Dutch scientist Gerard Mulder [4] of a common nitrogenous element in fibrin, egg albumin, and gluten, which he called "protein" (Greek προτευσ – "first") for its role as a "primary" nutritional element, and by more than 80 years the first chemical characterization of the amino acid composition of proteins by Kossel and Kutcher [5].

The availability of isotopically labeled amino acid tracers from the early 1950s onward, together with the development of radioimmunoassay methods and ion-exchange methods for automated amino acid analysis in the early 1960s, allowed the experimental study of protein and amino acid metabolism to enter the modern era. The explosion of experimental information that followed forms the basis of a current understanding of body protein metabolism.

Understanding the regulation of human protein metabolism requires a familiarity with the basic processes by which proteins are synthesized and degraded, as well as how these processes operate within individual cells and how tissues are integrated to serve the organism as a whole. Here we briefly review relevant aspects of the control of protein synthesis and degradation on a cellular level. We then review current understanding of the integration of these processes in healthy humans and how these

International Textbook of Diabetes Mellitus, Third Edition. Edited by R. A. DeFronzo, E. Ferrannini, H. Keen, and P. Zimmet.
 ISBN: 0-471-48655-8.

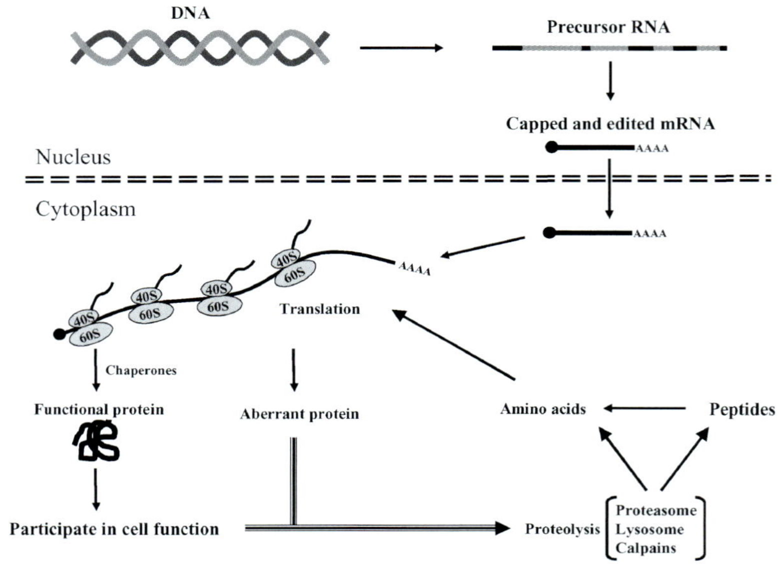

Figure 1 Schematic depiction of the pathway from DNA to protein in eukaryotes

processes become disordered with disease, particularly diabetes mellitus.

THE CELL BIOLOGY AND BIOCHEMISTRY OF PROTEIN SYNTHESIS

The year 2003 marks the 50th anniversary of the discovery of the double helical structure of DNA by Watson and Crick [6]. The decade that followed saw the unraveling of how the 40S and 60S eukaryotic ribosomal subunits accomplished the reading of sequence-specific nucleotides and accurately translated that into the primary structure of the protein. Simultaneously, first in bacteria and subsequently in eukaryotic systems, the control of gene expression began to be deciphered. The last two decades have been marked by ever more detailed characterization of the step-by-step processes by which the transcriptional and translational processes operate. This has included the discovery of multiple transcription factors as well as coactivators and corepressors that modulate the transcription of genes and the discovery of translational initiation, elongation, and termination factors that regulate translation at the ribosomal level.

The detailed cellular mechanisms involved in the transcription of messenger RNA (mRNA) from DNA, the processing of the primary transcript to mature mRNA, and the transport of mRNA from the nucleus to cytosol for subsequent translation by cytosolic ribosomal complexes lie beyond the scope of the present work. The reader may consult one of several excellent texts [7]. However, some aspects of the regulation of both the transcriptional and translational processes are relevant to understanding insulin's action and that of other hormones to regulate protein synthesis. It is also necessary for our understanding of how some pharmaceutical agents exert their therapeutic actions in the treatment of insulin resistance and diabetes. Figure 1 provides an overall summary schematic for the process of protein synthesis.

Regulation of Gene Transcription

Messenger RNA transcription begins when RNA polymerase II identifies and binds to a transcriptional start site on DNA. However, two features of the eukaryotic DNA make this seemingly simple job enormously complex. The first is simply the amount of DNA present in the cell. Although we now know the entire sequence of the human genome, we do not yet know precisely how many genes there are, because we cannot identify all of the transcription start sites. We do know that the fraction of DNA that is actually transcribed into mRNA constitutes less than 5% of the genome. A much greater fraction of DNA is never transcribed and the function of much of this DNA is uncertain. In addition to RNA polymerase II needing to find the right transcriptional start site, it has to contend with a complex structure of eukaryotic DNA which is packaged in association with a variety of proteins, principally histones, into nucleosomes and then into higher order structures that prevent the long DNA double helix that forms each chromosome from becoming an impossibly tangled meshwork but at the same time allowing timely transcription of the necessary genes. To accomplish the task of transcribing DNA, eukaryotic cells have developed an elaborate system whereby the RNA polymerase II binding site is recognized based upon the association of generalized transcription factors typically at the promoter region of a

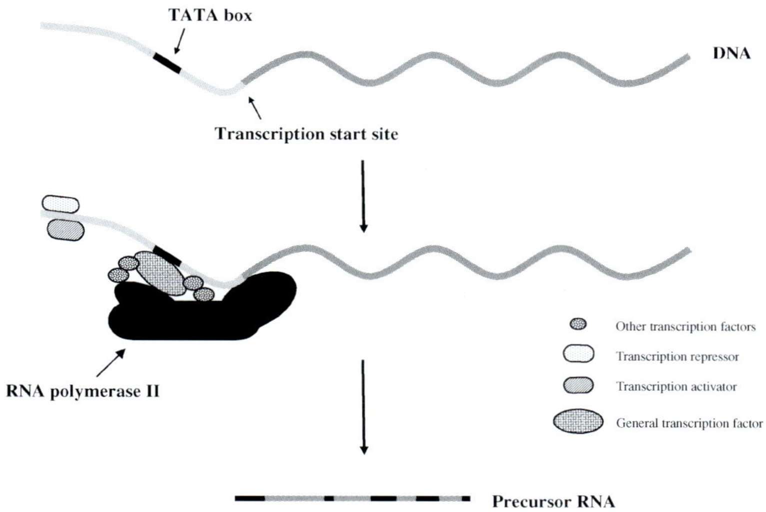

Figure 2 Initiation of gene transcription from DNA to RNA by RNA polymerase II and other transcription factors in eukaryocytes

gene (Figure 2). For RNA polymerase II the promoters are typically AT-rich regions called TATA boxes that are several dozen bases upstream of the initiation start site. This transcription initiation complex is large (containing over 100 proteins) and functions to allow RNA polymerase II to initiate transcription and facilitate the unwinding of the DNA helices, thereby opening it to base pairing to allow complementary ribonucleotides to pair with the template bases in the DNA strand being transcribed. As this process begins the RNA polymerase II dissociates from the initiation complex and begins transcribing at the transcriptional start site, and then progressively moves along the unwinding DNA strand.

In addition to generalized transcription factors, there are transcriptional activators (as well as transcriptional repressors) that play a more specific role to enhance (or restrict) the transcription of specific genes. These are proteins that bind to the outer surface of specific DNA sequences. In general, they have specific structural characteristics (e.g. helix–loop–helix, leucine–zipper, helix–turn–helix, etc.) that are involved in their binding to the outer surface of the DNA double helix. While the generalized transcription factors are required for initiation of transcription at all sites that utilize RNA polymerase II, individual transcriptional activators and repressors will regulate the transcription of a restricted number of genes. A significant part of their function appears to be attracting the generalized transcription factor complex as well as RNA polymerase II to the promoter region of a specific gene. While the generalized transcription factors typically bind at a recognizable sequence of nucleotides (the promoter region) that is closely aligned with the transcriptional start site, transcriptional activators and repressors can bind at sites removed by 1000 nucleotides or more from the promoter and exert their action through changes in the secondary structure of DNA. In addition to the transcriptional activators and repressors, proteins called corepressors and coactivators also regulate transcription initiation. These proteins do not bind directly to DNA sequences but rather interact with repressor or activator proteins. Taken together, it is estimated that there are more than 1000 proteins in the human genome that function as transcriptional activators, repressors, coactivators, or corepressors. In effect, the rate at which a specific gene is transcribed is regulated by the integrated input of these multiple transcriptional regulators. In any one gene there may be simultaneously bound proteins from all four categories of transcriptional regulatory proteins. Effectively the balance among these dictates the rate of transcription. As we will see below, hormones like insulin, glucocorticoids, glucagon (via cAMP) as well as glucose *per se* can influence the rate at which genes are transcribed based upon their effects on these transcriptional regulators.

Insulin, or insulin deficiency, can profoundly influence the transcription of mRNA. For example, in muscle tissue insulin deficiency provokes a significant change in the expression of over 230 genes as determined by microarray methods [8]. While mRNA coding for proteins that are involved in a variety of cellular functions is changed, a pattern is seen with coordinated increases in the expression of the mRNA of enzymes and transport proteins involved in fatty acid metabolism and in ubiquitin-mediated protein degradation (see below), with simultaneous decreases in mRNA coding for enzymes involved in carbohydrate metabolism as well as some mitochondrial oxidative enzymes. Whether these changes were mediated directly by genomic actions of insulin or secondarily from changes that occurred as a result of insulin-deficient diabetes is not certain. The findings emphasize, however, that transcription changes involving a large number of proteins occur as a result of decreases in insulin availability and these changes mediate some of the basic metabolic abnormalities seen with type 1 diabetes mellitus.

These changes are by no means restricted to muscle; the liver offers more specific example of the transcriptional action of insulin involved in the regulation of transcription of two key gluconeogenic enzymes in liver. These enzymes, phosphoenolpyruvate carboxykinase and glucose-6-phosphatase, appear to be principal sites at which insulin acts to limit glucose production by the liver. It has been known for some time that insulin can potently down-regulate the transcription of genes coding for these proteins [9]. Quite recently this has been further clarified with the demonstration that insulin, acting through its receptor and the lipid kinase phosphatidylinositol 3 kinase (PI3 kinase), phosphorylates a member of the forkhead family of transcription factors (foxo-1). This action leads to the exclusion of foxo-1 from the nucleus and a decrease in the transcription of the genes for these gluconeogenic enzymes [10].

Another example of transcriptional regulation occurs in the treatment of patients with type 2 diabetes using *insulin sensitizers* of the thiazolidinedione class. These agents bind to and activate a transcriptional factor, the γ isoform of the peroxisomal proliferation activator receptor or PPAR-γ, which in turn controls the expression of several hundred genes in different tissues. An outcome of this pleiotropic action is the increase in insulin sensitivity of skeletal muscle to glucose disposal. Other actions occur as well, which include an increase in the recruitment of preadipocytes to adipocytes, and an increase in sodium reabsorption in the kidney. The direct pathway(s) by which PPARγ activation accomplishes these effects is still being unraveled [11].

Regulation of mRNA Translation

Following transcription of mRNA almost immediately, a complex processing step begins that splices introns (non-translated RNA sequences) out from the mRNA. In addition, depending upon the specific mRNA, there may be alternative splicing that can generate more than one gene product as the final protein. This RNA processing is generally complete by the time the RNA exits the nucleus via the nuclear pore apparatus (Figure 1). It bears mention that some of the transcribed RNA codes ribosomal RNA (rRNA), which is assembled with ribosomal proteins in the nucleolus and is then exported as the intact ribosomal subunit. The mRNA for ribosomal proteins is translated in the cytosol but the end products return to the nucleus for assembly. The assembled ribosomal subunits then exit the nucleus via the nuclear pore apparatus.

The translation of mRNA proceeds in the direction from the 5′ to the 3′ end of the mRNA molecule (Figure 3). In most eukaryotic cells the 5′ end of mRNA is “capped” by a methyl-substituted guanosine that signals it as a translational start site. Other RNAs transcribed in eukaryotic cells (e.g. rRNA) lack this “cap,” which limits both their export from the nucleus and translation. A specific translation initiation factor, eukaryotic initiation factor 4E (eIF-4E), binds to the methylated guanosine at the 5′ end of mRNA. This, together with two other eukaryotic initiation factors (eIF-4G and eIF-4A), joins with the small (40S) ribosomal subunit and the initiator transfer RNA (tRNA; met-tRNA).

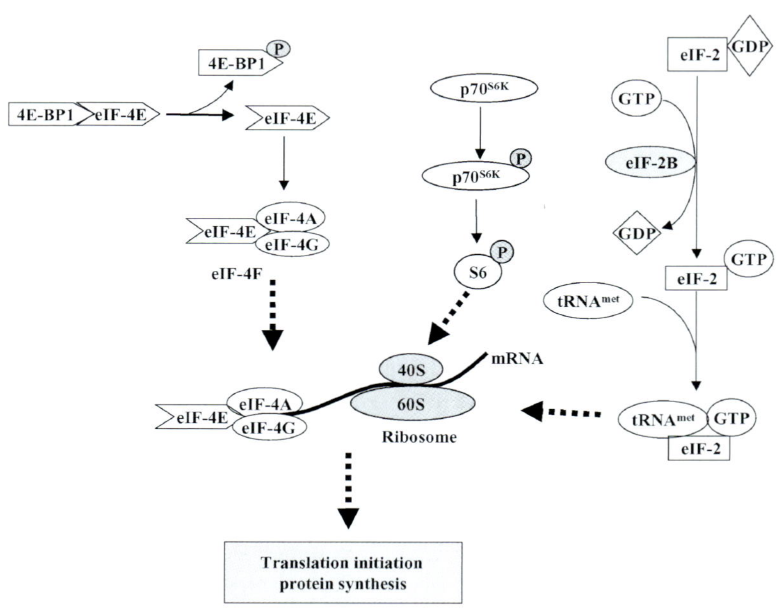

Figure 3 The translational control of protein synthesis

Together with several other initiation factors these form an initiation complex and allow the methionyl-tRNA to begin to move along the mRNA until it finds the correct triplet codon (AUG) match. At that point there is a joining of the large ribosomal subunit and cleavage of guanosine triphosphate (GTP). The complete ribosomal particle (large and small subunits) will now facilitate adding additional aminoacyl-tRNA and begin the process of forming successive peptide bonds as the ribosome moves along the mRNA molecule. This will continue until it encounters a stop codon (UAG). As a single ribosome is moving along an mRNA molecule translating a new protein, a second round of initiation will occur and then the third and fourth round such that the mRNA molecule will have multiple ribosomes associated with it (forming a "polysome") at any one time, each translating a peptide chain. In this manner amplification of the information carried in a single mRNA molecule is accomplished. Within the past several years the crystal structure of the ribosome has been resolved [12] and this has led to the conclusion that the actual catalysis of peptide bond formation results from the catalytic activity of the rRNA, which forms the core of the ribosome. Hence, rRNA acts as a "ribozyme" to catalyze peptide bond formation [13].

Although a highly accurate process (it is estimated that the wrong amino acid is incorporated into the growing peptide chain approximately once in every 10 000), mistakes during translation. Translational elongation factors are thought to play a role in minimizing the number of mistakes; they may also play a role in allowing recognition of mistakenly synthesized peptides. Despite these systems, it is estimated that as many as 30% of newly synthesized proteins contain errors that result in their being rapidly degraded. These aberrant proteins are targeted by ubiquitination to the proteasome to be degraded by the cell [14].

This process of mRNA translation occurs within the cytosol and can be further targeted. For example, proteins destined for secretion are typically synthesized on ribosomes associated with the endoplasmic reticulum (ER) and are transported into the cisternae of the ER as they are being translated. Other proteins soon after being translated (or even as translation is occurring) encounter specialized cellular proteins (called *chaperones*), which assist the folding and packaging of these newly translated proteins [15, 16]. These chaperone proteins include several members of the "heat-shock" family of proteins (HSP 60's and HSP 70's). Any uncorrected errors in the latter process once again lead to the proteins being targeted for early degradation. The assisted folding of proteins consumes ATP energy, but inasmuch as the synthesis of an incorrectly folded protein might have required 4000 or more ATP equivalents (four high-energy phosphate bonds per peptide bond formed) the investment of a few additional ATP molecules for refolding of an incorrectly folded, but otherwise correctly translated protein appears energetically worthwhile.

We have referred heretofore to protein synthesis as occurring in the cytosol. It is worth remembering that in eukaryotic cells mitochondria are also a site of protein synthesis. Interestingly, mitochondria possess their own ribosomes that resemble the 50S and 30S subunits of prokaryotic ribosomes and contain rRNA similar to that of prokaryotes.

It is interesting to consider the overall rate at which eukaryotic ribosomes are able to translate mRNA. Estimates suggest that it requires approximately 1 min to form a peptide chain of 100 amino acids. Hence, translation of mRNA for a larger protein (e.g. 100–120 kDa) would require approximately 10 min. This time issue, as can be easily appreciated, puts some limitation on the rate at which cells can respond with changes in enzyme activity, signaling behavior, or other functions when based on incrementing the quantity of protein present.

Beginning in the late 1960s, it was recognized that insulin exerted a major action in regulation of mRNA translation. In early studies from several laboratories it was appreciated that the rate of protein synthesis in insulin-sensitive tissues (skeletal muscle, liver, heart, etc.) increased in the presence of insulin, with little or no change in total RNA content of the tissue [17–19], consistent with increased translational efficiency. Here *efficiency* was defined as the amount or rate of protein synthesis per mRNA molecule. As rRNA constitutes ~90% of cellular RNA, this corresponded in effect to an increase in the amount of protein synthesis per ribosome. Careful analysis of the fraction of ribosomes present as polysomes in tissues incubated in the presence or absence of insulin demonstrated that insulin favored polysome formation in a variety of insulin-sensitive tissues. The mechanism by which insulin stimulates translation is still under investigation. Currently there is compelling evidence for a direct action beginning with postreceptor activation of PI3-kinase and downstream signaling through protein kinase B (PKB/Akt) and mammalian target of rapamycin (mTOR) via a cascade of phosphorylation reactions that leads to several actions on the translation initiation complex [20, 21]. In particular, eIF-4E binding protein 1 (4E-BP1) is phosphorylated at multiple sites, leading to its dissociation from eIF-4E [22, 23] (Figure 4). Free eIF-4E, together with additional initiation factors, binds in an ordered sequence to mRNA that promotes translation initiation.

In addition to affecting the translational initiation process, by activating 70-kDa ribosomal protein S6 kinase ($p70^{S6K}$), insulin can influence the formation of new ribosomes. This kinase acts in part to phosphorylate ribosomal protein S6. In its phosphorylated state, S6 protein favors translation of mRNAs with oligopyrimidine sequences in the 5′ untranslated region [24]. This includes mRNAs

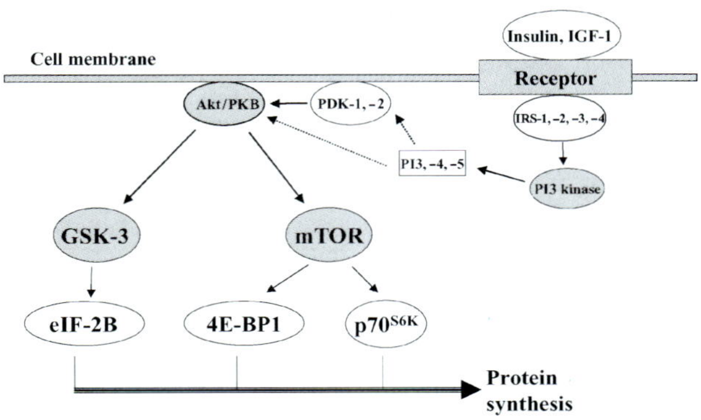

Figure 4 Insulin and IGF-1 stimulate protein synthesis through the PI3-kinase/Akt signaling pathway

coding for many ribosomal proteins as well as translational initiation and elongation factors. In this manner insulin can act specifically to increase the translational "machinery" to facilitate protein synthesis. In animal models of type 1 diabetes an early effect of insulin treatment is to induce ribosomal protein synthesis and this appears to precede generalized increases in protein synthesis.

Insulin also acts to increase the transport of amino acids into cells [25]. This effect appears to be due to the increase in the synthesis of some plasma membrane amino acid transporters. This can have a secondary dual effect to enhance mRNA translation, first by providing amino acid substrates for protein synthesis and second by enhancing further the activation of the translational initiation apparatus. This latter effect occurs by a direct action of amino acids to enhance mTOR phosphorylation and activity [26], which in turn leads to hyperphosphorylation of 4E-BP1 and p70^{S6K}. The details of how amino acids enhance mTOR phosphorylation are not currently known.

THE CELL BIOLOGY AND BIOCHEMISTRY OF PROTEIN DEGRADATION

We have seen that protein synthesis is a complex process. Unraveling its complexity has been a central theme of the molecular biology revolution of the second half of the twentieth century. Similarly important, but much less well studied, have been the processes involved in protein degradation. Although protein degradation has long been studied as a mechanism for recycling nutrients and as a general part of a cell or organism's protein economy, the role of proteolysis in the minute-to-minute regulation of metabolic pathways has come into focus only in the past 5–10 years. We can anticipate that this will be an area of more intense investigation in the coming decade.

There are at least three major pathways of proteolysis in eukaryotic cells. These include lysosomal proteolysis, the ubiquitin–proteasome pathway, and calcium-regulated cytosolic or calpain-mediated proteolysis. This does not include consideration of the numerous proteases that operate extracellularly and are involved in the regulation of clotting, the turnover of extracellular matrix, or protein digestion within the gastrointestinal tract.

Lysosomal breakdown of protein occurs in virtually all eukaryotic cells [27] (Figure 5). These cytoplasmic vesicular structures maintain an internal pH of approximately 5.0 that allows activity of a variety of acid hydrolases that would not operate at the general pH of the cytoplasm (~7.1). An ATP-driven proton pump in its membrane maintains the internal pH of the lysosome. Proteases are among the multiple hydrolases that are found in the lysosome. Enzymes involved in breakdown of nucleic acids, lipids, carbohydrates as well as phosphatases and sulfatases are also present. As such, the lysosome is an efficient, specialized organelle for degrading most biochemical compounds. There are three principal pathways by which proteins destined for destruction arrive within the lysosome. Lysosomes form by budding of vesicular material from the *trans*-Golgi. During the process of protein sorting that occurs as proteins move through the Golgi, hydrolytic enzymes are selected as a consequence of having mannose-6-phosphate attached to these proteins and being recognized by a mannose-6-phosphate receptor. These hydrolytic enzymes aggregate in a specific area of the *trans*-Golgi and small vesicles budding from the *trans*-Golgi and carry the hydrolytic enzymes to merge with late endosomal vesicles. The lysosomes that are thus formed can hydrolyze the contents of the endosomes. This material will have arrived from endocytosis at the plasma membrane, or from a process of autophagy whereby endosomes will have enveloped cytoplasmic structures (mitochondria, ribosomes, etc.) destined for degradation, or from some specialized cells (such as white blood cells), bacteria, or other foreign particles that have been taken up by phagocytosis. In all cases, the breakdown products of digested proteins are amino acids that exit the lysosome

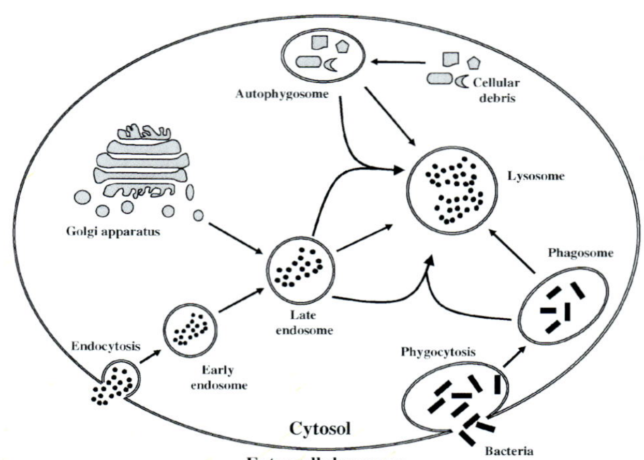

Figure 5 The lysosomal protein degradation pathways

and are available to the cell for another round of protein synthesis, or for use as an oxidative fuel.

A variation of the process of autophagy has been described in liver. In this process called *micro-autophagy* small vesicles are formed within the liver cytosol, which "pinch-off" bits of hepatic cytosol with the resident proteins and join with lysosomes where the internal proteins are digested. This process in liver appears to be regulated by both insulin and glucagon, as well as amino acids themselves [28, 29]. Details of how insulin (or amino acids) regulates this process, however, have not been defined in further detail. In recent years, there has been great excitement with regard to the identification of the ubiquitin–proteasomal pathway of protein degradation [30]. Unlike protein degradation within the lysosome, the ubiquitin-proteasomal pathway is a highly targeted pathway by which individual proteins can be selected for degradation. This is accomplished by a complex recognition process. It involves at least three steps (Figure 6). The first is the activation of ubiquitin (a highly conserved 5.8-kDa protein) by an ATP-dependent process, whereby ubiquitin is covalently attached to an *ubiquitin-activating enzyme*. Subsequently, this is transferred to one of a set of ubiquitin-conjugating enzymes. These latter proteins act in association with one of a family of accessory proteins that together transfer ubiquitin to a specific protein targeted for degradation. The ubiquitin is transferred to the ε-amino group of a lysine molecule in the targeted protein. Subsequently, the ubiquitin molecule itself has additional ubiquitin monomers attached again at the ε-amino group of lysine. It is this *polyubiquitin chain* that is recognized by the proteasome. The latter is a multicomponent cytosolic structure that is characterized by the presence of symmetric barrel-shaped structure with lid-like apparatus on either end [31, 32]. The polyubiquitinated protein is recognized by the proteasome and fed processively into the center of the barrel. Lining the interior are proteins with distinctive protease activities that degrade the ubiquitinated proteins into short peptides. The latter are released from the proteasome and subsequently degraded to amino acids, or in some cells enter the ER and subsequently associate with HLA class 1 molecules which present these peptides to the extracellular environment [33].

For some time it was believed that the ubiquitin–proteasomal system was principally involved in the degradation of proteins that were made aberrantly, i.e. with either errors in their primary sequence or folding errors that were not corrected by the chaperone proteins [14]. It is now clear that the ubiquitin–proteasome system is not restricted to cleaning up mistakes. An intriguing example has been the observation that cells entering mitosis selectively ubiquitinate cell-cycle-specific enzymes, thereby targeting them for degradation [34]. Proteins that are otherwise stable can likewise be targeted for degradation as a result of changes in conformation that result from phosphorylation or association with another protein.

It has recently been reported that proteasomal protein degradation can function to regulate insulin and insulin-like growth factor 1 (IGF-1) signaling by degrading the signaling protein insulin receptor substrate 2 (IRS-2) [35]. The latter undergoes tyrosine phosphorylation by the insulin receptor, and deficiency of IRS-2 (at least in mice) leads to development of diabetes secondary to insulin resistance and β-cell secretory failure. Within a few hours of insulin (or IGF-1) binding to its receptor the quantity of IRS-2 declines dramatically and this decline is inhibited by wortmanin (an inhibitor of PI3 kinase), rapamycin (an mTOR inhibitor), or lactacystin (a proteasome inhibitor). These findings are consistent with a phosphorylation-dependent degradation of IRS-2 by the ubiquitin-proteasomal pathway. In the presence of

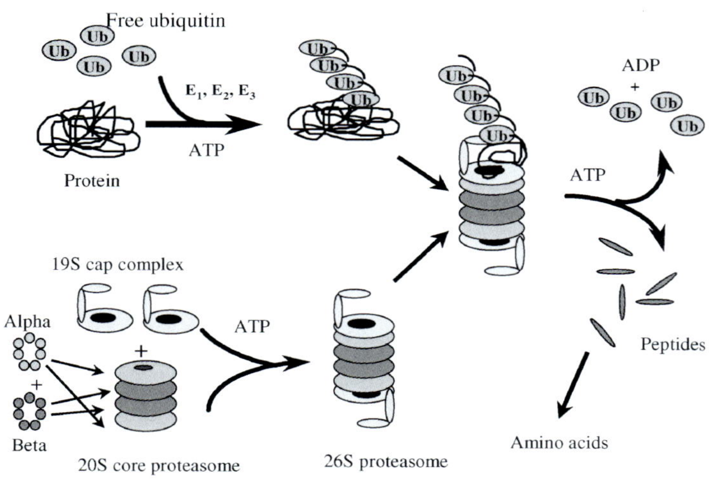

Figure 6 The ubiquitin–proteasome proteolytic pathway. Ub = ubiquitin

insulin, lactacystin produces a buildup of ubiquitinated IRS-2.

In skeletal muscle the ubiquitin-proteasomal pathway appears responsible for the majority of protein degradation [36–39]. However how proteasomal activity is regulated in a minute-to-minute way by insulin is not known. The synthesis of ubiquitin is enhanced by elevated levels of glucocorticoids. However, ubiquitin (a very abundant protein) availability is not likely rate-limiting for activity of the ubiquitin-proteasomal degradation pathway. It has been reported that in uncontrolled diabetes the expression of mRNA both for ubiquitin and for several subunits of the proteasomal complex are increased in muscle, heart, and liver tissue, suggesting a role for this process in the protein wasting that is characteristically seen in catabolic states like ketoacidosis or severely uncontrolled diabetes. However, the precise extent of the contribution of this pathway to the overall proteolytic process is not certain at this time.

Another family of cytosolic proteases is the calpains [40]. These are cysteine proteases that have a subunit with homology to calmodulin and when activated by Ca^{2+} display broad endopeptidase activity. There are multiple members in this family and they are hypothesized to play a role in processing signaling molecules (including insulin secretion by pancreatic islets) in a variety of species. Deficiency of one isoform of these proteases in muscle is responsible for one variant of limb-girdle muscular dystrophy. Clarification of their role in overall cellular protein economy has been hampered by the lack of good specific inhibitors of these proteases and by the fact that to be activated they require increases in cytoplasmic calcium to levels (micro or even millimolar ranges) generally higher than those seen physiologically. There is evidence that these proteases play a role in the degradation of proteins following tissue injury or even exercise in skeletal muscle [41].

The recent suggestion that calpain 10 is a candidate gene associated with increased risk of development of type 2 diabetes has heightened interest in defining the role of this and other calpains [42]. However, as disagreement persists regarding the latter association, it appears that it will require some time to resolve the role of this family of proteases in the regulation (or dysregulation) of glucose metabolism [43].

INTEGRATED PHYSIOLOGY OF PROTEIN METABOLISM IN HUMANS

Prior to the discovery of insulin, the wasting of body tissues that was seen with insulin deficiency in children and young adults diagnosed with diabetes only heightened the tragic circumstance faced by patients and families affected by this then uniformly fatal disease. Conversely, the remarkable restorative responses seen when insulin was first available as a therapy in 1922, and even today when given to individuals who have been experiencing weight loss and wasting prior to the diagnosis of diabetes, are a testament to the protein anabolic action of this hormone. Insulin's effects to stimulate protein synthesis and retard proteolysis were first described in experimental systems in the 1960s. Contemporaneously, extensive organ and whole body balance studies began to define the regulation of whole body metabolism and the interorgan exchange of amino acids in humans. It is here that methods for immunoassay, automated amino acid analysis, and tracer turnover methods have had their biggest impact to advance our understanding of normal physiology of human protein metabolism and how it is affected by diabetes [44].

Methods for Measurement of Whole-Body- and Tissue-specific Protein Metabolism

A variety of methods have been developed to quantify whole-body- and tissue-specific protein turnover *in vivo*. These include whole body and organ balance methods, isotopic turnover techniques, and tissue biopsy methods. Each has advantages and limitations [45]. The complexity of the processes of protein synthesis and degradation defy, by their very nature, efforts at quantitative description using simple measures available for clinical investigation [46]. Despite this, remarkable progress has allowed seemingly reasonable description of how the processes of protein synthesis and degradation are regulated *in vivo*.

Currently the most commonly used methods to measure parameters of whole body protein metabolism *in vivo* are (1) simple whole body nitrogen balance and (2) tracer methods that utilize either a stable or a radioactive essential amino acid (most commonly leucine or phenylalanine). To assess tissue-specific protein balances, organ balances for amino acids (arterial minus venous differences coupled with measurements of blood flow) are used. This relies on accurate measurement of amino acids and hormone concentrations and methods to accurately quantify blood flow to an organ. Tracer methods can be coupled with arterial–venous sampling to provide information on protein turnover within a specific tissue or organ. Estimates of tissue protein synthesis are also obtained when incorporation of a labeled amino acid into tissue protein is measured directly using biopsy methods [47]. Finally, biopsy methods have also been applied to investigate aspects of the regulation of translation initiation process in skeletal muscle using Western blotting methods [48]. These latter measurements do not quantify rates of either protein synthesis or degradation, but can clarify changes in regulatory processes that affect synthesis, degradation, or both.

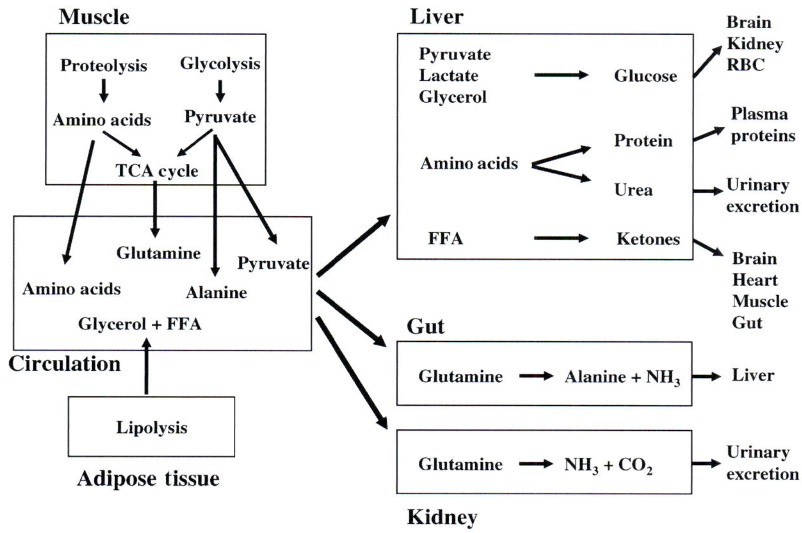

Figure 7 The net flux of fuels and metabolites between organs in fasting humans

Whole Body Protein Metabolism in the Fasting State

In considering the integrated physiology of protein metabolism in humans it is convenient to examine first the fasting state, then the transition to the fed state, and finally how diabetes affects these processes. In that context the abnormalities that accompany uncontrolled diabetes can be better understood. In healthy humans after an overnight fast plasma insulin concentration ranges from 25 to 60 pM. The body is in overall negative protein balance as evidenced by ongoing nitrogen excretion in the absence of dietary intake. This urinary nitrogen excretion is principally in the form of urea and ammonia, the former being produced from amino acids in the liver and the latter principally from glutamine in the kidney. In both cases it is the ongoing breakdown of body protein to amino acids at rates that exceed simultaneously occurring protein synthesis that supplies the urinary nitrogen (Figure 7).

Otherwise healthy young adults lose approximately 9–10 g nitrogen/day during the first day of fasting. This corresponds to a net protein loss of approximately 60 g. While the nitrogen is excreted principally as urea and ammonia, the carbon backbone of the amino acids is either converted to glucose in the liver and kidney (approximately 60%) or oxidized as fuels (approximately 40%). The synthesis of glucose from amino acids via gluconeogenesis is facilitated by a decline in the plasma insulin concentration and a rise in glucagon secretion. This combined hormonal shifts serves to enhance the transcription and translation of several key regulatory enzymes in liver (e.g. glucose-6-phosphatase, fructose bisphosphatase, and phosphoenolpyruvate carboxykinase) while simultaneously diminishing the expression of glucokinase, an early step in hepatic glycolysis. The control of transcription within the liver favors synthesis of proteins that facilitate the handling of amino acids derived from the degradation of other proteins. The extent to which these regulatory processes contribute to hepatic glucose production during simple fasting versus their role in states of more profound insulin deficiency such as insulin-deprived type 1 diabetes has not been quantified in clinical studies.

It is possible to set an upper limit to the contribution of body protein to total gluconeogenic glucose production from measures of urinary nitrogen excretion. In overnight fasting humans this comes to approximately at 60 g protein/day or at most 0.3–0.4 mg glucose/kg/min in a 70-kg subject. From this, one can estimate that gluconeogenesis from protein will account for at most 20% of endogenous glucose production (the latter being typically 1.8–2.0 mg/kg/min) [49], the remainder of glucose production being derived from glycogen metabolism and lactate/pyruvate/glycerol-derived gluconeogenesis. Estimates of amino acid driven gluconeogenesis derived in this manner are comparable to those obtained using splanchnic or hepatic balance methods in humans and canine species, respectively [49, 50].

It was earlier appreciated that giving insulin or simply feeding a high-carbohydrate meal decreased urinary nitrogen excretion. It also decreases the plasma concentrations of a number of amino acids. With the introduction of the insulin-clamp technique it became possible to demonstrate that under euglycemic conditions infusions of insulin to fasting humans that raised plasma insulin within the physiologic range caused progressive declines in plasma amino acid concentrations [51]. These declines occurred promptly after beginning the insulin infusion and most dramatically affected the branched chain amino acids

(BCAAs). The concentrations of these latter amino acids would frequently fall by 30–40% with physiologic hyperinsulinemia. When the insulin-clamp technique was coupled with measures of leucine turnover (using $1\text{–}^{14}C$-leucine) and a simple stochastic model for estimating the turnover of plasma leucine, it became apparent that the major effect of insulin was to diminish whole body protein degradation [52]. Whole body protein synthesis (estimated as the nonoxidative disposal of leucine labeled in the carbon 1 position) did not increase under these conditions [53–55]. Indeed, several laboratories demonstrated that increments of insulin concentration within the physiologic range in humans did not stimulate protein synthesis estimated using whole body isotopic turnover methods. Nearly simultaneously, however, it was appreciated that increasing the plasma concentrations of amino acids had a rather marked effect to increase whole body nonoxidative leucine disposal (an index of protein synthesis) [53, 56]. The observation that insulin had little or no stimulatory effect on protein synthesis in these clinical investigations contrasted with the previously noted, well-demonstrated effect of insulin in a variety of *in vitro* systems. Studies in whole animals yielded results somewhat intermediate; i.e., in young or juvenile animals a stimulatory effect of insulin *in vivo* was apparent [57]. However, this appeared to be lost as the animals reached adult age. Whether this indicates a developmental process or some difficulty with the application of the tracer turnover methods in either young or adult animals has not been resolved.

Interestingly, with more prolonged fasting (up to 72 h) protein degradation remains very insulin sensitive while during this time insulin's ability to stimulate glucose disposal wanes progressively [58]. This may in part accounts for the observation that the rate of whole body nitrogen excretion begins to decline after the first several days of fasting. The protein degradation and ammonia release that occurs during continued fasting provides the kidney with necessary precursors to increase the excretion of titratable acid. In this manner they serve to limit the extent of systemic acidosis that occurs during fasting. Glutamine appears particularly important in this regard as it directly donates its nitrogen to ammonia production in the kidney [59, 60]. As fasting progresses the kidney becomes an increasingly important site of gluconeogenic glucose production. The amino nitrogen is available for tubular excretion as ammonia. Although by no means resolved at the current time, estimates are that the kidney may contribute between 10 and 25% of total body glucose production in humans during an overnight fast and may increase as fasting persists.

It is important to recognize that throughout the period of time during a fast while body nitrogen balance is of necessity negative, there continues to be active protein synthesis in virtually all tissues. In some tissues synthesis becomes more selective and is directed toward enzymes that assist in the adaptation to fasting (for example the enzymes involved with glucose production in liver and kidney).

Whole Body Protein Metabolism in the Fed State

When feeding occurs in postabsorptive humans, the relative content of carbohydrate and protein in the meal is expected to determine changes in protein turnover. With ingestion of glucose alone the exaggerated rise in plasma insulin that follows causes a prompt decline in the plasma concentrations of many amino acids. Measures of whole body leucine turnover indicate a decline in both protein synthesis and degradation. Overall, there is a protein sparing effect of this nutritional intervention. However, with a pure carbohydrate load whole body nitrogen balance remains negative. With a high protein meal there is a prompt rise in the concentrations of both amino acids and insulin in plasma [61]. Although the insulin rise is less dramatic than with a high carbohydrate meal, the net anabolic effect is greater and whole body protein balance becomes positive.

The rise in both insulin and amino acids presumably each contributes to the net anabolic effect. Interestingly, feeding a high-protein meal causes a greater increase in caloric expenditure than is seen with a high-carbohydrate or high-fat meal. This is referred to as the *specific dynamic action of protein*. Presumably, this relates to the greater energy expenditure required for the digestion, transport, and synthesis of new proteins (discussed earlier) relative to that required for storage of carbohydrates or fats. The postprandial interval is also an important time for the synthesis of proteins that are exported into plasma. These include albumin and clotting factors, whose synthesis appears to be dependent upon nutritional status [62].

Whole Body Protein Metabolism in Diabetes

In uncontrolled human type 1 diabetes, urinary nitrogen excretion can increase two- to threefold; inasmuch as the liver in that setting is being strongly stimulated by counterregulatory hormones (glucagon, epinephrine, and cortisol particularly) it is reasonable to assume that the carbon skeleton of the gluconeogenic amino acids will be quantitatively converted to glucose. However, if the liver and the kidneys are to support higher rates of overall glucose production there must also be substantial increases in Cori cycle and glycerol-derived gluconeogenesis. This is particularly true as hepatic glycogen stores are generally depleted early in the development of ketoacidosis (Figure 8).

Withdrawal of insulin from patients with type 1 diabetes leads to a rise in circulating concentrations of the BCAAs and a decline in the plasma concentrations of most gluconeogenic amino acids. At the same time urinary nitrogen excretion increases and whole body leucine

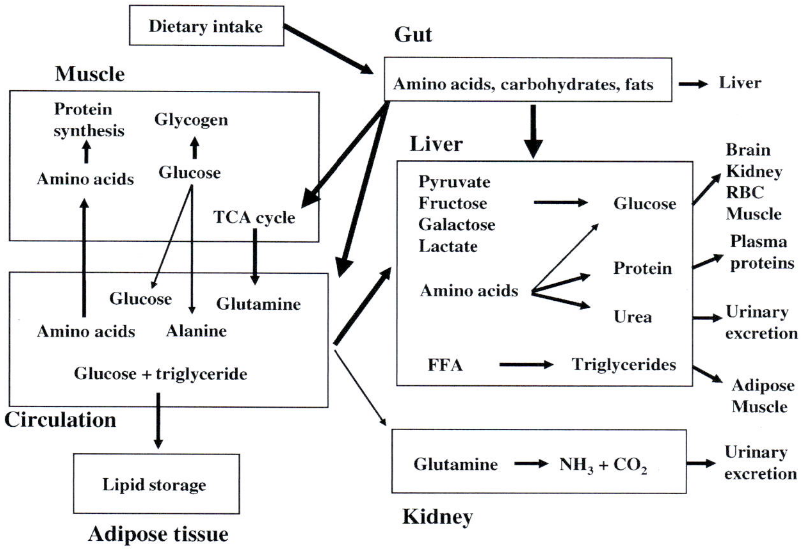

Figure 8 The net flux of fuels and metabolites between organs in the postprandial state

turnover likewise rises. This overall pattern indicates an increase in protein degradation that accounts for the increase in plasma BCAA concentration. The decline in circulating gluconeogenic amino acids is attributable to a marked increase in the fractional extraction of these amino acids by the liver (and perhaps the kidneys). While insulin deficiency appears to be the primary regulator of these changes, secondary rises in plasma glucagon and cortisol that occur at this time can contribute as well. The entire pattern—of increase in whole body protein degradation, increased urinary nitrogen wasting, and falling plasma gluconeogenic amino acids—is consistent with the wasting of lean body mass that accompanied insulin deficiency in the pre-insulin era and is frequently seen at the initial presentation of patients with type 1 diabetes even today. Somewhat surprising has been the observation that estimates of whole body nonoxidative leucine disposal in insulin-withdrawnt type 1 diabetic patients suggest that protein synthesis may be increased in this setting [63]. This contrasts with studies in experimental animals where insulin deficiency leads to a prompt decline in protein synthesis and a particular dramatic decline in ribosome number and synthesis with an accompanying decline in the activation of translational initiation factors [64, 65]. Whether this apparent discrepancy reflects a limitation of the leucine turnover method, species differences, or other factors has not yet been satisfactorily resolved.

Unlike type 1, type 2 diabetes does not (at least in its earlier stages) dramatically affect body protein metabolism. Plasma concentrations of most amino acids are not different in age- and weight-matched normal subjects, and urinary nitrogen wasting does not occur. However, protein metabolism appears to share with glucose and lipid metabolism an "insensitivity" to circulating insulin [66, 67]. Despite higher basal insulin concentrations, protein turnover (measured with 1–^{14}C-leucine) is similar in type 2 diabetes and matched controls, suggesting an element of insulin resistance. The ongoing release of amino acids from protein degradation may, by providing substrates, contribute to the hepatic insulin resistance manifest as a failure of suppression of gluconeogenesis. However, this insulin resistance is not sufficient in magnitude to promote protein wasting, and unlike insulin-withdrawn type 1 diabetes, subjects with type 2 diabetes achieve that protein metabolism in the fed state and effectively maintain body protein mass.

Inasmuch as insulin signaling of glucose disposal and protein synthesis share early steps in the insulin-signaling cascade, the maintenance of near-normal protein metabolism when glucose metabolism is markedly disturbed in type 2 diabetes suggests that vis-á-vis glucose less insulin action is required to maintain protein metabolism near-normal. In part this may result from amino acids themselves, especially the BCAAs, subsuming some of the role of insulin to regulate protein synthesis and degradation by regulating the phosphorylation of proteins in the insulin-signaling cascade.

Protein Metabolism in Human Muscle

Muscle is the largest tissue in the body, with the combined skeletal muscles contributing approximately 40% of body mass in the normal-weight adult. Muscle tissue has a protein content of ~200-mg/g wet weight, such that for the 70-kg individual, ~5.6 kg is muscle protein. Muscle protein, like all body protein, constantly turns over. Estimates of fractional turnover rate are 1.0–2.0%/day. Other tissues turn over more rapidly with fractional turnover rates estimated as high as 25–50%/day for liver and gut tissue. As a result, although muscle contains >50% of body protein it accounts for only approximately 30–40% of total body protein turnover.

Protein synthesis in skeletal muscle has been estimated using a combined limb balance and isotope infusion method [68] and by direct measurement of stable isotope incorporation into tissue protein using biopsy methods. While both methods are useful, both are limited by assumptions related to the extent of labeling of the amino acyl-tRNA pool used for protein synthesis. Recent studies, first *in vitro*, then in animals, and recently in humans, have demonstrated increases in the phosphorylation of several proteins downstream of PKB (Akt) in the insulin-signaling pathway in response to either amino acids or insulin infusions. This suggests that in human muscle regulation of protein synthesis at the translational level may be quite important.

Early studies in the laboratory of Cahill and colleagues demonstrated that after an overnight fast human skeletal muscle was in negative nitrogen balance [44]. The majority of the nitrogen leaving muscle was released as the amino acids alanine and glutamine [69]. Each amino acid was released in disproportionately greater amounts than was their contribution to the composition of muscle proteins [70]. Overall, these two amino acids contributed approximately 50–60% of amino acid nitrogen release. The net amino acid release from muscle is promptly reversed by even very small increments of plasma insulin concentration under euglycemic conditions. Isotopic turnover studies clearly demonstrated that this shift in balance is secondary to a prompt decline in protein degradation within the muscle. These measurements are obtained by combining arterial–venous difference methods with steady-state infusion of labeled essential amino acids (most frequently phenylalanine). As was seen for the whole body, the process of protein degradation appears more sensitive than synthesis to modest physiologic increments of plasma insulin [68]. Protein synthesis is clearly stimulated when higher insulin concentrations are used [71]. The effect of insulin to diminish the net loss of amino acid nitrogen from muscle likely contributes to the overall decline in whole body protein turnover (and plasma amino acid concentrations) inasmuch as splanchnic tissues appear to be less sensitive to the protein sparing effect of incremental increases of plasma insulin [72].

As muscle is a major source for amino acids that are used by the liver for gluconeogenesis, the decline in amino acid release that accompanies increases in plasma insulin appears to contribute to decreases in hepatic glucose production. A decline in amino acid nitrogen release from muscle also occurs with more prolonged fasting as an adaptation to prevent excessive muscle wasting. Simultaneously, during prolonged fasting other adaptations, principally increasing circulating ketone concentrations, diminish the rate of body glucose utilization, thereby avoiding hypoglycemia. The ketones may also function (although this is not certain) to signal muscle to decrease the rate of protein degradation.

In transitioning from fasting to the fed state, the rise in plasma amino acids may play a particularly important role. Amino acids can both provide substrates for protein synthesis and share with insulin a signaling role to indicate that feeding has occurred. Recognition that amino acids *per se* directly promote the phosphorylation of regulatory proteins downstream of mTOR may explain, at least in part, why insulin given under euglycemic conditions fails to stimulate whole body protein synthesis [56]. The concentrations of many amino acids in both plasma and intracellular fluid fall under conditions of euglycemic hyperinsulinemia. This decline may interdict any action of insulin to increase protein synthesis. Among amino acids it appears that the BCAAs are particularly important in activating mRNA translation [26, 73]. These amino acids (valine, leucine, and isoleucine) contribute ~18% of the amino acids in muscle protein. Insulin's action to reduce proteolysis has a more marked effect to lower the plasma and cellular concentrations of the BCAAs than any other amino acids. The BCAAs enter and leave the myocytes (and other cells) using a facilitative transporter ("L-system") that does not move these amino acids against a concentration gradient. Thus, there is no significant intracellular to extracellular BCAA concentration gradient in most tissues. The gut and renal epithelium are exceptions as these epithelia also express a sodium–amino acid cotransporter with a broad substrate specificity that includes the BCAAs and allows the active absorption and resorption of these amino acids against a significant concentration gradient.

With meal ingestion the rise in plasma insulin and plasma amino acid concentrations serves to signal muscle to slow the rate of proteolysis and increase protein synthetic processes. The increase of insulin stimulates the uptake of amino acids by muscle (especially for amino acids transported by the A or ASC transport systems, which appear most insulin sensitive). This effect to promote amino acid transport may be particularly important inasmuch as insulin stimulates the translational process and decreases protein degradation in muscle. Both of these actions would have an effect to lower the intracellular concentrations of amino acids in the myocytes.

Following a meal the BCAA concentration in plasma rises more dramatically than those of other amino acids [61]. This results from the relatively poor first-pass hepatic extraction of the BCAAs (<5% for each) in contrast to some gluconeogenesis amino acids that are efficiently removed (30–40% extraction) with each pass through the liver. The amplitude in the swing of BCAA concentration in the face of a carbohydrate (where their concentrations decline the greatest) or high-protein (where their concentrations rise the greatest) meals has some obvious implications for these amino acids signaling to synthetic and degradative processes in skeletal muscle. It is therefore quite interesting that the BCAAs are the most effective in stimulating the translational apparatus within skeletal muscle. Whether this signaling property of BCAAs extends to other peripheral tissues (bone, skin, fat, etc.) is not known.

Early studies demonstrated an increase of amino acid release from muscle in insulin-withdrawn type 1 diabetic subjects [44]. In addition, uncontrolled diabetes is accompanied by increased urinary excretion of 3-methyl histidine [74]. This amino acid derives principally from post-transcriptional methylation of actin (and to a lesser extent myosin) and muscle is the principal source of this amino acid in humans. Recent studies, combining tracer and limb-balance techniques, have demonstrated an exaggerated release of amino acids from muscle tissue consistent with an increase in proteolysis [75]. While measures of whole body nonoxidative leucine disposal suggest that this index of protein synthesis is either unchanged or increased with insulin deficiency, in skeletal muscle protein synthesis declines, a finding that is consistent with the muscle wasting typically seen. In animal models type 1 diabetes has been observed to dramatically diminish protein synthesis. More specifically ribosomal protein synthesis declines dramatically and simultaneously there is an increase in ribosomal proteolysis. This occurs even during a brief period of insulin deficiency. As a result restoration of protein synthesis requires resynthesis of the ribosomal pool [64].

Protein Metabolism in Liver and Splanchnic Tissues

The liver has long been recognized as a major site of regulation of body protein metabolism. In addition to its roles as the major organ of gluconeogenic glucose production and ureagenesis from amino acids, it is a major site for synthesis of plasma proteins. The turnover of proteins within the liver is significantly more rapid than for skeletal muscle. In animal studies (which are essentially the only data available) the fractional daily rate of protein synthesis of liver proteins is approximately 25%/day. Although its mass is only 1/20th that of skeletal muscle, its higher turnover allows it to contribute perhaps as much as 50% as skeletal muscle to whole body protein turnover measurements [76]. Liver, or more appropriately splanchnic, protein metabolism in humans was studied extensively using regional catheterization techniques in the 1970s. More recently, this method has been coupled with isotope turnover measurements using stable isotopes to allow more complete assessment of protein synthesis and degradation in splanchnic tissues.

Essentially simultaneous with the recognition that alanine and glutamine are the principal amino acids exported from muscle came the observation that alanine was the most avidly extracted amino acid by splanchnic tissues in humans [77]. These observations, again made using hepatic vein catheterization methods, led to the proposal of a glucose–alanine cycle, whereby alanine released from muscle was used by splanchnic tissues as a major substrate for glucose production. Subsequently, it was shown that the carbon backbone of alanine derives principally from pyruvate produced glycolytically in muscle [78]. Thus, the glucose–alanine cycle is very analogous to the Cori cycle, with the additional twist that it shuttles amino acid derived nitrogen from muscle to splanchnic tissues.

Organ balance studies of this sort suggested that in fasting humans amino acid extraction by the liver could provide approximately 10–15% of the carbon for postabsorptive glucose production. From studies in animals it was known that within the splanchnic bed liver and intestinal tissues handle amino acids differently. The gut uses glutamine as an oxidative fuel and disposes of amino nitrogen by producing additional alanine, which is again efficiently extracted by the liver. Hepatic glutamine extraction is quite modest ($<10\%$ extraction ratio) [59]. Thus, even within the splanchnic tissues alanine serves as a nitrogen shuttle providing amino groups that originate from other amino acids to the liver for ureagenesis.

In the fasting state the overall nitrogen balance of liver is strongly positive. As much of this nitrogen is directed toward ureagenesis (with the carbon skeleton of amino acids used for the gluconeogenesis) these balance measurements alone cannot provide any indication of tissue protein balance. When isotope turnover measurements are performed in combination with hepatic catheterization, current estimates would suggest that the liver protein balance (unlike muscle) is approximately neutral in the postabsorptive state. This includes all proteins made by the liver, even those like albumin that are immediately exported. The observation that with continued fasting liver volume declines (as much as 25% in 48 h) suggests that structural proteins within the liver progressively decline in mass during fasting. This would indicate a negative protein balance for these intrinsic hepatic proteins.

With the onset of feeding the liver removes a significant fraction of amino acid nitrogen that enters portal blood following the meal [79]. Presumably, this facilitates the repletion of hepatic structural proteins that may have been catabolized during an antecedent fast. During this time there is an increased synthesis of albumin and other plasma proteins [62]. Presumably, the rise in portal insulin concentration, coupled with the increase in amino acid concentrations, is the principal driving forces for this increased protein synthesis. Whether this occurs at all following a simple carbohydrate meal without inclusion of significant amino acid/protein substrate is not certain.

In patients with insulin-deficient diabetes that is out of control, extraction of amino acids by hepatic tissues is enhanced simultaneously with the increase in hepatic glucose production. This is also seen, to a less extreme extent, in individuals with type 2 diabetes. These increases in amino acid removal by the liver are consistent with an increased fractional contribution of gluconeogenic substrates to overall glucose production in these clinical circumstances.

Protein Metabolism in Kidney

The kidney, like the liver, converts the carbon backbone of some amino acids to glucose via the gluconeogenic pathway and can synthesize urea (although to a much lesser extent than liver). Rather than ureagenesis, the kidney directs amino acid derived nitrogen, particularly that which originates from glutamine, to ammonia production. This occurs principally in the proximal tubular cells and the ammonia is excreted into the tubular fluid. In postabsorptive humans different laboratories have estimated that between 10 and 25% of endogenous glucose production occurs in the kidney. If inasmuch as the kidney stores much less glycogen than does the liver, this renal glucose production is presumed essentially all derived from gluconeogenesis. To date, careful balance studies examining renal uptake of gluconeogenic precursors are most consistent with the 10% figure. Again as discussed earlier, based upon urinary nitrogen excretion rates, it appears that gluconeogenesis from amino acids overall (liver and kidney combined) will only support approximately 10–20% of total endogenous glucose production in postabsorptive subjects.

Interestingly, the endogenous protein pool of the kidney turns over at a rate similar or more rapid than that of liver and much more rapidly than muscle. The limited information on this process in clinical studies [80] suggests that the kidney accounts for ~10% of whole body leucine (protein) turnover. It is, of course, of interest that early in the course of either type 1 or type 2 diabetes there appears to be an increase in renal size, occasionally by as much as 50%. There is evidence from animal studies for an important role of IGF-1 in this process. However in humans whether this is attributable to changes in protein synthesis, protein degradation, or both is not currently known.

Renal amino acid and protein metabolic responses to feeding have not been studied in humans. Increases in plasma amino acids do appear to cause a rise in renal blood flow. Glucagon may mediate this process as it is released in response to a high protein meal.

Protein Metabolism in Fat

Inasmuch as the changing patterns of nutrition in many developed nations have resulted in adipose tissue mass rivaling that of skeletal muscle in humans (and in some individuals exceeding that of muscle), some comment on protein handling in this tissue seems appropriate. Unfortunately, very little attention has been given to the physiologic regulation of the protein mass in adipose tissue. In part this relates to the relatively low contribution of protein to overall adipose tissue mass. While liver, kidney, and skeletal muscle are composed of approximately 20% protein on a weight basis, for adipose tissues this is less than 5%. In addition, because adipose tissue generally fails to form a discrete organ but is distributed in many different depots, it has not been as amenable to sampling using balance techniques. Interestingly, the little data that is available would suggest that protein turnover in adipose tissue might be comparable to that of skeletal muscle [81]. If true, this would suggest that the adipose tissue might be a previously unappreciated significant contributor to whole body protein turnover. This, however, will require considerably more investigation before it can be integrated into our understanding of body protein metabolism.

Acknowledgment

This work was supported by grants from the US PHS DK-38578, RR-15540, and RR-0847.

REFERENCES

1. Munro H, Allison J. *Mammalian Protein Metabolism*, 1st edn Vol 1. New York: Academic Press, 1964.
2. Magendie F. *Precis elementaire de physiologie*. Paris: Meguinon-Mervais, 1817.
3. Schoenheimer R. *The Dynamic State of Body Constituents*. Cambridge, MA: Harvard University Press, 1942.
4. Mulder G. *Bul. Sci Phys Nat Neederland* 1838; 104.
5. Kossel A, Kutcher F. *Z Physiol Chem* 1900; 31: 165.
6. Watson JD, Crick FH. Molecular structure of nucleic acids: a structure for deoxyribose nucleic acid. *Nature*, No 4356, April 25, 1953. *Reprinted in Nature* 1974; 248 (5451): 765.
7. Alberts B, Johnson A, Lewis J, Raff M, Roberts K, Walter P. *Molecular Biology of the Cell*, 4th edn. New York: Garland Scienc, 2002.
8. Yechoor VK, Patti ME, Saccone R, Kahn CR. Coordinated patterns of gene expression for substrate and energy metabolism in skeletal muscle of diabetic mice. *Proc Natl Acad Sci USA* 2002; 99 (16): 10587–92.
9. O'Brien RM, Granner DK. Regulation of gene expression by insulin. *Biochem J* 1991; 278: 609–19.
10. Nakae J, Kitamura T, Silver DL, Accili D. The forkhead transcription factor Foxo1 (Fkhr) confers insulin sensitivity onto glucose-6-phosphatase expression. *J Clin Invest* 2001; 108 (9): 1359–67.
11. Olefsky JM, Saltiel AR. PPARgamma and the treatment of insulin resistance. *Trends Endocrinol Metab* 2000; 11 (9): 362–8.
12. Cate JH, Yusupov MM, Yusupova GZ, Earnest TN, Noller HF. X-ray crystal structures of 70S ribosome functional complexes. *Science* 1999; 285 (5436): 2095–104.
13. Ramakrishnan V. Ribosome structure and the mechanism of translation. *Cell* 2002; 108 (4): 557–72.

14. Schubert U, Anton LC, Gibbs J, Norbury CC, Yewdell JW, Bennink JR. Rapid degradation of a large fraction of newly synthesized proteins by proteasomes. *Nature* 2000; 404 (6779): 770–4.
15. Bohen SP, Kralli A, Yamamoto KR. Hold 'em high and fold 'em: chaperones and signal transduction. *Science* 1995; 268: 1303–65.
16. Sommer T, Wolf DH. Endoplasmic reticulum degradation—reverse protein flow of no return. *FASEB J* 1997; 11 (14): 1227–33.
17. Morgan HE, Rannels DE, McKee EE. Protein metabolicm of the heart. *Handbook of Physiology, The Cardiovascular System*. Bethesda: American Physiological Society, 1979; pp 845–71.
18. Rannels DE, Pegg AE, Rannels SR, Jefferson LS. Effect of starvation on initiation of protein synthesis in skeletal muscle and heart. *Am J Physiol* 1978; 235 (2): E126–33.
19. Jefferson LS. Role of insulin in the regulation of protein synthesis. *Diabetes* 1980; 29: 487–96.
20. Kimball SR, Horetsky RL, Jefferson LS. Signal transduction pathways involved in the regulation of protein synthesis by insulin by L6 myoblasts. *Am J Physiol Cell Physiol* 1998; 43 (1): C221–8.
21. Proud CG, Denton RM. Molecular mechanisms for the control of translation by insulin. *Biochem J* 1997; 328 (pt 2): 329–41.
22. Brunn GJ, Hudson CC, Sekulic A, Williams JM, Hosoi H, Houghton PJ, Lawrence JC, Abraham RT. Phosphorylation of the translational repressor PHAS-I by the mammalian target of rapamycin. *Science*, 1997; 277 (5322): 99–101.
23. Kimball SR, Jurasinski CV, Lawrence JC, Jefferson LS. Insulin stimulates protein synthesis in muscle by enhancing the association of eIF-4E and eIF-4G. *Am J Physiol Cell Physiol* 1997; 41 (2): C754–9.
24. Rhoads RE, Lamphear BJ. Cap-independent translation of heat shock messenger RNAs. *Curr Top Microbiol Immunol* 1995; 203: 131–53.
25. Bonadonna RC, Saccomani MP, Cobelli C, DeFronzo RA. Effect of insulin on System A amino acid transport in human skeletal muscle. *J Clin Invest* 1993; 91: 514–21.
26. Campbell LE, Wang X, Proud CG. Nutrients differentially regulate multiple translation factors and their control by insulin. *Biochem J* 1999; 344 (pt 2): 433–41.
27. Dice JF. Molecular determinants of protein half-lives in eukaryotic cells. *FASEB J* 1987; 1: 349–57.
28. Mortimore GE, Ward WF. Internalization of cytoplasmic protein by hepatic lysosomes in basal and deprivation-induced proteolytic states. *J Biol Chem* 1981; 256: 7659–65.
29. Mortimore GE, Lardeux BR, Adams CE. Regulation of microautophagy and basal protein turnover in rat liver. *J Biol Chem* 1988; 263: 2506–12.
30. Hershko A, Ciechanover A. The ubiquitin system. *Ann Rev Biochem* 1998; 67: 425–79.
31. Coux O, Tanaka K, Goldberg AL. Structure and function of the 20S and 26S proteasomes. *Annu Rev Biochem* 1996; 65: 801–26.
32. Groll M, Ditzel L, Lowe J, Stock D, Bochtler M, Bartunik H, Huber R. Structure of 20S proteasome from yeast at 2.4A resolution. *Nature* 1997; 386: 463–71.
33. Craiu A, Gaczynska M, Akopian T, Gramm CF, Fenteany G, Goldberg AL, Rock KL. Lactacystin and clasto-lactacystin beta-lactone modify multiple proteasome beta-subunits and inhibit intracellular protein degradation and major histocompatibility complex class I antigen presentation. *J Biol Chem* 1997; 272 (20): 13437–45.
34. Pagano M. Cell cycle regulation by the ubiquitin pathway. *FASEB J* 1997; 11 (13): 1067–75.
35. Rui L, Fisher TL, Thomas J, White MF. Regulation of insulin/insulin-like growth factor-1 signaling by proteasome-mediated degradation of insulin receptor substrate-2. *J Biol Chem* 2001; 276 (43): 40362–7.
36. Baracos VE, DeVivo C, Hoyle DHR, Goldberg AL. Activation of the ATP–ubiquitin–proteasome pathway in skeletal muscle of cachectic rats bearing a hepatoma. *Am J Physiol* 1995; 268: E996–1006.
37. Solomon V, Goldberg A. Importance of the ATP–ubiquitin–proteasome pathway in the degradation of soluble and myofibrillar proteins in rabbit muscle extracts. *J Biol Chem* 1996; 271: 26690–7.
38. Price SR, Bailey JL, Wang X, Jurkovitz C, England BK, Ding X, Phillips LS, Mitch WE. Muscle wasting in insulinopenic rats results from activation of the ATP-dependent, ubiquitin–proteasome proteolytic pathway by a mechanism including gene transcription. *Am Soc Clin Invest* 1996; 98 (8): 1703–8.
39. Tawa NE Jr, Odessey R, Goldberg AL. Inhibitors of the proteasome reduce the accelerated proteolysis in atrophying rat skeletal muscles. *J Clin Invest* 1997; 100 (1): 197–203.
40. Sorimachi H, Ishiura S, Suzuki K. Structure and physiological function of calpains. *Biochem J* 1997; 328 (pt 3): 721–32.
41. Fang CH, Tiao G, James H, Ogle C, Fischer JE, Hasselgren PO. Burn injury stimulates multiple proteolytic pathways in skeletal muscle, including the ubiquitin-energy-dependent pathway. *J Am Coll Surg* 1995; 180 (2): 161–70.
42. Horikawa Y, Oda N, Cox NJ, Li X, Orho-Melander M, Hara M, Hinokio Y, Lindner TH, Mashima H, Schwarz PE, et al. Genetic variation in the gene encoding calpain-10 is associated with type 2 diabetes mellitus. *Nat Genet* 2000; 26 (2): 163–75.
43. Elbein SC. Perspective: the search for genes for type 2 diabetes in the post-genome era. *Endocrinology* 2002; 143 (6): 2012–8.
44. Cahill GF Jr. Physiology of insulin in man. *Diabetes* 1971; 20: 785–99.
45. Liu Z, Barrett EJ. Human protein metabolism: its measurement and regulation. *Am J Physiol Endocrinol Metab* 2002; 283 (6): E1105–12.
46. Bier DM. Intrinsically difficult problems – The kinetics of body proteins and amino acids in man. *Diabetes Metab Rev* 1989; 5 (2): 111–32.
47. Nair KS, Halliday D, Griggs RC. Leucine incorporation into mixed skeletal muscle protein in humans. *Am J Physiol* 1988; 254: E208–13.
48. Liu Z, Jahn LA, Wei L, Long W, Barrett EJ. Amino acids stimulate translation initiation and protein synthesis through an Akt-independent pathway in human skeletal muscle. *J Clin Endocrinol Metab* 2002; 87 (12): 5553–8.
49. Barrett EJ, Liu Z. Hepatic glucose metabolism and insulin resistance in NIDDM and obesity. *Bailliere's Clinical Endocrinology and Metabolism, Vol 7, No 4*. London, England: BailliŠre Tindall, 1993; pp 875–901.
50. Felig P, Owen OE, Wahren J, Cahill GF Jr. Amino acid metabolism during prolonged starvation. *J Clin Invest*, 1969; 48: 584–94.

51. Fukagawa NK, Minaker KL, Young VR, Rowe JW. Insulin dose-dependent reductions in plasma amino acids in man. *Am J Physiol* 1986; 250: E13–7.
52. Tessari P, Trevisan R, Inchiostro S, Bioli G, Nosadini R, De Kreutzenberg SV, Duner E, Tiengo A, Crepaldi G. Dose–response curves of effects of insulin on leucine kinetics in humans. *Am J Physiol*, 1986; 251: E334–42.
53. Tessari P, Inchiostro S, Biolo G, Trevisan R, Fantin G, Marescotti MC, Iori E, Tiengo A, Crepaldi G. Differential effects of hyperinsulinemia and hyperaminoacidemia on leucine- carbon metabolism *in vivo*—evidence for distincr mechanisms in ragulation of net amino acid deposition. *J Clin Invest* 1987; 79: 1062–9.
54. Fukagawa NK, Minaker KL, Rowe JW, Googman MN, Matthews DW, Bier DM, Young VR. Insulin-mediated reduction of whole body protein breakdown—dose–response effects on leucine metabolism in postabsorptive man. *J Clin Invest* 1985; 76: 2306–11.
55. Pacy PJ, Nair KS, Ford C, Halliday D. Failure of insulin infusion to stimulate fractional muscle protein synthesis in type I diabetic patients. *Diabetes* 1989; 38: 618–24.
56. Castellino P, Luzi L, Simonson DC, Haymond M, DeFronzo RA. Effect of insulin and plasma amino acid concentrations on leucine metabolism in man. *J Clin Invest* 1987; 80: 1784–93.
57. Wraycahen D, Nguyen HV, Burrin DG, Beckett PR, Fiorotto ML, Reeds PJ, Wester TJ, Davis TA. Response of skeletal muscle protein synthesis to insulin in suckling pigs decreases with development. *Am J Physiol Endocrinol Metab* 1998; 38 (4): E602–9.
58. Jensen MD, Miles JM, Gerich JE, Cryer PE, Haymond MW. Preservation of insulin effects on glucose production and proteolysis during fasting. *Am J Physiol* 1988; 254: E700–7.
59. Meyer C, Dostou J, Nadkarni V, Gerich J. Effects of physiological hyperinsulinemia on systemic, renal, and hepatic substrate metabolism. *Am J Physiol* 1998; 275 (6, pt 2): F915–21.
60. Stumvoll M, Perriello G, Meyer C, Gerich J. Role of glutamine in human carbohydrate metabolism in kidney and other tissues. *Kidney Int* 1999; 55 (3): 778–92.
61. Wahren J, Felig P, Hagenfeldt L. Effect of protein ingestion on splanchnic and leg metabolism in normal man and in patients with diabetes mellitus. *J Clin Invest* 1976; 57: 987–99.
62. DeFeo P, Horber FF, Haymond MW. Meal stimulation of albumin synthesis: a significant contributor to whole body protein synthesis in humans. *Am J Physiol* 1992; 263: E794–9.
63. Pacy P, Nair K, Ford C, Halliday D. Failure of insulin infusion to stimulate fractional muscle protein synthesis in type I diabetic patients, anabolic effect of insulin and decreased proteolysis. *Diabetes* 1989; 38: 618–24.
64. Ashford AJ, Pain VM. Insulin stimulation of growth in diabetic rats—synthesis and degradation of ribosomes and total tissue protein in skeletal muscle and heart. *J Biol Chem* 1986; 261: 4066–70.
65. Ashford AJ, Pain VM. Effect of diabetes on the rates of synthesis and degradation of ribosomes in rat muscle and liver *in vivo*. *J Biol Chem* 1986; 261: 4059–65.
66. Staten MA, Matthews DE, Bier DM. Leucine metabolism in type II diabetes mellitus. *Diabetes* 1986; 35: 1249–53.
67. Luzi L, Petrides AS, DeFronzo RA. Different sensitivity of glucose and amino acid metabolism to insulin in NIDDM. *Diabetes* 1993; 42: 1868–77.
68. Gelfand RA, Barrett EJ. Effect of physiologic hyperinsulinemia on skeletal muscle protein synthesis and breakdown in man. *J Clin Invest* 1987; 80: 1–6.
69. Aoki TT, Brennan MF, Muller WA, Cahill GF. Amino acid levels across normal forearm muscle, whole blood vs plasma. *Adv Enzyme Regul* 1977; 12: 157–65.
70. Marliss EB, Aoki TT, Pozefsky T, Most AS, Cahill GF Jr. Muscle and splanchnic glutamine and glatamate metabolism in postabsoptive and starved man. *J Clin Invest* 1971; 50: 814–7.
71. Hillier T, Fryburg D, Jahn L, Barrett E. Extreme hyperinsulinemia unmasks insulin's effect to stimulate protein synthesis in the human forearm. *Am J Physiol* 1998; 274: E1067–74.
72. Meek SE, Fersson M, Ford GC, Nair KS. Differential regulation of amino acid exchange and protein dynamics across splanchnic and skeletal muscle beds by insulin in healthy human subjects. *Diabetes* 1998; 47 (12): 1824–35.
73. Wang X, Campbell LE, Miller CM, Proud CG. Amino acid availability regulates p70 S6 kinase and multiple translation factors. *Biochem J* 1998; 334: 261–7.
74. Huszar G, Koivisto V, Davis E, Felig P. Urinary 3-methyhistidine excretion in juvenile-onset diabetics, evidence of increased protein catabolism in the absence of ketoacidosis. *Metabolism* 1982; 31: 188–91.
75. Nair KS, Ford GC, Ekberg K, Fernqvist-Forbes E, Wahren J. Protein dynamics in whole body and in splanchnic and leg tissues in type I diabetic patients. *J Clin Invest* 1995; 95 (6): 2926–37.
76. Tessari P, Garibotto G, Inchiostro S, Robaudo C, Saffioti S, Vettore M, Zanetti M, Russo R, Deferrari G. Kidney, splanchnic, and leg protein turnover in humans—insight from leucine and phenylalanine kinetics. *J Clin Invest* 1996; 98 (6): 1481–92.
77. Felig P. The glucose–alanine cycle. *Metabolism* 1973; 22: 179–207.
78. Garber AJ, Karl IE, Kipnis DM. Alanine and glutamine synthesis and release from skeletal muscle. *J Biol Chem* 1976; 251: 851–7.
79. Barrett EJ, Gusberg R, Ferrannini E, Tepler J, DFelig P, Jacob R, Smith D, DeFronzo RA. Amino acid and glucose metabolism in the postabsorptive state and following amino acid ingestion in the dog. *Metabolism* 1986; 35: 709–17.
80. Tessari P, Pehling G, Nissen SL, Gerich JE, Service FJ, Rizza RA, Haymond MOW. Regulation of whole-body leucine metabolism with insulin during mixed-meal absorption in normal and diabetic humans. *Diabetes* 1988; 37: 512–9.
81. Coppack S, Persson M, Miles J. Phenylalanine kinetics in human adipose tissue. *J Clin Invest* 1996; 98: 692–7.

18

Lipid and Lipoprotein Metabolism

Giacomo Ruotolo and Barbara V. Howard

MedStar Research Institute, Washington, DC, USA

LIPIDS, LIPOPROTEINS, APOLIPOPROTEINS

Lipoproteins are large macromolecular complexes composed of a hydrophobic lipid core (cholesteryl esters, triglycerides, and fat-soluble vitamins) and a hydrophilic shell [phospholipids, free cholesterol, and specialized proteins known as apolipoproteins (apos)]. The lipid core is surrounded by a monolayer of phospholipids, with the polar heads facing out. Apolipoproteins are positioned into the phospholipid monolayer, and play a central role in regulating lipid transport and lipoprotein metabolism. Besides their lipid-binding ability, apos provide structural stability to lipoproteins, bind to cell receptors, and activate or inhibit key enzymes or transfer proteins.

The major function of lipoprotein particles is essentially the transport of lipids in the bloodstream and their redistribution among cells. Cholesterol is an essential component of cell membranes and a metabolic precursor of bile acids and steroid hormones (e.g., adrenocortical and sex hormones). It is obtained from the diet and synthesized in the liver, intestinal mucosa, and other cells. Approximately three quarters of the cholesterol in the bloodstream are esterified to a fatty acid to form cholesteryl ester. The rate-limiting step in cholesterol synthesis involves the enzyme 3-hydroxy-3-methylglutaryl coenzyme A (HMG-CoA) reductase, which converts HMG-CoA to mevalonic acid. Triglycerides consist of three fatty acid molecules esterified to one glycerol molecule. They are the most abundant complex lipids, and are mostly of dietary origin. Triglycerides serve as a storage form of fatty acids and, therefore, represent a major source of energy in humans. Phospholipids are the basic structural unit of virtually all cell membranes (phospholipid bilayer) and have an important role in brain tissue and fetal development. Because of its high phospholipid content, myelin can electrically insulate the nerve cell from its environment. Phospholipids consist of a hydrophobic tail, the phosphatidic acid, esterified to a hydrophilic head represented by molecules such as choline, serine, or ethanolamine, forming phosphatidylcholine, phosphatidylserine, and phosphatidylethanolamine, respectively. The phosphatidic acid is similar to a triglyceride molecule, the only difference being the presence of a phosphate instead of a fatty acid. The combination of hydrophilic and hydrophobic molecules makes phospholipids a perfect water–lipid interface.

The classification of lipoproteins is based on their diameter, density in preparative ultracentrifugation, electrophoretic mobility, and composition (Table 1). According to their major structural apo (Table 2), lipoproteins can be divided into three main broad classes: apoB48-, apoB100-, and apoAI-containing lipoproteins.

ApoB48-containing lipoproteins are chylomicrons and their by-products, namely chylomicron remnants. Chylomicrons are the largest and lightest lipoprotein particles, have no electrophoretic mobility, and are normally not found in plasma, during fasting. They appear in the bloodstream in the postprandial state and are mainly composed of triglycerides.

ApoB100-containing lipoproteins are very low-density lipoprotein (VLDL) particles and their by-products, namely intermediate-density lipoprotein (IDL) and low-density lipoprotein (LDL) particles. VLDL particles are quite large and light lipoproteins rich in triglycerides, with a pre-β electrophoretic mobility. They comprise two main subclasses: the larger and lighter VLDL1 (Sf 60–400) and the smaller and heavier VLDL2 (Sf 20–60). LDL particles transport most of plasma cholesterol, are smaller and heavier than VLDL particles, and have β-electrophoretic mobility. IDL particles have intermediate density, composition, and electrophoretic mobility between that of VLDL

International Textbook of Diabetes Mellitus, Third Edition. Edited by R. A. DeFronzo, E. Ferrannini, H. Keen, and P. Zimmet.
 ISBN: 0-471-48655-8.

Table 1 Characteristics of major lipoproteins

Lipoprotein	Diameter (nm)	Density (g/ml)	Electrophoretic mobility	Major lipids	Major apolipoproteins	Major sources
Chylomicrons	75–1200	<0.95	Origin	Triglycerides	B48, AIV (E and Cs by transfer from HDL)	Intestine
Chylomicron remnants	30–80	<1.006	Slow pre-β	Triglycerides, cholesterol	B48, E	Chylomicrons
VLDL	30–80	0.95–1.006	Pre-β	Triglycerides	B100, E, Cs	Liver
IDL	25–35	1.006–1.019	Slow pre-β	Triglycerides, cholesterol	B100, E	VLDL
LDL	18–25	1.019–1.063	β	Cholesterol	B100	IDL
HDL_2	8–12	1.063–1.125	α	Phospholipids, cholesterol	AI, AII, Cs	HDL_3
HDL_3	5–9	1.125–1.21	α	Phospholipids	AI, AII, E	Intestine, liver, chylomicrons, VLDL
Lp(a)	25–30	1.055–1.085	Pre-β	Cholesterol	B100, (a)	Liver

and LDL particles, and are equally rich in triglycerides and cholesterol. Each apoB100-containing lipoprotein is surrounded by a single molecule of apoB100, which constitutes the backbone of the particle from its hepatic synthesis as VLDL until its clearance from the circulation as IDL or LDL. After secretion into the plasma, VLDL particles (as well as chylomicrons) acquire apoCs and apoE by transfer from other lipoproteins, especially high-density lipoprotein (HDL) particles. Lipoprotein(a) [Lp(a)] is also an apoB100-containing lipoprotein. It is a cholesterol ester-rich, LDL-like lipoprotein containing the characteristic apo(a), which is coded by one of the most polymorphic genes known in humans.

ApoAI-containing lipoproteins are represented by HDL particles, which are the smallest and heaviest particles. HDL particles contain the least amount of lipid per protein, and have mostly an α-electrophoretic mobility. A small fraction of HDL particles has a pre-β mobility and is synthesized by the intestine as discoidal particles called pre-β LpAI. The protein component of HDL particles consists of several apos, about 90% being apoAI and apoAII. apoAIV and apoCs are also standard components of HDL particles. A minority of HDL particles, also called HDL_1 or HDL_c (where HDL_c is HDL induced by cholesterol feeding), contains apoE and is rich in cholesteryl esters [1]. These are larger particles (13–25 nm) floating at a density of 1.03–1.10 g/ml. HDL particles can be separated into two main subfractions by density-gradient centrifugation, HDL_2 (1.063–1.125 g/ml) and HDL_3 (1.125–1.210 g/ml), and are rich in phospholipids. The apoAI/apoAII molar ratio is 9:1 in HDL_2, and only 2:1 in HDL_3.

OVERVIEW OF LIPOPROTEIN METABOLISM

Metabolism of ApoB48-containing Lipoproteins

Chylomicrons are produced by the intestinal epithelial cells, particularly those of the proximal jejunum,

Table 2 Characteristics of major apolipoproteins

Apolipoprotein	Major sites of synthesis	Molecular mass (daltons)	Lipoprotein association	Major known functions
AI	Intestine, liver	28 100	HDL	LCAT activation
AII	Liver	17 400	HDL	Unknown
AIV	Intestine	43 000	HDL, chylomicrons	Triglyceride transport in chylomicrons
B48	Intestine	~246 000	Chylomicrons	Chylomicron formation
B100	Liver	~513 000	VLDL, IDL, LDL, Lp(a)	VLDL formation; ligand for LDLR
CI	Liver	6 600	VLDL, HDL, chylomicrons	Modulation of TRL receptor-mediated uptake
CII	Liver	8 800	VLDL, HDL, chylomicrons	LPL activation
CIII	Liver	8 750	VLDL, HDL, chylomicrons	Inhibition of TRL receptor-mediated uptake
E	Liver, macrophages, astrocytes, keratinocytes	34 200	Chylomicron remnants, IDL, HDL	Ligand for LDLR, LRP, and other apoE receptors
(a)	Liver	~400 000–800 000	Lp(a)	Unknown

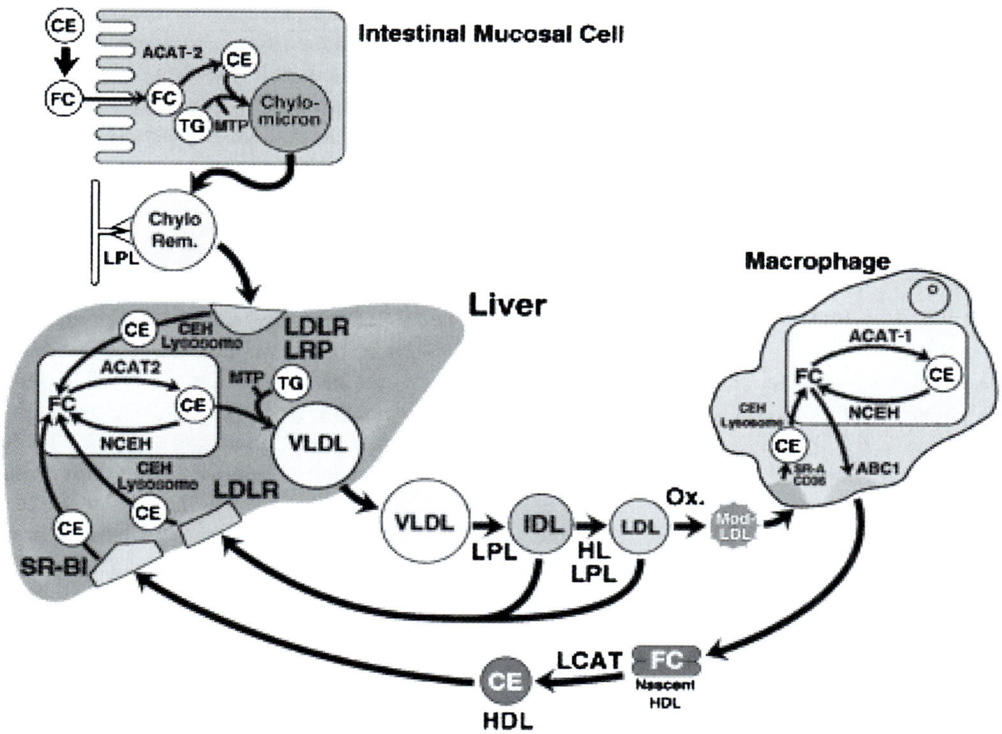

Figure 1 Overview of lipoprotein metabolism. Chylomicrons are secreted by the enterocyte, following the absorption of dietary lipids. Cholesteryl esters (CEs) are converted to free cholesterol (FC) before being absorbed. Acyl-coenzyme A:cholesterol-acyltransferase 2 (ACAT-2) reesterifies FC to CE intracellularly, whereas MTP facilitates the intracellular transfer of triglycerides (TGs). Both events are very important for the formation of chylomicrons and VLDLs. After secretion, chylomicron TGs are hydrolyzed by LPL and the resulting CE-rich chylomicron remnants (rem.) are taken up by hepatic LDLR and LRP. VLDL assembly in the hepatocyte is quite similar to chylomicron assembly in the enterocyte. Hepatocyte CE content is derived by the uptake of different lipoproteins (chylomicron remnants, IDLs, LDLs, and HDLs) by specific receptors (LDLR, LRP, and SR-BI). CE is hydrolyzed by cholesteryl ester hydrolase (CEH) to FC in lysosomes. FC can be easily reesterified to CE by ACAT-2, and CE can also be rehydrolyzed to FC by neutral cholesteryl ester hydrolase (NCEH) in a cycle. After secretion, VLDL TGs are hydrolyzed by LPL, and the resulting CE-rich IDLs are further converted to LDLs by LPL and HL or taken up by liver receptors (LDLR and LRP). LDLs return a good portion of CE to the liver via LDLR. However, some LDLs can undergo oxidation (Ox.) or other kinds of modification (Mod-LDL), and the Mod-LDLs are then taken up by macrophage scavenger receptors (CD36 and SR-A). Macrophage CE is converted to FC by NCEH, and FC can be re-esterified to CE by ACAT-1. Excess FC is removed from the macrophage by apoAI-mediated efflux through the ABC1 (or ABCA1) transporter. Nascent HDLs are discoidals since are mainly composed of apoAI, FC, and phospholipids. As soon as FC is converted to CE by LCAT, HDLs become spherical like all other lipoproteins. HDL can also return CE back to the liver via SR-BI receptor. See the text for all other abbreviations. (From reference 2)

following absorption of dietary fat (Figure 1). Short-chain fatty acids are absorbed directly into the portal circulation. Triglycerides utilized in the formation of chylomicron particles are synthesized from the absorbed long-chain fatty acids (those with more than 12–14 carbons) and monoglycerides, whereas phospholipids and cholesterol are derived from either direct absorption or synthesis by enterocytes. Lipids are assembled with apoB48 in a process that requires the microsomal triglyceride transfer protein (MTP). ApoB48 is derived from the same gene on chromosome 2 responsible for the production of apoB100. In the intestine, the apoB mRNA is edited by a complex that introduces a stop codon sequence giving rise to apoB48, whereas the full-length apoB mRNA is translated to produce apoB100 in the liver. Newly synthesized chylomicrons also possess apoAIV. After secretion into the mesenteric lymph, chylomicrons proceed through the thoracic duct, and finally enter the general circulation. Here, they acquire apoC and apoE primarily by exchange from HDLs. Once in the general circulation, chylomicrons bind to the enzyme lipoprotein lipase (LPL), which is anchored to capillary endothelial cells via heparan sulfate proteoglycans (HSPGs). LPL is activated by apoCII molecules emerging from the chylomicron surface. Triglycerides situated in the core of chylomicrons are therefore hydrolyzed to free fatty acids (FFAs), which are taken into different tissues for various purposes. FFA can be stored as triglycerides in the adipose tissue, oxidized as energy source in the muscle, or reutilized by the liver for lipoprotein synthesis. After most of the triglycerides are hydrolyzed, the particles are released from LPL as cholesterol-enriched chylomicron remnants. The remnant particles are rapidly cleared from the plasma by the LDL receptor (LDLR) and the LDL receptor-related protein (LRP), and ultimately degraded by the hepatocytes. Plasma clearance includes sequestration within the space of Disse by HSPGs, the involvement of LPL and hepatic lipase (HL) in further processing and cell-surface binding, and internalization through apoE–HSPGs–LDLR/LRP interaction.

Metabolism of ApoB100-containing Lipoproteins

VLDLs are smaller and denser than chylomicrons and are produced by hepatocytes (Figure 1). The first stages of VLDL metabolism are very similar to those of chylomicron metabolism. Triglycerides and cholesterol are assembled with apoB100 within the endoplasmic reticulum in a process that also requires MTP. After secretion into the plasma, VLDLs acquire apoC and apoE too by transfer primarily from HDLs. Like chylomicrons, VLDL triglycerides are hydrolyzed by LPL, producing remnant particles called IDLs. These particles may be taken up by hepatic LDLR or LRP or converted further to LDL by a process that involves HL. The main function of LDL particles is to supply cholesterol to essentially all cells. LDLRs are found in most tissues throughout the body, and apoB100 serves as the ligand for the LDLR. The great majority of LDL particles are cleared by the liver.

Lp(a) can be described as a LDL particle characterized by the presence of a unique protein, apo(a). Lp(a) assembly involves multiple interactions between apo(a) and apoB100 of LDL, as well as a disulfide linkage of two free cysteine residues on both proteins. Apo(a) shows a strong resemblance to plasminogen and varies substantially in its molecular weight, among different persons. Apo(a) is synthesized by the liver, and both transcriptional and posttranslational mechanisms have been identified as regulating Lp(a) production. The assembly of Lp(a) seems to occur extracellularly from newly synthesized apo(a) and circulating LDL, even though *in vivo* kinetic studies have revealed the possibility of an intracellular assembly. Lp(a) has a longer half-life than that of LDL and is not removed from the plasma by the LDLR. However, the site and mechanism of its catabolism are unknown. Plasma concentrations of Lp(a) vary enormously between individuals and considerably across populations, and are determined by synthesis and not by degradation.

Metabolism of ApoAI-containing Lipoproteins

HDLs are responsible for reverse cholesterol transport, a process in which excess peripheral cholesterol is returned to the liver for excretion into the bile (Figure 2). ApoAI is synthesized by both the intestine and the liver. Nascent HDLs are thought to be discoidal particles that acquire unesterified cholesterol from peripheral tissues, a process facilitated by a cellular protein called ATP-binding cassette protein A1 (ABCA1). Unesterified cholesterol is esterified on HDLs by the enzyme lecithin:cholesterol acyltransferase (LCAT), a plasma enzyme associated with HDLs. As LCAT activity generates more cholesteryl ester, nascent HDLs evolve into spherical particles, which enlarge further as they acquire additional lipid and protein constituents from chylomicrons and VLDLs when the triglyceride core of these lipoproteins is hydrolyzed. The HDL cholesteryl esters can be transferred to the liver through at least two pathways. First, HDL cholesteryl esters can be transferred to apoB-containing lipoproteins in exchange for triglyceride, through the action of cholesteryl ester transfer protein (CETP). Some of these apoB-containing lipoproteins are then removed from the plasma by the liver via LDLR or LRP. Triglyceride-enriched HDL is a substrate for hepatic lipase, which hydrolyzes HDL triglycerides and phospholipids and generates smaller HDL particles. Second, HDL cholesteryl esters can be taken up directly by the liver in a process termed selective cholesterol uptake. This process is mediated by scavenger receptor class B type I (SR-BI), a cell surface receptor that facilitates uptake of HDL cholesteryl ester but not of the entire lipoprotein particle. Thus, the metabolism of HDL cholesteryl ester and HDL apoAI are dissociated. Eventually, apoAI is removed from the circulation by a process that is not well understood but seems to involve primarily the kidney. Cubilin, the receptor for the intrinsic factor-vitamin B_{12}, has been shown to bind small HDLs and lipid-free apoAI in the epithelial cells of the proximal tubulus of the kidney [4, 5]. The endocytic receptor megalin, another member of the LDLR family, has been reported to bind cubilin and seems to act in conjunction with cubilin to mediate HDL endocytosis. Suppression of megalin activity or expression results in inhibition of cubilin-mediated endocytosis of HDL [6]. Lipid-free apoAI and small HDL are then degraded into lysosomes after internalization.

LIPOPROTEIN METABOLISM IN INSULIN RESISTANCE

The metabolic syndrome is characterized by a constellation of abnormalities that represent major risk factors for both type 2 diabetes mellitus and cardiovascular disease (CVD). The resistance to insulin-mediated glucose disposal and compensatory hyperinsulinemia are central to both the metabolic syndrome and diabetes, and seem to be responsible for most, if not all, of the associated abnormalities. The atherogenic dyslipidemia is an important component of the cluster of abnormalities characteristic of the metabolic syndrome, which also consists of abdominal obesity, insulin resistance (with or without

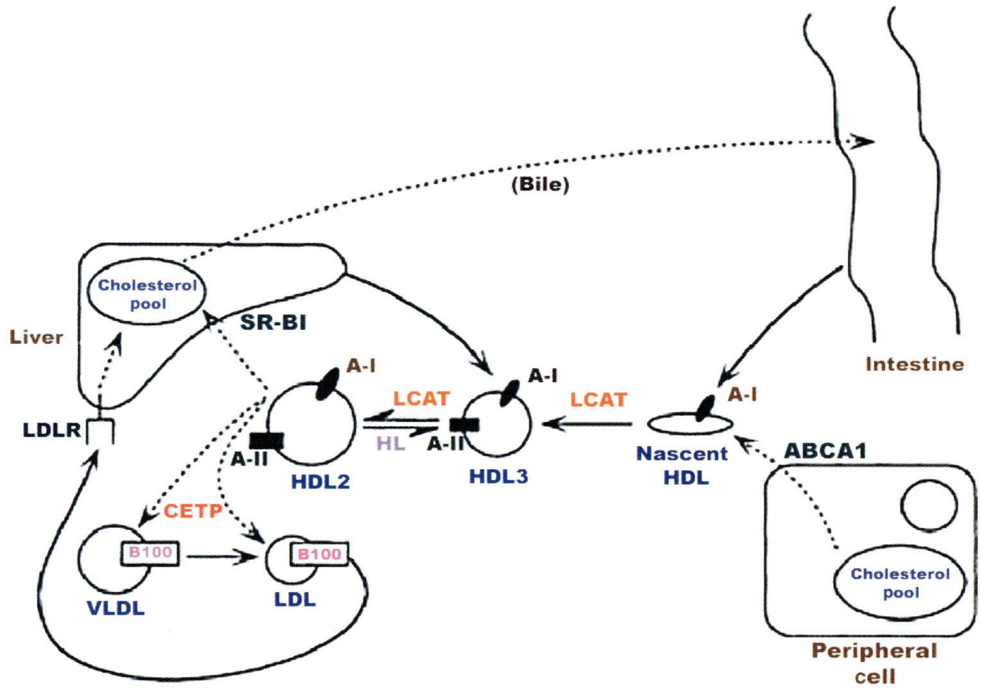

Figure 2 HDL metabolism. HDLs originate from different sources. ApoAI, the major protein component, is produced by intestine and liver, whereas apoAII, the second main protein is only produced by the liver. HDLs have many interactions with all other lipoproteins, and are responsible for reverse cholesterol transport. HDLs exchange lipids (through the action of CETP and phospholipid transfer protein, PLTP) and apos (mainly apoCs and apoE) with apoB-containing lipoproteins. LCAT, HL, CETP, and PLTP play an important role in HDL remodeling (HDL_2 and HDL_3). HDL CE is transported back to the liver by HDL itself through the action of SR-BI receptor. It can also be transported to apoB-containing lipoproteins by CETP (in exchange for triglycerides), and then these lipoproteins are taken up by LDLR and LRP. Part of cholesterol returned to the liver is secreted into the bile (enterohepatic circulation). B100, AI, and AII indicate specific apos. See text for all abbreviations. (From reference 3, slightly modified)

glucose tolerance), raised blood pressure, and prothrombotic and proinflammatory states. There are three major components of the dyslipidemia that occur in insulin resistance: increased fasting and postprandial triglyceride-rich lipoproteins (TRLs), decreased HDL, and increased small, dense LDL particles. Since the metabolism of all lipoproteins is highly interrelated, it is likely that an initial crucial defect triggers all of the lipoprotein changes occurring in the insulin-resistant state (Figure 3). It is indeed rare that these lipoprotein abnormalities are found separately in insulin-resistant individuals.

Population-based studies have universally and consistently found positive associations of measures of insulin resistance with plasma total or VLDL triglyceride, and negative associations with HDL cholesterol concentration. These associations have remained significant when adjusted for main covariates, like obesity, age, smoking, and physical activity, for example, and appear to be consistent in both genders and among various populations, such as Whites (Framingham Heart Study [7], Paris Prospective Study [8], Quebec Cardiovascular Study [9]), Blacks (Coronary Artery Risk Development in Young Adults, CARDIA [10]), Hispanics (San Antonio Heart Study [11]), Asians [12], and American Indians (Pima Indians [13], Strong Heart Study [14, 15]).

PATHOGENESIS

Elevated Fasting Triglycerides

The hepatic overproduction of VLDL appears to be the primary and crucial defect accompanying insulin resistance and compensatory hyperinsulinemia (Figure 4). Inability to suppress hepatic glucose production, impaired muscle glucose uptake and oxidation, and inability to suppress release of FFA from adipose tissue are the most important consequences of insulin resistance in liver, muscle, and adipose tissue, respectively. These events give rise to increased FFA and glucose flux to the liver, an important regulator of hepatic VLDL production [17].

Another key site in the regulation of VLDL secretion is the rate of apoB100 degradation. Newly synthesized apoB100 remains associated with the rough endoplasmic reticulum (RER) and is degraded by the ubiquitin/proteasome system, or is translocated into the lumen and incorporated into lipid-poor VLDL precursors. Next,

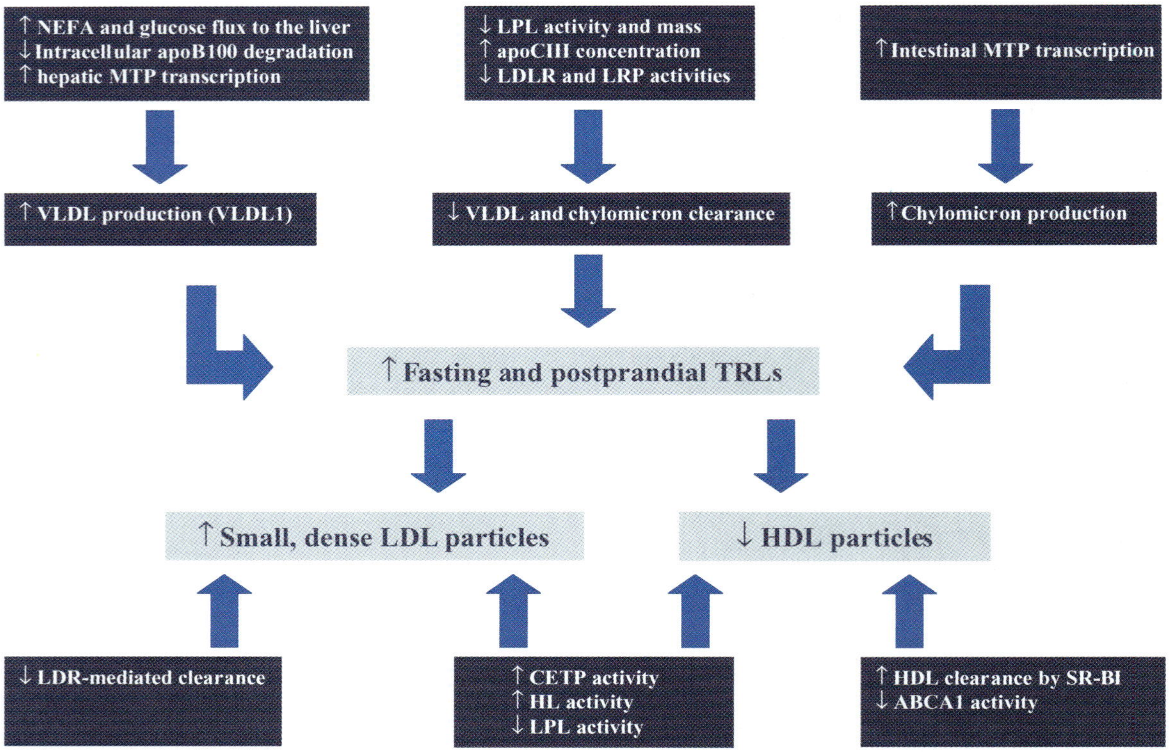

Figure 3 Pathogenesis of dyslipidemia in the insulin-resistant state. See the text for explanation and abbreviations

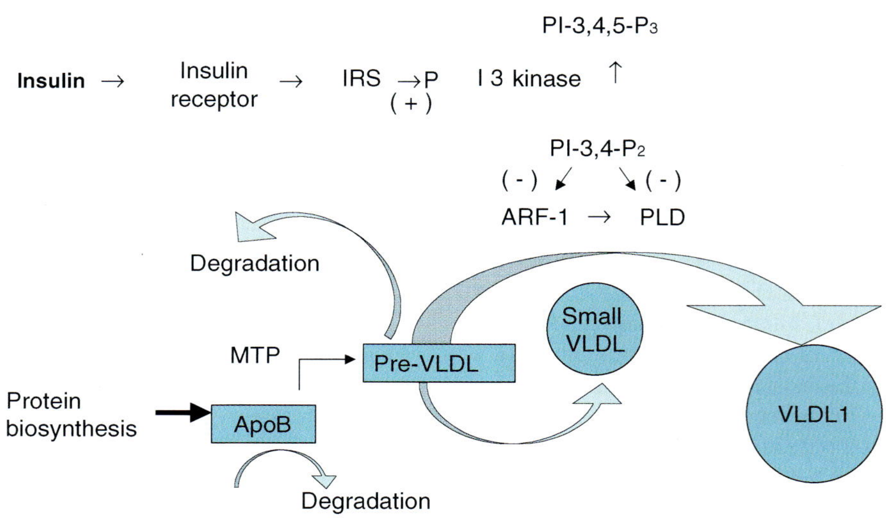

Figure 4 Assembly and secretion of VLDL particles in the insulin-resistant state. The assembly of VLDL is a two-step process that occurs in the lumen of the secretory pathway. Initially, two independent VLDL precursors, a partially lipidated apoB-containing VLDL, and a lipid droplet are formed at the same time. Subsequently, the two precursors fuse to form a mature VLDL particle. The formation of both VLDL precursors is dependent on MTP, whereas their fusion appears to be independent of MTP. The conversion of VLDL precursors to mature VLDL seems to be dependent on the ADP ribosylation factor 1 (ARF-1) and its activation of phospholipase D (PLD). Nascent apoB is sorted cotranslationally during the formation of the apoB-containing precursor. This process involves cytosolic chaperons and ubiquitination that targets apoB to proteasomal degradation. Insulin plays an important role in the intracellular degradation of freshly translated apoB100, as well as in the inhibition of ARF-1 and PLD. The binding of insulin to insulin receptor is followed by the activation of insulin receptor substrate (IRS) and phosphatidylinositol (PI) 3 kinase and generation of the lipid products, phosphatidylinositol-3,4-bisphosphate (PI-3,4-P_2), and phosphatidylinositol-3,4,5-trisphosphate (PI-3,4,5-P_3). PI-3,4-P_2 inhibits ARF-1 and, consequently, PLD. See the text for other abbreviations. (From reference 16)

the lumenal apoB100 is either degraded or advances, acquiring the remaining VLDL lipids in the smooth endoplasmic reticulum (SER)/cis-Golgi. ApoB100 is stabilized and protected from degradation by the heat shock protein 70 (HSP-70). Lipids and MTP, a heterodimeric lipid transfer protein that is required for the assembly of apoB-containing lipoproteins, play a major role in the translocation of apoB100. If it does not occur, then the apoB100 is degraded (Figure 4). Insulin seems to be an important factor for the intracellular degradation of freshly translated apoB100. Therefore, in the insulin-resistant state there is inability to suppress apoB100 degradation, and consequent imbalance between secretion and degradation in favor of the former [18]. Hepatic VLDL-apoB overproduction in the fructose-fed hamster, a novel animal model of insulin resistance, appears to result from both increased intracellular stability of nascent apoB and enhanced expression of MTP [19]. In fact, insulin also negatively regulates MTP gene expression, resulting in a decrease of MTP transcription, even though sustained changes in MTP mRNA levels would be required to affect MTP protein levels in humans [20, 21]. In addition, neither MTP nor newly synthesized triglycerides seems necessary for the later stages of apoB100-lipoprotein assembly and secretion in either HepG2 or McA-RH7777 cells [22]. Therefore, the end result in insulin-resistance states is an increased assembly and secretion of VLDL.

Insulin is a stimulator of LPL activity, by increasing LPL mRNA, and therefore enhancing its rate of synthesis. LPL activity in skeletal muscle of insulin-resistant subjects has been shown to be lower, suggesting a defective insulin regulation of LPL. Therefore, the decreased LPL activity and mass in insulin resistance slow down the normal lipoprotein metabolic cascade, resulting in decreased clearance of VLDL [23, 24]. The concentrations of apoC III, an important inhibitor of TRL receptor-mediated uptake, are also increased in insulin-resistant states [25].

VLDL particles are mainly cleared from circulation by the LDLR, also referred to as apoB/E receptor. The transcription of the LDLR gene is regulated by intracellular cholesterol concentration, hormones, and growth factors. Sterol regulatory element binding protein 1 (SREBP-1) is selectively involved in the signal transduction pathway of insulin and insulin-like growth factor 1 (IGF-1) leading to LDLR gene activation [26] (Figure 5). Insulin resistance may also impair LDLR activity, thus contributing to the delayed VLDL particle clearance accompanying this condition. On the other hand, insulin induces the expression of *SREBP-1c* gene in the liver [28–31], and insulin receptor substrate 1 (IRS-1)/phosphatidylinositol 3 kinase (PI 3-kinase) pathway is essential for this insulin-induced expression [32]. The concurrent hyperinsulinemia accompanying insulin resistance leads to increased expression of *SREBP-1c* gene, which is followed by activation of enzymes for *de novo* lipogenesis, like fatty acid synthase (FAS) and acetyl-CoA carboxylase (ACC), and, therefore, again increased hepatic triglyceride availability for VLDL assembly.

Insulin acutely suppresses the total production rate of VLDL particles by decreasing mainly the production of large, VLDL1 (Sf 60–400), without affecting that of small TRLs, VLDL2 (Sf 20–60) [33]. This effect seems to be independent of the availability of FFA [34]. In type 2 diabetes insulin appears unable to inhibit acutely the release of VLDL1 from the liver, despite efficient suppression of serum FFA [35]. However, the decrease in circulating VLDL particles, following acute insulin action in insulin-sensitive individuals appears to be the result not only of a decreased hepatic production [36], but also of an increased clearance.

VLDL particles have been shown to increase plasminogen activator inhibitor type 1 (PAI-1) biosynthesis in endothelial cells by inducing transcription of the *PAI-1* gene promoter. Similarly, VLDLs increase PAI-1 synthesis by stabilizing PAI-1 mRNA transcripts. The induction of PAI-1 by VLDL particles is dependent on the interaction of the lipoprotein with LDLR and correlates with intracellular triglyceride accumulation. VLDL-induced PAI-1 biosynthesis results from a principal signaling pathway involving protein-kinase-C-mediated mitogen-activated protein kinase activation [37]. The concurrent compensatory hyperinsulinemia of insulin resistance contributes to the increase of PAI-1 levels in this condition, since insulin also has been shown to increase *PAI-1* gene transcription through interaction with its receptor [38].

Elevated Postprandial Lipemia

Less is known about the mechanisms responsible of the association of insulin resistance with increased postprandial lipemia. During the postprandial state, dietary fatty acids are transported from the intestine to peripheral tissues as chylomicron triglycerides. In the capillary beds of peripheral tissues, chylomicron triglycerides are lipolyzed by LPL, allowing the delivery of FFA to cells and resulting in production of smaller, cholesteryl-ester-enriched chylomicron remnants. These particles are rapidly removed from the blood primarily by the liver through two receptors, LDLR and LRP, acting in association with HSPGs and/or HL [39].

Some investigators have examined the relation between postprandial lipemia and insulin resistance, plasma glucose, and insulin response to a meal, in healthy nondiabetic subjects [40]. Postprandial triglyceride levels, as an indirect measure of chylomicron remnant particles, were found to be significantly related to insulin action. A significant relation of triglyceride levels to postheparin plasma LPL activity was also demonstrated. Since LPL is an insulin-sensitive enzyme, which is suppressed in insulin-resistant individuals, its deficiency might

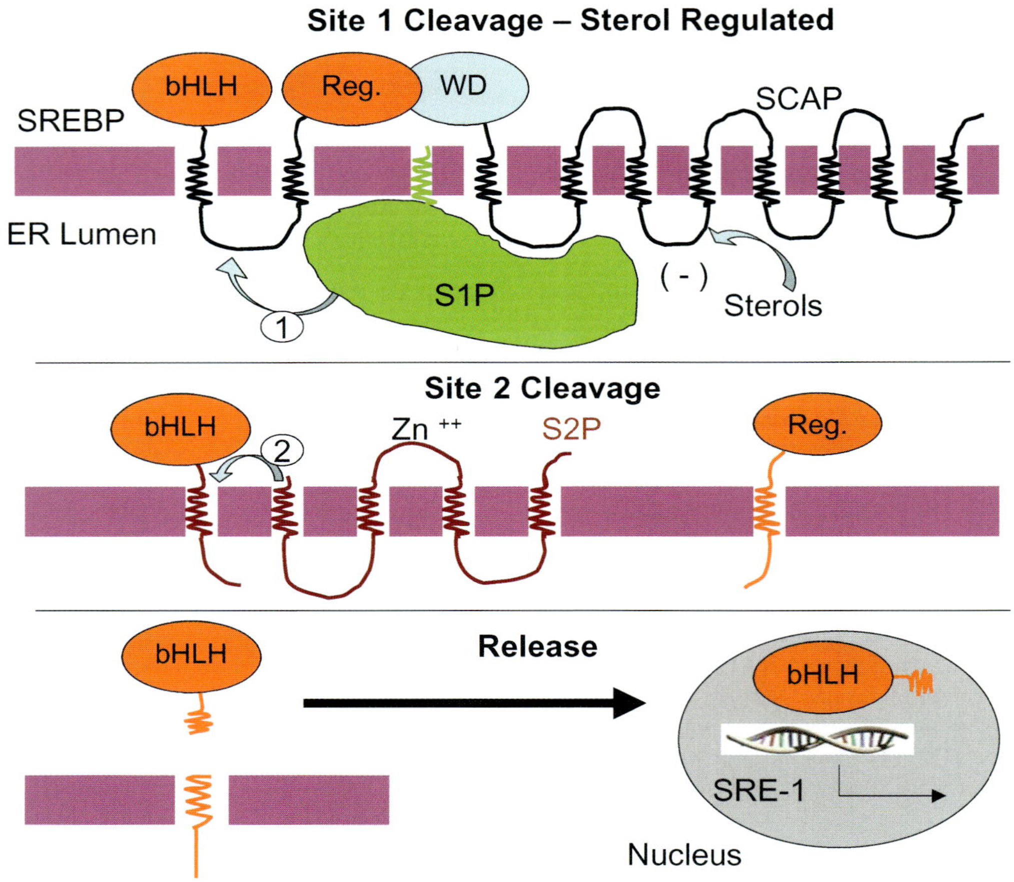

Figure 5 Model for the two-step sterol-mediated proteolytic release of SREBPs from membranes. Top: When cells are deprived of sterols, Site 1 protease (S1P), a sterol-regulated protease, binds to the SREBP cleavage-activating protein (SCAP)/SREBP complex and cleaves the SREBPs into the lumen of the endoplasmic reticulum (ER). This process is inhibited when sterols are abundant. Middle: Once the two halves of SREBP are separated, a second protease, Site 2 protease (S2P), cleaves the basic-loop-helix-leucine-Zip domain (bHLH) of SREBP within the membrane. Bottom: After the second cleavage, the bHLH-Zip domain of SREBP enters the nucleus, binds to sterol regulatory elements (SREs), and finally activates genes controlling lipid synthesis and uptake. See the text for other abbreviations. (From reference 27)

contribute to the abnormal levels of remnant particles, in insulin resistance. HL is also sensitive to portal insulin [41]. The relation of fasting insulin concentrations to postprandial lipoproteins has also been evaluated in a population-based study of healthy middle-aged men with apoE3/3 genotype [42]. Besides postprandial triglycerides, postprandial TRL apoB48 and apoB100 concentrations were also determined as a measure of chylomicron and VLDL remnant particle concentrations. Fasting plasma insulin was associated with the triglyceride response to the test meal, independently of obesity measures, blood glucose, and fasting triglyceride concentrations. Exaggerated and prolonged postprandial lipemia in subjects in the upper quartile of the plasma insulin distribution was largely accounted for by large TRLs (Sf >60). However, insulin relations to large postprandial TRLs exclusively reflected the association between plasma insulin and the fasting plasma concentrations of these lipoprotein species. On the other hand, plasma insulin and late postprandial plasma concentrations of small TRLs (Sf 20–60) were related independent of insulin influences on fasting concentrations. Indeed this slow removal of chylomicron remnants is a common observation in insulin-resistant individuals. This study concluded that the degree of insulin sensitivity is a major determinant of postprandial lipemia, and supports the hypothesis that the preferential clearance of chylomicron triglycerides by LPL leads to accumulation of hepatogenous VLDL during the alimentary period [43]. Because postprandial particles may play an important role in the pathogenesis of CVD, the increased postprandial lipemia in insulin resistance may contribute to increased CVD risk [44].

Insulin does not seem to influence LRP mRNA and protein expression acutely, while it does stimulate recycling of LRP from an endosomal pool to the plasma membrane, thus increasing the cell surface presentation of LRP

[45, 46]. The diminished insulin action on both receptors, LDLR and LRP, could theoretically contribute to the increased postprandial lipemia of insulin resistance, even though this process is far from saturable in normal functioning receptors.

It is not clear yet if an overproduction of intestinal TRLs (chylomicrons) has a role in causing the postprandial lipemia of diabetes in humans. Animal studies (obese Zucker rats and diabetic New Zealand white rabbits) have shown a higher secretion of lymph chylomicron particles in the insulin-resistant animals compared with the controls (lean rats and nondiabetic rabbits) [47, 48]. These animal studies suggest that intestinal MTP could play some role in the postprandial dyslipidemia of diabetes in humans.

Increased Small, Dense Low-Density Lipoprotein Particles

Elevated LDL cholesterol is not a characteristic of the dyslipidemia of insulin resistance. In the insulin-resistant state, the composition and distribution of LDL particles are altered, resulting in a preponderance of small, dense LDL. The association between LDL subclass patterns and plasma insulin, as a measure of insulin resistance, has been demonstrated in many population-based studies, even independently of plasma triglycerides and HDL cholesterol [49, 50].

As previously stated, the LDL particle is characterized by a core consisting primarily of cholesteryl ester surrounded by apoB100. In insulin resistance, the lipid content of the core changes since cholesteryl ester decreases and triglyceride increases relatively, leading to a decreased number of cholesterol molecules per apoB100 (or LDL) particle. Fasting triglyceride and small, dense LDL concentration are positively correlated, since the formation of small, dense LDL depends largely on the metabolism of VLDL particles. In insulin-resistant states, the increased concentration and delayed clearance of VLDL particles induce an increased exchange between cholesteryl esters in LDL and triglycerides in VLDL, mediated by CETP. This exchange produces LDL particles enriched in triglycerides, which are rapidly lipolyzed by HL leaving smaller, denser LDL particles. The activities of both CETP and HL appear to be increased in insulin resistance. This exchange process also leads to highly atherogenic cholesteryl-ester-enriched VLDL particles. Small, dense LDL particles seem to be more prone to modifications, such as oxidation and glycation (increased in the presence of high glucose levels), which could lead to increased production of antibodies against the modified apoB100 and formation of immunocomplexes. All these modifications might result in a decreased LDLR-mediated clearance of small, dense LDL particles [51], which could contribute to their elevated plasma levels in the insulin resistance syndrome, and particularly in uncontrolled type 2 diabetes.

It is well known that insulin resistance has profound effects on the composition of all lipoproteins, not only LDLs. Recently, the novel nuclear magnetic resonance (NMR) methodology has confirmed significant changes in lipoprotein size and subclass particle concentrations for VLDL, LDL, and HDL. In this study [52], insulin resistance was associated with an increase in VLDL size, and a decrease in LDL and HDL size. The increased VLDL size was due to an increase in large VLDL particle concentrations, whereas the decrease in LDL size was the result of a marked increase in small LDL particles and reduced large LDL. The decrease in HDL size was due to the depletion of large HDL particles and a modest increase in small HDL. These insulin-resistance-induced changes in the NMR lipoprotein subclass profile are most likely associated with an increased risk of CVD.

The modified LDL is mostly taken up by macrophage scavenger receptors, rather than the normal LDLR pathway, thus initiating the cascade of events leading to the formation of foam cells and, then, atherosclerotic plaques. Class A scavenger receptors (SR-A) are transmembrane glycoproteins that mediate both ligand internalization and cell adhesion. SR-A was originally identified on macrophages as the receptor that binds and internalizes modified lipoproteins via clathrin-coated pit-mediated endocytosis. However, it also binds and internalizes other polyanionic ligands, like bacterial products, and extracellular matrix proteins. Recent data suggest that the SR-A could also contribute to the adhesion of macrophages to the extracellular matrix of atherosclerotic plaques [53]. Scavenger receptors recognize not only modified LDL, such as acetylated LDL and oxidized LDL (OX-LDL) but also advanced glycation end products (AGEs). AGEs are nonenzymatically glycosylated proteins, which are generated through long-term exposure of proteins to glucose and accumulate in vascular tissues in aging and diabetes. Receptors for AGEs include scavenger receptors, which recognize acetylated LDL (Ac-LDL) such as SR-A, cell surface glycoprotein CD36, SR-BI, lectin-like oxidized LDLR-1, and newly discovered receptors, like the scavenger receptor expressed by endothelial cells I (SREC-I), the fasciclin EGF-like, laminin-type EGF-like, and link domain-containing scavenger receptor 1 (FEEL-1), and and its paralogous protein, FEEL-2 [54–57]. SR-BI, the first identified HDL receptor, plays key roles in reverse cholesterol transport by promoting selective uptake of HDL cholesteryl esters by hepatocytes, and cholesterol efflux of unesterified cholesterol from peripheral cells to HDL. However, it has been shown that a complex AGE-albumin can bind to SR-BI, and, therefore inhibit both processes, i.e., selective uptake of HDL cholesteryl esters as well as cholesterol efflux, suggesting potential roles of AGEs in diabetic dyslipidemia and accelerated atherosclerosis in diabetes.

Data on the role of Lp(a) in diabetes are still conflicting, even though a large, population-based study has failed to show elevated Lp(a) levels in type 2 diabetes. In this study, part of the San Antonio Heart Study, 260 patients with type 2 diabetes and 366 nondiabetic subjects had similar Lp(a) concentrations [58]. A recent sudy in American Indians has actually demonstrated that diabetic participants had significantly lower Lp(a) levels than did nondiabetic participants for both genders [59]. This study has also shown a lower concentration of Lp(a) in American Indians (almost half of that in Whites and one sixth in Blacks) and a high correlation of Lp(a) concentration with Indian heritage, confirming the concept that Lp(a) concentration is in large part genetically determined.

Decreased High-Density Lipoprotein Cholesterol

HDL particles are the smallest lipoprotein particles, with cholesteryl esters in the central core and a variety of apos that govern their metabolism. Although the mechanisms that regulate HDL are not completely understood, the atherogenic potential of low HDL levels is well known. Several mechanisms can contribute to the decreased HDL in insulin resistance, and as in the formation of small, dense LDL particles, TRL metabolism plays an important role. Most studies of lipoproteins have shown an inverse relationship between VLDL triglycerides and HDL cholesterol. Impaired TRL lipolysis leads to reduced HDL concentration, by decreasing the transfer of apos and phospholipids from TRL to the HDL compartment. In addition, the delayed cleareance of TRLs facilitates the CETP-mediated exchange between cholesteryl esters in HDL and triglycerides in VLDL. The increased activity of HL in insulin-resistant states produces smaller HDL particles and facilitates HDL clearance. An increased clearance of HDL particles might also occur in poor-controlled type 2 diabetes, following the increased glycation of the major apo of HDL, apoAI. Finally, insulin could also have a direct effect on the production of apoAI or hepatic secretion of nascent HDL. Therefore, in insulin resistance there is a substantial decrease of HDL particles, especially the larger HDL_2 (compared to the smaller HDL_3) and HDL containing mostly apoAI (referred to as LpAI particles). The LpAI particles are more effective than LpAI:AII particles in the reverse cholesterol process, and therefore are considered more antiatherogenic. The function of the other major apos of HDL, apoAII, is not clear yet. Recent data have suggested a possible role of apoAII in visceral fat accumulation, even though no direct relationship with insulin resistance has been demonstrated in humans [60]. However, studies on knockout and transgenic human apoAII mice have shown a clear role of this apo in insulin sensitivity.

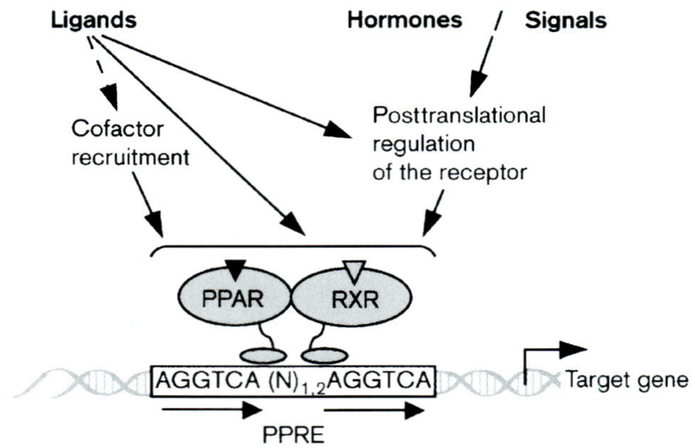

Figure 6 Mechanism of transcriptional regulation of PPARs. Ligands activate PPAR, which heterodimerize with RXR. The heterodimer binds to PPAR response element (PPRE) of target genes, resulting in regulation of their expression. PPAR activity can also be modulated by cofactors or posttranslational modifications. See the text for other abbreviations. (From reference 61)

Role of Peroxisome Proliferator-activated Receptors

Peroxisome proliferator-activated receptors (PPARs) are transcription factors that act as dietary lipid sensors regulating fatty acid, carbohydrate, and lipid metabolism (Figure 6). PPARs regulate gene expression upon heterodimerization with the retinoid X receptor (RXR) and subsequent binding to PPAR-response elements (PPREs), which are located in the promoter region of target genes. The hypolipidemic effects of the fibrates and the antidiabetic effects of the thiazolidinediones (TZDs) in humans are known, and are due to activation of PPAR-α and PPAR-γ subtypes, respectively.

PPAR-α is predominantly expressed in liver, kidney, heart, and skeletal muscle, where it controls fatty acid catabolism [61]. Fibrates efficiently lower plasma concentrations of cholesterol and triglycerides and increase HDL-cholesterol levels. PPAR-α enhances the transcription of the apoAI and apoAII, thereby increasing HDL production (Table 3). Fibrates lower triglycerides (and fasting and postprandial lipoproteins) as a result of enhanced lipolysis, by increasing LPL and reducing apoCIII gene expression, induction of fatty acid uptake and

Table 3 Role of activated PPAR-α and PPAR-γ on gene expression and protein secretion in lipoprotein metabolism

Activated PPAR-α effects	Activated PPAR-γ effects
↑ LPL	↑ LPL
↑ ApoAI, apoAII	↑ ABCA1
↓ ApoCIII	↑ CD36
↑ SR-BI	
↑ ABCA1	

catabolism, and reduced fatty acid synthesis and VLDL production by the liver. Moreover, fibrates increase the removal of LDL particles by modifying LDL composition, which increases the affinity of LDL for the LDLR. PPAR-α has also an effect on gene expression and protein secretion in fatty acid metabolism. Its activation results into increased concentrations of fatty acid transport protein (FATP), acyl-CoA synthetase (ACS), and carnitine palmitoyltransferase (CPT), leading to increased mitochondrial β-oxidation.

PPAR-γ is highly expressed in brown and white adipose tissue and the intestine, and triggers cellular differentiation, promotes lipid storage, and modulates the action of insulin. TZDs mainly exert hypotriglyceridemic effects by increasing lipolysis and clearance of TRLs in adipose tissue (Table 3). The lipolytic action of PPAR-α and PPAR-γ agonists may also contribute to increased HDL levels, accompanying their activation.

PPAR-α and PPAR-γ are also expressed in macrophages and foam cells that are resident in atherosclerotic lesions, where they exert antiatherogenic activities. The activation of PPAR-γ by TZDs in macrophages also induces ABCA1 expression and cholesterol removal from macrophages through a transcriptional cascade mediated by the nuclear receptor liver X receptor α (LXR-α) [62, 63] (Figure 7). Ligand activation of PPAR-γ leads to primary induction of LXR-α and to coupled induction of ABCA1. Therefore, PPAR-γ coordinates a complex physiologic response to ox-LDL that involves particle uptake, processing, and cholesterol removal through ABCA1. A recent study has shown that ABCA1 gene expression is severely decreased in the liver and peritoneal macrophages of diabetic mice, and treatment with insulin is able to restore this deficit [65]. PPAR-γ is also implicated in the regulation of CD36 expression and macrophage uptake of ox-LDL.

PPAR-δ, another member of the PPAR family, is ubiquitously expressed and controls brain lipid metabolism and fatty-acid-induced adipogenesis and preadipocyte proliferation. The function of PPAR-δ subtype is less known, even though recent data suggest a role in reverse cholesterol transport. PPAR-δ seems to increase the expression of ABCA1 in macrophages, thus inducing apoAI-specific cholesterol efflux. When a PPAR-δ ligand was given to insulin-resistant middle-aged obese rhesus monkeys, it produced a significant dose-dependent increase in serum HDL cholesterol, and a decrease in small, dense LDL, fasting triglycerides, and fasting insulin concentrations [66]. Interestingly, PPAR-δ also increases HDL cholesterol plasma concentrations in insulin-resistant mice.

While PPAR-γ promotes lipid uptake and efflux in macrophages, PPAR-δ seems to control the inflammatory status of these atherogenic cells [67] through its association and disassociation with transcriptional repressors. In addition, PPAR-δ activation seems to be required for the direct regulation of gene expression in atherosclerotic lesions by components of TRLs [68]. PPAR-δ and its ligands may thus also serve as therapeutic targets to slow the progression of atherosclerosis.

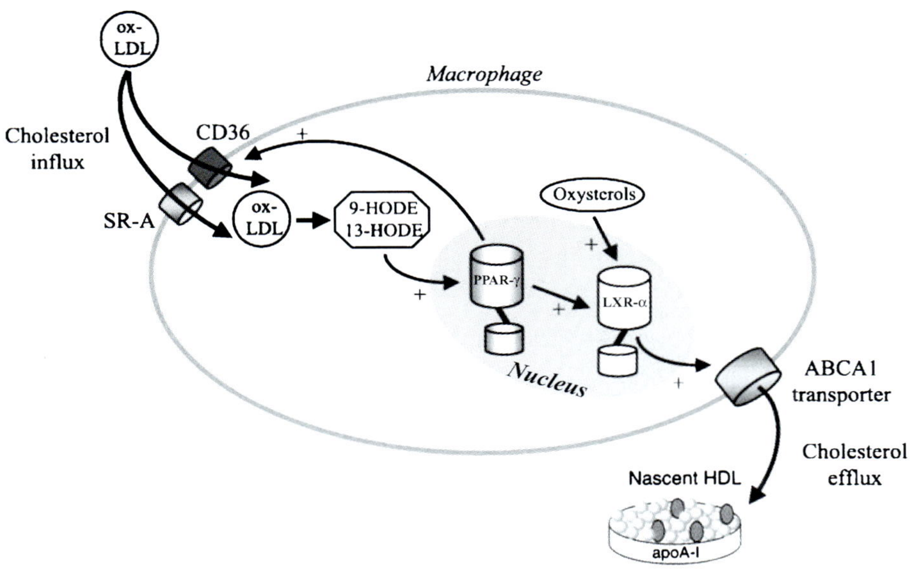

Figure 7 Central role of PPAR-γ activation in reverse cholesterol transport from macrophages. The uptake of oxidized LDL (ox-LDL) by the macrophage scavenger receptors SR-A and CD36 leads to the generation of PPAR-γ ligands, 9-hydroxyoctadecadienoic acid (HODE), and 13-HODE. The activation of PPAR-γ finally induces ABCA1 expression and cholesterol removal from macrophages through a transcriptional cascade mediated by the nuclear receptor LXR-α. See the text for other abbreviations. (From reference 64, slightly modified)

SUMMARY

The three major components of the dyslipidemia associated with insulin resistance are increased fasting and postprandial TRLs, decreased HDL, and increased small, dense LDL particles. The insulin resistance and compensatory hyperinsulinemia lead to overproduction of VLDL particles, an early abnormality of insulin resistance. A relative defective LPL-mediated lipolysis has also an important role in the dyslipidemia, since largely contributes to the decreased clearance of fasting and postprandial TRLs and to the decreased production of HDL particles. The resulting increased concentration of cholesteryl-ester-rich fasting and postprandial TRLs (IDL and chylomicron remnants, respectively) is a central lipoprotein abnormality of insulin resistance. The increase of small, dense LDL particles, and decrease of large, buoyant HDL particles seem to be consequential events of the delayed metabolism of TRLs. The dyslipidemia associated with insulin resistance plays a major role in the development of atherosclerosis, and contributes largely to the increased CVD risk in individuals with insulin resistance. PPARs (α, γ, and δ) are ligand-activated transcription factors belonging to the nuclear receptor family. PPARs agonists seem to improve the dyslipidemia of insulin resistance, by regulating the expression of important genes involved in the deranged lipoprotein metabolism associated with insulin resistance. New compounds with multiple PPAR-agonist activity are currently under investigation, and could represent a possible solution to the radical treatment of the dyslipidemia of insulin resistance.

REFERENCES

1. Koo C, Innerarity TL, Mahley RW. Obligatory role of cholesterol and apolipoprotein E in the formation of large cholesterol-enriched and receptor-active high density lipoproteins. *J Biol Chem* 1985; 260: 11934–43.
2. Brewer HB Jr. The lipid-laden foam cell: an elusive target for therapeutic intervention. *J Clin Invest* 2000; 105: 703–5.
3. Rader DJ. Disorders of lipid metabolism. In Kelly WN (ed), *Textbook of Internal Medicine*. Philadelphia: Lippincott-Raven; 1996; pp 72–89.
4. Kozyraki R, Fyfe J, Kristiansen M, Gerdes C, Jacobsen C, Cui S, Christensen EI, Aminoff M, de la CA, Krahe R, Verroust PJ, Moestrup SK. The intrinsic factor-vitamin B12 receptor, cubilin, is a high-affinity apolipoprotein A-I receptor facilitating endocytosis of high-density lipoprotein. *Nat Med* 1999; 5: 656–61.
5. Hammad SM, Stefansson S, Twal WO, Drake CJ, Fleming P, Remaley A, Brewer HB Jr, Argraves WS. Cubilin, the endocytic receptor for intrinsic factor-vitamin B(12) complex, mediates high-density lipoprotein holoparticle endocytosis. *Proc Natl Acad Sci USA* 1999; 96: 10158–63.
6. Hammad SM, Barth JL, Knaak C, Argraves WS. Megalin acts in concert with cubilin to mediate endocytosis of high density lipoproteins. *J Biol Chem* 2000; 275: 12003–8.
7. Castelli WP. Epidemiology of triglycerides: a view from Framingham. *Am J Cardiol* 1992; 70: 3H–9H.
8. Balkau B, Eschwege E. Insulin resistance: an independent risk factor for cardiovascular disease? *Diabetes Obes Metab* 1999; 1 (suppl 1): S23–31.
9. Lamarche B, Tchernof A, Mauriege P, Cantin B, Dagenais GR, Lupien PJ, Despres JP. Fasting insulin and apolipoprotein B levels and low-density lipoprotein particle size as risk factors for ischemic heart disease. *JAMA* 1998; 279: 1955–61.
10. Manolio TA, Savage PJ, Burke GL, Liu KA, Wagenknecht LE, Sidney S, Jacobs DR Jr, Roseman JM, Donahue RP, Oberman A, for the CARDIA Study. Association of fasting insulin with blood pressure and lipids in young adults. *Arteriosclerosis* 1990; 10: 430–6.
11. Haffner SM, Mykkanen L, Stern MP, Valdez RA, Heisserman JA, Bowsher RR. Relationship of proinsulin and insulin to cardiovascular risk factors in nondiabetic subjects. *Diabetes* 1993; 42: 1297–302.
12. Bhopal R, Unwin N, White M, Yallop J, Walker L, Alberti KG, Harland J, Patel S, Ahmad N, Turner C, Watson B, Kaur D, Kulkarni A, Laker M, Tavridou A. Heterogeneity of coronary heart disease risk factors in Indian, Pakistani, Bangladeshi, and European origin populations: cross sectional study. *BMJ* 1999; 319: 215–20.
13. Howard BV, Knowler WC, Vasquez B, Kennedy AL, Pettitt DJ, Bennett PH. Plasma and lipoprotein cholesterol and triglyceride in the Pima Indian population. Comparison of diabetics and nondiabetics. *Arteriosclerosis* 1984; 4: 462–71.
14. Gray RS, Fabsitz RR, Cowan LD, Lee ET, Howard BV, Savage PJ, for the Strong Heart Study. Risk factor clustering in the insulin resistance syndrome. *Am J Epidemiol* 1998; 148: 869–78.
15. Resnick HE, Jones K, Ruotolo G, Jain AK, Henderson J, Lu W, Howard BV. Insulin resistance, the metabolic syndrome, and risk of incident cardiovascular disease in nondiabetic american indians: the strong heart study. *Diabetes Care* 2003; 26: 861–7.
16. Taskinen M-R. Diabetic dyslipidemia: from basic research to clinical practice. Claude Bernard Lecture presented at the *38th Claude Bernard Lecture of European Association for the Study of Diabetes*, Budapest, Hungary, September 1–5, 2002.
17. Sparks JD, Sparks CE. Insulin regulation of triacylglycerol-rich lipoprotein synthesis and secretion. *Biochim Biophys Acta* 1994; 1215: 9–32.
18. Kendrick JS, Wilkinson J, Cartwright IJ, Lawrence S, Higgins JA. Regulation of the assembly and secretion of very low density lipoproteins by the liver. *Biol Chem* 1998; 379: 1033–40.
19. Taghibiglou C, Carpentier A, Van Iderstine SC, Chen B, Rudy D, Aiton A, Lewis GF, Adeli K. Mechanisms of hepatic very low density lipoprotein overproduction in insulin resistance. Evidence for enhanced lipoprotein assembly, reduced intracellular ApoB degradation, and increased microsomal triglyceride transfer protein in a fructose-fed hamster model. *J Biol Chem* 2000; 275: 8416–25.
20. Lin MC, Gordon D, Wetterau JR. Microsomal triglyceride transfer protein (MTP) regulation in HepG2 cells: insulin negatively regulates MTP gene expression. *J Lipid Res* 1995; 36: 1073–81.

21. Sato R, Miyamoto W, Inoue J, Terada T, Imanaka T, Maeda M. Sterol regulatory element-binding protein negatively regulates microsomal triglyceride transfer protein gene transcription. *J Biol Chem* 1999; 274: 24714–20.
22. Pan M, Liang J, Fisher EA, Ginsberg HN. The late addition of core lipids to nascent apolipoprotein B100, resulting in the assembly and secretion of triglyceride-rich lipoproteins, is independent of both microsomal triglyceride transfer protein activity and new triglyceride synthesis. *J Biol Chem* 2002; 277: 4413–21.
23. Taskinen MR. Lipoprotein lipase in diabetes. *Diabetes Metab Rev* 1987; 3: 551–70.
24. Miyashita Y, Shirai K, Itoh Y, Sasaki H, Totsuka M, Murano T, Watanabe H. Low lipoprotein lipase mass in preheparin serum of type 2 diabetes mellitus patients and its recovery with insulin therapy. *Diabetes Res Clin Pract* 2002; 56 (3): 181–7.
25. Manzato E, Zambon A, Lapolla A, Zambon S, Braghetto L, Crepaldi G, Fedele D. Lipoprotein abnormalities in well-treated type II diabetic patients. *Diabetes Care* 1993; 16: 469–75.
26. Streicher R, Kotzka J, Muller-Wieland D, Siemeister G, Munck M, Avci H, Krone W. SREBP-1 mediates activation of the low density lipoprotein receptor promoter by insulin and insulin-like growth factor-I. *J Biol Chem* 1996; 271: 7128–33.
27. Brown MS, Goldstein JL. A proteolytic pathway that controls the cholesterol content of membranes, cells, and blood. *Proc Natl Acad Sci USA* 1999; 96: 11041–8.
28. Foretz M, Guichard C, Ferre P, Foufelle F. Sterol regulatory element binding protein-1c is a major mediator of insulin action on the hepatic expression of glucokinase and lipogenesis-related genes. *Proc Natl Acad Sci USA* 1999; 96: 12737–42.
29. Foretz M, Pacot C, Dugail I, Lemarchand P, Guichard C, Le L, X, Berthelier-Lubrano C, Spiegelman B, Kim JB, Ferre P, Foufelle F. ADD1/SREBP-1c is required in the activation of hepatic lipogenic gene expression by glucose. *Mol Cell Biol* 1999; 19: 3760–8.
30. Shimomura I, Matsuda M, Hammer RE, Bashmakov Y, Brown MS, Goldstein JL. Decreased IRS-2 and increased SREBP-1c lead to mixed insulin resistance and sensitivity in livers of lipodystrophic and *ob/ob* mice. *Mol Cell* 2000; 6: 77–86.
31. Foufelle F, Ferre P. New perspectives in the regulation of hepatic glycolytic and lipogenic genes by insulin and glucose: a role for the transcription factor sterol regulatory element binding protein-1c. *Biochem J* 2002; 366: 377–91.
32. Matsumoto M, Ogawa W, Teshigawara K, Inoue H, Miyake K, Sakaue H, Kasuga M. Role of the insulin receptor substrate 1 and phosphatidylinositol 3-kinase signaling pathway in insulin-induced expression of sterol regulatory element binding protein 1c and glucokinase genes in rat hepatocytes. *Diabetes* 2002; 51: 1672–80.
33. Malmstrom R, Packard CJ, Watson TD, Rannikko S, Caslake M, Bedford D, Stewart P, Yki-Jarvinen H, Shepherd J, Taskinen MR. Metabolic basis of hypotriglyceridemic effects of insulin in normal men. *Arterioscler Thromb Vasc Biol* 1997; 17: 1454–64.
34. Malmstrom R, Packard CJ, Caslake M, Bedford D, Stewart P, Yki-Jarvinen H, Shepherd J, Taskinen MR. Effects of insulin and acipimox on VLDL1 and VLDL2 apolipoprotein B production in normal subjects. *Diabetes* 1998; 47: 779–87.
35. Malmstrom R, Packard CJ, Caslake M, Bedford D, Stewart P, Yki-Jarvinen H, Shepherd J, Taskinen MR. Defective regulation of triglyceride metabolism by insulin in the liver in NIDDM. *Diabetologia* 1997; 40: 454–62.
36. Ruotolo G, Micossi P, Galimberti G, Librenti MC, Petrella G, Marcovina S, Pozza G, Howard BV. Effects of intraperitoneal versus subcutaneous insulin administration on lipoprotein metabolism in type I diabetes. *Metab Clin Exp* 1990; 39: 598–604.
37. Banfi C, Mussoni L, Ris P, Cattaneo MG, Vicentini L, Battaini F, Galli C, Tremoli E. Very low density lipoprotein-mediated signal transduction and plasminogen activator inhibitor type 1 in cultured HepG2 cells. *Circulat Res* 1999; 85: 208–17.
38. Banfi C, Eriksson P, Giandomenico G, Mussoni L, Sironi L, Hamsten A, Tremoli E. Transcriptional regulation of plasminogen activator inhibitor type 1 gene by insulin: insights into the signaling pathway. *Diabetes* 2001; 50: 1522–30.
39. Yu KC, Cooper AD. Postprandial lipoproteins and atherosclerosis. *Front Biosci* 2001; 6: D332–54.
40. Jeppesen J, Hollenbeck CB, Zhou MY, Coulston AM, Jones C, Chen YD, Reaven GM. Relation between insulin resistance, hyperinsulinemia, postheparin plasma lipoprotein lipase activity, and postprandial lipemia. *Arterioscler Thromb Vasc Biol* 1995; 15: 320–4.
41. Ruotolo G, Parlavecchia M, Taskinen MR, Galimberti G, Zoppo A, Le NA, Ragogna F, Micossi P, Pozza G. Normalization of lipoprotein composition by intraperitoneal insulin in IDDM. Role of increased hepatic lipase activity. *Diabetes Care* 1994; 17: 6–12.
42. Boquist S, Hamsten A, Karpe F, Ruotolo G. Insulin and non-esterified fatty acid relations to alimentary lipaemia and plasma concentrations of postprandial triglyceride-rich lipoproteins in healthy middle-aged men. *Diabetologia* 2000; 43: 185–93.
43. Schneeman BO, Kotite L, Todd KM, Havel RJ. Relationships between the responses of triglyceride-rich lipoproteins in blood plasma containing apolipoproteins B-48 and B-100 to a fat-containing meal in normolipidemic humans. *Proc Nat Acad Sci USA* 1993; 90: 2069–73.
44. Boquist S, Ruotolo G, Tang R, Bjorkegren J, Bond MG, de Faire U, Karpe F, Hamsten A. Alimentary lipemia, postprandial triglyceride-rich lipoproteins, and common carotid intima-media thickness in healthy, middle-aged men. *Circulation* 1999; 100: 723–8.
45. Descamps O, Bilheimer D, Herz J. Insulin stimulates receptor-mediated uptake of apoE-enriched lipoproteins and activated alpha 2-macroglobulin in adipocytes. *J Biol Chem* 1993; 268: 974–81.
46. Ko KW, Avramoglu RK, McLeod RS, Vukmirica J, Yao Z. The insulin-stimulated cell surface presentation of low density lipoprotein receptor-related protein in 3T3-L1 adipocytes is sensitive to phosphatidylinositide 3-kinase inhibition. *Biochemistry* 2001; 40: 752–9.
47. Phillips C, Bennett A, Anderton K, Owens D, Collins P, White D, Tomkin GH. Intestinal rather than hepatic microsomal triglyceride transfer protein as a cause of postprandial dyslipidemia in diabetes. *Metab Clin Exp* 2002; 51 (7): 847–52.
48. Phillips C, Owens D, Collins P, Tomkin GH. Microsomal triglyceride transfer protein: does insulin resistance

play a role in the regulation of chylomicron assembly? *Atherosclerosis* 2002; 160: 355–60.

49. Haffner SM, Mykkanen L, Valdez RA, Paidi M, Stern MP, Howard BV. LDL size and subclass pattern in a biethnic population. *Arterioscler Thromb* 1993; 13: 1623–30.
50. Howard BV, Robbins DC, Sievers ML, Lee ET, Rhoades D, Devereux RB, Cowan LD, Gray RS, Welty TK, Go OT, Howard WJ. LDL cholesterol as a strong predictor of coronary heart disease in diabetic individuals with insulin resistance and low LDL: The Strong Heart Study. *Arterioscler Thromb Vasc Biol* 2000; 20: 830–5.
51. Lund-Katz S, Laplaud PM, Phillips MC, Chapman MJ. Apolipoprotein B-100 conformation and particle surface charge in human LDL subspecies: implication for LDL receptor interaction. *Biochemistry* 1998; 37: 12867–74.
52. Garvey WT, Kwon S, Zheng D, Shaughnessy S, Wallace P, Hutto A, Pugh K, Jenkins AJ, Klein RL, Liao Y. Effects of insulin resistance and type 2 diabetes on lipoprotein subclass particle size and concentration determined by nuclear magnetic resonance. *Diabetes* 2003; 52: 453–62.
53. Santiago-Garcia J, Kodama T, Pitas RE. The class A scavenger receptor binds to proteoglycans and mediates adhesion of macrophages to the extracellular matrix. *J Biol Chem* 2003; 278: 6942–6.
54. Ohgami N, Nagai R, Ikemoto M, Arai H, Kuniyasu A, Horiuchi S, Nakayama H. Cd36, a member of the class b scavenger receptor family, as a receptor for advanced glycation end products. *J Biol Chem* 2001; 276: 3195–202.
55. Ohgami N, Nagai R, Miyazaki A, Ikemoto M, Arai H, Horiuchi S, Nakayama H. Scavenger receptor class B type I-mediated reverse cholesterol transport is inhibited by advanced glycation end products. *J Biol Chem* 2001; 276: 13348–55.
56. Jono T, Miyazaki A, Nagai R, Sawamura T, Kitamura T, Horiuchi S. Lectin-like oxidized low density lipoprotein receptor-1 (LOX-1) serves as an endothelial receptor for advanced glycation end products (AGE). *FEBS Lett* 2002; 511: 170–4.
57. Tamura Y, Adachi H, Osuga J, Ohashi K, Yahagi N, Sekiya M, Okazaki H, Tomita S, Iizuka Y, Shimano H, Nagai R, Kimura S, Tsujimoto M, Ishibashi S. FEEL-1 and FEEL-2 are endocytic receptors for advanced glycation end products. *J Biol Chem* 2003; 278: 12613–7.
58. Haffner SM, Morales PA, Stern MP, Gruber MK. Lp(a) concentrations in NIDDM. *Diabetes* 1992; 41: 1267–72.
59. Wang W, Hu D, Lee ET, Fabsitz RR, Welty TK, Robbins DC, Yeh JL, Howard BV, for the Strong Heart Study. Lipoprotein(a) in American Indians is low and not independently associated with cardiovascular disease. *Ann Epidemiol* 2002; 12: 107–14.
60. van't Hooft FM, Ruotolo G, Boquist S, de Faire U, Eggertsen G, Hamsten A. Human evidence that the apolipoprotein a-II gene is implicated in visceral fat accumulation and metabolism of triglyceride-rich lipoproteins. *Circulation* 2001; 104: 1223–8.
61. Torra IP, Chinetti G, Duval C, Fruchart JC, Staels B. Peroxisome proliferator-activated receptors: from transcriptional control to clinical practice. *Curr Opin Lipidol* 2001; 12: 245–54.
62. Hsueh WA, Law RE. PPARgamma and atherosclerosis: effects on cell growth and movement. *Arterioscler Thromb Vasc Biol* 2001; 21: 1891–5.
63. Chawla A, Boisvert WA, Lee CH, Laffitte BA, Barak Y, Joseph SB, Liao D, Nagy L, Edwards PA, Curtiss LK, Evans RM, Tontonoz P. A PPAR gamma-LXR-ABCA1 pathway in macrophages is involved in cholesterol efflux and atherogenesis. *Mol Cell* 2001; 7: 161–71.
64. Gurnell M. PPAR gamma and metabolism. Insights from the study of human genetic variants. *Clin Endocrinol* 2003; 59: 267–77.
65. Uehara Y, Engel T, Li Z, Goepfert C, Rust S, Zhou X, Langer C, Schachtrup C, Wiekowski J, Lorkowski S, Assmann G, von Eckardstein A. Polyunsaturated fatty acids and acetoacetate downregulate the expression of the ATP-binding cassette transporter A1. *Diabetes* 2002; 51: 2922–8.
66. Oliver WR Jr, Shenk JL, Snaith MR, Russell CS, Plunket KD, Bodkin NL, Lewis MC, Winegar DA, Sznaidman ML, Lambert MH, Xu HE, Sternbach DD, Kliewer SA, Hansen BC, Willson TM. A selective peroxisome proliferator-activated receptor delta agonist promotes reverse cholesterol transport. *Proc Nat Acad Sci USA* 2001; 98: 5306–11.
67. Lee CH, Chawla A, Urbiztondo N, Liao D, Boisvert WA, Evans RM. Transcriptional repression of atherogenic inflammation: modulation by PPAR{delta}. *Science* 2003; 302: 453–7.
68. Chawla A, Lee CH, Barak Y, He W, Rosenfeld J, Liao D, Han J, Kang H, Evans RM. PPARdelta is a very low-density lipoprotein sensor in macrophages. *Proc Natl Acad Sci USA* 2003; 100: 1268–73.

19

Insulin Regulation of Ketone Body Metabolism

Theodore P. Ciaraldi and Robert R. Henry

University of California San Diego, San Diego, CA, USA

INTRODUCTION

The energy needs of the body are met by multiple systems maintaining an exquisite balance between storage and utilization of metabolic substrates. In the fed state, dietary fats and ingested glucose provide sufficient energy for all tissues. Adipose tissue triglyceride (TG) represents the major storage form of energy producing substrate, accounting for >100 000 kcal of energy in a 70 kg person, compared to only ∼1600 kcal as glucose, the latter predominantly in the form of glycogen [1]. Most tissues can utilize either glucose or free fatty acid (FFA) to meet their energy needs, but not the brain, as FFA cannot cross the blood–brain barrier. With an overnight fast there is major depletion of glycogen stores. In that circumstance, muscle switches to oxidation of FFA, sparing circulating glucose for use by the brain, and providing glycerol, the other product of lipolysis, for hepatic gluconeogenesis. The acetyl-CoA produced by FFA oxidation is also used to synthesize the ketone bodies (ketogenesis), 3-hydroxybutyrate, and acetoacetate. Ketones are utilized by multiple tissues, but, most importantly, by the brain in the partial replacement of glucose. After an overnight fast, when glucose stores are still available, circulating levels of ketones are in the range 0.1–0.4 mM, but can increase with prolonged fasting to as high as 7–10 mM.

OVERVIEW OF INTEGRATED METABOLISM

Figure 1 displays a schematic representation of the major processes and tissues involved in ketogenesis. The initiating event is a change in the ratio of the concentrations of insulin and glucagon (see next section), resulting in stimulation of lipolysis [1] and the release of FFA from tissue stores, predominantly adipose tissue, though there is also a lesser mobilization of FFA from the TG stores of skeletal muscle and liver. FFAs are delivered from the circulation to the liver [2], the major site of ketone body production, though production can also occur in the intestine. Once in the liver, FFAs are either stored as TGs or enter the mitochondria to undergo β-oxidation, producing acetyl-CoA, which is either completely oxidized via the tricarboxylic acid (TCA) cycle or converted into ketone bodies [3]. Ketone bodies are then released into the circulation and utilized by tissues [4], primarily brain.

The possibility exists for regulation of ketone body production to occur at any, or all, of these processes. Indeed, the identity of the rate-determining step can shift, depending on a number of factors. Figure 2 outlines the key steps in adipose tissue regarding the provision of substrate for ketogenesis and indicates the first level of the relationship between glucose and FFA/TG metabolism. FFAs provided by the diet circulate in the form of chylomicrons and very low-density lipoprotein (VLDL) triglyceride. Lipoprotein lipase in the endothelium releases FFA from transfer particles for uptake by the adipocyte. While glucose in the adipocyte is not directly converted to FFA to any significant extent, glucose provides the glycerol-3-phosphate backbone for esterification with FFA to produce TG, the major storage form of lipid. TGs in the adipocyte are usually collected in one large storage droplet that is surrounded by the lipid-organizing molecule perilipin. One role of perilipin is to protect TG from lipolysis by excluding or limiting access of hormone-sentitive

International Textbook of Diabetes Mellitus, Third Edition. Edited by R. A. DeFronzo, E. Ferrannini, H. Keen, and P. Zimmet, 2004.
 ISBN: 0-471-48655-8.

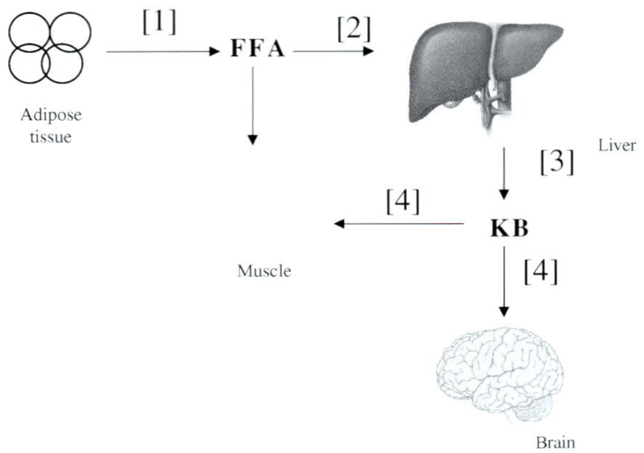

Figure 1 Key tissue and processes in ketone body metabolism. [1] – lipolyisis, [2] – hepatic FFA uptake, [3] – ketogenesis, [4] – utilization

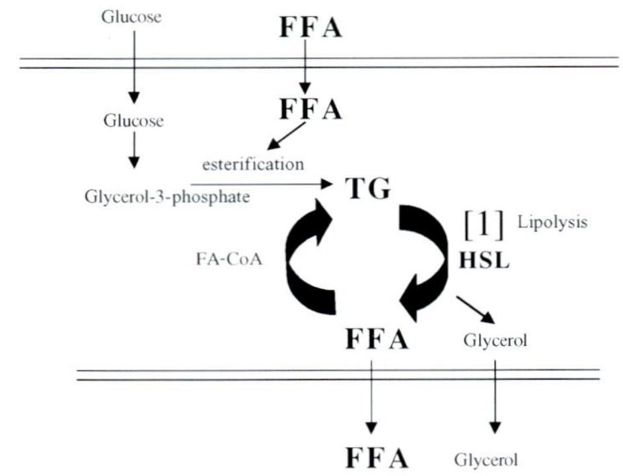

Figure 2 Pathways of FFA production and utilization in adipose tissue. Key process [1] taken from Figure 1. HSL – hormone-sensitive lipase; FA-CoA – fatty acyl-CoA

lipase (HSL) from the lipid droplet. The stimulus–response sequence in adipocytes initiated by lipolytic stimuli, such as epinephrine (Table 1), includes activation of adenylate cyclase, stimulation of protein kinase A (reviewed in reference 2) and phosphorylation of both HSL and perilipin (reviewed in reference 3). Phosphorylation of perilipin disrupts the structure surrounding the lipid droplet, while phosphorylation of HSL both activates the enzyme and results in redistribution of HSL from the cytosol to the lipid droplet [2], where lipolysis occurs. The two products of lipolysis, FFA and glycerol, are released from the adipocyte into the circulation; FFA is directed to the liver and muscle for oxidation and/or incorporation into TG, while glycerol is taken up by the liver to serve as a substrate for gluconeogenesis. FFA can also be reesterified back to TG in the adipocyte. It has been previously thought that, because of the absence of glycerol kinase in adipose tissue, glycerol could not be reutilized by that tissue. However, a recent study in cultured adipose cells indicates that glycerol kinase expression can be induced in adipocytes under certain conditions [4], providing additional glycerol-3-phosphate for reesterification beyond that provided by glucose, sparing glucose for other fates.

A second potential regulatory process is hepatic uptake of FFA. However, studies measuring arteriovenous differences across the liver *in vivo*, as well as in isolated perfused livers, have indicated that the major determinant of hepatic FFA uptake is the circulating concentration of FFA [5, 7]. Hepatic FFA uptake also appears to be unaltered by either hormones [5] or physiological state [5, 8, 9].

There are two major fates for FFAs once they enter the liver: esterification with glycerol-3-phosphate back into TG or entry into the mitochondria with subsequent β-oxidation, resulting in either total oxidation to CO_2 and H_2O or ketone body production (Figure 3).

While medium-chain fatty acids (MCFAs) can easily enter the mitochondria, long-chain fatty acyl-CoA (FA-CoA) esters are not freely permeable across the inner mitochondrial membrane. Rather, entry of long-chain fatty acid (LCFA) into the mitochondrial matrix occurs via a carnitine-CoA shuttle, a two-step process. Under most conditions it is the action of this system that is rate-limiting for LCFA entry into the mitochondria. The first step in this process, esterification of the LCFA to carnitine, with release of CoA into the cytoplasm, is catalyzed by carnitine palmitoyl transferase I (CPT-I). Once inside the mitochondria, long-chain FA-CoA is regenerated by a reversal of the CPT-I reaction, a process mediated by carnitine palmitoyltransferase II (CPT-II).

Table 1 Hormonal regulation of ketone body metabolism

Process	Insulin	Glucagon	Growth hormone	Epinephrine	Thyroid hormone
[1] Lipolysis	↓	↑	↑	↑	↑
HSL	↓	↑		↑	↑
[2] Fatty acid uptake	→	→		→	
[3] Ketogenesis	↓	↑*	↑ (?)	↑	↑ (?)
CPT-I	↓	↑		↑ (?)	↑
HMG-CoA synthase	↓			↑	
[4] Ketone body clearance	↑				↑ (?)

Note: Numbers in square brackets refer to processes presented in Figure 1. (?) indicates conflicting data in literature. HSL = hormone-sensitive lipase; CPT-I = carnitine palmitoyltransferase-I; HMG-CoA = hydroxymethylglutaryl-CoA.
* Response occurs only with a relative or profound deficiency of insulin.

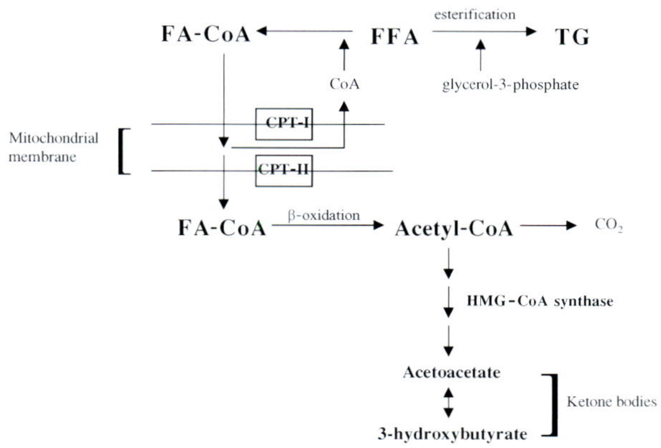

Figure 3 Pathways of hepatic FFA metabolism and ketogenesis

Entry of FAs into the mitochondrial matrix occurs through the concerted efforts of CPT-I and CPT-II. The proteins are products of different genes (reviewed in reference 10). CPT-II is a 658 AA protein in humans, with several crucial differences between it and CPT-I. The most important is that CPT-II is insensitive to malonyl-CoA, placing acute regulation at CPT-I. CPT-II is also only loosely associated with the inner mitochondrial membrane and retains its activity upon solubilization [11].

Several lines of evidence point to uptake of LCFA into the mitochondria via CPT-I as a control point in ketogenesis. One potentially useful tool is the fact that, unlike LCFA, medium chain (MC) FA-CoA esters can freely cross the mitochondrial membrane without esterification to carnitine, obviating the need for CPT-I [12]. McGarry and Foster exploited this property by comparing the metabolism of the LCFA oleic acid and the MCFA octanoate. Isolated livers from fasted rats displayed elevated (five- to sevenfold) ketogenesis, compared to livers from fed rats, when oleic acid was presented as substrate. However, when the livers were perfused with octanoate the extent of ketone formation was similar for both fed and fasted livers [13]. Thus, the ultimate ketogenic capacity of the liver was the same in the fed and fasted state; it was the delivery of the LCFA substrate to the mitochondrial matrix that was upregulated with fasting.

Given its importance as the key control point in FA oxidation and ketogenesis, CPT-1 has been a topic of considerable research interest. Two forms of CPT-I have been identified; the liver (L or α) and muscle (M or β) isoforms. Although quite similar in amino acid (AA) sequence (773 AA for L-CPT-I, 772 AA for M-CPT-I) they are products of different genes (10). The major difference between L- and M-CPT-I is that the latter is far more sensitive to malonyl-CoA ($IC_{50} = 0.03$ μM vs 2.5 mM for the liver form) [14]. The original designations of L- and M-CPT-I came from the tissues in which they were first identified. However, their distribution is not limited to those tissues. L-CPT-I is broadly distributed, present at high levels in kidney, intestine, pancreas, and ovary, amongst others, as well as liver; expression is low in heart, white adipose tissue, brown adipose tissue, skeletal muscle, and testis. Conversely, M-CPT-I is most abundant in those tissues with little L-CPT-I: skeletal muscle, brown and white adipocytes, and testis [15]. While M-CPT-I is the predominant form in heart, there is sufficient L-CPT-I in that tissue to contribute to overall CPT-I activity [10]. For a consideration of ketogenesis, attention must necessarily focus on L-CPT-1. One property of CPT-I that has hindered study is that the protein is tightly associated with the outer mitochondrial membrane; solubulization of the membrane results in a near total loss of activity [11].

Regulation of CPT-I occurs at several levels. Most important is the inhibition of activity by malonyl-CoA. In the fed state, when the insulin/glucagon ratio is high, there is increased flux through glycolysis and the provision of substrate for lipogenesis [16]. Insulin also activates acetyl-CoA carboxylase (ACC), the enzyme driving the production of malonyl-CoA from acetyl-CoA. The net result is an increase in the level of this lipogenic precursor. Malonyl-CoA inhibition of CPT-I then reduces FA oxidation, preventing a futile cycle of synthesis and degradation (lipogenesis/oxidation). Malonyl-CoA inhibition of CPT-I activity is mixed in nature, both allosteric and partially competitive [13]. This inhibition is also subject to regulation, as insulin increases the affinity of CPT-I for malonyl-CoA, making it a more effective inhibitor [17, 18].

In addition to acute regulation of CPT-I activity, the expression of CPT-I and -II are also under tight control. The mRNA for CPT-I is increased with fasting, just as the needs for FFA oxidation and ketogenesis increase [19]. CPT-I expression is also under substrate regulation, as LCFAs upregulate CPT-I mRNA [20–22]. This latter effect is thought to occur through the α form of the peroxisome-proliferator-activated receptor (PPARα) [22]. The PPARs are a family of nuclear receptors (α, β, and γ) that play crucial roles in the control of lipid metabolism [23]. The lipid-lowering fibrate drugs, which are selective ligands for PPARα, also increase the expression of both CPT-I and CPT-II [24]. Consistent with these observations, a PPAR response element (PPRE) has been identified on the promoter region of the CPT-I gene [25]. This PPRE is activated by ligands for both the α and γ members of the PPAR subfamily [25]. Conversely, insulin decreases gene expression of CPT-I [18].

Following transfer of FAs into the mitochondria, β-oxidation of FAs proceeds, generating acetyl-CoA. This acetyl-CoA proceeds through the series of reactions termed the hydroxymethylglutaryl-CoA (HMG-CoA) cycle, to produce acetoacetate and 3-hydroxybutyrate.

$$\text{2 acetyl-CoA} \xleftrightarrow{\text{acetoacetyl-CoA thiolase}} \text{acetoacetyl-CoA} + \text{CoA} \tag{1}$$

$$\text{acetoacetyl-CoA} + \text{acetyl-CoA} \xrightarrow{\text{HMG-CoA synthase}} \text{hydromethylglutaryl-CoA} + \text{CoA} \tag{2}$$

$$\text{Hydromethylglutaryl-CoA} \xrightarrow{\text{HMG-CoA lyase}} \text{acetoacetate} + \text{acetyl-CoA} \tag{3}$$

$$\text{acetoacetate} + \text{NADH} + \text{H}^+ \xleftrightarrow{\text{D-3-hydroxybutyrate DH}} \text{3-hydroxybutyrate} + \text{NAD}^+ \tag{4}$$

Equations 1 and 4 represent equilibrium reactions, while equations 2 and 3 are irreversible. The second reaction, and first committed step in ketogenesis, is catalyzed by HMG-CoA synthase, taken to be the rate-limiting enzyme for this process. Specifically, it is the mitochondrial form of HMG-CoA synthase that is important in ketogenesis, as another isoform, nonmitochondrial in localization, is pivotally involved in cholesterol biosynthesis [26]. As the next key control point in ketogenesis, regulation of HMG-CoA synthase, can occur at several levels. Activity of the enzyme is inversely correlated with cellular concentrations of succinyl-CoA. It turns out that the enzyme can be succinylated (reviewed in reference 26), providing acute inhibition of activity that is related to the balance of substrate fluxes. Control of the expression of HMG-CoA synthase can also be quite rapid. While starvation leads to increased mRNA levels for hepatic HMG-CoA synthase, upon refeeding there is a rapid reduction in mRNA, returning to baseline within 2.5 h [26]. Similarly, weaning is accompanied by a reduction in HMG-CoA synthase expression [26], as part of the transition from fatty acids as the primary exogenous substrate to an emphasis on glucose utilization. Conversely, specific dietary inputs can impact this system as well. Both 3-thia fatty acids [27] and saturated fats elevate HMG-CoA synthase mRNA, indicating another direct linkage between substrate availability and the capacity for ketogenesis. The reason for this relationship was revealed when it was discovered that the HMG-CoA synthase promoter also contains a PPRE [26, 28]. The major form of PPAR present in the liver, PPARα, can bind fatty acids and fibrate drugs, both of which upregulate HMG-CoA synthase mRNA [26, 29]. This indicates that sensing of FFA levels occurs at both the substrate and transcriptional levels. Interestingly, it has also been shown that HMG-CoA synthase can physically associate with PPARα in the liver and translocate into the nucelus [28], possibly regulating, in a feedback manner, its own transcription.

Consistent with the response to fasting, activation of protein kinase A, or dibutryl cAMP addition, upregulates HMG-CoA synthase mRNA. This occurs through cAMP response element (CRE) binding protein binding sites in the promoter of the HMG-CoA synthase gene [26]. Conversely, insulin can act acutely to downregulate mitochondrial HMG-CoA synthase mRNA in both liver and intestine while chronic hyperinsulinemia results in a further reduction in enzyme activity. The insulin effect on HMG-CoA synthase transcription could possibly occur through inhibition of the forkhead transcription factor (forkhead in rhabdosarcoma) (FKHRL1) [30].

IMPACT OF PATHOPHYSIOLOGICAL CONDITIONS ON KETOGENESIS

Ketone body levels increase with prolonged fasting, 2–20 days in duration, rising as high as 5–7 mM and usually peaking by 3 days of starvation [31]. This ketosis results from the concerted action of several responses: increased lipolysis, augmented hepatic ketogenesis beyond that due to the mass–action effect of increased substrate delivery, and reduced ketone body utilization in peripheral tissues, preserving the ketones for use by the brain [31, 32] (Table 2). All of these processes are opposed by insulin. Thus an initiating event in the adaptation to starvation is a reduction in the insulin/glucagon ratio [11]. The key role of insulin is further supported by the observation that the development of ketosis is delayed or reduced in hyperinsulinemic conditions such as obesity and type 2 diabetes (T2D) [11]. It is the lack of this constraining action of insulin that permits the development of ketoacidosis in insulin-deficient situations. A further limitation on the system is provided by the ability of circulating ketone bodies to inhibit both lipolysis and endogenous production of ketones [33].

Table 2 Ketone body metabolism in pathophysiological conditions

	Insulin-dependent diabetes	Type 2 diabetes	Starvation	Hyperthyroidism
[1] Lipolysis	↑	↑	↑	↑
[2] Fatty acid uptake	↑	↑ (?)	→	→
[3] Ketogenesis	↑	↑*	↑	↑
[4] Ketone body utilization	↓			

Note: Numbers in square brackets refer to processes in Figure 1. (?) indicates conflicting data in literature.
*Occurs in the presence of severe stress (e.g., sepsis).

Fasting FFA and ketone body levels are elevated in obese individuals, independent of the presence of normal or impaired glucose tolerance [34]. The higher ketone levels in obesity are most likely due to the higher substrate availability, as obese and non-obese subjects display similar β-hydroxybutyrate responses to changes in circulating FFA levels [31]. Suppression of FFA and ketone levels following an oral glucose load is also normal in obese individuals [35]. Several differences in ketone metabolism are apparent in obesity. Ketone body release into the blood in response to acetoacetate or β-hydroxybutyrate infusion is twofold greater in obese compared to non-obese individuals [32], indicating that ketone body clearance is decreased in obesity. Ketogenesis is also reduced in obese individuals with fatty liver [36].

Fasting FFA and ketone body levels are also elevated in insulin-dependent diabetic subjects [37]. This pattern is the result of several changes, one of which is increased substrate delivery due to reduced suppression of lipolysis as a consequence of insulin deficiency [32]. In this way the hormonal environment in the insulin-dependent diabetic is like that of starvation in the nondiabetic individual. In addition, FFA uptake across the splanchnic bed is higher in type 1 diabetics (T1D) [37]. The fraction of this FFA that is converted to ketones is threefold higher in diabetic subjects [32, 37]. One contributor to increased ketogenesis is a decreased affinity of CPT-1 for malonyl-CoA. In streptozotocin-treated rats this defect can be reversed with insulin treatment [18]. While sensitivity for the antilipolytic action of insulin is normal in T1D, the ketogenic response to epinephrine infusion is augmented at low insulin levels [38]. However higher insulin levels are able to suppress this response normally [37]. In addition to increased ketogenesis, clearance of ketones, especially β-hydroxybutyrate, is reduced in T1D [32]. This defect must occur at peripheral tissues because the transport and utilization of ketone bodies in the brain is normal in T1D patients [39].

The impact of T2D on ketone metabolism differs somewhat from that in T1D. In most T2D patients, both circulating FFA and total ketone body levels are elevated compared to those in normal individuals [40–43] and there is a strong correlation between FFA and ketone body levels [42]. However, non-obese T2D individuals have elevated (threefold) circulating ketone levels even in the presence of normal FFA levels [42, 43], suggesting greater conversion of FFA to ketones, albeit at a lower rate than observed in patients with T1D [43]. This increased ketogenesis occurs in the presence of elevated insulin levels [42], unlike the situations in starvation and T1D; yet glucagon levels are also elevated, leading to a lower than normal insulin/glucagon ratio. In addition, insulin sensitivity for reducing total ketone body levels, the balance of production and utilization, is reduced in T2D, independent of changes in insulin sensitivity for antilipolysis [44]. The regulation of hyperglycemia and ketosis in T2D is discordant in response to oral sulfonylurea agents. Sulfonylurea treatment reduces ketone body levels to a greater extent do than insulin or diet therapy, yet has a lesser effect on glucose levels [41]. A potential reason for this difference is that sulfonylureas have been shown to inhibit CPT-I, impairing fat oxidation and ketogenesis, at least in rat liver [45]. However, when FFA levels in sulfonylurea-treated patients with T2D are restored to pretreatment values, by heparin + intralipid infusion, total ketone body levels return to those seen in the absence of treatment [43], indicating that the sulfonylurea effect in humans may primarily involve FFA fluxes and not a direct effect on ketogenesis.

Hyperthyroid individuals display increases in circulating levels of glycerol, FFA, and ketone bodies [46, 47]. The primary contributor to this hyperlipidemia is elevated lipolysis from multiple adipose tissue depots [46]. A number of investigators have reported that hyperthyroid individuals also have an impaired ability of insulin to suppress lipolysis [46]. The induction of moderate hyperthyroidism in healthy individuals by thyroxine treatment did not replicate this behavior except in the presence of hypoinsulinemia [48], supporting the important role of basal insulin levels in counterbalancing thyroid hormone action. One cause of the increased circulating ketone body levels in hyperthyroidism is the augmented substrate delivery to the liver due to elevated lipolysis. Lipid oxidation is also increased in hyperthyroidism [49]. One reason for this is the fact that the expression of L-CPT-I is elevated in the liver of hyperthyroid rats, driven by thyroid response elements on the promoter of the L-CPT-I gene [50]. The effects of hyperthyroidism on ketogenesis itself are less clear. The percentage of FFA flux that is directed to ketone body production is higher in hyperthyroid individuals [47], compared to euthyroid subjects. However, when a TG infusion is used to elevate FFA levels in euthyroid subjects to the same levels as seen in the hyperthyroid subjects, this difference disappears [51], indicating that increased lipolysis and FFA delivery to the liver are the major reason for elevated ketone body levels in hyperthyroidism, and not a direct effect on ketogenesis [52].

CONCLUSION

The key to hormonal control of ketone body metabolism is the insulin level. In circumstances of relatively higher insulin levels, such as in the fed state, FFAs are directed toward storage, with glucose utilized to meet the energy needs of the body. When insulin levels are decreased, such as with fasting or starvation and T1D, FFA oxidation is increased and ketone bodies produced to fill that role. Insulin acts at three key processes in ketone metabolism: substrate availability (lipolysis), ketone body production (ketogenesis), and disposal (utilization). Insulin control of the exquisite balance between FFA storage and utilization, including conversion to ketone bodies, occurs at many levels including regulation of gene expression and posttranslational modulation of enzyme activity, with CPT-I being a crucial control point. Indeed, regulation of hepatic CPT-I expression or activity holds potential significance as an approach for controlling hyperglycemia and insulin resistance.

REFERENCES

1. Shulman GI, Barrett EJ, Sherwin RS. Integrated fuel metabolism. In Porte D, Sherwin RS, Baron A (eds), *Ellenberg & Rifkin's Diabetes Mellitus*. New York: McGraw-Hill, 2003; pp 1–13.
2. Holm C, Osterlund T, Laurell H, Contreras JA. Molecular mechanisms regulating hormone-sensitive lipase and lipolysis. *Annu Rev Nutr* 2000; 20: 365–93.
3. Londos C, Brasaemle DL, Schultz CJ, Adler-Wailes DC, Levin DM, Kimmel AR, Rondinone CM. On the control of lipolysis in adipocytes. *Ann NY Acad Sci* 1999; 892: 155–68.
4. Guan H-P, Li Y, Jensen MV, Newgard CB, Steppan CM, Lazar MA. A futile metabolic cycle activated in adipocytes by antidiabetic agents. *Nat Med* 2002; 8: 1122–8.
5. Fine MB, Williams RH. Effect of fasting, epinephrine and glucose and insulin on hepatic uptake on non-esterified fatty acids. *Am J Physiol* 1961; 199: 403–6.
6. Van Marken DR, Dixon CW, Heimberg M. Hepatic lipid metabolism in experimental diabetes, I: the effect of concentration of oleate on metabolism of triglycerides and on ketogenesis. *J. Biol Chem* 1969; 244: 2278–85.
7. Huang M. Saturating concentration for the uptake of free fatty acids and release of ketone bodies in vivo (in rat liver. *Life Sci* 1997; 60: 1915–22.
8. Hagenfeldt L, Wennlung A, Felig P, Wahren J. Turnover and splanchnic metabolism of free fatty acids in hyperthyroid patients. *J Clin Invest* 1981; 67: 1672–7.
9. Sorrentin D, Stump DD, Zhou SL, Van Ness K, Isola LM, Berk PD. The hepatocellular uptake of free fatty acids is selectively preserved during starvation. *Gastroenterology* 1994; 107: 1415–24.
10. McGarry JD, Brown NF. The mitochondrial carnitine palmitoyltransferase system. *Eur J Biochem* 1997; 244: 1–14.
11. Woeltje KF, Kuwajima M, Foster DW, McGarry JD. Characterization of the mitochondrial carnitine palnitoyltransferase enzyme system, II: Use of detergents and antibodies. *J Biol Chem* 1987; 262: 9822–7.
12. McGarry JD, Foster DW. Ketogenesis. In Porte D, Sherwin RS, Baron A (eds), *Ellenberg & Rifkin's Diabetes Mellitus*. New York: McGraw-Hill, 2003; pp 15–22.
13. McGarry JD, Foster DW. The regulation of ketogenesis from octanoic acid. The role of the tricayboxylic acid cycle and fatty acid synthesis. *J Biol Chem* 1971; 246: 1149–59.
14. Declercq PE, Falck JR, Kuwajima M, Tyminski H, Foster DW, McGarry JD. Characterization of the mitochondrial carnatine palmitoyltransferase enzyme system, I: use of inhibitors. *J Biol Chem* 1987; 262: 9812–21.
15. Weis BC, Esser DW, Foster DW, McGarry JD. Rat heart expresses two forms of mitochondrial carnitine palmitoyltransferase I. The minor component is identical to the liver enzyme. *J Biol Chem* 1994; 69: 18712–5.
16. Randle PJ. Regulatory interactions between lipids and carbohydrates: the glucose fatty acid cycle after 35 years. *Diabetes/Metab Rev* 1998; 4: 263–83.
17. Gamble MS, Cook GA. Alteration of the apparent K_i of carnitine palmitoyltransferase for malonyl-CoA by the diabetic state and reversal by insulin. *J Biol Chem* 1985; 60: 9516–9.
18. Park EA, Mynatt RL, Cook GA, Kashfi K. Insulin regulates enzyme activity, malonyl-CoA sensitivity and mRNA abundance of hepatic carnitine palmitoyltransferase-1. *Biochem J* 1995; 310: 853–8.
19. Arias G, Asins G, Hegardt FG, Serra D. The effect of fasting/refeeding and insulin treatment on the expression of the regulatory gene of ketogenesis in intestine and liver of suckling rats. *Arch Biochem Biophys* 1997; 349: 287–98.
20. Assimacopoulos-Jeannet F, Thumelin S, Roche E, Esser V, McGarry JD, Prentki M. Fatty acids rapidly induce the carnitine palmitoyltransferase I gene in the pancreatic β-cell line INS-1. *J Biol Chem* 1997; 72: 1659–64.
21. Brandt JM, Djouadi F, Kelly DP. Fatty acids activate transcription of the muscle carnitine palmitoyltransferase I gene in cardiac myocytes via the peroxisome proliferator-activated receptor alpha. *J Biol Chem* 1998; 273: 23786–92.
22. Chatelain F, Kohl C, Esser V, McGarry JD, Girard J, Pegorier JP. Cyclic AMP and fatty acids increase carnitine palmitoyltransferase I gene transcription in cultured fetal rat hepatocytes. *Eur J Biochem* 1996; 35: 789–98.
23. Spiegelman BM. PPAR-gamma: adipogenic regulator and thiazolidinedione receptor. *Diabetes* 1998; 47: 507–14.
24. Minnic A, Tian N, Byan L, Bilder G. A potent PPARalpha agonist stimulates mitochondrial fatty acid beta-oxidation in liver and skeletal muscle. *Am J Physiol Endocrinol Metab* 2001; 280: E270–9.
25. Mascaro C, Acosta E, Ortiz JA, Marrero PF, Hegardt FG, Haro D. Control of human muscle-type carnitine palmitoyltransferase I gene transcription by peroxisome proliferator-activated receptor. *J Biol Chem* 1998; 273: 8560–3.
26. Hegardt FG. Mitochondrial 3-hydroxy-3-methylglutaryl-CoA synthase: a control enzyme in ketogenesis. *Biochem J* 1999; 338: 569–82.
27. Madsen L, Garras A, Asins G, Serra D, Hegardt FG, Berge RK. Mitochondrial 3-hydroxy-3-methylglutaryl coenzyme a synthase and carnitine palmitoyltransferase II as potential control sites for ketogenesis during mitochondrion and peroxisome proliferation. *Biochem Pharmacol* 1999; 57: 1011–9.
28. Meertens LM, Miyata KS, Cechetto JD, Rachubinski RA, Capone JP. A mitochondrial ketogenic enzyme regulates its gene expression by association with the nuclear hormone receptor PPARalpha. *EMBO J* 1998; 17: 6972–8.
29. Cullingford TE, Dolphin CT, Sato H. The peroxisome proliferator-activated receptor alpha-selective activator ciprofibrate upregulates expression of genes encoding fatty acid oxidation and ketogenesis enzymes in rat brain. *Neuropharmacology* 2002; 42: 724–30.
30. Nadal A, Marrero PF, Haro D. Down-regulation of the mitochondrial 3-hydroxy-3-methylglutaryl-CoA synthase gene by insulin: the role of the forkhead transcription factor FKHRL1. *Biochem J* 2002; 366: 289–97.

31. Grey NJ, Karl I, Kipnis DM. Physiologic mechanisms in the development of starvation ketosis in man. *Diabetes* 1975; 24: 10–6.
32. Hall SE, Wastney ME, Bolton TM, Braaten JT, Berman M. Ketone body kinetics in humans: the effects of insulin-dependent diabetes, obesity, and starvation. *J Lipid Res* 1984; 25: 1184–94.
33. Keller U, Gerber PP, Stauffacher W. Stimulatory effect of norepinephrine on ketogenesis in normal and insulin-deficient humans. *Am J Physiol* 1984; 247: E732–9.
34. Krentz AJ, Singh BM, Hale PJ, Robertson DA, Nattrass M. Basal intermediary metabolism in impaired glucose tolerance and morbid obesity. *Diabetes Res* 1992; 20: 51–60.
35. Robertson DA, Singh BM, Nattrass M. Effect of obesity on circulating intermediary metabolite concentrations in the absence of impaired glucose tolerance. *Int J Obes* 1991; 15: 635–45.
36. Inokuchi T, Orita M, Imamura K, Takao T, Isogai S. Resistance to ketosis in moderately obese patients: influence of fatty liver. *Intern Med* 1992; 31: 978–83.
37. Wahren J, Sato Y, Ostman J, Hagenfeldt L, Felig P. Turnover and splanchnic metabolism of free fatty acids and ketones in insulin-dependent diabetics at reat and in response to exercise. *J Clin Invest* 1984; 73: 1367–76.
38. Avogaro A, Valerio A, Gnudi L, Maran A, Miola M, Duner E, Marescotti C, Iori E, Tiengo A, Nosadini R. The effects of different plasma insulin concentrations on lipolytic and ketotic responses to epinephrine in normal and type 1 (insulin-dependent) diabetic humans. *Diabetologia* 1992; 35: 129–38.
39. Blomqvist G, Alvarsson M, Grill V, Von Heijne G, Ingvar M, Thorell JO, Stone-Elander S, Widen L, Ekberg K. Effect of acute hyperketonemia on the cerebral uptake of ketone bodies in nondiabetic subjects and IDDM patients. *Am J Physiol Endocrinol Metab* 2002; 283: E20–8.
40. Okuda Y, Kawai K, Murayama Y, Yamashita K. Postprandial changes in plasma ketone body and carnitine levels in normal and non-insulin-dependent diabetic subjects. *Endocrinol Japanica* 1987; 34: 415–22.
41. Suzuki M, Kosegawa I, Miura S, Negishi K, Itabashi A, Katayama S, Ishii J, Kamata S, Fujita C. Blood ketone bodies in NIDDM: relationship with diabetic control and endogenous insulin secretion. *Diabetes Res* 1991; 18: 11–7.
42. Avogaroi A, Crepaldi C, Miola M, Maran A, Pengo V, Tiengo A, Del Prato S. High blood ketone body concentration in type 2 non-insulin dependent diabetic patients. *J Endocrinol Invest* 1996; 19: 99–105.
43. Avogaro A, Valerio A, Gnudi L, Maran A, Zolli M, Duner E, Riccio A, Del Prato S, Tiengo A, Nosadini R. Ketone body metabolism in NIDDM. Effect of sulfonylurea treatment. *Diabetes* 1992; 41: 968–74.
44. Singh BM, Krentz AJ, Nattrass M. Insulin resistance in the regulation of lipolysis and ketone body metabolism in non-insulin dependent diabetes is apparent at very low insulin concentrations. *Diabetes Res Clin Pract* 1993; 20: 55–62.
45. Cook GA. The hypoglycemic sulfonylureas glyburide and tolbutamide inhibit fatty acid oxidation by inhibiting carnitine palmitoyltransferase. *J Biol Chem* 1987; 262: 4968–72.
46. Riis ALD, Gravholt CH, Djurhuus CB, Norrelund H, Jorgensen JOL, Weeke J, Moller N. Elevated regional lipolysis in hyperthyroidism. *J Clin Endocrinol Metab* 2002; 87: 4747–53.
47. Beylot M, Martin C, Laville M, Riou JP, Cohen R, Mornex R. Lipolytic and ketogenic fluxes in human hyperthyroidism. *J Clin Endocrinol Metab* 1991; 3: 42–9.
48. Muller MJ, Acheson KJ, Jequier E, Burger AG. Thyroid hormone action on lipid metabolism in humans: a role for endogenous insulin. *Metabolism* 1990; 39: 480–5.
49. Randin JP, Scazziga B, Jequier E, Felber JP. Study of glucose and lipid metabolism by continuous indirect calorimetry in Graves's disease: effect of an oral glucose load. *J Clin Endocrinol Metab* 1985; 61: 1165–71.
50. Jansen MS, Cook GA, Song S, Park EA. Thyroid hormone regulates carnitine palmitoyltransferase Ia gene expression through elements in the promoter and first intron. *J Biol Chem* 2000; 275: 34989–97.
51. Beylot M, Martin C, Laville M, Riou JP, Cohen R, Mornex R. Lipolytic and ketogenic fluxes in human hyperthyroidism. *J Clin Endocrinol Metab* 1991; 73: 42–9.
52. Beylot M. Regulation of in vivo ketogenesis: role of free fatty acids and control by epinephrine, thyroid hormones, insulin and glucagon. *Diabetes Metab* 1996; 22: 299–304.

Pathogenesis

20

The Insulin Resistance Syndrome

Hannele Yki-Järvinen

Helsinki University, Helsinki, Finland

INTRODUCTION

Insulin resistance denotes the inability of insulin to produce its usual biological effects at circulating concentrations that are effective in normal subjects. Resistance can develop to all aspects of insulin action for many different reasons to degrees that vary between and within individuals. However, the most common condition associated with insulin resistance is that at least in part attributable to an increasingly sedentary lifestyle. In such individuals, multiple risk factors (hyperinsulinemia, dysglycemia, high triglycerides and low high-density-lipoprotein (HDL) cholesterol, hypertension, often obesity particularly of the abdominal type, and various other metabolic abnormalities) co-occur more often than would be expected by chance alone. This condition is associated with a two- to threefold increased risk of developing type 2 diabetes and cardiovascular disease and has been variously referred to as *the insulin resistance syndrome, syndrome X, or the metabolic syndrome* [1]. Insulin resistance is the key pathophysiologic feature of the syndrome, since its components are either causes or consequences of impaired insulin action. To help identification of the syndrome, the World Health Organization (WHO) [2] and the National Cholesterol Education Program (NCEP) [3] expert panel have published formal definitions (Table 1). According to these definitions the insulin resistance syndrome has been estimated to affect 25% of adults [4, 5]. This chapter discusses the definition, components, and significance of the insulin resistance syndrome. Candidate genes of insulin resistance are discussed in Chapter 24 and lessons from genome scans in Chapter 23. A detailed discussion on the relationship between obesity, location of fat depots, and insulin resistance can be found in Chapter 33. The impact of insulin resistance on lipid and lipoprotein metabolism is discussed in detail in Chapter 18.

INSULIN RESISTANCE, GENERAL

As discussed in detail elsewhere, insulin has a wide variety of effects on glucose (see Chapter 16), lipid (see Chapter 18), protein (see Chapter 17), and ketone body (see Chapter 19) metabolism. In addition, insulin regulates vascular and platelet function, electrolyte balance, and the activity of the autonomic nervous system. A defect in any of these multiple actions of insulin could be defined as insulin resistance. The tissues and actions that are resistant to insulin display marked interindividual variation due to physiological, environmental, and genetic causes. Table 2 lists some of the known causes of physiological variation in insulin sensitivity and causes of insulin resistance [34], as assessed by the euglycemic clamp technique, which provides a golden standard measure of insulin action on whole-body glucose metabolism [35]. These causes need to be considered in the differential diagnosis before attributing insulin resistance to "the insulin resistance syndrome," which, albeit clinically useful, represents an oversimplification of a heterogeneous, biologically continuous, and complex phenomenon.

THE INSULIN RESISTANCE SYNDROME HISTORY, DEFINITION, AND PREVALENCE

History

The history of the insulin resistance syndrome dates back to postmortem descriptions by Morgagni of both atherosclerosis and visceral obesity in noble persons whose lifestyle was characterized by "literary studies, sedentary life-style and abundant meals" [36]. In more modern times, an important landmark in the history of the insulin resistance syndrome was classification of obese subjects according to the degree of "masculine differentiation" into

International Textbook of Diabetes Mellitus, Third Edition. Edited by R. A. DeFronzo, E. Ferrannini, H. Keen, and P. Zimmet.
 ISBN: 0-471-48655-8.

Table 1 Modified NCEP and WHO definitions of the metabolic syndrome in men

NCEP definition	Modified WHO definition
At least 3 of the following: Fasting plasma glucose ≥110 mg/l Abdominal obesity Definition 1: Metabolic syndrome, NCEP definition with waist girth >102 cm Definition 2: Metabolic syndrome, NCEP definition with waist girth > 94 cm Serum triglycerides ≥150 mg/dl Serum HDL cholesterol <40 mg/dl Blood pressure ≥ 130/85 mmHg or medication	Hyperinsulinemia (upper quartile of the nondiabetic population) or fasting plasma glucose ≥110 mg/dl AND At least 2 of the following: Abdominal obesity Definition 1: Metabolic syndrome, WHO definition with waist-to-hip ratio > 0.90 or BMI ≥ 30 kg/m^2 Definition 2: Metabolic syndrome, WHO definition with waist girth ≥ 94 cm Dyslipidemia (serum triglycerides ≥150 mg/dl or HDL cholesterol <35 mg/dl) Hypertension (blood pressure ≥ 140/90 mmHg or medication)

Note: NCEP = National Cholesterol Education Program; WHO = World Health Organization; BMI = body mass index (calculated as weight in kilograms divided by the square of height in meters); HDL = high-density lipoprotein. To convert plasma glucose from mg/dl to mmol/ml, multiply by 0.0555; to convert serum triglycerides from mg/dl to mmol/l, multiply by 0.0113; and to convert serum HDL cholesterol from mg/dl to mmol/l, multiply by 0.0259. From references 2 and 3.

those with "gynoid" and those with "android" obesity by Vague in 1947 [37]. Gynoid obesity was characterized by lower-body deposition of fat (around the thighs and buttocks) and relative underdevelopment of the musculature, while android obesity defined upper-body (truncal) adiposity, greater muscular development and a tendency to develop hypertension, diabetes, atherosclerosis, and gout. These observations have subsequently been confirmed in prospective studies [38–41]. Other important contributions were development of methods to determine free fatty acid (FFA) [42] and insulin concentrations, the finding of hyper- rather than hypoinsulinemia in patients with type 2 diabetes [43], and development of the euglycemic insulin clamp technique as a golden standard method for

Table 2 Causes of Variation in Insulin Action

Factor	Change in insulin sensitivity	Reference
Physiological variations		
• Physical training, increased muscle mass	↑	[6, 7]
• Increased fat mass	↓	[8]
• Puberty	↓	[9]
• Pregnancy	↓	[10]
• Gender	Female > male	[11]
• Menstrual cycle	No effect	[12, 13]
Diet-induced changes		
• Overfeeding	↓	[14]
• Starvation	↓	[15]
• Alcohol (acutely)	↓	[16]
• Saturated vs. monounsaturated fat	↓	[17]
Metabolite and electrolyte disturbances		
• High free fatty acid concentrations	↓	[18]
• Chronic hyperglycemia	↓	[19]
• Hypoglycemia	↓	[20]
• Acidosis	↓	[21]
• Hyperosmolality	↓	[22]
• Hypophosphatemia	↓	
Other causes		
• Excessive secretion of counterregulatory hormones		
– Physical and mental stress	↓	[23, 24]
– Hypoglycemic counterregulation	↓	[25]
– Acromegaly, Cushing's, phaeochromocytoma	↓	[26–28]
• Growth hormone deficiency	↓	[29]
• Hypo- and hyperthyroidism	↑	[30]
• Nonalcoholic fatty liver disease	↓	[31]
• Uremia	↓	[32]
• Many infections	↓	[33]

quantification of whole-body insulin sensitivity [35]. Discovery of the glucose–fatty acid cycle [44] and of hyperinsulinemia [45] in patients with an acute myocardial infarction also added to the understanding of components of the syndrome. Several cases suggesting a close correlation between obesity, dysglycemia, and hyperlipidemia were described long before formal definition of the insulin resistance syndrome [46]. Finally, formal naming the co-occurrence of resistance to insulin-stimulated glucose uptake, glucose intolerance, hyperinsulinemia, increased very low density lipoprotein (VLDL) triglycride, decreased HDL cholesterol, and hypertension "syndrome X" was an important practical step [1].

Definition and Prevalence

The WHO initially proposed a definition of the metabolic syndrome in 1998 as described in Table 1 [2]. Later, the Third Report of the National Cholesterol Education Program Expert Panel on Detection, Evaluation and Treatment of High Blood Cholesterol in Adults (Adult Treatment Panel III, ATP III) provided another working definition of the syndrome [3]. In the United States in the Third National Health and Nutrition Examination Survey performed between 1988 and 1994, the age-adjusted prevalence in individuals aged 20 or older was 25% using the WHO and 24% using the ATP III definition [4, 5]. Among all participants in this survey, 86% were similarly classified under the two definitions. Defined by ATP III criteria, the prevalence increased from 6.7% among participants aged 20–29 years to 43.5% for those aged 60–69 years [4] (Figure 1). The prevalence differed little between men and women. It was highest among Mexican Americans (31.9%) and lowest among Whites (23.8%). In the Third National Health and Nutrition Examination Survey (NHANES III), in adults older than 50, 44% of the US population met the NCEP criteria [47]. In patients with diabetes, the prevalence of the insulin resistance syndrome was 86%. The prevalence of

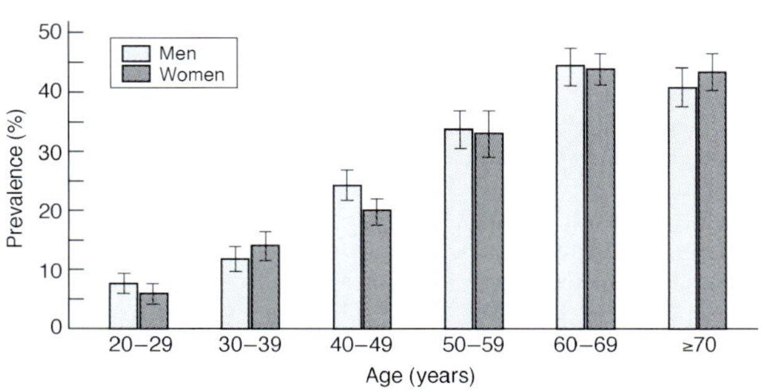

Figure 1 Age-specific prevalence of the metabolic syndrome among 8814 US adults aged at least 20 years, by gender, NHANES III 1988–1994. (Reproduced with permission from reference 4)

coronary heart disease (CHD) was increased only in patients with diabetes and the syndrome, not in those without it [47]. In Europe, the frequency of the WHO syndrome was reported to be between 7 and 36% for men 40–55 years, and for women of the same age, between 5 and 22% [48]. There was large variation in the frequency of the syndrome between different populations, due to the differing frequencies of the components and possibly differing methodologies of measurement.

COMPONENTS OF THE INSULIN RESISTANCE SYNDROME

Lessons from Epidemiology

Factors Analyses of Components Included in the Definition of Insulin Resistance Syndrome

The term insulin resistance syndrome implies that insulin resistance indeed is a unifying underlying abnormality, i.e. that the components are either causes or consequences of insulin resistance. This unity hypothesis has been formally tested by use of factor analysis in epidemiological studies [49–65]. Factor analysis allows a confusingly large number of apparently related risk variables to be reduced to a simpler set of underlying physiologic phenotypes. Finding more than one factor contradicts the unity hypothesis. In studies trying to define relations among metabolic risk variables using factor analysis, the number of factors identified in different populations has ranged from two to four. The most commonly observed phenotypes in the factor analyses listed above have been an "obesity–hyperinsulinemia–dysglycemia" factor, a lipid factor, and a blood pressure factor. Of these the blood pressure factor has consistently been very loosely associated with other features of the insulin resistance syndrome. These data suggest that while components of the insulin resistance co-occur, factors other than insulin resistance regulate some components of the insulin resistance syndrome, especially blood pressure.

Other Possible Components of the Insulin Resistance Syndrome

In addition to the components included in the definition of the insulin resistance syndrome (Table 1), *uric acid* was found to correlate with or "load on" the same factor as body mass index (BMI) and insulin/glucose in three studies [53, 55, 62], *plasminogen activator inhibitor 1* (PAI-1) with BMI in the Cardiovascular Health Study [62], *small LDL size* with high triglycerides–low HDL cholesterol in the Kaiser Permanente Women Twins Study [58]. In the Quebec Cardiovascular Study, fasting *plasma FFA* levels correlated with triglyceride concentrations and low-density-lipoprotein (LDL) size but did not improve the ability to predict cardiovascular disease after adjustment for other components of insulin resistance [66].

Microalbuminuria is characterized by an increase in the urinary albumin rate or the urinary albumin/creatinine ratio in the absence of clinically significant renal disease, and predicts overt diabetic nephropathy in patients with type 1 diabetes [67, 68]. In type 2 diabetes, microalbuminuria predicts cardiovascular rather than renal disease [69]. Insulin resistance has been associated with microalbuminuria in relatives of type 2 diabetes [70] and in nondiabetic subjects [71]. In the latter study, which included 982 subjects, this relationship was attenuated after adjustment for age, sex, ethnicity, hypertension, fasting glucose, and BMI, but it still remained significant. In a sample of Finnish nondiabetic men, however, the urinary albumin/creatinine ratio was closely correlated with blood pressure and not an independent component of the insulin resistance syndrome [57]. The mechanisms mediating the association between microalbuminuria and insulin resistance are poorly understood and the data still perhaps insufficient to justify inclusion of microalbuminuria in the insulin resistance syndrome.

Serum C-reactive protein, a marker of the acute-phase reaction, has been shown to correlate with multiple features of the insulin resistance. Serum C-reactive protein correlated with weight, waist circumference, glucose, insulin, and HDL cholesterol in the Cardiovascular Health Study [62], and with body fat, waist circumference, the amount of visceral adipose tissue and insulin in adult men in Quebec [72]. Comparable relationships were reported for both men and women in a large Japanese population [73], and in healthy middle-aged women in the Netherlands [74]. In the Third National Health and Nutrition Examination Survey (1988–1994), elevated C-reactive protein was associated with higher insulin among men and women after adjustment for several confounding variables [75].

Low birth weight is suggested to predict the subsequent occurrence of insulin resistance and associated conditions including hypertension, dyslipidemia, type 2 diabetes, and CHD [76]. The associations were initially described in the United Kingdom but have subsequently been confirmed by studies from the United States, Australia, Asia, and elsewhere in Europe [77]. Long-term "programming" of tissue in early-life metabolism has been proposed to explain these findings [78, 79]. Fetal overexposure to glucocorticoids has specifically been suggested to play a role in the early-life programming of insulin resistance and perhaps hypertension [80].

Abnormalities in the Autonomic Nervous System

In insulin-resistant, obese subjects, basal sympathetic tone is increased and the subsequent response to insulin blunted [81]. This defect is also observed in nonobese but insulin-resistant subjects [82], and in patients with type 2 diabetes [83]. Lower heart rate variability has been associated with higher normetanephrine excretion in men drawn from the Whitehall II cohort [84].

Mechanistic Links Between the Components

Hyperinsulinemia, Dysglycemia

In cross-sectional and prospective studies, fasting and postload glucose and insulin concentrations are positively correlated in nondiabetic subjects [85, 86] (Figure 2). The increase in insulin concentrations is paralleled by a decrease in whole-body insulin sensitivity of glucose metabolism (Figure 2). Such resistance of glucose metabolism to insulin reflects defects in both the ability of insulin to inhibit hepatic glucose production and to stimulate glucose uptake in peripheral tissues (Figure 3). Increased FFA concentrations and resistance to the antilipolytic effect of insulin may contribute to worsening of hyperglycemia because of multiple interactions between FFA and glucose metabolism both in the liver and in skeletal

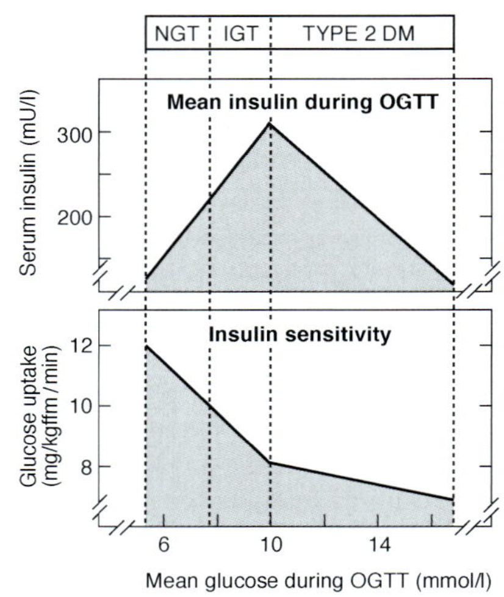

Figure 2 Natural history of type 2 diabetes. Upper panel: the relationship between mean glucose and mean insulin concentrations during an oral glucose tolerance test (OGTT), in individuals with normal (NGT), impaired (IGT), and diabetic (type 2 DM) glucose tolerance. There is a linear positive correlation between glucose and insulin concentrations during an OGTT in individuals with NGT and IGT. However, type 2 diabetes is characterized by worsening relative insulin deficiency; i.e., insulin concentrations decline with rising glucose concentrations. Bottom panel: the relationship between glucose concentrations during the OGTT and insulin sensitivity (determined by the euglycemic clamp technique). Insulin sensitivity decreases linearly as glucose tolerance worsens and, in patients with type 2 diabetes, insulin sensitivity worsens as glucose concentrations increase. This could be due to effects of chronic hyperglycemia *per se* on glucose uptake, or of relative insulin deficiency coupled with increases in FFA concentrations. kgffm = kilogram fat free mass. (Reproduced with permission from reference 85)

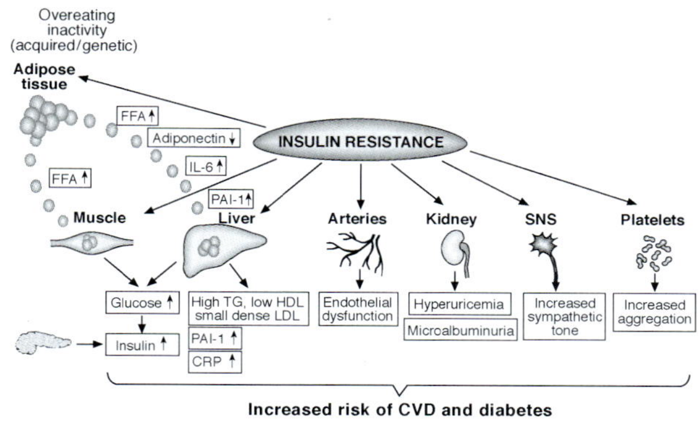

Figure 3 Causes and consequences of the insulin resistance syndrome. Overeating and inactivity are common and important but even among obese subjects, insulin resistance shows large interindividual variation. Subjects with triglyceride deposited within insulin-sensitive tissues such as liver and skeletal muscle are particularly insulin resistant. Insulin stimulates glucose uptake in skeletal muscle and inhibits hepatic glucose production; defects in these actions contribute to mild hyperglycemia and hyperinsulinemia, presumably because small increases in glucose concentrations stimulate β-cells to overproduce insulin to restore normoglycemia; failure of the β-cells to compensate in this way leads to worsening hyperglycemia and type 2 diabetes. Insulin has many other actions, including lowering of serum triglycerides via inhibition of hepatic VLDL production, inhibition of platelet aggregation and uric acid excretion in the kidney, stimulation of sympathetic nervous system activity, and possibly direct beneficial effects on endothelial function (via stimulation of nitric oxide production). In insulin-resistant individuals, many of these mostly antiatherogenic actions of insulin (lowering of glucose, triglycerides, inhibition of platelet aggregation) are blunted while some potentially harmful appear to be preserved (stimulation of sympathetic nervous system activity, inhibition of uric acid excretion). These alterations could explain why insulin resistance predisposes to atherothrombotic vascular disease. TG = triglyceride; HDL = high-density lipoprotein; LDL = low-density lipoprotein; CRP = C-reactive protein; FFA = free fatty acid; IL-6 = interleukin 6; PAI-1 = plasminogen activator inhibitor 1

muscle (see Chapter 16). The molecular mechanisms underlying insulin resistance of glucose uptake and production and the mechanisms through which FFA might interfere with these defects are discussed in Chapter d0310.

Obesity and Abdominal Obesity

Obesity is related to insulin resistance, although BMI accounts for only part of the variance in insulin sensitivity in the normal population. Nonetheless, insulin resistance generally increases in parallel with increasing body-fat mass. Obesity is associated with impaired insulin stimulation of glucose uptake and defect in the ability of insulin to inhibit endogenous glucose production and lipolysis in adipose tissue [8, 87] (see Chapter 34 obesity). These defects appear more severe in individuals with android (abdominal fat distribution) as compared to gynoid obesity. The enlarged adipose tissue mass in obesity is accompanied by changes in circulating levels of many hormones and metabolites. These include an increase in serum leptin (see Chapter 33) levels, which correlate closely with the size of the subcutaneous adipose tissue depot, a decrease in adiponectin (Chapter 34) and increases in serum IL-6 (interleukin 6) and FFA (see Chapter 34) concentrations. Adiponectin deficiency and increases in FFA induce insulin resistance in target tissues such as the liver and skeletal muscle [18, 88].

The mechanisms linking abdominal obesity to features of insulin resistance are controversial. It has been suggested that truncal obesity is harmful because it is accompanied by visceral fat accumulation within the abdomen; omental and mesenteric adipocytes have a higher rate of lipolysis than subcutaneous, and could liberate excessive amounts of FFA into the portal vein, thus causing the liver to become insulin-resistant. However, this "portal theory" lacks firm mechanistic evidence *in vivo* [89]. First, the limited data suggest that concentrations of FFA and glycerol in the portal vein are close to those in arterial plasma, and tracer studies have shown that FFA released within the splanchnic (visceral) bed contribute only about 10% of total FFA delivery to the liver [90]. Furthermore, although the turnover rate of FFA is higher in women with upper-body compared with lower-body obesity, the excess FFA originates from subcutaneous fat in the upper body rather than from the splanchnic bed [91].

Severe insulin resistance is a striking feature of several human lipodystrophy syndromes as well as certain mouse models that lack subcutaneous fat [92]. The absence of subcutaneous fat is accompanied by excessive triglyceride accumulation in insulin-sensitive tissues such as skeletal muscle and liver, and by typical defects in insulin signaling in the same tissues. The importance of confining triglyceride to its "appropriate" location within adipose tissue is graphically illustrated by the effects of transplanting normal adipose tissue subcutaneously into "fatless" transgenic mice: triglyceride is cleared from muscle and liver and redistributed into adipose tissue and insulin sensitivity is normalized [93].

In patients with type 2 diabetes, hepatic insulin sensitivity is closely correlated with hepatic triglyceride content [94], and skeletal muscle insulin sensitivity with intramyocellular fat [95–98]. The amount of fat in insulin-sensitive tissues also varies considerably in nondiabetic subjects, it increases as a function of overall and abdominal obesity but the relationship is weak [31, 95–99]. The amount of fat deposited in liver and muscle may thus explain why insulin sensitivity varies considerably at a given BMI. Low adiponectin production in adipose tissue may contribute to especially hepatic insulin resistance [88, 100]. The amount of fat in the liver is also correlated with other features of the insulin resistance syndrome, such as hypertriglyceridemia and increased plasma PAI-1 concentrations [31, 101].

Physical inactivity is not part of the definition of the insulin resistance syndrome but it should still be emphasized that physical training can greatly enhance insulin action, and there is a close and highly significant correlation between whole-body insulin sensitivity of glucose metabolism and maximal aerobic capacity (Vo_{2max}) [6, 102].

Hypertriglyceridemia and Low HDL Cholesterol

Evidence from both *in vitro* [103, 104] and *in vivo* [105] studies has suggested that insulin normally suppresses the production of VLDL particles from the liver (see Chapters 18 and 55). This effect is due not only to decreases in FFA availability following insulin inhibition of lipolysis in adipose tissue, but also to a direct hepatic effect of insulin, inhibiting the assembly and production of VLDL particles [106]. In contrast to normal subjects, insulin fails to suppress VLDL apoB production in type 2 diabetes, even though it profoundly suppresses FFA concentrations [107]. This intrahepatic defect appears to be a major contributory mechanism underlying the increase in serum triglycerides in insulin-resistant type 2 diabetic patients [108].

HDL levels are reduced in insulin-resistant patients with high serum triglycerides. Under hypertriglyceridemic conditions, there is excessive exchange of cholesterol esters and triglycerides between HDL and the expanded pool of triglyceride-rich lipoproteins, mediated by cholesterol ester transfer protein (CETP) [109]. HDL particles become enriched with triglycerides (and therefore separate in the lighter HDL_3 density range), and act as a good substrate for hepatic lipase, which now removes HDL particles at an accelerated rate. Subnormal activity of lipoprotein lipase (LPL), an enzyme that hydrolyzes circulating chylomicrons and VLDL triglyceride, and provides adipocytes with fatty acids, may further decrease levels of HDL cholesterol by decreasing the conversion of HDL_3 to HDL_2 particles [109]. Elevated concentrations of VLDL particles in the serum of patients with type 2 diabetes also increase the CETP-mediated exchange of cholesterol ester and triglyceride between VLDL and LDL particles [110]. This increases the triglyceride content of LDL particles and makes them a better substrate for hepatic lipase [111], which hydrolyzes triglycerides in the LDL particles and so decreases their size.

This sequence of events explains, at least in part, why subjects with the insulin resistance syndrome have a preponderance of small dense LDL particles [112, 113]. The small dense LDL particles are known to be highly atherogenic and provide a plausible link between insulin resistance and cardiovascular disease (*vide infra*) [114–116]. Men characterized by insulin resistance of glucose uptake, hypertriglyceridemia, and small dense LDL particles also have endothelial dysfunction, as determined from the blood flow response to an endothelium-dependent vasodilatary agent, compared to equally old and obese men with similar total LDL cholesterol concentrations [117].

Hypertension

As evidenced by the findings by factor analyses searching for components of the insulin resistance syndrome (*vide supra*), the association between insulin resistance and hypertension is perhaps the most controversial. Hypertension and insulin resistance have been shown to be linked, independently of confounding factors such as obesity [118], but the relationship appears inconsistent [119–121]. Numerous mechanisms have been postulated to explain this association, but it is currently unclear which (if any) are relevant. In insulin-resistant patients with essential hypertension, basal intracellular Ca^{2+} levels have been shown to be elevated, and the normal ability of insulin to attenuate angiotensin II-induced increases in intracellular Ca^{2+} is blunted in skin fibroblasts [122]. The renal action of insulin to reabsorb sodium is similar in normo- and hypertensive insulin-resistant subjects [123, 124]. Such a preserved action of insulin could contribute to an increase in blood pressure in hyperinsulinemic subjects but its quantitative significance is unknown. The suggestion that insulin sensitivity influences salt sensitivity is controversial [125–128]. Insulin resistance has consistently been found to correlate with high sodium–lithium counter–transport in erythrocyte membranes; this is thought to parallel increased activity of the Na^+–H^+ pump in the cell membrane of other tissues, which could raise intracellular Na^+ and Ca^{2+} concentrations and enhance vascular smooth muscle contractility. Such action could also contribute to the development of hypertension in nondiabetic, insulin-resistant subjects (see Chapter 97).

In theory, an increase in peripheral vascular resistance (which would raise diastolic blood pressure) could be a consequence of impaired insulin-induced vasodilatation. However, insulin is a weak and slowly acting vasodilatator and defects in insulin stimulation of blood flow in hypertensive subjects have not been documented under

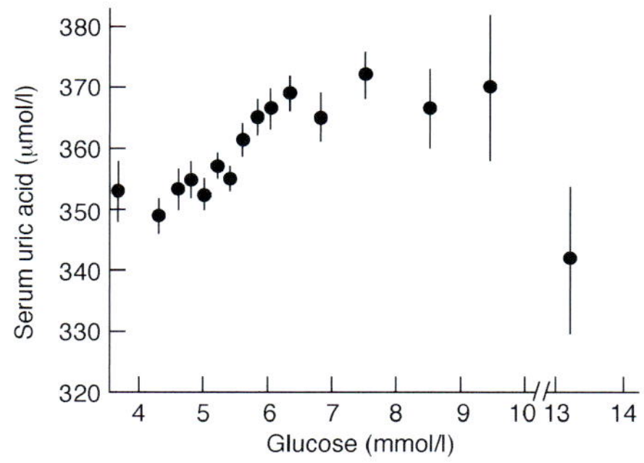

Figure 4 The relationship between blood glucose and serum uric acid in a survey of 7735 middle-aged men drawn at random from general practices in 24 British towns. The relationship resembles the inverted U-shaped relationship depicted in Figure 2. Worsening of insulin resistance and increasing hyperinsulinemia is associated with increases in uric acid concentrations until glucosuria occurs after fasting glucose exceeds 10–13 mmol/l. (Reproduced with permission from BMJ Publishing Group, Postgrad Medical Journal 1986; 62: 1001–6)

physiological conditions [129]. It is also unclear whether defects in insulin-induced vasodilatation observed at very high insulin concentrations are specific to insulin or are a consequence of a more generalized defect in endothelial or smooth-muscle function, or of structural changes in arteries secondary to hypertension [129].

Hyperuricemia

Within the nondiabetic range of glucose tolerance, serum uric acid concentrations are positively correlated with glucose [130] and insulin [131] concentrations and inversely with insulin resistance [132, 133] (Figure 4). In normal subjects, insulin acutely reduces the renal clearance of both sodium and uric acid [134]. These actions are preserved in insulin-resistant states such as obesity, diabetes, and essential hypertension, and so provide a potential mechanistic link for the clustering of insulin resistance with hyperuricemia [133–135]. Once glucose tolerance becomes diabetic, glucosuria inhibits reabsorption of uric acid, which therefore is excreted in the urine, together with glucose and serum uric acid levels decrease as a function or worsening hyperglycemia (Figure 4). These data imply that uric acid is a marker of insulin resistance in nondiabetic but not diabetic subjects. The co-occurrence of hyperuricemia and the insulin resistance syndrome also explains why the incidence of gout is increased in individuals with hypertriglyeridemia and why patients with hypertension may be particularly prone to hyperuricemia induced by diuretics.

Alterations in Coagulation, Fibrinolysis, and Platelet Function

Procoagulant changes such as impaired fibrinolysis and increased levels of PAI-1 and defects in platelet function are frequently associated with insulin resistance. Such abnormalities could predispose to atherothrombotic vascular disease. PAI-1 is an inhibitor of fibrinolysis, and raised plasma levels predict an increased risk of a coronary event [136]. Plasma levels of PAI-1 antigen are frequently elevated in obesity-associated insulin resistance [136]. The exact mechanisms underlying the increase are unknown. PAI-1 levels and activity are increased in the fatty liver of both lipodystrophic and obese subjects [100, 137] and in adipose tissue of obese subjects [138]. Plasma concentrations of tissue-type plasminogen activator (tPA) antigen, which represent mainly inactive tPA/PAI-1 complexes, are strongly correlated with those of PAI-1 (and thus are also frequently increased in obese, insulin-resistant subjects) and negatively correlated with overall fibrinolytic or tPA activity [136]. Insulin normally inhibits platelet aggregation, and this action is blunted both *in vitro* [139] and *in vivo* [140] in insulin-resistant obese nondiabetic subjects.

Changes in Inflammatory Markers

IL-6 is the main regulator of the synthesis of C-reactive protein in the liver [141]. Catheterization studies in human adipose tissue have documented that IL-6 is produced and released into the systemic circulation [142]. Up to one third of circulating IL-6 may originate from subcutaneous and visceral adipose tissue depots and circulating levels are increased in obese subjects [143, 144]. Tumor necrosis factor α (TNF-α) is a cytokine whose production is increased in adipose tissue from obese subjects and which stimulates production of IL-6. TNFα does not appear to be secreted into the systemic circulation and thus is likely to act as a local regulator of IL-6 production [142] and possibly lipolysis via inhibition of LPL activity [144].

Microalbuminuria

The mechanisms underlying the clustering of insulin resistance and microalbuminuria are poorly understood. Insulin has been shown to increase urinary excretion of albumin and protein markers of proximal tubular function in patients with type 2 diabetes but not in nondiabetic healthy volunteers [145]. Whether subjects with the insulin resistance syndrome respond to insulin like patients with type 2 diabetes or like healthy volunteers has not been studied. Microalbuminuria may also be a sign of preclinical endothelial or vascular damage [146–149].

Abnormalities in the Autonomic Nervous System

Regarding the increase in sympathetic activity in insulin-resistant subjects, insulin can enter the hypothalamus and other parts of the brain, where insulin receptors are expressed at high levels, and it acts centrally to stimulate the sympathetic nervous system. Manifestations include increases in muscle sympathetic nervous activity [150] and in noradrenaline spillover rate (a measure of noradrenaline release from sympathetic nerve endings in the tissues) [151]. Insulin also regulates the autonomic control of heart rate by decreasing vagal tone, and increasing sympathetic drive [82].

CLINICAL SIGNIFICANCE: INSULIN RESISTANCE SYNDROME AS A PREDICTOR OF TYPE 2 DIABETES AND CARDIOVASCULAR DISEASE

Components of the Insulin Resistance Syndrome as Predictors of Type 2 Diabetes

There has been much debate as to whether insulin resistance is the primary defect that precedes β-cell failure in the evolution of hyperglycemia in type 2 diabetes, or vice versa. Cross-sectional studies show a close relationship between the attenuation of first-phase insulin secretion, insulin resistance affecting glucose uptake, and the increase in postload glucose insulin concentrations; indeed, none of these abnormalities consistently appears to precede the others when examined over the full range of glucose tolerance [152]. Instead, there is a linear decrease in both first-phase insulin release and insulin sensitivity in individuals who progress from normal to impaired glucose tolerance. Once the plasma glucose concentration reaches the upper limit for impaired glucose tolerance (11.1 mmol/l, 200 mg/dl), postload glucose insulin concentrations fall and glucose then rises into the diabetic range (Figure 3). A similar picture emerges from prospective studies. Thus, even in extremely insulin-resistant populations such as the Pima Indians, low insulin sensitivity and impaired first-phase insulin release both predict the onset of type 2 diabetes [86]. Nevertheless, even if insulin resistance is not the only defect preceding type 2 diabetes, several prospective studies have documented that insulin resistance, measured (for methods used to assess insulin action in general, see Chapter 15) by direct quantification of insulin action of whole-body glucose metabolism, or indirectly by determining fasting insulin concentrations precedes and predicts type 2 diabetes [153]. In addition to such measures of insulin resistance, causes of insulin resistance such as obesity, abdominal fat distribution, and physical inactivity, and putative consequences of insulin resistance such as high triglycerides–low HDL cholesterol, and hypertension have all been shown to be predictors of type 2 diabetes [153]. If defined according to the WHO or ATP III criteria, the insulin resistance syndrome increases the risk of developing type 2 diabetes 5.0–8.8-fold (Figure 5). As discussed below, some of the more recently introduced components of the insulin resistance syndrome, which are not included in the ATP III or

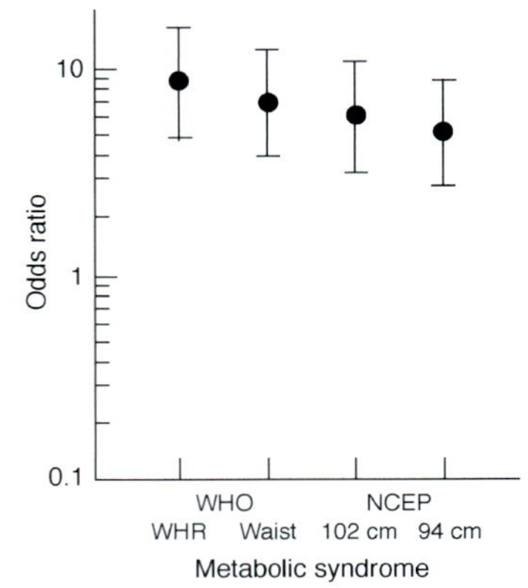

Figure 5 Relative risk of developing diabetes in a prospective study in a Finnish population-based cohort of 1005 middle-aged men subjects with the metabolic syndrome according to WHO and NCEP criteria. (Reproduced with permission from reference 154)

WHO definitions, have also been shown to predict type 2 diabetes.

Other Markers of Insulin Resistance as Predictors of Type 2 Diabetes

Almost all features that have been linked to the insulin resistance syndrome have been shown to predict type 2 diabetes. These include, in addition to the features discussed above, positive family history (for genetic causes of insulin resistance, see Chapter 23), hyperuricemia [153], nonalcoholic fatty liver disease [155], low adiponectin concentrations in Japanese [156] but not in Pima Indians [157], and high IL-6 [158, 159] concentrations. In the Atherosclerosis Risk in Communities Study, serum IL-6 remained a significant predictor of type 2 diabetes even after adjusting for BMI, waist-to-hip ratio and glucose and insulin [159]. Serum C-reactive protein was found to enhance the predictive value of the insulin resistance syndrome, defined as suggested by NCEP, for diabetes in men participating in the West of Scotland Coronary Prevention Study [160] and in women but not men in the Mexico City Diabetes Study [161]. Serum C-reactive protein also predicted diabetes in Caucasian women [162] and in elderly subjects [163]. In a large cohort of German men, those with C-reactive protein in the highest quartile had a 2.7 times higher risk of developing diabetes. The predictive value became, however, nonsignificant after adjustment for BMI, smoking, and systolic blood pressure [164].

Components of the Insulin Resistance Syndrome as Predictors of Cardiovascular Disease

All the components of the insulin resistance syndrome, with the possible exception of hyperinsulinemia itself, have been shown to predict cardiovascular disease. Two studies have hitherto reported data on the risk of cardiovascular disease using the definitions of insulin resistance syndrome listed in Table 2. In men participating in the West of Scotland Coronary Prevention Study, the insulin resistance syndrome defined according to NCEP criteria (Table 2) increased the risk for a CHD event by 1.76-fold. The syndrome continued to predict CHD events in a multivariate model incorporating conventional risk factors. Men with four to five features of the syndrome had a 3.7-fold increase in risk for CHD. Regarding hyperinsulinemia, the possibility that it itself may damage arteries, and specifically that it might be atherogenic, has long been controversial. The uncertainty surrounding the relationship between circulating insulin levels and arterial disease in type 2 diabetes was highlighted by the findings of the United Kingdom Prospective Diabetes Study [165]. Here, the incidence of macrovascular disease (notably myocardial infarction and stroke) was not increased by 9 years of insulin or sulfonylurea treatment, although both significantly raised plasma insulin levels [165]. The decrease in the incidence of myocardial infarction (a 16% decrease for a 0.9% decrease in HbA_{1c}) corresponded exactly to that predicted from cross-sectional epidemiological analysis of the relationship between HbA_{1c} and the incidence of myocardial infarction (14% decrease for a 1% decrease in HbA_{1c}) [166]. This landmark study thus implied that hyperinsulinemia has no harmful effects on cardiovascular disease.

Other Markers of Insulin Resistance as Predictors of Cardiovascular Disease

Inflammatory processes are involved in the pathogenesis of atherosclerosis [167]. Serum levels of C-reactive protein have been shown to predict CHD in several prospective studies including apparently healthy men in the US Physicians Health Study [168], the MONICA-Augsburg Cohort Study in Germany [152], and the MRFIT Study [169]. Similar data have also been reported for apparently healthy women [170]. In these studies, C-reactive protein has predicted cardiovascular disease independent of other risk factors. In the Hoorn Study, which is a population-based cohort study in a White population aged 50–75 years in the Netherlands, C-reactive protein levels in the upper tertile were associated with a twofold increase in cardiovascular mortality after adjustment for age, sex, and glucose tolerance status. After further adjustment for components of the insulin resistance syndrome (obesity hypertension, levels of HDL cholesterol and triglyceride), smoking, and preexisting cardiovascular disease, C-reactive protein no longer predicted and increased risk [171].

Hyperuricemia was associated with increased mortality from all causes and from cardiovascular disease in the NHANES I epidemiologic survey in women but not in men [172]. These associations persisted after adjustment for use of antihypertensive medications, blood pressure, and obesity [172]. In the Framingham Heart Study, hyperuricemia was similarly predictive of CHD, mortality from cardiovascular diseases, and death from all causes in women but these associations became nonsignificant after adjustment for cardiovascular risk factors [173]. It is thus unclear whether uric acid has a causal role in the development of CHD or whether the associations are due to correlations between uric acid and other risk factors.

PAI-1 has been found predictive for cardiovascular disease in several studies but as for uric acid, data are conflicting regarding its independent predictive capacity. Its predictive capacity thus seems to depend on the choice of variables that are controlled for [174].

Microalbuminuria and Markers of Endothelial Activation

Microalbuminuria, which has not as yet firmly secured its position as a component of the insulin resistance syndrome, appears to be a rather independent predictor of CHD. For example, in elderly nondiabetic subjects in Kuopio, hyperinsulinemic microalbuminuria increased the relative risk of CHD death eightfold and of all CHD events threefold even after adjusting for gender, smoking, waist-to-hip ratio, systolic blood pressure, and HDL cholesterol [149]. Similar data were found in the Islington Diabetes Survey in nondiabetic subjects in whom microalbuminuria predicted vascular disease independent of systolic and diastolic blood pressures, smoking, age, sex, ethnic origin, and BMI.

CONCLUSION

From the abundant data discussed above, it seems safe to conclude that recognition of the insulin resistance syndrome is clinically important as it predicts both type 2 diabetes and cardiovascular disease. Weight loss and exercise have proven effective in ameliorating insulin resistance and can prevent type 2 diabetes [175, 176] (see Chapter 117). In those who fail, insulin-sensitizing drugs such as metformin may become an accepted indication for diabetes prevention in the future [176]. Given the large variation of the prevalence and features of the insulin resistance syndrome listed as in Table 1, the definitions are oversimplifications as they attempt to define a biological continuous phenomenon by fixed numbers, which are unlikely to be equally useful in risk prediction in different ethnic groups. Clinical judgement therefore remains essential in assessing individuals at risk. Such risk assessment obviously also include cardiovascular risk factors such as gender, ethnicity, LDL cholesterol, smoking, and family history of cardiovascular disease.

REFERENCES

1. Reaven G. Banting Lecture 1988: role of insulin resistance in human disease. *Diabetes* 1988; 37: 1595–607.
2. Alberti KGMM, Zimmet PZ, for the WHO Consultation. Definition, diagnosis and classification of diabetes mellitus and its complications. Part 1: Diagnosis and classification of diabetes mellitus. Provisional Report of a WHO consultation. *Diabet Med* 1998; 15: 539–53.
3. Executive Summary of the Third Report of the National Cholesterol Education Program (NCEP) Expert Panel on Detection, Evaluation, and Treatment of High Blood Cholesterol in Adults (Adult Treatment Panel III). *JAMA* 2001; 285: 2486–97.
4. Ford ES, Giles WH, Dietz WH. Prevalence of the metabolic syndrome among US adults: findings from the third National Health and Nutrition Examination Survey. *JAMA* 2002; 287: 356–9.
5. Ford ES, Giles WH. A comparison of the prevalence of the metabolic syndrome using two proposed definitions. *Diabetes Care* 2003; 26: 575–81.
6. Yki-Järvinen H, Koivisto VA. Effect of body composition on insulin sensitivity. *Diabetes* 1983; 32: 965–9.
7. Dela F, Mikines KJ, Galbo H. Physical activity and insulin resistance in man. In Reaven G, Laws A (eds), Contemporary Endocrinology. *Insulin Resistance*. Totowa, NJ: Humana Press Inc, 1998; p 97.
8. Kolterman OG, Insel J, Saekow M, Olefsky JM. Mechanisms of insulin resistance in human obesity: evidence for receptor and postreceptor defects. *J Clin Invest* 1980; 65: 1272–84.
9. Amiel SA, Sherwin RS, Simonson DC, Lauritano AA, Tamborlane WV. Impaired insulin action in puberty. A contributing factor to poor glycemic control in adolescents with diabetes. *N Engl J Med* 1986; 315: 215–9.
10. Butte NF. Carbohydrate and lipid metabolism in pregnancy: normal compared with gestational diabetes mellitus. *Am J Clin Nutr* 2000; 71: 1256S–61S.
11. Yki-Järvinen H. Sex and insulin sensitivity. *Metabolism* 1984; 33: 1011–5.
12. Yki-Järvinen H. Insulin sensitivity during the menstrual cycle. *J Clin Endocrinol Metab* 1984; 59: 350–3.
13. Toth EL, Suthijumroon A, Crockford PM, Ryan EA. Insulin action does not change during the menstrual cycle in normal women. *J Clin Endocrinol Metab* 1987; 64: 74–80.
14. Mott DM, Lillioja S, Bogardus C. Overnutrition induced changes decrease in insulin action for glucose storage: in vivo and in vitro in man. *Metab Clin Exp* 1986; 35: 160–5.
15. Bjorkman O, Eriksson LS. Influence of a 60-hour fast on insulin-mediated splanchnic and peripheral glucose metabolism in humans. *J Clin Invest* 1985; 76: 87–92.
16. Yki-Järvinen H, Nikkilä EA. Ethanol decreases glucose utilization in healthy man. *J Clin Endocrinol Metab* 1985; 61: 941–5.
17. Vessby B, Uusitupa M, Hermansen K, Riccardi G, Rivellese A, Tapsell LC, Nälsen C, Berglund L, Louheranta A, Rasmussen BM, Calvert GD, Maffetone A, Pedersen E, Gustafsson I-B, Storlien LH. Substituting dietary saturated for monounsaturated fat impairs insulin sensitivity in helathy men and women: the KANWU Study. *Diabetologia* 2001; 44: 312–9.
18. Ferrannini E, Barrett EJ, Bevilacqua S, DeFronzo RA. Effect of fatty acids on glucose production and utilization in man. *J Clin Invest* 1983; 72: 1737–47.
19. Yki-Järvinen H, Helve E, Koivisto VA. Hyperglycemia decreases glucose uptake in type 1 diabetes. *Diabetes* 1987; 36: 892–6.
20. DeFronzo RA, Beckles AD. Glucose metabolism following chronic metabolic acidosis in man. *Am J Physiol* 1979; 236: E328–34.
21. Bratusch-Marrain PR, DeFronzo RA. Impairment of insulin mediated glucose metabolism by hyperosmolality in man. *Diabetes* 1983; 32: 1028–34.
22. DeFronzo RA, Lang R. Hypophosphatemia and glucose intolerance: evidence for tissue insensitivity to insulin. *N Engl J Med* 1980; 303: 1259–63.
23. Brandi LS, Santoro D, Natali A, Altomonte F, Baldi S, Frascerra S, Ferrannini E. Insulin resistance of stress: sites and mechanisms. *Clin Sci (Colch)* 1993; 85: 525–35.
24. Del Aguila LF, Krishnan RK, Ulbrecht JS, Farrell PA, Correll PH, Lang CH, Zierath JR, Kirwan JP. Muscle damage impairs insulin stimulation of IRS-1, PI 3-kinase, and Akt-kinase in human skeletal muscle. *Am J Physiol Endocrinol Metab* 2000; 279: E206–12.
25. Attvall S, Eriksson BM, Fowelin J, von Schenck H, Lager I, von Smith U. Early posthypoglycemic insulin resistance in man is mainly an effect of β-adrenergic stimulation. *J Clin Invest* 1987; 80: 437–42.
26. Moller N, Schmitz O, Joorgensen JO, Astrup J, Bak JF, Christensen SE, Alberti KG, Weeke J. Basal- and insulin-stimulated substrate metabolism in patients with active acromegaly before and after adenomectomy. *J Clin Endocrinol Metab* 1992; 74: 1012–9.
27. Nosadini R, Del Prato S, Tiengo A, Valerio A, Muggeo M, Opocher G, Mantero F, Duner E, Marescotti C, Mollo F, Belloni F. Insulin resistance in Cushing's syndrome. *J Clin Endocrinol Metab* 1983; 57: 529–36.
28. Bluher M, Windgassen M, Paschke R. Improvement of insulin sensitivity after adrenalectomy in patients with pheochromocytoma. *Diabetes Care* 2000; 23: 1591–2.
29. Hwu CM, Kwok CF, Lai TY, Shih KC, Lee TS, Hsiao LC, Lee SH, Fang VS, Ho LT. Growth hormone (GH) replacement reduces total body fat and normalizes insulin sensitivity in GH-deficient adults: a report of one-year clinical experience. *J Clin Endocrinol Metab* 1997; 82: 3285–92.
30. Pedersen O, Richelsen B, Bak J, Arnfred J, Weeke J, Schmitz O. Characterization of the insulin resistance of glucose utilization in adipocytes from patients with hyper- and hypothyroidism. *Acta Endocrinol (Copenh)* 1988; 119: 228–34.
31. Seppala-Lindroos A, Vehkavaara S, Hakkinen AM, Goto T, Westerbacka J, Sovijarvi A, Halavaara J, Yki-Järvinen H. Fat accumulation in the liver is associated with defects in insulin suppression of glucose production and serum free fatty acids independent of obesity in normal men. *J Clin Endocrinol Metab* 2002; 87: 3023–8.
32. DeFronzo RA, Alvestrand A, Smith D, Hendler R, Hendler E, Wahren J. Insulin resistance in uremia. *J Clin Invest* 1981; 67: 563–8.
33. Sammalkorpi K. Glucose intolerance in acute infections. *J Intern Med* 1989; 225: 15–9.
34. Yki-Järvinen H. Insulin resistance in type 2 diabetes. In Pickup JC, Williams G (eds) *Textbook of Diabetes*. Oxford: Blackwell, 2003; p 22.1.
35. DeFronzo RA, Tobin JD, Andres R. Glucose clamp technique: a method for quantifying insulin secretion and resistance. *Am J Physiol* 1979; 237: E214–23.
36. Enzi G, Busetto L, Inelmen EM, Coin A, Sergi G. Historical perspective: visceral obesity and related comorbidity in Joannes Baptista Morgagni's "De sedibus et

causis morborum per anatomen indagata." *Int J Obes Relat Metab Disord* 2003; 27: 534–5.
37. Vague J. La differentiation sexuelle. Facteur determinant des formes de l'obésite. *Presse Med* 1947; 55: 339–41.
38. Fontbonne A, Thibult N, Eschwege E, Ducimetiere P. Body fat distribution and coronary heart disease mortality in subjects with impaired glucose tolerance or diabetes mellitus: the Paris Prospective Study, 15-year follow-up. *Diabetologia* 1992; 35: 464–8.
39. Folsom AR, Kaye SA, Sellers TA, Hong CP, Cerhan JR, Potter JD, Prineas RJ. Body fat distribution and 5-year risk of death in older women. *JAMA* 1993; 269: 483–7.
40. Lapidus L, Bengtsson C, Larsson B, Pennert K, Rybo E, Sjöström L. Distribution of adipose tissue and risk of cardiovascular disease and death: a 12 year follow up of participants in the population study of women in Gothenburg, Sweden. *Br Med J* 1984; 289: 1257–61.
41. Kalmijn S, Curb JD, Rodriguez BL, Yano K, Abbott RD. The association of body weight and anthropometry with mortality in elderly men: the Honolulu Heart Program. *Int J Obes Relat Metab Disord* 1999; 23: 395–402.
42. Dole VP. A relation between non-esterified fatty acids in plasma and the metabolism of glucose [abstract]. *J Clin Invest* 1956; 35: 150–4.
43. Yalow R, Berson SA. Immunoassay of endogenous plasma insulin in man [abstract]. *J Clin Invest* 1960; 39: 1157–75.
44. Randle PJ, Hales CN, Garland PB, Newsholme EA. The glucose–fatty acid cycle. Its role in insulin sensitivity and the metabolic disturbances of diabetes mellitus. *Lancet* 1963; 1: 785–9.
45. Nikkilä EA, Miettinen TA, Vesenne M-R. Plasma insulin in coronary heart disease. *Lancet* 1965; 2: 508–11.
46. Avogaro P, Crepaldi G, Enzi G, Tiengo A. Associazone di iperlipemia, diabete mellito e obesita' di medio grado [abstract]. *Acta Diabetol Lat* 1967; IV: 571–90.
47. Alexander CM, Landsman PB, Teutsch SM, Haffner SM. NCEP-defined metabolic syndrome, diabetes, and prevalence of coronary heart disease among NHANES III participants age 50 years and older. *Diabetes* 2003; 52: 1210–4.
48. Balkau B, Charles MA, Drivsholm T, Borch-Johnsen K, Wareham N, Yudkin JS, Morris R, Zavaroni I, van Dam R, Feskins E, Gabriel R, Diet M, Nilsson P, Hedblad B. Frequency of the WHO metabolic syndrome in European cohorts, and an alternative definition of an insulin resistance syndrome. *Diabetes Metab* 2002; 28: 364–76.
49. Lindblad U, Langer RD, Wingard DL, Thomas RG, Barrett-Connor EL. Metabolic syndrome and ischemic heart disease in elderly men and women. *Am J Epidemiol* 2001; 153: 481–9.
50. Gray RS, Fabsitz RR, Cowan LD, Lee ET, Howard BV, Savage PJ. Risk factor clustering in the insulin resistance syndrome: the Strong Heart Study. *Am J Epidemiol* 1998; 148: 869–78.
51. Meigs JB, D'Agostino RBS, Wilson PW, Cupples LA, Nathan DM, Singer DE. Risk variable clustering in the insulin resistance syndrome: the Framingham Offspring Study. *Diabetes* 1997; 46: 1594–600.
52. Chen CH, Lin KC, Tsai ST, Chou P. Different association of hypertension and insulin-related metabolic syndrome between men and women in 8437 nondiabetic Chinese. *Am J Hypertens* 2000; 13: 846–53.
53. Shmulewitz D, Auerbach SB, Lehner T, Blundell ML, Winick JD, Youngman LD, Skilling V, Heath SC, Ott J, Stoffel M, Breslow JL, Friedman JM. Epidemiology and factor analysis of obesity, type II diabetes, hypertension, and dyslipidemia (syndrome X) on the Island of Kosrae, Federated States of Micronesia. *Hum Hered* 1903; 51: 8–19.
54. Donahue RP, Bean JA, Donahue RD, Goldberg RB, Prineas RJ. Does insulin resistance unite the separate components of the insulin resistance syndrome? Evidence from the Miami Community Health Study. *Arterioscler Thromb Vasc Biol* 1997; 17: 2413–7.
55. Snehalatha C, Sivasankari S, Satyavani K, Vijay V, Ramachandran A. Insulin resistance alone does not explain the clustering of cardiovascular risk factors in southern India. *Diabet Med* 2000; 17: 152–7.
56. Godsland IF, Leyva F, Walton C, Worthington M, Stevenson JC. Associations of smoking, alcohol and physical activity with risk factors for coronary heart disease and diabetes in the first follow-up cohort of the Heart Disease and Diabetes Risk Indicators in a Screened Cohort study (HDDRISC-1). *J Intern Med* 1998; 244: 33–41.
57. Lempiainen P, Mykkanen L, Pyorala K, Laakso M, Kuusisto J. Insulin resistance syndrome predicts coronary heart disease events in elderly nondiabetic men. *Circulation* 1999; 100: 123–8.
58. Hanley AJ, Karter AJ, Festa A, D'Agostino RJ, Wagenknecht LE, Savage P, Tracy RP, Saad MF, Haffner S. Factor analysis of metabolic syndrome using directly measured insulin sensitivity: the Insulin Resistance Atherosclerosis Study. *Diabetes* 2002; 51: 2642–7.
59. Edwards KL, Austin MA, Newman B, Mayer E, Krauss RM, Selby JV. Multivariate analysis of the insulin resistance syndrome in women. *Arterioscler Thromb* 1994; 14: 1940–5.
60. Edwards KL, Burchfiel CM, Sharp DS, Curb JD, Rodriguez BL, Fujimoto WY, LaCroix AZ, Vitiello MV, Austin MA. Factors of the insulin resistance syndrome in nondiabetic and diabetic elderly Japanese-American men. *Am J Epidemiol* 1998; 147: 441–7.
61. Shen BJ, Todaro JF, Niaura R, McCaffery JM, Zhang J, Spiro A, Ward KD. Are metabolic risk factors one unified syndrome? Modeling the structure of the metabolic syndrome X. *Am J Epidemiol* 2003; 157: 701–11.
62. Sakkinen PA, Wahl P, Cushman M, Lewis MR, Tracy RP. Clustering of procoagulation, inflammation, and fibrinolysis variables with metabolic factors in insulin resistance syndrome. *Am J Epidemiol* 2000; 152: 897–907.
63. Leyva F, Godsland IF, Worthington M, Walton C, Stevenson JC. Factors of the metabolic syndrome: baseline interrelationships in the first follow-up cohort of the Heart Disease and Diabetes Risk Indicators in a Screened Cohort (HDDRISC) Study (HDDRISC-1). *Arterioscler Thromb Vasc Biol* 1998; 18: 208–14.
64. Kekalainen P, Sarlund H, Pyorala K, Laakso M. Hyperinsulinemia cluster predicts the development of type 2 diabetes independently of family history of diabetes. *Diabetes Care* 1999; 22: 86–92.
65. Pyorala M, Miettinen H, Halonen P, Laakso M, Pyorala K. Insulin resistance syndrome predicts the risk of coronary heart disease and stroke in healthy middle-aged men: the 22-year follow-up results of the Helsinki Policemen Study. *Arterioscler Thromb Vasc Biol* 2000; 20: 538–44.
66. Pirro M, Mauriege P, Tchernof A, Cantin B, Dagenais GR, Despres JP, Lamarche B. Plasma free fatty acid levels and the risk of ischemic heart disease in men:

prospective results from the Quebec Cardiovascular Study. *Atherosclerosis* 2002; 160: 377–84.

67. Hall SEH, Braaten JT, McKendry JBR, Bolton T, Foster D, Berman M. Normal alanine–glucose relationships and their changes in diabetic patients before and after insulin treatment. *Diabetes* 1979; 28: 737–45.
68. Mogensen CE, Christensen CK. Predicting diabetic nephropathy in insulin-dependent patients. *N Engl J Med* 1984; 311: 89–93.
69. Mattock MB, Morrish NJ, Viberti G, Keen H, Fitzgerald AP, Jackson G. Prospective study of microalbuminuria as predictor of mortality in NIDDM. *Diabetes* 1992; 41: 736–41.
70. Forsblom CM, Eriksson JG, Ekstrand AV, Teppo AM, Taskinen MR, Groop LC. Insulin resistance and abnormal albumin excretion in nondiabetic first-degree relatives of patients with NIDDM. *Diabetologia* 1995; 38: 363–9.
71. Mykkanen L, Zaccaro DJ, Wagenknecht LE, Robbins DC, Gabriel M, Haffner SM. Microalbuminuria is associated with insulin resistance in nondiabetic subjects: the insulin resistance atherosclerosis study. *Diabetes* 1998; 47: 793–800.
72. Lemieux I, Pascot A, Prud'homme D, Almeras N, Bogaty P, Nadeau A, Bergeron J, Despres JP. Elevated C-reactive protein: another component of the atherothrombotic profile of abdominal obesity. *Arterioscler Thromb Vasc Biol* 2001; 21: 961–7.
73. Yamada S, Gotoh T, Nakashima Y, Kayaba K, Ishikawa S, Nago N, Nakamura Y, Itoh Y, Kajii E. Distribution of serum C-reactive protein and its association with atherosclerotic risk factors in a Japanese population: Jichi Medical School Cohort Study. *Am J Epidemiol* 2001; 153: 1183–90.
74. Hak AE, Stehouwer CD, Bots ML, Polderman KH, Schalkwijk CG, Westendorp IC, Hofman A, Witteman JC. Associations of C-reactive protein with measures of obesity, insulin resistance, and subclinical atherosclerosis in healthy, middle-aged women. *Arterioscler Thromb Vasc Biol* 1999; 19: 1986–91.
75. Wu T, Dorn JP, Donahue RP, Sempos CT, Trevisan M. Associations of serum C-reactive protein with fasting insulin, glucose, and glycosylated hemoglobin: the Third National Health and Nutrition Examination Survey, 1988–1994. *Am J Epidemiol* 2002; 155: 65–71.
76. Barker DJ, Osmond C, Golding J, Kuh D, Wadsworth ME. Growth in utero, blood pressure in childhood and adult life, and mortality from cardiovascular disease. *BMJ* 1989; 298: 564–7.
77. Seckl JR. Glucocorticoid programming of the fetus: adult phenotypes and molecular mechanisms. *Mol Cell Endocrinol* 2001; 185: 61–71.
78. Barker DJ, Gluckman PD, Godfrey KM, Harding JE, Owens JA, Robinson JS. Fetal nutrition and cardiovascular disease in adult life. *Lancet* 1993; 341: 938–41.
79. Edwards CR, Benediktsson R, Lindsay RS, Seckl JR. Dysfunction of placental glucocorticoid barrier: link between fetal environment and adult hypertension? *Lancet* 1993; 341: 355–7.
80. Seckl JR, Cleasby M, Nyirenda MJ. Glucocorticoids, 11beta-hydroxysteroid dehydrogenase, and fetal programming. *Kidney Int* 2000; 57: 1412–7.
81. Vollenweider P, Randin D, Tappy L, Jequier E, Nicod P, Scherrer U. Impaired insulin-induced sympathetic neural activation and vasodilatation in skeletal muscle in obese humans. *J Clin Invest* 1994; 93: 2365–71.
82. Bergholm R, Westerbacka J, Vehkavaara S, Seppala-Lindroos A, Goto T, Yki-Järvinen H. Insulin sensitivity regulates autonomic control of heart rate variation independent of body weight in normal subjects. *J Clin Endocrinol Metab* 2001; 86: 1403–9.
83. Paolisso G, Manzella D, Rizzo MR, Barbieri M, Varricchio G, Gambardella A, Varricchio M. Effects of insulin on the cardiac autonomic nervous system in insulin-resistant states. *Clin Sci (Colch)* 2000; 98: 129–36.
84. Brunner EJ, Hemingway H, Walker BR, Page M, Clarke P, Juneja M, Shipley MJ, Kumari M, Andrew R, Seckl JR, Papadopoulos A, Checkley S, Rumley A, Lowe GD, Stansfeld SA, Marmot MG. Adrenocortical, autonomic, and inflammatory causes of the metabolic syndrome: nested case-control study. *Circulation* 2002; 106: 2659–65.
85. Lillioja S, Mott DM, Howard BV, Bennett PH, Yki-Järvinen H, Freymond BL, Nyomba F, Zurlo B, Swinburn B, Bogardus C. Impaired glucose tolerance as a disorder of insulin action: longitudinal and cross-sectional studies in Pima indians. *N Engl J Med* 1988; 318: 1217–25.
86. Lillioja S, Mott DM, Spraul M, Ferraro R, Foley JE, Ravussin E, Knowler WC, Bennett PH, Bogardus C. Insulin resistance and insulin secretory dysfunction as precursors of non-insulin-dependent diabetes mellitus. *N Engl J Med* 1993; 329: 1988–1992.
87. Bonadonna RC, Groop L, Kraemer N, Ferrannini E, Del Prato S, DeFronzo RA. Obesity and insulin resistance in humans: a dose–response study. *Metabolism* 1990; 39: 452–9.
88. Berg AH, Combs TP, Du X, Brownlee M, Scherer PE. The adipocyte-secreted protein Acrp30 enhances hepatic insulin action. *Nat Med* 2001; 7: 947–53.
89. Frayn KN. Visceral fat and insulin resistance—causative or correlative? *Br J Nutr* 2000; 83 (suppl 1): S71–7.
90. Havel RJ, Kane JP, Balasse EO, Segel N, Basso LV. Splanchnic metabolism of free fatty acids and production of triglyserides of very low density lipoproteins in normotriglyceridemic and hypertriglyceridemic humans. *J Clin Invest* 1970; 49: 2017–35.
91. Martin ML, Jensen MD. Effects of body fat distribution on regional lipolysis in obesity. *J Clin Invest* 1991; 88: 609–13.
92. Reitman ML, Arioglu E, Gavrilova O, Taylor SI. Lipoatrophy revisited. *Trends Endocrinol Metab* 2000; 11: 410–6.
93. Gavrilova O, Marcus-Samuels B, Graham D, Kim JK, Shulman GI, Castle AL, Vinson C, Eckhaus M, Reitman ML. Surgical implantation of adipose tissue reverses diabetes in lipoatrophic mice. *J Clin Invest* 2000; 105: 271–8.
94. Ryysy L, Hakkinen AM, Goto T, Vehkavaara S, Westerbacka J, Halavaara J, Yki-Järvinen H. Hepatic fat content and insulin action on free fatty acids and glucose metabolism rather than insulin absorption are associated with insulin requirements during insulin therapy in type 2 diabetic patients. *Diabetes* 2000; 49: 749–58.
95. Levin K, Daa SH, Alford FP, Beck-Nielsen H. Morphometric documentation of abnormal intramyocellular fat storage and reduced glycogen in obese patients with Type II diabetes. *Diabetologia* 2001; 44: 824–33.
96. Krssak M, Falk PK, Dresner A, DiPietro L, Vogel SM, Rothman DL, Roden M, Shulman GI. Intramyocellular lipid concentrations are correlated with insulin sensitivity

in humans: a ^{1}H NMR spectroscopy study. *Diabetologia* 1999; 42: 113–6.

97. Pan DA, Lillioja S, Kriketos AD, Milner MR, Baur LA, Bogardus C, Jenkins AB, Storlien LH. Skeletal muscle triglyceride levels are inversely related to insulin action. *Diabetes* 1997; 46: 983–8.
98. Virkamaki A, Korsheninnikova E, Seppala-Lindroos A, Vehkavaara S, Goto T, Halavaara J, Hakkinen AM, Yki-Järvinen H. Intramyocellular lipid is associated with resistance to in vivo insulin actions on glucose uptake, antilipolysis, and early insulin signaling pathways in human skeletal muscle. *Diabetes* 2001; 50: 2337–43.
99. Tiikkainen M, Tamminen M, Hakkinen AM, Bergholm R, Vehkavaara S, Halavaara J, Teramo K, Rissanen A, Yki-Järvinen H. Liver-fat accumulation and insulin resistance in obese women with previous gestational diabetes. *Obes Res* 2002; 10: 859–67.
100. Sutinen J, Korsheninnikova E, Funahashi T, Matsuzawa Y, Nyman T, Yki-Järvinen H. Circulating concentration of adiponectin and its expression in subcutaneous adipose tissue in patients with highly active antiretroviral therapy-associated lipodystrophy. *J Clin Endocrinol Metab* 2003; 88: 1907–10.
101. Yki-Järvinen H, Sutinen J, Silveira A, Korsheninnikova E, Fisher RM, Kannisto K, Ehrenborg E, Eriksson P, Hamsten A. Regulation of Plasma PAI-1 Concentrations in HAART-Associated Lipodystrophy During Rosiglitazone Therapy. *Arterioscler Thromb Vasc Biol* 2003; 23: 688–94.
102. Nuutila P, Knuuti MJ, Heinonen OJ, Ruotsalainen U, Teräs M, Bergman J, Solin O, Yki-Järvinen H, Voipio-Pulkki L-M, Wegelius U, Koivisto VA. Different alterations in the insulin-stimulated glucose uptake in the athlete's heart and skeletal muscle. *J Clin Invest* 1994; 93: 2267–74.
103. Durrington PN, Newton RS, Weinstein DB, Steinberg D. Effects of insulin and glucose on very low density lipoprotein triglyceride secretion by cultured rat hepatocytes. *J Clin Invest* 1982; 70: 63–73.
104. Sparks JD, Sparks CE. Insulin modulation of hepatic synthesis and secretion of apolipoprotein B by rat hepatocytes. *J Biol Chem* 1990; 265: 8854–62.
105. Malmström R, Packard CJ, Watson TDG, Rannikko S, Caslake M, Bedford D, Stewart P, Yki-Järvinen H, Shepherd J, Taskinen M-R. Metabolic basis of hypotriglyceridemic effects of insulin in normal men. *Arterioscler Thromb Vasc Biol* 1997; 17: 1454–64.
106. Malmström R, Packard CJ, Caslake M, Bedford D, Stewart P, Yki-Järvinen H, Shepherd J, Taskinen MR. Defective regulation of triglyceride metabolism by insulin in the liver in NIDDM. *Diabetologia* 1997; 40: 454–62.
107. Malmström R, Packard CJ, Caslake M, Bedford D, Stewart P, Yki-Järvinen H, Shepherd J, Taskinen MR. Effects of insulin and acipimox on VLDL1 and VLDL2 apolipoprotein B production in normal subjects. *Diabetes* 1998; 47: 779–87.
108. Syvanne M, Taskinen MR. Lipids and lipoproteins as coronary risk factors in non-insulin-dependent diabetes mellitus. *Lancet* 1997; 350 (suppl 1): SI20–3.
109. Eisenberg S. High-density lipoprotein metabolism. In Betteridge DJ, Illinfworth DR, Shepherd J (eds), *Lipoproteins in Health and Disease*. London: Arnold, 1999; p 71.
110. Deckelbaum RJ, Granot E, Oschry Y, Rose L, Eisenberg S. Plasma triglyceride determines structure–composition in low and high density lipoproteins. *Arteriosclerosis* 1984; 4: 225–31.
111. Zambon A, Austin MA, Brown BG, Hokanson JE, Brunzell JD. Effect of hepatic lipase on LDL in normal men and those with coronary artery disease. *Arterioscler Thromb* 1993; 13: 147–53.
112. Lahdenpera S, Syvanne M, Kahri J, Taskinen MR. Regulation of low-density lipoprotein particle size distribution in NIDDM and coronary disease: importance of serum triglycerides. *Diabetologia* 1996; 39: 453–61.
113. Gray RS, Robbins DC, Wang W, Yeh JL, Fabsitz RR, Cowan LD, Welty TK, Lee ET, Krauss RM, Howard BV. Relation of LDL size to the insulin resistance syndrome and coronary heart disease in American Indians: the Strong Heart Study. *Arterioscler Thromb Vasc Biol* 1997; 17: 2713–20.
114. Austin MA, Rodriguez BL, McKnight B, McNeely MJ, Edwards KL, Curb JD, Sharp DS. Low-density lipoprotein particle size, triglycerides, and high-density lipoprotein cholesterol as risk factors for coronary heart disease in older Japanese-American men. *Am J Cardiol* 2000; 86: 412–6.
115. Coresh J, Kwiterovich POJ, Smith HH, Bachorik PS. Association of plasma triglyceride concentration and LDL particle diameter, density, and chemical composition with premature coronary artery disease in men and women. *J Lipid Res* 1993; 34: 1687–97.
116. Gardner CD, Fortmann SP, Krauss RM. Association of small low-density lipoprotein particles with the incidence of coronary artery disease in men and women. *JAMA* 1996; 276: 875–81.
117. Vakkilainen J, Mäkimattila S, Seppälä-Lindroos A, Vehkavaara S, Lahdenperä S, Groop P-H, Taskinen M-R, Yki-Järvinen H. Endothelial dysfunction in men with small LDL particles. *Circulation* 2000; 102: 716–21.
118. Ferrannini E, Buzzigoli G, Bonadonna R, Giorico MA, Oleggini M, Gradiadei L, Pedrinelli R, Brandi L, Bevilacqua S. Insulin resistance in essential hypertension. *N Engl J Med* 1987; 317: 350–7.
119. Dowse GK, Collins VR, Alberti KG, Zimmet PZ, Tuomilehto J, Chitson P, Gareeboo H, for The Mauritius Non-communicable Disease Study Group. Insulin and blood pressure levels are not independently related in Mauritians of Asian Indian, Creole or Chinese origin. *J Hypertens* 1993; 11: 297–307.
120. Liese AD, Mayer-Davis EJ, Chambless LE, Folsom AR, Sharrett AR, Brancati FL, Heiss G, for Atherosclerosis Risk in Communities Study Investigators. Elevated fasting insulin predicts incident hypertension: the ARIC Study. *J Hypertens* 1999; 17: 1169–77.
121. Modan M, Halkin H. Hyperinsulinemia or increased sympathetic drive as links for obesity and hypertension. *Diabetes Care* 1991; 14: 470–87.
122. Ceolotto G, Valente R, Baritono E, Reato S, Iori E, Monari A, Trevisan R, Semplicini A. Effect of insulin and angiotensin II on cell calcium in human skin fibroblasts. *Hypertension* 2001; 37: 1486–91.
123. Shimamoto K, Hirata A, Fukuoka M, Higashiura K, Miyazaki Y, Shiiki M, Masuda A, Nakagawa M, Iimura O. Insulin sensitivity and the effects of insulin on renal sodium handling and pressor systems in essential hypertensive patients. *Hypertension* 1994; 23: I29–33.
124. Skott P, Vaag A, Bruun NE, Hother-Nielsen O, Gall MA, Beck-Nielsen H, Parving HH. Effect of insulin on renal sodium handling in hyperinsulinaemic type 2

(non-insulin-dependent) diabetic patients with peripheral insulin resistance. *Diabetologia* 1991; 34: 275–81.
125. Dengel DR, Hogikyan RV, Brown MD, Glickman SG, Supiano MA. Insulin sensitivity is associated with blood pressure response to sodium in older hypertensives. *Am J Physiol* 1998; 274: E403–9.
126. Lind L, Lithell H, Gustafsson IB, Pollare T, Ljunghall S. Metabolic cardiovascular risk factors and sodium sensitivity in hypertensive subjects. *Am J Hypertens* 1992; 5: 502–5.
127. Fuenmayor N, Moreira E, Cubeddu LX. Salt sensitivity is associated with insulin resistance in essential hypertension. *Am J Hypertens* 1998; 11: 397–402.
128. Galletti F, Strazzullo P, Ferrara I, Annuzzi G, Rivellese AA, Gatto S, Mancini M. NaCl sensitivity of essential hypertensive patients is related to insulin resistance. *J Hypertens* 1997; 15: 1485–91.
129. Yki-Järvinen H, Utriainen T. Insulin-induced vasodilatation: physiology or pharmacology? *Diabetologia* 1998; 41: 369–79.
130. Cook DG, Shaper AG, Thelle DS, Whitehead TP. Serum uric acid, serum glucose and diabetes: relationships in a population study. *Postgrad Med J* 1986; 62: 1001–6.
131. Modan M, Halkin H, Karasik A, Lusky A. Elevated serum uric acid: a facet of hyperinsulinemia. *Diabetologia* 1987; 30: 713–8.
132. Facchini FS, Hollenbeck CB, Jeppesen J, Chen YD, Reaven GM. Insulin resistance and cigarrette smoking. *Lancet* 1992; 339: 1128–30.
133. Vuorinen-Markkola H, Yki-Järvinen H. Hyperuricemia and insulin resistance. *J Clin Endocrinol Metab* 1994; 78: 25–8.
134. Quinones GA, Natali A, Baldi S, Frascerra S, Sanna G, Ciociaro D, Ferrannini E. Effect of insulin on uric acid excretion in humans. *Am J Physiol* 1995; 268: E1–5.
135. Quinones-Galvan A, Ferrannini E. Renal effects of insulin in man. *J Nephrol* 1997; 10: 188–91.
136. Juhan-Vague I, Alessi MC, Vague P. Thrombogenic and fibrinolytic factors and cardiovascular risk in non-insulin-dependent diabetes mellitus. *Ann Med* 1996; 28: 371–80.
137. Alessi MC, Bastelica D, Mavri A, Morange P, Berthet B, Grino M, Juhan-Vague I. Plasma PAI-1 levels are more strongly related to liver steatosis than to adipose tissue accumulation. *Arterioscler Thromb Vasc Biol* 2003; 23: 1262–8.
138. Eriksson P, Reynisdottir S, Lonnqvist F, Stemme V, Hamsten A, Arner P. Adipose tissue secretion of plasminogen activator inhibitor-1 in non-obese and obese individuals. *Diabetologia* 1998; 41: 65–71.
139. Anfossi G, Mularoni EM, Burzacca S, Ponziani MC, Massucco P, Mattiello L, Cavalot F, Trovati M. Platelet resistance to nitrates in obesity and obese NIDDM, and normal platelet sensitivity to both insulin and nitrates in lean NIDDM. *Diabetes Care* 1998; 21: 121–6.
140. Westerbacka J, Yki-Järvinen H, Turpeinen A, Rissanen A, Vehkavaara S, Syrjälä M, Lassila R. Inhibition of platelet–collagen interaction: a novel in vivo action of insulin abolished by insulin resistance in obesity. *Arterioscler Thromb Vasc Biol* 2002; 22: 167–72.
141. Heinrich PC, Castell JV, Andus T. Interleukin-6 and the acute phase response. *Biochem J* 1990; 265: 621–36.
142. Mohamed-Ali V, Goodrick S, Rawesh A, Katz DR, Miles JM, Yudkin JS, Klein S, Coppack SW. Subcutaneous adipose tissue releases interleukin-6, but not tumor necrosis factor-alpha, in vivo. *J Clin Endocrinol Metab* 1997; 82: 4196–200.
143. Yudkin JS, Kumari M, Humphries SE, Mohamed-Ali V. Inflammation, obesity, stress and coronary heart disease: is interleukin-6 the link? *Atherosclerosis* 2000; 148: 209–14.
144. Kawakami M, Pekala PH, Lane MD, Cerami A. Lipoprotein lipase suppression in 3T3-L1 cells by an endotoxin-induced mediator from exudate cells. *Proc Natl Acad Sci USA* 1982; 79: 912–6.
145. Catalano C, Muscelli E, Quinones GA, Baldi S, Masoni A, Gibb I, Torffvit O, Seghieri G, Ferrannini E. Effect of insulin on systemic and renal handling of albumin in nondiabetic and NIDDM subjects. *Diabetes* 1997; 46: 868–75.
146. Berton G, Citro T, Palmieri R, Petucco S, De Toni R, Palatini P. Albumin excretion rate increases during acute myocardial infarction and strongly predicts early mortality. *Circulation* 1997; 96: 3338–45.
147. Yudkin JS, Forrest RD, Jackson CA. Microalbuminuria as predictor of vascular disease in nondiabetic subjects. Islington Diabetes Survey. *Lancet* 1998; 2: 530–3.
148. Damsgaard EM, Froland A, Jorgensen OD, Mogensen CE. Microalbuminuria as predictor of increased mortality in elderly people. *BMJ* 1990; 300: 297–300.
149. Kuusisto J, Mykkanen L, Pyorala K, Laakso M. Hyperinsulinemic microalbuminuria. A new risk indicator for coronary heart disease. *Circulation* 1995; 91: 831–7.
150. Berne C, Fagius J, Pollare T, Hjemdahl P. The sympathetic response to euglycemic hyperinsulinaemia. *Diabetologia* 1992; 35: 873–9.
151. Lembo G, Napoli R, Capaldo B, Rendina V, Iaccarino G, Volpe M, Trimarco B, Sacca L. Abnormal sympathetic overactivity evoked by insulin in the skeletal muscle of patients with essential hypertension. *J Clin Invest* 1992; 90: 24–9.
152. Koenig W, Sund M, Frohlich M, Fischer HG, Lowel H, Doring A, Hutchinson WL, Pepys MB. C-reactive protein, a sensitive marker of inflammation, predicts future risk of coronary heart disease in initially healthy middle-aged men: results from the MONICA (Monitoring Trends and Determinants in Cardiovascular Disease) Augsburg Cohort Study, 1984 to 1992. *Circulation* 1999; 99: 237–42.
153. Yki-Järvinen H. Prediction and prevention of non-insulin-dependent diabetes mellitus. In Williams G, Pickup J (eds) *Textbook of Diabetes*. Oxford: Blackwell, 2001; p 83.1.
154. Laaksonen DE, Lakka HM, Niskanen LK, Kaplan GA, Salonen JT, Lakka TA. Metabolic syndrome and development of diabetes mellitus: application and validation of recently suggested definitions of the metabolic syndrome in a prospective cohort study. *Am J Epidemiol* 2002; 156: 1070–7.
155. Vozarova B, Stefan N, Lindsay RS, Saremi A, Pratley RE, Bogardus C, Tataranni PA. High alanine aminotransferase is associated with decreased hepatic insulin sensitivity and predicts the development of type 2 diabetes. *Diabetes* 2002; 51: 1889–95.
156. Daimon M, Oizumi T, Saitoh T, Kameda W, Hirata A, Yamaguchi H, Ohnuma H, Igarashi M, Tominaga M, Kato T. Decreased serum levels of adiponectin are a risk factor for the progression to type 2 diabetes in the Japanese Population: the Funagata study. *Diabetes Care* 2003; 26: 2015–20.

157. Krakoff J, Funahashi T, Stehouwer CD, Schalkwijk CG, Tanaka S, Matsuzawa Y, Kobes S, Tataranni PA, Hanson RL, Knowler WC, Lindsay RS. Inflammatory markers, adiponectin, and risk of type 2 diabetes in the Pima Indian. *Diabetes Care* 2003; 26: 1745–51.
158. Spranger J, Kroke A, Mohlig M, Hoffmann K, Bergmann MM, Ristow M, Boeing H, Pfeiffer AF. Inflammatory cytokines and the risk to develop type 2 diabetes: results of the prospective population-based European Prospective Investigation into Cancer and Nutrition (EPIC)-Potsdam Study. *Diabetes* 2003; 52: 812–7.
159. Duncan BB, Schmidt MI, Pankow JS, Ballantyne CM, Couper D, Vigo A, Hoogeveen R, Folsom AR, Heiss G. Low-grade systemic inflammation and the development of type 2 diabetes: the Atherosclerosis Risk in Communities Study. *Diabetes* 2003; 52: 1799–805.
160. Sattar N, Gaw A, Scherbakova O, Ford I, O'Reilly DS, Haffner SM, Isles C, Macfarlane PW, Packard CJ, Cobbe SM, Shepherd J. Metabolic syndrome with and without C-reactive protein as a predictor of coronary heart disease and diabetes in the West of Scotland Coronary Prevention Study. *Circulation* 2003; 108: 414–9.
161. Han TS, Sattar N, Williams K, Gonzalez-Villalpando C, Lean ME, Haffner SM. Prospective study of C-reactive protein in relation to the development of diabetes and metabolic syndrome in the Mexico City Diabetes Study. *Diabetes Care* 2002; 25: 2016–21.
162. Pradhan AD, Manson JE, Rifai N, Buring JE, Ridker PM. C-reactive protein, interleukin 6, and risk of developing type 2 diabetes mellitus. *JAMA* 2001; 286: 327–34.
163. Barzilay JI, Abraham L, Heckbert SR, Cushman M, Kuller LH, Resnick HE, Tracy RP. The relation of markers of inflammation to the development of glucose disorders in the elderly: the Cardiovascular Health Study. *Diabetes* 2001; 50: 2384–9.
164. Thorand B, Lowel H, Schneider A, Kolb H, Meisinger C, Frohlich M, Koenig W. C-reactive protein as a predictor for incident diabetes mellitus among middle-aged men: results from the MONICA Augsburg cohort study, 1984–1998. *Arch Intern Med* 2003; 163: 93–9.
165. The UK Prospective Diabetes Study (UKPDS) Group. Intensive blood-glucose control with sulphonylureas or insulin compared with conventional treatment and risk of complications in patients with type 2 diabetes (UKPDS 33). *Lancet* 1998; 352: 837–52.
166. Stratton IM, Adler AI, Neil HA, Matthews DR, Manley SE, Cull CA, Hadden D, Turner RC, Holman RR. Association of glycaemia with macrovascular and microvascular complications of type 2 diabetes (UKPDS 35): prospective observational study [see comments]. *BMJ* 2000; 321: 405–12.
167. Ross R. The pathogenesis of atherosclerosis: a perspective for the 1990s. *Nature* 1993; 362: 801–9.
168. Ridker PM, Cushman M, Stampfer MJ, Tracy RP, Hennekens CH. Inflammation, aspirin, and the risk of cardiovascular disease in apparently healthy men. *N Engl J Med* 1997; 336: 973–9.
169. Kuller LH, Tracy RP, Shaten J, Meilahn EN. Relation of C-reactive protein and coronary heart disease in the MRFIT nested case-control study: Multiple Risk Factor Intervention Trial. *Am J Epidemiol* 1996; 144: 537–47.
170. Ridker PM, Buring JE, Shih J, Matias M, Hennekens CH. Prospective study of C-reactive protein and the risk of future cardiovascular events among apparently healthy women. *Circulation* 1998; 98: 731–3.
171. Jager A, van HV, Kostense PJ, Emeis JJ, Yudkin JS, Nijpels G, Dekker JM, Heine RJ, Bouter LM, Stehouwer CD. von Willebrand factor, C-reactive protein, and 5-year mortality in diabetic and nondiabetic subjects: the Hoorn Study. *Arterioscler Thromb Vasc Biol* 1999; 19: 3071–8.
172. Freedman DS, Williamson DF, Gunter EW, Byers T. Relation of serum uric acid to mortality and ischemic heart disease: the NHANES I Epidemiologic Follow-up Study. *Am J Epidemiol* 1995; 141: 637–44.
173. Culleton BF, Larson MG, Kannel WB, Levy D. Serum uric acid and risk for cardiovascular disease and death: the Framingham Heart Study. *Ann Intern Med* 1999; 131: 7–13.
174. Juhan-Vague I, Alessi MC, Morange PE. Hypofibrinolysis and increased PAI-1 are linked to atherothrombosis via insulin resistance and obesity. *Ann Med* 2000; 32 (suppl 1): 78–84.
175. Tuomilehto J, Lindstrom J, Eriksson JG, Valle TT, Hamalainen H, Ilanne-Parikka P, Keinanen-Kiukaanniemi S, Laakso M, Louheranta A, Rastas M, Salminen V, Uusitupa M. Prevention of type 2 diabetes mellitus by changes in lifestyle among subjects with impaired glucose tolerance. *N Engl J Med* 2001; 344: 1343–50.
176. Knowler WC, Barrett-Connor E, Fowler SE, Hamman RF, Lachin JM, Walker EA, Nathan DM. Reduction in the incidence of type 2 diabetes with lifestyle intervention or metformin. *N Engl J Med* 2002; 346: 393–403.

21

β-Cell Dysfunction in Type 2 Diabetes

Kristina M. Utzschneider and Steven E. Kahn

VA Puget Sound Health Care System and University of Washington, Seattle, WA, USA

INTRODUCTION

Type 2 diabetes is reaching epidemic proportions in concert with the increasing prevalence of obesity in many regions of the world [1]. Both type 2 diabetes and its precursor, impaired glucose tolerance (IGT), are also becoming more prevalent among children and adolescents who are obese [2]. The pathogenesis of the disease is complex, typically involving both insulin resistance and β-cell dysfunction, with both defects being present well before the development of frank hyperglycemia and the clinical diagnosis of diabetes. This chapter reviews the abnormalities in β-cell function observed in IGT and type 2 diabetes and elucidates some of the hypotheses regarding possible mechanisms responsible for the progressive failure of the β-cell over time.

ALTERATIONS IN THE PATTERNS OF PULSATILE AND OSCILLATORY INSULIN RELEASE IN THE BASAL STATE

In the basal state in healthy human subjects, insulin is secreted into the portal vein in both a rapid pulsatile pattern as well as a longer superimposed ultradian oscillatory pattern. Insulin pulses occur with a frequency of 6–10 min [3, 4] with this rapid pulsatile release appearing to be intrinsic to the β-cell as it has been demonstrated in human islets *in vitro* [5] and following pancreas transplantation [6]. In subjects with type 2 diabetes however, there is increased disorderliness of basal insulin release [7]. Studies examining subjects with IGT and a family history of type 2 diabetes have also demonstrated the loss of this regular rapid pulsatile pattern of insulin release, highlighting that this abnormality occurs early in the natural history of the disease [8]. In addition to this disorderly pattern of insulin release in type 2 diabetes, an inability to entrain these high-frequency pulses with glucose also occurs [9]. As in many other endocrine systems, this pulsatile release of insulin appears to be physiologically important. Simulation of a nonpulsatile pattern of insulin release is associated with impaired insulin action [10, 11].

In addition to these rapid pulses, a pattern of ultradian oscillatory insulin release is normally observed. These ultradian oscillations occur every 80–150 min and closely follow glucose oscillations of similar periodicity [12–15]. While the number of oscillations per 24 h is similar in healthy subjects and those with type 2 diabetes, the ultradian oscillations in individuals with type 2 diabetes are smaller in amplitude, are less regular, and typically not concomitant with a glucose pulse as observed in subjects with normal glucose tolerance (NGT) [12, 16]. Further, as with the high frequency pulses in healthy subjects, these ultradian insulin oscillations can also be entrained by administration of an oscillating glucose infusion. In contrast however, in subjects with IGT or type 2 diabetes, oscillatory glucose infusions fail to control the periodicity of the ultradian oscillations in insulin release [16]. These findings suggest that the β-cell in type 2 diabetes is unable to adequately sense or respond to fluctuations in glucose.

ALTERATIONS IN THE ABILITY OF GLUCOSE TO STIMULATE AND MODULATE THE INSULIN RESPONSE

Not only is the basal pattern of insulin release disrupted in type 2 diabetes, but the quantity of insulin released in response to a stimulus is inadequate, leading to the development of hyperglycemia. The oral glucose tolerance test is typically used to assess glucose tolerance, frequently in order to make the diagnosis of diabetes. In addition to

International Textbook of Diabetes Mellitus, Third Edition. Edited by R. A. DeFronzo, E. Ferrannini, H. Keen, and P. Zimmet, 2004.
This is a US Government Work and is in the public domain in the United States of America. ISBN: 0-471-48655-8.

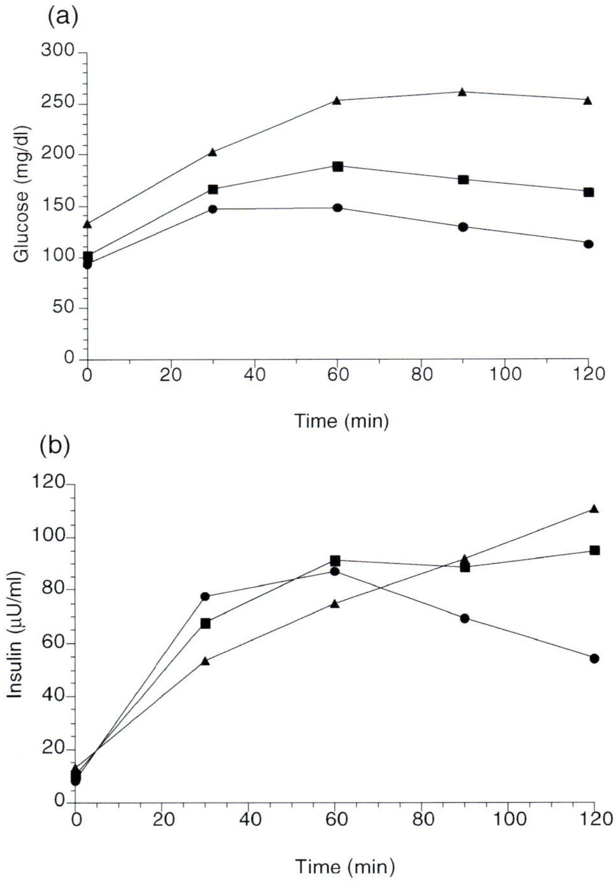

Figure 1 (a) Plasma glucose and (b) insulin responses to a 75-g oral glucose load in 531 first-degree relatives of type 2 diabetes with NGT (●, $n = 240$), IGT (■, $n = 191$), and diabetes (▲, $n = 100$). The early (0–30 min) insulin response is reduced in IGT and further reduced in subjects with diabetes. The elevated plasma glucose concentration at the end of the test stimulated insulin release, thus resulting in insulin levels in the subjects with diabetes approximating those in the individuals with NGT

assessment of the glucose response, it is possible to use this test to obtain measures of insulin release. Using this approach, it has been demonstrated that insulin release is diminished in type 2 diabetes, with this being clearly discernible when examining the early insulin response that occurs within 30 min of glucose ingestion [17–19] (Figure 1). Later following glucose ingestion, insulin levels may be similar or even higher than that in subjects with NGT because the plasma glucose level is elevated at these later time points [17, 18]. The critical nature of this early insulin response to glucose tolerance has been clearly demonstrated [20, 21]. As illustrated in Figure 2, the relationship between this early insulin response and glucose tolerance is nonlinear in nature [19]. Thus, small decreases in this early insulin response will have little effect on glucose tolerance in individuals in whom glucose tolerance is normal but reductions of a similar magnitude will have dramatic effects on the glucose excursion in individuals with type 2 diabetes. Individuals with IGT are intermediate, with the decreased insulin response being a critical determinant of their reduced glucose tolerance [19]. A similar situation exists when considering the consumption of a mixed meal [23].

The generation of the insulin response following ingestion of glucose or a meal is complex involving many different functions. These include the nature of the stimulus [24, 25], the release of incretin hormones by the gastrointestinal tract [26–28] (also see Chapter 12), neural input to the islet [29], and the rate of nutrient absorption [30]. Delineation of the importance of these different factors has been determined in part by intravenous testing.

When glucose is administered intravenously, the dynamics of insulin release comprise two distinct phases: an immediate first-phase response and a second-phase response. The first-phase response occurs within 2–5 min following glucose administration and lasts approximately 10 min. This response is felt to represent the release of insulin-containing granules from a readily releasable pool docked at the cell membrane [31]. This first-phase response delivers insulin rapidly to the liver and is important in inhibiting hepatic glucose production [32]. The second phase starts just after the glucose bolus and is related to the prevailing glucose level [33]. This second-phase response is believed to represent in large part the mobilization of insulin-containing granules from a large reserve pool [31].

In individuals with type 2 diabetes, both the first- and second-phase responses to glucose are diminished

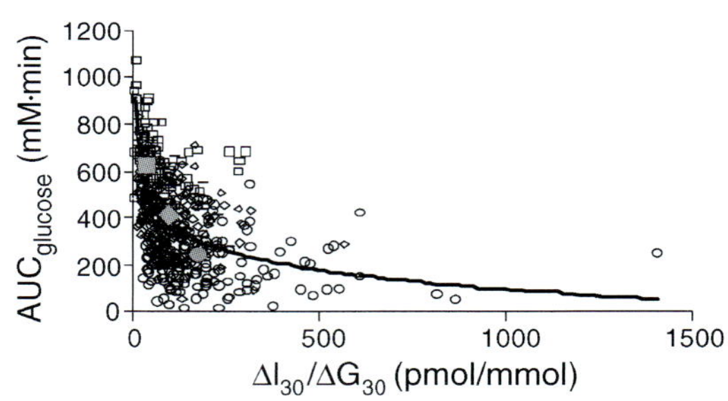

Figure 2 Relationship between the early insulin response quantified as the ratio of the incremental insulin and glucose responses over the first 30 min of the oral glucose tolerance test ($\triangle I_{30}/\triangle G_{30}$) and overall glucose metabolism determined as the incremental glucose response above baseline ($AUC_{glucose}$) in 531 first-degree relatives of type 2 diabetes. The mean value for each glucose tolerance category is represented as NGT (○, $n = 240$), IFG/IGT (◇, $n = 191$; IFG = impaired fasting glucose), and type 2 diabetes (□, $n = 100$). The relationship is nonlinear in nature, meaning that small differences in the insulin response in subjects with reduced glucose tolerance will have marked effects on the efficiency of glucose metabolism compared to a similar magnitude difference in those with NGT (reprinted with permission from reference 22)

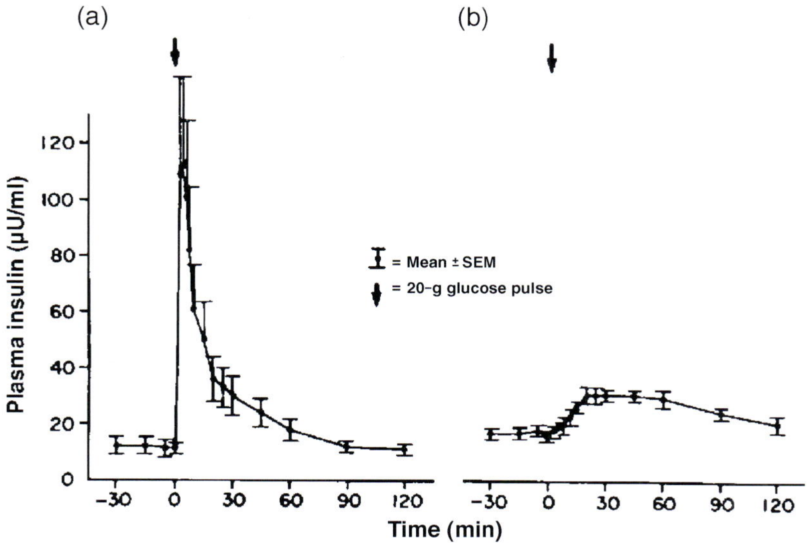

Figure 3 Plasma insulin response to a 20-g intravenous glucose bolus in (a) normal (mean fasting glucose 85 ± 3 mg/dl) and (b) type 2 diabetic subjects (mean fasting glucose 160 ± 10 mg/dl). The first-phase (acute) insulin response is absent in the subjects with diabetes while the second-phase response is relatively preserved because of the elevated plasma glucose following glucose injection. (Reprinted from American Journal of Medicine 1981 [34], with permission from Excerpta Medica Inc.)

(Figure 3). In fact, the lack of a first-phase response is a sina quo non for diabetes being absent in all individuals who are hyperglycemic [17, 35, 36]. This loss of the first-phase response can also be demonstrated in individuals whose fasting glucose level is above 6.4 mmol/l (115 mg/dl) but who do not yet have diabetes [36] (Figure 4a). While the second-phase response may seem to be relatively normal in subjects with type 2 diabetes, this "normal" response occurs as a result of the hyperglycemia that follows glucose administration in subjects with type 2 diabetes. Thus, when healthy and diabetic subjects are matched for the degree of glucose elevation, it is clear that the second-phase response is reduced in type 2 diabetes [35, 37]. The magnitude of the second-phase response declines as the fasting plasma glucose level increases [34] (Figure 4b).

In addition to its effect to directly stimulate the release of insulin, glucose is also able to modulate the magnitude of the insulin response to other secretagogues. This effect is known as *glucose potentiation* and is observed when insulin release is stimulated by the amino acid arginine [37], the peptide secretin [38], the β-adrenergic agonist isoproterenol [38], and sulfonylureas such as tolbutamide [39]. This potentiation effect of glucose results in an enhanced insulin response when the prevailing glucose level is elevated [40, 41]. This ability of glucose to potentiate the insulin response of the β-cell is also reduced in type 2 diabetes [37, 40]. Thus, when subjects with type 2 diabetes are matched for age and obesity with controls, their responses to non-glucose secretagogues may appear "normal." However, when the glucose level at which the assessment is being performed is matched in healthy and type 2 diabetic subjects, it is clear that the responses in the individuals with type 2 diabetes are diminished [40]. Assessing the insulin response to a non-glucose secretagogue when the glucose level is above 25.0 mmol/l (450 mg/dl) results in a maximal potentiated response. This maximal response has been termed AIR_{max}; and represents the secretory capacity of the β-cell [37]. In type 2 diabetes, AIR_{max}; is reduced in keeping with a reduction in the maximal secretory capacity of the β-cell, while the sensitivity of the β-cell to glucose is unchanged [37] (Figure 5). The severity of this reduction in β-cell secretory capacity is related to the fasting glucose level in an inverse, nonlinear manner [42] (Figure 6). The nature of this relationship suggests that a significant proportion (50–75%) of the secretory capacity of the β-cell is lost by the time fasting hyperglycemia appears. However, because fasting hyperglycemia is a late phenomenon in the pathogenesis of type 2 diabetes and β-cell dysfunction is progressive, lesser reductions in β-cell secretory capacity will be associated with reduced glucose tolerance before fasting hyperglycemia is manifest. The finding of reductions in β-cell secretory capacity has implications for the pathogenesis of type 2 diabetes as it has been demonstrated to occur in experimental models in which generalized reductions in islet mass have been produced [43, 44].

INEFFICIENT CONVERSION OF PROINSULIN TO INSULIN

In addition to the alterations in the release of insulin that characterize type 2 diabetes, abnormalities in the insulin

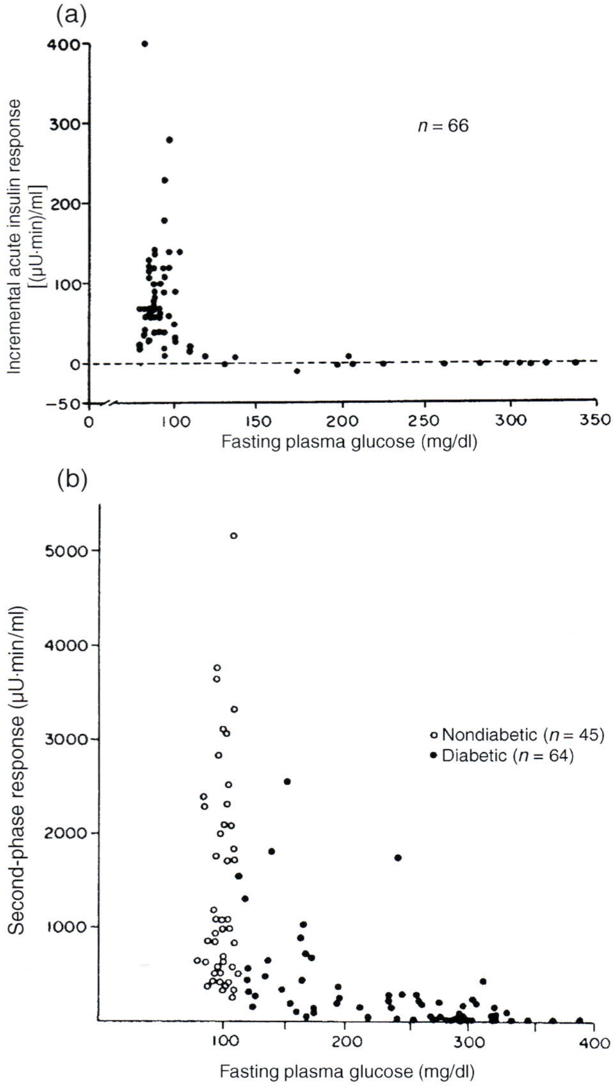

Figure 4 (a) Relationship between the incremental first-phase (acute) insulin response to intravenous glucose and fasting plasma glucose level in subjects with varying degrees of glucose tolerance. The acute insulin response is essentially absent in subjects with a fasting glucose level ≥110 mg/dl, the diagnostic cut point for impaired fasting glucose (The Journal of Clinical Endocrinology and Metabolism [34], © 1976. The Endocrine Society.) (b) Relationship between the incremental second-phase insulin response to intravenous glucose and the fasting plasma glucose levels in normal and type 2 diabetic subjects. The magnitude of the second-phase response is broad in the normal subjects, because of differences in insulin sensitivity. In subjects with type 2 diabetes this response decreases progressively with increasing fasting glucose, in keeping with progressively worse β-cell function. (Reprinted from American Journal of Medicine [34], 1981 with permission from Excerpta Medica Inc.)

biosynthetic process also occur. Insulin production requires the cleavage of the precursor peptide proinsulin into insulin and C-peptide by the endoproteases PC1/3 and PC2 [45]. This process occurs almost exclusively within the secretory granule that contains newly synthesized proinsulin [46, 47] and is regulated by strict pH and calcium requirements [48–50]. In healthy subjects, approximately 2% of the immunoreactive insulin released in response to β-cell stimulation is proinsulin and its cleavage intermediates des-31,32-split proinsulin and des-64,65-split proinsulin [51, 52]. This observation suggests that under normal circumstances proinsulin processing is incomplete. In type 2 diabetes however, the percentage of proinsulin released following acute stimulation is increased to between 5 and 8% of all insulin-like products [51, 52], reflecting a reduction in the efficiency of proinsulin processing. Because of the slower metabolic clearance rate of proinsulin, in the fasting state the proportion of proinsulin to immunoreactive insulin in healthy subjects is 15%, but is increased two- to threefold in those with type 2 diabetes [51–57]. As hyperglycemia worsens, the proportion

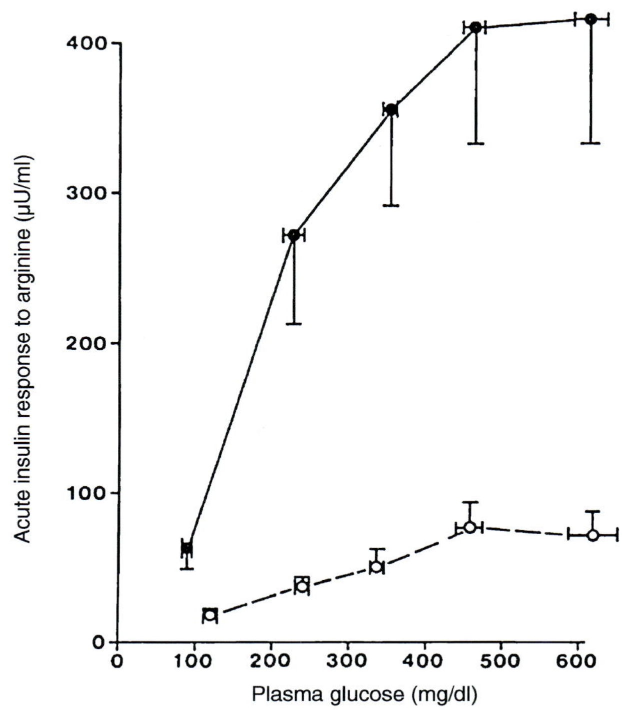

Figure 5 Comparison of the acute insulin response to a 5-g intravenous arginine injection (mean 2–5 min insulin increment) at different glucose levels in normal subjects (●) compared to those with type 2 diabetes (○) of similar age and body weight. The slope of potentiation is the linear portion of the curve relating plasma glucose between 5.5 and 13.9 mmol/l (100–250 mg/dl) and the acute insulin response. It is much flatter in the group with type 2 diabetes. The maximal insulin response occurs at a glucose level of >25 mmol/l (450 mg/dl) and is a measure of β-cell secretory capacity. It is also much lower in the diabetic group. However, the half-maximal glucose level, a measure of glucose sensitivity of the β-cell, is unchanged in the diabetic group and remains between 8.3 mmol/l (150 mg/dl) and 11.1 mmol/l (200 mg/dl) (reprinted with permission from reference 37)

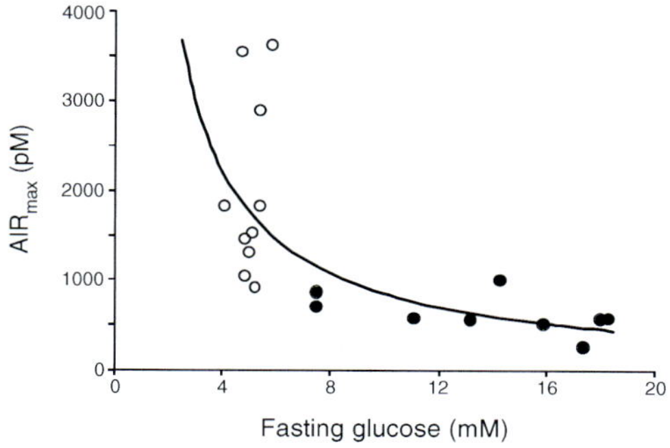

Figure 6 Relationship between β-cell secretory capacity (AIR_{max}) and fasting plasma glucose in 9 subjects with type 2 diabetes (●) and 10 subjects with NGT (○). There is a broad range of β-cell secretory capacity in the healthy subjects because of large differences in insulin sensitivity, while in subjects with type 2 diabetes the range is narrower as a manifestation of the impaired islet function. The nonlinear relationship between these two parameters ($r = -0.76$; $p < 0.0001$) demonstrates that the degree of β-cell function is a determinant of the fasting glucose level. In subjects with type 2 diabetes, β-cell secretory capacity is reduced by approximately 75% (The Journal of Clinical Endocrinology and Metabolism [42], © 1998. The Endocrine Society.)

of proinsulin as well as the ratio of fasting proinsulin to immunoreactive insulin (PI/IRI) increases (Figure 7). The PI/IRI also correlates inversely with AIR_{max}, in keeping with an increased PI/IRI ratio reflecting the magnitude of the decrease in β-cell secretory capacity [42].

Two main hypotheses have been advanced regarding the mechanism underlying the increased PI/IRI ratio seen in type 2 diabetes. The first hypothesis is that the increase in β-cell secretory demand that occurs in the face of hyperglycemia and insulin resistance results in the release of more immature secretory granules [45]. Release of immature granules would then be associated with increased proinsulin release, as insufficient time would have elapsed to allow normal processing of the propeptide. The alternative hypothesis states that the disproportionate release of proinsulin is a manifestation of an intrinsic defect in β-cell function [58]. The basis for this hypothesis is the observation that increased β-cell secretory demand imposed by insulin resistance in the absence of hyperglycemia is not associated with an increased PI/IRI ratio [57, 59] and that a glucose infusion in healthy subjects does not result in an increase in the ratio [60, 61]. While it is still unclear which of these hypotheses is correct, release of disproportionately increased amounts of proinsulin is a feature of type 2 diabetes [52, 57] and also predicts the subsequent development of diabetes in those at high risk [62–65].

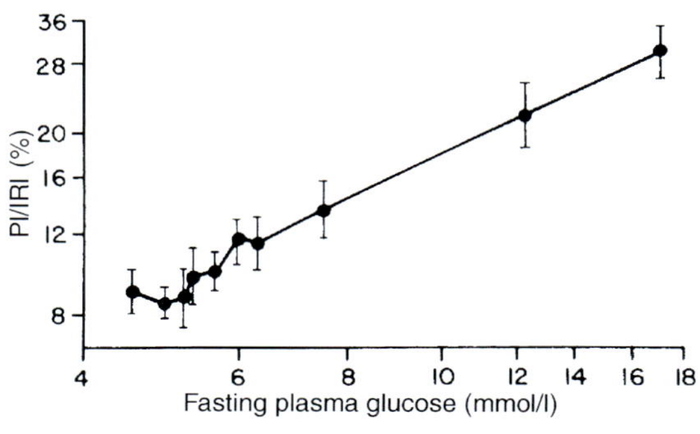

Figure 7 The relationship between the PI/IRI and fasting plasma glucose in obese Pima Indian subjects. Each point represents the mean ± SEM for 12–19 subjects (median 15). Subjects were ranked by fasting plasma glucose and divided into consecutive groups of approximately 15 subjects each. An increase in the PI/IRI ratio is seen very early with mild elevations in the fasting plasma glucose [57]. (The Journal of Clinical Endocrinology and Metabolism [57], © 1990. The Endocrine Society.)

THE EARLY PRESENCE AND PROGRESSIVE NATURE OF β-CELL DYSFUNCTION IN TYPE 2 DIABETES

It is well recognized that insulin sensitivity is an important factor modulating the insulin response of the β-cell [66, 67]. If insulin sensitivity is high, a smaller amount of insulin is released for a given stimulus compared to when insulin sensitivity is low. The ability of the β-cell to respond to changes in secretory demand imposed by insulin resistance is highlighted by the fact that while almost all subjects with diabetes have insulin resistance, the majority of obese individuals who are insulin resistant do not develop IGT or type 2 diabetes. This adaptive response occurs as a result of the presence of a feedback loop between the insulin-sensitive tissues and the β-cell. The interaction between these two systems is such that insulin sensitivity and insulin secretion are inversely and proportionally related (Figure 8). Appreciation of the nature of this relationship has highlighted the fact that evaluation of insulin responses as a measure of β-cell function requires knowledge of the prevailing insulin sensitivity. Thus, individuals with similar insulin responses who differ for the degree of insulin sensitivity will differ in terms of β-cell function.

Understanding the nature of the relationship between insulin sensitivity and insulin release has helped highlight the fact that β-cell function is markedly diminished in type 2 diabetes [68] and that β-cell dysfunction is an early and critical component of the pathophysiology of type 2 diabetes. Even before the development of fasting hyperglycemia and the clinical diagnosis of diabetes, evidence of β-cell dysfunction manifest as abnormalities in insulin secretion can be detected in groups at high risk for developing diabetes at a time when they do not have hyperglycemia and many still have NGT. Thus, cross-sectional studies have demonstrated that first-degree relatives of individuals with type 2 diabetes [69, 70], women with a history of either gestational diabetes [71–73] or polycystic ovarian disease [69, 74], older subjects

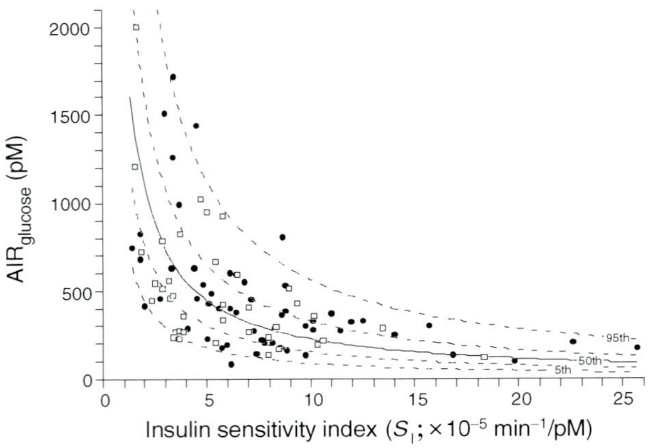

Figure 8 Relationship between insulin sensitivity and insulin release quantified as the first-phase insulin response ($AIR_{glucose}$) in 93 [55 males (●), 38 females (□)] apparently healthy, nondiabetic subjects under the age of 45 years. The cohort demonstrates a broad range of insulin sensitivity and insulin release. The solid line depicts the best-fit relationship (50th percentile) while the broken lines represent the 5th, 25th, 75th, and 95th percentiles. The relationship is best described by a hyperbolic function ($S_I \times$ AIRglucose is a constant) so that any change in insulin sensitivity is balanced by a reciprocal and proportionate change in insulin release (reprinted with permission from reference 66)

[75–77], and individuals with IGT [78] all have a reduced first-phase insulin response to intravenous glucose (Figure 9).

The approach of assessing β-cell function by interpreting insulin responses in the context of insulin sensitivity has clearly demonstrated the critical role of the β-cell. Assessments have shown that β-cell dysfunction is global, affecting not only the first-phase response, but also the second-phase insulin response to intravenous glucose [82], glucose potentiation [83], pulsatile insulin secretion [8], and the ultradian oscillatory pattern of insulin release including an inability of glucose to entrain insulin secretion [16, 69, 72]. In addition to these secretory defects, an inefficiency of proinsulin processing has also been demonstrated in individuals at increased risk, including women with a history of gestational diabetes [63], Japanese Americans with NGT or IGT at baseline who develop diabetes over a 5-year follow-up period [62], nondiabetic Mexican Americans with a parental history of diabetes [64], and older subjects who by virtue of their age develop diabetes more frequently [65]. It is also of interest that β-cell function, assessed as the insulin response relative to insulin sensitivity, is not only decreased in nondiabetic members of familial type 2 diabetes kindreds, but is also highly heritable demonstrating heritability of 67% when members with NGT and IGT were included and 70% when only family members with NGT were evaluated. This degree of heritability cannot be demonstrated when either first-phase insulin release or even insulin sensitivity is examined in isolation [84].

The loss of β-cell function appears to be progressive, with this outcome apparently occurring in most, if not all, population groups. This observation is based on both cross-sectional and longitudinal data obtained following either oral or intravenous glucose administration. Progressively decreasing β-cell function has been demonstrated in four different ethnic groups in the United States when the early insulin response after oral glucose ingestion has been evaluated [22] (Figure 10). Similarly, a longitudinal study in Pima Indians showed that the natural history of insulin secretion and insulin sensitivity in the pathogenesis of type 2 diabetes involves a decline in both these parameters [85]. In subjects who progressed from NGT to IGT and then on to diabetes over a 5-year period, β-cell function declined dramatically when the magnitude of the insulin response was examined relative to insulin sensitivity, whereas insulin sensitivity declined only slightly (Figure 11). In contrast, in those subjects who were followed over the same time period but who maintained NGT, insulin sensitivity declined similarly to that in the individuals who progressed to diabetes, but in this instance insulin secretion increased compatible with a compensatory change in β-cell function. Thus, a progressive loss of β-cell function appears to be a critical component in the pathogenesis of type 2 diabetes and appears to be a feature of the process of diabetes development in most, if not all, population groups.

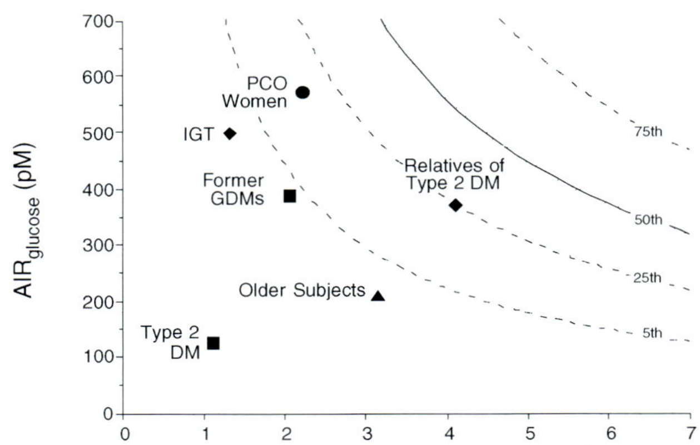

Figure 9 Percentile lines for the relationship between insulin sensitivity (S_I) and the first-phase insulin response ($AIR_{glucose}$) on the basis of data from 93 normal subjects [66]. Mean data from six other studies are plotted. The 10 subjects with type 2 diabetes are insulin resistant and have markedly impaired insulin secretion [79]. Groups at increased risk for the development of type 2 diabetes also exhibit reduced β-cell function including 13 healthy older subjects [75], 8 women with a history of gestational diabetes (GDM) [71], 11 women with polycystic ovarian disease (PCO) and a family history of type 2 diabetes [69], 21 subjects with IGT [78], and 14 subjects with a first-degree relative with type 2 diabetes mellitus [80] (reprinted with permission from reference 81)

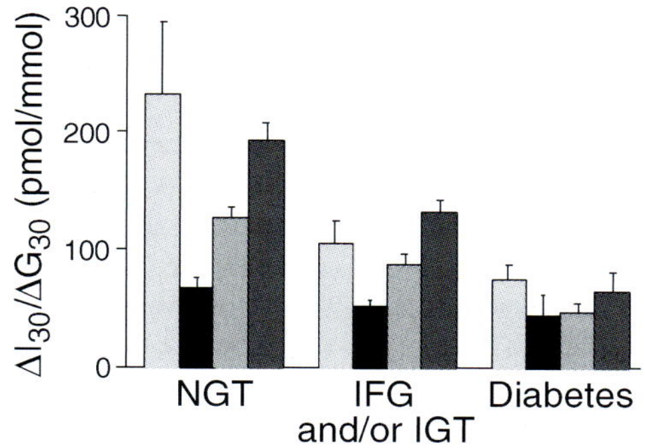

Figure 10 β-Cell function as quantified by $\Delta I_{30}/\Delta G_{30}$ during an oral glucose tolerance test in 531 first-degree relatives of subjects with type 2 diabetes from four different ethnic groups [55 African Americans (■), 66 Asian Americans (■), 217 Caucasians (■), and 193 Hispanic Americans (■)]. Individuals with IFG or IGT who had diabetes by the 2-h or fasting glucose criteria respectively were classified as having diabetes. A progressive loss of the early-phase response is seen between subjects who have NGT, IGT, and type 2 diabetes. The variability in the magnitude of the responses between ethnic groups within a glucose tolerance category is the result of differences in insulin sensitivity, with the greater responses being observed in the subjects that are more insulin resistant (reprinted with permission from reference 22)

This progressive decline in β-cell function not only predates the development of hyperglycemia, but also continues unabated after the diagnosis of diabetes. This change seems to occur even when different therapeutic modalities are used. This has been clearly demonstrated in the United Kingdom Prospective Diabetes Study (UKPDS) where β-cell function declined similarly in groups receiving different therapies [86, 87].

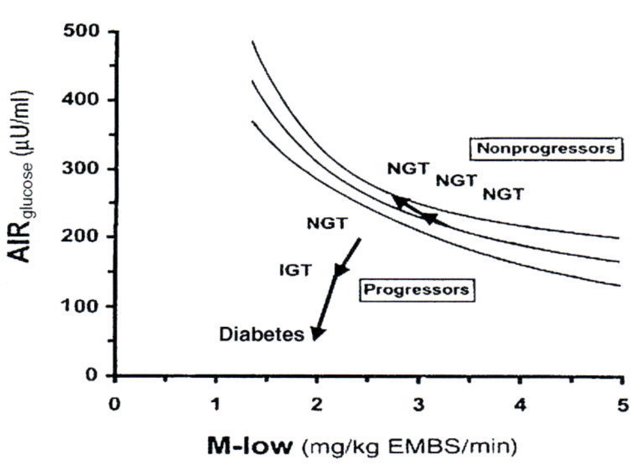

Figure 11 Changes in β-cell function measured as the acute insulin response to glucose ($AIR_{glucose}$) relative to changes in insulin sensitivity measured by the clamp technique at a low insulin concentration (M-low) in 11 Pima Indians in whom glucose tolerance deteriorated from NGT to IGT to diabetes (progressors), and in 23 subjects who maintained NGT throughout (nonprogressors). The lines represent the prediction line and the lower and upper limits of the 95% confidence interval of the regression between the AIR and M-low as determined from a population of 277 Pima Indians with NGT (reprinted with permission from reference 85)

POTENTIAL MECHANISMS FOR β-CELL DYSFUNCTION

Although β-cell dysfunction, manifest in part as defects in insulin secretion, is present early in the development of type 2 diabetes and is progressive, the exact nature of the underlying mechanism(s) leading to these defects is unclear. In addition to demonstrating dysfunction of the β-cells, it has been well documented that there is a decrease in β-cell mass in diabetes. The defects in insulin secretion that characterize type 2 diabetes are likely to be a result of the combination of both cellular dysfunction and a reduction in β-cell mass.

Examination of islet size and morphological characteristics of the islet in autopsy specimens has demonstrated that the overall islet mass in individuals with type 2 diabetes is reduced by 40–60% compared to matched nondiabetic subjects [88–90]. Quantification of β-cell mass has also shown this to be reduced by up to 30% in patients with type 2 diabetes compared with controls [91, 92]. Although islet mass is reduced, no significant reduction in α-, δ- and PP-cells has been documented in type 2 diabetes [92]. Since α-cell mass is not decreased while β-cell mass is reduced, α-cell mass is therefore disproportionately increased in type 2 diabetes [91, 92]. While the precise etiology of the reduction in β-cell mass is debated, changes in islet morphology have been noted in type 2 diabetes including the almost universal finding of amyloid deposits [88, 91]. On the basis of studies in humans who have undergone a partial pancreatectomy [93], this degree of reduction in β-cell mass is probably not enough to cause diabetes on its own. While surgical reduction of β-cell mass in humans and animals does not result in diabetes even when β-cell mass is reduced by 50% [43, 44, 94], this approach also results in a reduction in the mass of the other islet endocrine cells so that the imbalance of α- and β-cells observed in type 2 diabetes does not exist. However, it certainly appears that in type 2 diabetes, in addition to any reduction in β-cell mass, a functional defect in β-cell function has also to be present.

The etiology of this reduction in β-cell mass in type 2 diabetes is unclear. It may be related to an increase in programmed cell death known as *apoptosis*, a decrease in replication or a lack of adequate neogenesis, or a combination of increased loss and decreased regeneration. An analysis of autopsy specimens in both lean and obese subjects with NGT, IGT, or type 2 diabetes found that the frequency of apoptosis was higher in those with diabetes and that the frequency of neogenesis, while being higher in obese subjects, was no different in those with diabetes compared to their weight-matched NGT controls. They also reported that the frequency of regeneration appears to be very low and may not contribute significantly to β-cell mass in humans [90]. These changes in rates of cell turnover resulting in a reduction in β-cell mass could be primary or may be related to toxic factors such as islet amyloid polypeptide (IAPP) and subsequent amyloid fibril formation, increased glucose levels, or elevated lipid concentrations. Alternatively, a reduction in factors such as glucagon-like peptide 1 as observed in type 2 diabetes [95], may play a role as they are capable of stimulating β-cell proliferation and regeneration [27] (see Chapter 12).

IAPP AND ISLET AMYLOID

Islet amyloid deposits have been found at autopsy in up to 90% of individuals with type 2 diabetes [88, 96], and contain the normal β-cell secretory product IAPP as their unique peptide component. IAPP, also known as amylin, is a 37-amino acid peptide synthesized by the β-cell, co-localized with insulin in secretory granules within the β-cell, and released along with insulin in response to both oral and intravenous stimulation [97, 98]. The release of the peptide typically occurs in parallel with insulin in a molar ratio of approximately 1:100, with insulin being the abundant peptide [19, 97, 99]. In keeping with the fact that it is co-released with insulin, IAPP release has been demonstrated to be diminished in individuals with type 2 diabetes[19, 100]. Furthermore, a parallel reduction in both insulin and IAPP release has also been shown in individuals at high risk of developing diabetes by virtue of the fact that they have IGT [19, 100] or are first-degree relatives of individuals with type 2 diabetes [99].

The mechanism by which IAPP forms amyloid and potentially reduces β-cell mass does not appear to be due to the simple overproduction of the peptide, as obese individuals without diabetes are not more likely to have amyloid deposits than do lean subjects [90]. Studies using transgenic mice that overexpress the human amyloidogenic form of IAPP failed to demonstrate amyloid formation [101] until the mice were fed a high-fat diet for a year [102] or were made markedly insulin resistant by cross-breeding them with lines of genetically modified insulin-resistant mice and again following them for a prolonged period of time [103, 104]. It is of interest that islet amyloid is also found in humans with insulinomas, β-cell tumors that are characterized by an inefficiency of peptide processing and secretory defects, including increased release of propeptides through the constitutive secretory pathway [105, 106]. While the cellular changes responsible for the initiation and promulgation of amyloid fibril formation by IAPP remain unclear, it is apparent based on *in vitro* studies that these fibrils are toxic to β-cells and induce apoptosis [58, 107, 108]. Further, it is of interest that freshly formed fibrils are more cytotoxic than are the aggregates of amyloid, the latter likely representing the end stage of a process that is associated with β-cell dysfunction and death [109].

GLUCOSE DESENSITIZATION

Glucose desensitization, also known as glucose toxicity, has been proposed as a mechanism whereby chronic hyperglycemia induces dysfunction of the β-cell, resulting in a loss of responsiveness to glucose stimulation [110–112]. Assessments of these deleterious effects have commonly been made in cell culture following prolonged exposure to high glucose concentrations [112–114] or in rodents made markedly hyperglycemic by infusion of large quantities of glucose [115]. This desensitization to glucose-stimulated insulin release in rodents appears to be rapidly reversible, occurring within 6 h of initiation of an insulin infusion, a time course suggesting reversal of a defect in processing, activation, or regulation of a key protein rather than new gene transcription [115].

Balancing these findings in cell culture and rodents are observations that have been made in healthy humans infused with glucose. In these studies, enhanced responsiveness of the β-cell can be demonstrated after just 12 h of intravenous glucose administration and this increased responsiveness can still be shown to be present following 53 h of hyperglycemia [116–118]. This enhancement of insulin release during experimental hyperglycemia in humans would appear to prevent a dramatic rise in the plasma glucose concentration so that the maximum glucose concentration reached at the end of these studies was 7.2 mmol/l (130 mg/dl) [117]. In patients with type 2 diabetes, weight loss [119–125], sulfonylureas [123], and insulin therapy [123, 126–131] have all been shown to improve insulin secretion, possibly as a consequence of decreased hyperglycemia, suggesting that a portion of the deleterious effect of hyperglycemia on insulin secretion is reversible. However, while glucose desensitization may be playing a role in a portion of the β-cell dysfunction in established type 2 diabetes, on the basis of studies in healthy subjects and the fact that diminished β-cell function can be demonstrated in high-risk individuals when they do not yet have hyperglycemia, it is not likely to be a major factor in the early pathogenesis of the disease. Further, on the basis of findings in the intensively treated group in the UKPDS, it does not appear to be a major factor in the continued progression of β-cell dysfunction in established type 2 diabetes. In this treatment group, despite normalization of the fasting glucose and HbA_{1c} levels and the continuation of the intensive therapy that had achieved this near perfect level of control, β-cell function continued to decline progressively over time resulting in a gradual increase in both fasting glucose and HbA_{1c} [132].

Thus, while glucose desensitization may be a factor in the pathogenesis of human type 2 diabetes, its role appears to be largely one of impairing β-cell responsiveness once β-cell dysfunction is established rather than being an initiating factor in the development of the secretory abnormalities associated with the disease.

LIPOTOXICITY

Consumption of a high-fat diet is associated with an increased risk of developing diabetes. This increased risk is in part related to the increase in obesity, and particularly intra-abdominal fat, and the attendant insulin resistance that occur along with changes in β-cell function [133, 134].

One potential mechanism by which increased dietary fat may lead to impaired β-cell function is through an increase in free fatty acids (FFAs) that then may accumulate within and be toxic to the β-cell. *In vitro* studies suggest that excess FFAs in non-adipose tissue undergo nonoxidative metabolism to toxic substances such as ceramide, that then ultimately lead to apoptosis [135, 136]. Interestingly, studies examining the effects of different fatty acids in cultured rat islets suggest that saturated fatty acids such as palmitic acid increase apoptosis, reduce the proliferative capacity of β-cells, and impair insulin secretion [136]. On the other hand, the monounsaturated fatty acid palmitoleic acid does not affect apoptosis and in fact promotes β-cell proliferation at low glucose levels [136]. FFAs have also been shown to inhibit insulin release in animals and in *in vitro* islet preparations [137–139] and to impair proinsulin processing in both human and rodent islets [138]. Recent data suggest that hyperglycemia may be necessary for elevated fatty acids to have their deleterious effects on β-cell function [140, 141]. In humans, the effect of FFAs on β-cell function has been harder to discern because of the coexistent development of insulin resistance. However, data would suggest that the prolonged elevation of FFA levels is associated with a reduction in β-cell function [142]. Finally, while these changes have been observed with FFAs, the potential accumulation and role of triglycerides within islets is uncertain. Such a change has been observed in older adults, but these morphological changes have not been specifically studied in subjects with type 2 diabetes [143].

CONCLUSIONS

It is apparent that the development of type 2 diabetes is a complex and multifactorial process involving a combination of a genetic predisposition and environmental factors. Type 2 diabetes involves both insulin resistance and functional impairments of the β-cell that can be demonstrated to involve both processing and secretory components of insulin production and release. These β-cell abnormalities are present well before the diagnosis of diabetes and can even be identified in subjects at risk for developing diabetes who still exhibit NGT. There are a number of possible mechanisms that may account for these changes in β-cell function, including the effects of amyloid fibril formation by IAPP, hyperglycemia itself, and the effects of elevated FFAs. Understanding the pathophysiology of the β-cell dysfunction that is characteristic of type 2 diabetes should in the future allow for the development of new approaches that may be useful in both the prevention and treatment of this disorder.

REFERENCES

1. King H, Aubert RE, Herman WH. Global burden of diabetes, 1995–2025: prevalence, numerical estimates, and projections. *Diabetes Care* 1998; 21: 1414–31.
2. Sinha R, Fisch G, Teague B, Tamborlane WV, Banyas B, Allen K, Savoye M, Rieger V, Taksali S, Barbetta G, Sherwin RS, Caprio S. Prevalence of impaired glucose tolerance among children and adolescents with marked obesity. *N Engl J Med* 2002; 346: 802–10.
3. Porksen N, Munn S, Steers J, Vore S, Veldhuis J, Butler P. Pulsatile insulin secretion accounts for 70% of total insulin secretion during fasting. *Am J Physiol* 1995; 269: E478–88.
4. Song SH, McIntyre SS, Shah H, Veldhuis JD, Hayes PC, Butler PC. Direct measurement of pulsatile insulin secretion from the portal vein in human subjects. *J Clin Endocrinol Metab* 2000; 85: 4491–9.
5. Hellman B, Gylfe E, Bergsten P, Grapengiesser E, Lund PE, Berts A, Tengholm A, Pipeleers DG, Ling Z. Glucose induces oscillatory Ca^{2+} signalling and insulin release in human pancreatic beta cells. *Diabetologia* 1994; 37 (suppl 2): S11–20.
6. Sonnenberg GE, Hoffmann RG, Johnson CP, Kissebah AH. Low- and high-frequency insulin secretion pulses in normal subjects and pancreas transplant recipients: role of extrinsic innervation. *J Clin Invest* 1992; 90: 545–53.
7. Schmitz O, Juhl CB, Hollingdal M, Veldhuis JD, Porksen N, Pincus SM. Irregular circulating insulin concentrations in type 2 diabetes mellitus: an inverse relationship between circulating free fatty acid and the disorderliness of an insulin time series in diabetic and healthy individuals. *Metabolism* 2001; 50: 41–6.
8. O'Rahilly S, Turner RC, Matthews DR. Impaired pulsatile secretion of insulin in relatives of patients with non-insulin-dependent diabetes. *N Engl J Med* 1988; 318: 1225–30.
9. Hollingdal M, Juhl CB, Pincus SM, Sturis J, Veldhuis JD, Polonsky KS, Porksen N, Schmitz O. Failure of physiological plasma glucose excursions to entrain high-frequency pulsatile insulin secretion in type 2 diabetes. *Diabetes* 2000; 49: 1334–40.
10. Paolisso G, Sgambato S, Torella R, Varricchio M, Scheen A, D'Onofrio F, Lefebvre PJ. Pulsatile insulin delivery is more efficient than continuous infusion in modulating islet cell function in normal subjects and patients with type 1 diabetes. *J Clin Endocrinol Metab* 1988; 66: 1220–6.
11. Marangou AG, Weber KM, Boston RC, Aitken PM, Heggie JC, Kirsner RL, Best JD, Alford FP. Metabolic consequences of prolonged hyperinsulinemia in humans. Evidence for induction of insulin insensitivity. *Diabetes* 1986; 35: 1383–9.
12. Polonsky KS, Given BD, Hirsch LJ, Tillil H, Shapiro ET, Beebe C, Frank BH, Galloway JA, Van Cauter E. Abnormal patterns of insulin secretion in non-insulin-dependent diabetes mellitus. *N Engl J Med* 1988; 318: 1231–9.

13. Sturis J, Polonsky KS, Shapiro ET, Blackman JD, O'Meara NM, van Cauter E. Abnormalities in the ultradian oscillations of insulin secretion and glucose levels in type 2 (non-insulin-dependent) diabetic patients. *Diabetologia* 1992; 35: 681–9.
14. Scheen AJ, Sturis J, Polonsky KS, Van Cauter E. Alterations in the ultradian oscillations of insulin secretion and plasma glucose in aging. *Diabetologia* 1996; 39: 564–72.
15. Shapiro ET, Tillil H, Polonsky KS, Fang VS, Rubenstein AH, Van Cauter E. Oscillations in insulin secretion during constant glucose infusion in normal man: relationship to changes in plasma glucose. *J Clin Endocrinol Metab* 1988; 67: 307–14.
16. O'Meara NM, Sturis J, Van Cauter E, Polonsky KS. Lack of control by glucose of ultradian insulin secretory oscillations in impaired glucose tolerance and in non-insulin-dependent diabetes mellitus. *J Clin Invest* 1993; 92: 262–71.
17. Perley MJ, Kipnis DM. Plasma insulin responses to oral and intravenous glucose: studies in normal and diabetic subjects. *J Clin Invest* 1967; 46: 1954–62.
18. Bagdade JD, Bierman EL, Porte D Jr. The significance of basal insulin levels in the evaluation of the insulin response to glucose in diabetic and nondiabetic subjects. *J Clin Invest* 1967; 46: 1549–57.
19. Kahn SE, Verchere CB, Andrikopoulos S, Asberry PJ, Leonetti DL, Wahl PW, Boyko EJ, Schwartz RS, Newell-Morris L, Fujimoto WY. Reduced amylin release is a characteristic of impaired glucose tolerance and type 2 diabetes in Japanese Americans. *Diabetes* 1998; 47: 640–5.
20. Calles-Escandon J, Robbins DC. Loss of early phase of insulin release in humans impairs glucose tolerance and blunts thermic effect of glucose. *Diabetes* 1987; 36: 1167–72.
21. Pratley RE, Weyer C. The role of impaired early insulin secretion in the pathogenesis of Type II diabetes mellitus. *Diabetologia* 2001; 44: 929–45.
22. Jensen CC, Cnop M, Hull RL, Fujimoto WY, Kahn SE. Beta-cell function is a major contributor to oral glucose tolerance in high-risk relatives of four ethnic groups in the U.S. *Diabetes* 2002; 51: 2170–8.
23. Butler PC, Rizza RA. Contribution to postprandial hyperglycemia and effect on initial splanchnic glucose clearance of hepatic glucose cycling in glucose-intolerant or NIDDM patients. *Diabetes* 1991; 40: 73–81.
24. Gutniak M, Grill V, Efendic S. Effect of composition of mixed meals—low- versus high-carbohydrate content—on insulin, glucagon, and somatostatin release in healthy humans and in patients with NIDDM. *Diabetes Care* 1986; 9: 244–9.
25. Spiller GA, Jensen CD, Pattison TS, Chuck CS, Whittam JH, Scala J. Effect of protein dose on serum glucose and insulin response to sugars. *Am J Clin Nutr* 1987; 46: 474–80.
26. Perfetti R, Merkel P. Glucagon-like peptide-1: a major regulator of pancreatic beta-cell function. *Eur J Endocrinol* 2000; 143: 717–25.
27. Doyle ME, Egan JM. Glucagon-like peptide-1. *Recent Prog Horm Res* 2001; 56: 377–99.
28. Meier JJ, Nauck MA, Schmidt WE, Gallwitz B. Gastric inhibitory polypeptide: the neglected incretin revisited. *Regul Pept* 2002; 107: 1–13.
29. Ahren B. Autonomic regulation of islet hormone secretion—implications for health and disease. *Diabetologia* 2000; 43: 393–410.
30. Bjorck I, Granfeldt Y, Liljeberg H, Tovar J, Asp NG. Food properties affecting the digestion and absorption of carbohydrates. *Am J Clin Nutr* 1994; 59: 699S–705S.
31. Bratanova-Tochkova TK, Cheng H, Daniel S, Gunawardana S, Liu YJ, Mulvaney-Musa J, Schermerhom T, Straub SG, Yajima H, Sharp GW. Triggering and augmentation mechanisms, granule pools, and biphasic insulin secretion. *Diabetes* 2002; 51 (suppl 1): S83–90.
32. Luzi L, DeFronzo RA. Effect of loss of first-phase insulin secretion on hepatic glucose production and tissue glucose disposal in humans. *Am J Physiol* 1989; 257: E241–6.
33. Toschi E, Camastra S, Sironi AM, Masoni A, Gastaldelli A, Mari A, Ferrannini E, Natali A. Effect of acute hyperglycemia on insulin secretion in humans. *Diabetes* 2002; 51 (suppl 1): S130–3.
34. Pfeifer MA, Halter JB, Porte D Jr. Insulin secretion in diabetes mellitus. *Am J Med* 1981; 70: 579–88.
35. Porte D Jr. Banting lecture 1990. Beta-cells in type II diabetes mellitus. *Diabetes* 1991; 40: 166–80.
36. Brunzell JD, Robertson RP, Lerner RL, Hazzard WR, Ensinck JW, Bierman EL, Porte D, Jr, Relationships between fasting plasma glucose levels and insulin secretion during intravenous glucose tolerance tests. *J Clin Endocrinol Metab* 1976; 42: 222–9.
37. Ward WK, Bolgiano DC, McKnight B, Halter JB, Porte D Jr. Diminished B cell secretory capacity in patients with noninsulin-dependent diabetes mellitus. *J Clin Invest* 1984; 74: 1318–28.
38. Halter JB, Porte D Jr. Mechanisms of impaired acute insulin release in adult onset diabetes: studies with isoproterenol and secretin. *J Clin Endocrinol Metab* 1978; 46: 952–60.
39. Varsano-Aharon N, Echemendia E, Yalow RS, Berson SA. Early insulin responses to glucose and to tolbutamide in maturity-onset diabetes. *Metabolism* 1970; 19: 409–17.
40. Halter JB, Graf RJ, Porte D Jr. Potentiation of insulin secretory responses by plasma glucose levels in man: evidence that hyperglycemia in diabetes compensates for imparied glucose potentiation. *J Clin Endocrinol Metab* 1979; 48: 946–54.
41. Cerasi E. Potentiation of insulin release by glucose in man, II: role of the insulin response, and enhancement of stimuli other than glucose. *Acta Endocrinol (Copenh)* 1975; 79: 502–10.
42. Roder ME, Porte D Jr, Schwartz RS, Kahn SE. Disproportionately elevated proinsulin levels reflect the degree of impaired B cell secretory capacity in patients with noninsulin-dependent diabetes mellitus. *J Clin Endocrinol Metab* 1998; 83: 604–8.
43. Leahy JL, Bonner-Weir S, Weir GC. Abnormal glucose regulation of insulin secretion in models of reduced B-cell mass. *Diabetes* 1984; 33: 667–73.
44. Ward WK, Wallum BJ, Beard JC, Taborsky GJ Jr, Porte D Jr. Reduction of glycemic potentiation. Sensitive indicator of beta-cell loss in partially pancreatectomized dogs. *Diabetes* 1988; 37: 723–9.
45. Rhodes CJ, Alarcon C. What beta-cell defect could lead to hyperproinsulinemia in NIDDM? Some clues from recent advances made in understanding the proinsulin-processing mechanism. *Diabetes* 1994; 43: 511–7.
46. Rhodes CJ, Lucas CA, Mutkoski RL, Orci L, Halban PA. Stimulation by ATP of proinsulin to insulin conversion in isolated rat pancreatic islet secretory granules.

Association with the ATP-dependent proton pump. *J Biol Chem* 1987; 262: 10712–7.
47. Orci L, Ravazzola M, Storch MJ, Anderson RG, Vassalli JD, Perrelet A. Proteolytic maturation of insulin is a post-Golgi event which occurs in acidifying clathrin-coated secretory vesicles. *Cell* 1987; 49: 865–8.
48. Rhodes CJ, Lincoln B, Shoelson SE. Preferential cleavage of des-31,32-proinsulin over intact proinsulin by the insulin secretory granule type II endopeptidase. Implication of a favored route for prohormone processing. *J Biol Chem* 1992; 267: 22719–27.
49. Bailyes EM, Bennett DL, Hutton JC. Proprotein-processing endopeptidases of the insulin secretory granule. *Enzyme* 1991; 45: 301–13.
50. Davidson HW, Rhodes CJ, Hutton JC. Intraorganellar calcium and pH control proinsulin cleavage in the pancreatic beta cell via two distinct site-specific endopeptidases. *Nature* 1988; 333: 93–6.
51. Kahn SE, Halban PA. Release of incompletely processed proinsulin is the cause of the disproportionate proinsulinemia of NIDDM. *Diabetes* 1997; 46: 1725–32.
52. Ward WK, LaCava EC, Paquette TL, Beard JC, Wallum BJ, Porte D Jr. Disproportionate elevation of immunoreactive proinsulin in type 2 (non-insulin-dependent) diabetes mellitus and in experimental insulin resistance. *Diabetologia* 1987; 30: 698–702.
53. Kahn SE, Leonetti DL, Prigeon RL, Boyko EJ, Bergstrom RW, Fujimoto WY. Relationship of proinsulin and insulin with noninsulin-dependent diabetes mellitus and coronary heart disease in Japanese-American men: impact of obesity—clinical research center study. *J Clin Endocrinol Metab* 1995; 80: 1399–406.
54. Temple RC, Clark PM, Nagi DK, Schneider AE, Yudkin JS, Hales CN. Radioimmunoassay may overestimate insulin in non-insulin-dependent diabetics. *Clin Endocrinol (Oxf)* 1990; 32: 689–93.
55. Yoshioka N, Kuzuya T, Matsuda A, Taniguchi M, Iwamoto Y. Serum proinsulin levels at fasting and after oral glucose load in patients with type 2 (non-insulin-dependent) diabetes mellitus. *Diabetologia* 1988; 31: 355–60.
56. Mako ME, Starr JI, Rubenstein AH. Circulating proinsulin in patients with maturity onset diabetes. *Am J Med* 1977; 63: 865–9.
57. Saad MF, Kahn SE, Nelson RG, Pettitt DJ, Knowler WC, Schwartz MW, Kowalyk S, Bennett PH, Porte D, Jr, Disproportionately elevated proinsulin in Pima Indians with noninsulin-dependent diabetes mellitus. *J Clin Endocrinol Metab* 1990; 70: 1247–53.
58. Porte D Jr, Kahn SE. Hyperproinsulinemia and amyloid in NIDDM. Clues to etiology of islet beta-cell dysfunction? *Diabetes* 1989; 38: 1333–6.
59. Koivisto VA, Yki-Jarvinen H, Hartling SG, Pelkonen R. The effect of exogenous hyperinsulinemia on proinsulin secretion in normal man, obese subjects, and patients with insulinoma. *J Clin Endocrinol Metab* 1986; 63: 1117–20.
60. Hartling SG, Roder ME, Dinesen B, Binder C. Proinsulin, C-peptide, and insulin in normal subjects during an 8-h hyperglycemic clamp. *Eur J Endocrinol* 1996; 134: 197–200.
61. Nauck MA, Siegel EG, Creutzfeldt W. Prolonged maximal stimulation of insulin secretion in healthy subjects does not provoke preferential release of proinsulin. *Pancreas* 1991; 6: 645–52.
62. Kahn SE, Leonetti DL, Prigeon RL, Boyko EJ, Bergstrom RW, Fujimoto WY. Proinsulin as a marker for the development of NIDDM in Japanese-American men. *Diabetes* 1995; 44: 173–9.
63. Persson B, Hanson U, Hartling SG, Binder C. Follow-up of women with previous GDM. Insulin, C-peptide, and proinsulin responses to oral glucose load. *Diabetes* 1991; 40 (suppl 2): 136–41.
64. Haffner SM, Stern MP, Miettinen H, Gingerich R, Bowsher RR. Higher proinsulin and specific insulin are both associated with a parental history of diabetes in nondiabetic Mexican-American subjects. *Diabetes* 1995; 44: 1156–60.
65. Fritsche A, Madaus A, Stefan N, Tschritter O, Maerker E, Teigeler A, Haring H, Stumvoll M. Relationships among age, proinsulin conversion, and beta-cell function in nondiabetic humans. *Diabetes* 2002; 51 (suppl 1): S234–9.
66. Kahn SE, Prigeon RL, McCulloch DK, Boyko EJ, Bergman RN, Schwartz MW, Neifing JL, Ward WK, Beard JC, Palmer JP, et al. Quantification of the relationship between insulin sensitivity and beta-cell function in human subjects. Evidence for a hyperbolic function. *Diabetes* 1993; 42: 1663–72.
67. Olefsky J, Farquhar JW, Reaven G. Relationship between fasting plasma insulin level and resistance to insulin-mediated glucose uptake in normal and diabetic subjects. *Diabetes* 1973; 22: 507–13.
68. Kahn SE. Clinical review 135: the importance of beta-cell failure in the development and progression of type 2 diabetes. *J Clin Endocrinol Metab* 2001; 86: 4047–58.
69. Ehrmann DA, Sturis J, Byrne MM, Karrison T, Rosenfield RL, Polonsky KS. Insulin secretory defects in polycystic ovary syndrome. Relationship to insulin sensitivity and family history of non-insulin-dependent diabetes mellitus. *J Clin Invest* 1995; 96: 520–7.
70. Elbein SC, Wegner K, Kahn SE. Reduced beta-cell compensation to the insulin resistance associated with obesity in members of Caucasian familial type 2 diabetic kindreds. *Diabetes Care* 2000; 23: 221–7.
71. Ward WK, Johnston CL, Beard JC, Benedetti TJ, Halter JB, Porte D Jr. Insulin resistance and impaired insulin secretion in subjects with histories of gestational diabetes mellitus. *Diabetes* 1985; 34: 861–9.
72. Ryan EA, Imes S, Liu D, McManus R, Finegood DT, Polonsky KS, Sturis J. Defects in insulin secretion and action in women with a history of gestational diabetes. *Diabetes* 1995; 44: 506–12.
73. Buchanan TA, Xiang AH, Kjos SL, Trigo E, Lee WP, Peters RK. Antepartum predictors of the development of type 2 diabetes in Latino women 11–26 months after pregnancies complicated by gestational diabetes. *Dia-betes* 1999; 48: 2430–6.
74. Bergman RN. Toward physiological understanding of glucose tolerance: minimal-model approach. *Diabetes* 1989; 38: 1512–27.
75. Kahn SE, Larson VG, Beard JC, Cain KC, Fellingham GW, Schwartz RS, Veith RC, Stratton JR, Cerqueira MD, Abrass IB. Effect of exercise on insulin action, glucose tolerance, and insulin secretion in aging. *Am J Physiol* 1990; 258: E937–43.
76. Kahn SE, Larson VG, Schwartz RS, Beard JC, Cain KC, Fellingham GW, Stratton JR, Cerqueira MD, Abrass IB. Exercise training delineates the importance of B-cell dysfunction to the glucose intolerance of human aging. *J Clin Endocrinol Metab* 1992; 74: 1336–42.

77. Chen M, Bergman RN, Pacini G, Porte D Jr. Pathogenesis of age-related glucose intolerance in man: insulin resistance and decreased beta-cell function. *J Clin Endocrinol Metab* 1985; 60: 13–20.
78. Cavaghan MK, Ehrmann DA, Byrne MM, Polonsky KS. Treatment with the oral antidiabetic agent troglitazone improves beta cell responses to glucose in subjects with impaired glucose tolerance. *J Clin Invest* 1997; 100: 530–7.
79. Welch S, Gebhart SS, Bergman RN, Phillips LS. Minimal model analysis of intravenous glucose tolerance test-derived insulin sensitivity in diabetic subjects. *J Clin Endocrinol Metab* 1990; 71: 1508–18.
80. Kahn SE. Regulation of B-cell function *in vivo*: from health to disease. *Diabetes Rev* 1996; 4: 372–89.
81. Vidal J, Kahn SE. Regulation of insulin secretion *in vivo*. In WL Lowe Jr (ed), *Genetics of Diabetes Mellitus*. Boston: Kluwer, 2001; pp 109–31.
82. Pimenta W, Korytkowski M, Mitrakou A, Jenssen T, Yki-Jarvinen H, Evron W, Dailey G, Gerich J. Pancreatic beta-cell dysfunction as the primary genetic lesion in NIDDM. Evidence from studies in normal glucose-tolerant individuals with a first-degree NIDDM relative. *JAMA* 1995; 273: 1855–61.
83. Larsson H, Ahren B. Failure to adequately adapt reduced insulin sensitivity with increased insulin secretion in women with impaired glucose tolerance. *Diabetologia* 1996; 39: 1099–107.
84. Elbein SC, Hasstedt SJ, Wegner K, Kahn SE. Heritability of pancreatic beta-cell function among nondiabetic members of Caucasian familial type 2 diabetic kindreds. *J Clin Endocrinol Metab* 1999; 84: 1398–403.
85. Weyer C, Bogardus C, Mott DM, Pratley RE. The natural history of insulin secretory dysfunction and insulin resistance in the pathogenesis of type 2 diabetes mellitus. *J Clin Invest* 1999; 104: 787–94.
86. Matthews DR, Cull CA, Stratton IM, Holman RR, Turner RC, for the United Kingdom Prospective Diabetes Study (UKPDS) Group. UKPDS 26: sulphonylurea failure in non-insulin-dependent diabetic patients over six years. *Diabet Med* 1998; 15: 297–303.
87. Holman RR. Assessing the potential for alpha-glucosidase inhibitors in prediabetic states. *Diabetes Res Clin Pract* 1998; 40 (suppl): S21–5.
88. Westermark P, Wilander E. The influence of amyloid deposits on the islet volume in maturity onset diabetes mellitus. *Diabetologia* 1978; 15: 417–21.
89. Kloppel G, Lohr M, Habich K, Oberholzer M, Heitz PU. Islet pathology and the pathogenesis of type 1 and type 2 diabetes mellitus revisited. *Surv Synth Pathol Res* 1985; 4: 110–25.
90. Butler AE, Janson J, Bonner-Weir S, Ritzel R, Rizza RA, Butler PC. Beta-cell deficit and increased beta-cell apoptosis in humans with type 2 diabetes. *Diabetes* 2003; 52: 102–10.
91. Clark A, Wells CA, Buley ID, Cruickshank JK, Vanhegan RI, Matthews DR, Cooper GJ, Holman RR, Turner RC. Islet amyloid, increased A-cells, reduced B-cells and exocrine fibrosis: quantitative changes in the pancreas in type 2 diabetes. *Diabetes Res* 1988; 9: 151–9.
92. Sakuraba H, Mizukami H, Yagihashi N, Wada R, Hanyu C, Yagihashi S. Reduced beta-cell mass and expression of oxidative stress-related DNA damage in the islet of Japanese Type II diabetic patients. *Diabetologia* 2002; 45: 85–96.
93. Kendall DM, Sutherland DE, Najarian JS, Goetz FC, Robertson RP. Effects of hemipancreatectomy on insulin secretion and glucose tolerance in healthy humans. *N Engl J Med* 1990; 322: 898–903.
94. Seaquist ER, Kahn SE, Clark PM, Hales CN, Porte D Jr, Robertson RP. Hyperproinsulinemia is associated with increased beta cell demand after hemipancreatectomy in humans. *J Clin Invest* 1996; 97: 455–60.
95. Vilsboll T, Krarup T, Deacon CF, Madsbad S, Holst JJ. Reduced postprandial concentrations of intact biologically active glucagon-like peptide 1 in type 2 diabetic patients. *Diabetes* 2001; 50: 609–13.
96. Clark A, Saad MF, Nezzer T, Uren C, Knowler WC, Bennett PH, Turner RC. Islet amyloid polypeptide in diabetic and non-diabetic Pima Indians. *Diabeto-logia* 1990; 33: 285–9.
97. Kahn SE, D'Alessio DA, Schwartz MW, Fujimoto WY, Ensinck JW, Taborsky GJ, Jr, Porte D, Jr, Evidence of cosecretion of islet amyloid polypeptide and insulin by beta-cells. *Diabetes* 1990; 39: 634–8.
98. Lukinius A, Wilander E, Westermark GT, Engstrom U, Westermark P. Co-localization of islet amyloid polypeptide and insulin in the B cell secretory granules of the human pancreatic islets. *Diabetologia* 1989; 32: 240–4.
99. Knowles NG, Landchild MA, Fujimoto WY, Kahn SE. Insulin and amylin release are both diminished in first-degree relatives of subjects with type 2 diabetes. *Diabetes Care* 2002; 25: 292–7.
100. Enoki S, Mitsukawa T, Takemura J, Nakazato M, Aburaya J, Toshimori H, Matsukara S. Plasma islet amyloid polypeptide levels in obesity, impaired glucose tolerance and non-insulin-dependent diabetes mellitus. *Diabetes Res Clin Pract* 1992; 15: 97–102.
101. D'Alessio DA, Verchere CB, Kahn SE, Hoagland V, Baskin DG, Palmiter RD, Ensinck JW. Pancreatic expression and secretion of human islet amyloid polypeptide in a transgenic mouse. *Diabetes* 1994; 43: 1457–61.
102. Verchere CB, D'Alessio DA, Palmiter RD, Weir GC, Bonner-Weir S, Baskin DG, Kahn SE. Islet amyloid formation associated with hyperglycemia in transgenic mice with pancreatic beta cell expression of human islet amyloid polypeptide. *Proc Natl Acad Sci USA* 1996; 93: 3492–6.
103. Soeller WC, Janson J, Hart SE, Parker JC, Carty MD, Stevenson RW, Kreutter DK, Butler PC. Islet amyloid-associated diabetes in obese A(vy)/a mice expressing human islet amyloid polypeptide. *Diabetes* 1998; 47: 743–50.
104. Hoppener JW, Oosterwijk C, Nieuwenhuis MG, Posthuma G, Thijssen JH, Vroom TM, Ahren B, Lips CJ. Extensive islet amyloid formation is induced by development of Type II diabetes mellitus and contributes to its progression: pathogenesis of diabetes in a mouse model. *Diabetologia* 1999; 42: 427–34.
105. Halban PA, Irminger JC. Sorting and processing of secretory proteins. *Biochem J* 1994; 299 (pt 1): 1–18.
106. Nagamatsu S, Steiner DF. Altered glucose regulation of insulin biosynthesis in insulinoma cells: mouse beta TC3 cells secrete insulin-related peptides predominantly via a constitutive pathway. *Endocrinology* 1992; 130: 748–54.
107. Janson J, Ashley RH, Harrison D, McIntyre S, Butler PC. The mechanism of islet amyloid polypeptide toxicity is membrane disruption by intermediate-sized toxic amyloid particles. *Diabetes* 1999; 48: 491–8.

108. Lorenzo A, Razzaboni B, Weir GC, Yankner BA. Pancreatic islet cell toxicity of amylin associated with type-2 diabetes mellitus. *Nature* 1994; 368: 756–60.
109. Hiddinga HJ, Eberhardt NL. Intracellular amyloidogenesis by human islet amyloid polypeptide induces apoptosis in COS-1 cells. *Am J Pathol* 1999; 154: 1077–88.
110. Leahy JL, Bonner-Weir S, Weir GC. Beta-cell dysfunction induced by chronic hyperglycemia. Current ideas on mechanism of impaired glucose-induced insulin secretion. *Diabetes Care* 1992; 15: 442–55.
111. Yki-Jarvinen H. Glucose toxicity. *Endocr Rev* 1992; 13: 415–31.
112. Robertson RP, Olson LK, Zhang HJ. Differentiating glucose toxicity from glucose desensitization: a new message from the insulin gene. *Diabetes* 1994; 43: 1085–9.
113. Ling Z, Kiekens R, Mahler T, Schuit FC, Pipeleers-Marichal M, Sener A, Kloppel G, Malaisse WJ, Pipeleers DG. Effects of chronically elevated glucose levels on the functional properties of rat pancreatic beta-cells. *Diabetes* 1996; 45: 1774–82.
114. Purrello F, Rabuazzo AM, Anello M, Patane G. Effects of prolonged glucose stimulation on pancreatic beta cells: from increased sensitivity to desensitization. *Acta Diabetol* 1996; 33: 253–6.
115. Leahy JL, Weir GC. Beta-cell dysfunction in hyperglycaemic rat models: recovery of glucose-induced insulin secretion with lowering of the ambient glucose level. *Diabetologia* 1991; 34: 640–7.
116. Dimitriadis G, Cryer P, Gerich J. Prolonged hyperglycaemia during infusion of glucose and somatostatin impairs pancreatic A- and B-cell responses to decrements in plasma glucose in normal man: evidence for induction of altered sensitivity to glucose. *Diabetologia* 1985; 28: 63–9.
117. Ward WK, Halter JB, Beard JC, Porte D Jr. Adaptation of B and A cell function during prolonged glucose infusion in human subjects. *Am J Physiol* 1984; 246: E405–11.
118. Flax H, Matthews DR, Levy JC, Coppack SW, Turner RC. No glucotoxicity after 53 hours of 6.0 mmol/l hyperglycaemia in normal man. *Diabetologia* 1991; 34: 570–5.
119. Bogardus C, Ravussin E, Robbins DC, Wolfe RR, Horton ES, Sims EA. Effects of physical training and diet therapy on carbohydrate metabolism in patients with glucose intolerance and non-insulin-dependent diabetes mellitus. *Diabetes* 1984; 33: 311–8.
120. Zawadzki JK, Bogardus C, Foley JE. Insulin action in obese non-insulin-dependent diabetics and in their isolated adipocytes before and after weight loss. *Diabetes* 1987; 36: 227–36.
121. Henry RR, Wallace P, Olefsky JM. Effects of weight loss on mechanisms of hyperglycemia in obese non-insulin-dependent diabetes mellitus. *Diabetes* 1986; 35: 990–8.
122. Stanik S, Marcus R. Insulin secretion improves following dietary control of plasma glucose in severely hyperglycemic obese patients. *Metabolism* 1980; 29: 346–50.
123. Kosaka K, Kuzuya T, Akanuma Y, Hagura R. Increase in insulin response after treatment of overt maturity-onset diabetes is independent of the mode of treatment. *Diabetologia* 1980; 18: 23–8.
124. Savage PJ, Bennion LJ, Bennett PH. Normalization of insulin and glucagon secretion in ketosis-resistant diabetes mellitus with prolonged diet therapy. *J Clin Endocrinol Metab* 1979; 49: 830–3.
125. Eriksson KF, Lindgarde F. Prevention of type 2 (non-insulin-dependent) diabetes mellitus by diet and physical exercise. The 6-year Malmö feasibility study. *Diabetologia* 1991; 34: 891–8.
126. Garvey WT, Olefsky JM, Griffin J, Hamman RF, Kolterman OG. The effect of insulin treatment on insulin secretion and insulin action in type II diabetes mellitus. *Diabetes* 1985; 34: 222–34.
127. Yki-Jarvinen H, Nikkila E, Helve E, Taskinen M-R. Clinical benefits and mechanisms of a sustained response to intermittent insulin therapy in type 2 diabetic patients with secondary drug failure. *Am J Med* 1988; 84: 185–92.
128. Vague P, Moulin JP. The defective glucose sensitivity of the B cell in non insulin dependent diabetes. Improvement after twenty hours of normoglycaemia. *Metabolism* 1982; 31: 139–42.
129. Andrews WJ, Vasquez B, Nagulesparan M, Klimes I, Foley J, Unger R, Reaven GM. Insulin therapy in obese, non-insulin-dependent diabetes induces improvements in insulin action and secretion that are maintained for two weeks after insulin withdrawal. *Diabetes* 1984; 33: 634–42.
130. Hidaka H, Nagulesparan M, Klimes I, Clark R, Sasaki H, Aronoff SL, Vasquez B, Rubenstein AH, Unger RH. Improvement of insulin secretion but not insulin resistance after short term control of plasma glucose in obese type II diabetics. *J Clin Endocrinol Metab* 1982; 54: 217–22.
131. Ginsberg H, Rayfield EJ. Effect of insulin therapy on insulin resistance in type II diabetic subjects. Evidence for heterogeneity. *Diabetes* 1981; 30: 739–45.
132. The UKPDS Group. Intensive blood-glucose control with sulphonylureas or insulin compared with conventional treatment and risk of complications in patients with type 2 diabetes (UKPDS 33). *Lancet* 1998; 352: 837–53.
133. Kaiyala KJ, Prigeon RL, Kahn SE, Woods SC, Porte D, Jr, Schwartz MW. Reduced beta-cell function contributes to impaired glucose tolerance in dogs made obese by high-fat feeding. *Am J Physiol* 1999; 277: E659–67.
134. Mittelman SD, Van Citters GW, Kim SP, Davis DA, Dea MK, Hamilton-Wessler M, Bergman RN. Longitudinal compensation for fat-induced insulin resistance includes reduced insulin clearance and enhanced beta-cell response. *Diabetes* 2000; 49: 2116–25.
135. Shimabukuro M, Zhou YT, Levi M, Unger RH. Fatty acid-induced beta cell apoptosis: a link between obesity and diabetes. *Proc Natl Acad Sci USA* 1998; 95: 2498–502.
136. Maedler K, Spinas GA, Dyntar D, Moritz W, Kaiser N, Donath MY. Distinct effects of saturated and monounsaturated fatty acids on beta-cell turnover and function. *Diabetes* 2001; 50: 69–76.
137. Zhou YP, Grill VE. Long-term exposure of rat pancreatic islets to fatty acids inhibits glucose-induced insulin secretion and biosynthesis through a glucose fatty acid cycle. *J Clin Invest* 1994; 93: 870–6.
138. Zhou YP, Grill V. Long term exposure to fatty acids and ketones inhibits B-cell functions in human pancreatic islets of Langerhans. *J Clin Endocrinol Metab* 1995; 80: 1584–90.
139. Sako Y, Grill VE. A 48-hour lipid infusion in the rat time-dependently inhibits glucose-induced insulin secretion and B cell oxidation through a process likely coupled to fatty acid oxidation. *Endocrinology* 1990; 127: 1580–9.

140. Briaud I, Harmon JS, Kelpe CL, Segu VB, Poitout V. Lipotoxicity of the pancreatic beta-cell is associated with glucose-dependent esterification of fatty acids into neutral lipids. *Diabetes* 2001; 50: 315–21.
141. Poitout V, Robertson RP. Secondary beta-cell failure in type 2 diabetes—a convergence of glucotoxicity and lipotoxicity [minireview]. *Endocrinology* 2002; 143: 339–42.
142. Carpentier A, Mittelman SD, Lamarche B, Bergman RN, Giacca A, Lewis GF. Acute enhancement of insulin secretion by FFA in humans is lost with prolonged FFA elevation. *Am J Physiol* 1999; 276: E1055–66.
143. Cnop M, Grupping A, Hoorens A, Bouwens L, Pipeleers-Marichal M, Pipeleers D. Endocytosis of low-density lipoprotein by human pancreatic beta cells and uptake in lipid-storing vesicles, which increase with age. *Am J Pathol* 2000; 156: 237–44.

22

Metabolic and Molecular Pathogenesis of Type 2 Diabetes Mellitus

Ralph A. DeFronzo*, Lawrence Mandarino*, and Ele Ferrannini†

**University of Texas Health Science Center, San Antonio, TX, USA, and †Department of Internal Medicine, University of Pisa School of Medicine, Pisa, Italy*

NORMAL GLUCOSE HOMEOSTASIS

Following an overnight fast (postabsorptive state), the majority of total-body glucose utilization takes place in insulin-dependent tissues [1]. Under basal conditions approximately 50% of all glucose disposal occurs in the brain, which becomes saturated at a plasma glucose concentration of about 40 mg/dl and which is insulin independent [2]. Another 25% of glucose uptake occurs in the splanchnic area (liver plus gastrointestinal tissues) and also is insulin independent [3]. The remaining 25% of glucose metabolism in the postabsorptive state occurs in insulin-dependent tissues, primarily muscle [4, 5]. Basal glucose utilization, which averages ~2.0 mg/kg/min, is precisely matched by the rate of endogenous glucose production [1, 3–7] (Figure 1). The majority of endogenous glucose production is derived from the liver (~85%), and the remaining amount is produced by the kidney [8, 9]. Under basal, postabsorptive conditions, approximately half of hepatic glucose production (HGP) is derived from glycogenolysis and half from gluconeogenesis [9, 10].

Following the ingestion of a glucose-containing meal, the delicate balance between endogenous glucose production and tissue glucose uptake is disrupted. The rise in plasma glucose concentration stimulates the release of insulin from the pancreatic β-cells, and the resultant hyperinsulinemia and hyperglycemia serve [1] to stimulate glucose uptake by splanchnic (liver and gut) and peripheral (primarily muscle) tissues (Table 1) and [2] to suppress endogenous glucose production [1, 3–7, 11–15]. Hyperglycemia, in the absence of hyperinsulinemia, exerts its own independent effect to stimulate muscle glucose uptake [15] and to suppress endogenous glucose production [16, 17] in a dose-dependent fashion. Of the glucose that is taken up by peripheral tissues, the majority (~80–85%) is disposed of in muscle [1, 3–7, 11–15], with only a small amount (~4–5%) being metabolized in fat tissue [18, 19]. Although fat tissue is responsible for only a small amount of total body glucose disposal, it plays a very important role in the maintenance of total body glucose homeostasis (see below). Insulin is a potent antilipolytic hormone and even small increments in the plasma insulin concentration exert a potent antilipolytic effect, leading to a marked reduction in the plasma free falty acid (FFA) level [20, 21]. The decline in plasma FFA concentration results in increased glucose uptake in muscle [22, 23] and contributes to the inhibition of HGP [17, 24]. Thus, changes in the plasma FFA concentration in response to increased plasma levels of insulin and glucose play an important role in the maintenance of normal glucose homeostasis [25, 26].

Glucagon, the forgotten hormone, also plays a central role in the maintenance of normal glucose homeostasis [17, 27]. Under postabsorptive conditions approximately half of total hepatic glucose output is dependent upon the maintenance of normal basal glucagon levels and inhibition of basal glucagon secretion with somatostatin leads to a profound reduction in endogenous glucose production and decline in plasma glucose concentration [17, 27]. Following a glucose-containing meal, α-cell secretion of glucagon is inhibited by hyperinsulinemia [27]. The resultant hypoglucagonemia plays an important role in the suppression of hepatic glucose production

International Textbook of Diabetes Mellitus, Third Edition. Edited by R. A. DeFronzo, E. Ferrannini, H. Keen, and P. Zimmet.
 ISBN: 0-471-48655-8.

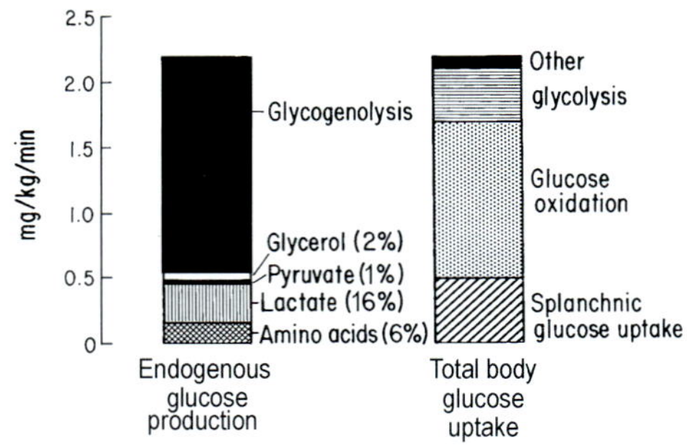

Figure 1 Schematic representation of glucose production and glucose utilization in the normal human in the postabsorptive state. (Reproduced by permission of the American Diabetes Association [1])

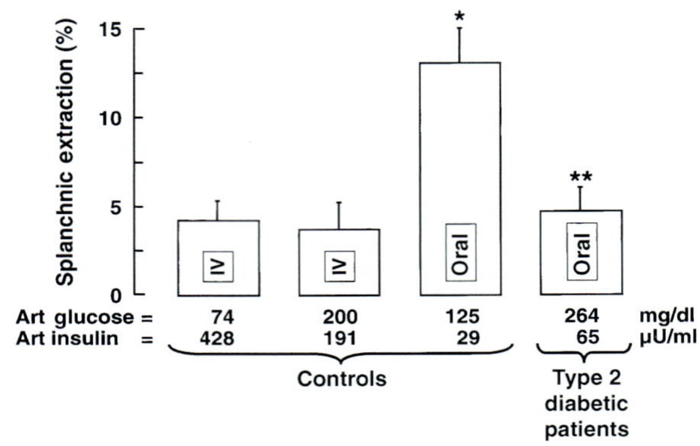

Figure 2 Effect of intravenous insulin, intravenous glucose, and oral route of glucose administration on splanchnic (primarily hepatic) glucose uptake. $^{*}p < 0.01$ vs. IV glucose; $^{**}p < 0.01$ vs. oral glucose in controls (from references 29 and 30, with permission)

and maintenance of normal postprandial glucose tolerance [17, 28].

The route of glucose administration also exerts a major influence on the distribution of administered glucose and overall glucose homeostasis [1, 4, 6, 7, 11–14, 17, 29–31] (Figure 2). Intravenous administration of insulin has no stimulatory effect on splanchnic (liver plus gut) glucose uptake, while hyperglycemia enhances splanchnic glucose uptake in direct proportion to the increase in plasma glucose concentration [3, 29, 30]. In contrast, oral glucose administration markedly enhances splanchnic glucose uptake [1, 4, 17, 29–31]. Cherrington et al. have shown that the portal signal that stimulates hepatic glucose uptake is closely related to the negative hepatic artery-portal vein glucose concentration gradient [31]. Widening of this gradient stimulates the splanchnic nerves, activating a neural reflex, which enhances vagal activity and inhibits sympathetic nerves that innervate the liver [17, 32, 33]. These neural changes enhance glucose uptake by the hepatocyte and stimulate hepatic glycogen synthase, while simultaneously inhibiting glycogen phosphorylase. In contrast to the intravenous administration of glucose/insulin, where muscle accounts for the majority (∼80–85%) of glucose disposal, the splanchnic tissues are responsible for the removal of approximately 30–40% of an ingested glucose load [6, 7, 11–14].

The oral route of glucose administration also has a potentiating effect on insulin secretion [34, 35]. It has long been recognized that the plasma insulin response following glucose ingestion is approximately twice as great as that created by intravenous glucose despite equivalent increases in the plasma glucose concentration. This potentiating effect of oral glucose administration is related to the release of glucagon-like peptide 1 (GLP-1) and glucose-dependent insulinotropic polypeptide (previously called gastric inhibitory polypeptide) (GIP) from the gastrointestinal tissues [36, 37].

Table 1 Factors responsible for the maintenance of normal glucose tolerance in healthy subjects

(1)	Insulin secretion
(2)	Tissue glucose uptake
	(a) Peripheral (primarily muscle)
	(b) Splanchnic (liver plus gut)
(3)	Suppression of HGP
	(a) Decreased FFA
	(b) Decreased glucagon
(4)	Route of glucose administration

GLUCOSE HOMEOSTASIS IN TYPE 2 DIABETES MELLITUS

Type 2 diabetic individuals are characterized by [1] defects in insulin secretion; [2] insulin resistance involving muscle, liver, and the adipcoyte; and [3] abnormalities in splanchnic glucose uptake [1, 3–6, 26, 29, 38].

Insulin Secretion

Numerous studies have demonstrated that insulin secretion is impaired in type 2 diabetic patients and the evolution of β-cell dysfunction has been well characterized in diverse ethnic populations [1, 4, 38–50]. Early in the natural history of type 2 diabetes, insulin resistance is well established [1, 4, 43, 45–49, 51–56] but glucose tolerance remains normal because of a compensatory increase in insulin secretion [1, 4, 40–43, 45–49, 52–55, 57–59]. This dynamic interaction between insulin secretion and insulin resistance has been well documented [60]. Within the normal-glucose-tolerant population, approximately 20–25% of individuals are severely resistant to the action of insulin [60–62] (Figure 3a). Using the euglycemic insulin clamp to quantitate insulin-mediated glucose disposal, Diamond et al. [60] divided healthy, nondiabetic

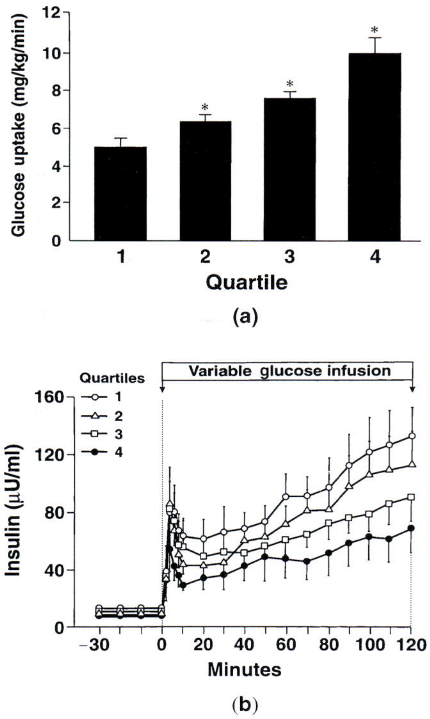

Figure 3 (a) Whole-body rate of glucose disposal during euglycemic insulin clamps in 32 women divided according to quartiles of insulin sensitivity. $^*p < 0.001$ for each quartile vs. the adjacent quartile. (b) Time course of plasma insulin response during the hyperglycemic clamp in the same 32 women divided into quartiles of insulin sensitivity. Insulin secretion rose progressively from the highest to the lowest quartile of insulin sensitivity ($p < 0.01$). (Reproduced by permission of Elsevier [60])

individuals into four quartiles. The subjects in the lowest quartile were as insulin resistant as type 2 diabetic patients (Figure 3b). When insulin secretion in these insulin-resistant, normal-glucose-tolerant individuals was measured with the hyperglycemic (+125 mg/dl) clamp technique, both the early (0–10 min) and late (10–120 min) phases of insulin release, as well as the fasting plasma insulin concentration, were increased in proportion to the severity of the insulin resistance ($r = 0.79$, $p < 0.001$). Thus, the pancreas in people with a normal-functioning beta cell is able to "read" the severity of insulin resistance and adjust its secretion of insulin to maintain normal glucose tolerance.

In type 2 diabetic patients, the fasting plasma insulin concentration invariably has been found to be normal or increased [1, 4, 38, 40–42, 49, 52, 59] and basal insulin secretion, measured from C-peptide kinetics, is elevated [1, 3, 4, 63, 64]. DeFronzo et al. [65] measured the fasting plasma insulin concentration and performed oral glucose tolerance tests (OGTTs) in 77 normal-weight type 2 diabetic patients and over 100 lean subjects with normal or impaired glucose tolerance (IGT). As can be seen in Figure 4, the relationship between the fasting plasma glucose concentration and the fasting plasma insulin concentration resembles an inverted U or horseshoe. Because this curve closely resembles Starling's curve of the heart, DeFronzo and colleagues have referred to it as Starling's curve of the pancreas. As the fasting plasma glucose concentration rises from 80 to 140 mg/dl, the fasting plasma insulin concentration increases progressively, peaking at a value that is 2–2.5-fold greater than in normal weight, non-diabetic, age-matched controls (Figure 4). The progressive rise in fasting plasma insulin level can be viewed as an adaptive response of the pancreas to offset the progressive deterioration in glucose homeostasis. However, when the fasting plasma glucose concentration exceeds 140 mg/dl, the beta cell no longer can maintain its elevated rate of insulin secretion and the fasting insulin concentration declines precipitously. This decrease in fasting insulin level has important physiologic implications, since it is at this point that hepatic glucose production (the primary determinant of the fasting plasma glucose concentration) begins to rise [65].

The relationship between the plasma insulin response during an OGTT and the fasting plasma insulin concentration also resembles an inverted U-shaped curve (Figure 5). However, the inflection point, ~120 mg/dl, at which the beta cell no longer can maintain its accelerated rate of insulin secretion is shifted to the left compared to the basal insulin secretory rate. A type 2 diabetic patient with a fasting plasma glucose concentration of 150–160 mg/dl

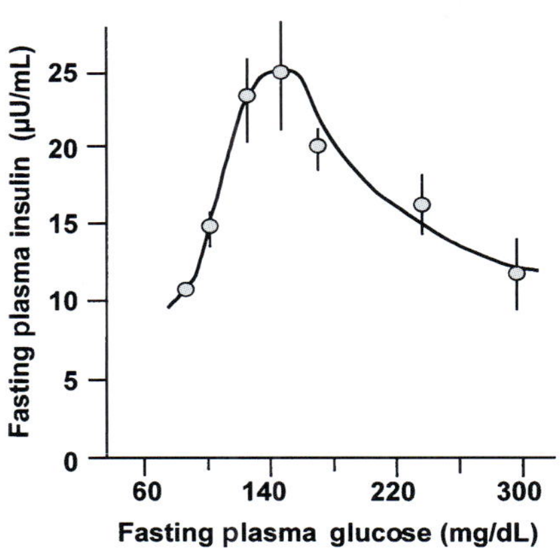

Figure 4 Relationship between the fasting plasma glucose concentration and the fasting plasma insulin concentration in normal-weight control subjects, in individuals with IGT, and in type 2 diabetic subjects with varying degrees of fasting hyperglycemia. As the fasting plasma glucose concentration rises from baseline to 140 mg/dl, there is a progressive increase in the fasting insulin concentration. Thereafter, further rises in the fasting glucose level are associated with a progressive decline in fasting insulin concentration. In diabetic subjects with fasting glucose concentrations in excess of 200–220 mg/dl, the fasting insulin level declines to values observed in control subjects. (Reproduced by permission of Elsevier [65])

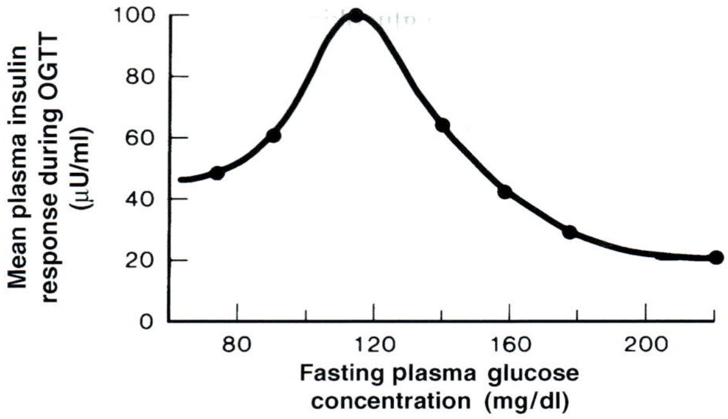

Figure 5 Starling's curve of the pancreas for insulin secretion. In normal-weight patients with IGT and mild diabetes, the plasma insulin response to ingested glucose (OGTT) increases progressively until the fasting glucose reaches 120 mg/dl. Thereafter, further increases in the fasting glucose concentration are associated with a progressive decline in insulin secretion. (Reproduced by permission of the American Diabetes Association [4])

secretes an amount of insulin that is similar to that in a healthy, non-diabetic individual. However, a "normal" insulin response in the presence of this degree of hyperglycemia and underlying insulin resistance is markedly abnormal. When the fasting plasma glucose concentration exceeds 150–160 mg/dl, the plasma insulin response, when viewed in absolute terms, becomes insulinopenic. Finally, when the fasting glucose exceeds 200–220 mg/dl, the plasma insulin response to a glucose challenge is markedly blunted. Nonetheless, the postabsorptive rate of insulin secretion remains elevated and fasting hyperinsulinemia persists, even with fasting plasma glucose concentrations as high as 250–300 mg/dl [1, 4, 38, 40–45, 52, 54–56, 59, 62, 65–67]. Despite severe fasting hyperglycemia, 24-h integrated plasma insulin and C-peptide profiles in lean type 2 diabetic patients remain normal [68, 69]. These normal day-long values result from the combination of elevated fasting and decreased postprandial insulin and C-peptide secretory rates.

The natural history of type 2 diabetes, starting with normal glucose tolerance, insulin resistance, and compensatory hyperinsulinemia with progression to IGT and overt diabetes mellitus, has been observed in a variety of populations (Caucasians, Native Americans, Mexican Americans, and Pacific Islanders) [4, 40–49, 54–58, 70] and in the rhesus monkey [59, 71], an animal model that closely resembles type 2 diabetes in humans. It is noteworthy that in all of these population studies, as well as in the rhesus monkey, the development of type 2 diabetes is closely associated with the presence of obesity and the close association of these two common metabolic disorders has been referred to as *diabesity*. In these populations at high risk to develop type 2 diabetes mellitus, as normal-glucose-tolerant subjects progress to IGT, there is a marked increase in both fasting and glucose-stimulated plasma insulin levels [4, 42, 70, 72] and a decrease in the body's sensitivity to insulin [1, 4, 43] (Figure 6). It should be emphasized, however, that even though the plasma insulin response is increased two- to threefold above that in normal-glucose-tolerant subjects, glucose intolerance does not develop unless a concomitant defect in insulin secretion is present. The defect in insulin secretion can be appreciated when β-cell function is viewed relative to the prevailing severity of insulin resistance. The progression from IGT to type 2 diabetes with mild fasting hyperglycemia (120–140 mg/dl, 6.7–7.8 mmol/l) is heralded by an inability of the β-cell to maintain its previously high rate of insulin secretion in response to a glucose challenge [4, 38, 42, 43, 55, 72] without any further or minimal deterioration in tissue sensitivity to insulin. It should be noted, however, that increased basal insulin secretion and fasting hyperinsulinemia are maintained until fasting plasma glucose levels exceed 140 mg/dl (Figure 4). A similar picture of insulin secretion is observed in the rhesus monkey [59, 71]. As monkeys age, they become obese and a high percentage develop typical type 2 diabetes. In monkeys, as in humans, both longitudinal and cross-sectional studies have documented that the earliest detectable abnormality that precedes the onset of diabetes mellitus is an increase in the fasting and glucose-stimulated plasma insulin concentration and a decrease in the body's sensitivity to insulin

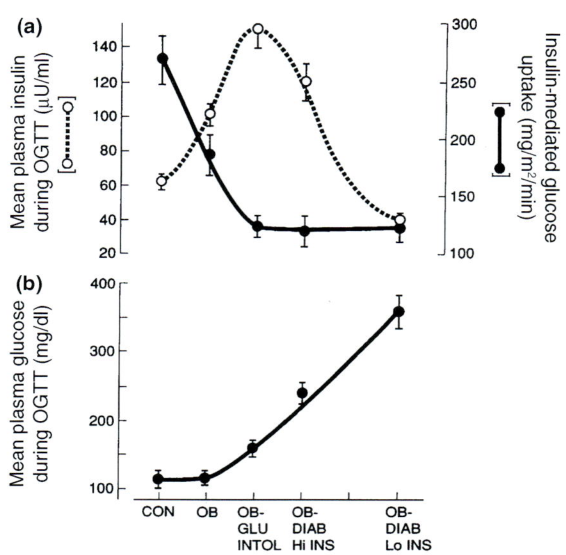

Figure 6 Summary of the plasma insulin (a, ○) and plasma glucose (b) responses during a 100-g OGTT and tissue sensitivity to insulin (a, ●) in control(CON), obese nondiabetic (OB), obese glucose-intolerant (OB-GLU INTOL), obese hyperinsulinemic diabetic (OB-DIAB Hi INS), and obese hypoinsulinemic diabetic subjects (OB-DIAB Lo INS). See text for a detailed discussion (from reference 4, with permission)

[59, 71]. With time, this high rate of insulin secretion cannot be maintained and the downward slope of Starling's curve commences (Figure 5). At this point, marked fasting hyperglycemia and glucose intolerance ensue. These studies [4, 42–45, 70, 72, 73] clearly demonstrate that hyperinsulinemia precedes the development of type 2 diabetes. Consistent with this depiction of the natural history, a number of studies in high-risk ethnic groups [40–42, 45–49, 70, 74–77] and in other populations [51, 54, 55, 78–80] have demonstrated that hyperinsulinemia predicts the development of IGT and type 2 diabetes. However, these studies [41, 45–49, 57–59, 72–76, 79] also demonstrate that overt type 2 diabetes (fasting glucose $>$126 mg/dl) does not develop in the absence of a significant defect in β-cell function. The nature of this β-cell defect is considered in subsequent sections.

Type 2 Diabetes with Hypoinsulinemia

Despite an impressive body of evidence that implicates the presence of hyperinsulinemia and insulin resistance as the antecedents of type 2 diabetes, a number of studies have documented that absolute insulin deficiency, with or without impaired tissue sensitivity to insulin, can lead to the development of type 2 diabetes. This is best exemplified by patients with maturity-onset diabetes of youth (MODY), which represents a familial subtype of type 2 diabetes characterized by an early age of onset, autosomal dominant inheritance with high penetrance, mild to moderate fasting hyperglycemia, and impaired insulin secretion [81–84].

The initial description of MODY was made by Fajans et al. [85]. Subsequently, Bell et al. [86] demonstrated MODY1 was related to a nonsense mutation in exon 7 of the hepatic nuclear factor 4α (HNF-4α) gene. Froguel and colleagues [81, 87, 88] demonstrated that MODY in French families was associated with mutations in the glucokinase gene on chromosome 7p (MODY2), and over 25 mutations in the glucokinase gene have since been described, although many of these are unlikely to cause a defect in insulin secretion. At present, six specific mutations in different genes have been shown to be responsible for the MODY profile, including glucokinase and five transcription factors: MODY1 = HNF-4α; MODY2 = glucokinase; MODY3 = HNF-1α; MODY4 = insulin promoter factor 1; MODY5 = HNF-1β; MODY6 = neurogenic differentiation 1/β-cell E-box transactivator 2 [83–91]. MODY individuals are characterized by impaired insulin secretion in response to glucose and other stimuli [38, 81, 82, 92–94]. Although diminished insulin secretion is clearly the primary defect in MODY, a number of studies have demonstrated that peripheral tissue resistance to insulin [81, 95, 96] and disturbances in hepatic glucose metabolism [81, 97] also play some role in the development of impaired glucose homeostasis. Although glucokinase mutations, leading to impaired insulin secretion, are well-established features of MODY2, intensive investigations in typical older-onset type 2 diabetic individuals in a variety of ethnic populations have demonstrated that a mutation in the glucokinase gene can account for no more than 1% of the common forms of type 2 diabetes [98–100].

The view that insulin deficiency represents the primary defect responsible for glucose intolerance in individuals who present with typical type 2 diabetes and who do not have a glucokinase or other MODY mutations has been championed by Cerasi, Luft, Hales, and coworkers [39, 66, 101–103]. These investigators argue that a defect in early insulin secretion leads to an excessive rise in plasma glucose levels and that the resultant hyperglycemia is responsible for late hyperinsulinemia. Hales and colleagues [66, 103] have demonstrated that many lean Caucasian individuals with mild fasting hyperglycemia ($<$140 mg/dl, 7.8 mmol/l) are characterized by insulin deficiency at all time points during an OGTT. An impaired early insulin response also has been a characteristic finding in Japanese Americans who progress to type 2 diabetes [104]. Unfortunately, none of these studies provided information about insulin sensitivity. Arner et al. [105] and the European Group for the Study of Insulin Resistance (EGIR) [106] have demonstrated normal insulin sensitivity in a minority of type 2 diabetic individuals, and Banerji and colleagues [107, 108] have suggested that up to 50% of African American type 2 diabetic patients who reside in New York City are characterized by severely impaired insulin secretion and normal insulin sensitivity. A similar defect in insulin secretion has been described in Black African type 2 diabetic patients living in Cameroon [109].

In summary, it is clear that impaired insulin secretion—in the absence of insulin resistance—can lead to the development of full-blown type 2 diabetes. However, it is unclear how frequently a pure β-cell defect results in typical type 2 diabetes.

First-Phase Insulin Secretion

In humans [110] and animals [111], insulin secretion in response to intravenous glucose is biphasic, with an early burst of insulin release within the first 10 min followed by a gradually increasing phase of insulin secretion that persists as long as the hyperglycemic stimulus is present. This biphasic insulin response is not easily identifiable after oral glucose, most likely because of the more gradual rise in plasma glucose concentration following oral glucose administration. It has been suggested that loss of first-phase insulin secretion is an early abnormality in patients who are destined to develop type 2 diabetes [38, 39, 82, 102, 112]. As reviewed by DeFronzo [1, 4], the early phase of insulin secretion during the OGTT (0– 30 min) and during the IVGTT intravenous glucose

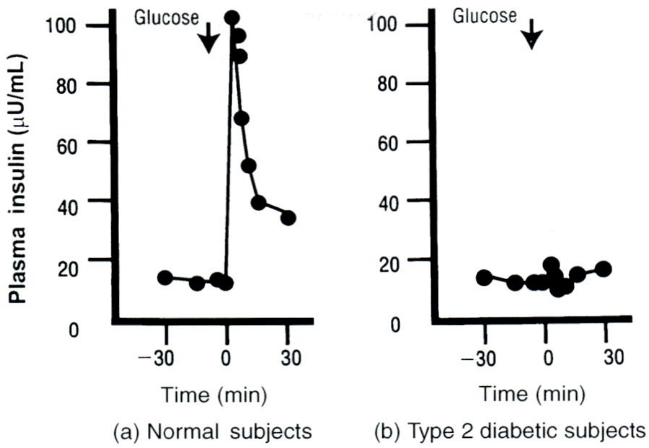

Figure 7 Acute insulin response to intravenous glucose: normal and type 2 diabetic subjects. The acute (0–10 min) insulin response represents the release of stored insulin from granules within the β-cell. Type 2 diabetic individuals are characterized by the loss of the acute phase insulin secretion. In subjects with IGT, it is common to observe a diminished or absent acute phase insulin response when the fasting plasma glucose concentration exceeds 115 mg/dl. (Reproduced by permission of the Endocrinol Society [114])

tolerance test (0–10 min) tends to be reduced in most type 2 diabetic subjects with fasting plasma glucose levels >110–120 mg/dl (6.1–6.7 mmol/l). During the OGTT, the defect in early insulin secretion is most readily detected if one calculates incremental plasma insulin response at 30 min divided by the incremental plasma glucose response at 30 min ($\Delta I_{30}/\Delta G_{30}$) [38, 39, 45–49, 66, 74, 82, 101, 103, 113]. Although the first-phase insulin secretory response is characteristically lost in type 2 diabetes, this defect is not consistently observed until the fasting plasma glucose concentration rises to 115–120 mg/dl (6.4–6.7 mmol/l) [114] (Figure 7). Moreover, tight metabolic control partially restores the defect in first-phase insulin response [115–117], indicating that at least part of the defect is acquired, most likely secondary to glucotoxicity [118] or liptoxicity [26, 119–121] (see subsequent discussion). The loss of the first phase of insulin secretion has important pathogenetic consequences since this early burst of insulin release primes insulin target tissues, especially the liver, that are responsible for the maintenance of normal glucose homeostasis [122–125].

Etiology of Impaired Insulin Secretion in Type 2 Diabetes Mellitus

The progression from normal to IGT to type 2 diabetes with mild fasting hyperglycemia (<120–140 mg/dl, 6.7–7.8 mmol/l) is characterized by hyperinsulinemia (Figures 3 and 4). However, when the fasting glucose concentration exceeds ~120 mg/dl (6.7 mmol/l) and ~140 mg/dl (7.8 mmol/l), respectively, there is a progressive decline in fasting and glucose-stimulated plasma insulin levels. These observations suggest that the decline in β-cell function is acquired. This conclusion is supported by the studies of Polonsky [38, 82], using more sophisticated techniques to evaluate insulin secretion. A number of pathogenic factors, both genetic and acquired, have been implicated in the progressive impairment in insulin secretion (Figure 8). A growing body of evidence indicates that pancreatic β-cells are in a constant state of dynamic change, with continued regeneration and apoptosis [126]. Islet neogenesis occurs from ductal endothelial cells of the exocrine pancreas [126]. In adults there is continued renewal and loss of β-cells and a number of factors have shown to disturb the delicate balance between beta cell replication and apoptosis (see subsequent discussion).

Investigations performed in first-degree relatives of type 2 diabetic patients [50, 127–131] and in twins [132, 133] have provided strong evidence for the genetic basis of beta cell dysfunction. In a recent study, Watanabe et al. [134] demonstrated that impaired insulin secretion was an inherited trait in Finnish families with type 2 diabetes mellitus, with evidence for a susceptibility locus on chromosome 12 [135].

Of the acquired defects leading to impaired insulin secretion, *glucotoxicity* [118] and *lipotoxicity* [26, 119–121] have received the most attention. Evidence in support of the glucotoxicity hypothesis in humans derives from the observation that improved glycemia, however achieved (diet, insulin therapy, sulfonylureas, metformin), leads to enhanced insulin secretion [115–117] (Figure 9). A more rigorous test of the glucotoxicity hypothesis requires that the plasma glucose concentration be reduced without altering other circulating substrate levels and without administering an agent (i.e., such as insulin or metformin) that has direct effects on cellular glucose metabolism. This can be accomplished by utilizing phlorizin, a potent inhibitor of renal tubular glucose transport. When phlorizin was administered to partially pancreatectomized, chronically hyperglycemic diabetic rats, restoration of normoglycemia was associated with a dramatic improvement in both the first and second phases of insulin

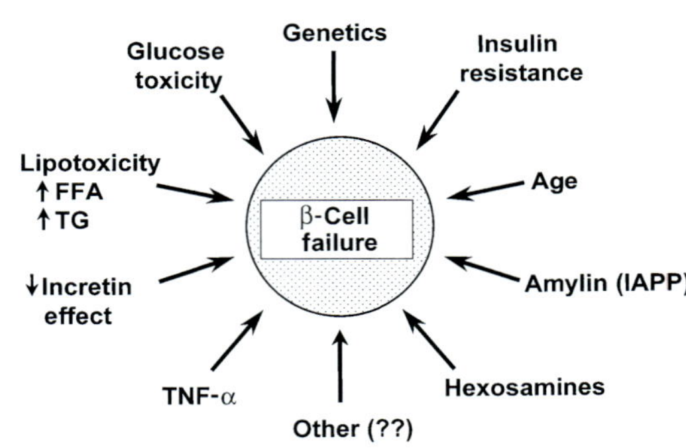

Figure 8 Pathogenetic factors implicated in the progressive impairment in insulin secretion in type 2 diabetes mellitus

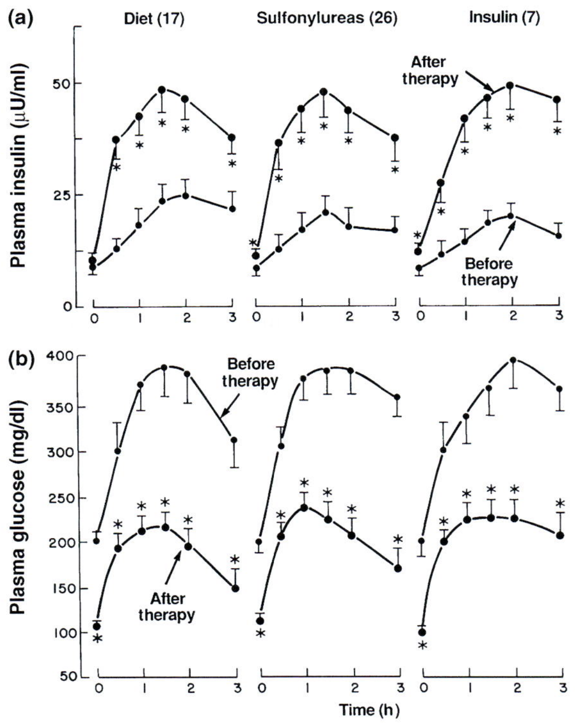

Figure 9 Effect of glycemic control on insulin secretion. Plasma insulin (a) and glucose (b) concentrations during OGTTs in type 2 diabetic patients before and after treatment with diet, sulfonylureas, or insulin. Improved glycemic control, regardless of the means by which it was achieved, uniformly led to an improvement in insulin secretion. $^*p < 0.01$ vs. before therapy. Numbers in parentheses indicate number of subjects (from reference 117, with permission)

secretion [136] (Figure 10). Weir and colleagues [137–139] have used both partially pancreatectomized and neonatal streptozotocin-induced diabetic rat models to produce a state of mild chronic hyperglycemia. When the pancreatic remnant was perfused *in vitro*, the insulin response to hyperglycemia was markedly impaired in diabetic compared with control animals. A rise in the plasma glucose concentration of as little as 15 mg/dl caused a 75% inhibition of insulin secretion by the pancreas perfused *in vitro* [140]. These results provide support for the concept that a minimal elevation in mean plasma glucose concentration, in the presence of a reduced β-cell mass, can lead to a major impairment in insulin secretion by the remaining pancreatic tissue [118, 136–140]. Additional support for a deleterious effect of hyperglycemia on β-cell function comes from chronic (72-h) glucose infusions in normal rats [141]. Robertson et al. [142] and Weir et al. [143] have provided evidence that prolonged β-cell exposure to high glucose concentrations impairs insulin gene transcription, leading to decreased insulin synthesis and secretion. The potential mechanisms responsible for the downregulation of insulin secretion have been reviewed by Rossetti et al. [118], Simonson et al. [144], and Weir et al. [143].

Lipotoxicity also has been implicated as an acquired cause of the progressive decline in beta cell function as individuals progress from IGT to overt type 2 diabetes mellitus. Short-term exposure of the beta cell to physiologic increases in FFAs stimulates insulin secretion [26] (Figure 11). Within the beta cell, long-chain fatty acids are converted to their fatty acyl-CoA derivates [119–121, 146], which lead to the increased formation of phosphatidic acid and diacylglycerol (DAG). These lipid intermediates activate specific protein kinase C (PKS) isoforms, which stimulate the exocytosis of insulin [119, 146–148]. Long-chain fatty acyl-CoA derivates also directly enhance exocytosis [119], cause closure of the K^+-ATPase channel [119], and stimulate Ca^{2+}-ATPase and increase intracellular calcium, thus augmenting insulin secretion [119, 146–148]. However, chronic exposure of β-cells to elevated FFA levels inhibits insulin secretion via operation of the Randle cycle [149], in which increased β-oxidation increases acetyl-CoA, leading to an inhibition of pyruvate dehydrogenase (PDH) and elevated citrate levels, which inhibit phosphofructokinase (PFK) and subsequently glycolysis [119–121, 146, 149, 150]. Since metabolism of glucose via the glycolytic pathway and the subsequent oxidation of pyruvate in the Krebs cycle to generate ATP is required for glucose-stimulated insulin

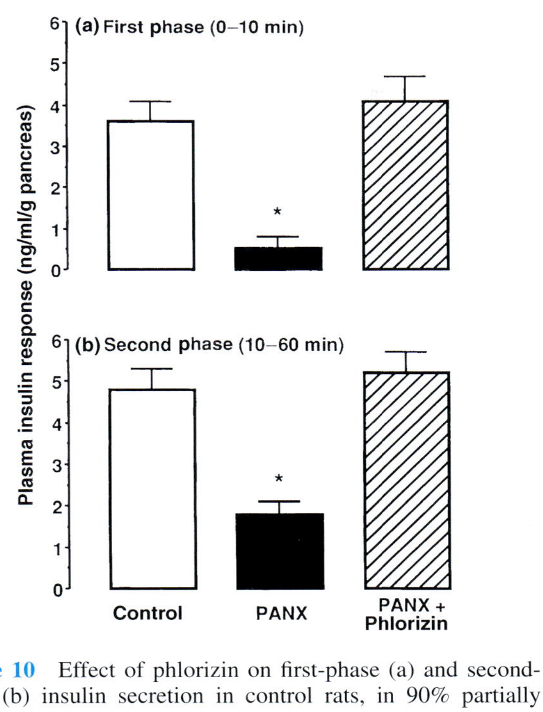

Figure 10 Effect of phlorizin on first-phase (a) and second-phase (b) insulin secretion in control rats, in 90% partially pancreatectomized rats (PANX), and in pancreatectomized rats treated with phlorizin. Phlorizin completely corrected the defects in fist- and second-phase insulin secretion (drawn from data presented in reference 136, with permission)

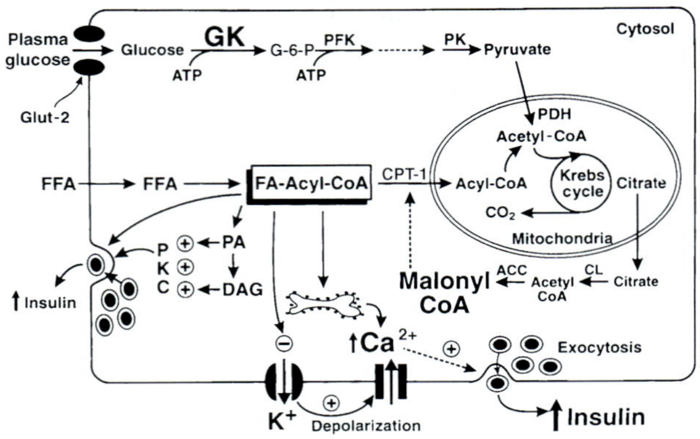

Figure 11 Relationship between lipid metabolism and insulin secretion in the β-cell. An increase in fatty acid acyl-CoA (FA-Acyl-CoA) can augment insulin secretion by (1) increasing intracellular calcium, which stimulates exocytosis of insulin-containing granules, and/or (2) enhancing exocytosis directly or through PKC. The later mechanism involves generation of phoshatidic acid (PA) and DAG. Note that malonyl-CoA generated from the metabolism of glucose is a potent inhibitor of carnitine palmitoyl transferase 1 (CPT-1). Inhibition of CPT-1 increases fatty acyl-CoA, which contributes to the stimulation of insulin secretion. Thus, a mechanism exists via which increased lipid metabolism within the β-cell potentiates glucose-stimulated insulin secretion. (Adapted by permission of the American Diabetes Association [145])

secretion, chronic exposure to elevated plasma FFA levels leads to an inhibition of insulin secretion. Increased fatty acyl-CoA levels within the beta cell also stimulate ceramide synthesis, which stimulates inducible nitric oxide synthase [121, 151]. The resultant increase in nitric oxide increases the expression of inflammatory cytokines, including interleukin-1 and tumor necrosis factor α, which impair beta cell function and cause apotosis of β-cells.

Recent studies suggest that "incretin" deficiency and/or "incretin" resistance play an important role in the pathogenesis of beta cell dysfunction in type 2 diabetic patients [36, 37, 152, 153]. It has long been recognized that glucose administered via the gastrointestinal route causes a much greater stimulation of insulin secretion than a comparable glucose challenge given intravenously [34, 35]. This prompted a search for the responsible "incretins" or gut-derived hormones that enhance glucose-stimulated insulin secretion. It is now clear that two gastrointestinal hormones, GIP and GLP-1, are responsible for more than 90% of the incretin effect observed following glucose or mixed meal ingestion [36, 37, 152–154]. Both peptide hormones are released from endocrine cells of the duodenum and jejunum in response to intraluminal carbohydrate but not in response to circulating glucose, and their release is proportional to the oral glucose load and dependent upon absorption of glucose across the intestinal mucosa [37, 152, 153]. The effectiveness of both GIP and GLP-1 to stimulate insulin secretion is dependent upon the plasma glucose concentration [36, 37, 152, 153]. Because of this, GIP has been renamed glucose-dependent insulinotropic polypeptide (GIP). Antibodies that neutralize GIP and GLP-1 [155] and GLP-1 antagonists [156] impair glucose tolerance in a variety of animal species, including primates. Although the quantities of GLP-1 released are considerably less than those of GIP, GLP-1 is such a potent glucose-sensitive potentiator of insulin secretion that it is thought to be the major incretin [37, 152, 153, 157]. In human type 2 diabetes the GIP response to glucose ingestion has consistently been shown to be normal, indicating the presence of beta cell resistance to the incretin effect of GIP [37, 157]. In contrast, the GLP-1 response to oral glucose has been shown to be reduced [37, 152, 153, 158]. Intravenous administration of GLP-1 in type 2 diabetic patients markedly enhances the postprandial insulin secretory response in type 2 diabetic patients [157, 159] and chronic continuous GLP-1 administration restores near-normal glycemia in type 2 diabetic patients [160]. GLP-1 also has been shown to augment islet regeneration in rodents [161].

Amylin (islet amyloid polypeptide, IAPP) also has been implicated in the progressive beta cell failure that is characteristic of type 2 diabetes mellitus [162]. IAPP is produced by the β-cell, packaged with insulin in secretory granules, and co-secreted into the sinusoidal space [163, 164]. This peptide has been shown to be the precursor for the amyloid deposits frequently observed in patients with type 2 diabetes [163, 164]. At very high doses, amylin inhibits insulin secretion by the perfused rat pancreas *in vitro* [165], and pancreatic amylin depots have been shown to precede the appearance of glucose intolerance in spontaneously diabetic monkeys [166]. Elevated plasma IAPP levels have been demonstrated in type 2 diabetic subjects [164], in obese glucose-intolerant subjects [167], in glucose-intolerant first-degree relatives of type 2 diabetic patients [168], and in animal models of diabetes [164, 169]. Using immunohistochemical and *in situ* hybridization techniques, amyloid polypeptide mRNA has been demonstrated within the islet [170]. Following secretion, amylin accumulates extracellularly in close contact with the β-cell, and it has been suggested that these amylin deposits might cause β-cell dysfunction and eventually death by impairing the transport of nutrients from the plasma to the beta cell or by interfering with the glucose-sensing and/or insulin-secreting apparatus of the β-cell [164–166]. Although attractive, this theory has been seriously challenged by Bloom and coworkers [171, 172], who failed to find any inhibitory effect of amylin on insulin secretion when the peptide was infused in pharmacological doses in rats, rabbits, and humans.

Hoppener et al. [173] have generated transgenic mice, with the gene encoding either human or rat IAPP under control of an insulin promoter. Although pancreatic and plasma amyloid polypeptide levels were significantly elevated in these transgenic mice, hyperglycemia and hyperinsulinemia were not observed. A recent provocative review suggests that IAPP in the islets of Langerhans may serve a protective role under conditions of increased insulin secretion [174]. In summary, at present, definitive evidence that amylin is responsible for the defect in β-cell dysfunction in type 2 diabetes in humans remains elusive, although recent evidence suggests that the combination of elevated plasma FFA levels and hypersecretion of amylin may interact synergistically to impair insulin secretion and cause injury to the pancreatic β-cells [162].

The number of β-cells is a critical determinant of the amount of insulin that is secreted by the pancreas. Most [175–180] but not all [181, 182] studies have demonstrated a modest reduction [20–40%] in β-cell mass in patients with long-standing type 2 diabetes. By routine histology, the islets of Langerhans appear normal morphologically, with the exception of beta cell degranulation. Insulitis is not observed. At present, the cause of decrease in β-cell mass remains undefined and cannot be explained simply by advancing age. A recent study suggests that new islet formation from exocrine ducts is markedly reduced in type 2 diabetic individuals [183]. Obesity, another insulin-resistant state, is characterized by a significant increase in β-cell mass [178]. Thus, the finding of even a modest reduction in β-cell mass in any insulin-resistant state is most impressive. Although recent studies with well matched for age, gender, and obesity suggest that β-cell mass is reduced even during the early stages of the development of type 2 diabetes [180], it seems likely that factors in addition to β-cell loss must be responsible for the impairment in insulin secretion.

Numerous studies in a variety of populations have demonstrated an association between low birth weight and the development of IGT and type 2 diabetes later in life [184–186]. Developmental studies in animals and humans have provided evidence that poor nutrition and impaired growth are associated with reduced insulin secretion and/or reduced β-cell mass [187]. Some studies have suggested that fetal malnutrition may also lead to the development of insulin resistance later in life [188]. One could postulate that an environmental influence, e.g., impaired fetal nutrition leading to an acquired defect in insulin secretion or reduced β-cell mass, when superimposed on an inherited defect in insulin action, could eventuate in type 2 diabetes later in life. Thus, with the normal aging process, the onset of obesity, or a worsening of the genetic component of the insulin resistance, the β-cell would be called on to augment its secretion of insulin to offset the defect in insulin action. If β-cell mass or function were reduced by an environmental insult during fetal life, the result would be the emergence of IGT or overt type 2 diabetes. Note that although such a defect may place a limit on the maximum amount of insulin that is secreted, it would not explain the progressive decline in the amount of insulin that is secreted in response to physiologic stimuli as individuals progress from IGT to mild-moderately severe type 2 diabetes (Figure 1).

Insulin Resistance and Type 2 Diabetes

Longitudinal and cross-sectional studies have documented conclusively that hyperinsulinemia precedes the development of type 2 diabetes in most ethnic populations with a high incidence of type 2 diabetes [40–49, 51, 53–55, 70–77, 127, 189, 190]. Studies employing the euglycemic insulin clamp, minimal model, and insulin suppression techniques have provided direct quantitative evidence that the progression from normal to IGT is associated with the development of severe insulin resistance [1, 4, 42, 45–49, 51, 53–56, 70–73, 191, 192], whereas plasma insulin concentrations, both in the fasting state and in response to a glucose load (Figures 4 and 5), are increased (see above discussion about insulin secretion).

Himsworth and Kerr [193], using a combined oral glucose and intravenous insulin tolerance test, were the first to demonstrate that tissue sensitivity to insulin was diminished in diabetic patients. In 1975 Reaven and colleagues [194, 195], using the insulin suppression test, found that the ability of insulin to promote tissue glucose uptake in type 2 diabetes was severely reduced. A defect in insulin action in type 2 diabetes also has been demonstrated with limb infusion of insulin using the forearm and leg catheterization techniques [3–5, 196, 197], as well as with radioisotope turnover studies [198, 199], the modified IVGTT [200], and the minimal model technique [201, 202].

DeFronzo et al. using the more physiologic euglycemic insulin clamp technique [110], have provided the most conclusive documentation that insulin resistance is a characteristic feature of *lean* type 2 diabetic individuals [1, 3, 4, 20, 21, 80, 203–205] (Figure 12). Because diabetic patients with severe fasting hyperglycemia (>180–200 mg/dl, 10.0–11.1 mmol/l) are known to be insulinopenic (Figure 4), and insulin deficiency is associated with the emergence of a number of intracellular defects in insulin action [206–208], only diabetic patients with mild to modest elevations in the fasting plasma glucose concentration (mean = 150 ± 8 mg/dl, 8.3 ± 0.4 mmol/l) were included in these studies in order to focus on the early stages of the evolution of type 2 diabetes in normal-weight subjects. Insulin-mediated whole-body glucose disposal was reduced by ~40–50% in type 2 diabetic subjects, conclusively demonstrating the presence of moderate to severe insulin resistance. Three additional points are noteworthy:

(1) In lean type 2 diabetic patients with more severe fasting hyperglycemia (198 ± 10 mg/dl), the severity of insulin resistance is only slightly (10–20%) greater

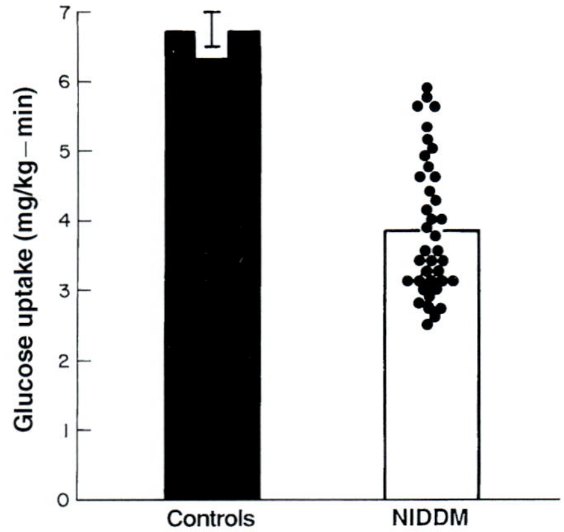

Figure 12 Insulin-mediated whole-body glucose uptake in 38 normal-weight type 2 diabetic patients (NIDDM) and in 33 control subjects matched for age and weight. Tissue sensitivity to insulin was reduced by ~40% in the type 2 diabetic group; each individual diabetic subject is represented by a solid circle. (Reproduced by permission of the American Diabetes Association [1])

than that in diabetic patients with mild fasting hyperglycemia [1, 4, 209–211].

(2) The defect in insulin action is observed at all plasma insulin concentrations, spanning the physiologic and pharmacologic range [1, 4, 20, 212, 213] (Figure 13).

(3) In diabetic patients with overt fasting hyperglycemia, even maximally stimulating plasma insulin concentrations are not capable of eliciting a normal glucose metabolic response under euglycemic conditions [1, 4, 20, 212, 213].

With a few exceptions [105, 107, 108], the great majority of investigators have demonstrated that lean type 2 diabetic subjects are resistant to the action of insulin [1, 3, 4, 20, 21, 45–49, 51, 52, 58, 62, 71–73, 80, 127, 192, 194, 195, 199, 201, 203–205, 212–214]. The ability of glucose to stimulate its own uptake, i.e. hyperglycemia, is also impaired in type 2 diabetic subjects [16, 215, 216].

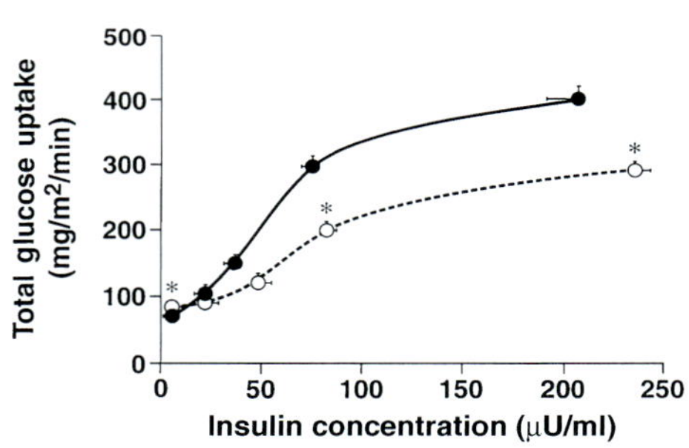

Figure 13 Dose–response curve relating the plasma insulin concentration to the rate of insulin-mediated whole-body glucose uptake in control (●) and type 2 diabetic (○) subjects. $^{*}p < 0.01$ vs. control subjects (from reference 20, with permission)

SITE OF INSULIN RESISTANCE IN TYPE 2 DIABETES

Maintenance of whole-body glucose homeostasis is dependent upon a normal pancreatic insulin secretory response and normal tissue sensitivity to the independent effects of hyperinsulinemia and hyperglycemia (i.e., the mass-action effect of glucose) to augment glucose uptake. In turn, the combined effects of insulin and hyperglycemia to promote glucose disposal are dependent on three tightly coupled mechanisms (Table 1): (1) suppression of HGP; (2) stimulation of glucose uptake by the splanchnic (hepatic plus gastrointestinal) tissues; and (3) stimulation of glucose uptake by peripheral tissues, primarily muscle [1, 4, 15]. Tissue glucose uptake is regulated by flux through two major metabolic pathways: glycolysis (of which ~90% represents glucose oxidation) and glycogen synthesis.

Hepatic Glucose Production

In the overnight fasted state the liver of healthy subjects produces glucose at the rate of ~1.8–2.0 mg/kg/min [1, 3, 4, 6, 20, 65]. This glucose flux is critical to meet the needs of the brain and other neural tissues, which utilize glucose at a constant rate of ~1–1.2 mg/kg/min [2, 217]. Brain glucose uptake accounts for ~50–60% of glucose disposal during the postabsorptive state and this uptake is insulin independent. Therefore, brain glucose uptake occurs at the same rate during absorptive and postabsorptive periods and is not altered in type 2 diabetes [217]. Following ingestion of a mixed meal or glucose, insulin is released into the portal vein and carried to the liver, where its primary function is to suppress hepatic glucose output. If the liver does not perceive this insulin signal and continues to produce glucose, there will be two inputs of glucose into the body, one from the liver and another from the gastrointestinal tract, and marked hyperglycemia will ensue.

In type 2 diabetic subjects with mild to moderate fasting hyperglycemia (140–200 mg/dl, 7.8–11.1 mmol/l), hepatic glucose production is increased by ~0.5 mg/kg/min (Figure 14). Thus, during the overnight sleeping hours (2200 to 0800), the liver of a 80-kg diabetic individual with modest fasting hyperglycemia would be expected to add an additional 35 g of glucose to the systemic circulation. Important, the increase in basal HGP is closely correlated ($r = 0.847$, $p < 0.001$) with the degree of fasting hyperglycemia [1, 3, 4, 6, 20, 65, 203–205, 209] (Figure 14). These findings indicate that in type 2 diabetic individuals with overt fasting hyperglycemia (>140 mg/dl, 7.8 mmol/l), an excessive rate of hepatic glucose output is the major factor responsible for the elevated fasting plasma glucose concentration. The close relationship between fasting plasma glucose concentration and HGP is

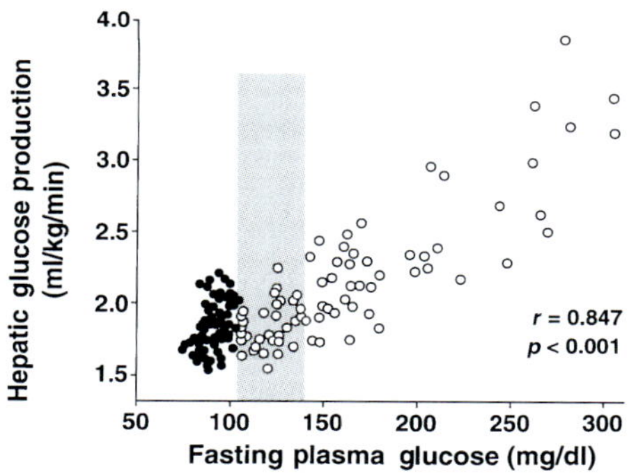

Figure 14 Summary of HGP in 77 normal-weight type 2 diabetic subjects (○) with fasting plasma glucose concentrations ranging from 105 to >300 mg/dl; 72 control subjects matched for age and weight are shown by solid circles (●). In the 33 diabetic subjects with fasting plasma glucose levels < 140 mg/dl (shaded area), the mean rate of HGP was identical to that of control subjects. In diabetic subjects with fasting plasma glucose concentrations > 140 mg/dl, there was a progressive rise in HGP that correlated closely ($r = 0.847$, $p < 0.001$) with the fasting plasma glucose concentration. (Reproduced by permission of Elsevier [65])

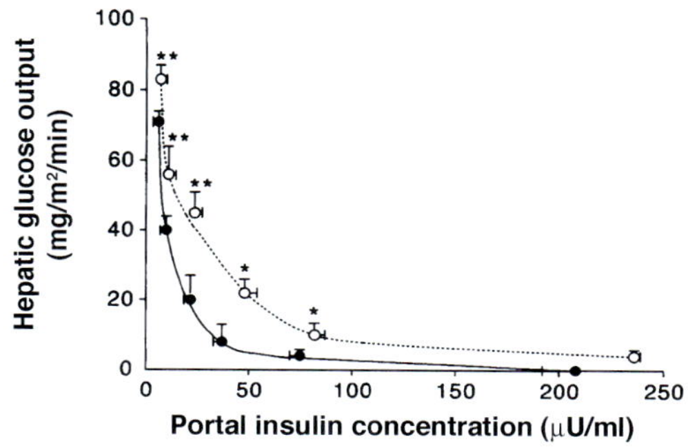

Figure 15 Dose–response curve relating the plasma insulin concentration to the suppression of HGP in control (●) and type 2 diabetic (○) subjects with moderately severe fasting hyperglycemia. $^*p < 0.05$, $^{**}p < 0.01$ vs. control subjects (from reference 20, with permission)

consistent with results that have been published by a number of other investigators [71, 212–214, 218–224].

In the postabsorptive state, type 2 diabetic subjects also manifest elevated plasma insulin concentrations that are two- to fourfold greater than in control subjects (Figure 4). Because hyperinsulinemia is a potent inhibitor of HGP [1, 3, 4–6, 17, 20, 212, 213, 225], hepatic resistance to the action of insulin must be present in the postabsorptive state to explain the excessive output of glucose by the liver. Hyperglycemia *per se* also exerts a powerful suppressive action on HGP [16, 215, 225–228]. Therefore, there also must be glucose resistance with respect to the inhibitory effect of hyperglycemia on hepatic glucose output, and this has been well documented [16, 215, 229, 230].

Using the euglycemic insulin clamp technique in combination with tritiated glucose, the dose–response relationship between hepatic glucose production and the plasma glucose concentration has been defined by Groop et al. [20] (Figure 15). The following points should be emphasized:

(1) The dose–response curve relating inhibition of HGP to the plasma insulin concentration is quite steep, with an effective dose for half-maximal concentration (ED_{50}) of ~30–40 μU/ml. Similar findings have been reported by Campbell et al. [213];

(2) Second, in type 2 diabetic individuals the dose–response curve is shifted to the right, indicating the presence of hepatic resistance to the action of insulin to inhibit glucose production. However, at plasma insulin concentrations within the high physiologic range (~100 μU/ml), the hepatic insulin resistance can be largely overcome and a near-normal suppression of HGP can be achieved;

(3) The severity of the hepatic insulin resistance is related to the severity of the diabetic state. In type 2 diabetic individuals with mild fasting hyperglycemia, an increment in plasma insulin concentration of 100 μU/ml causes a complete suppression of HPG. However, in diabetic subjects with more severe fasting hyperglycemia, the ability of the same plasma insulin concentration to suppress HGP is impaired [20]. These results suggest that there is an acquired component of hepatic insulin resistance and that this defect becomes progressively worse as the diabetic state decompensates over time.

The glucose released by the liver can be derived from either glycogenolysis or gluconeogenesis [6, 17, 227] (Figure 16). Studies by Waldhausl et al. [233] have shown that uptake of gluconeogenic precursors, especially lactate, is increased in type 2 diabetic subjects. Consistent with this observation, Consoli and coworkers [234, 235],

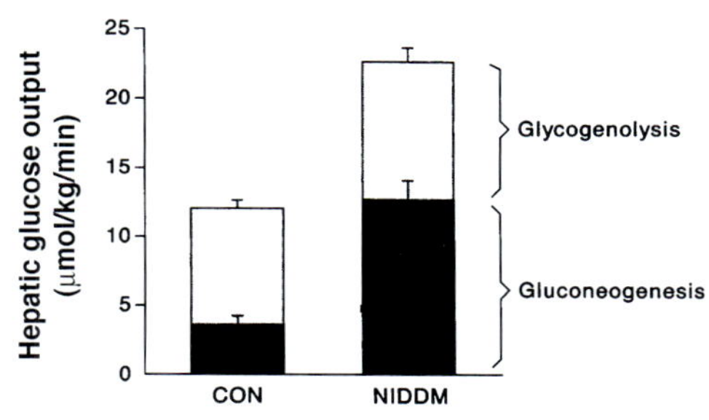

Figure 16 Contribution of gluconeogenesis and glycogenolysis in control (CON) and type 2 diabetic (NIDDM) subjects. All of the increase in total HGP in type 2 diabetes is accounted for by an excessive rate of gluconeogenesis. Schematic representation of the data presented in references 231 and 232. (Reproduced by permission of the American Diabetes Association)

using radiolabeled lactate, alanine, and glycerol, have shown that ∼90% of the increase in HGP above baseline can be accounted for by accelerated gluconeogenesis. More recent studies employing ^{13}C MRI (magnetic resonance imaging) [231] and D_2O [232, 233] have confirmed the important contribution of accelerated gluconeogenesis to the increase in HGP. An increased rate of conversion of glutamine to glucose also has been shown to contribute to the elevated rate of gluconeogenesis in type 2 diabetic subjects [237]. The mechanisms responsible for the increase in hepatic gluconeogenesis include hyperglucagonemia [238, 239], increased circulating levels of gluconeogenic precursors (lactate, alanine, glycerol) [234, 240], increased FFA oxidation [20, 21, 23, 241], enhanced sensitivity to glucagon [242], and decreased sensitivity to insulin [20, 21, 212, 213, 243].

Although the majority of evidence supports increased gluconeogenesis as the major cause of the increase in HGP in type 2 diabetic subjects [231, 232, 234–237], it is likely that accelerated glycogenolysis also contributes [234, 244]. Because of the inaccessibility of the liver in humans, it has been difficult to assess the role of key enzymes involved in the regulation of gluconeogenesis [pyruvate carboxylase, phosphoenol pyruvate carboxykinase (PEPCK)], glycogenolysis (glycogen, phosphorylase), and net hepatic glucose output [glucokinase, glucose-6-phosphatase (G-6-Pase)]. However, considerable evidence from both animal and human studies have implicated increased activity of PEPCK and G-6-Pase in the accelerated rate of hepatic glucose production in a variety of diabetic states [245–247].

The kidney also has been shown to be an important source of glucose, and estimates of the renal contribution to total endogenous glucose production have varied from 5 to 20% [8, 9, 248]. These varying estimates of the contribution of renal gluconeogenesis to total glucose production are largely related to methodology employed to measure glucose production by the kidney [249]. One unconfirmed study suggests that the rate of renal gluconeogenesis is increased in type 2 diabetic patients with fasting hyperglycemia [250]. Arguing against this possibility are studies by DeFronzo et al. [3] that have shown that all of the increase in endogenous glucose production (measured with [3-^{3}H]glucose) could be accounted for by increased hepatic glucose output (measured by hepatic vein catheter technique).

Peripheral (Muscle) Glucose Uptake

Muscle represents the major site of glucose disposal in humans [1, 3–5, 15]. Under euglycemic hyperinsulinemic conditions, approximately 80% of total body glucose uptake occurs in skeletal muscle [1, 3–5]. Using the euglycemic insulin clamp in combination with femoral artery/vein catheterization, the effect of insulin on leg glu-

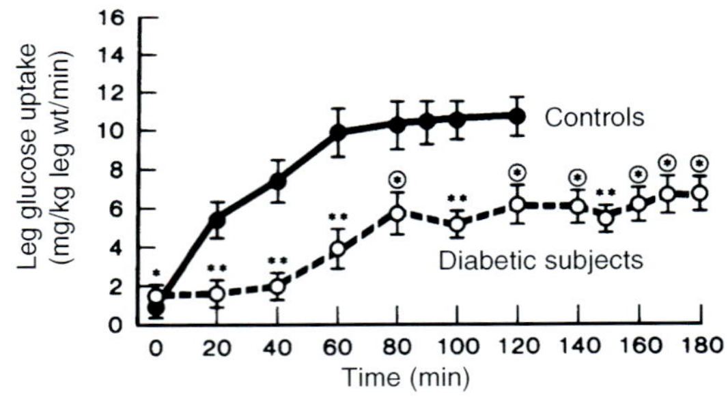

Figure 17 Time course of change in leg glucose uptake in type 2 diabetic (○) and control (●) subjects. In the postabsorptive state, glucose uptake in the diabetic group was significantly greater than that in control subjects. However, the ability of insulin (euglycemic insulin clamp) to stimulate leg glucose uptake was reduced by 50% in the diabetic subjects. $^{**}p < 0.05$ vs. controls; (⊙) $p < 0.01$ vs. controls (from reference 3, with permission)

cose uptake has been examined in type 2 diabetic and control subjects (3) (Figure 17). Since bone is metabolically inert and adipose tissue takes up less than 5% of an infused glucose load [18, 19, 251, 252], muscle represents the major tissue responsible for leg glucose uptake.

In response to a physiologic increase in plasma insulin concentration (∼80–100 μU/ml), leg (muscle) glucose uptake increases linearly, reaching a plateau value of 10 mg/kg leg wt/min (3) (Figure 17). In contrast, in lean type 2 diabetic subjects, the onset of insulin action is delayed for ∼40 min and the ability of the hormone to stimulate leg glucose uptake is markedly blunted, even though the study was carried out for an additional 60 min in the type 2 diabetic group to allow insulin to more fully express its biological effects (3). During the last hour of the insulin clamp study, the rate of glucose uptake was reduced by 50% in the diabetic group. These results provide conclusive evidence that the primary site of insulin resistance during euglycemic insulin clamp studies performed in type 2 diabetic subjects resides in muscle tissue (3). Using the forearm and leg catheterization techniques, a number of investigators [14, 196, 197, 253–256] also have demonstrated a decreased rate of insulin-mediated glucose uptake by peripheral tissues. The use of positron emission tomography (PET) scanning to quantitate leg glucose uptake in type 2 diabetic subjects has provided additional support for the presence of severe muscle resistance to insulin in diabetic subjects [257].

Splanchnic (Hepatic) Glucose Uptake

In humans, it is difficult to catheterize the portal vein, and glucose disposal by the liver has not been examined directly. Using the hepatic vein catheterization technique in combination with the euglycemic insulin clamp, DeFronzo et al. (3) examined the contribution of the splanchnic (liver plus gastrointestinal) tissues to overall

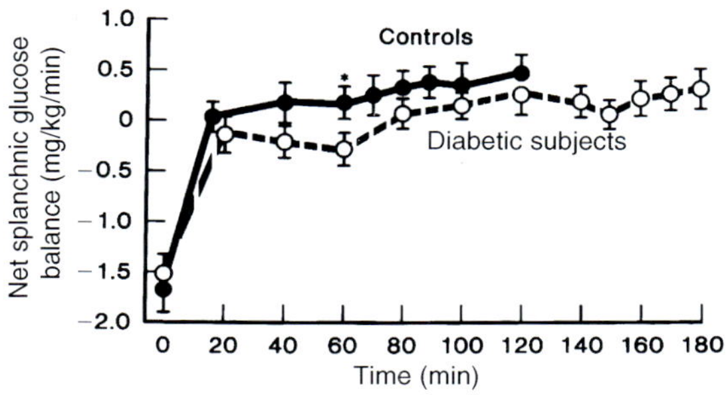

Figure 18 Time course of change in the net splanchnic glucose balance in type 2 diabetic (○) and control (●) subjects. The difference between diabetic and control subjects is small, is statistically insignificant, and cannot account for the marked impairment in total-body glucose metabolism observed during the euglycemic insulin clamp study. Also note that the total amount of glucose disposed of by the splanchnic area represents <10% of the infused glucose load in both groups (from reference 3, with permission)

glucose homeostasis in lean type 2 diabetic subjects with mild to moderate fasting hyperglycemia. In the postabsorptive state, there was a net release of glucose from the splanchnic area (i.e., negative balance) in both control and type 2 diabetic subjects (Figure 18), reflecting glucose production by the liver. In response to insulin, there was a prompt suppression of splanchnic glucose output (reflecting the inhibition of HGP), and by 20 min, the net glucose balance across the splanchnic region was zero (i.e., there was no net uptake or release). After 2 h of sustained hyperinsulinemia, there was a small net uptake of glucose by the splanchnic area (i.e., positive balance), which averaged ~0.5 mg/kg/min. This uptake was virtually identical to the rate of splanchnic glucose uptake observed in the basal state, indicating that the splanchnic tissues, like the brain, are insensitive to insulin at least with respect to the stimulation of glucose uptake [3, 5, 6, 225]. There was no difference between diabetic and control subjects in the amount of glucose taken up by the splanchnic tissues at any time during the insulin clamp study (3).

The results of these studies (see Figure 18) illustrate another important point: namely, that under conditions of euglycemic hyperinsulinemia, very little of the infused glucose is taken up by the splanchnic (and therefore hepatic) tissues [3, 5, 6, 225]. During the insulin clamp, the rate of whole-body glucose uptake averaged 7 mg/kg/min, and of this, only 0.5 mg/kg/min, or 7%, was disposed of by the splanchnic region. Because the difference in insulin-mediated total body glucose uptake between the type 2 diabetic and control groups during the euglycemic insulin clamp study was 2.5 mg/kg/min, from a purely quantitative standpoint it is clear that a defect in splanchnic (hepatic) glucose removal never could account for the magnitude of impairment in total body glucose uptake following intravenous glucose/insulin administration. However, after glucose ingestion, the oral route of administration and the resultant hyperglycemia conspire to enhance splanchnic (hepatic) glucose uptake [6, 7, 11, 12, 17, 31, 225], and, under these conditions, diminished hepatic glucose uptake contributes to the impairment in glucose tolerance in type 2 diabetes (see discussion below) [6, 258, 259].

Summary: Whole-Body Glucose Utilization

Insulin-mediated whole-body glucose utilization during the euglycemic insulin clamp is summarized in Figure 19. The height of each bar represents the total amount of glucose taken up during the insulin clamp in control and type 2 diabetic subjects. Net splanchnic glucose uptake, quantitated by the hepatic venous catheterization technique, was similar in both groups and averaged 0.5 mg/kg/min. Adipose tissue glucose uptake, which was not directly measured, was assumed to represent 2–3% of total glucose disposal [18, 19, 251, 252]. Brain glucose uptake, estimated to be 1.0–1.2 mg/kg/min in the postabsorptive state [2, 217, 260, 261], is unaffected by hyperinsulinemia [217]. Muscle glucose uptake (extrapolated from leg catheterization data) in control subjects accounted for ~75–80% of the total glucose uptake. In type 2 diabetic subjects, it is apparent that the largest part of the impairment in insulin-mediated glucose uptake can be accounted for by a defect in muscle glucose disposal. Even if adipose tissue of type 2 diabetic subjects took up absolutely no glucose, it could, at best, explain only a small fraction of the defect in whole-body glucose metabolism.

Glucose Disposal During OGTT

The gastrointestinal tract represents the normal route via which glucose enters the body. However, the assessment

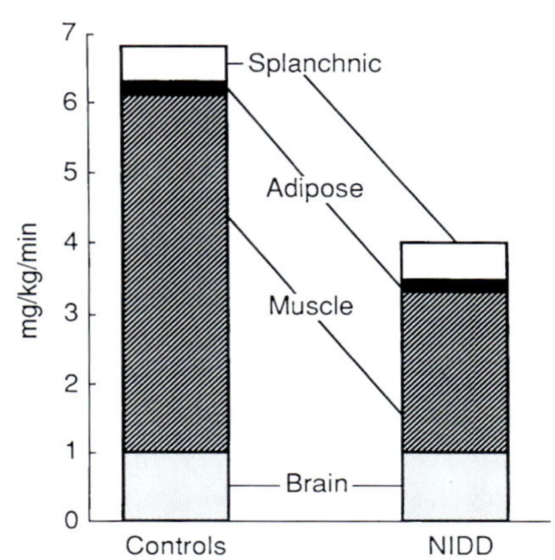

Figure 19 Summary of glucose metabolism during euglycemic insulin (100 μU/ml) clamp studies performed in normal-weight type 2 diabetic and control subjects. See text for a more detailed discussion. (Reproduced by permission of the American Diabetes Association [1])

Table 2 Balance sheet for the disposition of an oral glucose load in normal subjects*

	Mean ± SE (g)	Range (g)
Glucose		
Ingested	68 ± 3	55 to 93
Appearing in peripheral plasma (oral)	50 ± 4	32 to 56
Released by the liver	15 ± 2	5 to 20
Taken up by splanchnic tissues	19 ± 4	0.7 to 34
Taken up by peripheral tissues	48 ± 6	28 to 83
Remaining in the glucose space	2 ± 2	−2 to 15
Unrecovered	18 ± 3	8 to 31
"Saved" by the liver	18 ± 2	12 to 26
True net splanchnic balance (D − C)	4 ± 3	−17 to 17
Splanchnic "conversation" (D + H)	37 ± 4	20 to 62
Splanchnic overall contribution to glucose homeostasis (D + H − C)	22 ± 4	1 to 42

*Data are summarized from reference 11. (Reproduced by permission of the American Diabetes Association)

of tissue glucose disposal presents a challenge because of the difficulties in quantitating the rate of glucose absorption, suppression of hepatic glucose production, and organ (liver and muscle) glucose uptake. Moreover, because the plasma glucose and insulin concentrations are changing simultaneously, it is difficult to draw conclusions about insulin secretion or insulin sensitivity.

To address these issues, Ferrannini and colleagues [7, 11, 12, 259] administered an oral glucose load to healthy control subjects (Table 2) in combination with hepatic vein catheterization to quantitate the net splanchnic glucose balance. The oral glucose load and endogenous glucose pool were labeled with [1-^{14}C]glucose and [3-^{3}H]glucose, respectively, to quantitate total body glucose disposal (from tritiated glucose turnover) and endogenous HGP (difference between the total rate of glucose appearance, as measured with tritiated glucose, and the rate of oral glucose appearance, as measured with [1-^{14}C]glucose).

During the 3.5 h after glucose (68 g) ingestion (1) 19 g, or 28%, of the oral load was taken up by splanchnic tissues; (2) 48 g, or 72%, was disposed of by peripheral (non-splanchnic) tissues; (3) of the 48 g taken up by peripheral tissues, the brain (an insulin-independent tissue) accounted for ~15 g (~>1 mg/kg/min), or 22%, of the total glucose load [12]; (4) basal HGP declined by 53% (Table 2). Similar percentages for splanchnic glucose uptake [24–29%] and suppression of HGP [50–60%] in normal subjects have been reported by other investigators [14, 258, 262–264]. The contribution of skeletal muscle to the disposal of an oral glucose load has been reported to vary from a low of 26% [262] to a high of 56% [264], with a mean of 45% [11, 14, 262–264]. These results emphasize several important differences between oral versus intravenous glucose administration. After glucose ingestion (1) HGP is less completely suppressed; this may be related to activation of local sympathetic nerves that innervate the liver [265]; (2) peripheral tissue [primarily muscle] glucose uptake is quantitatively less important; (3) splanchnic glucose uptake is quantitatively much more important.

In type 2 diabetic individuals [14, 258, 259, 266, 267] the disposition of an oral glucose load is significantly altered. As originally demonstrated by Ferrannini et al. [259], the disturbance in glucose metabolism is accounted for by two factors: (1) decreased tissue glucose uptake and (2) impaired suppression of HGP (Figure 20). Splanchnic glucose uptake was similar in diabetic and control groups [259]. Inappropriate suppression of HGP accounted for approximately one third of the defect in total-body glucose homeostasis, while reduced peripheral (muscle) glucose uptake accounted for the remaining two thirds. Similar results have been reported by others [14, 219, 259, 266, 267]. One additional point should be emphasized. Since hyperglycemia *per se* enhances splanchnic (hepatic) glucose uptake [29, 225] in proportion to the increase in plasma glucose concentration, the splanchnic glucose clearance (splanchnic glucose uptake divided by plasma glucose concentration) is markedly reduced in all type 2 diabetic

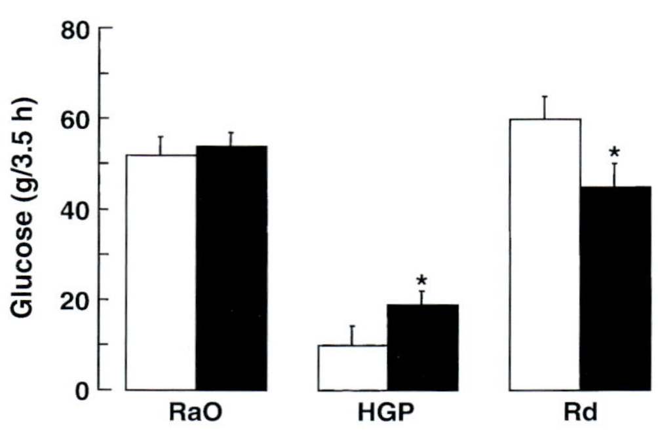

Figure 20 Disposal of an oral glucose load in type 2 diabetic subjects (solid bars) and control (open bars). Decreased peripheral tissue (muscle) glucose uptake and impaired suppression of HGP are responsible for the excessive rise in plasma glucose concentration. *$p < 0.01$, diabetic vs. controls. (Reproduced by permission of Elsevier [259])

subjects following glucose ingestion. Using a combined insulin clamp technique /OGTT, an impairment in glucose uptake by the splanchnic tissues in type 2 diabetic subjects has been demonstrated directly [268].

When viewed in absolute terms, most studies have demonstrated that the total amount of glucose taken up by all tissues of body over the 4-h period following the ingestion of an oral glucose load is normal [14] or slightly decreased [219, 258, 259, 266]. However, the efficiency of glucose disposal, i.e., the glucose clearance (tissue glucose uptake divided by plasma glucose concentration), is severely reduced. Most important, it is not the absolute glucose disposal rate, but rather the increment in glucose disposal above baseline that determines the rise in plasma glucose concentration above the fasting value. In every published study [14, 219, 258, 259, 266], the incremental response in whole-body glucose uptake has been shown to be moderately to severely reduced in type 2 diabetic individuals. Similar results have been reported for forearm muscle glucose uptake [14, 255, 256, 263, 264]. Thus, all published results are very consistent and point out the important contribution of diminished muscle glucose disposal to impaired oral glucose tolerance in type 2 diabetes.

In summary, results of the OGTT indicate that both impaired suppression of HGP and decreased tissue (muscle) glucose uptake contribute approximately equally to the glucose intolerance in type 2 diabetes. The efficiency of the splanchnic (hepatic) tissues to take up glucose (as reflected by the splanchnic glucose clearance) also is impaired in type 2 diabetic individuals.

Summary of Insulin Resistance in Type 2 Diabetes

Insulin resistance involving both muscle and liver is a characteristic feature of the glucose intolerance in type 2 diabetic individuals. In the basal state, the liver represents a major site of insulin resistance, and this is reflected by overproduction of glucose despite the presence of both fasting hyperinsulinemia and hyperglycemia. This accelerated rate of hepatic glucose output is the primary determinant of fasting hyperglycemia in type 2 diabetic individuals. Although tissue (muscle) glucose uptake in the postabsorptive state is increased when viewed in absolute terms, the efficiency with which glucose is taken up (i.e., the glucose clearance) is diminished. After glucose infusion or ingestion (i.e., the insulin-stimulated state), both decreased muscle glucose uptake and impaired suppression of HGP contribute to the insulin resistance. Following glucose ingestion, the defects in insulin-mediated glucose uptake by muscle and the suppression of HGP by insulin contribute approximately equally to the disturbance in whole-body glucose homeostasis in type 2 diabetes. However, under euglycemic hyperinsulinemic conditions, HPG is largely suppressed and impaired muscle glucose uptake is primarily responsible for the insulin resistance.

DYNAMIC INTERACTION BETWEEN INSULIN SENSITIVITY AND INSULIN SECRETION IN TYPE 2 DIABETES

Type 2 diabetic subjects manifest abnormalities both in tissue (muscle and liver) sensitivity to insulin and in pancreatic insulin secretion. To understand how these two metabolic disturbances interact to produce the full-blown diabetic condition, it is necessary to quantitate insulin action and insulin secretion in the same individual over a wide range of insulin sensitivity. This dynamic interaction is demonstrated graphically by results obtained in healthy, lean, young, normal-glucose-tolerant women who received a euglycemic insulin clamp (1 mU/kg/min) and were stratified into quartiles based upon the rate of insulin-mediated glucose disposal [60] (Figure 3a). Insulin secretion was measured independently on a separate day with a +125 mg/dl hyperglycemic clamp (Figure 3b). Insulin resistance and insulin secretion were strongly and positively correlated ($r = 0.79$, $p < 0.001$). Women who were the most insulin resistant (quartile 1) had the highest fasting plasma insulin concentrations and highest early- and late-phase plasma insulin responses (Figure 3b). Similar results relating the plasma insulin response and the severity of insulin resistance have been reported in normal-glucose-tolerant subjects with the minimal model technique [57, 58] and the insulin suppression test [269].

A number of groups have examined the dynamic interaction between insulin secretion and insulin sensitivity in type 2 diabetic subjects [1, 4, 42, 43, 46–49, 52, 57–59, 70, 72–74, 192, 209]. DeFronzo [4] studied lean (ideal body weight < 120%) and obese (ideal body weight > 125%) subjects with varying degrees of glucose tolerance as follows: group I – obese subjects ($n = 24$) with normal glucose tolerance; group II – obese subjects ($n = 23$) with IGT; group III – obese subjects ($n = 35$) with overt diabetes, subdivided into those with a hyperinsulinemic response and those with a hypoinsulinemic response during a 100-g OGTT; group IV – normal-weight type 2 diabetic subjects ($n = 26$); group V – normal-weight subjects ($n = 25$) with normal glucose tolerance. All subjects ingested 100 g glucose to provide a measure of glucose tolerance and insulin secretion. Whole-body insulin sensitivity was quantitated with the euglycemic insulin (~100 μU/ml) clamp technique, which was performed with indirect calorimetry to quantitate rates of glucose oxidation and nonoxidative glucose disposal, which primarily reflects glycogen synthesis [270].

In normal-weight type 2 diabetic subjects, insulin-mediated whole-body glucose uptake was reduced by 40–50% and the impairment in insulin action resulted from defects in both oxidative and nonoxidative glucose

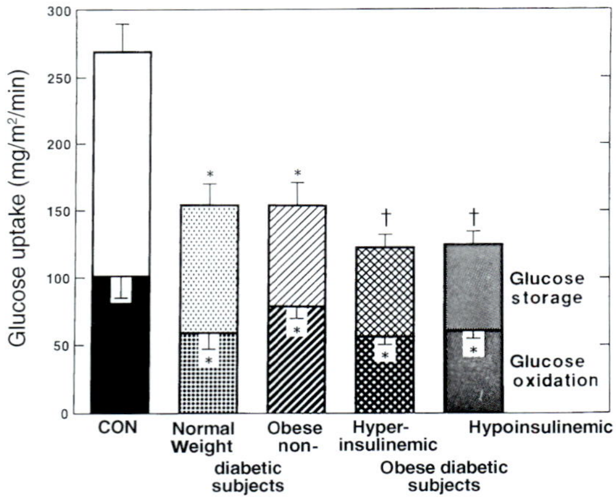

Figure 21 Insulin-mediated rates (100 μU/ml euglycemic insulin clamp) of whole-body glucose uptake (total height of bar), glucose oxidation (lower portion of each bar), and nonoxidative glucose disposal (upper part of each bar) in control, normal-weight diabetic, obese nondiabetic, and obese diabetic subjects. Obese diabetic patients were further subdivided into hyperinsulinemic and hypoinsulinemic groups based on their plasma insulin response during a 100-g OGTT. $^*p < 0.001$ vs control subjects. $^\dagger p < 0.05$ vs. nondiabetic subjects. (Reproduced by permission of the American Diabetes Association [1])

metabolism (Figure 21). Obese nondiabetic individuals were as insulin resistant as the normal-weight diabetic subjects (Figure 21). Defects in both glucose oxidation and glucose storage contributed to the insulin resistance in the obese nondiabetic group (Figure 21). From the metabolic standpoint, therefore, obesity and type 2 diabetes closely resemble each other. Similar results concerning reduced whole-body insulin sensitivity in obese and type 2 diabetic individuals have been reported by other investigators [207, 209, 214, 243, 271–275]. Despite nearly identical degrees of insulin resistance, normal-weight diabetic subjects (Figure 22) manifested fasting hyperglycemia and marked glucose intolerance, whereas the obese nondiabetic individuals had normal or only minimally impaired oral glucose tolerance. This apparent paradox is explained by the plasma insulin response during the OGTT (Figure 22). Compared with control subjects, the obese nondiabetic group secreted more than twice as much insulin, and this was sufficient to offset the insulin resistance. In contrast, in normal-weight diabetic subjects, the pancreas, when faced with the same challenge, was not able to augment its secretion of insulin sufficiently to compensate for the insulin resistance. This imbalance between insulin supply by the β-cells and the insulin requirement by tissues resulted in a frank diabetic state, with fasting hyperglycemia and marked glucose intolerance.

When obesity and diabetes coexist in the same individual, the severity of insulin resistance was only slightly greater than that in either the normal-weight diabetic or nondiabetic obese groups (Figure 21), and the magnitude of the defects in glucose oxidation and nonoxidative glucose disposal was similar in all obese and diabetic groups (Figure 21). Although hyperinsulinemic and hypoinuslinemic obese diabetic subjects were equally insulin resistant, the severity of glucose intolerance was worse in the hypoinsulinemic group, and this was related to the presence of severe insulin deficiency (Figure 22).

An integrated summary of insulin action and insulin secretion in obese, diabetic, and lean groups is presented in Figure 6. The plasma insulin response during the OGTT is shown in the top panel, along with the rate of insulin-mediated glucose disposal. In the obese nondiabetic subjects, tissue sensitivity to insulin is markedly reduced, but glucose tolerance remains perfectly normal because the β-cells are able to augment their insulin secretory capacity appropriately to offset the defect in insulin action. As the obese individual develops impaired glucose tolerance, there is a further reduction in insulin-mediated glucose disposal, which is primarily due to a decrease in glycogen synthesis. However, there is only a small additional impairment in glucose tolerance, because the β-cells are able to augment further their secretion of insulin to counteract the deterioration in insulin sensitivity. The progression of the obese glucose-intolerant person to overt diabetes is heralded by a decline in insulin secretion without any worsening of insulin resistance (Figure 6). The obese diabetic subject has tipped over the top of Starling's curve of the pancreas and is now on the descending portion (Figures 4 and 5). Even though the plasma insulin response is increased compared to

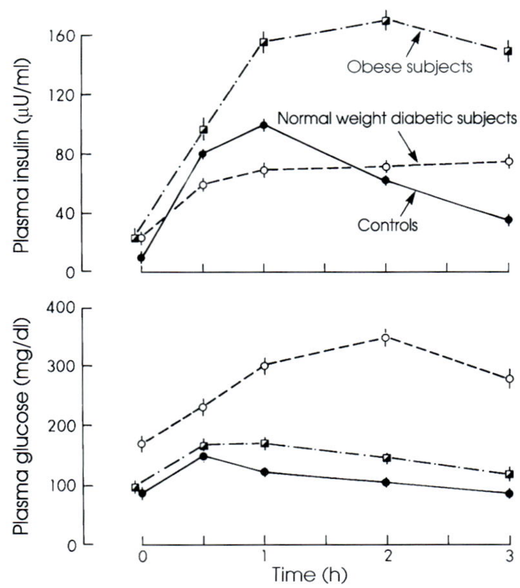

Figure 22 Plasma glucose and insulin concentrations during a 100-g OGTT in control (●), normal-weight diabetic (○), and obese nondiabetic (■) subjects whose tissue sensitivity to insulin is shown in Figure 21 (from reference 1, with permission)

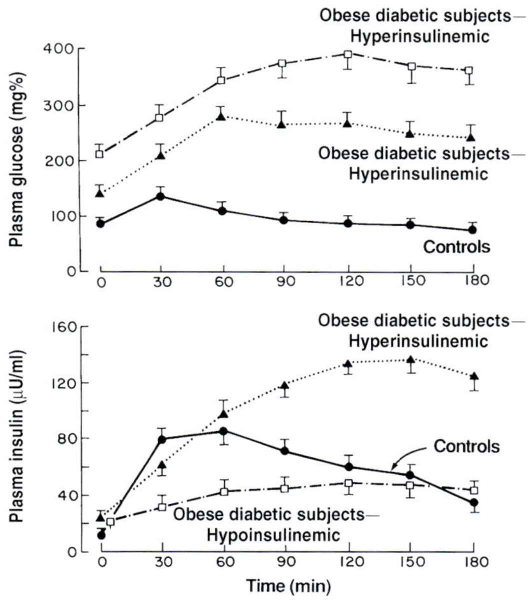

Figure 23 Plasma glucose and insulin concentrations in control (●), obese hyperinsulinemic diabetic (▲), and obese hypoinsulinemic diabetic (■) subjects whose tissue sensitivity to insulin is shown in Figure 21. (Reproduced by permission of the American Diabetes Association [1])

nondiabetic control subjects, it is not elevated appropriately for the degree of insulin resistance. In the normal-weight diabetic group, there is a further decline in glucose tolerance, which results from a greater impairment in insulin secretion without any additional deterioration in insulin sensitivity. Lastly, the obese diabetic group with a low insulin response manifests the greatest glucose intolerance, due to the presence of marked insulin deficiency without any further worsening of insulin sensitivity (Figure 23). The preceding sequence of events, leading from obesity with normal glucose tolerance to obesity with IGT and eventually to obesity with diabetes, has been confirmed in a 6-year prospective study [2] involving follow-up of the same subjects who previously participated in the cross-sectional study [1, 205, 209, 276].

The natural history of type 2 diabetes described above (see Figure 6) is consistent with results in humans and monkeys published by other investigators [41–49, 52, 53, 71–74, 127, 192]. Reaven et al. [52] studied five groups of lean subjects with a wide range of glucose tolerance, varying from normal to severely impaired. The progression from normal to IGT was marked by the development of severe insulin resistance, which was counterbalanced by a marked increase in insulin secretion (Figure 24). The onset of type 2 diabetes was associated with no (or only slight) deterioration in tissue sensitivity to insulin (Figure 24). Rather, there was a stepwise decline in insulin secretion that paralleled the decrease in glucose tolerance (Figure 24). In a prospective study in Pima Indians [42–

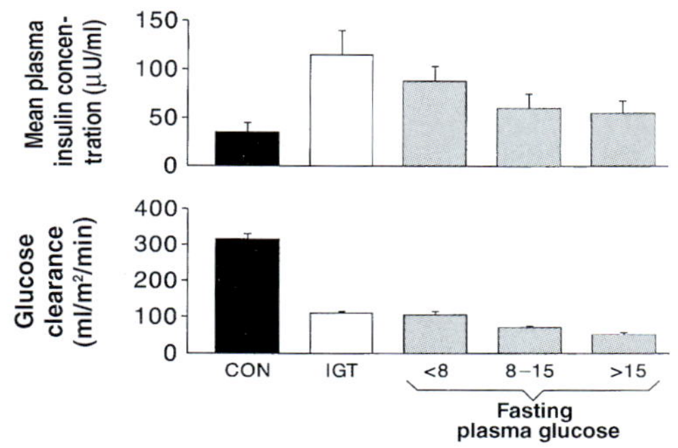

Figure 24 Insulin-mediated glucose clearance (measured with the insulin suppression test) and the plasma insulin response (measured with an OGTT) in controls (■), in subjects with IGT (□), and in type 2 diabetic individuals (■) with varying severity of glucose intolerance; see text for a more detailed discussion (drawn from data presented in reference 52)

45, 47, 49, 70, 73, 275], a similar sequence of events has been documented (Figure 25). The sequence of events described in Caucasians [1, 4, 46, 48, 51, 52, 54, 58, 72, 209], Pima Indians [42–45, 47, 49, 70, 73, 275], and Pacific Islanders [41, 75, 277] is consistent with the development of type 2 diabetes in the rhesus monkey [59, 71]. As the monkey grows older, it becomes obese and develops a diabetic condition closely resembling human type 2 diabetes. The earliest detectable abnormality in this primate model is a decrease in tissue sensitivity to insulin; because of a compensatory increase in insulin secretion, the fasting plasma glucose concentration and glucose tolerance remain normal.

The studies detailed above indicate that insulin resistance is an early and characteristic feature of the natural history of type 2 diabetes in high-risk populations. Overt diabetes develops only in those individuals whose β-cells are unable to appropriately augment their secretion of insulin to compensate for the defect in insulin

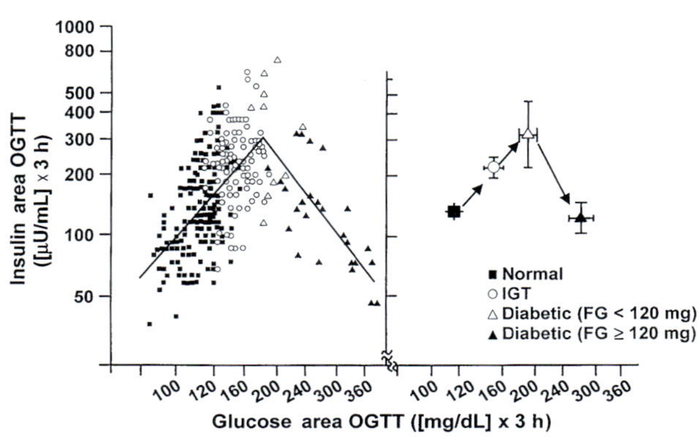

Figure 25 Natural history of β-cell dysfunction during the development of IGT and type 2 diabetes mellitus in Pima Indians (Reprinted with permission from Elsevier Science. (The Lancet, 1989, Vol; 1536–1539) [42])

action. It should be recognized, however, that there are well-described type 2 diabetic populations in whom insulin sensitivity is normal at the onset of diabetes, whereas insulin secretion is severely impaired [105–108]. How frequently this occurs in typical type 2 diabetic patients remains to be determined. This insulinopenic variety of type 2 diabetes appears to be more common in African Americans, elderly subjects, and lean Caucasians. In this later group, it is important to exclude type 1 diabetes, since ~10% of Caucasian individuals with older-onset diabetes are islet cell antibody and/or GAD positive [277].

ROLE OF THE ADIPOCYTE IN THE PATHOGENESIS OF TYPE 2 DIABETES MELLITUS: THE HARMONIOUS QUARTET

The majority (>80%) of type 2 diabetic subjects in the United States are overweight [278] and both lean and especially obese type 2 diabetic subjects are characterized by day-long elevations in the plasma FFA concentration, which fail to suppress normally following ingestion of a mixed meal or oral glucose load [279] (Figure 26). FFAs are stored in the form of triglycerides within adipocytes and serve as an important source of energy during conditions of fasting. Insulin is a potent inhibitor of lipolysis, and restrains the release of FFA from the adipocyte by inhibiting the hormone-sensitive lipase. In type 2 diabetic individuals the ability of insulin to inhibit lipolysis (as reflected by impaired suppression of radioactive palmitate turnover) and reduce the plasma FFA concentration is markedly reduced [18] (Figure 27). It is now recognized that chronically elevated plasma FFA concentrations can lead to insulin resistance in muscle and liver [1, 4, 22, 23, 25, 26, 62, 209, 280, 281] and impair insulin secretion [26, 282, 283] (Figure 28). Thus, elevated plasma FFA levels can cause/aggravate the three major pathogenic disturbances that are responsible for impaired glucose homeostasis in type 2 diabetic individuals and the time has arrived for the "triumvirate" (muscle, liver, β-cell) [1, 4] to be joined by the "fourth musketeer" [23] to form the "harmonious quartet" (Figure 29). In addition to FFAs that circulate in plasma in increased amounts, type 2 diabetic and obese patients have been shown to have increased stores of triglycerides in muscle [284, 285] and liver [286, 287], which correlate closely with the presence of insulin resistance in these tissues (Figure 30). It is now recognized that the triglycerides in liver and muscle

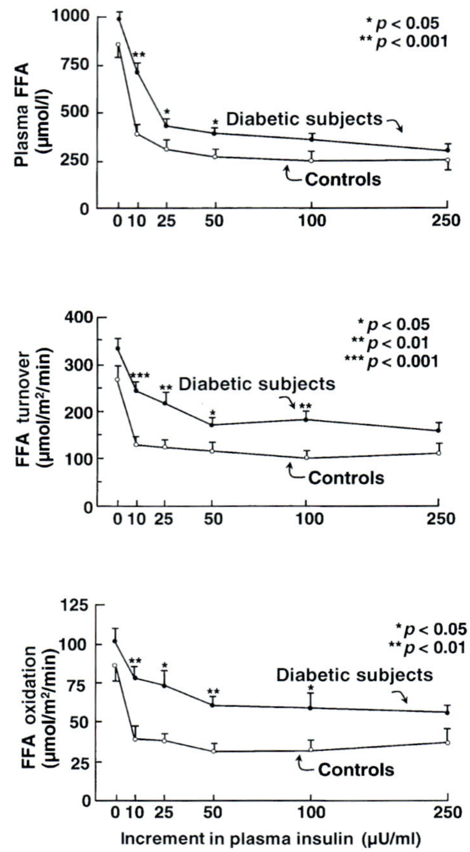

Figure 27 Dose—response relationship between the plasma insulin concentration and suppression of plasma FFA concentration, FFA turnover, and FFA oxidation in type 2 diabetic and nondiabetic control subjects (from refernce 20)

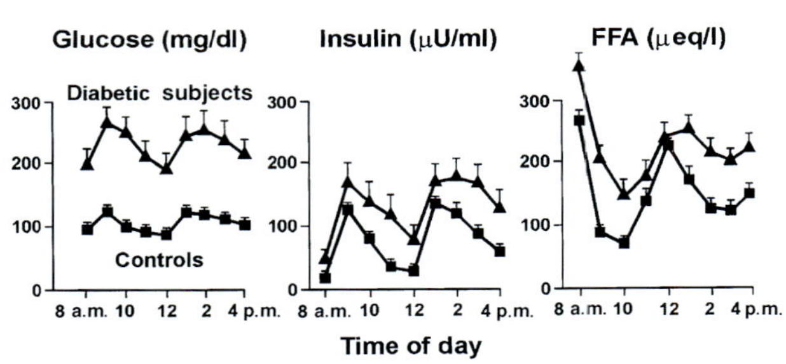

Figure 26 Plasma FFA, glucose, and insulin concentrations in type 2 diabetic and nondiabetic control subjects following standardized mixed meals given to 15 diabetic (▲) and control (■) subjects at 8 a.m. and 12 p.m. (Reproduced by permission of the American Diabetes Association [279])

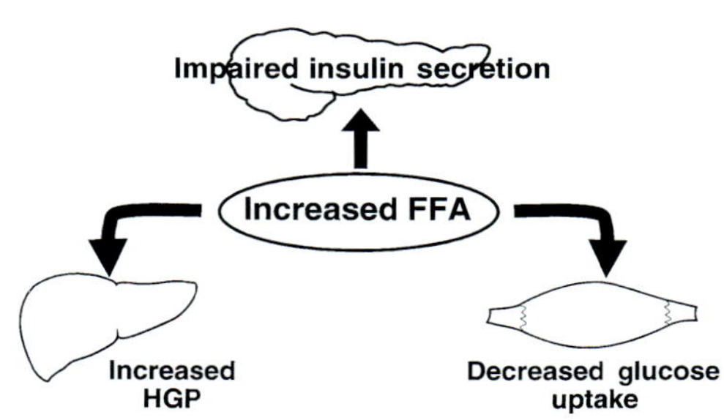

Figure 28 Schematic representation of the deleterious effect of chronically elevated plasma FFA concentrations on basal/insulin-suppressed rate of HGP, insulin-stimulated glucose uptake in muscle, and glucose-stimulated insulin secretion

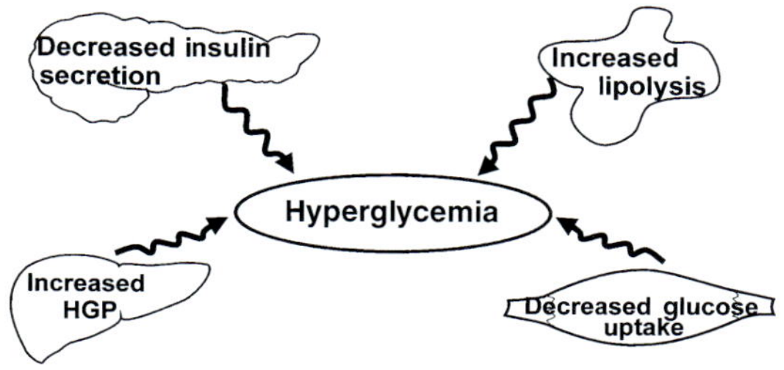

Figure 29 The "harmonious quartet." Insulin resistance in adipocytes, muscle, and liver, in combination with impaired insulin secretion by the pancreatic β-cells represent the four major organ system abnormalities that play a central role in the pathogenesis of type 2 diabetes mellitus

are in a state of constant turnover and that the metabolites (i.e., fatty acyl-CoAs) of intracellular FFA metabolism can impair insulin action in both liver and muscle [1, 4, 119]. This sequence of events has been referred to as *lipotoxicity* [1, 4, 26, 120]. Evidence also has accumulated to implicate lipotoxicity as an important cause of beta cell dysfunction [26, 120] (see earlier discussion).

FFA and Muscle Glucose Metabolism

Four decades ago, Randle and colleagues [289] proposed that increased FFA oxidation restrains glucose oxidation in muscle by altering the redox potential of the cell and by inhibiting key glycolytic enzymes (Figure 31). The excessive FFA oxidation (1) leads to the intracellular accumulation of acetyl-CoA, which is a potent inhibitor of PDH; (2) increases the NADH/NAD ratio, causing a slowing of the Krebs cycle; and (3) results in the accumulation of citrate, a powerful inhibitor of PFK. Inhibition of the enzyme PFK causes product inhibition of the early steps involved

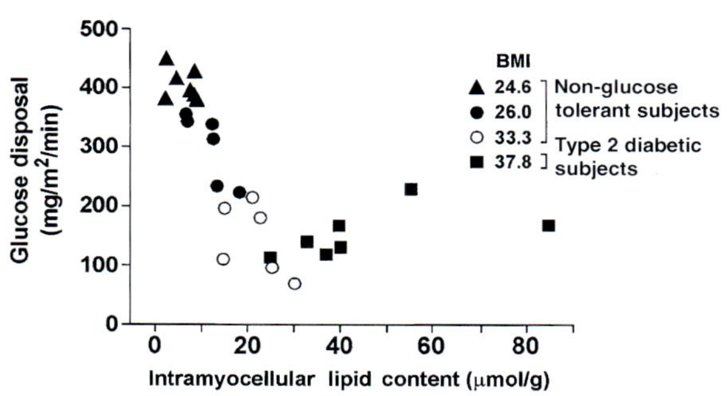

Figure 30 Relationship between intramyocellular lipid content (measured by MRI) and whole-body insulin-mediated glucose disposal (which primarily reflects muscle) measured by the euglycemic insulin clamp technique in lean and obese nondiabetic and obese type 2 diabetic subjects. Insulin resistance is strongly correlated with increase intramyocellular lipid content and reaches a maximum with muscle lipid concentrations of approximately 20 μmol/g tissue. (Reproduced by permission of the American Diabetes Association [288])

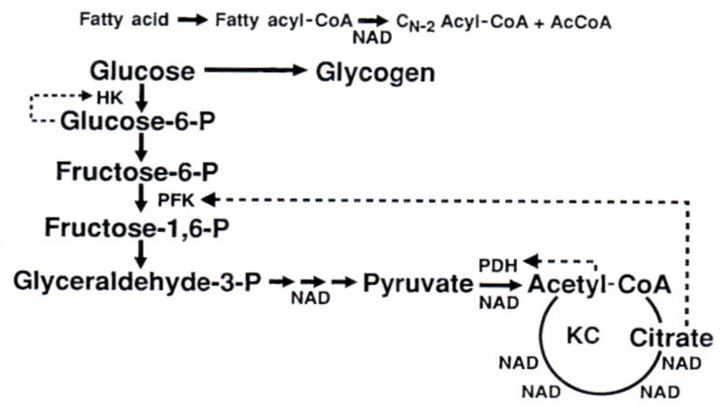

Figure 31 The Randle cycle. Enhanced FFA oxidation depletes NAD stores, leading to an inhibition of the Krebs cycle (KC) and a resultant increase in intracellular citrate and acetyl-CoA concentrations. Accumulation of acetyl-CoA and citrate leads to the inhibition of PDH and PFK, respectively. Build-up of G-6-P inhibits HK, leading to an inhibition of glucose transport into the cell. The decrease in glucose transport, in combination with an inhibitory effect of fatty acetyl-CoA on glycogen synthase, results in diminished glycogen formation. Dashed and interrupted lines represent sites of inhibition of glucose metabolism. See text for a more detailed description

in glucose metabolism, leading to the accumulation of glucose-6-phosphate (G-6-P), which in turn inhibits hexokinase II (HK-II). The block in glucose phosphorylation causes a build-up of intracellular free glucose, which restrains glucose transport into the cell via the GLUT-4 transporter. The resultant decrease in glucose transport would be expected to impair glycogen synthesis, although a direct inhibitory effect of fatty acyl-CoAs on glycogen synthase also has been demonstrated [290]. This sequence of events via which accelerated plasma FFA oxidation inhibits muscle glucose transport, glucose oxidation, and glycogen synthesis is referred to as the *Randle cycle* [289]. It should be noted that the same scenario would ensue if the FFA were derived from triglycerides stored in muscle [284, 285] or from plasma [279].

Felber and coworkers [72, 205, 209, 211, 291–293] were amongst the first to demonstrate that in obese non-diabetic and diabetic humans, basal plasma FFA levels and lipid oxidation (measured by indirect calorimetry) are increased and fail to suppress normally after glucose ingestion. The elevated basal rate of lipid oxidation was strongly correlated with a decreased basal rate of glucose oxidation, as well as with reduced rates of glucose oxidation and nonoxidative glucose disposal (glycogen synthesis) following ingestion of a glucose load. Further validation of the Randle cycle in humans has come from studies employing the euglycemic insulin clamp. In normal subjects, physiologic hyperinsulinemia (80–100 μU/ml) causes a 60–70% decline in plasma FFA concentration and a parallel decline in plasma FFA and total-body lipid oxidation [20, 21]. When Intralipid is infused concomitantly with insulin to maintain or increase the plasma FFA concentration/oxidation, both glucose oxidation and nonoxidative glucose disposal are inhibited

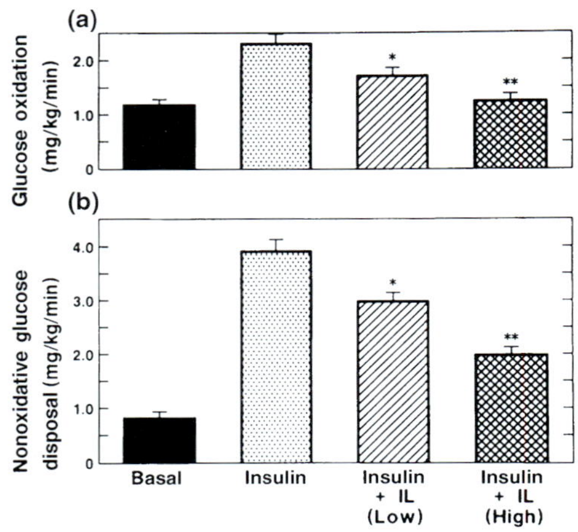

Figure 32 Inhibitory effect of Intralipid infusion and enhanced lipid oxidation on insulin-mediated rates of glucose oxidation (a) and nonoxidative glucose disposal (glycogen synthesis) (b) in healthy subjects during the basal state (■), and during a $+100\ \mu$U/ml euglycemic insulin clamp performed without (stippled bars) and with Intralipid. The Intralipid was infused at a low dose designed to maintain the plasma FFA concentration constant at the basal level (slashed bars) and at a high dose to increase plasma FFA concentrations two- to threefold (double diagonally slashed bars). $^{*}p < 0.01$ vs. insulin; $^{**}p < 0.01$ vs. insulin + IL (low) (drawn from data presented in reference 280. (Reproduced by permission of Elsevier)

in a dose-dependent fashion [280] (Figure 32). Using MRI, Roden et al. [294] have shown that the FFA-induced inhibition of nonoxidative glucose disposal reflects impaired glycogen synthesis. The inhibitory effect of elevated plasma FFA levels can be observed at all plasma insulin concentrations, spawning the physiologic and pharmacologic range [280].

The inhibitory effect of an acute elevation in plasma FFA concentration on muscle glucose metabolism is time dependent. Thus, the earliest (within 2 h) observed abnormality is a defect in glucose oxidation [295, 296], as would be predicted by operation of the Randle cycle [289]. This is followed (between 2 and 3 h) by defects in glucose transport and phosphorylation and eventually (after 3–4 h) by impaired glycogen synthesis.

Randle Cycle Revisited: Biochemical/Molecular Basis of FFA-induced Insulin Resistance

The original description of the Randle cycle was formulated based upon experiments performed in rat diaphragm and heart muscle [289]. More recent studies performed in human skeletal muscle implicate mechanisms, in addition to those originally proposed by Randle, in the FFA-induced insulin resistance. Thus, both Roden et al. [294] and Boden et al. [296, 297] have failed to observe a rise in G-6-P when insulin-stimulated glucose metabolism was inhibited by a lipid infusion to elevate the plasma FFA concentration, while the later group failed to demonstrate an increase in muscle citrate levels or an inhibition of PFK. Thus, while increased FFA/lipid and decreased glucose oxidation are closely coupled, as originally demonstrated by Randle, mechanisms other than product (i.e., elevated intracellular G-6-P and free glucose concentrations) inhibition of the early steps of glucose metabolism must be invoked to explain the defects in glucose transport, glucose phosphorylation, and glycogen synthesis.

Studies in humans and animals have shown a strong negative correlation between insulin-stimulated glucose metabolism and increased intramuscular lipid pools, including triglyceride [298–301], DAG [302, 303], and long-chain fatty acyl-CoAs [304]. An acute elevation in plasma FFA concentration leads to an increase in muscle fatty acyl-CoA and DAG concentrations. Both long-chain fatty acyl-CoAs and DAG activate PKC θ [302], which increases serine phosphorylation with subsequent inhibition of insulin receptor substrate 1 (IRS-1) tyrosine phosphorylation [305–307]. Consistent with this observation, two groups have shown that in human muscle, elevated plasma FFA levels inhibit insulin-stimulated tyrosine phosphorylation of IRS-1, the association of the p85 subunit of phosphatidylinositol 3 (PI3) kinase with IRS-1, and activation of PI3 kinase [308, 309] (Figure 33). Direct effects of long-chain fatty acyl-CoAs on glucose transport [310], glucose phosphorylation [311], and glycogen synthase [290] also have been demonstrated in muscle (Figure 33). Lastly, increased muscle ceramide levels (secondary to increased long-chain fatty acyl-CoAs) have been shown to interfere with glucose transport and to inhibit glycogen synthase in muscle via activation of PKB [312]. In summary, elevated plasma FFA concentrations can induce insulin resistance in muscle via multiple mechanisms involving alterations in a variety of intracellular lipid signaling molecules that exert their inhibitory effects on multiple steps (insulin signal transduction system, glucose transport, glucose

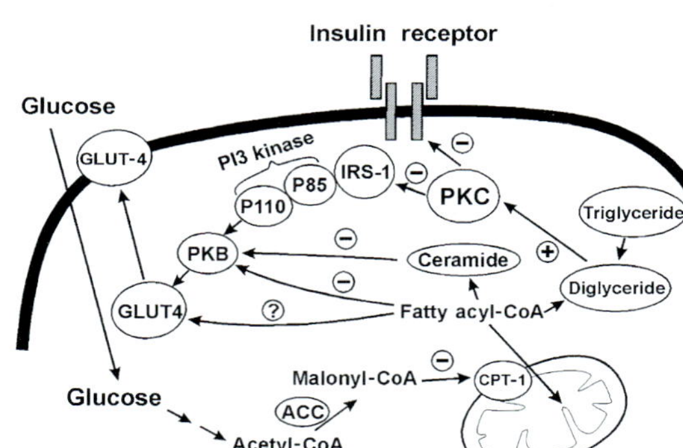

Figure 33 Schematic representation of the intracellular biochemical and molecular events that are inhibited by fatty acyl-CoAs and their intracellular metabolites. See text for a more detailed discussion

phosphorylation, glycogen synthase, PDH, Krebs cycle) involved in glucose metabolism.

FFA and Blood Flow

Insulin is a vasodilatory hormone and the stimulatory effect of insulin on muscle glucose metabolism has been shown to result from (1) direct action of insulin to augment muscle glucose metabolism, and (2) increased blood flow to muscle [313, 314]. The vasodilatory effect of insulin is mediated via the release of nitric oxide from the vascular endothelium [315]. In insulin-resistant conditions, such as obesity and type 2 diabetes, Baron et al. have provided evidence that as much as half of the impairment in insulin-mediated whole-body and leg muscle glucose uptake is related to a defect in insulin's vasodilatory action [313, 314] (Figure 34), although the link between insulin-mediated vasodilation and increased blood flow has been challenged by other investigators [316].

Because type 2 diabetes and obesity are insulin-resistant states characterized by day-long elevation in the plasma FFA concentration [279] and impaired endothelium-dependent vasodilation [313], investigators have examined the effect of increased plasma FFA levels on limb blood flow and muscle glucose uptake [317, 318]. In healthy, non-diabetic subjects an acute physiologic increase in plasma FFA concentration (brought about by

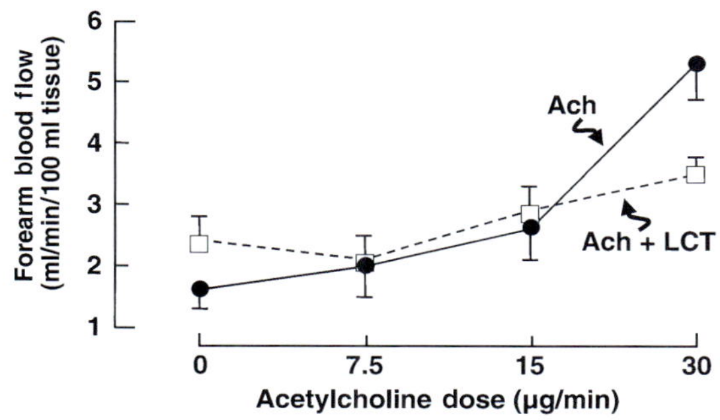

Figure 35 Effect of elevated plasma FFA concentrations on methacholine- (endothelium-dependent-) and nitroprusside- (endothelium-independent-) stimulated blood flow and insulin-stimulated leg muscle glucose uptake. LCT = long-chain triglyceride. (Reproduced by permission of the Endocrinol Society)

lipid infusion) inhibited methacholine- (endothelium-dependent) but not nitroprusside- (endothelium-independent) stimulated blood flow in association with an impairment in insulin-stimulated muscle glucose disposal (Figure 35). In subsequent studies, the inhibitory effect of FFA on insulin-stimulated leg blood flow was shown to be associated with decreased nitric oxide production [317]. FFA elevation also has been shown to inhibit nitric oxide production in endothelial cell cultures by decreasing nitric oxide synthase activity [319, 320]. Since the IRS-1/PI3-kinase signal transduction pathway is involved in the regulation of nitric oxide synthase activity [321, 322], one could hypothesize that FFA-induced inhibition of the insulin signal transduction pathway is responsible for the blunted vasodilatory response to the hormone.

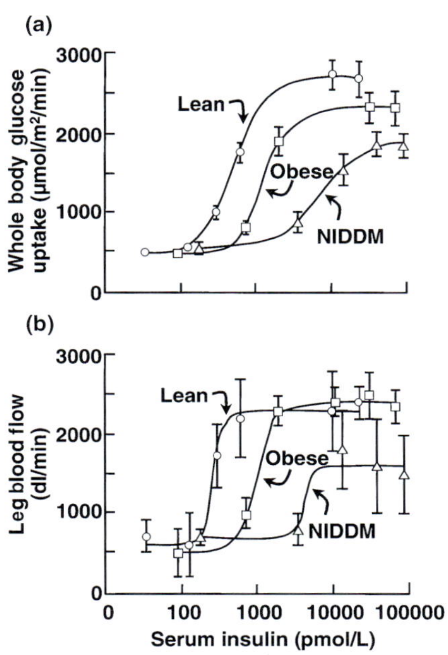

Figure 34 Dose–response curve relating whole-body glucose uptake (a) and leg blood flow (b) to the plasma insulin concentration during euglycemic insulin clamp studies performed in lean control subjects, normal-glucose-tolerant obese subjects, and type 2 diabetic subjects. To convert insulin concentrations from picomoles per liter to microunits per milliliter, divide by 7.175 (from reference 313)

FFA and Hepatic Glucose Metabolism

The liver plays a central role in the regulation of glucose metabolism [1, 4, 6, 11, 17, 259]. Following ingestion of a carbohydrate meal, it is essential that the liver suppresses its basal rate of glucose production [12]. In addition, the liver takes up approximately one third of the glucose in the ingested carbohydrate meal [12, 29, 30, 259]. Collectively, suppression of hepatic glucose production and augmentation of hepatic glucose uptake account for the maintenance of about half of the rise in plasma glucose concentration following ingestion of a carbohydrate meal [1, 4, 6, 12, 259].

The regulation of hepatic glucose production is controlled by a number of factors (Figure 36), of which insulin (inhibits HGP) and glucagon and FFA (stimulate HGP) are the most important. *In vitro* studies have demonstrated that plasma FFAs are potent stimulators of HGP and do so by increasing the activity of pyruvate carboxylase and PEPCK, the rate-limiting enzymes for gluconeogenesis [323–325]. FFAs also enhance the activity of G-6-Pase,

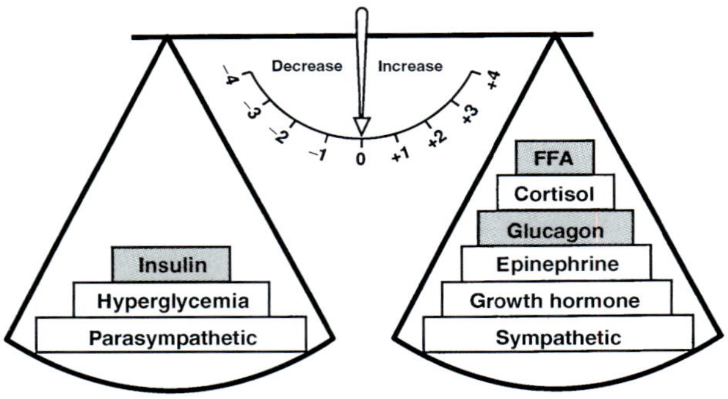

Figure 36 Regulation of HGP. Factors that increase HGP are shown to the right and factors that inhibit HGP are shown to the left

the enzyme that ultimately controls the release of glucose by the liver [326] (Figure 37).

In normal subjects, an increase in plasma FFA concentration stimulates gluconeogenesis [327, 328], while a decrease in plasma FFA concentration reduces gluconeogenesis [327]. With regard to the later, Bergman, Cherrington, and colleagues have shown that a significant portion of the suppressive effect of insulin on hepatic glucose production is mediated via inhibition of lipolysis and a reduction in circulating plasma FFA concentrations [17, 329, 330]. Moreover, FFA infusion in normal humans under conditions that simulate the diabetic state [331] and in obese insulin-resistant subjects [332] enhances hepatic glucose production, most likely secondarily to stimulation of gluconeogenesis.

In type 2 diabetic subjects, the fasting plasma FFA concentration and lipid oxidation rate are increased and are strongly correlated with the elevated fasting plasma glucose concentration/basal HGP rate [20, 21, 23, 62, 72, 209, 211, 333]. The relationship between elevated plasma FFA concentration, FFA oxidation, and hepatic glucose production in obesity and type 2 diabetes can be explained as follows:

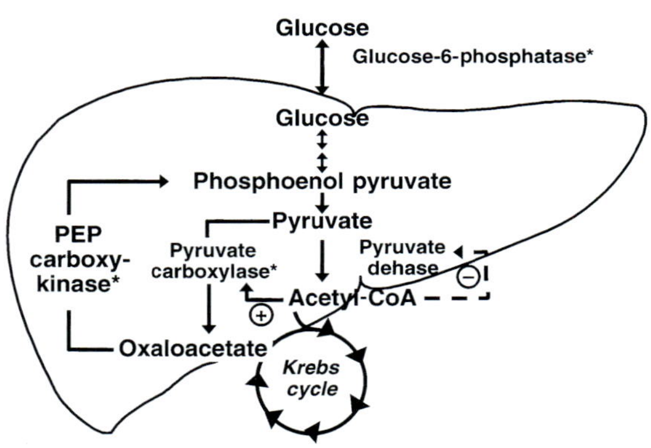

Figure 37 Schematic representation of the regulation of HGP and hepatic gluconeogenesis. Sites of stimulation by FFA are shown by the asterisk. See text for a more detailed discussion

(1) Increased plasma FFA levels, by mass action, augment FFA uptake by hepatocytes, leading to accelerated lipid oxidation and accumulation of acetyl-CoA. The increased concentration of acetyl-CoA stimulates pyruvate carboxylase, the rate-limiting enzyme in gluconeogenesis [323–325], as well as G-6-Pase, the rate-controlling enzyme for glucose release from the hepatocyte [326] (Figure 37).
(2) The increased rate of FFA oxidation provides a continuing source of energy (in the form of ATP) and reduced nucleotides (NADH) to drive gluconeogenesis.
(3) Elevated plasma FFA induce hepatic insulin resistance by inhibiting the insulin signal transduction system [303–308]. In type 2 diabetic patients these deleterious effects of elevated plasma FFA concentrations occur in concert with increased plasma glucagon levels [234, 242, 334], increased hepatic sensitivity to glucagon [242], and increased hepatic uptake of circulating gluconeogenic precursors [233].

Summary: FFA and the Pathogenesis of Obesity and Type 2 Diabetes Mellitus

In obese individuals and in the majority (>80%) of type 2 diabetic subjects, there is an expanded fat cell mass and the adipocytes are resistant to the antilipolytic effects of insulin [20, 21]. Most obese and diabetic individuals are characterized by visceral adipocity [335] and the visceral fat cells have a high lipolytic rate, which is especially refractory to insulin [336]. Not surprisingly, both type 2 diabetes and obesity are characterized by an elevation in the mean day-long plasma FFA concentration [62, 209, 279]. Elevated plasma FFA concentrations, as well as increased triglyceride/fatty acyl-CoA content in muscle, liver, and beta cell, lead to the development of muscle/hepatic insulin resistance and impaired insulin secretion (Figure 28).

CELLULAR MECHANISMS OF INSULIN RESISTANCE

In order for insulin to exert its biologic effects on glucose metabolism, it must first bind to specific receptors that are present on the cell surface of all insulin target tissues [1, 337–343]. After insulin has bound to and activated its receptor, "second messengers" are generated and these second messengers initiate a series of events involving a cascade of phosphorylation–dephosphorylation reactions [1, 337–343] that eventually result in the stimulation of intracellular glucose metabolism. The initial step

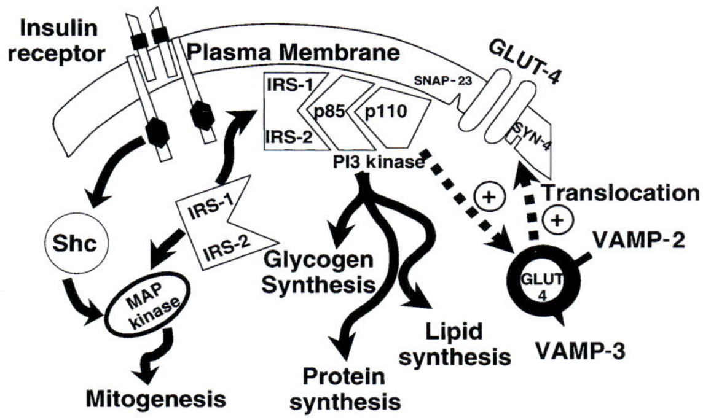

Figure 38 Schematic representation of the insulin receptor and the cascade of intracellular signaling molecules that have been implicated in insulin action. See text for a more detailed discussion

in glucose metabolism involves activation of the glucose transport system, leading to influx of glucose into insulin target tissues, primarily muscle [1, 344–347]. The free glucose, which has entered the cell, is subsequently metabolized by a series of enzymatic steps that are under the control of insulin. Of these, the most important are glucose phosphorylation (catalyzed by hexokinase), glycogen synthase (which controls glycogen synthesis), and PFK and PDH (which regulate glycolysis and glucose oxidation, respectively).

Insulin Receptor/Insulin Receptor Tyrosine Kinase

The insulin receptor is a glycoprotein consisting of two α-subunits and two β-subunits linked by disulfide bonds [1, 337–343, 346, 347] (Figure 38). The α-subunit of the insulin receptor is entirely extracellular and contains the insulin-binding domain. The β-subunit has an extracellular domain, a transcellular domain, and an intracellular domain that expresses insulin-stimulated kinase activity directed toward its own tyrosine residues [1, 337–340]. Insulin receptor phosphorylation of the β-subunit, with subsequent activation of insulin receptor tyrosine kinase, represents the first step in the action of insulin on glucose metabolism [337–343]. Mutagenesis experiments have shown that insulin receptors devoid of tyrosine kinase activity are completely ineffective in mediating insulin stimulation of cellular metabolism [348, 349]. Similarly, mutagenesis of any of the three major phosphorylation sites (at residues 1158, 1163, and 1162) impairs the insulin receptor kinase activity, and this is associated with a marked decrease in the acute metabolic and growth promoting effects of insulin [348, 350].

Insulin Receptor Signal Transduction

Following activation, insulin receptor tyrosine kinase phosphorylates specific intracellular proteins, of which at least nine have been identified [337] (Figure 38). Four of these belong to the family of insulin-receptor substrate proteins: IRS-1, IRS-2, IRS-3, IRS-4 (the others include Shc, Cbl, Gab-1, p60^{dok}, and APS). In muscle, IRS-1 serves as the major docking protein that interacts with the insulin receptor tyrosine kinase and undergoes tyrosine phosphorylation in regions containing amino acid sequence motifs (YXXM or YMXM) that, when phosphorylated, serve as recognition sites for proteins containing *src* homology 2 (SH2) domains [337, 338]. Mutation of these specific tyrosines severely impairs the ability of insulin to stimulate glycogen and DNA synthesis, establishing the important role of IRS-1 in insulin signal transduction [351]. In liver, IRS-2 serves as the primary docking protein that undergoes tyrosine phosphorylation and mediates the effect of insulin on hepatic glucose production, gluconeogenesis, and glycogen formation [352]. In adipocytes, *Cbl* represents another substrate which is phosphorylated following its interaction with the insulin receptor tyrosine kinase and which is required for stimulation of GLUT-4 translocation. Phosphorylation of *Cbl* occurs when the CAP/*Cbl* complex associates with flotillin in caveolae, or lipid rafts, containing insulin receptors [353, 354].

In muscle, the phosphorylated tyrosine residues on IRS-1 mediate an association between the SH2 domains of the 85-kDa regulatory subunit of PI3 kinase, leading to activation of the enzyme [337–349, 355, 356] (Figure 38). PI3 kinase is a heterodimeric enzyme composed of an 85-kDa regulatory subunit and a 110-kDa catalytic subunit. The latter catalyzes the 3′ phosphorylation of PI, PI-4-phosphate, and PI-4,5-diphosphate, resulting in the stimulation of glucose transport [337–340, 357]. Activation of PI3 kinase by phosphorylated IRS-1 also leads to activation of glycogen synthase [337, 338], via a process that involves activation of PKB/Akt and subsequent inhibition of kinases such as glycogen synthase kinase 3 (GSK-3) [358] and activation of protein phosphatase 1 (PP-1) [359]. Inhibitors of PI3 kinase impair glucose transport [337–340, 360, 361] by interfering with the translocation of GLUT-4 transporters from their intracellular location [345–347] and block the activation of glycogen synthase [362, 363] and HK-II expression [364]. The action of insulin to increase protein synthesis and inhibit protein synthesis also is mediated by PI3 kinase and involves the activation of mammalian target of rapamycin (mTOR) [365, 366]. mTOR controls translation machinery by phosphorylation and activation of p70 ribosomal S6 kinase (p70^{rsk}) [365] and phosphorylation of initiation factors [367, 368]. Insulin also promotes hepatic triglyceride synthesis via increasing the transcription factor steroid regulatory element-binding protein 1c [368] and this lipogenic effect of insulin also appears to be mediated via the PI3 kinase pathway [337].

Other proteins with SH2 domains, including the adapter protein Grb2 and *Shc*, also interact with IRS-1 and become phosphorylated following exposure to insulin [337–339, 369]. Grb2 and *Shc* serve to link IRS-1/IRS-2 to the mitogen-activated protein (MAP) signaling pathway (Figure 38), which plays an important role in the generation of transcription factors [337, 338]. Following the interaction between IRS-1/IRS-2 and *Grb2* and *Shc*, *Ras* is activated, leading to the stepwise activation of *Raf*, MEK, and ERK. Activated ERK than translocates into the nucleus of the cell where it catalyzes the phosphorylation of transcription factors that promote cell growth, proliferation, and differentiation [337–339, 369–372]. Blockade of the MAP-kinase pathway prevents the stimulation of cell growth by insulin but has no effect on the metabolic actions of the hormone [373–375].

Under anabolic conditions insulin stimulates glycogen synthesis by simultaneously activating glycogen synthase and inhibiting glycogen phosphorylase [376–378]. The effect of insulin is mediated via the PI3-kinase pathway that inactivates kinases such as GSK-3 and activates phosphatases, particularly PP-1. It is believed that PP-1 is the primary regulator of glycogen metabolism [376–379]. In skeletal muscle, PP-1 associates with a specific glycogen-binding regulatory subunit, causing dephosphorylation (activation) of glycogen synthase. PP-1 also phosphorylates (inactivates) glycogen phosphorylase. The precise steps that link insulin receptor tyrosine kinase/PI3-kinase activation to stimulation of PP-1 have yet to be defined. Some evidence suggests that p90 ribosomal S6 kinase may be involved in the activation of glycogen synthase [337]. Akt also has been shown to phosphorylate and thus inactivate GSK-3 [358]. This decreases glycogen synthase phosphorylation, leading to activation of the enzyme [358]. A number of studies have convincingly demonstrated that inhibitors of PI3 kinase inhibit glycogen synthase and abolish glycogen synthesis [337, 359, 379]. From the physiological standpoint, it makes sense that activation of glucose transport and glycogen synthase should be linked to the same signaling mechanism in order to provide a coordinated and efficient stimulation of intracellular glucose metabolism.

Insulin Signal Transduction Defects in Type 2 Diabetes

Insulin Receptor Number and Affinity

Both receptor and postreceptor defects have been shown to contribute to insulin resistance in type 2 diabetic individuals. Some studies, but not all, have demonstrated that insulin binding to monocytes and adipocytes from type 2 diabetic patients is modestly reduced, by ~20–30% [1, 380–386]. The reduction in insulin binding is due to a decrease in the number of insulin receptors without change in insulin receptor affinity. In addition to the decreased number of cell-surface receptors, a variety of defects in insulin receptor internalization and processing have been described [384, 385]. However, some caution should be employed in interpreting these studies. Muscle and liver, not adipocytes, are the major tissues responsible for the regulation of glucose homeostasis *in vivo*, and insulin binding to solubilized receptors obtained from skeletal muscle biopsies and liver has been shown to be normal in obese and lean diabetic individuals when expressed per milligram of protein [382, 383, 386–390]. Moreover, a decrease in insulin receptor number cannot be demonstrated in as many as half of all type 2 diabetic subjects [391, 392], and several groups have been unable to find a correlation between insulin binding and severity of insulin resistance in type 2 diabetic patients [393, 394]. The insulin receptor gene has been sequenced in a large number of type 2 diabetic patients from a wide diversity of ethnic populations using denaturing-gradient gel electrophoresis or single-stranded conformational polymorphism analysis, and with very rare exceptions [395], physiologically significant mutations in the insulin receptor gene were not observed [396–398]. This excludes a structural gene abnormality in the insulin receptor as a cause of common type 2 diabetes.

Insulin Receptor Tyrosine Kinase Activity

Insulin receptor tyrosine kinase activity has been examined in a variety of cell types (skeletal muscle, adipocytes, hepatocytes, and erythrocytes) from normal-weight and obese diabetic subjects. Most [341, 369, 381–383, 387, 392, 399–402] but not all [388, 403] investigators have found a significant reduction in insulin-stimulated tyrosine kinase activity (Figure 39) that cannot be explained by alterations in insulin receptor number or insulin receptor binding. The study of Freidenberg et al. [404] is

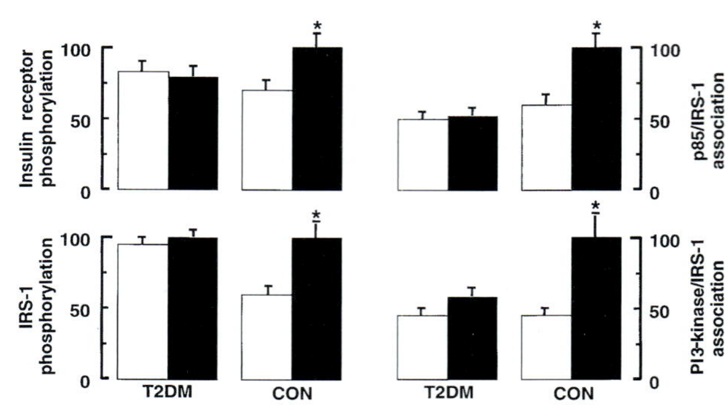

Figure 39 Effect of insulin on insulin receptor and IRS-1 tyrosine phosphorylation and the association of IRS-1 with p85 regulatory subunit of PI3 kinase and PI3-kinase activity in muscle from type 2 diabetic (T2DM) and control (CON) subjects. Data are expressed as percentage of the mean insulin-stimulated values in the control groups. Open bars = basal state; solid bars = insulin-stimulated state; $^{*}p < 0.05$, T2DM versus CON (from reference 369)

particularly informative. In this study weight loss with near-normalization of the fasting plasma glucose concentration led to a correction of the defect in insulin receptor tyrosine kinase activity. This observation suggests that the defect in tyrosine kinase is acquired and results from some combination of hyperglycemia, defective intracellular glucose metabolism, hyperinsulinemia, and insulin resistance—all of which improved after weight loss. A glucose-induced reduction in insulin receptor tyrosine kinase activity has been demonstrated in rat fibroblasts culture *in vitro* [405]. Insulin receptor tyrosine kinase activity assays are performed *in vitro*, and the results of these assays could provide misleading information with regard to insulin receptor function *in vivo*. To circumvent this problem, Cusi et al. [369] used the euglycemic hyperinsulinemic clamp in combination with muscle biopsies and anti-phosphotyrosine immunoblot analysis. Such analysis yields a "snapshot" of the insulin-stimulated tyrosine phosphorylation state of the receptor, which presumably would reflect its tyrosine kinase activity. They found a substantial decrease in insulin receptor tyrosine phosphorylation in obese nondiabetic and type 2 diabetic subjects [369]. Krook et al. [402] reported the same finding. When insulin-stimulated insulin receptor tyrosine phosphorylation was examined in normal-glucose-tolerant or impaired-glucose-tolerant individuals at high risk of developing type 2 diabetes, a normal increase in tyrosine phosphorylation of the insulin receptor has been observed [406] (Figure 40). These observations are consistent with the concept that impaired insulin receptor tyrosine kinase activity in type 2 diabetic patients is acquired secondarily to hyperglycemia or some other metabolic disturbance.

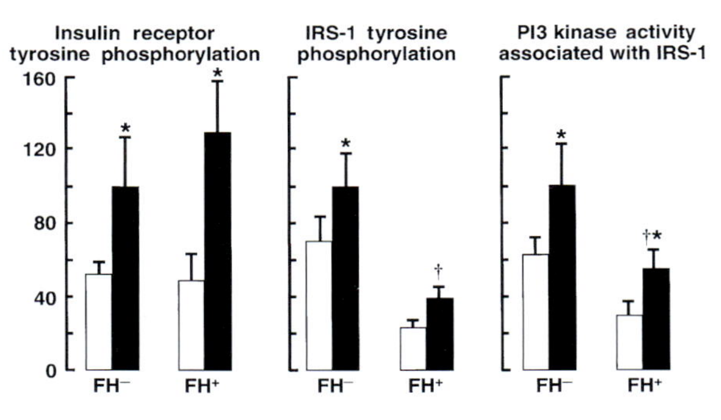

Figure 40 Effect of insulin on insulin receptor and IRS-1 tyrosine phosphorylation and the association of PI3-kinase activity with IRS-1 in insulin-resistant individuals with a strong family history of type 2 diabetes (FH^+) and in control individuals without any history of diabetes (FH^-). Data are presented as percentage of the mean insulin-stimulated values in the control (FH^-) group. Open bars = basal state; solid bars = insulin-stimulated state; $^*p < 0.05$ vs. basal; $\dagger p < 0.05$, FH^+ vs. FH^-. (Reproduced by permission of the American Diabetes Association [406])

Insulin Signaling (IRS-1 and PI3 Kinase) Defects

Physiologic hyperinsulinemia increases tyrosine phosphorylation of the insulin receptor and IRS-1 in lean, healthy subjects to 150–200% of basal values (Figure 39) [343, 369, 402, 406, 407]. In obese nondiabetic subjects, the ability of insulin to activate these two early insulin receptor signaling events in muscle is reduced, while in type 2 diabetic subjects insulin had no significant stimulatory effect on either insulin receptor or IRS-1 tyrosine phosphorylation [369] (Figure 39). The association of p85 protein and PI3-kinase activity with IRS-1 also is greatly reduced in obese non-diabetic and type 2 diabetic subjects compared to lean, healthy subjects [369, 402, 408] (Figure 39). Insulin stimulation also failed to increase the association of p85 with IRS-2 in muscle, indicating that type 2 diabetes is characterized by a combined defect in IRS-1 and IRS-2 function [369, 402]. The decrease in insulin stimulation of the association of the p85 regulatory subunit of PI3 kinase with IRS-1 is closely correlated with the impairment in muscle glycogen synthase activity and *in vivo* insulin-stimulated glucose disposal [369]. Defective regulation of PI3-kinase gene expression by insulin also has been demonstrated in skeletal muscle and adipose tissue of type 2 diabetic subjects [409]. In animal models of diabetes, an 80% decrease in IRS-1 phosphorylation and a greater than 90% reduction in insulin-stimulated PI3-kinase activity have been reported [410].

In the insulin-resistant, normal-glucose-tolerant offspring of two type 2 diabetic parents, IRS-1 tyrosine phosphorylation and the association of p85 protein and PI3-kinase activity with IRS-1 are markedly decreased despite normal tyrosine phosphorylation of the insulin receptor (Figure 40); these insulin signaling defects are correlated closely with the severity of insulin resistance, measured with the euglycemic insulin clamp technique [406]. In summary, a defect in the association of PI3 kinase with IRS-1 and its subsequent activation appears to be a characteristic abnormality in type 2 diabetic subjects, is closely correlated with *in vivo* muscle insulin resistance, and is unrelated to a disturbance in insulin receptor tyrosine phosphorylation. Several investigators [411, 412] have reported that a common mutation in the IRS-1 gene (Gly972Arg) is associated with type 2 diabetes, insulin resistance, and obesity, but the physiologic significance of this mutation remains to be established. Interestingly, the location of the IRS-1 gene on chromosome 2q36 is close to a linkage peak for insulin action in Pima Indians [413].

The profound insulin resistance of the PI3-kinase signaling pathway contrasts markedly with the ability of insulin to stimulate MAP-kinase pathway activity in insulin-resistant type 2 diabetic and obese non-diabetic individuals [369, 402] (Figure 41). Hyperinsulinemia increases MEK-1 activity and ERK-1/2 phosphorylation and activity to the same extent in lean, healthy as in

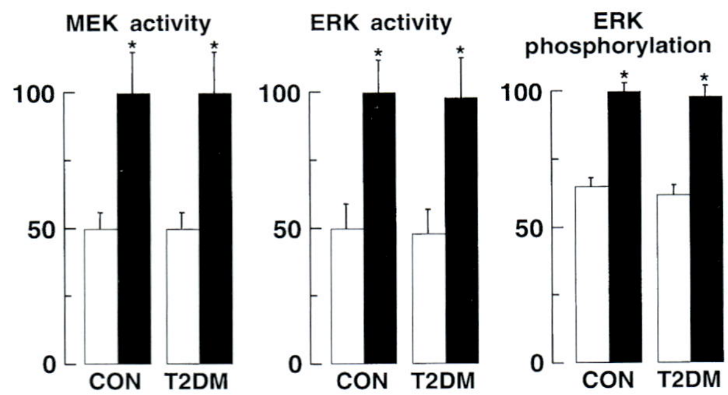

Figure 41 Effect of insulin on ERK and MEK activity and ERK phosphorylation in muscle of type 2 diabetic (T2DM) and control (CON) subjects. Data are presented as percentage of the mean insulin-stimulated values in the control group. Open bars = basal state; solid bars = insulin-stimulated state; $^{*}p < 0.05$ vs. baseline (from reference 369)

insulin-resistant, obese nondiabetic and type 2 diabetic patients [369, 402]. This finding of selective insulin resistance is similar to that recently observed in vasculature of Zucker fatty rats [414]. Two possible reasons for this difference are alternate insulin signaling pathways and differential signal amplification. With regard to the former, the MAP-kinase pathway can be activated through *Grb2/Sos* interaction either with IRS-1/IRS-2 or with *Shc*. Because IRS-1 tyrosine phosphorylation is dramatically reduced in the diabetic patients, it is possible that insulin activation of the MAP-kinase pathway *in vivo* primarily occurs through *Shc* activation. Evidence from *in vitro* studies supports this concept [415]. Like ERK and MEK activity, insulin increased *Shc* phosphorylation to the same extent in lean and obese nondiabetic and type 2 diabetic subjects [369]. These results indicate that in type 2 diabetes, insulin induces sufficient activation of the insulin receptor tyrosine kinase to increase Shc phosphorylation normally. It also is possible that differential signal amplification in the PI3-kinase and MAP-kinase pathways can explain their differing susceptibilities to the effects of insulin resistance.

Maintenance of insulin stimulation of the MAP-kinase pathway in the presence of insulin resistance in the PI3-kinase pathway may be important in the development of insulin resistance. ERKs can phosphorylate IRS-1 on serine residues [416], and serine phosphorylation of IRS-1 and the insulin receptor itself has been implicated in desensitization insulin receptor signaling [417]. Continued ERK activity, when IRS-1 function already is impaired, could lead to a worsening of insulin resistance. Thus, diabetic and obese subjects have inappropriately high MAP-kinase activity. One also could postulate that insulin resistance in the metabolic (PI3-kinase) pathway, with its compensatory increase in beta cell function and hyperinsulinemia, leads to excessive stimulation of the MAP-kinase pathway in vascular tissue [369, 370]. This would result in the proliferation of vascular smooth muscle cells, increased collagen formation, and increased production of growth factors and inflammatory cytokines, possibly explaining the accelerated rate of atherosclerosis in type 2 diabetic individuals.

Glucose Transport

Activation of the insulin signal transduction system in insulin target tissues leads to the stimulation of glucose transport. The effect of insulin is brought about by the translocation of a large intracellular pool of glucose transporters (associated with low-density microsomes) to the plasma membrane [344–347, 418]. There are five major, different facilitative glucose transporters with distinctive tissue distributions [345–347, 419, 420] (Table 3). GLUT-4, the insulin regulatable transporter, is found in insulin-sensitive tissues (muscle and adipocytes), has a K_m of ~5 mmol/l, which is close to that of the plasma glucose concentration, and is associated with HK-II [421–423]. In adipocytes and muscle, its concentration in the plasma membrane increases markedly after exposure to insulin, and this increase is associated with a reciprocal decline in the intracellular GLUT-4 pool. GLUT-1 represents the predominant glucose transporter in the insulin-independent tissues (brain and erythrocytes), but is also found in muscle and adipocytes. It is located primarily in the plasma membrane, where its concentration changes little after the addition of insulin. It has a low K_m (~1 mmol/l) and is well suited for its function, which is to mediate basal glucose uptake. It is found in association with HK-I

Table 3 Classification of glucose transport and HK activity according to their tissue distribution and functional regulation*

Organ	Glucose transporter	HK computer	Classification
Brain	GLUT-1	HK-I	Glucose dependent
Erythrocyte	GLUT-1	HK-I	Glucose dependent
Adipocyte	GLUT-4	HK-II	Insulin dependent
Muscle	GLUT-4	HK-II	Insulin dependent
Liver	GLUT-2	HK-IVL	Glucose sensor
GK β-cell	GLUT-2	HK-IVB (glucokinase)	Glucose sensor
Gut	GLUT-3 symporter	—	Sodium dependent
Kidney	GLUT-3 symporter	—	Sodium dependent

(Reproduced by permission of the American Diabetes Association [1]).

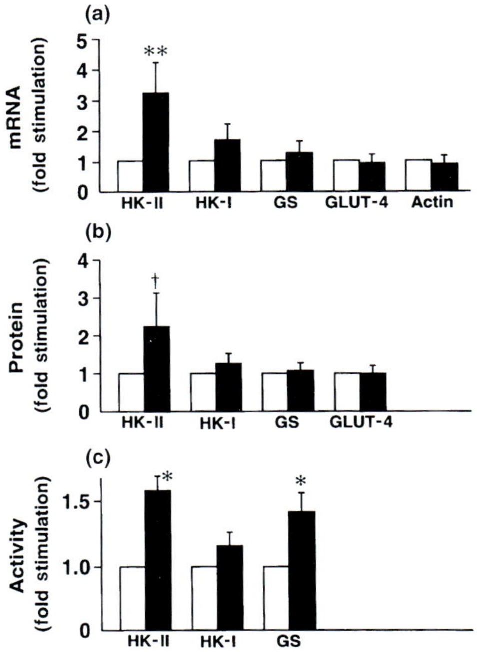

Figure 42 Effect of euglycemic hyperinsulinemia (63 μU/ml) for 4 h on HK, glycogen synthase (GS), and GLUT-4 mRNA levels (a), protein content (b), and activity (c) in healthy, young subjects. $^*p < 0.01$, $^{**}p < 0.05$, $\dagger p = 0.10$ (from reference 438)

[421–423]. GLUT-2 predominates in the liver and pancreatic β-cells, where it is found in association with a specific hexokinase, HK-IV [421–424]. In the β-cell, HK-IV is referred to as glucokinase [145, 424]. GLUT-2 has a high K_m (~15–20 mmol/l) and, as a consequence, the glucose concentration in cells expressing this transporter rises in direct proportion to the increase in plasma glucose concentration. This characteristic allows these cells to respond as glucose sensors. In summary, each tissue has a specific glucose transporter and associated hexokinase, which allow it uniquely to carry out its specialized function to maintain whole-body glucose economy.

Glucose transport activity in type 2 diabetic individuals has been found to be uniformly decreased in both adipocytes [345–347, 392, 425, 426] and muscle [345–347, 427–432]. In adipocytes from type 2 diabetic human and rodent models of diabetes there is a severe reduction in GLUT-4 mRNA and protein, and the ability of insulin to elicit a normal translocation response and to activate the GLUT-4 transporter after its insertion into the cell membrane is impaired [345–347, 392, 426, 433]. In contrast, muscle tissue obtained from lean and obese type 2 diabetic subjects exhibits normal or increased levels of GLUT-4 mRNA expression and normal levels of GLUT-4 protein [434–437]. Moreover, acute (2–4-h) physiologic hyperinsulinemia does not increase the number of GLUT-4 transporters in muscle in either healthy or type 2 diabetic subjects [434–437] (Figure 42). Several studies have demonstrated an increase in muscle GLUT-4 mRNA levels in response to insulin in controls [407, 436], but not in diabetic subjects [436], suggesting insulin resistance at the level of gene transcription. However, the physiologic significance of the blunted increase in muscle GLUT-4 mRNA levels in type 2 diabetic subjects is unclear, since both basal and insulin-stimulated GLUT-4 protein levels were normal. Large populations of type 2 diabetic subjects have been screened for mutations in the GLUT-4 gene [439, 440]. Such mutations are very uncommon and, when detected, have been of questionable physiologic significance.

The results summarized above indicate that the gene encoding the major insulin-responsive glucose transporter (GLUT-4), and its transcriptional and translational regulation gene in muscle, is not impaired in type 2 diabetes. However, in contrast to the normal expression of GLUT-4 protein and mRNA in muscle of type 2 diabetic subjects, every study that has examined adipose tissue has reported reduced basal and insulin-stimulated GLUT-4 mRNA levels, decreased GLUT-4 transporter number in all subcellular fractions, diminished GLUT-4 translocation, and impaired intrinsic activity of GLUT-4 [345–347, 426, 437, 441]. These observations demonstrate that GLUT-4 expression in humans is subject to tissue-specific regulation. Although insulin does not increase GLUT-4 expression in muscle, it stimulates the translocation of GLUT-4 transporters from their intracellular location to the cell membrane [429, 442, 443]. In type 2 diabetic humans, the ability of insulin to stimulate GLUT-4 translocation in muscle is impaired [429, 444, 445]. Using a novel triple-tracer technique [446], Bonadonna and colleagues have defined the *in vivo* dose–response curve for the action of insulin on glucose transport in forearm skeletal muscle of healthy human subjects [447] and have demonstrated that insulin-stimulated inward muscle glucose transport is severely impaired in type 2 diabetic subjects studied under euglycemic conditions [448, 449] (Figure 43). The

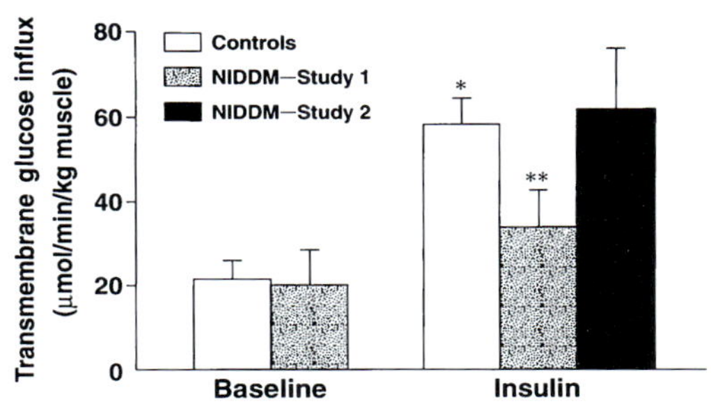

Figure 43 Rates of transmembrane glucose influx into forearm muscle at baseline and during the insulin clamp (~65 μU/ml). Study 1 was performed in the type 2 diabetic patients at euglycemia (~5.0 mmol/l) as in the control subjects, whereas study 2 was performed at hyperglycemia (~13 mmol/l). $^*p < 0.01$, insulin clamp vs. baseline in control subjects; $^*p < 0.05$, type 2 diabetic vs. control subjects. (Reproduced by permission of the American Diabetes Association [449])

defect in glucose transport could be overcome by repeating the insulin clamp at each subject's normal fasting glucose (hyperglycemia) level (Figure 43). Since the number of GLUT-4 transporters in the muscle of diabetic subjects is normal [434–437], impaired GLUT-4 translocation [345, 429, 444, 445] and decreased intrinsic activity of the glucose transporter [443, 450] are responsible for the defect in muscle glucose transport. Diminished *in vivo* muscle glucose transport in type 2 diabetic subjects also has been demonstrated using MRI [451] and PET [445, 452].

Glucose Phosphorylation

Glucose phosphorylation and glucose transport are tightly coupled phenomena [453]. Isoenzymes of hexokinase (HK-I to HK-IV) catalyze the first committed intracellular step of glucose metabolism—the conversion of glucose to G-6-P [421–424, 454] (Table 3). HK-I, HK-II, and HK-III are single-chain peptides that have a number of properties in common, including a very high affinity for glucose and product inhibition by G-6-P. HK-IV, also called glucokinase, has a lower affinity for glucose and is not inhibited by G-6-P. Glucokinase (HK-IVB) is believed to be the glucose sensor in the β-cell, while HK-IVL plays an important role in the regulation of hepatic glucose metabolism.

In both rat [454–456] and human [407, 422, 438, 457–458] skeletal muscle, HK-II transcription is regulated by insulin. HK-I also is present in human skeletal muscle, but it is not regulated by insulin [438]. In response to physiologic euglycemic hyperinsulinemia, HK-II cytosolic activity, protein content, and mRNA levels increase by 50–200% in healthy, non-diabetic subjects [438, 458] and this is associated with the translocation of HK-II from the cytosol to the mitochondria [459]. In contrast, insulin has no effect on HK-I activity, protein content, or mRNA levels [438].

In forearm muscle, insulin-stimulated glucose transport (measured with the triple-tracer technique) has been shown to be markedly impaired in lean type 2 diabetic subjects [449] (Figure 43). However, since the rate of intracellular glucose phosphorylation was impaired to an even greater extent (Figure 44), insulin caused an increase in the intracellular free glucose concentration. By performing the insulin clamp at each diabetic subject's normal level of fasting hyperglycemia, normal rates of whole-body glucose disposal and a normal rate of glucose influx into muscle were elicited (Figure 43). However, the rate of intracellular glucose phosphorylation increased only modestly (Figure 44); consequently, there was a dramatic rise in the free glucose concentration within the intracellular space that is accessible to glucose. These observations indicate that in type 2 diabetic individuals, while both glucose transport and glucose phosphorylation are severely

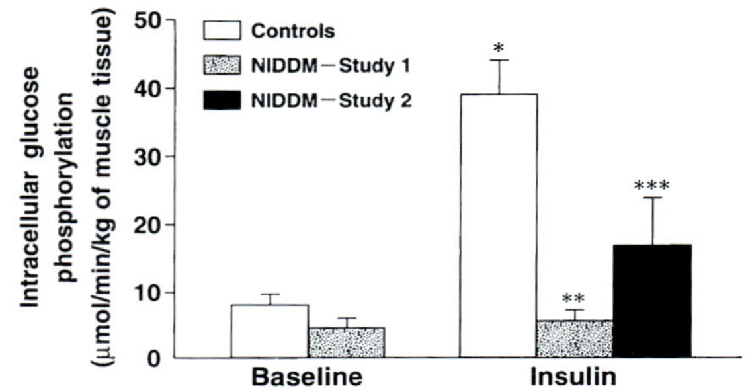

Figure 44 Rates of intracellular glucose phosphorylation in forearm muscle at baseline and during the insulin clamp (~65 μU/ml) study. Study 1 was performed in type 2 diabetic patients at euglycemia (~5 mmol/l) as in control subjects, whereas study 2 was performed at hyperglycemia (~13 mmol/l). *$p < 0.05$, insulin clamp vs. baseline in controls; ***$p < 0.05$, type 2 diabetic vs. control subjects during insulin clamp. **$p < 0.01$, type 2 diabetic vs. control subjects during insulin clamp. (Reproduced by permission of the American Diabetes Association [449])

resistant to the action of insulin, impaired glucose phosphorylation (HK-II) appears to be the rate-limiting step for insulin action. A similar pattern of impaired muscle glucose phosphorylation and transport is present in the insulin-resistant, normal-glucose-tolerant offspring of two diabetic parents [460]. These results are consistent with dose–response studies using PET to evaluate glucose phosphorylation and transport in skeletal muscle of type 2 diabetic subjects [452]. They also are consistent with ^{31}P NMR studies [461], which demonstrate that, during hyperinsulinemia, muscle G-6-P concentrations decline in type 2 diabetic versus control subjects. However, subsequent studies using ^{31}P NMR in combination with [1-^{14}C]glucose suggested that the defect in insulin-stimulated muscle glucose transport exceeds the defect in glucose phosphorylation and is responsible for the decline in muscle G-6-P concentration [451]. Because of methodologic differences, the results of the triple-tracer [449] and MRI studies [451] cannot be reconciled at present. Nonetheless, observations from these studies are consistent in demonstrating that the defects in glucose phosphorylation and glucose transport in muscle are established early in the natural history of type 2 diabetes and cannot be explained by glucose toxicity [118]. However, clear evidence that HK-II activity is crucial for glucose uptake derives from studies in transgenic mice who overexpress HK-II. In this model, HK-II overexpression increased both insulin- and exercise-stimulated muscle glucose uptake [462].

In healthy, nondiabetic subjects, physiologic hyperinsulinemia for as little as 2–4 h increases muscle HK-II activity, gene transcription, and translation [407, 438]. In lean type 2 diabetic subjects, insulin-stimulated HK-II activity and mRNA levels are markedly reduced compared

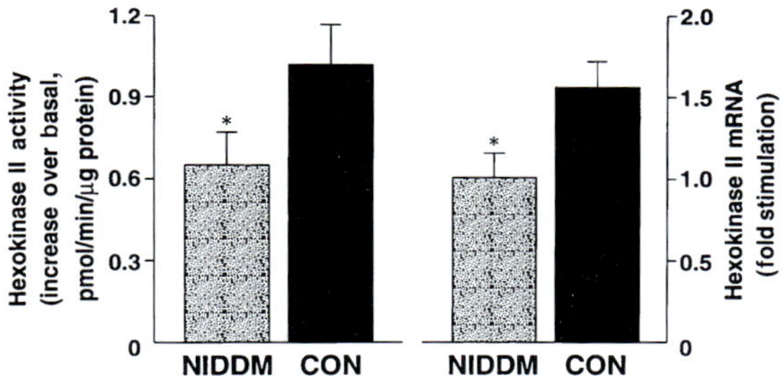

Figure 45 Muscle HK-II activity, mRNA level, and protein concentration before and after a 4-h euglycemic insulin clamp performed in control and type 2 diabetic subjects. $^{*}p < 0.01$ vs. controls (drawn from the data presented in reference 463). (Reproduced by permission of the American Diabetes Association)

to controls [461, 463] (Figure 45). Reduced basal muscle HK-II activity and mRNA levels [463] and decreased insulin-stimulated HK-II activity [457, 458, 464, 465] in type 2 diabetic subjects have been reported by other investigators. Impaired insulin-stimulated muscle HK-II activity has been described in subjects with IGT [466]. Because of its central role in insulin-mediated muscle glucose metabolism, several groups have looked for point mutations in the HK-II gene in individuals with type 2 diabetes [466–468]. Although a number of nucleotide substitutions have been found, none have been located close to the glucose and ATP binding sites and none have been associated with insulin resistance. Thus, an abnormality in the HK-II gene is unlikely to explain the inherited insulin resistance in common variety type 2 diabetes mellitus.

Glycogen Synthesis

After glucose enters the cell and is phosphorylated, it either can be converted to glycogen or enter the glycolytic pathway. Of the glucose that enters the glycolytic pathway, ~90% is oxidized. In the low physiologic range of hyperinsulinemia, glycogen synthesis and glucose oxidation are of approximately equal quantitative importance. With increasing plasma insulin concentrations, glycogen synthesis becomes predominant [20, 469]. If the rate of glucose oxidation is subtracted from the rate of whole-body insulin-mediated glucose disposal (determined from the insulin clamp), the difference represents nonoxidative glucose disposal (or glucose storage) [18, 436], which primarily reflects glycogen synthesis [1, 4, 209, 271, 470]. Glucose conversion to lipid accounts for <5% of total glucose disposal [20, 251, 252] and <5–10% of the glucose taken up by muscle is released as lactate [5, 471–473]. A major defect in insulin-stimulated glycogen synthesis is a characteristic finding in all insulin-resistant states, including obesity, diabetes, and the combination of obesity plus diabetes [1, 4, 20, 53, 72, 205, 209, 274–276, 456, 471–474]. Impaired glycogen synthesis also represents the major cause of insulin resistance in obese subjects with normal or only slightly IGT [1, 4, 209, 274, 472, 475]. Thus, the inability of insulin to promote glycogen synthesis represents a characteristic and early defect in the development of insulin resistance in both obesity and type 2 diabetes. The emergence of overt diabetes with fasting hyperglycemia is associated with a major reduction in insulin-mediated nonoxidative glucose disposal (glycogen synthesis) in all ethnic groups [1, 4, 20, 209, 211, 275, 456, 475]. Impaired nonoxidative glucose disposal has also been demonstrated in the normal-glucose-tolerant offspring of two diabetic parents [53, 476], in the first-degree relatives of type 2 diabetic individuals [51, 477, 478], and in the normoglycemic twin of a monozygotic twin pair in which the other twin has type 2 diabetes [132].

Using NMR imaging spectroscopy, Shulman et al. [270] have directly demonstrated decreased insulin-stimulated incorporation of [^{1}H,^{13}C]glucose into muscle glycogen of type 2 diabetic subjects (Figure 46). In all subjects, the rate of nonoxidative glucose disposal (glucose storage) correlated closely with the rate of glycogen synthesis, as determined by NMR ($r = 0.89$, $p < 0.001$). In type 2 diabetic subjects, there was a marked lag in the onset of insulin-stimulated glycogen synthesis (Figure 46), that was similar to the delay in insulin-mediated leg muscle glucose uptake [3] (see Figure 17). The rate of glycogen synthesis in type 2 diabetic subjects was decreased by ~50%, paralleling the decrease in total glucose uptake by leg muscle (Figure 17), and impaired muscle glycogen synthesis accounted for essentially all of the defect in whole-body glucose disposal.

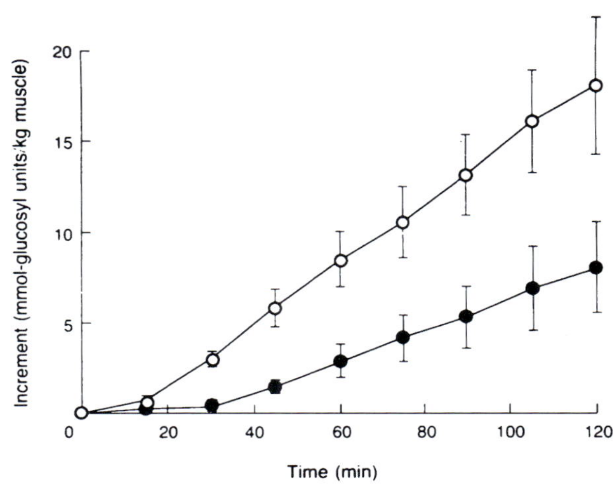

Figure 46 Effect of combined hyperinsulinemia (100 µU/ml) and hyperglycemia (200 mg/dl) on muscle glycogen synthesis in control (○) and type 2 diabetic (●) subjects. The ability of insulin to stimulate glycogen formation was delayed and markedly decreased in diabetic patients. The time course and magnitude of the decrease in leg muscle glycogen formation closely parallel those of total leg glucose uptake (from reference 270)

In summary, the results reviewed above provide convincing evidence that impaired glycogen synthesis represents the major metabolic defect in normal-glucose-tolerant obese subjects, in individuals with IGT, and in patients with overt diabetes. Moreover, studies by Gulli et al. [53] and others [4, 51, 53, 132, 460, 470, 478–480] indicate that the earliest detectable metabolic abnormality responsible for the insulin resistance in normal-glucose-tolerant individuals who are destined to develop type 2 diabetes is impaired glycogen synthesis.

Glycogen synthase is the key insulin-regulated enzyme that controls the rate of muscle glycogen formation [376, 377, 379, 457, 481, 482]. Insulin enhances glycogen synthase activity by stimulating a cascade of phosphorylation-dephosphorylation reactions [376, 377, 437, 439, 440, 483] (see above discussion of insulin receptor signal transduction), which ultimately lead to the activation of PP-1 (also called glycogen synthase phosphatase) [376, 377, 379, 482]. The regulatory subunit (G) of PP-1 has two serine phosphorylation sites, called site 1 and site 2. Phosphorylation of site 2 by cAMP-dependent kinase (PKA) inactivates PP-1, while phosphorylation of site 1 by insulin activates PP-1, leading to the stimulation of glycogen synthase [376, 377, 482, 484, 485]. Phosphorylation of site 1 of PP-1 by insulin in muscle is catalyzed by insulin-stimulated protein kinase 1 (ISPK-1) [378, 486], which is part of a family of serine/threonine protein kinases termed ribosomal S6 kinases. Because of their central role in muscle glycogen formation, considerable attention has been focused on the three enzymes glycogen synthase, PP-1, and ISPK-1 in the pathogenesis of insulin resistance in individuals with type 2 diabetes.

Glycogen synthase exists in an active (dephosphorylated) and an inactive (phosphorylated) form [376–379]. Under basal conditions, total glycogen synthase activity in type 2 diabetic subjects is reduced and the ability of insulin to activate glycogen synthase is severely impaired [369, 462, 487–493]. A similar defect in the ability of insulin to activate glycogen synthase has been demonstrated in the normal-glucose-tolerant relatives of type 2 diabetic individuals [479, 480]. Insulin-mediated activation of glycogen synthase and insulin-stimulated glycogen synthase gene expression also have been shown to be impaired in cultured myocytes and fibroblasts from type 2 diabetic subjects [494–496]. Studies in insulin-resistant nondiabetic and diabetic Pima Indians have demonstrated that the ability of insulin to activate muscle PP-1 (glycogen synthase phosphatase) is severely impaired [497]. PP-1 dephosphorylates glycogen synthase, leading to its activation. Therefore, a defect in PP-1 appears to play an important role in muscle insulin resistance [378].

The effect of insulin on glycogen synthase gene transcription and translation *in vivo* has been studied by employing the euglycemic insulin clamp in combination with muscle biopsies. Most [438, 498, 499] but not all [407] studies have shown that insulin does not increase glycogen synthase mRNA or protein expression in human muscle *in vivo*. However, basal glycogen synthase activity is decreased in muscle of type 2 diabetic patients [496, 499, 500], explaining in part the decrease in glycogen synthase activity in this disease. However, the major abnormality in glycogen synthase regulation in type 2 diabetes mellitus and other insulin-resistant conditions is its lack of dephosphorylation and activation by insulin as a result of insulin receptor signaling abnormalities (see previous discussion). The glycogen synthase gene [501] has been the subject of intensive investigation. An association between glycogen synthase gene markers and type 2 diabetes has been demonstrated in Japanese [502], French [503], Finnish [504], and Pima Indian [467] populations. However, DNA sequencing has revealed either no mutations [505] or rare nucleotide substitutions [506, 507] that cannot explain the defect in insulin-stimulated glycogen synthase. Nonetheless, the association between glycogen synthase and type 2 diabetes [502–505] suggests that another gene close to the glycogen synthase gene may be involved in the development of type 2 diabetes. The genes encoding the catalytic subunits of PP-1 [508, 509] and ISPK-1 [510] have been examined in insulin-resistant Pima Indians and Danes with type 2 diabetes. Several silent nucleotide substitutions were found in the PP-1 and ISPK-1 genes in the Danish population; the mRNA levels of both genes were normal in skeletal muscle [508, 509]. No structural gene abnormalities in the catalytic subunit of PP-1 were detected in Pima Indians [510]. Thus, neither abnormalities in the PP-1 and ISPK-1 genes nor abnormalities in their translation can explain the impaired enzymatic activities of glycogen synthase and PP-1 that have been observed *in vivo*. Similarly, there is no evidence that an alteration in glycogen phosphorylase plays any role in the abnormality in glycogen formation in type 2 diabetes [480].

In summary, glycogen synthase activity is severely impaired in type 2 diabetic patients and in insulin-resistant, normal-glucose-tolerant individuals who are predisposed to develop type 2 diabetes. However, the defect cannot be explained by an abnormality in the genes encoding glycogen synthase or its promoter, or by other key genes—PP-1 or ISPK-1—involved in the regulation of glycogen synthase activity.

Glycolysis/Glucose Oxidation

Glucose oxidation accounts for ~90% of total glycolytic flux, while anaerobic glycolysis accounts for the other 10% [472, 473]. Two enzymes, PFK and PDH, play central roles in the regulation of glycolysis and glucose oxidation, respectively. In type 2 diabetic individuals the glycolytic/glucose oxidative pathway has been shown to be impaired in many individuals with type 2 diabetes [80, 472, 473]. Although one study suggested that the activity of PFK is modestly reduced in muscle biopsies from type 2 diabetic subjects [511], the majority of evidence indicates that the activity of PFK is normal [489, 495, 501]. Insulin has no effect on muscle PFK activity, mRNA levels, or protein content in either nondiabetic or diabetic individuals [501]. PDH is a key insulin-regulated enzyme whose activity in muscle is acutely stimulated by a physiologic increment in the plasma insulin concentration [499]. Three previous studies have examined PDH activity in type 2 diabetic patients. Insulin-stimulated PDH activity was decreased in isolated subcutaneous human adipocytes [512] and in skeletal muscle from type 2 diabetic subjects undergoing euglycemic hyperinsulinemic clamps [513]. However, when type 2 diabetic patients had muscle biopsies during hyperglycemic hyperinsulinemic clamps, activation of PDH by insulin was normal [491], in concert with normalized rates of muscle glucose uptake. These results suggest that insulin stimulation of PDH activity is influenced by glycolytic flux.

Both obesity and moderate to severe diabetes are associated with accelerated FFA turnover and oxidation [1, 4, 20, 21, 209], which would be expected, according to the Randle cycle [289], to inhibit PDH and consequently glucose oxidation (see prior discussion). Thus, any observed defect in glucose oxidation or PDH activity could be acquired secondarily to increased FFA oxidation and feedback inhibition of PDH by elevated intracellular levels of acetyl-CoA and reduced availability of NAD. Consistent with this observation, the rate of basal and insulin-stimulated glucose oxidation has been shown to be normal in the normal-glucose-tolerant offspring of two diabetic parents [53] and in the first-degree relatives of type 2 diabetic subjects [51, 480], while it is decreased in overtly diabetic subjects [1, 4, 211, 276, 472, 473]. Studies examining PHD activity in muscle tissue from lean diabetic subjects with mild fasting hyperglycemia are needed before the role of this enzyme in the development of insulin resistance in type 2 diabetes can be established or excluded.

PATHOGENESIS OF TYPE 2 DIABETES: SUMMARY AND SYNTHESIS

The maintenance of normal glucose homeostasis is dependent on a finely balanced dynamic interaction between tissue (muscle and liver) sensitivity to insulin and insulin secretion. Even in the presence of severe insulin resistance, a perfectly normal β-cell is capable of secreting sufficient amounts of insulin to offset the defect in insulin action. Thus, the evolution of type 2 diabetes requires the presence of defects in both insulin secretion and insulin action, and both of these defects can have a genetic as well as an acquired component. When type 2 diabetic patients initially present to the physician, they will have had their diabetes for many years, and defects in insulin action and insulin secretion will be well established [1, 4]. At this stage, it is not possible to define which defect came first in the natural history of the disease. Nevertheless, it is now clear that in any given diabetic patient, whatever defect (insulin resistance or impaired insulin secretion) initiates the disturbance in glucose metabolism, it will eventually be followed by the emergence of its counterpart. Figure 47 represents an attempt to integrate the principal pathogenetic factors responsible for the development of type 2 diabetes, as we currently understand them. Note that the sequence of events outlined in Figure 47, like the development of type 2 diabetes, is still in a state of dynamic

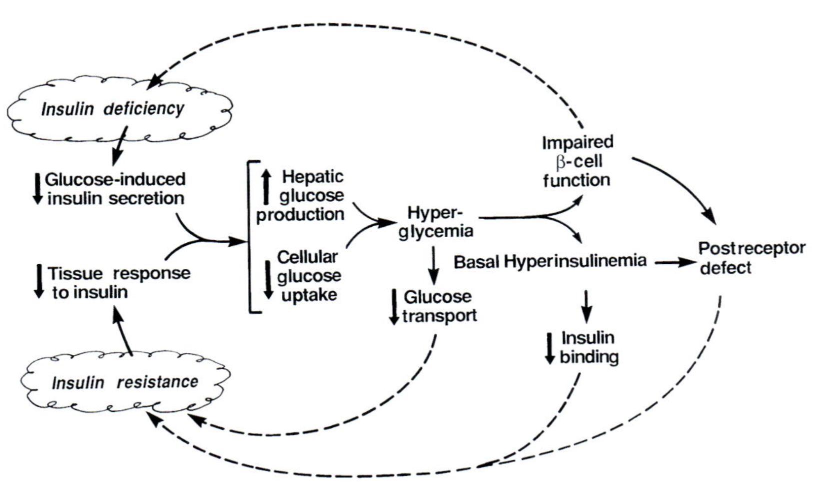

Figure 47 Pathogenetic sequence of events leading to the development of insulin resistance in type 2 diabetes. Note that whether the primary defect initiating the glucose intolerance resides in the β-cell or in peripheral tissues, development of insulin resistance will eventually ensue or become aggravated, respectively. By the time that overt fasting hyperglycemia (>140 mg/dl) develops, both impaired insulin secretion and severe insulin resistance are present. Broken arrows represent positive feedback loops, which result in self-perpetuation of primary defects. (Reproduced by permission of the American Diabetes Association [4])

evolution that is meant to be altered as new data become available. However, this hypothesis has as its foundation a large body of existing experimental evidence. The following discussion emphasizes three points:

(1) Individuals who are destined to develop type 2 diabetes inherit a gene (or set of genes) that confers insulin resistance and a propensity for progressive beta cell failure.

(2) Acquired abnormalities, especially obesity and altered FFA/lipid metabolism, accentuate the defects in insulin action and insulin secretion.

(3) The full blown diabetic syndrome with overt fasting hyperglycemia develops only in those subjects in whom a concomitant insulin secretory defect, be it acquired (as through glucolipotoxicity) or inherited, also is present.

Primary Defect in Insulin Sensitivity

Insulin resistance is a nearly universal finding in patients with established type 2 diabetes. In normal-weight and obese individuals with IGT and in type 2 diabetic subjects with mild fasting hyperglycemia (110–140 mg/dl, 6.1–7.8 mmol/l), both the basal and glucose-stimulated plasma insulin levels are increased. Although the first-phase insulin response may be decreased in some of these subjects, the total insulin response is increased. In each of these groups, tissue sensitivity to insulin, measured with the insulin clamp technique, has been shown to be diminished. Prospective studies have demonstrated that hyperinsulinemia and insulin resistance precede the development of IGT in high-risk populations and that IGT represents the forerunner of type 2 diabetes. This scenario has been well documented in Pima Indians, Mexican Americans, and Pacific Islanders. It is noteworthy that all of these populations are characterized by obesity and a younger age at onset of diabetes. Such results provide conclusive evidence that insulin resistance is the inherited defect that initiates the diabetic condition in the majority of type 2 diabetic patients. Studies in normal-glucose-tolerant first-degree relatives of diabetic individuals and in the normal-glucose-tolerant offspring of two diabetic parents indicate that the inherited defect in insulin action most likely results from an abnormality in the glycogen synthetic pathway in muscle. Defects in the insulin-signaling cascade are characteristically observed in these insulin resistant, genetically predisposed, normal-glucose-tolerant individuals. Hepatic glucose production also is resistant to the suppressive action of fasting hyperinsulinemia in these groups. Because of the compensatory increase in insulin secretion, initially the insulin resistance by itself is not sufficient to impair glucose uptake by muscle or to cause an increase in HGP. As the insulin resistance progresses and muscle glucose uptake becomes further impaired, the postprandial rise in plasma glucose concentration becomes excessive, but the increase in basal hyperinsulinemia is sufficient to maintain the fasting plasma glucose concentration and HGP within the normal range. Nonetheless, there is an excessive postprandial rise in plasma glucose concentration, and a longer time is required to restore normoglycemia after each meal. Eventually, however, the insulin resistance becomes so severe that the compensatory hyperinsulinemia no longer is sufficient to maintain the fasting glucose concentration at the basal level.

The development of hyperglycemia further stimulates β-cell secretion of insulin, and the resultant hyperinsulinemia causes a downregulation of insulin receptor number and of the intracellular events involved in insulin action, thus exacerbating the insulin resistance. Initially, the hyperglycemia-induced increase in insulin secretion serves a compensatory function to maintain normal or near-normal glucose tolerance. In some individuals, the persistent stimulus to the β-cell to oversecrete insulin leads to a progressive demise in β-cell function. Both chronic hyperglycemia (glucotoxicity) and disturbances in lipid metabolism (lipotoxicity) contribute to the defect in insulin secretion. It is likely that those individuals in whom "glucolipotoxicity" leads to a progressive impairment in insulin secretion have an underlying genetic defect in β-cell function that is unmasked by the persistent hyperglycemia and/or derangement in lipid metabolism. The resultant insulinopenia leads to the emergence or exacerbation of postreceptor defects in insulin action. Many of the intracellular events involved in glucose metabolism are dependent on the surge of insulin that occurs three or four times per day in response to nutrient ingestion. When the insulin response becomes deficient, the activity of the glucose transport system becomes severely impaired and a number of key intracellular enzymatic steps involved in glucose metabolism become depressed. Additionally, when severe insulinopenia ensues, plasma FFA levels rise and fatty acid oxidation increases, further contributing to the defects in intracellular glucose disposal. There is also compelling evidence that hyperglycemia *per se* can downregulate the glucose transport system, as well as a number of other intracellular events involved in insulin action (glucotoxicity), and a similar argument can be made concerning the intracellular derangement in lipid metabolism. This pathogenetic sequence can explain all of the clinical and laboratory features observed in type 2 diabetic patients. Insofar as the cellular defect is generalized, both hepatic and peripheral tissues, and possibly the β-cells themselves, would manifest alterations that are characteristic of the diabetic state and that could be related to one of the same primary defect.

At present, the basic defect responsible for insulin resistance remains unknown. Although diabetologists traditionally have tended to focus their attention on intracellular defects involved in glucose metabolism (i.e.,

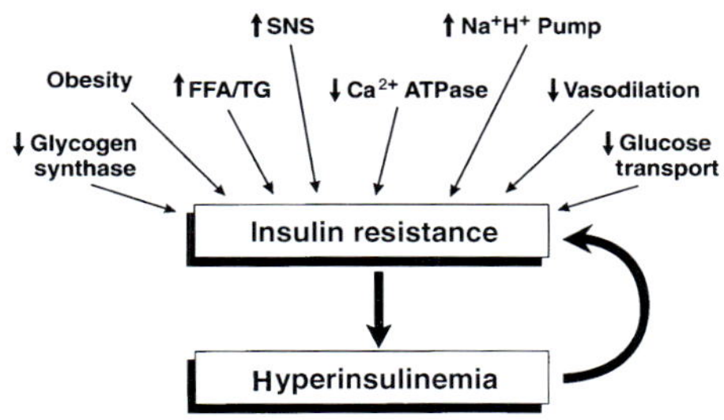

Figure 48 Schematic representation of potential defects that can lead to the development of insulin resistance in type 2 diabetes. Regardless of the etiology of the insulin resistance, the β-cell will enhance its secretion of insulin in an attempt to offset the defect in insulin action. The resultant compensatory hyperinsulinemia will downregulate a variety of intracellular events involved in insulin action and thus serve as a self-perpetuating cause of the insulin resistance

insulin receptor signal transduction, glucose transport, glucose phosphorylation, glycogen synthase), a number of other explanations are equally plausible (Figure 48). Thus, abnormalities in intracellular lipid metabolism, enhanced sympathetic nervous system activity, alterations in muscle blood flow or fiber type, disturbances in ion-pump activity, and others could represent the primary or inherited (genetic) defect in type 2 diabetes. The β-cell would respond to the insulin resistance by augmenting its secretion of insulin regardless of the etiology of the insulin resistance. The resultant hyperinsulinemia, in turn, would serve as a self-amplifying factor to further worsen the insulin resistance. Eventually, β-cell exhaustion would ensue, reproducing the sequence of events outlined in Figure 48.

Primary Defect in Insulin Secretion

Most evidence indicates that hyperinsulinemia precedes the development of IGT and type 2 diabetes in populations with a high prevalence of type 2 diabetes mellitus. In populations that are genetically predisposed to develop type 2 diabetes, hyperinsulinemia is a common finding. Such observations argue strongly against insulinopenia as the initiating cause of type 2 diabetes in the majority of individuals. However, there clearly are some diabetic subjects in whom the first and/or second phases of insulin secretion are impaired in the earliest stages of development of type 2 diabetes (Figure 47). In such individuals, the defect in insulin secretion will result in an excessive, prolonged rise in plasma glucose concentration. The postprandial hyperglycemia will present a persistent stimulus to the β-cell, and the total amount of insulin secreted in response to the meal actually may be increased early in the development of diabetes (Figure 47). Initially, this postprandial hyperinsulinemia may even be sufficient to return the fasting plasma glucose concentration to normal. As the diabetes become more severe (as a consequence of the progressive nature of the β-cell defect), the plasma insulin response (although still increased in absolute terms) will become insufficient to return the plasma glucose concentration to its basal level and fasting hyperglycemia will ensue. Fasting hyperglycemia will present a persistent stimulus to the pancreas to oversecrete insulin throughout the day, and fasting hyperinsulinemia will result. The elevated fasting insulin concentration will lead to a decrease in the number of insulin receptors on insulin target tissues and a downregulation of the intracellular events involved in insulin action. This pathogenetic sequence of events could explain all of the laboratory features observed in patients with IGT (fasting euglycemia, an impaired but not overtly diabetic glucose tolerance test, fasting hyperinsulinemia, an increased insulin response to glucose) and in patients with early diabetes (mild fasting hyperglycemia, a diabetic glucose tolerance test, fasting hyperinsulinemia, normal or increased plasma insulin response to glucose). In such an individual, the basal rate of HGP would remain within the normal range because of the restraining effects of fasting hyperglycemia and fasting hyperinsulinemia on glucose release by the liver, whereas the efficiency of tissue glucose uptake would be markedly reduced.

As the plasma insulin response becomes progressively more impaired as a result of the genetic β-cell defect, "pancreatic exhaustion," or glucose toxicity, both the early and late phases of insulin secretion will become absolutely deficient. However, the basal plasma insulin level will remain elevated because of the persistent stimulus presented to the β-cell by the fasting hyperglycemia. With the onset of insulinopenia, be it relative or absolute, marked fasting hyperglycemia will ensue because of excessive glucose production by the liver and a further reduction in tissue glucose clearance. Another important pathogenetic disturbance that emerges with the development of insulinopenia is a postreceptor defect in insulin action. The eventual clinical picture would be that of a typical type 2 diabetic patient.

In summary, the sequence of events, starting with a defect in insulin secretion and leading to the emergence of insulin resistance, appears to be quite plausible on the basis of the information currently available. What remains to be determined is how commonly a primary β-cell defect and resultant insulinopenia initiate the sequence of events leading to the development of type 2 diabetes in humans.

Combined Defects in Insulin Sensitivity and Insulin Secretion

Lastly, it is possible that the defects in insulin action (involving both muscle and liver) and insulin secretion result from the same, as yet unidentified genetic abnormality, and that insulin resistance and impaired β-cell function evolve in parallel.

REFERENCES

1. DeFronzo RA. Pathogenesis of type 2 diabetes mellitus: metabolic and molecular implications for identifying diabetes genes. *Diabetes* 1997; 5: 117–269.
2. Grill V. A comparison of brain glucose metabolism in diabetes as measured by positron emission tomography or by arteriovenous techniques. *Ann Med* 1990; 22: 171–5.
3. DeFronzo RA, Gunnarsson R, Bjorkman O, Olsson M, Wahren J. Effects of insulin on peripheral and splanchnic glucose metabolism in non-insulin dependent diabetes mellitus. *J Clin Invest* 1985; 76: 149–55.
4. DeFronzo RA. Lilly Lecture. The triumvirate: beta cell, muscle, liver. A collusion responsible for NIDDM. *Diabetes* 1988; 37: 667–87.
5. DeFronzo RA, Jacot E, Jequier E, Maeder E, Wahren J, Felber JP. The effect of insulin on the disposal of intravenous glucose: results from indirect calorimetry. *Diabetes* 1981; 30: 1000–7.
6. DeFronzo RA, Ferrannini E. Regulation of hepatic glucose metabolism in humans. *Diabetes Metab Rev* 1987; 3: 415–59.
7. Mari A, Wahren J, DeFronzo RA, Ferrannini E. Glucose absorption and production following oral glucose: comparison of compartmental and arteriovenous-difference methods. *Metabolism* 1994; 43: 1419–25.
8. Gerich JE, Meyer C, Woerle HJ, Stumvoll M. Renal gluconeogenesis. Its importance in human glucose homeostasis. *Diabetes Care* 2001; 24: 382–91.
9. Ekberg K, Landau BR, Wajngot A, Chandramouli V, Efendic S, Brunengraber H, Wahren J. Contributions by kidney and liver to glucose production in the postabsorptive state and after 60 h of fasting. *Diabetes* 1999; 48: 292–8.
10. Magnusson I, Katz LD, Shulman RG, Shulman GI. Quantitation of hepatic glycogenolysis and gluconeogenesis in fasting humans with ^{13}C NMR. *Science* 1991; 254: 573–6.
11. Katz LD, Glickman MG, Rapoport S, Ferrannini E, DeFronzo RA. Splanchnic and peripheral disposal of oral glucose in man. *Diabetes* 1983; 32: 675–9.
12. Ferrannini E, Bjorkman O, Reichard GA Jr., Pilo A, Olsson M, Wahren J, DeFronzo RA. The disposal of an oral glucose load in healthy subjects. *Diabetes* 1985; 34: 580–8.
13. Basu A, Basu R, Shah P, Vella A, Johnson CM, Nair KS, Jensen MD, Schwenk WF, Rizza RA. Effects of type 2 diabetes on the ability of insulin and glucose to regulate splanchnic and muscle glucose metabolism: evidence for a defect in hepatic glucokinase activity. *Diabetes*. 2000; 49: 272–83.
14. Mitrakou A, Kelley D, Veneman T, Jensen T, Pangburn T, Reilly J, Gerich J. Contribution of abnormal muscle and liver glucose metabolism to postprandial hyperglycemia in NIDDM. *Diabetes* 1990; 39: 1381–90.
15. Mandarino L, Bonadonna R, McGuinness O, Wasserman D. Regulation of muscle glucose uptake in vivo. In Jefferson LS, Cherrington AD (eds) *Handbook of Physiology, Section 7: The Endocrine System. Vol II: The Endocrine Pancreas and Regulation of Metabolism*, Oxford: Oxford University Press, 2001; pp 803–48.
16. Del Prato S, Riccio A. Vigili de Kreutzenberg S. Dorella M. Tiengo A. DeFronzo RA. Basal plasma insulin levels exert a qualitative but notquantitative effect on glucose-mediated glucose uptake. *Am J Physiol* 1995; 268: E1089–95.
17. Cherrington AD. Control of glucose uptake and release by the liver *in vivo*. *Diabetes* 1999; 48: 1198–214.
18. Jansson P-A, Larsson A, Smith U, Lonroth P. Lactate release from the subcutaneous tissue in lean and obese men. *J Clin Invest* 1994; 93: 240–6.
19. Virtanen KA, Peltoniemi P, Marjamaki P, Asola M, Strindberg L, Parkkola R, Huupponen R, Knuuti J, Lonnroth P, Nuutila P. Human adipose tissue glucose uptake determined using [^{18}F]-fluro-dexoy-glucose ([^{18}F]FDG) and PET in combination with microdialysis. *Diabetologia* 2001; 44: 2171–9.
20. Groop LC, Bonadonna RC, Del Prato S Ratheiser K, Zych K, Ferrannini E, DeFronzo RA. Glucose and FFA metabolism in non-insulin dependent diabetes mellitus. Evidence for multiple sites of insulin resistance. *J Clin Invest* 1989; 84: 205–15.
21. Groop L, Saloranta C, Shank M, Bonadonna RC, Ferrannini E, DeFronzo RA. The role of FFA metabolism in the pathogensis of insulin resistance inobesity and non-insulin dependent diabetes mellitus. *J Clin Endocrinol Metab* 1991; 72: 96–107.
22. Santomauro A, Boden G, Silva M, Rocha DM, Santos RF, Ursich MJM, Strassman PG, Wajchenberg BL. Overnight lowering of FFAs with acipimox improves insulin resistance andglucose tolerance in obese diabetic and non-diabetic subjects. *Diabetes* 1999; 48: 1836–41.
23. Reaven GM. The fourth Musketeer—from Alexandre Dumas to Claude Bernard. *Diabetologia* 1995; 38: 3–13.
24. Bergman RN. Non-esterified fatty acids and the liver: why is insulin secreted into the portal vein? *Diabetologia* 2000; 43: 946–52.
25. Boden G. Role of fatty acids in the pathogenesis of insulin resistance and NIDDM. *Diabetes* 1997; 46: 3–10.
26. McGarry JD. Banting Lecture 2001. Dysregulation of fatty acid metabolism in the etiology of type 2 diabetes. *Diabetes* 2002; 51: 7–18.
27. Baron AD, Schaeffer L, Shragg P, Kolterman OG. Role of hyperglucagonemia in maintenance of increased rates of hepatic glucose output in type II diabetics. *Diabetes* 1987; 36: 274–83.
28. Frank JW, Camilleri M, Thomforde GM, Dinneen SF, Rizza RA. Effects of glucagon on postprandial carbohydrate metabolism in nondiabetic humans. *Metabolism* 1998; 47: 7–12.
29. DeFronzo RA, Ferrannini E, Hendler R, Wahren J, and Felig P. Influence of hyperinsulinemia, hyperglycemia, and the route of glucose administration on splanchnic glucose exchange. *Proc Natl Acad Sci* 1978; 75: 5173–7.
30. Ferrannini E, Wahren J, Felig P, DeFronzo RA. Role of fractional glucose extraction in the regulation of splanchnic glucose metabolism in normal and diabetic man. *Metabolism* 1980; 29: 28–35.
31. Adkins, Myers SR, Hendrik GK, Stevenson RW, Williams PE, Cherrington AD. Importance of the route of glucose delivery to hepatic glucose uptake in the conscious dog. *J Clin Invest* 1987; 79: 557–65.
32. Hsieh P-S, Moore MC, Neal DW, Cherrington AD. Hepatic glucose uptake rapidly decreases after removal of the portal signal in conscious dogs. *Am J Physiol* 1998; 275: E987–92.
33. Adkins-Marshall B, Pagliassotti MJ, Asher JR, Connolly CC, Neal DW, Williams PE, Myers SR, Hendrick GK, Adkins RB Jr, Cherrington AD. Role of

hepatic nerves in response of liver to intraportal delivery in dogs. *Am J Physiol* 1992; 262: E679–86.

34. Perley MJ, Kipnis DM. Plasma insulin responses to oral and intravenous glucose: studies in normal and diabetic subjects. *J Clin Invest* 1967; 46: 1954–62.
35. Creutzfeldt W. The incretin concept today. *Diabetologia* 1979; 16: 75–85.
36. Drucker DJ. Glucagon-like peptides. *Diabetes* 1998; 47: 159–69.
37. Holst JJ, Gromada J, Nauck MA. The pathogenesis of NIDDM involves a defective expression of the GIP receptor. *Diabetologia* 1997; 40: 984–6.
38. Polonsky KS, Sturis J, Bell GI. Non-insulin-dependent diabetes mellitus—a genetically programmed failure of the beta cell to compensate for insulin resistance. *N Engl J Med* 1996; 334: 777–83.
39. Cerasi E. Insulin deficiency and insulin resistance in the pathogenesis of NIDDM: is a divorce possible? *Diabetologia* 1995; 38: 992–7.
40. Zimmet P, Whitehouse S, Kiss J. Ethnic variability in the plasma insulin response to oral glucose in Polynesian and Micronesian subjects. *Diabetes* 1979; 28: 624–8.
41. Sicree RA, Zimmet P, King HO, Coventry JO. Plasma insulin response among Nauruans. Prediction of deterioration in glucose tolerance over 6 years. *Diabetes* 1987; 36: 179–86.
42. Saad MF, Knowler WC, Pettitt DJ, Nelson RG, Mott DM, Bennett PH. Sequential changes in serum insulin concentration during development of non-insulin-dependent diabetes. *Lancet* 1989; i: 1356–9.
43. Saad MF, Knowler WC, Pettitt DJ, Nelson RG, Mott DM, Bennett PH. The natural history of IGT in the Pima Indians. *New Engl J Med* 1988; 319: 1500–5.
44. Haffner SM, Miettinen H, Gaskill SP, Stern MP. Decreased insulin secretion and increased insulin resistance are independently related to the 7-year risk of NIDDM in Mexican-Americans. *Diabetes* 1995; 44: 1386–91.
45. Weyer C, Hanson RL, Tataranni PA, Bogardus C, Pratley RE. A high fasting plasma insulin concentration predicts type 2 diabetes independent of insulin resistance. Evidence for a pathogenic role of relative hyperinsulinemia. *Diabetes* 2000; 49: 2094–101.
46. Tripathy D, Carlsson M, Almgren P, Osomaa B, Raskinen M-R, Tuomi T, Groop LC. Insulin secretion and insulin sensitivity in relation to glucose tolerance. Lessons from the Botnia Study. *Diabetes* 2000; 49: 975–80.
47. Weyer C, Bogardus C, Pratley RE. Metabolic characteristics of individuals with impaired fasting glucose and/or IGT. *Diabetes* 1999; 48: 2197–203.
48. Tripathy D, Carlsson A-L, Lehto M, Isomaa B, Tuomi T, Groop L. Insulin secretion and insulin sensitivity in diabetic subgroups: studies in the prediabetic and diabetic state. *Diabetologia* 2000; 43: 1476–83.
49. Weyer C, Tataranni PA, Bogardus C, Pratley RE. Insulin resistance and insulin secretory dysfunction are independent predictors of worsening of glucose tolerance during each stage of type 2 diabetes development. *Diabetes Care* 2000; 24: 89–94.
50. Pimenta W, Korytkowski M, Mitrakou A, Jenssen T, Yki-Jarvinen H, Evron W, Dailey G, Gerich J. Pancreatic beta-cell dysfunction as the primary genetic lesion in NIDDM. Evidence from studies in normal glucose-tolerant individuals with a first degree NIDDM relative. *JAMA* 1995; 273: 1855–61.
51. Eriksson J, Franssila-Kallunki A, Ekstrand A, Saloranta C, Widen E, Schalin C, Groop L. Early metabolic defects in persons at increased risk for non-insulin-dependent diabetes mellitus. *New Engl J Med* 1989; 321: 337–43.
52. Reaven GM, Hollenbeck CB, Chen YDI. Relationship between glucose tolerance, insulin secretion, and insulin action in non-obese individuals with varying degrees of glucose tolerance. *Diabetologia* 1989; 32: 52–5.
53. Gulli G, Ferrannini E, Stern M, Haffner S, DeFronzo RA. The metabolic profile of NIDDM is fully established in glucose-tolerant offspring of two Mexican-American NIDDM parents. *Diabetes* 1992; 41: 1575–86.
54. Martin BC, Warram JH, Krolewski AS, Bergman RN, Soeldner JS, Kahn RC. Role of glucose and insulin resistance in development of type 2 diabetes mellitus: results of a 25-year follow-up study. *Lancet* 1992; 340: 925–9.
55. Warram JH, Martin BC, Krolewski AS, Soeldner JS, Kahn CR. Slow glucose removal rate and hyperinsulinemia precede the development of type II diabetes in the offspring of diabetic parents. *Ann Intern Med* 1990; 113: 909–15.
56. Lillioja S, Mott DM, Zawadzki JK, Young AA, Abbott WG, Knowler WC, Bennett PH, Moll P, Bogardus C. In vivo insulin action is familial characteristic in nondiabetic Pima Indians. *Diabetes* 1987; 36: 1329–35.
57. Kahn SE. Clinical Review 135. The importance of ß-cell failure in the development and progression of type 2 diabetes. *J Clin Endocrinol Metab* 2001; 86: 4047–58.
58. Bergman RN, Finegood DT, Kahn SE. The evolution of ß-cell dysfunction and insulin resistance in type 2 diabetes. *Eur J Clin Invest* 2002; 32: 35–45.
59. Hansen BC, Bodkin NH. Heterogeneity of insulin responses: phases leading to type 2 (noninsulin-dependent) diabetes mellitus in the rhesus monkey. *Diabetologia* 1986; 29: 713–9.
60. Diamond MP, Thornton K, Connolly-Diamond M, Sherwin RS, DeFronzo RA. Reciprocal variations in insulin-stimulated glucose uptake and pancreatic insulin secretion in women with normal glucose tolerance. *J Soc Gynecol Invest* 1995; 2: 708–15.
61. Hollenbeck CB, Reaven GM. Variations in insulin-stimulated glucose uptake in healthy individuals with normal glucose tolerance. *J Clin Endocrinol Metab* 1987; 64: 1169–73.
62. Reaven GM. Banting Lecture. Role of insulin resistance in human disease. *Diabetes* 1988; 37: 595–607.
63. Faber OK, Damsgaard EM. Insulin secretion in type II diabetes. *Acta Endocrinol* 1984; 262 (suppl): 47–50.
64. Faber OK, Hagen C, Binder C, Markussen J, Naithani VK, Blix PM, Kuzuya H, Horwitz DL, Rubenstein AH, Rossing N. Kinetics of human connecting peptide in normal and diabetic subjects. *J Clin Invest* 1978; 62: 197–203.
65. DeFronzo RA, Ferrannini E, Simonson DC. J Fasting hyperglycemia in non-insulin-dependent diabetes mellitus: contributions of excessive hepatic glucose production and impaired tissue glucose uptake. *Metabolism* 1989; 38: 387–95.
66. Hales CN. The pathogenesis of NIDDM. *Diabetologia* 1994; 37: S162–8.
67. Kingston ME, Skoog WC. Maintenance of basal insulin secretion in severe non-insulin dependent diabetes. *Diabetes Care* 1986; 9: 232–5.

68. Reaven GM, Hollenbeck C, Jeng C-Y, Wu MS, Chen Y-DI. Measurement of plasma glucose, FFA, lactate, and insulin for 24 hours in patients with NIDDM. *Diabetes* 1988; 37: 1020–4.
69. Garvey WT, Olefsky JM, Rubenstein AH, Kolterman OG. Day-long integrated urinary C-peptide excretion. *Diabetes* 1988; 37: 590–9.
70. Lillioja S, Mott DM, Howard BV, Bennett PH, Yki-Jarvinen H, Freymond D, Nyomba BL, Zurlo F, Swinburn B, Bogardus C. IGT as a disorder of insulin action. Longitudinal and cross-sectional studies in Pima Indians. *New Engl J Med* 1988; 318: 1217–25.
71. Bodkin NL, Metzger BL, Hansen BC. Hepatic glucose production and insulin sensitivity preceding diabetes in monkeys. *Am J Physiol* 1989; 256: E676–81.
72. Jallut D, Golay A, Munger R, Frascarolo P, Schutz Y, Jequier E, Felber JP. IGT and diabetes in obesity: a 6 year follow-up study of glucose metabolism. *Metabolism* 1990; 39: 1068–75.
73. Lillioja S, Mott DM, Spraul M, Ferraro R, Foley JE, Ravussin E, Knowler WC, Bennett PH, Bogardus C. Insulin resistance and insulin secretory dysfunction as precursors of non-insulin-dependent diabetes mellitus. *N Engl J Med* 1993; 329: 1988–92.
74. Jensen CC, Cnop M, Hull RL, Fujimoto WY, Kahn SE, the American Diabetes Association GENNID Study Group. ß-Cell function is a major contributor to oral glucose tolerance in high-risk relatives of our ethnic groups in the U.S. *Diabetes* 2002; 51: 2170–8.
75. Dowse GK, Zimmet PZ, Collins VR. Insulin levels and the natural history of glucose intolerance in Nauruans. *Diabetes* 1996; 45: 1367–72.
76. Haffner SM, Stern MP, Hazuda HP, Pugh JA, Patterson JK. Hyperinsulinemia in a population at high risk for non-insulin-dependent diabetes mellitus. *New Engl J Med* 1986; 315: 220–4.
77. Balkau B, King H, Zimmet P, Raper LR. Factors associated with the development of diabetes in the Micronesian population of Nauru. *Am J Epidemiol* 1985; 122: 594–605.
78. Efendic S, Luft R, Wajngot A. Aspects of the pathogenesis of type 2 diabetes. *Endocr Rev* 1984; 5: 395–419.
79. Ho LT, Chang ZY, Wang JT, Li SH, Liu YF, Chen Y-DI, Reaven GM. Insulin insensitivity in offspring of parents with type 2 diabetes mellitus. *Diabet Med* 1990; 7: 31–4.
80. DeFronzo RA. Pathogenesis of type 2 (non-insulin dependent) diabetes mellitus: a balanced overview. *Diabetologia* 1992; 35: 389–97.
81. Clement K, Pueyo ME, Vaxillaire M, Rakotoambinina B, Thuillier F, Passa PH, Froguel PH, Robert JJ, Velho G. Assessment of insulin sensitivity in glucokinase-deficient subjects. *Diabetologia* 1996; 39: 82–90.
82. Polonsky KS. Lilly Lecture 1994. The beta cell in diabetes: from molecular genetics to clinical research. *Diabetes* 1995; 44: 705–17.
83. Bell GI, Polonsky KS. Diabetes mellitus and genetically programmed defects in ß-cell function. *Nature* 2001; 414: 788–91.
84. McCarthy MI, Froguel P. Genetic approaches to the molecular understanding of type 2 diabetes. *Am J Physiol* 2002; 283: E217–25.
85. Fajans SS. Maturity-onset diabetes of the young (MODY). *Diabetes Metab Rev* 1989; 5: 579–606.
86. Bell GI, Zian K, Newman M, Wu S, Wright L, Fajans S, Spielman RS, Cox NJ. Gene for non-insulin-dependent diabetes mellitus (maturity-onset diabetes of the young subtype) is linked to DNA polymorphism on human chromosome 20q. *Proc Natl Acad Sci* 1991; 88: 1484–8.
87. Froguel Ph, Vaxillaire M, Sun F, Velho G, Zouali H, Butel MO, Lesage S, Vionnet N, Clement K, Fougerousse F, Tanizawa Y, Weissenbach J, Beckmann JS, Lathrop GM, Passa Ph, Permutt MA, Cohen D. Close linkage of glucokinase locus on chromosome 7p to early-onset non-insulin-dependent diabetes mellitus. *Nature* 1992; 356: 162–614.
88. Froguel PH, Zouali H, Vionnet N, Velho G, Vaxillaire M, Sun F, Lesage S, Stoffel M, Takeda J, Passap P. Familial hyperglycaemia due to mutations in glucokinase: definition of a subtype of diabetes mellitus. *N Engl J Med* 1993; 328: 697–702.
89. Menzel S, Yamagata K, Trabb JB, Nerup J, Permutt MA, Fajans SS, Menzel R, Iwasaki N, Omori Y, Cox N, Bell GI. Localization of MODY3 to a 5-cM region of human chromosome 12. *Diabetes* 1995; 44: 1408–13.
90. Zhang Y, Warren-Perry M, Saker PJ, Hattersley AT, Mackie ADR, Baird JD, Greenwood RH, Stoffel M, Bell GI, Turner RC. Candidate gene studies in pedigrees with maturity-onset diabetes of the young not lined with glucokinase. *Diabetologia* 1995; 38: 1055–66.
91. Weng J, Macfarlane WM, Lehto M, Gu HF, Shepherd LM, Ivarsson SA, Wibell L, Smith T, Groop LC. Functional consequences of mutations in the MODY4 gene (IPF1) and coexistence with MODY3 mutations. *Diabetologia* 2001; 44: 249–58.
92. Bynre MM, Sturis J, Fajans SS, Ortiz FJ, Stoltz A, Stoffel M, Smith MJ, Bell GI, Halter JB, Polonsky KS. Altered insulin secretory responses to glucose in subjects with a mutation in the MODY1 gene on chromosome 20. *Diabetes* 1995; 44: 699–704.
93. Sturis J, Kurland IJ, Byrne MM, Mosekilde E, Froguel P, Pilkis SJ, Bell GI, Polonsky KS. Compensation in pancreatic ß-cell function in subjects with glucokinase mutations. *Diabetes* 1994; 43: 718–23.
94. Herman WH, Fajans SS, Ortiz FJ, Smith MJ, Sturis J, Bell GI, Polonsky KS, Halter JB. Abnormal insulin secretion, not insulin resistance, is the genetic or primary defect of MODY in the RW pedigree. *Diabetes* 1994; 43: 40–6.
95. Beck-Nielsen H, Nielsen OH, Pedersen O, Bak J, Faber O, Schmitz O. Insulin action and insulin secretion in identical twins with MODY: evidence for defects in both insulin action and insulin secretion. *Diabetes* 1988; 37: 730–5.
96. Mohan V, Sharp PS, Aber VR, Mather HM, Kohner EM. Insulin resistance in maturity-onset diabetes of the young. *Diabetes Metab* 1988; 13: 193–7.
97. Velho G, Petersen K, Perseghin G, Hwang J-H, Pueyo ME, Rothman DL, Pueyo ME, Cline GW, Froguel P, Shulman GI. Impaired hepatic glycogen synthesis in glucokinase-deficient (MODY-2) subjects. *J Clin Invest* 1996; 98: 1755–61.
98. Kazuhiro E, Sakura H, Shimokawa K, Kadowaki H, Hagura R, Akanuma Y, Yazaki Y, Kadowaki T. Sequence variations of the glucokinase gene in Japanese subjects with NIDDM. *Diabetes* 1994; 43: 730–3.
99. Zouali H, Vaxillaire M, Lesage S. , Sun F, Velho G, Vionnet N, Chiu K, Passa P, Permutt A, Demenais F, Cohen D, Beckmann S, Froguel P. Linkage analysis and molecular scanning of glucokinase gene in NIDDM families. *Diabetes* 1993; 42: 1238–45.
100. Elbein SC, Hoffman M, Qin H, Chiu K, Tanizawa Y, Permutt MA. Molecular screening of the glucokinase

gene in familial type 2 (non-insulin-dependent) diabetes mellitus. *Diabetologia* 1994; 37: 182–7.

101. Temple RC, Carrington Ca, Luzio SD, Owens DR, Schneider AE, Sobey WJ, Hales CN. Insulin deficiency in non-insulin-dependent diabetes. *Lancet* 1989; 1: 293–5.
102. Efendic S, Grill V, Luft R, Wajngot A. Low insulin response: a marker of pre-diabetes. *Adv Exp Med Biol* 1988; 246: 167–74.
103. Davies MJ, Metcalfe J, Gray IP, Day JL, Hales CN. Insulin deficiency rather than hyperinsulinaemia in newly diagnosed type 2 diabetes mellitus. *Diabet Med* 1993; 10: 305–12.
104. Chen K-W, Boyko EJ, Bergstrom RW, Leonetti DL, Newell-Morris L, Wahl PW, Fujimoto WY. Earlier appearance of impaired insulin secretion than of visceral adiposity in the pathogenesis of NIDDM. 5-year follow-up of initially nondiabetic Japanese-American men. *Diabetes Care* 1995; 18: 747–53.
105. Arner P, Pollare T, Lithell H. Different etiologies of Type 2 (non-insulin-dependent) diabetes mellitus in obese and non-obese subjects. *Diabetologia* 1991; 34: 483–7.
106. Ferrannini E, Natali A, Bell P, Cavallo-Perin P, Lalic N, for the European Group for the Study of Insulin Resistance (EGIR). Mingrone G. Insulin resistance and hypersecretion in obesity. *Journal of Clinical Investigation*. 1997; 100(5): 1166–73.
107. Banjeri MA, Lebovitz HE. Insulin action in black Americans with NIDDM. *Diabetes Care* 1992; 15: 1295–1302.
108. Banerji MA, Chaiken RL, Gordon D, Kral JG, Lebovitz HE. Does intra-abdominal adipose tissue in black men determine whether NIDDM is insulin-resistant or insulin-sensitive? *Diabetes* 1995; 44: 141–6.
109. Mbanya J-CN, Pani LN, Mbanya DNS, Sobngwi E, Ngogang J. Reduced insulin secretion in offspring of African type 2 diabetic patients. *Diabetes Care* 2000; 23: 1761–5.
110. DeFronzo RA, Tobin JD, Andres R. Glucose clamp technique: a method for quantifying insulin secretion and resistance. *Am J Physiol* 1979; 6: E214–23.
111. Curry DL, Bennett LL, Grodsky GM. Dynamics of insulin secretion by the perfused rat pancreas. *Endocrinology* 1968; 83: 572–84.
112. Cerasi E, Luft R, Efendic S. Decreased sensitivity of the pancreatic beta cells to glucose in pre-diabetic and diabetic subjects. *Diabetes* 1972; 21: 224–34.
113. Temple R, Clark PMS, Hales CN. Measurement of insulin secretion in type 2 diabetes: problems and pitfalls. *Diabet Med* 1992; 9: 503–12.
114. Brunzell JD, Robertson RP, Lerner RL, Hazzard WR, Ensinck JW, Bierman EL, Porte D. Relationships between fasting plasma glucose levels and insulin secretion during intravenous glucose tolerance tests. *J Clin Endocrinol* 1976; 46: 222–9.
115. Vague P, Moulin J-P. The defective glucose sensitivity of the B cell in insulin dependent diabetes. Improvement after twenty hours of normoglycaemia. *Metabolism* 1982; 31: 139–42.
116. Savage PJ, Bennion LJ, Flock EV. Diet-induced improvement of abnormalities in insulin and glucagon secretion and in insulin receptor binding in diabetes mellitus. *J Clin Endocrinol Metab* 1979; 48: 999–1007.
117. Kosaka K, Kuzuya T, Akanuma Y, Hagura R. Increase in insulin response after treatment of overt maturity onset diabetes mellitus is independent of the mode of treatment. *Diabetologia* 1980; 18: 23–8.
118. Rossetti L, Giaccari A, DeFronzo RA. Glucose toxicity. *Diabetes Care* 1990; 13: 610–30.
119. Prentki M, Corkey BE. Are the beta cell signaling molecules malonyl-CoA and cytosolic long-chain acyl-CoA implicated in multiple tissue defects of obesity and NIDDM? *Diabetes* 1996; 45: 273–83.
120. Unger RH. Lipotoxicity in the pathogenesis of obesity-dependent NIDDM. Genetic and clinical implications. *Diabetes* 1995; 44: 863–70.
121. Shimabukuro M, Zhou Y-T, Levi M, Unger RH. Fatty acid induced ß-cell apoptosis: a link between obesity and diabetes. *Proc Natl Acad Sci* 1998; 95: 2498–502.
122. Bruce DG, Chisholm DJ, Storlien LH, Kraegen EW. Physiological importance of deficiency in early prandial insulin secretion in non-insulin dependent diabetes. *Diabetes* 1988; 37: 736–44.
123. Steiner KE, Bowles CR, Mouton SM, Williams PE, Cherrington AD. The relative importance of first and second phase insulin secretion in countering the action of glucagon on glucose turnover in the conscious dog. *Diabetes* 1982; 31: 964–72.
124. Luzi L. Effect of the loss of first phase insulin secretion on glucose production and disposal in man. *Am J Physiol* 1989; 257: E241–6.
125. Calles-Escandon J, Robbins DC. Loss of early phase of insulin release in humans impairs glucose tolerance and blunts thermic effect of glucose. *Diabetes* 1987; 36: 1167–72.
126. Bonner-Weir S. ß-cell turnover. Its assessment and implications. *Diabetes* 2001; 50: S20–4.
127. Haffner SM, Miettinen H, Stern MP. Insulin secretion and resistance in nondiabetic Mexican Americans and non-Hispanic whites with a parental history of diabetes. *J Clin Endocrinol Metab* 1996; 81: 1846–51.
128. Gautier J-F, Wilson C, Weyer C, Mott D, Knowler WC, Cavaghan M, Polonsky KS, Bogardus C, Pratley RE. Low acute insulin secretory responses in adult offspring of people with early onset type 2 diabetes. *Diabetes* 2001; 50: 1828–33.
129. Janssen RC, Bogardus C, Takeda J, Knowler WC, Thompson DB: Linkage analysis of acute insulin secretion with GLUT2 and glucokinase in Pima Indians and the identification of a missense mutation in GLUT2. *Diabetes* 1994; 43: 558–63.
130. Sakul H, Pratley R, Cardon L, Ravussin E, Mott D, Bogardus C: Familiarity of physical and metabolic characteristics that predict the development of non-insulin-dependent diabetes mellitus in Pima Indians. *Am J Hum Genet* 1997; 60: 651–6.
131. Vauhkonen N, Niskanen L, Vanninen E, Kainulainen S, Uusitupa M, Laakso M. Defects in insulin secretion and insulin action in non-insulin-dependent diabetes mellitus are inherited. Metabolic studies on offspring of diabetic probands. *J Clin Invest* 1997; 100: 86–96.
132. Vaag A, Henriksen JE, Madsbad S, Holm N, Beck-Nielsen H. Insulin secretion, insulin action, and hepatic glucose production in identical twins discordant for non-insulin-dependent diabetes mellitus. *J Clin Invest* 1995; 95: 690–8.
133. Barnett AH, Spilipoulos AJ, Pyke DA, Stubbs WA, Burrin J, Alberti KGMM. Metabolic studies in unaffected co-twins of non-insulin-dependent diabetics. *Brit Med J* 1981; 282: 1656–8.

134. Watanabe RM, Valle T, Hauser ER, Ghosh S, Eriksson J, Kohtamaki K, Ehnholm C, Tuomilehto J, Collins FS, Bergman RN, Boehnke M, for the Finland-United States Investigation of NIDDM Genetics (FUSION) Study Investigators. Familiality of quantitative metabolic traits in Finnish families with non-insulin-dependent diabetes mellitus. *Hum Hered* 1999; 49(3): 159–68.
135. Mahtani MM, Widen E, Lehto M, Thomas J, McCarthy M, Brayer J, Bryant B, Chan G, Daly M, Forsblom C, Kanninen T, Kirby A, Kruglyak L, Munnelly K, Parkkonen M, Reeve-Daly MP, Weaver A, Brettin T, Duyk G, Lander ES, Groop LC. Mapping of a gene for type 2 diabetes associated with an insulin secretion defect by a genome scan in Finnish families. *Nat Genet* 1996; 14: 90–4.
136. Rossetti L, Shulman Gi, Zawalich W, DeFronzo RA. Effect of chronic hyperglycemia on in vivo insulin secretion in partially pancreatectomized rats. *J Clin Invest* 1987; 80: 1037–44.
137. Leahy JL, Bonner-Weir S, Weir GC. Abnormal glucose regulation of insulin secretion in models of reduced beta-cell mass. *Diabetes* 1984; 33: 667–73.
138. Bonner-Weir S, Trent DF, Weir GC. Partial pancreatectomy in the rat and subsequent defect in glucose-induced insulin release. *J Clin Invest* 1983; 71: 1544–53.
139. Leahy JL, Bonner-Weir S, Weir GC. Minimal chronic hyperglycemia is a critical determinant of impaired insulin secretion after an incomplete pancreatectomy. *J Clin Invest* 1988; 81: 1407–14.
140. Leahy JL, Cooper HE, Weir GC. Impaired insulin secretion associated with near normoglycemia. *Diabetes* 1987; 36: 459–64.
141. Leahy JL, Weir GC. Evolution of abnormal insulin secretory responses during 48-h *in vivo* hyperglycemia. *Diabetes* 1988; 37: 217–22.
142. Robertson RP, Olson IK, Zhang H-J. Differentiating glucose toxicity from glucose desensitization: a new message from the insulin gene. *Diabetes* 1994; 43: 1085–9.
143. Weir GC, Laybutt DR, Kaneto H, Bonner-Weir S, Sharma A. ß-Cell adaptation and decompensation during the progression of diabetes. *Diabetes* 2001; 50 (suppl 1): S154–9.
144. Simonson DC, Rossetti L, Giaccari A, DeFronzo RA. Glucose toxicity. In Alberti KGMM, DeFronzo RA, Keen H, Zimmet P (eds). *International Textbook of Diabetes Mellitus*, Wiley, Chichester, England, 1997; pp 713–44.
145. Matchinsky FM. Banting Lecture 1995. A lesson in metabolic regulation inspired by the glucokinase glucose sensor paradigm. *Diabetes* 1996; 45: 223–41.
146. Newgard CB, McGarry JD. Metabolic coupling factors in pancreatic beta cell signal transduction. *Annu Rev Biochem* 1995; 64: 689–719.
147. Nishizuka Y. Intracellular signaling by hydrolysis of phospholipids and activation of protein kinase C. *Science* 1992; 258: 607–14.
148. Corkey BE, Deeney JT. Acyl CoA regulation of metabolism and signal transduction. *Prog Clin Biol Res* 1990; 321: 217–32.
149. Zhou YP, Grill VE. Long-term exposure of rat pancreatic islets to fatty acids inhibits glucose-induced insulin secretion and biosynthesis through a glucose fatty acid cycle. *J Clin Invest* 1994; 93: 870–6.
150. Yaney GC, Schultz V, Cunningham BA, Dunaway GA, Corkey BE, Tornheim K. Phosphofructokinase isozymes in pancreatic islets and clonal beta-cells (INS-1). *Diabetes* 1995; 44: 1285–9.
151. Shimabukuro M, Higa M, Zhou YT, Wang MY, Newgard CB, Unger RH. Lipoapoptosis in beta-cells of obese prediabetic *fa/fa* rats. Role of serine palmitoyltransferase overexpression. *J Biol Chem* 1998; 273: 32487–90.
152. Fehmann HC, Goke R, Goke B. Cell and molecular biology of the incretin hormones glucagon-like peptide-I and glucose-dependent insulin releasing polypeptide. *Endocr Rev* 1995; 16: 390–410.
153. Drucker DJ. Minireview: the glucagon-like peptides. *Endocrinology* 2001; 142: 521–7.
154. Nauck MA, Bartels E, Orskov C, Ebert R, Creutzfeldt W. Additive insulinotropic effects of exogenous synthetic human gastric inhibitory polypeptide and glucagon-like peptide-1-(7-36) amide infused at near-physiological insulinotropic hormone and glucose concentrations. *J Clin Endocrinol Metab* 1993; 76: 912–7.
155. D'Alessio DA, Vogel R, Prigeon R, Laschansky E, Koerker D, Eng J, Ensinck JW. Elimination of the action of glucagon-like peptide 1 causes an impairment of glucose tolerance after nutrient ingestion by healthy baboons. *J Clin Invest* 1996; 97: 133–8.
156. Schirra J, Sturm K, Leicht P, Arnold R, Goke B, Katschinski M. Exendin(9-39)amide is an antagonist of glucagon-like peptide-1(7-36)amide in humans. *J Clin Invest* 1998; 101: 1421–30.
157. Nauck MA, Heimesaat MM, Orskov C, Holst JJ, Ebert R, Creutzfeldt W. Preserved incretin activity of glucagon-like peptide 1 [7-36 amide] but not of synthetic human gastric inhibitory polypeptide in patients with type 2 diabetes mellitus. *J Clin Invest* 1993; 91: 301–7.
158. Vilsboll T, Krarup T, Deacon CF, Madsbad S, Holst JJ. Reduced postprandial concentrations of intact biologically active glucagon-like peptide 1 in type 2 diabetic patients. *Diabetes* 2001; 50: 609–13.
159. Ahren B, Larsson H, Holst JJ. Effects of glucagon-like peptide-1 on islet function and insulin sensitivity in noninsulin-dependent diabetes mellitus. *J Clin Endocrinol Metab* 1997; 82: 473–8.
160. Nanauck MA, Kleine N, Orskov C, Holst JJ, Willms B, Creutzfeldt W. Normalization of fasting hyperglycaemia by exogenous glucagon-like peptide 1 (7-36 amide) in type 2 (non-insulin-dependent) diabetic patients. *Diabetologia* 1993; 36: 741–4.
161. Xu G, Stoffers DA, Habener JF, Bonner-Weir S. Exendin-4 stimulates both beta-cell replication and neogenesis, resulting in increased beta-cell mass and improved glucose tolerance in diabetic rats. *Diabetes* 1999; 48: 2270–6.
162. Kahn SE, Andrikopoulos S, Verchere CB. Islet amyloid. A long-recognized but underappreciated pathological feature of type 2 diabetes. *Diabetes* 1999; 48: 241–53.
163. Lukinius A, Willander E, Westermark GT, Engstrom U, Westermark P. Co-localization of IAPP and insulin in the beta cell secretory granules of the human pancreatic islets. *Diabetologia* 1989; 32: 240–4.
164. Johnson KH, O'Brien TD, Betysholtz C, Westermark P. Islet amyloid, islet-amyloid polypeptide, and diabetes mellitus. *New Engl J Med* 1989; 321: 513–8.
165. Ohsawa H, Kanatsuka A, Yamaguchi T, Makino H, Yoshida S. IAPP inhibits glucose-stimulated insulin secretion from isolated rat pancreatic islets. *Biochem Biophys Res Comm* 1989; 160: 961–7.

166. Howard CF. Longitudinal studies on the development of diabetes in individual *Macaca nigra*. *Diabetologia* 1986; 29: 301–6.
167. Hartter E, Svoboda T, Ludvik B, Schuller M, Lell B, Kuenburg E, Brunnbauer M, Woloszczuk W, Prager R. Basal and stimulated plasma levels of pancreatic amylin indicate its co-secretion with insulin in humans. *Diabetologia* 1991; 34: 52–4.
168. Eriksson J, Nakazato M, Miyazato M, Shiomi K, Matsukura S, Groop L. IAPP: plasma-concentrations in individuals at increased risk of developing type 2 (non-insulin-dependent) diabetes mellitus. *Diabetologia* 1992; 35: 292–3.
169. Bretherton-Watt D, Ghatei MA, Bloom SR, Jamal H, Ferrier GJ, Girgis SI, Legon S. Altered IAPP (amylin) gene expression in rat models of diabetes. *Diabetologia* 1989; 32: 881–3.
170. Westermark GT, Christmanson L, Terenghi G, Permerth J, Betsoltz C, Larsson J, Polak JM. Westermark P. IAPP: demonstration of mRNA in human pancreatic islets by in situ hybridization in islets with and without amyloid deposits. *Diabetologia* 1993; 36: 323–8.
171. Ghatei MA, Datta HK, Zaidi M, BrethertonWatt D, Wimalawansa SJ, Maclntyre L, Bloom SR. Amylin and amylin-amide lack an acute effect on blood glucose and insulin. *J Endocrinol* 1990; 124: R9–11.
172. Bretherton-Watt D, Gilbey SG, Ghatei MA, Beacham J, Bloom SR. Failure to establish IAPP (amylin) as a circulating beta cell inhibiting hormone in man. *Diabetologia* 1990; 33: 115–7.
173. Hoppener JWM, Verbeek JS, de Koning EJP, Oosterwijk C, van Hulst KL, Visser-Vernooy HJ, Hofhuis FMA, van Gaalen S, Berends MJH, Hackeng WHL, Jansz HS, Morris JF, Clark A, Capel PJA, Lipis CJM. Chronic overproduction of IAPP-amylin in transgenic mice: lysosomal localization of human IAPP and lack of marked hyperglycaemia or hyperinsulinaemia. *Diabetologia* 1993; 36: 1258–65.
174. Gebre-Medhin S, Olofsson C, Mulder H. IAPP in the islets of Langerhans: friend or foe? *Diabetologia* 2000; 43: 687–95.
175. Westermark P, Wilander E. The influence of amyloid deposits on the islet volume in maturity onset diabetes mellitus. *Diabetologia* 1978; 15: 417–21.
176. Gepts W, Lecompte PM. The pancreatic islets in diabetes. *Am J Med* 1981; 70: 105–14.
177. Saito K, Yaginuma N, Takahashi T. Differential volumetry of alpha, beta, and delta cells in the pancreatic islets of diabetic and nondiabetic subjects. *Tohoku J Exp Med* 1979; 129: 273–83.
178. Kloppel G, Lohr M, Habich K, Oberholzer M, Heitz PU. Islet pathology and the pathogenesis of type I and type 2 diabetes mellitus revisited. *Surv Synth Path Res* 1985; 4: 110–25.
179. Clark A, Wells CA, Buley ID, Cruickshank JK, Vanhegan RI, Matthews DR, Cooper GJ, Holman RR, Turner RC. Islet amyloid, increased alpha-cells, reduced beta-cells and exocrine fibrosis: quantitative changes in the pancreas in type 2 diabetes. *Diabetes Res* 1988; 9: 151–9.
180. Butler AE, Janson J, Bonner-Weir S, Ritzel RA, Butler PC. Decreased b-cell mass inpatients with type-2 diabetes mellitus. *Diabetes* 2002; 51 (suppl 2): A367.
181. Stefan Y, Orci L, Malaisse-Lagae F, Perrelet A, Patel Y, Unger R. Quantitation of endocrine cell content in the pancreas of non-diabetic and diabetic humans. *Diabetes* 1982; 31: 694–700.
182. Rahier J, Sempoux C, Moulin P, Guiot Y. No decrease of the B cell mass in type 2 diabetic patients. *Diabetologia* 2000; 43 (suppl 1): A65.
183. Janson J, Butler AE, Bonner-Weir S, Ritzel RA, Sultana C, Butler PC. Failure of compensatory increase in new islet formation in humans with type-2 diabetes mellitus. *Diabetes* 2002; 51 (suppl 2): A377.
184. Hales CN, Barker DJP, Clark PM, Cox J, Fall C, Osmond C, Winter PD. Fetal and infant growth and IGT at age 64 years. *BMJ* 1991; 303: 1019–22.
185. McCance DR, Pettitt DJ, Hanson RL, Jacobson LT, Knowler WC, Bennett PH. Birth weight and non-insulin dependent diabetes: thrifty genotype, thrifty phenotype, or surviving small baby genotype? *BMJ* 1994; 308: 942–5.
186. Eriksson UJ. Lifelong consequences of metabolic adaptations in utero? *Diabetologia* 1996; 39: 1123–5.
187. Hales CN, Barker DJP. Type 2 (non-insulin-dependent) diabetes mellitus: the thrifty phenotype hypothesis. *Diabetologia* 1993; 35: 595–601.
188. Phillips DIW. Insulin resistance as a programmed response to fetal under nutrition. *Diabetologia* 1996; 39: 1119–22.
189. Strauss W, Hales C. Plasma insulin in minor abnormalities of glucose tolerance: a 5 year follow-up. *Diabetologia* 1974; 10: 237–43.
190. Hara H, Egusa G, Yamakido M, Kawate R. The high prevalence of diabetes mellitus and hyperinsulinemia among the Japanese-Americans living in Hawaii and Los Angeles. *Diabetes Res Clin Pract* 1994; 24 (suppl 1): S37–42.
191. Berrish TS, Hetherington CS, Alberti KGMM, Walker M. Peripheral and hepatic insulin sensitivity in subjects with IGT. *Diabetologia* 1995; 38: 699–704.
192. Lillioja S, Nyomba BL, Saad MF, Ferraro R, Castillo C, Bennett PH, Bogardus C. Exaggerated early insulin release and insulin resistance in a diabetes-prone population: a metabolic comparison of Pima Indians and Caucasians. *J Clin Endocrinol Metab* 1991; 73: 866–76.
193. Himsworth HP, Kerr RB. Insulin-sensitive and insulin-insensitive types of diabetes mellitus. *Clin Sci* 1939; 4: 120–52.
194. Ginsberg H, Kimmerling G, Olefsky JM, Reaven GM. Demonstration of insulin resistance in untreated adult-onset diabetic subjects with fasting hyperglycemia. *J Clin Invest* 1975; 55: 454–61.
195. Kimmerling G, Javorski C, Olefsky JM, Reaven GM. Locating the site(s) of insulin resistance in patients with nonketotic diabetes mellitus. *Diabetes* 1976; 25: 673–8.
196. Butterfield WJH, Whichelow MJ. Peripheral glucose metabolism in control subjects and diabetic patients during glucose, glucose-insulin, and insulin sensitivity tests. *Diabetologia* 1965; 1: 43–53.
197. Zierler KL, Rabinowitz D. Roles of insulin and growth hormone, based on studies of forearm metabolism in man. *Medicine* 1963; 42: 385–402.
198. Bowen HF, Moorhouse JA. Glucose turnover and disposal in maturity-onset diabetes. *J Clin Invest* 1973; 52: 3033–45.
199. Katz H, Homan M, Jensen M, Caumo A, Cobelli C, Rizza R. Assessment of insulin action in NIDDM in the presence of dynamic changes in insulin and glucose concentration. *Diabetes* 1994; 43: 289–96.

200. Wangot A, Roovete A, Vranic M. Luft R, Efendic S. Insulin resistance and decreased insulin response to glucose in lean type II diabetes. *Proc Natl Acad Sci USA* 1982; 79: 4432–7.
201. Bergman RN. Lilly Lecture. Toward physiological understanding of glucose tolerance—minimal-model approach. *Diabetes* 1989; 38: 1512–26.
202. Welch S, Gebhart SSP, Bergman RN, Phillips LS. Minimal models analysis of intravenous glucose tolerance test-derived insulin sensitivity in diabetic subjects. *J Clin Endocrinol Metab* 1990; 71: 1508–18.
203. DeFronzo RA, Deibert D, Hendler R, Felig P. Insulin sensitivity and insulin binding to monocytes in maturity-onset diabetes. *J Clin Invest* 63: 1982; 939–46.
204. DeFronzo RA, Simonson D, Ferrannini E. Hepatic and peripheral insulin resistance: a common feature in non-insulin-dependent and insulin-dependent diabetes. *Diabetologia* 1982; 23: 313–9.
205. Golay A, DeFronzo RA, Ferrannini E, Simonson DC, Thorin D, Acheson K, Thiebaud D, Curchod B, Jequier E, Felber JP. Oxidative and nonoxidative glucose metabolism in non-obese Type 2 (non-insulin dependent) diabetic patients. *Diabetologia* 1988; 31: 585–91.
206. Karnieli E, Armoni, M, Cohen P, Kanter Y, Rafaeloff R. Reversal of insulin resistance in diabetic rat adipocytes by insulin therapy. *Diabetes* 1987; 36: 925–31.
207. Dall'Aglio E, Chang H, Hollenbeck CB, Mondon CE, Sims C, Reaven GM. In vivo and in vitro resistance to maximal insulin-stimulated glucose disposal in insulin deficiency. *Am J Physiol* 1985; 249: E312–6.
208. Vuorinen-Markkola H, Koivisto VA, Yki-Järvinen H: Mechanisms of hyperglycemia-induced insulin resistance in whole-body and skeletal muscle of type 1 diabetic patients. *Diabetes* 1992; 41: 571–80.
209. Golay A, Felber JP, Jequier E, DeFronzo RA, Ferrannini E. Metabolic basis of obesity and noninsulin-dependent diabetes mellitus. *Diabetes Metab Rev* 1988; 4: 727–47.
210. DeFronzo RA, Sherwin RS, Hendler R, and Felig P. Insulin binding to monocytes and insulin action in human obesity, starvation, and refeeding. *J Clin Invest* 1978; 62: 204–13.
211. Felber JP, Golay A, Jequier E, Curchod B, Temler E, DeFronzo RA, Ferrannini E. The metabolic consequences of long-term human obesity. *Int J Obesity* 1988; 12: 377–89.
212. Firth R, Bell P, Rizza R. Insulin action in non-insulin-dependent diabetes mellitus: the relationship between hepatic and extrahepatic insulin resistance and obesity. *Metabolism* 1987; 36: 1091–5.
213. Campbell PJ, Mandarino LJ, Gerich JE. Quantification of the relative impairment in actions of insulin on hepatic glucose production and peripheral glucose uptake in non-insulin dependent diabetes mellitus. *Metabolism* 1988; 37: 15–21.
214. Bogardus C, Lillioja S, Howard BV, Reaven G, Mott D. Relationships between insulin secretion, insulin action, and fasting plasma glucose concentration in non-diabetic and noninsulin-dependent subjects. *J Clin Invest* 1984; 74: 1238–46.
215. Del Prato S, Simonson DC, Sheehan P, Cardi F, DeFronzo RA. Studies on the mass effect of glucose in diabetes. Evidence for glucose resistance. *Diabetologia* 1997; 40: 687–97.
216. Nielsen MF, Basu R, Wise S, Caumo A, Cobelli C, Rizza RA. Normal glucose-induced suppression of glucose production but impaired stimulation of glucose disposal in type 2 diabetes. Evidence for a concentration-dependent defect in uptake. *Diabetes* 1998; 47: 1735–47.
217. Huang SC, Phelps ME, Hoffman EJ, Sideris K, Selin CJ, Kuhl DE. Non-invasive determination of local cerebral metabolic rate of glucose in man. *Am J Physiol* 1980; 238: E69–82.
218. Henry RR, Wallace P, Olefsky JM. Effects of weight loss on mechanisms of hyperglycemia in obese non-insulin dependent diabetes mellitus. *Diabetes* 1986; 35: 990–8.
219. Firth RG, Bell PM, Rizza RA. Effects of tolazamide and exogenous insulin on insulin action in patients with non-insulin-dependent diabetes mellitus. *New Engl J Med* 1986; 314: 1280–6.
220. Best JD, Judzewitsch RG, Pfeiffer MA, Beard JC, Halter JB, Porte D. The effect of chronic sulfonylurea therapy on hepatic glucose production in non-insulin-dependent diabetes mellitus. *Diabetes* 1982; 31: 333–8.
221. Garvey WT, Olefsky JM, Griffin J, Hamman RF, Kolterman OG. The effect of insulin treatment on insulin action in type II diabetes mellitus. *Diabetes* 1985; 34: 222–34.
222. Tayek JA, Katz J. Glucose production, recycling, and gluconeogenesis in normals and diabetics: a mass isotopomer [U-^{13}C] glucose study. *Am J Physiol* 1996; 270: E709–17.
223. Fery F. Role of hepatic glucose production and glucose uptake in the pathogenesis of fasting hyperglycemia in Type 2 diabetes: normalization of glucose kinetics by short-term fasting. *J Clin Endocrinol Metab* 1994; 78: 536–42.
224. Jeng C-Y, Sheu WHH, Fuh MM-T, Chen I, Reaven GM. Relationship between hepatic glucose production and fasting plasma glucose concentration in patients with NIDDM. *Diabetes* 1994; 43: 1440–4.
225. DeFronzo RA, Ferrannini E, Hendler R, Felig P, Wahren J, Regulation of splanchnic and peripheral glucose uptake by insulin and hyperglycemia. *Diabetes* 1983; 32: 35–45.
226. DeFronzo RA, Ferrannini E. Influence of plasma glucose and insulin concentration on plasma glucose clearance in man. *Diabetes* 1982; 31: 683–8.
227. Cherrington AD, Stevenson RW, Steiner KE, Davis MA, Myers SR, Adkins BA, Abumrad NN, Williams PE. Insulin, glucagon, and glucose as regulators of hepatic glucose uptake and production in vivo. *Diabetes Metab Rev* 1987; 3: 307–32.
228. Bergman RN, Bucolo RJ. Interaction of insulin and glucose in the control of hepatic glucose balance. *Am J Physiol* 1974; 227: 1314–22.
229. Mevorach M, Giacca A, Aharon Y, Hawkins M, Shamoon H, Rossetti L. Regulation of endogenous glucose production by glucose per se is impaired in type 2 diabetes mellitus. *J Clin Invest* 1998; 102: 744–53.
230. Basu R, Basu A, Nielsen M, Shah P, Rizza RA. Effect of overnight restoration of euglycemia on glucose effectiveness in type 2 diabetes mellitus. *J Cin Endocrinol Metab* 1999; 84: 2314–9.
231. Magnusson I, Rothman D, Katz L, Shulman R, Shulman G. Increased rate of gluconeogenesis in type II diabetes: a ^{13}C nuclear magnetic resonance study. *J Clin Invest* 1992; 90: 1323–7.
232. Gastaldelli A, Baldi S, Pettiti M, Toschi E, Camastra S, Natali A, Landau BR, Ferrannini E. Influence of obesity and type 2 diabetes on gluconeogenesis and glucose

output in humans: a quantitative study. *Diabetes* 2000; 49: 1367–73.

233. Waldhausl W, Bratusch-Marrain P, Gasic S, Korn A, Nowotny P. Insulin production rate, hepatic insulin retention, and splanchnic carbohydrate metabolism after oral glucose ingestion in hyperinsulinemic type II (non-insulin dependent) diabetes mellitus. *Diabetologia* 1982; 23: 6–15.
234. Consoli A, Nurjahn N, Capani F, Gerich J. Predominant role of gluconeogenesis in increased hepatic glucose production in NIDDM. *Diabetes* 1989; 38: 550–6.
235. Nurjhan N, Consoli A, Gerich J. Increased lipolysis and its consequences on gluconeogenesis in noninsulin-dependent diabetes mellitus. *J Clin Invest* 1992; 89: 169–75.
236. Gastaldelli A, Toschi E, Pettiti M, Frascerra S, Qinones-Galvan A, Sironi AM, Natali A, Ferrannini E. Effect of physiological hyperinsulinemia on gluconeogenesis in nondiabetic subjects and in type 2 diabetic patients. *Diabetes* 2001; 50: 1807–12.
237. Stumvoll M, Perriello G, Nurjhan N, Bucci A, Welle S, Jansson P-A, Dailey G, Bier D, Jenssen T, Gerich J. Glutamine and alanine metabolism in NIDDM. *Diabetes* 1996; 45: 863–8.
238. Unger RH, Aguilar-Parada E, Mueller WA, Eisentraut AM. Studies of pancreatic alpha-cell function in normal and diabetic subjects. *J Clin Invest* 1970; 49: 837–45.
239. Baron AD, Schaeffer L, Shragg P, Kolterman OG. Role of hyperglucagonemia in maintenance of increased rates of hepatic glucose output in type II diabetics. *Diabetes* 1987; 36: 274–83.
240. Felig P, Wahren J, Hendler R. Influence of maturity-onset diabetes on splanchnic balance after oral glucose ingestion. *Diabetes* 1978; 27: 121–6.
241. Foley JE. Rationale and application of fatty acid oxidation inhibitors in treatment of diabetes mellitus. *Diabetes Care* 1992; 15: 773–84.
242. Matsuda M, DeFronzo RA, Glass L, Consoli A, Giordano M, Bressler P, DelPrato S. Glucagon dose–response curve for hepatic glucose production and glucose disposal in type 2 diabetic patients and normal individuals. *Metabolism* 2002; 51: 1111–9.
243. Kolterman OG, Gray RS, Griffin J, Burstein P. Insel J, Scarlett JA, Olefsky JM. Receptor and postreceptor defects contribute to the insulin resistance in non-insulin-dependent diabetes mellitus. *J Clin Invest* 1981; 68: 957–69.
244. Cusi K, Consoli A, DeFronzo RA. Metabolic effects of metformin on glucose and lactate metabolism in NIDDM. *J Clin Endocrinol Metab* 1996; 81: 4059–67.
245. Clore JN, Stillman J, Sugerman H. G-6-Pase flux in vitro is increased in type 2 diabetes. *Diabetes* 2000; 49: 969–74.
246. O'Brien RM, Granner DK. PEPCK gene as model of inhibitory effects of insulin on gene transcription. *Diabetes Care* 1990; 13: 327–39.
247. Sutherland C, O'Brien RM, Granner DK. New connections in the regulation of PEPCK gene expression by insulin. *Philos Trans R Soc Lond, B: Biol Sci* 1996; 351: 191–9.
248. Cersosimo E, Garlick P, Ferretti J. Regulation of splanchnic and renal substrate supply by insulin in humans. *Metabolism* 2000; 49: 676–83.
249. Moller N. Rizza RA. Ford GC. Nair KS. Assessment of postabsorptive renal glucose metabolism in humans with multiple glucose tracers. *Diabetes* 2001; 50: 747–51.
250. Meyer C, Stumvoll M, Nadkarni V, Dostou J, Mitrakou A, Gerich J. Abnormal renal and hepatic glucose metabolism in type 2 diabetes mellitus. *J Clin Invest* 1998; 102: 619–24.
251. Bjorntorp P, Berchtold P, Holm J. The glucose uptake of human adipose tissue in obesity. *Eur J Clin Invest* 1971; 1: 480–5.
252. Frayn KN, Coppack SW, Humphreys SM, Whyte PL. Metabolic characteristics of human adipose tissue in vivo. *Clin Sci* 1989; 76: 509–16.
253. Revers R, Fink R, Griffin J, Olefsky J, Kolterman O. Influence of hyperglycemia in insulin's *in vivo* effects in type II diabetes. *J Clin Invest* 1984; 73: 664–72.
254. Campbell P, Mandarino L, Gerich J. Quantification of the relative impairment in actions of insulin on hepatic glucose production and peripheral glucose intake in non-insulin-dependent diabetes mellitus. *Metabolism* 1988; 37: 15–22.
255. Capaldo B, Napoli R, Dimarino L, Picardi A, Riccardi G, Sacca L. Quantitation of forearm glucose and FFA (FFA) disposal in normal subjects and type 2 diabetic patients: evidence against an essential role for FFA in the pathogenesis of insulin resistance. *J Clin Endocrinol Metab* 1988; 67: 893–8.
256. Jackson RA, Perry G, Rogers J, Advoni U, Pilkington TRE. Relationship between the basal glucose concentration, glucose tolerance, and forearm glucose uptake in maturity onset diabetes. *Diabetes* 1973; 22: 751–61.
257. Utriainen T, Takala T, Luotolahti M, Ronnemaa T, Laine H, Ruotsalainen U, Haaparanta M, Nuutila P, Yki-Jarvinen H. Insulin resistance characterizes glucose uptake in skeletal muscle but not in the heart in NIDDM. *Diabetologia* 1998; 41: 555–9.
258. Firth RG, Bell PM, Marsh HM, Hansen I, Rizza RA. Postprandial hyperglycemia in patients with non-insulin-dependent diabetes mellitus. *J Clin Invest* 1986; 77: 1525–32.
259. Ferrannini E, Simonson DC, Katz LD, Reichard G Jr, Bevilacqua S, Barrett EJ, Olsson M, DeFronzo RA. The disposal of an oral glucose load in patients with non-insulin dependent diabetes. *Metabolism* 1988; 37: 79–85.
260. Reinmuth OM, Schienberg P, Bourne B. Total cerebral blood flow and metabolism. *Arch Neurol* 1965; 12: 49–66.
261. Huang SC, Phelps ME, Hoffman EJ, Sideris K, Selin CJ, Kuhl DE. Non-invasive determination of local cerebral metabolic rate of glucose in man. *Am J Physiol* 1980; 238: E69–82.
262. Kelley D, Mitrakou A, Marsh H, Schwenk F, Benn J, Sonnenberg G, Arcangeli M, Aoki T, Sorensen J, Berger M, Sonksen P, Gerich J. Skeletal muscle glycolysis oxidation. and storage of an oral glucose load. *J Clin Invest* 1988; 81: 1563–71.
263. Jackson RA, Roshania RD, Hawa MI, Sim BM, DiSilvio L. Impact of glucose ingestion on hepatic and peripheral glucose metabolism in man: an analysis based on simultaneous use of the forearm and double isotope techniques. *J Clin Endocrinol Metab* 1986; 63: 541–9.
264. Jackson RA, Perry G, Rogers J, Advoni U, Pilkington TRE. Relationship between the basal glucose concentration, glucose tolerance, and forearm glucose uptake in maturity onset diabetes. *Diabetes* 1973; 22: 751–61.

265. Shimazu T. Neuronal regulation of hepatic glucose metabolism in mammals. *Diabetes Metab Rev* 1987; 3: 185–206.
266. McMahon V, Marsh HM, Rizza RA. Effects of basal insulin supplementation on disposition of mixed meal in obese patients with NIDDM. *Diabetes* 1989; 38: 291–303.
267. Basu A, Basu R, Shah P, Vella A, Johnson M, Nair KS, Jensen MD, Schwenk WF, Rizza RA. Effects of type 2 diabetes on the ability of insulin and glucose to regulate splanchnic and muscle glucose metabolism. Evidence for a defect in hepatic glucokinase activity. *Diabetes* 2000; 49: 272–83.
268. Ludvik B, Nolan JJ, Roberts A, Baloga J, Joyce M, Bell Jo M, Olefsky JM. Evidence for decreased splanchnic glucose uptake after oral glucose administration in non-insulin-dependent diabetes mellitus. *J Clin Invest* 1997; 100: 2354–61.
269. Reaven GM, Brand RJ, Chen Y-DI, Mathur AK, Goldfine I. Insulin resistance and insulin secretion are determinants of oral glucose tolerance in normal individuals. *Diabetes* 1993; 42: 1324–32.
270. Shulman GI, Rothman DL, Jue T, Stein P, DeFronzo RA, Shulman RG. Quantitation of muscle glycogen synthesis in normal subjects and subjects with non-insulin-dependent diabetes by ^{13}C nuclear magnetic resonance spectroscopy. *New Engl J Med* 1990; 322: 223–8.
271. Bonadonna RC, Bonora E. Glucose and FFA metabolism in human obesity: relationships to insulin resistance. *Diabetes Rev* 1997; 5: 21–51.
272. Reaven GM, Chen Y-DI, Donner CC, Fraze E, Hollenbeck CB. How insulin resistant are patients with non-insulin-dependent diabetes mellitus? *J Clin Endocrinol Metab* 1985; 61: 32–6.
273. Bogardus C, Lillioja S, Mott D, Reaven GR, Kashiwagi A, Foley J. Relationship between obesity and maximal insulin-stimulated glucose uptake in vivo and in vitro in Pima Indians. *J Clin Invest* 1984; 73: 800–5.
274. Lillioja A, Mott DM, Zawadzki JK, Young AA, Abbott WG, Bogardus C. Glucose storage is a major determinant of in vivo "insulin resistance" in subjects with normal glucose tolerance. *J Clin Endocrinol Metab* 1986; 62: 922–7.
275. Lillioja S, Bogardus C. Obesity and insulin resistance: lessons learned from the Pima Indians. *Diabetes Metab Rev* 1988; 4: 515–40.
276. Felber JP, Ferrannini E, Golay A, Meyer HV, Theibaud D, Curchod B, Maeder E, Jequier E, DeFronzo RA. Role of lipid oxidation in the pathogenesis of the insulin resistance of obesity and type II diabetes. *Diabetes* 1987; 36: 1341–50.
277. Zimmet PZ. The pathogenesis and prevention of diabetes in adults. *Diabetes Care* 1995; 18: 1050–64.
278. Mokdad AH, Ford ES, Bowman BA, Nelson DE, Engelgau MM, Vinicor F, Marks JS: Diabetes trends in the United States, 1990–1998. *Diabetes Care* 2000; 23: 1273–83.
279. Reaven GM, Hollenbeck C, Jeng C-Y, Wu MS, Chen Y-DI: Measurement of plasma glucose, FFA, lactate, and insulin for 24 hours in patients with NIDDM. *Diabetes* 1988; 37: 1020–4.
280. Thiebaud D, DeFronzo RA, Jacot E, Golay A, Acheson K, Maeder E, Jequier E, Felber JP. Effect of long-chain triglyceride infusion on glucose metabolism in man. *Metabolism* 1982; 31: 1128–36.
281. Kelley De, Mandarino LJ. Fuel selection in human skeletal muscle in insulin resistance. A reexamination. *Diabetes* 2000; 49: 677–83.
282. Kashyap S, Belfort R, Pratipanawatr T, Berria R, Pratipanawatr W, Bajaj M, Mandarino L, DeFronzo R, Cusi K: Chronic elevation in plasma FFAs impairs insulin secretion in non-diabetic offspring with a strong family history of T2DM. *Diabetes* 2002; 51 (suppl 2): A12.
283. Carpentier A, Mittelman SD, Bergman RN, Giacca A, Lewis GF. Prolonged elevation of plasma FFAs impairs pancreatic beta-cell function in obese nondiabetic humans but not in individuals with type 2 diabetes. *Diabetes* 2000; 49: 399–408.
284. Goodpaster BH, Thaete FL, Kelley BE. Thigh adipose tissue distribution is associated with insulin resistance in obesity and in type 2 diabetes mellitus. *Am J Clin Nutr* 2000; 71: 885–92.
285. Greco AV, Mingrone G, Giancaterini A, Manco M, Morroni M, Cinti S, Granzotto M, Vettor R, Camastra S, Ferrannini E. Insulin resistance in morbid obesity. Reversal with intramyocellular fat depletion. *Diabetes* 2002; 51: 144–51.
286. Ryysy L, Hakkinen AM, Goto T, Vehkavaara S, Westerbacka J, Halavaara J, Yki-Jarvinen H: Hepatic fat content and insulin action on FFAs and glucose metabolism rather than insulin absorption are associated with insulin requirements during insulin therapy in type 2 diabetic patients. *Diabetes* 2000; 49: 749–58.
287. Miyazaki Y, Mahankali A, Matsuda M, Mahankali S, Hardies J, Cusi K, Mandarino LJ, DeFronzo RA. Effect of pioglitazone on abdominal fat distribution and insulin sensitivity in type 2 diabetic patients. *J Clin Endocrinol Metab* 2002; 87: 2784–91.
288. Stein DT, Szczepanik L, Dobbins R, McGarry JD. Increasing intramyocellular triglyceride stores are associated with impaired glucose tolerance and NIDDM, *Diabetes* 1999; 48 (suppl 1): A287.
289. Randle PJ, Garland PB, Hales CN, Newsholme EA. The glucose fatty acid cycle. Its role in insulin sensitivity and the metabolic disturbances of diabetes mellitus. *Lancet* 1963; 1785–9.
290. Wititsuwannakul D, Kim K. Mechanism of palmityl coenzyme A inhibition or liver glycogen synthase. *J Biol Chem* 1977; 252: 7812–17.
291. Meyer HU, Curchod B, Maeder E, Pahud P, Jequier E, Felber JP. Modifications of glucose storage and oxidation in non-obese diabetics, measured by continuous indirect calorimetry. *Diabetes* 1980; 29: 752–6.
292. Golay A, Felber JP, Meyer HU, Curchod B, Maeder E, Jequier E. Study on lipid metabolism in obesity diabetes. *Metabolism* 1984; 33: 111–6.
293. Felber JP, Meyer HU, Curchod B, Iselin HU, Rousselle J, Maeder E, Pahud P, Jequier E. Glucose storage and oxidation in different degrees of human obesity measured by continuous indirect calorimetry. *Diabetologia* 1981; 20: 39–44.
294. Roden M, Krssak M, Stingl H, Gruber S, Hofer A, Furnsinn C, Moser E, Waldhausl W. Rapid impairment of skeletal muscle glucose transport/phosphorylation by FFAs in humans. *Diabetes* 1999; 48: 358–64.
295. Bonadonna RC, Groop LC, Zych K, Shank M, and DeFronzo RA. Dose dependent effect of insulin on plasma FFA turnover and oxidation in humans. *Am J Physiol* 1990; 22: 736–50.

296. Boden G. FFAs, insulin resistance, and type 2 diabetes mellitus. *Proc Assoc Am Physicians* 1999; 111: 241–8.
297. Boden G, Chen X, Ruiz J, White JV, Rossetti L. Mechanisms of fatty acid-induced inhibition of glucose uptake. *J Clin Invest* 1994; 93: 2438–46.
298. Pan DA, Lillioja S, Kriketos AD, Milner MR, Baur LA, Bogardus C, Jenkins AB, Storlien LH. Skeletal muscle triglyceride levels are inversely related to insulin action. *Diabetes* 1997; 46: 983–8.
299. Krssak M, Falk Petersen K, Dresner A, DiPietro L, Vogel SM, Rothman DL, Roden M, Shulman GI. Intramyocellular lipid concentrations are correlated with insulin sensitivity in humans: a ^{1}H NMR spectroscopy study. *Diabetologia* 1999; 42: 113–6.
300. Jacobs S, Machann J, Rett K, Brechtel K, Volk A, Renn W, Maerker E, Matthaei S, Schick F, Claussen CD, Hearing H-U. Association of increased intramyocellular lipid content with insulin resistance in lean non-diabetic offspring of type 2 diabetic subjects. *Diabetes* 1999; 48: 1113–9.
301. Kelley De, Goodpaster BH. Skeletal muscle triglyceride. An aspect of regional adiposity and insulin resistance. *Diabetes Care* 2001; 24: 933–41.
302. Kelley DE, Mandarino LJ. Fuel selection in human skeletal muscle in insulin resistance. *Diabetes* 2000; 49: 677–83.
303. Itani SI, Ruderman NB, Schmieder F, Boden G. Lipid-induced insulin resistance in human muscle is associated with changes in diacylglycerol, protein kinase C, and Iκ B-α. *Diabetes* 2002; 51: 2005–11.
304. Ellis BA, Poynten A, Lowy AJ, Furler SM, Chisholm DJ, Kraegen EW, Cooney GJ. Long-chain acyl-CoA esters as indicators of lipid metabolism and insulin sensitivity in rat and human muscle. *Am J Physiol* 2000; 279: E554–560.
305. De Fea K, Roth RA. Protein kinase C modulation of insulin receptor substrate-1 tyrosine phosphorylation requires serine 612. *Biochemistry* 1997; 36: 12939–47.
306. Ravichandran LV, Esposito DL, Chen J, Quon MJ. PKC-zeta phosphorylates IRS-1 and impairs its ability to activate P-3-kinase in response to insulin. *J Biol Chem* 2001; 276: 3543–9.
307. Faergeman NJ, Knudsen J. Role of long-chain fatty acyl-CoA esters in the regulation of metabolism and in cell signaling. *Biochem J* 1997; 323: 1–12.
308. Kruszynska YT, Worrall DS, Ofrecio J, Frias JP, Macaraeg G, Olefsky JM. Fatty acid-induced insulin resistance: decreased muscle PI3K activation but unchanged Akt phosphorylation. *J Clin Endocrinol Metab* 2002; 87: 226–34.
309. Dresner A, Laurent D, Marcucci M, Griffin ME, Dufour S, Cline SW, Slezak LA, Andersen DK, Hundal RS, Rothman DL, Petersen KF, Shulman GI. Effects of FFAs on glucose transport and IRS-1 associated phosphatidylinositol 3-kinase activity. *J Clin Invest* 1999; 103: 253–9.
310. Thompson AL, Cooney GJ. Acyl-CoA inhibition of hexokinase in rat and human skeletal muscle is a potential mechanism of lipid-induced insulin resistance. *Diabetes* 2000; 49: 1761–4.
311. Tippett PS, Neet KE. An allosteric model for the inhibition of glucokinase by long chain acyl coenzyme A. *J Biol Chem* 1982; 257: 14846–52.
312. Schmitz-Peiffer C, Craig DL, Biden TJ. Ceramide generation is sufficient to account for the inhibition of the insulin-stimulated PKB pathway in C_2C_{12} skeletal muscle cells pretreated with palmitate. *J Biol Chem* 1999; 274: 24202–10.
313. Baron AD. Hemodynamic actions of insulin. *Am J Physiol* 1994; 267: E187–202.
314. Mather K, Laakso M, Edelman S, Hook G, Baron A. Evidence for physiological coupling of insulin-mediated glucose metabolism and limb blood flow. *Am J Physiol Endocrinol Metab* 2000; 279: E1264–70.
315. Steinberg HO, Brechtel G, Johnson A, Fineberg N, Baron AD. Insulin-mediated skeletal muscle vasodilation is nitric oxide dependent. A novel action of insulin to increase nitric oxide release. *J Clin Invest* 1994; 94: 1172–9.
316. Utriainen T, Nuutila P, Takala T, Vicini P, Ruotsalainen U, Ronnemaa T, Tolvanen T, Raitakari M, Haaparanta M, Kirvela O, Cobelli C, Yki-Jarvinen H. Intact stimulation of skeletal muscle blood flow, its heterogeneity and redistribution, but not of glucose uptake in non-insulin-dependent diabetes mellitus. *J Clin Invest* 1997; 100: 777–85.
317. Steinberg HO, Paradisi G, Hook G, Crowder K, Cronin J, Baron AD. FFA elevation impairs insulin-mediated vasodilation and nitric oxide production. *Diabetes* 2000; 49: 1231–8.
318. Kreutzenberg SV, Crepaldi C, Marchetto S, Calo L, Tiengo A, Del Prato S, Avogaro A. Plasma FFAs and endothelium-dependent vasodilation: effect of chain-length and cyclooxygenase inhibition. *J Clin Endocrinol Metab* 2000; 85: 793–8.
319. Davda RK, Chandler LJ, Guzman NJ. Protein kinase C modulates receptor-independent activation of endothelial nitric oxide synthase. *Eur J Pharmacol* 1994; 266: 237–44.
320. Morrison KJ, Pollock D. Impairment of relaxations to acetylcholine and nitric oxide by a phorbol ester in rat isolated aorta. *Br J Pharmacol* 1990; 101: 432–6.
321. Fulton D, Gratton JP, McCabe TJ, Fontana J, Fujio Y, Walsh K, Franke TF, Papapetropoulos A, Sessa WC. Regulation of endothelium-derived nitric oxide production by the protein kinase Akt. *Nature* 1999; 399: 597–601.
322. Zeng G, Quon MJ. Insulin stimulated production of nitric oxide is inhibited by wortmannin: direct measurement in vascular endothelial cells. *J Clin Invest* 1996; 98: 894–8.
323. Exton JH, Corbin JG, Park CR. Control of gluconeogenesis in liver, IV: differential effects of fatty acids and glucagon on ketogenesis and gluconeogenesis in the perfused rat liver. *J Biol Chem* 1969; 244: 4095–102.
324. Bahl JJ, Matsuda M, DeFronzo RA, Bressler R. In vitro and in vivo suppression of gluconeogenesis by inhibition of pyruvate carboxylase. *Biochem Pharmacol* 1997; 53: 67–74.
325. Williamson JR, Kreisberg RA, and Felts PW. Mechanisms for the stimulation of gluconeogenesis by fatty acids in perfused rat liver. *Proc Natl Acad Sci USA* 1966; 56: 247–54.
326. Massillon D, Barzailai N, Hawkins M, Prus-Wetheimer D, Rossetti L. Induction of hepatic G-6-Pase gene expression by lipid infusion. *Diabetes* 1997; 46: 153–7.
327. Chen X, Iqbal N, Boden G. The effect of FFAs on gluconeogenesis and glycogenolysis in normal subjects. *J Clin Invest* 1999; 103: 365–72.
328. Roden M, Stingl H, Chandramouli V, Schumann WC, Hofer A, Landau BR, Nowotny P, Waldhausl W, Shulman GI. Effects of FFA elevation on postabsorptive

endogenous glucose production and gluconeogenesis in humans. *Diabetes* 2000; 49: 701–7.
329. Lewis GF. Vranic M. Harley P. Giacca A. Fatty acids mediate the acute extrahepatic effects of insulin on hepatic glucose production in humans. *Diabetes* 1997; 46: 1111–9.
330. Rebrin K. Steil GM. Getty L. Bergman RN. FFA as a link in the regulation of hepatic glucose output by peripheral insulin. *Diabetes* 1995; 44: 1038–45.
331. Ferrannini E, Barrett EJ, Bevilacqua S, DeFronzo RA. Effect of fatty acids on glucose production and utilization in man. *J Clin Invest* 1983; 72: 1737–47.
332. Bevilacqua S, Bonadonna R, Buzzigoli G, Boni C, Ciociaro D, Maccari F, Giorico MA, Ferrannini E: Acute elevation of FFA levels leads to hepatic insulin resistance in obese subjects. *Metabolism* 1987; 36: 502–6.
333. Golay A, Swislocki ALM, Chen Y-DI, Reaven GM: Relationships between plasma FFA concentration, endogenous glucose production, and fasting hyperglycemia in normal and non-insulin-dependent diabetic individuals. *Metabolism* 1987; 36: 692–6.
334. Baron AD, Schaeffer L, Shragg P, Kolterman OG: Role of hyperglucagonemia in maintenance of increased rates of hepatic glucose output in type II diabetics. *Diabetes* 1987; 36: 274–83.
335. Bjorntorp P. Metabolic implications of body fat distribution. *Diabetes Care* 1991; 14: 1132–43.
336. Arner P. Regional adipocity in man. *J Endocrinol* 1997; 155: 191–2.
337. Saltiel AR, Kahn CR. Insulin signaling and the regulation of glucose and lipid metabolism. *Nature* 2001; 414: 799–806.
338. Virkamaki A, Ueki K, Kahn CR. Protein–protein interaction in insulin signaling and the molecular mechanisms of insulin resistance. *J Clin Invest* 1999; 103: 931–43.
339. Pessin JE, Saltiel AR. Signaling pathways in insulin action: molecular targets of insulin resistance. *J Clin Invest* 2000; 106: 165–9.
340. Whitehead JP, Clark SF, Urso B, James DE. Signalling through the insulin receptor. *Curr Opin Cell Biol* 2000; 12: 222–8.
341. Wilden PA, Kahn CR. The level of insulin receptor tyrosine kinase activity modulates the activities of phosphatidylinositol 3-kinase, microtubule-associated protein, and S6 kinases. *Mol Endocrinol* 1994; 8: 558–67.
342. Haring HU, Mehnert H. Pathogenesis of type 2 (non-insulin-dependent) diabetes mellitus: candidates for a signal transmitter defect causing insulin resistance of the skeletal muscle. *Diabetologia* 1993; 36: 176–82.
343. Wajtaszewski JFP, Hansen BF, Kiens B, Richter EA. Insulin signaling in human skeletal muscle. Time course and effect of exercise. *Diabetes* 1997; 46: 1775–81.
344. Cushman SW, Wardzala LJ. Potential mechanism of insulin action on glucose transport in the isolated rat adipose cell. Apparent translocation of intracellular transport systems to the plasma membrane. *J Biol Chem* 1980; 255: 4758–62.
345. Shepherd PR, Kahn BB. Glucose transporters and insulin action. Implications for insulin resistance and diabetes mellitus. *N Engl J Med* 1999; 341: 248–57.
346. Holman GD, Kasuga M. From receptor to transporter: insulin signaling to glucose transport. *Diabetologia* 1997; 40: 991–1003.
347. Garvey WT. Insulin action and insulin resistance: diseases involving defects in insulin receptors, signal transduction, and the glucose transport effector system. *Am J Med* 1998; 105: 331–45.
348. Chou DK, Dull TJ, Russell DS, Gherzi R, Lebwohl D, Ullrich A, Rosen OM. Human insulin receptors mutated at the ATP-binding site lack protein tyrosine kinase activity and fail to mediate postreceptor effects of insulin. *J Biol Chem* 1987; 262: 1842–7.
349. Ebina Y, Araki E, Tiara F, Shimada F, Mari M, Craik CS, Siddle K, Pierce SB, Roth RA, Rutter WJ. Replacement of lysine residue 1030 in the putative ATP-binding region of the insulin receptor abolishes insulin and antibody-stimulated glucose uptake and receptor kinase activity. *Proc Natl Acad Sci USA* 1987; 84: 704–8.
350. Ellis LE, Clauser E, Morgan ME, Roth RA, Rutter WJ. Replacement of insulin receptor tyrosine residues 1162 and 1163 compromises insulin-stimulated kinase activity and uptake of 2-dexoyglucose. *Cell* 1986; 45: 721–32.
351. White MF, Livingston JN, Backer JM, Lauria V, Duli TJ, Ullrich A, Kahn DR. Mutation of the insulin receptor at tyrosine 960 inhibits signal transmission but does not affect its tyrosine kinase activity. *Cell* 1992; 54: 641–9.
352. Kerouz NJ, Horsch D, Pons S, Kahn CR. Differential regulation of insulin receptor substrates-1 and -2 (IRS-1 and IRS-2) and phosphatidylinositol 3-kinase isoforms in liver and muscle of the obese diabetic (*ob*/*ob*) mouse. *J Clin Invest* 1997; 100: 3164–72.
353. Baumann CA, Ribon V, Kanzaki M, Thurmond DC, Mora S, Shigematsu S, Bickel PE, Pessin JE, Saltiel AR. CAP defines a second signalling pathway required for insulin-stimulated glucose transport. *Nature* 2000; 407: 202–7.
354. Chiang SH, Baumann CA, Kanzaki M, Thurmond DC, Watson RT, Neudauer CL, Macara IG, Pessin JE, Saltiel AR. Insulin-stimulated GLUT-4 translocation requires the CAP-dependent activation of TC10. *Nature* 2001; 410: 944–8.
355. Backer JM, Myers MG Jr, Shoelson SE, Chin DJ, Sun XJ, Miralpeix M, Hu P, Margolis B, Skoinik EY, Schlessinger J, White MF. The phosphatidylinositol-3 kinase is activated by association with IRS-1 during insulin stimulation. *EMBO J* 1992; 11: 3469–79.
356. Sun XJ, Miralpeix M, Myers Jr MG, Glasheen EM, Backer JM, Kahn CR, White MF. The expression and function of IRS-1 in insulin signal transmission. *J Biol Chem* 1992; 267: 22662–72.
357. Ruderman N, Kapeller R, White MF, Cantley LC. Activation of phosphatidylinositol-3-kinase by insulin. *Proc Natl Acad Sci USA* 1990; 87: 1411–15.
358. Cross DA, Alessi DR, Cohen P, Andjelkovich M, Hemmings BA. Inhibition of glycogen synthase kinase-3 by insulin mediated by protein kinase B. *Nature* 1995; 378: 785–9.
359. Brady MJ, Nairn AC, Saltiel AR. The regulation of glycogen synthase by protein phosphatase 1 in 3T3-L1 adipocytes. Evidence for a potential role for DARPP-32 in insulin action. *J Biol Chem* 1997; 272: 29698–703.
360. Okada T, Sakuma L, Fukui Y, Hazeki O, Ui M. Essential role of phosphatidylinositol 3-kinase in insulin-induced glucose transport and antilipolysis in rat adipocytes. *J Biol Chem* 1994; 269: 3568–73.
361. Cheatham B, Viohos CJ, Cheatham L, Wang L, Blenis J, Kahn CR. Phosphatidylinositol 3-kinase activation is required for insulin stimulation of pp70 56 kinase, DNA synthesis and glucose transporter translocation. *Mol Cell Biol* 1994; 14: 4902–11.

362. Cross D, Alessi D, Vandenheed J, McDowell H, Hundal H, and Cohen P. The inhibition of glycogen synthase kinase-3 by insulin or insulin-like growth factor 1 in the rat skeletal muscle cell line L6 is blocked by wortmannin but not rapamycin. *Biochem J* 1994; 303: 21–6.
363. Sheperd P, Nave B, and Siddle K. Insulin stimulation of glycogen synthesis and glycogen syntase activity is blocked by wortmannin and rapamycin in 3T3L1 adipocytes. *Biochem J* 1995; 305: 25–8.
364. Osawa H, Sutherland C, Robey R, Printz R, Granner D. Analysis of the signaling pathway involved in the regulation of hexokinase II gene transcription by insulin. *J Biol Chem* 1996; 271: 16690–4.
365. Thomas G, Hall MN. TOR signalling and control of cell growth. *Curr Opin Cell Biol* 1997; 9: 782–7.
366. Nave BT, Ouwens M, Withers DJ, Alessi DR, Shepherd PR. Mammalian target of rapamycin is a direct target for protein kinase B: identification of a convergence point for opposing effects of insulin and amino-acid deficiency on protein translation. *Biochem J* 1999; 344 (pt 2): 427–31.
367. Miron M. Verdu J, Lachance PE, Birnbaum MJ, Lasko PF, Sonenberg N. The translational inhibitor 4E-BP is an effector of PI(3)K/Akt signalling and cell growth in Drosophila. *Nat Cell Biol* 2001; 3: 596–601.
368. Shimomura I. Bashmakov Y. Ikemoto S. Horton JD. Brown MS. Goldstein JL. Insulin selectively increases SREBP-1c mRNA in the livers of rats with streptozotocin-induced diabetes. *Proc Nat Acad Sci USA* 1999; 96: 13656–61.
369. Cusi K, Maezono K, Osman A, Pendergrass M, Patti ME, Pratipanawatr T, DeFronzo RA, Kahn CR, Mandarino LJ. Insulin resistance differentially affects the PI 3-kinase and MAP kinase-mediated signaling in human muscle. *J Clin Invest* 2000; 105: 311–20.
370. Hsueh WA, Law RE. Insulin signaling in the arterial wall. *Am J Cardiol* 1999; 84: 21J–4J.
371. Xi X-P, Graf K, Goetze S, HsuehWA, Law RE. Inhibition of MAP kinase blocks insulin-mediated DNA synthesis and transcriptional activation of c-*fos* by Elk-1 in vascular smooth muscle cells. *FEBS Lett* 1997; 417: 283–6.
372. Banskota NK, Taub R, Zellner K, King GL. Insulin, insulin-like growth factor I and platelet-derived growth factor interact additively in the induction of the protonocogene c-*myc* and cellular proliferation in cultured bovine aortic smooth muscle cells. *Mol Endocrinol* 1989; 3: 1183–90.
373. Boulton TG, Nye SH, Robbins DJ, Ip NY, Radziejewska E, Morgenbesser SD, DePinho RA, Panayotatos N, Cobb MH, Yancopoulos GD. ERKs: a family of protein-serine/threonine kinases that are activated and tyrosine phosphorylated in response to insulin and NGF. *Cell* 1991; 65: 663–75.
374. Lazar DF, Wiese RJ, Brady MJ, Mastick CC, Waters SB, Yamauchi K, Pessin JE, Cuatrecasas P, Saltiel AR. Mitogen-activated protein kinase kinase inhibition does not block the stimulation of glucose utilization by insulin. *J Biol Chem* 1995; 270: 20801–7.
375. Dorrestijn J, Ouwens DM, Van den Berghe N, Box JL, Maassen JA. Expression of dominant-negative *Ras* mutant does not affect stimulation of glucose uptake and glycogen synthesis by insulin. *Diabetologia* 1996; 39: 558–63.
376. Dent P, Lavoinne A, Nakielny S, Caudwell FB, Watt P, Cohen F. The molecular mechanisms by which insulin stimulates glycogen synthesis in mammalian skeletal muscle. *Nature* 1990; 348: 302–7.
377. Cohen P. The structure and regulation of protein phosphatases. *Annu Rev Biochem* 1989; 58: 453–508.
378. Newgard CB, Brady MJ, O'Doherty RB, Saltiel AR. Organizing glucose disposal. Emerging roles of the glycogen targeting subunits of protein phosphatase-1. *Diabetes* 2000; 49: 1967–77.
379. Sheperd PR, Nave BT, Siddle K. Insulin stimulation of glycogen synthesis and glycogen synthase activity is blocked by wortmannin and rapamycin in 3T3L1 adipocytes: evidence for the involvement of phosphoinositide 3 kinase and p70 ribosomal protein S6 kinase. *Biochem J* 1995; 305: 25–8.
380. Freidenberg GR, Henry RR, Klein HH, Reichart DR, Olefsky JM. Decreased kinase activity of insulin receptors from adipocytes of non-insulin-dependent diabetic studies. *J Clin Invest* 1987; 79: 240–50.
381. Thies RS, Molina JM, Ciaraldi TP, Freidenberg GR, Olefsky JM, Insulin-receptor autophosphorylation and endogenous substrate phosphorylation in human adipocytes from control, obese, and NIDDM subjects. *Diabetes* 1990; 39 (2): 250–9.
382. Caro JF, Sinha MK, Raju SM, Ittoop O, Pories WJ, Flickinger EG, Meelheim D, Dohm GL. Insulin receptor kinase in human skeletal muscle from obese subjects with and without non-insulin dependent diabetes. *J Clin Invest* 1987; 79: 1330–7.
383. Caro JF, Ittoop O, Pories WJ, Meelheim D, Flickinger EG, Thomas F, Jenquin M, Silverman JF, Khazanie PG, Sinha MK. Studies on the mechanism of insulin resistance in the liver from humans with non-insulin-dependent diabetes. Insulin action and binding in isolated hepatocytes, insulin receptor structure, and kinase activity. *J Clin Invest* 1986; 78: 249–58.
384. Molina JM, Ciaraldi TP, Brady D, Olefsky JM. Decreased activation rate of insulin-mediated glucose transport in adipocytes from obese and NIDDM subjects. *Diabetes* 1989; 38: 991–5.
385. Trichitta V, Brunetti A, Chiavetta A, Benzi L, Papa V, Vigneri R. Defects in insulin-receptor internalization and processing in monocytes of obese subjects and obese NIDDM patients. *Diabetes* 1989; 38: 1579–84.
386. Comi RJ, Grunberger G, Gorden P. Relationship of insulin binding and insulin-stimulated tyrosine kinase activity is altered in type II diabetes. *J Clin Invest* 1987; 79: 453–62.
387. Arner P, Pollare T, Lithell H, Livingston JN. Defective insulin receptor tyrosine kinase in human skeletal muscle in obesity and type II (non-insulin-dependent) diabetes mellitus. *Diabetologia* 1987; 30: 437–40.
388. Klein HH, Vestergaard H, Kotzke G, Pedersen O. Elevation of serum insulin concentration during euglycemic hyperinsulinemic clamp studies leads to similar activation of insulin receptor kinase in skeletal muscle of subjects with and without NIDDM. *Diabetes* 1995; 344: 1310–7.
389. Grasso G, Frittitta L, Anello M, Russo P, Sesti G, Trischitta V. Insulin receptor tyrosine-kinase activity is altered in both muscle and adipose tissue from non-obese normoglycaemic insulin-resistant subjects. *Diabetologia* 1995; 38: 55–61.
390. Obermaier-Kusser B, White MF, Pongratz DE, Su Z, Ermel B, Muhlbacher C, Haring HU. A defective intramolecular autoactivation cascade may cause the reduced kinase activity of the skeletal muscle insulin

receptor from patients with non-insulin-dependent diabetes mellitus. *J Biol Chem* 1989; 264: 9497–503.

391. Arner P, Einarsson K, Ewerth S, Livingston J. Studies on the human liver insulin receptor in non-insulin-dependent diabetes mellitus. *J Clin Invest* 1986; 77: 1716–8.
392. Kashiwagi A, Verso MA, Andrews J, Vasquez B, Reaven G, Foley JE. *In vitro* insulin resistance of human adipocytes isolated from subjects with non-insulin-dependent diabetes mellitus. *J Clin Invest* 1983; 72: 1246–54.
393. Lonnroth P, Digirolamo M, Krotkiewski M, Smith U. Insulin binding and responsiveness in fat cells from patients with reduced glucose tolerance and type II diabetes. *Diabetes* 1983; 32: 748–54.
394. Olefsky JM, Reaven GM. Insulin binding in diabetes. Relationships with plasma insulin levels and insulin sensitivity. *Diabetes* 1977; 26: 680–8.
395. Cocozza S, Procellini A, Riccardi G, Monticelli A, Condorelli G, Ferrara A, Pianese L, Miele C, Capaldo B, Beguinot F, Varrone S. NIDDM associated with mutation in tyrosine kinase domain of insulin receptor gene. *Diabetes* 1992; 41: 521–6.
396. Moller DE, Yakota A, Flier JS. Normal insulin receptor cDNA sequence in Pima Indians with non-insulin-dependent diabetes mellitus. *Diabetes* 1989; 38: 1496–500.
397. O'Rahilly S, Choi WH, Patel P, Turner RC, Flier JS, Moller DE. Detection of mutations in insulin-receptor gene in NIDDM patients by analysis of single-stranded conformation polymorphisms. *Diabetes* 1991; 40: 777–82.
398. Kusari J, Verma US, Buse JB, Henry RR, Olefsky JM. Analysis of the gene sequences of the insulin receptor and the insulin-sensitive glucose transporter (GLUT-4) in patients with common-type non-insulin-dependent diabetes mellitus. *J Clin Invest* 1991; 88: 1323–30.
399. Nyomba BL, Ossowski VM, Bogardus C, Mott DM. Insulin-sensitive tyrosine kinase relationship with in vivo insulin action in humans. *Am J Physiol* 1990; 258: E964–74.
400. Maegwa H, Shigeta Y, Egawa K, Kobayshai M. Impaired autophosphorylation of insulin receptors from abdominal skeletal muscles in non-obese subjects with NIDDM. *Diabetes* 1993; 40: 815–9.
401. Nolan JJ, Friedenberg G, Henry R, Reichart D, Olefsky JM. Role of human skeletal muscle insulin receptor kinase in the in vivo insulin resistance of noninsulin-dependent diabetes and obesity. *J Clin Endocrinol Metab* 1994; 78: 471–7.
402. Krook A, Bjornholm M, Galuska D, Jiang XJ, Fahlman R, Myers MG, Wallberg-Henriksson H, Zierath JR. Characterization of signal transduction and glucose transport in skeletal muscle from type 2 diabetic patients. *Diabetes* 2000; 49: 284–92.
403. Bak JF, Moller N, Schmitz O, Saaek A, Pedersen O. *In vivo* insulin action and muscle glycogen synthase activity in type 2 (non insulin dependent) diabetes mellitus: effects of diet treatment. *Diabetologia* 1992; 35: 777–94.
404. Freidenberg GR, Reichart D, Olefsky JM, Henry RR. Reversibility of defective adipocyte insulin receptor kinase activity in non-insulin dependent diabetes mellitus. Effect of weight loss. *J Clin Invest* 1988; 82: 1398–406.
405. Kellerer M, Kroder G, Tippmer S, Berti L, Kiehn L, Mosthaf L, Haring H. Troglitazone prevents glucose-induced insulin resistance of insulin receptor in rat-1 fibroblasts. *Diabetes* 1994; 43: 447–53.
406. Pratipanawatr W, Pratipanawatr T, Cusi K, Berria R, Adams JM, Jenkinson CP, Maezono K, DeFronzo RA, Mandarino LJ. Skeletal muscle insulin resistance in normoglycemic subjects with a strong family history of type 2 diabetes is associated with decreased insulin-stimulated insulin receptor substrate-1 tyrosine phosphorylation. *Diabetes* 2001; 50: 2572–8.
407. Laville M, Auboeuf D, Khalfallah Y, Vega N, Riou JP, Vidal H. Acute regulation by insulin of phosphatidylinositol-3-kinase, Rad, Glut 4. and lipoprotein lipase in mRNA levels in human muscle. *J Clin Invest* 1996; 98: 43–9.
408. Kim Y-B, Nikoulina S, Ciaraldi TP, Henry RR, Kahn BB. Normal insulin-dependent activation of Akt/protein kinase B, with diminished activation of phosphoinositide 3-kinase, in muscle in type 2 diabetes. *J Clin Invest* 1999; 104: 733–41.
409. Andreelli F, Laville M, Ducluzeau P-H, Vega N, Vallier P, Khalfallah Y, Riou J-P, Vidal H. Defective regulation of phosphatidylinositol-3-kinase gene expression in skeletal muscle and adipose tissue of non-insulin-dependent diabetes mellitus patients. *Diabetologia* 1999; 42: 358–64.
410. Folli F, Saad JA, Backer JM, Kahn CR. Regulation of phosphatidylinositol 3-kinase activity in liver and muscle of animal models of insulin-resistant and insulin-deficient diabetes mellitus. *J Clin Invest* 1993; 92: 1787–94.
411. Imai Y, Philippe N, Accili D, Taylor SI. Expression of variant forms of insulin receptor substrate-1 identified in patients with noninsulin dependent diabetes mellitus. *J Clin Endocrinol Metab* 1997; 82: 4201–7.
412. Hitman GA, Hawrammi K, McCarthy MI, Viswanathan M, Snehalatha C, Ramachandran A, Tuomilehto J, Tumilehto-Wolf E, Nissenen A, Pedersen O. Insulin receptor substrate-1 gene mutations in NIDDM: implication for the study of polygenic disease. *Diabetologia* 1995; 38: 481–6.
413. Pratley RE, Thompson DB, Prochazka M, Baier L, Mott D, Ravussin E, Sakul H, Ehm MG, Burns DK, Foroud T, Garvey WT, Hanson RL, Knowler WC, Bennett PH, Bogardus C. An autosomal genomic scan for loci linked to prediabetic phenotypes in Pima Indians. *J Clin Invest* 1998; 101: 1757–64.
414. Jiang ZY, Lin YW, Clemont A, Feener EP, Hein KD, Igarashi M, Yamauchi T, White MF, King GL. Characterization of selective resistance to insulin signaling in the vasculature of obese Zucker (*fa/fa*) rats. *J Clin Invest* 1999; 104: 447–57.
415. Sasaoka T, Draznin B, Leitner JW, Langlois WJ, Olefsky JM. Shc is the predominant signaling molecule coupling insulin receptors to activation of guanine nucleotide releasing factor and p21ras-GTP formation. *J Biol Chem* 1994; 269: 10734–8.
416. De Fea K, Roth RA. Modulation of insulin receptor substrate-1 tyrosine phosphorylation and function by mitogen-activated protein kinase. *J Biol Chem* 1997; 272: 31400–6.
417. Dunaif A, Xia J, Book CB, Schenker E, Tang Z. Excessive insulin receptor serine phosphorylation in cultured fibroblasts and in skeletal muscle. A potential mechanism for insulin resistance in the polycystic ovary syndrome. *J Clin Invest* 1995; 96: 801–10.
418. Kono T, Robinson FW, Blevins TL, Ezaki O. Evidence that translocation of the glucose transport activity is the

major mechanism of insulin action on glucose transport fat cells. *J Biol Chem* 1982; 257: 10942–7.

419. Bell GI, Kayano T, Buse JB, Burant CF, Takeda J, Lin D, Fikomoto H, Seino S. Molecular biology of mammalian glucose transporters. *Diabetes Care* 1990; 13: 198–200.
420. Joost H-G, Bell GI, Best JD, Birnbaum MJ, Charron MJ, Chen YT, Doege H, James DE, Lodish HF, Moley KH, Moley JF, Mueckler M, Rogers S, Schurmann A, Seino S, Thorens B. Nomenclature of the GLUT/SLC2A family of sugar/polyol transport facilitators. *Am J Physiol Endocrinol Metab* 2002; 282: E974–6.
421. Colowick SP. The hexokinases. In Boyer PD (ed) *The Enzymes, Vol 9.* New York: Academic Press, 1973; pp 1–48.
422. Printz RL, Koch S, Potter LR, O'Doherty RM, Tiesinga JJ, Moritz S, Granner DK. Hexokinase II mRNA and gene structure, regulation by insulin, and evolution. *J Biol Chem* 1993; 268: 5209–19.
423. Rogers PA, Fisher RA, Harris H. An electrophoretic study of the distribution and properties of human hexokinases. *Biochem Genet* 1975; 13: 857–66.
424. Magnuson MA, Andreone IL, Printz RL, Koch S, Granner DK. The glucokinase gene: structure and regulation by insulin. *Proc Natl Acad Sci USA* 1989; 86: 4838–42.
425. Mandarino LJ, Campbell PJ, Gottesman IS, Gerich JE. Abnormal coupling of insulin receptor binding in non-insulin-dependent diabetes. *Am J Physiol* 1984; 247: E688–92.
426. Garvey WT, Hueckstead TP, Mattaei S, Olefsky JM. Role of glucose transporters in the cellular insulin resistance of type II non-insulin dependent diabetes mellitus. *J Clin Invest* 1988; 81: 1528–36.
427. Carey JO, Azevedo JL Jr, Morris PG, Pories WJ, Dohn GL. Okadaic acid, vanadate and phenylarsine oxide stimulate 2-deoxyglucose transport in insulin-resistant human skeletal muscle. *Diabetes* 1995; 44: 682–8.
428. Jackson S, Bagstaff SM, Lynn S, Yeaman SJ, Turnbull DM, Walker M. Decreased insulin responsiveness of glucose uptake in cultured human skeletal muscle cells from insulin-resistant nondiabetic relatives of type 2 diabetic families. *Diabetes* 2000; 49: 1169–77.
429. Zierath JR, He L, Guma A, Odegoard Wahlstrom E, Klip A, Wallenberg-Henriksson H. Insulin action on glucose transport and plasma membrane GLUT-4 content in skeletal muscle from patients with NIDDM. *Diabetologia* 1996; 39: 1180–9.
430. Krook A, Bjornholm M, Galuska D, Jiang XJ, Fahlman R, Myers MG, Wallenberg-Henriksson H, Zierath JR. Characterization of signal transduction and glucose transport in skeletal muscle from type 2 diabetic patients. *Diabetes* 2000; 49: 284–2.
431. Andreasson K, Galuska D, Thorne T, Sonnenfeld T, Wallberg-Henriksson H. Decreased insulin-stimulated 3-*O*-methylglucose transport in *in vitro* incubated muscle strips from type II diabetic subjects. *Acta Physiol Scan* 1991; 142: 255–60.
432. Ciaraldi TP, Abrams L, Nikoulina S, Mudaliar S, Henry RR. Glucose transport in cultured human skeletal muscle cells. *J Clin Invest* 1995; 96: 2820–7.
433. Kahn BB, Shulman GI, DeFronzo RA, Cushman SW, Rossetti L. Normalization of blood glucose in diabetic rats with phlorizin treatment reverses insulin-resistant glucose transport in adipose cells without restoring glucose transporter gene expression. *J Clin Invest* 1991; 87: 561–70.
434. Pedersen O, Bak J, Andersen P, Lund S, Moller DE, Flier JS, Kahn BB. Evidence against altered expression of GLUT-1 or GLUT-4 in skeletal muscle of patients with obesity or NIDDM. *Diabetes* 1990; 39: 865–70.
435. Eriksson J, Koranyi L, Bourey R, Schalin-Jantti C, Widen E, Mueckler M, Permutt AM, Groop LC. Insulin resistance in type 2 (non-insulin-dependent) diabetic patients and their relatives is not associated with a defect in the expression of the insulin-responsive glucose transporter (GLUT-4) gene in human skeletal muscle. *Diabetologia* 1992; 35: 143–7.
436. Schalin-Jantti C, Yki-Jarvinen H, Koranyi L, Bourey R, Lindstrom J, Nikula-Ijas P, Franssila-Kallunki A, Groop LC. Effect of insulin on GLUT-4 mRNA and protein concentrations in skeletal muscle of patients with NIDDM and their first-degree relatives. *Diabetologia* 1994; 37: 401–7.
437. Garvey WT, Maianu L, Hancock JA, Golichowski AM, Baron A. Gene expression of GLUT-4 in skeletal muscle from insulin-resistant patients with obesity, IGT, GDM, and NIDDM. *Diabetes* 1992; 41: 465–75.
438. Mandarino LJ, Printz RL, Cusi KA, Kinchington P, O'Doherty RM, Osawa H, Sewell C, Consoli A, Granner DK, DeFronzo RA. Regulation of hexokinase II and glycogen synthase mRNA, protein, and activity in human muscle. *Am J Physiol* 1995; 269: E701–8.
439. Kusari J, Verma US, Buse JB, Henry RR, Olefsky JM. Analysis of the gene sequences of the insulin receptor and the insulin-sensitive glucose transporter (GLUT-4) in patients with common type non insulin dependent diabetes mellitus. *J Clin Invest* 1991; 88: 1323–30.
440. Choi WH, O'Rahilly S, Rees A, Morgan R, Flier JS, Moller DE. Molecular scanning of the insulin-responsive glucose transporter (GLUT 4) gene in patients with non-insulin dependent diabetes mellitus. *Diabetes* 1991; 40: 1712–8.
441. Sinha M, Raineri-Maldonado C, Buchanan C, Pories W, Carter-Su C, Pilch P, Caro J. Adipose tissue glucose transporters in NIDDM: decreased levels of muscle/fat isoform. *Diabetes* 1991; 40: 474–7.
442. Guma A, Zierath JR, Wallberg-Henriksson H, Klip A. Insulin induces translocation of GLUT-4 glucose transporters in human skeletal muscle. *Am J Physiol* 1995; 268: E613–22.
443. Goodyear LJ, Hirschman MF, Napoli R, Calles J, Markuns JF, Ljungqvist O, Horton ES. Glucose ingestion causes GLUT-4 translocation in human skeletal muscle. *Diabetes* 1996; 45: 1051–6.
444. Kelley DE, Mintun MA, Watkins SC, Simoneau J-A, Jadali F, Fredrickson A. The effect of non-insulin-dependent diabetes mellitus and obesity on glucose transport and phosphorylation in skeletal muscle. *J Clin Invest* 1996; 97: 2705–13.
445. Kelley DE, Mintun MA, Watkins SC, Simoneau J-A, Jadali F, Fredrickson A, Beattie J, Theriault R. The effect of non-insulin-dependent diabetes mellitus and obesity on glucose transport and phosphorylation in skeletal muscle. *J Clin Invest* 1996; 97: 2705–13.
446. Saccomani MP, Bonadonna RC, Bier DM, DeFronzo RA, Cobelli C. A model to measure insulin effects on glucose transport and phosphorylation in muscle: a three-tracer study. *Am J Physiol 270 Endocrinol Metab* 1996; 33: E170–85.
447. Bonadonna RC, Saccomani MP, Seely L, Zych KS, Ferrannini E, Cobelli C, DeFronzo RA. Glucose transport

in human skeletal muscle. The *in vivo* response to insulin. *Diabetes* 1993; 42: 191–8.
448. Bonadonna RC, Del Prato S, Saccomani MP, Bonora E, Gulli G, Ferrannini E, Bier D, Cobelli C, DeFronzo RA. Transmembrane glucose transport in skeletal muscle of patients with non-insulin-dependent diabetes. *J Clin Invest* 1993; 92: 486–94.
449. Bonadonna RC, Del Prato S, Bonora E, Saccomani MP, Gulli G, Natali A, Frascerra S, Pecro N, Ferrannini E, Bier D, Cobelli C, DeFronzo RA. Roles of glucose transport and glucose phosphorylation in muscle insulin resistance of NIDDM. *Diabetes* 1996; 45: 915–25.
450. Napoli R, Hirschman MF, Horton FS. Mechanisms of increased skeletal muscle glucose transport activity after an oral glucose load in rats. *Diabetes* 1995; 44: 1362–8.
451. Cline GW, Petersen KF, Krssak M, Shen J, Hundal RS, Trajanoski Z, Inzucchi S, Dresner A, Rothman DL, Shulman GI. Impaired glucose transport as a cause of decreased insulin stimulated muscle glycogen synthesis in type 2 diabetes. *N Engl J Med* 1999; 341: 240–6.
452. Williams KV, Price JC, Kelley DE. Interactions of impaired glucose transport and phosphorylation in skeletal muscle insulin resistance. A dose–response assessment using positron emission tomography. *Diabetes* 2001; 50: 2069–79.
453. Perriott LM, Kono T, Whitesell RR, Knobel SM, Piston DW, Granner DK, Powers AC, May JM. Glucose uptake and metabolism by cultured human skeletal muscle cells: rate-limiting steps. *Am J Physiol Endocrinol Metab* 2001; 281: E72–80.
454. Printz RL, Ardehali H, Koch S, Granner DK. Human hexokinase II mRNA and gene structure. *Diabetes* 1995; 44: 290–4.
455. Postic CA, Leturque A, Rencurel F, Printz R, Forest C, Granner D, Girard J. The effects of hyperinsulinemia and hyperglycemia on GLUT-4 and hexokinase II mRNA and protein in rat skeletal muscle and adipose tissue. *Diabetes* 1993; 42: 922–9.
456. Jones JP, Dohn GL. Regulation of glucose transporter GLUT-4 and hexokinase II gene transcription by insulin and epinephrine. *Am J Physiol: Endocrinol Metab* 1997; 36: E682–7.
457. Kruszynska YT, Mulford MI, Baloga J, Yu JG, Olefsky JM. Regulation of skeletal muscle hexokinase II by insulin in nondiabetic and NIDDM subjects. *Diabetes* 1998; 47: 1107–13.
458. Vogt C, Ardehali H, Iozzo P, Yki-Jarvinen H, Koval J, Maezono K, Pendergrass M, Printz R, Granner D, DeFronzo R, Mandarino L. Regulation of hexokinase II expression in human skeletal muscle *in vivo*. *Metabolism* 2000; 49: 814–8.
459. Vogt C, Yki-Jarvinen H, Iozzo P, Pipek R, Pendergrass M, Koval J, Ardehali H, Printz R, Granner D, DeFronzo RA, Mandarino L. Effects of insulin on subcellular localization of hexokinase II in human skeletal muscle *in vivo*. *J Clin Endocrinol Metab* 1998; 83: 230–4.
460. Pendergrass M, Fazioni E, Saccomani MP, Collins D, Bonadonna R, Gulli G. *In vivo* glucose transport and phosphorylation in skeletal muscle is impaired in insulin resistant, normal glucose tolerant offspring of two NIDDM parents. *Diabetes* 1995; 44 (suppl 1): 197A.
461. Rothman DL, Shulman RG, Shulman GI. ^{31}P nuclear magnetic resonance measurements of muscle glucose-6-phosphate. Evidence for reduced insulin-dependent muscle glucose transport or phosphorylation activity in non-insulin-dependent diabetes mellitus. *J Clin Invest* 1992; 89: 1069–75.
462. Halseth AE, Bracy DP, Wasserman DH. Overexpression of hexokinse II increases insulin- and exercise-stimulated muscle glucose uptake in vivo. *Am J Physiol* 1999; 276: E70–7.
463. Pendergrass M, Koval J, Vogt C, Yki-Jarvinen H, Iozzo P, Pipek R, Ardehali H, Printz R, Granner D, DeFronzo RA, Mandarino L. Insulin-induced hexokinase II expression is reduced in obesity and NIDDM. *Diabetes* 1998; 47: 387–94.
464. Vestergaard H, Bjorbaek C, Hansen T, Larsen FS, Granner DK, Pedersen O. Impaired activity and gene expression of hexokinase II in muscle from non-insulin-dependent diabetes mellitus patients. *J Clin Invest* 1995; 96: 2639–45.
465. Ducluzeau P-H, Perretti N, Laville M, Andreelli F, Vega N, Riou J-P, Vidal H. Regulation by insulin of gene expression in human skeletal muscle and adipose tissue. Evidence for specific defects in type 2 diabetes. *Diabetes* 2001; 50: 1134–42.
466. Lehto M, Huang X, Davis EM, Le Beau MM, Laurila E, Eriksson KF, Bell GI, Groop L. Human hexokinase II gene: exon–intron organization, mutation screening in NIDDM, and its relationship to muscle hexokinase activity. *Diabetologia* 1995; 38: 1466–74.
467. Laakso M, Malkki M, Kekalainen P, Kuusito J, Deeb SS. Polymorphisms of the human hexokinase II gene: lack of association with NIDDM and insulin resistance. *Diabetologia* 1995; 38: 617–22.
468. Echwald SM, Bjorbaek C, Hansen T, Clausen JO, Vestergaard H, Zierath JR, Printz RL, Granner DK, Pedersen O. Identification of four amino acid substitutions in hexokinase II and studies of relationships to NIDDM, glucose effectiveness, and insulin sensitivity. *Diabetes* 1995; 44: 347–53.
469. Thiebaud D, Jacot E, DeFronzo RA, Maeder E, Jequier E, Felber JP. The effect of graded doses of insulin on total glucose uptake, glucose oxidation, and glucose storage in man. *Diabetes* 1982; 31: 957–63.
470. Young A, Bogardus C, Wolfe-Lopez D, Mott D. Muscle glycogen synthesis and disposition of infused glucose in humans with reduced rates of insulin-mediated carbohydrate storage. *Diabetes* 1988; 37: 303–7.
471. Natali A, Buzzigoli G, Taddei S, Santoro D, Cerri M, Pedrinelli R, Ferrannini E. Effects of insulin on hemodynamics and metabolism in human forearm. *Diabetes* 1990; 39: 490–8.
472. Avogaro A, Toffolo G, Miola M, Valerio A, Tiengo A, Cobelli C, Del Prato S. Intracellular lactate- and pyruvate-interconversion rates are increased in muscle tissue of non-insulin-dependent diabetic individuals. *J Clin Invest* 1996; 98: 108–15.
473. Del Prato S, Bonadonna RC, Bonora E, Gulli G, Solini A, Shank M, DeFronzo RA. Characterization of cellular defects of insulin action in type 2 (non-insulin-dependent) diabetes mellitus. *J Clin Invest* 1993; 91: 484–94.
474. Bonadonna RC, Groop L, Kraemer N. Ferrannini E, Del Prato S, DeFronzo RA. Obesity and insulin resistance in man. A dose response study. *Metabolism* 1990; 39: 452–9.
475. Mandarino LJ, Consoli A, Kelley DE, Reilly JP, Nurjhan N. Fasting hyperglycemia normalizes oxidative and nonoxidative pathways of insulin-stimulated glucose

metabolism in non-insulin-dependent diabetes mellitus. *J Clin Endocrinol Metab* 1990; 71: 1544–51.

476. Kelley DE, Mandarino LJ. Hyperglycemia normalizes insulin-stimulated skeletal muscle glucose oxidation and storage in noninsulin-dependent diabetes mellitus. *J Clin Invest* 1990; 86: 1999–2007.
477. Bogardus C, Lillioja A, Stone K, Mott D. Correlation of muscle glycogen synthase activity and in vivo insulin action in man. *J Clin Invest* 1984; 73: 1185–90.
478. Rothman DL, Magnusson I, Cline G, Gerard D, Kahn CR, Shulman RG, Shulman GI. Decreased muscle glucose transport/phosphorylation is an early defect in the pathogenesis of non-insulin-dependent diabetes mellitus. *Proc Natl Acad Sci USA* 1995; 92: 983–7.
479. Vaag A, Henriksen JE, Beck-Nielsen. Decreased insulin activation of glycogen synthase in skeletal muscles in young non-obese Caucasian first-degree relatives of patients with non-insulin-dependent diabetes mellitus. *J Clin Invest* 1992; 89: 782–8.
480. Schalin-Jantti C, Harkonen M, Groop LC. Impaired activation of glycogen synthase in people at increased risk for developing NIDDM. *Diabetes* 1992; 41: 598–604.
481. Yki-Jarvinen H, Mott D, Young AA, Stone K, Bogardus C. Regulation of glycogen synthase and phosphorylase activity by glucose and insulin in human skeletal muscle. *J Clin Invest* 1987; 80: 95–100.
482. Frame S, Cohen P. GSK3 takes centre stage more than 20 years after its discovery. *Biochem J* 2001; 359 (pt 1): 1–16.
483. Cohen P. The Croonian Lecture 1999. Identification of a protein kinase cascade of major importance in insulin signal transduction. *Philos Trans R Soc Lond, Ser B: Biol Sci* 1999; 354: 485–95.
484. Stralfors P, Hiraga A, Cohen P. The protein phosphatases involved in cellular regulation: purification and characterization of the glycogen-bound form of protein phosphatase-1 from rabbit skeletal muscle. *Eur J Biochem* 1985; 149: 295–303.
485. Hubbard MJ, Cohen P. Regulation of protein phosphatase-1G from rabbit skeletal muscle. *Eur J Biochem* 1989; 186: 711–6.
486. Sutherland C, Campbell DG, Cohen P. Identification of insulin-stimulated protein kinase-1 as the rabbit equivalent of rsk-mo-2. *Eur J Biochem* 1993; 212: 581–8.
487. Vestergaard H, Lund S, Bjorbaek C, Pedersen O. Unchanged gene expression of glycogen synthase in muscle from patients with NIDDM following sulfonylurea-induced improvement of glycaemic control. *Diabetologia* 1995; 38: 1230–8.
488. Damsbo P, Vaag A, Hother-Nielsen O, Beck-Nielsen H. Reduced glycogen synthase activity in skeletal muscle from obese patients with and without type 2 (non-insulin-dependent) diabetes mellitus. *Diabetologia* 1991; 34: 239–45.
489. Mandarino LJ, Wright KS, Verity LS, Nichols J, Bell JM, Kolterman OG, Beck-Nielsen H. Effects of insulin infusion on human skeletal muscle pyruvate dehydrogenase, phosphofructokinase, and glycogen synthase. Evidence for their role in oxidative glucose metabolism. *J Clin Invest* 1987; 80: 655–63.
490. Thorburn AW, Gumbiner B, Bulacan F, Wallace P, Henry RR. Intracellular glucose oxidation and glycogen synthase activity are reduced in non-insulin-dependent (type II) diabetes independent of impaired glucose uptake. *J Clin Invest* 1990; 85: 522–9.
491. Mandarino LJ, Consoli A, Jain A, Kelley DE. Interaction of carbohydrate and fat fuels in human skeletal muscle: impact of obesity and NIDDM. *Am J Physiol* 1996; 270: E463–70.
492. Johnson AB, Argraki M, Thow JC, Jones IR, Broughton D, Miller M, Taylor R. Impaired activation of skeletal muscle glycogen synthase in non-insulin-dependent diabetes mellitus is unrelated to degree of obesity. *Metabolism* 1991; 40: 252–60.
493. Nikoulina SE, Ciaraldi TP, Mudaliar S, Mohideen P, Carter L, Henry RR. Potential role of glycogen synthase kinase-3 in skeletal muscle insulin resistance of type 2 diabetes. *Diabetes* 2000; 49: 263–71.
494. Henry RR, Ciaraldi TP, Abrams-Carter L, Mudaliar S, Park KS, Nikoulina SE. Glycogen synthase activity is reduced in cultured skeletal muscle cells of non-insulin-dependent diabetes mellitus subjects. *J Clin Invest* 1996; 98: 1231–6.
495. Wells AM, Sutcliffe IC, Johnson AB, Taylor R. Abnormal activation of glycogen synthesis in fibroblasts from NIDDM subjects. Evidence for an abnormality specific to glucose metabolism. *Diabetes* 1993; 42: 583–9.
496. Huang X, Vaag A, Hansson M, Weng J, Laurila E, Groop L. Impaired insulin-stimulate expression of the glycogen synthase gene in skeletal muscle of type 2 diabetic patients is acquired rather than inherited. *J Clin Endocrinol Metab* 2000; 85: 1584–90.
497. Nyomba BL, Freymond D, Raz I, Stone K, Mott DM, Bogardus C. Skeletal muscle glycogen synthase activity in subjects with non-insulin-dependent diabetes mellitus after glyburide therapy. *Metabolism* 1990; 39: 1204–10.
498. Pratipanawatr T, Cusi K, Ngo P, Pratipanawatr W, Mandarino LJ, DeFronzo RA. Normalization of plasma glucose concentration by insulin therapy improves insulin-stimulated glycogen synthesis in type 2 diabetes. *Diabetes* 2002; 51: 462–8.
499. Vestergaard H, Lund S, Larsen FS, Bjerrum OJ, Pedersen O. Glycogen synthase and phosphofructokinase protein and mRNA levels in skeletal muscle from insulin-resistant patients with non-insulin-dependent diabetes mellitus. *J Clin Invest* 1993; 91: 2342–50.
500. Vestergaard H, Bjocbaek C, Andersen PH, Bak JF, Pedersen O. Impaired expression of glycogen synthase mRNA in skeletal muscle of NIDDM patients. *Diabetes* 1991; 40: 1740–5.
501. Browner MF, Nakano K, Bang AG, Fleffenzk RJ. Human muscle glycogen synthase with DNA sequence: a negatively charged protein with asymmetric charge distribution. *Proc Natl Acad Sci USA* 1989; 86: 1443–7.
502. Kuroyama H, Sanke T, Ohagi S, Furuta M, Nanjo K. Simple tandem repeat DNA polymorphism in the human glycogen synthase gene is associated with NIDDM in Japanese subjects. *Diabetologia* 1994; 37: 536–9.
503. Zouali H, Velho G, Froguel P. Polymorphism of the glycogen synthase gene and non-insulin-dependent diabetes mellitus. *N Engl J Med* 1993; 328: 1568.
504. Groop LC, Kankuri M, Schalin-Jantti, Ekstrand A, Nikul-Ijas P, Widen E, Kusimanen E, Eriksson J, Franssila-Kallunki A, Saloranta C, Koskimies S. Association between polymorphism of the glycogen synthase gene and non-insulin-dependent diabetes mellitus. *N Engl J Med* 1993; 328: 10–4.
505. Majer M, Mott DM, Mochizuki H, Rowles JC, Pederson O, Knowler WC, Bogardus C, Prochazka M. Association

of the glycogen synthase locus on 19q13 with NIDDM in Pima Indians. *Diabetologia* 1996; 39: 314–21.

506. Orho M, Nikua-Ijas P, Schalin-Jantti C, Permutt MA, Groop LC. Isolation and characterization of the human muscle glycogen synthase gene. *Diabetes* 1995; 44: 1099–105.

507. Bjorbaek C, Echward SM, Hubricht P, Vestergaard H, Hansen T, Zierath J, Pedersen O. Genetic variants in promoters and coding regions of the muscle glycogen synthase and the insulin-responsive GLUT4 genes in NIDDM. *Diabetes* 1994; 43: 976–83.

508. Bjorbaek C, Fik TA, Echward SM, Yang P-Y, Vestergaard H, Wang JP, Webb GC, Richmond K, Hansen T, Erikson RL, Miklos GLG, Cohen PTW, Pedersen O. Cloning of human insulin-stimulated protein kinase (ISPK-1) gene and analysis of coding regions and mRNA levels of the ISPK-1 and the protein phosphatase-1 genes in muscle from NIDDM patients. *Diabetes* 1995; 44: 90–7.

509. Chen YH, Hansen L, Chen MX, Bjorbaek C, Vestergaard H, Hansen T, Cohen PTW, Pederson O. Sequence of the human glycogen-associated regulatory subunit of type 1 protein phosphatase and analysis of its coding region and mRNA level in muscle from patients with NIDDM. *Diabetes* 1994; 43: 1234–41.

510. Procharzka M, Michizuki H, Baier LJ, Cohen PTW, Bogardus C. Molecular and linkage analysis of type-1 protein phosphatase catalytic beta-subunit gene: lack of evidence for its major role in insulin resistance in Pima Indians. *Diabetologia* 1995; 38: 461–6.

511. Falholt K, Jensen I, Lindkaer Jensen S, Mortensen HB, Volund A, Heding LG, Norskov Petersen P, Falholt W. Carbohydrate and lipid metabolism of skeletal muscle in type 2 diabetic patients. *Diabet Med* 1988; 5: 27–31.

512. Mandarino LJ, Madar Z, Kolterman OG, Bell JM, Olefsky JM. Adipocyte glycogen synthase and pyruvate dehydrogenase in obese and type II diabetic patients. *Am J Physiol* 1986; 251: E489–96.

513. Kelley D, Mokan M, Mandarino L. Intracellular defects in glucose metabolism in obese patients with non-insulin-dependent diabetes mellitus. *Diabetes* 1992; 41: 698–706.

23

Genome Scans of Type 2 Diabetes Mellitus

Sue Rutherford, Alan R. Shuldiner, and Braxton D. Mitchell

University of Maryland School of Medicine, Baltimore, MD, USA

INTRODUCTION

A genetic susceptibility to type 2 diabetes is well recognized on the basis of twin studies showing higher concordance rates for the disease in monozygotic compared to dizygotic twin pairs [1, 2] and family studies showing a higher than expected prevalence of disease among family members of affected index cases [3–5]. However, identifying the specific mutations that are associated with diabetes is a formidable challenge. It is believed that mutations in several (many) different genes can influence susceptibility to the disease, both singly and in combination. Moreover, the expression of these mutations is likely to be influenced by the presence of nongenetic risk factors. The critical role of environment is illustrated by the fact that diabetes incidence is increasing sharply throughout the world [6], a trend that appears to be the result of changing dietary patterns and an increasingly sedentary lifestyle. These lifestyle changes are believed to produce a metabolic milieu that is conducive to the development of diabetes in genetically susceptible individuals.

Because there is no one-to-one correspondence between genotype and phenotype for diabetes, multiple strategies are used to identify specific diabetes susceptibility mutations. One commonly used approach (the *candidate gene approach*) is to concentrate on variants within candidate genes chosen based upon their known or presumed relevance to glucose metabolism. To date, numerous candidate genes have been identified and analyzed, but with the possible exception of the Pro12Ala variant of peroxisome proliferator activated receptor-γ2 (*PPAR*γ*2*) [7–10], none so far have been shown to confer substantial risk on the common forms of type 2 diabetes [11] (also see Chapter 24).

The emerging availability of large-scale genotyping technologies and more sophisticated statistical models has led in recent years to analytic approaches that are genome-wide (as opposed to candidate gene-wide) in scope. Because coverage of the genome is complete, the analysis proceeds without an *a priori* hypothesis regarding the location, function, or number of susceptibility gene(s). These strategies involve the use of 300–500 highly polymorphic short tandem repeat markers that are dispersed throughout the genome in known locations to enable a systematic analysis across the entire genome. Current strategies are geared toward detecting linkage of one or more of these genetic markers with a putative disease-causing mutation. Such genome-wide linkage studies (also referred to as *genome-wide scans*) are carried out in families since there exists established statistical approaches for systematically evaluating distances between genetic markers spaced at 5–10 megabase (Mb) intervals along the same chromosome. From this perspective, linkage analysis can be viewed as a method for tracking co-segregation within families between two genetic markers, one whose location is known (the *marker* locus) and the other whose location is unknown (the *disease* locus). If co-segregation is observed (as evidenced by the absence of recombination), this is taken to be evidence that the putative disease susceptibility locus must be located in physical proximity (or linked) to the genetic marker. Only by being in close physical proximity would the two loci be transmitted together from parents to offspring.

In this chapter we will provide a summary of these results. But first, we will present a brief description of linkage analysis and genome-wide scans and offer a few guidelines on their interpretation.

International Textbook of Diabetes Mellitus, Third Edition. Edited by R. A. DeFronzo, E. Ferrannini, H. Keen, and P. Zimmet.
 ISBN: 0-471-48655-8.

Approaches to Linkage Analysis

There are two general approaches to linkage analysis, and both have been used in studies of type 2 diabetes to localize disease susceptibility genes. The first of these approaches is the traditional parametric approach, for which the hypothesis of linkage is evaluated in the context of a fairly explicit set of assumptions regarding the transmission of diabetes and the penetrance of the disease. In contrast to this heavily model-based approach, is one based on allele-sharing methods, which require far fewer assumptions about the genetic model. A brief description of each follows.

The traditional parametric approach to linkage analysis is based on estimating the number of recombinations between alleles at an observed marker locus and a putative allele at the disease locus, whose presence is inferred. A very specific genetic model must be assumed so that the transmission probabilities of the putative disease gene can be inferred conditional on the observed phenotype. The simplest genetic models require knowledge of the penetrance of the disease given the transmitted genotype. Sometimes the validity of these model assumptions can be evaluated by statistical modeling of the pattern of disease transmission in families without consideration of genetic marker information (a modeling approach known as *segregation analysis*). Regardless, for parametric linkage analysis, one calculates the likelihood of the pedigree data given linkage (i.e., co-segregation between the disease and marker loci) and compares that to the likelihood of the data assuming no linkage (i.e., no co-segregation). More complex models (e.g., mixed models) allow for residual genetic effects, over and above that of the linked disease locus. When the estimates of model parameters are accurate, parametric methods may provide great statistical power to detect linkage.

The classical penetrance model–based approach has worked well for simple Mendelian diseases for which it is relatively easy to make assumptions about the disease penetrance. However, this approach has in general worked less well for complex genetic diseases, such as diabetes, cardiovascular disease, hypertension, and obesity, which are likely to be influenced by multiple genetic loci, and that have complex modes of inheritance.

Allele-sharing approaches to linkage analysis, in contrast, are much simpler in concept than the parametric-based approaches and are based on the simple idea that under linkage, there will be a correspondence between similarity of the phenotypes and genotypes between related individuals. The similarity in genotypes is assessed by the number of alleles that a pair of related individuals will share at a particular genetic locus. Thus, unlike parametric analysis, no assumptions regarding the mode of inheritance or penetrance are required. There are essentially two flavors of linkage analysis that utilize this allele-sharing principle: one that is based on analysis of affected pedigree members (APM); and the second that is based on all pedigree members (affected and unaffected). In APM analysis (of which affected sib pair analysis is a subset), one tests the hypothesis that affected individuals share more alleles with each other than would be expected on the basis of their biological relationship. For example, for an unlinked locus, affected (diabetic) sib pairs should share 50% of their alleles in common by chance. Allele-sharing at a particular locus that is in excess of 50% would provide evidence for linkage. Analysis of all pedigree members is typically performed either by regression or by variance component approaches. Under the latter, one partitions the variance in the trait (measured on either a discrete or a quantitative scale) into components attributable to environmental factors, excess allele sharing at a specific genetic locus (e.g., linkage), and residual familial factors. The hypothesis of linkage is tested by evaluating, by likelihood ratio test, whether inclusion of the linkage component significantly improves the likelihood of the data.

To obtain a better estimate of the probability that two relatives share both alleles identical by descent, information across a vector of genetic markers is typically used. Use of marker information at flanking loci can help to clarify whether the two relatives have identical genotypes at a particular loci because they have inherited the same allele(s) from a common ancestor (in which case the relatives are also likely to have identical copies of any [untyped] genes in this region), or whether the two relatives merely have the same variant of the marker (in which case the relative pair will be identical by state and will not necessarily be genetically identical for flanking genes in the region). Use of information across multiple markers to establish the probabilities at any single locus of being identical by descent is the principle underlying multipoint linkage analysis.

Regardless of the linkage method used, evidence for linkage is typically expressed as a logarithm of the odds (LOD) score, which corresponds to the odds of the data in support of linkage compared to the odds of the data not supporting linkage, with this ratio expressed as base 10 logarithm. Thus, a LOD score of 3 indicates that support for linkage is 1000 times better than support for no linkage. There continues to be considerable debate regarding what level of LOD score should be required as support of linkage, particularly for complex genetic diseases and in the context of a genome scan since multiple linkage tests are performed. Some experts have argued that for genome scans, LOD scores of 3.6 (corresponding to a p value of 2.2×10^{-5}) be required as evidence for significant linkage, on the basis that one would expect a LOD score this high by chance alone in only 1 out of every 20 full genome scans [12]. However, owing to the heterogeneous nature of complex diseases like diabetes, LOD scores in the range of 2–3 may be indicative of relevant susceptibility loci, especially when the linkage is replicated in one or more independent genome scans (see below).

Issues in Interpreting Genome Scans

The genome scan approach is a powerful one for localizing disease susceptibility loci, although this approach, as with any statistical method, has its limitations that must be appreciated before meaningful interpretation of genome scan results can ensue. A few of the major issues to be considered are described briefly below.

Resolution of Linkage Location

Linkage analysis is designed to identify regions along the chromosome that are likely to harbor disease susceptibility genes; it does identify the actual disease susceptibility loci within these regions. Unfortunately, the resolution of areas of linkage can be quite broad, particularly for the more commonly used nonparametric allele-sharing methods, for which the regions of linkage typically extend from 15 to as much as 30 cM (1 cM equals approximately 1 million base pairs). Regions of this size may include hundreds of different genes. Thus while the detection of linkage may provide evidence for the existence of a disease susceptibility mutation, the procedure does not provide a very precise localization of where this mutation is. Many researchers, in fact, report the location of their peak LOD score along with the locations encompassed by the 1–LOD unit support interval, a region bounded by the chromosomal positions that correspond to locations at (LOD score −1) and (LOD score +1) from the location of the peak LOD score. This region should not strictly be interpreted as a location confidence interval, because a statistical probability cannot be assigned to the likelihood that the actual mutation falls within this interval. In fact, simulation studies suggest that even when the linked locus has a strong genetic effect, the chromosomal position corresponding to the location of the peak LOD score can occur up to 20 cM away from the true location of the disease susceptibility locus [13, 14].

Power of Linkage Analysis

In general, linkage analysis does not have great statistical power for identifying loci influencing disease susceptibility. Power to detect linkage is a function of several factors, including the number of families or relative pairs studied and the magnitude of the genetic effect. Most studies in which genome scans have been carried out have sufficient statistical power to detect loci with fairly large effects only on disease susceptibility. Although segregation analysis studies have suggested that, at least in some populations, the transmission of diabetes through families may be consistent with the presence of a co-segregating major gene [15–17], such a pattern has not been observed in many other populations, and the magnitude of single gene effects remains debatable. Given that many loci influencing diabetes susceptibility are likely to have relatively modest effects, one should not interpret the absence of linkage to mean that a disease susceptibility locus does not exist in this population. To enhance the possibility of detecting linkage, many researchers have attempted to "stack the deck" by selecting families with a high burden of diabetes (to increase the likelihood of a strong genetic etiology) and having relatively homogeneous ethnic backgrounds (to minimize genetic heterogeneity). Another approach to minimize genetic heterogeneity and thus boost power to detect linkage is to exclude individuals with diabetes due to causes other than typical type 2 diabetes. This can typically be done by obtaining a detailed medical history (e.g., to exclude secondary causes of diabetes such as cystic fibrosis or chronic pancreatitis), or through specialized laboratory evaluation (e.g., to exclude subjects with type 1 diabetes or latent autoimmune diabetes of adults by measuring glutamic acid decarboxylase antibodies).

Replication of Linkage Signals

The relative paucity of linkages that replicate across different populations is a common finding for type 2 diabetes, as it is with many other complex diseases. There are several explanations that have been invoked by a failure to replicate linkage. For example, the initial linkage reported could represent a false positive result, or alternatively, the initial linkage could represent a true linkage, but one due to the presence of a population-specific genetic variant. Yet a third possibility is that failure to replicate could be a consequence of the relatively low power of linkage analysis to detect genetic effects of modest sizes in the first place. As described in the following section, linkages to diabetes have been reported to many different chromosomes, with most linkages being observed in only a single or very few studies. However, there are several chromosomal regions (most notably on chromosomes 1 and 20) for which linkage has been reported from multiple studies.

Analysis of Subsets

Following the completion of a genome scan in their overall study population, many investigators may go on to perform a series of secondary analyses in subsets of their study population (e.g., older/younger people with diabeties, obese/lean people with diabeties, people with young/old-onset diabetes). These secondary analyses have the advantage of possibly reducing heterogeneity of the phenotype and thus boosting power to detect a linkage, but have the disadvantage of smaller numbers of "affected" individuals and thus reduced power. In addition, to the extent that such analyses generate many additional sets of linkage results, they should be interpreted cautiously and in the context of the many additional comparisons generated.

GENOME SCANS OF TYPE 2 DIABETES AND RELATED QUANTITATIVE TRAITS

To date, genome-wide scans of type 2 diabetes have been conducted in over 20 different populations of varying ethnic backgrounds, including European and US Caucasian, Mexican American, native American Indian, African American, and Asian. From such studies, linkages have been identified in a number of regions, including some for which linkage has been detected across multiple studies. A summary of the different populations and results is presented in Table 1. In this section, we summarize results published to date, and attempt to synthesize areas of concordant (and discordant) findings. We will focus our attention primarily on genome scans based on the diabetes phenotype. However, it should be noted that a number of genome scans have been conducted on intermediate metabolic traits that are precursors of the diabetes endpoint, such as glucose, insulin, or C-peptide concentrations, or more sophisticated measures of insulin sensitivity or β-cell function. Indeed, evidence supports a heritable component to these traits [36–39]. A full discussion of genome scan results of the diabetes-precursor traits is beyond the scope of this chapter; however, we will discuss results of some of these scans to the extent that linkages coincide with regions also linked to the diabetes phenotype.

Chromosome 1

The most consistent evidence for linkage to type 2 diabetes mellitus is found for a region on chromosome 1 in the vicinity of 1q21-q25, with linkage to this region now reported in at least seven different populations (see Figure 1). The initial report of linkage to this region was in Pima Indians in which suggestive linkage to marker *D1S1677* on chromosome 1q23.3 was detected (LOD = 2.48) based on analysis of sib pairs concordant and discordant for early onset diabetes (onset before age 45) [40]. These investigators conducted a subanalysis of 55 affected sib pairs with age of diabetes onset ≤25 years and found that evidence for linkage increased to a LOD of 4.1, with the location of the peak linkage signal shifting approximately 20 cM telomeric to marker *D1S2127* at 1q25.3. In a later analysis of 295 Pima Indians with and without diabetes, suggestive evidence for linkage (LOD = 1.73) was also observed to the region of 1q21-q23 with the large subcutaneous abdominal adipocyte size trait, a risk factor for future development of diabetes [41].

Further support for the presence of a locus influencing susceptibility to diabetes, in this region on chromosome 1q, was reported from a study conducted in 19 extended Utah (USA) Caucasian families of Northern European ancestry. Strongest evidence for linkage was detected using a parametric analysis that assumed a common susceptibility allele with recessive mode of inheritance with peak linkage occurring with markers near the *CRP* and *APOA2* genes on 1q21-q23 (LOD = 4.3), although evidence for linkage was also found using a less model-dependent analytic approach based on APM analysis (LOD = 2.96) [3]. Modest evidence for linkage to this same region (APOA2-*D1S484*) was then detected in an analysis carried out in 143 French families (LOD = 1.23), although evidence for linkage increased substantially (LOD = 3.04) when the analysis was restricted to lean people with diabetes (defined as BMI [body mass index] < 27 kg/m^2) and with additional markers added to the region (maximum LOD score [MLS] = 3.04) [23]. Evidence for linkage to this region was next reported in a large set of sib pairs collected through the Diabetes UK Warren 2 Repository, with an initial LOD of 1.50 detected near marker *D1S218*, but increasing to 1.98 with the addition of more markers, and further increasing to 3.07 if conditioning the analysis on linkage detected at a second locus at 10q23.3 [25].

Several additional genome scan studies have also reported evidence for linkage to markers in this region. In an Amish population from southern Pennsylvania in the United States, evidence for linkage (LOD = 2.35, $p = 0.0008$) was observed for the diabetes or impaired glucose homeostasis trait [26], with the peak linkage signal occurring at marker *D1S2715* located approximately 6–12 cM from the peak linkage signals reported in the Utah Caucasian and French families. Linkage of diabetes to chromosome 1q21-q23 has also been recently reported from a genome scan of diabetes in a Chinese population, with a peak LOD of 5.4 occurring near marker *D1S2815* in families with early onset disease [42]. Meigs and colleagues performed a genome scan of the glycated hemoglobin levels trait in diabetic and nondiabetic subjects from the Framingham Offspring Study and reported suggestive evidence for linkage (LOD = 2.81) to *D1S1589*, which also falls in this region (see Figure 1).

Chromosome 2

The first published genome-wide scan of type 2 diabetes was based on a study of 330 affected sib pairs from Mexican American families in southern Texas, a genetically admixed population notable for its relatively high prevalence of type 2 diabetes [29]. Initial analyses revealed significant evidence for linkage to marker *D2S125* in the 2q37 region (two-point LOD = 4.1, multipoint LOD = 2.6) [29], although the linkage was substantially strengthened

Table 1 Published genome scans of type 2 diabetes

Population	Reference	Sample	Trait	LOD or p value (chromosome, location; linked marker)
European Caucasians				
Western Finland (Botnia)	[18]	Extended families (26 fams/120 affected individs)	Diabetes	3.65 (chr 12q24.31; *D12S1349*)
Western Finland (Botnia)	[19]	Extended families (58 fams/229 affected individs)	Diabetes	$p < 0.0002$ (chr 9q21.12; *D9S166/D9S301*)
Finland (FUSION Study)	[20]	Affected sib pairs ($n = 719$)	Diabetes	1.99 (chr 20p12.3, 18 cM; *D20S905*) 2.04 (chr 20q12, 56 cM; *D20S107*) 2.15 (chr 20q13.12, 69 cM; *D20S197*)
Finland/Sweden	[21]	Nuclear families (353 fams/959 affected individs)	Diabetes	1.41 (chr4q21.23; *D4S2361*) 1.29 (chr 17q25.1; *D17S1301*)
Mormon (Utah)	[3]	Extended families (19 fams/119 affected individs)	Diabetes	4.30 (chr 1q21-q23, 204 cM; *CRP/APOA2*) 2.18 (chr 2q37.2, 253 cM; *D2S336*)
U.S. (GENNID Study)	[22]	Families (77 fams/288 affected individs)	Diabetes or IGH	2.99 (chr X, 14 cM; *GATA172D05*) 2.81 (chr 12q21.23, 82 cM; *D12S853*) 2.80 (chr 5q31.1, 77 cM; *D5S1404*)
French	[23]	Nuclear families (143 fams/432 affected individs)	Diabetes	2.28 (ch 2p21, 75 cM; *D2S2259/D2S391*) 1.59 (chr 10q26.11, 175 cM; *D10S1655*)
French	[24]	Extended family (1 fam/37 affected)	Diabetes	2.4 (chr 5q14.4, 99 cM; *D5S428*)
UK	[25]	Affected sib pairs ($n = 743$)	Diabetes	2.55 (chr 8p21.3-p22, 42 cM; *D8S258*) 1.99 (chr 10q23.31-q23.2, 125 cM; *D10S1765*) 1.98 (chr 1q24.2-q23.2, 206 cM; *D1S2799/D1S452*)
Amish (Pennsylvania)	[26]	Extended families (31 fams/140 affected individs)	Diabetes or IGH	2.35 (chr 1q21-q23, 166 cM; *D1S2715*) 3.48 (chr 14q11.2, 7 cM; *D14S1023*)
Ashkenazi Jews	[27]	Extended families (267 fams/624 affected individs)	Diabetes	1.26 (chr 4q34.3; *D4S1505*)
Native American Indian				
Pima Indians	[5]	Nuclear families (264 fams/667 affected individs)	Age-adjusted Diabetes	$p = 0.0004$ (chr 1q23.3, 171 cM; *D1S1677*) $p = 0.003$ (chr 11q24.2, 137 cM; *D11S4464*)
Canandian Oji-Cree	[28]	Affected sib pairs ($n = 49$)	Diabetes	$p < 10^{-4}$ (chr 6q16.1; *D6S1056*) $p < 10^{-4}$ (chr 16p13.3; *D16S2616*)
Mexican American				
Starr County, TX, USA	[29]	Nuclear families (246 fams/440 ASP)	Diabetes	4.10 (chr 2q37; *D2S125*)
San Antonio, TX, USA (SAFDS)	[30]	Extended families (27 fams/116 affected individs)	Diabetes	2.88 (chr 10q26.13, 145 cM; *D10S587*) 2.67 (chr 3p13-p12.1, 71 cM; *D3S1566/GATA128C02*) 2.38 (chr 9p24.2-p22.2, 15 cM; *D9S288/D9S925*) 1.99 (chr 4q28, 172 cM; *D4S1615/D4S175*)
U.S. (GENNID Study)	[22]	Families (53 fams/233 affected individs)	Diabetes or IGH	3.91 (chr 3p24.1, 51 cM; *D3S2432*)
African American				
U.S. (GENNID Study)	[22]	Families (65 fams/152 affected individs)	Diabetes or IGH	2.39 (chr 10p14, 14 cM; *D10S1412*)
Indo-Asian				
Japanese	[31]	Nuclear families (159 fams/359 affected individs)	Diabetes	3.08 (chr 11p13-p12, 54 cM; *D11S935*) 2.19 (chr 15q13-q21, 43 cM; *D15S994*)
Japanese	[32]	Extended families (164 fams/368 affected individs)	Diabetes	1.92 (chr 21q22.3, 48 cM; *D21S266/D21S1446*) 1.40 (chr 9q33.3; 140 cM; *D9S282*)
Chinese Hans	[33]	Extended families (102 fams/282 affected individs)	Diabetes	$p = 1.19 \times 10^{-4}$ (chr 9p21, 42 cM; *D9S171*) $p = 4.47 \times 10^{-4}$ (chr 9q13-q21, 68 cM; *D9S175*)
Indo-Mauritians	[34]	Nuclear families (67 fams/198 ASP)	Diabetes	2.14 (chr 1q44, 319 cM; *D1S2836*) 2.06 (chr 3q22; 165 cM; *D3S1292*) 1.73 (chr 8q23, 132 cM; *D8S1784*)
Indigenous Australians				
North Stradbroke Island, Queensland	[35]	Extended family (138 individs/49 affected individs)	Diabetes	3.9 (chr 2q24.3, 177 cM; *D2S2345*) 1.8 (chr 3q29; *D3S1311*) 1.77 (chr 8p22; *D8S549*)

Note: IGH = impaired glucose homeostasis; ASP = affected sib pairs.

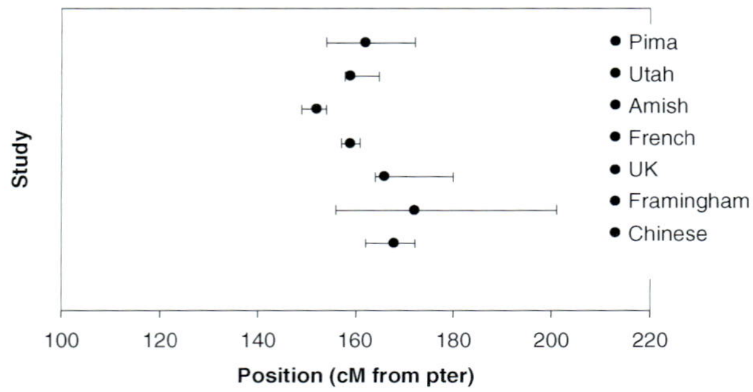

Figure 1 Regions on chromosome 1q showing linkage to diabetes in seven different populations. Lines represent the 1−LOD support intervals and points represent the position of peak linkage. Traits analyzed are diabetes (Pima, Utah, French, UK, Chinese), diabetes or impaired glucose homeostasis (Amish), and glycated hemoglobin (Framingham)

when an interaction with a locus on chromosome 15 was taken into account [43]. Suggestive evidence for linkage has since been observed in a French [44] and Indo-Mauritius population, although in the latter, the linkage to *D2S125* was replicated (LOD = 3.03) only in a subset analysis consisting of the leanest families [34]. Modest evidence for linkage (LOD = 1.87) has subsequently been reported between glycated hemoglobin levels and markers in a region 10 cM telomeric to *D2S125* in the Old Order Amish [26].

Subsequent linkage disequilibrium mapping efforts have revealed the linkage to be attributable to variation in or around the calpain 10 gene (*CAPN10*; MIM 605286) [45]. The single nucleotide polymorphism (SNP) with the greatest evidence for association and linkage lay within intron 3 (UCSNP-43) of *CAPN10*, with homozygosity for the G allele (allele frequency 0.80 in Mexican Americans) conferring a greater risk for type 2 diabetes. Further evidence for association was obtained by analysis of haplotypes consisting of three SNPs within *CAPN10*, UCSNP-43, -19, and -63. Interestingly, the haplotype combination 112/121 was associated with a 2.80-fold increased risk of diabetes (95% CI 1.23–6.34), while homozygotes for either of the two haplotypes showed no increased risk of diabetes. Similar results were obtained in German and Finnish samples, although the "at-risk" haplotype combination was much less common in these populations than in Mexican Americans.

The calpain family are calcium-activated neutral proteases that cause activation or inactivation of proteins involved in intracellular signaling, proliferation, and differentiation, including adipocyte differentiation and possibly insulin action and insulin secretion. However, how altered function or expression (or both) of calpain 10 affects glucose metabolism is presently unknown. DNA-binding studies using nuclear extracts from human pancreatic islets and HepG2 cells suggest that the more common "1" or G allele of UCSNP-43 may decrease binding of nuclear proteins, and *in vitro* reporter gene studies suggest that the G allele of UCSNP-43 may decrease transcription as compared to the "Z" or A allele [45]. In a study of Pima Indians, subjects homozygous for the G allele of UCSNP-43 had lower mRNA levels of calpain 10 in muscle and decreased rates of postabsorptive and insulin-stimulated glucose turnover, suggesting insulin resistance [46].

A linkage to diabetes has also been reported to the region of chromosome 2q24.3 based on a parametric analysis conducted in a very large pedigree consisting of 138 indigenous Australians from a large multigenerational family [35]. The linked marker was *D2S2345* (LOD = 3.9), located approximately 90 cM centromeric from *D2S125*. Interestingly, suggestive evidence for linkage of *D2S141*, located approximately 10 cM away (LOD = 2.7), to specific insulin concentrations has been reported in Mexican Americans [47].

Chromosome 3

Several studies have reported linkages of diabetes to the long arm of chromosome 3. Suggestive evidence for linkage was observed at marker *D3S1311* (two-point LOD = 1.8) on 3q24.3 in a large pedigree of indigenous Australians [35]. Strong evidence for linkage has been reported telomeric (3q27-qter near *D3S1580*) to this marker in French families (MLS = 3.56), but only when the analysis was restricted to 92 affected sib pairs with age of onset <45 years [23]. Noting that fasting insulin levels adjusted for insulin resistance predicted 6-year incidence of diabetes and were correlated with acute insulin response, Weyer and colleagues conducted a genome scan of this adjusted insulin trait in Pima Indians and detected suggestive evidence for linkage (LOD = 1.77) to the region harboring the *GLUT2* gene on 3q26.1 [48]. Also in Pima Indians, a genome scan of fasting insulin concentrations unadjusted for insulin resistance revealed suggestive evidence for linkage to *D3S1764* residing at 3q23 (multipoint LOD = 1.5–1.7) [49]. In the Mauritians, nominal evidence for linkage to type 2 diabetes mellitus was found on chromosome 3q22, near *D3S1292* (LOD = 2.06, $p = 0.0019$) [34]. These researchers then obtained modest evidence replicating this linkage in an analysis of 35 Tamil Indian families, where they observed a LOD of 1.36 to this same marker [34].

Strong evidence for linkage to diabetes has also been observed on the short arm of chromosome 3. In an analysis of Mexican Americans from the GENNID Study, Ehm et al. reported significant evidence for linkage (LOD = 3.91) to diabetes or impaired glucose homeostasis at 3p24.1, near *D3S243* [22]. In Caucasian families from western Finland, modest evidence of linkage of diabetes to markers *D3S1561* and *D3S1768* was observed in the region 3p24-p22 [19], with the peak linkage signal occurring only 4–5 cM centromeric from that found in Mexican Americans.

Linkage of diabetes has also been reported to *D3S4529* in the region of 3p12.1 in Mexican Americans (LOD = 2.67), with additional analyses revealing linkage of diabetes age of onset to the same marker (LOD = 2.51) [30]. In a different and nonoverlapping set of Mexican American families from this same area (San Antonio, TX, USA), Mitchell et al. conducted a genome scan of fasting insulin levels and observed significant evidence for linkage (multipoint LOD = 3.07, $p < 0.0001$) near markers *D3S1600* and *D3S2406* located nearby at 3p14.2-p13 [50].

Chromosome 4

Modest evidence for linkage has been reported to several different regions on chromosome 4q, including 4q32-q33 in Finnish Caucasians ($p < 0.01$) between *D4S3015* and *D4S2951* [19] and 4q35.1 in Ashkenazi Jews (LOD = 1.26) near *D4S1501* [27], located 5 cM from *D4S3015* and *D4S2951*. In addition, linkage of diabetes has been reported at 4q28 in Mexican Americans, with a LOD of 1.99 observed between markers *D4S1615* and *D4S175* [30]. Interestingly, linkages to serum insulin concentrations have also been reported in this region (4q28) in Native Americans ($p = 0.0005$ near FABP2 and ANX5 [51]) and in a different Mexican American population (LOD = 2.80) between FABP2 and 2-h insulin levels [52].

Chromosome 9

Linkage of diabetes to several different regions on chromosome 9 has been reported, although there appears to be little overlap between linkage signals. Linkages to diabetes have been reported on the short arm of chromosome 9 in Mexican Americans in the region of 9p24.2-p22.2 (LOD = 2.38 with markers *D9S288* and *D9S925*) [30] and in Chinese Hans at 9p21 near *D9S171* ($p = 1.2 \times 10^{-4}$) [33]. Modest evidence for linkage has also been reported on the long arm of chromosome 9 at 9q21.12, where Lindgren et al. observed linkages with markers *D9S166* and *D9S301* ($p < 0.0002$) in Caucasian families from western Finland [19].

Chromosome 10

Evidence for linkage to chromosome 10 was first reported in Mexican Americans where peak linkage at 10q26.13 was observed near *D10S587* for diabetes (LOD = 2.88), with the LOD increasing to 3.75 at the same location when diabetes age of onset was analyzed [30]. Modest evidence for linkage has been reported in French families to a region approximately 15 cM pter from *D10S587* at 10q26.3 near *D10S1655* (MLS = 1.59) [23].

Linkages to chromosome 10q have subsequently been reported centromeric to *D10S587* in the region of 10q22-q23. In the Diabetes UK Warren 2 Repository Study, Wiltshire et al. reported suggestive evidence (LOD = 1.99) for linkage of diabetes to *D10S1765* [25], while Meigs et al. reported linkage of fasting glucose levels to *D10S1432* (located ~15 cM away from *D10S1765*) in the Framingham Offspring Study (LOD = 2.81) [53].

At least one linkage of diabetes has been reported on the p arm of chromosome 10. In a collection of African American families studied as part of the GENNID Study, Ehm et al. observed linkage to *D10S1412* with the combined diabetes or impaired glucose homeostasis trait with a LOD of 2.39 [22].

Chromosome 11

Strong evidence for linkage to a quantitative trait locus on 11q24 influencing susceptibility to diabetes and obesity has been reported in the Pima Indians. In an analysis of 966 siblings from 264 families, Hanson et al. detected modest evidence for linkage of markers *D11S4464* and *D11S91* to diabetes (LOD = 1.7), but strong evidence for linkage of these markers to BMI (LOD = 3.6) [40]. Moreover, this linkage was considerably strengthened when a bivariate analysis was conducted utilizing both traits simultaneously. Adding further support for the presence of a diabetes susceptibility locus in this region is the subsequent finding of linkage of fasting-specific insulin concentrations, albeit modestly (LOD = 1.8), in Mexican Americans to another marker in this region, *D11S934* [47].

There is some support for a second locus influencing diabetes susceptibility on the p arm of chromosome 11, although the region is not well localized. Linkage of diabetes to the 11p15.2 region has been reported from Finnish Caucasians (LOD = 1.75) near marker *D11S899* [20], with additional evidence for linkage of 2-h postload glucose levels (LOD = 3.37) to nearby markers *D11S899/D11S1324* in this region [54]. Slightly centromeric to this region, evidence for linkage to diabetes has been reported in Utah Caucasians ($p = 0.00057$) [55] and to both diabetes (MLS = 2.35) and BMI (LOD = 3.0) in Japanese families [31]. Modest evidence for linkage to both fasting-specific insulin (LOD = 1.6) and 2-h glucose (LOD = 2.77) concentrations has also been reported telomeric to these regions at 11p15.4 near marker *D11S988* in Mexican Americans [47, 54].

Chromosome 12

Several Caucasian studies have observed evidence for a type 2 diabetes susceptibility locus on chromosome 12. An initial study conducted by Mahtani et al. found no strong evidence for linkage to chromosome 12 in the overall sample of 26 Caucasian families recruited from a relatively homogenous population in western Finland, but in a subanalysis of 6 families having the lowest levels of circulating insulin, found evidence for linkage to markers near *D12S1349* on chromosome 12q24.31 (LOD = 3.65) [18]. Located 9 cM centromeric from *D12S304* is marker *D12S321*, which has been linked to late-onset diabetes in an analysis of a single pedigree with 21 affected individuals from Australia (LOD = 3.65) [56]. Interestingly, the MODY3/HNF-1α gene locus has been mapped within the vicinity of this chromosome 12 region [57, 58]. Although a study in a UK population excluded this locus [59], a study in 53 Caucasian sib pairs affected with diabetic nephropathy showed evidence for linkage with MODY3-linked markers, *D12S349* ($p = 0.04$) and *D12S86* ($p = 0.006$) located less than 3 cM from *D12S321* [60].

Linkage to diabetes has also been reported to a region of chromosome 12q15 centromeric to that described above. Initial evidence was based on an analysis of 32 Caucasian families segregating for a form of early onset diabetes with strongest evidence for linkage detected near marker *D12S375* [61]. Additional support for this result was observed in an analysis of Caucasian families from the GENNID Study, where Ehm et al. reported evidence for linkage (LOD = 2.81) to marker *D12S853* in this same region [22].

Chromosome 20

There is substantial evidence for the existence of at least one locus influencing susceptibility to diabetes on chromosome 20. Two initial studies published simultaneously have provided suggestive evidence for linkage of diabetes with markers in the region of *D20S197*. In a small study of 53 sib pairs, Bowden et al. detected modest evidence for linkage of diabetes (LOD = 1.48) in Caucasian families to 20q13.12 in the *D20S197*/*D20S178* interval [60]. At about the same time Ji et al. reported very modest evidence for linkage ($p < 0.05$) to these markers in an analysis of 29 large Caucasian pedigrees, although evidence for linkage increased substantially ($p < 0.009$) when analysis was restricted to older-onset families [62]. In a later analysis of these data that included 14 additional families, evidence for linkage increased substantially ($p = 1.8 \times 10^{-5}$), peaking at marker *D20S197* in this region [63]. Additional populations showing evidence for linkage of diabetes to markers in this region include Caucasians from Finland (FUSION Study), where a LOD of 2.15 was reported [20], Japanese, in whom linkage was detected in a secondary analysis restricted to subjects with BMI < 30 kg/m^2 (MLS = 2.32) [31], and Mexican Americans, for which an LOD of 1.9 was reported for the fasting-specific insulin concentrations trait [47]. A subanalysis conducted in Chinese Hans also revealed evidence for linkage, but only when families with lower BMI were analyzed alone ($p = 6.5 \times 10^{-4}$) [33].

Evidence for linkage to the p arm of chromosome 20 has also been reported. In the FUSION Study, linkage to diabetes was observed at 20p12.3 near *D20S905*, with an MLS of 2.04 [20].

Other Chromosomes

Linkages to diabetes and/or other related traits have also been reported at several additional chromosomal regions. Linkage to diabetes in the 7p15.3 region (LOD = 1.31) of chromosome 7 was detected in 58 Caucasian families from western Finland [19], with this result loosely supported by studies in Japanese sib pairs showing suggestive linkage to maximal BMI on chromosome 7p22-p21 near *D7S517* (MLS = 3.51) [31] and in Pima Indians where suggestive evidence for linkage to diabetes (LOD = 1.8) was observed near *D7S1799* [40].

Evidence for a locus on chromosome 8 comes from two studies, one from the Diabetes UK Warren 2 Repository Study reporting linkage to 8p21.3 near *D8S258* (LOD = 2.55) [25] and the other in an indigenous Australian population showing linkage to diabetes at 8p22 near *D8S549* (two-point LOD = 1.77) located 10 cM pter from *D8S258* [35].

Only two genome scans, both conducted in Caucasian populations, have identified linkages of diabetes to regions on chromosome 5. The first study, based on an analysis of 77 Caucasian families from the GENNID Study, reported a LOD of 2.8 at 5q31.1 near *D5S1404* [22], while the second, conducted in a single large French family, reported a LOD of 2.4 at 5q14.4 near *D5S428* [24].

In a subanalysis of Japanese families with diabetes onset before age 45 years, Mori et al. reported suggestive evidence for linkage of diabetes to chromosome 14q11-q13 near *D14S275* (MLS = 2.37) [31]. This result is supported by another Japanese study showing nominal evidence for linkage to diabetes or impaired glucose homeostasis (LOD = 1.53) at *D14S608*, a marker that co-localizes to *D14S275* [22]. Diabetes has also been linked (LOD = 3.5) to the 14q11 region in an Amish population [26].

FUTURE PROSPECTS

Ultimately, the success of genome-wide linkage analysis depends on the positional cloning of the genes (and mutations) that generated the linkage. Although positional cloning through linkage disequilibrium (LD) mapping is straightforward for monogenic diseases, it is much more difficult for complex diseases like type 2 diabetes. Nonetheless, positional cloning through a combination of approaches including LD mapping and positional candidate gene sequencing, as was performed for NIDDM1 to identify variants in calpain 10, is actively being pursued at several linked loci, most notably on chromosomes 1 and 20.

Recently, the idea of performing genome-wide association studies to identify disease susceptibility mutations has been proposed. Compared to the genome-wide linkage approach, a systematic genome-wide association strategy would utilize up to 1 million or more SNPs that cover the genome at very high density (say every 10–50 kb) [64]. An advantage of this approach is that association analyses have greater power than linkage analysis to discern loci with more modest effects on the phenotype. However, the multiple comparison issue associated with performing millions of association tests for each SNP are formidable, not to mention the high cost of genotyping so many SNPs. Nevertheless, the genome-wide association approach is likely to play a role in identifying disease susceptibility mutations in the future as the SNP database becomes more complete and patterns of linkage disequlibrium between markers becomes better characterized at the population level.

SUMMARY

Genome scans for type 2 diabetes have been carried out in a number of populations. Because of the low power of genome scans to detect genes that have modest effects on disease susceptibility, replications of linkage across populations occur relatively infrequently. At the present time, it is unclear whether locus heterogeneity is likely to be greater within ethnic groups or across ethnic groups (i.e., if disease susceptibility loci are significantly more likely to vary across ethnic groups than within ethnic groups). Despite these issues, there is mounting evidence from multiple studies that diabetes susceptibility loci reside on a number of different chromosomes, including 1, 2, 3, 10, 11, and 20. The *NIDDM1* locus, first localized to chromosome 2q through a genome scan, has subsequently been identified as calpain 10. The most strongly replicated linkages appear to be for regions on chromosomes 1q and 20q. Evidence for a diabetes susceptibility gene points most persuasively now to a region on chromosome 1q21-q25, where linkages to diabetes or related traits have been detected in at least seven different populations. Linkage to this region in Pima Indians, Caucasians, and Chinese indicate that the diabetes susceptibility gene in this region is likely to be relevant to several diverse populations. Alternatively, more than one gene may be located in this region. There is also strong evidence supporting a diabetes susceptibility locus on chromosome 20q. Efforts to fine map the putative susceptibility genes in these regions are currently underway in a number of different populations.

REFERENCES

1. Barnett AH, Eff C, Leslie RD, Pyke DA. Diabetes in identical twins. A study of 200 pairs. *Diabetologia* 1981; 20: 87–93.
2. Newman B, Selby JV, King MC, Slemenda C, Fabsitz R, Friedman GD. Concordance for type 2 (non-insulin-dependent) diabetes mellitus in male twins. *Diabetologia* 1987; 30: 763–8.
3. Elbein SC, Hoffman MD, Teng K, Leppert MF, Hasstedt SJ. A genome-wide search for type 2 diabetes susceptibility genes in Utah Caucasians. *Diabetes* 1999; 48: 1175–82.
4. Hsueh W-C, Mitchell BD, Aburomia R, Pollin T, Sakul H, Ehm MG, Michelsen BK, Wagner MJ, St Jean PL, Knowler WC, Burns DK, Bell CJ, Shuldiner AR. Diabetes in the old order Amish: characterization and heritability analysis of the Amish Family Diabetes Study. *Diabetes Care* 2000; 23: 595–601.
5. Hanson RL, Knowler WC. Analytic strategies to detect linkage to a common disorder with genetically determined age of onset: diabetes mellitus in Pima Indians. *Genet Epidemiol* 1998; 15: 299–315.
6. King H, Aubert RE, Herman WH. Global burden of diabetes, 1995–2025: prevalence, numerical estimates, and projections. *Diabetes Care* 1998; 21: 1414–31.
7. Yen CJ, Beamer BA, Negri C, Silver K, Brown KA, Yarnall DP, Burns DK, Roth J, Shuldiner AR. Molecular scanning of the human peroxisome proliferator activated receptor gamma (hPPAR gamma) gene in diabetic Caucasians: identification of a Pro12Ala PPAR gamma 2 missense mutation. *Biochem Biophys Res Commun* 1997; 241: 270–4.
8. Deeb SS, Fajas L, Nemoto M, Pihlajamaki J, Mykkanen L, Kuusisto J, Laakso M, Fujimoto W, Auwerx J. A Pro12Ala substitution in PPARgamma2 associated with decreased receptor activity, lower body mass index and improved insulin sensitivity. *Nat Genet* 1998; 20: 284–7.
9. Altshuler D, Hirschhorn JN, Klannemark M, Lindgren CM, Vohl MC, Nemesh J, Lane CR, Schaffner SF, Bolk S, Brewer C, Tuomi T, Gaudet D, Hudson TJ, Daly M, Groop L, Lander ES. The common PPARgamma Pro12Ala polymorphism is associated with decreased risk of type 2 diabetes. *Nature Genet* 2000; 26: (1) 76–80.
10. Terrett J, Chamberlain J, Rastan S, Marshall R, McGinnis R, Spurr N, O'Brien E, Evans C, Rut A. The Pro-115Gln mutation in peroxisome-proliferator-activated receptor (PPAR) gamma2 is extremely rare in a large cohort of US Caucasians. *Clin Sci* 2000; 99 (1): 89–90.
11. Silver K, Shuldiner AR. Candidate genes for type 2 diabetes mellitus. In LeRoith D, Olefsky JM, Taylor SL (eds), *Diabetes Mellitus: a Fundamental and Clinical Text*, 2nd edn. Philadelphia: Lippincott Co, 2000; pp 705–19.
12. Lander E, Kruglyak L. Genetic dissection of complex traits: guidelines for interpreting and reporting linkage results. *Nat Genet* 1995; 11: 241–7.
13. Roberts SB, MacLean CJ, Neale MC, Eaves LJ, Kendler KS. Replication of linkage studies of complex traits: an examination of variation in location estimates. *Am J Hum Genet* 1999; 65: 876–84.
14. Hsueh WC, Goring HH, Blangero J, Mitchell BD. Replication of linkage to quantitative trait loci: variation in location and magnitude of the lod score. *Genet Epidemiol.* 2001; 21 (Suppl 1): S473–8.
15. Hanson RL, Elston RC, Pettitt DJ, Bennett PH, Knowler WC. Segregation analysis of non-insulin-dependent

diabetes mellitus in Pima Indians: evidence for a major-gene effect. *Am J Hum Genet* 1995; 57 (1): 160–70.
16. Elston RC, Namboodiri KK, Nino HV, Pollitzer WS. Studies on blood and urine glucose in Seminole Indians: indications for segregation of a major gene. *Am J Hum Genet* 1974; 26: 13–34.
17. Stern MP, Mitchell BD, Blangero J, Reinhart L, Krammerer CM, Harrison CR , Shipman PA, O'Connell P, Frazier ML, MacCluer JW. Evidence for a major gene for type II diabetes and linkage analyses with selected candidate genes in Mexican-Americans. *Diabetes* 1996; 45 (5): 563–8.
18. Mahtani MM, Widen E, Lehto M, Thomas J, McCarthy M, Brayer J, Bryant B, Chan G, Daly M, Forsblom C, Kanninen T, Kirby A, Kruglyak L, Munnelly K, Parkkonen M, Reeve-Daly MP, Weaver A, Brettin T, Duyk G, Lander ES, Groop LC. Mapping of a gene for type 2 diabetes associated with an insulin secretion defect by a genome scan in Finnish families. *Nat Genet* 1996; 14: 90–4.
19. Lindgren CM, Mahtani MM, Widen E, McCarthy MI, Daly MJ, Kirby A, Reeve MP, Kruglyak L, Parker A, Meyer J, Almgren P, Lehto M, Kanninen T, Tuomi T, Groop LC, Lander ES. Genomewide search for type 2 diabetes mellitus susceptibility loci in Finnish families: the Botnia study. *Am J Hum Genet* 2002; 70 (2): 509–16.
20. Ghosh S, Watanabe RM, Valle TT, Hauser ER, Magnuson VL, Langefeld CD, Ally DS, Mohlke KL, Silander K, Kohtamaki K, Chines P, Balow JJ, Birznieks G, Chang J, Eldridge W, Erdos MR, Karanjawala ZE, Knapp JI, Kudelko K, Martin C, Morales-Mena A, Musick A, Musick T, Pfahl C, Porter R, Rayman JB, Rha D, Segal L, Shapiro S, Sharaf R, Shurtleff B, So A, Tannenbaum J, Te C, Tovar J, Unni A, Welch C, Whiten R, Witt A, Blaschak-Harvan J, Douglas JA, Duren WL, Epstein MP, Fingerlin TE, Kaleta HS, Lange EM, Li C, McEachin RC, Stringham HM, Trager E, White PP, Eriksson J, Toivanen L, Vidgren G, Nylund SJ, Tuomilehto-Wolf E, Ross EH, Demirchyan E , Hagopian WA, Buchanan TA, Tuomilehto J, Bergman RN, Collins FS, Boehnke M. The Finland–United States Investigation of Non-Insulin-Dependent Diabetes Mellitus Genetics (FUSION) Study, I: An Autosomal Genome Scan for Genes That Predispose to Type 2 Diabetes. *Am J Hum Genet* 2000; 67 (5): 1174–85.
21. Parker A, Meyer J, Lewitzky S, Rennich JS, Chan G, Thomas JD, Orho-Melander M, Lehtovirta M, Forsblom C, Hyrkko A, Carlsson M, Lindgren C, Groop LC. A gene conferring susceptibility to type 2 diabetes in conjunction with obesity is located on chromosome 18p11. *Diabetes* 2001; 50 (3): 675–80.
22. Ehm MG, Karnoub MC, Sakul H, Gottschalk K, Holt DC, Weber JL, Vaske D, Briley D, Briley L, Kopf J, McMillen P, Nguyen Q, Reisman M, Lai EH, Joslyn G, Shepherd NS, Bell C, Wagner MJ, Burns DK. Genomewide search for type 2 diabetes susceptibility genes in four American populations. *Am J Hum Genet* 2000; 66: 1871–81.
23. Vionnet N, Hani E, Dupont S, Gallina S, Francke S, Dotte S, De Matos F, Durand E, Lepretre F, Lecoeur C, Gallina P, Zekiri L, Dina C, Froguel P. Genomewide search for type 2 diabetes-susceptibility genes in French whites: evidence for a novel susceptibility locus for early-onset diabetes on chromosome 3q27-qter and independent replication of a type 2-diabetes locus on chromosome 1q21-q24. *Am J Hum Genet* 2000; 67 (6): 1470–80.
24. Martin LJ, Comuzzie AG, Dupont S, Vionnet N, Dina C, Gallina S, Houari M, Blangero J, Froguel P. A quantitative trait locus influencing type 2 diabetes susceptibility maps to a region on 5q in an extended French family. *Diabetes* 2002; 51 (12): 3568–72.
25. Wiltshire S, Hattersley AT, Hitman GA, Walker M, Levy JC, Sampson M, O'Rahilly S, Frayling TM, Bell JI, Lathrop GM, Bennett A, Dhillon R, Fletcher C, Groves CJ, Jones E, Prestwich P, Simecek N, Rao PV, Wishart M, Foxon R, Howell S, Smedley D , Cardon LR, Menzel S, McCarthy MI. A genomewide scan for loci predisposing to type 2 diabetes in a U.K. population (the Diabetes UK Warren 2 Repository): analysis of 573 pedigrees provides independent replication of a susceptibility locus on chromosome 1q. *Am J Hum Genet* 2001; 69 (3): 553–69.
26. Hsueh WC, St Jean PL, Mitchell BD, Pollin TI, Knowler WC, Ehm MG, Bell CJ, Sakul H, Wagner MJ, Burns DK, Shuldiner AR. Genome-wide and fine-mapping linkage studies of type 2 diabetes and glucose traits in the Old Order Amish: evidence for a new diabetes locus on chromosome 14q11 and confirmation of a locus on chromosome 1q21-q24. *Diabetes* 2003; 52 (2): 550–7.
27. Permutt MA, Wasson JC, Suarez BK, Lin J, Thomas J, Meyer J, Lewitzky S, Rennich JS, Parker A, DuPrat L, Maruti S , Chayen S, Glaser B. A genome scan for type 2 diabetes susceptibility loci in a genetically isolated population. *Diabetes* 2001; 50 (3): 681–5.
28. Hegele RA, Sun F, Harris SB, Anderson C, Hanley AJ, Zinman B. Genome-wide scanning for type 2 diabetes susceptibility in Canadian Oji-Cree, using 190 microsatellite markers. *J Hum Genet* 1999; 44: 10–4.
29. Hanis CL, Boerwinkle E, Chakraborty R, Ellsworth DL, Concannon P, Stirling B, Morrison VA, Wapelhorst B, Spielman RS, Gogolin-Ewens KJ, Shepard JM, Williams SR, Risch N, Hinds D, Iwasaki N, Ogata M, Omori Y, Petzold C, Rietzch H, Schroder HE, Schulze J, Cox NJ, Menzel S, Boriraj VV, Chen X. A genome-wide search for human non-insulin-dependent (type 2) diabetes genes reveals a major susceptibility locus on chromosome 2. *Nat Genet* 1996; 13: 161–6.
30. Duggirala R, Blangero J, Almasy L, Dyer TD, Williams KL, Leach RJ, O'Connell P, Stern MP. Linkage of type 2 diabetes mellitus and of age at onset to a genetic location on Chromosome 10q in Mexican Americans. *Am J Hum Genet* 1999; 64: 1127–40.
31. Mori Y, Otabe S, Dina C, Yasuda K, Populaire C, Lecoeur C, Vatin V, Durand E, Hara K, Okada T, Tobe K, Boutin P, Kadowaki T, Froguel P. Genome-wide search for type 2 diabetes in Japanese affected sib-pairs confirms susceptibility genes on 3q, 15q, and 20q and identifies two new candidate Loci on 7p and 11p. *Diabetes* 2002; 51 (4): 1247–55.
32. Iwasaki N, Cox NJ, Wang YQ, Schwarz PE, Bell GI, Honda M, Imura M, Ogata M, Saito M, Kamatani N, Iwamoto Y. Mapping genes influencing type 2 diabetes risk and BMI in Japanese subjects. *Diabetes* 2003; 52 (1): 209–13.
33. Luo TH, Zhao Y, Li G, Yuan WT, Zhao JJ, Chen JL, Huang W, Luo M. A genome-wide search for type II diabetes susceptibility genes in Chinese Hans. *Diabetologia* 2001; 44 (4): 501–6.
34. Francke S, Manraj M, Lacquemant C, Lecoeur C, Lepretre F, Passa P, Hebe A, Corset L, Yan SL, Lahmidi S,

Jankee S, Gunness TK, Ramjuttun US, Balgobin V, Dina C, Froguel P. A genome-wide scan for coronary heart disease suggests in Indo-Mauritians a susceptibility locus on chromosome 16p13 and replicates linkage with the metabolic syndrome on 3q27. *Hum Mol Genet* 2001; 10 (24): 2751–65.

35. Busfield F, Duffy DL, Kesting JB, Walker SM, Lovelock PK, Good D, Tate H, Watego D, Marczak M, Hayman N, Shaw JT. A genomewide search for type 2 diabetes-susceptibility genes in indigenous Australians. *Am J Hum Genet* 2002; 70 (2): 349–57.
36. Lillioja S, Mott DM, Zawadzki JK, Young AA, Abbott WG, Knowler WC, Bennett PH, Moll P, Bogardus C. In vivo insulin action is familial characteristic in non-diabetic Pima Indians. *Diabetes* 1987; 36 (11): 1329–35.
37. Watanabe RM, Valle T, Hauser ER, Ghosh S, Eriksson J, Kohtamaki K, Ehnholm C, Tuomilehto J, Collins FS, Bergman RN, Boehnke M, for the Finland–United States Investigation of NIDDM Genetics (FUSION) Study Investigators. Familiarity of quantitative metabolic traits in Finnish families with non-insulin-dependent diabetes mellitus. *Hum Hered* 1999; 49: 159–68.
38. Elbein SC, Hasstedt SJ, Wegner K, Kahn SE. Heritability of pancreatic beta-cell function among nondiabetic members of Caucasian familial type 2 diabetic kindreds. *J Clin Endocrinol Metab* 1999; 84: 1398–403.
39. Sakul H, Pratley R, Cardon L, Ravussin E , Mott D, Bogardus C. Familiality of physical and metabolic characteristics that predict the development of non-insulin-dependent diabetes mellitus in Pima Indians. *Am J Hum Genet* 1997; 60: 651–6.
40. Hanson RL, Ehm MG, Pettitt DJ, Prochazka M, Thompson DB, Timberlake D, Foroud T, Kobes S, Baier L, Burns DK, Almasy L, Blangero J, Garvey WT, Bennett PH, Knowler WC. An autosomal genomic scan for loci linked to type II diabetes mellitus and body mass index in Pima Indians. *Am J Hum Genet* 1998; 63 (4): 1130–8.
41. Weyer C, Wolford JK, Hanson RL, Foley JE, Tataranni PA, Bogardus C, Pratley RE. Subcutaneous abdominal adipocyte size, a predictor of type 2 diabetes, is linked to chromosome 1q21-q23 and is associated with a common polymorphism in LMNA in Pima Indians. *Mol Genet Metab* 2001; 72 (3): 231–8.
42. Xiang K, Wang Y, Zheng T, Shen K, Jia W, Li J, Lin X, Wu S, Zhang G, Wang S, Lu H. Genome wide scan for type 2 diabetes susceptibility loci in Chinese [abstract]. *Diabetes* 2002; 51 (suppl 2): A262.
43. Cox NJ, Frigge M, Nicolae DL, Concannon P, Hanis CL, Bell GI, Kong A. Loci on chromosomes 2 (NIDDM1) and 15 interact to increase susceptibility to diabetes in Mexican Americans. *Nat Genet* 1999; 21: 213–5.
44. Hani EH, Hager J, Philippi A, Demenais F, Froguel P, Vionnet N. Mapping NIDDM susceptibility loci in French families: studies with markers in the region of NIDDM1 on chromosome 2q. *Diabetes* 1997; 46: 1225–6.
45. Horikawa Y, Oda N, Cox NJ, Li X, Orho-Melander M, Hara M, Hinokio Y, Lindner TH, Mashima H, Schwarz PE, Bosque-Plata L, Horikawa Y, Oda Y, Yoshiuchi I, Colilla S, Polonsky KS, Wei S, Concannon P, Iwasaki N, Schulze J, Baier LJ, Bogardus C, Groop L, Boerwinkle E, Hanis CL, Bell GI. Genetic variation in the gene encoding calpain-10 is associated with type 2 diabetes mellitus. *Nat Genet* 2000; 26: 163–75.
46. Baier LJ, Permana PA, Yang X, Pratley RE, Hanson RL, Shen GQ, Mott D, Knowler WC, Cox NJ, Horikawa Y, Oda N, Bell GI, Bogardus C. A calpain-10 gene polymorphism is associated with reduced muscle mRNA levels and insulin resistance. *J Clin Invest* 2000; 106: R69–73.
47. Duggirala R, Blangero J, Almasy L, Arya R, Dyer TD, Williams KL, Leach RJ, O'Connell P, Stern MP. A major locus for fasting insulin concentrations and insulin resistance on chromosome 6q with strong pleiotropic effects on obesity-related phenotypes in nondiabetic Mexican Americans. *Am J Hum Genet* 2001; 68 (5): 1149–64.
48. Weyer C, Hanson RL, Tataranni PA, Bogardus C, Pratley RE. A high fasting plasma insulin concentration predicts type 2 diabetes independent of insulin resistance: evidence for a pathogenic role of relative hyperinsulinemia. *Diabetes* 2000; 49 (12): 2094–101.
49. Pratley RE, Thompson DB, Prochazka M, Baier L, Mott D, Ravussin E, Sakul H, Ehm MG, Burns DK, Foroud T, Garvey WT, Hanson RL, Knowler WC, Bennett PH, Bogardus C. An autosomal genomic scan for loci linked to prediabetic phenotypes in Pima Indians. *J Clin Invest* 1998; 101 (8): 1757–64.
50. Mitchell BD, Cole SA, Hsueh WC, Comuzzie AG, Blangero J, MacCluer JW, Hixson JE. Linkage of serum insulin concentrations to chromosome 3p in Mexican Americans. *Diabetes* 2000; 49: 513–6.
51. Prochazka M, Lillioja S, Tait JF, Knowler WC, Mott DM, Spraul M, Bennett PH, Bogardus C. Linkage of chromosomal markers on 4q with a putative gene determining maximal insulin action in Pima Indians. *Diabetes* 1993; 42 (4): 514–9.
52. Mitchell BD, Kammerer CM, O'Connell P, Harrison CR, Manire M, Shipman P, Moyer MP, Stern MP, Frazier ML. Evidence for linkage of postchallenge insulin levels with intestinal fatty acid-binding protein (FABP2) in Mexican-Americans. *Diabetes* 1995; 44 (9): 1046–53.
53. Meigs JB, Panhuysen CI, Myers RH, Wilson PW, Cupples LA. A genome-wide scan for loci linked to plasma levels of glucose and HbA(1c) in a community-based sample of Caucasian pedigrees: the Framingham Offspring Study. *Diabetes* 2002; 51 (3): 833–40.
54. Stern MP, Duggirala R, Mitchell BD, Reinhart LJ, Shivakumar S, Shipman PA, Uresandi OC, Benavides E, Blangero J, O'Connell P. Evidence for linkage of regions on chromosomes 6 and 11 to plasma glucose concentrations in Mexican Americans. *Genome Res.* 1996; 6 (8): 724–34.
55. Elbein SC, Bragg KL, Hoffman MD, Mayorga RA, Leppert MF. Linkage studies of NIDDM with 23 chromosome 11 markers in a sample of whites of northern European descent. *Diabetes* 1996; 45: 370–5.
56. Shaw JT, Lovelock PK, Kesting JB, Cardinal J, Duffy D, Wainwright B, Cameron DP. Novel susceptibility gene for late-onset NIDDM is localized to human chromosome 12q. *Diabetes* 1998; 47: 1793–6.
57. Yamagata K, Takeda J, Menzel S, Chen X, Eng S, Lim LR, Concannon P, Hanis CL, Spielman RS, Cox NJ, Bell GI. Searching for NIDDM susceptibility genes: studies of genes with triplet repeats expressed in skeletal muscle. *Diabetologia* 1996; 39: 725–30.
58. Vaxillaire M, Boccio V, Philippi A, Vigouroux C, Terwilliger J, Passa P, Beckmann JS, Velho G, Lathrop GM, Froguel P. A gene for maturity onset diabetes of the young (MODY) maps to chromosome 12q. *Nat Genet* 1995; 9: 418–23.

59. Frayling TM, McCarthy MI, Walker M, Levy JC, O'Rahilly S, Hitman GA, Rao PVS, Bennett AJ, Jones EC, Menzel S, Ellard S, Hattersley AT. No evidence for linkage at candidate type 2 diabetes susceptibility loci on chromosomes 12 and 20 in United Kingdom Caucasians. *J Clin Endocrinol Metab* 2000; 85 (2): 853–7.
60. Bowden DW, Sale M, Howard TD, Qadri A, Spray BJ, Rothschild CB, Akots G, Rich SS, Freedman BI. Linkage of genetic markers on human chromosomes 20 and 12 to NIDDM in Caucasian sib pairs with a history of diabetic nephropathy. *Diabetes* 1997; 46: 882–6.
61. Bektas A, Suprenant ME, Wogan LT, Plengvidhya N, Rich SS, Warram JH, Krolewski AS, Doria A. Evidence of a novel type 2 diabetes locus 50 cM centromeric to *NIDDM2* on chromosome 12q. *Diabetes* 1999; 48 (11): 2246–51.
62. Ji L, Malecki M, Warram JH, Yang Y, Rich SS, Krolewski AS. New susceptibility locus for NIDDM is localized to human chromosome 20q. *Diabetes* 1997; 46: 876–81.
63. Klupa T, Malecki M, Hanna L, Sieradzka J , Frey J, Warram JH, Sieradzki J, Krolewski AS. Amino acid variants of the vitamin D-binding protein and risk of diabetes in white Americans of European origin. *Eur J Endocrinol* 1999; 141 (5): 490–3.
64. Risch N, Merikangas K. The future of genetic studies of complex human diseases. *Science* 1996; 273: 1516–7.

24

Molecular Genetics of Type 2 Diabetes—Candidate Genes

Leif Groop and Martin Ridderstråle

Lund University, Malmö, Sweden

About 150 million people suffer from type 2 diabetes in the world today and it has been predicted that this number will be doubled within 15 years [1]. It is no longer a disease of the elderly; age at onset has decreased with the epidemic increase in prevalence. There are large ethnic and geographic variations in the prevalence of type 2 diabetes. In Scandinavia, where type 1 diabetes is common, type 2 diabetes accounts for about 85% of all cases with diabetes. However, the distinction between type 1 and type 2 diabetes may not be as clear as hitherto thought. In addition, the disease seems to be quite heterogeneous [2]. There is plenty of evidence that type 2 diabetes is inherited: the lifetime risk in offspring of one diabetic parent is about 40% and the relative risk (λs) for a sibling to a patient with type 2 diabetes is about 3. It is though unlikely that the cause of the explosion of diabetes is found in our genes. It is rather the rapid change of the environment with an affluent westernized society that triggers the epidemic in genetically predisposed individuals.

What then makes up this genetic predisposition? In general, the chronic hyperglycemia characteristic of type 2 diabetes requires both insulin resistance in muscle and liver and impaired insulin secretion in pancreatic β-cells. Insulin resistance by itself cannot cause diabetes. As long as the β-cell can compensate for the degree of insulin resistance, glucose tolerance remains normal. Accumulation of abdominal fat often predates the manifestation of these defects. It has therefore been suggested that the normal function of the subcutaneous adipose tissue is to serve as a buffer for excess intake of fat [3]. When this buffer capacity is exceeded the body starts to deposit fat in places where it normally does not belong, e.g., muscle, liver, and β-cells. According to this hypothesis a common defect could explain all defects. There is, however, no proof for this and it is likely that the genetic predisposition involves several pathways in different organs (Figure 1).

Type 2 diabetes is considered a paradigm for a multifactorial polygenic disease where common variations in several genes interact (epistasis) to cause the disease when exposed to the affluent environment of too much food and too little exercise. In the following we discuss potential candidates that could contribute to this genetic predisposition to type 2 diabetes.

THE SEARCH FOR SUSCEPTIBILITY GENES

Several approaches are being used in the search for thrifty genes, or genes predisposing to type 2 diabetes and related traits. The *candidate gene approach* aims at the identification of genes based upon information of their function. While this approach has been successful in a number of monogenic disorders with known biochemical defects (e.g., phenylketonuria), our knowledge about the underlying defects causing type 2 diabetes is limited (Figure 1).

The *random gene search* assumes no knowledge of the underlying defects. Instead, positional cloning aims at localizing the disease gene on the basis of its position in the genome. If a chromosomal region has been linked to the disease, the next step would be the search for attractive candidate genes in the region or narrowing the region by linkage disequilibrium mapping. Using this approach the first gene in a polygenic disease like type 2 diabetes was identified, calpain 10 (see Chapter 23).

International Textbook of Diabetes Mellitus, Third Edition. Edited by R. A. DeFronzo, E. Ferrannini, H. Keen, and P. Zimmet.
 ISBN: 0-471-48655-8.

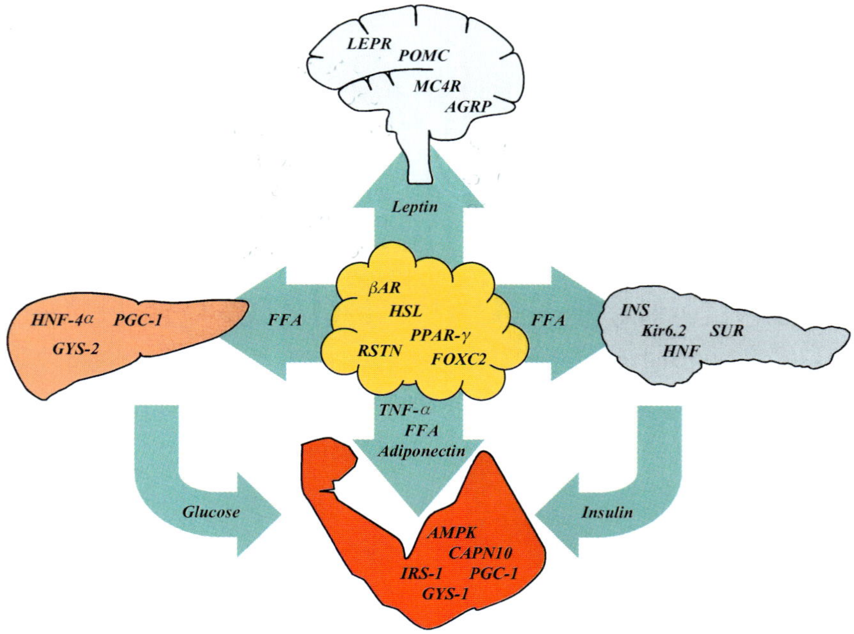

Figure 1 Schematic view of putative candidate genes for type 2 diabetes, their expression in different organs, and interaction

Expression profiling of a large number of gene transcripts (mRNA) or proteins is becoming increasingly popular with the availability of high-density microarrays containing more than 20 000 gene transcripts. Although appealing, the methods still have a lot of inherent problems mostly related to how to define what is different and how to handle the large amount of data. These methods have proven very useful in distinguishing between malignant and benign tissues, but it is still an open question whether the modest differences in gene expression that can be expected in complex disorders like type 2 diabetes can be detected by these methods. A recent paper, however, demonstrated that genes involved in oxidative phosphorylation and fat oxidation were downregulated in muscle from human subjects with type 2 diabetes and impaired glucose tolerance [4]. PGC-1, the coactivator of peroxisome proliferator-activated receptor γ (PPAR-γ), which is a master determinant of oxidative fibers, was also downregulated. Overexpression of PGC-1 in a muscle cell line normalized the expression of the oxidative genes. Several papers have been published in the past months, suggesting a pathogenic role for PGC-1 and mitochondrial oxidative genes in type 2 diabetes [5].

Transgenic animals are needed to prove that a genetic variant has any bearing on physiology. This can rarely be overcome by using cell systems as most cell lines represent nonphysiological clonal expansions of a cell. Another problem is that these cells usually have a normal copy of the gene to be tested, which means that only dominant negative effects of a mutation would be detected. The only way to overcome this is to either disrupt or overexpress a gene in mice. Many knockout experiments have yielded surprisingly negative results, probably because there are redundant mechanisms to overcome a germ-line disruption of a gene. Methods are available to temporally direct the disruption after birth or to restrict it to a certain tissue using the Cre-Lox system.

ASSOCIATION STUDIES

To identify the role of variants in candidate genes for contribution to type 2 diabetes risk one usually compares the frequency of the variant between cases and controls, i.e. whether the variant is associated with the disease. Association studies offer a potentially powerful approach to identifying genetic variants that influence susceptibility to disease but are often plagued by the impression that they are not consistently reproducible. In principle, the inconsistencies may be due to false positive studies, false negative studies, or heterogeneity between studied populations. Despite all these problems a surprisingly large number of candidate genes studies have been replicated and considered positive in meta-analyses [6]. The thrifty gene hypothesis proposes that efficient storage and saving of energy could have been associated with survival advantage during the evolution [7, 8]. Efficient storage of energy must include storage of fat and weight gain. Genes affecting body weight and fat distribution, lipolysis, fuel oxidation, or skeletal muscle glucose metabolism could predispose to the metabolic syndrome and thereby to type 2 diabetes.

GENES REGULATING LIPOLYSIS AND FREE FATTY ACID METABOLISM

β-Adrenergic Receptors

Catecholamines stimulate lipolysis through the β-adrenergic receptors and inhibit lipolysis through α-adrenergic receptors. The β_1- and β_2-adrenergic receptors (β_1-AR and β_2-AR) are expressed in several tissues and are the predominant β-receptor subtypes in cardiac myocytes and adipocytes, respectively. The β_3-adrenergic receptor (β_3-AR) is expressed in brown adipose tissue of rodents and considered responsible for thermogenesis [9]. It was long disputed whether the β_3-AR exists in humans, who do not show brown adipose tissue. The demonstration of mRNA from the β_3-AR in visceral fat changed this view [10]. Subsequently it was demonstrated that catecholamine-induced lipolysis was increased in visceral fat from subjects with abdominal obesity due to increased β_3-AR function [11]. The β_3-AR thereby became a prime candidate gene for abdominal obesity [11].

β_3-Adrenergic Receptor

A few years ago, we and others reported a mutation in the first intracellular loop of the receptor changing a tryptophan in position 64 to arginine [12–14]. Mutation carriers showed more abdominal obesity, higher insulin concentrations, more insulin resistance, and higher blood pressure than did individuals homozygous for the wild-type allele (Trp64Trp), i.e. features of the metabolic syndrome [13]. Furthermore, they had a lower metabolic rate [15] and lower resting sympathetic nervous system activity [16], features one would expect of a "thrifty" gene. This finding was later on replicated in Mexican American sibling pairs discordant for the Trp64Arg variant but concordant for the chromosome 2p21-p23 locus linked to leptin levels (close to proopiomelanocortin gene *POMC*) [17]. A number of negative population association studies have been reported [18, 19], but given the inherent problems in selecting the control group such association studies must be interpreted with caution.

β_2-Adrenergic Receptor

Using a case-control design, we have recently found that the homozygous carriers of the Arg16 allele of the β_2-AR gene had a significantly increased risk for hypertension, particularly among individuals with both hypertension and type 2 diabetes [20]. In addition, our results suggest the haplotype Cys19–Arg16–Gln27 as a risk haplotype for hypertension and obesity, the Gln27 as a risk-allele for elevated free fatty acid levels, and the combination of *β_2-AR* and *β_3-AR* genotypes with increased risk for type 2 diabetes. Thus, variations in the *β_2-AR* and *β_3-AR* genes may form an important part of the thrifty genotype.

β_1-Adrenergic Receptor

The third β-adrenergic receptor is encoded by the *β_1-AR* gene on chromosome 10q24-q26. β-Blocking agents are commonly used to treat elevated blood pressure and the antihypertensive effect is mediated by the β_1-AR, leading to lower cardiac output. Recently, an Arg389Gly polymorphism in the intracellular cytoplasmic tail near the seventh transmembrane domain of the receptor was described and the Arg389 allele was associated with higher basal and isoproterenol-stimulated adenylyl cyclase activity than did the Glu389 allele [21]. Individuals homozygous for the Arg389 allele had an increased risk for hypertension as well as higher heart rate and diastolic blood pressure compared to those without this genotype [22], but no clear association with type 2 diabetes was shown.

Hormone-sensitive Lipase

β-Adrenergic agonists stimulate lipolysis by activating the hormone-sensitive lipase (HSL) by covalent modification (serine phosphorylation). A decrease in the lipolytic effect of catecholamines, possibly through a lesser degree of activation of HSL, has repeatedly been demonstrated in obesity and it has been suggested that impaired expression of the HSL gene may at least in part explain this enzymatic defect [23]. Interestingly, a C-60G HSL promoter variant exhibits a 40% reduction in *in vitro* promoter activity [24] and variation in the HSL gene has been linked to both features of the metabolic syndrome and type 2 diabetes [25].

GENES AFFECTING INSULIN SENSITIVITY

Tumor Necrosis Factor α

Tumor necrosis factor α (TNF-α) is a cytokine that is overexpressed in adipose tissue of obese animals and humans [26, 27]. TNF-α can induce insulin resistance by inhibition of tyrosine phosphorylation of the insulin receptor β-chain and insulin receptor substrate 1 (IRS-1). A positive correlation has also been demonstrated between the level of TNF-α mRNA in fat tissue and the level of hyperinsulinemia, suggesting a role for this cytokine in the pathogenesis of insulin resistance in mice [26]. Although we have recently demonstrated a negative correlation between the plasma concentration of TNF-α and insulin-stimulated glucose metabolism in humans [28], it is more likely that this only represents a spillover and that TNF-α exerts a paracrine rather than an endocrine effect in humans. It has also been suggested that another cytokine, interleukin 6, is more important than TNF-α in humans [29]. Two polymorphisms have been identified in the 5′-untranslated region of the human TNF-α gene (chromosome 6p21.3), one G→A polymorphism at position 308 and another at position 238. Although these polymorphisms seem to influence the host response to infections, discrepant results have been obtained regarding a possible association with human obesity and insulin resistance [30, 31]. We were not able to replicate the findings of an association between the 238 polymorphism and type 2 diabetes using a family-based approach in which we studied transmission of the "disease" allele to affected offspring [32]. It may therefore be premature to ascribe the TNF-α gene a role in the pathogenesis of human obesity and the metabolic syndrome.

Peroxisome Proliferator-activated Receptor γ

There are three forms of peroxisome proliferator-activated receptors (PPARs), α, β (=δ), and γ, which heterodimerize with the retinoid X receptor (RXR) to induce transcription of a number of target genes in adipose tissue [33]. Fatty acids or their derivatives are naturally occurring ligands of PPARs, in addition to drugs like thiazolidinediones (TZDs, for PPAR-γ) and fibrates (for PPAR-α). The human *PPAR-γ* gene maps to chromosome 3p24, a region implicated in several genome-wide scans for type 2 diabetes. A rare Pro115Gln mutation in the N-terminal domain of *PPAR-γ* was described in four morbidly obese subjects [34]. This mutation leads to inhibition of phosphorylation of the protein at Ser114 and thereby to a constitutively active PPAR-γ, resulting in increased adipocyte differentiation and greater cellular accumulation of triglycerides. A more common variant, Pro12Ala, has been associated with lower body mass index (BMI), increased insulin sensitivity, and lower risk for diabetes [35]. *In vitro*, this mutation leads to decreased PPAR-γ activity. Recently, 16 gene variants that had earlier been reported to be associated with diabetes were studied within the Botnia study using a family-based association design [32]. Only one of the earlier findings was confirmed, the association of the PPAR-γ Pro12Ala with type 2 diabetes (Figure 2). A meta-analysis including 3000 individuals from earlier studies reporting evidence both for and against association, indicated a 15% risk reduction for diabetes associated with the Ala allele (allele frequency ~15%). Although the individual risk reduction associated with the Ala allele is moderate, the high frequency of the Pro12 risk allele in the population translates into a rather large population attributable risk of about 25% [32]. Whether individuals with different *PPAR-γ* genotypes respond differently to TZD treatment still needs to be demonstrated.

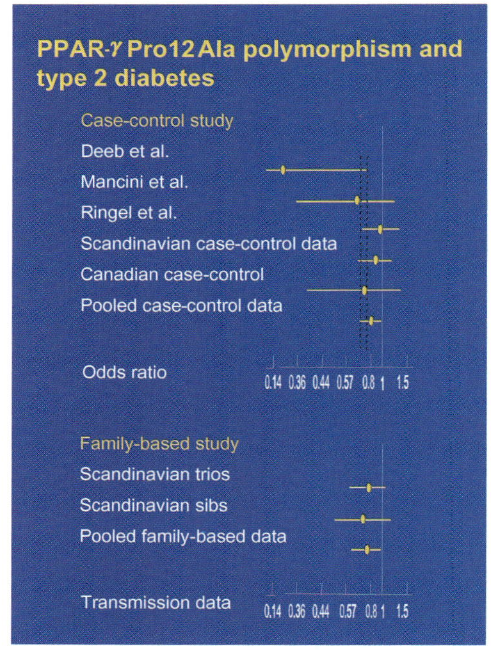

Figure 2 Meta-analysis of the effect of a Pro12Ala variant in the PPAR-γ gene on risk of type 2 diabetes (from reference 32)

Adiponectin

The adipose tissue has been ascribed a more central role in the pathogenesis of insulin resistance than previously thought. One of the main reasons for this is the identification of several hormones/cytokines secreted from adipose tissue that exert effects on insulin saction in other tissues. It has recently been shown that the adipocyte-derived hormone *adiponectin* [36] reduces glucose levels through activation of 5′ AMP kinase [37], an enzyme that also is central to the actions of leptin [38] and antidiabetic drugs such as metformin [39] and TZDs [40]. The plasma levels of adiponectin are decreased in both obesity and type 2 diabetes [41] and low levels of adiponectin predict type 2 diabetes [42, 43]. This may be important as adiponectin can counteract insulin resistance [44] and enhance insulin action [45]. Genetic variants in the adiponectin gene (*APM1*; chromosome 3q27) seem to predispose to both obesity and type 2 diabetes [46–49]. This chromosomal region has also been linked to type 2 diabetes in a genome-wide scan [50].

Forkhead Box C2

Another interesting adipocyte molecule is FOXC2 (forkhead box C2), a winged helix transcription factor that protects from diet-induced obesity and insulin resistance when transgenically overexpressed in the adipose tissue of mice [51]. A polymorphism in the 5′-untranslated region of the *FOXC2* gene seems to be associated with decreased expression of the gene in adipose tissue as well as insulin resistance in humans [52].

Resistin

Contrary to adiponectin and FOXC2, data obtained in mice for another adipocyte-derived hormone, *resistin*, that impairs insulin action and the plasma levels of which are increased in models of obesity [53], have not been readily confirmed in humans [54–56]. So far there has only been marginal evidence for association between genetic variation in the human resistin gene (*RSTN*; chromosome 19p13) and insulin resistance, obesity or type 2 diabetes [57–61].

Calpain 10

The gene encoding calpain 10 (*CAPN10*) on chromosome 2 illustrates the first successful positional cloning of a gene for a polygenic disease like type 2 diabetes [62, 63]. The diabetes-associated *CAPN10* single nucleotide polymorphism 43 G/G genotype has further been associated with reduced muscle CAPN10 mRNA expression in skeletal muscle and impaired insulin-stimulated glucose metabolism, mainly impaired glucose oxidation [64], as well as elevated free fatty acid levels [65]. The precise function of this cysteine protease in glucose metabolism or type 2 diabetes remains to be defined. It has been shown that calpain inhibitors increase the insulin secretory response to glucose in mouse pancreatic islets but reduce insulin-mediated glucose transport in muscle strips and adipocytes as well as incorporation of glucose into glycogen in muscle from rat [66].

Glycoprotein PC-1 (ENPP1)

The membrane glycoprotein PC-1 (prohormone convertase 1) was isolated from a patient with extreme insulin resistance and found to inhibit insulin receptor tyrosine kinase activity [67]. A Lys121Gln (K121Q) variant in exon 4 of the *PC-1* gene (chromosome 6q22-23) has been associated with insulin resistance and features of the metabolic syndrome [68, 69]. *In vitro*, this variant is associated with impaired autophosphorylation of the insulin receptor tyrosine kinase. This is in concert with our findings in genotype discordant sibling pairs; siblings with the Gln allele had higher fasting glucose and impaired insulin action to glucose during an oral glucose tolerance test [69]. Similarly, carriers of the Gln121 allele had impaired insulin-stimulated glucose uptake compared with carriers of the Lys121 allele [70].

Insulin Receptor Substrates

The docking protein IRS-1 links the tyrosine phosphorylated insulin receptor to the downstream part of the insulin signaling pathway [71]. IRS-1 is phosphorylated on multiple tyrosine residues, and could be a candidate for genetic insulin resistance. Two amino acid polymorphisms, Gly972Arg and Ala513Pro, have been described in the IRS-1 gene [72]. These amino acid substitutions, located close to tyrosine phosphorylation motifs, were slightly more frequent in type 2 diabetic patients than in control subjects. In obese nondiabetic Danish subjects, the presence of the codon 972 polymorphism was associated with insulin resistance and clustering of several other features of the metabolic syndrome [73]. Later on, several other insulin receptor substrates (*IRS2* [chromosome 13q34], *IRS3* and *IRS4* [chromosome Xq22]) have been discovered but no consistent variations in these genes have been found. It seems that the different IRS proteins play very different roles in the insulin signaling pathway. While *IRS1* knockout mice suffer from embryonal and postnatal growth retardation and muscle insulin resistance, *IRS2* knockout animals are normal in size but develop diabetes due to liver insulin resistance and lack of pancreatic β-cell compensation [74, 75]. In fact, the *IRS1* knockout mice maintained normoglycemia by compensatory β-cell hyperplasia, while the amount of β-cells was reduced in the *IRS2* knockout mouse underlining the importance of *IRS2* as a regulator of β-cell mass [75]. Moreover, the IRS-2 gene (but not *IRS1*) was recently reported as a target for TZDs. In differentiated 3T3-L1 adipocytes as well as in human adipose tissue cultures, the TZDs had a rapid and marked stimulatory effect on *IRS2* expression [76].

Glycogen Synthase

Impaired insulin stimulation of glycogen synthesis is a hallmark of insulin resistance in feature of type 2 diabetes and impaired glucose tolerance [8, 77]. The key enzyme of this pathway, the skeletal muscle glycogen synthase (GS), could therefore be an important candidate for a genetic defect causing insulin resistance. We have described the genomic structure of the human GS gene (*GYS1*) and assigned it to chromosome 19q13.3 [78, 79]. An *Xba*I polymorphism of the *GYS1* gene has been associated with type 2 diabetes and insulin resistance, particularly impaired insulin-stimulated glycogen synthesis in skeletal muscle [80, 81]. We applied the genotype discordant sibling pair approach to explore this association further. The sibling with the rare A2 allele had more features of the metabolic syndrome (obesity, hypertension, and microalbuminuria) and an increased risk of myocardial infarction compared to siblings with the A1 allele [82]. In addition, diabetic A2 carriers were more severely dyslipidemic and insulin resistant compared to those without A2 allele. Recently, similar results were reported in a Danish twin study; the twins with the A2 allele were significantly more insulin resistant, and had higher diastolic blood pressure compared to their genotype discordant dizygotic twin [83]. A recent study provides some evidence for how this variant may lead to insulin resistance. Neuromuscular electrical stimulation of muscle (and most likely exercise) increases the amount of GS protein in carriers of the A1 variant whereas this increase is impaired in carriers of the A2 allele [84].

In a meta-analysis, the *GYS1* gene showed evidence of ethnic heterogeneity [6]. A plausible explanation is that multiple alleles are contributing to the GYS1 association.

GENES AFFECTING β-CELL FUNCTION

Kir6.2 (KCNJ11) and SUR1 (ABCC8)

In pancreatic β-cells, ATP-sensitive potassium (K_{ATP}) channels control insulin secretion by coupling metabolism to changes in electrical activity. The K_{ATP} channels are composed of two subunits, the sulfonylurea receptor (SUR1 or ABCC8) and the inwardly rectifying potassium channel Kir6.2 [85]. The two genes are located 5 kb from each other on the short arm of chromosome 11. Sulfonylureas stimulate insulin secretion by closing K_{ATP} channels, which in turn results in opening of voltage-gated Ca^{2+} channels. An E23K variant in the Kir6.2 gene has in several studies been associated with type 2 diabetes and suggested to explain about 12% of the population attributable risk of type 2 diabetes [86–89]. This variant seems to induce spontaneous overactivity of the pancreatic β-cells, thereby decreasing the sensitivity of the β-cells to ATP [90].

Mutations in the *SUR1* gene cause decreased K_{ATP}-channel activity and congenital hyperinsulinemia [91, 92]. Recently it was shown that a dominant mutation, E1506K in the *SUR1* gene, which causes neonatal hypoglycemia in its heterozygous form, increases susceptibility to type 2 diabetes later in life [93]. It can thus be assumed that continuous overstimulation of insulin secretion might lead to subsequent insulin deficiency and diabetes. Several other variants (e.g., exon 16-3 t/c, exon 18 t/c) have been identified in the *SUR1* gene but none has been consistently associated with type 2 diabetes [88, 94].

Insulin Gene VNTR

The insulin gene is located close to the SUR1/Kir6.2 on chromosome 12. A variable number tandem repeat (INS-VNTR) 0.5-kb upstream of the gene has received a lot of attention over the past year as a potential susceptibility gene for both type 1 and type 2 diabetes and also obesity and low birth weight [95–99]. Depending on the number of repeats, INS-VNTR can be divided into class I (26–63 repeats), II (64–104 repeats), and III (141–209 repeats). The number of repeats is considered to influence expression of the insulin gene in both the thymus and the pancreas [100–103]. While the class I allele has been associated with increased risk of type 1 diabetes the class III allele has been suggested to increase risk for type 2 diabetes. Several studies have shown that the class I allele results in elevated insulin concentrations in children and juvenile obesity [98, 104]. A parent of origin effect has also been proposed in that this is particularly due to paternal expression of the class I allele [97, 105]. The association with type 2 diabetes is, however, less consistent and might be secondary to hyperinsulinemia and obesity.

Type 1 diabetes genes

In Scandinavia, there are about 10% of persons with type 1 diabetes in families with type 2 diabetes [106]. A family history of type 1 diabetes seems to influence the phenotype of patients with type 2 diabetes: there is an earlier onset of the disease, they have a lower BMI, lower C-peptide levels, and do require insulin more often. While HLA-DQB*0201/0302 is clearly associated with type 1 diabetes, DQB*0302/X also increases the risk of type 2 diabetes. Also, protective HLA genotypes are common among type 2 diabetic patients.

CONCLUSIONS

The genetics of type 2 diabetes is still a puzzle although no longer a nightmare. It has become evident that the disease is much more heterogeneous than hitherto. The interplay between common variants in candidate genes and an affluent environment seems to explain most of the genetic component of the disease. Many of these genes influence energy metabolism and regulation of insulin secretion.

At moment, two genes, one influencing insulin sensitivity (PPAR-γ) and another influencing β-cell function (Kir6.2), seem to be the most reproducible candidate genes for type 2 diabetes across the world. But certainly many more are out there to be identified.

REFERENCES

1. Zimmet P, Alberti KG, Shaw J. Global and societal implications of the diabetes epidemic. *Nature* 2001; 414: 782–7
2. Groop L, Tuomi T. Non-insulin-dependent diabetes mellitus—a collision between thrifty genes and an affluent society. *Ann Med* 1997; 29: 37–53.
3. Frayn KN, Karpe F, Fielding BA, Macdonald IA, Cppack SW. Integrative physiology of human adipose tissue. *Int J Obes* 2003; 27: 875–88.
4. Mootha VK, Lindgren CM, Eriksson K-F, Subramanian A, Sihag S, Lehar J, Puigserver P, Carlsson E, Ridderstråle M, Laurila E, Daly MJ, Patterson N, Mesirov JP, Todd RG, Tamayo P, Spiegelman B, Lander ES, Hirschhorn J, Altshuler DM, Groop LC. PGC-1 responsive genes involved in oxidative phosphorylation are coordinately downregulated in human diabetes. *Nat Genet* 2003; 34: 267–73.
5. Patti ME, Butte AJ, Crunkhorn S, Cusi K, Berria R, Kashyap S, Miyazaki Y, Kohane I, Costello M, Saccone R, Landaker EJ, Goldfine AB, Mun E, DeFRonzo R, Finlayson J, Kahn CR, Mandarino LJ. Coordinated reduction of genes of oxidative metabolism in humans with insulin resistance and diabetes: potential role of PGC-1 and NRF1. *Proc Natl Acad Sci USA* 2003; 100: 8466–71,
6. Lohmueller KE, Pearce CL, Pike M, Lander ES, Hieschhorn JN, Meta-analysis of genetic association studies supports a contribution of common variants to susceptibility to common disease. *Nat Genet* 2003; 33: 177–82.

7. Neel V. Diabetes mellitus: a "thrifty" genotype rendered detrimental by progress? *Am J Hum Genet* 1962; 14: 352–62.
8. Beck-Nielsen H, Groop L. Metabolic and genetic characterization of prediabetic states. Sequence of events leading to non-insulin-dependent diabetes mellitus. *J Clin Invest* 1994; 94: 1714–21.
9. Emorine L, Marullo S, Briend-Sutren M, Patey G, Tate K, Delavier-Klutchko C, Strosberg A. Molecular characterization of the human beta-3-adrenergic receptor. *Science* 1989; 245: 1118–21.
10. Krief S, Lönnqvist F, Raimbault S, Baude B, Van Spronsen A, Arner P, Strosberg A, Ricquier D, Emorine L. Tissue distribution of beta-3-adrenergic receptor mRNA in man. *J Clin Invest* 1993; 91: 344–9.
11. Lönnqvist F, Thörne A, Nilsell K, Hoffstedt J, Arner P. A pathogenetic role of visceral fat beta-3-adrenoreceptors in obesity. *J Clin Invest* 1995; 95: 1109–16.
12. Walston J, Silver K, Bogardus C, Knowler W, Celi F, Austin S, Manning B, Strosberg D, Stern M, Raben N, Sorkin J, Roth J, Shuldiner A. Time of onset of non-insulin-dependent diabetes mellitus and genetic variation in the beta3-adrenergic-receptor gene. *N Engl J Med* 1995; 333: 343–7.
13. Widén E, Lehto M, Kanninen T, Walston J, Shuldiner A, Groop L. Association of a polymorphism in the beta-3-adrenergic-receptor gene with features of the insulin resistance syndrome in Finns. *N Engl J Med* 1995; 333: 348–51.
14. Clément K, Vaisse C, Manning B, Basdevant A, Guy-Grand B, Ruiz J, Silver K, Shuldiner A, Froguel P, Strosberg A. Genetic variation in the beta3-adrenergic receptor and an increased capacity to gain weight in patients with morbid obesity. *New Engl J Med* 1995; 333: 352–4.
15. Sipiläinen R, Uusitupa M, Heikkinen S, Rissanen A, Laakso M. Polymorphism of the beta-3-adrenergic receptor gene affects basal metabolic rate in obese Finns. *Diabetes* 1997; 46: 77–80.
16. Shihara N, Yasuda K, Moritani T, Ue H, Adachi T, Tanaka H, Tsuda K, Seino Y. The association between Trp64Arg polymorphism of the beta-3-adrenergic receptor and autonomic nervous system activity. *J Clin Endocrinol Metab* 1999; 84: 1623–7.
17. Mitchell B, Blangero J, Comuzzie A, Almasy L, Shuldiner A, Silver K, Stern M, MacCluer J, Hixson J. A paired sibling analysis of the beta-3 adrenergic receptor and obesity in Mexican Americans. *J Clin Invest* 1998; 101: 584–7.
18. Gagnon J, Mauriege P, Roy S, Sjöström D, Chagnon Y, Dionne F, Oppert J-M, Perussé L, Sjöström L, Bouchard C. The Trp64Arg mutation of the beta-3-adrenergic receptor gene has no effect on obesity phenotypes in the Quebec family study and Swedish obese subjects cohort. *J Clin Invest* 1996; 98: 2086–93.
19. Fujisawa T, Ikegami H, Kawaguchi Y, Ogihara T. Meta-analysis of the association of the Trp64Arg polymorphism of the beta-3-adrenergic receptor gene with body mass index. *J Clin Endocrinol Metab* 1998; 83: 2441–4.
20. Bengtsson K, Orho-Melander M, Melander O, Lindblad U, Ranstam J, Rastam L, Groop L. Beta(2)-adrenergic receptor gene variation and hypertension in subjects with type 2 diabetes. *Hypertension* 2001; 37: 1303–8.
21. Mason DA, Moore JD, Green SA, Liggett SB. A gain-of-function polymorphism in a G-protein coupling domain of the human beta-1-adrenergic receptor. *J Biol Chem* 1999; 274: 12670–4.
22. Bengtsson K, Melander O, Orho-Melander M, Lindblad U, Ranstam J, Rastam L, Groop L. Polymorphism in the beta(1)-adrenergic receptor gene and hypertension. *Circulation* 2001; 104: 187–90.
23. Large V, Reynisdottir S, Langin D, Fredby D, Klannemark M, Holm C, Arner P. Decreased expression and function of adipocyte hormone-sensitive lipase in subcutaneous fat cells of obese subjects. *J Lipid Res* 1999; 40: 2059–65.
24. Talmud PJ, Palmen J, Walker M. Identification of genetic variation in the human hormone-sensitive lipase gene and 5′ sequences: homology of 5′ sequences with mouse promoter and identification of potential regulatory elements. *Biochem Biophys Res Commun* 1998; 252: 661–8.
25. Klannemark M, Orho M, Langin D, Laurell H, Holm C, Reynisdottir S, Arner P, Groop L. The putative role of the hormone-sensitive lipase gene in the pathogenesis of type II diabetes mellitus and abdominal obesity. *Diabetologia* 1998; 41: 1516–22.
26. Hotamisligil G, Shargill N, Spiegelman B. Adipose expression of tumor necrosis factor-α: direct role in obesity-linked insulin resistance. *Science* 1993; 259: 87–91.
27. Hotamisigil G, Arner P, Caro J, Atkinson R, Spiegelman B. Increased adipose tissue expression of tumor necrosis factor-α in human obesity and insulin resistance. *J Clin Invest* 1995; 95: 2409–15.
28. Kellerer M, Rett K, Renn W, Groop L, Häring H. Circulating TNF-alpha and leptin levels in offspring of NIDDM patients do not correlate to individual insulin sensitivity. *Horm Metab Res* 1996; 28: 737–43.
29. Mohamed-Ali V, Goodrick S, Rawesh A, Katz DR, Miles JM, Yudkin JS, Klein S, Coppack SW. Subcutaneous adipose tissue secretes interleukin-6 but not tumor necrosis factor-α in vivo. *J Clin Endocrinol Metab* 1997; 82: 4196–200.
30. Fernandéz-Real J, Gutierrez C, Ricart W, Casamitjana R, Fernandéz-Castanér M, Vendrell J, Richart C, Soler J. The TNF-alpha gene *Nco*I polymorphism influences the relationship among insulin resistance, percent body fat, and increased serum leptin levels. *Diabetes* 1997; 46: 1468–72.
31. Walston J, Seibert M, Jen-Yen C, Cheskin L, Andersen R. Tumor necrosis factor-alpha-238 and -308 polymorphisms do not associate with traits related to obesity and insulin resistance. *Diabetes* 1999; 48: 2096–8.
32. Altshuler D, Hirschorn JN, Klannemark M, Lindgren CM, Vohl M-C, Nemesh J, Lane CR, Schaffner SF, Bolk S, Brewer C, Tuomi T, Gaudet D, Hudson TJ, Daly M Groop L, Lander ES. The common PPARγ Pro12Ala polymorphism is associated with decreased risk of type 2 diabetes. *Nat Genet* 2000; 26: 76–80.
33. Auwerx J. PPARgamma, the ultimate thrifty gene. *Diabetologia* 1999; 42: 1033–49.
34. Ristow M, Muller-Wieland D, Pfeiffer A, Krone W, Kahn C. Obesity associated with a mutation in a genetic regulator of adipocyte differentiation. *N Engl J Med* 1998; 339: 953–9.
35. Deeb S, Fajas L, Nemoto M, Laakso M, Fujimoto W, Auwerx J. A Pro 12Ala substitution in the human peroxisome proliferator-activated receptor gamma2 is associated with decreased receptor activity, improved insulin sensitivity and lowered body mass index. *Nat Genet* 1998; 20: 284–7.

36. Scherer PE, Williams S, Fogliano M, Baldini G, Lodish HF. A novel serum protein similar to C1q, produced exclusively in adipocytes. *J Biol Chem* 1995; 270: 26746–9.
37. Yamauchi T, Kamon J, Minokoshi Y, Ito Y, Waki H, Uchida S, Yamashita S, Noda M, Kita S, Ueki K, Eto K, Akanuma Y, Froguel P, Foufelle F, Ferre P, Carling D, Kimura S, Nagai R, Kahn BB, Kadowaki T. Adiponectin stimulates glucose utilization and fatty-acid oxidation by activating AMP-activated protein kinase. *Nat Med* 2002; 8: 1288–95.
38. Minokoshi Y, Kim YB, Peroni OD, Fryer LG, Muller C, Carling D, Kahn BB. Leptin stimulates fatty-acid oxidation by activating AMP-activated protein kinase. *Nature* 2002; 415: 339–43.
39. Zhou G, Myers R, Li Y, Chen Y, Shen X, Fenyk-Melody J, Wu M, Ventre J, Doebber T, Fujii N, Musi N, Hirshman MF, Goodyear LJ, Moller DE. Role of AMP-activated protein kinase in mechanism of metformin action. *J Clin Invest* 2001; 108: 1167–74.
40. Fryer LG, Parbu-Patel A, Carling D. The anti-diabetic drugs rosiglitazone and metformin stimulate AMP-activated protein kinase through distinct signaling pathways. *J Biol Chem* 2002; 277: 25226–32.
41. Arita Y, Kihara S, Ouchi N, Takahaschi M, Maeda K, Miyagawa J, Hotta K, Shimomura I, Nakamura T, Miyaoka K, Kuriyama H, Nishida M, Yamashita S, Okubo K, Matsubara K, Muraguchi M, Ohmoto Y, Funahashi T, Matsuzawa Y. Paradoxical decrease of an adipose-specific protein, adiponectin, in obesity. *Biochem Biophys Res Commun* 1999; 275: 79–83.
42. Lindsay RS, Funahashi T, Hanson RL, Matsuzawa Y, Tanaka S, Tataranni PA, Knowler WC, Krakoff J. Adiponectin and development of type 2 diabetes in Pima Indian population. *Lancet* 2002; 360: 57–8.
43. Spranger J, Kroke A, Möhlig M, Bergmann MM, Ristow M, Boening H, Pfeiffer AFH. Adiponectin and protection against type 2 diabetes mellitus. *Lancet* 2003; 361: 226–8.
44. Yamauchi T, Kamon J, Waki H, Terauchi Y, Kubota N, Hara K, Mori Y, Ide T, Murakami K, Tsuboyama-Kasaoka N, Ezaki O, Akanuma Y, Gavrilova O, Vinson C, Reitman ML, Kagechika H, Shudo K, Yoda M, Nakano Y, Tobe K, Nagai R, Kimura S, Tmoita M, Froguel P, Kadowaki T. The fat-derived hormone adiponectin reverses insulin resistance associated with both lipoatrophy and obesity. *Nat Med* 2001; 7: 941–6.
45. Berg AH, Combs TP, Du X, Brownlee M, Scherer PE. The adipocyte-secreted protein Arp30 enhances hepatic insulin action. *Nat Med* 2001; 7: 947–53.
46. Stumvoll M, Tschritter O, Fritsche A, Staiger H, Renn H, Weisser M, Machicao F, Häring H. Association of the T-G polymorphism in adiponectin (exon 2) with obesity and insulin sensitivity. *Diabetes* 2002; 51: 37–41.
47. Hara K, Boutin P, Mori Y, Tobe K, Dina C, Yasada K, Yamauchi T, Otabe S, Okada T, Eto K, Kadowaki H, Hagura R, Akanuma Y, Yazaki Y, Nagai R, Taniyama M, Matsubara K, Yoda M, Nakano Y, Kimura S, Tomita M, Kimura S, Ito C, Froguel P, Kadowaki T. Genetic variation in the gene encoding adiponectin is associated with an increased risk of type 2 diabetes in the Japanese population. *Diabetes* 2002; 51: 536–40.
48. Menzaghi C, Ercolino T, Di Paola R, Berg AH, Warram JH, Scherer PE, Trischitta V, Doria A. A haplotype at the adiponectin locus is associated with obesity and other features of the insulin resistance syndrome. *Diabetes* 2002; 51: 2306–12.
49. Vasseur F, Helbecque N, Dina C, Lobbens S, Delannoy V, Gaget S, Boutin P, Vaxillaire M, Leprêtre F, Dupont S, Hara K, Clément K, Bilhain B, Kadowaki T, Froguel P. Single-nucleotide polymorphism haplotypes in both the proximal promoter and exon 3 of the *APM1* gene modulate adipocyte-secreted adiponectin hormone levels and contribute to the genetic risk for type 2 diabetes in French Caucasians. *Hum Mol Gen* 2002; 11: 2607–24.
50. Vionnet N, Hani El-H, Dupont S, Gallina S, Francke S, Dotte S, De Matos F, Durand E, Leprêtre F, Lecoeur C, Gallina P, Zekiri L, Dina Froguel P. Genome wide search for type 2 diabetes-susceptibility genes in French whites: evidence for a novel susceptibility locus for early-onset diabetes on chromosome 3q27-qter and independent replication of a type 2-diabetes locus on chromosome 1q21-q24. *Am J Hum Genet* 2000; 67: 1470–80.
51. Cederberg A, Grönning LM, Ahrén B, Taskén K, Carlsson P, Enerbäck S. *FOXC2* is a winged helix gene that counteracts obesity, hypertriglyceridemia, and diet-induced insulin resistance. *Cell* 2001; 106: 563–73.
52. Ridderstråle M, Carlsson E, Klannemark M, Cederberg M, Kösters C, Tornqvist H, Storgaard H, Vaag A, Enerbäck S, Groop L. *FOXC2* mRNA and a 5′UTR polymorphism of the gene are associated with insulin resistance. *Diabetes* 2002; 51: 3554–60.
53. Steppan CM, Bailey ST, Bhat S, Brown EJ, Banerjee RR, Wright CM, Patel HR, Ahima RS, Lazar MA. The hormone resistin links obesity to diabetes. *Nature* 2001; 409: 307–12.
54. Nagaev I, Smith U. Insulin resistance and type 2 diabetes are not related to resistin expression in human fat cells or skeletal muscle. *Biochem Biophys Res Commun* 2001; 285: 561–4.
55. Savage DB, Sewter CP, Klenk ES, Segal DG, Vidal-Puig A, Considine RV, O'Rahilly S. Resistin/Fizz3 expression in relation to obesity and peroxisome proliferator-activated receptor-γ action in humans. *Diabetes* 2001; 50: 2199–202.
56. Janke J, Engeli S, Gorzelniak K, Luft FC, Sharma AM. Resistin gene expression in human adipocytes is not related to insulin resistance. *Obes Res* 2002; 10: 1–5.
57. Sentinelli F, Romeo S, Arca M, Filippi E, Leonetti F, Banchieri M, Di Mario U, Baroni MG. Human resistin gene, obesity, and type 2 diabetes. *Diabetes* 2002; 51: 860–2.
58. Osawa H, Onuma H, Murakami A, Ochi M, Nishimiya T, Kato K, Shimizu I, Fujii Y, Ohashi J, Makino H. Systematic search for single nucleotide polymorphisms in the resistin gene: the absence of evidence for the association of three identified single nucleotide polymorphisms with Japanese type 2 diabetes. *Diabetes* 2002; 51: 863–6.
59. Engert JC, Vohl M-C, Williams SM, Lepage P, Loredo-Osti JC, Faith J, Doré C, Renaud Y, Burtt NP, Villeneuve A, Hirschhorn JN, Altshuler D, Groop LC, Després J-P, Gaudet D, Hudson TJ. 5′ flanking variants of resistin are associated with obesity. *Diabetes* 2002; 51: 1629–34.
60. Wang H, Chu WS, Hemphill C, Elbein SC. Human resistin gene: molecular scanning and evaluation of association with insulin sensitivity and type 2 diabetes in Caucasians. *J Clin Endocrinol Metab* 2002; 87: 2520–4.
61. Pizzuti A, Argiolas A, Di Paola R, Baratta R, Rauseo A, Bozzali M, Vigneri R, Dallapiccola B, Trischitta V, Frittitta L. An ATG repeat in the 3′-untranslated region

of the human resistin gene is associated with decreased risk of insulin resistance. *J Clin Endocrinol Metab* 2002; 87: 4403–6.

62. Hanis C, Boerwinkle E, Chakraborty R, Ellsworth D, Concannon P, Stirling B, Morrison V, Wapelhorst B, Spielman R, Goglin-Ewens K, Shephard J, Williams S, Risch N, Hinds D, Iwasaki N, Ogata M, Omori Y, Petzold C, Rietsch H, Schröder H-E, Schulze J, Cox N, Menzel S, Boriraj V, Chen X, Lim L, Lindner T, Mereu L, Wang Y-Q, Xiang K, Yamagata K, Yang Y, Bell G. A genome-wide search for human non-insulin-dependent (type 2) diabetes genes reveals a major susceptibility locus on chromosome 2. *Nat Genet* 1996; 13: 161–6.
63. Horikawa Y. Oda N, Cox NJ, Li X, Orho-Melander M, Hara M, Hinokio Y, Lindner TH, Mashima H, Schwarz PE, del Bosque-Plata L, Horikawa Y, Oda Y, Yoshiuchi I, Colilla S, Polonsky KS, Wei S, Concannon P, Iwasaki N, Schulze J, Baier LJ, Bogardus C, Groop L, Boerwinkle E, Hanis CL, Bell GI. Genetic variation in the gene encoding calpain-10 is associated with type 2 diabetes mellitus. *Nat Genet* 2000; 26: 163–75.
64. Baier LJ, Permana PA, Yang X, Pratley RE, Hanson RL, Shen G-Q, Mott D, Knowler WC, Cox NJ, Horikawa Y, Oda N, Bell GI, Bogardus C. A calpain-10 gene polymorphism is associated with reduced muscle mRNA levels and insulin resistance. *J Clin Invest* 2000; 106: R69–73.
65. Orho-Melander M, Klannemark M, Svensson M, Ridderstråle M, Lindgren C, Groop L. Variants in the calpain-10 gene predispose to insulin resistance and elevated free fatty acid levels. *Diabetes* 2002; 51: 2658–64.
66. Sreenan SK, Zhou Y-P, Otani K, Hansen PA, Currie KPM, Pan C-Y, Lee J-P, Ostrega DM, Pugh W, Horikawa Y, Cox NJ, Hanis CL, Burant CF, Fox AP, Bell GI, Polonsky KS. Calpains play a role in insulin secretion and action. *Diabetes* 2001; 50: 2013–20.
67. Maddux B, Sbraccia P, Kumakura S, Sasson S, Youngren J, Fisher A, Spemcer S, Grupe A, Henzel W, Stewart T, Reaven G, Goldfine I. Membrane glycoprotein PC-1 and insulin resistance in non-insulin dependent diabetes mellitus. *Nature* 1995; 273: 448–51.
68. Pizzuti A, Frititta L, Argiolas A, Baratta R, Goldfine I, Bozzali M, Ercolino T, Scarlato G, Iacovello L, Vigneri R, Tassi V, Trischitta V. A polymorphism (K121Q) of the human glycoprotein PC-1 gene coding region is strongly associated with insulin resistance. *Diabetes* 1999; 48: 1881–4.
69. Gu HF, Almgren P, Lindholm E, Frittitta L, Pizzuti A, Trischitta V, Groop LC. Association between the human glycoprotein *PC*-1 gene and elevated glucose and insulin levels in a paired-sibling analysis. *Diabetes* 2000; 49: 1601-3.
70. Kubaszek A, Pihlajamäki J, Karhapää P, Vauhkonen I, Laakso M. The K121Q polymorphism of the PC-1 gene is associated with insulin resistance but not with dyslipidemia. *Diabetes Care* 2003; 26: 464–7.
71. Sun X, Rothenberg P, Kahn R, Backer J, Arakai E, Wilden P, Cahill D, Goldhill B, White M. Structure of the insulin receptor substrate IRS-1 defines a unique signal transduction protein. *Nature* 1991; 352: 73–7.
72. Almind K, Bjoerbaek C, Vestergaard H, Hansen T, Echwald S, Pedersen O. Aminoacid polymorphism of the insulin receptor substrate-1 in non-insulin-dependent diabetes mellitus. *Lancet* 1993; 342: 828–32.
73. Clausen J, Hansen T, Bjoerbaek C, Echwald S, Urhammer S, Rasmussen S, Andersen C, Hansen L, Almind K, Winther K, Haraldsdottir J, Borch-Johnsen K, Pedersen O. Insulin resistance: interactions between obesity and a common variant of the insulin receptor substrate-1. *Lancet* 1995; 346: 397–402.
74. Abe H, Yamada N, Kamata K, Kuwaki T, Shimada M, Osuga J, Shionoiri F, Yahagi N, Kadowaki T, Tamemoto H, Ishibashi S, Yazaki Y, Makuuchi M. Hypertension, hypertriglyceridemia, and impaired endothelium-dependent vascular relaxation in mice lacking insulin receptor substrate-1. *J Clin Invest* 1998; 101: 1784–8.
75. Kubota N, Tobe K, Terauchi Y, Eto K, Yamauchi T, Suzuki R, Tsubamoto Y, Komeda K, Nakano R, Miki H, Satoh S, Sekihara H, Sciacchitano S, Lesniak M, Aizawa S, Nagai R, Kimura S, Akanuma Y, Taylor SI, Kadowaki T. Disruption of insulin receptor substrate 2 causes type 2 diabetes because of liver insulin resistance and lack of compensatory beta-cell hyperplasia. *Diabetes* 2000; 40: 1880–9.
76. Smith U, Gogg S, Johansson A, Olausson T, Rotter V, Svalstedt B. Thiazolidinediones (PPARgamma agonists) but not PPARalpha agonists increase IRS-2 gene expression in 3T3-L1 and human adipocytes. *FASEB J* 2001; 15: 215–20.
77. Eriksson J, Franssila-Kallunki A, Ekstrand A, Saloranta C, Widen E, Schalin C, Groop L. Early metabolic defects in persons at increased risk for non-insulin-dependent diabetes mellitus. *N Engl J Med* 1989; 321: 337–43.
78. Lehto M, Stoffel M, Groop L, Espinosa R, III, LeBeau M, Bell G. Assignment of the gene encoding glycogen synthase to human chromosome 19, band q13.3. *Genomics* 1993; 15: 460–1.
79. Orho M, Nikula-Ijäs P, Schalin-Jäntti C, Permutt M, Groop L. Isolation and characterization of the human muscle glycogen synthase gene. *Diabetes* 1995; 44: 1099–105.
80. Groop L, Kankuri M, Schalin-Jäntti C, Ekstrand A, Nikula-Ijäs P, Widén E, Kuismanen E, Eriksson J, Franssila-Kallunki A, Saloranta C, Koskimies S. Association between polymorphism of the glycogen synthase gene and non-insulin-dependent diabetes mellitus. *N Engl J Med* 1993; 328: 10–14.
81. Majer M, Mott D, Mochizuki H, Rowles J, Pedersen O, Knowler W, Bogardus C, Prochazka M. Association of the glycogen synthase locus 19q13 with NIDDM in Pima Indians. *Diabetologia* 1996; 39: 314–21.
82. Orho-Melander M, Almgren P, Kanninen T, Forsblom C, Groop L. A paired sibling analysis of the XbaI polymorphism in the muscle glycogen synthase gene. *Diabetologia* 1999; 42: 1138–45.
83. Fenger M, Poulsen P, Beck-Nielsen H, Vaag A. Impact of the *Xba*1 polymorphism of the human muscle glycogen synthase gene on parameters of the insulin resistance syndrome in a Danish twin population. *Diabet Med* 2000; 17: 735–40.
84. St-Onge J, Joanisse DR. Simoneau JA. The stimulation-induced increase in skeletal muscle glycogen synthase content is impaired in carriers of the glycogen synthase *Xba*I gene polymorphism. *Diabetes* 2001; 50: 195–8.
85. Aguilar-Bryan L, Bryan J. Molecular biology of triphosphate-sensitive potassium channels. *Endocr Rev* 1999; 20: 101–35.
86. Hani EH, Boutin P, Durand E, Inoue H, Permutt MA, Velho G, Froguel P. Missense mutations in the pancreatic islet beta cell inwardly rectifying K+ channel gene (KIR6.2/BIR): A meta-analysis suggests a role in

the polygenic basis of Type II diabetes mellitus in Caucasians. *Diabetologia* 1998; 41: 1511–5.

87. Love-Gregory L, Wasson J, Lin J, Skolnick G, Suarez B, Permutt MA. An E23K single nucleotide polymorphism in the islet ATP-sensitive potassium channel gene (Kir6.2) contributes as much to the risk of type II diabetes in Caucasians as the PPARγPro12Ala variant. *Diabetologia* 2003; 46: 136–7.
88. Gloyn AL, Weedon MN, Owen KR, Turner MJ, Knight BA, Hitman G, Walker M, Levy JC, Sampson M, Halford S, McCarthy M, Hattersley AT, Frayling TM. Large scale association studies of variants in genes encoding the pancreatic β-cell KATP channel subunits Kir 6.2 (KCNJ11) and SUR1 (ABCC8) confirm that the KCNJ11 E23K variant is associated with type 2 diabetes. *Diabetes* 2003; 52: 568–72.
89. Nielsen EM, Hansen L, Carstensen B, Echwald SM, Drivsholm T, Gulmer C, Thorsteinsoon B, Borch-Johnsen K, Hansen T, Pedersen O. The E23K variant of Kir6.2 associates with impaired post-OGTT serum insulin response and increased risk of type 2 diabetes. *Diabetes* 2003; 52: 573–7.
90. Schwanstecher C, Meyer U, Schwanstecher M. K(IR)6.2 polymorphism predisposes to type 2 diabetes by inducing overactivity of pancreatic beta-cell ATP-sensitive K(+) channels. *Diabetes* 2002; 51: 875–9.
91. Thomas PM, Cote GJ, Wohllk N, Haddad B, Mathew PM, Rabl W, Aguilar-Bryan L, Gagel RF, Bryan J. Mutations in the sulfonylurea receptor gene in familial persistent hyperinsulinemic hypoglycemia of infancy. *Science* 1995; 268: 426–9.
92. Huopio H, Reimann F, Ashfield R, Komulainen J, Lenko H-L, Rahier J, Vauhkonen I, Kere J, Laakso M, Aschcroft F, Otonkoski T. Dominantly inherited hyperinsulinism caused by a mutation in the sulfonylurea receptor type 1. *J Clin Invest* 2000; 106: 897–906.
93. Huopio H, Otonkoski T, Vauhkonen I, Reimann F, Aschcroft FM, Laakso M. A new subtype of autosomal dominant diabetes attributable to a mutation in the gene for sulfonylurea receptor 1. *Lancet* 2003; 361: 301–7.
94. Harsen T, Ambye L, Grarup N, Hansen L, Echwald SM, Ferrer J, Pedersen O. Genetic variability of the SUR1 promoter in relation to beta-cell function and Type II diabetes mellitus. *Diabetologia* 2001. 44: 1330–4.
95. Bell GI, Selby MJ, Rutter WJ. The highly polymorphic region near the human insulin gene is composed of simple tandemly repeating sequences. *Nature* 1982; 295: 31–5.
96. Lucassen AM, Juloer C, Beressi J-P, Boitard C, Froguel P, Lathrop M, Bell JI. Susceptibility to insulin dependent diabetes mellitus maps to a 4.1 kb segment of DNA spanning the insulin gene and associated VNTR. *Nat Genet* 1993; 4: 305–10.
97. Bennett ST, Wilson AJ, Esposito L, Bouzekri N, Undlien DE, Cucca F, Nistico L, Buzzetti R, the IMDIAB Group, Bosi E, Pociot F, Nerup J, Cambon-Thomsen A, Pugliese A, Shield JPH, Kinney PA, Bain SC, Polychronakos C, Todd JA. Insulin VNTR allele-specific effect in type 1 diabetes depends on identity of untransmitted paternal allele. *Nat Genet* 1997; 17: 350–52.
98. LeStunff C, Fallin D, Schork NJ, Bougnères P. Paternal transmission of the very common class I INS VNTR alleles predisposes to childhood obesity. *Nat Genet* 2001; 29: 96–9.
99. Lindsay RS, Hanson RL, Wiedrich C, Knowler WC, Bennett PH, Baier LJ. The insulin gene variable number tandem repeat class I/III polymorphism is in linkage disequilibrium with birth weight but not type 2 diabetes in the Pima population. *Diabetes* 2003; 52: 187–93.
100. Kennedy GC, German MS, Rutter WJ. The minisatellite in the diabetes susceptibility locus IDDM2 regulates insulin transcription. *Nat Genet* 1995; 9: 293–8.
101. Lucassen AM, Screaton GR, Julier C, Elliott TJ, Lathrop M, Bell JI. Regulation of insulin gene expression by the IDDM associated, insulin locus haplotype. *Hum Mol Genet* 1995; 4: 501–6.
102. Vafiadis P, Bennett ST, Colle E, Grabs R, Goodyer CG, Polychronakos C. Imprinted and genotype-specific expression of genes at the IDDM2 locus in pancreas and leucocytes. *J Autoimmun* 1996; 9: 397–403.
103. Pugliese A, Zeller M, Fernandez A, Jr, Zalcberg LJ, Bartlett RJ, Ricordi C, Pietropaolo M, Eisenbarth GS, Bennett ST, Patel DD. The insulin gene is transcribed in the human thymus and transcription levels correlated with allelic variation at the INS VNTR-IDDM2 susceptibility locus for type 1 diabetes. *Nat Genet* 1997; 15: 293–7.
104. Le Stunff C, Fallin D, Schork NJ, Bourgneres P. The insulin gene VNTR is associated with fasting insulin levels and development of juvenile obesity. *Nat Genet* 2000: 26: 444–6. Erratum in: *Nat Genet* 2001; 28: 97.
105. Huxtable SJ, Saker PJ, Haddad L, Walker M, Frayling TM, Levy JC, Hitman GA, O'Rahilly S, Hattersley AT, McCarthy MI. Analysis of parent–offspring trios provides evidence for linkage and association between the insulin gene and type 2 diabetes mediated exclusively through paternally transmitted class III variable number tandem repeat alleles. *Diabetes* 2000; 49: 126–30.
106. Li H, Isomaa B, Almgren P, Taskinen M-R, Groop L, Tuomi T: Consequences of a family history of type 1 or Type 2 diabetes on the phenotype of patients with type 2 diabetes. *Diabetes Care* 2000; 23: 589–94.

25

Glucose Toxicity

Hannele Yki-Järvinen

Helsinki University, Helsinki, Finland

INTRODUCTION

Clinical trials such as the Diabetes Control and Complications Trial (DCCT) and the United Kingdom Prospective Diabetes Study (UKPDS) have firmly established that hyperglycemia is the most important cause of diabetic microvascular complications [1, 2]. Chronic hyperglycemia also seems to be a significant and independent, albeit weak risk factor for macrovascular disease [3]. Other adverse consequences of hyperglycemia include an increased susceptibility to infections [4]. These complications affect tissues, where glucose utilization is predominantly non-insulin-dependent. However, since 1986, it has been clear, based on *in vivo* experiments in both rats [5–7] and humans [8], that chronic hyperglycemia is itself a regulator of both insulin secretion and action. In contrast to acute hyperglycemia, which stimulates insulin secretion and glucose utilization, chronic hyperglycemia inhibits both and thereby self-perpetuates the diabetic state. These harmful metabolic effects of chronic hyperglycemia have been referred to as *glucose toxicity* [9–11]. The ensuing discussion is focused on reviewing our present understanding of the occurrence, pathophysiology, and significance of this phenomenon on the basis of both clinical and experimental data.

HYPERGLYCEMIA AND GLUCOSE UTILIZATION

Acute Hyperglycemia

The Mass-Action Effect of Glucose

In virtually all tissues except the brain, glucose, at a fixed insulin concentration, promotes its own utilization in a concentration-dependent manner [12] (Figure 1). In insulin-sensitive tissues, the glucose-induced increase in glucose utilization is dependent upon the insulin concentration. For example, an increase in the blood glucose concentration from a fasting concentration from 5 to a peak postprandial concentration of 8.9 mmol/l (from 90 to 160 mg/dl) increases the rate of whole-body glucose utilization two- to threefold more in the presence of postprandial (serum insulin 50–160 mU/l) than fasting (insulin 10–20 mU/l) serum insulin concentrations [12]. This mass-action effect of glucose is quite significant if one compares it to the rate of whole-body glucose utilization, which averages ~2 mg/kg/min after an overnight fast, and increases two- to threefold to ~5–7 mg/kg/min after a meal [9]. As discussed below, the mass-action effect of glucose has important implications for the understanding of the mechanisms underlying glucose toxicity.

Consequences of the Acute Stimulatory Effect of Hyperglycemia on Postprandial Glucose Disposal in Patients with Type 1 and 2 Diabetes

Whole-body glucose uptake can be accurately quantitated, using the insulin clamp technique [10] during maintenance of similar glucose and insulin concentrations in normal subjects and diabetic patients. Under such conditions, insulin resistance is observed: i.e., the rate of glucose uptake is, on the average, reduced in both patients with type 1 and 2 diabetes [11]. If, however, the rate of glucose uptake is measured in patients with type 1 [13] or type 2 [14] diabetes under conditions simulating the actual glucose and insulin concentrations found in these patients postprandially, the rate of whole-body glucose uptake is normal. This is explained by the ability of hyperglycemia, via glucose mass-action, to compensate for the reduction in glucose utilization caused by insulin resistance. In the absence

International Textbook of Diabetes Mellitus, Third Edition. Edited by R. A. DeFronzo, E. Ferrannini, H. Keen, and P. Zimmet.
 ISBN: 0-471-48655-8.

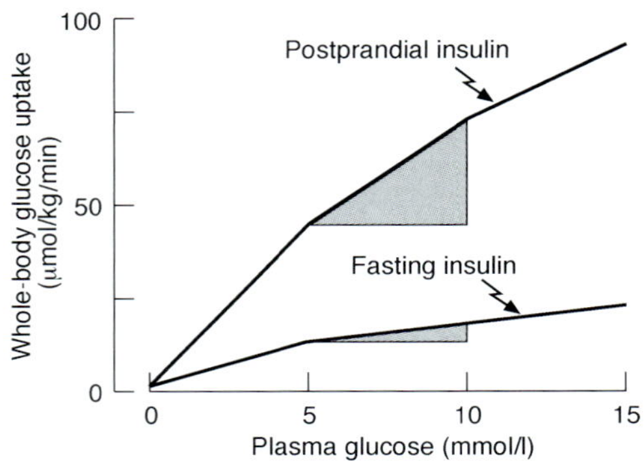

Figure 1 The mass-action effect of glucose. These dose–response curves were found in humans by inhibiting endogenous insulin secretion with somatostatin in healthy volunteers and by then increasing glucose and insulin concentrations to desired levels on separate days. Doubling the plasma glucose concentration from 5 to 10 mmol/l significantly increases the rate of glucose uptake. The mass-action effect of glucose is dependent upon the ambient insulin concentration and is much greater at postprandial than fasting insulin concentrations. (Reproduced with permission from reference 12)

of any insulin resistance, the mass-action effect of glucose would lead to overutilization of glucose not only in non-insulin-dependent but also in insulin-dependent tissues. In non-insulin-dependent tissues not protected by the blood–brain barrier, such as peripheral nerves, the kidney, and retina, the rate of glucose utilization is chronically elevated under hyperglycemic conditions, and is a key pathophysiologic abnormality leading to diabetic microvascular complications [15]. The normal glucose flux to insulin-sensitive tissues, such as skeletal muscle, spares them from hyperglycemia-induced damage.

Development of the Glucose Toxicity Concept: Chronic Hyperglycemia as a Cause of Insulin Resistance

Insulin Resistance in Patients with Type 1 Diabetes—A Consequence of Glucose Toxicity?

Insulin resistance characterizes not only patients with type 2 diabetes but also moderately and poorly controlled patients with type 1 diabetes [16–18]. Insulin resistance in patients with type 1 diabetes is an acquired and reversible phenomenon since insulin sensitivity is completely normalized during remission of the disease [17, 19]. In these patients, insulin resistance of glucose utilization is predominantly localized to skeletal muscle [20]. Since in insulin-treated patients the peripheral (although not the portal) insulin concentration is usually similar to that in normal subjects [21], insulin deficiency cannot explain insulin resistance in skeletal muscle. In a comprehensive analysis of clinical and laboratory parameters that potentially could explain insulin resistance in patients with type 1 diabetes, a significant correlation has often been found between the glycosylated hemoglobin concentrations and the degree of insulin resistance [18, 20]. This association has been independent of body weight, insulin dose, and residual C-peptide secretion. These data suggest that hyperglycemia *per se* or some associated metabolic alteration might be a cause of insulin resistance in these patients. Further support for this idea was obtained from studies where patients with type 1 diabetes were treated with continuous subcutaneous insulin infusion (CSII) therapy. With this physiologic mode of insulin administration, glycemic control and insulin sensitivity could be improved without increasing the total insulin dose [22, 23].

Induction of In Vivo Insulin Resistance by Hyperglycemia

In type 1 diabetic patients lacking endogenous insulin secretion, effects of hyperglycemia *per se* on insulin action can be examined. In the first of such studies, insulin-stimulated glucose uptake was measured on two occasions in patients treated with CSII, after 24 h of hyperglycemia induced by an intravenous glucose infusion (mean diurnal blood glucose 16 mmol/l) and after 24 h of normoglycemia (6 mmol/l) [8]. After 24 h of hyperglycemia, the rate of whole-body glucose uptake, when measured under standardized conditions, was consistently lower than that after normoglycemia, demonstrating that short-term hyperglycemia can cause insulin resistance in humans [8]. Subsequently, an identical study design was used to further locate glucose-induced insulin resistance to glucose extraction rather than blood flow [20] (Figure 2). This resistance could not be explained by circulating free fatty acid (FFA) or counterregulatory hormone concentrations [20]. These observations have subsequently been confirmed [24–26].

In the rat, removal of 90% of the pancreas causes insulin deficiency, hyperglycemia, and a 30% reduction in insulin-stimulated glucose utilization in skeletal muscle [5]. Selective correction of hyperglycemia with phlorizin, which induces glucosuria via inhibition of glucose reabsorption in the proximal tubuli, normalizes glycemia without changing serum insulin concentrations [5] (Figure 3). These studies together with the human data provided the first evidence of the ability of the blood glucose concentration itself to regulate insulin sensitivity, a phenomenon then referred to as *glucose toxicity* [28, 29]. Additional support for this concept has been obtained in studies using isolated skeletal muscle from patients with type 2 diabetes [30]. In the latter study, insulin-stimulated glucose transport in muscle strips of hyperglycemic type 2 diabetic patients was similar to that in normoglycemic subjects but impaired when measured after short-term exposure to normoglycemia. Prolonged exposure to normoglycemia completely normalized the defect in

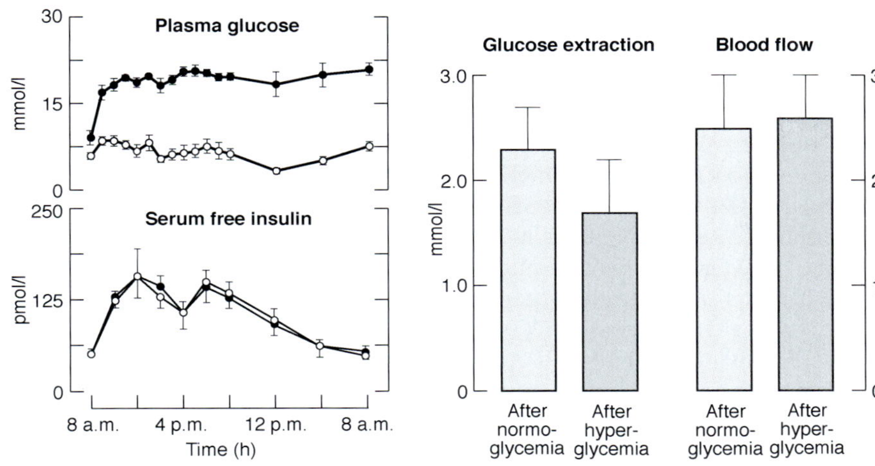

Figure 2 Induction of insulin resistance by hyperglycemia in C-peptide negative patients with type 1 diabetes. Plasma glucose and serum-free insulin concentrations during a normoglycemic day (-○-) and during a hyperglycemic day (-●-) induced by infusion of glucose. On both study days, the subjects received identical diets and insulin doses. After each study day, the rate of glucose uptake across the forearm was measured under standardized conditions of glycemia and insulinemia to quantitate insulin sensitivity. Preceding hyperglycemia significantly decreased glucose extraction but had no effect on blood flow. (Reproduced with permission from reference 20)

insulin-stimulated glucose transport [30]. In mice, hyperglycemia resulting from deletion of the insulin-sensitive glucose transporter 4 (GLUT-4) from skeletal muscle induces insulin resistance in both adipose tissue and the liver, since insulin resistance in these tissues can be reversed with phlorizin, which normalizes glycemia without changing insulin concentrations [31].

Location of Glucose-induced Insulin Resistance

Studies at the Level of the Whole Body In Vivo

In insulin-treated patients with type 1 diabetes, in whom glucose toxicity appears to be the major cause of insulin resistance, direct quantitation of tissue glucose uptake during insulin stimulation using positron emission tomography has demonstrated that skeletal muscle is the predominant tissue responsible for the defect in insulin-stimulated glucose utilization [32]. In contrast to skeletal muscle, glucose uptake in the heart is not affected by insulin resistance [32, 33]. Whether this is explained by differences in rate-limiting steps for insulin-stimulated glucose uptake in the heart and skeletal muscle, or by other factors such as greater dependence of glucose uptake in the heart as compared to skeletal muscle on insulin's antilipolytic effect than direct stimulation of glucose transport, is unknown. Indirect calorimetry can be used to determine the rate of glucose oxidation during hyperinsulinemia [34]. Since a substantial fraction of whole-body glucose oxidation either is independent of insulin or is not affected by insulin resistance (glucose oxidation in the heart), rates of whole-body glucose oxidation have to corrected for the estimated contribution of these components of glucose oxidation [35]. When this is done in patients with type 1 [13] or type 2 [36] diabetes, the fractions of glucose oxidized and disposed of nonoxidatively (the sum of glycogen synthesis and nonoxidative glycolysis) are similar to those in normal subjects. These data suggest that regardless of the primary cellular process causing insulin resistance, the ultimate gatekeeper for cellular glucose uptake is located at the level of glucose transport or phosphorylation. In support of this, muscle glucose-6-phosphate concentrations are similar in insulin-resistant patients with type 1 diabetes under conditions where glucose flux is acutely normalized by hyperglycemia under hyperinsulinemic conditions as under conditions of normoglycemic hyperinsulinemia [13]. Since both GLUT-4-mediated glucose transport [37]

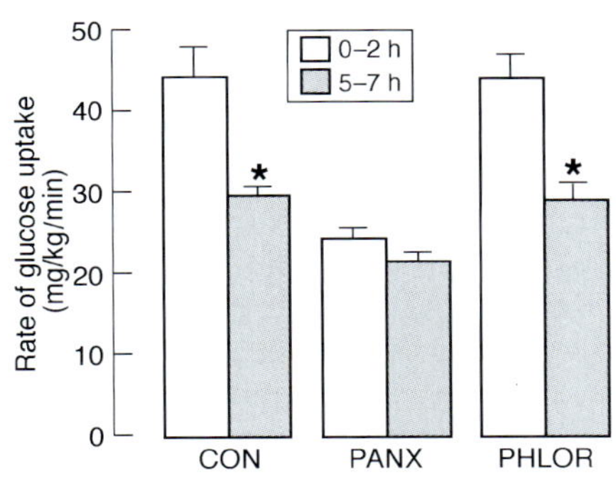

Figure 3 The rate of whole-body glucose disposal measured under similar euglycemic hyperinsulinemic conditions in control rats (CON), 90% pancreatectomized rats (PANX), and in phlorizin-treated diabetic rats (PHLOR). Normalization of plasma glucose concentrations with phlorizin did not change insulin concentrations but was still able to reverse insulin resistance in the PANX rats. * indicates significant difference between rates at 5–7 and 0–2 h. (Reproduced with permission from reference 27)

and glucose phosphorylation by hexokinase II [38] are regulated by insulin, either transport or phosphorylation could be rate-limiting for glucose disposal. Another hypothetical possibility is that glucose delivery could be rate-limiting for glucose disposal. Insulin, at physiological concentrations, increases blood flow, depending on factors such as limb muscularity [39] and physical fitness [40] from –10 to 80% (mean in 75 studies around 20% [41]). During a similar time period and at similar insulin concentrations, glucose extraction, as determined from the AV-glucose difference across a limb, increased 1000–2000% within 30–60 min [39]. Although defects in blood flow may be observed at supraphysiological insulin concentrations in patients with type 1 diabetes [42], studies performed at physiological insulin concentrations locate impaired insulin action exclusively to glucose extraction [13, 20, 43, 44]. Taken together, these data localize hyperglycemia-induced insulin resistance of glucose utilization in patients with type 1 diabetes to early steps in glucose uptake in skeletal muscle. This defect is accompanied by similar relative reductions in glucose oxidation and storage.

Cellular Mechanisms

Although the tissue and even cellular localization of glucose-induced insulin resistance has been rather well characterized in *in vivo* studies since 1987 [5, 8], the biochemical mechanism(s) sensing the extracellular glucose concentration, or glucose flux, and the mechanism coupling this putative sensing mechanism to glucose transport or phosphorylation remained an enigma for a long time.

The Hexosamine Pathway

Discovery of the pathway In 1991, Marshall and colleagues described a novel pathway that mediates glucose-induced insulin resistance in primary cultured rat adipocytes [45]. Downregulation of the insulin-responsive glucose transport system was observed to require three components—glucose, insulin, and glutamine. Inactivation of the glutamine-requiring enzyme, glutamine: fructose-6-amidotransferase (GFA), the rate-limiting enzyme of the hexosamine pathway, by glutamine analogues, prevented glucose-induced desensitization of glucose transport [45]. GFA catalyzes the interconversion of glutamine and fructose-6-phosphate to form glucosamine-6-phosphate (GlcN-6-P) and glutamate (Figure 4). GFA is widely expressed in insulin-sensitive tissues such as skeletal muscle, adipose tissue, the liver, heart, and the submandibular gland (greatest expression of all tissues) [46]. GFA is also expressed in other than classic insulin target tissues such as the endothelium and mesangium, where excessive activation of the hexosamine pathway may be involved in the pathogenesis of endothelial dysfunction [possibly via increased O-glycosylation of endothelial nitric oxide synthase (eNOS)] [47–49] and diabetic nephropathy [by increasing mesangial production of transforming growth factor β1 (TGF-β1) [50, 51]. The end product of the GFA reaction, GlcN-6-P, is subsequently, after a few intermediate steps, converted to UDP-*N*-acetylglucosamine (UDP-GlcNAc), which is a feedback inhibitor of GFA in the rat liver [52] and human skeletal muscle [36]. The GlcNAc moiety of UDP-GlcNAc is subsequently O-linked to serine and threonine residues of cytosolic and nuclear proteins by a UDP-GlcNAc:polypeptide β-acetylglucosaminyltransferase [53], which does not appear to be sensitive to insulin or glucose flux and is not altered in type 2 diabetes [54]. An O-GlcNAc selective *N*-acetyl-β-D-glucosaminidase selectively removes O-GlcNAc residues from proteins [55]. The molecular mechanism underlying glucose-induced changes in GFA activity and the coupling between altered activity of the hexosamine pathway, insulin signaling, and glucose transport/phosphorylation have recently been studied intensively, as discussed below.

Studies using glucosamine In rat adipocytes, glucosamine, which bypasses the rate-limiting step in the hexosamine pathway (Figure 4), completely abolishes insulin-stimulated glucose transport in 5 [45]. In cells, which express GLUT-1 and not GLUT-4, glucosamine has no effect on basal or insulin-stimulated glucose transport [56], suggesting that glucosamine-induced insulin resistance of glucose transport is restricted to GLUT-4-expressing cells. Since skeletal muscle is the major tissue responsible for insulin-stimulated glucose uptake [57], the role of the hexosamine pathway in mediating glucose-induced insulin resistance in this tissue is of particular interest. In isolated rat diaphragms, pre-exposure to high concentrations of glucosamine (5–22 mmol/l), inhibits, within 1 h, insulin-stimulated glucose transport and glycogen synthesis [56]. In rats, *in vivo* infusion of glucosamine (plasma glucosamine $\sim$1.3 mmol/l [27], for 2 [58] to 4 [27] h) significantly decreases insulin-stimulated glucose utilization via glycolytic and glycogen synthetic pathways. In the same model, glucosamine also induces a defect in the ability of GLUT-4 to translocate to the plasma membrane (see Chapter 13) [59]. While these studies demonstrate that glucosamine induces insulin resistance, they provide no information regarding the role of the hexosamine pathway in mediating glucose toxicity. The finding that infusion of glucosamine induces insulin resistance in normoglycemic, but not hyperglycemic, mildly insulin-deficient rats suggests that increased hexosamine metabolism may play a role in glucose toxicity, at least in rats [27].

Use of glucosamine as an experimental tool to activate the hexosamine pathway has limitations. During

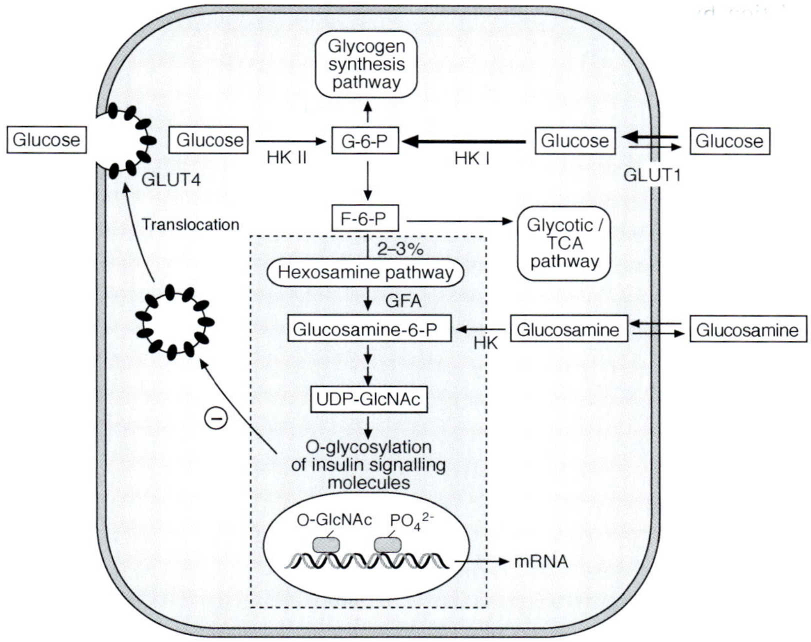

Figure 4 The hexosamine metabolic pathway proposed by Marshall et al. to explain glucose toxicity [45]. A small fraction (2–3%) of glucose, which enters insulin-sensitive tissues either using the insulin-independent glucose transporter GLUT-1 and glucose phosphorylating enzyme hexokinase I (HK-I) or with the help of the insulin-sensitive glucose transporter GLUT-4 and hexokinase II (HK-II), is metabolized to hexosamine products in the presence of glutamine. GFA is the rate-limiting enzyme of the pathway. The end product of the pathway is UDP-GlcNAc, which can be covalently linked to serine and threonine residues on specific proteins (O-glycosylation) such as insulin signaling molecules and GLUT-4. O-Glycosylation seems to decrease insulin action and GLUT-4 translocation, thus resulting in insulin resistance. Initial activation of the pathway is thought to occur via glucose mass-action, at low insulin concentrations (after an overnight fast), which is increased under hyperglycemic conditions. G-6-P = glucose-6-phosphate, F-6-P = fructose-6-phosphate. Glucosamine can bypass the rate-limiting step of the pathway and can therefore be used as a tool to study consequences of activation of the hexosamine pathway. (Reproduced with permission from The American Society for Biochemistry and Molecular Biology; and reprinted with permission from Nature 414; 813–20 (2001) Macmillan Magazines limited)

glucosamine infusions at doses used in most of the *in vivo* studies in rats [27, 60, 61], glucosamine-6-phosphate concentrations increase dramatically in skeletal muscle and the heart [62] to levels that are sufficient to stimulate glycogen synthase and inhibit hexokinase [62, 63]. Similar data have been reported in adipocytes [63, 64]. This effect appears responsible for the paradoxical combination of diminished glycogen synthesis and increased insulin-stimulated glycogen synthase activity during glucosamine infusions [56, 61, 63, 65]. In adipocytes, accumulation of glucosamine was found to be very closely correlated with insulin resistance of glucose transport [64]. Trapping of high-energy phosphate as glucosamine-6-phosphate has also been linked to ATP depletion in adipocytes [64, 66]. The doses of glucosamine used have not, however, altered ATP levels in skeletal muscle or the heart [62] but accumulation of glucosamine-6 phosphate may have contributed to the observed insulin resistance. These problems limit the usefulness of glucosamine as a tool to examine consequences of activation of the hexosamine pathway. Furthermore, two studies in normal volunteers suggested that glucosamine infusions, increasing glucosamine concentrations as much as in the rat [27], have no effect on insulin action or secretion [67, 68].

Overexpression of GFA in cell lines and animals Stable overexpression of the cDNA for GFA by 51–95% in rat-1 fibroblasts decreases insulin sensitivity of both glycogen synthase activity and glycogen synthesis [69]. In transgenic mice, which overexpress GFA in their skeletal muscles and adipose tissue, a 1.9-fold increase in GFA activity is accompanied by insulin resistance [70], and an unchanged total GLUT-4 content but disruption in the translocation of GLUT-4. In transgenic mice overexpressing GLUT-1 but with normal levels of GLUT-4 expression, GFA activity and the concentration of UDP-*N*-acetylhexosamines are increased in skeletal muscle [71]. The latter data are consistent with the idea that activation of the hexosamine pathway is a consequence of increased basal glucose uptake via GLUT-1. This activation then leads to maintenance of normal glucose flux in insulin-sensitive tissues at the expense of insulin resistance.

Consequences of tissue-specific overexpression of GFA have supported the idea that sensing of excessive glucose fuel via the hexosamine pathway has adverse metabolic consequences, although the pathway could be regarded as protective against excess glucose utilization in insulin-sensitive tissues. GFA overexpression in the liver results in obesity, glucose intolerance, and insulin resistance and increases in circulating triglyceride and FFA concentrations [72], while overexpression in β-cells leads to hyperinsulinemia [73]. These changes were observed with approximately twofold changes in hexosamine flux and were not accompanied by changes in ATP concentrations [74].

Studies in patients with type 2 diabetes GFA is expressed in multiple human tissues including adipose tissue and skeletal muscle [36, 54, 75] but data regarding the possible functional significance of the hexosamine pathway in diabetic patients are sparse. GFA activity has been found to be increased in skeletal muscle of patients with type 2 diabetes, in proportion to the degree of chronic hyperglycemia [36]. Exposure of cultured human skeletal muscle cells to chronic hyperglycemia also increases GFA activity [76]. Muscle hexosamine metabolite concentrations have been found to remain unchanged when measured in patients with type 2 diabetes before and after restoration of normoglycemia with 28 days of intravenous insulin [77]. Taken together, there are, in contrast to extensive data in animals, too few human data to allow conclusions to be drawn regarding the contribution of the hexosamine pathway to glucose-induced insulin resistance.

How do hexosamines impair glucose uptake? Despite the limitations of glucosamine as an experimental tool, the other data convincingly link overactivity of the hexosamine pathway to impaired insulin-stimulated glucose uptake, at least in animals. Activation of the pathway is likely to occur via glucose mass-action under basal (low insulin) conditions, when glucose flux is increased [71, 78]. This also occurs in patients with type 2 diabetes [78]. Hyperglycemia activates GFA [69] and increases levels of hexosamine metabolites, especially UDP-GlcNAc [71], which is then attached, in a reaction regulated by O-GlcNAc transferase (addition of GlcNAc) and O-GlcNAcase (removal of GlcNAc) to serine and threonine residues on proteins (O-GlcNAcylation) [79]. An increase in glucose flux increases O-GlcNAcylation [80, 81]. O-GlcNAcylation has, under some circumstances, been shown to be reciprocal with phosphorylation [79, 82] which could have important consequences on insulin signaling. Proteins relevant to insulin resistance, which have been shown to undergo O-GlcNAcylation, include phosphatidylinositol 3 kinase insulin receptor substrate 1 (IRS-1), and IRS-2 in skeletal muscle in rats infused with glucosamine and insulin [60, 61], IRS-1 in 3T3-L1 adipocytes [83], the transcription factor Sp1 in L6 myotubes [84], and GLUT-4 [80, 85]. Hexosamine-mediated O-GlcNAcylation has also been linked with stimulation of TGF-β expression in mesangial cells [86], plasminogen activator inhibitor 1 expression and activity in adipose tissue [87], and inhibition of the activity of eNOS in endothelial cells [48, 88]. The latter data raise the possibility that activation of the hexosamine pathway may also be involved in mediating harmful effects of hyperglycemia on diabetic nephropathy and atherothrombotic vascular disease.

Malonyl-CoA, Diacylglycerol, Protein Kinase C, and Insulin Resistance

In patients with type 2 diabetes, several investigators have found defects in insulin receptor kinase activity in adipocytes [89, 90] and skeletal muscle [91, 92]. This kinase defect is reversible with improvement of glycemic control by weight loss [90]. The decrease in insulin receptor kinase activity has been suggested to be mediated via glucose-induced activation of protein kinase C (PKC) [93]. PKC can cause insulin resistance via serine phosphorylation of the insulin receptor [94]. PKC also phoshorylates, independent of its effect on the insulin receptor kinase, glycogen synthase, a change that impairs glycogen synthesis [95]. Hyperglycemia activates PKC by stimulating the *de novo* synthesis of diacylglycerol (DAG) in many tissues, including skeletal muscle [96]. In rat fat cells [93] and rat-1 fibroblasts [94], PKC inhibitors prevent glucose-induced decreases in insulin receptor kinase activity and insulin resistance.

De novo synthesis of DAG requires glycerol-3-phosphate and long-chain fatty acyl CoA [96]. Recent studies in isolated rat soleus muscle preparations have showed that hyperglycemia, both in the absence and in the presence of insulin, increases the concentration of malonyl-CoA, a precursor of long-chain fatty acyl CoA [97]. Malonyl-CoA inhibits carnitine palmitoyl transferase 1, the rate-limiting enzyme for fatty acid entry to mitochondria, where they are oxidized. The latter effect could contribute to glucose-induced increases in DAG synthesis by channeling long-chain fatty acid CoA toward DAG synthesis rather than oxidation. The PKC and hexosamine pathways may not necessarily be alternative or parallel pathways regulating glucose utilization. In rat adipocytes, flux through the hexosamine pathway seems to activate PKC and the contribution of the hexosamine pathway seems even greater than PKC activation by *de novo* DAG synthesis [98]. Except for the studies addressing insulin receptor kinase activity, no human data are currently available to prove or disprove the role of PKC activation as a mechanism of glucose toxicity.

HYPERGLYCEMIA AND INSULIN SECRETION

Chronic Hyperglycemia as a Cause of Impaired Insulin Secretion

In 1948, Lukens and Dohan administered large doses of glucose to normal cats and induced permanent hyperglycemia, hydropic degeneration of the islet of Langerhans, and ketonuria in 4 out of 35 cats studied [99]. These investigators proposed that hyperglycemia could play a role in the pathogenesis of diabetes. In recent years, several approaches have been used to directly examine the harmful effects of chronic hyperglycemia on insulin secretion. These studies have established that chronic hyperglycemia impairs β-cell responsiveness to glucose although the exact biochemical mechanism(s) mediating this effect remain to be clearly defined.

Insulin Secretion During Experimental Hyperglycemia

In normal subjects, β-cell hyperresponsiveness and α-cell hyporesponsiveness are observed after mild hyperglycemia induced by glucose infusions [100–102]. However, exposure to higher glucose concentrations (12.6 mmol/l) for 68 h has been reported to be associated with significant reduction in insulin secretion [26]. As discussed under Clinical Significance below, treatment studies in patients with type 2 diabetes have provided additional support for the idea that chronic hyperglycemia impairs insulin secretion also in humans.

Since the early experiments [99], the ability of chronic hyperglycemia to desensitize the β-cell to glucose has been convincingly documented in animal models. In the partially pancreatectomized dog, maintenance of plasma glucose at greater than or equal to 14 mmol/l for 2 weeks induces persistent hyperglycemia, loss of glucose-induced insulin secretion, ketonuria, and weight loss [103]. Morphometric analysis of the endocrine pancreas revealed a profound reduction in the number and size of islets. These changes were not observed in portions of pancreases removed prior to the glucose infusions or in pancreases of similarly pancreatectomized dogs not subjected to hyperglycemia [103]. Leahy et al. infused normal rats *in vivo* with various concentrations of glucose and measured the insulin response thereafter *in vitro* using the isolated perfused pancreas [7]. Rats infused with 35% glucose showed a severely blunted insulin response to glucose after 48 h, and in rats infused with 50% glucose for 48 h, the glucose-induced insulin response was totally lost [104]. Further experiments revealed that addition of phlorizin to the 50% glucose infusion after 48 h for an additional 48-h period completely restored the insulin response [105]. Similar results were obtained by Rossetti

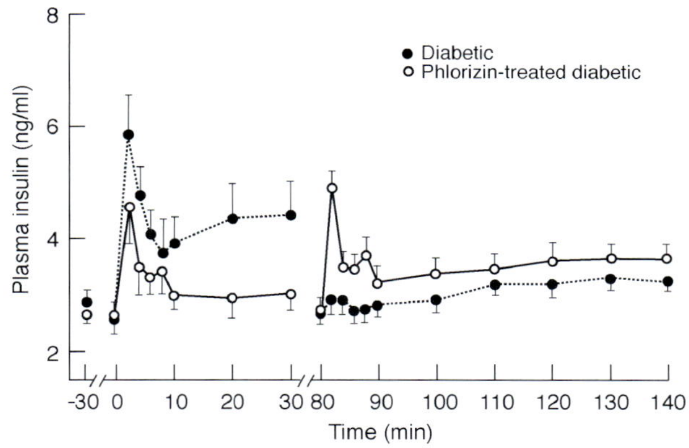

Figure 5 Effects of selective normalization of glucose concentrations, without changing insulin concentrations, on insulin responses to arginine (0–30 min) and glucose (80–140 min). The insulin response to arginine was exaggerated in diabetic animals while both first (80–90 min) and second (90–140 min) phase responses to glucose were blunted before treatment in the diabetic (90% pancreatectomized) animals. Phlorizin treatment restored both responses to arginine and glucose to normal. (Reproduced with permission from reference 6)

et al. who treated mildly hyperglycemic rats with a continuous infusion of phlorizin for 4 weeks [6]. The insulin responses to arginine, glucose, and arginine plus glucose were determined *in vitro* using the hyperglycemic clamp technique. Normalization of glycemia by phlorizin normalized all aspects of abnormal insulin secretion, i.e. the subnormal first and second phase insulin responses to glucose, the increased insulin response to arginine, and the potentiation of insulin secretion by hyperglycemia during infusion of arginine [6] (Figure 5). Correction of hyperglycemia with phlorizin also has been shown to restore glucose-induced suppression of glucagon release in insulin-deficient alloxan diabetic dogs [106].

Measurement of the secretory function of islets transplanted under the kidney capsule of normal and diabetic mice provides another model to study glucose toxicity on β-cell function *in vivo*. Collier et al. transplanted islets cultured in high and low glucose containing media to the kidney capsule of syngeneic mice made diabetic with streptozotocin [107]. Glycemia was normalized in the mice grafted with islets grown in low glucose whereas mice grafted with islets grown in high glucose never became normoglycemic [107]. Korsgren et al. measured insulin release by means of a kidney perfusion technique in islets grafted under the kidney capsule of normoglycemic and alloxan-induced diabetic mice [108]. Glucose stimulated insulin release from the grafted islets of normoglycemic but not diabetic mice [108]. The implanted islets isolated from hyperglycemic animals contained significantly less insulin, and exhibited reduced rates of proinsulin biosynthesis [108].

Chronic Hyperglycemia and Insulin Secretion, Cellular Mechanisms

Exposure of the β-cell to experimental chronic hyperglycemia induces specific desensitization to glucose whereas the insulin response to other secretagogues such as arginine [6, 105], leucine [104, 109], isoproterenol [110], and 3-isobutyl-1-methylxanthine [111] is either preserved or exaggerated. In keeping with this, the insulin content of the islet is not reduced by hyperglycemia to an extent that would account for the degree of glucose-induced desensitization [105]. Such selective desensitization to glucose but not other secretagogues like arginine has also been observed during the early phase of type 1 [112] and type 2 [113] diabetes. This desensitization is considered entirely reversible by restoration of normal glucose concentrations [114]. The term *glucose toxicity* has been used by some authors to characterize such reversible insulin secretory defects [6], while others have limited use of the term *toxicity* to irreversible damage of insulin content and secretion [114].

Regarding the cellular mechanisms of glucose toxicity on insulin secretion, increasing evidence links oxidative stress provoked by hyperglycemia to β-cell damage [114–116]. The initial events, i.e. formation of reactive oxygen species such as superoxide in mitochondria as a consequence of hyperglycemia and inhibition of glycolysis closely, resemble those characterizing glucose effects in non-insulin-dependent tissues (see Chapter 92) [15]. β-Cells are particularly susceptible to oxidative stress because they contain intrinsically low concentrations of antioxidant enzymes. In animals and cell lines, hyperglycemia induces a gradual loss of insulin gene expression and gene and protein expression levels pancreas duodenum homeobox 1 (PDX-1) transcription factor, which is a critical regulator of the insulin gene [114]. Insulin secretory defects and the changes in genes controlling insulin secretion in several experimental models of glucose toxicity have been prevented by various antioxidant treatments such as *N*-acetylcysteine, troglitazone, and aminoguanidine [114]. The hexosamine pathway is one of the pathways that can be activated by oxidative stress [15], and activation of the pathway *per se* may increase oxidative stress [116]. Overexpression of GFA in β-cells suppresses PDX-1 DNA binding and activity, and glucose-stimulated insulin secretion. These changes can also be prevented by antioxidant treatment and appear to be a consequence of oxidative stress rather than increased O-glycosylation [116]. Overexpression of GFA *in vivo* in β-cells in mice also decreases insulin gene expression [73]. Thus, as in insulin-sensitive tissues, increased glucose flux sensed by the hexosamine pathway could contribute to glucose toxicity in β-cells.

CLINICAL SIGNIFICANCE OF GLUCOSE TOXICITY

Type 1 Diabetes

After diagnosis of type 1 diabetes, initiation of insulin therapy induces partial clinical remission in ~30% of the patients during the first year [117]. This honeymoon period is characterized by normoglycemia, recovery of endogenous insulin secretion, and by improved insulin sensitivity [19]. Although correction of several alterations secondary to insulin deficiency, such as increased counterregulatory hormone secretion [118], hyperosmolarity [119], acidosis [120], electrolyte changes [121], and high free fatty acids [122], could contribute to normalization of insulin secretion and sensitivity, reversal of glucose toxicity might also be of importance for the occurrence of remission. In the DCCT, 855 patients had had type 1 diabetes for 1–5 years at baseline and of these 303 were considered C-peptide responders (C-peptide level 0.20–0.50 pmol/ml after ingestion of a standardized, mixed meal). Responders receiving intensive therapy maintained a higher stimulated C-peptide level and a lower likelihood of becoming nonresponders than did responders receiving conventional therapy (relative risk reduction 57%) [123].

As discussed above, in type 1 patients with long-standing disease, chronic hyperglycemia can be regarded as the key factor responsible for insulin resistance. Therefore and in contrast to the results obtained in patients with type 2 diabetes (*vide infra*), insulin sensitivity can be markedly improved and even normalized in type 1 diabetic patients by optimizing insulin therapy [29]. The enhanced insulin sensitivity explains why glycemic control can be improved without necessarily having to increase the daily dose [22, 23]. Thus, although the loss of insulin secretion is irreversible in type 1 diabetes, insulin sensitivity is amenable to marked modification by alterations in glycemic control.

Type 2 Diabetes

Data from both several cross-sectional and prospective studies have documented that hyperinsulinemia and insulin resistance both precede and predict the subsequent development of type 2 diabetes (see Chapter 22). The etiology of insulin resistance is multifactorial and involves familiar/genetic and acquired components (see Chapter 22). Consequently, one would not expect normalization of insulin sensitivity by improved glycemic control. In keeping with this, insulin resistance has been a uniform finding in patients with type 2 diabetes (see Chapter 22) and has only been partially reversed by, e.g., aggressive insulin therapy [28, 29, 124–127].

Both weight loss [128–134], and sulfonylureas [131] and insulin therapy [125, 127, 131, 135–137] improve insulin secretion. Since neither insulin therapy nor weight loss have any direct stimulatory effects on insulin secretion, their effects could be mediated indirectly via diminution of glucose toxicity on β-cell secretion. Indeed, the "extrapancreatic effect" (improved insulin sensitivity) of sulfonylureas has been entirely attributed to amelioration of insulin resistance via lowering of the plasma glucose concentration [138].

CLINICAL CONCLUSIONS

Chronic hyperglycemia is not only a marker of the diabetes state but also a factor that itself worsens the diabetic state by impairing glucose-induced insulin secretion and insulin sensitivity. In patients with type 1 diabetes, maintenance of excellent glycemic control early in the course of the disease prolongs remission by preserving insulin secretion and normalizing insulin sensitivity. In these patients, chronic hyperglycemia is the major cause for peripheral insulin resistance. When compared to age- and weight-related nondiabetic subjects. Consequently, if excellent glycemic control is achieved, insulin sensitivity is normal. In patients with type 2 diabetes, glucose toxicity concept is likely to explain at least part of the beneficial effects of exogenous insulin therapy and weight loss on endogenous insulin secretion and insulin sensitivity.

Acknowledgment

This study was supported by grants from the Finnish Academy of Science.

REFERENCES

1. The Diabetes Control and Complications Trial research Group. The effect of intensive treatment of diabetes on the development and progression of long-term complications in insulin-dependent diabetes mellitus. *N Engl J Med* 1993; 329: 977–86.
2. The UK Prospective Diabetes Study (UKPDS) Group. Intensive blood-glucose control with sulphonylureas or insulin compared with conventional treatment and risk of complications in patients with type 2 diabetes (UKPDS 33). *Lancet* 1998; 352: 837–52.
3. Laakso M. Hyperglycemia and cardiovascular disease in type 2 diabetes. *Diabetes* 1999; 48: 937–42.
4. Rayfield EJ, Ault MJ, Keusch GT, Brothers MJ, Nechemias C, Smith H. Infection and diabetes: the case for glucose control. *Am J Med* 1982; 72: 439–50.
5. Rossetti L, Smith D, Shulman GI, Papachristou D, DeFronzo RA. Correction of hyperglycemia with phlorizin normalizes tissue sensitivity to insulin in diabetic rats. *J Clin Invest* 1987; 79: 1510–5.
6. Rossetti L, Shulman G, Zawalich W, DeFronzo RA. Effect of chronic hyperglycemia on in vivo insulin secretion in partially pancreatectomized rats. *J Clin Invest* 1987; 80: 1037–44.
7. Leahy JL, Cooper HE, Deal DA, Weir GC. Chronic hyperglycemia is associated with impaired glucose influence on insulin secretion. A study in normal rats using chronic in vivo glucose infusions. *J Clin Invest* 1986; 77: 908–15.
8. Yki-Järvinen H, Helve E, Koivisto VA. Hyperglycemia decreases glucose uptake in type 1 diabetes. *Diabetes* 1987; 36: 892–6.
9. Kelley DE, Mandarino LJ. Hyperglycemia normalizes insulin-stimulated skeletal muscle glucose oxidation and storage in non-insulin-dependent diabetes mellitus. *J Clin Invest* 1990; 86: 1999–2007.
10. DeFronzo RA, Tobin JD, Andres R. Glucose clamp technique: a method for quantifying insulin secretion and resistance. *Am J Physiol* 1979; 237: E214–23.
11. DeFronzo RA, Simonson D, Ferrannini E. Hepatic and peripheral insulin resistance: a common feature of type 2 (non-insulin-dependent) and type 1 (insulin-dependent) diabetes mellitus. *Diabetologia* 1982; 23: 313–9.
12. Yki-Järvinen H, Young AA, Lamkin C, Foley JE. Kinetics of glucose disposal in whole body and across the forearm in man. *J Clin Invest* 1987; 79: 1713–9.
13. Yki-Järvinen H, Sahlin K, Ren JM, Koivisto VA. Localization of the rate-limiting defect for glucose disposal in skeletal muscle of insulin-resistant type 1 diabetic patients. *Diabetes* 1990; 39: 157–67.
14. Henry RR, Gumbiner B, Flynn T, Thorburn AW. Metabolic effects of hyperglycemia and hyperinsulinemia on fate of intracellular glucose in NIDDM. *Diabetes* 1990; 39: 149–56.
15. Brownlee M. Biochemistry and molecular cell biology of diabetic complications. *Nature* 2001; 414: 813–20.
16. DeFronzo RA, Hendler R, Simonson D. Insulin resistance is a prominent feature of insulin-dependent diabetes. *Diabetes* 1982; 31: 795–801.
17. Yki-Järvinen H, Koivisto VA. Natural course of insulin resistance in type 1 diabetes. *N Engl J Med* 1986; 315: 224–30.
18. Yki-Järvinen H, Taskinen M-R, Kiviluoto T, Hilden H, Helve E, Koivisto VA, Nikkila E. Site of insulin resistance in type 1 diabetes: insulin-mediated glucose disposal in vivo in relation to insulin binding and action in adipocytes in vitro. *J Clin Endocrinol Metab* 1984; 59: 1183–92.
19. Yki-Järvinen H, Koivisto VA. Insulin sensitivity in newly diagnosed type I diabetics following ketoacidosis and after a 3 month insulin therapy. *J Clin Endocrinol Metab* 1984; 59: 371–8.
20. Vuorinen-Markkola H, Koivisto VA, Yki-Järvinen H. Mechanisms of hyperglycemia-induced insulin resistance in whole body and skeletal muscle of type 1 diabetic patients. *Diabetes* 1992; 41: 571–80.
21. Rizza RA, Gerich JE, Haymond MW, Westland RE, Hall LD, Clemens AH, Service FJ. Control of blood sugar in insulin-dependent diabetes: comparison of an artificial endocrine pancreas, continuous subcutaneous insulin infusion, and intesified conventional insulin therapy. *N Engl J Med* 1980; 303: 1313–8.
22. Yki-Järvinen H, Koivisto VA. Continuous subcutaneous insulin infusion therapy decreases insulin resistance in type 1 diabetes. *J Clin Endocrinol Metab* 1984; 58: 659–66.
23. Lager I, Lonnroth P, Von Shenck H, Smith U. Reversal of insulin resistance in type 1 diabetes after treament with continuous subcutaneous insulin infusion. *Br Med J* 1983; 287: 1001–4.
24. Fowelin J, Attvall S, von Schenk H, Bengtsson B-Å, Smith U, Lager I. Effect of prolonged hyperglycemia on growth hormone levels and insulin sensitivity in

insulin-dependent diabetes mellitus. *Metabolism* 1993; 42: 387–94.
25. Fanelli C, Pampanelli S, Calderone S, Lepore M, Annibale B, Compagnucci P, Brunetti P, Bolli GB. Effects of recent, short-term hyperglycemia on responses to hypoglycemia in humans. Relevance to the pathogenesis of hypoglycemia unawareness and hyperglycemia-induced insulin resistance. *Diabetes* 1995; 44: 513–9.
26. Boden G, Ruiz J, Kim CJ, Chen X. Effects of prolonged glucose infusion on insulin secretion, clearance, and action in normal subjects. *Am J Physiol* 1996; 270: E251–8.
27. Rossetti L, Hawkins M, Gindi J, Barzilai N. In vivo glucosamine infusion induces insulin resistance in normoglycemic but not in hyperglycemic conscious rats. *J Clin Invest* 1995; 96: 132–40.
28. Rossetti L, Giaccari A, DeFronzo RA. Glucose toxicity. *Diabetes Care* 1990; 13: 610–30.
29. Yki-Järvinen H. Glucose toxicity. *Endocr Rev* 1992; 13: 415–31.
30. Zierath JR, Galuska D, Nolte LA, Thörne A, Smedegaard Kristensen J, Wallberg-Henriksson H. Effect of glycaemia on glucose transport in isolated skeletal muscle from patients with NIDDM: in vitro reversal of muscular insulin resistance. *Diabetologia* 1994; 37: 270–7.
31. Kim JK, Zisman A, Fillmore JJ, Peroni OD, Kotani K, Perret P, Zong H, Dong J, Kahn CR, Kahn BB, Shulman GI. Glucose toxicity and the development of diabetes in mice with muscle-specific inactivation of GLUT4. *J Clin Invest* 2001; 108: 153–60.
32. Nuutila P, Knuuti J, Ruotsalainen U, Koivisto VA, Eronen E, Teräs M, Bergman J, Haaparanta M, Voipio-Pulkki L-M, Viikari J, Rönnemaa T, Wegelius U, Yki-Järvinen H. Insulin resistance is localized to skeletal but not heart muscle in type 1 diabetes. *Am J Physiol* 1993; 264: E756–62.
33. Utriainen T, Takala T, Luotolahti M, Ronnemaa T, Laine H, Ruotsalainen U, Haaparanta M, Nuutila P, Yki-Järvinen H. Insulin resistance characterizes glucose uptake in skeletal muscle but not in the heart in NIDDM. *Diabetologia* 1998; 41: 555–9.
34. Ferrannini E. The theoretical bases of indirect calorimetry: a review. *Metab Clin Exp* 1988; 37: 287–301.
35. Yki-Järvinen H. Fate of glucose in insulin resistant states. In Crepaldi G, Tiengo A, Manzato E (eds), *Diabetes, Obesity and Hyperlipidemia: V. The Plurimetabolic Syndrome*. Amsterdam: Elsevier Science, 1993; pp 75–82.
36. Yki-Järvinen H, Daniels MC, Virkamäki A, Mäkimattila S, DeFronzo RA, McClain D. Increased glutamine: fructose-6-phosphate amidotransferase activity in skeletal muscle of patients with NIDDM. *Diabetes* 1996; 45: 302–7.
37. Mueckler M. Facilitative glucose transporters. *Eur J Biochem* 1994; 219: 713–25.
38. Printz RL, Koch S, Potter LR, O'Doherty R, Tiesinga JJ, Moritz S, Granner DK. Hexokinase II messenger RNA and gene structure, regulation by insulin, and evolution. *J Biol Chem* 1993; 268: 5209–19.
39. Utriainen T, Malmström R, Mäkimattila S, Yki-Järvinen H. Methodological aspects, dose–response characteristics and causes of interindividual variation in insulin stimulation of limb blood flow in normal subjects. *Diabetologia* 1995; 38: 555–64.
40. Utriainen T, Holmäng A, Björntorp P, Mäkimattila S, Sovijärvi A, Lindholm H, Yki-Järvinen H. Physical fitness, muscle morphology, and insulin-stimulated limb blood flow in normal subjects. *Am J Physiol* 1996; 270: E905–11.
41. Yki-Järvinen H, Utriainen T. Insulin-induced vasodilatation: physiology or pharmacology? *Diabetologia* 1998; 41: 369–79.
42. Baron AD, Laakso M, Brechtel G, Edelman SV. Mechanism of insulin resistance in insulin-dependent diabetes mellitus: a major role for reduced skeletal muscle blood flow. *J Clin Endocrinol Metab* 1991; 73: 637–43.
43. Mäkimattila S, Virkamäki A, Groop P-H, Cockcroft J, Utriainen T, Fagerudd J, Yki-Järvinen H. Chronic hyperglycemia impairs endothelial function and insulin sensitivity via different mechanisms in insulin-dependent diabetes mellitus. *Circulation* 1996; 94: 1276–82.
44. Mäkimattila S, Virkamäki A, Malmström R, Utriainen T, Yki-Järvinen H. Insulin resistance in type I diabetes mellitus: a major role for reduced glucose extraction. *J Clin Endocrinol Metab* 1996; 81: 707–12.
45. Marshall S, Bacote V, Traxinger RR. Discovery of a metabolic pathway mediating glucose-induced desensitization of the glucose transport system. Role of hexosamine biosynthesis in the induction of insulin resistance. *J Biol Chem* 1991; 266: 4706–12.
46. Virkamäki A, Daniels MC, Hämäläinen S, Utriainen T, McClain D, Yki-Järvinen H. Activation of the hexosamine pathway by glucosamine in vivo induces insulin resistance in multiple insulin sensitive tissues. *Endocrinology* 1997; 138: 2501–7.
47. Wu G, Haynes TE, Yan W, Meininger CJ. Presence of glutamine:fructose-6-phosphate amidotransferase for glucosamine-6-phosphate synthesis in endothelial cells: effects of hyperglycaemia and glutamine. *Diabetologia* 2001; 44: 196–202.
48. Du XL, Edelstein D, Dimmeler S, Ju Q, Sui C, Brownlee M. Hyperglycemia inhibits endothelial nitric oxide synthase activity by posttranslational modification at the Akt site. *J Clin Invest* 2001; 108: 1341–8.
49. Salt IP, Morrow VA, Brandie FM, Connell JM, Petrie JR. High glucose inhibits insulin-stimulated nitric oxide production without reducing endothelial nitric-oxide synthase Ser1177 phosphorylation in human aortic endothelial cells. *J Biol Chem* 2003; 278: 18791–7.
50. Kolm-Litty V, Sauer U, Nerlich A, Lehmann R, Schleicher ED. High glucose-induced transforming growth factor beta1 production is mediated by the hexosamine pathway in porcine glomerular mesangial cells. *J Clin Invest* 1998; 101: 160–9.
51. Nerlich AG, Sauer U, Kolm-Litty V, Wagner E, Koch M, Schleicher ED. Expression of glutamine:fructose-6-phosphate amidotransferase in human tissues: evidence for high variability and distinct regulation in diabetes. *Diabetes* 1998; 47: 170–8.
52. Kornfeld R. Studies on L-glutamine D-fructose 6-phophate amidotransferase, I: Feedback inhibition by uridine diphosphate-*N*-acetylglucosamine. *J Biol Chem* 1967; 242: 3135–41.
53. Haltiwanger RS, Blomber MA, Hart GW. Glycosylation of nuclear and cytoplasmic proteins. Purification and characterization of a uridine diphospho-*N*-acetylglucosamine: polypeptide *N*-acetyltransferase. *J Biol Chem* 1992; 267: 9005–13.
54. Yki-Järvinen H, Vogt C, Iozzo P, Pipek R, Daniels MC, Virkamäki A, Mäkimattila S, Mandarino L, DeFronzo RA, McClain D, Gottschalk WK. UDP-N-acetylglucosamine transferase and glutamine: fructose

6-phosphate amidotransferase activities in insulin-sensitive tissues. *Diabetologia* 1997; 40: 76–81.
55. Dong D, Hart GW. Purification and characterization of an *O*-GlcNAc selective *N*-acetyl-b-D-glucosaminidase from rat spleen cytosol. *J Biol Chem* 1994; 269: 19231–330.
56. Robinson KA, Sens DA, Buse MG. Pre-exposure to glucosamine induces insulin resistance of glucose transport and glycogen synthesis in isolated rat skeletal muscles. *Diabetes* 1993; 42: 1333–46.
57. DeFronzo RA, Jacot E, Jequier E, Maeder E, Wahren J, Felber JP. The effect of insulin on the disposal of intravenous glucose. Results from indirect calorimetry and hepatic and femoral venous catheterization. *Diabetes* 1981; 30: 1000–7.
58. Giaccari A, Morviducci L, Zorretta D, Bonadonna R. Glucosamine infusion induces insulin resistance. *Diabetes* 1994; 42 (suppl 1): 68A.
59. Baron AD, Zhu J-S, Zhu J-H, Weldon H, Maianu L, Garvey WT. Glucosamine induces insulin resistance in vivo by affecting GLUT4 translocation in skeletal muscle. *J Clin Invest* 1995; 96: 2792–801.
60. Patti ME, Virkamaki A, Landaker EJ, Kahn CR, Yki-Järvinen H. Activation of the hexosamine pathway by glucosamine in vivo induces insulin resistance of early postreceptor insulin signaling events in skeletal muscle. *Diabetes* 1999; 48: 1562–71.
61. Hawkins M, Hu M, Yu J, Eder H, Vuguin P, She L, Barzilai N, Leiser M, Backer JM, Rossetti L. Discordant effects of glucosamine on insulin-stimulated glucose metabolism and phosphatidylinositol 3-kinase activity. *J Biol Chem* 1999; 274: 31312–9.
62. Virkamaki A, Yki-Järvinen H. Allosteric regulation of glycogen synthase and hexokinase by glucosamine-6-phosphate during glucosamine-induced insulin resistance in skeletal muscle and heart. *Diabetes* 1999; 48: 1101–7.
63. Brady MJ, Kartha PM, Aysola AA, Saltiel AR. The role of glucose metabolites in the activation and translocation of glycogen synthase by insulin in 3T3-L1 adipocytes. *J Biol Chem* 1999; 274: 27497–504.
64. Nelson BA, Robinson KA, Buse MG. High glucose and glucosamine induce insulin resistance via different mechanisms in 3T3-L1 adipocytes. *Diabetes* 2000; 49: 981–91.
65. Ciaraldi TP, Carter L, Nikoulina S, Mudaliar S, McClain DA, Henry RR. Glucosamine regulation of glucose metabolism in cultured human skeletal muscle cells: divergent effects on glucose transport/phosphorylation and glycogen synthase in non-diabetic and type 2 diabetic subjects. *Endocrinology* 1999; 140: 3971–80.
66. Hresko RC, Heimberg H, Chi MM, Mueckler M. Glucosamine-induced insulin resistance in 3T3-L1 adipocytes is caused by depletion of intracellular ATP. *J Biol Chem* 1998; 273: 20658–68.
67. Pouwels MJ, Jacobs JR, Span PN, Lutterman JA, Smits P, Tack CJ. Short-term glucosamine infusion does not affect insulin sensitivity in humans. *J Clin Endocrinol Metab* 2001; 86: 2099–103.
68. Monauni T, Zenti MG, Cretti A, Daniels MC, Targher G, Caruso B, Caputo M, McClain D, Del Prato S, Giaccari A, Muggeo M, Bonora E, Bonadonna RC. Effects of glucosamine infusion on insulin secretion and insulin action in humans. *Diabetes* 2000; 49: 926–35.
69. Daniels MC, Ciaraldi TP, Nikoulina S, Henry RR, McClain DA. Glutamine:fructose-6-phosphate amidotransferase activity in cultured human skeletal muscle cells: relationship to glucose disposal rate in control and non-insulin-dependent diabetes mellitus subjects and regulation by glucose and insulin. *J Clin Invest* 1996; 97: 1235–41.
70. Hebert LF, Daniels MC, Zhou J, Crook ED, Turner RL, Simmons ST, Neidigh JL, Zhu J-S, Baron AD, McClain DA. Overexpression of glutamine:fructose-6-phosphate amidotransferase in skeletal muscle of transgenic mice leads to insulin resistance. *J Clin Invest* 1996; 98: 930–6.
71. Buse MG, Robinson KA, Marshall BA, Mueckler M. Differential effects of GLUT1 or GLUT4 overexpression on hexosamine biosynthesis by muscles of transgenic mice. *J Biol Chem* 1996; 38: 23197–202.
72. Veerababu G, Tang J, Hoffman RT, Daniels MC, Hebert LFJ, Crook ED, Cooksey RC, McClain DA. Overexpression of glutamine:fructose-6-phosphate amidotransferase in the liver of transgenic mice results in enhanced glycogen storage, hyperlipidemia, obesity, and impaired glucose tolerance. *Diabetes* 2000; 49: 2070–8.
73. Tang J, Neidigh JL, Cooksey RC, McClain DA. Transgenic mice with increased hexosamine flux specifically targeted to beta-cells exhibit hyperinsulinemia and peripheral insulin resistance. *Diabetes* 2000; 49: 1492–9.
74. Cooksey RC, McClain DA. Transgenic mice overexpressing the rate-limiting enzyme for hexosamine synthesis in skeletal muscle or adipose tissue exhibit total body insulin resistance. *Ann N Y Acad Sci* 2002; 967: 102–11.
75. Considine RV, Cooksey RC, Williams LB, Fawcett RL, Zhang P, Ambrosius WT, Whitfield RM, Jones R, Inman M, Huse J, McClain DA. Hexosamines regulate leptin production in human subcutaneous adipocytes. *J Clin Endocrinol Metab* 2000; 85: 3551–6.
76. Crook AD, Zhou J, Daniels M, Neidigh JL, McClain DA. Regulation of glycogen synthase by glucose, glucosamine, and glutamine:frucotse-6-phosphate amidotransferase. *Diabetes* 1995; 44: 314–20.
77. Pouwels MJ, Span PN, Tack CJ, Olthaar AJ, Sweep CG, van Engelen BG, de Jong JG, Lutterman JA, Hermus AR. Muscle uridine diphosphate-hexosamines do not decrease despite correction of hyperglycemia-induced insulin resistance in type 2 diabetes. *J Clin Endocrinol Metab* 2002; 87: 5179–84.
78. Gerich JE, Mitrakou A, Kelley D, Mandarino L, Nurjhan N, Reilly J, Jenssen T, Veneman T, Consoli A. Contribution of impaired muscle glucose clearance to reduced postabsorptive systemic glucose clearance in NIDDM. *Diabetes* 1990; 39: 211–6.
79. Hart GW, Greis KD, Dong D, Blomberg MA, Chou T-Y, Jiang M-S, Roquemore EP, Snow DM, Kreppel LK, Cole RN, Comer FI, Arnold CS, Hayes BK. O-Linked *N*-acetylglucosamine: the "Yin-Yang" of Ser/Thr phosphorylation? Nuclear and cytoplasmic glycosylation. New York: Plenum, In Alavi A, Axford JS (eds), *Glycoimmunology*. 1995; pp 115–23.
80. Buse MG, Robinson KA, Marshall BA, Hresko RC, Mueckler MM. Enhanced *O*-GlcNAc protein modification is associated with insulin resistance in GLUT1-overexpressing muscles. *Am J Physiol Endocrinol Metab* 2002; 283: E241–50.
81. Yki-Järvinen H, Virkamäki A, Daniels MC, McClain D, Gottschalk K. Insulin and glucosamine infusions increase O-linked *N*-acetyl-glucosamine in skeletal muscle proteins in vivo. *Metabolism* 1998; 47: 449–55.
82. Vosseller K, Sakabe K, Wells L, Hart GW. Diverse regulation of protein function by *O*-GlcNAc: a nuclear and

cytoplasmic carbohydrate post-translational modification. *Curr Opin Chem Biol* 2002; 6: 851–7.
83. Vosseller K, Wells L, Lane MD, Hart GW. Elevated nucleocytoplasmic glycosylation by *O*-GlcNAc results in insulin resistance associated with defects in Akt activation in 3T3-L1 adipocytes. *Proc Natl Acad Sci USA* 2002; 99: 5313–8.
84. Walgren JL, Vincent TS, Schey KL, Buse MG. High glucose and insulin promote *O*-GlcNAc modification of proteins, including alpha-tubulin. *Am J Physiol Endocrinol Metab* 2003; 284: E424–34.
85. Hawkins M, Angelov I, Liu R, Barzilai N, Rossetti L. The tissue concentration of UDP-*N*-acetylglucosamine modulates the stimulatory effect of insulin on skeletal muscle glucose uptake. *J Biol Chem* 1997; 272: 4889–95.
86. Schleicher ED, Weigert C. Role of the hexosamine biosynthetic pathway in diabetic nephropathy. *Kidney Int Suppl* 2000; 77: S13–8.
87. Du XL, Edelstein D, Rossetti L, Fantus IG, Goldberg H, Ziyadeh F, Wu J, Brownlee M. Hyperglycemia-induced mitochondrial superoxide overproduction activates the hexosamine pathway and induces plasminogen activator inhibitor-1 expression by increasing Sp1 glycosylation. *Proc Natl Acad Sci USA* 2000; 97: 12222–6.
88. Federici M, Menghini R, Mauriello A, Hribal ML, Ferrelli F, Lauro D, Sbraccia P, Spagnoli LG, Sesti G, Lauro R. Insulin-dependent activation of endothelial nitric oxide synthase is impaired by O-linked glycosylation modification of signaling proteins in human coronary endothelial cells. *Circulation* 2002; 106: 466–72.
89. Freidenberg GR, Henry RR, Klein HH, Reichart DR, Olefsky JM. Decreased kinase activity of insulin receptors from adipocytes of non-insulin-dependent diabetic subjects. *J Clin Invest* 1987; 79: 240–50.
90. Freidenberg GR, Reichart D, Olefsky JM, Henry RR. Reversibility of defective adipocyte insulin receptor kinase activity in non-insulin-dependent diabetic subjects. *J Clin Invest* 1988; 82: 1398–406.
91. Obermaier-Kusser B, White MF, Pongratz DE, Su Z, Ermel B, Mulbacher C, Häring HU. A defective intramolecular autoactivation cascade may cause the reduced kinase activity of skeletal muscle insulin receptor from patients with non-insulin-dependent diabetes mellitus. *J Biol Chem* 1989; 264: 9497–504.
92. Maegawa H, Shigeta Y, Egawa K, Kobayashi M. Impaired autophosphorylation of insulin receptors from abdominal skeletal muscles in non-obese subjects with NIDDM. *Diabetes* 1991; 40: 815–9.
93. Muller HK, Kellerer M, Ermel B, Muhlhofer A, Obermaier-Kusser B, Vogt B, Haring HU. Prevention by protein kinase C inhibitors of glucose-induced insulin receptor tyrosine kinase resistance in rat fat cells. *Diabetes* 1991; 40: 1440–8.
94. Berti L, Mosthaf L, Kroder G. Glucose induced translocation of protein kinase C isoforms in rat-1 fibroblasts is paralled by inhibition of the insulin receptor tyrosine kinase. *J Biol Chem* 1994; 269: 3381–6.
95. Ahmad A, Lee FT, De Paoli-Roach A, Roach PJ. Phosphorylation of glycogen synthase by the Ca^{2+} and phospholipid-activated protein kinase (protein kinase C). *J Biol Chem* 1984; 259: 8743–7.
96. Chen KS, Heydrick S, Kurowski T, Ruderman NB. Diacylglycerol-protein kinase C signaling in skeletal muscle: a possible link to insulin resistance. *Trans Assoc Am Physicians* 1991; 104: 206–12.
97. Saha AK, Kurowski TG, Ruderman NB. A malonyl-CoA fuel-sensing mechanism in muscle: effects of insulin, glucose and denervation. *Am J Physiol* 1995; 269: E283–9.
98. Filippis A, Clark S, Proietto J. Increased flux through the hexosamine biosynthesis pathway inhibits glucose transport acutely by activation of protein kinase C. *Biochem J* 1997; 324 (pt 3): 981–5.
99. Dohan FC, Lukens FDW. Experimental diabetes produced by the administration of glucose. *Endocrinology* 1948; 42: 244–62.
100. Dimitriadis G, Cryer P, Gerich J. Prolonged hyperglycaemia during infusion of glucose and somatostatin impairs pancreatic A- and B-cell responses to decrements in plasma glucose in normal man: evidence for induction of altered sensitivity to glucose. *Diabetologia* 1985; 28: 63–9.
101. Ward WK, Halter JB, Beard JC, Porte DJ. Adaptation of B and A cell function during prolonged glucose infusion in human subjects. *Am J Physiol* 1984; 246: E405–11.
102. Flax H, Matthews DR, Levy JC, Coppack SW, Turner RC. No glucotoxicity after 53 hours of 6.0 mmol/l hyperglycaemia in normal man. *Diabetologia* 1991; 34: 570–5.
103. Imamura T, Koffler M, Helderman JH, Prince D, Thirlby R, Inman L, Unger RH. Severe diabetes induced in subtotally depancreatized dogs by sustained hyperglycemia. *Diabetes* 1988; 37: 600–9.
104. Leahy JL, Weir GC. Evolution of abnormal insulin secretory responses during 48-h in vivo hyperglycemia. *Diabetes* 1988; 37: 217–22.
105. Leahy JL, Cooper HE, Weir GC. Impaired insulin secretion associated with near normoglycemia. Study in normal rats with 96-h in vivo glucose infusions. *Diabetes* 1987; 36: 459–64.
106. Starke A, Grundy S, McGarry JD, Unger RH. Correction of hyperglycemia with phloridzin restores the glucagon response to glucose in insulin-deficient dogs: implications for human diabetes. *Proc Natl Acad Sci USA* 1985; 82: 1544–6.
107. Collier SA, Mandel TE, Carter WM. Detrimental effect of high medium glucose concentration on subsequent endocrine function of transplanted organ-cultured foetal mouse pancreas. *Aust J Exp Biol Med Sci* 1982; 60 (pt 4): 437–45.
108. Korsgren O, Jansson L, Andersson A. Effects of hyperglycemia on function of isolated mouse pancreatic islets transplanted under kidney capsule. *Diabetes* 1989; 38: 510–5.
109. Giroix MH, Portha B, Kergoat M, Bailbe D, Picon L. Glucose insensitivity and amino-acid hypersensitivity of insulin release in rats with non-insulin-dependent diabetes. A study with the perfused pancreas. *Diabetes* 1983; 32: 445–51.
110. Weir GC, Clore ET, Zmachinski CJ, Bonner-Weir S. Islet secretion in a new experimental model for non-insulin-dependent diabetes. *Diabetes* 1981; 30: 590–5.
111. Weir GC, Bonner-Weir S, Leahy JL. Islet mass and function in diabetes and transplantation. *Diabetes* 1990; 39: 401–5.
112. Ganda OP, Srikanta S, Brink SJ, Morris MA, Gleason RE, Soeldner JS, Eisenbarth GS. Differential sensitivity to beta-cell secretagogues in "early," type I diabetes mellitus. *Diabetes* 1984; 33: 516–21.

113. Ward WK, Beard JC, Halter JB, Porte DJ. Pathophysiology of insulin secretion in diabetes mellitus. *Adv Exp Med Biol* 1985; 189: 137–58.
114. Robertson RP, Harmon J, Tran PO, Tanaka Y, Takahashi H. Glucose toxicity in beta-cells: type 2 diabetes, good radicals gone bad, and the glutathione connection. *Diabetes* 2003; 52: 581–7.
115. Evans JL, Goldfine ID, Maddux BA, Grodsky GM. Are oxidative stress-activated signaling pathways mediators of insulin resistance and beta-cell dysfunction? *Diabetes* 2003; 52: 1–8.
116. Kaneto H, Xu G, Song KH, Suzuma K, Bonner-Weir S, Sharma A, Weir GC. Activation of the hexosamine pathway leads to deterioration of pancreatic beta-cell function through the induction of oxidative stress. *J Biol Chem* 2001; 276: 31099–104.
117. Madsbad S. Prevalence of residual B cell function and its metabolic consequences in Type 1 (insulin-dependent) diabetes. *Diabetologia* 1983; 24: 141–7.
118. Ginsberg HN. Investigation of insulin resistance during diabetic ketoacidosis: role of counterregulatory substances and effect of insulin therapy. *Metabolism* 1977; 26: 1135–46.
119. Bratusch-Marrain PR, DeFronzo RA. Impairment of insulin mediated glucose metabolism by hyperosmolality in man. *Diabetes* 1983; 32: 1028–34.
120. DeFronzo RA, Beckles AD. Glucose metabolism following chronic metabolic acidosis in man. *Am J Physiol* 1979; 236: E328–34.
121. DeFronzo RA, Lang R. Hypophosphatemia and glucose intolerance: evidence for tissue insensitivity to insulin. *N Engl J Med* 1980; 303: 1259–63.
122. Randle PJ, Hales CN, Garland PB, Newsholme EA. The glucose–fatty acid cycle. Its role in insulin sensitivity and the metabolic disturbances of diabetes mellitus. *Lancet* 1963; 1: 785–9.
123. The Diabetes Control and Complications Trial Research Group. Effect of intensive therapy on residual beta-cell function in patients with type 1 diabetes in the diabetes control and complications trial. A randomized, controlled trial. *Ann Intern Med* 1998; 128: 517–23.
124. Firth RG, Bell PM, Rizza RA. Effects of tolazamide and exogenous insulin on insulin action in patients with non-insulin-dependent diabetes mellitus. *N Engl J Med* 1986; 314: 1280–6.
125. Garvey WT, Olefsky JM, Griffin J, Hamman RF, Kolterman OG. The effect of insulin treatment on insulin secretion and insulin action in type II diabetes mellitus. *Diabetes* 1985; 34: 222–34.
126. Scarlett JA, Gray RS, Griffin J, Olefsky JM, Kolterman OG. Insulin treatment reverses the insulin resistance in type II diabetes mellitus. *Diabetes Care* 1982; 5: 353–63.
127. Yki-Järvinen H, Nikkilä E, Helve E, Taskinen M-R. Clinical benefits and mechanisms of a sustained response to intermittent insulin therapy in type 2 diabetic patients with secondary drug failure. *Am J Med* 1988; 84: 185–92.
128. Bogardus C, Ravussin E, Robbins DC, Wolfe RR, Horton ES, Sims EA. Effects of physical training and diet therapy on carbohydrate metabolism in patients with glucose intolerance and non-insulin-dependent diabetes mellitus. *Diabetes* 1984; 33: 311–8.
129. Henry RR, Wallace P, Olefsky JM. Effects of weight loss on mechanisms of hyperglycemia in obese non-insulin-dependent diabetes mellitus. *Diabetes* 1986; 35: 990–8.
130. Stanik S, Marcus R. Insulin secretion improves following dietary control of plasma glucose in severely hyperglycemic obese patients. *Metabolism* 1980; 29: 346–50.
131. Kosaka K, Kuzuya T, Akanuma Y, Hagura R. Increase in insulin response after treatment of overt maturity-onset diabetes is independent of the mode of treatment. *Diabetologia* 1980; 18: 23–8.
132. Savage PJ, Bennion LJ, Bennett PH. Normalization of insulin and glucagon secretion in ketosis-resistant diabetes mellitus with prolonged diet therapy. *J Clin Endocrinol Metab* 1979; 49: 830–3.
133. Eriksson K-F, Lindgärde F. Prevention of type 2 (non-insulin-dependent) diabetes mellitus by diet and physical exercise. *Diabetologia* 1991; 34: 891–8.
134. Zawadzki JK, Bogardus C, Foley JE. Insulin action in obese non-insulin-dependent diabetics and in their isolated adipocytes before and after weight loss. *Diabetes* 1987; 36: 227–36.
135. Andrews WJ, Vasquez B, Nagulesparan M, Klimes I, Foley J, Unger R, Reaven GM. Insulin therapy in obese, non-insulin-dependent diabetes induces improvements in insulin action and secretion that are maintained for two weeks after insulin withdrawal. *Diabetes* 1984; 33: 634–42.
136. Hidaka H, Naugulesparan M, Klimes I. Improvement of insulin secretion but not insulin resistance after short term control of plasma glucose in obese type II diabetics. *J Clin Endocrinol Metab* 1982; 54: 217–22.
137. Ginsberg H, Rayfield EJ. Effect of insulin therapy on insulin resistance in type II diabetic subjects. Evidence for heterogeneity. *Diabetes* 1981; 30: 739–45.
138. Gerich JE. Oral hypoglycemic agents. *N Engl J Med* 1989; 321: 1231–45.

26

Monogenic Disorders of the β-Cell

Ewan R. Pearson and Andrew T. Hattersley

Peninsula Medical School, Exeter, UK

INTRODUCTION

The pancreatic β-cell is a finely tuned system that primarily ensures appropriate insulin secretion in order to maintain blood glucose levels in a physiological range. Defects in this glucose–insulin secretion coupling can cause undersecretion of insulin and hence diabetes, or more rarely oversecretion of insulin and hypoglycemia. The most common cause of β-cell dysfunction in humans is seen in type 2 diabetes. However, type 2 diabetes is a complex polygenic disorder, and the nature of the β-cell defects have yet to be defined. In the general population, monogenic disorders, of the β-cell account for 3–4% of diabetes. They are therefore an important cause of diabetes in their own right, and recognition of a monogenic etiology of diabetes has clinical management implications. In addition to this clinical importance, the discovery and study of monogenic disorders has given further insight into the physiology and pathophysiology of the β-cell.

To understand the pathophysiology of the β-cell in monogenic diabetes, it is important to outline the process whereby the β-cell senses glucose and translates this into an appropriate release of insulin. Figure 1 shows a schematic representation of the β-cell and the legend describes the process of glucose–insulin secretion coupling. The sites of monogenic defects (indicated on the figure) that cause diabetes or hypoglycemia are as follows:

Glut-2	Glut-2 mutations cause Fanconi–Bickel syndrome. The phenotype is predominantly due to defects in hepatic Glut-2 causing glycogen storage disease, rather than pancreatic Glut-2. This will not be discussed in this chapter
GCK	Loss of function mutations in glucokinase gene (*GCK*) are a cause of maturity-onset diabetes of the young (MODY) whereas activating mutations of *GCK* are a cause of familial hyperinsulinemia
Glycolysis	Defects in glycolysis are described under Transcription Factor MODY (TF-MODY) due to mutations in hepatocyte nuclear factor 1α (*HNF-1α*), *HNF-4α*, *HNF-1β*, *IPF-1* (insulin promoter factor 1), and *NeuroD1*
Mitochondria	Mitochondrial defects are described under Maternally Inherited Diabetes and Deafness (MIDD), Thiamine Responsive Megaloblastic Anemia syndrome (TRMA), TF-MODY
KATP channel	Mutations in *SUR-1* and *Kir 6.2* (components of the KATP channel) have been shown to cause hyperinsulinemia of infancy (HI)
Endoplasmic reticulum	Wolfram syndrome (*WFS-1*) and Wolcott–Rallison syndrome (*EIF2-AK3*) genes encode proteins that localize to the endoplasmic reticulum
Insulin	Insulin gene mutations cause mutant insulins, and familial hyperprolinsulinemia

This chapter will focus on MODY and MIDD, as these are by far the most prevalent of the monogenic disorders of the β-cell. TRMA, HI, Wolfram syndrome, Wolcott–Rallison syndrome, mutant insulins, and familial hyperproinsulinemia will be briefly discussed.

International Textbook of Diabetes Mellitus, Third Edition. Edited by R. A. DeFronzo, E. Ferrannini, H. Keen, and P. Zimmet.
 ISBN: 0-471-48655-8.

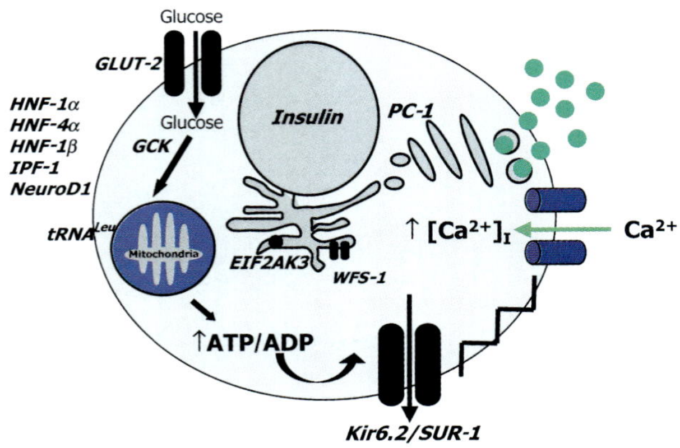

Figure 1 Glucose enters the β-cell via the Glut-2 transporter where it is phosphorylated to glucose-6-phosphate (G6P) by the enzyme glucokinase (GCK). G6P is metabolized via the glycolytic pathway to pyruvate. Pyruvate enters the mitochondria and is metabolized via the citric acid cycle to produce a rise in intracellular ATP and a fall in ADP. This increase in ATP/ADP acts to close ATP-dependent K channels (Kir6.2/SUR-1), allowing a rise in the membrane resting potential, which triggers a voltage-gated calcium channel to open, allowing calcium influx. It is this calcium influx that is the trigger for insulin exocytosis. Diabetes can be caused by mutations in Glut-2; *GCK* (Glucokinase); the transcription factors *HNF-1α* (Hepatocyte Nuclear Factor 1α), *HNF-1β*, *HNF-4α*, *IPF-1* (Insulin Promoter Factor 1), and *NeuroD1*; *tRNA*^{Leu} (the mitochondrial gene encoding leucine transfer RNA); *WFS1* (Wolfram syndrome 1 gene), *EIF2AK3* (encoding translation initiation factor 2 α); Insulin gene; Prohormone Convertase 1 (*PC-1*). Sites of monogenic defects causing hypoglycemia include *GCK*, *SUR-1* (encoding the sulfonylurea receptor 1), and *Kir6.2* (encoding the K^+ inward rectifying channel)

MATURITY-ONSET DIABETES OF THE YOUNG

Maturity-onset diabetes of the young (MODY) is a monogenic subtype of diabetes characterized by young onset (usually before 25 years) of non-insulin-dependent diabetes, β-cell dysfunction, and autosomal dominant inheritance. Mutations in six genes have been found to cause MODY: *GCK, HNF-1α, HNF-4α, HNF-1β, IPF-1, and NeuroD1*. The definition of the underlying genes has resulted in the recognition of distinct clinical and physiological subgroups of MODY with varying clinical course, prognosis, and treatment requirements. Recent classifications of diabetes by the American Diabetes Association (ADA) and the World Health Organization (WHO) [1] have recognized these discrete subtypes.

Definition of MODY

For a family to meet the strict criteria for MODY, successfully applied to genetic studies, they must fulfill the following:

(1) Young age of onset of diabetes. At least one, and ideally two, family members should have diabetes diagnosed before the age of 25.
(2) Non-insulin-dependent diabetes. They are not on insulin treatment or have significant circulating C-peptide 5 years after diagnosis.
(3) Autosomal dominant inheritance. There should be two generations with affected family members although most MODY families have three or more generations affected.

Most but not all families shown to have a mutation in one of the known MODY genes fulfill these criteria. However, patients can be diagnosed with MODY over the age of 25; they may be treated with insulin from diagnosis, and they may not have a family history of diabetes, as spontaneous mutations have been described. MODY subjects tend to be (but are not exclusively) nonobese, lack features of the insulin resistance syndrome, and are usually GAD (glutamic acid decarboxylase) antibody negative. Other clinical features that may be useful in the diagnosis of MODY are discussed later. A molecular genetic diagnosis is now possible in 80% of Caucasian families who fulfill strict MODY criteria.

Prevalence of MODY Subtypes

MODY accounts for 1–2% of non-insulin-dependent diabetes in Europe [2]. Large national collections allow assessment of the relative prevalence of the different subgroups of MODY as shown in Figure 2 (based on the UK collection of 125 families). [3] This prevalence is typical for European series that recruit from adult diabetic clinics but the relative prevalence does depend on how patients are recruited. *GCK* mutations are common (≅0.1% population) but most patients are asymptomatic and undiagnosed (see below). Therefore, series that include a large proportion of children with asymptomatic, mild fasting hyperglycemia found on screening will have a higher proportion of GCK-MODY patients [4, 5]. Allowing for this,

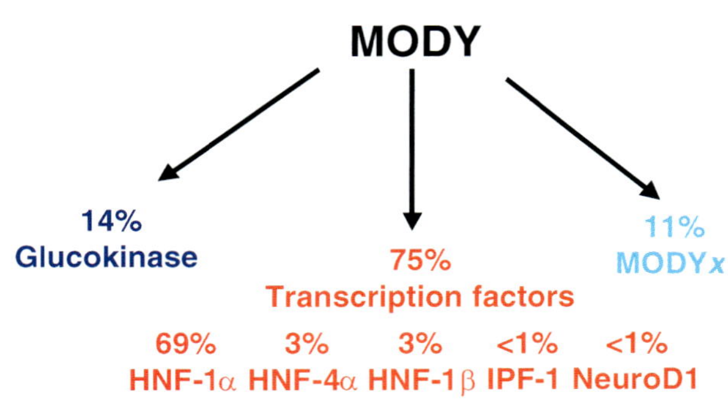

Figure 2 Subtypes and prevalence of MODY based on the UK population. MODY*x* refers to families that fulfill MODY criteria, but in whom a genetic cause has not been found [3]

the prevalence of the known MODY genes is considerably lower in Japanese and Chinese series when compared to European Caucasians.

The MODY Phenotypes

Despite the genetic heterogeneity in MODY, with mutations in at least six genes identified, the phenotypes of MODY can essentially be divided into two distinct groups: glucokinase MODY (GCK-MODY) and TF-MODY [6] (which includes mutations in *HNF-4α*, *HNF-1α*, *IPF-1*, *HNF-1β*, and *NeuroD1*). The phenotypes in these two groups are completely different, and it is confusing that they both fall under the same group name of MODY. GCK-MODY is characterized by stable fasting hyperglycemia that is present from birth, is nonprogressive, does not require treatment (except in pregnancy), and is rarely associated with microvascular complications. TF-MODY, on the other hand, is not present at birth but develops in children/young adults, is progressive with increasing treatment requirements, and is associated with the full range of microvascular complications [7].

Glucokinase MODY

GCK catalyzes the phosphorylation of glucose to glucose-6-phosphate. Unlike other hexokinases, it has a low affinity for glucose (high K_m) and is not inhibited by its product, glucose-6-phosphate. These unique kinetic properties result in the rate of glucose phosphorylation being proportional to the physiological glucose concentration, allowing the β-cell and hepatocyte to respond appropriately to the degree of glycemia [8]. In the pancreatic β-cell, GCK is the rate-limiting enzyme in glycolysis and acts as "the glucose sensor" [8], ensuring insulin release is appropriate to the glucose concentration. These features made *GCK* an ideal candidate gene for MODY.

Molecular Genetics of Glucokinase MODY

The first descriptions of linkage to a microsatellite polymorphism near the *GCK* gene were in French and English MODY pedigrees in early 1992 [9, 10]. These were rapidly followed by descriptions of a large number of mutations in the coding region or intron/exon boundaries of the 12 exons of the *GCK* gene [11–13] (MODY2). Over 100 different heterozygous mutations have now been described in French, English, Japanese, Swedish, Italian, and Afro-Caribbean families [4, 5, 11–16]. Expression studies show that the mutations in MODY families may alter the enzyme's affinity or activity for glucose metabolism or phosphorylation or alter structure or stability [17–19].

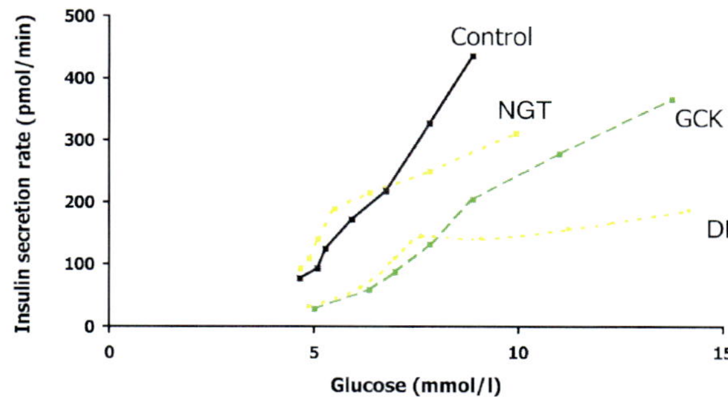

Figure 3 Insulin secretion rate vs. glucose in controls, G-CK mutation carriers, normoglycemic HNF-1α mutation carriers (NGT), and diabetic HNF-1α mutation carriers (DM) (data taken from references 22 and 23)

The Phenotype of Glucokinase MODY

Subjects with GCK-MODY have fasting hyperglycemia that is present from birth [20] and show very little deterioration with age [21]. The phenotype of GCK-MODY can be predicted from the kinetics of the GCK enzyme and its role as a "pancreatic glucose sensor." Byrne and colleagues have shown, using graded glucose infusions, that heterozygous mutations in *GCK* cause a right shift in the insulin response curve, leading to a resetting of the fasting glucose set point (Figure 3) [22]. So the majority of GCK-MODY subjects have a high fasting plasma glucose within a tight range (5.5–8 mmol/l).

The proinsulin/insulin (PI/I) ratio is elevated in type 2 diabetes and is thought to represent a β-cell "under stress" with oversecretion of insulin precursors. In GCK-MODY the PI/I ratio is not elevated (Figure 4a). This is consistent with the defect being one of glucose sensing, with the downstream glucose metabolism and insulin release mechanisms being intact.

GCK-MODY subjects are able to maximally stimulate their β-cells given enough of a glucose challenge [22], and this explains their small increment in plasma glucose 2 h following oral glucose load [24]. This ability to respond to a carbohydrate challenge also explains the near normal HbA_{1c} in subjects with GCK-MODY and the rarity of microvascular complications [15, 25]. The rare cases of proliferative retinopathy and diabetic retinopathy reported in the French series may represent coincidental conventional type 2 diabetes in patients who also have a *GCK* mutation.

It is hard to assess whether GCK-MODY subjects have significant macrovascular complications, as only approximately 500 patients have been described in the literature. In the Whitehall Study an increased risk of macrovascular disease was seen in patients with impaired glucose tolerance (IGT) and so an increase might be expected in GCK-MODY subjects [26]. However, in contrast to IGT, patients with *GCK* mutations have normal fasting lipids

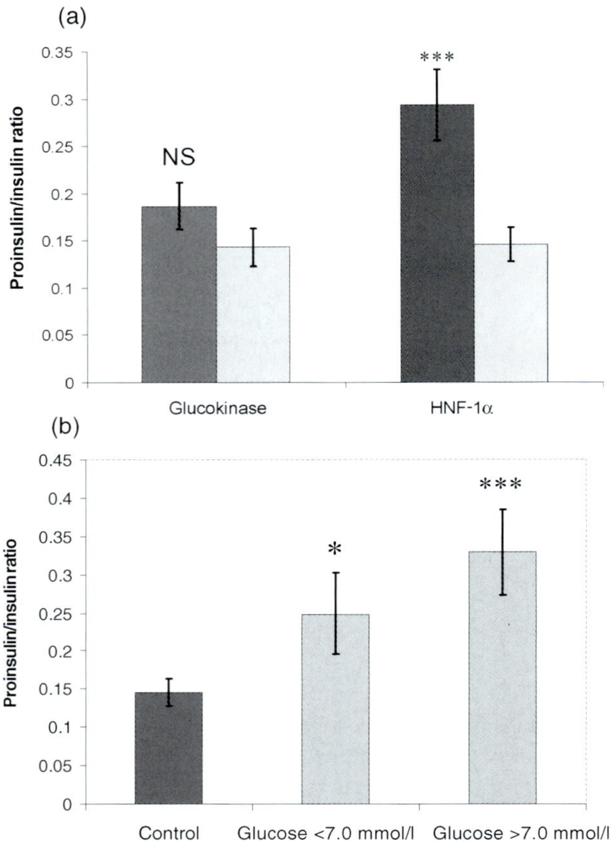

Figure 4 (a) Proinsulin/insulin ratio in control subjects ■, GCK-MODY ■, and HNF-1α-MODY subjects □. (b) The HNF-1α-MODY group is subdivided into those with a fasting plasma glucose less than 7 mmol/l and those with a fasting plasma glucose greater than 7 mmol/l. NS = not significant, $^{*}p < 0.05$, $^{***}p < 0.001$ (reproduced with permission from reference 7)

[25], are not significantly insulin resistant [9], and have less postprandial hyperglycemia [24, 27].

In addition to the important role of GCK in the β-cell, it is also expressed in hepatocytes, pancreatic α-cells, and the hypothalamus. GCK-MODY subjects have reduced glycogen synthesis consistent with GCK being a rate-limiting enzyme in hepatocytes, and the glucagon secretion to hypoglycemia occurs at a higher glucose threshold than in matched type 2 diabetic subjects (G Spyer, KM MacLeod, and AT Hattersley, personal communication, 2000).

Diagnosis and Treatment

As *GCK* mutations cause mild asymptomatic hyperglycemia, most cases of GCK-MODY are diagnosed following incidental testing of blood glucose, or following routine screening in pregnancy. Supporting clinical evidence for GCK-MODY can be obtained from an oral glucose tolerance test (OGTT), when the glucose increment at 2 h is usually <3 mmol/l [24]. A fasting plasma glucose below 5.5 mmol/l is extremely rare in GCK-MODY [24]. As the age of diagnosis depends on the age of testing, many GCK-MODY families do not meet MODY criteria until asymptomatic children and other relatives are tested.

Patients with GCK-MODY do not usually require treatment except in pregnancy (see below) [4]. If a patient is being treated with insulin or oral hypoglycemics, it is usually possible to stop treatment when a diagnosis of GCK-MODY is made. However, this should be done with caution, as it is theoretically possible for someone to have both a *GCK* mutation and type 1 or type 2 diabetes.

GCK-MODY and Pregnancy

Patients with *GCK* mutations are frequently found to have hyperglycemia during screening in pregnancy and represent approximately 3% of Caucasian patients with gestational diabetes [28]. Their identification is important because they have a different clinical course both within and outside pregnancy compared to other subjects with gestational diabetes.

The aim of treatment during diabetic pregnancy is to minimize fetal risk. This is usually achieved by strict control of the mother's blood glucose to prevent fetal macrosomia. However, in GCK-MODY pregnancies the need to reduce maternal blood glucose is not absolute. This is because the fetus has a 50% chance of inheriting the *GCK* mutation from the mother, and the presence of the *GCK* mutation in the fetus influences the fetus' sensing of maternal glucose. Therefore, if the fetus does not inherit the *GCK* mutation it will respond to maternal hyperglycemia by excess insulin production and therefore excess growth, whereas if the fetus does inherit the *GCK* mutation it will sense the maternal hyperglycemia as normal, produce normal amounts of insulin, and have normal growth [16, 29]. In this latter setting, aggressively lowering maternal glycemia may adversely affect fetal growth [30]. As it is not usually possible to determine the fetal genotype, decision on whether to treat the mother should be based on fetal growth.

A mother with a *GCK* mutation will need no pharmacological treatment postpartum even if she has received very high insulin doses in pregnancy. This is in contrast to subjects with non-GCK gestational diabetes where deterioration to type 2 diabetes is usually seen over the following 10–20 years.

Transcription Factor MODY

All MODY genes except *GCK* encode transcription factors (TFs). TFs have an important role in regulating the expression of genes. They play a critical role in the variations in gene expression in the different stages of embryological development, and in different tissues. TFs can also regulate expression of other TFs, thus establishing a complex regulatory network controlling gene expression.

Molecular Genetics of TF-MODY

HNF-1α was the first identified TF gene to cause MODY (MODY3) [31]. *HNF-1α* is found on the long arm of chromosome 12 (12q), and mutations in *HNF-1α* are the most common cause of MODY in the UK and most of Europe [3]. Over 100 mutations have been found scattered throughout the gene and consist of frameshift, missense, nonsense, and splice-site mutations.

The collection of DNA samples and careful longitudinal study of the extensive RW pedigree by Fajans resulted in MODY1 being the first genetic loci to be defined in MODY [32, 33]. However the identification of the gene *HNF-4α* at this locus occurred only after identification of *HNF-1α* mutations as a cause of MODY3 [34]. Mutations in *HNF-4α* are a much less common cause of MODY than are *HNF-1α* mutations, accounting for only 3% of MODY in the United Kingdom, with only 12 mutations being described in the first 4 years following description of the gene.

Following the discovery of *HNF-1α* as a MODY gene, *HNF-1β* became a logical candidate gene as HNF-1α and HNF-1β form heterodimers with one another. The first description of an *HNF-1β* mutation in a subject with MODY (MODY5) was in a Japanese family [35]. The fact that over 60 subjects were screened to find this one individual was an indication that such mutations were relatively rare and certainly considerably less frequent than *HNF-1α* mutations. No mutations in *HNF-1β* were found in strictly defined MODY in the UK population [36]. Mutations in *HNF-1β* have been described in 12 families and are usually truncating mutations [35, 37–44].

The unexpected finding of TF mutations as a cause of MODY focused work on other β-cell TFs, resulting in the identification of rare mutations causing MODY in *IPF-1* (MODY4) [45] and *NeuroD1* (MODY6). Stoffers and colleagues [45] studied a child with pancreatic agenesis and found a homozygous frameshift mutation in *IPF-1* that had dominant negative characteristics *in vitro* [46]. They noticed that there were multiple generations of diabetes on both sides of the family and went on to show that the heterozygous frameshift mutation co-segregated with non-insulin-dependent diabetes in both parents' families, with a significant total LOD (logarithm of the odds) score of 3.43 [45]. This is the only published report of a family with IPF-1 MODY (MODY4). *NeuroD1* mutations have been described in two families that fitted MODY criteria [47, 48], although only the Icelandic family showed complete co-segregation [48].

The Common Pancreatic Phenotype

The pancreatic phenotypes in HNF-1α MODY and HNF-4α MODY have been the most studied of the TF-MODYs. It is striking that the different TFs causing MODY can have

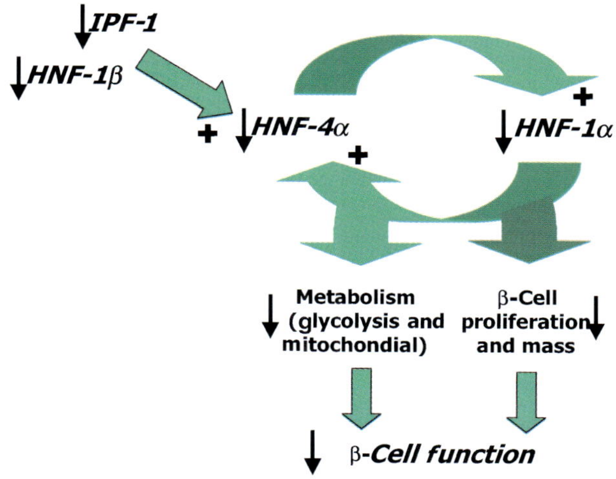

Figure 5 The β-cell transcription factor network. HNF-1α and HNF-4α positively regulate each other, forming a pancreatic switch. In MODY, loss of function in IPF-1, HNF-1α, HNF-1β, or HNF-4α has a common effect of reducing β-cell function by impaired glucose metabolism, and reduced β-cell proliferation and β-cell mass

such differing nonpancreatic phenotypes (e.g., abnormal lipids, renal cysts) but have essentially the same pancreatic phenotype. The TFs causing MODY all form part of a regulatory network (Figure 5). Recently, a pancreatic-specific alternative promoter of HNF-4α [49, 50] has been identified. Through binding sites in this alternative promoter, HNF-1α, HNF-4β, and IPF-1 can increase HNF-4α expression, and conversely HNF-4α can increase expression of HNF-1α through a binding site in the HNF-1α promoter [51]. Therefore, in the pancreas (but not in other tissues where the alternative HNF-4α promoter is not used) there is a positive feedback loop established between HNF-1α and HNF-4α. It has been hypothesized that this feedback loop acts as a bistable switch that is stable only when fully on or fully off. Therefore loss of function of HNF-1α or HNF-4α directly, or indirectly via *HNF-1β* and *IPF-1* mutations, will turn the switch fully off, thereby causing the same pancreatic phenotype irrespective of the TF mutated in this network [52]. The lack of this positive feedback switch in other tissues means that the nonpancreatic phenotype is determined by the role of the specific TF involved.

The pancreatic phenotype in TF-MODY is characterized by the following:

(1) *β-Cell dysfunction.* A β-cell defect was demonstrated in HNF-1α [23] and HNF-4α MODY [53] using graded glucose infusions (Figure 3a). Other studies have confirmed severe β-cell defects with marked loss of the first-phase response in diabetic HNF-1α subjects by using hyperglycemic clamps [54, 55], intravenous glucose tolerance tests [56], and homeostatic

model assessment (HOMA) [7]. In the one family described with IPF-1 MODY, glucose tolerance tests in apparently unaffected individuals with the *IPF-1* mutations who had a normal fasting blood glucose and HBA1c levels showed either diabetes or IGT on the basis of 2-h glucose values. Insulin secretion, particularly first-phase insulin secretion, was markedly reduced [57]. Of the two MODY families described with *NeuroD1* mutations, one has been shown to have low insulin and C-peptide levels. A third family is phenotypically more like type 2 diabetes, with a later age of diagnosis and higher basal and 2-h insulin levels at OGTT [47].

(2) *Progressive deterioration with time.* A cross-sectional study of 40 HNF-1α MODY subjects showed a progressive deterioration in fasting plasma glucose with age, which can be explained by progressive loss of β-cell function [7, 58]. This deterioration with time explains the increasing treatment requirements with time. Most patients can initially be managed with diet, before requiring oral hypoglycemic agents, and often in the later stages with insulin. The mechanism for this deterioration with time is unclear. It may relate to a progressive metabolic defect; however, two recent studies in mice overexpressing a dominant negative HNF-1α mutation in the β-cell have shown decreased β-cell proliferation and increased nonapoptotic cell death [59, 60], suggesting that the deterioration is due to a decrease in β-cell mass with time. There is no evidence of an autoimmune etiology for β-cell loss as GAD antibodies and other pancreatic autoantibodies are rarely detected (AT Hattersley, unpublished data, 1997).

(3) *Elevated PI/I ratio.* The PI/I ratio is elevated in HNF-1α MODY in contrast to GCK-MODY (Figure 4a) [7]. An elevated PI/I ratio is seen in type 2 diabetes and is associated with a "stressed" β-cell producing immature insulin precursors. Interestingly the PI/I ratio was elevated in prediabetic HNF-1α subjects, suggesting that the metabolic defect in HNF-1α precedes the onset of diabetes (Figure 4b).

It is still not entirely clear how the TF mutations cause diabetes. However, studies in *HNF-1α* transgenic mice and INS-1 cell lines overexpressing a dominant negative *HNF-1α* mutation have highlighted two potential mechanisms for the diabetes. First, a number of β-cell genes encoding glycolytic and mitochondrial enzymes are downregulated in these models. These include Glut-2, pyruvate kinase, and α-ketoglutarate dehydrogenase genes [61, 62]. These genes bear a striking similarity to the downregulated genes found to be targets of HNF-4α [63]. The resulting decrease in flux through glycolysis and/or mitochondrial metabolism causes decreased ATP production, and subsequent reduction in closure of the KATP channel, leading to decreased insulin release [64]. Second, studies in transgenic mice have shown decreased β-cell proliferation, increased β-cell death, and abnormal islet architecture [60]. Therefore, the development of diabetes and its deterioration with time is likely to be due to a metabolic defect in β-cell glycolysis and progressive loss of β-cell mass.

Specific Features of HNF-1α MODY

Insulin sensitivity HNF-1α MODY is a disease of the β-cell and is certainly not characterized by insulin resistance. Patients with *HNF-1α* mutations are considerably more insulin sensitive than BMI (body mass index)- and glycemia-matched type 2 patients. One study using HOMA showed elevated insulin sensitivity in diabetic HNF-1α mutation carriers compared with control subjects [7]. Another study using euglycemic clamps showed increased insulin sensitivity in diabetic HNF-1α subjects compared with first-degree relatives of type 2 diabetic subjects [55]. It is not possible to draw definite conclusion from either of these studies as they are comparing across different levels of glycemia. However, the finding of a normal hepatic glucose output despite overt hyperglycemia and insulinopenia in one study [65] and the fact that one of the *HNF-1α* knockout mouse models shows an increase insulin sensitivity compared with wild type [66] provides supportive evidence for an increased insulin sensitivity in HNF-1α MODY.

Sulfonylurea sensitivity Extreme sensitivity to the hypoglycemic effects of sulfonylurea medication was first described in 1989 [67] in a family that subsequently was found to have HNF-1α MODY [68]. This sulfonylurea sensitivity has subsequently been shown to be a consistent phenotype of *HNF-1α* mutations [69]. The mechanism is likely to be due to the increased insulin sensitivity compared with type 2 diabetes, and an increased insulin secretory response to sulfonylureas relative to the near absence of response to glucose in diabetic HNF-1α MODY [70]. While in most subjects with type 2 diabetes metformin and sulfonylureas are equally effective in reducing glycemia in patients with *HNF-1α* mutations, there have been reports of marked deterioration in glycemic control on transferring from sulfonylureas to metformin, with an improvement of HbA_{1c} of 4–5% on returning to sulfonylureas [69]. Therefore low-dose sulfonylureas are the appropriate first-line medication for patients with *HNF-1α* mutations although they must be introduced with caution. This is a clear example of pharmacogenetics and is a clear reason for establishing the etiology of young-onset non-insulin-dependent diabetes.

Renal glycosuria HNF-1α MODY patients, like the *HNF-1α* knockout animals, are characterized by a low renal threshold and hence glycosuria. This low renal threshold was in Robert Tattersall's original description of MODY [71] and has recently been characterized in HNF-1α [72–74]. Renal glycosuria has been shown to precede the development of diabetes and makes the screening of at-risk children by urinary screening for glycosuria an appropriate and sensitive screening test. In knockout mice, glycosuria is due to reduced expression of the high-capacity/low-affinity sodium–glucose transporter 2 (SGLT-2) and hence reduced glucose reabsorption in the proximal tubule [74]. The aminoaciduria seen in the transgenic mouse is present in HNF-1α MODY subjects but is a nonspecific feature of glycosuria [72].

Specific Features of HNF-4α MODY

HNF-4α mutations result in reduced transcription of hepatic target genes where hepatic TFs are abundantly expressed. In keeping with HNF binding sites in some lipoprotein promoters, patients with MODY1 have reduced concentrations of the apolipoproteins apoAII, apoCIII, and possibly apoB, which is not seen in patients with type 2 diabetes [75, 76]. Triglyceride levels are reduced in patients with MODY1 and probably reflect reduced lipoprotein lipase activity as a result of the reduced apolipoproteins [75]. This finding in HNF-4α MODY has recently been supported by the finding of low cholesterol, HDL, triglycerides, apoAII, apoAIV, apoCI, and apoCIII in a liver-specific *HNF-4α* knockout mouse [77].

Specific Features of HNF-1β MODY: Renal Cysts and Diabetes

HNF-1β forms heterodimers with HNF-1α, is present in similar tissues although at different levels, and binds to the same DNA consensus sequence. It is not surprising, therefore, that *HNF-1β* mutations cause MODY. What is surprising is that the predominant phenotype in *HNF-1β* mutations is that of nondiabetic renal disease, most noticeably renal cysts, and that diabetes is a less consistent finding, whereas nondiabetic renal disease is no more prevalent in HNF-1α MODY than in the normal population. The reason for this difference in phenotypes with mutations in two such similar TFs remains unclear, but is likely to be due in part to the earlier expression of HNF-1β in embryogenesis and its role in renal development.

The fact that renal disease predominates means that most cases of *HNF-1β* mutations present to the renal physicians. The renal phenotype is varied, but usually precedes the onset of diabetes. Three discreet renal histologies have been described: oligomeganephronia, cystic dysplasia, and familial hypoplastic glomerulocystic kidney disease [39]. However, renal cysts have been a consistent finding in some members of all families with *HNF-1β* mutations. Renal cysts are present in >75% of patients with *HNF-1β* mutations and are frequently seen on antenatal scanning [37, 39]. The association of renal cysts with diabetes in *HNF-1β* mutations has led to the description of a clinical syndrome—Renal Cysts and Diabetes (RCAD) [40]. There are varying degrees of renal dysfunction, with approximately 50% of patients ultimately requiring dialysis or transplantation for end-stage renal failure.

The other specific features of *HNF-1β* mutations are uterine and genital abnormalities, which have been described in approximately 30% of patients [38, 44]. In marked contrast to HNF-1α MODY, subjects with HNF-1β MODY have insulin resistance with hypertriglyceridemia (C Bingham and AT Hattersley, personal communication, 2002). Hyperuricemia has also been described [78] and may reflect the insulin resistance or a specific defect in renal tubular transport of urate.

Specific Features of IPF-1 Mutations

It is difficult to comment on the phenotype of IPF-1 MODY as a mutation has only been found in one family [45]. The age of onset of diabetes and treatment requirements of this family are similar to other TF-MODY families. The most striking feature of the IPF-1 MODY family was that a family member with a homozygous mutation developed pancreatic agenesis and hence had marked hyperglycemia and dysfunction of the non-endocrine pancreas from birth [79].

Specific Features of NeuroD1 MODY

One MODY family has been described with *NeuroD1* mutations. No specific features other than diabetes have been reported in these families.

Differential Diagnosis and Treatment of TF-MODY

A diagnosis of MODY needs to be considered in any person who develops diabetes at a young age. The differential diagnosis is between type 1 diabetes, type 2 diabetes, and more rarely other monogenic or secondary causes of diabetes mellitus. Table 1 outlines useful clinical features of type 1 diabetes, type 2 diabetes, MODY, and MIDD that can be used to distinguish between them.

Once MODY is suspected, a molecular genetic diagnosis should be sought. Clinical features can be used to target focused molecular genetic analysis. Table 2 summarizes the clinical features of GCK-MODY and TF-MODY and those features that can be used to differentiate between different TF mutations.

Clinical Features and Treatment of TF-MODY Diabetes

In subjects with TF-MODY mutations, diabetes usually develops in adolescence or early adult life. The youngest age of onset of diabetes in HNF-1α MODY reported is 4 years, with 63% of patients having developed diabetes by the age of 25.

Table 1 Differential diagnosis of MODY

	Number of parents usually affected	Inheritance	Obesity	Associated features	Initial treatment
MODY	1	Dominant	Rarely	See Table 2	Diet
Type 1	0	Polygenic	Rarely	Pancreatic autoantibodies	Insulin
MIDD	1	Maternal	Rarely	Deafness or neurological features (see text)	Diet
Early-onset type 2 diabetes	1–2	Polygenic	Usually	Acanthosis nigricans	Diet

It is usually sufficient to make the diagnosis of diabetes on a fasting plasma glucose. However, in young HNF-1α mutation carriers (<20 years), the fasting plasma glucose is often normal, but following an oral glucose load they have a 2-h value similar to that in diabetics, with a large increment between the fasting and 2-h plasma glucose [24]. This probably reflects the finding that nondiabetic subjects were shown to have normal insulin secretion until the glucose was elevated above a threshold of 8 mmol/l when the increase in insulin secretory rate was reduced [23]. This normal fasting glucose but abnormal response to an oral glucose load has implications for screening of family members, and current recommendation is that they should be screened with OGTT [24].

Diabetes usually presents with osmotic symptoms, or is found on screening of asymptomatic family members. The diabetes is usually non-insulin dependent at diagnosis, although there are rare case reports of presentation with ketoacidsosis.

Most patients can be managed initially with dietary control before requiring oral agents. When commencing oral agents the extreme sensitivity to sulfonylureas (cf. specific features of HNF-1α MODY) means that these are the treatment of choice but can often be difficult to initiate owing to hypoglycemia. Sulfonylureas should be started at *very* low dose, e.g. 20 mg gliclazide, before gradually increasing. Metformin and other insulin-sensitizing agents are relatively ineffective, as TF-MODY subjects are not insulin resistant. Experience of other insulin secretagogues is limited, but as most of these act via the sulfonylurea receptor then sensitivity would be expected and similar precautions observed. Once established on sulfonylurea treatment, many patients can be well controlled for many years. However, the inexorable decline in β-cell mass means that insulin is often needed in later life. The lipid profile is often favorable in TF-MODY. This relates largely to the lack of the insulin resistance phenotype that is seen in type 2 diabetes, but also specifically to the role of the HNF TFs in hepatic lipoprotein synthesis.

Diabetes-Related Complications in TF-MODY

Microvascular complications have been described in HNF-1α MODY [80], HNF-1β MODY [35], HNF-4α MODY [81], and NeuroD1 MODY [48]. This means that it is important to strive for excellent glycemic control. The pattern of complications and vascular dysfunction is similar to that seen in type 1 diabetes.

MITOCHONDRIAL DIABETES

Mitochondria are intracellular organelles present in almost each mammalian cell. They are responsible for the energy supply of the cell. They are intimately involved in the process of glucose–insulin secretion coupling, as they metabolize pyruvate (and other substrates) to produce the increase in the cellular ATP/ADP ratio that closes KATP channels to trigger insulin release. Defects in mitochondrial function would therefore be predicted to cause diabetes. Indeed, pancreatic-specific disruption of mitochondrial function in a transgenic mouse causes diabetes because of decreased β-cell insulin secretion [82].

Mitochondria are the only intracellular organelles (other than the nucleus) to contain their own DNA. The DNA is circular and 16 569 bp in length, and contains 37 genes encoding 22 types of transfer RNA (tRNA), 2 types of ribosomal RNA, and 13 enzymes of oxidative phosphorylation. However, the majority of mitochondrial components are encoded by the nucleus [83], and therefore, defective mitochondrial function could result from mutations in either mitochondrial or nuclear DNA.

Each mitochondrion contains a few copies of mitochondrial DNA (mtDNA), and on average each cell contains several hundred mitochondria. Individual cells often contain a mixture of mutated and normal mtDNA and this is termed *heteroplasmy*. The degree of heteroplasmy can vary between tissues and within families, and this explains the varied phenotypes seen with the same mitochondrial mutation. Mitochondrial mutations are inherited maternally, as during fertilization the mitochondria in the tail of the sperm do not enter the oocyte, and therefore the developing embryo has mitochondria inherited only from the mother. Diabetes due to mitochondrial dysfunction is described in a number of syndromes. MIDD is the most common and will be discussed in detail. Mitochondrial DNA deletions, and more rarely duplications, have been described in Kearns–Sayre syndrome (sporadic disorder with retinal dystrophy, progressive external

Table 2 Comparison of the different subtypes of maturity-onset diabetes of the young

		Transcription factors				
	GCK MODY2	*HNF-1α* MODY3	*HNF-4α* MODY1	*IPF-1* MODY4	*HNF-1β* MODY5	*NeuroD1* MODY6
Chromosomal location	7p	12q	20q	13q	17q	2q
Frequency (%)	14	69	3	1 family described	3	1 family described
Pathophysiology	Glucose sensing defect		Defect in mitochondrial ATP production; progressive β-cell loss			
Presentation	Usually detected at screening		Osmotic symptoms			
Onset of hyperglycemia	Birth		Adolescence/early adulthood			
Nature of hyperglycemia	Mild; Minimal deterioration with age		Marked hyperglycemia; progressive deterioration with age; may be severe (FPG frequently >14 mmol/l off treatment)			
Pattern in Oral glucose tolerance test	FPG > 5.5 mmol/l; increment at 2 h <3.5 mmol/l		Increment at 2 h usually >3.5 mmol/l			
Microvascular complications	Rare		Often present			
Extrapancreatic manifestations	Decreased hepatic glycogen stores	Insulin sensitive; renal glycosuria; sulfonylurea sensitive	Reduced plasma triglycerides	None described	Renal disease (esp. cysts) predominates; genital abnormalities	None described
Treatment	Not required except in pregnancy (see text)		Initially managed with diet but often need increasing treatment with OHA or insulin			

Note: GCK = glucokinase, MODY = maturity-onset diabetes of the young, HNF = hepatocyte nuclear factor, IPF = insulin promoter factor, FPG = fasting plasma glucose, OHA = oral hypoglycemic agent.

opthalmoplegia, heart block, cerebellar ataxia [84]) and Pearson syndrome (sideroblastic anemia, exocrine pancreatic dysfunction, and lactic acidosis [85]). Both Pearson syndrome and Kearns–Sayre syndrome can be associated with insulin-requiring diabetes developing in infancy and childhood.

Maternally Inherited Diabetes and Deafness

In 1989, Lemkes described a large family in which all nine children of a mother with diabetes developed non-insulin-dependent diabetes. Deafness of variable severity was also described in those members with diabetes. Subsequent analysis of the mt DNA in this family showed a heteroplasmic G→A substitution at nucleotide pair (np) 3243 in one of the two $tRNA^{(Leu)}$ genes [86]. The name of maternally inherited diabetes and deafness (MIDD) was proposed to describe this syndrome [86]. The association of this np3243 mutation with diabetes and deafness has been confirmed in a number of populations [87–89]. Since the description of the np3243 mutation a number of other mitochondrial mutations have been described in families with maternally inherited diabetes (with or without deafness) (reviewed in reference 90).

It is interesting that the same mutation that causes MIDD (np3243) also causes a syndrome of severe neuromuscular disease called MELAS (mitochondrial myopathy, encephalopathy, lactic acidosis, and stroke). Within a family there is usually a dominant phenotype, although occasionally some members develop MIDD while others develop MELAS [91, 92]. Most subjects with MELAS do not develop diabetes, but the association of diabetes with MELAS has been described. It is not clear why some np3243 mutation carriers develop diabetes whereas others develop MELAS, but it would appear that they are two distinct but overlapping syndromes.

In the Netherlands, in a study taking a cross section through the diabetic population, the prevalence of MIDD was 1.3% [93]. Almost all children of a mother with a np3243 mutation inherited the mutation; however, only 60% of 3243 mutation carriers developed diabetes, and the remainder seemed to have normal glycemic profiles during OGTT [93]. There is no obvious relationship between the degree of heteroplasmy of the 3243 mutation and severity or age of onset of diabetes. Spontaneous 3243 mutations have been described, and so a lack of family history of diabetes or deafness does not exclude MIDD.

The Phenotype of MIDD

Diabetes usually develops in the third to the fifth decade, although the age of presentation is variable. In one study the age of onset varied from 10 to 65 years [91]. Diabetes has been variously described as insulin-dependent, slow-onset insulin dependent, and non-insulin-dependent. The classification essentially depends on the rapidity of onset of the diabetes. The current WHO classification [94] classifies MIDD as a "genetic disorder of β-cell function," distinct from type 1 or type 2 diabetes. Ketoacidosis has been described although rarely [95]. Pancreatic autoantibodies are generally not a feature of MIDD, although islet-cell antibodies have been described [93]. Diabetes that is not insulin-requiring at outset can usually be managed with dietary treatment or oral hypoglycemic agents, although there is a fairly rapid conversion to insulin requirement.

Physiological studies of subjects with MIDD are scarce. The majority of studies demonstrate impaired insulin secretory capacity with poor insulin response following an OGTT, and low C-peptide response to glucagon [91, 96]. Alcolado reports an increased proinsulin plus des-32,33-proinsulin/total insulin ratio [97]. Postmortem specimens show loss of β-cell mass, without evidence of insulitis or apoptosis [98, 99]. Progressive β-cell loss is also seen in a transgenic mouse model with β-cell mitochondrial disruption [82]. Interestingly, this transgenic mouse showed increased insulin sensitivity, which is described in HNF-1α MODY and the *HNF-1α* knockout mouse. Most studies report normal insulin sensitivity in MIDD.

Sensorineural deafness is seen in the majority of patients who have diabetes. In a Japanese cohort, 61% of diabetic 3243 mutation carriers had hearing loss [91]. The deafness often presents after the diabetes, and so deafness may not be apparent at presentation; however, it is usually present in other family members to raise suspicion of MIDD. The hearing loss is usually loss of high frequency perception and may be severe enough to require use of a hearing aid [93]. Speech is not usually affected as the hearing loss is of adult onset. Other features of MIDD reflect the overlap of this syndrome with MELAS. A high serum lactate or lactate/pyruvate ratio, neuromuscular signs, nephropathy, cardiac problems with ECG abnormalities, and spontaneous abortions are described [93]. Many patients with np3243 mutations have pigmentary retinal dystrophy, although this does not usually affect vision [100]. In view of the young age of onset and often marked hyperglycemia, it is not surprising that diabetes-related microvascular complications are frequently reported. Some studies have suggested that diabetic nephropathy is relatively common in MIDD; however, this may reflect a nephropathy associated with the mitochondrial mutation rather than true diabetic nephropathy [90].

Diagnosis and Treatment of MIDD

The suspicion of MIDD should be raised in any family with diabetes, deafness, cerebellar ataxia, or other unusual neurological features. Diagnosis is made by confirmation of a mt DNA defect, usually a 3243 mutation. The low heteroplasmy levels in peripheral blood can, however, mean that a mitochondrial mutation is missed. If clinical suspicion is high then the molecular diagnosis should be repeated on DNA from oral mucosa or ideally from a muscle biopsy, where the heteroplasmy rates are higher.

Occasionally treatment with insulin is needed at diagnosis, but more often diabetes can be treated with diet or oral agents initially; however, there is usually a fairly rapid progression to insulin requirement. In a Japanese cohort of 44 subjects with mt3243 diabetes, 30% were treated with diet alone, 15% with oral agents, and 55% with insulin [91].

Coenzyme Q10 is an electron carrier of the respiratory chain in mitochondria, and has been shown to improve respiratory chain function in mitochondria with the np3243 mutation. There are some studies using coenzyme Q10 in MIDD. Most studies show some improvement in muscle function and lactic acid accumulation on exercise, but no studies have reported on the effects on glycemic control. However, in one study 50 patients with the np3243 mutation were treated with coenzyme Q10 for 3 years, and this study showed increased glucagon-stimulated insulin secretion in the diabetic group (but not those with impaired glucose tolerance or normal glucose tolerance) compared with untreated np3243 subjects [101].

WOLFRAM SYNDROME

Wolfram and Wagener [102] described a family with juvenile diabetes mellitus and optic atrophy in four out of eight siblings in 1938. Wolfram syndrome is also referred to as DIDMOAD because of the usual occurrence of *D*iabetes *I*nsipidus, *D*iabetes *M*ellitus, *O*ptic *A*trophy, and *D*eafness, although only the presence of diabetes mellitus and bilateral progressive optic atrophy (OA) are necessary to make the diagnosis of Wolfram syndrome. In addition, Wolfram syndrome is characterized by progressive neurodegeneration, with many patients developing urinary-tract atony, ataxia, peripheral neuropathy, and psychiatric illness. The syndrome is rare, with a prevalence of 1.3 per million population in the United Kingdom [103].

Molecular Genetics

Wolfram syndrome is an autosomal recessive disorder with consanguinity in about 25% of patients. Genetic linkage studies linked Wolfram syndrome to the short arm of chromosome 4 (4p16) [104, 105], and in 1998 two groups identified the gene as *WFS1* [106] or Wolframin [107]. In a screening of 19 British kindreds, 24 *WFS1* mutations were identified (8 nonsense, 8 missense, 3 in-frame deletions, 1 in-frame insertion, and 4 frameshift mutations). No mt DNA mutations were found [108]. A recent study found *WFS1* gene mutations in 90% of patients with Wolfram syndrome [109].

There is evidence for the existence of a second locus for Wolfram syndrome, 4q22-q24 (*WFS2*) [110]. There are also a few case reports of mitochondrial gene defects causing Wolfram syndrome. In one case a spontaneous 7.6-kb heteroplasmic mtDNA deletion was described in a girl with features of DIDMOAD and hyperlactatemia. [111]. Other reports describe within a family the presence of linkage to 4p16 and multiple mitochondrial deletions [112].

Pathophysiology

The identification of the *WFS1* gene, biochemical studies, and the use of a specific antibody to the C-terminus of the *WFS1* protein have shown that WFS1 is a membrane glycoprotein that localizes in the endoplasmic reticulum. The WFS1 protein does not co-localize with mitochondria, suggesting that the primary defect in Wolfram syndrome is not mitochondrial as was initially thought.

On the basis of postmortem examination it is believed that there is progressive loss of the β-cell with time. Histological examination of the pancreas showed atrophic islets with a selective loss of β-cells and preservation of α- and δ-cells. The lack of autoantibodies (GAD) suggests that β-cell loss is not autoimmune, but is more likely to be genetically determined. It has been hypothesized that *WFS1* is involved in pancreatic β-cell and neuronal cell survival.

Clinical Features

The best data on the clinical features of Wolfram syndrome are from a series of 45 UK patients with Wolfram syndrome [103]. Diabetes mellitus and OA by definition, were present in all subjects. Other features were diabetes insipidus (73%), deafness (62%), renal tract abnormality (58%), and neurological abnormality (62%). These develop at different ages (see Figure 6). The majority presented initially with diabetes mellitus. However, 13% presented with OA and 7% with diabetes insipidus. No patient presented with deafness.

Diabetes presented at a median age of 6 years (range 3 weeks to 16 years). Ninety-five percent were treated

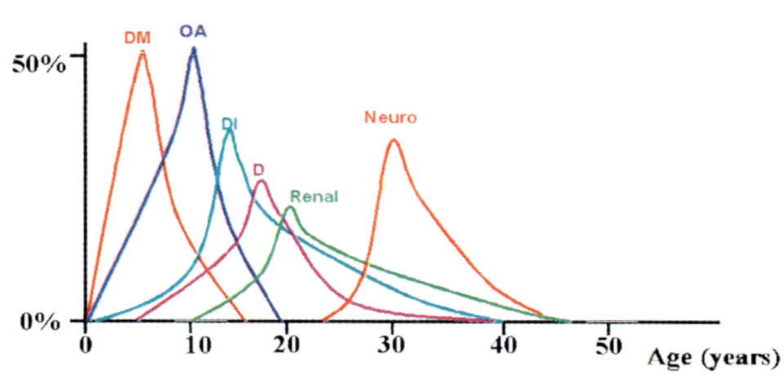

Figure 6 A schematic representation of timing and incidence of symptoms in Wolfram syndrome. DM = diabetes mellitus; OA = optic atrophy; DI = diabetes insipidus; D = deafness; renal = renal tract abnormalities; Neuro = neurological abnormalities (reproduced with permission from reference 103)

with insulin at outset, and C-peptide where measured was low (<165 pmol/l). Ketonuria was detected at presentation in 17 out of 45 patients, with 3 presenting with ketoacidosis. Diabetic retinopathy and autonomic neuropathy were present in approximately 10%. Nephropathy (as determined by a raised creatinine) was not detected.

Optic atrophy presented with reduced color vision and visual acuity with progression to blindness in most patients.

The deafness was a bilateral high frequency sensorineural loss, with 10 patients requiring hearing aids. Interestingly, heterozygous mutations in *WFS1* have been shown to be a common cause of autosomal dominant low frequency sensorineural hearing loss [113]. Neurological complications are varied, but the most common are truncal ataxia (33%), areflexia in lower limbs (20%), startle myoclonus (20%), and horizontal nystagmus (15%). MRI scan was abnormal in 18% with generalized atrophy, especially in the cerebellum or pons, and absence of signal from the posterior pituitary.

Depression and psychiatric illness is described in Wolfram syndrome, although in the UK series, depression was only seen in 4% [103]. A study of 68 Wolfram syndrome patients revealed 60% had episodes of severe depression, dementia, and compulsive verbal and physical aggression [114]. Heterozygous carriers of Wolfram syndrome (parents of subjects with Wolfram syndrome) had an eightfold increased risk of hospital admission for psychiatric illness or suicide [115].

Other clinical features include dilated renal outflow tracts, shown on urodynamic tests to be due to incomplete bladder emptying or complete bladder atony [102]; central apneas; gastrointestinal dysmotility. Primary gonadal atrophy was present in 7 out of 10 men in the UK series. Females had menstrual irregularity and delayed menarche; however, successful pregnancies with unaffected children were reported [103].

The median age of death in the UK series (10 deaths) was 30 years (range 25–49). Cause of death varied, but the most common was central respiratory failure.

Diagnosis and Treament

Diagnostic criteria of Wolfram syndrome require the presence of both diabetes mellitus and OA. The development of OA in a young person with insulin-treated diabetes mellitus should raise suspicion of Wolfram syndrome. A differential diagnosis of diabetes and OA is listed in Table 3. Other clinical features should be sought and the diagnosis confirmed by molecular genetic analysis, with direct sequencing of the *WFS1* gene, as mutations in this account for 90% of Wolfram cases.

There is no curative treatment, or treatment to slow progression of the disease. Diabetes invariably requires insulin treatment, hearing loss may require a hearing aid, and bladder atony may require either intermittent self-catheterization or siting of an indwelling catheter.

Table 3 Differential diagnosis of diabetes mellitus and optic atrophy

Wolfram syndrome
Lebers hereditary optic atrophy
Thiamine responsive megaloblastic anemia syndrome
Friedrichs ataxia
Refsum disease
Alstrom syndrome
Laurence–Beedle syndrome
Kearns–Sayre syndrome

THIAMINE RESPONSIVE MEGALOBLASTIC ANEMIA SYNDROME

The thiamine responsive megaloblastic anemia (TRMA) syndrome is an autosomal recessive condition that is characterized by megaloblastic anemia responsive to thiamine, diabetes mellitus, and sensorineural deafness [116, 117]. Other characteristics described include aminoaciduria, cardiac and neurological abnormalities, and one case of an ischemic stroke aged 20. The original description of TRMA was made by Rogers in 1969 and inheritance was confirmed as autosomal recessive by Mandel et al. in 1984.

The TRMA syndrome is due to mutations in the novel gene *SLC19A2* [118]. The gene encodes a thiamine transporter protein but little more is known of its function.

Pathogenesis

Thiamine is a coenzyme for pyruvate dehydrogenase, α-ketoglutarate dehydrogenase (oxo-glutarate dehydrogenase), and branched-chain ketoacid dehydrogenase complexes. Therefore, a defect in thiamine transport that causes decreased availability of thiamine will cause defective pyruvate dehdrogenase (glycolytic enzyme) and decreased α-ketoglutarate dehydrogenase (a mitochondrial citric acid cycle enzyme). This will cause decreased cellular ATP, which in the β-cell will cause an impaired insulin secretory response to glucose (similar to that seen in TF-MODY and MIDD). Muscle and skin biopsies in subjects with TRMA syndrome show decreased pyruvate dehydogenase and α-ketoglutarate. Presumably a similar defect is found in sensory neurons and bone marrow to cause deafness and anemia but a mechanism for this is not clear.

Clinical Features

Eighteen cases of TRMA syndrome have been reported in the literature since 1969. Characteristically these patients have a megaloblastic anemia with bone marrow showing megaloblastic erythropoiesis and ringed sideroblasts. These cases are reversible on treatment with thiamine (the usual dose being 50 mg a day). Two cases of thiamine responsive pancytopenia have also been described [119]. Sensorineural deafness is often picked up on screening when other features of the syndrome are present. No cases of hearing improvement with thiamine treatment have been described. Other characteristics described include aminoaciduria, cardiac and neurological abnormalities, and one case of an ischemic stroke aged 20.

The diabetes in TRMA syndrome is often the presenting symptom (10 out of 18 cases), with 15 cases being diagnosed before the age of 3 years. Most cases were commenced on insulin at diagnosis although a number were able to stop insulin, or at least reduce their dose, on commencing thiamine treatment. Ketoacidosis has been described on presentation [120]. Diabetes has not been that extensively studied, and reported response to thiamine is variable. Valerio et al. [121] present two cases who have had sequential OGTTs, an intravenous glucose tolerance test, and a glucagon stimulatory test. These two cases aged less than 3 years were diagnosed with TRMA syndrome and were commenced on a lipophilic thiamine treatment from this age (50 mg/day). Each subject was able to stop insulin and diabetes was controlled by diet alone until the onset of puberty. At this stage a deterioration in glycemic control necessitated the introduction of sulfonylurea medication. In both cases there was a good initial response to glibenclamide, but a deterioration in glycemic control led to the introduction of insulin within 2 years. OGTTs performed at puberty showed hyperinsulinemia, with a subsequent marked loss of fasting and stimulated insulin levels in the OGTT performed 4 years (in one case) or 9 years later. Both subjects showed evidence of β-cell dysfunction with a loss of first-phase insulin response to intravenous glucose, and glucagon stimulation showed an impaired but present C-peptide response.

WOLCOTT–RALLISON SYNDROME

Wolcott–Rallison syndrome is a rare, autosomal recessive disorder characterized by multiple epiphyseal dysplasia with early-onset diabetes. The diabetes usually presents in the neonatal period or early infancy and is insulin-requiring from diagnosis. Pancreatic histology shows a reduced β-cell mass [121]. Epiphyseal dsyplasia, osteoporosis, and growth retardation occur later. Hepatomegaly and renal dysfunction have been reported [122].

Mutations in *EIF2AK3* (eukaryotic translation initiation factor 2-α kinase 3) on chromosome 2p were recently found in patients with Wolcott–Rallison syndrome [123]. *EIF2AK3* has a role in protein translation and is highly expressed in pancreatic β-cells, and it is hypothesized that it has a role in maintaining β-cell growth and apotosis.

MUTANT INSULINS AND INSULIN PROCESSING DEFECTS

Mutations have been described in the insulin gene that cause either defective insulin (mutant insulin) or interfere with the cleavage of proinsulin to insulin and therefore cause familial hyperproinsulinemia.

Insulin consists of two dissimilar polypeptide chains, A and B, that are linked by two disulfide bonds. The insulin gene encodes the insulin precursor molecule proinsulin that is processed posttranslationally to produce the insulin A and B chains, and C-peptide. The majority of insulin is produced first by cleavage at Arg^{31},Arg^{32} by prohormone convertase (PC-1) to produce split-32,33-proinsulin, and subsequent cleavage at Lys^{64},Arg^{65} by PC-2 to produce insulin.

Three mutant insulins have been described: Insulin Chicago was the first described and is caused by substitution of a leucine for phenylalanine at position 25 in the B chain [124]. Insulin Los Angeles is due to a substitution of a serine for phenylalanine at position 24 in the B chain [125, 126]; Insulin Wakayama is due to a substitution of a leucine for valine at position 3 of the A chain [126]. These mutant insulins have decreased binding to the insulin receptor and decreased biological activity. Subjects with mutant insulin have diabetes with hyperinsulinemia but they remain sensitive to exogenous (nonmutant) insulin.

Familial hyperproinsulinemia is caused by insulin gene mutations that affect proinsulin cleavage. The most commonly described mutation is histidine for arginine at position 65 of proinsulin [127] and other mutations have been described at this site. This is the site of action of PC-2. Mutations have been described in family members with an autosomal dominant mode of inheritance. A number of reports describe subjects with normal glucose tolerance, but massively raised proinsulin levels. Proinsulin has about 5% of the biological activity of insulin, and hence normoglycemia can be achieved by a compensatory overproduction of proinsulin. Diabetes is described, and may reflect β-cell dysfunction but is more likely to reflect selection bias.

O'Rahilly et al. described a woman with extreme obesity, abnormal glucose homeostasis, hypogonadotrophic hypogonadism, hypocortisolism, and elevated plasma proinsulin, and pro-opiomelanocortin but very low insulin levels [128]. These features are in keeping with a generalized deficiency in prohormone processing, and a compound heterozygous mutation in PC-1 was described [129].

MONOGENIC DEFECTS CAUSING HYPERINSULINEMIA OF INFANCY

The monogenic β-cell defects discussed to this point cause impaired β-cell dysfunction leading to diabetes. However, some defects cause overproduction of insulin and subsequent hypoglycemia. This usually presents in infancy and is termed *hyperinsulinemia of infancy* (HI). HI is a heterogeneous disorder with an incidence of between 1 in 37 000 and 1 in 50 000. The most common cause of HI are recessively inherited mutations in the sulfonylurea receptor subunit gene (*SUR-1*). To date, more than 40 mutations have been identified [130]. Other described mutations are in *Kir-6.2* (the other component of the sulfonylurea receptor) [131], *GCK* [132, 133], and glutamate dehydrogenase (*GDH*) [134].

SUR-1 and *Kir6.2* mutations result in loss of operational channels (due to impaired assembly or impaired regulation of channel activity), causing persistent depolarization of the β-cell and therefore oversecretion of insulin. In a recent review of 175 cases of HI [135], almost all patients with *SUR-1* or *KIR6.2* mutations were unresponsive to diazoxide, a KATP channel opener. Treatment with a subtotal (95%) pancreatectomy is often required.

GDH mutations are a cause of HI that is particularly characterized by the presence of hyperammonemia. Glutamate dehydrogenase is activated by the amino acid leucine, and oxidizes glutamate to α-ketoglutarate (a mitochondrial enzyme). High concentrations of glutamate are needed for the synthesis of *N*-acetylglutamate, which is required for conversion of ammonia to urea. Excessive activity of GDH might therefore be expected to cause over stimulation of the β-cell, but depleted glutamate and therefore hyperammonemia. HI due to *GDH* mutations tend to respond to diazoxide.

As described previously, GCK acts as the glucose sensor, and nonfunctioning mutations are a cause of MODY characterized by a raised set point at which the β-cell responds to glucose. Activating mutations of *GCK* would therefore be expected to lower the set point at which the β-cell responds causing inappropriate insulin release. Dominantly inherited activating *GCK* mutations were first identified as a cause of familial hypoglycemia by Glaser et al. in 1998 [132], and subsequently only two further mutations have been described. In these families, treatment with diazoxide has been successful. This is to be expected, as diazoxide acts on the KATP channel, which is downstream from GCK and is therefore bypassed by diazoxide.

CONCLUSIONS

(1) Monogenic defects of β-cells can cause diabetes and HI.
(2) MODY accounts for 1–2% of diabetes.
(3) MODY can be divided into two groups: one due to mutations in Glucokinase gene (GCK-MODY) and another due to mutations in the TFs HNF-1α, HNF-1β, HNF-4α, IPF-1, NeuroD1 (TF-MODY).
(4) The phenotype of GCK-MODY is that of stable hyperglycemia (5.5–8 mmol/l) present from birth and is rarely associated with microvascular complications. Treatment is usually not required (except in pregnancy—see text).
(5) The phenotype of TF-MODY is of diabetes that develops in childhood/early adult life, which deteriorates with time, requiring increasing treatment. Microvascular complications do occur.
(6) MIDD accounts for 1–2% of diabetes. It is caused by a mitochondrial gene mutation (np3243) and is characterized by maternally inherited diabetes that is initially non-insulin-requiring, and a later onset sensorineural deafness.
(7) Other forms of monogenic diabetes discussed include Wolfram syndrome, thiamine response megaloblastic anemia syndrome, Wolcott–Rallison syndrome, mutant insulins, and familial hyperproinsulinemia.
(8) HI is most commonly caused by autosomal recessively inherited mutations in *SUR-1*. Other causes of HI include mutations in *Kir6.2, GCK,* and *GDH*.

REFERENCES

1. Alberti K, Zimmet P. Definition, diagnosis and classification of diabetes mellitus and its complications, part 1: Provisional report of a WHO consultation. *Diabet Med* 1998; 15: 539–53.
2. Lenderman HM. Is maturity onset diabetes at young age (MODY) more common in Europe than previously assumed? *Lancet* 1995; 345: 648.
3. Frayling TM, Evans JC, Bulman MP, Pearson E, Allen L, Owen K, Bingham C, Hannemann M, Shepherd M, Ellard S, Hattersley AT. Beta-cell genes and diabetes: molecular and clinical characterization of mutations in transcription factors. *Diabetes* 2001; 50: S94–100.
4. Froguel P, Zouali H, Vionnet N, Velho G, Vaxillaire M, Sun F, Lesage S, Stoffel M, Takeda J, Passa P, Permutt MA, Beckmann JS, Bell GI, Cohen D. Familial hyperglycemia due to mutations in glucokinase. Definition of a subtype of diabetes mellitus. *N Engl J Med* 1993; 328: 697–702.
5. Massa O, Meschi F, Cuesta-Munoz A, Caumo A, Cerutti F, Toni S, Cherubini V, Guazzarotti L, Sulli N, Matschinsky FM, Lorini R, Iafusco D, Barbetti F, for the Diabetes Study Group of the Italian Society of Paediatric Endocrinology and Diabetes (SIEDP). High prevalence of glucokinase mutations in Italian children with MODY. Influence on glucose tolerance, first-phase insulin response, insulin sensitivity and BMI. *Diabetologia* 2001; 44: 898–905.
6. Stride A, Hattersley AT. Different genes, different diabetes: lessons from maturity-onset diabetes of the young [review]. *Ann Med* 2002; 34 (3): 207–16.
7. Pearson ER, Velho G, Clark P, Stride A, Shepherd M, Frayling TM, Bulman MP, Ellard S, Froguel P, Hattersley AT. Beta-cell genes and diabetes: quantitative and qualitative differences in the pathophysiology of hepatic nuclear factor-1alpha and glucokinase mutations. *Diabetes* 2001; 50: S101–107.

8. Matschinsky F, Liang Y, Kesavan P, Wang L, Froguel P, Velho G, Cohen D, Permutt MA, Tanizawa Y, Jetton TL, et al. Glucokinase as pancreatic beta cell glucose sensor and diabetes gene [review]. *J Clin Invest* 1993; 92: 2092–8.
9. Hattersley AT, Turner RC, Permutt MA, Patel P, Tanizawa Y, Chiu KC, O'Rahilly S, Watkins PJ, Wainscoat JS. Linkage of type 2 diabetes to the glucokinase gene. *Lancet* 1992; 339: 1307–10.
10. Froguel P, Vaxillaire M, Sun F, Velho G, Zouali H, Butel MO, Lesage S, Vionnet N, Clement K, Fougerousse F, Tanizawa Y, Weissenbach J, Beckmann JS, Lathrop GM, Passa P, Permutt MA, Cohen D. Close linkage of glucokinase locus on chromosome 7p to early-onset non-insulin-dependent diabetes mellitus. *Nature* 1992; 356: 162–4.
11. Vionnet N, Stoffel M, Takeda J, Yasuda K, Bell GI, Zouali H, Lesage S, Velho G, Iris F, Passa P, et al. Nonsense mutation in the glucokinase gene causes early-onset non-insulin-dependent diabetes mellitus. *Nature* 1992; 356: 721–2.
12. Stoffel M, Froguel P, Takeda J, Zouali H, Vionnet N, Nishi S, Weber IT, Harrison RW, Pilkis SJ, Lesage S, et al. Human glucokinase gene: isolation, characterization, and identification of two missense mutations linked to early-onset non-insulin-dependent. *Proc Nat Acad Sci USA* 1992; 89: 7698–702.
13. Stoffel M, Patel P, Lo YM, Hattersley AT, Lucassen AM, Page R, Bell JI, Bell GI, Turner RC, Wainscoat JS. Missense glucokinase mutation in maturity-onset diabetes of the young and mutation screening in late-onset diabetes. *Nat Genet* 1992; 2: 153–6.
14. Eto K, Sakura H, Shimokawa K, Kadowaki H, Hagura R, Akanuma Y, Yazaki Y, Kadowaki T. Sequence variations of the glucokinase gene in Japanese subjects with NIDDM. *Diabetes* 1993; 42: 1133–7.
15. Velho G, Blanche H, Vaxillaire M, Bellanne-Chantelot C, Pardini VC, Timsit J, Passa P, Robert JJ, Weber IT, Marotta D, Pilkis SJ, Lipkind GM, Bell GI, Froguel P. Identification of 14 new glucokinase mutations and description of the clinical profile of 42 MODY-2 families. *Diabetologia* 1997; 40: 217–24.
16. Hattersley AT, Beards F, Ballantyne E, Appleton M, Harvey R, Ellard S. Mutations in the glucokinase gene of the fetus in reduced birthweight. *Nat Genet* 1998; 19: 268–70.
17. Gidh-Jain M, Takeda J, Xu LZ. Glucokinase mutations associated with non-insulin dependent (type 2) diabetes melltius have decreased enzymatic activity: implications for structure/function relationships. *Proc Nat Acad Sci USA* 1993; 90: 1932–6.
18. Burke CV, Buettger CW, Davis EA, McClane SJ, Matschinsky FM, Raper SE. Cell-biological assessment of human glucokinase mutants causing maturity-onset diabetes of the young type 2 (MODY-2) or glucokinase-linked hyperinsulinaemia (GK-HI). *Biochem J* 1999; 342: 345–52.
19. Liang Y, Kesavan P, Wang LQ, Niswender K, Tanizawa Y, Permutt MA, Magnuson MA, Matschinsky FM. Variable effects of maturity-onset-diabetes-of-youth (MODY)-associated glucokinase mutations on substrate interactions and stability of the enzyme. *Biochem J* 1995; 309: 167–73.
20. Prisco F, Iafusco D, Franzese A, Sulli N, Barbetti F. MODY 2 presenting as neonatal hyperglycaemia: a need to reshape the definition of "neonatal diabetes"? *Diabetologia* 2000; 43: 1331–2.
21. Hattersley AT. Maturity-onset diabetes of the young: clinical heterogeneity explained by genetic heterogeneity. *Diabet Med* 1998; 15: 15–24.
22. Byrne MM, Sturis J, Clement K, Vionnet N, Pueyo ME, Stoffel M, Takeda J, Passa P, Cohen D, Bell GI, et al. Insulin secretory abnormalities in subjects with hyperglycemia due to glucokinase mutations. *J Clin Invest* 1994; 93: 1120–30.
23. Byrne MM, Sturis J, Menzel S, Yamagata K, Fajans SS, Dronsfield MJ, Bain SC, Hattersley AT, Velho G, Froguel P, Bell GI, Polonsky KS. Altered insulin secretory responses to glucose in diabetic and nondiabetic subjects with mutations in the diabetes susceptibility gene MODY3 on chromosome 12. *Diabetes* 1996; 45: 1503–10.
24. Stride A, Vaxillaire M, Tuomi T, Barbetti F, Njolstad PR, Hansen T, Costa A, Conget I, Pedersen O, Sovik O, Lorini R, Groop L, Froguel P, Hattersley AT. The genetic abnormality in the beta cell determines the response to an oral glucose load. *Diabetologia* 2002; 45: 427–35.
25. Page RC, Hattersley AT, Levy JC, Barrow B, Patel P, Lo D, Wainscoat JS, Permutt MA, Bell GI, Turner RC. Clinical characteristics of subjects with a missense mutation in glucokinase. *Diabet Med* 1995; 12: 209–17.
26. Jarrett RJ, McCartney P, Keen H. The Bedford Survey: ten year mortality rates in newly diagnosed diabetics, borderline diabetics and normoglycaemic controls and risk indices for coronary heart disease in borderline diabetics. *Diabetologia* 1982; 22: 79–84.
27. O'Rahilly S, Hattersley A, Vaag A, Gray H. Insulin resistance as the major cause of impaired glucose tolerance: a self-fulfilling prophesy? *Lancet* 1994; 344: 585–9.
28. Ellard S, Beards F, Allen LIS, Shepherd M, Ballantyne E, Harvey R, Hattersley AT. A high prevalence of glucokinase mutations in gestational diabetic subjects selected by clinical criteria. *Diabetologia* 2000; 43: 250–3.
29. Velho G, Hattersley AT, Froguel P. Maternal diabetes alters birth weight in glucokinase-deficient (MODY2) kindred but has no influence on adult weight, height, insulin secretion or insulin sensitivity. *Diabetologia* 2000; 43: 1060–3.
30. Spyer G, Hattersley AT, Sykes JE, Sturley RH, MacLeod KM. Influence of maternal and fetal glucokinase mutations in gestational diabetes. *Am J Obstet Gynecol* 2001; 185: 240–1.
31. Yamagata K, Oda N, Kaisaki PJ, Menzel S, Furuta H, Vaxillaire M, Southam L, Cox RD, Lathrop GM, Boriraj VV, Chen X, Cox NJ, Oda Y, Yano H, Le Beau MM, Yamada S, Nishigori H, Takeda J, Fajans SS, Hattersley AT, Iwasaki N, Pedersen O, Polonsky KS, Turner RC, Velho G, Chevre J-C, Froguel P, Bell GI. Mutations in the hepatic nuclear factor 1 alpha gene in maturity-onset diabetes of the young (MODY3). *Nature* 1996; 384: 455–8.
32. Bell GI, Xiang KS, Newman MV. Gene for non-insulin dependent diabetes mellitus (maturity-onset diabetes of the young subtype) is linked to DNA polymorphism on human chromosome 20q. *Proc Nat Acad Sci USA* 1991; 88: 1484–8.
33. Cox NJ, Xiang KS, Fajans SS, Bell GI. Mapping diabetes-susceptibility genes. Lessons learned from search for DNA marker for maturity-onset diabetes of the young [review]. *Diabetes* 1992; 41: 401–7.

34. Yamagata K, Furuta H, Oda N, Kaisaki PJ, Menzel S, Cox NJ, Fajans SS, Signorini S, Stoffel M, Bell GI. Mutations in the hepatocyte nuclear factor 4 alpha gene in maturity-onset diabetes of the young (MODY1). *Nature* 1996; 384: 458–60.
35. Horikawa Y, Iwasaki N, Hara M, Furuta H, Hinokio Y, Cockburn B, Lindner T, Yamagata K, Ogata M, Tomonaga O, Kuroki H, Kasahar T, Iwamoto Y, Bell GI. Mutation in hepatocyte nuclear factor-1b gene (TCF2) associated with MODY. *Nat Genet* 1997; 17: 384–5.
36. Beards F, Frayling T, Bulman M, Horikawa Y, Allen L, Appleton M, Bell GI, Ellard S, Hattersley AT. Mutations in hepatocyte nuclear factor 1 beta are not a common cause of maturity-onset diabetes of the young in the UK *Diabetes* 1998; 47: 1152–4.
37. Nishigori H, Yamada S, Kohama T, Tomura H, Sho K, Horikawa Y, Bell GI, Takeuchi T, Takeda J. Frameshift mutation, A263fsinsGG, in the hepatocyte nuclear factor-1 beta gene associated with diabetes and renal dysfunction. *Diabetes* 1998; 47: 1354–5.
38. Lindner TH, Njolstad PR, Horikawa Y, Bostad L, Bell GI, Sovik O. A novel syndrome of diabetes mellitus, renal dysfunction and genital malformation associated with a partial deletion of the pseudo-POU domain of hepatocyte nuclear factor-1beta. *Hum Mol Genet* 1999; 8: 2001–8.
39. Bingham C, Ellard S, Allen L, Bulman M, Shepherd M, Frayling T, Berry PJ, Clark PM, Lindner T, Bell GI, Ryffel GU, Nicholls AJ, Hattersley AT. Abnormal nephron development associated with a frameshift mutation in the transcription factor hepatocyte nuclear factor-1 beta. *Kidney Int* 2000; 57 (3): 898–907.
40. Bingham C, Bulman M, Ellard S, Allen L, Lipkin G, van't Hoff W, Woolf A, Rizzoni G, Novelli G, Nicholls A, Hattersley A. Mutations in the HNF1-beta gene are associated with familial hypoplastic glomerulocystic kidney disease. *Am J Hum Genet* 2001; 68: 219–24.
41. Kolatsi-Joannou M, Bingham C, Ellard S, Bulman MP, Allen LI, Hattersley AT, Woolf AS. Hepatocyte nuclear factor-1beta: a new kindred with renal cysts and diabetes and gene expression in normal human development. *J Am Soc Nephrol* 2001; 12: 2175–80.
42. Iwasaki N, Okabe I, Momoi MY, Ohashi H, Ogata M, Iwamoto Y. Splice site mutation in the hepatocyte nuclear factor-1 beta gene, IVS2nt + 1G > A, associated with maturity-onset diabetes of the young, renal dysplasia and bicornuate uterus. *Diabetologia* 2001; 44: 387–8.
43. Yoshiuchi I, Yamagata K, Zhu Q, Tamada I, Takahashi Y, Onigata K, Takeda J, Miyagawa J, Matsuzawa Y. Identification of a gain-of-function mutation in the HNF-1 beta gene in a Japanese family with MODY. *Diabetologia* 2002; 45: 154–5.
44. Bingham C, Ellard S, Cole TR, Jones KE, Allen LI, Goodship JA, Goodship TH, Bakalinova-Pugh D, Russell GI, Woolf AS, Nicholls AJ, Hattersley AT. Solitary functioning kidney and diverse genital tract malformations associated with hepatocyte nuclear factor-1beta mutations. *Kidney Int* 2002; 61: 1243–51.
45. Stoffers DA, Ferrer J, Clarke WL, Habener JF. Early-onset type-II diabetes mellitus (MODY4) linked to IPF1. *Nat Genet* 1997; 17: 138–9.
46. Stoffers DA, Stanojevic V, Habener JF. Insulin promoter factor-1 gene mutation linked to early-onset type 2 diabetes mellitus directs expression of a dominant negative isoprotein. *J Clin Invest* 1998; 102: 232–41.
47. Malecki MT, Jhala US, Antonellis A, Fields L, Doria A, Orban T, Saad M, Warram JH, Montminy M, Krolewski AS. Mutations in NEUROD1 are associated with the development of Type 2 diabetes mellitus. *Nat Genet* 1999; 23: 323–8.
48. Kristinsson SY, Thorolfsdottir ET, Talseth B, Steingrimsson E, Thorsson AV, Helgason T, Hreidarsson AB, Arngrimsson R. MODY in Iceland is associated with mutations in HNF-1alpha and a novel mutation in NeuroD1. *Diabetologia* 2001; 44: 2098–103.
49. Boj SF, Parrizas M, Maestro MA, Ferrer J. A transcription factor regulatory circuit in differentiated pancreatic cells. *Proc Natl Acad Sci USA* 2001; 98: 14481–6.
50. Thomas H, Jaschkowitz K, Bulman M, Frayling TM, Mitchell SMS, Roosen S, Lingott-Frieg A, Tack CJ, Ellard S, Ryffel GU, Hattersley AT. A distant upstream promoter of the HNF-4alpha gene connects the transcription factors involved in maturity-onset diabetes of the young. *Hum Mol Genet* 2001; 10: 2089–97.
51. Shih DQ, Stoffel M. Dissecting the transcriptional network of pancreatic islets during development and differentiation. *Proc Natl Acad Sci USA* 2001; 98: 14189–91.
52. Ferrer J. A Genetic switch in pancreatic beta-cells: implications for differentiation and haploinsufficiency. *Diabetes* 2002; 51 (8): 2355–62.
53. Byrne MM, Sturis J, Fajans SS, Ortiz FJ, Stoltz A, Stoffel M, Smith MJ, Bell GI, Halter JB, Polonsky KS. Altered insulin secretory responses to glucose in subjects with a mutation in the MODY1 gene on chromosome 20. *Diabetes* 1995; 44: 699–704.
54. Vaxillaire M, Pueyo ME, Clement K, Fiet J, Timsit J, Philippe J, Robert J-J, Tappy L, Froguel P, Velho G. Insulin secretion and insulin sensitivity in diabetic and non-diabetic subjects with hepatic nuclear factor-1 alpha (maturity-onset diabetes of the young-3) mutations. *Eur J Endocrinol* 1999; 141: 609–18.
55. Tripathy D, Carlsson AL, Lehto M, Isomaa B, Tuomi T, Groop L. Insulin secretion and insulin sensitivity in diabetic subgroups: studies in the prediabetic and diabetic state. *Diabetologia* 2000; 43: 1476–83.
56. Lehto M, Tuomi T, Mahtani MM, Widen E, Forsblom C, Sarelin L, Gullstrom M, Isomaa B, Lehtovirta M, Hyrkko A, Kanninen T, Orho M, Manley S, Turner RC, Brettin T, Kirby A, Thomas J, Duyk G, Lander E, Taskinen M-R, Groop L. Characterization of the MODY3 phenotype. Early-onset diabetes caused by an insulin secretion defect. *J Clin Invest* 1997; 99: 582–91.
57. Clocquet AR, Egan JM, Stoffers DA, Muller DC, Wideman L, Chin GA, Clarke WL, Hanks JB, Habener JF, Elahi D. Impaired insulin secretion and increased insulin sensitivity in familial maturity-onset diabetes of the young 4 (insulin promoter factor 1 gene). *Diabetes* 2000; 49: 1856–64.
58. Hattersley AT. Maturity-onset diabetes of the young: clinical heterogeneity explained by genetic hetergeneity. *Diabet Med* 1998; 15: 15–24.
59. Hagenfeldt K, Herrera P, Wang H, Gjinovci A, Ishihara H, Wollheim C. B-cell-targeted expression of a dominant-negative hepatocyte nuclear factor-1a induces a maturity-onset diabetes of the young (MODY)3-like phenotype in transgenic mice. *Endocrinology* 2001; 142: 5311–20.
60. Yamagata K, Nammo T, Moriwaki M, Ihara A, Iizuka K, Yang Q, Satoh T, Li M, Uenaka R, Okita K, Iwahashi H, Zhu Q, Cao Y, Imagawa A, Tochino Y, Hanafusa T, Miyagawa J, Matsuzawa Y. Overexpression of dominant-negative mutant hepatocyte nuclear factor-1 alpha in pancreatic beta-cells causes abnormal islet architecture with decreased expression of E-cadherin, reduced

beta-cell proliferation, and diabetes. *Diabetes* 2002; 51: 114–23.

61. Shih DQ, Screenan S, Munoz KN, Philipson L, Pontoglio M, Yaniv M, Polonsky KS, Stoffel M. Loss of HNF-1alpha function in mice leads to abnormal expression of genes involved in pancreatic islet development and metabolism. *Diabetes* 2001; 50: 2472–80.
62. Hegele RA, Anderson CM, Wang J, Jones DC, Cao H. Association between nuclear lamin A/C R482Q mutation and partial lipodystrophy with hyperinsulinemia, dyslipidemia, hypertension, and diabetes. *Genome Res* 2000; 10: 652–8.
63. Stoffel M, Duncan SA. The maturity-onset diabetes of the young (MODY1) transcription factor HNF-4 alpha regulates expression of genes required for glucose transport and metabolism. *Proc Natl Acad Sci USA* 1997; 94: 13209–14.
64. Dukes ID, Sreenan S, Roe MW, Levisetti M, Zhou YP, Ostrega D, Bell GI, Pontoglio M, Yaniv M, Philipson L, Polonsky KS. Defective pancreatic beta-cell glycolytic signaling in hepatocyte nuclear factor-1alpha-deficient mice. *J Biol Chem* 1998; 273: 24457–64.
65. Surmely JF, Guenat E, Philippe J, Dussoix P, Schneiter P, Temler E, Vaxillaire M, Froguel P, Jequier E, Tappy L. Glucose utilization and production in patients with maturity-onset diabetes of the young caused by a mutation of the hepatocyte nuclear factor-1alpha gene. *Diabetes* 1998; 47: 1459–63.
66. Lee Y-H, Sauer B, Gonzalez FJ. Laron dwarfism and non-insulin-dependent diabetes mellitus in the Hnf-1α knockout mouse. *Mol Cell Biol* 1998; 18: 3059–68.
67. Heiervang E, Folling I, Sovik O, Sandnes T, Myrmael T, Moen T, Myking O. Maturity-onset diabetes of the young: studies in a Norwegian family. *Acta Paediatr Scand* 1989; 78: 74–80.
68. Sovik O, Njolstad P, Folling I, Sagen J, Cockburn BN, Bell GI. Hyperexcitability to sulphonylurea in MODY3. *Diabetologia* 1998; 41: 607–8.
69. Pearson ER, Liddell WG, Shepherd M, Corrall RJ, Hattersley AT. Sensitivity to sulphonylureas in patients with hepatocyte nuclear factor 1 alpha gene mutations: evidence for pharmacogenetics in diabetes. *Diabet Med* 2000; 17: 543–5.
70. Pearson ER, Starkey BJ, Powell RJ, Gribble FM, Clark PM, Hattersley AT. Genetic cause of hyperglycaemia determines response to treatment in diabetes: a randomised crossover trial. *Lancet* (in press).
71. Tattersall RB. Mild familial diabetes with dominant inheritance. *Q J Med* 1974; 43: 339–57.
72. Bingham C, Ellard S, Nicholls AJ, Pennock CA, Allen J, James AJ, Satchell SC, Salzmann MB, Hattersley AT. The generalized aminoaciduria seen in patients with hepatocyte nuclear factor-1alpha mutations is a feature of all patients with diabetes and is associated with glucosuria. *Diabetes* 2001; 50: 2047–52.
73. Menzel R, Kaisaki PJ, Rjasanowski I, Heinke P, Kerner W, Menzel S. A low renal threshold for glucose in diabetic patients with a mutation in the hepatocyte nuclear factor-1alpha (HNF-1alpha) gene. *Diabet Med* 1998; 15: 816–20.
74. Pontoglio M, Prie D, Cheret C, Doyen A, Lero C, Froguel P, Velho G, Yaniv M, Friedlander G. HNF1 alpha controls renal glucose reabsorption in mouse and man. *EMBO Rep* 2000; 1: 359–65.
75. Lehto M, Bitzen PO, Isomaa B, Wipemo C, Wessman Y, Forsblom C, Tuomi T, Taskinen MR, Groop L. Mutation in the HNF-4 alpha gene affects insulin secretion and triglyceride metabolism. *Diabetes* 1999; 48: 423–5.
76. Shih DQ, Dansky HM, Fleisher M, Assmann G, Fajans SS, Stoffel M. Genotype/phenotype relationships in HNF-4alpha/MODY1: haploinsufficiency is associated with reduced apolipoprotein (AII), apolipoprotein (CIII), lipoprotein(a), and triglyceride levels. *Diabetes* 2000; 49: 832–7.
77. Hayhurst GP, Lee YH, Lambert G, Ward JM, Gonzalez FJ. Hepatocyte nuclear factor 4alpha (nuclear receptor 2A1) is essential for maintenance of hepatic gene expression and lipid homeostasis. *Mol Cell Biol* 2001; 21: 1393–403.
78. Bingham C, Ellard S, Van't Hoff WG, Simmonds HA, Marinaki AM, Badman MK, et al. Atypical familial juvenile hyperuricemic nephropathy associated with a hepatocyte nucler factor-1beta gene mutation. *Kidney Int* 2003; 63 (5): 1645–51.
79. Stoffers DA, Zinkin NT, Stanojevic V, Clarke WL, Habener JF. Pancreatic agenesis attributable to a single nucleotide deletion in the human IPF1 gene coding sequence. *Nat Genet* 1997; 15: 106–10.
80. Velho G, Vaxillaire M, Boccio V, Charpentier G, Froguel P. Diabetes complications in NIDDM kindreds linked to the MODY3 locus on chromosome 12q. *Diabetes Care* 1996; 19: 915–9.
81. Fajans SS. Scope and heterogeneous nature of MODY [review]. *Diabetes Care* 1990; 13: 49–64.
82. Silva JP, Kohler M, Graff C, Oldfors A, Magnuson MA, Berggren PO, Larsson NG. Impaired insulin secretion and beta-cell loss in tissue-specific knockout mice with mitochondrial diabetes. *Nat Genet* 2000; 26: 336–40.
83. Wallace DC. Mitochondrial genetics: a paradigm for aging and degenerative diseases? *Science* 1992; 256: 628–32.
84. Kearns TP. External ophthalmoplegia, pigmentary degeneration of the retina, and cardiomyopathy: a newly recognized syndrome. *Trans Ophthal Soc UK* 1965; 63: 559–625.
85. Pearson HA, Lobel JS, Kocoshis SA, Naiman JL, Windmiller J, Lammi AT, Hoffman R, Marsh JC. A new syndrome of refractory sideroblastic anemia with vacuolization of marrow precursors and exocrine pancreatic dysfunction. *J Pediatr* 1979; 95: 976–84.
86. van den Ouweland JM, Bruining GJ, Lindhout D, Wit JM, Veldhuyzen BF, Maassen JA. Mutations in mitochondrial tRNA genes: non-linkage with syndromes of Wolfram and chronic progressive external ophthalmoplegia. *Nucleic Acids Res* 1992; 20: 679–82.
87. Reardon W, Ross RJ, Sweeney MG, Luxon LM, Pembrey ME, Harding AE, Trembath RC. Diabetes mellitus associated with a pathogenic point mutation in mitochondrial DNA. *Lancet* 1992; 340: 1376–9.
88. Sue CM, Holmes-Walker DJ, Morris JG, Boyages SC, Crimmins DS, Byrne E. Mitochondrial gene mutations and diabetes mellitus [letter]. *Lancet* 1993; 341: 437–8.
89. Awata T, Matsumoto T, Iwamoto Y, Matsuda A, Kuzuya T, Saito T. Japanese case of diabetes mellitus and deafness with mutation in mitochondrial tRNA(Leu(UUR)) gene [letter]. *Lancet* 1993; 341: 1291–2.
90. Alcolado JC, Laji K, Gill-Randall R. Maternal transmission of diabetes. *Diabet Med* 2002; 19: 89–98.
91. Kadowaki T, Kadowaki H, Mori Y. A subtype of diabetes mellitus associated with a mutation of mitochondrial DNA. *N Engl J Med* 1994; 330: 962–8.

92. Onishi H, Inoue K, Osaka H, Nagatomo H, Ando N, Yamada Y, Suzuki K, Hanihara T, Kawamoto S, Okuda K, et al. MELAS associated with diabetes mellitus and point mutation in mitochondrial DNA [Japanese]. *Brain Nerve* 1992; 44: 259–64.
93. Maassen JA, Kadowaki T. Maternally inherited diabetes and deafness: a new diabetes subtype. *Diabetologia* 1996; 39 (4): 375–82.
94. The WHO Study Group. Report of a WHO Consultation, Part 1: Diagnosis and Classification of Diabetes Mellitus. Geneva: WHO, 1999.
95. Smith PR, Dronsfield MJ, Mijovic CH, Hattersley AT, Yeung VT, Cockram C, Chan JC, Barnett AH, Bain SC. The mitochondrial tRNA[Leu(UUR)] A to G 3243 mutation is associated with insulin-dependent and non-insulin-dependent diabetes in a Chinese population. *Diabet Med* 1997; 14: 1026–31.
96. Kadowaki H, Tobe K, Mori Y, Sakura H, Sakuta R, Nonaka I, Hagura R, Yazaki Y, Akanuma Y, Kadowaki T. Mitochondrial gene mutation and insulin-deficient type of diabetes mellitus [letter]. *Lancet* 1993; 341: 893–4.
97. Alcolado JC, Clark PM, Rees A, Hales CN. Insulin resistance and impaired glucose tolerance. *Lancet* 1994; 344: 1293–4.
98. Kobayashi T, Nakanishi K, Nakase H, Kajio H, Okubo M, Murase T, Kosaka K. In situ characterization of islets in diabetes with a mitochondrial DNA mutation at nucleotide position 3243. *Diabetes* 1997; 46: 1567–71.
99. Otabe S, Yasuda K, Mori Y, Shimokawa K, Kadowaki H, Jimi A, Nonaka K, Akanuma Y, Yazaki Y, Kadowaki T. Molecular and histological evaluation of pancreata from patients with a mitochondrial gene mutation associated with impaired insulin secretion. *Biochem Biophys Res Commun* 1999; 259: 149–56.
100. Smith PR, Bain SC, Good PA, Hattersley AT, Barnett AH, Gibson JM, Dodson PM. Pigmentary retinal dystrophy and the syndrome of maternally inherited diabetes and deafness caused by the mitochondrial DNA 3243 tRNA(Leu) A to G mutation. *Ophthalmology* 1999; 106: 1101–8.
101. Suzuki S, Hinokio Y, Ohtomo M, Hirai M, Hirai A, Chiba M, Kasuga S, Satoh Y, Akai H, Toyota T. The effects of coenzyme Q10 treatment on maternally inherited diabetes mellitus and deafness, and mitochondrial DNA 3243 (A to G) mutation. *Diabetologia* 1998; 41: 584–8.
102. Wolfram DJ, Wagener HP. Diabetes mellitus and simple optic atrophy among siblings: report of four cases. *Mayo Clin Proc* 1938; 13: 715–8.
103. Barrett TG, Bundey SE, Macleod AF. Neurodegeneration and diabetes: UK nationwide study of Wolfram (DIDMOAD) syndrome. *Lancet* 1995; 346: 1458–63.
104. Polymeropoulos MH, Swift RG, Swift M. Linkage of the gene for Wolfram syndrome to markers on the short arm of chromosome 4. *Nat Genet* 1994; 8: 95–7.
105. Collier DA, Barrett TG, Curtis D, Macleod A, Arranz MJ, Maassen JA, Bundey S. Linkage of Wolfram syndrome to chromosome 4p16.1 and evidence for heterogeneity. *Am J Hum Genet* 1996; 59: 855–63.
106. Inoue H, Tanizawa Y, Wasson J, Behn P, Kalidas K, Mizrachi EB, Mueckler M, Marshall H, Donis-Keller H, Crock P, Rogers D, Mikuni M, Kumashiro H, Higashi K, Sobue G, Oka Y, Permutt MA. A gene encoding a transmembrane protein is mutated in patients with diabetes mellitus and optic atrophy (Wofram syndrome). *Nat Genet* 1998; 20: 143–8.
107. Strom TM, Hortnagel K, Hofmann S, Gekeler F, Scharfe C, Rabl W, Gerbitz KD, Meitinger T. Diabetes insipidus, diabetes mellitus, optic atrophy and deafness (DIDMOAD) caused by mutations in a novel gene (wolframin) coding for a predicted transmembrane protein. *Hum Mol Genet* 1998; 7 (13): 2021–8.
108. Hardy C, Khanim F, Torres R, Scott-Brown M, Seller A, Poulton J, Collier D, Kirk J, Polymeropoulos M, Latif FTB. Clinical and molecular genetic analysis of 19 Wolfram syndrome kindreds demonstrating a wide spectrum of mutations in WFS1. *Am J Hum Genet* 1999; 65: 1279–90.
109. Khanim F, Kirk J, Latif F, Barrett TG. WFS1/wolframin mutations, Wolfram syndrome, and associated diseases. *Hum Mutat* 2001; 17: 357–67.
110. El-Shanti H, Lidral AC, Jarrah N, Druhan L, Ajlouni K. Homozygosity mapping identifies an additional locus for Wolfram syndrome on chromosome 4q. *Am J Hum Genet* 2000; 66: 1229–36.
111. Rotig A, Cormier V, Chatelain P, Francois R, Saudubray JM, Rustin P, Munnich A. Deletion of mitochondrial DNA in a case of early-onset diabetes mellitus, optic atrophy, and deafness (Wolfram syndrome, MIM 222300). *J Clin Invest* 1993; 91: 1095–8.
112. Barrientos A, Volpini V, Casademont J, Genis D, Manzanares JM, Ferrer I, Corral J, Cardellach F, Urbano-Marquez A, Estivill X, Nunes V. A nuclear defect in the 4p16 region predisposes to multiple mitochondrial DNA deletions in families with Wolfram syndrome. *J Clin Invest* 1996; 97 (7): 1570–6.
113. Bespalova IN, Van Camp G, Bom SJ, Brown DJ, Cryns K, DeWan AT, Erson AE, Flothmann K, Kunst HP, Kurnool P, Sivakumaran TA, Cremers CW, Leal SM, Burmeister M, Lesperance MM. Mutations in the Wolfram syndrome 1 gene (WFS1) are a common cause of low frequency sensorineural hearing loss. *Hum Mol Genet* 2001; 10: 2501–8.
114. Swift RG, Sadler DB, Swift M. Psychiatric findings in Wolfram syndrome homozygotes. *Lancet* 1990; 336: 667–9.
115. Swift RG, Perkins DO, Chase CL, Sadler DB, Swift M. Psychiatric disorders in 36 families with Wolfram syndrome. *Am J Psychiatry* 1991; 148: 775–9.
116. Porter FS, Rogers LE, Sidbury JB Jr. Thiamine-responsive megaloblastic anemia. *J Pediatr* 1969; 74: 494–504.
117. Mandel H, Berant M, Hazani A, Naveh Y. Thiamine-dependent beriberi in the "thiamine-responsive anemia syndrome." *N Engl J Med* 1984; 311: 836–8.
118. Labay V, Raz T, Baron D, Mandel H, Williams H, Barrett T, Szargel R, McDonald L, Shalata A, Nosaka K, Gregory S, Cohen N. Mutations in SLC19A2 cause thiamine-responsive megaloblastic anaemia associated with diabetes mellitus and deafness. *Nat Genet* 1999; 22: 300–4.
119. Bazarbachi A, Muakkit S, Ayas M, Taher A, Salem Z, Solh H, Haidar JH. Thiamine-responsive myelodysplasia. *Br J Haematol* 1998; 102: 1098–100.
120. Valerio G, Franzese A, Poggi V, Tenore A. Long-term follow-up of diabetes in two patients with thiamine-responsive megaloblastic anemia syndrome. *Diabetes Care* 1998; 21: 38–41.
121. Weinzimer SA, Stanley CA, Berry GT, Yudkoff M, Tuchman M, Thornton PS. A syndrome of congenital hyperinsulinism and hyperammonemia. *J Pediatr* 1997; 130: 661–4.

122. Stoss H, Pesch HJ, Pontz B, Otten A, Spranger J. Wolcott-Rallison syndrome: diabetes mellitus and spondyloepiphyseal dysplasia. *Eur J Pediatr* 1982; 138: 120–9.
123. Delepine M, Nicolino M, Barrett T, Golamaully M, Lathrop GM, Julier C. EIF2AK3, encoding translation initiation factor 2-alpha kinase 3, is mutated in patients with Wolcott-Rallison syndrome. *Nat Genet* 2000; 25: 406–9.
124. Tager H, Given B, Baldwin D, Mako M, Markese J, Rubenstein A, Olefsky J, Kobayashi M, Kolterman O, Poucher R. A structurally abnormal insulin causing human diabetes. *Nature* 1979; 281: 122–5.
125. Haneda M, Chan SJ, Kwok SC, Rubenstein AH, Steiner DF. Studies on mutant human insulin genes: identification and sequence analysis of a gene encoding [SerB24]insulin. *Proc Natl Acad Sci USA* 1983; 80: 6366–70.
126. Nanjo K, Sanke T, Miyano M, Okai K, Sowa R, Kondo M, Nishimura S, Iwo K, Miyamura K, Given BD, et al. Diabetes due to secretion of a structurally abnormal insulin (insulin Wakayama). Clinical and functional characteristics of [LeuA3] insulin. *J Clin Invest* 1986; 77: 514–9.
127. Shibasaki Y, Kawakami T, Kanazawa Y, Akanuma Y, Takaku F. Posttranslational cleavage of proinsulin is blocked by a point mutation in familial hyperproinsulinemia. *J Clin Invest* 1985; 76: 378–80.
128. O'Rahilly S, Gray H, Humpreys PJ. Impaired processing of prohormones associated with glucose homeostasis and adrenal function. *N Engl J Med* 1995; 33: 1386–90.
129. Jackson RS, Creemers JW, Ohagi S, Raffin-Sanson ML, Sanders L, Montague CT, Hutton JC, O'Rahilly S. Obesity and impaired prohormone processing associated with mutations in the human prohormone convertase 1 gene. *Nat Genet* 1997; 16: 303–6.
130. Glaser B, Thornton PS, Otonkoski T, Junien C. The genetics of neonatal hyperinsulinism. *Arch Dis Child* 2000; 82: 79–86.
131. Thomas PM, Yuyang Y, Lightner E. Mutation of the pancreatic islet inward rectifier, Kir6.2 also leads to familial persistent hyperinsulinemic hypoglycemia of infancy. *Hum Mol Genet* 1996; 5: 1809–12.
132. Glaser B, Kesavan P, Haymen M, Davies E, Cuesta A, Buchs A, Stanley CA, Thornton PS, Permutt MA, Matschinsky FM, Herold KC. Familial hyperinsulinism caused by an activating glucokinase mutation. *N Engl J Med* 1998; 338: 226–30.
133. Christesen HB, Jacobsen BB, Odili S, Buettger C, Cuesta-Munoz A, Hansen T, Brusgaard K, Massa O, Magnuson MA, Shiota C, Matschinsky FM, Barbetti F. The second activating glucokinase mutation (A456V): implications for glucose homeostasis and diabetes therapy. *Diabetes* 2002; 51: 1240–6.
134. Stanley CA, Lieu YK, Hsu BY, Burlina AB, Greenberg CR, Hopwood NJ, Perlman K, Rich BH, Zammarchi E, Poncz M. Hyperinsulinism and hyperammonemia in infants with regulatory mutations of the glutamate dehydrogenase gene. *N Engl J Med* 1998; 338: 1352–7.
135. de LP, Fournet JC, Touati G, Groos MS, Martin D, Sevin C, Delagne V, Mayaud C, Chigot V, Sempoux C, Brusset MC, Laborde K, Bellane-Chantelot C, Vassault A, Rahier J, Junien C, Brunelle F, Nihoul-Fekete C, Saudubray JM, Robert JJ. Heterogeneity of persistent hyperinsulinaemic hypoglycaemia. A series of 175 cases. *Eur J Pediatr* 2002; 161: 37–48.

27

Immunopathogenesis of Type 1 Diabetes in Western Society

Johanna Paronen*† and George S. Eisenbarth*

**Barbara Davis Center for Childhood Diabetes, University of Colorado Health Sciences Center, Denver, CO, USA, and †University of Helsinki, Helsinki, Finland*

INTRODUCTION

The classical type 1A diabetes or insulin-dependent diabetes mellitus is a chronic immune-mediated disease that leads to selective loss of insulin-secreting β-cells in the pancreas. This results in a series of complex metabolic aberrations that produce micro- and macrovascular complications, increasing morbidity and mortality. It is a common disease, currently affecting about 0.5% of the population in developed countries and increasing in incidence (3.0% per year) [1]. Thus, type 1 diabetes is a great financial burden to the society, but even more a burden to an individual and to his/her family. Despite decades of intense study of both humans and animal models [the bio-breeding (BB) rat and nonobese diabetic (NOD) mouse] to characterize the pathogenesis of type 1 diabetes, there is at present no demonstrated safe and effective preventive therapy. Once considered a disease of acute onset, there is now compelling evidence that type 1 diabetes is a genetically determined chronic autoimmune disorder with a long subclinical prodromal phase [2, 3]. The prodromal phase, which begins in genetically susceptible individuals, can last for years and is associated with series of immunologic and metabolic abnormalities. Some of these abnormalities can be used to detect those individuals at risk of developing type 1 diabetes. There has been a dramatic increase in the biochemical identification of islet autoantigens and in the definition of alleles of genes associated with diabetes susceptibility. With increasing ability to predict the disorder, trials for the prevention of diabetes have begun.

ANIMAL MODELS OF TYPE 1 DIABETES

The BB rat and NOD mouse both develop spontaneous immune-mediated diabetes. Several similarities to human type 1 diabetes exist in these animal models, i.e. lymphocytic infiltration of islets and disease association with alleles of the major histocombatibility complex (MHC). In addition, NOD mice develop anti-insulin autoantibodies similar to individuals progressing to type 1 diabetes [4]. Genetic predisposition is necessary for the disease to occur, but environmental factors like viral infections and diet may influence disease risk. From the NOD mouse model we have learned that both CD4 and CD8 T-cells play a central role in the destruction of pancreatic β-cells [5]. In adoptive transfer experiments both CD4 and CD8 clones reacting with different islet cell peptides and molecules can produce β-cell destruction and diabetes [6], and apoptosis seems to play a central role in this process [7]. Data also suggest that Th-1 (T helper 1) immunity predisposes to diabetes (normally Th-1 responses represent cell-mediated immunity and are linked to many autoimmune diseases), while Th-2 (Th-3)-type responses may be protective (Th-2 responses comprise antibody-mediated immunity and are often associated with allergic diseases, whereas Th-3 responses represent mucosal immune activity and are linked to oral tolerance mechanisms) [8, 9]. Recent findings suggest that this classification is oversimplified, and that Th-2, Th-1 cellular, and even B-cell/antibody-mediated immune responses may contribute to type 1 diabetes [10–12]. What is now suggested for

International Textbook of Diabetes Mellitus, Third Edition. Edited by R. A. DeFronzo, E. Ferrannini, H. Keen, and P. Zimmet.
 ISBN: 0-471-48655-8.

Table 1 Classification of diabetes mellitus

Class of diabetes	Previous terminology	Etiological distinctions
Type 1 diabetes mellitus		
Immune-mediated	Juvenile-onset diabetes, IDDM	Autoimmunity
Idiopathic		Unknown
Type 2 diabetes mellitus	Adult-onset diabetes, NIDDM	Insulin resistance and/or relative insulin deficiency
Other specific types	Secondary diabetes	Specific genetic defects (e.g., MODY)
		Pancreatic disease
		Endocrinopathies
		Chemical-induced
		Infection-related
		Immune-mediated forms
		Genetic syndromes
Gestational diabetes mellitus		Onset during pregnancy

Note: IDDM = insulin-dependent diabetes mellitus; NIDDM; = non-insulin-dependent diabetes mellitus; MODY = maturity-onset diabetes of the youth.

the pathogenic model of NOD diabetes is that there are two checkpoints in the disease process: checkpoint 1—controlling the initiation of autoimmunity and onset of insulitis, and checkpoint 2—determining the progression to islet β-cell destruction and diabetes. There is indirect evidence that this maybe the case in humans, as well; i.e., there are individuals having long-term persisting anti-islet cell antibodies with little progression to diabetes, though the great majority expressing multiple autoantibodies do develop the disease [13]. The mechanisms contributing to diabetes in the NOD mouse model include lack of central tolerance (i.e., escape of autoreactive T-cells from the thymus), enhanced antigen presentation in the periphery by right ("wrong") MHC, and defective regulatory mechanisms (e.g., reduction or functional deficit of regulatory cells such as CD4CD25+ cells, NKT cells, and CD8 suppressor cells), all of which have been implicated in human type 1 diabetes, as well.

Through the use of transgenic technology, several new mouse models of human type 1 diabetes have been generated and are now extensively used to understand the complex nature of this disease. Most recently, insulin autoantibodies, insulitis, and even diabetes were successfully induced in non-autoimmune-prone mouse strains following immunization with islet autoantigens. Administration of the insulin peptide B9:23 to normal Balb/c mice induced insulin autoantibodies [14], and if combined with poly-IC, insulitis [15]. In addition, if these mice expressed the co-stimulatory molecule B7-1 on the islets (RIP-B7-1: rat insulin promoter transgene inducing B7-1 molecule expression on the β-cells), insulitis and diabetes could be induced even with the B9:23 peptide alone.

CLASSIFICATION OF DIABETES

Previous classifications of diabetes were mainly based on the requirement of exogenous insulin [insulin-dependent diabetes mellitus (IDDM) vs. non-insulin-dependent diabetes mellitus (NIDDM)] and on the age of onset (juvenile-onset vs. adult-onset diabetes). Diabetes caused by other known specific factors like pancreatitis and genetic syndromes was called *secondary diabetes*. Now, with characterization of mutations associated with diabetes and with the realization that insulin treatment may be indicated at some point in patients with any form of diabetes and that age of onset does not necessarily indicate the type of diabetes (i.e. immune-mediated diabetes can start at any age, and all children diagnosed with diabetes do not have an insulin-dependent form of diabetes), the American Diabetes Association Expert Committee on the Diagnosis and Classification of Diabetes Mellitus created a new classification based on etiology [16] (Table 1). The differentiation of diabetes types is based on genetic typing, presence or absence of immunologic markers and clinical presentation (ketosis- vs. non-ketosis-prone diabetes, dependence on insulin therapy). *Type 1 diabetes* is characterized by β-cell loss and by dependence on insulin therapy. It can be either immune-mediated (the typical diabetes of childhood – type 1A) or idiopathic with no relation to diabetes HLA risk alleles and lack of autoimmunity (type 1B). *Type 2 diabetes* may range from predominantly insulin resistance to predominantly insulin secretory defect with insulin resistance, with treatment varying from diet to insulin therapy. Genetically defined subtypes of type 2 diabetes include maturity-onset diabetes of the youth (MODY) that are now classified as other specific types of diabetes. *Other specific types of diabetes* include specific genetic defects (e.g., as mentioned MODY), pancreatic diseases, endocrinopathies, drug- or chemical-induced, infection-related, rare-immune-mediated forms of diabetes [e.g., autoimmune polyendocrine syndrome type I (APS-I) [17], stiff man syndrome], and other genetic syndromes. Lastly, *gestational diabetes* is defined as diabetes with onset during pregnancy.

Type 1A Diabetes

Type 1A diabetes represents the typical immune-mediated form of diabetes, with the majority of patients presenting

Table 2 Common autoimmune disorders associated with type 1A diabetes

Disorder	% in patients with type 1A diabetes	Screening recommended
Celiac disease	≅10% autoab+, ≅5% disease	TG autoantibodies
Addison's disease	2% autoab+, 0.5% disease	21-OH autoantibodies
Autoimmune thyroiditis	≅20% thyroid autoabs+, 5–10% disease	TSH sensitive assay
Graves's disease	≅0.5% disease	TSH-sensitive assay
Pernicious anemia (older patients)	≅20% PCA+, 10% disease	Vitamin B_{12}

Note: PCA = parietal cell autoantibodies; TG = tissue transglutaminase.

classic symptoms of insulin-dependent diabetes, including polyuria, polydipsia, ketonuria, and rapid weight loss. The majority of these patients also have HLA-related risk alleles for diabetes and express antibodies to islet cell antigens. Sudden onset of severe hyperglycemic symptoms often occurs in childhood. However, type 1A diabetes can present at any age [18, 19], and a significant fraction (5–10%) of adults presenting with diabetes after age 40 have an autoimmune etiology of their disorder [20]. Patients typically show an inadequate C-peptide response to stimulation, signaling a reduction in β-cell mass and need for insulin treatment. Immediate or eventual insulin therapy is required to maintain normoglycemia; however, at onset many patients experience a temporary clinical remission (the "honeymoon" phase). Type 1A diabetes is frequently associated with other autoimmune diseases, including Addison's disease, Graves' disease, autoimmune thyroiditis, celiac disease, and autoimmune gastritis, and routine screening for these disorders is recommended (Table 2). Latent autoimmune diabetes of adults describes a special disorder that is clinically similar to type 2 diabetes but with positivity for islet cell antibodies and progression to insulin requirement in most patients within 3 years of diagnosis [21, 22].

Type 1B Diabetes

Type 1B diabetes describes a form of diabetes with β-cell loss, but lack of autoimmunity and no relation to high-risk HLA alleles. The etiology of this disorder is unknown and at present is difficult to define. Approximately one half of African American and Hispanic American children with diabetes show no evidence of autoimmunity, but most appear to have type 2 diabetes. About 25% of these children have a body mass index exceeding 25 kg/m^2 and many carry HLA alleles associated with protection from autoimmune diabetes. Ketoacidosis may be present among these children, but many are able to discontinue insulin for prolonged periods of time [23]. More recent studies suggest though that many of these patients are variants of MODY [24]. Recently a form of diabetes was described among Japanese adult patients with abrupt onset of the disease (normal HbA_{1c} but marked hyperglycemia at onset), but lack of insulitis and islet-related antibodies. Interestingly, patients displayed exocrine pancreatic infiltrates [25]. These patients, however, have HLA alleles similar to those in patients in Japan with type 1A diabetes and may represent fulminant autoimmune diabetes. Although most patients with purported type 1B diabetes are from ethnic minorities, patients who present with the clinical characteristics typical of type 1 diabetes, but without evidence of autoimmunity, have also been reported in Caucasians [26].

STAGES IN THE DEVELOPMENT OF TYPE 1 DIABETES

Progression to overt type 1 diabetes can be divided into distinct stages starting with genetic susceptibility (Figure 1). In genetically susceptible individuals, a precipitating event (either intrinsic or environmental factor) presumably triggers the autoimmune attack against pancreatic β-cells. The presence at this stage of antibodies directed against islet-related antigens, including islet cell antibodies (ICA) [27], anti-insulin autoantibodies (IAA) [28], anti-GAD (glutamic acid decarboxylase) antibodies [29], and anti-IA-2 antibodies [30] can be used for the detection of individuals at high risk of developing the disease. T-cell reactivity (measured, for example, by a proliferation test) to these islet cell antigens has been measured, but the low frequency of antigen-specific T-cells in the blood, and the difficulties in standardizing these assays, has made it difficult to use such tests clinically [31]. Much hope is thus put on new T-cell assays [enzyme-linked immunospot assay (ELISPOT) [32], intracellular cytokine staining, and tetramer analysis]. The best approach would be to study the actual target tissue (i.e. pancreas), but in the case of human beings there is obvious lack of accessibility to this tissue. A few studies on pancreases from a small number of children identified at the time of death at onset of type 1 diabetes have indicated the presence of insulitis [33, 34], and a recent study carried out on patients with recent-onset type 1 diabetes could relate the presence of insulitis to the presence of autoantibodies [35].

With the progression of the destructive process, besides immune abnormalities, individuals show a progressive loss of first-phase insulin release (as shown by intravenous glucose tolerance testing). During the early phases of loss of insulin secretion individuals are still euglycemic, but in the 18 months preceding the clinical onset of the disease, a subclinical rise of blood glucose is frequently detected

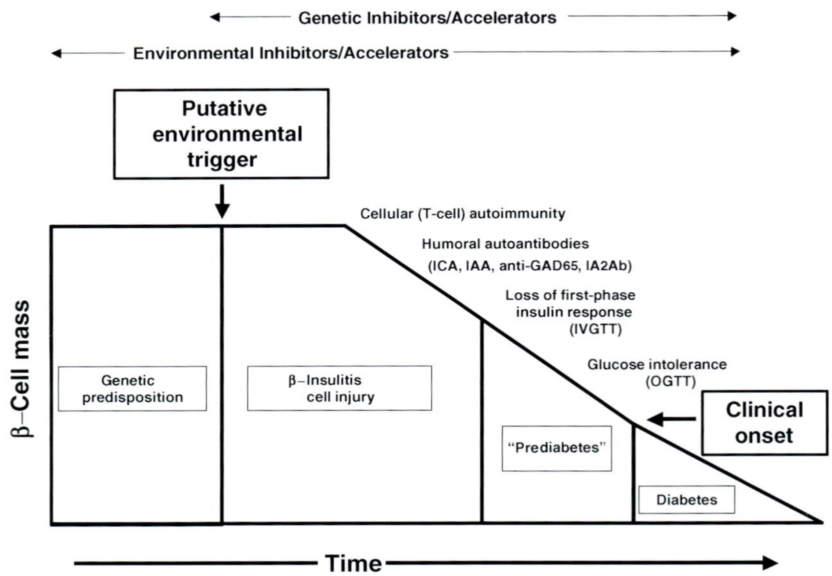

Figure 1 Putative natural history of type 1A diabetes. The progression to type 1A diabetes is staged according to genetic background of the host and immunological/metabolic abnormalities. In a genetically predisposed subject, an immune-mediated destruction of the β-cells starts possibly to an environmental trigger. This is accompanied with the development of islet cell autoantibodies and followed by progressive β-cell loss with loss of first-phase insulin response and abnormal glucose tolerance. The disease onset occurs when a critical mass of β-cells is destroyed. Environmental factors can act as initiators or accelerators of the "autoimmune" process, but may also provide an opposite effect on the disease process by inhibiting/regulating it. Moreover, genes may also act as inhibitors or accelerators of the "diabetic process"

[36]. In those individuals progressing to type 1 diabetes, there is also a slight progressive increase in glycosylated hemoglobin and deterioration on serial glucose-tolerance tests [37]. Progression to diabetes occurs at a faster rate among subjects (ICA+ first- or second-degree relatives of patients with type 1 diabetes) with abnormal baseline glucose tolerance than among those with normal baseline glucose tolerance [36, 37]. Consequently, the development of type 1 diabetes seems to be a chronic metabolic process. A debate continues on whether β-cell destruction in prediabetic relatives is a progressive, linear process with more β-cells destroyed overtime or if the disease actually accelerates at onset. Studies of cyclosporine therapy and recent data showing an effect of anti-CD3 antibody therapy on the preservation of β-cell function in new-onset patients implies that at diagnosis there are β-cells to be preserved [38]. In either case, the loss of first-phase insulin release is followed by hyperglycemia and the clinical onset of the disease. C-peptide secretion is usually present for a period following the onset of diabetes, but is progressively lost and ends once the autoimmune process destroys the remaining β-cells.

GENETIC FACTORS

Type 1 diabetes is either an oligogenic heterogeneous or polygenic disease (or both), in which genetic predisposition plays a necessary role for the disease to occur. In relatives of patients with type 1 diabetes the risk for the disease is increased. Studies with long follow-up times and/or good representation of older-aged patients and relatives suggest that the lifetime risk for type 1 diabetes in relatives of patients is higher than previously reported, i.e. about 50–70% for a monozygotic co-twin of a patient [13, 39] and about 5–15% for dizygotic co-twins or siblings of patients [13, 39, 40] compared to a 0.3–0.5% risk in the general population. The presence of high-risk HLA alleles increases the risk of diabetes in the co-twin or sibling. In addition, groups of initially disconcordant monozygotic twins of patients with type 1 diabetes differ in their risk of progression to diabetes. For example, if the first twin manifests with type 1 diabetes at the age of 25 or after, the risk of progression of the co-twin is around 5%, but if the first twin develops the disease before the age of 25, the disease risk of the co-twin is nearly 40% [41] (Figure 2). The greatest susceptibility to type 1 diabetes is determined by genes of the MHC or the HLA complex gene region in the short arm of chromosome 6. This region determines about 40% of the familial clustering of the disease [42]. HLA molecules play a major role in controlling immune responses by binding antigenic peptides of foreign and endogenous origin and presenting them to T-lymphocytes. The speculated effects of diabetes-related HLA risk alleles on the immunopathogenesis of type 1 diabetes include (1) lack of central tolerance due to poor binding capacity of self-peptides of certain HLA class II

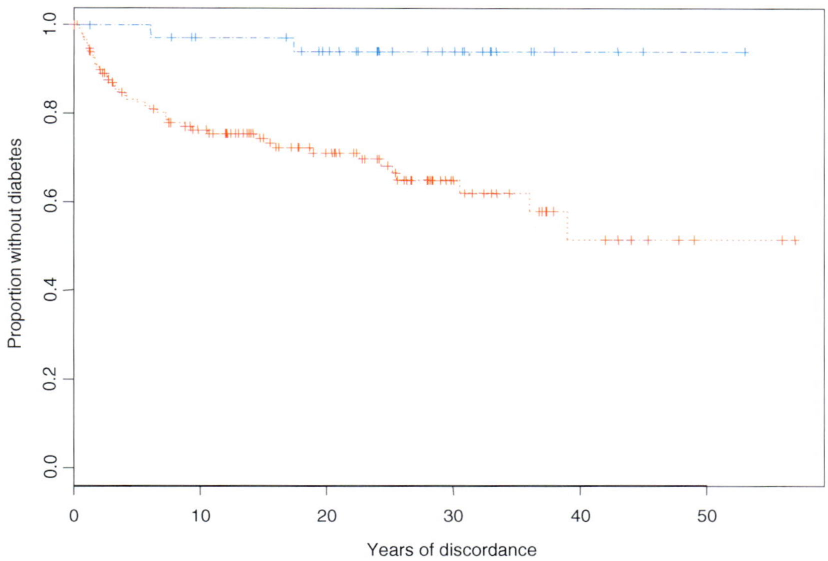

Figure 2 Diabetes-free survival of monozygotic twins of patients with type 1A diabetes for a UK and US cohort, by age at diagnosis in the index twin. Ages 0 to 24 years ($n = 150$) in dotted line (·····), 25 years and older ($n = 37$) in dashed line (-·-·-). Cross-lines represent censored subjects. P value = 0.004 (log-rank) (from reference 41)

(namely DR and DQ) molecules [43–45], (2) failure to maintain tolerance in the periphery through defective deletion/anergy of T-cells or inadequate stimulation of regulatory cells [44], (3) enhanced binding of islet cell peptides by diabetes-protective HLA class II alleles or diabetes-associated alleles [45, 46], and (4) inappropriate immune responses to cross-reactive environmental stimuli leading to initiation or sustenance of autoimmunity [47, 48].

The Major Histocombatibility Complex

The first evidence of an association of HLA coding genes with type 1 diabetes came from studies reporting that the HLA class I alleles B8 and B15 were more frequent in patients with diabetes than in controls [49, 50]. Since then it has become evident that class II alleles of the HLA complex confer the major susceptibility to type 1A diabetes. The highest risk alleles, DR3 with DQ2 or DR4 with DQ8, are present in about 95% of Caucasian type 1 diabetic patients compared to 50% of normal controls. The highest risk is associated with the heterozygous DR3/4 genotype, which is found in over one third of patients, but only in 2–3% of healthy individuals. The DR2 allele with DQB1*0602 is rarely seen in type 1 diabetic patients, suggesting that this allele confers protection against diabetes [51, 52]. With the serologic characterization of antigens corresponding to HLA-DQ and HLA-DP, it was found that the association between type 1 diabetes and the DQ2 (DQA1*0501, DQB1*0201) and DQ8 (DQA1*0301, DQB1*0302) alleles is even stronger than that for DR3 and DR4 [53, 54]. HLA-DQ8 was shown to be a susceptibility allele together with DQ2, and heterozygosity for these alleles confers the highest risk (approximately 1/15 in general population). The DQB1*0602 allele present in DR2-DQA1*0102-DQB1*0602 haplotype is the most common protective haplotype [55, 56] (Figure 3). Two other protective HLA alleles are DRB1*1401 and DQA1*0201,

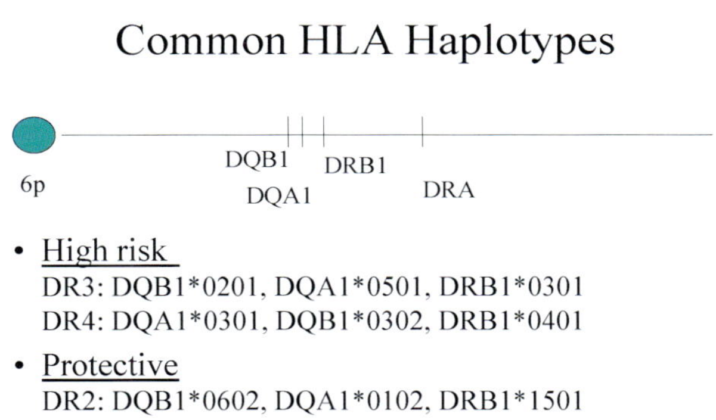

Figure 3 HLA associated risk/protection in type 1A diabetes. HLA alleles are designed according to gene locus (e.g., DRB1, DQA1, DQB1) and sequence variant (e.g., DRB1*0401, DQA1*0301, DQB1*0302), with the first two digits corresponding to previously serologically defined alleles (e.g., variants of DR4 are represented as DRB1*04xx) and the last two digits corresponding to a sequence-defined subtype. If five digits are given, the last digit represents silent nucleotide polymorphisms that do not change amino acid. Alleles on a single chromosome create a haplotype and the two haplotypes inherited from the mother and father compose a genotype of the individual. From teaching slides for Type 1 Diabetes: Cellular, Molecular & Clinical Immunology, 2002. Available at: www.barbaradaviscenter.org

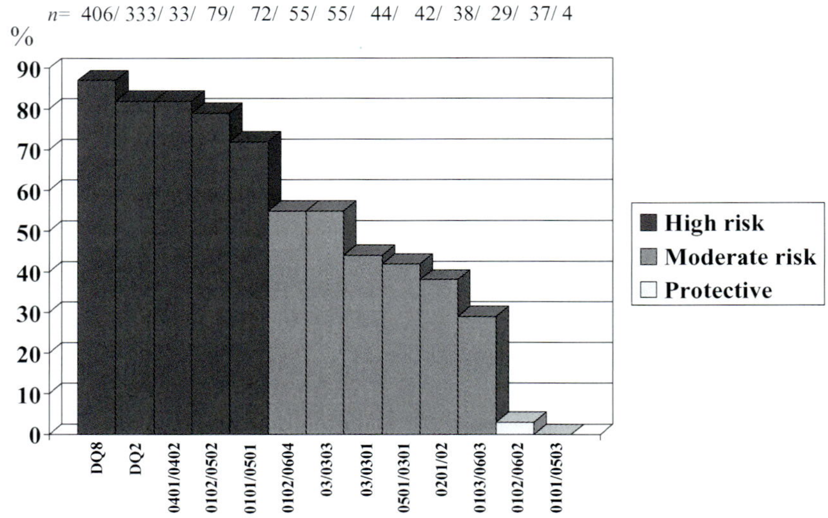

Figure 4 Transmission of DQ haplotypes to affected offsprings from parents with second haplotype not DQ2 or DQ8 (the HBDI family collection typed by Ehrlich et al.). n = the number of parents with a given allele for which transmission to diabetic offspring could be calculated. From teaching slides for Type 1 Diabetes: Cellular, Molecular & Clinical Immunology, 2002. Available at: www.barbaradaviscenter.org

DQB1*0303. Moreover, it has been suggested that the ability to confer susceptibility or resistance to type 1 diabetes resides with single amino acid residues of the HLA-DQ β-chain [57] and/or in the DQ α-chain [58], a rule with too many exceptions to be useful (e.g., DQB1*0401, DQB1*0402 associated with high risk). The initial associations between type 1 diabetes and the B8 and B15 alleles are now seen to result from linkage disequilibrium (nonrandom association of alleles) among HLA-B, HLA-DR, and HLA-DQ, leading to an increased frequency of the extended haplotypes B15-DR4-DQ8 and B8-DR3-DQ2 in patients with diabetes. HLA class I alleles seem to have, though, an independent effect on the pathogenesis of type 1 diabetes, as recently it was reported that in heterozygous DR3/4 siblings of patients with type 1 diabetes having class I HLA-A1, 2, there is increased risk of diabetes [59]. The HLA-encoded risk of diabetes is determined by the HLA genotype (HLA haplotypes of both chromosomes) and there is a spectrum of risk (Figure 4).

Insulin Gene Region

Of other genes associated with the risk for type 1 diabetes, polymorphisms of the insulin gene region (termed IDDM2) located on chromosome 11 clearly influences disease susceptibility [60, 61]. Insulin gene polymorphisms account for approximately 10% of the familial aggregation of type 1A diabetes. The marker showing strongest association with the disease is a variable nucleotide tandem repeat located in the proximal promoter of the insulin gene. The number of repeat units varies from individual to individual (i.e., variable number of tandem repeats – VNTR). Alleles at the VNTR near the insulin gene can be subgrouped into three classes: a common small class I allele, a rare intermediate class II allele, and a large class III allele. In Caucasians, a strikingly higher frequency of class I alleles are observed in patients with type 1 diabetes compared to controls, whereas the frequencies of the longest (class III) alleles are decreased in patients compared to controls [60–62]. In that insulin is a major autoantigen associated with type 1 diabetes, the insulin gene VNTR may influence risk by altering expression of insulin. In human thymus insulin expression is modulated by the VNTR alleles so that, in contrast to pancreas, protective class III alleles are associated with higher insulin mRNA levels than are predisposing class I alleles [63, 64]. This may affect central tolerance induction, because higher antigen levels in the thymus can be associated with negative selection and tolerance [65]. Direct evidence supporting this hypothesis comes from a mouse model in which there is graded thymic insulin deficiency in correlation with insulin gene copy numbers (i.e., one to four alleles of mouse insulin 1 and 2 genes), while pancreatic insulin remains unaltered [66]. The mice expressing low thymic insulin levels present detectable peripheral reactivity to insulin, whereas mice with normal levels show no response. Concerning the relevance of the insulin gene region affecting peripheral tolerance to insulin, the level of transcription of insulin mRNA in the pancreas correlates with the allelic variation within the VNTR, as well, so that the disease-associated haplotype (class I) produces higher insulin mRNA levels than does the negatively associated (class III) haplotype [67, 68]. The persistently higher rate of insulin transcription and translation may make the β-cells more vulnerable.

Although according to some studies relative risk for insulin-gene-region polymorphism is increased in HLA DR4 positive patients [69, 70], insulin-gene-region-encoded susceptibility can also play an independent role in disease risk [71]. In addition, there are conflicting reports about whether there is imprinting of the insulin gene (i.e., differential influence of maternal vs. paternal inheritance). Studies from the United States and France (but not United Kingdom) indicate that "protective" insulin gene alleles are not protective if inherited from the mother. In that there is no clear evidence of imprinting of insulin gene expression in the islets [67], genetic effect of the insulin gene may relate to expression of insulin in the thymus. Alternatively, maternally imprinted interleukin growth factor 2 gene may contribute to insulin-gene-region-encoded diabetes susceptibility as this gene lies next to the insulin gene.

Other Genes

About 15–20 candidate regions for diabetes susceptibility genes have been reported in linkage studies of affected sib pairs [42, 72], but evidence as to the role of these loci in diabetes risk is low or absent when compared to that of the HLA molecules and the insulin gene. However, reports of complex interactions of these loci with HLA and other factors, including each other, make it difficult to identify small effects on susceptibility conferred by each locus individually. Many of these candidate genes have not been identified yet, but the suspected ones encode immunologically relevant molecules such as cytotoxic T lymphocyte-associated antigen 4 (CTLA 4, IDDM12), IL-12B (IDDM18), vitamin D receptor, TNF-α (within the MHC region), and estrogen receptor (IDDM5). Unlike most of the putative diabetes susceptibility loci reported to date, which have been identified by genetic linkage studies in large samples of affected sib pairs from genetically heterogeneous populations, IDDM17 (chromosome 10q) was found by studying a large Bedouin Arab family with 20 relatives affected with type 1 diabetes [73]. All of the 19 affected relatives tested were found to carry at least one of two HLA-DR3 susceptibility haplotypes, each of which was rarely present in other family members. The large number of affected relatives, together with highly homogeneous genetic background and environment, made it possible to identify linkage between diabetes and markers on chromosome 10q25.1. It remains to be seen, if any of these other IDDM loci (other than HLA and insulin) are real, but as mentioned above it is likely that these loci may have different effects depending on alleles of the MHC and that they may well play a role in individual cases or ethnic groups.

IMMUNE-MEDIATED DISORDERS ASSOCIATED WITH TYPE 1 DIABETES

Immune-mediated tissue destruction or disregulation is the cause of multiple common "autoimmune" disorders including type 1 diabetes, celiac disease, Addison's disease, and autoimmune thyroid disease. A common genetic susceptibility is suggested by the clustering of a series of disorders in the same individual or in members of the same family. A major portion of the genetic susceptibility lies in the HLA region, but for several well-defined autoimmune syndromes mutations of transcription factors underlie disease susceptibility [e.g., APS-I, also known as APECED, and X-linked autoimmunity-allergic disregulation syndrome (XLAAD or XPID)].

Celiac Disease

Celiac disease is characterized by marked lymphocytic infiltration of the small bowel mucosa and destruction of the mucosa following gluten ingestion, and this results in malabsorption and gastrointestinal symptoms. Gluten avoidance reverses the condition. HLA-DQ2 strongly predisposes to this disease. Recently tissue transglutaminase was identified as a major autoantigen in celiac disease [74], and transglutaminase antibodies can be used for disease screening. Approximately 1/10 patients (11.6%) with type 1A diabetes express transglutaminase IgA autoantibodies and more than 1/2 of these individuals have celiac disease upon intestinal biopsy [75, 76]. Because of the known risks of celiac disease (e.g., osteoporosis, anemia, gastrointestinal malignancy, infertility) screening for celiac-disease-related autoantibodies is recommended for patients with type 1A diabetes.

Addison's Disease

Autoimmune Addison's disease results in hypoadrenalism and is characterized by autoimmunity to adrenal cortex. The highest risk genotype for Addison's disease is similar to type 1 diabetes (DR3/4, DQ2/DQ8) except that Addison's disease is more associated with DRB1*0404 than type 1A diabetes DRB1*0401 and 0405. Therapy consists of oral steroid replacement. Approximately 1/50 patients with type 1A diabetes have 21-hydroxylase autoantibodies and of those individuals approximately 1/4 progress to overt Addison's disease. Because it is not uncommon for patients with Addison's disease to suffer from hypoadrenalism for years prior to diagnosis or even die in adrenal crisis, 21-hydroxylase autoantibody screening is suggested for patients with type 1 diabetes.

Autoimmune Thyroiditis

Autoimmune or Hashimoto's thyroiditis is one of the most common autoimmune disorders of the endocrine system and is frequently associated with type 1A diabetes. Chronic progressive thyroiditis leads to hypothyroidism and can present as goiter. T-cells interacting with thyroid follicular cells and extracellular matrix are present and induce destruction of the thyroid tissue similar to the destruction of β-cells in type 1A diabetes. In addition, most patients with this disease have autoantibodies to thyroglobulin and thyroid peroxidase and occasionally to the thyroid-stimulating hormone receptor (TSHR). Certain HLA haplotypes predispose to autoimmune thyroiditis, but lack of consistency of HLA associations exists between different populations. According to a recent study the prevalence of thyroid peroxidase autoantibodies is 22% in patients with type 1A diabetes [77]. Measurement of thyroid-stimulating hormone (TSH) levels is recommended as a cost-effective screen in patients with type 1A diabetes.

Graves' Disease

Graves' disease is associated in Caucasians with HLA-DR3 and HLA-DQA1*0501, whereas HLA-DRB1*0701 is reported to be protective. It is also associated with polymorphism of the CTLA-4 gene, which is also associated with type 1 diabetes. A sensitization to a number of thyroid antigens, particularly thyroid peroxidase, TSHR, thyroglobulin, and the sodium–iodine co-transporter in thyroid tissue, occurs in Graves' disease. Unlike type 1A diabetes Graves' disease is an autoantibody-mediated disease, in which TSHR autoantibodies determine the clinical phenotype. If thyroid-stimulating antibodies (TSAb) predominate in the circulation, clinical hyperthyroidism develops. If thyroid inhibitory antibodies prevail, this may lead to hypothyroidism. Sensitive TSH assays are used to screen patients with type 1A diabetes and the disease is treated with antithyroid drugs, radioactive iodine, and/or surgery. The treatment of Graves' disease ophthalmopathy remains unsatisfactory, although use of corticosteroids provides some benefit.

Autoimmune Polyendocrine Syndrome Type 1

Autoimmune polyendocrine syndrome type 1 (APS-I), also called autoimmune polyendocrinopathy–candidasis–ectodermal dystrophy (APECED), is a rare autosomal recessive disorder characterized by an immune-mediated destruction of endocrine tissues, chronic candidasis, and additional ectodermal disorders. The major components of APS-I—chronic mucocutaneous candidasis, hypoparathyroidism, and autoimmune adrenal insufficiency—manifest typically during childhood, whereas other accompanying diseases continue to appear until adulthood. Single gene mutations of the AIRE gene (autoimmune regulator) have been identified on chromosome 21 (21q22.3), and gene sequencing can now contribute to diagnosis [78–80]. AIRE is not expressed in the target tissues of autoimmune destruction in APS-I, but expression has been found in medullary epithelial cells, monocyte-derived cells of the thymus, in cells of lymph nodes and spleen, and in fetal liver [81]. This expression pattern and the predicted protein function may indicate that AIRE is capable of playing a role in the induction and maintenance of immune tolerance. Lifetime frequency of type 1 diabetes is 18% in patients with APS-I, although more patients show autoimmunity to GAD (an important autoantigen in type 1 diabetes) without progression to diabetes [82, 83]. Interestingly, a higher frequency of the diabetes protective DQB1*0602 allele was found in nondiabetic APS-I patients in comparison to diabetic APS-I patients [84].

Autoimmune Polyendocrine Syndrome Type II

Autoimmune polyendocrine syndrome type 2 (APS-II) is usually defined by the occurrence in the same individual of two or more of the following: autoimmune Addison's disease, type 1A diabetes, and autoimmune thyroid disease. In addition, other endocrine and non-endocrine autoimmune disorders exist in APS-II, such as celiac disease, vitiligo, and hypogonadism. In contrast to APS-I, APS-II is commonly diagnosed in adulthood (between 20 and 40 years of age). Many of the disorders of this disease are associated with HLA-extended haplotype formed by HLA-A1, HLA-B8, MICA-5.1, HLA-DR3, DQA1*0501, DQB1*0201 alleles, which also are implicated in type 1 diabetes. Lifetime frequency of type 1 diabetes is approximately 50% in patients with APS-II. In addition, MICA and CTLA-4 gene polymorphisms have been associated with APS-II component disorders.

X-linked Autoimmunity-Allergic Disregulation Syndrome

X-linked autoimmunity-allergic disregulation syndrome (XLAAD), also termed as X-linked polyendocrinopathy, immune deficiency, and diarrhea (XPID), arises from a mutation in a single gene encoding a transcription factor (Foxp3, JM2, or scurfin). The same gene is mutated in humans and in Scurfy mice, and mutations produce overwhelming autoimmunity (including type 1A diabetes), allergic manifestations, and failure to thrive, resulting in death early in life. It has been shown that Scurfy mice have defects both in central and peripheral tolerance; i.e., Scurfy T-cells are hyperresponsive to antigenic stimuli, have defective peripheral tolerance, and cannot appropriately downregulate immune responses [85]. The gene appears to downregulate the threshold for T-cell activation.

Insulin Autoimmune Syndrome, Insulin Resistance, and Insulin Allergy

Two rare autoimmune metabolic disorders are the insulin autoimmune syndrome (Hirata disease) and the type B insulin resistance syndrome. The insulin autoimmune syndrome results from autoantibodies reacting with insulin and can be subdivided by whether the autoantibodies are monoclonal or polyclonal. Patients with this syndrome have recurrent hypoglycemia. A monoclonal response is associated with B lymphocyte tumors, whereas the polyclonal disorder is strongly associated with DRB1*0406, and usually follows therapy with sulfhydryl-containing medications such as methimizole. Essentially everyone treated with subcutaneous insulin (including human insulin) produce anti-insulin antibodies, but only rare patients treated with insulin (more common in case of animal insulin use) show immediate (IgE antibodies) or delayed type hypersensitivity reactions to insulin. In the case of extremely high levels of insulin antibodies, insulin resistance can develop, requiring therapy with >200 units of insulin/day. Changing the preparation of insulin and insulin desensitization often alleviate the latter two conditions [86]. The type B insulin resistance syndrome is due to autoantibodies reacting with insulin receptors, and this can cause marked insulin resistance. However, patients can also have severe hypoglycemia.

TRIGGERING EVENTS

Environmental factors are thought to play a role in the pathogenesis of immune-mediated diabetes in addition to genetic factors. The strongest evidence for environmental factors influencing diabetes susceptibility comes from an observation that in several countries the incidence of type 1A diabetes in childhood has more than doubled during the past two decades [87]. Viral infections and diet have been suggested as these environmental factors [88], but despite decades of searching for these factors only congenital rubella infection has been conclusively associated with the disease. Several different mechanisms by which viral infections may mediate β-cell destruction include direct β-cell lysis [89–91], persistent infection [92], and/or initiation and sustenance of the autoimmune reaction against β-cells [93, 94], activation of innate immunity [15], and molecular mimicry [95, 96]. Coxsackie viruses (namely Coxsackie B virus – CBV) have been associated with initiation of autoimmunity or destruction of β-cells. Some studies show direct evidence that CBV infections can induce β-cell damage; however, other mechanisms by which CBV infections may affect the disease process, like molecular mimicry or bystander activation of autoreactive cells [97, 98], are plausible [99]. Early epidemiological reports relating enterovirus infections to type 1 diabetes showed a high frequency of CBV-specific IgM responses in patients with newly diagnosed type 1A diabetes [100, 101]. An association between enterovirus infections and type 1A diabetes has been reported in some but not all prospective studies that have evaluated a role for enteroviruses in initiation and/or acceleration of the disease process (i.e., enterovirus infections coinciding with islet antibody seroconversion, enterovirus RNA in serum being a risk factor for β-cell autoimmunity and diabetes, and autoantibody-positive children having higher antibody titers to enteroviruses than do children without β-cell-related autoimmunity) [102–107]. Another hypothesis suggests that childhood vaccinations could play a role in diabetes [108], but two large case-control studies [109, 110] and two prospective studies following infants from birth for development of autoimmunity and diabetes [111, 112] do not support an association between any of the recommended childhood vaccinations and increased risk for type 1 diabetes (neither triggering nor protective).

Diet is another environmental factor suggested to influence the risk for type 1A diabetes. In animal models of immune-mediated diabetes (NOD mouse and BB rat) both cow's milk and plant (soy, cereals) proteins can increase diabetes incidence [113–116]. Opposite findings exist, showing no effect from cow's milk proteins on diabetes incidence [117, 118]. In humans conflicting evidence exists, as well, as to the role of milk proteins in β-cell autoimmunity and type 1 diabetes [112, 119–122]. Less data is available on the association between cereal proteins and type 1 diabetes in humans [123, 124]. Another potential dietary substance related to type 1 diabetes is vitamin D; i.e., vitamin D deficiency has been reported to predispose to type 1 diabetes [125, 126], but this may be of relevance only in countries with less sunshine (e.g., northern European countries). At present, given the conflicting epidemiologic data we do not recommend any change in infant diet for diabetes prevention and await the results of additional prospective studies and the important TRIGR Study where an experimental diet lacking cow's milk intact proteins will be studied.

TARGET ANTIGENS

A little more than a decade ago, screening for autoantibodies associated with type 1A diabetes was limited to measuring cytoplasmic ICA and insulin autoantibodies. Currently, sequenced autoantigens with recombinant autoantibody assays are available and include insulin, GAD, ICA512/IA-2, IA-2b (phogrin), and carboxypeptidase H. These biochemical autoantibody assays, especially insulin, GAD, and ICA512/IA-2, can for the most part replace the ICA test. In addition to utility in predicting type 1A diabetes, islet autoantibodies aid in the diagnosis of diabetes etiology.

Islet Cell Antibodies

The first autoantibodies described in type 1 diabetes were ICA, which were first discovered in patients with polyendocrine autoimmunity, including type 1 diabetes [127]. These patients had high titers of antibodies that reacted with frozen sections of human pancreas. The discovery of ICAs in this population facilitated their identification in patients with the more common form of diabetes, type 1A. However, Immunology of Diabetes Workshops rapidly demonstrated a large variation between laboratories in terms of sera called ICA positive. Following standardization of the assay and the use of JDF (Juvenile Diabetes Foundation) units, it became apparent that greater than 20 JDF units of ICAs were highly predictive of diabetes among first-degree relatives. However, prognostically significant heterogeneity of ICAs has been appreciated and there exist first-degree relatives of patients with type 1A diabetes or patients with polyendocrine autoimmunity with high titers of ICAs with a very low progression to overt diabetes. With identification of the antigens contributing to ICA reactivity, it became apparent that in the last two patient groups (with low progression to disease) ICA consisted of solely GAD autoantibodies. These restricted/selective cytoplasmic islet cell autoantibodies are also unique in that they fail to react with mouse islets (with extremely low GAD expression) and give a β-cell-specific pattern on rat but not human pancreas. Of note, other patient groups, such as patients with APS-I and stiff man syndrome, also can express high titers of GAD autoantibodies without other autoantibodies and progression to type 1 diabetes, indicating that GAD (and restricted ICA) reactivity do not always associate with type 1 diabetes. Other defined autoantigens accounting for a subset of ICA staining are antibodies reacting to ICA512/IA-2 and glycolipids. Along with GAD65 autoantibodies, these antibodies appear to be the bulk of ICA reactivity in individuals progressing to diabetes. Variability and limitations of the ICA test and availability of the new biochemical autoantibody assays have resulted in less use of this ICA assay.

Insulin

Insulin is a 51-amino acid protein hormone with disulfide-linked A- and B-chains. C-peptide is cleaved from the precursor proinsulin during processing in the β-cells. To date, insulin is the only known β-cell-specific antigen (all other putative autoantigens are produced by other islet cells, as well, or other neuroendocrine tissues than pancreas). Of note, both in humans and mice, proinsulin mRNA and proinsulin are present in the thymus [63], and self-antigen-presenting cells synthesizing proinsulin also exist in peripheral lymphoid organs [128]. The loss of tolerance to insulin in type 1A diabetes was first described as insulin autoantibodies (IAA) in new-onset patients prior to administration of exogenous insulin [28]. Subsequently, a large number of studies have demonstrated that IAA are present for years before the development of type 1A diabetes and can be used for prediction of the disease. IAA are most frequent in young children affected with type 1A diabetes [129], and most often appear as the first autoantibodies in children with β-cell autoimmunity [4, 130, 131], pointing to a primary role for insulin in the pathogenesis of immune-mediated diabetes. Presence of IAA and their levels are to some extent genetically influenced; for example, they are associated with HLA-DR4 [132]. Initially, two different assay formats were utilized to detect IAA (an ELISA format with insulin immobilized on plates and fluid-phase radioassays). The two different assay formats gave very different results relative to the positive predictive value for development of type 1A diabetes. A series of international workshops led to the observation that the two assay formats measure different antibodies, and that only antibodies detected with the radioassays are associated with risk for type 1A diabetes [133]. IAAs associated with disease risk are of high affinity and very low capacity, and react with a conformational epitope of insulin, making ELISA assays more difficult. Initial insulin autoantibody radioassays used polyethylene glycol for precipitation of antibodies. These used large volumes of serum and produced false-positive values for cord blood and hemolyzed sera. Both of these problems are now eliminated when the new micro-insulin autoantibody assay is used (small volumes of serum and protein A for precipitation of IAA) [134]. A further modification of this micro-IAA assay using 96-well filtration plates allows semiautomated determination of IAA in format similar to that for GAD65 and ICA512 autoantibody assays [4].

Glutamic Acid Decarboxylase

Sera from newly diagnosed diabetic children were found to immunoprecipitate a protein having a molecular mass of 64 000 Da (64K) from detergent lysates of human islet cells [135], and these anti-64K antibodies preceded the clinical onset of type 1A diabetes [136]. The 64K autoantigen was later characterized as the smaller isoform of GAD65, an enzyme that catalyzes the synthesis of the major inhibitory neurotransmitter γ-aminobutyric acid [29]. GAD exists in two distinct isoforms, as GAD65 and GAD67 with molecular masses of 65 and 67 kDa. This enzyme is synthesized in islets, neurons, and testes/ovaries. In humans GAD65 is not β-cell-specific, but is synthesized in non-β islet cells. Several different radioassays for anti-GAD autoantibodies have been developed. Radioassays utilizing endogenously labeled GAD produced by *in vitro* transcription and translation of GAD cDNA or I^{125}-labeled recombinant human GAD65 can give equivalent results with high sensitivity and specificity. The

Combinatorial Autoantibody International Workshop of the Immunology of Diabetes Society indicated that most laboratories (but not all) concordantly measured anti-GAD65 autoantibodies [137]. Autoantibodies to GAD are found in the majority (over 80%) of patients with newly diagnosed type 1A diabetes, with predominance in older children and adolescents ($\geq$10 years) [138], and are predictive of disease [139]. In diabetic children, anti-GAD antibodies are more prevalent in subjects with HLA-DR3 [140]. Anti-GAD autoantibodies (GADA) are not restricted to type 1A diabetes, but also appear in patients initially diagnosed with type 2 diabetes [141] and in women with gestational diabetes [142]. However, in these patients GADA predict insulin-dependency, as well. Interestingly, GADA also occur in patients with two rare autoimmune disorders, stiff man syndrome and APS-I. Although both these two disorders are associated with type 1 diabetes, patients with stiff man syndrome and APS-I exist having very high titer of autoantibodies without progression to diabetes [82, 143]. Most of sera from patients with type 1A diabetes target multiple different autoantigens, target only GAD65 protein epitopes dependent on protein conformation, and do not bind GAD65 proteins fragments or react with denatured GAD65 protein in immunoblotting, nor inhibit the enzymatic activity of GAD65. Furthermore, anti-GAD autoantibodies in patients with new-onset type 1A diabetes recognize different epitopes in contrast to the GADA usually found in patients with stiff man syndrome [82]. Comparisons of the autoimmune repertoires may provide insight why some individuals develop one disease while others develop another disease.

IA-2 (ICA512) and IA-2β (Phogrin)

A second islet membrane-associated autoantigen, distinct from GAD65, was found after trypsin treatment of immunoprecipitates from islet membrane detergent lysates. The majority of patients with type 1A diabetes have antibodies to these 37/40 tryptic fragments of an islet cell antigen [144, 145]. An islet cell antigen, ICA512 (also known as IA-2), was independently identified by two groups as an autoantigen in type 1A diabetes by the following methods: (1) screening a human islet cDNA expression library with a pool of sera from type 1 diabetic patients [30] and (2) by searching for clones enriched in a human insulinoma cDNA library obtained by subtracting glucaconoma cDNAs [146]. The next year ICA512/IA-2 was identified as the diabetes-related 37/40K autoantigen [147–149] and the 40K fragment was related to IA-2 and the 37K fragment to the molecule IA-2β [150, 151]. These two protein tyrosine phosphatase like molecules are most homologous in their C-terminal intra-cytoplasmic domains to which essentially all of the autoantibodies are directed. Because of strong cross-reactivity between autoantibodies to IA-2 and IA-2β and because autoantibodies to IA-2 are slightly more common in patients with type 1A diabetes, only IA-2 autoantibodies are routinely used for screening. These IA-2 autoantibodies can be used for prediction of the disease [152], and have higher predictive value for type 1A diabetes than GADA, but in general the best predictive value is reached with a combination of antibodies (IAA, GADA, and IA-2 autoantibodies) [153, 154].

Other Putative Autoantigens in Type 1A Diabetes

Candidate glycolipid autoantigens include gangliosides GT3 and GM2-1 and sulfatides. Antibodies directed against islet glycolipids give an ICA pattern of staining and show the same stability to acetone but removal by organic solvents as most ICA. In addition, binding of cytoplasmic ICA is blocked by human pancreatic glycolipid extract, thus showing that antibodies reacting to islet glycolipids contribute to ICA reactivity [155]. Antibodies to GT3, GM2-1, and sulfatides have been detected in prediabetic patients or in patients with type 1A diabetes, but the role of the antigens in the pathogenesis of type 1A diabetes remains to be determined. Carboxypeptidase H is another autoantigen discovered by the screening of islet expression libraries with prediabetic sera. It is localized in the insulin secretory granule and takes parts in the processing of proinsulin to insulin. The role of this autoantigen is in immune-mediated diabetes is unknown, as well.

Caveats of Antibody Testing

Because ICA assays vary in sensitivity/specificity, we recommend that the cytoplasmic ICA not be used but instead measure "biochemical autoantibodies." It should be noted that exogenous insulin therapy induces insulin antibodies, which will interfere with IAA results. Because at different ages, different autoantibodies are predominantly expressed in immune-mediated diabetes (IAA in children, GADA in adults) and because antibodies can appear at any age, it is recommended to screen for multiple antibodies and measure them over time. Combitorial autoantibody assays are also recommended because detection of a single antibody has a low predictive value for type 1A diabetes. Transient autoantibodies are possible and because borderline positive values maybe false positive, it is recommended to check the positive values more than once and over time. Lastly, islet cell autoantibody negative subjects (both prediabetic and diabetic subjects) exist; i.e., negativity does not always exclude diabetes risk or autoimmunity.

PREDICTION OF TYPE 1A DIABETES

Despite uncertainty about the pathogenic importance of autoantibodies, the ability to biochemically detect these autoantibodies greatly facilitates the prediction of type 1A

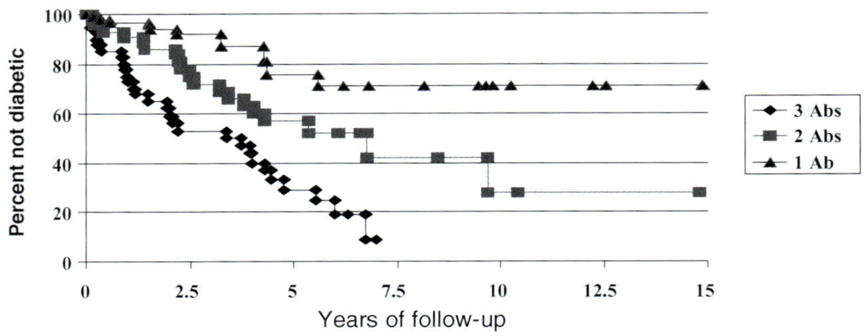

3 Abs *n* =	41	17	8	1		
2 Abs *n* =	44	27	15	4	2	1
1 Ab *n* =	93	23	14	10	6	4

Figure 5 Progression to diabetes vs. number of autoantibodies (insulin, GAD, and IA-2). Ab = antibody (from reference 154)

diabetes. Utilizing only three radioasssays for autoantibodies (insulin, GAD65, and IA-2) 95% of prediabetic or recent-onset diabetic children express one or more antibodies (versus 3 out of 100 controls). Eighty percent express two or more antibodies (versus less than 1/300 controls), and 25% of diabetic and prediabetic subjects express all three of the above autoantibodies. The expression of autoantibodies assorts independently in prediabetic individuals and thus, by screening for these autoantibodies, a high positive predictive value for disease is possible while retaining disease sensitivity (combitorial autoantibody prediction) [137] (Figure 5). Such autoantibody screening will likely have its largest impact for the prediction for type 1A diabetes in the general population where the positive predictive value of ICA positivity is less than 10%, while presence of two or more of three autoantibodies should give positive predictive values greater than 70%. Screening of high-risk individuals from the general population is important, because approximately 90% of individuals who develop type 1A diabetes have no first-degree relative with the disease. When genetic screening for HLA risk haplotypes is combined with autoantibody detection, high-risk children can be followed from birth. For example, in the highest risk children (DR3/4 heterozygotes) anti-islet autoantibodies often appear before 1 year of age [59, 156, 157]. On the other hand, subjects with the protective haplotypes rarely progress to the disease even when positive for β-cell autoimmunity [52]. These strategies help to identify people eligible for prevention trials. The identification of individuals developing type 1A diabetes can be important for other reasons, as well. If risk for type 1A diabetes is detected, mortality at onset should be preventable (approximately 1 in 200 children die at onset of the disease in the United States). A series of trials to preserve β-cell capacity at diabetes onset such as anti-CD3 treatment [38] are underway. The Diabetes Control and Complications Trial (DCCT) has identified that residual insulin secretion results in better glucose control with less hypoglycemia and slower progression to vascular complication, and the better glucose control in turn leads to prolonged β-cell function [158].

PREVENTION OF TYPE 1A DIABETES

Trials using immunosuppressive medication such as cyclosporin have showed some effect in slowing progression to clinical disease [159] or inducing transient remission in new-onset patients [160], but the toxic effects of such drugs [161], risk of immunosuppression, and the need for continuous treatment limit the use of these agents. In experimental models, antibodies against T-cells (anti-CD3) or CD4+ T-cells have been effective in preventing immune-mediated diabetes. A nonactivating humanized monoclonal antibody against CD3 eliminates some of the acute side effects of anti-CD3 therapy and in new-onset patients this therapy restored β-cell function, which was detected as maintained or improved insulin production and reduced HbA_{1c} levels and lower insulin doses [38]. It is, however, unlikely that a single course of the antibody will preserve β-cell function for more than 2 years. Another approach in preventing/delaying type 1A diabetes manifestation is to make β-cells more resistant to destruction. Treatment with high doses of nicotinamide prevents or delays immune-mediated diabetes in several animal models and protects islet cells against cytotoxic actions *in vitro*. In recent-onset type 1 diabetes, nicotinamide administration reportedly improved β-cell function without significantly decreased insulin requirements, but with no effect in children [162]. Nicotinamide may also have some other beneficial effects, i.e. altering immunonoregulatory balance [163]. Trials on nicotinamide in prevention of human type 1A diabetes are underway, and results from the European–Canadian Nicontinamide Diabetes Intervention Trial will be presented in 2003. A promising alternative is antigen-specific therapy, which suppresses diabetes in the two experimental models of immune-mediated diabetes.

Especially insulin or insulin peptides, given by various routes, prevent diabetes in NOD mice [164, 165]. This research has led to clinical trials. Although parenteral insulin delayed the progression to type 1A diabetes in two separate small pilot studies [166, 167], the large US Diabetes Prevention Trial – Type 1 (DPT-1) found no effect of parenterally administered insulin in delaying diabetes development in high-risk subjects with a projected 5-year risk of more than 50% [37]. This lack of effect may relate to starting the therapy too late (loss of first-phase insulin response present and/or abnormal oral glucose tolerance tests) or to the dose used. In animal models, effective insulin therapy has been started earlier and at a much higher dose. A second trial of DPT-1 studying the effect of oral insulin therapy in relatives with a projected 5-year risk of 26–50% is ongoing. In addition, the effect of nasal insulin in prevention of human type 1A diabetes is being studied in Finland, where high-risk individuals (DR3/4 or DR4) are screened from the general population at birth and followed for the development of anti-islet autoantibodies and diabetes. Persistently autoantibody-positive children are randomized to receive either nasal insulin therapy or placebo (Diabetes Prediction and Prevention Study). A word of caution is needed when antigen-specific therapies are used though, because they may, in theory, accelerate disease progression or even induce hypersensitivity reactions [168, 169]. The search for safer preventive therapies are underway, for example a clinical trial using altered peptide ligand of insulin in new-onset patients [170]. The NIH (National Institutes of Health) is committed to a large clinical North American trials program (TrialNet) with the task of testing the efficacy and safety of immunomodulatoy therapy in human type 1A diabetes (International collaboration is planned with Juvenile Diabetes Foundation support). Another network testing immunomodulation, is the Immune Tolerance Network (ITN org). Thus, although there is at present no effective and safe preventive therapy yet, collaborative studies with screening individuals at high risk for progression to type 1A diabetes are important. This could result in early diagnosis and better management of the disease. In addition, the community (physicians, researchers, and families with diabetes) will obtain important data on the natural course of type 1A diabetes, leading to better understanding of the pathogenesis of this disease, and hopefully its eventual prevention.

SUMMARY

Type 1A diabetes: Immune-mediated and associated with autoimmune disorders

Genes (HLA, insulin) and environmental factors affecting risk

Prediction with autoantibodies

Prevention by immunomodulatory agents under study

www.barbaradaviscenter.org: Immunology Diabetes Text with Teaching Slides

Acknowledgments

Research was supported by grants from the National Institutes of Health (DK32082, AI39213, DK55969, DK62718, AI508664, AI95380, DK32493, DK50970, AI46374), a Diabetes Endocrine Research Center (P30 DK57516), and Clinical Research Centers (MO1 RR00069, MO1 RR00051), the American Diabetes Association, the Juvenile Diabetes Foundation and the Children's Diabetes Foundation (GSE); and the Academy of Finland, The Finnish Cultural Foundation, and the Foundation of Pediatric Research (JP).

REFERENCES

1. Onkamo P, Vaananen S, Karvonen M, Tuomilehto J. Worldwide increase in incidence of Type I diabetes—the analysis of the data on published incidence trends. *Diabetologia* 1999; 42: 1395–403.
2. Eisenbarth G. Type I diabetes mellitus: a chronic autoimmune disease. *N Engl J Med* 1986; 314: 1360–8.
3. Eisenbarth GS. Natural history of type 1 diabetes. From *Type 1 Diabetes: Cellular, Molecular & Clinical Immunology*, 2002 (webbook). Available at: www.barbaradaviscenter.org.
4. Yu L, Robles DT, Abiru N, Kaur P, Rewers M, Kelemen K, Eisenbarth GS. Early expression of antiinsulin autoantibodies of humans and the NOD mouse: evidence for early determination of subsequent diabetes. *Proc Natl Acad Sci USA* 2000; 97: 1701–6.
5. Wong FS, Janeway CA Jr. The role of CD4 vs. CD8 T cells in IDDM. *J Autoimmun* 1999; 13: 290–5.
6. Kelemen K. The role of T cells in beta cell damage in NOD mice and humans. From *Type 1 Diabetes: Cellular, Molecular & Clinical Immunology*, 2002 (webbook). Available at: www.barbaradaviscenter.org.
7. Mathis D, Vence L, Benoist C. Beta-cell death during progression to diabetes. *Nature* 2001; 414: 792–8.
8. Healey D, Ozegbe P, Arden S, Chandler P, Hutton J, Cooke A. In vivo activity and in vitro specificity of CD4+ Th1 and Th2 cells derived from the spleens of diabetic NOD mice. *J Clin Invest* 1995; 95: 2979–85.
9. Katz JD, Benoist C, Mathis D. T helper cell subsets in insulin-dependent diabetes. *Science* 1995; 268: 1185–8.
10. Serreze DV, Fleming SA, Chapman HD, Richard SD, Leiter EH, Tisch RM. B lymphocytes are critical antigen-presenting cells for the initiation of T cell-mediated autoimmune diabetes in nonobese diabetic mice. *J Immunol* 1998; 161: 3912–8.
11. Weaver DJ Jr, Liu B, Tisch R. Plasmid DNAs encoding insulin and glutamic acid decarboxylase 65 have distinct effects on the progression of autoimmune diabetes in nonobese diabetic mice. *J Immunol* 2001; 167: 586–92.
12. Greeley SA, Katsumata M, Yu L, Eisenbarth GS, Moore DJ, Goodarzi H, Barker CF, Naji A, Noorchashm H. Elimination of maternally transmitted autoantibodies prevents diabetes in nonobese diabetic mice. *Nat Med* 2002; 8: 399–402.

13. Redondo MJ, Rewers M, Yu L, Garg S, Pilcher CC, Elliott RB, Eisenbarth GS. Genetic determination of islet cell autoimmunity in monozygotic twin, dizygotic twin, and non-twin siblings of patients with type 1 diabetes: prospective twin study. *BMJ* 1999; 318: 698–702.
14. Abiru N, Maniatis AK, Yu L, Miao D, Moriyama H, Wegmann D, Eisenbarth GS. Peptide and major histocompatibility complex-specific breaking of humoral tolerance to native insulin with the B9-23 peptide in diabetes-prone and normal mice. *Diabetes* 2001; 50: 1274–81.
15. Moriyama H, Wen L, Abiru N, Liu E, Yu L, Miao D, Gianani R, Wong FS, Eisenbarth GS. Induction and acceleration of insulitis/diabetes in mice with a viral mimic (polyinosinic-polycytidylic acid) and an insulin self-peptide. *Proc Natl Acad Sci USA* 2002; 99: 5539–44.
16. The Expert Committee on the diagnosis and classification of diabetes mellitus. Report of the Expert Committee on the Diagnosis and Classification of Diabetes Mellitus. *Diabetes Care* 2003; 26 (suppl 1): S5–20.
17. Perheentupa J. APS-I/APECED: the clinical disease and therapy. *Endocrinol Metab Clin North Am* 2002; 31: 295–320.
18. Laakso M, Pyorala K. Age of onset and type of diabetes. *Diabetes Care* 1985; 8: 114–7.
19. Tuomi T, Groop LC, Zimmet PZ, Rowley MJ, Knowles W, Mackay IR. Antibodies to glutamic acid decarboxylase reveal latent autoimmune diabetes mellitus in adults with a non-insulin-dependent onset of disease. *Diabetes* 1993; 42: 359–62.
20. Molbak AG, Christau B, Marner B, Borch-Johnsen K, Nerup J. Incidence of insulin-dependent diabetes mellitus in age groups over 30 years in Denmark. *Diabet Med* 1994; 11: 650–5.
21. Tuomi T, Carlsson A, Li H, Isomaa B, Miettinen A, Nilsson A, Nissen M, Ehrnstrom BO, Forsen B, Snickars B, Lahti K, Forsblom C, Saloranta C, Taskinen MR, Groop LC. Clinical and genetic characteristics of type 2 diabetes with and without GAD antibodies. *Diabetes* 1999; 48: 150–7.
22. Landin-Olsson M. Latent autoimmune diabetes in adults. *Ann N Y Acad Sci* 2002; 958: 112–6.
23. Winter WE, Maclaren NK, Riley WJ, Clarke DW, Kappy MS, Spillar RP. Maturity-onset diabetes of youth in Black Americans. *N Engl J Med* 1987; 316: 285–91.
24. Winter WE, Nakamura M, House DV. Monogenic diabetes mellitus in youth. The MODY syndromes. *Endocrinol Metab Clin North Am* 1999; 28: 765–85.
25. Imagawa A, Hanafusa T, Miyagawa J, Matsuzawa Y, for the Osaka IDDM Study Group. A novel subtype of type 1 diabetes mellitus characterized by a rapid onset and an absence of diabetes-related antibodies. *N Engl J Med* 2000; 342: 301–7.
26. Tiberti C, Buzzetti R, Anastasi E, Dotta F, Vasta M, Petrone A, Cervoni M, Torresi P, Vecci E, Multari G, Di Mario U. Autoantibody negative new onset type 1 diabetic patients lacking high risk HLA alleles in a caucasian population: are these type 1b diabetes cases? *Diabetes Metab Res Rev* 2000; 16: 8–14.
27. Bottazzo GF, Dean BM, Gorsuch AN, Cudworth AG, Doniach D. Complement-fixing islet-cell antibodies in type I diabetes: possible monitors of active beta-cell damage. *Lancet* 1980; 1: 668–72.
28. Palmer JP, Asplin CM, Clemons P, Lyen K, Tatpati O, Raghu PK, Paquette TL. Insulin antibodies in insulin-dependent diabetics before insulin treatment. *Science* 1983; 222: 1337–9.
29. Baekkeskov S, Aanstoot H-J, Christgau S, Reetz A, Solimena M, Cascalho M, Folli F, Richter-Olesen H, De Camilli P, Camilli PD. Identification of the 64K autoantigen in insulin-dependent diabetes as the GABA-synthesizing enzyme glutamic acid decarboxylase. *Nature* 1990; 347: 151–6.
30. Rabin DU, Pleasic SM, Shapiro JA, Yoo-Warren H, Oles J, Hicks JM, Goldstein DE, Rae PM. Islet cell antigen 512 is a diabetes-specific islet autoantigen related to protein tyrosine phosphatases. *J Immunol* 1994; 152: 3183–8.
31. Roep BO. Standardization of T-cell assays in Type I diabetes. Immunology of Diabetes Society T-cell Committee. *Diabetologia* 1999; 42: 636–7.
32. Kotani R, Nagata M, Moriyama H, Nakayama M, Yamada K, Chowdhury SA, Chakrabarty S, Jin Z, Yasuda H, Yokono K. Detection of GAD65-reactive T-cells in type 1 diabetes by immunoglobulin-free ELISPOT assays. *Diabetes Care* 2002; 25: 1390–7.
33. Gepts W. Pathologic anatomy of the pancreas in juvenile diabetes mellitus. *Diabetes* 1965; 14: 619–33.
34. Bottazzo GF, Dean BM, McNally JM, MacKay EH, Swift PG, Gamble DR. In situ characterization of autoimmune phenomena and expression of HLA molecules in the pancreas in diabetic insulitis. *N Engl J Med* 1985; 313: 353–60.
35. Imagawa A, Hanafusa T, Tamura S, Moriwaki M, Itoh N, Yamamoto K, Iwahashi H, Yamagata K, Waguri M, Nanmo T, Uno S, Nakajima H, Namba M, Kawata S, Miyagawa JI, Matsuzawa Y. Pancreatic biopsy as a procedure for detecting in situ autoimmune phenomena in type 1 diabetes: close correlation between serological markers and histological evidence of cellular autoimmunity. *Diabetes* 2001; 50: 1269–73.
36. Bleich D, Jackson RA, Soeldner JS, Eisenbarth GS. Analysis of metabolic progression to type I diabetes in ICA+ relatives of patients with type I diabetes. *Diabetes Care* 1990; 13: 111–8.
37. Diabetes Prevention Trial-Type 1 Diabetes Study Group. Effects of insulin in relatives of patients with type 1 diabetes mellitus. *N Engl J Med* 2002; 346: 1685–91.
38. Herold KC, Hagopian W, Auger JA, Poumian-Ruiz E, Taylor L, Donaldson D, Gitelman SE, Harlan DM, Xu D, Zivin RA, Bluestone JA. Anti-CD3 monoclonal antibody in new-onset type 1 diabetes mellitus. *N Engl J Med* 2002; 346: 1692–8.
39. Kyvik KO, Green A, Beck-Nielsen H. Concordance rates of insulin dependent diabetes mellitus: a population based study of young Danish twins. *BMJ* 1995; 311: 913–7.
40. Lorenzen T, Pociot F, Hougaard P, Nerup J. Long-term risk of IDDM in first-degree relatives of patients with IDDM. *Diabetologia* 1994; 37: 321–7.
41. Redondo MJ, Yu L, Hawa M, Mackenzie T, Pyke DA, Eisenbarth GS, Leslie RD. Heterogeneity of type 1 diabetes: analysis of monozygotic twins in Great Britain and the United States. *Diabetologia* 2001; 44: 354–62.
42. Davies JL, Kawaguchi Y, Bennett ST, Copeman JB, Cordell HJ, Pritchard LE, Reed PW, Gough SC, Jenkins SC, Palmer SM, Balfour KM, Rowe BR, Farrall M, Barnett AH, Bain SC, Todd JA. A genome-wide search for human type 1 diabetes susceptibility genes. *Nature* 1994; 371: 130–6.

43. Altmann DM, Sansom D, Marsh SG. What is the basis for HLA-DQ associations with autoimmune disease? *Immunol Today* 1991; 12: 267–70.
44. Sheehy MJ. HLA and insulin-dependent diabetes. A protective prospective. *Diabetes* 1992; 41: 123–9.
45. Nepom GT, Kwok WW. Perspectives in diabetes: molecular basis for HLA-DQ associations with IDDM. *Diabetes* 1998; 47: 1177–84.
46. Nepom GT. A unified hypothesis for the complex genetics of HLA associations with IDDM. *Diabetes* 1990; 39: 1153–7.
47. Behar SM, Porcelli SA. Mechanisms of autoimmune disease induction. The role of the immune response to microbial pathogens. *Arthritis Rheum* 1995; 38: 458–76.
48. Vreugdenhil GR, Geluk A, Ottenhoff TH, Melchers WJ, Roep BO, Galama JM. Molecular mimicry in diabetes mellitus: the homologous domain in coxsackie B virus protein 2C and islet autoantigen GAD65 is highly conserved in the coxsackie B-like enteroviruses and binds to the diabetes associated HLA-DR3 molecule. *Diabetologia* 1998; 41: 40–6.
49. Singal DP, Blajchman MA. Histocompatibility (HLA) antigens, lymphocytotoxic antibodies and tissue-specific antibodies in patients with diabetes mellitus. *Diabetes* 1973; 22: 429–32.
50. Nerup J, Platz P, Anderson OO, Christy M, Lyngsoe J, Poulsen JE, Ryder LP, Nielsen LS, Thomsen M, Svejgaard A. HLA antigens and diabetes mellitus. *Lancet* 1974; 2: 864–6.
51. Ilonen J, Herva E, Tiilikainen A, Akerblom HK, Koivukangas T, Kouvalainen K. HLA-Dw3 as a marker of resistance against juvenile diabetes mellitus. *Tissue Antigens* 1978; 11: 144–6.
52. Thomson G, Robinson WP, Kuhner MK, Joe S, MacDonald MJ, Gottschall JL, Barbosa J, Rich SS, Bertrams J, Baur MP, Partanen J, Tait BD, Schober E, Mayr WR, Ludvigsson J, Lindholm B, Farid NR, Thompson C, Deschamps I. Genetic heterogeneity, modes of inheritance, and risk estimates for a joint study of Caucasians with insulin-dependent diabetes mellitus. *Am J Hum Genet* 1988; 43: 799–816.
53. Owerbach D, Lernmark Å, Platz P, Ryder LP, Rask L, Peterson PA, Ludvigsson J. HLA-D region β-chain DNA endonuclease fragments differ between HLA-DR identical healthy and insulin-dependent diabetic individuals. *Nature* 1983; 303: 815–7.
54. Nepom BS, Palmer J, Kim SJ, Hansen JA, Holbeck SL, Nepom GT. Specific genomic markers for the HLA-DQ subregion discriminate between DR4+ insulin-dependent diabetes mellitus and DR4+ seropositive juvenile rheumatoid arthritis. *J Exp Med* 1986; 164: 345–50.
55. Kockum I, Wassmuth R, Holmberg E, Michelsen B, Lernmark A. HLA-DQ primarily confers protection and HLA-DR susceptibility in type I (insulin-dependent) diabetes studied in population-based affected families and controls. *Am J Hum Genet* 1993; 53: 150–67.
56. Pugliese A, Gianani R, Moromisato R, Awdeh ZL, Alper CA, Erlich HA, Jackson RA, Eisenbarth GS. HLA-DQB1*0602 is associated with dominant protection from diabetes even among islet cell antibody-positive first-degree relatives of patients with IDDM. *Diabetes* 1995; 44: 608–13.
57. Todd JA, Bell JI, McDevitt HO. HLA-DQB gene contributes to susceptibility and resistance to insulin-dependent diabetes mellitus. *Nature* 1987; 329: 599–604.
58. Khalil I, D'Auriol L, Gobet M, Morin L, Lepage V, Deschamps I, Park MS, Degos L, Galibert F, Hors J. A combination of HLA-DQ beta Asp 57-negative and HLA-DQα Arg 52 confers susceptibility to insulin-dependent diabetes mellitus. *J Clin Invest* 1990; 85: 1315–9.
59. Robles DT, Eisenbarth GS, Wang T, Erlich HA, Bugawan TL, Babu SR, Barriga K, Norris JM, Hoffman M, Klingensmith G, Yu L, Rewers M; Diabetes Autoimmunity Study in the Young. Millennium award recipient contribution. Identification of children with early onset and high incidence of anti-islet autoantibodies. *Clin Immunol* 2002; 102: 217–24.
60. Owerbach D, Nerup J. Restriction fragment length polymorphism of the insulin gene in diabetes mellitus. *Diabetes* 1982; 31: 275–7.
61. Bell GI, Horita S, Karam JH. A polymorphic locus near the human insulin gene is associated with insulin-dependent diabetes mellitus. *Diabetes* 1984; 33: 176–83.
62. Hitman GA, Tarn AC, Winter RM, Drummond V, Williams LG, Jowett NI, Bottazzo GF, Galton DJ. Type 1 (insulin-dependent) diabetes and a highly variable locus close to the insulin gene on chromosome 11. *Diabetologia* 1985; 28: 218–22.
63. Pugliese A, Zeller M, Fernandez A, Zalcberg LJ, Bartlett RJ, Ricordi C, Pietropaolo M, Eisenbarth GS, Bennett ST, Patel DD. The insulin gene is transcribed in the human thymus and transcription levels correlate with allelic variation at the INS VNTR-IDDM2 susceptibility locus for type I diabetes. *Nat Genet* 1997; 15: 293–7.
64. Vafiadis P, Bennett ST, Todd JA, Nadeau J, Grabs R, Goodyer CG, Wickramasinghe S, Colle E, Polychronakos C. Insulin expression in human thymus is modulated by INS VNTR alleles at the IDDM2 locus. *Nat Genet* 1997; 15: 289–92.
65. Sebzda E, Wallace VA, Mayer J, Yeung RS, Mak TW, Ohashi PS. Positive and negative thymocyte selection induced by different concentrations of a single peptide. *Science* 1994; 263: 1615–8.
66. Chentoufi AA, Polychronakos C. Insulin expression levels in the thymus modulate insulin-specific autoreactive T-cell tolerance: the mechanism by which the IDDM2 locus may predispose to diabetes. *Diabetes* 2002; 51: 1383–90.
67. Bennett ST, Lucassen AM, Gough SCL, Powell EE, Undlien DE, Pritchard LE, Merriman ME, Kawaguchi Y, Dronsfield MJ, Pociot F, Nerup J, Bouzekri N, Gambon-Thompsen A, Ronningen KS, Barnett AH, Bain SC, Todd JA. Susceptibility to human type I diabetes at IDDM2 is determined by tandem repeat variation at the insulin gene minisatellite locus. *Nat Genet* 1995; 9: 284–92.
68. Lucassen AM, Screaton GR, Julier C, Elliott TJ, Lathrop M, Bell JI. Regulation of insulin gene expression by the IDDM associated, insulin locus haplotype. *Hum Mol Genet* 1995; 4: 501–6.
69. Julier C, Hyer RN, Davies J, Merlin F, Soularue P, Briant L, Cathelineau G, Deschamps I, Rotter JI, Froguel P, Boitard C, Bell JI, Lathrop GM. Insulin-IGF2 region on chromosome 11p encodes a gene implicated in HLA-DR4-dependent diabetes susceptibility. *Nature* 1991; 354: 155–9.
70. Lucassen AM, Julier C, Beressi J-P, Boitard C, Froguel P, Lathrop M, Bell JI. Susceptibility to insulin dependent diabetes mellitus maps to a 4.1 kb segment of DNA spanning the insulin gene and associated VNTR. *Nat Genet* 1993; 4: 305–10.

71. Metcalfe KA, Hitman GA, Fennessy MJ, McCarthy MI, Tuomilehto J, Tuomilehto-Wolf E. In Finland insulin gene region encoded susceptibility to IDDM exerts maximum effect when there is low HLA-DR associated risk. DiMe (Childhood Diabetes in Finland) Study Group. *Diabetologia* 1995; 38: 1223–9.
72. Concannon P, Gogolin-Ewens KJ, Hinds DA, Wapelhorst B, Morrison VA, Stirling B, Mitra M, Farmer J, Williams SR, Cox NJ, Bell GI, Risch N, Spielman RS. A second-generation screen of the human genome for susceptibility to insulin-dependent diabetes mellitus. *Nat Genet* 1998; 19: 292–6.
73. Verge CF, Vardi P, Babu S, Bao F, Erlich HA, Bugawan T, Tiosano D, Yu L, Eisenbarth GS, Fain PR. Evidence for oligogenic inheritance of type 1A diabetes in a large Bedouin Arab family. *J Clin Invest* 1998; 102: 1569–75.
74. Molberg O, McAdam SN, Körner R, Quarsten H, Kristiansen C, Madsen L, Fugger L, Scott H, Noren O, Roepstorff P, Lundin KE, Sjostrom H, Sollid LM. Tissue transglutaminase selectively modifies gliadin peptides that are recognized by gut-derived T cells in celiac disease. *Nat Med* 1998; 4: 713–7.
75. Bao F, Yu L, Babu S, Wang T, Hoffenberg EJ, Rewers M, Eisenbarth GS. One third of HLA DQ2 homozygous patients with type 1 diabetes express celiac disease associated transglutaminase autoantibodies. *J Autoimmunity* 1999; 13: 143–8.
76. Hoffenberg EJ, Bao F, Eisenbarth GS, Uhlhorn C, Haas JE, Sokol RJ, Rewers M. Transglutaminase antibodies in children with a genetic risk for celiac disease. *J Pediatr* 2000; 137: 356–60.
77. De Block CE, De Leeuw IH, Van Gaal LF. High prevalence of manifestations of gastric autoimmunity in parietal cell antibody-positive type 1 (insulin-dependent) diabetic patients. The Belgian Diabetes Registry. *J Clin Endocrinol Metab* 1999; 84: 4062–7.
78. Aaltonen J, Bjorses P, Sandkuijl L, Perheentupa J, Peltonen L. An autosomal locus causing autoimmune disease: autoimmune polyglandular disease type I assigned to chromosome 21. *Nat Genet* 1994; 8: 83–7.
79. The Finnish–German APECED Consortium. An autoimmune disease, APECED, caused by mutations in a novel gene featuring two PHD-type zinc-finger domains. Autoimmune polyendocrinopathy–candidiasis–ectodermal dystrophy. *Nat Genet* 1997; 17: 399–403.
80. Nagamine K, Peterson P, Scott HS, Kudoh J, Minoshima S, Heino M, Krohn KJ, Lalioti MD, Mullis PE, Antonarakis SE, Kawasaki K, Asakawa S, Ito F, Shimizu N. Positional cloning of the APECED gene. *Nat Genet* 1997; 17: 393–8.
81. Heino M, Peterson P, Kudoh J, Nagamine K, Lagerstedt A, Ovod V, Ranki A, Rantala I, Nieminen M, Tuukkanen J, Scott HS, Antonarakis SE, Shimizu N, Krohn K. Autoimmune regulator is expressed in the cells regulating immune tolerance in thymus medulla. *Biochem Biophys Res Commun* 1999; 257: 821–5.
82. Bjork E, Velloso LA, Kampe O, Karlsson FA. GAD autoantibodies in IDDM, stiff-man syndrome, and autoimmune polyendocrine syndrome type I recognize different epitopes. *Diabetes* 1994; 43: 161–5.
83. Tuomi T, Bjorses P, Falorni A, Partanen J, Perheentupa J, Lernmark A, Miettinen A. Antibodies to glutamic acid decarboxylase and insulin-dependent diabetes in patients with autoimmune polyendocrine syndrome type I. *J Clin Endocrinol Metab* 1996; 81: 1488–94.
84. Gylling M, Tuomi T, Bjorses P, Kontiainen S, Partanen J, Christie MR, Knip M, Perheentupa J, Miettinen A. β-Cell autoantibodies, human leukocyte antigen II alleles, and type 1 diabetes in autoimmune polyendocrinopathy-candidiasis-ectodermal dystrophy. *J Clin Endocrinol Metab* 2000; 85: 4434–40.
85. Patel DD. Escape from tolerance in the human X-linked autoimmunity-allergic disregulation syndrome and the Scurfy mouse. *J Clin Invest* 2001; 107: 155–7.
86. Devendra D, Eisenbarth GS. 17: Immunologic endocrine disorders. *J Allergy Clin Immunol* 2003; 111 (2, suppl): S624–36.
87. The EURODIAB ACE Study Group. Variation and trends in incidence of childhood diabetes in Europe. *Lancet* 2000; 355: 873–6.
88. Akerblom HK, Knip M. Putative environmental factors in type 1 diabetes. *Diabetes Metab Rev* 1998; 14: 31–67.
89. Yoon JW, Austin M, Onodera T, Notkins AL. Virus-induced diabetes mellitus: isolation of a virus from the pancreas of a child with diabetic ketoacidosis. *N Engl J Med* 1979; 300: 1173–9.
90. Jenson AB, Rosenberg HS, Notkins AL. Pancreatic islet-cell damage in children with fatal viral infections. *Lancet* 1980; 2: 354–8.
91. Roivainen M, Rasilainen S, Ylipaasto P, Nissinen R, Ustinov J, Bouwens L, Eizirik DL, Hovi T, Otonkoski T. Mechanisms of coxsackievirus-induced damage to human pancreatic beta-cells. *J Clin Endocrinol Metab* 2000; 85: 432–40.
92. Chehadeh W, Kerr-Conte J, Pattou F, Alm G, Lefebvre J, Wattre P, Hober D. Persistent infection of human pancreatic islets by coxsackievirus B is associated with alpha interferon synthesis in beta cells. *J Virol* 2000; 74: 10153–64.
93. Ludvigsson J, Forsberg P, Fryden A, Lindblom B, Marshall MO, von Schenck H. Mumps with laboratory signs of subclinical pancreatitis may cause a disturbed beta-cell function. *Diabetes Res* 1988; 9: 193–5.
94. Horwitz MS, Bradley LM, Harbertson J, Krahl T, Lee J, Sarvetnick N. Diabetes induced by Coxsackie virus: initiation by bystander damage and not molecular mimicry. *Nat Med* 1998; 4: 781–5.
95. Kaufman DL, Erlander MG, Clare-Salzler M, Atkinson MA, Maclaren NK, Tobin AJ. Autoimmunity to two forms of glutamate decarboxylase in insulin-dependent diabetes mellitus. *J Clin Invest* 1992; 89: 283–92.
96. Honeyman MC, Stone NL, Harrison LC. T-cell epitopes in type 1 diabetes autoantigen tyrosine phosphatase IA-2: potential for mimcry with rotavirus and other environmental agents. *Mol Med* 1998; 4: 231–9.
97. Horwitz MS, Fine C, Ilic A, Sarvetnick N. Requirements for viral-mediated autoimmune diabetes: beta-cell damage and immune infiltration. *J Autoimmun* 2001; 16: 211–7.
98. Horwitz MS, Ilic A, Fine C, Rodriguez E, Sarvetnick N. Presented antigen from damaged pancreatic beta cells activates autoreactive T cells in virus-mediated autoimmune diabetes. *J Clin Invest* 2002; 109: 79–87.
99. Foulis AK, McGill M, Farquharson MA, Hilton DA. A search for evidence of viral infection in panreases of newly diagnosed patients with IDDM. *Diabetologia* 1997; 40: 53–61.
100. Banatvala JE, Bryant J, Schernthaner G, Borkenstein M, Schober E, Brown D, De Silva LM, Menser MA, Silink M. Coxsackie B, mumps, rubella, and cytomegalovirus

specific IgM responses in patients with juvenile-onset insulin-dependent diabetes mellitus in Britain, Austria, and Australia. *Lancet* 1985; 1: 1409–12.

101. Friman G, Fohlman J, Frisk G, Diderholm H, Ewald U, Kobbah M, Tuvemo T. An incidence peak of juvenile diabetes. Relation to Coxsackie B virus immune response. *Acta Paediatr Scand Suppl* 1985; 320: 14–9.
102. Hyoty H, Hiltunen M, Knip M, Laakkonen M, Vahasalo P, Karjalainen J, Koskela P, Roivainen M, Leinikki P, Hovi T, Akerblom HK, for the Childhood Diabetes in Finland (DiMe) Study Group. A prospective study of the role of coxsackie B and other enterovirus infections in the pathogenesis of IDDM. *Diabetes* 1995; 44: 652–7.
103. Hiltunen M, Hyoty H, Knip M, Ilonen J, Reijonen H, Vahasalo P, Roivainen M, Lonnrot M, Leinikki P, Hovi T, Akerblom HK, for the Childhood Diabetes in Finland (DiMe) Study Group. Islet cell antibody seroconversion in children is temporally associated with enterovirus infections. *J Infect Dis* 1997; 175: 554–60.
104. Lonnrot M, Korpela K, Knip M, Ilonen J, Simell O, Korhonen S, Savola K, Muona P, Simell T, Koskela P, Hyoty H. Enterovirus infection as a risk factor for beta-cell autoimmunity in a prospectively observed birth cohort: the Finnish Diabetes Prediction and Prevention Study. *Diabetes* 2000; 49: 1314–8.
105. Lonnrot M, Salminen K, Knip M, Savola K, Kulmala P, Leinikki P, Hyypia T, Akerblom HK, Hyoty H, for the Childhood Diabetes in Finland (DiMe) Study Group. Enterovirus RNA in serum is a risk factor for beta-cell autoimmunity and clinical type 1 diabetes: a prospective study. *J Med Virol* 2000; 61: 214–20.
106. Sadeharju K, Lonnrot M, Kimpimaki T, Savola K, Erkkila S, Kalliokoski T, Savolainen P, Koskela P, Ilonen J, Simell O, Knip M, Hyoty H. Enterovirus antibody levels during the first two years of life in prediabetic autoantibody-positive children. *Diabetologia* 2001; 44: 818–23.
107. Graves PM, Rotbart HA, Nix WA, Pallansch MA, Erlich HA, Norris JM, Hoffman M, Eisenbarth GS, Rewers M. Prospective study of enteroviral infections and development of beta-cell autoimmunity. Diabetes Autoimmunity Study in the Young (DAISY). *Diabetes Res Clin Pract* 2003; 59: 51–61.
108. Classen JB, Classen DC. Vaccines modulate IDDM. *Diabetologia* 1996; 39: 500–2.
109. The EURODIAB Substudy 2 Study Group. Infections and vaccinations as risk factors for childhood type I (insulin-dependent) diabetes mellitus: a multicentre case-control investigation. *Diabetologia* 2000; 43: 47–53.
110. DeStefano F, Mullooly JP, Okoro CA, Chen RT, Marcy SM, Ward JI, Vadheim CM, Black SB, Shinefield HR, Davis RL, Bohlke K; Vaccine Safety Datalink Team. Childhood vaccinations, vaccination timing, and risk of type 1 diabetes mellitus. *Pediatrics* 2001; 108: E112.
111. Graves PM, Barriga KJ, Norris JM, Hoffman MR, Yu L, Eisenbarth GS, Rewers M. Lack of association between early childhood immunizations and beta-cell autoimmunity. *Diabetes Care* 1999; 22: 1694–7.
112. Hummel M, Fuchtenbusch M, Schenker M, Ziegler AG. No major association of breast-feeding, vaccinations, and childhood viral diseases with early islet autoimmunity in the German BABYDIAB Study. *Diabetes Care* 2000; 23: 969–74.
113. Elliott RB, Martin JM. Dietary protein: a trigger of insulin-dependent diabetes in the BB rat? *Diabetologia* 1984; 26: 297–9.
114. Daneman D, Fishman L, Clarson C, Martin JM. Dietary triggers of insulin-dependent diabetes in the BB rat. *Diabetes Res* 1987; 5: 93–7.
115. Hoorfar J, Scott FW, Cloutier HE. Dietary plant materials and development of diabetes in the BB rat. *J Nutr* 1991; 121: 908–16.
116. Hoorfar J, Buschard K, Dagnaes-Hansen F. Prophylactic nutritional modification of the incidence of diabetes in autoimmune non-obese (NOD) mice. *Br J Nutr* 1993; 69: 597–607.
117. Malkani S, Nompleggi D, Hansen JW, Greiner DL, Mordes JP, Rossini AA. Dietary cow's milk protein does not alter the frequency of diabetes in the BB rat. *Diabetes* 1997; 46: 1133–40.
118. Paxson JA, Weber JG, Kulczycki A Jr. Cow's milk-free diet does not prevent diabetes in NOD mice. *Diabetes* 1997; 46: 1711–7.
119. Norris JM, Beaty B, Klingensmith G, Yu Liping, Hoffman M, Chase HP, Erlich HA, Hamman RF, Eisenbarth GS, Rewers M. Lack of association between early exposure to cow's milk protein and β-cell autoimmunity: Diabetes Autoimmunity Study in the Young (DAISY). *JAMA* 1996; 276: 609–14.
120. Couper JJ, Steele C, Beresford S, Powell T, McCaul K, Pollard A, Gellert S, Tait B, Harrison LC, Colman PG. Lack of association between duration of breast-feeding or introduction of cow's milk and development of islet autoimmunity. *Diabetes* 1999; 48: 2145–9.
121. Kimpimaki T, Erkkola M, Korhonen S, Kupila A, Virtanen SM, Ilonen J, Simell O, Knip M. Short-term exclusive breastfeeding predisposes young children with increased genetic risk of Type I diabetes to progressive beta-cell autoimmunity. *Diabetologia* 2001; 44: 63–9.
122. Akerblom HK, Virtanen SM, Hamalainen A, et al. Emergence of diabetes associated autoantibodies in the nutritional prevention of IDDM (TRIGR) project. *Diabetes* 1999; 48: A45.
123. Klemetti P, Savilahti E, Ilonen J, Akerblom HK, Vaarala O. T-cell reactivity to wheat gluten in patients with insulin-dependent diabetes mellitus. *Scand J Immunol* 1998; 47: 48–53.
124. Norris JM, Barriga K, Rewers M. Does cereal protein in the infant diet play a role in the etiology of beta-cell autoimmunity? The Diabetes Autoimmunity Study in the Young (DAISY). *Diabetes* 2002; 51 (suppl 2): A234.
125. The EURODIAB Substudy 2 Study Group. Vitamin D supplement in early childhood and risk for Type I (insulin-dependent) diabetes mellitus. *Diabetologia* 1999; 42: 51–4.
126. Hypponen E, Laara E, Reunanen A, Jarvelin MR, Virtanen SM. Intake of vitamin D and risk of type 1 diabetes: a birth-cohort study. *Lancet* 2001; 358: 1500–3.
127. Bottazzo GF, Florin-Christensen A, Doniach D. Islet-cell antibodies in diabetes mellitus with autoimmune polyendocrine deficiencies. *Lancet* 1974; 2: 1279–83.
128. Pugliese A, Brown D, Garza D, Murchison D, Zeller M, Redondo M, Diez J, Eisenbarth GS, Patel DD, Ricordi C. Self-antigen presenting cells expressing islet cell molecules in human thymus and peripheral lymphoid organs: phenotypic characterization and implications for immunological tolerance and type 1 diabetes. *J Clin Invest* 2001; 107: 555–64.

129. Arslanian SA, Becker DJ, Rabin B, Atchison R, Eberhardt M, Cavender D, Dorman J, Drash AL. Correlates of insulin antibodies in newly diagnosed children with insulin-dependent diabetes before insulin therapy. *Diabetes* 1985; 34: 926–30.
130. Ziegler AG, Hummel M, Schenker M, Bonifacio E. Autoantibody appearance and risk for development of childhood diabetes in offspring of parents with type 1 diabetes. The 2-year analysis of the German BABYDIAB study. *Diabetes* 1999; 48: 460–8.
131. Kimpimaki T, Kupila A, Hamalainen AM, Kukko M, Kulmala P, Savola K, Simell T, Keskinen P, Ilonen J, Simell O, Knip M. The first signs of beta-cell autoimmunity appear in infancy in genetically susceptible children from the general population: the Finnish Type 1 Diabetes Prediction and Prevention Study. *J Clin Endocrinol Metab* 2001; 86: 4782–8.
132. Ziegler R, Alper CA, Awdeh ZL, Castano L, Brink SJ, Soeldner JS, Jackson RA, Eisenbarth GS. Specific association of HLA-DR4 with increased prevalence and level of insulin autoantibodies in first-degree relatives of patients with type I diabetes. *Diabetes* 1991; 40: 709–14.
133. Greenbaum C, Palmer JP, Kuglin B, Kolb C. Insulin autoantibodies measured by radioimmunoassay methodology are more related to insulin-dependent diabetes mellitus than those measured by enzyme-linked immunosorbent assay: results of the Fourth International Workshop on the Standardization of Insulin Autoantibody Measurement. *J Clin Endocrinol Metab* 1992; 74: 1040–4.
134. Williams AJ, Bingley PJ, Bonifacio E, Palmer JP, Gale EA. A novel micro-assay for insulin autoantibodies. *J Autoimmun* 1997; 10: 473–8.
135. Baekkeskov S, Nielsen JH, Marner B, Bilde T, Ludvigsson J, Lernmark A. Autoantibodies in newly diagnosed diabetic children immunoprecipitate specific human pancreatic islet cell proteins. *Nature* 1982; 298: 167–9.
136. Baekkeskov S, Landin M, Kristensen JK, Srikanta S, Bruining GJ, Mandrup-Poulsen T, de Beaufort C, Soeldner JS, Eisenbarth G, Lindgren F, et al. Antibodies to a 64,000 Mr human islet cell antigen precede the clinical onset of insulin-dependent diabetes. *J Clin Invest* 1987; 79: 926–34.
137. Verge CF, Stenger D, Bonifacio E, Colman PG, Pilcher C, Bingley PJ, Eisenbarth GS. Combined use of autoantibodies (IA-2 autoantibody, GAD autoantibody, insulin autoantibody, cytoplasmic islet cell antibodies) in type 1 diabetes: Combinatorial Islet Autoantibody Workshop. *Diabetes* 1998; 47: 1857–66.
138. Sabbah E, Kulmala P, Veijola R, Vahasalo P, Karjalainen J, Tuomilehto-Wolf E, Akerblom HK, Knip M, for the Childhood Diabetes in Finland Study Group. Glutamic acid decarboxylase antibodies in relation to other autoantibodies and genetic risk markers in children with newly diagnosed insulin-dependent diabetes. *J Clin Endocrinol Metab* 1996; 81: 2455–9.
139. Greenbaum CJ, Sears KL, Kahn SE, Palmer JP. Relationship of beta-cell function and autoantibodies to progression and nonprogression of subclinical type 1 diabetes: follow-up of the Seattle Family Study. *Diabetes* 1999; 48: 170–5.
140. Hagopian WA, Sanjeevi CB, Kockum I, Landin-Olsson M, Karlsen AE, Sundkvist G, Dahlquist G, Palmer J, Lernmark A. Glutamate decarboxylase-, insulin-, and islet cell-antibodies and HLA typing to detect diabetes in a general population-based study of Swedish children. *J Clin Invest* 1995; 95: 1505–11.
141. Littorin B, Sundkvist G, Hagopian W, Landin-Olsson M, Lernmark A, Ostman J, Arnqvist HJ, Blohme G, Bolinder J, Eriksson JW, Lithner F, Schersten B, Wibell L. Islet cell and glutamic acid decarboxylase antibodies present at diagnosis of diabetes predict the need for insulin treatment. A cohort study in young adults whose disease was initially labeled as type 2 or unclassifiable diabetes. *Diabetes Care* 1999; 22: 409–12.
142. Fuchtenbusch M, Ferber K, Standl E, Ziegler AG. Prediction of type 1 diabetes postpartum in patients with gestational diabetes mellitus by combined islet cell autoantibody screening: a prospective multicenter study. *Diabetes* 1997; 46: 1459–67.
143. Solimena M, Folli F, Aparisi R, Pozza G, De Camilli P. Autoantibodies to GABA-ergic neurons and pancreatic beta cells in stiff-man syndrome. *N Engl J Med* 1990; 322: 1555–60.
144. Christie MR, Vohra G, Champagne P, Daneman D, Delovitch TL. Distinct antibody specificities to a 64-kD islet cell antigen in Type 1 diabetes as revealed by trypsin treatment. *J Exp Med* 1990; 172: 789–94.
145. Christie MR, Hollands JA, Brown TJ, Michelsen BK, Delovitch TL. Detection of pancreatic islet 64,000 M_r autoantigens in insulin-dependent diabetes distinct from glutamate decarboxylase. *J Clin Invest* 1993; 22: 240–8.
146. Lan MS, Lu J, Goto Y, Notkins AL. Molecular cloning and identification of a receptor-type protein tyrosine phosphatase, IA-2, from human insulinoma. *DNA Cell Biol* 1994; 13: 505–14.
147. Bonifacio E, Lampasona V, Genovese S, Ferrari M, Bosi E. Identification of protein tyrosine phosphatase-like IA2 (islet call antigen 512) as the insulin-dependent diabetes-related 37/40K autoantigen and a target of islet-cell antibodies. *J Immunol* 1995; 155: 5419–26.
148. Passini N, Larigan JD, Genovese S, Appella E, Sinigaglia F, Rogge L. The 37/40-kilodalton autoantigen in insulin-dependent diabetes mellitus is the putative tyrosine phosphatase IA-2. *Proc Natl Acad Sci USA* 1995; 92: 9412–6.
149. Payton MA, Hawkes CJ, Christie MR. Relationship of the 37,000- and 40,000-M_r tryptic fragments of islet antigens in insulin-dependent diabetes to the protein tyrosine phosphatase-like molecule IA-2 (ICA512). *J Clin Invest* 1995; 96: 1506–11.
150. Lu J, Li Q, Xie H, Chen ZJ, Borovitskaya AE, Maclaren NK, Notkins AL, Lan MS. Identification of a second transmembrane protein tyrosine phosphatase, IA-2β, as an autoantigen in insulin-dependent diabetes mellitus: precursor of the 37-kDa tryptic fragment. *Proc Natl Acad Sci USA* 1996; 93: 2307–11.
151. Hawkes CJ, Wasmeier C, Christie MR, Hutton JC. Identification of the 37-kDa antigen in IDDM as a tyrosine phosphatase-like protein (phogrin) related to IA-2. *Diabetes* 1996; 45: 1187–92.
152. Hawa M, Rowe R, Lan MS, Notkins AL, Pozzilli P, Christie MR, Leslie RD. Value of antibodies to islet protein tyrosine phosphatase-like molecule in predicting type 1 diabetes. *Diabetes* 1997; 46: 1270–5.
153. Bingley PJ, Christie MR, Bonifacio E, Bonfanti R, Shattock M, Fonte MT, Bottazzo GF, Gale EA. Combined analysis of autoantibodies improves prediction of IDDM in islet cell antibody-positive relatives. *Diabetes* 1994; 43: 1304–10.

154. Verge CF, Gianani R, Kawasaki E, Yu L, Pietropaolo M, Jackson RA, Chase HP, Eisenbarth GS. Prediction of type I diabetes in first-degree relatives using a combination of insulin, GAD, and ICA512bdc/IA-2 autoantibodies. *Diabetes* 1996; 45: 926–33.
155. Colman PG, Nayak RC, Campbell IL, Eisenbarth GS. Binding of cytoplasmic islet cell antibodies is blocked by human pancreatic glycolipid extracts. *Diabetes* 1988; 37: 645–52.
156. Schenker M, Hummel M, Ferber K, Walter M, Keller E, Albert ED, Janka HU, Kastendiek C, Sorger M, Louwen F, Ziegler AG. Early expression and high prevalence of islet autoantibodies for DR3/4 heterozygous and DR4/4 homozygous offspring of parents with Type I diabetes: the German BABYDIAB study. *Diabetologia* 1999; 42: 671–7.
157. Kupila A, Keskinen P, Simell T, Erkkila S, Arvilommi P, Korhonen S, Kimpimaki T, Sjoroos M, Ronkainen M, Ilonen J, Knip M, Simell O. Genetic determines the emergence of diabetes-associated autoantibodies in young children. *Diabetes* 2002; 51: 646–51.
158. The Diabetes Control and Complications Trial Research Group. Effect of intensive therapy on residual beta-cell function in patients with type 1 diabetes in the diabetes control and complications trial. A randomized, controlled trial. *Ann Intern Med* 1998; 128: 517–23.
159. Carel JC, Boitard C, Eisenbarth G, Bach JF, Bougneres PF. Cyclosporine delays but does not prevent clinical onset in glucose intolerant pre-type 1 diabetic children. *J Autoimmun* 1996; 9: 739–45.
160. De Filippo G, Carel JC, Boitard C, Bougneres PF. Long-term results of early cyclosporin therapy in juvenile IDDM. *Diabetes* 1996; 45: 101–4.
161. Parving HH, Tarnow L, Nielsen FS, Rossing P, Mandrup-Poulsen T, Osterby R, Nerup J. Cyclosporine nephrotoxicity in type 1 diabetic patients. A 7-year follow-up study. *Diabetes Care* 1999; 22: 478–83.
162. Chase HP, Butler-Simon N, Garg S, McDuffie M, Hoops SL, O'Brien D. A trial of nicotinamide in newly diagnosed patients with type 1 (insulin-dependent) diabetes mellitus. *Diabetologia* 1990; 33: 444–6.
163. Kolb H, Burkart V. Nicotinamide in type 1 diabetes. Mechanism of action revisited. *Diabetes Care* 1999; 22 (suppl 2): B16–20.
164. Zhang ZJ, Davidson L, Eisenbarth G, Weiner HL. Suppression of diabetes in nonobese diabetic mice by oral administration of porcine insulin. *Proc Natl Acad Sci USA* 1991; 88: 10252–6.
165. Daniel D, Wegmann DR. Protection of nonobese diabetic mice from diabetes by intranasal or subcutaneous administration of insulin peptide B-(9-23). *Proc Natl Acad Sci USA* 1996; 93: 956–60.
166. Keller RJ, Eisenbarth GS, Jackson RA. Insulin prophylaxis in individuals at high risk of type I diabetes. *Lancet* 1993; 341: 927–8.
167. Fuchtenbusch M, Rabl W, Grassl B, Bachmann W, Standl E, Ziegler AG. Delay of type I diabetes in high risk, first degree relatives by parenteral antigen administration: the Schwabing Insulin Prophylaxis Pilot Trial. *Diabetologia* 1998; 41: 536–41.
168. Pedotti R, Mitchell D, Wedemeyer J, Karpuj M, Chabas D, Hattab EM, Tsai M, Galli SJ, Steinman L. An unexpected version of horror autotoxicus: anaphylactic shock to a self-peptide. *Nat Immunol* 2001; 2: 216–22.
169. Liu E, Moriyama H, Abiru N, Miao D, Yu L, Taylor RM, Finkelman FD, Eisenbarth GS. Anti-peptide autoantibodies and fatal anaphylaxis with insulin self-peptides B:9-23 and B:13-23. *J Clin Invest* 2002; 110: 1021–7
170. Alleva DG, Gaur A, Jin L, Wegmann D, Gottlieb PA, Pahuja A, Johnson EB, Motheral T, Putnam A, Crowe PD, Ling N, Boehme SA, Conlon PJ. Immunological characterization and therapeutic activity of an altered-peptide ligand, NBI-6024, based on the immunodominant type 1 diabetes autoantigen insulin B-chain (9-23) peptide. *Diabetes* 2002; 51: 2126–34.

28

Molecular Genetics of Type 1 Diabetes

M. Ann Kelly*, Anthony H. Barnett*†, and Stephen C. Bain*†

**University of Birmingham, Birmingham, UK, and* †*Birmingham Heartlands Hospital, Birmingham, UK*

Type 1 diabetes mellitus is a T-cell-mediated autoimmune disease, which results from the selective destruction of the insulin-producing β-cells of the pancreas. The disease has a complex etiology, with both genetic and environmental factors influencing the risk of pancreatic autoimmunity and its subsequent progression to clinically overt diabetes. In White Caucasian populations, the lifetime risk of type 1 diabetes is approximately 0.4%. This is substantially increased, however, among subjects with a family history of the disease; and up to 5–6% among the siblings of a diabetic patient [1, 2]. Such familial clustering could be indicative of a genetic contribution to the disease or may reflect exposure to common environmental determinants. The difference in concordance rates between monozygotic twins (21–70%) and dizygotic twins (0–13%) is consistent with a significant inherited predisposition [3, 4]. As the majority of monozygotic twins are discordant for the disease, however, this indicates that the susceptibility genes have low penetrance—that is, many individuals who are "genetically at-risk" of type 1 diabetes will not develop the disease. This highlights the importance of environmental factors, which may account for up to two thirds of disease susceptibility.

A large number of genes may contribute to the genetic component of type 1 diabetes. These are termed *susceptibility genes* as they modify the risk of developing the disease but are not causative. A particular susceptibility gene is neither necessary nor sufficient for disease to develop. This is a significant problem for studies aiming to identify disease genes, as there is no simple correlation between genotype and phenotype.

Over the past three decades, several different approaches have been taken to investigate the genetic basis of type 1 diabetes. Early studies used population-based case/control analyses to investigate disease associations with candidate susceptibility genes: i.e., those genes whose products were believed to participate in the pathogenesis of type 1 diabetes. The first susceptibility locus to be identified in this way was the human leukocyte antigen (HLA) gene region on chromosome 6p [5]. Subsequent studies demonstrated an association between type 1 diabetes and the insulin gene region on chromosome 11p [6]. With the advent of high-throughput genotyping methodologies in the early 1990s, it became possible to screen the whole human genome to identify susceptibility markers for complex diseases. A number of complete and partial genome screens of families with two or more siblings with type 1 diabetes have since been reported [7–10]. These studies have identified more than 20 chromosomal regions that show varying degrees of evidence for linkage to the disease. Although there are inconsistencies between the studies, all have unequivocally confirmed linkage to the HLA gene region, which is now designated *IDDM1*. Several of the genome screens also showed evidence of linkage to the insulin gene region, designated *IDDM2* [7, 8, 10]. Although the studies mapped the approximate chromosomal locations of other susceptibility loci, the precise identity of the disease genes at these locations remains to be determined. Case/control and family-based association studies of candidate genes within these regions are currently being used to identify further susceptibility determinants for type 1 diabetes.

The HLA gene region (*IDDM1*) is the most powerful determinant of genetic susceptibility to type 1 diabetes, accounting for 42% of familial inheritance [7]. The contributions of the other susceptibility loci are minor, probably accounting for only a few percent of the total genetic predisposition.

International Textbook of Diabetes Mellitus, Third Edition. Edited by R. A. DeFronzo, E. Ferrannini, H. Keen, and P. Zimmet.
 ISBN: 0-471-48655-8.

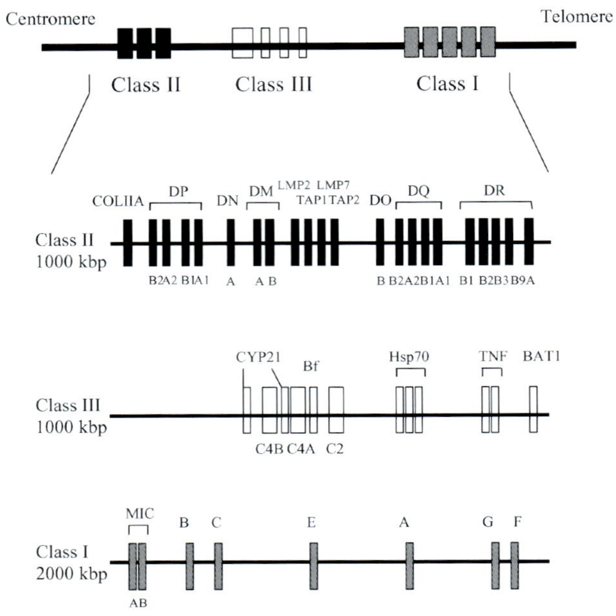

Figure 1 A simplified map of the major histocompatibility complex showing the major genes of the class I, class II, and class III regions

HLA-ENCODED SUSCEPTIBILITY TO TYPE 1 DIABETES

The HLA genes are located within the major histocompatibility complex (MHC) on chromosome 6 (6p21). The MHC spans a 3.5 Mb region and consists of over 200 genes arranged into three subclasses (see Figure 1). Genes in the class I and class II subregions encode the HLA antigens, which are complex, cell-surface glycoproteins.

Each class I gene encodes an α peptide chain, composed of three domains ($\alpha 1$, $\alpha 2$, and $\alpha 3$). The α chains associate with β_2-microglobulin, encoded by a gene on chromosome 15, to form the HLA class I molecules (Figure 2a). These include the transplantation antigens, HLA-A, -B, and -C. The class I molecules are expressed on the surface of all nucleated cell types, where they play a crucial role in the restriction of cytotoxic T-cell activity. CD8+ T-lymphocytes are only able to recognize peptide fragments derived from endogenous antigens when these are presented in the antigen-binding cleft of the appropriate HLA class I molecule (Figure 3b).

The class II (*HLA-D*) loci are subdivided into at least one A and one B gene. These encode respectively the α and β peptide chains that combine to form the heterodimeric class II antigens (Figure 2b). The expression of these molecules is normally restricted to professional antigen-presenting cells, B-lymphocytes, and activated T-lymphocytes. The HLA-DR, -DQ, and -DP antigens are involved in the activation of helper T-lymphocytes. The $\alpha 1$ and $\beta 1$ domains of these molecules form a cleft into which peptide fragments derived from exogenous antigens can bind. These peptides are then presented for recognition by the T-cell receptors (TCRs) of CD4-positive T-cells (Figure 3a).

Many of the HLA genes are highly polymorphic. The class I and class II antigens encoded by the allelic variants therefore show great variability in their three-dimensional structure, particularly in the antigen-binding regions of the molecules. This has important functional consequences as the structure of the antigen-binding site determines the way in which the molecule interacts with a particular antigenic peptide and TCR. Early studies of the HLA system defined the gene polymorphisms by serological typing, using antibodies that recognized specific epitopes of the HLA molecules. Modern molecular biology techniques now allow gene variation to be studied at the nucleotide level.

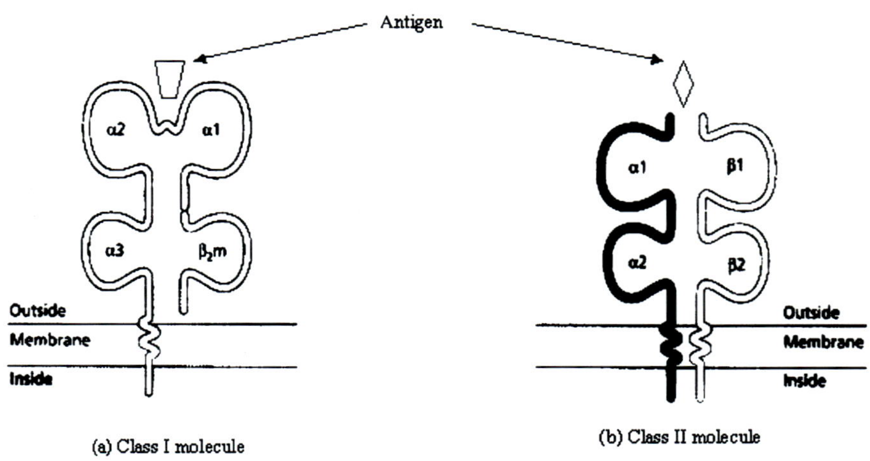

Figure 2 Structures of the HLA class I and class II molecules showing the peptide domains and the antigen-binding clefts (adapted from reference 11)

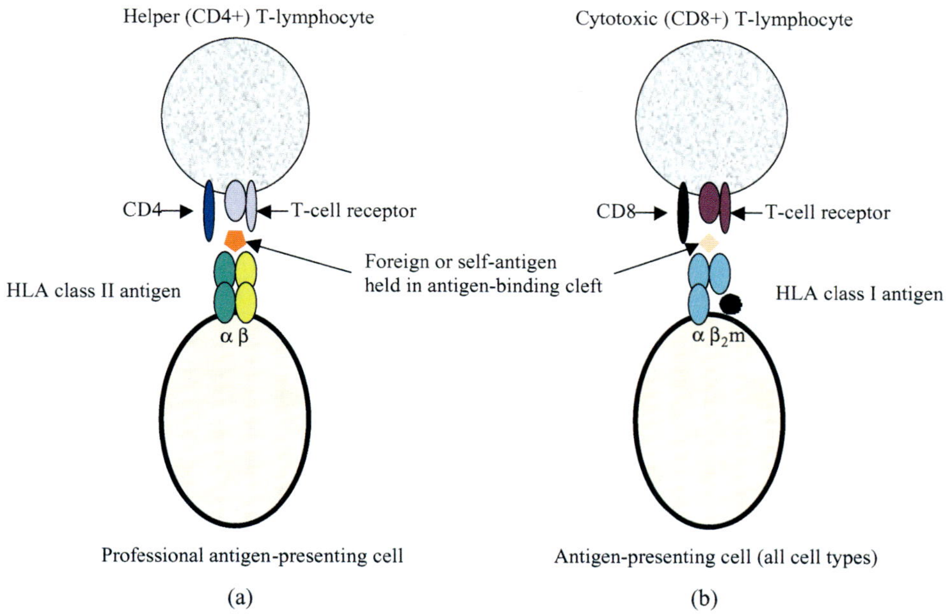

Figure 3 Antigen presentation by HLA class I and class II molecules. (a) Antigen associated with an HLA class II molecule is recognized by the T-cell receptor/CD4 complex of helper T-lymphocytes, (b) Antigen bound to an HLA class I molecule is recognized by cytotoxic T-lymphocytes, via the T-cell receptor/CD8 complex

The identification of disease susceptibility determinants within the MHC is complicated by strong linkage disequilibrium between the genes. Recombination during meiosis is relatively infrequent across the MHC. Particular alleles at distinct loci are therefore inherited together more frequently than would be expected by chance. The combination of alleles inherited *en bloc* is known as a *haplotype*. Because of linkage disequilibrium, it is difficult to distinguish a primary disease susceptibility gene from a gene that is only associated with disease because it is co-inherited with a susceptibility determinant at a different locus.

HLA Associations with Type 1 Diabetes—A Historical Perspective

The search for associations between antigens of the HLA system and disease was originally stimulated by the discovery of genetic linkage between the murine MHC (termed H-2) and resistance to virus-induced leukemia [12]. A role for these genes in autoimmunity was suggested when the H-2 complex was shown to include immune response genes. Singal and Blajchman [5] reported the first HLA association with type 1 (insulin-dependent) diabetes in 1973. This association, with the HLA-B15 antigen, was subsequently confirmed by Nerup et al. [13] and Cudworth and Woodrow [14]. The latter studies also reported an association with the HLA-B8 antigen. The class I genes were not thought to be primary susceptibility determinants, however; rather these polymorphisms were in linkage disequilibrium with true susceptibility alleles lying nearby within the HLA region.

With the development of antisera specific for class II molecules, it became clear that population associations between type 1 diabetes and the class II antigens were much stronger than those between type 1 diabetes and the class I antigens [15]. Subsequent studies of the segregation of HLA haplotypes in families with type 1 diabetes also implicated a disease susceptibility gene (or genes) closely linked to the class II region [2, 16]. The nomenclature used to refer to the HLA class II polymorphisms in these studies differs according to the methodology used to define the variations. Early studies defined differences at the molecular level; these polymorphisms are referred to by the name of the HLA antigen followed by a unique number, for example, DR3, DR4, DQ7, DQ8, etc. In later studies, advances in DNA sequence analysis allowed polymorphisms to be defined at the nucleotide level. This gave rise to a new nomenclature in which individual alleles were named according to the gene locus, followed by an asterisk and a unique code number, for example *DRB1*03*, *DRB1*04*, *DQA1*0301*, *DQB1*0302*, etc. The DR3 and DR4 antigens, encoded by the HLA class II loci *DRA* and *DRB1* (*DRB1*03* and *DRB1*04* alleles, respectively), were reported to be associated with an increased risk of type 1 diabetes. Over 95% of type 1 diabetic patients of White Caucasian origin were shown to carry one or both of these molecules, compared with 50% of healthy subjects [17]. The disease risk associated with DR4 was later shown to be dependent on the *DQB1* allele present. A restriction fragment length polymorphism (RFLP) of the *DQB1* gene was reported to split DR4 (*DRB1*04*) haplotypes into low-risk and high-risk [18]. This RFLP was subsequently shown to distinguish two DQ molecules, termed HLA-DQ7 (encoded by *DQA1*0301-DQB1*0301*) and -DQ8 (encoded by *DQA1*0301-DQB1*0302*) [19]. These molecules are found equally frequently among DR4-positive healthy subjects. Among DR4-positive diabetic individuals, however, the DQ8 molecule predominates, occurring in 90% of subjects, while the DQ7 molecule is uncommon [20]. These findings suggest that susceptibility to type 1 diabetes is more closely associated with the *DQB1* locus than the *DRB1* gene. This is consistent with observations in the nonobese diabetic (NOD) mouse, a spontaneous animal model of autoimmune type 1 diabetes, in which disease susceptibility is conferred primarily by the *IA* gene, a murine homologue of *HLA-DQ* [21].

The HLA-DQ2 molecule is also associated with susceptibility to type 1 diabetes [22]. The alleles encoding DQ2 (*DQA1*0501-DQB1*0201*) are in linkage disequilibrium with DR3 (*DRB1*03*). Heterozygosity for both the *DRB1*03.DQA1*0501. DQB1*0201* (*DR3.DQ2*) and *DRB1*04.DQA1*0301.DQB1*0302* (*DR4.DQ8*) haplotypes is associated with the highest risk of type 1 diabetes.

HLA Genes and Type 1 Diabetes—Current Understanding

The *DRB1* and *DQB1* loci were confirmed as the major determinants of HLA-encoded genetic susceptibility to type 1 diabetes by a recent fine-mapping study of the *IDDM1* locus in the UK population [23]. Although the *DQ* locus has been suggested to be more strongly associated with the disease than the *DRB1* gene [24], it is clear from recent studies that both loci are important for determining overall disease risk. For example, the *DQB1*0302* allele is reported to be the dominant risk factor on the *DRB1*04.DQ8* haplotype, but its influence may be modified by the *DRB1*04* subtype carried [25]. The *DRB1*0401*, **0402*, and **0405* alleles predispose to diabetes, independent of *DQB1*0302*, in several ethnic groups [24, 25]. In contrast, *DRB1*0403* and **0406* confer protection against the disease [26, 27]. The protective effect of *DRB1*0403* is able to override susceptibility conferred by *DQB1*0302*, even among subjects carrying the high-risk *DRB1*03.DQ2/DRB1*04.DQ8* genotype [28, 29]. On the *DRB1*03.DQ2* haplotype, the *DRB1*03* allele is generally considered to be the principal susceptibility determinant [25]. There is evidence to suggest that the *DQB1*0201* allele may have a direct effect on disease risk when carried on other haplotypes, however. In White Caucasian populations, the *DRB1*07.DQA1*0201. DQB1*0303* haplotype confers protection against diabetes, whereas the *DRB1*07.DQA1*0201.DQB1*0201* haplotype is neutral (i.e., it has no influence on disease risk) [30]. The *DRB1*07.DQA1*0301.DQB1*0201* haplotype, which is rare in Caucasians, predisposes to diabetes in Afro-Caribbeans [31]. These data clearly indicate that the *DQB1*0201* allele contributes to disease risk, but its effect is modified by the *DQA1* allele.

Disease risk conferred by the *DR* and *DQ* genes may be further modified by other HLA genes, including *HLA-B* and *-DPB1*. For example, the predisposing effect of *DRB1*03.DQ2* is increased if the *DPB1*0202* allele is carried on the same haplotype. In contrast, the *DPB1*0402* allele reduces the risk conferred [32]. Alleles of the *HLA-B* locus have been reported to influence the risk associated with both *DRB1*03.DQ2* and *DRB1*04.DQ8* haplotypes. For the former haplotype, the highest risk is conferred in the presence of the *HLA-B8* or *-B18* alleles [2], while the predisposing influence of the *DRB1*0404.DQ8* haplotype in Russian, Latvian, and Estonian populations is seen only in the presence of the *HLA-B39* allele [33]. This clearly shows that it is not possible to predict the overall disease risk conferred by an allele without considering the extended haplotype on which it is carried.

Although the *DRB1*03.DQ2* and *DRB1*04.DQ8* haplotypes are the major determinants of disease risk, a minority of diabetic patients possess neither of these markers. This subgroup constitutes approximately 10% of White Caucasian diabetic individuals, but a considerably larger proportion of non-Caucasoid diabetic subjects (up to 30%). In these individuals, disease risk is conferred by other HLA haplotypes, including *DRB1*01.DQA1*0101.DQB1*0501* (*DRB1*01.DQ5*), *DRB1*04.DQA1*0301.DQB1*0401* (*DRB1*04.DQ4*), *DRB1*07.DQA1*0301.DQB1*0201*, *DRB1*08.DQA1*0401.DQB1*0402* (*DRB1*08.DQ4*), *DRB1*09.DQA1*0301.DQB1*0303* (*DRB1*09.DQ9*), and *DRB1*13.DQA1*0102.DQB1*0604* [31, 34, 35]. The significance of these markers as disease determinants differs between different ethnic groups. For example, the association with the *DRB1*07.DQA1*0301.DQB1*0201* haplotype is usually seen only in Negroid populations, as this haplotype is uncommon in other racial groups [24, 31]. In contrast, the disease associations with the *DRB1*04.DQ4* and *DRB1*09.DQ9* haplotypes are most evident among subjects of Oriental Asian origin [24, 36]. It is not clear whether the non-*DRB1*03*/non-*DRB1*04* individuals develop the same form of type 1 diabetes as do subjects with one or both of the high-risk markers. The different HLA associations may reflect an interaction with different environmental triggers of the disease.

HLA haplotypes are also determinants of genetic protection from type 1 diabetes. Strong protection from the disease is conferred by the *DRB1*1501.DQA1*0102. DQB1*0602* (*DRB1*1501.DQ6*) haplotype; this marker occurs in approximately 20% of the healthy European or North American Caucasian population, whereas less than

1% of diabetic subjects carry the haplotype [37]. Analysis of the transmission of these alleles from unaffected parents to diabetic offspring suggests that the protective influence is associated with the *DQ6* alleles rather than *DRB1*1501*. Rare haplotypes carrying *DRB1*1501* in the absence of *DQ6* are transmitted significantly more frequently than the *DQA1*0102.DQB1*0602* allelic combination alone [37]. The protection provided by the *DQ6* alleles appears to be dominant over susceptibility conferred by other HLA markers, as individuals heterozygous for *DQA1*0102.DQB1*0602* and a high-risk HLA haplotype, such as *DRB1*03.DQ2* or *DRB1*04.DQ8*, do not usually develop diabetes [38]. The *DQ6* alleles can prevent progression to overt diabetes even after the onset of islet autoimmunity, suggesting that the molecule encoded by these alleles may have an immunomodulatory role [39]. The protective effect is not absolute, however, as diabetic subjects positive for *DQA1*0102.DQB1*0602* have been reported [40, 41]. A number of other HLA alleles/haplotypes have also been shown to reduce the risk of developing type 1 diabetes. These include the *DRB1*0403* and **0406* alleles, which have been reported to exert dominant protection over *DQ8* [24, 26, 27], *DRB1*07.DQA1*0201.DQB1*0303*, *DRB1*11.DQA1*0501.DQB1*0301*, *DRB1*13.DQA1*0103.DQB1*0603*, and *DRB1*1401.DQA1*0101.DQB1*0503* [24, 30, 34, 37]. The protective influence of the latter haplotype is probably mediated by the *DRB1*1401* allele [37].

The HLA contribution to susceptibility to type 1 diabetes is clearly complex, with many alleles influencing disease risk. These form a hierarchy from strongly protective (*DQ6*, *DRB1*0403*, *DRB1*0406*) to strongly predisposing (*DQ2* and *DQ8*). DR and DQ heterodimers encoded on the same haplotype or on different haplotypes can enhance or counteract the effects of one another. For example, on the *DRB1*0405.DQA1*0301.DQB1*0301* haplotype, the risk conferred by the *DRB1*0405* allele is decreased by the presence of *DQB1*0301*. Similarly, the predisposing effect of *DQB1*0302* on the *DRB1*0403.DQA1*0301.DQB1*0302* haplotype is completely masked by the protective *DRB1*0403* allele [24]. It is also important to consider genotypic combinations when assessing disease risk. This is illustrated by a recent study of Asian families, which suggested that the risk associated with DR4 haplotypes and their transmission to diabetic offspring may be dependent on the haplotype carried on the homologous chromosome. *DRB1*04.DQ8* haplotypes were transmitted more frequently to diabetic offspring with *DRB1*03* compared to those without *DRB1*03*, while *DRB1*04.DQ4* haplotypes were transmitted more often to *DRB1*03*-negative offspring [42]. Furthermore, high-risk *DRB1*04* subtypes were predominant among *DRB1*04/X* individuals (where X is not *DRB1*03*), whereas protective *DRB1*04* subtypes were observed mainly among *DRB1*03/*04* heterozygotes. This suggests that the contribution to disease risk of the *DRB1* locus may be greater in *DRB1*04/X* genotypes compared with *DRB1*03/*04* genotypes. The overall HLA-linked risk of disease is therefore determined by the complex interaction of all the HLA molecules in a given genotype. As discussed above, the highest risk of type 1 diabetes is conferred by the *DRB1*03.DQ2/DRB1*04.DQ8* genotype. In White Caucasians, high risk is also associated with the *DRB1*04.DQ8/DRB1*01.DQ5* and *DRB1*04.DQ8/DRB1*08.DQ4* genotypes, homozygosity for *DRB1*04.DQ8*, and homozygosity for *DRB1*03.DQ2*. The *DRB1*03.DQ2/DRB1*09.DQ9* genotype was recently reported to confer susceptibility to diabetes in a Dutch population [43], although this allelic combination is more frequently found as a risk factor in Oriental Asian populations [44]. Additional high-risk genotypes reported in Negroid and Oriental Asian populations include *DRB1*03.DQ2/DRB1*07.DQA1*0301.DQB1*0201*, *DRB1*03.DQ2/DRB1*09.DQA1*0301.DQB1*0201*, *DRB1*08.DQ8/DRB1*09.DQ9*, and *DRB1*04.DQ8/DRB1*08.DQ8* [24]. In contrast, any genotype that includes *DQ6* confers a low risk of disease, irrespective of the other alleles present.

The incidence of type 1 diabetes varies considerably between ethnic groups and between different geographical locations around the world. One possible explanation for this is the difference in frequency of high-risk HLA haplotypes in the background populations. For example, the high frequencies of *DRB1*0301*, *DRB1*0401*, *DQ2*, and *DQ8* correlate with the high incidence of the disease in the Scandinavian population (approximately 40 new cases per 100 000 person-years in Finland) [45]. Similarly, the incidence of the disease in Sardinians (35 cases per 100 000 person-years) is attributed to the high frequency of *DRB1*0301* [24, 46]. In contrast, lower frequencies of these alleles are observed in European populations with a low incidence of type 1 diabetes (3–8 cases per 100 000 person-years) [45–47]. Although the distribution of HLA susceptibility markers may account for some of the differences in disease incidence, it is likely that other genetic and environmental factors are also important [48]. Indeed, different *DR-DQ* linkage disequilibrium relationships may contribute to the interracial differences in diabetes incidence. This is particularly apparent in Chinese and Japanese populations, where it is common for a protective *DRB1*04* allele to be in linkage disequilibrium with a predisposing *DQB1* allele, while neutral/protective *DQB1* alleles are associated with predisposing *DRB1*04* subtypes. This counterbalance between predisposing and protective alleles may contribute to the low incidence of diabetes in these Asian populations [24, 49].

The association of type 1 diabetes with the HLA genes has been shown to be age-dependent. The high-risk *DRB1*03.DQ2/DRB1*04.DQ8* genotype is more frequently found among subjects who develop the disease at an early age, but its influence is attenuated with increasing age of onset [50]. Similarly, the protective influence of the *DQ6* haplotype is reduced with increasing age; patients positive for this marker tend, therefore, to have a much older age of disease onset compared with subjects carrying other HLA types [51]. A study of sibling pairs, however, suggested that the age at which diabetes develops is not determined wholly by *DR-DQ* haplotypes; other HLA genes, such as *HLA-A* and *-DPB1*, may also be involved [52].

The Molecular Basis of HLA-DR and -DQ Associations

As HLA-linked genetic susceptibility to type 1 diabetes is very complex, with many different *DR* and *DQ* alleles influencing disease risk, a simple unifying hypothesis has been sought to explain the observed associations. It has been postulated that the alleles associated with an increased risk of disease may encode HLA molecules with common molecular features that influence their ability to interact with diabetogenic antigens; these features would be absent from protective HLA molecules. In 1987, Michelsen and Lernmark [53] showed that the *DQ7* molecule (*DQA1*0301.DQB1*0301*) and the *DQ8* molecule (*DQA1*0301.DQB1*0302*) differed at only six amino acid residues in the β peptide chain, four of which (residues 13, 26, 45, and 57) lie within the polymorphic N-terminal domain. It was suggested that one or more of these amino acid substitutions might be responsible for the contrasting disease associations of the *DRB1*04.DQ7* (protective) and *DRB1*04.DQ8* (predisposing) haplotypes. Subsequent investigations suggested that the amino acid residue at position β57 might be the major determinant. Diabetogenic haplotypes were reported to carry *DQB1* alleles encoding an uncharged amino acid (particularly alanine, serine, or valine) at this position, whereas the *DQB1* alleles on protective haplotypes encoded the charged amino acid, aspartate, at residue β57 [54, 55].

A significant role for residue β57 in determining susceptibility to diabetes is supported by observations in animal models of the disease. The biobreeding (BB) rat, which develops a type 1 diabetes-like syndrome with autoimmune insulitis, carries a serine residue at position 57 in its homologous class II β-chain. The NOD mouse also possesses an *I-A*β allele (the murine homologue of *DQB1*) that encodes serine at residue 57. In contrast, diabetes-resistant mouse strains possess an *I-A*β allele encoding aspartate at this position [56]. Substitution of the Ser57 and His56 residues in the I-Aβ chain with Asp57 and Pro56 was shown to protect NOD mice from developing diabetes [57, 58].

The functional significance of the amino acid residue at position β57 has been investigated in some detail. In the crystal structure of the DR1 molecule, the aspartate residue at β57 forms a salt bridge with a conserved arginine (Arg) residue at position 76 of the DR α-chain [59]. An analogous situation in the DQ molecule would create a salt bridge between Asp57 on the β-chain and a conserved Arg79 residue on the α-chain (Figure 4). These interactions influence the structure of the antigen-binding cleft in the class II αβ heterodimers. Substitutions at this site could therefore affect the binding and presentation of peptides derived from β-cell autoantigens to diabetogenic T-cells. Indeed, amino acid substitutions at residue β57 have been shown to directly affect antigen-binding affinity and selectivity and recognition of HLA/peptide complexes by T-cell clones [61–63]. These functional consequences could underlie the disparate disease associations observed between Asp57- and non-Asp57-encoding *DQB1* alleles.

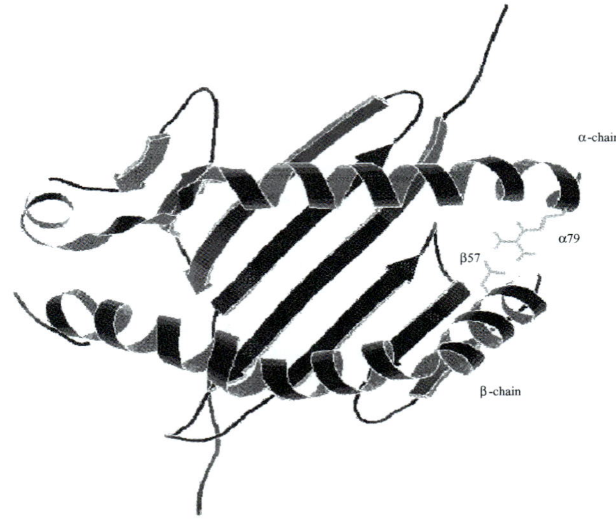

Figure 4 A diagrammatic representation of an HLA-DQ molecule showing the salt bridge between residues α79 (Arg) and β57 (Asp) (adapted from reference 60)

The identity of the amino acid at residue β57 cannot, however, fully account for susceptibility to diabetes. Transgenic studies in the NOD mouse have shown that the development of overt diabetes is influenced by the amino acid residue at position 57 in the I-Aβ chain, but certain non-Asp57 I-Aβ chains are protective [21, 58]. Furthermore, in humans the Asp/non-Asp β57 dimorphism does not explain all the observed associations with the *DQB1* locus. For example, in the Japanese population, a high risk of disease is associated with the Asp57-encoding alleles *DQB1*0401* and *DQB1*0303* [64]; 72% of Japanese and 27% of Chinese diabetic subjects are homozygous for Asp57-encoding *DQB1* alleles compared with <7% of Caucasian diabetic patients [65, 66]. In addition, HLA-encoded susceptibility to diabetes is not an "all-or-none" phenomenon, but depends on the complex interaction of multiple alleles on a genotype. It is, therefore, unlikely to be determined simply by the presence or absence of a single amino acid residue. Several studies have suggested that susceptibility is most strongly associated with DQαβ heterodimers composed of a non-Asp57 DQβ peptide chain and a DQα chain carrying arginine at residue 52 (Arg52) [67]. Although more predictive of disease risk than DQβ57 alone, this combination is still insufficient to account for all the *HLA-DQ* associations observed.

Recent studies have used more complex statistical approaches to identify the combinations of DR/DQ amino acid residues involved in determining the risk of diabetes. Using the haplotype method, Valdes et al. [68] suggested that a combination of seven residues (DRβ67, DRβ86, DQα47, DQβ9, DQβ26, DQβ57, and DQβ70) predicts the HLA class II susceptibility component. In contrast, Djoulah et al. [69] suggested that disease susceptibility could be explained by the absence of aspartate at DQβ57, combined with the presence of a positive or negative charge created by residues 70, 71, and 74 of the DRβ and DQβ peptide chains. Although these residues may not necessarily have functional importance in the pathogenesis of diabetes, they may be useful for predicting disease risk.

The Functional Basis for HLA Class II Associations with Type 1 Diabetes

A direct role for HLA-DR and -DQ molecules in the pathogenesis of type 1 diabetes was recently demonstrated in studies of HLA-transgenic mice. B10 mice expressing human DR3 (*DRB1*03*) or DQ8 (*DQB1*0302*), singly or in combination, were shown to develop spontaneous insulitis and loss of tolerance to glutamic acid decarboxylase (GAD65), a potential β-cell autoantigen [70, 71]. No T-cell response to GAD65 was seen if DR3 or DQ8 was co-expressed with the DQ6 (*DQB1*0602*) molecule [71]. This finding is consistent with the dominant protective role reported previously for DQ6. In a separate study of C57BL/6 HLA transgenic mice, expression of DQ8 or DR4 (*DRB1*0401*) was not sufficient to induce insulitis. When these animals were crossed with transgenic mice expressing the co-stimulatory molecule, B7.1, on their pancreatic β-cells, however, the double transgenic offspring were no longer tolerant to islet autoantigens and developed spontaneous diabetes [72, 73]. Although both HLA molecules could promote disease development, DQ8 was found to be more diabetogenic than DR4, whereas DR4 expression could downregulate the effect of DQ8 [73].

The influence of a particular HLA molecule on the risk of diabetes is largely determined by the three-dimensional structure of its antigen-binding cleft. This will dictate the way in which the molecule interacts with peptides derived from β-cell autoantigens and the TCRs of pathogenically relevant T-cells. Diabetogenic HLA molecules, such as DQ2, DQ8, and the I-A^{g7} molecule found in NOD mice, have been reported to share similar chemical and geometric properties at their antigen-binding sites [74, 75]. Likewise, there is marked structural similarity between the diabetes-protective molecules, such as DQ6, DQ7 (*DQA1*0501.DQB1*0301*), DR4 (*DRB1*0403*), and the murine I-A^b molecule [74]. The molecular features differ markedly between the two groups, however. The structural characteristics of three peptide-binding "pockets" (P1, P4, and P9) appear to be important determinants of disease susceptibility [74]. Consistent with this hypothesis, the P9 pocket contains residue 57 of the DR/DQ β-chain. The identity of the amino acid at this position has been shown to influence antigen-binding ability and possibly molecular stability [62, 76, 77].

The structural differences between the diabetogenic and protective molecules are reflected by differences in antigen peptide selectivity and binding affinity. Different HLA molecules favor distinct peptide-binding "motifs," dictated by the shape of specific pockets in the antigen-binding cleft [78, 79]. Structurally distinct molecules may therefore interact differently with a given autoantigenic peptide. Furthermore the structure of the protective DQ6 molecule has been suggested to confer greater stability on the cell surface compared with the predisposing DQ2 and DQ8 molecules [80]. The affinity of antigen binding and the half-life of the HLA/peptide complex will influence the strength of interactions with TCRs and ultimately determine the activation status of responding T-cells. Particular amino acid residues in the HLA molecules may also interact directly with TCRs to influence T-cell activation. Several hypotheses have been proposed to explain how these functional differences might influence the risk of type 1 diabetes (reviewed in reference 81).

(1) *Antigen binding in the periphery*. Predisposing HLA molecules may bind well to diabetogenic antigens in the periphery and hence activate an autoimmune T-cell response, whereas protective HLA molecules may not. Alternatively, the protective molecules may bind to the autoantigens with higher affinity, thus competing with the predisposing molecules. In this latter case, the threshold of binding required for T-cell activation by the predisposing molecules may not be reached.

(2) *Molecular stability and deletion of autoreactive T-cells*. Protective HLA molecules may form stable complexes with self-antigens in the thymus, leading to efficient deletion of potentially autoreactive T-cells. In contrast, the less stable complexes formed with the predisposing HLA molecules may result in inefficient T-cell removal and the release of diabetogenic T-cells into the periphery. Negative selection of autoreactive T-cells by protective class II molecules has been demonstrated in one transgenic NOD mouse model [82], but not in another [83].

(3) *Influence on T-cell phenotype*. Predisposing and protective HLA molecules may interact differently with the TCRs of diabetogenic T-cells, thereby affecting

the phenotype of the T-cells (proinflammatory vs. regulatory) or their activation status (proliferative vs. anergized). This immunomodulatory hypothesis is supported by the observation that DQ6 can protect against the development of type 1 diabetes, even after the onset of islet autoimmunity [39].

Other MHC-encoded Susceptibility Loci

Several studies have indicated that the *HLA-DRB1* and *-DQ* genes cannot account for all the *IDDM1*-encoded susceptibility to type 1 diabetes. It has been suggested that the molecules encoded by the *DR* and *DQ* genes determine the specificity of the antigen-driven autoimmune response, whereas the products of other genes act as nonspecific immune regulators to control the magnitude of the response. The contribution of other MHC loci is uncertain, however, and their precise location is unknown, owing to the strong linkage disequilibrium that extends across this region.

Several MHC genes have been proposed as candidate susceptibility genes for type 1 diabetes. Some are associated secondary to linkage disequilibrium with predisposing *HLA-DR* and *-DQ* alleles, for example, the transporter associated with antigen processing (*TAP*) genes and the large multifunctional protease (*LMP*) genes [84, 85]. Others, such as the *HLA-DPB1* gene, influence disease risk independently of *DR* and *DQ*. The overall contribution of *DPB1* to *IDDM1*-encoded susceptibility appears to be small [86], although its role may be more significant in subjects who do not carry the high-risk *DRB1*03.DQ2/DRB1*04.DQ8* genotype [87].

Fine mapping studies of recombinant MHC haplotypes have identified several regions that may contain additional disease susceptibility determinants. Lie et al. [88] showed that alleles of the *D6S2223* microsatellite, located 2.5 Mb telomeric to *HLA-F*, modify the risk conferred by the *DRB1*03.DQ2* haplotype, suggesting that a gene telomeric of the HLA class I region may contribute to susceptibility to diabetes. In contrast, other studies favor a role for central MHC genes. Moghaddam et al. [89] reported a significant disease association with the region encompassing the *HSP70* and *TNF* gene clusters (marked by the *D6S273* and *TNF*-α microsatellites). A number of studies have supported a role for the *TNF* genes as susceptibility determinants for type 1 diabetes, although it is unclear whether they act independently of *HLA-DR* and *-DQ* [90–92]. A recent study testing for associations conditional on the *DQB1-DRB1* haplotype found no evidence for a major role of either *D6S273* or *HLA-TNF* in *IDDM1*-encoded susceptibility [93].

An investigation of the ancestral HLA 8.1 haplotype (*HLA-A1*, *-B8*, *-DR3*, *-DQ2*) by Cheong et al. [94] suggested that a central MHC susceptibility locus for type 1 diabetes might lie between the *BAT1* gene and the *MIB* microsatellite, located between the *TNF* and *HLA-B* loci. This region encompasses the MHC class I chain-related (*MIC*) genes, *MIC-A* and *MIC-B*. A trinucleotide repeat microsatellite in exon 5 of the *MIC-A* gene has been associated with type 1 diabetes in several studies, although the alleles implicated in disease vary between different ethnic groups. A strong association with allele 5 was reported in Italian subjects [95]. In contrast, allele 9 showed the strongest association in Taiwanese [96], whereas allele 4 was positively associated and allele 6 negatively associated with diabetes in Korean subjects [97]. In both the Italian and Korean cohorts, the *MIC-A* gene was associated with the disease independent of the *DR/DQ* genes. A study of the diabetogenic *HLA-B39*, *-DR4* haplotype in Finns suggested that a gene in the 240 kb central MHC region surrounding *HLA-B* might also provide an additional predisposing effect to the *DRB1*04* and *DQB1*0302* alleles [98]. The *MIC-A* exon 5 microsatellite was excluded as a possible candidate polymorphism, however.

Three additional MHC loci have been identified as independent modifiers of disease risk on the *DRB1*03.DQ2* haplotype. Alleles of single nucleotide polymorphisms (SNPs) at the *DMB* and *DOB* loci and the microsatellite locus *TNFc* were shown to identify non-predisposing *DRB1*03.DQ2* haplotypes in a Sardinian population [99]. Consistent with these findings, the *DMB*0101* allele has been reported to be negatively associated with type 1 diabetes in subjects with the high-risk *DQA1*0501* allele [100].

In conclusion, susceptibility to diabetes conferred by *IDDM1* represents the combined effects of several genes within the MHC. At least three major loci are involved—*HLA-DRB1*, *-DQA1*, and *-DQB1*—but other genes may also contribute. The precise identity of these minor susceptibility loci remains to be determined.

THE INSULIN GENE REGION

The insulin gene on chromosome 11p was proposed as a candidate susceptibility gene for type 1 diabetes, as insulin and its precursors are uniquely produced by pancreatic β-cells and hence are potential target antigens for autoimmune β-cell destruction. In support of this hypothesis, circulating autoantibodies specific for insulin have been demonstrated in newly diagnosed diabetic individuals, prior to the start of insulin therapy [101]. In 1984, a case/control study reported a significant association between the disease and alleles of a polymorphic region flanking the insulin gene (*INS*) [6]. This was confirmed in subsequent case/control studies and the primary disease-associated polymorphism was identified as a variable number of tandem repeats (*VNTR*) region, located 596bp upstream of the insulin gene translational start site [102–104]. Alleles of the *INS-VNTR* are divided into three classes based on the number of repeats of a 14–15-bp sequence: class I (26–63 repeats), class II (64–139 repeats), and class III (140–210 repeats). The class I alleles are generally associated with susceptibility to type 1 diabetes, with homozygosity for class I conferring the highest risk, whereas the class III alleles generally confer dominant protection against the disease [104, 105]. There are exceptions to this pattern, however, as some class I alleles are not predisposing (for example, alleles 814 and 698) [104, 106]. It has now been shown that the class I alleles can be subdivided into three lineages, IC+, ID+, and ID–, on the basis of the combination of variant repeat distributions and flanking haplotypes. All class I alleles are equally predisposing to type 1 diabetes except the ID– alleles, which are protective when transmitted from ID–/III heterozygous fathers [107]. The ID– alleles, which include the non-predisposing 814 allele reported previously, can be distinguished from the other class I alleles by an Msp1(–) variant within the downstream *IGF2* locus. The class III alleles can be subdivided into two highly diverged lineages, protective haplotypes (IIIA) and very protective haplotypes (IIIB), on the basis of linkage disequilibrium with a microsatellite close to the upstream tyrosine hydroxylase gene [104, 107]. A recent study also identified a subgroup of rare class III alleles that appear to predispose to diabetes [108].

Although population-based association studies provided strong evidence for a role for the insulin gene in diabetes susceptibility, early attempts to show linkage of the disease with this locus in family studies were unsuccessful [109, 110]. Recent genome screens have also reported inconsistent findings regarding the role of the *INS* locus in type 1 diabetes. Reasonable evidence for linkage has been reported in some data sets, but not in others [7–9]. It has been suggested that these paradoxical findings may result from interactions with HLA susceptibility determinants or from parent-of-origin effects, which may differ between different populations [104, 105, 111–113]. Alternatively, the discrepancies may be due to the limited power of the linkage analysis approach to detect susceptibility alleles with a modest effect on disease risk, but with a high background frequency in the relatively small study populations. Indeed, when the data from three genome screens were combined for analysis, the larger data set of 831 affected sibling pairs showed significant evidence for linkage to the *INS* locus [10]. Furthermore, linkage in the presence of association has been confirmed at this locus using the transmission disequilibrium test (TDT), which tests for excess transmission of *INS* haplotypes from heterozygous parents to diabetic offspring [114, 115]. This approach has greater statistical power than classical linkage analysis, which tests for excess allele sharing in affected sib pairs. The *INS* locus is now designated *IDDM2* and has been reported to contribute approximately 10% of the familial clustering of type 1 diabetes [7].

The mechanism by which the *INS-VNTR* polymorphisms influence the risk of type 1 diabetes is unclear. This locus, however, has been shown to regulate the expression of two downstream genes that may be relevant to disease pathogenesis; the insulin gene and the insulin-like growth factor 2 (*IGF2*) gene. Insulin gene transcripts have been demonstrated in the human thymus as well as pancreatic tissue, and the levels of mRNA correlate with allelic variation at the *INS-VNTR* locus. Class I *VNTR* alleles are associated with a higher level of insulin gene transcription in the pancreas compared with the class III alleles [104, 116]. The reverse pattern is observed in the thymus, with higher insulin mRNA levels occurring in the presence of the class III alleles [117, 118]. Elevated levels of preproinsulin expressed in the thymus may promote the efficient deletion of autoreactive T-cells specific for this protein, leading to immune tolerance to a key autoantigen in the pathogenesis of diabetes. This mechanism may explain the dominant protective effect of the class III *VNTR* alleles. In subjects homozygous for the class I alleles, the combination of lower intrathymic insulin expression and higher expression in the pancreas would be expected to increase the risk of insulin-driven pancreatic autoimmunity. The immune tolerance hypothesis is supported by the finding of two rare class III alleles, which are associated with complete silencing of thymic *INS* transcripts and are reported to predispose to type 1 diabetes [108]. Furthermore, a recent study of a mouse model with graded thymic insulin deficiency showed an inverse correlation between thymic insulin levels and peripheral T-cell reactivity to insulin [119]. To date, however, there is no evidence of a correlation between *INS-VNTR* class and induction of tolerance to insulin in humans [120].

The *IGF2* gene may also contribute to *IDDM2*-associated susceptibility to diabetes. In most tissues, *IGF2* is expressed only from the paternally inherited gene, as the maternally inherited copy is transcriptionally silent [121]. This genomic imprinting may explain the parent-of-origin effects on the transmission of *VNTR* alleles seen in some populations [104, 105, 111]. The product of the *IGF2* gene (IGF-II) is a ubiquitously expressed mitogenic peptide with autocrine/paracrine signalling actions. Thymic IGF-II has been suggested to influence the risk of pancreatic autoimmunity, as it plays a significant role in T-cell development and negative selection. It may also act as a selecting peptide for insulin-reactive T-cells, because of its homology to proinsulin [122]. This mechanism cannot account for the disease associations observed with the *INS-VNTR* alleles, however, as the class I and class III alleles are associated with similar levels of *IGF2* expression in the pancreas and thymus [122, 123]. It is likely that the influence of the *IGF2* gene on disease risk is mediated by a less direct mechanism. For example, the class I *VNTR* alleles are associated with increased *IGF2* expression in the placenta [124]. This may affect intrauterine growth rate and birth weight, which have both been reported to influence the risk of developing type 1 diabetes [125].

GENOME SCREENS

Genome-wide linkage mapping to identify susceptibility genes for complex diseases was made possible by a number of technological advances in the late 1980s and early 1990s. These included the development of high-throughput genotyping methodologies, the identification of microsatellite DNA markers, and the construction of human genetic linkage maps. Using these advances, Davies et al. [7] performed the first complete genome screen to identify susceptibility genes for type 1 diabetes. In the initial phase of the study, 290 DNA markers were genotyped in 96 UK White Caucasian multiplex families (families with two or more affected siblings). Linkage between diabetes and these markers was investigated using the non-parametric affected sib pair method. This requires no prior knowledge of disease gene frequencies or the mode of inheritance. A significant excess of marker alleles shared identical-by-descent (IBD) in affected sibpairs suggests that the region containing the marker locus also contains a disease susceptibility locus [1]. The loci identified in the preliminary study were subsequently examined in two further data sets, comprising 102 UK and 84 US families. The study confirmed the importance of the HLA gene region (designated *IDDM1*) to disease susceptibility and excluded at least 97% of the genome from containing any susceptibility gene with an effect equivalent to that of *IDDM1*. Linkage to the *INS* region on chromosome 11p (designated *IDDM2*) was also observed, while an additional 18 chromosomal region showed some positive evidence of linkage to diabetes (Table 1). Among the most convincing susceptibility intervals were regions on chromosomes 11q and 6q (designated *IDDM4* and *IDDM5* respectively), which were confirmed by replication in the additional data sets. Linkage to *IDDM4* was particularly marked in subjects with low-risk HLA status (sharing zero or one HLA haplotype), whereas *IDDM5* was most tightly linked to disease in families with high-risk HLA status (sharing both HLA haplotypes).

Further genome screens of affected sibpairs confirmed linkage to some but not all of the loci identified by Davies et al. [7] and reported additional chromosomal regions that may contain susceptibility genes for type 1 diabetes (Table 1) [8–10, 115]. Linkage to *IDDM1* (the HLA gene region), *IDDM2* (the insulin gene region), *IDDM4* (chromosome 11q13), *IDDM5* (chromosome 6q25), *IDDM7*, *IDDM12*, *IDDM13* (all located on chromosome 2q31-35), *IDDM8* (chromosome 6q27), *IDDM10* (chromosome 10p11-q11), and *IDDM15* (chromosome 6q21) was replicated in independent data sets, but linkage to other intervals was not [8–10, 115, 126, 127]. The *IDDM6* locus on chromosome 18q was not identified in all the linkage studies, but shows evidence for association with type 1 diabetes in affected-family-based studies [128]. The discrepancies between the studies may be due to a number of factors, including sample size, genetic and phenotypic heterogeneity between data sets (for example, ethnic differences in the frequency of susceptibility alleles, differences in age at disease onset), and gender-specific effects (such as the sex of the affected offspring and the parental origin of shared alleles) [129–131]. Genetic epistasis may also be a confounding factor, and linkage to some loci may only be revealed after suitable stratification of the data sets. For example, significant linkage to the *DXS1068* marker was observed only in *HLA-DR3*-positive sibpairs [132]. The problem of linkage heterogeneity between studies is discussed comprehensively by Field [126].

Table 1 Susceptibility intervals implicated in type 1 diabetes*

Locus	Chromosomal location	Markers
IDDM1	6p21.3	*HLA-DRB1, DQB1, DQA1*
IDDM2	11p15	*INS-VNTR*
IDDM3	15q26	*D15S107*
IDDM4	11q13	*FGF3, D11S1337*
IDDM5	6q25	*ESR*
IDDM6	18q21	*JK, D18S487*
IDDM7	2q31	*HOXD8, D2S152*
IDDM8	6q27	*D6S264, D6S446*
IDDM9	3q21-q25	*D3S1576*
IDDM10	10p11-q11	*D10S193*
IDDM11	14q24.3-q31	*D14S67*
IDDM12	2q33	*CTLA4*
IDDM13	2q35	*D2S164*
IDDM14	Unpublished	Unpublished
IDDM15	6q21	*D6S283*
IDDM16	14q32.3	*D14S542, IGH*
IDDM17	10q25	*D10S554*
IDDM18	5q33-q34	*IL12B*
Unnamed	1q42	*D1S1617*
Unnamed	16q22-q24	*D16S3098*
Unnamed	19p13	*D19S247*
Unnamed	19q13	*D19S225*
Unnamed	Xp13-p11	*DXS1068*
Unnamed	7p13	*GCK*
Unnamed	12q14-q15	*IFNG*

* Adapted from reference 126.

Fine mapping studies have allowed the boundaries of some of the IDDM susceptibility intervals to be more precisely defined [133–136]. Several of these regions contain interesting candidate genes for type 1 diabetes.

(1) *IDDM4* contains the galanin (*GALN*) and Fas-associated death domain (*FADD*) genes. Galanin is a neuropeptide that is believed to inhibit insulin secretion from the pancreas, while FADD is involved in the apoptosis of peripheral T-cells and the homeostasis of mature lymphocytes.
(2) *IDDM5* is located close to the gene encoding manganese superoxide dismutase, which may influence

the sensitivity of pancreatic β-cells to damage by oxygen free radicals.

(3) *IDDM11* lies close to the *SEL1L* gene, which encodes a negative regulator of the Notch signalling pathway in the islets of Langerhans.

(4) *IDDM13* is located close to the natural-resistance-associated macrophage protein (*NRAMP1*) gene, a host resistance locus with an important role in macrophage function, and the *IA-2* gene, which encodes the tyrosine phosphatase, IA-2, a key autoantigen in type 1 diabetes.

Although the products of these genes could potentially participate in the pathogenesis of type 1 diabetes, none of the loci have shown significant association or linkage with the disease [135, 137–140].

IDDM7 maps close to the *NeuroD/BETA2* gene, which encodes an insulin gene transcription factor important for the development of pancreatic β-cells. Heterozygosity for the Ala45Thr variant of this gene has been associated with type 1 diabetes in some studies, but not in others [141, 142]. The effect of *NeuroD/BETA2* may be independent of *IDDM7*, however [143].

IDDM12 is thought to be the cytotoxic T-lymphocyte associated-4 (*CTLA-4*) gene. This susceptibility marker was mapped by linkage and by association with the *CTLA-4* locus in Spanish and Italian families. An SNP (A/G) in exon 1 of the gene was reported to be significantly associated with diabetes in these data sets, although this was not observed in British or American families [144]. An association with this marker was also reported in subsequent family-based and case/control studies, although marked population heterogeneity was again observed. The association was found to be stronger in Spanish, French, Italian, Mexican, Korean, and Japanese populations, whereas data from British, Sardinian, Chinese, and European American cohorts suggested a minor role for *CTLA-4* in disease susceptibility [145–147]. A microsatellite in the 3′ untranslated region of the gene has also been associated with diabetes in a number of data sets [139, 146–148]. The *CTLA-4* gene product is expressed by T-lymphocytes and acts as a negative regulator of T-cell activation by mediating T-cell apoptosis. *CTLA-4* is therefore a strong candidate gene for type 1 diabetes and other T-cell-mediated autoimmune diseases. Indeed, it has been implicated in susceptibility to autoimmune thyroid disease (both Graves' disease and Hashimoto's thyroiditis), celiac disease, multiple sclerosis, and rheumatoid arthritis [149–152].

COMPARATIVE MAPPING OF THE NOD MOUSE GENOME

The identification of loci associated with susceptibility to diabetes in the NOD mouse has provided useful insights into the genetic basis of the human condition. The NOD mouse is an inbred strain that spontaneously develops a disease with similar characteristics to type 1 diabetes in humans, including autoimmune destruction of the pancreatic β-cells, the presence of circulating autoantibodies to islet antigens, defects in T-cell activity, and an MHC-linked genetic susceptibility component [153]. Comparative mapping of the mouse and human genomes has revealed extensive regions of homology. This has allowed certain susceptibility loci in humans to be predicted from their location in the NOD mouse genome.

At least 17 loci have been suggested to influence the development of type 1 diabetes in the NOD mouse [154]. One of these, termed *Idd-5*, has been mapped to mouse chromosome 1, which shares a homologous 33-cM region with human chromosome 2q31–q35 [155]. This region contains three candidate genes for autoimmune disease, namely the interleukin-1 receptor gene (*IL-1R1*), the *Lsh/Ity/Bcg* locus and the *NRAMP1* gene, which influence macrophage activation and resistance to infection. Investigations of allele sharing at microsatellite markers within this region in family data sets led to the localization of two susceptibility intervals for type 1 diabetes, *IDDM7* and *IDDM13* [156, 157]. Fine mapping of this region, however, has yet to identify any diabetogenic polymorphisms.

Genetic studies of animal models have also identified functional candidate genes for type 1 diabetes. These include the *Il12b* gene, which encodes the p40 subunit of interleukin-12. This proinflammatory cytokine drives the differentiation of T-lymphocytes into the Th1 subset. *Il12b* alleles have been reported to differ between diabetes-prone and diabetes-resistant mouse strains, suggesting that the locus might influence disease susceptibility. These findings prompted an investigation of the human homologue (*IL12B*) in sibpairs with type 1 diabetes, which showed a significant disease association with polymorphisms in intron 4 and the 3′ untranslated region of the gene [158]. Although these associations were not replicated in subsequent case/control and family studies [159, 160], this susceptibility locus has been designated as *IDDM18*.

Overall the comparative mapping strategy has been somewhat disappointing, as it has identified few new susceptibility loci for human type 1 diabetes. Furthermore, despite considerable mapping work in different mouse strains, it is discouraging to note that the specific murine genes that influence the risk of diabetes have not yet been identified.

OTHER CANDIDATE GENES

A number of other genes have been implicated in susceptibility to type 1 diabetes using the candidate gene approach (the selection of genes whose products may be involved in immune modulation and the pathogenesis of β-cell destruction). These include the TCR genes, immunoglobulin genes, CD4 gene, the chemokine receptor CCR2 gene, vitamin D receptor gene, and nitric oxide synthase gene [161–166]. Disease association with some of these loci has not been replicated in independent data sets, while others have produced conflicting results. Their contribution to disease risk therefore remains to be established.

CONCLUSION

Type 1 diabetes is a complex, polygenic disease. The *HLA-DQB1* and *-DRB1* genes are the strongest genetic susceptibility factors identified to date, although their influence may be modified by other MHC genes, including *HLA-B* and *-DPB1*. The insulin gene *VNTR* also provides a significant contribution to disease risk. Although many other loci have been implicated in diabetes susceptibility, considerable work is still required to identify all the genetic factors involved. Such studies may be hampered, however, by the multifactorial nature of diabetes and by complex interactions between susceptibility loci. Large international collaborative studies will be necessary to provide data sets of sufficient size for the fine dissection of the genetic components. This work may be aided by improvements in high-throughput genotyping methodologies and better definition of the disease phenotype. For example, it may be necessary to stratify study subjects according to phenotypic characteristics, such as age of disease onset or the presence of islet cell antibodies, in order to demonstrate linkage and/or association with some susceptibility loci. The application of cross-ethnic studies will facilitate the mapping of susceptibility genes in regions that exhibit race-specific differences in the patterns of linkage disequilibrium between markers. Once the boundaries of the susceptibility intervals have been more precisely defined, suitable candidate genes for type 1 diabetes can be identified using information from animal models of the disease and the Human Genome Project. As environmental factors also have a major impact on the risk of diabetes, it is vital that genetic and environmental components are studied in tandem.

Fine-mapping of all the susceptibility loci will aid the development of screening strategies to identify individuals with a high genetic risk of type 1 diabetes. If these subjects could be identified before the onset of autoimmunity (preferably at birth), they would provide an ideal study group for the prospective assessment of environmental influences on diabetes development. Furthermore, these subjects would facilitate the testing of novel therapeutic strategies aimed at preventing the onset or progression of β-cell autoimmunity. The identification of susceptibility genes and studies of their function will allow new insights into the pathophysiology of type 1 diabetes, which will aid in the development of these therapeutic approaches. To that end, the HLA genes, as the major susceptibility determinants, should be further investigated at a functional level to elucidate the molecular mechanisms by which they influence disease risk.

REFERENCES

1. Risch N. Assessing the role of HLA-linked and unlinked determinants of disease. *Am J Hum Genet* 1987; 40: 1–14.
2. Thomson G, Robinson WP, Kuhner MK, Joe S, MacDonald MJ, Gottschall JL, Barbosa J, Rich SS, Bertrams J, Baur MP, Partanen J, Tait BD, Schober E, Mayr WR, Ludvigsson J, Lindblom B, Farid NR, Thompson C, Deschamps I. Genetic heterogeneity, modes of inheritance, and risk estimates for a joint study of Caucasians with insulin-dependent diabetes mellitus. *Am J Hum Genet* 1988; 43: 799–816.
3. Redondo MJ, Rewers M, Yu L, Garg S, Pilcher CC, Elliott RB, Eisenbarth GS. Genetic determination of islet cell autoimmunity in monozygotic twin, dizygotic twin, and non-twin siblings of patients with type 1 diabetes: prospective twin study. *BMJ* 1999; 318: 698–702.
4. Redondo MJ, Yu L, Hawa M, MacKenzie T, Pyke DA, Eisenbarth GS, Leslie RDG. Heterogeneity of type 1 diabetes: analysis of monozygotic twins in Great Britain and the United States. *Diabetologia* 2001; 44: 354–62.
5. Singal DP, Blajchman MA. Histocompatibility (HL-A) antigens, lymphocytotoxic antibodies and tissue antibodies in patients with diabetes mellitus. *Diabetes* 1973; 22: 429–32.
6. Bell GI, Horita S, Karam JH. A polymorphic locus near the human insulin gene is associated with insulin-dependent diabetes mellitus. *Diabetes* 1984; 33: 176–83.
7. Davies JL, Kawaguchi Y, Bennett ST, Copeman JB, Cordell HJ, Pritchard LE, Reed PW, Gough SCL, Jenkins SC, Palmer SM, Balfour KM, Rowe BR, Farrall M, Barnett AH, Bain SC, Todd JA. A genome-wide search for human type 1 diabetes susceptibility genes. *Nature* 1994; 371: 130–6.
8. Mein CA, Esposito L, Dunn MG, Johnson GCL, Timms AE, Goy JV, Smith AN, Sebag-Montefiore L, Merriman ME, Wilson AJ, Pritchard LE, Cucca F, Barnett AH, Bain SC, Todd JA. A search for type 1 diabetes susceptibility genes in families from the United Kingdom. *Nat Genet* 1998; 19: 297–300.
9. Concannon P, Gogolin-Ewens KJ, Hinds DA, Wapelhorst B, Morrison VA, Stirling B, Mitra M, Farmer J, Williams SR, Cox NJ, Bell GI, Risch N, Spielman RS. A second-generation screen of the human genome for susceptibility to insulin-dependent diabetes mellitus. *Nat Genet* 1998; 19: 292–6.
10. Cox NJ, Wapelhorst B, Morrison VA, Johnson L, Pinchuk L, Spielman RS, Todd JA, Concannon P. Seven regions of the genome show evidence of linkage to type 1 diabetes in a consensus analysis of 767 multiplex families. *Am J Hum Genet* 2001; 69: 820–30.
11. Bain SC, Kelly MA, Mijovic CH, Barnett AH. Genetic factors in the pathogenesis of type 1 diabetes. In Pickup JC, Williams G (eds) *Textbook of Diabetes*, 3rd edn. Oxford: Blackwell Science, 2003.
12. McDevitt HO, Bodmer WF. HLA-A, immune response genes and disease. *Lancet* 1974; i: 1269–75.
13. Nerup J, Platz P, Andersen OO, Christy M, Lyngsoe J, Poulsen JE, Ryder LP, Nielsen LS, Thomsen M, Svejgaard A. HL-A antigens and diabetes mellitus. *Lancet* 1974; ii: 864–6.

14. Cudworth AG, Woodrow JC. HL-A antigens and diabetes mellitus. *Lancet* 1974; ii: 1153.
15. Nerup J, Cathelineau C, Seignalet J, Thomsen M. HLA and endocrine disease. In Dausset J, Svejgaard A (eds), *HLA and Disease*. Copenhagen: Munksgaard, 1977; pp 149–67.
16. Spielman RS, Baur MP, Clerget-Darpoux F. Genetic analysis of IDDM: summary of the GAW5 IDDM results. *Genet Epidemiol* 1989; 6: 43–58.
17. Svejgaard A, Ryder LP. HLA and insulin-dependent diabetes: an overview. *Genet Epidemiol* 1989; 6: 1–14.
18. Owerbach D, Lernmark A, Platz P, Ryder LP, Rask L, Peterson PA, Ludvigsson J. HLA-D region β-chain DNA endonuclease fragments differ between HLA-DR identical healthy and insulin-dependent diabetic individuals. *Nature* 1983; 303: 815–7.
19. Nepom BS, Palmer J, Kim SJ, Jansen JA, Holbeck SL, Nepom GT. Specific genomic markers for the HLA-DQ subregion discriminate between DR4+ insulin dependent diabetes mellitus and DR4+ seropositive juvenile rheumatoid arthritis. *J Exp Med* 1986; 164: 345–50.
20. Kim SJ. Identification of a polymorphic variant associated with HLA-DQw3 and characterised by specific restriction sites within the DQ β-chain gene. *Proc Natl Acad Sci USA* 1985; 82: 8139–43.
21. Miyazaki T, Uno M, Uehira M, Kikutani H, Kishimoto T, Kimoto M, Nishimoto H, Miyazaki J, Yamamura K. Direct evidence for the contribution of the unique I-A^{NOD} to the development of insulitis in non-obese diabetic mice. *Nature* 1990; 345: 722–4.
22. Cavan DA, Jacobs KH, Penny MA, Kelly MA, Mijovic C, Jenkins D, Fletcher JA, Barnett AH. Both DQA1 and DQB1 genes are implicated in HLA-associated protection from type 1 (insulin-dependent) diabetes mellitus in a British Caucasian population. *Diabetologia* 1993; 36: 252–7.
23. Herr M, Dudbridge F, Zavattari P, Cucca F, Guja C, March R, Campbell RD, Barnett AH, Bain SC, Todd JA, Koeleman BPC. Evaluation of fine mapping strategies for a multifactorial disease locus: systematic linkage and association analysis of *IDDM1* in the HLA region on chromosome 6p21. *Hum Mol Genet* 2000; 9: 1291–301.
24. She JX. Susceptibility to type 1 diabetes: HLA-DQ and DR revisited. *Immunol Today* 1996; 17: 323–9.
25. Kockum I, Sanjeevi CB, Eastman S, Landin-Olsson M, Dahlquist G, Lernmark A. Complex interaction between HLA DR and DQ in conferring risk for childhood type 1 diabetes. *Eur J Immunogenet* 1999; 26: 361–72.
26. Donner H, Seidl C, van der Auwera B, Braun J, Siegmund T, Herwig J, Weets I, the Belgian Diabetes Registry, Usadel KH, Badenhoop K. HLA-DRB1*04 and susceptibility to type 1 diabetes mellitus in a German/Belgian family and German case/control study. *Tissue Antigens* 2000; 55: 271–4.
27. Undlien DE, Friede T, Rammensee HG, Joner G, Dahl-Jorgensen K, Sovik O, Akselsen HE, Knutsen I, Ronningen KS, Thorsby E. HLA-encoded genetic predisposition in IDDM. DR4 subtypes may be associated with different degrees of protection. *Diabetes* 1997; 46: 143–9.
28. Roep BO, Schipper R, Verduyn W, Bruining GJ, Schreuder GMT, de Vries RRP. HLA-DRB1*0403 is associated with dominant protection against IDDM in the general Dutch population and subjects with high-risk DQA1*0301-DQB1*0302/DQA1*0501-DQB1*0201 genotype. *Tissue Antigens* 1999; 54: 88–90.
29. Van der Auwera B, van Waeyenberge C, Schuit F, Heimberg H, Vandewalle C, Gorus F, Flament J. DRB1*0403 protects against IDDM in Caucasians with the high-risk heterozygous DQA1*0301-DQB1*0302/DQA1*0501-DQB1*0201 genotype. Belgian Diabetes Registry. *Diabetes* 1995; 44: 527–30.
30. Cavan DA, Bain SC, Barnett AH. The genetics of type 1 (insulin-dependent) diabetes mellitus. *J Med Genet* 1992; 29: 441–6.
31. Mijovic C, Jenkins D, Jacobs K, Penny MA, Fletcher J, Barnett AH. HLA-DQA1 and DQB1 alleles are associated with genetic susceptibility to type 1 diabetes in a Black population. *Diabetes* 1991; 40: 748–53.
32. Noble JA, Valdes AM, Thomson G, Erlich HA. The HLA class II locus DPB1 can influence susceptibility to type 1 diabetes. *Diabetes* 2000; 49: 121–5.
33. Nejentsev S, Reijonen H, Adojaan B, Kovalchuk L, Sochnevs A, Schwartz EI, Akerblom HK, Ilonen J. The effect of HLA-B allele on the IDDM risk defined by DRB1*04 subtypes and DQB1*0302. *Diabetes* 1997; 46: 1888–92.
34. Undlien DE, Kockum I, Ronningen KS, Lowe R, Sanjeevi CB, Graham J, Lie BA, Akselsen HE, Lernmark A, Thorsby E. HLA associations in type 1 diabetes among patients not carrying high-risk DR3-DQ2 or DR4-DQ8 haplotypes. *Tissue Antigens* 1999; 54: 543–51.
35. Kawasaki E, Noble J, Erlich H, Mulgrew CL, Fain PR, Eisenbarth GS. Transmission of DQ haplotypes to patients with type 1 diabetes. *Diabetes* 1998; 47: 1971–3.
36. Kawabata Y, Ikegami H, Kawaguchi Y, Fujisawa T, Shintani M, Ono M, Nishino M, Uchigata Y, Lee I, Ogihara T. Asian-specific HLA haplotypes reveal heterogeneity of the contribution of HLA-DR and -DQ haplotypes to susceptibility to type 1 diabetes. *Diabetes* 2002; 51: 545–51.
37. Redondo MJ, Kawasaki E, Mulgrew CL, Noble JA, Erlich HA, Freed BM, Lie BA, Thorsby E, Eisenbarth GS, Undlien DE, Ronningen KS. DR- and DQ-associated protection from type 1A diabetes: comparison of DRB1*1401 and DQA1*0102-DQB1*0602. *J Clin Endocrinol Metab* 2000; 85: 3793–7.
38. Baisch JM, Weeks T, Giles R, Hoover M, Stastny P, Capra JD. Analysis of HLA-DQ genotypes and susceptibility in insulin-dependent diabetes mellitus. *N Engl J Med* 1990; 322: 1836–41.
39. Pugliese A, Gianani R, Moromisato R, Awdeh ZL, Alper CA, Erlich HA, Jackson RA, Eisenbarth GS. HLA-DQB1*0602 is associated with dominant protection from diabetes even among islet cell antibody-positive first-degree relatives of patients with IDDM. *Diabetes* 1995; 44: 608–13.
40. Pugliese A, Kawasaki E, Zeller M, Yu L, Babu S, Solimena M, Moraes CT, Pietropaolo M, Friday RP, Trucco M, Ricordi C, Allen M, Noble JA, Erlich HA, Eisenbarth GS. Sequence analysis of the diabetes-protective human leukocyte antigen-DQB1*0602 allele in unaffected, islet cell antibody-positive first-degree relatives and in rare patients with type 1 diabetes. *J Clin Endocrinol Metab* 1999; 84: 1722–8.
41. Rayner ML, Kelly MA, Mijovic CH, Barnett AH. Sequencing of the second exon of the MHC class II DQ6 alleles in patients with type 1 diabetes. *Autoimmunity* 2002; 35: 155–7.
42. Park YS, She JX, Noble JA, Erlich HA, Eisenbarth GS. Transracial evidence for the influence of the homologous HLA DR-DQ haplotype on transmission of HLA DR4

haplotypes to diabetic children. *Tissue Antigens* 2001; 57: 185–91.

43. Schipper RF, Koeleman BPC, Bruining GJ, Schreuder GMT, Verduijn W, de Vries RRP, Roep BO. HLA class II associations with type 1 diabetes mellitus: a multivariate approach. *Tissue Antigens* 2001; 57: 144–50.
44. Chuang LM, Wu HP, Tsai WY, Lin BJ, Tai TY. Transcomplementation of HLA DQA1-DQB1 in DR3/DR4 and DR3/DR9 heterozygotes and IDDM in Taiwanese families. *Diabetes Care* 1995; 18: 1483–6.
45. Ronningen KS, Keiding N, Green A for the EURODIAB ACE Study Group. Europe and Diabetes. Correlations between the incidence of childhood-onset type 1 diabetes in Europe and HLA genotypes. *Diabetologia* 2001; 44 (suppl 3): B51–9.
46. Ionescu-Tirgoviste C, Guja C, Herr M, Cucca E, Welsh K, Bunce M, Marshall S, Todd JA. Low frequency of HLA DRB1*03-DQB1*02 and DQB1*0302 haplotypes in Romania is consistent with the country's low incidence of type 1 diabetes. *Diabetologia* 2001; 44 (suppl 3): B60–6.
47. Petrone A, Bugawan TL, Mesturino CA, Nistico L, Galgani A, Giorgi G, Cascino I, Erlich HA, Di Mario U, Buzzetti R. The distribution of HLA class II susceptible/protective haplotypes could partially explain the low incidence of type 1 diabetes in continental Italy (Lazio region). *Tissue Antigens* 2001; 58: 385–94.
48. Hermann R, Mijovic CH, Rayner M, Croft N, Kelly MA, Jenkins D, Soltesz G, Barnett AH. HLA alleles and IDDM in children in Hungary: a comparison with Finland. *Hum Immunol* 2001; 62: 391–8.
49. Park Y, Eisenbarth GS. Genetic susceptibility factors of type 1 diabetes in Asians. *Diabetes Metab Res Rev* 2001; 17: 2–11.
50. Caillat-Zucman S, Garchon H-J, Timsit J, Assan R, Boitard C, Djilali-Saiah I, Bougneres P, Bach JF. Age dependent HLA genetic heterogeneity of type 1 insulin-dependent diabetes mellitus. *J Clin Invest* 1992; 90: 2242–50.
51. Graham J, Kockum I, Sanjeevi CB, Landin-Olsson M, Nystrom L, Sundkvist G, Arnqvist H, Blohme G, Lithner F, Littorin B, Schersten B, Wibell L, Ostman J, Lernmark A, Breslow N, Dahlquist G, the Swedish Childhood Diabetes Study Group. Negative association between type 1 diabetes and HLA DQB1*0602-DQA1*0102 is attenuated with age at onset. *Eur J Immunogenet* 1999; 26: 117–27.
52. Valdes AM, Thomson G, Erlich HA, Noble JA. Association between type 1 diabetes age of onset and HLA among sibling pairs. *Diabetes* 1999; 48: 1658–61.
53. Michelsen B, Lernmark A. Molecular cloning of a polymorphic DNA endonuclease fragment that associates insulin-dependent diabetes with HLA-DQ. *J Clin Invest* 1987; 79: 1144–52.
54. Todd JA, Bell JI, McDevitt HO. HLA-DQβ gene contributes to susceptibility and resistance to insulin-dependent diabetes mellitus. *Nature* 1987; 329: 599–604.
55. Horn GT, Bugawan TL, Long CM, Erlich HA. Allelic sequence variation of the HLA-DQ loci. Relationship to serology and to insulin-dependent diabetes susceptibility. *Proc Natl Acad Sci USA* 1988; 85: 6012–6.
56. Acha-Orbea H, McDevitt HO. The first external domain of the nonobese diabetic mouse class II I-A beta chain is unique. *Proc Natl Acad Sci USA* 1987; 84: 2435–9.
57. Lund T, O'Reilly L, Hutchings P, Kanagawa O, Simpson E, Gravely R, Chandler P, Dyson J, Picard JK, Edwards A, Kioussis D, Cooke A. Prevention of insulin-dependent diabetes mellitus in non-obese diabetic mice by transgenes encoding modified I-A beta-chain or normal I-E alpha-chain. *Nature* 1990; 345: 727–9.
58. Singer SM, Tisch R, Yang XD, Sytwu HK, Liblau R, McDevitt HO. Prevention of diabetes in NOD mice by a mutated I-Aβ transgene. *Diabetes* 1998; 47: 1570–7.
59. Brown JH, Jardetzky TS, Gorga JC, Stern LJ, Urban RG, Strominger JL, Wiley DC. Three-dimensional structure of the human class II histocompatibility antigen HLA-DR1. *Nature* 1993; 364: 33–9.
60. Kelly MA, Rayner ML, Mijovic CH, Barnett AH. Molecular aspects of type 1 diabetes. *Mol Pathol* 2003; 56: 1–10.
61. Lundin KEA, Gaudernack G, Qvigstad E, Sollid LM, Thorsby E. T-lymphocyte clones recognising an HLA-DQw3.2-associated epitope involving residue 57 on the DQβ chain. *Hum Immunol* 1988; 22: 235–46.
62. Nepom BS, Nepom GT, Coleman M, Kwok WW. Critical contribution of β chain residue 57 in peptide binding ability of both HLA-DR and -DQ molecules. *Proc Natl Acad Sci USA* 1996; 93: 7202–6.
63. Reichstetter S, Papadopoulos GK, Moustakas AK, Swanson E, Liu A, Beheray S, Ettinger RA, Nepom GT, Kwok WW. Mutational analysis of critical residues determining antigen presentation and activation of HLA-DQ0602 restricted T-cell clones. *Hum Immunol* 2002; 63: 185–93.
64. Yamagata K, Nakajima H, Hanafusa T, Noguchi T, Miyazaki A, Miyagawa J, Sada M, Amemiya H, Tanaka T, Kono N, Tarui S. Aspartic acid at position 57 of DQ beta chain does not protect against type 1 (insulin-dependent) diabetes mellitus in Japanese subjects. *Diabetologia* 1989; 32: 762–4.
65. Awata T, Kuzuya T, Matsuda A, Iwamoto Y, Kanazawa Y, Okuyama M, Juji T. High frequency of aspartic acid at position 57 of HLA-DQβ chain in Japanese IDDM patients and non-diabetic subjects. *Diabetes* 1990; 39: 266–9.
66. Penny MA, Jenkins D, Mijovic CH, Jacobs KH, Cavan DA, Yeung VTF, Cockram CS, Hawkins BR, Fletcher JA, Barnett AH. Susceptibility to insulin-dependent diabetes in a Chinese population: role of HLA class II alleles. *Diabetes* 1992; 41: 914–9.
67. Khalil I, d'Auriol L, Gobet M, Morin L, Lepage V, Deschamps I, Park MS, Degos L, Galibert F, Hors J. A combination of HLA-DQ beta Asp57-negative and HLA-DQ alpha Arg52 confers susceptibility to insulin-dependent diabetes mellitus. *J Clin Invest* 1990; 85: 1315–9.
68. Valdes AM, McWeeney S, Thomson G. HLA class II DR-DQ amino acids and insulin-dependent diabetes mellitus: application of the haplotype method. *Am J Hum Genet* 1997; 60: 717–28.
69. Djoulah S, Busson M, Sasazuki T, Maillere B, Yasunaga S, Kimura A, Charron D, Hors J. A new predictive model for insulin-dependent diabetes mellitus susceptibility based on combinations of molecular HLA-DRB1 and HLA-DQB1 pockets. *Tissue Antigens* 1999; 54: 341–8.
70. Abraham RS, Kudva YC, Wilson SB, Strominger JL, David CS. Co-expression of HLA DR3 and DQ8 results in the development of spontaneous insulitis and loss of tolerance to GAD65 in transgenic mice. *Diabetes* 2000; 49: 548–54.

71. Abraham RS, Wen L, Marietta EV, David CS. Type 1 diabetes-predisposing MHC alleles influence the selection of glutamic acid decarboxylase (GAD) 65-specific T cells in a transgenic model. *J Immunol* 2001; 166: 1370–9.
72. Wen L, Wong FS, Tang J, Chen NY, Altieri M, David C, Flavell R, Sherwin R. *In vivo* evidence for the contribution of human histocompatibility leukocyte antigen (HLA)-DQ molecules to the development of diabetes. *J Exp Med* 2000; 191: 97–104.
73. Wen L, Chen N-Y, Tang J, Sherwin R, Wong FS. The regulatory role of DR4 in a spontaneous diabetes DQ8 transgenic model. *J Clin Invest* 2001; 107: 871–80.
74. Cucca F, Lampis R, Congia M, et al. A correlation between the relative predisposition of MHC class II alleles to type 1 diabetes and the structure of their proteins. *Hum Mol Genet* 2001; 10: 2025–37.
75. Lee KH, Wucherpfennig KW, Wiley DC. Structure of a human insulin peptide-HLA-DQ8 complex and susceptibility to type 1 diabetes. *Nat Immunol* 2001; 2: 501–7.
76. Sato AK, Sturniolo T, Sinigaglia F, Stern LJ. Substitution of aspartic acid at β57 with alanine alters MHC class II peptide binding activity but not protein stability: HLA-DQ(α1*0201,β1*0302) and (α1*0201,β1*0303). *Hum Immunol* 1999; 60: 1227–36.
77. Ettinger RA, Liu AW, Nepom GT, Kwok WW. β57-Asp plays an essential role in the unique SDS stability of HLA-DQA1*0102/DQB1*0602 αβ protein dimer, the class II MHC allele associated with protection from insulin-dependent diabetes mellitus. *J Immunol* 2000; 165: 3232–8.
78. Ettinger RA, Kwok WW. A peptide binding motif for HLA-DQA1*0102/DQB1*0602, the class II MHC molecule associated with dominant protection in insulin-dependent diabetes mellitus. *J Immunol* 1998; 160: 2365–73.
79. Vartdal F, Johansen BH, Friede T, Thorpe CJ, Stevanovic S, Eriksen JE, Sletten K, Thorsby E, Rammensee HG, Sollid LM. The peptide binding motif of the disease associated HLA-DQ (alpha 1*0501, beta 1*0201) molecule. *Eur J Immunol* 1996; 26: 2764–72.
80. Ettinger RA, Liu AW, Nepom GT, Kwok WW. Exceptional stability of the HLA-DQA1*0102/DQB1*0602 αβ protein dimer, the class II MHC molecule associated with protection from insulin-dependent diabetes mellitus. *J Immunol* 1998; 161: 6439–45.
81. Nepom GT, Kwok WW. Molecular basis for HLA-DQ associations with IDDM. *Diabetes* 1998; 47: 1177–84.
82. Schmidt D, Verdaguer J, Averill N, Santamaria P. A mechanism for the major histocompatibility complex-linked resistance to autoimmunity. *J Exp Med* 1997; 186: 1059–75.
83. Luhder F, Katz J, Benoist C, Mathis D. Major histocompatibility complex class II molecules can protect from diabetes by positively selecting T cells with additional specificities. *J Exp Med* 1998; 187: 379–87.
84. Cucca F, Congia M, Trowsdale J, Powis SH. Insulin-dependent diabetes mellitus and the major histocompatibility complex peptide transporters TAP1 and TAP2: no association in a population with a high disease incidence. *Tissue Antigens* 1994; 44: 234–40.
85. Undlien DE, Akselsen HE, Joner G, Dahl-Jorgensen K, Sovik O, Ronningen KS, Thorsby E. No independent associations of LMP2 and LMP7 polymorphisms with susceptibility to develop IDDM. *Diabetes* 1997; 46: 307–12.
86. Cucca F, Dudbridge F, Loddo M, Mulargia AP, Lampis R, Angius E, De Virgiliis S, Koeleman BPC, Bain SC, Barnett AH, Gilchrist F, Cordell H, Welsh K, Todd JA. The HLA-DPB1-associated component of the IDDM1 and its relationship to the major loci HLA-DQB1, -DQA1 and -DRB1. *Diabetes* 2001; 50: 1200–5.
87. Valdes AM, Noble JA, Genin E, Clerget-Darpoux F, Erlich HA, Thomson G. Modeling of HLA class II susceptibility to type 1 diabetes reveals an effect associated with DPB1. *Genet Epidemiol* 2001; 21: 212–23.
88. Lie BA, Todd JA, Pociot F, Nerup J, Akselsen HE, Joner G, Dahl-Jorgensen K, Ronningen KS, Thorsby E, Undlien DE. The predisposition to type 1 diabetes linked to the human leukocyte antigen complex includes at least one non-class II gene. *Am J Hum Genet* 1999; 64: 793–800.
89. Moghaddam PH, de Knijf P, Roep BO, van der Auwera B, Naipal A, Gorus F, Schuit F, Giphart MJ, the Belgian Diabetes Registry. Genetic structure of IDDM1. Two separate regions in the major histocompatibility complex contribute to susceptibility or protection. *Diabetes* 1998; 47: 263–9.
90. Pociot F, Briant L, Jongeneel CV, Molvig J, Worsaae H, Abbal M, Thomsen M, Nerup J, Cambon-Thomsen A. Association of tumor necrosis factor (TNF) and class II major histocompatibility complex alleles with the secretion of TNF-alpha and TNF-beta by human mononuclear cells: a possible link to insulin-dependent diabetes mellitus. *Eur J Immunol* 1993; 23: 224–31.
91. Moghaddam PH, Zwinderman AH, de Knijf P, Roep BO, Schipper RF, van der Auwera B, Naipal A, Gorus F, Schuit F, Giphart MJ, for the Belgian Diabetes Registry. TNFa microsatellite polymorphism modulates the risk of IDDM in Caucasians with the high-risk genotype HLA DQA1*0501-DQB1*0201/DQA1*0301-DQB1*0302. *Diabetes* 1997; 46: 1514–5.
92. Monos DS, Kamoun M, Udalova IA, Csanky E, Cizman B, Turetskaya RL, Smirnova JB, Zharkov VG, Gasser D, Zmijewski CM, Spielman RS, Nedospasov SA. Genetic polymorphism of the human tumor necrosis factor region in insulin-dependent diabetes mellitus. Linkage disequilibrium of TNFab microsatellite alleles with HLA haplotypes. *Hum Immunol* 1995; 44: 70–9.
93. Koeleman BP, Herr MH, Zavattari P, Dudbridge F, March R, Campbell D, Barnett AH, Bain SC, Mulargia AP, Loddo M, Amos W, Cucca F, Todd JA. Conditional ETDT analysis of the human leukocyte antigen region in type 1 diabetes. *Ann Hum Genet* 2000; 64: 215–21.
94. Cheong KY, Allcock RJN, Eerligh P, Witt CS, Christiansen FT, McCann V, Price P. Localization of central MHC genes influencing type 1 diabetes. *Hum Immunol* 2001; 62: 1363–70.
95. Gambelunge G, Ghaderi M, Cosentino A, Falorni Ad, Brunetti P, Falorni Al, Sanjeevi CB. Association of MHC Class I chain-related A (MIC-A) gene polymorphism with type 1 diabetes. *Diabetologia* 2000; 43: 507–14.
96. Lee YJ, Huang FY, Wang CH, Lo FS, Tsan KW, Hsu CH, Huang C, Chang SC, Chang JG. Polymorphism in the transmembrane region of the MICA gene and type 1 diabetes. *J Pediatr Endocrinol Metab* 2000; 13: 489–96.
97. Park Y, Lee H, Sanjeevi CB, Eisenbarth GS. MICA polymorphism is associated with type 1 diabetes in the Korean population. *Diabetes Care* 2001; 24: 33–8.
98. Nejentsev S, Gombos Z, Laine A-P, Veijola R, Knip M, Simell O, Vaarala O, Akerblom HK, Ilonen J. Non-class II HLA gene associated with type 1 diabetes maps to the

240-kb region near HLA-B. *Diabetes* 2000; 49: 2217–21.

99. Zavattari P, Lampis R, Motzo C, Loddo M, Mulargia A, Whalen M, Maioli M, Angius E, Todd JA, Cucca F. Conditional linkage disequilibrium analysis of a complex disease superlocus, IDDM1 in the HLA region, reveals the presence of independent modifying gene effects influencing the type 1 diabetes risk encoded by the major HLA-DQB1, -DRB1 disease loci. *Hum Mol Genet* 2001; 10: 881–9.
100. Siegmund T, Donner H, Braun J, Usadel KH, Badenhoop K. HLA-DMA and HLA-DMB alleles in German patients with type 1 diabetes mellitus. *Tissue Antigens* 1999; 54: 291–4.
101. Palmer JP, Asplin CM, Clemons P, Lyen K, Tatpati O, Raghu PK, Paquette TL. Insulin antibodies in insulin-dependent diabetics before insulin treatment. *Science* 1983; 222: 1337–9.
102. Hitman GA, Tarn AC, Winter RM, Drummond V, Williams LG, Jowett NI, Bottazzo GF, Galton DJ. Type 1 (insulin-dependent) diabetes and a highly variable locus close to the insulin gene on chromosome 11. *Diabetologia* 1985; 28: 218–22.
103. Lucassen AM, Julier C, Beressi JP, Boitard C, Froguel P, Lathrop M, Bell JI. Susceptibility to insulin dependent diabetes mellitus maps to a 4.1kb segment of DNA spanning the insulin gene and associated VNTR. *Nat Genet* 1993; 4: 305–10.
104. Bennett ST, Lucassen AM, Gough SCL, Powell EE, Undlien DE, Pritchard LE, Merriman ME, Kawaguchi Y, Dronsfield MJ, Pociot F, Nerup J, Bouzekri N, Cambon-Thomsen A, Ronningen KS, Barnett AH, Bain SC, Todd JA. Susceptibility to human type 1 diabetes at IDDM2 is determined by tandem repeat variation at the insulin gene minisatellite locus. *Nat Genet* 1995; 9: 284–92.
105. Bennett ST, Wilson AJ, Cucca F, Nerup J, Pociot F, McKinney PA, Barnett AH, Bain SC, Todd JA. IDDM2-VNTR-encoded susceptibility to type 1 diabetes: dominant protection and parental transmission of alleles of the insulin gene-linked minisatellite locus. *J Autoimmun* 1996; 9: 415–21.
106. Bennett ST, Wilson AJ, Esposito L, Bouzekri N, Undlien DE, Cucca F, Nistico L, Buzzetti R, Bosi E, Pociot F, Nerup J, Cambon-Thomsen A, Pugliese A, Shield JP, McKinney PA, Bain SC, Polychronakos C, Todd JA, for the IMDIAB Group. Insulin VNTR allele-specific effect in type 1 diabetes depends on identity of untransmitted paternal allele. *Nat Genet* 1997; 17: 350–2.
107. Stead JD, Buard J, Todd JA, Jeffreys AJ. Influence of allele lineage on the role of the insulin minisatellite in susceptibility to type 1 diabetes. *Hum Mol Genet* 2000; 9: 2929–35.
108. Vafiadis P, Ounissi-Benkalha H, Palumbo M, Grabs R, Rousseau M, Goodyer CG, Polychronakos C. Class III alleles of the variable number of tandem repeat insulin polymorphism associated with silencing of thymic insulin predispose to type 1 diabetes. *J Clin Endocrinol Metab* 2001; 86: 3705–10.
109. Cox NJ, Baker L, Spielman RS. Insulin gene sharing in sib pairs with insulin-dependent diabetes mellitus: no evidence for linkage. *Am J Hum Genet* 1988; 42: 167–72.
110. Field LL. Genes predisposing to IDDM in multiplex families. *Genet Epidemiol* 1989; 6: 101–6.
111. Julier C, Hyer RN, Davies J, Merlin F, Soularue P, Briant L, Cathelineau G, Deschamps I, Rotter JI, Froguel P, Boitard C, Bell JI, Lathrop GM. Insulin-IGF2 region on chromosome 11p encodes a gene implicated in HLA-DR4-dependent diabetes susceptibility. *Nature* 1991; 354: 155–9.
112. Bain SC, Prins JB, Hearne CM, Rodrigues NR, Rowe BR, Pritchard LE, Ritchie RJ, Hall JRS, Undlien DE, Ronningen KS, Dunger DB, Barnett AH, Todd JA. Insulin gene region-encoded susceptibility to type 1 diabetes is not restricted to HLA-DR4-positive individuals. *Nat Genet* 1992; 2: 212–5.
113. Van der Auwera BJ, Heimberg H, Schrevens AF, Waayenberge CV, Flament J, Schuit FC. 5′ insulin gene polymorphism confers risk to IDDM independently of HLA-class II susceptibility. *Diabetes* 1993; 42: 851–4.
114. Spielman RS, McGinnis RE, Ewens WJ. Transmission test for linkage disequilibrium: the insulin gene region and insulin-dependent diabetes mellitus (IDDM). *Am J Hum Genet* 1993; 52: 506–16.
115. The European Consortium for IDDM Genome Studies. A genomewide scan for type 1-diabetes susceptibility in Scandinavian families: identification of new loci with evidence of interaction. *Am J Hum Genet* 2001; 69: 1301–13.
116. Vafiadis P, Bennett ST, Colle E, Grabs R, Goodyer CG, Polychronakos C. Imprinted and genotype-specific expression of genes at the *IDDM2* locus in pancreas and leucocytes. *J Autoimmun* 1996; 9: 397–403.
117. Vafiadis P, Bennett ST, Todd JA, Nadeau J, Grabs R, Goodyer CG, Wickramasinghe S, Colle E, Polychronakos C. Insulin expression in human thymus is modulated by *INS VNTR* alleles at the *IDDM2* locus. *Nat Genet* 1997; 15: 289–92.
118. Pugliese A, Zeller M, Fernandez A Jr, Zalcberg LJ, Bartlett RJ, Ricordi C, Pietropaolo M, Eisenbarth GS, Bennett ST, Patel DD. The insulin gene is transcribed in the human thymus and transcription levels correlated with allelic variation at the *INS VNTR-IDDM2* susceptibility locus for type 1 diabetes. *Nat Genet* 1997; 15: 293–7.
119. Chentoufi AA, Polychronakos C. Insulin expression levels in the thymus modulate insulin-specific autoreactive T-cell tolerance: the mechanism by which the *IDDM2* locus may predispose to diabetes. *Diabetes* 2002; 51: 1383–90.
120. Sarugeri E, Dozio N, Belloni C, Meschi F, Pastore MR, Bonifacio E. Autoimmune responses to the β-cell autoantigen, insulin, and the *INS VNTR-IDDM2* locus. *Clin Exp Immunol* 1998; 114: 370–6.
121. Giannoukakis N, Deal C, Paquette J, Goodyer CG, Polychronakos C. Parental genomic imprinting of the human IGF2 gene. *Nat Genet* 1993; 4: 98–101.
122. Vafiadis P, Grabs R, Goodyer CG, Colle E, Polychronakos C. A functional analysis of the role of *IGF2* in *IDDM2*-encoded susceptibility to type 1 diabetes. *Diabetes* 1998; 47: 831–6.
123. Vafiadis P, Bennett ST, Todd JA, Grabs R, Polychronakos C. Divergence between genetic determinants of *IGF2* transcription levels in leukocytes and of *IDDM2*-encoded susceptibility to type 1 diabetes. *J Clin Endocrinol Metab* 1998; 83: 2933–9.
124. Paquette J, Giannoukakis N, Polychronakos C, Vafiadis P, Deal C. The INS 5′ variable number of tandem repeats is associated with *IGF2* expression in humans. *J Biol Chem* 1998; 273: 14158–63.
125. Dahlquist G, Bennich SS, Kallen B. Intrauterine growth pattern and risk of childhood onset insulin dependent

(type 1) diabetes: population based case-control study. *BMJ* 1996; 313: 1174–7.

126. Field LL. Genetic linkage and association studies of type 1 diabetes: challenges and rewards. *Diabetologia* 2002; 45: 21–35.
127. Luo DF, Buzzetti R, Rotter JI, Maclaren NK, Raffel LJ, Nistico L, Giovannini C, Pozzilli P, Thomson G, She JX. Confirmation of three susceptibility genes to insulin-dependent diabetes mellitus: *IDDM4*, *IDDM5* and *IDDM8*. *Hum Mol Genet* 1996; 5: 693–8.
128. Merriman T, Twells R, Merriman M, Eaves I, Cox R, Cucca F, McKinney P, Shield J, Baum D, Bosi E, Pozzilli P, Nistico L, Buzzetti R, Joner G, Ronningen K, Thorsby E, Undlien D, Pociot F, Nerup J, Bain S, Barnett A, Todd J. Evidence by allelic association-dependent methods for a type 1 diabetes polygene (*IDDM6*) on chromosome 18q21. *Hum Mol Genet* 1997; 6: 1003–10.
129. Paterson AD, Petronis A. Age and sex based genetic locus heterogeneity in type 1 diabetes. *J Med Genet* 2000; 37: 186–91.
130. Paterson AD, Petronis A. Sex of affected sibpairs and genetic linkage to type 1 diabetes. *Am J Med Genet* 1999; 84: 15–9.
131. Paterson AD, Naimark DM, Petronis A. The analysis of parental origin of alleles may detect susceptibility loci for complex disorders. *Hum Hered* 1999; 49: 197–204.
132. Cucca F, Goy JV, Kawaguchi Y, Esposito L, Merriman ME, Wilson AJ, Cordell HJ, Bain SC, Todd JA. A male-female bias in type 1 diabetes and linkage to chromosome Xp in MHC HLA-DR3-positive patients. *Nat Genet* 1998; 19: 301–2.
133. Owerbach D. Physical and genetic mapping of *IDDM8* on chromosome 6q27. *Diabetes* 2000; 49: 508–12.
134. Nakagawa Y, Kawaguchi Y, Twells RCJ, Muxworthy C, Hunter KMD, Wilson A, Merriman ME, Cox RD, Merriman T, Cucca F, McKinney PA, Shield JPH, Tuomilehto J, Tuomilehto-Wolf E, Ionesco-Tirgoviste C, Nistico L, Buzzetti R, Pozzilli P, San-Raffaele Family Study, Joner G, Thorsby E, Undlien DE, Pociot F, Nerup J, Ronningen KS, Bart's-Oxford Family Study Group, Bain SC, Todd JA. Fine mapping of the diabetes-susceptibility locus, *IDDM4*, on chromosome 11q13. *Am J Hum Genet* 1998; 63: 547–56.
135. Eckenrode S, Marron MP, Nicholls R, Yang MCK, Yang JJ, Guida Fonseca LC, She JX. Fine-mapping of the type 1 diabetes locus (*IDDM4*) on chromosome 11q and evaluation of two candidate genes (*FADD* and *GALN*) by affected sibpair and linkage-disequilibrium analyses. *Hum Genet* 2000; 106: 14–8.
136. Marron MP, Zeidler A, Raffel LJ, Eckenrode SE, Yang JJ, Hopkins DI, Garchon HJ, Jacob CO, Serrano-Rios M, Martinez Larrad MT, Park Y, Bach JF, Rotter JI, Yang MC, She JX. Genetic and physical mapping of a type 1 diabetes susceptibility gene (*IDDM12*) to a 100-kb phagemid artificial chromosome clone containing D2S72-CTLA4-D2S105 on chromosome 2q33. *Diabetes* 2000; 49: 492–9.
137. Pociot F, Lorenzen T, Nerup J. A manganese superoxide dismutase (SOD2) gene polymorphism in insulin-dependent diabetes mellitus. *Dis Markers* 1993; 11: 267–74.
138. Pociot F, Larsen ZM, Zavattari P, Deidda E, Nerup J, Cattaneo M, Chiaramonte R, Comi P, Sabbadini M, Zollo M, Biunno I, Cucca F. No evidence for SEL1L as a candidate gene for *IDDM11*-conferred susceptibility. *Diabetes Metab Res Rev* 2001; 17: 292–5.
139. Esposito L, Hill NJ, Pritchard LE, Cucca F, Muxworthy C, Merriman ME, Wilson A, Julier C, Delepine M, Tuomilehto J, Tuomilehto-Wolf E, Ionesco-Tirgoviste C, Nistico L, the IMDIAB Group, Buzzetti R, Pozzilli P, Ferrari M, Bosi E, Pociot F, Nerup J, Bain SC, Todd JA. Genetic analysis of chromosome 2 in type 1 diabetes. Analysis of putative loci *IDDM7*, *IDDM12*, and *IDDM13* and candidate genes *NRAMP1* and *IA-2* and the interleukin-1 gene cluster. *Diabetes* 1998; 47: 1797–9.
140. Nishino M, Ikegami H, Kawaguchi Y, Fujisawa T, Kawabata Y, Shintani M, Ono M, Horiki M, Kawasaki E, Ogihara T. Polymorphism in gene for islet autoantigen, IA-2, and type 1 diabetes in Japanese subjects. *Hum Immunol* 2001; 62: 518–22.
141. Iwata I, Nagafuchi S, Nakashima H, Kondo S, Koga T, Yokogawa Y, Akashi T, Shibuya T, Umeno Y, Okeda T, Shibata S, Kono S, Yasunami M, Ohkubo H, Niho Y. Association of polymorphism in the NeuroD/BETA2 gene with type 1 diabetes in the Japanese. *Diabetes* 1999; 48: 416–9.
142. Dupont S, Dina C, Hani EH, Froguel P. Absence of replication in the French population of the association between beta2/NEUROD-A45T polymorphism and type 1 diabetes. *Diabetes Metab* 1999; 25: 516–7.
143. Hansen L, Jensen JN, Urioste S, Petersen HV, Pociot F, Eiberg H, Kristiansen OP, Hansen T, Serup P, Nerup J, Pedersen O. NeuroD/BETA2 gene variability and diabetes: no associations to late-onset type 2 diabetes but an A45-allele may represent a susceptibility marker for type 1 diabetes among Danes. *Diabetes* 2000; 49: 876–8.
144. Nistico L, Buzzetti R, Pritchard LE, Giovannini C, Bosi E, Larrad MT, Rios MS, Chow CC, Cockram CS, Jacobs K, Mijovic C, Bain SC, Barnett AH, Vandewalle CL, Schuit F, Gorus FK, Tosi R, Pozzilli P, Todd JA. The CTLA-4 gene region of chromosome 2q33 is linked to, and associated with, type 1 diabetes. Belgian Diabetes Registry. *Hum Mol Genet* 1996; 5: 1075–80.
145. Marron MP, Raffel LJ, Garchon HJ, Jacob CO, Serrano-Rios M, Martinez Larrad MT, Teng WP, Park Y, Zhang ZX, Goldstein DR, Tao YW, Beaurain G, Bach JF, Huang HS, Luo DF, Zeidler A, Rotter JI, Yang MC, Modilevsky T, Maclaren NK, She JX. Insulin-dependent diabetes mellitus (IDDM) is associated with CTLA4 polymorphisms in multiple ethnic groups. *Hum Mol Genet* 1997; 6: 1275–82.
146. Ihara K, Ahmed S, Nakao F, Kinukawa N, Kuromaru R, Matsuura N, Iwata I, Nagafuchi S, Kohno H, Miyako K, Hara T. Association studies of *CTLA-4*, *CD28*, and *ICOS* gene polymorphisms with type 1 diabetes in the Japanese population. *Immunoge-netics* 2001; 53: 447–54.
147. McCormack RM, Maxwell AP, Carson D, Patterson CC, Bingham A, Savage DA. Possible association between CTLA4 DNA polymorphisms and early onset type 1 diabetes in a UK population. *Genes Immun* 2001; 2: 233–5.
148. Lowe RM, Graham J, Sund G, Kockum I, Landin-Olsson M, Schaefer JB, Torn C, Lernmark A, Dahlquist G. The length of the CTLA-4 microsatellite (AT)n-repeat affects the risk for type 1 diabetes. *Autoimmunity* 2000; 32: 173–80.
149. Awata T, Kurihara S, Iitaka M, Takei S, Inoue I, Ishii C, Negishi K, Izumida T, Yoshida Y, Hagura R, Kuzuya N, Kanazawa Y, Katayama S. Association of *CTLA-4* gene A-G polymorphism (*IDDM12* locus) with

acute-onset and insulin-depleted IDDM as well as autoimmune thyroid disease (Graves' disease and Hashimoto's thyroiditis) in the Japanese population. *Diabetes* 1998; 47: 128–9.

150. Naluai AT, Nilsson S, Samuelsson L, Gudjonsdottir AH, Ascher H, Ek J, Hallberg B, Kristiansson B, Martinsson T, Nerman O, Sollid LM, Wahlstrom J. The CTLA4/CD28 gene region on chromosome 2q33 confers susceptibility to celiac disease in a way possibly distinct from that of type 1 diabetes and other chronic inflammatory disorders. *Tissue Antigens* 2000; 56: 350–5.
151. Harbo HF, Celius EG, Vartdal F, Spurkland A. CTLA4 promoter and exon 1 dimorphisms in multiple sclerosis. *Tissue Antigens* 1999; 53: 106–10.
152. Gonzalez-Escribano MF, Rodriguez R, Valenzuela A, Garcia A, Garcia-Lozano JR, Nunez-Roldan A. CTLA4 polymorphisms in Spanish patients with rheumatoid arthritis. *Tissue Antigens* 1999; 53: 296–300.
153. Todd JA, Aitman TJ, Cornall RJ, Ghosh S, Hall JRS, Hearne CM, Knight AM, Love JM, McAleer MA, Prins JB, Rodrigues N, Lathrop M, Pressey A, DeLarato NH, Peterson LB, Wicker LS. Genetic analysis of autoimmune type 1 diabetes mellitus in mice. *Nature* 1991; 351: 542–7.
154. Lyons PA, Armitage N, Lord CJ, Phillips MS, Todd JA, Peterson LB, Wicker LS. Mapping by genetic interaction: high-resolution congenic mapping of the type 1 diabetes loci Idd10 and Idd18 in the NOD mouse. *Diabetes* 2001; 50: 2633–7.
155. Cornall RJ, Prins JB, Todd JA, Pressey A, DeLarato NH, Wicker LS, Peterson LB. Type 1 diabetes in mice is linked to the interleukin-1 receptor and Lsh/Ity/Bcg genes on chromosome 1. *Nature* 1991; 353: 262–5.
156. Copeman JB, Cucca F, Hearne CM, Cornall RJ, Reed PW, Ronningen KS, Undlien DE, Nistico L, Buzzetti R, Tosi R, Pociot F, Nerup J, Cornelis F, Barnett AH, Bain SC, Todd JA. Linkage disequilibrium mapping of a type 1 diabetes susceptibility gene (*IDDM7*) to chromosome 2q31-q33. *Nat Genet* 1995; 9: 80–5.
157. Morahan G, Huang D, Tait B, Colman P, Harrison L. Markers on distal chromosome 2q linked to insulin-dependent diabetes mellitus. *Science* 1996; 272: 1811–3.
158. Morahan G, Huang D, Ymer SI, Cancilla MR, Stephen K, Dabadghao P, Werther G, Tait BD, Harrison LC, Colman PG. Linkage disequilibrium of a type 1 diabetes susceptibility locus with a regulatory *IL12B* allele. *Nat Genet* 2001; 27: 218–21.
159. Nistico L, Giorgi G, Giordano M, Galgani A, Petrone A, D'Alfonso S, Federici M, Di Mario U, Pozzilli P, Buzzetti R, Cascino I. IL12B polymorphism and type 1 diabetes in the Italian population: a case-control study. *Diabetes* 2002; 51: 1649–50.
160. Dahlman I, Eaves IA, Kosoy R, Morrison VA, Heward J, Gough SCL, Allahabadia A, Franklyn JA, Tuomilehto J, Tuomilehto-Wolf E, Cucca F, Guja C, Ionescu-Tirgoviste C, Stevens H, Carr P, Nutland S, McKinney P, Shield JP, Wang W, Cordell HJ, Walker N, Todd JA, Concannon P. Parameters for reliable results in genetic association studies in common disease. *Nat Genet* 2002; 30: 149–50.
161. Millward BA, Welsh KI, Leslie RDG, Pyke DA. T-cell receptor beta chain polymorphisms are associated with insulin-dependent diabetes. *Clin Exp Immunol* 1987; 70: 152–7.
162. Field LL. Non-HLA region genes in insulin-dependent diabetes mellitus. *Bailliere's Clin Endocrinol Metab* 1991; 5: 413–38.
163. Kristiansen OP, Zamani M, Johannesen J, Mandrup-Poulsen T, Cassiman JJ, Nerup J, Pociot F, for the Danish IDDM Epidemiology and Genetics Group and the Danish Study Group of Diabetes in Childhood. Linkage and association between a CD4 gene polymorphism and IDDM in Danish IDDM patients. *Diabetes* 1998; 47: 281–3.
164. Szalai C, Csaszar A, Czinner A, Szabo T, Panczel P, Madacsy L, Falus A. Chemokine receptor CCR2 and CCR5 polymorphisms in children with insulin-dependent diabetes mellitus. *Pediatr Res* 1999; 46: 82–4.
165. Pani MA, Knapp M, Donner H, Braun J, Baur MP, Usadel KH, Badenhoop K. Vitamin D receptor allele combinations influence genetic susceptibility to type 1 diabetes in Germans. *Diabetes* 2000; 49: 504–7.
166. Johannesen J, Pie A, Pociot F, Kristiansen OP, Karlsen AE, Nerup J, for the Danish Study Group of Diabetes in Childhood and the Danish Insulin-dependent Diabetes Mellitus Epidemiology and Genetics Group. Linkage of the human inducible nitric oxide synthase gene to type 1 diabetes. *J Clin Endocrinol Metab* 2001; 86: 2792–6.

29

Diabetes Secondary to Acquired Disease of the Pancreas

Stefano Del Prato*, Alberto Coppelli*, and Antonio Tiengo†

**University of Pisa, Pisa, Italy and †University of Padova, Padova, Italy*

INTRODUCTION

Secondary diabetes is a condition of persistent disturbance of glucose metabolism (hyperglycemia), which develops after the destruction of the pancreatic tissue by an acquired disease with subsequent impairment of exocrine and endocrine pancreatic functions. This condition is well recognized in the recent etiologic classification of diabetes mellitus proposed by the Expert Committee on the Diagnosis and Classification of Diabetes Mellitus of the American Diabetes Association [1] and reported in Table 1. The new classification includes the fibrocalculous pancreatopathy, a condition previously identified as a form of malnutrition-related diabetes.

The American Diabetes Association (ADA) [1] and World Health Organization (WHO) [2] Expert Committees have recently agreed on new diagnostic criteria for the diagnosis of diabetes. These changes are likely to influence the prevalence of diabetes in patients with diseases of the exocrine pancreas, but direct assessment using the new criteria is still too scanty. When the 1979 NDDG (National Diabetes Data Group) [3] and 1985 WHO [4] criteria are used, it can be calculated that diabetes secondary to disease of the exocrine pancreas represents, approximately, 0.5% of all cases of diabetes mellitus. Its frequency is likely to be twice as high in populations with heavy alcohol consumption. In the tropics, the prevalence of diabetes secondary to fibrocalculous pancreatitis can be as high as 10–20% [5].

In general, any pathologic process of the pancreatic acinar tissue results in an insult to its endocrine diffuse component, leading to some degree of hormone insufficiency. The main causes of pancreatic diabetes are listed in Table 1, while Table 2 summarizes the frequency of association between the various pathologic conditions and diabetes mellitus. The epidemiology and the hormonal, metabolic, and clinical implications of these forms of diabetes will be presented and discussed below, with the exception of fibrocalculous diabetes.

HISTORICAL NOTES

Secondary diabetes was first described in 1788, when Sir Thomas Cawley reported the case of a man "aged 34 years, strong, healthy and corpulent, accustomed to free living and strong corporeal exertions in the pursuit of country amusements ... in December 1787, he was seized with diabetes." The patient gradually became emaciated and, despite treatment, eventually died. At necropsy "the pancreas was full of calculi, which were firmly impacted in its substance. They were of various sizes, not exceeding that of a pea ... which made their surface rough, like mulberry stones. The right extremity of the pancreas was very hard, and appeared to be scirrhous" [6]. However, more than 100 years passed before Minkowski's [7] demonstration that experimental pancreatectomy in dogs caused diabetes. With this discovery, the association between glycosuria and acute pancreatitis became clear, and in 1940 Schumacker [8] estimated that at least 2% of all cases of acute pancreatitis were followed by overt clinical diabetes. In spite of the appreciation that acute pancreatitis was infrequently followed by overt diabetes, clinicians began to recognize chronic pancreatitis or relapsing acute pancreatitis as a common cause of glucose intolerance. Total

International Textbook of Diabetes Mellitus, Third Edition. Edited by R. A. DeFronzo, E. Ferrannini, H. Keen, and P. Zimmet.
 ISBN: 0-471-48655-8.

Table 1 Diabetes mellitus secondary to diseases of the exocrine pancreas

(1) Pancreatitis
(a) Acute
(b) Chronic
(2) Trauma/pancreatectomy
(3) Neoplasia
(4) Cystic fibrosis
(5) Hemochromatosis
(a) Primary
(b) Secondary
(6) Fibrocalculous pancreatopathy
(7) Others

pancreatectomy in humans was first performed in 1942 [9] and has since been used for the surgical treatment of various pancreatic lesions. Extensive use of this procedure proved that more than 80–90% of the pancreas had to be removed before overt diabetes mellitus would ensue. An association between hemochromatosis and diabetes was also recognized at the beginning of the century, and the high incidence of diabetes in this rare metabolic disorder was subsequently confirmed [10].

PANCREATITIS

Acute Pancreatitis

Acute pancreatitis is an acute inflammatory process of the pancreas, with variable involvement of peripancreatic tissues and remote organ systems [11]. Gallstones are the leading cause of acute pancreatitis (more than 90% of cases worldwide). Alcohol abuse, drug reaction, hypertriglyceridemia, hypercalcemia (due to hyperparatyroidism), trauma, and infections are other, mostly infrequent, causes of the disease [12]. The pathogenesis of acute pancreatitis is not clearly understood, but it appears to be influenced and/or mediated by systemic inflammatory response [13, 14]. In humans, an increase in plasma concentration of cytokines, enhanced free radical activity, and increased lipid peroxide concentration in plasma and tissues in both early and late stage of acute pancreatitis has been reported [15]. Most patients with this disorder have minimum organ dysfunction. However, 10–15% of affected individuals develop a systemic inflammatory response leading to fulminant pancreatic necrosis and multiorgan failure. Systemic inflammatory response is supported by the activation of an inflammatory cascade mediated by cytokines, immunocytes, and complement system [12].

Table 2 Frequency of diabetes secondary to pancreatic diseases

Total pancreatectomy	100%
Partial pancreatectomy	
Pancreatoduodenectomy	20–40%
Distal pancreatectomy	20–40%
40–80% resection	40%
80–90% resection	>60%
Pancreatitis	
Acute	2%
Chronic calcifying	60–70%
Chronic noncalcifying	15–30%
Hemochromatosis	
Primary	75%
Secondary	16%
Carcinoma of the pancreas	40–50%
Cystic fibrosis	5–10%

Transient hyperglycemia and glycosuria are found in about 50% of patients with acute pancreatitis. The degree of glucose intolerance is an indicator of the severity of pancreatitis [16]. The incidence of glucose intolerance in acute pancreatitis ranges from 9 to 70% [17]. This wide range is related to the definition of impaired glucose tolerance used in different surveys, as well as to the cause of the acute inflammatory process. Alcohol, for example, is associated with more severe injury of pancreatic tissue, and alcoholic pancreatitis is complicated by higher incidence of glucose intolerance [18]. Hyperglycemia accompanying the bout of pancreatitis is influenced by the pancreatic damage and concomitant severe stress condition. Both the severity and the duration of the disturbance in carbohydrate metabolism are related to the extent of pancreatic tissue damage [19]. Hyperglycemia and glycosuria usually subside within 3–6 weeks, but about 10% of patients will continue to present impaired glucose tolerance [20]. Several studies have reported incidences of diabetes after severe acute pancreatitis ranging from 24 to 92%, with the highest incidences if pancreatic resection had been performed [21, 22].

Hormone Secretion

In patients with acute pancreatitis, plasma insulin concentration is lower than in healthy individuals with or without comparable degree of stress [23]. Insulin secretion in response to glucose or glucagon is impaired [19], whereas alanine infusion results in a normal increase in plasma insulin levels. With the amelioration of the acute process, normal insulin response is usually recovered [24]. In acute pancreatitis, plasma glucagon concentration is increased and tends to remain high for at least 1 week [25]. The combination of hyperglucagonemia and hypoinsulinemia is sufficient to account for the development of ketoacidosis and the rare occurrence of diabetic coma. Experimental studies have revealed increased basal levels of plasma pancreatic polypeptide (PP), suggesting a possible role for the peptide in the diagnosis of the disease [26]. Nonetheless, plasma PP levels in human studies are within normal values in the early phase of acute pancreatitis, and fail to increase in response to hyperglycemia or secretin infusion. In a severely damaged pancreas, however, basal PP release may be impaired and could be helpful in grading the severity of the disease [27].

Metabolic aspects Besides elevation in plasma glucose levels, in a minority of patients with acute pancreatitis and no previous history of hyperlipidemia, serum concentration of lipids may be elevated. Following an attack of acute pancreatitis, however, the rise in plasma triglyceride and cholesterol does not always occur [23], and a reduction in the cholesterol levels may be observed. Whether hypertriglyceridemia is primary or secondary to acute pancreatitis can be difficult to ascertain since high triglyceride levels can be a cause for acute pancreatitis. Plasma free fatty acid (FFA) concentrations are elevated following acute pancreatitis as a consequence of both impaired insulin secretion and concomitant increase in glucagon and cortisol secretion [23]. Although the hormonal milieu that follows acute pancreatitis may account for ketoacidosis, this is an unusual metabolic event [20], due to the persistence of residual endogenous insulin secretion sufficient to inhibit lipolysis and ketogenesis, and to deficient glucagon secretion.

Therapeutic aspects Acute pancreatitis is associated with significant hyperglycemia in 50% of patients with secondary diabetes and occasionally ketosis or diabetic coma may develop [20, 23]. In these cases, close monitoring of the plasma glucose concentration, electrolytes, ketones, and other aspects of metabolism is required, along with intravenous insulin infusion according to classic guidelines for treatment of diabetic ketoacidosis. Glucose tolerance should be assessed 3–6 months after an episode of acute pancreatitis. In the treatment of patients with acute fulminant pancreatitis conservative therapy rather than tissue resection should be advised, as the latter is associated with much higher incidence of diabetes.

Chronic Pancreatitis

Chronic pancreatitis is an inflammatory disease characterized by progressive and irreversible destruction primarily of the exocrine and, at a later stage, of the endocrine pancreatic parenchyma [12]. Fibrotic replacement of the exocrine parenchyma and inflammatory cell infiltration are the main histological characteristics of the disease [28]. There are several forms of chronic pancreatitis. Chronic calcifying pancreatitis (or pancreatic lithiasis) is by far the most frequent form. Chronic obstructive pancreatitis, recurrent acute pancreatitis, and idiopathic pancreatitis represent less frequent subsets of inflammatory processes of the pancreas [29]. Alcohol consumption is the major etiological factor in the Western world, accounting for at least 80% of all cases of chronic pancreatitis. Major predisposing risk factors to chronic pancreatitis have been recently categorized as (1) toxic-metabolic, (2) idiopathic, (3) genetic, (4) autoimmune, (5) recurrent, and severe acute pancreatitis, or (6) obstructive (TIGAR-O system) [30]. There is no general accepted concept explaining the pathophysiology of the disease, as primary intraductal obstruction, direct toxic-metabolic effects from alcohol, oxidative stress, necrosis–fibrosis sequence have been all proposed. Recently, it has been reported that cyclooxygenase 2 (COX-2)—a dominant regulator of prostaglandine production—plays a major role in the pathogenesis of exocrine and endocrine damage in chronic pancreatitis [31].

The frequency of diabetes secondary to chronic pancreatitis depends on the regional frequency of chronic pancreatitis, the type of lesion, and the duration of the disease [29]. In a series collected at the Mayo Clinic in 1947, Sprague [32] found that diabetes secondary to chronic pancreatitis represented 0.5% of all cases of diabetes. A higher incidence of diabetes mellitus is associated with fibrocalculous pancreatitis in the tropics.

Tropical pancreatitis is a well-recognized clinical entity [33]. It is a form of chronic calcific pancreatitis observed mainly among children and young adults in rural, tropical countries of Asia and Africa. Since its description in 1955 [34], several reports have appeared describing its prevalence in countries such as Nigeria, Uganda, Zaire, and Malawi. In 1985, this form of diabetes was classified by WHO as a subclass of malnutrition-related diabetes mellitus [4]. A few years ago, the evidence for and the features of malnutrition-related diabetes have been reviewed in an international meeting [35]. While it appeared that malnutrition could influence the metabolic control of diabetes, the evidence that malnutrition and protein deficiency could directly cause diabetes was not convincing. Therefore, diabetes secondary to fibrocalculous pancreatopathy has been recently more appropriately classified as a disease of the exocrine pancreas [1]. Its prevalence is variable, ranging from 0.5 to 16% of all diabetic patients in India, and perhaps up to 80% of young insulin-treated patients in Nigeria [36]. These patients present with abdominal pain and, commonly, a wasting syndrome. Most patients have extensive intraductal calculi at the time of presentation. Diabetes develops within a decade after onset of pancreatitis. Etiologies include a protein-calorie malnourished state, a variety of exogenous food toxins, pancreatic duct anomalies, and a possible genetic predisposition. Diabetes is usually severe and insulin-requiring [37], although histopathology and immunohistochemistry studies have documented partial preservation of insulin positivity in pancreata of patients with fibrocalculous pancreatitis [38]. The residual insulin secretion likely accounts for the rare development of ketoacidosis in patients with fibrocalculous pancreatitis.

In 1961, Sarles et al. [39] described a particular type of pancreatitis with hypergammaglobulinemia. It was suggested that an autoimmune mechanism may be involved, at least in some patients, with pancreatitis. In the TIGAR-O risk factor classification system proposed in 2001, autoimmunity was categorized as one out of six main risk factors [30]. Autoimmune pancreatitis has been occasionally observed in association with Sjögren's syndrome, primary sclerozing cholangitis, or primary biliary cirrhosis. Autoimmune chronic pancreatitis is characterized by diffuse swelling and severe fibrosis associated with mononuclear cell infiltration of the exocrine pancreas [40]. The disorder can induce severe pancreatic swelling or tumor formation, with malabsorption and often cholestasis, and is sometimes misdiagnosed as pancreatic carcinoma or lymphoma. Patients with autoimmune chronic pancreatitis are sometimes subjected to pancreatectomy or chemotherapy. In these individuals, diabetes is caused by T-cell-mediated mechanisms involving islet β-cells as well as pancreatic ductal cells [41]. Recent data indicate that corticosteroid therapy can result in normal or mild glucose intolerance with improved insulin response [42].

Diabetes is an almost universal late complication of chronic calcifying pancreatitis, and it correlates better with the patient's age than with duration of the disease [43]. In these patients the prevalence of impaired glucose tolerance or diabetes has been reported in 40–70% of the cases [44, 45].

The risk of diabetes mellitus in chronic pancreatitis does not seem to be influenced by elective pancreatic surgical procedures [46]; rather it is more strongly associated with the progression of the disease. Actuarial studies show that after 15 years, 80% of patients with chronic pancreatitis have diabetes [47]. Specific precipitating etiological factors contribute to carbohydrate intolerance. Hypertriglyceridemia, for instance, is associated with insulin resistance and commonly leads to overt diabetes mellitus. Alcohol impairs insulin action and leads to glucose intolerance through direct effects on the liver. Chronic pancreatitis secondary to alcohol and/or malnutrition is more often associated with diabetes mellitus [18]. By contrast, the idiopathic form of chronic pancreatitis is associated with a lower incidence of diabetes. In hereditary pancreatitis, a rare autosomal dominant disease [48], diabetes may develop at a late stage and long-term diabetic complications may ensue.

Whatever the cause, it can be calculated that in the western hemisphere, 60–70% of patients with calcific pancreatitis develop overt diabetes mellitus; 20% have impaired glucose tolerance and a further 5–8% exhibit abnormalities in insulin secretion. Among patient without pancreatic calcification, 30% are affected by diabetes mellitus, 25% show impaired glucose tolerance, and 25% present a defect in insulin secretion [49].

A positive family history of diabetes might predispose patients with chronic pancreatitis to develop diabetes at younger age [29]. The prevalence of diabetes without any association with pancreatitis is, indeed, higher in families of those patients who develop diabetes. However, no apparent increase in the frequency of HLA antigens B8, DR3, DR4, and DR3/DR4 has been demonstrated in patients with diabetes secondary to chronic pancreatitis [50–52]. It has been suggested that autoimmunity may contribute to the development of diabetes secondary to chronic pancreatitis, because islet cell antibodies (ICA) were found in some patients before the onset of diabetes [53]. However, this is a controversial issue. Other investigators were unable to demonstrate ICA in patients with either acute or chronic pancreatitis [51, 52, 54–56]. In our own series, ICA could be detected in only 1 of 88 patients, and the presence of organ-specific antibodies did not differ from that in the general population [50].

Pathology

As indicated by the definition of chronic pancreatitis, involvement of the endocrine tissue represents a late stage of the disease. The islets of Langerhans are, indeed, relatively well preserved as compared with the acinar cell destruction [57]. Sometimes the pancreas can assume an adenomatous aspect due to the complete loss of exocrine tissue as opposed to persistence of its endocrine component. Within the remaining islets, a rearrangement of the endocrine cell population takes place, with a proportionally greater loss of B-cells than of A-cells, leading to a reversal of the normal 2:1 ratio. The number of D-cells is usually normal and there is some increase in PP-cells. Islets surrounded by normal acinar tissue tend to exhibit a normal cytological composition, suggesting a trophic effect of the exocrine pancreas.

Hormone Secretion

In chronic pancreatitis, fibrosis leads to reduction of the B-cell mass. The fibrotic process may alter pancreatic capillary circulation, leading to diminished islet perfusion, which may account for impaired delivery of secretagogues to the B-cells and reduced outflow of pancreatic hormones. Chronic pancreatitis is associated with a loss of functioning B-cells, which accounts for reduced insulin secretion: the greater the loss of pancreatic endocrine tissue, the greater the impairment in insulin secretion and the greater the degree of glucose intolerance [49]. In patients with diabetes secondary to chronic pancreatitis with mild-to-moderate fasting hyperglycemia, the basal plasma insulin concentration is either normal or moderately elevated [58, 59].

Fasting insulin level tends to decrease as a function of the duration of the pancreatic process, and it is deficient whenever pancreatic calcification and steatorrhea are apparent [20, 60–67]. Exocrine and endocrine functions are correlated, suggesting a direct cause–effect relationship

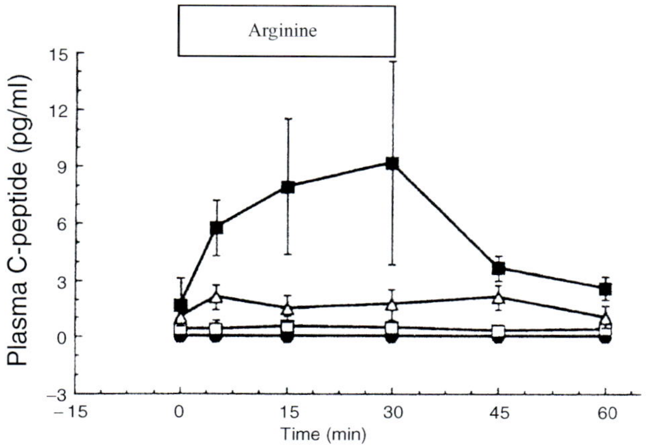

Figure 1 Plasma C-peptide concentration following IV infusion of L-arginine (25 g/30 min) in normal subjects (■) and individuals with impaired glucose tolerance (△) or diabetes mellitus secondary to chronic pancreatitis (□), and diabetic subjects with total pancreatectomy (●)

between the inflammatory process of the exocrine pancreas and the development of diabetes. A good correlation has been found between insulin response to oral glucose and the concentration of pancreatic enzymes in the duodenal juice after intravenous cholecystokinin-pancreozymin (CCK-PZ) [66, 67]. Patients with steatorrhea have lower C-peptide secretion than do patients with less severe impairment of the exocrine function [67]. Although fasting plasma insulin concentration may be normal or even increased, there is an almost universal impairment in insulin secretion following an oral glucose load [58–67]. A reduction in the maximal insulin secretory capability [61] is readily demonstrated in these patients, indicating reduced insulin reserve. When plasma glucose levels exceed 10 mmol/l (180 mg/dl), plasma insulin and C-peptide concentrations are often undetectable [62]. The B-cell response to amino acids is also reduced as a function of the degree of pancreatic B-cell destruction and severity of glucose intolerance [49]. Arginine-stimulated C-peptide secretion (Figure 1) can be normal in patients with chronic pancreatitis and impaired glucose tolerance, but is always reduced in patients with fasting hyperglycemia [62, 68].

In normal subjects, glucose ingestion elicits a greater insulin secretion than does the intravenous infusion of an equivalent amount of glucose as a consequence of the activation of the enteropancreatic axis. In chronic pancreatitis, the secretion of the incretin factors—CCK-PZ, gastrin, enteroglucagon, gastric inhibitory polypeptide (GIP), and vasoactive intestinal polypeptide (VIP)—is impaired. On the contrary, recent studies have reported an exaggerated glucagon-like peptide 1 (GLP-1) release in response to glucose ingestion in patients with diabetes secondary to pancreatitis as compared to patients who still retain normal or have impaired glucose tolerance [69]. In patients with diabetes secondary to chronic pancreatitis, the insulin response to CCK-PZ is proportional to the degree of hyperglycemia [70]. In contrast, insulin secretion in response to GIP is reduced. Nonetheless, GLP-1 infusion in diabetic patients with diabetes secondary to chronic pancreatitis was associated with a reduction in blood glucose and an increase in plasma C-peptide concentration, a response not different from that observed in normal subjects [71]. It remains unclear whether, in diabetes secondary to chronic pancreatitis, there is an unbalanced enteropancreatic axis or a simultaneous alteration in the secretion of gut and pancreatic hormones. The plasma concentration of GIP is elevated in diabetic patients with chronic pancreatitis, particularly following insulin withdrawal [72]. On the other hand, the meal-related increase in plasma CCK is reduced when compared with nondiabetic subjects or nondiabetic individuals with chronic pancreatitis [73].

In patients with chronic pancreatitis the greater the loss of pancreatic endocrine tissue, the greater the impairment in insulin secretion and the greater the degree of glucose intolerance. It is likely that these factors are linked in a vicious cycle through the negative effect of chronic hyperglycemia, a phenomenon also known as "glucose toxicity" [74]. Figure 2 summarizes the changes in plasma insulin and glucose concentrations as a function of residual B-cell mass [49]. In patients with chronic pancreatitis, normal fasting plasma glucose concentration is maintained until

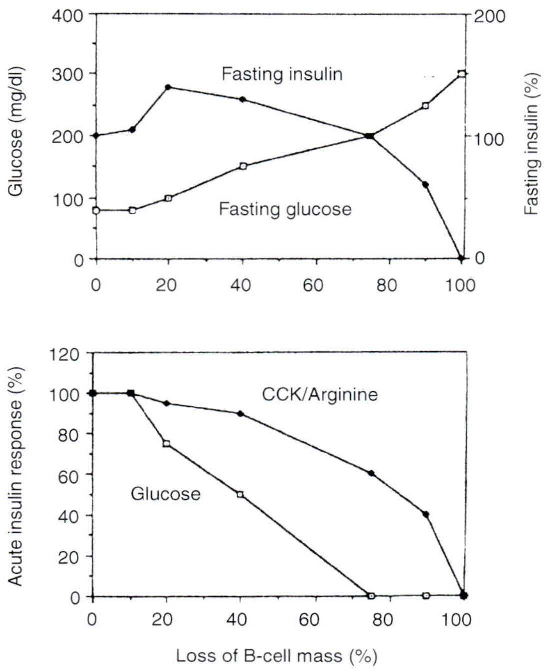

Figure 2 Diagram of changes in the plasma concentration of insulin and glucose, and insulin secretory response to glucose, gastrointestinal factors, and arginine expressed as a function of residual B-cell mass in patients with chronic pancreatitis. (From reference 49, with permission)

20–40% of the B-cell mass has been lost. Nonetheless, this degree of loss of B-cell mass is associated with a marked impairment in glucose-mediated insulin release [59], even though the response to CCK and arginine is still normal. An altered response to incretin factors and amino acids becomes apparent when 40–60% of B-cell mass has been lost. Finally, when the B-cell mass is reduced by more than 80–90%, both fasting hyperglycemia and impaired insulin secretion in response to all secretagogues develop. From a clinical point of view, B-cell function in diabetes secondary to chronic pancreatitis can be evaluated using the glucagon test [24, 67, 75].

Glucagon secretion in these patients is heterogeneous, and two main conditions are recognized [76]. While some patients present a combined defect in insulin and glucagon secretion, others may exhibit severe hypoinsulinemia and high plasma glucagon concentrations. Similarly, the glucagon response to arginine or alanine stimulation is blunted in only 50% of patients with impaired glucose tolerance (Figure 3). With the progression of the pancreatic disease, the ability of A-cells to respond to insulin-induced hypoglycemia wanes [77]. Nevertheless, the ingestion of an oral glucose load can be followed by a paradoxical rise in plasma glucagon levels, whereas the glucagon response to secretin and CCK-PZ is either normal or increased [61].

Controversy exists about the molecular nature and source of circulating glucagon in patients with diabetes secondary to chronic pancreatitis [78]. At least four varieties of immunoreactive glucagon ($M_r > 50000$, 9000, 3500, and 2000, respectively) have been identified in the plasma of normal individuals [79]. The 3500 M_r glucagon is of pancreatic origin and possesses full biological activity. This is the only form that responds to stimulation by arginine and suppression by somatostatin. Functional studies and gel chromatography analysis support the pancreatic origin of the circulating glucagon in chronic pancreatitis [80, 81], but a major contribution of enteropancreatic glucagon to the circulating plasma concentration measured by radioimmunoassay is also likely. Consistent with this, the basal concentration of gastrointestinal glucagon is increased in patients with pancreatic diabetes [82].

In chronic pancreatitis patients with residual insulin secretion, fasting plasma levels of PP are normal [24]. However, when residual B-cell function is severely impaired, a marked PP secretory defect is evident, as shown by the inability of arginine infusion, meal ingestion, or insulin-induced hypoglycemia to evoke any rise in plasma PP concentration [24, 83]. A strong relationship between pancreatic enzyme secretion and stimulated plasma PP concentration has been reported [84, 85]. In patients with chronic pancreatitis without steatorrhea, PP response to CCK is reduced, but when steatorrhea ensues this response is no longer elicited [86]. Therefore, evaluation of PP secretion represents a reliable index of endocrine function in these patients [24]. Plasma somatostatin concentration is increased both in the basal state and following stimulation by glucagon, arginine, mixed meal, and hyperglycemia [24].

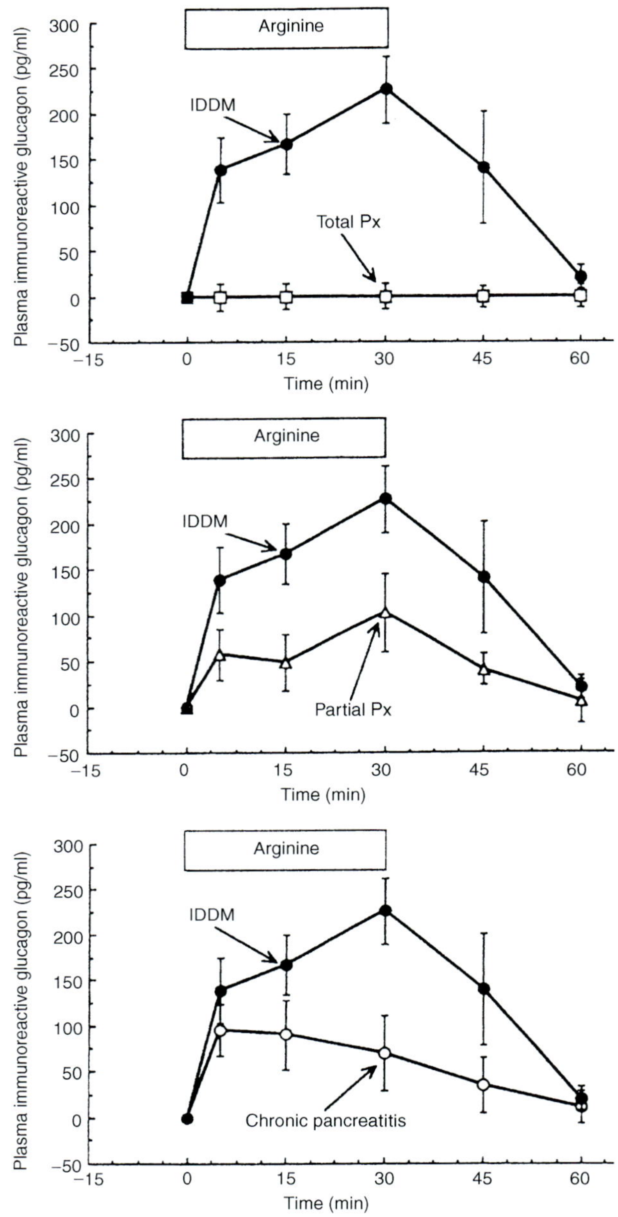

Figure 3 Increment above baseline of plasma immunoreactive glucagon following IV infusion of L-arginine (25 g/30 min) in type 1 diabetic patients (●) and individuals with diabetes secondary to total pancreatectomy (□), partial pancreatectomy (△), and chronic pancreatitis (○). IDDM = insulin-dependent diabetes mellitus; Px = pancreatectomy

Metabolic aspects In contrast to type 1 diabetes, all endocrine cell types are involved in the inflammatory

Table 3 Clinical differences between diabetes secondary to chronic pancreatitis/pancreatectomy and type 1 diabetes

	Secondary diabetes	Type 1 diabetes
Glycemic instability	++++	++
Insulin requirement	+	+++
Hypoglycemia	++++	++
Ketoacidosis	+	+++
Vascular complications	++	+++

process in pancreatic diabetes, and defects in both B- and A-cell function are characteristic. Impairment in insulin secretion is a function of the destruction of B-cells and it accounts for the different degree of fasting and postprandial hyperglycemia. It is the concomitant impairment in glucagon secretion that is mainly responsible for the peculiar metabolic and clinical features of diabetes secondary to pancreatic diseases (Tables 3 and 4): the more profound the defect in A-cell function, the more pronounced these features [87]. Therefore, the description of metabolic features, clinical manifestation, diabetic complications, and therapeutic approaches will be discussed together with diabetes secondary to pancreatectomy.

PANCREATECTOMY

In 1889, Minkowski demonstrated that ablation of the pancreas in dogs was associated with development of diabetes mellitus [7]. In humans, after sporadic attempts, total pancreatectomy was not performed until insulin became available. That early experience showed that more than 80–90% of the pancreas had to be removed to produce diabetes. Nevertheless, the postoperative onset of diabetes can be unpredictable and is not always directly related to the extent of pancreatic ablation. Preceding history of chronic pancreatitis is, indeed, associated with greater incidence of diabetes mellitus. Generally speaking, the development of diabetes mellitus after subtotal pancreatectomy is directly related to the amount of pancreatic tissue that is removed (Table 2). In the initial weeks following pancreaticoduodenectomy, the prevalence of diabetes mellitus ranges from 20 to 40%, while it approaches 70%

Table 4 Hormonal and metabolic differences between diabetes secondary to chronic pancreatitis/pancreatectomy and type 1 diabetes

	Secondary diabetes	Type 1 diabetes
Insulin secretion	↓	↓
Glucagon secretion	↓	↑
Hepatic glucose production	↓	↑
Gluconeogenic amino acids	↑	↓
Lactate and pyruvate	↑	↑↓
Ketone bodies	↓	↑
Insulin sensitivity	↑↓	↓

with longer follow-ups [88–91]. These figures are comparable with the incidence of diabetes (about 60%) observed in patients with chronic pancreatitis who received medical treatment alone [92]. Some differences exist between distal and proximal pancreatectomy [93]. Distal pancreatectomy is not followed by appreciable changes in exocrine function although it may result in an insulin-dependent diabetic condition. By contrast, after proximal pancreatectomy there is a sharp decline in the exocrine secretion without significant impairment of the endocrine function [93]. Preservation of the duodenum has been claimed to preserve hormone secretion and glucose tolerance [94]. Total pancreatectomy is invariably followed by diabetes.

Hormone Secretion

As already discussed, insulin secretory response is a function of residual B-cell mass, with the exception of pancreatectomy performed for chronic pancreatitis, because of preextensive disruption of the pancreatic parenchyma. In patients undergoing pancreatic resection for carcinoma of the pancreas, secretion of pancreatic hormones closely resembles that observed in patients with chronic pancreatitis receiving medical treatment (Figure 2). Medial pancreatectomy in patients with tumors of the neck of the pancreas has been reported not to be associated with diabetes mellitus [95]. Similarly, when hemipancreatectomy is carried out in healthy individuals for the purpose of donation to a family member with type 1 diabetes, a deterioration of insulin and glucagon secretion is evident in spite of persistent normal glucose homeostasis [96, 97]. It has been suggested that in otherwise normal, healthy individuals, undefined mechanisms must compensate for diminished insulin secretion following hemipancreatectomy [98].

Total pancreatectomy is always followed by complete insulin deficiency, as evidenced by the absence of insulin or C-peptide in the circulation (Figure 1). Measurement of stimulated plasma C-peptide concentration can be used to confirm completeness of the surgical removal of the pancreas [76]. In totally pancreatectomized patients arginine infusion does not elicit any insulin secretion, while a blunted response can be evoked in patients with chronic pancreatitis and partial pancreatectomy (Figure 1).

Basal concentration of immunoreactive glucagon can be normal or even increased [99]. The source and nature of measurable immunoreactive glucagon has been a matter of argument for many years. In pancreatectomized dogs and other animal species, including humans, total pancreatectomy does not lead to the disappearance of circulating glucagon molecules. In dogs, A-cells have been identified in the gastrointestinal tract and these cells secrete glucagon molecules that are biologically and immunologically indistinguishable from 3500 M_r, pancreatic glucagon [100]. In rats, salivary glands produce biologically active glucagon [101]. In humans, no such alternative sites of glucagon production are operative, so that total pancreatectomyl might be expected to result in a complete loss of pancreatic glucagon and thus leading to aglucagonemic diabetes [102–104]. Nevertheless, even when specific antisera are used, normal or increased levels of circulating glucagon have been reported in pancreatectomized patients [24, 82, 99, 103–112]. However, challenging glucagon secretion by stimulatory or suppressive maneuvers is never followed by appreciable changes in plasma immunoreactive glucagon concentration [99, 105–107, 110, 113], suggesting absolute lack of active pancreatic or extrapancreatic sources of 3500 M_r glucagon in humans after total pancreatectomy. Persistence of measurable basal levels of immunoreactive glucagon depends on the cross-reactivity, even with supposedly specific antibodies, of glucagon-like molecules of uncertain biological activity. Secretion of gastrointestinal glucagon-like polypeptides is increased after total pancreatectomy [114], and glucagon-related peptides arising from the gut are responsible for the paradoxical response to oral glucose load reported in some pancreatectomized subjects [112]. Standard chromatographic analysis could not demonstrate significant amounts of circulating 3500 M_r glucagon in the plasma of patients with total pancreatectomy. By further improvement in the sensitivity of the method of analysis, some pancreatic glucagon activity in patients with total pancreatectomy was detected [111]. Nevertheless, the magnitude of the ectopic 3500 M_r glucagon secretion is trivial compared with the pancreatic secretion of healthy subjects. Thus, chromatographic analysis of plasma taken from the portal vein in patients undergoing total pancreatectomy demonstrated negligible amounts of pancreatic glucagon, even after arginine infusion [115] (Figure 4). In summary, it is likely that, after total pancreatectomy, some

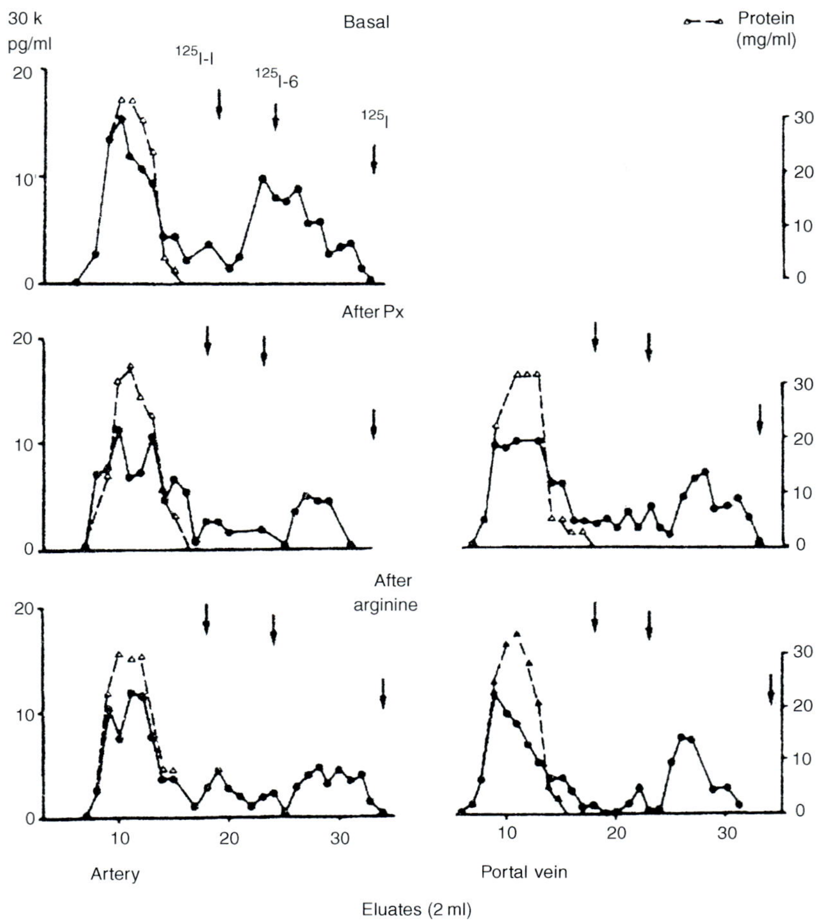

Figure 4 Chromatographic analysis (gel filtration on BioGel P30) of the plasma immunoreactive glucagon assessed by C-terminal antibody (30 K) in a subject who underwent total pancreatectomy. Blood specimens were collected at different phases of the surgical procedure from a radial artery and portal vein. Broken line indicates protein concentration in eluates. Elution times for ^{125}I-labeled insulin (^{125}I-I), ^{125}I-labeled glucagon (^{125}I-G), and ^{125}I are indicated by the arrows. Arterial basal profile of glucagon immunoreactivity obtained 60 min before pancreas removal is shown in the upper panel. Fifteen minutes after pancreatectomy, the peak of pancreatic glucagon (3500 M_r) eluting with ^{125}I-labeled glucagon is markedly reduced both in the arterial and portal circulation (middle panel). Injection of 12.5 g L-arginine does not elicit any change in the chromatographic glucagon profile. (From reference 115, with permission)

"pancreatic" glucagon may be measured in the circulation, but pancreatectomy does result in a chronic deficiency of 3500 M_r glucagons.

Basal plasma levels of somatostatin are normal or slightly increased following pancreatectomy, and the response to a mixed meal is normal [116], whereas no PP is detectable in plasma [114]. Among other gastrointestinal hormones, gastrin is increased, while plasma levels of neurotensin and motilin are within the normal range [114]. Both gastrointestinal inhibitory polypeptide and enteroglucagon concentrations are normal in pancreatectomized individuals; their response to glucose is preserved, while a supranormal increase follows a mixed meal [82].

The absence of significant amounts of pancreatic glucagon may account for diabetes "brittleness." In patients with diabetes secondary to total pancreatectomy, insulin sensitivity is diminished when compared to normal subjects but higher than in type 1 diabetic individuals[115] (Figure 5).

This observation has been confirmed by some [117–119] but not all [120, 121] investigators. Conversely, in normal subjects, long-term physiologic hyperglucagonemia induces a modest degree of insulin resistance [122]. Similarly in pancreatectomized patients, replacement of basal glucagon concentration leads to a worsening of the insulin resistance [121]. The liver, in particular, seems to be more sensitive to insulin in the absence of glucagon. Thus, in pancreatectomized patients the rate of hepatic glucose production is similar to that of type 1 diabetic subjects, even though plasma insulin concentrations are much lower [120], whereas, when comparable plasma insulin levels are attained, individuals with total pancreatectomy have a much lower rate of hepatic glucose production [123].

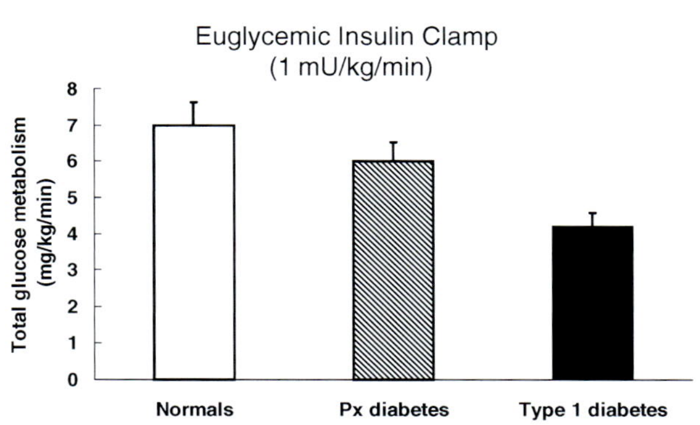

Figure 5 Whole-body glucose utilization during euglycemic (90 mg/dl, 5.0 mmol/l) insulin (1 mU/kg/min) clamp studies in 16 normal subjects (open column), 10 patients with diabetes secondary to total pancreatectomy (cross-hatched column), and 12 type 1 diabetic individuals (closed column). (From reference 115, with permission)

Table 5 Mean 24-h blood concentration (μmol/l) of gluconeogenic precursors during intensive subcutaneous insulin therapy in diabetes secondary to chronic pancreatitis/pancreatectomy and type 1 diabetes

	Totally pancreatectomized patients	Partially pancreatectomized patients	Type 1 diabetic patients
Lactate	1073 ± 105	792 ± 76	707 ± 49
Pyruvate	82 ± 8	47 ± 5	56 ± 5
Alanine	437 ± 62	226 ± 14	216 ± 10
Glycerol	60 ± 8	33 ± 6	35 ± 4

Metabolic Aspects

The metabolic picture is the consequence of the concomitant reduction of A- and B-cells of the pancreatic islet. Thus, chronic pancreatitis and pancreatectomy are more likely to develop the full picture of pancreatogenic diabetes (Table 4). In the extreme condition of diabetes secondary to total pancreatectomy or insulin-deficient pancreatitis, the blood levels of alanine, lactate, pyruvate, and glycerol are 50–100% higher than in type 1 diabetic patients (Table 5). This metabolic pattern is not affected by insulin therapy [124] or its withdrawal [109, 110, 115, 125]. Furthermore, in these patients, blood concentrations of gluconeogenic precursors and glucose are not affected by infusion of somatostatin (an inhibitor of glucagon secretion) or arginine (a stimulant of glucagon secretion) [110]. Conversely, exogenous glucagon infusion causes a significant drop in blood lactate, pyruvate, and alanine levels [115, 123]. Patients with diabetes secondary to chronic pancreatitis or partial pancreatectomy with residual glucagon secretion, exhibit blood levels of gluconeogenic substrates that are similar to those of type 1 diabetic patients, but much lower than those of patients with total pancreatectomy [115, 124] (Figure 6 and Table 5). Among the gluconeogenic precursors, alanine is particularly elevated in patients with pancreatectomy (Figure 6). Such metabolic specificity is supported by the immediate increase in blood alanine concentration that follows pancreatic resection [126]. Glucagon, indeed, plays a major stimulatory action on hepatic glucose production and gluconeogenesis [127].

In the absence of significant amounts of pancreatic glucagon, insulin exerts an enhanced inhibitory effect on the liver, causing a marked reduction in post-absorptive plasma glucose concentration [105]. The combined increase in hepatic [120, 123, 128] and peripheral [115, 117–119] insulin sensitivity may contribute to frequent hypoglycemic episodes in patients with total pancreatectomy or severe pancreatitis. When evaluating the overall metabolic status of a patient with total pancreatectomy, factors other than glucagon and insulin lack should be

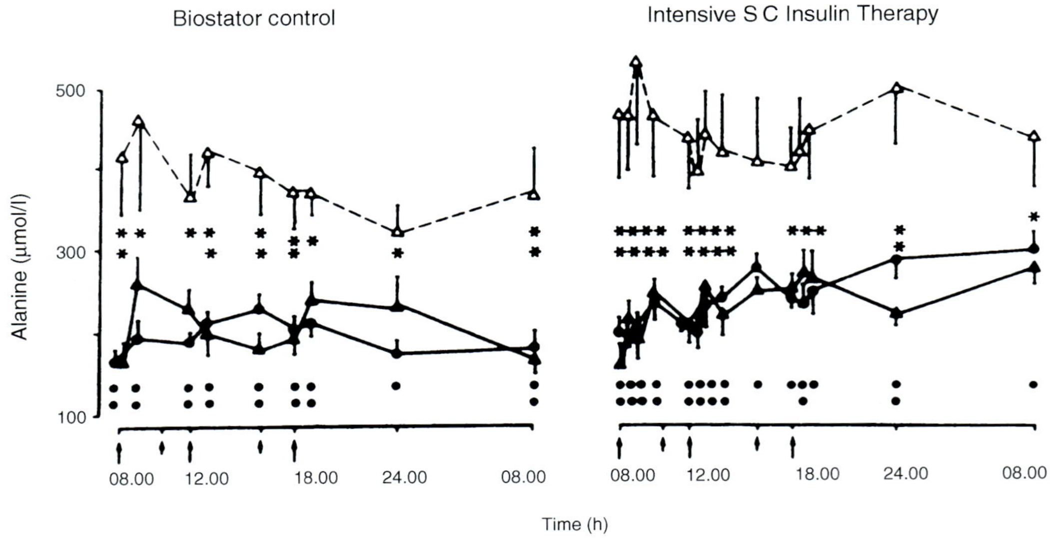

Figure 6 Blood alanine concentration during 24-h glucose-controlled insulin infusion (artificial endocrine pancreas – Biostator GCIIS) and intensive SC insulin therapy in patients with diabetes secondary to total pancreatectomy (△-△) compared with patients with diabetes secondary to partial pancreatectomy (▲-▲) (*$p < 0.05$; **$p < 0.005$) and with type 1 diabetic individuals (•-•) (•$p < 0.05$; ••$p < 0.005$). (Reproduced from reference 124 by permission of Springer-Verlag)

considered. Nutrition, malabsorption, changes in dietary behavior, abnormalities in gastrointestinal hormone secretion, local recurrence of tumor, and distant metastases can affect intermediary metabolism. Nevertheless, the available data suggest that a major metabolic difference exists between type 1 diabetic patients, who retain the ability to secrete glucagon (i.e. who have either absolute or relative hyperglucagonemia), and glucagon-deficient totally pancreatectomized patients. This difference is explained by a diminished rate of hepatic gluconeogenesis [123], and progressive accumulation in blood of gluconeogenic precursors, especially alanine.

In patients with total pancreatectomy and marked glucagon deficiency, insulin withdrawal is followed by a significant increment in plasma FFA and blood ketone body concentrations (Figure 7). However, the rise above baseline is less pronounced than in type 1 diabetic individuals [88–90]. By contrast, the rate of increase in blood

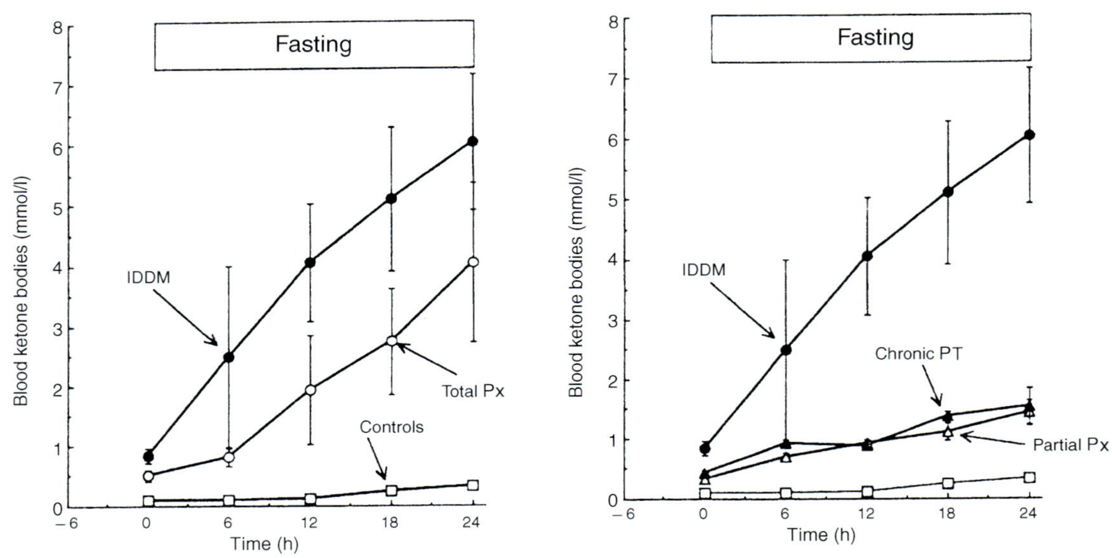

Figure 7 Blood ketone body concentration after insulin withdrawal and 24-h fasting in normal individuals (□), patients with type 1 diabetes (●), and patients with diabetes secondary to total (o) and partial (△) pancreatectomy, and chronic pancreatitis (▲). IDDM = insulin-dependent diabetes mellitus; Px = pancreatectomy; PT = pancreatitis

ketones in patients with diabetes secondary to chronic pancreatitis or partial pancreatectomy with residual insulin secretion, is lower than in pancreatectomized and type 1 diabetic patients [65, 89] (Figure 7). These observations suggest that insulin deficiency is the primary factor in promoting ketogenesis, whereas hyperglucagonemia is an accelerator of the process.

In type 1 diabetic patients, especially those with poor glycemic control, high plasma levels of FFA and triglycerides are common. Although raised fasting plasma FFA concentrations have been reported in insulin-treated pancreatectomized patients, this elevation occurs in the presence of much lower plasma-free-insulin concentrations [120]. In diabetes secondary to acquired disease of the pancreas, plasma lipid levels are variable. Low serum levels of cholesterol, phospholipids, and triglycerides have been reported in patients with diabetes secondary to chronic pancreatitis [91]. More recent surveys have found normal serum triglycerides and cholesterol [129]. In particular, plasma lipid concentrations do not seem to be related to duration of disease, the patient's age, or type of therapy. Conflicting results have been reported in patients with total pancreatectomy [128, 130, 131]. In these patients, glucagon replacement is not associated with significant effects on plasma lipid levels [130]. It is likely that this variability reflects the impact of other factors that affect lipid metabolism, including changes in the nutritional status, diet, malabsorption, and alcohol intake.

Alteration in the plasma amino acid profile seems to be a characteristic of diabetes secondary to total pancreatectomy, whereas less information is available for other forms of pancreatogenic diabetes. Glucagon deficiency that follows total pancreatectomy is associated with elevation in blood concentrations of gluconeogenic and urea cycle amino acids [132]. In particular, alanine, asparagine, cystine, aspartate, glycine, proline, serine, citrulline, ornithine, phenylalanine, taurine, threonine, and tyrosine are all increased in patients with glucagon deficiency (Figure 8). Similar changes in amino acid levels can be induced by inhibition of glucagon secretion with somatostatin [109], whereas restoration of physiologic plasma glucagon concentrations in pancreatectomized patients returns the plasma amino acid profile to normal [108, 109, 123, 130]. In contrast to the elevated plasma concentrations of gluconeogenic amino acids, plasma levels of branched-chain amino acids are not altered in pancreatectomized individuals [109, 130, 133]. In patients with chronic pancreatitis or partial pancreatectomy under strict metabolic control, blood alanine concentration is similar to that observed in type 1 diabetic patients [124]. The available data suggest that glucagon deficiency causes an impairment in the rates of both gluconeogenesis and ureagenesis, with secondary increases in the plasma concentrations of gluconeogenic but not branched-chain amino acids.

Clinical Manifestations

In general, patients with secondary forms of diabetes develop symptoms similar to those exhibited by patients with primary diabetes. The diabetic condition develops immediately after total pancreatectomy, whereas in patients with chronic diseases of the pancreas it tends to develop gradually over several (1–12) years.

Patients with chronic pancreatitis may experience hypoglycemia either after the initial dose of insulin or, unexpectedly, after maintenance insulin or oral antidiabetic therapy [20] has been established. These episodes tend to be severe and prolonged, and represent a frequent cause of hospital admission for coma, and of death in these patients [134, 135]. Hypoglycemia is even more frequent after pancreatectomy [136–141], being a cause of death in 20–50% of the patients [137, 142, 143]. The severity of these hypoglycemic episodes is the consequence of impaired counterregulation and glucose recovery [144, 145]. The inability of the organism to respond promptly to a drop in plasma glucose concentration is due to deficient glucagon secretion and blunted catecholamine response [146, 147] associated with impaired activation of hepatic glucose production [148]. Increased frequency of hypoglycemic episodes is associated with metabolic instability characterized by erratic fluctuation of plasma glucose concentrations [149, 150]. Thus, it is not uncommon to observe early postprandial hyperglycemic peaks followed by severe hypoglycemia even after small doses of regular insulin (Figure 9).

Chronic alcohol consumption is a frequent cause of pancreatitis, and it is associated with an increased frequency of carbohydrate intolerance [29]. Persistence of ethanol abuse after medical or surgical therapy of pancreatitis may affect the metabolic control of diabetic patients. Alcohol inhibits gluconeogenesis [151], affects hypothalamic–pituitary secretion of adrenocorticotropic hormone and growth hormone [152, 153], and induces insulin resistance [154, 155]. Hypoglycemia may be particularly troublesome if nutrient intake is reduced and liver glycogen stores are depleted. Alcohol abuse after pancreatectomy is a major factor in hypoglycemia and death [140, 142]. In these patients, poor compliance with the insulin regimen frequently contributes to metabolic instability. Finally, ethanol-induced liver disease will affect both hepatic glucose production and peripheral glucose metabolism [156]. In contrast to the frequent occurrence of hypoglycemia and the wide fluctuations in plasma glucose levels, development of ketoacidosis and diabetic coma in pancreatic diabetes is uncommon [20, 140, 142, 157]. When these problems do occur, they are almost always associated with stress, such as infection or surgery. The persistence of insulin secretion largely accounts for the resistance to ketosis [89]. However, even in patients without residual C-peptide secretion, ketoacidosis is quite rare. The rarity

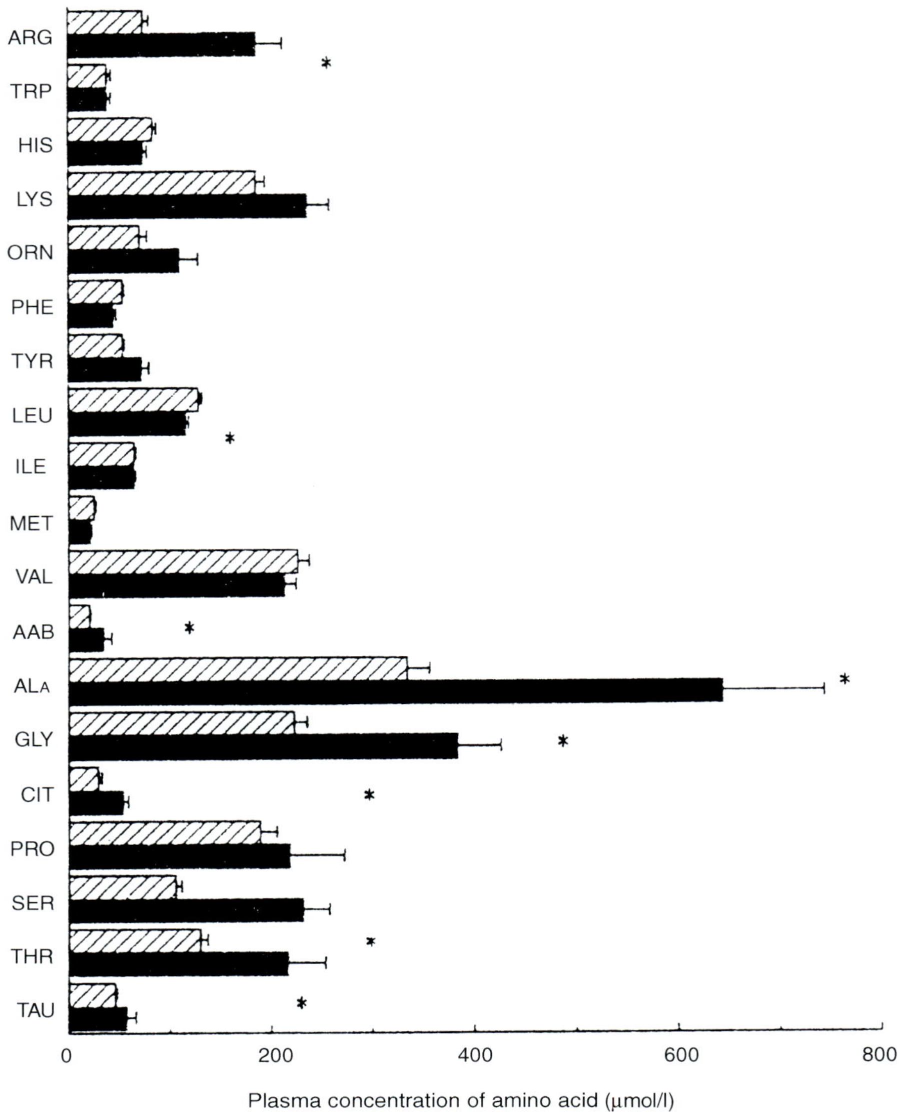

Figure 8 Basal plasma concentration of amino acids in patients with diabetes secondary to total pancreatectomy (closed columns) and normal individuals (cross-hatched columns) (*$p < 0.05$ vs. normal individuals). (Adapted from reference 132, with permission)

of diabetic ketoacidosis may be related to depletion of fat stores and to decreased rate of lipolysis [20]. A similar resistance to ketosis has been observed in diabetes of the tropics, where malnutrition and very low intake of unsaturated fat contribute to the rarity of ketoacidosis [158].

The role of glucagon deficiency in protecting pancreatectomized diabetic patients from ketoacidosis is controversial. Barnes et al. [88] suggested that glucagon lack in these subjects mitigates against the development of ketoacidosis. In type 1 diabetic patients, suppression of glucagon secretion with somatostatin prevents a rise in blood ketone concentrations [159]. Although insulin withdrawal in pancreatectomized patients causes a rise in plasma FFA and ketone bodies, this increase is significantly lower than in type 1 diabetic subjects [88, 89]. Therefore, it is likely that, even though glucagon may not be essential for the development of ketosis, its deficiency can delay or slow down progression toward diabetic ketoacidosis.

The difficulty in maintaining satisfactory, stable metabolic control in patients with diabetes secondary to acquired disease of the pancreas has prompted the inclusion of this group of disorders under the category of "brittle diabetes" [150]. Several factors are responsible for the unstable control in pancreatogenic diabetes (Table 6). The effects of glucagon deficiency have been discussed. Exocrine pancreatic insufficiency with malabsorption can contribute to the instability of glucose control [160]. Steatorrhea may cause glucose malabsorption, thus

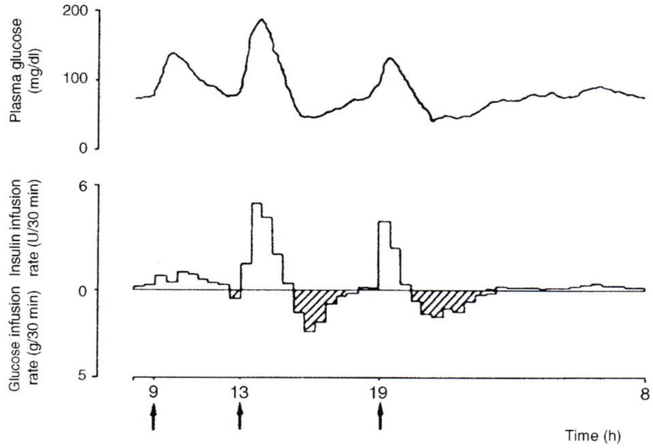

Figure 9 The 24-h plasma glucose profile and insulin/dextrose requirement in a patient with diabetes secondary to total pancreatectomy under control with a glucose-controlled insulin infusion system (artificial endocrine pancreas – Biostator GCIIS) illustrating postprandial tendency to hypoglycemia. (From reference 115, with permission)

contributing to postprandial hypoglycemic reactions and altered insulin secretion [156]. The development of diabetes in patients with pancreatic disease can be associated with dramatic weight loss, which is difficult to correct even with appropriate insulin therapy. Furthermore, weight loss *per se* can markedly alter insulin sensitivity.

Diabetic Complications

Since the late 1950s, the general idea has been that diabetes secondary to chronic pancreatitis was not associated with vascular complications [161–164]. Several factors have been claimed for this apparent reduced frequency of diabetic complications in pancreatogenic diabetes, including absent or less penetrant genetic predisposition, exocrine pancreatic insufficiency, low serum cholesterol levels, and low caloric intake. However, with the improved life expectancy of these patients, more and more cases of diabetic angiopathy have been reported [50, 129, 165, 166]. During the past few years a similar prevalence of retinopathy and microalbuminuria has been described in pancreatic and

Table 6 Factors contributing to excessive glucose fluctuation

(1) Hypoglycemia
- (a) Glucagon deficiency
- (b) Impaired catecholamine secretion
- (c) Malabsorption
- (d) Low carbohydrate intake
- (e) Alcohol consumption
- (f) Poor compliance with therapy and diet
- (g) Increased/preserved insulin sensitivity

(2) Hyperglycemia
- (a) Antral resection
- (b) Poor compliance with therapy and diet

type 1 diabetes mellitus. Caution is required in drawing conclusions on the unique role of hyperglycemia, because patients with pancreatogenic diabetes frequently have a family history of diabetes, and because the duration of their disease is still relatively short [22].

The prevalence of diabetic retinopathy in patients with diabetes secondary to chronic pancreatitis or pancreatectomy was initially reported to vary considerably (Table 7). During the last 10 years a more accurate assessment of diabetic lesions of the retina has yielded an incidence of 30–40%, a figure similar to that found in type 1 diabetic subjects [129, 172, 175, 176, 179]. Incidence of retinopathy is correlated with the duration of the hyperglycemia [50, 129] (Figure 10). By contrast, no apparent relationship exists between the presence of retinopathy and positive family history of diabetes, frequency of HLA antigens, presence of islet cell antibodies, or plasma C-peptide level [50, 129].

There is still controversy about the incidence of diabetic nephropathy in secondary diabetes. Calwell et al. [161] stated that they were "unable to find any one who knows about a case, verified at autopsy, of intercapillary glomerulosclerosis due to hemochromatosis or pancreatitis." However, more and more cases of nodular glomerulosclerosis in patients with diabetes secondary to pancreatitis [169] have been described. Sporadic cases of diabetic glomerulopathy have been reported in patients with total pancreatectomy [50]. The overall lower prevalence of diabetic nephropathy may be due to the shorter duration of diabetes, which does not allow the full appearance of clinically significant nephropathy. Furthermore, most of the studies have looked for patients with late-stage diabetic kidney involvement, but early functional alterations can be detected several years before the appearance of albuminuria. In a series of 86 patients with diabetes secondary to pancreatopathy [50], urinary albumin excretion >40 mg/24 h was found in 23% of the patients (Figure 11). Albuminuria is related to diabetes duration and arterial blood pressure, but not to family history of diabetes mellitus, HLA antigens, or plasma C-peptide levels [50, 176, 180]. Incidence of retinopathy was almost twice as high in patients with microalbuminuria, suggesting that the oculorenal syndrome described in type 1 diabetic patients may occur in pancreatogenic diabetes as well. Glomerular hyperfiltration, another early sign of renal dysfunction, can be detected in pancreatogenic diabetes [181] with a prevalence that is similar to that of type 1 diabetic individuals [177]. In spite of the demonstration of diabetic kidney involvement in these patients, albumin excretion rate >0.5 g/day or overt renal failure is unusual, in agreement with the rarity of reports of glomerulosclerosis in secondary diabetes.

A recent study [179] compared the prevalence, associations, and severity of retinopathy and nephropathy in patients with pancreatic diabetes (40 patients) and type 1

Table 7 Prevalence of microangiopathy in pancreatic diabetes

Author	Year		No. of patients	Diabetes duration (years)	Retinopathy No.	Retinopathy %	Nephropathy No.	Nephropathy %
Sprague [32]	1947	Pancreatitis	24		1/24	4	1/24	4
Deckert [165]	1960	Pancreatitis	26	0–12	7/26	26		
Dettwyler [157]	1964	Pancreatitis–cancer–hemochromatosis	28		2/28	7	2/28	7
Tutin [166]	1966	Pancreatitis	31		4/31	12		
Ennis [167]	1969	Pancreatitis	14	>3	5/14	35		
Sevel [168]	1971	Pancreatitis	27	3–15	2/27	7		
Verdonk [169]	1975	Pancreatitis	168	0–36	24/168	14	2/168	2
Maekawa [170]	1978	Pancreatitis	47	0–15	8/47	17		
Moinade [171]	1979	Pancreatitis	20	2–17	8/20	40	3/20	1.5
Tiengo [129]	1983	Pancreatitis–pancreatectomy	54	0–15	17/54	31		
Couet [172]	1985	Pancreatitis–pancreatectomy	88	1–26	36/88	41		
Rodman [173]	1986	Cystic fibrosis	24		2/24	8		
Tiengo [50]	1988	Pancreatitis–pancreatectomy	86	0–25	32/86	37	19/86	22*
Sullivan [174]	1989	Cystic fibrosis	19		3/19	15	3/19	15
Gullo [175]	1990	Pancreatitis	40	1–15	19/40	47		
Larsen [176]	1990		25	10†	5/25	20	1/25	4*
Tiengo [177]	1992	Pancreatitis–pancreatectomy	33	11†	9/33	27	10/33	30*
Lanng [178]	1994	Cystic fibrosis	41	0–17	2/41	4	1/41	2
Levitt [179]	1995	Pancreatitis	30		10/30	33	7/30	23

* >40 mg/24 h.
† Mean value.

diabetes (30 patients). The prevalence of microalbuminuria, glomerular hyperfiltration, reduced glomerular filtration rate (GFR), and overt nephropathy was similar in the two groups. Albumin excretion rate (AER) was directly correlated with retinopathy and indirectly with GFR in the pancreatic diabetes groups. Neuropathy is a common complaint in pancreatogenic diabetes. A 10–20% incidence of distal polyneuropathy or mononeuropathy is reported [169], and electrophysiological signs of impaired motor conduction velocity are found in >80% of patients with diabetes secondary to pancreatic disease [50]. Vibration threshold was found to be similar to that of matched type 1 diabetic patients [176]. At variance with both retinopathy and nephropathy, there is no relationship with the duration of diabetes. This may be because diabetic neuropathy is an early complication of diabetes mellitus, and/or factors

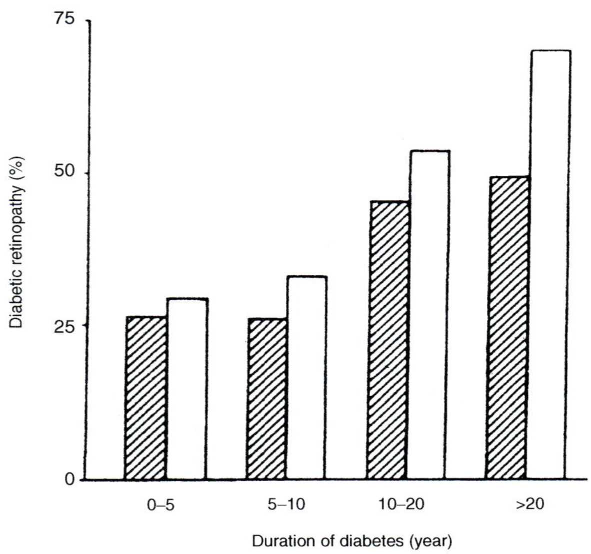

Figure 10 Prevalence of diabetic retinopathy in a cohort of 88 patients with pancreatogenic diabetes (cross-hatched columns) and in a population of type 1 diabetic individuals (open columns). (From reference 50, with permission)

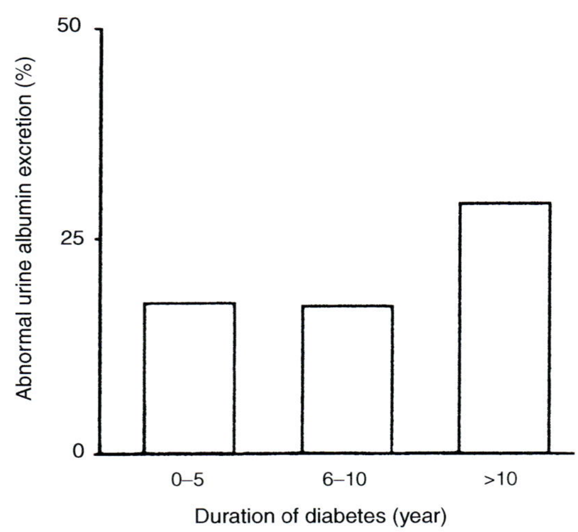

Figure 11 Prevalence of abnormal rate of urine albumin excretion (>40 mg/24 h) in pancreatogenic diabetes expressed as a function of duration of hyperglycemia. (From reference 50, with permission)

Table 8 Insulin requirement (U/day) in patients with diabetes secondary to chronic pancreatitis/pancreatectomy and type 1 diabetes during intensive subcutaneous insulin therapy and glucose-controlled insulin infusion*†

	Total pancreatectomy patients	Partial pancreatectomy patients	Type 1 diabetic patients
Intensive insulin therapy	47 ± 7	60 ± 1	66 ± 6
Artificial endocrine pancreas	44 ± 12	70 ± 8	62 ± 5

* Adapted from reference 124, with permission.
† Artificial endocrine pancreas – Biostator GCIIS.

other than hyperglycemia (smoking, alcohol, malabsorption) may contribute to its development.

Alterations of autonomic nervous function occur as well. Impaired cardiovascular reflexes have been found in 8% of a population with diabetes secondary to chronic pancreatitis, while a borderline defect was observed in an additional 13% of these patients [50]. However, some caution should be exercised in relating hyperglycemia to diabetic somatic and autonomic neuropathy, because alcohol consumption is common in these individuals. Therefore, the true pathogenetic mechanism(s) of neuropathy in diabetic patients with pancreatic disease is difficult to define.

Macroangiopathy, in particular myocardial infarction, is uncommon in pancreatogenic diabetes, although in one report [143] 25% of patients with diabetes secondary to chronic pancreatitis were found to be affected by vascular complications, and some required amputations or vascular bypass operations. The relatively short duration of diabetes and the underlying disease of the pancreas make it difficult to estimate the prevalence of macrovascular complications in pancreatogenic diabetes. When long enough follow-up has proved possible, cardiovascular complications have been found to account for 16% of deaths in chronic pancreatitis patients [92].

Therapeutic Aspects

The treatment of diabetes secondary to chronic pancreatitis or pancreatectomy is complex. In patients with chronic pancreatitis or partial pancreatectomy, oral hypoglycemic agents may be introduced in those individuals who still retain a satisfactory C-peptide response to glucagon or a meal [20]. Short- rather than long-acting sulfonylureas are preferred, in order to minimize the risk of severe hypoglycemia [182]. Nevertheless, care should be taken when employing sulfonylurea agents in patients with altered liver function tests, and biguanides should be avoided in such patients. More recently, a possible use of GLP-1 has been postulated [71] because its lowering effect on plasma glucose is apparently free of hypoglycemic risk [183]. Insulin therapy is mandatory following total pancreatectomy, although insulin requirements are lower than in type 1 diabetic patients, particularly at night [184]. In contrast, postprandial insulin requirement may be more pronounced. This is particularly true in patients with total pancreatectomy, while insulin-dependent patients with chronic pancreatitis or partial pancreatectomy usually have insulin requirements which are similar to those of type 1 diabetic individuals [124] (Table 8). Whatever the chosen therapy, hypoglycemia remains the main concern [149, 150]. The increased frequency and severity of hypoglycemic events is the likely consequence of the concurrence of several factors, including insulin excess, insulin sensitivity, impaired counterregulation, deficient diet or nutrient absorption, alcohol intake, and liver diseases [20, 150, 160]. The risk of lethal hypoglycemia is particularly high in totally pancreatectomized patients, and this has prompted the search for safer surgical and medical approaches. Thus, preservation of the duodenum and pylorus seems to ensure more stable metabolic control and fewer hypoglycemic episodes [185]. Finally, islet autotransplantation may be an effective adjunct to extensive pancreatic resection [186]. Intrahepatic autoislet transplantation could successfully maintain stable β-cell function and normal glucose and HbA_{1c} for up to 13 years after total pancreatectomy as treatment for chronic painful pancreatitis [187].

Rigorous home glucose monitoring and multiple administration of small doses of insulin, along with intensive education programs, may result in good, stable metabolic control in these patients as well [141, 182]. However, this must be associated with a number of specific steps (Table 9). Correction of the patient's nutritional status

Table 9 Therapeutic approaches to the patient with diabetes secondary to pancreatic disease

(1) Diet
  (a) High-energy diet (2200–3000 kcal/day)
  (b) Small and frequent meals
  (c) Alcohol withdrawal
  (d) Low intake of neutral fat
  (e) Increased intake of complex carbohydrates
(2) Pancreatic digestive enzyme replacement
(3) Electrolytes, calcium, vitamins D and K
(4) Sulfonylureas
  (a) If stimulated C-peptide >2 ng/ml
(5) Insulin
  (a) Small doses of regular insulin before each meal
  (b) Caution in the use of long-acting insulin preparations
  (c) Continuous subcutaneous infusion only in highly motivated and educated patients

must be pursued. Alcohol withdrawal is essential; often, it is the primary cause of the pancreatic inflammation, and it may precipitate hypoglycemia [151–153]. Excessive alcohol intake also causes progressive liver damage, which *per se* may worsen metabolic control [156]. Malabsorption with steatorrhea contributes to the development of hypoglycemic events. Steatorrhea may also impair insulin secretion through derangement of the enteropancreatic axis [160]. In patients with pancreatic diabetes, pancreatic digestive enzymes should be replaced to reduce stool fat excretion below 20 g/day. Concomitant treatment with H2-receptor antagonists should be considered, because reduction in gastric acid output may reduce pancreatic enzyme degradation. Acid-resistant preparations of pancreatic enzymes are recommended. A high-energy diet (>2500 kcal/day) with a high complex carbohydrate and low fat content is advisable. In patients with chronic pancreatitis, high-fat meals may increase the frequency and intensity of abdominal pain. Therefore, limitation of fat calories to 20–25% of total calorie intake is recommended. Meals should be small and frequent, with three principal meals and two or three intervening snacks. If needed, the diet should be supplemented with electrolytes, calcium, vitamin D, and potassium. The accelerated intestinal transit and dumping syndrome that occurs after gastrectomy may also contribute to malabsorption and unstable metabolic control. In defining a strategy for insulin treatment in patients with marked glycemic fluctuations, it is necessary to be cognizant of the lower insulin requirements in such patients, as well as the lower incidence and slower progression of diabetic complications (Table 10). A nighttime dose of intermediate insulin should be employed to control overnight and fasting hyperglycemia. The use of two injections per day of long-acting insulin has been advocated to achieve better glycemic stability [17]. In highly motivated and educated patients, insulin treatment by continuous subcutaneous infusion has been successfully employed to achieve meticulous metabolic control while avoiding hypoglycemia and ketosis.

Hypoglycemic reactions, if they occur, must be treated aggressively and their cause(s) and mechanism(s) carefully evaluated and explained to the patient. Even though ketoacidosis is uncommon in pancreatogenic diabetes, it can develop under conditions of stress (infection, surgery, etc.) and it requires appropriate adjustment of the insulin dose. Because of the extreme brittleness of patients with pancreatogenic diabetes, patient education and self-monitoring of blood glucose are extremely important. Lastly, in some patients with diabetes secondary to acquired disease of the pancreas it may be difficult to achieve optimal metabolic control because of the high risk of hypoglycemia. The maintenance of plasma glucose levels slightly above the normal range may be necessary to avoid frequent hypoglycemic reactions and to improve the quality of life. It should be remembered that many of these patients have a reduced life expectancy and are at lower risk of developing diabetic complications.

Table 10 Management goals in diabetes secondary to pancreatic disease

- Improve nutritional condition
- Avoid steatorrhea and malabsorption
- Maintain an adequate diet and energy intake
- Avoid excessive fluctuations in blood glucose
- Avoid hypoglycemia

NEOPLASIA

In 1833, Bright reported the case of a 49-year-old marked man who initially presented chronic symptoms of diabetes and subsequently suffered from jaundice. Twelve months following the onset of diabetes he died from complications of cancer of the head of the pancreas [188]. Following this original description, an association between carcinoma of the pancreas and diabetes mellitus was recognized. Pancreatic cancer has a high incidence worldwide and poor prognosis. In the United States, the disease presently accounts for 3% of all cancers responsible for 5% of all cancer deaths. It is the fourth most common cause of cancer death in men after lung, colorectal, and prostatic cancers, and the fifth cause of cancer death in women after breast, colorectal, lung, and ovarianuterine cancers [189].

Hyperglycemia and pancreatic neoplasia are usually diagnosed within 1–2 years of each other [190], suggesting that the neoplastic process may directly affect the endocrine pancreas. The incidence of hyperglycemia at the time of diagnosis of the pancreatic cancer ranges between 40 and 50% [191]. However, when challenged by oral glucose tolerance test (OGTT), impaired glucose tolerance can be diagnosed in about 80% of the patients [192, 193]. Although it has been suggested that carcinoma of the pancreas tends to be more prevalent in the diabetic population [106], a recent survey has concluded that diabetes in patients with pancreatic cancer is probably caused by the tumor, and that diabetes is not a risk factor for neoplasia of the pancreas [194]. The mechanism of impaired glucose metabolism that develops in most patients with pancreatic cancer is obscure, and the association between pancreatic cancer and diabetes is controversial [195], but up to 60% of the patients with impaired glucose tolerance or diabetes show improvement in glucose metabolism after surgery.

The mechanism(s) involved in the pathogenesis of diabetes are likely to include disruption of the islets of Langerhans, occlusion of the pancreatic duct with consequent cell degeneration, tumor-related pancreatitis, and fibrosclerosis with compression of blood vessels and autonomic nerve fibers. More recently, it has been demonstrated that diabetogenic substances can be produced by the tumor [195, 196], though it is not clear if they are the product of neoplastic cells, or endocrine cells within the tumor, or functionally altered islets near the tumor. The chronic (40 days) injection of extracts of human pancreatic cancer cell line into immunodeficient mice was associated with the development of hyperglycemia [197, 198].

Plasma islet amyloid polypeptide (IAPP) concentration is increased in patients with pancreatic cancer [199, 200], but a pathogentic role for accompanying diabetes seems unlikely since IAPP levels are actually low in neoplastic diabetic patients [200]. Besides IAPP other pancreatic factors may be involved in metabolic disorders associated with pancreatic cancer. Expression of tumor necrosis factor α (TNF-α) gene is upregulated in patients with pancreatic cancer and it is normalized after the pancreatic tumor is removed [201]. A direct involvement of islet cells in the carcinogenesis and impaired hormonal secretion has been postulated as well. It is, indeed, possible that islet and neoplastic ductal cells might arise from a common precursor of the ductal epithelium [202, 203]. Finally, factors such as inactivity, stress, weight loss, and low caloric intake may contribute to impaired glucose tolerance and to insulin resistance.

Pathology

B-cell number can be as low as 50% in patients with diabetes secondary to pancreatic cancer [204]. The reduction of B-cell mass is a function of the degree of fibrosis, which affects the supply of trophic factors to islets. In spite of the reported increase in circulating IAPP in nondiabetic patients with pancreatic cancer, its islet concentration is reduced [199]. The number of A-cells may be normal or reduced, while D-cells tend to be reduced. Conversely, intra- as well as extrainsular PP-cell hyperplasia is often observed along the front line of the carcinoma. In the hamster pancreatic cancer model, a plausible model for the human disease as far as morphological, molecular biological, clinical, and immunological aspects are concerned [205], the participation of endocrine cells in the development of exocrine cancer occurs very early in the carcinogenetic process. In this model, various numbers and types of islet cells are found within the hyperplastic, preneoplastic, and neoplastic tissue forming ductal and ductular structures [206]. The phenomenon could explain the higher level of islet hormones measurable in the pancreatic juice of animals with pancreatic cancer [207].

Hormone Secretion

Both insulin and C-peptide responses to oral glucose are frequently decreased and/or delayed. High fasting plasma C-peptide has been reported in non-insulin-requiring diabetic patients with pancreatic cancer compared to controls. Non-insulin- and insulin-requiring diabetic patients also have elevated fasting levels of IAPP, glucagon, and somatostatin. Tumor resection is followed by normalization of plasma IAPP and glucagons levels, but not somatostatin. In response to hyperglycemia, plasma C-peptide and IAPP increase in pancreatic cancer patients with normal glucose tolerance, while diabetic individuals exhibit impairment in both first- and second-phase insulin secretion [200, 208]. In spite of low plasma C-peptide, post-OGTT proinsulin secretion is increased in patients with pancreatic cancer [209].

Peripheral insulin resistance has been reported [192, 199]. Fasting plasma glucagon concentration can be either normal or increased, while a paradoxical rise has been observed following an oral glucose load by some [192], but not all investigators [208].

Clinical Manifestations and Therapeutic Considerations

In a recent survey, diabetes mellitus was found at a high frequency (53.1%) in patients with invasive ductal pancreatic carcinoma, and was mostly considered as secondary to the neoplastic process (45.9%) [210]. Glycemic control can be difficult in spite of insulin treatment. Nonetheless, amelioration of metabolic control is considered important for the treatment of the pancreatic carcinoma. Diabetic complications are unusual, because the survival period of the patients is still limited, but the coexistence of diabetes is associated with worse prognosis.

CYSTIC FIBROSIS

Cystic fibrosis is an autosomic recessive genetic disorder. Gene defects on the long arm of chromosome 7 are responsible for defective production of a protein known as the cystic fibrosis transmembrane regulator (CFTR). CFTR is a cAMP-dependent chloride channel which control water and electrolyte composition of secretions from sweat glands, lung, liver, hepatobiliary ducts, pancreatic duct, and gastrointestinal tract [211]. Defective action of CFTR is responsible for accumulation of thick secretions associated with progressive obstruction, scarring and destruction. Respiratory disease with chronic bacterial infection is the main cause of death (84%) [212]. The pancreatic involvement in cystic fibrosis accounts for the concomitance of impaired glucose tolerance and cystic fibrosis related diabetes (CFRD). Recent figures show that overt hyperglycemia occurs in 4–10% of the patients with cystic fibrosis, whereas impaired glucose tolerance is found in 8–75% [213, 214]. These figures are likely to be underestimated because no systematic screening is performed yet. With the increase in life expectancy brought about by improved medical therapy, the prevalence of diabetes mellitus

Table 11 Percent prevalence of diabetes in patients with cystic fibrosis within age groups*

	5–9 years	10–19 years	20–29 years	>30 years
Total number	61	139	105	66
NGT (%)	57	36	23	30
IGT (%)	34	38	42	27
Diabetes (%)	9	26	35	42

Note. NGT = normal glucose tolerance; IGT = impaired glucose tolerance.
* Adapted from reference 211.

increases: 43% in patients older than 30 (Table 11). The development of CFRD has classically been looked upon as a complication of the fibrotic process of the pancreas. However, CFRD can occur at any age, and no correlation exists between the duration of disease and the severity of glucose intolerance [173]. This suggests that etiological factors other than pancreatic fibrosis may contribute to the development of glucose intolerance and diabetes. A genetic linkage between cystic fibrosis and diabetes mellitus is unlikely, since there is no increased incidence of cystic fibrosis in families with diabetes mellitus. Recent investigations have reported that diabetic patients with cystic fibrosis have an increased incidence of the HLA-DR3 and HLA-DR4 antigens [215], although this finding has not been confirmed by others [216–218]. An increased incidence of islet cell antibodies has been reported as well [215, 219]. These findings suggest that in genetically predisposed patients, cystic fibrosis may damage the pancreatic tissue and result in a mounting autoimmune response which contributes to B-cell destruction and development of diabetes mellitus. It is also possible that different genotypes may be associated with different clinical manifestations. Thus, patients with the R117H ΔF508 genotype are likely to maintain long-term pancreatic function so that development of CFRD is delayed [220]. Finally, it is possible that progression to overt diabetes may primarily reflect genetic predisposition to type 2 diabetes [221].

Pathology

The volume and weight of the pancreas is severely reduced in patients with CFRD and the pancreatic tissue is disrupted by thick, collagenous bands that surround and separate clusters of islets of Langerhans. The number of B-cells is reduced by 40–50% [222] even in patients with normoglycemia, and this reduction is sufficient to explain the impairment in insulin secretion. Islet cellular composition is also disrupted with a significant percentage reduction of B-, A-, and PP-cells and relative increase of D-cells [223, 224]. Islet amyloid deposition is characteristic in CFRD [221].

Hormone Secretion

Insulin deficiency is the main cause of CFRD [225]. Insulin and C-peptide responses to oral and intravenous glucose, arginine, tolbutamide, and glucagon are reduced in patients with or without overt fasting hyperglycemia [226, 227]. The reduction in insulin secretion is a function of the loss of B-cell mass. Patients with no exocrine insufficiency have normal insulin secretion, whereas exocrine-insufficient patients without diabetes present a significant impairment in insulin secretion and oral glucose intolerance [228]. Alteration of islet cell microcirculation by fibrosis, and/or inhibition of insulin secretion by a somatostatin paracrine effect, may contribute to hypoinsulinemia.

Impaired insulin action has been described in CFRD [229, 230]. This reduction of insulin sensitivity has been attributed to elevated circulating levels of TNF-α and impaired translocation of GLUT-4 (glucose transporter 4) in muscle cells [231]. Similarly, hepatic insulin resistance with increased liver glucose output has been reported [232]. However, the issue is controversial. Some studies have reported increased insulin sensitivity [233–235], whereas others have shown decreased or normal insulin action [236, 237].

Arginine-stimulated glucagon response is altered in CFRD [226, 238]. Following an oral glucose load, plasma glucagon concentrations decline in nondiabetic patients, whereas they fail to be suppressed in diabetic individuals. Pancreatic polypeptide secretion is also impaired [227, 239], while somatostatin levels may be elevated [240]. The GIP response following oral glucose is normal, suggesting that enteropancreatic axis function is preserved [241].

Metabolic Aspects

Cholesterol and triglyceride levels have been found normal in Canadian adult patients with CFRD [242]. In an American cohort of 195 patients with cystic fibrosis, isolated hypertriglyceridemia was commonly found, whereas cholesterol concentrations were generally low. Increased serum triglyceride concentration may be related to chronic inflammation and/or dietary micronutrient imbalance with excessive simple carbohydrate absorption relative to fat absorption.

In the absence of significant underlying infection, clinically stable adult with cystic fibrosis has normal amino acid turnover in the fasting state, even when severe alterations in insulin secretion and severe impairment in pulmonary function are present. However, physiologic hyperinsulinemia is not associated with normal inhibition of protein breakdown, contributing to net protein catabolism of these patients [243].

Clinical Manifestations

Average age at diagnosis of CFRD is 18–21 years, with a slight female predominance [244, 245]. The disease is more frequent in patients carrying the ΔF508 mutation [244]. Most of the patients have pancreatic exocrine insufficiency. In the minority retaining exocrine function, the risk of developing CFRD is lower [246].

Exaggerated hyperglycemic response can develop during exacerbation of pulmonary infections in patients with cystic fibrosis [173]. Nonetheless, ketoacidosis is rare [212] because of residual B-cell function and impaired glucagon secretion. Overall mortality is greater in patients with CFRD than in the general diabetic population [245].

CFRD can be complicated by retinopathy (5–16%), nephropathy (3–16%), and neuropathy (5–21%) [173, 174, 178] (Table 7). On the contrary, there is no evidence for increased cardiovascular complications in these patients, but this finding can be biased owing to limited survival.

Therapeutic Considerations

Maintenance of optimal nutritional status is of primary importance in the management of CFRD. Because of the defect in insulin secretion and reduction of β-cell mass, exogenous insulin administration remains the main therapeutic tool in CFRD [212]. Multiple daily injections of regular insulin before each meal and modest amount of long-acting insulin at bedtime are usually indicated. In these individuals insulin requirement ranges between 0.6 and 3.3 U/kg body weigh/day, with an average of 1.45 U/kg/day [247]. The high insulin requirement is likely to reflect intercurrent flogistic and infective conditions and/or an insulin-resistant status. Fast-acting insulin analogues (lispro, aspart) should be used at mealtime to prevent excessive glucose excursions and prevent hypoglycemia. For this reason, all patients should perform home blood glucose monitoring. Insulin is definitely needed during hyperglycemic exacerbation related to recurrent pulmonary infections [173]. Moreover, insulin treatment can improve anabolism, increase body weight [248, 249], and protect pulmonary function [250].

Although sulfonylurea therapy has been largely used in patients with moderate hyperglycemia [173], there are no solid trials in the literature. In the few studies available [251–254], the effect of sulfonylureas on insulin secretion was limited. It is possible that in specific CFRD subgroup, however, sulfonylurea treatment can be maintained for a number of years with clinical outcomes similar to those of insulin-treated patients [255]. Since they inhibit CFTR [256], caution should be exercised with sulfonylurea treatment in combination with drug designed to improve the defective action of the protein. Glibenclamide should be avoided because of prevalent bile excretion. More recently, repaglinide effects in CFRD have been assessed [257]. Since insulin resistance is not a primary pathogenetic defect in CFRD, insulin sensitizers have a very limited indication. Moreover, metformin is contraindicated in patients with hypoxia, while its possible gastrointestinal side effects can be a problem in malnourished patients. The role of thiazoledinediones remains unclear in the absence of specific studies. While impaired liver function in patients with CFRD may be seen as a limitation, recent work suggests glitazones may retard liver fibrosis [258]. Finally, the use of a drug such as acarbose that reduces energy absorption is questionable.

Finally, since 18–47% of patients with cystic fibrosis have impaired glucose tolerance [227, 259], a close follow-up should be established in order to provide prompt intervention.

HEMOCHROMATOSIS

Primary

In 1865 Trousseau first reported the association between diabetes mellitus and hemochromatosis [260]. Six years later, Troisier described the association of diabetes with pigmentation of the liver and pancreas. The pigment was subsequently identified as iron by von Recklinghausen, who coined the term "hemochromatosis." Hereditary hemochromatosis is an inherited disorder of iron metabolism and is one of the most common genetic diseases in individuals of Northern Europe, affecting approximately 1 in 200–300 individuals [261]. The familial nature of hemochromatosis was first characterized in 1935 by Sheldon [262]. It was more than 40 years later than the genetic basis of the disease was proposed by Simon [263], based on the linkage with HLA-A3 and HLA-B7. In 1996, using positional cloning, Feder et al. [264] described the HFE gene (located 4500 kb distal to HLA-A on the short arm of chromosome 6, encoding a 343-amino acid protein consisting of a short cytoplasmic segment, a transmembrane domain, and three extracellular MHC class 1-like domains) and two mutations responsible for most cases of hereditary hemochromatosis.

Individuals with hemochromatosis chronically absorb iron in excess, causing iron deposition in parenchymal cells of many organs and eventually diabetes mellitus, cardiomyopathy, and hepatic cirrhosis [265]. Diabetes mellitus occurs in over 75% of patients with hemochromatosis [266, 267]. Even though concomitant liver cirrhosis can affect glucose metabolism, this does not fully account for the diabetic condition. In contrast to chronic pancreatitis, in patients with hemochromatosis, diabetes mellitus is an early complication. Thus, more often than not, diabetes precedes the clinical recognition of hemochromatosis. On average, diabetes mellitus is diagnosed approximately 1 year before hemochromatosis [268]. It is rarely associated with obesity and it affects males 10 times more frequently than females.

In primary hemochromatosis, diabetes was initially explained as a classic infiltrative disorder with destruction of endocrine tissue. More recently, it has been recognized that diabetes and hemochromatosis have independent genetic transmission [267]. Thus, diabetes associated with primary hemochromatosis results from the interaction of a diabetic genetic predisposition and iron pancreas infiltration.

Pathophysiology

The deposition of iron is reflected biochemically by an increase in the serum ferritin level, which is linearly correlated with the degree of increased body iron stores. Elevation of transferrin saturation is the earliest phenotypic manifestation occurring in the first decade and before iron overload has occurred [265]. Inspection of the pancreas shows a firm light-brown tissue, with focal fibrotic lesions. Microscopic examination reveals atrophy of the acini, with a marked increase in interstitial collagen. The deposition of hemosiderin is extensive. The iron deposits are more evident in the acinar tissue rather than in the islets of Langerhans, many of which appear histologically normal.

In 1997, Moirand et al. [269] described a condition of primary hepatic iron overload (HIO), in which transferrin saturation and HLA A3 genotype frequency were normal, and serum and liver iron depot were raised disproportionately to the increase in serum ferritin. The vast majority of those patients (94%) met criteria for the insulin resistance syndrome [270]. The pathophysiologic link between HIO and insulin resistance syndrome is not readily apparent [271]. Although it has been suggested that HIO can promote oxidative stress, nonalcoholic steatohepatitis (NASH), and fibrosis, the relationship between HIO and NASH remains unclear [272].

Hormone Secretion

Basal plasma insulin concentration and the plasma insulin response to oral glucose are often altered, while plasma glucagon concentration is usually increased [273]. Most of the circulating glucagon, however, is represented by high M_r species that do not possess full biological activity. Hypoinsulinemia reflects a primary defect in B-cell function. Insulin resistance is common in hemochromatosis, possibly because of the coexisting hepatic cirrhosis. Impaired glucose uptake assessed by the euglycemic insulin clamp technique suggests insulin resistance in muscle tissue as well. Heterozygosity for the C282Y mutation in the HFE gene (the main one that cause hemochromatosis) has been associated with an increased risk for diabetes [274]. However, no difference in insulin sensitivity or β-cell function was observed in diabetic patients with or without the presence of monoallelic HFE mutations [275].

Secondary Hemochromatosis

Excessive iron deposition occurs in a variety of conditions (other than primary hemochromatosis) that are unlikely to be genetically linked to diabetes mellitus, including thalassemia major [276] and other hemoglobin disorders associated with iron overload [277]. In thalassemia major, frequent blood transfusions are required and this leads to massive iron overload. The duration of the disease and the number of transfusions are highly correlated with the degree of glucose intolerance [278]. Therefore, the relationship between iron excess and diabetes mellitus is even more striking than in primary hemochromatosis where quantification of iron overload is less accurate. The development of diabetes in individuals receiving multiple chronic blood transfusions is a negative prognostic sign and usually precedes death by about 2 years [278]. The reported prevalence of diabetes in treated thalassemia major is about 5%, while the incidence of impaired glucose tolerance is approximately 27% [279]. A marked impairment of insulin sensitivity has been documented in patients with secondary hemochromatosis due to thalassemia, although a concomitant early defect in insulin secretion could not be excluded [280]. Although insulin secretion may be only moderately impaired, hyperglucagonemia is almost universally encountered.

A different model of iron infiltration of the pancreas is found in rural male Bantus. Many Bantus ingest in excess of 100 mg of iron/day in alcoholic drinks that are brewed in iron containers. In such individuals, the prevalence of diabetes is 10 times higher than in Bantus who do not consume such alcoholic beverages [277].

Clinical Manifestations

In primary hemochromatosis, the diagnosis of diabetes is often made before the disturbance in iron metabolism is recognized. The mean age of diagnosis for diabetes in patients with primary hemochromatosis ranges between 47 and 50 years [268], which is much younger than for type 2 diabetes in Caucasian patients. A short interval usually occurs between the diagnosis of diabetes mellitus and that of carcinoma of the pancreas. In cystic fibrosis, the onset of diabetes can occur at any age and bears no relationship to the initial diagnosis of the primary disease.

In spite of early observations suggesting that diabetes associated with primary hemochromatosis was relatively complication-free [164], all diabetic complications have been shown to occur at a rate comparable to that for primary diabetes after a 5-year duration of diabetes [281] (Table 7). Similar findings have been reported in patients with diabetes secondary to cystic fibrosis [208]. It is noteworthy that retinopathy in secondary diabetes is usually "background" in nature, while proliferative lesions are more rarely described [50, 129, 172, 173].

Therapeutic Considerations

Most patients with diabetes secondary to hemochromatosis are treated with insulin [263]. Although oral antidiabetic agents can be successfully employed, the presence of concomitant liver cirrhosis requires caution in their use. The removal of excess iron deposits by phlebotomy is usually associated with an improvement in glucose tolerance and a reduction in insulin requirement.

REFERENCES

1. The Expert Committee on the Diagnosis and Classification of Diabetes Mellitus. Report of the Expert Committee on the Diagnosis and Classification of diabetes mellitus. *Diabetes Care* 1997; 20: 1183–97.
2. Alberti KGMM, Zimmet PZ. Definition, diagnosis and classification of diabetes mellitus and its complications, Part I: Diagnosis and classification of diabetes mellitus. Provisional report of a WHO Consultation. *Diabet Med* 1998; 15: 539–53.
3. National Diabetes Data Group. Classification and diagnosis of diabetes mellitus and other categories of glucose intolerance. *Diabetes* 1979; 28: 1039–57.
4. World Health Organization Diabetes mellitus: Report of a WHO Study Group. Technical Report Series 727. Geneva: WHO, 1985; pp 10–20.
5. Yajnik CS. Diabetes secondary to tropical calcific pancreatitis. *Bailliéres Clin Endocrinol Metab* 1992; 6: 777–96.
6. Cawley T. A singular case of diabetes, consisting entirely in the quality of the urine: with an inquiry into the different theories of that disease. *Lond Med J* 1788; 9: 286–308.
7. Minkowski O. De l'estirpation du pancreas chez les animaux et du diabéte expérimentale. *Semaine Med* 1889; 9: 175–80.
8. Schumacker HS Jr. Acute pancreatitis and diabetes. *Ann Surg* 1940; 112: 177–200.
9. Priestly JT, Comfort MW, Randcliff J. Total pancreatectomy for hyperinsulinism due to an islet cell adenoma. *Ann Surg* 1944; 199: 211–21.
10. Finch SC, Finch CA. Idiopathic hemochromatosis. An iron storage disease. *Medicine* 1955; 34: 361–430.
11. Dervenis C, Johnson CD, Bassi C, Bradley E, Imrie CW, McMahon MJ, Modlin I. Diagnosis, objective assessment of severity, and management of acute pancreatitis. Santorini consensus conference. *Int J Pancreatol* 1999; 25: 195–210.
12. Mitchell RM, Byrne MF, Baillie J. Pancreatitis. *Lancet* 2003; 361: 1447–55.
13. Sweiry JH, Mann GE. Role of oxidative stress in the pathogenesis of acute pancreatitis. *Scand J Gastroenterol Suppl.* 1996; 219: 10–5.
14. Qader SS, Ekelund M, Andersson R, Obermuller S, Salehi A. Acute pancreatitis, expression of inducible nitric oxide synthase and defective insulin secretion. *Cell Tissue Res* September 2003; 313 (3): 271–9.
15. Schulz HU, Niederau C, Klonowski-Stumpe H, Halangk W, Luthen R, Lippert H. Oxidative stress in acute pancreatitis. *Hepatogastroenterology* 1999; 46: 2736–50.
16. Schneider A, Suman A, Rossi L, Barmada MM, Beglinger C, Parvin S, Sattar S, Ali L, Khan AK, Gyr N, Whitcomb DC. SPINK1/PSTI mutations are associated with tropical pancreatitis and type II diabetes mellitus in Bangladesh. *Gastroenterology* 2002; 123: 1026–30.
17. Thow J, Samad A, Alberti KGMM. Epidemiology and general aspects of diabetes secondary to pancreatopathy. In Tiengo A, Alberti KGMM, Del Prato S, Vranic M (eds) *Diabetes Secondary to Pancreatopathy*. Amsterdam: Excerpta Medica, 1988; pp 7–20.
18. Sarles H, Cros RC, Bidart JM. International Group for the Study of Pancreatic Diseases: a multicenter inquiry on the etiology of pancreatic diseases. *Digestion* 1979; 19: 110–25.
19. Malecka-Panas E, Gasiorowska A, Kropiwnicka A, Zlobinska A, Drzewoski J. Endocrine pancreatic function in patients after acute pancreatitis. *Hepatogastroenterology* 2002; 49: 1707–12.
20. Bank S, Marks IN, Vinik AL. Clinical and hormonal aspects of pancreatic diabetes. *Am J Gastroenterol* 1975; 64: 13–22.
21. Warren KW, Fallis LS, Barron J. Acute pancreatitis and diabetes. *Ann Surg* 1950; 132: 1103–10.
22. Scuro LA, Angelini G, Cavallini G, Vantini I. The late outcome of acute pancreatitis. In Gyr KL, Singer MV, Saries H (eds) *Pancreatitis: Concepts and Classification*. Amsterdam: Excerpta Medica, 1984; pp 403–8.
23. Drew SI, Joffe B, Vinik AI, Seften H, Singer F. The first 24 hours of acute pancreatitis. Changes in biochemical and endocrine homeostasis in patients with pancreatitis compared with those in control subjects undergoing stress for reasons other than pancreatitis. *Am J Med* 1978; 64: 795–803.
24. Larsen S, Hilsted J, Tronier B, Woming H. Metabolic control and B cell function in patients with insulin-dependent diabetes mellitus secondary to chronic pancreatitis. *Metabolism* 1987; 36: 964–7.
25. Donowitz M, Hendler R, Spiro HM, Binder H, Felig P. Glucagon secretion in acute and chronic pancreatitis. *J Intern Med* 1975; 83: 778–81.
26. Murtaugh RJ, Jacobs RM, Sherding RG, O'Dorisio TM. Serum pancreatic polypeptide and amylase concentrations in dogs with experimentally induced acute pancreatitis. *Am J Vet Res* 1985; 46: 654–6.
27. Hennig R, Kekis PB, Friess H, Adrian TE, Buchler MW. Pancreatic polypeptide in pancreatitis. *Peptides* 2002; 23: 331–8.
28. Malfertheiner P, Buchler M, Stanescu A, Ditschuneit H. Pancreatic morphology and function in relationship to pain in chronic pancreatitis. *Int J Pancreatol* 1987; 2: 59–66.
29. Sarles H. Chronic pancreatitis and diabetes. *Bailliéres Clin Endocrinol Metab* 1992; 6: 745–75.
30. Etemad B, Whitcomb DC. Chronic pancreatitis: diagnosis, classification, and new genetic developments. *Gastroenterology* 2001; 120: 682–707.
31. Koliopanos A, Friess H, Kleeff J, Roggo A, Zimmermann A, Buchler MW. Cyclooxygenase 2 expression in chronic pancreatitis: correlation with stage of the disease and diabetes mellitus. *Digestion* 2001; 64: 240–7.
32. Sprague RG. Diabetes mellitus associated with chronic relapsing pancreatitis. *Proc Mayo Clin* 1947; 22: 553–8.
33. Petersen JM. Tropical pancreatitis. *J Clin Gastroenterol* July 2002; 35: 61–6.
34. Zuidema PJ. Calcification and cirrhosis of the pancreas in patients with deficient nutrition. *Doc Med Geograph Trop Amsterdam* 1955; 5: 229–34.

35. Hoet JJ, Tripathy BB. Report of the International Workshop on Types of Diabetes Peculiar to the Tropics. *Diabetes Care* September 1996; 19 (9): 1014.
36. Mohan V, Alberti KGMM. Diabetes in the tropics. In Alberti KGMM, Keen H, Zimmet P (eds) *International Textbook of Diabetes Mellitus*. Chichester: Wiley, 1992; pp 177–96.
37. Mohan V, Premalatha G, Pitchumoni CS. Tropical chronic pancreatitis: an update. *J Clin Gastroenterol* 2003; 36: 337–46.
38. Govindarajan M, Mohan V, Deepa R, Ashok S, Pitchumoni CS. Histopathology and immunohistochemistry of pancreatic islets in fibrocalculous pancreatic diabetes. *Diabetes Res Clin Pract* 2001; 51: 29–38.
39. Sarles H, Sarles JC, Muratore R. Chronic inflammatory sclerosis of the pancreas—an autonomous pancreatic disease? *Am J Dig Dis* 1961; 6: 688–98.
40. Taniguchi T, Seko S, Okamoto M, Hamasaki A, Ueno H, Inoue F, Nishida O, Miyake N, Mizumoto T. Association of autoimmune pancreatitis and type 1 diabetes: autoimmune exocrinopathy and endocrinopathy of the pancreas. *Diabetes Care* 2000; 23: 1592–4.
41. Okazaki K, Uchida K, Ohana M, Nakase H, Uose S, Inai M, Matsushima Y, Katamura K, Ohmori K, Chiba T. Autoimmune-related pancreatitis is associated with autoantibodies and a Th1/Th2-type cellular immune response. *Gastroenterology* 2000; 118: 573–81.
42. Tanaka S, Kobayashi T, Nakanishi K, Okubo M, Murase T, Hashimoto M, Takeuchi K. Corticosteroid-responsive diabetes mellitus associated with autoimmune pancreatitis. *Lancet* 2000; 356: 910–1.
43. Sarles H, Sahel J, Satub JL, Bourry J, Laugier R. Chronic pancreatitis. In Howatt HT, Sarles H (eds) *The Exocrine Pancreas*. London: WB Saunders, 1979; pp 402–39.
44. Lowenfels AB, Maisonneuve P, Cavallini G, Ammann RW, Lankisch PG, Andersen JR, DiMagno EP, Andren-Sandberg A, Domellof L, Di Francesco V, for the International Pancreatitis Study Group. Prognosis of chronic pancreatitis: an international multicenter study. *Am J Gastroenterol* 1994; 89: 1467–71.
45. Wakasugi H, Funakoshi A, Iguchi H. Clinical assessment of pancreatic diabetes caused by chronic pancreatitis. *J Gastroenterol* 1998; 33: 254–9.
46. Malka D, Hammel P, Sauvanet A, Rufat P, O'Toole D, Bardet P, Belghiti J, Bernades P, Ruszniewski P, Levy P. Risk factors for diabetes mellitus in chronic pancreatitis. *Gastroenterology* 2000; 119: 1324–32.
47. Berney T, Rudisuhli T, Oberholzer J, Caulfield A, Morel P. Long-term metabolic results after pancreatic resection for severe chronic pancreatitis. *Arch Surg* 2000; 135: 1106–11.
48. Gross JB. Hereditary pancreatitis. In Go VLN (ed), *The Exocrine Pancreas: Biology, Pathology and Diseases*. New York: Raven Press, 1986; pp 541–75.
49. Vinik AI. Insulin secretion in chronic pancreatitis. In Tiengo A, Alberti KGMM, Del Prato S, Vranic M (eds) *Diabetes Secondary to Pancreatopathy*. Amsterdam: Excerpta Medica, 1988; pp 35–50.
50. Tiengo A, Briani G, Riva F, Midena E, Sgnaolin E, Bellavere F, Iori E, Trevisan R, Fedele D, Segato T, Del Prato S. Microangiopathic complications in diabetes secondary to pancreatopathy. In Tiengo A, Alberti KGMM, Del Prato S, Vranic M (eds) *Diabetes Secondary to Pancreatopathy*. Amsterdam: Excerpta Medica, 1988; pp 245–57.
51. Rummesen JJ, Mamer B, Pedersen NT, Permin H. Autoantibodies in chronic pancreatitis. *Scand J Gastroenterol* 1985; 20: 966–70.
52. Larsen S, Hilsted J, Jacobsen BK, Svejgaard A, Marner B, Woming H. Insulin-dependent diabetes mellitus secondary to chronic pancreatitis is not associated with HLA or the occurrence of islet-cell antibodies. *J Immunogenet* 1990; 17: 189–93.
53. Scuro LA, Bovo P, Sandrini T, Angelini G, Cavellini G, Mirakian R. Autoimmunity and diabetes associated with chronic pancreatitis. *Lancet* 1983; 1: 424–7.
54. Marner B, Bille G, Christy M, Damsgaard EM, Game S, Heinze E, Larsen S, Lernmark A, Mandrup-Poulsen T, Nerup J. Islet cell cytoplasmic antibodies (ICA) in diabetes and disorders of glucose tolerance. *Diabet Med* 1991; 8: 812–6.
55. Colman PG, Begley CG, Tait BD, Roberts-Thompson IC, Harrison LC. Evidence against an immunogenetic basis for diabetes in chronic pancreatitis. *Aust NZ J Med* 1987; 17: 392–5.
56. Lendrum R, Walker G. Serum antibodies in human pancreatic disease. *Gut* 1975; 16: 365–71.
57. Lankisch PG. Diagnosis of chronic pancreatitis. *Lancet* 1998; 351: 599–600.
58. Keller P, Bank S, Marks IN, O'Reilly IG. Plasma insulin levels in pancreatic diabetes. *Lancet* 1965; 2: 1211–4.
59. Bonora E, Rizzi C, Lesi C, Berra P, Coscelli C, Butturini U. Insulin and C-peptide plasma levels in patients with severe chronic pancreatitis and fasting normoglycemia. *Dig Dis Sci* 1988; 33: 732–6.
60. Peters N, Dick AP, Hales CN, Orrell DH, Samer M. Exocrine and endocrine pancreatic function in diabetes mellitus and chronic pancreatitis. *Gut* 1966; 7: 277–81.
61. Vinik AE, Jackson WPU. Endocrine secretion in chronic pancreatitis. In Podolsky S, Viswanathan M (eds) *Secondary Diabetes: The Spectrum of the Diabetic Syndromes*. New York: Raven Press, 1980; pp 165–89.
62. Kalk WJ, Vinik AI, Bank S, Keller P, Jackson WPU. Selective loss of beta cell response to glucose in chronic pancreatitis. *Horm Metab Res* 1974; 6: 95–8.
63. Joffe BI, Bank S, Jackson WPU, Keller P, O'Reilly TG, Vinik AI. Insulin reserve in patients with chronic pancreatitis. *Lancet* 1968; 2: 121–4.
64. McKiddie MT, Buchanan KD, McBain GC, Bell G. The insulin response to glucose in patients with pancreatic disease. *Postgrad Med J* 1969; 45: 726–30.
65. Larsen S, Hilsted J, Philipsen EK, Tronier B, Nielsen MD, Woming H. The effect of insulin withdrawal on intermediary metabolism in patients with diabetes secondary to chronic pancreatitis. *Acta Endocrinol* 1991; 124: 510–5.
66. Kalk WJ, Vinik AI, Jackson WPU, Bank S. Insulin secretion and pancreatic exocrine function in patients with chronic pancreatitis. *Diabetologia* 1979; 16: 355–8.
67. Nyboe Andersen B, Krarup T, Thorsgaard Pedersen N, Faber OK, Hagen C, Woming H. B cell function in patients with chronic pancreatitis and its relation to exocrine pancreatic function. *Diabetologia* 1982; 23: 86–9.
68. Duckworth WC, Solomon SS, Jallepalli P, Iyer R, Bobal MA. Hormonal response to intravenous glucose and arginine in patients with pancreatitis. *Horm Res* 1983; 17: 65–73.
69. Hiroyoshi M, Tateishi K, Yasunami Y, Maeshiro K, Ono J, Matsuoka Y, Ikeda S. Elevated plasma levels of glucagon-like peptide-1 after oral glucose ingestion in

patients with pancreatic diabetes. *Am J Gastroenterol* 1999; 94: 976–81.
70. Kalk WJ, Vinik AI, Botha JL, Keller P, Jackson WPU. Insulin responses to crude cholecystokinin pancreozymin in normal subjects, in patients with chronic pancreatitis and patients with mild maturity onset diabetes. *J Clin Endocrinol Metab* 1975; 41: 172–6.
71. Hedetoft C, Sheikh SP, Larsen S, Holst JJ. Effect of glucagon-like peptide 1(7-36) amide in insulin-treated patients with diabetes mellitus secondary to chronic pancreatitis. *Pancreas* 2000; 20: 25–31.
72. Botha JL, Vinik AI, Child PT. GIP in acquired pancreatic diabetes: effects of insulin treatment. *J Clin Endocrinol Metab* 1978; 47: 543–9.
73. Nakano I, Funakoahi A, Shinozaki H, Sakai K. Plasma cholecystokinin and pancreatic polypeptide response after ingestion of a liquid test meal rich in medium-chain fatty acids in patients with chronic pancreatitis. *Am J Nutr* 1989; 49: 247–51.
74. Rossetti L, Shulman GI, Zawalich W, DeFronzo RA. Effect of chronic hyperglycemia on in vivo insulin secretion in partially pancreatectomised rats. *J Clin Invest* 1987; 80: 1037–44.
75. Tiengo A, Del Prato S, Meneghel A. C-peptide values in diabetes following pancreatectomy. *Giom Ital Chim Clin* 1979; 4 (suppl 1): 169–70.
76. Kalk WJ, Vinik AI, Bank S, Buchanan KD, Keller P, Jackson WPU. Glucagon responses to arginine in chronic pancreatitis: possible pathogenic significance in diabetes. *Diabetes* 1974; 23: 257–63.
77. Persson I, Gyntelberg F, Heding LG, Ross Nielsen J. Pancreatic glucagon-like immunoreactivity after IV insulin in normal and chronic pancreatitis patients. *Acta Endocrinol* 1971; 67: 401–4.
78. Holst JJ. Sources and molecular moieties of glucagon in diabetes secondary to pancreatopathy. In Tiengo A, Alberti KGMM, Del Prato S, Vranic M (eds) *Diabetes Secondary to Pancreatopathy*. Amsterdam: Excerpta Medica, 1988; pp 63–70.
79. Valverde I, Rigolopoulou D, Marco J, Faloona GR, Unger RH. Molecular size of extractable glucagon and glucagon-like immunoreactivity (GLI) in plasma. *Diabetes* 1970; 19: 624–9.
80. Assan R, Tiengo A. Comparaison des sécrétions de glucagon chez le diabéte sucré avec ou sans pathologie organique acquis. *Path Biol* 1973; 21: 17–24.
81. Larsen S. Pancreatic hormone secretion in diabetes mellitus secondary to chronic pancreatitis. In Tiengo A, Alberti KGMM, Del Prato S, Vranic M (eds) *Diabetes Secondary to Pancreatopathy*. Amsterdam: Excerpta Medica, 1988; pp 203–7.
82. Botha JL, Vinik AI, Child PT, Paul M, Jackson WPU. Pancreatic glucagon-like immunoreactivity in a pancreatectomised patient. *Horm Metab Res* 1977; 9: 199–205.
83. Nealon WH, Townsend CM, Thompson JC. The time course of beta cell dysfunction in chronic ethanol-induced pancreatitis: a prospective analysis. *Surgery* 1988; 104: 1074–9.
84. Adrian TE, Basferman HS, Mallison CN, Garalotis C, Bloom SR. Impaired pancreatic polypeptide release in chronic pancreatitis with steatorrhea. *Gut* 1979; 20: 98–101.
85. Owyang C, Scarpello JH, Vinik AI. Correlation between pancreatic enzyme secretion and plasma concentration of human pancreatic polypeptide in health and chronic pancreatitis. *Gastroenterology* 1982; 83: 55–62.
86. Anagnostides AA, Cox TM, Adrian TE, Christfides ND, Maton PN, Bloom SR, Chadwick VS. Pancreatic exocrine and endocrine response in chronic pancreatitis. *Am J Gastroenterol* 1984; 79: 206–12.
87. Del Prato S, Vigili de Kreutzenberg S, Lisato G, Maifreni L, Riccio A, Duner E, Marescotti MC, Valerio A, Tiengo A. Glucose and intermediary metabolism in diabetes following total pancreatectomy. In Tiengo A, Alberti KGMM, Del Prato S, Vranic M (eds) *Diabetes Secondary to Pancreatopathy*. Amsterdam: Excerpta Medica, 1988; pp 143–62.
88. Barnes AJ, Bloom SD, Alberti KGMM, Smythe P, Alford FP, Chisholm DJ. Ketoacidosis in pancreatectomised man. *N Engl J Med* 1977; 296: 1250–3.
89. Del Prato S, Nosadini R, Riva F, Fedele D, Devide A, Tiengo A. Glucagon levels and ketogenesis in human diabetes following total or partial pancreatectomy and severe chronic pancreatitis. *Acta Diabetol Lat* 1980; 117: 111–8.
90. Santeusanio F, Massi-Benedetti M, Angeletti G, Calabrese G, Bueti A, Brunetti P. Glucagon and carbohydrate disorder in a totally pancreatectomised man. A study with the aid of an artificial endocrine pancreas. *J Endocrinol Invest* 1981; 4: 93–6.
91. Joffe B, Kurt L, Bank S, Marks IN, Keller P. Serum lipid levels in diabetes secondary to chronic pancreatitis. *Metabolism* 1970; 19: 87–9.
92. Ammann RW, Akovbiantz A, Largiader G, Schueler G. Course and outcome of chronic pancreatitis. Longitudinal study of a mixed medical–surgical series of 245 patients. *Gastroenterology* 1984; 86: 820–8.
93. Jalleh RP, Williamson RCN. Pancreatic exocrine and endocrine function after operations for chronic pancreatitis. *Ann Surg* 1992; 216: 656–62.
94. Bittner R, Butters M, Buchler M, Nagele S, Roscher R, Beger HG. Glucose homeostasis and endocrine pancreatic function in patients with chronic pancreatitis before and after surgical therapy. *Pancreas* 1994; 9: 47–53.
95. Rotman N, Sastre B, Fagniez PL. Medial pancreatectomy for tumors of the neck of the pancreas. *Surgery* 1993; 113: 532–5.
96. Kendall DM, Sutherland DER, Najarian JS, Goetz FC, Robertson RP. Effects of hemipancreatectomy on insulin secretion and glucose tolerance in healthy humans. *N Engl J Med* 1990; 322: 898–903.
97. Seaquist ER, Robertson RP. Effects of hemipancreatectomy on pancreatic alpha and beta cell function in healthy human donors. *J Clin Invest* 1992; 89: 1761–6.
98. Seaquist ER, Pyzdrowski K, Moran A, Teuscher AU, Robertson RP. Insulin-mediated and glucose-mediated uptake following hemipancreatectomy in healthy human donors. *Diabetologia* 1994; 37: 1036–43.
99. Valverde I, Alercon C, Ruiz-Grande C, Rovira A. Plasma glucagon and glucagon-like immunoreactivity in totally pancreatectomised humans. In Tiengo A, Alberti KGMM, Del Prato S, Vranic M (eds) *Diabetes Secondary to Pancreatopathy*. Amsterdam: Excerpta Medica, 1988; 51–62.
100. Doi K, Prentki M, Yip C, Muller WA, Jeanrenaud B, Vranic M. Identical biological effects of pancreatic glucagon and a purified moiety of canine gastric immunoreactive glucagon. *J Clin Invest* 1979; 63: 525–31.

101. Lawrence AM, Kristins L, Hoguat S, Tan S. Submaxillary gland hyperglycemic factor in man and animals: an extrapancreatic glucagon. *Clin Res* 1976; 24: 364–7.
102. Barnes AJ, Bloom RS. Pancreatectomised man: a model for diabetes without glucagon. *Lancet* 1976; 1: 219–21.
103. Geric JE, Karam JH, Lorenzi M. Diabetes without glucagon [letter]. *Lancet* 1976; 1: 855.
104. Donowitz M, Felig P. Diabetes without glucagon [letter]. *Lancet* 1976; 1: 855–6.
105. Muller WA, Brennan MF, Tan MH, Aoki TT. Studies of glucagon secretion in pancreatectomised patients. *Diabetes* 1974; 23: 512–16.
106. Werner PL, Palmer JP. Immunoreactive glucagon response to oral glucose, insulin infusion and deprivation, and somatostatin in pancreatectomised man. *Diabetes* 1978; 27: 1005–12.
107. Bringer J, Mirouze J, Marchal G, Pham TC, Luyckx A, Lefebvre P, Orsetti A. Glucagon immunoreactivity and antidiabetic action of somatostatin in the totally pancreatectomised and gastrectomized human. *Diabetes* 1981; 30: 851–6.
108. Muller WA, Berger M, Suter P, Cuppers JH, et al. Glucagon immunoreactivities and amino acid profile in plasma of duodenopancreatectomized patients. *J Clin Invest* 1979; 63: 820–7.
109. Boden G, Master RW, Rezvani I, Palmer JP, Lobe TE, Owen OE. Glucagon deficiency and hyperaminoacidemia after total pancreatectomy. *J Clin Invest* 1980; 65: 706–16.
110. Tiengo A, Bessioud M, Valverde I, Tabbi-Anneni A, Del Prato S, Alexandre J, Assan R. Absence of alfa cell function in pancreatectomized patients. *Diabetologia* 1982; 22: 25–32.
111. Holst JJ, Pederson JH, Baldissera F, Stadil F. Circulating glucagon after total pancreatectomy in man. *Diabetologia* 1983; 25: 396–9.
112. Bajorunas DR, Fortner JG, Jaspan JB. Glucagon immunoreactivity and chromatography pattem in pancreatectomised humans. Paradoxical response to glucose. *Diabetes* 1986; 35: 886–93.
113. Villanueva ML, Hedo JA, Marco J. Plasma glucagon immunoreactivity in a totally pancreatectomized man. *Diabetologia* 1976; 12: 613–6.
114. Dammann HG, Bestirman HS, Bloom SR, Schreiber H, Gut-hormone profile in totally pancreatectomised patients. *Gut* 1981; 22: 103–7.
115. Del Prato S, Vigili de Kreutzenberg S, Lisato G, et al. Glucose and intermediary metabolism in diabetes following total pancreatectomy. In Tiengo A, Alberti KGMM, Del Prato S, Vranic M (eds) *Diabetes Secondary to Pancreatopathy*. Amsterdam: Excerpta Medica, 1988; pp 143–62.
116. Gutniac M, Grill V, Wiechel K-L, Efendic S. Basal and meal-induced somatostatin-like immunoreactivity in healthy subjects and IDDM and totally pancreatectomised patients. Effect of acute blood glucose normalization. *Diabetes* 1987; 36: 802–7.
117. Yasida H, Harano Y, Ohgaku S, Kosugi K, Hideka H, Kashiwagi A, Shigeta Y. Insulin sensitivity in pancreatitis, liver diseases, steroid treatment and hyperthyroidism assessed by glucose, insulin, and somatostatin infusion. *Horm Metab Res* 1984; 16: 3–6.
118. Ginsberg H, Kimmerling G, Olefsky JM, Reaven GM. Demonstration of insulin resistance in untreated adult onset diabetic subjects with fasting hyperglycemia. *J Clin Invest* 1975; 55: 454–61.
119. Nosadini R, Del Prato S, Tiengo A, Duner E, Toffolo G, Cobelli C, Faronato PP, Moghetti P, Muggeo M. Insulin sensitivity, binding and kinetics in pancreatogenic diabetes. *Diabetes* 1982; 31: 346–55.
120. Yki-Jarvinen H, Kiviluoto T, Taskinen M-R. Insulin resistance is a prominent feature of patients with pancreatogenic diabetes. *Metabohsm* 1986; 35: 718–27.
121. Bajorunas DR, Dressler CM, Horowitz GD, McDermott K, Jeevanandam M, Fortner JG, Brennan MF. Basal glucagon replacement in chromc glucagon-deficiency increases insulin resistance. *Diabetes* 1986; 35: 556–62.
122. Del Prato S, Castellino P, Simonson DC, DeFronzo RA. Hyperglucagonemia and insulin-mediated glucose metabolism. *J Clin Invest* 1987; 79: 547–56.
123. Vigili de Kreutzenberg S, Maifreni L, Lisato G, Riccio A, Trevisan R, Tiengo A, Del Prato S. Glucose turnover and recycling in diabetes secondary to total pancreatectomy: effect of glucagon infusion. *J Clin Endocrinol Metab* 1990; 70: 1023–9.
124. Del Prato S, Tiengo A, Baccaglini U, Tremolada C, Duner E, Marescotti MC, Avogaro A, Valverde I, Nosadini R, Assan R. Effect of insulin replacement on intermediary metabolism in diabetes secondary to pancreatectomy. *Diabetologia* 1983; 25: 252–9.
125. Barnes AJ, Bloom SR, Mashiter K, Alberti KGMM. Persistent metabolic abnormalities in diabetes in the absence of glucagon. *Diabetologia* 1977; 13: 71–5.
126. Del Prato S, Vigili de Kreutzenberg S, Trevisan R, Duner E, Avogaro A, Nosadini R, Baccaglini U, Tremolada C, Tiengo A. Hyperalaninemia is an early feature of diabetes secondary to total pancreatectomy. *Diabetologia* 1985; 28: 277–81.
127. Cherrington AD. Gluconeogenesis: its regulation by insulin and glucagon. In Brownlee M (ed), *Diabetes Mellitus, Vol 3*. New York: Sarland SPIM Press, 1981; pp 49–117.
128. Kiviluoto T, Yki-Jarvinen H, Taskinen M-R. Metabolic characteristics in patients with pancreatogenic diabetes. In Tiengo A, Alberti KGMM, Del Prato S, Vranic M (eds) *Diabetes Secondary to Pancreatopathy*. Amsterdam: Excerpta Medica, 1988; pp 137–42.
129. Tiengo A, Segato T, Briani G, Setti A, Del Prato S, Devide A, Padovan D, Virgili F, Crepaldi G. The presence of retinopathy in patients with secondary diabetes following pancreatectomy or chronic pancreatitis. *Diabetes Care* 1983; 6: 570–8.
130. Muller WA, Cuppers HJ, Zimmerman-Telschow H, Micheli H, Wyss T, Renold AE, Berger M. Aminoacid and lipoproteins in plasma of duodenopancreatectomized patients: effects of glucagon in physiological amounts. *Eur J Clin Invest* 1983; 13: 141–9.
131. Kiviluoto T, Schroder T Karonen S-L, Kuusi T, Lempinen M, Taskmen M-R. Glycemic control and lipoproteins after total pancreatectomy. *Ann Clin Res* 1985; 17: 1 10–5.
132. Boden G. Amino acid metabolism in diabetes secondary to pancreatopathy. In Tiengo A, Alberti KGMM, Del Prato S, Vranic M (eds) *Diabetes Secondary to Pancreatopathy*. Amsterdam: Excerpta Medica, 1988; pp 179–86.
133. Trevisan R, Marescotti C, Avogaro A, Tessari P, Del Prato S, Tiengo A. Effects of different insulin administrations

on plasma amino acid profile in insulin-dependent diabetic patients. *Diabetes Res* 1989; 12: 57–62.
134. Sinha SK. Pacreatic diabetes in man: clinical features and management. In Podolsky S, Viswanathan M (eds) *Secondary Diabetes*. New York: Raven Press, 1980; pp 197–214.
135. Linde J, Nilsson LH, Baramy F. Diabetes and hypoglycemia in chronic pancreatitis. *Scand J Gastroenterol* 1977; 12: 369–73.
136. Ishe I, Lilja P, Arnesjo B, Bengmark S. Total pancreatectomy for cancer. *Ann Surg* 1977; 186: 675–80.
137. Braasch JW, Vito L, Nugent FW. Total pancreatectomy for end-stage chronic pancreatitis. *Ann Surg* 1978; 188: 317–22.
138. Trede M, Schwall G. The complications of pancreatectomy. *Ann Surg* 1988; 207: 39–47.
139. Pliam MB, ReMine WH. Further evaluation of total pancreatectomy. *Arch Surg* 1975; 110: 506–12.
140. Frey C, Child CG, Fry W. Pancreatectomy for chronic pancreatitis. *Ann Surg* 1976; 184: 403–14.
141. Dressler CM, Fortner JG, McDennott K, Bajorunas DR. Metabolic consequences of (regional) total pancreatectomy. *Ann Surg* 1991; 214: 131–40.
142. Gall FP, Guhe E, Gebhardt C. Results of partial and total pancreaticoduodenectomy in 117 patients with chronic pancreatitis. *World J Surg* 1981; 5: 269–75.
143. Assan R, Alexander HH, Tiengo A, Marre M, Costauoilleres L, Lhomme C. Survival and rehabilitation after total pancreatectomy: a follow-up of 36 patients. *Diabéte Métab* 1983; 11: 303–9.
144. Joffe BI, Bank S, Marks IN. Hypoglycemia in pancreatitis. *Lancet* November 9, 1968; 2 (7576): 1038.
145. Larsen S, Hilsted J, Philipsen EK, Tronier B, Christensen NJ, Damkjear Nielsen M, Worning H. Glucose counterregulation in diabetes secondary to chronic pancreatitis. *Metabolism* 1990; 39: 138–43.
146. Horie H, Matsuyama T, Namba M, et al. Responses of catecholamines and other counterregulatory hormones to insulin-induced hypoglycemia in totally pancreatectomized patients. *J Clin Endocrinol Metab* 1984; 59: 1193–6.
147. Polonski KS, Herold KC, Gilden JL, Bergenstal RM, Faug US, Moossa AR, Jaspan JB. Glucose counterregulation in patients after pancreatectomy. *Diabetes* 1984; 33: 1112–9.
148. Del Prato S, Vigili de Kreutzenberg S, Riccio A, Duner E, Lisato G, Valerio A, Tiengo A. Insulin-induced hypoglycemia in patients with diabetes secondary to total pancreatectomy: mechanisms of impaired counterregulation. *Diabet Nutr Metab* 1990; 3: 111–21.
149. Bajorunas DR. Insulin action and sensitivity in diabetes secondary to pancreatopathy. In Tiengo A, Alberti KGMM, Del Prato S, Vranic M (eds) *Diabetes Secondary to Pancreatopathy*. Amsterdam: Excerpta Medica, 1988; pp 123–36.
150. Alberti KGMM. Diabetes secondary to pancreatopathy: an example of brittle diabetes. In Tiengo A, Alberti KGMM, Del Prato S, Vranic M (eds) *Diabetes Secondary to Pancreatopathy*. Amsterdam: Excerpta Medica, 1988; pp 211–4.
151. Avogaro A, Tiengo A. Alcohol, glucose metabolism, and diabetes. *Diabetes Metab Rev* 1993; 9: 129–46.
152. Emanuele MA, Kirsteins L, Reda D, Emanuele NV, Lawrence AM. The effect of in vivo ethanol exposure on basal growth hormone secretion. *Endocr Res* 1989; 14: 283–91.
153. Jenkins JS, Connolly J. Adrenocortical response to ethanol in man. *Br Med J* 1968; 2: 804–5.
154. Avogaro A, Fontana P, Valerio A, Trevisan R, Riccio A, Del Prato S, Nosadini R, Tiengo A, Crepaldi G. Alcohol impairs insulin sensitivity in normal subjects. *Diabetes Res* 1987; 5: 23–7.
155. Yki-Jarvinen H, Nikkila EA. Ethanol decreases glucose utilization in healthy man. *J Clin Endocrinol Metab* 1985; 61: 941–5.
156. Petrides A, DeFronzo RA. Glucose metabolism in cirrhosis: a review with some perspective for the future. *Diabetes Metab Rev* 1989; 5: 691–709.
157. Dettwyler W. Le diabete des pancreatopathies. *Sem Hop Paris* 1964; 40: 1676–82.
158. Mohan V, Ramachandran A, Viswanathan M. Diabetes secondary to pancreatopathy in the tropics. In Tiengo A, Alberti KGMM, Del Prato S, Vranic M (eds) *Diabetes Secondary to Pancreatopathy*. Amsterdam: Excerpta Medica, 1988; pp 215–26.
159. Gerich JE, Lorenzi M, Bier DM, Schneider V, Tsalikian E, Karam JH, Forsham J. Prevention of human ketoacidosis by somatostatin: evidence for an essential role of glucagon. *N Engl J Med* 1975; 292: 985–9.
160. Ebert R, Creutzfeldt W. Reversal of impaired GIP and insulin secretion in patients with pancreatogenic steatorrhea following enzyme substitution. *Diabetologia* 1980; 19: 198–204.
161. Calwell AR, Alpert LK, Becker B, Kendall FE, Le Compte PM. Vascular disease. Panel discussion. *Diabetes* 1957; 6: 180–6.
162. Bell ET. Pancreatitis. *Surgery* 1958; 43: 527–37.
163. Siperstein MD, Unger RH, Madison LL. Studies of muscle capillary basement membranes in normal subjects, diabetic and prediabetic patients. *J Clin Invest* 1968; 1973–99.
164. Pirart J, Barbier S. Effect protecteur de l'hemochromatose vis-á-vis des lésions vasculaires du diabétiques. *Diabetologia* 1971; 7: 227–36.
165. Deckert T. Late complications in pancreatogenic diabetes mellitus. *Acta Med Scand* 1960; 168: 439–44.
166. Tutin M, Bour H. Le diabete des pancreatites chroniques. *Rev Prat Paris* 1966; 16: 3355–63.
167. Ennis G, Miller M, Unger FM, Unger L. Intercapillary glomerulosclerosis in diabetes secondary to chronic relapsing pancreatitis [abstract]. *Diabetes* 1969; 18: 333.
168. Sevel D, Bristow JH, Bank S, Marks I, Jackson P. Diabetic retinopathy in chronic pancreatitis. *Arch Ophthalmol* 1971; 86: 245–50.
169. Verdonk CA, Palumbo PJ, Gharib H, Bartholomew LG. Diabetic microangiopathy in patients with pancreatic diabetes mellitus. *Diabetologia* 1975; 11: 395–400.
170. Maekawa N. Ohneda A, Kai Y, Saito Y, Koseki S. Secondary diabetic retinopathy in chronic pancreatitis. *Am J Ophthalmol* 1978; 85: 835–40.
171. Moinade S, Meyrand G. Diabéte et pancréatite chronique: á propos de 20 cas. *Sem Hop Paris* 1979; 55: 188 3–6.
172. Couet C, Genton P, Pointel JP, et al. The prevalence of retinopathy is similar in diabetes mellitus secondary to chronic pancreatitis with or without pancreatectomy and in idiopathic diabetes mellitus. *Diabetes Care* 1985; 8: 323–8.

173. Rodman HM, Doezshuk CF, Roland JM. The interaction of 2 diseases: diabetes mellitus and cystic fibrosis. *Medicine* 1986; 65: 389–97.
174. Sullivan MM, Denning CR. Diabetic microangiopathy in patients with cystic fibrosis. *Pediatrics* 1989; 84: 642–7.
175. Gullo L, Parenti M, Monti L, Pezzilli R, Barbara L. Diabetic retinopathy in chronic pancreatitis. *Gastroenterology* 1990; 98: 1577–81.
176. Larsen S, Hilsted J, Philipsen EK, Lund-Anderson H, Parving HH, Worning H. A comparative study of microvascular complications in patients with secondary and type 1 diabetes. *Diabet Med* 1990; 7: 815–8.
177. Tiengo A, Briani G, Scaldaferri E, Riva F, Jori E, Sgnaolin E, Fenato R, D'Ambrosio M, Fioretto P, Nosadini R. Renal hemodynamics and albumin excretion rate in patients with diabetes secondary to acquired pancreatic disease. *Diabetes Care* 1992; 15: 1591–7.
178. Lanng S, Thorsteinsson B, Lund-Andersen C, Nerup J, Schiotz PO, Koch C. Diabetes mellitus in Danish cystic fibrosis patients: prevalence and late diabetic complications. *Acta Paediatr* 1994; 83: 72–7.
179. Levitt NS, Adams G, Salmon J, Marks IN, Musson G, Swanepoel C, Levy M, Byrne MJ. The prevalence and severity of microvascular complications in pancreatic diabetes and IDDM. *Diabetes Care* 1995; 18: 971–4.
180. Briani G, Riva F, Midena E, Trevisan R, Sgnaolin E, Jori E, Munari R, Bruttomesso D, Segato T, Tiengo A. Prevalence of microangiopathic complications in hyperglycemia secondary to acqired pancreatic disease. *J Diabet Compl* 1988; 2: 50–2.
181. Marre M, Hallab M, Roy J, Lejeune JJ, Jallet P, Fressinaud P. Glomerular hyperfiltration in type I, type II, and secondary diabetes. *J Diabet Compl* 1992; 6: 19–24.
182. Starke AAR, Cuppers HJ, Berger M. Therapeutic problems. In Tiengo A, Alberti KGMM, Del Prato S, Vranic M (eds) *Diabetes Secondary to Pancreatopathy*. Amsterdam: Excerpta Medica, 1988; pp 227–33.
183. Knop FK, Vilsboll T, Larsen S, Madsbad S, Holst JJ, Krarup T. No hypoglycemia after subcutaneous administration of glucagon-like peptide-1 in lean type 2 diabetic patients and in patients with diabetes secondary to chronic pancreatitis. *Diabetes Care* 2003; 26: 2581–7.
184. Beyer J, Schulz G, Cordes U. A glucose-controlled insulin infusion system (Biostator) in pancreatectomised patients. In Brunetti P, Alberti KGMM, Albisser M, Hepp KD, Massi Benedetti M (eds) *Artificial Systems for Insulin Delivery*. New York: Raven Press, 1983; pp 535–42.
185. Easter DW, Cuschieri A. Total pancreatectomy with preservation of the duodenum and pylorus for chronic pancreatitis. *Ann Surg* 1990; 214: 575–80.
186. Farney AC, Najarian JS, Nakheleh RE, Loveras G, Field MJ, Gores PF, Sutherland DE. Autotransplantation of dispersed pancreatic islet tissue combined with total or near-total pancreatectomy for treatment of chronic pancreatitis. *Surgery* 1991; 110: 427–37.
187. Robertson RP, Lanz KJ, Sutherland DE, Kendall DM. Prevention of diabetes for up to 13 years by autoislet transplantation after pancreatectomy for chronic pancreatitis. *Diabetes* 2001; 50: 47–50.
188. Bright R. Cases and observations connected with disease of the pancreas and duodenum. *Med Chir Tr* 1833; 18: 1–16.
189. Ghadirian P, Lynch HT, Krewski D. Epidemiology of pancreatic cancer: an overview. *Cancer Detect Prev* 2003; 27: 87–93.
190. Karmody AJ, Kyle J. The association between carcinoma of the pancreas and diabetes mellitus. *Br J Surg* 1969; 56: 362–4.
191. Kessler II. Cancer and diabetes mellitus. A review of the literature. *J Chron Dis* 1971; 23: 579–600.
192. Schwartz SS, Zeidler A, Moossa AR, Kuku SF, Rubenstein AH. A prospective study of glucose tolerance, insulin, C-peptide, and glucagon responses in patients with pancreatic carcinoma. *Dig Dis Sci* 1978; 23: 1107–14.
193. Saruc M, Pour PM. Diabetes and its relationship to pancreatic carcinoma. *Pancreas* 2003; 26: 381–7.
194. Gullo L, Pezzilli R, Morselli-Labate AM. and the Italian Pancreatic Cancer Study Group. Diabetes and the risk of pancreatic cancer. *N Engl J Med* 1994; 331: 81–4.
195. Schmied BM, Ulrich AB, Friess H, Buchler MW, Pour PM. The patterns of extrainsular endocrine cells in pancreatic cancer. *Teratog Carcinog Mutagen* 2001; 21: 69–81.
196. Basso D, Valerio A, Seraglia R, Mazza S, Piva MG, Greco E, Fogar P, Gallo N, Pedrazzoli S, Tiengo A, Plebani M. Putative pancreatic cancer-associated diabetogenic factor: 2030 MW peptide. *Pancreas* 2002; 24: 8–14.
197. Basso D, Brigato L, Veronesi A, Panozzo MP, Amadori A, Plebani M. The pancreatic cancer cell line MIA PaCa2 produces one or more factors able to induce hyperglycemia in SCID mice. *Anticancer Res* 1995; 15: 2585–8.
198. Valerio A, Basso D, Brigato L, Ceolotto G, Baldo G, Tiengo A, Plebani M. Glucose metabolic alterations in isolated and perfused rat hepatocytes induced by pancreatic cancer conditioned medium: a low molecular weight factor possibly involved. *Biochem Biophys Res Commun* 1999; 257: 622–8.
199. Permert J, Larsson J, Westermark GT, Herrington MK, Christmanson L, Pour PM, Westermark P, Adrian TE. Islet amyloid polypeptide in patients with pancreatic cancer and diabetes. *New Engl J Med* 1994; 330: 313–8.
200. Makimattila S, Hietaniemi K, Kiviluoto T, Timonen T, Yki-Jarvinen H. In vivo glucose-stimulated amylin secretion is increased in nondiabetic patients with pancreatic cancer. *Metabolism* 2001; 50: 1036–42.
201. Ariapart P, Bergstedt-Lindqvist S, van Harmelen V, Permert J, Wang F, Lundkvist I. Resection of pancreatic cancer normalizes the preoperative increase of tumor necrosis factor alpha gene expression. *Pancreatology* 2002; 2: 491–4.
202. Pour PM. The role of langerhans islets in pancreatic ductal adenocarcinoma Front Biosci. 1997; 2: 271–82.
203. Pour PM, Weide L, Liu G, Kazakoff K, Scheetz M, Toshkov I, Ikematsu Y, Fienhold MA, Sanger W. Experimental evidence for the origin of ductal-type adenocarcinoma from the islets of Langerhans. *Am J Pathol* 1997; 150: 2167–80.
204. Hayashida CY, Suzuki K, Fujika H, Koizumi M, Toyota T, Goto Y. Morphometrical quantitation of pancreatic endocrine cells in patients with carcinoma of the pancreas. *Tohoku J Exp Med* 1983; 141: 311–22.
205. Standop J, Schneider MB, Ulrich A, Pour PM. Experimental animal models in pancreatic carcinogenesis: lessons for human pancreatic cancer. *Dig Dis* 2001; 19: 24–31.

206. Schmied B, Liu G, Moyer MP, Hernberg IS, Sanger W, Batra S, Pour PM. Induction of adenocarcinoma from hamster pancreatic islet cells treated with *N*-nitrosobis(2-oxopropyl)amine in vitro. *Carcinogenesis* 1999; 20: 317–24.
207. Permert J, Herrington M, Kazakoff K, Pour PM, Adrian TE. Early changes in islet hormone secretion in the hamster pancreatic cancer model. *Teratog Carcinog Mutagen* 2001; 21: 59–67.
208. Permert J, Larsson J, Fruin AB, Tatemoto K, Herrington MK, von Schenck H, Adrian TE. Islet hormone secretion in pancreatic cancer patients with diabetes. *Pancreas* 1997; 15: 60–8.
209. Nakamori S, Ishikawa O, Ohigashi H, Sasakuma F, Shimizu T, Nakaizumi A, Furukawa H, Sasaki Y, Imaoka S. Increased blood proinsulin and decreased C-peptide levels in patients with pancreatic cancer. *Hepatogastroenterology* 1999; 46: 16–24.
210. Wakasugi H, Funakoshi A, Iguchi H. Clinical observations of pancreatic diabetes caused by pancreatic carcinoma, and survival period. *Int J Clin Oncol* 2001; 6: 50–4.
211. Cohn JA, Friedman KJ, Noone PG, Knowles MR, Silverman LM, Jowell PS. Relation between mutations of the cystic fibrosis gene and idiopathic pancreatitis. *New Engl J Med* 1998; 339: 653–8.
212. Moran A, Hardin D, Rodman D, Allen HF, Beall RJ, Borowitz D, Brunzell C, Campbell PW, Chesrown SE, Duchow C, Fink RJ, Fitzsimmons SC, Hamilton N, Hirsch I, Howenstine MS, Klein DJ, Madhun Z, Pencharz PB, Quittner AL, Robbins MK, Schindler T, Schissel K, Schwarzenberg SJ, Stallings VA, Tullis DE, Zipf WB. Diagnosis, screening and management of cystic fibrosis related diabetes mellitus: a consensus conference report. *Diabetes Res Clin Pract* 1999; 45: 61–73.
213. Dodge JA, Morrison G. Diabetes mellitus in cystic fibrosis: a review. *J R Soc Med* 1992; 85 (suppl 19): 25–8.
214. Hodson ME. Diabetes mellitus and cystic fibrosis. *Baillières Clin Endocrinol Metab* 1992; 6: 797–805.
215. Stutchfield PR, O'Halloran SM, Smith CS, Woodrow JC, Bottazzo GF, Heaf D. HLA type, islet cell antibodies and glucose intolerance in cystic fibrosis. *Arch Dis Child* 1988; 63: 1234–9.
216. Geffner ME, Lippe BM, Maclaren NK, Riley WJ. Role of autoimmunity in insulinopenia and carbohydrate derangements associated with cystic fibrosis. *J Pediatr* 1988; 112: 419–21.
217. De Luca F, Arrigo T, Conti Nibali S, Sferlazzas C, Gigante A, Di Cesare E, Cucinotta D. Insulin secretion, glycosylated haemoglobin and islet cell antibodies in cystic fibrosis children and adolescents with different degrees of glucose tolerance. *Horm Metab Res* 1991; 23: 495–8.
218. Lanng S, Thorsteinsson B, Pociot F, Marshall MO, Madsen HO, Schwartz M, Nerup J, Koch C. Diabetes mellitus in cystic fibrosis: genetic and immunological markers. *Acta Paediatr* 1993; 82: 150–4.
219. Nousia-Arvanitakis S, Galli-Tsinopoulou A, Dracoulacos D, Karamouzis M, Demitriadou A. Islet autoantibodies and insulin dependent diabetes mellitus in cystic fibrosis. *J Pediatr Endocrinol Metab* 2000; 13: 319–24.
220. The cystic fibrosis genotype-phenotype consortium. Correlation between genotype and phenotype in patients with cystic fibrosis. *N Engl J Med* 1993; 329: 1308–13.
221. Couce M, O'Brien TD, Moran A, Roche PC, Butler PC. Diabetes mellitus in cystic fibrosis is characterized by islet amyloidosis. *J Clin Endocrinol Metab* 1996; 81: 1267–72.
222. Lohr M, Goertchen P, Nizze H, Gould NS, Gould VE, Oberholzer M, Heitz PU, Kloppel G. Cystic fibrosis associated islet changes may provide a basis for diabetes. An immunocytochemical and morphometrical study. *Virchows Arch A Pathol Anat Histopathol* 1989; 414: 179–85.
223. Kopito LE, Shwachman H. The pancreas in cystic fibrosis: chemical composition and comparative morphology. *Pediatr Res* 1976; 10: 742–9.
224. Iannucci A, Mukai K, Johnson D, Burke B. Endocrine pancreas in cystic fibrosis: an immunohistochemical study. *Hum Pathol* 1984; 15: 278–84.
225. Lombardo F, De Luca F, Rosano M, Sferlazzas C, Lucanto C, Arrigo T, Messina MF, Crisafulli G, Wasniewska M, Valenzise M, Cucinotta D. Natural history of glucose tolerance, beta-cell function and peripheral insulin sensitivity in cystic fibrosis patients with fasting euglycemia. *Eur J Endocrinol* 2003; 149: 53–9.
226. Stahl M, Girard J, Rutishauser M, Nars PW, Zuppinger K. Endocrine function of the pancreas in cystic fibrosis: evidence for an impaired glucagon and insulin response following arginine infusion. *J Pediatr* 1974; 84: 821–4.
227. Moran A, Diem P, Klein DJ, Levitt MD, Robertson RP. Pancreatic endocrine function in cystic fibrosis. *J Pediatr* 1991; 118: 715–23.
228. Moran A, Pyzdrowski KL, Weinreb J, Kahn BB, Smith SA, Adams KL, Seaquist ER. Insulin sensitivity in cystic fibrosis. *Diabetes* 1994; 43: 1020–6.
229. Lanng S, Thorsteinsson F, Erichsen G, Nerup J, Koch C. Glucose tolerance in cystic fibrosis. *Arch Dis Child* 1991; 66: 612–6.
230. Holl RW, Wolf A, Rank N, Heinze E. Reduced pancreatic release and impaired insulin sensitivity contribute to high incidence of diabetes mellitus in young adults with cystic fibrosis. *Diabetes* 1993; 42: 60A.
231. Hardin DS, Leblanc A, Marshall G, Seilheimer DK. Mechanisms of insulin resistance in cystic fibrosis. *Am J Physiol Endocrinol Metab* 2001; 281: E1022–8.
232. Hardin DS, LeBlanc A, Para L, Seilheimer DK. Hepatic insulin resistance and defects in substrate utilization in cystic fibrosis. *Diabetes* 1999; 48: 1082–7.
233. Wilmshurst EG, Soeldner JS, Holsclaw DS, Kaufmann RL, Shwachman H, Aoki TT, Gleason RE. Endogenous and exogenous insulin responses in patients with cystic fibrosis. *Pediatrics* 1975; 55: 75–82.
234. Lippe BM, Kaplan SA, Neufeld ND, Smith A, Scott M. Insulin receptors in cystic fibrosis: increased receptor number and altered affinity. *Pediatrics* 1980; 65: 1018–22.
235. Anderson O, Game S, Heilmann C, Petersen KE, Petersen W, Koch C. Glucose tolerance and insulin receptor binding to monocytes and erythrocytes in patients with cystic fibrosis. *Acta Pediatr Scand* 1988; 77: 67–71.
236. Cucinotta D, Nibali SC, Arigo T, Di Benedetto A, Magazzu G, Di Cesare E, Costantino A, Pezzino V, De Luca F. Beta cell function and peripheral sensitivity to insulin and islet cell autoimmunity in cystic fibrosis patients with normal glucose tolerance. *Horm Res* 1990; 34: 33–8.
237. Austin A, Kalhan SC, Orenstein D, Nixon P, Arslanian S. Roles of insulin resistance and beta-cell dysfunction in

the pathogenesis of glucose intolerance in cystic fibrosis. *J Clin Endocrinol Metab* 1994; 79: 80–5.
238. Lippe BM, Sperling MA, Dooley RR. Pancreatic alpha and beta cell function in cystic fibrosis. *J Pediatr* 1977; 90: 751–5.
239. Lanng S, Thorsteinsson B, Roder ME, Orskov C, Holst JJ, Nerup J, Koch C. Pancreas and gut hormone responses to oral glucose and intravenous glucagon in cystic fibrosis patients with normal, impaired, and diabetic glucose tolerance. *Acta Endocrinol (Copenh)* 1993; 128: 207–14.
240. Meacham LR, McKean LP, Buchanan CN, Caplan DB, et al. Selective preservation of somatostatin secretion in cystic fibrosis patients with diabetes. *Pediatr Pulmonol* 1991; 11 (suppl 6): 333A.
241. Geffner ME, Lippe BM, Kaplan SA, Itami RM, Gaillard BK, Levin SR, Taylor IL. Carbohydrate tolerance in cystic fibrosis is closely linked to pancreatic exocrine function. *Pediatr Res* 1984; 18: 1107–11.
242. Stewart C, Wilson DC, Hanna AK, Corey M, et al. Lipid metabolism in adults with cystic fibrosis. *Pediatr Pulmonol* 1997; 24 (suppl 14): 366A.
243. Moran A, Milla C, Ducret R, Nair KS. Protein metabolism in clinically stable adult cystic fibrosis patients with abnormal glucose tolerance. *Diabetes* 2001; 50: 1336–43.
244. Rosenecker J, Eichler I, Kuhn L, Harms HK, von der Hardt H, for the Multicenter Cystic Fibrosis Study Group. Genetic determination of diabetes mellitus in patients with cystic fibrosis. *J Pediatr* 1995; 127: 441–3.
245. Finkelstein SM, Wielinski CL, Elliott GR, Warwick WJ, Barbosa J, Wu SC, Klein DJ. Diabetes mellitus associated with cystic fibrosis. *J Pediatr* 1988; 112: 373–7.
246. Stewart AK, Hanna M, Corey J, Zielenski J, Tsui LC, et al. Glucose tolerance in adults with cystic fibrosis: phenotype-genotype correlations. *Pediatr Pulmonol* 1997; 24 (suppl 14): 361A.
247. Rosnan RC, Shwachman H, Kulczycki L. Diabetes mellitus and cystic fibrosis of the pancreas. *Am J Dis Child* 1962; 104: 625–34.
248. Rolon MA, Benali K, Munck A, Navarro J, Clement A, Tubiana-Rufi N, Czernichow P, Polak M. Cystic fibrosis-related diabetes mellitus: clinical impact of prediabetes and effects of insulin therapy. *Acta Paediatr* 2001; 90: 860–7.
249. Nousia-Arvanitakis S, Galli-Tsinopoulou A, Karamouzis M. Insulin improves clinical status of patients with cystic-fibrosis-related diabetes mellitus. *Acta Paediatr* 2001; 90: 515–9.
250. Rosenecker J, Hofler R, Steinkamp G, Eichler I, Smaczny C, Ballmann M, Posselt HG, Bargon J, von der Hardt H. Diabetes mellitus in patients with cystic fibrosis: the impact of diabetes mellitus on pulmonary function and clinical outcome. *Eur J Med Res* 2001; 6: 345–50.
251. Culler FL, McKean LP, Buchanan CJ, Caplan DB, Meacham LR, et al. Glipizide treatment of patients with cystic fibrosis and impaired glucose tolerance. In *Endocrine Society Program and Abstracts*, San Antonio, TX, 1992. San Antonio, TX: Endocrine Society, 1992; p 45A.
252. Hinds A, Sheehan AG, Parsons HG. Tolbutamide causes a modest increase in insulin secretion in cystic fibrosis patients with impaired glucose tolerance. *Metabolism* 1995; 44: 13–8.
253. Horswill CA, Zipf WB, Kien CL, McCoy KS, O'Dorisio T, et al. Glipizide increased insulin secretion but not growth of children with cystic fibrosis. *FASEB J* 1990; 4: 3272A.
254. Zipf WB, Kien CL, Horswill CA, McCoy KS, O'Dorisio T, Pinyerd BL. Effects of tolbutamide on growth and body composition of nondiabetic children with cystic fibrosis. *Pediatr Res* 1991; 30: 309–14.
255. Rosenecker J, Eichler I, Barmeier H, von der Hardt H. Diabetes mellitus and cystic fibrosis: comparison of clinical parameters in patients treated with insulin versus oral glucose-lowering agents. *Pediatr Pulmonol* 2001; 32: 351–5.
256. Sheppard DN, Welsh MJ. Effect of ATP-sensitive K^+ channel regulators on cystic fibrosis transmembrane conductance regulator chloride currents. *J Gen Physiol* 1992; 100: 573–91.
257. Moran A, Phillips J, Milla C. Insulin and glucose excursion following premeal insulin lispro or repaglinide in cystic fibrosis-related diabetes. *Diabetes Care* 2001; 24: 1706–10.
258. Galli A, Crabb DW, Ceni E, Salzano R, Mello T, Svegliati-Baroni G, Ridolfi F, Trozzi L, Surrenti C, Casini A. Antidiabetic thiazolidinediones inhibit collagen synthesis and hepatic stellate cell activation in vivo and in vitro. *Gastroenterology* 2002; 122: 1924–40.
259. Lanng S, Hansen A, Thorsteinsson B, Nerup J, Koch C. Glucose tolerance in patients with cystic fibrosis: five year prospective study. *BMJ* 1995; 311: 655–9.
260. Trosseau A. Glycosurie, diabète, sucré. In *Clinique Médicale de l'Hotel Dieu de Paris*, 2nd edn. Vol 2. Balliere, Paris, 1865; p 663.
261. Lyon E, Frank EL. Hereditary hemochromatosis since discovery of the HFE gene. *Clin Chem* 2001; 47: 1147–56.
262. Sheldon JH. *Haemochromatosis*. London. Oxford University, 1935.
263. Simon M, Bourel M, Genetet B, Fauchet R. Idiopathic hemochromatosis. Demonstration of recessive transmission and early detection by family HLA typing. *New Engl J Med* 1977; 297: 1017–21.
264. Feder JN, Gnirke A, Thomas W, Tsuchihashi Z, Ruddy DA, Basava A, Dormishian F, Domingo R Jr, Ellis MC, Fullan A, Hinton LM, Jones NL, Kimmel BE, Kronmal GS, Lauer P, Lee VK, Loeb DB, Mapa FA, McClelland E, Meyer NC, Mintier GA, Moeller N, Moore T, Morikang E, Wolff RK. A novel MHC class I-like gene is mutated in patients with hereditary haemochromatosis. *Nat Genet* 1996; 13: 399–408.
265. Gochee PA, Powell LW. What's new in hemochromatosis. *Curr Opin Hematol* 2001; 8: 98–104.
266. Saudek CD. Diabetes and diseases of iron excess. In Podolsky S, Viswanathan M (eds) *Secondary Diabetes: The Spectrum of the Diabetic Syndrome*. New York: Raven Press, 1980; pp 165–89.
267. Milman N. Hereditary haemochromatosis in Denmark 1950–1985. Clinical, biochemical, and histological features in 179 patients and 13 preclinical cases. *Dan Med Bull* 1991; 38: 385–93.
268. Saddi R, Feingold J. Idiopathic haemochromatosis and diabetes mellitus. *Clin Genet* 1974; 5: 242–7.
269. Moirand R, Mortaji AM, Loreal O, Paillard F, Brissot P, Deugnier Y. A new syndrome of liver iron overload with normal transferrin saturation. *Lancet* 1997; 349: 95–7.
270. Mendler MH, Turlin B, Moirand R, Jouanolle AM, Sapey T, Guyader D, Le Gall JY, Brissot P, David V, Deugnier

Y. Insulin resistance-associated hepatic iron overload. *Gastroenterology* 1999; 117: 1155–63.

271. Ferrannini E. Insulin resistance, iron, and the liver. *Lancet* 2000; 355: 2181–2.
272. Marchesini G, Brizi M, Bianchi G, Tomassetti S, Bugianesi E, Lenzi M, McCullough AJ, Natale S, Forlani G, Melchionda N. Nonalcoholic fatty liver disease: a feature of the metabolic syndrome. *Diabetes* 2001; 50: 1844–50.
273. Nelson LR, Baldus WP, Rubenstein AH, Gov LW, Service FJ. Pancreatic cell function in diabetic hemochromatic subjects. *J Clin Endocrinol Metab* 1979; 48: 412–5.
274. Moczulski DK, Grzeszczak W, Gawlik B. Role of hemochromatosis C282Y and H63D mutations in HFE gene in development of type 2 diabetes and diabetic nephropathy. *Diabetes Care* 2001; 24: 1187–91.
275. Van Lerberghe S, Hermans MP, Dahan K, Buysschaert M. Clinical expression and insulin sensitivity in type 2 diabetic patients with heterozygous mutations for haemochromatosis. *Diabetes Metab* 2002; 28: 33–8.
276. Ellis JT, Schulman I, Smith CH. Generalized siderosis with fibrosis of liver and pancreas in Cooley's (Mediterranean) anemia. With observations on the pathogenesis of the siderosis and fibrosis. *Am J Pathol* 1953; 30: 287–309.
277. Isaacson C, Seftel SC, Keeley KJ, Bothwell TH. Siderosis in the Bantu: the relationship between iron overload and cirrhosis. *J Lab Clin Med* 1961; 58: 845–53.
278. Saudek CD, Hemm RM, Peterson CM. Abnormal glucose tolerance in B-thalassemia major. *Metabolism* 1977; 26: 43–52.
279. Cario H, Holl RW, Kohne E. Glucose intolerance in patients with thalassemia major: insulin resistance and hyperproinsulinemia. *J Pediatr Endocrinol Metab* 1998; 11 (suppl 3): 953–5.
280. Cario H, Holl RW, Debatin KM, Kohne E. Insulin sensitivity and beta-cell secretion in thalassaemia major with secondary haemochromatosis: assessment by oral glucose tolerance test. *Eur J Pediatr* 2003; 162: 139–46.
281. Griffiths JD, Dymock IW, Davies EWG, Hill DW, Williams R. Occurrence and prevalence of diabetic retinopathy in hemochromatosis. *Diabetes* 1971; 20: 766–70.

Obesity

30

The Relationship Between Obesity and Type 2 Diabetes—The Role of Neuroendocrine and Autonomic Factors

Per Björntorp*

Formerly of the University of Göteborg, Göteborg, Sweden

**Sadly, Professor Bjorntorp, an outstanding contributor to the obesity field, died prematurely in late 2003.*

INTRODUCTION

Type 2 diabetes mellitus develops when pancreatic β-cells cannot secrete sufficient amounts of insulin to compensate for peripheral insulin resistance. The development toward a clinically manifest diabetic state probably describes a curve, where insulin resistance is the primary factor generating increasingly elevated insulin secretion, keeping insulin effects on the periphery adequate until a breaking point at which glucose homeostasis can no longer be maintained. This first results in impaired glucose tolerance and then in diabetes. This breaking point is often characterized by a diminished insulin secretion as a sign of pancreatic β-cell insufficiency. This time point depends on several factors, such as the capacity of the β-cells, the severity and duration of insulin resistance, and hormonal activity, which are in turn based on a combination of genetic and environmental factors.

The genetic factors are well illustrated by the highly varying predisposition to develop diabetes among animal models ranging from the Israeli sand rat (*Psammomys obesus*), which develops diabetes after a short exposure to nutrients with a high-energy density, to other laboratory rat strains, which require partial pancreatectomy to induce diabetes [1]. The genetic effect in humans is illustrated by contrasting some Asian populations with high susceptibility to develop diabetes to Caucasians with low susceptibility to the disease [2].

Among predisposing factors, obesity is most prominently associated with a state of insulin resistance, although this is not always the case. The degree of insulin resistance is roughly proportional to body fat mass but very much influenced by the localization of body fat in obesity subgroups. Studies of these subgroups may provide a better understanding of the nature of insulin resistance in obesity.

TYPES OF OBESITY AND INSULIN RESISTANCE

What is the trigger of insulin resistance in obesity? It seems unlikely to be the obese state as such, simply because of the large variations in insulin resistance among equally obese subjects. This is apparent in the subgroups of obesity, characterized by differences in the distribution of the excess stored fat. These subgroups include the central, abdominal, the visceral, and the peripheral or gluteo-femoral obesities.

Central, abdominal obesity has enlarged abdominal fat depots. Visceral obesity is localized to the fat depots within the abdominal cavity among intestinal organs, mostly in the omentum and in the mesenteric region as well as retroperitoneally. Omental and mesenteric adipose tissue regions are, in contrast to all other adipose tissue regions, drained via the portal vein. Another subgroup of obesity has the major fat depots in the proximal parts of the extremities and is labeled peripheral or gluteo-femoral obesity.

These obesities have a highly varying degree of insulin resistance, peripheral obesity being much less

International Textbook of Diabetes Mellitus, Third Edition. Edited by R. A. DeFronzo, E. Ferrannini, H. Keen, and P. Zimmet.
 ISBN: 0-471-48655-8.

insulin-resistant than central obesity, particularly the visceral obesity subtype, independently of total body fat. Subjects, usually women, with very little visceral fat, have been found to have essentially normal insulin sensitivity in spite of elevated total fat mass [3, 4]. These differences are likely to contain the explanation to the insulin resistance of obesity most frequently preceding diabetes. This review summarizes work that has taken the advantage of seeking clues from such observations.

The difference between the subgroups of human obesity needs to be reemphasized. Epidemiological studies, clinical evaluations, and treatments as well as studies of the origin of obesity and the pathogenesis of the associated comorbidities clearly show that central obesity is the deleterious form of obesity. For example in a number of prospective epidemiological studies, central obesity is associated with the highest risk to develop type 2 diabetes and cardiovascular disease [5].

In addition, evidence suggests that peripheral obesity might not be an abnormal condition, at least not in moderate degrees. It may in fact be a condition resulting from evolutionary selections. Those who could store sufficient fat to meet periods of food deficiency and starvation were the survivors. In our current environment with energy-dense food easily available, combined with decreased need for physical activity, these genetically based selections are able to fully express themselves [6].

There is now sufficient background information to consider central and peripheral obesities as two separate diseases or conditions with a common symptom, accumulation of excess body fat mass. Other similar examples are found in clinical medicine, for example anemia, which is a common symptom for many diseases with totally different pathogenesis. Pernicious anemia is due to lack of vitamin B_{12} and sideropenia due to lack of iron. Like central and peripheral obesities, these two conditions with the same main symptom, anemia, have different causes and consequences, and require different treatments.

In addition to the difference in comorbidities and risks, central and peripheral obesities show clear gender differences. Central obesity is more prevalent among men than in women. Jean Vague almost 50 years ago [7] therefore labeled these obesities android (male-like) and gynoid (female-like). The significance of centralization of body fat stores and gender differences can be illustrated by the following observation. The incidence of myocardial infarction is three to six times higher in middle-aged men than in women. This difference is explained by gender variations in fat distribution as measured by the ratio of the waist and hip circumference ratio (WHR) [8]. Such observations again emphasize the importance of fat distribution, although the explanation is probably not the localization of fat as such, but rather a factor closely associated with fat distribution, as will be discussed below.

WHY IS EXCESS FAT DIRECTED TO ABDOMINAL VISCERAL DEPOTS?

A central problem then is, what directs excess fat predominantly to central fat depots.This problem has been reviewed in detail previously [9]. In brief, genetic and endocrine factors are involved. Among the latter, cortisol clearly increases visceral fat accumulation. This local specificity of fat storage by cortisol is probably due to the high density of glucocorticoid receptors (GRs) in this adipose tissue. Adrenal androgens seem more important than cortisol in women although the mechanism of this effect has not been clarified. Gender-specific sex-steroid hormones (androgens in men, estrogens in women) as well as growth hormone exert opposite effects, again probably more pronounced in visceral fat owing to higher specific receptor density. When the balance between the adrenal hormones on the one hand and sex-steroid and growth hormones on the other is shifted to the advantage of the former, visceral fat accumulates. Such hormonal dysbalance is seen in Cushing's syndrome, after glucocorticoid treatment, androgen exposure in women, and growth hormone and, in men, testosterone deficiency such as in aging, all associated with visceral fat accumulation. In all these conditions the excess of visceral fat is partly or fully reversible by appropriate hormonal interventions. These observations indicate cause–effect relationships between a hormonal dysbalance and the distribution of fat toward abdominal visceral depots.

A combination of these endocrine abnormalities is seen after chronic activation of the hypothalamic–pituitary–adrenal (HPA) axis [10]. There is evidence for such an activation in abdominal, visceral obesity [5] as reviewed below. It therefore seems likely that selective accumulation of abdominal, visceral fat is often due to a frequent or chronic activation of the HPA axis via the hormonal dysbalance mentioned above and its peripheral effects via specific receptors with high density in visceral depots. These observations indicate that central fat accumulation is a secondary phenomenon due to neuroendocrine abnormalities. Although genetic susceptibility is most likely involved, studies in monozygotic twins show that environmental factors can be solely responsible [11]. This is summarized schematically in Figure 1.

ABDOMINAL OBESITY, FREE FATTY ACIDS, AND LIPID OXIDATION

Central body fat distribution estimated by WHR, waist circumference only, or sagittal abdominal diameter is a more powerful risk factor than body mass index (BMI) [5] for the development of diabetes and cardiovascular disease in both men and women. Such observations clearly indicate that centralization of fat is the crucial factor rather than total fat mass.

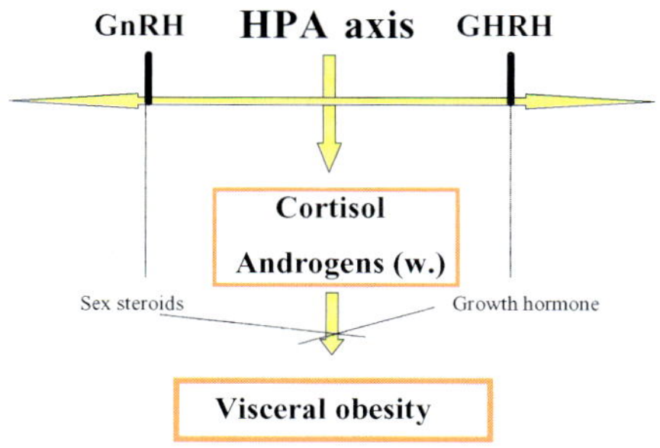

Figure 1 The neuroendocrine reactions leading to visceral obesity. Elevated activity of the HPA axis leads to increased cortisol and adrenal androgen production, the latter of significance in women (w.). These hormones generate accumulation of visceral fat due to high density of specific receptors in this adipose tissue. Secondarily, the hypothalamic–pituitary–gonadal (GnRH: gonadotropic-releasing hormone) and the growth hormone (GHRH: growth hormone-releasing hormone) axes are inhibited, leading to low sex-steroid and growth hormone secretions. Since these hormones have opposite effects than cortisol on visceral fat accumulation, low levels will amplify redistribution of storage fat to visceral depots

Fat oxidation is a powerful inducer of insulin resistance [12]. Recent experiments have shown a hierarchy of potential generators of insulin resistance in obesity, including, with increasing importance, obesity, abdominal obesity, plasma free fatty acids (FFAs), and muscle triglycerides, particularly lipids within the muscle cell [13, 14]. This indicates that the immediately available triglycerides in the muscle cell are the primary source of oxidative substrate, and that increased oxidation from elevated intramyocellular contents causes insulin resistance.

This area has recently been reviewed and the importance of fat oxidation for insulin resistance reemphasized [13]. In addition to inhibition of pyruvate oxidation [15] and glucose phosphorylation [16], the inhibitory step in fat oxidation is glucose transport [17] as shown in first-degree relatives of diabetics patients [18]. Long-chain fatty acid acyl-CoA seems to be critical [19], by disrupting the transport of glucose transporter 4 to the cell surface where phosphorylation of the insulin receptor substrate 1 is inhibited [14]. Generation of a pool of diacylglycerol might be involved [20].

In addition to these effects on insulin sensitivity there is considerable evidence of interference with insulin secretion by an impaired β-cell function after exposure to elevated triglyceride concentrations [13]. Taken together, this information clearly pinpoints the importance of the involvement of lipids in the pathogenesis of insulin resistance as well as in the capacity of insulin production. It appears likely that an increased availability of fat might be responsible in raising the important question of how and in which quantities lipids are delivered to these local oxidation sites.

Both circulating FFAs and very low density lipoproteins are elevated in abdominal obesity [1]. The elevated FFAs in abdominal obesity suggest that the fat cells have an increased sensitivity to lipolytic agents and/or that factors inducing fat mobilization are turned on. There is evidence for both. Lipolytic sensitivity varies in different regions of adipose tissue, with high sensitivity of adipocytes in central depots, particularly in the visceral region. In contrast adipocytes in peripheral depots, those enlarged in peripheral obesity, show a low lipolytic sensitivity resulting in low circulating FFA concentrations [9].

Factors stimulating lipolysis or blunting the antilipolytic effect of insulin are of major importance for the net outflux of FFAs from the adipocytes. In humans, the sympathetic nervous system (SNS) is the immediate trigger of lipolytic activity [21] and is activated in abdominal obesity [11, 22]. There is also evidence for increased HPA axis activity [5, 9, 11, 22, 23], expressing itself as higher cortisol secretion and, of importance in women, increased androgens. Cortisol and androgens exert “permissive” actions on lipolysis stimulation by the SNS, thereby facilitating the release of FFAs [9]. The nature and background of these neuroendocrine and autonomic abnormalities are further discussed.

The antilipolytic effect of insulin is a major factor in controlling outflux of FFAs from adipocytes. This control seems to be diminished in the course of the development toward diabetes [24]. Adipocytes in visceral depots are less sensitive to the antilipolytic effect of insulin, apparently because of less density of insulin receptors [25]. Furthermore, cortisol blunts the antilipolytic effect of insulin [26]. Cortisol may then have a key role not only as a permissive hormone for lipolysis, but also for blunting the antilipolytic effect of insulin.

Taken together, the elevated SNS and HPA axis activity in abdominal obesity facilitates lipolysis and blunts the antilipolytic effect of insulin causing elevated circulating FFAs. This in turn probably leads to enlarged local substrate pools of lipids with a high turnover and to increased fat oxidation followed by insulin resistance.

Are adipocytes different in different regions? Clearly, there are differences in the density of various lipolytic and antilipolytic receptors. For example, visceral fat cells have a higher density of β3, lipolytic receptors and lower density of insulin, antilipolytic receptors [25]. Are these genetic differences or are they due to adaptations to host factors? Adipocyte precursor cells from different regions seem to develop similar characteristics when exposed to the same environment in cell culture studies [27], suggesting that the host environment is of major importance for the development of adipocyte characteristics. This question has, however, not been resolved.

In summary, the role of abdominal obesity in the pathogenesis of insulin resistance appears to be related to an increased mobilization of FFAs, derived from excess of

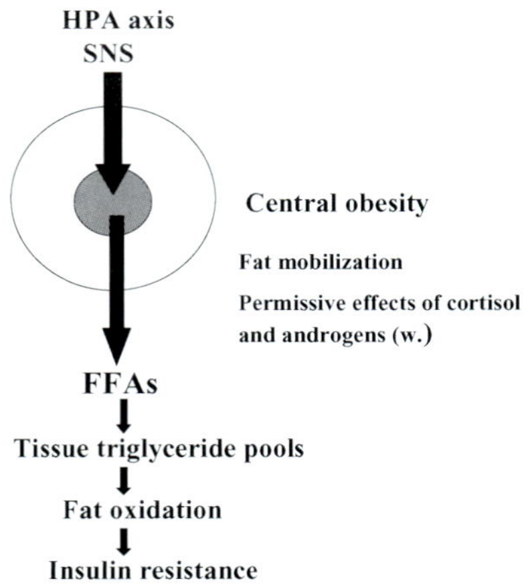

Figure 2 Fat oxidation as a pathogenetic factor for insulin resistance in central obesity. Elevated SNS activity stimulates lipid mobilization from central depots. By a concomitant elevation of the activity of the HPA axis, cortisol and adrenal androgens are elevated, the latter of importance for women (w.). These hormones have "permissive" actions on lipolysis as well as inhibitory effects on the antilipolytic effect of insulin. The result will be elevation of circulating FFAs, increasing local tissue triglyceride pools. This in turn increases fat oxidation, leading to insulin resistance and diabetes

adipose tissues, which are sensitive to lipolytic stimuli via "permissive" endocrine effects, combined with elevated activity of the SNS. Furthermore, a blunted antilipolytic effect of insulin is a contributing factor and may have a similar endocrine background. By furnishing excess substrate to fat oxidation, insulin resistance follows (Figure 2).

THE NEUROENDOCRINE AND AUTONOMIC ABNORMALITIES

In the previous section the importance of elevated FFA and very low density lipoprotein in abdominal obesity was pointed out as generators of substrate for local fat oxidation. The explanation to this increase is likely to be a combination of neuroendocrine, endocrine, and autonomic nervous system dysregulations.

Regulation of the HPA Axis

Because of the potentially significant role of the HPA axis activity in the development of abdominal obesity and diabetes, the regulation of this axis is considered. HPA axis activation is affected by a number of environmental factors that act with different impact depending on personal coping ability. The inherent sensitivity of the HPA axis may also vary. Furthermore, the controlling feedback system of the HPA axis has to be taken into account.

Central, Stimulating Factors

A number of different groups of factors are known to activate the HPA axis. These include various perceived stressors such as a poor socioeconomic status and the psychosocial milieu. Furthermore, infections and inflammation, chronic pain, or surgery activates the axis. Another factor is depression. Recently anxiety and the panic syndrome have been found to be associated with increased cortisol secretion. Sleep disturbances and stimulants such as alcohol and smoking are also involved [10].

In several studies utilizing saliva cortisol measurements, androgens in women, or surrogate measurements of the neuroendocrine disturbances, it has been possible to show that various socioeconomic handicaps are indeed present in men and women with abdominal obesity. These include low social class, low education, poorly paid jobs, and low housing standards. (For review, see references 5, 28, and 29.) This has also been clearly shown in the Whitehall studies where there is an inverse gradient between socioeconomic status and the WHR with associated metabolic aberrations [30].

There are also psychosocial handicaps, particularly in men, where factors such as living alone and divorce are found more frequently in men with central fat distribution. This is less pronounced in women. Lonely men often drink more alcohol, which might be a confounder [5, 28, 29].

Depressive and anxiety traits are often found in both men and women with central body fat. This is not fully expressed clinical melancholia but rather some increase in the scores of various depression measuring instruments such as Hamilton, Beck, or Montgomery-Åsberg scales, without reaching the scores for definition of depression [31]. Sleeping problems are often reported and could be a part of the psychological problems. These are factors such as difficulties falling asleep, waking up during night, and frequent use of sleeping pills [5, 28, 29]. Alcohol consumption is notoriously difficult to register in a reliable way. Using the AUDIT questionnaire it seems clear, however, that subjects with central fat distribution are often high alcohol consumers. Alcohol abuse might be followed by a pseudo-Cushing condition including high cortisol secretion and a habitus similar to that of Cushing's syndrome. It is known that cortisol is elevated after one or two drinks. Smoking is also involved, and elevates HPA axis activity [5, 28, 29].

Interestingly, similar factors have been found to be associated with primary hypertension via stimulation of the central SNS [32]. This may explain why the central SNS and the HPA axis are both activated in abdominal obesity, resulting not only in metabolic abnormalities, but also in hypertension [33].

It seems then that several environmental factors are associated with abdominal obesity and that the common link is the stimulation of the HPA axis. It should be noticed that the correlations between these environmental factors and measurements of centralization of body fat are present but disappear when BMI is used for expressing obesity. These observations suggest that the associations are more pronounced with distribution of body fat rather than with the total mass of body fat.

A recent study [11] has elegantly shown that environmental factors can be associated with abdominal obesity without genetic influence. Homozygous twin pairs were studied, where one twin had more pronounced abdominal obesity than the other. Visceral fat mass, measured with computerized tomography technique, was directly associated with cortisol and noradrenaline secretion. The abdominal obese twin with elevated cortisol and noradrenaline secretion also had the psychosocial problems described above. These results clearly show that the environment can be responsible alone, without genetic influence.

Sensitization of the HPA Axis

The response by the HPA axis to a challenge depends, in principle, on central signals as a result of the balance between input and coping, as well as on the controlling feedback system. The sensitivity of this system can probably be programmed perinatally.

Evidence for this came originally from Barker's group who found that subjects born small for gestational age, as adults developed abdominal obesity with its associated comorbidities, including risk to develop diabetes [34]. Recent work has now shown that such subjects are likely to have a sensitive HPA axis with overproduction of cortisol including an exaggerated response of cortisol after corticotropin administration [35]. This probably means that abdominal obesity develops via environmental challenges, but in this case activating a sensitized system for the control of cortisol secretion. It appears probable that exposure to intrauterine starvation during critical periods of the development of the central nervous system results in a defense to adapt to the prevailing situation, and that this programming to a higher sensitivity remains in adulthood.

Studies in experimental animals are now starting to open up this area. Several factors are involved in the programming mechanism, including the synthetic glucocorticoid dexamethasone, which passes the placenta barrier, androgens, cytokines, and simply maternal stress [36]. The resulting programming seems to be sensitive to the time point during pregnancy as well as to the power of the impact.

The question then becomes, how prevalent is this pathway toward abdominal obesity. Preliminary figures from Swedish men born in 1944 suggest that only a small part of abdominal obesity originates from the fetal programming pathway via intrauterine starvation (unpublished data). Maternal starvation or malnutrition was not very frequent in Sweden when these men were born. There are, however, other possibilities for recruitment via this type of mechanism by the agents mentioned above, including perhaps severe infections during pregnancy. This is obviously an important area for further exploration.

The Feedback Control System

The HPA axis is controlled by a feedback system localized to several parts of the brain, where the hippocampus area is particularly important. The regulatory system senses circulating cortisol levels via GRs in these brain areas. The efficiency of the system is usually tested by administration of the synthetic glucocorticoid dexamethasone, which normally shuts off cortisol secretion.

This system has been repeatedly studied in obesity. The results are varying with results of normal, high, or low efficiency of the system [23]. The inconsistencies of these results are probably explainable by methodological factors including doses of dexamethasone, type of obese subjects, and calculations of results. In diagnosing Cushings disease 1 mg dexamethasone should normally produce a certain defined inhibition. With this dose of 1 mg, very few obese subjects are abnormal. The method can, however, be refined by diminishing the dexamethasone dose, performing repeated measurements including the escape from the suppression as well as to use the absolute decrease in cortisol rather than a fixed upper suppression value of cortisol. This area of research needs improvements to assess the degree of suppressibility of the HPA axis activity.

In population studies [37, 38] 0.5 mg dexamethasone was used for suppression, and the difference between the average of two basal morning cortisol values and the value the morning after taking dexamethasone was used for evaluation. If these absolute cortisol values are used to measure the efficiency of the feedback system, the subgroups with an abnormal day curve seem to have comparably poor inhibition, particularly a group with a low, flat day curve of cortisol [37]. These results are, however, difficult to interpret, as discussed above.

A dose–response curve of dexamethasone suppression is another approach to the problem [39]. This was performed in a group of men with moderate obesity. Subjects were separated on the basis of the WHR. On average, the centrally obese group showed less suppression, which seemed to be most pronounced at the smallest doses, below 0.25 mg [39], while 1.0 mg showed total suppression [40]. These data suggest that there is no difference in maximal inhibition but there might be a difference in sensitivity. This would mean that much lower concentrations of dexamethasone than those used routinely may have to be used for the diagnosis of HPA axis regulation in abdominal obesity.

In parallel the function of the peripheral GR in adipose tissue was examined [39]. In these experiments the dose–response to cortisol of the expression of lipoprotein lipase was tested, a reaction mediated via the GR. There was no sign of differences in sensitivity, but a downregulation of activity across concentrations, suggesting a decreased density of GR—a known consequence of prolonged exposure to cortisol.

Although conducted in only a limited number of men, these experiments suggest the possibility that the central but not peripheral GR function is desensitized. This is further supported by the recent findings that the GR gene seems to have tissue-specific promoter domains, suggesting different regulation of GR density and function in different tissues [41].

Escape from dexamethasone suppression has also been tried. Cortisol was measured not only the next morning after taking dexamethasone but also several times during that day as well as next day. With the dose of 0.5 mg there was a fairly rapid escape, with no differences between abdominal obesity and controls (unpublished observations). There might be other more indirect methods to evaluate the feedback control. An increased elevation of cortisol after lunch, seen in abdominal obesity [42], might be a sign of poor control, but also of course a sign of a sensitive central facilitation mechanism. Cortisol secretion shows a peak activity immediately upon awakening. This peak is associated with abdominal obesity and its comorbidities, and might also be a sign of a poor control [43].

In summary, the currently available information does not allow any definite conclusions about the status of the feedback control of cortisol secretion in obesity, mainly because the methods used have to be refined for the purpose of measuring minor abnormalities in the feedback control system. However, some evidence suggests a desensitized central feedback regulation in abdominal obesity. This is a particularly exciting possibility because such an error has the potential to explain the abnormal neuroendocrine cascade seen in abdominal obesity.

Peripheral Consequences of Neuroendocrine Abnormalities

Cortisol, Testosterone, and Growth Hormone

The major products of stimulation of the HPA axis are cortisol and adrenal androgens, triggered by adrenocorticotropic hormone. Cortisol in obesity in humans is a much-studied problem, probably because several animal models of obesity have clearly elevated glucocorticoid secretion and enlarged adrenals, and obesity disappears after adrenalectomy. This field has recently been reviewed in detail [23] and is therefore only briefly summarized here.

In humans, elevated cortisol exposure is followed by obesity of the abdominal subtype, insulin resistance, and risk for diabetes. The most dramatic example is Cushing's syndrome. A recent study on homozygotic twins with a large difference of obesity and abdominal fat distribution within the pair shows that the twin with a larger visceral fat mass has an increased cortisol secretion [11], demonstrating the importance of the environment for this phenomenon. Such observations suggest that elevated cortisol secretion might play a role in the pathogenesis of abdominal obesity.

The problem does not, however, seem to be this simple and straightforward in the obese population at large. First, the kinetics of cortisol secretion seems to be as important as cortisol levels in plasma or total urinary excretion. Second, the peripheral metabolism of cortisol might be involved.

Saliva cortisol is a very useful tool in population studies because saliva can easily be collected during an ordinary working day, mirroring real life conditions. With this technique it has been found that in men, reporting stress in their life situation, morning cortisols are lower than those in a control group. However, cortisol levels do not "unwind" normally during the early part of the day, resulting in elevated total cortisol secretion over the day [23, 37]. Approximately 25% of the population showed these abnormalities (see Figure 3). In this group there was a correlation between total cortisol and the abdominal sagittal diameter, an estimate of visceral fat mass, as well as with insulin and fasting blood glucose, but not with BMI. Furthermore, other risk factors such as lipids and blood pressure were proportional to cortisol values. The same picture seemed to emerge after the physiological stimulus of cortisol secretion by a standardized meal [42]. In these subjects, it

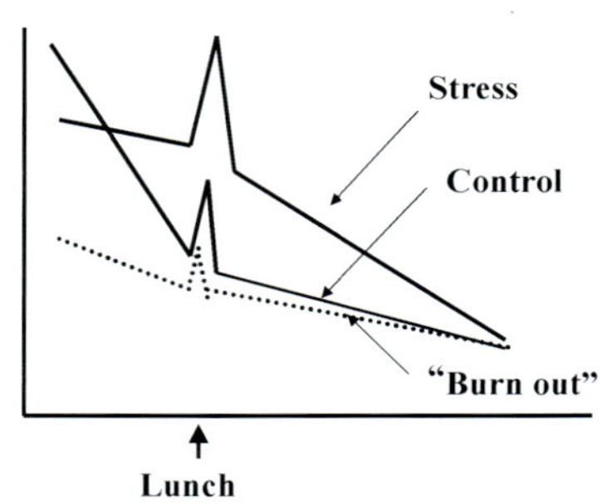

Figure 3 Saliva cortisol curves in men during an ordinary working day. Men with normal cortisol secretion (controls, about two thirds of the population examined) have high morning values, rapidly decreasing before a standardized lunch and then remaining low during the afternoon–evening. Men reporting stress during the test day and in their ordinary environment (about 25% of the population examined) have lower morning cortisol values, not decreasing before lunch and a higher lunch peak, resulting in an increased total cortisol secretion over the day. Less than 10% of the men showed a flat, low day curve ("burnout"). (Reproduced by permission of the American Society for Nutritional Sciences [23, 27])

seems likely that cortisol is responsible for both visceral fat distribution and insulin resistance. The insulin resistance could also result from FFA mobilization and fat oxidation, where cortisol is an efficient permissive hormone for lipolysis induced by the SNS as previously described.

A recent report from the Whitehall studies confirms these findings. Subjects with the metabolic syndrome display elevated cortisol secretion as well as evidence of increased activity of the SNS [44].

These observations are thus in accordance with what is known from excess exposure of cortisol in Cushing's syndrome or after treatment with glucocorticoids as well as after increased endogenous "functional" cortisol secretion [11] and may be explainable by increased exposure to the perceived stress reported by these men [23, 37].

In contrast, in another smaller subgroup (<10%) cortisol levels were low all over the day. There were strong associations not only to measurements of central fat but also to BMI, insulin, glucose, lipids, and blood pressure [37]. It is difficult to imagine that such low cortisols would be the trigger for the metabolic and hemodynamic abnormalities in this group. Other possibilities have therefore to be sought.

A low cortisol secretion might be a consequence of prolonged, severe stress. This has been shown in controlled animal experiments, where there is a development from an activated to a "burned out" HPA axis [45]. It is therefore possible that there is a time axis involved during stressful conditions from normal to activated to a "burned out" HPA axis. There are, however, no indications that this group of men with low cortisol levels were exposed to more stressors than the group with elevated cortisol.

A striking difference between the men who had elevated total cortisol secretion over the day (25%, see above) and the smaller (<10%) group with low cortisol levels is that the latter were obese while the former showed no associations between cortisol and BMI, only to sagittal diameter [23, 37]. In fact, men with a BMI $> 30\ \mathrm{kg/m^2}$ in this cohort have lower cortisols on most measured points over the day (unpublished). These observations then indicate that obesity is the major difference between these two groups. Elevated body fat mass has been shown to be associated with increased cortisol turnover. This is followed by a compensatory oversecretion of cortisol to maintain circulating levels at normal or even slightly lower than normal levels [36, 46, 47]. It is thus possible that obesity is the crucial factor responsible for the low cortisols in the subgroup in question. (See section on Cortisol Metabolism below.)

What is the origin of the metabolic and blood pressure abnormalities in this group with low levels of cortisol? Testosterone and insulin-like growth factor I (a surrogate measurement of growth hormone secretion) were also remarkably low. In men a low testosterone value is associated with abdominal obesity, and administration of testosterone to raise it to normal level decreases the mass of the visceral depot. Furthermore, insulin resistance is markedly improved, indicating a cause–effect relationship between low testosterone and abdominal obesity with insulin resistance [9, 48].

These effects of testosterone can apparently be explained by the mechanisms involved [9, 48]. First, testosterone exerts a pronounced lipolytic effect, particularly on visceral adipose tissue because of the high density of androgen receptors. This is amplified by growth hormone. Low levels of both hormones then would be expected to be followed by accumulation of visceral fat, something often seen in elderly men as these hormones tend to diminish with age. Similarly, testosterone in males exerts clear stimulating effects on insulin sensitivity of the nonoxidative pathway of glucose metabolism, more specifically the insulin-sensitive fraction of the glycogen synthase in muscle [48, 49]. Low testosterone would consequently be followed by insulin resistance. Surprisingly, low growth hormone also seems to be followed by insulin resistance, which can be improved by supplementary dosages, although here the mechanism is not known. Testosterone and growth hormone amplify each other's effects in several systems, and this might also be the case here [48].

Thus it is likely that low levels of testosterone and growth hormone might explain abdominal obesity and insulin resistance in this group, probably in a cause–effect manner, a statement based particularly on intervention studies and on the results of mechanistic studies [9, 48]. The low testosterone and growth hormone secretions might be mediated via increased activity of the HPA axis, well known to inhibit other central hormonal axes [10].

Other striking findings in this group with low levels of cortisol, testosterone, and growth hormone are elevated blood pressure and heart rate [37]. Such findings indicate that the SNS system is activated, supported by direct measurements in other studies [11, 22]. This in turn would be expected to be followed by increased mobilization of FFAs, worsening the insulin resistance.

In summary, men, who are exposed to perceived stress, oversecrete cortisol over the day, causing insulin resistance and centralization of body fat—both established effects of cortisol via known mechanisms. Another, smaller group had low saliva cortisol values all over the day. These men are obese and might have an increased cortisol turnover in the periphery. They also have low testosterone and growth hormone values, which probably generate insulin resistance and distribution of excess fat to central regions. In addition, a marked activation of the SNS probably stimulates adipose tissue lipolysis and worsens insulin resistance via elevated levels of FFAs.

Cortisol Metabolism

Peripheral cortisol metabolism might explain some of the inconsistencies in the studies of circulating cortisol levels in obesity [22]. Such metabolism seems to be tissue specific. Cortisone is transformed to cortisol by the enzyme 11β-hydroxysteroid dehydrogenase 1 (HSD-1), while the reaction in the other direction is catalyzed by HSD-2. In adipose tissue of the obese, the HSD-1 activity is dominating, increasing the formation of cortisol [46, 47, 50]. In obesity there is also an increased activity of pathways inactivating cortisol in the liver [46, 47]. The net result is low circulating levels of cortisol, which are compensated for by elevated central secretion to maintain normal cortisol levels. This may at least partly explain the elevated cortisol turnover in obesity as well as the fact that circulating levels are not elevated [23, 46, 47, 50].

The significance of the HSD system for obesity and its complications has recently been demonstrated in a transgenic mouse, which overexpresses the HSD-1 in adipose tissue [51]. The results were abdominal obesity and insulin resistance, which are the expected effects of increased cortisol secretion, and emphasize the potential role of adipose tissue in cortisol homeostasis.

The question then arises as to which is the most important pathway for increased cortisol secretion in abdominal obesity. There seems to be several possibilities for explanation. First, a primary elevation of secretion has been demonstrated in the population studies of men [23, 37] characterized mainly by central distribution of body fat. Another possibility is an increased peripheral turnover of cortisol, followed secondarily by a compensatory increase of central cortisol secretion as seen in obesity [46, 47].

Finally adipose tissue might contribute to peripheral cortisol levels via the HSD 1 pathway [50], again associated with obesity [47] (see Figure 4).

The activity of the HSD enzymes are modified by hormones [50], some of which are abnormal, particularly in abdominal obesity. Therefore, it cannot be excluded that changes in HSD activity in obesity are secondary to the prevailing endocrine changes of that condition. This area needs further clarifying studies.

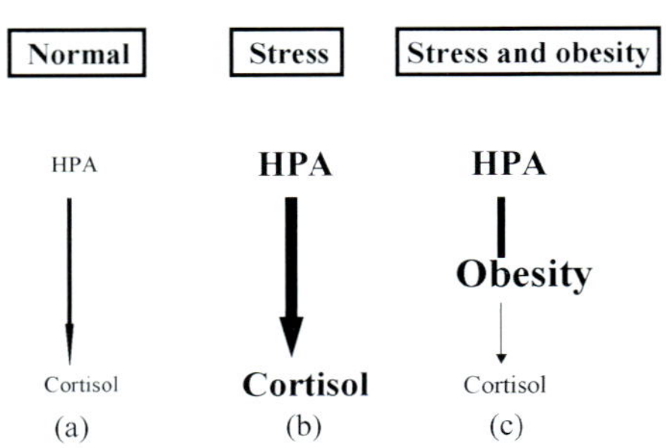

Figure 4 The influence of stress and obesity on circulating cortisol levels. (a) Normal condition. (b) Stress increases the activity of the HPA axis, resulting in increased circulating cortisol levels. (c) Obesity modifies circulating cortisol levels by increased conversion of stress-related cortisol to inactive metabolites

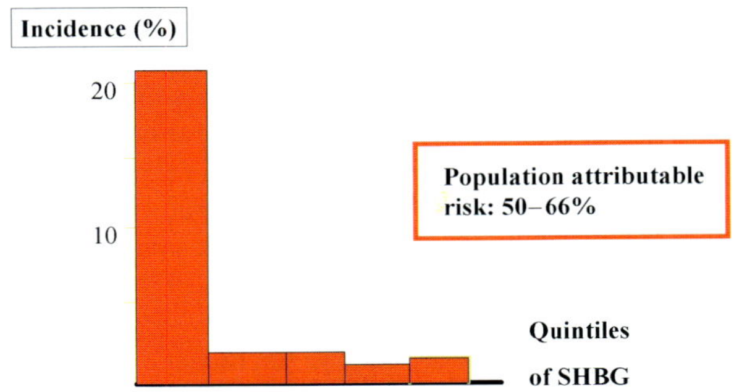

Figure 5 Low SHBG as a prospective risk factor for the development of diabetes in women (from reference 52). Almost all risk is confined to the lowest quintile, indicating a relative hyperandrogenicity. The population attributable risk in this quintile is in the order of 50–66% of all diabetes developing during the observation period of 12 years

ANDROGENS IN WOMEN

A new player in the discussion of insulin resistance in women is androgens. Prospective population studies demonstrate clearly that a low sex hormone binding globulin (SHBG) is a powerful risk factor for the development of type 2 diabetes among both pre- and postmenopausal women [52, 53]. Essentially all the risk is confined to the lowest quintile of SHBG, with very little risk in the rest of the population. From this information it is possible to estimate that the population attributable risk with a low SHBG could explain as much as between 50 and 66% of the diabetes appearing during a 12-year observation period (see Figure 5). The other major risk factors for diabetes in women, the WHR and insulin, correlate tightly and inversely with SHBG [52].

Low levels of SHBG are usually a sign of elevated androgens and/or low estrogens, because androgens inhibit and estrogens stimulate the hepatic synthesis of SHBG [54]. Population studies, in premenopausal women, all at the age of 40 years, show that insulin resistance is negatively associated with SHBG and positively with androgens. There are also strong correlations with measurements of centralization of body fat, triglycerides, total and low lipoprotein cholesterol, and blood pressure [38]. Free, active testosterone shows particularly strong correlations (see Table 1). These associations were also found with diurnal saliva cortisol measurements, but with less power than the androgens [38] (not shown in the table). Increase of risk factors was found in the highest quartile of free testosterone, within conventionally normal levels of free testosterone. This does not seem to be associated with polycystic ovaries in these women (unpublished observations), but is simply the highest levels in the normal female population, and is therefore a problem of particular importance.

In summary, prospective studies indicate that insulin resistance, abdominal obesity, and androgens, particularly

Table 1 Relationship between androgens and risk factors in women*

	T	Free T	SHBG	DHEAS
BMI	ns	0.448†	0.523†	0.140‡
WHR	ns	0.416†	−0.470†	0.221§
Sag.diam.	0.135‡	0.469†	−0.541†	0.200§
Insulin	ns	0.328†	−0.431†	ns
Glucose	ns	0.311†	0.269†	ns
Trig.	ns	0.352†	−0.410†	0.135‡
Chol.	ns	0.176§	ns	ns
LDL	ns	0.178§	−0.156§	ns
HDL	ns	−0.206†	0.415†	−0.136‡
Syst. BP	ns	0.275†	−0.172§	0.157‡
Diast. BP	ns	0.164§	−0.106‡	0.126‡

Note. T = testosterone; SHBG = sex hormone binding globulin; DHEAS = dihydroepiandrosterone sulfate; BMI = body mass index; WHR = waist/hip circumference ratio; Sag.diam = abdominal sagittal diameter; Trig. = triglycerides; Chol. = cholesterol; LDL, HDL = low-, high-density lipoprotein cholesterol; BP = blood pressure.
* From reference 38.
† $p < 0.001$.
‡ $p < 0.05$.
§ $p < 0.01$.

free testosterone, are clearly the most powerful risk factors for the development of diabetes in women.

Attempts to Integrate the Major Risk Factors for Diabetes in Women into a Mechanistic Chain

The question then is how these three most powerful risk factors for development of diabetes in women—insulin resistance, abdominal obesity, free testosterone—can be integrated, and how potential mechanistic pathways can be visualized.

A first possibility is that abdominal obesity with elevated FFAs is the primary factor, followed by increased fat oxidation, insulin resistance, and elevated free testosterone. SHBG is an important transporter of sex-steroid hormones [54]. Insulin lowers SHBG by inhibition of hepatic synthesis. Such inhibition would be expected to be followed by less binding capacity of testosterone and consequently leave a larger fraction of the hormone unbound [54]. It therefore seems possible to understand why insulin elevation causes increased free testosterone. However, this pathway does not explain why excess body fat has been specifically localized to central depots.

A second alternative is that elevated insulin is the primary factor, followed by elevated free testosterone, as described above. But it is difficult to understand how central obesity might develop from insulin resistance.

A third alternative is that elevated androgens are the primary factor. Androgens are powerful inducers of insulin resistance in women. Women and female rats given androgens develop severe insulin resistance, because of lower activity of the insulin-sensitive fraction of the glycogen synthase in muscle [55–58]. Furthermore, androgen administration to women is followed by visceral fat accumulation [55, 58] although the mechanisms have not been fully clarified. Thus androgen elevation may in fact be the primary factor in this chain of events, because androgens cause both insulin resistance and visceral obesity. Free testosterone may be more closely associated with insulin resistance than total testosterone because the prevailing elevated insulin levels may lower SHBG levels, thus increasing the physiologically most active androgen, free testosterone, as described above.

This pathway seems to gain credibility when the higher FFA levels of abdominal obesity are included in the picture. Androgens not only force excess fat to central depots in women, they also have a powerful permissive effect on lipolysis at several levels, from androgen receptor density through several steps in the lipolytic cascade [9]. The increased activity of the SNS in abdominal obesity [11, 22] then results in a marked elevation of lipolysis. The net results will be enlarged central adipose tissues with rapid turnover and increased circulating FFAs, leading to insulin resistance via elevated fat.

In summary, in women it seems likely that elevated androgen levels are a primary event causing muscular insulin resistance and generating large visceral depots with an elevated turnover via increased SNS activity. This results in increased concentrations of FFA, followed by insulin resistance via elevated fat oxidation. This seems to be the most plausible explanation to the prediabetic insulin resistance in women, because it embraces all powerful risk factors in a chain where the mechanisms of each step are known. This is schematically illustrated in Figure 6.

There are thus apparent differences in the action of testosterone in men and women. Increased levels of testosterone cause muscular insulin resistance in both genders, although in men at about 10 times higher levels than in women. Similarly a low testosterone also causes insulin resistance in men, while there might not be a critically low level in women. In other words, there seem to be gender-specific windows for the effects of testosterone on insulin

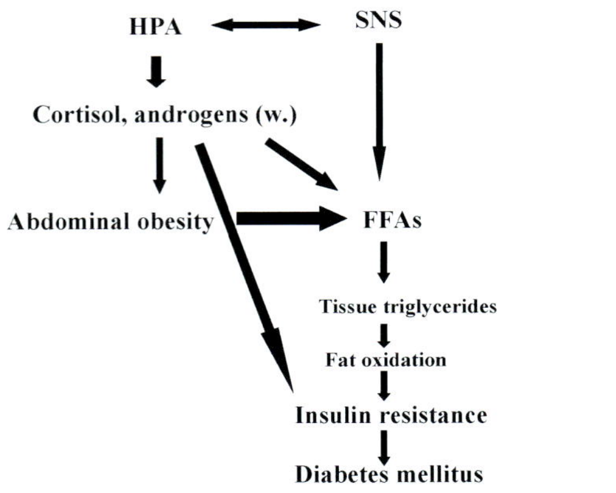

Figure 6 The contributions of increased activity of the HPA axis and the SNS to the development of diabetes. Various factors (see Figure 10) activate the HPA axis and the central SNS. The HPA axis activation is followed by adrenal secretions of cortisol and androgens (of particular importance in women, w.), which are followed by insulin resistance in muscle and direct excess fat to central depots. These hormones also provide permissive effects on lipolysis, induced by elevated activity of the SNS. The result is insulin resistance by direct hormonal effects and via elevated levels of FFAs. Local tissue pools of triglycerides accumulate, fat oxidation increases, and insulin resistance is amplified with increased risk to develop diabetes

sensitivity with optimal levels between about 15 and 40 nmol/l in men and between 0 and 5 nmol/l in women.

Origin of Androgens in Women

Environmental Factors Regulating Androgen Secretion

An important question then becomes, what is the origin of the elevated androgens in women with a high susceptibility to develop diabetes. Increased androgen secretion in women with abdominal obesity has been demonstrated in direct measurements, and is derived mainly from two sources, the ovaries and the adrenals. Adrenal origin of these androgens is suggested by the strong correlations between the concentration of testosterone or free testosterone and hormones secreted from the adrenals, namely dihydroepiandrosterone sulfate (DHEAS) and cortisol [38].

Another link to adrenal origin is the evidence of presence of stressors that activate the HPA axis, which regulates the secretion of adrenal hormones, including cortisol and androgens. These stressors include socioeconomic handicaps and resulting difficulties, traits of depression, and sleep problems. Similar correlations were also found largely with DHEAS and various cortisol measurements [38, 59]. Taken together, these observations suggest a hypersecretion of androgens of adrenal origin. Ovarian origin can not, however, be excluded, although recent studies, including ultrasound measurements of ovarian topography in relation to androgens do not suggest that the ovaries are involved (unpublished observations).

Androgen Removal

Circulating androgens are dependent not only on secretion but also on removal. A major pathway for this process is aromatization of androgens to estrogens. This process is catalyzed by the enzyme aromatase, which is widespread in the body and also present in adipose tissue [60].

The findings of a high androgen/estrogen ratio suggest indirectly a poor aromatase activity [38, 60]. We have recently examined aromatase activity in adipose tissue in a cohort of women, all 40 years of age. There was a lower activity of aromatase, negatively related to androgens, when abdominal obesity was statistically adjusted for (J. Öhrn and coworkers, unpublished data). These findings suggest the possibility that deficient aromatase function might be a factor for the chain of events linking elevated androgens, insulin resistance, abdominal obesity, and diabetes. The reason for the poor aromatase activity is not known. Among environmental factors smoking is not involved, because only nonsmoking women were examined. Genetic factors may well play a role as discussed in the next section.

Polymorphisms in the Aromatase Gene

The indications of poor aromatase activity have led to studies of the aromatase gene. This gene contains several polymorphisms of which those in a microsatellite in the fourth intron have attracted particular attention. This microsatellite contains seven tetranucleotide (TTTA) repeats with an upstream TCT deletion/insertion. Previous studies have shown that polymorphisms in this microsatellite are associated with increased risk to develop mammary and endometrial carcinomas as well as osteoporosis in women [38, 61, 62]. These diseases are thought to be dependent of or associated with abnormalities in sex-steroid hormones [60, 61].

The average length of the satellite stretches of this microsatellite has an interesting distribution, which clearly forms three subgroups with short, intermediate, or long stretches with little overlap between these three groups, particularly the extremes, the short and long microsatellite subgroups, which are totally separated [63] (see Figure 7).

The women with high androgens (testosterone, free testosterone, or androstenedione)/17β-estradiol ratios were characterized by the TCT deletion in the microsatellite of the gene [38]. In sharp contrast, women with the longest allele showed low androgens and high 17β-estradiol concentrations [64]. Consequently these genetic subgroups have totally different hormonal pattern of sex-steroid concentrations, and alleles in the aromatase gene [38, 64].

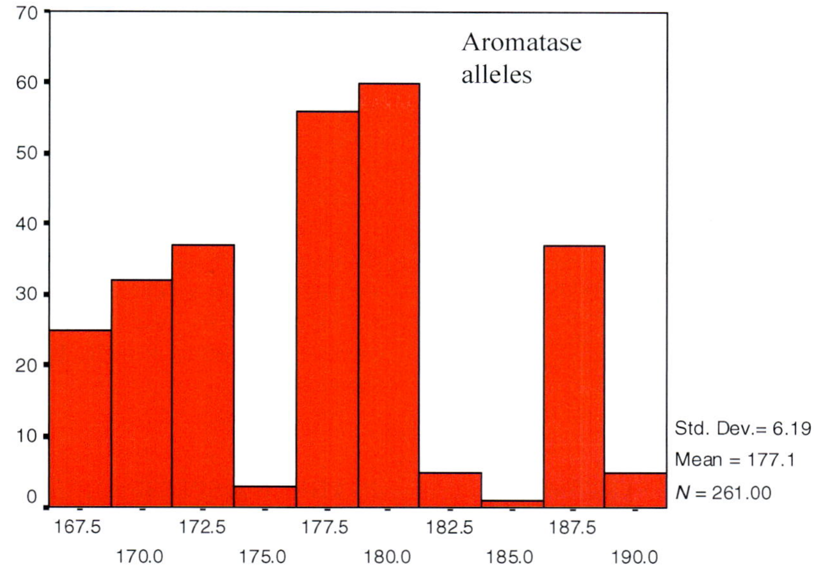

Figure 7 The distribution of average length of alleles in the tetranucleotide (TTTA) microsatellite in the fourth intron of the aromatase gene in women. Note the subgrouping with short, intermediate, and long alleles. The abscissa shows the average number of base pairs from the forward primer used [63] and the ordinate shows the frequencies. (Reproduced by permission of Oxford University Press)

There are other striking differences between these two groups. Women with the high androgen/estrogen ratio are abdominally obese, insulin resistant, and have several other risk factors not only for diabetes but also for cardiovascular disease. Prospective studies have shown that women with elevated androgens have a 10-fold increased risk to develop diabetes in comparison with the rest of the population [52, 53]. In dramatic contrast, women with the long allele not only have a normal sex-steroid hormone profile, but are also lean and without metabolic and hemodynamic risk factors for diabetes [64].

Despite these striking differences between these two molecular genetic subgroups, the functional significance of the aromatase gene polymorphism, if any, is not known. However, the importance for the aromatase enzyme for maintaining normal endocrine and metabolic functions has recently been demonstrated by knockout of the aromatase gene [65]. Female animals not only became hyperandrogenic with low estrogen values, they also developed increased masses of visceral fat and insulin resistance, a prediabetic condition, similar to that in women with elevated androgens. One may therefore speculate that the deletion of the TCT fragment in the microsatellite in the fourth intron of the aromatase gene is associated with poor aromatase function, with similar consequences as in the gene knockout model. Studies in cellular models and genetically manipulated animals have indicated that variations in microsatellite stretches might influence gene transcription or RNA splicing, particularly in genes involved in steroid hormone actions [61, 62]. Whether one of these alternatives may be involved or not in a potential functional significance of polymorphisms of the aromatase gene microsatellite in question remains to be determined.

Summary of Androgen Effects in Women

It seems reasonable from available data to suggest that a moderate elevation of androgens in women can be the consequence of a frequent activation of the HPA axis with increased secretion of androgens from the adrenals. This phenomenon may embrace as much as the highest quartile of the distribution of androgens in the population, which are within conventional normal limits. The consequences will be insulin resistance in muscle via inhibition of the insulin-sensitive fraction of the glycogen synthase. Furthermore, excess fat will be directed to central fat depots with a high turnover and facilitate fat mobilization via the SNS. The results are elevated FFAs and increased fat oxidation amplifying the insulin resistance exerted by androgens directly on muscle.

There is a possibility that a genetic susceptibility for a poor function of the aromatase enzyme amplifies the androgen elevation by a slow conversion of androgens to estrogens. A polymorphism characterized by a TCT deletion in the 5′ end of a microsatellite of the fourth intron of the aromatase gene is associated with elevated androgens. In contrast, women with a long microsatellite stretch in this gene locus show a totally different, perfectly normal phylogenetic status in endocrine, anthropometric, and metabolic variables. Aromatase gene polymorphisms may thus be important for health and disease in women (Figure 8).

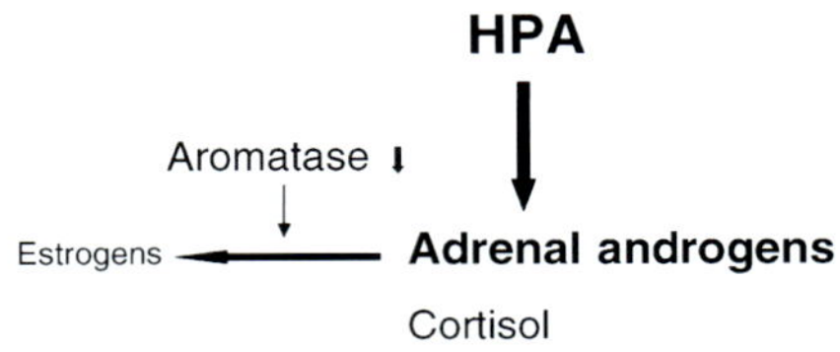

Figure 8 The origin of elevated androgens in the population of women. Adrenal androgens are increased via an elevated activity of the HPA axis. With a suboptimal activity of the aromatase with a slow removal of these androgens by conversion to estrogens, androgens will be further elevated. This is associated with a polymorphism in the aromatase gene, with a deletion of a TCT trinucleotide at the 5′ end of a microsatellite in the fourth intron (see Figure 7) (from reference 38)

THE SYMPATHETIC NERVOUS SYSTEM

As mentioned above, several psychosocial and socioeconomic "stress" factors can be traced in abdominal obesity in relation to activation of the HPA axis. Similar factors are known to activate the SNS and generate primary hypertension [66]. In fact it is difficult to activate one of these stress axis without activating the other [10]. This might be the explanation to the fact that hypertension is strongly statistically associated with abdominal obesity, where activation of the HPA axis has been shown. The abnormally low cortisol secretion found in a small fraction ($<10\%$) of men [23, 37] might be due to a "burn out" of the HPA axis after severe, repeated challenges, as discussed above. In such cases the SNS is activated, perhaps as a compensation in an attempt to maintain homeostasis [67]. This may explain the hypertension and increased heart rate in this group of men. These observations suggest activation mainly of the cardiovascular branches of the SNS.

Other studies indicate a generalized activation of the SNS specifically in abdominal obesity by findings of elevated excretion of noradrenaline or its metabolites [11, 22, 44]. This amplifies fat mobilization and is likely to be an important background factor for the elevated FFAs in abdominal obesity [1].

Leptin might also be involved in blood pressure regulation via the SNS. Leptin was primarily found to be a hormone regulating satiety, and is produced mainly from adipose tissue [68]. Additional effects were found to be stimulation of the SNS, followed by elevated blood pressure in several experimental models, provided that the function of the leptin receptor is intact [69]. Since leptin is overproduced in obesity, this may well be an additional pathway for the pathogenesis of hypertension in obesity, via leptin receptor signals to the SNS.

All obese subjects are not hypertensive. In addition to the difference between central and peripheral obesities, with hypertension mainly in the former subgroup, associated with central activation of the SNS by various stress factors, leptin might play a role. The leptin receptor gene has several polymorphisms. The presence of amino acid substitution in exon 4 (Lys109Arg) and 6 (Gln223Arg) is associated with considerably lower blood pressure than with the wild type of the gene. Furthermore, among 61 obese hypertensives ($>140/>90$ mmHg) only one had the polymorphisms mentioned, suggesting that these polymorphisms are protective against hypertension in obesity [70]. There is a possibility that such polymorphisms indicate a malfunction of the leptin receptor specifically in the pathway toward the SNS, but not toward satiety regulation, because the men examined who were carrying the polymorphisms had actually lower BMI than the rest of the men [70].

IS THERE A SPECIFIC FUNCTIONAL ROLE OF THE VISCERAL FAT DEPOT?

Most visceral fat masses are drained via the portal vein, implying that the liver is directly exposed to products from this adipose tissue. When visceral adipose tissue increases, one might expect an increased flow of FFAs to the liver. (For review, see reference 71.) This may be amplified because of the sensitive lipolytic system of visceral adipocytes as well as a dense innervation and a high blood flow. Elevated exposure of FFAs has several consequences for hepatic metabolism. First, FFAs are the rate-limiting substrate for the synthesis of very low density lipoproteins. Furthermore, FFA and lipid oxidation in the liver induce gluconeogenesis. In addition, experiments with the perfused rat liver show that FFAs inhibit hepatic clearance of insulin. The human relevance of this finding is uncertain because this phenomenon is only seen clearly in young rats but not in older, which might be due to fat deposits in the liver in the latter. If these consequences are indeed following hepatic exposure to excess FFAs from an enlarged visceral fat depot, then one would expect elevated triglycerides, glucose, and insulin in systemic circulation, in other words the metabolic pattern frequently preceding diabetes.

The major problem with this hypothesis is that it is very difficult to measure substrate concentrations in the human portal vein. Calculations from *in vitro* data of adipose tissue from the visceral fat depot clearly indicate that FFA release would be elevated in the portal vein in visceral obesity [71]. Such information does not, however, provide any information on important factors such as blood flow and innervation, which are crucial for *in situ* lipolysis.

It is possible with tracer dilution techniques to measure hepatic uptake of FFAs, but this uptake is a mixture of FFAs from the portal vein and the hepatic artery. This technique has provided information suggesting that the liver is exposed to elevated FFA in abdominal obesity, but it seems that this is explained by a mixture of portal and systemic fatty acids and may consequently not necessarily be a contribution by visceral adipose tissue itself [72]. Such an increased exposure of the liver to FFA may result in elevated hepatic glucose production, another sign of peripheral insulin resistance [13, 25].

Information is also obtained from another type of tracer technique [73]. When labeled oleic acid is given orally in a bolus of fat, the label is found after about a day mainly in adipose tissue and provides an estimate of total uptake when the masses of various fat depots are taken into account. With this technique it is clear that lipid uptake per unit of adipose tissue is higher in visceral than any other measured depot. Provided there is a steady state in energy balance, then the fat mobilization should be proportional to uptake. The turnover rate of femoral, subcutaneous abdominal, and visceral fat can, by this method, be estimated to be in the order of 8, 6, and 3 months. This means that visceral fat releases FFA at a higher rate per unit mass than the other depots. However, because of the small mass of the visceral depot it is questionable if FFAs from visceral fat contribute to a significant degree to an increase in portal FFA concentration.

In summary, the portal FFA hypothesis is interesting but lacks important information to be established. If the diabetogenic traits found in abdominal obesity are originating from this mechanism, then one is still missing the explanation to why certain subjects collect fat in the visceral depots in the first place. Although elevated exposure of the liver to portal FFAs from visceral fat remains an unproven mechanism for the generation of a prediabetic condition, other factors released from this depot might be responsible, because removal of part of visceral fat (the omentum) seems to improve insulin resistance [74].

GENETIC ASPECTS

There are obviously a number of possibilities for a genetic susceptibility to develop obesity and insulin resistance, leading to diabetes. The search for clues has not been very successful so far, probably because of the many genes in which polymorphisms of significance might be combined.

The above discussion has been focusing on abnormalities in central neuroendocrine regulatory factors leading to the combination of abdominal obesity and insulin resistance. There are also numerous possible genetic abnormalities in these pathways. Current knowledge of the details in the phylogenetic expression of insulin resistance through such pathways allows a focusing on points where abnormalities have been found. Such studies have just begun and are ongoing. Some examples of results will be mentioned here.

Genes regulating the activity of the HPA axis are of course of interest. Although there is still an uncertainty of whether or not the feedback regulation is abnormal in abdominal obesity, the GR gene locus is of obvious interest. The GR gene has nine exons where the last exon is doubled. The first exon has been considered to be silent; however, it appears that this part of the gene contains several tissue-specific promoter domains [41].

The enzyme *Bcl*I has a restriction site within the 5′ domain of the GR gene and cleaves the gene into two alleles of 4.5 and 2.9 kb. Several studies have shown the less common longer allele to be associated with abdominal obesity and insulin resistance [75–78]. Most important, there is also an association with stimulated cortisol secretion [78], suggesting the possibility that this polymorphism has the functional consequence of producing a GR without full effect in the HPA axis control. Homozygotes with the long allele constitute about 13% of men in the Swedish population, and are consequently rather frequent [78].

Further potential importance of this *Bcl*I polymorphism has been found in recent prospective studies in men. The longer, less frequent 4.5-kb allele was associated with worsening of a prediabetic state, including elevated glucose and insulin values. Appearance of clinical diabetes was 80% higher with this allele, which, however, did not reach statistical significance because of small number of events (Wallerius and coworkers, submitted).

With the restriction enzyme *Tth*III 1, cleaving the GR gene in the promoter area, associations have been found between resulting alleles and basal cortisol secretion [79]. There is thus some molecular genetic evidence of abnormalities in the 5′ end, perhaps promoter region of the gene. The *Bcl*I findings are most consistent. This polymorphism is localized to the first intron increasing the possibilities of a functional consequence for gene transcription. With the recently described multiple, apparently tissue-specific promoters for the GR gene [41], this will be a complex area to clarify but certainly worth the effort.

In the discussion of the potential significance of the microsatellite length in the aromatase gene, the potential significance of this type of polymorphisms was mentioned [61, 62]. The GR gene has a CAG repeat in the first exon, but the length of this microsatellite is not different in abdominal obesity as compared with controls [39].

There are obviously other possibilities of genetic abnormalities in the regulation of the HPA axis. The central regulation involves adrenergic, serotoninergic, and dopaminergic systems, presenting a challenging problem for the future.

STRESS-EATING

There is an interesting new development in the relationship between stress and obesity. The review above has dealt with the distribution of adipose tissue mass and the role of endocrine abnormalities, particularly cortisol, to direct excess fat primarily to abdominal depots. There is now growing evidence that cortisol may also interfere with food intake regulation and therefore with total body fat mass, irrespective of localization. This is the problem of "stress-eating".

The literature on stress-eating is very confusing reporting increased, decreased, or no change in food intake [80, 81]. The reason for this discrepancy might be individually different responses and/or the use of subjective methods.

Clinical experience clearly indicates that patients exposed to elevated levels of cortisol, such as in Cushing's syndrome and treatment with exogenous steroids, often get a voracious appetite and get obese with abdominal fat distribution. In contrast, patients with cortisol deficiency, such as in Addison's disease, become anorectic and lean.

Recent animal experiments are informative as to the mechanisms involved. Adrenalectomized rats show a decreased food intake and are extremely sensitive to the effects of leptin. When corticosterone is substituted gradually, food intake increases in parallel, and so does leptin. With excess corticosterone administration overeating is developed, followed by obesity and this is occurring in spite of an elevation of leptin, suggesting that a "leptin resistant" obesity is developing [82]. Human obesity is also characterized by elevated leptin levels [83].

Several reports show that after administration of glucocorticoids to humans, leptin levels are rising [84, 85]. In short-term experiments, food consumption, measured with an automatic food dispenser, is increased [86]. Prednisolone administration during a week (25 mg/day) is followed by overeating in spite of clearly elevated leptin concentrations [87]. This can also be seen in studies of patients with mild pulmonary sarcoidosis, treated up to 1 year with glucocorticoids. These patients consume more energy in spite of elevated leptin levels and accumulate central fat. The eating kinetics, measured by an eating monitor, show a slower decelerating phase, indicating delayed satiation [88]. It can consequently be concluded that glucocorticoid administration is followed by overeating in spite of elevated leptin levels, as well as abdominal obesity. The elevated leptin levels indicate a decreased efficiency of the satiety system, which then has been directly demonstrated by studies of eating kinetics.

The above results suggest that when exposed to elevated cortisol levels, subjects increase their food intake as a result of influence on satiety mechanisms. This does not, however, necessarily mean that "stress-eating" exists. Recent studies have shown that when subjects are exposed to laboratory stress, food intake is increased in parallel to the cortisol response during the stress [89]. In other words, stress-eating occurs only when there is a neuroendocrine response to the challenge, but not when there is no increase in cortisol secretion. This probably explains why only some subjects eat more upon stress exposure, and that the results in literature are highly varying. This problem is summarized schematically in Figure 9.

In addition to this biological mechanism stressful conditions might of course lead to development of obesity by eating rushed meals and not allowing time to experience normal satiety, which may result in consuming too much energy.

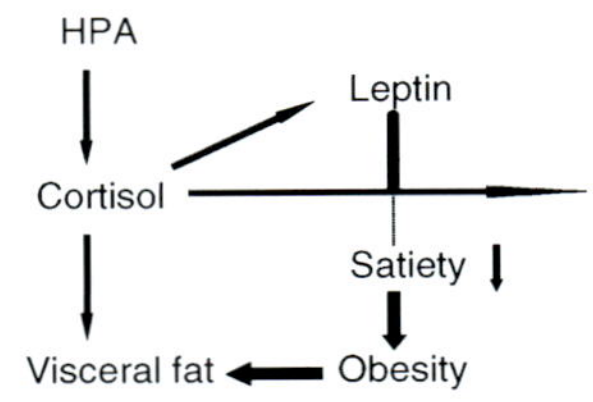

Figure 9 The associations between the activity of the HPA axis with cortisol secretion and the leptin system, inhibition of satiety, resulting in abdominal obesity

STRESS AND DIABETES

With the background provided above it is of course pertinent to inquire into the question of whether stressful conditions are indeed followed by increased risk to develop diabetes. Animal data clearly suggest a connection [90]. Particularly informative are studies with controlled psychosocial stress in primates, followed by insulin resistance and impaired glucose tolerance [91]. Human data are, however, scarce and nonconclusive [92]. Recent studies indicate, however, that work stress is followed by increased risk to develop diabetes [93, 94]. In established diabetes it is clear that stressful conditions worsen control and that stress management is followed by improvement [95, 96].

Taken together, current literature does not seem to allow a safe conclusion that stressful conditions are followed by increased risk for the development of diabetes in humans, but the problem does not seem to have been examined in adequately designed studies. Such studies require long-term observations relying on subjective reports of perceived stress and may therefore be difficult to perform in man. In addition, abdominal obesity is such an overwhelmingly strong risk factor for diabetes that other, "softer" risk factors may be hidden.

Repeated depressive periods are leading to increased risk to develop diabetes [97]. Depression might be considered as a long-term stressful condition, at least from a neuroendocrine point of view with similar, prolonged increases of cortisol secretion as in other psychological stress conditions. There is no doubt that frequent or chronic activation of the HPA axis is followed by increased secretion of cortisol and low sex-steroid and growth hormones [10], an endocrine constellation leading to insulin resistance, the major precursor to diabetes. Therefore, various stress factors that activate the HPA axis leading to these endocrine abnormalities should also be expected to be followed by increased risk to develop diabetes, although data supporting such a proposition are not conclusive.

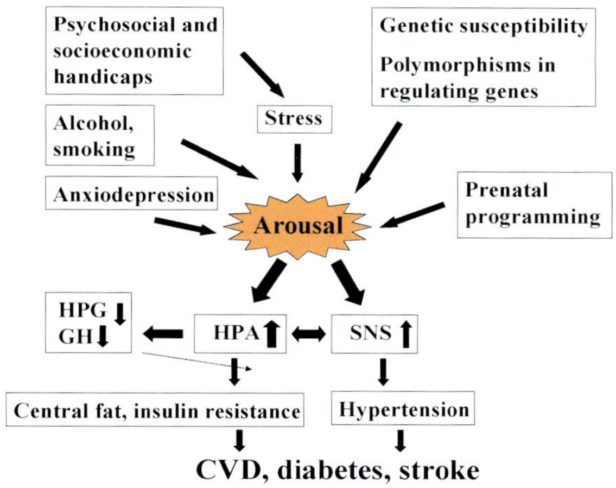

Figure 10 General summary of central factors resulting in an arousal syndrome with activation of the both stress axes, the HPA axis and the central SNS. HPG = hypothalamic–pituitary–gonadal axis; GH = growth hormone; CVD = cardiovascular disease. For detailed explanation, see text

SUMMARY AND CONCLUSIONS

Figure 10 provides a schematic summary of this review. Based on consistent results, it is suggested that obesity may develop into type 2 diabetes mellitus through the following chain of events. Several factors are involved in an "arousal syndrome," activating both stress axes, i.e. the HPA axis and the SNS. These include psychosocial and socioeconomic handicaps, which presumably lead to frequent stress reactions. Furthermore, alcohol, smoking, and anxiodepressive reactions, known activators of the HPA axis and the SNS, are involved. This is probably facilitated by genetic susceptibility but can be induced by environmental factors only. Prenatal programming to increase the sensitivity of the HPA axis may also be involved. The peripheral consequences of such arousal are summarized in Figures 2 and 6.

The HPA axis activation causes elevations of adrenal secretions, including cortisol, and of particular importance in women, adrenal androgens, resulting in accumulation of central visceral fat. Insulin resistance is induced by these hormonal disturbances directly and by their permissive actions on lipolysis via a concomitant activation of the SNS, causing elevated FFA. This in turn may explain the current view of the importance of increased fat oxidation to generate insulin resistance, because it provides the background to how excess fat may be directed to the locus of increased oxidation of fat.

This chain of events then includes the major risk factors for the development of diabetes via insulin resistance. Genetic factors are probably involved at several levels of this chain of events. A prerequisite for the precipitation of clinical diabetes is also strongly dependent on the genetic capacity of the pancreatic β-cells to produce insulin. There are indications that elevated FFA might impair insulin production by the β-cells, making central obesity with its elevated production particularly vulnerable.

The significance of a primary defect in lipid rather than glucose metabolism has attracted increased attention recently in the pathogenesis of type 2 diabetes. The primary problem then becomes to find out where such a defect is originating. In this overview it is suggested that abdominal obesity, with evidence of elevated fat mobilization through primary elevated neuroendocrine and autonomic dysregulations, leads to diabetes via increased fat oxidation in muscle as well as effects on hepatic metabolism and β-cell function. A number of important environmental factors include among others overeating, low physical activity, stress factors, abuse, and mood changes. The currently marked increase of incidence of type 2 diabetes may then be considered as a consequence of lifestyle changes, part of a "civilization syndrome," based on genetic susceptibility at different levels [5].

REFERENCES

1. Shafrir E. Diabetes in animals. In Porte D Jr, Sherwin RS (eds) *Diabetes Mellitus*. Stamford, CO: Appleton & Lange, 1997; pp 301–48.
2. Bennet PH, Rewers MJ, Knowler WC. Epidemiology of diabetes mellitus. In Porte D Jr, Sherwin RS (eds) *Diabetes Mellitus*. Stamford, CO: Appleton & Lange, 1997; pp 373–400.
3. Kissebah AH, Krakower GR, Sonnenberg G, Hennes MMI. Clinical manifestations of the metabolic syndrome. In Bray GA, Bouchard C, James PCT (eds) *Handbook of Obesity*. New York: Marcel Dekker, 1998; pp 601–36.
4. Despres JP, Moorjani S, Lupien PJ, Tremblay A, Nadeau A, Bouchard C. Regional distribution of body fat. *Arterioscler Thromb Vasc Biol* 1990; 10: 497–511.
5. Björntorp P. Visceral obesity: a "civilization syndrome." *Obes Res* 1993; 1: 206–22.
6. Björntorp P. Thrifty genes and human obesity. Are we chasing ghosts? *Lancet* 2001; 358: 1006–8.
7. Vague J. The degree of masculine differentiation of obesity—a factor determining predisposition to diabetes, atherosclerosis, gout and uric calculus. *Am J Clin Nutr* 1956; 4: 20–34.
8. Larsson B, Bengtsson C, Björntorp P, Lapidus L, Sjöström L, Svärdsudd K, Tibblin G, Wedel H, Wilhelmsen L. Is abdominal fat distribution a major explanation for the sex difference in the incidence of myocardial infarction? The study of men born 1913 and the study of women, Göteborg, Sweden. *Am J Epidemiol* 1992; 135: 266–73.
9. Björntorp P. The regulation of adipose tissue distribution in humans. *Int J Obes Relat Metab Disord* 1996; 20: 291–302.
10. Chrousos GP, Gold PW. The concepts of stress and stress system disorders. Overview of physical and behavioral homeostasis. *JAMA* 1992; 267: 1244–52.
11. Marniemi J, Kronholm E, Aunola S, Toikka T, Mattlar C-E, Koskenvuo M, Rönnemaa T. Visceral fat and psychosocial stress in identical twins discordant for obesity. *J Int Med* 2002; 251: 35–43.

12. Pan DA, Lillioja S, Kriketos AD, Milner MR, Baur LA, Bogardus C, Jenkins AB, Storlien LH. Skeletal muscle triglyceride levels are inversely related to insulin action. *Diabetes* 1997; 46: 983–8.
13. McGarry JD. Banting Lecture 2001. Dysregulation of fatty acid metabolism in the etiology of type 2 diabetes. *Diabetes* 2002; 51: 7–18.
14. Schick F, Eisman B, Jung WI, Bongers H, Bunse M, Lutz O. Comparison of localized proton NMR signals of skeletal muscle and fat tissue *in vivo*. Two lipid compartments in muscle tissue. *Magn Reson Med* 1993; 29: 158–67.
15. Randle PJ, Garland PB, Hales CN, Newsholme E. The glucose–fatty acid cycle. Its role in insulin sensitivity and the metabolic disturbances of diabetes mellitus. *Lancet* 1963; 1: 785–9.
16. Kelley DE, Mintun MA, Watkins SC, Simoneau JA, Jadali F, Fredrickson A, Beattle J, Theriault R. The effects of non-insulin-dependent diabetes mellitus and obesity on glucose transport and phosphorylation in muscle. *J Clin Invest* 1996; 97: 2705–13.
17. Dresner A, Laurent D, Marcucci M, Griffin ME, Dufour S, Cline GW, Slezak LA, Andersen DK, Hundal RS, Rothman DL, Petersen KF, Shulman GI. Effects of free fatty acids on glucose transport and IRS-1-associated phosphatidylinositiol 3-kinase activity. *J Clin Invest* 1999; 103: 253–9.
18. Rothman DL, Magnusson I, Cline G, Gerard D, Kahn CR, Shulman RG, Shulman GI. Decreased muscle glucose transport/phosphorylation is an early defect in the pathogenesis of non-insulin-dependent diabetes mellitus. *Proc Natl Acad Sci USA* 1995; 92: 983–7.
19. Ellis BA, Poynten A, Lowy AJ, Furtler SM, Chisholm DJ, Kraegen EW, Cooney GJ. Long-chain acyl-CoA esters as indicators of lipid metabolism and insulin sensitivity in rat and human muscle. *Am J Physiol* 2000; 279: E554–60.
20. Griffin ME, Marcucci MJ, Cline GW, Bell K, Barucci N, Lee D, Goodyear LJ, Kraegen EW, White MF, Shulman GI. Free fatty-acid induced insulin resistance is associated with activation of protein kinase C and alterations in the insulin signaling cascade. *Diabetes* 1999; 48: 1270–4.
21. Björntorp P, Östman J. Human adipose tissue. Dynamics and regulation. *Adv Metab Dis* 1971; 5: 277–327.
22. Ljung T, Holm G, Friberg P, Andersson B, Bengtsson BÅ, Svensson J, Dallman M, McEwen B, Björntorp P. The activity of the hypothalamic–pituitary–adrenal axis and the SNS in relation to the waist/hip circumference in men. *Obes Res* 2000; 8: 487–95.
23. Björntorp P, Rosmond R. Obesity and cortisol. *Nutrition* 2000; 16: 924–36.
24. Reaven GM, Hollenbeck C, Jeng CY, Wu MS, Chen Y DL. Measurement of plasma glucose, free fatty acids, lactate, and insulin for 24 h in patients with NIDDM. *Diabetes* 1988; 37: 1020–4.
25. Arner P, Bolinder J, Engfeldt P, Östman J. The antilipolytic effect of insulin in human adipose tissue in obesity, diabetes mellitus, hyperinsulinemia and starvation. *Metabolism* 1981; 30: 753–60.
26. Cigolini M, Smith U. Human adipose tissue in culture, VIII: studies on the insulin-antagonistic effect of glucocorticoids. *Metabolism* 1979; 28: 502–10.
27. Yang S, Xu X, Björntorp P. Effects of dexamethasone on primary cultured newly differentiated rat adipocytes from different adipose tissue regions. *Obes Res* 1993; 2: 99–105.
28. Björntorp P. Hypothesis: visceral fat accumulation. The missing link between psychosocial factors and cardiovascular disease? *J Intern Med* 1991; 230: 195–201.
29. Björntorp P. Do stress reactions cause abdominal obesity and comorbidities? *Obes Rev* 2001; 2: 73–86.
30. Brunner E, Marmot MG, Nanchatal K, Shipley MJ, Stansfield SA, Juneja M. Social inequality in coronary risk: central obesity and the Metabolic Syndrome. Evidence from the Whitehall II study. *Diabetologia* 1997; 40: 1341–9.
31. Ahlberg AC, Ljung T, Rosmond R, McEwen B, Holm G, Åkesson HO, Björntorp P. Depression and anxiety symptoms in relation to anthropometry and metabolism in men. *Psychiatry Res* 2002; 112: 101–10.
32. Folkow B. Physiological aspects of primary hypertension. *Physiol Rev* 1982; 62: 384–504.
33. Björntorp P, Holm G, Rosmond R, Folkow B. Hypertension and the metabolic syndrome: closely related central origin? *Blood Press* 2000; 9: 71–82.
34. Barker, DJP, Hales CN, Fall CHD, Osmond C, Phipps K, Clark PMS. Type 2 (non-insulin dependent) diabetes mellitus, hypertension and hyperlipidemia (syndrome X): relation to reduced fetal growth. *Diabetologia* 1993; 36: 62–7.
35. Phillips DIW, Barker DJP, Fall CHD, Seckl JR, Whorwood CB, Wood PJ, Walker BR. Elevated plasma cortisol concentrations: a link between low birth weight and the insulin resistance syndrome? *J Clin Endocr Metab* 1998; 83: 757–60.
36. Seckl J. Glucocorticoids, feto-placental 11β-hydroxysteroid dehydrogenase type 2, and early life origins of adult disease. *Steroids* 1997; 62: 89–94.
37. Rosmond R, Dallman MF, Björntorp P. Stress-related cortisol secretion in men: relationships with abdominal obesity and endocrine, metabolic and hemodynamic abnormalities. *J Clin Endocrinol Metab* 1998; 83: 1853–9.
38. Baghaei F, Rosmond R, Westberg L, Hellstrand M, Eriksson E, Holm G, Björntorp P. Polymorphism in the CYP 19 aromatase gene and associations with risk factors for type II diabetes mellitus in premenopausal women. *Obes Res* (in press).
39. Ljung T, Ottosson M, Ahlberg AC, Edén S, Odén A, Okret S, Brönnegård M, Stierna P, Björntorp P. Central and peripheral glucocorticoid receptor function in abdominal obesity. *J Endocr Invest* 2002; 25: 229–35.
40. Mårin P, Darin N, Amemeiya T, Andersson B, Jern S, Björntorp P. Cortisol secretion in relation to body fat distribution in obese premenopausal women. *Metabolism* 1992; 41: 882–6.
41. McCormick J, Lyons V, Jacobson MD, Noble J, Diorio J, Nyirenda M, Weaver S, Ester W, Yau JLW, Meaney MJ, Seckl JR, Chapman KE. 5′-Heterogeneity of glucocorticoid receptor messenger ribonucleic acid is tissue-specific: differential regulation of variant transcripts by "early life" events. *Mol Endocr* 2000; 14: 506–17.
42. Rosmond R, Holm G, Björntorp P. Food-induced cortisol secretion in relation to anthropometric, metabolic and haemodynamic variables in men. *Int J Obes* 2000; 24: 416–22.
43. Wallerius S, Rosmond R, Ljung T, Holm G, Björntorp P. Rise in morning cortisol is associated with abdominal obesity in men. *J Endocr Invest* (in press).
44. Brunner EJ, Hemingway H, Walker BR, Page M, Clarke P, Juneja M, Shipley MJ, Kumari M, Andrew R, Seckl JR,

Papadopoulos A, Checkley S, Rumley A, Lowe GD, Stansfeld SA, Marmot MG. Adrenocortical, autonomic, and inflammatory causes of the metabolic syndrome: nested case-control study. *Circulation* 2002; 106: 2659–65.
45. McEwen BS. Protective and damaging effects of stress mediators. *N Engl J Med* 1998; 338: 171–9.
46. Edwards CRW, Benediktsson R, Lindsay RS, Seckl JR. 11β-Hydroxysteroid dehydrogenases: key enzymes in determining tissue-specific glucocorticoid effects. *Steroids* 1996; 61: 263–9.
47. Rask E, Olsson T, Söderberg S, Andrew R, Livingstone DEW, Johnson O, Walker BR. Tissue-specific dysregulation of cortisol metabolism in human obesity. *J Clin Endocr Metab* 2001; 86: 1418–21.
48. Björntorp P. Hyperandrogenicity in women—a prediabetic condition. *J Int Med* 1993; 234: 579–84.
49. Holmäng A, Björntorp P. The effects of testosterone on insulin sensitivity in male rats. *Acta Physiol Scand* 1992; 146: 505–10.
50. Seckl JR, Chapman KE. Medical and physiological aspects of the 11β-hydroxysteroid dehydrogenase system. *Eur J Biochem* 1997; 249: 361–4.
51. Masuzaki H, Paterson J, Shinyama H, Morton NM, Mullins JJ, Seckl JR, Flier JS. A transgenic model of visceral obesity and the metabolic syndrome. *Science* 2001; 294: 2166–70.
52. Lindstedt G, Lundberg PA, Lapidus L, Lundgren H, Bengtsson C, Björntorp P. Low sex-hormone-binding globuline concentration as independent risk factor for development of NIDDM. 12-yr follow-up of population study of women in Gothenburg, Sweden. *Diabetes* 1991; 40: 123–8.
53. Haffner SM. Sex hormone-binding protein, hyperinsulinemia, insulin resistance and noninsulin-dependent diabetes. *Horm Res* 1996; 45: 233–7.
54. Partridge WM. Bioavailability of sex steroid hormones. *J Clin Endocr Metab* 1986; 15: 259–78.
55. Lovejoy JC, Bray GA, Bourgeois MO, Macchiavelli R, Rood JC, Greeson C, Partington C. Exogenous androgens influence on body composition and regional body fat distribution in obese postmenopausal women—a clinical research center study. *J Clin Endocrinol Metab* 1996; 81: 2189–203.
56. Polderman KH, Gooren LJG, Asschemann H. Induction of insulin resistance by androgens and estrogens. *J Clin Endocrinol Metab* 1994; 79: 265–71.
57. Holmäng A, Svedberg J, Jennische E, Björntorp P. Effects of testosterone on muscle insulin sensitivity and morphology in female rats. *Am J Physiol* 1990; 259: E555–60.
58. Elbers JMH, Asschemann H, Seidell JC, Megens JA, Gooren LJG. Long-term testosterone administration increases visceral fat in female to male transsexuals. *J Clin Endocrinol Metab* 1997; 82: 2044–7.
59. Rosmond R, Baghaei F, HolmG, Björntorp P. Relationships between personality disorders and anthropometry, hormones and metabolism in women. *J Endocr Invest* 2001; 24: 159–65.
60. Simpson ER. Role of aromatase in sex steroid action. *J Mol Endocr* 2000; 25: 149–56.
61. Riggins GJ, Lokey LK, Chastain JL. Human genes containing polymorphic trinucleotide repeats. *Nat Genet* 1992; 2: 186–91.
62. Comings DE. Polygenic inheritance and micro/minisatellites. *Mol Psychiatry* 1998; 3: 21–31.
63. Polymeropoulos MH, Xiao H, Rath DS, Merril CR. Tetranucleotide repeat polymorphism at the human aromatase cytochrome P450 gene (CYP 19). *Nucleic Acids Res* 1991; 19: 195.
64. Baghaei F, Rosmond R, Westberg L, Hellstrand M, Landén M, Eriksson E, Holm G, Björntorp P. The lean woman. *Obes Res* 2002; 10: 115–21.
65. Jones MEE, Thorburn AW, Britt KL, et al. Aromatase-deficient (ArKO) mice have a phenotype of increased adiposity. *Proc Natl Acad Sci USA* 2000; 97: 12735–40.
66. Folkow B. Physiological organization of neurohormonal responses to psychosocial stimuli: implications for health and disease. *Ann Behav Med* 1993; 15: 236–44.
67. Plotsky PM. Regulation of hypophysiotropic factors mediating ACTH secretion. *Ann N Y Acad Sci* 1987; 512: 205–17.
68. Friedman JM. Leptin, leptin receptors, and the control of body weight. *Nutr Rev* 1998; 56: 38–46.
69. Haynes WG, Morgan DA, Walsh SA, Mark AL, Sivitz WI. Receptor-mediated regional sympathetic nerve activation by leptin. *J Clin Invest* 1997; 100: 270–8.
70. Rosmond R, Chagnon YC, Holm G, Chagnon M, Pérusse L, Lindell K, Carlsson B, Bouchard C, Björntorp P. Hypertension in obesity and the leptin receptor gene locus. *J Clin Endocr Metab* 2000; 85: 3126–31.
71. Björntorp P. "Portal" adipose tissue as a generator of risk factors for cardiovascular disease and diabetes. *Arterioscl Thromb Vasc Biol* 1990; 10: 493–6.
72. Martin ML, Jensen MD. Effect of body fat distribution on regional lipolysis in obesity. *J Clin Invest* 1991; 88: 609–13.
73. Mårin P, Lönn L, Andersson B, Odén O, Olbe L, Bengtsson BÅ, Björntorp P. Assimilation of triglycerides in subcutaneous and intraabdominal adipose tissues in vivo in men: effects of testosterone. *J Clin Endocr Metab* 1996; 81: 1018–22.
74. Thorne A, Lönnqvist F, Apelman J, Hellers G, Arner P. A pilot study of long-term effects of a novel obesity treatment: osmentectomy in connection with adjustable gastric binding. *Int J Obes Relat Metab Disord* 2002; 26: 193–9.
75. Weaver JU, Hitman GA, Kopelman PG. An association between a *Bcl*I restriction fragment length polymorphism of the glucocorticoid receptor gene locus and hyperinsulinemia in obese women. *J Mol Endocrinol* 1992; 9: 295–300.
76. Buemann B, Vohl MC, Chagnon M, Chagnon YC, Gagnon J, Pérusse L, Dionne F, Despres JP, Tremblay A, Nadeau A, Bouchard C. Abdominal visceral fat is associated with a *Bcl*I restriction fragment length polymorphism at the glucocorticoid receptor gene locus. *Obes Res* 1997; 5: 186–92.
77. Watt GCM, Harrap SB, Foy CJW, Holton DW, Edwards HV, Davidson HR. Abnormalities of glucocorticoid metabolism and the renin–angiotensin system: a four corners approach to identification of genetic determinants of blood pressure. *J Hypertens* 1992; 10: 473–82.
78. Rosmond R, Chagnon YC, Holm G, Chagnon M, Pérusse L, Lindell K, Carlsson B, Bouchard C, Björntorp P. A glucocorticoid receptor gene marker is associated with abdominal obesity, leptin, and dysregulation of the hypothalamic–pituitary–adrenal axis. *Obes Res* 2000; 8: 211–8.
79. Rosmond R, Chagnon YC, Chagnon M, Perusse L, Bouchard C, Björntorp P. A polymorphism on the 5′-flanking region of the glucocorticoid receptor gene locus

is associated with basal secretion of cortisol in men. *Metabolism* 2000; 49: 1197–9.

80. Grenoo CG, Wing RR. Stress-induced eating. *Psychol Bull* 1994; 115: 444–64.
81. Allison DB, Heshka S. Emotion and eating in obesity? A critical analysis. *Int J Eat Disord* 1993; 13: 289–95.
82. Zakrzewska KE, Cusin I, Sainsbury A, Rohner-Jeanrenaud F, Jeanrenaud B. Glucocorticoids as counter-regulatory hormones of leptin. Toward an understanding of leptin resistance. *Diabetes* 1997; 46: 717–9.
83. Considine RV, Sinha NK, Heiman ML, Kriauciunas A, Stephens TW, Nyce MR, Ohannesian JP, Marco CC, McKee LJ, Bauer TL, Caro JF. Serum immunoreactive leptin concentrations in normal weight and obese humans. *N Engl J Med* 1996; 334: 292–5.
84. Newcomer JKW, Selke G, Melson AK, Gross J, Vogler GP, Dagogo-Jack S. Dose-dependent cortisol-induced increases of plasma leptin concentrations in healthy humans. *Arch Gen Psychiatry* 1998; 55: 995–1000.
85. Dagogo-Jack S, Selke L, Melson AK, Newcomer JW. Effect of dexamethasone on plasma leptin concentration in lean and obese humans: a randomized placebo-controlled study. *J Clin Endocr Metab* 1997; 82: 3230–3.
86. Tattarani PA, Larson DE, Snitker S, Young JB, Flatt JB, Ravussin E. Effects of glucocorticoids on energy metabolism and food intake in humans. *Am J Physiol* 1996; 271: 317–25.
87. Uddén J, Björntorp P, Arner P, Barkeling B, Meurling L, Hill M, Rössner S. Effects of glucocorticoids on leptin levels and eating behaviour in women. *Intern Med* 2003; 253: 225–31.
88. Uddén J, Barkeling B, Brismar TB, Björntorp P, Berlin M, Berinder K, Rössner S. Effects of long-term prednisolone treatment on leptin levels, eating behaviour and body composition. (Submitted).
89. Epel E, Lapidus R, McEwen B, Brownell K. Stress may add a bite to appetite in women: a laboratory study of stress-induced cortisol and eating behavior. *Psychoneuroendocrinology* 2001; 26: 37–49.
90. Surwit RS, Feinglos MN, Livingston EG, Kuhn CM, McCubbin JA. Behavioral manipulation of the diabetic phenotype in *ob/ob* mice. *Diabetes* 1984; 33: 616–8.
91. Shively CA, Laber-Laird K, Anton RF. Behavior and physiology of social stress and depression in female cynomolgus monkeys. *Biol Psychiatry* 1997; 41: 871–82.
92. Surwit RS, Schneider MS, Feinglos MN. Stress and diabetes mellitus. *Diabetes Care* 1992; 15: 1413–22.
93. Kawakami N, Araki S Takatsuka N, Shimizu H, Ishibashi H. Overtime, psychosocial working conditions, and occurrence of non-insulin dependent diabetes mellitus in Japanese men. *J Epidemiol Community Health* 1999; 53: 359–63.
94. Kawakami N, Haratani T. Epidemiology of job stress and health in Japan: review of current evidence and future direction. *Ind Health* 1999; 37: 174–86.
95. Lane JD, McCaskill CC, Williams PG, Parekh PI, Feinglos MN. Personalty correlates and glycemic control in type 2 diabetes. *Diabetes Care* 2000; 23: 1321–5.
96. Surwit RS, van Tilburg MA, Zucker N, McCaskill CC, Parekh P, Feinglos MN, Edwards CL, Williams P, Lane JD. Stress management improves long-term glycemic control in type 2 diabetes. *Diabetes Care* 2002; 25: 30–4.
97. Eaton WW, Armenian H, Gallo J, Pratt L, Ford DE. Depression and risk for onset of type II diabetes mellitus. A prospective population study. *Diabetes Care* 1996; 19: 1097–102.

31

Is Type 2 Diabetes the Result of a "Thrifty Genotype" or a "Thrifty Phenotype"?

Robert S. Lindsay

MedStar Research Institute, Washington, DC, USA

INTRODUCTION

Type 2 diabetes is a common, complex disease. It is described in all ethnic groups and prevalence is increasing worldwide, representing a major health burden [1]. While a number of important risk factors for development of type 2 diabetes have been described—most notably overweight and obesity—much of the detail of the etiology of the disease remains unknown. Both genetic and environmental factors will be important and disease risk is likely to reflect a complex interaction of both. Certain aspects of the epidemiology of type 2 diabetes, the widespread predisposition to the disease, increased prevalence in certain ethnic groups, and more recently, well-described associations of diabetes risk and lower birth weight have prompted a number of hypotheses. These hypotheses attempt to explain these important epidemiological features of type 2 diabetes but also place our understanding of the etiology of type 2 diabetes in a wider context. A unifying theme of the thrifty genotype and thrifty phenotype hypotheses is the concept that predisposition to type 2 diabetes may reflect previous nutritional conditions. In the case of the thrifty genotype the nutritional history of populations favors genetic polymorphisms, which also render individuals diabetes prone [2]. By contrast the thrifty phenotype proposes that adverse nutritional conditions in the early environment predispose to later disease in individuals [3]. Both hypotheses are connected by a further underlying aim—to aid our understanding of the causes of type 2 diabetes and thus find ways to prevent, treat, and ultimately cure the disease.

Three main areas are reviewed in this chapter: first, the notion of the thrifty Genotype—the hypothesis first proposed by Neel in 1962 [2]; second, the Thrifty Phenotype—the suggestion made in 1992 by Hales and Barker, partly prompted by their observations of associations of birth weight and type 2 diabetes, that undernutrition in early life predisposes to adult type 2 diabetes [3]; third, an alternative explanation for some of the observations that prompted the thrifty phenotype hypothesis—the proposal of Hattersley and Tooke [4] that genetic (rather than environmental) factors underpin the associations of birth weight and type 2 diabetes.

TYPE 2 DIABETES AND THE THRIFTY GENOTYPE

The Thrifty Genotype

In 1962 Professor JV Neel introduced the thrifty genotype hypothesis, addressing the etiology of diabetes (the distinctions between type 1 and type 2 diabetes had not been clearly defined at that time) and obesity from the perspective of evolutionary biology [2]. Neel proposed that predisposition to diabetes might arise because of genetic variations, which were advantageous in historical environments but were rendered disadvantageous—and disease causing—in modern environments. In this he drew the analogy with genetic variation responsible for sickle cell hemoglobin—advantageous to the population when the environment contains a high risk of malaria. By contrast if risk of malaria is removed, the polymorphism is

International Textbook of Diabetes Mellitus, Third Edition. Edited by R. A. DeFronzo, E. Ferrannini, H. Keen, and P. Zimmet.
 ISBN: 0-471-48655-8.

disadvantageous because of the detrimental effects of sickle cell anemia in homozygotes. More specifically he proposed that human variations that were favorable in populations facing challenges of episodic undernutrition (feast or famine) might be disadvantageous when food supplies became abundant: in Neel's words "a thrifty genotype rendered detrimental by 'progress' " [2].

Ironically, given the associations of lower birth weight and type 2 diabetes risk that later prompted the hypothesis of Hales and Barker, the thinking of Neel was, in part, prompted by *increased* birth weight in offspring of diabetic mothers. Subsequent data (in part reviewed below) suggest that this increase in birth weight likely represented effects of maternal diabetes acting on the fetal environment *in utero* rather than a genetic effect [5]. Nevertheless, it prompted Neel to hypothesize that, before onset of disease, diabetic patients had a "thrifty" genotype favoring increased intake or particularly efficient utilization of food.

There are a number of interesting elements of this hypothesis. As type 2 diabetes is such a common condition it seems both plausible and intriguing that genetic variation predisposing to diabetes might have been associated with selective advantage at some point over the course of human evolution. The disease itself is unlikely to have been heavily selected against previously. Although historical records suggest that diabetes is likely to have been present for many thousands of years, type 2 diabetes was almost certainly a rare disease historically. It is also likely to have occurred after child bearing, type 2 diabetes in children being a very recent phenomenon. It follows that morbidity and mortality relating to type 2 diabetes would probably have had limited impact on transmission and evolutionary success of predisposing polymorphisms. The hypothesis has also been used to try to explain why different ethnic groups might have different propensities to type 2 diabetes. Varying environmental selection pressures between human populations, for example with regard to nutrition, might therefore explain differing ethnic propensities to diseases like type 2 diabetes.

Mechanisms of the Thrifty Genotype

For Neel the critical genetic polymorphisms driving the thrifty genotype were predicted to increase either appetite or energy "efficiency." Following prevailing physiological paradigms of the time, Neel proposed that the thrifty gene would result in *increased* insulin secretion in early life (which he later termed a *fast insulin trigger* [6]) coupled to a later increase in circulating "anti-insulins." In the model, increased insulin action in the early years would contribute to increased survival by favoring fat deposition. Anti-insulins would lead to later development of diabetes. As detailed by Neel himself, much of the physiological thinking of his original paper has been superseded [6]; however, the critical central notion that diabetes-causing polymorphisms might have exerted beneficial effects in historical environments has informed many researchers since.

In considering the thrifty genotype it is useful to consider three further issues. First, how might disease polymorphisms increase risk of type 2 diabetes? Second, what physiological advantages could they have posed in previous environments? Third, what were the critical environments that encouraged selection of the diabetes-causing polymorphisms?

Neel favored genetic polymorphisms, which would favor increased early growth and energy efficiency. While many of the proponents of the thrifty gene have favored effects on fat deposition or energy metabolism, the critical polymorphism could act in a variety of ways. In the broadest terms, it might increase propensity to obesity, reduce insulin sensitivity, or reduce β-cell secretion in the modern "diabetes prone" environment.

A thrifty gene would also act to increase reproductive fitness. This could occur by a variety of mechanisms—not necessarily by increasing either fat deposition or early growth. Indeed, as much modern evidence suggests a reduction of growth (at least at birth) in association with later type 2 diabetes it might now be supposed that such diabetes-causing polymorphisms would either be neutral or even impede early growth. Discussion of this area is expanded in our consideration of the thrifty phenotype of Hales and Barker [3] and fetal insulin hypothesis of Hattersley and Tooke [4]. Further, with the description of leptin—a critical mediator of appetite and energy metabolism [7], it has become apparent that there is considerable cross talk between physiological systems involved in appetite and energy storage with reproductive and immune axes. When we consider how a thrifty gene might have increased reproductive fitness in the past, this cross talk increases the range of possibilities. Indeed, later, several authors have questioned whether a gene need not be "thrifty" at all in the narrow sense of increasing growth or energy efficiency, or acting to increase propensity to adiposity. Reaven, expanding upon the work of Cahill [8] and others, hypothesized that genetic polymorphisms that decrease insulin action in muscle might have been favored as they allowed conservation of muscle protein in times of starvation [9].

More recently it has become apparent that there are numerous cross-sectional relationships between insulin resistance and obesity, both important predictors of later risk of type 2 diabetes [10], and markers of inflammation and endothelial dysfunction [11]. As argued by Pickup and Crook, activation of inflammation and the innate immune system appear characteristic of insulin resistance and type 2 diabetes [11]. Fernandez-Real and coworkers have suggested the elegant hypothesis that genes predisposing to insulin resistance might thus have been historically advantageous because of an enhanced innate immune response [12]. In this they posit that the major selection pressure in the past might have been infectious disease and trauma [12]. Polymorphisms favoring an enhanced immune response would be advantageous for survival in this environment but, for example by reducing sensitivity to insulin, increase risk of diabetes in modern environments. Investigation in this field is at a relatively early stage, but it is of interest that markers of inflammation are also predictive of type 2 diabetes in a variety of populations [13–17]. Fernandez-Real et al. have also reported that polymorphisms of the interleukin-6 (IL-6) gene are associated with both crude markers of an increased immune response as evidenced by higher IL-6 concentrations and insulin resistance in studies in European populations [18]. Clearly, even if infection or trauma were an additional selective mechanism, nutrition may still play a critical role as proposed by Neel.

Finally, one has to consider the selecting environment. Neel suggested that the thrifty gene would increase early growth in environments subject to episodic undernutrition [2]. Conceivably, a thrifty gene could have been selected by particular advantage during chronic or episodic undernutrition. The presence of excess versus only adequate nutrition at the end of periods of undernutrition might also be important in which polymorphisms were selected. In addition, a range of other environmental insults, importantly, noting the theories of Fernandez-Real, trauma and infection, might also be critical in creating the selective environment either independently of or in interaction with particular nutritional environments. It becomes clear that defining the critical environment is difficult and attempts in animal models to test thrifty genes are difficult to interpret, particularly if negative.

The Thrifty Genotype and Prevalence of Diabetes in Human Populations

Consideration of the selecting environment leads us to another important point. The thrifty genotype is often also invoked as an explanation for the reason that certain populations are more prone to type 2 diabetes than others [6]. It is clear that the prevalence of type 2 diabetes is profoundly different in different ethnic groups. The highest known prevalence of type 2 diabetes occurs in the Pima Indian population of Arizona, among whom over 60% of adults develop the disease [19]. Other American Indian groups as well as Polynesian and Micronesian populations also have very high prevalence of type 2 diabetes, followed by migrant Asian Indians [1]. Neel suggested that selection of thrifty genes would have occurred in the long period when humans followed a hunter-gatherer existence [2]. In turn, diabetes-prone populations have been characterized as those who have most recently changed from a hunter-gatherer economy. Notably, however, the evidence that "hunter-gatherer" societies are less well nutritioned than those following agricultural economies is scanty. Indeed, there is some evidence that hunter-gatherers, both in modern times and in the archeological record, were relatively well nutritioned compared to agriculture based peers [20]. Interestingly, the Pima are also believed to have had a largely agriculture-based lifestyle for hundreds, and perhaps thousands of years. The precise nature of the selecting environment may never be known and there may be subtle effects of the periodicity of undernutrition or lack of key nutritional components common to the Pima and other groups but not obvious to us today. Alternatively, following the hypotheses of Fernandez Real et al. [12] we have suggested that the increased propensity of groups such as the Pima might not relate to selection by undernutrition but rather the infectious disease histories of such population groups. It is well described that following contact with Europeans in the sixteenth century the predominant cause of death in Native American populations was imported infection including measles, mumps, and rubella [21]. Native American populations fell to a fraction of their previous numbers, perhaps declining by up to 95% [22]. Given the proposal of Fernandez-Real that polymorphisms give increased protection in the face of infectious or traumatic insults, one might speculate that increased diabetes propensity in these populations reflects selection of individuals resistant to infectious disease who also have increased diabetes propensity [14].

Thrifty Genes

Do thrifty genes exist? In recent years it has become apparent that genetic variation can result in increased propensity to both type 2 diabetes and obesity. Currently, in humans this mainly refers to the effects of very rare mutations, with fewer descriptions of functional polymorphisms common enough to affect propensity to type 2 diabetes or obesity at the population level.

Leptin has been proposed as a putative thrifty gene. Defects in the leptin gene account for rare obesity syndromes in humans [23]. Further, animal models of defective leptin action—the *ob/ob* and *db/db* mouse with genetic defects in the leptin gene and leptin receptor respectively—have a phenotype of both increased weight gain and increased survival in the face of undernutrition [24]. It seems unlikely, however, that either leptin or the leptin receptor is Neel's thrifty gene. In general, polymorphisms of these two genes do not appear to account for major variation in adiposity in human populations [25–29]. In addition the fact that hypogonadism is part of the phenotype of the rare leptin gene mutations in humans [23] has been taken as an argument against leptin being a thrifty gene, as the obesity causing mutation is associated with a reduction in reproductive ability. While true, this would not exclude other polymorphisms having a combination of obesity-promoting and reproductively advantageous effects. The leptin system remains an attractive target for putative thrifty genes.

Defects of central melanocortin signaling also influence human adiposity. Mutations of the proopiomelanocortin gene result in a rare syndrome of human obesity [30]. Perhaps of more interest in light of the thrifty genotype hypothesis is the observation that common variations of the melanocortin 4 receptor (MC4R) may account for up to 4% of severe obesity in some human populations even if this observation has recently been challenged [31, 32]. These mutations do not appear to affect reproductive function [31, 32] and may influence obesity by actions on food intake [31]. MC4R mutations do not appear to be responsible for greater propensity to obesity in other populations such as the Pima Indians [33].

Variation in 24-h energy expenditure is predictive of weight gain in humans [34]. This suggests that genetic polymorphisms of genes in pathways influencing energy expenditure might be both candidate genes for obesity and putative thrifty genes. In this context both the β_3-adrenergic receptor and uncoupling proteins (UCP-1, -2, -3) have been proposed as candidate genes, although associative studies have not provided consistent results across populations [35].

TYPE 2 DIABETES AND THE THRIFTY PHENOTYPE

The Thrifty Phenotype

The thrifty phenotype hypothesis was proposed in 1992 by Hales and Barker [3]. The term *thrifty phenotype* alludes to the *thrifty genotype* but proposes a very different cause of type 2 diabetes. In their model undernutrition acts not as a selection pressure acting over many generations to alter the genetic make up of the population as proposed by Neel, but rather as an early environmental influence acting in an individual to increase risk of type 2 diabetes [3]. In Neel's hypothesis entire populations have an increased predisposition to type 2 diabetes—because of genetic selection they are better adapted to different nutritional circumstances than those they experience today. In the thrifty phenotype hypothesis disease risk increases as a result of environmentally induced alteration of physiology in the early life of the individual. In part, the thrifty phenotype arises in response to observations that lower birth weight is associated with later risk of metabolic disease and in particular type 2 diabetes. [3] It is therefore useful to consider some of this evidence.

The Epidemiology of Birth Weight and Metabolic Disease

The Birth Weight Hypothesis

Birth weight has been used as an important epidemiologic indicator of well-being in childhood for some time. It is well known that lower birth weight is associated with a range of adverse events *in utero* and in addition is associated with a range of adverse environmental conditions pertaining to the mother. In particular lower birth weight is associated with poorer socioeconomic conditions as well as more obvious adverse events in the *in utero* experience including placental failure and relative hypoxia either due to placental malfunction or altitude.

In this context Barker noted interesting historical patterns of disease [36]. Historically, a range of diseases could be considered diseases of affluence. Thus, ischemic heart disease, gastric ulceration, hypertension, and type 2 diabetes are all increased in societies considered more affluent and westernized. Paradoxically however, the burden of these diseases appeared to fall predominantly on the poorer members of these societies. Further, immigrants from developing to developed countries also appear to be at increased risk of these "Western" diseases. Barker noted that experiences in early life either in the context of relative poverty in Western societies or the experience of immigration into these societies were determining propensity to these diseases [36]. In particular he proposed that relative undernutrition *in utero* might be critical in determining later risk of cardiovascular disease [36]. In support of this they observed in large population series that lower birth weight was associated with later cardiovascular disease [37, 38].

Birth Weight and Type 2 Diabetes

The relation of birth weight to cardiovascular disease and hypertension has been extensively reviewed. We here concentrate on some of the evidence for associations of birth weight and type 2 diabetes. The first series suggesting an association between birth weight and type 2 diabetes was published in 1991 [39]. Hales and Barker reported an inverse association between birth weight and type 2 diabetes (Figure 1). In subsequent years this initial finding has been confirmed in several populations. A number of

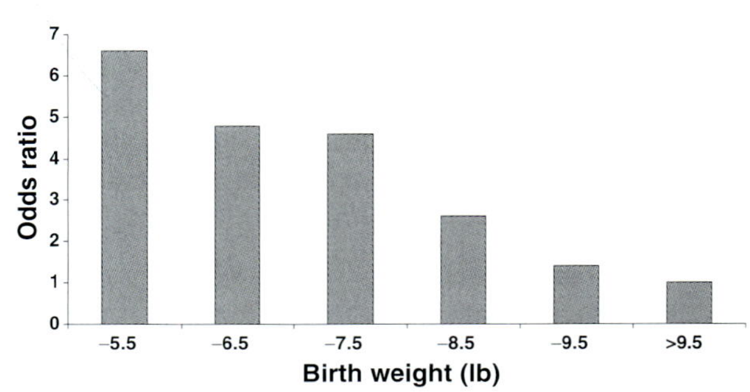

Figure 1 Odds ratio for impaired glucose tolerance or type 2 diabetes by birth weight in 370 men aged 64 years born in Hertfordshire (odds ratio adjusted for BMI). (Reproduced by permission of the British Medical Journal [39])

points are worth stressing. First, in general the influence of birth weight is striking. In the Preston study [40] the odds ratio for the risk of diabetes or impaired glucose tolerance fell from 3.5 for birth weight less than 2.5 kg to 1.0 for birth weight greater than 3.4 kg in men, and from 12.1 for birth weight less than 2.5 kg to 1.0 for birth weight greater than 3.4 kg in women. In the combined data from the Preston and Hertfordshire studies there is an even more marked effect for syndrome X (defined as 2-h plasma glucose greater than 7.8 mmol/l, fasting triglycerides greater than 1.4 mmol/l^{-1}, systolic blood pressure greater than 160 mmHg), with a fall from 22% of the population positive for syndrome X if birth weight had been less than 2.95 kg to under 2% if birth weight had been greater than 4.31 kg [41].

Second, the relation of birth weight to type 2 diabetes appears consistent. A number of later studies have followed, almost all of which have corroborated the original findings and ranging over a variety of populations and ethnic groups including those in the United Kingdom (Hertfordshire [39, 41] Preston [41, 42], Southampton [43]) as well as in the United States [44, 45], Sweden [46], and India [47]. The relation of birth weight to type 2 diabetes has also been reported in two large series, together examining over 90 000 subjects [48, 49]. While the majority of the data are in predominantly Caucasian populations, similar relationships have been observed in diverse ethnic groups including South Asians [47], Native Americans [45], African, and Jamaican populations.

While it is reassuring that the relationship of birth weight and type 2 diabetes has been found in several studies, differing in populations and age of participants, it is also possible that these studies have used a broadly similar study design, having similar inherent biases [50]. It is therefore important then that other confirmatory evidence using different designs is published. In particular, twin studies have examined birth weight in monozygotic and dizygotic twins discordant for type 2 diabetes and found that in both sets of twins birth weight was significantly lower in those with later type 2 diabetes [51]. These data further support the role of the early environment in the relation of birth weight and type 2 diabetes.

Birth Weight and Risk Phenotypes for Type 2 Diabetes

Both β-cell failure and altered insulin sensitivity are present when type 2 diabetes is clinically apparent [52] and both have been implicated as predictors of type 2 diabetes [10, 53]. It is now generally accepted that abnormalities of both insulin secretion and action are important in the pathogenesis of type 2 diabetes [54]. The role of birth weight in later development of type 2 diabetes might therefore be mediated through intermediate effects on insulin sensitivity, β-cell function, or both. It is worth noting that obesity, a further important risk factor for development of type 2 diabetes, is not an immediately obvious intermediary in the relation of birth weight and type 2 diabetes. Indeed, where sufficiently powered, studies show a *positive* relationship of birth weight and later adiposity [48].

There are few studies that have measured both insulin sensitivity and insulin secretion by accepted gold standard techniques. For assessment of insulin sensitivity in large size studies, insulin sensitivity has been assessed by indirect measures, such as fasting insulin, or derived measures from fasting glucose and insulin. Fasting insulin correlates well with such gold standard measures of insulin sensitivity as do derived measures [55]. In the main, measures of fasting insulin would support the hypothesis that low birth weight is associated with relative insulin resistance in later life [46, 56, 57]. A study of mono- and dizygotic twins has also been interpreted as favoring a role of insulin resistance as a consequence of lower birth weight [51]. Studies using other methodologies including insulin tolerance test [56] and intravenous glucose tolerance with minimal modeling [58–60] and the euglycemic hyperinsulinemic glucose clamp [61] also support the hypothesis that lower birth weight is associated with relative insulin resistance.

Lower birth weight might also act by affecting either β-cell mass or β-cell function. Notably, the technical assessment of β-cell function is less satisfactory than measures of insulin resistance. A number of dynamic measures are used that are likely to reflect different aspects of β-cell physiology without clear evidence that any single measure is superior [62, 63]. An older study suggests that low birth weight is associated with abnormalities of pancreatic β-cell development in humans [64]. More recent studies tend to be conflicting. Cook et al. suggested that lower birth weight was associated with impaired insulin secretion as estimated by the homeostatic model [65]. Similarly Crowther et al. reported decreased insulin secretion with lower birth weight in 7-year-old children [66]. By contrast, a variety of studies have reported no or even an inverse relationship of birth weight and insulin secretion in population. [56, 58, 59, 67, 68].

Taken together, the above evidence would broadly support a relationship of reduced insulin action with lower birth weight. A role of lower birth weight in association with defects in insulin secretion is as yet unclear. The simpler measures of β-cell function that have been used in many epidemiological studies correlate relatively poorly to these measures and importantly may even show similar correlation to measures of insulin sensitivity [55]. Importantly, even mild degrees of hyperglycemia appear to have secondary effects on insulin secretion, and there are clear relationships between insulin resistance and secretion [62, 63], which most studies do not take into account. It is perhaps not surprising that the relation of birth weight to β-cell function remains unclear although whether this reflects biology or simply less satisfactory physiological measures is undetermined at present.

Low or Lower? Small or Small-for-Dates?

It is worth noting two other features of the epidemiologic data relating birth weight and type 2 diabetes. Studies have varied in whether they examine birth weight as a continuous variable or by predefined criteria of "low" birth weight—generally using accepted definitions of low birth weight as <2.5 kg. Importantly, the majority of studies that have examined birth weight as a continuous rather than a dichotomous variable suggest that there is a continuous relationship of birth weight and later diabetes risk—lower birth weight increases risk even above thresholds for "low" birth weight. In keeping with this, both the causes and consequences of lower birth weight appear to extend across the spectrum of birth weight and are not confined to only low birth weight offspring [36]. Second, birth weight may be reduced secondary to either shortened gestation or restricted growth *in utero*. Not all studies were able to make this distinction as information on length of gestation at delivery was not always available. When available, data suggest that the important relationship of birth weight and type 2 diabetes arises in offspring who are small for dates (i.e. small for the expected birth dates) rather than of shortened gestation (who are small for dates rather than born prematurely) [36].

Ponderal Index and Other Anthropometric Indices at Birth

It has been suggested that patterns of fetal morphology might be of importance, potentially representing the impact of different intrauterine insults on growth patterns and later disease. For example, in the case of hypertension, patterns based on ponderal index at birth (weight/height^3—used as a measure of adiposity at birth), head and abdominal circumference as well as placental weight have been proposed as being of potential importance [36]. In the majority of studies such detailed morphological information to allow this assessment is not available. For relationships with glycemia, low ponderal index has been more strongly related than birth weight to impaired glucose tolerance in adults [42, 46, 56]. A relationship of diabetes to small head circumference relative to length has also been noted [41, 42, 46, 56]. In the main, these additional measures have not been examined in sufficient number of studies to ascertain whether these patterns will be consistent or more valuable than birth weight. They illustrate an important point, however. Given the nature of the large epidemiological series examining these questions, more information is available on birth weight than other measures. Even with adjustment for gestational age and gender, birth weight is likely a relatively crude measure of the types of programming effects *in utero*, which Hales and Barker propose. By analogy, in the Pima population, maternal diabetes results in increased birth weight and exerts an intrauterine effect to increase later risk of type 2 diabetes and obesity (discussed below). Despite this, as noted by Pettitt et al., birth weight is a relatively poor indicator of the risk conferred by being the offspring of a diabetic mother in the Pima population [69]. It is likely that lower birth weight is also acting as an equally limited indicator of the genetic and/or environmental effects that predispose to type 2 diabetes.

Birth Weight and Catch-up Growth

Previous studies have also examined the relationship of "catch-up" growth to later disease. In the case of hypertension, investigators suggested some time ago that the phenomenon of catch up might be critical rather than the original reduction in weight for hypertension [70]. Similarly there is some evidence that accelerated growth in childhood acts as a risk factor for development of type 2 diabetes. The analysis of such data is complex, and untangling the effects of reduced birth weight, increased current weight, and catch up is difficult. In particular, given that birth weight and later weight are likely to be correlated, the importance of systematically examining relationships of birth weight, current weight, and interactions between these has been stressed [71].

Examining data from the Finnish population, Barker and coworkers have suggested that accelerated weight gain in childhood [72] is particularly associated with increased risk of type 2 diabetes. They propose that it is this accelerated weight gain through childhood, with crossing of expected centile scores for age, that is critical to later development of type 2 diabetes. Interestingly in the Pima Indians, a population markedly prone to type 2 diabetes and obesity, weight gain also begins early, with increases in standard deviation (Z) scores for weight and body mass index (BMI) from 2 to 11 years [73].

Determinants of Birth Weight

Birth weight has been the subject of extensive epidemiological investigation, partly as it has proven to be a powerful predictor of perinatal mortality. The weight of the newborn might be influenced by many factors: both the products of fetal genes and the fetal environment may be of importance and the latter will in turn be determined by maternal genotype, phenotype, and influences in the maternal environment.

If one examines certain specialized situations then both environmental and genetic factors clearly have some influence. Birth weight is reduced with multiple births—an effect of the fetal environment usually attributed to the physical constraint of the uterus [74]. This is also seen in classic, often quoted, animal studies where offspring of crossbreeding between Shetland and Shire horses have a size closer to maternal than paternal size [75]. Effects of fetal genes are seen in the growth-inhibiting effects of chromosomal abnormalities [76], and of influences of the sex chromosomes: males are observed to grow faster after the 28th week and are born on average 150 g heavier [74].

In part reflecting such effects, examination of the extremes of the distribution curve for birth weight reveals a number of causes. Intrauterine growth retardation is said to affect 3–10% of all pregnancies, depending on diagnostic criteria used, arising secondary to causes such as chronic uteroplacental insufficiency, drug exposure, congenital infection, and genetic abnormalities (reviewed in reference 77). In the UK population, obstetric studies pick out maternal height, smoking in pregnancy, parity, and history of preeclampsia as the most important determinants of birth weight in surveys. While some of these factors (smoking, pre-eclampsia, congenital abnormalities) are estimated to account for up to 60% of the occurrence of very low birth weight (below 2 standard deviations) [78], their influence on weight away from the extreme appears to be less marked.

There is a strong familial aggregation of birth weight [79]. Studies examining the importance of the genetic and environmental influences on birth weight across the whole population vary widely in their estimation [80–86] but in the main favor a low influence of the fetal genotype [80, 84–86] and stress the importance of environmental factors derived from the mother [80, 85, 86]. It should be pointed out that all such studies are poor at picking out environmental factors, which might be shared across generations, from genetic factors [82] and as such will tend to underestimate environmental factors. Further caution is necessary as the relative influences of genetic and environmental factors may differ depending on the population studied. There is a large international variation in birth weight, with frequency of births weighing less than 2500 g varying between 3 and 43% in different populations [87], with undoubted effects of poverty and undernutrition at the extremes of these figures [87].

While bearing these caveats in mind, in Western populations, factors such as parity, pre-pregnancy weight, weight gain in pregnancy, maternal and paternal birth weights, maternal smoking, and fetal gender are all associated with birth weight but account for only 10–20% of the variance [82, 84], with gestational age accounting for a further 10% [84]. Even in those studies that add measures of maternal glycemia, only 30% of the total variance in birth weight is accounted for [88]. The available data then would leave much of the variance of birth weight unexplained.

It is also possible that the association of lower birth weight and metabolic disease is not cause-specific—that any growth-restraining insult might result in later risk, perhaps as has been proposed for high blood pressure, as a result of catch-up growth [70]. This, however, does not seem to be the case. When one considers twin births, the physical restraints of the uterus result in a reduction in birth weight [74] but this does not seem to be reflected in a later increase in cardiovascular mortality compared to the singleton population [89]. Similarly, maternal smoking, which reduces birth weight [82, 84], is not associated with an increase in type 2 diabetes.

The Thrifty Phenotype: Environmental Influences on Later Type 2 Diabetes

Environmental Factors in Early Life and Later Disease Before the Thrifty Phenotype

The basic concept advanced by the thrifty phenotype hypothesis is that human disease may arise because of early environmental effects whose influence to cause disease is expressed only much later in life. Thus the influences of the environmental exposure are not confined to the time frame in which they are experienced but may continue to act throughout the life of the organism and long after an adverse exposure has ended. As a further refinement of this hypothesis it is proposed that certain key developmental windows exist during which exposures "set" physiological systems and thus lead to long-term consequences. This concept has been termed environmental programming [90].

When the thrifty phenotype hypothesis was proposed, this concept was not new to the field of metabolic disease in humans. The importance of the early environment had already been invoked as an explanation of increased propensity to diabetes in offspring of diabetic mothers, a very different early nutritional model to that proposed in the thrifty phenotype hypothesis. As early as 1960, White made fundamental observations regarding the high prevalence of abnormal glucose tolerance in offspring of diabetic mothers [91]. Around the same time, Pedersen developed the hypothesis that early *over*exposure to glucose *in utero* resulted in organomegaly and excessive growth that might then predispose to subsequent diabetes [92]. Freinkel then extended this hypothesis to propose that overexposure to a range of intermediary metabolites, most importantly glucose and amino acids, might act in the long term to alter metabolism and lead to human disease [5], a concept he termed fuel-mediated teratogenesis [5]. Pettitt and coworkers subsequently showed that both obesity [93] and type 2 diabetes [94] were more prevalent in the offspring of mothers who had diabetes during pregnancy, suggesting that predisposition to these conditions had arisen as a consequence of the intrauterine environment. Similar findings have been reported in the US Nurse's Study [49].

In the field of obesity it had already been proposed that influences in early life might be important. In 1972 Brook proposed that obesity might be influenced by events *in utero* [95], following the concept of the time that adipocyte differentiation occurred primarily in the intrauterine period. Ravelli et al. explored the influence of early undernutrition, due to exposure to wartime famine, on later predisposition to obesity, finding that exposure to famine early in intrauterine life was associated with an increase in later obesity [96].

A variety of observations and hypotheses regarding long-term influences of hormonal exposure to endocrine axes had also been established in experimental animals. The best known of these is the example of plasticity in the hypothalamic–pituitary–gonadal axis. Since the 1960s it had been recognized that there is a "window" in the first 10 days of life in which exposure of a newborn female rat to a single pulse of testosterone leads to reduced fertility in adult life [97]. This arises because androgen exposure or nonexposure at this stage of development permanently alters hypothalamic responses to a male or female pattern respectively [97, 98], a phenomenon the authors also termed imprinting.

The thrifty phenotype hypothesis has also been important in stimulating later hypotheses addressing how the environment in early life might act to influence later disease. The presence or absence of breastfeeding in early life has been proposed to influence later development and predisposition to disease. Pettitt et al. observed that breastfeeding in the first 2 months of life was associated with a lower risk of development of type 2 diabetes in the Pima population [99]. Such a protective effect of breastfeeding has also been observed for childhood obesity [100].

Undernutrition and Later Type 2 Diabetes

The concept that birth weight is associated with later type 2 diabetes has been debated and is subject to a number of explanations. The thrifty phenotype hypothesis proposes that nutrition *in utero* is critical in this relationship [3]. As detailed below, explanations based on genetic effects have also been proposed [4]. Others have suggested that early environmental insults other than nutrition *in utero*, for example by exposure to glucocorticoids, might be important [101–103].

What is the evidence that nutrition *in utero* influences later metabolic disease? The role of nutrition in altering pancreatic insulin secretion and insulin resistance had been addressed by a large number of studies in animal models. Broadly, two major paradigms have been followed, hypothesizing that either protein and calorie undernutrition or isolated protein deficiency will be critical. It is clear that in the extreme either manipulation may result in decreases in birth weight. Interestingly however, more subtle manipulations may provoke surprising results. For example it is a well-established practice in animal husbandry to expose sheep to poor pasture in mid-gestation, with resulting *increases* in the size of the lambs [104]. Classic studies of McCance and Widdowson displayed that caloric deprivation in early life can reduce birth weight and produce permanent alterations in body composition at least in terms of relative organ weights [105], with the effects of such under nutrition appearing to be less reversible the earlier they occur in life [105]. Animal models also suggest that the pancreas is sensitive particularly to protein malnutrition in development and that the effects of this under nutrition vary depending on the timing of restriction. Malnourishment of dams results in lower offspring birth weight [106] along with impaired development of the fetal endocrine pancreas [106]. Protein malnutrition during pregnancy alone [107], and in the first postnatal weeks of life alone [108, 109], has also been shown to result in permanent deficits in insulin secretion in such animal models. Protein malnutrition during pregnancy and up to weaning has been associated with evidence of muscle insulin resistance in the absence of insulin secretory defects [110].

In humans previous under-nutrition, although not necessarily occurring *in utero*, had also been proposed as an important factor in the development of diabetes. In the 1950s workers in the tropics described tropical or type J diabetes [111]. Such patients had a mixture of the features of type 1 and type 2 diabetes. The disease developed at a young age, patients were insulin requiring but not insulin dependent, being resistant to ketoacidosis after insulin withdrawal, and in all cases previous malnutrition was involved [111]. Insulin secretory responses were found to be acutely reduced by severe malnutrition in childhood [112] and the study of some populations who had been exposed to severe childhood under-nutrition supported a continued effect on glucose tolerance [113] and on the incidence of type 2 diabetes [114]. The observation that Ethiopian Jews migrating after famine from Ethiopia to Israel experienced a 9% rate of diabetes in those younger than 30 within 4 years of migration, was also taken to support an important role for prior under-nutrition in development of type 2 diabetes [114]. Clearly dissecting the effects of undernutrition from preexisting genetic risks in a population experiencing a large change in adult environment is difficult. In recent years the place of malnutrition as an etiological factor in tropical diabetes has also weakened however, with evidence of tropical diabetes in individuals never exposed to malnutrition and low rates of such diabetes in previously malnourished African populations [115] (and reviewed in reference 116). Malnutrition may, however, play a role as a contributory factor in some individuals [116].

More recently, the influences of nutrition *in utero* on birth weight and metabolic outcomes have also been examined in human populations. Again the timing and nature of altered nutrition may be critical. For example, Godfrey et al. reported that *higher* carbohydrate intake in early pregnancy and *lower* protein intake in late pregnancy were associated with lower birth weights [117]. The long-term effects of undernutrition have been examined in two human populations exposed to severe wartime famine. Children born during famine in Holland during World War II (survivors of "the Dutch Hunger Winter") were found to have significantly higher 2-h plasma glucose concentrations [96]. By contrast, children whose mothers survived the siege of Leningrad appeared to have no long-term effect on blood glucose, although the authors comment on the difficulty of ascertaining the extent of exposure to famine in this group, especially when pregnant women may have had preferential access to food [118]. While the observations in the Dutch population would support the hypothesis that under-nutrition during pregnancy can lead to metabolic consequences, the second raises doubts as to whether such effects may only be exerted in the most extreme circumstances, making under-nutrition unlikely to be instrumental in the etiology of most cases of type 2 diabetes. It has been argued that characteristics of the histories of these two populations might explain the differing results. In particular, exposure to famine in the Dutch Hunger Winter was of relatively sudden onset and adequate nutrition was restored soon thereafter. By contrast, the siege of Leningrad resulted in famine over a longer historical period, without a return to adequate nutrition for some years after the "end" of the famine. If the later metabolic effects of lower birth weight are dependent on the presence of accelerated growth during childhood years, as proposed by Barker, then this is one potential explanation of the discrepant findings.

The population exposed to the Dutch Hunger Winter has also been examined with relation to later obesity. In 1976 Ravelli et al. reported an increase in obesity in those individuals who were as children exposed to famine in the first two trimesters of pregnancy, whereas exposure to famine in the last trimester and the first 3–5 months postnatally resulted in a reduction in the frequency of obesity [96]. They concluded that factors in early life affect adiposity later in life, a hypothesis previously proposed, with some experimental evidence, by Brook [95]. In examining the relationship of this data to the birth weight and thrifty phenotype hypotheses it is interesting to consider the birth weights of these cohorts. The group exposed to famine in the first two trimesters in the original study had no reduction in birth weight but did have an increase in later obesity [96]. In contrast, the group with exposure to famine in the last trimester and the first 3–5 months postnatally suffered both a reduction in birth weight and a *reduction* in later obesity. Interestingly, higher 2-h glucose concentrations were described in association both with lower birth weight and in those exposed to famine late in gestation. In all, these data can be used to support the contention that maternal under-nutrition might influence later obesity and predisposition to type 2 diabetes. These effects appear to be taking part at different times in pregnancy and associations with lower birth weight are found only in the case of the relations with blood glucose.

Genes, birth weight and type 2 diabetes

As detailed, the evidence for the thrifty phenotype rests upon the observation of associations of later human disease and lower birth weight. More recently, others have explored whether that association might arise not because of environmental insults *in utero*, but because of a genetic connection between lower birth weight and later diabetes [4]. Maturity-onset diabetes of the young (MODY) was originally described as a syndrome of early-onset non-insulin-dependent diabetes, with clinical features more typical of type 2 than type 1 diabetes and with an autosomal dominant pattern of inheritance [119]. It is now known that MODY is caused by a range of genetic mutations [120]. Hattersley and coworkers demonstrated that one of the causes of MODY—mutation of the glucokinase gene—when present in the fetus is also associated with lower birth weight as well as later diabetes [121]. While the frequency of this mutation is too low to explain the associations seen in the populations described by Barker and Hales, it does demonstrate the potential for genetic mechanisms to underpin associations of birth weight and later disease. Insulin is a major promoter of growth *in utero* [4]. Consequently, genes that affect either insulin secretion or insulin resistance might well influence both fetal growth and subsequently development of diabetes [4]. Indeed, disruption of a variety of genes involved in insulin secretion or signaling, such as insulin receptor substrate 2 (IRS-2), is known in animal models to result in alteration of fetal growth [122]. Does variation in such genes result in alteration of birth weight in human populations? At present the evidence is limited, although in a single study common variants of several candidates genes did not appear to influence birth weight [123].

The Pima population of Arizona have an extremely high prevalence of obesity and type 2 diabetes, an increase that is believed to reflect both current environmental influences (such as reduced levels of exercise and inappropriately high caloric intake) as well as genetic predisposition to both type 2 diabetes and obesity. As described previously, both low and high birth weight are associated with an increased risk of type 2 diabetes in Pima Indians (Figure 2) [45]. Higher birth weight principally reflects influences of maternal diabetes in pregnancy both to increase birth weight and to increase likelihood of type 2 diabetes in later life [69]. More recently relationships of parental diabetes to low birth weight have been examined. If the association between low birth weight and later diabetes is due to genetic effects, then the parents of low birth weight offspring should themselves be at a greater risk of diabetes [124]. Conversely, the absence of such effects would be more consistent with the notion that early environmental

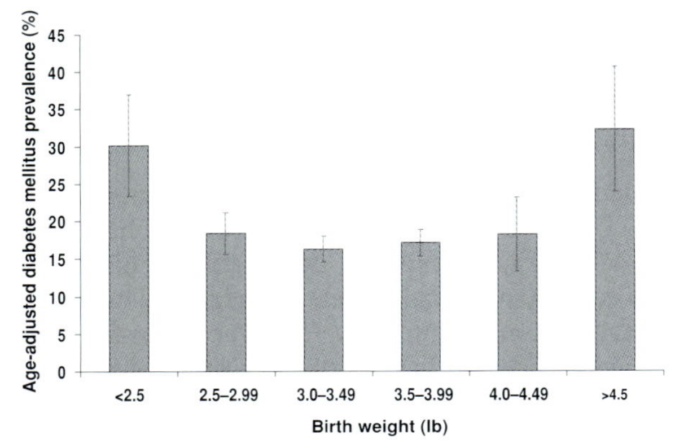

Figure 2 The relation of birth weight and later prevalence of type 2 diabetes in the Pima population. Prevalence of type 2 diabetes is adjusted for age using the direct method using the age distribution of 1179 subjects, and presented as mean and 68% confidence intervals. (Reproduced by permission of the British Medical Journal [45])

influences are a cause of diabetes in these lower birth weight offspring. In the Pima, lower birth weight is indeed associated with parental diabetes, but in fact solely with diabetes in fathers (Figure 3). Furthermore, the ability of low birth weight to predict later diabetes in offspring appears to depend on the presence of diabetes in fathers [124]. These observations appear to strengthen the case for a genetic link between low birth weight and type 2 diabetes. The particular association with paternal diabetes has also led to consideration of whether genomic imprinting—differential expression of genes depending on parent of origin—might be a determining factor in the low birth weight/diabetes relationship [124]. Imprinting is known to act in syndromic causes of obesity and diabetes, such as Prader-Willi syndrome and transient neonatal diabetes mellitus (OMIM 610410). Intriguingly, the majority of currently recognized imprinted genes appear to influence pathways involving fetal growth or placental development [125, 126]. If low birth weight is associated with type 2 diabetes secondary to genetic influences, might this arise through actions of imprinted genes on both fetal growth and glucose homeostasis? In support of this, type 2 diabetes has been associated with a genetic polymorphism on chromosome 11p found close to the insulin gene (*INS* VNTR III), but only if the associated allele was transmitted from the father [127]. The authors concluded that an imprinted gene in this region might increase the risk of type 2 diabetes [127].

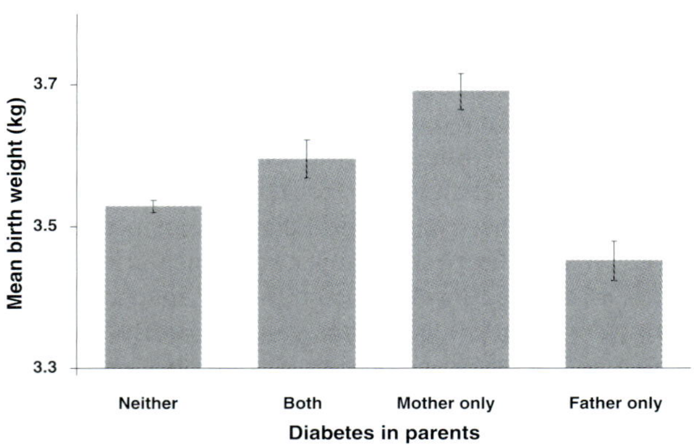

Figure 3 Mean birth weight of children divided by last known diabetes status of their parent. Groups: Neither = neither parent ever diagnosed with diabetes; Both = both parents diagnosed with diabetes; Mother only and Father only = mother or father diabetic, respectively, second parent nondiabetic. Values are expressed as mean ± SEM. General linear model consistent with a significant effect of parental diabetes diagnosis on birth weight ($P < 0.001$) and independent effects of both maternal (*post hoc* Student Newman-Keuls: $P < 0.0001$) and paternal (Student Newman-Keuls: $P < 0.001$) diabetes status (redrawn with permission from reference 124)

The role of genes and environment in determining associations of low birth weight with later disease is by no means settled. The strictly genetic interpretation is challenged by twin studies of Poulsen et al. who have demonstrated that in identical twins the smaller twin is more likely to develop type 2 diabetes [128]. Given that identical twins share all of their genes, the authors interpret this as evidence that an environmental effect acting on the smaller twin is increasing risk of metabolic disease, lending support to the environmental hypothesis of Hales and Barker. On the other hand a recent report of a considerably larger series of monozygotic twins (together with a contemporary series of dizygotic twins) failed to find any relationship between birth weight and either blood pressure or glucose intolerance among the twin pairs [129]. This report casts doubt on the hypothesis that environmental effects on intra-uterine growth *per se* are important determinants of low birth weight/blood pressure and low birth weight/glucose intolerance relationships.

CONCLUSIONS

So is type 2 diabetes the result of a thrifty genotype or a thrifty phenotype? At time of writing the question remains unresolved. The thrifty gene or genes have not been identified and the role of long-term programming of disease by under-nutrition in human populations remains controversial. Somewhat paradoxically, one can trace a path from Neel's suggestion of a genetic explanation for associations of diabetes and *increased* early growth via the entirely environmental explanations of the thrifty phenotype to the fetal insulin hypothesis—the suggestion that *lower* birth weight and type 2 diabetes are connected by genetic effects. There can be no doubt, however, that these hypotheses have been enormously influential in stimulating progress in our understanding of type 2 diabetes. It seems likely that when we understand the cause of type 2 diabetes both the thrifty genotype and the thrifty phenotype will be proven at least partially correct. The cause of type 2 diabetes will be multifactorial and roles for physiological adaptation of individuals and genetic adaptation of populations to adverse environments will be found to account in part for the current high prevalence of the disease. Finally, both hypotheses hold a further promise for the future—that by understanding type 2 diabetes we will not only help to prevent and cure this destructive disease but we will also shed light on pathways critical to human growth, development, and survival.

REFERENCES

1. Amos AF, McCarty DJ, Zimmet P. The rising global burden of diabetes and its complications: estimates and projections to the year 2010. *Diabet Med* 1997; 14 (suppl 5): S1–85.
2. Neel JV. Diabetes mellitus: a thrifty genotype rendered detrimental by "progress". *Am J Hum Genet* 1962; 14: 353–62.
3. Hales CN, Barker DJ. Type 2 (non-insulin-dependent) diabetes mellitus: the thrifty phenotype hypothesis. *Diabetologia* 1992; 35: 595–601.
4. Hattersley AT, Tooke JE. The fetal insulin hypothesis: an alternative explanation of the association of low birthweight with diabetes and vascular disease. *Lancet* 1999; 353: 1789–92.
5. Freinkel N. Banting Lecture 1980. Of pregnancy and progeny. *Diabetes* 1980; 29: 1023–35.
6. Neel JV. The "thrifty genotype" in 1998. *Nutr Rev* 1999; 57: S2–S9.
7. Friedman JM, Halaas JL. Leptin and the regulation of body weight in mammals. *Nature* 1998; 395: 763–70.
8. Owen OE, Felig P, Morgan AP, Wahren J, Cahill GF Jr. Liver and kidney metabolism during prolonged starvation. *J Clin Invest* 1969; 48: 574–83.
9. Reaven GM. Hypothesis: muscle insulin resistance is the ("not-so") thrifty genotype. *Diabetologia* 1998; 41: 482–4.
10. Lillioja S, Mott DM, Spraul M, Ferraro R, Foley JE, Ravussin E, Knowler WC, Bennett PH, Bogardus C. Insulin resistance and insulin secretory dysfunction as precursors of non-insulin-dependent diabetes mellitus. Prospective studies of Pima Indians. *N Engl J Med* 1993; 329: 1988–92.
11. Pickup JC, Crook MA. Is type II diabetes mellitus a disease of the innate immune system? *Diabetologia* 1998; 41: 1241–8.
12. Fernandez-Real JM, Ricart W. Insulin resistance and inflammation in an evolutionary perspective: the contribution of cytokine genotype/phenotype to thriftiness. *Diabetologia* 1999; 42: 1367–74.
13. Festa A, D'Agostino RB, Tracy RP, Haffner SM. Elevated levels of acute phase proteins and plasminogen activator inhibitor-1 (PAI-1) predict the development of type 2 diabetes mellitus: the Inslin Resistance Atherosclerosis Study (IRAS). *Diabetes* 2002; 51: 1131–7.
14. Lindsay RS, Krakoff J, Hanson RL, Bennett PH, Knowler WC. Gamma globulin levels predict type 2 diabetes in the Pima Indian population. *Diabetes* 2001; 50: 1598–603.
15. Pradhan AD, Manson JE, Rifai N, Buring JE, Ridker PM. C-reactive protein, interleukin 6, and risk of developing type 2 diabetes mellitus. *JAMA* 2001; 286: 327–34.
16. Ford ES. Leukocyte count, erythrocyte sedimentation rate, and diabetes incidence in a national sample of US adults. *Am J Epidemiol* 2002; 155: 57–64.
17. Vozarova B, Weyer C, Lindsay RS, Pratley RE, Bogardus C, Tataranni PA. High white blood cell count is associated with a worsening of insulin sensitivity and predicts the development of type 2 diabetes. *Diabetes* 2002; 51: 455–61.
18. Fernandez-Real JM, Broch M, Vendrell J, Gutierrez C, Casamitjana R, Pugeat M, Richart C, Ricart W. Interleukin-6 gene polymorphism and insulin sensitivity. *Diabetes* 2000; 49: 517–20.
19. Knowler WC, Pettitt DJ, Saad MF, Bennett PH. Diabetes mellitus in the Pima Indians: incidence, risk factors and pathogenesis. *Diabetes Metab Rev* 1990; 6: 1–27.
20. Cordain L, Miller J, Mann N. Scant evidence of periodic starvation among hunter-gatherers. *Diabetologia* 1999; 42: 383–4.
21. McNeill W. *Plagues and Peoples*. Garden City, NY: Doubleday, 1976.
22. Dobyns H. *Their Numbers Became Thinned*. Knoxville: University of Tennessee Press, 1983.
23. Montague CT, Farooqi IS, Whitehead JP, Soos MA, Rau H, Wareham NJ, Sewter CP, Digby JE, Mohammed SN, Hurst JA, Cheetham CH, Earley AR, Barnett AH, Prins JB, O'Rahilly S. Congenital leptin deficiency is associated with severe early-onset obesity in humans. *Nature* 1997; 387: 903–8.
24. Coleman DL. Obesity genes: beneficial effects in heterozygous mice. *Science* 1979; 203: 663–5.
25. Li WD, Reed DR, Lee JH, Xu W, Kilker RL, Sodam BR, Price RA. Sequence variants in the 5′ flanking region of the leptin gene are associated with obesity in women. *Ann Hum Genet* 1999; 63: 227–34.
26. Hager J, Clement K, Francke S, Dina C, Raison J, Lahlou N, Rich N, Pelloux V, Basdevant A, Guy-Grand B, North M, Froguel P. A polymorphism in the 5′ untranslated region of the human ob gene is associated with low leptin levels. *Int J Obes Relat Metab Disord* 1998; 22: 200–5.
27. Mammes O, Betoulle D, Aubert R, Herbeth B, Siest G, Fumeron F. Association of the G-2548A polymorphism in the 5′ region of the LEP gene with overweight. *Ann Hum Genet* 2000; 64: 391–4.
28. Mammes O, Betoulle D, Aubert R, Giraud V, Tuzet S, Petiet A, Colas-Linhart N, Fumeron F. Novel polymorphisms in the 5′ region of the LEP gene: association with leptin levels and response to low-calorie diet in human obesity. *Diabetes* 1998; 47: 487–9.
29. Heo M, Leibel RL, Boyer BB, Chung WK, Koulu M, Karvonen MK, Pesonen U, Rissanen A, Laakso M, Uusitupa MI, Chagnon Y, Bouchard C, Donohoue PA, Burns TL, Shuldiner AR, Silver K, Anderson RE, Pedersen O, Echwald S, Sorensen TI, Behn P, Permutt MA, Jacobs KB, Elston RC, Hoffman DJ, Allison DB. Pooling analysis of genetic data: the association of leptin receptor (LEPR) polymorphisms with variables related to human adiposity. *Genetics* 2001; 159: 1163–78.
30. Krude H, Biebermann H, Luck W, Horn R, Brabant G, Gruters A. Severe early-onset obesity, adrenal insufficiency and red hair pigmentation caused by POMC mutations in humans. *Nat Genet* 1998; 19: 155–7.
31. Farooqi IS, Yeo GS, Keogh JM, Aminian S, Jebb SA, Butler G, Cheetham T, O'Rahilly S. Dominant and recessive inheritance of morbid obesity associated with

melanocortin 4 receptor deficiency. *J Clin Invest* 2000; 106: 271–9.
32. Vaisse C, Clement K, Durand E, Hercberg S, Guy-Grand B, Froguel P. Melanocortin-4 receptor mutations are a frequent and heterogeneous cause of morbid obesity. *J Clin Invest* 2000; 106: 253–62.
33. Norman RA, Permana P, Tanizawa Y, Ravussin E. Absence of genetic variation in some obesity candidate genes (GLP1R, ASIP, MC4R, MC5R) among Pima indians. *Int J Obes Relat Metab Disord* 1999; 23: 163–5.
34. Ravussin E, Lillioja S, Knowler WC, Christin L, Freymond D, Abbott WG, Boyce V, Howard BV, Bogardus C. Reduced rate of energy expenditure as a risk factor for body-weight gain. *N Engl J Med* 1988; 318: 467–72.
35. Groop L, Orho-Melander M. The dysmetabolic syndrome. *J Intern Med* 2001; 250: 105–20.
36. Barker DJ. *Fetal and Infant Origins of Adult Disease*. London: British Medical Journal, 1992.
37. Barker DJ, Osmond C, Golding J, Kuh D, Wadsworth ME. Growth in utero, blood pressure in childhood and adult life, and mortality from cardiovascular disease. *BMJ* 1989; 298: 564–7.
38. Osmond C, Barker DJ, Winter PD, Fall CH, Simmonds SJ. Early growth and death from cardiovascular disease in women. *BMJ* 1993; 307: 1519–24.
39. Hales CN, Barker DJ, Clark PM, Cox LJ, Fall C, Osmond C, Winter PD. Fetal and infant growth and impaired glucose tolerance at age 64. *BMJ* 1991; 303: 1019–22.
40. Phipps K, Barker DJ, Hales CN, Fall CH, Osmond C, Clark PM. Fetal growth and impaired glucose tolerance in men and women. *Diabetologia* 1993; 36: 225–8.
41. Barker DJ, Hales CN, Fall CH, Osmond C, Phipps K, Clark PM. Type 2 (non-insulin-dependent) diabetes mellitus, hypertension and hyperlipidaemia (syndrome X): relation to reduced fetal growth. *Diabetologia* 1993; 36: 62–7.
42. Phipps K, Barker DJ, Hales CN, Fall CH, Osmond C, Clark PM. Fetal growth and impaired glucose tolerance in men and women. *Diabetologia* 1993; 36: 225–8.
43. Robinson S, Walton RJ, Clark PM, Barker DJ, Hales CN, Osmond C. The relation of fetal growth to plasma glucose in young men. *Diabetologia* 1992; 35: 444–6.
44. Valdez R, Athens MA, Thompson GH, Bradshaw BS, Stern MP. Birthweight and adult health outcomes in a biethnic population in the USA. *Diabetologia* 1994; 37: 624–31.
45. McCance DR, Pettitt DJ, Hanson RL, Jacobsson LT, Knowler WC, Bennett PH. Birth weight and non-insulin dependent diabetes: thrifty genotype, thrifty phenotype, or surviving small baby genotype? *BMJ* 1994; 308: 942–5.
46. Lithell HO, McKeigue PM, Berglund L, Mohsen R, Lithell UB, Leon DA. Relation of size at birth to non-insulin dependent diabetes and insulin concentrations in men aged 50–60 years. *BMJ* 1996; 312: 406–10.
47. Yajnik CS, Fall CH, Vaidya U, Pandit AN, Bavdekar A, Bhat DS, Osmond C, Hales CN, Barker DJ. Fetal growth and glucose and insulin metabolism in four-year-old Indian children. *Diabet Med* 1995; 12: 330–6.
48. Curhan GC, Willett WC, Rimm EB, Spiegelman D, Ascherio AL, Stampfer MJ. Birth weight and adult hypertension, diabetes mellitus, and obesity in US men. *Circulation* 1996; 94: 3246–50.
49. Rich-Edwards JW, Colditz GA, Stampfer MJ, Willett WC, Gillman MW, Hennekens CH, Speizer FE, Manson JE. Birthweight and the risk for type 2 diabetes mellitus in adult women. *Ann Intern Med* 1999; 130: 278–84.
50. Kramer MS, Joseph KS. Enigma of fetal/infant-origins hypothesis. *Lancet* 1996; 348: 1254–5.
51. Poulsen P, Vaag AA, Kyvik KO, Moller JD, Beck-Nielsen H. Low birth weight is associated with NIDDM in discordant monozygotic and dizygotic twin pairs. *Diabetologia* 1997; 40: 439–46.
52. Cahill GF Jr. Beta-cell deficiency, insulin resistance, or both? *N Engl J Med* 1988; 318: 1268–70.
53. Skarfors ET, Selinus KI, Lithell HO. Risk factors for developing non-insulin dependent diabetes: a 10 year follow up of men in Uppsala. *BMJ* 1991; 303: 755–60.
54. DeFronzo RA, Bonadonna RC, Ferrannini E. Pathogenesis of NIDDM. A balanced overview. *Diabetes Care* 1992; 15: 318–68.
55. Hanson RL, Pratley RE, Bogardus C, Narayan KM, Roumain JM, Imperatore G, Fagot-Campagna A, Pettitt DJ, Bennett PH, Knowler WC. Evaluation of simple indices of insulin sensitivity and insulin secretion for use in epidemiologic studies. *Am J Epidemiol* 2000; 151: 190–8.
56. Phillips DI, Barker DJ, Hales CN, Hirst S, Osmond C. Thinness at birth and insulin resistance in adult life. *Diabetologia* 1994; 37: 150–4.
57. Dabelea D, Pettitt DJ, Hanson RL, Imperatore G, Bennett PH, Knowler WC. Birth weight, type 2 diabetes, and insulin resistance in Pima Indian children and young adults. *Diabetes Care* 1999; 22: 944–50.
58. Clausen JO, Borch-Johnsen K, Pedersen O. Relation between birth weight and the insulin sensitivity index in a population sample of 331 young, healthy Caucasians. *Am J Epidemiol* 1997; 146: 23–31.
59. Flanagan DE, Moore VM, Godsland IF, Cockington RA, Robinson JS, Phillips DI. Fetal growth and the physiological control of glucose tolerance in adults: a minimal model analysis. *Am J Physiol Endocrinol Metab* 2000; 278: E700–E706.
60. Hofman PL, Cutfield WS, Robinson EM, Bergman RN, Menon RK, Sperling MA, Gluckman PD. Insulin resistance in short children with intrauterine growth retardation. *J Clin Endocrinol Metab* 1997; 82: 402–6.
61. McKeigue PM, Lithell HO, Leon DA. Glucose tolerance and resistance to insulin-stimulated glucose uptake in men aged 70 years in relation to size at birth. *Diabetologia* 1998; 41: 1133–8.
62. Ferrannini E. Insulin resistance versus insulin deficiency in non-insulin-dependent diabetes mellitus: problems and prospects. *Endocr Rev* 1998; 19: 477–90.
63. Pratley RE, Weyer C. The role of impaired early insulin secretion in the pathogenesis of Type II diabetes mellitus. *Diabetologia* 2001; 44: 929–45.
64. Van Assche FA, De Prins F, Aerts L, Verjans M. The endocrine pancreas in small-for-dates infants. *Br J Obstet Gynaecol* 1977; 84: 751–3.
65. Cook JT, Levy JC, Page RC, Shaw JA, Hattersley AT, Turner RC. Association of low birth weight with beta cell function in the adult first degree relatives of non-insulin dependent diabetic subjects. *BMJ* 1993; 306: 302–6.
66. Crowther NJ, Trusler J, Cameron N, Toman M, Gray IP. Relation between weight gain and beta-cell secretory activity and non-esterified fatty acid production in 7-year-old African children: results from the Birth to Ten study. *Diabetologia* 2000; 43: 978–85.

67. Alvarsson M, Efendic S, Grill VE. Insulin responses to glucose in healthy males are associated with adult height but not with birth weight. *J Intern Med* 1994; 236: 275–9.
68. Wills J, Watson JM, Hales CN, Phillips DI. The relation of fetal growth to insulin secretion in young men. *Diabet Med* 1996; 13: 773–4.
69. Pettitt DJ, Knowler WC, Bennett PH, Aleck KA, Baird HR. Obesity in offspring of diabetic Pima Indian women despite normal birth weight. *Diabetes Care* 1987; 10: 76–80.
70. Lever AF, Harrap SB. Essential hypertension: a disorder of growth with origins in childhood? *J Hypertens* 1992; 10: 101–20.
71. Lucas A, Fewtrell MS, Cole TJ. Fetal origins of adult disease-the hypothesis revisited. *BMJ* 1999; 319: 245–9.
72. Forsen T, Eriksson J, Tuomilheto J, Reunanen A, Osmond C, Barker D. The fetal and childhood growth of persons who develop type 2 diabetes. *Ann Intern Med* 2000; 133: 176–82.
73. Lindsay RS, Cook V, Hanson RL, Salbe AD, Tataranni A, Knowler WC. Early excess weight gain of children in the Pima Indian population. *Pediatrics* 2002; 109: E33.
74. Kline J, Stein ZA, Susser M. *Conception to Birth: Epidemiology of Prenatal Development*. New York: Oxford University Press, 1989.
75. Walton A, Hammond J. The maternal effects on growth and conformation in Shire-Shetland Crosses. *Proc R Soc Ser B* 1938; 125: 311–35.
76. Ratcliffe SG. The effect of chromosome abnormalities on growth. *Br Med Bull* 1981; 37: 291–5.
77. Seeds JW. Impaired fetal growth: definition and clinical diagnosis. *Obstet Gynecol* 1984; 64: 303–10.
78. Ounsted M, Moar VA, Scott A. Risk factors associated with small-for-dates and large-for-dates infants. *Br J Obstet Gynaecol* 1985; 92: 226–32.
79. Wang X, Zuckerman B, Coffman GA, Corwin MJ. Familial aggregation of low birth weight among whites and blacks in the United States. *N Engl J Med* 1995; 333: 1744–9.
80. Morton NE. The inheritance of human birth weight. *Ann Hum Genet* 1955; 20: 125–34.
81. Robson EB. Birth weight in cousins. *Ann Hum Genet* 1955; 19: 262–8.
82. Magnus P, Berg K, Bjerkedal T, Nance WE. Parental determinants of birth weight. *Clin Genet* 1984; 26: 397–405.
83. Magnus P. Further evidence for a significant effect of fetal genes on variation in birth weight. *Clin Genet* 1984; 26: 289–96.
84. Langhoff-Roos J, Lindmark G, Gustavson KH, Gebre-Medhin M, Meirik O. Relative effect of parental birth weight on infant birth weight at term. *Clin Genet* 1987; 32: 240–8.
85. Carr-Hill R, Campbell DM, Hall MH, Meredith A. Is birth weight determined genetically? *Br Med J* 1987; 295: 687–9.
86. Brooks AA, Johnson MR, Steer PJ, Pawson ME, Abdalla HI. Birth weight: nature or nurture? *Early Hum Dev* 1995; 42: 29–35.
87. Villar J, Belizan JM. The relative contribution of prematurity and fetal growth retardation to low birth weight in developing and developed societies. *Am J Obstet Gynecol* 1982; 143: 793–8.
88. Breschi MC, Seghieri G, Bartolomei G, Gironi A, Baldi S, Ferrannini E. Relation of birthweight to maternal plasma glucose and insulin concentrations during normal pregnancy. *Diabetologia* 1993; 36: 1315–21.
89. Christensen K, Vaupel JW, Holm NV, Yashin AI. Mortality among twins after age 6: fetal origins hypothesis versus twin method. *BMJ* 1995; 310: 432–6.
90. Lucas A. Programming by early nutrition in man. In Bock G, Whelan J (eds). *The Childhood Environment and Adult Disease*, Chichester, UK: Wiley, 1991; pp 38–55.
91. White PW. Childhood diabetes: its course and influence in the second and third generations. *Diabetes* 1960; 9: 345–55.
92. Pedersen J. Weight and length at birth in infants of diabetic mothers. *Acta Endocrinol* 1954; 16: 330–42.
93. Pettitt DJ, Baird HR, Aleck KA, Bennett PH, Knowler WC. Excessive obesity in offspring of Pima Indian women with diabetes during pregnancy. *N Engl J Med* 1983; 308: 242–5.
94. Pettitt DJ, Aleck KA, Baird HR, Carraher MJ, Bennett PH, Knowler WC. Congenital susceptibility to NIDDM. Role of intrauterine environment. *Diabetes* 1988; 37: 622–8.
95. Brook CG. Evidence for a sensitive period in adipose-cell replication in man. *Lancet* 1972; 2: 624–7.
96. Ravelli GP, Stein ZA, Susser MW. Obesity in young men after famine exposure in utero and early infancy. *N Engl J Med* 1976; 295: 349–53.
97. Gorski RA, Barraclough CA. Effects of low dosages of androgens on the differentiation of hypothalamic regulatory control of ovulation in the rat. *Endocrinology* 1963; 73: 210–6.
98. Harris G. Sex hormones, brain development and brain function. *Endocrinology* 1964; 75: 627–48.
99. Pettitt DJ, Forman MR, Hanson RL, Knowler WC, Bennett PH. Breastfeeding and incidence of non-insulin-dependent diabetes mellitus in Pima Indians. *Lancet* 1997; 350: 166–8.
100. von Kries R, Koletzko B, Sauerwald T, von Mutius E, Barnert D, Grunert V, von Voss H. Breast feeding and obesity: cross sectional study. *BMJ* 1999; 319: 147–50.
101. Benediktsson R, Lindsay RS, Noble J, Seckl JR, Edwards CR. Glucocorticoid exposure in utero: new model for adult hypertension. *Lancet* 1993; 341: 339–41.
102. Edwards CR, Benediktsson R, Lindsay RS, Seckl JR. Dysfunction of placental glucocorticoid barrier: link between fetal environment and adult hypertension? *Lancet* 1993; 341: 355–7.
103. Lindsay RS, Lindsay RM, Waddell BJ, Seckl JR. Prenatal glucocorticoid exposure leads to offspring hyperglycaemia in the rat: studies with the 11 beta-hydroxysteroid dehydrogenase inhibitor carbenoxolone. *Diabetologia* 1996; 39: 1299–305.
104. Barker DJ. The malnourished baby and infant. *Br Med Bull* 2002; 60: 69–88.
105. Widdowson E, McCance R. The effect of finite periods of undernutrition at different ages on the composition and subsequent development of the rat. *Proc R Soc Ser B* 1963; 158: 329–42.
106. Girard JR, Ferre P, Gilbert M, Kervran A, Assan R, Marliss EB. Fetal metabolic response to maternal fasting in the rat. *Am J Physiol* 1977; 232: E456–63.
107. Dahri S, Snoeck A, Reusens-Billen B, Remacle C, Hoet JJ. Islet function in offspring of mothers on low-protein

diet during gestation. *Diabetes* 1991; 40 (suppl 2): 115–20.

108. Eriksson UJ, Swenne I. Diabetes in pregnancy: fetal macrosomia, hyperinsulinism, and islet hyperplasia in the offspring of rats subjected to temporary protein-energy malnutrition early in life. *Pediatr Res* 1993; 34: 791–5.
109. Swenne I, Crace CJ, Milner RD. Persistent impairment of insulin secretory response to glucose in adult rats after limited period of protein-calorie malnutrition early in life. *Diabetes* 1987; 36: 454–8.
110. Holness MJ, Sugden MC. Suboptimal protein nutrition in early life later influences insulin action in pregnant rats. *Diabetologia* 1996; 39: 12–21.
111. Hugh-Jones P. Diabetes in Jamaica. *Lancet* 1955; ii: 891–7.
112. Rao RH. The role of undernutrition in the pathogenesis of diabetes mellitus. *Diabetes Care* 1984; 7: 595–601.
113. Cook GC. Glucose tolerance after kwashiorkor. *Nature* 1967; 215: 1295–6.
114. Cohen MP, Stern E, Rusecki Y, Zeidler A. High prevalence of diabetes in young adult Ethiopian immigrants to Israel. *Diabetes* 1988; 37: 824–8.
115. Swai AB, Kitange HM, Masuki G, Kilima PM, Alberti KG, McLarty DG. Is diabetes mellitus related to undernutrition in rural Tanzania? *BMJ* 1992; 305: 1057–62.
116. Rao RH. Is tropical pancreatic diabetes malnutrition related? *Diabetes Care* 1993; 16: 941–5.
117. Godfrey KM, Robinson S, Hales CN, Barker DJ, Osmond C, Taylor KP. Nutrition in pregnancy and the concentrations of proinsulin, 32–33 split proinsulin, insulin, and C-peptide in cord plasma. *Diabet Med* 1996; 13: 868–73.
118. Stanner SA, Bulmer K, Andres C, Lantseva OE, Borodina V, Poteen VV, Yudkin JS. Does malnutrition in utero determine diabetes and coronary heart disease in adulthood? Results from the Leningrad siege study, a cross sectional study. *BMJ* 1997; 315: 1342–8.
119. Fajans SS, Floyd JC, Tattersall RB, Williamson JR, Pek S, Taylor CI. The various faces of diabetes in the young: changing concepts. *Arch Intern Med* 1976; 136: 194–202.
120. Hattersley AT. Maturity-onset diabetes of the young: clinical heterogeneity explained by genetic heterogeneity. *Diabet Med* 1998; 15: 15–24.
121. Hattersley AT, Beards F, Ballantyne E, Appleton M, Harvey R, Ellard S. Mutations in the glucokinase gene of the fetus result in reduced birth weight. *Nat Genet* 1998; 19: 268–70.
122. Tamemoto H, Kadowaki T, Tobe K, Yagi T, Sakura H, Hayakawa T, Terauchi Y, Ueki K, Kaburagi Y, Satoh S. Insulin resistance and growth retardation in mice lacking insulin receptor substrate-1. *Nature* 1994; 372: 182–6.
123. Rasmussen SK, Urhammer SA, Hansen T, Almind K, Moller AM, Borch-Johnsen K, Pedersen O. Variability of the insulin receptor substrate-1, hepatocyte nuclear factor-1alpha (HNF-1alpha), HNF-4alpha, and HNF-6 genes and size at birth in a population-based sample of young Danish subjects. *J Clin Endocrinol Metab* 2000; 85: 2951–3.
124. Lindsay RS, Dabelea D, Roumain J, Hanson RL, Bennett PH, Knowler WC. Type 2 diabetes and low birth weight: the role of paternal inheritance in the association of low birth weight and diabetes. *Diabetes* 2000; 49: 445–9.
125. Fall JG, Pulford DJ, Wylie AA, Jirtle RL. Genomic imprinting: implications for human disease. *Am J Pathol* 1999; 154: 635–47.
126. Morison IM, Reeve AE. A catalogue of imprinted genes and parent-of-origin effects in humans and animals. *Hum Mol Genet* 1998; 7: 1599–609.
127. Huxtable SJ, Saker PJ, Haddad L, Walker M, Frayling TM, Levy JC, Hitman GA, O'Rahilly S, Hattersley AT, McCarthy MI. Analysis of parent-offspring trios provides evidence for linkage and association between the insulin gene and type 2 diabetes mediated exclusively through paternally transmitted class III variable number tandem repeat alleles. *Diabetes* 2000; 49: 126–30.
128. Poulsen P, Vaag AA, Kyvik KO, Moller JD, Beck-Nielsen H. Low birth weight is associated with NIDDM in discordant monozygotic and dizygotic twin pairs. *Diabetologia* 1997; 40: 439–46.
129. Baird J, Osmond C, MacGregor A, Sneider H, Hales CN, Phillips DIW. Testing the fetal origins hypothesis in twins: the Birmingham twin study. *Diabetologia* 2001; 44: 33–9.

32

The Genetics of Human Obesity

Claude Bouchard* **and Louis Pérusse†**

**Louisiana State University, Baton Rouge, LA, USA, and †Laval University, Québec, Canada*

INTRODUCTION

There are about 250 million adults who are obese and at least 500 million who are overweight in the world at the moment [1]. Given these numbers, it is not surprising that the genetics of human obesity is receiving increasing attention. The interest in the causes of the present epidemic of obesity and the promise of finding potentially new prophylactic and therapeutic means are largely responsible for this new interest. Excess weight has also become the most important public health problem as it is associated with increases in type 2 diabetes mellitus and other morbidities as well as premature death rates.

Obesity is characterized by excess body mass or body fat without any particular reference to the concentration of fat in a given area of the body. Many obese individuals are characterized by an excess amount of subcutaneous fat on the trunk, particularly in the abdominal area, the so-called android obesity or male type of fat deposition. Another type is characterized by an excessive amount of fat in the abdominal visceral area and has been labeled abdominal visceral obesity. The last is known as gluteofemoral obesity and is observed primarily in women (gynoid obesity). Thus, excess fat can be stored primarily in the truncal-abdominal area or in the gluteal and femoral area. This implies that a given relative body fat content, say 30%, or absolute fat mass, say 20 kg, may exhibit different anatomical distribution characteristics. Thus, obesity can no longer be seen as a homogeneous phenotype.

But the situation is even more complex as the phenotypes are not of the simple Mendelian kind. Segregation of the genes is not readily perceived and whatever the role of the genotype in the etiology, it is generally attenuated or exacerbated by nongenetic factors. In other words, variation in human body fat is caused by a complex network of genetic, nutritional, metabolic, energy expenditure, psychological, and social variables, all playing a role in the modulation of energy balance and nutrient partitioning. Figure 1 depicts the key determinants and suggests that the impact of genetic differences on food intake, energy expenditure, energy partitioning, and adipogenesis can lead to obesity over time.

In clinical settings, the body mass index (BMI), measured in kg/m^2, is commonly used to assess the normality of body weight in patients. This is perfectly reasonable as most of the evidence from large-scale prospective studies that have associated obesity with morbidities and premature death is based on the BMI. The correlation between the BMI and total body fat or percent body fat is high in large and heterogeneous samples. The predictive value of the BMI is, however, much less impressive in a given individual, especially when the BMI is below 30 kg/m^2 or so. Thus, the BMI is an indicator of heaviness and only indirectly of body fat [2, 3]. Any estimate of the genetic effect on BMI should not necessarily be considered valid for adiposity as it is influenced in unknown proportions by the contribution of the genotype to fat mass, muscle mass, skeletal mass, and other components as well. Nevertheless, the BMI is worth considering because of its clinical validity, simplicity to measure, and widespread use.

The same point can be made for regional fat distribution phenotypes. The most important phenotype here is probably total abdominal fat. Abdominal fat is reasonably well approximated by waist circumference. However, a more direct measure of total abdominal fat level can only be obtained by imaging technologies such as CT (computed tomography) and MRI (magnetic resonance imaging). In the case of type 2 diabetes, abdominal visceral fat level may

International Textbook of Diabetes Mellitus, Third Edition. Edited by R. A. DeFronzo, E. Ferrannini, H. Keen, and P. Zimmet.
 ISBN: 0-471-48655-8.

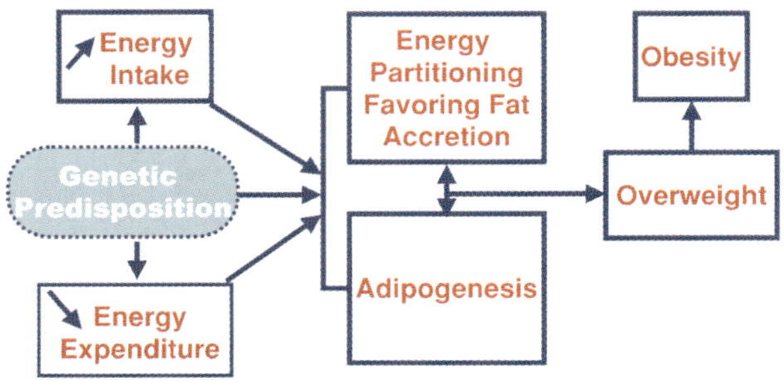

Figure 1 Diagram of the determinants of positive energy balance and fat deposition, with indication about the sites of action of a genetic predisposition

be of particular importance. Here again, surrogate measures such as abdominal girth or sagittal diameter may be clinically useful but only CT and MRI technologies can provide an accurate measure of visceral adiposity. It is important to realize that the relationship between total and visceral adiposity is characterized by a high degree of heterogeneity. As shown in Table 1, when BMI and percent body fat are constrained to narrow ranges, one finds generally a threefold range for the amount of CT-assessed abdominal visceral fat in adult males. Thus in 16 men with BMI values of 30 or 31 kg/m^2 and a percentage of body fat ranging from 30 to 33, mean abdominal visceral fat was 153 cm^2 with a range from 77 to 261 cm^2. Again, the same poor coupling between BMI, percent body fat, and abdominal visceral fat was observed in adult women.

The above data suggest that even though it may be necessary to use BMI or waist circumference in clinical settings, such practice is not desirable in the context of scientific research designed to understand the causes and metabolic consequences of variation in body fat content or in fat topography.

GENETIC EPIDEMIOLOGY

Obesity is not a homogeneous trait stemming from a unique gene or set of genes. Genetic epidemiological methods are useful for addressing specific questions in human obesity, such as determining if there are genetic factors underlying an obesity phenotype, characterizing the sources of the genetic influence through maternal vs. paternal transmission, and whether the trait is sex-limited or age-dependent, or if there is assortative mating, etc.

While most multifactorial studies of the BMI show significant familial resemblance, the relative importance of genes and common familial environments varies. Some studies place more importance on the familial environment as compared to polygenic effects [5–9] and others suggest that genetic effects outweigh those of the familial environment [10–18]. For example, in monozygotic (MZ) twins reared apart [13, 16, 19], the correlations were very similar to those for MZ twins reared together, suggesting that the shared familial environment had little or no effect. Two of the larger studies of the BMI (Norwegian sample of about 75 000 individuals [20] and over 9000 individuals in Tecumseh, MI [9]) suggest that the total additive familial effect may be between 30 and 40% in families. A somewhat higher estimate (69%) was reported in the large Virginia study of adult twins and their families (nearly 30 000 individuals) [21]. Table 2 describes the trends in the heritability levels based upon a large number of studies [22]. The results are generally quite heterogeneous. The heritability level is highest with twin studies, intermediate with nuclear family data, and lowest when derived from adoption data. When several types of relatives are used jointly in the same design, the heritability estimates typically cluster around 25–40% of the age- and gender-adjusted phenotype variance. There is no clear evidence for a specific maternal or paternal effect, and the common familial environmental effect is marginal. In most of these studies, the BMI was the phenotype considered. In some cases, skinfolds or estimates of percent body fat or fat mass were used.

Age effects in the familial resemblance for BMI have also been explored [23]. Two studies using path analysis techniques [24, 25] suggested that the familiality increased from birth to adulthood, which Cardon [24], using adoptive and biological families measured longitudinally, attributed to genetic rather than environmental factors. In studies assessing familiality in adults [26–29], there was a general decrease in the genetic heritability during adulthood. Fabsitz et al. [27] suggested that there were two major genetic effects in male twins, one increasing at or prior to age 20, and the other decreasing after age 20. Similarly, a longitudinal analysis of Polish twins suggested a peak additive genetic effect at about age 18 in males and

Table 1 Variation in amount of abdominal visceral fat for given BMI and percent body fat classes in males, 35–54 years of age*

			Visceral fat in cm^2		
N	BMI	% Fat	Mean	Min	Max
15	21–22	14–18	58	31	84
19	24–25	19–24	89	50	140
18	27–28	25–29	133	63	199
16	30–31	30–33	153	77	261

* Abdominal visceral fat measured by CT scan at the L4-L5 level. Percent fat derived from underwater weighing. From reference 4.

Table 2 Overview of the genetic epidemiology of human body fat/obesity*

	Heritability/transmission	Maternal/paternal	Familial environment
Nuclear families	30–50%	No	Minor
Adoption studies	10–30%	Mixed results	Minor
Twin studies	50–80%	No	No
Combined strategies	25–40%	No	Minor

* From reference 22.

about age 14 in females [30]. These and other studies (e.g., see reference 31) suggest that although some of the same genes are active across ages, there are unique genetic factors active as well.

Different genes may also be responsible for adiposity in the normal or moderate range as versus those leading to massive obesity (see reference 32 for review). A common observation is that the obese cases in familial studies of obesity is, on the average, 10–15 BMI units heavier than his or her mother, father, brothers, or sisters [33–35]. Such a large difference between a proband and his or her first-degree relative is suggestive of the contribution of a recessive gene having a large effect. In further support, the risk for obesity when a first-degree relative is extremely obese (BMI $\geq$ 40 kg/m^2) is higher than when a relative is moderately obese (BMI $\geq$ 30 kg/m^2).

This risk can be quantified using a statistic called the lambda coefficient (λ_R), defined as the ratio of the risk of being obese when a biological relative is obese compared to the risk in the population at large, i.e., the prevalence of obesity [36]. Estimates of λ_R based on BMI data have been reported [37, 38]. Figure 2 presents an example of these age- and gender-standardized risk ratios obtained from 2349 first-degree relatives of 840 obese probands and 5851 participants of the National Health and Nutrition Examination Survey III (NHANES III). The fig ure shows that the prevalence of obesity (BMI $\geq$ 30 kg/m^2) is about two times higher in families of obese individuals than in the population at large. Moreover, the risk increases with

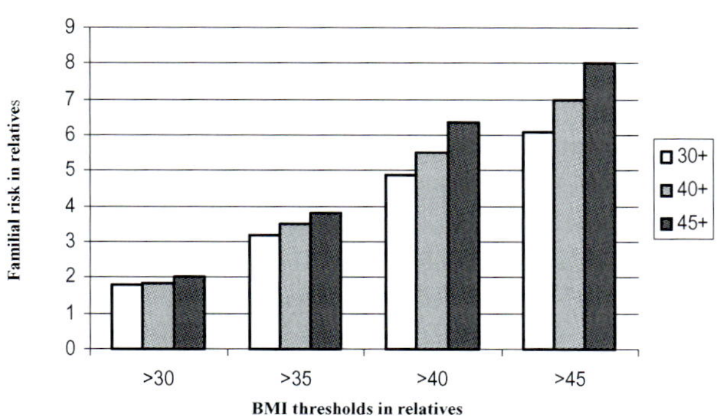

Figure 2 Familial risk of obesity in relatives of obese probands. Values are age- and sex-standardized risk ratios of the prevalence rate of obesity in relatives of probands to the population prevalence (adapted with permission from reference 38)

the severity of obesity in the proband as well as with the BMI threshold used to define the obesity. Thus, the risk of extreme obesity (BMI $\geq$ 45 kg/m^2) is about eight times higher in families of extremely obese (BMI $\geq$ 45 kg/m^2) subjects [38]. These data clearly illustrate that obesity aggregates in families at a level that tends to increase with the severity of the condition.

Less is known about direct measures of general adiposity [i.e., fat mass (FM) and percent body fat (%BF)] than about BMI. In Utah families, Ramirez [39] reported that the familiality for %BF (measured with bioelectrical impedance) was about 25%. In the Québec Family Study (QFS), the familiality for %BF (measured with underwater weighing) was 40% and dropped slightly to 36% after adjusting for energy intake and energy expenditure [40, 41]. In Québec twins and adopted and biological families, the genetic heritability for each of %BF and FM was about 25%, with an additional 30% due to familial environmental effects [42]. Together, these studies suggest that between 25 and 40% of the variance in total fat mass may be genetic because of additive genetic effects. Somewhat more variance in total fat is accounted for when both multifactorial and major gene effects are included in the models.

Upper Body Fat (Android Obesity)

For the waist-to-hip ratio (WHR), familiality estimates varied from 28% in adoptive and biological families [43] to 40–50% in traditional nuclear families [44, 45] to over 60% in longitudinal family data (Fels Longitudinal Study) [46]. Two family studies have also indicated that total abdominal fat level adjusted for fat mass is characterized by heritability coefficients of the order of 50% [47, 48].

These results suggest that there is a significant familial influence on abdominal fat and upper body obesity. Thus for a given level of fatness, some individuals store fat on the trunk or abdominal area (android) while others store primarily on the lower body (gynoid). This pattern is consistent with a hypothesis of both genetic pleiotropy (i.e., similar genes affecting both fat distribution and total body fat) and oligogenic (an additional major genetic system specific to fat distribution).

Abdominal Visceral Fat

We are aware of only two family studies that have investigated abdominal visceral fat, the Québec Family Study

(QFS) and the HERITAGE Family Study. Familial correlations in the QFS [47] for abdominal visceral and abdominal subcutaneous fat tissues were about 0.35, with somewhat lower spouse correlations for subcutaneous fat (0.21) but higher spouse correlations for abdominal visceral fat (0.36). The heritability was about 70% for each of the three measures. The effect of adjusting each of these measures for total body fat was to reduce the magnitude of the familial correlations and thus the heritability estimates (greater than 55% for abdominal visceral fat and 42% for subcutaneous abdominal fat). This suggests that some of the same multifactorial factors (polygenic and/or familial environmental) impact similarly on total body fat and visceral fat. Similar results were obtained in the HERITAGE Family Study [48].

A cross-trait study conducted between fat mass and abdominal visceral fat [49] supported a pleiotropy hypothesis. The bivariate (cross-trait) familiality was 29–50% (with sex differences), indicating genetic pleiotropy. Moreover, since the univariate familiality for each trait was even higher (55–77% for fat mass and 55–65% for abdominal visceral fat), each trait was assumed influenced by additional familial factors that were specific to each (i.e., oligogenic). Given the significant spouse cross-trait correlations, at least some of the bivariate familial effect may be environmental in origin.

GENES AND MOLECULAR MARKERS OF HUMAN OBESITY

The yearly updates of the obesity gene map published since 1996 [50–57] provide a good indication of the progress accomplished in the past 15 years in the search for genes and DNA sequence variations associated and/or linked with human obesity or variation in body fat content. This section of the chapter reviews the data accumulated so far from three lines of evidence: (1) human obesity cases caused by single-gene deficiencies, (2) association studies, and (3) human linkage studies. All the gene symbols, names, and chromosomal locations of the genes are given in the Appendix.

Single-Gene Deficiencies

Strong evidence that genes could be involved in determining human obesity comes from molecular studies that have identified cases of human obesity due to deficiencies in single genes. These monogenic forms of human obesity include mutations in the leptin (*LEP*), leptin receptor (*LEPR*), proopiomelanocortin (*POMC*), Proprotein convertase subtilisin/kexin type 1 (*PCSK1*), single-minded homologue 1 (*SIM1*), melanocortin-3 receptor (*MC3R*), and melanocortin-4 receptor (*MC4R*) genes. Although these monogenic forms of obesity are rare, they have contributed to our understanding of the metabolic pathways involved in the regulation of energy balance and body weight. These seven genes and related mutations are listed in Table 3.

The first cases were reported in 1997 and involved mutations in the *PCSK1* [58] and *LEP* [59] genes. The case with the mutation in the *PCSK1* gene involved a 43-year-old obese woman with elevated levels of proinsulin and very low levels of insulin suggestive of an impaired processing of proinsulin by the prohormone convertase-1. A screening of the patient's *PCSK1* gene revealed that she was a compound heterozygote for two mutations in the gene: an A→C transversion at position +4 of the intron 5 donor splice site, leading to a premature stop codon; and a G→A substitution in exon 13, leading to a Gly483Arg missense mutation [58].

The first mutation in the *LEP* gene was reported in two obese cousins of Pakistani origin [59]. A 2-year-old boy and an 8-year-old girl with congenital leptin deficiency resulting in severe early-onset obesity were found to be homozygous for a frameshift mutation at codon 133 of the *LEP* gene, resulting from a guanine deletion at nucleotide 398 [59]. A second mutation in the *LEP* gene, a C→T change in the first base of codon 105 in exon 3, was described in 4 obese subjects (3 females; 1 male) of a Turkish family [60, 61]. The latter mutation of the *LEP* gene, which results in an Arg→Trp replacement in the mature protein, is equivalent to that observed in the *ob/ob* mouse. It is known to result in a protein synthesized but not secreted, suggesting that the mutation alters the maturation of the protein. A G→A base substitution in the splice donor site of exon 16 of the *LEPR* gene was also reported in 3 morbidly obese (BMI ranging from 52 to 71 kg/m^2) female subjects who also exhibited pituitary dysfunction [62]. The homozygotes exhibited a deletion of exon 16, leading to a truncated protein lacking both the transmembrane and intracellular domains of the receptor.

Mutations in the *POMC* gene were also found in two patients with severe obesity, adrenal insufficiency, and red hair pigmentation [63]. The first patient was a 3-year-old female weighing 30 kg who was a compound heterozygote for two mutations in exon 3, a G→T substitution at nucleotide 7013 and a 1-bp deletion at nucleotide 1733, leading to a premature termination at codons 79 and 131, respectively. The second patient was a 5-year-old male weighing 50 kg and homozygous for a C→A transversion at nucleotide 3804 in exon 2 of the *POMC* gene. The latter mutation was located 11-bp upstream of the start codon within the 5′ untranslated region of the gene and resulted in the addition of a start codon, abolishing the translation of the protein. Other mutations in the *POMC* gene were described in obese children and adolescents, but were not implicated as the cause of obesity in these subjects [76]. Another case involved a 6-year-old girl with a weight of 47.5 kg and a BMI of 29 kg/m^2 who was found to carry a *de novo* balanced translocation between chromosomes 1p22.1 and 6q16.2 [64]. The chromosomal anomaly was

Table 3 Cases of human obesity caused by single-gene mutations

Gene	Location	Subjects	Age (years)	BMI (kg/m^2)	Mutation: Base change	Mutation: Effect on amino acid sequence	Reference
PCSK1	5q15-q21	One British obese woman with impaired processing of proinsulin	43	34	A→C^{+4} (intron 5) G→A (exon 13)	Stop codon Gly483Arg	[58]
LEP	7q31.3	Two obese (1 male; 1 female) subjects from a Pakistani pedigree	2–8	37–46	G398Δ	Frameshift mutation codon 133	[59]
		Four obese (3 females; 1 male) subjects from a Turkish pedigree	6–34	33–56	C→T (exon 3)	Arg105Trp	[60, 61]
LEPR	1p31	Three obese female subjects from a French family of Kabilian origin	13–19	53–71	G→A (exon 16)	Skipping of exon 16 leading to a truncated protein	[62]
POMC	2p23.3	One obese female patient from Germany	3	N/A	G7013T nt7133(del C)	Stop codon 79 Stop codon 131	[63]
		One obese male patient from Germany	5	N/A	C3804A (exon 2)	Addition of a initiation codon	
SIM1	6q16.3-q21		6	29	C1328T (exon 9)	Loss of function	[64]
MC4R	18q22	10 cases from British ($n = 2$) and German ($n = 8$) families	4–30	28–41	nt631(del CTCT) at codon 211	Stop codon 5-aa downstream	[65–67]
		6 cases from a French Family	11–58	30–57	nt732 (insGATT) at codon 246	Truncated protein	[68]
		8 morbidly obese French subjects	20 (F)	42	47–48insG	16 + 12 a.a.	[69]
			47 (F)	45	A31G	Thr11Ser	
			44 (F)	53	C52T	Arg18Cys	
			52 (M)	50	C449T	Thr150Ile	
			28 (F)	50	A508G	Ile170Val	
			49 (F)	65	C493T	Arg165Trp	
			50 (F)	59	T749A	Leu250Gln	
			30 (F)	55	T902C	Ile301Thr	
		7 cases from 4 French families	6–39	2.8–5.4 (z score)	G148A	Val50Met	[70]
			13–39		A172T	Ser58Cys	
			16	2.1–4.2 (z score)	T305G	Ile102Ser	
			13–45	4.1 (z score)	A508G	Ile170Val	
				3.8–44 (z score)			
		11 cases from German families	8–64	26–57	C105A	Tyr35X	[66, 67]
		5 cases from Caucasian American family	15–51	27-57	T410C	Ile137Thr	[71]
		13 cases from British families	5–46	27–48	GTins codon 279 Cdel		[72]
						N62S T112M R165Q V253I C271Y	
		Two female cases from a Turkish family	52–55	42–43		N274S	[73]
		One Japanese woman	40	62	G292A	Gly98Arg	[74]
MC3R	20q13.2-q13.3	Two obese cases from a Singaporean family	13–40	33–37	T548A	Ile183Asn	[75]

found to disrupt the *SIM1* gene on 6q, a critical transcription factor for the formation of paraventricular hypothalamic nuclei in mice. The patient carried a C→T substitution at nucleotide 1328 in exon 9, presumably associated with a loss of function of *SIM1* [64].

The other cases described in Table 3 include mutations in the *MC3R* and *MC4R* genes. The melanocortin pathway plays an important role in the regulation of feeding behavior and energy balance, particularly through the MC3R and MC4R, which are highly expressed in the brain and which have been involved in the development of obesity in mice [77, 78]. Since the demonstration that targeted disruption of the *MC4R* gene in mice produces hyperphagia and obesity, the *MC4R* gene has been the object of intense mutation screening in various human populations. The first cases of single-gene obesity syndromes due to mutations in the *MC4R* gene were reported in October 1998 in a British family [65] and a French family [68]. In a screening of 63 severely obese British children, Yeo et al. [65] identified a 4-year-old boy (BMI = 28 kg/m^2) heterozygous for 4-bp deletion (CTCT) at codon 211 of the gene, resulting in the introduction of a stop codon 5 amino acids downstream the mutation leading to a truncated protein of 215 residues. The proband's father was also found to be heterozygous for the mutation [65]. At the same time, a screening of 43 obese adult subjects from French families led to the identification of a 35-year-old women (BMI = 57 kg/m^2) heterozygous for a 4-bp insertion (GATT) at codon 246 of the gene, leading to the expression of a truncated receptor lacking the sixth and seventh transmembrane domains [68]. Five members of the proband's family were also found to be heterozygous for the mutation. Other studies performed in the French population led to the identification of other obesity cases due to mutations in the *MC4R* gene. In one of these studies, 209 severely obese (BMI > 40 kg/m^2) subjects were screened for mutations in the *MC4R* gene and eight different mutations not detected in 366 normal weight controls, were observed among 8 obese subjects [69]. Finally, in a report based on severely obese French children, 7 subjects (4 probands with 3 family members) were found with four mutations (Val50Met, Ser58Cys, Ile102Ser, and Ile170Val) not observed in control subjects (70). Mutation screening of the *MC4R* gene undertaken in 512 severely obese German children revealed the presence of nine different mutations that were found only in obese individuals, but only two mutations cosegregated with obesity [66, 67]. One of these mutations was the 4-bp deletion at codon 211, previously identified in French obese subjects and observed in 8 obese subjects (one female proband and 7 other subjects of her extended family), while the other was C→A nonsense mutation at codon 35, leading to a premature stop codon (Tyr35-X) and generating a truncated protein, identified in 11 obese subjects (3 index cases and 8 of their family members). In another study [71], *MC4R* sequence variants were examined in 94 subjects from families ascertained through a proband which was a member of the TOPS (Take Off Pounds Sensibly, a weight loss support group) Club and in 96 subjects from a cohort of extremely obese (BMI ≥ 50 kg/m^2) individuals recruited at the Obesity Research Center in St. Lukes/Roosevelt hospital in New York. Among the 190 individuals that were screened, a total of 9 subjects were found to be heterozygous for three MC4R variants: a Val103Ile variant found in 7 subjects (including 2 lean subjects), a Thr112Met variant found in a nonobese woman, and a Ile137Thr variant identified in an extremely obese (BMI = 57 kg/m^2) 43-year-old woman. *In vitro* functional analyses revealed that only the Ile137Thr variant showed impaired ligand binding and signaling [71]. Screening of 9 additional members of the proband's extended family revealed that 4 subjects (2 males and 2 females with BMI values from 27 to 51 kg/m^2) were heterozygous for the Ile137Thr variant. In a study of a large British cohort of subjects with severe early-onset obesity, nine mutations were described in 18 probands [72]. However, only seven mutations were observed in 8 obese probands and not in controls (see Table 3). Among family members who were available for study, 5 other obese subjects were found, for a total 13 individuals. In particular, the N62S variant was present in the homozygous state in 5 severely obese children from a highly consanguineous family of Pakistani origin [72]. In another report, screening of 40 morbidly obese subjects from Turkish families led to the identification of a novel heterozygous mutation (N274S) carried in 2 sisters, one aged 52 years with a BMI of 41.7 kg/m^2 and another aged 55 years with a BMI of 43 kg/m^2 [73]. A novel homozygous missense mutation in the *MC4R* gene was recently identified in a nondiabetic 40-year-old Japanese woman with severe (BMI = 62 kg/m^2) obesity [74]. The Gly98Arg mutation, which was not detected in 100 healthy controls, was associated with no discernable agonist ligand binding, suggesting a severe loss-of-function mutation. Finally, an analysis of the *MC3R* gene in 41 morbidly obese children and adolescents led to the identification of a heterozygous Ile183Asn missense mutation in a 13-year-old girl (BMI = 37 kg/m^2) and her 40-year-old father (BMI = 33 kg/m^2) [75]. The *MC3R* sequence variant observed in a Singaporean family was not found in 121 control subjects.

In summary, a total of 78 published obesity cases due to mutations in seven different genes have now been reported. The majority of these cases are found in severely obese subjects with early onset of obesity. The mutations in the *MC4R* gene are the most frequent and are responsible for 63 out of the 78 cases published so far. The majority of the obesity cases due to mutations in the *MC4R* gene are characterized by a dominant pattern of inheritance, compared to other single-gene deficiencies, which are mainly recessive.

Association Studies

The search for genes influencing overweight and obesity in humans is mostly based on association and/or linkage studies with candidate genes. Candidate genes refer to genes that are metabolically or physiologically relevant for the phenotype under study (functional candidate genes) or to genes that have been targeted primarily because of their physical position in a region of the genome (positional candidate gene), as defined by a Mendelian obesity syndrome, a quantitative trait locus, or other strategies. A quantitative trait locus (QTL) refers to a locus at which segregation contributes to a quantitative trait, such as BMI. The genes showing positive evidence of association with obesity-related phenotypes are listed in Table 4. The table provides the chromosomal location of the gene, the phenotypes that were shown to be associated with the gene, and the range of p values from the various studies. It should be noted that the table does not include the results of early association studies performed with the ABO (9q34) blood group and the human leukocyte antigen system on chromosome 6p21.3. A review of these studies [238] reveals that the results of these early studies are rather ambiguous, some studies finding associations with obesity, while others did not.

Despite the large number of positive findings reported in this table, it is important to keep in mind that for most of these genes, very few replications in independent populations have been reported. Moreover, for many of these genes, there are as many negative as positive studies. A good example of this is the results obtained with the β3-adrenergic receptor gene (*ADRB3*). The *ADRB3* gene is probably the candidate gene that has been the most widely tested for association with obesity-related phenotypes, with positive findings reported for weight gain [164–167], obesity, body mass index and/or body fatness [134, 168–175, 177–183], various indicators of abdominal fat [134, 167, 173–176], and changes in BMI during pregnancy [164]. Despite these positive findings, several negative studies, reviewed elsewhere [55, 239, 240], have also been reported for the *ADRB3* gene. Three independent meta-analyses yielded contradictory results, one concluding that the *ADRB3* gene has no effect on obesity [241], while the others concluded for the presence of an effect [242, 243].

Among the genes listed in Table 4, a few have been shown to be associated with obesity-related phenotypes in at least five different studies. These include the *LEPR*, *PPARG*, *ADRB2*, *TNFA*, *LEP*, *UCP2*, *UCP3*, *GNB3*, and *LDLR* genes. The studies summarized in Table 4 reveal that a total of 59 candidate genes have been shown to be associated with obesity-related phenotypes. These genes are found on all chromosomes, except chromosomes 6, 17, 21, 22, and Y. Chromosome 11 is the chromosome harboring the largest number of genes associated with obesity; a total of seven genes (*APOA4*, *DRD2*, *GNB3*, *IGF2*, *INS*, *SUR1*, *UCP2*, and *UCP3*) were associated with obesity-related phenotypes in at least one study.

Linkage Studies

Several linkage studies have been performed with obesity-related phenotypes [57]. The majority of the linkage studies were genome-wide scans that were undertaken with the aim of detecting obesity QTLs. The obesity QTLs uncovered in such scans define chromosomal regions or, in some cases, positional candidate genes that can be further investigated for their role in the phenotype of interest. The methodology underlying the identification of these obesity QTLs and a review of some of the findings in this area can be found elsewhere [244]. The evidence of linkage is assessed by a statistic called the Lod score (Lod = Logarithm of the odds); a Lod score ≥ 1.75 or a p value < 0.0023 is considered as suggestive evidence of linkage [245]. Because of their importance in the identification of putative obesity genes, the results of the genome scans for obesity are reviewed in detail in this section (see the next section and Table 5).

Linkages from Genome-wide Scans of Obesity

To the best of our knowledge, a total of 24 genomic scans for obesity, performed in 14 different populations with various obesity phenotypes, have been published so far. The obesity QTLs uncovered in these genome-wide linkage analyses are listed in Table 5 by chromosomal location. Only QTLs uncovered from genome-wide linkage screens are reported in this table; linkage studies with markers covering only one chromosome are not reviewed here. The studies that have led to the identification of these QTLs are described below.

Pima Indians A total of five genomic scans have been performed in this population known for its high prevalence of obesity and diabetes. The first genome-wide scan for obesity was performed in this population and used percent body fat as the phenotype [263]. A total of 674 genetic markers with an average intermarker distance of 8.3 cM were tested for linkage with percent body fat measured by underwater weighing in 283 sibling pairs from 88 Pima Indian families. Significant evidence of linkage was reported at 11q21-q22, with a peak Lod score of 2.8 between markers D11S2000 and D11S2366. Another second scan for obesity (451 sibpairs from 127 families) and energy metabolism (236 sibpairs from 82 families) phenotypes was performed using 576 markers [248]. The phenotypes investigated included, in addition to percent body fat, the ratio of waist to thigh circumference, 24-h energy expenditure (EE) and 24-h respiratory quotient (RQ) measured in a respiratory chamber. For percent body fat, the strongest linkages were detected at 11q21-q22 and

Table 4 Evidence for the presence of an association between markers of candidate genes with BMI, body fat, and other obesity-related phenotypes

Gene	Location	Phenotype	p value	Reference
TNFRSF1B	1p36.3-p36.2	BMI, overweight, leptin	<0.05	[79, 80]
NR0B2	1p36.1	Early-onset obesity	0.0094	[81]
LEPR	1p31	%Fat, abdominal fat, BMI, fat-free mass, fat mass, hip girth, leptin, obesity, weight loss	$0.003 < p < 0.05$	[82–89]
HSD3B1	1p13.1	Subcutaneous fat	0.04	[90]
LMNA	1q21.2-q21.3	Leptin, BMI, WHR, lipodystrophy	$0.0001 < p < 0.05$	[91–93]
ATP1A2	1q21-q23	%Fat, respiratory quotient	$0.0001 < p < 0.05$	[94, 95]
AGT	1q42-q43	WHR, fat mass	$0.007 < p < 0.02$	[96, 97]
ACP1	2p25	BMI	$0.002 < p < 0.02$	[98, 99]
APOB	2p24-p23	BMI, %fat, abdominal fat	$0.005 < p < 0.05$	[100, 101]
POMC	2p23.3	Leptin, early-onset obesity	<0.01	[102, 103]
ADRA2B	2p13-q13	Basal metabolic rate	0.01	[104]
IRS1	2q36	BMI, leptin	$0.03 < p < 0.05$	[105–107]
GHRL	3p26-p25	Obesity in women	<0.05	[108]
PPARG	3p25	BMI, leptin, body weight, fat-free mass, fat mass, waist and hip girths, obesity, overweight	$0.001 < p < 0.05$	[109–118]
APOD	3q26.2-qter	BMI	0.006	[119]
APM1	3q27	BMI in subjects with family history of type 2 diabetes	0.02	[120]
CCKAR	4p15.2-p15.1	%Fat, leptin	0.003–0.041	[121]
FABP2	4q28-q31	Abdominal fat, BMI, %fat, fat oxidation	$0.008 < p < 0.01$	[122–124]
UCP1	4q28-q31	High fat gainers, weight, BMI	$0.001 < p < 0.05$	[125–127]
NPY5R	4q31-q32	Morbid obesity	<0.05	[128]
CART	5q	WHR in men, BMI, obesity	$0.0021 < p < 0.04$	[129, 130]
GRL	5q31-q32	Abdominal visceral fat, BMI, WHR, leptin	$0.001 < p < 0.039$	[131–133]
ADRB2	5q31-q32	BMI, fat mass, fat cell volume, body weight, waist and hip girths, WHR,obesity, leptin, body weight gain and subcutaneous fat accumulation in response to overfeeding	$0.001 < p < 0.05$	[115, 134–143]
TNFA	6p21.3	%Fat, BMI, obesity	$0.004 < p < 0.035$	[80, 144–148]
ESR1	6q25.1	Android obesity	0.0001	[149]
GCK	7p15.3-p15.1	Birth weight	0.002	[150]
NPY	7p15.1	Birth weight, BMI, WHR	$0.03 < p < 0.04$	[151, 152]
PON2	7q21.3	Birth weight	<0.05	[153]
LEP	7q31.3	Weight loss, body weight, leptin, BMI, obesity, overweight	$0.005 < p < 0.05$	[154–161]
LPL	8p22	BMI (leanness), training-induced changes in BMI, fat mass and percent body fat	$0.01 < p < 0.05$	[162, 163]
ADRB3	8p12-p11.2	Weight gain, weight, WHR, BMI, obesity, abdominal fat, fat mass, hip and waist girths, fat mass	$0.002 < p < 0.05$	[134, 164–183]
CBFA2T1	8q22	%Fat, BMI, waist and hip girths	$0.0002 < p < 0.02$	[184]
SH3D5	10q23.3-q24.1	Obesity	<0.05	[185]
ADRA2A	10q24-q26	Abdominal fat, trunk-to-extremity skinfolds ratio	$0.002 < p < 0.012$	[134, 186]
IGF2	11p15.5	BMI	0.02	[187]
INS	11p15.5	Birth weight, WHR, BMI	$0.0002 < p < 0.009$	[187–189]
SUR1	11p15.1	Morbid obesity	0.02	[190]
UCP2	11q13	Obesity, BMI, body weight, energy expenditure, fat oxidation, respiratory quotient, percent fat, fat mass	$0.001 < p < 0.05$	[191–197]

Table 4 (*continued*)

Gene	Location	Phenotype	p value	Reference
UCP3	11q13	BMI, body weight, fat oxidation, respiratory quotient, WHR, fat mass, percent body fat, leptin, training-induced changes in subcutaneous fat	$0.0004 < p < 0.04$	[198–204]
APOA4	11q23	BMI, WHR, %fat	$0.004 < p < 0.023$	[205, 206]
DRD2	11q23	Relative weight, subcutaneous fat, obesity, BMI	$0.002 < p < 0.05$	[207–210]
GNB3	12p13	BMI, body weight, waist and hip girths, subcutaneous fat, birth-weight,training-induced changes in fat mass and percent body fat	$0.001 < p < 0.05$	[211–216]
VDR	12q12-q14	BMI in patients with early-onset type 2 diabetes	0.0058	[217]
IGF1	12q22-q23	%Fat, fat mass, fat-free mass, changes in fat-free mass after 20-week endurance training	<0.05	[218]
CD36L1	12q24.1-q24.3	BMI in lean women	0.004–0.03	[219]
HTR2A	13q14-q21	Total energy, carbohydrate and alcohol intakes in obese subjects	0.028–0.047	[220]
HSPA2	14q21	Obesity	$<10^{-6}$	[221]
NMB	15q22-qter	Obesity, body weight	0.03	[222]
SAH	16p13.11	BMI, WHR	0.03	[223]
MC5R	18p11.2	BMI in females	0.003	[224]
MC4R	18q22	Fat mass, %fat, fat-free mass in females	$0.002 < p < 0.004$	[224]
INSR	19p13.3-p.13.2	Obesity (BMI > 26) in hypertensives	0.05	[225]
LDLR	19p13.3	BMI in hypertensives and normotensives, obesity, subcutaneous fat	$0.001 < p < 0.04$	[226–230]
LIPE	19q13.1-q13.2	Obesity, BMI, subcutaneous fat, percent body fat	$0.0009 < p < 0.005$	[231, 232]
APOE	19q13.2	Leptin	0.020	[233]
GYS1	19q13.3	Obesity	0.03	[234]
ADA	20q12-q13.11	BMI in diabetic subjects	0.0004–0.01	[235]
PPARA	22q12-q13.1	BMI in type 2 diabetics	0.02	[236]
HTR2C	Xq24	BMI > 28 kg/m^2	0.009–0.02	[237]

18q21. For 24-h EE, the strongest linkage was observed at 11q23 with marker D11S976 (Lod = 2.0), while for 24-h RQ, linkages were found at 1p31-p21 (Lod = 2.8 with D1S550) and 20q11.2 (Lod = 3.0 with D20S601). A third scan for loci linked to phenotypes related to diabetes revealed evidence of linkage to BMI (Lod = 3.6) between markers D11S4464 and D11S912 at 11q24 [264] near the dopamine D2 receptor gene. A fourth genomic scan based on 770 subjects from 239 families revealed evidence of linkage between plasma leptin levels near marker D6S271 (Lod = 2.1) at 6p21-p12 [258]. Finally, a fifth study was performed to assess the evidence of linkage of BMI to loci derived from either father or mother in 860 individuals from 235 nuclear families genotyped for 516 autosomal markers [257]. Evidence of linkage of BMI to maternally and paternally derived alleles was found on chromosomes 5p12 (Lod = 1.7) and 10p15 (Lod = 1.7), respectively. In the combined model (non-parent-specific linkage), evidence of linkage to BMI was found on 11q23 (Lod = 2.7) [257].

San Antonio Family Heart Study The results of the genome scans for obesity-related phenotypes in the San Antonio Family Heart Study (SAFHS) have been reported in three studies [102, 250, 261]. The phenotypes investigated include BMI, body fat mass measured by bioelectric impedance, and plasma leptin levels measured in a sample of up to 470 Mexican Americans from 10 large multigenerational families. The first study based on a 20-cM map [250] revealed evidence of linkage at 2p21 between marker D2S1788 and fat mass (Lod = 2.8) as well as plasma leptin levels (Lod = 4.9). Evidence of linkage with leptin was also observed at 8q11.1. In a second study in which six additional markers were typed around the peak linkage for leptin at 2p21, in addition to the 15 that were already available in the first study, the Lod score for leptin was increased to 7.5 [102]. The QTL for leptin identified in SAFHS at 2p21 was weakly replicated in a study performed in African Americans [267]. Finally, a genome scan for BMI performed using a 10-cM map revealed evidence of linkage

Table 5 Summary of genome scan studies for obesity-related phenotypes*

QTL location	Phenotype†	Markers	Lod score	Population‡	Reference
Chromosome 1					
1p36	BMI	D1S468	4.4	CUOFS	[246]
1p31	Leptin	D1S3728–D1S1665	3.4	DF	[247]
1p31-p21	24-h RQ	D1S550	2.8	PIMAS	[248]
1p11.2	ASF	D1S534	2.3	QFS	[249]
Chromosome 2					
2p21	FM, leptin	D2S1788, 165, 367	2.4–7.5	SAFHS, PLFS	[250, 251]
2p14	ASF	D2S411	1.9	HERITAGE	[252]
2q14	BMI, FM, %FAT	D2S347	2.1–4.4	CUOFS	[246]
2q22.1	AVF	D2S1399, 1334	2.0–2.3	HERITAGE	[252]
2q36	AVF	D2S434, IRS1	1.9–2.5	HERITAGE	[252]
Chromosome 3					
3p26.3	ASF	D3S2387	2.2	HERITAGE	[252]
3q27	BMI, WC	D3S2427	1.8–3.3	AAF, TOPS	[253, 254]
3q29	ASF	D3S1311	2.5	HERITAGE	[252]
Chromosome 4					
4p15.1	ASF	D4S2397	2.3	QFS	[249]
4p15-p14	BMI females	D4S2632, 3350	6.1–9.1	UF	[255]
4q12	BMI	D4S1592	2.1	CUOFS	[246]
4q31.22-q32.1	ASF	D4S2431, 2417	1.8–2.3	HERITAGE, QFS	[249, 252]
Chromosome 5					
5p15.3	BMI, adiponectin	D5S827	1.9–4.1	AAF, TOPS	[254, 256]
5p12	BMI	D5S2489–D5S2500	1.7	PIMAS	[257]
5p11	Leptin	D5S426	2.9	PLFS	[251]
5q31	ASF, ATF	D5S658, 1480	1.9–2.1	HERITAGE	[252]
Chromosome 6					
6p21-p12	Leptin	D6S271	2.1	PIMAS	[258]
6p21.3	%FAT	D6S1959	2.7	AAF	[254]
Chromosome 7					
7p15.3	FFM	D7S1808	2.7	QFS	[259]
7q31	ASF	D7S1875	2.0	QFS	[249]
7q31-q36	Leptin-BMI	D7S640, 636	1.8	OOA	[109]
7q32.3	BMI	D7S1804	4.9	NHLBIFHS	[260]
Chromosome 8					
8p12-p11.2	BMI	D8S1121	3.2	SAFHS	[261]
8q11.1	Leptin	D8S1110	2.2	SAFHS	[250]
8q23.3	BMI	D8S556	2.0	HERITAGE	[262]
Chromosome 9					
9q22.1	ASF	D9S1122, 257	2.1–2.3	QFS	[249]
9q34.3	BMI	D9S158	2.3	HERITAGE	[252]
Chromosome 10					
10p15	BMI, FM	D10S1435, 189	1.7–2.7	PIMAS, HERITAGE	[257, 262]
10p12	Obesity	D10S197	4.9	PLFS	[251]
10p12-p11	Leptin-BMI	D10S220	2.7	OOA	[109]
10qter	BMI	AFM198ZB	3.3	DF	[247]
Chromosome 11					
11p15.2	ASF	CP11P15_3	1.9	HERITAGE	[252]
11p14.1	ASF	GATA34E08	1.8	HERITAGE	[252]
11q21-q22	%FAT	D11S200–D11S2366	2.8	PIMAS	[263]
11q23-q24	24-h EE, BMI	D11S976, 1998, 4464, 912	2.0–3.6	PIMAS	[248, 257, 264]
Chromosome 12					
12p12.1	BMI, FM	D12S1042	2.1–2.2	HERITAGE	[262]
12q22-q23	ASF	IGF1	1.9	QFS	[249]
12q24.3	ASF	D12S1045	2.9	QFS	[249]

Table 5 (*continued*)

QTL location	Phenotype†	Markers	Lod score	Population‡	Reference
Chromosome 13					
13q14	BMI	D13S257	3.2	NHLBIFHS	[260]
13q34	ASF	D13S285	1.9	QFS	[249]
Chromosome 14					
14q11-q11.2	BMI, FM, FFM, Adiponectin	D14S283, 742, 1280, 608, 599	1.8–3.2	HERITAGE, TOPS	[256, 262]
14q22-q31	WC, Leptin-BMI	D14S276, 74, 280	1.8–2.5	OOA	[109]
14q24.1	ASF	D14S588	2.4	HERITAGE	[252]
Chromosome 15					
15q25-q26	FFM	IGF1R	3.6	QFS	[259]
Chromosome 16					
16q21	Leptin	D16S265	2.0	PIMAS	[258]
Chromosome 17					
17p12	Leptin	D17S947	5.0	TOPS	[253]
17q11	BMI	D17S1293	2.3	SAFHS	[261]
17q21.1-q21.3	ASF	D17S2180, 1301	2.2	QFS	[249]
Chromosome 18					
18q12	FFM	D18S535	3.6	QFS	[259]
18q21	%FAT, obesity	D18S877, 535	2.3–3.6	PIMAS, FF	[248, 265]
Chromosome 19					
19p13	Leptin	LDLR	$P = 0.0009$	HERITAGE	[262]
Chromosome 20					
20q11.2	24-h RQ	D20S601	3.0	PIMAS	[248]
20q13	Obesity	D20S476, 211	3.2	UPFS	[266]
Chromosome X					
Xq24	Obesity	DX6799–DX6804	3.5	FF	[265]

* Only QTLs from genome-wide scans and with Lod scores ≥ 1.75 are reported.

† Phenotypes abbreviations: BMI = body mass index; RQ = respiratory quotient; FM = fat mass; FFM = fat-free mass; %FAT = percent body fat; ASF = abdominal subcutaneous fat; AVF = abdominal visceral fat; ATF = total abdominal fat; WC = waist circumference; Leptin-BMI = leptin adjusted for BMI.

‡ Population abbreviations: AAF = African American families; CUOFS = Creighton University Osteoporosis Family Study; DF = Dutch families; FF = Finish families; HERITAGE = HERITAGE Family Study; NHLBIFHS = NHLBI Family Heart Study; OOA = Old Order Amish; PIMAS = Pima Indians; PLFS = Paris-Lille French Study; QFS = Quebec Family Study; SAFHS = San Antonio Family Heart Study; TOPS = TOPS Family Study; UF = Utah families; UPFS = University of Pensylvania Family Study.

at 6q25, 8p12-p11.2 near the *ADRB3* gene, and 17q11 [102].

Paris-Lille French Study In a study based on 158 morbidly obese (BMI ≥ 40 kg/m^2) French families from the Hôtel-Dieu Hospital in Paris and the Institut Pasteur in Lille, strong evidence of linkage with obesity (defined as a BMI > 27 kg/m^2) was found at 10p12 (Lod = 4.9 with marker D10S197) [251]. Linkages with plasma leptin levels were also found at 2p21 (Lod = 2.7) and 5p11 (Lod = 2.9). Two independent studies attempted to replicate the linkage (10p12 with obesity) found in the French population. The first study was performed in 386 subjects from 93 German families with at least 2 obese children, using 11 markers spanning a 23-cM region on chromosome 10 [268]. Although the linkage with marker D10S197 was not as strong (Lod = 1.7) as in the French families, evidence of linkage with obesity was observed with four other markers (Lods ranging from 1.1 to 2.4) located within 5 cM of the peak linkage found in the French population. The second study investigated linkage between obesity and 13 markers spanning about 110 cM on chromosome 10 in two cohorts: one comprising 862 subjects from 170 Caucasian families and the other comprising 212 individuals from 43 African American families [269]. Evidence of linkage was found with markers located on 10p in both Caucasians ($p = 0.03$ with marker D10S208) and African Americans ($p = 0.01$ with marker D10S582) as well as in the combined cohort ($p = 0.0005$ with D10S197).

University of Pennsylvania Family Study The fourth published genomic scan for obesity was undertaken in 513 individuals from 92 families ascertained through a morbidly obese proband as part of an ongoing linkage study at the University of Pennsylvania [266]. Several obesity phenotypes were measured in these subjects including BMI, percent body fat measured by bioelectric impedance, the waist-to-hip circumference ratio, and plasma leptin levels. The strongest evidence of linkage reported in that study was between obesity, defined as a BMI $\geq 30\ kg/m^2$, and three markers spanning 12 cM on chromosome 20q13 [266].

The Quebec Family Study Two genomic scans for phenotypes related to obesity were published from data of the Quebec Family Study. One investigated linkage with fat-free mass (FFM) derived from body density measurements obtained from underwater weighing in 748 subjects from 194 families [259], while the other investigated linkage with abdominal fat assessed by CT in 521 subjects from 156 families [249]. Results of the study with FFM revealed evidence of linkage on three different regions: 7p15.3 with marker D7S1808 (Lod = 2.7), 15q25-q26 with a polymorphism within the insulin-like growth factor 1 receptor (Lod = 3.6), and 18q12 with marker D18S535 (Lod = 3.6). In the other genome scan, a total of nine QTLs affecting abdominal subcutaneous fat adjusted for total body fatness were uncovered [249]. Two of these QTLs were found close to genes involved in the regulation of food intake (4q32 and 17q21), while three others (1p11.2, 9q22, and 17q21) were found in the vicinity of genes influencing sex steroid metabolism.

The Finnish Families Another genome scan performed in 367 obese individuals from 166 Finnish families revealed evidence of two QTLs influencing obesity, defined as a BMI $\geq 30\ kg/m^2$ [265]. The strongest evidence of linkage was uncovered on Xq24, between markers DX6799 and DX6804 (Lod = 3.5), in a region where the serotonin 2C receptor gene (*HTR2C*) is located. Evidence of linkage with obesity was also observed in a region of chromosome 18q21 (Lod = 2.4 with D18S1155) flanking the *MC4R* gene. Another study based on 614 subjects from 247 families (from combining data from five study groups) found no evidence of linkage with BMI [270].

The TOPS Family Study In an attempt to identify QTLs influencing phenotypes associated with the metabolic syndrome, Kissebah et al. [253] tested 2209 individuals distributed over 507 Caucasian families recruited from the TOPS membership. A total of 387 markers, including 17 X-linked and 4 Y-linked markers, with an average genetic spacing of 10 cM were tested for linkage with seven phenotypes including the following obesity phenotypes: BMI, waist circumference, and plasma leptin levels. Plasma leptin levels showed its strongest linkage signal on chromosome 17p12 (Lod = 5.0) near marker D17S947 in a region where the glucose transporter 4 (*GLUT4*) and the peroxisome proliferative-activated receptor-alpha (*PPARA*) genes are located. The peak Lod scores for BMI (Lod = 3.3) and waist circumference (Lod = 2.4) were found on the same region of chromosome 3 (3q27) close to the marker D3S2427. The candidate genes located in this region of chromosome 3 include glucose transporter 2 (*GLUT2*) and the adipose tissue secreted protein adiponectin (*APM1*). Plasma adiponectin levels were measured in 1100 individuals from 170 families and tested for linkage with the same panel of markers [256]. Two QTLs for adiponectin were found on chromosomes 5p15.3 (Lod = 4.1 near marker D5S817) and 14q11.2 (Lod = 3.2 between markers D14S608 and D14S599).

The HERITAGE Family Study The HERITAGE Family Study is a study designed to investigate the role of genetic factors in determining cardiovascular, metabolic, and hormonal responses to exercise training. Two genome-wide scans of obesity-related traits were reported in this population, using a panel of 344 autosomal markers with a mean spacing of 9.7 cM and obesity-related phenotypes measured before and after 20 weeks of endurance training in Caucasian and Black families [252, 262]. Only linkage results from pretraining phenotypes are presented below. In the first study [262], BMI, subcutaneous fat, percent body fat, FM, FFM, and plasma leptin levels were measured in 522 subjects from 99 families of Whites and tested for linkage. The strongest multipoint linkages were found on chromosomes 8q23.3 (BMI), 9q34.3 (BMI), 10p15.3-p15.1 (BMI and FM), 12p12.1 (BMI and FM), and 14q11-q11.2 (BMI, FM, and FFM). For plasma leptin levels, evidence of linkage was found on chromosome 19p13 with the LDL receptor gene ($p = 0.0009$). In the second study, based on abdominal fat measures obtained by CT in 668 subjects from White and Black families, several QTLs affecting abdominal fat were identified [252]. For total abdominal fat, the regions providing evidence of linkage include 5q31.2, and 5q31.3. For abdominal subcutaneous fat (ASF), the regions providing evidence of linkage include 2p14, 5q31.2 and 22q11.23 in Whites and 3p26.3, 3q29, 4q31.22, 11p15.2, 11p14.1, and 14q24.1 in Blacks. Finally, for abdominal visceral fat, linkages were found on 2q22.1, 2q36.1, and 2q36.3 in Whites. Some of the regions showing linkage with ASF (4q31.22, 11p14.1) replicated the results of the Quebec Family Study [249].

The Old Order Amish Population A genome-wide scan of obesity-related traits was also performed in the Old Order Amish population, a rural-living population characterized by considerable homogeneity in lifestyle [109]. BMI, waist circumference, percent body fat estimated by bioelectric impedance, and serum leptin concentrations were measured in 672 individuals from 28 extended families. The obesity phenotypes and leptin concentrations adjusted for BMI (leptin-BMI) were tested for linkage with 357 autosomal markers with average intermarker distance of 10.2 cM. Peak linkages were found on chromosomes 3p25.2 for percent body fat, 7q31-q36 and 10p12-p11 for leptin-BMI, 14q22-q31 for waist circumference and leptin-BMI, and 16p for BMI and leptin concentrations. The strongest linkage for leptin-BMI on 10p12-p11 (Lod = 2.7) was approximately 10–20 cM telomeric to the obesity QTL reported on 10p12 in the French population [251] and other studies [268, 269].

The Dutch Families A search for obesity QTLs was also undertaken in 198 subjects from 18 Dutch pedigrees with familial combined hyperlipidemia [247]. Linkage to BMI and plasma leptin levels was tested using a panel of 399 markers distributed over all autosomes and the X and Y chromosomes. The strongest evidence of linkage for leptin was found on 1p31 in a 10-cM region flanking the *LEPR* gene and defined by markers D1S3728 and D1S1665 (Lod = 3.4). After adjustment for age and sex, the Lod score decreased to 1.8. For BMI, the peak linkage was observed on 10q-ter (Lod = 3.3 with marker AFM198ZB).

NHLBI Family Heart Study A genome scan for BMI was recently reported in two samples of families participating in the National Heart, Lung, and Blood Institute (NHLBI) Family Heart Study [260]. The first sample included 1184 individuals from 317 sibships genotyped for 243 markers, while the second included 3027 subjects from 401 three-generation families genotyped for 404 markers. Linkage analyses were performed in each sample as well as in the combined sample by putting the markers from each sample on a common genetic map. Strong evidence of linkage with BMI was found in each sample as well as in the combined sample on 7q32.3 (Lod = 4.9 with D7S1804) and 13q14 (Lod = 3.2 with D13S257).

African American Families A genome-wide scan for obesity was also conducted in 618 Black subjects from 202 African American families living in the suburb of Chicago [254]. Evidence of linkage with BMI and percent body fat measured by bioelectric impedance was assessed using 387 markers with an average intermarker distance of 10 cM. Evidence of linkage for BMI was found on chromosomes 3q27 (Lod = 1.8 with marker D3S2427) and 5p15.3 (Lod = 1.9 with marker D5S817). For percent body fat, the only significant evidence of linkage was found on chromosome 6p21.3 (Lod = 2.7 with marker D6S1959).

Utah Family Study A genome-wide scan for genes affecting severe obesity (BMI $\geq 40\ kg/m^2$) was recently performed in multigenerational Utah pedigrees [255]. In this study, linkages were investigated using 628 markers (average spacing of 5.8 cM) and three different BMI phenotypes: a sex-nonspecific phenotype (BMI), a female-only phenotype (BMIf), and a male-only phenotype (BMIm). A total of 64 pedigrees with 1687 subjects were included in the analysis of BMI, 37 pedigrees with 994 subjects in the analysis of BMIf, and 14 pedigrees with 479 subjects in the analysis of BMIm. A strong evidence of linkage with BMIf was found on chromosome 4p15-p14 in a 10-cM interval centered around marker D4S2632 (Lod = 6.1). After increasing the marker density around the marker and the size of the data set by adding 14 pedigrees, the evidence of linkage increased to a Lod score of 9.2 at marker D4S3350. No evidence of significant linkage (after adjustment for multiple testing) was observed for BMIm [255]. A previous study undertaken in the same population tested evidence of linkage of BMI to 48 chromosome 20 markers genotyped on 1711 individuals from 103 extended pedigrees [271]. The results provided evidence of linkage with BMI (Lod = 3.5 with D20S438) on 20p11.1-q11.1, a 10-cM region around the centromere of chromosome 20.

Creighton University Osteoporosis Family Study Using a sample of pedigrees collected to identify genes underlying the risk of osteoporosis, a genome-wide linkage scan for BMI and body composition assessed by DXA (dual-energy X-ray absorptiometry) was performed in 630 subjects from 53 Caucasian pedigrees ascertained through a proband with low bone mineral density [246]. Linkage with BMI, percent body fat, FM, and lean body mass was tested with 380 autosomal markers, with an average intermarker distance of 8.6 cM. Significant evidence of linkage was found at the terminal end of the short arm of chromosome 1 (1p36) for BMI (Lod = 2.1 with marker D1S468), on 2q14 for BMI (Lod = 4.4), fat mass (Lod = 2.2), and percent body fat (Lod = 2.1) with marker D2S247, and on 4q12 for BMI (Lod = 2.1 with marker D4S1592).

In summary, the genome-wide linkage studies summarized in Table 5 have led to the identification of 60 obesity QTLs distributed on all chromosomes except 21, 22, and Y. Chromosome 2 is the chromosome harboring the largest number of obesity QTLs with five of them. Despite the large number of obesity QTLs identified thus far, only a few were replicated in a different population. These include the QTLs on chromosome 2p21, 3q27, 4q31-q32, 5p13.3, 10p15, 14q11-q11.2, and 18q21. Moreover, the QTL on chromosome 2p was replicated in one study, while the chromosome 10p QTL was replicated in three different populations.

GENE–ENVIRONMENT AND GENE–GENE INTERACTIONS

Genotype–environment interaction (G $\times$ E) arises when the response of a phenotype to environmental changes depends on the genotype of the individual. Although it is well known that there are interindividual differences in the responses to various dietary interventions, very few attempts have been made to test whether these differences are genotype-dependent for adiposity phenotypes.

We have proposed that one way to test for the presence of a G $\times$ E effect in humans is to challenge several genotypes in a similar manner by submitting both members of MZ twin pairs to a standardized treatment (environment) and compare the within- and the between-pair variances of the response to the treatment [272]. This comparison can be done using a two-way analysis of variance (ANOVA) for repeated measures on one factor (the treatment effect), in which the genotype effect is random, the treatment effect is fixed, and twins are nested within pairs. Using this ANOVA, F ratios for the treatment effect and for genotype-treatment effect can be easily obtained. The intraclass correlation can be computed from the within- and between-pair mean squares. The finding of a significantly higher variance in the response between pairs than within pairs suggests that the changes induced by the treatment are more heterogeneous in genetically dissimilar individuals, which will translate into a higher intrapair resemblance in the response.

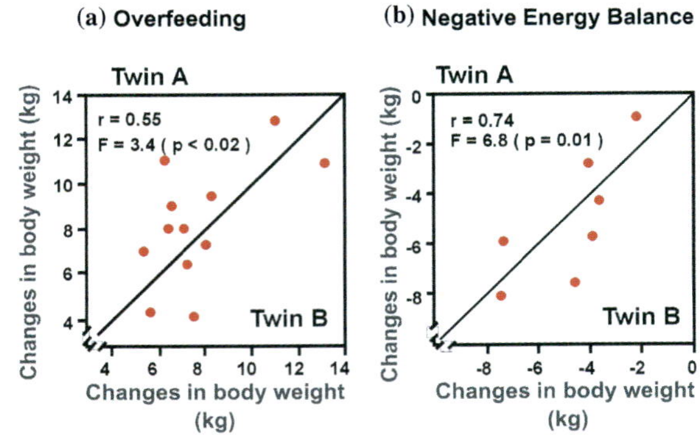

Figure 3 Intrapair resemblance in the response of identical twins to long-term changes in energy balance. (A) 12 pairs of identical twins were submitted to an 84 000-kcal energy-intake surplus over 100 days. (B) 7 pairs were subjected to a negative energy balance protocol caused by exercise. The energy deficit was 58 000 kcal over 93 days (reproduced with permission from references 273 and 275)

The Positive Energy Balance Experiments

It is generally recognized that there are some individuals prone to excessive accumulation of fat, for whom losing weight represents a continuous battle, and others who seem relatively well protected against such a menace. We studied the role of the genotype in determining the response to changes in energy balance by submitting both members of MZ twin pairs to either positive energy balance induced by overfeeding [273, 274] or negative energy balance induced by exercise training [275–277]. The objective of these studies was to determine whether the sensitivity of individuals to gain fat when exposed to positive energy balance or to lose fat when exposed to negative energy balance was modulated by the genotype.

Twelve pairs of male MZ twins ate a 2.4 MJ/day (1000 kcal/day) caloric surplus, 6 days a week, during a period of 100 days [273]. At the beginning of the overfeeding treatment, almost all the daily caloric surplus was recovered as body energy gain, but the proportion decreased to 60% at the end of the 100-day protocol [278]. The weight gain pattern followed an exponential with a half-duration of about 86 days. We have estimated that the weight gain attained in the experiment would have reached about 55% of the anticipated maximal weight gain had the overfeeding protocol been continued indefinitely [278]. The mean body mass gain for the 24 subjects of the 100-day overfeeding experiment was 8.1 kg, of which 5.4 kg was FM and 2.7 kg was FFM. Assuming that the energy content of body fat is about 22 MJ/kg (9300 kcal/kg, assuming a 100% triglyceride content) and that of fat-free tissue is 2.42 MJ/kg (1020 kcal/kg), about 63% of the excess energy intake was recovered on the average as body mass changes. This proportion is of the same order as that reported by other investigators [279, 280], i.e., between 60 and 75% of total excess energy intake. There were, however, individual differences among the 24 subjects with respect to the amount of fat and fat-free tissue gained.

However, the variation observed was not randomly distributed, as indicated by the significant within pair resemblance in response. For instance, there was at least three times more variance in response between pairs than within pairs for the gains in body weight, FM, and FFM (Figure 3A). These data demonstrate that some individuals are more at risk than others to gain fat when energy-intake surplus is clamped at the same level for everyone and when all subjects are confined to a sedentary lifestyle. The within-identical-twin-pair response to the standardized caloric surplus suggests that the amount of fat stored is likely influenced by the genotype. Similar results were essentially obtained in a shorter (22 days) overfeeding experiment [274]. The long-term overfeeding study also revealed that there was six times more variance between pairs than within pairs for the changes in upper body fat and in CT-determined abdominal visceral fat when both were adjusted for the gain in total fat mass [273]. These observations indicate that some individuals are storing fat predominantly in selected fat depots primarily as a result of undetermined genetic characteristics.

Attempts have been made to identify genetic variants that could account for the differences in response to overfeeding among the 12 pairs of twins. No associations were seen between markers in *UCP1*, *UCP2*, and *UCP3* genes, and body weight or body fatness increases [281]. On the other hand, the Gln223Arg polymorphism in the *LEPR* gene was related to plasma leptin induced changes in response to the long-term overfeeding protocol, with the Gln/Gln genotypes experiencing the largest increases, but it was not associated with body mass and adiposity changes [282]. In contrast, Gln27Gln twins at the *ADRB2* gene gained more weight and subcutaneous fat than other genotypes, with exposure to 100 days of overfeeding [135]. Finally, twins with the GG genotype at an

*Apa*I (restriction enzyme) polymorphism in the *IGF2* gene gained more fat mass and subcutaneous fat with overfeeding than the twins with the AA and AG genotypes [283]. These exploratory studies with a small sample size suggest that it may be possible in larger studies to eventually identify the genes and sequence variants responsible for genotype–overfeeding interaction effects.

The Negative Energy Balance Experiment

Seven pairs of young adult male identical twins completed a negative energy balance protocol during which they exercised on cycle ergometers twice a day, 9 out of 10 days, over a period of 93 days while being kept on a constant daily energy and nutrient intake [275]. The mean total energy deficit caused by exercise above the estimated energy cost of body weight maintenance reached 244 MJ. Baseline energy intake was estimated over a period of 17 days preceding the negative energy balance protocol. Mean body weight loss was 5 kg and was entirely accounted for by the loss of fat mass. FFM was unchanged. Body energy losses reached 191 MJ, which represented about 78% of the estimated energy deficit. Decreases in metabolic rates and in the energy expenditure of activity not associated with the cycle ergometer protocol must have occurred to explain the difference between the estimated energy deficit and the body energy losses. Subcutaneous fat loss was slightly more pronounced on the trunk than on the limbs as estimated from skinfolds, circumferences, and CT. The reduction in abdominal visceral fat area was quite striking, from 81 to 52 cm^2. At the same submaximal power output level, subjects oxidized more lipids than carbohydrates after the program as indicated by the changes in the respiratory exchange ratio. Intrapair resemblance was observed for the changes in body weight (Figure 3b), fat mass, percent fat, body energy content, sum of 10 skinfolds, abdominal visceral fat, and respiratory exchange ratio during submaximal work. Even though there were large individual differences in response to the negative energy balance and exercise protocol, subjects with the same genotype were more alike in responses than subjects with different genotypes, particularly for body fat, body energy, and abdominal visceral fat changes. High lipid oxidizers and low lipid oxidizers during submaximal exercise were also seen despite the fact that all subjects had experienced the same exercise and nutritional conditions for about 3 months.

Thus, changes in body mass, body fat, and body energy content were characterized by more heterogeneity between twin pairs than within pairs. These results are remarkably similar to those that we reported for body mass, body fat, and body energy gains, with 12 pairs of twins subjected to a 100-day overfeeding protocol.

CONCLUSIONS

The evidence reviewed herein suggests a significant genetic component in human obesity. However, the nature of the evidence and the magnitude of the genetic component varied a great deal depending on the phenotype and the analytical method used. A picture that is clearly emerging from the diverse findings is that multiple genetic loci are involved in the common forms of human obesity.

The ultimate goal of the studies designed to understand the genetic and molecular basis of human variation in a trait such as obesity is to resolve the issue in terms of the specific genes and DNA sequence variants.

Advances in the genome sequence together with the progress in the development of large panels of single-nucleotide polymorphisms, the availability of efficient high-throughput sequencing technologies, and the large repertoire of mapped expressed sequences have increased the ability of investigators to resolve genetic effects in terms of genes and sequence differences. However, the success of this complex process is highly dependent on the quality and informativeness of the populations of normal weight and obese subjects upon which the project is anchored. Finally, detailed phenotypic characterization and studies of additional covariates will enable characterization of the gene effects and investigations of gene–gene and gene–environment interactions.

APPENDIX

Symbols, full names, and cytogenetic location of genes and loci listed in this chapter*

Gene or locus	Name	Location
A		
ACP1	Acid phosphatase 1, soluble	2p25
ADA	Adenosine deaminase	20q12-q13.11
ADRA2A	Adrenergic, α-2A-, receptor	10q24-q26
ADRA2B	Adrenergic, α-2B-, receptor	2p13-q13
ADRB2	Adrenergic, β-2-, receptor, surface	5q31-q32
ADRB3	Adrenergic, β-3-, receptor	8p12-p11.2
AGT	Angiotensinogen	1q42-q43
AK1	Adenylate kinase 1	9q34.1

APPENDIX (*continued*)

Gene or locus	Name	Location
ANG	Angiogenin, ribonuclease, RNase A family, 5	14q11.1-q11.2
APM1	Adipose most abundant gene transcript 1, adiponectin	3q27
APOA4	Apolipoprotein A-IV	11q23
APOB	Apolipoprotein B (including Ag (×) antigen)	2p24-p23
APOD	Apolipoprotein D	3q26.2-qter
APOE	Apolipoprotein E	19q13.2
ATP1A2	ATPase, Na^+/K^+ transporting, α-2-(+)-polypeptide	1q21-q23
B/C		
BF	B-factor, properdin	6p21.3
CART	Cocaine- and amphetamine-regulated transcript	5q
CBFA2T1	Core-binding factor, runt domain, alpha subunit 2; translocated to, 1; cyclin D-related	8q22
CCKAR	Cholecystokinin A receptor	4p15.2-p15.1
CD36L1	CD36 antigen (collagen type I receptor, thrombospondin receptor)-like 1	12q24.1-q24.3
D/F		
DRD2	Dopamine receptor D2	11q23
ESR1	Estrogen receptor 1	6q25.1
FABP2	Fatty acid binding protein 2, intestinal	4q28-q31
G to K		
GCK	Glucokinase (hexokinase 4, maturity onset diabetes of the young 2)	7p15.3-p15.1
GHRL	Ghrelin precursor	3p26-p25
GLUT2	Glucose transporter 2	3q26.1-q26.2
GLUT4	Glucose transporter 4	17p13
GNB3	Guanine nucleotide binding protein (G protein), β-polypeptide 3	12p13
GPC4	Glypican 4	Xq26.1
GRL	Glucocorticoid receptor	5q31-q32
GYS1	Glycogen synthase 1 (muscle)	19q13.3
HSD3B1	Hydroxy-δ-5-steroid dehydrogenase, 3-β- and steroid δ-isomerase 1	1p13.1
HSPA2	Heat shock 70 kD protein 2	14q21
HTR2A	5-Hydroxytryptamine (serotonin) receptor 2A	13q14-q21
HTR2C	5-Hydroxytryptamine (serotonin) receptor 2C	Xq24
IGF1	Insulin-like growth factor 1 (somatomedin C)	12q22-q23
IGF1R	Insulin-like growth factor 1 receptor	15q25-q26
IGF2	Insulin-like growth factor 2 (somatomedin A)	11p15.5
INS	Insulin	11p15.5
INSR	Insulin receptor	19p13.3-p13.2
IRS1	Insulin receptor substrate 1	2q36
L		
LDLR	Low density lipoprotein receptor (familial hypercholesterolemia)	19p13.3
LEPR	Leptin receptor	1p31
LEP	Leptin (murine obesity homologue)	7q31.3
LIPE	Lipase, hormone sensitive	19q13.1-q13.2
LMNA	Lamin A/C	1q21.2-q21.3
LPL	Lipoprotein lipase	8p22
M to O		
MC3R	Melanocortin 3 receptor	20q13.2-q13.3
MC4R	Melanocortin 4 receptor	18q22
MC5R	Melanocortin 5 receptor	18p11.2
NMB	Neuromedin B	15q22-qter
NPY	Neuropeptide Y	7p15.1
NPY5R	Neuropeptide Y receptor Y5	4q31-q32
NR0B2	Nuclear receptor subfamily 0, group B, member 2	1p36.1
P/S		
PCSK1	Proprotein convertase subtilisin/kexin type 1	5q15-q21
POMC	Proopiomelanocortin	2p23.3
PON2	Paraoxonase 2	7q21.3
PPARA	Peroxisome proliferative activated receptor, α	22q13.31
PPARG	Peroxisome proliferative activated receptor, γ	3p25

APPENDIX (*continued*)

Gene or locus	Name	Location
SAH	SA hypertension-associated homologue	16p13.11
SH3D5	Src homologue 3 domain protein 5 (ponsin)	10q23.3-q24.1
SIM1	Single-minded (Drosophila) homologue 1	6q16.3-q21
SUR1	Sulfonylurea receptor 1	11p15.1
T to W		
TNFA	Tumor necrosis factor	6p21.3
TNFRSF1B	Tumor necrosis factor receptor superfamily member 1B	1p36.3-p36.2
UCP1	Uncoupling protein 1 (mitochondrial, proton carrier)	4q28-q31
UCP2	Uncoupling protein 2 (mitochondrial, proton carrier)	11q13
UCP3	Uncoupling protein 3 (mitochondrial, proton carrier)	11q13
VDR	Vitamin D receptor	12q12-q14

* The gene symbols, names, and cytogenetic locations are from the Locus Link Web site (http://www.ncbi.nlm.nih.gov/LocusLink) available from the National Center for Biotechnology Information (NCBI), which provides the official nomenclature of genetic loci.

REFERENCES

1. Seidell JC. Obesity: a growing problem. *Acta Paediatr Suppl* 1999; 88 (428): 46–50.
2. Bouchard C. Human obesities: chaos or determinism. In Ailhaud G, Guy-Grand B, Lafontan M, Ricquier C (eds) *Obesity in Europe 91, Proceedings of the 3rd European Congress of Obesity*. Paris: John Libbey & Co Ltd, 1992; pp 7–14.
3. Garn SM, Leonard WR, Hawthorne VM. Three limitations of the body mass index. *Am J Clin Nutr* 1986; 44 (6): 996–7.
4. Bouchard C. Genetics of human obesities: Introductory Notes. In Bouchard C (ed) *The Genetics of Obesity*. Boca Raton, FL: CRC Press, 1994; pp 1–15.
5. Annest JL, Sing CF, Biron P, Mongeau JG. Familial aggregation of blood pressure and weight in adoptive families, III: analysis of the role of shared genes and shared household environment in explaining family resemblance for height, weight and selected weight/height indices. *Am J Epidemiol* 1983; 117 (4): 492–506.
6. Garn SM, Bailey SM, Cole PE. Similarities between parents and their adopted children. *Am J Phys Anthropol* 1976; 45 (3, pt 2): 539–43.
7. Hartz A, Giefer E, Rimm AA. Relative importance of the effect of family environment and heredity on obesity. *Ann Hum Genet* 1977; 41 (2): 185–93.
8. Khoury P, Morrison JA, Laskarzewski P, Glueck CJ. Parent–offspring and sibling body mass index associations during and after sharing of common household environments: The Princeton School District Family Study. *Metabolism* 1983; 32: 82–9.
9. Longini IM Jr, Higgins MW, Hinton PC, Moll PP, Keller JB. Genetic and environmental sources of familial aggregation of body mass in Tecumseh, Michigan. *Hum Biol* 1984; 56 (4): 733–57.
10. Biron P, Mongeau JG, Bertrand D. Familial resemblance of body weight and weight/height in 374 homes with adopted children. *J Pediatr* 1977; 91 (4): 555–8.
11. Heller R, Garrison RJ, Havlik RJ, Feinleib M, Padgett S. Family resemblances in height and relative weight in the Framingham Heart Study. *Int J Obes* 1984; 8 (5): 399–405.
12. Price RA, Cadoret RJ, Stunkard AJ, Troughton E. Genetic contributions to human fatness: an adoption study. *Am J Psychiatry* 1987; 144 (8): 1003–8.
13. Price RA, Gottesman II. Body fat in identical twins reared apart: roles for genes and environment. *Behav Genet* 1991; 21 (1): 1–7.
14. Sorensen TI, Price RA, Stunkard AJ, Schulsinger F. Genetics of obesity in adult adoptees and their biological siblings. *BMJ* 1989; 298 (6666): 87–90.
15. Stunkard AJ, Foch TT, Hrubec Z. A twin study of human obesity. *JAMA* 1986; 256 (1): 51–4.
16. Stunkard AJ, Harris JR, Pedersen NL, McClearn GE. The body-mass index of twins who have been reared apart. *N Engl J Med* 1990; 322 (21): 1483–7.
17. Stunkard AJ, Sorensen TI, Hanis C, Teasdale TW, Chakraborty R, Schull WJ, Schulsinger F. An adoption study of human obesity. *N Engl J Med* 1986; 314 (4): 193–8.
18. Vogler GP, Sorensen TI, Stunkard AJ, Srinivasan MR, Rao DC. Influences of genes and shared family environment on adult body mass index assessed in an adoption study by a comprehensive path model. *Int J Obes Relat Metab Disord* 1995; 19 (1): 40–5.
19. MacDonald A, Stunkard A. Body-mass indexes of British separated twins. *N Engl J Med* 1990; 322 (21): 1530.
20. Tambs K, Moum T, Eaves L, Neale M, Midthjell K, Lund-Larsen PG, et al. Genetic and environmental contributions to the variance of the body mass index in Norwegian sample of first- and second-degree relatives. *Am J Hum Biol* 1991; 3: 257–67.
21. McLaughlin JA. The inheritance of body-mass index in the Virginia 30,000. *Behav Genet* 1991; 21: 581.
22. Bouchard C. Genetics of obesity: overview and research directions. In Bouchard C (ed) *The Genetics of Obesity*. Boca Raton, FL: CRC Press, 1994; pp 223–33.
23. Borecki IB, Rice T, Perusse L, Bouchard C, Rao DC. Major gene influence on the propensity to store fat in trunk versus extremity depots: evidence from the Quebec Family Study. *Obes Res* 1995; 3 (1): 1–8.
24. Cardon LR. Developmental analysis of the body mass index in the Colorado Adoption Project. *Behav Genet* 1991; 21: 563–4.
25. Province MA, Rao DC. Path analysis of family resemblance with temporal trends: applications to height, weight, and Quetelet index in northeastern Brazil. *Am J Hum Genet* 1985; 37 (1): 178–92.
26. Fabsitz R, Feinleib M, Hrubec Z. Weight changes in adult twins. *Acta Genet Med Gemellol (Roma)* 1980; 29 (4): 273–9.

27. Fabsitz RR, Carmelli D, Hewitt JK. Evidence for independent genetic influences on obesity in middle age. *Int J Obes Relat Metab Disord* 1992; 16 (9): 657–66.
28. Fabsitz RR, Sholinsky P, Carmelli D. Genetic influences on adult weight gain and maximum body mass index in male twins. *Am J Epidemiol* 1994; 140 (8): 711–20.
29. Korkeila M, Kaprio J, Rissanen A, Koskenvuo M. Effects of gender and age on the heritability of body mass index. *Int J Obes* 1991; 15 (10): 647–54.
30. Huggins RM, Hoang NH, Loesch DZ. Analysis of longitudinal data from twins. *Genet Epidemiol* 2000; 19 (4): 345–53.
31. Rice T, Perusse L, Bouchard C, Rao DC. Familial aggregation of body mass index and subcutaneous fat measures in the longitudinal Quebec family study. *Genet Epidemiol* 1999; 16 (3): 316–34.
32. Perusse L, Chagnon YC, Bouchard C. Etiology of massive obesity: role of genetic factors. *World J Surg* 1998; 22 (9): 907–12.
33. Adams TD, Hunt SC, Mason LA, Ramirez ME, Fisher AG, Williams RR. Familial aggregation of morbid obesity. *Obes Res* 1993; 1: 261–70.
34. Lissner L, Sjostrom L, Bengtsson C, Bouchard C, Larsson B. The natural history of obesity in an obese population and associations with metabolic aberrations. *Int J Obes Relat Metab Disord* 1994; 18 (6): 441–7.
35. Reed DR, Bradley EC, Price RA. Obesity in families of extremely obese women. *Obes Res* 1993; 1: 167–72.
36. Risch N. Linkage strategies for genetically complex traits, I: multilocus models. *Am J Hum Genet* 1990; 46 (2): 222–8.
37. Allison DB, Faith MS, Nathan JS. Risch's lambda values for human obesity. *Int J Obes Relat Metab Disord* 1996; 20 (11): 990–9.
38. Lee JH, Reed DR, Price RA. Familial risk ratios for extreme obesity: implications for mapping human obesity genes. *Int J Obes Relat Metab Disord* 1997; 21 (10): 935–40.
39. Ramirez ME. Familial aggregation of subcutaneous fat deposits and the peripheral fat distribution pattern. *Int J Obes Relat Metab Disord* 1993; 17 (2): 63–8.
40. Bouchard C. Inheritance of fat distribution and adipose tissue metabolism. In Vague J, Bjorntorp P, Guy-Grand B, Rebuffe-Scrive M, Pague P (eds) *Metabolic Complications of Human Obesities*. Amsterdam: Elseveir Science, 1985; pp 87–96.
41. Savard R, Bouchard C, Leblanc C, Tremblay A. Familial resemblance in fatness indicators. *Ann Hum Biol* 1983; 10 (2): 111–8.
42. Bouchard C, Perusse L, Leblanc C, Tremblay A, Theriault G. Inheritance of the amount and distribution of human body fat. *Int J Obes* 1988; 12 (3): 205–15.
43. Perusse L, Leblanc C, Bouchard C. Inter-generation transmission of physical fitness in the Canadian population. *Can J Sport Sci* 1988; 13 (1): 8–14.
44. Donahue RP, Prineas RJ, Gomez O, Hong CP. Familial resemblance of body fat distribution: the Minneapolis Children's Blood Pressure Study. *Int J Obes Relat Metab Disord* 1992; 16 (3): 161–7.
45. Sellers TA, Drinkard C, Rich SS, Potter JD, Jeffery RW, Hong CP, et al. Familial aggregation and heritability of waist-to-hip ratio in adult women: the Iowa Women's Health Study. *Int J Obes Relat Metab Disord* 1994; 18 (9): 607–13.
46. Towne B, Roche A, Chumlea W, Guo S, Sievogel R. No evidence of pleiotropy for either body mass index or waist/hip circumference ratio and plasma cholesterol concentration. *Obes Res* 1993; 1: 1105.
47. Perusse L, Despres JP, Lemieux S, Rice T, Rao DC, Bouchard C. Familial aggregation of abdominal visceral fat level: results from the Quebec family study. *Metabolism* 1996; 45 (3): 378–82.
48. Rice T, Despres JP, Daw EW, Gagnon J, Borecki IB, Perusse L, et al. Familial resemblance for abdominal visceral fat: the HERITAGE family study. *Int J Obes Relat Metab Disord* 1997; 21 (11): 1024–31.
49. Rice T, Perusse L, Bouchard C, Rao DC. Familial clustering of abdominal visceral fat and total fat mass: the Quebec Family Study. *Obes Res* 1996; 4 (3): 253–61.
50. Bouchard C, Perusse L. Current status of the human obesity gene map. *Obes Res* 1996; 4 (1): 81–90.
51. Perusse L, Bouchard C. Identification of genes contributing to excess body fat and fat distribution. In Angel A, Anderson H, Bouchard C, Lau D, Leiter L, Mendelson R (eds) *Progress in Obesity Research, 7th International Congress on Obesity*. London: John Libbey & Co Ltd, 1996; pp 281–9.
52. Perusse L, Chagnon YC, Dionne FT, Bouchard C. The human obesity gene map: the 1996 update. *Obes Res* 1997; 5 (1): 49–61.
53. Chagnon YC, Perusse L, Bouchard C. The human obesity gene map: the 1997 update. *Obes Res* 1998; 6 (1): 76–92.
54. Perusse L, Chagnon YC, Weisnagel J, Bouchard C. The human obesity gene map: the 1998 update. *Obes Res* 1999; 7 (1): 111–29.
55. Chagnon YC, Perusse L, Weisnagel SJ, Rankinen T, Bouchard C. The human obesity gene map: the 1999 update. *Obes Res* 2000; 8 (1): 89–117.
56. Perusse L, Chagnon YC, Weisnagel SJ, Rankinen T, Snyder E, Sands J, et al. The human obesity gene map: the 2000 update. *Obes Res* 2001; 9 (2): 135–69.
57. Rankinen T, Perusse L, Weisnagel SJ, Snyder EE, Chagnon YC, Bouchard C. The human obesity gene map: the 2001 update. *Obes Res* 2002; 10 (3): 196–243.
58. Jackson R, Creemers J, Ohagi S, Raffin-Sanson M, Sanders L, Montague C, et al. Obesity and impaired prohormone processing associated with mutations in the human prohormone convertase 1 gene. *Nat Genet* 1997; 16: 303–6.
59. Montague CT, Farooqi IS, Whitehead JP, Soos MA, Rau H, Wareham NJ, et al. Congenital leptin deficiency is associated with severe early-onset obesity in humans. *Nature* 1997; 387: 903–8.
60. Strobel A, Issad T, Camoin L, Ozata M, Strosberg A. A leptin missense mutation associated with hypogonadism and morbid obesity. *Nat Genet* 1998; 18: 213–5.
61. Ozata M, Ozdemir IC, Licinio J. Human leptin deficiency caused by a missense mutation: multiple endocrine defects, decreased sympathetic tone, and immune system dysfunction indicate new targets for leptin action, greater central than peripheral resistance to the effects of leptin, and spontaneous correction of leptin-mediated defects. *J Clin Endocrinol Metab* 1999; 84 (10): 3686–95.
62. Clément K, Vaisse C, Lahlou N, Cabrol S, Pelloux V, Cassuto D, et al. A mutation in the human leptin receptor gene causes obesity and pituitary dysfunction. *Nature* 1998; 392: 398–401.
63. Krude H, Biebermann H, Luck W, Horn R, Brabant G, Gruters A. Severe early-onset obesity, adrenal insufficiency and red hair pigmentation caused by POMC mutations in humans. *Nat Genet* 1998; 19 (2): 155–7.

64. Holder JL Jr, Butte NF, Zinn AR. Profound obesity associated with a balanced translocation that disrupts the *SIM1* gene. *Hum Mol Genet* 2000; 9 (1): 101–8.
65. Yeo GSH, Farooqi IS, Aminian S, Halsall DJ, Stanhope RG. A frameshift mutation in MC4R associated with dominantly inherited human obesity. *Nat Genet* 1998; 20: 111–2.
66. Sina M, Hinney A, Ziegler A, Neupert T, Mayer H, Siegfried W, et al. Phenotypes in three pedigrees with autosomal dominant obesity caused by haploinsufficiency mutations in the melanocortin-4 receptor gene. *Am J Hum Genet* 1999; 65 (6): 1501–7.
67. Hinney A, Schmidt A, Nottebom K, Heibult O, Becker I, Ziegler A, et al. Several mutations in the melanocortin-4 receptor gene including a nonsense and a frameshift mutation associated with dominantly inherited obesity in humans. *J Clin Endocrinol Metab* 1999; 84 (4): 1483–6.
68. Vaisse C, Clement K, Guy-Grand B, Froguel P. A frameshift mutation in human MC4R is associated with a dominant form of obesity. *Nat Genet* 1998; 20: 113–4.
69. Vaisse C, Clement K, Durand E, Hercberg S, Guy-Grand B, Froguel P. Melanocortin-4 receptor mutations are a frequent and heterogeneous cause of morbid obesity. *J Clin Invest* 2000; 106 (2): 253–62.
70. Dubern B, Clement K, Pelloux V, Froguel P, Girardet JP, Guy-Grand B, et al. Mutational analysis of melanocortin-4 receptor, agouti-related protein, and alpha-melanocyte-stimulating hormone genes in severely obese children. *J Pediatr* 2001; 139 (2): 204–9.
71. Gu W, Tu Z, Kleyn PW, Kissebah A, Duprat L, Lee J, et al. Identification and functional analysis of novel human melanocortin-4 receptor variants. *Diabetes* 1999; 48 (3): 635–9.
72. Farooqi IS, Yeo GS, Keogh JM, Aminian S, Jebb SA, Butler G, et al. Dominant and recessive inheritance of morbid obesity associated with melanocortin 4 receptor deficiency. *J Clin Invest* 2000; 106 (2): 271–9.
73. Mergen M, Mergen H, Ozata M, Oner R, Oner C. A novel melanocortin 4 receptor (MC4R) gene mutation associated with morbid obesity. *J Clin Endocrinol Metab* 2001; 86 (7): 3448.
74. Kobayashi H, Ogawa Y, Shintani M, Ebihara K, Shimodahira M, Iwakura T, et al. A novel homozygous missense mutation of melanocortin–4 receptor (MC4R) in a Japanese woman with severe obesity. *Diabetes* 2002; 51 (1): 243–6.
75. Lee YS, Poh LK, Loke KY. A novel melanocortin 3 receptor gene (*MC3R*) mutation associated with severe obesity. *J Clin Endocrinol Metab* 2002; 87 (3): 1423–6.
76. Hinney A, Becker I, Heibult O, Nottebom K, Schmidt A, Ziegler A, et al. Systematic mutation screening of the pro-opiomelanocortin gene: identification of several genetic variants including three different insertions, one nonsense and two missense point mutations in probands of different weight extremes. *J Clin Endocrinol Metab* 1998; 83 (10): 3737–41.
77. Chen AS, Marsh DJ, Trumbauer ME, Frazier EG, Guan XM, Yu H, et al. Inactivation of the mouse melanocortin-3 receptor results in increased fat mass and reduced lean body mass. *Nat Genet* 2000; 26 (1): 97–102.
78. Huszar D, Lynch CA, Fairchild-Huntress V, Dunmore JH, Fang Q, Berkemeier LR, et al. Targeted disruption of the melanocortin-4 receptor results in obesity in mice. *Cell* 1997; 88 (1): 131–41.
79. Benjafield AV, Wang XL, Morris BJ. Tumor necrosis factor receptor 2 gene (*TNFRSF1B*) in genetic basis of coronary artery disease. *J Mol Med* 2001; 79 (2–3): 109–15.
80. Fernandez-Real JM, Gutierrez C, Ricart W, Casamitjana R, Fernandez-Castaner M, Vendrell J, et al. The TNF-alpha gene *Nco*I polymorphism influences the relationship among insulin resistance, percent body fat, and increased serum leptin levels. *Diabetes* 1997; 46 (9): 1468–72.
81. Nishigori H, Tomura H, Tonooka N, Kanamori M, Yamada S, Sho K, et al. Mutations in the small heterodimer partner gene are associated with mild obesity in Japanese subjects. *Proc Natl Acad Sci USA* 2001; 98 (2): 575–80.
82. Chagnon YC, Chung WK, Perusse L, Chagnon M, Leibel RL, Bouchard C. Linkages and associations between the leptin receptor (LEPR) gene and human body composition in the Quebec Family Study. *Int J Obes Relat Metab Disord* 1999; 23 (3): 278–86.
83. Chagnon YC, Wilmore JH, Borecki IB, Gagnon J, Perusse L, Chagnon M, et al. Associations between the leptin receptor gene and adiposity in middle-aged Caucasian males from the HERITAGE family study. *J. Clin Endocrinol Metab* 2000; 85 (1): 29–34.
84. Mammes O, Aubert R, Betoulle D, Pean F, Herbeth B, Visvikis S, et al. LEPR gene polymorphisms: associations with overweight, fat mass and response to diet in women. *Eur J Clin Invest* 2001; 31 (5): 398–404.
85. Rosmond R, Chagnon YC, Holm G, Chagnon M, Perusse L, Lindell K, et al. Hypertension in obesity and the leptin receptor gene locus. *J Clin Endocrinol Metab* 2000; 85 (9): 3126–31.
86. Roth H, Korn T, Rosenkranz K, Hinney A, Ziegler A, Kunz J, et al. Transmission disequilibrium and sequence variants at the leptin receptor gene in extremely obese German children and adolescents. *Hum Genet* 1998; 103 (5): 540–6.
87. Thompson DB, Ravussin E, Bennett PH, Bogardus C. Structure and sequence variation at the human leptin receptor gene in lean and obese Pima Indians. *Hum Mol Genet* 1997; 6 (5): 675–9.
88. Wauters M, Mertens I, Chagnon M, Rankinen T, Considine RV, Chagnon YC, et al. Polymorphisms in the leptin receptor gene, body composition and fat distribution in overweight and obese women. *Int J Obes Relat Metab Disord* 2001; 25 (5): 714–20.
89. Yiannakouris N, Yannakoulia M, Melistas L, Chan JL, Klimis-Zacas D, Mantzoros CS. The Q223R polymorphism of the leptin receptor gene is significantly associated with obesity and predicts a small percentage of body weight and body composition variability. *J Clin Endocrinol Metab* 2001; 86 (9): 4434–9.
90. Vohl MC, Dionne FT, Pérusse L, Dériaz O, Chagnon M, Bouchard C. Relation between *Bgl*II polymorphism in 3beta-hydroxysteroid dehydrogenase gene and adipose-tissue distribution in human. *Obes Res* 1994; 2: 444–9.
91. Hegele RA, Cao H, Harris SB, Zinman B, Hanley AJ, Anderson CM. Genetic variation in LMNA modulates plasma leptin and indices of obesity in aboriginal Canadians. *Physiol Genomics* 2000; 3 (1): 39–44.
92. Hegele RA, Cao H, Huff MW, Anderson CM. LMNA R482Q mutation in partial lipodystrophy associated with reduced plasma leptin concentration. *J Clin Endocrinol Metab* 2000; 85 (9): 3089–93.

93. Hegele RA, Anderson CM, Wang J, Jones DC, Cao H. Association between nuclear lamin A/C R482Q mutation and partial lipodystrophy with hyperinsulinemia, dyslipidemia, hypertension, and diabetes. *Genome Res* 2000; 10 (5): 652–8.
94. Deriaz O, Dionne F, Perusse L, Tremblay A, Vohl MC, Cote G, et al. DNA variation in the genes of the Na,K-adenosine triphosphatase and its relation with resting metabolic rate, respiratory quotient, and body fat. *J Clin Invest* 1994; 93 (2): 838–43.
95. Katzmarzyk PT, Rankinen T, Perusse L, Deriaz O, Tremblay A, Borecki I, et al. Linkage and association of the sodium potassium-adenosine triphosphatase alpha2 and beta1 genes with respiratory quotient and resting metabolic rate in the Quebec Family Study. *J Clin Endocrinol Metab* 1999; 84 (6): 2093–7.
96. Hegele RA, Brunt JH, Connelly PW. Genetic variation on chromosome 1 associated with variation in body fat distribution in men. *Circulation* 1995; 92 (5): 1089–93.
97. Rankinen T, Gagnon J, Perusse L, Rice T, Leon AS, Skinner JS, et al. Body fat, resting and exercise blood pressure and the angiotensinogen M235T polymorphism: the HERITAGE Family Study. *Obes Res* 1999; 7 (5): 423–30.
98. Lucarini N, Finocchi G, Gloria-Bottini F, Macioce M, Borgiani P, Amante A, et al. A possible genetic component of obesity in childhood. Observations on acid phosphatase polymorphism. *Experientia* 1990; 46 (1): 90–1.
99. Lucarini N, Antonacci E, Bottini N, Gloria BF. Low-molecular-weight acid phosphatase (ACP1), obesity, and blood lipid levels in subjects with non-insulin-dependent diabetes mellitus. *Hum Biol* 1997; 69 (4): 509–15.
100. Rajput-Williams J, Knott TJ, Wallis SC, Sweetnam P, Yarnell J, Cox N, et al. Variation of apolipoprotein-B gene is associated with obesity, high blood cholesterol levels, and increased risk of coronary heart disease. *Lancet* 1988; 2 (8626–8627): 1442–6.
101. Saha N, Tay JS, Heng CK, Humphries SE. DNA polymorphisms of the apolipoprotein B gene are associated with obesity and serum lipids in healthy Indians in Singapore. *Clin Genet* 1993; 44 (3): 113–20.
102. Hixson JE, Almasy L, Cole S, Birnbaum S, Mitchell BD, Mahaney MC, et al. Normal variation in leptin levels in associated with polymorphisms in the proopiomelanocortin gene, *POMC*. *J Clin Endocrinol Metab* 1999; 84 (9): 3187–91.
103. del Giudice EM, Cirillo G, Santoro N, D'Urso L, Carbone MT, Di TR, et al. Molecular screening of the proopiomelanocortin (POMC) gene in Italian obese children: report of three new mutations. *Int J Obes Relat Metab Disord* 2001; 25 (1): 61–7.
104. Heinonen P, Koulu M, Pesonen U, Karvonen MK, Rissanen A, Laakso M, et al. Identification of a three-amino acid deletion in the alpha2B-adrenergic receptor that is associated with reduced basal metabolic rate in obese subjects. *J Clin Endocrinol Metab* 1999; 84 (7): 2429–33.
105. Celi FS, Negri C, Tanner K, Raben N, De Pablo F, Rovira A, et al. Molecular scanning for mutations in the insulin receptor substrate-1 (IRS-1) gene in Mexican Americans with Type 2 diabetes mellitus. *Diabetes Metab Res Rev* 2000; 16 (5): 370–7.
106. Krempler F, Hell E, Winkler C, Breban D, Patsch W. Plasma leptin levels: interaction of obesity with a common variant of insulin receptor substrate-1. *Arterioscler Thromb Vasc Biol* 1998; 18 (11): 1686–90.
107. Lei HH, Coresh J, Shuldiner AR, Boerwinkle E, Brancati FL. Variants of the insulin receptor substrate-1 and fatty acid binding protein 2 genes and the risk of type 2 diabetes, obesity, and hyperinsulinemia in African Americans: the Atherosclerosis Risk in Communities Study. *Diabetes* 1999; 48 (9): 1868–72.
108. Ukkola O, Ravussin E, Jacobson P, Snyder EE, Chagnon M, Sjostrom L, et al. Mutations in the preproghrelin/ghrelin gene associated with obesity in humans. *J Clin Endocrinol Metab* 2001; 86 (8): 3996–9.
109. Hsueh WC, Mitchell BD, Schneider JL, St Jean PL, Pollin TI, Ehm MG, et al. Genome-wide scan of obesity in the Old Order Amish. *J Clin Endocrinol Metab* 2001; 86 (3): 1199–205.
110. Cole SA, Mitchell BD, Hsueh WC, Pineda P, Beamer BA, Shuldiner AR, et al. The Pro12Ala variant of peroxisome proliferator-activated receptor-gamma2 (PPAR-gamma2) is associated with measures of obesity in Mexican Americans. *Int J Obes Relat Metab Disord* 2000; 24 (4): 522–4.
111. Deeb SS, Fajas L, Nemoto M, Pihlajamaki J, Mykkanen L, Kuusisto J, et al. A Pro12Ala substitution in PPARgamma2 associated with decreased receptor activity, lower body mass index and improved insulin sensitivity. *Nat Genet* 1998; 20 (3): 284–7.
112. Ek J, Urhammer SA, Sorensen TI, Andersen T, Auwerx J, Pedersen O. Homozygosity of the Pro12Ala variant of the peroxisome proliferation-activated receptor-gamma2 (PPAR-gamma2): divergent modulating effects on body mass index in obese and lean Caucasian men. *Diabetologia* 1999; 42 (7): 892–5.
113. Lei HH, Chen MH, Yang WS, Chiu MC, Chen MC, Tai TY, et al. Peroxisome proliferator-activated receptor gamma2 Pro12Ala gene variant is strongly associated with larger body mass in the Taiwanese. *Metabolism* 2000; 49 (10): 1267–70.
114. Meirhaeghe A, Fajas L, Helbecque N, Cottel D, Lebel P, Dallongeville J, et al. A genetic polymorphism of the peroxisome proliferator-activated receptor gamma gene influences plasma leptin levels in obese humans. *Hum Mol Genet* 1998; 7 (3): 435–40.
115. Meirhaeghe A, Fajas L, Helbecque N, Cottel D, Auwerx J, Deeb SS, et al. Impact of the peroxisome proliferator activated receptor gamma2 Pro12Ala polymorphism on adiposity, lipids and non-insulin-dependent diabetes mellitus. *Int J Obes Relat Metab Disord* 2000; 24 (2): 195–9.
116. Ristow M, Muller-Wieland D, Pfeiffer A, Krone W, Kahn CR. Obesity associated with a mutation in a genetic regulator of adipocyte differentiation. *N Engl J Med* 1998; 339 (14): 953–9.
117. Vaccaro O, Mancini FP, Ruffa G, Sabatino L, Colantuoni V, Riccardi G. Pro12Ala mutation in the peroxisome proliferator-activated receptor gamma2 (PPARgamma2) and severe obesity: a case-control study. *Int J Obes Relat Metab Disord* 2000; 24 (9): 1195–9.
118. Valve R, Sivenius K, Miettinen R, Pihlajamaki J, Rissanen A, Deeb SS, et al. Two polymorphisms in the peroxisome proliferator-activated receptor-gamma gene are associated with severe overweight among obese women. *J Clin Endocrinol Metab* 1999; 84 (10): 3708–12.
119. Vijayaraghavan S, Hitman GA, Kopelman PG. Apolipoprotein-D polymorphism: a genetic marker for obesity and hyperinsulinemia. *J Clin Endocrinol Metab* 1994; 79 (2): 568–70.

120. Stumvoll M, Tschritter O, Fritsche A, Staiger H, Renn W, Weisser M, et al. Association of the T-G polymorphism in adiponectin (exon 2) with obesity and insulin sensitivity: interaction with family history of type 2 diabetes. *Diabetes* 2002; 51 (1): 37–41.
121. Funakoshi A, Miyasaka K, Matsumoto H, Yamamori S, Takiguchi S, Kataoka K, et al. Gene structure of human cholecystokinin (CCK) type-A receptor: body fat content is related to CCK type-A receptor gene promoter polymorphism. *FEBS Lett* 2000; 466 (2–3): 264–6.
122. Hegele RA, Harris SB, Hanley AJ, Sadikian S, Connelly PW, Zinman B. Genetic variation of intestinal fatty acid-binding protein associated with variation in body mass in aboriginal Canadians. *J Clin Endocrinol Metab* 1996; 81 (12): 4334–7.
123. Kim CH, Yun SK, Byun DW, Yoo MH, Lee KU, Suh KI. Codon 54 polymorphism of the fatty acid binding protein 2 gene is associated with increased fat oxidation and hyperinsulinemia, but not with intestinal fatty acid absorption in Korean men. *Metabolism* 2001; 50 (4): 473–6.
124. Yamada K, Yuan X, Ishiyama S, Koyama K, Ichikawa F, Koyanagi A, et al. Association between Ala54Thr substitution of the fatty acid-binding protein 2 gene with insulin resistance and intra-abdominal fat thickness in Japanese men. *Diabetologia* 1997; 40 (6): 706–10.
125. Fumeron F, Durack-Bown I, Betoulle D, Cassard-Doulcier AM, Tuzet S, Bouillaud F, et al. Polymorphisms of uncoupling protein (UCP) and beta3 adrenoreceptor genes in obese people submitted to a low calorie diet. *Int J Obes Relat Metab Disord* 1996; 20 (12): 1051–4.
126. Heilbronn LK, Kind KL, Pancewicz E, Morris AM, Noakes M, Clifton PM. Association of -3826 G variant in uncoupling protein-1 with increased BMI in overweight Australian women. *Diabetologia* 2000; 43 (2): 242–4.
127. Kogure A, Yoshida T, Sakane N, Umekawa T, Takakura Y, Kondo M. Synergic effect of polymorphisms in uncoupling protein 1 and beta3-adrenergic receptor genes on weight loss in obese Japanese. *Diabetologia* 1998; 41 (11): 1399.
128. Jenkinson CP, Cray K, Walder K, Herzog H, Hanson, Ravussin E. Novel polymorphisms in the neuropeptide–Y Y5 receptor associated with obesity in Pima Indians. *Int J Obes Relat Metab Disord* 2000; 24 (5): 580–4.
129. Challis BG, Yeo GS, Farooqi IS, Luan J, Aminian S, Halsall DJ, et al. The CART gene and human obesity: mutational analysis and population genetics. *Diabetes* 2000; 49 (5): 872–5.
130. Yamada K, Yuan X, Otabe S, Koyanagi A, Koyama W, Makita Z. Sequencing of the putative promoter region of the cocaine- and amphetamine-regulated-transcript gene and identification of polymorphic sites associated with obesity. *Int J Obes Relat Metab Disord* 2002; 26 (1): 132–6.
131. Buemann B, Vohl MC, Chagnon M, Chagnon YC, Gagnon J, Perusse L, et al. Abdominal visceral fat is associated with a *BcI*I restriction fragment length polymorphism at the glucocorticoid receptor gene locus. *Obes Res* 1997; 5 (3): 186–92.
132. Dobson MG, Redfern CP, Unwin N, Weaver JU. The N363S polymorphism of the glucocorticoid receptor: potential contribution to central obesity in men and lack of association with other risk factors for coronary heart disease and diabetes mellitus. *J Clin Endocrinol Metab* 2001; 86 (5): 2270–4.
133. Rosmond R, Chagnon YC, Holm G, Chagnon M, Perusse L, Lindell K, et al. A glucocorticoid receptor gene marker is associated with abdominal obesity, leptin, and dysregulation of the hypothalamic–pituitary–adrenal axis. *Obes Res* 2000; 8 (3): 211–8.
134. Ukkola O, Rankinen T, Weisnagel SJ, Sun G, Perusse L, Chagnon YC, et al. Interactions among the alpha2-, beta2-, and beta3-adrenergic receptor genes and obesity-related phenotypes in the Quebec Family Study. *Metabolism* 2000; 49 (8): 1063–70.
135. Ukkola O, Tremblay A, Bouchard C. Beta-2 adrenergic receptor variants are associated with subcutaneous fat accumulation in response to long-term overfeeding. *Int J Obes Relat Metab Disord* 2001; 25 (11): 1604–8.
136. Bengtsson K, Orho-Melander M, Melander O, Lindblad U, Ranstam J, Rastam L, et al. Beta(2)-adrenergic receptor gene variation and hypertension in subjects with type 2 diabetes. *Hypertension* 2001; 37 (5): 1303–8.
137. Ehrenborg E, Skogsberg J, Ruotolo G, Large V, Eriksson P, Arner P, et al. The Q/E27 polymorphism in the beta2-adrenoceptor gene is associated with increased body weight and dyslipoproteinaemia involving triglyceride-rich lipoproteins. *J Intern Med* 2000; 247 (6): 651–6.
138. Ishiyama-Shigemoto S, Yamada K, Yuan X, Ichikawa F, Nonaka K. Association of polymorphisms in the beta2-adrenergic receptor gene with obesity, hypertriglyceridaemia, and diabetes mellitus. *Diabetologia* 1999; 42 (1): 98–101.
139. Large V, Hellstrom L, Reynisdottir S, Lonnqvist F, Eriksson P, Lannfelt L, et al. Human beta-2 adrenoceptor gene polymorphisms are highly frequent in obesity and associate with altered adipocyte beta-2 adrenoceptor function. *J Clin Invest* 1997; 100 (12): 3005–13.
140. Meirhaeghe A, Helbecque N, Cottel D, Amouyel P. Beta2-adrenoceptor gene polymorphism, body weight, and physical activity. *Lancet* 1999; 353 (9156): 896.
141. Mori Y, Kim–Motoyama H, Ito Y, Katakura T, Yasuda K, Ishiyama-Shigemoto S, et al. The Gln27Glu beta2-adrenergic receptor variant is associated with obesity due to subcutaneous fat accumulation in Japanese men. *Biochem Biophys Res Commun* 1999; 258 (1): 138–40.
142. Rosmond R, Ukkola O, Chagnon M, Bouchard C, Bjorntorp P. Polymorphisms of the beta2-adrenergic receptor gene (*ADRB2*) in relation to cardiovascular risk factors in men. *J Intern Med* 2000; 248 (3): 239–44.
143. Yamada K, Ishiyama-Shigemoto S, Ichikawa F, Yuan X, Koyanagi A, Koyama W, et al. Polymorphism in the 5′-leader cistron of the beta2-adrenergic receptor gene associated with obesity and type 2 diabetes. *J Clin Endocrinol Metab* 1999; 84 (5): 1754–7.
144. Herrmann SM, Ricard S, Nicaud V, Mallet C, Arveiler D, Evans A, et al. Polymorphisms of the tumour necrosis factor-alpha gene, coronary heart disease and obesity. *Eur J Clin Invest* 1998; 28 (1): 59–66.
145. Hoffstedt J, Eriksson P, Hellstrom L, Rossner S, Ryden M, Arner P. Excessive fat accumulation is associated with the TNF alpha-308 G/A promoter polymorphism in women but not in men. *Diabetologia* 2000; 43 (1): 117–20.
146. Kamizono S, Yamada K, Seki N, Higuchi T, Kimura A, Nonaka K, et al. Susceptible locus for obese type 2 diabetes mellitus in the 5′-flanking region of the tumor necrosis factor-alpha gene. *Tissue Antigens* 2000; 55 (5): 449–52.

147. Norman RA, Bogardus C, Ravussin E. Linkage between obesity and a marker near the tumor necrosis factor-alpha locus in Pima Indians. *J Clin Invest* 1995; 96 (1): 158–62.
148. Pausova Z, Deslauriers B, Gaudet D, Tremblay J, Kotchen TA, Larochelle P, et al. Role of tumor necrosis factor-alpha gene locus in obesity and obesity-associated hypertension in French Canadians. *Hypertension* 2000; 36 (1): 14–9.
149. Speer G, Cseh K, Winkler G, Vargha P, Braun E, Takacs I, et al. Vitamin D and estrogen receptor gene polymorphisms in type 2 diabetes mellitus and in android type obesity. *Eur J Endocrinol* 2001; 144 (4): 385–9.
150. Hattersley AT, Beards F, Ballantyne E, Appleton M, Harvey R, Ellard S. Mutations in the glucokinase gene of the fetus result in reduced birth weight. *Nat Genet* 1998; 19 (3): 268–70.
151. Bray MS, Boerwinkle E, Hanis CL. Sequence variation within the neuropeptide Y gene and obesity in Mexican Americans. *Obes Res* 2000; 8 (3): 219–26.
152. Karvonen MK, Koulu M, Pesonen U, Uusitupa MI, Tammi A, Viikari J, et al. Leucine 7 to proline 7 polymorphism in the prepроneuropeptide Y is associated with birth weight and serum triglyceride concentration in preschool aged children. *J Clin Endocrinol Metab* 2000; 85 (4): 1455–60.
153. Busch CP, Ramdath DD, Ramsewak S, Hegele RA. Association of PON2 variation with birth weight in Trinidadian neonates of South Asian ancestry. *Pharmacogenetics* 1999; 9 (3): 351–6.
154. Butler MG, Hedges L, Hovis CL, Feurer ID. Genetic variants of the human obesity (OB) gene in subjects with and without Prader–Willi syndrome: comparison with body mass index and weight. *Clin Genet* 1998; 54 (5): 385–93.
155. Hager J, Clement K, Francke S, Dina C, Raison J, Lahlou N, et al. A polymorphism in the 5′ untranslated region of the human ob gene is associated with low leptin levels. *Int J Obes Relat Metab Disord* 1998; 22 (3): 200–5.
156. Le Stunff C, Le Bihan C, Schork NJ, Bougneres P. A common promoter variant of the leptin gene is associated with changes in the relationship between serum leptin and fat mass in obese girls. *Diabetes* 2000; 49 (12): 2196–200.
157. Li WD, Reed DR, Lee JH, Xu W, Kilker RL, Sodam BR, et al. Sequence variants in the 5′ flanking region of the leptin gene are associated with obesity in women. *Ann Hum Genet* 1999; 63 (pt 3): 227–34.
158. Mammes O, Betoulle D, Aubert R, Giraud V, Tuzet S, Petiet A, et al. Novel polymorphisms in the 5′ region of the *LEP* gene: association with leptin levels and response to low-calorie diet in human obesity. *Diabetes* 1998; 47 (3): 487–9.
159. Mammes O, Betoulle D, Aubert R, Herbeth B, Siest G, Fumeron F. Association of the G-2548A polymorphism in the 5′ region of the *LEP* gene with overweight. *Ann Hum Genet* 2000; 64 (pt 5): 391–4.
160. Oksanen L, Ohman M, Heiman M, Kainulainen K, Kaprio J, Mustajoki P, et al. Markers for the gene *ob* and serum leptin levels in human morbid obesity. *Hum Genet* 1997; 99 (5): 559–64.
161. Shintani M, Ikegami H, Yamato E, Kawaguchi Y, Fujisawa T, Nakagawa Y, et al. A novel microsatellite polymorphism in the human OB gene: a highly polymorphic marker for linkage analysis. *Diabetologia* 1996; 39 (11): 1398–401.
162. Garenc C, Perusse L, Bergeron J, Gagnon J, Chagnon YC, Borecki IB, et al. Evidence of LPL gene-exercise interaction for body fat and LPL activity: the HERITAGE Family Study. *J Appl Physiol* 2001; 91 (3): 1334–40.
163. Jemaa R, Tuzet S, Portos C, Betoulle D, Apfelbaum M, Fumeron F. Lipoprotein lipase gene polymorphisms: associations with hypertriglyceridemia and body mass index in obese people. *Int J Obes Relat Metab Disord* 1995; 19 (4): 270–4.
164. Festa A, Krugluger W, Shnawa N, Hopmeier P, Haffner SM, Schernthaner G. Trp64Arg polymorphism of the beta3-adrenergic receptor gene in pregnancy: association with mild gestational diabetes mellitus. *J Clin Endocrinol Metab* 1999; 84 (5): 1695–9.
165. Nagase T, Aoki A, Yamamoto M, Yasuda H, Kado S, Nishikawa M, et al. Lack of association between the Trp64Arg mutation in the beta3-adrenergic receptor gene and obesity in Japanese men: a longitudinal analysis. *J Clin Endocrinol Metab* 1997; 82 (4): 1284–7.
166. Clement K, Vaisse C, Manning BS, Basdevant A, Guy-Grand B, Ruiz J, et al. Genetic variation in the beta3-adrenergic receptor and an increased capacity to gain weight in patients with morbid obesity. *N Engl J Med* 1995; 333 (6): 352–4.
167. Widen E, Lehto M, Kanninen T, Walston J, Shuldiner AR, Groop LC. Association of a polymorphism in the beta3-adrenergic-receptor gene with features of the insulin resistance syndrome in Finns. *N Engl J Med* 1995; 333 (6): 348–51.
168. Ongphiphadhanakul B, Rajatanavin R, Chanprasertyothin S, Piaseu N, Chailurkit L, Komindr S, et al. Relation of beta3-adrenergic receptor gene mutation to total body fat but not percent body fat and insulin levels in Thais. *Metabolism* 1999; 48 (5): 564–7.
169. Kadowaki H, Yasuda K, Iwamoto K, Otabe S, Shimokawa K, Silver K, et al. A mutation in the beta3-adrenergic receptor gene is associated with obesity and hyperinsulinemia in Japanese subjects. *Biochem Biophys Res Commun* 1995; 215 (2): 555–60.
170. Urhammer SA, Clausen JO, Hansen T, Pedersen O. Insulin sensitivity and body weight changes in young white carriers of the codon 64 amino acid polymorphism of the beta3-adrenergic receptor gene. *Diabetes* 1996; 45 (8): 1115–20.
171. Fujisawa T, Ikegami H, Yamato E, Takekawa K, Nakagawa Y, Hamada Y, et al. Association of Trp64Arg mutation of the beta3-adrenergic-receptor with NIDDM and body weight gain. *Diabetologia* 1996; 39 (3): 349–52.
172. Oksanen L, Mustajoki P, Kaprio J, Kainulainen K, Janne O, Peltonen L, et al. Polymorphism of the beta3-adrenergic receptor gene in morbid obesity. *Int J Obes Relat Metab Disord* 1996; 20 (12): 1055–61.
173. Sakane N, Yoshida T, Umekawa T, Kondo M, Sakai Y, Takahashi T. Beta3-adrenergic-receptor polymorphism: a genetic marker for visceral fat obesity and the insulin resistance syndrome. *Diabetologia* 1997; 40 (2): 200–4.
174. Kim-Motoyama H, Yasuda K, Yamaguchi T, Yamada N, Katakura T, Shuldiner AR, et al. A mutation of the beta3-adrenergic receptor is associated with visceral obesity but decreased serum triglyceride. *Diabetologia* 1997; 40 (4): 469–72.
175. Mitchell BD, Blangero J, Comuzzie AG, Almasy LA, Shuldiner AR, Silver K, et al. A paired sibling analysis of the beta-3 adrenergic receptor and obesity in Mexican Americans. *J Clin Invest* 1998; 101 (3): 584–7.

176. Strazzullo P, Iacone R, Siani A, Cappuccio FP, Russo O, Barba G, et al. Relationship of the Trp64Arg polymorphism of the beta3-adrenoceptor gene to central adiposity and high blood pressure: interaction with age. Cross-sectional and longitudinal findings of the Olivetti Prospective Heart Study. *J Hypertens* 2001; 19 (3): 399–406.
177. Endo K, Yanagi H, Hirano C, Hamaguchi H, Tsuchiya S, Tomura S. Association of Trp64Arg polymorphism of the beta3-adrenergic receptor gene and no association of Gln223Arg polymorphism of the leptin receptor gene in Japanese schoolchildren with obesity. *Int J Obes Relat Metab Disord* 2000; 24 (4): 443–9.
178. Higashi K, Ishikawa T, Ito T, Yonemura A, Shige H, Nakamura H. Association of a genetic variation in the beta 3-adrenergic receptor gene with coronary heart disease among Japanese. *Biochem Biophys Res Commun* 1997; 232 (3): 728–30.
179. Hoffstedt J, Poirier O, Thorne A, Lonnqvist F, Herrmann SM, Cambien F, et al. Polymorphism of the human beta3-adrenoceptor gene forms a well-conserved haplotype that is associated with moderate obesity and altered receptor function. *Diabetes* 1999; 48 (1): 203–5.
180. Jeyasingam CL, Bryson JM, Caterson ID, Yue DK, Donnelly R. Expression of the beta 3-adrenoceptor gene polymorphism (Trp64Arg) in obese diabetic and non-diabetic subjects. *Clin Exp Pharmacol Physiol* 1997; 24 (9–10): 733–5.
181. McFarlane-Anderson N, Bennett F, Wilks R, Howell S, Newsome C, Cruickshank K, et al. The Trp64Arg mutation of the beta3-adrenergic receptor is associated with hyperglycemia and current body mass index in Jamaican women. *Metabolism* 1998; 47 (5): 617–21.
182. Shima Y, Tsukada T, Nakanishi K, Ohta H. Association of the Trp64Arg mutation of the beta3-adrenergic receptor with fatty liver and mild glucose intolerance in Japanese subjects. *Clin Chim Acta* 1998; 274 (2): 167–76.
183. Thomas GN, Tomlinson B, Chan JC, Young RP, Critchley JA. The Trp64Arg polymorphism of the beta3-adrenergic receptor gene and obesity in Chinese subjects with components of the metabolic syndrome. *Int J Obes Relat Metab Disord* 2000; 24 (5): 545–51.
184. Wolford JK, Bogardus C, Prochazka M. Polymorphism in the 3′ untranslated region of MTG8 is associated with obesity in Pima Indian males. *Biochem Biophys Res Commun* 1998; 246 (3): 624–6.
185. Lin WH, Chiu KC, Chang HM, Lee KC, Tai TY, Chuang LM. Molecular scanning of the human sorbin and SH3-domain-containing-1 (SORBS1) gene: positive association of the T228A polymorphism with obesity and type 2 diabetes. *Hum Mol Genet* 2001; 10 (17): 1753–60.
186. Oppert JM, Tourville J, Chagnon M, Mauriege P, Dionne FT, Perusse L, et al. DNA polymorphisms in the alpha2- and beta2-adrenoceptor genes and regional fat distribution in humans: association and linkage studies. *Obes Res* 1995; 3 (3): 249–55.
187. O'Dell SD, Bujac SR, Miller GJ, Day IN. Associations of IGF2 ApaI RFLP and INS VNTR class I allele size with obesity. *Eur J Hum Genet* 1999; 7 (7): 821–7.
188. Dunger DB, Ong KKL, Huxtable SJ, Sherriff A, Woods KA, Ahmed ML, et al. Association of the INS VNTR with size at birth. *Nat Genet* 1998; 19: 98–100.
189. Weaver JU, Kopelman PG, Hitman GA. Central obesity and hyperinsulinaemia in women are associated with polymorphism in the 5′ flanking region of the human insulin gene. *Eur J Clin Invest* 1992; 22 (4): 265–70.
190. Hani EH, Clement K, Velho G, Vionnet N, Hager J, Philippi A, et al. Genetic studies of the sulfonylurea receptor gene locus in NIDDM and in morbid obesity among French Caucasians. *Diabetes* 1997; 46 (4): 688–94.
191. Astrup A, Toubro S, Dalgaard LT, Urhammer SA, Sorensen TI, Pedersen O. Impact of the v/v 55 polymorphism of the uncoupling protein 2 gene on 24-h energy expenditure and substrate oxidation. *Int J Obes Relat Metab Disord* 1999; 23 (10): 1030–4.
192. Cassell PG, Neverova M, Janmohamed S, Uwakwe N, Qureshi A, McCarthy MI, et al. An uncoupling protein 2 gene variant is associated with a raised body mass index but not Type II diabetes. *Diabetologia* 1999; 42 (6): 688–92.
193. Esterbauer H, Schneitler C, Oberkofler H, Ebenbichler C, Paulweber B, Sandhofer F, et al. A common polymorphism in the promoter of UCP2 is associated with decreased risk of obesity in middle-aged humans. *Nat Genet* 2001; 28 (2): 178–83.
194. Evans D, Minouchehr S, Hagemann G, Mann WA, Wendt D, Wolf A, et al. Frequency of and interaction between polymorphisms in the beta3-adrenergic receptor and in uncoupling proteins 1 and 2 and obesity in Germans. *Int J Obes Relat Metab Disord* 2000; 24 (10): 1239–45.
195. Nordfors L, Heimburger O, Lonnqvist F, Lindholm B, Helmrich J, Schalling M, et al. Fat tissue accumulation during peritoneal dialysis is associated with a polymorphism in uncoupling protein 2. *Kidney Int* 2000; 57 (4): 1713–9.
196. Walder K, Norman RA, Hanson RL, Schrauwen P, Neverova M, Jenkinson CP, et al. Association between uncoupling protein polymorphisms (UCP2–UCP3) and energy metabolism/obesity in Pima Indians. *Hum Mol Genet* 1998; 7 (9): 1431–5.
197. Yanovski JA, Diament AL, Sovik KN, Nguyen TT, Li H, Sebring NG, et al. Associations between uncoupling protein 2, body composition, and resting energy expenditure in lean and obese African American, white, and Asian children. *Am J Clin Nutr* 2000; 71 (6): 1405–20.
198. Argyropoulos G, Brown AM, Willi SM, Zhu J, He Y, Reitman M, et al. Effects of mutations in the human uncoupling protein 3 gene on the respiratory quotient and fat oxidation in severe obesity and type 2 diabetes. *J Clin Invest* 1998; 102 (7): 1345–51.
199. Cassell PG, Saker PJ, Huxtable SJ, Kousta E, Jackson AE, Hattersley AT, et al. Evidence that single nucleotide polymorphism in the uncoupling protein 3 (UCP3) gene influences fat distribution in women of European and Asian origin. *Diabetologia* 2000; 43 (12): 1558–64.
200. Halsall DJ, Luan J, Saker P, Huxtable S, Farooqi IS, Keogh J, et al. Uncoupling protein 3 genetic variants in human obesity: the c-55t promoter polymorphism is negatively correlated with body mass index in a UK Caucasian population. *Int J Obes Relat Metab Disord* 2001; 25 (4): 472–7.
201. Lanouette CM, Giacobino JP, Perusse L, Lacaille M, Yvon C, Chagnon M, et al. Association between uncoupling protein 3 gene and obesity-related phenotypes in the Quebec Family Study. *Mol Med* 2001; 7 (7): 433–41.
202. Lanouette CM, Chagnon YC, Rice T, Perusse L, Muzzin P, Giacobino JP, et al. Uncoupling protein 3 gene is associated with body composition changes with training in HERITAGE study. *J Appl Physiol* 2002; 92 (3): 1111–8.

203. Otabe S, Clement K, Dubois S, Lepretre F, Pelloux V, Leibel R, et al. Mutation screening and association studies of the human uncoupling protein 3 gene in normoglycemic and diabetic morbidly obese patients. *Diabetes* 1999; 48 (1): 206–8.
204. Otabe S, Clement K, Dina C, Pelloux V, Guy-Grand B, Froguel P, et al. A genetic variation in the 5′ flanking region of the UCP3 gene is associated with body mass index in humans in interaction with physical activity. *Diabetologia* 2000; 43 (2): 245–9.
205. Fisher RM, Burke H, Nicaud VV, Ehnholm C, Humphries SE. Effect of variation in the apo A-IV gene on body mass index and fasting and postprandial lipids in the European Atherosclerosis Research Study II. *J Lipid Res* 1999; 40 (2): 287–94.
206. Lefevre M, Lovejoy JC, DeFelice SM, Keener JW, Bray GA, Ryan DH, et al. Common apolipoprotein A-IV variants are associated with differences in body mass index levels and percentage body fat. *Int J Obes Relat Metab Disord* 2000; 24 (8): 945–53.
207. Jenkinson CP, Hanson R, Cray K, Wiedrich C, Knowler WC, Bogardus C, et al. Association of dopamine D2 receptor polymorphisms Ser311Cys and *Taq*IA with obesity or type 2 diabetes mellitus in Pima Indians. *Int J Obes Relat Metab Disord* 2000; 24 (10): 1233–8.
208. Spitz MR, Detry MA, Pillow P, Hu YH, Amos CI, Hong WK, et al. Variant alleles of the D2 dopamine receptor gene and obesity. *Nutr Res* 2000; 20: 371–80.
209. Thomas GN, Tomlinson B, Critchley JA. Modulation of blood pressure and obesity with the dopamine D2 receptor gene *Taq*I polymorphism. *Hypertension* 2000; 36 (2): 177–82.
210. Thomas GN, Critchley JA, Tomlinson B, Cockram CS, Chan JC. Relationships between the *Taq*I polymorphism of the dopamine D2 receptor and blood pressure in hyperglycaemic and normoglycaemic Chinese subjects. *Clin Endocrinol (Oxf)* 2001; 55 (5): 605–11.
211. Gutersohn A, Naber C, Muller N, Erbel R, Siffert W. G protein beta3 subunit 825 TT genotype and post-pregnancy weight retention. *Lancet* 2000; 355 (9211): 1240–1.
212. Hegele RA, Anderson C, Young TK, Connelly PW. G-protein beta3 subunit gene splice variant and body fat distribution in Nunavut Inuit. *Genome Res* 1999; 9 (10): 972–7.
213. Hocher B, Slowinski T, Stolze T, Pleschka A, Neumayer HH, Halle H. Association of maternal G protein beta3 subunit 825T allele with low birthweight. *Lancet* 2000; 355 (9211): 1241–2.
214. Rankinen T, Rice T, Leon AS, Skinner JS, Wilmore JH, Rao DC, et al. G protein beta 3 polymorphism and hemodynamic and body composition phenotypes in the HERITAGE Family Study. *Physiol Genomics* 2002; 8 (2): 151–7.
215. Siffert W, Forster P, Jockel KH, Mvere DA, Brinkmann B, Naber C, et al. Worldwide ethnic distribution of the G protein beta3 subunit 825T allele and its association with obesity in Caucasian, Chinese, and Black African individuals. *J Am Soc Nephrol* 1999; 10 (9): 1921–30.
216. Siffert W, Naber C, Walla M, Ritz E. G protein beta3 subunit 825T allele and its potential association with obesity in hypertensive individuals. *J Hypertens* 1999; 17 (8): 1095–8.
217. Ye WZ, Reis AF, Dubois-Laforgue D, Bellanne-Chantelot C, Timsit J, Velho G. Vitamin D receptor gene polymorphisms are associated with obesity in type 2 diabetic subjects with early age of onset. *Eur J Endocrinol* 2001; 145 (2): 181–6.
218. Sun G, Gagnon J, Chagnon YC, Perusse L, Despres JP, Leon AS, et al. Association and linkage between an insulin-like growth factor-1 gene polymorphism and fat free mass in the HERITAGE Family Study. *Int J Obes Relat Metab Disord* 1999; 23 (9): 929–35.
219. Acton S, Osgood D, Donoghue M, Corella D, Pocovi M, Cenarro A, et al. Association of polymorphisms at the SR-BI gene locus with plasma lipid levels and body mass index in a white population. *Arterioscler Thromb Vasc Biol* 1999; 19 (7): 1734–43.
220. Aubert R, Betoulle D, Herbeth B, Siest G, Fumeron F. 5-HT2A receptor gene polymorphism is associated with food and alcohol intake in obese people. *Int J Obes Relat Metab Disord* 2000; 24 (7): 920–4.
221. Chouchane L, Danguir J, Beji C, Bouassida K, Camoin L, Sfar H, et al. Genetic variation in the stress protein hsp70-2 gene is highly associated with obesity. *Int J Obes Relat Metab Disord* 2001; 25 (4): 462–6.
222. Oeffner F, Bornholdt D, Ziegler A, Hinney A, Gorg T, Gerber G, et al. Significant association between a silent polymorphism in the neuromedin B gene and body weight in German children and adolescents. *Acta Diabetol* 2000; 37 (2): 93–101.
223. Iwai N, Katsuya T, Mannami T, Higaki J, Ogihara T, Kokame K, et al. Association between SAH, an acyl-CoA synthetase gene, and hypertriglyceridemia, obesity, and hypertension. *Circulation* 2002; 105 (1): 41–7.
224. Chagnon YC, Chen WJ, Perusse L, Chagnon M, Nadeau A, Wilkison WO, et al. Linkage and association studies between the melanocortin receptors 4 and 5 genes and obesity-related phenotypes in the Quebec Family Study. *Mol Med* 1997; 3 (10): 663–73.
225. Zee RYL, Lou YK, Morris BJ. Insertion variant in intron 9, but not microsatellite in intron 2, of the insulin receptor gene is associated with essential hypertension. *J Hypertens* 1994; 12 (suppl): S13–22.
226. Griffiths LR, Nyholt DR, Curtain RP, Gaffney PT, Morris BJ. Cross-sectional study of a microsatellite marker in the low density lipoprotein receptor gene in obese normotensives. *Clin Exp Pharmacol Physiol* 1995; 22 (6–7): 496–8.
227. Mattevi VS, Coimbra CE Jr, Santos RV, Salzano FM, Hutz MH. Association of the low-density lipoprotein receptor gene with obesity in Native American populations. *Hum Genet* 2000; 106 (5): 546–52.
228. Rutherford S, Nyholt DR, Curtain RP, Quinlan SR, Gaffney PT, Morris BJ, et al. Association of a low density lipoprotein receptor microsatellite variant with obesity. *Int J Obes Relat Metab Disord* 1997; 21 (11): 1032–7.
229. Zee RYL, Griffiths LR, Morris BJ. Marked association of a RFLP for the low density lipoprotein receptor gene with obesity in essential hypertensives. *Biochem Biophys Res Commun* 1992; 189: 965–71.
230. Zee RYL, Schrader AP, Robinson BG, Griffiths LR, Morris BJ. Association of *Hinc*II RFLP of low density lipoprotien receptor gene with obesity in essential hypertensives. *Clin Genet* 1995; 47: 118–21.
231. Garenc C, Perusse L, Chagnon YC, Rankinen T, Gagnon J, Borecki IB, et al. The hormone-sensitive lipase gene and body composition: the HERITAGE Family Study. *Int J Obes Relat Metab Disord* 2002; 26 (2): 220–7.

232. Magré J, Delepine M, Khallouf E, Gedde-Dahl T Jr, Van Maldergem L, Sobel E, et al. Identification of the gene altered in Berardinelli–Seip congenital lipodystrophy on chromosome 11q13. *Nat Genet* 2001; 28 (4): 365–70.
233. Yanagisawa Y, Hasegawa K, Dever GJ, Otto CT, Sakuma M, Shibata S, et al. Uncoupling protein 3 and peroxisome proliferator-activated receptor gamma2 contribute to obesity and diabetes in palauans. *Biochem Biophys Res Commun* 2001; 281 (3): 772–8.
234. Orho-Melander M, Almgren P, Kanninen T, Forsblom C, Groop LC. A paired-sibling analysis of the *Xba*I polymorphism in the muscle glycogen synthase gene. *Diabetologia* 1999; 42 (9): 1138–45.
235. Bottini E, Gloria-Bottini F. Adenosine deaminase and body mass index in non-insulin-dependent diabetes mellitus. *Metabolism* 1999; 48 (8): 949–51.
236. Evans D, Aberle J, Wendt D, Wolf A, Beisiegel U, Mann WA. A polymorphism, L162V, in the peroxisome proliferator-activated receptor alpha (PPARalpha) gene is associated with lower body mass index in patients with non-insulin-dependent diabetes mellitus. *J Mol Med* 2001; 79 (4): 198–204.
237. Yuan X, Yamada K, Ishiyama-Shigemoto S, Koyama W, Nonaka K. Identification of polymorphic loci in the promoter region of the serotonin 5-HT2C receptor gene and their association with obesity and type II diabetes. *Diabetologia* 2000; 43 (3): 373–6.
238. Perusse L, Chagnon YC. Summary of human linkage and association studies. *Behav Genet* 1997; 27 (4): 359–72.
239. Mauriège P, Bouchard C. Trp64Arg mutation in β3-adrenoceptor gene of doubtful significance for obesity and insulin resistance. *Lancet* 1996; 348: 698–9.
240. Chagnon YC, Perusse L, Bouchard C. Familial aggregation of obesity, candidate genes and quantitative trait loci. *Curr Opin Lipidol* 1997; 8 (4): 205–11.
241. Allison DB, Heo M, Faith MS, Pietrobelli A. Meta-analysis of the association of the Trp64Arg polymorphism in the beta3 adrenergic receptor with body mass index. *Int J Obes Relat Metab Disord* 1998; 22 (6): 559–66.
242. Fujisawa T, Ikegami H, Kawaguchi Y, Ogihara T. Meta-analysis of the association of Trp64Arg polymorphism of beta3-adrenergic receptor gene with body mass index. *J Clin Endocrinol Metab* 1998; 83 (7): 2441–4.
243. Kurokawa N, Nakai K, Kameo S, Liu ZM, Satoh H. Association of BMI with the beta3-adrenergic receptor gene polymorphism in Japanese: meta-analysis. *Obes Res* 2001; 9 (12): 741–5.
244. Comuzzie AG, Williams JT, Martin LJ, Blangero J. Searching for genes underlying normal variation in human adiposity. *J Mol Med* 2001; 79 (1): 57–70.
245. Rao DC. CAT scans, PET scans, and genomic scans. *Genet Epidemiol* 1998; 15 (1): 1–18.
246. Deng HW, Deng H, Liu YJ, Liu YZ, Xu FH, Shen H, et al. A genomewide linkage scan for quantitative-trait loci for obesity phenotypes. *Am J Hum Genet* 2002; 70 (5): 1138–51.
247. van der Kallen CJ, Cantor RM, van Greevenbroek MM, Geurts JM, Bouwman FG, Aouizerat BE, et al. Genome scan for adiposity in Dutch dyslipidemic families reveals novel quantitative trait loci for leptin, body mass index and soluble tumor necrosis factor receptor superfamily 1A. *Int J Obes Relat Metab Disord* 2000; 24 (11): 1381–91.
248. Norman RA, Tataranni PA, Pratley R, Thompson DB, Hanson RL, Prochazka M, et al. Autosomal genomic scan for loci linked to obesity and energy metabolism in Pima Indians. *Am J Hum Genet* 1998; 62 (3): 659–68.
249. Perusse L, Rice T, Chagnon YC, Despres JP, Lemieux S, Roy S, et al. A genome-wide scan for abdominal fat assessed by computed tomography in the Quebec Family Study. *Diabetes* 2001; 50 (3): 614–21.
250. Comuzzie AG, Hixson JE, Almasy L, Mitchell BD, Mahaney MC, Dyer TD, et al. A major quantitative trait locus determining serum leptin levels and fat mass is located on human chromosome 2. *Nat Genet* 1997; 15 (3): 273–6.
251. Hager J, Dina C, Francke S, Dubois S, Houari M, Vatin V, et al. A genome-wide scan for human obesity genes reveals a major susceptibility locus on chromosome 10. *Nat Genet* 1998; 20 (3): 304–8.
252. Rice T, Chagnon YC, Perusse L, Borecki IB, Ukkola O, Rankinen T, et al. A genomewide linkage scan for abdominal subcutaneous and visceral fat in black and white families: the HERITAGE Family Study. *Diabetes* 2002; 51 (3): 848–55.
253. Kissebah AH, Sonnenberg GE, Myklebust J, Goldstein M, Broman K, James RG, et al. Quantitative trait loci on chromosomes 3 and 17 influence phenotypes of the metabolic syndrome. *Proc Natl Acad Sci USA* 2000; 97 (26): 14478–83.
254. Zhu X, Cooper RS, Luke A, Chen G, Wu X, Kan D, et al. A genome-wide scan for obesity in African Americans. *Diabetes* 2002; 51 (2): 541–4.
255. Stone S, Abkevich V, Hunt SC, Gutin A, Russell DL, Neff CD, et al. A major predisposition locus for severe obesity, at 4p15-p14. *Am J Hum Genet* 2002; 70 (6): 1459–68.
256. Comuzzie AG, Funahashi T, Sonnenberg G, Martin LJ, Jacob HJ, Black AE, et al. The genetic basis of plasma variation in adiponectin, a global endophenotype for obesity and the metabolic syndrome. *J Clin Endocrinol Metab* 2001; 86 (9): 4321–5.
257. Lindsay RS, Kobes S, Knowler WC, Bennett PH, Hanson RL. Genome-wide linkage analysis assessing parent-of-origin effects in the inheritance of type 2 diabetes and BMI in Pima Indians. *Diabetes* 2001; 50 (12): 2850–7.
258. Walder K, Hanson RL, Kobes S, Knowler WC, Ravussin E. An autosomal genomic scan for loci linked to plasma leptin concentration in Pima Indians. *Int J Obes Relat Metab Disord* 2000; 24 (5): 559–65.
259. Chagnon YC, Borecki IB, Perusse L, Roy S, Lacaille M, Chagnon M, et al. Genome-wide search for genes related to the fat-free body mass in the Quebec family study. *Metabolism* 2000; 49 (2): 203–7.
260. Feitosa MF, Borecki IB, Rich SS, Arnett DK, Sholinsky P, Myers RH, et al. Quantitative-trait loci influencing body-mass index reside on chromosomes 7 and 13: the National Heart, Lung, and Blood Institute Family Heart Study. *Am J Hum Genet* 2002; 70 (1): 72–82.
261. Mitchell BD, Cole SA, Comuzzie AG, Almasy L, Blangero J, MacCluer JW, et al. A quantitative trait locus influencing BMI maps to the region of the beta-3 adrenergic receptor. *Diabetes* 1999; 48 (9): 1863–7.
262. Chagnon YC, Rice T, Perusse L, Borecki IB, Ho-Kim MA, Lacaille M, et al. Genomic scan for genes affecting body composition before and after training in Caucasians from HERITAGE. *J Appl Physiol* 2001; 90 (5): 1777–87.

263. Norman RA, Thompson DB, Foroud T, Garvey WT, Bennett PH, Bogardus C, et al. Genome wide search for genes influencing percent body fat in Pima Indians: suggestive linkage at chromosome 11q21-q22. *Am J Hum Genet* 1997; 60: 166–73.
264. Hanson RL, Ehm MG, Pettitt DJ, Prochazka M, Thompson DB, Timberlake D, et al. An autosomal genomic scan for loci linked to type II diabetes mellitus and body-mass index in Pima Indians. *Am J Hum Genet* 1998; 63 (4): 1130–8.
265. Ohman M, Oksanen L, Kaprio J, Koskenvuo M, Mustajoki P, Rissanen A, et al. Genome-wide scan of obesity in Finnish sibpairs reveals linkage to chromosome Xq24. *J Clin Endocrinol Metab* 2000; 85 (9): 3183–90.
266. Lee JH, Reed DR, Li WD, Xu W, Joo EJ, Kilker RL, et al. Genome scan for human obesity and linkage to markers in 20q13. *Am J Hum Genet* 1999; 64 (1): 196–209.
267. Rotimi CN, Comuzzie AG, Lowe WL, Luke A, Blangero J, Cooper RS. The quantitative trait locus on chromosome 2 for serum leptin levels is confirmed in African Americans. *Diabetes* 1999; 48 (3): 643–4.
268. Hinney A, Ziegler A, Oeffner F, Wedewardt C, Vogel M, Wulftange H, et al. Independent confirmation of a major locus for obesity on chromosome 10. *J Clin Endocrinol Metab* 2000; 85 (8): 2962–5.
269. Price RA, Li WD, Bernstein A, Crystal A, Golding EM, Weisberg SJ, et al. A locus affecting obesity in human chromosome region 10p12. *Diabetologia* 2001; 44 (3): 363–6.
270. Perola M, Ohman M, Hiekkalinna T, Leppavuori J, Pajukanta P, Wessman M, et al. Quantitative-trait locus analysis of body-mass index and of stature, by combined analysis of genome scans of five Finnish study groups. *Am J Hum Genet* 2001; 69 (1): 117–23.
271. Hunt SC, Abkevich V, Hensel CH, Gutin A, Neff CD, Russell DL, et al. Linkage of body mass index to chromosome 20 in Utah pedigrees. *Hum Genet* 2001; 109 (3): 279–85.
272. Bouchard C, Perusse L, Leblanc C. Using MZ twins in experimental research to test for the presence of a genotype–environment interaction effect. *Acta Genet Med Gemellol (Roma)* 1990; 39 (1): 85–9.
273. Bouchard C, Tremblay A, Despres JP, Nadeau A, Lupien PJ, Theriault G, et al. The response to long-term overfeeding in identical twins. *N Engl J Med* 1990; 322 (21): 1477–82.
274. Poehlman ET, Tremblay A, Despres JP, Fontaine E, Perusse L, Theriault G, et al. Genotype-controlled changes in body composition and fat morphology following overfeeding in twins. *Am J Clin Nutr* 1986; 43 (5): 723–31.
275. Bouchard C, Tremblay A, Despres JP, Theriault G, Nadeau A, Lupien PJ, et al. The response to exercise with constant energy intake in identical twins. *Obes Res* 1994; 2: 400–10.
276. Poehlman ET, Tremblay A, Nadeau A, Dussault J, Theriault G, Bouchard C. Heredity and changes in hormones and metabolic rates with short-term training. *Am J Physiol* 1986; 250 (6, pt 1): E711–7.
277. Poehlman ET, Tremblay A, Marcotte M, Perusse L, Theriault G, Bouchard C. Heredity and changes in body composition and adipose tissue metabolism after short-term exercise-training. *Eur J Appl Physiol Occup Physiol* 1987; 56 (4): 398–402.
278. Deriaz O, Tremblay A, Bouchard C. Non-linear weight gain with long term overfeeding in man. *Obes Res* 1993; 1: 179–85.
279. Norgan NG, Durnin JV. The effect of 6 weeks of overfeeding on the body weight, body composition, and energy metabolism of young men. *Am J Clin Nutr* 1980; 33 (5): 978–88.
280. Ravussin E, Schutz Y, Acheson KJ, Dusmet M, Bourquin L, Jequier E. Short-term, mixed-diet overfeeding in man: no evidence for "luxuskonsumption." *Am J Physiol* 1985; 249 (5, pt 1): E470–7.
281. Ukkola O, Tremblay A, Sun G, Chagnon YC, Bouchard C. Genetic variation at the uncoupling protein 1, 2 and 3 loci and the response to long-term overfeeding. *Eur J Clin Nutr* 2001; 55 (11): 1008–15.
282. Ukkola O, Tremblay A, Despres JP, Chagnon YC, Campfield LA, Bouchard C. Leptin receptor Gln223Arg variant is associated with a cluster of metabolic abnormalities in response to long-term overfeeding. *J Intern Med* 2000; 248 (5): 435–9.
283. Ukkola O, Sun G, Bouchard C. Insulin-like growth factor 2 (IGF2) and IGF-binding protein 1 (IGFBP1) gene variants are associated with overfeeding-induced metabolic changes. *Diabetologia* 2001; 44 (12): 2231–6.

33

The Role of Energy Expenditure in the Regulation of Energy Balance

Eric Ravussin and Leslie P. Kozak

Pennington Biomedical Research Center, Baton Rouge, LA, USA

Throughout evolution, humans and animals have evolved redundant mechanisms promoting accumulation of fat (minimal energy expenditure and maximal food intake) during periods of feast to survive periods of famine [1–3]. With the recent abrupt change in environmental conditions in which high fat food is constantly available and in which there is little need for physical activity (the current "pathoenvironment" or "toxic environment"), obesity has reached epidemic proportions in both industrialized countries and in urbanized populations around the world [4, 5].

Obesity results from a chronic imbalance between energy intake and energy expenditure. Hyperphagia, a low metabolic rate, low rates of fat oxidation, and an impaired sympathetic nervous activity characterize animal models of obesity. Similar metabolic factors have been found to characterize humans susceptible to weight gain. Despite the discovery of leptin more than 8 years ago and an unprecedented expansion of research efforts, our knowledge about the molecular mechanisms underlying obesity remains rudimentary. The cloning of genes corresponding to several mouse monogenic obesity syndromes and the subsequent characterization of the pathways involved have however shed some light, mostly on the regulation of food intake but much less on energy metabolism. This chapter will first state the premises of the regulation of energy balance, then review the variability of physiological mechanisms underlying the variability in energy balance, and finally summarize some of the important recent discoveries of the molecular mechanisms of energy expenditure.

ENERGY BALANCE EQUATIONS

The balance between energy intake and energy expenditure determines energy stores. Since living organisms must obey the first law of thermodynamics, the energy balance equation has been used to predict changes in body weight when energy intake or expenditure is changed. However, the classic equation of energy balance, which states that the body energy store is equal to energy intake minus energy expenditure, has provided both insight and confusion in the understanding of energy balance in humans. Much of the confusion comes from inappropriate energy calculations using the static equation of energy balance as described below.

Equation During Weight Maintenance

Energy Intake = Energy Expenditure

This equation is self-evident and quite accurate under conditions of weight maintenance as only limited changes in body composition are possible without changing body weight. It has been most useful in uncovering problems with reported energy intake. For example, most dietary intake studies show either no correlation or a negative correlation between energy intake and body weight [6, 7]. Even more confounding, obese subjects usually report only one half to two thirds of their total energy intake when compared with lean subjects who report 80–100% [8]. This gap between the food that obese people perceive themselves eating and what they actually eat has been termed the *eye–mouth gap* and represents a major challenge for

International Textbook of Diabetes Mellitus, Third Edition. Edited by R. A. DeFronzo, E. Ferrannini, H. Keen, and P. Zimmet.
 ISBN: 0-471-48655-8.

psychologists and psychiatrists interested in obesity and food intake [9]. The inverse correlation between self-reported intake and body weight is in marked contrast to studies of energy expenditure where there is a positive relationship. In addition to their greater fat mass, obese individuals have a greater fat-free mass, which is the main determinant of both resting and 24-h metabolic rate as measured in a respiratory chamber [10]. Many studies involving free-living individuals report measured energy expenditure using the doubly labeled water technique and energy intake using continuous recording of diet diaries [8, 11, 12].

Static Energy Balance Equation

Change in Energy Stores = Energy Intake − Energy Expenditure

This is the most common equation used in discussions and calculations of energy balance. Intuitively, it seems valid, but Alpert [13] has elegantly demonstrated that this equation is inadequate for calculations on living organisms, because it does not take into account the increasing energy expenditure with increasing weight [10, 14, 15]. Thus, a small initial increase in energy intake sustained over a number of years cannot lead to a large weight gain, as is often claimed. For example, if someone would increase energy intake by 100 kcal/day over baseline energy requirement for 40 years, this increase would result in a 160 kg weight gain using the above equation. Of course nobody would believe such a potential weight gain, but a lot of scientists would however still do this kind of calculation over a year period. In the above example, one can safely claim that a weight gain of the order of 2–3 kg is sufficient to offset the excess energy intake (100 kcal/day) and therefore stabilize the weight gain curve.

Dynamic Energy Balance Equation

Rate of Change of Energy Stores = Rate of Energy Intake − Rate of Energy Expenditure

The use of "rates" in this equation introduces time dependency thereby allowing the effect of changing energy stores on energy expenditure to enter into the calculation [13]. This explains why a small initial positive energy balance (for example, from an increased energy intake or a lower thermic effect of food) will not lead to large weight increases over a number of years. After a short period of positive energy balance, the energy stores (fat mass and fat-free mass) will increase and cause an increase in energy expenditure, which will balance the increased energy intake. The individual will then once again be in energy balance, but with a higher energy intake, higher energy expenditure, and higher energy stores. Weight gain can therefore be viewed not only as the consequence of an initial positive energy balance but also as the mechanism by which energy balance is eventually restored. How is intake balanced against expenditure, and how might a chronic mismatch between the two occur? A fruitful approach to these questions has been to dissect the energy balance equation into its various nutrient balance equations, i.e., protein, lipid and, carbohydrate.

Nutrient Balance

If the origins of a positive energy balance lie in the chronic imbalance of energy intake and expenditure, a key question is "What conditions allow a long-lasting imbalance between intake and expenditure?" An examination of each nutrient balance equation to determine if a chronic imbalance between nutrient intake and oxidation exists is only valid if each nutrient has a separate balance equation, implying separate regulation (Figure 1). In practical terms: Is each nutrient either oxidized or stored in its own compartment (separate regulation), or does it get converted into another compartment for storage? This applies particularly to the issue of whether dietary carbohydrate is stored as fat (*de novo* lipogenesis). In contrast to animals [16], *de novo* lipogenesis is very limited in humans, and occurs only when large excess of carbohydrate is ingested [17–21]. Because *de novo* lipogenesis does not occur in humans under physiological conditions, it seems reasonable to consider each nutrient balance equation as a separate entity.

Protein Balance

Protein intake is usually about 15% of calories and the protein stores in the body represent about one third of

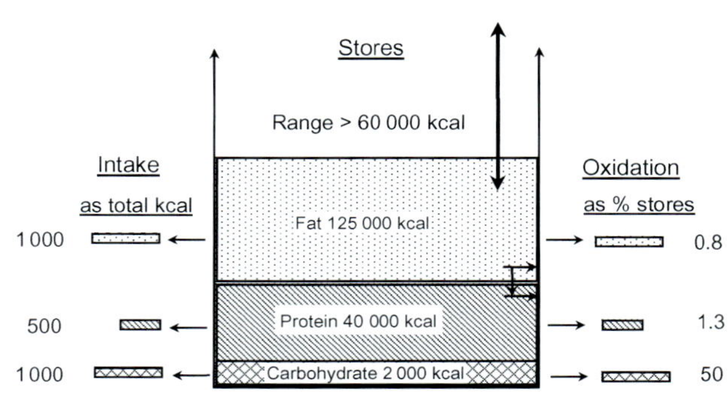

Figure 1 The daily nutrient balance of a 70-kg (20% body fat) man in relationship to nutrient stores, macronutrient intake, and macronutrient oxidation. Each nutrient intake and oxidation on a 2500 kcal/day diet (40% fat, 40% carbohydrate, 20% protein) is shown on the left as absolute calorie intake and on the right as a percentage of its respective nutrient store. The ranges for each of the nutrient stores are shown and are based on values for a 70-kg man (20% body fat) and a 150-kg man (50% body fat). The fat stores for a 150-kg man are more than five times that of a 70-kg man and extend far beyond the top of the diagram

the total stored calories in a 70-kg man. The daily protein intake amounts to a little over 1% of the total protein stores [22, 23] (Figure 1). The protein stores increase in size in response to such growth stimuli as growth hormone, androgens, physical training, and weight gain, but do not increase simply from increased dietary protein. Protein stores are, therefore, tightly controlled and on a day-to-day basis protein balance is achieved [24]. Therefore, protein imbalance cannot be implicated as a direct cause of obesity although, as with the other nonfat nutrients, protein intake may affect the fat balance equation [22].

Carbohydrate Balance

Carbohydrate is usually the main source of dietary calories, yet the body stores of glycogen are very limited: 500–1000 g on average [21]. Daily intake of carbohydrate corresponds to about 50–100% of the carbohydrate stores compared to about 1% for protein and fat [25] (Figure 1), so that over a period of hours and days, the carbohydrate stores fluctuate markedly compared with those of protein and fat. However, as with protein stores, they are tightly controlled [26]. Whether this control is based on humoral and/or nervous signals exchanged between the muscle and liver and the brain remains to be established. Dietary carbohydrate stimulates both glycogen storage and glucose oxidation and suppresses fat oxidation [27]. That which is not stored as glycogen, is oxidized (not converted to fat), and carbohydrate balance is achieved [24, 27]. Therefore, as with the other nonfat nutrients, a chronic imbalance between carbohydrate intake and oxidation cannot be the basis of weight gain because storage capacity is limited and controlled.

Fat Balance

In marked contrast to the other nutrients, body fat stores are large and fat intake has no influence on fat oxidation [25, 27]. As with protein, the daily fat intake represents less than 1% of the total energy stored as fat, but the fat stores contain about six times the energy of the protein stores [23] (Figure 1). These fat stores are the energy buffer for the body and daily surplus or deficit in energy intake is directly translated into surplus or deficit in fat mass [24]. A deficit of 200 kcal of energy over 24 h means 200 kcal comes from the fat stores, and the same holds true for an excess of 200 kcal of energy, which ends up in the fat stores. Even in conditions of spontaneous overfeeding, the entire excess fat intake is stored as body fat [26]. Ingestion of a mixed meal is followed by an increase in carbohydrate oxidation and a decrease in fat oxidation and the addition of extra fat does not alter that mix of nutrient oxidation [25, 27]. What promotes fat oxidation if it is not dietary fat intake? The amount of total body fat exerts a small, but significant, effect on fat oxidation and this promotion of fat oxidation at higher body fat levels may represent a mechanism for attenuating the rate of weight gain [28]. Besides some genetic predisposition [28–30] energy balance is the driving force for fat oxidation [24, 28]: when it is negative (i.e., energy expenditure exceeding intake), fat oxidation increases.

In summary, when one considers energy balance in humans under physiological conditions, fat is the only nutrient capable of maintaining a chronic imbalance between intake and oxidation, thus directly contributing to the increase in adipose tissue. The other nutrients will indirectly influence adiposity by their contribution to overall energy balance and thus fat balance as emphasized by Frayn [31]. The use of the fat balance equation instead of the energy balance equation offers a new framework for understanding the pathogenesis of obesity.

Alcohol Balance

There is an inconsistent relationship between reported alcohol intake and body mass index (BMI), with many studies showing a negative relationship [32, 33]. However, it has been shown that in healthy individuals the fate of ingested alcohol is oxidation and not storage (as fat), and therefore perfect alcohol balance is achieved [34]. In the same manner as dietary carbohydrate and protein, alcohol diverts dietary fat away from oxidation and toward storage and therefore indirectly promotes fat deposition.

ENERGY EXPENDITURE

Several methods have been developed to measure daily energy expenditure. The most accurate methods involve continuous measurements of heat output (direct calorimetry) or gas exchange (indirect calorimetry) in subjects confined in metabolic chambers. Because confined subjects are unable to pursue habitual activities, a number of field methods have been developed to measure energy expenditure in free-living conditions, including factorial methods, heart rate monitoring, body weight clamping, and the doubly labeled water method.

Components of energy expenditure and their relevance to obesity: Knowledge of daily energy requirements in humans is a prerequisite for understanding how obesity might develop from a chronic energy imbalance [35]. Sedentary daily energy requirements can be accurately measured in a respiratory chamber. Since 1985 we have performed measurements of 24-h sedentary energy expenditure on more than 900 individuals using a respiratory chamber [15]. These data firmly establish that sedentary daily energy expenditure is a linear function of body size, i.e., heavier people have higher metabolic rates than do lighter people. Because a higher body weight can only be maintained by matching energy expenditure with intake, this data also gives little credence to studies showing no

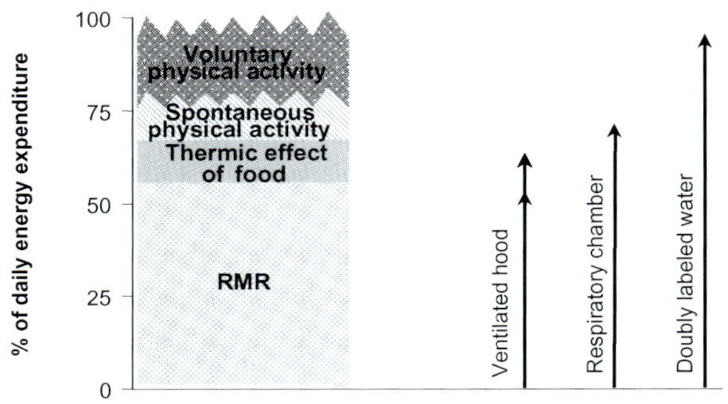

Figure 2 Components of daily energy expenditure in humans. Daily energy expenditure can be divided into three major components: the resting metabolic rate, which represents 50–70% of daily energy expenditure; the thermic effect of food, which represents ~10% of daily energy expenditure; and the energy cost of physical activity [sum of spontaneous physical activity (fidgeting) and unrestricted/voluntary physical activity], which represents 20–40% of daily energy expenditure

correlation or negative correlation between energy intake and body weight [36]. The variability in daily energy requirements is related to the variability in energy expended for the four major components of daily energy expenditure, i.e., resting metabolic rate, thermogenesis, spontaneous physical activity, and voluntary physical activity (Figure 2).

Resting Metabolic Rate

The resting metabolic rate (RMR) is the energy expended by a subject resting in the fasting state under comfortable ambient conditions. RMR includes the cost of maintaining the integrated systems of the body and the homeothermic temperature at rest. In most sedentary adults, RMR accounts for approximately 60–70% of daily energy expenditure [10]. The close correlation between RMR and body size has been known for many years and has formed the basis for the development of widely used equations to predict RMR from height and weight [37–41].

Fat-free mass, fat mass, age, and sex are the major determinants of RMR, explaining ~80% of its variance [10, 42]. However, some of the remaining variance is explained by family membership, suggesting that RMR is at least partly genetically determined [43]. Further support for a genetic determinant of RMR comes from studies of twins by Bouchard et al. [44]. In our search for the possible mechanisms underlying the intersubject variability in RMR, we have explored the impact of body composition, gender, physical training, age, muscle metabolism, sympathetic nervous system (SNS) activity, and body temperature on RMR. Independent of differences in fat-free mass, fat mass, and age, females have lower RMR when compared to males (~100 kcal/day less) [45]. This might be due to the effect of sex hormones on metabolic rate. Whether the levels of physical activity and training are determinants of the RMR remain controversial [46–54]. Cross-sectional studies of RMR indicate significant age-related declines [55–57]. On the basis of longitudinal data, Keys et al. [58] estimated that the decline in RMR was less than 1–2% per decade from the second to the seventh decade of life. Subsequent work has supported Keys' conclusion that the decrease in RMR seen in elderly people can be explained largely by decreases in fat-free mass [59–61].

Data from studies using indirect assessment of SNS activity suggest that the SNS may be involved in the regulation of RMR under eucaloric conditions [62, 63]. Using a more direct measurement (microneurography), we found that the variability in energy expenditure was related to the variability of muscle sympathetic nerve activity [64]. Resting skeletal muscle metabolism also seems to be a significant determinant of whole-body metabolism [65, 66], and studies suggest that uncoupling protein 3 (UCP-3) expression may underlie some of this variability [67]. However more recent studies in humans do not seem to provide support for an important role of UCP-3 as a mitochondrial uncoupler [68]. Finally, the variability in RMR after adjustment for differences in fat-free mass, fat mass, and age, is related to the variability in body temperature, indicating that body temperature could be a marker for a high or low relative metabolic rate [69]. Later in this chapter, we describe some of the new molecular mechanisms underlying the variability in metabolic rate in rodents.

Thermic Effect of Food

The thermic effect of food (TEF) is the increase in energy expenditure observed after the administration of a meal. TEF accounts for approximately 5–15% of the daily energy expenditure [70, 71]. Many factors influence the TEF: meal size and composition, palatability of the food, time of the meal as well as the subject's genetic background, age, physical fitness, and sensitivity to insulin. Brundin et al. have shown that TEF is also a function of the heat leakage across the abdominal wall, which is inversely related to the thickness of the abdominal adipose tissue layer [72]. These influences, plus technical aspects such as the position of the subject and the duration of measurement, make TEF the most difficult to measure and the least reproducible component of daily energy expenditure [70, 71]. TEF has long been regarded as a component of daily energy expenditure that could cause significant variations in daily energy balance and therefore predispose individuals to obesity. TEF may have evolved as a mechanism for enriching protein-poor diets by disposing of the excess nonessential energy [73–76]. Consequently, Stock [73] and Dulloo [74] have argued that large interindividual differences in TEF can only be uncovered under conditions of overfeeding with protein-depleted diets. However, given adequate protein and other essential nutrients in the diet, one can safely state that individual differences in TEF can account for only small differences in daily energy expenditure. While a review of the published literature suggests that obesity may be associated with an impaired TEF [77], it is important to note that numerous studies have provided support to an impaired TEF in obese vs. lean subjects [20, 75, 76, 78–102] whereas others did not [98, 103–117]. Importantly, in a prospective study in more than 100 subjects, we could not find any relationship between the TEF and weight change [70]. Decreased thermogenesis is, therefore, a very unlikely explanation for significant degrees of obesity.

Physical Activity

Physical activity, the most variable component of daily energy expenditure, can account for a significant amount of calories in very active people. However, sedentary adult individuals exhibit a range of physical activity that represents only 20–30% of total energy expenditure.

Reduced physical activity as a cause of obesity is an obvious and attractive hypothesis. The energy expended in physical activity is quite variable and the secular increase in obesity parallels the increase in sedentary lifestyles. In the United Kingdom, the prevalence of obesity has increased dramatically over the past three to four decades despite a marked decrease in energy intake, suggesting that physical activity has decreased even more during the same period [118]. There is no doubt that physical activity has decreased dramatically in many populations over the past few decades with the increase number of cars per household and the increase in the numbers of hours spent in front of television sets or personal computers. However, until the very recent introduction of the doubly labeled water method for measuring energy expenditure in free-living condition [119, 120], there had been no satisfactory method by which to assess the impact of physical activity on daily energy expenditure. Schulz and Schoeller [121] have provided data on more than 200 subjects and have evidenced a wide variability in total energy expenditure and, therefore, in physical activity. Using the ratio between total energy expenditure and RMR as an index of the level of physical activity, they have also shown that physical activity is decreased in heavier or fatter subjects. In a review of 574 doubly labeled water measurements, Black et al. compiled data to (1) establish the limits of sustainable human energy expenditure, (2) establish the average and range of habitual energy expenditure in relationship to age and sex, and (3) describe the lifestyles and activity patterns associated with different levels of physical activity [122]. From this review, Black et al. concluded that levels of energy expenditure were similar to the recommendations for energy requirements adopted by FAO/WHO/UNU (1985) and the UK Department of Health (1991). Prentice et al. described the relationship between graded levels of obesity and free-living energy expenditure in men and women of affluent societies and confirmed that habitual total energy expenditure is increased with obesity because of concomitant increase in fat-free mass [123]. They also suggest that except in massive obesity, the level and cost of physical activity is quite similar at different levels of body weight and BMI.

This, however, does not exclude the possibility that an inactive lifestyle may be an important risk factor for the development of obesity. Whether a low level of physical activity is a cause or a consequence of obesity can only be tested in prospective studies. An elegant prospective study now provides evidence that differences in nonvolitional muscle activity (i.e., fidgeting, muscle tone, maintenance of posture) may be important in determining predisposition to obesity and/or resistance to diet-induced weight gain [124].

METABOLIC RISK FACTORS FOR BODY WEIGHT GAIN

An understanding of the etiology of human obesity demands longitudinal studies. Cross-sectional studies have added little to our understanding of the physiological mechanisms predisposing to weight gain [125]. Cross-sectional studies can only provide associations, whereas longitudinal studies reveal predictors or risk factors. Several studies have examined these predictors in Pima Indians, a population prone to obesity [126].

Low Metabolic Rate

A low absolute metabolic rate cannot cause obesity since obese individuals have high metabolic rate, both in resting and sedentary conditions [10, 15]. Many investigators who have studied energy expenditure in humans have suggested that in the absence of a clear defect in energy expenditure in obese subjects, obesity can only be the result of excessive energy intake. However, the scatter around the regression line between metabolic rate and body size suggests that at any given body size, individuals can have a "high," "normal," or "low" relative metabolic rate. From our own studies in adult nondiabetic Pima Indians, we found that a low relative metabolic rate, adjusted for differences in fat-free mass, fat-mass, age, and sex, was a risk factor for body weight gain [127]. After 4 years of follow-up, the risk of gaining 10 kg was approximately eight times greater in subjects with the lowest RMR (lower tertile) compared with those with the highest RMR (higher tertile) (Figure 3). According to a recent meta-analysis of published studies, formerly obese subjects have a 3–5% lower mean relative RMR than do control subjects, which likely contributes to the high rate of weight regain in formerly obese persons [128]. Nevertheless, these data need

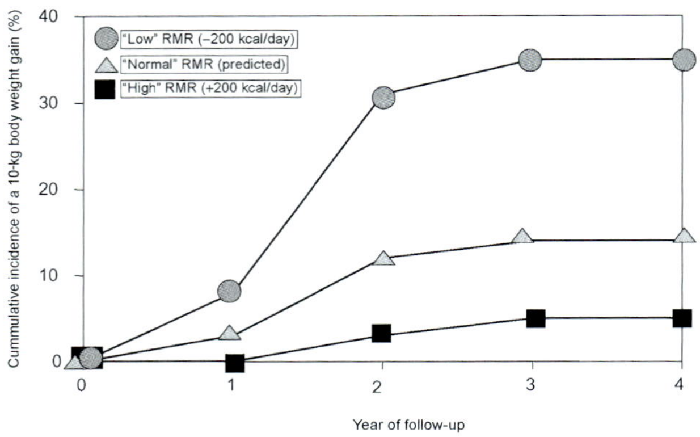

Figure 3 Cumulative incidence of a 10-kg body weight gain in subjects with a "high" relative metabolic rate (200 kcal/day above that predicted for body size and body composition), for a subject with a "normal" relative RMR (equal to that predicted), and for a subject with a "low" RMR (200 kcal/day below that predicted). The cumulative incidence was calculated on the basis of follow-up data obtained in 126 Pima Indians followed for an average of 3 years using a survival analysis (proportional hazard linear model). Note that subjects with a "low" metabolic rate have approximately eight times the risk of gaining weight as compared to those with a "high" metabolic rate. (Reproduced by permission of the New England Journal of Medicine [127])

to be interpreted with caution since the variability of baseline energy expenditure accounted for only 16% of the variability of weight gain. Second, theoretical estimates suggest that only 30–40% of the increase in body energy stores in people who gained weight can be attributed to the baseline deficit in energy expenditure. Third, relatively low energy expenditure does not seem to be a predictor of weight gain in other adult populations [129, 130]. Together, the results may suggest that a low metabolic rate may not only be a direct risk factor for body weight gain but also be a marker for hyperphagia or inactivity.

Low Physical Activity

Another component of 24-h energy expenditure is the energy cost of spontaneous physical activity, which accounts for 8–15% of total daily expenditure [10]. Consistent with the cross-sectional observation of a decrease in spontaneous physical activity in obese subjects, our longitudinal studies showed that even in the confined environment of a respiratory chamber, spontaneous physical activity is a familial trait and that a low level of spontaneous physical activity is associated with subsequent weight gain in males, but not in females [131]. A recent study found that resistance to the development of obesity might be due to the ability of increasing spontaneous physical activity (also defined as non-exercise activity thermogenesis or NEAT) in response to overfeeding [124]. Prospective studies in which free-living physical activity is measured (doubly labeled water technique) are absolutely needed to objectively assess what most scientists believe, i.e., that a low level of physical activity is a major predisposing factor for weight gain in individuals and in populations [132]. Studies from Schoeller's group indicate that patients successful at maintaining weight loss are those engaging in considerable amount of physical activity up to 80 min/day [133].

Low Rates of Fat Oxidation

The composition of nutrient intake has been shown to be an important factor in the genesis of obesity, and consequently, one might expect that the composition of nutrient oxidation would also play a role. The nonprotein respiratory quotient is an index of the ratio of carbohydrate to fat oxidation, ranging from a value of about 0.80 after an overnight fast when fat is the main oxidative substrate [134] to values close to 1.00 after a large carbohydrate meal when glucose is the major substrate [135]. Apart from the effect of diet composition, the respiratory quotient is also influenced by recent energy balance (negative balance causing more fat oxidation), sex (females tend to have reduced fat oxidation), adiposity (higher fat mass leads to higher fat oxidation), and family membership, suggesting genetic determinants [28, 136].

In a longitudinal study in Pima Indians, a high 24-h respiratory quotient predicted weight gain [28]. Those in the 90th percentile for respiratory quotient ("low fat oxidizers") had a 2.5 times greater risk of gaining 5 kg or more body weight than those in the 10th percentile ("high fat oxidizers"). This effect was independent of a relatively low or high 24-h metabolic rate. Similar results were found in Caucasian volunteers participating in the Baltimore Longitudinal Study on Aging [137]. In support of these observations, others have demonstrated that weight-reduced obese volunteers have high respiratory quotients, i.e., low rates of fat oxidation [138, 139], and those who are able to maintain weight loss have lower respiratory quotients compared to those experiencing weight relapse [140].

Insulin Sensitivity

Insulin sensitivity is measured as the total glucose disposal stimulated by insulin during a glucose clamp and is the sum of oxidative and nonoxidative (mainly storage) glucose disposal. Since higher rates of carbohydrate oxidation predict weight gain, we investigated whether insulin sensitivity would also predict weight gain in Pima Indians. Subjects in the 90th percentile (most insulin sensitive) were approximately four times more likely to gain 10 kg or more body weight compared with those in the 10th percentile (most insulin resistant), and this effect was more closely related to the oxidative than the nonoxidative component of glucose metabolism [141]. Thus, insulin sensitivity predicts weight gain, or conversely, insulin resistance is associated with significantly lower rates of weight gain. Similar observations were reported in Mexican Americans [142] and Caucasians from the San Luis Valley Study [143]. Yost et al. also reported that increased insulin sensitivity predicts weight regain following sustained weight loss [144]. At least in adults, it appears that insulin resistance is a mechanism counteracting further weight gain [145].

Low Sympathetic Nervous Activity

The activity of the SNS is positively related to the three major components of energy expenditure (RMR [64], the TEF [63], spontaneous physical activity [146]) and negatively to 24-h respiratory quotient [147]. Further indications of the possible role of SNS activity in the regulation of energy balance in humans comes from a study showing that a low SNS activity is associated with a poor weight loss outcome in obese subjects treated with diet [135]. Furthermore, Pima Indians, who are prone to obesity, have low rates of muscle sympathetic nerve activity compared to weight-matched Caucasians [64]. In a prospective study, we found that baseline urinary excretion rate of norepinephrine, a global index of SNS activity, was negatively correlated with body weight gain in male Pima Indians [148]. Thus, a low activity of the SNS is associated with the development of obesity.

Low Plasma Concentration of Leptin

Leptin, the product of the *OB* gene, is a hormone produced by the adipose tissue that inhibits food intake and increases energy expenditure [149]. To investigate whether individuals prone to weight gain are hypoleptinemic, we measured fasting plasma leptin concentrations in two groups of weight-matched, nondiabetic Pima Indians followed for approximately 3 years, 19 of whom subsequently gained weight (average weight gain 23 kg) and 17 of whom maintained their weight within 0.5 kg. After adjustment for initial percent body fat, mean plasma leptin concentration was lower in those who gained weight than in those whose weight was stable [150]. Despite the leptin resistance apparent in obesity [151], this data indicates that relatively low plasma leptin concentrations may play a role in the development of obesity. However, relative hypoleptinemia was not a risk factor for obesity in other studies [152, 153].

METABOLIC ADAPTATION TO DEFICIT OR SURFEIT OF CALORIES

Metabolic risk factors for body weight gain such as a relatively low metabolic rate, a low energy cost of spontaneous physical activity, a low activity of the SNS, and a high respiratory quotient are shown to change in response to weight gain. Upon gaining weight, the original abnormal state becomes normalized, and because the change in metabolic risk factors is greater than the cross-sectional data would predict, this may be a mechanism to counteract further weight gain (Figure 4).

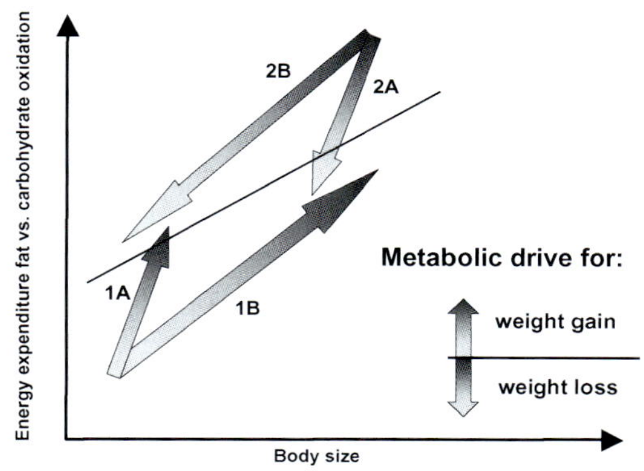

Figure 4 On the basis of our cross-sectional, prospective, and longitudinal studies in Pima Indians, we have developed a theoretical model to explain the possible role of energy metabolism in the long-term regulation of body weight. Cross-sectionally, energy expenditure and the rate of fat-to-carbohydrate oxidation increase with increasing body size (prediction line), but at any given body size both measures vary considerably among individuals. Prospectively, relatively low rates of energy expenditure or fat oxidation predispose to weight gain. In longitudinal analyses, a relatively low rate of energy expenditure or fat oxidation tend to normalize but again there is large variability in this response among individuals. Thus, the metabolic drive to weight gain may soon diminish in some individuals (limited weight gain, arrow 1A), whereas it may be more sustained in others (larger weight gain, arrow 1B). Opposite considerations apply to weight loss (arrows 2A and 2B). (Reproduced by permission of the Endocrine Society [153])

Changes in metabolic factors, which are not explained by changes in body weight and composition, are the hallmark of metabolic adaptation. The concept of metabolic adaptation was introduced by the pioneering work of Keys et al. who defined the drop in energy expenditure observed in healthy men in response to semistarvation "a useful adjustment to altered circumstances" [155]. A more recent definition of adaptation has been proposed in the 1985 FAO/WHO/UNU report [156] as "a process by which a new or different steady state is reached in response to a change or difference in the intake of food and nutrients." Results from most overfeeding studies indicate that short-term experimental weight gain is accompanied by an overcompensatory increase in energy expenditure [157–159]. A recent study indicates that most of the overcompensatory response may be due to an increase in nonexercise activity thermogenesis, i.e. fidgeting [124]. Similarly most underfeeding studies reveal that in the short term, intentional weight loss leads to a decrease in energy expenditure beyond predicted values [155, 160–162]. Therefore, there is substantial evidence that metabolic adaptation occurs in response to large perturbations in body weight over a relatively short period of time, but it is unknown whether similar adaptive mechanisms also operate in response to long-term weight changes in free-living conditions.

We recently examined longitudinal changes in energy expenditure and respiratory quotient associated with spontaneous long-term weight change in Pima Indians [154]. Results indicated that metabolic adaptation does occur in response to spontaneous long-term weight change, but the magnitude of the adaptive changes is small and the interindividual variability is large. On the basis of these and other data, we have developed a theoretical model to explain how metabolic propensity to obesity (or resistance to weight loss) might thus depend not only on initial rates of energy expenditure and fat oxidation, but also on how these measures change in response to weight change (Figure 4).

MOLECULAR MECHANISMS OF ENERGY METABOLISM

Knowing that obesity increases susceptibility to the development of type 2 diabetes, it is therefore important to understand the molecular mechanisms of the factors favoring the development of obesity if one wants to develop strategies aimed at preventing or curing diabetes. As described above, the positive energy balance that leads to the excessive deposition of fat results from excessive food consumption together with reduced total energy expenditure. Understanding the mechanisms by which variation in energy expenditure contributes to the development of obesity has been an elusive goal. Energy expenditure includes many components such as physical activity, fidgeting, the TEF, ambient temperature, fever, shivering, and the efficiency of basal metabolism. The effects of some of these factors such as physical exercise and ambient temperature are obvious; however, what determines "metabolic efficiency" is extremely complex. All components of energy expenditure, whether simple or complex, are most likely influenced by variations in the genetic constitution of an individual.

Upon the basis of the "thrifty gene" hypothesis, one would predict that mutations changing the efficiency of energy metabolism should exist. Yet biochemical spontaneous or induced mutations in the mouse or humans that can cause obesity without increased food consumption are not known. In both mouse and humans, single gene mutations in the genes for leptin, leptin receptor, or melanocortin receptors are acting both directly on the CNS to affect food intake and indirectly on peripheral tissues to affect energy expenditure [163]. There is recent evidence that leptin administered to mice can stimulate directly lipid oxidation in skeletal muscle [164] and the expression of genes of lipid oxidation in the liver [165]. It is known that peripheral metabolism, including adipocyte, muscle, and liver metabolism, accounts for a major portion of the obesity phenotype of *ob/ob* mice. In other words, food-restricted *ob/ob* mice remain fatter even though total body weight is diminished to the level of wild-type controls [166, 167]. Whether genetic variations that modulate but do not totally inactivate leptin signaling system exist among obese individuals is not known. An obesity genetic model in which the primary effect is on the "efficiency of energy expenditure" alone would therefore improve our understanding of how variations in energy expenditure contribute to the development of obesity. This part of the review will examine the genetic evidence related to obesity phenotypes that appear to be acting at the level of energy expenditure.

We are here considering mutations related to energy metabolism at two levels: those that affect the generation of fuels for thermogenesis and those that directly affect the thermogenic mechanisms themselves. The goal in this categorization is to determine at which level lie the rate-limiting steps for a given energy homeostasis. Put another way, it is conceivable that the capacity for thermogenesis, that is, those mechanisms that consume ATP by substrate cycling or generate heat by uncoupling respiration from ATP synthesis, is not limiting and is always in excess. In this case, simply increasing the availability of oxidizable fuel, preferentially lipids, would reduce obesity. Alternatively, if thermogenic mechanisms are rate limiting, then no matter how active fatty acid oxidation may be, the low mitochondrial uncoupling or ATPase will prevent the combustion of calories and obesity cannot be reduced.

Examples of substrate cycling that could function as futile ATPases to "waste" energy include the phoshpofructokinase/fructose diphosphatase cycle, the glycerol phosphate cycle, and the Cori cycle. Variants for the fructose phosphate cycle have not been reported, but spontaneous and induced mutations for the cytoplasmic and mitochondrial glycerol 3-phosphate dehyrogenases have been characterized [168, 169]. Mice deficient in the cytoplasmic enzyme have no obesity phenotype even though muscle ATP levels are reduced during exercise. Mice deficient in the mitochondrial enzyme are slightly smaller, but not obese. Similarly, mutations to a putative substrate cycle, which is also inducible in liver by thyroid hormone [170], have no significant effects on obesity. There is also evidence supporting the existence of a substrate cycling system, formed by lipolysis of triacylglycerol and reesterification of fatty acids, that can be stimulated by leptin [171].

Genetic variation can alter energy expenditure not only at the level of substrate cycles, ATPases, or uncoupling proteins, but at any of the steps at which the organism manages its nutrients. Can genetic studies (gene knockout or gene overexpression) help in elucidating the thermogenic mechanisms underlying the interindividual variability in energy expenditure? For example, mice with an inactive long- or short-chain acyl-CoA dehydrogenase gene are cold sensitive like mice with an inactive *Ucp-1* gene. The acyl-CoA dehydrogenases are not thermogenic *per se*, but their absence affects the ability of the mouse to provide fuel for thermogenesis through fatty acid oxidation. Thus, either modulations of the thermogenic mechanism itself (i.e. UCP-1 inactivation) or the supportive mechanisms can have significant effects on the thermogenic mechanisms. This distinction between true thermogenic mechanisms and those that are supportive is important for understanding the mechanisms controlling energy expenditure. We have therefore attempted to review variations in genes believed to be directly associated with thermogenic mechanisms as well as some that are closely associated with fuel partitioning.

Insulin Receptor

Through its effects on the mobilization of cellular fuels at the metabolite, enzymatic, and gene expression levels, the insulin pathway plays a pivotal role in the control of fuels available for thermogenesis. Although unexpectedly normal at birth (only slight growth retardation), mice homozygous for a deletion of the insulin receptor quickly develop severe hyperglycemia and hyperinsulinemia and die shortly after of β-cell failure, severe diabetes, and ketosis [172, 173]. Therefore, to define the function of the insulin receptor in different insulin responsive tissues and its contribution to both type 1 and type 2 diabetes, a strategy was developed based upon Cre/lox technology for conditional inactivation of the insulin receptor gene in specific tissues [174]. This experimental approach was expected to provide a clear, unambiguous picture of the role of selective insulin responsive tissues in glucose and fat homeostasis. In contrast, a very confusing picture has emerged that has become difficult to interpret. The muscle-specific knockout causes dyslipidemia with no effects on glucose metabolism [175]. On the other hand, muscle/adipose knockout mice have impaired glucose tolerance whereas the adipose-specific knockout mice are lean and have improved glucose tolerance with no insulin resistance [174]. Even more surprising, brown fat insulin receptor knockout mice have defective β-cells insulin secretion [176]. In summary, this experimental approach designed to identify the contribution of the insulin receptor in insulin responsive tissues has not been conclusive. It will be necessary to repeat such experiments in mice on congenic backgrounds to explain these unpredicted results. In addition the analyses of new independent lines are necessary to eliminate possible chromosomal positional effects of the Cre transgenic mice used to generate tissue-specific gene inactivation.

Adrenergic receptor activation of nonshivering thermogensis

Adrenergic activation of the nonshivering thermogenesis in adult animals is mediated by the fat-specific β_3-adrenergic receptor via induction of *Ucp-1* expression [177]. The inactivation of the *Ucp-1* gene causes cold sensitivity in mice and a targeted inactivation of dopamine β-hydroxylase (Dbh) preventing the animal from synthesizing catecholamines makes the mice even more sensitive to the cold [178]. Furthermore, neither the $Ucp\text{-}1^{-/-}$ mice nor the $Dbh^{-/-}$ mice show any evidence of increased obesity compared to the wild-type mice despite reduced capacity for thermogenesis [179]. Accordingly, neither the inability to synthesize catecholamines nor the absence of UCP-1 causes obesity in mice. Lowell and colleagues have approached this problem of thermogenesis and susceptibility to obesity by the selective inactivation of the β-adrenergic receptors by gene targeting [180]. They first inactivated the β_3-adrenergic receptor and found that the mice had normal levels of *Ucp-1* mRNA, normal cold sensitivity, but showed only a mild obesity with increasing age [180]. The normal levels of *Ucp-1* expression in β_3-deficient mice indicated that other β-adrenergic receptors might be compensatory. The mild obesity, even though *Ucp-1* expression was unaffected, suggested that a reduction in adrenergically stimulated lipolysis occurred, probably in the white fat. Mice with an inactivated β_1-adrenergic receptor died perinatally but some survived depending on the background genotype [181]. On the contrary, β_2-adrenergic-receptor-deficient mice appeared normal, but weighed about 10% less than wild-type mice [182]. Thus, none of the three β-adrenergic receptor mutants produced significant obesity. However, Lowell and his colleagues carried this analysis further by inactivating all three β-adrenergic receptor genes in the same mouse [183]. Remarkably, these animals survived and had the very intriguing phenotype of being sensitive to cold exposure and very prone to diet-induced obesity. Thus, we are faced with the conundrum that UCP-1 and Dbh-deficient mice have a phenotype of cold sensitivity but resistance to obesity, whereas the β-adrenergic receptor deficient mice are also cold sensitive, but susceptible to diet-induced obesity. Taken together, these results suggest that other adrenergic receptors, i.e., the α receptors are important in the etiology of obesity. Indeed, β_3-adrenergic-receptor-deficient mice expressing the human α_2-adrenergic receptor as a transgene are obese because of adipocyte hyperplasia [184]. In addition, the presence of the β-adrenergic receptors in the *Ucp-1*-deficient mice may enable the mice to utilize alternative mechanisms of thermogenesis [185].

Mutations in Fatty Acid Oxidation pathways

Acetyl-CoA Carboxylase

Acetyl-CoA carboxylase 2 (ACC-2) catalyzes the rate-limiting step in fatty acid biosynthesis from acetyl-CoA. Mice deficient in ACC-2 are fertile, have a normal life span, but weigh less and have smaller fat depots than do wild-type mice [186]. These mice consume up to 30% more food, suggesting increased energy expenditure. In the absence of ACC-2, malonyl-CoA is elevated and fatty acid oxidation is stimulated in muscle to serve as a sink for fatty acids that would normally be deposited in the liver and adipose tissue. While the effects of ACC-2 deficiency on adiposity are striking, there are some important unanswered questions. In face of a major increase in β-oxidation in muscle, what is the heat-producing mechanism, since there is a reduction in fat depots in the mice despite increased food intake? The enhanced generation of NADH and FADH2 by fatty acid oxidation is dissipated by mitochondrial respiration as long as there is a continual supply of ADP or the muscle mitochondria are uncoupled by one of the uncoupling proteins. If the mitochondria are coupled to ATP synthesis, then energy must be expended by either a futile ATPase or by muscle activity. This would become evident experimentally by increased oxygen consumption at rest or through increased physical activity. Similarly, if the mitochondria were dissipating the membrane potential by an uncoupling mechanism then increases in oxygen consumption and heat production would be observed. It is hoped that these determinations will be reported in the near future.

An encouraging aspect of this model is that the capacity for increased energy expenditure exists in response to increased fuel oxidation due to a shift in metabolism caused by blocking fatty acid synthesis and reducing malonyl-CoA levels, an inhibitor of fatty acid uptake by the mitochondria. Whether the mice are generating heat or have increased physical activity remains to be shown.

Acyl-CoA Dehydrogenase Deficiency

A spontaneous mutation that occurs in the short chain of the acyl-CoA dehydrogenase gene (*Acads*) of BALB/cByJ mice and a targeted mutation in the long chain of the acyl-CoA dehydrogenase gene (*Acadl*), both cause a phenotype characterized by extreme cold sensitivity [187]. Although *Ucp-1* mRNA levels are similar in mutant and wild-type controls maintained at an ambient temperature of 23°C, the rate of induction of *Ucp-1* and type 2 deiodinase levels lags in the mutant mice when housed at near thermoneutrality. The basis for this difference in mRNA inductions for these two genes is unknown. Although not proven, it has been hypothesized that the inability of the mice to mount a thermogenic response that would maintain body temperature is due to the deficiency in β-oxidation of fatty acids in the brown fat. Histological examination of interscapular brown fat shows an accumulation of fat in the *Acads*-deficient mice similar to that previously found in *Ucp-1*-deficient mice. The effects of acyl-CoA dehydrogenase deficiency on adiposity and other parameters of energy metabolism have not been fully studied.

Diacylglycerol Transferase

Mice with the targeted inactivation of the *Dgat* gene are leaner than wild-type mice when fed a high fat diet [188]. In addition, diacylglycerol transferase (DAGT) deficiency causes reduced obesity in Ay mice but not in *ob/ob* mice. The reduced obesity in both fat-fed mice and Ay mice leads to improved glucose tolerance and insulin sensitivity in *Dgat*$^{-/-}$ mice [189]. The authors propose that *Dgat*$^{-/-}$ mice have increased energy expenditure; however, the evidence for this is not strong yet. It is possible that the difference in oxygen consumption would not be apparent if the data had been calculated on the basis of lean body mass, rather than body weight. Furthermore, the authors failed to express their results using the appropriate way of normalizing energy expenditure data using regression analysis instead of ratios [190, 191]. Since the *Dgat*$^{-/-}$ mice are more active physically, it is necessary to consider the increased energy expenditure from activity before concluding about "energy efficiency." A more recent publication from this group is proposing that increased leptin sensitivity in *Dgat*$^{-/-}$ is associated with a mechanism for increased energy expenditure [189]. At this time one can conclude that *Dgat*$^{-/-}$ mice are leaner than wild-type controls probably because of the reduced capacity of triglyceride synthesis, but the energy expenditure phenotype needs to be better studied. Indeed, it is important to normalize correctly the energy expenditure data of animals with different body size [191, 192]. Since DGAT could be part of a thermogenic substrate cycle of triacyglycerol and fatty acids (see above), it is puzzling that the absence of DGAT would stimulate energy expenditure.

The Mitochondria Uncoupling Protein UCP-l and Brown Fat Thermogenesis

It is well established from analysis of transgenic mice that an increase in *Ucp-1* expression or an increase in the number of brown adipocytes (induced by the conversion of white adipocytes to brown adipocytes) can reduce obesity, insulin resistance, and diabetes. Transgenic mice have been created in which the *Ucp-1* gene has been placed under the control of a promoter that causes ectopic expression in tissues such as white adipose and skeletal muscle [193–196]. In addition, genetic variation among inbred strains of mice causes a variation in the induction of brown fat in traditional white fat depots [197, 198]. These mice provide some of the strongest experimental proof of principle for the idea that increased uncoupling of mitochondria by genetic manipulation can reduce obesity and the development of type 2 diabetes [195, 199]. However, practical application of this experimental approach to humans by pharmacological activation of the *UCP-1* gene seems remote. It is less far fetched to think that induction of brown adipocytes in white fat depots of humans can be achieved pharmacologically [200, 201]. Given the effectiveness of increased brown adipocyte number in white fat depots on reducing obesity in rats and mice, such an approach clearly represents a promising strategy in humans. Much evidence has accumulated showing that UCP-1 is present in white adipose depots of adult humans [202]; however, whether the expression of UCP-1 can achieve a level sufficient to reduce obesity remains to be answered.

Excluding the obvious difference that mice have major depots of brown fat around several vital organs and in the interscapular region, there are important features of brown adipocyte expression in white fat depots that are relevant to the characteristics of the brown adipocyte phenotype in humans:

(1) In the absence of sympathetic stimulation (cold or adrenergic agonists), mice 2 months of age or older have very low levels of *Ucp-1* expression in traditional white fat [198]. Chronic exposure to cold is a rare occurrence among humans since we use behavioral strategies rather than physiological adaptative thermogenesis to protect ourselves from the cold.
(2) The amount of *Ucp-1* that can be induced by adrenergic stimulation varies by approximately 2 orders of magnitude in different white fat depots of the same animal [198]. Although several morphological and a few molecular studies have identified small numbers of brown adipocytes in humans under standard conditions [203], none of these studies have attempted to map out relative expression among different fat depots.
(3) Large genetic variation in the induction of brown adipocytes is found among inbred strains of mice, with some strains being highly resistant to induction and others showing that the majority of adipocytes in a white fat depot have acquired brown adipocyte morphology [198].

To confidently assess the potential for brown adipocyte induction in humans, it will be necessary to establish appropriate environmental conditions, sample the right fat depots, and determine genetic haplotypes that carry variant genes for induction. We propose that genetic studies should be undertaken to identify the range of haplotypes for regulatory genes implicated in brown adipocyte induction from genetic studies in mice.

Mechanisms Controlling the Induction of Brown Adipocytes

There are two ways of identifying the mechanisms controlling the induction of brown adipocytes. The first is based upon transgenic and gene knockout models that cause an increase in the number of brown adipocytes in white fat depots [196, 204, 205]. The discovery of these genes (including the FoxC2 transcription factor [196], 4BP translation inhibitor [205], and the protein kinase A RIIβ regulatory subunit [206]) has been largely serendipitous, since the initial phenotype of the genetically altered mouse was reduced body weight and only subsequent analysis revealed increased number of brown adipocytes in white fat and increased *Ucp-1* expression. Overexpression of the β_1-adrenergic receptor also increases brown adipocytes in white fat depots [204]. The mechanism of the induction of new brown adipocytes is unknown but in most cases, the genetic manipulations cause an increase in cAMP levels in the white adipocytes, which seems to be essential for the subsequent induction of brown adipocytes.

Other Potential Thermogenic Mechanisms: UCP-2 and UCP-3

Following the discovery of two genes with homology to brown-fat-specific *Ucp-1*, there was great excitement that these genes could become targets for the induction of thermogenesis in the human. Their structural similarity to UCP-1 also suggested that they could serve an uncoupling function in the mitochondria. Indeed expression of UCP-2 and UCP-3 in yeast and in reconstituted proteoliposomes supports an uncoupling function. Moreover, these genes are broadly expressed in humans, and in particular, UCP-3 is abundantly expressed in skeletal muscle, an important tissue for thermogenesis [65]. As evidenced by recent literature [207, 208], a huge effort has been made to establish a function for UCP-2 and UCP-3 in the regulation of body weight. However, the phenotypes of mice in which the *Ucp-2* and *Ucp-3* genes have been inactivated do not indicate that these homologues have a function in regulating either body temperature or body weight [209–212]. In one study in which *Ucp-3* was overexpressed in skeletal muscle of transgenic mice, mice showed a resistance to diet-induced obesity and an improvement in insulin sensitivity [199]. Since the amount of UCP-3 in the muscle of the transgenic mice was at a level that had been shown previously, by the same group of investigators, to be toxic to the mitochondria of mammalian cells, it is possible that the mitochondria of the transgenic mice were leaky because of toxicity from the high levels of UCP-3 [213]. Consequently, the effects of the *UCP-3* transgene expression were not indicative of a normal physiological function. A recent study in which *Ucp-3* was induced in human muscle by a high fat diet and then the rate of recovery of energy stores, i.e. creatine phosphate, was determined, failed to find an effect, suggesting that UCP-3 in humans does not uncouple muscle mitochondria [68].

Although there is no genetic evidence for variation in genes encoding ion transporters other than the UCPs, the human genome project has revealed a huge number of genes that could function in thermogenic mechanisms.

The known possibilities for energy dissipation by ion-transport-related processes are huge and becoming even larger as we continue with the mining of human and mouse genomic databases (see databases being compiled by the Alliance for Cellular Signalling, http://www.signaling-gateway.org). However, evidence that these mechanisms actually limit the development of obesity by stimulating energy expenditure must be demonstrated. Ultimately, proof that a putative mechanism of energy expenditure actually has a role in maintaining caloric homeostasis must come through genetic studies in animal models and then through the discovery of genetic variability for these mechanisms in humans.

CONCLUSIONS

One of the major strategies for reducing obesity in humans is to develop drugs that act on the central nervous system to control appetite and at the periphery to stimulate the expenditure of calories. However, is it possible that the only "effective" mechanism available to humans for burning off excessive calories is physical exercise? An answer to this question is critical for future research on the design of drugs that can stimulate energy expenditure to reduce excess body weight. There is however hope that novel thermogenic mechanisms can be discovered from genetic studies in mice as reviewed here. Such pathways after full validation will be used to develop new drugs for obesity.

REFERENCES

1. Neel JV. Diabetes mellitus: a "thrifty" genotype rendered detrimental by progress? *Am J Hum Genet* 1962; 14: 353–63.
2. Neel JV. The "thrifty genotype" in 1998. *Nutr Rev* 1999; 57 (5, pt 2): S2–9.
3. Pickup JC, Crook MA. Is type II diabetes mellitus a disease of the innate immune system? *Diabetologia* 1998; 41 (10): 1241–8.
4. WHO. Obesity: Preventing and Managing the Global Epidemic. Report of a WHO Consultation on Obesity. World Health Organization: Geneva, June 3–5, 1997.
5. Ravussin E. Obesity in Britain. Rising trend may be due to "pathoenvironment." *BMJ* 1995; 311 (7019): 1569.
6. Heymsfield SB, Darby PC, Muhlheim LS, Gallagher D, Wolper C, Allison DB. The calorie: myth, measurement, and reality. *Am J Clin Nutr* 1995; 62 (5, suppl): 1034S–41S.
7. Romieu I, Willett WC, Stampfer MJ, Colditz GA, Sampson L, Rosner B, Hennekens CH, Speizer FE. Energy intake and other determinants of relative weight. *Am J Clin Nutr* 1988; 47 (3): 406–12.
8. Mertz W, Tsui JC, Judd JT, Reiser S, Hallfrisch J, Morris ER, Steele PD, Lashley E. What are people really eating? The relation between energy intake derived from estimated diet records and intake determined to maintain body weight. *Am J Clin Nutr* 1991; 54 (2): 291–5.
9. Stunkard AJ, Wadden TA. *Obesity: Theory and Therapy*, 2nd edn. New York: Raven Press, 1993.
10. Ravussin E, Lillioja S, Anderson TE, Christin L, Bogardus C. Determinants of 24-hour energy expenditure in man. Methods and results using a respiratory chamber. *J Clin Invest* 1986; 78 (6): 1568–78.
11. Prentice AM, Black AE, Coward WA, Davies HL, Goldberg GR, Murgatroyd PR, Ashford J, Sawyer M, Whitehead RG. High levels of energy expenditure in obese women. *Br Med J (Clin Res Ed)* 1986; 292 (6526): 983–7.
12. Bandini LG, Schoeller DA, Cyr HN, Dietz WH. Validity of reported energy intake in obese and nonobese adolescents. *Am J Clin Nutr* 1990; 52 (3): 421–5.
13. Alpert SS. Growth, thermogenesis, and hyperphagia. *Am J Clin Nutr* 1990; 52 (5): 784–92.
14. Jequier E, Acheson K, Schutz Y. Assessment of energy expenditure and fuel utilization in man. *Annu Rev Nutr* 1987; 7: 187–208.
15. Weyer C, Snitker S, Rising R, Bogardus C, Ravussin E. Determinants of energy expenditure and fuel utilization in man: effects of body composition, age, sex, ethnicity and glucose tolerance in 916 subjects. *Int J Obes Relat Metab Disord* 1999; 23 (7): 715–22.
16. Zelewski M, Swierczynski J. Comparative studies on lipogenic enzyme activities in the liver of human and some animal species. *Comp Biochem Physiol B* 1990; 95 (3): 469–72.
17. Chascione C, Elwyn DH, Davila M, Gil KM, Askanazi J, Kinney JM. Effect of carbohydrate intake on *de novo* lipogenesis in human adipose tissue. *Am J Physiol* 1987; 253 (6, pt 1): E664–9.
18. Just B, Messing B, Darmaun D, Rongier M, Camillo E. Comparison of substrate utilization by indirect calorimetry during cyclic and continuous total parenteral nutrition. *Am J Clin Nutr* 1990; 51 (1): 107–11.
19. Manji S, Shikora S, McMahon M, Blackburn GL, Bistrian BR. Peritoneal dialysis for acute renal failure: overfeeding resulting from dextrose absorbed during dialysis. *Crit Care Med* 1990; 18 (1): 29–31.
20. Acheson KJ, Schutz Y, Bessard T, Flatt JP, Jequier E. Carbohydrate metabolism and *de novo* lipogenesis in human obesity. *Am J Clin Nutr* 1987; 45 (1): 78–85.
21. Acheson KJ, Schutz Y, Bessard T, Anantharaman K, Flatt JP, Jequier E. Glycogen storage capacity and *de novo* lipogenesis during massive carbohydrate overfeeding in man. *Am J Clin Nutr* 1988; 48 (2): 240–7.
22. Snyder WS, Cook NJ, Nasset ES, Karhausen LR, Howells GP, Tipton IH. Report of the Task Group on Reference Man. The International Commission on Radiological Protection, No. 23 ed. New York: Pergamon Press, 1974.
23. Bray GA. Treatment for obesity: a nutrient balance/nutrient partition approach. *Nutr Rev* 1991; 49 (2): 33–45.
24. Abbott WG, Howard BV, Christin L, Freymond D, Lilloja S, Boyce VL, Anderson TE, Bogardus C, Ravussin E. Short-term energy balance: relationship with protein, carbohydrate, and fat balances. *Am J Physiol* 1988; 255 (3, pt 1): E332–7.
25. Schutz Y, Flatt JP, Jequier E. Failure of dietary fat intake to promote fat oxidation: a factor favoring the development of obesity. *Am J Clin Nutr* 1989; 50 (2): 307–14.
26. Rising R, Alger S, Boyce V, Seagle H, Ferraro R, Fontvieille AM, Ravussin E. Food intake measured

by an automated food-selection system: relationship to energy expenditure. *Am J Clin Nutr* 1992; 55 (2): 343–9.

27. Flatt JP, Ravussin E, Acheson KJ, Jequier E. Effects of dietary fat on postprandial substrate oxidation and on carbohydrate and fat balances. *J Clin Invest* 1985; 76 (3): 1019–24.
28. Zurlo F, Lillioja S, Esposito-Del Puente A, Nyomba BL, Raz I, Saad MF, Swinburn BA, Knowler WC, Bogardus C, Ravussin E. Low ratio of fat to carbohydrate oxidation as predictor of weight gain: study of 24-h RQ. *Am J Physiol* 1990; 259 (5, pt 1): E650–7.
29. Smith SR, de Jonge L, Zachwieja JJ, Roy H, Nguyen T, Rood J, Windhauser M, Volaufova J, Bray GA. Concurrent physical activity increases fat oxidation during the shift to a high-fat diet. *Am J Clin Nutr* 2000; 72 (1):131–8.
30. Smith SR, de Jongel L, Zachwieja JJ, Roy H, Nguyen T, Rood JC, Windhauser MM, Bray GA. Fat and carbohydrate balances during adaptation to a high-fat. *Am J Clin Nutr* 2000; 71 (2): 450–7.
31. Frayn KN. Physiological regulation of macronutrient balance. *Int J Obes Relat Metab Disord* 1995; 19 (suppl 5): S4–10.
32. Hellerstedt WL, Jeffery RW, Murray DM. The association between alcohol intake and adiposity in the general population. *Am J Epidemiol* 1990; 132 (4): 594–611.
33. Colditz GA, Giovannucci E, Rimm EB, Stampfer MJ, Rosner B, Speizer FE, Gordis E, Willett WC. Alcohol intake in relation to diet and obesity in women and men. *Am J Clin Nutr* 1991; 54 (1): 49–55.
34. Shelmet JJ, Reichard GA, Skutches CL, Hoeldtke RD, Owen OE, Boden G. Ethanol causes acute inhibition of carbohydrate, fat, and protein oxidation and insulin resistance. *J Clin Invest* 1988; 81 (4): 1137–45.
35. Durnin JV, Edholm OG, Miller DS, Waterlow JC. How much food does man require? *Nature* 1973; 242 (5397): 418.
36. Lichtman SW, Pisarska K, Berman ER, Pestone M, Dowling H, Offenbacher E, Weisel H, Heshka S, Matthews DE, Heymsfield SB. Discrepancy between self-reported and actual caloric intake and exercise in obese subjects. *N Engl J Med* 1992; 327 (27): 1893–8.
37. Boothby WM, Sandiford I. Summary of the basal metabolism data on 8,614 subjects with special reference to the normal standards for the estimation of the basal metabolic rate. *J Biol Chem* 1922; 54: 783–803.
38. Harris JA, Benedict FG. *A Biometric Study of Basal Metabolism in Man*. Washington, DC: The Carnegie Institute, 1919.
39. Roza AM, Shizgal HM. The Harris Benedict equation reevaluated: resting energy requirements and the body cell mass. *Am J Clin Nutr* 1984; 40 (1): 168–82.
40. Schofield WN. Predicting basal metabolic rate, new standards and review of previous work. *Hum Nutr Clin Nutr* 1985; 39 (suppl 1): 5–41.
41. Cunningham JJ. Body composition as a determinant of energy expenditure: a synthetic review and a proposed general prediction equation. *Am J Clin Nutr* 1991; 54 (6): 963–9.
42. Jequier E, Schutz Y. Long-term measurements of energy expenditure in humans using a respiration chamber. *Am J Clin Nutr* 1983; 38 (6): 989–98.
43. Bogardus C, Lillioja S, Ravussin E, Abbott W, Zawadzki JK, Young A, Knowler WC, Jacobowitz R, Moll PP. Familial dependence of the resting metabolic rate. *N Engl J Med* 1986; 315 (2): 96–100.
44. Bouchard C, Tremblay A, Nadeau A, Despres JP, Theriault G, Boulay MR, Lortie G, Leblanc C, Fournier G. Genetic effect in resting and exercise metabolic rates. *Metabolism* 1989; 38 (4): 364–70.
45. Ferraro R, Lillioja S, Fontvieille AM, Rising R, Bogardus C, Ravussin E. Lower sedentary metabolic rate in women compared with men. *J Clin Invest* 1992; 90 (3): 780–4.
46. Tremblay A, Fontaine E, Poehlman ET, Mitchell D, Perron L, Bouchard C. The effect of exercise-training on resting metabolic rate in lean and moderately obese individuals. *Int J Obes* 1986; 10 (6): 511–7.
47. Poehlman ET, Melby CL, Badylak SF. Resting metabolic rate and postprandial thermogenesis in highly trained and untrained males. *Am J Clin Nutr* 1988; 47 (5): 793–8.
48. Tremblay A, Nadeau A, Fournier G, Bouchard C. Effect of a three-day interruption of exercise-training on resting metabolic rate and glucose-induced thermogenesis in training individuals. *Int J Obes* 1988; 12 (2): 163–8.
49. Schulz LO, Nyomba BL, Alger S, Anderson TE, Ravussin E. Effect of endurance training on sedentary energy expenditure measured in a respiratory chamber. *Am J Physiol* 1991; 260 (2, Pt 1): E257–61.
50. Davis JR, Tagliaferro AR, Kertzer R, Gerardo T, Nichols J, Wheeler J. Variations of dietary-induced thermogenesis and body fatness with aerobic capacity. *Eur J Appl Physiol Occup Physiol* 1983; 50 (3): 319–29.
51. Hill JO, Sparling PB, Shields TW, Heller PA. Effects of exercise and food restriction on body composition and metabolic rate in obese women. *Am J Clin Nutr* 1987; 46 (4): 622–30.
52. Stern JS, Schutz C, Mole P. Effect of caloric restriction and exercise on basal metabolism and thyroid hormone. *Aliment Nutr Metab* 1980; 1: 361.
53. Lennon D, Nagle F, Stratman F, Shrago E, Dennis S. Diet and exercise training effects on resting metabolic rate. *Int J Obes* 1985; 9 (1): 39–47.
54. Donahoe CP Jr, Lin DH, Kirschenbaum DS, Keesey RE, Metabolic consequences of dieting and exercise in the treatment of obesity. *J Consult Clin Psychol* 1984; 52 (5): 827–36.
55. Boothby WM, Berkson J, Dunn HL. Studies of the energy metabolism of normal individuals: a standard for basal metabolism with a nomogram for clinical application. *Am J Physiol* 1936; 116: 468–84.
56. Shock NW, Yiengst MJ. Age changes in basal respiratory measurements and metabolism in males. *J Gerontol* 1955; 10: 31–40.
57. Vaughan L, Zurlo F, Ravussin E. Aging and energy expenditure. *Am J Clin Nutr* 1991; 53 (4): 821–5.
58. Keys A, Taylor HL, Grande F. Basal metabolism and age of adult man. *Metabolism* 1973; 22 (4): 579–87.
59. Calloway DH, Zanni E. Energy requirements and energy expenditure of elderly men. *Am J Clin Nutr* 1980; 33 (10): 2088–92.
60. Tzankoff S, Norris A. Effect of muscle mass decrease on age related BMR changes. *J Appl Physiol* 1977; 43 (6): 1001–6.
61. Cohn SH, Vartsky D, Yasumura S, Sawitsky A, Zanzi I, Vaswani A, Ellis KJ. Compartmental body composition

based on total-body nitrogen, potassium, and calcium. *Am J Physiol* 1980; 239 (6): E524–30.

62. Saad MF, Alger SA, Zurlo F, Young JB, Bogardus C, Ravussin E. Ethnic differences in sympathetic nervous system-mediated energy expenditure. *Am J Physiol* 1991; 261 (6, pt 1): E789–94.
63. Schwartz RS, Jaeger LF, Veith RC. Effect of clonidine on the thermic effect of feeding in humans. *Am J Physiol* 1988; 254 (1, pt 2): R90–4.
64. Spraul M, Ravussin E, Fontvieille AM, Rising R, Larson DE, Anderson EA. Reduced sympathetic nervous activity. A potential mechanism predisposing to body weight gain. *J Clin Invest* 1993; 92 (4): 1730–5.
65. Zurlo F, Larson K, Bogardus C, Ravussin E. Skeletal muscle metabolism is a major determinant of resting energy expenditure. *J Clin Invest* 1990; 86 (5): 1423–7.
66. Kirkwood SP, Zurlo F, Larson K, Ravussin E. Muscle mitochondrial morphology, body composition, and energy expenditure in sedentary individuals. *Am J Physiol* 1991; 260 (1, pt 1): E89–94.
67. Schrauwen P, Xia J, Walder K, Snitker S, Ravussin E. A novel polymorphism in the proximal UCP-3 promoter region: effect on skeletal muscle UCP-3 mRNA expression and obesity in male nondiabetic Pima Indians. *Int J Obes Relat Metab Disord* 1999; 23 (12): 1242–5.
68. Hesselink MK, Greenhaff PL, Constantin-Teodosiu D, Hultman E, Saris WH, Nieuwlaat R, Schaart G, Kornips E, Schrauwen P. Increased uncoupling protein 3 content does not affect mitochondrial function in human skeletal muscle in vivo. *J Clin Invest* 2003; 111 (4): 479–86.
69. Rising R, Keys A, Ravussin E, Bogardus C. Concomitant interindividual variation in body temperature and metabolic rate. *Am J Physiol* 1992; 263 (4, pt 1): E730–4.
70. Tataranni PA, Larson DE, Snitker S, Ravussin E. Thermic effect of food in humans: methods and results from use of a respiratory chamber. *Am J Clin Nutr* 1995; 61 (5): 1013–9.
71. Weststrate JA. Resting metabolic rate and diet-induced thermogenesis: a methodological reappraisal. *Am J Clin Nutr* 1993; 58 (5): 592–601.
72. Brundin T, Thorne A, Wahren J. Heat leakage across the abdominal wall and meal-induced thermogenesis in normal-weight and obese subjects. *Metabolism* 1992; 41 (1): 49–55.
73. Stock MJ. Gluttony and thermogenesis revisited. *Int J Obes Relat Metab Disord* 1999; 23 (11): 1105–17.
74. Dulloo AG, Jacquet J. Low-protein overfeeding: a tool to unmask susceptibility to obesity in humans. *Int J Obes Relat Metab Disord* 1999; 23 (11): 1118–21.
75. Ravussin E, Bogardus C, Schwartz RS, Robbins DC, Wolfe RR, Horton ES, Danforth E Jr, Sims EA. Thermic effect of infused glucose and insulin in man. Decreased response with increased insulin resistance in obesity and noninsulin-dependent diabetes mellitus. *J Clin Invest* 1983; 72 (3): 893–902.
76. Segal KR, Gutin B. Thermic effects of food and exercise in lean and obese women. *Metabolism* 1983; 32 (6): 581–9.
77. de Jonge L, Bray GA. The thermic effect of food and obesity: a critical review. *Obes Res* 1997; 5 (6): 622–31.
78. Kaplan ML, Leveille GA. Calorigenic response in obese and nonobese women. *Am J Clin Nutr* 1976; 29 (10): 1108–13.
79. Pittet P, Chappuis P, Acheson K, De Techtermann F, Jequier E. Thermic effect of glucose in obese subjects studied by direct and indirect calorimetry. *Br J Nutr* 1976; 35 (2): 281–92.
80. Zahorska-Markiewicz B. Thermic effect of food and exercise in obesity. *Eur J Appl Physiol Occup Physiol* 1980; 44 (3): 231–5.
81. Shetty PS, Jung RT, James WP, Barrand MA, Callingham BA. Postprandial thermogenesis in obesity. *Clin Sci (Lond)* 1981; 60 (5): 519–25.
82. Golay A, Schutz Y, Meyer HU, Thiebaud D, Curchod B, Maeder E, Felber JP, Jequier E. Glucose-induced thermogenesis in nondiabetic and diabetic obese subjects. *Diabetes* 1982; 31 (11): 1023–8.
83. Schwartz RS, Halter JB, Bierman EL. Reduced thermic effect of feeding in obesity: role of norepinephrine. *Metabolism* 1983; 32 (2): 114–7.
84. Bessard T, Schutz Y, Jequier E. Energy expenditure and postprandial thermogenesis in obese women before and after weight loss. *Am J Clin Nutr* 1983; 38 (5): 680–93.
85. Segal KR, Presta E, Gutin B. Thermic effect of food during graded exercise in normal weight and obese men. *Am J Clin Nutr* 1984; 40 (5): 995–1000.
86. Schutz Y, Golay A, Felber JP, Jequier E. Decreased glucose-induced thermogenesis after weight loss in obese subjects: a predisposing factor for relapse of obesity? *Am J Clin Nutr* 1984; 39 (3): 380–7.
87. Schutz Y, Bessard T, Jequier E. Diet-induced thermogenesis measured over a whole day in obese and nonobese women. *Am J Clin Nutr* 1984; 40 (3): 542–52.
88. Bogardus C, Lillioja S, Mott D, Zawadzki J, Young A, Abbott W. Evidence for reduced thermic effect of insulin and glucose infusions in Pima Indians. *J Clin Invest* 1985; 75 (4): 1264–9.
89. Swaminathan R, King RF, Holmfield J, Siwek RA, Baker M, Wales JK. Thermic effect of feeding carbohydrate, fat, protein and mixed meal in lean and obese subjects. *Am J Clin Nutr* 1985; 42 (2): 177–81.
90. Segal KR, Gutin B, Nyman AM, Pi-Sunyer FX. Thermic effect of food at rest, during exercise, and after exercise in lean and obese men of similar body weight. *J Clin Invest* 1985; 76 (3): 1107–12.
91. Golay A, Schutz Y, Felber JP, de Fronzo RA, Jequier E. Lack of thermogenic response to glucose/insulin infusion in diabetic obese subjects. *Int J Obes* 1986; 10 (2):107–16.
92. Devlin JT, Horton ES. Potentiation of the thermic effect of insulin by exercise: differences between lean, obese, and noninsulin-dependent diabetic men. *Am J Clin Nutr* 1986; 43 (6): 884–90.
93. Zed C, James WP. Dietary thermogenesis in obesity. Response to carbohydrate and protein meals: the effect of beta-adrenergic blockade and semistarvation. *Int J Obes* 1986; 10 (5): 391–405.
94. Steiniger J, Karst H, Noack R, Steglich HD. Diet-induced thermogenesis in man: thermic effects of single protein and carbohydrate test meals in lean and obese subjects. *Ann Nutr Metab* 1987; 31 (2): 117–25.
95. Segal KR, Gutin B, Albu J, Pi-Sunyer FX. Thermic effects of food and exercise in lean and obese men of similar lean body mass. *Am J Physiol* 1987; 252 (1, pt 1): E110–7.
96. Schutz Y, Bessard T, Jequier E. Exercise and postprandial thermogenesis in obese women before and after weight loss. *Am J Clin Nutr* 1987; 45 (6): 1424–32.
97. Golay A, Schutz Y, Felber JP, Jallut D, Jequier E. Blunted glucose-induced thermogenesis in "overweight" patients:

a factor contributing to relapse of obesity. *Int J Obes* 1989; 13 (6): 767–75.

98. Thorne A, Naslund I, Wahren J. Meal-induced thermogenesis in previously obese patients. *Clin Physiol* 1990; 10 (1): 99–109.
99. Katzeff HL, Danforth E Jr. Decreased thermic effect of a mixed meal during overnutrition in human obesity. *Am J Clin Nutr* 1989; 50 (5): 915–21.
100. Tremblay A, Sauve L, Despres JP, Nadeau A, Theriault G, Bouchard C. Metabolic characteristics of postobese individuals. *Int J Obes* 1989; 13 (3): 357–66.
101. Segal KR, Lacayanga I, Dunaif A, Gutin B, Pi-Sunyer FX. Impact of body fat mass and percent fat on metabolic rate and thermogenesis in men. *Am J Physiol* 1989; 256 (5, pt 1): E573–9.
102. Segal KR, Edano A, Blando L, Pi-Sunyer FX. Comparison of thermic effects of constant and relative caloric loads in lean and obese men. *Am J Clin Nutr* 1990; 51 (1): 14–21.
103. Felber JP, Meyer HU, Curchod B, Iselin HU, Rousselle J, Maeder E, Pahud P, Jequier E. Glucose storage and oxidation in different degrees of human obesity measured by continuous indirect calorimetry. *Diabetologia* 1981; 20 (1): 39–44.
104. Sharief NN, Macdonald I. Differences in dietary-induced thermogenesis with various carbohydrates in normal and overweight men. *Am J Clin Nutr* 1982; 35 (2): 267–72.
105. Welle SL, Campbell RG. Normal thermic effect of glucose in obese women. *Am J Clin Nutr* 1983; 37 (1): 87–92.
106. Nair KS, Halliday D, Garrow JS. Thermic response to isoenergetic protein, carbohydrate or fat meals in lean and obese subjects. *Clin Sci (Lond)* 1983; 65 (3): 307–12.
107. Blaza S, Garrow JS. Thermogenic response to temperature, exercise and food stimuli in lean and obese women, studied by 24 h direct calorimetry. *Br J Nutr* 1983; 49 (2): 171–80.
108. Felig P, Cunningham J, Levitt M, Hendler R, Nadel E. Energy expenditure in obesity in fasting and postprandial state. *Am J Physiol* 1983; 244 (1): E45–51.
109. Welle, S. Metabolic responses to a meal during rest and low-intensity exercise. *Am J Clin Nutr* 1984. 40 (5): 990–4.
110. Schwartz RS, Ravussin E, Massari M, O'Connell M, Robbins DC. The thermic effect of carbohydrate versus fat feeding in man. *Metabolism* 1985; 34 (3): 285–93.
111. Ravussin E, Acheson HJ, Vernet O, Danforth E, Jequier E. Evidence that insulin resistance is responsible for the decreased thermic effect of glucose in human obesity. *J Clin Invest* 1985; 76 (3): 1268–73.
112. Anton-Kuchly B, Laval M, Choukroun ML, Manciet G, Roger P, Varene P. Postprandial thermogenesis and hormonal release in lean and obese subjects. *J Physiol (Paris)* 1985; 80 (5): 321–9.
113. Owen OE, Kavle E, Owen RS, Polansky M, Caprio S, Mozzoli MA, Kendrick ZV, Bushman MC, Boden G. A reappraisal of caloric requirements in healthy women. *Am J Clin Nutr* 1986; 44 (1): 1–19.
114. Nair KS, Webster J, Garrow JS. Effect of impaired glucose tolerance and type II diabetes on resting metabolic rate and thermic response to a glucose meal in obese women. *Metabolism* 1986; 35 (7): 640–4.
115. Vernet O, Christin L, Schutz Y, Danforth E Jr, Jequier E. Enteral versus parenteral nutrition: comparison of energy metabolism in lean and moderately obese women. *Am J Clin Nutr* 1986; 43 (2): 194–209.
116. D'Alessio DA, Kavle EC, Mozzoli MA, Smalley KJ, Polansky M, Kendrick ZV, Owen LR, Bushman MC, Boden G, Owen OE. Thermic effect of food in lean and obese men. *J Clin Invest* 1988; 81 (6): 1781–9.
117. Scalfi L, Coltorti A, Contaldo F. Postprandial thermogenesis in lean and obese subjects after meals supplemented with medium-chain and long-chain triglycerides. *Am J Clin Nutr* 1991; 53 (5): 1130–3.
118. Prentice AM, Jebb SA. Obesity in Britain: gluttony or sloth? *BMJ* 1995; 311 (7002): 437–9.
119. Schoeller DA, van Santen E. Measurement of energy expenditure in humans by doubly labeled water method. *J Appl Physiol* 1982; 53 (4): 955–9.
120. Schoeller DA, Fjeld CR. Human energy metabolism: what have we learned from the doubly labeled water method? *Annu Rev Nutr* 1991; 11: 355–73.
121. Schulz LO, Schoeller DA. A compilation of total daily energy expenditures and body weights in healthy adults. *Am J Clin Nutr* 1994; 60 (5): 676–81.
122. Black AE, Coward WA, Cole TJ, Prentice AM. Human energy expenditure in affluent societies: an analysis of 574 doubly-labelled water measurements. *Eur J Clin Nutr* 1996; 50 (2): 72–92.
123. Prentice AM, Black AE, Coward WA, Cole TJ. Energy expenditure in overweight and obese adults in affluent societies: an analysis of 319 doubly-labelled water measurements. *Eur J Clin Nutr* 1996; 50 (2): 93–7.
124. Levine JA, Eberhardt NL, Jensen MD. Role of nonexercise activity thermogenesis in resistance to fat gain in humans. *Science* 1999; 283 (5399): 212–4.
125. Ravussin E, Swinburn BA. Metabolic predictors of obesity: cross-sectional versus longitudinal data. *Int J Obes Relat Metab Disord* 1993; 17 (suppl 3): S28–31, S41–2.
126. Knowler WC, Pettitt DJ, Saad MF, Charles MA, Nelson RG, Howard BV, Bogardus C, Bennett PH. Obesity in the Pima Indians: its magnitude and relationship with diabetes. *Am J Clin Nutr* 1991; 53 (6, suppl): 1543S–51S.
127. Ravussin E, Lillioja S, Knowler WC, Christin L, Freymond D, Abbott WG, Boyce V, Howard BV, Bogardus C. Reduced rate of energy expenditure as a risk factor for body-weight gain. *N Engl J Med* 1988; 318 (8): 467–72.
128. Astrup A, Gotzsche PC, van de Werken K, Ranneries C, Toubro S, Raben A, Buemann B. Meta-analysis of resting metabolic rate in formerly obese subjects. *Am J Clin Nutr* 1999; 69 (6): 1117–22.
129. Weinsier RL, Nelson KM, Hensrud DD, Darnell BE, Hunter GR, Schutz Y. Metabolic predictors of obesity. Contribution of resting energy expenditure, thermic effect of food, and fuel utilization to four-year weight gain of post-obese and never-obese women. *J Clin Invest* 1995; 95 (3): 980–5.
130. Amatruda JM, Statt MC, Welle SL. Total and resting energy expenditure in obese women reduced to ideal body weight. *J Clin Invest* 1993; 92 (3): 1236–42.
131. Zurlo F, Ferraro RT, Fontvielle AM, Rising R, Bogardus C, Ravussin E. Spontaneous physical activity and obesity: cross-sectional and longitudinal studies in Pima Indians. *Am J Physiol* 1992; 263 (2, pt 1): E296–300.
132. Sundquist J, Johansson SE. The influence of socioeconomic status, ethnicity and lifestyle on body mass index in a longitudinal study. *Int J Epidemiol* 1998; 27 (1): 57–63.
133. Schoeller DA, Shay K, Kushner RF. How much physical activity is needed to minimize weight gain in

previously obese women? *Am J Clin Nutr* 1997; 66 (3): 551–6.
134. McNeill G, Bruce AC, Ralph A, James WP. Inter-individual differences in fasting nutrient oxidation and the influence of diet composition. *Int J Obes* 1988; 12 (5): 455–63.
135. Astrup A, Buemann B, Gluud C, Bennett P, Tjur T, Christensen N. Prognostic markers for diet-induced weight loss in obese women. *Int J Obes Relat Metab Disord* 1995; 19 (4): 275–8.
136. Toubro S, Sorensen TI, Hindsberger C, Christensen NJ, Astrup A. Twenty-four-hour respiratory quotient: the role of diet and familial resemblance. *J Clin Endocrinol Metab* 1998; 83 (8): 2758–64.
137. Seidell JC, Muller DC, Sorkin JD, Andres R. Fasting respiratory exchange ratio and resting metabolic rate as predictors of weight gain: the Baltimore Longitudinal Study on Aging. *Int J Obes Relat Metab Disord* 1992; 16 (9): 667–74.
138. Astrup A, Buemann B, Christensen NJ, Toubro S. Failure to increase lipid oxidation in response to increasing dietary fat content in formerly obese women. *Am J Physiol* 1994; 266 (4, pt 1): E592–9.
139. Larson DE, Ferraro RT, Robertson DS, Ravussin E. Energy metabolism in weight-stable postobese individuals. *Am J Clin Nutr* 1995; 62 (4): 735–9.
140. Froidevaux F, Schutz Y, Christin L, Jaquier E. Energy expenditure in obese women before and during weight loss, after refeeding, and in the weight-relapse period. *Am J Clin Nutr* 1993; 57 (1): 35–42.
141. Swinburn BA, Nyomba BL, Saad MF, Zurlo F, Raz I, Knowler WC, Lillioja S, Bogardus C, Ravussin E. Insulin resistance associated with lower rates of weight gain in Pima Indians. *J Clin Invest* 1991; 88 (1): 168–73.
142. Valdez R, Mitchell BD, Haffner SM, Hazuda HP, Morales PA, Monterrosa A, Stern MP. Predictors of weight change in a bi-ethnic population. The San Antonio Heart Study. *Int J Obes Relat Metab Disord* 1994; 18 (2): 85–91.
143. Hoag S, Marshall JA, Jones RH, Hamman RF. High fasting insulin levels associated with lower rates of weight gain in persons with normal glucose tolerance: the San Luis Valley Diabetes Study. *Int J Obes Relat Metab Disord* 1995; 19 (3): 175–80.
144. Yost TJ, Jensen DR, Eckel RH. Weight regain following sustained weight reduction is predicted by relative insulin sensitivity. *Obes Res* 1995; 3 (6): 583–7.
145. Eckel RH. Insulin resistance: an adaptation for weight maintenance. *Lancet* 1992; 340 (8833): 1452–3.
146. Christin L, O'Connell M, Bogardus C, Danforth E Jr, Ravussin E. Norepinephrine turnover and energy expenditure in Pima Indian and white men. *Metabolism* 1993; 42 (6): 723–9.
147. Snitker S, Tataranni PA, Ravussin E. Respiratory quotient is inversely associated with muscle sympathetic nerve activity. *J Clin Endocrinol Metab* 1998; 83 (11): 3977–9.
148. Tataranni PA, Young JB, Bogardus C, Ravussin E. A low sympathoadrenal activity is associated with body weight gain and development of central adiposity in Pima Indian men. *Obes Res* 1997; 5 (4): 341–7.
149. Caro JF, Sinha MK, Kolaczynski JW, Zhang PL, Considine RV. Leptin: the tale of an obesity gene. *Diabetes* 1996; 45 (11): 1455–62.
150. Ravussin E, Pratley RE, Maffei M, Wang H, Friedman JM, Bennett PH, Bogardus C. Relatively low plasma leptin concentrations precede weight gain in Pima Indians. *Nat Med* 1997; 3 (2): 238–40.
151. Caro JF, Kolaczynski JW, Nyce MR, Ohannesian JP, Opentanova I, Goldman WH, Lynn RB, Zhang PL, Sinha MK, Considine RV. Decreased cerebrospinal-fluid/serum leptin ratio in obesity: a possible mechanism for leptin resistance. *Lancet* 1996; 348 (9021): 159–61.
152. Lissner L, Karlsson C, Lindroos AK, Sjostrom L, Carlsson B, Carlsson L, Bengtsson C. Birth weight, adulthood BMI, and subsequent weight gain in relation to leptin levels in Swedish women. *Obes Res* 1999; 7 (2): 150–4.
153. McNeely MJ, Boyko EJ, Weigle DS, Shofer JB, Chessler SD, Leonnetti DL, Fujimoto WY. Association between baseline plasma leptin levels and subsequent development of diabetes in Japanese Americans. *Diabetes Care* 1999; 22 (1): 65–70.
154. Weyer C, Pratley RE, Salbe AD, Bogardus C, Ravussin E, Tataranni PA. Energy expenditure, fat oxidation, and body weight regulation: a study of metabolic adaptation to long-term weight change. *J Clin Endocrinol Metab* 2000; 85 (3): 1087–94.
155. Keys A, Brozek J, Henschel A, Mickelson O, Taylor H. *The Biology of Human Starvation.* Minneapolis, MN: University of Minnesota Press, 1950.
156. WHO. Energy and Protein Requirements. Report of a Joint FAO/WHO/UNU Expert Consultation. World Health Organ Technical Report Series, WHO Technical Report Series No. 724. Geneva: WHO, 1985; pp 1–206.
157. Sims EA, Danforth E Jr, Horton ES, Bray GA, Glennon JA, Salans LB. Endocrine and metabolic effects of experimental obesity in man. *Recent Prog Horm Res* 1973; 29: 457–96.
158. Norgan NG, Durnin JV. The effect of 6 weeks of overfeeding on the body weight, body composition, and energy metabolism of young men. *Am J Clin Nutr* 1980; 33 (5): 978–88.
159. Tremblay A, Despres JP, Theriault G, Fournier G, Bouchard C. Overfeeding and energy expenditure in humans. *Am J Clin Nutr* 1992; 56 (5): 857–62.
160. Elliot DL, Goldberg L, Kuehl KS, Bennett WM. Sustained depression of the resting metabolic rate after massive weight loss. *Am J Clin Nutr* 1989; 49 (1): 93–6.
161. Heshka S, Yang MU, Wang J, Burt P, Pi-Sunyer FX. Weight loss and change in resting metabolic rate. *Am J Clin Nutr* 1990; 52 (6): 981–6.
162. Leibel RL, Rosenbaum M, Hirsch J. Changes in energy expenditure resulting from altered body weight. *N Engl J Med* 1995; 332 (10): 621–8.
163. Friedman JM, Halaas JL. Leptin and the regulation of body weight in mammals. *Nature* 1998; 395 (6704): 763–70.
164. Minokoshi Y, Kim YB, Peroni OD, Fryer LG, Muller C, Carling D, Kahn BB. Leptin stimulates fatty-acid oxidation by activating AMP-activated protein kinase. *Nature* 2002; 415 (6869): 339–43.
165. Zhou Y-T, Shimabukuro M, Koyama K, Lee Y, Wang M-Y, Trieu F, Newgard CB, Unger RH. Induction by leptin of uncoupling protein-2 and enzymes of fatty acid oxidation. *Proc Natl Acad Sci USA* 1997; 94: 6386–90.
166. Alonso LG, Maren TH. Effect of food restriction on body composition of hereditary obese mice. *Am J Physiol* 1955; 183: 284–90.

167. Levin N, Nelson C, Gurney A, Vandlen R, De Sauvage F. Decreased food intake does not completely account for adiposity reduction after ob protein infusion. *Proc Natl Acad Sci USA* 1996; 93: 1726–30.
168. Prochazka M, Kozak UC, Kozak LP. A glycerol-3-phosphate dehydrogenase null mutant in BALB/cHeA mice. *J Biol Chem* 1989; 264 (8): 4679–83.
169. Brown LJ, Koza RA, Everett C, Reitman ML, Marshall L, Fahien LA, Kozak LP, MacDonald MJ. Normal thyroid thermogenesis, but reduced viability and adiposity in mice lacking the mitochondrial glycerol phosphate dehydrogenase. *J Biol Chem* 2002; 277: 32892–8.
170. Lee Y-P, Lardy HA. Influence of thyroid hormones on L-α-glycerophosphate dehydrogenases and other dehydrogenases in various organs of the rat. *J Biol Chem* 1965; 240: 1427–36.
171. Reidy SP, Weber JM. Accelerated substrate cycling: a new energy-wasting role for leptin in vivo. *Am J Physiol Endocrinol Metab* 2002; 282 (2): E312–7.
172. Joshi RL, Lamothe B, Cordonnier N, Mesbah K, Monthioux E, Jami J, Bucchini D. Targeted disruption of the insulin receptor gene in the mouse results in neonatal lethality. *EMBO J* 1996; 15 (7): 1542–7.
173. Accili D, Drago J, Lee EJ, Johnson MD, Cool MH, Salvatore P, Asico LD, Jose PA, Taylor SI, Westphal H. Early neonatal death in mice homozygous for a null allele of the insulin receptor gene. *Nat Genet* 1996; 12 (1): 106–9.
174. Kitamura T, Kahn CR, Acilli D. Insulin receptor knockout mice. *Annu Rev Physiol* 2003; 65: 8.120.
175. Bruning JC, Michael MD, Winnay JN, Hayashi T, Horsch D, Accili D, Goodyear LJ, Kahn CR. A muscle-specific insulin receptor knockout exhibits features of the metabolic syndrome of NIDDM without altering glucose tolerance. *Mol Cell* 1998; 2 (5): 559–69.
176. Guerra C, Navarro P, Valverde AM, Arribas M, Bruning J, Kozak LP, Kahn CR, Benito M. Brown adipose tissue-specific insulin receptor knockout shows diabetic phenotype without insulin resistance. *J Clin Invest* 2001; 108 (8): 1205–13.
177. Arch JRS, Ainsworth AT, Cawthorne MA, Piercy V, Senitt MV, Thody VE, Wilson C, Wilson S. Atypical β-adrenoreceptor on brown adipocytes as targets for anti-obesity drugs. *Nature* 1984; 309: 163–5.
178. Enerback S, Jacobsson A, Simpson EM, Guerra C, Yamashita H, Harper ME, Kozak LP. Mice lacking mitochondrial uncoupling protein are cold-sensitive but not obese [see comments]. *Nature* 1997; 387 (6628): 90–4.
179. Thomas SA, Palmiter RD. Thermoregulatory and metabolic phenotypes of mice lacking noradrenaline and adrenaline. *Nature* 1997; 387 (6628): 94–7.
180. Susulic VS, Frederich RC, Lawitts J, Tozzo E, Kahn BB, Harper M-E, Himms-Hagen J, Flier JS, Lowell BB, Targeted disruption of the β_3-adrenergic receptor gene. *J Biol Chem* 1995; 270: 29483–92.
181. Rohrer DK, Desai KH, Jasper JR, Stevens ME, Regula DP Jr, Barsh GS, Bernstein D, Kobilka BK. Targeted disruption of the mouse beta1-adrenergic receptor gene: developmental and cardiovascular effects. *Proc Natl Acad Sci USA* 1996; 93 (14): 7375–80.
182. Chruscinski AJ, Rohrer DK, Schauble E, Desai KH, Bernstein D, Kobilka BK. Targeted disruption of the beta2 adrenergic receptor gene. *J Biol Chem* 1999; 274 (24): 16694–700.
183. Bachman ES, Dhillon H, Zhang CY, Cinti S, Bianco AC, Kobilka BK, Lowell BB. betaAR signaling required for diet-induced thermogenesis and obesity resistance. *Science* 2002; 297 (5582): 843–5.
184. Valet P, Grujic D, Wade J, Ito M, Zingaretti MC, Soloveva V, Ross SR, Graves RA, Cinti S, Lafontan M, Lowell BB. Expression of human alpha 2-adrenergic receptors in adipose tissue of beta3-adrenergic receptor-deficient mice promotes diet-induced obesity. *J Biol Chem* 2000; 275 (44): 34797–802.
185. Liu X, Rossmeisl M, McClaine J, Kozak LP. Paradoxical resistance to diet-induced obesity in UCP-1-deficient mice. *J Clin Invest* 2003; 111 (3): 399–407.
186. Abu-Elheiga L, Matzuk MM, Abo-Hashema KA, Wakil SJ. Continuous fatty acid oxidation and reduced fat storage in mice lacking acetyl-CoA carboxylase 2. *Science* 2001; 291 (5513): 2613–6.
187. Guerra C, Koza RA, Walsh K, Kurtz DM, Wood PA, Kozak LP. Abnormal nonshivering thermogenesis in mice with inherited defects of fatty acid oxidation. *J Clin Invest* 1998; 102 (9): 1724–31.
188. Smith SJ, Cases S, Jensen DR, Chen HC, Sande E, Tow B, Sanan DA, Raber J, Eckel RH, Farese RV Jr. Obesity resistance and multiple mechanisms of triglyceride synthesis in mice lacking Dgat [see comments]. *Nat Genet* 2000; 25 (1): 87–90.
189. Chen HC, Smith SJ, Ladha Z, Jensen DR, Ferreira LD, Pulawa LK, McGuire JG, Pitas RE, Eckel RH, Farese RV Jr. Increased insulin and leptin sensitivity in mice lacking acyl CoA:diacylglycerol acyltransferase 1. *J Clin Invest* 2002; 109 (8): 1049–55.
190. Ravussin E, Bogardus C. Relationship of genetics, age, and physical-fitness to daily energy-expenditure and fuel utilization. *Am J Clin Nutr* 1989; 49 (5): 968–75.
191. Poehlman ET. Reduced metabolic rate after caloric restriction—can we agree on how to normalize the data? *J Clin Endocrinol Metab* 2003; 88 (1): 14–5.
192. Ravussin E, Bogardus C. A brief overview of human energy metabolism and its relationship to essential obesity. *Am J Clin Nutr* 1992; 55 (1, suppl): 242S–5S.
193. Kopecky J, Clarke G, Enerback S, Spiegelman B, Kozak LP. Expression of the mitochondrial uncoupling protein gene from the aP2 gene promoter prevents genetic obesity. *J Clin Invest* 1995; 96 (6): 2914–23.
194. Kopecky J, Hodny Z, Rossmeisl M, Syrovy I, Kozak LP. Reduction of dietary obesity in aP2–Ucp transgenic mice: physiology and adipose tissue distribution. *Am J Physiol* 1996; 270 (5, pt 1): E768–75.
195. Li B, Nolte LA, Ju JS, Han DH, Coleman T, Holloszy JO, Semenkovich CF. Skeletal muscle respiratory uncoupling prevents diet-induced obesity and insulin resistance in mice. *Nat Med* 2000; 6 (10): 1115–20.
196. Cederberg A, Gronning LM, Ahren B, Tasken P, Carlsson P, Enerback S. *FOXC2* is a winged helix gene that counteracts obesity, hypertriglceridemia, and diet-induced insulin resistance. *Cell* 2001; 106: 563–73.
197. Koza RA, Hohmann SM, Guerra C, Rossmeisl M, Kozak LP. Synergistic gene interactions control the induction of the mitochondrial uncoupling protein (Ucp-1) gene in white fat tissue. *J Biol Chem* 2000; 275 (44): 34486–92.
198. Guerra C, Koza RA, Yamashita H, Walsh K, Kozak LP. Emergence of brown adipocytes in white fat in mice is under genetic control. Effects on body weight and adiposity. *J Clin Invest* 1998; 102 (2): 412–20.

199. Clapham JC, Arch JR, Chapman H, Haynes A, Lister C, Moore GB, Piercy V, Carter SA, Lehner I, Smith SA, Beeley LJ, Godden RJ, Herrity N, Skehel M, Changani KK, Hockings PD, Reid DG, Squires SM, Hatcher J, Trail B, Latcham J, Rastan S, Harper AJ, Cadenas S, Buckingham JA, Brand MD. Mice overexpressing human uncoupling protein-3 in skeletal muscle are hyperphagic and lean. *Nature* 2000; 406 (6794): 415–8.
200. Champigny O, Ricquier D, Blondel O, Mayers RM, Briscoe MG, Holloway BR. Beta 3-adrenergic receptor stimulation restores message and expression of brown-fat mitochondrial uncoupling protein in adult dogs. *Proc Natl Acad Sci USA* 1991; 88 (23): 10774–7.
201. Himms-Hagen J, Cui J, Danforth E Jr, Taatjes DJ, Lang SS, Waters BL, Claus TH. Effect of CL-316, 243, a thermogenic beta 3-agonist, on energy balance and brown and white adipose tissues in rats. *Am J Physiol* 1994; 266 (4, pt 2): R1371–82.
202. Lean M. Evidence for brown adipose tissue in humans. In Bjorntrop P, Brodoff BN. (eds) *Obesity*. Philadelphia: J.B. Lippincott, 1992; pp 117–29.
203. Esterbauer H, Oberkofler H, Liu YM, Breban D, Hell E, Krempler F, Patsch W. Uncoupling protein-1 mRNA expression in obese human subjects: the role of sequence variations at the uncoupling protein-1 gene locus. *J Lipid Res* 1998; 39 (4): 834–44.
204. Soloveva V, Graves RA, Rasenick MM, Spiegelman BM, Ross SR. Transgenic mice overexpressing the β1-adrenergic receptor in adipose tissue are resistant to obesity. *Mol Endocrin* 1997; 11: 27–38.
205. Tsukiyama-Kohara K, Poulin F, Kohara M, DeMaria CT, Cheng A, Wu Z, Gingras AC, Katsume A, Elchebly M, Spiegelman BM, Harper ME, Tremblay ML, Sonenberg N. Adipose tissue reduction in mice lacking the translational inhibitor 4E- BP1. *Nat Med* 2001; 7 (10): 1128–32.
206. Cummings DE, Brandon EP, Planas JV, Motamed K, Idzerda RL, McKnight GS. Genetically lean mice result from targeted disruption of the RII beta subunit of protein kinase A [see comments]. *Nature* 1996; 382 (6592): 622–6.
207. Ricquier D, Bouillaud F. The uncoupling protein homologues: UCP-1, UCP-2, UCP-3, StUCP and AtUCP. *Biochem J* 2000; 345 (pt 2): 161–79.
208. Kozak, LP, Harper M-E. Mitochondrial uncoupling proteins in energy expenditure. *Annu Rev Nutr* 2000; 20: 339–63.
209. Gong DW, Monemdjou S, Gavrilova O, Leon LR, Marcus-Samuels B, Chou CJ, Everett C. Kozak LP, Li C, Deng C, Harper ME, Reitman ML. Lack of obesity and normal response to fasting and thyroid hormone in mice lacking uncoupling protein-3. *J Biol Chem* 2000; 275: 26251–7.
210. Vidal-Puig AJ, Grujic D, Zhang CY, Hagen T, Boss O, Ido Y, Szczepanik A, Wade J, Mootha V, Cortright R, Muoio DM, Lowell BB. Energy metabolism in uncoupling protein 3 gene knockout mice. *J Biol Chem* 2000; 275: 16258–66.
211. Arsenijevic D, Onuma H, Pecqueur C, Raimbault S, Manning BS, Miroux B, Couplan E, Alves-Guerra MC, Goubern M, Surwit R, Bouillaud F, Richard D, Collins S, Ricquier D. Disruption of the uncoupling protein-2 gene in mice reveals a role in immunity and reactive oxygen species production [In Process Citation]. *Nat Genet* 2000; 26 (4): 435–9.
212. Zhang CY, Baffy G, Perret P, Krauss S, Peroni O, Grujic D, Hagen T, Vidal-Puig AJ, Boss O, Kim YB, Zheng XX, Wheeler MB, Shulman GI, Chan CB, Lowell BB. Uncoupling protein-2 negatively regulates insulin secretion and is a major link between obesity, beta cell dysfunction, and type 2 diabetes. *Cell* 2001; 105 (6): 745–55.
213. Stuart JA, Harper JA, Brindle KM, Jekabsons MB, Brand MD. Physiological levels of mammalian uncoupling protein 2 do not uncouple yeast mitochondria. *J Biol Chem* 2001; 276 (21): 18633–9.

34

Role of the Adipocyte in Type 2 Diabetes

Stephen R. Farmer and Deepanwita Prusty

Boston University School of Medicine, Boston, MA, USA

TYPE 2 DIABETES AND INSULIN RESISTANCE

Type 2 diabetes mellitus is characterized by two primary defects: a reduced sensitivity of insulin-responsive tissues to insulin (insulin resistance) and a progressive decline in the secretion of insulin from pancreatic β-cells [1]. Insulin resistance develops in the early stages of the disease and is a major contributor to the eventual loss of β-cell function. In prediabetic individuals, the reduced sensitivity of liver, muscle, and adipose tissues to insulin lead to an elevation in plasma insulin levels (hyperinsulinemia) in order to maintain euglycemia. In addition to the effects on the pancreas, the combination of insulin resistance and hyperinsulinemia contributes to other metabolic abnormalities that together constitute the insulin resistance (metabolic) syndrome. Individuals with metabolic syndrome are at risk for developing pathophysiological defects, including dyslipidemia, hypertension, and cardiovascular disease [2, 3].

The development of insulin resistance is closely associated with an increase in adipose tissue, particularly in central visceral depots [4, 5]. Understanding the mechanisms that link obesity to insulin resistance is presently an area of active research in both basic and clinical establishments, with the goal of identifying targets for possible therapeutics. The conclusions drawn from this research implicate the adipocyte as a central player in the development of insulin resistance, affecting muscle and liver of individuals with excess adipose tissue. In fact, the role of the adipocyte in regulating overall energy balance has been significantly redefined. Specifically, in addition to storing excess energy as triglycerides, adipocytes secrete many biologically active molecules (Figure 1) that regulate mechanisms related to energy balance in other metabolically active tissues including the brain, muscle, and liver [6]. These bioactive molecules include hormones and several cytokines, collectively referred to as *adipocytokines*, which include leptin, tumor necrosis factor α (TNF-α), adiponectin/ACRP30/adipoQ/apM1, and resistin [7]. Certain adipocytokines have been directly linked to insulin resistance in obese humans as well as in various animal models. An approach to combating type 2 diabetes mellitus, therefore, is to understand the molecular and physiological mechanisms that regulate the formation and function of adipocytes in specific adipose tissue depots.

An increase in regional adiposity is believed to involve both adipocyte hyperplasia and an increase in adipocyte size (hypertrophy) due to the accumulation of stored triglycerides. A balance of fundamental biological processes including proliferation, differentiation, and cell death (apoptosis) regulates the number of adipocytes within adipose tissue. In fact, all of these processes have been shown to be involved either in the development of obesity or in the treatment of obesity-associated insulin resistance in various animal models. The formation of adipocytes involves expansion of a population of precursor stem cells that become committed to the adipogenic lineage, followed by terminal differentiation of the resulting preadipocytes into mature insulin-responsive adipocytes. Adipogenic stem cells are most likely localized to the stromal vascular component of adipose tissue, together with other mesenchymal cells that have the potential to differentiate into different cell types. Consequently, understanding the physiologic events that selectively induce the differentiation of these cells into fat cells may serve as an approach in regulating adiposity and controlling insulin resistance. In addition, however, it is likely that the

International Textbook of Diabetes Mellitus, Third Edition. Edited by R. A. DeFronzo, E. Ferrannini, H. Keen, and P. Zimmet.
 ISBN: 0-471-48655-8.

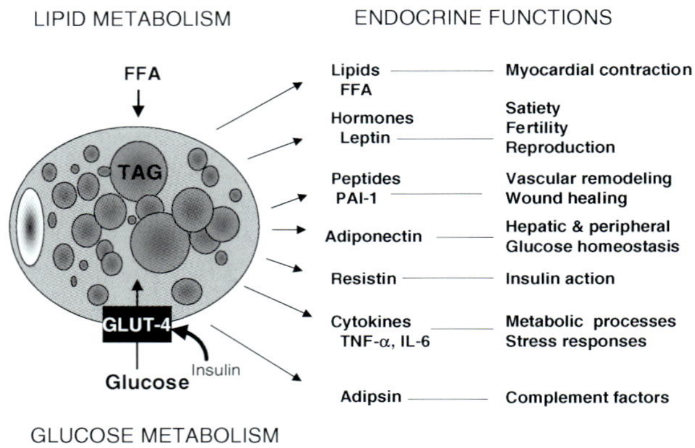

Figure 1 Functions of the adipocyte in regulating energy balance. Adipocytes play important roles in lipid metabolism by storing free fatty acids (FFA) as triacylglycerol (TAG) and in glucose metabolism by absorbing glucose in response to insulin via the insulin-dependent glucose transporter (GLUT-4). Adipocytes also secrete many molecules including hormones and cytokines involved in energy balance

various functions of the adipocyte in secreting bioactive molecules and controlling glucose and lipid homeostasis are regulated by events operating in the mature fat cell, which may also serve as therapeutic targets.

REGULATION OF THE FORMATION AND FUNCTION OF ADIPOCYTES

Adipogenesis

Most of our understanding of the mechanisms regulating the differentiation of mesenchymal precursor cells into adipocytes has come from studies performed in various cell culture models. Notable among these models are the 3T3-L1 and 3T3-F422A mouse preadipocyte cell lines originally isolated and characterized by Green and collaborators [8, 9]. Using these cell lines, investigators during the last two decades have demonstrated that adipogenesis involves the interplay between many extracellular effectors that regulate a complex transcriptional cascade orchestrating the expression of the entire adipogenic program [10–12]. Although the nature of the extracellular effectors varies from one model to the other, their effect on a select number of adipogenic transcription factors appears to be similar. These adipogenic transcription factors have been shown to function as key regulators of differentiation in transgenic animals. In the case of the 3T3-L1 model of adipogenesis, exposure of a confluent population of preadipocytes to insulin, glucocorticoids, and agents that stimulate cyclic adenosine monophosphate (cAMP) signaling pathways induces differentiation as characterized by progressive morphological changes of a fibroblastic cell to large round cells laden with multiple fat droplets [10]. Adipogenic differentiation involves reentry of quiescent, confluent cells into the cell cycle, followed by at least two rounds of cell division. This growth event is often referred to as clonal expansion and has been considered to be a prerequisite for differentiation [13]. Recent findings suggest, however, that cell division may not be required to render the mature adipogenic phenotype; instead, cell cycle related events that accompany clonal expansion appear to be directly involved in regulating the differentiation process. One of the earliest events during adipogenesis is a change in the expression and/or activity of a family of retinoblastoma-related pocket proteins, including p105RB, p107, and p130, as the preadipocytes progress through the cell cycle. These pocket proteins likely regulate the activity of the E2F family of transcription factors that control the expression of adipogenic genes [14]. Coincident with these cell cycle associated events is the induction of expression of two members of the CCAAT/enhancer binding protein family, C/EBPβ and C/EBPδ, by mechanisms that involve glucocorticoids, cAMP [15], and possibly the cAMP regulatory element binding protein CREB [16]. An important role of C/EBPβ and C/EBPδ appears to be activation of PPAR-γ [17, 18], a member of the peroxisome proliferator-activated receptor family of nuclear hormone receptors [19]. It is generally considered that PPAR-γ is the master regulator of adipogenesis since its overexpression and activation in nonadipogenic fibroblasts is sufficient to initiate the entire program responsible for the development of mature fat cells [20]. In fact, PPAR-γ induces the transcription of a series of target genes that encode proteins which regulate several of the different biological processes occurring in the adipocyte. As expected, these proteins include many enzymes, as well as other components involved in lipid and glucose metabolism [21]. Induction of another key transcription factor involved in terminal adipogenesis is C/EBPα whose expression appears to coincide with that of PPAR-γ and may also be regulated by C/EBPβ and C/EBPδ [12, 22]. Once PPAR-γ and C/EBPα are expressed, they cooperate to orchestrate the full expression of the adipogenic gene program (Figure 2) that includes induction of additional transcription factors such as STAT-5A and STAT-5B [23], suppression of growth-associated genes [24, 25], as well as stimulation of insulin-dependent glucose transport [26].

Regulation of PPAR-γ Expression and Activity

PPAR-γ has become the focus of many studies aimed at understanding the mechanisms regulating glucose homeostasis since it is a direct target of the thiazolidinedione (TZD) family of oral insulin sensitizers [21]. The transcriptional activity of PPAR-γ depends on several structural features contained within the molecule [19]. The DNA-binding domain is the most conserved domain among all members of the nuclear hormone receptor

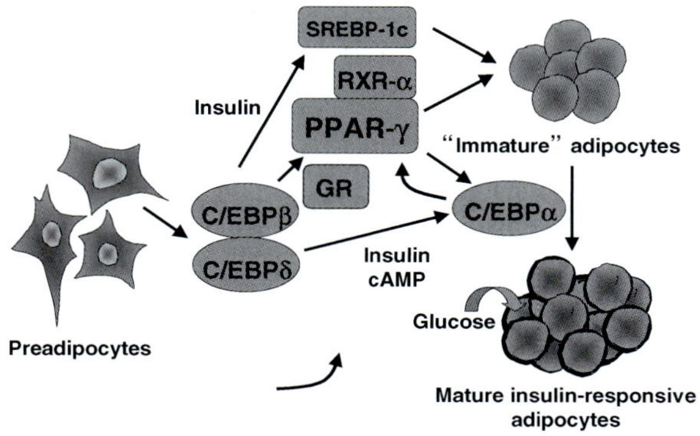

Figure 2 Regulation of adipogenesis by a cascade of transcription factors. Exposure of preadipocytes to adipogenic hormones (glucocorticoids, insulin, and inducers of intracellular cAMP) activates C/EBPβ, C/EBPδ, and SREBP-1c expression. These transcription factors along with glucocorticoid receptors (GRs) induce both PPAR-γ and C/EBPα, which enhance each other's expression as well as the many genes involved in the development of fat cells. PPAR-γ is required for differentiation, while C/EBPα plays a critical role in converting immature adipocytes into mature insulin-responsive adipocytes

superfamily that facilitates docking of PPAR-γ to specific DNA sequences referred to as PPAR response elements (PPREs) in the promoters and enhancers of its target genes. PPREs consist of two copies of a core hexanucleotide motif AGGTCA arranged as direct repeats and separated by either one nucleotide or two nucleotides, giving rise to direct repeat elements DR-1 or DR-2, respectively [19, 27]. PPAR-γ binds as a heterodimer to its respective PPRE where the heterodimeric partner is a member of the retinoid X receptor (RXR) family [28]. The PPAR/RXR complex can associate with a variety of coactivators and corepressors through direct protein–protein interactions involving specific transactivation domains, thereby imparting a more sophisticated level of control on gene expression. The ability of these domains to associate with co-activators and promote subsequent transcription is dependent upon the binding of an appropriate ligand to the ligand-binding domain within the PPAR-γ molecule [29]. Several long-chain polyunsaturated fatty acids (PUFAs) and their derivatives have the ability to bind PPAR-γ with varying affinities and, in some cases, can act as functional ligands to enhance transcriptional activity [19, 30, 31]. This is particularly true of the eicosinoids, which are a class of lipids derived from PUFAs by the enzymatic action of lipoxygenases or cyclooxygenases, giving rise to leukotrienes, hydroxyoctadenoic acids (13S-HODE), or prostaglandins (15-deoxy-D12,14-prostaglandin J2) [32–34]. There is a growing list of synthetic compounds currently being developed as therapeutic agents that are potent PPAR-γ ligands, including members of the TZD family of insulin sensitizers that activate PPAR-γ, i.e. troglitazone, pioglitazone, and rosiglitazone [35]. Like PPAR-γ, RXR also associates with a specific ligand, 9-*cis*-retinoic acid, and in so doing contributes to the transcriptional activity of the PPAR/RXR heterodimer.

Factors other than C/EBPβ and C/EBPδ have been proposed to stimulate PPAR-γ expression and facilitate terminal differentiation. Support for this notion stems from observations in mice deficient in both C/EBPβ and C/EBPδ that still express PPAR-γ and are capable of developing adipose tissue, albeit to a significantly lower extent when compared to control littermates [36]. One of these factors is the adipocyte determination and differentiation factor 1 (ADD-1) [37], which is a member of the basic helix–loop–helix family of sterol regulatory element binding proteins (SREBPs) [38]. SREBPs are known to regulate cholesterol metabolism in the liver and other tissues [39], but it appears that ADD-1 (SREBP-1c) also contributes to the transcriptional induction of the PPAR-γ gene by binding SREBP response elements in its promoter [40]. Yet other factors acting early during adipogenesis may include glucocorticoid receptors, which demonstrates that glucocorticoids can induce both PPAR-γ1 and PPAR-γ2 gene expression in the presence or absence of the C/EBPs [17, 41].

These positive mechanisms are certainly not the only means by which PPAR-γ gene expression is activated during adipogenesis. Recent investigations demonstrate a role for the suppression of inhibitory factors that maintain preadipocytes in an undifferentiated state. Most notable among these negative regulators are members of the GATA and TCF/LEF families of transcription factors. In the former case, studies demonstrate that constitutive expression of GATA-2 or GATA-3 in preadipocytes blocks adipogenesis in part by inhibiting PPAR-γ expression through the interaction of these proteins with GATA response elements in the PPAR-γ2 gene [42]. Moreover, GATA-3-deficient embryonic stem cells exhibit an enhanced ability to undergo adipogenesis, and GATA 2 and GATA 3 expression is downregulated in obese mice. The antiadipogenic activity of TCF/LEF factors, on the other hand, is accomplished by activation of the Wnt signaling pathway in preadipocytes upon secretion of Wnt proteins, in particular Wnt 10b [43]. In fact, ectopic expression of Wnt in preadipocytes blocks adipogenesis by inhibiting PPAR-γ gene expression, the precise mechanism of which is not known.

To date, only a limited number of genes expressed during the terminal stages of adipogenesis have been shown to contain PPREs. It is likely, therefore, that PPAR-γ induces the expression of many adipogenic genes through the activation of intermediary *trans*-acting factors. In this regard, our recent investigations suggest that PPAR-γ can directly transactivate the C/EBPα gene and may induce C/EBPα expression during adipogenesis [41]. In fact, PPAR-γ and C/EBPα can cross-regulate each other in order to maintain their high level of expression required for orchestrating the pleiotrophic functions of the adipocyte [44]. Additional intermediary factors may include the STAT family of transcription factors, specifically STAT-1, STAT-5A, and STAT-5B, whose differentiation-dependent induction during adipogenesis is regulated by PPAR-γ [23]. Although achievement of the mature adipocyte phenotype in mice requires STAT-5 [45], the precise function of these transcription factors during adipogenesis is yet to be determined.

It is clear that PPAR-γ is an indispensable component of the network of factors regulating adipogenesis; therefore, production of its ligand may contribute significantly to the differentiation of preadipocytes. In fact, one reason that various fibroblasts are unable to differentiate into mature adipocytes following their exposure to adipogenic inducers may be their inability to produce PPAR-γ ligands. For example, ectopic expression of PPAR-γ in nonadipogenic fibroblasts requires a potent PPAR-γ ligand such as a thiazolidinedione to activate the adipogenic program and induce the expression of C/EBPα [46]. If, however, both PPAR-γ and C/EBPα are co-expressed in these fibroblasts, differentiation ensues in a ligand-independent manner, suggesting that C/EBPα plays a role in activating a pathway that leads to PPAR-γ ligand production [47]. Moreover, recent studies suggest that C/EBPβ may also participate in this process, since ectopic expression of a dominant negative isoform of C/EBPβ (LIP) renders 3T3-L1 preadipocytes ligand-dependent [41]. Whether or not these C/EBPs directly transactivate the genes that code for enzymes controlling ligand synthesis is not known; however, one might postulate the involvement of a possible intermediary factor in this process, such as ADD-1 (SREBP-1c). In fact, ectopic expression of ADD-1 in non-adipogenic fibroblasts has been shown to induce the secretion of lipids that are able to activate PPAR-γ in *in vitro* assays [48].

PPAR-γ and Transcriptional Control of the Pleiotropic Functions of the Adipocyte

Until very recently, the results from both *in vivo* and *in vitro* investigations positioned PPAR-γ and C/EBPα as co-master regulators of adipogenesis. For instance, mice deficient in either transcription factor are compromised with regard to their ability to develop adipose tissue [49–51]. In addition, ectopic expression of either C/EBPα or PPAR-γ in non-adipogenic fibroblasts has been shown to induce adipogenesis [47, 52], and the expression of one can be induced by the ectopic expression of the other [44]. It is possible therefore that either of these factors may be capable of acting independently to promote fat cell differentiation. Since both C/EBPα and PPAR-γ can cross-regulate each other's expression, definitive analysis of their independent roles requires the use of both C/EBPα- and PPAR-γ-deficient cell lines. In this regard, recent studies demonstrate that mouse embryonic fibroblasts lacking either C/EBPα or PPAR-γ have limited adipogenic potential upon exposure to a cocktail of adipogenic hormones. Ectopic expression of PPAR-γ in the C/EBPα-deficient cells in the presence of a potent exogenous ligand could induce adipogenesis [44]. The converse experiment, however, demonstrated that ectopic expression of C/EBPα could not induce adipogenesis in the PPARγ-deficient fibroblasts [53]. Taken together, these observations provide strong evidence to suggest that there is a unified pathway of transcriptional events that leads to the development of adipocytes. Accordingly, a model based on these data identifies PPAR-γ as the direct regulator of adipogenesis, while C/EBPα provides additional functions that are dependent on PPAR-γ activity. One of the functions of C/EBPα may include maintaining PPAR-γ expression through its ability to transactivate the PPAR-γ gene, which consequently maintains the mature adipocyte phenotype [44, 46]. An example of this is demonstrated in studies addressing the mechanisms responsible for expression of the β_3-adrenergic receptor [54] and the insulin-dependent glucose transport system [55]. Specifically, activation of PPAR-γ alone in C/EBPα-deficient fibroblasts under potent adipogenic conditions induces the formation of lipid droplets and the expression of several genes associated with adipocyte differentiation. These C/EBPα-deficient *adipocytes* do not express all the functions of a mature adipocyte since they do not express the β_3-adrenergic receptor nor are they capable of taking up glucose in response to insulin [44, 46, 54]. This defect can be overcome, however, by co-expressing C/EBPα together with PPAR-γ in the C/EBPα-deficient fibroblasts, thereby implicating a positive cooperative role for C/EBPα in conjunction with PPAR-γ during terminal adipocyte differentiation (Figure 2).

THE ADIPOCYTE AND INSULIN RESISTANCE

The Role of Free Fatty Acids

In normoglycemic individuals, adipose tissue only accounts for ~10% of the insulin-stimulated whole body glucose disposal, whereas skeletal muscle accounts for at least 70% of this function [56]. This fact has led to the notion that muscle is the principal tissue responsible for the development of insulin resistance in type 2 diabetes. It is becoming apparent though that adipose tissue also plays a fundamental role in glucose homeostasis [57] (Figure 3). In fact, mice and humans with significantly reduced amounts of fat, as is the case in familial lypodystrophy or genetic ablation of adipose tissue, are extremely insulin resistant [58–62]. Moreover, some investigators suggest that insulin resistance may in fact be initiated in adipose tissue, which may later lead to impairments in insulin signaling in both muscle and liver [63]. Insulin is known to regulate other biological processes besides glucose uptake in responsive tissues. In adipose tissue, insulin

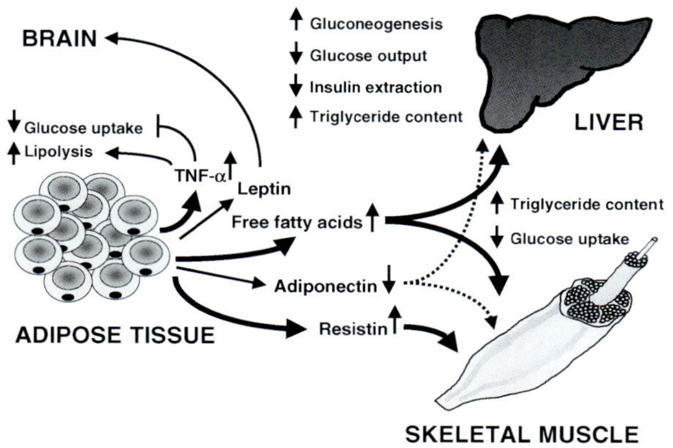

Figure 3 Central role of adipose tissue in the insulin-resistant syndrome. The effect of elevated levels of circulating free fatty acids and the change in secretion of important hormones and adipocytokines positions the adipocyte as a central mediator of the insulin-resistant syndrome in obese individuals

suppresses lipolysis; consequently, defects in insulin action in adipocytes lead to an enhanced release of free fatty acids from various fat depots. In fact, one of the hallmarks of obesity is an elevated level of circulating free fatty acids, despite an increase in triglyceride storage in adipose tissue [64]. Moreover, visceral fat appears to release significantly higher amounts of fatty acids than subcutaneous depots, probably because visceral fat cells are less sensitive to suppression of lipolysis by insulin [65]. High fatty acid concentrations in the circulation are believed to attenuate insulin responsiveness in muscle and liver [66]. The mechanisms responsible for the effect of fatty acids on insulin action are presently being elucidated. In the case of muscle, Randle and collaborators demonstrated that fatty acids compete with glucose for substrate oxidation, which led to the hypothesis that the metabolism of fatty acids results in an increased ratio of intramitochondrial acetyl-CoA/CoA and NADH/NAD^+, with subsequent inhibition of pyruvate dehydrogenase. This leads to an elevation of citrate levels and consequently an inhibition of phosphofructokinase activity, resulting in an accumulation of glucose-6-phosphate. Since glucose-6-phosphate negatively feeds back on hexokinase II, the overall effect of elevated free fatty acids would be increased intracellular glucose concentrations, resulting in subsequent prevention of glucose uptake [67–69]. The results from a series of recent studies by Shulman and colleagues [70–72], however, are not consistent with the Randle hypothesis. They show that elevated levels of fatty acids in plasma caused a significant reduction in intracellular glucose concentration. Moreover, the studies go on to demonstrate that the rate-controlling step for fatty acid induced insulin resistance in human muscle is glucose uptake. Specifically, it appears that the effect of fatty acids is to increase the levels of diacylglycerol, long-chain fatty acyl-CoA, and ceramides, which leads to activation of a serine/threonine kinase cascade (likely initiated by protein kinase C theta), resulting in phosphorylation of the insulin receptor substrates IRS-1 and IRS-2. The phosphorylated forms of IRS-1/2 are incapable of associating with phosphatidylinositol 3 kinase (PI3K), resulting in decreased activation of glucose transport.

An increase in hepatic uptake of fatty acids leads to triglyceride synthesis and formation of fat droplets, which in some obese individuals can eventually lead to steatosis of the liver. Other effects of elevated levels of fatty acids is to enhance gluconeogenesis and inhibit extraction of insulin from the circulation, contributing, therefore, to the hyperglycemia, hyperinsulinemia, and dyslipidemia associated with insulin resistance [66, 73].

The Role of Adipocytokines

As mentioned above, adipose tissue is not only a store for excess energy in the form of triglycerides, but it also actively secretes a variety of biologically active molecules that act at distant sites to regulate several different physiological functions, including energy balance, bone formation, and reproduction [74, 75]. At present, several dozen secreted molecules have been identified, and some of which are considered to play a role in regulating glucose and lipid homeostasis (Figure 3). The most notable among this group of molecules is leptin, TNF-α, adiponectin/Acrp30/AdipoQ/apM, and resistin.

Leptin

Leptin, the obese (ob) gene product, is a hormone secreted primarily by adipose tissue in response to a variety of stimuli including insulin. It acts both in the brain and periphery to regulate the appetite as well as overall energy balance [76–78]. The various target cells of leptin express one or more isoforms of the leptin receptor, in which the long splice variant (OB-Rb) is the key signaling form expressed most abundantly in the arcuate nucleus and paraventricular nucleus of the hypothalamus [79]. These regions of the brain are associated with the central control of energy balance. In the hypothalamus, leptin interacts with several neuroendocrine systems by activating specific target cells that lead to suppression of food intake [78]. Other studies suggest that leptin may also act in peripheral tissues to regulate insulin sensitivity in skeletal muscle. Recent studies by Kahn and associates suggest that leptin stimulates the oxidation of fatty acids and the uptake of glucose in muscle via 5′-AMP-activated protein kinase (AMPK), which has been identified as a principal mediator of these effects [80].

Tumor Necrosis Factor α

TNFα secretion from adipose tissue is increased in obese and insulin-resistant individuals [81]. Various *in vitro* studies have demonstrated that TNFα inhibits insulin-dependent glucose transport in adipocytes by stimulating the phosphorylation of IRS-1, which in turns blocks the transmission of signals from the insulin receptor to the glucose transport machinery [82–85]. The role of TNFα in glucose homeostasis has been supported by studies on mice mutated either for TNFα or for both isoforms of its receptor. TNFα-deficient mice develop slightly less pronounced insulin resistance when treated with a high-fat diet than their wild-type counterparts [86]. Similarly, mice lacking both TNFα receptors are protected from insulin resistance and hyperglycemia when crossed with *ob*/*ob* mice [86, 87].

Adiponectin/Acrp30/AdipoQ

Four separate groups using different approaches originally identified adiponectin as a protein expressed primarily in adipose tissue. Human adiponectin was isolated by large-scale random sequencing of a 3′-directed, human adipose tissue cDNA library [88]. The mouse counterparts referred to as Acrp30 and AdipoQ were cloned by differential display using preadipocytes and adipocytes corresponding to the 3T3-L1 and 3T3-F422 cell lines, respectively [89, 90]. Adiponectin is an adipocyte-specific secreted protein, which displays sequence homology with C1q, the first component of the classical complement activation pathway. Its gene expression is enhanced manyfold during adipogenesis and it is regulated by various effectors including insulin [89, 90]. Moreover, adiponectin mRNA expression is dysregulated in obesity, being significantly downregulated in adipose tissue from obese mice and humans [89]. Furthermore, plasma concentrations of adiponectin are much lower in obese individuals than in lean controls, consistent with the more recent observations, demonstrating that this adipocytokine is involved in regulating energy balance [91]. In fact, adiponectin decreases insulin resistance by increasing fatty acid oxidation in muscle and liver of obese and insulin-resistant mice [92]. It also suppresses hepatic glucose production by sensitizing the hepatocytes to insulin [93, 94]. The signaling pathway involved in these insulin-sensitizing processes appears to involve activation of AMPK [95]. Interestingly, the gene encoding adiponectin has been mapped to a locus of the human chromosome 3q27, which is associated with susceptibility to diabetes and the metabolic syndrome [96]. In fact, a series of recent studies present evidence of an association between single nucleotide polymorphisms in the adiponectin gene and type 2 diabetes in humans [97–100]. Moreover, disruption of the adiponectin gene leads to insulin resistance and atherosclerosis *in vivo* [101, 102].

Resistin

Resistin is a novel 12.5-kDa, cysteine-rich, adipocyte-derived secreted protein, which belongs to a murine family that includes two other members called RELM (resistin-like molecule) and FIZZ (found in inflammatory zone) proteins [103–105]. It is also known as ADSF (adipocyte secreted factor) [106] and FIZZ-3, and is the only member of the RELM family to be expressed primarily in adipose tissue [105]. Its discovery was made during a search for genes that are downregulated by the insulin sensitizers, TZDs, in mouse adipocytes [104, 107]. Resistin has been shown to circulate at increased levels in obese mice and counteracts the actions of insulin on glucose homeostasis. Administration of the recombinant protein to wild-type mice caused an impairment in glucose tolerance and insulin action, and resistin levels were reported to be increased in genetic and diet-induced forms of obesity [107]. When an antibody against resistin was administered to obese mice, a concomitant increase in systemic insulin sensitivity was noted [104].

ROLE OF PPAR-γ LIGANDS (TZDS) IN TREATING TYPE 2 DIABETES

The thiazolidinediones are a new class of oral therapeutics for the treatment of type 2 diabetes that improve glycemic control by increasing insulin sensitivity in target tissues: muscle, adipose tissue, and liver [108]. During the last few years, three TZDs have been approved for clinical use: troglitazone (Rezulin™), rosiglitazone (Avandia™), and pioglitazone (Actos™). While the latter two are still in use, troglitazone has been withdrawn from the market because of its association with hepatotoxicity [109, 110]. TZDs are a valuable addition to the group of antidiabetic drugs because they improve insulin resistance in insulin-responsive tissues. This activity, therefore, leads to a correction of hyperinsulinemia and an improvement in many of the secondary features of the metabolic syndrome, without causing hypoglycemia [111].

The TZDs were originally developed through screening of compounds for antilipidemic and antihyperglycemic activity in rodent models of dyslipidemia and diabetes [112]. It was several years after these initial studies that the TZDs were shown to stimulate PPAR-γ activity. As discussed above, TZDs are potent ligands for PPAR-γ [113] and their antidiabetic effects are considered to be mediated through their activation of PPAR-γ [21]. In fact, the clinical potency of each of the TZDs closely correlates with their affinity for binding PPAR-γ [114].

Mechanism of Action of TZDs in Type 2 Diabetes

The fact that TZDs stimulate PPAR-γ activity raised the notion that these drugs act by effecting PPAR-γ gene expression in tissues that express this nuclear hormone receptor. PPAR-γ is expressed at high levels in adipose tissue, colon, and activated macrophages, and at lower levels in other tissues [115, 116]. The TZDs have been shown to sensitize subjects to insulin by increasing glucose utilization in muscle and suppressing glucose production in the liver [21]. These highly metabolic tissues, however, express relatively low levels of PPARγ; therefore, adipose tissue is considered to be the principal target of TZDs since it is the only insulin-responsive tissue with a high level of PPAR-γ expression. Support for this idea has come from studies using lipoatrophic A-ZIP/F1 mice that have virtually no adipose tissue; consequently, these mice are markedly insulin resistant, hyperglycemic, hyperinsulinemic, hyperlipidemic, and exhibit steatosis of the liver [60]. Transplantation of fat into these mice reversed the metabolic manifestations of lipodystrophy, demonstrating that the lack of adipose tissue contributes significantly to their insulin resistance [117]. Moreover, treatment of the mice with rosiglitazone or troglitazone did not reduce glucose or insulin levels compared to wild-type controls, demonstrating that adipose tissue is required for the antidiabetic effects of the TZDs [118]. With this in mind, several investigators have suggested that TZDs may modulate key communication signals between fat, muscle, and liver via fatty acids and adipocytokines.

TZDs and Circulating Fatty Acids

The improvement in insulin responsiveness in rats treated with TZDs was associated with a repartitioning of fatty acids toward adipose tissue rather than muscle and liver [119, 120]. Furthermore, treatment of subjects with rosiglitazone also resulted in an improvement in peripheral adipocyte insulin responsiveness, as indicated by increased insulin suppression of lipolysis in adipocytes and decreased plasma fatty acid concentrations [121]. This effect likely improves insulin sensitivity because fatty acid accumulation leads to an attenuation of insulin-dependent glucose uptake in muscle and an increase in gluconeogenesis in liver. Studies strongly suggest that the drop in circulating free fatty acids is due to a direct effect of the TZDs on adipogenesis in specific adipose tissue depots. In fact, prolonged treatment of subjects with TZDs leads to an increased fat mass that seems to involve redistribution of adipose tissue from the visceral depot to the subcutaneous compartment [122]. Along with this remodeling process is a shift in the cell population within each depot in which the enlarged, mature adipocytes appear to be replaced by small, newly differentiated adipocytes [123]. The reduction in the mature adipocyte population is thought to be caused by a PPAR-γ-associated induction of apoptosis [124].

Stimulation of adipogenesis by PPAR-γ in adipose tissue may be one reason why TZDs promote fatty acid uptake and storage in the adipocytes of insulin-resistant individuals. In fact, expression of several genes involved in fatty acid metabolism have been shown to be enhanced by TZD-dependent activation of PPAR-γ during adipocyte differentiation, such as genes coding for the fatty acid transporter [125], fatty acid binding protein [20], lipoprotein lipase [126], acyl-CoA synthetase [127], and phosphoenolpyruvate carboxykinase [128]. As stated above, another effect of TZDs is the sensitization of adipose tissue to insulin, an event that should contribute to the enhanced accumulation of lipids in the adipocyte. Specifically, insulin should be more effective at suppressing lipolysis and inducing insulin-dependent glucose transport in TZD-treated subjects compared to untreated individuals. In fact, studies have shown that activation of PPAR-γ by TZDs during adipogenesis induces the expression of several genes associated with insulin-responsive glucose uptake, such as the insulin-dependent glucose transporter (GLUT-4) [26], the insulin receptor substrate 2 (IRS-2) [129], the p85 subunit of PI3K [130], and the Cbl-associated protein (CAP) [131, 132]. Since adipose tissue only contributes to $\sim$10% of the total body glucose disposal in normoglycemic individuals, it is still unclear whether there is a role for the enhanced PPAR-γ-associated insulin-dependent glucose uptake in adipocytes. Recent studies by Kahn and associates, however, demonstrate that mice with adipose-selective reduction of GLUT-4 (G4A$^{-/-}$) have normal growth and adipose tissue mass despite markedly impaired insulin-stimulated glucose uptake in adipocytes [133]. Although GLUT-4 expression is preserved in muscle, these mice are insulin resistant in muscle and liver, and develop glucose intolerance and hyperinsulinemia. The role of adipocyte-specific GLUT-4 in glucose homeostasis is not known, but one possible role of the enhanced glucose uptake into adipocytes in response to TZDs may serve to provide glycerol phosphate for triglyceride production from fatty acids. In this regard, Lazar and coworkers [134] have recently discovered that adipocytes are capable of producing glycerol kinase in response to treatment with TZDs. It has generally been considered that adipocytes lack glycerol kinase and thereby avoid futile cycles of triglyceride breakdown and resynthesis from glycerol and fatty acids. By inducing glycerol kinase, TZDs can markedly stimulate glycerol incorporation into triglyceride and, consequently, reduce the secretion of fatty acids into the circulation.

TZDs and Adipocytokines

Several recent studies suggest that TZDs may act by modulating the expression and secretion of particular adipocytokines from adipose tissue in insulin-resistant individuals (Figure 4). For instance, studies in obese and diabetic animals and humans demonstrate that TZDs suppress TNFα expression under conditions that also improve insulin sensitivity [135, 136]. TZDs may also act to block the inhibitory effects of TNFα on insulin signaling and lipolysis [137, 138]. Leptin and resistin also belong to the group of secreted proteins whose expression is attenuated by TZDs.

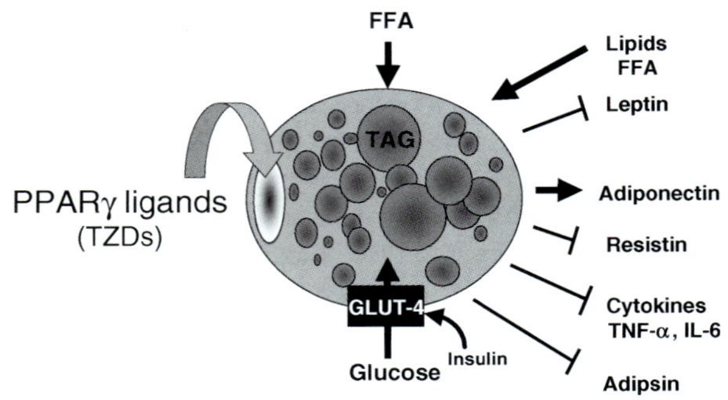

Figure 4 The effect of PPAR-γ ligands on adipocyte function. Activation of PPAR-γ in adipocytes by exposure to the TZD family of insulin sensitizers enhances glucose uptake and the storage of free fatty acids (FFA) as triacylglycerol (TAG). Additionally, TZDs modulate expression and secretion of a variety of adipocytokines in a manner consistent with their role in sensitizing individuals to insulin (see text for details)

Whether these molecules are responsible for the insulin-sensitizing activity of TZDs is presently the topic of significant debate. In the case of leptin, most *in vivo* studies demonstrate that this hormone increases insulin sensitivity [139, 140], and therefore, its suppression by TZDs would be counteractive. In fact, such a TZD-associated decrease in circulating leptin levels may contribute to the increased adiposity observed in patients treated with TZDs [122, 141].

Resistin was initially identified as being one of the proteins whose expression in 3T3-L1 adipocytes is suppressed by the TZD-associated activation of PPAR-γ [104]. Its role as a mediator of PPAR-γ activity, however, remains to be clarified as other reports suggest that PPAR-γ agonists stimulate rather than decrease its expression [142]. In the case of adiponectin, its expression and secretion has been shown to be increased in humans and insulin-resistant mice *in vivo* in response to treatment with TZDs [143–145].

THE ADIPOCYTE AS A TARGET FOR FUTURE ANTIDIABETIC THERAPIES

Based on the successful use of the thiazolidinediones in sensitizing diabetic patients to insulin, there is an intensive research effort to develop more potent and selective agonists of PPAR-γ. The outcome of this effort is the development of a series of *N*-(2-benzoylphenyl)-L-tyrosine derivatives that bind PPAR-γ with higher affinity than thiazolidinediones and are effective in the treatment of insulin resistance associated with type 2 diabetes. It is interesting, however, that the higher potency with regard to activation of PPAR-γ does not translate into improved antidiabetic efficacy. Moreover, the L-tyrosine-based PPAR-γ ligands also share the same side effects of the TZDs. Consequently, an alternative approach has been adopted, which is based on a strategy used for the development of chemotherapeutic agents targeting estrogen receptors. Specifically, evidence from recent research suggests that selective PPAR-γ modulators and antagonists may serve as promising antidiabetic drug candidates. For instance, a PPAR-γ antagonist, LG100641, was shown to inhibit TZD-induced gene expression in 3T3-L1 adipocytes, yet it stimulated glucose uptake [146]. Similarly, a new thiazolidinedione, NC-2100, is a weak PPAR-γ activator, but it has potent antidiabetic activities in obese mice [147]. These observations are consistent with the effects of the partial loss of PPAR-γ function caused by mutations in both the human and mice PPAR-γ genes [148, 149], which suggest that an attenuation of PPAR-γ activity can also lead to insulin sensitivity. As discussed earlier, the transcriptional activity of PPAR-γ depends on its ability to form a complex with the 9-*cis*-retinoic acid receptor RXR. Consequently, additional therapeutic approaches have considered using RXR agonists and/or antagonists to modulate PPAR-γ activity. In this regard, injection of an RXR antagonist into high-fat-fed mice improved insulin sensitivity, and was associated with decreased triglyceride content in adipose tissue and skeletal muscle [150].

In considering alternative therapies, one must also consider targeting other receptors and/or transcription factors that influence the formation of adipose tissue. It is well established that excess glucocorticoids results in visceral obesity and diabetes [151] (also see chapter 32). In humans with Cushing's syndrome, the increased visceral obesity is accompanied by an increased secretion of glucocorticoids into the plasma [151]; however, obese individuals not suffering from Cushing's syndrome have normal circulating levels of glucocorticoids [152]. An explanation for this apparent paradox has come from a series of studies targeting the enzyme 11β-hydroxysteroid dehydrogenase type 1 (11β-HSD-1), which converts inactive glucocorticoids (cortisone in humans, 11-dehydrocortisone in rodents) to the active forms (cortisol and corticosterone, respectively) in liver, lung, brain, and adipose tissue. In fact, mice homozygous for a targeted deletion of the 11β-HSD-1 gene cannot regenerate active corticosterone from inert 11-dehydrocorticosterone *in vivo*, demonstrating that 11β-HSD-1 is the sole 11β-reductase in the rodent. Moreover, these 11β-HSD-1-deficient mice could be made obese if fed a high-fat diet, yet they were resistant to diabetes [153]. Furthermore, adipose tissue from obese humans and rats has been shown to express an increase in 11β-HSD-1 activity. These observations are consistent with the notion that intracellular levels of glucocorticoids are determined not only by plasma hormone levels, but also by activation of the inactive hormone within target tissues. In fact, Flier and collaborators recently tested the hypothesis that increased production of glucocorticoids exclusively in adipose tissue would lead to visceral obesity and metabolic syndrome by targeted overexpression of 11β-HSD-1 in adipose tissue [154]. The resulting transgenic mice had increased adipose levels of corticosterone and developed visceral obesity that was exaggerated by a high-fat diet. The mice also exhibited pronounced insulin resistance and hyperlidemia, suggesting that adipocyte 11β-HSD-1 may be a potential target for combating visceral obesity and its associated metabolic disorders.

Acknowledgment

This work was supported by National Institutes of Health Grant DK51586 and DK58825.

REFERENCES

1. Reaven GM. Insulin resistance: a chicken that has come to roost. *Ann N Y Acad Sci* 1999; 892: 45–57.
2. Reaven GM. Banting lecture 1988. Role of insulin resistance in human disease. *Diabetes* 1988; 37:1595–607.
3. Reaven GM. Pathophysiology of insulin resistance in human disease. *Physiol Rev* 1995; 75: 473–86.
4. Evans DJ, Hoffmann RG, Kalkhoff RK, Kissebah AH. Relationship of body fat topography to insulin sensitivity and metabolic profiles in premenopausal women. *Metabolism* 1984; 33: 68–75.
5. Golay A, Chen N, Chen YD, Hollenbeck C, Reaven GM. Effect of central obesity on regulation of carbohydrate metabolism in obese patients with varying degrees of glucose tolerance. *J Clin Endocrinol Metab* 1990; 71: 1299–304.
6. Kahn BB, Flier JS. Obesity and insulin resistance. *J Clin Invest* 2000; 106: 473–81.
7. Shuldiner AR, Yang R, Gong DW. Resistin, obesity and insulin resistance—the emerging role of the adipocyte as an endocrine organ. *N Engl J Med* 2001; 345: 1345–6.
8. Green H, Kehinde O. Sublines of mouse 3T3 cells that accumulate lipid. *Cell* 1974; 1: 113–6.
9. Green H, Kehinde O. An established preadipose cell line and its differentiation in culture, II: factors affecting the adipose conversion. *Cell* 1975; 5: 19–27.
10. Gregoire FM, Smas CM, Sul HS. Understanding adipocyte differentiation. *Physiol Rev* 1998; 78: 783–809.
11. Morrison RF, Farmer SR. Hormonal signaling and transcriptional control of adipocyte differentiation. *J Nutr* 2000; 130: 3116–21.
12. Rosen ED, Walkey CJ, Puigserver P, Spiegelman BM. Transcriptional regulation of adipogenesis. *Genes Dev* 2000; 14: 1293–307.
13. Scott RE, Florine DL, Wille JJJ, Yun K. Coupling of growth arrest and differentiation at a distinct state in the G_1phase of cell cycle: G_D. *Proc Natl Acad Sci* 1982; 79: 845–9.
14. Fajas L, Landsberg RL, Huss-Garcia Y, Sardet C, Lees JA, Auwerx J. E2Fs regulate adipocyte differentiation. *Dev Cell* 2002; 3: 39–49.
15. Cao Z, Umek RM, McKnight SL. Regulated expression of three C/EBP isoforms during adipose conversion of 3T3-L1 cells. *Genes Dev.* 1991; 5: 1538–52.
16. Reusch JE, Colton LA, Klemm DJ. CREB activation induces adipogenesis in 3T3-L1 cells. *Mol Cell Biol* 2000; 20: 1008–20.
17. Wu Z, Bucher NLR, Farmer SR. Induction of peroxisome proliferator-activated receptor gamma during conversion of 3T3 fibroblasts into adipocytes is mediated by C/EBPβ, C/EBPδ and glucocorticoids. *Mol Cell Biol* 1996; 16: 4128–36.
18. Wu Z, Xie Y, Bucher NLR, Farmer SR. Conditional ectopic expression of C/EBPβ in NIH-3T3 cells induces PPAR-γ and stimulates adipogenesis. *Genes Dev* 1995; 9: 2350–63.
19. Desvergne B, Wahli W. Peroxisome proliferator-activated receptors: nuclear control of metabolism. *Endocr Rev* 1999; 20: 649–88.
20. Tontonoz P, Hu E, Graves RA, Budavari AI, Spiegelman BM. mPPARγ2: tissue-specific regulator of an adipocyte enhancer. *Genes Dev* 1994; 8: 1224–34.
21. Picard F, Auwerx J. PPAR(gamma) and glucose homeostasis. *Annu Rev Nutr* 2002; 22: 167–97.
22. Morrison RF, Farmer SR. Insights into the transcriptional control of adipocyte differentiation. *J Cell Biochem* 1999; (suppl 32–33): 59–67.
23. Stephens JM, Morrison RF, Wu Z, Farmer SR. PPARgamma ligand-dependent induction of STAT1, STAT5A, and STAT5B during adipogenesis. *Biochem Biophys Res Commun* 1999; 262: 216–22.
24. Altiok S, Xu M, Spiegelman BM. PPARgamma induces cell cycle withdrawal: inhibition of E2F/DP DNA-binding activity via down-regulation of PP2A. *Genes Dev* 1997; 11: 1987–98.
25. Morrison RF, Farmer SR. Role of PPAR-γ in regulating a cascade expression of cyclin-dependent kinase inhibitors, p18(INK4c) and p21(Waf/Cip1), during adipogenesis. *J Biol Chem* 1999; 274: 17088–97.
26. Wu Z, Xie Y, Morrison RF, Bucher NLR, Farmer SR. PPAR-γ induces the insulin-dependent glucose transporter GLUT-4 in the absence of C/EBPα during the conversion of 3T3 fibroblasts into adipocytes. *J Clin Invest* 1998; 101: 22–32.
27. Gervois P, Chopin-Delannoy S, Fadel A, Dubois G, Kosykh V, Fruchart JC, Najib J, Laudet V, Staels B. Fibrates increase human REV-ERBalpha expression in liver via a novel peroxisome proliferator-activated receptor response element. *Mol Endocrinol* 1999; 13: 400–9.
28. Kliewer SA, Umesono K, Noonan DJ, Heyman RA, Evans RM. Convergence of 9-*cis*-retinoic acid and peroxisome proliferator signalling pathways through heterodimer formation of their receptors. *Nature* 1992; 358: 771–4.
29. Nolte RT, Wisely GB, Westin S, Cobb JE, Lambert MH, Kurokawa R, Rosenfeld MG, Willson TM, Glass CK, Milburn MV. Ligand binding and co-activator assembly of the peroxisome proliferator- activated receptor-gamma. *Nature* 1998; 395: 137–43.
30. Forman BM, Chen J, Evans RM. Hypolipidemic drugs, polyunsaturated fatty acids, and eicosanoids are ligands for peroxisome proliferator-activated receptors. *Proc Natl Acad Sci USA* 1997; 94: 4312–7.
31. Xu HE, Lambert MH, Montana VG, Parks DJ, Blanchard SG, Brown PJ, Sternbach DD, Lehmann JM, Wisely GB, Willson TM, Kliewer SA, Milburn MV. Molecular recognition of fatty acids by peroxisome proliferator-activated receptors. *Mol Cell* 1999; 3: 397–403.
32. Forman BM, Tontonoz P, Chen J, Brun RP, Spiegelman BM, Evans RM. 15-Deoxy-D12,14-prostaglandin J2 is a ligand for the adipocyte determination factor PPAR-γ. *Cell* 1995; 83: 803–12.

33. Kliewer SA, Lenhard JM, Wilson TM, Patel I, Morris DC, Lehmann JM. A prostaglandin J2 metabolite binds peroxisome proliferator-activated receptor γ and promotes adipocyte differentiation. *Cell* 1995; 83: 813–9.
34. Nagy L, Tontonoz P, Alvarez JG, Chen H, Evans RM. Oxidized LDL regulates macrophage gene expression through ligand activation of PPARgamma. *Cell* 1998; 93: 229–40.
35. Kliewer SA, Xu HE, Lambert MH, Willson TM. Peroxisome proliferator-activated receptors: from genes to physiology. *Recent Prog Horm Res* 2001; 56: 239–63.
36. Tanaka T, Yoshida N, Kishimoto T, Akira S. Defective adipocyte differentiation in mice lacking the C/EBPbeta and/or C/EBPdelta gene. *EMBO J* 1997; 16: 7432–43.
37. Tontonoz P, Kim JB, Graves RA, Spiegelman BM. ADD1: a novel helix-loop-helix transcription factor associated with adipocyte determination and differentiation. *Mol Cell Biol* 1993; 13: 4753–9.
38. Kim JB, Spotts GD, Halvorsen YD, Shih HM, Ellenberger T, Towle HC, Spiegelman BM. Dual DNA binding specificity of ADD1/SREBP1 controlled by a single amino acid in the basic helix–loop–helix domain. *Mol Cell Biol* 1995; 15: 2582–8.
39. Brown MS,Goldstein JL. The SREBP pathway: regulation of cholesterol metabolism by proteolysis of a membrane-bound transcription factor. *Cell* 1997; 89: 331–40.
40. Fajas L, Schoonjans K, Gelman L, Kim JB, Najib J, Martin G, Fruchart JC, Briggs M, Spiegelman BM, Auwerx J. Regulation of peroxisome proliferator-activated receptor gamma expression by adipocyte differentiation and determination factor 1/sterol regulatory element binding protein 1: implications for adipocyte differentiation and metabolism. *Mol Cell Biol* 1999; 19: 5495–503.
41. Hamm JK, Park BH, Farmer SR. A role for C/EBPbeta in regulating peroxisome proliferator-activated receptor gamma activity during adipogenesis in 3T3-L1 preadipocytes. *J Biol Chem* 2001; 276: 18464–71.
42. Tong Q, Dalgin G, Xu H, Ting CN, Leiden JM, Hotamisligil GS. Function of GATA transcription factors in preadipocyte-adipocyte transition. *Science* 2000; 290: 134–8.
43. Ross SE, Hemati N, Longo KA, Bennett CN, Lucas PC, Erickson RL, MacDougald OA. Inhibition of adipogenesis by Wnt signaling. *Science* 2000; 289: 950–3.
44. Wu Z, Rosen ED, Brun R, Hauser S, Adelmont G, Troy AE, McKeon C, Darlington GJ, Spiegelman BM. Cross-regulation of C/EBPα and PPAR-γ controls the transcriptional pathway of adipogenesis and insulin sensitivity. *Mol Cell* 1999; 3: 151–8.
45. Teglund S, McKay C, Schuetz E, van Deursen JM, Stravopodis D, Wang D, Brown M, Bodner S, Grosveld G, Ihle JN. Stat5a and Stat5b proteins have essential and nonessential, or redundant, roles in cytokine responses. *Cell* 1998; 93: 841–50.
46. El-Jack AK, Hamm JK, Pilch PF, Farmer SR. Reconstitution of insulin-sensitive glucose transport in fibroblasts requires expression of both PPAR-γ and C/EBPα. *J Biol Chem* 1999; 274: 7946–51.
47. Tontonoz P, Hu E, Spiegelman BM. Stimulation of adipogenesis in fibroblasts by PPAR-γ, a lipid-activated transcription factor. *Cell* 1994; 79: 1147–56.
48. Kim JB, Wright HM, Wright M, Spiegelman BM. ADD1/SREBP1 activates PPAR gamma through the production of endogenous ligand. *Proc Natl Acad Sci USA* 1998; 95: 4333–7.
49. Barak Y, Nelson MC, Ong ES, Jones YZ, Ruiz-Lozano P, Chien KR, Koder A, Evans RM. PPAR gamma is required for placental, cardiac, and adipose tissue development. *Mol Cell* 1999; 4: 585–95.
50. Linhart HG, Ishimura-Oka K, DeMayo F, Kibe T, Repka D, Poindexter B, Bick RJ, Darlington GJ. C/EBPalpha is required for differentiation of white, but not brown, adipose tissue. *Proc Natl Acad Sci USA* 2001; 98: 12532–7.
51. Wang ND, Finegold MJ, Bradley A, Ou CN, Abdelsayed SV, Wilde MD, Taylor LR, Wilson Dr, Darlington GJ. Impaired energy homeostasis in C/EBP alpha knockout mice. *Science* 1995; 269: 1108–12.
52. Freytag SO, Paielli DL, Gilbert JD. Ectopic expression of the CCAAT/enhancer-binding protein alpha promotes the adipogenic program in a variety of mouse fibroblastic cells. *Genes Dev* 1994; 8: 1654–63.
53. Rosen ED, Hsu CH, Wang X, Sakai S, Freeman MW, Gonzalez FJ, Spiegelman BM. C/EBPalpha induces adipogenesis through PPARgamma: a unified pathway. *Genes Dev* 2002; 16: 22–6.
54. Dixon TM, Daniel KW, Farmer SR, Collins S. CCAAT/enhancer-binding protein alpha is required for transcription of the beta 3-adrenergic receptor gene during adipogenesis. *J Biol Chem* 2001; 276: 722–8.
55. Hamm JK, el Jack AK, Pilch PF, Farmer SR. Role of PPAR gamma in regulating adipocyte differentiation and insulin-responsive glucose uptake. *Ann N Y Acad Sci* 1999; 892: 134–45.
56. Kraegen EW, James DE, Jenkins AB, Chisholm DJ. Dose-response curves for in vivo insulin sensitivity in individual tissues in rats. *Am J Physiol* 1985; 248: E353–62.
57. Colditz GA, Willett WC, Stampfer MJ, Manson JE, Hennekens CH, Arky RA, Speizer FE. Weight as a risk factor for clinical diabetes in women. *Am J Epidemiol* 1990; 132: 501–13.
58. Burant CF, Sreenan S, Hirano K, Tai TA, Lohmiller J, Lukens J, Davidson NO, Ross S, Graves RA. Troglitazone action is independent of adipose tissue. *J Clin Invest* 1997; 100: 2900–8.
59. Ganda OP. Lipoatrophy, lipodystrophy, and insulin resistance. *Ann Intern Med* 2000; 133: 304–6.
60. Moitra J, Mason MM, Olive M, Krylov D, Gavrilova O, Marcus-Samuels B, Feigenbaum L, Lee E, Aoyama T, Eckhaus M, Reitman ML, Vinson C. Life without white fat: a transgenic mouse. *Genes Dev* 1998; 12: 3168–81.
61. Reue K, Xu P, Wang XP, Slavin BG. Adipose tissue deficiency, glucose intolerance, and increased atherosclerosis result from mutation in the mouse fatty liver dystrophy (fld) gene. *J Lipid Res* 2000; 41: 1067–76.
62. Shimomura I, Hammer RE, Richardson JA, Ikemoto S, Bashmakov Y, Goldstein JL, Brown MS. Insulin resistance and diabetes mellitus in transgenic mice expressing nuclear SREBP-1c in adipose tissue: model for congenital generalized lipodystrophy. *Genes Dev* 1998; 12: 3182–94.
63. Smith U. Impaired ("diabetic") insulin signaling and action occur in fat cells long before glucose intolerance—is insulin resistance initiated in the adipose tissue? *Int J Obes Relat Metab Disord* 2002; 26: 897–904.
64. Arner P. Free fatty acids—do they play a central role in type 2 diabetes? *Diabetes Obes Metab* 2001; 3 (suppl 1): 11–9.

65. Zierath JR, Livingston JN, Thorne A, Bolinder J, Reynisdottir S, Lonnqvist F, Arner P. Regional difference in insulin inhibition of non-esterified fatty acid release from human adipocytes: relation to insulin receptor phosphorylation and intracellular signalling through the insulin receptor substrate-1 pathway. *Diabetologia* 1998; 41: 1343–54.
66. Arner P. Insulin resistance in type 2 diabetes: role of fatty acids. *Diabetes Metab Res Rev* 2002; 18 (suppl 2): S5–9.
67. Randle PJ. Regulatory interactions between lipids and carbohydrates: the glucose fatty acid cycle after 35 years. *Diabetes Metab Rev* 1998; 14: 263–83.
68. Randle PJ, Garland PB, Hales CN, Newsholme EA. The glucose-fatty acid cycle. Its role in insulin sensitivity and the metabolic disturbances of diabetes mellitus. *Lancet* 1963; i: 785–9.
69. Randle PJ, Garland PB, Newsholme EA, Hales CN. The glucose fatty acid cycle in obesity and maturity onset diabetes mellitus. *Ann N Y Acad Sci* 1965; 131: 324–33.
70. Dresner A, Laurent D, Marcucci M, Griffin ME, Dufour S, Cline GW, Slezak LA, Andersen DK, Hundal RS, Rothman DL, Petersen KF, Shulman GI. Effects of free fatty acids on glucose transport and IRS-1-associated phosphatidylinositol 3-kinase activity. *J Clin Invest* 1999; 103: 253–9.
71. Griffin ME, Marcucci MJ, Cline GW, Bell K, Barucci N, Lee D, Goodyear LJ, Kraegen EW, White MF, Shulman GI. Free fatty acid-induced insulin resistance is associated with activation of protein kinase C theta and alterations in the insulin signaling cascade. *Diabetes* 1999; 48: 1270–4.
72. Roden M, Price TB, Perseghin G, Petersen KF, Rothman DL, Cline GW, Shulman GI. Mechanism of free fatty acid-induced insulin resistance in humans. *J Clin Invest* 1996; 97: 2859–65.
73. Shulman GI. Cellular mechanisms of insulin resistance. *J Clin Invest* 2000; 106: 171–6.
74. Ahima RS, Flier JS. Adipose tissue as an endocrine organ. *Trends Endocrinol Metab* 2000; 11: 327–32.
75. Trayhurn P, Beattie JH. Physiological role of adipose tissue: white adipose tissue as an endocrine and secretory organ. *Proc Nutr Soc* 2001; 60: 329–39.
76. Ahima RS, Flier JS. Leptin. *Annu Rev Physiol* 2000; 62: 413–37.
77. Friedman JM. Obesity in the new millennium. *Nature* 2000; 404: 632–4.
78. Friedman JM, Halaas JL. Leptin and the regulation of body weight in mammals. *Nature* 1998; 395: 763–70.
79. Friedman JM. Leptin, leptin receptors, and the control of body weight. *Nutr Rev* 1998; 56: s38–46, s54–75.
80. Minokoshi Y, Kim YB, Peroni OD, Fryer LG, Muller C, Carling D, Kahn BB. Leptin stimulates fatty-acid oxidation by activating AMP-activated protein kinase. *Nature* 2002; 415: 339–43.
81. Peraldi P, Spiegelman B. TNF-alpha and insulin resistance: summary and future prospects. *Mol Cell Biochem* 1998; 182: 169–75.
82. Aguirre V, Uchida T, Yenush L, Davis R, White MF. The c-Jun NH(2)-terminal kinase promotes insulin resistance during association with insulin receptor substrate-1 and phosphorylation of Ser(307). *J Biol Chem* 2000; 275: 9047–54.
83. Hotamisligil GS, Peraldi P, Budavari A, Ellis R, White MF, Spiegelman BM. IRS-1-mediated inhibition of insulin receptor tyrosine kinase activity in TNF-alpha- and obesity-induced insulin resistance. *Science* 1996; 271: 665–8.
84. Peraldi P, Hotamisligil GS, Buurman WA, White MF, Spiegelman BM. Tumor necrosis factor (TNF)-alpha inhibits insulin signaling through stimulation of the p55 TNF receptor and activation of sphingomyelinase. *J Biol Chem* 1996; 271: 13018–22.
85. Rui L, Aguirre V, Kim JK, Shulman GI, Lee A, Corbould A, Dunaif A, White MF. Insulin/IGF-1 and TNF-alpha stimulate phosphorylation of IRS-1 at inhibitory Ser307 via distinct pathways. *J Clin Invest* 2001; 107: 181–9.
86. Uysal KT, Wiesbrock SM, Marino MW, Hotamisligil GS. Protection from obesity-induced insulin resistance in mice lacking TNF- alpha function. *Nature* 1997; 389: 610–4.
87. Hotamisligil GS. The role of TNFalpha and TNF receptors in obesity and insulin resistance. *J Intern Med* 1999; 245: 621–5.
88. Maeda K, Okubo K, Shimomura I, Funahashi T, Matsuzawa Y, Matsubara K. cDNA cloning and expression of a novel adipose specific collagen-like factor, apM1 (AdiPose Most abundant Gene transcript 1). *Biochem Biophys Res Commun* 1996; 221: 286–9.
89. Hu E, Liang P, Spiegelman BM. AdipoQ is a novel adipose-specific gene dysregulated in obesity. *J Biol Chem* 1996; 271: 10697–703.
90. Scherer PE, Williams S, Fogliano M, Baldini G, Lodish HF. A novel serum protein similar to C1q, produced exclusively in adipocytes. *J Biol Chem* 1995; 270: 26746–9.
91. Arita Y, Kihara S, Ouchi N, Takahashi M, Maeda K, Miyagawa J, Hotta K, Shimomura I, Nakamura T, Miyaoka K, Kuriyama H, Nishida M, Yamashita S, Okubo K, Matsubara K, Muraguchi M, Ohmoto Y, Funahashi T, Matsuzawa Y. Paradoxical decrease of an adipose-specific protein, adiponectin, in obesity. *Biochem Biophys Res Commun* 1999; 257: 79–83.
92. Yamauchi T, Kamon J, Waki H, Terauchi Y, Kubota N, Hara K, Mori Y, Ide T, Murakami K, Tsuboyama-Kasaoka N, Ezaki O, Akanuma Y, Gavrilova O, Vinson C, Reitman ML, Kagechika H, Shudo K, Yoda M, Nakano Y, Tobe K, Nagai R, Kimura S, Tomita M, Froguel P, Kadowaki T. The fat-derived hormone adiponectin reverses insulin resistance associated with both lipoatrophy and obesity. *Nat Med* 2001; 7: 941–6.
93. Berg AH, Combs TP, Du X, Brownlee M, Scherer PE. The adipocyte-secreted protein Acrp30 enhances hepatic insulin action. *Nat Med* 2001; 7: 947–53.
94. Combs TP, Berg AH, Obici S, Scherer PE, Rossetti L. Endogenous glucose production is inhibited by the adipose-derived protein Acrp30. *J Clin Invest* 2001; 108: 1875–81.
95. Yamauchi T, Kamon J, Minokoshi Y, Ito Y, Waki H, Uchida S, Yamashita S, Noda M, Kita S, Ueki K, Eto K, Akanuma Y, Froguel P, Foufelle F, Ferre P, Carling D, Kimura S, Nagai R, Kahn BB, Kadowaki T. Adiponectin stimulates glucose utilization and fatty-acid oxidation by activating AMP-activated protein kinase. *Nat Med* 2002; 8: 1288–95.
96. Kissebah AH, Sonnenberg GE, Myklebust J, Goldstein M, Broman K, James RG, Marks JA, Krakower GR, Jacob HJ, Weber J, Martin L, Blangero J, Comuzzie AG. Quantitative trait loci on chromosomes 3 and 17 influence phenotypes of the metabolic syndrome. *Proc Natl Acad Sci USA* 2000; 97: 14478–83.

97. Hara K, Boutin P, Mori Y, Tobe K, Dina C, Yasuda K, Yamauchi T, Otabe S, Okada T, Eto K, Kadowaki H, Hagura R, Akanuma Y, Yazaki Y, Nagai R, Taniyama M, Matsubara K, Yoda M, Nakano Y, Tomita M, Kimura S, Ito C, Froguel P, Kadowaki T. Genetic variation in the gene encoding adiponectin is associated with an increased risk of type 2 diabetes in the Japanese population. *Diabetes* 2002; 51: 536–40.
98. Kondo H, Shimomura I, Matsukawa Y, Kumada M, Takahashi M, Matsuda M, Ouchi N, Kihara S, Kawamoto T, Sumitsuji S, Funahashi T, Matsuzawa Y. Association of adiponectin mutation with type 2 diabetes: a candidate gene for the insulin resistance syndrome. *Diabetes* 2002; 51: 2325–8.
99. Menzaghi C, Ercolino T, Di Paola R, Berg AH, Warram JH, Scherer PE, Trischitta V, Doria A. A haplotype at the adiponectin locus is associated with obesity and other features of the insulin resistance syndrome. *Diabetes* 2002; 51: 2306–12.
100. Vasseur F, Helbecque N, Dina C, Lobbens S, Delannoy V, Gaget S, Boutin P, Vaxillaire M, Lepretre F, Dupont S, Hara K, Clement K, Bihain B, Kadowaki T, Froguel P. Single-nucleotide polymorphism haplotypes in the both proximal promoter and exon 3 of the APM1 gene modulate adipocyte-secreted adiponectin hormone levels and contribute to the genetic risk for type 2 diabetes in French Caucasians. *Hum Mol Genet* 2002; 11: 2607–14.
101. Kubota N, Terauchi Y, Yamauchi T, Kubota T, Moroi M, Matsui J, Eto K, Yamashita T, Kamon J, Satoh H, Yano W, Froguel P, Nagai R, Kimura S, Kadowaki T, Noda T. Disruption of adiponectin causes insulin resistance and neointimal formation. *J Biol Chem* 2002; 277: 25863–6.
102. Maeda N, Shimomura I, Kishida K, Nishizawa H, Matsuda M, Nagaretani H, Furuyama N, Kondo H, Takahashi M, Arita Y, Komuro R, Ouchi N, Kihara S, Tochino Y, Okutomi K, Horie M, Takeda S, Aoyama T, Funahashi T, Matsuzawa Y. Diet-induced insulin resistance in mice lacking adiponectin/ACRP30. *Nat Med* 2002; 8: 731–7.
103. Holcomb IN, Kabakoff RC, Chan B, Baker TW, Gurney A, Henzel W, Nelson C, Lowman HB, Wright BD, Skelton NJ, Frantz GD, Tumas DB, Peale FV Jr, Shelton DL, Hebert CC. FIZZ1, a novel cysteine-rich secreted protein associated with pulmonary inflammation, defines a new gene family. *Embo J* 2000; 19: 4046–55.
104. Steppan CM, Bailey ST, Bhat S, Brown EJ, Banerjee RR, Wright CM, Patel HR, Ahima RS, Lazar MA. The hormone resistin links obesity to diabetes. *Nature* 2001; 409: 307–12.
105. Steppan CM, Brown EJ, Wright CM, Bhat S, Banerjee RR, Dai CY, Enders GH, Silberg DG, Wen X, Wu GD, Lazar MA. A family of tissue-specific resistin-like molecules. *Proc Natl Acad Sci USA* 2001; 98: 502–6.
106. Kim KH, Lee K, Moon YS, Sul HS. A cysteine-rich adipose tissue-specific secretory factor inhibits adipocyte differentiation. *J Biol Chem* 2001; 276: 11252–6.
107. Steppan CM, Lazar MA. Resistin and obesity-associated insulin resistance. *Trends Endocrinol Metab* 2002; 13: 18–23.
108. Mudaliar S, Henry RR. New oral therapies for type 2 diabetes mellitus: the glitazones or insulin sensitizers. *Annu Rev Med* 2001; 52: 239–57.
109. Scheen AJ. Hepatotoxicity with thiazolidinediones: is it a class effect?*Drug Saf* 2001; 24: 873–88.
110. Scheen AJ. Thiazolidinediones and liver toxicity. *Diabetes Metab* 2001; 27: 305–13.
111. Stumvoll M, Haring HU. Glitazones: clinical effects and molecular mechanisms. *Ann Med* 2002; 34: 217–24.
112. Fujita T, Sugiyama Y, Taketomi S, Sohda T, Kawamatsu Y, Iwatsuka H, Suzuoki Z. Reduction of insulin resistance in obese and/or diabetic animals by 5-[4-(1-methylcyclohexylmethoxy)benzyl]-thiazolidine-2,4-dione (ADD-3878, U-63,287, ciglitazone), a new antidiabetic agent. *Diabetes* 1983; 32: 804–10.
113. Lehmann JM, Moore LB, Smith-Oliver TA, Wilkison WO, Willson TM, Kliewer SA. An antidiabetic thiazolidinedione is a high affinity ligand for peroxisome proliferator-activated receptor gamma (PPAR gamma). *J Biol Chem* 1995; 270: 12953–6.
114. Goldstein BJ. Differentiating members of the thiazolidinedione class: a focus on efficacy. *Diabetes Metab Res Rev* 2002; 18 (suppl 2): S16–22.
115. Auboeuf D, Rieusset J, Fajas L, Vallier P, Frering V, Riou JP, Staels B, Auwerx J, Laville M, Vidal H. Tissue distribution and quantification of the expression of mRNAs of peroxisome proliferator-activated receptors and liver X receptor-alpha in humans: no alteration in adipose tissue of obese and NIDDM patients. *Diabetes* 1997; 46: 1319–27.
116. Loviscach M, Rehman N, Carter L, Mudaliar S, Mohadeen P, Ciaraldi TP, Veerkamp JH, Henry RR. Distribution of peroxisome proliferator-activated receptors (PPARs) in human skeletal muscle and adipose tissue: relation to insulin action. *Diabetologia* 2000; 43: 304–11.
117. Kim JK, Gavrilova O, Chen Y, Reitman ML, Shulman GI. Mechanism of insulin resistance in A-ZIP/F-1 fatless mice. *J Biol Chem* 2000; 275: 8456–60.
118. Chao L, Marcus-Samuels B, Mason MM, Moitra J, Vinson C, Arioglu E, Gavrilova O, Reitman ML. Adipose tissue is required for the antidiabetic, but not for the hypolipidemic, effect of thiazolidinediones. *J Clin Invest* 2000; 106: 1221–8.
119. Oakes ND, Camilleri S, Furler SM, Chisholm DJ, Kraegen EW. The insulin sensitizer, BRL 49653, reduces systemic fatty acid supply and utilization and tissue lipid availability in the rat. *Metabolism* 1997; 46: 935–42.
120. Oakes ND, Kennedy CJ, Jenkins AB, Laybutt DR, Chisholm DJ, Kraegen EW. A new antidiabetic agent, BRL 49653, reduces lipid availability and improves insulin action and glucoregulation in the rat. *Diabetes* 1994; 43: 1203–10.
121. Mayerson AB, Hundal RS, Dufour S, Lebon V, Befroy D, Cline GW, Enocksson S, Inzucchi SE, Shulman GI, Petersen KF. The effects of rosiglitazone on insulin sensitivity, lipolysis, and hepatic and skeletal muscle triglyceride content in patients with type 2 diabetes. *Diabetes* 2002; 51: 797–802.
122. Kelly IE, Han TS, Walsh K, Lean ME. Effects of a thiazolidinedione compound on body fat and fat distribution of patients with type 2 diabetes. *Diabetes Care* 1999; 22: 288–93.
123. Okuno A, Tamemoto H, Tobe K, Ueki K, Mori Y, Iwamoto K, Umesono K, Akanuma Y, Fujiwara T, Horikoshi H, Yazaki Y, Kadowaki T. Troglitazone increases the number of small adipocytes without the change of white adipose tissue mass in obese Zucker rats. *J Clin Invest* 1998; 101: 1354–61.

124. Yamauchi T, Kamon J, Waki H, Murakami K, Motojima K, Komeda K, Ide T, Kubota N, Terauchi Y, Tobe K, Miki H, Tsuchida A, Akanuma Y, Nagai R, Kimura S, Kadowaki T. The mechanisms by which both heterozygous peroxisome proliferator-activated receptor gamma (PPARgamma) deficiency and PPARgamma agonist improve insulin resistance. *J Biol Chem* 2001; 276: 41245–54.
125. Frohnert BI, Hui TY, Bernlohr DA. Identification of a functional peroxisome proliferator-responsive element in the murine fatty acid transport protein gene. *J Biol Chem* 1999; 274: 3970–7.
126. Schoonjans K, Peinado-Onsurbe J, Lefebvre AM, Heyman RA, Briggs M, Deeb S, Staels B, Auwerx J. PPARalpha and PPARgamma activators direct a distinct tissue-specific transcriptional response via a PPRE in the lipoprotein lipase gene. *EMBO J* 1996; 15: 5336–48.
127. Schoonjans K, Watanabe M, Suzuki H, Mahfoudi A, Krey G, Wahli W, Grimaldi P, Staels B, Yamamoto T, Auwerx J. Induction of the acyl-coenzyme A synthetase gene by fibrates and fatty acids is mediated by a peroxisome proliferator response element in the C promoter. *J Biol Chem* 1995; 270: 19269–76.
128. Tontonoz P, Hu E, Devine J, Beale EG, Spiegelman BM. PPAR gamma 2 regulates adipose expression of the phosphoenolpyruvate carboxykinase gene. *Mol Cell Biol* 1995; 15: 351–7.
129. Smith U, Gogg S, Johansson A, Olausson T, Rotter V, Svalstedt B. Thiazolidinediones (PPARgamma agonists) but not PPARalpha agonists increase IRS-2 gene expression in 3T3-L1 and human adipocytes. *Faseb J* 2001; 15: 215–20.
130. Rieusset J, Auwerx J, Vidal H. Regulation of gene expression by activation of the peroxisome proliferator-activated receptor gamma with rosiglitazone (BRL 49653) in human adipocytes. *Biochem Biophys Res Commun* 1999; 265: 265–71.
131. Baumann CA, Chokshi N, Saltiel AR, Ribon V. Cloning and characterization of a functional peroxisome proliferator activator receptor-gamma-responsive element in the promoter of the CAP gene. *J Biol Chem* 2000; 275: 9131–5.
132. Ribon V, Johnson JH, Camp HS, Saltiel AR. Thiazolidinediones and insulin resistance: peroxisome proliferatoractivated receptor gamma activation stimulates expression of the CAP gene. *Proc Natl Acad Sci USA* 1998; 95: 14751–6.
133. Abel ED, Peroni O, Kim JK, Kim YB, Boss O, Hadro E, Minnemann T, Shulman GI, Kahn BB. Adipose-selective targeting of the GLUT-4 gene impairs insulin action in muscle and liver. *Nature* 2001; 409: 729–33.
134. Guan HP, Li Y, Jensen MV, Newgard CB, Steppan CM, Lazar MA. A futile metabolic cycle activated in adipocytes by antidiabetic agents. *Nat Med* 2002; 8: 1122–8.
135. Hofmann C, Lorenz K, Braithwaite SS, Colca JR, Palazuk BJ, Hotamisligil GS, Spiegelman BM. Altered gene expression for tumor necrosis factor-alpha and its receptors during drug and dietary modulation of insulin resistance. *Endocrinology* 1994; 134: 264–70.
136. Katsuki A, Sumida Y, Murata K, Furuta M, Araki-Sasaki R, Tsuchihashi K, Hori Y, Yano Y, Gabazza EC, Adachi Y. Troglitazone reduces plasma levels of tumour necrosis factor-alpha in obese patients with type 2 diabetes. *Diabetes Obes Metab* 2000; 2: 189–91.
137. Peraldi P, Xu M, Spiegelman BM. Thiazolidinediones block tumor necrosis factor-alpha-induced inhibition of insulin signaling. *J Clin Invest* 1997; 100: 1863–9.
138. Souza SC, Yamamoto MT, Franciosa MD, Lien P, Greenberg AS. BRL 49653 blocks the lipolytic actions of tumor necrosis factor-alpha: a potential new insulin-sensitizing mechanism for thiazolidinediones. *Diabetes* 1998; 47: 691–5.
139. Halaas JL, Gajiwala KS, Maffei M, Cohen SL, Chait BT, Rabinowitz D, Lallone RL, Burley SK, Friedman JM. Weight-reducing effects of the plasma protein encoded by the obese gene. *Science* 1995; 269: 543–6.
140. Kamohara S, Burcelin R, Halaas JL, Friedman JM, Charron MJ. Acute stimulation of glucose metabolism in mice by leptin treatment. *Nature* 1997; 389: 374–7.
141. Gorson DM. Significant weight gain with rezulin therapy. *Arch Intern Med* 1999; 159: 99.
142. Way JM, Gorgun CZ, Tong Q, Uysal KT, Brown KK, Harrington WW, Oliver WR Jr, Willson TM, Kliewer SA, Hotamisligil GS. Adipose tissue resistin expression is severely suppressed in obesity and stimulated by peroxisome proliferator-activated receptor gamma agonists. *J Biol Chem* 2001; 276: 25651–3.
143. Combs TP, Wagner JA, Berger J, Doebber T, Wang WJ, Zhang BB, Tanen M, Berg AH, O'Rahilly S, Savage DB, Chatterjee K, Weiss S, Larson PJ, Gottesdiener KM, Gertz BJ, Charron MJ, Scherer PE, Moller DE. Induction of adipocyte complement-related protein of 30 kilodaltons by PPARgamma agonists: a potential mechanism of insulin sensitization. *Endocrinology* 2002; 143: 998–1007.
144. Maeda N, Takahashi M, Funahashi T, Kihara S, Nishizawa H, Kishida K, Nagaretani H, Matsuda M, Komuro R, Ouchi N, Kuriyama H, Hotta K, Nakamura T, Shimomura I, Matsuzawa Y. PPARgamma ligands increase expression and plasma concentrations of adiponectin, an adipose-derived protein. *Diabetes* 2001; 50: 2094–9.
145. Yang WS, Jeng CY, Wu TJ, Tanaka S, Funahashi T, Matsuzawa Y, Wang JP, Chen CL, Tai TY, Chuang LM. Synthetic peroxisome proliferator-activated receptor-gamma agonist, rosiglitazone, increases plasma levels of adiponectin in type 2 diabetic patients. *Diabetes Care* 2002; 25: 376–80.
146. Mukherjee R, Hoener PA, Jow L, Bilakovics J, Klausing K, Mais DE, Faulkner A, Croston GE, Paterniti JR Jr. A selective peroxisome proliferator-activated receptor-gamma (PPARgamma) modulator blocks adipocyte differentiation but stimulates glucose uptake in 3T3-L1 adipocytes. *Mol Endocrinol* 2000; 14: 1425–33.
147. Fukui Y, Masui S, Osada S, Umesono K, Motojima K. A new thiazolidinedione, NC-2100, which is a weak PPAR-gamma activator, exhibits potent antidiabetic effects and induces uncoupling protein 1 in white adipose tissue of KKAy obese mice. *Diabetes* 2000; 49: 759–67.
148. Deeb SS, Fajas L, Nemoto M, Pihlajamaki J, Mykkanen L, Kuusisto J, Laakso M, Fujimoto W, Auwerx J. A Pro12Ala substitution in PPARgamma2 associated with decreased receptor activity, lower body mass index and improved insulin sensitivity. *Nat Genet* 1998; 20: 284–7.
149. Miles PD, Barak Y, He W, Evans RM, Olefsky JM. Improved insulin-sensitivity in mice heterozygous for

PPAR-gamma deficiency. *J Clin Invest* 2000; 105: 287–92.

150. Yamauchi T, Waki H, Kamon J, Murakami K, Motojima K, Komeda K, Miki H, Kubota N, Terauchi Y, Tsuchida A, Tsuboyama-Kasaoka N, Yamauchi N, Ide T, Hori W, Kato S, Fukayama M, Akanuma Y, Ezaki O, Itai A, Nagai R, Kimura S, Tobe K, Kagechika H, Shudo K, Kadowaki T. Inhibition of RXR and PPARgamma ameliorates diet-induced obesity and type 2 diabetes. *J Clin Invest* 2001; 108: 1001–13.
151. Bjorntorp P, Rosmond R. Obesity and cortisol. *Nutrition* 2000; 16: 924–36.
152. Wajchenberg BL. Subcutaneous and visceral adipose tissue: their relation to the metabolic syndrome. *Endocr Rev* 2000; 21: 697–738.
153. Kotelevtsev Y, Holmes MC, Burchell A, Houston PM, Schmoll D, Jamieson P, Best R, Brown R, Edwards CR, Seckl JR, Mullins JJ. 11β-Hydroxysteroid dehydrogenase type 1 knockout mice show attenuated glucocorticoid-inducible responses and resist hyperglycemia on obesity or stress. *Proc Natl Acad Sci USA* 1997; 94: 14924–9.
154. Masuzaki H, Paterson J, Shinyama H, Morton NM, Mullins JJ, Seckl JR, Flier JS. A transgenic model of visceral obesity and the metabolic syndrome. *Science* 2001; 294: 2166–70.

35

Lipodystrophies and Diabetes

Abhimanyu Garg and Anoop Misra

The University of Texas Southwestern Medical Center at Dallas, Dallas, TX, USA

INTRODUCTION

Lipodystrophies are among one of the many rare etiologies of diabetes mellitus. Lipodystrophies are heterogeneous disorders characterized by selective loss of adipose tissue either due to genetic defects or due to acquired causes. The extent of fat loss varies depending on the type of lipodystrophy, and determines the severity of the metabolic complications [1]. Diabetes in these disorders is usually ketosis-resistant and requires sometimes extremely large doses of insulin and other hypoglycemic drugs for management. Patients with lipodystrophies are also predisposed to other complications of insulin resistance, such as hypertriglyceridemia, hepatic steatosis, and hyperuricemia [1]. Recently, significant advances have been made in characterization of the phenotypes on the basis of clinical features as well as in study of body fat distribution using anthropometry and magnetic resonance imaging (MRI). Furthermore, the genetic basis of several inherited lipodystrophies has recently been elucidated. This chapter thus reviews current knowledge of understanding of the metabolic and pathophysiologic basis of these disorders.

These disorders can be broadly classified into genetic or acquired disorders; each of these categories can be further subclassified into several distinct varieties (Table 1).

The prevalence of diabetes varies and is extremely high in patients with congenital and acquired generalized lipodystrophies (Figure 1). Patients with familial partial lipodystrophies also have high prevalence of diabetes but those with acquired partial lipodystrophy do not show such increased prevalence.

GENETIC LIPODYSTROPHIES

Congenital Generalized Lipodystrophy (Berardinelli–Seip Syndrome)

Congenital generalized lipodystrophy (CGL; Online Mendelian Inheritance in Man [OMIM] # 269700) was first described in 1954 by Berardinelli and later by Seip [1]. It is transmitted in an autosomal recessive manner. Approximately 200 cases have been reported in scientific literature from all ethnic groups; however, it is more prevalent in populations where consanguinity is common. It appears that CGL1 type due to 1-acylglycerol-3-phosphate *O*-acyltransferase 2 gene (*AGPAT2*) mutations is more common in people of African origin. The prevalence of CGL has been estimated to be 1 in 12.5 million people.

Genetic Basis for CGL

Two CGL loci have been reported till now: *CGL1* on human chromosome 9q34, and *CGL2* on chromosome 11q13. It is likely that there may be other loci as well. Our group reported *CGL1* locus on chromosome 9q34 by linkage analysis of 17 pedigrees [2]. By positional cloning, we recently discovered mutations in *AGPAT2* gene in CGL patients linked to 9q34 [3]. The AGPAT2 enzyme belongs to acyltransferase family and acylates lysophosphatidic acid (1-acylglycerol-3 phosphate) at sn-2 position to form phosphatidic acid (1,2-diacylglycerol-3-phosphate), a key step in glycerophospholipids and triacylglycerol biosynthesis [4, 5] (Figure 2).

Of the five known AGPAT isoforms, which are encoded by five different genes, *AGPAT2* is highly expressed in the

International Textbook of Diabetes Mellitus, Third Edition. Edited by R. A. DeFronzo, E. Ferrannini, H. Keen, and P. Zimmet.
 ISBN: 0-471-48655-8.

Table 1 Classification of lipodystrophies

- (A) Genetic lipodystrophies
  - (1) Congenital generalized lipodystrophy (CGL; Berardinelli–Seip syndrome)
    - (a) CGL1: *AGPAT2* (1-acylglycerol-3-phosphate *O*-acyltransferase 2) mutations
    - (b) CGL2: *BSCL2* (Berardinelli–Seip congenital lipodystrophy 2) mutations
    - (c) Other varieties
  - (2) Familial partial lipodystrophy (FPL)
    - (a) Dunnigan variety (FPLD): *LMNA* (lamin A/C) mutations
    - (b) FPL associated with *PPARG* (peroxisome proliferator-activated receptor γ) mutations
    - (c) Kobberling variety
    - (d) Other varieties
  - (3) Mandibuloacral dysplasia variety
    - (a) Partial lipodystrophy (type A pattern): *LMNA* (lamin A/C) mutation
    - (b) Generalized lipodystrophy (type B pattern)
  - (4) SHORT syndrome
  - (5) Neonatal progeroid syndrome
  - (6) Late-onset generalized lipodystrophy associated with *LMNA* mutation
- (B) Acquired lipodystrophies
  - (1) Acquired generalized lipodystrophy (AGL, Lawrence syndrome)
    - (a) Type 1: The panniculitis variety
    - (b) Type 2: The autoimmune disease variety
    - (c) Type 3: Idiopathic variety
  - (2) Acquired partial lipodystrophy (APL, Barraquer–Simons syndrome)
  - (3) Lipodystrophy in HIV-infected patients
  - (4) Localized lipodystrophies

omental adipose tissue [4, 6, 7], which suggests that the mutations in *AGPAT2* may affect triglyceride and phospholipid biosynthesis in adipocytes.

Mutations in Berardinelli–Seip Congenital Lipodystrophy 2 (*BSCL2*) gene have been reported in CGL pedigrees linked to 11q13 [8]. *BSCL2* encodes a protein, seipin, of 398 amino acid, which has no known function. The gene is highly expressed in the brain and testis [8]. The mechanism by which *BSCL2* mutations cause CGL remains unclear.

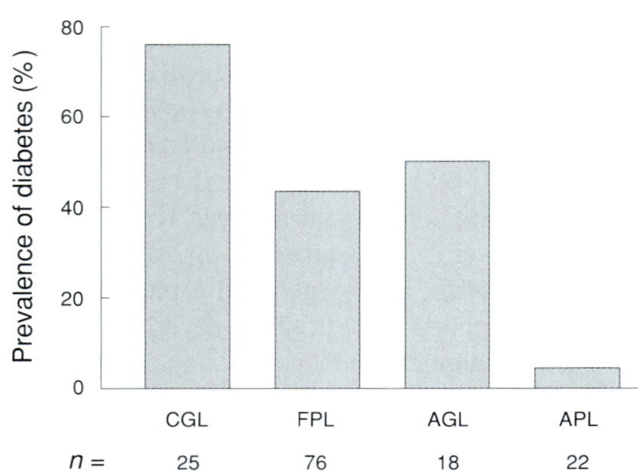

Figure 1 Prevalence of diabetes mellitus in our patients with various types of lipodystrophies. CGL: congenital generalized lipodystrophy; FPL: familial partial lipodystrophy, Dunnigan variety; AGL: acquired generalized lipodystrophy; APL: acquired partial lipodystrophy

Clinical Features

Affected neonates have a striking "muscular appearance" at birth or soon thereafter due to almost complete absence of adipose tissue. The affected children have voracious appetite, increased linear growth, advanced bone age, slight enlargement of the hands, feet, and mandible ("acromegaloid" features), and increased basal metabolic rate. Acanthosis nigricans occurs late in childhood or adolescence and may involve neck, axillae, groin, and occasionally trunk (Figure 3). Patients with CGL commonly have umbilical hernia, and enlargement of the liver and spleen. Excessive body hair and sweating may occur rarely.

Fatty infiltration of the liver occurs early and may lead to cirrhosis and its complications. Clitoromegaly, mild hirsutism, oligoamenorrhea, and polycystic ovaries have been reported in postpubertal females. Successful pregnancy is uncommon in females. Some patients have hypertrophic cardiomyopathy [9]. Focal lytic lesions in the appendicular bones have been reported in postpubertal patients [10].

Phenotypic differences in patients with *AGPAT2* and *BSCL2* mutations remain to be fully elucidated. It appears that cardiomyopathy and mild intellectual impairment may be more common in CGL patients with *BSCL2* mutations [3, 11].

Body Fat Distribution

Patients with CGL show almost complete absence of metabolically active adipose tissue located in most

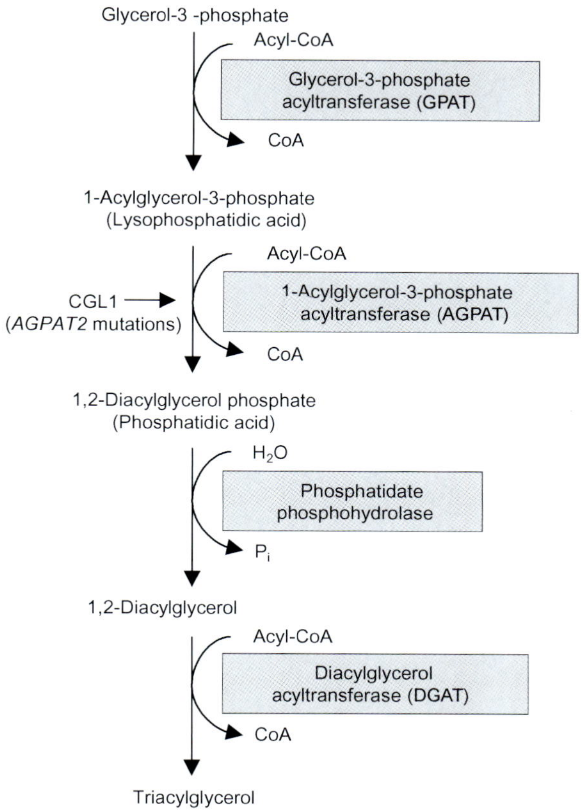

Figure 2 The pathway showing biosynthesis of triacylglycerol from glycerol-3-phosphate. Initially, glycerol-3-phosphate acyltransferase (GPAT) acylates glycerol-3-phosphate at sn-1 position to form lysophosphatidic acid. 1-Acylglycerol-3-phosphate *O*-acyltransferases (AGPATs, including AGPAT2, which is mutated in CGL1) catalyze acylation of lysophosphatidic acid at sn-2 position to form phosphatidic acid. Phosphatidic acid is then dephosphorylated to form 1,2-diacylglycerol, which is further acylated to form triacylglycerol using diacylglycerol acyltransferases (DGATs)

subcutaneous areas, intraabdominal and intrathoracic regions, and bone marrow. Interestingly, mechanical adipose tissue located in the palms, soles, under the scalp, retro-orbital and periarticular regions are well preserved [12, 13].

Diagnostic Criteria

(A) Essential criteria:

- (1) Generalized lack of body fat and extreme muscularity at birth
- (2) Autosomal recessive inheritance

(B) Supportive Criteria

- (1) Clinical
  - (a) Acanthosis nigricans
  - (b) Acromegaloid features
  - (c) Umbilical hernia
  - (d) Hepatomegaly or fatty liver
  - (e) Clitoromegaly and mild hirsutism in women
  - (f) Onset of impaired glucose tolerance or diabetes during teenage years
- (2) Laboratory
  - (a) Severe fasting or postprandial hyperinsulinemia
  - (b) Hypertriglyceridemia with low levels of serum high-density lipoprotein (HDL) cholesterol
  - (c) Extremely low serum levels of leptin and adiponectin
  - (d) Characteristic body fat distribution on MRI, including absence of bone marrow fat (confirmatory)

Metabolic Features

Patients have marked hyperinsulinemia, suggesting extreme insulin resistance. Hypertriglyceridemia and low levels of HDL cholesterol are universally noted. Diabetes usually appears during the pubertal years. Serum leptin and adiponectin concentrations are extremely low, consistent with the near total absence of body fat [14].

Although the precise mechanism(s) for extreme insulin resistance in patients with CGL is not known, it is likely that marked limitation in triglyceride deposition in the adipose tissue may divert triglycerides to the liver and skeletal muscle (Figure 4). This may result in hepatic steatosis and high intramyocellular triglyceride content, resulting in hepatic and peripheral insulin resistance, respectively. In CGL patients with *AGPAT2* mutations, triglyceride biosynthesis in the liver and muscle may not be interrupted because of higher mRNA expression of *AGPAT1* in these tissues as compared to *AGPAT2* [3]. The underlying pancreatic pathology is similar to that observed in the patients with type 2 diabetes. On autopsy of a young female with CGL and diabetes, we reported marked islet amyloidosis and β-cell atrophy [15]. Thus, it is likely that extreme insulin resistance induces islet amyloidosis and β-cell atrophy early in life and causes diabetes during teenage years in CGL (Figure 4).

Familial Partial Lipodystrophy, Dunnigan Type

In 1973, Ozer et al. [16] described a family with lipodystrophy with distinctive adipose tissue distribution, and subsequently, Dunnigan et al. [17] provided detailed description of the phenotype in two families. Nearly 200 patients have been described in the literature. It is an autosomal dominant disorder (OMIM # 151660) with estimated prevalence of 1 in 15 million. Familial partial lipodystrophy, Dunnigan type (FPLD) is mostly seen in Caucasians but has been reported in other ethnic groups.

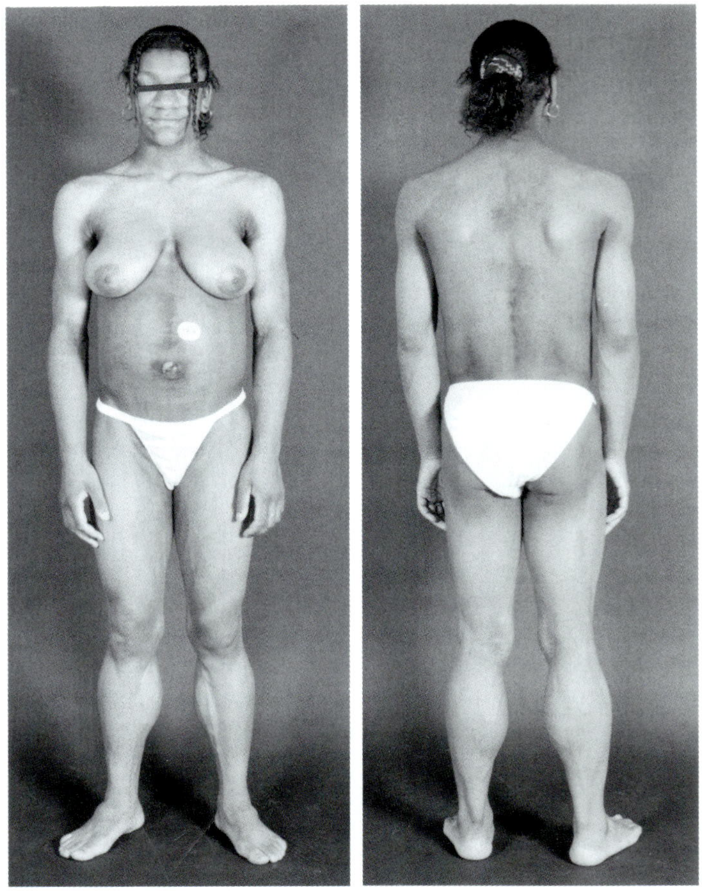

Figure 3 Anterior and posterior views of a 16-year-old African American girl with congenital generalized lipodystrophy due to *AGPAT2* mutation. The patient has almost complete absence of subcutaneous body fat, muscular appearance, and prominent superficial veins. Marked acanthosis nigricans is seen over the axillae and midline anteriorly over the abdomen. She also has slight enlargement of lower jaw, hands, and feet ("acromegaloid" features) and umbilical hernia (reprinted with permission from The Endocrine Society, *Journal of Clinical Endocrinology and Metabolism*)

Genetic Basis of FPLD

We initially found a locus for FPLD on chromosome 1q21-22 using a genome-wide linkage analysis [18]. Mutational analysis of several candidate genes in the critical region led to identification of mutations in the lamins A/C (*LMNA*) in the affected subjects [19–21]. Lamins A and C are alternatively spliced products of *LMNA* gene. Lamins form hetero- or homo-dimeric coiled-coil structures that are components of the nuclear lamina, a polymeric structure intercalated between chromatin and the inner membrane of the nuclear envelope. Most of the missense mutations causing FPLD have been reported in exon 8 encoding the globular C-terminal portion of the protein [20]. We have also reported phenotypic heterogeneity and an atypical, less severe form of lipodystrophy in a family with mutation in exon 11, which affects lamin A and not lamin C [22]. Mutations in *LMNA* have also been reported in many other disorders such as dilated cardiomyopathy and conduction-system disease [23, 24], autosomal dominant variety of Emery-Dreifuss muscular dystrophy [25], limb-girdle muscular dystrophy [26], and Charcot-Marie-Tooth disorder type 2 [27]. In two families with FPLD who had mutations in *LMNA* exon 1, we found evidence of cardiomyopathy and proximal muscle weakness, which had led us to propose a multisystem dystrophy syndrome in patients with *LMNA* mutations [28] (Figure 5).

Loss of adipocytes in FPLD may be due to defective interactions of lamins A/C with chromatin during the cell division, leading to apoptosis and cell death.

Clinical Features

Affected subjects have normal adipose tissue distribution at birth and during childhood. With the onset of puberty, subcutaneous adipose tissue is gradually lost from the extremities and variably from the trunk, causing "increased muscularity" appearance (Figure 6). Excess fat may get deposited in the regions not affected by lipodystrophy,

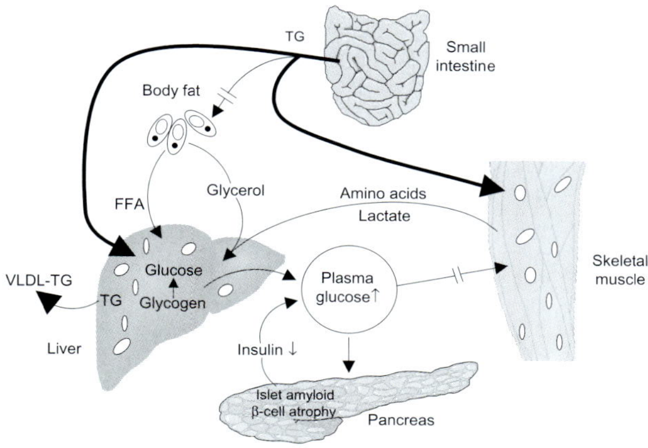

Figure 4 Proposed pathophysiological mechanisms of insulin resistance, glucose intolerance, and diabetes mellitus in patients with lipodystrophies. Patients with lipodystrophies are able to store triglycerides only in the adipose tissues not affected by lipodystrophy. Depending upon the extent of lipodystrophy, the amount of triglycerides that can be stored in the non-lipodystrophic adipose tissue may be limited and thus may be deposited in excess amounts in the liver (hepatic steatosis) and skeletal muscles (intramyocellular triglycerides) and results in hepatic and peripheral insulin resistance. Hepatic insulin resistance causes overproduction of hepatic glucose. Skeletal muscles are unable to utilize blood glucose owing to peripheral insulin resistance. Compensatory hyperinsulinemia is initially able to keep blood glucose in the normal range. Finally, persistence of severe insulin resistance leads to decrease in the production of insulin due to amyloid deposition in the pancreatic islets and β-cell exhaustion and atrophy, thus causing severe hyperglycemia. Excess fat in the liver and skeletal muscle is shown as white structures

resulting in double chin, excess supraclavicular fat, and a round face ("cushingoid appearance"). Rare patients develop excess fat in dorsocervical region ("buffalo hump"). Phenotype can be recognized easily in affected women; however, in men it can be misconstrued as "muscular appearance." Acanthosis nigricans, hirsutism, menstrual abnormalities, and polycystic ovaries occur in 20–33% of the patients.

Body Fat Distribution

The hallmark of FPLD is severe loss of subcutaneous fat from all the extremities after puberty. The neck, submental area, and face may have excess fat. On MRI, preservation of intermuscular fat and bone marrow fat is usually noted [29]. Subcutaneous fat loss occurs more in the anterior truncal region. Intraabdominal and intrathoracic fat are not reduced and may be present in excess.

Diagnostic Criteria

(A) Essential criteria:

- (1) Loss of subcutaneous fat from all the extremities, commencing at puberty with normal physical appearance at birth
- (2) Autosomal dominant inheritance

(B) Supportive Criteria

- (1) Clinical
  - (a) Excessive or normal amount of adipose tissue in the face, neck, and supraclavicular region
  - (b) Acanthosis nigricans
  - (c) Onset of impaired glucose tolerance or diabetes after 20 years of age
- (2) Laboratory
  - (a) Mild to moderate fasting or postprandial hyperinsulinemia

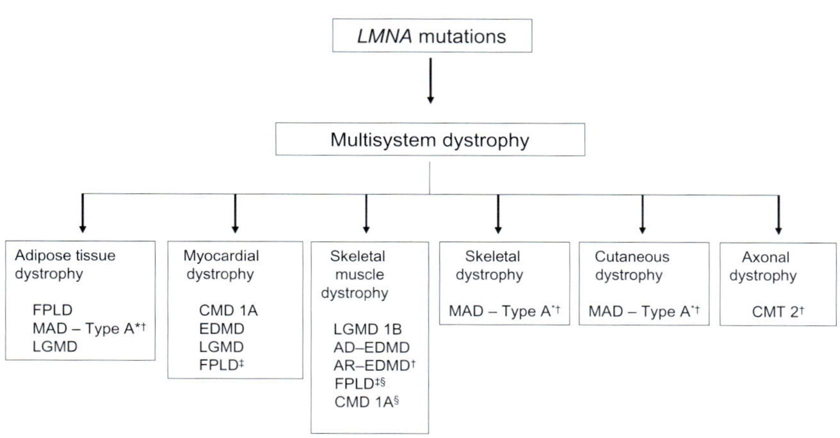

Figure 5 Multisystem dystrophy due to mutations in the lamin A/C gene (*LMNA*). As shown, several patients may have evidence of multisystem involvement. *: Refers to *type A* lipodystrophy pattern; †: these disorders are due to homozygous missense mutations, autosomal recessive; ‡: exon 1 mutations; §: mild phenotypic features; FPLD: familial partial lipodystrophy, Dunnigan variety; MAD: mandibuloacral dysplasia; LGMD: limb-girdle muscular dystrophy; CMD 1A: dilated cardiomyopathy; EDMD: Emery-Dreifuss muscular dystrophy; AD: autosomal dominant; AR: autosomal recessive; CMT 2: Charcot-Marie-Tooth disorder type 2

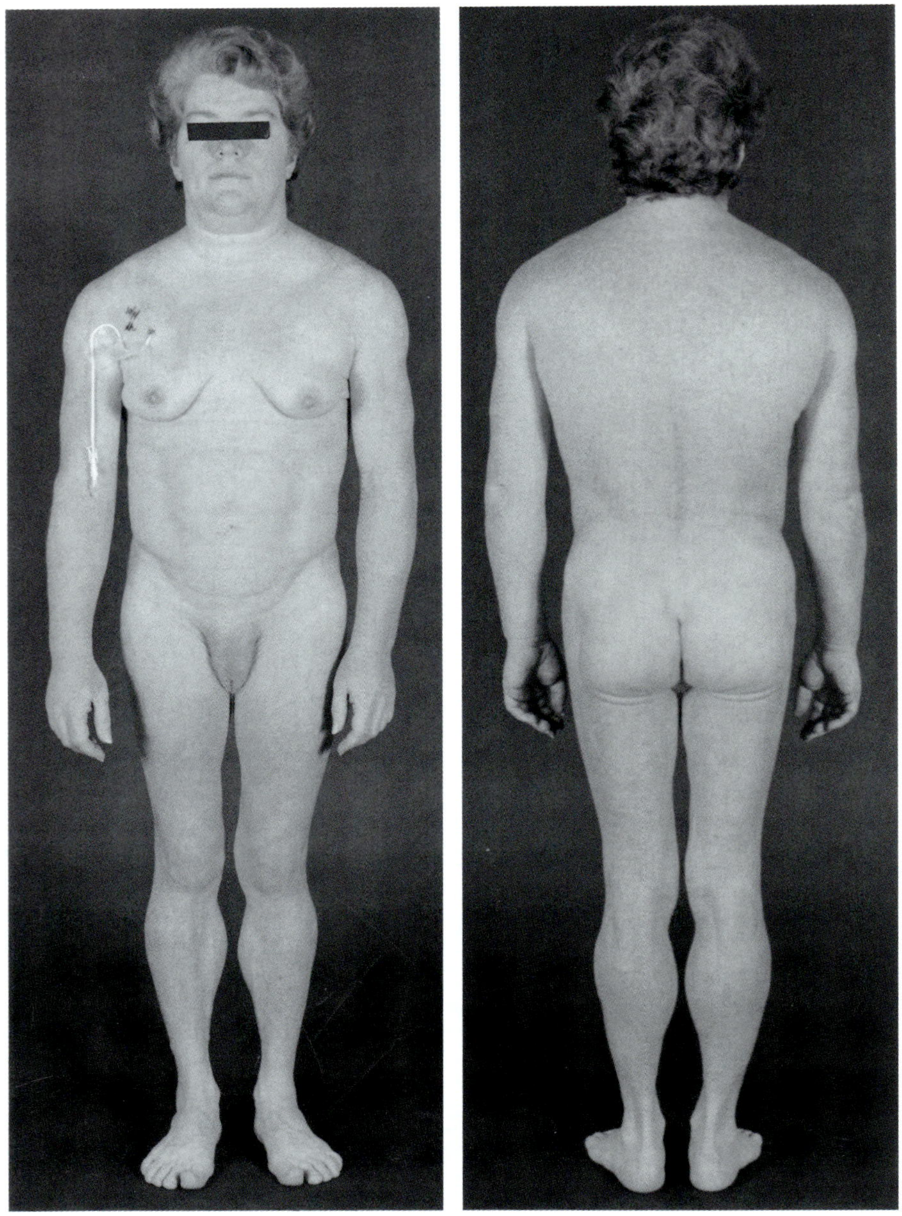

Figure 6 Anterior and posterior views of 37-year-old Caucasian woman with familial partial lipodystrophy, Dunnigan type due to *LMNA* mutation. She has almost complete absence of subcutaneous fat from the extremities and trunk with prominence of muscles and veins. There is excess fat deposition over the face, chin, supraclavicular region, neck, and labia majora

(b) Hypertriglyceridemia with low serum levels of HDL cholesterol
(c) Characteristic body fat distribution on MRI (confirmatory)

Metabolic Features

Women with FPLD have more severe metabolic complications of insulin resistance as compared to men [30]. More than 50% of women develop diabetes mellitus compared to ~20% of men. Women also develop extreme hypertriglyceridemia and low serum HDL-cholesterol concentrations. In general insulin-mediated glucose disposal is severely reduced and fasting plasma and free fatty acids are high, and not suppressed by an oral glucose load [31].

We have noted amyloidosis of pancreatic islets in a woman with FPLD and diabetes, suggesting similarity in the mechanism of development of diabetes to that noted in CGL [32].

Familial Partial Lipodystrophy, Köbberling Variety

In this variety, the adipose tissue loss is confined to the extremities [33–35]. Facial subcutaneous fat may be normal; however, there may be excessive amounts of subcutaneous truncal fat. The published reports are limited to a few affected women from two small pedigrees and four sporadic cases. Hypertriglyceridemia and diabetes mellitus occurred in most of the affected subjects. The age of onset, mode of inheritance, and diagnostic features of adipose tissue distribution are not known. Although this variety of lipodystrophy has been described in women so far, it cannot be concluded that men are exempt. Whether the Köbberling variety is a distinct entity or a variant of the Dunnigan phenotype is unknown.

Familial Partial Lipodystrophy Associated with PPARG Mutation

Recently, we reported a heterozygous mutation C $\rightarrow$ T at nucleotide 1273 in exon 6 of peroxisome proliferator-activator receptor γ gene (*PPARG*) in a patient with FPL [36]. The proband, a 64-year-old woman, developed diabetes mellitus and hypertriglyceridemia at the age of 32 years and noted gradual loss of subcutaneous fat from the arms and legs at the age of 50 years. This patient had marked loss of subcutaneous fat from the distal regions of the extremities and the face but truncal region was spared. She had hypertriglyceridemia and low levels of serum HDL cholesterol. The transmission was consistent with autosomal dominant inheritance although the mutation may have appeared *de novo* in the proband. Thus, a unique type of FPL was observed in this patient, which was distinct from FPLD and Kobberling variety. Since PPARG plays a key role in adipocyte differentiation [37], the mutation may cause lipodystrophy by reducing development of adipocytes from preadipocytes.

Mandibuloacral Dysplasia

Mandibuloacral dysplasia (MAD) is a rare autosomal recessive disorder (OMIM # 248370) characterized by abnormalities such as mandibular hypoplasia, dental overcrowding, bird-like facies with prominent eyes and beaked nose, progressive osteolysis of the clavicles and terminal phalanges (acro-osteolysis), delayed closure of the cranial sutures, mottled hyperpigmentation over the trunk, and skin atrophy over the hands and feet. Two patterns of lipodystrophy have been reported by us in patients with MAD; type A pattern is characterized by loss of subcutaneous fat from the extremities with normal or slight excess in the face, neck, and truncal regions similar to that seen in the patients with FPL, Dunnigan variety [38]. Homozygous R527H *LMNA* (lamin A/C) mutation was recently noted in affected subjects from five consanguineous Italian pedigrees and type A lipodystrophy [39]. Type B pattern is characterized by more generalized loss of subcutaneous fat involving the face, trunk, and extremities. Patients with MAD are predisposed to insulin resistance, diabetes, and hypertriglyceridemia.

SHORT Syndrome-associated Lipodystrophy

Gorlin et al. [40] and Sensenbrenner et al. [41] first described this rare syndrome (OMIM # 269880 and 151680). Both autosomal recessive and autosomal dominant inheritance patterns have been described [42]. Approximately 22 patients with SHORT syndrome have been reported till now. The clinical features of SHORT syndrome include *s*hort stature, *h*yperextensibility of joints and/or inguinal hernia, *o*cular depression, *R*eiger anomaly (iris and teeth abnormalities), and teething delay. A common feature of this syndrome is lipodystrophy affecting the face, upper extremities, and trunk. The lower extremities are usually spared. Some patients develop insulin-resistant diabetes. The genetic basis of SHORT syndrome-associated lipodystrophy remains to be determined.

Neonatal Progeroid Syndrome (Wiedemann–Rautenstrauch Syndrome)

This syndrome was first described by Rautenstrauch and coworkers [43] in 1977 and subsequently in 1979, by Wiedemann [44]. Inheritance appears to be autosomal recessive. Nine more cases with this rare syndrome have been reported till now. The clinical features include a progeroid face (triangular, old-looking face with relatively large skull, prominent veins especially of the scalp, sparse scalp hair, large anterior fontanel) and near total absence of subcutaneous fat with prominent veins and muscles. Subcutaneous fat is preserved in the gluteal region.

ACQUIRED LIPODYSTROPHIES

Acquired Generalized Lipodystrophy

Initial description of acquired generalized lipodystrophy (AGL) was provided by Ziegler in 1928 [45], followed by detailed description by Lawrence [46] in 1946. It is a rare disease characterized by loss of adipose tissue from large areas of the body, which occurs during childhood and adolescence. Nearly 80 patients have been reported in the literature till now.

Clinical Features

Females are affected approximately three times more as compared to males. The disease usually begins insidiously in the childhood and adolescence, and onset after 30 years of age is rare. The onset can be quite rapid in some patients. Children may have voracious appetite and increased linear growth [9, 47]. Acromegaloid features are rarely seen in contrast to CGL. Acanthosis nigricans is observed in approximately one third of the patients. Mild hirsutism may be seen in women. Most of the patients have hepatomegaly [9, 45, 46, 48, 49]. Hepatic steatosis or steatohepatitis may occur, which can progress to cirrhosis and its complications [50, 51]. Although menstrual irregularity is common, normal reproduction in women has been reported. Polycystic ovaries may also occur. Accelerated development of coronary heart disease has been reported in some patients.

AGL patients have been subclassified into three varieties on the basis of clinical presentation and possible etiopathogenetic mechanisms as follows: the panniculitis variety (type 1), the autoimmune diseases variety (type 2), and the idiopathic variety (type 3) [52]. Panniculitis may precede or accompany fat loss in patients with AGL. In acute stage, tender and inflamed subcutaneous nodules develop. Upon healing, localized atrophy of subcutaneous fat and subsequently generalized lipodystrophy may occur. Pathologically, panniculitis is characterized by an infiltration of adipose tissue with lymphocytes and histiocytes with granulomatous reaction and multinucleated giant cells [53, 54].

Patients with autoimmune variety of AGL have associated autoimmune diseases such as juvenile dermatomyositis, Sjogren's syndrome, chronic active hepatitis, Hashimoto's thyroiditis, and juvenile rheumatoid arthritis [55–57]. Patients with idiopathic variety of AGL have no evidence of panniculitis or autoimmune diseases.

Body Fat Distribution

There is heterogeneity in the magnitude of fat loss. Fat loss in most patients is extensive, affecting the head, face, trunk, abdomen, gluteal regions, and extremities; however, some patients have patchy fat loss, particularly in the panniculitis variety (Figure 7). Subcutaneous fat loss

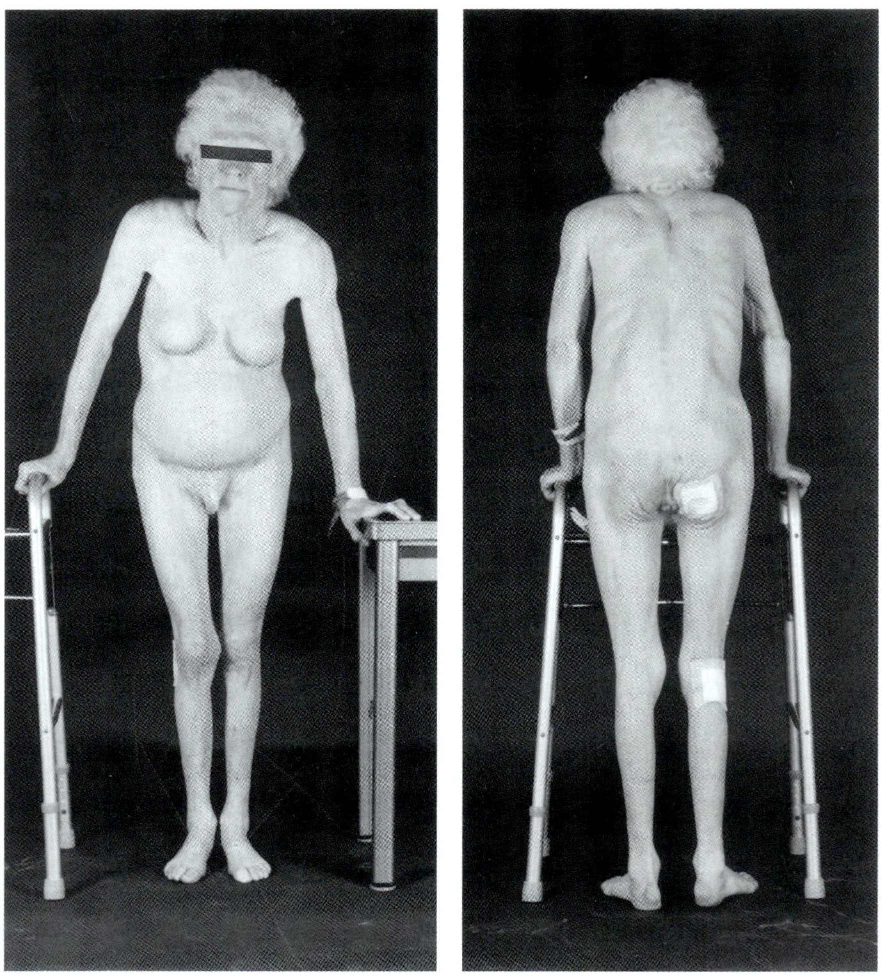

Figure 7 Anterior and posterior views of 59-year-old Caucasian woman with acquired generalized lipodystrophy. She has near complete absence of subcutaneous fat. The lipodystrophy started at $2^{1/2}$ years of age following "lumpy" subcutaneous swellings over the extremities and abdomen, suggestive of panniculitis. She developed diabetes mellitus and severe hypertriglyceridemia at 15 years of age. She had vitiligo and pernicious anemia. She had long-standing hepatic steatosis and died of hepatocellular carcinoma at age 63 years

from the palms and soles may also be evident in some patients. Intraperitoneal and perirenal fat may also be lost in some patients, and in others it may be preserved or even be excessive. All patients have preserved retro-orbital fat and bone marrow fat.

Pathogenesis

Destruction of adipocytes could be due to either cell-mediated or antibody-mediated autoimmune processes or both in all varieties of AGL, though the target autoantigen(s) have not been identified.

Diagnostic Criteria

(A) Essential criteria: Loss of body fat from extensive areas of body, occurring after birth, in childhood, adolescence, or later in life

(B) Supportive criteria:

 (1) Clinical

  (a) Loss of subcutaneous fat from the palms and soles
  (b) Acanthosis nigricans
  (c) Hepatosplenomegaly
  (d) History of subcutaneous tender nodular swellings suggestive of panniculitis preceding the onset of lipodystrophy or histological confirmation of biopsied lesions
  (e) Presence of other autoimmune diseases

 (2) Laboratory

  (a) Impaired glucose tolerance or diabetes mellitus
  (b) Severe fasting and/or postprandial hyperinsulinemia
  (c) Hypertriglyceridemia and/or low levels of serum HDL cholesterol
  (d) Reduced serum concentrations of leptin and/or adiponectin
  (e) MRI documentation of;

   (i) Loss of fat from large regions of the body
   (ii) Preservation of bone marrow fat.

Metabolic Features

The pathogenesis of diabetes mellitus may be related to extreme insulin resistance [58]. However, in some patients, diabetes mellitus develops before the onset of lipodystrophy and it is likely that some of them may have type 1 diabetes mellitus. Patients have marked hyperglycemia, which requires extremely high doses of insulin [59, 60]. Hypertriglyceridemia is usually severe and accompanied by low levels of HDL cholesterol. Diabetes mellitus and hypertriglyceridemia are less prevalent in the panniculitis variety of AGL as compared to the other varieties [52]. Patients have low serum levels of leptin and adiponectin [14].

Acquired Partial Lipodystrophy (Barraquer–Simons Syndrome)

Approximately 250 patients with acquired partial lipodystrophy (APL) of various ethnicities have been reported. There is no predilection for any ethnic group. Females are affected approximately four times more often than males [61]. The onset occurs during childhood or adolescence, usually before 16 years of age.

Pathogenesis

A polyclonal immunoglobulin G, complement 3 nephritic factor (C3NeF) is present in ~90% of the patients [62–64]. Serum C3 is low and suggests alternative complement pathway activation. It is hypothesized that the fat loss is caused by C3NeF-induced lysis of adipocytes, which express factor D [64]. C3NeF also binds to C3 convertase, C3b, Bb and stabilizes it, making it resistant to the action of factor H. This process may contribute to the development of mesangio-capillary glomerulonephritis.

Clinical Features

Fat loss is gradual over several months to years. Initially, the face is affected, followed by the upper regions of the body. Acanthosis nigricans, hirsutism, and menstrual abnormalities are usually not observed.

A specific feature of APL is development of mesangio-capillary glomerulonephritis in 20–33% of the patients ~10 years after the diagnosis of lipodystrophy. Some patients have associated systemic lupus erythematosus and other autoimmune diseases [65].

Body Fat Distribution

Fat loss affects the face, neck, upper limbs, thorax, and upper abdomen, sparing the hips and lower extremities [66] (Figure 8). Occasionally, fat loss is observed from the inguinal region or thighs. Some patients, particularly women, deposit excess fat over the lower extremities after puberty. The intrathoracic, intraabdominal, bone marrow, and mechanical adipose tissues are usually spared.

Metabolic Features

Insulin resistance and dyslipidemia are generally not seen and diabetes occurs rarely.

Lipodystrophy in HIV-infected Patients

In the last few years lipodystrophy has been reported in HIV-infected patients being treated with highly active

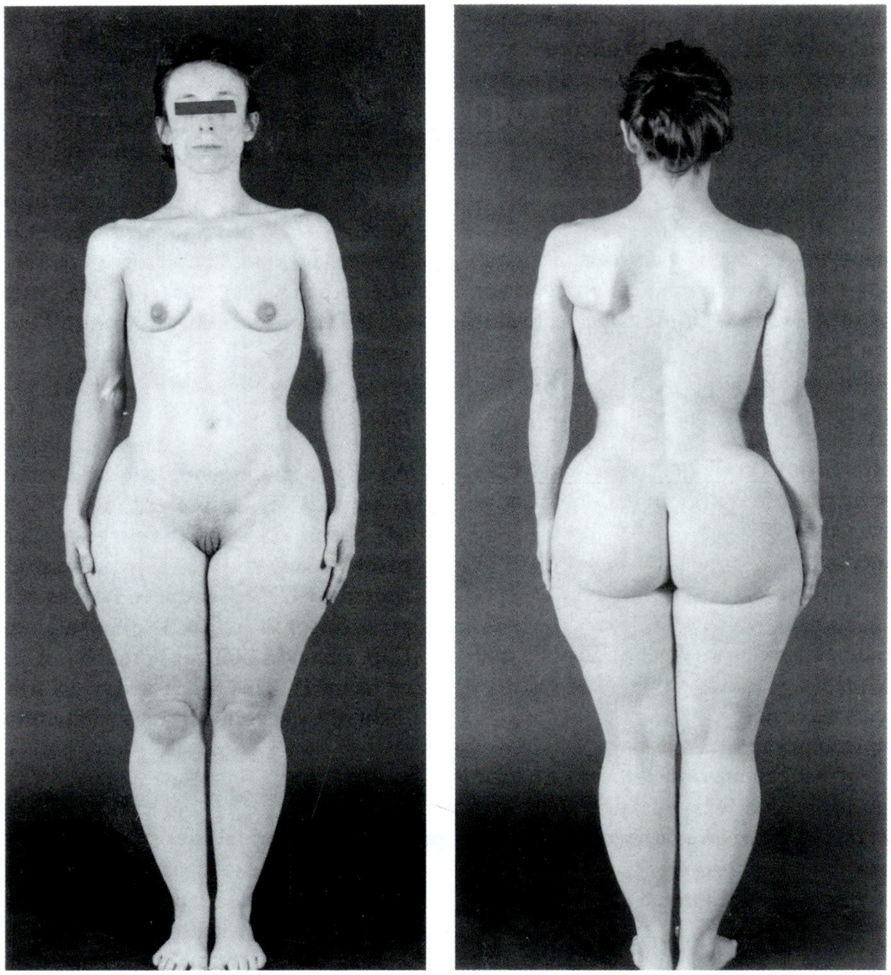

Figure 8 A 28-year-old Caucasian woman with acquired partial lipodystrophy. The onset of the lipodystrophy occurred at 12 years of age. There is almost complete absence of subcutaneous fat from the face, neck, upper extremities, and trunk upto waist. She has excessive deposition of fat over the hips, buttocks, and lower extremities. She had no diabetes, dyslipidemia, or acanthosis nigricans. She had low serum levels of complement 3

antiretroviral therapy (HAART), which included HIV-1 protease inhibitors (PIs). This syndrome is characterized by the loss of subcutaneous fat from the face and extremities and excess fat deposition in the neck and abdomen [67, 68]. Insulin resistance and hypertriglyceridemia usually accompany it.

Prevalence

The data from various reports reveal an overall prevalence of 17% in patients treated with PI-containing HAART for less than 1 year and 43% in those treated for a year or more [69]. Although some investigators have reported body fat redistribution in patients treated with nucleoside analogue reverse transcriptase inhibitors (NRTIs) alone, however, for lack of associated metabolic changes and occurrence of weight loss, liver enlargement, and lactic acidosis [70], it does not deserve to be classified as a distinct type of lipodystrophy [69]. With the widespread use of PI-containing HAART, lipodystrophy in HIV-infected patients is currently the most common form of the lipodystrophy [69].

Clinical Features and Body Fat Distribution

Most of the HIV patients with lipodystrophy (LDHIV patients) have normal immune status, suppressed HIV viral load, and absence of AIDS-defining illnesses. The typical appearance of the patient consists of sunken cheeks and increased muscular extremities with prominence of superficial veins due to loss of fat. Excess fat may accumulate over the neck ("double chin"), dorsocervical spine ("buffalo hump"), over the upper torso, and intraabdominal region [71–73] (Figure 9). Compared to men, peripheral fat loss in women with LDHIV is often more subtle, whereas increased truncal adiposity may be

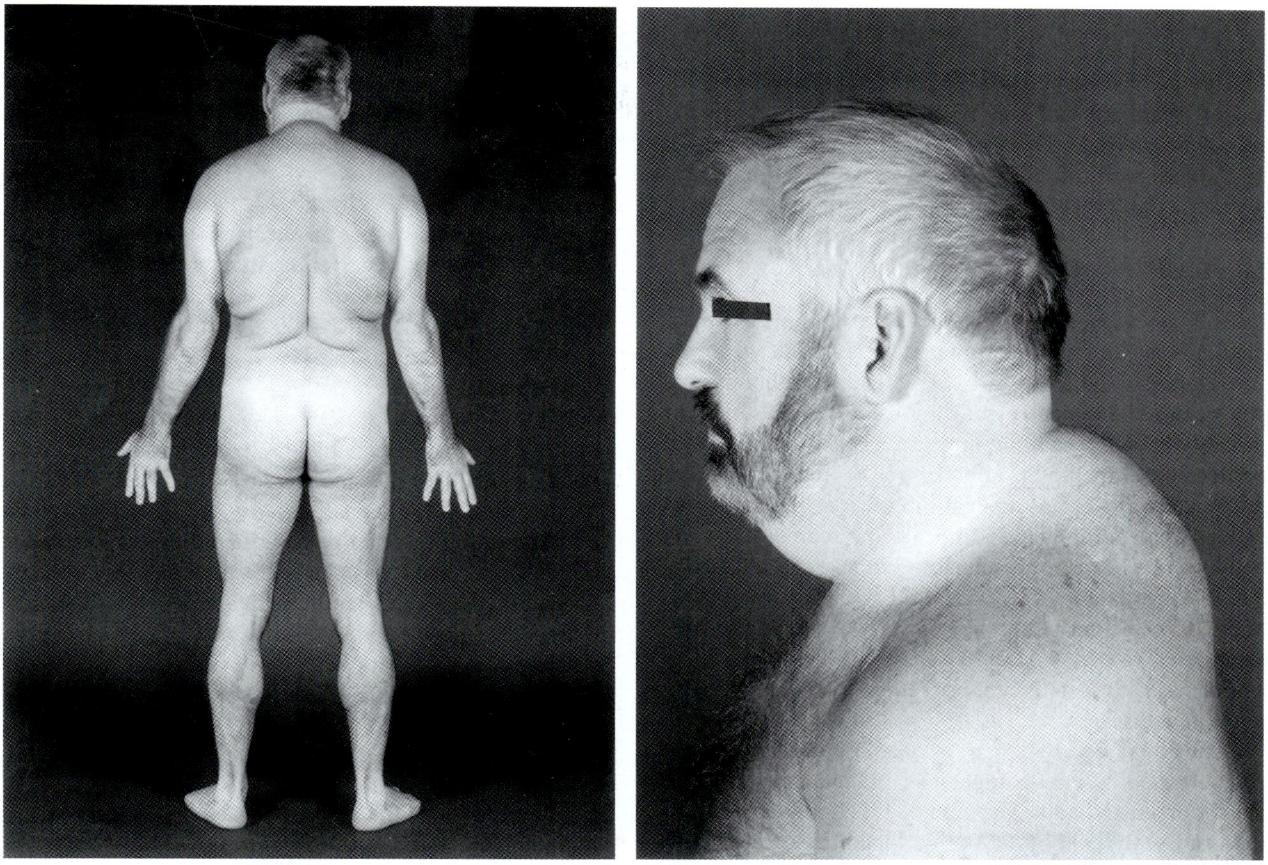

Figure 9 Anterior and left lateral views of a 47-year-old HIV-infected Caucasian man with lipodystrophy. He was being treated with protease-inhibitor-containing antiretroviral regimen for ~2 years. The patients had marked subcutaneous fat loss from the extremities including gluteal region and face. Fat transplantation of cheeks had been carried out. Excess fat deposition is seen at the chin ("double chin"), dorsocervical region ("buffalo hump"), and upper torso. The patients also had diabetes mellitus and hypertriglyceridemia and low levels of high-density lipoprotein cholesterol

more apparent. Breast enlargement has been reported in both women and men [74]. Acanthosis nigricans has not been reported. Women may have menstrual irregularities.

Diagnostic Criteria

Many investigators diagnose LDHIV based on either loss or excess of fat, or both. However, we believe that the fat loss from the face and extremities is the primary abnormality while excess deposition of fat over the neck and abdomen occurs secondarily as a compensatory phenomenon [69].

Risk Factors and Pathogenesis

There is a strong association between LDHIV and PI-containing HAART [75]. LDHIV has been reported with all PIs, particularly with the combination therapy of two PIs. LDHIV is particularly associated with the longer duration of PI therapy and with increasing age [69].

PIs have been reported to inhibit adipocyte differentiation and induce subcutaneous adipocyte apoptosis in the lipodystrophic areas, but it is not reversed on switching to non-PI therapy. In experimental studies, indinavir and saquinavir have been shown to selectively affect intrinsic transport activity of glucose transporter 4 (GLUT-4), thus inhibiting insulin-stimulated glucose uptake [76, 77]. Recently, altered levels of sterol regulatory element-binding protein 1 (SREBP-1) have been shown in the liver and adipose tissue in PI-treated experimental animals [78]. PI-induced alterations of SREBP-1 expression may be a mechanism for the pathogenesis of LDHIV since SREBP-1c overexpression in adipose tissue of mice has been shown to cause lipodystrophy [79].

Metabolic Features

In LDHIV patients treated with PIs, dyslipidemia is characterized by hypertriglyceridemia, hypercholesterolemia, and low levels sf serum HDL cholesterol, and has been reported in 50–70% of patients [75, 80]. Ritonavir and combination therapy with two PIs, in particular, increase risk of hypertriglyceridemia and hypercholesterolemia [81].

Fasting and/or postprandial hyperinsulinemia and insulin resistance in patients on PI therapies and with LDHIV is common [82, 83], particularly in those with prolonged treatment, and may be related to increased truncal adiposity and excessive visceral adipose tissue. New onset of diabetes mellitus and worsening of preexisting hyperglycemia on PI therapy are relatively uncommon [84].

Localized Lipodystrophies

Loss of subcutaneous adipose tissue from single or multiple areas causing well-demarcated, depressed areas characterize localized lipodystrophies. Localized lipodystrophy occurred frequently with the use of animal insulins possibly related to autoimmune mechanisms [85]. Local corticosteroid therapy is effective in the treatment. Other drugs, such as steroids and antibiotics, can also cause localized lipodystrophy [86]. Repeated pressure against any body part can cause subcutaneous adipose tissue atrophy due to microtrauma or reduced perfusion [87]. Avoidance of pressure results in improvement. Acute panniculitis can cause localized lipodystrophy besides AGL [88]. It can be associated with systemic lupus erythematosus or other autoimmune diseases.

Centrifugal lipodystrophy occurs in childhood and is characterized by a centrifugal loss of subcutaneous fat in the abdomen and adjacent region with slightly erythematous and scaly changes at the periphery associated with regional lymphadenopathy in $\sim$50% of the cases [89]. The centrifugal spread stops by 8 years of age and approximately half of the patients recover spontaneously. Corticosteroids therapy is not effective in this variety of localized lipodystrophy. It has been described in nearly 100 patients from Japan, Korea, and Singapore [90, 91]. Some patients who do not belong to any of the above categories are classified as having idiopathic localized lipodystrophy [92].

COMPLICATIONS IN PATIENTS WITH LIPODYSTROPHIES

Patients with lipodystrophies are predisposed to complications of diabetes mellitus such as nephropathy, retinopathy, and neuropathy. These may appear early in life in patients with generalized lipodystrophies, both CGL and AGL, as many of these develop diabetes during childhood and adolescence and despite hypoglycemic therapy may have severe and persistent hyperglycemia. Two of our CGL patients with *AGPAT2* mutations developed end-stage renal disease due to diabetes at ages 25 and 43 years. One of them has recently received a renal transplant. She is also legally blind due to proliferative diabetic retinopathy.

Extreme hypertriglyceridemia may result in recurrent attacks of acute pancreatitis, eruptive xanthomas, and lipemia retinalis. Patients with generalized lipodystrophy and FPLD commonly develop lipemia-induced pancreatitis. Occasional patient with LDHIV has also been reported to have acute pancreatitis and eruptive xanthomas.

Another important cause of morbidity and mortality in patients with lipodystrophies is related to long-standing fatty infiltration of the liver, which may cause steatohepatitis and cirrhosis. One of our patients with FPL developed cirrhosis and received hepatic transplantation [93]. One patient with panniculitis variety of AGL died of hepatocellular carcinoma at age 60 after longstanding hepatic steatosis [52]. Patients with AGL are also predisposed to develop autoimmune hepatitis.

Early onset and severe hyperglycemia and dyslipidemia may cause accelerated atherosclerosis, which has been documented in some patients with FPLD and AGL. Women with FPLD are particularly predisposed to develop atherosclerotic vascular disease including coronary heart disease, peripheral vascular disease, and cerebrovascular accidents [30, 94]. Even though patients with CGL have extreme metabolic abnormalities, accelerated atherosclerosis has not yet been documented. However, most of the reported cases with CGL have been children or young adults.

Other rare complications may be related to peculiar phenotypes of different disorders. For example, patients with FPLD having exon 1 mutations are predisposed to cardiomyopathy and conduction system disturbances. They may develop congestive heart failure and sudden death due to arrhythmias, particularly atrial fibrillation. Cardiac failure in CGL patients with *BSCL2* mutations may result in premature death [11]. Marked lack of fat in the soles in some patients with AGL may result in painful callosities. A few patients with APL have developed end-stage renal disease due to mesangioproliferative glomerulonephritis and have received renal transplantation.

DIFFERENTIAL DIAGNOSIS

Diagnosis of typical patient of lipodystrophy with severe and generalized fat loss does not pose much difficulty to a knowledgeable physician. However, the diagnosis of partial lipodystrophies may be missed unless there is a high index of suspicion.

Leprechaunism and Werner syndrome should be differentiated from CGL, neonatal progeroid syndrome, AGL, and MAD (type B pattern). FPLD should be differentiated from multiple symmetric lipomatosis, Cushing's syndrome, and LDHIV; and AGL and LDHIV from conditions that cause generalized and nonselective weight loss and cachexia (starvation, anorexia nervosa, cancer cachexia, wasting associated with acquired immunodeficiency syndrome, thyrotoxicosis, malabsorption syndromes, advanced tuberculosis, adrenal insufficiency, and uncontrolled diabetes mellitus). Many poorly nourished subjects may have extreme paucity of subcutaneous fat but they also have reduced muscle mass and do not manifest metabolic complications such as diabetes mellitus and hyperlipidemia and thus can be easily differentiated from patients with lipodystrophies.

MANAGEMENT

Management of lipodystrophies is a challenging task. Most of the patients are extremely concerned about the disfiguring cosmetic appearance. Persistent morbidities due to uncontrolled glycemia and hypertriglyceridemia may require repeated physician visits and hospitalizations and can be frustrating to the patients. However, judicious use of lifestyle management and pharmacotherapy for the management of metabolic complications can benefit most of the patients.

Management of Cosmetic Appearance

Cosmetic appearance is affected because of facial fat loss, acanthosis nigricans, xanthomas, hirsutism, and muscular prominence. Currently, there is no medical management to improve loss of subcutaneous body fat. Several cosmetic surgical procedures have been tried with varied success including free flaps transfer, transposition of facial muscle, silicone implants, and collagen injections [95, 96]. Excess fat deposition occurring in the patients with FPLD has been treated with liposuction or lipectomy. Decrease in the excess fat deposition parallels weight loss achieved with the lifestyle management. In some patients acanthosis nigricans has improved with the use of Etretinate and fish oil [97, 98]. Recently, subcutaneous recombinant human leptin replacement therapy has been shown to improve acanthosis nigricans. Effectiveness of thiazolidinediones in inducing body fat gain is unclear [99].

Physical Activity

Physical activity, particularly aerobic exercise, should be encouraged in all patients. Daily physical exercise may lead to decrease in insulin resistance and may also improve dyslipidemia. Aerobic and resistance exercises have been shown to improve insulin resistance and dyslipidemia, and reduce excess truncal fat in patients with LDHIV [100, 101].

Diet

The optimal diet for patients with lipodystrophy is not clear. Moreover the compliance of the patients is often poor because of their voracious appetite. Patients with severe hypertriglyceridemia and hyperglycemia should be prescribed decreased energy intake. Low-fat diet is beneficial in patients with extreme hypertriglyceridemia and chylomicronemia. In CGL patients with defective biosynthesis of triacylglycerol, low-fat diets should be advised. It is important to note that diets low in fat and high in carbohydrate can also exacerbate hypertriglyceridemia and decrease levels of HDL cholesterol. Particular attention should be given to the nutrition and calorie requirement of growing children. Medium chain triglycerides have been reported to be of benefit in anecdotal patients with AGL [102].

Pharmacological Therapy

In patients with CGL and AGL, control of hyperglycemia is often difficult and extremely high doses of insulin may be required. The efficacy of oral hypoglycemic drugs—sulfonylureas, biguanides, and thiazolidinediones—has not been systematically investigated in patients with CGL, AGL, and FPLD, though these drugs have been proved useful in some patients. Metformin has been shown to be beneficial in LDHIV by improving insulin resistance and decreasing visceral fat [103] but there may be an increased risk of lactic acidosis when used in combination with NRTIs. Optimal glycemic control also decreases serum triglyceride levels and if maintained, prevents and retards chronic microvascular and macrovascular diabetic complications.

Severe hypertriglyceridemia not controlled on diet and lifestyle measures should be managed with lipid-lowering drugs. Significant lowering of triglycerides levels can be achieved with the help of fibrates and/or high doses of ω-3 polyunsaturated fatty acids. Combination therapy with fibrates and statins has also been attempted; however, risk of myopathy may be a limitation. Many statins (simvastatin, lovastatin, atorvastatin) are metabolized by cytochrome P4503A4, which is inhibited by PIs. This drug interaction may elevate plasma levels of statins and can increase the risk of myopathy. Pravastatin and fibrates may be safer drugs since these drugs are not metabolized in the similar manner [104–106]. Plasma exchange can dramatically decrease serum triglyceride concentrations but the effect may be transient [51]. Niacin should be avoided since it can exacerbate hyperglycemia and decrease insulin sensitivity. It is prudent to avoid oral contraceptive drugs containing estrogens or postmenopausal hormone replacement therapy, since these drugs can raise serum levels of triglycerides. A few patients have developed acute pancreatitis with the use of estrogen-containing oral contraceptives for hirsutism, polycystic ovarian disease, and uncontrolled menstrual bleeding.

For management of hepatic steatosis, optimal control of hyperglycemia and hyperlipidemia is important. Preliminary data suggest some benefit with the use of fibrates, ursodeoxycholic acid, betaine, and α-tocopherol in patients with hepatic steatosis not having lipodystrophy. In patients

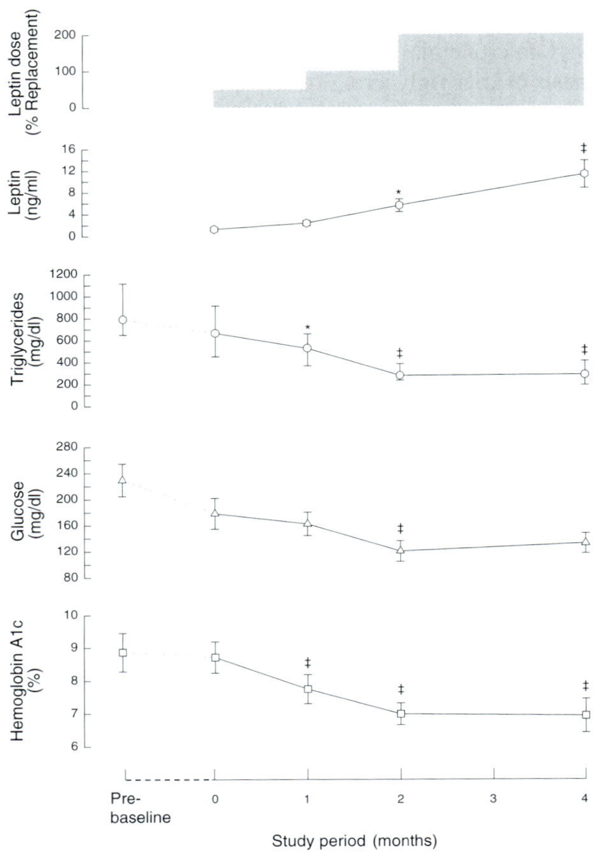

Figure 10 Effects of administration of recombinant methionyl human leptin administered over a period of 4 months on the levels of serum leptin, hemoglobin A1c, fasting plasma glucose, and serum triglycerides in nine patients with lipodystrophies. $^{*}p < 0.05$, $\ddagger\, p < 0.001$

with type 2 diabetes, metformin therapy has shown some beneficial effects on hepatic steatosis. Rosiglitazone has shown some efficacy in reducing liver triglycerides in patients with type 2 diabetes [107].

Steroid therapy has been shown to halt the progression of panniculitis in AGL but had minimal or no effect on lipodystrophy [53, 54]. It is unclear if significant improvement in subcutaneous fat loss occurs after withdrawal of PIs and switching to other antiretroviral drugs [108]. Dyslipidemia, insulin resistance, or hyperglycemia has been reported to improve in some studies after discontinuation of PIs [109].

Efficacy and safety of subcutaneous recombinant leptin has been shown in patients with CGL, AGL, and FPLD who had low concentrations of serum leptin [110]. Four-month therapy with recombinant leptin significantly decreased levels of fasting blood glucose, glycosylated hemoglobin, and serum triglycerides (Figure 10).

Additionally, leptin therapy also led to an improvement in the levels of serum transaminases and liver volume [110]. Leptin therapy also reduced intrahepatic and intramyocellular triglyceride concentrations, which could be related to improvement of insulin sensitivity in these patients [111, 112].

REFERENCES

1. Garg A. Lipodystrophies. *Am J Med* 2000; 108: 143–52.
2. Garg A, Wilson R, Barnes R, Arioglu E, Zaidi Z, Gurakan F, Kocak N, O'Rahilly S, Taylor SI, Patel SB, Bowcock AM. A gene for congenital generalized lipodystrophy maps to human chromosome 9q34. *J Clin Endocrinol Metab* 1999; 84: 3390–4.
3. Agarwal AK, Arioglu E, De Almeida S, Akkoc N, Taylor SI, Bowcock AM, Barnes Rl, Garg A. *AGPAT2* is mutated in congenital generalized lipodystrophy linked to chromosome 9q34. *Nat Genet* 2002; 31: 21–3.
4. West J, Tompkins CK, Balantac N, Nudelman E, Meengs B, White T, Bursten S, Coleman J, Kumar A, Singer JW, Leung DW. Cloning and expression of two human lysophosphatidic acid acyltransferase cDNAs that enhance cytokine-induced signaling responses in cells. *DNA Cell Biol* 1997; 16: 691–701.
5. Leung DW. The structure and functions of human lysophosphatidic acid acyltransferases. *Front Biosci* 2001; 6: d944–53.
6. Eberhardt C, Gray PW, Tjoelker LW. Human lysophosphatidic acid acyltransferase. cDNA cloning, expression, and localization to chromosome 9q34.3. *J Biol Chem* 1997; 272: 20299–305.
7. Eberhardt C, Gray PW, Tjoelker LW. cDNA cloning, expression and chromosomal localization of two human lysophosphatidic acid acyltransferases. *Adv Exper Med Biol* 1999; 469: 351–6.
8. Magre J, Delepine M, Khallouf E, Gedde-Dahl T Jr, Van Maldergem L, Sobel E, Papp J, Meier M, Megarbane A, Bachy A, Verloes A, d'Abronzo FH, Seemanova E, Assan R, Baudic N, Bourut C, Czernichow P, Huet F, Grigorescu F, de Kerdanet M, Lacombe D, Labrune P, Lanza M, Loret H, Matsuda F, Navarro J, Nivelon-Chevalier A, Polak M, Robert JJ, Tric P, Tubiana-Rufi N, Vigouroux C, Weissenbach J, Savasta S, Maassen JA, Trygstad O, Bogalho P, Freitas P, Medina JL, Bonnicci F, Joffe BI, Loyson G, Panz VR, Raal FJ, O'Rahilly S, Stephenson T, Kahn CR, Lathrop M, Capeau J; BSCL Working Group. Identification of the gene altered in Berardinelli–Seip congenital lipodystrophy on chromosome 11q13. *Nat Genet* 2001; 28: 365–70.
9. Seip M, Trygstad O. Generalized lipodystrophy, congenital and acquired (lipoatrophy). *Acta Paediatr Suppl* 1996; 413: 2–28.
10. Fleckenstein JL, Garg A, Bonte FJ, Vuitch MF, Peshock RM. The skeleton in congenital, generalized lipodystrophy: evaluation using whole-body radiographic surveys, magnetic resonance imaging and technetium-99m bone scintigraphy. *Skeletal Radiol* 1992; 21: 381–6.
11. Van Maldergem L, Magre J, Khallouf TE, Gedde-Dahl T Jr, Delepine M, Trygstad O, Seemanova E, Stephenson T, Albott CS, Bonnici F, Panz VR, Medina JL, Bogalho P, Huet F, Savasta S, Verloes A, Robert JJ, Loret H, De Kerdanet M, Tubiana-Rufi N, Megarbane A, Maassen J, Polak M, Lacombe D, Khan CR, Silveira EL, D'Abronzo FH, Grigorescu F, Lathrop M, Capeau J, O'Rahilly S.

Genotype–phenotype relationships in Berardinelli-Seip congenital lipodystrophy. *Med Genet* 2002; 39: 722–33.

12. Garg A, Fleckenstein JL, Peshock RM, Grundy SM. Peculiar distribution of adipose tissue in patients with congenital generalized lipodystrophy. *J Clin Endocrinol Metab* 1992; 75: 358–61.
13. Chandalia M, Garg A, Vuitch F, Nizzi F. Postmortem findings in congenital generalized lipodystrophy. *J Clin Endocrinol Metab* 1995; 80: 3077–81.
14. Haque WA, Shimomura I, Matsuzawa Y, Garg A. Serum adiponectin and leptin levels in patients with lipodystrophies. *J Clin Endocrinol Metab* 2002; 87: 2395–8.
15. Garg A, Chandalia M, Vuitch F. Severe islet amyloidosis in congenital generalized lipodystrophy. *Diabetes Care* 1996; 19: 28–31.
16. Ozer FL, Lichtenstein JR, Kwiterovich PO, McKusick VA. A new genetic variety of lipodystrophy. *Clin Res* 1973; 21: 533.
17. Dunnigan MG, Cochrane MA, Kelly A, Scott JW. Familial lipoatrophic diabetes with dominant transmission. A new syndrome. *Q J Med* 1974; 43: 33–48.
18. Peters JM, Barnes R, Bennett L, Gitomer WM, Bowcock AM, Garg A. Localization of the gene for familial partial lipodystrophy (Dunnigan variety) to chromosome 1q21-22. *Nat Genet* 1998; 18: 292–5.
19. Cao H, Hegele RA. Nuclear lamin A/C R482Q mutation in canadian kindreds with Dunnigan-type familial partial lipodystrophy. *Hum Mol Genet* 2000; 9: 109–12.
20. Speckman RA, Garg A, Du F, Bennett L, Veile R, Arioglu E, Taylor SI, Lovett M, Bowcock AM. Mutational and haplotype analyses of families with familial partial lipodystrophy (Dunnigan variety) reveal recurrent missense mutations in the globular C-terminal domain of *lamin A/C*. *Am J Hum Genet* 2000; 66: 1192–8.
21. Shackleton S, Lloyd DJ, Jackson SN, Evans R, Niermeijer MF, Singh BM, Schmidt H, Brabant G, Kumar S, Durrington PN, Gregory S, O'Rahilly S, Trembath RC. *LMNA*, encoding lamin A/C, is mutated in partial lipodystrophy. *Nat Genet* 2000; 24: 153–6.
22. Garg A, Vinaitheerthan M, Weatherall P, Bowcock A. Phenotypic heterogeneity in patients with familial partial lipodystrophy (Dunnigan variety) related to the site of mis-sense mutations in Lamin A/C (*LMNA*) gene. *J Clin Endocrinol Metab* 2001; 86: 59–65.
23. Fatkin D, MacRae C, Sasaki T, Wolff MR, Porcu M, Frenneaux M, Atherton J, Vidaillet HJ Jr, Spudich S, De Girolami U, Seidman JG, Seidman C, Muntoni F, Muehle G, Johnson W, McDonough B. Missense mutations in the rod domain of the lamin A/C gene as causes of dilated cardiomyopathy and conduction-system disease. *N Engl J Med* 1999; 341: 1715–24.
24. Brodsky GL, Muntoni F, Miocic S, Sinagra G, Sewry C, Mestroni L. Lamin A/C gene mutation associated with dilated cardiomyopathy with variable skeletal muscle involvement. *Circulation* 2000; 101: 473–6.
25. Bonne G, Di Barletta MR, Varnous S, Becane HM, Hammouda EH, Merlini L, Muntoni F, Greenberg CR, Gary F, Urtizberea JA, Duboc D, Fardeau M, Toniolo D, Schwartz K. Mutations in the gene encoding lamin A/C cause autosomal dominant Emery-Dreifuss muscular dystrophy. *Nat Genet* 1999; 21: 285–8.
26. Muchir A, Bonne G, van der Kooi AJ, van Meegen M, Baas F, Bolhuis PA, de Visser M, Schwartz K. Identification of mutations in the gene encoding lamins A/C in autosomal dominant limb girdle muscular dystrophy with atrioventricular conduction disturbances (LGMD1B). *Hum Mol Genet* 2000; 9: 1453–9.
27. De Sandre-Giovannoli A, Chaouch M, Kozlov S, Vallat JM, Tazir M, Kassouri N, Szepetowski P, Hammadouche T, Vandenberghe A, Stewart CL, Grid D, Levy N. Homozygous defects in LMNA, encoding lamin A/C nuclear-envelope proteins, cause autosomal recessive axonal neuropathy in human (Charcot-Marie-Tooth disorder type 2) and mouse. *Am J Hum Genet* 2002; 70: 1075.
28. Garg A, Speckman RA, Bowcock AM. Multisystem dystrophy syndrome due to novel missense mutations in the amino terminal head and alpha-helical rod domain of the lamin A/C (*LMNA*) gene. *Am J Med* 2002; 112: 549–55.
29. Garg A, Peshock RM, Fleckenstein JL. Adipose tissue distribution pattern in patients with familial partial lipodystrophy (Dunnigan variety). *J Clin Endocrinol Metab* 1999; 84: 170–4.
30. Garg A. Gender differences in the prevalence of metabolic complications in familial partial lipodystrophy (Dunnigan variety). *J Clin Endocrinol Metab* 2000; 85: 1776–82.
31. Garg A, Fleckenstein JL, Abate N. Insulin resistance and body fat distribution in a male patient with familial partial lipodystrophy (FPL). *Clin Res* 1994; 42: 199A.
32. Haque WA, Vuitch F, Garg A. Postmortem findings in familial partial lipodystrophy, Dunnigan variety. *Diabet Med* 2002; 19 (12): 1022–5.
33. Kobberling J, Willms B, Kattermann R, Creutzfeldt W. Lipodystrophy of the extremities. A dominantly inherited syndrome associated with lipatrophic diabetes. *Humangenetik* 1975; 29: 111–20.
34. Kobberling J, Schwarck H, Cremer P, Fiechtl J, Seidel D, Creutzfeldt W. Partielle Lipodystrophie mit lipatrophischem Diabetes und Hyperlipoproteinamie. *Verh Dtsch Ges Inn Med* 1981; 87: 958–61.
35. Kobberling J, Dunnigan MG. Familial partial lipodystrophy: two types of an X linked dominant syndrome, lethal in the hemizygous state. *J Med Genet* 1986; 23: 120–7.
36. Agarwal AK, Garg A. A novel heterozygous mutation in peroxisome proliferator-activated receptor-gamma gene in a patient with familial partial lipodystrophy. *J Clin Endocrinol Metab* 2002; 87: 408–11.
37. Rosen ED, Sarraf P, Troy AE, Bradwin G, Moore K, Milstone DS, Spiegelman BM, Mortensen RM. PPAR gamma is required for the differentiation of adipose tissue *in vivo* and *in vitro*. *Mol Cell* 1999; 4: 611–7.
38. Simha V, Garg A. Body fat distribution and metabolic derangements in patients with familial partial lipodystrophy associated with mandibuloacral dysplasia. *J Clin Endocrinol Metab* 2002; 87: 776–85.
39. Novelli G, Muchir A, Sangiuolo F, Helbling-Leclerc A, D'Apice MR, Massart C, Capon F, Sbraccia P, Federici M, Lauro R, Tudisco C, Pallotta R, Scarano G, Dallapiccola B, Merlini L, Bonne G. Mandibuloacral dysplasia is caused by a mutation in LMNA–encoding lamin A/C. *Am J Hum Genet* 2002; 71: 426–31.
40. Gorlin RJ, Cervenka J, Moller K, Horrobin M, Witkop J. Rieger anomaly and growth retardation (the S-H-O-R-T syndrome). *Birth Defects* 1975; 11: 46–48.
41. Sensenbrenner JA, Hussels IE, Levin LS. CC—A low birthweight syndrome, Reiger syndrome. *Birth Defects* 1975; 11: 423–6.

42. Aarskog D, Ose L, Pande H, Eide N. Autosomal dominant partial lipodystrophy associated with Rieger anomaly, short stature, and insulinopenic diabetes. *Am J Med Gen* 1983; 15: 29–38.
43. Rautenstrauch T, Snigula F, Krieg T, Gay S, Muller PK. Progeria: a cell culture study and clinical report of familial incidence. *Eur J Pediatr* 1971; 124: 101–11.
44. Wiedemann HR. An unidentified neonatal progeroid syndrome: follow-up report. *Eur J Pediatr* 1979; 130: 65–70.
45. Ziegler LH. Lipodystrophies: report of seven cases. *Brain* 1928; 51: 145–67.
46. Lawrence RD. Lipodystrophy and hepatomegaly with diabetes, lipemia, and other metabolic disturbances. *Lancet* 1946; 1: 724–31.
47. Senior B, Gellis SS. The syndromes of total lipodystrophy and of partial lipodystrophy. *Pediatrics* 1964; 33: 593–612.
48. Klein S, Jahoor F, Wolfe RR, Stuart CA. Generalized lipodystrophy: *in vivo* evidence for hypermetabolism and insulin-resistant lipid, glucose, and amino acid kinetics. *Metabolism* 1992; 41: 893–6.
49. Saito I, Saruta T, Iyori S, Sakaguchi H. The renal lesion associated with total lipodystrophy. *J Am Geriatr Soc* 1977; 25: 175–8.
50. Dolberg BK, Lenhard MJ. Successful outcome of pregnancy in a patient with generalized lipoatrophic diabetes mellitus. *Endocr Pract* 2000; 6 (1): 34–6.
51. Bolan C, Oral EA, Gorden P, Taylor S, Leitman SF. Intensive, long-term plasma exchange therapy for severe hypertriglyceridemia in acquired generalized lipoatrophy. *J Clin Endocrinol Metab* 2002; 87: 380–4.
52. Misra A, Garg A. Clinical features and metabolic derangements in acquired generalized lipodystrophy: case reports and review of literature. *Medicine* 2003; 82 (2): 129–46.
53. Edge J, Dunger DB, Dillon MJ. Weber-Christian panniculitis and chronic active hepatitis. *Eur J Pediatr* 1986; 145: 227–9.
54. Billings JK, Milgraum SS, Gupta AK, Headington JT, Rasmussen JE. Lipoatrophic panniculitis: a possible autoimmune inflammatory disease of fat. Report of three cases. *Arch Dermatol* 1987; 123: 1662–6.
55. Bourke B, Powell D. Progression from partial to generalised lipodystrophy—a case report. *Iri J Med Sci* 1992; 161: 458–9.
56. Hubler A, Abendroth K, Keiner T, Stocker W, Kauf E, Hein G, Stein G. Dysregulation of insulin-like growth factors in a case of generalized acquired lipoatrophic diabetes mellitus (Lawrence Syndrome) connected with autoantibodies against adipocyte membranes. *Exp Clin Endocrinol Diabetes* 1998; 106: 79–84.
57. Huemer C, Kitson H, Malleson PN, Sanderson S, Huemer M, Cabral DA, Chanoine JP, Petty RE. Lipodystrophy in patients with juvenile dermatomyositis–evaluation of clinical and metabolic abnormalities. *J Rheumatol* 2001; 28: 610–5.
58. Golden MP, Charles MA, Arquilla ER, Myers GL, Lippe BM, Duckworth WC, Zuniga OF, Tanner SM, Palmer AM, Spell M. Insulin resistance in total lipodystrophy: evidence for a pre-receptor defect in insulin action. *Metabolism: Clinical & Experimental* 1985; 34: 330–5.
59. Robbins DC, Sims EA. Recurrent ketoacidosis in acquired, total lipodystrophy (lipoatrophic diabetes). *Diabetes Care* 1984; 7: 381–5.
60. Vantyghem MC, Vigouroux C, Magre J, Desbois-Mouthon C, Pattou F, Fontaine P, Lefebvre J, Capeau J. Late-onset lipoatrophic diabetes. Phenotypic and genotypic familial studies and effect of treatment with metformin and lispro insulin analog. *Diabetes Care* 1999; 22: 1374–6.
61. Barraquer L. Histoire clinique d'un cas d'atrophie du tissu celluloadipeux. *Neurolog Zentralbl* 1907; 26: 1072.
62. Williams DG, Bartlett A, Duffus P. Identification of nephritic factor as an immunoglobulin. *Clin Exp Immunol* 1978; 33: 425–9.
63. Williams DG. C3 nephritic factor and mesangiocapillary glomerulonephritis. *Pediatr Nephrol* 1997; 11: 96–8.
64. Mathieson PW, Peters K. Are nephritic factors nephritogenic? *Am J Kidney Dis* 1994; 24: 964–6.
65. Jasin HE. Systemic lupus erythematosus, partial lipodystrophy and hypocomplementemia. *J Rheumatol* 1979; 6: 43–50.
66. Yuh WT, Collison JS, Sickels WJ, Barloon TJ, Brennan DC, Flanigan MJ. Partial lipodystrophy. Magnetic resonance findings in one case. *J Comput Tomogr* 1988; 12: 287–91.
67. Carr A, Samaras K, Burton S, Law M, Freund J, Chisholm DJ, Cooper DA. A syndrome of peripheral lipodystrophy, hyperlipidaemia and insulin resistance in patients receiving HIV protease inhibitors. *AIDS* 1998; 12: F51–8.
68. Carr A, Samaras K, Chisholm DJ, Cooper DA. Pathogenesis of HIV-1-protease inhibitor-associated peripheral lipodystrophy, hyperlipidaemia, and insulin resistance. *Lancet* 1998; 351: 1881–3.
69. Chen D, Misra A, Garg A. Lipodystrophy in HIV-infected patients. *J Clin Endocrinol Metab* 2002; 87 (11): 4845–56.
70. Carr A, Miller J, Law M, Cooper DA. A syndrome of lipoatrophy, lactic acidaemia and liver dysfunction associated with HIV nucleoside analogue therapy: contribution to protease inhibitor-related lipodystrophy syndrome. *AIDS* 2000; 14: F25–32.
71. Mercie P,Tchamgoue S, Thiebaut R, Viallard J, Faure II, Dancourt VV, Marimoutou C, Dabis F, Rispal P, Darmon Y, Leng B, Pellegrin J. Atherogenic lipid profile in HIV-1-infected patients with lipodystrophy syndrome. *Eur J Intern Med* 2000; 11: 11.
72. Miller KD, Jones E, Yanovski JA, Shankar R, Feuerstein I, Falloon J. Visceral abdominal-fat accumulation associated with use of indinavir. *Lancet* 1998; 351: 871–5.
73. Engelson ES, Kotler DP, Tan Y, Agin D, Wang J, Pierson RN Jr, Heymsfield SB. Fat distribution in HIV-infected patients reporting truncal enlargement quantified by whole-body magnetic resonance imaging. *Am J Clin Nutr* 1999; 69: 1162–9.
74. Madge S, Kinloch-de-Loes S, Mercey D, Johnson MA, Weller IV. Lipodystrophy in patients naive to HIV protease inhibitors. *AIDS* 1999; 13: 735–7.
75. Carr A, Samaras K, Thorisdottir A, Kaufmann GR, Chisholm DJ, Cooper DA. Diagnosis, prediction, and natural course of HIV-1 protease-inhibitor-associated lipodystrophy, hyperlipidaemia, and diabetes mellitus: a cohort study. *Lancet* 1999; 353: 2093–9.
76. Murata H, Hruz PW, Mueckler M. The mechanism of insulin resistance caused by HIV protease inhibitor therapy. *J Biol Chem* 2000; 275: 20251–4.
77. Murata H, Hruz PW, Mueckler M. Indinavir inhibits the glucose transporter isoform Glut4 at physiologic concentrations. *AIDS* 2002; 16: 859–63.

78. Riddle TM, Kuhel DG, Woollett LA, Fichtenbaum CJ, Hui DY. HIV protease inhibitor induces fatty acid and sterol biosynthesis in liver and adipose tissues due to the accumulation of activated sterol regulatory element-binding proteins in the nucleus. *J Biol Chem* 2001; 276: 37514–9.
79. Shimomura I, Hammer RE, Richardson JA, Ikemoto S, Bashmakov Y, Goldstein JL, Brown MS. Insulin resistance and diabetes mellitus in transgenic mice expressing nuclear SREBP-1c in adipose tissue: model for congenital generalized lipodystrophy. *Genes Dev* 1998; 12: 3182–94.
80. Thiebaut R, Dabis F, Malvy F, Jacqmin-Gadda H, Mercie P, Valentin VD. Serum triglycerides, HIV infection, and highly active antiretroviral therapy. *J Acquir Immune Defic Syndr* 2000; 23: 261–5.
81. Periard D, Telenti A, Sudre P, Cheseaux JJ, Halfon P, Reymond MJ, Marcovina SM, Glauser MP, Nicod P, Darioli R, Mooser V. Atherogenic dyslipidemia in HIV-infected individuals treated with protease inhibitors. *Circulation* 1999; 100: 700–5.
82. Walli R, Herfort O, Michl GM, Demant T, Jager H, Dieterle C, Bogner JR, Landgraf R, Goebel FD. Treatment with protease inhibitors associated with peripheral insulin resistance and impaired oral glucose tolerance in HIV-1-infected patients. *AIDS* 1998; 12: F167–73.
83. Mynarcik DC, McNurlan MA, Steigbigel RT, Fuhrer J, Gelato MC. Association of severe insulin resistance with both loss of limb fat and elevated serum tumor necrosis factor receptor levels in HIV lipodystrophy. *J Acquir Immune Defic Syndr* 2000; 25: 312–21.
84. Dube MP, Johnson DL, Currier JS, Leedom JM. Protease inhibitor-associated hyperglycaemia. *Lancet* 1997; 350: 713–4.
85. Reeves WG, Allen BR, Tattersall RB. Insulin-induced lipoatrophy: evidence for an immune pathogenesis. *BMJ* 1980; 280: 1500–3.
86. Andre P. Lipo-atrophie post-cortisonique traitee par greffe autologue d'ilots adipocytaires. *Ann Dermatol Venereol* 1990; 117: 733–4.
87. Hodak E, David M, Sandbank M. Semicircular lipoatrophy—a pressure-induced lipoatrophy? *Clin Exp Dermatol* 1990; 15: 464–5.
88. Tsuji T, Kosaka K, Terao J. Localized lipodystrophy with panniculitis: light and electron microscopic studies. *J Cutan Pathol* 1989; 16: 359–64.
89. Imamura S, Yamada M, Ikeda T. Lipodystrophia centrifugalis abdominalis infantilis. *Arch Dermatol* 1971; 104: 291–8.
90. Imamura S, Yamada M, Yamamoto K. Lipodystrophia centrifugalis abdominalis infantilis. A follow-up study. *J Am Acad Dermatol* 1984; 11: 203–9.
91. Caputo R. Lipodystrophia centrifugalis sacralis infantilis. A 15-year follow-up observation. *Acta Derm Venereol* 1989; 69: 442–3.
92. Dahl PR, Zalla MJ, Winkelmann RK. Localized involutional lipoatrophy: a clinicopathologic study of 16 patients. *J Am Acad Dermatol* 1996; 35: 523–8.
93. Cauble MS, Gilroy R, Sorrell MF, Mailliard ME, Sudan DL, Anderson JC, Wisecarver JL, Balakrishnan S, Larsen JL. Lipoatrophic diabetes and end-stage liver disease secondary to nonalcoholic steatohepatitis with recurrence after liver transplantation. *Transplantation* 2001; 71: 892–5.
94. Hegele RA. Premature atherosclerosis associated with monogenic insulin resistance. *Circulation* 2001; 103: 2225–9.
95. Hurwitz PJ, Sarel R. Facial reconstruction in partial lipodystrophy. *Ann Plast Surg* 1982; 8: 253–7.
96. Zafarulla MY. Lipodystrophy: a case report of partial lipodystrophy. *Br J Oral Maxillofac Surg* 1985; 23: 53–7.
97. Mork NJ, Rajka G, Halse J. Treatment of acanthosis nigricans with etretinate (Tigason) in a patient with Lawrence–Seip syndrome (generalized lipodystrophy). *Acta Derm Venereol* 1986; 66: 173–4.
98. Schretz E. Improved acanthosis nigricans with lipodystrophic diabetes during dietary fish oil supplementation. *Arch Dermatol* 1988; 124: 1094–96.
99. Arioglu E, Duncan-Morin J, Sebring N, Rother KI, Gottlieb N, Lieberman J, Herion D, Kleiner DE, Reynolds J, Premkumar A, Sumner AE, Hoofnagle J, Reitman ML, Taylor SI. Efficacy and safety of troglitazone in the treatment of lipodystrophy syndromes. *Ann Intern Med* 2000; 133: 263–74.
100. Jones SP, Doran DA, Leat PB, Maher B, Pirmohamed M. Short-term exercise training improves body composition and hyperlipidaemia in HIV-positive individuals with lipodystrophy. *AIDS* 2001; 15: 2049–51.
101. Roubenoff R, Weiss L, McDermott A, Heflin T, Cloutier GJ, Wood M, Gorbach S. A pilot study of exercise training to reduce trunk fat in adults with HIV-associated fat redistribution. *AIDS* 1999; 13: 1373–5.
102. Wilson DE, Chan IF, Stevenson KB, Horton SC, Schipke C. Eucaloric substitution of medium chain triglycerides for dietary long chain fatty acids in acquired total lipodystrophy: effects on hyperlipoproteinemia and endogenous insulin resistance. *J Clin Endocrinol Metab* 1983; 57: 517–23.
103. Hadigan C, Corcoran C, Basgoz N, Davis B, Sax P, Grinspoon S. Metformin in the treatment of HIV lipodystrophy syndrome: a randomized controlled trial. *JAMA* 2000; 284: 472–7.
104. Calza L, Manfredi R, Chiodo F. Use of fibrates in the management of hyperlipidemia in HIV-infected patients receiving HAART. *Infection* 2002; 30: 26–31.
105. Fichtenbaum CJ, Gerber JG, Rosenkranz SL, Segal Y, Aberg JA, Blaschke T, Alston B, Fang F, Kosel B, Aweeka F; Pharmacokinetic interactions between protease inhibitors and statins in HIV seronegative volunteers. *AIDS* 2002; 16: 569–77.
106. Amacher DE, Beck R, Schomaker SJ, Kenny CV. Hepatic microsomal enzyme induction, beta-oxidation, and cell proliferation following administration of clofibrate, gemfibrozil, or bezafibrate in the Cd rat. *Toxicol Appl Pharmacol* 1997; 142: 143–50.
107. Mayerson AB, Hundal RS, Dufour S, Lebon V, Befroy D, Cline GW, Enocksson S, Inzucchi SE, Shulman GI, Petersen KF. The effects of rosiglitazone on insulin sensitivity, lipolysis, and hepatic and skeletal muscle triglyceride content in patients with type 2 diabetes. *Diabetes* 2002; 51: 797–802.
108. Carr A, Hudson J, Chuah J, Mallal S, Law M, Hoy J, Doong N, French M, Smith D, Cooper DA; HIV protease inhibitor substitution in patients with lipodystrophy: a randomized, controlled, open-label, multicentre study. *AIDS* 2001; 15: 1811–22.
109. Martinez E, Conget I, Lozano L, Casamitjana R, Gatell JM. Reversion of metabolic abnormalities after switching

from HIV-1 protease inhibitors to nevirapine. *AIDS* 1999; 13: 805–10.

110. Oral EA, Simha V, Ruiz E, Andewelt A, Premkumar A, Snell P, Wagner AJ, DePaoli AM, Reitman ML, Taylor SI, Gorden P, Garg A. Leptin-replacement therapy for lipodystrophy. *N Engl J Med* 2002; 346: 570–8.

111. Simha V, Szczepaniak LS, Wagner A, DePaoli A, Garg A. Effect of leptin replacement on intrahepatic and intramyocellular lipid content in patients with generalized lipodystrophy. *Diabetes Care* 2003; 26 (1): 30–5.

112. Petersen KF, Oral EA, Dufour S, Befroy D, Ariyan C, Yu C, Cline GW, DePaoli AM, Taylor SI, Gorden P, Shulman GI. Leptin reverses insulin resistance and hepatic steatosis in patients with severe lipodystrophy. *J Clin Invest* 2002; 109: 1345–50.

36

Treatment of Obesity

Arne Astrup

The Royal Veterinary and Agricultural University, Frederiksberg, Denmark

INTRODUCTION AND OVERVIEW

The epidemic of type 2 diabetes is due to environmental factors, but the individuals developing the disease have a strong genetic predisposition. A number of recent observational surveys and intervention studies have shown that excess body fatness is the major environmental cause of type 2 diabetes, and that even a minor weight loss can prevent its development in high-risk subjects. Randomized trials using diet, weight loss agents, or surgical treatment of obesity have all clearly demonstrated that fat loss *per se* is crucial, whereas diet composition and physical activity play a minor role in improving insulin resistance and reducing the risk of overt diabetes. Weight loss improves glycemic control in type 2 diabetic patients and has a clinically relevant beneficial effect on all cardiovascular risk factors. Weight management programs are therefore a cornerstone in both the prevention and treatment of type 2 diabetes. A weight loss of 5–10% can be induced in almost all simple and diabetic obese patients, provided treatment is offered by a professional team consisting of a physician and dieticians or nurses trained to focus on weight loss and maintenance. Although increasing daily physical activity and regular exercise does not significantly affect the rate of weight loss in the induction phase, it plays an important role in the weight maintenance phase due to an important impact on daily energy expenditure and also to a direct enhancement of insulin sensitivity. Weight loss drugs have a role in patients in whom the lifestyle treatment is insufficient to produce the required weight control, and in obese subjects drugs like orlistat and sibutramine may both produce weight loss and reduce the risk of complications of obesity, such as type 2 diabetes. In obese individuals with impaired glucose tolerance (IGT), metformin and orlistat reduce the risk of developing type 2 diabetes, and in type 2 diabetic patients the drugs produce weight loss, improved glycemic control, and beneficial effects on cardiovascular risk factors. Bariatric surgery is a very effective means to produce a longer lasting weight loss, and may be an option in the severely obese patients who are difficult to treat with the other weight management tools.

PRINCIPLES TO ACHIEVE DIET-INDUCED WEIGHT LOSS

In almost every overweight and obese patient the diet must be adjusted to reduce energy intake. Dietary therapy consists of instructing patients on how to modify their dietary intake to achieve a decrease in energy intake while maintaining a nutritionally adequate diet. Obese patients have, because of their enlarged body size, higher energy requirements for a given level of physical activity than their normal-weight counterparts (Figure 1). Obese diabetic patients have slightly higher energy requirements than simple obese patients for a given body size and composition. Reducing the obese patient's total energy intake compared to that of a normal-weight individual will inevitably cause weight loss, consisting of about 75% fat and 25% lean tissue, until weight normalization occurs at a new energy equilibrium [1, 2]. For patients with class I obesity this requires an energy deficit of 300–500 kcal/day, and for patients with class III obesity, 500–1000 kcal/day.

There is no evidence to support that differences in diet composition exert clinically important effects on energy absorption and energy expenditure, and so the main mechanism of weight-reduction diets is to reduce total energy intake. This can be achieved by setting an upper limit for energy intake. The larger the daily deficit in energy balance, the more rapid the weight loss. A deficit of

International Textbook of Diabetes Mellitus, Third Edition. Edited by R. A. DeFronzo, E. Ferrannini, H. Keen, and P. Zimmet.
 ISBN: 0-471-48655-8.

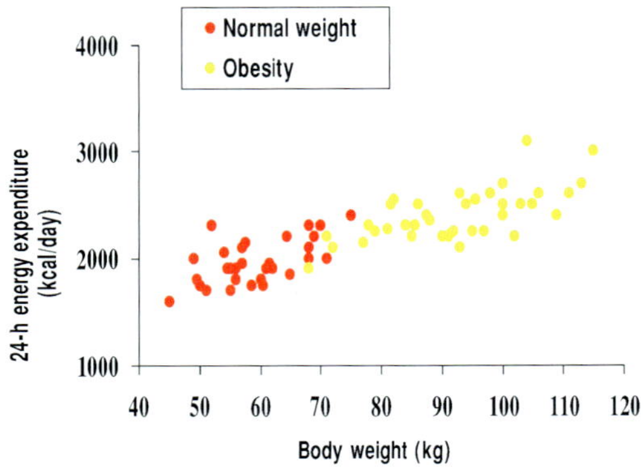

Figure 1 Energy expenditure (energy requirements) of normal weight, overweight, and obese subjects. Relationship between body weight and energy requirements assessed by measurement of energy expenditure or by apparent energy intake during weight stability. The growing underreporting with increasing body fatness makes the self-reported energy intake invalid for estimation of energy requirements in obese patients

300–500 kcal/day will produce a weight loss of 300–500 g/week, and a deficit of 500–1000 kcal/day will produce a weight loss of 500–1000 g/week [1]. Greater initial energy deficits may produce even larger weight loss rates. Total energy expenditure declines and normalizes along with weight loss, and total energy intake should therefore gradually be further reduced to maintain the energy deficit. An alternative approach is to take advantage of the differences in the satiating power of the various dietary components in order to cause a spontaneous reduction in energy intake. This is the principle of the *ad libitum* low-fat diet.

Choosing the Dietary Deficit

Initially, the target of a weight loss program should be to decrease body weight by 10% [1–4]. Once this is achieved a new target can be set. Patients will generally want to lose more weight, but it should be remembered that even a 5% weight reduction improves risk factors and risk of comorbidities. However, several factors should be taken into consideration, e.g. the patient's degree of obesity, previous weight loss attempts, risk factors, comorbidities, and personal and social capacity to undertake the necessary lifestyle changes. To prescribe a diet with a defined energy deficit, it is necessary to estimate the patient's actual energy requirements. It would seem natural to estimate the patient's habitual energy intake from self-reported diet registration over 3–7 days of weight stability, calculating the energy content of the diet by use of food table programs. However, these estimates are invalid because of systematic underreporting by obese individuals of energy intake amounting to 30–40%. Energy requirements should therefore be assessed indirectly by estimation of total energy expenditure. Resting metabolic rate (RMR) can be measured by indirect calorimetry, or be estimated with great accuracy using equations based on body weight, gender, and age [5] (Table 1) or, even better, estimated from information on the size of fat-free mass and fat mass [6]. Total energy expenditure (=energy requirement) is estimated by multiplication of RMR (kcal/day) by an activity factor (PAL, physical activity level) [5] (Table 1). The energy level of the prescribed diet is defined as the patient's energy requirement minus the prescribed daily energy deficit.

Theoretical Versus Clinical Outcome

Translating the physiologically based considerations regarding energy balance and weight loss into clinical practice requires a high degree of compliance, which can be difficult to obtain. Weight loss results tend to be much better in clinical trials conducted in specialized clinics than in trials conducted by nonspecialists without sufficient resources and access to auxiliary therapists (dieticians, psychologists, etc.). Compliance and adherence to the diet are the cornerstones of successful weight loss, and are the most complicated part of the dietary treatment of obesity. To improve adherence, consideration should be given to

Table 1 Estimating energy needs*

Revised WHO equations for estimating basal metabolic rate (BMR)	
Men	
18–30 years	=(0.0630 × actual weight in kg + 2.8957) × 240 kcal/day
31–60 years	=(0.0484 × actual weight in kg + 3.6534) × 240 kcal/day
Women	
18–30 years	=(0.0621 × actual weight in kg + 2.0357) × 240 kcal/day
31–60 years	=(0.342 × actual weight in kg + 3.5377) × 240 kcal/day
Estimated total energy expenditure = BMR × activity factor	

Activity level	Activity factor
Low (sedentary)	1.3
Intermediate (some regular exercise)	1.5
High (regular activity or demanding job)	1.7

* Reproduced by permission of Handbooks in Health Care Co. [5].

the patient's food preferences, as well as to personal, educational, and social factors. Great efforts should be made to see the patient frequently and regularly.

Furthermore, long-term weight reduction is unlikely to succeed unless the patient acquires new eating and physical activity habits. These behavioral changes should be an integral part of the treatment program.

OPTIONS FOR WEIGHT LOSS DIETS

Therapeutic obesity diets distinguish between several recognized weight reduction regimens. Low-energy diets (LEDs) usually provide 800–1500 kcal/day and use fat-reduced foods, though weight loss occurs independent of the diet composition. Diets providing 1200 kcal/day or more can be classified as *balanced-deficits diets* [4, 6], but this definition will not be used in this chapter. Very low energy diets (VLEDs) are "modified fasts", providing 200–800 kcal/day that replace normal foods. Examples of weight loss on such diets are shown in Figure 2 *Ad libitum* low-fat diets do not restrict energy intake directly, but target a restriction of *ad libitum* fat intake to 20–30% of total energy intake. Energy intake is spontaneously reduced because of the higher satiating effect of this diet and a modest weight loss occurs.

Very Low Energy Diets

Starvation (diet providing less than 200 kcal/day) is the ultimate dietary treatment of obesity, but it is no longer used because of the numerous and serious medical complications associated with prolonged starvation [8]. Starvation has been replaced by VLEDs (200–800 kcal/day), which aims to supply very little energy but all essential nutrients. Reducing the energy content of a diet requires an increased nutrient density. This can be difficult to obtain with natural foods if the diet is to be acceptable once the energy content of the diet becomes lower than 800 kcal/day. This has led to the commercial production of VLEDs, supplemented with all nutrients in RDA (recommended dietary allowance) amounts. For decades, 250–400 kcal/day formula diets were extremely popular. The first VLEDs were clearly nutritionally insufficient, but reports of adverse effects and results from research have brought about a gradual increase in energy level. Today the 800 kcal/day VLED is the only version recognized as being both effective and safe [8]. A number of studies have shown that VLEDs with energy levels of less than 800 kcal/day do not produce a greater weight loss and are less well accepted than those comprising 800 kcal/day [9]. VLEDs usually provide a ketogenic diet with an energy content of around 800 kcal/day in the form of nutrition powders, or in the form of protein-, mineral-, trace-element-, and vitamin-enriched meals or drinks. VLEDs can induce very rapid weight loss over a 2–3-month period (Figure 2), but do not seem to facilitate weight maintenance [9]. This is not because a rapid initial weight loss causes poorer long-term weight maintenance *per se* [10], as initial weight losses are positively, not negatively, associated with long-term weight loss [11]. However, VLEDs are not educational and do not facilitate the gradual modification of the patient's eating behavior, nutritional knowledge, and skills, which seems to be required for long-term weight maintenance. Some concern has been raised about the cardiac safety of the use of VLEDs with less than 800 kcal/day [3], and patients using VLEDs have an increased risk of developing gallstones (Table 2). Their use without medical supervision has generally been abandoned and should not be recommended [1, 3, 4, 8].

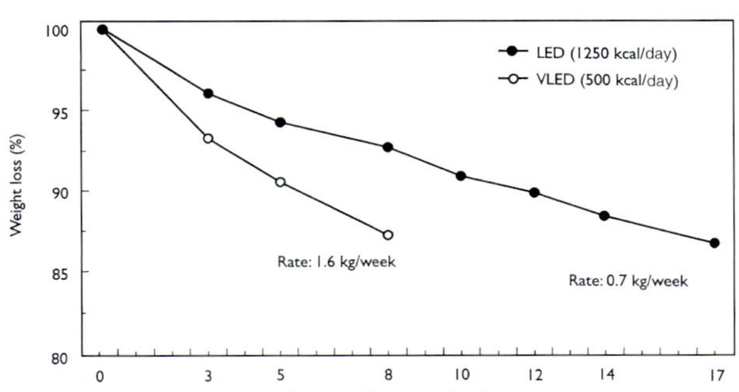

Figure 2 Weight loss in obese patients randomized to either an LED or a VLED. Initial mean body weight was nearly 100 kg and mean weight loss 12.6 kg in both groups. (Reproduced by permission of the British Medical Journal [7])

Table 2 Adverse effects and complications of VLEDs

Adverse effect	Occurrence
Cold intolerence	~50%
Dry skin	~50%
Fatigue, dizzines, muscle cramps, headache, gastrointestinal distress	10–20%
Hair loss	10%
Gallstones	10–30%
Bad breath	20–30%

Low-Energy Diets

LEDs usually provide 800–1500 kcal/day and normally consist of natural normal foods. LEDs are also called *traditional diets* and *calorie-counting diets*, because previously more emphasis was put on restricting the total energy level of the diet and less on the macronutrient composition. Although macronutrient composition of the diet is of less importance for short-term weight loss, it is now usually modified in order to maximize the beneficial effect on cardiovascular risk factors and insulin resistance, and to prevent cancers, perhaps also promoting long-term weight

Table 3 Example of the composition of an LED

Nutrient	Recommended intake
Calories	500–1000 kcal/day below energy requirements
Total fat	20–30% of total calories
Saturated fatty acids	<10% of total calories
Monunsaturated fatty acids	<15% of total calories
Polyunsaturated fatty acids	<10% of total calories
Protein	15–20% of total calories
Carbohydrate	>55% of total calories
Fiber	20–30 g/day
Calcium	1000–1500 mg/day
Other vitamins, minerals, and trace elements	RDA. Full coverage should be ensured by a vitamin/mineral supplement daily

maintenance. For practical reasons, LEDs are low-fat, carbohydrate-rich diets with a fixed energetic allowance. An example of an appropriate nutrient composition for an LED is given in Table 3. It should be supplemented with a daily vitamin and mineral tablet. A patient may choose an energy level of 1000–1200 kcal/day for women and 1200–1500 kcal/day for men. LEDs produce a lower rate of weight loss than VLEDs (Figure 2), but randomized clinical trials demonstrate that the long-term (>1 year) weight loss is not different from that of the LEDs [1]. Furthermore, using LEDs for weight loss induction introduces healthy eating habits early in the weight reduction program, giving a longer period in which to familiarize the patient with the dietary changes that are a central element in a weight maintenance program.

Based on 34 randomized clinical trials examining the impact of LED in obese subjects, it was concluded that LED produces weight loss regardless of duration of treatment, and body weight was reduced by an average of 8% over 3–12 months [1]. In trials lasting 3–6 months, and 6–12 months, LED produced mean weight losses of approximately 8% compared to controls [1]. Although they targeted the same energy deficit there was a large variation in mean weight loss between the studies. The variation is less owing to differences in patient selection than to the differences in efforts to promote a low-fat intake as a practical way to reduce energy intake, and owing to differences in the skills and efforts of the therapeutic teams. The same large variation exists within each cohort of patients, and the mean weight loss of 8% corresponds to approximately 80% of the patients losing >5% and 15% losing >10%. It is difficult to separate the impact of the dietary therapy because all trials included some elements of behavior modification, which clearly contributed to the results.

Prognostic Markers of Weight Loss Success and Reasons for Failure

There is considerable variation in the weight loss and weight maintenance achieved by patients enrolled in dietary treatment programs. Some variation can be attributed to physiological differences (RMR, age, gender, sympathetic activity) and some to differences in adherence (behavior), though combinations of and interactions between physiology and behavior may be the major factor. This variation is not seen from the mean weight loss of a group, which is difficult to translate into a clinically relevant success rate based on the intention-to-treat principle, i.e. how large a proportion of the patients entering a treatment achieve a certain weight loss, typically >5% and >10% of pretreatment body weight. It is difficult to identify clinically the patients who will benefit most before treatment is initiated. Positive predictors of weight loss are (1) high initial body weight, (2) high RMR and/or 24-h energy expenditure, (3) high fat oxidation rate, (4) high sympathetic activity, (5) high plasma dihydrotestosterone concentration, and (6) high perceived self-efficacy [4, 12]. However, these factors, separately or in combination, do not seem to explain enough of the variation to have a measurable clinical relevance.

Ad Libitum Low-Fat Diets (<30% Energy from Fat)

Efficacy

Data from animal and experimental research, observational studies, and numerous randomized clinical trials have shown that a high dietary fat content plays an important role in the development of obesity [13–15]. A high-fat diet promotes weight gain and obesity in sedentary individuals with little self-restraint, who have a genetic predisposition to obesity in particular. The main mechanisms are the passive overconsumption of energy promoted by the high energy density of fatty foods and a reduced fat oxidation capacity in susceptible individuals. Low-fat diets are more satiating because of the high content of complex carbohydrates and protein. Restricting intake of dietary fat should be seen as a means to reducing the diet's energy density and hence restricting the patient's total energy intake. Unfortunately, while the effect of fat-rich foods on weight gain and obesity is substantial, the ability of the *ad libitum* low-fat, carbohydrate-rich diet to induce weight loss is less pronounced. A systematic review of 28 *ad libitum* low-fat diet randomized clinical trials showed that a weight loss of 1.6 g/day was achieved per each percentage point reduction in energy from fat [14]. A realistic reduction in dietary fat can result in a weight loss of 20–100 g/week, which becomes clinically significant when the total exceeds 5% of body weight [14]. A meta-analysis of 34 *ad libitum* low-fat diet interventions lasting >2 months and 35 control groups found a statistically highly significant weight loss difference of 3.3 kg [16]. The size of the weight loss was mainly determined by the reduction in dietary fat energy, but pretreatment body weight was also positively associated with the weight loss. The analysis indicates that obese patients with a body weight of 95 kg who reduce dietary fat from 45 to 25 energy% under *ad libitum* conditions will reduce energy intake and will, on average, achieve a weight loss of 7.1 kg before a new equilibrium is reached. On the other hand, a normal-weight subject (60 kg) will loose only 0.5 kg with the same fat reduction. These weight loss predictions are probably underestimated because the analysis relies on the reductions in dietary fat as reported by the patients, which tend to be exaggerated. Moreover, patients with better adherence also achieved better weight loss than those with poorer adherence [17] (Figure 3). The systematic review [14] and the meta-analysis [16, 18] show that *ad libitum* low-fat, high-carbohydrate diet have a modest but predictable effect on weight loss. This is clinically relevant for obese patients habitually consuming a high-fat

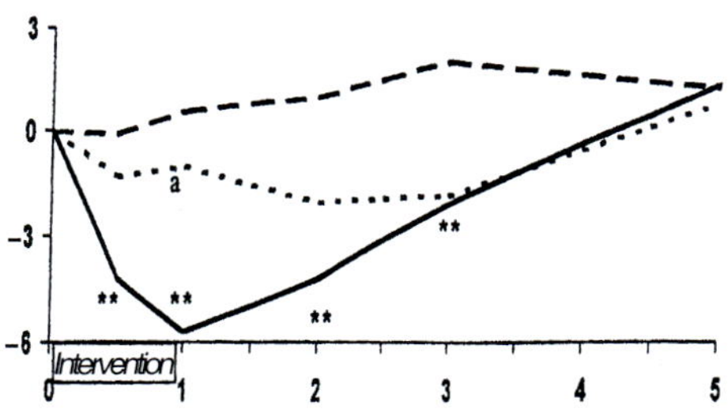

Figure 3 A 5-year follow-up of a 1-year randomized controlled trial of a reduced-fat *ad libitum* diet versus a usual diet. Obese patients with IGT were randomized to a reduced-fat diet or control, and participated in monthly small-group education sessions on reduced-fat eating for 1 year. Weight decreased significantly in the reduced-fat-diet group; the greatest difference was noted at 1 year (−3.3 kg), best in the most compliant group, but diminished at subsequent follow-up (** denotes differences between low-fat and normal-fat diets). Glucose tolerance also improved in patients on the reduced-fat diet; a lower proportion had type 2 diabetes or IGT at 1 year (47% vs. 67%). This difference disappeared in subsequent years, but the more compliant 50% of the intervention group maintained lower fasting and 2-h glucose at 5 years compared to control subjects. (Copyright © 2001 American Diabetes Association. From Diabetes Care, Vol 24, 2001; 619–624. Reprinted with permission from *The American Diabetes Association* [17])

diet, where an *ad libitum* low-fat, high-carbohydrate diet would be 15–20 percentage points lower in energy from fat than the habitual diet.

Safety

Under certain experimental conditions the change from a normal-fat to a low-fat, high-carbohydrate diet has been shown to induce hyperinsulinemia, hypertriglyceridemia, and low high-density lipoprotein (HDL) cholesterol concentrations [19, 20]. Such observations have prompted some researchers to advocate the implementation of healthier high-fat diets, i.e. emphasizing the replacement of saturated and *trans*-fats with unsaturated oils instead of with carbohydrates [20]. However, these studies replaced fat for carbohydrate under strictly isoenergetic conditions, not allowing the spontaneous weight loss with the accompanying beneficial changes in these risk factors to occur as in other studies [21–23]. This was stressed by Schaefer et al., who reduced dietary fat isoenergetically from 35 to 15% of total energy in hypercholesterolemic patients and found plasma reductions of 13% in total cholesterol and 17% in low-density lipoprotein (LDL) cholesterol, but a 23% decrease in HDL cholesterol. A rise of 47% in plasma triglycerides after 6 weeks was also seen [21]. The same diet was subsequently continued for 10–12 weeks under *ad libitum* conditions and it produced a mean weight loss of 3.6 kg, a further reduction in LDL cholesterol and a normalization of HDL cholesterol to total cholesterol ratio. Improvements in other risk factors, e.g. blood pressure [24], blood coagulation, and fibrinolysis, occurred independent of weight loss [18, 25].

Blood lipids should be monitored in obese patients with type 2 diabetes resistant to weight loss. This is the only precaution currently recommended. The use of *ad libitum* low-fat, high-carbohydrate diets in which carbohydrates are mainly of the complex and fiber-rich types have not given rise to safety concerns.

LED Versus Ad Libitum Low-Fat Diets?

Ad libitum low-fat diets produce a rate of weight loss of 100–200 g/week in unselected obese patients, whereas LEDs induce weight losses of 300–700 g/week. Four randomized clinical trials have compared LEDs (using low-fat diets) with *ad libitum* low-fat diets. Taken together, these studies show that the impact of the *ad libitum* low-fat diets on weight loss is increased if total energy intake is restricted to some extent [26–29].

LEDs using low-fat diets are more effective in inducing weight loss than *ad libitum* low-fat diets, and they allow a better adjustment of the reduction in energy intake. LEDs are therefore the preferred dietary treatment for obesity. However, in an individually tailored treatment the first step could be to prescribe an *ad libitum* low-fat diet to patients habitually consuming a high-fat diet, subsequently limiting energy intake if weight loss proves unsatisfactory.

Ad Libitum Low-Carbohydrate Diets (<25 g/day Carbohydrate)

Diets that promote very low-carbohydrate intakes have become very popular as part of a popular physiological concept that links surges in blood glucose and insulin to weight gain and obesity [30–32]. The *Atkins' New Diet Revolution* is the most popular and recommends a daily intake of <25 g carbohydrates [33]. It is likely that such a "ketogenic" diet possesses anorectic properties and produces weight loss in the short term, but it may be very problematic in the weight maintenance phase because of side effects, adverse effects on risk factor profile, and an increased risk of developing type 2 diabetes in overweight and obese subjects. Very few controlled studies testing the low-carbohydrate diet have been published. Westman et al. found, in an uncontrolled study, that an *ad libitum* low-carbohydrate diet (<25 g/day) produced a weight loss of 10.3% over 6 months in 51 obese subjects [34]. They also found positive changes in blood lipids and blood pressure, but 68% of the participants experienced constipation, probably because of the low fiber intake. Other studies have shown that a fat-rich diet impairs the beneficial effects of training on insulin resistance [35]. When the weight loss has subsided it is likely that the low-carbohydrate (high-fat) diet will have very negative effects on most cardiovascular risk factors, and despite the weight loss, may increase insulin resistance and risk of type 2 diabetes. Low-carbohydrate diets cannot therefore be recommended.

DIETARY WEIGHT MAINTENANCE PROGRAMS

In professional weight loss programs LEDs induce a 5% weight loss in almost all patients, and frequent clinical encounters during the initial 6 months of weight reduction appear to facilitate achievement of the therapy goals. Larger success criteria (>10% weight loss) can be met by the majority of patients if the treatment program also includes group therapy and behavior modification. The real challenge is to maintain the reduced body weight and prevent subsequent relapse (Figure 4). In a systematic review of long-term (>3-year follow-up) efficacy of dietary treatment of obesity, success was defined as maintenance of all weight initially lost or maintenance of at least 9 kg of initial weight loss [36]. Initial weight loss was 4–28 kg, and 15% of the followed-up patients fulfilled one of the criteria for success, and the success rate was stable for up to 14 years of observation. Diet combined with group therapy led to better long-term success rates (27%) than did diet alone

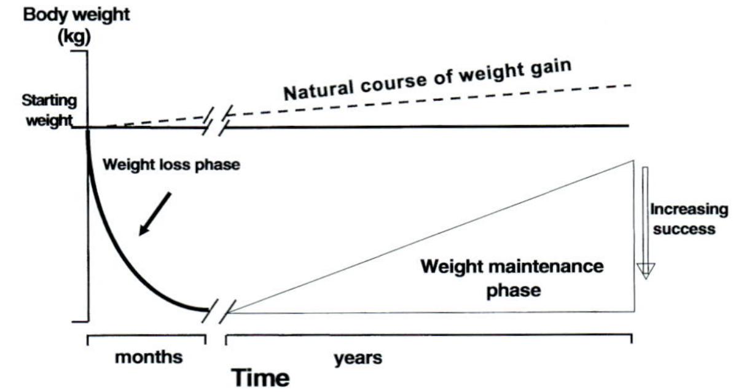

Figure 4 Weight loss outcomes for obese patients treated in weight management programs compared to predicted outcome of continued habitual lifestyle. It is noted that even weight stability may be a partial success and a goal in certain patients

(15%), or diet combined with behavior modification and active follow-up, though active follow-up produced better weight maintenance than passive follow-up (19% vs. 10%).

Although the principle of energy restriction (LED) is successful for weight loss induction independent of dietary composition, the low-fat, high-protein/carbohydrate diet seems to be more effective for long-term weight maintenance and preventing weight regain. In a study by Toubro and Astrup, patients were randomly assigned to two different weight maintenance groups, receiving either a low-fat diet *ad libitum* or a fixed-energy diet (LED) for 1 year after having lost a mean of 13.6 kg on energy restricted diets [7]. There was only a small weight regain during the weight maintenance program. However, 2 years after the weight loss the LED group had regained 11.3 kg whereas the low-fat group had regained only 5.4 kg. Forty percent of the patients in the LED group and 65% of the patients in the low-fat group had maintained a weight loss of >5 kg [7].

This and other studies show that the success rate may be improved by using the *ad libitum* low-fat diet for prevention of relapse, although it is not effective in all patients [1]. Whether long-term weight maintenance failure is due to lack of treatment efficacy or lack of compliance is unknown. Notably, the amount of time spent with the patient and frequent contact between the professional counselors and patients favorably affect weight maintenance.

DOES DIET COMPOSITION MATTER?

Numerous popular diet books promote changing diet compositions in accordance with principles that are claimed to have a particularly favorable impact on weight loss and maintenance. Generally these claims are unsubstantiated and scientifically improbable, and some may even promote nutritionally insufficient diets (for review see references 4 and 37). For LEDs there is little evidence to support that weight loss may be improved by diets different from that given in Table 2. For *ad libitum* diets, and for weight maintenance diets particularly, differences in the satiating effects of different macronutrients may have some importance.

Carbohydrate Types

The high carbohydrate content of low-fat diets stems mainly from the complex carbohydrates of different vegetables, fruits, and whole grains, which are more satiating for fewer calories than fatty foods and are a good source of vitamins, minerals, trace elements, and fiber. A high fiber content may further improve the satiating effect of the diet and a diet rich in soluble fiber, including oat bran, legumes, barley, and most fruits and vegetables, may be effective in reducing blood cholesterol and blood pressure levels. The recommended intake is 20–30 g of fiber daily. The role of simple carbohydrates in low-fat diets remains controversial, mainly because of the lack of proper randomized clinical trials. One large European multicenter trial has compared two different *ad libitum* low-fat diets, high in either complex or simple carbohydrates, with a normal-fat diet. The two low-fat diets induced similar fat loss in overweight and obese subjects over 6 months, and the diet high in simple carbohydrates had no detrimental effects on blood lipids [38]. However, more recent studies suggest that a high intake of sugar from soft drinks may have a special fattening property [39, 40].

Glycemic Index

Some scientists have warned against the fattening properties of high-GI (glycemic index) foods such as potatoes, white bread, bagels, and rice—foods that people are otherwise advised to eat more of as part of the currently recommended low-fat diet. Instead, the public is advised to eat more whole grain products, and types of rice and potatoes characterized by a low GI. Although low-GI foods are beneficial for glycemic control in diabetic patients [41] and have a modest beneficial effect on cardiovascular risk factors, its effect on body weight regulation is controversial [42]. The proponents of the GI hypothesis suggest that high-GI foods produce rapid and transient surges in blood glucose and insulin, which are in turn followed by rapidly returning hunger sensations and excessive caloric intake [31]. However, a recent systematic review of the different types of studies found that of the 31 studies that measured appetite sensations following low-GI vs. high-GI meals, low-GI meals produced greater satiety and reduced hunger in 15 studies, no difference was found in 14 studies, and in 2 studies the high-GI meals produced greatest satiety. Similarly, among the 20 longer term intervention studies identified, 4 studies found larger weight loss and 2 studies less weight loss on the low-GI diets, and 14 studies found no difference [32]. It was concluded that most of the studies were statistically underpowered to pick up clinically relevant differences in weight loss.

The lack of robust evidence prohibits issuing general dietary advice that low-GI foods are preferable to high-GI foods in preventing weight gain, although it appears likely that this dietary change will have beneficial effects on risk factors of cardiovascular disease and diabetes, and unlikely that it will exert any adverse effects. However, the GI concept is complicated for the patients and comprehensive tables are required in order to calculate the diet [43]. Newer research shows that GI of meals cannot accurately be calculated by the carbohydrate source alone, but requires information about the energy, fat, and protein contents as well [44]. There is a need for well-powered, randomized, long-term trials to show the potential for low-GI vs. high-GI diets to produce weight loss or maintenance, and for a more patient-friendly classification of carbohydrate foods (Figure 5).

Protein Content

A large body of experimental human data suggests that protein possesses a higher satiating power per calorie than do carbohydrate and fat [45]. The impact on weight loss of replacing carbohydrate with protein in *ad libitum* low-fat diets has been addressed in only one randomized clinical trials. Two fat-reduced diets (30% of energy) with either normal protein (12% of energy) or high protein content (25%) were compared with a normal fat diet in 65 obese patients. Weight loss after 6 months was 5.1 kg in the low-protein group and 8.9 kg in the high-protein group, and more subjects lost >10 kg in the high-protein group (35%) than in the low-protein group (9%). The protein-rich diet had no adverse effect on blood lipids, renal function, or bone mineral density, and seems to have a positive influence on the atherogenic risk factor profile in abdominally obese men [46]. Replacement of some dietary carbohydrate by protein in *ad libitum* low-fat diets may improve weight loss. More freedom to choose between protein-rich and complex-carbohydrate-rich foods may encourage obese subjects to choose more lean meat and dairy products and hence improve adherence to low-fat diets in weight reduction programs. Increased protein allowances in weight reduction diets should await confirmation of these results by other studies. The study results do not endorse the dietary principles promoted in recent popular diet books advocating high-protein, low-carbohydrate diets [47].

Fat Quality and High-Monounsaturated-Fat Diets

Although similar amounts of different fats contain nearly the same amount of energy, differences may exist in their satiating effects, which could influence total energy intake of *ad libitum* low-fat diets and weight maintenance diets.

From a biochemical and physiological view saturated fatty acids behave very differently from monounsaturated fats (MUFA), which seem to be more neutral than other fats in relation to cardiovascular disease, insulin resistance, and cancer. However, animal studies suggest that MUFA increase body weight more than polyunsaturated fatty acids (PUFA) do [48]. In a cross-sectional, observational study in 128 males the highest positive correlation was found between the intake of MUFA and body fat mass, whereas no significant association was found between PUFA and body fat, and only a weak association to saturated fat was seen [49]. Two experimental appetite studies have concordantly shown that meals/infusions with MUFA produce lower satiety, and that they suppress energy intake for the remainder of the day less than PUFA [50, 51]. These preliminary reports suggest that a high MUFA content in the diet may promote passive overconsumption and obesity. Two randomized trials have compared diets moderate in fat, high MUFA, with low-fat diet. The first trial failed to find any difference in weight loss after 18 months [52]. However, in this study, both groups were on energy restriction, the study was small, and it had a large dropout rate in the low-fat group. The other study randomized 257 obese subjects with IGT to *ad libitum* diets of reduced-fat, high-carbohydrate with either high- or low-GI, or a third normal-fat (35% energy from fat), high-MUFA, low-carbohydrate diet for 16 weeks [53] (Figure 5). The high-MUFA group gained more weight, increased insulin resistance and HbA_{1c}, and the high-carbohydrate, low-GI diet had the most positive effect on β-cell function and body weight.

The *ad libitum* normal-fat, high-MUFA diets might therefore have adverse effects on body weight, insulin sensitivity, and other risk factors as compared to fat-reduced, high-carbohydrate diets with low GI [53, 54]. Some caution should be exercised before recommending replacement of low-fat diets with higher-fat, MUFA-based diets for both simple obese and diabetic obese patients until

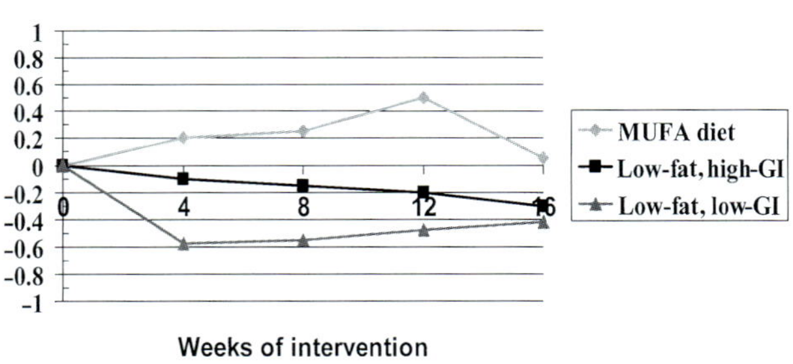

Figure 5 The only randomized trial compared *ad libitum* diets with either a low-carbohydrate, high-MUFA diet; high-carbohydrate, high-GI diet; or high-carbohydrate, low-GI diet. There was a statistically significant difference in weight loss between all three diets. Low-carbohydrate, high-MUFA diet also adversely influenced glucose homoestasis. (Reproduced by permission of The Nutrition Society [53])

more and better randomized clinical trials have been conducted.

Alcohol

Alcohol provides energy that displaces more nutritious foods. Alcohol suppresses fat oxidation, thereby allowing more dietary fat to be stored. The satiating effect of alcohol energy may be low and alcohol consumption has been shown to promote passive overconsumption of fat [55]. Alcohol has also been associated with obesity in epidemiological studies [56]. High alcohol consumption also increases the risk of losing control over otherwise restrained behavior. Consequently, energy from alcohol should be limited and needs to be assessed and appropriately controlled.

WEIGHT MANAGEMENT PROGRAMS FOR THE PREVENTION OF TYPE 2 DIABETES

The potential of intensive lifestyle treatment to induce and maintain weight loss has been evaluated in two recent major studies on the prevention of type 2 diabetes in obese subjects with IGT [57, 58]. In the Finnish Diabetes Prevention study, 522 overweight individuals with IGT were randomized to an intensive lifestyle intervention or to a control group [58]. The intervention aimed at a weight loss of >5% achieved by reduction of total fat to <30% of calories from fat (<10% from saturated fat), >15 g/1000 kcal fiber, and >30 min of exercise per day (walking, jogging, etc.). The subjects were instructed to have a frequent intake of whole grain products, vegetables, fruits, low-fat milk and meat products, and soft margarines, and vegetables oils rich in monounsaturated fatty acids. Subjects attended seven counseling sessions with nutritionists during the first year of the intervention, and one session every 3 months in the subsequent years. The weight loss after 1 year was 5%, and after 5 years the weight loss maintained was still 3 kg. This intervention produced a 58% reduction in the incidence of type 2 diabetes. In a subsequent analysis weight loss was the strongest predictor of the diabetes preventive effect, and a weight reduction of 5% was associated with a reduction in relative risk of 61%. Every 3 kg of additional weight loss doubled this effect. In the much larger, but very similar, American Diabetes Prevention Program, 3234 obese individuals (mean BMI, 34 kg/m^2) with IGT were randomized to intensive lifestyle, metformin, or a control group [57]. The goals of the lifestyle intervention were >7% weight loss, achieved by a diet providing <25% energy from fat and restricted to 1200–1800 kcal/day, and >150-min brisk walking per week [57]. The participants in the intervention group had 16 sessions with a nutritionist over the first 6 months, and subsequently one session per month for the remaining 2.5 years. After 1 year the weight loss was 7%, and 5% was maintained throughout the trial as compared to the placebo group. The relative risk reduction of diabetes was the same as in the Finnish study, 58% [57, 58]. These studies strengthen the evidence to support the low-fat diet in combination with physical activity as the superior strategy for diabetes prevention.

Achieving and maintaining a desirable body weight is a major goal in management of type 2 diabetes. Weight loss dramatically improves glycemic control, lipid profile, and blood pressure in obese individuals with type 2 diabetes (ADA recommendations). Although it is more difficult to produce and maintain weight loss in type 2 diabetic patients than in simple obese patients, it is possible, and the health benefits are more substantial [59]. In overweight and obese type 2 diabetic patients who have difficulty in losing weight on a conventional diet, a liquid-formula 800 kcal/day diet may be a safe alternative. Irrespective of whether an intensive 800 kcal/day diet consists of normal foods or of a liquid-formula diet, weight loss after 3 months is 14–15% of initial body weight. This also produces substantial improvements in glycemic control, blood lipids, and blood pressure [60]. Most of the weight loss is maintained after 1 year. These studies show that it is possible to obtain substantial benefits in the treatment of type 2 diabetic patients through intensive diet therapy and lifestyle modification. The major problem in the execution of this treatment is that most diabetologists do not give it the priority it deserves, and resources are not allocated to staff with the necessary skills.

Physical Activity in Type 2 Diabetes

Physical activity alone may have a modest, but nevertheless important, effect on glycemic control. Favorable changes in glucose tolerance and insulin sensitivity usually deteriorate within 72 h of the last exercise session. Consequently, regular physical activity is imperative to sustain glucose-lowering effects and improved insulin sensitivity [61].

According to a meta-analysis of intervention studies (>8 weeks) addressing the effect of exercise on glycemic control and body weight in type 2 diabetic patients, aerobic and resistance training produced a beneficial effect on HbA_{1c} of −0.66%, whereas they failed to find any effect on body weight [62]. However, training may reduce body fat and increase lean tissue mass, so that body mass index (BMI) is unchanged. In addition, physical activity has other important beneficial effects in type 2 diabetes, such as those on cardiovascular risk factors and general well-being.

CURRENT DRUGS FOR TREATMENT OF OBESITY

This section focuses solely on drugs currently available for the treatment of obesity, or drugs with weight-reducing properties used for the treatment of type 2 diabetes or for smoking cessation. These will be grouped within each of the following three categories: those that shift nutrient metabolism; those that reduce food intake; and those that increase energy expenditure. For more recent reviews covering most of the current drugs, including new potential compounds, the reader is referred to references 63 and 64.

Amylase Inhibitors (Acarbose)

Inhibition of digestion of starch and disaccharides reduces absorption of di- and monosaccharides and may produce a negative energy balance, providing that energy intake is not increased because of counterregulatory mechanisms. Theoretically, the efficacy with respect to body weight regulation is modest, as starch that is not digested in the small intestine is fermented in the colon and finally absorbed as short-chain fatty acids. It is estimated that fermentation of carbohydrates in the colon is associated with a 50% reduction of energy content available for the body, thus reducing the energetic value of carbohydrates from 4 to 2 kcal/g.

Acarbose is an antidiabetic drug that lowers blood glucose by inhibition of α-glucosidase in the gastrointestinal tract, thereby delaying the hydrolysis of ingested disaccharides and complex carbohydrates. However, the effect of acarbose on glycemic control in diabetic patients is modest, and the effect on body weight is negligible in simple obese [65], obese with IGT [66], and in type 2 diabetic [67] patients. In a weight maintenance study in obese subjects, Hauner et al. failed to find any effect of 6-month acarbose treatment on body weight after an initial diet-induced weight loss of 10 kg [65]. About 50% more patients reported side effects on treatment with acarbose than with placebo, these being mainly flatulence, abdominal pain, and diarrhea. In the STOP-NIDDM trial, 1429 overweight and obese patients with IGT were randomized to a 3-year treatment with acarbose or placebo [66]. After 3 years acarbose produced a weight loss of 0.8 kg compared to placebo, and the risk of progression to diabetes over 3.3 years was reduced by 25%. The risk reduction was partially attributable to the weight loss [66]. However, 31% of the patients in the acarbose group, compared to 19% in placebo group, discontinued treatment early, mainly owing to gastrointestinal side effects [66]. The effects of acarbose in type 2 diabetes are equally unpromising. In the UK Prospective Diabetes Study (UKPDS), 1946 type 2 diabetic patients randomized to acarbose or placebo were followed for 3 years [67]. Fifty-eight percent of the included patients discontinued acarbose versus 39% dropouts in the placebo group. In an intention-to-treat analysis acarbose produced only a 0.2% lower HbA_{1c} than did placebo, while in those who remained on the allocated therapy HbA_{1c} was 0.5% lower. Mean body weight was lower by 0.4 kg in the acarbose group after 1 year, but no difference was seen after 2 or 3 years [66].

In conclusion, acarbose produces only a very modest weight loss (<1 kg), if any, and taken together with its low tolerability due to prevalent gastrointestinal side effects, has no place in the treatment of obesity. Acarbose may, however, have some role in type 2 diabetic patients with a capacity to tolerate the compound [63].

Lipase Inhibitors (Orlistat)

Mechanism of Action and Use

Malabsorption of dietary fat is an obvious drug target as high dietary fat intake plays a special role in promoting weight gain and obesity. A number of compounds that act as intestinal lipase inhibitors are currently being investigated for use in the treatment of obesity and related disorders, but only orlistat is currently approved and freely available.

Orlistat is a specific inhibitor of intestinal lipase, the enzyme secreted from the exocrine pancreas and responsible for enzymatic fat digestion [68, 69]. Within the small intestine, lipase and colipase hydrolyze ingested triglyceride, and produce fatty acids and mono- and diglycerides that interact with bile to form micelles, enabling absorption of ingested fat. Orlistat inhibits lipase activity through formation of a covalent bond with serine within the catalytic site of gastric and pancreatic lipase. At the recommended therapeutic dose (120 mg) taken immediately prior to or within 1 h of each of the three daily main meals, the absorption of dietary fat is reduced by ~30%. Fecal energy loss is not fully compensated by an increased total caloric intake, and so orlistat produces a negative energy balance resulting in weight loss. Moreover, the reduced absorption of saturated fatty acids and *trans*-fatty acids has, independent of weight loss, a beneficial effect on plasma total and LDL cholesterol and triglycerides. Furthermore, there is some evidence to support that the reduction in total fat uptake exerts a similar positive effect on thrombotic factors.

Orlistat is recommended for use as the pharmacological support for a nutritional strategy of a modest caloric restriction and a diet providing less than 30% of energy from fat. An obese patient with a typical energy requirement of 2600 kcal/day will, on a 600 kcal deficit diet with 30% of calories from fat, experience an extra loss of 220 kcal fat in fecal energy. Systemic absorption of orlistat and its metabolites is negligible, and so adverse effects of orlistat are a consequence of the partial reduction of fat absorption, leading to an increased proportion of undigested fat in the bowel. The most frequent adverse effects of orlistat are flatulence, flatulence with discharge, oily spotting, fecal urgency and incontinence, oily stools, and steatorrhea. In the majority of patients these adverse effects are self-limiting and mostly transient, generally occurring within the first months of treatment and often triggered by the ingestion of high-fat meals. The unabsorbed fat binds some fat-soluble vitamins (A, D, and E) and secondary nutrients (β-carotene, lycopene, flavanoids, etc.). A simple vitamin supplement and increased intake of fruit and vegetables counteracts this effect. Pharmacodynamic studies suggest that orlistat does not affect the pharmacokinetic properties of lipid-soluble drugs such as digoxin, phenytoin, warfarin, glyburide, furosemide, captopril, nifedipine, atenolol, or oral contraceptives [64].

Efficacy and safety in adolescents have so far only been examined in an open-labeled pilot study [70], and remain to be demonstrated in pregnant women.

Treatment in Simple Obese Subjects

The efficacy and safety of orlistat have been documented in several short- and long-term double-blind trials lasting for up to 4 years, involving a total of more than 30 000 patients, making orlistat the most well-investigated drug for the treatment of obesity. In most trials, orlistat induces a dose-dependent reduction in body weight, and the recommended dose induces a mean weight loss that typically exceeds that of the placebo group by 3–5 kg, to some extent independent of the degree of dietary energy restriction or other ancillary treatment (Figure 6). The weight loss typically continues for the first 3–6 months of treatment and then plateaus, and the patients may subsequently remain weight stable or regain some weight, depending on the intensity of the dietary treatment. However, the weight difference between the orlistat and placebo groups is sustained over 1–4 years, which indicates that efficacy is maintained. The weight loss may not seem large viewed in relation to the patients' excessive body fat, but it has important clinical implications. Typically, orlistat doubles the proportion of patients achieving >5% and >10% weight loss, and it also doubles the proportion maintaining this goal after 1 and 2 years. The immediate weight regain

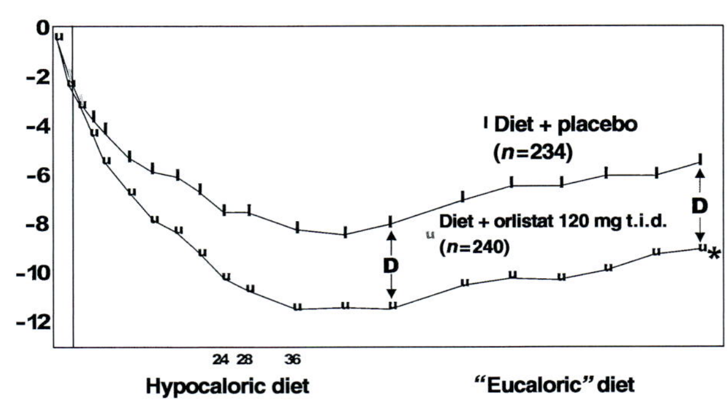

Figure 6 Weight loss and maintenance of simple obese patients treated with energy-restricted diet and randomized to orlistat or placebo. $^*P < 0001$; least-squares mean difference from placebo. (Reproduced by permission of Elsevier [71])

Table 4 Changes in body weight and HbA_{1C} in overweight type 2 diabetes during long-term orlistat treatment*

Medication	Baseline HbA_{1C} (%)	Change in HbA_{1C}[†] (%)	Change in Body weight[†] (%)
Sulfonylurea	7.5	−0.46	−1.9
Insulin	9.0	−0.35	−2.6
Metformin	8.9	−0.29	−2.9

[†] Placebo subtracted.

is greater in orlistat-treated patients after discontinuation of treatment than in placebo-treated patients which indicates that orlistat maintains its pharmacological efficacy. However, the total weight loss and maintenance is greater after orlistat than after placebo.

In obese subjects with metabolic syndrome (insulin-resistance syndrome) orlistat produces weight loss of the same magnitude as in simple obese subjects, and the weight loss is associated with significant decreases in fasting insulin, triglycerides, and the LDL/HDL cholesterol ratio and increase in HDL cholesterol [72].

Treatment in Obese Subjects with IGT

Treatment of obese subjects with IGT by orlistat as an adjuvant to diet and lifestyle modification has been shown to decrease the incidence of conversion to type 2 diabetes. In a retrospective analysis of obese adults with IGT treated with orlistat, the additional weight loss produced by orlistat reduced the 1-year incidence of type 2 diabetes from 7.6% in the placebo group to 3.0% [73]. Moreover, while 49% converted from IGT to normal glucose tolerance in the lifestyle (plus placebo) group, 72% did so in the orlistat group [73]. In a recent multicenter trial, 3304 nondiabetic obese subjects underwent intensive lifestyle modification with a dietary energy deficit of 800 kcal/day, and were randomized to either orlistat or placebo for 4 years [71]. They attended reinforcement sessions every fortnight for the first 6 months, and subsequently every month for the following 3.5 years. More orlistat-treated than placebo-treated patients completed the trial (52% vs. 34%). The mean weight loss was greater by 4 kg in the orlistat group after 1 year, and most of this weight loss was maintained throughout the rest of the study period. The weight loss was 6.9 kg in the orlistat group and 4.1 kg in the placebo group after 4 years. About 50% more patients treated with orlistat achieved and maintained >5% and >10% weight loss after 1 and 4 years. Nine percent in the placebo group and only 6.2% in the orlistat group had developed type 2 diabetes after 4 years (relative risk reduction = 37%, $P = 0.003$). In addition, orlistat patients obtained greater reductions in waist circumference, LDL cholesterol, and systolic and diastolic blood pressures than did placebo patients. The study clearly shows that the additional weight loss achieved by orlistat is sufficient to reduce the incidence of diabetes, even among more nonselected obese subjects where 80% had normal glucose tolerance. In the 20% of patients with IGT, at enrollment the intensive lifestyle change alone resulted in a similar absolute diabetes incidence as the lifestyle treatment in the Diabetes Prevention Program [57]. The addition of orlistat further improved the preventive effect.

Treatment in Obese Diabetic Patients

One-year multicenter trials have been conducted with the use of orlistat in addition to each of the treatments of type 2 diabetic patients: sulfonylurea, insulin, and metformin. Whatever medication the diabetic patients received at baseline, orlistat produced weight loss above that produced by diet and placebo (of 2–5 kg) [68], and reductions in HbA_{1c} of 0.46% (sulfonylurea), 0.35% (insulin) [63, 74], and 0.29% (metformin) (Table 4). Greater reductions were also seen in LDL cholesterol and blood pressure in the orlistat groups. Consequently, orlistat can be used as first drug of choice in type 2 diabetic patients when diet and lifestyle is not sufficient to achieve glycemic control, and it can be used safely in combination with the second drug of choice, metformin.

Metformin

Metformin is a biguanide that is approved for the treatment of type 2 diabetes. It lowers plasma glucose by reducing the intestinal absorption of glucose, suppressing hepatic glucose production and increasing peripheral insulin sensitivity. It has long been known to induce a slight weight loss not only in diabetic patients but also in obese subjects with metabolic syndrome or IGT. The size of the placebo-subtracted weight loss induced by metformin in diabetic patients varies from 0.5 to 8 kg, probably depending on BMI, age, and glycemic control [63]. In the Diabetes Prevention Program of obese subjects with IGT, metformin produced a 2 kg weight loss and reduced the incidence of diabetes by 31% above placebo after 3 years [57]. A subgroup analysis revealed no difference in efficacy across gender and ethnicity, but the effect was mainly seen in subjects aged 25–59 years with a BMI above 30 kg/m^2, whereas it was largely ineffective in nonobese (BMI < 30 kg/m^2) and those above 60 years [57]. In this trial, more than 1000 patients entered each treatment arm and the resulting high statistical power gives more credit to the outcome than to that of smaller trials.

It is not known how metformin produces weight loss, but it is possible that the improvement in insulin sensitivity increases the central effect of insulin where it acts as a satiety hormone [75]. Another possibility is that reduced food intake is caused by nausea and other gastrointestinal effects. There are no indications of any thermogenic effect of metformin.

Sibutramine

Sibutramine is a serotonin and norepinephrine reuptake inhibitor with only a weak inhibitory action on dopamine reuptake. Unlike amphetamine, sibutramine does not stimulate locomotor activity, and unlike dexfenfluramine and fenfluramine, it does not induce serotonin release, and has not been implicated in the development of valvular disease [76].

Sibutramine decreases food intake in humans by increasing meal-induced satiety [77, 78]. It also exerts a weak thermogenic effect both acutely and during long-term use [78, 79].

Controlled trials in simple obesity have consistently shown dose-related weight loss, and optimal weight loss with a dose of 10–15 mg sibutramine once daily. Typically, weight loss was 3–5 kg greater than with placebo at 24 weeks, and weight loss was sustained for 2 years. The proportion of patients losing at least 5% of body weight over 12 months was 29% with placebo, 56% with sibutramine 10 mg, and 65% with sibutramine 15 mg/day [80]. Intermittent and continuous sibutramine therapies are similar in regard to effectiveness and safety [81]. Wadden et al. found that patients treated with sibutramine alone achieved a weight loss of 4% after 12 months, but the drug plus lifestyle intervention produced a weight loss of 11% and better outcomes in terms of risk factor reductions [82].

In the STORM trial, sibutramine was assessed for the potential to both induce and maintain weight loss [83]. Six-hundred five obese individuals were treated with a 600 kcal/day deficit diet and sibutramine 10 mg daily for 6 months (Figure 7). The 467 participants who lost more than 5% were randomly assigned to continue to receive sibutramine or placebo for 18 months. The mean weight loss after 6 months was 12 kg, and whereas weight was gradually regained in the placebo group during the second year of follow-up, the sibutramine group essentially maintained the weight lost during the initial 6 months [83]. Although sibutramine had positive effects on blood lipids as expected from the weight loss, it seems to have an HDL-cholesterol increasing effect that is independent of weight loss [83], and it has been shown to be appropriate for correction of lipid abnormalities in obese patients having high-serum triglyceride levels and low HDL-cholesterol levels [84]. Sibutramine also increases weight loss and improves maintenance of reduced weight in obese patients

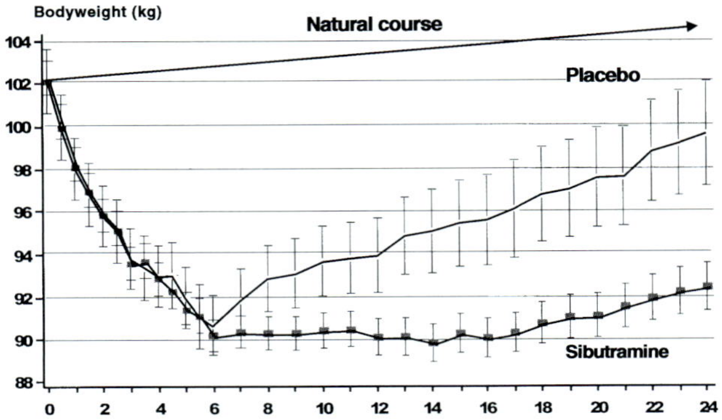

Figure 7 The STORM trial. Mean body weight changes during weigh-loss and weight-maintenance phases. During the first 6 months all patients received −600 kcal/day diet and sibutramine. Those who lost >5% were randomized to continue on sibutramine or placebo. (Reprinted with permission from Elsevier Science (The Lancet, 2000, 356; 2119–2125) [83])

who have previously lost weight on a very low calorie diet [85].

Sibutramine is generally well tolerated and has few side effects. These include dry mouth, headache, insomnia, and constipation. The adverse effects of sibutramine include increase in blood pressure and heart rate. Although these increases are generally mild and without clinical relevance, blood pressure should be monitored on a regular basis. Increases in blood pressure may lead to discontinuation of treatment in about 5% of patients.

Obese patients with well-controlled hypertension (calcium-channel blockers, β-blocking agents, angiotensin-converting enzyme inhibitors, thiazide diuretics) do not experience any rise in blood pressure with sibutramine therapy, and their overall risk factor profile will benefit from the induced weight loss [86–88].

Sibutramine has been shown to produce a substantial weight loss above that of placebo (~9 kg) and a 2% decrease in HbA_{1c} over 6 months in type 2 diabetic patients with poor glycemic control despite maximum doses of sulfonylureas and metformin [89]. In a 12-month study Rissanan et al. found sibutramine to produce a weight loss of 7.1 kg in diet-treated type 2 diabetic patients vs. 2.6 kg in the placebo group. Overall, there was no benefit of sibutramine therapy on glycemic control (−0.3% vs. −0.2%), but in a subgroup with $HbA_{1c}>8\%$ the improvement was superior in the sibutramine group (−1.4% vs. −0.6%). Longer term studies and studies in other groups of diabetic patients have not been published.

Bupropion

Bupropion has dual neurotransmitter properties working as norepinephrine and dopamine reuptake inhibitors, which may both have relevance for body weight regulation. Sustained-release bupropion is approved for the treatment of smoking cessation and for major depression. In depressed patients with normal weight, bupropion seems to have a weight neutral profile, whereas there are suggestions of weight-reducing properties in overweight and obese depressed patients [90, 91]. Moreover, weight gain after smoking cessation is less in bupropion-treated subjects than in placebo-treated subjects [92, 93]. Two randomized, placebo-controlled trials have been conducted in nondiabetic obese subjects. Both found that bupropion was superior to placebo in reducing body weight when given together with an energy-restricted diet [94, 95]. In the largest trial, 327 simple obese patients were treated with diet and lifestyle modification and randomized to bupropion SR 300 mg/day, SR 400 mg/day, or placebo for 24 weeks. In completers, weight loss was greater than with placebo by 2.2 kg in the SR 300 mg/day group, and by 5.1 kg in the SR 400 mg/day group [95]. In a 24-week extension of the study, weight loss was essentially maintained. Bupropion has little, if any, effect on heart rate and blood pressure, but should be used with caution in patients with a history of seizures.

These studies suggest that bupropion may be of particular relevance for smoking cessation in obese and diabetic patients, and perhaps even for weight reduction in nonsmoking obese individuals.

Nicotine

Cigarette smoking is recognized as one of the most important preventable causes of premature death, but still 20–35% of the population in the affluent world continue to smoke. One of the most important barriers to quit smoking is the subsequent weight gain, and the weight control properties of smoking reinforce the decision to continue smoking.

Anorectic and thermogenic properties produced by nicotine are considered to be factors responsible for the lower body weight of smokers compared with nonsmokers. Nicotine gum has been shown to relieve withdrawal symptoms and to double the success rates over placebo in trials of smoking cessation, and has been shown to diminish weight gain after smoking cessation. The use of nicotine gum is therefore an accepted tool to treat withdrawal symptoms and prevent weight gain in a vulnerable phase after smoking cessation. Dale et al. [96] demonstrated that 100% replacement does not completely prevent weight gain. To determine whether attempts to prevent weight gain will increase success rates for stopping smoking, 287 female weight-concerned smokers were enrolled into a combination of a standard smoking cessation program with nicotine gum and a behavioral weight control program including a low-energy diet [97]. A control group was treated with the identical program but without the diet. After 16 weeks, 50% of the women had stopped smoking in the diet group versus 35% in the control group. Among these women, weight fell by mean 2.1 kg in the diet group but increased by 1.6 kg in the control group ($P < 0.001$). After 1 year the success rates in the diet and control groups were 28 and 16% respectively ($P < 0.05$), but there was no statistical difference in weight gain. Combining the smoking cessation program with an intervention to control body weight helped women to stop smoking and control weight; nicotine replacement alone is insufficient to prevent weight gain when quitting smoking. No weight loss trials have been conducted with the use of nicotine.

Ephedrine/Caffeine

Ephedrine is both an indirect sympathomimetic, causing release of norepinephrine from the sympathetic nerve endings, and a direct agonist on β-receptors. Numerous studies have shown that ephedrine (E) as monotherapy decreases body fat in obese subjects by a combined action of suppression of appetite and stimulation of energy expenditure. Adenosine antagonists such as caffeine (C) potentiate the thermogenic and clinical effects. Combinations of E+C have been shown to be effective for treatment of obesity for up to 50 weeks. In a study including 180 obese patients it was found that E+C (20 mg/200 mg t.i.d.) produced a larger weight loss than did placebo, C, or E, in combination with a hypoenergetic diet over 24 weeks [98]. After 24 weeks the placebo group had lost 13.2 kg, and E+C further increased the weight loss by 3.4 kg to a total of 16.6 kg. Also, more patients in the E+C group than in the placebo group lost more than 5% and 10% of initial body weight. Breum et al. tested E+C against dexfenfluramine in a double-blind, placebo-controlled trial, and found that E+C produced a greater weight loss than did dexfenfluramine in subjects with a BMI of more than 30 kg/m^2 [99]. The reductions in pulse rate and blood pressure were similar with the two treatments. E+C has also been evaluated for prevention of weight gain after smoking cessation. The double-blind, placebo-controlled trial included 225 subjects and after 12 weeks weight gain was less in the E+C group than in placebo group [100]. However, after 1 year there was no difference in the proportion of subjects not smoking.

Molnar reported a 20-week, randomized double-blind, placebo-controlled trial of E+C in adolescents aged 16 years and in Tanner stage III–V, and found that E+C produced more substantial weight loss than did placebo (14.4 vs. 2.2%) [101]. Subjects dropped out only in the placebo group, and adverse effects were mild and not different from those in the placebo group after 4 weeks.

Notably, E+C increases blood pressure and heart rate slightly with the first exposure [102]. However, during chronic treatment tachyphylaxis develops to the cardiovascular effects of the compound, but not to the anorectic and thermogenic [98]. In the largest trial of E+C, only a slight increase in blood pressure and heart rate could be detected when the treatment was initiated, but after 12 weeks of dietary treatment, the reductions in blood pressure were similar in the E+C group to those in the placebo group [98]. A hypothetical cardiovascular safety concern could be raised by the combination of E+C and exercise. With more extensive measurement of cardiovascular function by thoracic impedance, automatic sphygmomanometry, and continuous electrocardiographic recording, Waluga et al. concluded that E+C had no undesirable effects on cardiovascular function in obese subjects [103]. E+C has also been tested in overweight subjects with controlled hypertension [104]. Treatment with E+C produced a larger weight loss and a greater reduction in systolic blood pressure (5.5 mmHg) than did treatment with placebo; moreover the antihypertensive effect of β-blockers was not reduced by E+C [104]. E+C does not seem to have any long-term effect on glucose and lipid metabolism apart from the beneficial changes in risk factors secondary to weight loss. Buemann et al. reported that E+C prevented the decline in HDL cholesterol associated with weight loss, and it increased the ratio of HDL cholesterol to total cholesterol, whereas no effect on fasting glucose metabolism was observed [105].

The clinical studies of E+C clearly show that the compound is effective in the treatment of obesity for up to 1 year [10]. However, because of the limited number of patients treated in the trials, the total evidence does not meet the efficacy and safety requirements of the American FDA or the European CPMP for licensing E+C as a prescription compound.

Various herbal combinations of E+C based on Ma Huang, guarana, and aspirin are sold over the counter in the United States and the total sales reached about 950 million dollars in 1999. The pharmacokinetics of these herbal preparations may vary, and they contain many other ingredients such as minerals and herbs that might alter or interact with E or C [106].

As concluded by Greenway [106],

> These herbal products containing ephedrine and caffeine should be tested in controlled clinical trials to confirm their presumed efficacy and safety which cannot truly be extrapolated from the peer-reviewed scientific literature using pharmaceutical grade caffeine and ephedrine in isolation.

No studies exist in obese subjects with IGT or type 2 diabetes, and the use of E/C compounds in these conditions is not substantiated.

SURGICAL TREATMENT OF OBESITY

Weight management programs fail in a substantial proportion of the severely obese patients, and to ensure a better long-term outcome, bariatric surgery is the treatment of choice for well-informed and well-motivated obese patients with acceptable operative risks [107]. Patients should be obese for at least 5 years and have a strong desire for a substantial weight loss, or have severe impairments because of their obesity. Surgery is indicated for patients with a BMI greater than 40 kg/m^2, or for those with serious medical comorbidities and a BMI greater than 35 kg/m^2. A number of different procedures are available: (1) adjustable silicone gastric banding, (2) vertical gastric banding, and (3) gastric bypass, which should be reserved for the heavier patients. The malabsorptive intestinal bypass (jejuno-ileal) has a high rate of complications and cannot be recommended.

Effect in Simple Obesity

In a series of 100 obese patients gastric bypass was shown to prevent the progression of IGT to frank type 2 diabetes [108]. In the Swedish Obese Subjects (SOS) study, 2000 matched morbidly, but simple obese patient pairs will be followed for 10 years each, one pair member is surgically treated, while the other serves as a control group [109]. The 2-year mean weight reduction was 28 kg in the operated patients and 0.5 kg in the controls. After 8 years the weight loss was 20 kg in the surgical group, while the controls had gained 0.7 kg. The average weight loss for gastric bypass and vertical banded gastroplasty was 16% after 10 years. These weight reductions were sufficient to reduce the 2-year incidence of type 2 diabetes 32 times as compared to the controls. After 5 years the relative risk reduction was 80%, and after 10 years, 67%. However, while the incidence of hypertension was markedly reduced the first years, after 8 years the incidence of hypertension was almost equal in the two study groups. The weight loss achieved by surgery has pronounced effects on cardiac structure and function, quality of life, rates of employment, and health care costs.

Gastric Surgery in Type 2 Diabetes

The weight loss achieved by surgical procedures in obese type 2 diabetic patients has marked effects on glycemic control, cardiovascular risk factors, progression of the disease, and mortality [110, 111]. In a study of 154 type 2 diabetic patients followed for up to 10 years, the proportion of control subjects being treated with oral hypoglycemics or insulin increased from 56.4% at initial contact to 87.5% at last contact, whereas the percentage of surgical patients requiring medical management fell from 31.8% preoperatively to 8.6% at last contact. The mortality rate in the control group was 28% compared to 9% in the surgical group. The improvement in the mortality rate in the surgical group was primarily due to a decrease in the number of cardiovascular deaths.

Laparoscopic adjustable gastric banding is a minimally invasive and reversible surgical procedure that yields a significant reduction in gastric volume and hunger sensation. This procedure has been shown to be a very effective treatment of grade 3 obesity, inducing long-lasting reduction of body weight and arterial blood pressure, modifying body fat distribution, and improving glucose and lipid metabolism, especially in type 2 diabetic patients [112, 113].

These data show that surgical treatment of obesity has a place in the prevention and treatment of severely obese patients with type 2 diabetes, and with the less invasive techniques this treatment should be used in more obese type 2 diabetic patients resistant to other treatment programs [114].

REFERENCES

1. National Institutes of Health (NIH). Clinical guidelines on the identification, evaluation and treatment of overweight and obesity in adults—The Evidence Report. *Obes Res* 1998; 6 (suppl 2): 1S–209S.
2. Van Gaal LF. Dietary treatment of obesity. In Bray GA, Bouchard C, James WPT (eds) *Handbook of Obesity*. New York: Marcel Dekker, 1998; pp 875–90.
3. WHO. Obesity: preventing and managing the global epidemic. WHO Consultation on Obesity, Geneva, 3–5 June 1997. Geneva: WHO, 1998. Report WHO/NUT/NCD/98.1.
4. Thomas PR (ed). *Weighing the Options*. Washington: National Academy Press, 1995.
5. Bray GA. *Comtemporary Diagnosis and Management of Obesity*. Newton: Handbooks in Health Care Co, 1998.
6. Astrup A, Hansen DL, Lundsgaard C, Toubro S. Sibutramine and energy balance. *Int J Obes* 1998; 22 (suppl 1): S30–5.
7. Toubro S, Astrup A. Randomised comparison of diets for maintaining obese subjects' weight after major weight loss: ad lib, low fat, high carbohydrate diet vs. fixed energy intake. *BMJ* 1997; 314: 29–34.
8. National Task Force on the Prevention and Treatment of Obesity, National Institutes of Health. Very low-calorie diets. *JAMA* 1993; 270: 967–74.
9. Wadden TA, Foster GD, Letizia KA. One-year behavioral treatment of obesity: comparison of moderate and severe caloric restriction and the effects of weight maintenance therapy. *J Consult Clin Psychol* 1994; 62: 165–17.
10. Toubro S, Astrup A, Breum L, Quaade F. Safety and efficacy of long-term treatment with ephedrine, caffeine and an ephedrine/caffeine mixture. *Int J Obes* 1993; 17: S69–72.
11. Jeffery RW, Wing RR, Mayer RR. Are smaller weight losses or more achievable weight loss goals better in the long term for obese patients. *J Consult Clin Psychol* 1998; 66: 641–5.
12. Astrup A, Lundsgaard C. What do pharmacological approaches to obesity management offer? Linking pharmacological mechanisms of obesity management agents to clinical practice. *Exp Clin Endocrinl Diabetes* 1998; 106 (suppl 2): 29–34.
13. Astrup A, Toubro S, Raben A, Skov AR. The role of low-fat diets and fat substitutes in body weight management: what have we learnt from clinical studies? *J Am Diet Assoc* 1997; 27 (suppl): S82–7.
14. Bray GA, Popkin BM. Dietary fat intake does affect obesity! *Am J Clin Nutr* 1998; 68: 1157–73.
15. Hill JO, Peters JC, Reed GW, Schlundt DG, Sharp T, Greene HL. Nutrient balance in humans: effects of diet composition. *Am J Clin Nutr* 1991; 54: 10–7.
16. Astrup A, Grunwald GK, Melanson EL, Saris WHM, Hill JO. The role of low-fat diets in body weight control: a meta-analysis of *ad libitum* intervention studies. *Int J Obes* 2000; 24: 1545–52.
17. Swinburn BA, Metcalf PA, Ley SJ. Long-term (5-year) effects of a reduced-fat diet intervention in individuals with glucose intolerance. *Diabetes Care* 2001; 24: 619–24.
18. Yu-Poth S, Zhao G, Etherton T, Naglak M, Jonnalagadda S, Kris-Etherthon PM. Effects of the National Cholesterol Education Programs step I and step II dietary intervention programs on cardiovascular disease risk factors: a meta-analysis. *Am J Clin Nutr* 1999; 69: 632–46.
19. Jeppesen J, Schaaf P, Jones G, Zhou MY, Chen YD, Reaven GM. Effects of low-fat, high-carbohydrate diets on risk factors for ischemic heart disease in postmenopausal women. *Am J Clin Nutr* 1997; 65: 1027–33.
20. Katan MB, Grundy SM, Willett WC. Should a low-fat. High-carbohydrate diet be recommended for everyone? Beyond low-fat diets. *N Engl J Med* 1997; 337: 563–6.
21. Schaefer EJ, Lichtenstein AH, Lamon-Fava S, McNamara JR, Schaefer MM, Rasmussen H, Ordovas JM. Body weight and low-density lipoprotein cholesterol changes after consumption of a low-fat *ad libitum* diet. *JAMA* 1995; 274: 1450–5.
22. Westrate JA, van het Hof KH, van den Berg H, Velthuis-te-Wierik EJM, de Graaf C, Zimmermanns NJ, Westerterp KR, Westerterp-Plantenga MS, Verboeket-van de Venne WP. A comparison of the effect of free access to reduced fat products or their full fat equivalents on food intake, body weight, blood lipids and fat-soluble antioxidants levels and haemostasis variables. *Eur J Clin Nutr* 1998; 52: 389–95.
23. Turley ML, Skeaff CM, Mann JI, Cox B. The effect of a low-fat, high-carbohydrate diet on serum high density lipoprotein cholesterol and triglyceride. *Eur J Clin Nutr* 1998; 52: 728–32.
24. Appel LJ, Moore TJ, Obarsanek E, Vollmer WM, Svetkey LP, Sacks FM, Bray GA, Vogt TM, Cutler JA, Windhauser MM, Lin PH, Karanja N, for the DASH Collaborative Research Group. A clinical trial of the effects of dietary patterns on blood pressure. *N Engl J Med* 1997; 336 (16): 1117–24.
25. Marckmann P, Sandström B, Jespersen J. Favorable long-term effect of a low-fat/high fiber diet on human blood coagulation and fibrinolysis. *Arterioscler, Thromb Vasc Biol* 1993; 13: 505–11.
26. Hammer RL, Barrier CA, Roundy ES, Bradford JM, Fisher AG. Calorie-restricted low-fat diet and exercise in obese women. *Am J Clin Nutr* 1989; 49: 77–85.
27. Jeffery RW, Hellerstedt WL, French SA, Baxter JE. A randomised controlled trial of counseling for fat restriction versus calorie restriction in the treatment of obesity. *Int J Obes* 1995; 19: 132–7.
28. Schlundt DG, Hill JO, Pope-Cordle J, Arnold D, Virst KL, Hatahn M. Randomized evaluation of a low fat *ad libitum* carbohydrate diet for weight reduction. *Int J Obes* 1993; 17: 623–9.
29. Shah M, McGovern P, French S, Baxter J. Comparison of a low-fat, *ad libitum* complex-carbohydrate diet with

a low-energy diet in moderately obese women. *Am J Clin Nutr* 1994; 59: 980–4.

30. Astrup A. The role of the glycaemic index of foods in body weight regulation and obesity. Is more evidence needed? *Obes Rev* 2002; 3: 233.
31. Pawlak DB, Ebbeling CB, Ludwig DS. Should obese patients be counselled to follow a low glycaemic index diet? Yes. *Obes Rev* 2002; 3: 235–43.
32. Raben A. Should obese patients be counselled to follow a low glycaemic index diet? No. *Obes Rev* 2002; 3: 245–56.
33. Atkins RC. *Dr. Atkins' New Diet Revolution*. New York: Simon & Schuster, 1998.
34. Westman EC, Yancy WS, Edman JS, Tomlin KF, Perkins CE. Effect of 6-month adherence to a very low carbohydrate diet program. *Am J Med* 2002; 113: 30–6.
35. Helge JW. Prolonged adaptation to fat-rich diet and training; effects on body stores and insulin resistance in man. *Int J Obes* 2002; 26: 1118–24.
36. Ayyad C, Andersen T. Long-term efficacy of dietary treatment of obesity: a systematic review of studies published between 1931 and 1999. *Obes Rev* 2000; 1: 113–9.
37. Dwyer JT, Lu D. Popular diets for weight loss. From nutritionally hazardous to healthful. In Stunkard AJ, Wadden TA (eds) *Obesity—Theory and Therapy*, 2nd edn. New York: Raven Press, 1993; pp 231–52.
38. Saris WHM, Astrup A, Prentice AM, Zunft HJH, Formiguera X, Verboeket-van de Venne WPHG, Raben A, Poppitt SD, Seppelt B, Johnston S, Vasilaras TH, Keogh GF. Randomized controlled trial of changes in dietary carbohydrate/fat ratio and simple vs. complex carbohydrates on body weight and blood lipids: the CARMEN study. *Int J Obes* 2000; 24: 1310–8.
39. Ludvig DS, Peterson KE, Gortmaker SL. Relation between consumption of sugar-sweetened drinks and childhood obesity: a prospective, observational analysis. *Lancet* 2001; 357: 505–8.
40. Raben A, Vasilaras TH, Møller AC, Astrup A. Sucrose compared artificial sweeteners: different effects on *ad libitum* food intake and body weight after 10 wk supplementation in overweight subjects. *Am J Clin Nutr* (in press).
41. Wolever TMS, Jenkins DJA, Vuksan V, Jenkins AL, Wong GS, Josse RG. Beneficial effect of low-glycemic index diet in overweight NIDDM subjects. *Diabetes Care* 1992; 15: 562–4.
42. Hu FB, van Dam RM, Liu S. Diet and risk of type II diabetes: the role of types of fat and carbohydrate. *Diabetologia* 2001; 44: 805–7.
43. Foster-Powell K, Miller JB. International tables of glycemic index. *Am J Clin Nutr* 1995; 62: 871S–93S.
44. Pedersen D, Raben A, Flint A, Møller BK, Tetens I, Astrup A. Glycemic index—is it a useful tool? *Int J Obes* 2002; 26 (suppl 1): S132.
45. Skov AR, Toubro S, Rønn B, Holm L, Astrup A. Randomized trial on protein versus carbohydrate in *ad libitum* fat reduced diet for the treatment of obesity. *Int J Obes* 1999; 23: 528–36.
46. Dumesnil JG, Turgeon J, Tremblay A, Poirier P, Gilbert M, Gagnon L, St-Pierre S, Garneau C, Lemieux I, Pascot A, Bergeron J, Després J-P. Effect of a low-glycaemic index-low-fat-high protein diet on atherogenic metabolic risk profile of abdominally obese men. *Br J Nutr* 2001; 86: 557–68.
47. Eades MRE, Eades MDE. *Protein Power*. New York: Bantam Books; 1996.
48. Dulloo AG, Mensi N, Seydoux J, Girardier L. Differential effects of high-fat diets varying in fatty acid composition on the efficiency of lean and fat tissue deposition during weight recovery after low food intake. *Metabolism* 1995; 44: 273–9.
49. Doucet E, Alméras N, White MD, Després J-P, Bouchard C, Tremblay A. Dietary fat compostion and human adiposity. *Eur J Clin Nutr* 1998; 52: 2–6.
50. Lawton C, Delargy H, Smith F, Blundell J. Does the degree of saturation of fatty acids affect post-ingenstive satiety? *Int J Obes* 1997; 21: S35.
51. French S, Mutuma S, Francis J, Read N, Meijer G. The effect of fatty acid composition on intestinal satiety in man. *Int J Obes* 1998; 22 (suppl 3): S82.
52. McManus K, Antinoro L, Sacks F. A randomized controlled trial of a moderate-fat, low-energy diet compared with a low fat, low-energy diet for weight loss in overweight adults. *Int J Obes* 2001; 25: 1503–11.
53. Wolever TMS, Mehling C. High-carbohydrate-low-glycaemic index dietary advice improves glucose disposition index in subjects with impaired glucose tolerance. *Br J Nutr* 2002; 87: 477–87.
54. Tsihlias EB, Gibbs AL, McBurney MI, Wolever TMS. Comparison of high- and low-glycemic-index breakfast cereals with monounsaturated fat in the long-term dietary management of type 2 diabetes. *Am J Clin Nutr* 2000; 72: 439–49.
55. Tremblay A, Wouters E, Wenker M, St-Pierre S, Bouchard C, Despres JP. Alcohol and a high-fat diet: a combination favoring overfeeding. *Am J Clin Nutr* 1995; 62: 639–44.
56. Tremblay A, St-Pierre S. The hyperphagic effect of a high-fat diet and alcohol intake persists after control for energy density. *Am J Clin Nutr* 1996; 63: 479–82.
57. Knowler WC, Barrett-Connor E, Fowler SE, Hamman RF, Lachin JM, Walker EA, Nathan M, for the Diabetes Prevention Program Research Group. Reduction in the incidence of type 2 diabetes with lifestyle intervention or metformin. *N Engl J Med* 2002; 346: 393–403.
58. Toumilehto J, Lindström J, Eriksson JG, Valle TT, Hamalainen H, Ilanne-Parikka P, Keinanen-Kiukaanniemi S, Laakso M, Louheranta A, Rastas M, Salminen V, Uusitupa M; Finnish Diabetes Prevention Study Group. Prevention of type 2 diabetes mellitus by changes in lifestyle among subjects with impraired glucose tolerance. *N Engl J Med* 2001; 344: 1343–50.
59. Wing RR, Anglin K. Effectiveness of a behavioral weight control program for blacks and whites with NIDDM. *Diabetes Care*. 1996; 19 (5): 409–13.
60. Anderson JW, Brinkman-Kaplan V, Hamilton CC, Logan JEB, Collins RW, Gustafson NJ. Food-containing hypocaloric diets are as effective as liquid-supplement diets for obese individuals with NIDDM. *Diabetes Care* 1994; 17: 602–4.
61. Albright A, Franz M, Hornsby G, Kriska A, Marrero D, Ulrigh I, Verity LS. American College of Sports Medicine position stand. Exercise and type 2 diabetes. *Med Sci Sports Exer* 2000; 7: 1345–60.
62. Boulé NG, Haddad E, Kenny GP, Wells GA, Sigal RJ. Effects of exercise on glycemic control and body mass in type 2 diabetes mellitus. A meta-analysis of controlled clinical trials. *JAMA* 2001; 286: 1218–27.
63. Bray GA, Greenway FL. Current and potential drugs for treatment of obesity. *Endocr Rev* 1999; 20: 805–75.
64. Bray GA. Pharmacological treatment of obesity. In Bray GA, Bouchard C, James WPT (eds) *Handbook of Obesity*. New York: Marcel Dekker, 1998; pp 953–75.

65. Hauner H, Petzinna D, Sommerauer B, Toplak H. Effect of acarbose on weight maintenance after dietary weight loss in obese subjects. *Diabetes Obes Metab* 2001; 3: 423–7.
66. Chiasson J-L, Josse RG, Gomis R, Hanefeld M, Karasik A, Laakso M, for the STOP-NIDDM Trial Research Group. Acarbose for prevention of type 2 diabetes mellitus: the STOP-NIDDM randomised trial. *Lancet* 2002; 359; 2072–7.
67. Holman RR, Turner RC, Cull CA, on behalf of the UKPDS Study Group. A randomized double-blind trial of acarbose in type 2 diabetes shows improved glycemic control over 3 years (U.K. Prospective Diabetes Study 44). *Diabetes Care* 1999; 22: 960–4.
68. Kelley DE, Jneidi M. Orlistat in the treatment of type 2 diabetes mellitus. *Exp Opin Pharmacother* 2002; 3: 599–605.
69. Snider LJ, Malone M. Orlistat use in type 2 diabetes. *Ann Pharmacother* 2002; 36: 1210–8.
70. McDuffie JR, Calis KA, Uwaifo GI, Sebring NG, Fallon EM, Hubbard VS, Yanovski JA. Three-month tolerability of orlistat in adolescents with obesity-related comorbid conditions. *Obes Res* 2002; 10: 642–50.
71. Sjöström L, Togerson JS, Hauptman J, Boldrin M. XENDOS—a landmark study: xenical in the prevention of diabetes in obese subjects. In *Abstracts from the Satellite Symposium New Frontiers in Weight Management, 9th International Congress on Obesity*, Sao Paolo, Brazil, 2002.
72. Reaven P, Segal K, Hauptman J, Boldrin M, Lucas C. Effect of orlistat-assisted weight loss in decreasing coronary heart disease risk in patients with syndrome X. *Am J Cardiol* 2001; 87: 827–31.
73. Heymsfield SB, Segal KR, Hauptman J, Lucas CP, Boldrin MN, Rissanen A, Wilding JP, Sjostrom L. Effects of weight loss with orlistat on glucose tolerance and progression to type 2 diabetes in obese adults. *Arch Intern Med* 2000; 160: 1321–6.
74. Kelley DE, Hill J, Bray GA, Miles J, Pi-Sunyer FX, Hollander P, Klein S. Clinical efficacy of orlistat therapy in overweight and obese patients with insulin-treated type 2 diabetes. *Diabetes Care* 2002; 25: 1033–41.
75. Schwartz MB, Puhl R. Childhood obesity: a societal problem to solve. *Obes Rev* 2003; 4: 57–71.
76. Kilpatrick IC, Traut M, Heal DJ. Monoamine oxidase inhibition is unlikley to be relevant to the risks associated with phentermine and fenfluramine: a comparison with their abilities to evoke monoamine release. *Int J Obes* 2001; 25: 1454–8.
77. Rolls BJ, Thorwart ML, Shide DJ, Ulbrecht JS. Sibutramine reduces food intake in non-dieting women with obesity. *Obes Res* 1998; 9: 1–11.
78. Hansen DL, Toubro S, Stock MJ, Macdonald IA, Astrup A. The effect of sibutramine on energy expenditure and appetite during chronic treatment without dietary restriction. *Int J Obes* 1999; 23: 1016–24.
79. Hansen DL, Toubro S, Stock MJ, Macdonald IA, Astrup A. Thermogenic effects of sibutramine in humans. *Am J Clin Nutr* 1998; 68: 1180–6.
80. Bray GA, Ryan DH, Gordon D, Heidingsfelder S, Cerise F, Wilson K. Double-blind randomized placebo-controlled trial of sibutramine. *Obes Res* 1996; 4: 263–70.
81. Wirth A, Krause J. Long-term weight loss with sibutramine. A randomized controlled trial. *JAMA* 2001; 286: 1331–9.
82. Wadden TA, Berkowitz RI, Sarwer DB, Prus-Wisniewski R, Steinberg C. Benefits of lifestyle modification in the pharmacological treatment of obesity. A randomized trial. *Arch Intern Med* 2001; 161: 218–27.
83. James WPT, Astrup A, Finer N, Hilsted J, Kopelman P, Rössner S, Saris WHM, van Gaal LF. Effect of sibutramine on weight maintenance after weight loss: a randomised trial. *Lancet* 2000; 356: 2119–25.
84. Dujovne CA, Zavoral JH, Rowe E, Mendel CM, for the Sibutramine Study Group. Effects of sibutramine on body weight and serum lipids: a double-blind, randomized, placebo-controlled study in 322 overweight and obese patients with dyslipidemia. *Am Heart J* 2001; 142: 489–97.
85. Apfelbaum M, Vague P, Ziegler O, Hanotin C, Thomas F, Leutenegger E. Long-term maintenance of weight loss after a very-low-calorie diet: a randomized blinded trial of the efficacy and tolerability of sibutramine. *Am J Med.* 1999; 106: 179–84.
86. McMahon FG, et al. Efficacy and safety of sibutramine in obese white men and African American patients with hypertension: a 1-year, double-blind, placebo controlled, multicenter trial. *Arch Intern Med* 2000; 160: 2185–91.
87. McMahon FG, Weinstein SP, Row E, ERnst KR, Johnson F, Fujioka K, and the Sibutramine in Hypertensives Clinical Study Group. Sibutramine is safe and effective for weight loss in obese patients whose hypertension is well controlled with angiotensin-converting enzyme inhibitors. *J Hum Hypertens* 2002; 16: 5–11.
88. Sramek JJ, Leibowitz MT, Weinstein SP, Rowe ED, Mendel CM, Levy B, McMahon FG, Mullican WS, Toth PD, Cutler NR. Efficacy and safety of sibutramine for weight loss in obese patients with hypertension well controlled by β-adrenergic blocking agents: a placebo-controlled, double-blind, randomised trial. *J Hum Hypertens* 2002; 16: 13–9.
89. Gokcel A, Karakose H, Ertorer EM, Tanaci N, Tutuncu NB, Guvener N. Effects of sibutramine in obese female subjects with type 2 diabetes and poor blood glucose control. *Diabetes Care* 2001; 24: 1957–60.
90. Settle E, Stahl S, Batey S, Johnson J, Ascher J. Safety profile of sustained-release bupropion in depression: results of three clinical trials. *Clin Ther* 1999; 21: 455–63.
91. Croft H, Houser TL, Jamerson BD, Leadbetter R, Bolden-Watson C, Donahue R, Metz A. Effect on body weight of bupropion sustained-release in patients with major depression treated for 52 weeks. *Clin Ther* 2002 Apr; 24 (4): 662–72.
92. Jorenby DE, Leischow SJ, Nides MA, Rennard SI, Johnston JA, Hughes AR, Smith SS, Muramoto ML, Daughton DM, Doan K, Fiore MC, Baker TB. A controlled trial of sustained-release bupropion, a nicotine patch, or both for smoking cessation. *N Engl J Med* 1999; 340: 685–92.
93. Ahluwalia JS, Harris KJ, Catley D, Okuyemi KS, Mayo MS. Sustained-release bupropion for smoking cessation in African Americans. A randomized controlled trial. *JAMA* 2002; 288: 468–74.
94. Gadde K, Parker CB, Maner LG, Wagner HR, Drezner MK, Krishann KRR. Bupropion for weight loss: an investigation of efficacy and tolerability in overweight and obese women. *Obes Res* 2001; 9: 544–51.
95. Anderson JW, Greenway FL, Fujioka K, Gadde KM, McKenney J, O'Neil P. Bupropion SR enhances weight

loss: a 48-week double-blind, placebo-controlled trial. *Obes Res* 2002; 10: 633–41.

96. Dale LC, Schroeder DR, Wolter TD, Croghan IT, Hurt RD, Offord KP. Weight change after smoking cessation using variable doses of transdermal nicotine replacement. *J Gen Intern Med* 1998; 13: 9–15.
97. Danielsson T, Rossner S, Westin A. Open randomised trial of intermittent very low energy diet together with nicotine gum for stopping smoking in women who gained weight in previous attempts to quit. *BMJ* 1999; 319: 490–4.
98. Astrup A, Breum L, Toubro S, Hein P, Quaade F. The effect and safety of an ephedrine/caffeine compound compared to ephedrine, caffeine and placebo in obese subjects on an energy restricted diet. A double blind trial. *Int J Obes* 1992; 16: 269–77.
99. Breum L, Pedersen JK, Ahlstrom F, Frimodt-Moller J. Comparison of an ephedrine/caffeine combination and dexfenfluramine in the treatment of obesity. A double-blind multi-centre trial in general practice. *Int J Obes* 1994; 18: 99–103.
100. Norregaard J, Jorgensen S, Mikkelsen KL, Tonnesen P, Iversen E, Sorensen T, Soeberg B, Jakobsen HB. The effect of ephedrine plus caffeine on smoking cessation and postcessation weight gain. *Clin Pharmacol Ther* 1996; 60 (6): 679–86.
101. Molnar D. Effects of ephedrine and aminophylline on resting energy expenditure in obese adolescents. *Int J Obes Metab Disord* 2000; 24: 1573–8.
102. Astrup A, Toubro S. Thermogenic, metabolic and cardiovascular responses to ephedrine and caffeine in man. *Int J Obes* 1993; 17: S41–3.
103. Waluga M. Janusz M, Karpel E, Hartleb M, Nowak A. Cardiovascular effects of ephedrine, caffeine and yohimbine measured by thoracic electrical bioimpedance in obese women. *Clin Physiol* 1998; 18: 69–76.
104. Svendsen TL, Ingerslev J, Mork A. Is Letigen contraindicated in hypertension? A double-blind, placebo controlled multipractice study of Letigen administered to normotensive and adequately treated patients with hypersensitivity. *Ugeskr Laeger* 1998; 160: 4073–5.
105. Buemann B, Astrup A, Marckmann P, Christensen NJ. The effect of ephedrine + caffeine on plasma lipids and lipoproteins during a 4.2-MJ/d diet. *Int J Obes* 1994; 18: 329–32.
106. Greenway FL. The safety and efficacy of pharmaceutical and herbal caffeine and ephedrine use as a weight loss agent. *Obes Rev* 2001; 2: 199–211.
107. Albrecht RJ, Pories WJ. Surgical intervention for the severely obese. *Bailliéres Clin Endocrinol Metab* 1999; 13: 149–72.
108. Pories WJ, Swanson MS, MacDonald KG, Long SB, Morris PG, Brown BM, Barakat HA, deRamon RA, Israel G, Dolezal JM, et al. Who would have thought it? An operation proves to be the most effective therapy for adult-onset diabetes mellitus. *Ann Surg*. 1995 September; 222 (3): 339–52.
109. Torgerson JS, Sjostrom L. The Swedish Obese Subjects (SOS) study—rationale and results. *Int J Obes Relat Metab Disord* 2001; 25 (suppl 1): S2–4.
110. Lean ME, Powrie JK, Anderson AS, Garthwaite PH. Obesity, weight loss and prognosis in type 2 diabetes. *Diabet Med* 1990; 7: 228–33.
111. MacDonald KG Jr, Long SD, Swanson MS, Brown BM, Morris P, Dohm GL, Pories WJ. The gastric bypass operation reduces the progression and mortality of non-insulin-dependent diabetes mellitus. *J Gastrointest Surg* 1997; 1: 213–20.
112. Evans JD, Scott MH, Brown AS, Rogers J. Laparoscopic adjustable gastric banding for the treatment of morbid obesity. *Am J Surg* 2002; 184: 97–102.
113. Pontiroli AE, Pizzocri P, Librenti MC, Vedani P, Marchi M, Cucchi E, Orena C, Paganelli M, Giacomelli M, Ferla G, Folli F. Laparoscopic adjustable gastric banding for the treatment of morbid (grade 3) obesity and its metabolic complications: a three-year study. *J Clin Endocrinol Metab* 2002; 87: 3555–61.
114. Pinkney JH, Sjostrom CD, Gale EA. Should surgeons treat diabetes in severely obese people? *Lancet* 2001; 357: 1357–9.

37

Animal Models of Obesity

David A. York

Louisiana State University, Baton Rouge, LA, USA

INTRODUCTION

Until the recent past, the animal models that were available for the study of obesity either were of spontaneous origin or were the result of experimental manipulation of the environment or the hypothalamic centers that regulate food intake and energy balance [1]. Over the last few years, there has been an explosion in the number of animal models available for studying the development of obesity and its comorbidities. This has resulted from the use of transgenic and gene-targeting approaches for proof of function of genes, some of which were thought to alter energy balance from prior knowledge of the gene but many of which had no previous known function on energy balance. Indeed, body weight change on a high-fat diet has become a standard phenotype to investigate for all new transgenic and gene knockout studies. These new models have complemented the information that has been gained over several decades from the studies of the spontaneous single gene mutation obesities, the experimental hypothalamic models, and from various dietary and endocrine manipulations [1].

Table 1 summarizes the wide range of genes that have now been shown to alter some aspects of energy balance: either food intake, energy expenditure, or substrate partitioning; physical activity; tissue metabolism; or adipose tissue differentiation. They include the genes for a range of hormones and peptides, receptors, transcriptional regulators, metabolic and structural genes, and others. These models have provided new insight into the complexity of the systems that regulate food intake, energy balance, and energy partitioning. Further important developments have come from the identity of the genes responsible for the spontaneous obesities of the obese mouse (leptin), the diabetes mouse, the fatty and koletsky rats (the leptin receptor), the tubby mouse (tub protein), and the fat mouse (carboxypeptidase E). The wide range of genes that have been shown to alter the susceptibility to develop obesity emphasize the multicausational nature of this disease.

To provide an overview of the many rodent models of obesity that are now available, they have been subdivided into loose etiological subgroups according to the function of the responsible gene. The reader should recognize that, for several models, there is significant overlap in the function of the gene product that would have allowed a specific model to be included in a number of groups.

ENDOCRINE MODELS

Genes of the Leptin Signaling Pathway

Mutations in both the leptin gene and the leptin receptor gene underlie the phenotype of three single gene obesity models. The obese mouse (lep^{ob}/lep^{ob}) inherits its obesity as a result of a C428T mutation of the leptin gene, which changes an arginine codon (CGA) to a stop codon (TGA) at codon 105, resulting in a shortened nonfunctional product [2]. Despite very high levels of expression of the lep^{ob} gene in adipose tissue of the lep^{ob}/lep^{ob} mouse, no leptin can be detected in the serum of these mice. A second mutation ob^{2j}/ob^{2j} has been mapped 7 kb upstream of the 4.5 kb ob RNA start site and is assumed to be the result of a structural alteration or a mutation in the promoter region.

As predicted from the classical parabiotic studies of Coleman [3] and Hervey et al. [4], the mutations responsible for the obesity phenotype of the diabetes mouse ($lepr^{db}/lepr^{db}$) and the Zucker fatty rat ($lepr^{fa}/lepr^{fa}$) are both in the leptin receptor. The long intracellular signaling domain of the leptin receptor is not translated

International Textbook of Diabetes Mellitus, Third Edition. Edited by R. A. DeFronzo, E. Ferrannini, H. Keen, and P. Zimmet.
 ISBN: 0-471-48655-8.

Table 1 Natural genetic, transgenic, and gene knockout models of obesity

Gene for	Name	Position (Chr, cM)	Natural (N), transgenic (Tg), or knockout (KO)	Comment	Effect
Endocrine models					
Leptin	*Lep*	6, 10.5	N	Obese mouse	Severe early-onset obesity
Leptin receptor	*Lepr*	4, 46.7	N	Diabetes mouse, fatty and Koletsky rats	Severe early-onset obesity
GRII antisense			Tg		Cushingoid-type obesity
GRII	*Nr3c1*	18, 20	KO	Targeted to brain	Cushingoid-type obesity
Insulin receptor	*Insr*	8, 1	KO	Neuron specific knockout	Obesity on a high-fat diet
Tub protein	*tub*	7, 51.45	N	Tubby mouse	Slow, late-onset development of obesity
CCK_A	*Cckar*	5, 34	KO		Natural – OLETF rats
Growth hormone	*Gh*	11, 65	KO		Obese "little" mice
Growth hormone	*Gh*	11,65	Tg	On metallothionein promoter	Cessation of expression leads to obesity
GHRH	*Ghrh*	2, 89	Tg		Obesity despite increased GH levels
CRH	*Crh*	3, 8	Tg	Metallothionein promoter	Cushingoid-type obesity
CRH binding protein	*Crhbp*	13, 52	Tg	Metallothionein promoter	Sexually dimorphic obesity
Aromatase	*Cyp19*	9, 31	KO		Increase in intraabdominal adipose tissue
11-β-hydroxysteroid dehydrogenase 1	*Hsd11b1*	1, syntenic	Tg	aP2 promoter	Central adiposity and syndrome X characteristics
Amylin	*Iapp*	6, 62	KO		Increase in body weight and fat
CCK_A receptor	*Cckar*	Unknown	N		OLETF rats become obese
Central nervous system models					
Agouti	*a*	2, 89	N and Tg	N-Yellow mouse; Tg on β-actin promoter	Severe obesity, Tg reproduces obesity syndrome of A^y/a mice
AgRP	*Agrp*	8	Tg	β-Actin promoter	Obesity without coat color changes
POMC	*Pomc*	12, 4	KO		Obesity
7B2	*Sgne1*	2, 64	KO	Necessary for synthesis of proconvertase 2	Cushingoid-type of obesity
MC3 receptor	*Mc3r*	2, 100	KO		Obesity without hyperphagia, hyperactivity
MC4 receptor	*Mc4r*	Unknown	KO		Hyperphagia and obesity
MC3/MC4			KO	Double knockout	Greater obesity than MC3 or MC4 knockouts
Syndecan 1	*Sdc1*	12, 1	Tg		Maturity-onset obesity that resembles agouti-related obesity
NPY1 receptor	*Npy1r*	8, 33	KO		Mild obesity with aging
NPY2 receptor	*Npy2r*	3, 36	KO		Obesity on high-fat diets
NPY5 receptor	*Npy5r*	8, 32.5	KO		Mild obesity with aging
MCH	*Pmch*	10, 47	Tg		Obesity on a high-fat diet; KO is lean
Bombesin receptor subtype 3 (BRS-3)	*Grpr*	X, 70	KO		Mild obesity, hypertension, and glucose intolerance
CRH	*Crh*	3, 8	Tg	Metallothionein, promoter	Cushingoid-type obesity
CRH binding protein	*Crhbp*	13, 52	Tg	Metallothionein, promoter	Sexually dimorphic obesity
Histamine H1	*H1r*	6, 49	KO		Increased weight gain on a high-fat diet
5HT2C	*Htr2c*	X, 66.15	KO		Obese on high-fat diet/attenuates response to D-fenfluramine
GABA transporter I	*Gabt1*	3, 50.4	Tg		Obesity with altered feeding patterns
Carboxypeptidase E	*Cpe*	8,	N		Fat mouse
Nhlh2	*Nhlh2*	3, syntenic	KO		Obesity at 10–15 weeks of age

Table 1 (*continued*)

Gene for	Name	Position (Chr, cM)	Natural (N), transgenic (Tg), or knockout (KO)	Comment	Effect
Adipose tissue models					
PPARα	*Ppara*	15, 48.8	KO		Sexually dimorphic late-onset obesity
Hormone-sensitive lipase	*Lipe*	7, 5.5	KO		Normal body weight, increased fat cell size but increased BAT mass
aP2	*Fabp4*	6, 56	KO	Fatty acid binding protein	Obesity when fed a high-fat diet
Glut4	*Slc2a4*	11, 40	Tg	Effect depends upon promoter used	Obesity on normal and high-fat diets
Acyl-CoA:diacylglycerol acyl transferase	*Dgat*		KO		KO has low body fat but gains excess fat on a high-fat diet
Gsα	*Gnas*	2, 104	KO	Homozygous lethal	Heterozygote with maternal null allele obese, paternal null allele lean
UCP1-Dta			KO	UCP1 promoter linked to diptheria toxin chain	Obesity and hyerphagia
Agouti	*a*	2, 89	Tg	On aP2 promotor	Mild obesity and increased sensitivity to insulin
Other models					
Glutamine:fructose-6-phosphate amino transferase	*Gfpt1*	6, 35.5	Tg	Increased hepatic exosamine flux	Obesity and insulin resistance in older mice
Metallothionein I and II	*Mt*	8, 45	KO		Moderate obesity and hyperphagia
ICAM-1	*Icam1*	9, 7	KO		Late-onset obesity

Note. References to all these models can be found within the text.

in $lepr^{db}/lepr^{db}$ mice since a G→T mutation [5] introduces a novel consensus splice donor site (AGGGAAA sequence to an AGGTAAA sequence). As a result of this mutation a 106 base sequence of the terminal exon of the short form of the receptor is spliced into the long form of the receptor mRNA. This introduces a stop codon that prevents translation of the long intracellular domain of the receptor. In contrast, the mutations in the Zucker rat [6] and the Koletsky rat [7] are both in the extracellular domain of the leptin receptor; in the $lepr^{fa}/lepr^{fa}$ rat an A880C (Gln269Pro) mutation reduces the localization of the receptor in the cell membrane [8] whereas in the Koletsky rats a T2349A nonsense mutation results in no expression of the gene [7].

It is thus not surprising that all these animals share a similar phenotype, the variation appearing to result mainly from the background genome on which the mutation is expressed. The phenotype is of an early-onset form of obesity associated with hyperphagia, impaired sympathetic activation of brown adipose tissue (BAT) thermogenesis and an enhanced insulin secretory activity, overactivity of the hypothalamic–pituitary–adrenal axis, decreased growth hormone secretion and stunted growth, impaired thyroid hormone metabolism, and infertility, together with some immune function deficits. The reader is referred to a previous review for a fuller description [9]. The phenotype of $lepr^{db}/lepr^{db}$ mice can be partially corrected by transgenic expression of the long form, but not the short form, of the leptin receptor [10].

The severity and temporal characteristics of diabetes varies with the background strain in these obese mice models; hyperglycemia and hypertension are significant phenotypic variations across the rat mutations with strain. By introducing the Koletsky gene (fa^{cp}) onto an inbred strain of rats derived from the hypertensive Okamoto strain (SHR/N) and further crossing onto other strains, e.g. LA/N, a variety of strains exhibiting various aspects of the syndrome X metabolic profile have been developed [11]. By transferring the $lepr^{fa}$ gene from its Brown-Norway background strain, on which diabetes is normally absent, to other backgrounds, long-lasting severe diabetes may become characteristic, e.g. Zucker diabetic fatty (ZDF/Drt-fa), the Wistar Kyoto fatty (WKY/NDrt-fa), or the Wistar Kyoto diabetic (WDF/TA-fa). Transgene insertion to prevent the expression of the long form of the leptin receptor in an outbred strain of mice led to wide divergence in the diabetes phenotype and provides another model for studies of the interactions of the leptin system with the background genome [12].

The other major difference across these models is the obvious one that those with mutations in the leptin receptor are partially or totally resistant to the effects of leptin whereas the obese mouse has a supersensitivity to exogenous leptin [13–15]. Treatment of the lep^{ob}/lep^{ob} mouse

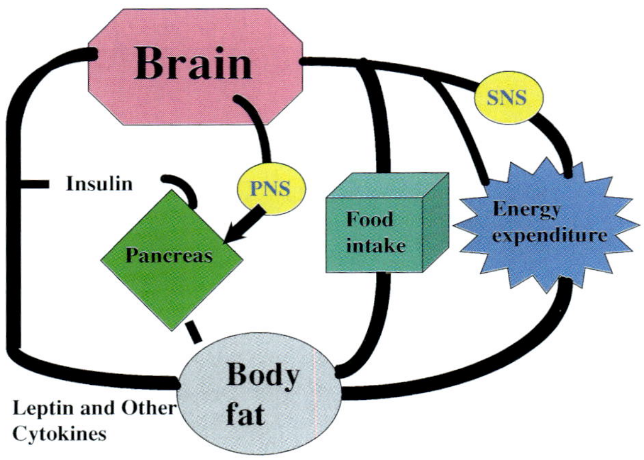

Figure 1 Leptin regulation of arcuate nucleus activity

with leptin reverses all of the phenotypic characteristics, reducing body fat, food intake, insulin secretion, and corticosterone levels and restoring sympathetic activity and BAT thermogenesis to yield a lean mouse that is also fertile [13–15]. Likewise, transgenic overexpression of leptin in normal mice leads to a very lean animal [16].

Leptin receptors are expressed in several regions of the brain, but most importantly for energy balance on the proopiomelanocortin/neuropeptide Y (POMC/NPY) and agouti-related protein/cocaine–amphetamine-related transcript (AgRP/CART) neurons in the arcuate nucleus (Figure 1). These neurons project to the paraventricular nucleus (PVN) and to the lateral hypothalamic melanin-concentrating hormone (MCH) and orexin neurons through which the leptin effects in modulating feeding and the autonomic nervous system are modulated. Several natural mutations and numerous experimental gene manipulations have been used for proof of function of these components. They are described in more detail under The Melanocortin Pathway.

Insulin

Insulin has also been shown to affect food intake and body weight through actions in the central nervous system (CNS), affecting similar signaling pathways to leptin. While diabetic mice are hyperphagic and show a preference for dietary fat, the physiological role of insulin in regulating food intake and energy expenditure has received less attention. However, its potential importance has been emphasized by the neuron-specific knockout of the insulin receptor. These mice become obese when given a high-fat diet and develop mild insulin resistance and hypertriglyceridemia. Hyperphagia was only evident in female mice [17].

The importance of insulin sensitivity in muscle for the prevention of obesity is emphasized by the observation that transgenic overexpression of dominant-negative insulin receptors in muscle, which causes muscle insulin resistance, results in a major increase in body fat (22–38%) and a loss of lean body mass [18].

Tubby (*tub/tub*) Mouse

The tubby mutation was first reported by Coleman and Eicher in 1990 [19]. It is an autosomal recessive mutation on mouse chromosome 7 in the gene coding for the tubby protein, one of a family of four proteins that also includes TULPs 1–3. A characteristic of these proteins is the ~260-amino acid domain at the carboxyl terminus that forms a helix barrel structure that binds avidly to DNA. The tubby mutation introduces a splice site at the junction of the 3′-coding sequence that leads to the loss of this carboxyl terminus domain [20]. Knockout of tub confirmed that the tubby gene mutation is a loss of function mutation [21].

The wild-type tub protein is expressed in the hypothalamus and other brain regions where it is localized to plasma membranes, released by activation of Gαq protein, and translocated into the nucleus [22]. This process may be activated by 5HT2c receptor activity. Studies of Chinese hamster ovary (CHO) cells expressing the human insulin receptor have shown an insulin-dependent phosphorylation of tyrosine residues on the tub protein. This has led to the suggestion that tub acts as an adapter protein linking the insulin receptor to protein tyrosine kinases and may function as part of a neural insulin signaling mechanism [23].

On the C57BL/6J background, Tubby mice are phenotypically very similar to 5HT2c receptor knockout mice and to fat mice, except that the obesity in fat mice develops more slowly, not being visually apparent until 9–12 weeks of age. All fat depots are enlarged. The tub mutation is associated with distinct sexual dimorphism in blood glucose, serum insulin, islet hypertrophy and hyperplasia, and β-cell degranulation, all changes being more pronounced in male mice. The hyperinsulinemia, mild at weaning, progressively increases with age. Morphological changes in the pancreatic islets occur earlier and are more pronounced in males. However, the tub mice remain mildly hypoglycemic, indicating the absence of the pronounced insulin resistance common to other mouse models of obesity. This insulin resistance appears to be centrally expressed since NPY mRNA levels are massively elevated in tubby mice [24]. Infertility is also a feature of this mouse when severe obesity develops.

Amylin

Amylin is a 361-amino acid protein cosecreted with insulin from pancreatic β-cells. It has been shown to have multiple effects including suppression of food intake and inhibition of gastric emptying. Amylin knockout mice of both sexes show an approximate 20% increase in body weight and body fat [25].

Growth Hormone

Both overexpression and knockout approaches have been used to study the effects of growth hormone (GH) on energy balance and body composition. GH deficiency, as in "little" mice, is associated with decreased somatic growth but increased body fat [26] despite normophagia (per gram body weight). In contrast, overexpression of GH is associated with increased somatic growth and decreased body fat [27], which has been related to a severe insulin resistance of adipose tissue [28]. Overexpression of an ovine GH transgene driven by a metallothionein promoter [29] leads as expected to larger mice. However, when expression of this transgene is switched off by removal of dietary zinc, significant obesity results, suggesting downstream effects in the GH pathway. Overexpression of growth hormone-releasing hormone (GHRH), which results in elevated GH levels, results in hyperphagic mice of increased body mass but unexpectedly also increased body fat [30]. The reason for the increased body fat is unclear but may be related to a dysregulation of the leptin receptor system in the hypothalamus.

The Carticotropin Releasing Hormone/ Urocortin-Glucocorticoid System

In addition to a role in regulation of pituitary–adrenal function, Carticotropin Releasing Hormone (CRH) and urocortin inhibit food intake and promote energy expenditure, particularly the sympathetically mediated BAT thermogenesis. Numerous models, targeting specific components of this system, have identified their ability to alter homeostasis. These models generally produce a cushingoid-type of central adiposity. The models include the transgenic overexpression of antisense cDNA to the brain type II glucocorticoid receptor (GR) [31], knockout of the brain type II GR, and transgenic expression of CRH [32]. The concentration of free CRH in the CNS is affected by the levels of the CRH-binding protein. Knockout of this gene results in a hypophagic small mouse whereas overexpression regulated by the metallothionein promoter caused obesity [33, 34]. Despite these effects, knockout of CRH1 and CRH2 receptors does not have any major phenotypic effects on body weight or food intake although the response to exogenous urocortin or CRH may be absent or diminished [35, 36].

A mouse model of syndrome X has been developed by the transgenic overexpression of 11β-hydroxysteroid dehydrogenase 1 (11-βHSD1) in adipose tissue [37]. This enzyme converts cortisone (humans) or 11-dehydrocorticosterone (rodents) into their active glucocorticoid forms of cortisol or corticosterone respectively. The increased adipose tissue production of corticosterone resulted in a visceral form of obesity that was further enhanced by high-fat diets. The mice were hyperglycemic, insulin resistant, hyperlipidemic, and hypertensive, the latter probably resulting from the resultant overexpression of angiotensinogen in the adipose tissue of the transgenic mice. The obesity was associated with a small increase in food intake, decreased BAT thermogenesis, and an enhanced partitioning of lipid into adipose tissue through lipoprotein lipase.

Gut Hormones

Cholecystokinin (CCK) is expressed both in the gastrointestinal (GI) tract and in the CNS. When given both peripherally and centrally, CCK inhibits food intake through actions mediated by CCK_A receptors [38]. A natural mutation that prevents the expression of CCK_A receptors has been identified in OLETF rats [39]. These are hyperphagic and heavier than the wild-type LETO rats. Further they fail to suppress food intake normally in response to a dietary supplement of fat [40]. In contrast, knockout of CCK_A receptors in mice does not appear to have any effects on energy balance [41].

Gastric inhibitory polypeptide (GIP), a hormone secreted by the duodenum in response to dietary fat, appears to be necessary for obesity to develop on this type of diet. Mice null for the GIP receptor ($Gipr^{-/-}$) are resistant to this form of obesity and do not develop insulin resistance, possibly because of their increased propensity to oxidize fatty acids [42]. In addition, the loss of GIP function protects mice from the effects of leptin deficiency.

Sex Steroids

Estrogens have been recognized to have significant effects in feeding behavior. Knockout of the estradiol α-receptor or the aromatase gene (responsible for conversion of C19 steroids to estrogen) is associated with increased adiposity, which appears to develop after the onset of puberty and also be associated with a decrease in energy expenditure rather than hyperphagia [43–45]. Similarly, knockout of the fillicle follicle stimulating hormone (FSH) receptor, which causes severe estrogen deficiency from an early age, induces obesity and skeletal abnormalities that give a hunchback appearance to the mice [46].

CNS MODELS

The neurochemical explanations for the hyperphagia and obesity that results from lesions of the VMH (ventromedial hypothalamus) and the PVN and for the aphagia and leanness that follows lesions of the lateral hypothalamus [1] have become apparent during the last few years. Studies with these models have illustrated the inextricable links between regulation of feeding behavior and autonomic regulation of peripheral metabolism and endocrine activity. The effects of these lesions may now be mimicked by infusions of specific neuropeptides or manipulations of the expression of specific genes. This provides the functional neurochemical links to the anatomical circuitry that had been previously identified. Much of the recent work has focused on the hypothalamic arcuate–PVN and lateral hypothalamic axes, particularly as they relate to the regulation of energy balance by leptin and insulin. The mechanisms through which endocrine, e.g. insulin and leptin, manipulations alter feeding behavior and body composition are also now becoming clearer as their interactions with the central neuropeptide circuits within the arcuate–PVN–lateral hypothalamic axes are identified.

Within the CNS, natural or experimental genetic changes that alter expression of neuropeptides, receptors for neuropeptides or aminergic transmitters, signaling proteins, processing enzymes, or transcriptional regulators have all been shown to affect body composition. The leptin receptor mutation has already been described (see under Genes of the Leptin Signaling Pathway) but others related to the CNS are discussed in the following sections.

The Melanocortin Pathway

The agouti gene of the Yellow (A^y/a) obese mouse was the first single gene mutation for obesity to be identified in mice (see reference 1 for review). The Yellow (A^y/a) obese mouse and the KK mouse [47] discussed below are the only models of dominant inheritance of obesity described so far. The obesity of the yellow mouse is inherited as a mutation in the agouti protein coded on chromosome 2 and is associated with moderate obesity and a high incidence of tumor growth. Although the homozygous (A^y/A^y) mouse is lethal *in utero*, there are a number of different alleles (A^{vy}/A^{vy}, A^{iy}/A^{iy}) at the agouti locus in which the defects are less severe and in which the degree of obesity is linked directly to the level of yellow pigmentation in the coat [48]. The obesity of the yellow mice is less pronounced than that of the obese and diabetic mice and is of later onset (8–12 weeks of age). While these animals share many of the characteristics common to all rodent obesities, they do differ in the clear sexual dimorphism of the associated hyperglycemia [49] and in the apparently normal activity of the hypothalamic–pituitary–adrenal axis [49, 50].

The agouti gene (a) encodes a 131-amino acid protein that is normally uniquely expressed in the hair follicle where it acts to inhibit eumelanin synthesis in response to stimulation by α-melanophore-stimulating hormone (α-MSH). In the yellow mouse, exon 1 of the agouti gene is replaced by a unique sequence but exons 2–4 that contain the full coding sequence are normal. The result of this mutation is the ubiquitous expression of the agouti gene in a wide range of tissues, including white adipose tissue and brain [51]. Transgenic mice expressing agouti unregulated and ubiquitously driven by the human β-actin promoter also develop yellow coat color and become obese [52, 53], confirming that ectopic expression of normal agouti protein results in the obese yellow phenotype.

Two potential actions of agouti protein have been identified. Its ability to increase intracellular calcium levels may promote insulin resistance [54]. Intracellular calcium levels are related to the level of expression of agouti protein and to body weight and degree of coat color. Using a murine melanoma cell line, Lu et al. [55] were able to demonstrate that agouti protein inhibited the stimulation of adenylyl cyclase by α-MSH, shifting the dose required for half-maximal stimulation from 1.7 to 13.4 nM by acting as a potent antagonist of the melanocortin-4 (MC4) receptor. However, agouti had no effects on MC1, MC2, MC3, or MC5 receptors.

Studies of the Yellow obese syndrome (A^y/a, A^{vy}/a, etc.) led to the identification of the important role of α-MSH, an anorectic peptide [56] derived from the precursor POMC, and the antagonist AgRP peptide as the major regulators of this system [57–60] that affects feeding behavior, energy expenditure, and insulin secretion. Several genetic models have been used to illustrate the functionality of this system. Transgenic mice ectopically expressing agouti recapitulate the obese yellow syndrome of the A^y/a mouse [53]. Likewise expression of the hypothalamic homologue protein AgRP produces a similar obesity but without the coat color changes associated with antagonism of the MC1 receptor [61] (Figure 2). α-MSH, a product cleaved from the POMC precursor protein, is an agonist for all melanocortin receptors except MC2. Knockout of the precursor POMC gene produces obesity [62]. The effect of α-MSH on energy balance appears to result from actions at both the MC4 and MC3 receptors. MC4 receptor knockout mice

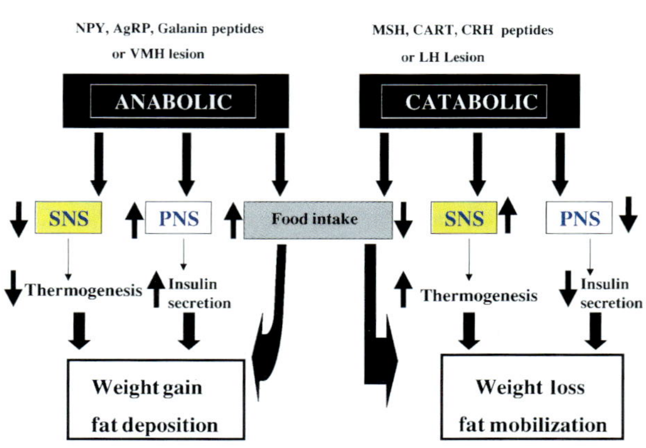

Figure 2 Actions of agouti and agouti-related peptide on melanocortin receptors. LH = lateral hypothalamus

[63] are hyperphagic and obese whereas MC3 receptor knockout mice become obese in the absence of significant hyperphagia [64], while exhibiting decreased locomotor activity and an atypical increase in respiratory quotient on a high-fat diet [65]. These observations suggest that α-MSH may primarily inhibit feeding through MC4 receptors and enhance energy expenditure and influence energy partitioning through MC3 receptors. Indeed, the double knockout $Mc3r^{-/-}/Mc4r^{-/-}$ becomes more obese than either of the individual receptor knockouts.

Neural tracing and immunohistochemical approaches have been used to identify the functional neuroanatomy of the melanocortin system. Two subsets of neurons in the arcuate nucleus, co-expressing either POMC and CART or NPY and AGRP, send axonal projections to both the PVN and lateral hypothalamus to synapse with cell bodies that express either MC3 or MC4 receptors and may regulate secretion of MCH and orexin (Figure 1). The presence of leptin receptors on the arcuate POMC and AgRP neurons provides the link between leptin, the melanocortin system, feeding behavior, and energy expenditure. Of all the animal models, the natural mutations and the experimental manipulations of this melanocortin system appear to be most relevant to human obesity where a number of mutations have also been linked to severe obesity and changes in hair color [66, 67].

In addition to the agouti mutation, two other genes—mahogany (*mg*) and mahoginoid (*md*) [68]—have effects on both body weight and coat color. Several mutations have been identified at the *mg* locus, giving total or partial loss of function, but, to date, only a single *md* mutation has been reported. The phenotypes of these mutant animals are similar, although the degree of obesity is variable. Both *md* and *mg* mutations inhibit agouti-related obesity and its associated changes in linear growth and insulin secretion, but do not alter the hyperphagia. *mg* and *md* (*Atrn*) mutations appear to enhance food intake and *mg* also increases physical activity.

Mahogany, a transmembrane protein, is a member of the Attractin (*Atrn*) gene family [69]. It is expressed widely in the CNS, including the major regions known to be important for the regulation of energy balance [70], but its site of action is unknown although it is thought to act upstream of the MC4 and MC1 receptors.

The Syndecans

Syndecans are a family of cell surface heparin sulfate proteoglycans that show differential tissue distribution. The extracellular domains of the syndecans are released from the cell surface and may act as either positive or negative paracrine regulators. Transgenic overexpression of Syndecan I (*Sdc*1) using the cytomegalovirus (CMV) promoter [71] led to a maturity-onset type of obesity that was phenotypically very similar to the obesities associated with agouti or agouti-related protein. Reizes et al. [71] propose that the released ectodomains of the syndecans modulate the interactions between α-MSH and agouti-related protein with the MC4 receptor, and that the hypothalamic Syndecan III levels are physiological modulators of feeding behavior.

The NPY System

Neuropeptide Y is recognized as the most powerful orexigenic peptide yet to be identified. Physiological and pharmacological evidence supports a role for NPY in the regulation of feeding behavior. However, experimental genetic manipulations of the NPY system have failed to show that it is essential for normal feeding. Recently, however, *Npy* knockout mice have been shown to have an attenuated response to fasting [72]. When *ob*/*ob* mice are made $Npy^{-/-}$ there is an attenuation of the level of obesity [73]. However $Npy^{-/-}$ mice grow normally and knockout of NPY1, NPY2, and NPY5 receptors does not attenuate food intake or weight gain as would have been predicted from pharmacological studies. Indeed, surprisingly, both NPY1- and NPY5-receptor-deficient mice develop a mild obesity with aging, and NPY2-receptor-deficient mice become obese when provided with a high-fat diet.

Melanin-concentrating Hormone

This peptide is synthesized in lateral hypothalamic neurons that are innervated by POMC/CART or NPY/AgRP axons from the arcuate nucleus. Although MCH has only a modest orexigenic effect when given intracerebroventricularly, *Mch* knockout mice have reduced body weight and are hypophagic and lean [74]. Absence of MCH release could explain the effects of lateral hypothalamic lesions. In contrast, transgenic overexpression of MCH increases body weight of mice fed a chow diet and induces obesity in mice fed a high-fat diet [75].

Orexin

Orexin is also expressed in the lateral hypothalamus. While orexin appears to have moderate orexigenic effects, mutations in this receptor appear to be related to narcolepsy [76], suggesting that orexin has a primary role in arousal rather than energy homeostatis. However, ablation of orexigenic neurons by specific expression of a truncated Machado-Joseph disease product Ataxin-3 produced a late-onset obesity in addition to a narcoleptic phenotype [77].

Bombesin

Bombesin is one member of a family of peptides that are also expressed widely in the CNS and GI tract. They inhibit food intake and stimulate sympathetic-related energy expenditure. Of the three receptors identified, the bombesin-receptor subtype 3 (BRS-3) appears to be important for energy balance since BRS-3 knockout mice develop mild obesity, hypertension, and impaired glucose tolerance [78].

Serotonergic Receptors

The anorectic response of 5HT is diminished in both 5HT2c and 5HT1b receptor knockout mice. This suggests that both receptor subtypes are necessary for this activity. The 5HT2c knockout mice become obese with age and show a greater sensitivity to high-fat diets than wild-type mice but 5HT1bR knockout mice have normal body weight [79, 80].

Histamine

Histamine appears to be an important neurotransmitter for feeding behavior. Knockout of the H1 receptor has no effect in mice fed a regular chow diet, but is associated with excessive weight gain on a high-fat diet and a reduced response to intracerebroventricular leptin [81].

Acetylcholine

Acetylcholine is widely distributed in the central and autonomic nervous systems. Mice that are deficient in the M3 muscarinic receptors are hypophagic and have a reduced body weight [82].

γ-Aminobutyric Acid

γ-Aminobutyric acid (GABA) is a major inhibitory neurotransmitter within the CNS. Ubiquitous overexpression of the GABA transporter I gene caused a moderate obesity that was characterized by an altered feeding pattern and a small reduction in physical activity [83].

Processing Enzymes

Carboxypeptidase E

Mutations in carboxypeptidase E, a peptide processing enzyme, also cause obesity, but of the late-onset form [19]. The obesity may be severe (60–70 g body weight at 24 weeks) and is expressed in all adipose depots. In this mutant the obesity is not normally evident until 8–12 weeks of age and is not pronounced until 16–20 weeks of age. The fat mouse is characterized by massive hyperproinsulinemia and normal insulin [84] without significant hyperglycemia from weaning, but does not display the pancreatic failure and severe diabetes that are evident in older lep^{ob}/lep^{ob} and $lepr^{db}/lepr^{db}$ mice [19]. When the mutation is transferred to the C57BLKS/J(HKS) background strain the *fat/fat* mouse is diabetic but the diabetes is still less severe than that seen with lep^{ob}/lep^{ob} and $lepr^{db}/lepr^{db}$ mice on the same background. Indeed, the mouse remains extremely sensitive to exogenous insulin.

The fat gene located on chromosome 8 codes for carboxypeptidase E [84]. A single base mutation that results in a ser202pro substitution severely reduces or completely abolishes the activity of carboxypeptidase E in the pancreatic islet, hypothalamus, pituitary, GI tract, and other tissues [85]. Immunoreactive carboxypeptidase E protein is undetectable in pancreas and pituitary of *fat/fat* mice, suggesting that the mutation affects either transcriptional or translational activity or stability of the mRNA or protein.

Carboxypeptidase E (also known as carboxypeptidase H) is required for cleavage of two arginine residues from the B-chain of insulin during its processing from proinsulin. The impairment in enzyme activity in Cpe^{fat}/Cpe^{fat} mice explains their 10-fold increased proinsulin to insulin ratios in the pancreas and the very high level of proinsulin rather than insulin in the circulation. The obesity, however, results from the role of carboxypeptidase E in the posttranslational processing of numerous neuropeptides (including POMC) to α-MSH, β-endorphin and β-lipotropin, proenkephalins, preproNPY, vasopressin, oxytocin, gastrin, and CCK. While Naggert et al. [84] suggest that the obesity of Cpe^{fat}/Cpe^{fat} mouse is likely to result from a complex pattern of alterations in neuropeptide activity and secretion within the hypothalamic–pituitary system rather than the hyperproinsulinemia, it is not surprising that it has many similarities to the obesity of the MC4 receptor knockout mouse [86].

The 7B2 Gene (Sgne1)

Knockout of this gene, which prevents the production of proconvertase 2 that is responsible for cleavage of ACTH and α-MSH, produces an obesity phenotype as might be expected [87].

Nhlh2

This transcription factor gene is expressed in neural tissue particularly in those hypothalamic areas that have been implicated in the regulation of energy balance, the arcuate nucleus, ventomedial, and lateral hypothalamus. Both homozygous and heterozygous knockout mice develop a severe maturity-onset obesity, yet do not develop diabetes on the 129 × C56BL/6J background.

Hypothalamic Damage

It has long been recognized that destruction of or damage to the VMH is associated with the development of obesity in a wide range of animal species including mice, rats, dogs, nonhuman primates, and humans [88, 89]. While the original studies suggested that the hyperphagia associated with major lesions in this area was the primary cause of the obesity, subsequent studies in weanling rats [90] and with chemically induced lesions [91–93] (see below) indicated that the hyperphagia was not necessary and was only evident when the lesions extended beyond the VMN, probably damaging the ventral noradrenergic bundle (VNAB) input to the PVN [94]. Lesions to the VNAB cause mild hyperphagia [95] but none of the other changes in feeding behavior normally associated with VMH lesions [96].

VMH lesions can be caused by electrical, chemical (gold thioglucose, bipiperidyl mustard, monosodium glutamate, ibotenic acid), or viral (scrapie and coxassie virus) routes. Bipiperidyl mustard damages the VMH and dorsal vagal complex to produce obesity without hyperphagia [90, 97], whereas monosodium glutamate, which damages the arcuate nucleus, induces hyperinsulinemia and obesity without hyperphagia [97, 98]. When these drugs are combined the full hypothalamic syndrome of hyperphagia, hyperinsulinemia, and obesity is produced [98]. However, ibotenic acid, which only damages neuronal cell bodies, does produce the full syndrome of hyperphagia and obesity after injection into the VMH [99]. Thus, there appear to be two distinct syndromes of hypothalamic obesity. Damage restricted to the VMN normally produces obesity without hyperphagia as a result of changes in autonomic control of thermogenesis and insulin. In contrast, damage to neural pathways innervating the PVN or to the PVN itself predominantly causes a hyperphagic syndrome that may be related to changes in the melanocortin and/or NPY pathways (Figure 3).

Electrical lesions of the PVN or selective knife cuts in the hypothalamus may also induce an immediate increase in food intake and rapid development of severe obesity [88, 89, 100, 101]. Unlike VMH obesity, PVN obesity is prevented by restriction of food intake [100]. These studies suggest that damage to the arcuate–PVN

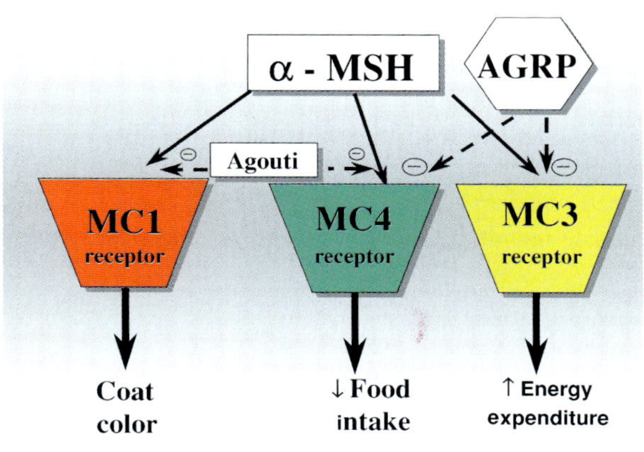

Figure 3 Neuropeptides and hypothalamic lesions that regulate food intake and the autonomic nervous system

axis and the autonomic VMH center is required for the development of the full hypothalamic obesity syndrome including hyperphagia, hyperinsulinemia, impaired sympathetic drive to BAT, and obesity. The involvement of these centers is further supported by the observations that chronic infusions of norepinephrine into the VMH but not the PVN and repeated injections of NPY into the PVN induce the rapid development of obesity [102–105]. Indeed, overexpression and secretion of NPY may be a major stimulus to the development of obesity that is common to several models [106]. Blockade of serotonin receptors [107] and damage to the ventral noradrenergic bundle by 6-hydroxydopamine [95, 108] will also induce obesity.

Changes in autonomic activity that result from VMH lesions are primarily responsible for the alterations in peripheral metabolism [88, 89, 106]. After VMH lesions, there is an increase in the activity of the afferent vagus innervation from the GI tract [109] and the efferent vagal drive to the endocrine pancreas promoting insulin secretion [109].

Initially a VMH-lesioned rat is very sensitive to this hyperinsulinemia and both hepatic and adipose tissue lipogenesis and fat deposition are increased substantially [106]. This, together with the reduced sympathetic drive to BAT and the consequent reduced level of thermogenesis [88, 89, 106, 110], leads to a rapid increase in fat deposition and body weight. This is followed by the development of insulin resistance, initially in muscle and subsequently in adipose tissue and liver, that slows the weight gain until body weight plateaus at a much higher level.

VMH lesions reduce and VMH stimulation increases the sympathetic drive to BAT [88, 89, 111, 112]. The VMH lesion apparently blocks selectively the ability of BAT to respond to signals associated with feeding and nutrient status since the BAT thermogenic response to hypothermia remains intact. However, the sympathetic drive to other tissues, e.g. liver and adrenal, may also be impaired since VMH-lesioned rats show a blunted increase in non-esterified fatty acids (NEFA) after glucoprivation and stress [113]. The metabolic, anthropometric, endocrine, and CNS changes observed in obesity that develops after VMH lesions are very similar to those observed in the genetic obesities of the *fa*/*fa* rat and *ob*/*ob* and *db*/*db* mice [88, 89, 106].

Virally Induced Obesity

Four animal viruses and one human virus have been shown to induce obesity or some degree of additional adiposity in animal models. These are the canine distemper virus in mice, the Rous associated virus in chickens, the Borna-disease virus in rats, the adenovirus SMAM-1 in chickens, and the related human adenovirus Ad-36 in chicken and mice [114]. In general, there is variability in the level of obesity and the metabolic changes that are dependent upon the age of infection and the animal model. The demonstration that a human adenovirus can induce obesity has raised interest particularly since antibodies to the virus have been reported to be linked to higher body weight in small numbers of humans [115]. However, the effect size is small, and has been linked with an atypical reduction in serum cholesterol, making it unlikely to be a major cause of human obesity. Similarly, in mice and chicken the increase in body fat in response to adenoviral infection is small, less than 10%. While the mechanisms of action of all of the viruses have not been demonstrated, evidence of neuronal damage supports the hypothesis that the virus may have their effects through changes in the activity of the hypothalamic neuropeptide circuits that are modulated by leptin [116].

The hypothalamic models of obesity have led to the recognition of the different but overlapping functions of specific hypothalamic regions in the control of energy balance. The VMH is recognized as a primary center regulating the autonomic outflow in response to dietary related signals [88, 89, 106]. The lateral hypothalamus has opposing actions to the VMH on the autonomic nervous system but also is responsible for feeding behavior. In contrast the PVN region has less to do with sympathetic regulation of BAT and vagal regulation of insulin secretion but is a powerful site for the regulation of feeding behavior. It is only in recent years, with the benefit of molecular and genetic studies, that the neurochemical basis for the activities of these centers has been identified. In particular, the identification of leptin and the recognition that leptin, insulin, and other circulatory factors affect two subpopulations of neurons in the arcuate–PVN pathway (NPY/AGRP neurons and POMC/CART neurons) and the MCH and orexin (hypocretin) neurons in the lateral hypothalamus have provided neurochemical basis for the observed responses to hypothalamic stimulation and/or damage (Figure 4).

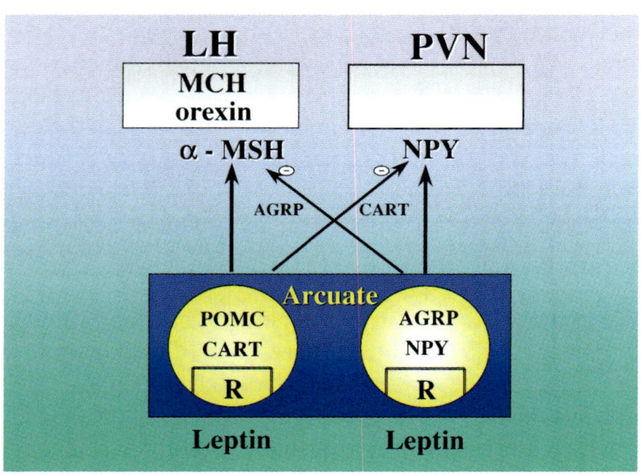

Figure 4 Role of leptin and insulin in regulation of energy balance through their actions in the CNS

ADIPOSE TISSUE MODELS

It is now recognized that the adipose tissue is a major endocrine organ in addition to the major storage site for energy in the form of triacylglycerol deposits. Animal models of obesity have been developed in relation to both functions. The important role of adipose tissue as the primary source of leptin has already been described (see Genes of the Leptin Signaling Pathway).

Adipose Tissue Metabolism

There have been multiple genetic manipulations that reduce adipose tissue mass, including knockout of Perilipin A, PKARIIβ, Lipin, and FOXC2 and transgenic overexpression of SREBP-1c and A-ZIP/P-1. These are not considered in this chapter, which focuses on increasing adipose tissue mass, but have been reviewed previously [117].

Adrenergic Receptors

β_3AR (β_3-adrenergic receptor) and α_2AR (α_2-adrenergic receptor) regulate both lipolysis and thermogenesis in adipose tissue. While α_3AR knockout mice do not become obese [118] despite the role of this receptor in signaling sympathetically mediated BAT thermogenesis, overexpression of α_2AR in β_3AR null mice leads to obesity and adipocyte hyperplasia in mice fed a high-fat diet [119], emphasizing the importance of α_2ARs in the stimulation of adipocyte hyperplasia.

G-protein Alpha Subunit

This is a stimulatory G-protein linked with receptor-mediated activation of adenyl cyclase and other membrane-related proteins. The phenotype associated with knockout of the G-protein alpha subunit (GSα) gene (*Gnas*) depends upon the parental origin of the mutation. Homozygous null mice die *in utero*. Obesity is associated with maternal origin of the heterozygote null allele, but leanness is the result with paternal origin of the mutation. The changes in body composition are related to alterations in energy expenditure rather than food intake. Male *Gnas*$^{-/+}$ mice have high basal metabolic rate and increased physical activity whereas female *Gnas*$^{-/+}$ mice have low metabolic rate and decreased physical activity [120].

Hormone-sensitive Lipase (Lipe)

Mice null for this gene do not become obese although fat cells in white and brown adipose tissues were significantly enlarged by two- to fivefold respectively [121], and brown adipose tissue mass was increased.

Adipocyte Binding Protein (aP2; Fabp4)

This gene is expressed mainly in adipose tissue and binds intracellular fatty acids. Its promoter is frequently used to target gene expression to adipose tissue. Knockouts of the *Fabp4* gene produce the unusual syndrome of an exaggerated high-fat diet induced obesity in the absence of any insulin resistance [122]. Transfer of the *Fabp4* null allele onto the lep^{ob}/lep^{ob} mouse increases its level of obesity yet enhances the insulin sensitivity compared to lep^{ob}/lep^{ob} mice expressing the *Fabp4* gene [123].

Acyl-CoA:diacylglycerol Acyl Transferase (Dgat)

This enzyme transfers a fatty acid to convert diglycerides into triglycerides. While *Dgat* null mice have normal body weight and lower body fat when fed a standard chow diet they gain significant weight and body fat when fed a high-fat diet to reach levels similar to those in wild-type mice [124].

Glucose Transporters

Glut4 is an insulin-regulated glucose transporter expressed in adipose tissue and muscle. In adipose tissue, glucose carbon is required for glyceride synthesis and for fatty acid synthesis. Overexpression of the Glut4 gene (*Slc2a4*) in adipose tissue using the aP_2 promoter results in an obese mouse with enhanced glucose clearance that is not further exaggerated by feeding a high-fat diet [125]. In contrast Glut4 (*Slc2a4*) null mice have little white adipose tissue and have a lower body weight but decreased sensitivity to insulin [126].

Adipocyte Differentiation

PPARα

It is a member of the peroxisome proliferator-activated receptors (PPARs) that are transactivating proteins related to the steroid/thyroid/retinoid receptors. PPARα gene (*Ppara*) null mice develop a late-onset obesity that shows a sexual dimorphism in the temporal development, females becoming obese at a much younger age than males [127, 128]. The cause of this obesity remains unclear since investigators have been unable to identify changes in either food intake [127] or metabolic rate [128].

Agouti (a)

The expression of the agouti gene in humans differs from that in mice where it is only transiently expressed in hair follicles. In humans agouti is also expressed in a variety of peripheral tissues including adipose tissue. In order to develop a model of human agouti, Mynatt and colleagues [129, 130] have created transgenic mice expressing agouti in adipose tissue. These transgenic mice develop a mild obesity and show an enhanced sensitivity of adipose tissue to insulin.

Uncoupling Proteins

Multiple approaches have been used to alter the expression of genes coding for uncoupling proteins (UCPs). Targeted expression of a diptheria toxin A-chain gene has been used to selectively knock out tissue functional activity. By coupling the gene to uncoupling protein gene expression, BAT thermogenic function was abolished and mice became obese [131] and developed hyperphagia. This model not only illustrates the importance of BAT thermogenesis to energy balance in rodents but also emphasizes that BAT may reciprocally affect food intake [110] probably through a sympathetically mediated signal, e.g. heat. This approach appears to be more successful than knockout of the β_3-adrenergic receptor gene in white and brown adipose tissues [132] as this yields only a moderate form of obesity in which BAT remained morphologically normal and responded normally to cold acclimation. Surprisingly, however, *Ucp1* knockouts do not induce obesity although they do induce an impaired thermogenic response to a cold environmental stimulus [133]. This suggests that other thermogenic mechanisms can replace the dietary thermogenic needs but not the greater thermogenic requirement imposed by cold temperatures.

Targeted overexpression of *Ucp1* to adipose tissue using the aP_2 promoter had no phenotypic effect until mice were placed on a high-fat diet on which they were resistant to becoming obese [134]. Likewise, targeting *Ucp1* gene expression to muscle with the rat myosin light chain 2 promoter reduces body size and confers resistance to high-fat dietary obesity [135] but the physiological significance of high expression of this gene in muscle has to be questioned. Knockout of the genes encoding UCP2 and UCP3 likewise does not produce an obesity phenotype.

OTHER MODELS

Intercellular Adhesion Molecule 1

Intercellular Adhesion Molecule 1 (ICAM-1) is a membrane protein that interacts with β-integrins to facilitate the migration of leukocytes. ICAM-1 gene (*Icam1*) null mice develop a late-onset moderate form of obesity, where excess adipose tissue is predominantly deposited in subcutaneous depots [136]. Food intake appears to be similar to that of wild-type mice.

Glutamine:fructose-6-phosphate Amidotransferase

Glutamine:fructose-6-phosphate amidotransferase (GFAT) is the rate-limiting enzyme for hexosamine synthesis in the liver. Transgenic overexpression of the GFAT gene (*Gfpt1*) using the phosphoenolpyruvate carboxykinase (PEPCK) promoter resulted in mice that appear to have enhanced or normal insulin sensitivity and elevated hepatic glycogen when young, but which become obese when old [137].

Other Obesity Models of Unknown Etiology

Several different strains of KK mice have been identified (see references 7 and 24 for review). The obesity and diabetes of this mouse is inherited as a dominant gene with low (25%) penetrance [47]. The obesity and hyperinsulinemia are relatively mild, although the hyperglycemia may be severe, and may be prevented by dietary restriction. The temporal changes in this mouse are also very different from the other mouse models in that changes to or toward normality of body composition, insulin secretion, and insulin resistance may be evident in older (>6 months) animals.

The polygenic forms of obesity provide a particular challenge to identify the individual genes and their contributions to the phenotype. In general polygenic obesity has been related to those rodent strains that will develop obesity either spontaneously or in response to a dietary influence, although this also applies to primate and other large animal models [138]. The Sand Rat (*Psammomys obesus*) becomes obese when it is transferred from its usual herbivorous desert diet to a high carbohydrate laboratory chow. A similar murine obesity and diabetes has been reported in the Spiny Mouse (*Acomys caharinus*) [139]. The NZO mouse develops a moderate form of obesity from early life and has many of the features of the metabolic syndrome (hypertension, elevated blood lipids, hyperglycemia) [140]. While these mice have a variant leptin receptor (A720T/T1044I) it alone does not explain the obesity. However interactions with other genes (e.g., *Nob1* on chromosome 5) may be a significant contributor to the obesity [141].

More recently, the variation in susceptibility to become obese in the offspring of crosses of individual inbred strains that differed in their propensity to become obese, has become a popular form of polygenic obesity to study. BSB mice, derived from a backcross of *Mus spretus* and C57BL/6J strains have a body fat content that shows individual variation from 1 to 50% [142, 143]. Backcrosses between AKR/J and C57BL/J mice likewise give a variation in body fat that has allowed the identification of linked chromosomal regions [144]. The full range of linkages gained from genome-wide scans in crosses of different mouse strains has been summarized elsewhere [66, 67].

Several laboratories have mapped quantitative trait loci that influence body fat, particularly after feeding a high-fat diet. Numerous linkages on multiple chromosomes have been identified, many in regions not known to contain an obesity gene [142–147]. Congenic mice or radiation-induced chromosomal deletions have been used to try to narrow the DNA region and identify the specific gene. This approach has successfully identified a novel ATPase coded on chromosome 7 as a potential obesity-related gene [148] although no functional studies have yet been made for proof of function.

Finally, while this chapter has concentrated on rodent models of obesity, there are also models in larger animals and primates. These have been reviewed previously [67].

REFERENCES

1. Bray GA, York DA. Obesity. *Handbook of Physiology*, Vol II. Oxford: Oxford University Press, 2001; sect 7, chap 34, pp 1015–56.
2. Zhang Y, Proenca R, Maffei M, Barone M, Leopold L, Friedman JM. Positional cloning of the mouse obese gene and its human homologue. *Nature (Lond)* 1994; 372: 425–32.
3. Coleman DL. Obesity and diabetes: two mutant genes causing diabetes-obesity syndromes in mice. *Diabetologia* 1978; 14: 141–8.
4. Harris RB, Hervey E, Hervey GR, Tobin G. Body composition of lean and obese Zucker rats in parabiosis. *Int J Obesity* 1987; 11: 275–83.
5. Chen H, Charlat O, Tartaglia LA, Woolf EA, Weng X, Ellis SJ, Lakey ND, Culpepper J, Moore KJ, Breitbart RE, Duyk GM, Tepper RI, Morgenstern JP. Evidence that the diabetes gene encodes the leptin receptor: identification of a mutation in the leptin receptor gene in *db/db* mice. *Cell* 1996; 84: 491–5.
6. Iida M, Muraakami T, Ishida K, Mizuno A, Kuwajima M, Shima K. Phenotype-linked amino acid alteration in leptin receptor cDNA from Zucker fatty *(fa/fa) rat. Biochem Biophys Res Commun* 1996; 222: 19–26.
7. Takaya K, Ogawa Y, Hiraoka J, Hosoda K, Yamori Y, Nakao K, Koletsky R.J. Nonense mutation of leptin receptor in the obese spontaneously hypertensive Koletsky rat. *Nat Genet* 1996; 14: 130–1.
8. Crouse JA, Elliott GE, Burgess TL, Chiu L, Bennett L, Moore J, Nicolson M, Pacifici RE. Altered cell surface expression and signaling of leptin receptors containing the fatty mutation. *J Biol Chem* 1998; 273: 18365–73.
9. York DA, Hansen B. Animal models of obesity. In Bray GA, Bouchard C, James WP (eds) *Handbook of Obesity*. New York: Marcel Dekker, 1997; pp 191–221.
10. Kowalski TJ, Liu SM, Leibel RL, Chua SC Jr. Transgenic complementation of leptin-receptor deficiency, I: rescue of the obesity/diabetes phenotype of LEPR-null mice expressing a LEPR-B transgene. *Diabetes* 2001; 50: 425–35.
11. Shafrir E. Animal models of non-insulin-dependent diabetes. *Diab Metab Revs* 1992; 8: 179–208.
12. Reichart U, Renner-Muller I, Hoflich A, Muller OJ, Franz WM, Wolf E, Muller M, Brem G, Aigner B. Contrasting obesity phenotypes uncovered by partial leptin receptor gene deletion in transgenic. *Biochem Biophy Res Commun* 2000; 269: 502–7.
13. Campfield LA, Smith FJ, Guisez Y, Devos R, Burn P. Recombinant mouse ob protein: evidence for a

peripheral signal linking adiposity and central neural networks. *Science* 1995; 269: 546–9.

14. Halaas JL, Gajiwala KS, Maffei M, Cohen SL, Chait BT, Rabinowitz D, Lallone RL, Burley SK, Friedman JM. Weight-reducing effects of the plasma protein encoded by the obese gene. *Science* 1995; 269: 543–6.
15. Pelleymounter MA, Cullen MJ, Baker MB, Hecht R, Winters D, Boone T, Collins F. Effects of the obese gene product on body weight regulation in *ob/ob* mice. *Science* 1995; 269: 540–3.
16. Masuzaki H, Ogawa Y, Aizawa-Abe M, Hosoda K, Suga J, Ebihara K, Satoh N, Iwai H, Inoue G, Nishimura H, Yoshimasa Y, Nakao K. Glucose metabolism and insulin sensitivity in transgenic mice overexpressing leptin with lethal yellow agouti mutation: usefulness of leptin for the treatment of obesity-associated diabetes. *Diabetes* 1999; 48: 1615–22.
17. Bruning JC, Gautam D, Burks DJ, Gillette J, Schubert M, Orban PC, Klein R, Krone W, Muller-Wieland D, Kahn CR. Role of brain insulin receptor in control of body weight and reproduction. *Science* 2000; 289: 2122–5.
18. Moller DE, Change PY, Yaspelkis BB III, Flier JS, Wallberg-Henriksson H, Ivy JL. Transgenic mice with muscle-specific insulin resistance develop increased adiposity, impaired glucose tolerance, and dyslipidemia. *Endocrinology* 1996; 137: 2397–405.
19. Coleman DL, Eicher EM. Fat (fat) and tubby (tub): two autosomal recessive mutations causing obesity syndromes in the mouse. *J Hered* 1990; 81: 424–7.
20. Kleyn PW, Fan W, Kovats SG, Lee JJ, Pulido JC, Wu Y, Berkemeier LR, Misumi DJ, Holmgren L, Charlat O, Woolf EA, Tayber O, Brody T, Shu P, Hawkins F, Kennedy B, Baldini L, Ebeling C, Alperin GD, Deeds J, Lakey ND, Culpepper J, Chen H, Glucksmann-Kuis MA, Carlson GA, Duyk GM, Moore KJ. Identification and characterization of the mouse obesity gene tubby: a member of a novel gene family. *Cell* 1996; 85: 281–90.
21. Stubdal H, Lynch CA, Moriarty A, Fang Q, Chickering T, Deeds JD, Fairchild-Huntress V, Charlat O, Dunmore JH, Kleyn P, Huszar D, Kapeller R. Targeted deletion of the tub mouse obesity gene reveals that tubby is a loss-of-function mutation. *Mol Cell Biol* 2000; 20: 878–82.
22. Santagata S, Boggon TJ, Baird CL, Gomez CA, Zhao J, Shan WS, Myszka DG, Shapiro L. G-protein signaling through tubby proteins. *Science* 2001; 292: 2041–50.
23. Kapeller R, Moriarty A, Strauss A, Stubdal H, Theriault K, Siebert E, Chickering T, Morgenstern JP, Tartaglia LA, Lillie J. Tyrosine phosphorylation of tub and its association with Src homogy 2 domain-containing proteins implicate tub in intracellular signaling by insulin. *J Biol Chem* 1999; 274: 24980–6.
24. Guan XM, Yu H, Van der Ploeg LH. Evidence of altered hypothalamic proopiomelanocortin/neuropeptideY mRNA expression in tubby mice. *Brain Res* 1998; 59: 273–9.
25. Devine E, Young AA. Weight gain in male and female mice with amylin gene knockout [abstract]. *Diabetes* 1998; 47: A317.
26. Donahue LR, Beamer WG. Growth hormone deficiency in "little" mice results in aberrant body composition, reduced insulin-like growth factor-I and insulin-like grown factor-binding protein-3 (IGFBP-3), but does not affect IGFBP-2, -1 or -4. *J Endocrinology* 1993; 136: 91–104.
27. Searle TW, Murray JD, Baker PJ. Effect of increased production of growth hormone on body composition in mice: transgenic versus control. *J Endocrinol* 1992; 132: 285–91.
28. Chen XL, Lee K, Hartzell DL, Dean RG, Hausman GJ, McGraw RA, Della-Ferra MA, Baile CA. Adipocyte insensitivity to insulin in growth hormone-transgenic mice. *Biochem Biophys Res Comm* 2001; 283: 933–7.
29. Oberbauer AM, Runstadler JA, Murray JD, Havel PJ. Obesity and elevated plasma leptin concentration in oMT1A-o growth hormone transgenic mice. *Obes Res* 2001; 9: 51–8.
30. Cai A, Hyde JF. The human growth hormone-releasing hormone transgenic mouse as a model of modest obesity: differential changes in leptin receptor (OBR) gene expression in the anterior pituitary and hypothalamus after fasting and OBR localization in somatotrophs. *Endocrinology* 1999; 140: 3609–14.
31. Richard D, Chapdelaine S, Deshaies Y, Pepin M-C, Barden N. Energy balance and lipid metabolism in transgenic mice bearing an antisense GCR gene construct. *Am J Physiol* 1993; R146–50.
32. Stenzel-Poore MP, Cameron VA, Vaughan J, Sawchenko PE, Vale W. Development of Cushing's syndrome in corticotropin-releasing factor transgenic mice. *Endocrinology* 1992; 130: 3378–86.
33. Karolyi IJ, Burrows HL, Ramesh TM, Nakajima M, Lesh JS, Seong E, Camper SA, Seasholtz AF. Altered anxiety and weight gain in corticotropin-releasing hormone-binding protein-deficient mice. *Proc Natl Acad Sci USA* 1999; 96: 11595–600.
34. Lovejoy DA, Aubry JM, Turnbull A, Sutton S, Potter E, Yehling J, Rivier C, Vale WW. Ectopic expression of the CRF-binding protein: minor impact on HPA axis regulation but induction of sexually dimorphic weight gain. *J Neuroendocrinol* 1998; 10: 483–91.
35. Bale L, Contarino A, Smith GW, Chan R, Gold LH, Sawchenko PE, Koob GF, Vale WW, Lee KF. Mice deficient for corticotropin-releasing hormone receptor-2 display anxiety-like behaviour and are hypersensitive to stress. *Nat Genet* 2000; 24: 410–4.
36. Bradbury MJ, McBurnie MI, Denton DA, Lee KF, Vale WW. Modulation of urocortin-induced hypophagia and weight loss by corticotropin-releasing factor receptor 1 deficiency in mice. *Endocrinology* 2000; 141: 2715–24.
37. Masuzaki H, Paterson J, Shinyama H, Morton NM, Mullins JJ, Seckl JR, Flier JS. A transgenic model of visceral obesity and the metabolic syndrome. *Science* 2001; 294: 2166–9.
38. Baldwin BA, Parrott RF, Ebenezer IS. Food for thought: a critique on the hypothesis that endogenous cholecystokinin acts as a physiological satiety factor. *Prog Neurobiol* 1998; 55: 477–507.
39. Fumakoshi A, Miyassaka K, Shinozaki H, Masada M, Kawanami T, Takata Y, Komo A. An animal model of congenital defect of gene expression of cholecystokinin (CCK)-A receptor. *Biochem Biophy Res Commun* 1993; 210: 787–96.
40. Schwartz GJ, Whitney A, Skoglund C, Castonguay TW, Moran TH. Decreased responsiveness to dietary fat in Otsuka Long-Evans Tokushima fatty rats lacking CCK-A receptors. *Am J Physiol* 1999; 277: R1144–51.
41. Kopin AS, Mathes WF, McBride EW, Nguyen M, Al-Haider W, Schmitz F, Bonner-Weir S, Kanarak S, Beinbom M. The cholecystokinin-A receptor mediates

inhibition of food intake yet is not essential for the maintenance of body weight. *J Clin Invest* 1999; 103: 383–91.

42. Miyawaki K, Yamada Y, Ban N, Ihara Y, Tsukiyama K, Zhou H, Fujimoto S, Oku A, Tsuda K, Toyokuni S, Hiai H, Mizunoya W, Fushiki T, Holst JJ, Makino M, Tashita A, Kobara Y, Tsubamoto Y, Jinnouchi T, Jomori T, Seino Y. Inhibition of gastric inhibitory polypeptide signaling prevents obesity. *Nat Med July* 2002; 8(7): 738–42.
43. Heine PA, Taylor JA, Iwamoto GA, Lubahn DB, Cooke PS. Increased adipose tissue in male and female estrogen receptor-knockout mice. *Proc Natl Acad Sci USA* 2000; 97: 12729–34.
44. Cooke PS, Heine PA, Tyalor JA, Lubahn DB. The role of estrogen and estrogen receptor-alpha in male adipose tissue. *Mol Cell Endocrinol* 2001; 178: 147–54.
45. Jones MEE, Thorburn AW, Britt KL, Hewitt KN, Wreford NG, Proietto J, Oz OK, Leury BJ, Robertson KM, Yao S, Simpson ER. Aromatase-deficient (ArKO) mice have a phenotype of increased adiposity. *Proc Nat Acad Sci USA* 2000; 97: 12735–40.
46. Danilovich N, Babu PS, Xing W, Gerdes M, Krishnamurthy H, Sairam MR. Estrogen deficiency, obesity, and skeletal abnormalities in follicle-stimulating hormone receptor knockout (FORKO) female mice. *Endocrinology* 2000; 141: 4295–308.
47. Butler L, Gerritsen GC. A comparison of the modes of inheritance of diabetes in the Chinese hamster and KK mouse. *Diabetologia* 1970; 6: 163–7.
48. Wolff GC. Body composition and coat colour correlation in different phenotypes of "viable yellow" mice. *Science* 1965; 147: 1145–7.
49. Gill AM, Leiter EH, Powell JG, Chapman HD, Yen TT. Dexamethasone-induced hyperglycemia in obese A^{vy}/a (viable yellow) female mice entails preferential induction of hepatic estrogen sulfotransferase. *Diabetes* 1994; 43: 999–1004.
50. Wolff GL, Flack JD. Genetic regulation of plasma corticosterone concentration and its response to castration and allogenic tumor growth in the mouse. *Nat New Biol* 1971; 232: 181–2.
51. Bultman SJ, Michaud EJ, Woychik RP. Molecular characterization of the mouse agouti locus. *Cell* 1992; 71: 1195–204.
52. Perry W, Hustad C, Swing D, Jenkins N, Copeland N. A transgenic mouse assay for agouti protein activity. *Genetics* 1995; 140: 267–74.
53. Klebig ML, Wilkinson JE, Geisler JG, Woychik RP. Ectopic expression of the agouti gene in transgenic mice causes obesity, features of type II diabetes, and yellow fur. *Proc Natl Acad Sci USA* 1995; 92: 4728–32.
54. Zemel MB, Kim JH, Woychik RP, et al. Agouti regulation of intracellular calcium: role in the insulin resistance of viable yellow mice. *Proc Natl Acad Sci USA* 1995; 92: 4733–7.
55. Lu D, Willard D, Patel IR, Kadwell S, Overton L, Kost T, Luther M, Chen W, Woychik RP, Wilkison WO, Cone RD. Agouti protein is an antagonist of the melanocyte-stimulating-hormone receptor. *Nature (Lond)* 1994; 371: 799–802.
56. Shimizu H, Shargill NS, Bray GA, Yen FT, Geselchen PD. Effects of MSH on food intake, body weight and coat color of the yellow obese mouse. *Life Sci* 1989; 45: 543–52.
57. Ollman MM, Wilson BD, Yang Y-K, Kerns JA, Chen Y, Gantz I, Barsh GS. Antagonism of central melanocortin receptors in vitro and in vivo by agouti-related protein. *Science* 1997; 278: 135–8.
58. Fan W, Boston BA, Kesterson RA, Hruby VJ, Cone RD. Role of melanocortinergic neurons in feeding and the agouti obesity syndrome. *Nature* 1997; 385: 165–8.
59. Fan W, Dinulescu DM, Butler AA, Zhou J, Marks DL, Cone RD. The central melanocortin system can directly regulate serum insulin levels. *Endocrinology* 2000; 141: 3072–9.
60. Flier JS, Harris M, Hollenberg AN. Leptin, nutrition, and the thyroid: the why, the wherefore, and the wiring. *J Clin Invest* 2000; 105: 859–61.
61. Graham M, Shutter JR, Sarmiento U, Sarosi I, Stark KL. Overexpression of Agrt leads to obesity in transgenic mice. *Nat Genet* 1997; 17: 273–4.
62. Yaswen L, Diehl N, Brennan MB, Hochgeschwender U. Obesity in the mouse model of proopiomelanocortin deficiency responds to peripheral melanocortin. *Nat Med* 1999; 5: 1066–117.
63. Huszar D, Lynch CA, Fairchild-Huntress V, Dunmore JH, Fang Q, Berkemeier L, Gu W, Kesterson RA, Boston BA, Cone RD, Smith FJ, Campfield LA, Burn P, Lee F. Targeted disruption of the melanocortin-4 receptor results in obesity in mice. *Cell* 1997; 88: 131–41.
64. Chen AS, Marsh DJ, Trumbauer ME, Frazier EG, Guan X-M, Yu H, Rosenblum CI, Vongs A, Feng Y, Cao L, Metzger JM, Strack AM, Camacho RE, Mellin TN, Nunes CN, Min W, Fisher J, Gopal-Truter S, MacIntyre DE, Chen HY, Van der Ploeg LHT. Inactivation of the mouse melanocortin-3 receptor results in increased fat mass and reduced lean body mass. *Nat Genet* 2000; 26: 97–102.
65. Butler AA, Kesterson RA, Khong K, Cullen MJ, Pelleymounter MA, Dekoning J, Baetscher M, Cone RD. A unique metabolic syndrome causes obesity in the melanocortin-3 receptor-deficient mouse. *Endocrinology* 2000; 141: 3518–21.
66. Barsh GS, Farooqi IS, O'Rahilly S. Genetics of body-weight regulation. *Nature* 2000; 404: 644–51.
67. Perusse L, Chagnon YC, Weisnagel SJ, Rankinen T, Snyder E, Sands J, Bouchard C. The human obesity gene map: the 2000 update. *Obes Res* 2001; 9(2): 135–69.
68. Miller KA, Gunn TM, Carrasquillo MM, Lamoreaux ML, Galbraith DB, Barsh GS. Genetic studies of the mouse mutations mahogany and mahoganoid. *Genetics* 1997; 146: 1407–15.
69. Gunn TM, Miller KA, He L, Hyman RW, Davis RW, Azarani A, Schlossman SF, Duke-Cohan JS, Barsh GS. The mouse mahogany locus encodes a transmembrane form of human attractin. *Nature* 1999; 398: 152–6.
70. Lu X, Gunn TM, Shieh K, Barsh GS, Akil H, Watson SJ. Distribution of mahogany/attractin mRNA in the rat central nervous system. *FEBS Lett* 1999, 462: 101–7.
71. Reizes O, Lincecum J, Wang Z, Goldberger O, Huang L, Kaksonen M, Ahima R, Hinkes MT, Barsh GS, Rauvala H, Bernfield M. Transgenic expression of syndecan-1 uncovers a physiological control of feeding behavior by syndecan-3. *Cell* 2001; 106: 105–16.
72. Bannon AW, Seda J, Carmouche M, Francis JM, Norman MH, Karbon B, McCaleb ML. Behavioral characterization of neuropeptide Y knockout mice. *Brain Res* 2000; 868: 79–87.
73. Erickson JC, Hollopeter G, Palmiter JD. Attenuation of the obesity syndrome of *ob/ob* mice by the loss of neuropeptide Y. *Science* 1996; 274: 1704–7.

74. Shimada M, Tritos NA, Lowell BB, Flier JS, Maratos-Flier E. Mice lacking melanin-concentrating hormone are hypophagic and lean. *Nature* 1998; 396: 670–4.
75. Ludwig DS, Tritos NA, Mastaitis JW, Kulkarni R, Kokkotou E, Elmquist J, Lowell B, Flier JS, Maratos-Flier E. Melanin-concentrating hormone overexpression in transgenic mice leads to obesity and insulin resistance. *J Clin Invest* 2001; 107: 379–86.
76. Chemelli RM, Willie JT, Sinton CM, Elmquist JK, Scammell T, Lee C, Richardson JA, Williams SC, Xiong Y, Kisanuki Y, Fitch TE, Nakazato M, Hammer RE, Saper CB, Yanagisawa M. Narcolepsy in orexin knockout mice: molecular genetics of sleep regulation. *Cell* 1999; 98: 437–51.
77. Hara J, Beuckmann CT, Nambu T, Willie JT, Chemelli RM, Sinton CM, Sugiyama F, Yagami K, Goto K, Yanagisawa M, Sakurai T. Genetic ablation of orexin neurons in mice results in narcolepsy, hypophagia, and obesity. *Neuron* 2001; 30: 345–54.
78. Ohki-Hamazaki H, Watase K, Yamamoto K, Ogura H, Yamano M, Yamada K, Maeno H, Imaki J, Kikuyama S, Wada E, Wada K. Mice lacking bombesin receptor subtype-3 develop metabolic defects and obesity. *Nature* 1997; 390: 165–9.
79. Nonogaki K, Strack AM, Dallman MF, Tecott LH. Leptin-independent hyperphagia and type 2 diabetes in mice with a mutated serotonin 5-HT2C receptor gene. *Nat Med* 1998; 4: 1152–6.
80. Lucas JJ, Yamamoto A, Scearce-Levie K, Saudou F, Hen Rene. Absence of fenfluramine-induced anorexia and reduced c-*fos* induction in the hypothalamus and central amygdaloid complex of serotonin 1B receptor knock-out mice. *J Neuroscience* 1998; 18: 5537–44.
81. Masaki T, Yoshimatsu H, Chiba S, Watanabe T, Sakata T. Targeted disruption of histamine H1-receptor attenuates regulatory effects of leptin on feeding, adiposity, and UCP family in mice. *Diabetes* 2001; 50: 385–91.
82. Yamada M, Miyakawa T, Duttaroy A, Yamanaka A, Moriguchi T, Makita R, Ogawa M, Chou CJ, Xia B, Crawley JN, Felder CC, Deng CX, Wess J. Mice lacking the M3 muscarinic acetylcholine receptor are hypophagic and lean. *Nature* 2001; 410: 207–12.
83. Ma YH, Hu JH, Zhou XG, Zeng RW, Mei ZT, Fei J, Guo LH. Transgenic mice overexpressing gamma-aminobutyric acid transporter subtype I develop obesity. *Cell Res* 2000; 10: 303–10.
84. Naggert JK, Fricker LD, Varlamov O, Nishina PM, Rouille Y, Steiner DF, Carroll RJ, Paigen BJ, Leiter EH. Hyperproinsulinaemia in obese *fat/fat* mice associated with a carboxypeptidase E mutation which reduces enzyme activity. *Nat Genet* 1995; 10: 135–42.
85. Udupi V, Gomez P, Song L, Varlamov O, Reed JT, Leiter EH, Fricker LD, Greeley GH Jr. Effect of carboxypeptidase E deficiency on progastrin processing and gastrin messenger ribonucleic acid expression in mice with the fat mutation. *Endocrinology* 1997; 138: 1959–63.
86. Huszar D, Lynch CA, Fairchild-Huntress V, Dunmore JH, Fang Q, Berkemeier L, Gu W, Kesterson RA, Boston BA, Cone RD, Smith FJ, Campfield LA, Burn P, Lee F. Targeted disruption of the melanocortin-4 receptor results in obesity in mice. *Cell* 1997; 88: 131–41.
87. Westphal CH, Muller L, Zhou A, Zhu X, Bonner-Weir S, Schambelan M, Steiner DF, Lindberg I, Leder P. The neuroendocrine protein 7B2 is required for peptide hormone processing in vivo and provides a novel mechanism for pituitary Cushing's disease. *Cell* 1999; 96: 689–700.
88. Bray GA, York DA, Fisler JS. Experimental obesity: a homeostatic failure due to defective nutrient stimulation of the sympathetic nervous system. *Vitam Horm* 1990; 45: 1–125.
89. Bray GA, Fisler JS, York DA. Neuroendocrine control of the development of obesity: understanding gained from studies of experimental models of obesity. *Prog Neuroendocrinol* 1990; 4: 128–81.
90. Bernardis LL. Ventromedical and dorsomedial hypothalamic syndromes in the weaning rat: is the "center" concept really outmoded? Brain Res Bull 1985; 14: 537–49.
91. Laughton W, Powley TL. Bipiperidyl mustard produced brain lesions and obesity in the rat. Brain Res 1981; 221: 415–20.
92. Brecher G, Waxler SH. Obesity in albino mice due to single injections of gold thioglucose. *Proc Soc Exp Biol Med* 1949; 70: 498–501.
93. Rutman RJ, Lewis FS, Bloomer WD. Bipiperidyl mustard, a new obesifying agent in the mouse. *Science* 1966; 153: 1000–2.
94. Parkinson WL, Weingarten HP. Dissociative analysis of ventromedial hypothalamic syndrome. *Am J Physiol* 1990; 259: R829–35.
95. Ahlskog JE, Randall PK, Hoebel BG. Hypothalamic hyperphagia: dissociation from hyperphagia following destruction of noradrenergic neurons. *Science* 1975; 190: 399–401.
96. Sahakian BJ, Winn P, Robbins TW, Deeley RJ, Everitt BJ, Dunn LT, Wallace M, James WPT. Changes in body weight and food-related behavior induced by destruction of the ventral or dorsal noradrenergic bundle in the rat. *Neuroscience* 1983; 10: 1405–20.
97. Scallet AC, Olney JW. Components of hypothalamic obesity: bipiperidyl-mustard lesions add hyperphagia to monosodium glutamate-induced hyperinsulinemia. *Brain Res* 1986; 374: 380–4.
98. Tanaka K, Shimada M, Nakao K, Kusonoki T. Hypothalmic lesion induced by injection of monosodium glutamate in suckling period and subsequent development of obesity. *Exp Neurol* 1978; 62: 191–9.
99. Shimizu N, Oomura Y, Plata-Salaman CR, Morimoto M. Hyperphagia and obesity in rats with bilateral ibotenic acid-induced lesions of the ventromedial hypothalamic nucleus. *Brain Res* 1987; 416: 153–6.
100. Weingarten HP, Change PK, McDonald TJ. Comparison of the metabolic and behavioral disturbances following paraventricular and ventromedial hypothalamic lesions. *Brain Res Bull* 1985; 14: 551–9.
101. Sclafani A, Grossman SP. Hyperphagia produced by knife cuts between the medial and lateral hypothalamus in the rat. *Physiol Behav* 1969; 4: 533–7.
102. Beck B, Sticker-Krongrad A, Nicolas JP, Burlet C. Chronic and continuous intracerebroventricular infusion of neuropeptide Y in Long-Evans rats mimics the feeding behavior of obese Zucker rats. *Int J Obes* 1992; 16: 295–302.
103. Zarjevskin, Cusin I, Vettor R, Rohner-Jeanrenaud F, Jeanrenaud B. Chronic intracerebroventricular neuropeptide-Y/administration to normal rats mimics hormonal and metabolic change of obesity. *Endocrinology* 1993; 133: 1753–8.

104. Shimazu T, Noma M, Saito M. Chronic infusion of norepinephrine into the ventromedial hypothalamus induces obesity in rats. *Brain Res* 1986; 369: 215–23.
105. Stanley BG, Kyrkouli SE, Lampert S, Leibowitz SF. Neuropeptide Y chronically injected into the hypothalamus; a powerful neurochemical inducer of hyperphagia and obesity. *Peptides* 1986; 7: 1189–92.
106. Rohner-Jeanrenaud F. A neuroendocrine reappraisal of the dual-center hypothesis: its implications for obesity and insulin resistance. *Int J Obes* 1995; 19: 517–34.
107. Breisch ST, Zemlan FP, Hoebel BG. Hyperphagia and obesity following serotonin depletion by intraventricular *p*-chlorophenylalanine. *Science* 1976; 192: 382–5.
108. Ahlskog JE, Hoebel BG. Overeating and obesity from damage to a noradrenergic system in the brain. *Science* 1982; 182: 166–9.
109. Berthoud H-R. Cephalic phase insulin response as a prediction of body weight gain and obesity induced by a palatable cafeteria diet. *J Obes Weight Regul* 1985; 4: 120–8.
110. Bray GA. Reciprocal relation between the sympathetic nervous system and food intake. *Brain Res Bull* 1991; 27: 517–20.
111. Niijima A, Rohner-Jeanrenaud F, Jeanrenaud B. Role of the ventromedial hypothalamus on sympathetic efffer-ents of brown adipose tissue. *Am J Physiol* 1984; 247: R650–4.
112. Holt SJ, Wheal H, York DA. Response of brown adipose tissue to electrical stimulation of hypothalamic centers in intact and adrenalectomized Zucker rats. *Neurosci Lett* 1988; 84: 63–7.
113. Nishizawa Y, Bray GA. Ventromedial hypothalamic lesions and mobilization of fatty acids. *J Clin Invest* 1978; 61: 714–21.
114. Dhurandhar NV, Atkinson RL. Viruses and obesity. Curr *Opin Endocrinol Diabetes* 2000; 7: 247–51.
115. Dhurandhar NV, Kulkarni PR, Ajinkya SM, Sherikar AA, Atkinson RL. Association of adenovirus infection with human obesity. *Obes Res* 1997; 5: 464–9.
116. Bernard A, Cohen R, Khuth ST, Vedrine B, Verlaeten O, Akaoka H, Giraudon P, Belin MF. Alteration of the leptin network in late morbid obesity induced in mice by brain infection with canine distemper virus. *J Virol* 1999; 73: 7317–27.
117. York DA, Hansen B. Animal models of obesity. In Bray GA, Bouchard C, James WP (eds) *Handbook of Obesity*. New York: Marcel Dekker, 1997; pp 191–221.
118. Susulic VS, Frederich RC, Lawitts J, Tozzo E, Kahn BB, Harper ME, Himms-Hagen J, Flier JS, Lowell BB. Targeted disruption of the beta 3-adrenergic receptor gene. *J Biol Chem* 1995; 270: 29483–92.
119. Valet P, Grujic D, Wade J, Ito M, Zingaretti MC, Soloveva V, Ross SR, Graves RA, Cinti S, Lafontan M, Lowell BB. Expression of human alpha2-adrenergic receptors in adipose tissue of beta3-adrenergic receptor-deficient mice promotes diet-induced obesity. *J Biol Chem* 2000; 275: 34797–802.
120. Yu S, Gavrilova O, Chen H, Lee R, Liu J, Pacak K, Parlow AF, Quon MJ, Reitman ML, Weinstein LS. Paternal versus maternal transmission of a stimulatory G-protein alpha subunit knockout produces opposite effects on energy metabolism. *J Clin Invest* 2000; 105: 615–23.
121. Osuga J, Ishibashi S, Oka T, Yaguy H, Tozawa R, Fujimoto A, Shionoiri F, Yahagi N, Kraemer FB, Tsutsumi O, Yamada N. Targeted disruption of hormone-sensitive lipase results in male sterility and adipocyte hypertrophy, but not in obesity. *Proc Natl Acad Sci USA* 2000; 97: 787–92.
122. Hotamisligil GS, Johnson RS, Distel RJ, Ellis R, Papaioannou VE, Spiegelman BM. Uncoupling of obesity from insulin resistance through a targeted mutation in aP2, the adipocyte fatty acid binding protein. *Science* 1996; 274: 1377–9.
123. Uysal KT, Scheja L, Wiesbrock SM, Bonner-Weir S, Hotamisligil GS. Improved glucose and lipid metabolism in genetically obese mice lacking aP_2. *Endocrinology* 2000; 141: 3388–96.
124. Smith SJ, Cases S, Jensen DR, Chen HC, Sande E, Tow B, Sanan DA, Raber J, Eckel RH, Farese RV Jr. Obesity resistance and multiple mechanisms of triglyceride synthesis in mice lacking *Dgat. Nat Genet* 2000; 25: 87–90.
125. Shepherd PR, Gnudi L, Tozzo E, Yang H, Leach F, Kahn BB. Adipose cell hyperplasia and enhanced glucose disposal in transgenic mice overexpressing GLUT4 selectively in adipose tissue. *J Biol Chem* 1993; 268: 22243–6.
126. Stenbit AE, Tsao TS, Li J, Burcelin R, Geenen DL, Factor SM, Houseknecht K, Katz EB, Charron MJ. GLUT4 heterozygous knockout mice develop muscle insulin resistance and diabetes. *Nat Med* 1997; 3: 1080–1.
127. Costet P, Legendre C, More J, Edgar A, Galtier P, Pineau T. Peroxisome proliferator-activated receptor alpha-isoform deficiency leads to progressive dyslipidemia with sexually dimorphic obesity and steatosis. *J Biol Chem* 1998; 273: 29577–85.
128. Kersten S, Seydoux J, Peters JM, Gonzalez FJ, Desvergne B, Wahli W. Peroxisome proliferator-activated receptor alpha mediates the adaptive response to fasting. *J Clin Invest* 1999; 103: 1489–98.
129. Mynatt RL, Stephens JM. Agouti regulates adipocyte transcription factors. *Am Physiol Cell Physiol* 2001; 280: C954–61.
130. Mynatt RL, Miltenberger RJ, Klebig ML, Zemel MB, Wilkinson JE, Wilkinson WO, Woychick RP. Combined effects of insulin treatment and adipose tissue-specific agouti expression on the development of obesity. *Proc Natl Acad Sci USA* 1997; 94: 919–22.
131. Lowell BB, S-Susulic V, Hamann A, Lawitts JA, Himms-Hagen J, Boyers BB, Kozak LP, Flier JS. Development of obesity in transgenic mice after genetic ablation of brown adipose tissue. *Nature (Lond)* 1993; 366: 740–2.
132. Ross SR, Graves RA, Spiegelman BM. Targeted expression of a toxin gene to adipose tissue: transgenic mice resistant to obesity. *Genes Dev* 1993; 7: 1318–24.
133. Enerback S, Jacobsson A, Simpson EM, Guerra C, Yamashita H, Harper M-E, Kozak LE. Mice lacking mitochondrial uncoupling protein are cold-sensitive but not obese. *Nature* 1997; 387: 90–4.
134. Kopecky J, Hodny Z, Rossmeisl M, Syrovy I, Kozak LP. Reduction of dietary obesity in aP2-Ucp transgenic mice: physiology and adipose tissue distribution. *Am J Physiol* May 1996; 270(5, pt 1): E768–75.
135. Li B, Nolte LA, Ju JS, Han DH, Coleman T, Holloszy JO, Semenkovich CF. Skeletal muscle respiratory uncoupling prevents diet-induced obesity and insulin resistance in mice. *Nat Med* October 2000; 6(10): 1115–20.
136. Dong ZM, Gutierrez-Ramos JC, Coxon A, Mayadas TN, Wagner DD. A new class of obesity genes encodes

leukocyte adhesion receptors. *Proc Natl Acad Sci USA* 1997; 4: 7526–30.
137. Veerababu G, Tang J, Hoffman RT, Daniels MC, Hebert LF Jr, Crook ED, Cooksey RC, McClain DA. Overexpression of gluatamine: fructose-6-phosphate amidotransferase in the liver of transgenic mice results in enhanced glycogen storage, hyperlipidemia, obesity, and impaired glucose tolerance. *Diabetes* 2000; 49: 2070–8.
138. Pomp D. Animal models of obesity. *Mol Med Today* 1999; 5: 459–60.
139. Gonet AE, Stauffacher W, Pictet R, Renold AE. Obesity and diabetes mellitus with striking congenital hyperplasia of the islets of Langerhans in spiny mice (*Acomys cahirinus*), I: histological findings and preliminary metabolic observations. *Diabetologia* 1965; 1: 162–71.
140. Ortlepp JR, Kluge R, Giesen K, Plum L, Radke P, Hanrath P, Joost HG. A metabolic syndrome of hypertension, hyperinsulinaemia and hypercholesterolaemia in the New Zealand obese mouse. *Eur J Clin Invest* 2000; 30: 195–202.
141. Kluge R, Giesen K, Bahrenberg G, Plum L, Ortlepp JR, Joost HG. Quantitative trait loci for obesity and insulin resistance (Nob1, Nob2) and their interaction with the leptin receptor allele (LeprA720T/T1044I) in New Zealand obese mice. *Diabetologia* 2000; 43: 1565–72.
142. Warden CH, Fisler JS, Shoemaker SM, Ping-Zi W, Svenson KL, Pace M, Lusis AJ. Identification of four chromosomal loci determining obesity in a multifactorial mouse model. *J Clin Invest* 1995; 95: 1545–52.
143. Warden CH, Fisler JS, Pace MJ, Svenson L, Lusis AJ. Coincidence of genetic loci for plasma cholesterol levels and obesity in a multifactorial mouse model. *J Clin Invest* 1993; 92: 773–9.
144. Taylor BA, Phillips SA. Detection of of obesity QTLs on mouse chromosomes 1 and 7 by selective DNA pooling. *Genomics* 1996; 34: 389–98.
145. West DB, Waguespack J, York B, Goudey-Lefevre J, Price RA. Genetics of dietary obesity in AKR/J × SWR/J mice: segregation of the trait and identification of a linked locus on chromosome 4. *Mamm Genome* 1994; 5: 546–52.
146. West DB, Goudey-Lefevre J, York B, Truett GE. Dietary obesity linked to genetic loci on chromosomes 9 and 15 in a polygenic mouse model. *J Clin Invest* 1994; 94: 1410–6.
147. York B, Truett AA, Monteiro MP, Barry SJ, Warden CH, Naggert JK, Maddatu TP, West DB. Gene–environment interaction: a significant diet-dependent obesity locus demonstrated in a congenic segment on mouse chromosome 7. *Mamm Genome* 1999; 10: 457–62.
148. Dhar M, Webb LS, Smith L, Hauser L, Johnson D, West D. A novel ATPase on mouse chromosome 7 is a candidate gene for increased body fat. *Physiol Genomics* 2000; 4: 93–100.

38

The Role of the Hypothalamus in the Maintenance of Energy Balance and Peripheral Glucose Control

Randy J. Seeley*, Deborah J. Clegg*, Michael W. Schwartz†, and Stephen C. Woods*

**University of Cincinnati, Cincinnati, OH, USA, and †Harborview Medical Center and University of Washington, Seattle, WA, USA*

INTRODUCTION AND HISTORICAL PERSPECTIVE

Introduction

A wealth of evidence indicates that one important function of the hypothalamus is to participate in the control of energy balance. While there is little debate as to whether the hypothalamus contributes to the control of feeding behavior, the precise nature of its role has been a topic of intense experimentation for more than 50 years. In particular, the last 8 years have seen an enormous effort to understand the role of specific hypothalamic nuclei and neurotransmitter systems to control food intake. There are multiple reasons for this increase in interest in hypothalamic control systems. First, the clinical need to understand the control of food intake and body weight has increased in concert with the growing prevalence of obesity and obesity-related health problems in the developed world. Second, the discovery of the adipocyte hormone leptin and the subsequent finding that its receptors are concentrated in the hypothalamus have made the understanding of these hypothalamic circuits critical to a complete understanding and appreciation of the potent effects that leptin has to influence food intake and body weight. Finally, powerful new molecular tools have been profitably applied to the study of these hypothalamic circuits. From this work, a number of new systems have emerged and systems not previously thought to be important in the control of food intake now appear to play critical roles.

While the enormous expansion of literature on the hypothalamic control of food intake and body weight makes this an exciting time to study these systems, its fast-moving pace makes a comprehensive review nearly impossible. Consequently, this chapter does not provide an exhaustive list of the hypothalamic systems proposed to be involved in the control of food intake. Rather, the central theme of this chapter is to describe an evolving conceptual framework for the role of the hypothalamus and highlight some of the key advances. Needless to say, this means that many important aspects of hypothalamic control of food intake are not covered. When possible, we try point the reader to other reviews that cover these topics.

The Dual-Centers Hypothesis

Historically, the conceptual framework that dominated thinking about the role played by the hypothalamus in the control of food intake was the Dual-Centers Hypothesis proposed by Stellar in a very influential article appearing in *Psychological Review* in 1954 [1]. In the same year that the discovery of leptin focused additional attention on the role of the hypothalamus, *Psychological Review* honored Stellar's article as one of the 10 most influential articles it had published in a century of publications. Stellar eloquently argued that the hypothalamus is the

International Textbook of Diabetes Mellitus, Third Edition. Edited by R. A. DeFronzo, E. Ferrannini, H. Keen, and P. Zimmet.
 ISBN: 0-471-48655-8.

central neural structure involved in "motivation" generally and in the control of food intake more specifically. This control is divided into two conceptual categories controlled by two separate hypothalamic structures. The first category was "satiety" and was thought to be controlled by the ventromedial hypothalamus (VMH). Among the data that contributed to this hypothesis was evidence that bilateral lesions of the VMH resulted in rats that ate more than controls and became obese. Such rats were thought to have a defect in satiety and thus the function of the VMH was deemed to be a "satiety" center. Second, electrical stimulation of the VMH caused animals to stop eating, i.e., to demonstrate enhanced satiety. In contrast to the VMH, lesions of the lateral hypothalamic area (LHA) resulted in rats that underate and lost body weight and electrical stimulation of the LHA caused eating in sated animals. As a consequence, the LHA was proposed to be the brain's hunger center. This Dual-Centers Hypothesis was the dominant conceptualization of how the central nervous system (CNS) controlled food intake for almost 30 years.

Challenges to the Dual-Centers Hypothesis

Several challenges gradually emerged to the Dual-Centers Hypothesis. One was the growing realization of the limitations of lesions as an approach to understanding CNS function. In particular, the concept that what an animal no longer does after a lesion of a specific nucleus encapsulates the function of that nucleus is no longer widely accepted. The central problem is that it is difficult to move from the symptom that is produced by making a lesion to the function that the destroyed tissue had under normal circumstances. For example, although lesions of the VMH result in hyperphagic and obese rats, they also result in rapid and dramatic increases in insulin secretion from pancreatic β-cells [2]. It has been well demonstrated that exogenous peripheral insulin administration will result in increased food intake and that repeated administration can result in rapid weight gain [3]. Hence, one explanation for the increased body weight of VMH-lesioned rats is not that the VMH is a "satiety" center, but rather that it is important in the control of insulin secretion. The obesity resulting from VMH lesions may arise not so much from a loss of "satiety" but rather from excessive insulin secretion [2]. In fact, the story is even more complicated because the typical electrolytic lesion destroys not only cell bodies but also neuronal fibers that simply pass through the VMH. In particular, later data indicated that it was not cell bodies in the VMH but rather fibers running from the paraventricular nucleus (PVN) to the brainstem that were critical for the effect of VMH lesions on insulin secretion [4, 5]. So not only did it appear that changes in insulin secretion were potentially responsible for the effects of VMH lesions on food intake and body weight, but that even the control of insulin secretion was not directly mediated by the VMH.

A second major challenge to Stellar's formulation is that it, by necessity, focused upon how specific anatomical locations mediated functions rather than how specific neurochemical pathways might mediate functions. While it is clear that the CNS is organized into regions that can be defined by careful neuroanatomical analysis, the functional unit for the CNS is specific neurochemicals interacting with populations of specific receptors. Hence, it seems unlikely that a large and complex nuclear area like the VMH, which contains multiple neurotransmitters and receptors, would serve a single unified function related to the control of food intake. Therefore labeling the VMH as the "satiety" center would seem inappropriate in that it ignores many other potential functions of the cells located there.

Another challenge to Stellar's view of the hypothalamus arose from transection of the neuraxis at different levels. Grill and his colleagues studied the competencies of the chronic decerebrate rat in terms of its ingestive behavior. The chronic decerebrate rat has a complete transection of the neuraxis at the meso-diencephalic junction that completely isolates the brainstem, severing all neural input from more rostral structures like the hypothalamus. Hence, neither the VMH nor LHA (nor any other hypothalamic nuclei for that matter) can exert direct influence on the motor neurons in the brainstem critical for executing ingestive behavior. The strategy of studying the chronic decerebrate rat is quite different from that of the focal lesion [6]. The basic premise of a focal lesion is to eliminate the contribution of a specific area of the brain and then to figure out what an animal can no longer do. Presumably, the area of the brain that has been compromised then subserves the function that is no longer present. In Grill's strategy, the idea is to simplify the CNS by eliminating all inputs rostral to the meso-diencephalic juncture and then determine what the animal still *can* do. Whatever remaining function the chronic decerebrate rat retains are those that can be accomplished entirely by the caudal brainstem.

Despite a complete loss of neural input from the hypothalamus, the chronic decerebrate animal has the ability to engage in consummatory behavior and to adjust that behavior in response to both external and internal stimuli. For example, chronic decerebrate rats respond appropriately to taste stimuli [6–9]. Chronic decerebrate rats reject bitter tastes and consume sweet tastes in a manner that is almost indistinguishable from that of normal rats. This indicates that the integration of sensory taste information into the rat's ongoing motor behavior can be done within the caudal brainstem. More important, chronic decerebrate rats demonstrate satiety and the size of the meals taken by decerebrate rats is influenced in the same manner by several factors that influence meal size in the normal rat [6, 8]. The caudal brainstem is therefore sufficient to integrate internal regulatory signals that limit meal size into ongoing ingestive behavior independent of the hunger and satiety centers of the hypothalamus. These data provide a strong challenge to the Dual-Centers Hypothesis and indicate that a distributed neural network mediates the control of food intake and that no single brain area constitutes either a "hunger" or "satiety" center.

BEYOND THE DUAL-CENTERS HYPOTHESIS: ADIPOSITY SIGNALS AND EFFECTOR PATHWAYS

These challenges to the Dual-Centers Hypothesis led to new models for understanding the role of the hypothalamus in the control of food intake. Rather than emphasizing factors that initiate and terminate individual bouts of ingestion, the focus has shifted to the signals and pathways that control long-term energy balance. Adult mammals typically match their caloric intake to their caloric expenditure with remarkable precision. Gordon Kennedy postulated in the 1950s that such regulation could be accomplished by monitoring the major form of energy storage in the body, adipose mass [10]. When caloric intake exceeds caloric expenditure, fat stores are expanded and when caloric expenditure exceeds caloric intake, fat stores are reduced. Hence if the size of the adipose mass could be monitored, energy intake and energy expenditure could be adjusted to keep adipose mass constant and thereby keep the energy equation balanced over long periods of time.

Adiposity Signals

A key issue is therefore to understand how total body adipose mass is monitored by the CNS. While many fat pads are innervated, there are few data to suggest that total fat mass is monitored by afferent neural information. However, a large body of evidence indicates that circulating factors related to body adipose mass can potently influence energy balance [11, 12]. A great deal of effort has been directed at identifying these circulating factors that might influence food intake and energy expenditure in order to maintain energy balance. Historically, the first such hormone that was hypothesized as a potential afferent signal concerning energy balance was the pancreatic hormone insulin [13, 14]. While insulin is released from the pancreas as a result of glucose stimulation of the β-cell, the magnitude of this secretory response is tightly coupled to total adipose mass [15, 16]. Importantly, circulating insulin also crosses the blood–brain barrier [17] where it can interact with specific receptors for insulin that are found in many locations in the CNS but prominently in the arcuate nucleus (ARC) of the hypothalamus [18, 19]. While peripheral administration of insulin results in increased food intake and increased deposition of fat tissue because of insulin's hypoglycemic and metabolic actions, when delivered in small amounts directly into the CNS it decreases food intake and body weight without causing nonspecific aversive effects [13, 20, 21]. Moreover, reduced insulin signaling produced either by administration of insulin antibodies [22] or by selective genetic disruption of the insulin receptor in the CNS [23] produces increased food intake and increased body weight.

The hormone that has received the most attention as a potential afferent signal to the CNS about the status of peripheral adipose mass is leptin. Leptin is made primarily in adipocytes and circulates in proportion to total body fat [24]. Like insulin, however, leptin's relationship with total body fat is complex. During periods of negative energy balance, plasma leptin levels fall much faster than body fat is mobilized to provide energy. During a 48-h fast, leptin levels fall by 90% in both rodents and humans yet far less than 90% of the body fat has been burned [25–28]. Hence, plasma leptin levels convey information not only about body adipose mass but also about current energy balance. Like insulin, leptin crosses the blood–brain barrier with kinetics that are consistent with active transport by a saturable, receptor-mediated process [29, 30]. Leptin receptors exist in several splice variants and the long form of the leptin receptor (LepRb) is most strongly implicated in intracellular signal transduction. LepRb is found in several areas of the CNS but is most concentrated in the hypothalamus and particularly in the ARC [31, 32]. Leptin receptors are also found prominently in the dorsomedial (DMH) and VMH hypothalamic nuclei [32]. Finally, leptin administration either peripherally or directly into the CNS reduces food intake and body weight, and as occurs following exogenous insulin into the brain, this response cannot be attributed to nonspecific aversive effects [33, 34]. Reduced leptin signaling produced by genetic disruption of the leptin receptor, as in the *db/db* mouse or *fa/fa* rat, results in dramatic increases in food intake and body weight. A few individual humans have recently been identified to have a leptin receptor mutation and these individuals suffer from morbid obesity, indicating that leptin signaling also plays an important inhibitory role in humans [35]. For a more complete review of the CNS system engaged by leptin see reference 36.

While leptin and insulin have received considerable attention as afferent adiposity signals to the CNS, other potential humoral factors exist as well. For example, some evidence points to the possibility that amylin, a peptide hormone which is co-secreted with insulin from pancreatic β-cells, also acts as a negative feedback signal to the CNS [37]. Considerable evidence also implicates a role for adrenal glucocorticoids as potential positive feedback signals in the control of food intake and energy balance [38, 39]. However, the precise role of glucocorticoids in the control of energy homeostasis is complex and controversial. The important point is that while leptin continues to receive a tremendous amount of attention as an adiposity signal, the ultimate picture of how several circulating

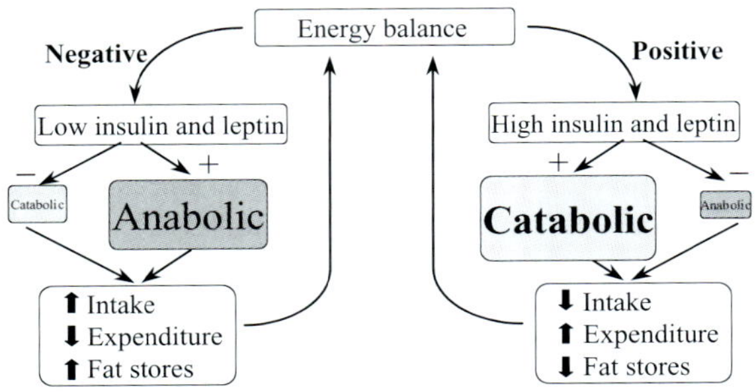

Figure 1 Theoretical model of how adiposity signals interact with two classes of hypothalamic neurotransmitter systems in order to regulate energy homeostasis

factors contribute to the CNS regulation of energy homeostasis is far from complete and will likely involve complex interactions between many hormones and their receptors.

Hypothalamic effector systems that respond to hormonal adiposity signals have been identified, and several of these are capable of potently influencing food intake and energy balance [40–42]. On functional grounds, relevant hypothalamic effector systems can be partitioned into two categories: anabolic and catabolic (see Figure 1). Anabolic effectors elicit increased food intake, decrease energy expenditure, and consequently increase stored energy in the form of adipose tissue. They are hypothesized to be activated when energy stores are low (negative energy balance), as signaled by reduced levels of insulin and leptin. Catabolic effectors do just the opposite and are activated by positive energy balance as signaled by elevated insulin and leptin. These circuits decrease food intake, increase energy expenditure, and result in decreased adipose tissue mass. A critical aspect of this negative feedback model is that hormones responsive to increasing levels of adiposity are proposed to inhibit anabolic pathways while activating catabolic pathways, and it is the balance between these pathways that ultimately determines the animal's ingestive behavior and defended level of adiposity [40, 42, 43].

Anabolic Effector Systems

Neuropeptide Y

Neuropeptide Y (NPY) is a highly expressed peptide in the mammalian CNS [44, 45] and is well conserved across species. This peptide received tremendous experimental attention following the demonstration that when administered into the CNS, NPY induces a robust feeding response [46–48]. Repeated central administration of NPY results in sustained hyperphagia and rapid body weight gain [49, 50]. Hence, NPY is proposed to be an anabolic effector that induces positive energy balance when body fat is depleted. Moreover, activity of the hypothalamic NPY system is in turn regulated by energy balance. Hypothalamic NPY neurons are found primarily in the ARC and DMH. In the arcuate, food deprivation, food restriction, or exercise-induced negative energy balance each results in upregulation of NPY mRNA in the ARC and increased NPY peptide content in targets of these neurons, such as the PVN [51–56]. Activation of the NPY system in response to negative energy balance is mediated, at least in part, by the accompanying fall of both insulin and leptin levels that accompany negative energy balance since central insulin or central or peripheral leptin infusion attentuates this NPY response [57–60].

While the ARC NPY system has received the most attention, evidence implicates an important role for the DMH NPY system as well. In several genetic murine obesity models, NPY mRNA in the DMH is elevated whereas it is normal in the ARC (such as in tubby and agouti mice [61–63]). Rats that do not make a specific receptor for the classic gut-satiety factor, cholecystokinin (CCK), have elevated body fat mass [64]. Accompanying this obesity is elevated NPY mRNA in the DMH but not the ARC. Moreover, Moran and his colleagues recently reported that there are CCK receptors on NPY neurons [64], opening the possibility that CCK directly regulates NPY signaling via the DMH. The point here is that until recently the primary emphasis on NPY signaling in the hypothalamus has been on activity of ARC NPY neurons and their regulation by leptin. However, growing evidence points to the hypothesis that there are multiple inputs that determine NPY activity in both the ARC and DMH.

Considerable controversy surrounds several aspects of the NPY system. First, mice with targeted deletion of the NPY gene do not show a dramatic phenotype in terms of their regulation of energy balance [65]. When NPY-deficient mice are crossed with obese *ob*/*ob* mice, the resultant mice with both absent NPY and leptin deficiency weigh less than *ob*/*ob* mice that have an intact NPY system indicating that the NPY system contributes significantly to the obesity of *ob*/*ob* mice [66]. However, a number of other murine models of genetic obesity have no apparent difference when crossed with NPY-deficient mice [67]. Thus, one conclusion from experiments on NPY-deficient mice suggests that NPY's importance may not be as great as the pharmacological evidence has indicated. Alternatively, NPY-deficient mice may compensate for developing in the absence of NPY signaling over the course of development [68, 69].

A second controversy concerns the identity of the critical receptor that mediates NPY's effects on food intake. Both the Y1 and Y5 receptors have significant expression in areas of the hypothalamus that are sensitive to the orexigenic effects of NPY. Conflicting data exist from both pharmacological [70–75] and transgenic approaches to assessing the relative contributions of Y1 and Y5 receptors. There remains some speculation that an as yet unidentified NPY receptor exists that contributes significantly to the feeding response [76].

Melanin-concentrating Hormone

As reviewed in Stellar's original paper, evidence dating back to the 1940s and 1950s indicates that the LHA contributes significantly to excitatory influences on food intake. Recently, two LHA peptide systems have been identified that appear to mediate these excitatory effects in the LHA. The first of these is melanin-concentrating hormone (MCH). MCH was originally identified as being relevant to the control of food intake when its expression was found to be increased in *ob/ob* mice [77]. Hence, MCH is inhibited by leptin and is elevated by food deprivation. Consistent with a proposed role as an anabolic effector transmitter in the CNS, when delivered into the lateral ventricle MCH increases food intake [78, 79]. However, unlike what happens with NPY, repeated administration of MCH does not result in increased body weight [80]. Also unlike NPY, mice with targeted deletion of MCH have reduced food intake and decreased body weight and body adiposity [81]. Recent evidence indicates that MCH is potently regulated by estrogen and may be an important component of mediating the effects of estrogen on food intake and energy balance [82]. Because MCH projections and MCH receptors are broadly distributed throughout the neuraxis, this peptide likely has a broader role than simply the control of food intake.

Hypocretin–Orexin

Another LHA peptide system was simultaneously identified by two groups of investigators. One group termed these peptides "hypocretins" [83] and the other "orexins" [84]. Both terms continue to be used but hypocretins are the more common name in circles studying sleep/waking cycles while orexin is more commonly used when referring to the control of food intake. The orexins are composed of two peptides (ORX-A and ORX-B) and two receptors, and while the cell bodies are located in close proximity to MCH-expressing neurons in the LHA, the two peptides do not co-localize to any significant extent [85]. Considerable evidence indicates that like MCH, central administration of ORX-A increases food intake [86, 87]. Like MCH, orexins also have a broad distribution pattern of axonal projections, and a variety of evidence links the ORX system directly to the control of arousal [88, 89]. ORX mRNA in the LHA is inhibited by leptin [84] and increased by decreased glucose utilization [90], suggesting that it is tied to energy homeostasis as well.

Interestingly, there appears to be significant interactions between the ARC and the LHA involving these neuropeptide systems. Projections from the ARC synapse on both MCH and ORX neurons in the LHA [91]. Hence, while there is little in the way of leptin receptors in the LHA, information concerning the levels of adiposity signals can be transmitted to the LHA via these projections from the ARC. Additionally, there is functional evidence that NPY and melanocortin neurons from the ARC interact in a specific way with MCH and ORX systems in the LHA [86, 87, 92, 93].

Ghrelin

The endogenous ligand for the growth hormone secretagogue receptor was recently identified and termed "ghrelin" [94, 95]. Ghrelin is made primarily in endocrine cells of the stomach and circulating ghrelin levels are increased during fasting and rapidly decline after nutrients are provided to the stomach [94, 95]. Consistent with a role as an anabolic effector, peripheral ghrelin infusion results in increased food intake in both rats [96] and humans [97] and sustained ghrelin infusions results in dramatic obesity. The growth hormone secretagogue receptor is found in the ARC of the hypothalamus and central administration of ghrelin results in increased food intake at doses much lower than in peripheral administration [96, 98, 99]. Evidence points to a significant role for NPY-producing cells in the ARC as critical mediators of the orexigenic effect of ghrelin [100–103]. Finally, clinical evidence points to elevated levels of ghrelin in weight-reduced patients [104], with the notable exception of patients who have been successfully treated for obesity by gastric bypass where circulating ghrelin levels are close to undetectable [105].

Catabolic Effector Systems

As opposed to the anabolic systems described above, catabolic systems are those that are activated during positive rather than negative energy balance. Hence, the activity of these systems can be best ascertained by feeding animals calories in excess of their normal caloric need. When animals are overfed in this manner, voluntary food intake drops to near zero and the animals gain body weight. Additionally, for some time after the overfeeding regimen is terminated, spontaneous food intake remains low until body weight has returned to the level of control animals [106, 107]. Hence, animals not only have potent regulatory responses to being in negative energy balance, but they also possess regulatory responses to being in positive energy balance. Catabolic systems are defined here as those that are activated during positive energy balance and that act to reduce energy intake and/or to increase energy expenditure and thereby restore energy stores to its defended level.

Melanocortin System

Considerable evidence implicates the CNS melanocortin system as an important catabolic effector system. The precursor molecule of hypothalamic melanocortins is proopiomelanocortin (POMC). In addition to several other important neuropeptides, POMC contains α-melanocyte-stimulating hormone (α-MSH), a melanocortin that is an agonist at several melanocortin receptors. POMC-expressing neurons are found primarily in the ARC and project strongly to the PVN and LHA. When given into the third ventricle, α-MSH and other nonselective melanocortin receptor agonists (including the synthetic analogue MTII) reduce food intake and body weight, whereas administration of melanocortin receptor antagonists (such as SHU-9119) increases food intake and body weight [108–111]. Several melanocortin receptor subtypes are found in the CNS, and attention has focused primarily on the MC4 and MC3 receptors since they are expressed in the hypothalamus. The observations that relatively selective MC4 receptor agonists inhibit and selective MC4 antagonists stimulate food intake [112] suggest a key role for this receptor in energy homeostasis. Consistent with this, MC4 receptor "knockout" mice have increased food intake and frank obesity, and they are insensitive to the actions of nonselective MC4 receptor agonists to reduce food intake [113, 114]. MC3 receptor knockouts also have increased body fat, but this occurs along with decreased lean body mass and no change in food intake [115, 116]. Hence while the evidence is clear that the MC4 receptor plays a role to inhibit food intake, the exact role of MC3 receptors remains open.

POMC gene expression is reduced in negative energy balance and in *ob/ob* and *db/db* mice [117, 118]. The effect of leptin to reduce food intake as well as to induce fos-like immunoreactivity in the PVN can be completely blocked by pretreatment with an melanocortin receptor antagonist [111]. POMC gene expression is increased in positive energy balance resulting from involuntary overfeeding [119]. Moreover, the potent reductions in food intake that follow periods of involuntary overfeeding are completely blocked by melanocortin receptor antagonists [119]. All of this evidence points to the endogenous POMC/α-MSH/MC4 hypothalamic system as being a key catabolic effector pathway capable of eliciting robust effects on food intake and body weight.

Interestingly, besides being stimulated by the agonist α-MSH, melanocortin signaling in the hypothalamus is also a function of an endogenous receptor antagonist termed agouti-related protein (AgRP). AgRP is expressed exclusively in the ARC in a population of neurons that is distinct from neurons that express POMC. However, AgRP neurons almost completely co-localize with neurons that express NPY [120, 121]. Like NPY, AgRP expression is elevated by food deprivation or genetic leptin deficiency [122–124]. Ventricular administration of an AgRP fragment (AgRP 83-132) potently increases food intake [125, 126]. In fact, the effect of a single injection of 1 nmol of this fragment increases incremental 24-h food intake for 6 days [126]. These results indicate that over periods greater than a few hours, AgRP is the most potent orexigenic peptide described to date. Curiously, these very long-term effects of AgRP appear not to be mediated by continued melanocortin receptor antagonism but rather to engage alternate mechanisms that include the recruitment of neurons in the nucleus accumbens, the LHA, and the central nucleus of the amygdala [127]. So, in a discrete population of leptin-sensitive neurons in the ARC, negative energy balance simultaneously results in increased NPY signaling and independently reduces melanocortin signaling. For more detailed reviews see references 128 and 129.

Cocaine–Amphetamine-related Transcript

Many of the POMC-expressing neurons in the ARC also express cocaine–amphetamine-related transcript (CART) [130]. As its name suggests, *CART* was first identified as a gene whose expression is regulated by cocaine and amphetamine. As with POMC, *CART* expression is reduced during negative energy balance and is stimulated by leptin [131]. Moreover, administration of CART peptide fragments into the ventricular system potently reduces food intake [131–133]. At these same doses, however, CART also produces a number of other behavioral actions that make its exact role in the control of food intake unclear [134]. Ventricular administration of antibodies to CART produce significant increases in intake, implicating a role for endogenous CART in the inhibition of food intake [131]. The role for this very prevalent peptide is further confused by data, indicating that when delivered specifically into the ARC, CART actually produces an increase in food intake [135].

Corticotropin-releasing Hormone and Urocortin

Corticotropin-releasing hormone (CRH) is a key controller of the hypothalmic–pituitary–adrenal (HPA) axis that regulates glucocorticoid secretion from the adrenal gland. CRH is synthesized in the PVN and LHA and is negatively regulated by levels of glucocorticoids. CRH mRNA in the PVN is also potently increased by involuntary overfeeding [107], and administration of CRH into the ventricular system potently reduces food intake, increases energy expenditure, and reduces body weight [136, 137]. In the LHA, CRH mRNA appears to be closely linked to anorexia that is produced by dehydration [138]. Understanding the CRH system is made more complicated by the presence of a binding protein within the CNS and evidence that inhibition of this binding protein results in decreased food intake [139].

Urocortin, a second peptide in the CRH family, is produced in the caudal brainstem and has prominent projections to the PVN [140]. Urocortin administration reduces food intake, but unlike what occurs following CRH, these reductions in food intake are not associated with other aversive effects [141]. Given the central importance of the CRH system to the activity of the HPA axis, the important role of peripheral glucocorticoids in controlling metabolic processes, and the inverse relationship between peripheral leptin and glucocorticoid levels, unraveling the complicated relationship of the CRH/urocortin systems in control of energy balance remains a critical but elusive goal. For a more thorough review of the CRH system and energy balance see references 142 and 143.

Proglucagon-derived Peptides

Preproglucagon is a peptide made both in the periphery and in the CNS. In addition to glucagons, preproglucagon encodes two peptides with described central activity: glucagon-like-peptide 1 (GLP-1) and glucagon-like-peptide 2 (GLP-2). Both peptides are made in the L-cells of the distal intestine and have well-described functions in the periphery, with GLP-1 critical for enhancing nutrient-induced insulin secretion [144] and GLP-2 playing an important role in maintenance of the gut mucosa [145]. Preproglucagon is also made in a distinct population of neurons in the nucleus of the solitary tract with prominent projections to the PVN and DMH [146, 147] as well as to the spinal cord. Preproglucagon neurons appear to be targets of leptin since peripheral leptin administration induces fos expression in them [148, 149]. Both GLP-1 and GLP-2 have distinct receptors, with the GLP-1 receptor found predominantly in the PVN and the GLP-2 receptor in the DMH. When administered into the ventricular system, GLP-1 produces a profound reduction in food intake and antagonists to the GLP-1 receptor increase food intake [150, 151]. However, exogenous GLP-1 administration is also associated with a number of the symptoms of visceral illness [152, 153], and GLP-1 receptor antagonists can block the visceral illness effects of the toxin LiCl [154, 155]. GLP-2 administration is associated with a less potent anorexic response but one that appears not to be accompanied by the symptoms of visceral illness associated with GLP-1 [156]. The interaction of these two co-secreted peptides is yet to be determined.

THE ROLE OF THE HYPOTHALAMUS IN PERIPHERAL GLUCOSE METABOLISM

In addition to the control of energy balance, growing evidence points to very specific roles for the hypothalamus in the control of peripheral glucose homeostasis. Neural control of insulin secretion was demonstrated by a number of investigators, with several hypothalamic nuclei including the VMH, PVN, and LHA being implicated [157–159]. The activity of efferent fibers to glucoregulatory organs including pancreas, liver, and adrenal medulla is modulated by both central glucose-responsive neurons and peripheral (gustatory, intestinal, portal vein, and hepatic) glucose sensors. It is well known that induction of hyperglycemia facilitates efferent activity of the pancreatic and hepatic branches of the vagus nerve. This in turn increases insulin secretion from the pancreas and glycogen synthesis in the liver. Hypoglycemia activates efferent activity of the pancreatic, hepatic, and adrenal branches of the splanchnic nerve, and this results in increased glucagon secretion from the pancreas, release of glucose from the liver, and secretion of catecholamines from the adrenal medulla. Thus, the picture that emerges is one in which nutrient sensing in the hypothalamus results in altered neural tone to key peripheral organs involved in glucose homeostasis. These central controls are critical to normal glucose homeostasis in a varied environment and represent a critical problem in using strategies such as pancreatic transplant, islet transplant, or insulin gene therapy as sole therapies to control diabetes.

More recent evidence implicates many of the same hypothalamic systems that control energy balance in the control of peripheral glucose homeostasis. For example, central NPY administration increases insulin secretion while melanocortin agonists decrease insulin secretion [160, 161]. Not only can central melanocortin signaling alter insulin secretion but both melanocortin agonists and leptin can also alter insulin sensitivity in the liver via actions in the CNS [162]. Leptin replacement in genetically leptin-deficient mice reduces the dramatic hyperglycemia in these animals and several lines of evidence point to this being an effect that is at least partially mediated by leptin actions in the hypothalamus to alter insulin sensitivity in peripheral tissues. Rossetti and his colleagues have also shown that decreasing insulin signaling in the medial hypothalamus not only increases food intake but reduces the ability of peripheral insulin to reduce glucose output from the liver [163]. The implication that derangements in hypothalamic signaling pathways can produce disruptions of both overall energy balance that favor development of obesity and disordered glucose homeostasis that can predispose to type 2 diabetes, provides potentially new insights into the etiology of both disorders. It is possible that the profound relationship between obesity and type 2 diabetes involves disorders related to these important hypothalamic pathways.

CONCLUSIONS

In this chapter we have tried to present a basic outline of hypothalamic systems that are involved in the control of food intake. One review can no longer capture even a small percentage of the current knowledge on the various hypothalamic systems that are involved in the regulation of food intake and body weight, let alone those also involved in peripheral glucose homeostasis. Hence, many other CNS systems including those utilizing serotonin, neurotensin [164], histamine [165], or norepinephrine

[166] (or many others) have not been discussed here. Likewise, hypothalamic neurons that are involved in direct nutrient sensing and that play a prominent role in the control of food intake have also been ignored (see reference 167 for a review). What has been included is a review of the pathways important in integrating body adiposity with food intake and energy expenditure since these pathways are the focus of so much ongoing research activity.

The pace of research on energy homeostasis has been extraordinary over the last decade. This explosion in our knowledge has been driven both by the multitude of new tools now available to investigators and by the crushing clinical need to address the epidemic of obesity that confronts the developed world. In many ways, the explosion of knowledge around these systems reflects the application of powerful molecular tools to pick the "lowest hanging fruit" by identifying peptide systems whose activity is somehow regulated by changes in energy balance. The hard work remains in front of us, which is to understand the interactions of these systems whose combined output doggedly defends the level of stored fuel in the body with incredible precision. The work of Grill and his colleagues using the chronic decerebrate rat to cast doubt on the Dual-Centers Hypothesis should continue to be a cautionary tale. As has been demonstrated for a number of these systems, the ligands and their receptors that control energy homeostasis are widely distributed throughout the CNS, including in specific regions of the caudal brainstem. In fact, several of these ligands, when administered in the fourth ventricle or directly into specific brainstem nuclei, produce robust changes in food intake. CRH, NPY, CART, melanocortin agonists, and antagonists, and most recently leptin itself are all capable of altering food intake when delivered to brainstem rather than hypothalamic sites [168, 169]. Hence, these control systems can no longer be considered to be merely hypothalamic. Rather, even these specific peptide systems and their interaction with adiposity signals must be thought of as functional circuits that transcend multiple levels of the nervous system.

A key challenge, therefore, is to understand the independent contribution of specific receptor populations to the maintenance of energy balance. To address this issue, we not only have to understand the neuroscience of how food intake and energy expenditure are controlled, but how the body weight regulatory system interfaces with other critical functions such as arousal, reward, sensation, emotion, and memory. The important point is that the control of energy balance is not an isolated function but rather an integrated part of how an animal survives. Hence, the hypothalamic systems that we have described in this chapter must also be understood in the context of how they interface with other CNS circuits inside and outside the hypothalamus.

Stellar's Dual-Centers Hypothesis dominated our view of how food intake is controlled for several decades. Building upon these pioneering insights, the conceptualization offered in this chapter emphasizes the regulation of long-term energy balance rather than the initiation and termination of individual bouts of ingestion. It also emphasizes neurochemical effector pathways over specific hunger and satiety centers. These changes in emphasis provide a new context in which to interpret the mountain of data concerning these hypothalamic systems. However, the new emphases outlined in this chapter can hardly be considered the final word. Our ability to meet the next challenges in understanding the regulation of energy balance and the interaction of multiple systems will not rest solely upon developing better tools for collecting data but will require that we advance our theoretical perspectives as well.

SUMMARY

(1) Maintenance of energy balance depends on several intertwined hypothalamic circuits.

(2) Adiposity signals such as leptin and insulin that signal to the CNS about the status of peripheral energy balance provide critical input to effector pathways, which in turn can influence both food intake and energy expenditure.

(3) These effector pathways can be divided into anabolic and catabolic. Anabolic pathways are inhibited by adiposity signals and increased activity results in increased energy intake and decreased energy expenditure. Catabolic pathways are stimulated by adiposity signals and increased activity results in decreased energy intake and increased energy expenditure.

(4) The adiposity signals and effector pathways implicated in the control of energy balance also have been implicated in the control of peripheral glucose homeostasis, opening up the possibility of common underlying etiologies for both obesity and diabetes involving hypothalamic dysregulation.

Acknowledgments

This work was supported by a number of grants from the NIH (DK54890, DK54080, DK-17844), and funds from the Procter & Gamble Co.

REFERENCES

1. Stellar E. The physiology of motivation. *Psychol Rev* 1954; 61: 5–22.
2. Powley TL. The ventromedial hypothalamic syndrome, satiety, and a cephalic phase hypothesis. *Psychol Rev* 1977; 84: 89–126.
3. Sclafani A. The role of hyperinsulinema and the vagus nerve in hypothalamic hyperphagia reexamined. *Diabetologia* 1981; 20 (suppl): 402–10.

4. Bray GA, Sclafani A, Novin D. Obesity-inducing hypothalamic knife cuts: effects on lipolysis and blood insulin levels. *Am J Physiol* 1982; 243 (3): R445–9.
5. Aravich PF, Sclafani A. Paraventricular hypothalamic lesions and medial hypothalamic knife cuts produce similar hyperphagia syndromes. *Behav Neurosci* 1983; 97 (6): 970–83.
6. Grill HJ, Norgren R. Chronically decerebrate rats demonstrate satiation but not bait shyness. *Science* 1978; 201 (4352): 267–9.
7. Grill HJ, Norgren R. The taste reactivity test, II: mimetic responses to gustatory stimuli in chronic thalamic and chronic decerebrate rats. *Brain Res* 1978; 143 (2): 281–97.
8. Grill HJ, Smith GP. Cholecystokinin decreases sucrose intake in chronic decerebrate rats. *Am J Physiol* 1988; 254: R853–6.
9. Flynn FW, Grill HJ. Intraoral intake and taste reactivity responses elicited by sucrose and sodium chloride in chronic decerebrate rats. *Behav Neurosci* 1988; 102 (6): 934–41.
10. Kennedy GC. The role of depot fat in the hypothalamic control of food intake in the rat. *Proc R Soc Lond (Biol)* 1953; 140: 579–92.
11. Coleman DL. Effects of parabiosis of obese with diabetes and normal mice. *Diabetologia* 1973; 9: 294–8.
12. Hervey GR. The effects of lesions in the hypothalalmus in parabiotic rats. *J Physiol* 1952; 145: 336–52.
13. Woods SC, Lotter EC, McKay LD, Porte D Jr. Chronic intracerebroventricular infusion of insulin reduces food intake and body weight of baboons. *Nature* 1979; 282: 503–5.
14. Woods SC, Nolan LJ. The insulin story: a 25-year perspective. *Appetite* 1997; 28: 281–2.
15. Polonsky BD, Given E, Carter V. Twenty-four-hour profiles and pulsatile patterns of insulin secretion in normal and obese subjects. *J Clin Invest* 1988; 81: 442–8.
16. Polonsky KS, Given BD, Hirsch L, Shapiro ET, Tillil H, Beebe C, Galloway JA, Frank BH, Karrison T, Van-Cauter E. Quantitative study of insulin secretion and clearance in normal and obese subjects. *J Clin Invest* 1988; 81: 435–41.
17. Baura G, Foster D, Porte D Jr, Kahn SE, Bergman RN, Cobelli C, Schwartz MW. Saturable transport of insulin from plasma into the central nervous system of dogs *in vivo*: a mechanism for regulated insulin delivery to the brain. *J Clin Invest* 1993; 92: 1824–30.
18. Baskin DG, Sipols AJ, Schwartz MW, White MF. Insulin receptor substrate-1 (IRS-1) expression in rat brain. *Endocrinology* 1994; 134: 1952–5.
19. Baskin DG, Marks JL, Schwartz MW, Figewicz DP, Woods SC, Porte D Jr. Insulin and insulin receptors in the brain in relation to food intake and body weight. In Lehnert H, Murison R, Weiner H, Hellhammer D, Beyer J (eds). *Endocrine and Nutritional Control of Basic Biological Functions*, Stuttgart: Hogrefe & Huber, 1990; pp 202–22.
20. Chavez M, Seeley RJ, Woods SC. A comparison between the effects of intraventricular insulin and intraperitoneal LiCl on three measures sensitive to emetic agents. *Behav Neurosci* 1995; 109: 547–50.
21. Chavez M, Kaiyala K, Madden LJ, Schwartz MW, Woods SC. Intraventricular insulin and the level of maintained body weight in rats. *Behav Neurosci* 1995; 109: 528–31.
22. McGowan MK, Andrews KM, Grossman SP. Chronic intrahyphothalamic infusions of insulin or insulin antibodies alter body weight and food intake in the rat. *Physol-Behav* 1992; 51: 753–66.
23. Brüning JC, Gautam D, Burks DJ, Gillette J, Schubert M, Orban PC, Klein R, Krone W, Müller-Wieland D, Kahn CR. Role of brain insulin receptor in control of body weight and reproduction. *Science* 2000; 289: 2122–5.
24. Zhang Y, Proenca R, Maffie M, Barone M, Leopold L, Friedman JM. Positional cloning of the mouse obese gene and its human homologue. *Nature* 1994; 372: 425–32.
25. Ahima RS, Prabakaran D, Mantzoros C, Qu D, Lowell B, Flier-Maratos E, Flier JS. Role of leptin in the neuroendocrine response to fasting. *Nature* 1996; 382: 250–2.
26. Kolaczynski JW, Considine RV, Ohannesian J, Marco C, Opentanova I, Nyce MR, Caro JF. Responses of leptin to short-term fasting and refeeding in humans: a link with ketogenesis but not ketones themselves. *Diabetes* 1996; 45: 1511–5.
27. Ahima RS, Kelly J, Elmquist JK, Flier JS. Distinct physiologic and neuronal responses to decreased leptin and mild hyperleptinemia. *Endocrinology* 1999; 140 (11): 4923–31.
28. Boden G, Chen X, Mozzoli M, Ryan I. Effect of fasting on serum leptin in normal human subjects. *J Clin Endocrinol Metab* 1996; 81: 3419–23.
29. Banks WA, Kastin AJ, Huang Wea. Leptin enters the brain by a saturable system independent of insulin. *Peptides* 1996; 17: 305–11.
30. Banks WA, DiPalma CR, Farrell CL. Impaired transport of leptin across the blood–brain barrier in obesity. *Peptides* 1999; 20: 1341–5.
31. Schwartz MW, Seeley RJ, Campfield LA, Burn P, Baskin DG. Identification of hypothalmic targets of leptin action. *J Clin Invest* 1996; 98: 1101–6.
32. Elmquist JK, Bjorbaek C, Ahima RS, Flier JS, Saper CB. Distributions of leptin receptor mRNA isoforms in the rat brain. *J Comp Neurol* 1998; 395 (4): 535–47.
33. van Dijk G, Thiele TE, Donahey JCK, Campfield LA, Smith FJ, Burn P, Bernstein IL, Woods SC, Seeley RJ. Central infusion of leptin and GLP-1 (7-36) amide differentially stimulate c-Fos-like immunoreactivity in the rat brain. *Am J Physiol* 1996; 271: R1096–100.
34. Thiele TE, van Dijk G, Campfield LA, Smith FJ, Burn P, Woods SC, Bernstein IL, Seeley RJ. Central administration of GLP-1, but not leptin, produce conditioned taste aversions in the rat. *Am J Physiol* 1997; 272: R726–30.
35. Clement K, Vaisse C, Lahlou N, Cabrol S, Pelloux V, Cassuto D, Gourmelen M, Dina C, Chambaz J, Lacorte JM, Basdevant A, Bougneres P, Lebouc Y, Froguel P, Guy-Grand B. A mutation in the human leptin receptor gene causes obesity and pituitary dysfunction [see comments]. *Nature* 1998; 392 (6674): 398–401.
36. Ahima RS, Saper CB, Flier JS, Elmquist JK. Leptin regulation of neuroendocrine systems. *Front Neuroendocrinol* 2000; 21: 263–307.
37. Rushing PA, Hagan MM, Seeley RJ, Lutz TA, Woods SC. Amylin: a novel action in the brain to reduce body weight. *Endocrinology* 2000; 141: 850–3.
38. Jeanrenaud B, Rohner-Jeanrenaud F. CNS-periphery relationships and body weight homeostasis: influence of the glucocorticoid status. *Int J Obes Relat Metab Disord* 2000; 24 (suppl 2): S74–6.

39. Strack AM, Sebastian RJ, Schwartz MW, Dallman MF. Glucocorticoids and insulin: reciprocal signals for energy balance. *Am J Physiol* 1995; 268: 142–9.
40. Schwartz MW, Woods SC, Porte DJ, Seeley RJ, Baskin DG. Central nervous system control of food intake. *Nature* 2000; 404: 661–71.
41. Seeley R, Schwartz M. Neuroendocrime regulation of food intake. *Acta Paediatrica Supplement* 1999; 88 (Feb): 58–61.
42. Woods SC, Seeley RJ, Porte DJ, Schwartz MW. Signals that regulate food intake and energy homeostasis. *Science* 1998; 280: 1378–83.
43. Seeley RJ, Woods SC. Leptin actions in the hypothalamus. Regulation of pituitary hormone secretion, 1999.
44. Allen YS, Adrian TE, Tatemoto K, Crow TJ, Bloom SR, Polak JM. Neuropeptide Y distribution in the rat brain. *Science* 1983; 221: 877–9.
45. Minth CD, Andrews PC, Dixon JE. Characterization, sequence and expression of the cloned human neuropeptide Y gene. *J Biol Chem* 1986; 261 (26): 11975–9.
46. Clark JT, Kalra PS, Crowley WR, Kalra SP. Neuropeptide Y and human pancreatic polypeptide stimulate feeding behavior in rats. *Endocrinology* 1984; 115 (1): 427–9.
47. Stanley BG, Leibowitz SF. Neuropeptide Y injected into the paraventricular hypothalamus: a powerful stimulant of feeding behavior. *Proc Natl Acad Sci USA* 1984; 82: 3940–3.
48. Seeley RJ, Payne CJ, Woods SC. Neuropeptide Y fails to increase intraoral intake in rats. *Am J Physiol* 1995; 268: R423–7.
49. Stanley BG, Kyrkouli SE, Lampert S, Leibowitz SF. Neuropeptide Y chronically injected into the hypothalamus: a powerful neurochemical inducer of hyperphagia and obesity. *Peptides* 1986; 7: 1189–92.
50. McMinn JE, Seeley RJ, Wilkinson CW, Havel PJ, Woods SC, Schwartz MW. NPY-induced overfeeding suppresses hypothalamic NPY mRNA expression: potential roles of plasma insulin and leptin. *Regul Pept* 1998; 75–76: 425–31.
51. Mizuno TM, Makimura H, Silverstein J, Roberts JL, Lopingco T, Mobbs CV. Fasting regulates hypothalamic neuropeptide Y, agouti-related peptide, and proopiomelanocortin in diabetic mice independent of changes in leptin or insulin. *Endocrinology* 1999; 140 (10): 4551–7.
52. Sahu A, Sninsky CA, Phelps CP, Dube MG, Kalra PS, Kalra SP. Neuropeptide Y release from the parventricular nucleus increases in association with hyperphagia in streptozotocin-induced diabetic rats. *Endocrinology* 1992; 131 (6): P2979–85.
53. Marks JL, Mu L, Schwartz MW, Porte D Jr, Baskin DG. Effect of fasting on regional levels of neuropeptide Y mRNA and insulin receptors in the rat hypothalamus: an autoradiographic study. *Mol Cell Neurosci* 1992; 3: 199–205.
54. Sahu A, Sninsky CA, Kalra PS, Kalra SP. Neuropeptide Y concentration in microdissected hypothalamic regions and *in vitro* release from the medial basal hypothalamus-preoptic area of streptozotocin-diabetic rats with and without insulin substitution therapy. *Endocrinology* 1990; 126: 192–8.
55. Kalra SP, Dube MG, Sahu A, Phelps CP, Kalra P. Neuropeptide Y secretion increases in the paraventricular nucleus in association with increased appetite for food. *Proc Natl Acad Sci USA* 1991; 88: 10931–5.
56. Sahu A, Kalra PS, Kalra SP. Food deprivation and ingestion induce reciprocal changes in neuropeptide Y concentrations in the paraventricular nucleus. *Peptides* 1988; 9: 83–6.
57. Sipols AJ, Baskin DG, Schwartz MW. Effect of intracerebroventricular insulin infusion on diabetic hyperphagia and hypothalamic neuropeptide gene expression. *Diabetes* 1995; 44: 147–51.
58. Sipols AJ, Baskin DG, Schwartz MW. The importance of central nervous system insulin deficiency to diabetic hyperphagia. *Diabetes* 1993; 42 (suppl 1): 152.
59. Stephens TW, Bashinski M, Bristow PK, Bue-Vallesky JM, Burgetti SG, Craft L, Prater J, Hoffman J, Huang HM, Kriasticinas A, Mackeltar W, Rostack PR, Schoner B, Smith D, Tinarley FC, Zhang XY, Metman M. The role of neuropeptide Y in the antiobesity action of the obese gene product. *Nature* 1995; 377: 530–4.
60. Schwartz MW, Baskin DG, Bukowski TR, Kuijper JL, Foster D, Lasser G, Prunkard DE, Porte D, Woods SC, Seeley RJ, Weigle DS. Specificity of leptin action on elevated blood glucose levels and hypothalamic neuropeptide Y gene expression in *ob*/*ob* mice. *Diabetes* 1996; 45: 531–5.
61. Bernardis LL, Bellinger LL. The dorsomedial hypothalamic nucleus revisited: 1998 update. *Proc Soc Exp Biol Med* 1998; 218 (4): 284–306.
62. Kesterson RA, Huszar D, Lynch CA, Simerly RB, Cone RD. Induction of neuropeptide Y gene expression in the dorsal medial hypothalamic nucleus in two models of the agouti obesity syndrome. *Mol Endocrinol* 1997; 11 (5): 630–7.
63. Guan XM, Yu H, Trumbauer M, Frazier E, Van der Ploeg LH, Chen H. Induction of neuropeptide Y expression in dorsomedial hypothalamus of diet-induced obese mice. *Neuroreport* 1998; 9 (15): 3415–9.
64. Bi S, Ladenheim EE, Moran TH. Elevated neuropeptide Y expression in the dorsomedial hypothalamic nucleus may contribute to the hyperphagia and obesity in OLETF rats with CCKA receptor deficit. Annual Meeting for the Society for Neuroscience 2000; New Orleans, LA.
65. Erickson JC, Clegg KE, Palmiter RD. Sensitivity to leptin and susceptibility to seizures of mice lacking neuropeptide Y. *Nature* 1996; 381: 415–8.
66. Erickson JC, Hollopeter G, Palmiter RD. Attenuation of the obesity syndrome of *ob*/*ob* mice by the loss of neuropeptide Y. *Science* 1996; 274 (5293): 1704–7.
67. Hollopeter G, Erickson JC, Palmiter RD. Role of neuropeptide Y in diet-, chemical- and genetic-induced obesity of mice. *Int J Obes Relat Metab Disord* 1998; 22 (6): 506–12.
68. Palmiter RD, Erickson JC, Hollopeter G, Baraban SC, Schwartz MW. Life without neuropeptide Y. *Recent Prog Horm Res* 1998; 53: 163–99.
69. Woods SC, Figlewicz DP, Madden L, Porte J, D., Sipols AJ, Seeley RJ. NPY and food intake: discrepancies in the model. *Regul Pept* 1998; 75–76: 403–8.
70. Criscione L, Rigollier P, Batzl-Hartmann C, Rueger H, Stricker-Krongrad A, Wyss P, Brunner L, Whitebread S, Yamaguchi Y, Gerald C, Heurich RO, Walker MW, Chiesi M, Schilling W, Hofbauer KG, Levens N. Food intake in free-feeding and energy-deprived lean rats is mediated by the neuropeptide Y5 receptor. *J Clin Invest* 1998; 102 (12): 2136–45.

71. Marsh D, Hollopeter G, Huszar D, Laufer R, Yagaloff K, Fisher S, Burn P, Palmiter R. Response of melanocortin-4 receptor-deficient mice to anorectic and orexigenic peptides. *Nat Genet* 1999; 21 (January): 119–22.
72. Kanatani A, Mashiko S, Murai N, Sugimoto N, Ito J, Fukuroda T, Fukami T, Morin N, MacNeil DJ, Van der Ploeg LH, Saga Y, Nishimura S, Ihara M. Role of the Y1 receptor in the regulation of neuropeptide Y-mediated feeding: comparison of wild-type, Y1 receptor-deficient, and Y5 receptor-deficient mice. *Endocrinology* 2000; 141 (3): 1011–6.
73. Tang-Christensen M, Kristensen P, Stidsen CE, Brand CL, Larsen PJ. Central administration of Y5 receptor antisense decreases spontaneous food intake and attenuates feeding in response to exogenous neuropeptide Y. *J Endocrinol* 1998; 159 (2): 307–12.
74. Larsen PJ, Tang-Christensen M, Stidsen CE, Madsen K, Smith MS, Cameron JL. Activation of central neuropeptide Y Y1 receptors potently stimulates food intake in male rhesus monkeys [In Process Citation]. *J Clin Endocrinol Metab* 1999; 84 (10): 3781–91.
75. Hellig M, Pich M, Koob GF, Yee F, Wahlestedt C. *In vivo* downregulation of neuropeptide Y (NPY) Y1-receptors by i.c.v. antisense oligodeoxynucleotide administration is associated with signs of anxiety in rats. *Soc Neruosci Abstr* 1992; 18: 1539.
76. O'Shea D, Morgan DG, Meeran K, Edwards CM, Turton MD, Choi SJ, Heath MM, Gunn I, Taylor GM, Howard JK, Bloom CI, Small CJ, Haddo O, Ma JJ, Callinan W, Smith DM, Ghatei MA, Bloom SR. Neuropeptide Y induced feeding in the rat is mediated by a novel receptor. *Endocrinology* 1997; 138 (1): 196–202.
77. Qu D, Ludwig DS, Gammeltoft S, Piper M, Pelleymounter MA, Cullen MJ, Mathes WF, Przypek R, Kanarek R, Maratos-Flier E. A role for melanin-concentrating hormone in the central regulation of feeding behaviour. *Nature* 1996; 380 (6571): 243–7.
78. Ludwig D, Mountjoy K, Tatro J, Gillette J, Frederich R, Flier J, Maratos-Flier E. Melanin-concentrating hormone: a functional melanocortin antagonist in the hypothalamus. *Am J Physiol* 1998; 274 (Apr): E627–33.
79. Sanchez M, Baker B, Celis M. Melanin-concentrating hormone (MCH) antagonizes the effects of alpha-MSH and neuropeptide E-I on grooming and locomotor activities in the rat. *Peptides* 1997; 18: 393–6.
80. Rossi M, Choi SJ, O'Shea D, Miyoshi T, Ghatei MA, Bloom SR. Melanin-concentrating hormone acutely stimulates feeding, but chronic administration has no effect on body weight. *Endocrinology* 1997; 138 (1): 351–5.
81. Shimada M, Tritos N, Lowell B, Flier J, Maratos-Flier E. Mice lacking melanin-concentrating hormone are hypophagic and lean. *Nature* 1998; 396 (December 17): 670–4.
82. Mystkowski P, Seeley RJ, Hahn TM, Baskin DG, Havel PJ, Matsumoto AM, Wilkinson CW, Peacock-Kinzig K, Blake KA, Schwartz MW. Hypothalamic melanin-concentrating hormone and estrogen-induced weight loss [In Process Citation]. *J Neurosci* 2000; 20 (22): 8637–42.
83. de Lecea L, Kilduff TS, Peyron C, Gao X, Foye PE, Danielson PE, Fukuhara C, Battenberg EL, Gautvik VT, Bartlett FS, Frankel WN, van den Pol AN, Bloom FE, Gautvik KM, Sutcliffe JG. The hypocretins: hypothalamus-specific peptides with neuroexcitatory activity. *Proc Nat Acad Sci USA* 1998; 95: 322–7.
84. Sakurai T, Amemiya A, Ishii M, Matsuzaki I, Chemelli RM, Tanaka H, Williams SC, Richardson JA, Kozlowski GP, Wilson S, Arch JR, Buckingham RE, Haynes AC, Carr SA, Annan RS, McNulty DE, Liu WS, Terrett JA, Elshourbagy NA, Bergsma DJ, Yanagisawa M. Orexins and orexin receptors: a family of hypothalamic neuropeptides and G protein-coupled receptors that regulate feeding behavior [see comments]. *Cell* 1998; 92 (4): 573–85.
85. Broberger C, De Lecea L, Sutcliffe JG, Hokfelt T. Hypocretin/orexin- and melanin-concentrating hormone-expressing cells form distinct populations in the rodent lateral hypothalamus: relationship to the neuropeptide Y and agouti gene-related protein systems. *J Comp Neurol* 1998; 402: 460–74.
86. Yamanaka A, Kunii K, Nambu T, Tsujino N, Sakai A, Matsuzaki I, Miwa Y, Goto K, Sakurai T. Orexin-induced food intake involves neuropeptide Y pathway. *Brain Res* 2000; 859 (2): 404–9.
87. Rauch M, Riediger T, Schmid HA, Simon E. Orexin A activates leptin-responsive neurons in the arcuate nucleus [In Process Citation]. *Pflugers Arch* 2000; 440 (5): 699–703.
88. Peyron C, Tighe DK, van den Pol AN, de Lecea L, Heller HC, Sutcliffe JG, Kilduff TS. Neurons containing hypocretin (orexin) project to multiple neuronal systems. *J Neurosci* 1998; 18: 9996–100015.
89. Kilduff TS, Peyron C. The hypocretin/orexin ligand–receptor system: implications for sleep and sleep disorders. *Trends Neurosci* 2000; 23 (8): 359–65.
90. Sergeyev V, Broberger C, Gorbatyuk O, Hokfelt T. Effect of 2-mercaptoacetate and 2-deoxy-D-glucose administration on the expression of NPY, AGRP, POMC, MCH and hypocretin/orexin in the rat hypothalamus. *Neuroreport* 2000; 11 (1): 117–21.
91. Elias CF, Saper CB, Maratos-Flier E, Tritos NA, Lee C, Kelly J, Tatro JB, Hoffman GE, Ollmann MM, Barsh GS, Sakurai T, Yanagisawa M, Elmquist JK. Chemically defined projections linking the mediobasal hypothalamus and the lateral hypothalamic area. *J Comp Neurol* 1998; 402 (4): 442–59.
92. Tritos NA, Vicent D, Gillette J, Ludwig DS, Flier ES, Maratos-Flier E. Functional interactions between melanin-concentrating hormone, neuropeptide Y, and anorectic neuropeptides in the rat hypothalamus. *Diabetes* 1998; 47: 1687–92.
93. Jain MR, Horvath TL, Kalra PS, Kalra SP. Evidence that NPY Y1 receptors are involved in stimulation of feeding by orexins (hypocretins) in sated rats. *Regul Pept* 2000; 87 (1–3): 19–24.
94. Kojima M, Hosoda H, Date Y, Nakazato M, Matsuo H, Kangawa K. Ghrelin is a growth-hormone-releasing acylated peptide from stomach. *Nature* 1999; 402 (6762): 656–60.
95. Kojima M, Hosoda H, Kangawa K. Purification and distribution of ghrelin: the natural endogenous ligand for the growth hormone secretagogue receptor. *Horm Res* 2001; 56 (suppl 1): 93–7.
96. Tschop M, Smiley DL, Heiman ML. Ghrelin induces adiposity in rodents. *Nature* 2000; 407 (6806): 908–13.
97. Wren AM, Seal LJ, Cohen MA, Brynes AE, Frost GS, Murphy KG, Dhillo WS, Ghatei MA, Bloom SR. Ghrelin enhances appetite and increases food intake in humans. *J Clin Endocrinol Metab* 2001; 86 (12): 5992.

98. Kamegai J, Tamura H, Shimizu T, Ishii S, Sugihara H, Wakabayashi I. Central effect of ghrelin, an endogenous growth hormone secretagogue, on hypothalamic peptide gene expression. *Endocrinology* 2000; 141 (12): 4797–800.
99. Wren AM, Small CJ, Ward HL, Murphy KG, Dakin CL, Taheri S, Kennedy AR, Roberts GH, Morgan DG, Ghatei MA, Bloom SR. The novel hypothalamic peptide ghrelin stimulates food intake and growth hormone secretion. *Endocrinology* 2000; 141 (11): 4325–8.
100. Asakawa A, Inui A, Kaga T, Yuzuriha H, Nagata T, Ueno N, Makino S, Fujimiya M, Niijima A, Fujino MA, Kasuga M. Ghrelin is an appetite-stimulatory signal from stomach with structural resemblance to motilin. *Gastroenterology* 2001; 120 (2): 337–45
101. Kamegai J, Tamura H, Shimizu T, Ishii S, Sugihara H, Wakabayashi I. Chronic central infusion of ghrelin increases hypothalamic neuropeptide Y and agouti-related protein mRNA levels and body weight in rats. *Diabetes* 2001; 50 (11): 2438–43.
102. Nakazato M, Murakami N, Date Y, Kojima M, Matsuo H, Kangawa K, Matsukura S. A role for ghrelin in the central regulation of feeding. *Nature* 2001; 409 (6817): 194–8.
103. Wang L, Saint-Pierre DH, Tache Y. Peripheral ghrelin selectively increases Fos expression in neuropeptide Y-synthesizing neurons in mouse hypothalamic arcuate nucleus. *Neurosci Lett* 2002; 325 (1): 47–51.
104. Tschop M, Weyer C, Tataranni PA, Devanarayan V, Ravussin E, Heiman ML. Circulating ghrelin levels are decreased in human obesity. *Diabetes* 2001; 50 (4): 707–9.
105. Cummings DE, Weigle DS, Frayo RS, Breen PA, Ma MK, Dellinger EP, Purnell JQ. Plasma ghrelin levels after diet-induced weight loss or gastric bypass surgery. *N Engl J Med* 2002; 346 (21): 1623–30.
106. Bernstein IL, Lotter EC, Kulkosky PJ. Effect of force-feeding upon basal insulin levels in rats. *Proc Soc Exp Biol Med* 1975; 150: 546–8.
107. Seeley RJ, Matson CA, Chavez M, Woods SC, Schwartz MW. Behavioral, endocrine and hypothalamic responses to involuntary overfeeding. *Am J Physiol* 1996; 271: R819–23.
108. Fan W, Boston B, Kesterson R, Hruby V, Cone R. Role of melanocortinergic neurons in feeding and the agouti obesity syndrome. *Nature* 1997; 385 (January 9): 165–8.
109. Tsujii S, Bray GA. Acetylation alters the feeding response to MSH and beta-endorphin. *Brain Res Bull* 1989; 23: 165–9.
110. Thiele T, van DG, Yagaloff K, Fisher S, Schwartz M, Burn P, Seeley R. Central infusion of melanocortin agonist MTII in rats: assessment of c-Fos expression and taste aversion. *Am J Physiol* 1998; 274 (January): R248–54.
111. Seeley R, Yagaloff K, Fisher S, Burn P, Thiele T, van DG, Baskin D, Schwartz M. Melanocortin receptors in leptin effects. *Nature* 1997; 390 (November 27): 349.
112. Benoit SC, Schwartz MW, Lachey JL, Hagan MM, Rushing PA, Blake KA, Yagaloff KA, Kurylko G, Franco L, Danhoo W, Seeley RJ. A novel selective melanocortin-4 receptor agonist reduces food intake in rats and mice without producing aversive consequences. *J Neurosci* 2000; 20 (9): 3442–8.
113. Huszar D, Lynch C, V. F-H, Dunmore J, Fang Q, Berkemeier L, Gu W, Kesterson R, Boston B, Cone R, Smith F, Campfield L, Burn P, Lee F. Targeted disruption of the melanocortin-4 receptor results in obesity in mice. *Cell* 1997; 88 (January 10): 131–41.
114. Marsh DJ, Hollopeter G, Kofer KE, Palmiter RD. Role of the Y5 neuropeptide Y receptor in feeding and obesity [see comments]. *Nat Med* 1998; 4 (6): 718–21.
115. Chen AS, Marsh DJ, Trumbauer ME, Frazier EG, Guan XM, Yu H, Rosenblum CI, Vongs A, Feng Y, Cao L, Metzger JM, Strack AM, Camacho RE, Mellin TN, Nunes CN, Min W, Fisher J, Gopal-Truter S, MacIntyre DE, Chen HY, Van Der Ploeg LH. Inactivation of the mouse melanocortin-3 receptor results in increased fat mass and reduced lean body mass [In Process Citation]. *Nat Genet* 2000; 26 (1): 97–102.
116. Butler AA, Kesterson RA, Khong K, Cullen MJ, Pelleymounter MA, Dekoning J, Baetscher M, Cone RD. A unique metabolic syndrome causes obesity in the melanocortin-3 receptor-deficient mouse. *Endocrinology* 2000; 141 (9): 3518–21.
117. Mizuno T, Kleopoulos S, Bergen H, Roberts J, Priest C, Mobbs C. Hypothalamic pro-opiomelanocortin mRNA is reduced by fasting and in *ob/ob* and *db/db* mice, but is stimulated by leptin. *Diabetes* 1998; 47 (February): 294–7.
118. Schwartz MW, Seeley RJ, Weigle DS, Burn P, Campfield LA, Baskin DG. Leptin increases hypothalamic proopiomelanocoritin (POMC) mRNA expression in the rostral arcuate nucleus. *Diabetes* 1997; 46: 2119–23.
119. Hagan M, Rushing P, Schwartz M, Yagaloff K, Burn P, Woods S, Seeley R. Role of the CNS melanocortin system in the response to overfeeding. *J Neurosci* 1999; 19 (March 15): 2362–7.
120. Hahn TM, Breininger JF, Baskin DG, Schwartz MW. Coexpression of Agrp and NPY in fasting-activated hypothalamic neurons. *Nat Neurosci* 1998; 1: 271–2.
121. Chen P, Li C, Haskell-Luevano C, Cone RD, Smith MS. Altered expression of agouti-related protein and its colocalization with neuropeptide Y in the arcuate nucleus of the hypothalamus during lactation. *Endocrinology* 1999; 140 (6): 2645–50.
122. Fong T, Mao C, MacNeil T, Kalyani R, Smith T, Weinberg D, Tota M, Van dPL. ART (protein product of agouti-related transcript) as an antagonist of MC-3 and MC-4 receptors. *Biochem Biophys Res Commun* 1997; 237 (August 28): 629–31.
123. Ollmann M, Wilson B, Yang Y, Kerns J, Chen Y, Gantz I, Barsh G. Antagonism of central melanocortin receptors *in vitro* and *in vivo* by agouti-related protein. *Science* 1997; 278 (October 3): 135–8.
124. Shutter J, Graham M, Kinsey A, Scully S, Luthy R, Stark K. Hypothalamic expression of ART, a novel gene related to agouti, is up-regulated in obese and diabetic mutant mice. *Genes Dev* 1997; 11 (March 1): 593–602.
125. Rossi M, Kim M, Morgan D, Small C, Edwards C, Sunter D, Abusnana S, Goldstone A, Russell S, Stanley S, Smith D, Yagaloff K, Ghatei M, Bloom S. A C-terminal fragment of agouti-related protein increases feeding and antagonizes the effect of alpha-melanocyte stimulating hormone *in vivo*. *Endocrinology* 1998; 139 (October): 4428–31.
126. Hagan MM, Rushing PA, Pritchard LM, Schwartz MW, Strack AM, Van der Ploeg HT, Woods SC, Seeley RJ. Long-term orexigenic effects of AgRP-(83-132) involve mechanisms other than melanocortin receptor blockade. *Am J Physiol* 2000; 279: R47–52.

127. Hagan MM, Benoit SC, Rushing PA, Pritchard LM, Woods SC, Seeley RJ. Immediate and prolonged patterns of agouti-related peptide-(83-132)-induced c-Fos activation in hypothalamic and extrahypothalamic sites. *Endocrinology* 2001; 142 (3): 1050–6.
128. Cone RD. The central melanocortin system and energy homeostasis. *Trends Endocrinol Metab* 1999; 10 (6): 211–6.
129. Benoit SC, Schwartz MW, Baskin DG, Woods SC, Seeley RJ. CNS melanocortin system involvement in the regulation of food intake and body weight. *Horm Behav* 2000; 37: 299–308.
130. Elias CF, Lee C, Kelly J, Aschkenasi C, Ahima RS, Couceyro PR, Kuhar MJ, Saper CB, Elmquist JK. Leptin activates hypothalamic CART neurons projecting to the spinal cord. *Neuron* 1998; 21: 1375–85.
131. Kristensen P, Judge ME, Thim L, Ribel U, Christjansen KN, Wulff BS, Clausen JT, Jensen PB, Madsen OD, Vrang N, Larsen PJ, Hastrup S. Hypothalamic CART is a new anorectic peptide regulated by leptin. *Nature* 1998; 393: 72–6.
132. Lambert PD, Couceyro PR, Mcgirr KM, Vechia SE, Smith Y, Kuhar MJ. CART peptides in the central control of feeding and interactions with neuropeptide Y. *Synapse* 1998; 29: 293–8.
133. Vrang N, Tang-Christensen M, Larsen PJ, Kristensen P. Recombinant CART peptide induces c-Fos expression in central areas involved in control of feeding behaviour. *Brain Res* 1999; 818: 499–509.
134. Kask A, Schioth HB, Mutulis F, Wikberg JE, Rago L. Anorexigenic cocaine- and amphetamine-regulated transcript peptide intensifies fear reactions in rats. *Brain Res* 2000; 857 (1–2): 283–5.
135. Abbott CR, Rossi M, Wren AM, Murphy KG, Kennedy AR, Stanley SA, Zollner AN, Morgan DG, Morgan I, Ghatei MA, Small CJ, Bloom SR. Evidence of an orexigenic role for cocaine- and amphetamine-regulated transcript after administration into discrete hypothalamic nuclei. *Endocrinology* 2001; 142 (8): 3457–63.
136. Krahn DD, Gosnell BA. Behavioral effects of corticotropin-releasing factor: localization and characterization of central effects. *Brain Res* 1988; 443: 63–9.
137. Arase K, York DA, Shimizu H, Shargil NS, Bray GA. Effects of corticotropin releasing factor on food intake and brown adipose tissue thermogenesis in rats. *Am J Physiol* 1988; 255: E255–9.
138. Watts AG, Sanchez-Watts G, Kelly AB. Distinct patterns of neuropeptide gene expression in the lateral hypothalamic area and arcuate nucleus are associated with dehydration- induced anorexia. *J Neurosci* 1999; 19 (14): 6111–21.
139. Heinrichs S, Lapsansky J, Behan D, Chan R, Sawchenko P, Lorang M, Ling N, Vale W, De SE. Corticotropin-releasing factor-binding protein ligand inhibitor blunts excessive weight gain in genetically obese Zucker rats and rats during nicotine withdrawal. *Proc Natl Acad Sci USA* 1996; 93 (December 24): 15475–80.
140. Vaughan J, Donaldson C, Bittencourt J, Perrin M, Lewis K, Sutton S, Chan R, Turnbull A, Lovejoy D, Rivier C, et al. Urocortin, a mammalian neuropeptide related to fish urotensin I and to corticotropin-releasing factor [see comments]. *Nature* 1995; 378 (November 16): 287–92.
141. Spina M, M-P E, Chan R, Basso A, Rivier J, Vale W, Koob G. Appetite-suppressing effects of urocortin, a CRF-related neuropeptide. *Science* 1996; 273 (September 13): 1561–4.
142. Richard D, Huang Q, Timofeeva E. The corticotropin-releasing hormone system in the regulation of energy balance in obesity. *Int J Obes Relat Metab Disord* 2000; 24 (suppl 2): S36–9.
143. Heinrichs SC, Richard D. The role of corticotropin-releasing factor and urocortin in the modulation of ingestive behavior. *Neuropeptides* 1999; 33 (5): 350–9.
144. D'Alessio DA, Vogel R, Prigeon R, Laschansky E, Koerker D, Eng J, Ensinck JW. Elimination of the action of glucagon-like peptide 1 causes an impairment of glucose tolerance after nutrient ingestion by healthy baboons. *J Clin Invest* 1996; 97 (1): 133–8.
145. Drucker DJ. Glucagon-like peptide 2. *Trends Endocrinol Metab* 1999; 10 (4): 153–6.
146. Drucker DJ. Glucagon-like peptides. *Diabetes* 1998; 47 (2): 159–69.
147. van Dijk G, Thiele TE. Glucagon-like peptide-1 (7-36) amide: a central regulator of satiety and interoceptive stress. *Neuropeptides* 1999; 33 (5): 406–14.
148. Goldstone AP, Morgan I, Mercer JG, Morgan DG, Moar KM, Ghatei MA, Bloom SR. Effect of leptin on hypothalamic GLP-1 peptide and brain-stem preproglucagon mRNA. *Biochem Biophys Res Commun* 2000; 269 (2): 331–5.
149. Elmquist JK, Ahima RS, Maratos-Flier E, Flier JS, Saper CB. Leptin activates neurons in ventrobasal hypothalamus and brainstem. *Endocrinology* 1997; 138: 839–42.
150. Turton MD, O'Shea D, Gunn I, Beak SA, Edwards CM, Meeran K, Choi SJ, Taylor GM, Heath MM, Lambert PD, Wilding JP, Smith DM, Ghatei MA, Herbert J, Bloom SR. A role for glucagon-like peptide-1 in the central regulation of feeding [see comments]. *Nature* 1996; 379 (6560): 69–72.
151. Tang-Christensen M, Larsen PJ, Goke R, Fink-Jensen A, Jessop DS, Moller M, Sheikh SP. Central administration of GLP-1-(7–36) amide inhibits food and water intake in rats. *Am J Physiol* 1996; 271 (4, pt 2): R848–56.
152. Van Dijk G, Thiele TE, Donahey JC, Campfield LA, Smith FJ, Burn P, Bernstein IL, Woods SC, Seeley RJ. Central infusions of leptin and GLP-1-(7-36) amide differentially stimulate c-FLI in the rat brain. *Am J Physiol* 1996; 271 (4, pt 2): R1096–100.
153. Thiele TE, Van Dijk G, Campfield LA, Smith FJ, Burn P, Woods SC, Bernstein IL, Seeley RJ. Central infusion of GLP-1, but not leptin, produces conditioned taste aversions in rats. *Am J Physiol* 1997; 272 (2, pt 2): R726–30.
154. Thiele TE, Seeley RJ, D'Alessio D, Eng J, Bernstein IL, Woods SC, van Dijk G. Central infusion of glucagon-like peptide-1-(7-36) amide (GLP-1) receptor antagonist attenuates lithium chloride-induced c-Fos induction in rat brainstem. *Brain Res* 1998; 801 (1–2): 164–70.
155. Seeley RJ, Blake K, Rushing PA, Benoit SC, Eng J, Woods SC, D'Alessio D. The role of CNS GLP-1-(7–36) amide receptors in mediating the visceral illness effects of lithium chloride. *J Neurosc* 2000; 20: 1616–21.
156. Tang-Christensen M, Larsen PJ, Thulesen J, Romer J, Vrang N. The proglucagon-derived peptide, glucagon-like peptide-2, is a neurotransmitter involved in the regulation of food intake. *Nat Med* 2000; 6 (7): 802–7.

157. Steffens AB, Scheurink AJ, Luiten PG, Bohus B. Hypothalamic food intake regulating areas are involved in the homeostasis of blood glucose and plasma FFA levels. *Physiol Behav* 1988; 44 (4–5): 581–9.
158. Storlien LH. The role of the ventromedial hypothalamic area in periprandial glucoregulation. *Life Sci* 1985; 36 (6): 505–14.
159. Weingarten HP, Chang PK, McDonald TJ. Comparison of the metabolic and behavioral disturbances following paraventricular- and ventromedial-hypothalamic lesions. *Brain Res Bull* 1985; 14 (6): 551–9.
160. Obici S, Feng Z, Tan J, Liu L, Karkanias G, Rossetti L. Central melanocortin receptors regulate insulin action. *J Clin Invest* 2001; 108 (7): 1079–85.
161. Baran K, Preston E, Wilks D, Cooney GJ, Kraegen EW, Sainsbury A. Chronic central melanocortin-4 receptor antagonism and central neuropeptide-Y infusion in rats produce increased adiposity by divergent pathways. *Diabetes* 2002; 51 (1): 152–8.
162. Mevorach M, Giacca A, Aharon Y, Hawkins M, Shamoon H, Rossetti L. Regulation of endogenous glucose production by glucose per se is impaired in type 2 diabetes mellitus. *J Clin Invest* 1998; 102 (4): 744–53.
163. Obici S, Feng Z, Karkanias G, Baskin DG, Rossetti L. Decreasing hypothalamic insulin receptors causes hyperphagia and insulin resistance in rats. *Nat Neurosci* 2002; 5 (6): 566–72.
164. Watts AG. Understanding the neural control of ingestive behaviors: helping to separate cause from effect with dehydration-associated anorexia. *Horm Behav* 2000; 37 (4): 261–83.
165. Sakata T, Yoshimatsu H, Kurokawa M. Hypothalamic neuronal histamine: implications of its homeostatic control of energy metabolism. *Nutrition* 1997; 13 (5): 403–11.
166. Wellman PJ. Norepinephrine and the control of food intake [In Process Citation]. *Nutrition* 2000; 16 (10): 837–42.
167. Levin BE, Dunn-Meynell AA, Routh VH. Brain glucose sensing and body energy homeostasis: role in obesity and diabetes. *Am J Physiol* 1999; 276: R1223–31.
168. Grill HJ, Kaplan JM. The neuroanatomical axis for control of energy balance. *Front Neuroendocrinol* 2002; 23 (1): 2–40.
169. Grill HJ, Schwartz MW, Kaplan JM, Foxhall JS, Breininger J, Baskin DG. Evidence that the caudal brainstem is a target for the inhibitory effect of leptin on food intake. *Endocrinology* 2002; 143 (1): 239–46.

Management of Diabetes: Diet, Exercise, and Drugs

39

Dietary Management of Diabetes Mellitus in Europe and North America

J.I. Mann*† and N.J. Lewis-Barned‡§

**University of Otago, Dunedin, New Zealand, †Diabetes Service, Dunedin Hospital, Dunedin, New Zealand, ‡University of Newcastle Medical School, Newcastle upon Tyne, UK, and §North Tyneside General Hospital, Tyne and Wear, UK*

INTRODUCTION

Dietary modification is the mainstay of treatment for type 2 diabetes (T2DM). Despite its usually progressive nature, many patients with T2DM who comply with dietary advice will show improvement in the major metabolic abnormalities associated with this condition to an extent that will obviate the need for oral agents and insulin. For those who cannot be managed without drug therapy, attention to dietary advice may modify blood lipids in a way that would be expected to reduce lipoprotein-mediated risk of coronary heart disease (CHD) and further improve glycemic control. In type 1 diabetes (T1DM) the role of diet is twofold: first, to help minimize the short-term fluctuations in blood glucose (especially to reduce any tendency toward hypoglycemia); second, to reduce risk of long-term complications by helping to achieve optimal glycemic control and satisfactory levels of blood lipids. Dietary advice in relation to choices about types of food for those with T2DM and T1DM is similar, and the major principles resemble those for entire populations at high risk of CHD. There is therefore no need for diabetic patients to be given meals that differ from those eaten by the rest of the family. Dietary recommendations for people with diabetes have been made in many countries. It is reassuring that those of the Diabetes and Nutrition Study Group of the European Association for the Study of Diabetes, representing the majority of European countries [1], and the American Diabetes Association [2, 3] are generally consistent. The points of difference between the two sets of recommendations are indicated in the text below. Table 1 summarizes the basic principles of diabetic dietary recommendations.

TOTAL ENERGY INTAKE

The majority of people with T2DM are overweight and usually have other metabolic features of the insulin resistance (or metabolic) syndrome [i.e., insulin resistance and raised levels of insulin, raised triglyceride and low high-density lipoprotein (HDL) levels, hypertension, high levels of uric acid, and elevated levels of plasminogen activator inhibitor 1 (PAI-1)] in addition to hyperglycemia. Successful weight reduction, at least in part because it results in reduced insulin resistance, will result in lowering of blood glucose, and an improvement in the other abnormalities associated with the syndrome. The reduction in triglyceride and very low-density lipoprotein (VLDL) and increase in HDL levels may particularly be important since levels are respectively elevated and reduced in T2DM and obesity, and in T2DM such dyslipidemia may be even more important as a risk indicator of CHD than in those without diabetes (Table 2). Even modest weight reduction is associated with a reduction in insulin resistance, a reduction in hepatic glucose production, and perhaps an improvement in islet β-cell function [4]. It is generally accepted that total energy should be reduced so that body mass index (BMI) moves toward the desirable range (20–25 kg/m^2). However, despite advice and support many people with T2DM are unable to achieve this target. It is important therefore to set realistic goals for weight

International Textbook of Diabetes Mellitus, Third Edition. Edited by R. A. DeFronzo, E. Ferrannini, H. Keen, and P. Zimmet.
 ISBN: 0-471-48655-8.

Table 1 Nutritional recommendations for people with diabetes, 2003

Recommendations	Comment
Energy	
Achieve or maintain optimum body weight (BMI < 25)*	Even modest weight reduction will improve glycemic control and reduce cardiovascular risk
Carbohydrate and dietary fiber 45–60% of total energy/day from carbohydrate	Prefer foods rich in fiber and with low glycemic load, e.g., legumes, green leafy and root vegetables, fresh fruit, wholegrain bread and cereals, parboiled rice, pasta
Sucrose and other added sugars <10% of total energy/day	Beverages with high sucrose/glucose content are suitable to treat hypoglycemia
Non-nutritive sweeteners can be taken if desired	Consider accepted daily intake (ADI) levels
Total fat 25–35% of total energy/day	
Saturated fatty acids plus *trans*-unsaturated fatty acids <10% of total energy/day	If LDL-cholesterol is elevated <7% of total energy/day
Polyunsaturated fatty acids up to 10% of total energy/day	
Consider *n*-3 unsaturated fatty acids	For example, in oily fish (at least 1–2 servings/week), rapeseed oil, soybean oil, nuts, green leafy vegetables
Monounsaturated fatty acids 10–20% of total energy/day	Prefer vegetable sources
Cholesterol <300 mg/day	If LDL-cholesterol is elevated <200 mg/day
Protein 10–20% of total energy/day	0.8 g/kg of body weight in incipient or overt nephropathy
Alcohol <30 g/day for male, <15 g/day for female	

Note. BMI = body mass index; ADI = accepted daily intake; LDL = low-density lipoprotein.
*For some populations (e.g., those with origins in the Indian subcontinent) a lower cut off may be appropriate.

reduction and to provide intermediate as well as long-term targets. Despite the strong evidence that central distribution of obesity is particularly associated with an increased risk of diabetes and a range of metabolic derangements associated with the condition [5], there is insufficient evidence to suggest that advice regarding energy intake should be influenced by distribution of body fat. There is now considerable evidence to support the suggestion that a diet low in fat and relatively high in wholegrains and fiber-rich carbohydrate is more appropriate for achieving and maintaining weight reduction than are other dietary prescriptions [6–8].

Very low calorie diets (VLCDs) have been the subject of considerable controversy that has centerd around concerns about reductions in resting metabolic rate and in lean body mass, and inconsistent evidence of their long-term effectiveness. They can be used either as total diet replacement for short periods (not usually more than 4 weeks) or as meal replacement incorporated into more conventional weight reduction regimens. There is no doubt that when used as total diet replacement they result in striking short-term improvements in the metabolic profile for T2DM patients [9–11]. These changes are attributed to improved insulin sensitivity [12]. The long-term benefits of these diets have been less certain. In some studies a high proportion of individuals show benefit after up to 18 months [13–15], especially when combined with behavior modification approaches. One study has suggested that the metabolic benefits of VLCD used for induction of weight loss are greater at 1 year than for a conventional weight reduction regimen, despite similar amounts of weight lost, and this requires further investigation; however, in at least one of these studies, after initial benefits at 1 year, a 5-year follow-up suggested that a conventional weight loss program achieved greater sustained weight loss, higher HDL-cholesterol levels, and lower blood pressure than VLCD. While some authorities believe that this approach has a place for some patients [16], such diets are not recommended for general use. When they are used by people with diabetes, it should always be under close medical supervision and with long-term dietary support.

Table 2 Lipid and lipoprotein-mediated risk of coronary heart disease in those with and without diabetes

	Nondiabetics	T1DM	T2DM
Total cholesterol	+++	+++	+++
LDL-cholesterol	+++	+++	+++
Triglyceride	+	+	+++
VLDL	+	+	+++
HDL-cholesterol (low levels)	++	+	+++
Remnant particles	++	+	++

Note. +++ = appreciable risk; ++ = moderate risk; + = some risk.

It is widely accepted that a sustained weight loss of 1–2 kg/month (which can usually be achieved by a reduction of about 500 kcal below that required for weight maintenance) is the preferred means of weight loss. Regular physical activity enhances weight loss and is particularly important in weight maintenance when targets have been achieved. In addition, exercise increases insulin action, the glucose transporter Glut4 in muscle, and HDL (especially HDL_2), whereas triglycerides, low-density lipoprotein (LDL)-cholesterol, and blood pressure are reduced [17, 18]. Further evidence for the benefit of exercise comes from a study demonstrating appreciable reduction in mortality in physically active compared with sedentary people with diabetes [19].

The most appropriate approach to achieving weight reduction depends upon the requirements of individual patients. For some it may be sufficient to advise the restriction of energy-dense foods and provide advice with regard to appropriate food types, as well as to provide some general guidance concerning increased physical activity. For those unable to lose weight, a more prescriptive approach based on calorie-counting as well as an exercise prescription may be helpful, especially when this approach is used in conjunction with behavioral modification techniques.

For those with T2DM who are not overweight, and for the majority of those with T1DM, self-selected energy intakes are appropriate. It is important to ensure that energy intake is sufficient to achieve growth and development in childhood and adolescence. The prescription of insulin in excess of requirements may lead to weight gain. Overweight patients with T1DM can often appreciably improve glycemic control and at the same time reduce insulin requirements if they are able to lose weight. With increasing rates of obesity in North America and most European countries it is hardly surprising that an increasing number of people with T1DM are also presenting with overweight and obesity and associated insulin resistance. It is important that this situation be recognized and managed with advice to lose weight.

QUANTITY AND NATURE OF DIETARY FAT

In most Western countries, fat provides 36–40% of total energy and saturated fatty acids (SAFA) 13–18%. The modification of quantity and nature can favorably influence several important lipoprotein-mediated predictors of CHD (Table 2). The recommendation that SAFA and *trans* isomers of unsaturated fatty acids be restricted is almost universal [1–3] and has a several-fold justification. Fat is the most energy-rich of all nutrients and reduction of fat intake helps to reduce total energy intake, which is important for many people with T2DM and some with T1DM. Much epidemiological evidence suggests that people with diabetes (as is the case with nondiabetics) in populations consuming a low saturated fat diet have reduced incidence and mortality from CHD, compared with those living in countries with a high intake of saturated fat. Reduced saturated fat intake is associated with reduced levels of LDL-cholesterol. These attributes may not be associated with all SAFA. Thus, in nondiabetics, stearic and lauric acids do not have as striking an effect on LDL as do myristic and palmitic acids [20]. However, because these fatty acids coexist in foods and it is difficult to disentangle separate effects, for the purpose of recommendations they are generally considered as a group. Recent evidence suggests that the *trans* isomers of unsaturated fatty acids, which are produced in a range of manufacturing processes, have a similar adverse effect to that of saturated fatty acids on LDL [21, 22]. In addition, they result in lowering of HDL [22] and an increase of lipoprotein (a), Lp(a), which may further contribute to the lipoprotein-mediated risk of CHD [23–25]. It is for all these reasons that restriction of saturated and *trans* unsaturated fatty acids to 10% or less of total energy has been advised. For those with elevated levels of LDL-cholesterol, a lower level of intake (i.e. 7% or less of total energy) may be advised.

n-6 Polyunsaturated fatty acids (chiefly linoleic acid) may help to reduce LDL-cholesterol, but in large quantities (i.e. more than 10% of total energy) can reduce HDL [26]. *n*-3 Polyunsaturated fatty acids (eicosapentaenoic and docosahexaenoic acids), chiefly derived from oily fish, can help to reduce triglycerides and VLDL, as well as reduce the risk of thrombosis as a result of reduced platelet aggregation [27–29]. However, these fatty acids have a variable effect on LDL [30, 31] and the most appropriate ratio of *n*-3 to *n*-6 unsaturated fatty acids has yet to be established. Total intake of polyunsaturated fatty acids is very low in most European countries and some increase may be appropriate, though total intake should not exceed 10% of total energy. Fish oil supplements are not advised, though increased intake of fish will facilitate the reduction of saturated fat as well as increase the intake of naturally occurring *n*-3 fatty acids, especially if oily fish is eaten regularly.

Monounsaturated fatty acids with a *cis* configuration (principally oleic acid from olive oil and the rapeseed oil derivative, canola) on the other hand, appear not only to facilitate the reduction of SAFA, but also help to decrease LDL-cholesterol, increase HDL-cholesterol, and may also have antioxidant properties that reduce oxidizability of LDL. When compared with high carbohydrate–low soluble fiber diets, diets high in monounsaturated fat are associated with improved peripheral insulin sensitivity and improved glycemic control [32–34]. A fairly wide range of intakes is considered acceptable. Indeed, it is these properties of *cis*-monounsaturated fatty acids that have facilitated the more flexible recommendation regarding the acceptable percentage intake of total fat, compared with previous recommendations. Degree of adiposity, metabolic characteristics, and personal and cultural preferences can all determine the extent to which appropriate fatty acids and appropriate carbohydrate-containing foods contribute to total energy intake (see Section Carbohydrates, Fiber, and Glycemic Index).

Substantial reduction of saturated fat will almost invariably be associated with a reduction of dietary cholesterol to 300 mg or less per day. There is no good evidence to suggest that a further reduction of dietary cholesterol confers additional benefit when intake of saturated fat is already low.

CARBOHYDRATE, FIBER, AND GLYCEMIC INDEX

Carbohydrate and Fiber

Traditionally in many affluent societies, low carbohydrate diets (i.e., carbohydrate providing 40% or less of total energy) were recommended for people with diabetes. It is now widely accepted that this was unnecessary and indeed undesirable when associated with a high intake of SAFA [35]. In the 1980s and 1990s it was generally recommended that carbohydrate provide at least 50% of total energy. The recent appreciation of the importance of insulin resistance in T2DM and that some such individuals have improved glycemic control on a somewhat lower carbohydrate intake have led to the recommendation that a wider range of intakes is appropriate. An intake of dietary fiber around 20 g/1000 kcal or, on average, about 40 g per day is generally regarded as ideal. It is acceptable for the amount of carbohydrates to be at the upper end of the recommended range or possibly even higher provided that the foods are also rich in soluble fiber and have a low *glycemic index* (GI). Such diets may be helpful in promoting satiety and facilitating weight loss, but when other metabolic features of insulin resistance are prominent somewhat lower intakes may be more appropriate.

High carbohydrate diets are certainly not new to diabetes. They have been recommended intermittently for at least 2000 years. However, recent interest stems from the work of Anderson who, in uncontrolled studies in the mid-1970s, showed that patients with T2DM, but treated with insulin, who were given a diet high in carbohydrate and fiber required less insulin [36] (Figure 1). At about the same time Jenkins and colleagues showed that the addition of guar, a viscous fiber, to a test meal reduced postprandial glucose and insulin responses [37] (Figure 2). In order to appreciate some of the subsequent, apparently conflicting, research findings, it is necessary to appreciate the complexity of the components of dietary fiber and that the so-called "complex" carbohydrates vary appreciably in their glycemic potential. For convenience, dietary fiber may be divided into two broad classes: soluble fiber, which includes gums, gels, mucilages, and pectic substances; and insoluble fiber including lignin, cellulose, and some of the hemicelluloses. Soluble fiber delays absorption of glycemic carbohydrate in the small intestine and in the large bowel to produce gas and short-chain fatty acids. Thus this type of fiber influences carbohydrate and lipid metabolism. Insoluble fiber increases fecal bulk and has less metabolic effect, though cereal-derived foods rich in this form of fiber have been shown to be associated with a reduced risk of developing diabetes. Two principal approaches have been used to study the effects of increasing carbohydrate and fiber in diabetes: in some studies purified forms of soluble fiber are given as a

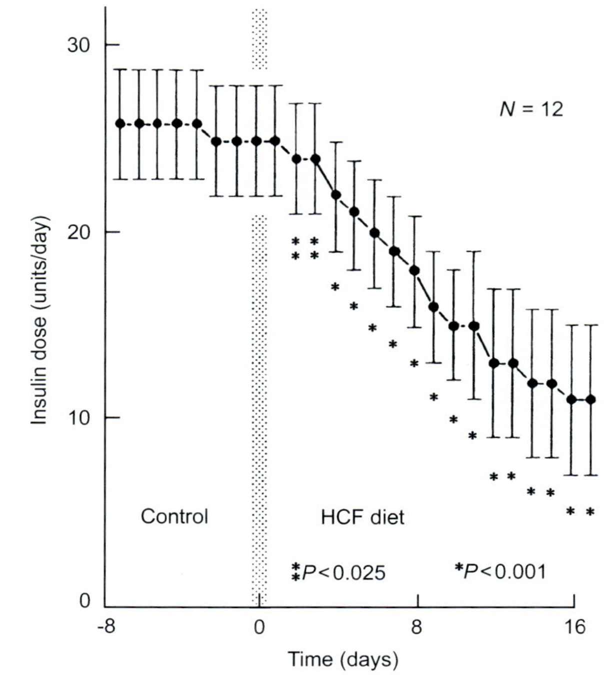

Figure 1 Insulin requirements of T2DM patients before and after the introduction of a high-carbohydrate, high-fiber (HCF) diet

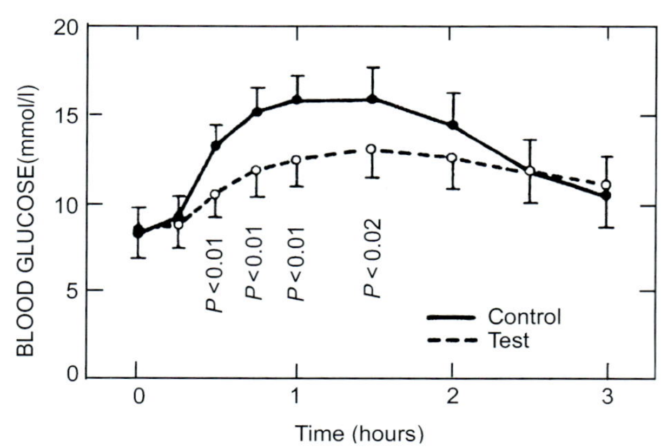

Figure 2 Mean blood glucose levels (mmol/l) of eight non-insulin-requiring diabetic patients after taking control and fiber-enriched test meals. (Reproduced from reference 37, with permission)

supplement; in others, foods high in dietary fiber have been increased.

Purified Forms of Soluble Fiber

Reports from Jenkins' group that the regular addition of guar, pectin, and other soluble fibers may improve glycemic control and in addition lower cholesterol levels have now been confirmed [38]. At first it was thought that the effect of these fibers was to reduce postprandial glycemia by slowing absorption. However, a Finnish study has suggested that when soluble fiber is regularly consumed over a prolonged period the apparent improvement in postprandial levels is explained by the fall in basal (fasting) glucose levels [39]. Failure of some researchers to confirm the beneficial effect of these substances has been a result of failure to appreciate that all fibers are not equally effective (those with the highest viscosity appear to be most potent in altering blood glucose and lipid profiles), that the fibers need to be incorporated into foods, and that the beneficial effect is only apparent when the substances are taken as part of a high-carbohydrate diet (carbohydrate providing at least 50% of total energy). These issues have been reviewed in detail by Vinik and Jenkins [40]. Equally important is the fact that until recently many of the commercially available preparations of soluble fiber have been unpalatable and were undoubtedly associated with poor compliance. Different preparations appear to have different potencies and a dose–response effect may operate. The effect of different preparations on glucose and cholesterol is shown in Figure 3. Relatively acceptable preparations are now available and these may have a role in patients with T2DM who have not responded adequately to dietary modification alone, as well as in those with T2DM or T1DM already on tablets or insulin whose glycemic control remains unsatisfactory [41]. However, in Europe and North America the preparations are not widely used and should be regarded as pharmacological treatment rather than forming a component of dietary management. Although it seems very unlikely that significant side effects will occur when used in the recommended doses, longer-term studies, continued for years rather than months, are desirable in order to establish safety as well as long-term benefits.

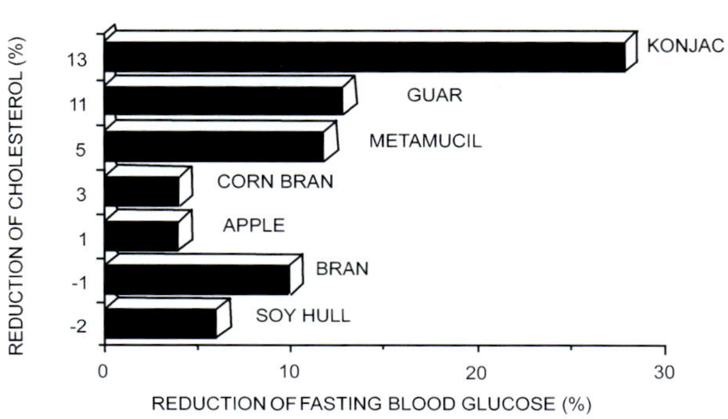

Figure 3 Effect of different types of fiber on cholesterol and glucose levels

Table 3 Indices of diabetes control in T2DM patients unsatisfactorily controlled on maximum doses of oral hypoglycemic agents*

	After 6 weeks on a reinforced low-carbohydrate diet	After 6 weeks on a high carbohydrate/ high-fiber diet
HbA_1 (%)	†10.3 ± 2.2	†8.5 ± 1.9
Fasting glucose (mmol/l)	†8.4 ± 2.8	†6.8 ± 2.8
Average preprandial blood glucose (mmol/l)	‡9.5 ± 2.9	‡7.5 ± 3.1
Average 2-h postprandial blood glucose (mmol/l)	11.4 ± 3.5	§10.8 ± 2.8
Mean 24-h blood glucose (mmol/l)	†10.8 ± 1.3	†9.3 ± 1.7

* From reference 42, with permission.
† $P < 0.01$.
‡ $P < 0.001$.
§ $P < 0.5$.

Dietary Fibers Fed as Part of a Mixed Diet

Studies to establish conclusively the benefit of increasing fiber in ordinary foods are more difficult to carry out than are studies of fiber supplementation. Carefully controlled studies have shown that increasing carbohydrate to the recommended level, by increasing the intake of foods high in soluble fiber (e.g., legumes, lentils, some fruits, oats, and barley), can produce an appreciable improvement in glycemic control and a reduction in LDL-cholesterol, without an increase in triglycerides or a reduction in the ratio of HDL to LDL. Table 3 shows the results of one study in which relatively poorly controlled patients with T2DM on maximum doses of oral therapy were randomized to receive either reinforced advice concerning their low-carbohydrate diets or advice to change to a high-carbohydrate/high-fiber diet. After 6 weeks a metabolic profile was carried out and the diets were reversed for a further 6-week period, before a final metabolic profile. The reinforced low-carbohydrate diet produced little benefit, whereas an appreciable improvement was observed on the experimental diet [42]. Similar findings have been reported in those with T1DM [43]. Some of the studies carried out in the 1980s were criticized on the grounds that total carbohydrate and fiber were increased simultaneously at the expense of fat and it is impossible to disentangle separate effects. However, recent studies using comparable experimental designs, but where total carbohydrate was kept constant, yielded virtually identical results [44]. Some of the experimental studies have also included substantial quantities of root and green leafy vegetables as well as grain cereals, and these foods may have conferred some additional benefit. In particular, recent interest has centered around the potential benefit of wholegrain cereals, which have been shown to be protective against the development of T2DM. The precise mechanism is unclear, especially as cereal-derived insoluble fiber appears to have little effect in controlled studies in people with diabetes. The intact structure of the wholegrain may be relevant.

There is no doubt that increasing carbohydrate *per se* without a parallel increase in dietary fiber gives no overall benefit and is associated with several potential disadvantages, despite a slight fall in fasting and overnight glucose levels on such dietary regimens. Glucose levels throughout the day are the same as, or higher than, on a low-carbohydrate diet, HDL-cholesterol levels fall, and there may be an increase in triglyceride levels. Thus, there is no merit in increasing carbohydrate without soluble fiber [45, 46].

Two potential problems remain with regard to extrapolating the findings of the various experimental studies of high-fiber diets into clinical practice. First, the majority of the studies have used extremely large quantities of dietary fiber, which are most unlikely to be acceptable in clinical practice. One study showing a most impressive effect of a diet high in soluble fiber involved participants taking up to 90 g/day [43]. However, other studies appear to show benefits with amounts ranging from 35 to 50 g/day. Vegetarians usually have an intake of around 40 g/day, and studies in Oxford suggest that well-instructed and reasonably well-motivated people with diabetes, attending outpatient clinics can achieve an intake in this range [47]. Second, it has been correctly argued that, as with the pharmacological preparations of guar and other soluble fibers, the experimental studies of high-fiber foods have been carried out over periods of months rather than years. One of the few relatively long-term studies to be carried out, which claims to show no benefit of a high-fiber diet in terms of glycemic control, had various flaws in experimental design; in particular, there was remarkably little difference in achieved intake of dietary fiber between experimental and control groups [48]. Appropriate long-term studies would clearly be of considerable benefit, but there is widespread acceptance that the present experimental data supported by epidemiological evidence are sufficient to justify the recommendations to increase fiber to around 20 g/1000 kcal to encourage the use of fiber-rich foods mentioned above and to justify the suggestion that carbohydrate restriction is generally unnecessary. Such advice is regarded as being appropriate for those with T2DM and T1DM, though the importance of not increasing fiber-depleted starchy foods, especially in the presence of hypertriglyceridemia or unsatisfactory glycemic control, must be emphasized.

Concerns have been expressed regarding the vitamin and mineral status of people who take large quantities of fiber-rich food. There is certainly no evidence that diets such as those recommended cause significant malabsorption of macronutrients or micronutrients. Such diets are not different from those traditionally eaten by some populations; however, it may be prudent to ensure adequate intakes of both macronutrients and micronutrients in the elderly as well as in growing children who are taking large quantities of fiber-rich foods.

Sugars

Mono- and disaccharides naturally present in milk and fruits have not usually been restricted provided they are included in the energy allowance, but sucrose has traditionally been restricted. A number of studies have now shown that at least under certain circumstances, monosaccharides and disaccharides do not result in deterioration of glycemic control or elevated lipid levels. The results of one study in which 45 g of sucrose replaced an isocaloric amount of carbohydrate (mostly bread and potato) are shown in Table 4 [49]. As a result of this and other similar studies the recommendations do not preclude the use of limited quantities (up to 30 g/day) of sucrose as a sweetener as a part of mixed meals, provided that the energy content is taken into account and it does not replace foods high in fiber.

Fructose is another naturally occurring sweetener, sweeter than sucrose, which has been widely used for people with diabetes in the past. However, fructose may increase fasting triglyceride and VLDL, and can cause gastrointestinal disturbances when taken in large amounts, and concerns have also been expressed regarding protein fructosylation. Thus, while there is no concern about fructose, which occurs naturally (e.g., in fruits), there is at present no strong case to suggest that fructose has advantages over sucrose as a nutritive sweetener for people with diabetes [50–53]. While sucrose intake is decreasing in some countries the use of corn syrup as a sweetener is increasing. It is therefore appropriate to suggest a maximum intake of total nutritive sweeteners to include all mono- and disaccharides (other than those in fruits, vegetables, and milk) as well as sugar alcohols such as sorbitol and xylitol, which have been recommended because they have lower glycemic responses than does sucrose, and a slightly lower energy value. The intake of oligosaccharides is also increasing in many countries, mainly as a component of

Table 4 Indices of glycemic control from diurnal profiles for T1DM patients

	Plasma glucose (mmol/l)	
	Control diet	Sucrose diet
Fasting	10.5 ± 1.8	10.3 ± 1.5
Preprandial mean	10.5 ± 1.3	10.0 ± 1.3
Incremental postprandial mean	3.3 ± 0.7	3.7 ± 0.8
Mean daily	11.4 ± 1.0	11.4 ± 1.2
HbA_1 (%)	9.9 ± 0.3	10.3 ± 0.6

Note: Similar results were observed in patients with T2DM.

functional foods. It has usually been recommended that sucrose plus other added sugars provide no more than 10% of total energy. However a recent recommendation in a World Health Organization (WHO) report suggests that total sugars should provide less than 10% of total energy.

Glycemic Index

One approach to looking at physiological responses to different types of ingested carbohydrate has been the use of the GI. Classifying foods according to their GI has been suggested as an appropriate means of identifying the optimal carbohydrate-containing foods [54]. The *glycemic index* has been defined as the ratio of the incremental blood glucose area after food to the corresponding area after a glucose load or portion of white bread containing an equal quantity of carbohydrate. It is usually expressed as a percentage. The suggestion is that foods with a low GI may be the most appropriate carbohydrate-containing foods for people with diabetes; regular use of such foods has also been shown to improve glycemic control over a period of several weeks.

The main objections to the GI approach were identified in a National Institutes of Health Consensus Conference on diet and exercise, and include the large individual variation in responses, lack of agreement among centers, lack of difference between mixed meals including foods of different GI, and lack of studies showing long-term benefits of low-GI foods [55]. To these might be added the fact that different researchers have used different mathematical approaches in the calculation of GI. These criticisms have been addressed in detail in three reviews [54, 56, 57]. While these criticisms are acknowledged, it does appear that many of the foods with low GIs (e.g. legumes, pasta, grains such as oats and barley, cracked wheat) when incorporated into diets are associated with reduction in LDL-cholesterol and improved glycemic control. Provided that it is conceded that acceptability of food should not be determined solely on the basis of having a low GI (e.g. many high-fat foods, undesirable for other reasons, have a low GI), it seems reasonable to use GI as a means of ranking carbohydrate-containing foods. The GIs of a range of foods are shown in Table 5. A recent meta-analysis of studies in which diets of overall high and low GI have been compared over weeks or months confirms the benefit of such an approach [58]. While some foods with a low GI are rich in soluble dietary fiber, others are not, the lower glycemic response being conferred by other properties resulting in reduced digestion and absorption in the small intestine. A particularly helpful study in this regard was carried out by Jarvi and colleagues who compared diets with identical fiber content but with varying GI achieved by altering the food structure [59]. It would seem that the intact structure of grains and particle size were the important determinants of the low GI that was associated with lower blood glucose and insulin levels, reduced total and LDL cholesterol, and reduced plasminogen activator-1 (PAI-1). The GI is also a useful indicator regarding choice of so-called complex carbohydrate foods. For example, white and wholemeal (wheat) bread, mashed potato, millet, and cornflakes all have a GI that is no different from that of glucose, the high glycemic load indicating that despite the carbohydrate being "complex" the foods are

Table 5 Mean *glycemic index* of a range of foods studied by various investigators and adjusted so that *glycemic index* of white bread = 100*

Food	Mean GI
Breads	
Rye	
Crispbread	95
Wholemeal	89
Pumpernickel (wholegrain)	68
Wheat	
White	100
Wholemeal	100 ± 2
Pasta	
Macaroni	64
Spaghetti	38–61
Cereal grains	
Barley	31
Buckwheat	74
Bulgar	65
Millet	103
Breakfast cereals	
All Bran	74 ± 1
Cornflakes	115 ± 4
Porridge oats	87 ± 6
Weetabix	109
Root vegetables	
Potatoes	
Mashed	100
Boiled (new)	80 ± 7
Sweet	70
Yam	74
Legumes	
Canned baked beans	60
Butter beans	46
Chick peas	49
Green peas	65
Haricot beans	57 ± 10
Kidney beans	45 ± 11
Red lentils	37 ± 6
Soybeans (dried)	20
Fruit	
Apple	53
Banana	84 ± 7
Orange	
Whole	59 ± 8
Juice	67
Dairy products	
Skimmed milk	46
Whole milk	49
Yoghurt	52

* From reference 54, with permission.

readily digested and absorbed in the small intestine and should not therefore be eaten in large amounts by people with diabetes, especially those with T2DM who are particularly insulin resistant. Studies of GI need to be carried out in different countries in order to investigate local foods, because processing as well as composition of foods, which can profoundly influence GI, differs from country to country.

DIETARY PROTEIN

The WHO recommends 0.6 g of protein per kilogram per day as a safe intake, although it is clear that measured intakes are frequently greater than this in diabetes (often exceeding 1 g of protein per kilogram per day). The low-carbohydrate dietary prescription (for diabetes) of the past was associated with relatively high intakes of protein (as much as 20% or more of total energy). There is now a consistent body of evidence to suggest that reducing protein intake to the levels recommended by the WHO can reduce albuminuria and improve renal hemodynamics in T1DM patients with incipient and established nephropathy [60–65]. These early studies have been supported by a recent meta-analysis. Such diets do not necessarily worsen blood glucose control [66], and protein undernutrition does not occur in the long term [67]. One small but well designed study has shown a significant reduction in the rate of progression to end stage renal failure or death, with 0.6 g of dietary protein intake per kilogram per day. In patients with advanced nephropathy the benefits of even very low-protein diets are more limited [68]. While there is limited evidence concerning the extent to which partial or total substitution of animal protein by vegetable protein may reduce proteinuria [69], vegetable proteins are generally less bioavailable, and more vegetarian-type diets may allow liberalization of overall protein intake in those with early nephropathy. Overall, while there is no confirmation of early suggestions that a high-protein diet contributes to the pathogenesis of early diabetic nephropathy, there is certainly no need for a high-protein diet among people with diabetes in general.

DISTRIBUTION OF ENERGY FROM MACRONUTRIENTS

The major dietary restriction is that of saturated and *trans*-unsaturated fatty acids to no more than 10% of total energy, or 7% if LDL-cholesterol is raised. If energy restriction is not required (i.e., if BMI is in the satisfactory range) the lost energy may be replaced by either an increase in *cis*-monounsaturated fatty acids from vegetable sources (e.g., olive oil, canola) or carbohydrates rich in soluble fiber and/or that have a low GI. Both these nutrients have a wide acceptable range of intakes: *cis*-monounsaturated fatty acid, 10–20% of total energy; total carbohydrates, 45–60% of total energy. This involves a restriction of fatty meat and meat products as well as high-fat dairy products, confectionery, cakes, and high-fat manufactured foods, which are replaced by monounsaturated vegetable oils and spreads and fiber-rich or low-GI carbohydrate derived from a range of lightly processed cereals, pulses, vegetables, and fruits. An apparent discrepancy between European and North American recommendations concerns the carbohydrate composition of the diet. The American Diabetes Association (ADA) recommendations acknowledge that "foods containing carbohydrate from whole grains, fruits and vegetables and low fat milk should be included in a healthy diet" and that "sucrose and sucrose-containing foods should be eaten in the context of a healthy diet." [2] However the advice to the effect that "the total amount of carbohydrate in meals or snacks is more important than the source of type" and that "sucrose does not increase glycemia to a greater extent than isocaloric amounts of starch, (thus) sucrose and sucrose-containing foods do not need to be restricted by people with diabetes" is in apparent conflict with the European recommendations [1]. The recommendations from the Diabetes and Nutrition Study Group of the European Association for the Study of Diabetes suggest that "carbohydrate-containing foods which [that] are rich in dietary fiber or have a low *glycemic index* should be preferred over other carbohydrate-containing foods and that vegetables, legumes, fruits and cereal-derived foods are the preferred source of carbohydrate." Furthermore the European recommendations include a note of caution concerning sucrose, which may be included within the diet for both types of diabetes but should not exceed 10% of total energy. Thus the European recommendations provide clear encouragement toward carbohydrate-containing foods that are associated with low glycemic loads and are not energy dense, whereas the ADA suggests less distinction between different carbohydrate-containing foods so that at least in theory a diet might be selected in which highly processed starchy foods and foods rich in sucrose and other sugars might provide the bulk of dietary carbohydrate. It is important to emphasize that the overall distribution of macronutrients is no different from that widely advised for the population as a whole in countries with high CHD risk. For those who are overweight it is appropriate to recommend only partial replacement of energy lost by reduced intake of saturated and *trans*-unsaturated fatty acids. A number of overweight patients have opted to try very low carbohydrate, high-fat dietary approaches to weight loss (e.g. the Atkins Diet). While such diets often achieve short-term weight loss and associated benefits, including dose reduction of hypoglycemic drug therapy, they should be discouraged at least until such a time as they have been subjected to further appropriate evaluation. At present there is no evidence that in the long term they are more efficacious than established dietary approaches, and there is at least a theoretical basis for believing that there may be deleterious long-term effects.

MICRONUTRIENTS: VITAMINS AND MINERALS

A whole range of micronutrients have at one time or another been the focus of attention in diabetes. In particular chromium, zinc, and magnesium have received special attention. However, apart from the possibility of chromium deficiency leading to glucose intolerance in association with inappropriate parenteral nutrition prescriptions, the occasional need for magnesium replacement in patients with persistently poor diabetes control (associated with osmotic diuresis) or those on diuretic therapy, and the possibility that zinc supplementation may occasionally aid the healing of venous leg ulcers, there is little evidence that those with diabetes have different requirements for vitamins and minerals than those who do not have diabetes [70]. Nonetheless, because of the increased frequency of hypertension and the increased cardiovascular risk in diabetes, advice concerning some micronutrients is especially relevant. As in the general population, people with diabetes should be advised to restrict sodium intake to under 6 g/day. Those with even modestly raised blood pressure should be encouraged to aim for an intake of 3 g/day or less [71]. Increased potassium intake and sometimes supplementation is particularly important when those with diabetes are treated with thiazide and loop-acting diuretics, whereas hyperkalemia requiring dietary restriction may occur in patients taking potassium-sparing diuretics or angiotensin converting enzyme (ACE) inhibitors, or in those with renal failure.

There is powerful epidemiological evidence that a range of antioxidant nutrients (e.g., tocopherols, carotenoids, vitamin C, flavenoids) protect against CHD and certain cancers in nondiabetic people. There is a disturbed equilibrium between pro- and antioxidants in diabetes and there is no doubt that increased oxidative stress can adversely influence cardiovascular risk (e.g., increased oxidation of LDL). In the past many people with diabetes may have had a low intake of dietary antioxidants as a result of restriction of fruit and some vegetables. Although no intervention studies have been carried out in people with diabetes, the circumstantial evidence is sufficiently strong to recommend an increase in foods rich in antioxidant nutrients (a wide range of vegetables and fruits). While pharmacological doses of some of these nutrients have been shown to influence risk indicators in diabetes [72–74], recent evidence has shown conclusively that supplementation of vitamins E, C, and β-carotene at least has no impact on cardiovascular outcomes.

ALCOHOL

The same caution regarding alcohol intake that applies to the general population applies to those with diabetes. Alcohol consumption should be eliminated as far as possible in those with hypertriglyceridemia, those who are overweight, and those with hypertension. When alcohol is taken by those on insulin or tablets, it should be taken with meals because of its potentially profound hypoglycemic effect, which can be prolonged or delayed. There is evidence, principally in people who do not have diabetes, that a modest intake of alcohol, in particular wine, may reduce cardiovascular risk because of a beneficial effect on HDL-cholesterol, reduced coagulability, and reduced lipid oxidation. For those who choose to drink alcohol and do not have the complications listed above, a quantity equivalent to two glasses of wine per day is acceptable [75, 76].

SWEETENERS

A range of nonnutritive sweeteners (including saccharin, aspartame, cyclamate, acesulphame K) are available and may be useful in drinks and for cooking. Aspartame may be considered in this category, although it is a dipeptide, because it is so intensely sweet that only minute quantities are required. These sweeteners provide a useful means of reducing energy intake.

Several nutritive sweeteners (notably fructose and sorbitol) have been recommended for use by people with diabetes when required in baking as an alternative to sucrose. They are also used extensively in so-called "diabetic foods." They generally have the same energy content as sucrose and may be associated with untoward effects (e.g., in large quantities fructose may cause hypertriglyceridemia and diarrhea). However, while they have no proven advantage over sucrose, moderate intakes (up to a maximum of 50 g/day) do not appear to have adverse gastrointestinal or metabolic effects.

"Diabetic foods" are not an essential part of the diet for people with diabetes. Some may be convenient, but they are usually expensive and often relatively high in energy. Low-calorie and sugar-free drinks usually contain no nutritive sweeteners and are useful for many people with diabetes.

IMPLEMENTATION OF DIET THERAPY

The dietary prescription for people with diabetes often involves a major change in lifestyle, and physicians are rarely competent to be the sole providers of appropriate advice, although there are relatively simple communication skills that can be acquired that are likely to be of help. Lessons can be also be learned from the high effectiveness of the programs used in the studies of T2DM

Table 6 Guidelines for optimal food choices*

Eat regularly (servings to aim for/serving size)	Eat in moderate amts		Avoid
	More often	Occasionally	
Pulses (2–3 per week/1 cup cooked) Beans (e.g., haricot, red kidney, soya, baked, black-eyed) Lentils Chick-peas	Peanuts (see under nuts below)		
Fruit—with skin where possible (2–4 per day/1 piece)	Fruit canned in water or fruit juice—as part of fruit recommendation (1/2 to 2/3 cup)	Dried fruit Fruit juice Crystallized fruit	Canned fruit in heavy syrup
Vegetables Colored vegetables (3–5 per day/1/2 to 1 cup) Fresh or frozen, cooked (e.g., carrots, cauliflower, cabbage, spinach, green beans, peas, corn, parsnip, beetroot, etc.) Salad or raw vegetables (e.g., tomato, lettuce, cucumber, radish, celery, capsicum)			
Starchy vegetables (1–2 per day/ 1 medium/1/2 cup) Potatoes (with skin)		Mashed or instant potetoes Crisps, potato cakes Potato scallops Baked chips Potato wedges	Hot chips or French fries Vegetables cooked in dripping, lard, or hardened coconut fat, or hard margarine
Sweet potatoes (baked)		Chips or roast vegetables cooked in a little mono- or polyunsaturated oil	
Breads and Cereals [6 servings/day (3 wholegrain)]; *Breads & rolls* (1 slice/ 1 small roll); *Cereals* (1/3–1 cup) Oats, barley			
Wholegrain breads and rolls Pumpernickle bread Low-fat wholemeal crispbreads		White bread, white flour	
Wholegrain cereals (e.g., All Bran™, Weetbix™, Porridge, Bircher muesli, oat-based unsweetened muesli)	Unsweetened breakfast cereals (e.g., Special K™, Cornflakes™)		Sugar-coated cereals (e.g. Sugar Puffs™, Frosties™, Coco Pops™)
Brown rice	Basmati rice		
Wholemeal pasta Wholemeal flour, rye flour		Pudding cereals (e.g., rice sago, custard powder White flour pasta)	
	Oatcakes		
Meat, poultry, and fish Meat & poultry (3–4 per week/50–120 g)	Lean meat or poultry		Meat fat Poultry fat Duck, goose Luncheon meat Salami Tinned, corned beef Fatty bacon
Fish (1–2 per week/75–120 g) White fish Some oily fish (50–75 g) (e.g., salmon, tuna, sardines tinned in water)	Shell fish		Fried fish, Fish & meat pate

Table 6 (*continued*)

Eat regularly (servings to aim for/serving size)	Eat in moderate amts		Avoid
	More often	Occasionally	
Eggs (1 egg or egg white)			
Egg whites	Whole eggs (up to 4 per week)		
Dairy products—low fat (LF) (2–3 per day/100–150 ml)			
LF/low sugar yoghurt			
Skimmed milk			
Cottage cheese (40 g) Curd cheese Low-fat quark	Medium fat cheeses (Serving size 20 g) (e.g. Mozzarella, Gouda, Edam cheese)	Cheddar cheese Whole milk Plain ice cream Blue cheeses, full fat sweetened yoghurt Lite sour cream Lite cream cheese	Cream Cream cheese Condensed milk Sour cream
Fats and oils (1–2 tsp)	Use in place of spreads high in animal fats *cis*-Monounsaturated (e.g. olive or canola) Oils or soft margarine Hydrogenated fats and oils *cis*-Polyunsaturated (e.g. sunflower, soya, grapeseed) Soft margarine Margarine butter mixture	Butter	Lard, suet, dripping Oils: coconut, palm (e.g., hard oils or margarine)
Nuts and seeds			
Nuts	Use in place of foods high in animal fats (3–5 per week/20–30 g) (e.g., almonds, pistachios, Brazil nuts, hazelnuts, cashews, macadamias, peanuts, pinenuts, walnuts, pecans (all nuts should be unsalted, & not roasted in other oils or fats)		Salted nuts and/or nuts roasted in unknown fats
Seeds	Use in place of foods high in animal fats 1tbsp (e.g. sunflower, seasame, pumpkin, flaxseed)		
Made-up dishes			
H/M Vegetable or clear soups	"Cream" soups made with skim milk Sauces made with skim milk	Filo pastry with oil made with wholemeal flour and MUFA or PUFA margarine	Cream soups Sauces with cream Puff pastry Flaky or short pastry Meat Pork pies Sausage rolls Sweet pastries High fat, high sugar desserts
		LF, low sugar, high fiber desserts, cakes, or biscuits made from special recipes, with wholemeal flour and MUFA or PUFA margarine	
Takeaways		Pasta (small serving with tomatoes, chicken, lean meat, seafood or pesto) Steamed rice or noodles, plus Chicken, fish or beef with vegetables	Deep fried takeaways Pasta with cream sauce
		Chicken or meat cooked in a savoury sauce without butter or cream	Cream or butter sauces

Table 6 (*continued*)

Eat regularly (servings to aim for/serving size)	Eat in moderate amts		Avoid
	More often	Occasionally	
		Burger grilled meat patty and salad Grilled chicken or meat with salad Oven baked chips, wedges Pizza (small) with tomato, vegetable, lean meat, chicken or fish, very little cheese	Thin crisps Salami, extra cheese
Spreads and preserves	Marmite™, Vegemite™	Jam, marmalade	Sugar, glucose, honey, syrup, treacle, Sweets, chocolates, fudges, butterscotch Mincemeat Lemon curd
Drinks Water, tea, coffee, tomato juice, sugar free drinks (e.g., soda water, sugar free squash)		Spirits, beer, dry wine, & sherry French champagne	Sweet wines Liqueurs Sweet sherry, sweetened fruit drink Sweetened fizzy drinks High fat drinks with alcohol and cream

* Table prepared by Alexandra Chisholm, Registered Dietitian, University of Otago.

prevention for people with diabetes. These involved the development of individual support, structured education, supervized physical activity sessions, flexible maintenance approaches, and a toolbox of adherence strategies. Packages of support have successfully included the use of Internet technology. At the same time where dietary change is concerned an experienced dietitian is important in order to give the individual practical help and to provide the relevant food knowledge required by patients. Where a dietitian is not available, a trained nurse specialist can provide valuable assistance. The diet must be tailored to suit individual and family food, culture, and economic and cooking conditions. The techniques of implementation differ from country to country. For example, in the United Kingdom, patients with T2DM are usually provided with dietary principles, guidelines as to how they might be implemented and key areas for change can be identified, and their importance to the patient established and prioritized. Sometimes precise energy intakes are advised, but frequently even this is achieved by the provision of lists including foods to be eaten regularly, to be taken in moderation, and to be avoided. Such lists also facilitate recommendations concerning the relative proportions of macronutrients, and an example is shown in Table 6.

Carbohydrate exchanges that in the past were the mainstay of treatment for T1DM are no longer invariably used. Newer approaches based on highly structured education that helps patients to estimate accurately the carbohydrate content of meals and to match insulin doses to these have recently been shown to achieve high rates of acceptability with patients, improve-quality-of-life measures and glucose control, and also to reduce hypoglycemia risk. While the extent to which these approaches can be introduced into mainstream care, and benefits can be maintained in long-term (more than a year) still needs to be tested there is some evidence to suggest that this can be achieved.

Those on oral therapy are simply advised to have regular meals. Precise energy intakes are prescribed and carbohydrate exchange lists are used for those on insulin as well as some T2DM patients on sulfonylureas. Unfortunately, there are few comparative studies of different techniques of implementing dietary advice.

While advice for older people may concentrate on energy balance and restriction of rapidly absorbed carbohydrate, younger people are encouraged to pay attention to all aspects of the recommendations. Exchange systems are still widely recommended for insulin-requiring patients who need to ensure consistency and regularity of carbohydrate intake to balance injected insulin and exercise. Exchange lists are at present being developed, which encourage patients to select the most beneficial carbohydrate-containing foods.

New techniques of food preparation often need to be learned. The provision of recipes and cookery demonstrations are helpful aids to compliance, and it is very helpful if other family members can be persuaded to eat the same meals. With appropriate and enthusiastic instruction, many diabetic patients can be persuaded to make the changes that are often more effective than is oral hypoglycemic therapy in improving glycemic control and blood lipids. A daily meal plan complying with current dietary recommendations is shown in Table 7.

Table 7 A sample eating plan for a patient requiring 2200 kcal/day*

Breakfast	
Porridge	200 g
Milk	200 ml
Sugar	10 g
Toast	80 g
Margarine	10 g
Mid-morning	
Bran muffin	×1
Margarine	5 g
Mid-day	
Home-made vegetable soup	250 ml
Barley	50 g
Bread roll	90 g
Margarine	10 g
Jam	10 g
Macaroni cheese	100 g
Lettuce	20 g
Orange	100 g
Mid-afternoon	
Fruit bread	60 g
Evening	
Beef stew	100 g
Haricot beans	50 g
Potatoes	140 g
Peas	75 g
Carrots	100 g
Apple charlotte	1 serving
Milk	400 ml
Before bed	
Banana	100 g
Bread	50 g
Margarine	5 g
Energy	2200 kcal
Carbohydrate	58% of total energy
Protein	16%
Fat	26%
Saturated fat	7%
Polyunsaturated fat	8%
Monounsaturated fat	11%
Fiber	20 g/1000 kcal
Sugar and jam	20 g total

Note. Carbohydrate provides 58%, protein 16%, and fat 26% of total energy.
* Sample diet prepared by Alex Chisholm, Registered Dietitian, Otago University.

REFERENCES

1. Diabetes and Nutrition Study Group of the European Association for the Study of Diabetes. Recommendations for the nutritional management of patients with diabetes mellitus. *Eur J Clin Nutr* 2000; 54: 353–5.
2. American Diabetes Association. Evidence-based nutrition principles and recommendations for the treatment and prevention of diabetes and related complications. *Diabetes Care* 2003; 26 (suppl 1): S51–61.
3. Franz MJ, Bantle JP, Beebe CA, Brunzell JD, Chiasson J-L, Garg A, Holzmeister LA, Hoogwerf B, Mayer-Davis E, Mooradian AD, Purnell JQ, Wheeler M. Evidence-based nutrition principles and recommendations for the treatment and prevention of diabetes and related complications. *Diabetes Care* 2002; 25: 148–98.
4. Goldstein DJ. Beneficial health effects of modest weight loss. *Int J Obes* 1992; 16: 397–415.
5. Yudkin JS. How can we best prolong life? The benefits of coronary risk factor reduction in non-diabetic and diabetic subjects. *BMJ* 1993; 306: 1313–8.
6. Prewitt TE, Schmeisser D, Bowen PE, Aye P, Dolecek TA, Langenberg P, Cole T, Brace L. Changes in body weight, body composition, and energy intake in women fed high- and low-fat diets. *Am J Clin Nutr* 1991; 54: 304–10.
7. Miller WC, Linderman AK, Wallace J, Niederpruem M. Diet composition, energy intake, and exercise in relation to body fat in men and women. *Am J Clin Nutr* 1990; 52: 426–30.
8. Dreon DM, Frey-Hewitt B, Ellsworth N, Williams PT, Terry RB, Wood PD. Dietary fat: carbohydrate ratio and obesity in middle-aged men. *Am J Clin Nutr* 1988; 47: 995–1000.
9. Henry RR, Wallace P, Olefsky JM. Effects of weight loss on mechanisms of hyperglycaemia in obese non-insulin dependent diabetes mellitus. *Diabetes* 1986; 35: 990–8.
10. Henry RR, Schaeffer L, Olefsky JM. Glycaemic effects of intensive calorie restriction and iso-caloric refeeding in non-insulin dependent diabetes mellitus. *J Clin Endocrinology* 1985; 61: 917–25.
11. Henry RR, Wiest-Kent TA, Schaeffer L, et al. Metabolic consequences of very-low-calorie diet therapy in obese non-insulin dependent diabetic and non-diabetic subjects. *Diabetes* 1986; 35: 155–64.
12. Olefsky J, Reaven GM, Farquhar JW. Effects of weight reduction on obesity: studies of lipid and carbohydrate metabolism in normal and hyperlipidaemic subjects. *J Clin Invest* 1974; 53: 64–76.
13. Kern PA, Trozzolino L, Wolfe G, Purdy L. Combined use of behavior modification and very-low-calorie diet in weight loss and weight maintenance. *Am J Med Sci* 1994; 307: 325–8.
14. Anderson JW, Hamilton CC, Brinkman-Kaplan V. Benefits and risks of an intensive very-low-calorie diet program for severe obesity. *Am J Gastroenterol* 1992; 87: 6–15.
15. Wing RR, Marcus MD, Blair EH, Burton LR. Psychological responses of obese type 2 diabetic subjects to very-low-calorie diet. *Diabetes Care* 1991; 14: 596–9.
16. Henry RR, Gumbiner B. Benefits and limitations of very-low-calorie diet therapy in obese NIDDM. *Diabetes Care* 1991; 14: 802–23.
17. Hughes VA, Fiatarone MA, Fielding RA, Kahn BB, et al. Exercise increases muscle Glut-levels and insulin action in subjects with impaired glucose tolerance. *Am J Physiol* 1993; 264: E855–62.
18. Barnard RJ, Ugianskis EJ, Martin DA, Inkeles SB. Role of diet and exercise in the management of hyperinsulinemia and associated atherosclerotic risk factors. *Am J Cardiol* 1992; 69: 440–4.
19. Moy CS, Songer TJ, LaPorte RE, et al. Insulin dependent diabetes mellitus, physical activity and death. *Am J Epidemiol* 1993; 137: 74–81.
20. Zock PL, de Vries HM, Katan MB. Impact of myristic acid versus palmitic acid on serum lipid and lipoprotein levels in healthy women and men. *Arterioscler Thromb* 1994; 14: 567–75.
21. Mensink RP, Katan MB. Effect of dietary *trans* fatty acids on high-density lipoprotein cholesterol levels in healthy subjects. *N Engl J Med* 1990; 323: 439–45.
22. Zock PL, Katan MB. Hydrogenation alternatives: effects of *trans* fatty acids and stearic acid versus linoleic acid on

serum lipids and lipoprotein in humans. *J Lipid Res* 1992; 33: 399–410.
23. Mensink RP, Zock PL, Katan MB, Hornstra G. Effect of dietary cis and *trans* fatty acids on serum lipoprotein(a) levels in humans. *J Lipid Res* 1992; 33: 1493–501.
24. Nestel P, Noakes M, Belling B, McArthur R, Clifton P, Janus E, Abbey M. Plasma lipoprotein lipid and Lp(a) changes with substitution of elaidic acid for oleic acid in the diet. *J Lipid Res* 1992; 33: 1029–36.
25. Willett WC, Stampfer MJ, Manson JE, Colditz GA, et al. Intake of *trans* fatty acids and risk of coronary heart disease among women. *Lancet* 1993; 341: 581–5.
26. Foley M, Ball M, Chisholm A, Duncan A, Spears G, Mann J. Should mono- or polyunsaturated fats replace saturated fat in the diet? *Eur J Clin Nutr* 1992; 46: 429–36.
27. Rillaerts EG, Engelmann GJ, van Camp KM, De Leeuw I. Effect of omega-3 fatty acids in diet of type 1 diabetic subjects on lipid values and haemorrheological parameters. *Diabetes* 1989; 38: 1412–6.
28. Popp-Snijders C, Schouten JA, Heine RJ, van der Meer J, van der Veen EA. Dietary supplementation of omega-3 polyunsaturated fatty acids improves insulin sensitivity in non-insulin dependent diabetes. *Diabetes Res* 1987; 4: 141–7.
29. Jones DB, Haitas B, Bown EG, Carter RD, Barker K, Jelfs R, Turner RC, Mann JI, Prescott RJ. Platelet aggregation in non-insulin dependent diabetes in association with platelet fatty acids. *Diabet Med* 1986; 3: 52–5.
30. Mori TA, Vandongen R, Masarei JR, Stanton KG, Dunbar D. Dietary fish oil increases serum lipids in insulin-dependent diabetes compared with healthy controls. *Metabolism* 1989; 38: 404–9.
31. Schetchman G, Kaul S, Kissebah AH. Effect of fish oil concentrate on lipoprotein composition in NIDDM. *Diabetes* 1988; 37: 1567–73.
32. Garg A, Bonanome A, Grundy SM, Zhang Z-J, Unger RH. Comparison of a high-carbohydrate diet with a high-monounsaturated-fat diet in patients with non-insulin dependent diabetes mellitus. *N Engl J Med* 1988; 391: 829–34.
33. Garg A, Reaven GM, Bantle JP, Griver K. Multi centre diet study group. Long-term effects of high carbohydrate versus high MUFA diets in NIDDM. *Diabetes* 1992; 41 (suppl 1): 72A.
34. Parillo M, Rivellese AA, Ciardullo AV, Capaldo B, Giacco A, Genovese S, Riccardi G. A high-monounsaturated-fat/low-carbohydrate diet improves peripheral insulin sensitivity in non-insulin dependent diabetic patients. *Metabolism* 1992; 41: 1373–8.
35. Mann JI. Diet and diabetes. *Diabetologia* 1980; 18: 89–95.
36. Kiehm TG, Anderson JW, Ward K. Beneficial effects of a high carbohydrate, high fibre diet on hyperglycaemic men. *Am J Clin Nutr* 1976; 29: 895–9.
37. Jenkins DJA, Wolever TMS, Haworth R, Leeds AR, Hockaday TDR. Guar gum in diabetes. *Lancet* 1976; 2: 1086–7.
38. Jenkins DJA, Leeds AR, Gassull MA, Cochet B, Alberti KGMM. Decrease in postprandial insulin and glucose concentrations for guar and pectin. *Ann Intern Med* 1977; 86: 20–3.
39. Aro A, Uusitupa M, Voutilainen E, et al. Improved diabetic control and hypocholesterolaemic effect induced by long-term supplementation with guar in type 2 diabetics. *Diabetologia* 1981; 21: 29–33.
40. Vinik AI, Jenkins DJA. Dietary fibre in the management of diabetes. *Diabetes Care* 1988; 11: 160–73.
41. Peterson DB, Mann JI. Guar: pharmacological fibre or food fibre? *Diabet Med* 1985; 2: 345–7.
42. Lousley SE, Jones DB, Slaughter P, Carter RD, Jelfs R, Mann JI. High carbohydrate/high fibre diets in poorly controlled diabetes. *Diabet Med* 1984; 1: 21–5.
43. Simpson HCR, Simpson RW, Lousley S, Carter RD, Geekie M, Hockaday TD, Mann JI. A high carbohydrate leguminous fibre diet improves all aspects of diabetic control. *Lancet* 1981; 1: 1–5.
44. Chandalia M, Garg A, Lutjohann D, von Bergmanm K, Grundy SM, Brinkley LJ. Beneficial effects of high dietary fibre intake in patients with type 2 diabetes. *N Engl J Med* 2000; 342 (19): 1392–8.
45. Riccardi G, Rivellese A, Pacioni D, Genovese D, Mastranzo P, Mancini M. Separate influence of dietary carbohydrate and fibre on the metabolic control in diabetes. *Diabetologia* 1984; 26: 116–21.
46. Simpson HCR, Carter RD, Lousley S, Mann JI. Digestible carbohydrate—an independent effect on diabetic control in type 2 (non-insulin dependent) diabetic patients? *Diabetologia* 1982; 23: 235–9.
47. Geekie MA, Porteous J, Hockaday TDR, Mann JI. Acceptability of high-fibre diets in diabetic patients. *Diabet Med* 1986; 3: 52–5.
48. McCulloch DK, Mitchell RD, Ambler J, Tattersall RB. A prospective comparison of ‘conventional’ and high carbohydrate/high fibre/low fat diets in adults with established type 1 (insulin-dependent) diabetes. *Diabetologia* 1985; 28: 208–12.
49. Peterson DB, Lambert J, Gerring S, Darling P, Carter RD, Jerfs R, Mann JI. *Diabetologia* 1986; 29: 216–20.
50. Anderson JW, Story LJ, Zettwoch NC, Gustafson NJ, Jefferson BS. Metabolic effects of fructose supplementation in diabetic individuals. *Diabetes Care* 1989; 12: 337–44.
51. Crapo PA, Kolterman OG, Henry RR. Metabolic consequence of two-week fructose feeding in diabetic subjects. *Diabetes Care* 1986; 9: 111–9.
52. Born P, Eimiller A, Paul F. High rate of gastrointestinal side effects in fructose-consuming patients. *Diabetes Care* 1987; 10: 376–7.
53. Dills WL. Protein fructosylation: fructose and the Maillard reaction. *Am J Clin Nutr* 1993; 58 (suppl): 779S–87S.
54. Jenkins DJA, Wolever TMS, Jenkins AL. Starchy foods and glycemic index. *Diabetes Care* 1988; 11: 149–59.
55. Kolata G. Diabetics should lose weight, avoid fad diets. *Science* 1987; 235: 163–4.
56. Thorburn AW, Brand JC, Truswell AS. The glycaemic index of foods. *Med J Aust* 1986; 144: 580–2.
57. Gannon MC, Nuttall FQ. Factors affecting interpretation of postprandial glucose and insulin areas. *Diabetes Care* 1987; 10: 754–63.
58. Brand-Miller J, Hayne S, Petocz, Colagiuri S, Low-glycemic index diets in the management of diabetes: a meta-analysis of randomized controlled diets. *Diabetes Care* 2003; 2261–7.
59. Järvi AE, Karlström BE, Granfeldt YE, Björck IE, Asp N-GL, Vessby BOH. Improved glycemic control and lipid profile and normalized fibrololytic activity on a low-glycemic index diet in type 2 diabetic patients. *Diabetes Care* 1999; 22: 10–8.
60. Dullaart RP, Beusekamp BJ, Meijer S, van-Doormaal JJ, Sluiter WJ. Long-term effects of protein-restricted diet on

albuminuria and renal function in IDDM patients without clinical nephropathy and hypertension. *Diabetes Care* 1993; 16: 483–92.

61. Jones SL, Kontessis P, Wiseman M, Dodds R, Bognetti E, Pinto J, Viberti G. Protein intake and blood glucose as modulators of GFR in hyperfiltering diabetic patients. *Kidney Int* 1992; 41: 1620–8.
62. Keller K, Whittaker E, Sullivan L, Raskin P, Jacobson HR. Effect of restricting dietary protein on the progression of renal failure in patients with insulin-dependent diabetes mellitus. *N Engl J Med* 1991; 324: 78–84.
63. Evanoff G, Thompson C, Brown J, Weinman E. Prolonged dietary protein restriction in diabetic nephropathy. *Arch Intern Med* 1989; 149: 1129–33.
64. Walker JD, Bending JJ, Dodds RA, Mattock MB, Murrells TJ, Keen H, Viberti GC. Restriction of dietary protein and progression of renal failure in diabetic nephropathy. *Lancet* 1989; 2 (8677): 1411–5.
65. Ciavarella A, Di Mizio G, Stefoni S, et al. Reduced albuminuria after dietary protein restriction in insulin dependent diabetic patients with clinical nephropathy. *Diabetes Care* 1987; 10: 407–13.
66. Pomerleau J, Verdy M, Garrel DR, Nadeau MH. Effect of protein intake on glycaemic control and renal function in type 2 (non-insulin dependent) diabetes mellitus. *Diabetologia* 1993; 36: 829–34.
67. Brodsky IG, Robbins DC, Hiser E, Fuller SP, Fillyaw M, Devlin JT. Effects of low-protein diets on protein metabolism in insulin-dependent diabetes mellitus patients with early nephropathy. *J Clin Endocrinol Metab* 1992; 75: 351–7.
68. Klahr S, Levey AS, Beck GJ, Caggiula AW, Hunsicker L, Kusek JW, Striker G, for the Modification of Diet in Renal Disease Study Group. The effects of dietary protein restriction and blood-pressure control on the progression of chronic renal disease. *N Engl J Med* 1994; 330: 877–84.
69. Jibani MM, Bloodworth LL, Foden E, Griffiths KD, Galpin OP. Predominantly vegetarian diet in patients with incipient and early clinical diabetic nephropathy: effects on albumin excretion rate and nutritional status. *Diabet Med* 1991; 8: 949–53.
70. Walter RM, Uriu-Hare JY, Lewis Olin K, Oster MH, Anawalt BD, Critchfield JW, Keen CL. Copper, zinc, manganese, and magnesium status and complications of diabetes mellitus. *Diabetes Care* 1991; 14: 1050–6.
71. American Diabetes Association. Treatment of hypertension in adults with diabetes. *Diabetes Care* 2003; 26 (suppl 1): S80–2.
72. Rimm EB, Stampfer MJ, Ascherio A, Giovannucci E, Colditz GA, Willett WC. Vitamin E consumption and risk of coronary heart disease in men. *N Engl J Med* 1993; 328: 1450–6.
73. Paolisso G, D'Amore A, Galzerano D, Balbi V, et al. Daily vitamin E supplements improve metabolic control but not insulin secretion in elderly type 2 diabetic patients. *Diabetes Care* 1993; 16: 1433–7.
74. Ceriello A, Guigliano D, Quatraro A, Donzella C, Dipalo G, Lefebvre PJ. Vitamin E reduction of protein glycosylation in diabetes. *Diabetes Care* 1991; 14: 68–72.
75. Christiansen C, Thomsen C, Rasmussen O, Balle M, Hauerslev C, Hansen C, Hermansen K. Wine for type 2 diabetic patients? *Diabet Med* 1993; 10: 958–61.
76. Koivisto VA, Tulokas S, Toivonen M, Haapa E, Pelkonen R. Alcohol with a meal has no adverse effects on postprandial glucose homeostasis in diabetic patients. *Diabetes Care* 1993; 16: 1612–4.

40

Dietary Management of Diabetes Mellitus in India and South East Asia

Ambady Ramachandran, Chamukuttan Snehalatha, and Vijay Viswanathan

Diabetes Research Centre, M.V. Hospital for Diabetes and WHO Collaborating Centre for Research Education and Training in Diabetes, Chennai, India

DIETARY THERAPY IN DIABETES MELLITUS—A HISTORICAL BACKGROUND

Attempts to alleviate diabetes mellitus by diet were first made by the Egyptians as early as 3500 BC. In India, about 2500 years ago, Susruta and Charaka had recognized the importance of dietary regulation in the treatment of diabetes and many of the principles suggested by these eminent physicians hold good even today. They adopted measures to correct obesity in subjects with diabetes, advised feeding of lean diabetic individuals, and prohibited the use of sugar, jaggery (unrefined cane sugar), wines, ghee (clarified butter), butter, and meat [1].

In the eighteenth century, it was observed that glycosuria could be decreased by moderation in the quantity of food taken by diabetic individuals and by restriction of the diet to animal foods [2]. In the twentieth century, prior to the discovery of insulin, the treatment of diabetes mellitus included intermittent fasting, under nutrition and carbohydrate restriction. With the advent of insulin and the oral hypoglycemic drugs, there was a tendency to prescribe liberal diets. Nevertheless, several long-term studies have unequivocally proved the prime importance of a calorie-restricted well-balanced diet in the treatment of diabetes.

DIETARY PATTERN IN INDIA AND SOUTH EAST ASIA

The acceptance of a diet and adherence to it by a diabetic individual is made easier if the diet advised resembles that to which the diabetic individual and his or her family are accustomed. A high degree of patient acceptability ensures long-term compliance and thus, better metabolic control. This helps in achieving the main objective of successful dietary therapy in diabetes. Fortunately, the food consumption patterns seen in India and other countries of South East Asia do not present any major obstacles to acceptance of the diet prescribed for a diabetic subject.

Data available from the National Nutritional Monitoring Bureau (NNMB) show that in recent years in India there has been a moderate increase in the average energy consumption of food which is mainly cereal-based, with rice and wheat being consumed as the staple items of food in the southern and northern states in India, respectively [3].

Determination of the proximate principles in the food indicates that 70–75% of the total energy intake is being derived from complex carbohydrates, 12% from proteins, and 14% from fats. The common Indian diet is made up of whole-grain cereals, pulses (legumes), leafy vegetables, fruits, milk, and milk products. The majority of the population in India is vegetarian, and even in so-called non-vegetarians the actual intake of meat, eggs, and poultry is restricted to once or twice a week. Vegetable oils are the main source of fat. The traditional diet of the majority of the population in India and South East Asia is rich in whole-grain cereals and complex carbohydrates, low in animal proteins and saturated fats, and rich in unsaturated fats from vegetable oils. The overall energy content is fairly restricted, with a high intake of fiber-rich food and a low intake of free sugar.

International Textbook of Diabetes Mellitus, Third Edition. Edited by R. A. DeFronzo, E. Ferrannini, H. Keen, and P. Zimmet.

Table 1 Break up of the dietary components* and anthropometric data in relation to glucose tolerance

	Mean ± SD		
	Nondiabetic cases ($n = 762$)	New diabetic cases ($n = 26$)	Known diabetic cases ($n = 55$)
Body mass index (kg/m^2)	22.8 ± 3.9	23.8 ± 2.6	23.5 ± 2.9
Waist-to-hip ratio	0.86 ± 0.09	0.92 ± 0.08†	0.94 ± 0.08†
Calories	1911 ± 425	1865 ± 446	1557 ± 338
Carbohydrate (g)‡	312 ± 82 (66.5 ± 17.5)	302 ± 85 (65.9 ± 18.1)	233 ± 65† (61.6 ± 17)
Fat (g)‡	39.8 ± 8.0 (19 ± 3.8)	37.7 ± 5.2 (18.5 ± 2.4)	37.7 ± 5.0† (22.4 ± 2.9)
Protein (g)‡	65.8 ± 23.0 (14 ± 4.9)	71.0 ± 23.4 (15.5 ± 5.1)	60.2 ± 19.9† (15.9 ± 5.2)

* Dietary components calculated per day.
† $p < 0.001$ versus nondiabetic.
‡ Values in parentheses represent percentages.

A study of urban population in Chennai, Tamil Nadu, India, showed that in general, there was a uniform pattern of diet among different social strata [3]. The total energy consumption in adults varied from 1028 to 3662 kcal. The mean percentages of carbohydrates, protein, and fats were 66.7 ± 17.7, 14.1 ± 4.9, and 19.2 ± 3.8, respectively, which showed little variations when analyzed with respect to age, gender, economic class, or physical activity. Calorie consumption was lower in women and older people. This could be partly related to the degree of physical activity as women and old people tend to be sedentary. As the energy consumption was directly proportionate to the physical activity, these changes were expected. Energy consumption was also proportional to the body weight.

Lower energy consumption among the high-income group could be related to (a) lower physical activity as most of them were engaged in sedentary occupation and (b) also to the awareness of healthy diet habits. Obesity was less common among them. Lower calorie consumption in women and older people could be related to lower physical activity.

The dietary analysis of urban south Indians collected in the epidemiological survey showed that all the dietary factors are similar in the nondiabetic and the newly diagnosed diabetic cases (Table 1). The calorie consumption and the composition of the diet varied only in known diabetic cases who were prescribed dietary modifications. The results indicated that dietary habits were generally uniform in the urban society and did not have a significant contributory role in the development of diabetes [4].

DIET IN THE MANAGEMENT OF DIABETES MELLITUS

The importance of the diet in the management of diabetes has been recognized for centuries. Diet is the main pillar in the treatment and control of diabetes, but successful dietary therapy depends as much on the patient as on the physician. Although dietary goals are often dismissed as impossible to achieve, intensive education and motivation of the diabetic patient has convinced us that dietary therapy can be successful. Furthermore, the traditional diets consumed in India offer specific advantages in the dietary management of diabetes.

THE EVOLUTION OF THE HIGH-CARBOHYDRATE, HIGH-FIBER DIET

In the late 1950s, the diet advised for diabetic patients was based on the Western-diet pattern, in which a marked reduction in carbohydrate content and a high-fat intake were advised. This restricted-carbohydrate diet provided only about 33% of the calories from carbohydrate. Such a diet was not suitable for the Indian diabetic patient, as the diet of an average Indian has very high carbohydrate content. For better and sustained dietary compliance, the Indian diabetic patient had to be given enough carbohydrate in his or her diet. The only advice given at that time was to avoid free sugar completely and reduce the total intake of calories in the diet. As early as 1958, Viswanathan and his coworkers evolved the ‘High Carbohydrate Diet’ which provided about 60% of the calories in the form of complex carbohydrates [5]. Contrary to existing beliefs, the diet did not worsen carbohydrate tolerance, neither was the control of diabetes difficult. Indeed, the dose of drugs required to control diabetes was very small [6]. The diet was further modified around 1968 by increasing the protein content to 20% and reducing the fat content to 13% [7]. As the traditional Indian diet is vegetarian, the protein content of the diabetic diet was increased by increasing the content of pulses and legumes. (Table 2 shows the proximate principles in some of the commonly used pulses and legumes, the most popular of which are Bengal gram, green gram, and black gram, (Table 2). This change further increased the fiber content of the diet. Analysis showed that the diet provided 52 g of fiber, which is almost double of that in the standard Americans Diabetes Association diet. Hence the diet is now called *the high-carbohydrate, high-fiber (HCHF) diet* (Table 3).

Our observations on a large number of patients in the Diabetes Research Center, Chennai, India, seen

Table 2 Proximate principles in the common pulses and legumes used in the Indian diet*

Foodstuff	Protein (N × 6.25) (g)	Fat (g)	Minerals (g)	Fiber (g)	Carbohydrates (g)	Energy (kcal)
Bengal gram, dhal	30.8	5.6	2.2	1.2	59.8	372
Black gram, dhal	24.0	1.4	3.2	0.9	59.6	347
Green gram, dhal	24.5	1.2	3.5	0.8	59.9	348
Lentil	25.1	0.7	2.1	0.7	59.0	343
Moth beans	23.6	1.1	3.5	4.5	56.5	330
Peas, green	7.2	0.1	0.8	4.0	15.9	93
Rajmah	22.9	1.3	3.2	4.8	60.6	346
Red gram, dhal	22.3	1.7	3.5	1.5	57.6	335
Soyabean	43.2	19.5	4.6	3.7	20.9	432

* All values are per 100 g of edible portion.

during the last four decades show that the diet is acceptable to the patients, which ensures long-term compliance [8, 9]. There is rapid and sustained control of hyperglycemia [6] with lowering of plasma cholesterol and triglycerides levels [10]. It does not reduce the level of high-density-lipoprotein cholesterol, the protective factor for cardiovascular complications [11], and it improves peripheral sensitivity of insulin [12].

PRINCIPLES OF THE HCHF DIET

The total calories advised will vary with each patient. The calories are restricted much more in the obese patient who is required to reduce his body weight. Carbohydrates are mainly derived from cereals like rice and wheat. Refined sugars are totally prohibited. Proteins prescribed are mainly vegetable proteins derived from pulses (legumes) like Bengal gram, green gram, and black gram, and fresh vegetables. The proteins of cereals and pulses have mutual supplementary effects, a deficiency of any particular amino acid in the one being made good by an excess in the other if both are consumed at the same time. The fat content of the diet is restricted to the oil used in cooking. By prescribing vegetables containing 3–4% carbohydrate, like greens, cucumber, drumstick, bitter gourd, banana flower, banana stem, cabbage, cauliflower, and ash pumpkin, the bulk of the meal is increased and the patient's hunger satisfied without appreciably increasing the total calories.

Table 3 Composition of the high-carbohydrate high-fiber diet of the Diabetes Research Center, Chennai, India, for a patient requiring 1800 kcal/day*

	Weight (g)	Energy (kcal)
Carbohydrate	301	1204 (67%)
Protein	86	344 (19%)
Fat	28	252 (14%)

*From reference 6, with permission.

THERAPEUTIC BENEFITS OF DIETARY FIBER IN THE INDIAN DIET

Dietary fiber comprises those components of plant cells that are present as part of the diet yet are resistant to digestive secretions of the gastrointestinal tract. It is not a single entity but includes a wide range of complex polysaccharides, consisting of a mixture of cellulose, lignin, hemicellulose, plant gums, pectins, and mucin. A number of studies [13, 14] have established that intake of high-fiber diet has definite therapeutic benefits for diabetic patients. A high-fiber diet can help the diabetic patient in reducing postprandial hyperglycemia [15] and insulin secretion [16], and in decreasing the raised plasma lipids (triglycerides and cholesterol, particularly low-density-lipoprotein (LDL) cholesterol), and also helps in the reduction of body weight. Although it is not entirely clear how all these effects are produced, possible mechanisms that have been suggested include (a) delayed gastric emptying time [17], (b) increased intestinal transit time, and (c) alterations in the rate and site of nutrient absorption in the gut, possibly as a result of a release of gut hormones [18].

The fact that an HCHF diet is an ideal diet for diabetic patients has gained acceptance all over the world and was substantiated by the recommendations made by the World Health Organization (WHO) study group in 1985 [19]. During the 1980s many Western diabetologists were recommending that high-carbohydrate diets for their patients be supplemented with artificial fibers in the form of bran, guar gum, and pectins. In India, since natural foods are rich in soluble fiber, addition of artificial fiber is rarely indicated or necessary. While artificial fibers are good for research purposes, the addition of fiber-containing natural foods to the diet in communities in the developing world is preferable for achieving better metabolic control and is also cost-effective.

DIETARY PROTEIN

Dietary protein should contribute about 15% of total energy intake and is mainly derived from vegetable sources. A high-protein diet may accelerate the progression of diabetic nephropathy. Currently, a protein intake of 0.6–0.8 g/kg body weight/day is recommended for the diabetic patient [20]. Diabetic nephropathy is a major complication of diabetes, causing severe morbidity and early mortality due to diabetes. Dietary protein restriction has been shown to help retard the progression of diabetic renal disease in humans and in experimentally induced renal disease in animals [20–22]. The recommended dietary allowance of protein intake is 0.8 g/kg body weight/day in patients with overt nephropathy. Once the glomerular filtration rate (GFR) falls, further restriction to 0.6 g/kg body weight/day may prove useful in slowing the decline of GFR. However, in a cross-sectional study conducted in 405 south Indian vegetarian and nonvegetarian type 2 diabetic subjects, it was shown that although the mean protein intake was significantly higher in nonvegetarians when compared with vegetarians (protein intake: 57.3 ± 16.1 vs. 52.2 ± 12.5 g/kg body weight/day, $p < 0.0008$) [23], it did not exceed the limit recommended for patients with diabetic nephropathy (i.e., 0.6–0.8 g/kg body weight/day). The prevalence of microalbuminuria (vegetarians = 18% and nonvegetarians = 26%) and proteinuria (vegetarians = 21% and nonvegetarians = 24%) did not vary between vegetarians and nonvegetarians.

Since the dietary intake of protein is found to be less than the recommended allowance in south Indian patients with diabetic nephropathy, it appears that marked reduction in proteins is unnecessary for these subjects. However in nonvegetarians restriction of animal protein may be necessary in stages of overt nephropathy.

Protein restrictions in the meal plan, if prescribed, should be designed by a dietitian familiar with all components of the dietary managements of diabetes to prevent nutritional deficiency.

DIETARY FAT

Sustained hyperglycemia and hyperlipidemia have been implicated as factors in the etiology of the long-term micro- and macrovascular complications of diabetes. Presence of diabetes in the absence of other risk factors have been linked to a two- to threefold increase in cardiovascular disease risk, and diabetic patients often have a mixed dyslipidemia [20]. The control of plasma lipids and lipoprotein profile is a prime objective when considering the dietary management of diabetes.

It is recommended that about 15% of the total calories allowed should be derived from fats. About one third of the total fat content of the diet can be in the form of saturated fats and the rest is to be contributed by polyunsaturated and monounsaturated fats (e.g. vegetable and fish oils). This has been found to improve the lipemic profile, reducing atherogenic LDL-cholesterol levels [20].

Several reports have indicated antiatherogenic benefits of omega-3-fatty acids in normal and hyperlipidemic individuals [24]. Increased intake of this type of fatty acid, which is widely present in some of the common food items of Indians (fish oil, wheat-germ oil, green leafy vegetables, common beans, etc.), is believed to exert a protective effect against cardiovascular diseases in diabetic individuals [25]. However, the clinical utility of omega-3-fatty acids has been questioned in relation to glucose metabolism following the demonstration of possible proatherogenic effects [20]. A number of reports have found that fish oil supplementation may impair overall glycemic control in type 2 diabetic subjects and thus negate the beneficial effects on plasma triglycerides and very low density lipoprotein cholesterol.

In a recent study from our center it was noted that type 2 diabetic patients who have been consuming HCHF diet for long periods did not have postprandial hypertriglyceridemia [26]. A group of patients (26%) who had postprandial elevation of serum triglycerides were consuming lower percentage of carbohydrate and higher percentage of fats than prescribed. Therefore the postprandial rise in triglycerides was probably due to the high-fat intake of the diet and also due to a lower insulin sensitivity.

MEAL PLANNING

Daily energy requirements are calculated taking into consideration the following points: (a) type of diabetes; (b) ideal body weight to be achieved and maintained; (c) special requirements such as optimal growth and development in children; and (d) pregnancy and lactation in women. The distribution of energy intake between carbohydrates, protein, and fats must closely match the distribution of these proximate principles in the traditional diet. The food exchange system practiced in Western societies helps to keep the diet varied to prevent monotony, while maintaining the daily pattern of food intake. However, exchanges based on whole meals are preferable to those concentrating on the carbohydrate content of different foods. The glycemic index may be useful as it takes into account factors that reduce absorption rate, such as the nature of the starch, fiber, and antinutrients (e.g., phytate, lectins, tannins, and saponins). At present, it may prove a useful addition to dietary management in identifying how particular foods might be used in the diabetic diet. A low glycemic index food forming the basic and major component of each meal may offer advantages. Thus, an approximately equivalent amount of cereal, bread, or rice may be suggested as a basis for a meal-planning approach to diabetic diets, together with appropriate guidelines about cooking and the use of fresh vegetables.

NUTRITIONAL COUNSELING AND PATIENT EDUCATION FOR DIETARY COMPLIANCE

Nutritional Counseling

Effective nutritional counseling must take into consideration the social, cultural, and religious aspects of food consumption. It is widely believed in the Orient that certain food items have to be restricted or totally avoided in diseases states. Therefore most patients do expect physicians to advise them regarding the food items that are to be restricted or prohibited. Physicians rarely have enough time to be the sole providers of appropriate and balanced advice on nutrition because of their heavy clinical workload. Hence, experienced dietitians are essential to provide individual guidance. Training programs and learning experiences for the health care providers constitute an essential strategy for diabetes care. Health care providers must render appropriate nutritional counseling so as to enable the diabetic patients to follow religious practices without unduly disturbing their metabolic control. Frequent intervals of follow-up, individualization of diet prescription, and family involvement are some of the factors that contribute to the success of diet therapy.

India is facing a grave burden because of the rising prevalence of diabetes in the urban areas. One of the major reasons for increased prevalence of diabetes worldwide is a rising trend in obesity among adults and also in children. Overweight in children is an antecedent of adult obesity. Modernization and urbanization cause changes in diet habits and reduce physical activity, which contributes to this phenomenon. A recent study in urban Indian adolescent school children showed that nearly 16.6% of children in the age group of 13–18 years were overweight [27]. Lifestyle factors especially low physical activity and high socioeconomic background favored overweight among the children. A diet score was not strongly associated with increasing body mass index but decreased physical activity showed a strong association with overweight. Recently, it has been shown by us that the healthy body mass index of an Indian is below 23 kg/m^2, above which the risk for diabetes becomes statistically significant [28]. Age at menarche was lower in the low economic group, probably reflecting a nutritional imbalance as a result of poverty. It is well known that social deprivation results in unavailability of sufficient food that causes nutritional deficiency.

Patient Education

Patient education regarding the dietary management of diabetes mellitus in developing countries poses a variety of difficulties. The two major handicaps that one faces in patient education are (a) the existence of a multilingual society, and (b) the large number of adults with low standards of literacy [29]. Printed pamphlets and materials are of only limited use. Teaching sessions that include the use of food models that exhibit the model diet plan for an entire day, simple pictorial charts, and other audiovisual aids, and demonstration of household measures for food exchanges do help in motivating the patients to achieve a high level of dietary compliance [30, 31]. Wherever possible the spouse and other family members must also take part in the education programs. Experience at the Diabetes Research Center, Chennai, India, has convinced us of the usefulness of this approach in Indian diabetic subjects.

CONCLUDING REMARKS

The objectives and goals of diet therapy in diabetes mellitus are (a) to achieve and maintain normal blood glucose levels, lipid profile, and ideal body weight; (b) to maintain optimal nutrition; and (c) to relieve obvious symptoms and minimize chronic degenerative vascular complications. Nutritional requirements and dietary recommendations to diabetic patients are not different from those of the general population, although the emphasis and practical approaches may be different. In our experience, as the diet in India and South East Asia is essentially cereal-based and rich in fiber, the prescription of an HCHF diet presents few practical difficulties and dietary compliance is easily achieved. However, constant motivation through nutrition counseling and education imparted in an appropriate way goes a long way in achieving these goals.

The younger generation should be given education regarding a healthy diet which will definitely have a role in reducing the occurrence of nutritional deficiencies, overweight, and also may probably be useful in delaying the onset of diabetes due to impaired insulin sensitivity.

REFERENCES

1. Frank LL. Diabetes mellitus in the texts of old Hindu medicine (Charaka, Susruta, Vaghbata). *Am J Gastroenterol* 1957; 27: 76.
2. Joslin EP. Development of the present treatment of diabetes. *J Am Diet Assoc* 1949; 25: 213.
3. ICMR. National Institute of Nutrition. Hyderabad – Annual Report 1985–86, pp 105–35.
4. Shobana R, Snehalatha C, Latha E, Vijay V, Ramachandran A. Dietary profile of urban south Indians and its relation with glycaemic status. *Diabetes Res Clin Prac* 1998; 42: 181–6.
5. Viswanathan M. High carbohydrate diet in diabetes. *J Diabetes Assoc India* 1968; 8: 353–60.
6. Viswanathan M, Snehalatha C, Ramachandran A, Mohan V. Rapid control of diabetes with high carbohydrate diet and combination of glibenclamide and phenformin. *J Diabetes Assoc India* 1978; 18: 119–23.

7. Viswanathan M, Ramachandran A, Mohan V, Snehalatha C. High-carbohydrate, high fiber diet in diabetes. *J Diabetes Assoc India* 1981; 21 (suppl): 90–6.
8. Viswanathan M, Mohan V, Ramachandran A, Snehalatha C, Anderson JW, Long-term experience with high carbohydrate high fiber diets in Indian diabetic patients. *Diabetologia Croat* 1984; 13: 163–74.
9. Viswanathan M, Snehalatha C, Ramachandran A, Mohan V. High-carbohydrate diet in diabetes: long-term experience. In *Proceedings of the International Diabetes Federation Congress*, Vienna. Amsterdam: Excerpta Medica, 1979; p 84.
10. Viswanathan M, Snehalatha C, Ramachandran A, Mohan V, Shobana R. Effect of a calorie-restricted, high carbohydrate, high protein, low fat diet on serum lipids: a follow-up study. *J Assoc Phys India* 1978; 26: 163–8.
11. Susheela L, Shyamsundar R, Ramachandran A, Mohan V, Viswanathan M. Favourable alterations in serum total/HDL and LDL/HDL cholesterol ratios after glucoregulation in newly diagnosed NIDDM. *Diabetologia Croat* 1983; 12: 17–33.
12. Viswanathan M, Snehalatha C, Ramachandran A, Mohan V. Effect of high-carbohydrate, high fiber diet on immunoreactive insulin level in diabetes. *J Diabetes Assoc India* 1983; 23: 45–8.
13. Carpo PA, Reaven G, Olefsky J. Postprandial plasma glucose and insulin responses to different complex carbohydrates. *Diabetes* 1977; 26: 1179–83.
14. Crapo PA, Kolterman OG, Waldeck N, Reaven GM, Olefsky JM. Postprandial hormonal responses to different types of complex carbohydrate in individuals with impaired glucose tolerance. *Am J Clin Nutr* 1980; 33: 1723–8.
15. Vinik AI, Jenkins DJA. Dietary fiber in management of diabetes. *Diabetes Care* 1988; 11: 160–72.
16. Viswanathan M, Ramachandran A, Mohan V, Snehalatha C. Effect of ingestion of natural food fiber on glucose tolerance and plasma immunoreactive insulin response. *Biomedicine* 1980; 1: 43–6.
17. Holt S, Heading RC, Carter DC, Prescott LF, Tothill P. Effect of gel fiber on gastric emptying and absorption of glucose and paracetamol. *Lancet* 1979; 1: 636–9.
18. Morgan LM, Goulder TJ, Tsiolakis D, Marks V. Alberti KGMM. The effect of unabsorbable carbohydrate on gut hormones: modification of postprandial GIP secretion by guar. *Diabetologia* 1979; 17: 85–9.
19. WHO Study Group. Diabetes Mellitus. Technical Report Series 727. Geneva: WHO, 1985; p77.
20. Boctor DL, Jenkins DJA. Trends in dietary management of diabetes mellitus: an update. In Alberti KGMM, Krall LP (eds), *The Diabetes Annual*, Vol 6. Amsterdam: Elsevier Science, 1991; pp 105–36.
21. Ihle BU, Becker GJ, Whitworth JA, Charlwood RA, Kincaid-Smith PS. The effect of protein restriction on the progression of renal insufficiency. *N Engl J Med* 1989; 321: 1733–77.
22. Rosman JB, Meijer S, Sluiter WJ, Ter Wee PM, Piers Becht TP, Donker AJ. Prospective randomized trial of early dietary protein restriction in chronic renal failure. *Lancet* 1984; ii: 1291–6.
23. Vijay V, Snehalatha C, Varadharani MP, Nair BM, Jayaraman M, Ramachandran A. Prevalence of albuminuria among vegetarian and nonvegetarian south Indian diabetic patients. *Indian J Nephrol* 2002; 12: 73–6.
24. Stacpoole PW, Alig J, Ammon L, Crockett SE. Dose–response effects of dietary marine oil on carbohydrate and lipid metabolism in normal subjects and patients with hypertriglyceridaemia. *Metabolism* 1989; 38: 946–56.
25. Raheja BS. Indian diet—diabetes and its complications. *IDF Bull* 1988; 33: 14–7.
26. Snehalatha C, Sivasankari S, Satyavani K, Vijay V, Ramachandran A. Postprandial hypertriglyceridaemia in treated type 2 diabetic subjects—the role of dietary components. *Diabetes Res Clin Pract* 2000; 48: 57–60.
27. Ramachandran A, Vinitha R, Megha Thayyil, Sathish kumar CK, Sheeba L, Joseph S, Vijay V. Prevalence of overweight in urban Indian adolescent school children. *Diabetes Res Clin Prac* 2002; 57: 185–90.
28. Snehalatha C, Vijay V, Ramachandran A, Cut-off values for normal anthropometric variables in Asian Indian Adults. *Diabetes Care* 2003; 26: 1380–84.
29. Shobana R, Indira P, Ramachandran A, Mohan V, Viswanathan M. Effectiveness of patient education in a multilingual, multiliterate population. *J Med Assoc Thai* 1987; 70 (suppl 2): 219–22.
30. Bajaj JS. Dietary therapy: principles and practice. *Diabetes Health Care: Trainers' Manual for Allied Health Professionals*. Srinagar: Vishwanatha Press, 1982; pp 34–7.
31. Shobana R, Premila L, Shyamala P, Mohan V, Ramachandran A, Viswanathan M. Assessment of background knowledge of diabetes mellitus in diabetic patients. *J Diabetes Assoc India* 1989; 29: 70–3.

This chapter is based in part on a chapter of the same title which was published in an earlier edition of the *International Textbook of Diabetes Mellitus*, by A Ramachandran and M Viswanathan.

41

Dietary Management of Diabetes Mellitus: Japanese Guidance and Methodology

Shigeaki Baba* **and Seiki Nambu**†

International Institute for Diabetes Education and Study, Kobe, Japan, and †Mukogawa Women's University, Nishinomiya, Japan

INTRODUCTION

Helping people understand the dietary value, the nutritional and energy, of the meals they eat content is important not only for those with diabetes, but also for achieving a healthy diet in general. The guidance provided must be easy to understand so that patients and their families can follow it. People quite often have very different tastes, likes, and dislikes as well as eating habits, making it difficult to obtain an accurate picture of their food intake. Frequently, the individual dieticians can also differ with respect to their recommendations concerning the most appropriate diet for an individual. We therefore suggest, that patients should continue to take advice from a single dietician where possible.

The dietician should use a patients' meal records as a basis to calculate the most appropriate amounts of food for each meal and to advise on suitable menus, ingredients, and cooking times. It is important to give comprehensive dietary instructions, with the patient's breakfast or daily meal as a starting point, rather than stand-alone numerical estimates of an ideal calorie intake and desirable proportions of macronutrients. Dietary recommendations and nutritional guidance should also be sensitive to other issues such as the patient's lifestyle, profession, or age and must be modified as necessary to take account of the patients current antidiabetic therapy. Dietary advice serves, of course, only as a template. Its potential success depends in part on the patient's psychological state, the completeness of the dietary records supplied, and the degree to which patients provide only that information that they think we would like to hear. With these provisos, dietary therapy can be very successful, helping to gain the patient's trust and cooperation and the opportunity to obtain more accurate dietary records. In other words, we should keep on encouraging patients and providing advice but interpret dietary feedback with caution.

In Japan there are many changes taking place in the food and catering industries and in society. Food imports are growing rapidly, there is a growing trend toward nuclear families, and many more women are now taking jobs outside the home. Westernization, globalization, simplification of meals, and the increased tendency toward dining out are but some of the many influences affecting meal patterns and the types of food eaten. Increasingly, many people now skip breakfast and do not eat set or balanced meals. People frequently take on trust the misleading dietary information they get from TV and media sources. This in turn leads to the adoption of inappropriate diet habits whose unbalanced nutritional composition may lead to lifestyle-related diseases [1].

These issues reflect daily life in Japan as a whole. We need to acquaint ourselves with them if we are to provide the most appropriate instructions with regard to a healthy and balanced diet for our patients.

DISTINCTIVE FEATURES OF JAPANESE CUISINE

The World Health Organization (WHO) has defined *health* as a state of good physical and mental well-being from a societal point of view [2]. However, it can also be said that *health* is a state of living daily life to the full, with the

International Textbook of Diabetes Mellitus, Third Edition. Edited by R. A. DeFronzo, E. Ferrannini, H. Keen, and P. Zimmet.
 ISBN: 0-471-48655-8.

feeling of self-actualization as a major factor. Accomplishing this new health policy is easier in a culture-based lifestyle, taking root and adjusted according to the local specifications, with an emphasis on societal factors than on improving the quality of life. This is what we would call the creation of a healthy society.

The Japanese approach to diet has evolved over the nation's history, reflecting its customs and many tradition, but, naturally, is not perfect from a nutritional viewpoint. Starting from the Meiji era, more and more meat ingredients have been included in Japanese foodstuffs, especially during and after the Second World War. The effects of adding meat to the Japanese diet have had unpredictable consequences, leading to an improvement in the physical constitution of people and prolongation of the average lifespan. However, along with other changes relating to Westernization, a number of new cardiovascular-related problems have appeared and arterial diseases have increased in general.

The essential feature of traditional Japanese cuisine, which is known worldwide to be healthy, is that staple foodstuffs and main dishes are principally vegetarian. This is historically rooted and provides the basis of most current Japanese cuisine, notwithstanding the influence of West.

A strong connection to nature has turned Japanese cuisine into a special culture that takes pleasure in taking advantage of opportunities provided by seasonal changes and places a great emphasis on the way food is presented. The reduced frequency of obesity among Japanese people and their lower death rate from cardiovascular diseases is the reason why the Japanese diet is so often called a healthy diet and is attracting more and more people's attention [3].

HOW TO APPLY THE FOOD GUIDE PYRAMID FOR JAPANESE PEOPLE WITH DIABETES

Using the information presented above, we have created a Food Guide Pyramid for Japanese people that focuses mainly on preventing lifestyle-related diseases and that can be used to recommend a medically approved diet. The pyramid was constructed primarily for Japanese people, with one of the essential design features being for it to be as comprehensive as possible. Some features are similar to the Food Guide Pyramid drawn up in 2000 by the United States Department of Agriculture [2, 3]. However, in the American Food Guide Pyramid, fat content is limited to 30% of total calorie intake, dietary fibre intake is greater, salt intake is smaller, and there is an emphasis on promotion of physical activity, with a primary intention being the prevention of cardiovascular diseases.

Figure 1 shows the pyramid adjusted for diet guidance based on daily Japanese meal, which can also apply for a healthy diet. The figure was composed mainly for daily allocation of food, and is intended to help in choosing the food ingredients.

The left side of the Pyramid indicates those foodstuffs that should be taken daily, while those on the right side should be consumed on a weekly basis. Importantly, the seasonings and spices are those that are used frequently in Japanese cuisine. Take two or three ingredients as a main dish from Block A [4], which might be rice or bread; zero to two snacks as refreshment between meals from Block A [5], but consider intake separately. Then take about three meals based on four to six kinds of vegetables and one or two kinds of seaweeds, mushrooms, or bamboo from the Block B. The antioxidant, vitamins, minerals, and fiber of green vegetables and proper seasoning of seaweeds and mushrooms while cooking will help better managing of calcium and polyphenol intake. Main products from Block D (take about three meals based on three to five ingredients) like meat, fish, chicken meat, beans, and eggs serve as body-building meterials. Then choose one or two ingredients from Block C. Choose about one or two products (milk, yogurt, cheese, etc.) from Block E. Add seasonings: sugar, soybean sauce, salt, oils, and fats, which are indispensable in Japanese cuisine. Seasonings should be consumed sparingly and not taken in excess.

Each block plays its own unique nutritional role, and cannot be judged as more or less than one other as they are of equal importance. The amount of food to be consumed from each block depends on total energy requirements. The proper intake of energy, nutrients, minerals, and vitamins can be achieved by consuming meals containing foodstuffs from all of the different blocks, with the ideal daily intake consisting of 30 food ingredients.

The principles outlined here allow for a varied dietary approach and provide a philosophy for a healthy diet. It uses a careful choice of food ingredients considering their nutritional value; limits oil, fat, and salt intake; emphasizes dietary fibre consumption; and promotes the proper balance of vitamins, minerals, and antioxidants.

BIORHYTHM IN LINE WITH DIET

Another key element for a healthy lifestyle is the adoption of a biorhythm-tailored diet. All human beings have daily, weekly, monthly, and annual biological rhythms. Accordingly, nutritional assessments should be judged considering these rhythms. Simply put, asking people to consider their energy intake and the nutritional value of their food on a daily basis, day after day, frequently takes an emotional toll. Asking that patients consider and calculate the nutritional value of their diet on a weekly basis makes it much easier for them to follow dietary recommendations. Correspondingly, evaluating the effectiveness of dietary guidance on a weekly basis is a more practical approach, more efficient, and likely to give improved results.

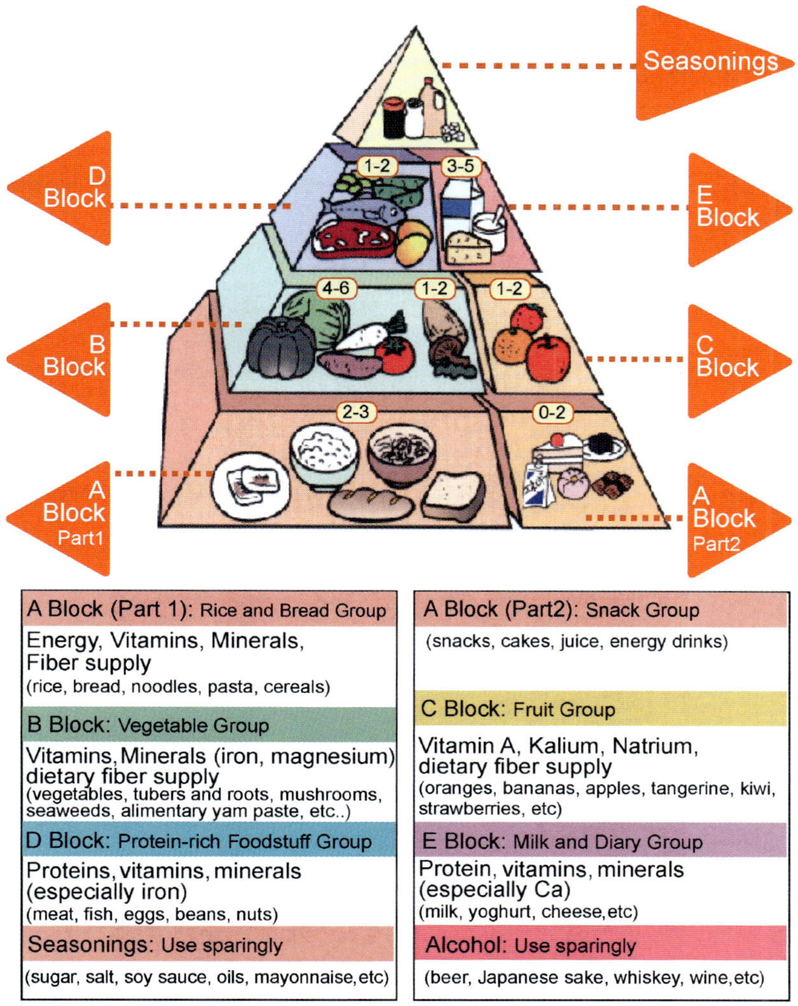

Figure 1 Food guide pyramid

Daily physical exercise is a good example of a way to adjust biorhythms functioning and to coordinate them in our everyday life. Thus, exercise can improve the effectiveness of dietary guidance by helping with the digestion of a meal.

Sporting activities and psychological rest following a meal, can be identified as main criteria of health. Dietary guidance provided in connection with biorhythm adjustments will definitely lead to creating a healthy constitution.

USING A MEAL LOG CHART FOR CHECKING DIETARY HABIT

Regular dietary checks and nutritional value assessments are key elements of good dietary guidance. The Food Guide Pyramid and the meal log chart are easy to understand, provide a visual approach to treatment evaluation, and incorporate the characteristic features of Japanese cuisine.

The main purpose of the Food Guide Pyramid and the meal log chart is to make it easier and less stressful for the patient and his family when completing the log chart based on the Food Guide Pyramid. The log chart provides the dietician with a clear picture of the patient's eating pattern. The dietician can present the data from the chart in a visual format, evaluating patients' eating habits and their nutritional balance. Dieticians with a good knowledge of local dietary customs are well placed to assess a patient's eating pattern, to identify anomalies in the log chart, and to obtain more complete information.

EVALUATION/ASSESSMENT FOR DIABETES PATIENTS

Two separate dietary guidance tables have been produced: one for dieticians and one, with easy to understand explanations, for the patient. The first evaluates nutrition and eating habits, while the other evaluates nutritional status of meal and its balance, as shown in Tables 1 and 2.

For effective evaluation of nutritional status it is necessary to interpret it in context. Improvement following previous guidance is scored as 0, while problematic issues from a nutritional balance and energy level point of view are scored as −1 or −2.

After the form is completed, we recommend that a copy be given to the patient as an aid to self-management. In the comments column, suggestions concerning the choice of food ingredients, preferred cooking methods, and advised eating habits should be written.

The dietician's nutritional evaluation should compare assessments before and after guidance has been given. The focus should be particularly on the degree to which improvements have been made and the decrease or increase in energy balance. For health care professionals a separate column for scientific notes is provided for more specific comments on particular deficits and advice about further modifications. These comments may prove usefully to more interested patients, acknowledging dietary therapy [6, 7].

CASE STUDIES

One method for promoting more effective dietary treatment of patients with diabetes is to make greater use of information technology (IT). We have undertaken clinical trials to evaluate the scoring system described and the diagrammatic depiction of the answers obtained.

The effectiveness of the treatment of diabetes mellitus depends to a great extent on the patient's lifestyle, eating habits, and nutritional balance of meals. Counseling, therefore, by a professional dietician on nutrition and eating habits should be undertaken in order to achieve better results of the treatment. We have used our scoring system to assess and indicate diagrammatically evaluation of clinical regimens as shown in Table 3.

Making the visuals simple to understand helps promote the patient's own will to manage the treatment and speed it up.

Case 1

A 74-year-old, obese, female patient was living alone. Her daily life was full of family-oriented stress, which led to

Table 1 Evaluation of eating habits

	Previous time	Present time	0	−1	−2	Notes
Distribution of meal/day			Regularly 3 meals	More than 4 times	Skipping meal	
Meal time			Almost well-ordered meals	Occasionally taking meal out of schedule	Always disordered meal intake	
Quantity of meal/day			Almost same amount	Always differ	Not settled at all	
Nutritional balance of the meal			Consider nutritional balance	Products' intake is biased	Not taken into consideration	
Eating manner			Slowly, chewing thoroughly and enjoying the taste	Sometimes eating fast enough	Always eating fast	
Frequency of dining out/box-lunches			Almost do not (0–2 times/week)	3–4 times/week	More than 5 times/week	
Alcohol intake			Adequate amount or no alcohol	Moderate amount	Much alcohol	
Self-satisfaction level			Satisfied	Almost satisfied	Always unsatisfied	

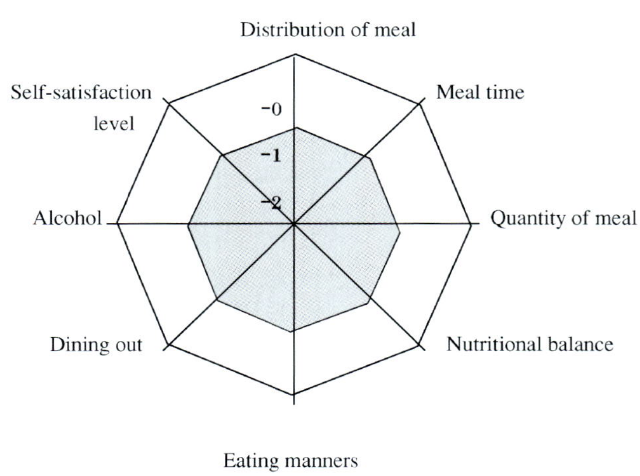

Table 2 Evaluation of nutritional status of meal

	Previous time	Present time	0	−1	−2	Notes
Quantity of staple foodstuff			Adequate	Not enough	Overeating	
Snacks			Adequate	Sometimes overeating	Overeating	
Vegetables amount			Adequate	Light deficit	Deficit	
Fruits			Adequate	Overeating	Deficit	
Milk and dairy products			Adequate	Overeating	Deficit	
Meat, fish, soybean, eggs, etc.			Adequate	Overeating	Deficit	
Spices, seasonings			Adequate	Deficit	Over seasoning	
Alcohol			Adequate	Drink averagely	Drink much	

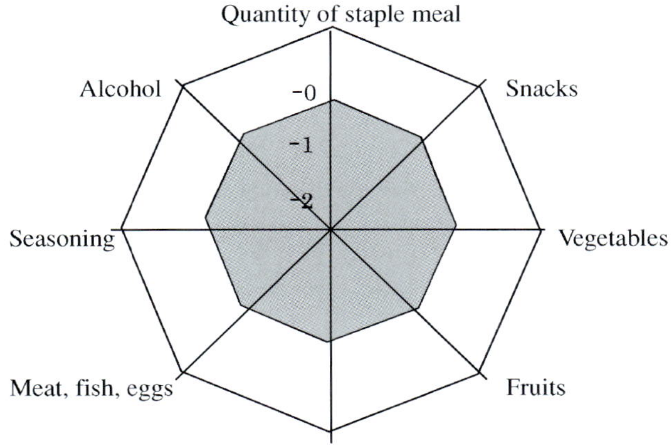

overeating, a large intake of fruits and snacks, as well as frequent extra meals before sleeping. Oral hypoglycemic drug therapy appeared to be ineffective at the time the patient contacted us. Counseling, lifestyle guidance, and advice concerning well-balanced nutrition proved difficult to implement initially. After 6 months, however, a personal relationship had been established, the patient became more cooperative, and within 2 years repeat assessment of dietary habits and nutrition (Figures 2 and 3) showed a major improvement.

Constant guidance provided by the dietician made possible the improvements shown in the two figures. The

Table 3 Evaluation of clinical regimens

	Previous time	Present time	0	−1	−2	−3	Notes
Treatment effectiviveness			Good	Fair improvement	Poor	Terminal care	
Body weight			Appropriate	Slight gain or underweight	Obesity (BMI $\geq$ 25)	Lean weight loss	
Cardiovascular diseases (CVD)			Appropriate	Hypertension, atherosclerosis, hyperlipidemia	Abnormal ECG, angina, arrhythmia	Myocardial infarct, stroke	
Nephropathy			Normal	Micro albuminuria	Proteinuria	Renal failure, hemodialysis	
Eyesight, retinopathy			No abnormalities	Simple retinopathy	Cataract, preproliferate retinopathy	Proliferate retinopathy, glaucoma, blindness	
Eyesight, retinopathy							
Diabetic neuropathy			No abnormalities	Numbness, dyshidrosis	Neuralgia	Foot gangrene, paralysis	
Physical ability			No abnormalities	Arthropathia, difficulties while walking	Joint deformity, charcoaljoint	Physical inability	
Nutritional value, eating habits			No abnormalities	Excess of nutrition intake	Slight nutrition deficit	Nutritional deficit	

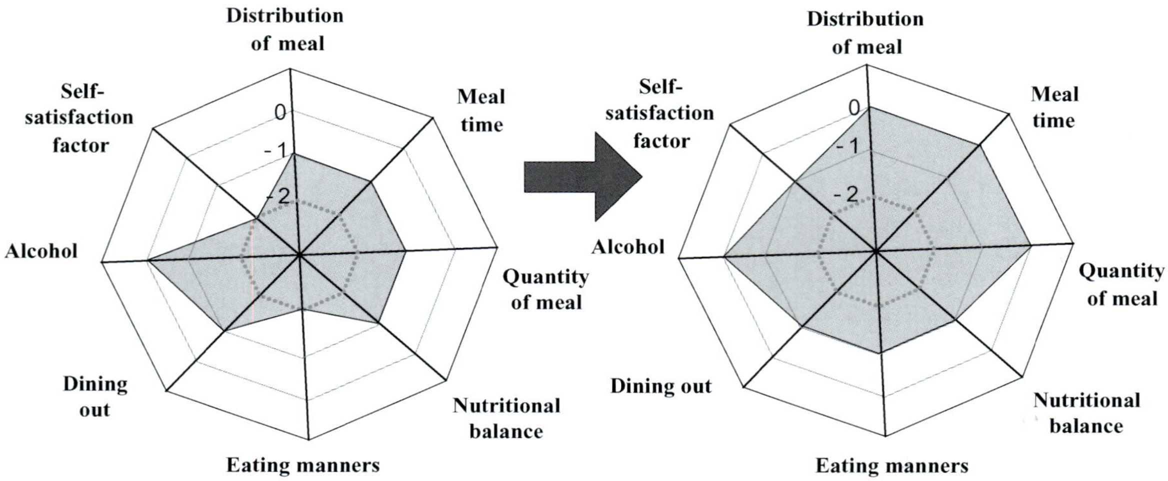

Figure 2 Evaluation of eating habits (Case 1)

advanced age and the factor of living alone did not decrease any snacking or late suppers, but in general a definite improvement in eating habits was noticed. Results generally indicated improvement, with HbA_{1c} lowered from 9.6 to 7.0%, and BMI from 27.6 to 24.8 kg/m^2, the patient cooperated well, and no complications occurred (as shown in Figure 4).

Visual representation of assessments means that patients can more easily follow the process, better understand the advice given, and are more able to cooperate. This IT for accurate evaluation and diagrammatical presentation proved to be useful and effective during the whole of the treatment process.

Case 2

A 48-year-old female patient with diabetes for 10 years, very cooperative to the physician in charge instructions and very disciplined with respect to meals (Figure 5). At

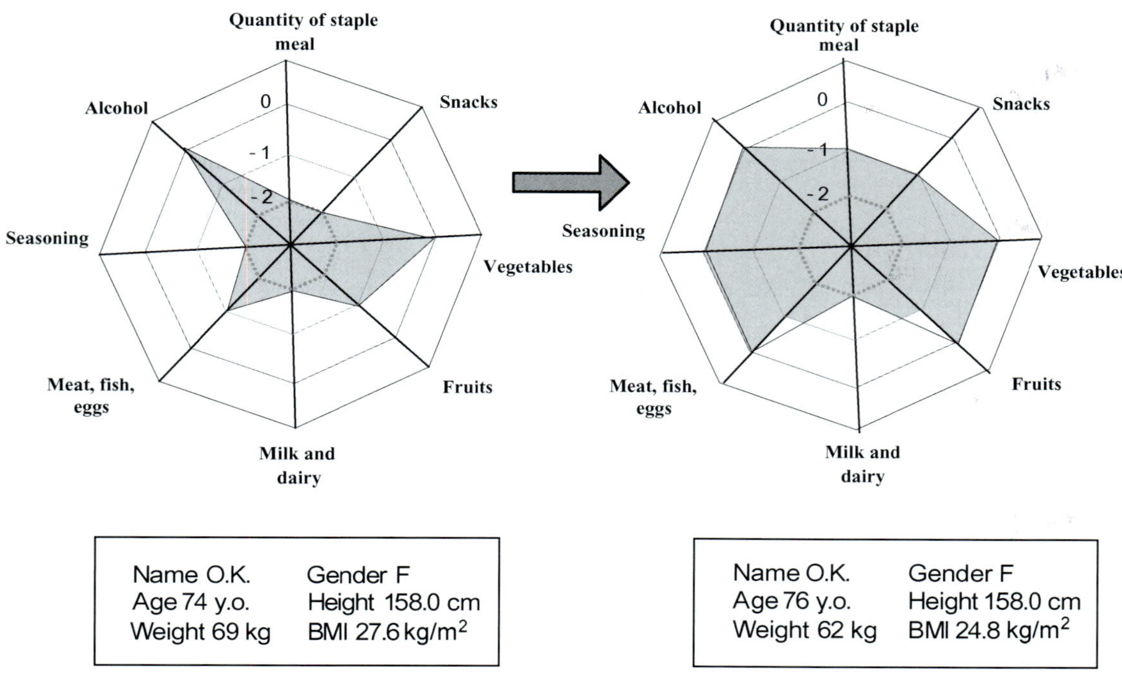

Figure 3 Evaluation of nutritional status of meal (Case 1)

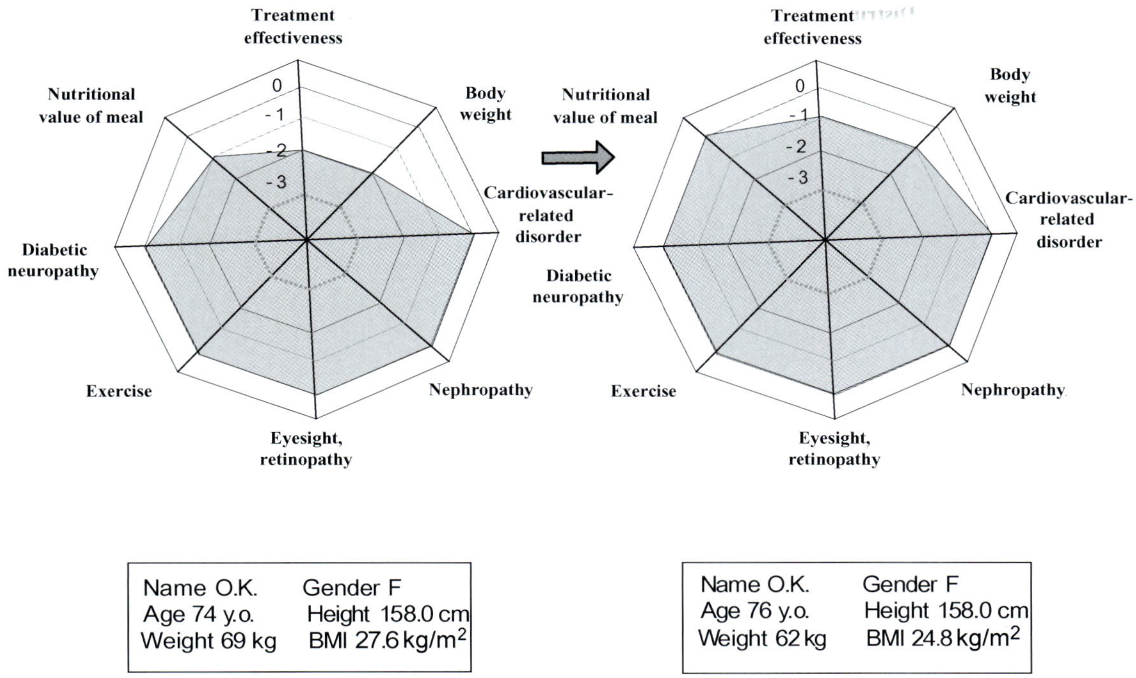

Figure 4 Diabetes Mellitus treatment evaluation (Case 1)

the assessment some diabetic retinopathy and numbness of the toes was present but no other complications. Analyzing the patient's meal showed an unbalanced food intake with, as described in Figure 5, a reduced intake of vegetables, milk, and dairy products. Following advice to increase the consumption of dietary fibre, calcium, and vitamins, continued observation of the patient has shown no further progression of complications. The patient remains on treatment with appropriate nutritional guidance.

The clinical features of the two cases described above are quite different but both show how the importance of continuous observation, the patience of dietician in developing a partnership with the patient, and the IT method in providing accurate evaluation and assessments promote improved understanding and achieve patient cooperation.

It was especially evident during the general assessment of many cases over time that helping patients to understand the importance of their diet is the key to obtaining their cooperation. We cannot foresee where the progress of IT can lead us, but it is definitely effective not only in prevention of diabetes, but can also contribute to rehabilitation and welfare in the future, providing us with some new methods for preventing the development of diabetes and its complications. Patients' education and mutual communication with physicians and health care professionals can also be predicted as IT's primary important role.

CONCLUSION

In order to adjust a patient's eating habits, lifestyle, and clinical state, nutritional guidance needs to be given repeatedly and a real attempt made to develop better relationships between patients and health care professionals.

To simplify explanation of our dietary guidance, we have separated it into evaluation of an individual's nutrition and eating habits, and evaluation of food nutritional balance by means of the Food Guide Pyramid for Japanese. Providing a visual representation of these, along with suggested changes, gives real understanding and elicits patient support.

During patient hospitalization, priority should be given to the critical treatment, and after consulting the physician in charge or dietician and diabetes counselor and getting their agreement for cooperation, dietary instructions should be issued as a part of the complete treatment package.

When the time for the patient to leave the hospital draws near, it is important to get the details of the patient's lifestyle, how active his or her life and profession are, etc., and provide him/her with the most appropriate advice based on the information collected. The best way to make the patient feel welcome is to continue to provide advice even long after they have left the hospital.

Using dietary guidance to help improve the quality of life and improve diabetic control can be an effective way to improve outcomes for people with diabetes.

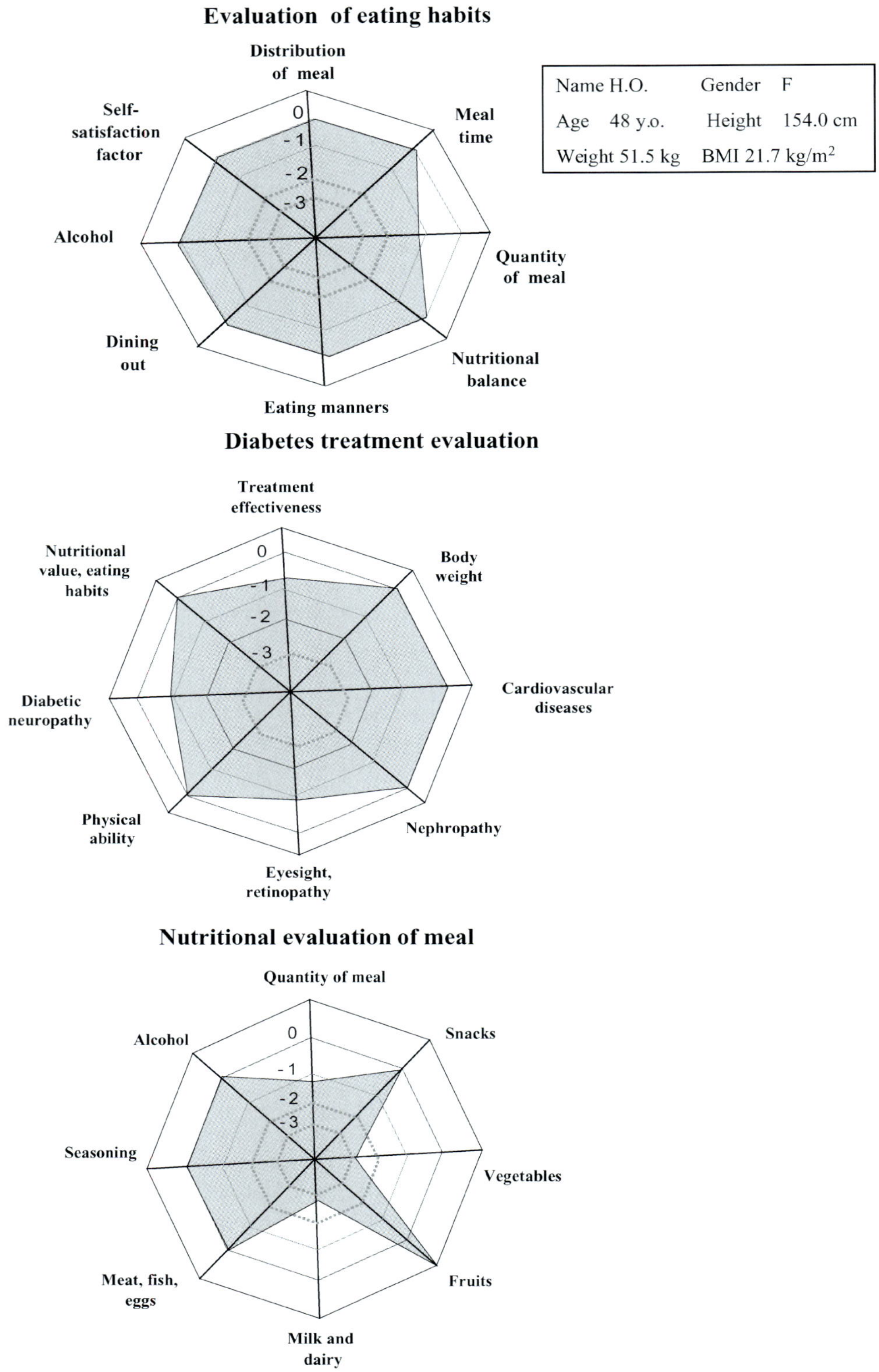

Figure 5 Evaluation of eating habits

REFERENCES

1. USDA. *The Pyramid.* Washington, DC: USDA, 2001; pp 1–29.
2. US Health News. Customizing Your Found Pyramid. Available at: http://www.kenkou.co.jp/147/food.htm, 2001.
3. Shigeaki Baba. The Philosophy of fighting the diabetes, the progress in medical research. 2001 Shindan To Chiryosha, Tokyo. Japanese Society for Diabetes Studies 35th issue, 2001, pp 1–7.
4. Shigeaki Baba. *"Belonging to Medical Science" and Creating a Healthy Culture for the 21st Century*. Osaka, Japan: Primedo Sha Co, 1997.
5. Shigeaki Baba. *WHO Preventing the Diabetes*. Tokyo: Nankodo, 1994.
6. Shigeaki Baba. *Nutrition Guide on Preventing the Diabetes Manual*, 2nd edn. Tokyo: Ishiyaku Publishers, 2001.
7. Shegeaki Baba. *Nutrition Guide on Diabetes-Related Complications Q&A*, 1st edn. Tokyo: Ishiyaku Publishers Inc, 2001.

42

Dietary Management of Diabetes Mellitus in Sub-Saharan Africa

Nelia P. Steyn* **and Naomi S. Levitt†**

South African Medical Research Council, Tygerberg, Cape Town, South Africa, and †University of Cape Town, Cape Town, South Africa

INTRODUCTION

Infectious diseases and malnutrition (undernutrition) remain major causes of morbidity and mortality in sub-Saharan Africa (SSA). However, in recent decades, noncommunicable diseases (NCDs) have increasingly become a significant player [1]. Indeed, the Global Burden of Disease Study has predicted that the prevalence of NCDs in this region will increase by 37–42% in adults aged 15–59 years by the year 2020 [2]. In the same vein, King et al. predicted that the prevalence of diabetes in adults in SSA would rise by 18%, from 1995 to 2025 (from 1.1 to 1.3%) and further, that this would translate into an increase in the number of people with diabetes from approximately 3 to 8 million [3]. Today, however, it is understood that the predicted diabetes burden was significantly underestimated. Increasing urbanization and related lifestyle changes in particular, dietary intake, lower levels of physical activity, higher stress levels, increasing nicotine and alcohol consumption, increases in weight, and subsequent obesity are believed to be responsible for the rise in prevalence of diabetes and associated NCDs [4].

SSA is not only faced with the burdens of the traditional infectious diseases, undernutrition, and emerging NCDs, it is also in the midst of the HIV-AIDS epidemic. In countries of the region that are characterized by considerably smaller gross national products and proportions of budget allocated to health than middle to high income countries, the multiple disease burdens are already placing major demands on the under-resourced health services and will continue to do so for decades to come [5]. Prevention and/or cost-effective management of diseases will become increasingly important. Diabetes mellitus is no exception and in this regard, dietary management is not only a cornerstone of therapy, it is a low-cost and relatively simple way of helping patients to manage their disease.

DIETARY INTAKE AND STAPLE FOODS IN SUB-SAHARAN AFRICA

Dietary management of diabetes in SSA cannot be considered in isolation; it has to be seen in the context of the prevailing dietary practices of people in the region. SSA is a geographically heterogeneous area, ranging from tropical forest to high mountain plains to desert. The region has experienced profound climatic changes over the past decades, with cycles of drought and irregular rainfall impacting upon the production of crops and food availability. There are differences in dietary patterns in the various subregions of SSA, as these depend largely on the crops grown locally. Yet overall the diet is a prudent one as reflected in Tables 1 and 2. These tables show the staple foods, the per capita calorie intake, and the contribution of macronutrients toward total daily energy intake of a number of countries in each of the subregions. The data in the tables have been calculated from the Food and Agricultural Organization's food balance sheets that are derived from combining all foodstuffs available for consumption in that particular country [6].

International Textbook of Diabetes Mellitus, Third Edition. Edited by R. A. DeFronzo, E. Ferrannini, H. Keen, and P. Zimmet.
 ISBN: 0-471-48655-8.

Table 1 Staple foods consumed in selected sub-Saharan countries according to FAO food balance sheets of 2000*

Country	Main staple foods†	Total kcal	Protein (g) (%E)	Fat (g) (%E)	Carbohydrate (g) (%E)
West coast					
Angola	Cassava, maize, wheat, rice, millet, sugar, beans, soy oil, palm oil, vegetables‡, fruit‡, meat‡	1902	41.3 (8.6)	38.1 (18)	349 (73.4)
Cameroon	Maize, cassava, sorghum, rice, wheat, sugar, beans, groundnuts, palm oil, vegetables‡, plantains	2254	57.2 (10.2)	50.7 (20.2)	392.2 (69.6)
Gabon	Wheat, cassava, rice, yams, maize, sugar, groundnuts, soybean oil, rape oil, palm oil, vegetables‡, plantains, barley beer, poultry, fish	2585	73.7 (11.4)	66.1 (23.0)	423.9 (65.6)
Central					
Central African Rep	Cassava, yams, maize, sorghum, wheat, pulses, sesame seed, sesame oil, groundnut oil, fruit‡, beef, & veal	1968	44.6 (9.1)	61.1 (27.9)	310.0 (63.0)
Congo	Cassava, maize, pulses, groundnuts, palm oil, fruit‡, vegetables‡	1557	24.1 (6.2)	23.6 (13.6)	312.2 (80.2)
Zambia	Maize, cassava, wheat, sugar, pulses, oilcrops‡, fruit‡, vegetables‡, meat‡	1901	47.1 (9.9)	33.1 (15.7)	353.6 (74.4)
East Coast					
Kenya	Maize, wheat, sugar, pulses, palm oil, vegetables‡, plantains, milk, beef, & veal	2037	53.2 (10.4)	48.9 (21.6)	346.3 (68)
Mozambique	Cassava, maize, wheat, rice, sorghum, sugar, oilcrops‡, pulses, fruit‡, meat‡	1939	38.0 (7.8)	26.9 (12.5)	386.3 (79.7)
Tanzania	Maize, cassava, rice, sorghum, sugar, beans, oilcrops‡, vegetable oil‡ vegetables‡, fruit‡, fermented beverages, meat‡	1958	47.6 (9.7)	30.0 (13.8)	374.5 (76.5)
South					
Botswana	Maize, wheat, sorghum, sugar, pulses, sunflower oil, vegetables‡, fruit‡, milk, meat‡	2256	71.2 (12.6)	55.1 (22.0)	368.9 (65.4)
South Africa	Maize, wheat, rice, potatoes, sugar, oilcrops‡, sunflower oil, vegetables‡, fruit‡, beef, poultry, milk	2908	76.6 (10.5)	73.0 (22.6)	486.4 (66.9)
Zimbabwe	Maize, wheat, starchy roots‡, sugar, pulses, groundnuts, soybean oil, fruit‡, vegetables‡	2104	49.9 (9.5)	54.9 (23.5)	352.4 (67)

Note. %E = percentage contributed to total daily energy intake.
* Adapted from reference 6.
† Individual food provides more than 50 kcal/day.
‡ is used when no single food in that group provides more than 50 kcal/day and this category contains a number of foods all less than 50 kcal/day.

Carbohydrates constitute 63–80% of total per capita energy intake of these countries, with maize, wheat, and sorghum being the major dietary sources together with starchy roots such as cassava and yams. Sugar is also a substantial contributor to energy intake. Potatoes are found as the only major staple food in South Africa.

Per capita protein intake varies from 6.2 to 12.6% of total energy. The bulk of protein comes from vegetable sources, particularly pulses such as peas and beans (26.3 g), and from nuts and seeds (15.3 g/day) (Table 2). Beef and veal are the most common sources of animal protein and the average intake is a mere 31 g per day. In countries along the eastern and western coastal areas, fish (22.2 g/day) is also an important source of protein unlike in the land-locked countries. Dairy products are not consumed in significant quantities in most SSA countries and with the exception of Kenya, Botswana, and South Africa, only 78.6 g (about 1/3 cup) of milk is drunk per person per day.

Not surprisingly, in view of the limited consumption of animal products, fat intake (particularly saturated fat) is low. The per capita fat intake is 12.5–27.9% of energy intake. Vegetable oils (20 g/day), the most commonly used of which are palm, groundnut, and soybean, are the major source of fat. Despite the fact that only a small amount of palm oil is used (8.5 g/day) it should be borne in mind that it is a saturated fat.

Table 2 Main food products consumed in sub-Saharan Africa in 2000*

Products	(Kg/year)	Grams/day	Kcals/day
Wheat	18.2	49.9	144
Rice	19.4	53.2	190
Barley	1.4	3.8	11
Maize	37.5	102.7	327
Millet	17.1	46.8	135
Sorghum	23.5	64.4	193
Cassava	104.9	287.4	277
Potatoes	7.5	20.5	15
Sweet potatoes	13.9	38.1	37
Yams	27.6	75.6	76
Other roots	11.5	31.5	36
Sugar	9.5	26.0	93
Pulses	9.6	26.3	89
Oilcrops	5.6	15.3	66
Vegetable oils	7.3	20	175
Vegetables	31.8	87.1	24
Fruit	50.0	136.9	88
Alcoholic beverages	34.7	95.1	42
Meat	11.3	31.0	55
Offal	1.3	3.6	4
Animal fats	0.6	1.6	12
Milk (excluding butter)	28.7	78.6	52
Eggs	1.4	3.8	5
Fish	8.1	22.2	16

*Adapted from reference 6.

Fruit and vegetable intake amounts to 136.9 and 87.1 g/day, respectively. The most commonly eaten fruits are plantains (tropical fruit similar to bananas) (61.9 g/day) and bananas (17.0 g/day). The most commonly eaten vegetables are starchy ones, such as cassava (287.4 g/day) and sweet potatoes (38.1 g/day). Tomatoes (13.2 g/day) and onions (7.4 g/day) too are frequent items in the diet. Furthermore it is known that people in rural areas make extensive use of naturally growing fruits and vegetables [7], which are not reflected on food balance sheets.

With urbanization there is a major shift in the composition of dietary staples as well as in the intake of fat and sugar [8]. This was clearly shown by Bourne [9] who found that consumption of dairy products and cereals by African adults declined markedly with increased duration of residence in Cape Town, while the intake of nonstaple (luxury) food items increased the most.

In urban areas of Tanzania it has been reported that traditional staple foods such as millet have been replaced in the diet by imported foods such as rice [10]. Further, a trend since the 1960s has been that a large percentage of foods consumed are processed and packaged, instead of being homegrown. Many of these items are high in fats and sugars. Popular snacks include donuts, cakes, and sugary drinks [10]. A recent study from Tanzania showed significant dietary urban–rural differences. Urban subjects from all age groups had higher intakes of cholesterol and sucrose and lower intakes of fiber than did their rural counterparts. Rural subjects, on the other hand, had a lower consumption of animal foods such as milk and meat [11].

Two further examples of urban–rural differences are provided. First, women undergraduate students from urban areas, attending a South African university consumed significantly more sugar (65.8 vs. 52.2 g) and confectionary (290.4 vs. 183.7 g) and significantly less legumes (6.3 vs. 18.9 g) than did undergraduate women from rural areas [12]. Second, in Cameroon, rural children whose level of physical activity was more than double that of urban children consumed a diet containing less fat and more fruits and vegetables than did urban children [13].

In addition to urban–rural differences, large dietary disparities between socioeconomic groups have been found in urban areas. This was shown in a study of high versus low-income participants in Dar es Salaam [14]. The low- and moderate-income groups consumed a diet comprising a fat intake of 15%, protein intake of 15%, and carbohydrate intake of 70% of total energy intake. By contrast, the smaller, elite group from a high-income category consumed a fat intake of 43%, protein intake of 17%, and carbohydrate intake of 40%.

The importance of knowing and understanding the dietary practices in SSA cannot be sufficiently emphasized, since these should form the foundation of the diet for people with diabetes in the region.

DIETARY RECOMMENDATIONS FOR PEOPLE WITH DIABETES MELLITUS

Individual Versus Ideal Regime

Internationally, dietary management of diabetes has undergone a paradigm shift over the past decade [15, 16]. Prior to 1994, nutrition recommendations were generally based on an *ideal* regimen, which would apply to everyone with diabetes. Since 1994 the American Diabetes Association's (ADA's) nutrition recommendations (Table 3) have focused on addressing individual nutritional needs within the context of the individual's personal and cultural preferences, willingness to change, and values, rather than a set prescription based only on ideal percentages of carbohydrate, protein, and fat relative to energy intake [18, 21]. Self-management as the cornerstone of therapy has also been stressed [22].

In view of the proven efficacy of dietitians in improving glycemic control and dyslipidemia in people with diabetes, the ADA have recommended that a registered dietitian should provide dietary therapy. Nevertheless, all health professionals involved in the care of diabetic patients should be knowledgeable about their dietary management.

Macronutrient Composition of the Diet

The dietary recommendations issued by the European Association for the Study of Diabetes (EASD) in 1995 [19]

Table 3 Dietary guidelines aimed at optimal dietary management of diabetes mellitus

	Guidelines		
	South Africa*	United States†	Europe 1995/98‡
Energy	To achieve or maintain a desirable/reasonable body weight	To bring about desired weight loss; older adults require less energy than younger ones	To achieve or maintain a desirable/ reasonable body weight
CHO	CHO 50–65% EI	CHO and MUF 60–70% EI. Total CHO more important than the source; type 1 patients to balance CHO intake according to insulin doses	Percentage not given; Fruits, vegetables, legumes, and cereals are the preferred sources of carbohydrate; type 1 patients to balance CHO according to insulin doses
Sucrose	Limited amounts (not specified)	Not restricted but should be substituted for other CHO	<10% EI. Preferably with meals
Fiber	6–8 g NSP/1000 kJ	Same as for all Americans	Not specified
Fat	Total fat <30% EI	Not given	Not specified
Type of fat	SFA<10%, PUS <10%	Saturated fat <10% and trans fat <7% EI; cholesterol <300 mg; <200 mg if LDL-C ≥100 mg/dl	SFA <10%, PUS <10% EI; cholesterol <300 mg/day
Protein	10–20% EI	15–20% EI; if microalbuminaria protein <0.8g/kg/day	10–20% EI; if microalbuminaria 0.7–0.9 g/kg/day
Micronutrients	No specific supplements recommended	According to the Dietary Reference Intakes	Encourage the use of dietary antioxidants (tocopherols, carotenoids, vitamin C, and possibly flavonoids)
Alcohol	Limited, not to exceed 6–10% EI	1 drink for women 2 drinks for men (maximum per day)	1–2 drinks/day maximum.; those on insulin or sulfonylureas to consume alcohol with CHO-containing foods
Sweeteners	A variety in moderate amounts allowed	Safe when staying within ADI levels	Not specified
Sodium	None given	Reduce to <6 g/day	Reduce to <6 g/day
Weight loss	No specific recommendations	Reduced energy intake in insulin-resistant patients; structured lifestyle programs; exercise and behavior modification strategies recommended	Decreased calories for those overweight; with exercise; first try reduction in fat intake. If this fails to achieve weight loss reduce energy intake by 500 kcal/day
Meal frequency	Minimum of 3 meals/day; snacks according to medication	Not specified	Not given

Note. CHO = carbohydrate; MUF = monounsaturated fat; LDL-C = low-density lipoprotein cholesterol; ADI = average daily intake; EI = energy intake; NSP = nonstarch polysaccharides; SFA = saturated fatty acids; PUS = polyunsaturated fatty acids.
*Reference 17.
†Reference 18.
‡Reference 19 and 20.

(Table 3) are similar to those of the ADA. They also emphasized that people with diabetes should eat foods similar to those consumed by the rest of the family and the general population, in addition to recommending that dietitians (if available) should provide the dietary advice, or failing this doctors. Furthermore, the 1995 recommendations emphasized the importance of a nutritional program being adapted to the specific needs of the individual.

More recently, the European Diabetes Policy Group (EDPG) published dietary guidelines for Europe. These placed great emphasis on self-management and provided an education framework within which health professionals should counsel patients [23]. This framework included basic information on healthy eating, physical activity, and smoking cessation, but little mention was made of caloric intake and the role of diet in weight management. Advice on meal planning and sodium intake was not provided.

There is not only a paucity of published data on dietary management of diabetes in SSA, but also a scarcity of published guidelines in the region. The sole published guidelines, in 1997 (Table 3), composed of a position paper on the dietary management of type 2 diabetes in South Africa [17]. In this the Association for Dietetics in South Africa (ADSA) recommended a diet that maintains a reasonable body weight, has a carbohydrate intake of 50–65% of total energy, fat intake of less than 30%, saturated fat intake less than 10% of energy, and protein intake of 10–20% of energy intake. Further, it recommended that fiber intake should comprise 6–8 g nonstarch polysaccharides (fiber) per 1000 kJ (240 cal) and that foods high in soluble fiber (legumes, lentils, oats) and insoluble fiber (vegetables and most grains) be eaten. A minimum of 3 meals/day with snacks according to the timing of medication was recommended. These guidelines also included specific recommendations for pregnancy and lactation.

In many respects the guidelines for South Africa are similar to those for Europe and the United States. One important exception is that the guidelines for South Africa recommend a lower range of carbohydrate intake than do the ADA guidelines. This may present a problem when planning a diet for diabetic patients in an African context, where a number of countries have an average carbohydrate intake between 70 and 80% of total energy intake (Table 1).

In South Africa, the National Department of Health has developed a program for management and control of diabetes mellitus at all levels of care [24]. This program has largely consisted of the development of national management guidelines that include recommendations relating to dietary management. For example, Step 1 of the program recommended that lifestyle modification be undertaken.

> This includes weight control/weight loss for overweight and obese patients, an exercise program and a healthy diet with 3 meals a day (5 for those on insulin), reduced fat intake, increased fiber intake, and restricted salt intake. Alcohol is limited to 2 drinks or less per day. [24].

Three studies conducted in different parts of South Africa found that development and dissemination of the guidelines did not improve care or outcomes [25–27]. Although none of the studies were designed to specifically evaluate the implementation of the dietary recommendations, it is unlikely that this aspect would any more be successfully implemented than would the remainder of the guidelines.

Meal Plans for People with Diabetes

It is well recognized that nutrition therapy will be unsuccessful if the diet prescription does not take the patients' culture, economic status, and literacy level into consideration [28]. Thus the challenge of developing a dietary regimen for a patient in SSA, that stands a reasonable chance of being followed, is to ensure that the meal plan includes available and affordable foods. Since many patients in the region may not have access to optimal pharmacotherapy for glycemic control, dietary self-management has particular relevance and importance.

Two examples of meal plans for people with diabetes managed by diet alone, or by diet and oral medication, appear in Tables 4 and 5. These meal plans have a protein and fat intake between 16 and 21% of energy intake each, and a carbohydrate and monounsaturated fat intake of 65–72% of energy intake; thus they comply with the current dietary practices in the region as well as with the most recent ADA nutritional recommendations [16, 18] (Table 6). The ADA guidelines are relevant to SSA as the high-carbohydrate (with monounsaturated fat) recommendation is a feature of the traditional African diet. The one exception to the typical African diet in the meal plans is the inclusion of two servings of milk. This represents a

Table 4 An example of a meal plan of about 2200 kcal for a diabetic adult in SSA, using exchange lists

Meal and time	Foods selected and amount
Breakfast (0700 h)	
Starch: 3	Soft maize porridge (3 × 1/2 cup)
Milk: 1	Whole milk (1 cup)
Fruit: 1	Papaya (1/2 fruit)
Snack (1000 h)	
Starch: 2	Brown bread (2 slices)
Fat: 2	Avocado (1/4)
Lunch (1300 h)	
Starch: 3	Stiff maize (3 × 1/2 cup)
Meat/substitute: 1	Split pea stew (1/2 cup)
Vegetable (starchy): 1	Plantains (1/2 cup)
Vegetable: 1	Tomato and onion gravy (1/2 cup)
Snack (1500 h)	
Starch: 2	Cold maize porridge (1 cup)
Fat: 1	Pumpkin seeds (1 T)
Dinner (1800 h)	
Starch: 4	Sorghum (4×1/2 cup)
Vegetable (starchy): 1	Sweet potatoes (1/2 cup)
Vegetable: 1	Green leafy vegetables (1/2 cup)
Meat: 1	Lentils (1/2 cup)
Snack (1900 h)	
Starch: 2	Brown bread (2 slices)
Milk: 1	Sour milk (1 cup)
Fruit: 1	Mango (1/2)

Note. Carbohydrate = 364 g; fat = 51 g; protein = 94 g.

Table 5 An example of a meal plan of about 1800 kcal for a diabetic adult in SSA, using exchange lists

Meal and time	Foods selected and amount
Breakfast (0700 h)	
Starch: 2	Soft sorghum porridge (2 × 1/2 cup)
Milk: 1	Milk (1 cup)
Fruit: 1	Banana (1 small)
Snack (1000 h)	
Starch: 1	Maize bread (1 slice)
Fat: 2	Peanuts (10)
Lunch (1300 h)	
Starch: 2	Samp (2 × 1/2 cup)
Meat/substitute: 1	Chicken stew (60 g white flesh)
Vegetable (starchy): 1	Sweet potato (1 small)
Vegetable: 1	Spinach (1/2 cup)
Snack (1500 h)	
Starch: 1	Boiled mealie (corn on cob) (1)
Fat: 2	Avocado (1/4)
Dinner (1800 h)	
Starch: 3	Maize porridge (3 × 1/2 cup)
Vegetable (starchy): 1	Cassava (1/3 cup)
Vegetable: 1	Boiled cabbage (1/2 cup)
Meat: 1	Dry bean stew (1/2 cup)
Snack (1900 h)	
Starch: 1	Cold maize porridge (1/2 cup)
Milk: 1	Sour milk (1 cup)
Fruit: 1	Wild plum (2 small)

Note. Carbohydrate = 259 g; fat = 52 g; protein = 73 g.

Table 6 A summary of the main nutrition recommendations for diabetes mellitus based on the evidence currently available, namely type A and type E evidence*

Carbohydrates (CHO)

- *Foods containing CHO from whole grains, fruits, vegetables, and milk should be included in the diet (A).* In SSA unsifted maize meal, sorghum, millet, cassava, yams are CHO sources. Milk may be expensive/not available in many areas. Use goats milk, soymilk, or powdered cow's milk, if available
- *The total amount of CHO in the meal is more important than the type of CHO food (A).*
- *Sugar*[†] *may be added* as table sugar to foods. If used it should be substituted for another CHO or covered by insulin or other glucose-lowering medication (A)
- *Non-nutritive sweeteners (saccharine, aspartame, acesulfame potassium, and sucralose) are allowed within acceptable daily intakes (A)*
- *CHO and monounsaturated fats (MUF) should together provide 65–70% of energy intake (E).* In SSA the usual diet of the population is at this level. MUF can be provided by soybean, canola, safflower, and peanut oils; also from peanuts, avocado, and cashews.
- *Sucrose may be eaten in the context of a healthy diet* (E)—small amounts added to foods to improve the taste. NOT soft drinks, candy, and confectionary

Protein

- *Intake of protein still recommended as 15–20% of total energy intake (E).* In SSA this can be done using pulses and nuts as protein sources
- Long-term effects of high protein diets unknown, therefore discouraged (E)

Fat

- *Less than 10% energy should be from saturated fats (SF). If LDL cholesterol is >100 mg/dl then SF should be <7% (A).*
- *Dietary cholesterol should be less than 300 mg/day. If LDL cholesterol is <100 mg/dl then lower cholesterol to <200 mg/day.* Cholesterol sources are eggs, meats, and dairy products (A). In most of SSA animal food intake is still fairly low

Energy balance and obesity

- *In insulin-resistant individuals, reduced energy intake and modest weight loss can improve insulin resistance and glycemia in the short-term (A)*
- *Reduced energy intake and modest weight loss improves insulin resistance and glycemia in the short-term (A)*
- *Structured programs that emphasize lifestyle changes (education, reduced fat intake (<30%), regular physical activity, and regular participant contact) can produce long-term weight loss (A)*
- *Exercise and behavior modification are most useful as adjuncts to other weight loss strategies (A)*

Alcohol

- *If persons choose to drink only one drink for women allowed and two for men and it should be drunk WITH food (B)*

Note. Text given in italic is taken from reference 16. Type A evidence is based on evidence from multiple supportive studies. Type E evidence is based on expert consensus. CHO = carbohydrate; SSA = sub-Saharan Africa.

*Adapted from reference 16.

†Here, sugar indicates sucrose.

substantial increase in milk intake in most of SSA, which is less than 100 ml compared to a recommended intake of 500 ml [29]. As milk may be unavailable and unaffordable for many, it is unclear how feasible the two servings are. In many areas, small fish may be included as a good alternative source of calcium while other options for improving calcium intake should be discussed. It is not essential for people with diabetes managed by diet alone or in combination with oral hypoglycemic agents to have snacks. However, it is simpler to spread the large amount of dietary carbohydrates across three meals and snacks during the day. Furthermore, patients with type 2 diabetes often manage their diets better when they have smaller meals and snacks [30].

Simple practical guidelines about *meal planning* are required to educate people with diabetes about dietary management. This is particularly pertinent in SSA where there are a limited number of dietitians, and other health professionals will be the main providers of dietary advice. Consequently, guidelines need to be simple to understand and implement. In the absence of such guidelines in SSA, it may be reasonable to follow the examples of meal planning approaches suggested by the ADA [30]. One approach provided in a low-literacy booklet developed by the International Diabetes Center in Minneapolis is based on the "plate method" of selecting foods. Another meal planning option is included in a pamphlet developed by the ADA and the American Dietetic Association. This provides guidelines for making healthy food choices and uses simplified exchange lists [30].

A further option is the use of "carbohydrate counting" that focuses on the total amount of carbohydrate eaten at meals and snacks. At Level 1, people with diabetes are taught about foods containing carbohydrate, the concept of choices, and how to use food lists to count carbohydrate. The target range for grams of carbohydrate at meals and snacks can be negotiated with the individual taking cognizance of his/her usual diet and culture [30].

Table 7 Foods allowed and foods to be avoided for the diabetic person living in Sub-Saharan Africa

Best choices for daily use	Reasonable choices for less frequent use	Foods to avoid	Reasons for avoidance
Starches			
Unrefined maize meal	Refined maize meal	White bread	Low in fiber
Unrefined sorghum	Refined sorghum	Cake flour	Low in fiber
Millet		White rice	Low in fiber
Brown bread and wheat flour			
Instant high fiber cereals			
Oats			
Brown rice			
Milk			
Low-fat sour milk	Full cream cow milk		
Low-fat/skim milk	Goat milk		
Low-fat yoghurt	Sour milk from whole milk		
	Soy milk		
Fruits			
Fresh fruit including wild fruit	Fruit canned in juice	Fruit canned in syrup	High in sugar
Dried fruit			
Fruit juice (pure)		Sweetened fruit juice	High in sugar
Vegetables			
Fresh and frozen vegetables	Tinned vegetables		
Starchy vegetables (e.g. cassava, yams)			
Indigenous vegetables			
Meat and substitutes			
Pulses-beans, lentils	Eggs (3 a week)	High fat meats (i.e. bacon, sausage)	High in saturated fats
Chicken, white meat without skin	Lean beef/game with fat trimmed	Fried meat and fish	High in fat
Fresh or frozen fish (cod/trout/haddock)	Lean pork with fat trimmed	Mutton and Lamb	High in fat
Cottage cheese	Chicken, dark meat without skin	Regular cheeses	High in fat
	Insects		
Fats			
MUF in restricted amounts: canola oil peanut oil, peanuts, avocado			
PUF in restricted amounts: corn, safflower, soybean oils, pumpkin and sunflower seeds, soft margarine		Bacon, butter, coconut, cream, lard, hard margarine, palm oil	High in saturated fats
Tea and coffee		Soft drinks, cordials, squashes, candy, cakes, pastries, pizza,	High in sugar and/or fat

Note. MUF = monounsaturated fat; PUF = polyunsaturated fat.

Some practical choices of foods allowed and those to be avoided for people with diabetes in SSA are given in Table 7. For people with type 1 diabetes there are a number of additional recommendations. These include that those using intensive insulin therapy understand that premeal insulin dosages should be adjusted for the carbohydrate content of the meal [16]. The majority will however require an evening snack to prevent overnight hypoglycemia, while those using morning intermediate-acting insulins require an afternoon snack. In contrast, those using rapidly acting insulin do not require snacks [30].

Dietary Management of Obesity

Numerous studies in SSA have shown that the majority of people with diabetes in urban areas, particularly women, are overweight or obese [31–36] (Table 8).

Weight loss in diabetic patients results in improved glycemic control, improved insulin sensitivity, decreased serum lipids, and lowering of blood pressure [37–41]. Consequently, one of the cornerstones of dietary management should be maintaining weight and/or weight loss in overweight patients optimally in conjunction with a physical activity program.

The ADA recommend that overweight patients should be treated by means of an intensive lifestyle program, encompassing a weight-reducing diet, increased physical activity, and behavior modification, with regular follow-up sessions [18]. This level of intervention is difficult to achieve and maintain in the context of a research study, let alone in busy routine clinical practice in well-resourced

Table 8 Weight status of diabetic adults screened in selected sub-Saharan countries*

Country	Setting	Age range (years)	Median age (years)	BMI ≥ 25 kg/m²		BMI ≥ 30 kg/m²	
				Male	Female	Male	Female
Cameroon							
Evodoula [32]	rural	24–74	46	11	16	2	3
Yaounde [32]	urban	24–74	37	46	61	10	25
South Africa [33]							
Cape Town	urban	>30	42	23	23.8	8.3	50.7
Mamre [34]	peri-urban	>15	35	24.8	24.4	9.3	31.6
Manguang [35]	urban	>25	46	18.7	43.4	13.2	27.3
Qwaqwa [35]	peri-urban	>25	48	18.8	28.4	12.0	37.5
Durban [36]	urban	>15	30	39.7	77.6	15.1	45.0
Tanzania							
Kilimanjaro [37]	rural	>15	35	3.2	8.0	0.1	1.5
Mara [37]	rural	>15		3.1	7.1	0.9	19.5
Morogo [37]	rural	>15	32	2.3	7.4	0.1	1.1
Dar-es-Salaam [37]	urban	>15	30	13.5	20.7	2.0	10.6

* Adapted from reference 31.

health systems. Such a program is not feasible for the majority of people with diabetes in SSA as there are insufficient resources—both expertise and manpower—to undertake such interventions. In addition the immediate urgency of life-threatening conditions in family members, the care of small children orphaned by the effects of HIV-AIDS, and food insecurity overshadow the long-term benefits of lifestyle modification for one of the remaining older members of the family.

As a realistic alternative, health professionals should encourage weight loss and increased physical activity on the basis of time and expertise available at the health care settings attended by diabetic patients. Weight loss should be encouraged by advocating a reduction in calories preferably from fat or carbohydrate or both, depending on the meal plan currently followed. Fat intake should be less than 30% of energy intake [18]. Ideally, weight loss should be achieved by means of a diet that provides 500–1000 cal less per day above what is required for normal maintenance. It should be recognized however that all of the weight lost may be regained by the end of 5 years and that weight-reducing diets alone are unlikely to produce long-term weight loss [18]. Although weight loss drugs appear to have modest beneficial outcomes in overweight people with diabetes [18], this once again is not a feasible option for the majority of the population in the region, due to cost constraints and unavailability.

Dietary Management of Dyslipidemia

The primary objective with regard to dietary fat intake in people with diabetes is to reduce the intake of saturated fat and dietary cholesterol (Table 6). People in SSA actually have an average fat intake less than 30% of energy intake (Table 1). In addition they have a low intake of animal fats, which are the primary sources of saturated fats and cholesterol. Perhaps this may be one of the reasons why coronary heart disease is still relatively uncommon in the region. However, with increasing urbanization and accompanying changes in lifestyle, this is likely to change. In this context it is important to reinforce a restricted fat intake, particularly saturated fats. Examples of these are given in the meal plans (Tables 4 and 5).

Dietary Management of Hypertension

In addition to keeping the diet low in energy and fat it is recommended that patients who have hypertension should reduce their salt intake. In this regard, health workers need to classify local foods according to the amount of sodium they contain. For example, in South Africa, many hypertensive patients have been found to decrease table salt intake, yet unknowingly use a large amount of flavor enhancers that contain monosodium glutamate. Because of the beneficial effect of potassium on blood pressure it is recommended that five to nine servings per day of fruit and vegetables be encouraged within the framework of planned meals and snacks [16]. In the SSA context some fruit and vegetables are generally available to most consumers [6].

Use of the Glycemic Index in Dietary Management

The use of the glycemic index (GI) in managing patients with diabetes is still controversial; it has not been universally accepted, nor included in the evidence-based ADA recommendations. On the basis of the strongest (A level) evidence, the ADA has indicated that the *total* carbohydrate in the meal is more important than the type of carbohydrate foods consumed (Table 6).

Despite this, there are many dietary practitioners who do use the GI index and principles, possibly based on the premise that low GI foods are generally healthy food

Table 9 Glycemic index of foods commonly consumed in sub-Saharan Africa

Reference	Food	Mean glycemic index using glucose as reference	Mean glycemic index, using white bread as reference
Indar-Brown et al. [42]	Rice	72	
	Lentils	29	
	Chick peas	36	
	Pumpkin	50	
Mbhenyane et al. [43]	Sorghum porridge, no sugar		123
	Sorghum porridge+ sugar		106
	Stiff mealiemeal + nkaka		105
	Fermented sorghum porridge		113
	Stiff maize porridge and dry green bean leaf stew		87
	Samp		130
	Samp and beans		98
	Dry bean stew		68
	Soft maize porridge		117
	Soft maize + sugar		123
Walker and Walker [44]	White bread	71	
	Brown bread	75	
	Unrefined maize porridge	71	
	Butter beans	32	
	Brown beans	27	
	Dhal	6	
	Sweetcorn	62	
	Potatoes mashed	71	
	Pumpkin	75	
	Marogo (green leafy vegetables)	68	
	Banana	70	
	Orange	33	
	Sugar	65	
Ayuo and Ettyang [45]	Brown bread		123.5
	White rice		159.9
	English potatoes		34.3
	Maize meal		156.0
	Millet		153.1
	Cassava		65.4

options as well as generally being traditional staple foods. As seen in Table 9, foods analyzed in SSA that have the lowest GI values are legumes such as dry beans and peas. These range from 6 (dhal) to 68 (dry bean stew), when using glucose as a reference food. By contrast, foods with a high GI value are staple starchy foods such as maize (156), millet (153), and rice (159) [45]. Potatoes and vegetables generally have an intermediate value (34–71). When legumes and/or green leafy vegetables are added to porridge this decreases the GI value of the meal [43]. Combinations of staple foods that make up traditional mixed meals have been shown to have low GI values of 34–52 [46].

Interestingly, temperature and gender appear to affect the GI of foods. For example, cold maize porridge (50) has a lower GI value than does either hot (66) or reheated maize porridge (56) [47]. The GI of a typical traditional African meal comprising maize, green vegetables, and legumes was found to be significantly lower in women (71) than in men (131), implying that there may be gender differences in the GI of certain foods [48].

DIETARY INTAKE AND PRACTICES OF PEOPLE WITH DIABETES IN SSA

There is little reported data on the dietary practices of people with diabetes in SSA and they are predominantly limited to type 2 patients. It appears that few are treated by diet alone. In Addis Ababa, 5% of patients were reportedly treated by diet alone, in Tanzania 8%, and in South Africa less than 7% [28, 49, 50].

Descriptive Studies

One of the most recent and comprehensive dietary studies undertaken in SSA assessed the dietary intake of 288 adults with diabetes in the Limpopo (Northern) Province of South Africa [28]. This is a rural area of South

Africa where a large proportion of the population is illiterate and there are accompanying high rates of unemployment and poverty. Interestingly, the energy distribution of the macronutrients described in this study was in keeping with the recommendations for a prudent diet as well as with those of the ADSA [17]. Fat, saturated fat, and protein intakes were respectively less than 30, 10, and 20% of energy intake, but nonstarch polysaccharide intake was lower (19–21 g) than expected in a rural area. More than 90% of the subjects ate three meals a day, 32–47% had a midmorning snack, and 19–27% had a late evening snack. Brown bread, chicken, maize porridge, tea, sorghum porridge, beef, apples, milk, cabbage, spinach, and oranges were the most commonly consumed food items, in descending order. These items comprise the staple foods of adults without diabetes in the same area [51].

An earlier study evaluated the dietary intake of 63 obese people with diabetes in Ga-Rankuwa, an urban area near Pretoria, South Africa [52]. Findings were that participants followed a three meals/day meal pattern. Fat intake (35%) exceeded the recommended intake of less than 30% of energy. Carbohydrate intake was lower (48%) than that recommended (50–55% of energy intake). The most commonly consumed foods in descending order were maize porridge, full cream milk, bread, apples, oranges, beef, carbonated "diet" cold drinks, tomato and onion relish, cabbage, and chicken. The dietary intakes of people in this urban sample were similar to those found by Nthangeni et al. [28] in the rural Limpopo province. The main difference noted between the two studies was the higher fat and lower carbohydrate intake in the urban area, which is typical of urban dwellers.

Recently the dietary patterns of 59 overweight (BMI > 25 kg/m^2) people with diabetes from northern Tanzania were described [53]. Two thirds of the patients consumed 4–6 meals/day, but 68% had less than 5 meals/day. Plantains, highly extracted maize meal, white bread, and polished rice were the sources of carbohydrates. The major vegetables eaten were cabbage, spinach, carrots, and amaranth leaves. The main pulses eaten were kidney beans, cow peas, soy beans, and groundnuts, and the most commonly reported fruits were bananas, orange, and papaya. Unusually for this subregion, the primary protein source was beef, followed by milk, fish, and eggs. Another surprising finding was that although fat intake in Tanzania is reported to be low at 12.5% of energy intake, the vast majority of the patients used oils or fat, predominantly sunflower oil, in preparation of food.

Experimental Studies

The effect of a traditional African diet compared to a typical "western" diet on glycemic control of overweight and obese (BMI = 27–35 kg/m^2) people with diabetes attending Ga-Rankuwa Hospital near Pretoria was evaluated [54]. A control group (n = 22) followed an adapted "western diet" and a test group (n = 43) followed a typical African diet comprising staple foods such as maize porridge, soya mince, and green leafy vegetables ("marogo"). The test diet was low in fat (24%) and high in plant protein and complex carbohydrate. There was a small but significant loss of weight in both men (1.6 kg) and women (1.1 kg) in the test group, compared to a small increase in weight in the control group. After 5 months, despite the weight loss, there was no significant improvement in glycemic control in the test group.

A study from Nigeria examined glycemic control of 160 newly diagnosed, non-obese people with type 2 diabetes on a traditional high carbohydrate diet combined with oral hypoglycemic agents over a period of 3 years [55]. The diet consisted of 250–300 g of carbohydrate and was low in fat and protein. As such the diet was similar to the traditional diet of Nigerians. At 3 years, 83% of patients achieved satisfactory glycemic control. This study illustrates that satisfactory glycemic control can be achieved when using a traditional diet in combination with oral agents.

BARRIERS TO DIETARY MANAGEMENT

Numerous factors within the health care system hamper optimal dietary management of diabetes in SSA. First, there is a paucity of trained nutrition experts, such as dietitians, who are able to give appropriate dietary advice, or failing this, to educate health workers who in turn would undertake patient education. This is illustrated by the finding that less than 16% of people with diabetes in a rural area of South Africa had received advice from a dietitian [28]. Apart from South Africa and Kenya, no countries in the region have a training program for dietitians. As a result many have been trained in the United States and Europe. Indeed, even in South Africa there are only 1450 registered dietitians to serve a population of 40 million people [56]. Furthermore, less than 30% of the dietitians work in the public sector [57] that provides health care to 80% of the population. If nutrition education is to take place at primary care level, which category of health workers' responsibility this will be, needs to be clearly defined and special training be implemented.

In South Africa, and we suspect elsewhere in the region, nurses are the primary source of dietary education for people with diabetes. As evidenced by the findings of a study [28] that evaluated patients' knowledge, perceptions, and feelings about the dietary advice they had received from nurses and doctors at primary care clinics in Limpopo Province, South Africa, this constitutes a problem. Patients in the study were generally unhappy or confused about the dietary advice they had received. They complained that the diet was too expensive, not tasty, poorly understood, and culturally inappropriate. In many instances it was also found that the dietary information reportedly given was also incorrect. For example, patients were told not to eat certain local foods such as pumpkin and red apples, which were important sources of nutrients in their diet.

Second, dietary management guidelines frequently originate in the United States or Europe. As a result they are constructed around typical Western foods and meal patterns. Adapting these guidelines to include local dietary practices requires additional research and expertise, both of which have cost implications.

Third, many health professionals do not understand or are unaware of the health belief system of their patients. In this regard Tripp-Reimer et al. [58] state,

> Common beliefs across ethnic groups are that health is a state of equilibrium, and illness is caused by excesses or deficiencies. Diabetes is often believed to be caused by eating excess sweets (particularly sugar), brought on by stress and worry, or as a form of punishment for immoral behavior.

The Pedi people [28] believed that diabetes could be cured, which led them to seek alternative curative medicines. Chicken bladders, aloes, boiled litchi leaves, herbal medicines, balsam kofifi, mopani worms, nngu, church tea, salt water, prayer water, and dancing rituals are examples of alternative cures. Traditional and faith healers play a large role in the management of diabetes in Africa, including as providers of dietary advice [59, 60]. A recent study found that 28.7% of people with diabetes relied exclusively on traditional medicine, 49.7% used conventional, medicine, and 21.5% used a combination of the two [61]. Interestingly, interviews with traditional healers have revealed that diet is one of the major causative factors of diabetes, specifically too much sugar, salt, alcohol or, perhaps unexpectantly, chillies. Clearly, it is essential to tailor dietary information to health beliefs.

A major challenge for the region is to overcome the barriers to providing optimal dietary therapy to people with diabetes. There are a number of possible solutions. The most logical of these may be to increase the number of trained dietitians, but this is unfeasible because of the lack of training facilities other than in South Africa. Another option may be to use nutritionists who could be trained to deal with specific dietary aspects of common conditions found in primary health care.

A third most feasible and sustainable solution is to provide specific dietary therapy training of nurses and community health workers, by dietitians. The training must include an awareness of local health beliefs.

CONCLUSION

In conclusion, dietary management clearly has a major role in the therapeutic armamentarium of health workers caring for people with diabetes in SSA, similar to the rest of the world. The major challenges lie in providing the health workers with the necessary knowledge, skill, and time to educate and motivate the patients and their families to undertake the adjustments to their lifestyle that will improve their outcome.

REFERENCES

1. Gwatkin D, Guillot M, Heuveline P. The burden of disease among the global poor. *Lancet* 1999; 354: 586–9.
2. Murray C, Lopez A (eds). *The Global Burden of Disease.* Boston, MA: Harvard University Press on behalf of WHO and the World Bank, 1996.
3. King H, Aubert RE, Herman WH. Global burden of diabetes. Prevalence numerical estimates and projections. *Diabetes Care* 1998; 21: 1414–31.
4. World Health Organisation. *Diet, Nutrition and the Prevention of Chronic Diseases.* Technical Report Series 196. Geneva: WHO, 2003.
5. Latham MC. *Human Nutrition in the Developing World.* FAO Food and Nutrition Series No 29. Rome: Food and Agriculture Organization of the United Nations, 1997.
6. Food Balance Sheets. FoodBalanceSheet & Domain. Available at: http://apps.fao.org/lim5000/wrap.pl? Accessed May 22, 2003.
7. Steyn NP, Olivier J, Winter P, Burger S, Nesamvuni C. A survey of wild, green, leafy vegetables and their potential in combating micronutrient deficiencies in rural populations. *S Afr J Sci* 2001; 97 (7/8): 276–8.
8. Marter A, Gordon A. The RNR sector in sub-Saharan Africa. *Food Policy* 1996; 21: 229–41.
9. Bourne L. Dietary intake of of urban Africans in Cape Town. *Med Res Counc Urbanisat Health Newslett* 1994; (22): 3–5.
10. Maletnlema TN. A Tanzanian perspective on the nutrition transition and its implications for health. *Public Health Nutr* 2002; 5 (1A): 163–8.
11. Mazengo MC, Simell O, Lukmanji Z, Shirima R, Karvetti RL. Food Consumption in rural and urban Tanzania. *Acta Trop* 1997; 68 (3): 313–26.
12. Steyn NP, Senekal M, Brits S, Nel J. Urban and rural differences in dietary intake, weight status and nutrition knowledge of black female students. *Asia Pacific J Clin Nutr* 2000; 9 (1): 53–9.
13. Proctor MH, Moore LL, Singer MR, Hood MY, Nguyen US, Ellison RC. Risk profiles for non-communicable diseases in rural and urban schoolchildren in the Republic of Cameroon. *Ethn Dis* 1996; 6: 235–43.
14. Tanner M, Lukmanji Z. Food consumption patterns in a rural Tanzanian community. *Acta Trop* 1987; 44: 229–44.
15. Franz MJ, Horton ES, Bantle JP, Beebe CA, Brunzell JD, Coulston AM, Henry RR, Hoogwey BJ, Stacpod PW. Nutrition principles for the management of diabetes and related complications. *Diabetes Care* 1994; 17: 490–518.
16. Franz MJ, Bantle JP, Beebe CA, Brunzell JD, Chiasson J-L, Garg A, Holzmeister LA, Hoogwerf B, Mayer-Davis P, Mooradian AD, Purnell JQ, Wheeler M. American diabetes association position statement: evidence-based nutrition principles and recommendations for the treatment and prevention of diabetes and related complications. *J Am Diet Assoc* 2002; 25: 148–98.

17. Association for Dietetics South Africa. Dietary management of type 11 diabetes. *South Afr Med J* 1997; 87: 503–5.
18. American Diabetes Association. Standards of medical care for patients with diabetes mellitus (position statement). *Diabetes Care* 2002; 25 (suppl 1) S33–49.
19. Diabetes and Nutrition Study Group (DSNG) of the European Association for the Study of Diabetes (EASD). Recommendations for the nutritional management of patients with diabetes mellitus. *Diabet Nutr Metab* 1995; 8: 186–9.
20. Ha TKK, Lean MM. Recommendations for the nutritional management of patients with diabetes mellitus. *Eur J Clin Nutr* 1998; 52: 467–81.
21. American Diabetes Association. Nutrition recommendations and principles for people with diabetes mellitus (position statement). *Diabetes Care* 1994; 17: 519–22.
22. Mensing C, Boucher J, Cypress M, Weinger K, Mulcahy K, Barta P, Hosey Cr, Kopher W, Lasichak A, Lamb B, Mangan M, Norman J, Tanja J, Yauk L, Wisdom K, Adams C. National standards for diabetes self-management education. *Diabetes Care* 2000; 23: 682–6.
23. European Diabetes Policy Group 1998–1999. A desktop guide to type 2 diabetes mellitus. *Diabet Med* (September) 1999; 16: 716–30.
24. Department of Health. *National Program for Management and Control of Diabetes Type 2 at primary level*. Pretoria, South Africa: DOH, 1997.
25. Mohamed E. The implementation of the national diabetes type 2 guidelines at primary level. *JEMDSA* 2001; 6 (1): 38.
26. Rotchford AP, Rotchford KM. Diabetes in rural South Africa—an assessment of care and complications. *JEMDSA* 2002; 7 (2): 60–5.
27. Levitt NS, Steyn K, Daniels AD, Patel M, Lombard C. Lack of impact of a national diabetes guideline-based intervention package on glycaemic and blood pressure control at primary care level in Cape Town. *JEMDSA* 2002; 7 (1): 21.
28. Nthangeni G, Steyn NP, Alberts M, Steyn K, Levitt NS, Laubscher R, Bourne L, Dick J, Temple N. Dietary intake and barriers to dietary compliance in black type 2 diabetic patients attending primary health-care services. *Public Health Nutr* 2002; 5 (2): 329–38.
29. Krauss RM, Eckel RH, Howard B, Appel LJ, Daniels SR, Deckelbaum RJ, Erdman JW Jr, Kris-Etherton P, Goldberg IJ, Kotchen TA, Lichtenstein AH, Mitch WE, Mullis R, Robinson K, Wylie-Rosett J, Sachiko St. J, Suttie J, Tribble DL, Bazzarre TL. AHA Dietary Guidelines: revision 2000: A statement for healthcare professionals from the Nutrition Committee of the American Heart Association. *Circulation* 2000; 102 (18): 2284–99.
30. Mahan LK, Escott-Stump S. *Krause's Food and Nutrition & Diet Therapy, 10th* edn. London: Saunders, 2000.
31. Levitt NS, Unwin NC, Bradshaw D, Kitange HM, Mbanya J-C, Mollentze WF, Omar MAK, Motala AA, Joubert G, Masuki G, Machibya H. Application of the new ADA criteria for the diagnosis of diabetes to population studies in sub-Saharan Africa. *Diabet Med* 2000; 17: 381–5.
32. Mbanya JCN, Ngogang J, Salah JN, Miukovlov E, Balkau B. Prevalence of NIDDM and impaired glucose tolerance in a rural and an urban population in Cameroon. *Diabetologia* 1997; 40: 824–9.
33. Levitt NS, Katzenellenbogen JM, Bradshaw D, Hoffman MN, Bonnici F. The prevalence of identification of risk factors for NIDDM in urban Africans in Cape Town, South Africa. *Diabetes Care* 1993; 16: 601–7.
34. Levitt NS, Steyn K, Lambert EV, Reagon G, Lombard CJ, Roussouw K, Fourie JM, Hoffman M. Modifiable risk factors for type 2 diabetes mellitus in a peri-urban community in South Africa. *Diabet Med* 1999; 16: 946–50.
35. Mollentze WF, Moore AJ, Steyn AF, Joubert G, Steyn K, Oosthuizen GM, Weich DJ. Coronary heart disease risk factors in a rural and urban Orange Free State black population. *S Afr Med J* 1995; 85: 90–6.
36. Omar MAK, Seedat MA, Motala AA, Dyer RP, Becker P. The prevalence of diabetes and impaired glucose tolerance in a group of urban South African Blacks. *S Afr Med J* 1993; 83: 641–3.
37. McLatty DG, Swai ABM, Kitange HM, Masuki G, Mtinangi BL, Kilima PM, et al. Prevalence of diabetes and impaired glucose tolerance in rural Tanzania. *Lancet* 1989; 1: 871–5.
38. Tuomilehto J, Lindstrom J, Eriksson JG, Valle TT, Hamalainen H, Ilanne-Parikka P, Keinanen-Kiukaanniemi S, Laakso M, Louheranta A, Rastas M, Salminen V, Uusitupa M, for the Finnish Diabetes Prevention Study Group. Prevention of type 2 diabetes mellitus by changes in lifestyle among subjects with impaired glucose tolerance. *N Engl J Med* 2001; 344: 1343–50.
39. Diet and exercise dramatically delay type 2 diabetes. Press release of the National Institute of Diabetes and Digestive and Kidney Diseases. August 8, 2001. Available at: httpp:/www.nih.gov/news/pr/aug2001/ niddk-08.htm. Accessed November 29, 2001.
40. Pan XR, Li GW, Hu YH, Wang JX, Yang WY, An ZX, Hu ZX, Lin J, Xiao JZ, Cao HB, Liu PA, Jiang XG, Jiang YY, Wang JP, Zheng H, Zhang H, Bennett PH, Howard BV. Effects of diet and exercise in preventing NIDDM in people with impaired glucose tolerance. The Da Qing IGT and Diabetes Study. *Diabetes Care* 1997; 20: 537–44.
41. Eriksson K-F, Lindgarde F. Prevention of type 2 (non-insulin-dependent) diabetes mellitus by diabetes mellitus by diet and physical exercise: the 6-Year Malmö Feasibility Study. *Diabetologia* 1991; 34: 891–8.
42. Indar-Brown K, Norenberg C, Madar Z. Glycemic and insulinemic responses after ingestion of ethnic foods by NIDDM and healthy subjects. *Am J Clin Nutr* 1992; 55: 89–95.
43. Mbhenyane XG, Venter CS, Vorster HH, Steyn HS. The glycaemic index of indigenous South Africa foods. *S Afr J Clin Nutr* 2001; 14 (3): 88–95.
44. Walker ARP, Walker BF. Glycaemic index of South African foods determined in rural blacks—a population at low risk of diabetes. *Hum Nutr Clin Nutr* 1984; 38C: 215–22.
45. Ayuo PO, Ettyang GA. Glycaemic responses after ingestion of some local foods by non-insulin dependent diabetic subjects. *East Afr Med J* 1996; 73 (12): 782–5.
46. Mbanya JC, Sobngwi E, Mbanya DN, Ngogang JY. Metabolic and hormonal effects of five common African diets eaten as mixed meals: The Cameroon Study. *Eur J Clin Nutr* 2003; 57 (4): 580–5.
47. Venter CS, Vorster HH, van Rooyen A, Kruger-Locke MM, Silvis N. Comparison of the effects of maize porridge consumed at different temperature on blood glucose, insulin and acetate levels in healthy volunteers. *S Afr J Food Sci Nutr* 1990; 2 (1): 2–5.
48. Gresse A, Vorster HH, Dauth J, Vermaak H, Welgemoed DJ. The long term effects of a traditional African diet on

the metabolic control of black patients with type II diabetes mellitus. *S Afr J Food Sci Nutr* 1991; 3 (4): 90.

49. Lester FT. Clinical features, complications and mortality in type 2 (non-insulin dependent) diabetic patients in Addis Ababa, Ethiopia, 1976–1990. *Ethiop Med J* 1993; 31 (2): 109–26.
50. Ahren B. Diabetes mellitus at a rural hospital in north western Tanzania. *Trop Geogr Med* 1984; 36 (3): 237–42.
51. Steyn NP, Burger S, Monyeki KM, Alberts M, Nthangeni G. Seasonal variation in dietary intake of the adult population of Dikgale. *S Afr J Clin Nutr* 2001; 14 (4): 140–5.
52. Gresse A, Vorster HH. Eating habits and nutrient intakes of black patients with diabetes mellitus. *S Afr J Food Sci Nutr* 1992; 4 (3): 76.
53. Hoffmeister M, Lyaruu I, Krawinkel MB. Nutritional management of diabetes in Northern Tanzania. *Diabetes Care* 2002; 8: 1486.
54. Gresse A, Vorster HH, Dauth J, Welgemoed DJ, Crowter G. Effects of a typical African diet on metabolic control of black non-insulin dependent diabetes mellitus patients. *S Afr J Food Sci Nutr* 1993; 5 (2): 43–8.
55. Oli JM, Ikeakor IP. High carbohydrate diet in the management non- obese non-insulin-dependent Nigerian diabetics. *Hum Nutr Appl Nutr* 1984; 38 (6): 479–86.
56. Statistics South Africa. *Statistics in brief 2000*. Pretoria, South Africa: Central Statistics Services, 2000.
57. Steyn NP. Dietitians Knowledge and Practices Regarding the Use of Dietary Supplements and Fortified Foods. MPH thesis, UCT, 2003.
58. Tripp-Reimer T, Choi E, Enslein JC. Cultural barriers to care: inverting the problem. *Diabetes Spectrum* 2001; 14 (1): 13–22.
59. Peltzer K. A community survey of traditional healers in South Africa (Northern Province). *S Afr J Ethnol* 1998; 21 (4): 191–7.
60. Peltzer K, Khoza LB, Lekhuleni ME, Madu SN, Cherian VI, Cherian L. Concepts and treatment for diabetes among traditional and faith healers in the Northern Province, South Africa. *Curationis* 2001; 24 (2): 42–7.
61. Ziqubu-Page TT, Dangor CM, Makubalo LE, Chetty M. Determinants of traditional medicine used by diabetic patients in the Northern Kwa Zulu-Natal Province. *Curare* 1984; 22: 49–61.

43

Exercise

Henrik Galbo and Erik A. Richter

University of Copenhagen, Copenhagen, Denmark

INTRODUCTION

A certain minimum of skeletal muscle activity in excess of that required for basal pulmonary ventilation is necessary for all people, including diabetic patients, for everyday activities such as smiling, dressing, cooking, and eating. House work and walking and bicycling for the purpose of transportation represent heavier exercise, and severe physical activity may be required in occupational activities in agriculture, forestry, fishing, industry, and obviously, professional sports and ballet. In addition to such obligatory exercise, many people also engage in sports to increase their physical, psychological, and social well-being.

However, the trend is that the advancing of modern technology promotes physical inactivity. This is unfortunate, because physical activity has a pivotal role in health promotion and prevention of disease, including type 2 diabetes [1]. For that reason it has become necessary for national health authorities to recommend planned, regular exercise [2]. The recommendation also applies to diabetic patients. Among the weighty arguments are that for both type 1 and type 2 diabetic pateints evidence exists that exercise reduces the risk of cardiovascular events [3, 4] and increases life expectancy [5, 6]. The recommendation of physical activity to patients with diabetes is supported by both national academic diabetes and sports associations, e.g. the American Diabetes Association [7, 8] and the American College of Sports Medicine [9, 10].

Because exercise is an essential part of life and, furthermore, is associated with potential health benefits, it is important to know the inherent risks and to know how it influences the body, with regard to organ function, dietary needs, and interaction with medicine and environment. This is of particular interest in people with diabetes, since many of the characteristics and manifestations of this disease would be expected to interfere with work performance and vice versa.

EXERCISE PHYSIOLOGY

In healthy humans who perform severe dynamic exercise with big muscle groups, oxygen uptake may increase 15–20-fold because of increased metabolic rate in the working muscles. In these, arterioles dilate, capillaries are recruited, and fluid accumulates intra- and extracellularly. Pulmonary ventilation may exceed 100 l/min and cardiac output increases to 20–30 l/min to meet the needs of the working muscles, while blood flow to resting muscles, the splanchnic area, and the kidneys decreases. Systolic and mean arterial blood pressure increase. Some of the heat produced is accumulated in the body, and the core temperature may exceed 40°C. Most of the heat is removed by evaporation, however, and the sweat rate during exercise in hot and humid air may be 2 l/h. The glomerular filtration rate decreases while potassium is released from contracting muscle and may attain a concentration in plasma of 8 mEq/l at maximum exercise.

During exercise in the postabsorptive state, the energy demand of the working muscles is met by breakdown of intramuscular glycogen and triglyceride stores as well as by an increased supply of glucose from the liver and free fatty acids (FFAs) from extramuscular triglyceride stores [11]. Protein oxidation does not increase significantly unless muscle glycogen stores are exhausted. The relative contribution of carbohydrate to overall energy delivery increases with exercise intensity, while fat oxidation in absolute terms peaks at 70% of V_{O_2}max and becomes negligible

International Textbook of Diabetes Mellitus, Third Edition. Edited by R. A. DeFronzo, E. Ferrannini, H. Keen, and P. Zimmet.
 ISBN: 0-471-48655-8.

at maximum exercise. Breakdown of intramuscular energy stores as well as overall carbohydrate oxidation wanes with time, during mild to moderate exercise. The increase in glucose production in response to exercise primarily reflects hepatic glycogenolysis, but contribution from gluconeogenesis increases with duration of mild exercise. At moderate workloads the plasma glucose concentration is usually well maintained (Figure 1). However, at high work intensities the glucose concentration increases [11, 12], while hypoglycemia may develop during prolonged exercise [13], these deviations being favored when prior to exercise carbohydrate stores are high and low, respectively [14, 15]. Because selection of fuel for oxidation is affected by substrate availability [11, 16], exogenous nutrients, e.g. glucose [17–19], administered prior to or during exercise influence muscle metabolism.

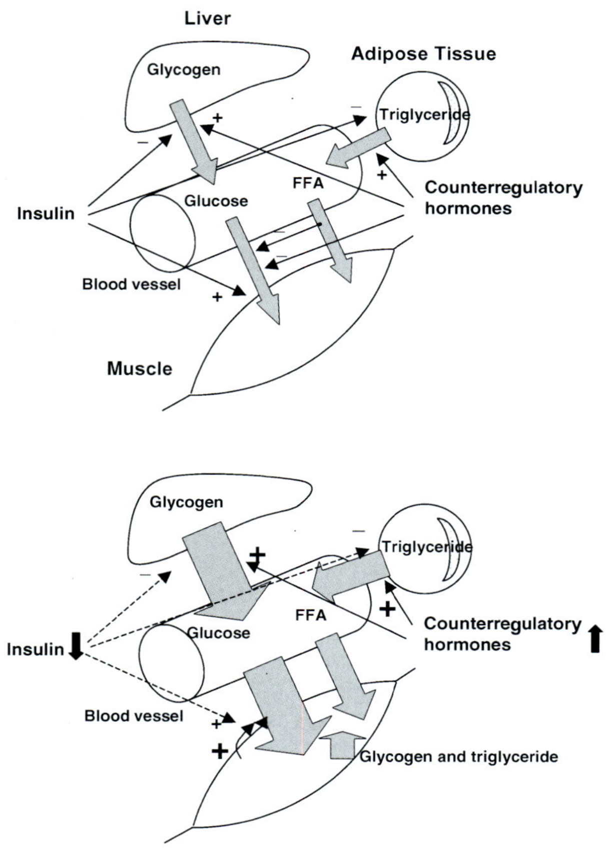

Figure 1 Simplified schemes of substrate fluxes and their hormonal regulation in healthy subjects in the postabsorptive state at rest (upper panel) and during moderate exercise (lower panel). FFA means free fatty acids; "+" and "−" indicate enhancing and inhibiting effects, respectively. During exercise a decrease in plasma insulin and an increase in concentrations of counterregulatory hormones are seen, while plasma glucose remains constant because an increase in glucose uptake in contracting muscles is matched by an increase in hepatic glucose output

Hormonal Regulation

The autonomic neuroendocrine system serves the coordination of the various functions of the body to allow coping with the physical challenges of life. Accordingly, it follows from the depicted multiple perturbations that depending on its intensity and duration, exercise may elicit extensive autonomic neuroendocrine responses. These adaptations resemble those seen in hypoglycemia, early fasting, hyperthermia, surgery, and hemorrhage, i.e. including a decrease in plasma insulin as well as an increase in sympathetic nervous activity, insulin counterregulatory hormones, and hormones retaining sodium and water in the kidneys [16].

The endocrine adaptations to exercise are based on the same fundamental regulatory principles that are thought to control circulatory, respiratory, and thermoregulatory responses in exercise, a fact guaranteeing that the responses of the major physiological systems are highly coordinated [16]. At the onset of exercise, nervous impulses from motor centers in the brain and from working muscles elicit an increase in sympathoadrenal activity and in the release of some pituitary hormones [e.g. growth hormone (GH), adrenocorticotropic hormone (ACTH), β-endorphin, prolactin and antidiuretic hormone (ADH)]. This exercise specific, "feedforward" stimulus is determined by workload relative to the individual's maximum capacity ($V_{O_2}/V_{O_2}max$) rather than by absolute workload. The primary neuroendocrine responses, in turn, change the secretion of subordinate endocrine cells, e.g. sympathetic nervous activity depresses insulin secretion by α-receptor-mediated mechanisms, while the renin–angiotensin–ADH system is stimulated by β-receptor mechanisms, and ACTH stimulates cortisol secretion.

The fast nervous mechanisms intimately related to contractile activity operate throughout exercise, but the hormonal responses may be gradually intensified according to feedback from metabolic error signals (among which a decrease in glucose availability is the most important) as well as from nonmetabolic error signals sensed by pressure, volume, osmolality, electrolyte, and temperature receptors. At high work rates, feedforward control dominates. At low exercise intensities, just as at rest, feedback regulation dominates the hormonal changes, and at least in humans, an increase in plasma glucagon concentration is always predominantly determined by a decrease in plasma glucose availability. The primary setting of the hormonal response to exercise depends on the state of the organism with respect to training, nutrition, hydration, phase of menstrual cycle, and state of health [16].

Hormonal Influence on Exercise Metabolism

The overall hormonal response to exercise appears to be geared to stimulation of hepatic glucose production. However, which components are the more important is, particularly in humans, not clear [16]. A decrease in plasma insulin concentration is always essential, because glucose production during exercise varies inversely with modest artificial changes in insulin levels [16]. In rats and dogs the exercise-induced increases in glucagon and epinephrine concentrations are the major determinants of the increase in glucose production [11, 16]. Furthermore, the potency of the rise in glucagon has been shown to be enhanced by the accompanying fall in insulin [20]. On the other hand, both in these species, in guinea pigs [21], and in humans [22, 23] sympathetic liver nerves do not influence glucose production in exercise. Strange to say, neither epinephrine [23, 24] nor glucagon [11, 23] or angiotensin [25] seems to be major stimuli in humans. In healthy man, arterial glucagon does not increase above basal levels until after more than 1 h of submaximal exercise; it even decreases during maximal exercise, when glucose production peaks [11].

It may seem surprising that during exercise the glucose uptake in muscle varies inversely with the rate of secretion and the plasma concentration of insulin [11]. However, muscle contractions *per se* enhance muscle glucose uptake by mechanisms that are independent of insulin [26, 27]. These mechanisms include feedforward components, which probably are Ca^{++} mediated [28], as well as feedback components, which may be mediated by AMP-activated protein kinase (AMPK) [29, 30]. In isolated skeletal muscle, contractions are a more powerful stimulus to glucose transport than is insulin, and the two stimuli are fully additive [31]. They translocate glucose transporting protein (GLUT-4) to the sarcolemma by at least partly different signaling mechanisms, and have different preference for recruitment from the various intracellular GLUT-4 stores [32].

During exercise the decrease in plasma insulin curbs glucose uptake in muscle, and the same is true for the increase in plasma epinephrine [24]. The effect is due to the direct actions of hormonal changes on glucose transport as well as inhibition of glucose uptake secondary to an enhancement of lipolysis and muscle glycogen breakdown [11, 33, 34]. In addition to the decrease in plasma insulin, both sympathetic nerve activity and epinephrine are major determinants of adipose tissue lipolysis in exercise [35].

The primary setting of substrate mobilization in exercise is simple. The same enzymes, i.e. glycogen phosphorylase and hormone-sensitive lipase (HSL), are flux-generating for glycogenolysis and lipolysis, respectively, in both muscle and extramuscular stores of glycogen (i.e. liver) and triglyceride (i.e. adipose tissue). Furthermore, the two enzymes are stimulated by the same neuroendocrine changes, and in muscle they are also stimulated in parallel by mechanisms accompanying contractions [34, 36, 37]. The autonomic neuroendocrine response to exercise includes increases in several components potentially enhancing the activity of glycogen phosphorylase and HSL, and, in addition, a decrease in insulin, a hormone inhibiting these enzymes. Metaphorically speaking, substrate mobilization in exercise is increased by stepping on the accelerator while releasing the brake (Figure 1).

METABOLISM DURING EXERCISE IN DIABETIC PATIENTS

Type 1

While the insulin concentration in the plasma of healthy people is automatically adjusted to any work condition, this adjustment does not take place in type 1 diabetic patients. Instead, they have to carry out the work during the influence of the given amount of insulin they have administered subcutaneously. Therefore, the changes in metabolism that take place in type 1 diabetic patients in response to exercise usually reflect either too much or too little insulin in plasma.

While plasma insulin is low during exercise in healthy people, that in diabetic patients is not low if they take the same dose of insulin as they use on nonexercise days. In diabetic patients, in contrast to healthy subjects, plasma insulin may even increase during exercise because absorption of insulin may be favored by exercise-induced movements of the site of administration in the skin and increases in skin blood flow [38, 39]. A high plasma insulin level implies risk of hypoglycemia because the normal increase in hepatic glucose production is inhibited, and insulin stimulates muscular glucose uptake both directly and by an inhibition of FFA release from triglyceride stores and, in turn, of fat combustion [38] (Figure 2).

If, then, type 1 diabetic patients reduce their dose of insulin, they risk getting too little insulin in plasma [40]. In this event, hepatic glucose production and the release of FFA from adipose tissue increase more than normally, while muscular glucose uptake is inhibited (Figure 2). The high plasma FFA level and an increased hepatic fractional extraction and conversion to ketone bodies of FFA result in an increased production of ketone acids and increased muscular fat oxidation [41]. In patients who have been insulin deficient prior to exercise too, increased fat oxidation during work also reflects increased stores of intramuscular triglycerides and that these stores are depleted during exercise [42–44]. In such patients the muscular glycogen concentration and exercise-induced glycogen depletion are reduced in comparison to those of healthy subjects [43]. Nevertheless, lactate accumulation is enhanced as a consequence of incomplete carbohydrate oxidation due to increased fat oxidation and diminished pyruvate dehydrogenase activity [42, 45, 46]. Furthermore, an increased production of lactic acid, glycerol, and glycogenic amino acids results in higher hepatic gluconeogenesis during exercise than in control subjects [42, 45]. Taken together,

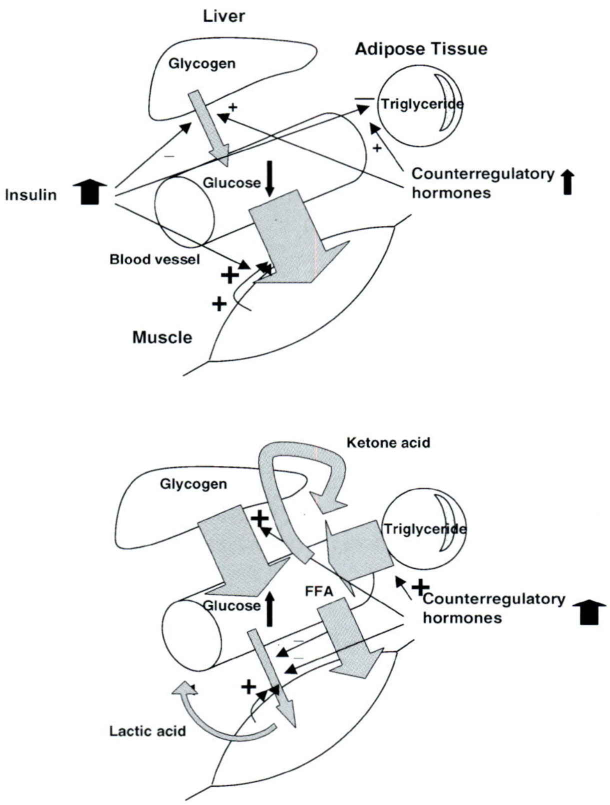

Figure 2 Simplified schemes of substrate fluxes and their hormonal regulation during moderate exercise in type 1 diabetes patients, who have taken a normal dose of insulin (upper panel) or are insulin deficient (lower panel). After insulin administration the uptake of glucose in contracting muscles increases more than the hepatic glucose output, and the plasma glucose concentration falls. In contrast, without insulin the plasma glucose concentration rises, because hepatic glucose output exceeds muscle glucose uptake. The increases in counterregulatory hormones and FFA are exaggerated and the production of ketones is increased

in insulin-deficient exercising individuals, the plasma glucose concentration increases and acid accumulates—the diabetic state deteriorates [40, 45].

It is evident that the physically active diabetic individual, like the sedentary one, balances between hyper- and hypoglycemia. However, exercise accelerates the rate at which both of these unpleasant alternatives develop (Figure 3). On the one hand, exercise increases sympathetic nervous activity and the plasma concentrations of counterregulatory hormones, a phenomenon that *per se* causes an accumulation of glucose and lactic acid and ketone bodies in plasma by enhancing glucose and FFA production and inhibiting glucose uptake in muscle [47, 48]. Moreover, in diabetic patients who have taken too little insulin the autonomic neuroendocrine response is exaggerated, and so are its effects. Therefore, these patients are especially prone to hyperglycemia and ketoacidosis [41, 46, 49–52]. The increase in plasma glucose during exercise may even in itself stimulate the counterregulatory hormonal response [52]. In other words, the type 1 diabetic patient, who exercises with a too low plasma insulin concentration, in terms of fuel mobilization, steps harder on the accelerator and less hard on the brake than healthy subjects do.

On the other hand, the plasma glucose concentration decreases more rapidly in diabetic patients, who take too much insulin, if they also exercise [53–55] (Figures 2 and 4). This phenomenon is due to the fact that glucose uptake in muscle becomes extra high because contractions *per se* increase glucose uptake in muscle cells and also increase the sensitivity to insulin of glucose uptake in these cells [56], and because delivery of insulin and glucose to the sarcolemma of contracting muscle cells is increased by increases in blood flow and capillary permeability surface area product in exercising muscle [57]. Furthermore, the indirect enhancing effect of insulin on glucose uptake in muscle, which is exerted via inhibition of fat cell lipolysis, may be augmented in exercise compared with rest, because insulin prevents the marked increase in lipolysis, which normally occurs during exercise. In addition, insulin can prevent the rise in hepatic glucose production during exercise. Because glucose turnover is accelerated during exercise, inhibition of hepatic glucose production leads to more marked hypoglycemia than at rest when glucose turnover is less. The risk of exercise-associated hypoglycemia in type 1 diabetic patients is probably increased after antecedent hypoglycemia. This is so, because previous-day hypoglycemia has been shown to reduce counterregulatory hormonal responses as well as glucose production and lipolysis during prolonged exercise, with clamped plasma glucose concentration [58].

Type 2

Type 2 diabetic patients, in contrast to type 1 diabetic patients, have some insulin secretory capacity, and their insulin secretion changes with needs in principle as it does in normal individuals. Accordingly, if they are not treated with exogenous insulin, they cannot respond as dramatically to exercise as type 1 diabetic patients. In other words, they do not run the same metabolic risks with exercise. Still, although insulin resistance is a major hallmark of type 2 diabetes, contraction-mediated glucose transport in muscle of type 2 diabetic patient is not reduced [57, 59, 60]. It has been claimed that its reliance on NO is higher than that seen in normal muscle [61], but exercise-induced increases in atypical protein kinase C (PKC) and AMPK-$\alpha 2$ activities in muscle are normal [62, 63].

So, in diet-treated type 2 diabetic patients, who perform prolonged mild to moderate exercise in the postabsorptive state, a marked reduction in hyperglycemia can be seen [64, 65]. This reflects that hyperglycemia enhances the exercise-induced increase in muscle glucose uptake and

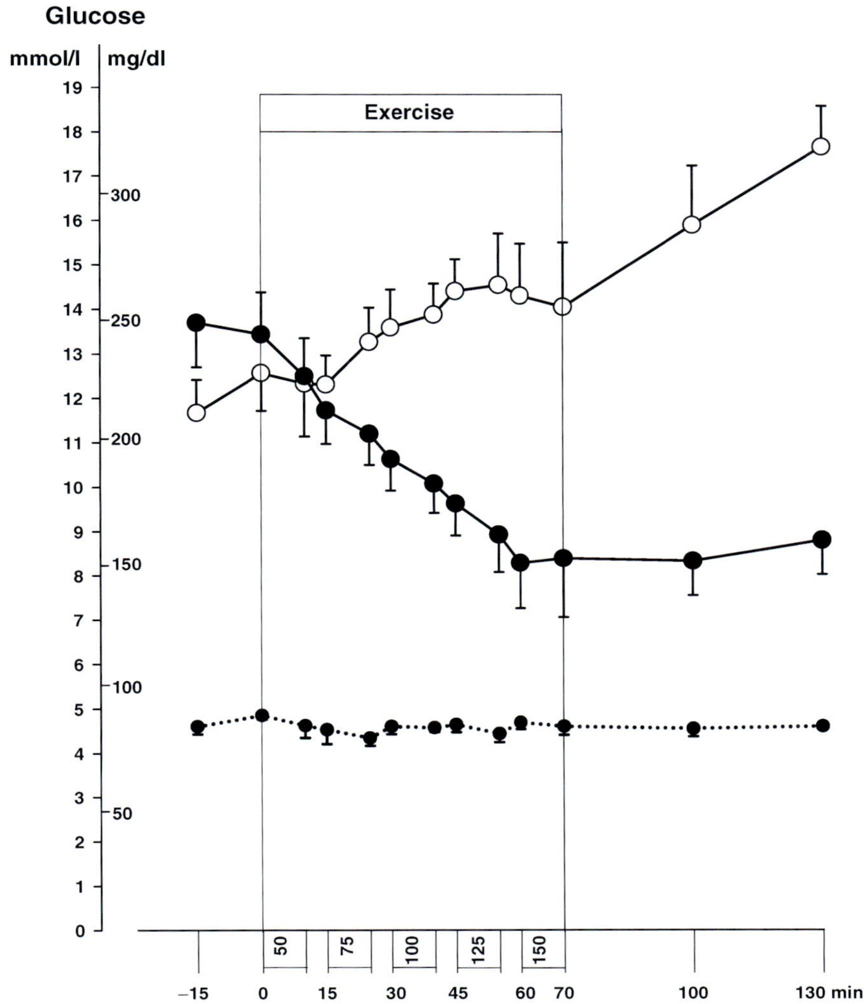

Figure 3 The figure illustrates the delicate balance between too little and too much insulin available during exercise. After an overnight fast, 24-year-old type 1 diabetes patients injected 4 IU of regular insulin either 3 h (white dots, $n = 11$) or 1 h (black dots, $n = 15$) before intermittent, graded, exhausting ergometer cycle exercise (5×10 min at 50–150 W with 5-min rest intervals). The plasma glucose concentration increased 5.1 mM and decreased 4.7 mM, respectively. The broken line represents data from six healthy subjects. (Adapted from reference 40)

inhibits the increase in hepatic glucose production, effects that are reinforced by the fact that the secretion and, in turn, plasma concentration of insulin, at least as long as hyperglycemia prevails, are not depressed as readily as in normal subjects [64, 66–69].

The rate of decrease in plasma glucose concentration is augmented if sulfonylurea drugs are taken shortly before exercise (Figure 5) [70]. Sulfonylureas stimulate insulin secretion, and although the secretion is depressed by exercise, the plasma insulin concentration remains higher than that during exercise without prior drug intake (Figure 5). This relative hyperinsulinemia explains that the exercise-induced rise in hepatic glucose production is lower, and accordingly, the hypoglycemic effect of exercise is larger than when exercise is performed without acute sulphonylurea intake. Interestingly, the hyperinsulinemia apparently overrides the effect of the augmented counterregulatory hormone response observed when sulphonylureas are taken (Figure 5) [70]. Abstaining from sulfonylurea treatment for 5 days does not result in an exaggerated counterregulatory hormone response and hyperglycemic reaction to exercise as seen in type 1 diabetic patients after insulin withdrawal. In contrast, during 60 min of moderate exercise the plasma glucose concentration decreases more after prolonged sulfonylurea abstention than after abstention only from the morning dose prior to exercise. This is because the basal plasma glucose level increases during the prolonged drug abstention, and, in turn, maintains the basal insulin secretion and impairs the exercise-induced depression of insulin secretion. The augmented hyperglycemia and relatively high insulin levels then blunt the exercise-induced increase in hepatic glucose output,

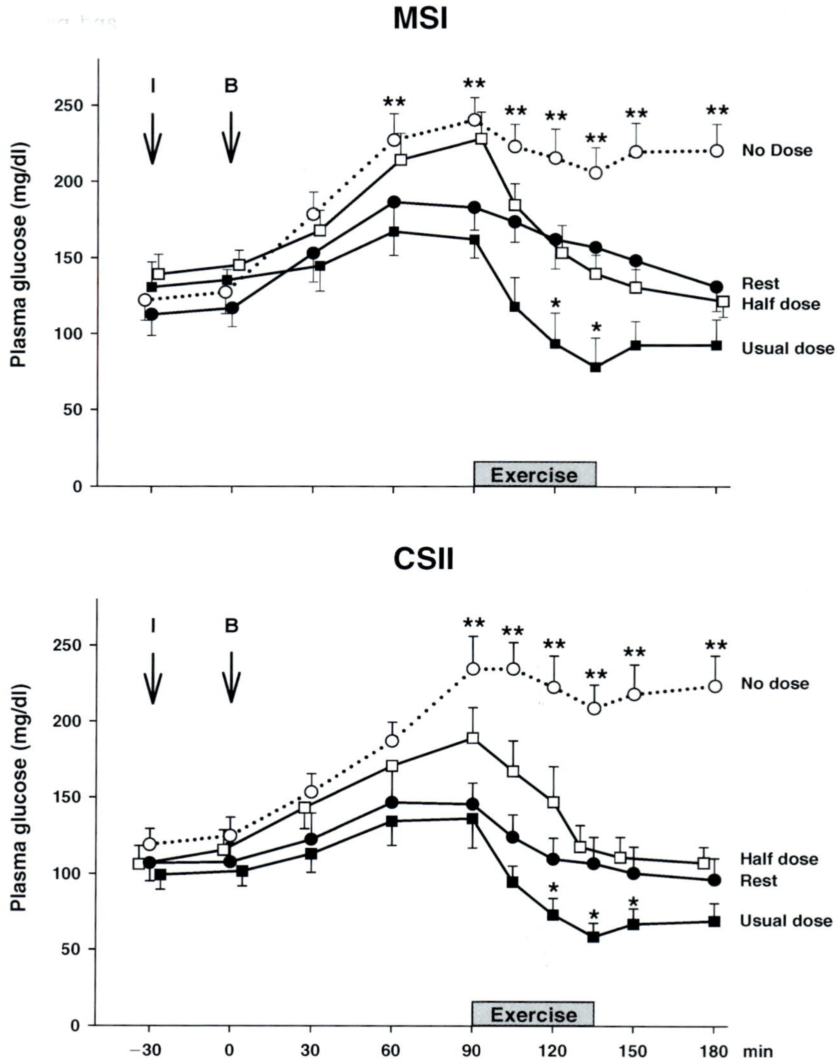

Figure 4 The interaction between breakfast (B), ergometer cycle exercise (45 min at 55% $\dot{V}O_2max$) and different doses of insulin (I) in 15–18-year-old type 1 diabetes patients treated with multiple subcutaneous insulin injections (MSI, upper panel, $n = 6$) or continuous subcutaneous insulin infusion [CSII (pump), lower panel, $n = 7$]. If premeal insulin dose is reduced, plasma glucose concentration increases before exercise but during exercise hypoglycemia is avoided. The two regimens allow similar coping with exercise. $^{*}p < 0.05$ and $^{**}p < 0.01$ vs. rest. (Adapted from reference 55).

thereby promoting a decrease in plasma glucose. Still, an exaggerated counterregulatory hormone response and glucose production, and an ensuing increase in plasma glucose is seen in type 2 diabetic patients performing brief intense exercise in the postabsorptive state [71].

The plasma glucose concentration also decreases markedly during prolonged moderate exercise in type 2 diabetic patients in the postprandial state (Figure 6) [72]. This is accompanied by reduced meal-induced increases in insulin and C-peptide concentrations and reflects an exercise-induced increase in glucose clearance, while glucose appearance in plasma is unchanged [72]. The plasma-glucose-lowering effect of exercise is higher after a meal than in the fasted state, even at a time at which only plasma insulin and not plasma glucose is increased in the former compared to the latter condition [73]. In contrast to findings in the postabsorptive state [71], in the postprandial state hyperglycemia is not aggravated during severe exercise [74]. This probably reflects that the counterregulatory hormonal response to exercise is lower in the latter compared with the former state, and that, furthermore, the high glucose and insulin concentrations accompanying food intake inhibit an exercise-induced increase in hepatic glucose production and enhance an increase in glucose uptake in muscle [74]. Repeated, high-intensity exercise in fact reduces both glucose concentrations and insulin secretion after a meal [74]. Interestingly, exercise-induced reductions in glucose, insulin, and C-peptide responses are

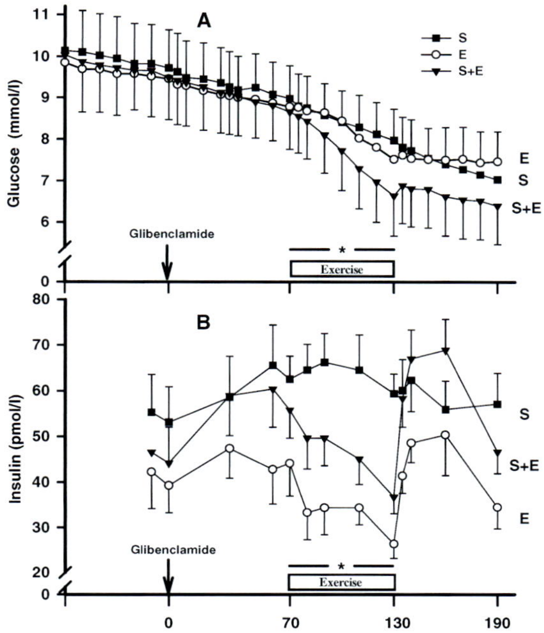

Figure 5 The interaction between sulfonylurea (S, 7 mg glibenclamide) and exercise (E, 60 min of ergometer cycle exercise at 57% $V_{O_2}max$) on plasma glucose and insulin concentrations in eight postabsorptive type 2 diabetic patients. * indicates that average concentrations from 70 to 130 min differed ($p < 0.05$) between thethree experiments. (Adapted from reference 70)

similar during repeated, high-intensity exercise compared with isocaloric but prolonged moderate postprandial exercise [74]. This indicates that in the postprandial state, overall energy expenditure is the major determinant of exercise-induced changes in overall glucose homeostasis and insulin secretion in type 2 diabetic patients. The peak exercise intensity is not of major importance in this respect. Apparently, in terms of reducing glucose levels and insulin secretion acute exercise has no effect beyond that of increasing energy expenditure. In line with this view, it has been shown that a reduction of energy content of a meal has the same lowering effect on postprandial glycemia and insulin secretion as an equivalent exercise-induced increase in energy expenditure (Figure 6) [72]. Neither prolonged moderate nor intermittent severe exercise performed in the postprandial state influences glucose and insulin responses to a subsequent meal [72, 74]. Besides postprandial hyperglycemia the meal-induced increase in chylomicron triglyceride concentrations is also reduced by postprandial exercise in type 2 diabetic patients.

Special Patient Groups

Children

$V_{O_2}max$ and physical work capacity are impaired in young people with type 1 diabetes [75]. Inactivity likely contributes to lower fitness and performance because when matched for age, body size, and physical activity, adolescents with type 1 diabetes have similar cardiac function and $V_{O_2}max$ as healthy adolescents [75]. Children often engage in spontaneous exercise the extent of which is little predictable, a fact that makes appropriate adjustments in insulin and diet difficult. Such adjustments are also rendered difficult by the fact that during similar conditions the variation in glycemic response to exercise is high in children both on the inter- and intraindividual level [76]. Furthermore, glycemic awareness seems to be poor in adolescents with type 1 diabetes [77], and their perceived exertion is high compared to findings in control subjects [78], while carbohydrate utilization may be impaired [79]. Hypoglycemia during prolonged moderate postprandial exercise is a particular threat due to prevailing

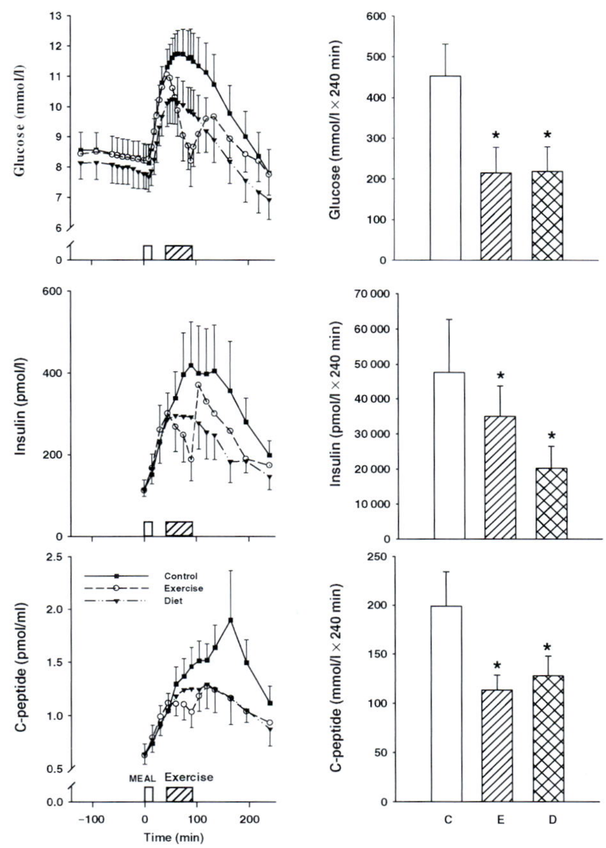

Figure 6 The effect of moderate exercise (45 min of ergometer cycle exercise at 53% $V_{O_2}max$) 45 min after start of breakfast, on plasma glucose, insulin, and C-peptide concentrations in nine diet-treated type 2 diabetes patients. The patients were studied at three occasions; control day without exercise (C), exercise day (E), and diet day without exercise (D). On D, breakfast was reduced corresponding to the extra energy expenditure during exercise on E. Incremental areas under the plasma concentration vs. time curves (AUC) calculated from 0 to 240 min are shown to the right. * indicates difference form C ($p < 0.05$). (Adapted from reference 72)

hyperinsulinemia, but intermittent ingestion of carbohydrate beverages matched with total carbohydrate utilization has been shown to markedly attenuate the drop in plasma glucose in exercising adolescents with type 1 diabetes [80]. The fact that severe postexercise late-onset hypoglycemia may be particularly prevalent in active diabetic children probably reflects that proper strategies are not adopted to replace muscle and liver glycogen stores [81]. If, on the other hand, brief high-intensity exercise is performed, a dramatic increase in plasma glucose along with marked increases in catecholamine concentrations may be seen even in well-insulinized diabetic children [82], just as it is the case in diabetic adults [83]. Because requirements for insulin and food change with growth and sexual maturation, the management of physical activity in youth with diabetes requires great care. In the case of an amenorrheic athletic girl with type 1 diabetes, dietary instruction is paramount as part of the exercise program, not only as treatment of the exercise-induced menstrual disorder, but also to maintain as near-normal plasma glucose level as is safe and feasible, because chronic hyperglycemia delays puberty and is associated with short stature [84].

Pregnant Women

Oligo- or amenorrhoea may, in both healthy and diabetic women, result from excessive physical training [16]. If these women want to become pregnant they must reduce or abstain from exercise. Even in normally menstruating, insulin-treated women, this step may be necessary to achieve a glucoregulation compatible with fertilization, because exercise adds an additional variable that may make glucose control difficult [84]. For the same reason it has been concluded that the utility of an exercise program as part of the glucose control program for the pregnant woman with pregestational diabetes, be it type 1 or type 2, is questionable [84]. The paramount management goal for the best outcome of pregnancy is to achieve and maintain normoglycemia. However, exercise-induced deterioration may only be associated with a risk of spontaneous abortion if plasma glucose levels exceed 4 SDs of the mean of the level in a healthy pregnant woman [84].

Insulin sensitivity declines progressively during the second half of gestation, and if insulin secretion is not increased appropriately, the previously nondiabetic pregnant woman develops gestational diabetes. Exercise of moderate intensity is recommended along with diet in the treatment of these patients, because exercise may lower their plasma glucose levels and insulin needs [85–87].

After menopause basal metabolic rate decreases. Exercise may help postmenopausal women with type 2 diabetes to avoid weight gain [84]. If postmenopausal women with diabetes undertake hormonal replacement therapy with estrogen and progesterone their insulin requirement increases. When an exercise program is combined with hormonal replacement therapy, the insulin regimen becomes especially challenging [84].

Autonomic Neuropathy

Diabetic autonomic neuropathy influences cardiovascular and hormonal responses to exercise. Exercise endurance as well as $V\text{O}_2$max are diminished by autonomic neuropathy [88, 89]. Vagal insufficiency results in an increased heart rate at rest, and impairment of both parasympathetic and sympathetic nervous function results in diminished increases in heart rate in response to exercise [88–91]. In patients with diabetic autonomic neuropathy stroke volume is diminished both at rest and during exercise [88]. This seems to reflect impaired cardiac contractility, which may be due to diminished cardiac adrenergic stimulation, impaired sympathetically mediated dilatation of coronary resistance vessels, and diabetic cardiomyopathy [88, 92]. The mentioned changes imply that in diabetic patients with autonomic neuropathy cardiac output increases less with exercise than in diabetic patients without neuropathy [88]. The exercise-induced increase in hepatosplanchnic vascular resistance too is diminished in patients with autonomic neuropathy [88]. Probably reflecting splanchnic sympathetic neuropathy and, in turn, reduced splanchnic vasoconstriction. Defective increases in cardiac output and hepatosplanchnic resistance explain that the arterial blood pressure response to exercise may also be reduced [88, 90]. The mentioned impairments in cardiovascular function are less pronounced in patients with diminished beat-to-beat variation in heart rate during deep breathing than in patients, who also have orthostatic hypotension, showing that the impairments are directly related to the degree of autonomic neuropathy [88, 89]. In patients with autonomic neuropathy the hypoxic ventilatory drive may be impaired [93]; nevertheless, these patients may show an exaggerated pulmonary ventilation during heavy exercise [94]. Impaired sympathetic function is accompanied by diminished catecholamine responses to exercise, and responses of GH, cortisol, renin, and pancreatic polypeptide too may be diminished in diabetic patients with autonomic neuropathy [95–97]. Nevertheless, metabolite responses may be only little influenced, a fact that probably reflects augmented sensitivity of target tissues to hormonal stimulation in these patients [98].

ADAPTATIONS TO TRAINING

Insulin Action and Secretion in Healthy Subjects

Insulin action on whole-body glucose disposal is reduced in the early recovery period after short-term maximal dynamic exercise in both untrained and trained subjects [12], and insulin action is also reduced after marathon running [99]. These findings have been ascribed to elevated levels of counterregulatory hormones as well as metabolic inhibition of glucose uptake in muscle, by accumulated glycolytic intermediates and increased fat metabolism, respectively. After a marathon the reduced insulin action is accompanied by impaired muscle glycogen resynthesis in the face of unaltered GLUT-4 content and increased glycogen synthase activity [99, 100]. Unaccustomed, severe exercise (e.g. eccentric exercise) that causes muscle damage also impairs insulin action [101, 102]. The reduced insulin action after eccentric exercise includes diminished insulin action on glucose uptake and glycogen synthesis in the recruited muscles, and is seen in the face of diminished total GLUT-4 content [103], decreased insulin signaling [104], but unaltered glycogen synthase activity [101, 102]. In accordance with these findings insulin-mediated glucose transport has been shown to be decreased in rat muscle after eccentric contractions, while glycogen synthase responded normally [105].

However, nonexhausting endurance-type exercise, which consists predominantly of concentric contractions, enhances the effect of insulin on glucose disposal [106, 107], and insulin action increases over the full range of activity levels from inactivity during bedrest to daily endurance training [102]. Also regular strength training enhances insulin action [102]. The exercise-induced increase in insulin effect is predominantly located in the recruited muscles and reflects local contraction-dependent mechanisms [102]. The enhancing effect of acute exercise, to a large extent, reflects muscle glycogen depletion and accompanying glycogen synthase activation, and includes an increase in insulin sensitivity of muscle glucose transport [102]. With increasing habitual physical activity level the muscle GLUT-4 content increases and so does insulin responsiveness of glucose transport [102]. Also muscle capillarization increases, and these changes may to some extent reflect conversion of muscle fibers from type II B/X to type II A and perhaps further on to type I [102]. The content of key enzymes in glucose storage and metabolism too increases with level of physical activity in muscles [102, 108]. The mentioned changes explain that muscle glucose extraction during insulin stimulation varies directly with activity level [102]. Because the ability of insulin to stimulate muscle blood flow also increases with activity level, insulin-mediated glucose uptake in muscle must vary directly with level of habitual activity [102]. After acute exercise glucose taken up in muscle is predominantly subjected to storage as glycogen while glycolysis is diminished [102]. In contrast, in the trained as well as in the inactive state, insulin-mediated glycogen storage and glycolysis essentially vary in parallel [57, 102].

Exercise may also enhance insulin action in extramuscular tissues. The hepatic glucose storage capacity is increased by training [102]. Furthermore, in trained subjects the suppressive effect of insulin on hepatic glucose production is increased, probably reflecting an effect of the last exercise bout [102, 108]. The suppressive action of insulin on pancreatic secretion of insulin and glucagon may also be enhanced by exercise, making it difficult to tell whether exercise-induced changes in hepatic sensitivity to insulin are direct or secondary to changes in glucagon secretion [102]. In line with the view that the insulin-sparing effect of training is more pronounced in peripheral tissues than in liver, studies carried out during ordinary living conditions have shown that a relatively smaller fraction of secreted insulin is delivered to "posthepatic" tissues in athletes, compared to healthy subjects [102]. This finding also points at a higher hepatic insulin extraction after training [102]. Microdialysis studies have shown that training enhances insulin-mediated glucose uptake in human subcutaneous adipose tissue [109], and studies in rats have shown a similar effect in several intra-abdominal adipose tissues [110]. In line with these findings, in adipocytes insulin-mediated glucose transport as well as GLUT-4 mRNA and protein are increased by training [102]. While such effects are not elicited by a single bout of exercise, insulin-mediated suppression of lipolysis is enhanced by both acute exercise and training [102, 109]. Training decreases basal concentrations of triglyceride, total cholesterol, and LDL cholesterol, in plasma, and increases the HDL fraction of total cholesterol [111]. Postprandial lipidemia is also reduced by both acute exercise and training. The effect of training probably reflects increased lipoprotein lipase activity in muscle [102, 112]. In addition to enhancing the effect of insulin on carbohydrate and fat metabolism, physical activity also enhances the protein anabolic effect of insulin in human muscle [102, 113, 114].

The insulin secretory capacity is not changed by a single bout of dynamic exercise [102], but otherwise an inverse relationship between glucose-stimulated pancreatic β-cell secretion and insulin sensitivity is seen over the whole range of physical activity levels, from inactivity during bedrest to elite training [102]. The training-induced decrease in insulin secretion capacity reflects adaptations within the β-cells, including increased glucose metabolism [102], but the mechanism for the development of the adaptations is not known. The training-induced reduction in insulin and C-peptide responses may be more pronounced during oral compared with intravenous glucose testing, a fact that may be due to diminished glucose-induced incretin secretion from the gut after exercise and training [102]. Comparison between trained, detrained, and untrained subjects has revealed that the training-induced decrease in β-cell secretory capacity may very accurately match the accompanying increase in insulin action, because during hyperglycemic clamping glucose disposal was identical in the groups despite widely differing plasma insulin concentrations [102]. However, upon extreme athletic training oral glucose tolerance is better than that in untrained subjects, indicating that enhancement of insulin action is not fully compensated by reduced β-cell function [102]. In the athletes the sparing of insulin secretion and reduction in plasma glucose concentration are only relative to food intake; during 24 h trained subjects have, compared with untrained subjects, the same overall insulin secretion and average plasma glucose concentration in the face of a higher food intake, and they also have similar blood HbA_{1C} concentrations [102]. Accordingly, the predominant health benefit of the adaptations in pancreas and insulin-sensitive tissues, resulting from intense training, is that the adaptations allow the necessary increase in food intake without potentially harmful hyperglycemia and overloading of β-cells. To this may be added lowering of arterial insulin concentrations in consequence of the training-induced increase in hepatic insulin extraction [102]. In the other end of the activity spectrum insulin secretion and action, respectively, are also not well matched. Thus, during bedrest glucose tolerance deteriorates and glucose disposal is diminished in the face of augmented insulinemia during hyperglycemic clamping, illustrating that reduction in insulin sensitivity is not fully overcome by enhancement of glucose-stimulated insulin secretion [102]. This indicates that a minimal level of physical activity is necessary for normal glucose homeostasis. In this context it should be noted that adaptations in insulin secretion and action develop rapidly upon an increase in habitual physical activity, but the adaptations disappear within less than 2 weeks, if the altered lifestyle is not upheld [102, 115]. The described relationships between physical activity and secretion and action of insulin also apply to old people [102, 115, 116]. Of note is the fact that the tendency for plasma insulin concentrations to increase with aging can be neutralized by a physically active lifestyle [115].

Adaptations to Training in Diabetic Patients

Type 1

If type 1 diabetic patients have a normal activity level and do not have long-term complications, they also have a normal oxidative capacity of skeletal muscle and normal physical work capacity [111]. However, their skeletal muscles are insulin resistant [111]. These patients generally respond to both endurance and strength training just as healthy subjects, e.g., by diminished heart rate and blood pressure during rest and exercise, and increased muscle force, respectively [38, 111, 117]. Insulin sensitivity increases and the activity of oxidative enzymes, glycogen synthase, and hexokinase increases in muscle [38, 75, 111, 118]. Also muscle capillarization increases but the increase may be less pronounced than in healthy subjects [38, 111]. A case report indicates that improvement in insulin sensitivity through physical training may help to induce and prolong remission at onset of type 1 diabetes [119]. However, after the honeymoon period a decrease in insulin requirements with training is not a universal finding, possibly because carbohydrate intake may increase [38, 111]. Since exercise makes diabetes more difficult to control, the daily fluctuations in blood glucose may increase, and the average plasma glucose concentration, which is reflected in the HbA_{1C} level, does not generally decline during training [38, 75, 111]. An improved glucoregulation is more likely to occur, if patients have been poorly controlled prior to training [111], probably because training then is accompanied by more attention to disease control [75]. However, type 1 diabetic patients who participate in competitive sports may even experience deterioration of glycemic control in spite of improvements in fitness [120]. This probably reflects an irregular schedule, high exercise intensities, and measures to avoid hypoglycemia in response to exercise, i.e. excessive reductions in insulin dose and excessive intake of carbohydrate. These patients also may not show increased insulin sensitivity [120]. Probably reflecting the variation seen in effect of training on metabolic homeostasis, some studies have, whereas other studies have not, found changes in plasma triglyceride and cholesterol levels upon training, similar to those seen in healthy subjects [38, 111].

Type 2

Patients with type 2 diabetes have a low $V_{O_2}max$, a low maximal peripheral O_2 extraction, and a reduced fraction of oxidative, highly insulin-responsive muscle fibers, compared with healthy subjects even when matched for levels of ambient activity [8, 108, 121, 122]. In agreement with this, also their nonobese, nondiabetic first-degree relatives have a low level of fitness and a high content of nonoxidative fibers in skeletal muscle [102, 123]. The myocardial phosphocreatine (PCr)/ATP ratio may be diminished in resting diabetic patients, while skeletal muscle PCr and pH decrease faster during exercise and recover more slowly afterwards [124].

In type 2 diabetic patients, $V_{O_2}max$ as well as the enzymatic potential for oxidation and fat combustion in muscle increase normally during endurance training [38, 111, 125, 126], whereas the increase in capillarization in muscle is impeded [38, 111]. Bedrest exacerbates the insulin resistance of obese individuals with preexisting impaired glucose tolerance [108]. Conversely, in the postabsorptive state a single bout of prolonged submaximal dynamic [127] or resistance [128] exercise improves whole-body insulin sensitivity in type 2 diabetic patients. The effect of dynamic exercise has been shown to be both in liver and peripheral tissues [127, 129]. Impairment of the activity of atypical protein kinase C in muscle is probably important for the reduced insulin-mediated glucose transport in type 2 diabetes, and this activity is increased by exercise [62]. In contrast to the response to submaximal exercise insulin sensitivity, in response to brief intense dynamic exercise, is reduced for the first 1–2 h postexercise but increased after 24 h [71]. Also in the postprandial state moderate exercise seems to increase insulin-mediated glucose disposal in the immediate postexercise period, but the effect does not persist during or after the next meal [72].

Regularly repeated exercise, i.e. training, may increase insulin sensitivity in elderly glucose-intolerant subjects [116], women with gestational diabetes [86], type 2 diabetic patients [125, 130], and their first-degree relatives [102] more than can be inferred from a single bout of exercise. However, the improvement may, in type 2 diabetic patients, be difficult to detect on the whole-body level [108, 131]. Studies in which type 2 diabetic patients had catheterization of leg vessels before and after bicycle training have shown that the effect of training is predominantly, but not entirely, due to an enhanced insulin-mediated glucose clearance in skeletal muscle [125] (Figure 7). The mechanisms include enhancement of the insulin-mediated increase in blood flow and glucose extraction in muscle [125]. The increase in extraction is in line with a training-induced increase in muscle GLUT-4 protein and mRNA [132]. The increase in glucose clearance reflects increases in both nonoxidative glycolysis and glucose storage [125]. Increases in fractional velocity of glycogen synthase and mRNA for this enzyme have been found after endurance training in diabetic muscle but total glycogen synthase, hexokinase, and lactate dehydrogenase activities were unaltered [125]. Interestingly, in type 2 diabetes patients this type of training may increase muscle glucose clearance to values seen in healthy untrained control subjects (Figure 7). It is of note, however, that training does not exactly revert the muscle defect in type 2 diabetes because training, at least partly, exerts its effect by enhancing blood flow and GLUT-4 concentrations, variables that are not subnormal in the untrained state. Furthermore, the improvement in insulin action on skeletal muscle are, in type 2 diabetic patients, lost within a week if training is discontinued [125]. Strength training has also been shown to increase insulin action on glucose clearance in skeletal muscle of type 2 diabetes patients [133]. The effect was independent of changes in muscle mass and reflected an enhanced insulin-mediated increase in muscle blood flow as well as increases in protein content of the insulin receptor, GLUT-4, protein kinase B α/β, and glycogen synthase.

In addition to the described effects that may be seen in weight-stable patients [125], training may increase diet-induced weight loss, and this occurrence may, in itself, increase insulin sensitivity [102, 134]. Regular exercise causes a preferential loss of intra-abdominal adipose tissue, and this correlates with improvement in insulin action

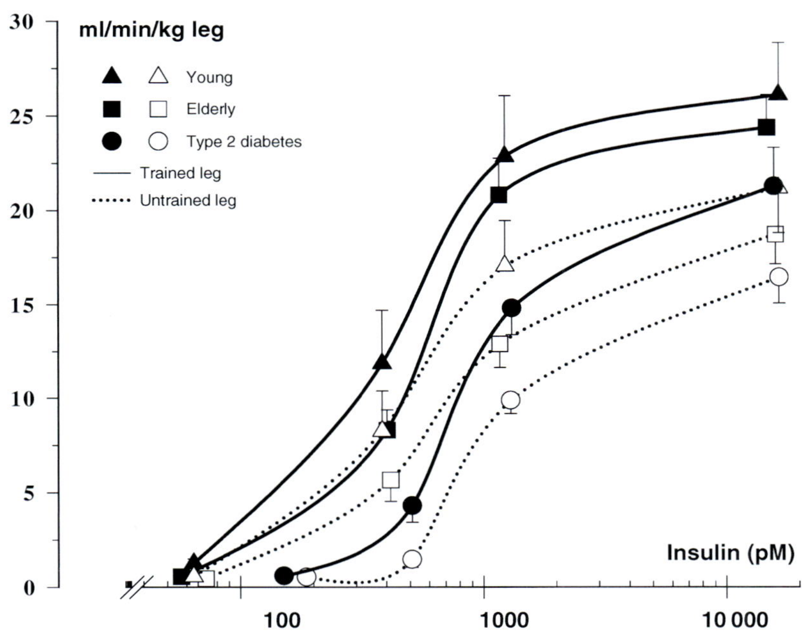

Figure 7 Insulin-mediated glucose clearance rates in trained and untrained legs in healthy young (23 years, $n = 7$) or elderly (59 years, $n = 8$) subjects, and in type 2 diabetic patients (58 years, $n = 7$). All subjects endurance trained one leg 30 min/day, 6 days/week for 10 weeks. Insulin was infused and glucose always clamped at the individual pretraining fasting concentration. Trained legs were studied 16 h after last exercise bout, at which time a preceding single exercise bout would have no effect in untrained legs. During insulin infusion glucose clearance was always higher in trained compared with untrained legs ($p < 0.05$) and always higher in control subjects compared with diabetic patients ($p < 0.05$). (Adapted from reference 102)

[130]. However, training *per se* does not generally result in lower body mass, a fact that may be explained by either changes in opposite directions of lean and fat body masses, respectively, reduced physical activity between training, periods, or increased food intake [135].

A training-induced reduction in glucose-stimulated β-cell secretion as seen in healthy subjects would appear less expedient in type 2 diabetes patients. However, some studies have, in fact, indicated improvement in β-cell function by training, in these patients [38, 102]. In a study using stimulation with hyperglycemic clamping and arginine bolus, increases in β-cell responses were seen in patients who prior to training had a moderate residual β-cell function, whereas no change was seen in patients with a low remaining secretory capacity [102]. One possible explanation might be that a diminished glucose stress resulting from an increase in target tissue insulin sensitivity might improve the secretory capacity of overloaded, yet recoverable, β-cells. However, in the mentioned hyperglycemic clamp study no change in insulin sensitivity and HbA_{1C} was seen. Interestingly, in agreement with the findings in humans, training has been shown to improve glucose-stimulated insulin secretion in rats made mildly or moderately diabetic by partial pancreatectomy, but training did not influence secretion in severely diabetic rats [136]. Also in that study other mechanisms than reduced glycemia apparently accounted for the positive β-cell adaptation to training [136].

The impact of the training-induced adaptations in both secretion and effect of insulin on glucose homeostasis during ordinary living conditions has been evaluated in a study in which type 2 diabetic patients had blood samples drawn around the clock. Areas under plasma concentration versus time curves were identical for glucose, while energy intake was at least as high after compared to that before training [102]. Integrated insulin and C-peptide levels were reduced after training, indicating that during physiological conditions insulin action is enhanced and insulin secretion spared by training [102]. The lack of change in integrated glucose levels is in accordance with the fact that a significant change in HbA_{1C} concentration is often not seen in training studies. However, meta-analyses have revealed that training may reduce HbA_{1C} by 0.66% [135], and that exercise intensity is a better predictor of improvement in HbA_{1C} than exercise volume is [126]. The improvement of glucose homeostasis by regular exercise may be more marked in younger patients with type 2 diabetes and in patients with short duration of disease [102].

A single bout of prolonged dynamic exercise reduces postprandial chylomicron triglyceridemia in type 2 diabetic patients. Furthermore, regular exercise has been shown to reduce fasting triglyceride concentrations in these patients, whereas total cholesterol and its subfractions are not consistently changed [8, 38, 131, 137, 138].

BENEFITS, RISKS, AND PRECAUTIONS ASSOCIATED WITH EXERCISE IN DIABETES

Benefits

In type 2 diabetes, training may improve overall glycemic control as indicated by a fall in HbA_{1C} concentration that should be sufficient to markedly reduce the risk of diabetic complications and death [135]. The underlying mechanism is a training-induced increase in insulin sensitivity, which is accompanied by beneficial relief of overloaded β-cells and diminished plasma insulin levels. Adding to the risk reduction, training also tends to favorably influence body fat [139], arterial blood pressure [140, 141], baroreflex sensitivity [142], endothelium-dependent vasodilation in both conduit and resistance vessels [143], skin blood flow [144], the heart rate × blood pressure product at rest and during exercise [139], hypertriglyceridemia, and fibrinolysis [140, 141, 145]. In line with these findings, cohort studies have in fact shown that in type 2 diabetic patients cardiovascular morbidity and mortality vary inversely with both physical fitness and level of physical activity and may be 50% lower in physically active compared with sedentary individuals [3, 5, 146].

In type 1 diabetic patients, exercise renders metabolic regulation difficult, and improvement of glycemic control should not be the aim of training [147]. However, endurance training has also been shown to improve vascular endothelial function in patients with type 1 diabetes [148]. Furthermore, both epidemiological prospective and retrospective studies indicate that in type 1 diabetic patients too regular physical activity protects against macrovascular as well as microvascular complications and increases life expectancy [4, 6, 148]. Additional proven benefits of regular physical activity are, in both types of diabetes, maintenance or improvement of aerobic exercise capacity and muscle strength and, accordingly, a better tolerance toward physical demands. Another benefit that has been shown in healthy subjects and that in all probability also applies to diabetic patients is protection against osteoporosis. Furthermore, it is a general experience that exercise and sports in diabetic patients, like in healthy subjects, may improve mental health (e.g. reducing depression and anxiety and enhancing well-being and self-esteem) and may promote social interaction and joy in a recreational environment [75, 149].

Metabolic Risks and Precautions

In type 1 diabetes patients the immediate risk inherent in exercise is development of hyperglycemia and ketosis or hypoglycemia. Both conditions will extend into the postexercise period. Hypoglycemia may even develop many hours after exercise, because enhancement of insulin sensitivity and replenishment of glycogen stores from plasma glucose may last more than 12 h [150, 151]. This means

Table 1 General advice to the physically active insulin-dependent diabetes patient

- Be educated in exercise physiology and diabetes
- Use frequent insulin injections or pump therapy
- Reduce insulin dose prior to significant exercise
- Monitor blood glucose
- Take extra carbohydrate before, during, or after exercise
- Always carry readily digested carbohydrate
- Have regular medical examinations
- Follow good exercise practice (e.g., regarding equipment, warm-up, technique, and hydration)
- Avoid extreme conditions or exercise with a healthy person

that particular caution has to be exerted when exercise is carried out in the evening. To meet these challenges the diabetic patient has to be in good metabolic control prior to exercise [8, 111]. Furthermore, the patient must imitate the normal response to exercise by reducing the insulin dose and/or increase the carbohydrate intake (Tables 1 and 2). The necessary adjustments depend on the exercise taken, the environment, and the individual, and accordingly, have to be individually tailored on the basis of frequent blood glucose measurements before, during, and after exercise. Extensive exercise should not be carried out earlier than 1–2 h after a main meal and accompanying insulin administration. The new, short-acting monomeric insulin analogues are absorbed faster than regular insulin, and accordingly, the risk of undesirable interaction between peak insulin concentrations and exercise is over soon after a meal if analogues are used, compared with regular insulin [152, 153]. The optimum insulin dosage depends on the intensity and duration of exercise, and less insulin is needed, if more energy is spent. In response to short-term strenuous exercise, transient hyperglycemia may develop in well-controlled type 1 diabetic patients [83]. If the diabetic patient is not aware of the passing nature of the hyperglycemia, the patient may be tempted to inject extra insulin and may, in turn, provoke hypoglycemia [154]. For a given amount of work, more insulin may be needed in the morning than in the evening. If the ambient temperature is high less insulin should be injected prior to exercise because absorption from the skin may be facilitated [154]. Neither in this nor in other situations can exercise-induced hypoglycemia be avoided by changing the insulin injection site [154].

Reductions in short-acting insulin dosage taken before exercise may amount to 30–80%, and postexercise reductions may also be necessary, e.g. to avoid nocturnal hypoglycemia [154, 155, 155]. Similarly, in order to perform long-term physical activity, patients treated with pump therapy may have to reduce the premeal insulin bolus by more than 50% and even to stop the basal infusion rate while exercising and to reduce it 25% for several hours afterwards [156, 157]. On the other hand, a necessary reduction in insulin dosage prior to less extensive exercise may cause a given meal taken after exercise to increase plasma glucose concentrations to more than those on nonexercise days when the full insulin dose is administered [38]. Accordingly, supplemental short-acting insulin may be required, particularly if food intake is increased after exercise. If before physical activity plasma glucose is below 5.5 mM extra, carbohydrate (e.g. a snack), should be eaten [8, 111]. It is also recommended that during exercise sessions of moderate intensity lasting more than 30 min, 15–25 g extra, readily absorbable carbohydrate should be taken by adult diabetic patients every 30 min [19]. Carbohydrate may be supplemented as 100 ml 5–8% sucrose solution every 10 min, whereby exercise-induced fluid losses too are substituted. After prolonged exhaustive exercise, 100–200 g additional carbohydrate may be needed to optimize glycogen repletion and prevent late hypoglycemia [111, 158]. Prevention of hypoglycemia by carbohydrate administration before, during, and after exercise may, particularly in youth, be more realistic than

Table 2 General guidelines for regulation of insulin-dependent diabetes in relation to exercise

Glucose

- Measure blood glucose before, during, and after exercise.
- If blood glucose is higher than 14 mM (250 mg/100 ml) measure ketones in urine and do not exercise in case of ketonuria.
- If blood glucose is higher than 16.5 mM (300 mg/100 ml) before exercise, be cautious even if no ketosis is present.
- If blood glucose is below 5.5 mM (100 mg/100 ml) ingest extra carbohydrate (e.g. 20 g) before exercise.
- Learn the glycemic response to various activity conditions.
- Remember that hypoglycemia may develop after exercise, e.g. during the night after evening exercise.

Insulin

- Reduce dose of short-acting (maybe also of intermediate- or long-acting) insulin before exercise.
- After exercise, supplemental insulin may be necessary, e.g. if meals are increased. However, after extensive exercise insulin dose may have to be reduced.

Diet

- Do not exercise until 1–2 h after a main meal.
- Take 15–25 g extra carbohydrate/30 min exercise before unplanned postprandial exercise, when it is too late to reduce insulin.
- Always carry readily digestible carbohydrate in case of hypoglycemia.

Note: Exact prescriptions cannot be given because of variation depending on the individual, the physical activity, and the environment.

adjustment of insulin dose, because activities may be spontaneous and of unforeseeable intensity and duration [75]. The total amount of carbohydrate ingested should match the carbohydrate expenditure [80], and tables exist with estimates of carbohydrate utilization during various activities in children of various body masses [75]. However, it is of note that people with type 1 diabetes tend to overeat with exercise [158].

As in type 1 diabetes patients, exercise should also be avoided in type 2 diabetes patients if metabolic control is poor [111]. However, alarming exercise-induced hyperglycemia and ketosis have not been observed in type 2 diabetes patients, and neither has exercise-induced hypoglycemia been noted in diabetic patients solely treated by diet [154]. If type 2 diabetes patients are treated with insulin they should take the same precautions as type 1 diabetes patients. Although frank hypoglycemia is rare, also for patients treated with oral hypoglycemic agents, antidiabetic medication, extent of exercise, and food intake should in principle be mutually adjusted [70]. This means that on exercise days the dosage of the drug may have to be reduced. Because weight loss usually is desirable in these patients, carbohydrate supplement is less expedient.

Long-term Complications

In both type 1 and type 2 diabetes patients the presence of long-term complications is of special concern. If the patient has coronary artery disease he or she should, just as the nondiabetic patient, have a supervised graded exercise test with electrocardiographic and blood pressure monitoring (Table 3). During the test the threshold for possible development of ischemia, arrhythmia, left ventricular failure, or anginal equivalents as nausea, profound dyspnea, or undue fatigue is defined [159, 160]. Exercise programs at intensities below the critical threshold can then be prescribed. For example, in patients with angina, aerobic training should be carried out at a heart rate at least 10 beats per min lower than the ischemic threshold. The patient will then benefit with gradually increasing functional capacity.

Table 3 The American Diabetes Association's criteria for graded exercise testing with ECG and blood pressure measurement before increase in physical activity*

Age >35 years
Age >25 years and type 2 diabetes for more than 10 years, or type 1 diabetes for more than 15 years
Any additional risk factor for or overt coronary heart disease
Peripheral arteriosclerosis
Proliferative retinopathy or nephropathy including microalbuminuria
Autonomic neuropathy

* From reference 8.

Cardiac disease may also be present in patients with diabetes in the absence of coronary artery disease. Even in the absence of clinical signs of cardiac impairment, left ventricular function may be impaired during exercise in both type 1 and type 2 diabetic patients by mechanisms that are not well understood [159, 161]. On the other hand, the increase in arterial blood pressure in response to exercise may be exaggerated in diabetic patients [159, 162] and, in particular, in hypertensive diabetic patients [163]. So, in hypertensive diabetic patients the blood pressure response to exercise should be monitored initially, and adjustments in therapy should be made accordingly. For hypertensive diabetic patients as well as for diabetic patients with stable coronary artery disease, dynamic, aerobic activity of 50–75% $\dot{V}O_2max$ is recommended, whereas high-intensity activities known to elicit high increases in blood pressure, e.g. heavy resistance exercises involving breath-holding, should be minimized [159].

Autonomic neuropathy is associated with increased mortality from myocardial infarction and sudden death, and it may be a marker for clinically unrecognized cardiac disease [159]. Thus, silent ischemia upon exertion is more frequent in this condition because the anginal perceptual threshold may be increased in the presence of autonomic neuropathy [164, 165]. Also diabetic cardiomyopathy with impaired left ventricular function at rest and during exercise is closely associated with cardiovascular autonomic neuropathy [166]. And so is prolonged QT interval in the electrocardiogram, and this predisposes to ventricular arrhythmias [167]. Because of the risk of an adverse cardiovascular event during exercise, a supervised graded exercise test is recommended prior to initiation of training programs in diabetic patients with autonomic neuropathy [8, 167]. It should always be remembered that because of impaired heart rate response, in these patients rate of perceived exertion is a safer guide for exercise intensity than is heart rate [167]. If the patients have orthostatic hypotension, which may be present in the absence of symptoms at rest, they may benefit from body stockings to increase venous return during exercise, and they will need long warm-up and cool-down periods of low-intensity exercise in relation to training sessions [159]. Another problem for patients with autonomic neuropathy may be reduced hypoglycemia awareness [167]. They may also have gastroparesis, which may delay the intestinal absorption of ingested carbohydrate. So, more careful glucose monitoring is appropriate in relation to exercise. These patients may also have difficulties in thermoregulation and be prone to dehydration and electrolyte disturbances. For these reasons they are generally advised to avoid exercise in hot or cold environments and to be vigilant about adequate hydration [8, 111, 167]. Taken together, diabetic patients with autonomic neuropathy need extensive examination prior to embarking on an exercise program, and subsequently progression should be slow and carefully monitored.

Autonomic neuropathy may be accompanied by anhidrosis of the lower body, resulting in dry, brittle skin that cracks easily. The tendency to fissures may be supported by compromised cutaneous vasomotion [167]. Also somatic neuropathy favors ulcer formation. Loss of protective sensation plays a major role allowing repeated trauma, the feet being in particular danger. However, motor neuropathy may also contribute by inducing interosseous muscle atrophy and, in turn, foot deformities [167, 168]. Ulcers become easily infected because of poor antimicrobial defense mechanisms in diabetic patients, and their healing may also be impeded by peripheral atherosclerosis, which is frequently present in these patients. Leg muscle atrophy secondary to motor neuropathy as well as reduced proprioception and ensuing reduced reflex stabilization and coordination of movements predispose to traumatic injuries. In addition to ulceration such injuries may provoke a Charcot foot (neuroarthropathy) and, in turn, osteopenia predisposing to fractures of the small bones in the foot [167, 169, 170]. In order to avoid the potential, serious consequences of peripheral neuropathy, e.g. amputation, the diabetic patient suffering from this condition should inspect his or her feet daily for calluses, blisters, cuts, and scratches. Furthermore, the patient should keep up good foot hygiene, avoid wet feet, and use polyester or cotton socks and comfortable shoes with good pressure absorption. Repetitive weight-bearing exercises, e.g. prolonged walking and jogging, should be avoided, and instead swimming or bicycling—on a stationary bicycle in case of severely impaired coordination—can be recommended [8, 168]. In addition to metabolic neuropathy, diabetes predisposes to nerve entrapment syndromes, e.g. including the medial or lateral plantar nerves or the median nerve in the carpal tunnel, and these syndromes also warrant exercise restrictions [167].

The potential acute ocular complications of exercise in diabetic retinopathy are intraretinal, preretinal, or vitreous hemorrhage from damaged retinal capillaries or fragile new vessels, as well as retinal detachment due to bleeding or traction mediated by newly formed fibrous tissue [8, 171]. Such events might be provoked by increases in arterial pressure in vascular beds with poor autoregulation and/or increases in venous pressure and by trauma, respectively. Furthermore, an exercise-induced increase in GH secretion has been speculated to contribute to development of diabetic retinopathy [171]. In agreement with this hypothesis, it has been found that GH rose during exercise in diabetic patients with retinopathy but not in those without retinopathy [172]. However, that difference may simply reflect that the former group was more heavily strained than the latter, because workloads were not adjusted to individual exercise capacities, which may very well have been lower in patients with retinopathy compared to those without [173, 174]. Anyhow, the best available studies indicate that at least exercise of moderate activity does not worsen diabetic retinopathy [111, 175, 176]. In both type 1 and type 2 diabetes, retinopathy is associated with impaired cardiac performance and reduced exercise capacity [173, 174], and also abnormal autoregulation of ophthalmic circulation during exercise has been described in diabetic patients [177]. However, studies of people with diabetic retinopathy have shown cardiovascular improvement with moderate physical training [178]. With appropriate hemodynamic and glucose monitoring, patients with diabetic retinopathy, who have regular eye examinations by a retinal specialist, can exercise safely [171]. According to a conservative estimate an acceptable maximum systolic blood pressure during exercise is 200 mmHg [171]. In case of untreated proliferative or very severe nonproliferative retinopathy severe exercise, e.g. including breath holding, pounding, or jarring, and activities that lower the head below waist level, should be avoided [8, 171]. Acceptable activities would be swimming, bicycling, and walking. Patients whose retinopathy has been adequately treated with laser therapy can probably undertake even strenuous exercise 6 weeks later, without undue risk.

In both type 1 and type 2 diabetic patients exercise may provoke transient microalbuminuria, and if abnormal albumin excretion is present at rest, exercise increases the albuminuria because of increased glomerular permeability [179, 180]. Exercise-induced increases in albumin excretion correlates with exercise-induced increases in systolic blood pressure, and the latter may be exaggerated in diabetic patients [162, 181]. The exercise-induced increase in albumin excretion can be ameliorated by both antihypertensive medical treatment and good metabolic control [180, 182]. It is a matter of concern whether diabetic patients, who exercise regularly and thus have more exercise-induced albuminuria and blood pressure increases, run a risk of more rapid progression of nephropathy. However, comparisons between diabetic patients with different activity levels do not confirm this suspicion [183]. Although no permanent adverse effects have been documented, diabetic patients with microalbuminuria or overt albuminuria are nevertheless often dissuaded from strenuous physical activity [8, 111, 180]. Prior to embarking on a moderate to high-intensity physical activity program these patients should be examined for macro- and microvascular disease, including a graded exercise test with blood pressure monitoring; and those who suffer from hypertension should be well treated for this disease. In end-stage renal disease, probably reflecting chronic uremia, inactivity, and accompanying autonomic neuropathy and heart disease, the aerobic exercise capacity is markedly reduced because of both reductions in oxygen carrying capacity of the blood (diminished maximal cardiac output and hemoglobin concentration) and in oxygen extraction by muscle [184, 185]. Also muscle strength is reduced [186, 187]. The influence of uremia is illustrated by the fact that kidney transplantation leads to increases in hemoglobin and aerobic capacity [185]. Patients with end-stage renal disease can benefit from training, which may take place either on off-dialysis days or during hemodialysis [188]. The latter option offers a number of advantages, such as improved compliance to exercise, monitoring of potassium and glucose concentrations, and less muscle cramping and hypotensive episodes during dialysis. Patients treated by continuous ambulatory peritoneal dialysis have also been successfully trained [189]. Before initiation of an exercise program diabetic patients with end-stage renal disease should be screened for macro- and microvascular disease, the examination including a supervised graded exercise test [188]. Because of their susceptibility to fluid and electrolyte disturbances these patients are advised to avoid exercising in extreme environmental conditions [188].

Other Conditions Requiring Special Precautions

Type 2 diabetic patients are mostly overweight and, accordingly, more prone to overload injuries. Degenerative joint disease is more common in these patients. For these reasons, swimming, bicycling, rowing, and walking are preferable to pounding weight-bearing exercise as jogging. During pregnancy the diabetic woman must abstain from more than mild exercise or even be prescribed bedrest if she develops medical complications as hypertension or albuminuria or obstetrical complications, e.g., those resulting in vaginal bleeding or evidence of intrauterine growth retardation [84, 190]. Stroke and amputation are common disabling conditions in diabetic individuals. Rehabilitation requires therapeutic exercise, during which caution should be exerted because of the high risk of concurring diabetic long-term complications [191]. Age and duration of diabetes are independent criteria for supervised graded exercise testing of diabetic patients prior to training, because these variables are related to the risk of unrecognized cardiovascular disease (Table 3) [8]. Finally, it has to be remembered that particularly older diabetic patients often take other drugs than insulin or oral hypoglycemic agents, and that these drugs may cause alterations in the metabolic and cardiovascular response to exercise and potentially limit physical performance [192]. For instance, β-adrenergic antagonists tend to reduce cardiac output and muscle blood flow and also promote development of hypoglycemia while masking the symptoms of this.

GUIDELINES FOR TRAINING IN DIABETES

For both type 1 and type 2 diabetic patients physical activity is accompanied by gains as well as risks. The physical hazards are generally higher and the metabolic profit lower in the type 1 than in the type 2 diabetic patients. On the other hand, the level of physical activity desirable for psychological and social reasons is higher for type 1 diabetic patients because they are younger. Before increasing usual patterns of physical activity all diabetes patients should undergo a medical evaluation consisting of a careful medical history and a physical examination focusing on symptoms and signs of disease affecting the heart and blood vessels, eyes, kidneys, feet, and the autonomic and peripheral somatic nervous systems. If the diabetic patient is older than 35 years, or has had the disease for more than 10 years (type 2 diabetic patients) or 15 years (type 1 diabetic patients), or has complications or any additional risk factor for coronary artery disease, he or she should also be subjected to a graded exercise test including ECG and blood pressure measurements (Table 3) [8]. Identification of areas of concern will allow appropriate treatment as well as individualized exercise prescription, minimizing risk to the patient. As the disease is not stationary, the diabetic patient ought to see the doctor regularly.

Particularly for the type 1 diabetic patient, who wants to be physically active, it is of utmost importance that he or she—or the parents if the diabetic patient is a child—has a sound knowledge of the disease with a profound understanding of the interaction between food, insulin, and exercise in the regulation of the plasma glucose concentration (Table 1). The patients should be taught how normal persons respond to exercise and how they differ from normal persons. Such knowledge will enable the diabetic patient to attempt to imitate the normal response by reducing the insulin dose prior to exercise, and/or to take extra carbohydrate. However, the patients should also be aware of the fact that the effect of exercise on glucose homeostasis during and after exercise is not accurately predictable and may differ between and even within subjects [193, 194]. This underlines the necessity of frequent blood glucose measurements as well as the need for readily available carbohydrate snacks. Furthermore, the diabetic patient should carry written information about him- or herself and his/her condition. It will appear that it is not possible to give exact recommendations on how to adjust insulin and diet for exercises that are broadly applicable. The diabetic patient must also individually tailor his or her regimen on the basis of experience. Combination of frequent blood glucose monitoring with multiple short-acting insulin injections or, even better, with insulin pump treatment offers the highest flexibility in relation to engaging in unplanned exercise, and the best glucose control. Provided that the patients have been properly educated, intensified insulin therapy is not accompanied by a high risk of exercise-induced hypoglycemia [195, 196]. Some rules are generally agreed upon [8]; if, before exercise, blood glucose is below 5.5 mM, then extra carbohydrate should be taken before initiation of exercise. If, conversely, blood glucose is above 14 mM urine ketones should be measured, and if they are positive insulin should be taken and exercise delayed until ketones are negative. Even if ketones are negative, caution must be exerted if blood glucose is higher than 16.5 mM (Table 2).

The best glucose control is achieved if exercise is fitted into a regular lifestyle in which insulin, food, and exercise are elements of a fixed schedule with the amount and timing of the components carefully adjusted. However, the more diabetic patients know about their disease, and the more familiar they become with their responses to exercise through blood glucose measurements, the greater a variation in physical activity from day to day they will be able to handle. From a medical point of view the recommended goal would be at least 30 min of exercise a day. For endurance-type exercises moderate intensity corresponding to 50–75% of individual maximum aerobic capacity (%$\dot{V}O_2$max, relative workload) is generally recommended. In subjects with a normal heart rate regulation, the relative workload can be estimated as (actual heart rate − resting heart rate) × 100/(maximum heart rate–resting heart rate). If the individual maximum heart rate is not known, it can be roughly estimated as 220 − age. Alternatively, perceived exertion may be evaluated from a scale ranging from 6 (*very mild*) to 20 (*extremely heavy*), and relative load be calculated as (actual level of exertion − 6) × 100/14. It is of note that exercise does not have to be strenuous; even regular walking has beneficial effects, e.g. on cardiovascular health [146, 197]. Much evidence indicates that the overall energy expenditure is more important than exercise intensity when it comes to health benefits [146, 197–199]. Within recent years it has been realized that resistance exercises with advantage can also be included, e.g. two times a week, in the training program of diabetic patients [116, 139, 200]. All the various skeletal muscle groups of the body may be engaged by this means. Just as for endurance exercises, the intensity of resistance exercises can be varied according to the fitness and health status of the diabetic patient, and responses to exercise can be monitored. Excessive blood pressure increases can be avoided by omitting any breath holding. In both type 1 and type 2 diabetic patients, strength training has been shown to elicit beneficial effects on insulin sensitivity and HbA_{1C} levels, similar to those seen with endurance exercise [117, 133, 135, 141, 201–203]. In addition, resistance training serves to maintain or improve muscle mass and strength, which is important, e.g. with aging [116, 202, 204, 205].

From analysis of the diabetic patients condition and the demands of exercise it is possible to predict the extent of a given physical activity the patient will be able to tolerate. Diabetic patients in good metabolic control and without long-term complications can exercise on equal terms with healthy subjects. Adjustment of the therapeutic regimen will allow safe participation in all forms of physical activity even during changing daily schedules and preferences. The fact that personal preferences can be complied with is important for maintenance of a physically active lifestyle. Activities that are felt enjoyable, varied, convenient in time and location, and that offer appreciable gains, are supervised and free, and can be performed in groups are likely to be associated with the best compliance. An exercise consultation combining motivational theory and cognitive behavioral strategies also promotes an increase in physical activity [206]. Appropriate exercise options for diabetic patients with long-term complications are suggested above, and are described in more detail elsewhere [176]. For all kinds of training, in order to prevent musculoskeletal injuries and dropout for other reasons too, progression in exercise intensity and duration should be slow, and each training session should begin and end with muscle stretching and contractions of low intensity. Furthermore, optimum equipment (e.g. shoes) should be used. Exercise that markedly increases cardiac output should be avoided in the incubation and fever phases of infectious diseases, and caution should also be exerted in other acute or unstable chronic medical disorders. In case of unusual sensations (e.g. chest pain) exercise must be interrupted.

It is comforting, reassuring, and motivating for the diabetic patients to know that other patients meet the same troubles as him/her and that the disease does not necessarily restrain desired activities. In this context, the existence of summer camps, where diabetic children meet, play, and learn to handle their disease, should be remembered. Sharing of experiences among physically active people with diabetes may also take place through organizations like the Diabetes Exercise and Sport Association (DESA, www.diabetes-exercise.org), the mission of which is to enhance the quality of life for people with diabetes, through exercise. Diabetic patients are involved in all kinds of sports, e.g. marathon running [207], competitive cross-country skiing [208], scuba diving [209], and mountain climbing [210], even at the professional level. There are examples from the past of diabetic athletes, who have become Olympic gold medalists and world champions [211, 212], and todays knowledge and technology within diabetes care allow this to become a more frequent event.

EXERCISE IN THE PREVENTION OF DIABETES

Notwithstanding the therapeutic effect of exercise in patients who have developed diabetes, exercise may be particularly efficacious if instituted earlier in life. This supposition is in line with the fact that in experimental studies physical activity increases insulin sensitivity and improves glucose tolerance in both healthy subjects and in people with obesity, gestational diabetes, and impaired glucose tolerance as well as in first-degree relatives of patients with type 2 diabetes. More support for the ability of exercise to prevent type 2 diabetes has come from a multitude of descriptive studies of societies undergoing a transition from traditional lifestyle patterns to more Westernized patterns, examinations of migrants from traditional to more urbanized environments and vice versa, comparisons of active rural versus more sedentary urban populations, case-control studies, retrospective cohort studies, and prospective studies of active compared with sedentary individuals [38, 108, 213]. The most powerful evidence has been provided by one nonrandomized [214] and three randomized [1, 215, 216], controlled interventional epidemiological studies. According to these studies the risk of getting type 2 diabetes within a 6-year period can be reduced by at least 40% with an active compared with a sedentary lifestyle. Weight loss is not necessary for a beneficial effect of exercise, and an effect can be obtained by mild or moderate exercise, the effect depending on overall energy expenditure rather than on intensity of exercise [197]. The most marked benefit of exercise in diabetes prevention has been observed in people with obesity or a family history of diabetes [217]. So, obvious target populations for training programs would be people at increased risk of type 2 diabetes, e.g. first-degree relatives, women with gestational diabetes, people with low birth weight or visceral obesity, and certain ethnic groups.

REFERENCES

1. Knowler WC, Barrett-Connor E, Fowler SE, Hamman RF, Lachin JM, Walker EA, Nathan DM. Reduction in the incidence of type 2 diabetes with lifestyle intervention or metformin. *N Engl J Med* 2002; 346: 393–403.
2. US Department of Health and Human Services. *Physical Activity and Health: A Report of the Surgeon General*. Centers for Disease Control and Prevention, National Center for Chronic Disease Prevention and Health Promotion, 1996.
3. Hu FB, Stampfer MJ, Solomon C, Liu S, Colditz GA, Speizer FE, Willett WC, Manson JE. Physical activity and risk for cardiovascular events in diabetic women. *Ann Intern Med* 2001; 134: 96–105.
4. Kriska AM, LaPorte RE, Patrick SL, Kuller LH, Orchard TJ. The association of physical activity and diabetic complications in individuals with insulin-dependent diabetes mellitus: the Epidemiology of Diabetes Complications Study – VII. *J Clin Epidemiol* 1991; 44: 1207–14.
5. Wei M, Gibbons LW, Kampert JB, Nichaman MZ, Blair SN. Low cardiorespiratory fitness and physical inactivity as predictors of mortality in men with type 2 diabetes. *Ann Intern Med* 2000; 132: 605–11.
6. Moy CS, Songer TJ, LaPorte RE, Dorman JS, Kriska AM, Orchard TJ, Becker DJ, Drash AL. Insulin-dependent diabetes mellitus, physical activity, and death. *Am J Epidemiol* 1993; 137: 74–81.
7. Sherwin RS, Anderson RM, Buse JB, Chin MH, Eddy D, Fradkin J, Ganiats TG, Ginsberg H, Kahn R, Nwankwo R, Rewers M, Schlessinger L, Stern M, Vinicor F, Zinman B. The prevention or delay of type 2 diabetes. *Diabetes Care* 2003; 26 (suppl 1): S62–9.
8. Zinman B, Ruderman N, Campaigne BN, Devlin JT, Schneider SH. Physical activity/exercise and diabetes mellitus. *Diabetes Care* 2003; 26 (suppl 1): S73–7.
9. Albright A, Franz M, Hornsby G, Kriska A, Marrero D, Ullrich I, Verity LS. for the American College of Sports Medicine position stand. Exercise and type 2 diabetes. *Med Sci Sports Exerc* 2000; 32: 1345–60.
10. American College of Sports Medicine and American Diabetes Association joint position statement. Diabetes mellitus and exercise. *Med Sci Sports Exerc* 1997; 29: i–vi.
11. Galbo H. *Hormonal and Metabolic Adaptation to Exercise*. New York: Georg Thieme, 1983.
12. Kjaer M, Farrell P, Christensen N, Galbo H. Increased epinephrine response and inaccurate glucoregulation in exercising athletes. *J Appl Physiol* 1986; 61: 1693–1700.
13. Felig P, Cherif A, Minagawa A, Wahren J. Hypoglycemia during prolonged exercise in normal men. *N Engl J Med* 1982; 306: 895–900.
14. Galbo H, Holst J, Christensen NJ. The effect of different diets and of insulin on the hormonal response to prolonged exercise. *Acta Physiol Scand* 1979; 107: 19–32.
15. Wojtaszewski JF, MacDonald C, Nielsen JN, Hellsten Y, Hardie DG, Kemp BE, Kiens B, Richter EA. Regulation of 5′AMP-activated protein kinase activity and substrate utilization in exercising human skeletal muscle. *Am J Physiol Endocrinol Metab* 2003; 284: E813–22.
16. Galbo H. Integrated endocrine responses and exercise. In De Groot LJ (ed), *Endocrinology*, 3rd edn. Philadelphia: Saunders, 1995; pp 2692–701.
17. Pirnay F, Crielaard J, Pallikarakis N, Lacroix M, Mosora F. Fate of exogenous glucose during exercise of different intensities in humans. *J Appl Physiol* 1982; 53: 1620–4.
18. Rehrer NJ, Wagenmakers AJM, Beckers EJ, Halliday D, Leiper JB, Brouns F, Maughan RJ, Westerterp K, Saris WHM. Gastric emptying, absorption and carbohydrate oxidation during prolonged exercise. *J Appl Physiol* 1992; 72: 468–75.
19. Ramires PR, Forjaz CL, Strunz CM, Silva ME, Diament J, Nicolau W, Liberman B, Negrao CE. Oral glucose ingestion increases endurance capacity in normal and diabetic (type I) humans. *J Appl Physiol* 1997; 83: 608–14.
20. Wasserman DH, Spalding JA, Lacy DB, Colburn CA, Goldstein RE, Cherrington AD. Glucagon is a primary controller of hepatic glycogenolysis and gluconeogenesis during muscular work. *Am J Physiol* 1989; 257: E108–17.
21. Wiersma MM, Vissing J, Mikines KJ, Steffens AB, Galbo H. Effect of liver denervation on glucose production during running in guinea pigs. *Am J Physiol* 1995; 268: R72–7.
22. Kjaer M, Keiding S, Engfred K, Rasmussen K, Sonne B, Kirkegård P, Galbo H. Glucose homeostasis during exercise in humans with a liver or kidney transplant. *Am J Physiol* 1995; 268: E636–44.
23. Kjaer M, Engfred K, Fernandes A, Secher NH, Galbo H. Regulation of hepatic glucose production during exercise in humans: role of sympathoadrenergic activity. *Am J Physiol* 1993; 265: E257–83.
24. Howlett K, Galbo H, Lorentsen J, Bergeron R, Zimmerman-Belsing T, Bulow J, Feldt-Rasmussen U, Kjaer M. Effect of adrenaline on glucose kinetics during exercise in adrenalectomised humans. *J Physiol* 1999; 519: 911–21.

25. Bergeron R, Kjaer M, Simonsen L, Bulow J, Skovgaard D, Howlett K, Galbo H. Splanchnic blood flow and hepatic glucose production in exercising humans: role of renin–angiotensin system. *Am J Physiol Regul Integr Comp Physiol* 2001; 281: R1854–61.
26. Ploug T, Galbo H, Richter EA. Increased muscle glucose uptake during contractions: no need for insulin. *Am J Physiol* 1984; 247: E726–31.
27. Richter EA, Ploug T, Galbo H. Increased muscle glucose uptake after exercise. *Diabetes* 1985; 34: 1041–8.
28. Ihlemann J, Ploug T, Hellsten Y, Galbo H. Effect of stimulation frequency on contraction-induced glucose transport in rat skeletal muscle. *Am J Physiol Endocrinol Metab* 2000; 279: E862–7.
29. Ihlemann J, Ploug T, Hellsten Y, Galbo H. Effect of tension on contraction-induced glucose transport in rat skeletal muscle. *Am J Physiol* 1999; 277: E208–14.
30. Richter EA, Nielsen JN, Jorgensen SB, Frosig C, Wojtaszewski JF. Signalling to glucose transport in skeletal muscle during exercise. *Acta Physiol Scand* 2003; 178: 329–35.
31. Ploug T, Galbo H, Vinten J, Jørgensen M, Richter EA. Kinetics of glucose transport in rat muscle: effects of insulin and contractions. *Am J Physiol* 1987; 253: E12–20.
32. Ploug T, van Deurs B, Ai H, Cushman SW, Ralston E. Analysis of GLUT4 distribution in whole skeletal muscle fibers: identification of distinct storage compartments that are recruited by insulin and muscle contractions. *J Cell Biol* 1998; 142: 1429–46.
33. Han XX, Handberg A, Petersen LN, Ploug T, Galbo H. Stability of GLUT-1 and GLUT-4 expression in perfused rat muscle stimulated by insulin and exercise. *J Appl Physiol* 1995; 78: 46–52.
34. Richter EA, Ruderman NB, Gavras H, Belur ER, Galbo H. Muscle glycogenolysis during exercise: dual control by epinephrine and contractions. *Am J Physiol* 1982; 242: E25–32.
35. Stallknecht B, Lorentsen J, Enevoldsen LH, Bulow J, Biering-Sorensen F, Galbo H, Kjaer M. Role of the sympathoadrenergic system in adipose tissue metabolism during exercise in humans. *J Physiol* 2001; 536: 283–294.
36. Langfort J, Donsmark M, Ploug T, Holm C, Galbo H. Hormone-sensitive lipase in skeletal muscle: regulatory mechanisms. *Acta Physiol Scand* 2003; 178: 397–403.
37. Connet RJ, Sahlin K. Control of glycolysis and glycogen metabolism. In Rowell LB, Shepherd JT (eds), *Handbook of Physiology, Section 12: Exercise: Regulation and Integration of Multiple Systems*. New York: Oxford University Press, 1996; pp 870–911.
38. Galbo H. Exercise and diabetes. *Scand J Sports Sci* 1988; 10: 89–95.
39. Ronnemaa T, Koivisto VA. Combined effect of exercise and ambient temperature on insulin absorption and postprandial glycemia in type I patients. *Diabetes Care* 1988; 11: 769–73.
40. Zander E, Bruns W, Wulfert P, Besch W, Lubs D, Chlup R, Schulz B. Muscular exercise in type I-diabetics, I: Different metabolic reactions during heavy muscular work in dependence on actual insulin availability. *Exp Clin Endocrinol* 1983; 82: 78–90.
41. Wahren J, Sato Y, Ostman J, Hagenfeldt L, Felig P. Turnover and splanchnic metabolism of free fatty acids and ketones in insulin-dependent diabetics at rest and in response to exercise. *J Clin Invest* 1984; 73: 1367–76.
42. Bjorkman O. Fuel metabolism during exercise in normal and diabetic man. *Diabetes Metab Rev* 1986; 1: 319–57.
43. Standl E, Lotz N, Dexel Th, Janka H, Kolb H. Muscle triglycerides in diabetic subjects. *Diabetologia* 1980; 18: 463–9.
44. Raguso CA, Coggan AR, Gastaldelli A, Sidossis LS, Bastyr EJ III, Wolfe RR. Lipid and carbohydrate metabolism in IDDM during moderate and intense exercise. *Diabetes* 1995; 44: 1066–74.
45. Wahren J, Hagenfeldt L, Felig P. Splanchnic and leg exchange of glucose, amino acids and free fatty acids during exercise in diabetes mellitus. *J Clin Invest* 1975; 55: 1303–14.
46. Wasserman DH, Lavina H, Lickley A, Vranic M. Role of β-adrenergic mechanisms during exercise in poorly controlled diabetes. *J Appl Physiol* 1985; 59: 1282–9.
47. Simonson DC, Koivisto V, Sherwin RS, Ferrannini E, Hendler R, Juhlin-Dannfelt A, DeFronzo RA. Adrenergic blockade alters glucose kinetics during exercise in insulin-dependent diabetics. *J Clin Invest* 1984; 73: 1648–58.
48. Tuttle K, Marker J, Dalsky G, Schwartz N, Shah S. Glucagon, not insulin, may play a secondary role in defense against hypoglycemia during exercise. *Am J Physiol* 1988; 254: E713–9.
49. Bjorkman O, Milles P, Wasserman D, Lickley L, Vranic M. Regulation of glucose turnover during exercise in pancreatectomized, totally insulin-deficient dogs. *J Clin Invest* 1988; 81: 1759–67.
50. Schneider SH, Vitug A, Ananthakrishnan R, Khachadurian AK. Impaired adrenergic response to prolonged exercise in type I diabetes. *Metabolism* 1991; 40: 1219–25.
51. Kemmer FW, Berger M. Exercise and diabetes mellitus. Physical activity as part of daily life and its role in the treatment of diabetic patients. *Int J Sports Med* 1983; 4: 77–88.
52. Wasserman DH, Lickley HL, Vranic M. Important role of glucagon during exercise in diabetic dogs. *J Appl Physiol* 1985; 59: 1272–81.
53. Nelson JD, Poussier P, Marliss EB, Albisser AM, Zinman B. Metabolic response of normal man and insulin-infused diabetics to postprandial exercise. *Am J Physiol* 1982; 242: E309–16.
54. Poussier P, Zinman B, Marliss EB, Albisser AM, Perlman K, Caron D. Open-loop intravenous insulin waveforms for postprandial exercise in type I diabetes. *Diabetes Care* 1983; 6: 129–34.
55. Schiffrin A, Parikh S. Accommodating planned exercise in type I diabetic patients on intensive treatment. *Diabetes Care* 1985; 8: 337–42.
56. Vergauen L, Hespel P, Richter EA. Adenosine receptors mediate synergistic stimulation of glucose uptake and transport by insulin and by contractions in rat skeletal muscle. *J Clin Invest* 1994; 93: 974–81.
57. Dela F, Mikines KJ, Larsen JJ, Galbo H. Glucose clearance in aged trained skeletal muscle during maximal insulin with superimposed exercise. *J Appl Physiol* 1999; 87: 2059–67.
58. Galassetti P, Tate D, Neill RA, Morrey S, Wasserman DH, Davis SN. Effect of antecedent hypoglycemia on counterregulatory responses to subsequent euglycemic exercise in type 1 diabetes. *Diabetes* 2003; 52: 1761–9.
59. Brozinick JT Jr, Etgen GJ Jr, Yaspelkis BB III, Ivy JL. Contraction-activated glucose uptake is normal in

insulin-resistant muscle of the obese Zucker rat. *J Appl Physiol* 1992; 73: 382–87.

60. Kennedy JW, Hirshman MF, Gervino EV, Ocel JV, Forse RA, Hoenig SJ. Aronson D, Goodyear LJ, Horton ES. Acute exercise induces GLUT4 translocation in skeletal muscle of normal human subjects and subjects with type 2 diabetes. *Diabetes* 1999; 48: 1192–7.
61. Kingwell BA, Formosa M, Muhlmann M, Bradley SJ, McConell GK. Nitric oxide synthase inhibition reduces glucose uptake during exercise in individuals with type 2 diabetes more than in control subjects. *Diabetes* 2002; 51: 2572–80.
62. Beeson M, Sajan MP, Dizon M, Grebenev D, Gomez-Daspet J, Miura A, Kanoh Y, Powe J, Bandyopadhyay G, Standaert ML, Farese RV. Activation of protein kinase C-zeta by insulin and phosphatidylinositol-3,4,5-$(PO_4)_3$ is defective in muscle in type 2 diabetes and impaired glucose tolerance: amelioration by rosiglitazone and exercise. *Diabetes* 2003; 52: 1926–34.
63. Musi N, Fujii N, Hirshman MF, Ekberg I, Froberg S, Ljungqvist O, Thorell A, Goodyear LJ. AMP-activated protein kinase (AMPK) is activated in muscle of subjects with type 2 diabetes during exercise. *Diabetes* 2001; 50: 921–7.
64. Minuk HL, Vranic M, Marliss EB, Hanna AK, Albisser AM, Zinman B. Glucoregulatory and metabolic response to exercise in obese noninsulin-dependent diabetes. *Am J Physiol* 1981; 240: E458–64.
65. Koivisto VA, DeFronzo RA. Exercise in the treatment of type II diabetes. *Acta Endocrinol* 1984; 105: 107–11.
66. Giacca A, Groenewoud Y, Tsui E, McClean P, Zinman B. Glucose production, utilization, and cycling in response to moderate exercise in obese subjects with type 2 diabetes and mild hyperglycemia. *Diabetes* 1998; 47: 1763–70.
67. Kang J, Kelley DE, Robertson RJ, Goss FL, Suminski RR, Utter AC, DaSilva SG. Substrate utilization and glucose turnover during exercise of varying intensities in individuals with NIDDM. *Med Sci Sports Exerc* 1999; 31: 82–9.
68. Krotkiewski M, Gorski J. Effect of muscular exercise on plasma C-peptide and insulin in obese nondiabetics and diabetics, type II. *Clin Physiol* 1986; 6: 499–506.
69. Martin IK, Wahren J. Glucose metabolism during physical exercise in patients with noninsulin-dependent (type II) diabetes. *Adv Exp Med Biol* 1993; 334: 221–33.
70. Larsen JJ, Dela F, Madsbad S, Vibe-Petersen J, Galbo H. Interaction of sulfonylureas and exercise on glucose homeostasis in type 2 diabetic patients. *Diabetes Care* 1999; 22: 1647–54.
71. Kjaer M, Hollenbeck C, Frey-Hewitt B, Galbo H, Haskell W, Reaven G. Glucoregulation and hormonal responses to maximal exercise in non-insulin-dependent diabetes. *J Appl Physiol* 1990; 68: 2067–74.
72. Larsen JJ, Dela F, Kjaer M, Galbo H. The effect of moderate exercise on postprandial glucose homeostasis in NIDDM patients. *Diabetologia* 1997; 40: 447–53.
73. Poirier P, Mawhinney S, Grondin L, Tremblay A, Broderick T, Cleroux J, Catellier C, Tancrede G, Nadeau A. Prior meal enhances the plasma glucose lowering effect of exercise in type 2 diabetes. *Med Sci Sports Exerc* 2001; 33: 1259–64.
74. Larsen JJ, Dela F, Madsbad S, Galbo H. The effect of intense exercise on postprandial glucose homeostasis in type II diabetic patients. *Diabetologia* 1999; 42: 1282–92.
75. Riddell MC, Bar-Or O. Children and adolescents. In Ruderman NB, Devlin JT, Kriska A (eds), *Handbook of Exercise in Diabetes*. Alexandria, VA: American Diabetes Association, 2002; pp 547–67.
76. Temple MY, Bar-Or O, Riddell MC. The reliability and repeatability of the blood glucose response to prolonged exercise in adolescent boys with IDDM. *Diabetes Care* 1995; 18: 326–32.
77. Nurick MA, Johnson SB. Enhancing blood glucose awareness in adolescents and young adults with IDDM. *Diabetes Care* 1991; 14: 1–7.
78. Riddell MC, Bar-Or O, Gerstein HC, Heigenhauser GJ. Perceived exertion with glucose ingestion in adolescent males with IDDM. *Med Sci Sports Exerc* 2000; 32: 167–73.
79. Riddell MC, Bar-Or O, Hollidge-Horvat M, Schwarcz HP, Heigenhauser GJ. Glucose ingestion and substrate utilization during exercise in boys with IDDM. *J Appl Physiol* 2000; 88: 1239–46.
80. Riddell MC, Bar-Or O, Ayub BV, Calvert RE, Heigenhauser GJ. Glucose ingestion matched with total carbohydrate utilization attenuates hypoglycemia during exercise in adolescents with IDDM. *Int J Sport Nutr* 1999; 9: 24–34.
81. Tupola S, Rajantie J, Maenpaa J. Severe hypoglycaemia in children and adolescents during multiple-dose insulin therapy. *Diabet Med* 1998; 15: 695–9.
82. Yasar SA, Tulassay T, Madacsy L, Korner A, Szucs L, Nagy I, Szabo A, Miltenyi M. Sympathetic-adrenergic activity and acid-base regulation under acute physical stress in type I (insulin-dependent) diabetic children. *Horm Res* 1994; 42: 110–5.
83. Purdon C, Brousson M, Nyveen SL, Miles PD, Halter JB, Vranic M, Marliss EB. The roles of insulin and catecholamines in the glucoregulatory response during intense exercise and early recovery in insulin-dependent diabetic and control subjects. *J Clin Endocrinol Metab* 1993; 76: 566–73.
84. Bornstein K, Jovanovic L. Women and Exercise. In Ruderman NB, Devlin JT, Kriska A (eds), *Handbook of Exercise in Diabetes*. Alexandria, VA: American Diabetes Association, 2002; pp 511–32.
85. Bung P, Artal R, Khodiguian N, Kjos S. Exercise in gestational diabetes. An optional therapeutic approach? *Diabetes* 1991; 40 (suppl 2): 182–5.
86. Jovanovic-Peterson L, Durak EP, Peterson CM. Randomized trial of diet versus diet plus cardiovascular conditioning on glucose levels in gestational diabetes. *Am J Obstet Gynecol* 1989; 161: 415–9.
87. Avery MD, Walker AJ. Acute effect of exercise on blood glucose and insulin levels in women with gestational diabetes. *J Matern Fetal Med* 2001; 10: 52–8.
88. Hilsted J, Galbo H, Christensen NJ, Parving HH, Benn J. Haemodynamic changes during graded exercise in patients with diabetic autonomic neuropathy. *Diabetologia* 1982; 22: 318–23.
89. Hilsted J, Galbo H, Christensen NJ. Impaired cardiovascular responses to graded exercise in diabetic autonomic neuropathy. *Diabetes* 1979; 28: 313–9.
90. Bottini P, Tantucci C, Scionti L, Dottorini ML, Puxeddu E, Reboldi G, Bolli GB, Casucci G, Santeusanio F, Sorbini CA. Cardiovascular response to exercise in diabetic patients: influence of autonomic neuropathy of different severity. *Diabetologia* 1995; 38: 244–50.

91. Kahn JK, Zola B, Juni JE, Vinik AI. Decreased exercise heart rate and blood pressure response in diabetic subjects with cardiac autonomic neuropathy. *Diabetes Care* 1986; 9: 389–94.
92. Di Carli MF, Bianco-Batlles D, Landa ME, Kazmers A, Groehn H, Muzik O, Grunberger G. Effects of autonomic neuropathy on coronary blood flow in patients with diabetes mellitus. *Circulation* 1999; 100: 813–9.
93. Sobotka PA, Liss HP, Vinik AI. Impaired hypoxic ventilatory drive in diabetic patients with autonomic neuropathy. *J Clin Endocrinol Metab* 1986; 62: 658–63.
94. Tantucci C, Bottini P, Dottorini ML, Puxeddu E, Casucci G, Scionti L, Sorbini CA. Ventilatory response to exercise in diabetic subjects with autonomic neuropathy. *J Appl Physiol* 1996; 81: 1978–86.
95. Hilsted J, Galbo H, Tronier B, Christensen NJ, Schwartz TW. Hormonal and metabolic responses to exercise in insulin-dependent diabetics with and without autonomic neuropathy and in normal subjects. *Int J Sports Med* 1981; 2: 216–19.
96. Hilsted J, Galbo H, Christensen N. Impaired responses of catecholamines, groth hormone and cortisol to grades exercise in diabetic autonomic neuropathy. *Diabetes* 1980; 29: 257–62.
97. Bottini P, Boschetti E, Pampanelli S, Ciofetta M, Del Sindaco P, Scionti L, Brunetti P, Bolli GB. Contribution of autonomic neuropathy to reduced plasma adrenaline responses to hypoglycemia in IDDM: evidence for a nonselective defect. *Diabetes* 1997; 46: 814–23.
98. Hilsted J, Richter E, Madsbad S, Tronier B, Christensen NJ, Hildebrandt P, Damkjaer M, Galbo H. Metabolic and cardiovascular responses to epinephrine in diabetic autonomic neuropathy. *N Engl J Med* 1987; 317: 421–6.
99. Tuominen JA, Ebeling P, Bourey R, Koranyi L, Lamminen A, Rapola J, Sane T, Vuorinen-Markkola H, Koivisto VA. Postmarathon paradox: insulin resistance in the face of glycogen depletion. *Am J Physiol* 1996; 270: E336–43.
100. Asp S, Rohde T, Richter EA. Impaired muscle glycogen resynthesis after a competetive marathon race is not caused by decreased muscle GLUT4 content. *J Appl Physiol* 1997; 83: 1482–5.
101. Asp S, Daugaard JR, Kristiansen S, Kiens B, Richter EA. Eccentric exercise decreases maximal insulin action in humans: muscle and systemic effects. *J Physiol (Lond)* 1996; 494: 891–8.
102. Dela F, Mikines K, Galbo H. Physical activity and insulin resistance in man. In Reaven G, Laws A (eds), *Insulin Resistance: The Metabolic Syndrome X*. Totowa, NJ: Humana Press 1999; pp 97–120.
103. Asp S, Daugaard JR, Richter EA. Eccentric exercise decreases glucose transporter GLUT4 protein in human skeletal muscle. *J Physiol (Lond)* 1995; 482: 705–12.
104. Del Aguila LF, Krishnan RK, Ulbrecht JS, Farrell PA, Correll PH, Lang CH, Zierath JR, Kirwan JP. Muscle damage impairs insulin stimulation of IRS-1, PI 3-kinase, and Akt-kinase in human skeletal muscle. *Am J Physiol Endocrinol Metab* 2000; 279: E206–12.
105. Asp S, Richter EA. Decreased insulin action on muscle glucose transport after eccentric contractions in rats. *J Appl Physiol* 1996; 81: 1924–8.
106. Richter EA, Mikines KJ, Galbo H, Kiens B. Effect of exercise on insulin action in human skeletal muscle. *J Appl Physiol* 1989; 66: 876–85.
107. Wojtaszewski JF, Nielsen JN, Richter EA. Invited Review: effect of acute exercise on insulin signaling and action in humans. *J Appl Physiol* 2002; 93: 384–92.
108. Ivy JL, Zderic TW, Fogt MS. Prevention and treatment of non-insulin-dependent diabetes mellitus. In Holloszy JO (ed), *Exercise and Sport Sciences Reviews*. Philadelphia: Lippincott, Williams & Wilkins, 1999; pp 1–34.
109. Stallknecht B, Larsen JJ, Mikines KJ, Simonsen L, Bulow J, Galbo H. Effect of training on insulin sensitivity of glucose uptake and lipolysis in human adipose tissue. *Am J Physiol Endocrinol Metab* 2000; 279: E376–85.
110. Enevoldsen LH, Stallknecht B, Fluckey JD, Galbo H. Effect of exercise training on in vivo insulin-stimulated glucose uptake in intra-abdominal adipose tissue in rats. *Am J Physiol Endocrinol Metab 2000; 278: E25–34.*
111. Wallberg-Henriksson H. Exercise and diabetes mellitus. In Holloszy JO (ed), *Exercise and Sport Sciences Reviews*. Baltimore, MD: Williams & Wilkins, 1992; pp 339–68.
112. Kiens B, Lithell H. Lipoprotein metabolism influenced by training-induced changes in human skeletal muscle. *J Clin Invest* 1989; 83: 558–64.
113. Biolo G, Williams BD, Fleming RY, Wolfe RR. Insulin action on muscle protein kinetics and amino acid transport during recovery after resistance exercise. *Diabetes* 1999; 48: 949–57.
114. Mikines K, Sonne B, Farrell P, Tronier B, Galbo H. Effect of physical exercise on sensitivity and responsiveness to insulin in humans. *Am J Physiol* 1988; 254: E248–59.
115. Galbo H. Influence of aging and exercise on endocrine function. *Int J Sport Nutr Exerc Metab* 2001; 11: S49–57.
116. Evans WJ. Exercise and aging. In Ruderman NB, Devlin JT, Kriska A (eds), *Handbook of Exercise in Diabetes*. Alexandria, VA: American Diabetes Association, 2002; pp 567–85.
117. Mosher PE, Nash MS, Perry AC, LaPerriere AR, Goldberg RB. Aerobic circuit exercise training: effect on adolescents with well-controlled insulin-dependent diabetes mellitus. *Arch Phys Med Rehabil* 1998; 79: 652–7.
118. Bak J, Jacobsen U, Jørgensen F, Pedersen O. Insulin receptor function and glycogen synthase activity in skeletal muscle biopsies from patients with insulin-dependent diabetes mellitus: effects of physical training. *J Clin Endocrinol Metab* 1989; 69: 158–64.
119. Koivisto VA, Leirisalo-Repo M, Ebeling P, Tuominen JA, Knip M, Turunen U, Mandrup-Poulsen T, Pelkonen R. Seven years of remission in a type I diabetic patient. *Diabetes Care* 1993; 16: 990–5.
120. Ebeling P, Tuominen JA, Bourey R, Koranyi L, Koivisto VA. Athletes with IDDM exhibit impaired metabolic control and increased lipid utilization with no increase in insulin sensitivity. *Diabetes* 1995; 44: 471–7.
121. Schneider SH, Khachadurian AK, Amorosa LF, Clemow L, Ruderman NB. Ten-year experience with an exercise-based outpatient life-style modification program in the treatment of diabetes mellitus. *Diabetes Care* 1992; 15: 1800–10.
122. Baldi JC, Aoina JL, Oxenham HC, Bagg W, Doughty RN. Reduced exercise arteriovenous O2 difference in Type 2 diabetes. *J Appl Physiol* 2003; 94: 1033–38.
123. Nyholm B, Qu Z, Kaal A, Pedersen SB, Gravholt CH, Andersen JL, Saltin B, Schmitz O. Evidence of an increased number of type IIb muscle fibers in insulin-resistant first-degree relatives of patients with NIDDM. *Diabetes* 1997; 46: 1822–8.

124. Scheuermann-Freestone M, Madsen PL, Manners D, Blamire AM, Buckingham RE, Styles P, Radda GK, Neubauer S, Clarke K. Abnormal cardiac and skeletal muscle energy metabolism in patients with type 2 diabetes. *Circulation* 2003; 107: 3040–6.
125. Dela F, Larsen JJ, Mikines KJ, Ploug T, Petersen LN, Galbo H. Insulin-stimulated muscle glucose clearance in patients with NIDDM. Effects of one-legged physical training. *Diabetes* 1995; 44: 1010–20.
126. Boule NG, Kenny GP, Haddad E, Wells GA, Sigal RJ. Meta-analysis of the effect of structured exercise training on cardiorespiratory fitness in Type 2 diabetes mellitus. *Diabetologia* 2003; 46: 1071–81.
127. Devlin JT, Hirshman M, Horton ED, Horton ES. Enhanced peripheral and splanchnic insulin sensitivity in NIDDM men after single bout of exercise. *Diabetes* 1987; 36: 434–9.
128. Fluckey JD, Hickey MS, Brambrink JK, Hart KK, Alexander K, Craig BW. Effects of resistance excercise on glucose tolerance in normal and glucose-intolerant subjects. *J Appl Physiol* 1994; 77: 1087–92.
129. Cusi KJ, Pratipanawatr T, Koval J, Printz R, Ardehali H, Granner DK, DeFronzo RA, Mandarino LJ. Exercise increases hexokinase II mRNA, but not activity in obesity and type 2 diabetes. *Metabolism* 2001; 50: 602–6.
130. Mourier A, Gautier JF, De Kerviler E, Bigard AX, Villette JM, Garnier JP, Duvallet A, Guezennec CY, Cathelineau G. Mobilization of visceral adipose tissue related to the improvement in insulin sensitivity in response to physical training in NIDDM. Effects of branched-chain amino acid supplements. *Diabetes Care* 1997; 20: 385–91.
131. Ligtenberg PC, Hoekstra JB, Bol E, Zonderland ML, Erkelens DW. Effects of physical training on metabolic control in elderly type 2 diabetes mellitus patients. *Clin Sci (Lond)* 1997; 93: 127–35.
132. Dela F, Ploug T, Handberg A, Petersen LN, Larsen JJ, Mikines KJ, Galbo H. Physical training increases muscle GLUT4 protein and mRNA in patients with NIDDM. *Diabetes* 1994; 43: 862–5.
133. Holten MK, Zacho M, Gaster M, Juel C, Wojtaszewski JFP, Dela F. Strength training increases insulin-mediated glucose uptake, GLUT4 content and insulin signaling in skeletal muscle in patients with Type 2 diabetes. *Diabetes* (in press).
134. Wing R. Exercise and weight control. In Ruderman NB, Devlin JT, Kriska A (eds), *Handbook of Exercise in Diabetes*. Alexandria, VA: American Diabetes Association, 2002; pp 355–64.
135. Boule NG, Haddad E, Kenny GP, Wells GA, Sigal RJ. Effects of exercise on glycemic control and body mass in type 2 diabetes mellitus: a meta-analysis of controlled clinical trials. *JAMA* 2001; 286: 1218–27.
136. Farrell PA, Caston AL, Rodd D. Changes in insulin response to glucose after exercise training in partially pancreatectomized rats. *J Appl Physiol* 1991; 70: 1563–8.
137. Dunstan DW, Mori TA, Puddey IB, Beilin LJ, Burke V, Morton AR, Stanton KG. The independent and combined effects of aerobic exercise and dietary fish intake on serum lipids and glycemic control in NIDDM. A randomized controlled study. *Diabetes Care* 1997; 20: 913–21.
138. Lehmann R, Engler H, Honegger R, Riesen W, Spinas GA. Alterations of lipolytic enzymes and high-density lipoprotein subfractions induced by physical activity in type 2 diabetes mellitus. *Eur J Clin Invest* 2001; 31: 37–44.
139. Maiorana A, O'Driscoll G, Goodman C, Taylor R, Green D. Combined aerobic and resistance exercise improves glycemic control and fitness in type 2 diabetes. *Diabetes Res Clin Pract* 2002; 56: 115–23.
140. Lehmann R, Vokac A, Niedermann K, Agosti K, Spinas GA. Loss of abdominal fat and improvement of the cardiovascular risk profile by regular moderate exercise training in patients with NIDDM. *Diabetologia* 1995; 38: 1313–9.
141. Castaneda C, Layne JE, Munoz-Orians L, Gordon PL, Walsmith J, Foldvari M, Roubenoff R, Tucker KL, Nelson ME. A randomized controlled trial of resistance exercise training to improve glycemic control in older adults with type 2 diabetes. *Diabetes Care* 2002; 25: 2335–41.
142. Loimaala A, Huikuri HV, Koobi T, Rinne M, Nenonen A, Vuori I. Exercise training improves baroreflex sensitivity in type 2 diabetes. *Diabetes* 2003; 52: 1837–42.
143. Maiorana A, O'Driscoll G, Cheetham C, Dembo L, Stanton K, Goodman C, Taylor R, Green D. The effect of combined aerobic and resistance exercise training on vascular function in type 2 diabetes. *J Am Coll Cardiol* 2001; 38: 860–6.
144. Colberg SR, Stansberry KB, McNitt PM, Vinik AI. Chronic exercise is associated with enhanced cutaneous blood flow in type 2 diabetes. *J Diabetes Complications* 2002; 16: 139–45.
145. Lindahl B, Nilsson TK, Jansson JH, Asplund K, Hallmans G. Improved fibrinolysis by intense lifestyle intervention. A randomized trial in subjects with impaired glucose tolerance. *J Intern Med* 1999; 246: 105–12.
146. Gregg EW, Gerzoff RB, Caspersen CJ, Williamson DF, Narayan KM. Relationship of walking to mortality among US adults with diabetes. *Arch Intern Med* 2003; 163: 1440–7.
147. Roberts L, Jones TW, Fournier PA. Exercise training and glycemic control in adolescents with poorly controlled type 1 diabetes mellitus. *J Pediatr Endocrinol Metab* 2002; 15: 621–7.
148. Fuchsjager-Mayrl G, Pleiner J, Wiesinger GF, Sieder AE, Quittan M, Nuhr MJ, Francesconi C, Seit HP, Francesconi M, Schmetterer L, Wolzt M. Exercise training improves vascular endothelial function in patients with type 1 diabetes. *Diabetes Care* 2002; 25: 1795–801.
149. Cohen ST, Jacobson AM. Psychological benefits of exercise. In Ruderman NB, Devlin JT, Kriska A (eds), *Handbook of Exercise in Diabetes*. Alexandria, VA: American Diabetes Association, 2002; pp 125–34.
150. Kemmer FW. Prevention of hypoglycemia during exercise in type I diabetes. *Diabetes Care* 1992; 15: 1732–5.
151. Meinders AE, Willekens FL, Heere LP. Metabolic and hormonal changes in IDDM during long-distance run. *Diabetes Care* 1988; 11: 1–7.
152. Tuominen JA, Karonen SL, Melamies L, Bolli G, Koivisto VA. Exercise-induced hypoglycaemia in IDDM patients treated with a short-acting insulin analogue. *Diabetologia* 1995; 38: 106–11.
153. Yamakita T, Ishii T, Yamagami K, Yamamoto T, Miyamoto M, Hosoi M, Yoshioka K, Sato T, Onishi S, Tanaka S, Fujii S. Glycemic response during exercise after administration of insulin lispro compared with that after administration of regular human insulin. *Diabetes Res Clin Pract* 2002; 57: 17–22.
154. Berger M. Adjustment of insulin and oral agent therapy. In Ruderman NB, Devlin JT, Kriska A (eds), *Handbook*

of Exercise in Diabetes. Alexandria, VA: American Diabetes Association, 2002; pp 365–76.

155. Rabasa-Lhoret R, Bourque J, Ducros F, Chiasson JL. Guidelines for premeal insulin dose reduction for postprandial exercise of different intensities and durations in type 1 diabetic subjects treated intensively with a basal-bolus insulin regimen (ultralente-lispro). *Diabetes Care* 2001; 24: 625–30.
156. Sonnenberg GE, Kemmer FW, Berger M. Exercise in type 1 (insulin-dependent) diabetic patients treated with continuous subcutaneous insulin infusion. Prevention of exercise induced hypoglycaemia. *Diabetologia* 1990; 33: 696–703.
157. Zinman B. Insulin pump therapy with continuous subcutaneous insulin infusion and exercise in patients with type 1 diabetes. In Ruderman NB, Devlin JT, Kriska A (eds), *Handbook of Exercise in Diabetes*. Alexandria, VA: American Diabetes Association, 2002; pp 377–81.
158. Franz MJ. Nutrition, physical activity, and diabetes. In Ruderman NB, Devlin J, Kriska A (eds), *Handbook of Exercise in Diabetes*. Alexandria, VA: American Diabetes Association, 2002; pp 321–37.
159. Waxman S, Nesto EW. Cardiovascular complications. In Ruderman NB, Devlin JT, Kriska A (eds), *Handbook of Exercise in Diabetes*. Alexandria, VA: American Diabetes Association, 2002; pp 415–31.
160. Yamagishi H, Yoshiyama M, Shirai N, Akioka K, Takeuchi K, Yoshikawa J. Impact of diabetes mellitus on worsening of the left ventricular ejection fraction in exercise-gated 201Tl myocardial single photon emission computed tomography in patients with coronary artery disease. *Circ J* 2003; 67: 839–45.
161. Mustonen JN, Uusitupa MI, Tahvanainen K, Talwar S, Laakso M, Lansimieş E, Kuikka JT, Pyorala K. Impaired left ventricular systolic function during exercise in middle-aged insulin-dependent and noninsulin-dependent diabetic subjects without clinically evident cardiovascular disease. *Am J Cardiol* 1988; 62: 1273–9.
162. Blake GA, Levin SR, Koyal SN. Exercise-induced hypertension in normotensive patients with NIDDM. *Diabetes Care* 1990; 13: 799–801.
163. Raber W, Raffesberg W, Waldhausl W, Gasic S, Roden M. Exercise induces excessive normetanephrine responses in hypertensive diabetic patients. *Eur J Clin Invest* 2003; 33: 480–7.
164. Ambepityia G, Kopelman PG, Ingram D, Swash M, Mills PG, Timmis AD. Exertional myocardial ischemia in diabetes: a quantitative analysis of anginal perceptual threshold and the influence of autonomic function. *J Am Coll Cardiol* 1990; 15: 72–7.
165. Umachandran V, Ranjadayalan K, Ambepityia G, Marchant B, Kopelman PG, Timmis AD. The perception of angina in diabetes: relation to somatic pain threshold and autonomic function. *Am Heart J* 1991; 121: 1649–54.
166. Zola B, Kahn JK, Juni JE, Vinik AI. Abnormal cardiac function in diabetic patients with autonomic neuropathy in the absence of ischemic heart disease. *J Clin Endocrinol Metab* 1986; 63: 208–14.
167. Vinik AI, Erbas T. Neuropathy. In Ruderman NB, Devlin JT, Kriska A (eds), *Handbook of Exercise in Diabetes*. Alexandria, VA: American Diabetes Association, 2002; pp 463–496.
168. Levin ME. The diabetic foot. In Ruderman NB, Devlin JT, Kriska A (eds), *Handbook of Exercise in Diabetes*. Alexandria, VA: American Diabetes Association, 2002; pp 385–400.
169. Young MJ, Marshall A, Adams JE, Selby PL, Boulton AJ. Osteopenia, neurological dysfunction, and the development of Charcot neuroarthropathy. *Diabetes Care* 1995; 18: 34–8.
170. Childs M, Armstrong DG, Edelson GW. Is Charcot arthropathy a late sequela of osteoporosis in patients with diabetes mellitus? *J Foot Ankle Surg* 1998; 37: 437–9.
171. Aiello LP, Wong J, Cavallerano JD, Bursell S-E, Aiello LM. Retinopathy. In Ruderman NB, Devlin JT, Kriska A (eds), *Handbook of Exercise in Diabetes*. Alexandria, VA: American Diabetes Association, 2002; pp 401–14.
172. Passa P, Gauville C, Canivet J. Influence of muscular exercise on plasma level of growth hormone in diabetics with and without retinopathy. *Lancet* 1974; 2: 72–4.
173. Margonato A, Gerundini P, Vicedomini G, Gilardi MC, Pozza G, Fazio F. Abnormal cardiovascular response to exercise in young asymptomatic diabetic patients with retinopathy. *Am Heart J* 1986; 112: 554–60.
174. Estacio RO, Regensteiner JG, Wolfel EE, Jeffers B, Dickenson M, Schrier RW. The association between diabetic complications and exercise capacity in NIDDM patients. *Diabetes Care* 1998; 21: 291–5.
175. Cruickshanks KJ, Moss SE, Klein R, Klein BE. Physical activity and the risk of progression of retinopathy or the development of proliferative retinopathy. *Ophthalmology* 1995; 102: 1177–82.
176. Graham C, Lasko-McCarthey P. Exercise options for persons with diabetic complications. *Diabetes Educ* 1990; 16: 212–20.
177. Albert SG, Gomez CR, Russell S, Chaitman BR, Bernbaum M, Kong BA. Cerebral and ophthalmic artery hemodynamic responses in diabetes mellitus. *Diabetes Care* 1993; 16: 476–82.
178. Bernbaum M, Albert SG, Cohen JD, Drimmer A. Cardiovascular conditioning in individuals with diabetic retinopathy. *Diabetes Care* 1989; 12: 740–2.
179. Fujita Y, Matoba K, Takeuchi H, Ishii K, Yajima Y. Anaerobic threshold can provoke microalbuminuria in non-insulin-dependent diabetics. *Diabetes Res Clin Pract* 1994; 22: 155–62.
180. Mogensen CE. Nephropathy: early. In Ruderman NB, Devlin JT, Kriska A (eds), *Handbook of Exercise in Diabetes*. Alexandria, VA: American Diabetes Association, 2002; pp 433–49.
181. Christensen CK. Abnormal albuminuria and blood pressure rise in incipient diabetic nephropathy induced by exercise. *Kidney Int* 1984; 25: 819–23.
182. Romanelli G, Giustina A, Agabiti-Rosei E, Bossoni S, Girelli A, Muiesan ML, Muiesan G, Giustina G. Short-term effect of captopril and nifedipine on microalbuminuria induced by exercise in hypertensive diabetic patients. *J Hypertens Suppl* 1989; 7: S312–3.
183. Matsuoka K, Nakao T, Atsumi Y, Takekoshi H. Exercise regimen for patients with diabetic nephropathy. *J Diabetes Complications* 1991; 5: 98–100.
184. Johansen KL. Physical functioning and exercise capacity in patients on dialysis. *Adv Ren Replace Ther* 1999; 6: 141–8.
185. Painter P. The importance of exercise training in rehabilitation of patients with end-stage renal disease. *Am J Kidney Dis* 1994; 24: S2–9.
186. Bohannon RW, Hull D, Palmeri D. Muscle strength impairments and gait performance deficits in kidney transplantation candidates. *Am J Kidney Dis* 1994; 24: 480–5.

187. Fahal IH, Bell GM, Bone JM. Edwards RH. Physiological abnormalities of skeletal muscle in dialysis patients. *Nephrol Dial Transplant* 1997; 12: 119–27.
188. Headley SA, Germain MJ, Braden GL. Nephropathy: advanced. In Ruderman NB, Devlin JT, Kriska A (eds), *Handbook of Exercise in Diabetes*. Alexandria, VA: American Diabetes Association, 2002; pp 451–62.
189. Lo CY, Li L, Lo WK, Chan ML, So E, Tang S, Yuen MC, Cheng IK, Chan TM. Benefits of exercise training in patients on continuous ambulatory peritoneal dialysis. *Am J Kidney Dis* 1998; 32: 1011–8.
190. Buchanan T. Exercise and gestational diabetes. In Ruderman NB, Devlin JT, Kriska A (eds), *Handbook of Exercise in Diabetes*. Alexandria, VA: American Diabetes Association, 2002; pp 533–46.
191. Stein J. Exercise in diabetic patients with disabilities. In Ruderman NB, Devlin JT, Kriska A (eds), *Handbook of Exercise in Diabetes*. Alexandria, VA: American Diabetes Association, 2002; pp 601–14.
192. Ganda OP. Patients on various drug therapies. In Ruderman NB, Devlin JT, Kriska A (eds), *Handbook of Exercise in Diabetes*. Alexandria, VA: American Diabetes Association, 2002; pp 587–600.
193. Campaigne BN, Wallberg-Henriksson H, Gunnarsson R. Glucose and insulin responses in relation to insulin dose and caloric intake 12 h after acute physical exercise in men with IDDM. *Diabetes Care* 1987; 10: 716–21.
194. Caron D, Poussier P, Marliss EB, Zinman B. The effect of postprandial exercise on meal-related glucose intolerance in insulin-dependent diabetic individuals. *Diabetes Care* 1982; 5: 364–9.
195. Bott S, Bott U, Berger M, Muhlhauser I. Intensified insulin therapy and the risk of severe hypoglycaemia. *Diabetologia* 1997; 40: 926–32.
196. Jorgens V, Grusser M, Bott U, Muhlhauser I, Berger M. Effective and safe translation of intensified insulin therapy to general internal medicine departments. *Diabetologia* 1993; 36: 99–105.
197. Hu FB, Sigal RJ, Rich-Edwards JW, Colditz GA, Solomon CG, Willett WC, Speizer FE, Manson JE. Walking compared with vigorous physical activity and risk of type 2 diabetes in women: a prospective study. *JAMA* 1999; 282: 1433–9.
198. Fletcher GF, Balady G, Blair SN, Blumenthal J, Caspersen C, Chaitman B, Epstein S, Sivarajan Froelicher ES, Froelicher VF, Pina IL, Pollock ML. Statement on exercise: benefits and recommendations for physical activity programs for all Americans. A statement for health professionals by the Committee on Exercise and Cardiac Rehabilitation of the Council on Clinical Cardiology, American Heart Association. *Circulation* 1996; 94: 857–62.
199. *American College of Sports Medicine Guidelines for Exercise Testing and Prescription*. Philadelphia: Lippincott Williams and Wilkins, 2000.
200. Hornsby WG, Chetlin RD. Resistance exercise. In Ruderman NB, Devlin J, Kriska A (eds), *Handbook of Exercise in Diabetes*. Alexandria, VA: American Diabetes Association, 2002; pp 311–20.
201. Durak EP, Jovanovic-Peterson L, Peterson CM. Randomized crossover study of effect of resistance training on glycemic control, muscular strength, and cholesterol in type I diabetic men. *Diabetes Care* 1990; 13: 1039–43.
202. Dunstan DW, Daly RM, Owen N, Jolley D, De Court, Shaw J, Zimmet P. High-intensity resistance training improves glycemic control in older patients with type 2 diabetes. *Diabetes Care* 2002; 25: 1729–36.
203. Ryan AS, Hurlbut DE, Lott ME, Ivey FM, Fleg J, Hurley BF, Goldberg AP. Insulin action after resistive training in insulin resistant older men and women. *J Am Geriatr Soc* 2001; 49: 247–53.
204. American College of Sports Medicine. American College of Sports Medicine Position Stand: exercise and physical activity for older adults. *Med Sci Sports Exerc* 1998; 30: 992–1008.
205. Brandon LJ, Gaasch DA, Boyette LW, Lloyd AM. Effects of long-term resistive training on mobility and strength in older adults with diabetes. *J Gerontol A Biol Sci Med Sci* 2003; 58: 740–5.
206. Kirk A, Mutrie N, MacIntyre P, Fisher M. Increasing physical activity in people with type 2 diabetes. *Diabetes Care* 2003; 26: 1186–92.
207. Tuominen JA, Ebeling P, Vuorinen-Markkola H, Koivisto VA. Post-marathon paradox in IDDM: unchanged insulin sensitivity in spite of glycogen depletion. *Diabet Med* 1997; 14: 301–8.
208. Sane T, Helve E, Pelkonen R, Koivisto V. The adjustment of diet and insulin dose during long-term endurance exercise in type 1 (insulin-dependent) diabetic men. *Diabetologia* 1988; 31: 35–40.
209. Lorber D. Scuba diving. In Ruderman NB, Devlin JT, Kriska A (eds), *Handbook of Exercise in Diabetes*. Alexandria, VA: American Diabetes Association, 2002; pp 639–48.
210. Grimm J-J. Mountain hiking. In Ruderman NB, Devlin JT, Kriska A (eds), *Handbook of Exercise in Diabetes*. Alexandria, VA: American Diabetes Association, 2002; pp 649–54.
211. Harper P. The diabetic athlete as a model. In Ruderman NB, Devlin JT, Kriska A (eds), *Handbook of Exercise in Diabetes*. Alexandria, VA: American Diabetes Association. 2002; pp. 615–24.
212. Peirce NS. Diabetes and exercise. *Br J Sports Med* 1999; 33: 161–72.
213. Skerret PJ, Manson JE. Reduction in risk of coronary heart disease and diabetes. In Ruderman NB, Devlin JT, Kriska A (eds), *Handbook of Exercise in Diabetes*. Alexandria, VA: American Diabetes Association, 2002; pp 155–82.
214. Eriksson KF, Lindgarde F. Prevention of type 2 (non-insulin-dependent) diabetes mellitus by diet and physical exercise. The 6-year Malmö feasibility study. *Diabetologia* 1991; 34: 891–8.
215. Pan XR, Li GW, Hu YH, Wang JX, Yang WY, An ZX, Hu ZX, Lin J, Xiao JZ, Cao HB, Liu PA, Jiang XG, Jiang YY, Wang JP, Zheng H, Zhang H, Bennett PH, Howard BV. Effects of diet and exercise in preventing NIDDM in people with impaired glucose tolerance. The Da Qing IGT and Diabetes Study. *Diabetes Care* 1997; 20: 537–44.
216. Tuomilehto J, Lindstrom J, Eriksson JG, Valle TT, Hamalainen H, Ilanne-Parikka P, Keinanen-Kiukaanniemi S, Laakso M, Louheranta A, Rastas M, Salminen V, Uusitupa M. Prevention of type 2 diabetes mellitus by changes in lifestyle among subjects with impaired glucose tolerance. *N Engl J Med* 2001; 344: 1343–50.
217. Helmrich SP, Ragland DR, Leung RW, Paffenbarger S. Physical activity and reduced occurrence of non-insulin-dependent diabetes mellitus. *N Engl J Med* 1991; 325: 147–52.

44

Should We Treat Impaired Glucose Tolerance and Impaired Fasting Glycemia?

Rury Holman

Diabetes Trials Unit, Radcliffe Infirmary, Oxford, UK

IMPAIRED GLUCOSE TOLERANCE AND IMPAIRED FASTING GLUCOSE

The term impaired glucose tolerance (IGT) was introduced first in 1979, replacing less well-defined dysglycemic categories such as "borderline," "chemical," or "latent" diabetes that were not thought to be associated with a risk of developing microvascular complications [1, 2]. The formal IGT definition by the World Health Organisation (WHO) in 1985 [3] was updated in 1999 [4], at which time the term impaired fasting glucose (IFG) was coined to denote elevated but not diabetic levels of fasting glycemia [4, 5]. Both IGT and IGF are thought to be stages in the evolution of dysglycemia from normal glucose tolerance to T2DM. Neither is regarded as a disease state but in many subjects will represent a "prediabetic" state with a high probability of progression to T2DM and/or the development of CVD. Subjects with IGT or IFG often will have normal or only minimally elevated HbA1c values but nonetheless frequently have other features of the metabolic or "insulin resistance" syndrome [6], explaining in part their increased risk of CVD. This dual risk relationship has been termed the "common soil" hypothesis [7].

The fasting plasma glucose (FPG) level is determined largely by the ability of β-cells to secrete sufficient insulin in the basal state to suppress appropriately hepatic glucose production for a given degree of hepatic insulin sensitivity. The plasma glucose level achieved 2 h after a standard oral glucose load (2hPG), however, depends not only on the FPG but also on the β-cells ability to respond to a sudden plasma glucose rise and the degree to which reduced insulin sensitivity impacts on the efficiency with which peripheral tissues can take up glucose. Not surprisingly, individual differences in these physiological processes mean that people may have predominantly an elevated FPG or an elevated 2hPG, which in turn means that many will be classified as having only IFG or IGT with a minority falling into both categories [8] (Figure 1). The FPG and 2hPG values used currently to define an individual's glycaemic status are shown in Table 1, although an ADA expert committee has recommended recently that the lower cut point for IFG should be reduced to 100 mg/dl, redefining IFG as an FPG of 100–125 mg/dl (5.6–6.9 mmol/l) [9]. The prevalence of IGT among adults varies between 3 and 10% in European populations and between 11 and 20% in North American populations [10]. Since the risk of developing T2DM or CVD would appear to be greater for those with IGT, compared to those with IFG, it is important to consider undertaking an oral glucose tolerance test (OGTT) in subjects with IFG to better define their glycaemic status, especially as their 2hPG may classify them as already having diabetes.

Progression from IGT or IGF to T2DM occurs when, as a result of increasing β-cell dysfunction [11], the pancreas is no longer able to meet the increased demand for insulin required because of decreased insulin sensitivity, which often can be present many years before diabetes is diagnosed [12, 13]. Rates of progression vary between 1.5 and 7.3% per year for different regions of the world and ethnic groups [14]. The T2DM epidemic is being driven by the projected growth in the world population, especially among the middle aged and elderly, although T2DM is increasingly being diagnosed in children and adolescents

International Textbook of Diabetes Mellitus, Third Edition. Edited by R. A. DeFronzo, E. Ferrannini, H. Keen, and P. Zimmet.
 ISBN: 0-471-48655-8.

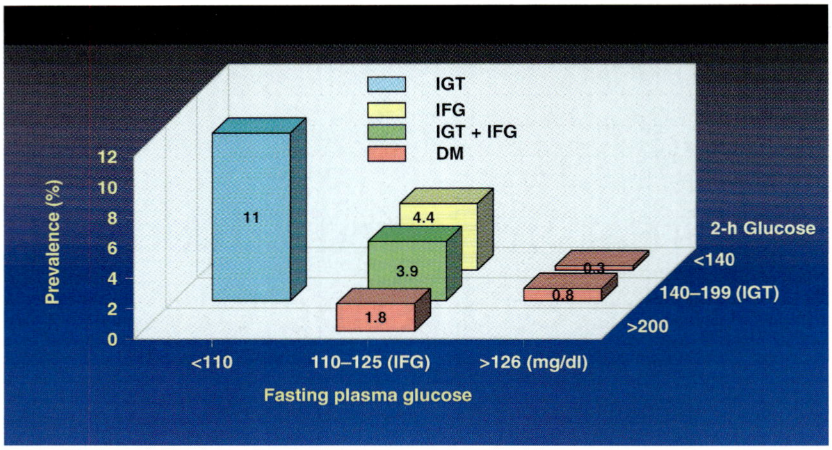

Figure 1 Prevalence of IGT and IFG in 2662 persons (aged 40–74 years) without diabetes by 1985 WHO criteria, NHANES III study [8]

[15, 16]. The development of diabetes in younger age groups reflects the tendency for people to adopt increasingly sedentary lifestyles with a dramatic increase in the proportion who become obese [15].

LIFESTYLE INTERVENTION

The Malmö Study [17] followed 217 middle-aged men with IGT who received treatment with diet and exercise advice or standard medical care, according to requirements rather than by randomization. Neither group was given antidiabetic therapy. Over a 5-year period the diet and exercise group reduced their weight and developed T2DM less frequently compared to the control group (10.6% vs. 28%). More recently, the Da Qing Study [18] examined the effect of diet, exercise, and diet plus exercise compared to conventional advice in preventing the development of type 2 diabetes in subjects with IGT. This cluster randomized trial of 577 subjects followed in 35 Chinese clinics showed that the risk over 6 years of progressing to T2DM was reduced from 15.7 to 10.0% with diet alone, 8.3% with exercise alone, and 9.6% with diet plus exercise, with relative risk reductions of 36, 47, and 39% respectively.

Table 1 Venous plasma glucose levels for the diagnosis of diabetes, IGT, and IFG [4]

Diabetes mellitus	
Fasting	$\geq$7.0 mmol/l ($\geq$126 mg/dl)
2-h 75-g post-glucose load	$\geq$11.1 mmol/l ($\geq$200 mg/dl)
IGT	
Fasting (if measured)	<7.0 mmol/l (<126 mg/dl)
2-h 75-g post-glucose load	7.8–11.0 mmol/l (140–199 mg/dl)
IFG	
Fasting	6.1–6.9 mmol/l (110–125 mg/dl)
2-h 75-g post-glucose load (if measured)	<7.8 mmol/l (<140 mg/dl)

THE FINNISH DIABETES PREVENTION STUDY

The Finnish Diabetes Prevention Study (DPS) enrolled 523 overweight [body mass index (BMI) $> 25\ kg/m^2$] subjects (aged 40–65 years) with IGT from five centers [19] between 1993 and 1998. The DPS examined the effect of randomized allocation to a diet and exercise program compared to a control group who received general verbal and written information about diet and exercise at baseline. The intervention group received individualized dietary counselling aimed at reducing weight, total fat, and saturated fat intake and increasing intake of fiber undertaken through face-to-face sessions with a dietitian seven times during the first year and three monthly thereafter. Physical activity counselling was individually designed and included both aerobic exercise and resistance training. Increased walking and exercise associated with routine daily activities was encouraged. Some of the activities were carried out and supervised in local health clubs or physical training facilities accessible to the participants. Subjects in the intervention group were monitored regularly during the study period. An OGTT was performed annually on all subjects. This study, which achieved a mean reduction in body weight of 4.7% in the intensive group during a mean follow-up of 3.2 years, showed a reduction in new-onset T2DM from 23 to 11%, with relative risk reduction of 58% ($p < 0.001$) (Figure 2). The reduced incidence of diabetes was associated directly with the degree of lifestyle change; those achieving more diet, exercise, and weight loss goals experience the largest risk reductions.

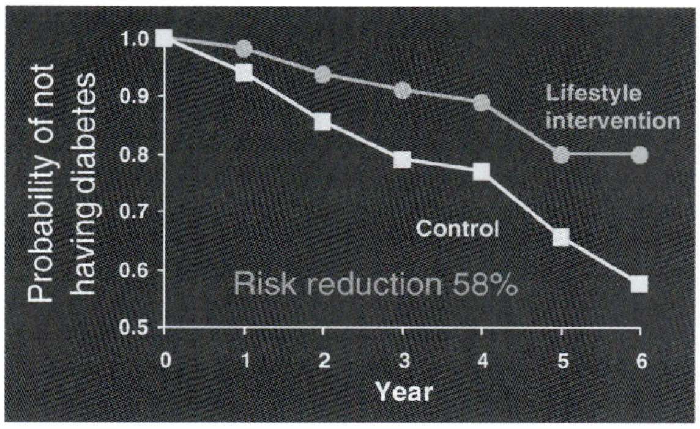

Figure 2 Cumulative incidence of T2DM according to study group in 523 IGT subjects randomized to standard or intensive lifestyle intervention in the Finnish Diabetes Prevention Study [19]

THE US DIABETES PREVENTION PROGRAM

The US Diabetes Prevention Program (DPP) [20, 21] assigned 3234 subjects with IGT and a FPG concentration in the range 5.3–7.0 mmol/l (95–125 mg/dl) in 27 centers to treatment with a placebo, metformin (850 mg twice daily), or to a lifestyle-modification program. This program included goals of a 7% weight reduction from initial body weight and at least 150 min of physical exercise per week with participants receiving training in diet, exercise, and behavior modification from case managers who met with each participant on a one-to-one basis for at least 16 sessions in the first 24 weeks and monthly thereafter. A further group was assigned to receive troglitazone but this arm was discontinued after 2 years because of the significant increased risk of liver damage, and in some instances fatal hepatic toxicity, caused by this agent. The mean age of the participants was 51 years and mean BMI was 34.0 kg/m^2, with 68% of the participants being female and 55% Caucasian. Ethnic minority groups included African American, Hispanic, American Indian, and Asian Americans. During an average follow-up period of 2.8 years the cumulative incidence of diabetes was 28.9, 21.7, and 14.4% in the placebo, the metformin, and the lifestyle intervention groups, respectively. The lifestyle intervention reduced the incidence of T2DM by 58% and metformin by 31% compared to placebo (Figure 3); the lifestyle intervention was significantly more effective than metformin. The nature of the lifestyle intervention was more intensive than in the Finnish DPS, with at least 16 clinic visits during the first 6 months. The effect of metformin was less with a lower BMI or a lower FPG concentration than with higher values for those variables. Neither interaction was explained by the other variable or by age. The advantage of the lifestyle intervention over metformin was greater in older persons and those with a lower BMI than in younger persons and those with a higher BMI.

THE STOP-NIDDM STUDY

The STOP-NIDDM Study, an international, multicenter, placebo-controlled, randomized diabetes prevention trial, randomly allocated 1429 patients with IGT to acarbose (100 mg three times a day) or to placebo [22]. After a mean of 3.3 years of follow-up, 211 (31%) of 682 patients in the acarbose group and 130 (19%) of 686 on placebo had discontinued treatment. A total of 221 (32%) patients randomized to acarbose and 285 (42%) randomized to placebo developed new-onset T2DM, a relative risk reduction of 25% attributable to acarbose (Figure 4). The drug appeared to be similarly effective irrespective of age, gender, and BMI. However, the benefit of treatment on prevention was reduced substantially when reassessed 3 months after cessation of active treatment. Acarbose in

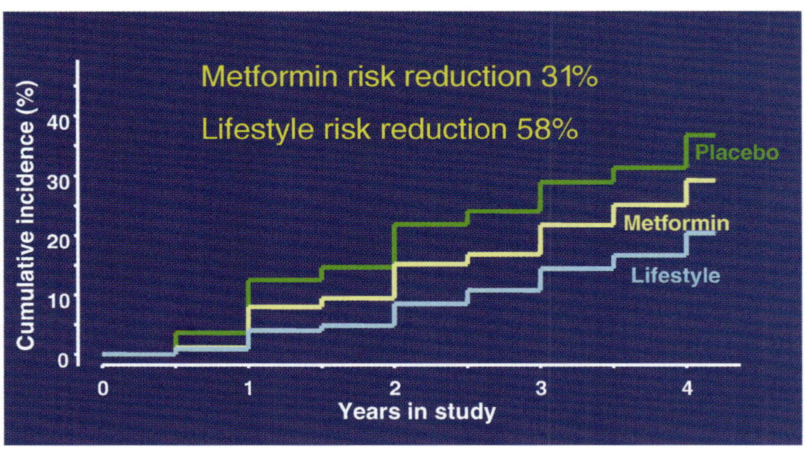

Figure 3 Cumulative incidence of T2DM according to study group in 3234 IGT subjects randomized to placebo, metformin (850 mg twice daily), or to a lifestyle-modification program in the US Diabetes Prevention Program [20, 21]

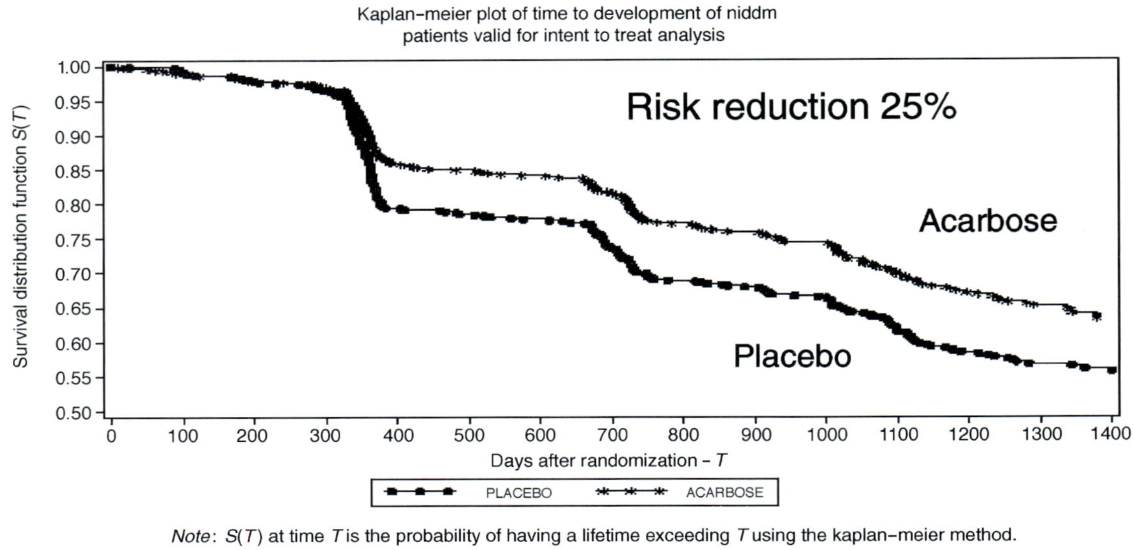

Figure 4 Cumulative incidence of T2DM according to study group in 1429 IGT subjects randomized to placebo or to acarbose (100 mg three times daily) in the STOP-NIDDM Study [22]

the STOP-NIDDM Study has also been reported to reduce the development of hypertension and the frequency of cardiovascular events, although the event rate was low [23].

THE TRIPOD STUDY

The TRIPOD Study randomized 250 Hispanic women with a previous history of gestational diabetes, approximately 70% of whom had IGT, to troglitazone or to placebo [24]. After a median follow-up period of 31 months there was a 56% reduction in new-onset T2DM with troglitazone compared to placebo, with a suggestion that the troglitazone effect persisted for 8.5 months after treatment ceased.

THE WENYING STUDY

A Chinese diabetes prevention study [25] randomized 321 subjects with IGT and mean BMI of 25 kg/m^2 to conventional education, a diet and exercise program, metformin (250 mg three times a day), or to acarbose (50 mg three times a day). Over a 3-year period 5.2% withdrew. New-onset T2DM occurred in 11.6% of the conventional group, 8.2% of the diet and exercise group, 4.1% of the metformin group, and 2.0% of the acarbose group, with relative risk reductions of 43, 87, and 88% respectively for the active interventions; 34.9, 12.4, and 6.0% of each group respectively progressed to diabetes. This represents a risk reduction of 76.8% for metformin and 87.8% for acarbose compared with the control group.

STUDIES IN PROGRESS

The DREAM Study

Ramipril, an ACE inhibitor, was shown in the HOPE trial to reduce the risk of cardiovascular disease in a broad range of diabetic and nondiabetic individuals [26]. In addition, during 4.5 years of follow-up, those subjects allocated to ramipril were 34% less likely to report new-onset T2DM [27] than those allocated to placebo ($p < 0.001$). The DREAM study is an international multicenter trial, in over 5269 subjects (aged 30 years or more) with IGT or IGF, designed to determine whether an ACE inhibitor (ramipril, titrated to 15 mg per day) or a thiazolidinedione (rosiglitazone, titrated to 8 mg per day) can prevent or delay the onset of T2DM. This double-blind, two-by-two, factorial-design study, based on an expected progression rate to diabetes in the targeted population of over 5% per year, is projected to report in 2006. The primary endpoint is clinical or biochemical development of new-onset T2DM, with secondary endpoints examining cardiorenal events, β-cell function, and insulin resistance.

THE NAVIGATOR STUDY

The NAVIGATOR Study is an international multicenter study in over 9523 subjects with IGT who are either aged more than 50 years with a history of cardiovascular disease or aged more than 55 years with one or more cardiovascular risk factors. This two-by-two, factorial-design trial is examining whether nateglinide (a fast-acting non-sulfonylurea insulin secretagogue) and/or valsartan (an angiotensin II receptor antagonist) can not only prevent or delay progression to T2DM but also reduce the risk of cardiovascular disease. It is expected to report in 2007.

CONCLUSIONS

T2DM is a common chronic disease that causes suffering to millions, is a major drain on health care resources, and is increasing rapidly worldwide. IGT and IGF not only represent stages in the natural history of T2DM but also identify subjects at substantially increased risk of macrovascular disease because of their association with other features of the metabolic syndrome, including hypertension, dyslipidemia, and central obesity [28]. The potential to minimize the epidemic of T2DM and its burdensome complications by primary prevention of the disease, is an attractive possibility. To be really successful, however, this is likely to require that intervention be commenced at an early age to encourage an active lifestyle and the adoption of a diet that does not promote obesity. While instigating an intensive diet and/or increased exercise at a later age can delay the onset of diabetes, considerable effort is needed to alter established behavioral patterns. It may also be a case of "too little, too late" if the progressive decline in β-cell function has moved into an irreversible phase, whereas intervention at a much earlier stage might be more effective at preventing, rather than delaying, T2DM. A community-wide approach is needed to encourage a healthy lifestyle from childhood but this will require major socioeconomic changes to implement.

Where lifestyle measures alone prove to be inadequate, a combined approach utilizing pharmacological interventions should be considered although the effect of combining these therapies with lifestyle interventions has yet to be formally evaluated. Therapy with both acarbose and metformin has been shown to reduce the risk of T2DM over 3 years by 25 and 31% respectively, although metformin was less successful in older and in less overweight subjects. Alternative pharmacological approaches, using a prandial glucose regulator (nateglinide), an angiotensin 2 receptor blocker (valsartan), a thiazolidinedione (rosiglitazone), and an ACE inhibitor (ramipril), are now being evaluated in the DREAM and in the NAVIGATOR Studies.

REFERENCES

1. National Diabetes Data Group. Classification and diagnosis of diabetes and other categories of glucose intolerance. *Diabetes* 1979; 28: 1039–57.
2. WHO Expert Committee on Diabetes Mellitus. Technical Report Series 646, Second report. Geneva: World Health Organisation, 1980.
3. WHO Study Group. Diabetes mellitus. Technical Report Series 727. Geneva: World Health Organisation, 1985.
4. World Health Organization. Definition, Diagnosis and Classification of Diabetes Mellitus and Its Complications; Part 1: Diagnosis and Classification of Diabetes Mellitus. Report No. WHO/NCD/NCS/99.2. Geneva: Department of Noncommunicable Disease Surveillance, World Health Organization, 1999.
5. The Expert Committee on the Diagnosis and Classification of Diabetes Mellitus. Report of the Expert Committee on the Diagnosis and Classification of Diabetes Mellitus. *Diabetes Care* 1997; 20: 1183–97.
6. Reaven GM. Banting Lecture: insulin resistance in human disease. *Diabetes* 1988; 37: 1595–607.
7. Stern MP. Diabetes and cardiovascular disease. The "common soil" hypothesis. *Diabetes* 1995; 44: 369–74.
8. Harris MI, Eastman RC, Cowie CC, Flegal KM, Eberhardt MS, Comparison of diabetes diagnostic categories in the U.S. population according to the 1997 American Diabetes Association and 1980–1985 World Health Organization diagnostic criteria. *Diabetes Care* 1997; 20: 1859–62.
9. The Expert Committee on the Diagnosis and Classification of Diabetes Mellitus. Follow-up report on the diagnosis of diabetes mellitus. *Diabetes Care* 2003; 26: 3160–7.
10. King H, Rewers M, WHO Ad Hoc Diabetes Reporting Group. Global estimates for prevalence of diabetes mellitus and impaired glucose tolerance in adults. *Diabetes Care* 1993; 16: 157–77.
11. Kahn SE. Clinical review 135. The importance of beta-cell failure in the development and progression of type 2 diabetes. *J Clin Endocrinol Metab* 2001; 86: 4047–58.
12. Warram JH, Martin BC, Krolewski AS, Soeldner JS, Kahn CR. Slow glucose removal rate and hyperinsulinemia precede the development of type II diabetes in the offspring of diabetic parents. *Ann Intern Med* 1990; 113: 909–15.
13. Martin BC, Warram JH, Rosner B, Rich SS, Soeldner JS, Krolewski AS. Familial clustering of insulin sensitivity. *Diabetes* 1992; 41: 850–4.
14. Harris MI. Impaired glucose tolerance: prevalence and conversion to NIDDM. *Diabet Med* 1996; 13 (suppl 2): S9–11.
15. Zimmet P, Alberti KG, Shaw J. Global and societal implications of the diabetes epidemic. *Nature* 2001; 414: 782–7.
16. Fagot-Campagna A, Narayan K. Type 2 diabetes in children. *BMJ* 2001; 322: 377–87.
17. Eriksson KF, Lindgärde F. Prevention of type 2 (noninsulin-dependent) diabetes mellitus by diet and physical exercise. The 6-year Malmö feasibility study, *Diabetologia* 1991; 34: 891–98.
18. Pan XR, Li GW, Hu YH, et al. Effects of diet and exercise in preventing NIDDM in people with impaired glucose tolerance: The Da Qing IGT and Diabetes Study, *Diabetes Care* 1997; 20: 537–44.
19. Tuomilehto J, Lindstrom J, Eriksson JG, et al. Prevention of type 2 diabetes mellitus by changes in lifestyle among subjects with impaired glucose tolerance, *N Engl J Med* 2001; 344: 1343–50.
20. The Diabetes Prevention Program: Design and methods for a clinical trial in the prevention of type 2 diabetes, *Diabetes Care* 1999; 22: 623–34.
21. Knowler WC, Barrett-Conner E, Fowler SE, et al. Diabetes Prevention Program Research Group. Reduction

in the incidence of type 2 diabetes with lifestyle intervention or metformin, *N Engl J Med* 2002; 346: 393–403.

22. Chiasson JL, Josse RG, Gomis R, Hanefeld M, Karasik A, Laakso M, for The STOP-NIDDM Trial Research Group. Acarbose for prevention of type 2 diabetes mellitus: the STOP-NIDDM randomized trial, *Lancet* 2002; 359: 2072–7.
23. Chiasson JL, Josse RG, Gomis R, Hanefeld M, Karasik A, Laakso M. Acarbose treatment and the risk of cardiovascular disease and hypertension in patients with impaired glucose tolerance: the STOP-NIDDM trial. *JAMA* 2003; 290 (4): 486–94.
24. Buchanann TA, Xiang AH, Peters RK, et al. Preservation of pancreatic B-cell function and prevention of type 2 diabetes by pharmacological treatment of insulin resistance in high-risk Hispanic women, *Diabetes* 2002; 51: 2796–803.
25. Wenying Y, Lixiang L, Jinwu Q, et al. The preventative effect of acarbose and metformin on the progression to diabetes mellitus in the IGT population: a 3-year multicentre prospective study, *Chin J Endocrinol Metab* 2001; 17: 131–5.
26. HOPE Study Investigators. Effects of an angiotensin-converting-enzyme inhibitor, ramipril, on cardiovascular events in high-risk patients. *N Engl J Med* 2000; 342 (3): 145–53.
27. Heart Outcome Prevention Evaluation (HOPE) Study Investigators. Effects of ramipril on cardiovascular and microvascular outcomes in people with diabetes mellitus: results of the HOPE study and MICRO HOPE substudy. *Lancet* 2000; 255: 253–9.
28. Isomaa B, Almgren P, Tuomi T, Forsen B, Lahti K, Nissen M, et al. Cardiovascular morbidity and mortality associated with the metabolic syndrome. *Diabetes Care* 2001; 24: 683–9.

45

Sulfonylureas: Basic Aspects and Clinical Uses

H.E. Lebovitz* **and Arne Melander†**

State University of New York, Brooklyn, NY, USA, and †The NEPI Foundation, Medical Research Centre, University Hospital, Malmö, Sweden

After more than 50 years of clinical use, and despite having been the subject of thousands of investigative studies, the role of sulfonylureas in the management of type 2 diabetes mellitus (NIDDM) remains enigmatic. Some clinicians are convinced that oral antidiabetic agents are drugs of convenience and would not be needed if patients were compliant with nonpharmacologic therapy. Others are certain that sulfonylureas help to ameliorate one of the basic defects of type 2 diabetes (deficient insulin secretion) and that most patients can benefit from their judicious use. The European Diabetes Policy Group of the International Diabetes Federation has recognized "that (except in emergency cases) if diet and exercise treatment fails, metformin or sulfonylureas are generally the first choice for additional treatment." The number of diabetic patients taking oral sulfonylureas has increased: the percentage taking sulfonylureas in the United States has increased from 29.5% in 1982 to 35.7% in 1986 to approximately 47% in 2000. [1]. In a recent analysis of type 2 diabetic patients starting oral antidiabetic treatment in the United States, 66% were given sulfonylureas [2].

Many questions concerning sulfonylurea therapy remain to be answered. Why do a few type 2 diabetic patients fail to respond to sulfonylureas initially, whereas the majority respond remarkably well? Why do many patients who respond well to sulfonylurea therapy initially later lose their responsiveness? Are the ATP-dependent potassium channels and the sulfonylurea receptor (SUR) subunit involved in the pathogenesis and progression of β-cell insufficiency? What mechanisms are responsible for the extrapancreatic effects of sulfonylureas and do these effects contribute to the therapeutic benefits of any of the sulfonylureas? Do any sulfonylurea drugs in ordinary therapeutic concentrations interact with sulfonylurea binding sites on ATP-dependent potassium channels in extrapancreatic tissues and cause clinically significant effects? Can intervention in prediabetic states with sulfonylureas prevent the development of type 2 diabetes and its complications? What role should combinations of sulfonylureas with other antidiabetic agents have in the current therapy of patients with type 2 diabetes?

This review examines the contemporary knowledge of these issues as well as current views on the relative merits and disadvantages of the various sulfonylureas and their clinical use.

PHARMACOLOGY AND CLINICAL PHARMACOLOGY

Chemistry and Structure of Sulfonylureas

The sulfonylureas are sulfonamide derivatives (Figure 1). Their hypoglycemic actions were discovered inadvertently when one of the initial agents was given to treat patients with typhoid fever. For many years it was believed that the hypoglycemic activities of sulfonylurea drugs were related to the presence of the sulfonylurea moiety. The demonstrations that non-sulfonylurea analogues of glibenclamide and gliquidone mimic the effects both *in vitro* and *in vivo* of their parent compounds on pancreatic B-cell function and insulin release indicated that the structural requirements for stimulating insulin secretion

International Textbook of Diabetes Mellitus, Third Edition. Edited by R. A. DeFronzo, E. Ferrannini, H. Keen, and P. Zimmet.
 ISBN: 0-471-48655-8.

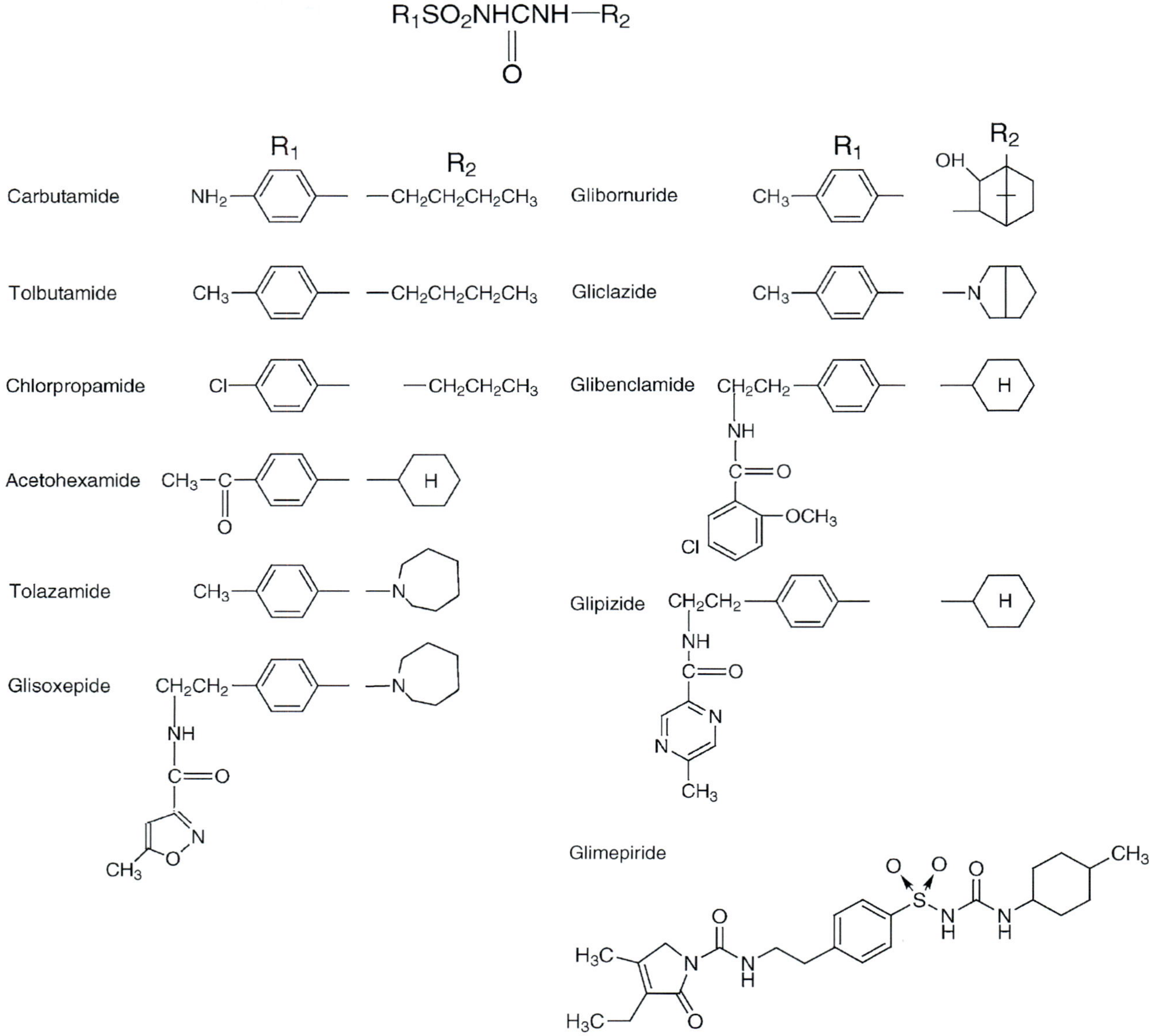

Figure 1 Chemical structures of sulfonylurea. (Adapted from reference 3, with permission)

did not necessarily require the sulfonylurea moiety [4, 5]. These findings have been explained by the recent characterizations of the pancreatic B-cell plasma membrane ATP-dependent potassium channel and its role in regulating insulin secretion [6, 7]. It seems likely that the sulfonylurea moiety facilitates the distribution of these drugs to the B-cell and is important for their specific binding to the SUR-1 subunit of the pancreatic B-cell plasma membrane ATP-dependent potassium channel [7, 8]. The "first generation" sulfonylureas such as tolbutamide and chlorpropamide have a phenyl ring with simple substituent groups at one end and an aliphatic side chain at the other end of the molecule (Figure 1). In "second generation" sulfonylureas such as glibenclamide (glyburide in the United States), glipizide, and glimepiride, the aliphatic side chain has been replaced by a cyclohexyl group and the substituent at the other end is a more complex structure than in the "first generation" agents (Figure 1). These substitutions have markedly increased the molecular affinity to binding sites on SUR-1 of the pancreatic B-cell plasma membrane ATP-dependent potassium channel. This explains the higher intrinsic activity and higher potency of these "second generation" sulfonylureas (see below). Detailed descriptions and comparisons of the different sulfonylureas are given later in the chapter.

The ATP-dependent Potassium Channel and Insulin Secretion

Glucose-stimulated insulin secretion is modulated by ion channels, which are located in the plasma membrane of the pancreatic B-cell [6, 9]. These ion channels are an ATP-sensitive potassium channel and a voltage-gated L-type calcium channel [10, 11].

As the ambient plasma glucose level changes, the quantity of glucose delivered to the mitochondria in the B-cell for oxidation is rapidly and quantitatively regulated by glucose transporter 2 (GLUT-2) and glucokinase activities. The intracellular ATP and ADP concentrations are therefore tightly coupled to the ambient plasma glucose concentrations. The plasma membrane ATP-dependent potassium channel in the presence of low ATP and high ADP concentrations (low plasma glucose) is open and is transporting potassium from the intracellular compartment to the extracellular compartment. This maintains the resting membrane potential. The voltage-gated calcium channel under such conditions is closed, the intracellular calcium concentration is low, and insulin secretion is minimal.

When the ambient plasma glucose rises, the intracellular ATP concentration increases and the ADP concentration decreases. This results in closure of ATP-dependent potassium channels. The membrane potential decreases, and the voltage-gated calcium channel opens. Calcium ion moves from the extracellular into the intracellular compartment, raising the cytosolic calcium ion concentrations and stimulating β-cell granule exocytosis and insulin secretion.

Pancreatic Effects of Sulfonylureas

The main effect of sulfonylureas is to improve glycemic control by reducing fasting and nonfasting blood glucose levels. This follows from their effects on insulin secretion, insulin action, and, possibly, on systemic availability of insulin.

Acute Effect on Insulin Secretions

Initial studies on the hypoglycemic actions of sulfonylureas indicated that a functional pancreas was necessary for this effect [12]. Sulfonylurea administration is without effect on blood glucose in pancreatectomized [13] or alloxan-diabetic [14] animals, or in persons with well-established type 1 diabetes [15] or pancreatic diabetes [16]. Acute intravenous or oral administration of sulfonylurea leads to a rapid rise in portal and then peripheral plasma insulin and C-peptide levels in normal or type 2 diabetic humans or animals [17]. Direct stimulation of insulin release by sulfonylureas has been demonstrated *in vitro* utilizing perifused pancreas preparations, isolated islets, and B-cell cultures [18, 19]. Sulfonylurea stimulation of insulin secretion from normal B-cells is usually weaker than nutrient stimulation, but the reverse is frequently true with diabetic B-cells.

A number of observations had suggested that the initial event in sulfonylurea stimulation of insulin secretion involved binding of the sulfonylurea molecule to a specific site on the B-cell plasma membrane. Early studies of the distribution of tolbutamide *in vivo* concluded that the drug was restricted to the extracellular compartment with the possible exception of the liver [20]. The uptake of [^{35}S]tolbutamide into microdissected pancreatic islets was found to be identical to that of markers known to equilibrate with the extracellular space [8]. When perfused through isolated rat pancreas, dextran-linked tolbutamide was shown to be as effective as tolbutamide in stimulating first-phase insulin release [21].

Pursuing the concept that sulfonylurea action involves drug interaction with the plasma membrane, several groups of investigators demonstrated that radiolabeled sulfonylureas such as [^{3}H]glipizide or [^{3}H]glibenclamide bind to purified plasma membranes from either rat insulinoma or transformed hamster tumor B-cells with characteristics that are compatible with specific receptor binding [11, 22, 23]. Displacement by sulfonylureas occurs in proportion to their activity (Figure 2). Table 1 lists the characteristics reported by some of the investigators for the presumed sulfonylurea B-cell binding site. Patch clamp techniques have shown a potency order of glibenclamide > glipizide > tolbutamide in the inhibition of the ATP-dependent potassium current in insulin secreting cells [22].

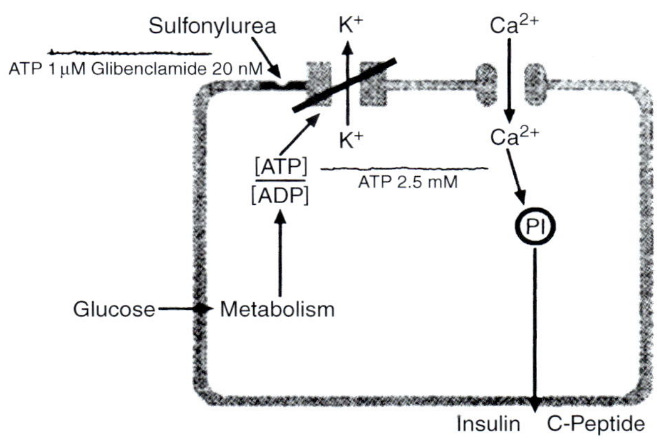

Figure 2 Scheme of a stimulated B-cell. Sulfonylureas stimulate by binding to plasma membrane receptors that are coupled to ATP-dependent K^+ channels. This inhibits efflux of K^+, causing depolarization of the plasma membrane. As a consequence, voltage-dependent Ca^{2+} channels open, causing influx of Ca^{2+} into the cytosol, which stimulates extrusion of both mature and immature insulin granules. ATP-dependent K^+ channels can also be inhibited by intracellular metabolic events that increase the ATP : ADP ratio. Typical recorded transmembrane voltage patterns from patch clamps from Schmid'-Antomarchi et al. [22] are illustrated. PI = proinsulin. (From reference 23, with permission)

Table 1 Studies demonstrating sulfonylurea plasma membrane binding sites

Ligand	Binding site	K_d (nmol/l)	R_0*(pmol/mg)
[^{3}H]Glipizide	Rat insulinoma purified plasma membranes	7.0	0.93
[^{3}H]Glibenclamide	RINm5F cell microsomes	0.3	0.15
[^{3}H]Glibenclamide	HIT cell membrane pellet	0.76	1.09
[^{3}H]Glibenclamide	Rat insulinoma crude membranes	0.01–0.05	0.29–0.52
		24–0.32	0.75–1.29
[^{3}H]Gliquidone	Rat brain crude membrane preparation	0.9	
[^{3}H]Glipizide	Rat cerebral cortex membranes	1.5	0.11
[^{3}H]Glibenclamide	Rat cerebral cortex membranes	0.041–0.1	0.013–0.024
		0.05–0.4	0.030–0.034

* R_0 = number of binding sites.

Within several years, the sulfonylurea binding site was cloned and identified as a component of one of the subunits of the B-cell plasma membrane ATP-dependent potassium channel [24, 25]. The ATP-dependent potassium channel is a hetero-octameric complex composed of two types of protein subunits [6, 9, 26]. Four Kir6.*x* subunits assemble as a tetramer and form the inwardly rectifying potassium channel. Four SUR subunits surround the Kir6.*x* subunits. SUR is a member of the ABC transporter family and has 17 transmembrane helices. ATP binds to the intracellular domains of the Kir6.*x* subunits and causes inhibition of the channel. The SUR subunits contain nucleotide binding domains and drug binding sites, which mediate channel activity. Several isoforms exist for both the Kir6.*x* and SUR subunits [6, 9, 27]. ATP-dependent channels are present in the membranes of many tissues including pancreatic B-cells, brain, heart, and skeletal muscle and vascular smooth muscle, and their isoform composition varies, which gives them different metabolic and drug sensitivities [9, 27]. Table 2 lists the characteristics of the different ATP-dependent potassium channels. Pancreatic B-cells and brain ATP-dependent potassium channels are made up of Kir6.2 and SUR-1 subunits. The SUR-1 has two known binding sites that when activated inhibit channel activity: a sulfonylurea binding site, which recognizes sulfonylureas, and a meglitinide binding site, which recognizes non-sulfonylurea components such as the non-sulfonylurea component of the glibenclamide structure and repaglinide [7]. As discussed later, SUR-2 has a somewhat different binding profile in that it does not bind tolbutamide or gliclazide and has lesser affinity for glimepiride and non-sulfonylurea insulin secretogogues than does SUR-1.

Sulfonylurea binding to the ATP-dependent potassium channel initiates events similar to those occurring with glucose stimulation (Figure 3). Sulfonylureas inhibit ^{86}Rb efflux (used as a tracer for K^+ movement) from islets incubated at basal glucose concentrations [19, 28]. The stimulatory effect of sulfonylureas on insulin secretion is abolished in Ca^{2+}-deprived media [22, 29], and blockage of Ca^{2+} entry by agents such as verapamil causes a dose-dependent inhibition of sulfonylurea-mediated insulin secretion [29]. Sulfonylureas cause a two- to threefold increase in B-cell cytosolic Ca^{2+} as determined by quin-2 fluorescence [19, 29]. Thus, the ion flux changes seen with sulfonylurea stimulation of B-cells are similar to those following glucose stimulation. In both instances the rise in cytosolic Ca^{2+} activates the microtubular–microfilamentous system in B-cells through one or more of several proposed mechanisms involving protein kinase phosphorylation [19].

While the delineation of the interaction between sulfonylureas and the B-cell plasma membrane ATP-dependent potassium channel explains much of the mechanism by which sulfonylureas stimulate insulin secretion, a number of questions and observations remain unanswered. Several studies have demonstrated that as much as 75% of glibenclamide that attaches to the B-cell is actually bound to B-cell granules [30, 31]. These data are consistent with an observed direct effect of sulfonylureas in stimulating the exocytotic process itself. Rorsman and his colleagues have presented data to support the hypothesis that sulfonylureas bind to a 65-kDa receptor in the B-cell granule membrane and activate granular CIC-3 chloride channels [32]. These channels are proposed to act in concert with v-type H^+-ATPase. The combined effect is postulated to

Table 2 ATP-dependent potassium channels and their physiologic functions

Tissue	Inward rectifier	Sulfonylurea receptor	Basal state	Stimulus	Effect
Pancreatic B-cell	Kir6.2	SUR-1	Open	↑ Glucose	↑ Insulin secretion
Neuronal cells	Kir6.2	SUR-1	?	?	?
Myocardial cells	Kir6.2	SUR-2A	Closed	Ischemia and hypoxia	↓ Energy consumption and ischemic preconditioning
Vascular smooth	Kir6.1	SUR-2B	Closed	Ischemia and hypoxia	Vasodilatation
	Kir6.2	SUR-2B			

Note. "?" indicates "not known."

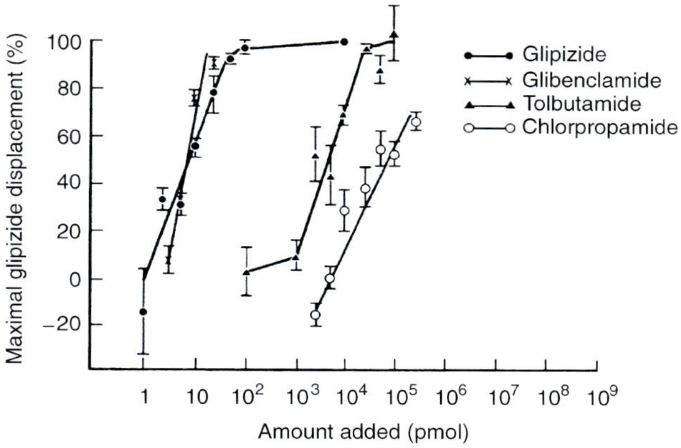

Figure 3 Displacement of [^{3}H]glipizide from purified plasma membranes from RINm5F-generated insulinomas by glipizide (●), glyburide (×), tolbutamide (▲), and chlorpropamide (○). Data are mean ± SE of three determinations. (From reference 23, with permission)

promote acidification of the granule interior, which is essential for the granule to gain release competence [32].

The ATP-dependent potassium channel model does not explain the known differences between nutrient-stimulated insulin secretion and sulfonylurea stimulation of insulin secretion. D-Glucose is thought to stimulate insulin secretion by increasing ATP and/or modifying other factors that close the ATP-sensitive K^+ channel from the cytoplasmic surface of the membrane [10, 19]. Sulfonylureas differ from D-glucose in that they do not increase intracellular ATP or increase the efflux of radioactive phosphate from prelabeled islets [19]. In contrast to glucose, sulfonylureas decrease K^+ inflow into islet cells, increase their Na^+ content, and lower their intracellular pH [19]. Similarly, they do not stimulate proinsulin biosynthesis, neither do they inhibit [2-^{3}H]-adenosine efflux from prelabeled islets [19]. Sulfonylureas only stimulate first-phase insulin secretion [19, 28]. Thus there are many differences between sulfonylurea-mediated and nutrient-mediated insulin secretion.

The presence of sulfonylurea and meglitinide binding sites on the SUR subunit raises the question of whether there are natural ligands for these binding sites? If so, what are they and are alterations in the ligands or in the ATP-dependent potassium channel playing a role in the pathogenesis of B-cell insufficiency in type 2 diabetes.

Chronic Effects on Insulin Secretion

In numerous clinical studies it was shown that chronic treatment with sulfonylureas, in contrast to acute treatment, resulted in improved glycemia but with less rather than more insulin secretion [33, 34]. Similarly when patients on chronic sulfonylurea therapy showed deteriorating glycemic control it was assumed that the sulfonylurea drugs had lost their insulin secretory activity. Assessments of the chronic effects of sulfonylureas on insulin secretion in patients with type 2 diabetes have been difficult to interpret because the magnitude of sulfonylurea stimulation of insulin secretion is influenced by many factors. Some of the factors that influence insulin secretion during chronic sulfonylurea therapy are (a) the intrinsic effect of sulfonylureas on B-cell insulin secretion; (b) the level of glycemia attained during the sulfonylurea stimulus for insulin secretion; (c) the degree of chronic fasting hyperglycemia, which itself may cause inhibition of insulin secretion (glucose toxicity); (d) the stage of glucose intolerance (the functional state of the β-cells); and (e) tachyphylaxis to sulfonylureas during chronic, continuous sulfonylurea therapy.

Many studies in type 2 diabetic patients indicate that chronic sulfonylurea treatment increases the ability of the B-cell to respond to a fixed stimulus. Porte and colleagues have defined the insulin secretory responses of non-glucose stimuli at different ambient glycemic levels in normal subjects and in patients with type 2 diabetes [35]. Normal individuals have an increase in insulin secretion stimulated by intravenous arginine or isoproterenol during an acute intravenous tolbutamide infusion, provided that the plasma glucose level is clamped, but not if it is allowed to fall [35]. It was also shown that 4 of 9 type 2 diabetic patients treated with chlorpropamide for 12–16 weeks had an increase in non-glucose-mediated insulin secretion when their pretreatment glycemic values were restored [36]. The same phenomenon may explain why type 2 diabetic patients on chronic sulfonylurea therapy will show a rise in nutrient-mediated insulin responses immediately following discontinuation of sulfonylurea therapy [37]. A chronic effect of sulfonylurea therapy to increase the insulin secretory capacity of laboratory animal pancreas to stimuli has not been observed; rather, nutrient-stimulated insulin secretion is decreased.

Studies in type 2 diabetic patients with normal or mildly elevated fasting plasma glucose concentrations show that the degree of the nutrient-evoked rise in plasma glucose is a major determinant of insulin secretion [38]: thus, a lesser rise such as that occurs during chronic sulfonylurea therapy will result in less secretion.

The chronic level of fasting hyperglycemia is as important as the nutrient-evoked rise in plasma glucose in determining insulin secretion. In this case, however, the higher the fasting plasma glucose value, the lower the nutrient-mediated insulin secretion. A reduction in fasting hyperglycemia by any form of therapy (diet, drugs, or insulin) results in increased glucose-mediated insulin secretion [39]. Exhaustive experimental and clinical data support the concept that chronic hyperglycemia itself inhibits glucose-mediated insulin secretion [40]. Apparently, reduction of fasting and postprandial hyperglycemia in type 2 diabetic patients by any modality can either increase or decrease glucose-mediated insulin secretion.

The question of sulfonylurea tachyphylaxis has been raised by Karam et al. [41], who studied the acute insulin secretory response to intravenous tolbutamide or glucagon in 10 type 2 diabetic patients, before, during, and after tolazamide therapy. They found that chronic tolazamide therapy abolished the insulin secretory response to tolbutamide but not to glucagon, and they also showed that the acute response to tolbutamide reappeared after cessation of tolazamide therapy. They concluded that chronic continuous sulfonylurea therapy may blunt the acute insulin secretory response to sulfonylurea. *In vitro* studies have shown that prolonged incubation of B-cells with sulfonylureas causes a disturbance in the assembly and functional activity of the ATP-dependent potassium channel [42]. It is unclear whether this mechanism is operative in humans. Another possibility is that this phenomenon could be explained by downregulation of the SUR-1 receptor. Support for this assumption can be obtained from two studies described below under Kinetic–Dynamic Relations, showing that increases of dosage and sulfonylurea steady-state concentrations over a certain level impaired rather than improved glucose and insulin responses.

This complexity explains why so much controversy exists as to whether the primary action of chronic sulfonylurea therapy is increased insulin secretion and why there has been continuing interest in whether extrapancreatic effects of sulfonylureas are clinically meaningful.

Effects on the Secretion of Insulin Precursors

There is increasing evidence that small amounts of insulin precursors, particularly intact proinsulin and 32/33 split proinsulin, are released along with insulin, and that the proportions of these precursors are increased in type 2 diabetic subjects [43]. In addition, the levels of 32/33 split proinsulin correlate more closely with cardiovascular risk factors in type 2 diabetes than do those of insulin itself. If the increased levels of 32/33 split proinsulin were to be causally related to the cardiovascular complications in type 2 diabetes, and if sulfonylurea treatment further enhanced the levels of 32/33 split proinsulin, sulfonylurea treatment could be detrimental. However, recent studies indicate that such treatment does not increase the concentrations of 32/33 split proinsulin in type 2 diabetic subjects, although insulin and proinsulin levels are enhanced [43]. The ratio of proinsulin to insulin in plasma is unaltered by sulfonylurea treatment [44].

Effects on Proinsulin Biosynthesis

A major difference between sulfonylurea-stimulated insulin secretion and nutrient-stimulated insulin secretion is that sulfonylureas cause only first-phase insulin release (preformed insulin) whereas nutrients stimulate both first-phase and second-phase insulin release [44]. Second-phase insulin release consists largely of newly synthesized insulin. The explanation for the failure of sulfonylureas to stimulate second-phase insulin release might be found in studies utilizing models *in vivo* and *in vitro* of animal perfused pancreas, isolated islets, or islet cell cultures, which have shown that sulfonylureas inhibit the biosynthesis of proinsulin [45, 46].

Effects on Glucagon and Somatostatin Secretion

Normal α-cells do not appear to have functional ATP-sensitive potassium channels and do not show significant *in vitro* effects of sulfonylureas in regulating glucagon secretion. However, several studies in humans show that glibenclamide treatment causes impairment of glucagon secretion in response to insulin-induced hypoglycemia [47–49]. The mechanism whereby sulfonylureas reduce glucagon secretion is thought to be an increase in intraislet insulin flow from B-cells to A-cells. D-cells contain ATP-dependent potassium channels with SURs. Sulfonylureas stimulate pancreatic D-cell somatostatin release [47, 50], but it is not clear whether this plays any part in their antidiabetic actions.

Extrapancreatic Effects of Sulfonylureas

Sulfonylurea drugs have been investigated extensively for extrapancreatic actions. Most studies demonstrating such actions have utilized organ perfusion, cell culture, or subcellular preparations from laboratory animals. Some have shown extrapancreatic effects with concentrations of sulfonylureas far in excess of ordinarily attainable therapeutic plasma levels. Studies *in vivo* have frequently failed to validate that the action is a primary one rather than a consequence of better glycemic regulation due to increased insulin secretion. The two sulfonylureas that have most recently been promoted as having clinically significant extrapancreatic effects in humans are gliclazide and glimepiride, as are discussed later in this chapter.

Table 3 summarizes some of the reported extrapancreatic effects. As sulfonylureas lower blood glucose only in the presence of a functioning pancreas, it is difficult to attribute a meaningful antidiabetic action to an extrapancreatic effect that occurs in the absence of insulin [54]. Thus, a primary action in increasing fructose 2,6-bisphosphate in the liver with subsequent stimulation of glycolysis and inhibition of gluconeogenesis, although of interest, is unlikely to explain the antidiabetic action [55]. A similar analysis can be made for primary actions on muscle or adipose tissue [55].

Effects on Insulin Action

The main extrapancreatic action of sulfonylureas that is likely to have a meaningful antidiabetic effect is involved in the potentiation of insulin action. Such an action was

Table 3 Extrapancreatic actions of sulfonylurea drugs*

Probably related to antidiabetic action:

(1) Potentiation of insulin stimulation of carbohydrate transport in skeletal muscle and adipose tissue
(2) Potentiation of insulin-mediated translocation of glucose transport molecules
(3) Potentiation of insulin-mediated activation of hepatic glycogen synthase and glycogen synthesis
(4) Potentiation of insulin-mediated hepatic lipogenesis
(5) Increase of insulin-stimulated glycogen synthesis in human muscle [51, 52]

Possibly related to antidiabetic action:

(1) Direct effects on the liver
  (a) Increase in fructose 2,6-biphosphate
  (b) Increase in glycolysis
  (c) Decrease in gluconeogenesis
  (d) Decrease in long-chain fatty acid oxidation
  (e) Increase intracellular sorting of the insulin–receptor complex toward the degradative route [53]
(2) Direct effects on skeletal muscle
  (a) Increase in amino acid transport
  (b) Increase in fructose 2,6-biphosphate
(3) Inhibition of insulinase

Unlikely to be related to antidiabetic action:

(1) Direct effects on adipose tissue
  (a) Increase in glycogen synthase
  (b) Activation of adenosine 3′,5′-monophosphate diesterase and inhibition of lipolysis
(2) Direct effects on myocardial tissue
  (a) Increase in contractility, oxygen consumption, and glycogenolysis and decrease in sarcolemmal Ca^{2+}-ATPase
  (b) Increase in glucose transport, glycolysis, phosphofructokinase activity, and pyruvate oxidation
(3) Increase in synthesis and secretion of plasminogen activator from endothelial cells

* Modified from reference 50, with permission.

described in 1955 and has been controversial ever since. The clearest demonstrations of sulfonylurea potentiation of insulin action have been carried out in animal models. Experiments on mouse diaphragm and on organ culture with rat adipose tissue have demonstrated that ordinary doses or concentrations of sulfonylureas will potentiate insulin-mediated 2-deoxy-D-glucose uptake after a latent period of about 12 h [56]. One study has suggested that this is attributable to sulfonylurea potentiation of insulin-mediated translocation of the glucose transporter from intracellular storage sites to the plasma membrane [57]. This needs to be confirmed and extended, as the genes for the insulin-sensitive and insulin-insensitive glucose transport molecules now have been cloned.

Putnam et al. [58] utilized the euglycemic insulin clamp at physiological insulin levels in normal dogs and showed that 2 weeks' treatment with glipizide caused a twofold increase in insulin-mediated glucose disposal. The chronic treatment caused no significant alterations in plasma glucose or insulin.

Studies in patients with type 2 diabetes that have attempted to demonstrate whether sulfonylureas potentiate insulin-mediated glucose disposal have reported diverse results. Some show that sulfonylurea treatment increased insulin-mediated glucose disposal, but only in patients who have increased insulin secretion [59, 60]; the improved glucose disposal is attributed to higher plasma insulin levels. In a study on insulin-treated type 2 diabetic subjects who had little or no remaining endogenous insulin, sulfonylurea failed to evoke any glucose reduction [61]. Other studies also show that sulfonylurea treatment increases insulin-mediated glucose disposal, but the improvement is attributed to the effect of better glycemic regulation. Finally, there are studies in which sulfonylurea treatment improves glycemic control, increases insulin-mediated glucose disposal, and yet does not correlate with improved insulin secretion, suggesting that true sulfonylurea-induced potentiation of insulin action does occur in some patients with type 2 diabetes [62–64].

Apart from muscle and adipose tissue, the liver may be a site of sulfonylurea potentiation of insulin action. Sulfonylureas have been reported to potentiate insulin-mediated glycogen and lipid synthesis. These effects have been well described in hepatic cell cultures [55]. Clinical studies suggest that the reduction in fasting hyperglycemia during sulfonylurea treatment can be attributed in large part to potentiation of insulin action on glycogen synthesis and gluconeogenesis [65]. Detailed discussions of the relative roles of pancreatic versus extrapancreatic mechanisms in the antidiabetic action of sulfonylureas are available in several recent reviews [55, 66, 67].

The mechanisms of the various extrapancreatic actions of sulfonylureas have not been defined. ATP-dependent potassium channels and specific plasma membrane sulfonylurea binding sites have been found in many tissues, as noted in Table 3. They have not been found in liver cells or are present in very minimal quantities in skeletal muscle cells. There is no evidence to suggest that ionic fluxes have any role in mediating the extrapancreatic effects desribed in Table 2. The insulin-potentiating action of sulfonylureas has a latent period of several hours, and this effect is blocked by cycloheximide, indicating that new protein synthesis may be necessary for that effect to occur [68].

The effect of sulfonylureas in potentiating insulin action on muscle, adipose tissue, and liver has raised the issue of whether these effects are mediated by a direct action in increasing insulin binding by the insulin receptor (an increase either in receptor number or in affinity) or through postreceptor mechanisms. Studies *in vivo* in which insulin binding is assessed are invalid to answer this question because changes in plasma insulin levels will influence the number of insulin receptors, and measurements of insulin binding to circulating monocytes or adipose tissues may not reflect what is occurring at liver and muscle cells. Assessment of insulin binding to fibroblasts in culture has little physiologic meaning. Several studies *in vitro* indicate that the effect occurs at a postreceptor site [50].

Effect on Systemic Availability of Insulin

One of the earliest extrapancreatic actions of sulfonylureas to be described was inhibition of insulinase, particularly in the liver [69]. Later studies disputed these data, and the idea was abandoned. However, several recent studies suggest that at least glipizide [70–73] and glibenclamide [74] may increase the systemic availability of insulin through reduction of the hepatic extraction of insulin secreted from the pancreas. It is not known whether the effect is a primary one, e.g. inhibition of hepatic insulinase [69] or displacement of insulin from hepatic binding sites, or is secondary to the increased rate of insulin secretion subsequent to sulfonylurea stimulation of the B-cells [73]. If the increased systemic availability were attributable to displacement of insulin from hepatic insulin receptors, it is also possible that such displacement might reduce the effect of insulin exerted on the liver and hence would lead to an increased hepatic output of glucose, provided that the displacement was extensive enough. Such a phenomenon would help to explain why high doses of sulfonylurea may impair instead of improve blood glucose control [75, 76].

Effects on Blood Lipids

Sulfonylurea treatment has been reported to have beneficial, neutral, or adverse effects on blood lipids [3]. It seems unlikely, therefore, that sulfonylureas have direct effects on very low-density lipid triglycerides, low-density lipid cholesterol, or high-density lipid cholesterol.

Effect on Fibrinolysis

A recent study on bovine aortic endothelial cells indicated that certain sulfonylureas may enhance fibrinolysis and that the fibrinolytic mechanism is associated with sulfonylurea-enhanced production of plasminogen activator [77].

Differences in Extrapancreatic Effects

Some extrapancreatic effects of sulfonylureas are related to parts of the molecule other than the sulfonylurea core and are therefore unrelated to the antidiabetic action. These extrapancreatic effects may confer unique advantages or disadvantages to a particular sulfonylurea. Chlorpropamide facilitates both the release and the tubular action of vasopressin, causing water retention and hyponatremia in certain patients [78]. Sulfonylureas increase the synthesis and secretion of plasminogen activator from bovine aortic endothelial cells, but the potency is unrelated to the blood glucose lowering activity [61]. The spectrum of action of glibenclamide on the myocardium differs from that of tolbutamide [55] and glimepiride, as discussed in a later section. The clinical potential of many of these differences has yet to be explored.

CLINICAL ASPECTS OF SULFONYLUREA THERAPY

Clinical Effects

Knowledge about the clinical effects of sulfonylurea drugs can be divided into that obtained prior to 1995 and that obtained after 1995. The early clinical studies that documented the beneficial effects of sulfonylurea drugs in type 2 diabetic patients were, for the most part, poorly designed and inadequately implemented. Frequently, they did not have a proper dietary run-in period. The large trials were rarely double blind and placebo controlled. The new era studies include large placebo-controlled, double-blind trials of the efficacy and safety of new or newly formulated sulfonylureas such as glimepiride or glipizide GITS, short-term clinical pharmacologic studies utilizing small numbers of patients, and the landmark United Kingdom Prospective Diabetes Study (UKPDS). All of the studies, both old and new, demonstrate that sulfonylurea drugs have their major effects in lowering the fasting plasma glucose levels [79–81]. They do so by decreasing hepatic glucose production as they stimulate the release of insulin from the B-cell into the portal vein and into the liver. The postprandial plasma glucose excursion is only slightly decreased because sulfonylurea drugs do not significantly improve the delay in meal-mediated insulin secretion, which is characteristic of type 2 diabetes [79–81]. They significantly increase late meal-mediated insulin secretion. As a result of the insulin secretory dynamics,

Table 4 Effect of sulfonylurea treatment on glycemic control in type 2 diabetic patients

Sulfonylurea (reference no.)	No. of patients	Duration of treatment (years)	Glycemic control*		
			Excellent	Good	Unsatisfactory
Tolbutamide [85]	1812	1–5	43	23	34
Chlorpropamide [86]	339	1–6	30	28	42
Glibenclamide [87]	3440	0.6†	37	32	31
Glipizide [88]	1015	0.6†	25	34	41

* Criteria for glycemic control are as follows:

Blood glucose levels	Excellent	Good
Fasting, mmol/l (mg/dl)	$\leq$5.6 (100)	$\leq$7.2 (130)
1-h postprandial, mmol/l (mg/dl)	$\leq$8.3 (150)	$\leq$10.0 (180)
2-h postprandial, mmol/l (mg/dl)	$\leq$7.2 (130)	$\leq$ 8.3 (150)

† Average duration of treatment.

sulfonylurea drugs have little impact on early postprandial glycemic excursions and a major impact on late excursions. The late postprandial effects of sulfonylurea drugs are mediated by an increased peripheral glucose disposal through enhanced insulin secretion and possibly some potentiation of insulin action [39, 62, 82–84]. Table 4 lists the results reported from several pre-1995 large open-labeled studies which examined the effects of different sulfonylureas on glycemic control in type 2 diabetic patients [85–88]. The criteria for glycemic control in these older studies varied a little, but generally "excellent control" signified that 70% of blood glucose measurements showed fasting, 1-h, and 2-h postprandial levels that did not exceed 5.6, 8.3, and 7.2 mmol/l (100, 150, and 130 mg/dl), respectively. In "good control," 70% of blood glucose measurements showed fasting, 1-h, and 2-h postprandial levels not exceeding 7.2, 10.0, and 8.3 mmol/l (130, 180, and 150 mg/dl), respectively. "Unsatisfactory control" meant values exceeding those for good control. The effects of the various sulfonylureas on glycemic control in these studies do not differ to any relevant extent, and they suggest that approximately 60–65% of type 2 diabetic patients might be expected to achieve excellent or good glycemic control on sulfonylurea therapy.

An initially successful therapeutic response to sulfonylurea treatment is often followed by secondary failure. The data on the frequency with which secondary failure occurs are limited, as few long-term data on sulfonylurea treatment have been reported [89]. Approximately 20% of patients treated with tolbutamide for 1–5 years develop secondary failure (4% in the first year and about 9% per year in years 2–5) [85]. Of patients taking the drug for 6–9 years, 26% develop secondary failure [90]. The secondary failure rates for chlorpropamide and other sulfonylureas are probably similar to that for tolbutamide [86, 89].

The new era studies have utilized the measurement of hemoglobin A_{1c} (HbA_{1c}) as the gold standard for defining glycemic control [79–81]. Evaluation of the efficacy of antihyperglycemic therapy is the absolute decrease in HbA_{1c} or the percentage of treated patients that achieve the target goal (usually $HbA_{1c} \leq 7.0\%$). In all recent clinical trials with antihyperglycemic agents it has been observed that the absolute decrease in HbA_{1c} is a function of the baseline HbA_{1c}: the higher the baseline HbA_{1c}, the greater the decrease; the lower the baseline HbA_{1c}, the less the decrease. In long-term studies decreasing sulfonylurea effect is recognized as sulfonylurea inadequacy rather than sulfonylurea failure since the patients still have some, albeit a small, response to the sulfonylurea drugs [91]. Table 5 lists the results of registration trials for several newer sulfonylurea drugs illustrating these points [79].

Sulfonylurea treatment has been shown to cause a near-euglycemic remission, which persists for at least several months and possibly years after the drugs have been discontinued. This was well documented by Singer and Hurwitz in 1967 [95] following tolbutamide (31% of patients) or chlorpropamide treatment (17% of patients), and later confirmed by Lev-Ran [96]. It is likely that the remission is related to excellent glycemic regulation rather

Table 5 Effects of new sulfonylurea drugs and new formulations on glycemic control in type 2 diabetic patients

Sulfonylurea (reference no.)	No. of patients	Duration of treatment	HbA_{1c} (%)	
			Baseline	Decrease compared to placebo
Glipizide GITS [92]	204	16 weeks	8.7	1.8
Glimepiride [93]	416	14 weeks	8.1	1.9
Glibenclamide* [94]	289	20 weeks	8.1	1.0

* From Glucovance trial.

than to a specific effect of sulfonylurea treatment, but this concept needs more verification.

Patients who are most likely to show an excellent or good glycemic response to sulfonylurea therapy are those who have relatively recently diagnosed type 2 diabetes, have mild to moderate fasting hyperglycemia (fasting plasma glucose levels below 12.5 mmol/l) on dietary management, have a good B-cell reserve as reflected by high C-peptide levels, have a normal weight or are moderately obese, and have either never been treated with insulin or are taking less than 30 U of insulin daily [79, 80].

One large, randomized, double-blind, placebo-controlled study of tolbutamide treatment for 8 years was the University Group Diabetes Program (UGDP) [97]. A total of 823 patients were randomly assigned initially to one of four treatments: placebo, tolbutamide 1.5 g/day, a fixed dose of insulin, or a variable insulin dose adjusted to achieve normal blood glucose levels. This controversial study indicated that the fixed dose of tolbutamide decreased fasting blood glucose levels by 20% in the first year of treatment. Over the ensuing 4 years the fasting blood glucose values increased, and by 5 years they were the same as before treatment and no different from those of the placebo-treated group. The significance of these data is obscured by the lack of intention to treat to a specific glycemic endpoint.

Our knowledge about sulfonylurea therapy of type 2 diabetes has been revolutionized by the results of the landmark UKPDS, which started in the late 1970s and concluded in 1997. This study recruited slightly more than 5000 newly diagnosed type 2 diabetic patients and after a 3-month diet modification randomized most of them to either continued lifestyle modification without drug addition ("conventional treatment") or continued lifestyle modification to which was added a sulfonylurea (glibenclamide, chlorpropamide, or glipizide) or insulin ("intensive control"). Some overweight patients were randomized to addition or no addition of metformin, and in a substudy, some normal-weight and overweight patients already on sulfonylurea were also randomized to addition or no addition of metformin, to enable assessment of combination treatment [98, 99]. The patients were followed for a mean of 11 years and the endpoints were the development of clinically significant diabetic complications. The aim was to achieve a fasting plasma glucose <6 mmol/l.

Sulfonylurea treatment achieved the same glycemic control over the 10 years as did insulin treatment, with less increase in body weight [99] (median HbA_{1c}: chlorpropamide 6.7%, glibenclamide 7.2%, insulin 7.1%, conventional 7.9%). These data are somewhat misleading since glycemic control in all groups deteriorated with time. For example in the intensively treated groups which included those randomized to sulfonylureas, median HbA_{1c} increased for each successive 5-year treatment period (6.6% in the first 5 years, 7.5% in the second 5 years, and 8.1% in the last 5 years) [100].

A detailed analysis of the UKPDS monotherapy data showed that the percentage of patients treated with sulfonylureas that achieved a HbA_{1c} $<7\%$ were 50% at 3 years, 34% at 6 years and 24% at 9 years [101]. An analysis of 1305 patients treated with glibenclamide or chlorpropamide over 6 years showed that loss of sulfonylurea responsiveness was related to higher initial plasma glucose concentrations at randomization, younger age of presentation of diabetes, lower initial B-cell reserve as measured by the HOMA model, and to those randomized to glibenclamide compared with chlorpropamide [102]. For example, 61% of patients with a fasting plasma glucose ≥ 10 mmol/l required additional antihyperglycemic therapy by 6 years. By contrast only 23% required additional therapy if the fasting plasma glucose was <7.8 mmol/l.

During the first 6 years of the UKPDS $<\beta$-cell function as estimated by the HOMA model was assessed in 511 patients allocated to sulfonylurea therapy and compared to that of 376 patients allocated to diet [103]. At randomization the patients on $_{1c}$ conventional" therapy (diet without drugs) had 51% of normal B-cell function and the sulfonylurea patients 46%. The B-cell function of the patients on diet decreased progressively over the 6 years to 28%. The mean B-cell function in the sulfonylurea-treated patients rose to 78% at 1 year but then decreased progressively and was 52% at 6 years. The data were interpreted as consistent with an inability of sulfonylureas to change the progressive B-cell loss that occurs in type 2 diabetes. Oral antidiabetic therapy failure most likely is the result of the progressive loss of B-cell function with time.

Similarities and Differences Between Sulfonylureas

It is generally assumed that all sulfonylureas have the same mechanism of action on the pancreatic B-cell, and that this relates to receptor binding to the B-cell plasma membrane ATP-dependent potassium channel (see above). Evidence that SUR-1 has at least two distinct binding sites and that some sulfonylureas bind at only one site while others bind at both sites [7] as well as the observations that sulfonylureas stimulate exocytosis independent of the ATP-dependent potassium channel [32] leave open the possibility that all sulfonylureas may not have exactly the same effects on B-cells. Additionally, as all sulfonylureas have not been tested or compared in similar pharmacodynamic systems *in vitro* and *in vivo*, it cannot be excluded that there may be qualitative pharmacodynamic differences between them. One such difference might reside in the ability of sulfonylureas to penetrate the B-cell; in contrast to most other sulfonylureas, glibenclamide may accumulate within the B-cells [30]. On the other hand, as both glibenclamide and other sulfonylureas seem to release insulin by an interaction with the plasma membrane ATP-sensitive potassium channel of the B-cell, the relevance of the B-cell penetrating ability of glibenclamide remains uncertain and may relate to direct effects on exocytosis.

All sulfonylureas are weak acids. Some of them are highly lipophilic, e.g. glibenclamide and glipizide, whereas chlorpropamide is rather hydrophilic. Most sulfonylureas seem to be extensively absorbed, some of them completely. However, the rates of absorption differ between agents, formulations, and individuals, and this may be clinically important (see below). All have a small distribution volume, signifying that most of the drug is contained within blood plasma; they are extensively bound to plasma albumin, the most lipophilic ones to the greatest extent [3]. All sulfonylureas are metabolized, the more lipophilic ones virtually completely, whereas the more hydrophilic chlorpropamide is partially excreted unchanged through the kidneys [3, 104]. All sulfonylureas have a low clearance [3, 104]. Some, but not all, sulfonylureas have active metabolites that may depend upon renal function for their elimination. There is no evidence of any relevant first-pass metabolism of any sulfonylurea [3, 104]. A detailed description of the pharmacokinetics of the different sulfonylureas is given later in the chapter.

Potency and Intrinsic Molecular Activity

Although the sulfonylureas may have identical or similar pharmacodynamics, they have different potencies and intrinsic activities related to the variations in chemical structure (see Figure 1). These structural variations are associated with differences in pharmacokinetics, which determine the concentration of the sulfonylurea achieved in the islets and in differences in sulfonylurea binding affinities to the SUR-1 subunit of the ATP-dependent potassium channel of the B-cell [6, 23] (Table 1, Figure 3). The highest affinity to B-cell binding sites has been observed for glibenclamide, glipizide, and glimepiride [23], and these three sulfonylureas also have the highest activity in terms of their minimum effective plasma concentrations, which are 50–100 nmol/l [3]. At the other end of the binding spectrum are tolbutamide and chlorpropamide, which have a B-cell affinity and intrinsic activity that are only about 1/1000 of that of glibenclamide and glipizide, as expressed by their minimum effective plasma concentrations (which are 50–100 μmol/l) [3]. Acetohexamide and tolazamide seem to be active in the latter range [104], whereas glibornuride, gliclazide, and gliquidone seem to have an intermediate activity [3, 104].

As the common daily dose of chlorpropamide is 250–500 mg, whereas that of tolbutamide is 1500–3000 mg, it may be said that chlorpropamide is more potent than tolbutamide. However, the reason why a lower daily dose of chlorpropamide can be used is that the elimination of this compound is very slow, allowing a high degree of accumulation of the drug. Indeed, at a similar degree of glucose control, the plasma levels of chlorpropamide are higher than those of tolbutamide, suggesting that the intrinsic activity of the chlorpropamide molecule is, in fact, lower than that of tolbutamide [23, 105].

The issue of potency and activity may be mainly academic, as no appropriately controlled study has shown that any sulfonylurea, in appropriate dosage, is clinically more effective than any other. However, the differences in potency and intrinsic activity may be relevant from the safety aspect, including the issues of hypoglycemia, side effects, and drug interactions (see later).

Rate of Onset and Duration of Action

The structural variations between the different sulfonylureas are associated with differences in pharmacokinetics, i.e. in the rate and extent of absorption, distribution, biotransformation, and excretion. These differences, in turn, lead to variations in the rate of onset and in the duration of action of the sulfonylureas, and these variations may be clinically more relevant than the differences in potency and intrinsic activity (pharmacodynamics).

Rate and timing of onset of sulfonylurea action The rate of onset is relevant as it relates to the capacity to improve the acute insulin release in response to meals, which is impaired in patients with type 2 diabetes as well as in subjects with impaired glucose tolerance (IGT) [3, 106–109]. Indeed, a recent study, employing a highly selective insulin assay, indicates that a delayed and reduced insulin response to glucose challenge is a dominant feature in both type 2 diabetes and IGT [109]. Accordingly, a rapid onset of sulfonylurea action may be important. The most rapidly acting sulfonylurea currently available is glipizide [3], and it has been shown that glipizide is able to increase the rate of insulin release in response to meals, both acutely and chronically [3, 110, 111]. Moreover, glipizide may rapidly enhance the systemic availability of insulin by reducing its first-pass hepatic clearance [70–73]. The importance of the rate of absorption and onset of action is also apparent from the fact that the efficacy of glipizide is directly dependent upon its absorption rate: the time to reach the threshold concentration of this drug correlates with the time to reach the nadir of blood glucose concentration [112].

Chlorpropamide is the most slowly absorbed sulfonylurea [3]. Glibenclamide is slower in onset than glipizide, partly because it is more slowly and incompletely absorbed, at least from the non-micronized formulation that has been available in North and South America, Asia, Australia, and in the tropical areas [3, 113]. In Germany, Scandinavia, and the United Kingdom, this formulation has been replaced by a micronized one from which glibenclamide is more rapidly and more completely absorbed [113]. The micronized form has become available in the United States and other countries. However, glibenclamide is slower in onset than glipizide even when infused at an equal rate and to a similar plasma level [114].

For several sulfonylureas, e.g. glibenclamide [104, 115], gliclazide [104, 116], and glipizide [104, 117], it has been shown that certain individuals are "slow absorbers," leading to extensive delays in their uptake of these drugs. This may be clinically important, but the long-term relevance has not been elucidated.

Another potentially important finding is the observation that hyperglycemia may delay sulfonylurea absorption [118]; indeed, this might help to explain some primary and secondary failures in type 2 diabetic patients who have pronounced hyperglycemia.

From the above it follows that the timing of sulfonylurea dosing relative to the time of meal intake would be important. It may, in fact, be more relevant than the dose size: 2.5 mg glibenclamide half an hour before breakfast was found to be more effective than 7.5 mg taken with breakfast [119]. Glipizide [120] and tolbutamide [121] are also more effective when given half an hour before, rather than with, a meal. These findings emphasize the relevance of developing optimum biopharmaceutic formulations of at least some of the sulfonylureas [113]. For a slow, long-acting agent such as chlorpropamide, which accumulates extensively, the timing of the dose would seem to be irrelevant.

Duration of sulfonylurea action The duration of action is important as it may relate to the probability of certain adverse effects, such as long-lasting hypoglycemia [3, 104, 122, 123], and also relates to the issue of discontinuous sulfonylurea exposure. As sulfonylureas act via B-cell receptors, it is possible that continuous exposure may desensitize the B-cells (see below).

The short-acting sulfonylureas include glipizide, which has the shortest half-life (1–5 h) and no active metabolites; other sulfonylureas with short half-lives are glibornuride (5–12 h), gliclazide (6–15 h), glimepiride (5–9 h), tolazamide (4–7 h), and tolbutamide (6–12 h), and these also have metabolites with little or no activity [3, 104].

Chlorpropamide has the longest elimination half-life (24–48 h, or longer in subjects with renal impairment) of all sulfonylureas currently in use, and is very long acting [3, 104]. This is a probable explanation of the fact that chlorpropamide is one of the sulfonylureas most likely to provoke long-lasting (and hence dangerous) hypoglycemic reactions [3, 104, 124]. Gliquidone has the next-longest elimination half-life (24 h) reported, but little is known of its clinical duration of action and the risk of long-lasting hypoglycemia, mainly because the use of this sulfonylurea has so far been very limited.

While previous studies have reported a short elimination half-life of glibenclamide (2–10 h), a recent study, employing a more sensitive HPLC method, showed that the elimination half-life is rather long, 15–20 h [125]. This is also in agreement with the impression that this drug seems to have a rather long duration of action and may have been implicated in more cases of long-lasting hypoglycemic reactions than other sulfonylureas [3, 104, 121, 122]. This is not only because glibenclamide is the most widely used sulfonylurea in many countries; the number of long-lasting cases is higher, even after correction for number of patients on the drug and the number of doses prescribed [122, 123, 126]. A possibility not yet examined is that glibenclamide is slowly distributed; another possibility is accumulation of polar, active metabolites [127]; a recent study shows that both metabolites of glibenclamide are active in humans [128]. Yet another possibility relates to the observation that glibenclamide, in contrast to other sulfonylureas, may accumulate within B-cells [30].

Kinetic–Dynamic Relations

The kinetic–dynamic relations of sulfonylureas are complex. First, as glucose is the major stimulator of insulin secretion, differences in dietary regimens, amount of food, and time of food intake hinder the establishment of a relation between the plasma level of the sulfonylurea in question and the reductions of blood glucose and HbA_{1c}. Second, differences in the severity of diabetes will further confound this relation; indeed, as most doctors assume that progressive dose increase will bring about a progressive reduction of blood glucose levels, the most severely hyperglycemic patients will be given the highest doses, with the result that high sulfonylurea levels will be associated with high glucose levels. In this context, it is of particular interest that pronounced hyperglycemia may delay the absorption of sulfonylurea [118]. Third, as blood glucose reduction by any therapeutic means will gradually improve B-cell function and insulin action [111, 129], there may not exist any stable relation between the plasma drug level and its effect. Fourth, a sulfonylurea with a long elimination half-life, such as chlorpropamide, will show little fluctuation in the diurnal concentration profile of the drug, whereas a sulfonylurea with a short half-life, e.g. glipizide, will not only show large fluctuations in its plasma concentration but the level may fall to zero before the next dose [3, 72, 117]. Finally, there is evidence to suggest that chronic, continuous sulfonylurea exposure over a certain level may lead to desensitization of the insulin-releasing effect [42], and there is also evidence that very high drug levels may impair instead of improve glucose control [75, 76]. What is needed in order to establish a relationship between possible dose, plasma drug level, and effect is long-term, strictly dietary regulated, placebo-controlled studies at several dose levels of the various sulfonylureas given to type 2 diabetic patients with a uniform degree of metabolic disturbance and of sulfonylurea sensitivity. Such studies are exceedingly difficult to perform. The same applies to appropriate comparisons between different sulfonylureas.

Characteristics and Comparisons of Different Sulfonylureas

In this section relevant pharmacokinetic and pharmacodynamic data are given for different sulfonylureas, and mention is also made of comparative studies.

Tolbutamide Having been available since 1955, tolbutamide is still in use in many countries, given in various formulations from different manufacturers. There are differences in absorption rate between formulations [104, 130] and this may be important, as more rapid absorption may signify a higher efficacy in reducing postprandial hyperglycemia (see above). Tolbutamide is more rapidly absorbed than chlorpropamide [3], but less rapidly than glipizide. Many, but not all, tolbutamide formulations have a high degree of absorption, but there are no appropriate estimates of the absolute bioavailability of this drug.

Concomitant food intake may not delay the absorption of tolbutamide, but its efficacy may be improved if the drug is given half an hour before meals rather than with meals [121].

The volume of distribution of tolbutamide is small, like that of all other sulfonylureas. It is highly bound to plasma albumin, but the extent of protein binding decreases with age, roughly in parallel with decreasing plasma albumin levels [104]. Tolbutamide is completely metabolized, mainly to hydroxytolbutamide and subsequently to carboxytolbutamide, both of which have little or no activity. Metabolism occurs by oxidation, and it has been suggested that the first oxidative step to hydroxytolbutamide is genetically polymorphic with a trimodal distribution [131]. Phenylbutazone [104] and cimetidine [104] may inhibit the metabolism of tolbutamide.

Little, if any, tolbutamide is excreted unchanged. The metabolites are excreted by the kidney [104].

The usual dosage of tolbutamide is 0.5–1.0 g three times daily. It has not been ascertained whether or not its efficacy may be maintained on a once-daily basis.

Chlorpropamide Chlorpropamide has been available almost as long as tolbutamide, and it has been extensively used all over the world. Chlorpropamide is more slowly absorbed than tolbutamide and has the longest elimination half-life of all sulfonylureas. This leads to pronounced accumulation with very small fluctuations over the day within the individual [105]. Therefore, the elimination rate is the major determinant of its effect, whereas variations in its rate of absorption are unimportant. Hence the timing of the daily dose is irrelevant, and it is also irrelevant whether chlorpropamide is ingested before or with breakfast. There are no data on the absolute bioavailability of chlorpropamide. Like that of all other sulfonylureas, the volume of distribution is small, but its binding to plasma albumin is less pronounced.

In contrast to widespread belief, chlorpropamide undergoes extensive, albeit slow, metabolic transformation. This occurs by oxidation to 2-hydroxychlorpropamide, 3-hydroxychlorpropamide, and *p*-chlorobenzene sulfonylurea [104]. It is not clear whether the hydroxylated metabolites are active; however, they are more rapidly eliminated than the parent drug, at least in subjects with normal renal function, and would hence add little to the overall activity except perhaps in patients with renal insufficiency.

A significant portion of chlorpropamide is excreted unchanged by the kidneys [104]; this proportion can be increased by alkalinization and reduced by acidification of the urine [3, 104, 132]. The elimination half-life of chlorpropamide is long but variable (24–48 h), partly because of variations in the excretion rate of the unchanged compound and partly because of variations in the metabolic turnover rate. This also helps to explain why there is a very large interindividual variation in the steady-state plasma concentrations of chlorpropamide during treatment [105].

The usual dosage of chlorpropamide is 250–500 mg once daily.

Given intravenously, tolbutamide and chlorpropamide have shown similar acute blood glucose reductions. As they differ in both rates of absorption and rates of elimination it is difficult to make appropriate comparisons during long-term treatment. This is also evident from the previously mentioned fact that, although a larger tolbutamide dose is needed to maintain the same degree of blood glucose control, the steady-state levels of chlorpropamide become higher than those of tolbutamide because of more extensive accumulation [105].

Chlorpropamide is more commonly associated with long-lasting hypoglycemic events than are most other sulfonylureas, possibly with the exception of glibenclamide (see below); this is probably related to the slow elimination and pronounced accumulation of the drug. On the other hand, chlorpropamide is the only sulfonylurea with elimination that can be enhanced by forced diuresis and urine alkalinization [3, 104, 132]. The pronounced accumulation may also help to explain why chlorpropamide, more often than other sulfonylureas, is involved in events of ethanol-provoked facial flushing (see below).

A major unique side effect of chlorpropamide treatment is water retention and hyponatremia. This is related to chlorpropamide, both stimulating the release of vasopressin from the posterior pituitary and potentiating vasopressin action on the renal tubule [78]. This side effect might explain the observation in the UKPDS that the patients randomized to chlorpropamide had significantly higher systolic and diastolic blood pressures throughout the study than those assigned to glibenclamide, insulin, or conventional treatment [100].

Comparisons between chlorpropamide and glibenclamide have given a variety of results, depending upon the design of the studies: in some of these, chlorpropamide has tended to promote lower fasting blood glucose levels but higher nonfasting ones; other studies have failed to show any difference [104]. The UKPDS, however, clearly showed that chronic chlorpropamide treatment achieves better glycemic control than does glibenclamide (median 10-year HbA_{1c}: 6.7% versus 7.2%, $p < 0.008$) [100]. Despite the better glycemic control the chlorpropamide-treated patients had less risk reduction for the progression of retinopathy than did the glibenclamide-treated group [100].

Acetohexamide The absorption of acetohexamide appears to be almost complete, but its absolute bioavailability is not known [104].

There are no reports on its volume of distribution or its degree of protein binding, but it may be assumed that the distribution volume is small and the extent of protein binding great, like those of all other sulfonylureas.

Acetohexamide undergoes metabolic reduction to hydroxyhexamide; this is an active metabolite responsible for a significant part of the clinical effect. Other metabolites are inactive, and part of acetohexamide is eliminated unchanged through the kidneys.

Acetohexamide has a very limited use nowadays. The recommended dosage is 125–750 mg twice daily.

Tolazamide Tolazamide is absorbed relatively slowly, and its absorption rate is formulation sensitive [104]. It is not known whether its effect is improved if the drug is taken before rather than with meals. There are no reported estimates of its absolute bioavailability, nor of its volume of distribution or degree of protein binding. However, the latter are probably similar to those of other sulfonylureas.

Tolazamide is almost completely metabolized, mainly by oxidative hydroxylation. The hydroxylated metabolite is active, but it is uncertain to what extent the metabolite adds to the clinical effect [104]. One may assume that it would accumulate in patients with renal impairment, as most of the tolazamide metabolites are eliminated by renal excretion. Little, if any, tolazamide is excreted unchanged. Its elimination rate is relatively high, with a half-life of about 4–7 h.

The common dose range is 250–500 mg once or twice daily.

A comparison between tolazamide and tolbutamide showed no difference in the effect on fasting blood glucose levels [104].

Glibenclamide The most extensively used sulfonylurea in many parts of the world is glibenclamide (called glyburide in the United States). It was the first "second-generation" sulfonylurea to be introduced in clinical practice, and it is one of the most potent.

The absorption of glibenclamide is rather slow and incomplete from the non-micronized formulation still used in the American continents and in Asia and Australia, whereas the rate and degree of absorption are higher from the micronized formulation available initially in Germany, the United Kingdom, and Scandinavia [113] but now available worldwide. Both non-micronized and micronized generic formulations have appeared, but it is not clear whether they are fully equivalent to the original products. Although concomitant food intake does not seem to delay the absorption of glibenclamide, its efficacy may be increased if given before meals, at least in the short term. Indeed, as previously mentioned, 2.5 mg given half an hour before breakfast was more effective than 7.5 mg given together with breakfast [119]. The rate of absorption varies extensively between individuals [115], and this may be important at least during short-term conditions.

Like other sulfonylureas, glibenclamide has a small volume of distribution, and it is very extensively bound to albumin.

Glibenclamide is completely metabolized, mainly by oxidation to two hydroxylated metabolites, both of which have blood glucose reducing activity [128].

About half of a given dose of glibenclamide is eliminated by renal excretion of metabolites, and a significant portion is excreted through the bile. Although renal insufficiency should not alter the elimination rate of this very lipophilic and completely metabolized drug, it may nevertheless increase the risk of hypoglycemia [104, 127]. This may be because renal insufficiency is associated with reduced drug binding to albumin; in addition, renal impairment may lead to accumulation of polar, active metabolites [127, 128]. Surprisingly, severe renal impairment in one subject has been associated with delayed elimination of glibenclamide itself [104].

Both clinical experience and various studies support the view that glibenclamide should be classified as a long-acting sulfonylurea. Indeed, glibenclamide has been associated with long-lasting (and hence dangerous) hypoglycemic reactions more often than other sulfonylureas except, perhaps, chlorpropamide [3, 104, 120, 123, 126]. There may be various reasons for this, including the now recognized fact that glibenclamide's elimination half-life is longer than previously assumed [125] and that both its main metabolites are active in humans [128] (see also above).

The usual daily dose of glibenclamide is 1.75–14 mg (micronized) or 2.5–20 mg (non-micronized), given in a single morning dose or split in a morning and an evening dose.

Studies comparing glibenclamide and chlorpropamide have been commented upon above. Glibenclamide and glipizide have also been compared, but the comparisons suffer from various problems. Some studies have used only one fixed-dose level; some have involved patients whose clinical responses have been minute and hence were unsuitable for study; some have been too short to allow for the progressive improvement of blood glucose levels that follows the improved B-cell function and insulin action secondary to the reduction of hyperglycemia. It appears quite certain, however, that glipizide releases insulin more rapidly than glibenclamide [72, 114, 133], and that glibenclamide suppresses hepatic glucose output more than does glipizide [114].

In a placebo-controlled study wherein glibenclamide and glipizide were given in a crossover fashion for 6 months, and in which most patients were continuously exposed to either drug, there was no difference in the final mean daily dose, nor in final mean blood glucose or hemoglobin levels. Moreover, although fasting blood glucose values tended to be lower in patients on glibenclamide and postprandial blood glucose values lower in those on glipizide, neither difference was significant [72].

In one short-term study with fixed doses (10 mg of each drug), fasting blood glucose values were lower after glibenclamide [133], whereas in another short-term study postprandial glucose was more reduced by glipizide [134]. Together with the findings in the long-term study [72], and in view of the different rates of onset and different durations of action of the two compounds, it is possible that glibenclamide is slightly more able to reduce fasting blood glucose levels and glipizide is slightly more able to reduce nonfasting blood glucose levels. This would also be in accord with the findings that glibenclamide suppresses hepatic glucose output more than glipizide does [114], and that glipizide is more able to enhance acute insulin release than does glibenclamide [114]. However, this would be clinically relevant only when the dosage is such that it generates discontinuous exposure to the sulfonylurea (see below).

Differences between glibenclamide and glipizide with regard to the risk of causing long-lasting hypoglycemia are discussed at the end of the chapter.

Latent autoimmune diabetes of adults is frequently confused with type 2 diabetes and treated initially with sulfonylureas. A recent report of 14 such patients treated with insulin and glibenclamide found that discontinuing glibenclamide partially decreased ICA positivity and improved metabolic control [135]. These data imply that glibenclamide treatment may accelerate the autoimmune process. Whether this effect is specific to glibenclamide or an effect of sulfonylureas in general is unknown.

A population-based case control study of 1.4 million inhabitants in Sweden found that glibenclamide treatment was associated with an odds ratio adjusted for covariates of 2.5 for the development of acute pancreatitis without previous gallbladder disease [136].

Despite concerns about the use of sulfonylurea drugs in pregnancy, a comparison of glibenclamide and insulin treatment of 404 women with gestational diabetes showed that both treatments gave equal glycemic control and no difference in maternal and neonatal complications. Thus glibenclamide may be a clinically effective alternative to insulin treatment in women with gestational diabetes [137].

Gliclazide Gliclazide is a rapid-acting and short-acting sulfonylurea that is widely used in some countries, among them France and the United Kingdom. It is rapidly absorbed, but its absolute bioavailability is not known. Absorption is slower in the elderly [138]. Like other sulfonylureas, gliclazide is extensively bound in plasma and has a small volume of distribution [104, 116]. It is not known whether intake before meals makes gliclazide more effective than does intake together with meals.

Gliclazide is almost completely metabolized, and the metabolites seem to be inactive [104].

Most gliclazide is eliminated by excretion of the inactive metabolites through the kidneys, but a small fraction is eliminated by the bile [104]. The elimination half-life is short but variable, between 6 and 15 h. Although this might not be expected for a completely metabolized drug, the elimination half-life might be increased in subjects with renal insufficiency [104].

It has been argued that gliclazide offers an advantage over other sulfonylureas in being able to reduce platelet aggregation [139]. However, it is most likely that all sulfonylureas are able to improve platelet aggregation as an indirect effect of improved blood glucose control [3]. There are no comparative studies showing that gliclazide is superior to other sulfonylureas in reducing platelet aggregation. In terms of blood glucose control, gliclazide seems to be as effective as other sulfonylureas [104].

The usual daily dose is 40–320 mg, given in a single morning dose or in morning and evening.

Glipizide Glipizide is widely used in the United States and in several European countries. It is the most rapidly acting sulfonylurea available, and is also one of the most short-acting [3, 104]. Its potency and intrinsic activity are in the same range as those of glibenclamide.

The absorption and bioavailability of glipizide are fast and complete [3, 117]. It is more rapidly absorbed when taken before breakfast than when ingested together with breakfast, and intake before breakfast is also associated with a more appropriate timing of insulin release relative to the meal, and with an enhanced efficacy of the drug [120]. Its absorption rate correlates with its efficacy [110, 112], and pronounced hyperglycemia may reduce the absorption rate [118].

Glipizide has been shown to improve the acute insulin release in response to a meal [110], and this capacity may be maintained during long-term therapy, at least when the exposure is discontinuous [111]. This is interesting in view of the possibility that chronic, continuous sulfonylurea exposure may desensitize the B-cell to sulfonylurea stimulation [3, 42, 81].

The volume of distribution of glipizide is small, like that of other sulfonylureas, and the binding to albumin is very extensive [104].

Glipizide is completely metabolized, mainly by oxidative hydroxylation [104]. The metabolites appear to be inactive [104].

Glipizide is rapidly eliminated with a half-life of 1–5 h. The half-life does not seem to increase with age [140]. Renal insufficiency does not seem to alter the elimination rate of glipizide. These facts may explain why glipizide seems to carry a lower risk of long-lasting hypoglycemia than do glibenclamide and chlorpropamide (see end of chapter).

Although glipizide is rapidly eliminated, a morning dose of 7.5 mg or more maintains effective plasma concentrations for more than 12 h [3, 123, 141]. This may help to explain why glipizide, despite its short half-life, can be equally effective when given once daily or three times daily [141]. On the basis of available documentation, dosage should be in the range of 2.5–10 mg daily, either as a single morning dose half an hour before breakfast or divided in a morning and an evening dose. In the United States, the official maximum dose is 40 mg, but there is very limited support for increased efficacy with daily doses over 10–15 mg. Instead, dose increase from 15 to 25 mg/day has been found to impair rather than improve glucose control [75], and a placebo-controlled study using 3-month periods of glipizide at 10, 20, and 40 mg daily showed impaired glucose and insulin responses above 10 mg daily [76]. On the other hand, ethnic differences may exist in the disposition and effect of sulfonylureas, and hence in appropriate dosage (see below).

Comparisons between glipizide and glibenclamide have been commented upon above.

Glipizide GITS Glipizide has been formulated in an extended-release tablet. This formulation provides steady-state constant plasma levels(5-mg tablet – 54 ng/ml). One might expect this type of formulation to lose the advantages of glipizide as a rapid- and short-acting oral hypoglycemic agent. A comparison of 10 mg twice a day of immediate-release glipizide to 20 mg once a day of the extended-release form showed that the immediate-release glipizide had significantly greater C_{max} (peak serum concentration) and shorter T_{max} (time taken to reach the maximum concentration) than did the extended-release glipizide [142]. In contrast, the C_{min} with the extended-release form was about 80% higher than with the immediate-release form. The two formulations had similar effects on serum concentrations of glucose, insulin, and C-peptide.

Clinical trials comparing the immediate-release form to the extended-release form for 8 and 16 weeks showed similar improvement in HbA_{1c} but a slightly lower fasting plasma glucose and lower plasma insulin levels with the extended-release form [92]. The mean decrease in HbA_{1c} with the extended-release form was 1.5–1.8% compared to placebo treatment. The extended-release form maintains relatively constant low plasma levels of glipizide. These levels appear to facilitate meal-mediated insulin secretion without much increase in basal insulin secretion. The suggestion that low-dose extended-release form improves insulin sensitivity more than does the immediate-release form needs further validation. Some data have been published to suggest that the extended-release form causes less hypoglycemia and weight gain than does the immediate-release form. These data need to be confirmed in large well-controlled studies. Glipizide extended-release is administered once a day in doses of 5–20 mg.

Gliquidone The absorption of gliquidone seems to be rapid but formulation-dependent [104]. Data on its absolute bioavailability have not been found. It is not known whether the efficacy of gliquidone is improved by intake before meals.

Gliquidone is extensively bound in plasma. Its volume of distribution is not known but is presumably small.

The drug is almost completely metabolized by oxidation to demethylated and hydroxylated products. One of the latter is active, but reaches only low plasma concentrations [104].

Gliquidone has a terminal elimination half-life of about 24 h; nevertheless, it is recommended that the daily dose (which may range from 15 to 180 mg) should be divided, being given two or even three times daily [104].

There are no controlled comparative studies showing any therapeutic advantage of gliquidone over more commonly used sulfonylureas such as tolbutamide, chlorpropamide, glibenclamide, gliclazide, or glipizide.

Glibornuride Glibornuride is rapidly absorbed, but there are no data on its absolute bioavailability. It is not known whether the efficacy of glibornuride is improved by intake before meals.

Like that of other sulfonylureas, its volume of distribution is small, and the drug is extensively bound in plasma.

Glibornuride is metabolized by oxidative processes to metabolites that seem to be inactive.

Its elimination is rapid, with an elimination half-life of 5–12 h [104].

The recommended dose is 12.5–25 mg, and it may be given once or twice daily.

Glisoxepide Glisoxepide is a high-potency sulfonylurea that is not well characterized from the pharmacokinetic point of view and is not much used.

Glimepiride Glimepiride is a second generation sulfonylurea that differs structurally from glibenclamide in its two side chains. It is rapidly and completely absorbed after oral administration. Peak serum concentrations (C_{max}) are achieved at 2–3 h [143]. When glimepiride is taken with meals the time to reach the maximum concentration and the concentration achieved are decreased by 10% [143]. Plasma protein binding of glimepiride is >99% and the volume of distribution is small. The elimination half-life is 5–9 h [143]. Glimepiride is completely biotransformed by oxidative metabolism (CYP2C9) in the liver and conversion to a carboxyl derivative by cytosolic enzymes [143]. The hydroxylated metabolite has hypoglycemic activity. The hydroxy-metabolite is excreted in the urine (60%) and the carboxy-metabolite in the feces (40%) [143].

Glimepiride has a 2.5–3-fold faster rate of association and an 8–9-fold faster rate of dissociation from the SUR-1 binding sites than does glibenclamide [80]. Glimepiride therefore has a rapid onset of action and is short acting. Glimepiride is equally as effective as glibenclamide and glipizide in improving glycemic control in type 2 diabetic patients [80]. Chronic treatment of type 2 diabetic patients with glimepiride for 3–12 months reduces HbA_{1c} by 1.5–2.0% [80, 93]. Glimepiride treatment is associated with far less hypoglycemia than does glibenclamide [80, 143]. A recent prospective population-based 4-year study in a region of Germany found severe hypoglycemia incidence of 0.86/1000 person-years for glimepiride and 5.6/1000 person-years for glibenclamide [144].

The presumed advantages of glimepiride over other sulfonylureas are (1) the demonstration that glimepiride has extrapancreatic effects in humans [51–53, 145], (2) the observations that glimepiride has relatively low binding to SUR-2A and SUR-2B and does not block ischemic preconditioning in the heart [146, 147], and (3) that glimepiride stimulates first-phase insulin secretion [148]. The extrapanceatic effects described in humans do not appear to be of sufficient magnitude to be clinically significant. The lack of altering ATP-dependent potassium channels in cardiovascular tissues may well be a considerable advantage but more clinical studies are needed. The recently demonstrated stimulation of first-phase insulin secretion is quite small and is of questionable clinical significance.

Glimepiride is started at 1 mg once daily. The usual maintenance dose is 1–4 mg once daily. The maximum recommended dose is 8 mg once daily.

Selection of Sulfonylureas for Therapeutic Use

As emphasized earlier, there is little or no evidence that one sulfonylurea is therapeutically more effective than another, at least not when used to promote continuous sulfonylurea exposure, and when dosage is adjusted on the basis of the individual control of blood glucose. A well-nourished, middle-aged individual with type 2 diabetes (but otherwise healthy) can be treated effectively with any one of the available sulfonylureas. A rapid-acting sulfonylurea may improve acute insulin release and promote better control of postprandial blood glucose, whereas a long-acting sulfonylurea may give better control of overnight glycemia. A short-acting agent may allow a better chance of maintaining the insulinotrophic effect through discontinuous exposure, and carries a lower risk of provoking long-lasting hypoglycemia. High-potency sulfonylureas may reduce the risk of drug–drug interactions compared with low-potency agents, because many fewer molecules are needed to achieve blood glucose control (see later). An old type 2 diabetic patient, particularly if poorly nourished and having other chronic ailments, is at considerable risk of developing long-lasting, severe hypoglycemia and should be treated (if at all) with a sulfonylurea with short action and inactive metabolites.

Type 2 diabetic patients with impaired renal function should be treated with a short-acting sulfonylurea, the elimination of which is entirely dependent upon hepatic metabolic degradation to inactive metabolites. The use of chlorpropamide might be discouraged because of its very long duration of action, high incidence of alcohol-induced flushing, considerable water retention with subsequent hyponatremia, dependence upon renal function for elimination, and high prevalence for long-lasting hypoglycemic reactions (see later).

WHEN AND HOW TO USE SULFONYLUREAS

Indications

The primary indication for sulfonylurea therapy is type 2 diabetes in which optimum blood glucose control has not been achieved by dietary regulation and exercise [149, 150]. Presumed advantages of oral sulfonylurea therapy are delivery of insulin through the physiologic route (portal vein), less hyperinsulinemia than that occurring from insulin treatment, and possible extrapancreatic actions. In rare instances, sulfonylurea therapy may be indicated because of insulin allergy or hypersensitivity, or severe insulin resistance [151].

Early Intervention

The chronic hyperglycemia of type 2 diabetes evolves slowly, and subjective symptoms of the disease usually occur only after several years. However, at least some complications may occur in the early phase of type 2 diabetes and the risk of cardiovascular complications is increased even in the prediabetic phase of IGT [152–157]. Retinopathy may be present in 20% of type 2 diabetic patients at the time of diagnosis [157, 158]. Accordingly, there is reason to assume that therapeutic intervention should be introduced in the early stages of glucose intolerance. Indeed, there is reason to argue that efforts should be made to find type 2 diabetic subjects before they experience symptoms that spontaneously bring them to medical care [83]. Detection programs can be made very simple: a random blood sample of nonfasting glucose may suffice for type 2 diabetes screening [111, 159].

A most important reason for early detection and intervention is the increasingly recognized fact that chronic hyperglycemia is a self-perpetuating condition: it not only results from, but may also exacerbate, impaired insulin secretion and impaired insulin action [41]; in other words, chronic hyperglycemia generates a vicious circle. Conversely, reduction of chronic hyperglycemia has been shown to improve both insulin secretion and insulin action [39, 40, 55, 129]. Hence, it seems logical that therapeutic intervention should start as soon as persistent hyperglycemia has been recorded, and, with due reservations for individual needs, euglycemia should be the principal goal of therapy (see below).

Therapeutic intervention should always start with dietary regulation, and the importance of persistence in dietary regulation should be emphasized at regular intervals (see Chapter 41). The same applies for regular exercise (see Chapter 47). If euglycemia is not achieved after 2–3 months of dietary regulation and increased regular exercise, addition of a sulfonylurea is usually indicated. However, sulfonylureas must not be used instead of dietary regulation but always as a supplement; otherwise, secondary sulfonylurea failure is likely to ensue, and even primary sulfonylurea failure may occur [3, 111] (see below).

Critics of the sulfonylureas often argue that sulfonylurea treatment could be counterproductive because it may lead to weight increase, chronic hyperinsulinemia, and more severe insulin resistance, and it has also been claimed that long-term sulfonylurea treatment might cause B-cell exhaustion. However, there is little scientific support for these views. On the contrary, early sulfonylurea introduction may be able to reverse the vicious circle of hyperglycemia and thereby improve insulin secretion and insulin action. There is even evidence to suggest that sulfonylurea treatment in combination with dietary restriction might delay the development of IGT to manifest type2 diabetes and reduce the increased risk of cardiovascular morbidity and mortality [160, 161]. As for B-cell exhaustion by sulfonylurea treatment, there is no support for this in the literature; instead, the blood glucose reduction subsequent to sulfonylurea treatment improves B-cell function [39, 40, 129]. Finally, even though chronic hyperinsulinemia might occur during treatment with long-acting sulfonylureas, treatment with a rapid-acting and short-acting sulfonylurea in combination with hypocaloric dietary regulation can attain and maintain near-normal blood glucose levels for years without provoking chronic hypersecretion of insulin or chronic hyperinsulinemia [111]. The concept of discontinuous sulfonylurea exposure is of particular interest in this context (see below).

Discontinuous Exposure

As sulfonylureas release insulin by activation of a receptor-mediated mechanism in the B-cell [5–11, 22, 23], it is possible that chronic, continuous exposure to sulfonylurea at or over a certain level may desensitize the B-cell by downregulation of the SUR or alteration in the function of the ATP-dependent potassium channel. This hypothesis may draw support from a recent study showing that the insulin-releasing effect of a single dose of sulfonylurea (tolbutamide) vanished during chronic treatment with another sulfonylurea (tolazamide), even though glucose levels were kept similar, and even though the response to another secretagogue, glucagons, was unaltered. In addition, the acute insulinotrophic effect of tolbutamide reappeared after cessation of the chronic tolazamide treatment [42]. Further support for this idea may be found in the fact that high concentrations of sulfonylureas inhibit proinsulin biosynthesis *in vitro* [45, 46] and attenuate insulin secretion *in vitro* [162]. Furthermore, dosage increase of glipizide from 15 to 25 mg daily has been associated with impaired instead of improved blood glucose control in type 2 diabetic subjects [75]. In addition, treatment with glipizide at 10, 20, and 40 mg daily for 3-month periods was accompanied by reduced instead of increased insulin and glucose responses at the 20 and 40 mg dose levels [76]. Conversely, acute insulin release could be maintained in type 2 diabetic patients during low-dose, once-daily glipizide treatment [111]. The validity of this concept remains to be proved. Numerous studies *in vitro* suggest that desensitization may occur with many different insulin secretagogues and that desensitization may also result from the insulin secreted in response to the secretagogues [162, 163]. The significance of desensitization therefore needs to be clarified, but it may add to the ar guments for low-dose sulfonylurea therapy (see below).

Therapeutic Goals in Practice

The management of patients with type 2 diabetes should have three major goals: to alleviate symptoms, to improve the sense of well-being, and to prevent the development of chronic complications.

The alleviation of symptoms such as polyuria, polydipsia, polyphagia, weight loss, and recurrent infections can usually be achieved by reducing the fasting plasma glucose level to, or below, 10 mmol/l (180 mg/dl). The sense of well-being of patients with non-insulin-dependent diabetes is usually maximal at a fasting plasma glucose value of 7.5–8.0 mmol/l (135–145 mg/dl). The prevention of chronic complications, however, requires achievement of near-euglycemia (fasting plasma glucose values below 7 mmol/l (125 mg/dl); HbA_{1c} at upper limit of normal) and maintenance of normal blood pressure and normal serum lipid levels [149, 150].

The goal for the management of the individual type 2 diabetic patient must be individually defined. The prevention of chronic complications can only occur in an individual who will live long enough to develop the complications and does not already have severe complications. Thus, in new-onset, elderly type 2 diabetic patients, or in those with a complicating life-threatening illness, control aimed at preventing chronic complications is unjustified. In contrast, a newly diagnosed 40-year-old type 2 diabetic patient with no other complications is an ideal candidate for intensive metabolic regulation. The therapeutic treatment program is developed for type 2 diabetic patients after the goals of treatment have been defined.

Dose and Dosage of Sulfonylureas

Dose Size and Dose Change

Regardless of the compound chosen, sulfonylurea therapy should always be started with the lowest effective dose. Moreover, as the blood glucose reduction evoked by this initial low dose may secondarily improve B-cell function and insulin action, the dosage should be only slowly increased. It is often recommended that dose increase be carried out after 1–2 weeks, but it is quite possible that monthly or even longer intervals are preferable. As a matter of fact, there are very few clinical dose–response studies that show any therapeutic improvement by dose increases within the dose intervals officially recommended for the various sulfonylureas. In addition, little is known about the different dosage needs between different ethnic groups and between lean, overweight, and grossly obese patients. As an illustration of the problem, one of the authors has the experience that very high doses of, for example, glipizide (up to 25 mg) may be needed in certain Black or Hispanic patients, whereas the other author has the experience that doses beyond 10–15 mg of glipizide add little benefit in Scandinavian patients; higher doses may actually impair blood glucose control [75, 76]. More studies are needed to define the appropriate dose range for sulfonylureas in different ethnic groups.

Dosage Intervals

It is well known that patient adherence to chronic pharmacotherapy improves if the medication is given only once or (at most) twice daily. Owing to its very long half-life, chlorpropamide can be given once daily without loss of efficacy. In fact, the half-life is long enough to suggest that the dosage interval should be longer than 24 h.

Glibenclamide can also be given once or twice daily, owing to its rather long duration of action, even though this has not seemed to correspond to its elimination half-life (see above). Glimepiride is very effective when given once daily. Gliclazide may also be given once or twice daily. Although glipizide is short-acting, it is so potent that a single dose of 5 mg maintains effective concentrations for 8–10 h, and a single dose of 7.5–15 mg maintains effective concentrations for 16 h or more [117, 141]. Once-daily glipizide at this dose level has also been shown to be as effective as dosage three times daily [141]. No such comparisons are known to exist for tolbutamide, but by inference from pharmacokinetic data this agent also might be given once or twice daily.

If after-breakfast or after-lunch hypoglycemic reactions occur during once-daily dosage of sulfonylureas, the daily dose should be split in two, the latter dose being given before dinner. A dose before lunch does not add effectiveness for any sulfonylurea.

SULFONYLUREA FAILURES

The concept of sulfonylurea failure arose from initial clinical observations which indicated that about 10–20% of patients initially treated with sulfonylureas failed to show a significant decrease in hyperglycemia (primary failure) and an additional 20–30% lost their initial satisfactory decrease in hyperglycemia after 6 months or more of treatment (secondary failure) [85–90].

The cause of primary failure, although not extensively studied, would seem most probably attributable to a marked deficiency in insulin secretory capacity. These individuals generally have fasting plasma glucose values in excess of 15 mmol/l (270 mg/dl), and some may prove to be slowly evolving patients with insulin-dependent diabetes [164].

Secondary failure has been attributed to a variety of causes. Groop *et al.* have divided the causes of secondary failure in type 2 diabetes into patient-related factors (failure to follow a reasonable dietary program, poor knowledge about diabetes, lack of exercise, stress, and intercurrent illnesses), disease-related factors (increasing insulin deficiency or increasing insulin resistance) and therapy-related factors (inadequate drug dosage, desensitization to chronic sulfonylurea exposure, impaired absorption of sulfonylurea due to hyperglycemia, concomitant therapy with diabetogenic drugs) [165, 166].

The practical questions raised by sulfonylurea failure are the following:

(1) How do we define failure in the 2000s?
(2) Can we predict sulfonylurea failures?
(3) Can we reverse or prevent secondary failures?

The definition of primary or secondary sulfonylurea failure has never been standardized. Previously it was arbitrarily defined by the level of glycemic control achieved. A positive response to therapy was considered to be the attainment of "excellent" or "good" control. When that level of control could no longer be maintained, the patient was defined as a sulfonylurea failure. In the 1990s, when the goal of treatment of type 2 diabetes was to minimize chronic complications (which means achieving near-euglycemia), the concept of sulfonylurea failure needed to be revised; a patient who fails to achieve any significant degree of glycemic control should be defined as a sulfonylurea failure; a patient who achieves near-euglycemia on diet and sulfonylureas should be defined as a sulfonylurea success; if diet and sulfonylureas achieve only partial restoration of glycemia to normal, this might be called sulfonylurea inadequacy [91, 167]. The cause of such "sulfonylurea inadequacy" should be evaluated, and appropriate measures added to achieve the appropriate glycemic goals defined for the specific individual. These might involve intensified dietary management with weight loss, treatment of an intercurrent illness, reduction of diabetogenic drugs, temporary treatment with insulin [168], or as is most common combination therapy with other antihyperglycemic agents such as insulin, biguanides, or thiazolidinediones. In the UKPDS, a substudy evaluated the effect of adding insulin to sulfonylurea-treated patients if the fasting plasma glucose remained >6.0 mmol/l despite maximal sulfonylurea doses. Over 6 years approximately 53% of sulfonylurea-treated patients required additional insulin treatment [167].

SULFONYLUREAS OR BIGUANIDES?

In most countries, biguanides are available as alternative antihyperglycemic oral agents. In many of these countries metformin is the only biguanide available. The doctor hence has the option of using either a sulfonylurea or a metformin as the first choice for pharmacologic therapy. Many studies have compared the therapeutic efficacy of sulfonylurea with that of metformin (see Chapter 30). However, many of these studies suffer from various flaws. In general, blood glucose control has been equal following the two treatments [169].

The advantages of sulfonylureas are that the mechanisms of action are better known, that sulfonylurea-induced enhancement of insulin release corrects one of the primary disturbances in type 2 diabetes in a physiologic manner, and that lactic acidosis and gastrointestinal distress are avoided. The advantages with metformin are that obese patients tend to lose weight during metformin treatment, that this drug seems to have beneficial effects on insulin resistance and plasma lipids, and that hypoglycemia can be avoided. Also, while both sulfonylureas and metformin reduced microvascular complications in the UKPDS, only metformin reduced macrovascular complications [170]. As sulfonylureas and metformin have different mechanisms of action, they may be therapeutically combined on a rational basis.

SULFONYLUREA AND BIGUANIDE IN COMBINATION

Several studies suggest that the combination of a sulfonylurea and a biguanide can be very effective [171–173], and recent findings from a placebo-controlled randomized study gives further support to this view. While sulfonylurea (glibenclamide) and biguanide (metformin) were equally effective in reducing glucose levels, primary or secondary combination of the two drugs promoted better control than single-drug treatment [172]. Mean fasting blood glucose levels following treatment with high-dose combination were reduced from 13.3 to 7.8 mmol/l (240 to 140 mg/dl) [172], and there was little or no weight increase and little or no accentuation of hyperinsulinemia [172]. The study also suggested that body weight is not a predictor of therapeutic outcome or an indicator of which drug to select [173]; however, low initial blood glucose and high initial C-peptide levels predicted successful treatment [173].

The advantage of combining metformin and a sulfonylurea as a single therapeutic intervention has been documented in recent clinical trials with glibenclamide and metformin (Glucovance) [94]. Better glycemic control was achieved in initial therapy with low doses of each in a combined pill than giving the maximally tolerated dose of either drug alone.

On the other hand, an analysis of the UKPDS data on mortality indicated that the combination of sulfonylurea and metformin in a 6-year substudy was associated with 96% higher mortality than was treatment with sulfonylurea alone [170]. While these findings have been disparaged by the UKPDS authors as well as by others, they should be borne in mind. Prospective studies are needed to substantiate or refute the observation.

SULFONYLUREAS OR INSULIN?

It is a common view that insulin therapy is able to achieve euglycemia in most, if not all, patients with type 2 diabetes. If this is correct, one may question the rationale in using xenobiotic antihyperglycemic drugs such as sulfonylureas or metformin. On the other hand, insulin therapy by subcutaneous injections in the arm or the leg administers insulin in a unphysiological manner: whereas the endogenous insulin levels following a meal normally are very much higher in the portal than in the systemic circulation, the situation is reversed following subcutaneous, systemic administration of exogenous insulin. Furthermore, it is well established that many type 2 diabetic patients require large doses of insulin and a daily multiple injection program if they are to achieve a satisfactory control of blood glucose by exogenous insulin [174]. Insulin therapy is frequently associated with increased body weight and an increased requirement of insulin. This may be due to decreased glucosuria or to an increased appetite (perhaps secondary to frequent episodes of hypoglycemia). Irrespective of the mechanism involved, insulin therapy must be accompanied by considerable dietary energy restriction if it is to be successful. Moreover, all patients with type 2 diabetes who are treated with insulin have chronic systemic hyperinsulinemia. This should be borne in mind because hyperinsulinemia has been postulated by some to be an independent risk factor for the development of atherosclerotic disease [156].

Sulfonylureas, on the other hand, enhance insulin secretion and improve insulin action in muscle tissue, adipose tissue, and the liver. If used appropriately, sulfonylureas may attain and maintain euglycemia without causing hyperinsulinemia [76].

Clinical studies indicate that in type 2 diabetic patients who respond to sulfonylureas, sulfonylurea therapy and insulin therapy are essentially equal in controlling blood glucose levels [97, 100]. This is particularly true during the first 5 years of clinical type 2 diabetes. Thus, unless a true sulfonylurea failure has developed, there is no apparent disadvantage in using a sulfonylurea, and sulfonylurea therapy may in fact be advantageous from both a practical and a physiological point of view.

SULFONYLUREAS AND INSULIN IN COMBINATION

Sulfonylurea–insulin therapy has been studied extensively [175, 176]. Simultaneous treatment with both agents can significantly improve glycemia in about 20–30% of mildly to moderately obese type 2 diabetic patients who have adequate endogenous insulin secretory reserves and are in poor glycemic control (fasting plasma glucose values above 11 mmol/l) despite twice-daily insulin administration of more than 70 U/day and a history of inadequate glycemic control on diet and sulfonylurea. Most patients on combination Sulfonylurea–insulin therapy will require 20–50% less insulin for the same level of glycemic control as when given insulin alone.

In the UKPDS substudy evaluating the effect of early addition of insulin to sulfonylurea therapy that failed to achieve fasting plasma glucose $\leq$6 mmol/l, the median HbA_{1c} was significantly lower in the sulfoylurea + insulin group (6.6%) than in the group taking insulin alone (7.1%). More individuals in the sulfonylurea + insulin group achieved a HbA_{1c} <7% (47% versus 35%) and less had hypoglycemia than in the insulin-alone group [167].

A Sulfonylurea–insulin combination that appears to be more effective in improving glycemic control in type 2 diabetic patients is the administration of NPH, Lente, or Glargine insulin at 10 p.m. to achieve normal fasting plasma glucose levels, and sulfonylurea therapy during the day to improve postprandial glycemia. This sequential therapy has been evaluated extensively in the last few years [177–181]. It results in decreases of glycosylated hemoglobin between 1.0 and 2.0% and fasting plasma glucose of 2 to 3 mmol/l (35–50 mg/dl) [133–135]. Bedtime insulin–sulfonylurea combinations are superior to daytime insulin–sulfonylurea combinations [177]. In short-term studies (3 months), bedtime insulin–sulfonylurea combination is as effective as multiple injections of insulin in controlling glycemia and does so with less hyperinsulinemia and less weight gain [177, 178]. Sequential insulin sulfonylurea therapy has been effective in controlled studies for more than 1 year [179–181]. One report claims that initial hypertriglyceridemia predicts a poor long-term outcome.

SULFONYLUREAS AND α-GLUCOSIDASE INHIBITORS IN COMBINATION

Combination sulfonylurea–α-glucosidase inhibitor therapy improves glycemic control in sulfonylurea-treated patients by a mean decrement of plasma glucose levels of about 1.5–2.0 mmol/l (27–36 mg/dl) and a mean decrease of HbA_{1c} of about 0.5 [182, 183]. The major effect of adding the α-glucosidase inhibitor is to decrease further the postprandial plasma glucose rise.

SULFONYLUREA AND THIAZOLIDINEDIONES IN COMBINATION

Thiazolidinedione drugs (pioglitazone and rosiglitazone) are PPAR-γ agonists that increase insulin action and decrease hyperglycemia in type 2 diabetic patients by making endogeneous insulin more effective on muscle, liver, and adipose tissue. Thiazolidinediones become less effective as antihyperglycemic agents as B-cell insufficiency progressives. The addition of sulfonylureas to thiazolidinediones improves glycemic control by a decrement in HbA_{1c} of approximately 1.0–1.4% since they increase endogenous insulin secretion [184].

ADVERSE EFFECTS OF SULFONYLUREAS

The overall frequency of adverse effects is low, in the range of 2–5%, and most adverse effects are mild and reversible upon withdrawal. The most serious side effect of sulfonylurea therapy is hypoglycemia, which though usually mild to moderate, can cause fatal complications. Moderate weight gain is a frequent occurrence during sulfonylurea therapy. The possibility that some sulfonylureas, and in particular glibenclamide, may cause unfavorable cardiovascular effects during episodes of myocardial ischemia has received considerable attention during the last several years.

Hypoglycemia

The incidence of any hypoglycemic symptoms during sulfonylurea therapy varies with the specific sulfonylurea and has been reported to be as high as 20–30% per year [185]. Documented severe hypoglycemia, usually defined as symptoms requiring assistance by a third party is far less frequent. In the UKPDS study [100] the rates of any hypoglycemic symptoms were 11.0% for chlorpropamide, 17.7% for glibenclamide, 36.5% for insulin, and 1.2% for lifestyle management. The rates of major (severe) hypoglycemia were 0.4% for chlorpropamide, 0.6% for glibenclamide, 2.3% for insulin, and 0.1% for lifestyle. A US population-based retrospective analysis of the incidence of severe hypoglycemia episodes requiring medical assistance in older individuals reported rates of 1.23/100 person-years with sulfonylurea use versus 2.76/100 person-years in insulin users [186]. A retrospective study of 33243 patients taking sulfonylureas in the United Kingdom reported the risk rate for hypoglycemia of 1.8% annually [187].

There is reason to suspect that long-lasting hypoglycemia in the elderly may be misdiagnosed as a cerebrovascular insult, and the number of sulfonylurea-induced hypoglycemic reactions is probably underreported. The prevalence of sulfonylurea-associated hypoglycemia requiring hospital treatment has been reported as 0.38 per 1000 treatment-years in Switzerland [123], 0.19 per 1000 treatment-years in Sweden [122] and 4.2 per 1000 treatment-years in the Swedish island of Gotland, where the use of sulfonylurea is particularly common [126]. The Swiss survey reported a fatality rate of 4.3% among the hospital-admitted patients [123]. In a US survey done in the middle 1970s, 10% of hypoglycemic patients referred to hospitals died, and 3% had permanent neurologic damage [186].

Long-lasting, and hence serious, hypoglycemia occurs more often with long-acting sulfonylureas, such as glibenclamide and chlorpropamide, than with short-acting ones, such as glipizide and tolbutamide [123, 126, 188, 189]. The numbers of serious cases in the Swiss review were 0.38, 0.34, 0.15, and 0.07 per 1000 treatment-years for glibenclamide, chlorpropamide, glipizide, and tolbutamide, respectively [123]. Figures from Sweden for the period 1975–1985 show that the number of long-lasting hypoglycemic cases per million defined daily doses were 0.195 for glibenclamide and 0.184 for chlorpropamide, but only 0.004 for glipizide and 0.072 for tolbutamide [126]. Data from the retrospective elderly type 2 diabetic population in the United States found an incidence of hypoglycemia requiring medical intervention to be greatest with glibenclamide (1.66 episodes/100 person-years) and least with tolbutamide (0.35 episodes/100 person-years) [190]. Chlorpropamide use was associated with an event rate similar to that for glibenclamide, and glipizide use had an event rate that was approximately half that of the glibenclamide. A recently reported Swiss study found the incidence of severe hypoglycemia to be threefold greater for long-acting sulfonylureas as compared to short-acting forms [189]. As noted earlier the incidence of severe hypoglycemia in type 2 diabetic patients treated with glimepiride is significantly less than those treated with glibenclamide (0.86 episodes/1000 person-years versus 5.6/1000 person-years) [144].

A predisposing factor for the development of sulfonylurea-induced hypoglycemia is age: most serious cases in Sweden were patients over 75 years old, 21% of whom were over 85 years old [122]. Other predisposing factors are reduced food intake, intercurrent illness, renal disease, hepatic disease and cardiovascular disease [122, 123, 191]. It is of note that patients with mutations in the hepatic nuclear factor 1 alpha gene which is the most common form of maturity-onset diabetes of the youth are exquitely sensitive to the hypoglycemic effects of sulfonylureas. Treatment of these patients with sulfonylureas is extremely effective; however, the risk of developing severe hypoglycemia is high [192]. Therefore treatment of these patients should be initiated with low doses of short-acting sulfonylureas There is no apparent dose relation to the development of severe sulfonylurea-induced hypoglycemia in type 2 diabetic patients: severe and fatal hypoglycemia may occur with low doses of the offending sulfonylurea. Drug interactions frequently may be involved, often involving aspirin, salicylate, or alcohol (see below).

The occurrence of severe sulfonylurea-induced hypoglycemia is minimized by avoiding sulfonylureas, particularly long-acting ones, in patients with predisposing conditions or who are taking potentially interacting drugs. When such cases do occur, the patients should be hospitalized. A bolus of 50% glucose should be given intravenously and should be followed by continuous infusion of 10% or 20% glucose. Blood glucose levels should be monitored for at least 3 days and maintained at 6–8 mmol/l (110–145 mg/dl). If intravenous glucose treatment is insufficient, hydrocortisone and/or glucagon administration may be useful. A somatostatin analogue (octreotide) has been shown to reverse sulfonylurea-induced hyperinsulinemia and hypoglycemia and has been shown to be very effective in severe or intractable cases of sulfonylurea-induced hypoglycemia [193–195].

Weight Gain

Weight gain is a frequent complication of sulfonylurea treatment. Older well-controlled studies found that on sulfonylurea treatment the mean increase in body weight was 2.8 kg [169]. This contrasted with a mean decrease of 1.2 kg that occurred with comparable improvements in glycemic control by metformin treatment. Patients receiving sulfonylurea therapy in the UKPDS had a net increase in body weight of 3 kg compared to the conventionally treated patients [103]. This weight gain occurred during the first 3–4 years of treatment and then stabilized.

There are several potential mechanisms that have been proposed to explain the weight gain associated with sulfonylurea treatment. Improvement in glycemic control decreases glycosuria and can increase caloric balance if food intake is not sufficiently decreased. Many patients taking sulfonylureas have episodes of mild hypoglycemia that manifest themselves as hunger and contribute to excess calorie intake. There is some evidence that hyperinsulinemia itself may increase appetite.

Sulfonylureas and Cardiovascular ATP-dependent Potassium Channels

The most frequently debated adverse effect of sulfonylureas is that of an alleged increase in cardiovascular mortality. This was reported in 1970 in subjects treated with tolbutamide in the UGDP study [196]. After extensive analyses and debate it seems likely that these data were based on a spuriously low mortality rate in the placebo group [197]. However, more recently, there is concern that sulfonylureas such as glibenclamide, which have significant binding to SUR-2A and SUR-2B subunits of the cardiovascular ATP-dependent potassium channels, may compromise adaptive responses to ischemia, as has been discussed previously.

As noted earlier, there are ATP-dependent potassium channels in the membranes of myocardial and vascular smooth muscle cells (Table 3). These channels have different isoforms of the SUR subunit than do pancreatic B-cells. These isoforms differ in their drug binding capacities from the SUR-1 [6, 26, 198]. With the exception of glibenclamide the sulfonylurea drugs have a much greater specificity for the SUR-1 than the SUR-2A and SUR-2B [198]. Therefore most sulfonylurea drugs in the doses used to treat type 2 diabetes have no demonstrable effects on myocardial and vascular smooth muscle ATP-dependent potassium channels [80]. Glibenclamide in ordinary doses does effect the cardiovascular ATP-dependent potassium channels.

Under normal conditions the cardiovascular ATP-dependent potassium channels are closed because of the high ATP concentrations generated by oxidative metabolism [80]. The voltage-gated calcium ion channels are open, the consequence being that calcium ion inflow increases and potassium ion outflow is reduced. During ischemia, the ATP concentration falls, the cardiovascular ATP-dependent potassium channel opens, calcium entry into the cell decreases, and potassium flux out of the cell is increased. In the myocardium this decreases contractility and reduces oxygen demand. In the coronary artery this facilitates vasodilatation. The net effect of these changes is to decrease the vulnerability of the heart to subsequent ischemic attacks. This phenomenum whereby an initial short ischemic attack reduces the consequences (size of the infarction) of a subsequent ischemic attack is known as ischemic preconditioning [80]. If the ATP-dependent potassium channel is prevented from opening, ischemic preconditioning does not occur [80].

Studies in normal and diabetic humans have clearly demonstrated that glibenclamide in ordinary antidiabetic doses abolishes ischemic preconditioning [146, 147]. Other sulfonylureas such as glimepiride do not adversely effect ischemic preconditioning [146, 147]. The controversy that exists is whether this effect of glibenclamide has clinical significance. A retrospective analysis of diabetic patients undergoing balloon angioplasty for myocardial infarction at the Mayo Clinic showed a 2.77-fold increased early mortality risk in patients taking sulfonylureas compared to other treatments [199]. Scognamiglio et al. showed that glibenclamide treatment in contrast to insulin treatment with comparable glycemic control decreased left ventricular ejection fraction and increased wall motion score index [200]. Several large clinical outcome studies of type 2 diabetic patients treated with sulfonylureas compared to other antihyperglycemic treatments have not shown any increase in cardiovascular events [201, 202]. Many of these studies included large cohorts treated with glibenclamide. It is unlikely that this controversy will be resolved. Riddle in a recent editorial reflected that there are no specific benefits that can be attributed to glibenclamide as an insulin secretogogue and many potential problems [203]. Perhaps it is best to avoid this controversial cardiovascular issue by using sulfonylureas that have no effects on ischemic preconditioning [204].

Interactions

Several drugs interfere with the efficacy of sulfonylureas, by influencing their pharmacokinetics or pharmacodynamics, or both. As the majority of type 2 diabetes patients are elderly subjects or are in late middle age, they are liable to be exposed to other medication in addition to sulfonylurea. Thus, the risk of interactions is considerable. Two of the most important interactions may occur with alcohol and with aspirin, both of which may provoke, prolong, and/or deepen a hypoglycemic reaction [3, 104, 112, 122]. Plausible and/or documented interactions are listed in Table 6. It should be noted that the degree and extent of a certain interaction may vary between the different sulfonylureas.

Table 6 Mechanisms of drug interactions with sulfonylureas

Agents that augment sulfonylurea action and may cause profound hypoglycemia:

(A) Displacers of sulfonylureas from albumin binding sites
- (1) Aspirin and salicylic acid
- (2) Other nonsteroidal anti-inflammatory drugs
- (3) Sulfonamides
- (4) Trimethoprim
- (5) Fibrates

(B) Competitive inhibitors of sulfonylurea metabolism
- (1) Alcohol
- (2) H_2-blockers
- (3) Sulfonamides
- (4) Anticoagulants
- (5) Pyrazolone derivatives (phenylbutazone, oxiphenbutazone, sulfinpyrazone)
- (6) Monoamine oxidase inhibitors

(C) Inhibitors of urinary excretion of sulfonylurea and active metabolites
- (1) Probenecid
- (2) Aspirin and salicylic acid
- (3) Other nonsteroidal anti-inflammatory drugs
- (4) Allopurinol
- (5) Sulfonamides

(D) Augmentors of the effect of sulfonylurea
- (1) Alcohol
- (2) Aspirin and salicylic acid
- (3) Guanethidine and betanidine
- (4) Monoamine oxidase inhibitors

(E) Antagonists of endogenous hyperglycemic hormones
- (1) β-Blockers
- (2) Sympatholytic drugs

Agents that attenuate sulfonylurea action and may counteract the antihyperglycemic effect:

(A) Enzyme inducers that increase sulfonylurea elimination
- (1) Alcohol (chronic, moderate use)
- (2) Barbiturates (chronic, moderate use)
- (3) Rifampicin

(B) Agents that antagonize sulfonylurea action
- (1) β-Blockers

(C) Inhibitors of insulin secretion or insulin action
- (1) Thiazides and loop diuretics
- (2) Diazoxide
- (3) β-Blockers
- (4) Phenytoin
- (5) Corticosteroids
- (6) Estrogens
- (7) Indomethacin
- (8) Isoniazid
- (9) Nicotinic acid

(D) Mechanism obscure
- (1) Phenothiazines
- (2) Acetazolamide

Toxicity

Hypoglycemic reactions have been commented upon above. Most other adverse effects are said to appear within the first 2 months of treatment, and they include the following:

Blood Agranulocytosis, thrombocytopenia, bone marrow aplasia, red cell aplasia, hemolytic anemia

Skin Rashes, pruritus, erythema nodosum, erythema multiforme, Stevens–Johnson syndrome, exfoliative dermatitis, purpura, photosensitivity

Gastrointestinal tract Nausea, vomiting, heartburn

Liver Abnormal function tests, jaundice, cholestasis, granulomatous hepatitis

Lung Possible diffuse pulmonary reaction

Thyroid Weak antithyroid activity

Kidney Antidiuresis, water retention (chlorpropamide)

Vasomotor Alcohol flush, tachycardia, headache (mainly chlorpropamide)
Cardiovascular Vasculitis

Contraindications

The following patients should not be treated with sulfonylureas

(1) patients with IDDM or "pancreatic" diabetes
(2) pregnant women
(3) patients with severe infections, stress or trauma
(4) patients with a history of severe adverse reactions to sulfonylureas
(5) patients particularly prone to develop hypoglycemia, e.g. with liver or kidney disease

CONCLUSION

Sulfonylureas have a definite and important role in the management of patients with type 2 diabetes. They are able to counteract several metabolic disturbances of this disease and may help to reduce the risk of certain complications, provided that they are introduced early in the course of type 2 diabetes. However, they must not be introduced until intense and persistent treatment with dietary regulation and regular exercise has proved to be insufficient, and they should never be used instead of such treatment. When used appropriately, sulfonylureas are safe, particularly the short-acting ones.

REFERENCES

1. Kennedy DL, Piper JM, Baum C. Trends in the use of oral hypoglycemic agents. *Diabetes Care* 1988; 11: 558–62.
2. Boccuzzi SJ, Sung JCY, Wogen J, Shah AB, Fox J, Kim J. Utilization of oral hypoglycemic agents in a drug-insured U.S. population. *Diabetes Care* 2001; 24: 1411–5.
3. Melander A, Bitzén P-O, Faber O, Groop L. Sulphonylurea antidiabetic drugs: an update of their clinical pharmacology and rational therapeutic use. *Drugs* 1989; 37: 58–72.
4. Ribes G, Trimble ER, Blayac JP, Wollheim CB, Puech R, Loubatières-Mariani MM. Effect of a new hypoglycaemic agent (HB 699) on the *in vivo* secretion of pancreatic hormones in the dog. *Diabetologia* 1981; 20: 501–5.
5. Garrino M-G, Meissner H-P, Henquin J-C. The non-sulphonylurea moiety of gliquidone mimics the effects of the parent molecule on pancreatic B-cells. *Eur J Pharmacol* 1986; 124: 309–16.
6. Proks P, Reimann F, Green N, Gribble F, Ashcroft F. Sulfonylurea stimulation of insulin secretion. *Diabetes* 2002; 51 (suppl 1): S368–76.
7. Hansen AM, Christensen IT, Hansen JB, Carr RD, Ashcroft FM, Wahl P. Differential interactions of nateglinide and repaglinide on the human beta-cell sulphonylurea receptor 1. *Diabetes* 2002; 51: 2789–95.
8. Hellman B, Sehlin J, Täljedal I-B. The pancreatic B-cell recognition of insulin secretagogues, II: sites of action of tolbutamide. *Biochem Biophys Res Comm* 1971; 45: 1384–8.
9. Aguilar-Bryan L, Bryan J. Molecular biology of adenosine triphosphate-sensitive potassium channels. *Endocr Rev* 1999; 20: 101–35.
10. Cook DL, Satin LS, Ashford MLJ, Hales CN. ATP-sensitive K^+ channels in pancreatic B-cells. Spare channel hypothesis. *Diabetes* 1988; 37: 495–8.
11. Boyd AE III. Sulfonylurea receptors, ion channels, and fruit flies. *Diabetes* 1988; 37: 847–50.
12. Levine R. Sulfonylureas: background development of the field. *Diabetes Care* 1984; 7 (suppl 1): 3–7.
13. Loubatières A. Analyse du mécanisme de l'action hypoglycemiante du *p*-aminobenzène-sulfamidothiodiazol. *Compt Rend Soc Biol* 1944; 138: 766–7.
14. Mirsky IA, Perisutti G, Jinks R. Ineffectiveness of sulfonylureas in alloxan diabetic rats. *Proc Soc Exp Biol Med* 1956; 91: 475–7.
15. Parker ML, Pildes RS, Chao K, Cornblath M, Kipnis DM. Juvenile diabetes mellitus. A deficiency in insulin. *Diabetes* 1968; 17: 27–32.
16. Joffe BI, Jackson WPU, Bank S, Vinik AI. Effect of oral hypoglycemic agents on glucose tolerance in pancreatic diabetes. *Gut* 1972; 13: 285–7.
17. Yalow RS, Black H, Villazon M, Berson SA. Comparison of plasma insulin levels following administration of tolbutamide and glucose. *Diabetes* 1960; 9: 356–62.
18. Hellman B, Täljedal I-B. Effects of sulphonylurea derivatives on pancreatic beta cells. In Dorzbach E (ed), *Insulin*, Part 2. Berlin: Springer, 1975: pp 175–94.
19. Malaisse WJ, Lebrun P. Mechanisms of sulfonylurea-induced insulin release. *Diabetes Care* 1990; 13 (suppl 3): 9–17.
20. Wick AN, Britton B, Gabowski R. The action of a sulfonylurea hypoglycemic agent (Orinase) in extrahepatic tissues. *Metabolism* 1956; 5: 739–43.
21. Bowen V, Lazarus NR. Insulin release from the perfused rat pancreas. *Biochem J* 1974; 142: 385–9.
22. Schmid-Antomarchi H, De Weille J, Fosset M, Lazdunski M. The receptor for antidiabetic sulphonylureas controls the activity of the ATP-modulated K^+ channel in insulin secreting cells. *J Biol Chem* 1987; 262: 15840–4.
23. Siconolfi-Baez L, Banerji MA, Lebovitz HE. Characterization and significance of sulfonylurea receptors. *Diabetes Care* 1990; 13 (suppl 3): 2–8.
24. Aguilar-Bryan L, Nichols CG, Wechsler SW, Clement IV JP, Boyd AE III, Gonzalez G, Herrera-Sosa H, Nguy K, Bryan J, Nelson DA. Cloning of the B-cell high affinity sulfonylurea receptor: a regulator of insulin secretion. *Science* 1995; 268: 423–6.
25. Inagaki N, Gonoi T, Clement IV JP, Namba N, Inazawa J, Gonzalez G, Aguilar-Bryan L, Seino S, Bryan J. Reconstition of I_{KATP} an inward rectifier subunit plus the sulfonylurea receptor. *Science* 1995; 270: 1166–70.
26. Ashcroft FM, Gribble FM. ATP-sensitive K^+ channels and insulin secretion: their role in health and disease. *Diabetologia* 1999; 42: 903–19.
27. Inagaki N, Gonoi T, Clement JP, Wang CZ, Aguilar-Bryan L, Bryan J, Seino S. A family of sulfonylurea receptors determines the properties of ATP-sensitive channel K^+ channels. *Neuron* 1996; 16: 1011–7.
28. Gylfe E, Hellman B, Sehlin J, Täljedal I-B. Interaction of sulphonylurea with the pancreatic B-cell. *Experientia* 1984; 40: 1126–34.

29. Boyd AE III, Hill RS, Oberwetter JM, Berg M. Calcium dependency and free calcium concentrations during insulin secretion in a hamster beta cell line. *J Clin Invest* 1986; 77: 774–81.
30. Hellman B, Sehlin J, Täljedal I-B. Glibenclamide is exceptional among hypoglycaemic sulphonylureas in accumulating progressively in B-cell rich pancreatic islets. *Acta Endocrinol* 1984; 385–90.
31. Carpentier J-L, Sawano F, Ravazzola M, Malaisse WJ. Internalization of [^{3}H] glibenclamide in pancreatic islet cells. *Diabetologia* 1986; 29: 259–61.
32. Renstrom E, Barg S, Thevenod F, Rorsman P. Sulfonylurea-mediated stimulation of insulin exocytosis via an ATP-sensitive K^+ channel-independent action. *Diabetes* 2002; 51 (suppl 1): S33–6.
33. Reaven G, Dray J. Effect of chlorpropamide on serum glucose and immunoreactive insulin concentrations in patients with maturity-onset diabetes mellitus. *Diabetes* 1967; 16: 487–92.
34. Feldman JM, Lebovitz HE. Endocrine and metabolic effects of glibenclamide: evidence for an extra-pancreatic mechanism of action. *Diabetes* 1971; 20: 745–51.
35. Pfeifer MA, Halter JB, Graf R, Porte D Jr. Potentiation of insulin secretion to non-glucose stimuli in normal man by tolbutamide. *Diabetes* 1980; 29: 335–40.
36. Judzewitsch RG, Pfeifer MA, Best JD, Beard JC, Halter JB, Porte D Jr. Chronic chlorpropamide therapy of non-insulin-dependent diabetes augments basal and stimulated insulin secretion by increasing islet sensitivity to glucose. *J Clin Endocrinol Metab* 1982; 55: 321–7.
37. Sumi S, Ichihara K, Nonaka K, Tauri S. Effect of the discontinuation of long-term sulfonylurea treatment on blood glucose and insulin secretion in non-insulin-dependent diabetes mellitus. *Endocrinol Jpn* 1982; 29: 41–7.
38. DeFronzo RA. The triumvirate: B-cell, muscle, liver. A collusion responsible for NIDDM. *Diabetes* 1988; 37: 667–87.
39. Kosaka K, Kuzuya T, Akanuma Y, Hagura R. Increase in insulin response after treatment of overt maturity onset diabetes mellitus is independent of the mode of treatment. *Diabetologia* 1980; 18: 23–8.
40. Unger RH, Grundy S. Hyperglycaemia as an inducer as well as a consequence of impaired islet cell function and insulin resistance: implication for the management of diabetes. *Diabetologia* 1985; 28: 119–21.
41. Karam JH, Sanz N, Salamon E, Nolte MS. Selective unresponsiveness of pancreatic B-cells to acute sulfonylurea stimulation during sulfonylurea therapy in NIDDM. *Diabetes* 1986; 35: 1314–20.
42. Kawaki J, Nagashima K, Tanaka J, Miki T, Miyazaki M, Gonio T, Mitsuhashi N, Nakajima N, Iwanaga T, Yano H, Seino S. Unresponsiveness to glibenclamide during chronic treatment induced by reduction of ATP-sensitive K^+ channel activity. *Diabetes* 1999; 48: 2001–6.
43. Davies MJ, Metcalf J, Day JL, Greenfell A, Hales CN, Gray IP. Effect of sulphonylurea therapy on plasma insulin, intact and 32/33 split proinsulin in subjects with type 2 diabetes mellitus. *Diabet Med* 1994; 11: 293–8.
44. Prigeon RL, Jacobson RK, Porte D Jr, Kahn SE. Effect of sulfonylurea withdrawal on proinsulin levels, B cell function, and glucose disposal in subjects with noninsulin-dependent diabetes mellitus. *J Clin Endocrinol Metab* 1996; 81: 3295–8.
45. Levy J, Malaisse WJ. The stimulus–secretion coupling of glucose-induced insulin release, XVII: effects of sulfonylureas and diazoxide on insular biosynthetic activity. *Biochem Pharmacol* 1975; 24: 235–9.
46. Duckworth WC, Solomon SS, Kitabchi AE. Effect of chronic sulfonylurea therapy on plasma insulin and proinsulin levels. *J Clin Endocrinol Metab* 1972; 35: 585–91.
47. Quesada I, Nadal A, Soria B. Different effects of tolbutamide and diazoxide in (α-, (β-, (δ-cells within intact islets of Langerhans induces impairment of glucagon and growth hormone responses during mild insulin-induced hypoglycemia. *Diabetes* 1999; 48: 2390–7.
48. Landstedt-Hallin L, Adamson U, Lins P-E. Oral glibenclamide suppresses glucagon secretion during insulin-induced hypoglycemia in patients with type 2 diabetes. *J Clin Endocrinol Metab* 1999; 84: 3140–5.
49. Ter Braak EW, Appelman, van der Tweel I, Erkelens DW, van Haeften TW. The sulfonylurea glyburide induces impairment of glucagon and growth hormone responses during mild insulin-induced hypoglycemia. *Diabetes Care* 2002; 25: 107–12.
50. Lebovitz HE. Oral hypoglycemic agents. In Rifkin H, Porte D Jr (eds), *Diabetes Mellitus: Theory and Practice*, 4th edn. New York: Excerpta Medica, 1990; pp 554–75.
51. Lebovitz HE, Feinglos MN. Sulfonylurea drugs: mechanism of antidiabetic action and therapeutic usefulness. *Diabetes Care* 1978; 1: 189–97.
52. Lebovitz HE. Oral hypoglycemic agents. In Alberti KGMM, Krall LP (eds), *Diabetes Annual 3*. Amsterdam: Elsevier, 1987; pp 72–93.
53. Haupt A, Kausch C, Dahl D, Bachmann O. Stumvoll M, Haring H-U, Matthaei S. Effect of glimepiride on insulin-stimulated glycogen synthesis in cultured human skeletal muscle cells. *Diabetes Care* 2002; 25: 2129–32.
54. Overkamp D, Volk A, Maerker E, Heide PE, Wahl HG, Rett K, Haring H-U. Acute effect of glimepiride on insulin-stimulated glucose metabolism in glucose-intolerant insulin-resistant offspring of patients with type 2 diabetes. *Diabetes Care* 2002; 25: 2065–73.
55. Hribal ML, D'Alfonso R, Giovannone B, Lauro D, Liu YY, Borboni P, Federici M, Lauro R, Sesti G. The sulfonylurea glimepiride regulates intracellular routing of the insulin-receptor complexes through their interaction with specific protein kinase C isoforms. *Mol Pharmacol* 2001; 59: 322–30.
56. Lebovitz HE. Cellular loci of sulfonylurea actions. *Diabetes Care* 1984; 7 (suppl 1): 67–71.
57. Jacobs DB, Hayes GR, Lockwood DH. *In vitro* effects of sulfonylurea on glucose transport and translocation of glucose transporters in adipocytes from streptozotocin-induced diabetic rats. *Diabetes* 1989; 38: 205–10.
58. Putnam WS, Andersen DK, Jones RS, Lebovitz HE. Selective potentiation of insulin-mediated glucose disposal in normal dogs by the sulfonylurea, glipizide. *J Clin Invest* 1981; 67: 1016–23.
59. Firth RG, Bell PM, Rizza RA. Effects of tolazamide and exogenous insulin on insulin action in patients with non-insulin-dependent diabetes mellitus. *N Engl J Med* 1986; 314: 1280–6.
60. Simonson DC, Delprato S, Castellino P, Groop L, DeFronzo RA. Effect of glyburide on glycemic control, insulin requirement, and glucose metabolism in insulin-treated diabetic patients. *Diabetes* 1987; 36: 136–46.
61. Sartor G, Ursing D, Nilsson-Ehle P, Wåhlin-Boll E, Melander A. Lack of primary effect of sulphonylurea (glipizide) on plasma lipoproteins and insulin action in

former type 2 diabetics with attenuated insulin secretion. *Eur J Clin Pharmacol* 1987; 33: 279–82.

62. Lebovitz HL, Feinglos MN, Bucholtz HK, Lebovitz FL. Potentiation of insulin action: a probable mechanism for the antidiabetic action of sulfonylurea drugs. *J Clin Endocrinol Metab* 1977; 45: 601–4.
63. Kolterman OG, Gray RS, Shapiro G, Scarlett JA, Griffin J, Olefsky JM. The acute and chronic effects of sulfonylurea therapy in type II diabetic subjects. *Diabetes* 1984; 33: 346–54.
64. Ward G, Harrison LC, Proietto J, Aitken P, Nankervis A. Gliclazide therapy is associated with potentiation of post-binding insulin action in obese, non-insulin-dependent diabetic subjects. *Diabetes* 1985; 34: 241–5.
65. Faber OK, Beck-Nielsen H, Binder C, Butzer P, Damsgaard EM, Froland F, Hjollund E, Lindskov HO, Melander A, Pedersen O, Petersen P, Schwarts Sorensen N, Wåhlin-Boll E. Acute actions of sulfonylurea drugs during long-term treatment of NIDDM. *Diabetes Care* 1990; 13 (suppl 3): 26–31.
66. Lebovitz HE. Oral hypoglycemic sulfonylureas: pancreatic vs extrapancreatic actions. In Shigeta Y, Lebovitz HE, Gerich JE, Malaisse WJ (eds), *Best Approach to Ideal Therapy of Diabetes Mellitus*. Amsterdam: Excerpta Medica, 1987; pp 21–6.
67. Beck-Nielsen H, Hother-Hielsen O, Pedersen O. Mechanism of action of sulphonylureas with special reference to the extrapancreatic effect: an overview. *Diabet Med* 1988; 5: 613–20.
68. Wang PH, Beguinot F, Smith RJ. Augmentation of the effects of insulin and insulin-like growth factors I and II on glucose uptake in cultured rat skeletal muscle cells by sulfonylureas. *Diabetologia* 1987; 30: 797–803.
69. Mirsky IA, Perisutti G, Diengatt D. The inhibition of insulinase by hypoglycemic sulfonamides. *Metabolism* 1956; 5: 138–43.
70. Almér L-O, Johansson E, Melander A, Wåhlin-Boll E. Influence of sulphonylureas on the secretion, disposal and effect of insulin. *Eur J Clin Pharmacol* 1982; 22: 27–32.
71. Scheen AJ, Lefebvre PJ, Luyckx AS. Glipizide increases plasma insulin but not C-peptide level after a standardized breakfast in type 2 diabetic patients. *Eur J Clin Pharmacol* 1984; 26: 471–4.
72. Groop L, Groop P-H, Stenman S, Saloranta C, Tötterman K-J, Fyhrquist F, Melander A. Comparison of pharmacokinetics, metabolic effects and mechanisms of action of glyburide and glipizide during long-term treatment. *Diabetes Care* 1987; 10: 671–8.
73. Groop L, Groop P-H, Stenman S, Saloranta C, Tötterman K-J, Fyhrquist F, Melander A. Do sulfonylureas influence hepatic insulin clearance? *Diabetes Care* 1988; 11: 689–90.
74. Beck-Nielsen H, Hother Nielsen O, Andersen PH, Pedersen O, Schmitz O. *In vivo* action of glibenclamide. *Diabetologia* 1986; 29: 515A (abstract 26).
75. Wåhlin-Boll E, Sartor G, Melander A, Scherstén B. Impaired effect of sulphonylurea following increased dosage. *Eur J Clin Pharmacol* 1982; 22: 21–5.
76. Stenman S, Melander A, Groop P-H, Groop L. What is the benefit of increasing the sulphonylurea dose? *Ann Int Med* 1993; 118: 169–72.
77. Kuo BS, Korner G, Bjornsson TD. Effects of sulfonylureas on the synthesis and secretion of plasminogen activator from bovine aortic endothelial cells. *J Clin Invest* 1988; 81: 730–7.
78. Moses AM, Numann P, Miller M. Mechanism of chlorpropamide-induced antidiuretics in man. Evidence for release of ADH and enhancement of peripheral action. *Metabolism* 1973; 22: 59–66.
79. Lebovitz HE. Oral therapies for diabetic hyperglycemia. *Endocrinol Metab Clin North Am* 2001; 30: 909–33.
80. Lebovitz HE. Insulin secretogogues: old and new. *Diabetes Rev* 1999; 7: 139–53.
81. Lindblad U, Melander A. Sulphonylurea dose–response relationships: relation to clinical practice. *Diabetes Obes Metab* 2000; 2: 25–31.
82. Greenfield MS, Doberne L, Rosenthal M, Schulz B, Widström A, Reaven GM. Effect of sulfonylurea treatment on *in vivo* insulin secretion and action in patients with non-insulin-dependent diabetes mellitus. *Diabetes* 1982; 31: 307–12.
83. Best JD, Judzewitsch RG, Pfeifer MA, Beard JC, Halter JB, Porte D Jr. The effect of chronic sulfonylurea therapy on hepatic glucose production in non-insulin-dependent diabetes mellitus. *Diabetes* 1982; 31: 333–8.
84. Lebovitz HE, Feinglos MN. Mechanism of action of the second generation sulfonylurea glipizide. *Am J Med* 1983; 75 (suppl 5B): 46–54.
85. Camerini-Davalos R, Lozano-Castaneda O, Marble A. Five years experience with tolbutamide. *Diabetes* 1962; 11 (suppl): 74–80.
86. Cervantes-Amezeua A, Naldjian S, Camerini-Davalos R, Marble A. Long-term use of chlorpropamide in diabetes. *JAMA* 1965; 193: 759–62.
87. Muller R, Bauer G, Schroder R, Saito S. Summary report of clinical investigation of the oral antidiabetic drug HB 419 (glibenclamide). *Horm Metab Res* 1969; 1 (suppl): 88–92.
88. Emanueli A, Molari E, Colombo A, Pirola L, Caputo G. Glipizide, a new sulfonylurea in the treatment of diabetes mellitus. *Arzneim Forsch (Drug Res)* 1972; 22: 1881–5.
89. Rizza RA. Is secondary failure inevitable? In Cameron D, Colagiuri S, Heding L, Kuhl C, Ma A, Mortimer R (eds), *Non-insulin-dependent Diabetes Mellitus*. Hong Kong: Excerpta Medica, 1989; pp 57–61.
90. Balodimos MC, Camerini-Davalos R, Marble A. Nine years experience with tolbutamide in the treatment of diabetes. *Metabolism* 1966; 11: 957–70.
91. Turner RC, Holman RR, Matthews DR. Sulfonylurea failure and inadequacy. In Cameron D, Colagiuri S, Heding L, Kuhl C, Ma A, Mortimer R (eds), *Non-insulin-dependent Diabetes Mellitus*. Hong Kong: Excerpta Medica, 1989; pp 52–6.
92. Simonson DC, Kourides IA, Feinglos M, Shamoon, Fishette CT. Efficacy, safety, and dose–response characteristics of glipizide gastrointestinal therapeutic system on glycemic control and insulin secretion in NIDDM. *Diabetes Care* 1997; 20: 597–606.
93. Rosenstock J, Samols E, Muchmore DB, Schneider J. Glimepiride, a new once-daily sulfonylurea. *Diabetes Care* 1996; 19: 1194–9.
94. Garber AJ, Larsen J, Schneider SH, Piper BA, Henry D. Simultaneous glyburide/metformin therapy is superior to component monotherapy as an initial pharmacological treatment for type 2 diabetes. *Diabetes Obes Metab* 2002; 4: 201–8.
95. Singer DL, Hurwitz D. Long-term experience with sulfonylureas and placebo. *N Engl J Med* 1967; 277: 450–6.

96. Lev-Ran A. Trial of placebo in long-term chlorpropamide-treated diabetics. *Diabetologia* 1974; 10: 197–200.
97. University Group Diabetes Program. Effects of hypoglycemic agents on vascular complication in patients with adult-onset diabetes, III: clinical implications of UGDP results. *JAMA* 1971; 218: 1400–10.
98. The United Kingdom Prospective Diabetes Study (UKPDS) Group. UK Prospective Study of Therapies of Maturity-onset Diabetes, I: effect of diet, sulphonylurea, insulin or biguanide therapy on fasting plasma glucose and body weight over one year. *Diabetologia* 1983; 24: 404–11.
99. The United Kingdom Prospective Diabetes Study (UKPDS) Group. UK Prospective Diabetes Study, II: reduction in HbA_{1c} with basal insulin supplement, sulfonylurea or biguanide therapy in maturity-onset diabetes. *Diabetes* 1985; 34: 793–8.
100. The United Kingdom Prospective Diabetes Study (UKPDS) Group. Intensive blood-glucose control with sulphonylureas or insulin compared with conventional treatment and risk of complications in patients with type 2 diabetes (UKPDS 33). *Lancet* 1998; 352: 837–53.
101. Turner RC, Cull CA, Frighi V, Holman RR. Glycemic control with diet, sulfonylurea, metformin, or insulin in patients with type 2 diabetes mellitus. Progressive requirement for multiple therapies (UKPDS 49). *JAMA* 1999; 281: 2005–12.
102. Matthews DR, Cull CA, Stratton IM, Holman RR, Turner RC. UKPDS 26: Sulphonylurea failure in non-insulin dependent diabetic patients over six years. *Diabet Med* 1998; 15: 297–303.
103. The UKPDS Group. UKPDS, 16: Overview of 6 years' therapy of type 2 diabetes: a progressive disease. *Diabetes* 1995; 44: 1249–58.
104. Ferner RE, Chaplin S. The relationship between the pharmacokinetics and pharmacodynamic effects of oral hypoglycaemic drugs. *Clin Pharmacokin* 1987; 12: 379–401.
105. Melander A, Sartor G, Wåhlin E, Schersten B, Bitzén P-O. Serum tolbutamide and chlorpropamide concentrations in patients with diabetes mellitus. *Br Med J* 1978; 1: 142–4.
106. Cerasi E, Efendic S, Luft R. Dose response relation between insulin and blood glucose levels during oral glucose loads in prediabetic and diabetic subjects. *Lancet* 1973; i: 794–7.
107. Luft R, Wajngot A, Efendic S. On the pathogenesis of maturity-onset diabetes. *Diabetes Care* 1981; 4: 58–63.
108. DeFronzo RA, Ferrannini E, Koivisto V. New concepts in the pathogenesis and treatment of noninsulin-dependent diabetes mellitus. *Am J Med* 1983; 74 (suppl 1A): 52–81.
109. Temple RC, Carrington CA, Luzio SD, Owens DR, Schneider AE, Sobey WJ, Hales CN. Insulin deficiency in non-insulin-dependent diabetes. *Lancet* 1989; i: 293–5.
110. Bitzén P-O, Melander A, Scherstén B, Wåhlin-Boll E. The influence of glipizide on early insulin release and glucose disposal before and after diet regulation in diabetic patients with different degrees of hyperglycaemia. *Eur J Clin Pharmacol* 1988; 35: 31–7.
111. Bitzén P-O. *On the Early Detection and Treatment of Non-insulin-dependent Diabetes Mellitus in Primary Health Care*, PhD Thesis. Sweden: University of Lund, 1988.
112. Hartling SG, Faber OK, Wegmann M-L, Wåhlin-Boll E, Melander A. Interaction of ethanol and glipizide in humans. *Diabetes Care* 1987; 10: 683–6.
113. Arnqvist HJ, Karlberg BE, Melander A. Pharmacokinetics and effects of glibenclamide in two formulations, HB419 and HB420, in type 2 diabetics. *Ann Clin Res* 1983; 15 (suppl 37): 21–5.
114. Groop L, Luzi L, Melander A, Groop P-H, Ratheiser K, Simonson DC, DeFronzo RA. Different effects of glyburide and glipizide on insulin secretion and hepatic glucose production in normal and NIDDM subjects. *Diabetes* 1987; 36: 1320–8.
115. Ikegawi H, Shima K, Tanaka A, Tahara Y, Hirota M, Kumahara Y. Interindividual variation in the absorption of glibenclamide in man. *Acta Endocrinol* 1986; 111: 528–32.
116. Campbell DB, Adriaenssens P, Hopkins YW, Gordon B, Williams JRB. Pharmacokinetics and metabolism of gliclazide: a review. In Keen H et al. (eds), *Gliclazide and the Treatment of Diabetes*. (International Congress and Symposium Series 20). London: Academic Press, 1980; pp 71–82.
117. Wåhlin-Boll E, Almér L-O, Melander A. Bioavailability, pharmacokinetics and effects of glipizide in type 2 diabetics. *Clin Pharmacokinet* 1982; 7: 363–72.
118. Eriksson J, Franssila-Kalluni A, Ekstrand A, Saloranta C, Widén E, Schalin C, Groop L. Early metabolic defects in persons at increased risk for non-insulin-dependent diabetes mellitus. *N Engl J Med* 1989; 321: 337–43.
119. Sartor G, Lundquist I, Melander A, Scherstén B, Wåhlin-Boll E. Improved effect of glibenclamide on administration before breakfast. *Eur J Clin Pharmacol* 1982; 21: 403–8.
120. Wåhlin-Boll E, Melander A, Sartor G, Scherstén B. Influence of food intake on the absorption and effect of glipizide in diabetics and in healthy subjects. *Eur J Clin Pharmacol* 1980; 18: 279–83.
121. Silins RA, Butcher MA, Marlin GE. Improved effect of tolbutamide when given before food in patients on long-term therapy [letter]. *Br J Clin Pharmacol* 1984; 18: 647–8.
122. Asplund K, Wiholm B-E, Lithner F. Glibenclamide-associated hypoglycaemia. A report on 57 cases. *Diabetologia* 1983; 24: 412–7.
123. Berger W, Cardiff F, Pasquel M, Rump A. Die relative Häufigkeit der schweren Sulfonylharnstoff-Hypoglykämie in den letzten 25 Jahren in der Schweiz. *Schweiz Med Wschr* 1986; 116: 145–51.
124. Seltzer HS. Severe drug-induced hypoglycemia. A review. *Comp Ther* 1979; 5: 21–9.
125. Jönsson A, Rydberg T, Ekberg G, Hallengren B, Melander A. Slow elimination of glyburide in NIDDM subjects. *Diabetes Care* 1994; 17: 142–5.
126. Statistics from the Department of Drugs. Uppsala, Sweden: Swedish Board of Health and Welfare, 1985.
127. Behrle M. *Untersuchung zur Pharmakokinetik von Glibenclamid bei nierengesunden und niereninsuffizienten Diabetikern*, Thesis. Heidelberg, Germany: Ruprecht-Karl-Universität, 1980.
128. Rydberg T, Jönsson A, Röder M, Melander A. Hypoglycemic activity of glyburide (glibenclamide) metabolites in man. *Diabetes Care* 1994; 17: 1026–30.
129. Ferner R, Rawlins MD, Alberti KGMM. Impaired B-cell responses improve when fasting blood glucose concentration is reduced in non-insulin-dependent diabetes. *Q J Med* 1988; 66: 137–46.

130. Olson SC, Ayres JW, Antal EJ, Albert KS. Effect of food and tablet age on relative bioavailability and pharmacodynamics of two tolbutamide products. *J Pharm Sci* 1985; 74: 735–9.
131. Scott J, Poffenbarger PL. Pharmacodynamics of tolbutamide metabolism in humans. *Diabetes* 1979; 28: 41–51.
132. Neuvonen PJ, Kärkkäinen S. Effects of charcoal, sodium bicarbonate and ammonium chloride on chlorpropamide kinetics. *Clin Pharmacol Ther* 1983; 33: 386–93.
133. Groop L, Wåhlin-Boll E, Groop P-H, Tötterman K-J, Melander A, Tolppanen E-M, Fyhrqvist F. Pharmacokinetics and metabolic effects of glibenclamide and glipizide in Type 2 diabetics. *Eur J Clin Pharmacol* 1985; 28: 697–704.
134. Taylor R, Isles TE, MacLaren S, Stevenson IH, Newton RW. Comparison of metabolic profiles in non-obese non-insulin-dependent diabetics receiving glipizide and glibenclamide. *Diabetologia Croatica* 1983; 12: 279–92.
135. Cabrera-Rode E, Perich P, Diaz-Horta O, Tiberti C, Molina G, Arranz C, Martin JM, Licea M, DeLeiva AD, Puig-Domingo M, Dimario U. Slowly progressing type 1 diabetes: persistence of islet cell autoantibodies is related to glibenclamide treatmenr. *Autoimmunity* 2002; 35: 469–74.
136. Blomgren KB, Sundstrom A, Steineck G, Wiholm BE. Obesity and treatment of diabetes with glyburide may both be risk factors for acute pancreatitis. *Diabetes Care* 2002; 25: 298–302.
137. Langer O, Conway DL, Berkus MD, Xenakis EMJ. Gonzales O. A comparison of glyburide and insulin in women with gestational diabetes mellitus. *New Engl J Med* 2000; 343: 1134–8.
138. Forette B, Rolland A, Hopkins Y, Gordon B, Campbell B. Gliclazide kinetics in the elderly. In Alberti KGMM, Ogada T, Aluoch JA, Mngola EN (eds), *11th Congress of the International Diabetes Federation*. Amsterdam: Excerpta Medica, 1982; p 9.
139. Holmes B, Heel RC, Brogden RN, Speight TM, Avery GS. Gliclazide. A preliminary review of its pharmacodynamic properties and therapeutic efficacy in diabetes mellitus. *Drugs* 1984; 27: 301–27.
140. Kradjian W, Kobayashi KA, Bauer LA, Horn JR, Opheim K, Wood F Jr. Glipizide pharmacokinetics: effects of age, diabetes and multiple dosing (in press).
141. Wåhlin-Boll E, Groop L, Karhumaa S, Groop P-H, Tötterman K-J, Melander A. Therapeutic equivalence of once- and thrice-daily glipizide. *Eur J Clin Pharmacol* 1986; 31: 95–9.
142. Berelowitz M, Fischette C, Cefalu W, Shade DS, Sutfin T, Kourides IA. Comparative efficacy of a once daily contolled-release type 2 diabetes. Formulation of glipizide and immediate-release glipizide in patients with NIDDM. *Diabetes Care* 1994; 17: 1460–4.
143. Campbell RK. Glimepiride: role of a new sulfonylurea in the treatment of type 2 diabetes mellitus. *Ann Pharmacother* 1998; 32: 1044–52.
144. Holstein A, Plaschke A, Egberts EH. Lower incidence of severe hypoglycaemia in patients with type 2 diabetes treated with glimepiride versus glibenclamide. *Diabetes Metab Res Rev* 2001; 17: 467–73.
145. Tsunekawa T, Hayashi T, Suzuki Y, Matsui-Hirai H, Kano H, Fukatsu A, Nomura N, Miyazaki A, Iguchi A. Plasma adiponectin plays an important role in improving insulin resistance with glimepiride in elderly type 2 diabetic subjects. *Diabetes Care* 2003; 26: 285–9.
146. Klepzig H, Kober G, Matter C, Luus H, Schneider H, Boedekert KH, Klowski W, Amann FW, Gruber D, Harris S, Burger W. Sulphonylureas and ischemic preconditioning. A double-blind, placebo-controlled evaluation of glimepiride and glibenclamide. *Eur Heart J* 1999; 20: 439–46.
147. Lee T-M, Chou T-F. Impairment of myocardial protection in type 2 diabetic patients. *J Clin Endocrinol Metab* 2003; 88: 531–7.
148. Korytkowski M, Thomas A, Reid L, Tedesco MB, Gooding WE, Gerich J. Glimepiride improves both first and second phases of insulin secretion in type 2 diabetes. *Diabetes Care* 2002; 25: 1607–11.
149. Alberti KGMM. A desktop guide to type 2 diabetes mellitus. European Diabetes Policy Group 1998–1999 International Diabetes Federation European Region. *Exp Clin Endocrinol Diabetes* 1999; 107: 390–420.
150. Lebovitz HE. Treating hyperglycemia in type 2 diabetes: new goals and strategies. *Cleve Clin J Med* 2002; 69: 809–20.
151. Rendell M, Slevin D, Meltz G, Simpson J, Barquet A. A case of maturity-onset diabetes mellitus resistant to insulin but responsive to tolbutamide. *Arch Int Med* 1979; 90: 195–7.
152. Persson G. Cardiovascular complications in diabetics and subjects with reduced glucose tolerance. *Acta Med Scand* 1977; (suppl 605).
153. Donahue RP, Abbott RD, Reed DM, Katsuhiko Y. Postchallenge glucose concentration and coronary heart disease in men of Japanese ancestry. Honolulu Heart Program. *Diabetes* 1987; 36: 689–92.
154. Fuller JH, Shipley MJ, Rose G, Jarrett RJ, Keen H. Coronary-heart-disease risk and impaired glucose tolerance. *Lancet* 1980; i: 1373–6.
155. Jarrett RJ, McCartney P, Keen H. The Bedford Survey. Ten year mortality rates in newly diagnosed diabetics, borderline diabetics and normoglycaemic controls and risk indices for coronary heart disease in borderline diabetics. *Diabetologia* 1982; 22: 79–84.
156. Eschwège E, Richard JL, Thibault N, et al. Coronary heart disease mortality in relation with diabetes, blood glucose and plasma insulin levels. The Paris prospective study, ten years later. *Horm Metab Res* 1985; 15 (suppl): 41–6.
157. The UKPDS Group. UKPDS 6: Complications in newly diagnosed type 2 diabetic patients and their association with different clinical and biochemical risk factors. *Diabetes Res* 1990; 13: 1–11.
158. Owens DR, Dolben J, Vora JP, et al. Retinopathy and nephropathy in relation to metabolic status in newly diagnosed NIDDM. In Cameron D, Colagiuri S, Heding L, Kuhl C, Ma A, Mortimer R (eds), *Non-insulin-dependent Diabetes Mellitus*. Hong Kong: Excerpta Medica, 1989; pp 11–9.
159. Bitzén P-O, Scherstén B. Assessment of laboratory methods for detection of unsuspected diabetes in primary health care. *Scand J Prim Health Care* 1986; 4: 85–95.
160. Sartor G, Scherstén B, Carlström S, Melander A, Nordén Å, Persson G. Ten-year follow-up of subjects with impaired glucose tolerance. Prevention of diabetes by tolbutamide and diet regulation. *Diabetes* 1980; 29: 41–9.
161. Knowler WC, Sartor G, Melander A, Scherstén B. Glucose tolerance and mortality, including a substudy of tolbutamide treatment. *Diabetologia* 1997; 40: 680–6.

162. Bailey TS, Lebovitz HE. Continuous sulfonylurea exposure desensitizes beta-cell insulin secretion at a distal site. *Diabetes* 1990; 39 (suppl 1): 137A (abstract 548).
163. Grodsky GM. A new phase of insulin secretion. How will it contribute to our understanding of B-cell function? *Diabetes* 1989; 38: 673–8.
164. Groop LC, Bottazzo GF, Doniach D. Islet cell antibodies identify latent type I diabetes in patients aged 35–75 years at diagnosis. *Diabetes* 1986; 35: 237–41.
165. Groop LC, Eriksson J, Schalin C, Ahola A. Does secondary oral failure represent slowly evolving type I diabetes? In Cameron D, Colagiuri S, Heding L, Kuhl C, Ma A, Mortimer R (eds), *Non-insulin-dependent Diabetes Mellitus*. Hong Kong: Excerpta Medica, 1989; pp 48–51.
166. Groop LC, Pelkonen R, Koskimies S, Bottazzo GF, Doniach D. Secondary failure to treatment with oral antidiabetic agents in non-insulin-dependent diabetes. *Diabetes Care* 1986; 9: 129–33.
167. Wright A, Burden AC, Paisey RB, Cull CA, Holman RR. Sulfonylurea inadequacy: efficacy of addition of insulin over 6 years in patients with type 2 diabetes in the UK Prospective Diabetes Study (UKPDS 57). 2002; 25: 330–6.
168. Sinagra D, Greco D, Amato MC, D'Acquisto G, Galluzzo A. A 12-h intravenous insulin infusion restores the B-cell response torpidity to sulfonylureas in patients affected by type 2 diabetes. *Diabetes Care* 2000; 23: 1857–8.
169. Campbell IW, Howlett HCS. Worldwide experience of metformin as an effective glucose-lowering agent: a meta-analysis. *Diabetes Metab Rev* 1995; 11: S57.
170. The UKPDS Group. Effect of intensive blood-glucose control with metformin on complications in overweight patients with type 2 diabetes (UKPDS 34). *Lancet* 1998; 353: 854–65.
171. DeFronzo RA, Goodman AM. Efficacy of metformin in patients with non-insulin-dependent diabetes mellitus. *New Engl J Med* 1995; 333: 541–9.
172. Hermann LS, Scherstén B, Bitzén P-O, Kjellström T, Lindgärde F, Melander A. Therapeutic comparison of metformin and sulfonylurea, alone and in various combinations: a double-blind controlled study. *Diabetes Care* 1994; 17: 1100–9.
173. Hermann LS, Scherstén B, Melander A. Antihyperglycaemic efficacy, response prediction and dose–response relations of treatment with metformin and sulphonylurea, alone and in primary combination. *Diabet Med* 1994; 11: 953–60.
174. Yu JG, Kruszynska YT, Mulford MI, Olefsky JM. A comparison of troglitazone and metformin on insulin requirements in euglycemic intensively insulin-treated type 2 diabetic patients. *Diabetes* 1999; 48: 2414–21.
175. Lebovitz HE, Pasmantier RM. Combination insulin–sulfonylurea therapy. *Diabetes Care* 1990; 13: 667–75.
176. Groop LC, Groop P-H, Stenman S. Combined insulin–sulfonylurea therapy in treatment of NIDDM. *Diabetes Care* 1990; 13 (suppl 3): 47–52.
177. Yki-Järvinen H, Kauppila M, Kusansuu E, et al. Comparisons of insulin regimens in patients with non-insulin-dependent diabetes mellitus. *N Engl J Med* 1992; 327: 1426–33.
178. Pugh JA, Wagner ML, Sawyer J, Ramirez G, Tuley M, Friedberg SJ. Is combination sulfonylurea and insulin therapy useful in NIDDM patients? A meta-analysis. *Diabetes Care* 1992; 15: 953–8.
179. Sane T, Helve E, Yki-Järvinen H, Taskinen MR. One year response to evening insulin therapy in non-insulin dependent diabetes. *J Int Med* 1992; 231: 253–60.
180. Yki-Jarvinen H, Dressler A, Zieman M. Study Group HOE 901/3002. Less nocturnal hypoglycemia and better post dinner glucose control with bedtime insulin glargine compared with bedtime NPH insulin during combination therapy in type 2 diabetes. *Diabetes Care* 2001; 23: 1130–6.
181. Yki-Jarvinen H, Ryysy L, Nikkila K, Tulokas T, Vanamo R, Heikkila M. Comparison of bedtime insulin regimens in patients with type 2 diabetes mellitus: a randomized, controlled trial. *Ann Intern Med* 1999; 130: 389–96.
182. Chiasson JL, Josse R, Hunt J, Palmason C, Rodger NW, Ross SA, et al. The efficacy of acarbose in the treatment of patients with non-insulin dependent diabetes mellitus. *Ann Intern Med (USA)* 1994; 121: 928–35.
183. Holman RR, Cull CA, Turner RC. A randomized double-blind trial of acarbose in type 2 diabetes shows improved glycemic control over 3 years. *Diabetes Care* 1999; 22: 960–4.
184. Raskin P, Rendell M, Riddle MC, Dole JF, Freed MI, Rosenstock J, for the Rosiglitazone Clinical Trials Study Group. A randomized trial of rosiglitazone therapy in patients with inadequately controlled insulin-treated type 2 diabetes. *Diabetes Care* 2001; 24: 1226–32.
185. Burge MR, Sood V, Sobhy TA, Rassam AG, Schade DS. Sulphonylurea-induced hypoglycaemia in type 2 diabetes melltus: a review. *Diabetes Obes Metab* 1999; 1: 199–206.
186. Shorr RI, Daugherty WA, Griffin MR. Incidence and risk factors for serious hypoglycemia in older persons using insulin or sulfonylureas. *Arch Int Med* 1997; 157: 1681–7.
187. van Staa T, Abenhaim L, Monette J. Rates of hypoglycemia in users of sulfonylureas. *J Clin Epidemiol* 1997; 50: 735–41.
188. Seltzer HS. Drug-induced hypoglycemia. *Endocrinol Metab Clin North Am* 1989; 18: 163–83.
189. Stahl M, Berger M. Higher incidence of severe hypoglycaemia leading to hospital admission in type 2 diabetic patients treated with long-acting versus short-acting sulphonylureas. *Diabet Med* 1999; 16: 586–90.
190. Shorr RI, Ray WA, Daugherty WA, Griffin MR. Individual sulfonylureas and serious hypoglycemia in older people. *J Am Geriatr Soc* 1996; 44: 751–5.
191. Krepinsky J, Ingram AJ, Clase CM. Prolonged sulfonylurea-induced hypoglycemia in diabetic patients with end stage renal disease. *Am J Kidney Dis* 2000; 35: 500–5.
192. Pearson ER, Liddle WG, Shepherd M, Corrall RJ, Hattersley AT. Sensitivity to sulphonylureas in patients with hepatic nuclear factor (HNF)-1 alpha gene mutations: evidence for pharmacogenetics in diabetes. *Diabet Med* 2000; 17: 543–5.
193. McLaughlin SA, Crandall CS, McKinney PE. Octreotide: an antidote for sulfonylurea-induced hypoglycemia. *Ann Emerg Med* 2001; 37: 417–8.
194. Nzerue CM, Thomas J, Volcy J, Edeki T. Use of octreotide to treat prolonged sulfonylurea-induced hypoglycemia in a patient with chronic renal failure. *Int J Artif Organs* 2003; 26: 86–9.
195. Boyle PJ, Justice K, Krentz AJ, Nagy RJ, Schade DS. Octreotide reverses hyperinsulinemia and prevents

hypoglycemia induced by sulfonylurea overdoses. *J Clin Endocrinol Metab* 1993; 76: 752–6.

196. University Group Diabetes Program. A study of the effects of hypoglycemic agents on vascular complications in patients with adult-onset diabetes. *Diabetes* 1970; 19 (suppl 2).
197. Williamson JR, Kilo C. Effect of tolbutamide (TOLB) treatment on cardiovascular (CV) mortality in the University Group Diabetes Program (UGDP). In *Abstracts of 10th Congress of the International Diabetes Federation No. 663F. Amsterdam: Exerpta Medica*, 1979; p 255.
198. Hu S, Wang S, Dunning BE: Tissue selectivity of antidiabetic agent nateglinide: study on cardiovascular and beta-cell KATP channels. *J Pharmacol Exp Ther* 1999; 291: 1372–9.
199. Garratt KN, Brady PA, Hassinger NL, Grill DE, Terzic A, Holmes DR Jr. Sulfonylurea drugs increase early mortality in patients with diabetes mellitus after direct angioplasty for acute myocardial infarction. *J Am Coll Cardiol* 1999; 33: 119–24.
200. Scognamiglio R, Avogaro A, Vigili De Kreutzenberg S, Negut C, Palisi M, Bagolin E, Tiengo A. Effects of treatment with sulfonylurea drugs or insulin on ischemia-induced myocardial dysfunction in type 2 diabetes. *Diabetes* 2002; 51: 808–12.
201. Jollis JG, Simpson RJ, Cascio WE, Chowdhury MK, Crouse JR, Smith SC Jr. Relation between sulfonylurea therapy, complications and outcome for elderly patients with acute myocardial infarction. *Am Heart J* 1999; 138: S376–80.
202. Klamann A, Sarfert P, Launhardt V, Schulte G, Schmiegel WH, Nauck MA. Myocardial infarction in diabetic vs non-diabetic subjects. Survival and infarct size following therapy with sulfonylureas (glibenclamide). *Eur Heart J* 2000; 21: 220.
203. Riddle MC, Schneider J. Beginning insulin treatment of obese patients with evening 70/30 insulin plus glimepiride versus insulin alone. *Diabetes Care* 1998; 21: 1052–7.
204. Ashcroft FM, Gribble FM, *J Diabetes Complications* 2000; 14 (4): 192–6.

46

Meglitinides: Basic Aspects and Clinical Uses

M.J. Davies and Sudesna Chatterjee

Leicester Royal Infirmary, University Hospitals of Leicester NHS Trust, Leicester

INTRODUCTION

General Background

Type 2 diabetes mellitus (T2DM) is one of the commonest chronic diseases in the world and the number of new cases continues to rise inexorably. It is estimated that the worldwide prevalence of all types of diabetes will rise from 100 million in 1994 to 220 million in 2010 [1]. The majority of cases will be of T2DM, especially in developing countries. Adolescents and even children are becoming more susceptible to this chronic condition, which is related to lifestyle factors such as obesity and reduced activity levels. In the United States, there has been a fivefold increase in the number of new patients with T2DM and approximately $100 billion of health care costs are currently spent annually on diabetes management [2]. The bulk of this cost is related to hospitalization and management of complications such as cardiovascular disease and nephropathy. There is a significant increase in mortality in patients with T2DM, particularly from cardiovascular causes. The need for agents that will provide effective control of glucose metabolism and lessen the development of macrovascular and microvascular complications is therefore a high priority.

Type 2 Diabetes and Glycemic Control

The United Kingdom Prospective Diabetes Study (UKPDS), a landmark study and the largest of its kind to date, looked at more than 5000 patients with T2DM who were followed for up to 20 years [3]. The aim of this study was to clarify whether more intensive management of glycemic control in T2DM lessened microvascular and macrovascular complications. In addition, various modes of therapy namely sulfonylureas, metformin, insulin, and latterly acarbose were also compared. This study clearly demonstrated that improved glycemic control resulted in fewer complications. For example a 0.9% reduction in glycosylated haemoglobin (HbA_{1c}) resulted in the benefits shown in Table 1.

However, despite showing initial improvement in HbA_{1c} with intensive treatment, glycemic control deteriorated progressively with time (Figure 1).

The key metabolic defects characterizing T2DM are β-cell dysfunction and insulin resistance. β-Cell dysfunction is progressive and leads to a rise in HbA_{1c}, necessitating management with higher doses and combinations of oral hypoglycemic agents (OHAs) and insulin. UKPDS showed that 3 years into the study about 50% of patients required combination therapy, and by 9 years this figure rose to 75%. The need for agents capable of sustaining improved glycemic control and maintaining or improving β-cell function has become clear from the findings of UKPDS.

Current Therapies

Since the 1950s, the biguanides and sulfonylureas have formed the mainstay of treatment of T2DM. Metformin, the only biguanide in routine clinical practice, targets insulin resistance probably by suppressing hepatic glucose output and possibly by reducing peripheral glucose uptake and utilization. It may have other mechanisms of actions that are not completely understood. UKPDS showed that metformin was effective in lowering HbA_{1c}, and in particular was the only agent to confer cardiovascular benefits. However, like sulfonylureas and insulin, metformin did not maintain good glycemic control. Metformin is also associated with significant gastrointestinal side effects (resulting in around 10% of patients being unable to

International Textbook of Diabetes Mellitus, Third Edition. Edited by R. A. DeFronzo, E. Ferrannini, H. Keen, and P. Zimmet.

Table 1 Effect of 1% reduction in HbA_{1c} on complications of type 2 diabetes*

An intensive vs. conventional glucose control policy, which achieved a median HbA_{1c} of 7.0% vs 7.9% (Æ = 0.9%) over 10 years, reduced risk by:		
12%	Any diabetes-related endpoint	$p = 0.029$
16%	Myocardial infarction	$p = 0.52$
25%	Microvascular disease	$p = 0.0099$
21%	Retinopathy at 12 years	$p = 0.015$
33%	Albuminuria at 12 years	$p = 0.000054$

* From reference 3.

tolerate therapy), however it may only rarely cause lactic acidosis.

The sulfonylureas such as gliclazide and glibenclamide (glyburide) are insulin secretagogues that bind to the sulfonylurea receptor of the pancreatic β-cell, promoting closure of ATP-dependent potassium channels. They are effective at improving glycemic control but are associated with weight gain and increased risk of hypoglycemia. The incidence of severe episodes of hypoglycemia with sulfonylurea therapy is approximately 0.2/1000 patient-years. About 20–25% of patients with T2DM are initially unresponsive to the sulfonylureas, and secondary failure of these agents occurs in 5–10% of individuals on an annual basis.

α-Glucosidase inhibitors such as acarbose are used either as monotherapy or in combination with metformin and sulfonylureas to reduce carbohydrate absorption from the small intestine. UKPDS showed that acarbose was less efficacious in lowering HbA_{1c} compared to other agents. The study to prevent non-insulin-dependent diabetes mellitus (STOP-NIDDM) trial showed that acarbose can delay progression to T2DM in impaired glucose tolerance (IGT) by 32% [4]. Although acarbose is not associated with any serious adverse effects, unfortunately many subjects have to discontinue the drug because of unpleasant gastrointestinal side effects. In the STOP-NIDDM trial, 31% of subjects had to discontinue the drug because of its side effects.

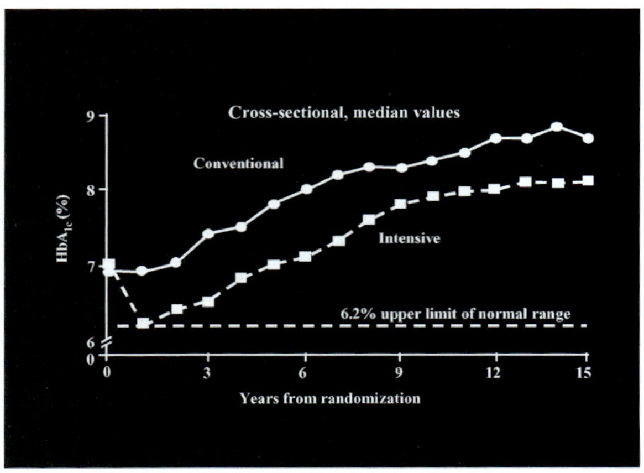

Figure 1 Progressive decline in glycemic control regardless of treatment intensity (from reference 3)

A summary of the characteristics of these oral hypoglycemic agents is given in Table 2.

New Therapeutic Options

Thiazolidinediones

More recent oral hypoglycemic agents include the thiazolidinediones or peroxisome proliferator-activated receptor γ(PPAR-γ) agonists, which enhance the effects of endogenous insulin on target organs, mainly skeletal muscle, liver, and adipose tissue. The first of these to be launched was troglitazone but had to be withdrawn because of hepatotoxicity. Rosiglitazone and pioglitazone are currently available and appear to have no such effects on the liver. They target insulin resistance, which is a major component of the metabolic syndrome. They potentially have other benefits (reduce cardiovascular risk) and these areas continue to be explored (see under Thiazolidinediones).

Meglitinides

A new class of drugs known as the meglitinides have recently been launched on the international market. These agents have been developed to improve early-phase insulin secretion, which is one of the earliest pathophysiological manifestations of T2DM. They are derived from the meglitinide portion of sulfonylureas. Currently available drugs of this group are repaglinide and nateglinide. Another meglitinide known as mitiglinide is still in clinical trials. Repaglinide is derived from the non-sulfonylurea moiety of glibenclamide whereas nateglinide is derived from an amino acid. The meglitinides are rapid-acting insulin secretagogues (also known as prandial glucose regulators) that have a fast onset and short duration of action resulting in more physiological secretion of insulin from the β-cell. The mechanism of action of the meglitinides is glucose-dependent and this has important implications for lessening the risk of hypoglycemia.

This chapter will begin by discussing the pathophysiology of T2DM and the importance of postprandial hyperglycemia (PPH). The mechanism of action and pharmacokinetics of repaglinide and nateglinide will then be described, followed by a review of their clinical use both as monotherapy and in combination with other agents.

PATHOPHYSIOLOGY OF T2DM

General Introduction

T2DM is a complex heterogeneous condition characterized by abnormalities of both insulin action (resistance) and secretion. The relative contribution of these

Table 2 Characteristics of current oral hypoglycemic agents

	Sulfonylureas	Biguanides	α-glucosidase inhibitors
Fasting plasma glucose	↓ 3–4 mmol/l	↓ 3–4 mmol/l	↓ 1–1.7 mmol/l
HbA_{1c}	↓ 1–2%	↓ 1–2%	↓ 0.2–1.0%
Triglycerides	—	(↓)	—
LDL cholesterol	—	(↓)	—
HDL cholesterol	—	(↑)	—
Body weight	(↑)	—	—
Plasma insulin	(↑)	(↓)	—
Side effects	Hypoglycemia	Gastrointestinal Lactic acidosis	Gastrointestinal

abnormalities may vary between populations, as exemplified by the Pima Indians of Arizona and Pacific Islanders of Nauru who are severely insulin resistant, compared to other populations such as White Caucasians. A number of factors appear to predispose to insulin resistance. A genetic contribution is likely although as yet specific genes remain unidentified. Obesity and insulin resistance are significantly related and central adiposity is of particular importance. A low-calorie, low-fat diet enhances insulin sensitivity possibly by promoting weight loss. Exercise has also been shown to increase insulin sensitivity.

β-Cell Dysfunction

The importance of β-cell dysfunction is increasingly recognized although earlier work has concentrated mainly on insulin resistance as the primary abnormality in T2DM. It is not clear which pathological condition develops first. It has been suggested that insulin resistance leads to relative insulin deficiency, whereas β-cell exhaustion means that insufficient insulin is produced to overcome the degree of insulin resistance. The combination of insulin resistance and insufficient insulin secretion lowers glucose uptake in insulin-sensitive tissues and reduces the suppression of hepatic glucose output.

The normal secretion of insulin is divided into two phases. Following an acute secretagogue challenge, there is an initial early-phase insulin response that peaks at 3–5 min and is complete by 10 min. This is followed by a late-phase insulin response that typically lasts for 2–3 h with a slow sustained rise in circulating insulin levels (Figure 2).

This dual-phase insulin response ensures normal glucose tolerance and primes tissues, especially the liver, to glucose levels. Early-phase insulin secretion also leads to a reduction in hepatic glucose output. Reduced suppression of hepatic glucose output exaggerates postchallenge hyperglycemia, promoting late hyperinsulinemia.

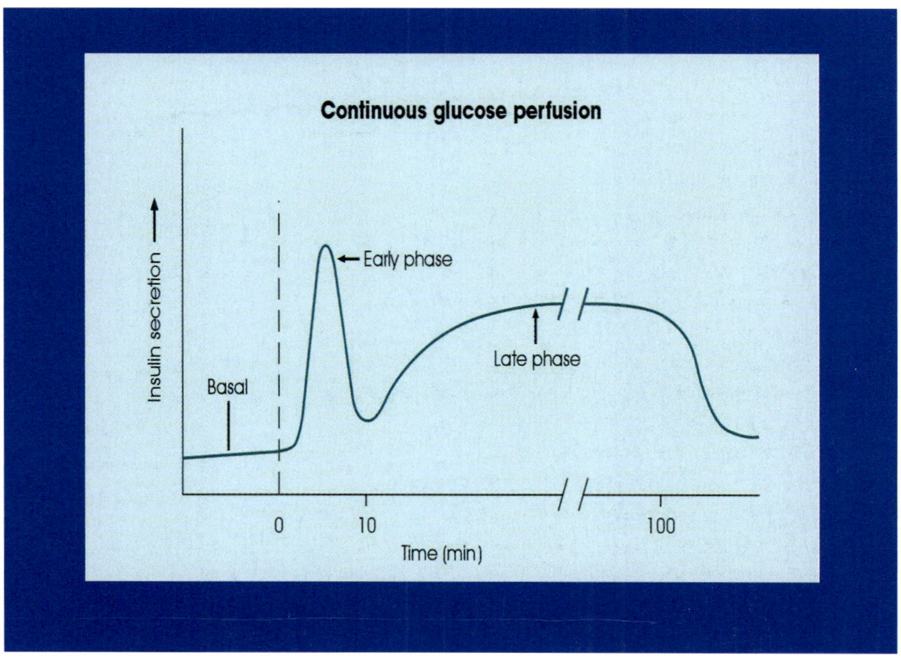

Figure 2 Physiological secretion of insulin. (Reproduced by permission of Elsevier)

Insulin secretion in the basal fasting state is pulsatile, occurring every 10–14 min with a slower superimposed cycle of secretion every 105–120 min. Biological activity is greater when insulin is secreted in a pulsatile fashion as opposed to continuous infusion. One of the earliest changes in the pathogenesis of T2DM is loss of the normal oscillatory pattern of insulin secretion.

Early-Phase Insulin Secretion

Loss or reduction of early-phase insulin secretion occurs early in subjects with T2DM and even in those with IGT (Figure 3).

Reduced early-phase insulin secretion has been discovered to be the most reliable predictor of subsequent development of T2DM even in the Pima Indians (Figure 4).

Insulin secretion is controlled by the membrane potential of the β-cell. This is dependent on the activity of ATP-sensitive $K^+(K_{ATP})$ channels in the plasma membrane. When there is an increase in the cytoplasmic ATP/ADP ratio, membrane depolarization occurs with opening of the voltage-gated Ca^{2+}channels, and the cytoplasmic Ca^{2+} rises. This leads to stimulation of Ca^{2+}-dependent exocytosis of the insulin-containing granules. These K_{ATP} channels are the site of action for both sulfonylureas and meglitinides.

Deterioration of β-Cell Function

UKPDS identified that β-cell function worsened from approximately 53% at diagnosis of diabetes to around 28% after 6 years of follow-up. Deterioration in blood glucose control was correlated with increasing loss of β-cell function. Extrapolation of these data suggests that β-cell dysfunction may have commenced about 12 years before T2DM was clinically diagnosed (Figure 5a).

In the past it has been suggested that sulfonylureas might increase β-cell demise. UKPDS showed that the rate of loss of β-cell function was similar regardless of body mass index or the type of therapy used to improve glycemic control (Figure 5b).

However, the sulfonylureas undergo prolonged binding with the β-cell receptor, leading to hyperinsulinemia and the potential for subsequent β-cell failure.

Significance of Postprandial Hyperglycemia

In today's westernized societies, little time while awake is spent in the fasting state. Patients with established T2DM have fasting and postprandial hyperglycemia both of which increase HbA_{1c} levels. At the present time, HbA_{1c} is considered the gold standard for monitoring and assessing long-term glycemic control. Some studies have shown that postprandial plasma glucose is a better predictor of glycemic control than is fasting plasma glucose. In one study, 66 patients with T2DM were asked to provide a glycemic profile consisting of plasma glucose measurements at prebreakfast, prelunch, postlunch (2 h), and extended postlunch (4 h) intervals between 8 a.m. and 5 p.m. [8]. Sixty-six percent of these patients were on combination therapy with

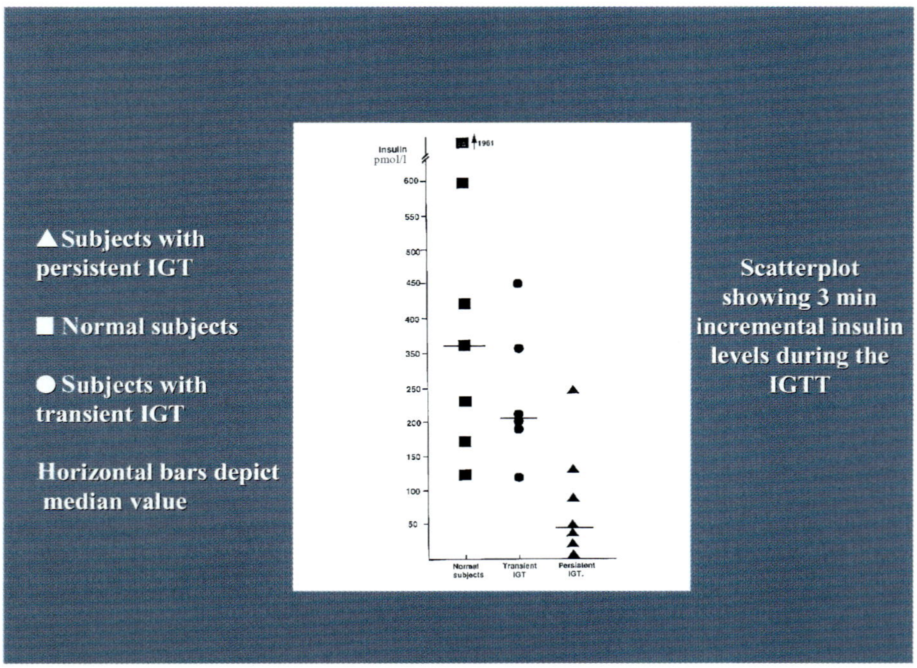

Figure 3 Loss of early-phase insulin secretion early in disease process (reproduced with permission from reference 5)

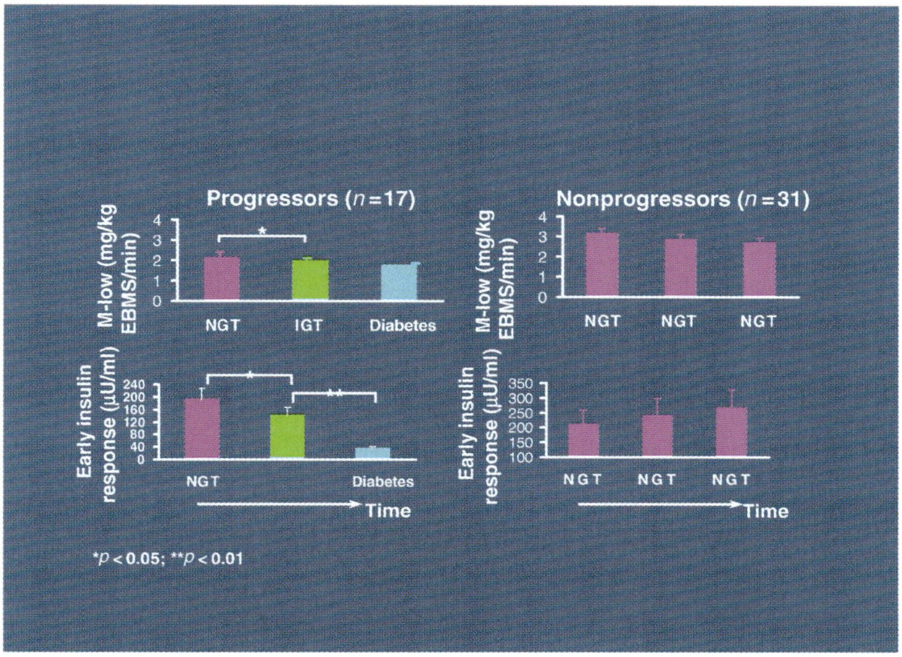

Figure 4 Natural history of type 2 diabetes in Pima Indians (NGT = normal glucose tolerance) (reproduced with permission from reference 6)

sulfonylureas and metformin. None were on insulin therapy. The results showed that extended postlunch plasma glucose was lower than prebreakfast plasma glucose in patients demonstrating good glycemic control (HbA_{1c} ≤7.0%). In addition, postlunch and extended postlunch plasma glucose demonstrated better sensitivity, specificity, and positive predictive value in predicting poor glycemic control than did prebreakfast or prelunch plasma glucose.

The extent of PPH was identified by a study in 218 patients with T2DM, aged between 40 and 74 years, and who were not on insulin [9]. This data was obtained from the Third National Health and Nutrition Examination Survey (NHANES III) conducted between 1988 and 1994 in the United States. In this cross-sectional analysis, PPH was determined by 2-h plasma glucose of >11 mmol/l after an oral glucose challenge. In patients on sulfonylurea therapy with HbA_{1c} >7%, PPH was present in 99% of cases. Even in those with HbA_{1c} <7%, PPH occurred in 39%. In the subgroup of patients taking sulfonylureas and with HbA_{1c} <7%, PPH was prevalent in 63%.

Association of Postprandial Hyperglycemia to Adverse Outcomes

In recent years, the American Diabetes Association (ADA) has moved away from the use of a postchallenge glucose or oral glucose tolerance test in favor of the exclusive use of fasting glucose in diagnosing diabetes. This has raised some concern with respect to the importance of postchallenge or postprandial hyperglycemia and its relationship to both diagnosis of T2DM and cardiovascular outcomes across the spectrum of glucose intolerance.

In the Diabetes Epidemiology: Collaborative Analysis of Diagnostic Criteria in Europe (DECODE) the relationship between fasting and postchallenge glucose to mortality and morbidity was analyzed in more than 25 000 subjects [9]. This large study identified that postchallenge glucose was more sensitive than fasting glucose at predicting risk of all-cause mortality.

Several other large epidemiological studies have provided data suggesting a link between postchallenge hyperglycemia and adverse cardiovascular outcomes that are consistent with the findings of DECODE (Table 3).

Potential Pathological Associations with Postprandial Hyperglycemia

In theory, there are a number of reasons for the association of adverse cardiovascular outcomes with PPH. PPH is linked to several deleterious pathological effects. PPH is associated with the production of increased free radicals with subsequent oxidative stress [15]. Other effects include increased insulin resistance and glucose autooxidation with decreased early-phase insulin secretion. In addition, there is increased blood coagulation and high density lipoprotein-cholesterol (HDL-C) catabolism. Free fatty acids and triglyceride-rich lipoproproteins and low density lipoprotein (LDL) removal are reduced. Effects on the arterial wall include decreased fibrinolysis, disturbed

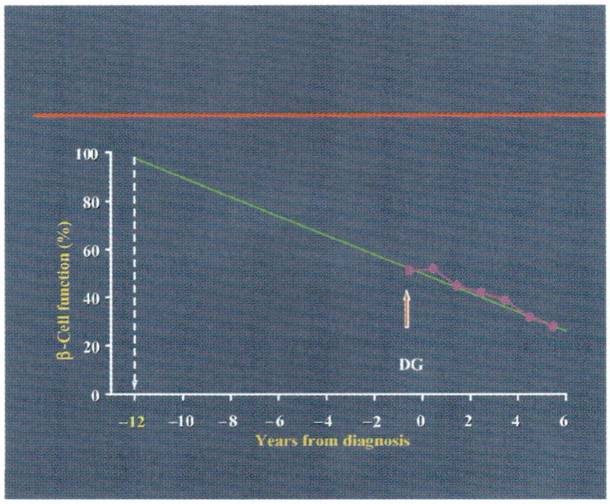

(a)

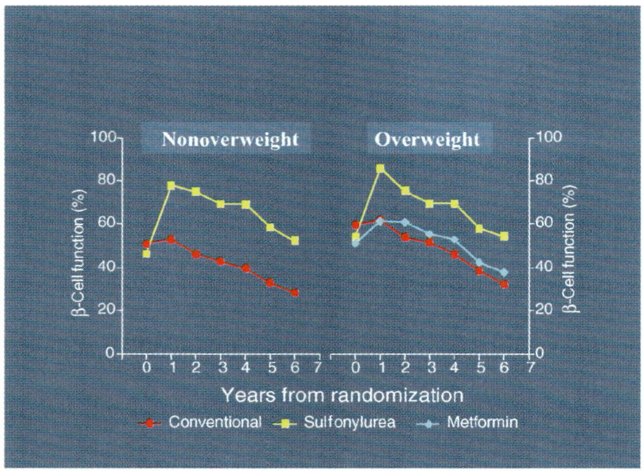

(b)

Figure 5 (a) Extrapolation of the time of deterioration of β-cell dysfunction (DG = diagnosis) (reproduced with permission from reference 6). (b) Progressive loss of β-cell function with different agents (from reference 7)

endothelial function with reduction in nitric oxide release, and reduced plaque stability (Figure 6).

The importance of circulating inflammatory markers such as cytokines and their role in the pathogenesis of vascular disease in T2DM is gradually emerging. A prospective study has found that the risk of development of T2DM in apparently healthy middle-aged women correlated with two circulating markers of systemic inflammation, namely C-reactive protein and the cytokine interleukin 6 (IL-6) [16]. Tumour necrosis factor α (TNF-α) has also been linked with the insulin resistance syndrome and clinically overt T2DM. Another recently published study has shown that subjects with IGT had higher fasting plasma IL-6 and TNF-α levels than did control subjects. Interleukin-18 (IL-18), which has been implicated in plaque destabilization, was also measured and its levels rose along with IL-6 and TNF-α in the control subjects but not in the subjects with IGT. Cytokine levels were affected more by oscillatory than continuous hyperglycemia, which correlates with postprandial glucose excursions. The different pattern of cytokine secretion with PPH may be of clinical relevance, since vascular risk increases with increased cytokine circulation, such as IL-6 and TNF-α [17].

Despite the wealth of epidemiological studies to date, none have investigated the direct relationship of PPH to cardiovascular outcomes. As a result, the link between PPH and adverse cardiovascular events remains an interesting hypothesis.

Postprandial Monitoring in Clinical Practice: Is it Justified?

Only one study to date has shown that monitoring and targeting postprandial blood glucose levels improves

Table 3 Association between postprandial glucose values and the risk of cardiovascular heart disease (CHD) across the spectrum of glucose tolerance

Study	Characteristics	Cardiovascular outcomes
DECODE Study Group [10]	18 408 men 7316 women 13 European centers 28-year follow-up	All-cause mortality is more related to 2-h postmeal glucose than fasting plasma glucose
Whitehall, Paris Prospective, and Helsinki Policeman Studies [11]	17 285 men 44–55 years 20-year follow-up	Men in upper 2.5% of 2-h postmeal glucose distribution had significantly higher CHD mortality
Hoorn Study [12]	2363 subjects 50–75 years 8-year follow-up	High plasma glucose levels especially 2-h postload glucose concentrations and to a lesser extent HbA_{1c} values indicate a risk of CHD mortality
Diabetes Intervention Study [13]	1139 subjects with type 2 diabetes 30–55 years 11-year follow-up	1-h postbreakfast blood glucose but not fasting blood glucose was associated with higher rates of myocardial infarction and death
Honolulu Heart Program [14]	6005 men 45–70 years 12-year follow-up	CHD incidence and mortality increase stepwise with increasing 1-h postchallenge glucose

outcomes. In a randomized study of 66 women with gestational diabetes, two glucose monitoring protocols were used to achieve glycemic control. In one group, the women were asked to perform preprandial monitoring before meals and at bedtime. The other group was assigned to capillary blood glucose monitoring before breakfast (fasting) and 1 h after each meal. This study showed that in the postprandial monitoring group, the mean change in HbA_{1c} was greater and there was less macrosomia. Also in this group, rate of neonatal hypoglycemia was reduced and infants were less often delivered by caesarean section due to cephalopelvic disproportion. There was also a fivefold reduction in HbA_{1c} (3% vs. 0.6%) [18].

The ADA has published a consensus statement with regard to which individuals should monitor postprandial glucose levels [19]. The recommendation includes all women with gestational diabetes. In addition, postprandial glucose monitoring should be carried out by patients who

- achieve preprandial targets but whose HbA_{1c} remains suboptimal
- are on treatments that specifically target PPH
- experience PPH.

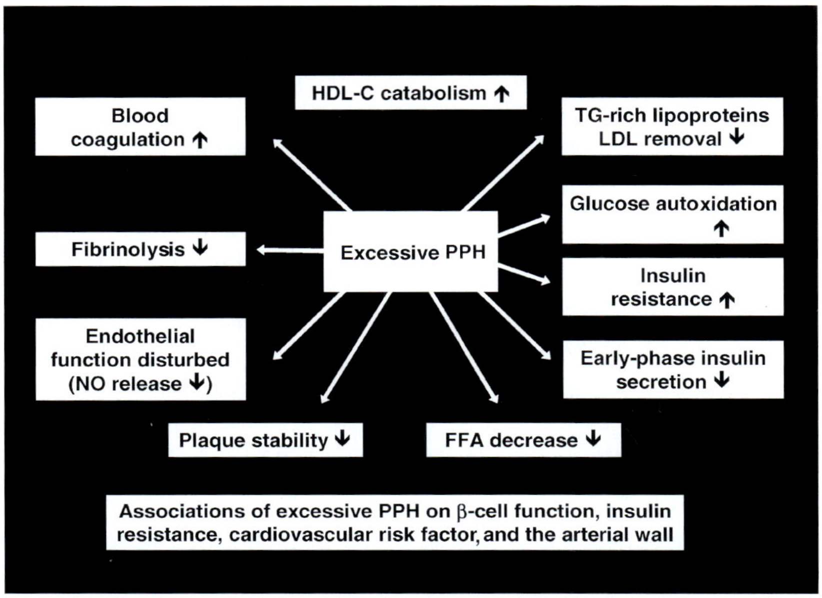

Figure 6 Pathological associations with postprandial hyperglycemia. (Reproduced by permission of the American Diabetes Association)

Table 4 Predominant targets of currently available hypoglycemic therapies

Target fasting plasma glucose	Target postprandial hyperglycemia
Sulfonylureas	Acarbose
Metformin	Meglitinides
Isophane and insulin glargine	Short-acting insulin analogues
Thiazolidinediones	

Current drug therapies in the management of T2DM can be divided into those that predominantly target fasting plasma glucose or PPH (Table 4).

Meglitinide—Basic Aspects

Chemical Structure of the Meglitinides

More than 20 years ago, the insulinotropic and antidiabetic properties of the non-sulfonylurea moiety of glibenclamide were identified. This chemical structure was subsequently referred to as meglitinide.

Repaglinide is an acylaminobenzoic acid derived from the non-sulfonylurea moiety of glibenclamide. It has a molecular formula of $C_{27}H_{36}N_2O_4$ and a molecular mass of 452.6 Da. Nateglinide is distinct from the sulfonylureas and is chemically derived from an amino acid. It consists of an acylamino moiety and D-phenylalanine. The structures of these compounds are shown in Figure 7.

Mechanism of Action of Repaglinide

Repaglinide (Novonorm, Prandin, Novo Nordisk) was the first meglitinide to be commercially available. It was launched in 1998.

Repaglinide is structurally different from the sulfonylurea group although it binds to a specific site of the sulfonylurea receptor on the pancreatic β-cell. This site is distinct from the sulfonylurea binding site. Binding with this site closes the K^+_{ATP} channel and this initiates insulin secretion (Figure 8).

It has been proposed that insulin-secreting cells have two or three distinct binding sites for glibenclamide and repaglinide with differing affinities for each drug [21]. It would appear that there are some common and some distinct cellular mechanisms of action between repaglinide and glibenclamide.

Repaglinide increases cytoplasmic Ca^{2+} concentration in β-TC3 insulinoma cells. Unlike glibenclamide, repaglinide does not enhance exocytosis in voltage-clamped β-cells or stimulate insulin secretion from β-TC3 insulinoma cells in the absence of glucose. Additionally, repaglinide has no direct biosynthetic activity and is not taken up by the β-cell despite its lipophilic nature. Repaglinide is five times more potent at stimulating insulin secretion than is glibenclamide. Repaglinide does not stimulate insulin secretion in the complete absence of glucose and its action is usually confined to intermediate concentrations of glucose. These characteristics may account for the reduced risk of hypoglycemia seen with repaglinide in contrast to the sulfonylureas.

A recently published randomized controlled open-label study of 46 patients with T2DM evaluated the effect of repaglinide on insulin secretion and oxidative stress as measured by reduced serum antioxidants and superoxide dismutase [22]. This study showed that first-phase insulin secretion was significantly increased in the repaglinide group, which is already well-established. More interestingly, a significant increase in total serum antioxidant

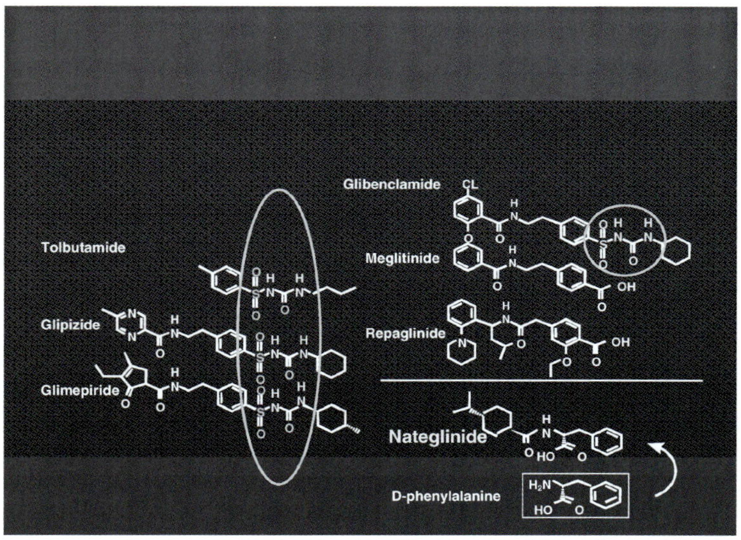

Figure 7 Chemical structures of the meglitinides

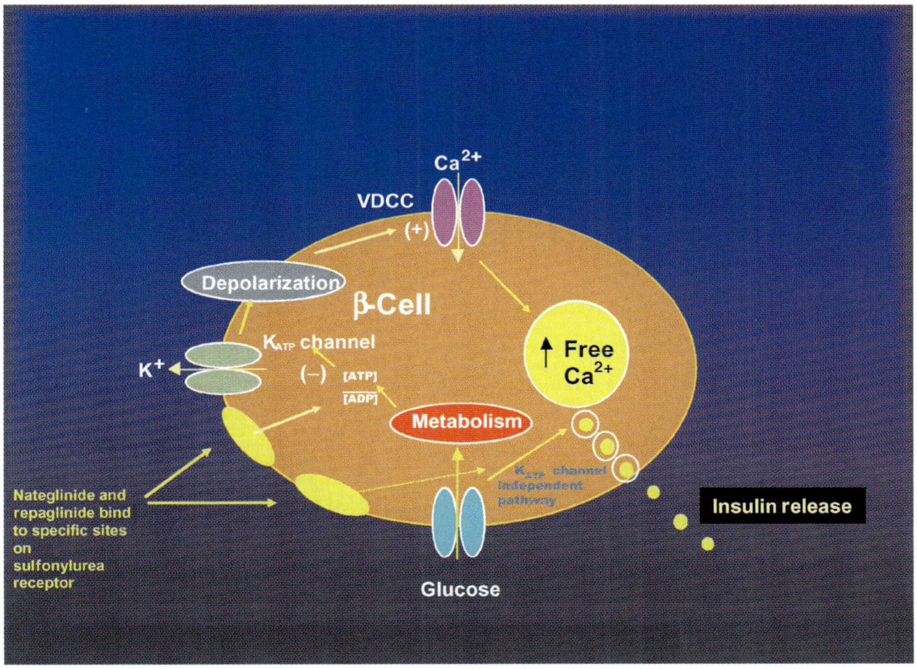

Figure 8 Mechanism of action of meglitinides at level of pancreatic β-cell (from reference 20)

capacity ($p < 0.05$) and serum superoxide dismutase ($p < 0.0004$) was discovered in the repaglinide group.

The S-enantiomer of repaglinide is the pharmacologically active part of the racemic molecule. In the rat model, this enantiomer has more than 100 times greater hypoglycemic potency than the R-enantiomer. Clinically available repaglinide is about 98% pure for the S-enantiomer.

Mechanism of Action of Nateglinide

Nateglinide (Starlix™, Novartis) is derived from D-phenylalanine and has no sulfonylurea moiety. It is biochemically and pharmacologically distinct from other hypoglycemic agents. Its mechanism of action is similar to that of repaglinide, involving inhibition of pancreatic β-cell K_{ATP}-sensitive channels (Figure 8). Studies have shown that nateglinide has significantly faster association/dissociation kinetics in the pancreatic β-cell, which results in a more rapid and transient increase in early-phase insulin secretion in normal healthy volunteers compared to that with [23] repaglinide (Figure 9).

Kinetic information from experiments on rat pancreatic cells has shown that time to 50% maximal inhibition was 4.1 min for nateglinide and 12 min for repaglinide. Time to 50% relief of inhibition was 35 min for nateglinide compared to 175 min for repaglinide. Overall insulin exposure is much less with nateglinide, and plasma insulin concentrations return to baseline 2 h after oral administration of the drug.

Isolated rat islet experiments have shown that there is 16-fold enhancement of nateglinide-induced inhibition of K^+_{ATP} current when the glucose concentration is raised from 3 to 16 mmol/l. Repaglinide potency is increased fourfold whereas glibenclamide potency is reduced under the same conditions. These observations may explain the low incidence of mild and severe hypoglycemia reported in clinical trials with nateglinide.

Pharmacokinetics of the Meglitinides

Pharmacokinetics of Repaglinide Repaglinide is rapidly absorbed after oral administration and appears in the bloodstream within 15 min. Maximum plasma levels (C_{max}) are reached within 30–60 min of oral administration of a 2 mg tablet of repaglinide. This occurs in healthy volunteers and in those with T2DM. Notably repaglinide does not accumulate with repeated dosing and has a rapid elimination half-life of approximately 1 h. These factors potentially lessen the risk of hypoglycemia. C_{max} and area under the curve (AUC) increase in a dose-dependent manner in healthy subjects and in those with T2DM. The absolute bioavailability of a 2 mg tablet of repaglinide is 62.5%, which is slightly affected by meal composition. In particular, a high fat meal decreases AUC and C_{max} from fasting levels by 20 and 12.4% respectively. Repaglinide is highly bound to plasma proteins in the circulation [25].

AUC and C_{max} are greater in elderly patients with T2DM. Mean half-life is slightly longer but elimination is

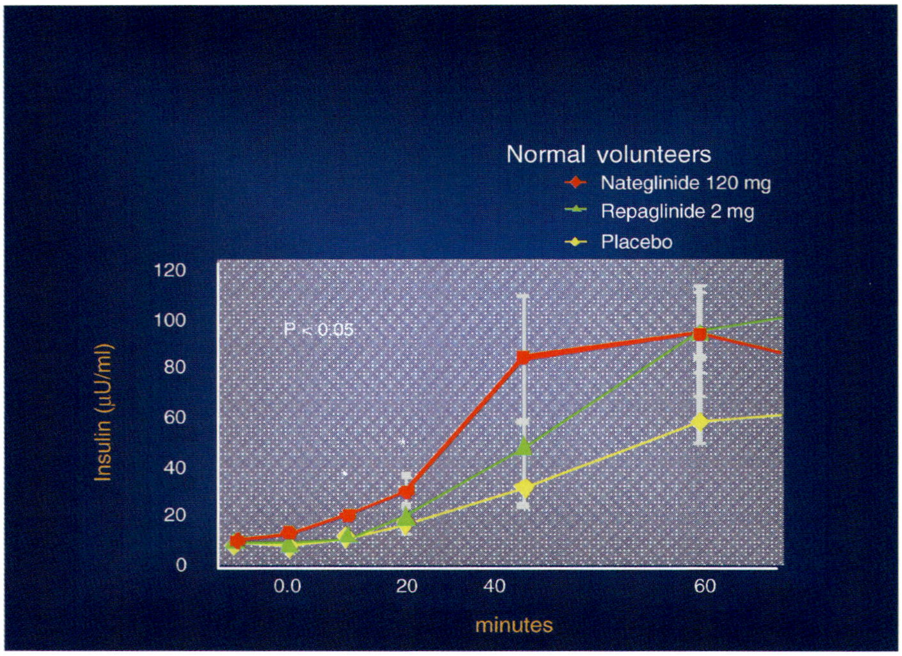

Figure 9 Comparison of repaglinide and nateglinide with placebo on early-phase insulin secretion (reproduced with permission from reference 24)

still rapid in elderly patients. Repaglinide is well-tolerated in the elderly, and dosage adjustment in this group is not necessary.

Approximately 98% of repaglinide is metabolized after oral administration with the remaining 2% excreted unchanged. Repaglinide undergoes hepatic metabolism by the CYP3A4 isoform of the P450 cytochrome enzyme and is mainly excreted via bile. AUC and C_{max} of repaglinide are increased in patients with moderate or severe hepatic impairment. In these patients half-life of the drug is prolonged compared to that in healthy volunteers (14.7 vs. 0.6–0.7 h).

Only 6% is excreted by the kidneys, and repaglinide is thus licensed for use in mild to moderate renal dysfunction. In severe renal impairment the plasma half-life of repaglinide is increased from 1.5 to 3.6 h and it is therefore not recommended in this situation.

Theoretically any compound inhibiting or inducing CYP3A4 isoenzyme might affect the metabolism of repaglinide. Ketoconazole and erythromycin both inhibit CYP3A4 but do not appear to cause clinically relevant changes in repaglinide plasma concentration.

Rifampicin, carbamazepine, and barbiturates induce CYP3A4 and may increase the metabolism of repaglinide. Higher doses of repaglinide would therefore be needed to maintain adequate plasma concentrations and an effective hypoglycemic effect.

Pharmacokinetics of Nateglinide Nateglinide has 75% systemic bioavailability and is mostly unaffected by first-pass hepatic metabolism. Only 10% is metabolized and excreted by the kidneys. Nateglinide and its metabolites are rapidly eliminated with a half-life of 1.5 h. Ninety-nine percent of nateglinide is bound to plasma proteins.

The CYP2C9 and CYP3A4 isoenzymes are thought to be involved in hepatic breakdown of nateglinide. No interactions between nateglinide and warfarin, diclofenac, or digoxin have been reported. A study of the pharmacokinetic profile and bioavailability of nateglinide in subjects with biopsy-proven hepatic cirrhosis compared to healthy individuals showed no statistically significant or clinically relevant differences between the two groups. Thus, nateglinide may be used without dose adjustment in patients with mild to moderate hepatic cirrhosis.

A recent open-label, two-center, controlled study of 40 subjects investigated the pharmacokinetics and safety of nateglinide in renal disease [26]. Patients with impaired renal function and those with renal failure on hemodialysis were compared with age-, sex-, height-, and weight-matched healthy controls. Plasma nateglinide concentrations increased rapidly in all subjects and there was no statistically significant difference in C_{max} or AUC between the groups. Nateglinide was eliminated rapidly in all groups ($t_{1/2} = 1.9–2.8$ h) with no correlation between the level of renal function and systemic exposure. The extent of renal excretion of nateglinide was low in healthy subjects (11%) and diabetic patients with renal impairment (3%). These data suggest that use of nateglinide may be safe in patients with impaired renal function.

CLINICAL USE OF THE MEGLITINIDES

Clinical Use of Repaglinide

Repaglinide is licensed as monotherapy in the treatment of T2DM and may be prescribed in combination with metformin when metformin alone is inadequate. It may also be used in combination with the thiazolidinediones. It is licensed for use between 18 and 75 years.

Repaglinide is usually given 15–30 min before meals up to three times daily at a starting dose of 500 μg. An initial dose of 1 mg can be used if the patient was previously on another oral hypoglycemic agent. The maximal single dose is 4 mg with a total daily dose of 16 mg. It is recommended that dose adjustments be made at intervals of 1–2 weeks according to response. In comparison to sulfonylureas, repaglinide is more expensive.

Repaglinide as Monotherapy

Studies have shown that repaglinide is effective at lowering HbA_{1c} when used as monotherapy in comparison with placebo-controlled trials (Table 5).

A multicenter, double-blind, randomized, placebo-controlled, parallel group study of 408 patients with T2DM assessed the safety and efficacy of repaglinide when used in a flexible mealtime dosing regimen [26]. Patients who were considered poorly controlled by diet were randomly assigned to receive either repaglinide 0.5 mg at mealtimes or placebo. The prandial dose of repaglinide was doubled to 1 mg after 4 weeks if fasting plasma glucose exceeded 7.8 mmol/l. This trial showed a reduction in HbA_{1c} of 1.14% from baseline ($p < 0.001$) and fasting plasma glucose of 1.8 mmol/l ($p < 0.001$). Nine patients (four on repaglinide and five on placebo) were withdrawn from the trial because of a deterioration of ≥1% in HbA_{1c}. No significant increase in body weight occurred. Hypoglycemia was the most frequent adverse event but did not appear related to meal pattern. Minor hypoglycemia occurred in 18% with 0.5 mg/meal of repaglinide and 11% with 1 mg/meal compared to placebo (3%). One percent reported a total of four major hypoglycemic events but none required hospitalization or intravenous glucose or glucagon.

Repaglinide in "Head-to-Head" Studies with Sulfonylureas

The efficacy and safety of repaglinide compared to glipizide was investigated in 256 patients with T2DM in a double-blind, multicenter, parallel-group trial (Table 6) [29]. Patients were randomized to receive either repaglinide 1–4 mg at mealtimes up to three times daily or glipizide 5–15 mg daily and were followed up for 12 months. HbA_{1c} fell by 1.5% in the repaglinide group and 0.3% in the glipizide group ($p < 0.05$ between groups) in those patients who were oral hyperglycemic agent (OHA)-naive. HbA_{1c} increased by 0.5% in the repaglinide group and 0.9% in the glipizide group in patients who were previously treated with OHAs ($p < 0.05$). Fasting blood glucose decreased with repaglinide but increased with glipizide. There were no major hypoglycemic episodes in either group. Minor hypoglycemia was equivalent in both groups (15% with repaglinide, 19% with glipizide).

Repaglinide in Combination with Metformin

The combination of metformin with repaglinide has been shown to be more effective than is repaglinide or metformin monotherapy. In a randomized study of 83 patients (Table 7) with T2DM, the combination group showed a significant reduction in HbA_{1c} of 1.4% and a fall in fasting plasma glucose of 2.2 mmol/l [31]. The mean weight gain in this group was 3 kg.

A much larger uncontrolled prospective study of 5985 patients with T2DM demonstrated the practical advantages of being able to dose flexibly with repaglinide in the everyday clinical setting [32]. The use of repaglinide as a prandial glucose regulator to be taken at the same time as a main meal was explored. The major subgroups in

Table 5 Studies of repaglinide as monotherapy

Study	Intervention	Outcomes	Adverse effects
Moses et al. [27] Double-blind, randomized, placebo-controlled; 408 T2DM	Repaglinide 0.5–1 mg or placebo, preprandially for 16 weeks	HbA_{1c} ↓ 1.14% ($p < 0.001$) FPG ↓ 1.8 mmol/l ($p < 0.001$)	Hypoglycemia Repaglinide 17% Placebo 3% Weight No significant difference ($p = 0.49$) between groups
Van Gaal et al. [28] Double-blind, randomized, placebo-controlled, parallel group; 25 T2DM sulfonylurea-naive	Repaglinide 0.5–4 mg bd; follow-up 10 weeks	HbA_{1c} ↓ 2.3% ($p = 0.018$) FPG ↓ 3.9 mmol/l PBG ↓ 6.2 mmol/l ($p < 0.001$)	Hypoglycemia Repaglinide 15 patients Placebo 20 patients (NS) Weight Repaglinide ↑ 2.1 kg ($p < 0.01$) Placebo ↓ 0.8 kg (NS)

Note: T2DM = type 2 diabetes mellitus; FPG = fasting plasma glucose; P3G = plasma blood glucose; NS = non significant.

Table 6 Summary of trials of repaglinide versus sulfonylureas

Study	Intervention	Outcomes	Adverse effects
Madsbad et al. [29] Double-blind, randomized, parallel-group, multicentre; 256 T2DM	Repaglinide 1–4 mg, premeals or glipizide 5–15 mg, daily; follow-up for 1 year	HbA_{1c} Repaglinide (mean baseline HbA_{1c} 7.3%) Therapy-naive ↓ 1.5% Previous therapy ↑ 0.5% Glipizide (mean baseline HbA_{1c} 7.2%) Therapy-naive ↓ 0.3% Previous therapy ↑ 0.9% FPG Repaglinide ↓ 2.4 mmol/l Glipizide ↑ 1.0 mmol/l $p < 0.05$ for all groups	Hypoglycemia No major events Minor hypoglycemia Repaglinide 15% Glipizide 19% Weight Repaglinide ↓ 0.7 kg Glipizide ↓ 0.9 kg (NS)
Marbury et al. [30] Double-blind, randomized, parallel-group, multicentre; 576 T2DM	Repaglinide 0.5–4 mg three times, preprandially or Glyburide 2.5–15 mg, daily; follow-up for 1 year	HbA_{1c} Repaglinide Therapy-naive ↓ 1.3% Previous therapy ↑ 0.3% ($p < 0.05$) Glyburide Therapy-naive ↓ 1.1% Previous therapy ↑ 0.3% ($p < 0.05$)	Hypoglycemia Repaglinide 15% Glyburide 19% Weight Repaglinide ↓ 0.22 kg Glyburide ↑ 0.05 kg (NS)

this study were 2091 therapy-naive patients, 2180 patients who had switched to repaglinide from another oral hypoglycemic agent, usually a sulfonylurea, and 1530 combination therapy (with metformin) patients. Overall mean HbA_{1c} decreased from 8.6 to 7.4% with reduction in fasting blood glucose from 10.2 to 7.4 mmol/l. Preprandial and 2-h postprandial blood glucose concentrations were also reduced. Body weight decreased slightly by 1.2 kg. Only 49 episodes of hypoglycemia were reported, the majority of which were mild, and in general, adverse drug reactions were rare. Psychosocial benefits were also identified and 80% of patients indicated a sense of relief at being able to miss meals. The need to take snacks for fear of hypoglycemia was also reduced.

Repaglinide in Combination with Insulin

The addition of repaglinide to insulin therapy has been investigated. Repaglinide in combination with bedtime NPH insulin was associated with lowering of HbA_{1c} to 1.68% over a 14-week period [33]. A statistically nonsignificant deterioration in HbA_{1c} was observed in a study comparing insulin combination with either metformin, or repaglinide. However, the additive effect of bedtime isophane insulin, metformin, and premeal repaglinide has been shown to significantly reduce HbA_{1c} and also lower the actual dose of subcutaneous insulin required, compared with the combination of twice daily insulin and metformin [34].

Table 7 Repaglinide in combination with metformin

Study	Intervention	Outcomes	Adverse effects	Comments
Moses et al. [31] Multicentre, double-blind, randomized; 83 T2DM	Metformin alone (1–3 g/d) or repaglinide alone (0.5–4 mg thrice daily) or metformin and repaglinide for 3 months	HbA_{1c} ↓ 1.4% ($p = 0.0016$) FPG ↓ 2.2 mmol/l ($p = 0.0003$) No significant difference in HbA_{1c} or FPG in either monotherapy group	Hypoglycemia Metformin 0% patients Repaglinide 10.7% patients Combination 33.3% patients Weight gain Repaglinide 2.4 ± 0.5 kg Combination 3.0 ± 0.5 kg Diarrhoea Headache	
Landgraf et al. [32] Uncontrolled prospective, 5985 T2DM; 2091 therapy naive, 2180 other OHA → repaglinide, 1530 combination with metformin	Prandial flexible dosing with repaglinide 0.5–2 mg/meal, Mean follow-up 46 days	Mean HbA_{1c} ↓ 1.2% ($p = 0.0001$) Mean FPG ↓ 2.8 mmol/l ($p = 0.0001$) Mean 2-h PG ↓ 3.7 mmol/l ($p = 0.0001$)	Hypoglycemia 38 mild 11 severe Weight ↓ 1.2 ± 2.7 kg	Fewer snacks on repaglinide Patients able to miss meals

Repaglinide in Combination with Other Agents

The combination of repaglinide with troglitazone (now withdrawn following hepatotoxicity) was investigated in 256 patients with T2DM inadequately controlled by monotherapy. In this multicenter open-label clinical trial, there was a fall of 1.7% in HbA_{1c} in the combination group. Repaglinide was also shown to be more effective as monotherapy compared to troglitazone (−0.8% vs. −0.4%, $p < 0.05$). It will be interesting to examine the results of current trials comparing and combining the use of repaglinide with either pioglitazone or rosiglitazone.

Clinical Use of Nateglinide

In the United Kingdom and Europe, nateglinide may be used in combination with metformin when metformin alone is inadequate. It is not licensed for use in the pediatric age group (below 18 years). It is more expensive than other oral hypoglycemic agents such as the sulfonylureas.

Several studies have reported the efficacy of nateglinide either as monotherapy or in combination with other oral hypoglycemic agents such as metformin or troglitazone. A number of trials have compared nateglinide with other sulfonylureas and there are some early reports comparing it with repaglinide.

The starting dose of nateglinide is usually 60 mg three times daily taken within 30 min of a main meal. The dose should subsequently be adjusted according to response, with a maximal dose of 180 mg three times daily.

Nateglinide as Monotherapy

As has been reported with other insulin secretagogues, nateglinide has a glucose-dependent action. A study in 24 patients with T2DM observed significantly greater insulin secretion when nateglinide was taken with a meal compared to when it was taken while fasting.

In a randomized, double-blind, placebo-controlled, multicenter study consisting of 289 patients with T2DM, patients were randomized to receive either nateglinide at doses of 30, 60, 120, or 180 mg, or placebo, before three main meals for 12 weeks (Table 8) [35]. Baseline HbA_{1c} was 8.3–8.5% across all groups. This trial showed a modest although statistically significant reduction of 0.45–0.64% in HbA_{1c} at study endpoint with nateglinide at doses of 60 mg upwards compared with placebo. In the 120-mg-nateglinide group only, the mean level of fasting plasma glucose was significantly reduced. Following a liquid meal challenge, the administration of nateglinide resulted in rapid onset of prandial insulin secretion with high insulin levels present 15 min postdose and maximal plasma concentrations observed 30–60 min postdose. This demonstrates the rapid action and short duration of nateglinide therapy. Nateglinide was well-tolerated. Mild symptoms suggestive of hypoglycemia were reported in the pooled nateglinide group although most of these were not confirmed biochemically.

Nateglinide in "Head-to-Head" Studies with Sulfonylureas

Nateglinide reduces postmeal glucose excursions more effectively than does glyburide (glibenclamide) as shown by a double-blind, placebo-controlled, parallel group study of 8 weeks' duration in 152 patients with T2DM (Table 9) [36]. Nateglinide 120 mg before meals was compared with glyburide 10 mg four times daily. It was shown that nateglinide primarily reduced mealtime glucose excursion (as measured by AUC) whereas glibenclamide reduced fasting glucose levels. Nateglinide did not increase fasting insulin levels and increased only the early insulin response to a liquid meal. This represents a more physiological release of insulin than that for glibenclamide. In patients with T2DM, nateglinide monotherapy for 12 weeks resulted in a dose-dependent reduction in HbA_{1c} and a very low risk of hypoglycemia (Figure 10).

A recently published small, double-blind study compared the efficacy of acute premeal administration of glipizide with nateglinide in 20 patients with T2DM. Patients were randomly assigned to glipizide monotherapy, nateglinide monotherapy, a combination of glipizide and nateglinide, or placebo. This study demonstrated that there was equal efficacy in controlling postbreakfast hyperglycemia with glipizide and nateglinide, in contrast to previous studies comparing these agents. It was suggested that this was due to administration of glipizide

Table 8 Nateglinide as monotherapy

Study	Intervention	Outcomes	Adverse effects
Hanefeld et al. [35] Randomized; double-blind, placebo-controlled, multicenter; 289 T2DM	Nateglinide (thrice daily), 30 mg ($n = 51$) or 60 mg ($n = 63$) or 120 mg ($n = 63$) or 180 mg ($n = 57$) or placebo; 12-week follow-up	HbA_{1c} 60 mg ↓ 0.45% 120 mg ↓ 0.62% 180 mg ↓ 0.64% ($p < 0.05$) FPG 120 mg ↓ 1.14 mmol/l ($p < 0.01$)	Mild symptoms suggestive of hypoglycemia confirmed in 1.3% Weight 120 mg ↑ 0.72 kg

Table 9 Summary of studies of nateglinide versus sulfonylureas

Study	Intervention	Outcomes	Adverse effects
Hollander et al. [36] Double-blind, randomized, placebo-controlled, multicentre; 152 T2DM	Nateglinide 120 mg tds or glyburide 5–10 mg qds or placebo; follow-up 8 weeks	AUC Nateglinide ↓−4.94 mmol/h/l Glyburide ↓ 2.71 mmol/h/l ($p < 0.05$) FPG Nateglinide ↓ 1.0 mmol/h/l Glyburide ↓ 2.9 mmol/h/l ($p < 0.001$)	Hypoglycemia Symptomatic Nateglinide 12 events Glyburide 53 events Placebo 2 events Confirmed Nateglinide 3 events Glyburide 14 events Placebo 1 event
Carroll et al. [37] Double-blind, randomized, placebo-controlled; 20 T2DM	Nateglinide 120 mg, premeal or Glipizide 10 mg, premeal or Nateglinide 120 mg + Glipizide 10 mg, premeal or placebo; follow-up 4 h	PPG excursion Glipizide + nateglinide 4.1 mmol/l Nateglinide 4.2 mmol/l ($p = 0.001$) Glipizide 4.3 mmol/l Placebo 6.1 mmol/l AUC Nateglinide + glipizide 5.6 mmol/h/l Nateglinide 9.7 mmol/h/l Glipizide 6.9 mmol/h/l Placebo 14 mmol/h/l	Hypoglycemia confirmed Glipizide 3 events Nateglinide + glipizide 3 events

30 min (rather than 10 min) before the meal. The combination of nateglinide and glipizide resulted in increased early insulin secretion compared with nateglinide alone but did not significantly change the postprandial glucose profile compared with monotherapy with either agent.

Despite some data that suggest that there may be benefits, there are no large- or medium-term data of head-to-head studies between nateglinide and sulfonylureas looking at weight gain, hypoglycemia, or glycemic control.

Nateglinide in Combination with Metformin

The efficacy of nateglinide in combination with metformin was demonstrated in a randomized double-blind study of 701 patients with T2DM (Table 10) [38].

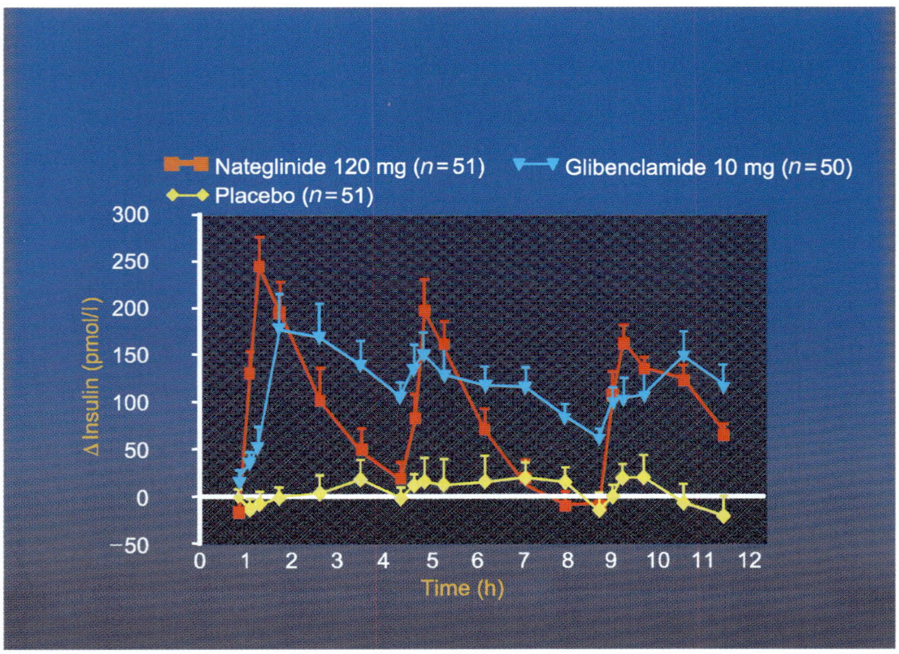

Figure 10 Comparison of nateglinide with glibenclamide and placebo. (Reproduced by permission of the American Diabetes Association [35])

Table 10 Nateglinide in combination with metformin

Study	Intervention	Outcomes	Adverse effects	Comments
Horton et al. [38] Randomized, double-blind, placebo-controlled; 701 T2DM	Nateglinide 120 mg tds or Metformin 500 mg tds or Combination therapy or placebo	HbA_{1c} Nateglinide ↓ 0.5% Metformin ↓ 0.8% Placebo ↑ 0.5% ($p \leq 0.0001$) Combination ↓ 1.4% ($p \leq 0.01$) FPG Nateglinide ↓ 0.7 mmol/l Metformin ↓ 1.6 mmol/l Placebo ↑ 0.4 mmol/l Combination ↓ 2.4 mmol/l AUC Nateglinide ↓ 2.1 mmol/h/l Metformin ↓ 1.1 mmol/h/l Combination ↓ 2.5 mmol/h/l	Hypoglycemia No severe episodes Confirmed episodes Nateglinide 3 patients Metformin 1 patients Combination 5 patients	
Marre et al. [39] Randomized, double-blind, placebo-controlled, parallel-group, multi-center; 467 T2DM on metformin	Nateglinide 60 mg tds or nateglinide 120 mg tds or placebo, Added to metformin 1 g bd; 24-week follow-up	HbA_{1c} Nateglinide 60 mg + metformin ↓ 0.36% ($p = 0.003$) Nateglinide 120 mg + metformin ↓ 0.59% ($p < 0.001$)	Hypoglycemia Metformin + placebo 3.9% Nateglinide 60 mg 8.4% Nateglinide 120 mg 15.6% Weight Nateglinide 120 mg ↑ 0.9 kg ($p < 0.001$)	Greater reduction in HbA_{1c} for combination with both nateglinide doses if baseline HbA_{1c} >9.5%

Patients were assigned to four different groups, namely placebo, nateglinide monotherapy metformin monotherapy, or a combination of nateglinide and metformin. After 24 weeks of therapy, HbA_{1c} and fasting plasma glucose was lowered by 1.9% and 2.4 mmol/l respectively in the combination group, which showed the greatest effect. This study also showed that nateglinide decreased mealtime glucose excursions after a liquid meal challenge, whereas metformin mainly had an effect on fasting plasma glucose.

In a multicenter, double-blind, parallel group trial, 467 metformin-treated patients were randomized to treatment with 60 mg or 120 mg nateglinide or placebo before three meals [39]. This was in combination with 1 g metformin twice daily for 24 weeks. The results showed a significant reduction in HbA_{1c} with nateglinide at either dose (-0.36%, $p = 0.003$; -0.59%, $p < 0.001$, respectively) compared with metformin alone. Hypoglycemic symptoms were more likely to occur if HbA_{1c} was less than 8% at baseline. Weight gain in the nateglinide 120 mg plus metformin group was 0.9 kg. There was no change in plasma lipids.

Nateglinide in Combination with Other Agents

A double-blind, randomized, multicenter study has compared the effects of monotherapy using nateglinide, the thiazolidinedione troglitazone, and the combination of these two agents on HbA_{1c} in patients with T2DM inadequately controlled by diet alone [40]. Monotherapy with nateglinide after 16 weeks resulted in 0.6% reduction in HbA_{1c} compared with 0.8% in the troglitazone monotherapy group. Combination therapy with nateglinide and troglitazone resulted in an even greater improvement of 1.7% in HbA_{1c}. Longer follow-up studies investigating the combination of nateglinide with either pioglitazone or rosiglitazone are needed.

Nateglinide and Impaired Glucose Tolerance

The Pharmacokinetics of nateglinide make it an ideal agent to address the loss of early-phase insulin secretion seen in IGT. Studies are underway to explore the effect of nateglinide in IGT.

A recently published multicenter, double-blind, randomized, parallel-group, fixed-dose study of 8 weeks' duration in 288 patients with IGT has assessed the effects of various doses of nateglinide and associated adverse events, including hypoglycemia. Patients received nateglinide (30, 60, and 120 mg) or placebo before main meals, and response to standardized meal challenges was recorded. The study showed that nateglinide increased early insulin response to a meal and reduced prandial glucose excursions in a dose-dependent manner with no significant effect on fasting plasma glucose or fasting insulin levels. Apart from hypoglycemia (28 cases in nateglinide group and 1 in placebo group), the overall incidence of adverse events was low. The study concluded that nateglinide was safe and effective in reducing PPH in subjects with IGT and recommended that the lower doses (30 mg and 60 mg) would be suitable for investigation in longer term studies.

A large, multicenter, randomized, double-blind, placebo-controlled trial known as NAVIGATOR is currently in progress. This has set out to explore the efficacy of nateglinide in combination with valsartan on glycemic control and cardiovascular outcomes in individuals with IGT. This 7-year study of 10 000 subjects with IGT is the largest ever diabetes prevention study and should provide data about whether targeting PPH will improve cardiovascular outcomes. By design, one third of patients recruited to the study have established cardiovascular disease, which should provide sufficient power to look at cardiovascular outcomes.

Safety of Meglitinides

Trials have shown that the safety of meglitinides is comparable with other oral hypoglycemic agents such as the sulfonylureas. Three large 1-year studies indicated that repaglinide has an adverse event profile similar to that of glibenclamide. The most common side effect is hypoglycemia but this is usually mild. The incidence of serious hypoglycemia was 0.6% with repaglinide and 1% with sulfonylureas. From pooled data from Phase III studies, the proportion of patients presenting with hypoglycemia was 16% for repaglinide, compared with 20% for glibenclamide, 19% for glipizide, and 15% for gliclazide.

In long-term clinical trials, incidence of serious adverse events was low with repaglinide (10%) and similar to the incidence reported with sulfonylureas (11.6%).

Similarly for nateglinide, studies have shown that the commonest adverse event is symptoms suggestive of mild hypoglycemia. A study of 152 patients showed that symptomatic hypoglycemia occurred in 12 patients randomized to nateglinide and 53 patients on glyburide. Confirmed hypoglycemia was documented in 3 patients on nateglinide and 14 patients on glyburide. Other studies suggest that the incidence of hypoglycemia is similar for both sulfonylureas and nateglinide.

Respiratory disorders are the next most frequently reported adverse events in long-term clinical trials, namely upper respiratory tract infection (10%), rhinitis (7%), and bronchitis (6%). However the incidence and severity of these events was similar in patients treated with sulfonylureas and most were not drug related.

Other reported side effects are hypersensitivity reactions, increased liver enzymes, gastrointestinal symptoms, and headache. These have been reported with similar incidence to placebo. Combination therapy does not appear to result in more adverse events compared to monotherapy.

According to national drug formulary guidelines (British National Formulary), in the presence of fever, trauma, infection, or surgery, the meglitinides should be substituted by insulin therapy. The risk of hypoglycemia is increased in patients with adrenal or pituitary insufficiency, in malnourished individuals, and in the elderly.

SUMMARY

The meglitinides offer an opportunity to target specifically the PPH that occurs commonly in patients with type 2 diabetes [41, 42]. Their rapid onset and short duration of action leads to more "physiological" release of insulin and partially restores the pattern of postprandial insulin secretion that is defective in type 2 diabetes mellitus. This potentially allows tighter glycemic control while reducing the risk of hypoglycemia. As prandial glucose regulators they allow flexible dosing such that a tablet need only be taken before a patient has a meal. Repaglinide in particular has been shown to reduce HbA_{1c} and is well-tolerated by patients both as monotherapy and in combination with other agents. It appears to have some advantages from head-to-head studies with sulfonylureas. Nateglinide appears to produce a faster early-phase insulin response that gives it the potential to produce less hypoglycemia, but randomized controlled trials in comparison with sulfonylureas are lacking. Both agents are more expensive than sulfonylureas. Formal data regarding cost-effectiveness are not currently available. However, their flexible administration may be of benefit in certain subgroups such as shift-workers and those with flexible lifestyles. Efficacy in early diabetes and impaired glucose tolerance is currently being investigated. The ability to flexibly dose with these agents makes them useful in patients with flexible lifestyles. Macrovascular and microvascular outcome data for the meglitinides are awaited.

REFERENCES

1. Amos AF, McCarty DJ, Zimmet P. The rising global burden of diabetes and its complications: estimates and projections to the year 2010. *Diabet Med* 1997; 14 (suppl 5): 1–85.
2. Takiya L, Chawla S. Therapeutic options for the management of type 2 diabetes. *Am J Manag Care* 2002; 8 (11): 1009–23.
3. The UK Prospective Diabetes Study (UKPDS) Group. Intensive blood-glucose control with sulphonylureas compared with conventional treatment and risks of complications in patients with type 2 diabetes (UKPDS 33). *Lancet* 1998; 352: 837–53.
4. Chiasson JL, Josse RG, Gomis R, Hanefeld M, Karasik A, Laakso M, for the STOP-NIDDM Trail Research Group. Acarbose for prevention of type 2 diabetes mellitus: the STOP-NIDDM randomised trial. *Lancet* June 2002; 359 (9323): 2072–7.
5. Davies MJ, Rajman G, Grenfell A, Gray IP, Day JL, Males CN. Loss of the first phase insulin response to intravenous

glucose in subjects with persistent impaired glucose tolerance. *Diabet Med* 1994; 11: 432–6.
6. Weyer C, Bogardus C, Mott DM, Pratley RE. The natural history of insulin secretory dysfunction and insulin resistance in the pathogenesis of type 2 diabetes Mellitus. *J Clin Invest* 1999; 104: 789–94.
7. The UKPDS group. UKPDS 16. Overview of 6 years therapy of Type II diabetes: a progressive disease. *Diabetes* 1995; 44: 1249–58.
8. Avignon A, Radauceanu A, Monnier L. Non-fasting glucose is a better marker of diabetes control than fasting plasma glucose in type 2 diabetes. *Diabetes Care* 1997; 20: 1822–6.
9. Erlinger TP, Brancati FL. Postchallenge hyperglycaemia in a national sample of US adults with type 2 diabetes. *Diabetes Care* 2001; 24: 1734–8.
10. DECODE Study Group on behalf of the European Diabetes Epidemiology Study Group. Glucose tolerance and mortality: comparison of WHO and American Diabetes Association diagnostic criteria. *Lancet* 1999; 354: 617–21.
11. Balkau B, Shipley M, Jarrett RJ, Pyorala K, Pyorala M, Forhan A, Eschwege E. High blood glucose concentration is a risk factor for mortality in middle-aged nondiabetic men. 20-year follow-up in the Whitehall Study, the Paris Prospective Study, and the Helsinki Policemen Study. *Diabetes Care* 1998; 21 (3): 360–7.
12. de Vegt F, Dekker JM, Ruhe HG, Stehouwer CD, Nijpels G, Bouter LM, Heine RJ. Hyperglycaemia is associated with all-cause and cardiovascular mortality in the Hoorn population: the Hoorn Study. *Diabetologia* 1999; 42 (8): 926–31.
13. Hanefeld M, Fischer S, Julius U, Schulze J, Schwanebeck U, Schmechel H, et al. Risk factors for myocardial infarction and death in newly detected NIDDM: The Diabetes Intervention Study (DIS), 11-year follow-up. *Diabetologia* 1996; 39: 1577–83.
14. Donahue RP, Abbot RD, Reed DM, Yano K. Postchallenge glucose concentration and coronary heart disease in men of Japanese ancestry. Honolulu Heart Program. *Diabetes* 1987; 36: 689–92.
15. Ceriello A. The emerging role of post prandial hyperglycaemic spikes in the pathogenesis of diabetic complications. *Diabet Med* 1998; 15: 188–93.
16. Pradhan AD, Manson JAE, Rifai N, et al. C-reactive protein, interleukin-6, and risk of developing T2DM. *JAMA* 2001; 286: 327–34.
17. Esposito K, Nappo F, Marfella R, et al. Inflammatory cytokine concentrations are acutely increased by hyperglycaemia in humans—role of oxidative stress. *Circulation* 2002; 106: 2067–72.
18. De Veciana M, Major CA, Morgan MA, Asrat T, Toohey JS, Lien JM, Evans AT. Postprandial versus preprandial blood glucose monitoring in women with gestational diabetes mellitus requiring insulin therapy. *N Engl J Med* 1995; 333: 1239–41.
19. American Diabetes Association. Postprandial blood glucose. *Diabetes Care* 2001; 24: 775–8.
20. Hu S, Wang S, Fanelli B, Bell PA, Dunning BE, Geisse S, Schmitz R, Boettcher BR. Pancreatic B-cell K-ATP channel activity and membrane-binding studies with nateglinide: a comparison with sulfonylurcas and repaglinide. *J Pharmacol Exp Ther* 2000; 293: 444–52.
21. Fuhlendorff J, Rorsman P, Kofod H, et al. Stimulation of insulin release by repaglinide and glibenclamide involves both common and distinct processes. *Diabetes* 1998; 47: 345–51.
22. Tankova T, Koev D, Dakovska L, Kirilov G. The effect of repaglinide on insulin secretion and oxidative stress in type 2 diabetic patients. *Diabetes Res Clin Pract* 2003; 59: 43–9.
23. Hu S, Wang S, Dunning BE. Glucose-dependent and glucose-sensitising insulinotropic effect of nateglinide: a comparison to sulfonylureas and repaglinide. *Int J Exp Diabetes Res* 2001; 2 (1): 63–72.
24. Kalbag J, Hirschberg Y, Mcleod JF, Garrefta S, Lassetes K. Comparison of Mealtime glucose regulation by nateglinide and repaglinide in healthy subjects. *Diabetes* 1999 (suppl 1): Abstract 106.
25. Massi-Benedetti M, Damsbo P. Pharmacology and clinical experience with repaglinide. *Exp Opin Invest Drugs* 2000; 9 (4): 885–98.
26. Devineni D, Walter YH, Smith HT, Lee JS, Prasad P, McLeod JF. Pharmacokinetics of nateglinide in renally impaired diabetic patients. *J Clin Pharmacol* 2003; 43 (2): 163–70.
27. Moses RG, Gomis R, Frandsen KB, et al. Flexible meal-related dosing with repaglinide facilitates glycaemic control in therapy-naive type 2 diabetes. *Diabetes Care* 2001; 24: 11–5.
28. Van Gaal LF, Van Acker KL, De Leeuw IH. Repaglinide improves blood glucose control in sulphonylurea-naïve type 2 diabetes. *Diab Res Clin Pract* 2001; 53: 141–8.
29. Madsbad S, Kilhovd B, Lager I, et al. Comparison between repaglinide and glipizide in type 2 diabetes mellitus: a 1 year multicenter study. *Diabet Med* 2001; 18: 395–401.
30. Marbury T, Huang WC, Strange P, Lebovitz H. Repaglinide versus glyburide: a one year comparison trial. *Diab Res Clin Pract* 1999; 43: 155–66.
31. Moses R, Siobodniuk R, Boyages S, Colagiuri S, et al. Effect of repaglinide addition to metformin monotherapy on glycaemic control in patients with type 2 diabetes. *Diabetes Care* 1999; 22 (1): 119–24.
32. Landgraf R, Frank M, Bauer C, Dieken ML. Prandial glucose regulation with repaglinide: it's clinical and lifestyle impact in a large cohort of patients with type 2 diabetes. *Int J Obes Relat Metab Disord* 2000; 24 (suppl 3): 38–44.
33. Yki-Jarvinen H, Ryysy L, Nikkila K, et al. Comparison of betime insulin regimens in patients with type 2 diabetes mellitus. A randomized controlled trial. *Ann Intern Med* 1999; 130: 389–96.
34. Davies MJ, Johnston V, Howe J, et al. Comparison of combination regimes of insulin, repaglinide and metformin in type 2 diabetes: an interim analysis. *Diabet Med* 2001; 18 (suppl 2): A44.
35. Hanefeld M, Bouter KP, Dickinson S, Guitard C. Rapid and short-acting mealtime insulin secretion with nateglinide controls both prandial and mean glycaemia. *Diabetes Care* 2000; 23: 202–7.
36. Hollander P, Schwartz SL, Gatlin MR, et al. Nateglinide but not glyburide, selectively enhances early insulin release and more effectively controls post-meal glucose excursions with less insulin exposure. *Diabetes* 2000; 49: 449.
37. Carroll F, Izard A, Riboni K, Burge MR, et al. Control of postprandial hyperglycaemia. Optimal use of short-acting insulin secretagogues. *Diabetes Care* 2002; 25: 2147–52.
38. Horton E, Clinkingbeard C, Gatlin M, et al. Nateglinide alone and in combination with metformin improves

glycaemic control by reducing mealtime glucose levels in type 2 diabetes. *Diabetes Care* 2000; 23: 1660–5.

39. Marre M, Van Gaal L, Usadel K-H, Ball M, Whatmough I, Guitard C. Nateglinide improves glycaemic control when added to metformin monotherapy: results of a randomized trial with type 2 diabetes. *Diabetes Obes Metab* 2002; 4: 177–86.

40. Rosenstock J, Shen SG, Gatlin MR, Foley JE. Combination therapy with nateglinide and a thiazolidinedione improves glycemic control in type 2 diabetes. *Diabetes Care* 2002; 25: 1529–33.

41. Davies MJ. Insulin secretagogues. *Curr Med Res Opin* 2002; 18 (suppl 1): S22–30.

42. Dornhorst A. Insulinotropic meglitinides analogues. *Lancet* 2001; 358: 1709–16.

47

Metformin and Other Biguanides: Pharmacology and Therapeutic Usage

Alan J. Garber

Baylor College of Medicine, Houston, TX, USA

INTRODUCTION

Historical information regarding the use of guanidine-containing compounds for medicinal purposes dates to medieval times in Europe. *Galega officinalis*—also known as French lilac, Italian fitch, or goat's rue—containing the active ingredient galegine, or isoamylene guanidine, was used to relieve urination associated with diabetes and for other disorders [1, 2]. The clinical observation that guanidines lower blood glucose was first recorded in 1928 [3]. Although the clinical utility of *G. officinalis* preparations was limited by gastrointestinal toxicity, their blood glucose-lowering effects ultimately led to the development of the diguanides (two guanidine molecules connected by an intermediate chain) in the early 20th century. However, their use was short-lived owing to hepatotoxicity and the discovery of insulin by Sir F.G. Banting.

Biguanides were introduced for clinical use in Europe in the 1950s. The biguanides phenformin, buformin, and metformin initially were widely used in treating type 2 diabetes for nearly 20 years. However, two significant events led to their removal in some countries or limited usage in others over the subsequent 20 years. Phenformin and buformin were withdrawn from the market in most countries, including the United States, by 1978 because of the large numbers of cases of fatal lactic acidosis associated with their use [3]. Additionally, in the late 1970s, the University Group Diabetes Program trial reported an increased risk for cardiovascular mortality with the prolonged use of oral hypoglycemic agents compared with the use of insulin [4, 5]. Metformin has a very low rate of lactic acidosis compared with phenformin. Furthermore, flaws in the design and conclusion of the University Group Diabetes Program trial later emerged. Nonetheless, these events precluded the appearance of metformin in the United States for nearly two decades.

A resurgence of interest in metformin occurred in the 1980s and 1990s based on numerous clinical studies demonstrating its considerable efficacy and safety in type 2 diabetes, especially the landmark United Kingdom Prospective Diabetes Study (UKPDS) [6]. These studies demonstrated that metformin improves insulin resistance, a major pathogenic component of type 2 diabetes [7]. Metformin was shown to have efficacy similar to that of sulfonylureas in reducing fasting plasma glucose (FPG) and postprandial glucose concentrations, but metformin did not cause weight gain or hypoglycemia in contrast to sulfonylurea therapy [6, 8–14]. Of greatest importance in the UKPDS was the finding that metformin, but not insulin or sulfonylurea therapy, was associated with significant reductions in diabetes-related macrovascular endpoints and all-cause mortality compared with conventional therapy, primarily with diet [15].

Although metformin has been used widely for many years in Europe, Latin America, and Canada, it only became available for use in the United States in 1995. Metformin usage has increased substantially worldwide, pursuant to the UKPDS findings and subsequent favorable recommendations regarding its use [16]. Although phenformin is still used in Italy and to a lesser extent in Mexico for control of type 2 diabetes, metformin currently is the biguanide of choice in Europe, Canada, and the United States. Recently completed studies have more thoroughly elucidated the pharmacodynamics and safety

International Textbook of Diabetes Mellitus, Third Edition. Edited by R. A. DeFronzo, E. Ferrannini, H. Keen, and P. Zimmet.
 ISBN: 0-471-48655-8.

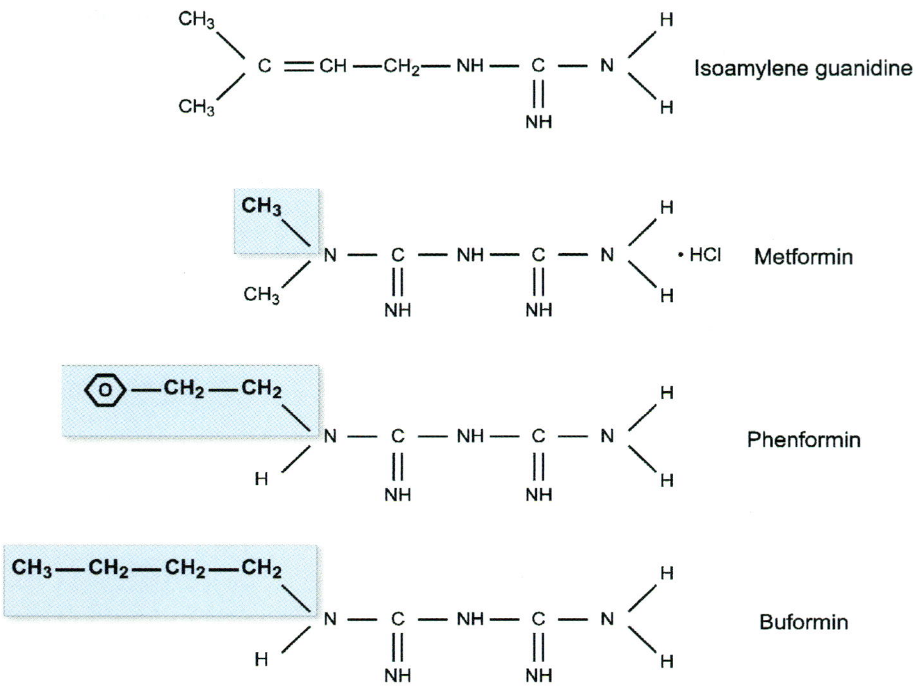

Figure 1 Chemical structures of isoamylene guanidine, phenformin, buformin, and metformin. The nonpolar hydrocarbon side chain in the biguanides (shaded area) determines the degree of lipophilicity of the molecule and binding to the biological membrane site

of metformin. This chapter focuses primarily on metformin and its recent clinical developments and applications.

CHEMISTRY

All biguanides are derived from guanidine and consist of two linked guanidine molecules minus an ammonia radical (Figure 1). Of the 300 synthesized biguanides, only a few exhibit a blood glucose-lowering effect in man, including metformin, phenformin, and buformin [3]. Biguanides bind to membrane phospholipids in biological and artificial structures. Consequently, the fundamental difference between individual biguanides lies in the type and length of the nonpolar hydrocarbon side chain, which determines membrane lipophilicity and binding affinity [3]. Phenformin is more lipophilic than metformin and has a greater affinity for mitochondrial membranes [17]. The same side chain determines pharmacologic differences between biguanides. For example, metformin (methyl side chain) is excreted unchanged by glomerular filtration, whereas phenformin requires hepatic hydroxylation.

MECHANISM OF ACTION

Type 2 diabetes is a complex, slowly evolving metabolic disorder, characterized by impaired insulin-stimulated glucose uptake and utilization (insulin resistance) in both the liver and muscle, impaired β-cell insulin secretory function, and enhanced glucagon and reduced glucagon-like peptide 1 secretion [18, 19]. Metformin appears to exert several antidiabetic pharmacodynamic actions through unclear molecular mechanisms in type 2 diabetes, although newly postulated mechanisms of action continue to be elucidated. In patients with type 2 diabetes, metformin significantly reduces FPG concentrations, glycosylated hemoglobin (A_{1c}), postprandial glucose concentrations, and 24-h plasma glucose concentrations independent of circulating insulin levels [7, 20–32]. Clinical data show that metformin improves insulin resistance in the liver, skeletal muscle, and adipose tissue by reducing excess basal hepatic glucose production and by increasing insulin-mediated and glucose-mediated whole-body glucose uptake by the peripheral tissues and liver [7, 22, 26, 27, 33–38]. Hepatic glucose production is reduced 25–40% with metformin in patients with type 2 diabetes [34, 35]. Additionally, metformin increases glucose utilization 20–50% [21, 24] and improves glucose metabolism primarily through nonoxidative pathways in the liver [23, 27, 31, 35, 36]. Metformin does not increase insulin secretion in type 2 diabetes [21, 22, 24, 26, 33], and does not cause hypoglycemia, as do insulin secretagogues and exogenous insulin. Consequently, metformin is more accurately described as an antihyperglycemic agent rather than as a hypoglycemic agent.

Other actions of metformin contribute to its effects on glycemic control and improved outcomes in patients with type 2 diabetes. Metformin decreases serum triglyceride and free fatty acid concentrations [21, 35, 39, 40], and slows the rate of lipid oxidation [20, 21, 23, 30, 35], actions that indirectly inhibit gluconeogenesis. Metformin treatment is associated with statistically and clinically significant reductions in body weight (primarily adipose tissue) in obese patients with type 2 diabetes. These are independent of its effects on glycemic control [26, 34]. The effects of metformin on insulin-binding affinity to insulin receptors on circulating blood cells are reported variously, as some clinical data show unchanged binding [21, 25, 41], increased binding that did not correlate to the level of glycemic control [29, 33, 42], and reduced binding of insulin to monocytes [31].

The molecular mechanisms of metformin action have only recently been partially elucidated at the cellular level, despite the fact that metformin has been used clinically for the management of type 2 diabetes for more than 40 years. Activation of the enzyme adenosine monophosphate (AMP)-activated protein kinase, a major cellular regulator of glucose and fat metabolism, plays a role in enhancing sensitivity to insulin by interacting with the insulin-signaling pathway [43, 44]. Activation of AMP protein kinase has been suggested as a potential target for the treatment of type 2 diabetes [43]. Metformin has been shown to activate AMP protein kinase in rat hepatocytes, and in this model AMP protein kinase activation was required for the inhibitory effect of metformin on hepatocyte glucose production [45]. In patients with type 2 diabetes, 10 weeks of treatment with therapeutic doses of metformin significantly increased the α-2 isoform of AMP protein kinase in skeletal muscle by 80%, as measured by biopsy, and increased AMP protein kinase phosphorylation by 80% [46]. It has recently been suggested that the beneficial effects of metformin on cardiovascular disease and insulin resistance may be related to its activation of AMP protein kinase [44].

Additionally, metformin stimulates tyrosine kinase activity of the intracellular β-subunit of the human insulin receptor and the intracellular epidermal growth factor receptor [47]. Additionally, metformin has been shown to stimulate glucose transport in human fibroblasts by increasing glucose transporter protein and gene expression *de novo* in a dose-dependent and time-dependent manner [48]. In human hepatocytes, metformin increased insulin receptor β-subunit tyrosine phosphorylation by 78% in the absence of insulin and increased insulin receptor substrate 2 (IRS-2) tyrosine phosphorylation by 60%. The increase in 2-deoxyglucose uptake was mediated via increased translocation of GLUT-1 to the plasma membrane. The addition of metformin to insulin did not result in an additive effect, and the effects of metformin were abolished in the presence of an insulin receptor tyrosine kinase inhibitor, strongly supporting the hypothesis that metformin may act through the insulin receptor to alter glucose metabolism. Metformin significantly increased basal insulin receptor kinase activity by 150%. Thus, the mechanism of action of metformin in the liver may involve a sequence of events from insulin receptor activation, followed by IRS-2 activation, and increased glucose uptake via GLUT-1 translocation [49].

Insulin resistance is accompanied by endothelial dysfunction, thereby resulting in disturbances of vasoregulatory and thrombosis-related substances secreted by endothelial cells. One of these substances is plasminogen activator inhibitor 1 (PAI-1), the principal antagonist of tissue plasminogen activator (tPA). The effects of metformin on the production of PAI-1, the main antifibrinolytic component in the circulatory system that is elevated in insulin-resistant states, was assessed *in vitro* using human adipose tissue obtained from individuals undergoing cosmetic surgery. At concentrations from 0.1 to 10 μM, metformin dose-dependently decreased PAI-1 production and PAI-1 mRNA from 43 to 100% over the dose range under both basal and interleukin-1β-stimulated conditions [50]. This action may explain the cardiovascular risk reduction with metformin therapy independent of its effects on glucose control. Additionally, recent analyses of the UKPDS data suggest that the macrovascular risk reduction associated with metformin may be independent of dose [51].

The Diabetes Prevention Program, initiated in 1996, assessed whether intensive lifestyle modification or metformin therapy reduced the development or delayed the onset of type 2 diabetes in at-risk patients with impaired glucose tolerance [52]. The incidence of diabetes was reduced 58% with intensive lifestyle modification and 31% with metformin treatment compared with the placebo treatment [53]. There were no differences in outcomes by sex or ethnic group, but metformin was most effective in patients 60 years of age or younger and in individuals with higher body mass index and higher FPG [53].

PRODUCT FORMULATIONS

Metformin is available in several product formulations (Table 1) [54–57].

CLINICAL EFFICACY OF METFORMIN

Insulin-Resistant Prediabetic States

In the Diabetes Prevention Program, therapeutic doses of metformin prevented the progression from impaired glucose tolerance to type 2 diabetes, presumably as the result of its insulin-sensitizing effects [53]. Similarly, in the Biguanides and Prevention of Risks in Obesity Study, 324 middle-aged, obese nondiabetic subjects with

Table 1 Metformin product formulations*

Active ingredient	Formulation	Strength (mg)	Usual dosage
Metformin	Immediate-release tablet	500, 850, 1000	• 500 or 850 mg daily with meals • Up to 2550 mg daily in divided doses with meals
Metformin	Extended-release tablet	500, 750	• 500 mg once daily with the evening meal • Up to a maximum of 2000 mg once daily
Glipizide/metformin	Combination tablet	2.5/250, 2.5/500, 5/500	• Initial diabetes pharmacotherapy: 2.5 mg/250 mg once daily • Up to 10 mg/2000 mg daily in divided doses • Second-line therapy: 20 mg/2000 mg
Glyburide/metformin	Combination tablet	1.25/250, 2.5/500, 5/500	• Initial diabetes pharmacotherapy: 1.25 mg/250 mg once or twice daily with meals • Increased every 2 weeks as need for maximal effects • Maximum first-line dose: 10 mg/2000 mg • Previously treated patients: 2.5/500 mg or 5/500 mg twice daily with meals • Maximum first-line dose: 20 mg/2000 mg
Rosiglitazone/metformin	Combination tablet	1/500, 2/500, 4/500	• For patients on metformin therapy: 4 mg rosiglitazone daily + current metformin dose • For patients already on rosiglitazone therapy: 1000 mg metformin daily + current rosiglitazone dose

* From references 54–57.

a high waist–hip ratio were randomly assigned to receive double-blind metformin 850 mg twice daily or placebo for 3 years [58]. Patients who received metformin had increased weight loss and lower mean concentrations of fasting serum insulin, low-density lipoprotein (LDL) cholesterol, and tPA (a measure of fibrinolytic impairment compared with patients given placebo). Treatment with metformin resulted in better FPG maintenance in the population of patients with impaired glucose tolerance at study entry. There were no significant changes in blood pressure, triglycerides, or high-density lipoprotein (HDL) cholesterol in metformin-treated patients.

Metformin also has been shown to have beneficial effects in other insulin-resistant states. The insulin resistance syndrome (also referred to as syndrome X or as the metabolic syndrome) is characterized by impairment of glucose tolerance or insulin-mediated glucose disposal, which may result in hyperglycemia, compensatory hyperinsulinemia, dyslipidemia, atherosclerosis, endothelial dysfunction, and hypertension [59, 60]. Metformin may be useful in improving outcomes in patients with the insulin resistance syndrome based on its proven efficacy in improving insulin sensitivity, delaying the development of type 2 diabetes, and potentially reducing cardiovascular risk [36, 53, 58, 61–64]. The latter is a particularly important point. Although untested experimentally, treatment with metformin may reduce the excess risk for coronary heart disease (three- to fourfold) in patients with the metabolic syndrome [65].

Polycystic ovary syndrome is a common endocrine disorder occurring among women of reproductive age (6% of menstruating women) and the predominant cause of chronic anovulation and infertility. Insulin resistance and compensatory hyperinsulinemia play a central role in the pathogenesis of polycystic ovary syndrome. In response to hyperinsulinemia, ovarian tissues in affected women overproduce testosterone, thereby lowering sex hormone binding globulin. Luteinizing hormone secretion is chronically increased, which stimulates follicles to further produce excess androgen. Insulin resistance also stimulates cytochrome P450c17-α activity, which catalyzes the conversion from testosterone to estradiol. Consequently, women with polycystic ovary syndrome overproduce testosterone and estradiol. Clinical features of the syndrome include laboratory findings of elevated luteinizing hormone, androgens, and insulin; hypertriglyceridemia; reduced HDL cholesterol; and elevated PAI-1 concentrations. Physical findings include obesity, hirsutism, oligomenorrhea, amenorrhea, and hypertension. Previously, the drugs of choice for the disorder have included metformin, clomiphene, and oral contraceptives. However, response rates to clomiphene are variable and low, and oral contraceptive use may exacerbate glucose intolerance and do not restore fertility.

Metformin has proved to be beneficial in polycystic ovary syndrome, improving metabolic features as well as restoring ovulation and fertility [66]. The effects of metformin on weight loss and insulin sensitivity have been inconsistent, with some studies showing a benefit and others not [67–73]. However, clinical trial data show that metformin reduces P450c17-α activity, serum free testosterone, luteinizing hormone concentrations, and PAI-1 concentrations; normalizes 17-α-hydroxyprogesterone concentrations; restores menstrual cycling and improves menstrual cycle regularity; and normalizes the serum ratio of luteinizing hormone to follicle-stimulating hormone

[67–70, 74–76]. Ovulation and fertility rates have been improved with metformin, either as monotherapy or in combination with clomiphene, in several clinical trials [66, 68, 69, 76, 77]. A trial involving 60 women with polycystic ovary syndrome desiring to become pregnant compared the efficacy and persistency rates of metformin and clomiphene with human menstrual gonadotropin [78]. The use of metformin 1500 mg/day for 6 months significantly improved menstrual cycles (40% of patients), and when followed by a combination of metformin plus clomiphene for at least 3 ovulation cycles, resulted in significant improvement in ovulation (46.7% ovulation rate) and an overall pregnancy rate of 16.7%. Metformin also significantly decreased fasting insulin levels. In the group receiving human gonadotropin, the ovulation rate (43.0%) and the pregnancy rate (23.3%) were similar to those in the metformin group, but the dropout rate and cost of therapy were higher. The lower cost and improved tolerability of metformin relative to other treatments for polycystic ovary syndrome and related infertility and comorbidities suggest that metformin is a useful treatment for the disorder.

In patients with acquired immunodeficiency syndrome (AIDS) treated with antiretroviral agents, hyperinsulinemia with lipodystrophy and abdominal obesity have resulted. In a small study of 11 patients, treatment with metformin produced sustained reductions in tPA levels, serum insulin levels, body mass index, and waist circumference over a 9-month treatment period, but had no effect on other cardiovascular markers [79]. Metformin reduces glucose production, increases glucose clearance, and increases insulinemia in severely burned (>60% of body surface area), hypermetabolic patients, suggesting a potential clinical utility of metformin in stress-induced hyperglycemia [80].

Treatment of Type 2 Diabetes: Glycemic Control

The efficacy of metformin in improving indices of glycemic control and reducing the risk for adverse diabetes outcomes has been well established through many well-controlled clinical trials with sample sizes ranging from several hundred to several thousand patients. Metformin is a first-line pharmacologic treatment option for patients with type 2 diabetes and is the agent of choice for those who are overweight [15, 54]. The dose response is log-linear to 2000 mg/day [81], allowing for incremental titration to effect. Additionally, metformin has been evaluated and proven useful in children with type 2 diabetes who are unable to achieve glycemic control with diet and exercise [82] and in overweight children with type 1 diabetes to reduce high insulin dosages [83]. The effects are additive when used in combination with other glucose-lowering agents, attributable to the simultaneous targeting of multiple physiologic defects in type 2 diabetes. This approach is preferable to the sequential addition of agents as needed for glycemic control, as type 2 diabetes is often present before being diagnosed, and data from UKPDS support the early, aggressive management of glycemic control to attenuate microvascular and macrovascular complications [84]. Thus, combination therapy with metformin represents a new paradigm for the initial treatment of type 2 diabetes. Table 2 summarizes data regarding metformin therapy derived from placebo- and active-controlled clinical trials [6, 14, 24, 28, 81, 85–115].

Metformin Monotherapy

Metformin immediate-release tablets can be administered twice daily with meals if ≤2000 mg is needed for blood glucose control or three times daily in divided doses with meals for daily dosages >2000 mg. Metformin extended-release tablets offer the advantage of once-daily administration at any dose and appear to have a better gastrointestinal tolerability profile. Metformin extended-release tablets contain a dual hydrophilic polymer matrix system in which the drug is released slowly once the tablet is ingested. After ingestion, fluid from the gastrointestinal tract enters the tablet and causes the polymers in the tablet to hydrate and swell [93]. Metformin is released through the process of diffusion and metered out over the dosing period. This process is independent of the pH of the gastrointestinal fluid and agitation. In healthy volunteers, peak plasma levels achieved are approximately 20% lower following a single dose of metformin extended-release than with the immediate-release formulation. Time to peak concentration is reached later (median, 7 h) with metformin extended-release than with metformin immediate-release (approximately 2–3 h), but the extent of absorption (as measured by area under the concentration–time curve [AUC]) is similar between the formulations [54]. In patients with type 2 diabetes, steady-state peak plasma concentrations were approximately 25% higher and time to peak concentration was delayed by 3–5 h with metformin extended-release compared with immediate-release metformin [116–118]. The overall AUC of metformin extended-release is similar in healthy volunteers and patients with type 2 diabetes [116–118].

Compared with immediate-release metformin, metformin extended-release is equally efficacious in reducing A_{1c}, FPG, postprandial glucose concentrations, and serum insulin [92]. In patients switching from immediate-release metformin 500 mg twice daily to metformin extended-release 1000 mg or 1500 mg once daily, comparable glycemic control was attained in a randomized, double-blind, 24-week trial, although metformin extended-release was better tolerated. Treatment-emergent gastrointestinal adverse events were reported by 29% of patients receiving metformin extended-release 1000 mg and by 39% of patients receiving immediate-release metformin 500 mg twice daily [93]. For patients who require a 1500-mg

Table 2 Efficacy of metformin in improving glycemic control in type 2 diabetes on the basis of clinical trial data

		Reference
Metformin monotherapy		
Patients uncontrolled on dietary changes alone*	• FPG reduced 52–92 mg/dl vs. placebo • A_{1c} reduced 1.4–2% vs. placebo • Basal metabolic glucose clearance increased 30–53%	[24, 81–87]
Compared with sulfonylurea therapy	• Comparable antihyperglycemic effects	[6, 14, 28, 87–91]
Immediate-release vs. extended-release formulations	• Similar effects on FPG, A_{1c}, and serum insulin between formulations and when switching from immediate- to extended-release metformin	[92, 93]
Children >10 years of age	• FPG reduced 42.9 mg/dl • A_{1c} reduced 1.0% vs. placebo ($P < 0.001$)	[94]
Metformin combination therapy		
Metformin + glipizide	First-line therapy • Additional reductions in A_{1c} in the range of 0.4–0.7% with combination tablets • Greater proportion of patients had A_{1c} <7% (57–60% vs. 35–44% for either agent used alone)	[95] [96]
	Second-line therapy (sulfonylurea failure) • A_{1c} reduced an additional 0.98–1.06% with combination tablets • FPG reduced an additional 37 mg/dl compared with either agent used alone • Greater proportion of patients had A_{1c} levels <7% (36.3 vs. 9–10% for either agent used alone)	
Metformin + glyburide	First-line therapy • A_{1c} reduced 1.7–3.4% with combination tablets • FPG reduced 61.5–129.2 mg/dl • Glyburide/metformin tablets provided superior glycemic control over sulfonylurea + metformin	[14, 97–100]
	Second-line therapy (sulfonylurea failure) • FPG reduced an additional 63 mg/dl (29%) with combination tablets • A_{1c} reduced an additional 1.7–1.9% vs. either agent used alone	[87, 101–104]
Metformin + rosiglitazone	First-line therapy: not studied Second-line therapy • The addition of rosiglitazone to metformin therapy produces an additional 1.0–1.2% reduction in A_{1c} and FPG by an additional 40–58 mg/dl vs. metformin monotherapy • The effects of adding rosiglitazone to metformin are most pronounced in obese patients	[105, 106]
Metformin + acarbose	• Adding acarbose to metformin therapy produces an additional 0.65–0.80% reduction in A_{1c} vs. metformin monotherapy	[107, 108]
Metformin + meglitinide	• Adding repaglinide or nateglinide to metformin therapy produces an additional 1.4% reduction in A_{1c} and 2.2 mmol/l reduction in FPG vs. metformin monotherapy	[109]
Metformin + insulin	• The combination reduces A_{1c} 1.5–2.5% and FPG 5.3–5.8 mmol/l compared with insulin monotherapy • Reduces insulin dosage 25–36%, or obviates the need for insulin entirely	[110–115]

Note: FPG = fasting plasma glucose; A_{1c} = glycosylated hemoglobin.
* The majority of studies were conducted in overweight or obese patients.

daily dose of metformin, once-daily optimal dosing can be achieved with either 500 mg or 750 mg tablets. Two metformin extended-release 750 mg tablets administered at one time are bioequivalent (i.e. equivalent rate and extent of absorption) to three metformin extended-release 500 mg tablets in both fasting and fed healthy subjects [119, 120].

In clinical trials, metformin monotherapy reduced FPG by 52–92 mg/dl and A_{1c} by 1.4–2.0% over the dose range of 1700 mg–3000 mg daily (Table 2) [6, 14, 24, 28, 81, 85–94, 114, 115]. The majority of these trials enrolled overweight or obese patients with type 2 diabetes in whom glycemic control was inadequate with dietary changes alone. Reductions in these glycemic parameters are

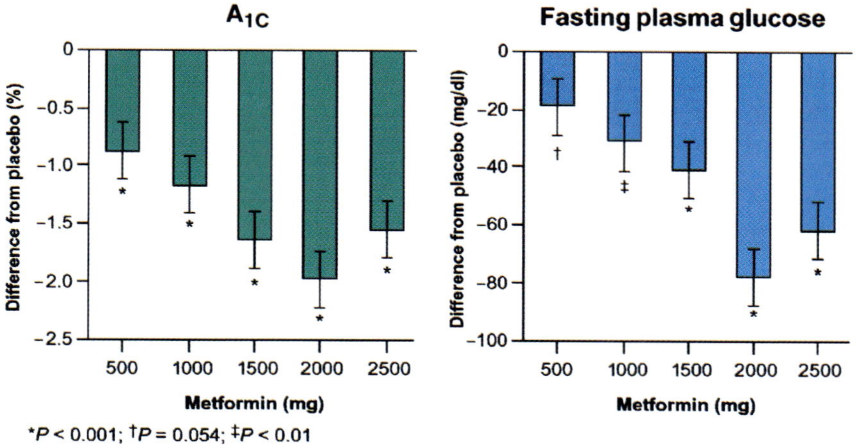

Figure 2 Dose-dependent changes in (a) glycosylated hemoglobin (A_{1c}) and (b) fasting plasma glucose (FPG) concentrations with metformin therapy in patients with type 2 diabetes. (Reprinted from reference 81, Copyright (1997), with permission from Excerpta Medica, Inc.)

log-linear and dose-dependent over the dose range of 500–2000 mg daily (Figure 2) [81]. Metformin is as effective as sulfonylureas or insulin in reducing FPG and A_{1c} levels in patients with type 2 diabetes [14, 15, 28, 87–91]. Fasting and postprandial serum insulin concentrations are unchanged or decreased with metformin, whereas they are increased with sulfonylureas [21, 28, 85].

Reductions in FPG and A_{1c} are comparable between metformin extended-release and immediate-release formulations [92]. Patients may be safely switched from immediate-release to extended-release metformin and maintain comparable glycemic control [93]. In a trial involving patients aged 10 years and older with type 2 diabetes, reductions in FPG and A_{1c} were significantly better than with placebo and slightly less than those observed in adult patients (Table 2) [92, 120].

Metformin in Combination with Other Glucose-Lowering Agents

The combination of metformin with either glyburide or glipizide has been evaluated as both a first-line and a second-line pharmacologic therapy for the management of type 2 diabetes (Table 2) [14, 87, 95–104]. The combination of metformin with a sulfonylurea is attractive as an option for first-line management of type 2 diabetes because it addresses the primary physiologic defects of type 2 diabetes (β-cell dysfunction and insulin resistance). This is particularly important in those patients with substantial hyperglycemia beyond that correctable with monotherapy. In comparative trials, metformin plus sulfonylurea, either as two tablets administered together or as glyburide/metformin tablets or glipizide/metformin tablets, provides significantly better glycemic control than either agent used alone.

The glyburide/metformin combination tablet contains metformin plus controlled particle-size glyburide ranging from 6 to 21 μm. A rapid release of glyburide occurs 2 to 3 h following oral administration, followed by a secondary peak 5–6 h postdose [56]. In contrast, glyburide tablets administered with metformin tablets produce a single peak serum concentration and a twofold lower glyburide delivery in the first 3 h, but the overall AUCs as a single dose and at steady state are similar [121]. The glyburide/metformin tablet with the controlled particle-size glyburide is associated with enhanced pharmacodynamics, compared with the coadministration of drugs as separate tablets. In a randomized, double-blind crossover study, 27 patients with type 2 diabetes received treatment with glyburide/metformin 2.5/500 mg tablets or the individual component tablets twice daily for 14 days. Treatments were separated by a 2-week washout period. Two-hour postprandial glucose excursion was significantly lower on day 14 after a mixed meal of solids and liquids with the combination tablet than with the individual drugs being coadministered (89.5 mg/dl vs. 117.4 mg/dl, respectively; $P = 0.011$) [121].

The combination tablet of glipizide/metformin is bioequivalent to the same doses of glipizide and metformin administered together as separate tablets [55]. Clinical data support its efficacy as a first- and second-line therapy for type 2 diabetes in randomized, double-blind comparative trials [95, 96].

Metformin also is available in combination with the thiazolidinedione rosiglitazone. Thiazolidinediones improve peripheral insulin sensitivity by interacting with peroxisome proliferator-activated receptor γ (PPAR-γ) nuclear receptors, which, when activated, stimulate the expression of insulin-responsive genes involved in glucose and lipid metabolism, primarily in muscle and adipose tissue.

Improvements in insulin sensitivity occur in skeletal muscle and whole-body adipose tissue with PPAR-γ agonists [122, 123], whereas metformin acts primarily in the liver and secondarily in the muscle. Although thiazolidinediones and metformin are both insulin sensitizers, their differing mechanisms for lowering insulin resistance, their site of action, and their lack of pharmacokinetic interaction when administered together provide rationale for the combination [124].

The development of the rosiglitazone/metformin combination tablet was based on bioequivalence data of the combination compared with each component administered together as separate tablets [57]. No clinical trials in diabetes have been published to date, regarding the efficacy or safety of the combination tablet.

In patients achieving a less than desirable response with metformin monotherapy, the addition of a thiazolidinedione (rosiglitazone or pioglitazone), acarbose, or a meglitinide (repaglinide or nateglinide) produces significant, additive reductions in A_{1c} and FPG, compared with the continuation of metformin monotherapy (Table 2) [105–109, 125]. The effects of adding a thiazolidinedione to metformin are more pronounced in the most obese patients [106]. Some evidence suggests that acarbose may reduce the bioavailability of metformin [126]; thus, this combination should be evaluated further to determine its value.

One study compared the efficacy of glyburide/metformin tablets with metformin plus rosiglitazone in patients with type 2 diabetes uncontrolled on metformin 1500 mg/day monotherapy [127]. The mean baseline A_{1c} was 8.4%. After 24 weeks of therapy titrated based on glycemic response, A_{1c} was reduced an additional 1.5% with glyburide/metformin combination tablet therapy and 1.1% with metformin plus rosiglitazone ($P < 0.001$). Decreases in FPG also were significantly greater with the glyburide/metformin regimen (–46 mg/dl) than with metformin plus rosiglitazone (–36 mg/dl) ($P = 0.03$). No patients receiving glyburide/metformin therapy discontinued because of lack of glycemic control, compared with 3.2% of patients receiving metformin plus rosiglitazone.

Given the availability of additional classes of oral antihyperglycemic agents, triple combination therapy is available for patients who cannot attain or maintain target glycemic control on dual therapy. The efficacy of glyburide/metformin tablets versus glyburide/metformin tablets plus rosiglitazone (dosage titrated to glycemic response) was compared in patients with long-standing type 2 diabetes [128]. After 24 weeks of therapy, A_{1c} values were reduced an additional 1.0% ($P < 0.001$) and FPG was reduced an additional 49 mg/dl ($P < 0.001$) with glyburide/metformin plus rosiglitazone versus glyburide/metformin tablets plus placebo. Although hypoglycemia occurred more frequently in the glyburide/metformin plus rosiglitazone group (22.1%) than in the glyburide/metformin tablets plus placebo group (3.3%), 65% of patients with hypoglycemia receiving glyburide/metformin tablets plus rosiglitazone also had final A_{1c} concentrations of 7.0% or lower. These results support the addition of rosiglitazone to an established regimen of glyburide/metformin in patients requiring additional glycemic control.

The addition of metformin to insulin therapy in patients with type 2 diabetes further improved FPG and A_{1c} and reduced insulin dosages by approximately 25–36% in some studies and obviated the need for insulin completely in other studies [110–115, 129]. Similarly, the use of metformin for 3 months in 27 adolescents with type 1 diabetes and high insulin dosage reduced A_{1c} values by 0.6% while lowering insulin dosages by 13%, compared with metformin plus placebo [83]. Additionally, metformin therapy does not induce hypoglycemia when added to insulin therapy, and compared with insulin monotherapy, metformin plus insulin is associated with weight loss and reductions in serum total and LDL cholesterol [110, 111, 113].

In addition to improved glycemic control, the use of metformin as an adjunct to other agents in the treatment of type 2 diabetes may allow patients to benefit from the macrovascular risk reductions associated with metformin therapy, which appear to be independent of glycemic effects [15].

Microvascular and Macrovascular Risk Reduction

The value of metformin monotherapy in reducing adverse microvascular and macrovascular endpoints in type 2 diabetes emerged in the UKPDS. This landmark trial was undertaken to determine the long-term effects of intensive glycemic control on complications of type 2 diabetes and whether any specific treatments (insulin, metformin, or sulfonylurea) were of particular benefit [130]. The study enrolled and followed 4075 patients with newly diagnosed type 2 diabetes. Patients had a mean age of 54 years and a mean baseline A_{1c} of 9.1%. Patients were randomly assigned to receive either conventional (mainly dietary) therapy with a goal FPG <270 mg/dl, or intensive therapy with sulfonylurea, insulin, or metformin (if >120% ideal body weight) with a target FPG <108 mg/dl. More than 80% of patients receiving conventional therapy ultimately required pharmacologic therapy to reach their glycemic target [6]. Predefined clinical endpoints were microvascular and macrovascular in nature and included any diabetes-related endpoint (i.e. sudden death, death from hypoglycemia, fatal or nonfatal myocardial infarction, angina, heart failure, stroke, renal failure, amputation of at least one digit, vitreous hemorrhage, retinopathy requiring photocoagulation, blindness in at least one eye, cataract extraction); diabetes-related death from myocardial infarction, stroke, peripheral vascular disease, renal disease, hyperglycemia, hypoglycemia, and sudden death; and all-cause mortality [6].

Over a mean of 10 years of follow-up, the intensively treated patients had a median A_{1c} concentration of 7.0% compared with 7.9% in conventionally treated patients [6]. The improvement in glycemic control in the intensive therapy relative to the conventional therapy group was associated with a 12% reduction in risk for any diabetes-related endpoint and a 25% reduction in the risk for microvascular complications. In a subsequent epidemiological analysis of the UKPDS data, it was shown that each 1% reduction in A_{1c} was associated with a 21% reduction in any diabetes-related endpoint, a 14% reduction in risk for myocardial infarction, and a 37% reduction in risk for microvascular complications [84].

Although a somewhat smaller A_{1c} difference was achieved in the intensive treatment group of overweight patients allocated to metformin therapy, a greater than expected benefit was observed [15]. Patients randomly assigned to metformin with a mean A_{1c} of 7.4% (compared with 8.0% in the conventional group) had significant reductions in risk for any diabetes-related endpoint, all-cause mortality, and stroke versus intensive therapy with sulfonylureas or insulin (Table 3, [8, 10, 15, 20, 21, 26, 34, 39, 58, 61, 85, 87, 88, 90, 114, 115, 131–152] Figure 3) [15]. The macrovascular risk reduction associated with metformin did not appear to be related to dose [51]. Among patients in whom metformin was added early following sulfonylurea failure, the risk for diabetes-related death was increased 96% compared with continued sulfonylurea monotherapy. However, it has been suggested that this unexpected finding is either the result of an unusually low death rate in the sulfonylurea monotherapy group or an increase in the event or mortality rate in the metformin plus sulfonylurea combination group or a chance occurrence [15, 153]. Indeed, a combined analysis of the main and supplementary UKPDS studies found a 19% reduction in risk in diabetes-related endpoints with metformin ($P = 0.033$). Additionally, a retrospective review of a large Saskatchewan database revealed no increase in cardiovascular endpoints with metformin [154]. To date, metformin is the only antidiabetic agent to show an independent benefit on the macrovascular complications of diabetes, by reducing the risk for myocardial infarction. Although the effects of metformin in this regard were independent of glucose-lowering effects (as all intensive therapies were similarly effective in achieving glycemic control as well as lipid-regulating effects), they are likely the result of the favorable effects of metformin on multiple nontraditional cardiovascular risk factors, in part, associated with insulin resistance, such as fibrinolysis, hyperinsulinemia, vascular inflammation, and endothelial dysfunction.

Lipid and Lipoprotein Parameters

Given the adverse cardiovascular outcomes associated with type 2 diabetes, risk factor management is critical to optimize patient outcomes. Indeed, serum lipid and blood pressure goals are more aggressive for individuals with type 2 diabetes than for nondiabetic individuals [155–157]. Metformin has well-documented favorable effects on serum lipid and lipoprotein parameters (Table 3) [20, 21, 39, 58, 61, 85, 87, 114, 115, 131–144, 146]. The most pronounced effects are reductions in serum triglycerides,

Table 3 Benefits of metformin on reducing microvascular and macrovascular complications of type 2 diabetes

Marker	Effect	References
Any diabetes-related endpoint	Reduced 31% compared with intensive sulfonylurea or insulin therapy in overweight patients ($P = 0.0034$); not evaluated in normal-weight patients	[15]
All-cause mortality	Reduced 36% compared with intensive sulfonylurea or insulin therapy in overweight patients ($P = 0.021$); not evaluated in normal-weight patients	[15]
Stroke	Reduced 41% compared with intensive sulfonylurea or insulin therapy in overweight patients ($P = 0.032$); not evaluated in normal-weight patients	[15]
Serum triglycerides	Decreased 15–45%; reductions correspond to baseline levels, with higher reductions in patients with higher baseline levels	[20, 21, 39, 58, 61, 85, 87, 114, 115, 131–139]
High-density lipoprotein cholesterol levels	Unchanged or slightly increased	[20, 21, 85, 87, 114, 138–143]
Low-density lipoprotein cholesterol levels	Decreased 8–10%	[87, 133, 142, 144]
Total serum cholesterol	Reduced 5–10%	[87, 134, 144–146]
Body weight	No weight loss reported in some studies, but most studies show mean weight loss ranging from 0.7 to 5 kg; greater magnitude of weight loss in heaviest patients	[8, 10, 26, 34, 58, 87, 88, 90, 147–150]
Fibrinolysis	Metformin significantly reduces PAI-1 concentrations 20%; also significantly reduces tPA concentrations and euglobin clot lysis time	[58, 85, 134, 151, 152]

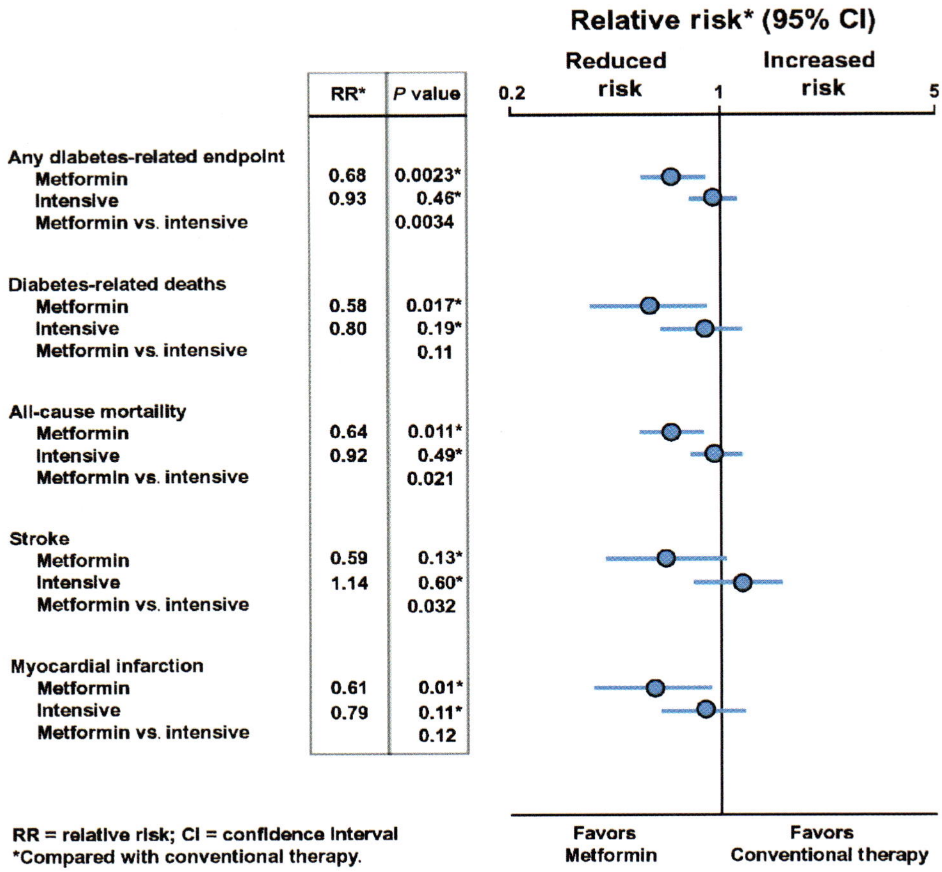

Figure 3 Clinical outcomes with metformin compared with other intensive therapy regimens. (Reprinted with permission from Elsevier (reference 15))

which range from 15 to 45%, depending on baseline serum triglycerides. Total and LDL cholesterol concentrations are also reduced, although to a lesser extent. HDL cholesterol concentrations are usually unchanged or slightly increased with metformin therapy. The lipid-improving effects of metformin occur in patients with type 2 diabetes as well as in those with prediabetic states (i.e. polycystic ovary syndrome and Syndrome X) and in nondiabetic individuals [61, 114, 137, 138, 146, 152]. Improvements occur when metformin is administered with sulfonylureas or insulin [87, 115, 158], but have not been observed when metformin is administered with a thiazolidinedione [105]. Withdrawal of metformin from combination therapy with sulfonylureas resulted in an increase in total and LDL cholesterol concentrations, which declined when metformin was reintroduced [133].

Possible mechanisms of action of metformin in reducing triglyceride concentrations include decreased synthesis of very low-density lipoprotein (VLDL) particles, which are lowered with metformin therapy [7, 20, 21, 138]; increased clearance of chylomicrons and remnants [40]; a direct inhibitory effect of metformin on hepatic VLDL secretion [20, 21, 141]; or modification of lipoprotein composition, such as a reduced amount of cholesterol in VLDL particles [141].

Body Weight

Metformin has been shown to reduce body weight independent of dosage. Mean weight loss in the range of 1–5 kg, or a 1–3% reduction from baseline, has been reported in clinical trials in both diabetic patients and nondiabetic individuals (Table 3) [8, 10, 26, 34, 58, 87, 88, 90, 147–150]. Weight loss is greatest in the most obese patients [26]. The majority of this effect is evident within 6 months of beginning metformin therapy [7]. The association between weight loss and metformin therapy is not clearly understood, but potential explanations include coincidentally reduced food consumption during therapy [149]; increased thermogenic activity of brown adipose tissue or increased futile substrate cycling [7]; enhanced carbohydrate utilization or carbohydrate malabsorption [135]; and reduced hyperinsulinemia [148]. Leptin concentrations do not appear to be affected by metformin [150].

The weight loss associated with metformin offers an additional advantage in terms of reducing adverse outcomes compared with other drug therapies for diabetes, which increase body weight, such as insulin, sulfonylurea therapy, and thiazolidinedione [6, 105, 106, 133, 144]. In the UKPDS, body weight increased by 4 kg in patients receiving insulin and by 1.7 kg in patients receiving glyburide [6]. In studies evaluating metformin plus rosiglitazone, patients receiving metformin monotherapy had mean weight losses from baseline of 0.9 kg (1% of body weight) in one study [106] and 1.2 kg in another study [105]. Corresponding mean weight gains with the rosiglitazone/metformin combination tablets in these respective studies were 2.5 kg (2.6% increase) [106] and 0.7–1.9 kg [105].

Fibrinolysis

Metformin enhances fibrinolytic response in patients with type 2 diabetes and in nondiabetic individuals [159]. PAI-1 concentrations are reduced approximately 20% with metformin therapy. tPA concentrations and euglobin clot lysis time also are significantly reduced with metformin therapy [134]. The effects of metformin on these parameters were dose-independent in a clinical trial, over the dose range of 1500–3000 mg daily [134]. The mechanism of action of metformin in increasing fibrinolytic activity is unknown.

PATIENT ADHERENCE

Good patient adherence is critical to the success of therapeutic regimens in chronic illnesses. However, it is difficult to achieve good adherence in the clinical setting, particularly when the disease being treated is typically asymptomatic, and drug administration does not result in symptom improvement. A factor that has consistently been shown to be associated with poor adherence is a complicated drug regimen, the need for numerous medications or frequent administration [160].

Adherence with antidiabetic regimens has received thorough study and supports a simplified dosing regimen [161–165]. In a national pharmacy claims database in the United States, patients who were prescribed glipizide extended-release had a mean adherence index of 60.5% versus a 52.0% adherence rate for patients receiving immediate-release glipizide twice daily ($P = 0.027$), even though patients receiving once-daily dosing required more pills per day than those receiving immediate-release glipizide (2.25 vs. 2.00, $P < 0.001$) [162]. Twelve months following initial prescription, 44.4% of patients receiving glipizide extended-release remained on therapy compared with 35.8% of those receiving immediate-release glipizide. In a US government insurer database, patients who received metformin or sulfonylurea monotherapy had approximately 65% more days of continuous treatment than did patients receiving therapy with multiple products [163]. In a Scottish population of 2920 patients with type 2 diabetes receiving a regimen consisting of a sulfonylurea plus metformin as individual tablets had a 13% lower adherence index compared with those receiving oral hypoglycemic monotherapy, which was statistically significant ($P < 0.01$) [164]. There was no difference in adherence rates between patients receiving sulfonylurea monotherapy or metformin monotherapy; however, once-daily dosing was associated with improved adherence, whereas each increase in daily dose frequency was associated with a 22% decrease in adherence. Among 1815 patients with type 2 diabetes prescribed metformin or glyburide monotherapy or the combination therapy for glycemic control, adherence rates were significantly lower, 54%, compared with 105 patients who were switched to the fixed-dose tablet (77%) [165]. Among patients previously receiving metformin and glyburide therapy as 2 tablets, adherence rates improved from 71 to 87% when they were switched to glyburide/metformin tablets. Thus, strategies to reduce dosing frequency of complicated regimens, such as extended-release formulations and combination products, are likely to improve long-term adherence and optimize patient outcomes.

SAFETY AND TOLERABILITY

Lactic Acidosis

The historical use of metformin since it became available more than 40 years ago has been greatly affected by the adverse safety profile of other biguanides. Lactic acidosis is the most severe reaction to biguanide therapy and is fatal in 50% of cases. Indeed, the excess risk for lactic acidosis was directly responsible for the withdrawal of phenformin from the market; this in turn precluded consideration of metformin for approval in the United States for many years. However, there are some important differences in the risk for developing lactic acidosis between phenformin and metformin. Metformin increases lactate oxidation, whereas phenformin alters the rate of serum lactate turnover [34]. Phenformin is partially metabolized in the liver through hydroxylation. Approximately 9% of the population has genetic polymorphisms that result in slow phenformin hydroxylation, which reduces drug clearance and predisposes individuals to the risk for developing lactic acidosis [145, 166, 167]. In contrast, metformin is excreted unchanged in the urine, primarily through tubular excretion [54]. The enhanced lipophilicity of phenformin relative to metformin may also play a role in the greater incidence of lactic acidosis with phenformin, as this biguanide can more readily penetrate lipid membranes and accumulate in the mitochondria [7]. The incidence of lactic acidosis with phenformin is estimated to be 10–20 times greater than with metformin [87].

Lactic acidosis is rare with metformin therapy. Evidence suggests that the overall incidence of lactic acidosis in patients with type 2 diabetes has decreased over time, presumably due to more prudent monitoring of patients. In the United States, lactic acidosis among patients with type 2 diabetes occurred at a rate of 9.7 episodes per 100 000 patient-years [168]; the incidence of lactic acidosis with metformin therapy is three cases per 100 000 patient-years [33, 168–171]. In Sweden, the incidence of metformin-associated lactic acidosis decreased from 1.5 cases per 10 000 patient-years during the years 1977 to 1981 to 0.24 cases per 10 000 patient-years from 1987 to 1991 [171]. In the vast majority of lactic acidosis cases occurring during metformin therapy, patients had concurrent illnesses that could have precipitated the reaction [168, 169, 171–174]. Moreover, in cases in which metformin was considered causally related to the development of lactic acidosis, patients had poor renal function (and thus were at risk for metformin accumulation) or were in hypoxic states (e.g. heart failure, surgical procedures), which increases the risk for developing lactic acidosis [54, 169, 175–177]. High plasma levels of metformin (>5 μg/ml) usually are found when metformin therapy is established as the cause of the reaction [54]. Only rarely has lactic acidosis occurred among patients receiving metformin without any other contributory causes or conditions [151, 169, 178, 179]. A recent large-scale study was undertaken to determine the long-term serious adverse event profile of metformin, either as monotherapy or as combination therapy with a sulfonylurea. The study was undertaken in patients with type 2 diabetes in a naturalistic, physician-based clinical practice setting [180]. A total of 8732 patients were randomly assigned in a 4:1 ratio to receive metformin therapy or usual care; 77% percent of patients completed the 1-year study. No hospitalizations or deaths due to lactic acidosis were reported in either group. A total of 445 patients (366 metformin and 79 usual care) participated in a substudy to evaluate the effects of therapy of plasma lactate levels [181]. After 12 months of treatment, mean plasma lactate levels were similar in the metformin and usual-care roups (1.76 mmol/lvs. 1.6 mmol/l, respectively; $P = 0.137$) These recent observations, together with the lack of increased incidence of lactic acidosis among metformin users versus patients with type 2 diabetes as a whole [168], support the opinion that lactic acidosis does not appear to be causally related to metformin therapy [176]. Relative to serious adverse reactions with other agents used for diabetes, the incidence of lactic acidosis in metformin-treated patients is lower than the incidence of hypoglycemic coma in patients treated with glyburide, although mortality rates with these conditions are comparable and notable [172].

The risk for developing lactic acidosis is increased in renal dysfunction, hepatic dysfunction, and with advanced age [54]. Metformin therapy is contraindicated in patients with renal dysfunction characterized by serum creatinine levels ≥ 1.5 mg/dl in men and ≥1.4 mg/dl in women; congestive heart failure requiring pharmacologic treatment; and acute or chronic metabolic acidosis, including diabetic ketoacidosis [54]. Additionally, since hepatic impairment has been associated with lactic acidosis, the use of metformin in patients with hepatic disease should be avoided. To further minimize the development of lactic acidosis, renal function, determined by creatinine clearance, should be monitored when metformin is used in patients aged 80 or older [54]. Metformin therapy should not be used in patients with evidence of hypoxemia, dehydration, or sepsis. Alcohol intake should also be avoided with metformin therapy, as alcohol may potentiate an effect of metformin on lactate metabolism [54]. When therapy with drugs that may interfere with renal function and have been associated with lactic acidosis, such as iodinated contrast materials, is necessary, metformin should be temporarily discontinued before or at the time of the contrast procedure and withheld for 48 h after the procedure to assess adequacy of renal function [54].

Other Adverse Events

The most common adverse events occurring with metformin therapy are gastrointestinal in nature and appear to be dose-independent (Table 4) [54]. Although gastrointestinal adverse events are notable, they rarely result

Table 4 Frequency (%) of adverse events occurring in more than 5% of patients receiving metformin immediate-release and extended-release therapy and occurring more frequently than with placebo in controlled clinical trials*

Adverse event	Metformin ($N = 141$)	Placebo ($N = 145$)	Metformin extended-release ($N = 781$)	Placebo ($N = 195$)
Diarrhea	53.5	11.7	9.6	2.6
Nausea/vomiting	25.5	8.3	6.5	1.5
Flatulence	12.1	5.5	—	—
Asthenia	9.2	5.5	—	—
Indigestion	7.1	4.1	—	—
Abdominal discomfort	6.4	4.8	—	—
Headache	5.7	4.8	—	—

* From reference 54.

in drug discontinuation. In clinical trials, only 4–6% of patients discontinued due to intolerable adverse events [54, 81, 101]. Gastrointestinal symptoms are usually transient and subside with continued treatment [101].

Gastrointestinal tolerability can be improved by initiating metformin therapy at low doses and slowly titrating to effect, taking metformin doses with meals, and using metformin extended-release tablets. As mentioned previously, treatment-emergent gastrointestinal adverse events have been reported less frequently by patients receiving metformin extended-release 1000 mg tablets daily (29%) than with immediate-release metformin 500 mg twice daily (39%) [93].

Reductions in serum vitamin B_{12} and folic acid have been observed in a small percentage of patients receiving metformin therapy (7%), presumably due to impaired gastric absorption of these vitamins with metformin [54, 87, 182, 183]. In a study of 60 nondiabetic male patients with cardiovascular disease, metformin treatment was associated with a reduction in serum vitamin B_{12} and folic acid concentrations and an increase in homocysteine concentrations [183]. A study involving 40 patients with type 2 diabetes found only slight differences in homocysteine concentrations between those who received metformin for 6 months compared with those who did not (11.5 μmol/l vs. 10.6 μmol/l, respectively) [184].

Serious adverse events with metformin (including those requiring hospitalizations and serious episodes of hypoglycemia) occur at a rate similar to other diabetic therapies and generally reflect the expected events in this population of patients. In the large-scale study involving 8732 patients mentioned previously [180], 10.3% of metformin-treated patients and 11.0% of usual-care patients reported at least one serious adverse event during the 1-year observation period. Cardiac disorders occurred in 3.3% of both metformin and usual-care groups. Vascular disorders were more common in usual-care patients (2.4%) than in metformin-treated patients (1.4%). A retrospective cohort study was performed to assess the incidence of serious acute liver injury with glucose-lowering pharmacotherapy [185]. In a cohort of 171 264 health insurance plan members receiving oral hypoglycemic agents or insulin, there were 35 cases of acute liver failure not attributable to causes other than the use of these agents. The incidence of liver injury per 1000 patient-years was 0.08 for sulfonylurea users, 0.10 for troglitazone users, 0.12 for metformin users, and 0.15 for insulin users. Thus, relative to other therapies, metformin use is not associated with increased serious adverse events, including acute hepatotoxicity.

There are no human data to support the use of metformin during pregnancy, although in animal studies metformin was not teratogenic at six times the maximum recommended human dosage [54]. However, aggressive glycemic control is warranted during pregnancy to reduce the risk for congenital abnormalities.

SUMMARY

Metformin is a valuable agent for the treatment of type 2 diabetes. Its ability to improve insulin sensitivity allows for broader use beyond the treatment of type 2 diabetes (i.e., prediabetic states, diabetes prevention, polycystic ovary syndrome, and metabolic syndrome). The efficacy of metformin in improving glycemic control and reducing microvascular complications of disease is similar to that of other oral agents used for the treatment of diabetes. However, unlike those agents, metformin has been shown to provide additional benefits in reducing macrovascular complications of type 2 diabetes in overweight patients, including any diabetes-related endpoint, all-cause mortality, and stroke [15]. Metformin also improves serum lipoprotein parameters, reduces body weight, and stimulates fibrinolysis, factors that likely contribute to reduced adverse macrovascular outcomes that are exclusive to metformin.

Metformin can be administered with insulin and other oral antihyperglycemic agents. Given the complementary actions of metformin and other classes of agents and the multiple metabolic defects in type 2 diabetes, improvements in glycemic parameters are additive when metformin is combined with other agents. Insulin dosages can be reduced with metformin therapy or obviated altogether. The recent availability of metformin in an extended-release formulation and in combination tablets (together with glyburide, glipizide, or rosiglitazone) allows for simplified dosage regimens. This is particularly attractive among a population of patients likely having comorbidities and requiring multiple medications.

REFERENCES

1. Witters LA. The blooming of the French lilac. *J Clin Invest* 2001; 108: 1105–7.
2. Bailey CJ, Day C. Traditional plant medicines as treatments for diabetes. *Diabetes Care* 1989; 12: 553–64.
3. Schafer G. Biguanides. A review of history, pharmacodynamics, and therapy. *Diabete Metab* 1983; 9: 148–63.
4. Meinart CL, Knatterud GL, Prout TE, Klimt CR. A study of the effects of hypoglycemic agents on vascular complications with adult-onset diabetes, II: Mortality results. *Diabetes* 1970; 19 (suppl): 789–830.
5. University Group Diabetes Program. A study of the effects of hypoglycemic agents on vascular complications in patients with adult-onset diabetes, V: Evaluation of phenformin therapy. *Diabetes* 1975; 24 (suppl 1): 65–184.
6. UK Prospective Diabetes Study (UKPDS) Group. Intensive blood-glucose control with sulfonylureas or insulin compared with conventional treatment and risk of complications in patients with type 2 diabetes (UKPDS 33). *Lancet* 1998; 352: 837–53.
7. Bailey CJ. Biguanides and NIDDM. *Diabetes Care* 1992; 15: 755–72.
8. Clarke BF, Duncan LJ. Comparison of chlorpropamide and metformin treatment on weight and blood-glucose

response of uncontrolled obese diabetics. *Lancet* 1968; 1: 123–6.
9. Hermann LS. Metformin: a review of its pharmacological properties and therapeutic use. *Diabete Metab* 1979; 5: 233–45.
10. Clarke BF, Campbell IW. Comparison of metformin and chlorpropamide in non-obese, maturity-onset diabetics uncontrolled by diet. *BMJ* 1977; 2: 1576–8.
11. Lim P, Khoo OT. Metformin compared with tolbutamide in the treatment of maturity-onset diabetes mellitus. *Med J Aust* 1970; 1: 271–3.
12. Nattrass M, Hinks L, Smythe P, Todd PG, Alberti KG. Metabolic effects of combined sulfonylurea and metformin therapy in maturity-onset diabetes. *Horm Metab Res* 1979; 11: 332–7.
13. Clarke BF, Duncan LJP. Biguanide treatment in the management of insulin dependent (maturity-onset) diabetes: clinical experience with metformin. *Res Clin Forums* 1979; 1: 53–63.
14. Campbell IW, Howlett HC. Worldwide experience of metformin as an effective glucose-lowering agent: a meta-analysis. *Diabetes Metab Rev* 1995; 11 (suppl 1): S57–62.
15. UK Prospective Diabetes Study (UKPDS) Group. Effect of intensive blood-glucose control with metformin on complications in overweight patients with type 2 diabetes (UKPDS 34). *Lancet* 1998; 352: 854–65.
16. Wandell PE, Gafvels C. Drug prescription in men and women with type-2 diabetes in Stockholm in 1995 and 2001: change over time. *Eur J Clin Pharmacol* 2002; 58: 547–53.
17. Hermann LS, Melander A. Biguanides: basic aspects and clinical uses. In Alberti KGMN, Zimmer P, DeFronzo RA, Keen H (eds), *International Textbook of Diabetes Mellitus*. Chichester, UK: Wiley 1997; pp 841–64.
18. Olefsky JM, Nolan JJ. Insulin resistance and non-insulin-dependent diabetes mellitus: cellular and molecular mechanisms. *Am J Clin Nutr* 1995; 61: 980S–6S.
19. Groop LC, Bonadonna RC, Del Prato S, Ratheiser K, Zyck K, Ferrannini E, DeFronzo RA. Glucose and free fatty acid metabolism in non-insulin-dependent diabetes mellitus: evidence for multiple sites of insulin resistance. *J Clin Invest* 1989; 84: 205–13.
20. Jeppesen J, Zhou MY, Chen YD, Reaven GM. Effect of metformin on postprandial lipemia in patients with fairly to poorly controlled NIDDM. *Diabetes Care* 1994; 17: 1093–9.
21. Wu MS, Johnston P, Sheu WH, Hollenbeck CB, Jeng CY, Goldfine ID, Chen YD, Reaven GM. Effect of metformin on carbohydrate and lipoprotein metabolism in NIDDM patients. *Diabetes Care* 1990; 13: 1–8.
22. Hother-Nielsen O, Schmitz O, Andersen PH, Beck-Nielsen H, Pedersen O. Metformin improves peripheral but not hepatic insulin action in obese patients with type II diabetes. *Acta Endocrinol* (*Copenh*) 1989; 120: 257–65.
23. Riccio A, Del Prato S, Vigili DK, Tiengo A. Glucose and lipid metabolism in non-insulin-dependent diabetes: effect of metformin. *Diabete Metab* 1991; 17: 180–4.
24. McIntyre HD, Ma A, Bird DM, Paterson CA, Ravenscroft PJ, Cameron DP. Metformin increases insulin sensitivity and basal glucose clearance in type 2 (non-insulin dependent) diabetes mellitus. *Aust NZ J Med* 1991; 21: 714–9.
25. Prager R, Schernthaner G. Insulin receptor binding to monocytes, insulin secretion, and glucose tolerance following metformin treatment: results of a double-blind cross-over study in type II diabetics. *Diabetes* 1983; 32: 1083–6.
26. DeFronzo RA, Barzilai N, Simonson DC. Mechanism of metformin action in obese and lean noninsulin-dependent diabetic subjects. *J Clin Endocrinol Metab* 1991; 73: 1294–301.
27. Johnson AB, Webster JM, Sum CF, Heseltine L, Argyraki M, Cooper BG, Taylor R. The impact of metformin therapy on hepatic glucose production and skeletal muscle glycogen synthase activity in overweight type II diabetic patients. *Metabolism* 1993; 42: 1217–22.
28. Hermann LS, Schersten B, Bitzen PO, Kjellstrom T, Lindgarde F, Melander A. Therapeutic comparison of metformin and sulfonylurea, alone and in various combinations: a double-blind controlled study. *Diabetes Care* 1994; 17: 1100–9.
29. Gregorio F, Ambrosi F, Marchetti P, Cristallini S, Navalesi R, Brunetti P, Filipponi P. Low-dose metformin in the treatment of type II non-insulin-dependent diabetes: clinical and metabolic evaluations. *Acta Diabetol Lat* 1990; 27: 139–55.
30. Abbasi F, Kamath V, Rizvi AA, Carantoni M, Chen YD, Reaven GM. Results of a placebo-controlled study of the metabolic effects of the addition of metformin to sulfonylurea-treated patients: evidence for a central role of adipose tissue. *Diabetes Care* 1997; 20: 1863–9.
31. Nosadini R, Avogaro A, Trevisan R, Valerio A, Tessari P, Duner E, Tiengo A, Velussi M, Del Prato S, De Kreutzenberg S. Effect of metformin on insulin-stimulated glucose turnover and insulin binding to receptors in type II diabetes. *Diabetes Care* 1987; 10: 62–7.
32. Fantus IG, Brosseau R. Mechanism of action of metformin: insulin receptor and postreceptor effects in vitro and in vivo. *J Clin Endocrinol Metab* 1986; 63: 898–905.
33. Cusi K, DeFronzo RA. Metformin: a review of its metabolic effects. *Diabetes Rev* 1998; 6: 89–131.
34. Stumvoll M, Nurjhan N, Perriello G, Dailey G, Gerich JE. Metabolic effects of metformin in non-insulin-dependent diabetes mellitus. *N Engl J Med* 1995; 333: 550–4.
35. Perriello G, Misericordia P, Volpi E, Santucci A, Santucci C, Ferrannini E, Ventura MM, Santeusanio F, Brunetti P, Bolli GB. Acute antihyperglycemic mechanisms of metformin in NIDDM: evidence for suppression of lipid oxidation and hepatic glucose production. *Diabetes* 1994; 43: 920–8.
36. Widen EI, Eriksson JG, Groop LC. Metformin normalizes nonoxidative glucose metabolism in insulin-resistant normoglycemic first-degree relatives of patients with NIDDM. *Diabetes* 1992; 41: 354–8.
37. Dunn CJ, Peters DH. Metformin: a review of its pharmacological properties and therapeutic use in non-insulin-dependent diabetes mellitus. *Drugs* 1995; 49: 721–49.
38. Lehtovirta M, Forsen B, Gullstrom M, Haggblom M, Eriksson JG, Taskinen MR, Groop L. Metabolic effects of metformin in patients with impaired glucose tolerance. *Diabet Med* 2001; 18: 578–83.
39. Zavaroni I, Dall'Aglio E, Bruschi F, Alpi O, Coscelli C, Butturini U. Inhibition of carbohydrate-induced hypertriglyceridemia by metformin. *Horm Metab Res* 1984; 16: 85–7.
40. Grosskopf I, Ringel Y, Charach G, Maharshak N, Mor R, Iaina A, Weintraub M. Metformin enhances clearance of chylomicrons and chylomicron remnants in nondiabetic mildly overweight glucose-intolerant subjects. *Diabetes Care* 1997; 20: 1598–602.

41. Prager R, Schernthaner G, Graf H. Effect of metformin on peripheral insulin sensitivity in non-insulin-dependent diabetes mellitus. *Diabete Metab* 1986; 12: 346–50.
42. Marena S, Tagliaferro V, Montegrosso G, Pagano A, Scaglione L, Pagano G. Metabolic effects of metformin addition to chronic glibenclamide treatment in type 2 diabetes. *Diabete Metab* 1994; 20: 15–9.
43. Musi N, Goodyear LJ. Targeting the AMP-activated protein kinase for the treatment of type 2 diabetes. *Curr Drug Targets Immune Endocr Metab Disord* 2002; 2: 119–27.
44. Ruderman NB, Cacicedo JM, Itani S, Yagihashi N, Saha AK, Ye JM, Chen K, Zou M, Carling D, Boden G, Cohen RA, Keaney J, Kraegen EW, Ido Y. Malonyl-CoA and AMP-activated protein kinase (AMPK): possible links between insulin resistance in muscle and early endothelial cell damage in diabetes. *Biochem Soc Trans* 2003; 31: 202–6.
45. Zhou G, Myers R, Li Y, Chen Y, Shen X, Fenyk-Melody J, Wu M, Ventre J, Doebber T, Fujii N, Musi N, Hirshman MF, Goodyear LJ, Moller DE. Role of AMP-activated protein kinase in mechanism of metformin action. *J Clin Invest* 2001; 108: 1167–74.
46. Musi N, Hirshman MF, Nygren J, Svanfeldt M, Bavenholm P, Rooyackers O, Zhou G, Williamson JM, Ljunqvist O, Efendic S, Moller DE, Thorell A, Goodyear LJ. Metformin increases AMP-activated protein kinase activity in skeletal muscle of subjects with type 2 diabetes. *Diabetes* 2002; 51: 2074–81.
47. Stith BJ, Woronoff K, Wiernsperger N. Stimulation of the intracellular portion of the human insulin receptor by the antidiabetic drug metformin. *Biochem Pharmacol* 1998; 55: 533–6.
48. Hamann A, Benecke H, Greten H, Matthaei S. Metformin increases glucose transporter protein and gene expression in human fibroblasts. *Biochem Biophys Res Commun* 1993; 196: 382–7.
49. Gunton JE, Delhanty PJ, Takahashi S, Baxter RC. Metformin rapidly increases insulin receptor activation in human liver and signals preferentially through insulin-receptor substrate-2. *J Clin Endocrinol Metab* 2003; 88: 1323–32.
50. He G, Pedersen SB, Bruun JM, Lihn AS, Richelsen B. Metformin, but not thiazolidinediones, inhibits plasminogen activator inhibitor-1 production in human adipose tissue in vitro. *Horm Metab Res* 2003; 35: 18–23.
51. Stratton IM, Holman RR. Is the cardioprotective effect of metformin in type 2 diabetes dose dependent? *Diabetes* 2003; 52 (suppl 1): A167.
52. The diabetes prevention program. Design and methods for a clinical trial in the prevention of type 2 diabetes. *Diabetes Care* 1999; 22: 623–34.
53. Knowler WC, Barrett-Connor E, Fowler SE, Hamman RF, Lachin JM, Walker EA, Nathan DM. Reduction in the incidence of type 2 diabetes with lifestyle intervention or metformin. *N Engl J Med* 2002; 346: 393–403.
54. *Glucophage® (metformin hydrochloride tablets) and Glucophage® XR (Metformin Hydrochloride Extended-Release Tablets) Prescribing Information*. Princeton, NJ: Bristol-Myers Squibb Company, 2001.
55. *Metaglip™ (Glipizide/Metformin Tablet) Prescribing Information*. Princeton, NJ: Bristol-Myers Squibb Company, 2002.
56. *Glucovance® (Glyburide/Metformin Tablets) Prescribing Information*. Princeton, NJ: Bristol-Myers Squibb Company, 2002.
57. *Avandamet™ (Rosiglitazone/Metformin Tablet) Prescribing Information*. King of Prussia, PA: GlaxoSmith-Kline 2002.
58. Fontbonne A, Charles MA, Juhan-Vague I, Bard JM, Andre P, Isnard F, Cohen JM, Grandmottet P, Vague P, Safar ME, Eschwege E., for the BIGPRO Study Group. The effect of metformin on the metabolic abnormalities associated with upper-body fat distribution. *Diabetes Care* 1996; 19: 920–6.
59. Baillie GM, Sherer JT, Weart CW. Insulin and coronary artery disease: is syndrome X the unifying hypothesis? *Ann Pharmacother* 1998; 32: 233–47.
60. Deedwania PC. The deadly quartet revisited. *Am J Med* 1998; 105: 1S–3S.
61. Landin K, Tengborn L, Smith U. Treating insulin resistance in hypertension with metformin reduces both blood pressure and metabolic risk factors. *J Intern Med* 1991; 229: 181–7.
62. Giugliano D, De Rosa N, Di Maro G, Marfella R, Acampora R, Buoninconti R, D'Onofrio F. Metformin improves glucose, lipid metabolism, and reduces blood pressure in hypertensive, obese women. *Diabetes Care* 1993; 16: 1387–90.
63. Scheen AJ, Letiexhe MR, Lefebvre PJ. Effects of metformin in obese patients with impaired glucose tolerance. *Diabetes Metab Rev* 1995; 11 (suppl 1): S69–80.
64. Scheen AJ, Letiexhe MR, Lefebvre PJ. Short administration of metformin improves insulin sensitivity in android obese subjects with impaired glucose tolerance. *Diabet Med* 1995; 12: 985–9.
65. Lakka HM, Laaksonen DE, Lakka TA, Niskanen LK, Kumpusalo E, Toumilehto J, Salonen JT. The metabolic syndrome and total and cardiovascular disease mortality in middle-aged men. *JAMA* 2002; 288: 2706–16.
66. Nestler JE, Stovall D, Akhter N, Iuorno MJ, Jakubowicz DJ. Strategies for the use of insulin-sensitizing drugs to treat infertility in women with polycystic ovary syndrome. *Fertil Steril* 2002; 77: 209–15.
67. Zarate A, Hernandez M, Fonseca ME, Ochoa R. Use of metformin in the management of adolescents with polycystic ovary syndrome. *Ginecol Obstet Mex* 1997; 65: 504–7.
68. Velazquez E, Acosta A, Mendoza SG. Menstrual cyclicity after metformin therapy in polycystic ovary syndrome. *Obstet Gynecol* 1997; 90: 392–5.
69. Velazquez EM, Mendoza S, Hamer T, Sosa F, Glueck CJ. Metformin therapy in polycystic ovary syndrome reduces hyperinsulinemia, insulin resistance, hyperandrogenemia, and systolic blood pressure, while facilitating normal menses and pregnancy. *Metabolism* 1994; 43: 647–54.
70. Velazquez EM, Mendoza SG, Wang P, Glueck CJ. Metformin therapy is associated with a decrease in plasma plasminogen activator inhibitor-1, lipoprotein(a), and immunoreactive insulin levels in patients with the polycystic ovary syndrome. *Metabolism* 1997; 46: 454–7.
71. Acbay O, Gundogdu S. Can metformin reduce insulin resistance in polycystic ovary syndrome? *Fertil Steril* 1996; 65: 946–9.
72. Crave JC, Fimbel S, Lejeune H, Cugnardey N, Dechaud H, Pugeat M. Effects of diet and metformin administration on sex hormone-binding globulin, androgens, and insulin in hirsute and obese women. *J Clin Endocrinol Metab* 1995; 80: 2057–62.
73. Ehrmann DA, Cavaghan MK, Imperial J, Sturis J, Rosenfield RL, Polonsky KS. Effects of metformin on

insulin secretion, insulin action, and ovarian steroidogenesis in women with polycystic ovary syndrome. *J Clin Endocrinol Metab* 1997; 82: 524–30.

74. Glueck CJ, Wang P, Fontaine R, Tracy T, Sieve-Smith L. Metformin-induced resumption of normal menses in 39 of 43 (91%) previously amenorrheic women with the polycystic ovary syndrome. *Metabolism* 1999; 48: 511–9.
75. Morin-Papunen LC, Koivunen RM, Ruokonen A, Martikainen HK. Metformin therapy improves the menstrual pattern with minimal endocrine and metabolic effects in women with polycystic ovary syndrome. *Fertil Steril* 1998; 69: 691–6.
76. Diamanti-Kandarakis E, Kouli C, Tsianateli T, Bergiele A. Therapeutic effects of metformin on insulin resistance and hyperandrogenism in polycystic ovary syndrome. *Eur J Endocrinol* 1998; 138: 269–74.
77. Nestler JE, Jakubowicz DJ, Evans WS, Pasquali R. Effects of metformin on spontaneous and clomiphene-induced ovulation in the polycystic ovary syndrome. *N Engl J Med* 1998; 338: 1876–80.
78. George SS, George K, Irwin C, Job V, Selvakumar R, Jeyaseelan V, Seshadri MS. Sequential treatment of metformin and clomiphene citrate in clomiphene-resistant women with polycystic ovary syndrome: a randomized, controlled trial. *Hum Reprod* 2003; 18: 299–304.
79. Hadigan C, Rabe J, Grinspoon S. Sustained benefits of metformin therapy on markers of cardiovascular risk in human immunodeficiency virus-infected patients with fat redistribution and insulin resistance. *J Clin Endocrinol Metab* 2002; 87: 4611–5.
80. Gore DC, Wolf SE, Herndon DN, Wolfe RR. Metformin blunts stress-induced hyperglycemia after thermal injury. *J Trauma* 2003; 54: 555–61.
81. Garber AJ, Duncan TG, Goodman AM, Mills DJ, Rohlf JL. Efficacy of metformin in type II diabetes: results of a double-blind, placebo-controlled, dose-response trial. *Am J Med* 1997; 103: 491–7.
82. American Diabetes Association. Type 2 diabetes in children and adolescents. *Diabetes Care* 2000; 23: 381–9.
83. Hamilton J, Cummings E, Zdravkovic V, Finegood D, Daneman D. Metformin as an adjunct therapy in adolescents with type 1 diabetes and insulin resistance: a randomized controlled trial. *Diabetes Care* 2003; 26: 138–43.
84. Stratton IM, Adler AI, Neil HA, Matthews DR, Manley SE, Cull CA, Hadden D, Turner RC, Holman RR on behalf of the UK Prospective Diabetes Study Group. Association of glycaemia with macrovascular and microvascular complications of type 2 diabetes (UKPDS 35): prospective observational study. *BMJ* 2000; 321: 405–12.
85. Nagi DK, Yudkin JS. Effects of metformin on insulin resistance, risk factors for cardiovascular disease, and plasminogen activator inhibitor in NIDDM subjects: a study of two ethnic groups. *Diabetes Care* 1993; 16: 621–9.
86. Hoffmann J, Spengler M. Efficacy of 24-week monotherapy with acarbose, metformin, or placebo in dietary-treated NIDDM patients: the Essen-II Study. *Am J Med* 1997; 103: 483–90.
87. DeFronzo RA, Goodman AM. Efficacy of metformin in patients with non-insulin-dependent diabetes mellitus: the Multicenter Metformin Study Group. *N Engl J Med* 1995; 333: 541–9.
88. Campbell IW, Menzies DG, Chalmers J, McBain AM, Brown IR. One year comparative trial of metformin and glipizide in type 2 diabetes mellitus. *Diabete Metab* 1994; 20: 394–400.
89. Turner R, Cull C, Holman R. United Kingdom prospective diabetes study 17: a 9-year update of a randomized, controlled trial on the effect of improved metabolic control on complications in non-insulin-dependent diabetes mellitus. *Ann Intern Med* 1996; 124: 136–45.
90. UKPDS Group. United Kingdom prospective diabetes study (UKPDS) 13: relative efficacy of randomly allocated diet, sulfonylurea, insulin, or metformin in patients with newly diagnosed non-insulin dependent diabetes followed for three years. *BMJ* 1995; 310: 83–8.
91. Calle-Pascual AL, Garcia-Honduvilla J, Martin-Alvarez PJ, Vara E, Calle JR, Munguira ME, Maranes JP. Comparison between acarbose, metformin, and insulin treatment in type 2 diabetic patients with secondary failure to sulfonylurea treatment. *Diabete Metab* 1995; 21: 256–60.
92. Niecestro R, Luckacsko P, Walters E, Sterman A, Friedhoff L, Isaacsohn J. Safety and efficacy of metformin XT to immediate-release metformin in patients with type 2 diabetes. *Diabetes* 2002; 51 (suppl 2): A131–2.
93. Fujioka K, Pans M, Joyal S. Glycemic control in patients with type 2 diabetes mellitus switched from twice-daily immediate-release metformin to a once-daily extended-release formulation. *Clin Ther* 2003; 25: 515–29.
94. Jones KL, Arslanian S, Peterokova VA, Park JS, Tomlinson MJ. Effect of metformin in pediatric patients with type 2 diabetes: a randomized controlled trial. *Diabetes Care* 2002; 25: 89–94.
95. Rubin CJ, Soufer J, Pieters A, Fiedorek FT. Glipizide/metformin tablets as first-line treatment in type 2 diabetes: efficacy, safety, and tolerability. *Diabetes* 2002; 51 (suppl 2): A113.
96. Rubin CJ, Meneghini L, Pans M, Fiedorek FT. Glipizide/metformin tablets as second-line therapy in type 2 diabetes: efficacy, safety, and tolerability. *Diabetes* 2002; 51 (suppl 2): A113.
97. Garber AJ, Larsen J, Schneider SH, Piper BA, Henry D. Simultaneous glyburide/metformin therapy is superior to component monotherapy as an initial pharmacological treatment for type 2 diabetes. *Diabetes Obes Metab* 2002; 4: 201–8.
98. Garber AJ, Bruce S, Fiedorek FT. Durability of efficacy and long-term safety profile of glyburide/metformin tablets in patients with type 2 diabetes mellitus: an open-label extension study. *Clin Ther* 2002; 24: 1401–13.
99. Bokhari SU, Gopal UM, Duckworth WC. Beneficial effects of a glyburide/metformin combination preparation in type 2 diabetes mellitus. *Am J Med Sci* 2003; 325: 66–9.
100. Duckworth M, Marcelli M, Padden M, Kellick K, Duhancik T, Wilhardt M, Colgan K, Romie A. Improvements in glycemic control in type 2 diabetes patients switched from sulfonylurea coadministered with metformin to glyburide-metformin tablets. *J Manag Care Pharm* 2003; 9: 256–62.
101. Haupt E, Knick B, Koschinsky T, Liebermeister H, Schneider J, Hirche H. Oral antidiabetic combination therapy with sulfonylureas and metformin. *Diabete Metab* 1991; 17: 224–31.
102. Blonde L, Rosenstock J, Mooradian AD, Piper BA, Henry D. Glyburide/metformin combination product is safe and efficacious in patients with type 2 diabetes failing sulfonylurea therapy. *Diabetes Obes Metab* 2002; 46: 368–75.

103. Marre M, Howlett H, Lehert P, Allavoine T. Improved glycemic control with metformin-glibenclamide combined tablet therapy (Glucovance®) in type 2 diabetic patients inadequately controlled on metformin. *Diabet Med* 2002; 19: 673–80.
104. Blonde L, Rosenstock J, Piper BA, Henry D. Durable antidiabetic effect of glyburide/metformin tablets as second-line therapy for type 2 diabetes. *Diabetes* 2001; 50 (suppl 2): A106.
105. Fonseca V, Rosenstock J, Patwardhan R, Salzman A. Effect of metformin and rosiglitazone combination therapy in patients with type 2 diabetes mellitus: a randomized controlled trial. *JAMA* 2000; 283: 1695–702.
106. Jones TA, Sautter M, Van Gaal LF, Jones NP. Addition of rosiglitazone to metformin is most effective in obese, insulin-resistant patients with type 2 diabetes. *Diabetes Obes Metab* 2003; 5: 163–70.
107. Rosenstock J, Brown A, Fischer J, Jain A, Littlejohn T, Nadeau D, Sussman A, Taylor T, Krol A, Magner J. Efficacy and safety of acarbose in metformin-treated patients with type 2 diabetes. *Diabetes Care* 1998; 21: 2050–5.
108. Chiasson JL, Josse RG, Hunt JA, Palmason C, Rodger NW, Ross SA, Ryan EA, Tan MH, Wolever TMS. The efficacy of acarbose in the treatment of patients with non-insulin-dependent diabetes mellitus: a multicenter controlled clinical trial. *Ann Intern Med* 1994; 121: 928–35.
109. Moses R, Slobodniuk R, Boyages S, Colagiuri S, Kidson W, Carter J, Donnelly T, Moffitt P, Hopkins H. Effect of repaglinide addition to metformin monotherapy on glycemic control in patients with type 2 diabetes. *Diabetes Care* 1999; 22: 119–24.
110. Bell DSH, Mayo MS. Outcome of metformin-facilitated reinitiation of oral diabetic therapy in insulin-treated patients with non-insulin-dependent diabetes mellitus. *Endocr Pract* 1997; 3: 73–6.
111. Bergenstal RM. Optimization of insulin therapy in patients with type 2 diabetes. *Endocr Pract* 2000; 6: 93–7.
112. Aviles-Santa L, Sinding J, Raskin P. The effects of metformin in poorly controlled insulin-treated type 2 diabetes mellitus. *Diabetes* 1998; 47 (suppl 1): A89.
113. Yki-Jarvinen H, Ryysy L, Nikkila K, Tulokas T, Vanamo R, Heikkila M. Comparison of bedtime insulin regimens in patients with type 2 diabetes mellitus: a randomized, controlled trial. *Ann Intern Med* 1999; 130: 389–96.
114. Giugliano D, Quatraro A, Consoli G, Minei A, Ceriello A, De Rosa N, D'Onofrio F. Metformin for obese, insulin-treated diabetic patients: improvement in glycemic control and reduction of metabolic risk factors. *Eur J Clin Pharmacol* 1993; 44: 107–12.
115. Robinson AC, Burke J, Robinson S, Johnston DG, Elkeles RS. The effects of metformin on glycemic control and serum lipids in insulin-treated NIDDM patients with suboptimal metabolic control. *Diabetes Care* 1998; 21: 701–5.
116. Marathe P, Turner K. Steady-state pharmacokinetics of the metformin extended-release tablet versus the immediate-release tablet of metformin in healthy subjects. *Diabetes* 2002; 51 (suppl 2): A474.
117. Donahue S, Marathe P, Guld T, Meeker J. The pharmacokinetics and pharmacodynamics of the metformin extended-release tablet versus immediate-release metformin in subjects with type 2 diabetes. *Diabetes* 2002; 51 (suppl 2): A468.
118. Lamson M, Niecestro RM, Luckacsko P, Sterman A, Howard C, Walters E, Friedhoff L, Isaacsohn J. Pharmacokinetics of metformin XT versus immediate-release metformin. *Diabetes* 2002; 51 (suppl 2): A131.
119. Gao X, Xie J, Moore KT, Uderman HD, Areeves RA, Turner KC. Glucophage® extended release (XR) 750-mg tablets and Glucophage® XR 500-mg tablets are bioequivalent in healthy fasting subjects. *Diabetes* 2003; 52 (suppl 1): A108.
120. Gao X, Xie J, Moore KT, Uderman HD, Reeves RA, Turner KC. Glucophage® extended release (XR) 750-mg tablets and Glucophage® XR 500-mg tablets are bioequivalent in healthy fed subjects. *Diabetes* 2003; 52 (suppl 1): A109.
121. Donahue SR, Turner KC, Patel S. Pharmacokinetics and pharmacodynamics of glyburide/metformin tablets (Glucovance®) versus equivalent doses of glyburide and metformin in patients with type 2 diabetes. *Clin Pharmacokinet* 2002; 41: 1301–9.
122. Hallsten K, Virtanen KA, Lonnqvist F, Sipila H, Oksanen A, Viljanen T, Ronnemaa T, Viikari J, Knuuti J, Nuutila P. Rosiglitazone but not metformin enhances insulin- and exercise-stimulated skeletal muscle glucose uptake in patients with newly diagnosed type 2 diabetes. *Diabetes* 2002; 51: 3479–85.
123. Virtanen KA, Hallsten K, Parkkola R, et al. Differential effects of rosiglitazone and metformin on adipose issue distribution and glucose uptake in type 2 diabetic subjects. *Diabetes Care* 2003; 52: 283–90.
124. Di Cicco RA, Allen A, Carr A, Fowles S, Jorkasky DK, Freed MI. Rosiglitazone does not alter the pharmacokinetics of metformin. *J Clin Pharmacol* 2000; 40: 1280–5.
125. Einhorn D, Rendell M, Rosenzweig J, Egan JW, Mathisen AL, Schneider RL, for the Pioglitazone 027 Study Group. Pioglitazone hydrochloride in combination with metformin in the treatment of type 2 diabetes mellitus: a randomized, placebo-controlled study. *Clin Ther* 2000; 22: 1395–409.
126. Scheen AJ, De Magalhaes AC, Salvatore T, Lefebvre PJ. Reduction of the acute bioavailability of metformin by the alpha-glucosidase inhibitor acarbose in normal man. *Eur J Clin Invest* 1994; 24 (suppl 3): 50–4.
127. Garber AJ, Sankoh S, Mohideen P, Bruce S. Glyburide/metformin tablets versus metformin plus rosiglitazone in type 2 diabetes patients uncontrolled on metformin: attaining glycemic goals. *Diabetes* 2003; 52 (suppl 1): A119.
128. Bruce S, Lee H, Goldstein BJ. Incidence of hypoglycemia following addition of rosiglitazone to glyburide/metformin tablets in patients with type 2 diabetes. *Diabetes* 2002; 51 (suppl 2): A466.
129. Chow CC, Tsang LW, Sorensen JP, Cockram CS. Comparison of insulin with or without continuation of oral hypoglycemic agents in the treatment of secondary failure in NIDDM patients. *Diabetes Care* 1995; 18: 307–14.
130. UKPDS Group. United Kingdom Prospective Diabetes Study (UKPDS) 13: Relative efficacy of randomly allocated diet, sulfonylurea, insulin, or metformin in patients with newly diagnosed non-insulin dependent diabetes followed for three years. *BMJ* 1995; 310: 83–8.
131. Montaguti U, Celin D, Ceredi C, Descovitch GC. Efficacy of the long-term administration of metformin in hyperlipidaemic patients. *Res Clin Forums* 1979; 1: 95–103.
132. Sirtori CR, Tremoli E, Sirtori M, Conti F, Paoletti R. Treatment of hypertriglyceridemia with metformin: effectiveness and analysis of results. *Atherosclerosis* 1977; 26: 583–92.

133. Rains SG, Wilson GA, Richmond W, Elkeles RS. The effect of glibenclamide and metformin on serum lipoproteins in type 2 diabetes. *Diabet Med* 1988; 5: 653–8.
134. Grant PJ. The effects of high- and medium-dose metformin therapy on cardiovascular risk factors in patients with type II diabetes. *Diabetes Care* 1996; 19: 64–6.
135. Palumbo PJ. Metformin: effects on cardiovascular risk factors in patients with non-insulin-dependent diabetes mellitus. *J Diabetes Complications* 1998; 12: 110–9.
136. Marchetti P, Benzi L, Cerri M, Cecchetti P, Giannarelli R, Giannecchini M, Di Cianni G, Cristofani R, Miccoli R, Bertolotto A. Effect of plasma metformin concentrations on serum lipid levels in type II diabetic patients. *Acta Diabetol Lat* 1988; 25: 55–62.
137. Carlsen SM, Rossvoll O, Bjerve KS, Folling I. Metformin improves blood lipid pattern in nondiabetic patients with coronary heart disease. *J Intern Med* 1996; 239: 227–33.
138. Pentikainen PJ, Voutilainen E, Aro A, Uusitupa M, Penttila I, Vapaatalo H. Cholesterol lowering effect of metformin in combined hyperlipidemia: placebo controlled double blind trial. *Ann Med* 1990; 22: 307–12.
139. Chan JC, Tomlinson B, Critchley JA, Cockram CS, Walden RJ. Metabolic and hemodynamic effects of metformin and glibenclamide in normotensive NIDDM patients. *Diabetes Care* 1993; 16: 1035–8.
140. Sirtori CR. Clinical experience with metformin in patients with peripheral vascular. *Diabete Metab* 1988; 14: 601–7.
141. Schneider J, Erren T, Zofel P, Kaffarnik H. Metformin-induced changes in serum lipids, lipoproteins, and apoproteins in non-insulin-dependent diabetes mellitus. *Atherosclerosis* 1990; 82: 97–103.
142. Dailey GE III, Mohideen P, Fiedorek FT. Lipid effects of glyburide/metformin tablets in patients with type 2 diabetes mellitus with poor glycemic control and dyslipidemia in an open-label extension study. *Clin Ther* 2002; 24: 1426–38.
143. American Diabetes Association. Standards of medical care for patients with diabetes mellitus. *Diabetes Care* 2001; 24: S33–43.
144. Aviles-Santa L, Sinding J, Raskin P. Effects of metformin in patients with poorly controlled, insulin-treated type 2 diabetes mellitus: a randomized, double-blind, placebo-controlled trial. *Ann Intern Med* 1999; 131: 182–8.
145. Bosisio E, Kienle MG, Galli G, Ciconali M, Negri A, Sessa A, Morosati S, Sirtori CR. Defective hydroxylation of phenformin as a determinant of drug toxicity. *Diabetes* 1981; 30: 644–9.
146. Chou KH, Von Eye CH, Capp E, Spritzer PM. Clinical, metabolic and endocrine parameters in response to metformin in obese women with polycystic ovary syndrome: a randomized, double-blind and placebo-controlled trial. *Horm Metab Res* 2003; 35: 86–91.
147. Fanghanel G, Sanchez-Reyes L, Trujillo C, Sotres D, Espinosa-Campos J. Metformin's effects on glucose and lipid metabolism in patients with secondary failure to sulfonylureas. *Diabetes Care* 1996; 19: 1185–9.
148. McCollough P, Glueck CJ, Lang J, Wang P, Tracy T, Sieve-Smith L. Metformin safely and effectively facilitates weight loss in obese non-diabetic and diabetic hyperlipidemic patients. *J Invest Med* 1998; 46.
149. Lee A, Morley JE. Metformin decreases food consumption and induces weight loss in subjects with obesity with type II non-insulin-dependent diabetes. *Obes Res* 1998; 6: 47–53.
150. Carlsen SM, Grill V, Folling I. Evidence for dissociation of insulin- and weight-reducing effects of metformin in nondiabetic male patients with coronary heart disease. *Diabetes Res Clin Pract* 1998; 39: 47–54.
151. Grant PJ. The effects of metformin on cardiovascular risk factors. *Diabetes Metab Rev* 1995; 11 (suppl 1): S43–50.
152. Vague P, Juhan-Vague I, Alessi MC, Badier C, Valadier J. Metformin decreases the high plasminogen activator inhibition capacity, plasma insulin and triglyceride levels in non-diabetic obese subjects. *Thromb Haemost* 1987; 57: 326–8.
153. Turner RC, Holman RR. Metformin and risk of cardiovascular disease. *Cardiology* 1999; 91: 203–4.
154. Johnson JA, Majumdar SR, Simpson SH, Toth EL. Decreased mortality associated with the use of metformin compared with sulfonylurea monotherapy in type 2 diabetes. *Diabetes Care* 2002; 25: 2244–8.
155. Executive Summary of the Third Report of the National Cholesterol Education Program (NCEP) Expert Panel on Detection, Evaluation, and Treatment of High Blood Cholesterol in Adults (Adult Treatment Panel III). *JAMA* 2001; 285: 2486–97.
156. National Institutes of Health, National Heart, Lung, and Blood Institute. *The Seventh Report of the Joint National Committee on Prevention, Detection, Evaluation, and Treatment of High Blood Pressure*, Vol. 7. Washington, DC: US Department of Health and Human Services, 2003; pp 1–34. NIH Publication No. 03-5233.
157. 1999 World Health Organization—International Society of Hypertension guidelines for the management of hypertension. Guidelines subcommittee. *J Hypertens* 1999; 17: 151–83.
158. Dailey GE, Mohideen P, Fiedorek FT. Lipid effects of glyburide/metformin tablets in patients with type 2 diabetes mellitus with poor glycemic control and dyslipidemia in an open-label extension study. *Diabetes Obes Metab* 2002; 24: 1426–38.
159. Bell PM, Hadden DR. Metformin. *Endocrinol Metab Clin North Am* 1997; 26: 523–37.
160. Dezii CM. Medication noncompliance: what is the problem? *Manag Care* 2000; 9: 7–12.
161. Dailey G, Kim MS, Lian JF. Patient compliance and persistence with anti-hyperglycemic therapy: evaluation of a population of type 2 diabetic patients. *J Int Med Res* 2002; 30: 71–9.
162. Dezii CM, Kawabata H, Tran M. Effects of once-daily and twice-daily dosing on adherence with prescribed glipizide oral therapy for type 2 diabetes. *South Med J* 2002; 95: 68–71.
163. Dailey G, Kim MS, Lian JF. Patient compliance and persistence with antihyperglycemic drug regimens: evaluation of a medicaid patient population with type 2 diabetes mellitus. *Clin Ther* 2001; 23: 1311–20.
164. Morris AD, Brennan GM, MacDonald TM, Donnan PT. Population-based adherence to prescribed medication in type 2 diabetes: a cause for concern. *Diabetes* 2000; 49 (suppl 1): A76.
165. Melikian C, White TJ, Vanderplas A, Dezii CM, Chang E. Adherence to oral antidiabetic therapy in a managed care organization: a comparison of monotherapy, combination therapy, and fixed-dose combination therapy. *Clin Ther* 2002; 24: 460–7.
166. Oates NS, Shah RR, Idle JR, Smith RL. Genetic polymorphism of phenformin 4-hydroxylation. *Clin Pharmacol Ther* 1982; 32: 81–9.

167. Shah RR, Evans DA, Oates NS, Idle JR, Smith RL. The genetic control of phenformin 4-hydroxylation. *J Med Genet* 1985; 22: 361–6.
168. Brown JB, Pedula K, Barzilay J, Herson MK, Latare P. Lactic acidosis rates in type 2 diabetes. *Diabetes Care* 1998; 21: 1659–63.
169. Misbin RI, Green L, Stadel BV, Gueriguian JL, Gubbi A, Fleming GA. Lactic acidosis in patients with diabetes treated with metformin. *N Engl J Med* 1998; 338: 265–6.
170. Stang MR, Lueck L, Wysowski DK, Downey W, Butler-Jones D. Metformin and lactic acidosis. *Can Pharmacoepidemiol Forum* 1997.
171. Wiholm BE, Myrhed M. Metformin-associated lactic acidosis in Sweden 1977–1991. *Eur J Clin Pharmacol* 1993; 44: 589–91.
172. Campbell IW. Metformin and the sulfonylureas: the comparative risk. *Horm Metab Res* 1985; 15 (suppl): 105–11.
173. Lalau JD, Race JM, Brinquin L. Lactic acidosis in metformin therapy: relationship between plasma metformin concentration and renal function. *Diabetes Care* 1998; 21: 1366–7.
174. Lalau JD, Mourlhon C, Bergeret A, Lacroix C. Consequences of metformin intoxication. *Diabetes Care* 1998; 21: 2036–7.
175. Gueriguian J, Green L, Misbin RI, Stadel B, Fleming GA. Efficacy of metformin in non-insulin-dependent diabetes mellitus. *N Engl J Med* 1996; 334: 269–70.
176. Stacpoole PW. Metformin and lactic acidosis: guilt by association? *Diabetes Care* 1998; 21: 1587–8.
177. Hulisz DT, Bonfiglio MF, Murray RD. Metformin-associated lactic acidosis. *J Am Board Fam Pract* 1998; 11: 233–6.
178. al Jebawi AF, Lassman MN, Abourizk NN. Lactic acidosis with therapeutic metformin blood level in a low-risk diabetic patient. *Diabetes Care* 1998; 21: 1364–5.
179. Pepper GM, Schwartz M. Lactic acidosis associated with Glucophage® use in a man with normal renal and hepatic function. *Diabetes Care* 1997; 20: 23 2–3.
180. Cryer DR, Mills DJ, Henry DH, Nicolas SP. Comparative outcomes study of metformin intervention versus conventional approach: the COSMIC Approach Study. *Diabetes* 2003; 52 (suppl 1): A115.
181. Cryer DR, Mills DJ, Henry DH, Nicholas SP. Comparative outcomes study of metformin intervention versus conventional approach (COSMIC): lactate level substudy. *Diabetes* 2003; 52 (suppl 1): A115.
182. Connolly V, Kesson CM. Metformin treatment in NIDDM patients with mild renal impairment. *Postgrad Med J* 1996; 72: 352–4.
183. Carlsen SM, Folling I, Grill V, Bjerve KS, Schneede J, Refsum H. Metformin increases total serum homocysteine levels in non-diabetic male patients with coronary heart disease. *Scand J Clin Lab Invest* 1997; 57: 521–7.
184. Hoogeveen EK, Kostense PJ, Jakobs C, Bouter LM, Heine RJ, Stehouwer CD. Does metformin increase the serum total homocysteine level in non-insulin-dependent diabetes mellitus? *J Intern Med* 1997; 242: 389–94.
185. Chan KA, Truman A, Gurwitz JH, Hurley JS, Martinson B, Platt R, Everhart JE, Moseley RH, Terrault N, Ackerson L, Selby JV. A cohort study of the incidence of serious acute liver injury in diabetic patients treated with hypoglycemic agents. *Arch Intern Med* 2003; 163: 728–34.

48

Thiazolidinediones as PPAR Agonists

Sunder Mudaliar and Robert R. Henry

VA San Diego Healthcare System, San Diego, CA, USA, and University of California at San Diego, San Diego, CA, USA

INTRODUCTION

Type 2 diabetes is a common, chronic disease characterized by hyperglycemia and numerous other metabolic abnormalities and complications. This disabling metabolic disorder is one of the leading causes of premature cardiovascular morbidity and mortality and currently affects more than 150 million people worldwide and is estimated to afflict nearly 200 million people by the year 2010 [1, 2]. Three major pathophysiologic abnormalities contribute toward the development of hyperglycemia in patients with type 2 diabetes: impaired insulin secretion, excessive hepatic glucose output, and insulin resistance in skeletal muscle, liver, and adipose tissue [3]. The oral pharmacologic agents available for the treatment of type 2 diabetes act primarily by increasing insulin availability (sulfonylureas (SUs) and meglitinides); delaying gastrointestinal glucose absorption (α-glucosidase inhibitors); suppressing excessive hepatic glucose output (metformin); and improving insulin sensitivity at target tissues, mainly adipose tissue, skeletal muscle, and liver [thiazolidinediones (TZDs) or glitazones]. Of these potential sites of action, targeting insulin resistance appears particularly promising because of growing evidence that insulin resistance is intricately involved in the development of not only hyperglycemia, but also dyslipidemia, hypertension, hypercoagulation, vasculopathy, and, ultimately, premature atherosclerotic cardiovascular disease [4, 5]. This cluster of metabolic abnormalities has been variously termed the "Insulin Resistance Syndrome," the "Cardiovascular Dysmetabolic syndrome", or simply the "Metabolic Syndrome" [4, 5]. Since the TZDs are potent insulin sensitizers, they appear to be ideally suited for treatment of not only hyperglycemia, but also perhaps the cardiovascular dysmetabolic syndrome.

The TZDs are chemically and functionally unrelated to the other classes of oral antidiabetic agents. A thiazolidine-2,4-dione structure is common to all agents of this class (Figure 1), but they differ in their side chains, which alter their pharmacologic and side effect profiles [6]. These drugs are highly selective and potent agonists for the peroxisome proliferator-activated receptor γ (PPAR-γ). Two compounds in this class are presently approved for use. Rosiglitazone (Avandia®) was first approved in the United States in May 1999, and pioglitazone (Actos®) was granted approval for marketing in the United States in July 1999. The first agent in this class, troglitazone (Rezulin®) was originally marketed in the United States from March 1997 until it was withdrawn in March 2000, when it was determined that the risk of idiosyncratic hepatotoxicity associated with troglitazone therapy outweighed its potential benefits. In clinical use so far, rosiglitazone and pioglitazone appear to be devoid of idiosyncratic, fulminant hepatotoxicity attributable to troglitazone use. Both the currently available TZDs are effective in lowering blood glucose and improving glycemic control when used as monotherapy and in combination with other oral agents. In the United States, rosiglitazone and pioglitazone are also approved for use in combination with insulin. In addition to their glucose-lowering properties, through their PPAR-γ agonist effects, the TZDs as "insulin sensitizers" also have significant beneficial effects on blood pressure (BP), lipid metabolism, vascular tone, and endothelial function. Here, we review the mechanism of action, pharmacology, and clinical applications of the newest antidiabetic agents, the TZDs—rosiglitazone and pioglitazone.

International Textbook of Diabetes Mellitus, Third Edition. Edited by R. A. DeFronzo, E. Ferrannini, H. Keen, and P. Zimmet, 2004.
 ISBN: 0-471-48655-8.

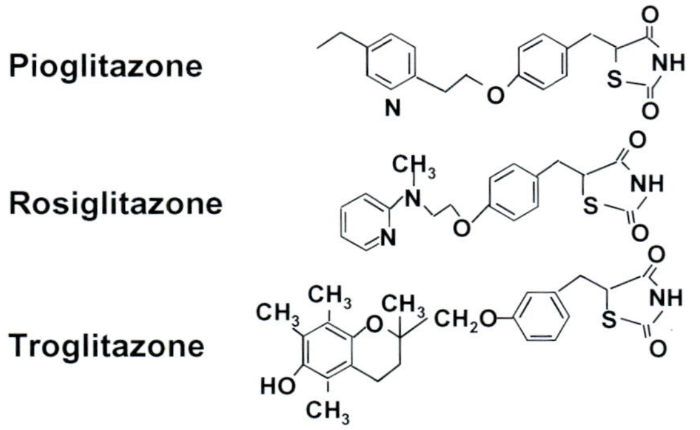

Figure 1 Structure of the thiazolidinediones

MECHANISM OF ACTION

A close relationship has been shown to exist between the potency of various TZDs to stimulate PPAR-γ and their antidiabetic action [7]. The PPARs are a family of nuclear receptors consisting of three subtypes designated PPAR-α, PPAR-γ, and PPAR-δ or -β [8] (Table 1). PPAR-γ receptors are found in key target tissues for insulin action such as adipose tissue, skeletal muscle, and liver, and there is strong evidence to indicate that these receptors may be important regulators of adipocyte differentiation, lipid homeostasis, insulin action, and vascular endothelial function [7–10]. Three different isomers of PPAR-γ have been identified—PPAR-γ1, PPAR-γ2 and PPAR-γ3. PPAR-γ1 and PPAR-γ3 mRNAs are regulated by different promoters but result in the production of identical proteins, whereas the PPAR-γ2 mRNA encodes a protein that has additional 30 amino acids at its N-terminus end [11]. Evidence from *in vitro* studies suggests that while PPAR-γ2 is a key regulator in adipose tissue, PPAR-γ1 is the dominant isoform in muscle tissue [12]. Further, there also appears to be differences in the relative distribution of PPAR-γ mRNA and protein in insulin-sensitive tissue. While the abundance of PPAR-γ mRNA in skeletal muscle is approximately 5% of that in adipose tissue on the basis of total RNA, the amount of PPAR-γ protein in muscle is on average about two thirds of that present in fat [12].

Irrespective of whether TZDs exert their primary effects directly on liver, muscle, and adipose tissue or indirectly improve insulin sensitivity through changes in circulating concentrations of adipocyte-derived free fatty acids (FFAs) and peptide hormones, a close relationship has been shown to exist between the potency of various TZDs to stimulate PPAR-γ and their antidiabetic action [6]. TZDs have been shown to favorably influence the expression of several genes involved in glucose metabolism, including GLUT-1, GLUT-4, leptin, tumor necrosis factor α (TNF-α), Akt (protein kinase B), and hepatic glucokinase [13] (Figure 2). In obese Zucker rats, treatment with troglitazone leads to a reduction in leptin and TNF-α expression that is associated with apoptosis of large adipocytes and an increase in the number of small adipocytes (with no net change in adipose tissue weight) [15]. Both TNF-α and leptin (an *ob* gene product) have been associated with insulin resistance and it is plausible that apoptosis of large adipocytes leads to lower TNF-α and leptin levels and consequent amelioration of insulin resistance. Moreover, the increase in the number of small adipocytes may also contribute to the reduction of insulin resistance. Small adipocytes take up more glucose than large adipocytes at submaximal insulin levels and are also more sensitive to the antilipolytic action of insulin [16]. These effects could result in lower FFA and triglyceride levels and improved insulin sensitivity.

In human studies, the TZDs improve glucose transport in subcutaneous adipocytes. In a recent study, adipocytes obtained from the abdominal subcutaneous fat of obese type 2 diabetic subjects who were treated with troglitazone for 3 months, exhibited increased glucose transport both in the absence and presence of insulin. This increased glucose uptake in human adipocytes after troglitazone treatment was associated with a significant increase in GLUT-4 expression and insulin-stimulated serine phosphorylation of Akt (protein kinase B) [17]. In the same study, adipocytes from metformin-treated subjects (who achieved similar glycemic control) showed none of the above changes. Surprisingly, in this study, the size of subcutaneous (SQ) adipocytes actually increased with troglitazone treatment, compared to a decrease in size after metformin treatment [17]. In another study in freshly isolated human adipocytes, rosiglitazone increased p85 α-phosphatidylinositol 3 kinase (p85α PI-3K) and

Table 1 Tissue expression profile and metabolic effects of the peroxisome proliferator-activated receptors

	PPAR-α	PPAR-β	PPAR-γ
Tissue expressin profile	Liver, kidney, adrenal, skeletal muscle, adipose tissue, vascular tissues	Ubiquitous	Adipose tissues, skeletal muscle, heart, liver, kidney, gut, macrophages, vascular tissues, islet cells γ1 dominant isoform in muscle γ2 key regulator in fat tissue
Metabolic effects	Vascular, anti-inflammatory, fat oxidation	Reverse cholesterol transport	Adipogenesis, fat redistribution, glucose metabolism, fat oxidation, vascular, anti-inflammatory

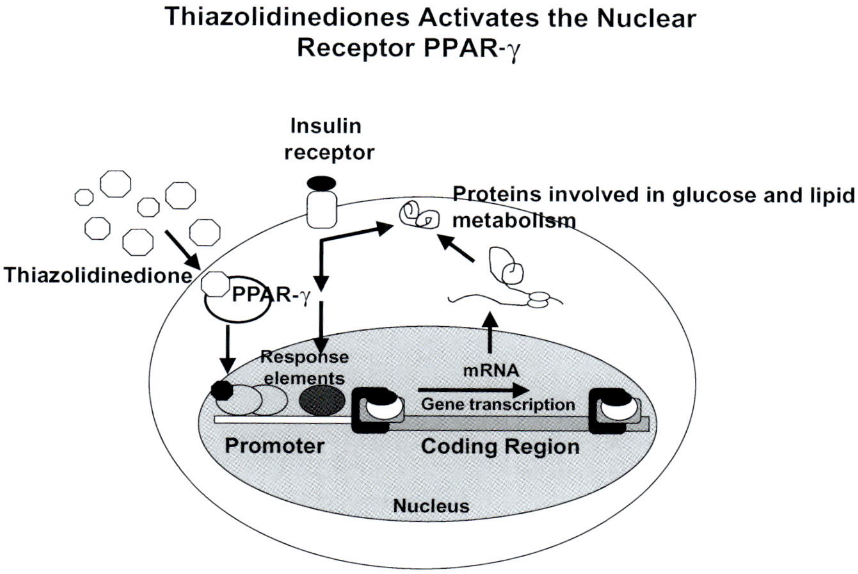

Figure 2 Cellular effects of the thiazolidinediones on the PPAR receptor. (Copyright © 1996 American Diabetes Association, from reference 14. Reprinted with permission from The American Diabetes Association)

uncoupling protein 2 (UCP-2) mRNA levels and decreased leptin expression. p85a PI-3K is a major component of the insulin signal transduction pathway and the induction of its expression might explain, at least in part, the insulin-sensitizing effect of the TZDs [18].

There is also some evidence from animal studies that some of the insulin-sensitizing effects of the TZDs may be mediated through PPAR-γ effects on UCPs in adipose tissue and skeletal muscle [19–21]. Some studies also suggest that the TZDs have direct effects in skeletal muscle. In human skeletal muscle culture systems, troglitazone treatment markedly increases PPAR-γ protein expression along with other genes involved in glucose and lipid metabolism [22]. In the same skeletal muscle culture system, troglitazone has been demonstrated to have acute effects on glucose uptake and chronic effects on glucose uptake and glycogen synthase (GS) activity [23]. Concomitantly there were increases in GLUT-1 mRNA and protein and no change in GLUT-4 or GS mRNA or protein. However, the clinical significance of these effects in humans remains to be determined.

Perhaps the most exciting development in the field of adipocyte biology and TZD action has been the identification and characterization of adiponectin, which is a novel adipocyte-derived hormone [also called apM1 (adipose most abundant gene transcript 1) and acrp30 or adipoQ for the murine homologue] [24, 25]. Adipose tissue expression of adiponectin is lower in insulin-resistant states, and lower plasma levels of adiponectin have been documented in human subjects with obesity, type 2 diabetes, or coronary artery disease [26, 27]. Plasma adiponectin levels have been shown to correlate negatively with plasma glucose, insulin, triglyceride levels, and body mass index (BMI) and positively with plasma levels of high-density lipoprotein (HDL) cholesterol [26]. In one study, plasma adiponectin levels were shown to correlate positively with insulin-stimulated glucose disposal (RD) as measured by the hyperinsulinemic-euglycemic clamp technique [27]. In both human subjects [28] and animal models of insulin resistance and type 2 diabetes [29–32], the TZDs, have been shown to enhance the expression of adiponectin mRNA and increase plasma levels of adiponectin protein.

In two recent studies, treatment with both rosiglitazone and pioglitazone was associated with increased adiponectin levels [33, 34]. In the study with rosiglitazone, multivariate linear regression analysis showed that the single variable significantly related to the changes of plasma adiponectin was whether rosiglitazone treatment was used. The amount of variance in changes of plasma adiponectin level explained by the treatment was ~24% ($r^2 = 0.24$) after adjusting for age, sex, and changes in fasting plasma glucose (FPG), HbA_{1c}, insulin resistance index, and BMI.

Although the above studies demonstrate a close correlation between changes in plasma levels of adiponectin after TZD treatment and measures of insulin-mediated glucose metabolism and adipose tissue distribution, the exact tissue and molecular mechanisms by which adiponectin mediates its effects in human beings still remains to be determined (Figure 3). Further, it is still not clear if adiponectin is predominantly secreted by SQ or omental adipose tissue. In a recent study, Motoshima et al. studied the secretion of adiponectin *in vitro* from paired samples of isolated human omental and SQ adipocytes and its regulation by

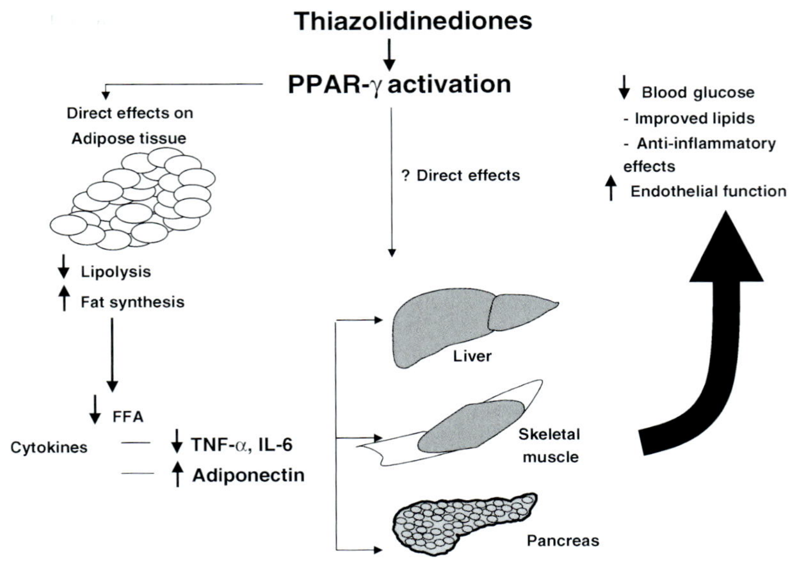

Figure 3 Possible sites of sensitizing actions of the thiazolidinediones. Here ? effects mean possible effects

insulin and rosiglitazone [35]. Secretion of adiponectin by omental cells was generally higher than SQ cells and showed a strong negative correlation with BMI ($r = -0.78$; $P = 0.013$). In contrast, secretion from the sc cells was unrelated to BMI. Compared with sc-derived adipocytes, adiponectin secretion from omental cells was increased by insulin or rosiglitazone alone and was up to 2.3-fold higher following combined treatment with insulin and rosiglitazone, whereas secretion from SQ adipose cells was unaffected by these treatments. These data suggest that reduced secretion from the omental adipose depot may account for the decline in plasma adiponectin observed in obesity. Furthermore, enhanced adiponectin secretion from fat cells derived from the visceral compartment in response to rosiglitazone alone or in combination with insulin may play a role in some of the systemic insulin-sensitizing and anti-inflammatory properties of the TZDs.

However, in contrast to the findings from this study, a recent study by Phillips et al. evaluated adipocytes from the abdominal SQ fat biopsies of obese type 2 diabetic subjects who were treated with troglitazone for 3 months. In this study the adiponectin protein content from the SQ abdominal adipocytes was increased following troglitazone treatment and unchanged in those who had been treated with metformin [36]. It remains unclear whether the differential response to troglitazone by SQ adipocytes in this study is related to the fact that these adipocytes were obtained after treatment of the diabetic subjects with troglitazone for 3 months, as compared to the SQ adipocytes in the previous study in which the adipocytes were obtained from nondiabetic subjects and were treated *in-vitro* with rosiglitazone. Also unclear so far, is the mechanism by which adiponectin improves insulin sensitivity. Postulated mechanisms include increases in muscle lipid metabolism through increased expression of genes encoding CD36, acyl-CoA oxidase, fatty acid transporters, and UCP-2, with consequent increases in fatty acid transport, fat combustion, and heat dissipation [37].

Of note, the antihypertensive and antiatherosclerotic effects of the TZDs may also occur through PPAR-γ agonism [38–40]. Human and rat vascular smooth muscle cells (VSMCs) express mRNA and nuclear receptors for PPAR-γ1 [38, 40]. These receptors are upregulated during vascular injury and are present in early human atheroma and precursor lesions. Pharmacological activation of PPAR-γ with troglitazone and rosiglitazone inhibits VSMC proliferation and migration, with the potential to limit restenosis and atherosclerosis. Also, both troglitazone and pioglitazone inhibit vasopressin and platelet-derived growth factor (PDGF)-induced Ca^{2+} entry and proliferation in rat VSMCs [38].

Thus, the TZDs act, at least in part, by binding with PPAR-γ in various tissues to influence the expression of a number of genes encoding proteins involved in glucose and lipid metabolism, endothelial function, and atherogenesis [38–41]. As regards the insulin-sensitizing effects, since the TZDs potently induce adipocyte differentiation, it is possible that the primary action of TZDs is in fat cells, with secondary effects on skeletal muscle to improve insulin-action, possibly through a TZD-mediated changes in circulating FFA levels, adiponectin secretion, or some other signal and/or there may be direct TZD effects on insulin-sensitive tissues (Figure 3). Further studies are necessary to delineate the physiologically important tissue sites and mechanisms of TZD-mediated PPAR agonist action on insulin sensitivity. The recent cloning of

Table 2 Relative efficacy of rosiglitazone and pioglitazone*

	Reduction in fasting plasma glucose (mg/dl) mean change from control group	Reduction in HbA_{1C} (%)
Monotherapy		
Rosiglitazone 4 mg	43–58	0.9–1.2
Rosiglitazone 8 mg	62–76	1.5
Pioglitazone 15 mg	39	1.0
Pioglitazone 30 mg	41–58	1.0–1.5
Pioglitazone 45 mg	65–68	1.5–1.6
Combination with SUs		
Rosiglitazone 4 mg	39–47	0.9–1.13
Pioglitazone 15 mg	39	0.9
Pioglitazone 30 mg	58	1.3
Combination with metformin		
Rosiglitazone 4 mg	40	1.0
Rosiglitazone 8 mg	53	1.5
Pioglitazone 30 mg	38	0.8
Combination with insulin		
Rosiglitazone 4 mg	41	0.7
Rosiglitazone 8 mg	45	1.3
Pioglitazone 15 mg	35	1.0
Pioglitazone 30 mg	40	1.3

Note. Since the above data was not obtained from simultaneous trials, the comparative data is only a rough approximation of the relative effectiveness, as stage, severity of hyperglycemia, and type of patients studied varied in the above studies.
* From references 43–54.

adiponectin receptors 1 (AdipoR-1) and 2 (AdipoR-1 is abundantly expressed in skeletal muscle and AdipoR-2 is predominantly expressed in the liver) is expected give further impetus to research in this field [42].

GLYCEMIC EFFECTS/CLINICAL INDICATIONS

As potent insulin sensitizers, the TZDs have major effects on glucose metabolism that result in significantly lower blood glucose levels in insulin-resistant patients with type 2 diabetes (Table 2). Several studies have documented the glucose-lowering effects of rosiglitazone and pioglitazone not only when used as monotherapy agents, but also in combination with SUs, metformin, and insulin. In this context, it must be pointed that although both rosiglitazone and pioglitazone are approved by the Food and Drug Administration (FDA) in the United States for use as monotherapy and in combination with the SUs, metformin, and with insulin, in Europe, the TZDs are not approved for use in combination with insulin.

Thaizolidinedione Monotherapy

In a large, multicenter study, Lebowitz et al. evaluated the efficacy and safety of rosiglitazone monotherapy in 493 patients with type 2 diabetes who were randomized to receive rosiglitazone 2 or 4 mg twice daily or placebo [43]. After 26 weeks, rosiglitazone 2 and 4 mg twice daily reduced FPG concentrations relative to placebo by 58 and 76 mg/dl and mean HbA_{1C} levels by 1.2 and 1.5% respectively. In addition, there were also beneficial changes in measures of insulin sensitivity, β-cell function, and microalbuminuria.

Similar to rosiglitazone, Aronof et al. demonstrated the efficacy and safety of four doses of pioglitazone monotherapy in a large multicenter, double-blind, placebo-controlled clinical trial with 408 patients with HbA_{1c} >7.0% and FPG >140 mg/dl [44]. After 26 weeks, patients treated with 15, 30, or 45 mg pioglitazone had significant mean decreases in HbA_{1c} (range −1.00 to −1.60% difference from placebo) and FPG (−39 to −65 mg/dl difference from placebo). The decreases in FPG were observed as early as the second week of therapy; maximal decreases occurred after 10–14 weeks and were maintained until the end of therapy (week 26). In addition, in all pioglitazone groups, there were significant mean decreases in triglycerides, significant mean increases in HDL cholesterol, and only small changes in total cholesterol and low-density lipoprotein (LDL). Of interest, the subset of patients naive to oral antidiabetic therapy had greater improvements in HbA_{1c} and FPG (difference from placebo of −2.55% and −80 mg/dl for the 45-mg group) compared with previously treated patients. The overall adverse event profile of pioglitazone was similar to that of placebo and there was no evidence of drug-induced hepatotoxicity or drug-induced elevations of liver enzymes in this study. Similar results were reported in a 23-week, placebo-controlled monotherapy trial by Rosenblatt et al. who demonstrated that compared with placebo, 30 mg of pioglitazone daily significantly reduced FPG by 58 mg/dl and HbA_{1c} by 1.37% [45]. In addition, as with rosiglitazone, there were significant improvements in measures of insulin sensitivity and β-cell function in this study.

In the context of monotherapy, it is noteworthy that there are few prospective clinical trials in patients with type 2 diabetes that have directly compared the impact of the various available antidiabetic agents on metabolic and clinical outcomes. The largest of these, the United Kingdom Prospective Diabetes Study (UKPDS) observed a progressive failure of the glucose-lowering therapies used (metformin, SUs, and insulin) to maintain glycemic control. Also, in this study, the stepwise addition of antihyperglycemic agents to achieve glycemic goals resulted in substantial therapeutic overlap between the groups, making it difficult to analyze the effects of individual therapies. More importantly, the only insulin sensitizer available at the time of the UKPDS was metformin. With the introduction of the TZDs, which increase insulin sensitivity of target peripheral tissues by a completely different mechanism, it would be important to conduct a long-term, blinded, prospective, randomized controlled trial to compare the three mechanistically distinct antidiabetic agents currently available for the first-line pharmacological treatment of type 2 diabetes (SUs, metformin, and TZDs), in terms of their effects on glycemic control, β-cell function, and cardiovascular risk factors. Such a study, A Diabetes Outcome Progression Trial (ADOPT) started in March 2000 and is ongoing [55]. The three agents in this study include rosiglitazone as the TZD agent to increase the sensitivity of target tissues to insulin; metformin as a biguanide whose primary mechanism is to reduce hepatic glucose output and glyburide; and a sulfonylurea as an insulin secretagogue. This study will assess treatment effects in terms of attainment of sustained glycemic control, time to monotherapy failure, prevention of β-cell deterioration, and effects on risk factors for the vascular complications of type 2 diabetes.

Combination Therapy with SUs

The addition of a TZD to existing sulfonylurea therapy has been shown to significantly improve glycemic control in several large studies. In one large international, 26-week, open-label study, 348 patients with type 2 diabetes from India, Brazil, Philippines, Thailand, Argentina, and Tunisia were randomized to receive 4 mg rosiglitazone or placebo daily in addition to existing sulfonylurea (SU) therapy [46]. Of the 348 patients, 175 received 2 mg rosiglitazone twice daily plus SU (RSG + SU) and 173 received SU alone. After 26 weeks, the RSG + SU group showed a significant reduction in mean HbA_{1c} from 9.05 to 7.92% (mean change, −1.13). Mean HbA_{1c} essentially remained unchanged in the control group (8.9–9.0%). The RSG + SU group also showed a significant decrease in mean FPG concentration from 199 to 160 mg/dl, while the controls showed a nonsignificant increase from 194 to 200 mg/dl. Although adverse events were similar in both groups, more patients in the RSG + SU group reported mild hypoglycemia. This study emphasizes that adding rosiglitazone to existing SU treatment improves glycemic control and is well tolerated in patients with type 2 diabetes from a wide range of non-Western countries. Similar improvements in glycemic control were obtained in another ethnic population in the United Kingdom (Asian Indians) in whom rosiglitazone 8 mg daily in combination with concurrent sulfonylurea therapy decreased mean HbA_{1C} levels by 1.15% as compared to an increase of 0.26% in the placebo group [47]. Thus the effects of the TZDs on glucose control appear to be consistent across populations.

The glucose-lowering effects of pioglitazone in combination with SUs were demonstrated by Kipnes et al. in a 16-week, double-blind study that included patients on a stable regimen of a sulfonylurea for at least 30 days and with HbA_{1C} levels >8.0% [48]. Patients were randomly assigned to receive sulfonylurea plus either once daily pioglitazone 15 mg ($n = 184$), pioglitazone 30 mg ($n = 189$), or placebo ($n = 187$). After 16 weeks, as compared with patients treated with placebo + sulfonylurea, those receiving pioglitazone + sulfonylurea had significant decreases from baseline in HbA_{1C} by 0.9% with pioglitazone 15 mg and 1.3% with pioglitazone 30 mg, respectively. FPG levels also decreased by 39 mg/dl and 58 mg/dl in the pioglitazone 15 mg and 30 mg, respectively. In addition, both pioglitazone + sulfonylurea groups had significant improvements in lipid levels. In this study, pioglitazone was well tolerated, and the rates of adverse events were similar in all groups.

Combination with Metformin

In obese type 2 diabetic patients inadequately controlled on metformin alone, it might be expected that addition of a TZD would further improve glycemic control, insulin sensitivity, and β-cell function to a clinically important extent. To evaluate the efficacy of metformin–rosiglitazone therapy in type 2 diabetes patients inadequately controlled with metformin alone, Fonseca et al. conducted a large, US multicenter, double-blind study in which 348 patients (mean BMI of 30.1 kg/m^2) with a mean FPG of 216 mg/dl and a mean HbA_{1C} level of 8.8% were randomized to receive 2.5 g/day of metformin plus either placebo, 4 mg/day of rosiglitazone, or 8 mg/day of rosiglitazone [49]. After 26 weeks, all measures of glucose control, insulin sensitivity, and β-cell function improved significantly with metformin–rosiglitazone therapy in a dose-dependent manner. The mean levels of HbA_{1C} decreased by 1.0% in the 4 mg/day metformin–rosiglitazone group and by 1.2% in the 8 mg/day metformin–rosiglitazone group, and FPG levels by 40 mg/dl and 53 mg/dl, compared with the metformin–placebo group ($P < 0.001$, for all). Interestingly, in this study, while those in the control group experienced a mean decrease in body mass of 1.2 kg from baseline, those in the rosiglitazone groups experienced a significant mean increase of 0.7 kg in the 4-mg/day and 1.9 kg in the 8-mg/day rosiglitazone groups. Also of interest, there were no significant differences in waist-to-hip ratios among groups.

In another study from Mexico, 116 obese patients (BMI ~28 kg/m^2) were randomized to metformin 2.5 g/day plus either placebo, rosiglitazone 2 mg b.i.d., or rosiglitazone 4 mg b.i.d. [50]. After 26 weeks, while HbA_{1C} levels increased in the placebo group by 0.3%, the mean HbA_{1c} levels decreased significantly from baseline by 0.7% and 1.2% in the rosiglitazone 2 mg and 4 mg b.i.d. groups, respectively. Further, C-peptide and immunoreactive insulin (IRI) levels were decreased from baseline in both the rosiglitazone groups. Thus in this study, the addition of rosiglitazone to metformin therapy improved glycemic control in Mexican patients whose type 2 diabetes was inadequately controlled by metformin alone.

As with rosiglitazone, the combination of pioglitazone and metformin also significantly improves HbA_{1c} and FPG levels, with positive effects on insulin sensitivity and no evidence of drug-induced hepatotoxicity. In a 16-week study (followed by an 1.5-year open-label extension), Einhorn et al. studied 328 patients with type 2 diabetes who had suboptimal control on maximum doses of metformin [51]. These patients were randomized to either pioglitazone + metformin or placebo + metformin. Two hundred forty-nine subjects completed the study. After 16 weeks, patients receiving pioglitazone 30 mg + metformin had significant decreases in FPG levels by 38 mg/dl and HbA_{1c} by −0.83% compared with the placebo + metformin group. One hundred fifty-four of the study subjects also entered the open-label phase where all patients were treated with open-label pioglitazone 30 mg + metformin for 72 weeks and had mean changes from baseline of −1.36% in HbA_{1c} and −63.0 mg/dl in FPG.

In the context of combination TZD and metformin therapy, it is interesting to note that in one analysis, the combination of metformin and TZDs appears to be more effective in more obese patients. Jones et al. undertook an analysis to evaluate the efficacy of rosiglitazone when added to the therapy of obese type 2 diabetes mellitus patients taking maximal doses (2.5 g/day) of metformin [52]. Data were pooled from two double-blind studies involving a total of 550 patients, in whom rosiglitazone was added to 2.5 g/day metformin. Patients were categorized as non-overweight, overweight, and obese according to their baseline BMI <25 kg/m^2, 25–30 kg/m^2, and >30 kg/m^2, respectively. Rosiglitazone improved glycemia to a clinically significant extent in all three subgroups but its effect was most pronounced in the more obese patients. Improvements in HOMA estimates of insulin resistance and β-cell function were also greatest in the obese patients (4 mg: −16% and +19%; 8 mg: −37% and +33% respectively), as were reductions in fasting insulin. The profile of adverse events was not demonstrably different in obese patients versus non-obese patients.

Combination with Insulin

At the outset, it must be stated that the use of TZDs in patients with type 2 diabetes who are on insulin treatment is not approved in Europe. In the United States, both pioglitazone and rosiglitazone are approved for use in combination with insulin. However, the FDA has cautioned that because combination TZD and insulin therapy is associated with an increased incidence of pedal edema and a potentially greater propensity for patients to develop congestive heart failure (CHF), rosiglitazone and pioglitazone should be used prudently in patients with pre-existing pedal edema, especially in those who have evidence of milder degrees of heart failure [New York Heart Association (NYHA) Class 1 and 2]. In patients with NYHA Class 3 and 4 cardiac status, treatment with rosiglitazone or pioglitazone is currently not recommended.

Two large, multicenter studies have evaluated the efficacy and safety of the TZDs in insulin-treated patients with type 2 diabetes [53, 54]. In one study, Raskin et al. studied 319 type 2 diabetic patients with mean baseline $HbA_{1c} >7.5\%$ on twice-daily insulin therapy (total daily dose >30 U) [54]. These patients were randomized to 26 weeks of additional treatment with rosiglitazone (RSG) 4 or 8 mg daily or placebo (PBO). By intent-to-treat analysis, treatment with RSG plus insulin (I) resulted in a significant mean reduction in HbA_{1c} from baseline of 0.6% and 1.2% in the 4- and 8-mg groups respectively, despite a 6% and 12% mean reduction of insulin dosage in the two groups. The most common adverse event was symptoms consistent with hypoglycemia, which was reported in 53% of the I + RSG 4-mg group and 67% of the I + RSG 8-mg group compared with 38% in the I + PBO group. A total of 36 patients (5, 14, and 17 in the I + PBO, I + RSG 4-mg, and I + RSG 8-mg treatment groups, respectively) had at least one episode of one type of edema during the double-blind treatment period. Four of these patients (two in each I + RSG treatment group) entered the study with edema. No case of edema was considered to be a serious and no patients were withdrawn from the study because of edema. Of note, although BP was unchanged in the I + PBO and I + RSG 4 mg/day groups, there was a decrease of 2.6 mmHg in diastolic pressure in the I + RSG 8-mg/day group ($P < 0.005$). As expected, body weight increased significantly in all treatment groups (mean increase 0.9, 4.0, and 5.3 kg in I + PBO, I + RSG 4-mg, and I+RSG 8-mg groups, respectively).

In the other large, multicenter study, Rosenstock et al. studied 566 patients with type 2 diabetes on stable insulin regimens for >30 days and $HbA_{1c} >8.0\%$ [54]. These subjects were randomized to receive either 15 or 30 mg pioglitazone, or placebo in a 16-week double-blind, placebo-controlled trial. Per study protocol, the insulin dose remained unchanged, but could be decreased in response to hypoglycemia. At the end of double-blind treatment, patients receiving pioglitazone (15 mg or 30 mg) showed statistically significant mean decreases relative to baseline HbA_{1c}, of −1.0 and −1.3%. As in the study with rosiglitazone and insulin, the incidence of weight increase, hypoglycemia, and edema were higher among patients receiving insulin plus pioglitazone.

Since treatment with the TZDs is at times associated with variable amounts of weight gain, an excessive weight-gaining potential might be expected when these agents are used in massively obese patients with type 2 diabetes who invariably require large quantities of insulin to maintain glucose control. Buch et al. conducted such a study to evaluate the influence of the addition of rosiglitazone to insulin therapy over a 24-week period in massively obese patients with poorly controlled type 2 diabetes taking large doses of insulin [56]. Eight massively obese patients (median BMI = 42 kg/m^2) with type 2 diabetes who were on large doses of insulin (median daily dose of 204 U) and had poor glycemic control (median HbA_{1c} of 8.1%) were treated with the combination of insulin and maximum doses of rosiglitazone. Outcomes monitored were changes in weight, BMI, HbA_{1c}, dose of insulin, and the development of side effects. At the end of 24 weeks there was a median weight gain of 3 kg ($P < 0.01$), a fall in median HbA_{1c} from 8.1 to 6.7% ($P < 0.01$), and a reduction in median insulin dose from 204 to 159 U/day ($P < 0.01$) (23% reduction from baseline). Peripheral edema was the only significant side effect and was seen in five of the eight patients. The authors concluded that the combination of insulin and rosiglitazone is effective in massively obese patients with type 2 diabetes, without excessive weight gain but a high incidence of peripheral edema.

Dosage

The usual starting dose of rosiglitazone is 4 mg p.o. given as either a single dose once daily or in divided doses twice daily. For patients who respond inadequately after 12 weeks of initial treatment with rosiglitazone, the dose may be increased to 8 mg p.o. given as a single dose once daily or in divided doses twice daily. For pioglitazone, initiate therapy may be initiated at 15 mg or 30 mg p.o. once daily. For patients who respond inadequately to the initial dose, the dose can be increased in 15-mg increments up to 45 mg p.o. once daily. Patients not responding adequately to monotherapy with either rosiglitazone or pioglitazone should be considered for combination therapy with other antidiabetic agents. The safety and efficacy of both drugs in adolescents and children has not yet been established.

Patients with Hepatic Impairment

If a patient exhibits clinical or laboratory evidence of active liver disease or increased serum transaminase levels [alanine transaminase (ALT) >2.5 times the upper limit of normal] at start of therapy, rosiglitazone or pioglitazone therapy should not be initiated (see contraindications below).

Patients with Renal Impairment

There are no clinically relevant differences in the pharmacokinetics of rosiglitazone or pioglitazone in patients with mild to severe renal impairment or in hemodialysis-dependent patients, compared to patients with normal renal function [57]. Hence dosage adjustments are not required in patients receiving these agents alone. However, since metformin is contraindicated in patients with renal impairment, concomitant administration of rosiglitazone or pioglitazone with metformin is also contraindicated in patients with renal impairment.

METABOLIC EFFECTS

The TZDs have been shown to have multiple beneficial effects not only on peripheral insulin sensitivity, hepatic glucose metabolism, and lipid metabolism, but also on endothelial function, atherogenesis, fibrinolysis, ovarian steroidogenesis, and immune function [13].

Effects on Insulin Sensitivity

Several studies have documented the *in vivo* effects of TZDs on peripheral insulin action not only in patients with type 2 diabetes, but also in other insulin-resistant states like impaired glucose tolerance (IGT), polycystic ovary disease, previous gestational diabetes, and Werner's syndrome [58–64]. Some of these studies have used the hyperinsulinemic-euglycemic clamp study that is currently considered the "gold standard" to evaluate peripheral insulin sensitivity, while others have used the frequently sampled intravenous glucose tolerance test (FSIGTT) and other less direct methods, including the insulin tolerance test, the intravenous or oral glucose tolerance test (OGTT), and the homeostatis model of assessment (HOMA)-S to assess TZD effects on insulin resistance. In all these studies, the TZDs have improved insulin-mediated peripheral glucose utilization in both obese and lean, insulin-resistant, type 2 diabetes patients by approximately 30 to 100%.

Miyazaki et al. used the two-step (40 and 160 mU/min/m^2) hyperinsulinemic clamp, indirect calorimetry, and hepatic tracer technology to evaluate hepatic and peripheral insulin sensitivity in 23 obese (BMI <36 kg/m^2) diabetic patients, who after being treated with a stable dose of sulfonylurea, were randomly assigned to the addition of either placebo or pioglitazone (45 mg/day) ($n = 12$) [65]. After 16 weeks, with pioglitazone treatment, there were significant decreases in FPG (184 to 135 mg/dl), HbA_{1C} (8.9 to 7.2%), and plasma FFA levels. In addition, before and after pioglitazone treatment, basal endogenous glucose production (EGP) and FPG were strongly correlated ($r = 0.67$, $P < 0.01$). Further, EGP during the first insulin clamp step was significantly decreased after pioglitazone treatment ($P < 0.05$), whereas insulin-stimulated total and nonoxidative glucose disposal during the second insulin clamp was increased by 38% ($P < 0.01$) (Figure 4) The change in FPG was related to the change in basal EGP, EGP during the first insulin clamp step, and total glucose disposal during the second insulin clamp step. These results suggest that pioglitazone therapy in type 2 diabetic patients decreases fasting and postprandial plasma glucose levels by improving hepatic and peripheral (muscle) tissue sensitivity to insulin.

In another recent large, international study, Pavo et al. studied the effect of 32 weeks of monotherapy with either pioglitazone or metformin on glycemic control and

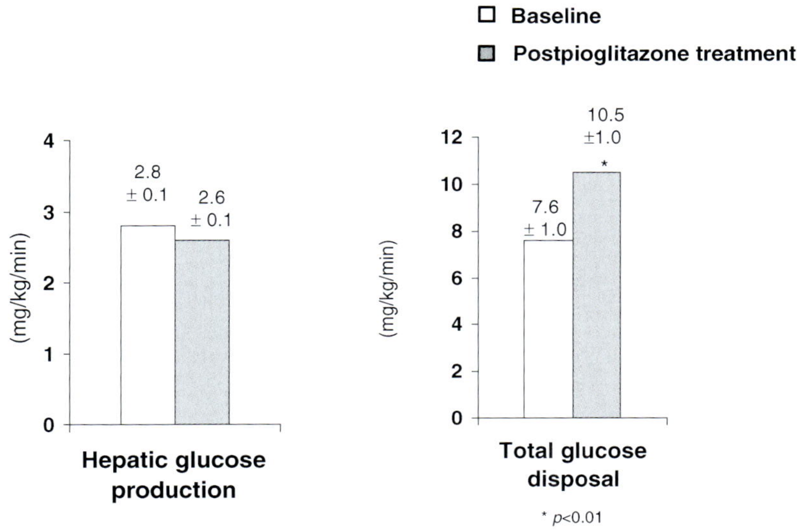

Figure 4 Effects of pioglitazone 45 mg daily for 4 months on hepatic glucose production (HGP) and glucose disposal rate (Rd) in patients with type 2 diabetes. (Data from reference 65; figure modified from reference 66)

insulin sensitivity in 205 patients with recently diagnosed type 2 diabetes who were naive to antidiabetic therapy [67]. Subjects were randomized to either 30 mg pioglitazone or 850 mg metformin daily, with titrations upward to 45 mg (77% of pioglitazone patients) and 2550 mg (73% of metformin patients), as indicated, to achieve FPG levels of <126 mg/dl. Although pioglitazone was comparable to metformin in improving glycemic control as measured by HbA_{1C} and FPG (decreases of $\sim$1.3% and 54 mg/dl respectively), after 24 weeks of treatment, insulin sensitivity (as assessed by HOMA-S) increased significantly in the pioglitazone group (17.4%; $P < 0.05$) as compared with an increase of only 8.9% in the metformin group ($P = 0.21$).

There are also two early studies from Japan that document the insulin-sensitizing effects of pioglitazone in Japanese patients with type 2 diabetes [68, 69]. In a double-blind, placebo-controlled clinical trial, Kawamori et al. evaluated the effect of pioglitazone on insulin resistance in patients with type 2 diabetes [68]. Insulin sensitivity (measured as Rd by the hyperinsulinemic clamp technique) and splanchnic glucose uptake (SGU) both increased significantly after 3 months of pioglitazone treatment. Placebo treatment produced no significant changes in either Rd or SGU. The authors concluded that pioglitazone is effective in ameliorating insulin resistance in type 2 diabetes by enhancing SGU as well as peripheral glucose uptake [68]. In the other Japanese study, Yamasaki et al. also evaluated the effect of pioglitazone on Rd in 20 patients with type 2 diabetes. After oral administration of pioglitazone (30 mg/day) for 3 months, together with improvements in glycemic control, fasting insulin, and C peptide as well as lipid levels, Rd significantly improved by more than 50%. In this study, the change in Rd before and after pioglitazone administration significantly correlated with baseline values of FPG, serum insulin, and BMI [69].

Similar to pioglitazone, there are several studies documenting the effects of rosiglitazone on peripheral insulin sensitivity in both diabetic and nondiabetic subjects. In one of the early studies, Miyazaki et al. studied 29 diet-treated diabetic patients who were randomly assigned to receive either rosiglitazone, 8 mg/day or placebo [70]. After 12 weeks, as expected, rosiglitazone not only improved the FPG (195–150 mg/dl) and HbA_{1c} (8.7–7.4%), but also significantly suppressed EGP by 13% and increased whole body glucose uptake (as measure by the insulin clamp technique) by 37% (Figure 5). These beneficial changes that also included a decrease in FFA levels occurred despite an increase in both body weight and total fat mass of 4 kg. Also as expected, there were significant correlations between measures of insulin sensitivity and plasma FFA levels. The authors concluded that rosiglitazone increases hepatic and peripheral (muscle) tissue insulin sensitivity and reduces FFA turnover despite increased total body fat mass and suggested that the beneficial effects of rosiglitazone on glycemic control are mediated, in part, by the drug's effect on FFA metabolism [70].

It does appear paradoxical that despite an increase in body fat mass, the TZDs improve insulin sensitivity. There is now evidence that this increase in fat mass occurs in the SQ but not visceral body regions. Furthermore, the TZDs redistribute intracellular lipid away from insulin-responsive organs (like skeletal muscle and liver, where their accumulation appears to be deleterious) and into peripheral SQ adipocytes that are rendered more insulin sensitive after TZD treatment. This concept is elegantly demonstrated in a study by Mayerson et al. who examined the effect of 3 months of rosiglitazone treatment

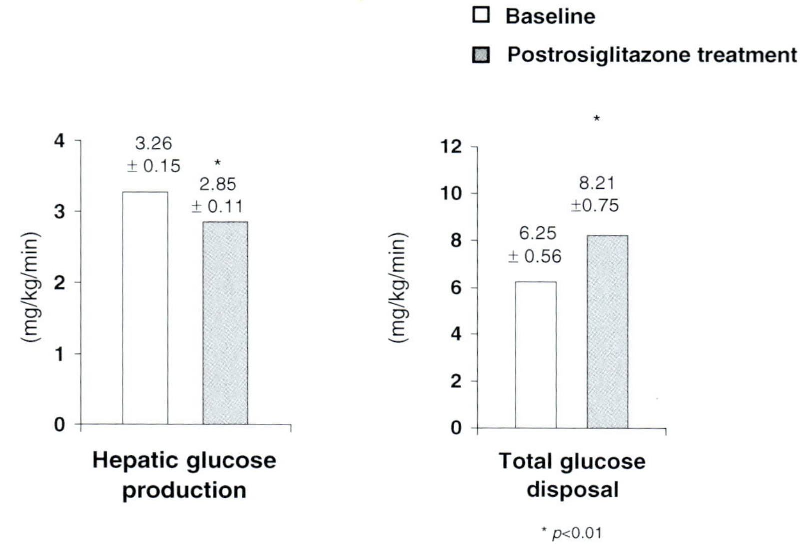

Figure 5 Effects of rosiglitazone 8 mg daily for 4 months on hepatic glucose production (HGP) and glucose disposal rate (Rd) in patients with type 2 diabetes. (Data from reference 70)

(4 mg b.i.d.) on whole-body insulin sensitivity and *in vivo* peripheral adipocyte insulin sensitivity (as assessed by a novel glycerol release in microdialysis from SQ fat) during a two-step hyperinsulinemic-euglycemic clamp in nine type 2 diabetic subjects [71]. Also measured were the effects of rosiglitazone on liver and muscle triglyceride content as assessed by ^{1}H-nuclear magnetic resonance spectroscopy. After rosiglitazone treatment, there were significant improvements in insulin-stimulated glucose metabolism by 68% and 20% during the low- and high-dosage insulin clamps, respectively. This was associated with significant reductions in plasma fatty acid concentration and hepatic triglyceride content, a 39% increase in extramyocellular lipid content and a 52% increase in the sensitivity of peripheral adipocytes to the inhibitory effects of insulin on lipolysis. These results support the hypothesis that TZDs enhance insulin sensitivity in patients with type 2 diabetes by promoting increased insulin sensitivity in peripheral adipocytes, which results in lower plasma fatty acid concentrations and a redistribution of intracellular lipid from insulin-responsive organs into peripheral adipocytes. Results from this study are reinforced by the findings from another recent study by Virtanen et al. from Finland who evaluated the effects of rosiglitazone (4 mg b.i.d.) and metformin (1 g b.i.d.) monotherapy for 26 weeks on adipose tissue insulin-stimulated glucose uptake in 41 patients with early type 2 diabetes (FPG ~140 mg/dl) [72]. Before and after the treatment, glucose uptake was measured using 2-[^{18}F]fluoro-2-deoxyglucose and positron emission tomography (PET), and adipose tissue masses were quantified using magnetic resonance imaging (MRI). After 6 months of treatment, rosiglitazone improved insulin-stimulated whole-body glucose uptake by 44%, as compared with no change with metformin treatment despite a decrease in body weight of 2.0 kg and no weight change in the rosiglitazone group. In visceral adipose tissue, glucose uptake increased by 29% in the rosiglitazone group and by 17% in the metformin group. Since the visceral adipose tissue mass simultaneously decreased with both treatments, no change was observed in total visceral glucose uptake. Rosiglitazone, but not metformin, significantly enhanced glucose uptake in the femoral SQ area. This study highlights the central role of adipose tissue in mediating the action of TZDs *in vivo* and also the role of SQ adipose tissue in improving whole-body insulin sensitivity.

The same investigators have also conducted another interesting study in which they compared the effects of rosiglitazone and metformin on skeletal muscle insulin responsiveness at rest and during exercise in patients with newly diagnosed type 2 diabetes [73]. Skeletal muscle glucose uptake was measured using fluorine-18-labeled fluorodeoxyglucose and PET during a euglycemic-hyperinsulinemic clamp and one-legged exercise before and after treatment with rosiglitazone or metformin for 3 months. Glucose uptake in skeletal muscle was increased by 38% and whole-body glucose uptake by 44% in the rosiglitazone group. Furthermore, the exercise-induced increment during insulin stimulation was significantly enhanced by 99% in the rosiglitazone group. Results from this study suggest that rosiglitazone improves the synergistic action of insulin and exercise.

All the above studies on insulin sensitivity have been performed in patients with type 2 diabetes. It is important to note that the TZDs also have insulin-sensitizing effects in nondiabetic subjects. Raji et al. examined the effect of rosiglitazone on insulin resistance and BP in 24 hypertensive nondiabetic patients (age 58 years, BMI = 30 kg/m^2) before and after rosiglitazone treatment (4 mg b.i.d.) [74]. After 16 weeks, although there was no change in FPG (83 vs. 82 mg/dl), fasting insulin levels decreased (16.1 vs. 12.5 μU/ml, $P < 0.01$). Total glucose disposal during an insulin clamp increased (5.0 vs. 5.9 mg/kg/min, $P < 0.001$), with no change in suppression of hepatic glucose output. There were also significant decreases in mean 24-h systolic (138 vs. 134 mmHg, $P < 0.02$) and diastolic (85 vs. 80 mmHg, $P < 0.0001$) BP, and the decline in systolic blood pressure (SBP) was correlated with the improvement in insulin sensitivity ($r = 0.59$, $P < 0.005$). Interestingly, there were decreases in all the lipid parameters—triglycerides (135 vs. 89 mg/dl, $P < 0.01$), LDL cholesterol (129 vs. 122 mg/dl, $P = 0.18$), and HDL cholesterol (51 vs. 46 mg/dl, $P < 0.02$), with no change in the LDL-to-HDL ratio. Plasminogen activator inhibitor 1 (PAI-1) and C-reactive protein also declined significantly. Thus rosiglitazone treatment of obese, nondiabetic, hypertensive patients improves insulin sensitivity, reduces systolic and diastolic blood pressure (DBP), and induces favorable changes in markers of cardiovascular risk [74].

Similar results were obtained in a study of 60 nondiabetic patients with arterial hypertension who were randomized to receive either pioglitazone (45 mg/day) or placebo for 16 weeks [75]. After 4 months, insulin sensitivity (*M*-value) increased by 1.2 mg/kg/min with pioglitazone, compared with 0.4 mg/kg/min ($P = 0.022$) with placebo. Decreases in fasting insulin and glucose were significantly greater with pioglitazone than placebo. Body weight did not change significantly with either treatment. HDL-cholesterol was increased and apolipoprotein B was decreased to a significantly greater extent with pioglitazone. There was also a significantly greater decrease from baseline in DBP, with pioglitazone. As with rosiglitazone, these changes suggest improved glucose metabolism and a possible reduction in risk of cardiovascular disease with pioglitazone treatment of nondiabetic patients with arterial hypertension.

Effects on β-Cell Function

Along with defects in action in target insulin-sensitive tissues, defects in insulin secretion from the pancreatic β-cells also play a major role in the pathogenesis of type 2 diabetes. Data from the UKPDS and other studies have suggested that β-cell function decreases with duration of type 2 diabetes whether treated with diet therapy or antihyperglycemic pharmacologic therapy [76, 77]. The recent demonstration that PPAR-γ is expressed in human islet endocrine cells, both at the mRNA and protein levels, supports the hypothesis of a direct influence of TZDs on human pancreatic endocrine cells [78]. Indeed, there is now preliminary data in humans that TZD therapy may improve β-cell function. In one 6-month study [43], patients treated with 2 and 4 mg rosiglitazone b.i.d. showed increases in estimated β-cell function of 49.5% and 60.0%, respectively ($P < 0.00001$, compared with placebo for both groups). By contrast, estimated β-cell function decreased 4.5% in the placebo group. The improvement in β-cell function may be secondary to the increased insulin sensitivity, the concomitant decrease in hyperglycemia, or direct effects of the TZDs on the pancreatic β-cell. It will be important to determine whether the improvement in β-cell function that occurs with TZD therapy persists over the long-term and prevents progressive pancreatic decompensation in patients with type 2 diabetes.

As compared to the above study in which HOMA was used to measure β-cell function, other investigators have used the plasma insulin response to a glucose load as a measure of β-cell insulin secretory capacity. Using this method, some studies have reported a decrease in plasma insulin response to a glucose challenge [79, 80], whereas others have failed to observe any significant change [81]. However, in a recent study, Miyazaki et al. [82] found an increase in plasma insulin response during OGTT in diabetic patients treated with 30 and 45 mg/day of pioglitazone. An increased or maintained plasma insulin response in the presence of a decreased plasma glucose concentration suggests an improvement in β-cell function. It is possible that the variable effect of TZDs on the plasma insulin response to a glucose challenge is explained by two opposing effects. First, a decrease in fasting and postprandial glucose concentrations, leading to reduced "glucose toxicity" on the β-cell and improved insulin secretion, and second, with the improvement in insulin sensitivity, there is a reduced requirement for insulin secretion [83, 84]. Another surrogate measure of β-cell function is the ratio of proinsulin (PI) to IRI. An elevated ratio of PI to IRI is often present in type 2 diabetes and may reflect dysfunctional β-cell processing of the prohormone and associated reduced β-cell secretory capacity [85]. Treatment with several TZDs has been shown to be associated with a decrease in PI/IRI ratio suggestive of direct effects on the β-cell [85, 86].

The exact mechanisms by which the TZDs influence pancreatic insulin secretion is still not known, but in animal studies, it has been shown that rosiglitazone has a potentiation effect on insulin secretion in the presence of glucose, which is mediated by the PI-3K pathway and is clearly distinct from that of glucose-stimulated insulin secretion [87].

Effects on Diabetes Prevention

It is well recognized that subjects with IGT (those with a plasma glucose between 140 and 199 mg/dl, 2 h after a

75-g oral glucose load) are not only insulin resistant, but also at high-risk to progress on to type 2 diabetes. Since the TZDs are potent insulin sensitizers, they have the potential to be used as agents to prevent type 2 diabetes in such high-risk populations. Indeed, in a recent study, Buchanan et al. observed that troglitazone at 400 mg daily for up to 5 years, reduced the incidence of type 2 diabetes by 50% in high-risk Hispanic women with a recent history of gestational diabetes mellitus (GDM) [88]. Also, in the landmark Diabetes Prevention Program, troglitazone along with metformin and intensive lifestyle intervention was one of the intervention arms [89]. However, the troglitazone arm was discontinued after reports of idiosyncratic hepatotoxicity associated with its use. Interestingly however, in the subjects who did receive troglitazone for a mean of 0.9 years (0.5–1.5 years), there was a robust 75% reduction in the incidence of diabetes compared to the placebo group [90]. In the same period, there was a 57% reduction in the intensive lifestyle group and a 44% reduction in the metformin group. Of note, after troglitazone withdrawal, the diabetes incidence rate increased to that of the placebo group, thereby indicating that the protective effect did not persist after the drug was stopped. This is in contrast to the findings from the study conducted by Buchanan et al. in Hispanic women with GDM, in whom the effects of troglitazone persisted for up to 8 months after discontinuation [88]. Clearly, long-term studies are needed to determine whether other drugs in the TZD class, when used for short or long periods, can safely delay or prevent diabetes.

Effects on Lipids

In type 2 diabetes, the major quantitative changes in lipid levels are an elevation in triglyceride-rich lipoproteins, and a decrease in HDL cholesterol concentrations and LDL cholesterol levels that are often quantitatively similar to those in the general population [91]. However, qualitative changes in the composition of the LDL molecule, including an increase in the proportion of small dense LDL (which is prone to glycation and oxidation), tend to make it more atherogenic [91]. This diabetic dyslipidemic profile is closely related to underlying insulin resistance and may, in part, be responsible for the increased cardiovascular morbidity and mortality in type 2 diabetic patients [92]. By improving glucose tolerance and reducing insulin resistance, the TZDs have the potential to favorably influence diabetic dyslipidemia.

In initial studies with pioglitazone, triglycerides were lowered by ~9% and HDL levels increased by ~12–19% [93, 94]. Earlier, troglitazone also was shown to lower the triglyceride levels ~15–20% [95] and increase HDL cholesterol levels ~5–8% [13]. Reduction in triglyceride levels appears to result from several mechanisms including reduced FFA substrate availability, decreased hepatic triglyceride synthesis, and enhanced peripheral clearance [13]. In the case of rosiglitazone, however, despite a significant decrease in FFA levels by up to 22%, studies have not demonstrated any significant lowering of triglycerides, although HDL levels do increase by up to 19%. The reasons for these differences are not clear at present. Recently, Freed et al. published results from a large study that evaluated the effects of rosiglitazone therapy on lipids and also the efficacy and safety of rosiglitazone in combination with atorvastatin in patients with type 2 diabetes mellitus [96]. Three-hundred thirty-two patients entered an 8-week, open-label, run-in treatment phase with rosiglitazone 8 mg/day, and 243 were randomized to a 16-week, double-blinded period of continued rosiglitazone plus placebo, atorvastatin 10 mg/day, or atorvastatin 20 mg/day. With rosiglitazone alone, at 8 weeks, there was a modest increase in LDL cholesterol (9%), a shift in LDL phenotype from dense to large buoyant subfractions (52% of patients), an increase in total HDL cholesterol levels (6%), and no significant change in triglyceride levels. After 24 weeks of rosiglitazone + placebo treatment, there was no change in LDL levels from baseline, and small nonsignificant 4.4% decrease in HDL levels and 2.2% increase in triglyceride levels. When atorvastatin was added to rosiglitazone, however, there was a further increase in HDL3 (5%) from week 8 and significant reductions in LDL cholesterol (−39%), apolipoprotein B (−35%), and triglyceride levels (−27%). Glycemic control achieved with rosiglitazone alone was not adversely affected by add-on atorvastatin. The combination was well tolerated, compared with placebo. Thus in this study, the LDL-cholesterol-lowering effect of atorvastatin was not influenced negatively by rosiglitazone.

At present, based on current available evidence, it is not possible to say which of the currently available TZDs is superior in improving lipid parameters. Although there have been two studies published so far showing differences in lipid parameters with pioglitazone and rosiglitazone, neither of these studies are head-to-head, randomized, double-blind studies in the same population [97, 98].

Of note, with all the TZDs studied so far, there is an increase in LDL cholesterol levels, which is concerning [13, 99]. However, data are emerging that this increase in LDL cholesterol with the TZDs is not accompanied with any changes in atherogenic apolipoprotein B levels [13, 67, 96]. Moreover, following TZD treatment, the LDL particles became larger, more buoyant, and less prone to oxidative modification [96, 100, 101]. However, long-term follow-up will be needed to see if the rise in LDL has a negative impact on atherosclerosis and cardiovascular mortality.

Another aspect of TZD effects on lipids that is not yet clear at present is their effect on the other atherogenic lipoprotein, lipoprotein(a) [Lp(a)]. There have been reports in the past that Lp(a) levels increase significantly after troglitazone treatment [102, 103]. However, in a recent report, Nagai et al. reported that unlike with troglitazone therapy, pioglitazone treatment was not associated with an increase in Lp(a) levels [104]. Since Lp(a) may be associated with the development of coronary artery disease, further larger, long-term studies are needed to confirm and evaluate the significance of changes in Lp(a) levels in TZD-treated diabetic patients.

Effects on Adipose Tissue

One of the intriguing aspects of treatment with the TZDs has been the observation that although patients treated with the TZDs significantly improve their insulin sensitivity and glucose and lipid profiles, they tend to gain weight and accumulate adipose tissue. Considerable research has focused on the sites and nature of this adipose tissue weight gain. It is well known that the TZDs, through PPAR-γ activation cause preadipocytes to differentiate into mature fat cells and also cause the induction of key enzymes involved in lipogenesis [105]. At the tissue level, however, *in vitro* studies have demonstrated that troglitazone specifically promotes the differentiation of preadipocytes into adipocytes only in SQ fat and not in omental fat [106]. Site differences in adipose tissue function appear to have implications for insulin-resistant conditions. In mature adipose tissue, SQ adipocytes have higher leptin secretion, similar tumor necrosis factor TNF-α secretion, and lower catecholamine-stimulated lipolysis as compared with omental adipocytes [107]. Thus it would appear that the accumulation of SQ fat rather that visceral (omental) fat might be beneficial in terms of promoting insulin sensitivity.

In vivo studies in human beings appear to confirm that the TZD treatment produces a shift in adipose tissue distribution from omental to the SQ compartment. In one of the early studies, Mori et al. demonstrated that in 30 mildly obese, Japanese patients with type 2 diabetes, troglitazone at 400 mg/day for 6 months not only improved glycemia and increased BMI, but also resulted in fat accumulation in the SQ rather than the visceral adipose tissue depot [108]. Similar findings were obtained by Kelley et al. in a Caucasian population. In this double-blind, randomized trial, troglitazone therapy for 12 weeks significantly decreased intraabdominal (visceral) fat mass as measured by MRI [109]. In this study, there were no significant changes in total body fat and body weight as compared to placebo.

As with the above studies using troglitazone, determinations of fat distribution after rosiglitazone and pioglitazone therapy have also confirmed that there is greater accumulation in the SQ adipose tissue compartment at the expense of visceral fat. Carey et al. investigated the effects of rosiglitazone on insulin sensitivity and regional adiposity (including intrahepatic fat) in 33 patients with type 2 diabetes who were randomized to either rosiglitazone 8 mg/day or placebo [110]. Measurements of insulin sensitivity (euglycemic hyperinsulinemic clamp), body fat [abdominal MRI and DEXA (dual energy X-ray absorptiometry)] and liver fat (magnetic resonance spectroscopy) were taken at baseline and repeated after 16 weeks of treatment. As compared with baseline, rosiglitazone treatment was associated with a significant improvement in glycemic control ($HbA_{1C} = -0.7\%$) and an 86% increase in insulin sensitivity. Total body weight and fat mass increased with rosiglitazone (2.1 ± 2.0 kg and 1.4 $\pm$1.6 kg, respectively) with 95% of the increase in adiposity occurring in nonabdominal regions. In the abdominal region, rosiglitazone increased SQ fat area by 8%, did not alter intraabdominal fat area, and reduced intrahepatic fat levels by 45%. Thus, in this study, improvements in insulin sensitivity were associated with an increase in adiposity only in SQ but not visceral depots.

Similar results were obtained after pioglitazone therapy, by Miyazaki and coworkers [111]. They examined the effect of pioglitazone on abdominal fat distribution in 13 type 2 diabetic patients (nine men and four women; age, 52 years; BMI = 29.0 kg/m^2), who were being treated with a stable dose of sulfonylurea ($n = 7$) or with diet alone ($n = 6$) and received pioglitazone (45 mg/day) for 16 weeks. Before and after pioglitazone treatment, subjects underwent a 75-g OGTT and an insulin clamp. Abdominal fat distribution was evaluated using MRI at L4-5. After 16 weeks of pioglitazone treatment, there were significant improvements in FPG (179 to 140 mg/dl, HbA_{1C} 8.6 to 7.2% along with decreases in EGP, and fasting plasma FFA levels. These improvement in hepatic and peripheral tissue insulin sensitivity occurred despite increases in body weight (82 to 85 kg; $P < 0.05$) and fat mass (27 to 30 kg; $P < 0.05$). After pioglitazone treatment, SQ fat area at L4-5 (301 to 342 cm^2; $P < 0.01$) increased, whereas visceral fat area at L4-5 (144 to 131 cm^2; $P < 0.05$) and the ratio of visceral to SQ fat (0.59 to 0.44; $P < 0.01$) decreased (Figure 6). In the postabsorptive state, hepatic insulin resistance (as measured by basal EGP $\times$ basal IRI) correlated positively with visceral fat area ($r = 0.55$; $P < 0.01$) and the glucose metabolic clearance rates (MCRs) during the insulin clamp steps were negatively correlated with the visceral fat area [111]. These results demonstrate that a shift in fat distribution from visceral to SQ adipose depots after pioglitazone treatment is associated with improvements in hepatic and peripheral tissue sensitivity to insulin.

CARDIOVASCULAR EFFECTS

The TZDs have multiple beneficial effects on the cardiovascular system, and these are detailed below and in Table 3.

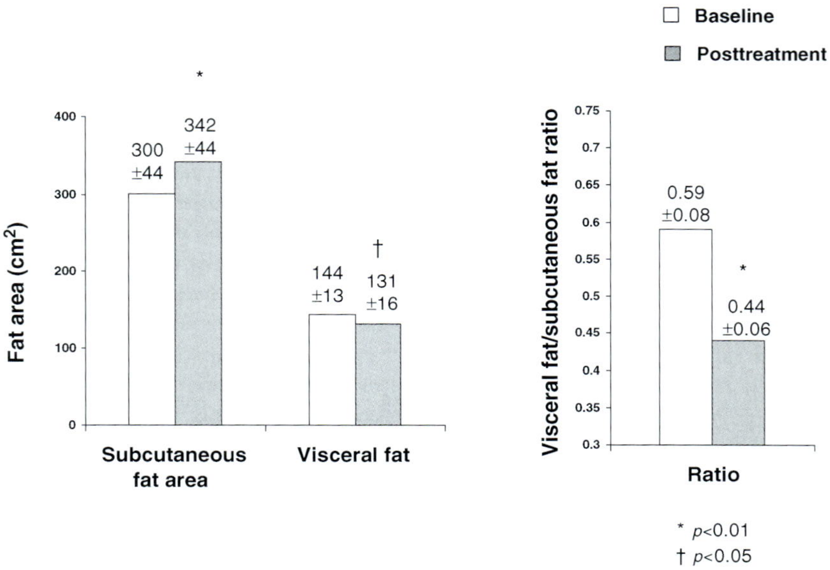

Figure 6 Effects of pioglitazone 45 mg daily for 4 months on abdominal fat distribution in patients with type 2 diabetes. (Data from reference 111)

Effects on Cardiac Structure and Function

Early in the course of development of the TZDs, it was noted that troglitazone caused reversible increases in heart weight in Wistar rats after chronic treatment with doses exceeding 10 times those recommended in human beings [112]. Subsequent studies, however, demonstrated that treatment of cultured murine cardiac myocytes with PPAR-γ ligands such as troglitazone, pioglitazone, and rosiglitazone actually inhibited angiotensin-II-induced upregulation of skeletal α-actin and atrial natriuretic peptide genes and an increase in cell surface area. Further, treatment of mice with pioglitazone inhibited pressure overload-induced increases in the heart-weight-to-body-weight ratio, wall thickness, and myocyte diameter in wild-type mice [113]. In human studies, it has been shown in a large randomized, double-blind study that treatment with troglitazone at 800 mg produced no significant changes in left ventricular mass index (LVMI) after 48 weeks of surveillance. In fact, as compared to the control glyburide group, significant increases in cardiac stroke volume and cardiac index and significant decreases in diastolic pressure and peripheral vascular resistance were observed in troglitazone-treated patients [112]. Thus in this study, not only did troglitazone-treated patients not show any cardiac mass increase or cardiac function impairment, they actually demonstrated improved cardiac function with enhanced cardiac output and stroke volume, possibly as a result of decreased peripheral vascular resistance. In another recent study, St. John Sutton et al. assessed the effect of long-term treatment with rosiglitazone on cardiac structure/function and glycemic control in patients with type 2 diabetes compared with a sulfonylurea (glyburide). After 52 weeks of treatment, small but significant increases from baseline in LVMI were observed in the rosiglitazone-treated group [114]. These changes occurred primarily by week 28 but did not progress further at week 52. However, the change in LVMI in the rosiglitazone group was not statistically significantly different to that in the glyburide group, with mean values in both groups staying within 1 SD of the mean value in healthy patient. In addition to the increase in LVMI, in this study, small increases in left ventricular end diastolic volume (LVEDV) were also observed in both treatment groups at weeks 28 and 52, but these were not considered clinically relevant because the final values did not exceed the mean normal value plus 1 SD. Of note and consistent with previous studies, there were small but significant decreases in DBP in the rosiglitazone group.

Table 3 Cardiovascular risk factor reduction with thaizolidinedione Treatment

- Improve dyslipidemia (↑ HDL-C, ↓ triglyceride (TG), ↓ LDL density)
- Decrease microalbuminuria, BP
- Reduce carotid intimal medial thickness
- Reduce neointimal/VSMC proliferation, macrophage migration
- Improve vascular reactivity, endothelial function
- Decrease vascular inflammation, CRP, Endothelin-1, MMP-9, MCP-1 levels
- Increase thrombolysis, decrease PAI-1 activity
- Increase adiponectin levels

Interestingly, in mice with post-MI heart failure, pioglitazone treatment has been shown to attenuate LV expression of inflammatory cytokines and chemokines, resulting in improved left ventricular remodeling and function [115, 116]. It remains to be determined whether similar effects occur in human beings.

In another interesting recent report, Rizvi et al. have described the successful use of a TZD agent for the treatment of diabetes diagnosed after heart transplantation [117]. In this case, rosiglitazone was used to treat a 51-year-old woman who underwent cardiac transplantation because of cardiomyopathy, and developed diabetes 6 months later and required high dose insulin to achieve glucose control during maintenance immunosuppressive therapy. After rosiglitazone therapy was instituted, the patient's insulin dose was gradually tapered and eventually stopped. Target glycemic control was maintained without apparent aggravation of cardiac function or volume overload. Further, no deleterious effects on other organ systems or interactions with the antirejection medications were noted during close follow-up.

It must be mentioned here that, notwithstanding the multiple beneficial effects on cardiac structure and function mentioned above, there appears to be a paradox that in clinical practice, use of the TZDs has been associated with a propensity toward increased fluid retention and possibly precipitation of congestive heart failure in a small minority of patients. In the United States the FDA cautions that during clinical use of rosiglitazone and pioglitazone, prescribers should closely evaluate for signs of edema and CHF in all patients; moreover, patients with advanced degrees of CHF (NYHA Class III and IV) should not be started on TZD treatment. The effects of the TZDs on fluid retention and CHF and possible mechanisms are discussed in detail under Side Effects.

Effects of BP

Hypertension is often associated with insulin resistance and several other components of the insulin resistance (metabolic) syndrome. Indeed, the prevalence of hypertension in diabetic patients is up to twofold higher than in nondiabetic individuals [118]. In type 2 diabetes and other insulin-resistant states there is impaired insulin-induced vasodilation [119] and it is possible that by enhancing insulin action, the TZDs may enhance the tonic vasodilator response to insulin and thereby reduce peripheral vascular resistance and BP. Further, by reducing hyperinsulinemia and plasma insulin levels, it is possible that the TZDs attenuate the potential blood-pressure-raising actions of insulin, such as renal sodium retention and increased sympathetic activity [118–121]. The data are now consistent that the TZDs have small, but beneficial effects on BP. In one study, compared to glyburide, rosiglitazone treatment at 4 mg b.i.d. over 52 weeks was associated with a significant decrease in SBP of 3.5 mmHg and DBP of 2.7 mmHg, despite similar glycemic control [122]. Similar results were obtained with pioglitazone in another study. In this study, as compared to placebo, pioglitazone 45 mg daily for 16 weeks reduced mean SBP by 6.7 mmHg and DBP by 7.9 mmHg as compared to a decrease of 3.1 and 1.8 mmHg with placebo [123]. In another study in Japanese patients with type 2 diabetes, pioglitazone at 30 mg daily for 3 months reduced mean BP from 109 to 101 mmHg [124]. Thus, although small, the effects of the TZDs on BP are consistent and may be beneficial in the long-term prevention of cardiovascular complications.

Effects on Glomerular Function and Albuminuria

Microalbuminuria, defined as a urinary albumin excretion (UAE) rate between 30 and 300 mg/24 h is widely considered to be a marker of impaired vascular integrity in type 2 diabetic patients and is also considered to be an early indicator of renal and cardiovascular disease risk as well as of an increased risk of all-cause mortality [125]. Thus, microalbuminuria is an indication for aggressive intervention to improve glycemic and BP control and to reduce cardiovascular risk factors. In early animal studies, the TZDs have been shown to reduce both BP and albuminuria [126, 127]. Beneficial effects in humans have been demonstrated with both pioglitazone and rosiglitazone. In a study from Japan [128], 45 type 2 diabetes patients with microalbuminuria were randomly assigned to treatment with pioglitazone at 30 mg/day, glibenclamide at 5 mg/day, or voglibose (an α-glucosidase inhibitor) at 0.6 mg/day. After 3 months, only pioglitazone 30 mg daily was effective in reducing not only UAE, but also urinary endothelin-1 (ET-1) concentrations (Figure 7). Urinary ET-1 excretion is present in type 2 diabetes patients with microalbuminuria, and an increase in circulating ET-1 precedes the microalbuminuric phase of renal injury related to diabetes.

Effects of rosiglitazone on microalbuminuria were demonstrated in a 26-week, randomized, placebo-controlled study in which rosiglitazone 2 mg b.i.d. and 4 mg b.i.d. was shown to significantly reduce UAE (as assessed by the urinary albumin/creatinine ratio [ACR]) [43] (Figure 8). These effects were confirmed in a larger, longer term 52-week, open-label, cardiac-safety study comparing rosiglitazone and glyburide. In this study, 203 patients were randomized to treatment with rosiglitazone 4 mg b.i.d. or glyburide [114]. At 52 weeks, despite similar control of blood glucose levels, rosiglitazone, but not glyburide, reduced UAE. Because both agents controlled blood glucose equally, it would seem that glycemic control *per se* is not sufficient to repair vascular damage and reduce albuminuria. Also of note, in this study rosiglitazone concomitantly lowered BP significantly more than did glyburide, as observed by ambulatory BP monitoring. Thus, it remains unclear, whether the beneficial effect of rosiglitazone in reducing microalbuminuria is mediated through

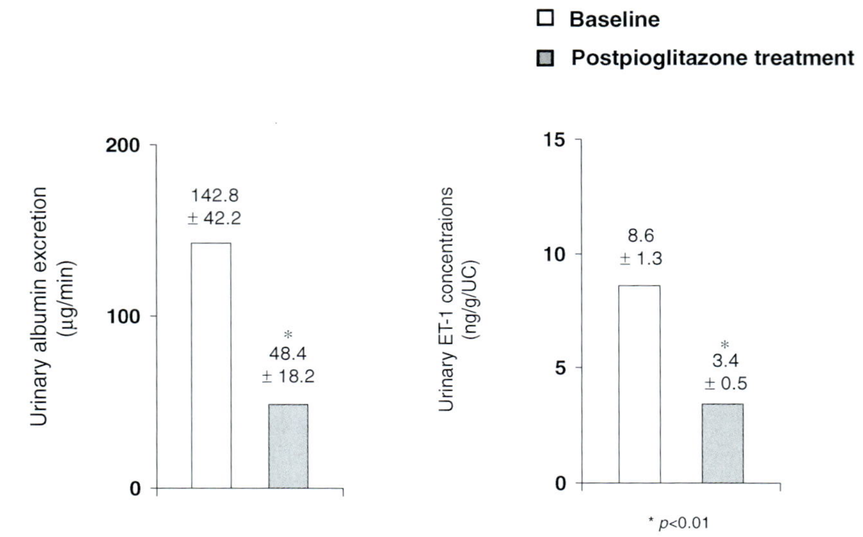

Figure 7 Effect of pioglitazone treatment for 3 months on urinary albumin excretion and endothelin-1 (ET-1) in normotensive patients with type 2 diabetes and microalbuminuria

BP reduction or via direct vasculoprotective mechanisms. Regardless of the mechanism, it is important to know that rosiglitazone not only controls blood glucose levels in patients with type 2 diabetes mellitus but also reduces BP and microalbuminuria.

Antiatherogenic Effects

Atherosclerosis is a progressive vascular disease initiated by the accumulation of plasma LDL cholesterol in the subintimal space of the vessels and culminating in plaque rupture with resultant thrombosis and acute occlusion, leading to a myocardial infarction or stroke [129].

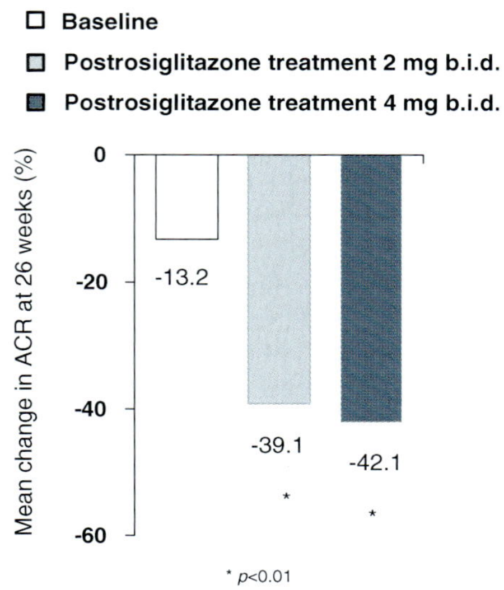

Figure 8 Effect of rosiglitazone treatment for 26 weeks on microalbuminuria in patients with type 2 diabetes

Three key components, the endothelial cells (ECs), the monocyte/macrophage cells, and the VSMCs all play a crucial role in the development of accelerated atherosclerosis [130]. There is growing evidence from both *in vitro* and animal studies that the TZDs as PPAR-γ agonists modify the risk of atherosclerosis progression. The ECs play a major role in the initiation of atherosclerosis through the secretion/activation of several proatherogenic groups of molecules including the cellular adhesion molecules, which promote recruitment and adhesion of monocytes/lymphocytes to the endothelium; ET-1, which is a powerful vasoconstrictor and promoter of VSMC proliferation; and PAI-1, which plays a major role in the inhibition of clot lysis. Several studies have documented that the PPAR agonists inhibit the expression of the cellular adhesion molecules [monocyte chemoattractant protein 1 (MCP-1), intracellular adhesion molecule (ICAM-1), and vascular cell adhesion molecule 1 (VCAM-1)] [131–133], repress thrombin-induced expression of ET-1 by interfering with the AP-1 pathway [134], and modulate the expression of PAI-1 [135]. The monocyte/macrophage cell system is another key component of the atherosclerosis cascade. These cells play a major role in several processes in this cascade through the secretion of inflammatory cytokines; the production of foam cells; the release of procoagulant proteins such as tissue factor (TF); and the release of matrix metalloproteinases (MMPs) (which promote plaque instability) [129, 136]. The TZDs have been shown to have significant effects in negatively regulating macrophage activation [137]; inhibiting the production of inflammatory cytokines (TNF-a, interleukin 1b (IL-1b), IL-6) [138]; regulating macrophage lipid homeostasis through activation of the ATP-binding cassette, subfamily A, member 1 (ABCA 1)-mediated reverse cholesterol

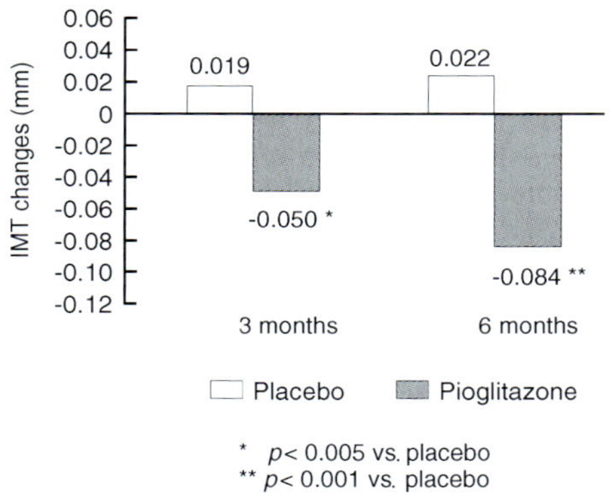

Figure 9 Effect of 3 and 6 months of pioglitazone treatment on carotid intimal media thickness (IMT) in 106 Japanese patients with type 2 diabetes

pathway [139]; and reducing the expression and release of MMP and TF [136, 140]. When stimulated, VSMCs proliferate and migrate from the media to the intima, with the formation of a fibrous cap. Further activation of these cells leads to the release of proinflammatory cytokines, which, combined with the secretion of MMPs and other procoagulant factors leads to plaque instability with the potential for rupture of the lipid laden plaque and acute occlusion by thrombosis, resulting in a myocardial infarction or stroke [130]. In human aortic smooth muscle cells (SMCs), the TZDs inhibit the proliferation and migration of vascular SMC [141, 142].

Thus, the PPAR agonists through their beneficial effects on endothelial, VSMC, and macrophage function may ameliorate the vascular pathology and thrombogenicity associated with atherosclerosis and improve the stability of the atherosclerotic plaque. So far the effects of these changes upon biochemical markers and surrogate markers of atherosclerosis progression [like carotid intimal–medial thickening (IMT)] appear to be favorable [140, 143, 144]. Intimal–medial thickness is a clinical measure of atherosclerotic progression and has been shown to be correlated with insulin levels in patients with and without type 2 diabetes [145]. In a small clinical study of 135 Japanese diabetic patients [146], troglitazone reduced intimal and medial complex thickening in carotid arteries by 0.08 ± 0.015 mm (control group: increase by $0.027 + 0.007$ mm) as determined by B-mode ultrasound over a surprisingly short time period of 3 months. Similar results were reported by the same group after pioglitazone therapy for 3 months [147] (Figure 9). However, since both these studies were not randomized, placebo-controlled, or double-blind, the results must be interpreted with caution. However, in a randomized study [148], Takagi et al. studied 62 coronary stented lesions in 52 patients with type 2 diabetes who were randomized into two groups: a troglitazone-treated group (400 mg) with 25 patients (29 stents), and a control group of 27 patients with 33 stents. Intravascular ultrasound studies (performed at baseline and at the 6-month follow-up) showed a significant reduction in neointimal tissue proliferation after coronary stent implantation in the diabetic patients treated with troglitazone. In a similar study, Choi et al. randomized 100 subjects with type 2 diabetes who had received coronary stents to treatment with either rosiglitazone 4 mg daily or placebo [149] (Figure 10). Follow-up angiography after 6 months revealed a significant reduction in restenosis in the rosiglitazone group (12% restenosis rate) versus a 37% restenosis rate in the placebo group. These

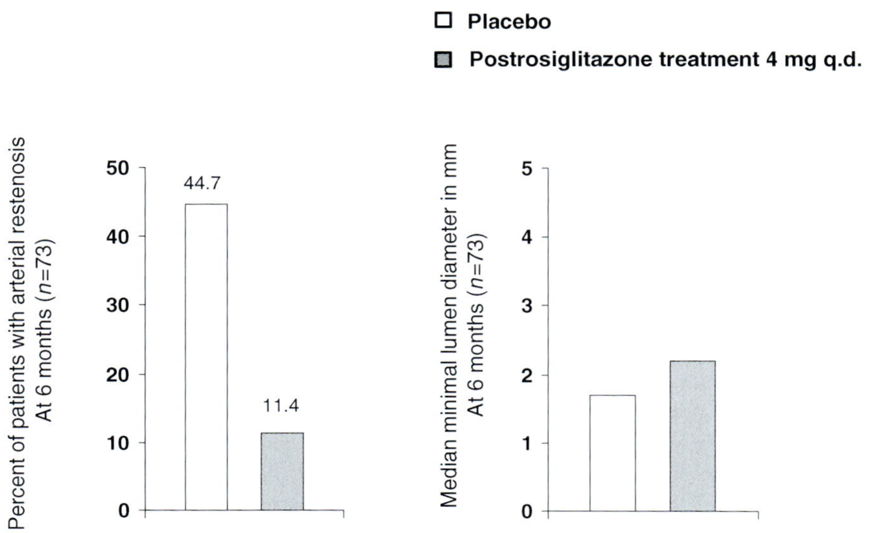

Figure 10 Effects of rosiglitazone treatment for 6 months treatment on the restenosis rate after coronary stent placement in 73 patients with type 2 diabetes ($n = 38$ on placebo, and 35 on rosiglitazone)

effects of the TZDs on IMT, both in the presence and absence of stents, if confirmed and shown to persist long-term, could be highly beneficial in delaying or preventing development of the accelerated atherosclerosis of diabetes.

OTHER BENEFICIAL NONGLYCEMIC EFFECTS

Effects on Cancer Cells

Although PPAR-γ is predominantly expressed in insulin-sensitive tissues, these receptors are also found to be expressed in several human cancer cell lines. Indeed, there is preliminary evidence that the TZDs through their action on PPAR-γ suppress the growth of several human cancer lines, including colon, breast, pancreatic, and prostate, *in vitro* and *in vivo* [150–154]. Interestingly, in a recent study, Panigrahy et al. have reported that not only is PPAR-γ expressed at high levels in tumor endothelium and activated in ECs by its ligands, but more importantly that the PPAR-γ ligands, rosiglitazone, inhibits primary tumor growth and metastasis by both direct and indirect antiangiogenic effects [155]. These results suggest that PPAR-γ ligands may be useful in treating angiogenic diseases such as cancer by inhibiting angiogenesis. However, these promising data from *in vivo* studies have not so far been borne out in clinical studies. In a recent phase II study, Kulke et al. treated 25 patients with metastatic colorectal cancer with oral troglitazone and followed them for evidence of toxicity, tumor response, and survival [156]. Although treatment was well tolerated, no objective tumor responses were noted, and all 25 patients had progressive disease as their best response to therapy. The authors concluded that troglitazone is not an active agent for the treatment of metastatic colorectal cancer.

In contrast to the antiproliferative effects described above, there is some evidence of tumor-inducing effects of the TZDs in a murine model for familial adenomatous polyposis and sporadic colon cancer [157]. Hence it is prudent that these drugs not be prescribed for people from families with adenomatous polyposis coli. Long-term studies are needed to monitor effects on the development of sporadic colon tumors.

Effects in PCOS

Polycystic Ovary Syndrome (PCOS) is the most common cause of hyperandrogenemia in women, and insulin resistance is a prominent feature of this syndrome. Consistent with their role as insulin sensitizers, the TZDs have been shown to have both insulin-sensitizing and ovulation-inducing effects in women with PCOS [158]. In a recent published 44-week, placebo controlled study in 305 patients with PCOS, Azziz et al. demonstrated that ovulatory rates were significantly greater for patients receiving 300 and 600 mg of troglitazone than for those receiving placebo (0.42 and 0.58 vs. 0.32; $P < 0.05$ and 0.0001, respectively) [159]. Notably, of PCOS patients treated with 600 mg of troglitazone, 57% ovulated over 50% of the time compared with only 12% of placebo-treated patients. Other beneficial effects included significant decreases in free testosterone and sex-hormone-binding globulin levels and concurrent improvements in hirsutism scores. Importantly, the total number and severity of adverse events (including elevations in liver enzymes) and the proportion of patients withdrawn from the study because of the development of adverse effects were similar between treatment groups. The authors concluded that troglitazone improves the ovulatory dysfunction, hirsutism, hyperandrogenemia, and insulin resistance of PCOS in a dose-related fashion, with a minimum of adverse effects. In a subsequent publication, the same authors have also reported that troglitazone treatment also decreased adrenal androgen levels in PCOS women [160]. The insulin-sensitizing effects of the TZDs have also been reported by Paradisi et al. in their study in which troglitazone treatment for 3 months not only improved insulin sensitivity as measured by the glucose clamp technique, but was also associated with significant decreases in serum free testosterone levels, serum triglyceride levels, and improvements in insulin-stimulated vasodilation [161].

Effects of the TZDs to induce ovulation have also been documented by Ghazeeri et al. who investigated the effect of rosiglitazone on ovulation induction in 25 overweight and obese, clomiphene-resistant women with PCOS in a double-blind, randomized, placebo-controlled trial [162]. These women were randomized into two treatment groups with subjects in Group I ($n = 12$) randomized to receive rosiglitazone 4 mg b.i.d., with a placebo on cycle days 5–9 and those in Group II ($n = 13$) randomized to receive rosiglitazone 4 mg b.i.d., with clomiphene citrate on cycle days 5–9. The duration of the study was 2 months. In this study, the authors demonstrated that short-term rosiglitazone therapy enhanced both spontaneous and clomiphene-induced ovulation in overweight and obese women with PCOS with one pregnancy occurring in Group I and two pregnancies in Group II. Concurrently, there were decreases in hyperandrogenemia primarily through increases in sex-hormone-binding globulin (SHBG).

It must be mentioned here that *in vitro* studies suggest that the beneficial effects of troglitazone in PCOS may not be due solely to improvement of peripheral insulin resistance and hyperinsulinemia, but also to a possible direct effect on ovarian steroidogenesis. In one study, troglitazone was found to directly inhibit 3β-hydroxy steroid dehydrogenase enzyme activity in steroidogenic cells in the ovary [163]. This effect could potentially lead to a decrease in secretion of C19 steroids, testosterone, and androstenedione.

Effects on HIV

In recent years, the use of highly active antiretroviral therapy (HAART) has greatly increased life expectancy and improved quality of life in patients with HIV disease. However, HAART is also associated with several metabolic complications including fat redistribution, insulin resistance, and increased incidence of diabetes mellitus, hyperlipidemia, and hypertension [164]. The insulin-sensitizing TZDs should, in theory, be a good option to improve insulin sensitivity and body fat distribution in HAART-treated AIDS patients. In a recent study [165], Gelato et al. evaluated the ability of rosiglitazone (8 mg/day) to improve insulin sensitivity and modulate body fat distribution in eight HIV-positive, HAART-treated patients. After rosiglitazone treatment of 6–12 weeks, insulin sensitivity as measured by the rate of glucose disposal during a hyperinsulinemic-euglycemic clamp increased significantly by 59% along with a 23% increase in SQ adipose tissue and a 21% decrease in visceral adipose tissue. There were no significant changes in blood counts, viral loads, or CD4 counts with rosiglitazone treatment. Similar results have earlier been shown with troglitazone therapy [166]. Clearly more studies are needed, but the preliminary data above suggest that the TZDs with their effects to improve insulin sensitivity, decrease visceral adipose tissue, and increase SQ adipose tissue have the potential as a therapeutic agent for the current metabolic complications of HAART.

Effects on Inflammation and Immunity

It is now clear that in addition to being present in the classic insulin-responsive tissues, PPAR-γ is also found in other cell types, including the white and red pulp of rat spleen, human bone-marrow precursors, and macrophages/monocytes [167]. *In vivo* and *in vitro* studies with numerous, different cell types have shown that the TZDs appear to exert largely anti-inflammatory effect through several mechanisms that include inhibition of proliferation of activated T-cells, inhibition of IL-2 secretion and/or the induction of apoptosis [168], and inhibition of the NF-κB pathway [169]. However, one problem in the interpretation of many of the studies of PPAR-γ, inflammation, and immunity is that ligands thought to be specific for PPAR-γ may have regulatory effects on inflammatory parameters that are PPAR-γ-independent. Nevertheless, in several animal models, the TZDs have been shown to modify autoimmune diseases. Su et al. [170] showed that in a mouse model of inflammatory bowel disease, pioglitazone and rosiglitazone markedly reduced colonic inflammation. These authors proposed that this effect might be a result of a direct effect on colonic epithelial cells, which express high levels of PPAR and can produce inflammatory cytokines. In another study, Kawahito et al. [171] demonstrated that intraperitoneal administration of the PPAR ligands, 15d-PGJ2 and troglitazone, ameliorated adjuvant-induced arthritis with suppression of pannus formation and mononuclear cell infiltration in rats. Even more exciting are the results of a study by Lewis that examined the potential efficacy of rosiglitazone, as a therapy for active ulcerative colitis [172]. Fifteen patients with mild to moderately active ulcerative colitis despite therapy with 5-aminosalicylic acid compounds were enrolled in an open-label study of rosiglitazone (4 mg b.i.d.) for 12 weeks. Thirteen of 15 patients were receiving concomitant therapy with corticosteroids and/or immunomodulator medications. After 12 weeks of therapy, four patients (27%) had achieved clinical remission, of whom three (20%) also had an endoscopic remission. Four additional patients (27%) had a clinical response without achieving remission. Two patients were hospitalized with worsened disease activity, and one patient was withdrawn for nephrotic syndrome. These data suggest that the TZDs may represent a novel therapy for ulcerative colitis. Clearly, however, there is a need to conduct a double blind, placebo-controlled, randomized trial in this patient population.

DRUG INTERACTIONS

There are significant differences in drug interactions among the TZDs. Both pioglitazone and troglitazone are metabolized by the cytochrome P450 isoform CYP3A4 [94, 173]. Thus, safety and efficacy could possibly be affected when pioglitazone is coadministered with other drugs metabolized by this enzyme. In contrast, at clinically relevant concentrations, rosiglitazone has no drug interactions with any drugs metabolized by any of the major cytochrome P450 enzymes. *In vitro* data demonstrate that rosiglitazone is predominantly metabolized by CYP2C8, and to a lesser extent, 2C9. Drugs metabolized by the cytochrome P450 isoform CYP3A4 include alfentanil, alprazolam, astemizole, carbamazepine, cisapride, some corticosteroids, cyclosporine, diazepam, diltiazem, donepezil, erythromycin, felodipine, fexofenadine, indinavir, lidocaine, lovastatin, midazolam, nifedipine, quinidine, saquinavir, simvastatin, sirolimus, tacrolimus, terfenadine, triazolam, trimetrexate, and verapamil. Blood glucose should be monitored more carefully in patients receiving pioglitazone in combination with the above drugs and also when administered with inhibitors of CYP3A4 such as ketoconazole or itraconazole. *In vitro*, ketoconazole appears to significantly inhibit the metabolism of pioglitazone. It is recommended that patients receiving both pioglitazone and ketoconazole be evaluated more frequently with respect to glycemic control and the potential for hepatotoxicity. Studies with itraconazole, which also inhibits CYP enzymes, have not been performed.

Oral contraceptive (OC) concentrations have been reduced by up to 30%, with the coadministration of troglitazone. Since pioglitazone is also metabolized by CYP3A4, it is possible that poglitazone may also reduce the bioavailability of OCs containing ethinyl estradiol and norethindrone by induction of CYP3A4, and hence coadministration of pioglitazone with oral contraceptives OCs may reduce the effectiveness of these agents. Higher dosage OCs formulations may be needed to increase contraceptive efficacy during pioglitazone use. Alternatively, the use of other methods of contraception is recommended. On the other hand, multiple dose studies have shown that rosiglitazone has no clinically relevant effect on the pharmacokinetics of OCs (ethinyl estradiol and norethindrone).

Repeat dosing with rosiglitazone had no clinically relevant effect on the steady-state pharmacokinetics of either warfarin, nifedipine, digoxin, or ranitidine in healthy volunteers, nor did the administration of these medications alter the pharmacokinetics of rosiglitazone. Also in healthy volunteers, coadministration of pioglitazone with either digoxin, glipizide, metformin, or warfarin for 7 days did not alter the steady-state pharmacokinetics of these medications. Coadministration of acarbose (100 mg three times daily) for 7 days in healthy volunteers had no clinically relevant effect on the pharmacokinetics of a single oral dose of rosiglitazone. A single administration of a moderate amount of alcohol did not increase the risk of acute hypoglycemia in type 2 diabetes mellitus patients treated with rosiglitazone.

Large doses of aspirin should be used cautiously in patients receiving TZDs. Salicylates inhibit prostaglandin E2 synthesis and indirectly increase insulin secretion and in large doses may cause hypoglycemia. Also in large doses, salicylates may uncouple oxidative phosphorylation, deplete hepatic and muscle glycogen, and cause hyperglycemia and glycosuria acutely. Bexarotene (used in the treatment of cutaneous manifestations of T-cell lymphoma [mycosis fungoides]) may enhance the action of pioglitazone. Patients should be closely monitored while receiving bexarotene in combination with pioglitazone.

SIDE EFFECTS

Both rosiglitazone and pioglitazone have now been in clinical use worldwide with several million patients treated with these drugs. The vast majority of these patients have tolerated these agents well and have shown clinical improvement in their glycemic status. During double-blind, clinical trials, the most frequently reported adverse reactions in nearly 2600 patients receiving rosiglitazone monotherapy included back pain, diarrhea, fatigue, headache, hyperglycemia, hypoglycemia, injury, sinusitis, and upper respiratory tract infection [173]. In pioglitazone-treated patients, the most frequently reported adverse reactions during placebo-controlled clinical trials were headache, hyperglycemia, myalgia, pharyngitis, sinusitis, tooth disorder, and upper respiratory tract infection [94]. Overall, the types of adverse experiences reported when rosiglitazone and pioglitazone were used either as monotherapy or in combination with SUs, metformin, and insulin were similar to placebo, except for hypoglycemia and edema. Importantly, the incidence of withdrawals from clinical trials due to an adverse event other than hyperglycemia was similar for patients receiving placebo or a TZD.

Edema with the TZDs

In clinical trials and postmarketing surveillance, the incidence of edema has varied from about 3 to 7.5% with the TZDs, compared to 1 to 2.2% with placebo or other oral antidiabetic agents [94, 173]. Of note, the highest incidence of edema has been reported when the TZDs are used in combination with insulin. In controlled clinical studies, these patients have an incidence of edema of 15.3% when treated with insulin plus pioglitazone and 14.7% when treated with insulin plus rosiglitazone, compared to 7.0% and 5.4% in the insulin plus placebo-treated patients, respectively. However, in a very small minority of patients, the TZDs lead to significant peripheral edema and in some patients possibly precipitation/worsening of congestive heart failure [174–177]. In two large, 26-week clinical trials in the United States with 611 patients with long-standing type 2 diabetes and a high prevalence of pre-existing medical conditions, an increased incidence of heart failure and other cardiovascular events was seen with rosiglitazone in combination with insulin, as compared to patients treated with insulin and placebo [173]. Patients who experienced heart failure in these studies were, on average, older, had a longer duration of diabetes, and were mostly on the higher 8 mg daily dose of rosiglitazone. In this population however, it was not possible to determine specific risk factors that could be used to identify all patients at risk of heart failure, on combination therapy with rosiglitazone and insulin. Of note, heart failure developed in some patients not known to have prior congestive heart failure or pre-existing cardiac conditions.

It is still not clear by what precise mechanism(s) the TZDs cause edema or whether the edema is related to decompensation of cardiac function [174]. In early studies in nondiabetic volunteers, the TZDs were found to increase plasma volume by about 6–7% [173]. Whether it is this increase in plasma volume that leads to edema, or other causes such as increased renal tubular sodium reabsorption, reflex sympathetic activation, alteration of intestinal ion transport, or increased production of vascular endothelial growth factor, VEGF (a potent tissue permeability factor) is not known (Figure 11). Studies into

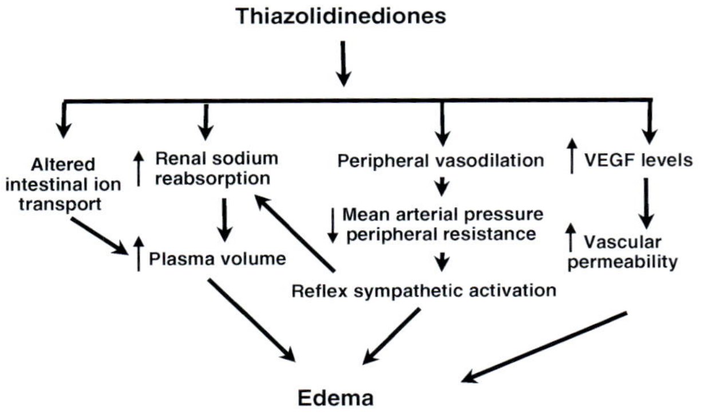

Figure 11 Multifactorial mechanisms of edema formation with thiazolidinediones. (Reproduced from reference 174)

the pathophysiology of edema associated with TZDs are ongoing, since it is important to elucidate the mechanism(s) responsible for the causation of edema in patients with type 2 diabetes treated with TZDs, and even more important to determine if it is possible to predict those patients susceptible to development of edema, and especially congestive heart failure. Knowledge of the mechanisms of edema formation could lead to effective preventative or therapeutic modalities.

Weight Gain

Weight gain has also been reported more frequently with glitazone therapy. In the 26-week rosiglitazone clinical trials, the mean weight gain in patients treated with rosiglitazone monotherapy was 1.2 kg (on 4 mg daily) and 3.5 kg (on 8 mg daily) [173]. When administered in combination with metformin, weight gain was blunted at 0.7 kg (on 4 mg daily) and 2.3 kg (on 8 mg daily). There was a mean weight loss of about 1 kg in both placebo and metformin-only groups in these studies [173]. In the 52-week glyburide-controlled study, there was a mean weight gain of 1.75 kg and 2.95 kg for patients treated with 4 mg and 8 mg of rosiglitazone daily, respectively, versus 1.9 kg in glyburide-treated patients [114]. Similarly, in clinical studies, pioglitazone treatment has been accompanied by weight gain in a dose-related manner [94]. The change in average weight in US placebo-controlled monotherapy trials ranged from 0.5–2.8 kg for pioglitazone-treated patients, compared to a weight loss of 1.3–1.9 kg in placebo-treated patients. In combination with a SU, the change in average weight was 1.9 kg and 2.9 kg for 15 mg and 30 mg of pioglitazone, respectively, and −0.8 kg for placebo. The change in average weight in combination with insulin was 2.3 kg and 3.7 kg for 15 mg and 30 mg of pioglitazone, respectively, and no weight change for placebo. Even in combination with metformin, the increase in average weight was 1.0 kg for 30 mg of pioglitazone versus −1.4 kg for placebo. Of note, at the present time, it is still not clear how much of the TZD-induced weight gain is due to fluid retention versus adipose tissue accumulation. Studies to determine the nature and components of this weight gain are in progress.

Anemia

As seen above, with an increase in plasma volume induced by the TZDs, it is to be expected that due to a dilutional effect, there will be decreases in hemoglobin and hematocrit. This has been shown to occur in a dose-related fashion in patients treated with rosiglitazone and pioglitazone alone or in combination [94, 173]. These changes occur primarily during the first 4–12 weeks of therapy and remain relatively constant thereafter. These changes have not been associated with any significant hematologic clinical effects. Reports of anemia (7.1%) were greater in patients treated with a combination of rosiglitazone and metformin; however, lower pretreatment hemoglobin/hematocrit levels in patients taking metformin concurrently may have contributed to the higher reporting rate of anemia in these studies. For pioglitazone, in US double-blind studies, anemia was reported in 0.3–1.6% of pioglitazone-treated patients and 0–1.6% of placebo-treated patients in monotherapy and combination studies. Rosiglitazone-treated patients also experience slight decreases in white blood cell counts, which may be related to the increased plasma volume.

Hypoglycemia

The TZDs do not stimulate insulin secretion and hence when used as monotherapy, are not expected to cause hypoglycemia. However, mild to moderate hypoglycemia can occur and has been reported during combination therapy with SUs or insulin [94, 173]. Hypoglycemia was reported for 1% of placebo-treated patients and 2% of patients receiving pioglitazone in combination with a SU. In combination with insulin, hypoglycemia was reported for 5% of placebo-treated patients, 8% for patients treated with pioglitazone 15 mg, and 15% for patients treated with pioglitazone 30 mg.

During required laboratory testing in the pioglitazone clinical trials, sporadic, transient elevations in creatine phosphokinase levels (CPK) without symptoms were observed [94]. A single, isolated elevation to greater than 10 times the upper limit of normal (values of 2150–8610) was noted in seven patients. Five of these patients continued to receive pioglitazone and the other two patients had completed receiving study medication at the time of the elevated value. These elevations resolved without any apparent clinical sequelae, and the relationship of these events to pioglitazone therapy is unknown.

MONITORING REQUIREMENTS/ PRECAUTIONS/CONTRAINDICATIONS

Liver Function

Currently in the United States, the FDA has mandated that during treatment with rosiglitazone or pioglitazone, liver function tests (LFTs) should be monitored every 2 months in the first year and periodically thereafter. This has resulted primarily because of the occurrence of severe hepatocellular failure with troglitazone. Troglitazone, the first glitazone marketed in the United States was associated with idiosyncratic hepatotoxicity and rare cases of liver failure, liver transplants, and death, which led to its recall from clinical use in March 2000. In clinical trials with rosiglitazone and pioglitazone, the incidence of hepatotoxicity and ALT elevations has been similar to placebo [94, 173]. In clinical use up-to-date, there have only been a few reports of hepatotoxicity associated with rosiglitazone and pioglitazone [178–183]. In a recent large analysis of data from several large studies of rosiglitazone use, no evidence of hepatotoxic effects was observed in studies that involved 5006 patients taking rosiglitazone as monotherapy or combination therapy for 5508 person-years [184]. These findings suggest that the idiosyncratic liver toxicity observed with troglitazone is unlikely to be a TZD or a PPAR-γ agonist class effect. In fact, poorly controlled patients with type 2 diabetes may even have moderate elevations of serum ALT that decrease with improved glycemic control, during treatment with rosiglitazone or other antihyperglycemic agents [184]. Despite this, it is still prudent that rosiglitazone and pioglitazone should be used cautiously in patients with hepatic disease, since both rosiglitazone and pioglitazone are structurally similar to troglitazone. Liver enzymes should be checked prior to the initiation of therapy with rosiglitazone or pioglitazone in all patients and therapy with TZDs should not be initiated in patients with increased baseline liver enzyme levels (ALT >2.5 times the upper limit of normal). In patients with normal baseline liver enzymes, following initiation of therapy with rosiglitazone or pioglitazone, it is recommended that liver enzymes be monitored every 2 months for the first 12 months, and periodically thereafter. If at any time ALT levels increase to >3 times the upper limit of normal in patients on therapy with rosiglitazone or pioglitazone, liver enzyme levels should be rechecked as soon as possible. If ALT levels remain >3 times the upper limit of normal, glitazone therapy should be discontinued.

Congestive Heart Failure

Although most patients tolerate TZD treatment well, a small minority of patients will develop clinically significant edema. Experience from clinical trials and widespread clinical use of the TZDs indicate that there is a slight expansion in plasma volume associated with TZD use, which might result in edema occurring in the peripheral interstitial space [174]. In susceptible patients, the edema starts early, usually within several weeks, and is mild. Occasionally, it can be severe with rapid weight gain. Although the fluid accumulation usually occurs in the lower extremities, occasionally it may be seen throughout the body and rarely even precipitate pulmonary edema. At present, the duration of the mild to moderate edema that may be seen with TZD therapy is not known and there is no evidence whether this edema is transient or not.

On the basis of the above, rosiglitazone and pioglitazone should be used with caution in patients with preexisting edema, especially in those who have milder degrees of heart failure (NYHA Class 1 and 2) [94, 173]. In patients with NYHA Class 3 and 4 cardiac status, treatment with rosiglitazone or pioglitazone is not recommended. In all other patients, rosiglitazone or pioglitazone therapy should be initiated with a low dose and patients should be evaluated early for edema (within several weeks) (Figure 12). If edema does occur, dose reduction may be attempted. In those who develop symptoms of CHF however, it may be prudent to discontinue the drug altogether, since in the published case reports of pulmonary edema, clinical improvement did not occur with diuretics and inotropes, while the TZD agent was still continued. Only after discontinuation of drug, there was diuresis and resolution of the heart failure and peripheral edema. In those with peripheral edema who do not respond to conventional doses of diuretics, it may be wise to discontinue the TZD agent permanently and use other oral agents or insulin. As yet, treatment of TZD-associated edema has not been systematically evaluated and treatment must be guided by clinical judgment.

Caution should also be exercised when using pioglitazone or rosiglitazone in premenopausal anovulatory

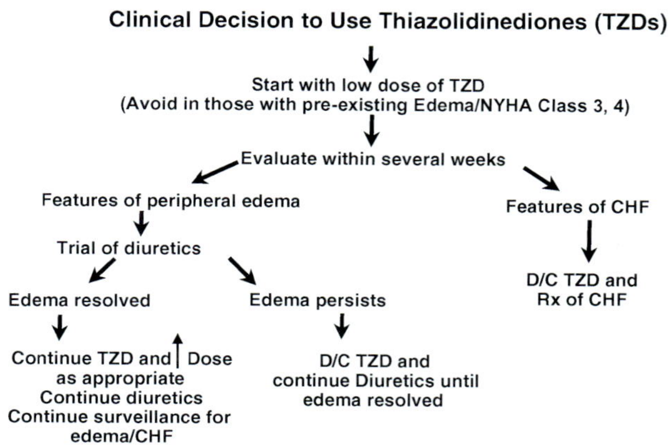

Figure 12 Proposed algorithm to treat edema associated with the use of thiazolidinediones. (Reproduced from reference 174)

females with insulin resistance who may resume ovulation as a result of glitazone therapy. These patients may be at risk of becoming pregnant if adequate contraception is not used. In the case of pioglitazone those who use OC therapy may also be at risk due to CYP3A4 enzyme induction; although in a recent study, administration of pioglitazone did not result in clinically significant effects on the pharmacokinetics of other CYP3A4 substrates [185].

Rosiglitazone and pioglitazone are contraindicated in pregnancy. Although animal data suggest no teratogenic effects, there are no adequate and well-controlled studies in pregnant women. Also it is unknown whether these drugs are secreted in human milk and hence they should not be administered to breast-feeding women.

CONCLUSION

The introduction of the TZDs has heralded a new era in the treatment of patients with type 2 diabetes. These agents constitute a unique new class of oral antidiabetic agents that exert direct effects on the mechanisms of insulin resistance, which is a major pathophysiologic abnormality in type 2 diabetes. As highly selective and potent agonists for PPAR-γ, the TZDs regulate the expression of numerous genes that affect carbohydrate and lipid metabolism and vascular function. This results not only in lower blood glucose levels and improved glycemia, but also amelioration of several components of the insulin resistance syndrome, including dyslipidemia, hypertension, and endothelial dysfunction, which lead to accelerated atherosclerosis and premature cardiovascular morbidity and mortality in patients with type 2 diabetes. Thus, the TZDs have the potential not only to reduce glycemia and insulin requirements in type 2 diabetics, but also to improve other components of the insulin resistance syndrome including dyslipidemia and hypertension and thereby may be able to prevent or delay premature atherosclerotic cardiovascular disease, morbidity, and death. Long-term studies are in progress to determine the consequences of these potential cardiovascular benefits. Notwithstanding the multiple beneficial effects of the TZDs, in a small minority of patients, weight gain and edema remain undesirable side effects of these agents. At present, these drugs should not be used in patients with advanced degrees of congestive heart failure. In the future, it is possible to envisage the availability of tailored TZD or even non-TZD compounds that through their selective agonist effects will have enhanced beneficial effects on glucose, lipid, and vascular endothelial metabolism, and through their partial agonist, or even selective antagonist effects, do not possess the unwanted side effects of weight gain and fluid retention. The ultimate goal, however, in the treatment of diabetes is the prevention of the disease. Preliminary evidence suggests that the TZDs have the potential to delay or even prevent the development of type 2 diabetes in high-risk individuals.

Acknowledgments

This work was supported by the Department of Veterans Affairs and the VA San Diego Healthcare System, San Diego, CA, Grant DK-58291 from the NIDDK, and Grant MO1 RR-00827 from the General Clinical Research Branch, Division of Research Resources, National Institutes of Health.

REFERENCES

1. Zimmet P, Alberti KG, Shaw J. Global and societal implications of the diabetes epidemic. *Nature* 2001; 414: 782–7.
2. King H, Aubert RE, Herman W. Global Burden of Diabetes, 1995–2025: Prevalence, numerical estimates, and projections. *Diabetes Care* 1998; 21: 1414–31.
3. DeFronzo RA, Bonadonna RC, Ferrannini E. Pathogenesis of NIDDM: a balanced overview. *Diabetologia* 1992; 35: 389–97.
4. Fagan TC, Deedwania PC. The cardiovascular dysmetabolic syndrome. *Am J Med* 1998; 105 (1A): 77S–82S.
5. Expert Panel on Detection, Evaluation and Treatment of High Blood Cholesterol in Adults. Executive summary of the Third Report of the National Cholesterol Education Program (NCEP) of High Blood Cholesterol in Adults (Adult Treatment Panel III). *JAMA* 2001; 285: 2486–97.
6. Willson TM, Cobb JE, Cowan DJ, Wiethe RW, Correa ID, Prakash SR, Beck KD, Moore LB, Kliewer SA, Lehmann JM. The structure–activity relationship between peroxisome-proliferator-activated receptor and agonism and the antihyperglycemic activity of thiazolidinediones. *J Med Chem* 1996; 39: 665–8.
7. Lemberger T, Desvergne B, Wahli W. Peroxisome proliferator-active receptors: a nuclear receptor signaling pathway in lipid physiology. *Annu Rev Cell Dev Biol* 1996; 12: 335–63.
8. Desvergne B, Wahli W. Peroxisome proliferator-activated receptors: nuclear control of metabolism. *Endocr Rev* 1999; 20 (5): 649–88.
9. Kersten S, Desvergne B, Wahli W. Role of PPARs in health and disease. *Nature* 2000; 405: 421–4.
10. Duez H, Fruchart JC, Staels B. PPARs in inflammation, atherosclerosis and thrombosis. *J Cardiovasc Risk* 2001; 8 (4): 187–94.
11. Zhu Y. Structural organization of mouse peroxisome proliferator-activated receptor g gene: alternative promoter use and different splicing yield two PPAR γ isoforms. *Proc Natl Acad Sci USA* 1995; 92: 7921–5.
12. Loviscach M, Rehman N, Carter L, Mudaliar S, Mohideen P, Ciaraldi TP, Veerkamp JH, Henry RR. Distribution of peroxisome proliferator-activated receptors (PPARs) in human skeletal muscle and adipose tissue: relation to insulin action. *Diabetologia* 2000; 43: 304–11.
13. Mudaliar S, Henry RR. New oral therapies for type 2 diabetes—the thiazolidinediones or insulin sensitizers. *Annu Rev Med* 2001; 52: 239–57.

14. Sattiel AR, Olefsky JM. Thiazolidinediones in the treatment of insulin resistance and type II diabetes. *Diabetes* 1996; 45: 1661–9.
15. Okuno A, Tamemoto H, Tobe K. Troglitazone increases the number of small adipocytes without the change of white adipose tissue mass in obese Zucker rats. *J Clin Invest* 1998; 101 (6): 1354–61.
16. Olefsky JM. The effects of spontaneous obesity on insulin binding, glucose transport and glucose oxidation of isolated rat adipocytes. *J Clin Invest* 1976; 57: 842–51.
17. Ciaraldi TP, Kong APS, Chu NV, Kim DD, Baxi S, Loviscach M, Plodkowski R, Reitz R, Caulfield M, Mudaliar S, Henry RR. Regulation of glucose transport and insulin signaling by troglitazone or metformin in adipose tissue of type 2 diabetic subjects. *Diabetes* 2002; 51 (1): 30–6.
18. Rieusset J, Auwerx J, Vidal H. Regulation of gene expression by activation of the peroxisome proliferator-activated receptor g with rosiglitazone (BRL 49653) in human adipocytes. *Biochem Biophys Res Commun* 1999; 265 (1): 265–71.
19. Matsuda J, Hosoda K, Itoh H, Son C, Doi K, Hanaoka I, Inoue G, Nishimura H, Yoshimasa Y, Yamori Y, Odaka H, Nakao K. Increased adipose expression of the uncoupling protein-3 gene by thiazolidinediones in Wistar fatty rats and in cultured adipocytes. *Diabetes* 1998; 47 (11): 1809–14.
20. Brun S, Carmona MC, Mampel T, Vinas O, Giralt M, Iglesias R, Villarroya F. Activators of peroxisome proliferator-activated receptor-a induce the expression of the uncoupling protein-3 gene in skeletal muscle: a potential mechanism for the lipid intake-dependent activation of uncoupling protein-3 gene expression at birth. *Diabetes* 1999; 48 (6): 1217–22.
21. Fukui Y, Masui S, Osada S, Umesono K, Motojima K. A new thiazolidinedione, NC-2100, which is a weak PPAR-g activator, exhibits potent antidiabetic effects and induces uncoupling protein 1 in white adipose tissue of KKAy obese mice. *Diabetes* 2000; 49 (5): 759–67.
22. Park KS, Ciaraldi TP, Lindgren K, Abrams-Carter L, Mudaliar S, et al. Troglitazone effects on gene expression in human skeletal muscle of type 2 diabetic subjects involve upregulation of PPAR gamma. *J Clin Endocrinol Metab* 1998; 83 (8): 2830–5.
23. Park KS, Ciaraldi TP, Carter LA, Mudaliar S, Nikoulina SE, et al. Troglitazone regulation of glucose metabolism in human skeletal muscle cultures from obese type 2 diabetic subjects. *J Clin Endocrinol Metab* 1998; 83 (5): 1636–43.
24. Hu E, Liang P, Spiegelman BM. AdipoQ is a novel adipose-specific gene dysregulated in obesity. *J Biol Chem* 1996; 271: 10697–703.
25. Scherer PE, Williams S, Fogliano M, Baldini G, Lodish HF. A novel serum protein similar to C1q, produced exclusively in adipocytes. *J Biol Chem* 1995; 270: 26746–9.
26. Hotta K, Funahashi T, Arita Y, Takahashi M, Matsuda M, Okamoto Y, Iwahashi H, Kuriyama H, Ouchi N, Maeda K, Nishida M, Kihara S, Sakai N, Nakajima T, Hasegawa K, Muraguchi M, Ohmoto Y, Nakamura T, Yamashita S, Hanafusa T, Matsuzawa Y. Plasma concentrations of a novel, adipose-specific protein, adiponectin, in type 2 diabetic patients. *Arteriosler Thromb Vasc Biol* 2000; 20: 1595–9.
27. Weyer C, Funahashi T, Tanaka S, Hotta K, Matsuzawa Y, Pratley RE, Tataranni PA. Hypoadiponectinemia in obesity and type 2 diabetes: close association with insulin resistance and hyperinsulinemia. *J Clin Endocrinol Metab* 2001; 86: 1930–5.
28. Maeda N, Takahashi M, Funahashi T, Kihara S, Nishizawa H, Kishida K, Nagaretani H, Matsuda M, Komuro R, Ouchi N, Kuriyama H, Hotta K, Nakamura T, Shimomura I, Matsuzawa Y. PPAR[gamma] ligands increase expression and plasma concentrations of adiponectin, an adipose-derived protein. *Diabetes* 2001; 50: 2094–9.
29. Moore GB, Chapman H, Holder JC, Lister CA, Piercy V, Smith SA, Clapham JC. Differential regulation of adipocytokine mRNAs by rosiglitazone in *db/db* mice. *Biochem Biophys Res Commun* 2001; 286: 735–41.
30. Yamauchi T, Kamon J, Waki H, Murakami K, Motojima K, Komeda K, Ide T, Kubota N, Terauchi Y, Tobe K, Miki H, Tsuchida A, Akanuma Y, Nagai R, Kimura S, Kadowaki T. Mechanisms by which both heterozygous peroxisome proliferator-activated receptor γ (PPAR γ) deficiency and PPAR γ agonist improve insulin resistance. *J Biol Chem* 2001; 276: 41245–54.
31. Combs TP, Wagner JA, Berger J, Doebber T, Wang WJ, Zhang BB, Tanen M, Berg AH, O'Rahilly S, Savage DB, Chatterjee K, Weiss S, Larson PJ, Gottesdiener KM, Gertz BJ, Charron MJ, Scherer PE, Moller DE. Induction of adipocyte complement-related protein of 30 kilodaltons by PPAR γ agonists: a potential mechanism of insulin sensitization. *Endocrinology* 2002; 143: 998–1007.
32. Halleux CM, Takahashi M, Delporte ML, Detry R, Funahashi T, Matsuzawa Y, Brichard SM. Secretion of adiponectin and regulation of apM1 gene expression in human visceral adipose tissue. *Biochem Biophys Res Commun* 2001; 288: 1102–7.
33. Yang WS, Jeng CY, Wu TJ, Tanaka S, Funahashi T, Matsuzawa Y, Wang JP, Chen CL, Tai TY, Chuang LM. Synthetic peroxisome proliferator-activated receptor-gamma agonist, rosiglitazone, increases plasma levels of adiponectin in type 2 diabetic patients. *Diabetes Care* 2002; 25 (2): 376–80.
34. Hirose H, Kawai T, Yamamoto Y, Taniyama M, Tomita M, Matsubara K, Okazaki Y, Ishii T, Oguma Y, Takei I, Saruta T. Effects of pioglitazone on metabolic parameters, body fat distribution, and serum adiponectin levels in Japanese male patients with type 2 diabetes. *Metabolism* 2002; 51 (3): 314–7.
35. Motoshima H, Wu X, Sinha MK, Hardy VE, Rosato EL, Barbot DJ, Rosato FE, Goldstein BJ. Differential regulation of adiponectin secretion from cultured human omental and subcutaneous adipocytes: effects of insulin and rosiglitazone. *J Clinical Endocrinol Metab* December 2002; 87 (12): 5662–7.
36. Phillips SA, Ciaraldi TP, Kong AP, Bandukwala R, Aroda V, Carter L, Baxi S, Mudaliar SR, Henry RR. Modulation of circulating and adipose tissue adiponectin levels by antidiabetic therapy. *Diabetes* 2003; 52 (3): 667–74.
37. Saltiel AR. You are what you secrete. *Nat Med* 2001; 7 (8): 887–8.
38. Law RE, Goetze S, Xi XP, et al. Expression and function of PPARgamma in rat and human vascular smooth muscle cells. *Circulation* 2000; 101 (11): 1311–8.
39. Asano M, Nakajima T, Iwasawa K. Troglitazone and pioglitazone attenuate agonist-dependent Ca^{2+} mobilization and cell proliferation in vascular smooth muscle cells. *Br J Pharmacol* 1999; 128 (3): 673–83.

40. Benson S, Wu J, Padmanabhan S. Peroxisome proliferator-activated receptor (PPAR)-gamma expression in human vascular smooth muscle cells: inhibition of growth, migration, and *c-fos* expression by the peroxisome proliferator-activated receptor (PPAR)-gamma activator troglitazone. *Am J Hypertens* 2000; 13 (1, pt 1): 74–82.
41. Saleh YM, Mudaliar SR, Henry RR. Metabolic and vascular effects of the thiazolidinedione, troglitazone. *Diabetes Rev* 2000; 7 (2): 55–76.
42. Yamauchi T, Kamon J, Ito K, Tsuchida A, Yokomizo T, Kita S, Sugiyama T, Miyagishi M, Kadowaki T. Cloning of adiponectin receptors that mediate antidiabetic metabolic effects. *Nature* 2003; 423 (6941): 762–7.
43. Lebovitz HE, Dole JF, Patwardhan R, Rappaport EB, Freed MI, for the Rosiglitazone Clinical Trials Study Group. Rosiglitazone monotherapy is effective in patients with type 2 diabetes. *J Clin Endocrinol Metab* 2001; 86 (1): 280–8. [erratum appears in *J Clin Endocrinol Metab* April 2001; 86 (4): 1659].
44. Aronoff S, Rosenblatt S, Braithwaite S, Egan JW, Mathisen AL, Schneider RL, for the Pioglitazone 001 Study Group. Pioglitazone hydrochloride monotherapy improves glycemic control in the treatment of patients with type 2 diabetes: a 6-month randomized placebo-controlled dose-response study. *Diabetes Care* 2000; 23 (11): 1605–11.
45. Rosenblatt S, Miskin B, Glazer NB, Prince MJ, Robertson KE, for the Pioglitazone 026 Study Group. The impact of pioglitazone on glycemic control and atherogenic dyslipidemia in patients with type 2 diabetes mellitus. *Coron Artery Dis* 2001; 12 (5): 413–23.
46. Vongthavaravat V, Wajchenberg BL, Waitman JN, Quimpo JA, Menon PS, Ben Khalifa F, Chow WH, for the 125 Study Group. An international study of the effects of rosiglitazone plus sulphonylurea in patients with type 2 diabetes. *Curr Med Res Opin* 2002; 18 (8): 456–61.
47. Barnett AH, Grant PJ, Hitman GA, Mather H, Pawa M, Robertson L, Trelfa A, for the Indo-Asian Trial Investigators. Rosiglitazone in type 2 diabetes mellitus: an evaluation in British Indo-Asian patients. *Diabet Med* 2003; 20 (5): 387–93.
48. Kipnes MS, Krosnick A, Rendell MS, Egan JW, Mathisen AL, Schneider RL. Pioglitazone hydrochloride in combination with sulfonylurea therapy improves glycemic control in patients with type 2 diabetes mellitus: a randomized, placebo-controlled study. *Am J Med* 2001; 111 (1): 10–7.
49. Fonseca V, Rosenstock J, Patwardhan R, Salzman A. Effect of metformin and rosiglitazone combination therapy in patients with type 2 diabetes mellitus: a randomized controlled trial. *JAMA* 2000; 283 (13): 1695–702.
50. Gomez-Perez FJ, Fanghanel-Salmon G, Antonio Barbosa J, Montes-Villarreal J, Berry RA, Warsi G, Gould EM. Efficacy and safety of rosiglitazone plus metformin in Mexicans with type 2 diabetes. *Diabetes Metab Res Rev* 2002; 18 (2): 127–34.
51. Einhorn D, Rendell M, Rosenzweig J, Egan JW, Mathisen AL, Schneider RL, for the Pioglitazone 027 Study Group. Pioglitazone hydrochloride in combination with metformin in the treatment of type 2 diabetes mellitus: a randomized, placebo-controlled study. *Clin Ther* 2000; 22 (12): 1395–409.
52. Jones TA, Sautter M, Van Gaal LF, Jones NP. Addition of rosiglitazone to metformin is most effective in obese, insulin-resistant patients with type 2 diabetes. *Diabetes Obes Metab* 2003; 5 (3): 163–70.
53. Raskin P, Rendell M, Riddle MC, Dole JF, Freed MI, Rosenstock J, for the Rosiglitazone Clinical Trials Study Group. A randomized trial of rosiglitazone therapy in patients with inadequately controlled insulin-treated type 2 diabetes. *Diabetes Care* 2001; 24 (7): 1226–32.
54. Rosenstock J, Einhorn D, Hershon K, Glazer NB, Yu S, for the Pioglitazone 014 Study Group. Efficacy and safety of pioglitazone in type 2 diabetes: a randomized, placebo-controlled study in patients receiving stable insulin therapy. *Int J Clin Pract* 2002; 56 (4): 251–7.
55. Viberti G, Kahn SE, Greene DA, Herman WH, Zinman B, Holman RR, Haffner SM, Levy D, Lachin JM, Berry RA, Heise MA, Jones NP, Freed MI. A diabetes outcome progression trial (ADOPT): an international multicenter study of the comparative efficacy of rosiglitazone, glyburide, and metformin in recently diagnosed type 2 diabetes. *Diabetes Care* 2002; 25 (10): 1737–43.
56. Buch HN, Baskar V, Barton DM, Kamalakannan D, Akarca C, Singh BM. Combination of insulin and thiazolidinedione therapy in massively obese patients with type 2 diabetes. *Diabet Med* 2002; 19 (7): 572–4.
57. Thompson-Culkin K, Zussman B, Miller AK, Freed MI. Pharmacokinetics of rosiglitazone in patients with end-stage renal disease. *J Int Med Res* 2002; 30 (4): 391–9.
58. Suter SL, Nolan JJ, Wallace P, Olefsky JM. Metabolic effects of new oral hypoglycemic agent CS-045 in NIDDM subjects. *Diabetes Care* 1992; 15: 193–203.
59. Nolan JJ, Ludvik B, Beerdsen P, et al. Improvement in glucose tolerance and insulin resistance in obese subjects treated with troglitazone. *N Eng J Med* 1994; 331: 1188–98.
60. Berkowitz K, Peters R, Kjos SL, et al. Effect of troglitazone on insulin sensitivity and pancreatic beta-cell function in women at high risk for NIDDM. *Diabetes* 1996; 45: 1572–9.
61. Dunaif A, Scott D, Finegood D, et al. The insulin-sensitizing agent troglitazone improves metabolic and reproductive abnormalities in the polycystic ovary syndrome. *J Clin Endocrinol Metab* 1996; 81: 3299–306.
62. Iuorno MJ, Nestler JE. Insulin-lowering drugs in polycystic ovary syndrome. *Obstet Gynecol Clin North Am* 2001; 28 (1): 153–64.
63. Takino H, Oghuni S, Uotani S, et al. Increased insulin responsiveness after C-045 treatment in diabetes associated with Werner's syndrome. *Diabetes Res Clin Pract* 1994; 24 (3): 167–72.
64. Iuorno MJ, Nestler JE. Insulin-lowering drugs in polycystic ovary syndrome. *Obstet Gynecol Clin North Am* 2001; 28 (1): 153–64.
65. Miyazaki Y, Mahankali A, Matsuda M, Glass L, Mahankali S, Ferrannini E, Cusi K, Mandarino LJ, DeFronzo RA. Improved glycemic control and enhanced insulin sensitivity in type 2 diabetic subjects treated with pioglitazone. *Diabetes Care* 2001; 24 (4): 710–9.
66. Mudaliar S, Henry RR. The oral hypoglycemic agents. In Porte D, Sherwin R, Baron A (eds), *Ellenberg and RifKin's Diabetes Mellitus*, 3rd edn. New York: McGraw-Hill, 2002; p 539.
67. Pavo I, Jermendy G, Varkonyi TT, Kerenyi Z, Gyimesi A, Shoustov S, Shestakova M, Herz M, Johns D, Schluchter BJ, Festa A, Tan MH. Effect of pioglitazone compared with metformin on glycemic control and indicators of insulin sensitivity in recently diagnosed patients with

type 2 diabetes. *J Clin Endocrinol Metab* 2003; 88 (4): 1637–45.

68. Kawamori R, Matsuhisa M, Kinoshita J, et al. for the AD-4833 Clamp-OGL Study Group. Pioglitazone enhances splanchnic glucose uptake as well as peripheral glucose uptake in non-insulin-dependent diabetes mellitus. *Diabetes Res Clin Pract* 1998; 41 (1): 35–43.
69. Yamasaki Y, Kawamori R, Wasada T, for the AD-4833 Glucose Clamp Study Group, Japan. Pioglitazone (AD-4833) ameliorates insulin resistance in patients with NIDDM. *Tohoku J Exp Med* 1997; 183 (3): 173–83.
70. Miyazaki Y, Glass L, Triplitt C, Matsuda M, Cusi K, Mahankali A, Mahankali S, Mandarino LJ, DeFronzo RA. Effect of rosiglitazone on glucose and non-esterified fatty acid metabolism in type II diabetic patients. *Diabetologia* 2001; 44 (12): 2210–9.
71. Mayerson AB, Hundal RS, Dufour S, Lebon V, Befroy D, Cline GW, Enocksson S, Inzucchi SE, Shulman GI, Petersen KF. The effects of rosiglitazone on insulin sensitivity, lipolysis, and hepatic and skeletal muscle triglyceride content in patients with type 2 diabetes. *Diabetes* 2002; 51 (3): 797–802.
72. Virtanen KA, Hallsten K, Parkkola R, Janatuinen T, Lonnqvist F, Viljanen T, Ronnemaa T, Knuuti J, Huupponen R, Lonnroth P, Nuutila P. Differential effects of rosiglitazone and metformin on adipose tissue distribution and glucose uptake in type 2 diabetic subjects. *Diabetes* 2003; 52 (2): 283–90.
73. Hallsten K, Virtanen KA, Lonnqvist F, Sipila H, Oksanen A, Viljanen T, Ronnemaa T, Viikari J, Knuuti J, Nuutila P. Rosiglitazone but not metformin enhances insulin- and exercise-stimulated skeletal muscle glucose uptake in patients with newly diagnosed type 2 diabetes. *Diabetes* 2002; 51 (12): 3479–85.
74. Raji A, Seely EW, Bekins SA, Williams GH, Simonson DC. Rosiglitazone improves insulin sensitivity and lowers blood pressure in hypertensive patients. *Diabetes Care* 2003; 26 (1): 172–8.
75. Fullert S, Schneider F, Haak E, Rau H, Badenhoop K, Lubben G, Usadel KH, Konrad T. Effects of pioglitazone in nondiabetic patients with arterial hypertension: a double-blind, placebo-controlled study. *J Clin Endocrinol Metab* 2002; 87 (12): 5503–6.
76. UK Prospective Diabetes Study Group. 1995 UK Prospective Diabetes Study 16. Overview of 6 years' therapy of type II diabetes: a progressive disease. *Diabetes* 1995; 44: 1249–58.
77. Levy J, Atkinson AB, Bell PM, McCance DR, Hadden DR. 1998 beta-cell deterioration determines the onset and rate of progression of secondary dietary failure in Type 2 diabetes mellitus: the 10-year follow-up of the Belfast diet study. *Diabet Med* 1998; 15: 290–6.
78. Dubois M, Pattou F, Kerr-Conte J, Gmyr V, Vandewalle B, Desreumaux P, Auwerx J, Schoonjans K, Lefebvre J. Expression of peroxisome proliferator-activated receptor gamma (PPARgamma) in normal human pancreatic islet cells. *Diabetologia* 2000; 43 (9): 1165–9.
79. Maggs DG, Buchanan TA, Burant CF, Cline G, Gumbiner B, Hsueh WA, Inzucchi S, Kelley D, Nolan J, Olefsky JM, Polonsky KS, Silver D, Valiquett TR, Shulman GI: Metabolic effects of troglitazone monotherapy in type 2 diabetes mellitus); a randomized, double-blind, placebo-controlled trial. *Ann Intern Med* 1999; 128: 176–85.
80. Patel J, Anderson RJ, Rappaport EB: Rosiglitazone monotherapy improve glycaemic control in patients with type 2 diabetes: a twelve-week, randomized, placebo-controlled study. *Diabetes Obes Metab* 1999; 1: 165–72.
81. Inzucchi SE, Maggs D, Spollet GR, Page SL, Rife FS, Walton V, Shulman GI: Efficacy and metabolic effects of metformin and troglitazone in type II diabetes mellitus. *N Engl J Med* 1998; 338: 867–72.
82. Miyazaki Y, Matsuda M, DeFronzo RA. Dose-response effect of pioglitazone on insulin sensitivity and insulin secretion in type 2 diabetes. *Diabetes Care* 2002; 25 (3): 517–23.
83. Rossetti L, Giacarri A, DeFronzo RA: Glucose toxicity. *Diabetes Care* 1990; 13: 610–30.
84. Diamond MP, Thornton K, Connoly-Diamond M, Sherwin RS, DeFronzo RA: Reciprocal variation in insulin-mediated glucose uptake and pancreatic insulin secretion in women with normal glucose tolerance. *J Soc Gynecol Invest* 1995; 2: 708–15.
85. Prigeon RL, Kahn SE, Porte D: Effect of troglitazone on B cell function, insulin sensitivity and glycemic control in subjects with type 2 diabetes mellitus. *J Clin Endocrinol Metab* 1998; 83 (3): 819–923.
86. Kubo K. Effect of pioglitazone on blood proinsulin levels in patients with type 2 diabetes mellitus. *Endocr J* 2002; 49 (3): 323–8.
87. Yang C, Chang TJ, Chang JC, Liu MW, Tai TY, Hsu WH, Chuang LM. Rosiglitazone (BRL 49653) enhances insulin secretory response via phosphatidylinositol 3-kinase pathway. *Diabetes* 2001; 50 (11): 2598–602.
88. Buchanan TA, Xiang AH, Peters RK, Kjos SL, Marroquin A, Goico J, Ochoa C, Tan S, Berkowitz K, Hodis HN, Azen SP. Preservation of pancreatic beta-cell function and prevention of type 2 diabetes by pharmacological treatment of insulin resistance in high-risk hispanic women. *Diabetes* 2002; 51 (9): 2796–803.
89. The Diabetes Prevention Program Research Group. The Diabetes Prevention Program. Reduction in the incidence of type 2 diabetes with lifestyle intervention or metformin. *N Engl J Med* 2002; 346 (6): 393–403.
90. The Diabetes Prevention Program Group. Prevention of type 2 diabetes with troglitazone in the Diabetes Prevention Program. *Diabetes* 2003; 52 (suppl 1): 251OR.
91. Garg A. Dyslipoproteinemia and diabetes. *Endocr Metab Clin North Am* 1998; 27 (3): 613–26.
92. Haffner SM, Miettinen H: Insulin resistance implications for type II diabetes and coronary artery disease. *Am J Med* 1997; 103: 152–62.
93. *Actos (Prescribing information).* Lincolnshire, IL: Takeda; Indianapolis, IN: Elli Lilly Company; July 2002.
94. Rosenblatt S, Miskin B, Glazer NB, Prince MJ, Robertson KE, for the Pioglitazone 026 Study Group. The impact of pioglitazone on glycemic control and atherogenic dyslipidemia in patients with type 2 diabetes mellitus. *Coron Artery Dis* 2001; 12 (5): 413–23.
95. Fonseca VA, Valiquett TR, Huang SM, Ghazzi MN, Whitcomb RW, for the Troglitazone Study Group. Troglitazone monotherapy improves glycemic control in patients with type 2 diabetes mellitus: a randomized, controlled study. *J Clin Endocrinol Metab* 1998; 83 (9): 3169–76.
96. Freed MI, Ratner R, Marcovina SM, Kreider MM, Biswas N, Cohen BR, Brunzell JD, for the Rosiglitazone Study 108 Investigators. Effects of rosiglitazone alone and in combination with atorvastatin on the metabolic

abnormalities in type 2 diabetes mellitus. *Am J Cardiol* 2002; 90 (9): 947–52.

97. Khan MA, St. Peter JV, Xue JL. A prospective, randomized comparison of the metabolic effects of pioglitazone or rosiglitazone in patients with type 2 diabetes who were previously treated with troglitazone. *Diabetes Care* 2002; 25: 708–11.
98. Boyle PJ, King AB, Olansky L, Marchetti A, Lau H, Magar R, Martin J. Effects of pioglitazone and rosiglitazone on blood lipid levels and glycemic control in patients with type 2 diabetes mellitus: a retrospective review of randomly selected medical records. *Clin Ther* 2002; 24 (3): 378–96.
99. Aronoff S, Rosenblatt S, Braithwaite S, Egan JW, Mathisen AL, Schneider RL, for the Pioglitazone 001 Study Group. Pioglitazone hydrochloride monotherapy improves glycemic control in the treatment of patients with type 2 diabetes: a 6-month randomized placebo-controlled dose-response study. *Diabetes Care* 2000; 23 (11): 1605–11.
100. Tack CJJ, Smits P, Demacker PNM. Troglitazone decreases the proportion of small dense LDL and increases the resistance of LDL to oxidation in obese subjects. *Diabetes Care* 1998; 21 (5): 796–9.
101. Hirano T, Yoshino G, Kazumi T. Troglitazone and small low-density lipoprotein in type 2 diabetes. *Ann Intern Med* 1998; 129 (2): 162–3.
102. Matsumoto K, Miyake S, Yano M, et al. Increase of lipoprotein (a) with troglitazone. *Lancet* 1997; 350: 1748–9.
103. Ovalle F, Bell DSH. Troglitazone's effect on lipoprotein(a) levels (Letter). *Diabetes Care* 1999; 22: 859–60.
104. Nagai Y, Abe T, Nomura G. Does pioglitazone, like troglitazone, increase serum levels of lipoprotein(a) in diabetic patients? *Diabetes Care* 2001; 24: 408–9.
105. Spiegelman BM. PPARγ: adipogenic regulator and thiazolidinedione receptor. *Diabetes* 1998; 47: 507–14.
106. Adams M, Montague CT, Prins JB, et al. Activators of peroxisome proliferator-activated receptor-γ have depot-specific effects on human preadipocyte differentiation. *J Clin Invest* 1997; 100: 3149–53.
107. van Harmelen V, Dicker A, Ryden M, Hauner H, Lonnqvist F, Naslund E, Arner P. Increased lipolysis and decreased leptin production by human omental as compared with subcutaneous preadipocytes. *Diabetes* 2002; 51 (7): 2029–36.
108. Mori Y, Murakawa Y, Okada K, et al. Effect of troglitazone on body fat distribution in type 2 diabetic patients. *Diabetes Care* 1999; 22 (6): 908–12.
109. Kelly IE, Han TS, Walsh K, et al. Effects of a thiazolidinedione compound on body fat and fat distribution of patients with type 2 diabetes. *Diabetes Care* 1999; 22 (2): 288–93.
110. Carey DG, Cowin GJ, Galloway GJ, Jones NP, Richards JC, Biswas N, Doddrell DM. Effect of rosiglitazone on insulin sensitivity and body composition in type 2 diabetic patients. *Obes Res* 2002; 10 (10): 1008–15.
111. Miyazaki Y, Mahankali A, Matsuda M, Mahankali S, Hardies J, Cusi K, Mandarino LJ, DeFronzo RA. Effect of pioglitazone on abdominal fat distribution and insulin sensitivity in type 2 diabetic patients. *J Clin Endocrinol Metab* 2002; 87 (6): 2784–91.
112. Ghazzi MN, Perez JE, Antonucci TK, Driscoll JH, Huang SM, Faja BW, Whitcomb RW, for the Troglitazone Study Group. Cardiac and glycemic benefits of troglitazone treatment in NIDDM. *Diabetes* 1997; 46: 433–9.
113. Asakawa M, Takano H, Nagai T, Uozumi H, Hasegawa H, Kubota N, Saito T, Masuda Y, Kadowaki T, Komuro I. Peroxisome proliferator-activated receptor gamma plays a critical role in inhibition of cardiac hypertrophy in vitro and in vivo. *Circulation* 2002; 105 (10): 1240–6.
114. St John Sutton M, Rendell M, Dandona P, Dole JF, Murphy K, Patwardhan R, Patel J, Freed M. A comparison of the effects of rosiglitazone and glyburide on cardiovascular function and glycemic control in patients with type 2 diabetes. *Diabetes Care* 2002; 25 (11): 2058–64.
115. Shiomi T, Tsutsui H, Hayashidani S, Suematsu N, Ikeuchi M, Wen J, Ishibashi M, Kubota T, Egashira K, Takeshita A. Pioglitazone, a peroxisome proliferator-activated receptor-gamma agonist, attenuates left ventricular remodeling and failure after experimental myocardial infarction. *Circulation* 2002; 106 (24): 3126–32.
116. Wayman NS, Hattori Y, McDonald MC, Mota-Filipe H, Cuzzocrea S, Pisano B, Chatterjee PK, Thiemermann C. Ligands of the peroxisome proliferator-activated receptors (PPAR-gamma and PPAR-alpha) reduce myocardial infarct size. *FASEB J* 2002; 16 (9): 1027–40.
117. Rizvi AA, Bowman MA. Thiazolidinedione therapy in a patient with diabetes after cardiac transplantation. *Endocr Pract* 2002; 8 (4): 287–91.
118. Simonson DC. Etiology and prevalence of hypertension in diabetic patients. *Am J Hypertens* 1995; 8: 316–20.
119. Baron AD. Hemodynamic actions of insulin. *Am J Physiol* 1994; 267: E187–202.
120. Laakso M, Edelman SV, Brechtel G, et al. Impaired insulin-mediated skeletal muscle blood flow in patients with NIDDM. *Diabetes* 1992; 41: 1076–83.
121. Anderson EA, Balon TW, Hoffman RP, et al. Insulin increases sympathetic activity but not blood pressure in borderline hypertensive humans. *Hypertension* 1992; 19: 621–7.
122. Bakris G, Viberti G, Weston WM, Heise M, Porter LE, Freed MI. Rosiglitazone reduces urinary albumin excretion in type II diabetes. *J Human Hypertens* 2003; 17 (1): 7–12.
123. Fullert S, Schneider F, Haak E, Rau H, Badenhoop K, Lubben G, Usadel KH, Konrad T. Effects of pioglitazone in nondiabetic patients with arterial hypertension: a double-blind, placebo-controlled study. *J Clin Endocrinol Metab* 2002; 87 (12): 5503–6.
124. Hirose H, Kawai T, Yamamoto Y, Taniyama M, Tomita M, Matsubara K, Okazaki Y, Ishii T, Oguma Y, Takei I, Saruta T. Effects of pioglitazone on metabolic parameters, body fat distribution, and serum adiponectin levels in Japanese male patients with type 2 diabetes. *Metabolism* 2002; 51 (3): 314–7.
125. American Diabetes Association. Position statement: diabetic nephropathy. *Diabetes Care* 2000; 23 (suppl 1): S69–72.
126. Yamashita H, Nagai Y, Takamura T, Nohara E, Kobayashi K. Thiazolidinedione derivatives ameliorate albuminuria in streptozotocin-induced diabetic spontaneous hypertensive rat. *Metabolism* 2002; 51 (4): 403–8.
127. Isshiki K, Haneda M, Koya D, Maeda S, Sugimoto T, Kikkawa R. Thiazolidinedione compounds ameliorate glomerular dysfunction independent of their insulin-sensitizing action in diabetic rats. *Diabetes* 2000; 49 (6): 1022–32.

128. Nakamura T, Ushiyama C, Shimada N, Hayashi K, Ebihara I, Koide H. Comparative effects of pioglitazone, glibenclamide, and voglibose on urinary endothelin-1 and albumin excretion in diabetes patients. *J Diabetes Complications* 2000; 14 (5): 250–4.
129. Lusis AJ. Atherosclerosis. *Nature* 2000; 407: 233–41.
130. Duez H, Fruchart JC, Staels B. PPARs in inflammation, atherosclerosis and thrombosis. *J Cardiovasc Risk* 2001; 8 (4): 187–94.
131. Hsueh WA, Javkson S, Law RE. Control of vascular cell proliferation and migration by PPARg. *Diabetes Care* 2001; 24 (2): 392–7.
132. Pasceri V, Wu HD, Willerson JT, Yeh ET. Modulation of vascular inflammation in vitro and in vivo by peroxisome proliferator-activated receptor-g activators. *Circulation* 2000; 101: 235–8.
133. Murao K, Imachi H, Momoi A, Sayo Y, Hosokawa H, Sato M, et al. Thiazolidinedione inhibits the production of monocyte chemoattractant protein-1 in cytokine-treated human vascular endothelial cells. *FEBS Lett* 1999; 454: 27–30.
134. Delerive P, Martin-Nizard F, Chinetti G, Trottein F, Fruchart JC, Najib J, et al. Peroxisome proliferator-activated receptor activators inhibit thrombin-induced endothelin-1 production in human vascular endothelial cells by inhibiting the activator protein-1 signaling pathway. *Circ Res* 1999; 85: 394–402.
135. Fonseca VA, Reynolds T, Hemphill D, et al. Effect of troglitazone on fibrinolysis and activated coagulation in patients with non-insulin-dependent diabetes mellitus. *J Diabetes Complications* 1998; 12: 181–6.
136. Marx N, Libby P, Plutzky. Peroxisome proliferator-activated receptors (PPARs) and their role in the vessel wall:possible mediators of cardiovascular risk? *J Cardiovasc Risk* 2001; 8 (4): 203–10.
137. Ricote M, Li AC, Willson TM, Kelly CJ, Glass CK. The peroxisome proliferator-activated receptor-g is a negative regulator of macrophage activation. *Nature* 1998; 391: 79–82.
138. Jiang C, Ting AT, Seed B. PPAR-g agonists inhibit production of monocyte inflammatory cytokines. *Nature* 2001; 391: 1998; 82–6.
139. Chawla A, Boisvert WA, Lee CH, Laffitte BA, Barak Y, Joseph SB, Liao D, Nagy L, Edwards PA, Curtiss LK, Evans RM, Tontonoz P. A PPAR g-LXR-ABCA1 pathway in macrophages is involved in cholesterol efflux and atherogenesis. *Mol Cell* 2001; 7 (1): 161–71.
140. Haffner SM, Greenberg AS, Weston WM, Chen H, Williams K, Freed MI. Effect of rosiglitazone treatment on nontraditional markers of cardiovascular disease in patients with type 2 diabetes mellitus. *Circulation* 2002; 106 (6): 679–84.
141. Marx N, Froehlich J, Siam L, Ittner J, Wierse G, Schmidt A, Scharnagl H, Hombach V, Koenig W. Antidiabetic PPAR gamma-activator rosiglitazone reduces MMP-9 serum levels in type 2 diabetic patients with coronary artery disease. *Arterioscler Thromb Vasc Biol* 2003; 23 (2): 283–8.
142. Ishibashi M, Egashira K, Hiasa K, Inoue S, Ni W, Zhao Q, Usui M, Kitamoto S, Ichiki T, Takeshita A. Antiinflammatory and antiarteriosclerotic effects of pioglitazone. *Hypertension* 2002; 40 (5): 687–93.
143. Hsueh WA, Javkson S, Law RE. Control of vascular cell proliferation and migration by PPARγ. *Diabetes Care* 2001; 24 (2): 392–7.
144. Marx N, Kehrle B, Kohlhammer K, Grub M, Koenig W, Hombach V, Libby P, Plutzky J. PPAR activators as anti-inflammatory mediators in human T lymphocytes: implications for atherosclerosis and transplantation-associated arteriosclerosis. *Circ Res* 2002; 90 (6): 703–10.
145. Folsom AR, Eckfeldt JH, Weitzman S. Relation of carotid artery wall thickness to diabetes mellitus, fasting glucose and insulin, body size, and physical activity. *Stroke* 1994; 25: 66–73.
146. Minamikawa J, Tanaka S, Yamauchi M, et al. Potent inhibitory effect of troglitazone on carotid arterial wall thickness in type 2 diabetes. *J Clin Endocrinol Metab* 1998; 83: 1818–20.
147. Koshiyama H, Shimono D, Kuwamura N, Minamikawa J, Nakamura Y. Inhibitory effect of pioglitazone on carotid arterial wall thickness in type 2 diabetes. *J Clin Endocrinol Metab* 2001; 86: 3452–6.
148. Takagi T, Akasaka T, Yamamuro A, Honda Y, Hozumi T, Morioka S, Yoshida K. Troglitazone reduces neointimal tissue proliferation after coronary stent implantation in patients with non-insulin dependent diabetes mellitus: a serial intravascular ultrasound study. *J Am Coll Cardiol* 2000; 36 (5): 1529–35.
149. Choi SH, Choi DH, KO YK, Chang YS, Cho Yl, Cha BS. Preventive effects of rosiglitazone on restenosis after coronary stenting in patients with type 2 diabetes. *Diabetes* 2003; 52 (suppl 1): 82OR.
150. Sasaki T, Fujimoto Y, Tsuchida A, Kawasaki Y, Kuwada Y, Chayama K. Activation of peroxisome proliferator-activated receptor gamma inhibits the growth of human pancreatic cancer. *Pathobiology* 2001; 69 (5): 258–65.
151. Sarraf P, Mueller E, Jones D, King FJ, DeAngelo DJ, Partridge JB, Holden SA, Chen LB, Singer S, Fletcher C, Spiegelman BM. Differentiation and reversal of malignant changes in colon cancer through PPAR[gamma]. *Nat Med* 1998; 4: 1046–52.
152. Elstner E, Muller C, Koshizuka K, Williamson EA, Park D, Asou H, Shintaku P, Said JW, Heber D, Koeffler HP. Ligands for peroxisome proliferator-activated receptor [gamma] and retinoic acid and receptor inhibit growth and induce apoptosis of human breast cancer cells in vitro and in BNX mice. *Proc Natl Acad Sci USA* 1998; 95: 8806–11.
153. Ohta K, Endo T, Haraguchi K, Hershman JM, Onaya T. Ligands for peroxisome proliferator-activated receptor γ inhibit growth and induce apoptosis of human papillary thyroid carcinoma cells. *J Clin Endocrinol Metab* 2001; 86: 2170–7.
154. Fujiwara T, Horikoshi H. Troglitazone and related compounds: therapeutic potential beyond diabetes. *Life Sci* 2000; 67 (20): 2405–16.
155. Panigrahy D, Singer S, Shen LQ, Butterfield CE, Freedman DA, Chen EJ, Moses MA, Kilroy S, Duensing S, Fletcher C, Fletcher JA, Hlatky L, Hahnfeldt P, Folkman J, Kaipainen A. PPARgamma ligands inhibit primary tumor growth and metastasis by inhibiting angiogenesis. *J Clin Invest* 2002; 110 (7): 923–32.
156. Kulke MH, Demetri GD, Sharpless NE, Ryan DP, Shivdasani R, Clark JS, Spiegelman BM, Kim H, Mayer RJ, Fuchs CS. A phase II study of troglitazone, an activator of the PPARgamma receptor, in patients with chemotherapy-resistant metastatic colorectal cancer. *Cancer J* 2002; 8 (5): 395–9.
157. Seed B. PPAR- and colorectal carcinoma: conflicts in a nuclear family. *Nat Med* 1998; 4: 1004–5.

158. Dunaif A, Scott D, Finegood D, Quintana B, Whitcomb R. The insulin-sensitizing agent troglitazone improves metabolic and reproductive abnormalities in the polycystic ovary syndrome. *J Clin Endocrinol Metab* 1996; 81 (9): 3299–306.
159. Azziz R, Ehrmann D, Legro RS, Whitcomb RW, Hanley R, Fereshetian AG, O'Keefe M, Ghazzi MN, for the PCOS/Troglitazone Study Group. Troglitazone improves ovulation and hirsutism in the polycystic ovary syndrome: a multicenter, double blind, placebo-controlled trial. *J Clin Endocrinol Metab* 2001; 86 (4): 1626–32.
160. Azziz R, Ehrmann DA, Legro RS, Fereshetian AG, O' Keefe M, Ghazzi MN, for the PCOS/Troglitazone Study Group. Troglitazone decreases adrenal androgen levels in women with polycystic ovary syndrome. *Fertil Steril* 2003; 79 (4): 932–7.
161. Paradisi G, Steinberg HO, Shepard MK, Hook G, Baron AD. Troglitazone therapy improves endothelial function to near normal levels in women with polycystic ovary syndrome. *J Clin Endocrinol Metab* 2003; 88 (2): 576–80.
162. Ghazeeri G, Kutteh WH, Bryer-Ash M, Haas D, Ke RW. Effect of rosiglitazone on spontaneous and clomiphene citrate-induced ovulation in women with polycystic ovary syndrome. *Fertil Steril* 2003; 79 (3): 562–6.
163. Gasic S, Nagamani M, Green A, Urban RJ. Troglitazone is a competitive inhibitor of 3beta-hydroxysteroid dehydrogenase enzyme in the ovary. *Am J Obstet Gynecol* 2001; 184 (4): 575–9.
164. Hadigan C, Miller K, Corcoran C. Fasting hyperinsulinemia and changes in regional body composition in human immunodeficiency virus-infected women. *J Clin Endocrinol Metab* 1999; 84: 1932–7.
165. Gelato MC, Mynarcik DC, Quick JL, Steigbigel RT, Fuhrer J, Brathwaite CE, Brebbia JS, Wax MR, McNurlan MA. Improved insulin sensitivity and body fat distribution in HIV-infected patients treated with rosiglitazone: a pilot study. *J Acquir Immune Defic Syndr JAIDS* 2002; 31 (2): 163–70.
166. Walli R, Michl GM, Muhlbayer D, Brinkmann L, Goebel FD. Effects of troglitazone on insulin sensitivity in HIV-infected patients with protease inhibitor-associated diabetes mellitus. *Res Exp Med* 2000; 199 (5): 253–62.
167. Clark RB. The role of PPARs in inflammation and immunity. *J Leukoc Biol* 2002; 71 (3): 388–400.
168. Chinetti G, Fruchart JC, Staels B. Peroxisome proliferator-activated receptors (PPARs): nuclear receptors at the crossroads between lipid metabolism and inflammation. *Inflamm Res* 2000; 49 (10): 497–505.
169. Shiojiri T, Wada K, Nakajima A, Katayama K, Shibuya A, Kudo C, Kadowaki T, Mayumi T, Yura Y, Kamisaki Y. PPAR gamma ligands inhibit nitrotyrosine formation and inflammatory mediator expressions in adjuvant-induced rheumatoid arthritis mice. *Eur J Pharmacol* 2002; 448 (2/3): 231–8.
170. Su CG, Wen X, Bailey ST, Jiang W, Rangwala SM, Keilbaugh SA, Flanigan A, Murthy S, Lazar MA, Wu GD. A novel therapy for colitis utilizing PPAR-ligands to inhibit the epithelial inflammatory response. *J Clin Invest* 1999; 104: 383–9.
171. Kawahito Y, Kondo M, Tsubouchhi Y, Hashiramoto A, Bishop-Bailey D, Inoue K, Kohno M,t Yamada R, Hla T, Sano H. 15-Deoxy-delta (12,14)-PGJ(2) induces synoviocyte apoptosis and suppresses adjuvant-induced arthritis in rats. *J Clin Invest* 2000; 106: 189–97.
172. Lewis JD, Lichtenstein GR, Stein RB, Deren JJ, Judge TA, Fogt F, Furth EE, Demissie EJ, Hurd LB, Su CG, Keilbaugh SA, Lazar MA, Wu GD. An open-label trial of the PPAR-gamma ligand rosiglitazone for active ulcerative colitis. *Am J Gastroenterol* 2001; 96 (12): 3323–8.
173. Avandia (Prescribing information). Philadelphia, PA: Smith Kline Beecham Pharmaceuticals, April 2000.
174. Mudaliar S, Henry RR. Thiazolidinediones, peripheral edema and type 2 diabetes: incidence, pathophysiology and clinical implications. *Endocr Pract* 2003; 9 (5): 406–16.
175. Wang F, Aleksunes LM, Reagan LA, Vergara CM. Management of rosiglitazone-induced edema: two case reports and a review of the literature. *Diabetes Technol Thera* 2002; 4 (4): 505–14.
176. Hirsch IB, Kelley J, Cooper S. Pulmonary edema associated with troglitazone therapy. *Arch Intern Med* 1999; 159 (5): 1811–2.
177. Thomas ML, Lloyd SJ. Pulmonary edema associated with rosiglitazone and troglitazone. *Ann Pharmacother* 2001; 35: 123–4.
178. Al-Salman J, Arjomand H, Kemp DG. Hepatocellular injury in a patient receiving rosiglitazone. A case report. *Ann Intern Med* 2000; 132 (2): 121–4.
179. Forman LM, Simmons DA, Diamond RH. Hepatic failure in a patient taking rosiglitazone. *Ann Intern Med* 2000; 132 (2): 118–21.
180. Chase MP, Yarze JC. Pioglitazone-associated fulminant hepatic failure. [Letter]. *Am J Gastroenterol* 2002; 97 (2): 502–3.
181. Pinto AG, Cummings OW, Chalasani N. Severe but reversible cholestatic liver injury after pioglitazone therapy. *Ann Intern Med* 2002; 137 (10): 857.
182. Maeda K. Hepatocellular injury in a patient receiving pioglitazone [Letter]. *Ann Intern Med* 2001; 135: 306.
183. May LD, Lefkowitch JH, Kram MT, Rubin DE. Mixed hepatocellular-cholestatic liver injury after pioglitazone therapy. *Ann Intern Med* 2002; 136: 449–52.
184. Lebovitz HE, Kreider M, Freed MI. Evaluation of liver function in type 2 diabetic patients during clinical trials: evidence that rosiglitazone does not cause hepatic dysfunction. *Diabetes Care* 2002; 25 (5): 815–21.
185. Nowak SN, Edwards DJ, Clarke A, Anderson GD, Jaber LA. Pioglitazone: effect on CYP3A4 activity. *J Clin Pharmacol* 2002; 42 (12): 1299–302.

49

α-Glucosidase Inhibitors

Rémi Rabasa-Lhoret and Jean-Louis Chiasson

Research Centre, Centre Hospitalier de l'Université de Montréal, Montréal, Canada, and Université de Montréal, Montréal, Canada

INTRODUCTION

Type 2 diabetes mellitus is a major health problem associated with excess morbidity and mortality, resulting in substantial health care costs [1]. Its prevalence worldwide will double over the next 25 years [2]. The UKPDS (United Kingdom Prospective Diabetes Study), DCCT (Diabetes Control and Complication Trial), and Kumamoto Study have provided excellent evidence that intensive glycemic treatment has a significant beneficial impact on microvascular complications [3–5]. These investigations also suggest that the incidence of macrovascular disease may be delayed by intensive glucose control, and this has recently been confirmed in two different trials in type 1 and type 2 diabetic patients [6, 7].

Dietary interventions still remain the cornerstone in the treatment of patients with type 2 diabetes mellitus. Although the focus is frequently on weight reduction, it is also aimed specifically at hyperglycemia management [8]. When diet and physical exercise fail, oral hypoglycemic agents such as sulfonylureas, biguanides, or, more recently, thiazolidinediones are added. These agents have been shown to decrease fasting plasma blood glucose, but postprandial hyperglycemia persists in more than 60% of patients, accounting in part for the sustained increase in HbA_{1c} [9]. Postprandial glycemic excursion contributes to the development of diabetes-specific complications (i.e. retinopathy and nephropathy) and could be involved in the development of macrovascular complications [10, 11]. Slowly absorbable carbohydrates and high-fiber diets blunt the postprandial increase in plasma glucose and insulin levels. Most patients, however, find these regimens difficult to follow in the long-term [12].

α-Glucosidase inhibitors have been developed specifically to delay the digestion of complex carbohydrates and decrease the postprandial rise in plasma glucose, thus reproducing the effect of a low glycemic index/high fiber diet. By their novel mechanism of action, α-glucosidase inhibitors significantly reduce postprandial glycemic and insulinemic excursion whether they are used as monotherapy or combined in the treatment of type 1 or type 2 diabetes. These drugs also have an excellent safety profile.

MECHANISM OF ACTION

α-Gucosidase inhibitors competitively block small intestine brush border enzymes that are necessary to hydrolyze oligo- and polysaccharides to monosaccharides [13]. Normally, carbohydrates are primarily and rapidly absorbed in the first half of the small intestine. With α-glucosidase inhibitions, carbohydrate absorption and digestion occur throughout the small intestine. This results in slower absorption of ingested carbohydrates and consequently, the postprandial plasma glucose rise is blunted [14].

Three α-glucosidase inhibitors have been developed: acarbose, miglitol, and voglibose (Figure 1), which have similar pharmacological profiles. Voglibose is currently marketed only in Japan with little clinical trial information [15, 16]. Acarbose, a pseudotetrasaccharide of microbial origin, is structurally analogous to an oligosaccharide derived from starch digestion. It is made up of a maltose unit link to an acarviosine unit, which represents the active part of the molecule [14]. The acarviosine unit has nitrogen linkage, which is responsible for its high affinity for the carbohydrate-binding site of various α-glucosidases, and exceeds the affinity (10- to 100 000-fold) of regular oligosaccharides from nutritional carbohydrates [13]. Because of this C—N linkage, acarbose cannot be cleaved and, therefore, enzymatic hydrolysis is

International Textbook of Diabetes Mellitus, Third Edition. Edited by R. A. DeFronzo, E. Ferrannini, H. Keen, and P. Zimmet.
 ISBN: 0-471-48655-8.

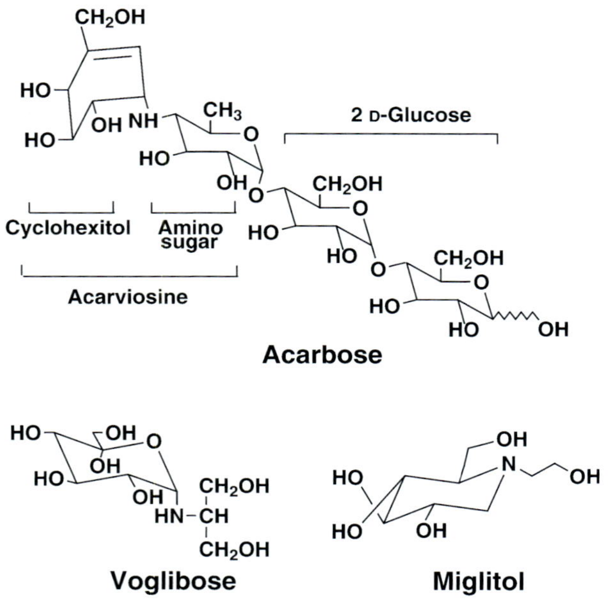

Figure 1 Structural formula of the α-glucosidase inhibitors acarbose, miglitol, and voglibose

blocked [13, 17]. Despite its high affinity for these enzymes, acarbose-binding is reversible, and its inhibition kinetics are competitive. Owing to its specificity for α-glucosidases, β-glucosidases (e.g. lactases) are not inhibited by acarbose, and so lactose digestion and absorption are not affected by it. Intestinal glucose absorption is also not impacted by α-glucosidase inhibitors [13, 14, 17]. Because acarbose is poorly absorbed (less than 1–2% of the active compound), it displays its inhibitory activity not only in the proximal jejunum but all along the small intestine up to the ileum [13, 17]. Acarbose is cleaved in the large intestine by bacterial enzymes into several metabolizable intermediates and 4-methylpyrogallol derivatives. Thus even though acarbose itself is poorly absorbed, 35% of an oral dose appears as metabolites in the urine [18].

Miglitol is not metabolized and is excreted quantitatively by the kidney [18]. However, because of its close resemblance to the glucose molecule, miglitol is significantly absorbed through a jejunal transport mechanism identical to that for glucose [18]. It then circulates and concentrates in enterocytes of the small intestine.

To be efficient, α-glucosidase inhibitors must be present at the site of enzymatic action at the same time as the oligosaccharide or disaccharide. Therefore, they should be taken with the first bite and not more than 15 min after starting the meal [19]. The delay in carbohydrate digestion and absorption in the small bowel increases the amount of fermentable carbohydrates reaching the colon. This results in gastrointestinal symptoms (flatulence, diarrhea).

CLINICAL EFFICACY OF α-GLUCOSIDASE INHIBITORS

Treatment of Diabetes Mellitus

Much experience has been gained with α-glucosidase inhibitors in the treatment of diabetes mellitus. The benefit of adding α-glucosidase inhibitors to the diet, sulfonylureas, metformin, combination of sulfonylureas and metformin as well as insulin-treatment in type 2 or type 1 patients has been investigated in various randomized, double-blind, placebo-controlled trials; open-labeled, controlled investigations; and postmarketing surveillance trials. More studies have been done and more experience has been acquired with acarbose than with miglitol or voglibose.

When α-glucosidase inhibitors are added to current treatment, published data routinely show a significant reduction in postprandial blood glucose levels (~3 mmol/l), but a decrease in fasting blood glucose occurs only in some studies. Nevertheless, there is a decline in HbA_{1c}, ranging from 0.5 to 1.5%, with a mean around 0.7% (Figure 2).

Large, controlled or open trials have revealed a number of constant features associated with acarbose therapy in diabetes [21–24]. The glucose-lowering effect of acarbose is observed from the first week of therapy, and is maintained throughout the treatment period, even after 3 years. Acarbose efficacy is present whatever the current treatment. However, a greater response to treatment has been reported in patients with recently diagnosed diabetes and/or naive to oral hypoglycemic agents. The drug is effective independent of sex or racial origin. The higher the initial HbA_{1c}, the larger its mean reduction with acarbose treatment. No weight gain occurs and most studies have shown small but consistent weight loss. Used as monotherapy, there is no risk of hypoglycemia. The main cause of treatment discontinuation is gastrointestinal side effects. The percentage of discontinuation related to side effects differs widely between studies, varying from 5 to 40%. However, no serious adverse effects are associated with α-glucosidase inhibitors, making it a particularly safe drug.

Dose–Response Relationship

The dose–response relationship has been studied in two large multicenter trials. In the European trial, doses ranging from 25 to 200 mg t.i.d. for 24 weeks were tested [25]. Even at a low dosage (25 mg t.i.d.), acarbose significantly reduced fasting and postprandial plasma glucose values as well as HbA_{1c}. The plasma glucose-lowering effect reached a plateau at the 50–100 mg t.i.d. dose-level and the greatest impact on these parameters was obtained with 200 mg t.i.d. An American trial investigated doses ranging from 100 to 300 mg t.i.d. in patients poorly controlled on diet alone [24]. Here again, the maximal dose

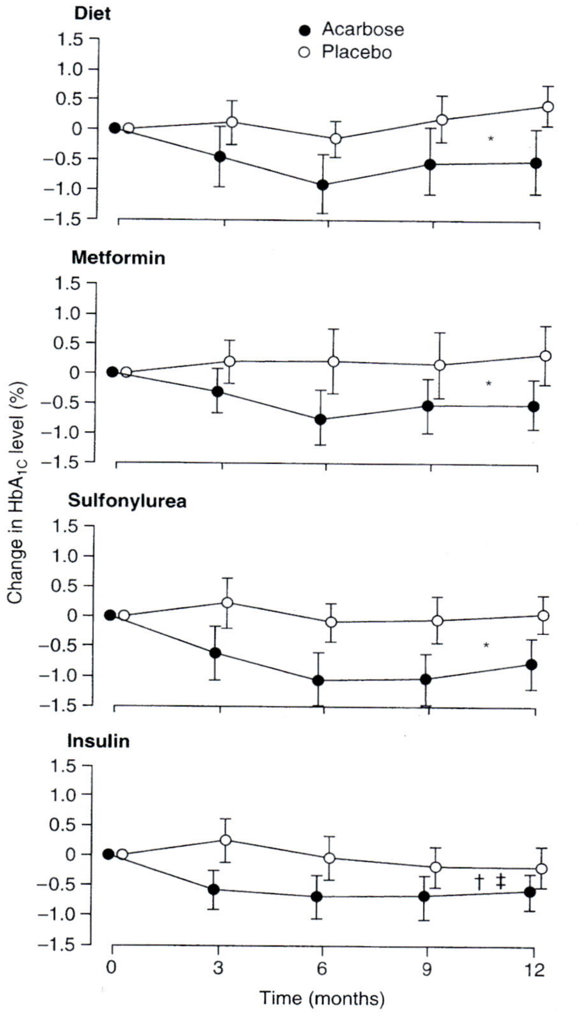

Figure 2 Effects of acarbose and placebo on HbA_{1c} levels throughout the 1-year study period in groups of patients treated with diet alone, metformin, sulfonylurea, or insulin. Data are expressed as means with 95% CIs. $^{*}p \leq 0.010$, $^{\dagger}p = 0.077$. p values represent differences between changes from baseline (time 0) to endpoint (time 12 months) for acarbose and placebo. $^{\ddagger}p = 0.01$ by covariance analysis. (From reference 22, With permission)

gave the best results, and there was a plateau effect between the 100 and 200 mg t.i.d. doses. These clinical trials indicate that the 100 mg t.i.d. dose evoked a near maximal response in glycemic control.

Comparative Studies Between α-Glucosidase Inhibitors

To the best of our knowledge, only two studies of α-glucosidase inhibitors have compared acarbose and voglibose [15, 16].

In the first one, acute investigation, pharmacological profiles were compared in nondiabetic subjects [16]. In that situation, voglibose seemed slightly less potent than acarbose, with no difference in gastrointestinal side effects.

In the second study, voglibose (0.2 mg t.i.d.) and acarbose (100 mg t.i.d.) were compared in type 2 diabetic subjects on diet therapy. The study design was a crossover trial of 8 weeks of active treatment versus placebo with 1 month of washout between the two treatment periods. Voglibose was associated with less gastrointestinal side effects, but was also less effective in reducing postprandial blood glucose excursion [15].

Efficacy of α-Glucosidase Inhibitors Combined with Diet Therapy in Type 2 Diabetic Patients

Seventeen major randomized trials, including patients insufficiently controlled by diet only and followed for at least 16 weeks, tested α-glucosidase inhibitors versus placebo in more than 1700 type 2 diabetic subjects [20, 21, 23, 24, 26–38]. Overall, these 17 studies confirmed drug efficacy in improving the glycemic control. They showed a mean reduction of 0.74% in HbA_{1c}, a 1.20 mmol/l decline in fasting hyperglycemia, and a 2.71 mmol/l fall in 1-h postprandial glycemia (Figures 2 and 3).

Efficacy of α-Glucosidase Inhibitors in Comparison to Sulfonylureas or Metformin

The efficacy of acarbose in type 2 diabetes has been compared to biguanides and sulfonylureas.

Six studies have directly compared, head to head, α-glucosidase inhibitors with sulfonylureas in type 2 diabetic patients on diet only [29, 30, 35, 39–41]. α-Glucosidase inhibitors appear to be slightly less potent, with mean HbA_{1c} reduction of 0.85% versus 1.02% with sulfonylureas (Figures 2 and 4).

Only two studies have compared acarbose [27] or miglitol [37] with metformin in diet failure. In the study by

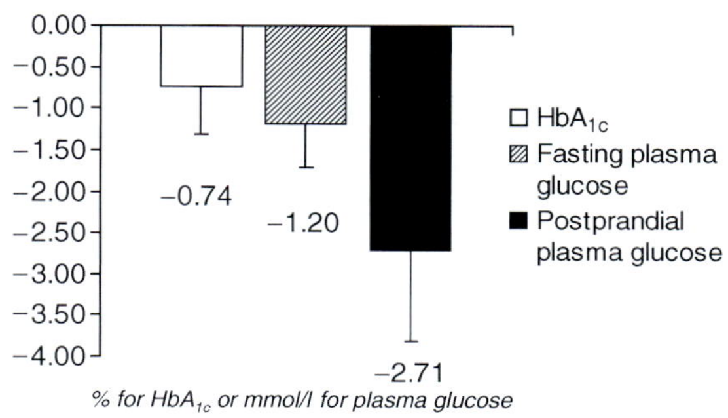

Figure 3 Effect of α-glucosidase inhibitors in type 2 diabetic patients treated with diet only (mean of 17 studies including 1704 subjects with a mean follow-up of 51 weeks). See text for references

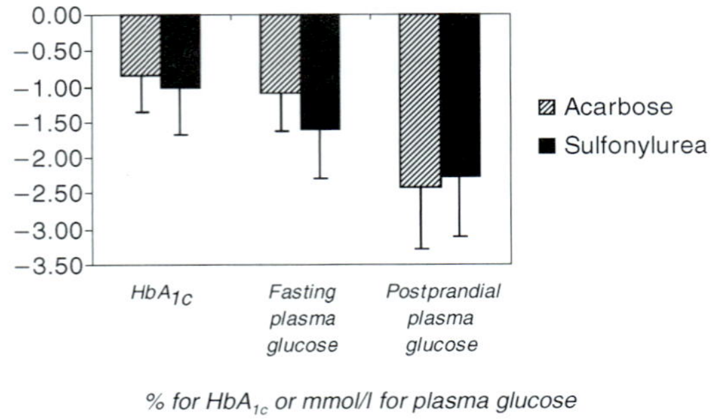

Figure 4 Comparison between α-glucosidase inhibitors and sulfonylurea in type 2 diabetic patients (mean of 6 studies including 704 subjects). See text for references

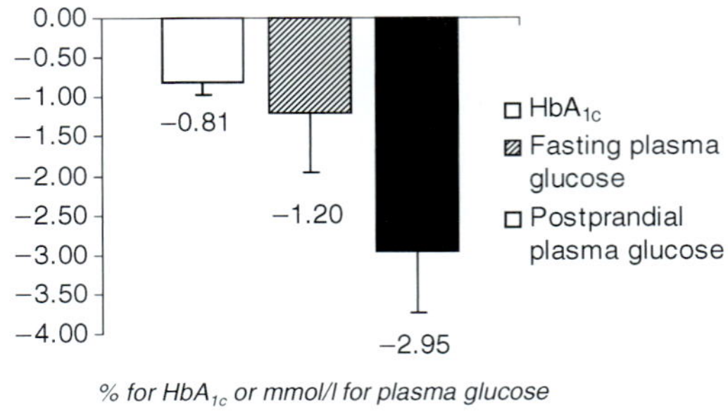

Figure 6 Effect of α-glucosidase inhibitors in diabetic patients previously treated with biguanides (mean of 5 studies including 512 subjects). See text for references

Hoffman and Spengler (26), acarbose (300 mg d.i.e.) had the same efficacy as metformin (1700 mg d.i.e.), with a mean HbA_{1c} reduction of 1% [27]. In Chiasson's work, miglitol (300 mg d.i.e.) had a lower efficacy (HbA_{1c}: −0.4%) than metformin (1500 mg d.i.e.; HbA_{1c}: −1.2%) [37], but there was a synergism effect when combining miglitol with metformin (HbA_{1c}: −1.8%) (see below).

Efficacy of α-Glucosidase Inhibitors as an Adjunct Treatment to Sulfonylureas and/or Metformin

Acarbose and miglitol have been tested in people with type 2 diabetes insufficiently controlled with sulfonylureas, as adjunct treatment in nine different studies [20, 21, 29, 41–45]. When added to sulfonylureas therapy, HbA_{1c} was decreased by −1.1%, fasting plasma glucose by −1.5 mmol/l, and postprandial plasma glucose by −2.4 mmol/l (Figures 2 and 5). In patients previously treated with sulfonylureas, the benefit of acarbose seemed comparable to the addition of metformin for lowering HbA_{1c} [42, 44].

In type 2 diabetic patients suboptimally controlled with metformin, the addition of acarbose produced a mean reduction of −0.8% in HbA_{1c}, −1.2 mmol/l in fasting plasma glucose, and −2.95 mmol/l in postprandial plasma glucose [20, 21, 46–49] (Figures 2 and 6).

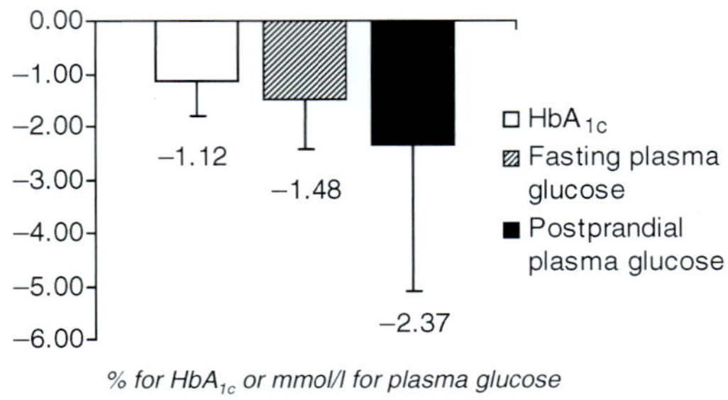

Figure 5 Effect of α-glucosidase inhibitors in diabetic patients previously treated with sulfamides (mean of 9 studies including 669 subjects). See text for references

When combined sulfonylurea and biguanide therapy fails to deliver adequate metabolic control, the addition of acarbose has been shown to result in significant glycemic improvement, with a mean HbA_{1c} decrease of 0.7% [21, 49–51] (Figure 7). In a large, open trial, diabetic patients failing with a combination of sulfonylureas and biguanides had a much smaller benefit than did patients treated previously with a single oral hypoglycemic agent [23]. Approximately one third of patients reached a good level of glucose control when a third oral hypoglycemic agent, either acarbose or a thiazolidinedione, was added [23, 52]. Thus, adding acarbose treatment to the failing combination of sulfonylureas and biguanides is usually a compromise for patients who refuse insulin injections.

Glitazone and α-Glucosidase Inhibitors

Few data are available for this combination. One publication indicates that acarbose produces a slight and clinically insignificant delay in rosiglitazone absorption [53]. Another suggests that HbA_{1c} is significantly improved 6 months after the addition of troglitazone to ongoing acarbose treatment [54].

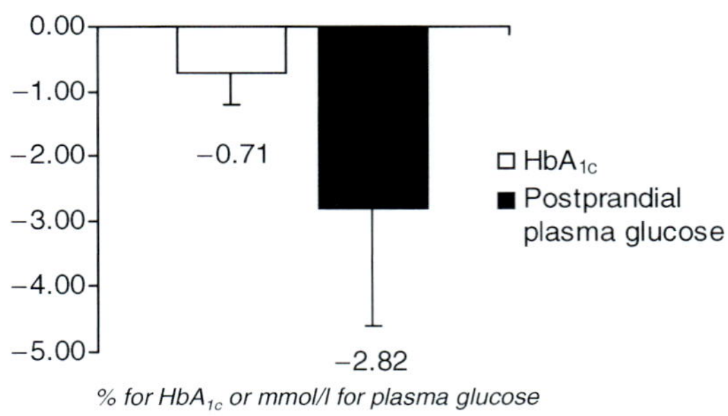

Figure 7 Effect of α-glucosidase inhibitors in diabetic patients previously treated with the combination of sulfonylureas and biguanides (mean of 6 studies including 374 subjects). See text for references

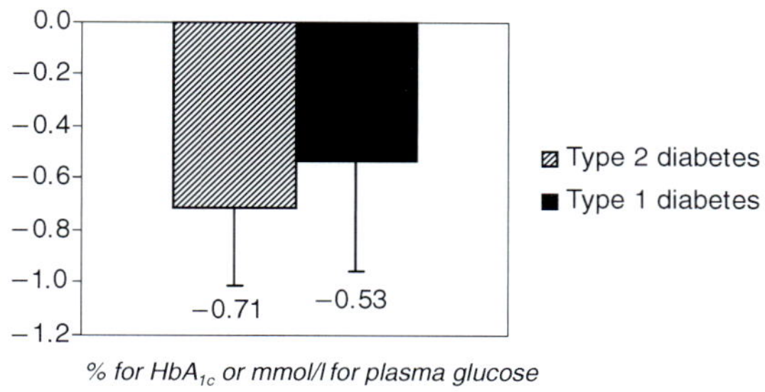

Figure 8 Effect of α-glucosidase inhibitors in diabetic patients previously treated with insulin (mean of 6 studies including 426 subjects). See text for references

Efficacy of α-Glucosidase Inhibitors in Insulin-treated Type 2 Diabetic Patients

The addition of bedtime NPH-insulin is a frequent option for type 2 diabetic patients insufficiently controlled with diet, exercise, and adequate doses of sulfonylureas and metformin. The addition of acarbose has been compared to the introduction of bedtime NPH. Although acarbose resulted in significant improvement of metabolic control compared to placebo, it was less effective than bedtime insulin [55]. Therefore, this strategy is generally an alternative for patients who refuse insulin injections.

When acarbose is combined with insulin therapy, however, it results in further metabolic improvement, with a mean reduction of −0.71 for HbA_{1c} [20, 56–59] (Figures 2 and 8). The addition of acarbose is usually associated with a decrease in insulin requirements [56, 58], but the significance of this diminution is controversial. Unlike sulfonylureas, the addition of acarbose to insulin therapy is not associated with weight gain [59].

Benefits of α-Glucosidase Inhibitors in Elderly Patients

Because of its mechanism of action and safety profile, acarbose could be a first-line drug for many elderly type 2 diabetic patients.

There have been two major trials in this group of patients. In the study by Johnston et al. [41] small doses of miglitol (25 or 50 mg t.i.d.) were compared to titrated doses of glyburide (1.25–20 mg, mean dose 9 mg/day) in elderly type 2 diabetic patients (mean age 68 years) inadequately controlled with diet alone. In this 56-week trial, all medications had a significant impact on HbA_{1c} but the two doses of miglitol were significantly less effective than glyburide on HbA_{1c} (−0.49% and −0.40% versus −0.92%). However, the higher benefit of glyburide on glycemic control was obtained at the cost of a significant increase in weight and in the incidence of clinical and subclinical hypoglycemia. There was also a significantly lower rate of cardiovascular adverse events (as a whole as well as serious) with miglitol compared to glyburide [41].

More recently, a Canadian trial compared acarbose with placebo in 182 elderly (mean age 70 years old) type 2 diabetic patients [38]. In that 1-year trial, acarbose was associated with a significant reduction in HbA_{1c} (−0.6%) as well as fasting (−0.7 mmol/l) and postprandial (−2.1 mmol/l) plasma glucose. Here again, the safety profile was excellent with side effects limited to mild gastrointestinal reactions. Acarbose was also associated with a significant decrease of insulin resistance evaluated in the total population ($n = 192$) with the HOMA model and confirmed in a subgroup ($n = 45$) with the euglycemic hyperinsulinemic clamp [38, 60].

Hypoglycemia is always a major concern in elderly patients who present and increase risk for this complications [60–67]. Hypoglycemic risk persist even with low dose or new generation sulfonylureas [68]. Thus the absence of hypoglycemic risk when α-glucosidase is used as monotherapy is a major advantage in this population [14].

In elderly diabetic patients in whom constipation is a major problem, gastrointestinal side effects reducing colonic transit time may be perceived as an advantage [41, 69].

The absence of drug interaction with acarbose is also an important advantage for elderly patients often on multitherapy [14]. Thus, acarbose should be considered as a first choice in this population [38, 41].

Impaired Glucose Tolerance and Prevention of Type 2 Diabetes

The STOP-NIDDM trial has investigated the potential of acarbose in preventing or delaying the development of type 2 diabetes in subjects with impaired glucose tolerance (IGT). One thousand four hundred twenty-nine subjects were randomized in a double-blind fashion to acarbose (up to 100 mg t.i.d.) or placebo. On the basis of a single OGTT (oral glucose tolerance test), acarbose reduced the risk of developing type 2 diabetes by 25% [70] (Figure 9). If

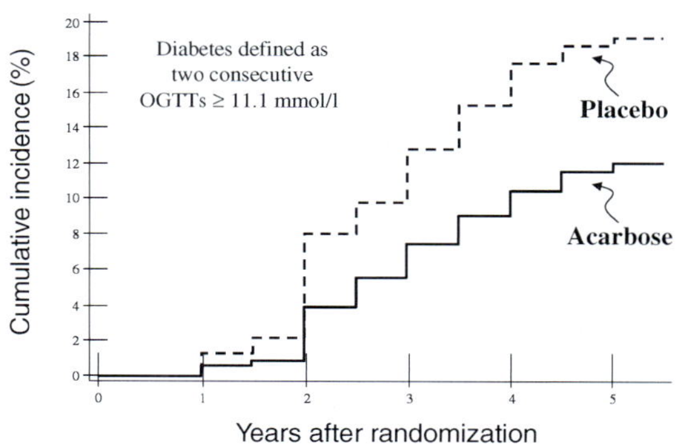

Figure 9 Effect of acarbose on the cumulative incidence of diabetes in the STOP-NIDDM trial [70]

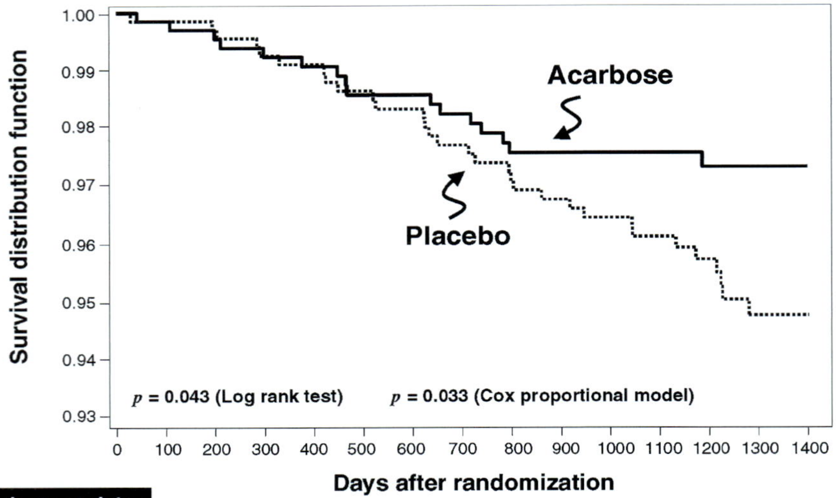

Patients at risk														
Acarbose	659	635	622	608	601	596	590	577	567	558	473	376	286	203
Placebo	675	667	658	643	638	633	627	615	611	604	519	424	332	232

Figure 10 Effect of acarbose on the probability of remaining free of cardiovascular events in the STOP-NIDDM trial [71]

two positive OGTTs were used to confirm the diagnosis of type 2 diabetes as recommended by the WHO (World Health Organization) and the Expert Committee of the ADA (American Diabetes Association), the relative risk reduction was 36.4% [70]. The beneficial effect of acarbose was independent of age, sex, and body mass index. The STOP-NIDDM trial also showed that acarbose treatment was associated with an increase in the reversion of IGT to normal glucose tolerance. These results indicate that 11 patients should be treated for 3.3 years to prevent or delay one case of type 2 diabetes. Subjects in the active treatment arm also experienced a significant reduction in the incidence of macrovascular events and new cases of hypertension [71] (Figure 10). Thus, for those with IGT, acarbose is effective in decreasing the risk of diabetes and potentially cardiovascular complications [71].

Other interventions using an intensive lifestyle modification program (diet and exercise) or pharmacological means (metformin or troglitazone) have also shown significant risk reduction for diabetes in subjects with IGT [72–74]. Lifestyle intervention had the highest efficacy with a risk reduction of 58%.

Efficacy of α-Glucosidase Inhibitors in Type 1 Diabetic Patients

Although, α-glucosidase inhibitors in type 1 diabetic patients have been tested in a number of studies, most of them were done on a small number of subjects and for a short duration.

All these investigations have shown acute and chronic reductions of postprandial plasma glucose [75–84]. In long-term treatment, the effect of acarbose on postprandial plasma glucose diminution resulted in a significant decrease of HbA_{1c} in all but one study [80]. Mean HbA_{1c} reduction in eight published trials including 471 patients was –0.53% when acarbose was added to insulin treatment (Figure 8). In most studies, acarbose improved the plasma glucose profile with lowered postprandial plasma glucose excursion and delayed nadir values [78, 82, 85]. Some showed that the smoother plasma glucose profile was associated with a reduced risk of hypoglycemia [82], but this was not observed in other trials [80, 83]. The possibility that acarbose might prevent nocturnal hypoglycemia has been studied in a double-blind crossover trial of 14 patients, 6 of whom suffered from recent nocturnal hypoglycemia [86]. The 100-mg dose taken with the evening meal was demonstrated to significantly reduce the number of hypoglycemic episodes [86, 87].

When combined with regular insulin, acarbose was found to have several advantages: insulin injection could be given immediately before the meal [85, 88], meal timing could be modified [88], and the need for between-meal snacks is optional [89]. The risk of hypoglycemia during postprandial exercise (moderate intensity) was reduced [82, 90, 91]. However, the usefulness of and the interest in these associations has decreased now that fast-acting insulin analogues are available.

Acute studies have also shown an insulin-sparing effect of acarbose (approximately 30%), especially for premeal insulin requirements [76, 81, 87, 92]. However, the largest placebo-controlled trial with type 1 diabetic patients could not confirm this sparing effect after 24 weeks of treatment [83].

Other Effects of α-Glucosidase Inhibitors

Gastrointestinal Peptide Secretion

α-Glucosidase inhibitors modify the secretion of *gastrointestinal peptides*, such as gastric inhibitory peptide (GIP) and glucagon-like peptide 1 (GLP-1). When α-glucosidase inhibitors are taken with a meal rich in carbohydrates, GIP secretion is decreased while GLP-1 is markedly increased, especially in the late postprandial period [18, 81, 93]. Whether these effects on GIP and GLP-1 play a role in the therapeutic effect of α-glucosidase inhibitors is unclear. It has been hypothesized that the impact of acarbose on glucose toxicity could be related to the combination of decreasing postprandial glucose excursion and its action on gastrointestinal hormones; this could theoretically explain the small (~−1.2 mmol/l) but frequently reported decrease in fasting plasma glucose [18].

Cardiovascular Risk Factors

In animal models of diabetes and/or dyslipidemia, α-glucosidase inhibitors reduces serum *triglycerides* in a dose-dependent manner [17]. In humans, the results are less clear. Acarbose has been shown to lower the postprandial triglyceride rise [94, 95], but its effect on fasting levels has been inconsistent with most studies reporting a small but significant diminution [17, 35, 44, 76, 96–99]. A more pronounced action has been reported in patients with familial hypertriglyceridemia [98, 100].

The effects of acarbose on fasting total cholesterol and HDL cholesterol are controversial, and appear to be minor or absent in the dose range used in clinical practice [99, 101]. The reported changes may reflect modifications in glycemic control more than a direct action of the drug [18, 101].

Because of their effect on postprandial plasma glucose and insulin excursion, α-glucosidase inhibitors can decrease insulin resistance [70]. Three studies of subjects with IGT have shown that acarbose and voglibose treatment for 8–16 weeks significantly reduce insulin resistance [102–104]. Comparable results have been reported in elderly type 2 diabetic patients after 1 year of treatment [38, 60] as well as in obese patients after 16 weeks [105]. An improvement in insulin secretion has also been documented in obese patients, as assessed by the C-peptide response to a glucagon challenge [105]. However, four studies conducted in younger type 2 diabetic patients in worse glycemic control failed to find any improvement in insulin sensitivity in spite of better glycemic control [96, 106–108].

Acarbose could have a favorable effect on blood pressure. In a trial in type 2 diabetic patients with mild hypertension, 6 months of treatment resulted in a 5.2 mmHg reduction of mean 24-h systolic blood pressure with acarbose compared to 1.6 mmHg with glibenclamide ($p = 0.0001$) [35]. Other studies suggest a slight but positive effect of acarbose on blood pressure [99]. Recent data of the STOP-NIDDM trial indicate that acarbose could delay the appearance of high blood pressure [71]. This positive outcome of acarbose on systolic blood pressure could be interesting, since there is a strong relationship between systolic blood pressure and cardiovascular mortality [109].

Because of its gastrointestinal side effects, acarbose could be associated with changes in dietary eating patterns and/or body weight. Two different studies have not documented any action of acarbose on energy intake, nutrient intake, or dietary patterns [110, 111]. Theoretically, carbohydrate malabsorption associated with acarbose could produce weight loss. However, it has been shown that carbohydrates that reach the colon are metabolized by bacteria into short chain fatty acids which are then absorbed, resulting in no or minimal caloric loss [26]. Clinical trials with acarbose found no [21] or minimum (~0.8 kg) weight loss after 24 weeks to 3 years of treatment [15, 22, 34, 35, 42, 49, 70, 110]. Combination of α-glucosidase inhibitors with sulfonylurea reduces the sulfonylurea-associated weight gain to minimal levels [29]. The moderate effect of acarbose on weight could occur through its action on postprandial triglyceride uptake by adipose tissue [112]. Using ^{14}C-radiolabeled triolein, Bischoff reported that if sulfonylureas increase triglyceride storage threefold compared to placebo, acarbose is able to reduce it by 40%. Furthermore, after combined administration of sulfonylureas and acarbose, sulfonylurea-induced triglyceride uptake was completely abolished [112].

Acarbose offers no benefit as an adjunct treatment in weight loss programs or to prevent weight regain after a very low-calorie diet in obese nondiabetic patients [113, 114].

Two studies have suggested a positive effect of acarbose on coagulation markers, which are increased in type 2 diabetic patients, especially in the postprandial state [99, 115].

Overall, α-glucosidase inhibitors exert neutral or slightly favorable actions on different cardiovascular risk factors: body weight, blood pressure, postprandial lipemia or coagulation markers, and insulin resistance. This potential benefit is supported by the reduction of atherosclerotic lesions in two animal models [116, 117] and the recent demonstration of a favorable effect of acarbose on cardiovascular events in IGT [71].

Potential Effects of α-Glucosidase Inhibitor on the Prevention of Long-term Diabetic Complications

Clinical studies (i.e. UKPDS or DCCT) have demonstrated that any level in improvement of glycemic control

Table 1 Comparison of adverse effects of different available antidiabetic oral agents

Adverse effects	Sulfonylureas	Metformin	Glitazone	Acarbose
Weight gain	+	−	+/++	−
Hypoglycemia	+/++	−	−	−
Hypersensitivity reactions	+	−	+	−
Drug interactions	+	−	−	−
Lactic acidosis	−	+	−	−
Gastrointestinal disturbance or hepatic reaction	+	++	++	++
Edema	−	−	+/++	−

Note: + Minor clinical problem; ++ major clinical problem; − not or rarely associated with this side effect.

is beneficial for the primary or secondary prevention of diabetic retinopathy, nephropathy, and neuropathy [3, 5]. Thus, acarbose, through its effect on glucose control, is expected to reduce long-term complications. However, this hypothesis has not been, and will probably not be, tested directly in humans.

Data from animal studies suggest that acarbose has significant beneficial actions on retinal, renal, and neural complications [118]. All of them indicate that acarbose has a positive effect through its influence on glycemic control. Some investigations also suggest that acarbose could have a positive outcome on macrovascular disease [118].

Four studies in different animal models of diabetes have shown that acarbose successfully reduces or prevents renal abnormalities associated with diabetes [119–122]. The same number of studies have investigated the effect of acarbose treatment on the prevention of diabetic retinopathy and cataract [123–126]. All of them have reported significant protection against the development of diabetes-associated eye problems. Similarly, acarbose efficacy has been examined in the field of diabetic neuropathy. It has been demonstrated to have a positive effect on models of peripheral polyneuropathy as well as autonomic neuropathy [123, 127, 128].

Finally, there is evidence from animal studies that acarbose could be useful in reducing macrovascular complications associated with diabetes. In a rodent model of obesity, diabetes, and macrovascular complications (the LA-corpulent rat), 8 months of acarbose treatment led to the significant regression of myocardial lesions [116]. Similar findings on aortic atherosclerosis have been obtained in a rabbit model fed an atherogenic diet [117]. These results are concordant with the recent report of a significant reduction in macrovascular events in patients with IGT treated with acarbose [71].

However, it is not known if the effect of α-glucosidase inhibitors on diabetic complications is related to a diminution of total integrated glucose concentrations or to a specific outcome in lowering postprandial glucose excursion. Some studies suggest that postprandial glycemic excursion could specifically contribute to diabetic complications through the polyol pathway [128] and lipid abnormalities [112] because enzymes involved in these changes require high glucose levels.

Treatment of Reactive Hypoglycemia

On the basis of their pharmacology, α-glucosidase inhibitors can be useful in the treatment of reactive hypoglycemia and/or dumping syndrome in nondiabetic patients [18, 129, 130].

TOLERABILITY OF ACARBOSE

Thousands of patients have been treated with this medication for several years without any major adverse effects (Table 1); acarbose is a safe drug [18, 22, 101].

Gastrointestinal Side Effects

The main side effects of acarbose are gastrointestinal symptoms consisting of abdominal distention, flatulence, diarrhea, and borborygmus in approximately 50% of patients. These adverse events are related to intracolonic fermentation and the consequent gas production of carbohydrates not absorbed in the small bowel. The symptoms are usually mild to moderate and tend to decrease with continued treatment [25, 26, 38]. With time, the α-glucosidase content of the distal small intestine will increase, and more carbohydrates can be digested and absorbed distally, reducing the spill way into the large bowel. That is why starting with a low dose of the inhibitor and increasing it slowly can help to minimize the side effects [18, 70, 131, 132]. The importance of this strategy is confirmed by the positive relationship between higher initial doses and higher discontinuation rates [132].

In contrast to initial reports [57], more recent work demonstrates no correlation between carbohydrate intake, fiber content of the diet or meal pattern (regular versus irregular), and side effects associated with acarbose [133, 134]. Beano, an over-the-counter α-galactosidase preparation, can decrease the gastrointestinal side effects if taken with acarbose, but also probably dilutes its glucose-lowering action [135].

The treatment discontinuation rate is mostly related to gastrointestinal side effects, but its true prevalence is unclear. In most large trials, the discontinuation rate is close to 25% [21, 37, 70]. Some studies including the UKPDS have reported much higher discontinuation rates (~40%) [18, 20, 21, 132]. However, others have found a much lower rate of patients unable to tolerate acarbose, which is comparable to that observed with biguanides (i.e. 5–7%) [25, 37, 42, 136]. No clear explanations are available for such discrepancies, but false evaluation of the gastrointestinal side effects can lead to unnecessary gastroenterologist consultations [132].

Despite these frequent gastrointestinal symptoms, the quality of life of patients on acarbose has been shown to be as good as, if not better, than with sulfonylurea or insulin therapy [38, 137].

Because of the importance of the problem, it is surprising that there are no published trials specifically designed to confirm that the "start low and go slow" strategy to titrate the medication is efficient in reducing the gastrointestinal side effects.

Hypoglycemia

Acarbose monotherapy does not cause hypoglycemia [21]. However, it may potentiate the hypoglycemic action of sulfonylureas and insulin. A reduction in dosage of concomitant hypoglycemic agents may be necessary when acarbose is introduced [22]. The acute effect of the combination of acarbose and glibenclamide resulted in an additive glucose-lowering effect and a reduced hypoglycemic risk [138]. Another acute study also suggested that this was true when acarbose was combined with insulin [82]. However, if a patient taking acarbose experiences hypoglycemia, it is recommended that it should be treated with glucose since the absorption of sucrose and complex carbohydrates could be delayed by the drug.

Other Potential and Demonstrated Side Effects Related to α-Glucosidase Inhibitor Therapy

Because of gastrointestinal side effects, there has been concern about the risk of colon cancer associated with α-glucosidase inhibitors [17]. There has been no increase of colon cancer in large cohorts followed for more than 1 year [20, 21, 70], and acarbose use is linked with serum and fecal butyrate as well as anatomopathological findings thought to reduce the risk of colon cancer [139, 140].

An elevation of liver enzyme has been reported in less than 2% of patients on high doses of acarbose (≥300 mg t.i.d.); the increase is moderate and always returns to normal after cessation of the drug [22, 83, 141]. In the Bayer database on worldwide trials with acarbose at doses of 100 mg t.i.d. or less, only 19 cases of transminase elevation over 500 UI/l have been documented in 500 000 patients [18]. In type 2 diabetic patients with liver cirrhosis, acarbose (100 mg t.i.d.) is well-tolerated [141, 142]. However, 2 cases of severe hepatotoxic reaction categorized as probable idiosyncratic reaction related to acarbose have been reported [143, 144]. Thus, hepatic reactions are extremely rare and unpredictable, and there are no specific recommendations to monitor liver enzymes with this therapy [141, 142].

A few reports associated ileus with acarbose treatment in Japanese patients [145, 146]. The occasional observation of anemia is controversial and probably not of clinical significance [26]. Finally, occasional reports indicate that acarbose could lower or increase digoxin levels, and thus plasma levels; plasma levels should probably be monitored when α-glucosidase inhibitor therapy is initiated or the dose is modified [147].

Overall, gastrointestinal side effects are the main clinical issue. To maximize treatment compliance, it is essential for clinicians to start patients on a low dose, titrating the dose gradually based on clinical efficacy and tolerance, and make sure to discuss the anticipated gastrointestinal side effects as well as their expected decrease over time during acarbose treatment.

CONTRAINDICATIONS TO α-GLUCOSIDASE INHIBITORS

Formal contraindications to acarbose therapy are intestinal malabsorption syndromes, inflammatory bowel disease, intestinal obstruction, and hepatic disease. It is also contraindicated in cases of severe renal impairment (creatinine clearance <25 ml/min), in pregnant or lactating women, and in children below 12 years of age, because of a lack of data in these patient groups. Since trials in diabetic cirrhotic patients have demonstrated a positive action of acarbose on glycemic control without adverse effects on liver function, restrictions related to hepatic function could be withdrawn in the future [141].

INDICATIONS FOR α-GLUCOSIDASE INHIBITORS

α-Glucosidase inhibitors exert their primary action on postprandial hyperglycemia. Therefore, they should be considered as first-line therapy in individuals in whom postprandial hyperglycemia is a dominant abnormality.

α-Glucosidase inhibitors should be considered as monotherapy in the following cases:

(1) *Patients with normal or slightly elevated fasting blood glucose and postprandial hyperglycemia*: In these patients, postprandial hyperglycemia contributes significantly to increased HbA_{1c} [9]. This population includes most recently diagnosed patients. When diet and exercise fails to normalize blood glucose,

α-glucosidase inhibitors can bring glycemic control into the desirable range for an important portion of these patients and should be considered as first-line treatment.

(2) *Elderly diabetic patients*: There is now much evidence that this patient population significantly benefits from α-glucosidase inhibitor treatment [38, 41, 60]. The absence of hypoglycemic risk is a major advantage in this subgroup, and moderately decreased kidney function is not a contraindication.

(3) *As an alternative to other oral hypoglycemic agents when they are contraindicated*: To avoid an existing or significant risk of hypoglycemia with sulfonylureas and the risk of lactic acidosis with biguanides.

α-Glucosidase inhibitors can also be prescribed in combination with other hypoglycemic agents in various situations:

(1) *As an adjunct* to other hypoglycemic agents that have not produced adequate glycemic control. Combination of α-glucosidase inhibitors with all other treatments has demonstrated a moderate but significant, constant, and sustained glycemic improvement.

(2) *As an alternative* for patients not controlled with a combination of oral hypoglycemic agents and who refuse insulin.

The proper use of α-glucosidase inhibitors requires attention on two major points:

- To be effective, they must be administered at the onset of meals with the first bite and not later than 15 min after meals.
- Therapy must be initiated with a low dose and titrated upward slowly based on 1-h postprandial glucose as well as gastrointestinal side effects.

Recommended doses are as follows:

- 25–100 mg t.i.d. for acarbose
- 25–100 mg t.i.d. for miglitol
- 0.2 mg t.i.d. for voglibose

CONCLUSIONS

α-Glucosidase inhibitors are drugs that delay the digestion of complex carbohydrates by acting as competitive inhibitors of intestinal α-glucosidase enzymes that hydrolyze oligosaccharides into monosaccharides, an essential step for absorption. Thus, these drugs decrease the rise in postprandial plasma glucose and insulin.

In subjects with impaired glucose tolerance, α-glucosidase inhibitors improve insulin sensitivity, delay the onset of type 2 diabetes mellitus and hypertension, and possibly reduce macrosvascular events. In type 2 diabetic patients, α-glucosidase inhibitors have shown moderate but constant and sustained reduction of hemoglobin A_{1c} (HbA_{1c}; ~0.7%) regardless of concomitant antidiabetic medication. In type 1 diabetic patients, α-glucosidase inhibitors have also been reported to decrease postprandial glycemic excursion.

Additional benefits of α-glucosidase inhibitors are the lack of hypoglycemia with monotherapy, no weight gain, and an excellent safety profile. Adverse events associated with α-glucosidase inhibitors' flatulence, abdominal discomfort, and bloating are the consequence of undigested carbohydrates reaching the colon, where they are fermented by bacteria. This explains the necessity of initiating treatment at a low dose and increasing the dosage slowly to minimize side effects.

Postprandial glycemic excursion contributes to the development of diabetes-specific complications (i.e. retinopathy and nephropathy) and could be involved in the etiology of macrovascular complications. Thus, α-glucosidase inhibitors are potentially important agents that help to improve plasma glucose control and potentially reduce diabetes-related complications.

REFERENCES

1. Harris MI. Diabetes in America: epidemiology and scope of the problem. *Diabetes Care* 1998; 21 (suppl 3): C11–4.
2. King H, Aubert RE, Herman WH. Global burden of diabetes, 1995–2025. *Diabetes Care* 1998; 21: 1414–31.
3. The Diabetes Control and Complication Trial Group. The effect of intensive treatment of diabetes on the development and progression of long-term complications in insulin-dependent diabetes mellitus. *New Engl J Med* 1993; 329: 977–86.
4. Shichiri M, Kishikawa H, Ohkubo Y, Wake N. Long-term results of the Kumamoto Study on optimal diabetes control in type 2 diabetic patients. *Diabetes Care* 2000; 23 (suppl 2): B21–9.
5. The United Kingdom Prospective Diabetes Study Group. UK Prospective Diabetes Study (UKPDS 33). Intensive blood-glucose control with sulfonylureas or insulin compared with conventional treatment and risk of complications in patients with type 2 diabetes. *Lancet* 1998; 352: 837–53.
6. Gaede P, Vedel P, Larsen N, Jensen GV, Parving HH, Pedersen O. Multifactorial intervention and cardiovascular disease in patients with type 2 diabetes. *New Engl J Med* 2003; 348: 383–93.
7. Nathan DM, Lachin JM, Cleary P, Orchard T, Brillon DJ, Backlund JY, O'Leary DH, Genuth S. Intensive diabetes therapy and carotid intima-media thickness in type 1 diabetes mellitus. *New Engl J Med* 2003; 348: 2294–303.
8. American Diabetes Association. Position statement. Nutrition recommandation and principle for people with diabetes mellitus. *Diabetes Care* 1998; 24 (suppl 1): S44–7.
9. Monnier L, Lapinski H, Colette C. Contributions of fasting and postprandial plasma glucose increments to the overall diurnal hyperglycemia of type 2 diabetic patients:

variations with increasing levels of HbA(1c). *Diabetes Care* 2003; 26: 881–5.
10. American Diabetes Association. Postprandial blood glucose. *Diabetes Care* 2001; 24: 775–8.
11. Davidson J. Should postprandial glucose be measured and treated to a particular target? Yes. *Diabetes Care* 2003; 26: 1919–21.
12. Wolever TMS. The glycemic index: flogging a dead horse? *Diabetes Care* 1997; 20: 452–6.
13. Bischoff H. The mechanism of α-glucosidase inhibition in the management of diabetes. *Clin Invest Med* 1995; 18: 303–11.
14. Rabasa-Lhoret R, Chiasson J-L. Potential of alpha-glucosidase inhibitors in elderly patients with diabetes mellitus and impared glucose tolerance. *Drug Aging* 1998; 13: 131–43.
15. Vichayanrat A, Ploybutr S, Tunlakit M, Watanakejorn P. Efficacy and safety of voglibose in comparison with acarbose in type 2 diabetic patients. *Diabetes Res Clin Pract* 2002; 55: 99–103.
16. Kageyama S, Nakamichi N, Sekino H, Nakano S. Comparison of the effects of acarbose and voglibose in healthy subjects. *Clin Ther* 1997; 19: 720–9.
17. Balfour JA, McTavish D. Acarbose: an update of its pharmacology and therapeutic use in diabetes mellitus [see erratum in *Drugs* 1994; 48: 929]. *Drugs* 1993; 46: 1025–54.
18. Lebovitz H. Alpha-glucosidase inhibitors as agents in the treatment of diabetes. *Diabetes Rev* 1998; 6: 132–45.
19. Rosak C, Nitzsche G, Konig P, Hofmann U. The effect of the timing and the administration of acarbose on postprandial hyperglycaemia. *Diabet Med* 1995; 12: 979–84.
20. Chiasson J-L, Josse RG, Hunt JA, et al. The efficacy of acarbose in the treatment of patients with non-insulin-dependent diabetes mellitus. *Ann Intern Med* 1994; 121: 928–35.
21. Holman RR, Cull C, Turner RC, UKPDS Study Group. A randomized double-blind trial of acarbose in type 2 diabetes shows improved glycemic control over 3 years (UKPDS 44). *Diabetes Care* 1999; 22: 960–4.
22. Buse J, Hart K, Minasi L. The PROTECT Study: final results of a large multicenter postmarketing study in patients with type 2 diabetes. Precose Resolution of Optimal Titration to Enhance Current Therapies. *Clin Ther* 1998; 20: 257–69.
23. Mertes G. Efficacy and safety of acarbose in the treatment of type 2 diabetes: data from a 2-year surveillance study. *Diabetes Res Clin Pract* 1998; 40: 63–70.
24. Coniff RF, Shapiro JA, Robbins D, et al. Reduction of glycosylated hemoglobin and postprandial hyperglycemia by acarbose in patients with NIDDM: a placebo controlled dose-comparison study. *Diabetes Care* 1995; 18: 817–24.
25. Fischer S, Hanefeld M, Spengler M, Boehme K, Temelkova-Kurktschiev T. European study on dose–response relationship of acarbose as a first-line drug in non-insulin-dependent diabetes mellitus: efficacy and safety of low and high doses. *Acta Diabetol* 1998; 35: 34–40.
26. Santeusanio F, Compagnucci P. A risk-benefit apparaisal of acarbose in the management of non-insulin-dependent diabetes mellitus. *Drug Saf* 1994; 11: 432–44.
27. Hoffmann J, Spengler M. Efficacy of 24-week monotherapy with acarbose, metformin, or placebo in dietary-treated NIDDM patients: the Essen-II Study. *Am J Med* 1997; 103: 483–90.
28. Braun D, Schönherr U, Mitzkat H-J. Efficacy of acarbose in monotherapy in patients with type 2 diabetes: a double-blind study conducted in general practice. *Endocrinol Metab* 1996; 3: 275–80.
29. Coniff RF, Shapiro JA, Seaton TB, Bray GA. Multicenter placebo-controlled trial comparing acarbose (Bay g 5421) with placebo, tolbutamide and tolbutamide-plus-acarbose in non-insulin-dependent diabetes mellitus. *Am J Med* 1995; 98: 443–51.
30. Hoffman J, Spengler M. Efficacy of 24-week monotherapy with acarbose, glibenclamide, or placebo in NIDDM patients. The Essen Study. *Diabetes Care* 1994; 17: 561–6.
31. Hotta N, Kakuta H, Sano T, et al. Long-term effect of acarbose on glycaemic control in non-insulin-dependent diabetes mellitus: a placebo-controlled double-blind study. *Diabet Med* 1993; 10: 134–8.
32. Hanefeld M, Fischer S, Schulze J, et al. Therapeutic potentials of acarbose as first-line drug in NIDDM insufficiently treated with diet alone. *Diabetes Care* 1991; 14: 732–7.
33. Coniff RF, Shapiro JA, Seaton TB. Long-term efficacy and safety of acarbose in the treatment of obese subjects with non-insulin-dependent diabetes mellitus. *Arch Intern Med* 1994; 154: 2442–8.
34. Chan JC, Chan KW, Ho LL, et al., the Asian Acarbose Study Group. An Asian multicenter clinical trial to assess the efficacy and tolerability of acarbose compared with placebo in type 2 diabetic patients previously treated with diet. *Diabetes Care* 1998; 1058–61.
35. Rosenthal JH, Mauerserger H. Effects on blood pressure of the alpha-glucosidase inhibitor acarbose compared with the insulin enhancer glibenclamide in patients with hypertension on type 2 diabetes mellitus. *Clin Drug Invest* 2002; 22: 695–701.
36. Hasche H, Mertes G, Bruns C, et al. Effects of acarbose treatment in Type 2 diabetic patients under dietary training: a multicentre, double-blind, placebo-controlled, 2-year study. *Diabetes Nutr Metab* 1999; 12: 277–85.
37. Chiasson J-L, Naditch L. The synergistic effect of miglitol plus metformin combination therapy in the treatment of type 2 diabetes. *Diabetes Care* 2001; 24: 989–94.
38. Josse RG, Chiasson JL, Ryan EA, et al. Acarbose in the treatment of elderly patients with type 2 diabetes. *Diabetes Res Clin Pract* 2003; 59: 37–42.
39. Segal P, Feig PU, Scherthaner G, et al. The efficacy and safety of miglitol therapy compared with glimenclamide in patients with NIDDM inadequatly controlled by diet alone. *Diabetes Care* 1997; 20: 687–91.
40. Salman S, Salman F, Satman I, et al. Comparison of acarbose and gliclazide as first-line agents in patients with type 2 diabetes. *Curr Med Res Opin* 2001; 16: 296–306.
41. Johnston PS, Lebovitz HE, Coniff RF, Simonson DC, Raskin P, Munera CL. Advantages of alpha-glucosidase inhibition as monotherapy in elderly type 2 diabetic patients. *J Clin Endocrinol Metab* 1998; 83: 1515–22.
42. Willms B, Ruge D. Comparison of acarbose and metformin in patients with Type 2 diabetes mellitus insufficiently controlled with diet and sulphonylureas: a randomized, placebo-controlled study. *Diabet Med* 1999; 16: 755–61.
43. May C. Efficacy and tolerability of stepwise increasing dosage of acarbosein patients with NIDDM treated with sulfonylurea. *Diabetes Stoffwechsel* 1995; 4: 3–7.
44. Bayraktar M, Van Thiel DH, Adalar N. A comparison of acarbose versus metformin as an adjuvant therapy

in sulfonylurea-treated NIDDM patients. *Diabetes Care* 1996; 19: 252–4.
45. Calle-Pascual A, Garcia-Honduvilla J, Martin-Alvarez PJ, et al. Comparison between acarbose, metformin and insulin treatment in type 2 diabetic patients with secondary failure to sulfonylurea treatment. *Diabete Metab* 1995; 21: 256–60.
46. Rosenstock J, Magner J, Krol T. Efficacy and safety of acarbose in patients with type 2 diabetes inadequtely controlled with metformin [abstract]. *Diabetes* 1998; 47 (suppl 1): 1357.
47. Phillips P, Karrasch J, Scott R, Wilson D, Moses R. Acarbose improves glycemic control in overweight type 2 diabetic patients insufficiently treated with metformin. *Diabetes Care* 2003; 26: 269–73.
48. Halimi S, Le Berre MA, Grange V. Efficacy and safety of acarbose add-on therapy in the treatment of overweight patients with Type 2 diabetes inadequately controlled with metformin: a double-blind, placebo-controlled study. *Diabetes Res Clin Pract* 2000; 50: 49–56.
49. Lam KS, Tiu SC, Tsang MW, Ip TP, Tam SC. Acarbose in NIDDM patients with poor control on conventional oral agents. A 24-week placebo-controlled study. *Diabetes Care* 1998; 21: 1154–8.
50. Soonthornpun S, Rattarasarn C, Thamprasit A, Leetanaporn K. Effect of acarbose in treatment of type II diabetes mellitus: a double-blind, crossover, placebo-controlled trial. *J Med Assoc Thai* 1998; 81: 195–200.
51. Kaye TB. Triple oral antidiabetic therapy. *J Diabetes Complications* 1998; 12: 311–3.
52. Yale JF, Valiquett TR, Ghazzi NM, Owens-Grillo JK, Whitcomb RW, Foyt HL. The effect of a thiazolidinedione drug, troglitazone, on glycemia in patients with type 2 diabetes mellitus poorly controlled with sulfonylurea and metformin. A multicenter randomized, double-blind, placebo-controlled trial. *Ann Intern Med* 2001; 134: 737–45.
53. Miller AK, Inglis AM, Culkin KT, Jorkasky DK, Freed MI. The effect of acarbose on the pharmacokinetics of rosiglitazone. *Eur J Clin Pharmacol* 2001; 57: 105–9.
54. Bando Y, Ushiogi Y, Okafuji K, Toya D, Tanaka N, Fujisawa M. Troglitazone combination therapy in obese type 2 diabetic patients poorly controlled with alpha-glucosidase inhibitors. *J Int Med Res* 1999; 27: 53–64.
55. Lopez J, Aguilar C, Velasco ML, Arita O, Guillen L, et al. Acarbose vs bedtime NPH insulin in the treament of secondary failures to sulfonylurea–metformin therapy in NIDDM. *Diabetes* 1997; 46 (suppl 1): 94A.
56. Standl E, Baumgartl HJ, Fuchtenbusch M, Stemplinger J. Effect of acarbose on additional insulin therapy in type 2 diabetic patients with late failure of sulphonylurea therapy. *Diabetes Obes Metab* 1999; 1: 215–20.
57. Hara T, Nakuamura J, Koh N, Sakakibara F, Takeuchi N, Hotta N. An importance of carbohydrate ingestion for the expression of the effect of α-glucosidase inhibitor in NIDDM. *Diabetes Care* 1996; 19: 642–6.
58. Coniff RF, Shapiro JA, Seaton TB, Hooggwerf BJ, Hunt JA. A double-blind placebo controlled trial evaluating the safety and efficacy of acarbose for the treatment of patients with insulin-requiring type II diabetes. *Diabetes Care* 1995; 18: 928–32.
59. Guvener N, Gedik O. Effects of combination of insulin and acarbose compared with insulin and gliclazide in type 2 diabetic patients. *Acta Diabetol* 1999; 36: 93–7.
60. Meneilly GS, Ryan EA, Radziuk J, et al. Effect of acarbose on insulin sensitivity in elderly patients with diabetes. *Diabetes Care* 2000; 23: 1162–7.
61. Marker JC, Cryer PE, Clutter WE. Attenuated glucose recovery from hypoglycemia in the elderly. *Diabetes* 1992; 41: 671–8.
62. Meneilly GS, Minaker KL, Young JB, Landsberg L, Rowe JW. Counterregulation response to insulin-induced glucose reduction in the elderly. *J Clin Endocrinol Metab* 1985; 61: 178–82.
63. Meneilly GS, Cheung E, Tuokko H. Counterregulatory hormone response to hypoglycemia in the elderly patient with diabetes. *Diabetes* 1994; 43: 403–10.
64. Heinsimer JA, Lefkowitz RJ. The impact of aging on adrenergic receptor function: clinical and biochemical aspects. *J Am Geriatr Soc* 1985; 33: 184–8.
65. Pulsinelli WA, Levy DE, Sigsbee B, Scherer P, Plum F. Increased damage after ischemic stroke in patients with hyperglycemia with or without established diabetes mellitus. *Am J Med* 1983; 74: 540–4.
66. Seltzer HS. Drug-induced hypoglycemia. A review based on 1418 cases. *Endocrinol Metab Clin* 1989; 18: 163–83.
67. Sonneblick A, Shilo S. Glibenclamide induced prolonged hypoglycaemia. *Age Ageing* 1986; 15: 185–9.
68. Hasslacher C. Safety and efficacy of repaglinide in type 2 diabetic patients with and without impaired renal function. *Diabetes Care* 2003; 26: 886–91.
69. Ron Y, Wainstein J, Leibovitz A, et al. The effect of acarbose on the colonic transit time of elderly long-term care patients with type 2 diabetes mellitus. *J Gerontol A Biol Sci Med Sci* 2002; 57: M111–4.
70. Chiasson JL, Josse RG, Gomis R, Hanefeld M, Karasik A, Laakso M. Acarbose for prevention of type 2 diabetes mellitus: the STOP-NIDDM randomised trial. *Lancet* 2002; 359: 2072–7.
71. Chiasson J-L, Josse R, Gomis R, et al. Acarbose treatment reduces the risk of cardiovascular disease and hypertension in subjects with impaired glucose tolerance: The STOP-NIDDM Trial. *JAMA* 2003; 290: 486–94.
72. Diabetes Prevention Programm Research Group. Reduction in the incidence of type 2 diabetes with lifestyle intervention or metformin. *New Engl J Med* 2002; 346: 393–403.
73. Tuomilehto J, Lindstrom J, Eriksson JG, et al. Prevention of type 2 diabetes mellitus by changes in lifestyle among subjects with impaired glucose tolerance. *New Engl J Med* 2001; 344: 1343–50.
74. Buchanan TA, Xiang AH, Peters RK, et al. Preservation of pancreatic beta-cell function and prevention of type 2 diabetes by pharmacological treatment of insulin resistance in high-risk Hispanic women. *Diabetes* 2002; 51: 2796–803.
75. Viviani GL, Camogliano L, Boroglio MG, et al. Acarbose treatment in insulin-dependent diabetics—a double blind crossover study. *Curr Ther Res Clin Exp* 1987; 42: 1–11.
76. Marena S, Tagliaferro V, Cavallero G, et al. Double-blind crossover study of acarbose in type 1 diabetic patients. *Diabet Med* 1991; 8: 674–8.
77. Austenat E. Neure therapiestudien mit Acarbose bei type-I-diabetikern. *Akt Endokr Stoffw* 1991; 12: 19–24.
78. Gerard J, Luyckx AS, Lefebvre PJ. Improvement of metabolic control in insulin dependent diabetics treated with the alpha-glucosidase inhibitor acarbose for two months. *Diabetologia* 1981; 21: 446–51.
79. Sels JP, Verdonk HE, Wolffenbuttel BH. Effects of acarbose (Glucobay) in persons with type 1 diabetes: a

multicentre study. *Diabetes Res Clin Pract* 1998; 41: 139–45.
80. Riccardi G, Giacco R, Parillo M, et al. Efficacy and safety of acarbose in the treatment of Type 1 diabetes mellitus: a placebo-controlled, double-blind, multicentre study. *Diabet Med* 1999; 16: 228–32.
81. Juntti-Berggren L, Pigon J, Hellstrom P, Holst JJ, Efendic S. Influence of acarbose on postprandial insulin requirements in patients with Type 1 diabetes. *Diabetes Nutr Metab* 2000; 13: 7–12.
82. Rabasa-Lhoret R, Burelle Y, Ducros F, et al. Use of an alpha-glucosidase inhibitor to maintain glucose homeostasis during post-prandial exercise in intensively treated type 1 diabetic subjects. *Diabete Med* 2001; 18: 739–44.
83. Hollander P, Pi-Sunyer X, Coniff RF. Acarbose in the treatment of type I diabetes. *Diabetes Care* 1997; 20: 248–53.
84. Escobar-Jimenez F, de Leiva A, Pinon F, et al. Clinical effectiveness and tolerance of acarbose in the treatment of insulin-dependent diabetic patients (type I). *Med Clin (Barc)* 1993; 100: 488–91.
85. Dimitriadis G, Hatziagellaki E, Alexopoulos E, et al. Effects of α-glucosidase inhibition on meal glucose tolerance and timing of insulin administration in patients with type 1 diabetes mellitus. *Diabetes Care* 1991; 14: 393–8.
86. McCulloch DK, Kurtz AB, Tattersall RB. A new approch to the treatment of noctural hypoglycaemia using alphaglucosidase inhibition. *Diabetes Care* 1983; 6: 48 3–7.
87. Tattersall R. Alpha-glucosidase inhibition as an adjunct to the treatment of type 1 diabetes. *Diabete Med* 1993; 10: 688–93.
88. Koch HH, Wudy A, Eberlein G, Quast C. Use of acarbose for eliminating the interval between meal consumption and insulin injection in patients with Type 1 diabetes. *Diabetes Nutr Metab* 1999; 12: 195–201.
89. Franck M, Sneige N, Koglmeier J. Acarbose can eliminate the need for between meal snacks in type I diabetes. *Diabetes* 1997; 46 (suppl 1): 92A.
90. Creutzfeldt W (ed). Comparative metabolic availability of glucose and sucrose and the effect of acarbose on sucrose utilisation during exercise in type I diabetic patients. In *Second International Symposium on Acarbose.* Berlin: Springer-Verlag, 1987.
91. Gerard G, Jandrain B, Pirnay F, et al. Utilisation of an oral sucrose load during exercise in humans. Effects of the α-glucosidase inhibitor acarbose. *Diabetes* 1986; 35: 1294–301.
92. Lecavallier L, Hamet P, Chiasson J-L. The effects of sucrose meal on insulin requirement in IDDM and its modulation by acarbose. *Diabete Metab* 2003; 12: 156–61.
93. Seifarth C, Bergmann J, Holst JJ, Ritzel R, Schmiegel W, Nauck MA. Prolonged and enhanced secretion of glucagon-like peptide 1 (7-36 amide) after oral sucrose due to alpha-glucosidase inhibition (acarbose) in Type 2 diabetic patients. *Diabet Med* 1998; 15: 485–91.
94. Leonhardt W, Hanefeld M, Fischer S, Schulze J. Efficacy of alpha-glucosidase inhibitors on lipids in NIDDM subjects with moderate hyperlipidaemia. *Eur J Clin Invest* 1994; 24 (suppl 3): 45–9.
95. Kado S, Murakami T, Aoki A, et al. Effect of acarbose on postprandial lipid metabolism in type 2 diabetes mellitus. *Diabetes Res Clin Pract* 1998; 41: 49–55.
96. Schnack C, Prager RJF, Winkler J, Klauser RM, Schneider BG, Schernthaner G. Effects of 8-week α-glucosidase inhibition on metabolic control, C-peptide secretion, hepatic glucose output, and peripheral sensitivity in poorly controlled type II diabetic patients. *Diabetes Care* 1989; 12: 537–43.
97. Mughal MA, Memon MY, Zardari MK, Tanwani RK, Ali M. Effect of acarbose on glycemic control, serum lipids and lipoproteins in type 2 diabetes. *J Pak Med Assoc* 2000; 50: 152–6.
98. Malaguarnera M, Giugno I, Ruello P, Maugeri D, Pistone G. Treatment of familial hypertriglyceridaemia with acarbose. *Diabetes Obes Metab* 2000; 2: 33–8.
99. Scott R, Lintott CJ, Zimmet P, Campbell L, Bowen K, Welborn T. Will acarbose improve the metabolic abnormalities of insulin-resistant type 2 diabetes mellitus? *Diabetes Res Clin Pract* 1999; 43: 179–85.
100. Malaguarnera M, Giugno I, Panebianco MP, Pistone G. Beneficial effects of acarbose on familiar hypertriglyceridemias. *Int J Clin Pharmacol Ther* 1998; 36: 441–5.
101. Scheen AJ. Clinical efficacy of acarbose in diabetes mellitus: a critical review of controlled trials. *Diabete Metab* 1998; 24: 311–20.
102. Chiasson J-L, Josse RG, Leitter L, et al. The effect of acarbose on insulin sensitivity in subjects with impaired glucose tolerance. *Diabetes Care* 1996; 19: 1190–3.
103. Shinozaki K, Suzuki M, Ikebuchi M, Hirose J, Hara Y, Harano Y. Improvement of insulin sensitivity and dyslipidemia with a new alpha-glucosidase inhibitor, voglibose, in nondiabetic hyperinsulinemic subjects. *Metabolism* 1996; 45: 731–7.
104. Laube H, Linn T, Heyen P. The effect of acarbose on insulin sensitivity and proinsulin in overweight subjects with impaired glucose tolerance. *Exp Clin Endocrinol Diabetes* 1998; 106: 231–3.
105. Delgado H, Lehmann T, Bobbioni-Harsch E, Ybarra J, Golay A. Acarbose improves indirectly both insulin resistance and secretion in obese type 2 diabetic patients. *Diabetes Metab* 2002; 28: 195–200.
106. Reaven GM, Lardinois CK, Greenfield MS, Schwartz HC, Vreman HJ. Effect of acarbose on carbohydrate and lipid metabolism in NIDDM patients poorly controlled by sulfonylureas. *Diabetes Care* 1990; 13 (suppl 3): 32–6.
107. Jenney A, Proietto J, O'Dea K, Nankervis A, Traianedes K, D'Embden H. Low-dose acarbose improves glycemic control in NIDDM patients without changes in insulin sensitivity. *Diabetes Care* 1993; 16: 499–502.
108. Johnson AB, Taylor R. Does suppression of postprandial blood glucose excursion by the α-glucosidase inhibitor miglitol improve insulin sensitivity in diet-treated type II diabetic patients. *Diabetes Care* 1996; 19: 559–63.
109. Staessen JA, Gasowski J, Wang JG, et al. Risks of untreated and treated isolated systolic hypertension in the elderly: meta-analysis of outcome trials. *Lancet* 2000; 355: 865–72.
110. Wolever TM, Chiasson JL, Josse RG, et al. Small weight loss on long-term acarbose therapy with no change in dietary pattern or nutrient intake of individuals with non-insulin-dependent diabetes. *Int J Obes Relat Metab Disord* 1997; 21: 756–63.
111. Lindstrom J, Tuomilehto J, Spengler M, The Finnish Acargbos Study Group. Acarbose treatment does not change the habitual diet of patients with Type 2 diabetes mellitus. *Diabete Med* 2000; 17: 20–5.
112. Bischoff H. Pharmacology of alpha-glucosidases inhibitors. *Eur J Clin Invest* 1994; 24 (suppl 2): 3–10.

113. Hauner H, Petzinna D, Sommerauer B, Toplak H. Effect of acarbose on weight maintenance after dietary weight loss in obese subjects. *Diabetes Obes Metab* 2001; 3: 42 3–7.
114. Bayraktar F, Hamulu F, Ozgen AG, Yilmaz C, Tuzun M, Kabalak T. Acarbose treatment in obesity: a controlled study. *Eat Weight Disord* 1998; 3: 46–9.
115. Ceriello A, Taboga C, Tonutti L, et al. Post-meal coagulation activation in diabetes mellitus: the effect of acarbose. *Diabetologia* 1996; 39: 469–73.
116. Russell J, Koeslag DG, Dolphin PJ, Amy RM. Beneficial effects of acarbose in the atherosclerosis-prone JCR: LA-corpulent rat. *Metabolism* 1993; 42: 218–23.
117. Kritchevsky D, Tepper SA, Davidson LM, Klurfeld DM. Influence of acarbose (a glucosidase inhibitor) on experimental atherosclerosis in the rabbit. *Artery* 1990; 17: 170–5.
118. Creutzfeldt W. Effects of the alpha-glucosidase inhibitor acarbose on the development of long-term complications in diabetic animals: pathophysiological and therapeutic implications. *Diabetes Metab Res Rev* 1999; 15: 289–96.
119. Cohen MP, Klepser H, Wu VY. Effect of alpha-glucosidase inhibition on the nonenzymatic glycation of glomerular basement membrane. *Gen Pharmacol* 1991; 22: 515–9.
120. Lee SM. The effect of chronic alpha-glycosidase inhibition on diabetic nephropathy in the *db/db* mouse. *Diabetes* 1982; 31: 249–54.
121. Cohen AM, Rosenmann E. Acarbose treatment and diabetic nephropathy in the Cohen diabetic rat. *Horm Metab Res* 1990; 22: 511–5.
122. Cohen MP, Vasselli JR, Neuman RG, Witt J. Treatment with acarbose, an alpha-glucosidase inhibitor, reduces increased albumin excretion in streptozotocin-diabetic rats. *Gen Pharmacol* 1995; 26: 1355–61.
123. Peterson RG. alpha-Glucosidase inhibitors in diabetes: lessons from animal studies. *Eur J Clin Invest* 1994; 24 (suppl 3): 11–8.
124. Cohen-Melamed E, Nyska A, Pollack A, Madar Z. Aldose reductase (EC 1.1.1.21) activity and reduced-glutathione content in lenses of diabetic sand rats (*Psammomys obesus*) fed with acarbose. *Br J Nutr* 1995; 74: 607–15.
125. Takagi C, King GL, Clermont AC, Cummins DR, Takagi H, Bursell SE. Reversal of abnormal retinal hemodynamics in diabetic rats by acarbose, an alpha-glucosidase inhibitor. *Curr Eye Res* 1995; 14: 741–9.
126. Chakrabarti S, Cherian PV, Sima AA. The effect of acarbose on diabetes- and age-related basement membrane thickening in retinal capillaries of the BB/W-rat. *Diabetes Res Clin Pract* 1993; 20: 123–8.
127. Katovich MJ, Meldrum MJ, Vasselli JR. Beneficial effects of dietary acarbose in the streptozotocin-induced diabetic rat. *Metabolism* 1991; 40: 1275–82.
128. Sima AAF, Chakrabarti S. Long-term suppression of postprandial hyperglycemia with acarbose retards the development of neuropathies in the BB/W-rat. *Diabetologia* 1992; 325–30.
129. Gerard J, Luyckx AS, Lefebvre PJ. Acarbose in reactive hypoglycemia: a double-blind study. *Int J Clin Pharmacol Ther Toxicol* 1984; 22: 25–31.
130. Lefebvre PJ, Scheen AJ. The use of acarbose in the prevention and treatment of hypoglycemia. *Eur J Clin Invest* 1994; 24 (suppl 3): 40–4.
131. Lebovitz HE. Alpha-glucosidase inhibitors. *Endocrinol Metab Clin North Am* 1997; 26: 539–51.
132. Catalan VS, Couture JA, LeLorier J. Predictors of persistence of use of the novel antidiabetic agent acarbose. *Arch Intern Med* 2001; 161: 1106–12.
133. Wolever TM, Chiasson JL, Josse RG, et al. No relationship between carbohydrate intake and effect of acarbose on HbA1c or gastrointestinal symptoms in type 2 diabetic subjects consuming 30–60% of energy from carbohydrate. *Diabetes Care* 1998; 21: 1612–8.
134. Harrower AD, Harrower A, Jack H. Effect of fiber intake and meal pattern on gastrointestinal symptoms with acarbose. *Diabetes Care* 1999; 22: 1227.
135. Lettieri JT, Dain B. Effects of beano on the tolerability and pharmacodynamics of acarbose. *Clin Ther* 1998; 20: 497–504.
136. Krentz AJ, Ferner RE, Bailey CJ. Comparative tolerability profiles of oral antidiabetic agents. *Drug Saf* 1994; 11: 223–41.
137. Deutschmann R, Moser G, Mertes G. Favourable quality of life for acarbose trated patients with type II diabetes when compared with other treatments. *Diabetes* 1997; 46 (suppl 1): 292A.
138. Rosak C, Haupt E, Walter T, Werner J. The effect of combination treatment with acarbose and glibenclamide on postprandial glucose and insulin profiles: additive blood glucose lowering effect and decreased hypoglycaemia. *Diabetes Nutr Metab* 2002; 15: 143–51.
139. Weaver GA, Tangel CT, Krause JA, et al. Biomarkers of human colonic cell growth are influenced differently by a history of colonic neoplasia and the consumption of acarbose. *J Nutr* 2000; 130: 2718–25.
140. Wolever TM, Chiasson JL. Acarbose raises serum butyrate in human subjects with impaired glucose tolerance. *Br J Nutr* 2000; 84: 57–61.
141. Gentille S, Turco S, Gurino G, et al. Aminotransferas activity and acarbose treatment in patients with type 2 diabetes. *Diabetes Care* 1999; 22: 1217–8.
142. Gentile S, Turco S, Guarino G, et al. Effect of treatment with acarbose and insulin in patients with non-insulin-dependent diabetes mellitus associated with non-alcoholic liver cirrhosis. *Diabetes Obes Metab* 2001; 3: 33–40.
143. Carrascosa M, Pascual F, Aresti S. Acarbose-induced acute severe hepatotoxicity. *Lancet* 1997; 349: 698–9.
144. Andrade RJ, Lucena MI, Rodriguez-Mendizabal M. Hepatic injury caused by acarbose. *Ann Intern Med* 1996; 124: 931.
145. Nishii Y, Aizawa T, Hashizume K. Ileus: a rare side effect of acarbose [letter]. *Diabetes Care* 1996; 19: 1033.
146. Odawara M, Bannai C, Saitoh T, Kawakami Y, Yamashita K. Potentially lethal ileus associated with acarbose treatment for NIDDM. *Diabetes Care* 1997; 20: 1210–1.
147. Magner J, Amatruda JM, Alpha-glucosidase inhibitors in the treatment of diabetes. In Olefsky JM, Taylor SI, Olefsky JM (eds), *Diabetes Mellitus: A Fundamental and Clinical Text*. Phlidelphia, PA: Lippincott Williams and Wilkins, 2000; pp 797–803.

50

Combination Therapy in Type 2 Diabetes

Mandeep Bajaj and Ralph A. DeFronzo

University of Texas Health Science Center at San Antonio, San Antonio, TX, USA

INTRODUCTION

In the United States, approximately 15.6 million persons have type 2 diabetes mellitus, and about 13.4 million have impaired fasting glucose. Over the last decade alone there has been a striking 33% increase in the prevalence of type 2 diabetes [2], which is largely attributed to the epidemic of obesity [3]. Worldwide, there are approximately 150 million type 2 diabetic individuals and it has been estimated that the number will increase to 300 million by the year 2025 [4]. Decreased physical activity, increasing obesity, and changes in food consumption have been implicated in this epidemic [3, 5].

Patients with diabetes experience significant morbidity and mortality from microvascular (retinopathy, nephropathy, and neuropathy) and macrovascular (heart attacks, stroke, and peripheral vascular disease) complications. Proliferative retinopathy, macular edema, or both occur in 40–50% of patients with type 2 diabetes, and diabetes is the leading cause of blindness in the United States [6]. The prevalence of renal disease varies considerably among ethnic populations, ranging from a low of 5–10% in Caucasians to 50% in Native Americans [7]. Diabetes is the leading cause of end-stage renal failure, accounting for one of every three patients who enter dialysis or transplantation programs [7]. Peripheral and autonomic neuropathy occur in 50–60% of patients with type 2 diabetes [8]. Heart attacks and stroke occur two to four times more frequently in persons with diabetes than in those without the disease [9, 10]. The cost of treating diabetes and associated microvascular and macrovascular complications exceeds $100 billion per year [11].

To provide a rational approach to therapy, we will briefly review the pathogenesis of type 2 diabetes mellitus and then consider the therapeutic agents that presently are available to reduce the hemoglobin A_{1c}(HbA_{1c}) to levels that have been shown to prevent/delay/minimize the development of microvascular complications [12–14]. We will focus on oral agents, as monotherapy and in combination with each other and with insulin, since insulin therapy is discussed in detail in Chapter 53. Indications for insulin therapy are discussed briefly, but the major emphasis is on therapy with oral agents, alone and in combination.

PATHOGENESIS OF TYPE 2 DIABETES MELLITUS

The appropriate treatment of any disease is based on an understanding of its pathophysiology [15–18]. The mechanisms responsible for impaired glucose homeostasis in type 2 diabetes mellitus (Figure 1) are discussed briefly to provide the foundation for discussion of currently available oral agents, including their mechanism of action, efficacy, and side effects.

After ingestion of glucose, maintenance of normal glucose tolerance depends on three events that must occur in a tightly coordinated fashion: (1) stimulation of insulin secretion; (2) insulin-mediated suppression of endogenous (primarily hepatic) glucose production by the resultant hyperinsulinemia; and (3) insulin-mediated stimulation of glucose uptake by peripheral tissues, primarily muscle [15–17]. Hyperglycemia also has its own independent effect to suppress hepatic glucose production and to enhance muscle glucose uptake, but these effects are modest compared to those of insulin [19].

In type 2 diabetic patients with established fasting hyperglycemia, the rate of basal hepatic glucose production is excessive, despite plasma insulin concentrations that are increased twofold to fourfold [20] (Figure 1). These

International Textbook of Diabetes Mellitus, Third Edition. Edited by R. A. DeFronzo, E. Ferrannini, H. Keen, and P. Zimmet.
 ISBN: 0-471-48655-8.

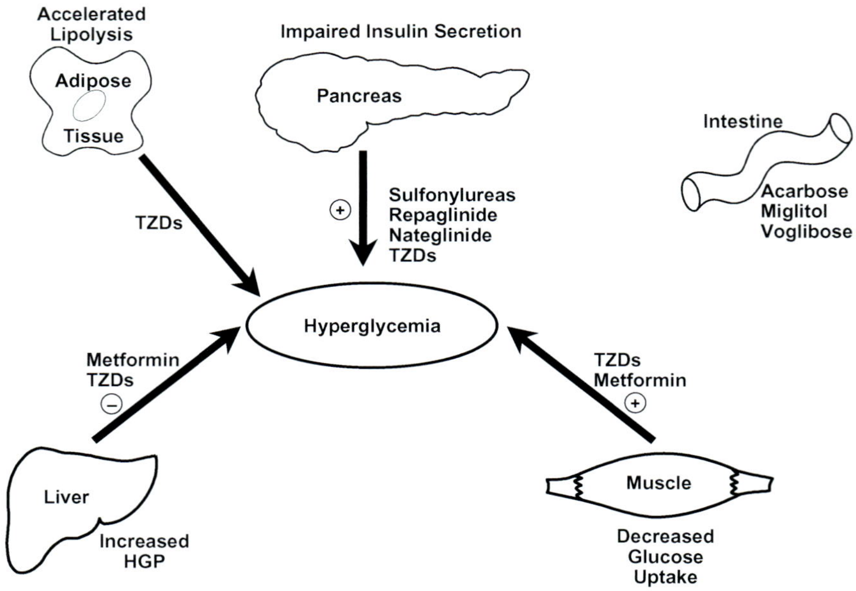

Figure 1 Pathogenesis of type 2 diabetes diabetes mellitus. Sites of action of oral agents are indicated. Acarbose, miglitol, and voglibose do not inhibit any specific pathogenic disturbance that is present in type 2 diabetes mellitus. Negative sign indicates inhibition; positive sign indicates stimulation. HGP = hepatic glucose production; TZDs = thiazolidinediones

findings provide unequivocal evidence for hepatic resistance to insulin, and this is substantiated by an impaired ability of insulin to suppress hepatic glucose output [21]. Accelerated gluconeogenesis is the major abnormality responsible for the increased rate of basal hepatic glucose production [22, 23]. The increased rate of basal hepatic glucose production is closely correlated with the increase in fasting plasma glucose level [20–23]. Because the fasting plasma glucose concentration is the major determinant of the mean daylong blood glucose level (which clinically is reflected by the HbA_{1c} value), it follows that agents that reduce the elevated basal rate of hepatic glucose production will be especially effective in improving glycemic control (Figure 1).

Muscle tissue in patients with type 2 diabetes also is resistant to insulin [15–17, 21, 24] (Figure 1). Defects in insulin receptor function, insulin receptor-signal transduction pathway, glucose transport and phosphorylation, glycogen synthesis, and glucose oxidation contribute to muscle insulin resistance [15–17]. In response to a meal, the ability of endogenously secreted insulin to augment muscle glucose uptake and to suppress hepatic glucose production is markedly impaired [25, 26], and muscle insulin resistance and impaired suppression of hepatic glucose production contribute approximately equally to the excessive postprandial increase in the plasma glucose level [26, 27]. It follows that drugs that improve muscle insulin sensitivity will be effective in decreasing the excessive increase in plasma glucose level after carbohydrate ingestion (Figure 1).

From a quantitative standpoint, however, in type 2 diabetic patients with established fasting hyperglycemia [glucose level > 7.8 mmol/l (>140 mg/dl)], the excessive increase in the plasma glucose level above baseline after a meal plays a much smaller role in determining the mean daylong plasma glucose concentration than does the elevated fasting plasma glucose level. This is clear from studies that have examined the mean daylong glycemic excursions in diabetic patients who consume typical mixed meals. For example, in a study by Jeppesen and colleagues [28], the fasting glucose level in type 2 diabetic patients was 10.6 mmol/l (190 mg/dl), indicating an increment of 5.6 mmol/l ($\Delta = 100$ mg/dl) in basal glucose level above that in nondiabetic controls [5 mmol/l (90 mg/dl)]. This increase above baseline was present 24 h/day, giving a hyperglycemic index of 2400 (100 mg/dl × 24 h). After each of three daily meals, the increase in plasma glucose concentration was greater by ~1.9 mmol/l (35 mg/dl) in diabetic patients than in controls but returned to the baseline value by 4–6 h. The hyperglycemic index accounted for by the excessive increase in plasma glucose level during all three meals is 525 (35 mg/dl × 3 meals × 5 h). Thus, the contribution of postprandial hyperglycemia to daylong hyperglycemia is only 22% (525/2400).

Impaired insulin secretion also plays a major role in the pathogenesis of glucose intolerance in patients with type 2 diabetes [29–32]. Although debate still continues about which defect—insulin resistance or impaired insulin secretion—initiates the cascade of events leading to overt diabetes mellitus, essentially all patients who have type 2 diabetes with elevated fasting plasma glucose levels have a defect in insulin secretion [29–34]. In diabetic patients with mild fasting hyperglycemia [glucose level < 7.8 mmol/l (<140 mg/dl)], plasma insulin levels during an oral glucose tolerance test (OGTT) or a mixed meal usually are elevated in absolute terms [16, 35]. However, relative to the severity of insulin resistance and prevailing hyperglycemia, even these elevated plasma insulin levels are deficient [16, 31, 32, 35]. As the fasting plasma glucose level increases to more than 7.8 mmol/l (>140 mg/dl), insulin secretion decreases progressively, and essentially all diabetic patients with a fasting plasma glucose level that exceeds 8.9–10 mmol/l (160–180 mg/dl) have a plasma insulin response that is deficient in absolute terms [16, 35]. It follows, therefore, that drugs that improve insulin secretion will be effective in treating type 2 diabetes as β-cell failure ensues and plasma glucose levels exceed 160–180 mg/dl (Figure 1).

More recently, the important contribution of adipocyte insulin resistance to the disturbance in glucose tolerance has become well established [36]. Fat cells are severely resistant to the antilipolytic effect of insulin [20] and patients with type 2 diabetes are characterized by daylong elevation in fasting and postprandial plasma free fatty acid (FFA) levels [37]. Elevated plasma FFA levels have been shown to induce insulin resistance in muscle [38, 39], to impair the suppression of hepatic glucose production [40, 41] and to inhibit insulin secretion [42, 43]. Thus, the adipocyte must be added to the triumvirate [16] to form the dysharmonious quartet (Figure 1).

In summary, patients with type 2 diabetes mellitus are characterized by defects in both insulin secretion and insulin action. Several recent extensive reviews [15, 17] provide more detailed discussion about the pathogenesis of type 2 diabetes mellitus at the whole body, organ, cellular, and molecular levels.

GLYCEMIC CONTROL AND COMPLICATIONS

The Diabetes Control and Complications Trial (DCCT) [44] established that, in type 1 diabetes mellitus, the risk for microvascular complications could be reduced by maintaining near-normal blood glucose levels with intensive insulin therapy. No glycemic threshold for the development of long-term microvascular complications was observed in the DCCT [45]. Microvascular complications decreased markedly as the HbA_{1c} decreased from 11–12% to 8% and continued to decrease as the HbA_{1c} declined from 8.0% to 6.0% [46]. On average a 1% decrement in HbA_{1c} was associated with a 30–35% reduction in diabetic retinopathy, nephropathy, and neuropathy. A similar decrease in microvascular complications was observed in Japanese patients with type 2 diabetes who were intensively treated with insulin [47].

More definitive information on the relationship between improved glycemic control and prevention of microvascular complications has been provided by the United Kingdom Prospective Diabetes Study (UKPDS) [48, 49]. In the main randomization group of the UKPDS [28], after a dietary run-in period of 3 months, 3867 patients with newly diagnosed type 2 diabetes were randomly assigned to intensive therapy with a sulfonylurea or insulin ($n = 2729$) or to conventional diet therapy ($n = 1138$). In the intensively treated group, the aim was to achieve a fasting plasma glucose level less than 6 mmol/l (108 mg/dl). In the sulfonylurea group, patients were switched to insulin therapy or metformin was added if the therapeutic goal was not achieved after maximum titration of the drug dose. In patients assigned to insulin treatment in whom the therapeutic goal was not met, the dose of ultralente insulin was increased progressively and regular insulin was added. In patients assigned to conventional diet treatment, the aim was to maintain a fasting plasma glucose level less than 15 mmol/l (270 mg/dl) without symptoms. If the fasting plasma glucose level exceeded 15 mmol/l (270 mg/dl) or symptoms occurred, patients were randomly assigned to receive therapy with a sulfonylurea or insulin. The median follow-up was 10.0 years, and during this period a difference of 0.9% (7.0% compared with 7.9%; $P < 0.001$) in HbA_{1c} value was maintained between the group assigned to intensive therapy and the group assigned to conventional therapy (Figure 2). This difference was associated with a 25% risk reduction ($P = 0.009$) in combined microvascular endpoints (eye, kidney, and nerve) compared with the conventionally treated group. No difference in combined macrovascular endpoints was observed between the two groups, although there was a tendency toward fewer myocardial infarctions in the group assigned to intensive therapy.

In addition to the 2729 patients with type 2 diabetes assigned to intensive therapy and the 1138 patients assigned to conventional therapy, 342 overweight patients were randomly assigned to intensive treatment with metformin [49]. These 342 patients were compared with 411 overweight diabetic patients receiving conventional therapy and with 951 overweight diabetic patients receiving intensive therapy (of whom 542 were receiving sulfonylureas and 409 were receiving insulin). The median follow-up in this group was 10.7 years and during this time a difference of 0.6% (7.4% compared with 8.0%; $P < 0.001$) in the HbA_{1c} value was maintained between the group assigned to metformin therapy and the group assigned to conventional therapy. The magnitude of reduction (29%) in the risk for microvascular complications in the metformin-treated group was similar to that in patients treated intensively with insulin or sulfonylureas (Figure 2). Patients assigned to intensive blood glucose control with metformin had a 32% lower risk ($P = 0.002$) for any diabetes-related endpoint, a 36% lower risk ($P = 0.021$)

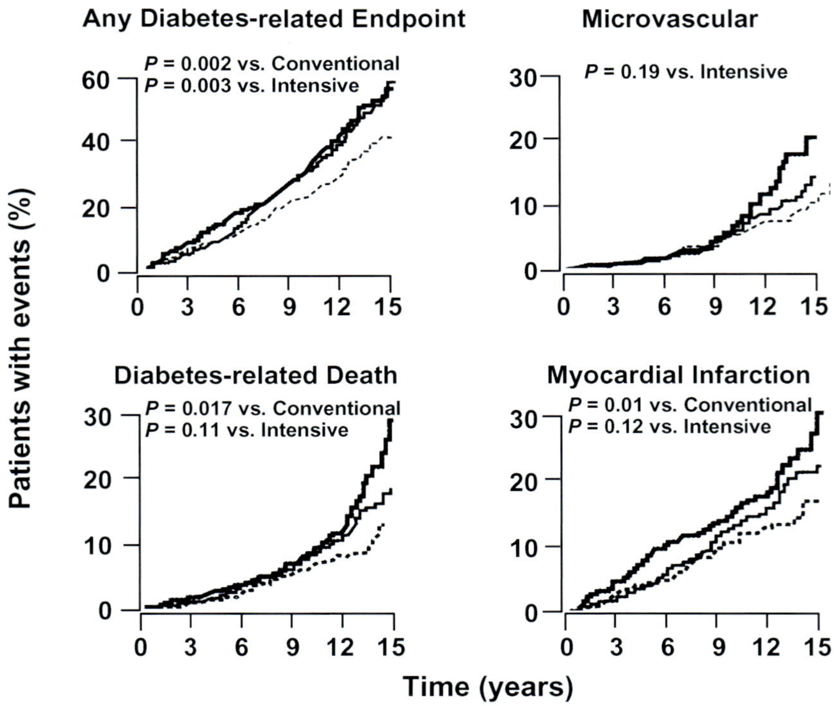

Figure 2 Effect of conventional treatment with diet (heavy bold line) versus intensive treatment with sulfonylureas or insulin (solid thin line) and metformin (interrupted line) on any diabetes-related endpoint (upper left), microvascular complications (upper right), diabetes-related death (lower left), and myocardial infarction (bottom right). *P* values represent differences between metformin and other therapies [48, 49]

for death from any cause, a 42% reduction in diabetes-related death ($P = 0.11$), a 39% lower risk ($P = 0.010$) for myocardial infarction, and a 41% lower risk ($P = 0.032$) for stroke compared with patients who received conventional treatment (Figure 2). The risk reduction for any diabetes-related endpoint ($P = 0.003$) and death from any cause ($P = 0.021$) in the metformin group was significantly greater than that in the group assigned to intensive therapy with insulin or sulfonylureas (Figure 2). Since the reduction in HbA_{1c} was similar in the metformin-treated ($\Delta = 0.6\%$) and sulfonylurea/insulin-treated ($\Delta = 0.9\%$) groups, the marked reduction in cardiovascular events and death cannot be related to better glycemic control (Figure 2). It is most likely that metformin's beneficial effect to prevent atherosclerotic cardiovascular events is related to the beneficial effects of biguanides to improve insulin sensitivity [50] and to improve many of the components of the insulin resistance syndrome [51]. This syndrome has also been referred to as the *metabolic syndrome*, *dysmetabolic syndrome*, or *syndrome X*.

In summary, the results of the UKPDS demonstrated that (1) the development of microvascular complications was similarly reduced in patients with type 2 diabetes treated with sulfonylureas, insulin, or metformin; (2) there was no threshold for the reduction in HbA_{1c} and the development of microvascular complications; (3) in patients with type 2 diabetes assigned to intensive therapy with sulfonylureas or insulin, the incidence of macrovascular complications was not decreased compared with the group assigned to conventional therapy; and (4) a decrease in macrovascular complications was seen only in patients with type 2 diabetes assigned to intensive therapy with metformin. Thus, the findings of the UKPDS are consistent with those of the DCCT [44] and the study by Ohkubo and associates [47].

On the basis of the results reviewed above, it seems most prudent to reduce blood glucose levels in patients with type 2 diabetes to or as close to normal as possible while avoiding symptomatic hypoglycemia. Consistent with this conclusion both the European Association for the Study of Diabetes (EASD) [13] and the American Association of Clinical Endocrinologists (AACE) [14] have adapted an HbA_{1c} goal of $\leq 6.5\%$ and the American Diabetes Association (ADA) has lowered their goal from 8% [52] to 7.0% [12] (Table 1). It is the authors' personal opinion that the HbA_{1c} should be reduced to $<6.5\%$ and ideally to $<6.0\%$. Moreover, since the UKPDS showed a very weak relationship between glycemic control and macrovascular complications, yet metformin, an insulin-sensitizing agent [50], markedly reduced the number of cardiovascular events and death, we believe that pharmacologic therapy should be initiated with an oral agent that

Table 1 2003 ADA recommendations for glycemic control in type 2 diabetes

	Goal
A_{1C}	<7%
Preprandial plasma glucose	90–130 mg/dl
Peak postprandial plasma glucose	<180 mg/dl

improves insulin resistance, preferably metformin or alternatively with a thiazolidinedione, in diabetic patients who cannot tolerate metformin (because of gastrointestinal side effects) or in whom metformin is contraindicated (individuals with impaired renal function). However, it is important to recognize that effective control of hyperglycemia will require the combined use of diet, exercise, oral agents (metformin, thiazolidinediones, sulfonylureas, meglitinides, α-glucosidase inhibitors), and insulin.

DIAGNOSTIC CRITERIA AND THERAPEUTIC GOALS

On the basis of results from long-term prospective epidemiologic studies showing that 10–15% of persons with a fasting plasma glucose level of 7 mmol/l (126 mg/dl) or more develop diabetic retinopathy within 10 years of follow-up, an expert committee convened by the ADA recommended that diabetes be diagnosed when the fasting plasma glucose level is 7 mmol/l or more (126 mg/dl) [53] or the 2-h plasma glucose concentration is ≥11.1 mmol/l (200 mg/dl) during an OGTT [54]. A fasting plasma glucose concentration of 126 mg/dl is approximately equivalent to a 2-h plasma glucose concentration (during the OGTT) of 200 mg/dl. These values correspond to an HbA_{1c} value of about 6.9% [53]. Similar criteria have been adopted by the World Health Organization [54]. The ADA also accepts a random plasma glucose level of ≥11 mmol/l (200 mg/dl) with symptoms to establish the diagnosis of type 2 diabetes mellitus. The authors do not advocate the use of this later criteria in adults, but this later criteria is helpful in pediatric patients in whom the OGTT may be difficult to perform. To definitively establish the diagnosis, one of the three previous diagnostic criteria (preferably the fasting plasma glucose concentration or the 2-h plasma glucose concentration during the OGTT) must be repeated.

TREATMENT STRATEGY

In developing a treatment strategy for patients with type 2 diabetes, it must be remembered that glucose intolerance occurs not in isolation but as part of a complex metabolic–cardiovascular syndrome that includes dyslipidemia, hypertension, obesity, clotting abnormalities, endothelial dysfunction, microalbuminuria, and accelerated atherosclerosis [45, 51, 55–57], although not every one of these disorders occurs in every diabetic patient. Although hyperglycemia has been implicated as a risk factor for coronary artery disease [58], it is a relatively weak cardiovascular risk factor [59] and dyslipidemia far outweighs all other risk factors [60]. Therefore, treatment of concomitant lipid abnormalities, hypertension, and other known risk factors for coronary artery disease is essential [9, 51, 60]. Long-term prospective studies have shown that treatment of hypertension [61] and dyslipidemia [62] reduces cardiac events in patients with type 2 diabetes. The UKPDS [63] showed that improved control of blood pressure reduced not only macrovascular complications (heart attacks, strokes, and death) but also the risk for microvascular endpoints by 37% ($P = 0.009$). Although the incidence of hypercholesterolemia in patients with type 2 diabetes is not any greater than the incidence in the general population, when the low-density lipoprotein cholesterol (LDL-cholesterol) is elevated, it represents a major risk factor and reduction of the LDL-cholesterol to ≤100 mg/dl has been shown to dramatically reduce the incidence of heart attacks [64]. Elevated plasma triglyceride and reduced plasma high-density lipoprotein cholesterol (HDL-cholesterol) also are major risk factors for cardiovascular disease and improvement in these circulating lipids has been shown to reduce cardiovascular events [65]. The recent Steno study [66] has demonstrated that a multiple interventional approach to reduce glycemia and to treat all cardiovascular risk factors reduced the incidence of macrovascular and microvascular complications by about 50% in type 2 diabetic patients. Given the preceding considerations, it is especially important that pharmacologic therapy does not aggravate associated cardiovascular risk factors and, preferably, leads to their improvement. Because obesity and physical inactivity are risk factors for coronary artery disease [67] as well as for diabetes [3], the need for weight loss and exercise must be stressed when diabetes is initially diagnosed and must be reinforced throughout the natural history of the disease. Many excellent reviews on diet and exercise have been published [68, 69]. If diet and exercise fail to achieve the desired level of glycemic control, pharmacologic intervention is indicated.

The UKPDS showed that type 2 diabetes mellitus is a progressive disorder [48, 49] (Figure 2). Although it was hoped that treatment with sulfonylureas, metformin, and/or insulin would halt the progressive deterioration of glycemic control, this has not turned out to be the case. After an initial and similar decrease in HbA_{1c} with metformin, sulfonylureas, or insulin, the rate of increase in HbA_{1c} was identical to that in the group treated with diet therapy. These results indicate that once overt fasting hyperglycemia has developed, the decline in glycemic control is relentless. What remains to be determined is the precise level of fasting hyperglycemia and duration of diabetes at which β-cell failure is unevitable. In the UKPDS, the progressive rise in HbA_{1c} in all treatment groups was related to the decline in β-cell function [48]. Numerous prospective and cross-sectional studies have demonstrated that insulin resistance is established early in the natural history of type 2 diabetes and that the progressive rise in mean daylong blood glucose level and HbA_{1c} is related to the deterioration in β-cell function [16, 70–72]. The results of the University Group Diabetes Program study [73, 74] also documented the progressive nature of type 2 diabetes mellitus. These important observations emphasize the need for constant reassessment of the diabetic patient and appropriate adjustment of the therapeutic regimen in order to maintain the desired level of glycemic control.

From these observations about the natural history of type 2 diabetes mellitus, the following treatment strategy can be proposed for diabetic patients whose disease is inadequately controlled with diet and exercise (Figure 3):

(1) Initiate pharmacologic therapy with an oral agent, preferably an insulin sensitizer. It is important that the oral agent which is chosen to initiate therapy has the potential to reduce HbA_{1c} to ≤6.5–7.0%. If not, initiation of therapy with two oral agents should be considered. If the blood glucose level is especially high [>280–300 mg/dl (15.6–16.7 mM)] and the patient is symptomatic, insulin should be considered as first-line therapy.

(2) Quickly increase the dose of oral agent or insulin until adequate glycemic control is achieved. We recommend that patients be seen or contacted via telephone at 1- to 2-week intervals or more frequently during this titration phase. Metformin and thiazolidinediones can be titrated every 2 weeks, sulfonylureas/meglitinides every week, and thiazolidinediones every 2–3 weeks. Insulin can be titrated every 3–5 days.

(3) In diabetic patients treated with an oral agent, the physician should choose a drug whose glucose-lowering potency can achieve the desired level of glycemic control (HbA_{1c} ≤6.5–7%) when used as monotherapy. Because most patients with type 2 diabetes are overweight and have associated cardiovascular risk factors, drugs that promote weight loss or are weight neutral (metformin) and improve cardiovascular risk factors are preferred.

(4) In diabetic patients whose disease is inadequately controlled with a single oral agent, we favor addition of a second oral agent with rapid dose titration until the desired level of glycemic control is achieved or the maximum dose is reached. Because multiple oral agents currently are available, the combination of a single oral agent with bedtime long-acting insulin has become uncommon.

(5) In diabetic patients in whom glycemic control is not achieved with two oral agents, several options are available: (1) addition of a third oral agent; (2) addition of bedtime insulin to oral agent therapy; if this option is chosen, we prefer to stop the sulfonylurea (if the patient is on one) and continue the insulin sensitizer [75]; (3) switching the patient to a mixed-split insulin regimen with or without an insulin sensitizer.

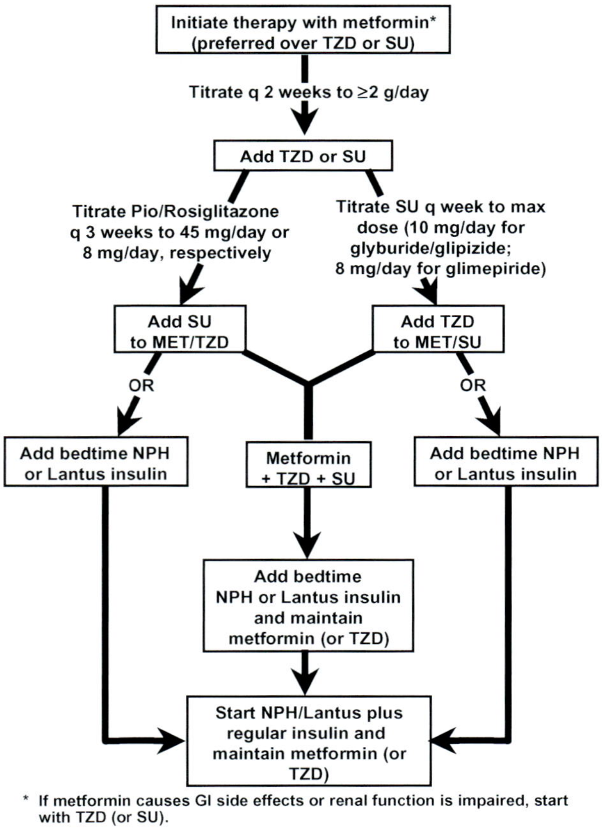

Figure 3 Pharmacologic algorithm for the treatment of type 2 diabetic patients who are inadequately controlled with diet and exercise

It is important to recognize that, ultimately, most patients with type 2 diabetes will require treatment with insulin, either alone or in combination with an oral agent.

INSULIN THERAPY

Although the primary focus of this review is combination therapy with oral agents, comment about insulin is indicated because some diabetologists prefer to initiate therapy with insulin in patients with newly diagnosed type 2 diabetes. Several comprehensive reviews of insulin therapy in type 2 diabetes mellitus have been published [76, 77]. Numerous studies have shown that excellent glycemic control can be obtained with intensive insulin therapy in patients with type 2 diabetes [78, 79]. An educated, compliant patient with an experienced physician can achieve excellent glycemic control with insulin therapy. However, most studies of intensive insulin therapy have been carried out in academic settings, using strict research protocols with specialty teams devoted to patient care. In such settings, one can expect decreases of about 2–3 percentage points in HbA_{1c} value. However, most primary care physicians do not have specialized training in insulin use and management of its complications, do not have sufficient time to follow up patients at frequent intervals to ensure appropriate adjustment of the insulin dose, and do not have diabetes specialty teams to assist them. Therefore, institution of intensive insulin therapy in the community setting by primary care physicians can be difficult.

Hayward and coworkers [80] examined insulin therapy prescribed by general practice physicians in a large staff-model health maintenance organization. In 1738 insulin-treated patients with type 2 diabetes, the mean decrease in HbA_{1c} value was 0.9%, and 60% of patients had an HbA_{1c} value that exceeded 8.0% at 2 years. In a parallel cohort, 43% of patients with type 2 diabetes who were taking sulfonylureas had an HbA_{1c} value that exceeded 8.0%. Although one can raise criticisms about this study [47], the results do not indicate any superiority of insulin over sulfonylureas or vice versa in the general practice setting. The UKPDS [48, 49] also failed to show any advantage of insulin over oral agents or vice versa (Figure 2). The most commonly used insulin regimen in general practice is a single dose of long-acting insulin in the morning. Dosages in excess of 80 U/day are rarely given [81]. Because most patients with type 2 diabetes require an insulin dosage of at least 80–100 U/day (usually well in excess of 100 U/day if the patient is obese) and a multiple, split-dose regimen [78, 79], it is not surprising that blood glucose levels are inadequately controlled in most of these patients [80].

Weight gain and hypoglycemia are common side effects of insulin therapy [48, 49, 79, 82–84]. Weight gain results from increased truncal fat [83] and is closely related to the mean daylong plasma insulin level and daily insulin dose [79]. In the UKPDS, insulin-treated obese patients with type 2 diabetes gained 4.0 kg more after 10 years than did patients assigned to diet therapy ($P < 0.001$) [48]. Patients assigned to sulfonylurea therapy (chlorpropamide or glibenclamide) gained 2.2 kg more, while those assigned to metformin therapy gained the same weight as did patients assigned to diet therapy [48, 49]. More pronounced weight gain has been observed in other studies where more intensive insulin therapy had been used to bring about a normalization or near-normalization of the blood glucose profile. Because obesity is a known cause of insulin resistance [85, 86] and represents an independent risk factor for coronary artery disease, hypertension, and dyslipidemia [5, 87], weight gain is an undesirable side effect of insulin therapy. Moreover, despite normalization of the blood glucose level, intensive insulin therapy does not improve insulin resistance [79].

Hypoglycemia is another potential side effect of insulin therapy in patients with type 2 diabetes [48, 49, 79, 82–84]. In the UKPDS [48, 49], after 10 years, percentages of diabetic patients with one or more major (requiring third-party assistance or hospitalization) hypoglycemic episodes were 0.5% in the sulfonylurea group, 2.3% in the insulin group ($P < 0.001$ for insulin compared with all other groups), 0% in the metformin group, and 0.1% in the diet group. The corresponding rates for any hypoglycemic reaction were 14% in the sulfonylurea group, 36% in the insulin group, 4% in the metformin group, and 1% in the diet group.

The authors of the 6-year summary of the UKPDS [84] stated that "In patients with primary diet failure, it may not be advantageous to proceed directly to insulin therapy. It is reasonable to initiate therapy with oral agents and proceed to insulin if the goal is not achieved." The 10-year summary of the UKPDS [49] concluded that metformin is an appropriate first-line therapy in overweight diabetic patients because, compared with insulin or sulfonylurea treatment, metformin therapy decreased the risk for both diabetes-related microvascular and macrovascular endpoints and resulted in less weight gain and fewer hypoglycemic attacks.

On the basis of the preceding discussion, we recommend initiating pharmacologic therapy with an oral agent (preferably metformin) in patients with newly diagnosed type 2 diabetes. However, insulin is indicated as initial therapy in specific patients, as follows:

(1) Any patient who has type 2 diabetes with a markedly elevated fasting plasma glucose level [>15.6–16.7 mmol/l (>280–300 mg/dl)], and ketonuria or ketonemia.
(2) Symptomatic patients (polyuria, polydipsia, nocturia, weight loss) who have type 2 diabetes with a markedly elevated fasting plasma glucose level [>15.6–16.7 mmol/l (>280–300 mg/dl)]. After 6–8 weeks of good glycemic control, these patients can be switched to an oral agent, or they can be continued on insulin therapy. A benefit of intensive insulin therapy with tight glycemic control is the reversal of glucose toxicity [88]. This will improve both insulin sensitivity and insulin secretion [88] and will enhance the subsequent response to oral agent therapy [89, 90].
(3) Any patient with type 2 diabetes who, after discussing the options with the primary care physician, wishes to receive insulin as initial therapy.
(4) Women with gestational diabetes mellitus whose disease is not controlled with diet alone. All oral agents are contraindicated during pregnancy.

Table 2 Comparison of metformin, thiazolidinediones, sulfonylureas, repaglinide, nateglinide, and acarbose when used as monotherapy

	Metformin	Rosiglitazone plus pioglitazone	Sulfonylureas	Repaglinide plus nateglinide	Acarbose
Mechanism of action	↓HGP; ↑muscle insulin sensitivity	↓HGP; ↑muscle insulin sensitivity	↑Insulin secretion	↑Insulin secretion	↓GI absorption
Decrease in FPG (mg/dl)	60–70	45–55	60–70	20–30	20–30
Decrease in HbA_{1c}	1.5–2.0	1.3–1.5	1.5–2.0	0.8–1.0	0.6–1.0
Triglycerides	↓↓	0,↓*	0	0	0
HDL-cholesterol	sl ↑	↑	0	0	0
LDL-cholesterol	sl ↓	0,↑†	0	0	0
Body weight	↓	↑	↑	sl↑	0
Plasma insulin	↓	↓	↑	↑	0
Adverse events	GI disturbances; lactic acidosis‡	Anemia, edema; abnormal LFTs§	Hypoglycemia	Hypoglycemia	GI disturbances

Note. HGP = hepatic glucose production; GI = gastrointestinal; FPG = fasting plasma glucose; HDL = high-density lipoprotein; LDL = low-density lipoprotein; LFTs = liver function tests.

*Only pioglitazone decreases plasma triglycerides; rosiglitazone has no consistent effect on plasma triglycerides.

†No consistent change in LDL-cholesterol is observed with pioglitazone; rosiglitazone often is associated with an increase in LDL-cholesterol.

‡The incidence of lactic acidosis is 3 cases per 100 000 patient-treatment years.

§Unequivocal cases of hepatotoxicity with rosiglitazone and pioglitazone are extremely rare; abnormal LFTs usually improve with thiazolidinedione therapy.

TREATMENT ALGORITHM FOR INITIATION OF ORAL THERAPY

In patients with newly diagnosed type 2 diabetes in whom insulin therapy is not indicated, we recommend that pharmacologic therapy with metformin, a thiazolodinedione, or a sulfonylurea be initiated as monotherapy, as long as no contraindications are present (Figure 3). This view, which is based on proven efficacy, safety, and long-term clinical experience with oral agents, is shared by other leading authorities on diabetes [48, 49, 84, 91, 92], is the approach used in the UKPDS [48, 49, 92], and is consistent with the guidelines of the ADA [93]. The meglitinides (repaglinide and nateglinide) [94, 95] and the α-glucosidase inhibitors [96] are less effective than metformin/thiazolidinediones/sulfonylureas in reducing the HbA_{1c} level and are less commonly used, at least in the United States, to initiate therapy.

When used as monotherapy, metformin, thiazolidinediones, and sulfonylureas are equally effective in decreasing plasma glucose levels [97, 98], and are more potent than other available oral agents (Table 2). Because metformin promotes weight loss and reduces lipid levels, it is preferred in overweight patients with type 2 diabetes and dyslipidemia. In lean patients with type 2 diabetes, therapy can be initiated with metformin, a thiazolidnedione, or a sulfonylurea. These recommendations are consistent with the findings of the UKPDS [48, 49]. Because insulin resistance with its accompanying metabolic–cardiovascular disorders is a characteristic feature of type 2 diabetes [45, 51, 55], whether diabetic individuals are lean or obese [16, 17], we prefer to initiate therapy with an insulin sensitizer—metformin—or a thiazolidinedione. The dose of the oral agent should be increased rapidly until the therapeutic goal [fasting plasma glucose level < 6.1 mmol/l (<110 mg/dl) and HbA_{1c} value $< 7\%$] is achieved or the maximum dose is reached. Diet and exercise must be emphasized even after pharmacologic therapy has begun.

If monotherapy with metformin, a thiazolidinedione, or a sulfonylurea fails to achieve the desired level of glycemic control, a second oral agent should be added, with dose escalation over 1–3 weeks to the maximum (Figure 3). Some diabetologists choose to initiate therapy with a combination of two oral agents. This approach may be necessary in patients with HbA_{1c} >9.0–9.5%, as monotherapy often fails to achieve the desired level of glycemic control (HbA_{1c} <7.0%). In the United States and Europe a number of oral agents combination tablets are available, including Metaglip (glipizide plus metformin) [99], Glucovance (glyburide plus metformin) [100], and Advandamet (rosiglitazone plus metformin) [101]. If combination therapy with two oral agents does not achieve the desired goal, three options are available: (1) add a third oral agent; (2) add bedtime insulin while maintaining therapy with one or both oral agents; and (3) switch the patient to a mixed-split (short-acting plus long-acting insulin given in two to four daily injections) insulin regimen (Figure 3). It is important to individualize therapy on the basis of patient and physician preferences.

Specific insulin regimens to treat type 2 diabetes are not discussed here. The reader is referred to several excellent reviews of this topic [76, 77] and to Chapter 53.

ORAL AGENTS

In the United States and Europe, five classes of oral agents are approved for the treatment of type 2 diabetes mellitus, and several new oral antidiabetic medications are being tested in humans. Oral agent therapy is indicated in any patient with type 2 diabetes in whom diet and exercise fail to achieve acceptable glycemic control [12]. In subsequent sections, we examine the mechanism of action, hypoglycemic efficacy, other beneficial effects, dosing schedule, cost, and safety of currently available antidiabetic drugs when used as monotherapy. This will be followed by a review of the use of these agents in combination with each other and with insulin.

Sulfonylureas

Mechanism of Action

Sulfonylureas have been the mainstay of antidiabetic therapy for many years. Their primary mechanism of action is enhancement of insulin secretion (Table 2, Figure 1). They initiate their action by binding to a specific sulfonylurea receptor (SUR) on pancreatic β-cells [102]. This closes a potassium-dependent adenosine triphosphate channel, leading to decreased potassium influx and depolarization of the β-cell membrane. This results in increased calcium flux into the β-cell, activating a cytoskeletal system that causes translocation of secretory granules to the cell surface and extrusion of insulin through exocytosis [103]. Insulin released by the pancreas enters the portal vein, and the resultant portal hyperinsulinemia suppresses the elevated basal rate of hepatic glucose production. Simonson [104] and Best [105] and their colleagues were the first to demonstrate that the decrease in fasting plasma glucose level with sulfonylurea therapy was closely related to inhibition of basal hepatic glucose production. In addition, the elevated arterial insulin concentration enhances muscle glucose uptake, leading to a reduction in postmeal plasma glucose levels [104, 105]. Although a direct effect of sulfonylureas to enhance tissue sensitivity to insulin has been suggested [106], most investigators believe that the small improvement in insulin action observed during sulfonylurea treatment [104, 105] is explained by the improvement in glucose toxicity [88].

Efficacy

The hypoglycemic potency of sulfonylureas (as well as all other oral hypoglycemic agents) is directly related to the starting fasting plasma glucose level [107, 108]. The higher the fasting plasma glucose level, the greater is its decrease from baseline. In the United States, the mean HbA_{1c} value in diabetic patients is approximately 8.5–9.0%, corresponding to a fasting plasma glucose level of approximately 10.0 mmol/l (~180 mg/dl) [109, 110]. This value is similar to that reported in recent large clinical trials of treatment of patients with type 2 diabetes with sulfonylureas [107, 108] and other oral agents [97, 111]. In such patients, one can expect the fasting plasma glucose level to decrease by 3.3–3.9 mmol/l (60–70 mg/dl) and the HbA_{1c} value to decrease by 1.5–2.0 percentage points [107, 108] (Table 1). Approximately 25% of such patients will achieve an HbA_{1c} level less than 7.0% (the current ADA goal) and fasting plasma glucose concentration less than 6.1–7.0 mmol/l (110–126 mg/dl) and should be considered complete responders [107, 108]. Factors that predict a good response include recently diagnosed diabetes, mild to moderate fasting hyperglycemia [<12.2–13.3 mmol/l (<220–240 mg/dl)], good β-cell function as reflected by a high fasting C-peptide level, no history of insulin therapy, and absence of islet cell or glutamic acid decarboxylase antibodies [109].

About 75% of patients with type 2 diabetes treated with a sulfonylurea will not reach the desired goal [HbA_{1c} <7.0% and fasting plasma glucose <6.1–7.0 mmol/l (110–126 mg/dl)] and will require addition of a second oral agent. Patients in whom sulfonylurea therapy fails can be subdivided into two groups. Ten percent to 20% will have a poor initial response [decrease in fasting plasma glucose level < 1.1 mmol/l (<20 mg/dl)] [105, 106] and these patients are considered to have primary failure [112]. Such patients usually have a low fasting C-peptide level and a fasting plasma glucose level that exceeds 15.5–16.6 mmol/l (280–300 mg/dl). In some of these patients, the disease represents slowly evolving type 1 diabetes [113]. Fifty percent to 60% of patients with type 2 diabetes have a good initial response to sulfonylurea therapy [decrease in fasting plasma glucose level > 1.7 mmol/l (>30 mg/dl)], but they do not reach the desired treatment goal (HbA_{1c} <7.0%). Such patients are considered to have a partial response.

After a good initial response to sulfonylurea therapy, the secondary failure rate is about 5–7% per year [48, 49, 84, 114, 115] and, after 10 years, most sulfonylurea-treated patients require a second oral agent [48, 49, 84, 116]. Secondary treatment failure is divided into patient-related factors (weight gain, lack of exercise, failure to comply with prescribed treatment regimen, or coexisting medial disorders), therapy-related factors (use of concomitant medications that antagonize insulin action or insulin secretion, β-cell desensitization secondary to long-term sulfonylurea exposure, inadequate drug dosage, or impaired sulfonylurea absorption secondary to hyperglycemia), and disease-related problems (progression of insulin resistance and increasing insulin deficiency). It is commonly stated (without experimental support) that the high rate of secondary failure is related to the pancreas's inability to maintain its augmented insulin secretory rate in response to long-term sulfonylurea stimulation. However, the UKPDS [48, 49, 84] negates this theory, because a similar rate of secondary failure was observed with metformin therapy. Metformin, by improving insulin sensitivity and decreasing plasma insulin levels, would have been expected to preserve β-cell function. The UKPDS results suggest that once the fasting plasma glucose level exceeds a certain value [>7.8–8.9 mmol/l

(>140–160 mg/dl)] for a prolonged period of time (yet to be defined), β-cell failure inexorably progresses.

Clinical trials have not demonstrated superiority of any one sulfonylurea over another when given in maximally effective doses [107, 108]. To the contrary, large prospective placebo-controlled trials have shown that glipizide, glyburide, and glimepiride exert equipotent glucose-lowering effects [107, 108, 112, 117]. Similar results have been reported in studies comparing first- and second-generation sulfonylureas [48, 49]. Although short-term studies indicate that glipizide releases insulin more rapidly than glyburide does and that glyburide suppresses hepatic glucose production more than glipizide does [118], both sulfonylureas produce similar mean daylong glycemic profiles when used long term in patients with type 2 diabetes [117].

Other Effects

Type 2 diabetes mellitus is part of a complex metabolic–cardiovascular cluster of disorders referred to as the insulin resistance syndrome (the metabolic syndrome or syndrome X) [45, 51, 55–57]. Because coronary artery disease represents the major cause of death in type 2 diabetes mellitus, it is desirable that any hypoglycemic agent favorably affect known cardiovascular risk factors. In most studies, sulfonylureas have been reported to have neutral or slightly beneficial effects on plasma lipid levels [107, 119] (Table 2). Plasma triglyceride levels decreased modestly in some studies. This hypolipidemic effect most likely represents both a direct effect of sulfonylurea on the metabolism of very low density lipoprotein (VLDL) and an indirect action of the drug secondary to reduced plasma glucose levels [77]. No consistent effect of sulfonylureas on the fibrinolytic system has been described [78]. Sulfonylurea therapy usually is associated with mild-modest weight gain [48], which has been implicated as a cause of secondary drug failure (Table 2). However, at least one study indicates that long-acting glipizide is not associated with weight gain [107].

Dosing Schedule

Sulfonylureas are divided into first-generation and second-generation drugs. First-generation sulfonylureas have a lower binding affinity to the SUR and must be given in higher doses than second-generation sulfonylureas [120]. Although short-acting glipizide has been approved at a dosage of 40 mg/day, the maximally effective dosage is 20 mg/day [120]. However, it is the author's personal experience that little, if any, additional benefit is observed by increasing the dose of glipizide or glyburide above 10 mg/day or glimepiride above 8 mg/day.

When initiating therapy, one should start with the lowest effective dose and titrate upward every 1–2 weeks until the desired level of glycemic control is achieved. Some diabetes experts use a 3–4-week titration interval, and there is no therapeutic advantage in waiting more than 4 weeks to increase the sulfonylurea dose.

Because sulfonylureas act by augmenting insulin secretion, their maximum hypoglycemic effect is seen within a week. Therefore, escalation of the sulfonylurea dose can be performed at weekly intervals, but must be based upon the fasting plasma glucose concentration, since the HbA_{1c} requires 2–3 months to reach its maximum decrement. All patients with type 2 diabetes should perform blood glucose monitoring at home. At the end of the week, the patient can tell the fasting plasma glucose values to his/her physician or nurse. If the fasting plasma glucose concentration is greater than 6.1 mmol/l (110 mg/dl), the physician or nurse should instruct the patient to increase the dose of glyburide or glipizide by 2.5 mg/day every week up to a maximum of 10 mg/day. For glimepiride the dose should be increased by 2 mg/day on a weekly basis up to a maximum of 8 mg/day. Using a nurse case manager with treatment algorithms (for sequential combination therapy with glipizide plus metformin), the HbA_{1c} was reduced by 3.2% (from 10.5% to 7.3%) in a community outpatient clinic [121]. Most (75%) of the hypoglycemic action of the sulfonylurea is observed with a daily dose that represents half of the maximally effective dose: that is, 5–7.5 mg of glyburide or glipizide and 4–6 mg of glimepiride. If no hypoglycemic effect is observed with half of the maximally effective dose, it is unlikely that further dose increases will have a clinically significant effect on blood glucose level. Other sulfonylureas (gliclazide, gliquidone, glibornuride, and glisoxepide) are available outside the United States.

Safety

The frequency of adverse effects in sulfonylurea-treated patients is low (2–5%), and side effects typically are mild and reversible on discontinuation of therapy [120]. The major adverse effect is hypoglycemia, which has been reported more commonly with the longer acting sulfonylureas, glyburide and chlorpropamide [48, 49, 84, 118, 120]. The greater suppression of hepatic glucose production with glyburide [118] has been offered as an explanation for the higher incidence of hypoglycemia. Mild hypoglycemic reactions occur in about 2–4% of patients, and severe hypoglycemic reactions requiring hospitalization occur with a frequency of 0.2–0.4 cases per 1000 patient-treatment years [116, 122], although the UKPDS reported a much higher incidence of sulfonylurea-related episodes of hypoglycemia [48]. Because patients older than 80 years of age are at high risk for hypoglycemia [114, 122, 123], short-acting sulfonylureas or a meglitinide (nateglinide or repaglinide) may be preferred. However, no published long-term prospective studies have compared short-acting sulfonylureas or repaglinide/nateglinide with long-acting sulfonylureas in elderly patients with type 2 diabetes. One prospective, short-term study [124] failed to find any difference in the occurrence of hypoglycemia in elderly diabetic patients (65 years of age) treated with either glyburide or glipizide, but the number of patients studied ($n = 52$) was relatively small.

Sulfonylurea therapy should be initiated with the lowest dose in patients with a reduced glomerular filtration rate, because the risk for hypoglycemia is increased. Therapy with chlorpropamide, which is renally excreted, should be avoided in individuals with impaired renal function.

Hypoglycemia also occurs more frequently in patients who have type 2 diabetes with mild fasting hyperglycemia [<7.0 mmol/l (<126 mg/dl)], typically occurring 2–3 h after breakfast or during exercise. Various drug interactions have been described, especially with first-generation sulfonylureas, and these are discussed in a review by Lebovitz and Melander [120].

The results of the University Group Diabetes Program study suggested that sulfonylureas may exacerbate coronary artery disease in patients with type 2 diabetes [73, 74]. However, that study has been widely criticized [125, 126], and subsequent clinical trials have not demonstrated increased cardiac mortality rates in diabetic patients treated with sulfonylureas [127–129]. Moreover, the UKPDS found no increased incidence of coronary artery disease in patients with type 2 diabetes assigned to intensive therapy with sulfonylureas compared with patients receiving diet therapy [48]. This topic was the subject of a recent review [130]. On the basis of currently available data—especially from the UKPDS—we believe that physicians should abide by the ADA's policy statement [131]: "We oppose any formal restrictions on use of the sulfonylurea agents that are based on the interpretations of the University Group Diabetes Program findings." No published clinical study demonstrates an advantage of one sulfonylurea, including glimepiride, over any other sulfonylurea with respect to coronary artery disease.

Sulfonylureas initiate their action by binding to the SUR, leading to closure of the potassium-ATP channel [102]. This has raised concern that sulfonylureas might cause arrhythmias and interfere with preischemic conditioning. However, closure of the K^+-ATPase channel would lead to a decrease in K^+ efflux from cardiac myocytes, causing a stabilization of the membrane potential and a decline in myocardial irritability. Consistent with this, patients with diabetes treated with sulfonylureas have been shown to have a reduced incidence of ventricular arrhythmias [132, 133]. There are three distinct SURs in the body: SUR-1 (β-cells), SUR-2A (cardiac), and SUR-2B (vasculature). Only sulfonylureas that possess a benzamido group bind to SUR-2A and SUR-2B. An impairment in preischemic conditioning could potentially lead to impaired vasodilation and, in diabetic patients who experience a myocardial infarction, it has been suggested that this could lead to necrosis of myocardial tissue with borderline perfusion. However, impaired preischemic conditioning occurs only with sulfonylureas that possess a benzamido group (second-generation sulfonylureas) and with nateglinide, which also possess a benzamido group [134, 135]. Moreover, based upon the binding affinity of the benzamido group to SUR-2A (cardiac), one would require a pharmacologic dose of glyburide, glipizide, glimepiride, or nateglinide to inhibit ischemic preconditioning and to impair arterial vasodilation. Such pharmacologic levels are well in excess of those achieved with standard oral sulfonylurea therapy in patients with type 2 diabetes [136]. Although pharmacologic doses of sulfonylureas can interfere with brachial arterial vasodilation [137], physiologic doses do not impair brachial arterial vasodilation [136] and neither an increased incidence of myocardial infarction [138] nor extension of infracted myocardial tissue [139] have been demonstrated in patients with type 2 diabetes who are being treated with sulfonylureas.

Summary

In summary, sulfonylureas are very effective glucose-lowering agents (decrease in HbA_{1c} value, 1.5–2.0 percentage points) that work by enhancing insulin secretion. They have no direct effect on plasma lipids, and mild-modest weight gain is common with their use. The only significant side effect associated with the sulfonylureas is hypoglycemia. The sulfonylureas, especially the generic ones, are inexpensive.

Metformin

Metformin, a biguanide that has been in clinical use for 45 years [140], was introduced in the United States in 1995 [98]. Although other biguanides, buformin and phenformin, are available outside the United States, their use has decreased dramatically. Phenformin was previously approved for use in the United States but was removed from the market because it caused lactic acidosis. Metformin, which differs structurally from phenformin, has low lipid solubility and, when used in diabetic patients with normal renal function, rarely causes lactic acidosis [141].

Mechanism of Action

Metformin enhances the sensitivity of both hepatic and peripheral tissues (primarily muscle) to insulin [50, 142–144] (Table 2, Figure 1). Metformin inhibits hepatic gluconeogenesis both *in vitro* [145] and *in vivo* [143]. Evidence for an inhibitory effect on hepatic glycogenolysis has also been provided [144]. The decline in basal hepatic glucose production is closely correlated with the reduction in fasting plasma glucose level [142–144]. Metformin also enhances muscle insulin sensitivity [50, 140, 142–144] through direct [146] and indirect effects [50]. At the cellular level, improved insulin action in muscle is explained by multiple actions, including increased insulin receptor tyrosine kinase activity [147], augmented GLUT-4 transporter number and activity [148], and enhanced glycogen synthesis [142, 144, 148]. In rat hepatocytes, metformin phosphorylates AMP kinase (AMPK) [149]. Once activated AMPK reduces the expression of sterol regulatory element-binding protein 1 (SREBP-1), a nuclear transcription factor that, when inhibited, reduces the expression of key enzymes involved in the stimulation of gluconeogenesis (phosphoenolpyruvate carboxykinase and glucose-6-phosphatase) and VLDL–triglyceride secretion [149]. The net result is a decrease in hepatic glucose production and fasting plasma glucose and triglyceride concentrations [149]. Metformin also increases AMPK activity in skeletal muscle, leading to the activation of the GLUT-4 transporter [149]. In patients with type 2 diabetes, metformin increases muscle AMPK activity, leading to enhanced insulin-mediated muscle glucose disposal, primarily by augmenting muscle glycogen synthesis [150]. Metformin has no direct effect on β-cell function. In metformin-treated patients with diabetes, fasting and postprandial insulin levels consistently decrease [140, 142–144], reflecting the normal compensatory response of the pancreas to enhanced insulin sensitivity.

Efficacy

Clinical trials [98, 140, 151–153] have documented that metformin therapy consistently decreases the fasting plasma glucose level by 3.3–3.9 mmol/l (60–70 mg/dl) and the HbA_{1c} value by 1.5–2.0 percentage points in patients with poorly controlled diabetes (Table 2). In a large double-blind, prospective study involving 289 diet-treated patients with type 2 diabetes [fasting plasma glucose level = 13.3 mmol/l (240 mg/dl)], metformin decreased the fasting plasma glucose level by 2.9 mmol/l (52 mg/dl) and the HbA_{1c} value by 1.4 percentage points from baseline [98]. These decreases were independent of age, ethnicity, duration of diabetes, body mass index, or fasting and glucose-stimulated plasma insulin or C-peptide levels. Approximately 25% of patients with type 2 diabetes treated with metformin monotherapy achieved a fasting plasma glucose level less than 7.8 mmol/l (<140 mg/dl) and an HbA_{1c} value less than 7% [98]. Similar results have been reported in a large dose-ranging study [153] and have been confirmed in a meta-analysis [154]. Thus, metformin and sulfonylureas are equally effective in reducing fasting plasma glucose and HbA_{1c} values in patients with type 2 diabetes, and both are indicated as primary therapy (Table 2).

As with sulfonylurea therapy, the decrease in fasting plasma glucose level from baseline with metformin therapy is highly correlated with the starting fasting plasma glucose level [98]. The hypoglycemic action of metformin increases linearly, even at very high fasting plasma glucose levels [>16.7 mmol/l (>300 mg/dl)]. In diabetic patients with a fasting plasma glucose level of 16.7 mmol/l or more (300 mg/dl), the mean decrease in the fasting plasma glucose level is about 6.7 mmol/l (120 mg/dl) [98]. This observation is predictable because metformin inhibits hepatic glucose production and the magnitude of fasting hyperglycemia is primarily determined by the increased basal rate of hepatic glucose production. In contrast, when the fasting plasma glucose level exceeds 16.7 mmol/l (>300 mg/dl), insulin secretion is severely impaired and the pancreatic response to sulfonylureas often is poor [112, 117].

Other Effects

When used as monotherapy or with a sulfonylurea, metformin decreases plasma triglyceride and LDL-cholesterol levels by 10–15% [28, 98, 140, 142, 149, 155] (Table 2), reduces postprandial hyperlipemia [28], decreases plasma free fatty acid levels [156], and decreases free fatty acid oxidation [28, 155, 157]. The magnitude of the decrease in plasma triglyceride concentration is related to the fasting triglyceride level [98] and is independent of changes in the plasma glucose level [28, 98, 155]. Consistent with this, metformin reduces triglyceride levels in nondiabetic patients with hypertriglyceridemia [158]. HDL-cholesterol levels either do not change or increase slightly after metformin therapy [28, 140, 142, 155, 159, 160]. Elevated plasminogen activator inhibitor-1 (PAI-1) levels are decreased with metformin therapy in patients with and without diabetes [159–161]. Weight gain does not occur in patients with type 2 diabetes who receive metformin alone or in combination with other oral agents or insulin [48, 49, 84, 98, 151–153]. Most studies show a modest weight loss of 2–3 kg during the first 6 months of treatment [98, 140, 142, 143, 151, 153, 159] (Table 2). In a 1-year randomized, double-blind trial in 457 nondiabetic patients with android (male type or abdominal) obesity, metformin also caused significant weight loss [162].

Dosing Schedule

The starting metformin dosage is 500 mg twice daily, given with the two largest meals to minimize gastrointestinal side effects. The fasting plasma glucose level begins to decrease within 3–5 days after therapy is started and reaches a nadir within 1–2 weeks. The dosage should be increased by 500 mg/day every 2 weeks until the desired therapeutic goal is achieved or a maximum dosage of 2000 mg/day is reached [98, 153]. Because the HbA_{1c} level does not reach equilibrium until 2–3 months, the metformin dose should be titrated upward every 2 weeks based upon a fasting plasma glucose concentration >110 mg/dl.

A long-acting metformin preparation, Glucophage-XL, is also available [163]. It can be taken once daily and has fewer gastrointestinal side effects than does generic metformin [163]. Eighty percent to 85% of the maximal glucose-lowering effect of metformin is observed with a daily dose of 1500 mg [103].

Safety

Gastrointestinal side effects, including abdominal discomfort and diarrhea, are the most common adverse events, occurring in 20–30% of patients [98, 153]. These side effects usually are mild and transient and can be minimized by slow titration. If symptoms occur during titration, one should return to the previous metformin dose at which no symptoms were encountered and wait at least 2 weeks before increasing the dose. Less than 5–10% of patients cannot tolerate metformin therapy [98]. The long-acting metformin (Glucophage-XL) has fewer gastrointestinal side effects than the short-acting metformin [163]. Metformin can interfere with vitamin B_{12} absorption, but this is rarely of clinical significance. Because metformin does not increase insulin secretion, biochemically documented hypoglycemia is rare in diabetic patients treated with metformin alone [48, 49, 84, 98].

Although uncommon, lactic acidosis has been reported with a frequency of 3 cases per 100 000 patient-years [140, 164, 165]. No cases of lactic acidosis with metformin therapy were observed in the UKPDS [49]. A similar incidence has been reported in US surveillance studies [98]. Lactic acidosis is rare in the absence of other serious medical disorders, including renal insufficiency, severe tissue hypoperfusion, cardiogenic or septic shock, pulmonary insufficiency with hypoxemia, or severe liver disease [98, 140, 164–166]. In these situations, it is difficult to discern whether the lactic acidosis is due to the severe underlying medical disorder or to metformin therapy.

Metformin therapy is contraindicated in patients with renal and hepatic disease, respiratory insufficiency, any hypoxemic condition, severe infection, and alcohol abuse. Impaired renal function is an especially important contraindication to metformin use, because the drug is excreted via the kidneys. If the serum creatinine concentration is more than 124 mol/l (1.4 mg/dl) in women or more than 133 mol/l (1.5 mg/dl) in men, metformin should not be administered. In patients with reduced muscle mass, such as elderly patients, the serum creatinine concentration may underestimate the glomerular filtration rate, and creatinine clearance rate should be determined. If the creatinine clearance rate is less than 70–75 ml/min metformin should not be given. Metformin should not be used in diabetic patients with congestive heart failure requiring pharmacologic therapy, because, in this situation, decreased renal perfusion and glomerular filtration rate can impair metformin excretion. In elderly patients, especially those older than 80 years, an age-related decrease in glomerular filtration rate is often seen. In such patients, it is advisable to measure the creatinine clearance rate before starting metformin therapy and to use the minimum dose required to achieve the desired level of glycemic control.

Diabetic patients, especially those with proteinuria and reduced glomerular filtration rate, are at increased risk for acute renal failure after administration of radiocontrast dye. If dye-induced renal failure is not recognized and metformin therapy is continued, plasma metformin levels will increase progressively, and lactic acidosis may occur. In diabetic patients who present with an acute medical illness that requires administration of radiocontrast dye, the study should be performed and further metformin doses should be withheld until normal renal function has been documented by serum creatinine measurement 24–48 h after the procedure.

In the UKPDS [49], metformin monotherapy was associated with a highly significant decrease in the risk for macrovascular complications, including myocardial infarction, stroke, and death. However, these results have been questioned because of findings in a substudy of 537 patients with poorly controlled type 2 diabetes who had been treated with sulfonylureas for 7.1 years and who were randomly assigned to receive either metformin with continued sulfonylurea treatment ($n = 268$) or continued sulfonylurea monotherapy ($n = 269$). After a mean follow-up of 4 years, the investigators reported a 96% increase in the risk for diabetes-related death ($P = 0.04$) in the group receiving sulfonylureas plus metformin compared with the group that continued receiving sulfonylurea monotherapy. Although the absolute number of heart attacks (33 and 31) and strokes (15 and 13) was very similar in the two groups, more patients in the sulfonylurea plus metformin group experienced a fatal heart attack or stroke. The authors pointed out that in the substudy, the number of patients and events was small and the duration of combination therapy was short. A more relevant question is whether the relative increase in heart attack and stroke mortality resulted from an increased number of deaths in the sulfonylurea plus metformin group or to a decrease in the number of deaths in the sulfonylurea monotherapy group. This question was addressed in a subsequent analysis by Turner and colleagues [167], who found that all of the relative increase in mortality observed in the patients who received sulfonylurea plus metformin compared with those who received sulfonylurea alone resulted from a significant reduction in the expected number of deaths in the latter group; there was no increase in mortality in the sulfonylurea plus metformin group. In absolute terms, the number of fatal heart attacks actually decreased in the sulfonylurea plus metformin group compared with the expected number of deaths [167]. The investigators also performed a meta-analysis of all patients receiving sulfonylurea plus metformin in the UKPDS and reported significant reductions in all diabetes-related endpoints and for myocardial infarction.

Summary

In summary, metformin is very effective in decreasing the plasma glucose level (decrease in HbA_{1c} value = 1.5–2.0 percentage points). It also reduces plasma triglyceride and LDL-cholesterol levels, lowers PAI-1 levels, and improves endothelial dysfunction. Metformin works by suppressing basal hepatic glucose production and enhancing insulin sensitivity in muscle. Metformin is the only oral antidiabetic agent that, when used as monotherapy, has been shown to reduce macrovascular complications. Most patients treated with metformin lose weight or fail to gain weight. The most common side effects are related to gastrointestinal disturbances. Lactic acidosis is a very rare complication of metformin therapy, and this biguanide is absolutely contraindicated in diabetic patients with impaired renal function. Generic less expensive preparations of metformin are now available in the United States and worldwide.

Because metformin reduces cardiovascular events and is as effective as any other oral hypoglycemic agent in reducing HbA_{1c} and microvascular events, we believe that, in the absence of some contraindication to its use, metformin should be used as first-line therapy in all type 2 diabetic patients.

Thiazolidinediones

The thiazolidinediones are now widely used to treat patients with type 2 diabetes mellitus in the United States. Two thiazolidinediones, pioglitazone (Actos, Takeda Pharmaceuticals North America, Lincolnshire, IL, USA) and rosiglitazone (Avandia, SmithKline Beecham, Philadelphia, PA, USA), currently are approved by the Food and Drug Administration (FDA) for the treatment of type 2 diabetes in the United States and are available in Europe, South America, and the Orient.

Mechanism of Action

Thiazolidinediones work by binding to the peroxisome proliferator activator receptor-γ (PPAR-γ), which primarily is located on adipocytes [168, 169], vascular cells [169], and circulating mononuclear cells [170]. Although PPAR-γ receptors can be found in muscle, they are present in very low levels [171]. The glucose-lowering effect of thiazolidinediones is related to the drugs' ability to enhance insulin sensitivity in liver and muscle [168–179] (Table 1, Figure 1). Since there are no PPAR-γ receptors in liver and only small numbers in muscle, it is very unlikely that the thiazolidinediones have direct insulin-sensitizing effects on these organs. A major effect of PPAR-γ activation is to cause preadipocytes in subcutaneous tissue depots to differentiate into mature fat cells, with the induction of all of the key enzymes involved in lipogenesis [168–174]. This results in smaller, more insulin-sensitive peripheral adipocytes [168, 172–174]. The newly formed small fat cells also are more sensitive to insulin with respect to inhibition of lipolysis and glucose uptake [172–175]. As the newly formed fat cells take up FFA from the plasma compartment, there is a marked reduction in plasma FFA concentration, which closely predicts the decrease in HbA_{1c} [175, 176]. As the plasma FFA declines, there is movement of FFA out of the visceral fat cells and liver [177–179]. The net result is a shift in fat topography, characterized by decline in visceral and hepatic fat content. PPAR-γ activation also causes apoptosis of large visceral fat cells [180]. The reduction in hepatic fat content is associated with improved hepatic sensitivity to insulin [175–177, 179], enhanced splanchnic glucose uptake [179] and improved hepatic liver function tests [179]. Muscle fat content (measured by magnetic resonance imaging) does not decline following thiazolidinedione therapy [178]. However, intracellular lipid molecules (fatty acyl-CoAs, diacylglycerol, ceramides), which inhibit the insulin signal system, decline, contributing to the improvement in muscle insulin sensitivity [181–184]. The preceding sequence of events explains the paradoxical observation that increased weight gain is closely correlated with improved muscle and hepatic insulin sensitivity [176, 180]. Although there is an increase in subcutaneous fat mass, there is a depletion of fat and insulin resistance producing fatty acid metabolites from all other tissues in the body. It should be noted that a simple redistribution of fat from muscle, liver, and visceral fat to subcutaneous fat would not cause a net increase in fat mass and weight gain. However, thiazolidinediones also inhibit expression of the leptin gene in adipocytes [168, 173]. The decline in plasma leptin (and perhaps other satiety factors) leads to the stimulation of appetite and increased food intake. Increased weight gain, reduced plasma FFA concentration, and improved insulin sensitivity all are strong predictors of the reduction in HbA_{1c}during thiazolidinedione therapy [176, 177, 178, 180] .

Recent studies also indicate that thiazolidinediones exert important effects to preserve β-cell function. In the insulin-resistant Zucker diabetic fatty rat, the onset of diabetes at 3–4 months of life is associated with a marked increase in β-cell fat fatty acyl-CoA levels [185, 186], which in turn leads to increased ceramide levels and the release of inflammatory cytokines, which impair insulin secretion and cause β-cell apoptosis. Treatment of these animals with a variety of thiazolidinediones reduces intracellular fatty acyl CoA and ceramide levels, prevents the release of inflammatory cytokines within the β-cells, and preserves β-cell function [187]. Despite significant weight gain associated with thiazolidinedione treatment, the Zucker diabetic fatty rat does not develop diabetes.

A number of studies in humans have demonstrated that thiazolidinediones, working either directly through PPAR-γ receptors on the β-cell [188] or more likely via a reduction in plasma FFA levels [189], or via presently undefined mechanisms, improve β-cell function. In subjects with impaired glucose tolerance (IGT), treatment with troglitazone improved β-cell function by 52% [190]. In the TRIPOD study [191] troglitazone also reduced the conversion rate to diabetes in women with a prior history of gestational diabetes by preserving β-cell function. A similar beneficial effect of pioglitazone on β-cell function has been observed in the PIPOD extension of the TRIPOD study [192]. In a dose-ranging study [193] pioglitazone was shown to increase both the early (0–30 min) and total (0–120 min) insulinogenic index ($\Delta I/\Delta G$) in type 2 diabetic subjects who were treated with the thiazolidinedione for 26 weeks. More recently, troglitazone in the Diabetes Prevention Program (DPP) [194] was shown to decrease the conversion rate of IGT to diabetes after 4 years even through subjects received treatment with troglitazone for only 10 months on average and had not received the drug for 3 years and 2 months. The long-term protective effect of troglitazone in the DPP was shown to be related to the preservation of β-cell function. What remains unclear is at what stage in the natural history of type 2 diabetes (i.e. at what level of hyperglycemia and at what duration of diabetes), do the thiazolidinediones become unable to afford protection against the progressive decline in β-cell function that is characteristic of patients with type 2 diabetes mellitus.

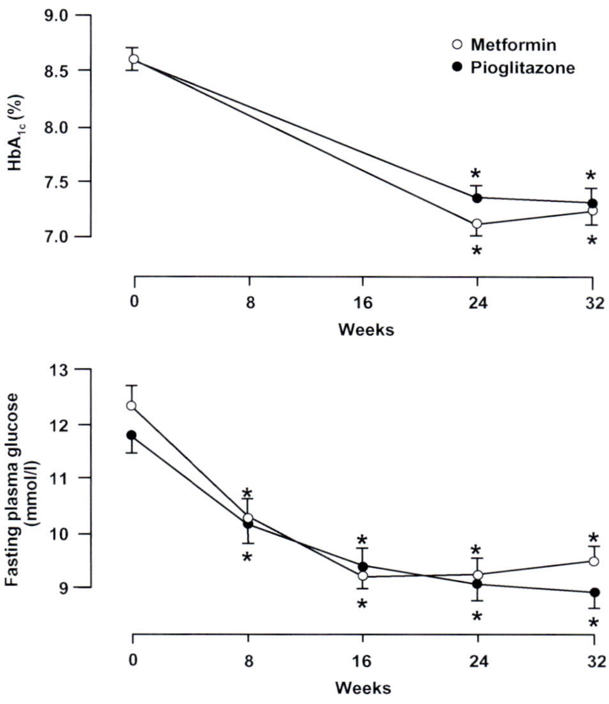

Figure 4 Top: Effect of pioglitazone (up to 45 mg/day) and metformin (up to 2550 mg/day) treatment on HbA_{1c}. $^*P < 0.0001$ vs. baseline. Bottom: Effect of pioglitazone (up to 45 mg/day) and metformin (up to 2550 mg/day) treatment on fasting plasma glucose. $^*P < 0.0001$ vs. baseline [97]. (Reproduced by permission of The Endocrine Society from Pavo I, Jermendy G, Varkonyi TT, Kerenyi Z, Gyimesi A, Shoustov S, Shestakova M, Herz M, Johns D, Schluchter BJ, Festa A, Tan MH. Effect of pioglitazone compared with metformin on glycemic control and indicators of insulin sensitivity in recently diagnosed patients with type 2 diabetes. *J Clin Endocrinol Metab* 2003; 88: 1637–45. Copyright © 2003 The Endocrine Society)

Efficacy

Several trials have examined the effect of thiazolidinedione monotherapy in patients with poorly controlled type 2 diabetes. Data on file with the FDA demonstrate that when pioglitazone and rosiglitazone are used as monotherapy in drug-naïve diabetic patients, the HbA_{1c} value decreases by about 1.2–1.6 percentage points after 26 weeks of treatment. In a placebo-controlled, dose–response study [195] carried out in 408 drug-naïve/drug-withdrawn type 2 diabetic patients who received 15, 30, and 45 mg of pioglitazone per day or placebo for 26 weeks, the mean decreases in fasting plasma glucose concentration and HbA_{1c} values at the highest dosage were 3.6 mmol/l (65 mg/dl) and 1.6 percentage points, respectively, compared to placebo. In a 26-week placebo-controlled study involving drug-naïve/drug-withdrawn diabetic patients, 8 mg of rosiglitazone per day decreased the fasting plasma glucose concentration and HbA_{1c} values by 4.2 mmol/l (76 mg/dl) and 1.5 percentage points, respectively [196]. There has been only one head-to-head, double-blind clinical trial comparing any thiazolidinedione (pioglitazone) with any other oral hypoglycemic agent (metformin) [97]. In 205 drug-naïve type 2 diabetic patients, 32 weeks of pioglitazone (45 mg/day) or metformin (2.55 g/day) produced comparable reductions in HbA_{1c} and fasting plasma glucose concentration (Figure 4). However, pioglitazone was significantly more effective than metformin in improving indices of insulin sensitivity, as determined by a reduction in the fasting serum insulin concentration ($P = 0.003$) and homeostasis model assessment (HOMA) for insulin sensitivity (HOMA-S; $P = 0.002$). Although there are no published trials comparing thiazolidinediones and sulfonylureas on glycemic control and since metformin and sulfonylureas produce a comparable reduction in fasting plasma glucose and HbA_{1c} levels [98], it is reasonable to conclude that the thiazolidinediones, metformin, and the sulfonylureas are approximately equally effective in improving glycemic control (Table 2) and all three are more efficacious than the other two classes of oral hypoglycemic agents (Table 2).

Other Effects

When used as monotherapy, pioglitazone consistently decreases the plasma triglyceride level by 10–20% [97, 195], whereas rosiglitazone either has no effect on or raises the plasma triglyceride concentration [111, 196, 197]. Most published studies have shown that pioglitazone does not affect the plasma LDL-cholesterol concentration [97, 195], whereas rosiglitazone tends to raise the plasma LDL-cholesterol level [111, 196, 197]. Both pioglitazone [97, 195] and rosiglitazone [111, 196, 197] increase the HDL-cholesterol by 3–9 mg/dl, with the greatest increments being seen in diabetic individuals with the lowest starting HDL-cholesterol levels. Both pioglitazone [198] and rosiglitazone [199] convert small dense LDL-cholesterol particles to larger, less dense, less atherogenic LDL particles. Thiazolidinediones cause small decreases in blood pressure [200, 201], reduce PAI-1 levels [202], and improve endothelial dysfunction [203, 204]. All thiazolidinediones inhibit the expression and release of insulin resistance-inducing [resistin, tumor necrosis factor α (TNF-α)] [205, 206], inflammatory (interleukin 6, TNF-α) [206, 207], and procoagulant (PAI-1) [208] cytokines from adipocytes, while increasing the expression and secretion of adiponectin [209, 210], an insulin-sensitizing antiatherosclerotic cytokine. Both pioglitazone and rosiglitazone cause weight gain, with increases of 1.5–3.5 kg typically being observed during the first 6–12 months after initiation of therapy [176–178, 180]. Of note, the greater the weight gain, the greater is the decline in HbA_{1c} [176, 178, 211]. More significant increases in body weight occur when rosiglitazone or pioglitazone is combined with insulin [212, 213].

Dosing Schedule

The recommended starting dosages of pioglitazone and rosiglitazone are 15 mg once daily and 2–4 mg once daily, respectively. The dosage should be increased every 2–4 weeks to a maximum of 45 mg once daily for pioglitazone and 8 mg once daily (or 4 mg twice daily) for rosiglitazone.

Safety

With troglitazone, the first thiazolidinedione introduced into the United States, 1.9% of diabetic patients experienced an increase in alanine aminotransferase (ALT) to levels that were more than three times the upper limit of normal. A number of cases of severe liver toxicity [214] with 28 reported deaths from liver failure in troglitazone-treated patients prompted the withdrawal of troglitazone from clinical use in March 2000. The incidence of elevated liver enzyme levels in diabetic patients treated with pioglitazone and rosiglitazone (0.25 and 0.2%, respectively) was similar to that in patients who received placebo [data on file with Food and Drug Administration (FDA)]. There have been only rare reports of hepatotoxicity associated with rosiglitazone and pioglitazone, since their introduction into the clinical marketplace [215–218]. However, no evidence of hepatotoxicity was observed in an analysis of more than 5000 patients who participated in clinical trials of rosiglitazone [219] or pioglitazone [220]. The US FDA has recommended that liver enzymes be checked prior to initiating therapy with rosiglitazone or pioglitazone. Thiazolidinedione therapy should not be initiated in patients with increased liver enzymes (ALT $>$2.5 times the upper limit of normal). After initiating therapy, the ALT level should be measured every 2 months for the first year and periodically (up to the discretion of the physician) thereafter.

Across all clinical trials, diabetic patients treated with pioglitazone and rosiglitazone experienced a decrease of 2–4% in the plasma hemoglobin level from baseline. This has been attributed to the dilutional effect of fluid retention and expansion of the plasma volume, but a direct marrow suppressant effect also seems likely, since modest decreases in the white blood cell count also have been reported during thiazolidinedione therapy [207]. Edema has been reported in about 4–5% of patients on pioglitazone or rosiglitazone monotherapy or in combination with metformin or a sulfonylurea; the incidence of edema is significantly higher in patients on combination therapy with insulin plus a thiazolidinedione (10–15%) [212]. The etiology of the edema has been poorly studied but peripheral arterial vasodilation with resultant renal hypoperfusion, sending a signal to the kidney to enhance sodium retention, is a likely contributing factor [221]. It is noteworthy that in this study of 154 patients with type 2 diabetes, who were randomized to treatment with troglitazone or glyburide for 48 weeks, the cardiac index increased appropriately in response to the decline in peripheral vascular resistance and decline in blood pressure in the troglitazone-treated patients [221]. Glyburide had no effect on peripheral vascular resistance, blood pressure, or cardiac index. Although leaky blood vessels with extravasation of salt and water into the interstitial space has been postulated, there is, at present, no experimental evidence to support this hypothesis. A direct effect of the thiazolidinedione on the kidney to enhance salt and water absorption seems very unlikely, since this would be expected to increase the intravascular volume, causing vasoconstriction and hypertension. In contrast, a decrease in peripheral vascular resistance [221] and reduced blood pressure, albeit modest [200, 201, 221], is the typical finding in thiazolidinedione-treated patients. The greater incidence of peripheral edema in insulin-treated type 2 diabetic patients may reflect an enhanced sensitivity of the renal tubule to the antinatriuretic effect of insulin [222]. Thiazolidinediones are contraindicated in diabetic patients with advanced congestive heart failure (New York

Heart Association (NYHA) class III or IV cardiac status) and they should be used cautiously in diabetic patients with lesser degrees of congestive heart failure.

Summary

Thiazolidinedione monotherapy is effective in reducing the HbA_{1c} value ($\Delta = \sim 1.5$ percentage points). Thiazolidinediones work by improving insulin sensitivity in muscle and liver, effects that are closely correlated with weight gain and a reduction in plasma FFA concentration and mobilization of FFA and triglyceride metabolities out of muscle and liver. The thiazolidinediones also have been shown to preserve β-cell function and prevent the development of type 2 diabetes in individuals with IGT. Pioglitazone, but not rosiglitazone, decreases plasma triglyceride levels and both drugs significantly increase HDL-cholesterol. Rosiglitazone is associated with a rise in LDL-cholesterol, whereas pioglitazone is LDL-cholesterol neutral. All thiazolidinediones are associated with weight gain, and the more the weight gain, the greater is the reduction in HbA_{1c}. Thiazolidinediones are considerably more expensive than the other first-line therapies, metformin and sulfonylureas, for which generic preparations are available.

Acarbose

Two α-glucosidase inhibitors, acarbose (Precose, Bayer, West Haven, CT, USA) and miglitol (Glyset, Pharmacia & Upjohn, Kalamazoo, MI, USA) are available in the United States. A third, voglibose (Basen, Takeda, Osaka, Japan), is available in Japan and Europe. There appears to be no particular advantage of any one α-glucosidase inhibitor over another with respect to their glucose reducing efficacy.

Mechanism of Action

α-Glucosidase inhibitors competitively inhibit the ability of enzymes (maltase, isomaltase, sucrase, and glucoamylase) in the small intestinal brush border to break down oligosaccharides and disaccharides into monosaccharides [223–225]. Acarbose has a slight (about 10%) inhibitory effect on lactase [224, 225]. By delaying digestion of carbohydrates, the α-glucosidase inhibitors shift their absorption to more distal parts of the small intestine and colon. They do not cause malabsorption. By slowing the digestive/absorptive process, the α-glucosidase inhibitors retard glucose entry into the systemic circulation, allowing the β-cells ample time to augment insulin secretion in response to the blunted increase in plasma glucose level. The α-glucosidase inhibitors do not reverse any pathophysiologic abnormalities in patients with type 2 diabetes (Figure 1).

Efficacy

Clinical trials [223–231] have shown that the hypoglycemic potency of acarbose and other α-glucosidase inhibitors is less than that of sulfonylureas, metformin, and thiazolidinediones (Table 2). As monotherapy, acarbose and other α-glucosidase inhibitors decrease the fasting plasma glucose level by 1.4–1.7 mmol/l (25–30 mg/dl) and the HbA_{1c} value by 0.7–1.0% [223–231]. The α-glucosidase inhibitors primarily affect the postprandial plasma glucose level, which is decreased by 2.2–2.8 mmol/l (40–50 mg/dl) after meal ingestion, although a small reduction in the fasting plasma glucose concentration is also observed [223–231]. The reduction in postprandial plasma glucose level occurs without change or with a slight decrease in the plasma insulin level. This hypoglycemic profile of the α-glucosidase inhibitors dictates their clinical indications. The drugs are most useful in patients with new-onset type 2 diabetes who have mild fasting hyperglycemia in whom the elevated HbA_{1c} primarily results from postprandial hyperglycemia. The α-glucosidase inhibitors also are indicated in type 2 diabetic patients who are taking a sulfonylurea or metformin or a thiazolidinedione and require an additional reduction of 1.4–1.7 mmol/l (25–30 mg/dl) in fasting plasma glucose level, because this is the typical decrease in fasting plasma glucose concentration reported in clinical trials [223–231]. Acarbose and other α-glucosidase inhibitors also are indicated in diabetic patients with predominant postprandial hyperglycemia. These patients can be recognized by measuring the postprandial glucose level under defined conditions or by documenting a mildly elevated fasting plasma glucose level [6.1–7.0 mmol/l (110–126 mg/dl)] with a disproportionately increased HbA_{1c} value (>7.0–7.5%).

Other Effects

Some studies have reported a modest decrease in plasma triglyceride levels [228, 229] without a change in LDL- or HDL-cholesterol levels with acarbose. Body weight does not change significantly when the α-glucosidase inhibitors are employed as monotherapy (Table 2). The recently completed STOP-NIDDM study demonstrated that acarbose decreased the conversion rate of IGT to type 2 diabetes [232] and reduced the incidence of cardiovascular events [233]. Because the close out OGTT in STOP-NIDDM was performed while the subjects were still taking acarbose, one cannot determine whether the drug truely "prevented" the development of diabetes or simply was "masking" the diabetic state by treating the postprandial plasma glucose excursion. Since hyperglycemia is a weak risk factor for cardiovascular disease (UKPDS) [59], the reduction in cardiovascular events in STOP-NIDDM is somewhat unexpected and suggests that there may be some unique benefit of treating postprandial hyperglycemia [234].

Dosing Schedule

Acarbose therapy should be initiated with a low dose, 25 mg once or twice daily, to minimize gastrointestinal side effects. It is our clinical experience that when acarbose therapy is being initiated, the drug is best given with the smallest meals to minimize gastrointestinal side effects. Acarbose must be ingested with the first bite of food because the drug must be present in the small bowel with food to be effective. It is recommended that the acarbose dose be increased by 25 mg/day every 2–4 weeks to minimize gastrointestinal side effects. The maximum dosage is 75–100 mg twice or three times daily, although many diabetic patients experience adverse gastrointestinal side effects at these doses. Because acarbose works by interfering with starch digestion and absorption, its effectiveness is diminished in patients with low carbohydrate intake.

Miglitol is initiated at a dose of 25 mg once or twice daily and increased by 25 mg/day every 2–4 weeks. The maximum dose is 100 mg twice or three times daily. Voglibose is initiated at a dose of 0.2 mg once or twice daily and increased by 0.1 mg/day every 2–4 weeks. The maximum dose is 0.3 mg three times daily.

Safety

Gastrointestinal side effects, including bloating, abdominal discomfort, diarrhea, and flatulence, occur in up to 30% of diabetic patients treated with acarbose and other α-glucosidase inhibitors, but these effects tend to diminish with continued drug use. Initiation of therapy with a low dose and slow titration helps to minimize these adverse effects. With very high doses of acarbose, 200–300 mg three times daily, elevated serum aminotransferase levels have been reported. Abnormal liver function tests return to normal when therapy with the drug is discontinued [223, 225]. Acarbose and other α-glucosidase inhibitors are contraindicated in patients with inflammatory bowel disease, a plasma creatinine concentration more than 177 mmol/l (>2.0 mg/dl), or cirrhosis.

Hypoglycemia does not occur in diabetic patients taking the α-glucosidase inhibitors. However, if hypoglycemia occurs when an α-glucosidase is used simultaneously with a sulfonylurea or insulin, recovery will be retarded, if carbohydrate is orally administered. Ingestion of pure glucose is advised in diabetic patients who experience hypoglycemia while taking an α-glucosidase inhibitor.

Summary

In summary, the major effect of the α-glucosidase inhibitors is to decrease postprandial glucose levels. The respective decreases in fasting plasma glucose and HbA_{1c} values are 25–30 mg/dl and 0.5–1.0 percentage points. Acarbose, miglitol, and voglibose work by interfering with carbohydrate digestion and delaying gastrointestinal absorption of glucose. They do not cause weight gain and do not significantly affect plasma lipid levels. The major side effects of the α-glucosidase inhibitors are related to the gastrointestinal tract.

Repaglinide and Nateglinide

Repaglinide (Prandin, Novo Nordisk, Princeton, NJ, USA) and nateglinide (Starlix, Novartis Pharmaceuticals, East Hanover, NJ, USA) are new, rapid-onset, short-acting insulin secretagogues that stimulate insulin secretion and reduce postprandial hyperglycemia. Repaglinide is a benzoic acid derivative and nateglinide is an amino acid derivative.

Mechanism of Action

Repaglinide and nateglinide are nonsulfonylurea insulin secretagogues (Figure 1) that require the presence of glucose for their action and work by closing an adenosine triphosphatase-dependent potassium channel, leading to an increase in insulin secretion [235]. Both nateglinide and repaglinide are fast-acting, short-duration, insulinotropic agents that improve postprandial hyperglycemia by enhancing insulin secretion [95, 236].

Efficacy

When used as monotherapy, both repaglinide and nateglinide are effective in decreasing postprandial hyperglycemia and HbA_{1c} values [94, 95, 236]. In diet-treated type 2 diabetic patients, not previously exposed to oral agents, 4 mg of repaglinide three times daily decreased the HbA_{1c} value by 1.0 percentage point from baseline [94]. In this double-blind, randomized, parallel-group study, glyburide produced a greater decrease in HbA_{1c} than did repaglinide (decrement = 2.4 vs. 1.0 percentage point) over a 1-year period [94]. In diet-treated type 2 diabetic patients, 120 mg of nateglinide three times daily decreased the HbA_{1c} value by 0.8% from baseline [95].

Other Effects

Neither repaglinide nor nateglinide have any significant effects on plasma lipid levels [237, 238]. In drug-naïve patients treated with repaglinide, body weight increased by about 2.4 kg [239]. Nateglinide monotherapy did not significantly increase body weight in drug-naïve patients with type 2 diabetes [95].

Dosing Schedule

Repaglinide is rapidly absorbed (0.5–1 h) and has a short plasma half-life (<1 h). Because of its pharmacokinetic behavior, its administration results in a rapid but brief release of insulin. The starting dosage of repaglinide is 0.5 mg three times daily, given 15 minutes before each meal. Dose increases can be made weekly to a maximum daily dose of 16 mg. A repaglinide dosage of 1 mg three times daily produces 90% of the maximal glucose-lowering effect [239]. Because 90% of repaglinide is recovered in the feces, it is not contraindicated in patients with renal insufficiency. In patients with liver disease, a slower titration schedule is recommended. The pharmacokinetics of nateglinide are similar to those of repaglinide, with an onset of action of 0.3–1 h. Nateglinide usually does not require dosage titration [240], and is dosed at 120 mg three times daily before each meal. In some studies nateglinide produced a more rapid postprandial increase in insulin secretion, and its duration of response was shorter than that of repaglinide [240]. Nateglinide is not contraindicated in patients with renal impairment or mild hepatic impairment [240]. However, it is contraindicated in diabetic patients with moderate to severe hepatic impairment, since appropriate dosage titration has not been studied.

Safety

Hypoglycemia was the only adverse effect noted with increased frequency in patients who received repaglinide compared with those who received placebo. In diabetic patients treated for 1 year with repaglinide or sulfonylurea, hypoglycemic episodes were slightly, although not significantly, less common in the former group (15% vs. 19%, $P = \text{NS}$) [241]. In type 2 diabetic patients receiving monotherapy with nateglinide versus sulfonylureas, the incidence of hypoglycemia was lower in the former group (3% vs. 14%, $P < 0.05$) [242].

Summary

Both repaglinide and nateglinide are effective in reducing the HbA_{1c} level. Their primary effect is on the postprandial plasma glucose level, with only a modest effect to decrease the fasting plasma glucose concentration. They work by augmenting insulin secretion. Repaglinide and nateglinide have no direct effect on plasma lipids. Weight gain and hypoglycemia may be observed with repaglinide, but appear to be less common with nateglinide. Repaglinide and nateglinide are considerably more expensive than the generic sulfonylureas.

COMBINATION THERAPY WITH ORAL AGENTS

Treatment Strategy

Combination therapy with oral hypoglycemic agents is indicated in two groups of type 2 diabetic patients: (1) individuals in whom monotherapy fails to achieve the recommended goal for glycemic control, HbA_{1c} <6.5–7.0%, and (2) drug-naïve diabetic patients in whom the starting HbA_{1c} is >9.0–9.5%. When the maximal dose of metformin [98] or a sulfonylurea [107, 108] is used as monotherapy, only ~20–25% of type 2 diabetic patients with a starting HbA_{1c} > 9.0% will achieve an HbA_{1c} level < 6.5–7.0%. Similarly, less than 20–25% of patients with type 2 diabetes with a starting HbA_{1c} >9.0% and who are treated with pioglitazone (45 mg/day) [243] or rosiglitazone (8 mg/day) [244] will achieve an acceptable level of glycemic control (HbA_{1c} <6.5–7.0%). An even smaller percentage of patients with type 2 diabetes will achieve acceptable glycemic control with acarbose [223, 226–229], or with nateglinide [245] or with repaglinide [246]. Therefore, most type 2 diabetic patients who present with an HbA_{1c} level > 9.0–9.5% will require combination therapy to reach recommended goals of glycemic control. Moreover, because type 2 diabetes mellitus is a progressive disease [48, 49, 73, 74, 84, 92] even patients with a good initial response to oral agents eventually will require a second (or third) medication.

Oral Combination Regimens

Metformin Plus Sulfonylurea

The most commonly used combination therapy in the United States and throughout the world is metformin plus a sulfonylurea [92, 152, 247, 248]. Addition of a sulfonylurea to metformin therapy gives a completely additive glucose-lowering effect [151, 152, 249]. Similarly, addition of metformin to sulfonylurea therapy gives a completely additive response, both with respect to the biguanide's glucose-lowering [152, 250–252] and lipid-lowering [98, 152] effects. Hermann and colleagues [152] (Figure 5) provided clinical validation of this approach in 144 poorly controlled [fasting plasma glucose level = 13.3 mmol/l (240 mg/dl)] diet-treated type 2 diabetic patients, who were randomly assigned to receive therapy with metformin, glyburide, or primary combination treatment with metformin plus glyburide. Doses were titrated upward to achieve a fasting plasma glucose level less than 6.7 mmol/l (121 mg/dl). All diabetic patients initially treated with monotherapy required addition of the second oral agent. After 6 months, decreases in HbA_{1c} and fasting blood glucose values were similar among patients who received metformin plus glyburide [$\Delta HbA_{1c} = 2.3$ percentage points; fasting plasma glucose = 6.1 mmol/l (110 mg/dl)], those who received glyburide plus metformin [$\Delta HbA_{1c} = 2.0$ percentage points; fasting plasma glucose = 4.8 mmol/l (86 mg/dl)], and those who received combination therapy from the onset [$\Delta HbA_{1c} = 2.2$ percentage points; fasting plasma glucose = 6.1 mmol/l (110 mg/dl)]. All patients had an HbA_{1c}

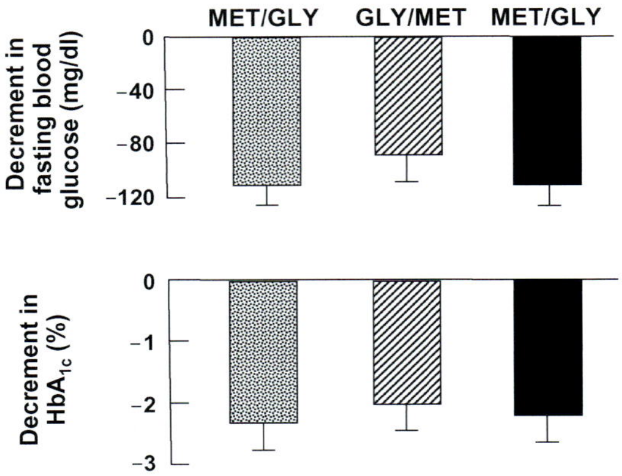

Figure 5 Comparison of initiating treatment with combined metformin-glyburide (MET/GLY) therapy (solid bars) versus monotherapy with glyburide (GLY/MET) (cross-hatched bars) or metformin (MET/GLY) (stippled bars) in poorly controlled type 2 diabetic patients. The goal of treatment was to reduce the fasting plasma glucose (FPG) concentration to <110 mg/dl. If the FPG remained above 110 mg/dl, patients who were started on metformin had glyburide added to their regimen, while patients who were started on glyburide had metformin added. After 6 months, all three groups achieved a similar level of glycemic control [152]. (Copyright © 1994 American Diabetes Association. Reprinted by permission of The American Diabetes Association from *Diabetes Care* 1994; 17: 1100–9)

value less than 7% and 50% of the entire group achieved a fasting blood glucose level less than 7 mmol/l (126 mg/dl). No weight gain was observed in any group.

In the largest published study of metformin plus sulfonylurea combination therapy, 422 type 2 diabetic patients who were poorly controlled [starting $HbA_{1c} = 8.7\%$ and fasting plasma glucose = 249 mg/dl (13.8 mmol/l)] with glyburide monotherapy were randomly assigned to have metformin or placebo added to their regimen [98] (Figure 6). In the placebo group, fasting plasma glucose and HbA_{1c} values increased by 14 mg/dl (0.8 mmol/l) and 0.2 percentage points, respectively, after 29 weeks. In the metformin-treated group, fasting plasma glucose and HbA_{1c} values decreased by 63 mg/dl (3.5 mmol/l) and 1.7 percentage points, respectively. Similar decreases were observed with metformin monotherapy in patients with poorly controlled diet-treated type 2 diabetes. About 25% of those patients who were poorly controlled achieved an HbA_{1c} value less than 7% with addition of metformin therapy. These results indicate that the hypoglycemic action of metformin is completely additive to that of sulfonylureas. In sulfonylurea-treated type 2 diabetic patients in whom the desired therapeutic goal is not reached or who experience secondary failure, it is important not to discontinue sulfonylurea therapy. The sulfonylurea is still working, but its hypoglycemic effect is too small to reduce the glucose level to the desired value. In such cases, sulfonylurea therapy should be continued and metformin should be added. Discontinuation of sulfonylurea therapy and substitution of metformin (or another oral agent) will not decrease the plasma glucose level below that observed with sulfonylurea monotherapy [98, 153].

A number of sulfonylurea metformin combination tablets currently are available in the United States and Europe. Of these Glucovance (metformin plus glyburide) has achieved the most widespread usage. When given to drug-naïve type 2 diabetic patients with a starting HbA_{1c} of 8.2%, Glucovance reduced the HbA_{1c} by 1.5 percentage points [253]. It is noteworthy that Glucovance decreased the HbA_{1c} by 0.5 percentage points more than when glyburide and metformin were administered as separate tablets [254]. The greater decrement in HbA_{1c} in Glucovance-treated patients resulted from an augmented insulin response [255] that resulted from increased bioavailability of glyburide in the Glucovance preparation [255]. Consistent with these observations, type 2 diabetic patients on chronic treatment with glyburide and metformin, as separate tablets, experienced an additional 0.6 percentage point reduction in HbA_{1c} when switched to Glucovance [256]. Metaglip, a combination tablet with metformin plus glipizide, also is available in the United States and is slightly less potent than Glucovance in reducing the HbA_{1c} [99], most likely because the Metaglip formulation does not result in increased glipizide bioavailability.

Metformin Plus Thiazolidinedione

The combination of a thiazolidinedione with metformin is another widely used combination for the treatment of

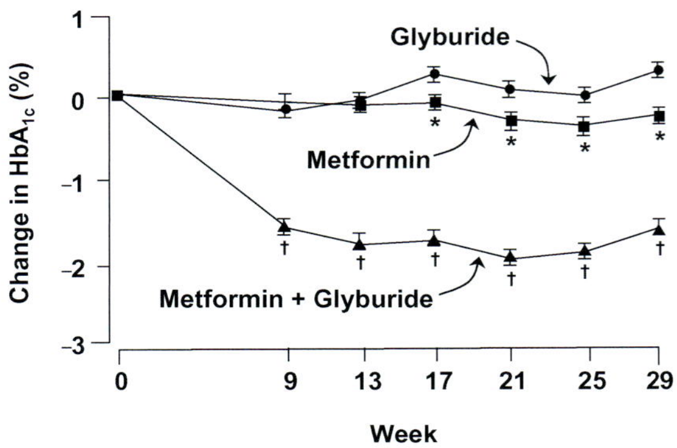

Figure 6 Time-related change in HbA_{1c} in sulfonylurea-treated patients who were (1) continued on glyburide therapy (solid circles), (2) switched to metformin therapy (solid squares), and (3) had metformin added to their glyburide treatment (solid triangles). $^*P < 0.01$ vs. glyburide. $^\dagger P < 0.001$ vs. both metformin and glyburide [98]. (Reproduced by permission of the Massachusetts Medical Society from DeFronzo RA, Goodman AM. Efficacy of metformin in patients with non-insulin-dependent diabetes mellitus. The Multicenter Metformin Study Group. *N Engl J Med* 1995; 333: 541–9. Copyright © 1995 Massachusetts Medical Society. All rights reserved)

type 2 diabetes [257] and is second only to metformin plus a sulfonylurea in the United States [258]. Because metformin has been shown to decrease myocardial infarction, stroke, and cardiovascular death in the UKPDS [49] and because the thiazolidinediones reverse multiple components of the insulin resistance syndrome [97], reduce carotid intimal thickness [259–261], and prevent restenosis of coronary artery stents [262, 263], the combination of metformin plus a thiazolidinedione might prove to be especially effective in preventing atherosclerotic cardiovascular disease in type 2 diabetic patients.

Einhorn and colleagues [264] studied the effects of pioglitazone plus metformin combination therapy in 328 poorly controlled ($HbA_{1c} > 8.0\%$), metformin-treated patients with type 2 diabetes in a 16-week, double-blind study with the option of enrollment into a continuing open-ended, open-label study. Patients were randomized to receive pioglitazone, 30 mg/day, plus metformin or placebo plus metformin. In the open-label extension all diabetic patients received pioglitazone, 30 mg/day (with optional titration to 45 mg/day), plus metformin. Patients receiving pioglitazone (30 mg/day) plus metformin had a significant decrease in HbA_{1c} ($\Delta = 0.83\%$) and fasting plasma glucose [38 mg/dl (2.1 mmol/l)] compared with metformin plus placebo treatment. Pioglitzone/metformin-treated patients experienced a greater reduction in plasma triglyceride concentration and a greater increase in HDL-cholesterol compared with metformin/placebo treatment. During the extension study, patients were treated with open-label pioglitazone (optional increase from 30 to 45 mg/day) plus metformin for 72 weeks, and the HbA_{1c} declined by 1.4% and the fasting plasma glucose by 63 mg/dl (3.5 mmol/l). The incidence of adverse events was similar in both groups. Similar results have been demonstrated with rosiglitazone plus metformin therapy in type 2 diabetic patients who were inadequately controlled with metformin alone [265]. In a randomized, double-blind, placebo-controlled trial of 348 poorly controlled type 2 diabetic patients [mean fasting plasma glucose = 12.0 mmol/l (216 mg/dl) and $HbA_{1c} = 8.8\%$], participants were randomized to receive metformin (2.5 g/day) plus placebo, metformin plus rosiglitazone (4 mg/day), or metformin plus rosiglitazone (8 mg/day) for 26 weeks. HbA_{1c} decreased by 1.0% in the metformin rosiglitazone (4 mg/day) group and by 1.2% in the metformin rosiglitazone (8 mg/day) group. The fasting plasma glucose concentration declined by 2.2 mmol/l (40 mg/dl) and 2.9 mmol/l (53 mg/dl), respectively. Of patients who received metformin rosiglitazone (8 mg/day), 28% achieved an HbA_{1c} value $\leq 7\%$. Insulin sensitivity and β-cell function, measured by HOMA, improved significantly with metformin rosiglitazone therapy in a dose-dependent manner. A rosiglitazone metformin combination tablet (Avandamet) is available in the United States and a pioglitazone metformin tablet currently is being evaluated.

Sulfonylurea Plus Thiazolidinedione

Two recently published studies have examined the effect of combination therapy with a thiazolidinedione plus a sulfonylurea in patients with poorly controlled type 2 diabetes [266, 267]. Five hundred seventy-six sulfonylurea-treated type 2 diabetic paitents ($HbA_{1c} \geq 8.0\%$) were randomly assigned to receive placebo, 15 mg/day of pioglitazone, or 30 mg/day of pioglitazone. Compared with placebo, HbA_{1c} decreased by 0.9% with 15 mg/d of pioglitazone and 1.3% with 30 mg/d of pioglitazone; fasting plasma glucose levels decreased by 39 mg/dl (2.2 mmol/l) and by 58 mg/dl (3.2 mmol/l), respectively. Both pioglitazone/sulfonylurea groups had significant decreases in plasma triglyceride levels (17 and 26% for the 15 mg/d and 30 mg/d groups, respectively) and increases in HDL-cholesterol levels (6 and 13%, respectively) compared with placebo/sulfonylurea. Pioglitazone was well tolerated, and the rates of adverse events were similar in all groups. Rosiglitazone has been examined in 574 poorly controlled [$HbA_{1c} = 9.2\%$ and fasting plasma glucose = 11.4 mmol/l (250 mg/dl)] sulfonylurea-treated type 2 diabetic patients who were randomized to receive placebo, 1 mg of rosiglitazone twice daily, or 2 mg of rosiglitazone twice daily for 26 weeks [267]. Rosiglitazone at doses of 2 and 4 mg/day plus sulphonylurea reduced HbA_{1c} by 0.6 and 1.0%, respectively, while the fasting plasma glucose declined by 24 mg/dl (1.4 mmol/l) and 44 mg/dl (2.4 mmol/l), respectively. Total cholesterol, LDL-cholesterol, and HDL-cholesterol increased in the rosiglitazone groups. The overall incidence of adverse experiences was similar in all three treatment groups, with no significant cardiac events, hypoglycemia, or hepatotoxicity.

Acarbose Plus Oral Hypoglycemic Agents

Numerous studies [268–270] have shown that addition of acarbose to sulfonylureas or to metformin therapy provides an additive effect. With acarbose monotherapy one observes decrements of 0.7–1.0% [226–232] in HbA_{1c} and similar decrements are observed when acarbose is added to the treatment regimen of metformin-treated or sulfonylurea-treated type 2 diabetic patients [268–270].

Nateglinide or Repaglinide Plus Oral Hypoglycemic Agents

Combined metformin plus repaglinide therapy has been shown to be effective in improving glycemic control in type 2 diabetic patients who are inadequately controlled with metformin alone [271]. Eighty-three metformin-treated patients with type 2 diabetes were randomly assigned to receive repaglinide in combination with metformin or to receive repaglinide or metformin monotherapy plus placebo. The HbA_{1c} value decreased by 1.4 percentage points, from 8.3 to 6.9% in the group that received repaglinide in combination with metformin; significant reductions in HbA_{1c} were not observed in patients receiving monotherapy with metformin or who were switched from metformin to repaglinide monotherapy. The glucose-lowering effect of nateglinide also has been shown to be additive to that of metformin [95]. In diet-treated patients with type 2 diabetes, combination therapy with metformin plus nateglinide resulted in significantly greater reductions in HbA_{1c} (1.4% vs. baseline) compared to that with nateglinide or metformin monotherapy.

The efficacy and safety of repaglinide versus nateglinide, when used in combination with metformin, has been examined in an open-label, parallel-group, randomized, multicenter trial of 192 type 2 diabetic patients [272]. After a 4-week metformin run-in period (doses escalated to 1000 mg b.i.d.), patients were randomized to receive the addition of repaglinide ($n = 96$) (1 mg/meal, maximum dose = 4 mg/meal) or nateglinide ($n = 96$) (120 mg/meal) for 16 weeks. Glucose, insulin, and glucagon were assessed after a liquid test meal at baseline and week 16. Treatment with repaglinide plus metformin produced significantly ($P < 0.001$) greater reductions in HbA_{1c} (1.3% vs. 0.7%) and fasting plasma glucose [39 mg/dl (2.2 mmol/l) vs. 21 mg/dl (1.2 mmol/l)]. Changes in the area under the curve of postprandial plasma glucose, insulin, and glucagon concentrations after a test meal were not significantly different between the two treatment groups.

The combination of repaglinide with thiazolidinediones also results in consistent decreases in the fasting plasma glucose concentration and HbA_{1c} [246]. A recent double-blind, placebo-controlled study [244] evaluated the efficacy of addition of nateglinide (120 mg prior to each meal) versus placebo in 402 poorly controlled (mean $HbA_{1c} = 8.4\%$) type 2 diabetic patients who were inadequately controlled with rosiglitazone, 8 mg/day. In patients randomized to receive nateglinide in combination with rosiglitazone, HbA_{1c} decreased by 0.8% versus placebo, and the fasting plasma glucose concentration decreased by 13 mg/dl (0.7 mmol/l). The 2-h postprandial glucose level declined by 49 mg/dl (2.7 mmol/l) in association with a 165 pmol/l (27 μU/ml) increase in the acute (30-min) plasma insulin concentration. These results demonstrate that by selectively augmenting the early insulin response and decreasing postprandial glucose excursions with nateglinide, a clinically meaningful improvement in overall glycemic control can be achieved in type 2 diabetic patients who are inadequately controlled with rosiglitazone monotherapy.

Treatment Failure with Two Oral Hypoglycemic Agents

If combination therapy with two oral hypoglycemic agents fails to produce acceptable glycemic control, several options are available (Figure 3): (1) addition of a third oral agent, (2) addition of bedtime long-acting neutral protamine Hagedorn (NPH) or Lantus insulin while maintaining therapy with one or two of the oral agents, and (3) institution of a mixed- (long- and short-acting) split (multiple injections) insulin regimen.

Two studies have examined the efficacy of triple oral agent therapy with metformin, sulfonylureas, and a thiazolidinedione. In poorly controlled type 2 diabetic patients (mean $HbA_{1c} = 9.6\%$), who were on maximum doses of metformin plus a sulfonylurea, addition of troglitazone versus placebo produced a 1.4% decrement in HbA_{1c}, indicating that the thiazolidinedione produced a completely additive effect when added to metformin/sulfonylurea combination therapy [273] (Figure 7). In a recent study addition of rosiglitazone (8 mg/day) to the treatment regimen of poorly controlled type 2 diabetic patients receiving maximum doses of glimepiride and metformin produced a decrement of 1.4 percentage points in HbA_{1c} [274].

Triple oral therapy (thiazolidinedione in combination with metformin plus sulfonylurea therapy) has not been compared with bedtime NPH or Lantus in combination with oral agents. However, a recent study [275] has shown that triple oral agent therapy is comparable in efficacy to treatment with a mixed-split insulin (70/30) regimen administered twice daily in combination with metformin in type 2 diabetic patients who were inadequately controlled with two oral agents. However, the failure rate, as well as the cost of treatment, was higher in patients receiving triple oral agent therapy compared to those receiving the mixed-split insulin regimen in combination with metformin. This result is not surprising, since one eventually reaches a maximum dose of oral agents, whereas the dose of insulin can continue to be titrated. We favor the use of triple oral agent combination therapy (metformin plus a sulfonylurea plus a thiazolidinedione) because of the potential antiatherogenic benefits of metformin and the thaizolidinedione, as long as the HbA_{1c}level can be maintained at less than 6.5–7.0%. In diabetic patients in whom triple oral agent therapy produces an initial good response, but the therapeutic efficacy begins to wane with time, the physician can add a long-acting bedtime insulin preparation. When adding bedtime insulin to triple oral agent therapy, we discontinue the sulfonylurea and continue only one of the insulin sensitizers. We prefer continuation of metformin over the thiazolidinedione, since insulin/thiazolidinedione-treated patients with type 2 diabetes are more likely to experience weight (fat) gain and edema [176–178]. It is important to reduce the dose of the thiazolidinedione slowly, while titrating up the dose of bedtime long-acting insulin, in order to maintain the HbA_{1c} at the desired goal (HbA_{1c} <6.5–7.0%). A large multicenter Veterans Administration trial [276] in the United States has shown that if bedtime insulin (generally, we do not exceed 60–70 U) plus metformin does not produce the requisite level of glycemic

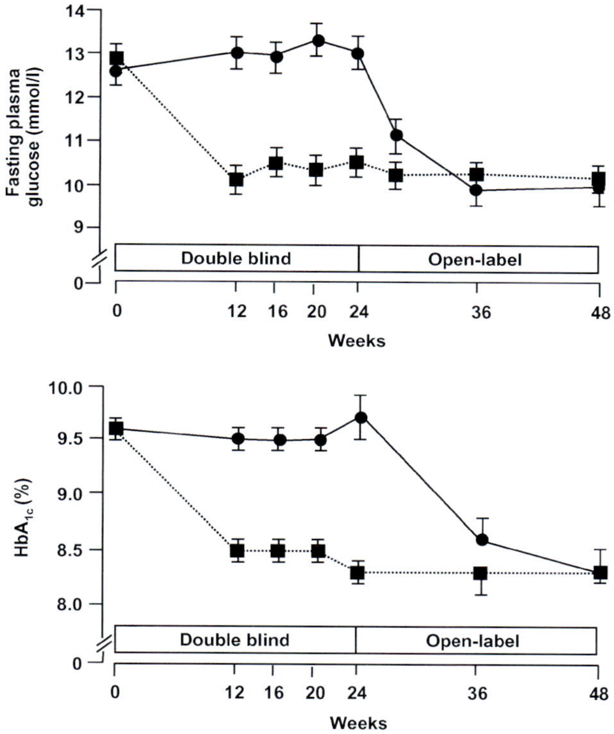

Figure 7 The effect of addition of troglitazone or placebo triple oral agent treatment in type 2 diabetic patients inadequately controlled on metformin/sulfonylurea combination therapy. Changes in fasting plasma glucose (Top) and HbA_{1c} (bottom) levels from baseline to 6 and 12 months. The troglitazone/troglitazone group (dotted-lines) received 400 mg/day of troglitazone for the entire 48 weeks; the placebo/troglitazone group (solid lines) received placebo for the first 24 weeks (double-blind period) and troglitazone, 400 mg/day, for the last 24 weeks (open-label period) Data are presented as the mean ± SE [273]. (Reproduced by permission of the American College of Physicians from Yale JF, Valiquett TR, Ghazzi MN, Owens-Grillo JK, Whitcomb RW, Foyt HL. The effect of a thiazolidinedione drug, troglitazone, on glycemia in patients with type 2 diabetes mellitus poorly controlled with sulfonylurea and metformin. A multicenter, randomized, double-blind, placebo-controlled trial. *Ann Intern Med* 2001; 134: 737–45. Copyright © 2001 American College of Physicians)

control, a thiazolidinedione (rosiglitazone) can be effectively combined with the bedtime insulin/metformin regimen. Alternatively, the physician can initiate a mixed-split insulin regimen while continuing the metformin.

If satisfactory glycemic control is not attained with combined metformin sulfonylurea (or other double oral agent) therapy many diabetes experts would recommend addition of bedtime insulin and continuation of metformin therapy (rather than triple oral agent therapy). This approach is supported by results from a study by Yki-Järvinen and colleagues [75]. Use of insulin as monotherapy requires large doses (>80–100 U/day) to achieve normoglycemia, and weight gain (10–20 lb) commonly occurs [48, 49, 75, 79, 82, 84, 85, 277, 278]. Because combination therapy with bedtime insulin plus metformin effectively reduces elevated plasma glucose levels, requires considerably less insulin, thereby minimizing weight gain [75, 277–280]), and often allows for fewer insulin injections per day [281], this approach has achieved widespread acceptance (see discussion below).

COMBINATION THERAPY WITH ORAL AGENTS PLUS BEDTIME INSULIN

The effectiveness of addition of bedtime insulin to the treatment regimen of type 2 diabetic patients in whom acceptable glycemic control is not attained with oral agents alone or in combination is well documented. In such patients, the elevated fasting plasma glucose level is caused by incomplete suppression of basal hepatic glucose production by sulfonylurea, metformin, and/or thiazolidinedione [104, 105, 146, 155]. Although the oral agent is still working, it is not producing the desired hypoglycemic effect. Bedtime insulin takes advantage of the differential sensitivity of hepatic compared with peripheral tissues to insulin [15–20]. Low doses of insulin effectively suppress hepatic glucose production and have a much smaller effect to stimulate muscle glucose uptake [282]. By giving a modest dose of intermediate long-acting insulin (such as NPH or Lantus insulin) at bedtime, the elevated basal rate of hepatic glucose production can be reduced to normal, and the likelihood of hypoglycemia will decrease because muscle glucose uptake is only minimally stimulated.

A meta-analysis of 16 randomized, placebo-controlled trials comparing sulfonylureas plus insulin with placebo plus insulin showed significantly lower fasting plasma glucose and HbA_{1c} values, a lower daily insulin dose, and absent or minimal weight gain in patients who received bedtime insulin plus daytime sulfonylurea [279]. Similar findings have been reported in other trials [282–284]. However, none of these studies were designed to examine the superiority of bedtime intermediate-acting insulin over a mixed-split insulin regimen. Two large, well-designed trials have addressed this question. In the Finnish Multicenter Insulin Study [278], 153 poorly controlled type 2 diabetic patients on sulfonylurea monotherapy were randomly assigned to treatment with sulfonylurea alone, sulfonylurea plus NPH insulin given at 7 a.m., sulfonylurea plus NPH insulin given at 9 p.m., NPH plus regular insulin given before breakfast and dinner, or NPH insulin given at 9 p.m. and regular insulin given with each meal. All insulin regimens improved glycemic control similarly, but the insulin dose was 50–60% lower in the two groups that received sulfonylurea plus once-daily NPH insulin. Bedtime insulin plus sulfonylurea caused significantly less weight gain and a 50% lower level of daylong serum-free insulin concentration. Similar results were reported in a

Swedish study of patients with type 2 diabetes who were poorly controlled with glyburide and subsequently were randomly assigned to receive bedtime NPH insulin or a multiple-dose insulin regimen [280]. In type 2 diabetic patients inadequately controlled with metformin alone, addition of bedtime NPH insulin compared with switching to a multiple-insulin injection regimen produced equivalent glycemic control [285]. However, the group that received metformin plus bedtime NPH insulin required 50% less insulin and experienced no weight gain.

In summary, addition of bedtime intermediate-acting insulin to either sulfonylurea or metformin monotherapy is a safe and effective way of normalizing the daylong glycemic profile, while minimizing weight gain and reducing the insulin dose by 50–60% compared with a multiple-injection insulin regimen. Because of metformin's insulin-sensitizing [50, 142–145] and antiatherogenic [50] effects, we prefer the combination of bedtime insulin plus metformin.

Several well-designed studies have compared the addition of a second oral agent with addition of bedtime insulin in patients with poorly controlled type 2 diabetes receiving oral agent monotherapy. Combined oral agent therapy (metformin plus sulfonylurea) was as effective in improving glycemic control as was the addition of bedtime NPH insulin to a sulfonylurea [284, 286–288]. An advantage of the metformin/sulfonylurea combination was less weight gain (or even weight loss) and improvement in dyslipidemia. Hermann and colleagues [152] have also shown that most newly diagnosed type 2 diabetic patients [fasting plasma glucose = 12.2–13.3 mmol/l (220–240 mg/dl)] can achieve the desired level of blood glucose control (HbA_{1c} < 7.0%) with combined sulfonylurea/metformin therapy and similar findings were reported in the UKPDS [48, 92]. In sulfonylurea/metformin-treated diabetic patients in whom the desired therapeutic goal is not reached, options include addition of a third oral agent (a thiazolidinedione or acarbose; since nateglinide and repaglinide work on the β-cell to augment insulin secretion, they would be expected to have no additive effect to sulfonylurea therapy), addition of bedtime NPH or Lantus insulin, or a switch to a multiple-injection insulin regimen. The last two options were explored in a study by Yki-Järvinen and colleagues [75] (Figure 8). Ninety-six type 2 diabetic patients who were poorly controlled with sulfonylureas, metformin, or both were assigned to receive (1) bedtime NPH insulin plus glibenclamide (glyburide) (15 mg/day), (2) bedtime NPH insulin plus metformin (2 g/day), (3) bedtime NPH insulin plus metformin plus sulfonylurea, or (4) bedtime NPH insulin plus morning NPH insulin. After 1 year, glycemic control was substantially better in the group receiving bedtime insulin plus metformin (mean decrement in HbA_{1c} = 2.5 percentage points) than in all other groups, including the group receiving bedtime insulin plus sulfonylurea plus

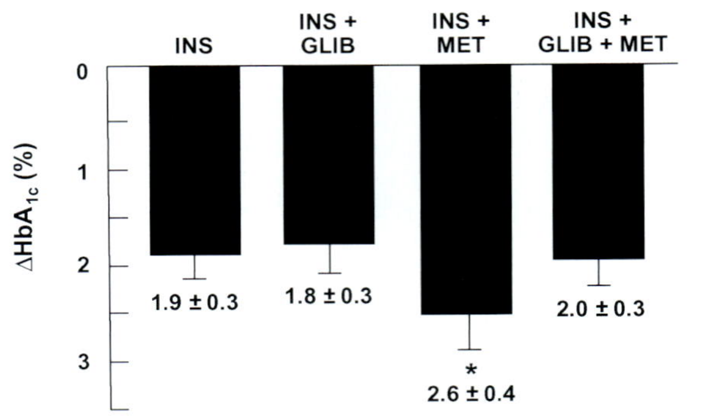

Figure 8 Effect of bedtime NPH insulin treatment on the decrement in HbA_{1c} in poorly controlled type 2 diabetic patients receiving metformin/sulfonylurea treatment (FINFAT study). After the start of bedtime NPH insulin, diabetic patients were randomized to receive: (1) metformin plus glibenclamide (glyburide), (2) metformin alone, (3) glibenclamide (glyburide) alone, (4) no oral agents [75]. $^*P < 0.05$ vs. all other groups. INS = insulin; GLIB = glibenclamide; MET = metformin. (Reproduced by permission of the American College of Physicians from Yki-Jarvinen H, Ryysy L, Nikkila K, Tulokas T, Vanamo R, Heikkila M. Comparison of bedtime insulin regimens in patients with type 2 diabetes mellitus. A randomized, controlled trial. *Ann Intern Med* 1999; 130: 389–96. Copyright © 1999 American College of Physicians)

metformin (mean decrement in HbA_{1c} = 1.9 percentage points). Better control in the group that received bedtime insulin plus metformin was attributed to less frequent hypoglycemia and the absence of significant weight gain (0.9 kg at 1 year). In contrast, mean weight gain was 3.9 kg in the insulin/sulfonylurea group, 3.6 kg in the insulin/sulfonylurea/metformin group, and 4.6 kg in the bedtime insulin/morning insulin group.

OVERALL SUMMARY

In summary, we recommend the following overall approach to therapy in patients with type 2 diabetes. Begin therapy with metformin because of its established efficacy [49, 98], proven antiatherogenic effects [49, 50], and insulin-sensitizing action [50, 142, 143]. If metformin cannot be tolerated (because of gastrointestinal side effects) or is contraindicated (because of impaired renal or hepatic function), we prefer to initiate therapy with a thiazolidinedione because of their proven efficacy [97, 111], established insulin-sensitizing action [176–180], beneficial effects on multiple components of the insulin resistance syndrome [97], potential antiatherogenic benefit [259–263], and ability to preserve β-cell function [191–194]. If the desired level of glycemic control (HbA_{1c} <6.5–7.0%) is not achieved with monotherapy, we would add a thiazolidinedione to metformin (Figure 3), although the most commonly employed combination in the United States and worldwide remains metformin plus a sulfonylurea

(Figure 3). If additional therapy is required, we prefer addition of a third oral agent (metformin plus thiazolidinedione plus sulfonylurea), although addition of bedtime NPH or Lantus insulin is an equally established and effective regimen (Figure 3). Alternately, the patient can be switched to a mixed-split insulin regimen. Because, in type 2 diabetic patients, insulin monotherapy requires very high doses (>100 U/day), which usually are associated with significant weight gain, we favor maintaining an insulin sensitzer, preferably metformin, when initiating a mixed-split insulin regimen (Figure 3).

ADDITION OF ORAL HYPOGLYCEMIC AGENTS IN INSULIN-TREATED TYPE 2 DIABETIC PATIENTS

It is common to encounter patients with poorly controlled type 2 diabetes who are taking large doses of insulin. Both thiazolidinediones and metformin have received FDA approval for use in these patients in the United States. The primary therapeutic goal is to improve the daylong glycemic profile (HbA_{1c} <6.5–7.0%). A secondary treatment goal is to reduce the insulin dose, the number of insulin injections, or both, but this should not be attempted until optimal glycemic control has been achieved. In a large multicenter trial [213], 566 poorly controlled (HbA_{1c} >8.0%), insulin-treated patients with type 2 diabetes were randomized to receive 15 mg/day of pioglitazone, 30 mg/day of pioglitazone, or placebo for 16 weeks. As per study protocol, the insulin dose was to remain unchanged, but could be decreased in response to hypoglycemia. Patients receiving pioglitazone (15 or 30 mg/day) showed statistically significant decreases (relative to baseline and placebo) in HbA_{1c} (1.0 and 1.3%, respectively) and fasting plasma glucose concentration [35 mg/dl (1.9 mmol/l) and 48 mg/dl (2.7 mmol/l)], respectively. Pioglitazone (both 15 mg/d and 30 mg/d) treatment was associated with significant increases in HDL-cholesterol (by 7 and 9%, respectively) The 30 mg/day dose also significantly reduced the plasma triglyceride concentration by 24%. No changes in total cholesterol or LDL-cholesterol levels were observed. Weight gain, hypoglycemia, and edema were more frequent among patients receiving insulin plus pioglitazone. No cases of congestive heart failure were reported in either of the pioglitazone-treated groups. Raskin et al. [212] studied the effect of addition of rosiglitazone to the treatment regimen of type 2 diabetic patients who were inadequately controlled on insulin monotherapy. After 8 weeks of insulin standardization and placebo run-in, 319 type 2 diabetic patients (baseline HbA_{1c} 9.0%) were randomized to 26 weeks of treatment with rosiglitazone (4 or 8 mg/day) or placebo. Insulin dose could be down-titrated for safety reasons only. The primary end point was reduction of HbA_{1c} from baseline. Rosiglitazone, both 4 and 8 mg/day, significantly improved glycemic control, which was unchanged in the placebo group. Rosiglitazone, 8 mg/day, plus insulin resulted in a mean reduction of 1.2% in HbA_{1c}, despite a 12% reduction in insulin dose. Mean total cholesterol, LDL-cholesterol, and HDL-cholesterol increased in both rosiglitazone-treatment groups, while the plasma triglyceride concentration did not change significantly from baseline. More patients in the insulin/rosiglitazone groups reported edema (13% with insulin/rosiglitazone, 4 mg/day, and 16% with insulin/rosiglitazone, 8 mg/day) than in the insulin/placebo group (4.7%). Congestive heart failure was reported in two patients in each insulin/rosiglitazone group. Body weight increased significantly in both rosiglitazone groups (mean increase = 4.0 and 5.3 kg, respectively) compared to the placebo group (mean increase = 0.9 kg). The US FDA has cautioned that both rosiglitazone and pioglitazone should be used cautiously in combination with insulin in patients with even mild degrees of congestive heart failure (NYHA classes 1 and 2). In patients with more severe congestive heart failure (NYHA class 3 or 4) thiazolidinedione therapy is contraindicated.

In a large prospective study of 234 patients with poorly controlled, insulin-treated type 2 diabetes, addition of 600 mg/day of troglitazone decreased the fasting plasma glucose level by 49 mg/dl (2.7 mmol/l), the HbA_{1c} value by 1.4 percentage points, and the insulin dose by 29% [289]. Similar observations were reported by Buse and associates [290]. However, in both of these studies, troglitazone therapy was associated with significant increases in body weight and LDL-cholesterol level.

Metformin also has been widely used to improve glycemic control in insulin-treated type 2 diabetic patients. In a study by Giuliano and coworkers [291], 50 insulin-treated patients with poorly controlled type 2 diabetes were randomly assigned to receive metformin or placebo for 6 months. In the metformin-treated group, HbA_{1c} values decreased by 1.9 percentage points, fasting plasma glucose levels decreased by 92 mg/dl (5.1 mmol/l), and the insulin dose was reduced by 24%. Two double-blind, placebo-controlled studies performed in insulin-treated patients with poorly controlled type 2 diabetes also showed significant improvements in glycemic control and reductions in the insulin dose and number of injections following the addition of metformin [281, 292]. In all three of these studies [281, 291–293], body weight decreased significantly or did not increase, and levels of LDL- and total cholesterol decreased. Bell et al. [293] initiated combination therapy with metformin plus a sulfonylurea in 55 poorly controlled, insulin-treated type 2 diabetic patients and were able to completely withdraw insulin therapy in 42 of 55 (76%) patients. After 1 year, HbA_{1c} values decreased by 1.3 percentage points in these 42 patients, and body weight declined by 2.3 kg. Collectively, these results [281, 291–293] indicate that addition of metformin to insulin therapy in patients with poorly controlled type 2 diabetes is very effective in improving glycemic control and reducing insulin requirements. Importantly, unlike thiazolidinediones, metformin does not cause weight (fat) gain or fluid retention/edema when added to insulin therapy. For these reasons, we prefer the combination of insulin/metformin over insulin/thiazolidinedione.

The safety and efficacy of 4 months of treatment with insulin alone, insulin plus metformin (2 g/day), and insulin plus troglitazone (600 mg/day) has been compared in 88 poorly controlled (HbA_{1c} 8.7%) type 2 diabetic patients [294]. HbA_{1c} levels decreased in all groups (insulin alone to 7.0%, insulin plus metformin to 7.1%, and insulin plus troglitazone to 6.4%). However, the insulin dose increased by 55 U/day in the insulin monotherapy group ($P < 0.0001$ vs. baseline, metformin, and troglitazone), remained unchanged in the insulin/metformin group, and decreased by 13 U/day in the insulin/troglitazone group. Similar increments in body weight were observed in the insulin monotherapy ($\Delta = 4.4$ kg) and troglitazone/insulin ($\Delta = 4.4$ kg) groups ($P < 0.0001$ baseline) compared to the absence of significant weight gain in the insulin/metformin group ($\Delta = 0.5$ kg). Diabetic subjects taking metformin experienced significantly fewer hypoglycemic episodes than did the insulin monotherapy and insulin/troglitazone groups. The investigators concluded that although troglitazone was the most effective combination in lowering HbA_{1c} levels and the total daily insulin dose, treatment with insulin plus metformin was advantageous in avoiding weight gain and hypoglycemia. On the basis of the results of these studies, we recommend adding metformin rather than a thiazolidinedione in poorly controlled patients with type 2 diabetes receiving insulin treatment.

Addition of acarbose in insulin-treated type 2 diabetic patients has been examined [119, 295] and the reduction in HbA_{1c} values (0.4–0.7 percentage points) and daily insulin dose (0–10%) is modest compared with that achieved with addition of either a thiazolidinedione or metformin. Slightly greater decrements in HbA_{1c} (1.0–1.2%) have been reported with the addition of repaglinide to insulin therapy in patients with type 2 diabetes [296]. However, there was no decrease in the patients' daily insulin dose.

REFERENCES

1. Harris MI, Flegal KM, Cowie CC, Eberhardt MS, Goldstein DE, Little RR, Wiedmeyer HM, Byrd-Holt DD. Prevalence of diabetes, impaired fasting glucose, and impaired glucose tolerance in U.S. adults. The Third National Health and Nutrition Examination Survey. 1988–1994 *Diabetes Care* 1998; 21: 518–24.
2. Narayan KM, Boyle JP, Thompson TJ, Sorensen SW, Williamson DF. Lifetime risk for diabetes mellitus in the United States. *JAMA* 2003; 290: 1884–90.
3. Mokdad AH, Ford ES, Bowman BA, Dietz WH, Vinicor F, Bales VS, Marks JS. The continuing epidemics of obesity and diabetes in the United States. *JAMA* 2001; 286: 1195–200.
4. Zimmet P. The burden of type 2 diabetes: are we doing enough? *Diabetes Metab* 2003; 29: 6S9–18.
5. Stern MP, Gonzalez C, Mitchell BD, Villalpando E, Haffner SM, Hazuda HP. Genetic and environmental determination of type II diabetes in Mexico City and San Antonio. *Diabetes* 1992; 41: 484–92.
6. Klein R. Hyperglycemia and microvascular and macrovascular disease in diabetes. *Diabetes Care* 1995; 18: 258–68.
7. Molitch ME, DeFronzo RA, Franz MJ, Keane WF, Mogensen CE, Parving HH, for American Diabetes Association. Diabetic nephropathy. *Diabetes Care* 2003; 26 (suppl 1): S94–8.
8. Vinik AI, Park TS, Stansberry KB, Pittenger GL. Diabetic neuropathies. *Diabetologia* 2000; 43: 957–73.
9. Kannel WB, McGee DL. Diabetes and cardiovascular risk factors: the Framingham Study. *Circulation* 1979; 59: 8–13.
10. Wei M, Gaskill SP, Haffner SM, Stern MP. Effects of diabetes and level of glycemia on all-cause and cardiovascular mortality: The San Antonio Heart Study. *Diabetes Care* 1998; 21: 1167–72.
11. Rubin RJ, Altman WM, Mendelson DN. Health care expenditures for people with diabetes mellitus, 1992. *J Clin Endocrinol Metab* 1994; 78: 809A–F.
12. American Diabetes Association. Standards of medical care for patients with diabetes mellitus. *Diabetes Care* 2003; 26: S33–50.
13. European Diabetes Policy Group. Guidelines for diabetes care: a desktop guide to type II diabetes mellitus. International Diabetes Federation (European Region). *Diabet Med* 1999; 16: 716–30.
14. American Association of Clinical Endocrinologists. The American Association of Clinical Endocrinologists Medical Guidelines for the Management of Diabetes Mellitus: the AACE system of intensive diabetes self-management—2000 update. *Endocr Pract* 2000; 6: 43–84.
15. Bajaj M, DeFronzo RA. Metabolic and molecular basis of insulin resistance. *J Nucl Cardiol* 2003; 10: 311–23.
16. DeFronzo RA. Lilly Lecture 1987. The triumvirate: beta-cell, muscle, liver. A collusion responsible for NIDDM. *Diabetes* 1988; 37: 667–87.
17. DeFronzo RA. Pathogenesis of type 2 diabetes: metabolic and molecular implications for identifying diabetes genes. *Diabetes Rev* 1997; 5: 177–269.
18. DeFronzo RA. Pharmacologic therapy for type 2 diabetes mellitus. *Ann Intern Med* 1999; 131: 281–303.
19. Del Prato S, Matsuda M, Simonson DC, Groop LC, Sheehan P, Leonetti F, Bonadonna RC, DeFronzo RA. Studies on the mass action effect of glucose in NIDDM and IDDM: evidence for glucose resistance. *Diabetologia* 1997; 40: 687–97.
20. DeFronzo RA, Ferrannini E, Simonson DC. Fasting hyperglycemia in non-insulin dependent diabetes mellitus: contributions of excessive hepatic glucose production and impaired tissue glucose uptake. *Metabolism* 1989; 38: 387–95.
21. Groop LC, Bonadonna RC, Del Prato S, Ratheiser K, Zyck K, DeFronzo RA. Glucose and free fatty acid metabolism in non-insulin-dependent diabetes mellitus.

Evidence for multiple sites of insulin resistance. *J Clin Invest* 1989; 84: 205–13.

22. Magnusson I, Rothman DL, Katz LD, Shulman RG, Shulman GI. Increased rate of gluconeogenesis in type II diabetes mellitus. A ^{13}C nuclear magnetic resonance study. *J Clin Invest* 1992; 90: 1323–7.
23. Gastaldelli A, Toschi E, Pettiti M, Frascerra S, Quinones-Galvan A, Sironi AM, Natali A, Ferrannini E. Effect of physiological hyperinsulinemia on gluconeogenesis in nondiabetic subjects and in type 2 diabetic patients. *Diabetes* 2001; 50: 1807–12.
24. Bonadonna RC, Del Prato S, Bonora E, Saccomani MP, Gulli G, Natali A, et al. Roles of glucose transport and glucose phosphorylation in muscle insulin resistance of NIDDM. *Diabetes* 1996; 45: 915–25.
25. Mitrakou A, Kelley D, Veneman T, Jenssen T, Pangburn T, Reilly J, Gerich J. Contribution of abnormal muscle and liver glucose metabolism to postprandial hyperglycemia in NIDDM. *Diabetes* 1990; 9: 1381–90.
26. Ferrannini E, Simonson DC, Katz LD, Reichard G Jr, Bevilacqua S, Barrett EJ, et al. The disposal of an oral glucose load in patients with non-insulin-dependent diabetes. *Metabolism* 1988; 37: 79–85.
27. DeFronzo RA, Ferrannini E, Simonson DC. Fasting hyperglycemia in non-insulin-dependent diabetes mellitus: contributions of excessive hepatic glucose production and impaired tissue glucose uptake. *Metabolism* 1989; 38: 387–95.
28. Jeppesen J, Zhou MY, Chen YD, Reaven GM. Effect of metformin on postprandial lipemia in patients with fairly to poorly controlled NIDDM. *Diabetes Care* 1994; 17: 1093–9.
29. Polonsky KS. Lilly Lecture 1994. The beta-cell in diabetes: from molecular genetics to clinical research. *Diabetes* 1995; 44: 705–17.
30. Ferrannini E, Gastaldelli A, Miyazaki Y, Matsuda M, Pettiti M, Natali A, Mari A, DeFronzo RA. Predominant role of reduced beta-cell sensitivity to glucose over insulin resistance in impaired glucose tolerance. *Diabetologia* 2003; 46: 1211–9.
31. Jensen C, Cnop M, Hull R, Fujimoto W, Kahn S, for the American Diabetes Association GENNID Study Group. ß-Cell function is a major contributor to oral glucose tolerance in high-risk relatives of four ethnic groups in the U.S. *Diabetes* 2002; 51: 2170–8.
32. Bergman RN, Finegood DT, Kahn SE. The evolution of beta-cell dysfunction and insulin resistance in type 2 diabetes. *Eur J Clin Invest* 2002; 32 (suppl 3): 35–45.
33. Weyer C, Bogardus C, Mott DM, Pratley RE. The natural history of insulin secretory dysfunction and insulin resistance in the pathogenesis of type 2 diabetes mellitus. *J Clin Invest* 1999; 104: 787–94.
34. Tripathy D, Carlsson M, Almgren P, Isomaa B, Taskinen MR, Tuomi T, Groop LC. Insulin secretion and insulin sensitivity in relation to glucose tolerance: lessons from the Botnia Study. *Diabetes* 2000; 49: 975–80.
35. Saad MF, Knowler WC, Pettitt DJ, Nelson RG, Mott DM, Bennett PH. Sequential changes in serum insulin concentration during development of non-insulin-dependent diabetes. *Lancet* 1989; 1: 1356–9.
36. McGarry J. Banting lecture 2001: dysregulation of fatty acid metabolism in the etiology of type 2 diabetes. *Diabetes* 2002; 51: 7–18.
37. Reaven GM. The fourth musketeer—from Alexandre Dumas to Claude Bernard. *Diabetologia* 1995; 38: 3–13.
38. Thiebaud D, DeFronzo RA, Jacot E, Golay A, Acheson K, Maeder E, Jequier E, Felber JP. Effect of long chain triglyceride infusion on glucose metabolism in man. *Metabolism* 1982; 31: 1128–36.
39. Boden G, Jadali F, White J, Liang Y, Mozzoli M, Chen X, Coleman E, Smith C. Effects of fat on insulin-stimulated carbohydrate metabolism in normal men. *J Clin Invest* 1991; 88: 960–6.
40. Chen X, Iqbal N, Boden G. The effects of free fatty acids on gluconeogenesis and glycogenolysis in normal subjects. *J Clin Invest* 1999; 103: 365–72.
41. Ferrannini E, Barrett EJ, Bevilacqua S, DeFronzo RA. Effect of fatty acids on glucose production and utilization in man. *J Clin Invest* 1983; 72: 1737–47.
42. Kashyap S, Belfort R, Gastaldelli A, Pratipanawatr T, Berria R, Pratipanawatr W, Bajaj M, Mandarino L, DeFronzo R, Cusi K. A sustained increase in plasma free fatty acids impairs insulin secretion in nondiabetic subjects genetically predisposed to develop type 2 diabetes. *Diabetes* 2003; 52: 2461–74.
43. Carpentier A, Mittelman S, Lamarche B, Bergman R, Giacca A, Lewis G. Acute enhancement of insulin secretion by FFA in humans is lost with prolonged FFA elevation. *Am J Physiol* 1999; 39: E1055–66.
44. The Diabetes Control and Complications Trial Research Group. The effect of intensive treatment of diabetes on the development and progression of long-term complications in insulin-dependent diabetes mellitus. *N Engl J Med* 1993; 329: 977–86.
45. Ferrannini E, Haffner SM, Mitchell BD, Stern MP. Hyperinsulinaemia: the key feature of a cardiovascular and metabolic syndrome. *Diabetologia* 1991; 34: 416–22.
46. The Diabetes Control and Complications Trial Research Group. The absence of a glycemic threshold for the development of long-term complications: the perspective of the Diabetes Control and Complications Trial. *Diabetes* 1996; 45: 1289–98.
47. Ohkubo Y, Kishikawa H, Araki E, Miyata T, Isami S, Motoyoshi S, Kojima Y, Furuyoshi N, Shichiri M. Intensive insulin therapy prevents the progression of diabetic microvascular complications in Japanese patients with non-insulin-dependent diabetes mellitus: a randomized prospective 6-year study. *Diabetes Res Clin Pract* 1995; 28: 103–17.
48. The UK Prospective Diabetes Study (UKPDS) Group. Intensive blood-glucose control with sulphonylureas or insulin compared with conventional treatment and risk of complications in patients with type 2 diabetes (UKPDS 33). *Lancet* 1998; 352: 837–53.
49. The UK Prospective Diabetes Study (UKPDS) Group. Effect of intensive blood-glucose control with metformin on complications in overweight patients with type 2 diabetes (UKPDS 34). *Lancet* 1998; 352: 854–65.
50. Cusi K, DeFronzo RA. Metformin: a review of its metabolic effects. *Diabetes Rev* 1998; 6: 89–131.
51. DeFronzo RA, Ferrannini E. Insulin resistance. A multifaceted syndrome responsible for NIDDM, obesity, hypertension, dyslipidemia, and atherosclerotic cardiovascular disease. *Diabetes Care* 1991; 14: 173–94.
52. American Diabetes Association. Standards of medical care for patients with diabetes mellitus. *Diabetes Care* 1998; 21 (suppl 1): S23–31.
53. Report of the Expert Committee on the diagnosis and classification of diabetes mellitus. *Diabetes Care* 1997; 20: 1183–97.

54. Report of a WHO Consultation. Definition, diagnosis and classification of diabetes mellitus and its complications. Part 1: Diagnosis and classification of diabetes mellitus. World Health Organization, Department of Noncommunicable Disease Surveillance: Geneva 1999.
55. Reaven GM, Laws A. Insulin resistance, compensatory hyperinsulinemia, and coronary heart disease. *Diabetologia* 1994; 37: 948–52.
56. Expert Panel on Detection, Evaluation, and Treatment of High Blood Cholesterol in Adults. Executive summary of the Third Report of the National Cholesterol Education Program (NCEP) Expert Panel on Detection, Evaluation, and Treatment of High Blood Cholesterol in Adults (Adult Treatment Panel III). *JAMA* 2001; 285: 2486–97.
57. Balkau B, Charles MA, Drivsholm T, Borch-Johnsen K, Wareham N, Yudkin JS, Morris R, Zavaroni I, van Dam R, Feskins E, Gabriel R, Diet M, Nilsson P, Hedblad B, for European Group for the Study of Insulin Resistance (EGIR). Frequency of the WHO metabolic syndrome in European cohorts, and an alternative definition of an insulin resistance syndrome. *Diabetes Metab* 2002; 28: 364–76.
58. Lehto S, Ronnemaa T, Haffner SM, Pyorala K, Kallio V, Laakso M. Dyslipidemia and hyperglycemia predict coronary heart disease events in middle-aged patients with NIDDM. *Diabetes* 1997; 46: 1354–9.
59. Turner RC, Millns H, Neil HA, Stratton IM, Manley SE, Matthews DR, Holman RR. Risk factors for coronary artery disease in non-insulin dependent diabetes mellitus: United Kingdom Prospective Diabetes Study (UKPDS: 23). *BMJ* 1998; 316: 823–8.
60. Assmann G, Schulte H. The Prospective Cardiovascular Munster (PROCAM) study: prevalence of hyperlipidemia in persons with hypertension and/or diabetes mellitus and the relationship to coronary heart disease. *Am Heart J* 1988; 116: 1713–24.
61. Curb JD, Pressel SL, Cutler JA, Savage PJ, Applegate WB, Black H, Camel G, Davis BR, Frost PH, Gonzalez N, Guthrie G, Oberman A, Rutan GH, Stamler J. Effect of diuretic-based antihypertensive treatment on cardiovascular disease risk in older diabetic patients with isolated systolic hypertension. Systolic Hypertension in the Elderly Program Cooperative Research Group. *JAMA* 1996; 276: 1886–92.
62. Pyorala K, Pedersen TR, Kjekshus J, Faergeman O, Olsson AG, Thorgeirsson G. Cholesterol lowering with simvastatin improves prognosis of diabetic patients with coronary heart disease. A subgroup analysis of the Scandinavian Simvastatin Survival Study (4S) Group. *Diabetes Care* 1997; 20: 614–20.
63. The UK Prospective Diabetes Study (UKPDS) Group. Tight blood pressure control and risk of macrovascular and microvascular complications in type 2 diabetes: UKPDS 38. *BMJ* 1998; 317: 703–13.
64. Goldberg RB, Mellies MJ, Sacks FM, Moye LA, Howard BV, Howard WJ, Davis BR, Cole TG, Pfeffer MA, Braunwald E, The Care Investigators. Cardiovascular events and their reduction with pravastatin in diabetic and glucose-intolerant myocardial infarction survivors with average cholesterol levels: subgroup analyses in the cholesterol and recurrent events (CARE) trial. *Circulation* 1998; 98: 2513–9.
65. Rubins HB, Robins SJ, Collins D, Nelson DB, Elam MB, Schaefer EJ, Faas FH, Anderson JW. Diabetes, plasma insulin, and cardiovascular disease: subgroup analysis from the Department of Veterans Affairs high-density lipoprotein intervention trial (VA-HIT). *Arch Intern Med* 2002; 162: 2597–604.
66. Gaede P, Vedel P, Larsen N, Jensen GV, Parving HH, Pedersen O. Multifactorial intervention and cardiovascular disease in patients with type 2 diabetes. *N Engl J Med* 2003; 348: 383–93.
67. Manson JE, Colditz GA, Stampfer MJ, Willett WC, Rosner B, Monson RR, Speizer FE, Hennekens CH. A prospective study of obesity and risk of coronary heart disease in women. *N Engl J Med* 1990; 322: 882–9.
68. Hensrud DD. Dietary treatment and long-term weight loss and maintenance in type 2 diabetes. *Obes Res* 2001; 9 (suppl 4): 348S–53S.
69. Wing RR, Goldstein MG, Acton KJ, Birch LL, Jakicic JM, Sallis JF Jr, Smith-West D, Jeffery RW, Surwit RS. Behavioral science research in diabetes: lifestyle changes related to obesity, eating behavior, and physical activity. *Diabetes Care* 2001; 24: 117–23.
70. Weyer C, Tataranni PA, Bogardus C, Pratley RE. Insulin resistance and insulin secretory dysfunction are independent predictors of worsening of glucose tolerance during each stage of type 2 diabetes development. *Diabetes Care* 2001; 24: 89–94.
71. Haffner SM, Miettinen H, Gaskill SP, Stern MP. Decreased insulin secretion and increased insulin resistance are independently related to the 7-year risk of NIDDM in Mexican-Americans. *Diabetes* 1995; 44: 1386–91.
72. Gastaldelli A, Ferrannini E, Miyazaki Y, Matsuda M, DeFronzo RA. Beta cell dysfunction and glucose intolerance: results from the San Antonio Metabolism (SAM) study. *Diabetologia* (in press).
73. Klimt CR, Knatterud GL, Meinert CL, Prout TE. A study of the effect of hypoglycemic agents on vascular complications in patients with adult-onset diabetes, I: Design, methods and baseline characteristics. The University Group Diabetes Program. *Diabetes* 1970; 19 (suppl): 747–88.
74. Meinert CL, Knatterud GL, Prout TE, Klimt CR. A study of the effects of hypoglycemic agents on vascular complications in patients with adult-onset diabetes, II: Mortality results. *Diabetes* 1970; 19 (suppl): 789–830.
75. Yki-Jarvinen H, Ryysy L, Nikkila K, Tulokas T, Vanamo R, Heikkila M. Comparison of bedtime insulin regimens in patients with type 2 diabetes mellitus. A randomized, controlled trial. *Ann Intern Med* 1999; 130: 389–96.
76. Edelman SV, Henry RR. Insulin therapy for normalizing glycosylated hemoglobin in type II diabetes. Application, benefits, and risks. *Diabetes Rev* 1995; 3: 308–34.
77. Sasali A, Leahy JL. Insulin therapy for type 2 diabetes. *Curr Diab Rep* 2003; 3: 378–85.
78. Abraira C, Colwell JA, Nuttall FQ, Sawin CT, Nagel NJ, Comstock JP, Emanuele NV, Levin SR, Henderson W, Lee HS. Veterans Affairs Cooperative Study on glycemic control and complications in type II diabetes (VA CSDM). Results of the feasibility trial. Veterans Affairs Cooperative Study in Type II Diabetes. *Diabetes Care* 1995; 18: 1113–23.
79. Henry RR, Gumbiner B, Ditzler T, Wallace P, Lyon R, Glauber HS. Intensive conventional insulin therapy for type II diabetes. Metabolic effects during a 6-mo outpatient trial. *Diabetes Care* 1993; 16: 21–31.
80. Hayward RA, Manning WG, Kaplan SH, Wagner EH, Greenfield S. Starting insulin therapy in patients with type 2 diabetes: effectiveness, complications, and resource utilization. *JAMA* 1997; 278: 1663–9.

81. Harris MI. Medical care for patients with diabetes. Epidemiologic aspects. *Ann Intern Med* 1996; 124: 117–22.
82. Kudlacek S, Schernthaner G. The effect of insulin treatment on HbA_{1c}, body weight and lipids in type 2 diabetic patients with secondary-failure to sulfonylureas. A five year follow-up study. *Horm Metab Res* 1992; 24: 478–83.
83. Sinha A, Formica C, Tsalamandris C, Panagiotopoulos S, Hendrich E, DeLuise M, Seeman E, Jerums G. Effect of insulin on body composition in patients with insulin-dependent and non-insulin-dependent diabetes. *Diabet Med* 1996; 13: 40–6.
84. The United Kingdom Prospective Diabetes Study (UKPDS) Group. UKPDS 24: a 6-year, randomized, controlled trial comparing sulfonylurea, insulin, and metformin therapy in patients with newly diagnosed type 2 diabetes that could not be controlled with diet therapy. *Ann Intern Med* 1998; 128: 165–75.
85. Yki-Jarvinen H, Ryysy L, Kauppila M, Kujansuu E, Lahti J, Marjanen T, Niskanen L, Rajala S, Salo S, Seppala P, Tulokas T, Viikari J, Taskinen MR. Effect of obesity on the response to insulin therapy in noninsulin-dependent diabetes mellitus. *J Clin Endocrinol Metab* 1997; 82: 4037–43.
86. DeFronzo RA, Soman V, Sherwin RS, Hendler R, Felig P. Insulin binding to monocytes and insulin action in human obesity, starvation, and refeeding. *J Clin Invest* 1978; 62: 204–13.
87. Pi-Sunyer FX. Medical hazards of obesity. *Ann Intern Med* 1993; 119: 655–60.
88. Rossetti L. Glucose toxicity: the implications of hyperglycemia in the pathophysiology of diabetes mellitus. *Clin Invest Med* 1995; 18: 255–60.
89. Ilkova H, Glaser B, Tunckale A, Bagriacik N, Cerasi E. Induction of long-term glycemic control in newly diagnosed type 2 diabetic patients by transient intensive insulin treatment. *Diabetes Care* 1997; 20: 1353–6.
90. Kayashima T, Yamaguchi K, Konno Y, Nanimatsu H, Aragaki S, Shichiri M. Effects of early introduction of intensive insulin therapy on the clinical course in non-obese NIDDM patients. *Diabetes Res Clin Pract* 1995; 28: 119–25.
91. Colwell JA. Should we use intensive insulin therapy after oral agent failure in type II diabetes? *Diabetes Care* 1996; 19: 896–8.
92. The UK Prospective Diabetes Study (UKPDS) Group. UKPDS 28: a randomized trial of efficacy of early addition of metformin in sulfonylurea-treated type 2 diabetes. *Diabetes Care* 1998; 21: 87–92.
93. American Diabetes Association. The pharmacologic treatment of hyperglycemia in NIDDM. *Diabetes Care* 1996; 19 (suppl 1): 553–61.
94. Wolffenbuttel BH, Landgraf R, for the Dutch and German Repaglinide Study Group. A 1-year multicenter randomized double-blind comparison of repaglinide and glyburide for the treatment of type 2 diabetes. *Diabetes Care* 1999; 22: 463–7.
95. Horton ES, Clinkingbeard C, Gatlin M, Foley J, Mallows S, Shen S. Nateglinide alone and in combination with metformin improves glycemic control by reducing mealtime glucose levels in type 2 diabetes. *Diabetes Care* 2000; 23: 1660–5.
96. Holman RR, Cull CA, Turner RC. A randomized double-blind trial of acarbose in type 2 diabetes shows improved glycemic control over 3 years (U.K. Prospective Diabetes Study 44). *Diabetes Care* 1999; 22: 960–4.
97. Pavo I, Jermendy G, Varkonyi TT, Kerenyi Z, Gyimesi A, Shoustov S, Shestakova M, Herz M, Johns D, Schluchter BJ, Festa A, Tan MH. Effect of pioglitazone compared with metformin on glycemic control and indicators of insulin sensitivity in recently diagnosed patients with type 2 diabetes. *J Clin Endocrinol Metab* 2003; 88: 1637–45.
98. DeFronzo RA, Goodman AM, for the Multicenter Metformin Study Group. Efficacy of metformin in patients with non-insulin-dependent diabetes mellitus. *N Engl J Med* 1995; 333: 541–9.
99. Goldstein BJ, Pans M, Rubin CJ. Multicenter, randomized, double-masked, parallel-group assessment of simultaneous glipizide/metformin as second-line pharmacologic treatment for patients with type 2 diabetes mellitus that is inadequately controlled by a sulfonylurea. *Clin Ther* 2003; 25: 890–903.
100. Marre M, Howlett H, Lehert P, Allavoine T. Improved glycaemic control with metformin–glibenclamide combined tablet therapy (Glucovance) in Type 2 diabetic patients inadequately controlled on metformin. *Diabet Med* 2002; 19: 673–80.
101. Bell DS. Why I initiate therapy with two insulin sensitizers in patients with type 2 diabetes. *Endocr Pract* 2003; 9: 98–101.
102. Proks P, Reimann F, Green N, Gribble F, Ashcroft F. Sulfonylurea stimulation of insulin secretion. *Diabetes* 2002; 51 (suppl 3): S368–76.
103. Rorsman P. The pancreatic beta-cell as a fuel sensor: an electrophysiologist's viewpoint. *Diabetologia* 1997; 40: 487–95.
104. Simonson DC, Ferrannini E, Bevilacqua S, Smith D, Barrett E, Carlson R, DeFronzo RA. Mechanism of improvement in glucose metabolism after chronic glyburide therapy. *Diabetes* 1984; 33: 838–45.
105. Best JD, Judzewitsch RG, Pfeifer MA, Beard JC, Halter JB, Porte D Jr. The effect of chronic sulfonylurea therapy on hepatic glucose production in non-insulin-dependent diabetes. *Diabetes* 1982; 31: 333–8.
106. Beck-Nielsen H, Hother-Nielsen O, Pedersen O. Mechanism of action of sulfonylureas with special reference to the extrapancreatic effect: an overview. *Diabet Med* 1988; 5: 613–20.
107. Simonson DC, Kourides IA, Feinglos M, Shamoon H, Fischette CT, for the Glipizide Gastrointestinal Therapeutic System Study Group. Efficacy, safety, and dose–response characteristics of glipizide gastrointestinal therapeutic system on glycemic control and insulin secretion in NIDDM. Results of two multicenter, randomized, placebo-controlled clinical trials. *Diabetes Care* 1997; 20: 597–606.
108. Rosenstock J, Samols E, Muchmore DB, Schneider J, for the Glimepiride Study Group. Glimepiride, a new once-daily sulfonylurea. A double-blind placebo-controlled study of NIDDM patients. *Diabetes Care* 1996; 19: 1194–9.
109. Blaum CS, Velez L, Hiss RG, Halter JB. Characteristics related to poor glycemic control in NIDDM patients in community practice. *Diabetes Care* 1997; 20: 7–11.
110. American Diabetes Association. Implications of the United Kingdom Prospective Diabetes Study. *Diabetes Care* 2003; 26: S28–32.
111. Lebovitz HE, Dole JF, Patwardhan R, Rappaport EB, Freed MI, for the Rosiglitazone Clinical Trials Study Group. Rosiglitazone monotherapy is effective in patients

with type 2 diabetes. *J Clin Endocrinol Metab* 2001; 86: 280–8.

112. Groop LC. Sulfonylureas in NIDDM. *Diabetes Care* 1992; 15: 737–54.
113. Turner R, Stratton I, Horton V, Manley S, Zimmet P, Mackay IR, Shattock M, Bottazzo GF, Holman R, for the UK Prospective Diabetes Study Group. UKPDS 25: autoantibodies to islet-cell cytoplasm and glutamic acid decarboxylase for prediction of insulin requirement in type 2 diabetes. *Lancet* 1997; 350: 1288–93.
114. Haupt E, Laube F, Loy H, Schoffling K. Secondary failures in modern therapy of diabetes mellitus with blood glucose lowering sulfonamides. *Med Klin* 1977; 72: 1529–36.
115. Camerini-Davalos R, CLozano-astaneda O, Marble A. Five year experience with tolbutamide. *Metabolism* 1962; 11 (suppl): 74–80.
116. Balodimos MC, Camerini-Davalos R, Marble A. Nine years' experience with tolbutamide in the treatment of diabetes. *Metabolism* 1966; 11: 957–70.
117. Groop L, Groop PH, Stenman S, Saloranta C, Totterman KJ, Fyhrquist F, Melander A. Comparison of pharmacokinetics, metabolic effects and mechanisms of action of glyburide and glipizide during long-term treatment. *Diabetes Care* 1987; 10: 671–8.
118. Groop L, Luzi L, Melander A, Groop PH, Ratheiser K, Simonson DC, DeFronzo RA. Different effects of glibenclamide and glipizide on insulin secretion and hepatic glucose production in normal and NIDDM subjects. *Diabetes* 1987; 36: 1320–8.
119. Jeppesen J, Zhou MY, Chen YD, Reaven GM. Effect of glipizide treatment on postprandial lipaemia in patients with NIDDM. *Diabetologia* 1994; 37: 781–7.
120. Lebovitz HE, Melander A. Sulfonylureas: basic aspects and clinical uses. In Alberti KG, Zimmet P, DeFronzo RA (eds), *International Textbook of Diabetes Mellitus*, 2d edn. New York: Wiley, 1997; pp 817–40.
121. Fanning EL, Selwyn BJ, Larme AC, DeFronzo RA. Efficacy of diabetes treatment with a nurse case manager following treatment algorithms versus primary care physicians. *Diabetes Care* 2003; 52 (suppl 1): A261.
122. Berger W, Caduff F, Pasquel M, Rump A. The relatively frequent incidence of severe sulfonylurea-induced hypoglycemia in the last 25 years in Switzerland. Results of 2 surveys in Switzerland in 1969 and 1984. *Schweiz Med Wochenschr* 1986; 116: 145–51.
123. van Staa T, Abenhaim L, Monette J. Rates of hypoglycemia in users of sulfonylureas. *J Clin Epidemiol* 1997; 50: 735–41.
124. Burge MR, Schmitz-Fiorentino K, Fischette C, Qualls CR, Schade DS. A prospective trial of risk factors for sulfonylurea-induced hypoglycemia in type 2 diabetes mellitus. *JAMA* 1998; 279: 137–43.
125. Schor S. The University Group Diabetes Program. A statistician looks at the mortality results. *JAMA* 1971; 217: 1673–5.
126. Kilo C, Miller L, Williamson J. The crux of the UGDP. Spurious results and biologically inappropriate data analysis. *Diabetologia* 1980; 18: 179–85.
127. Ohneda A, Maruhama Y, Itabashi H, Oikawa SI, Kobayashi T, Horigome K, Chiba M, Kai Y, Sakai T, Okuguchi F, Nihei J. Vascular complications and long-term administration of oral hypoglycemic agents in patients with diabetes mellitus. *Tohoku J Exp Med* 1978; 124: 205–22.
128. Jarrett RJ, McCartney P, Keen H. The Bedford survey: ten year mortality rates in newly diagnosed diabetics, borderline diabetics and normoglycaemic controls and risk indices for coronary heart disease in borderline diabetics. *Diabetologia* 1982; 22: 79–84.
129. Paasikivi J, Wahlberg F. Preventive tolbutamide treatment and arterial disease in mild hyperglycaemia. *Diabetologia* 1971; 7: 323–7.
130. Leibowitz G, Cerasi E. Sulphonylurea treatment of NIDDM patients with cardiovascular disease: a mixed blessing? *Diabetologia* 1996; 39: 503–14.
131. American Diabetes Association. Policy statement: the UGDP controversy. *Diabetes Care* 1979; 2: 1–3.
132. Aronson D, Mittleman MA, Burger AJ. Effects of sulfonylurea hypoglycemic agents and adenosine triphosphate dependent potassium channel antagonists on ventricular arrhythmias in patients with decompensated heart failure. *Pacing Clin Electrophysiol* 2003; 26: 1254–61.
133. Brady PA, Terzic A. The sulfonylurea controversy: more questions from the heart. *J Am Coll Cardiol* 1998; 31: 950–6.
134. Ashcroft FM, Gribble FM. Tissue-specific effects of sulfonylureas: lessons from studies of cloned K(ATP) channels. *J Diabetes Complications* 2000; 14: 192–6.
135. Hu S, Wang S, Dunning BE. Tissue selectivity of antidiabetic agent nateglinide: study on cardiovascular and beta-cell K(ATP) channels. *J Pharmacol Exp Ther* 1999; 291: 1372–9.
136. Spallarossa P, Schiavo M, Rossettin P, Cordone S, Olivotti L, Cordera R, Brunelli C. Sulfonylurea treatment of type 2 diabetic patients does not reduce the vasodilator response to ischemia. *Diabetes Care* 2001; 24: 738–42.
137. Bijlstra PJ, den Arend JA, Lutterman JA, Russel FG, Thien T, Smits P. Blockade of vascular ATP-sensitive potassium channels reduces the vasodilator response to ischaemia in humans. *Diabetologia* 1996; 39: 1562–8.
138. Brady PA, Jovanovic A. The sulfonylurea controversy: much ado about nothing or cause for concern? *J Am Coll Cardiol* 2003; 42: 1022–5.
139. Klamann A, Sarfert P, Launhardt V, Schulte G, Schmiegel WH, Nauck MA. Myocardial infarction in diabetic vs. non-diabetic subjects: survival and infarct size following therapy with sulfonylureas (glibenclamide). *Eur Heart J* 2000; 21: 220–9.
140. Bailey CJ, Turner RC. Metformin. *N Engl J Med* 1996; 334: 574–9.
141. Salpeter S, Greyber E, Pasternak G, Salpeter E. Risk of fatal and nonfatal lactic acidosis with metformin use in type 2 diabetes mellitus. *Cochrane Database Syst Rev* 2003; (2): CD002967.
142. DeFronzo RA, Barzilai N, Simonson DC. Mechanism of metformin action in obese and lean noninsulin-dependent diabetic subjects. *J Clin Endocrinol Metab* 1991; 73: 1294–301.
143. Stumvoll N, Nurjhan N, Perriello G, Dailey G, Gerich JE. Metabolic effects of metformin in non-insulin-dependent diabetes mellitus. *N Engl J Med* 1995; 333: 550–4.
144. Johnson AB, Webster JM, Sum CF, Heseltine L, Argyraki M, Cooper BG, Taylor R. The impact of metformin therapy on hepatic glucose production and skeletal muscle glycogen synthase activity in overweight type II diabetic patients. *Metabolism* 1993; 42: 1217–22.
145. Wollen N, Bailey CJ. Inhibition of hepatic gluconeogenesis by metformin. Synergism with insulin. *Biochem Pharmacol* 1988; 37: 4353–8.
146. Widen EI, Eriksson JG, Groop LC. Metformin normalizes nonoxidative glucose metabolism in insulin-resistant

normoglycemic first-degree relatives of patients with NIDDM. *Diabetes* 1992; 41: 354–8.
147. Rossetti L, DeFronzo RA, Gherzi R, Stein P, Andraghetti G, Falzetti G, Shulman GI, Klein-Robbenhaar E, Cordera R. Effect of metformin treatment on insulin action in diabetic rats: in vivo and in vitro correlations. *Metabolism* 1990; 39: 425–35.
148. Klip A, Leiter LA. Cellular mechanism of action of metformin. *Diabetes Care* 1990; 13: 696–704.
149. Zhou G, Myers R, Li Y, Chen Y, Shen X, Fenyk-Melody J, Wu M, Ventre J, Doebber T, Fujii N, Musi N, Hirshman MF, Goodyear LJ, Moller DE. Role of AMP-activated protein kinase in mechanism of metformin action. *J Clin Invest* 2001; 108: 1167–74.
150. Musi N, Hirshman MF, Nygren J, Svanfeldt M, Bavenholm P, Rooyackers O, Zhou G, Williamson JM, Ljunqvist O, Efendic S, Moller DE, Thorell A, Goodyear LJ. Metformin increases AMP-activated protein kinase activity in skeletal muscle of subjects with type 2 diabetes. *Diabetes* 2002; 51: 2074–81.
151. Campbell IW, Howlett HC. Worldwide experience of metformin as an effective glucose-lowering agent: a meta-analysis. *Diabetes Metab Rev* 1995; 11 (suppl 1): S57–62.
152. Hermann LS, Schersten B, Bitzen PO, Kjellstrom T, Lindgarde F, Melander A. Therapeutic comparison of metformin and sulfonylurea, alone and in various combinations. A double-blind controlled study. *Diabetes Care* 1994; 17: 1100–9.
153. Garber AJ, Duncan TG, Goodman AM, Mills DJ, Rohlf JL. Efficacy of metformin in type II diabetes: results of a double-blind, placebo-controlled, dose-response trial. *Am J Med* 1997; 103: 491–7.
154. Johansen K. Efficacy of metformin in the treatment of NIDDM. Meta-analysis. *Diabetes Care* 1999; 22: 33–7.
155. Reaven GM, Johnston P, Hollenbeck CB, Skowronski R, Zhang JC, Goldfine ID, Chen YD. Combined metformin-sulfonylurea treatment of patients with noninsulin-dependent diabetes in fair to poor glycemic control. *J Clin Endocrinol Metab* 1992; 74: 1020–6.
156. Riccio A, Del Prato S, Vigili de Kreutzenberg S, Tiengo A. Glucose and lipid metabolism in non-insulin-dependent diabetes. Effect of metformin. *Diabete Metab* 1991; 17: 180–4.
157. Perriello G, Misericordia P, Volpi E, Santucci A, Santucci C, Ferrannini E, Ventura MM, Santeusanio F, Brunetti P, Bolli GB. Acute antihyperglycemic mechanisms of metformin in NIDDM: evidence for suppression of lipid oxidation and hepatic glucose production. *Diabetes* 1994; 43: 920–8.
158. Gustafson A, Bjorntorp P, Fahlen M. Metformin administration in hyperlipidemic states. *Acta Med Scand* 1971; 190: 491–4.
159. Fontbonne A, Charles MA, Juhan-Vague I, Bard JM, Andre P, Isnard F, Cohen JM, Grandmottet P, Vague P, Safar ME, Eschwege E, for the BIGPRO Study Group. The effect of metformin on the metabolic abnormalities associated with upper-body fat distribution. *Diabetes Care* 1996; 19: 920–6.
160. Vague P, Juhan-Vague I, Alessi MC, Badier C, Valadier J. Metformin decreases the high plasminogen activator inhibition capacity, plasma insulin and triglyceride levels in non-diabetic obese subjects. *Thromb Haemost* 1987; 57: 326–8.
161. Nagi DK, Yudkin JS. Effects of metformin on insulin resistance, risk factors for cardiovascular disease, and plasminogen activator inhibitor in NIDDM subjects. A study of two ethnic groups. *Diabetes Care* 1993; 16: 621–9.
162. Charles MA, Eschwege E, Grandmottet P, Isnard F, Cohen JM, Bensoussan JL, Berche H, Chapiro O, Andre P, Vague P, Juhan-Vague I, Bard JM, Safar M. Treatment with metformin of non-diabetic men with hypertension, hypertriglyceridaemia and central fat distribution: the BIGPRO 1.2 trial. *Diabetes Metab Res Rev* 2000; 16: 2–7.
163. Fujioka K, Pans M, Joyal S. Glycemic control in patients with type 2 diabetes mellitus switched from twice-daily immediate-release metformin to a once-daily extended-release formulation. *Clin Ther* 2003; 25: 515–29.
164. Campbell IW. Metformin and the sulphonylureas: the comparative risk. *Horm Metab Res Suppl* 1985; 15: 105–11.
165. Wiholm BE, Myrhed M. Metformin-associated lactic acidosis in Sweden 1977–1991. *Eur J Clin Pharmacol* 1993; 44: 589–91.
166. Misbin RI, Green L, Stadel BV, Gueriguian JL, Gubbi A, Fleming GA. Lactic acidosis in patients treated with metformin. *N Engl J Med* 1998; 338: 265–6.
167. Turner RC, Holman R, Stratton I. Correspondence. The UK Prospective Diabetes Study. *Lancet* 1999; 352: 1934.
168. Spiegelman BM. PPAR-gamma: adipogenic regulator and thiazolizinedione receptor. *Diabetes* 1998; 47: 507–14.
169. Benson S, Wu J, Padmanabhan S, Kurtz TW, Pershadsingh HA. Peroxisome proliferator-activated receptor (PPAR)-gamma expression in human vascular smooth muscle cells: inhibition of growth, migration, and c-fos expression by the peroxisome proliferator-activated receptor (PPAR)-gamma activator troglitazone. *Am J Hypertens* 2000; 13: 74–82.
170. Ricote M, Li AC, Willson TM, Kelly CJ, Glass CK. The peroxisome proliferator-activated receptor-gamma is a negative regulator of macrophage activation. *Nature* 1998; 391: 79–82.
171. Brunmair B, Gras F, Neschen S, Roden M, Wagner L, Waldhausl W, Furnsinn C. Direct thiazolidinedione action on isolated rat skeletal muscle fuel handling is independent of peroxisome proliferator-activated receptor-gamma-mediated changes in gene expression. *Diabetes* 2001; 50: 2309–15.
172. Olefsky JM. Treatment of insulin resistance with peroxisome proliferator-activated receptor gamma agonists. *J Clin Invest* 2000; 106: 467–72.
173. Hallakou S, Doare F, Foufelle F, Kergoat M, Guerre-Millo M, Berthault MF, Dugail I, Morin J, Auwerx J, Ferre P. Pioglitazone induces in vivo adipocyte differentiation in obese Zucker *fa/fa* rat. *Diabetes* 1997; 46: 1393–9.
174. Lambe KG, Tugwood JD. A human peroxisome-proliferator-activated receptor-gamma is activated by inducers of adipogenesis, including thiazolidinedione drugs. *Eur J Biochem* 1996 239: 1–7.
175. Okuno A, Tamemoto H, Tobe K, Ueki K, Mori Y, Iwamoto K, Umesono K, Akanuma Y, Fujiwara T, Horikoshi H, Yazaki Y, Kadowaki T. Troglitazone increases the number of small adipocytes without the change of white adipose tissue mass in obese Zucker rats. *J Clin Invest* 1998; 101: 1354–61.
176. Miyazaki Y, Glass L, Triplitt C, Matsuda M, Cusi K, Mahankali A, Mahankali S, Mandarino LJ, DeFronzo RA. Effect of rosiglitazone on glucose and non-esterified

fatty acid metabolism in Type II diabetic patients. *Diabetologia* 2001; 44: 2210–9.

177. Miyazaki Y, Mahankali A, Matsuda M, Glass L, Mahankali S, Ferrannini E, Cusi K, Mandarino LJ, DeFronzo RA. Improved glycemic control and enhanced insulin sensitivity in type 2 diabetic subjects treated with pioglitazone. *Diabetes Care* 2001; 24: 710–9.
178. Miyazaki Y, Mahankali A, Matsuda M, Mahankali S, Hardies J, Cusi K, Mandarino LJ, DeFronzo RA. Effect of pioglitazone on abdominal fat distribution and insulin sensitivity in type 2 diabetic patients. *J Clin Endocrinol Metab* 2002; 87: 2784–91.
179. Mayerson AB, Hundal RS, Dufour S, Lebon V, Befroy D, Cline GW, Enocksson S, Inzucchi SE, Shulman GI, Petersen KF. The effects of rosiglitazone on insulin sensitivity, lipolysis, and hepatic and skeletal muscle triglyceride content in patients with type 2 diabetes. *Diabetes* 2002; 51: 797–802.
180. Bajaj M, Suraamornkul S, Pratipanawatr T, Hardies LJ, Pratipanawatr W, Glass L, Cersosimo E, Miyazaki Y, DeFronzo RA. Pioglitazone reduces hepatic fat content and augments splanchnic glucose uptake in patients with type 2 diabetes. *Diabetes* 2003; 52: 1364–70.
181. de Souza CJ, Eckhardt M, Gagen K, Dong M, Chen W, Laurent D, Burkey BF. Effects of pioglitazone on adipose tissue remodeling within the setting of obesity and insulin resistance. *Diabetes* 2001; 50: 1863–71.
182. Ye JM, Frangioudakis G, Iglesias MA, Furler SM, Ellis B, Dzamko N, Cooney GJ, Kraegen EW. Prior thiazolidinedione treatment preserves insulin sensitivity in normal rats during acute fatty acid elevation: role of the liver. *Endocrinology* 2002; 143: 4527–35.
183. Oakes ND, Camilleri S, Furler SM, Chisholm DJ, Kraegen EW. The insulin sensitizer, BRL 49653, reduces systemic fatty acid supply and utilization and tissue lipid availability in the rat. *Metabolism* 1997; 46: 935–42.
184. Solomon SS, Usdan LS, Palazzolo MR. Mechanisms involved in tumor necrosis factor-alpha induction of insulin resistance and its reversal by thiazolidinedione(s). *Am J Med Sci* 2001; 22: 75–8.
185. Lee Y, Hirose H, Ohneda M, Johnson JH, McGarry JD, Unger RH. Beta-cell lipotoxicity in the pathogenesis of non-insulin-dependent diabetes mellitus of obese rats: impairment in adipocyte–beta-cell relationships. *Proc Natl Acad Sci USA* 1994; 91: 10878–82.
186. Shimabukuro M, Zhou YT, Levi M, Unger RH. Fatty acid-induced beta cell apoptosis: a link between obesity and diabetes. *Proc Natl Acad Sci USA* 1998; 95: 2498–502.
187. Higa M, Zhou YT, Ravazzola M, Baetens D, Orci L, Unger RH. Troglitazone prevents mitochondrial alterations, beta cell destruction, and diabetes in obese prediabetic rats. *Proc Natl Acad Sci USA* 1999; 96: 11513–8.
188. Dubois M, Pattou F, Kerr-Conte J, Gmyr V, Vandewalle B, Desreumaux P, Auwerx J, Schoonjans K, Lefebvre J. Expression of peroxisome proliferator-activated receptor γ (PPARγ) in normal human pancreatic islet cells. *Diabetologia* 2000; 43: 1165–9.
189. Qvigstad E, Mostad IL, Bjerve KS, Grill VE. Acute lowering of circulating fatty acids improves insulin secretion in a subset of type 2 diabetes subjects. *Am J Physiol Endocrinol Metab* 2003; 284: E129–37.
190. Cavaghan MK, Ehrmann DA, Byrne MM, Polonsky KS. Treatment with oral antidiabetic agent troglitazone improves ß-cell responses to glucose in subjects with impaired glucose tolerance. *J Clin Invest* 1997; 100: 530–7.
191. Buchanan TA, Xiang AH, Peters RK, Kjos SL, Marroquin A, Goico J, Ochoa C, Tan S, Berkowitz K, Hodis HN, Azen SP. Preservation of pancreatic beta-cell function and prevention of type 2 diabetes by pharmacological treatment of insulin resistance in high-risk hispanic women. *Diabetes* 2002; 51: 2796–803.
192. Xiang A, Peters R, Kjos S, Goico J, Marroquin A, Ochoa C, Tan S, Buchanan T. Continued protection from diabetes during treatment of the TRIPOD cohort with pioglitazone. *Diabetes* 2003; 52 (suppl 1): A75.
193. Miyazaki Y, Matsuda M, DeFronzo RA. Dose–response effect of pioglitazone on insulin sensitivity and insulin secretion in type 2 diabetes. *Diabetes Care* 2002; 25: 517–23.
194. The DPP Research Group. Prevention of type 2 diabetes with troglitazone in the Diabetes Prevention Program (DPP). *Diabetes* 2003; 52 (suppl 1): A58.
195. Aronoff S, Rosenblatt S, Braithwaite S, Egan JW, Mathisen AL, Schneider RL, for the Pioglitazone 001 Study Group. Pioglitazone hydrochloride monotherapy improves glycemic control in the treatment of patients with type 2 diabetes: a 6-month randomized placebo-controlled dose-response study. *Diabetes Care* 2000; 23: 1605–11.
196. Phillips LS, Grunberger G, Miller E, Patwardhan R, Rappaport EB, Salzman A, for the Rosiglitazone Clinical Trials Study Group. Once- and twice-daily dosing with rosiglitazone improves glycemic control in patients with type 2 diabetes. *Diabetes Care* 2001; 24: 308–15.
197. van Wijk JPH, de Koning EJP, Martens EP, Rabelink TJ. Thiazolidinediones and blood lipids in type 2 diabetes. *Arterioscler Thromb Vasc Biol* 2003; 23: 1744–9.
198. Winkler K, Konrad T, Fullert S, Friedrich I, Destani R, Baumstark MW, Krebs K, Wieland H, Marz W. Pioglitazone reduces atherogenic dense LDL particles in nondiabetic patients with arterial hypertension: a double-blind, placebo-controlled study. *Diabetes Care* 2003; 26: 2588–94.
199. Freed MI, Ratner R, Marcovina SM, Kreider MM, Biswas N, Cohen BR, Brunzell JD, for the Rosiglitazone Study 108 Investigators. Effects of rosiglitazone alone and in combination with atorvastatin on the metabolic abnormalities in type 2 diabetes mellitus. *Am J Cardiol* 2002; 90: 947–52.
200. Shargorodsky M, Wainstein G, Gavish E, Leibovitz Z, Matas D, Zimlichman R. Treatment with rosiglitazone reduces hyperinsulinemia and improves arterial elasticity in patients with type 2 diabetes mellitus. *Am J Hypertens* 2003; 16: 617–22.
201. Gerber P, Lubben G, Heusler S, Dodo A. Effects of pioglitazone on metabolic control and blood pressure: a randomised study in patients with type 2 diabetes mellitus. *Curr Med Res Opin* 2003; 19: 532–9.
202. Kato K, Satoh H, Endo Y, Yamada D, Midorikawa S, Sato W, Mizuno K, Fujita T, Tsukamoto K, Watanabe T. Thiazolidinediones down-regulate plasminogen activator inhibitor type 1 expression in human vascular endothelial cells: a possible role for PPAR gamma in endothelial function. *Biochem Biophys Res Commun* 1999; 258: 431–5.
203. Watanabe Y, Sunayama S, Shimada K, Sawano M, Hoshi S, Iwama Y, Mokuno H, Daida H, Yamaguchi H. Troglitazone improves endothelial dysfunction in patients with insulin resistance. *J Atheroscler Thromb* 2000; 7: 159–63.
204. Natali A, Baldeweg S, Toschi E, Barbaro D, Capaldo B, Yudkin J, Ferrannini E. Rosiglitazone directly improves

endothelial function in type 2 diabetic patients. *Diabetes* 2002; 51 (suppl 2): A142.

205. Steppan CM, Bailey ST, Bhat S, Brown EJ, Banerjee RR, Wright CM, Patel HR, Ahima RS, Lazar MA. The hormone resistin links obesity to diabetes. *Nature* 2001; 409: 307–12.
206. Marx N, Froehlich J, Siam L, Ittner J, Wierse G, Schmidt A, Scharnagl H, Hombach V, Koenig W. Antidiabetic PPAR gamma-activator rosiglitazone reduces MMP-9 serum levels in type 2 diabetic patients with coronary artery disease. *Arterioscler Thromb Vasc Biol* 2003; 23: 283–8.
207. Haffner SM, Greenberg AS, Weston WM, Chen H, Williams K, Freed MI. Effect of rosiglitazone treatment on nontraditional markers of cardiovascular disease in patients with type 2 diabetes mellitus. *Circ* 2002; 106: 679–84.
208. Harte AL, McTernan PG, McTernan CL, Smith SA, Barnett AH, Kumar S. Rosiglitazone inhibits the insulin-mediated increase in PAI-1 secretion in human abdominal subcutaneous adipocytes. *Diabetes Obes Metab* 2003; 5: 302–10.
209. Phillips SA, Ciaraldi TP, Kong AP, Bandukwala R, Aroda V, Carter L, Baxi S, Mudaliar SR, Henry RR. Modulation of circulating and adipose tissue adiponectin levels by antidiabetic therapy. *Diabetes* 2003; 52: 667–74.
210. Bajaj M, Suraamornkul S, Piper P, Hardies LJ, Glass L, Cersosimo E, Pratipanawatr T, Miyazaki Y, DeFronzo RA. Decreased plasma adiponectin concentrations are closely related to hepatic fat content and hepatic insulin resistance in pioglitazone-treated type 2 diabetic patients. *J Clin Endocrinol Metab* 2004; 89: 200–6.
211. Akazawa S, Sun F, Ito M, Kawasaki E, Eguchi K. Efficacy of troglitazone on body fat distribution in type 2 diabetes. *Diabetes Care* 2000; 23: 1067–71.
212. Raskin P, Rendell M, Riddle MC, Dole JF, Freed MI, Rosenstock J, for the Rosiglitazone Clinical Trials Study Group. A randomized trial of rosiglitazone therapy in patients with inadequately controlled insulin-treated type 2 diabetes. *Diabetes Care* 2001; 24: 1226–32.
213. Rosenstock J, Einhorn D, Hershon K, Glazer NB, Yu S, for Pioglitazone 014 Study Group. Efficacy and safety of pioglitazone in type 2 diabetes: a randomised, placebo-controlled study in patients receiving stable insulin therapy. *Int J Clin Pract* 2002; 56: 251–7.
214. Gitlin N, Julie NL, Spurr CL, Lim KN, Juarbe HM. Two cases of severe clinical and histologic hepatotoxicity associated with troglitazone. *Ann Intern Med* 1998; 129: 36–8.
215. Maeda K. Hepatocellular injury in a patient receiving pioglitazone. *Ann Intern Med* 2001; 135: 306.
216. May LD, Lefkowitch JH, Kram MT, Rubin DE. Mixed hepatocellular-cholestatic liver injury after pioglitazone therapy. *Ann Intern Med* 2002; 136: 449–52.
217. Forman LM, Simmons DA, Diamond RH. Hepatic failure in a patient taking rosiglitazone. *Ann Intern Med* 2000; 132: 118–21.
218. Al-Salman J, Arjomand H, Kemp DG, Mittal M. Hepatocellular injury in a patient receiving rosiglitazone. *Ann Intern Med* 2000; 132: 121–4.
219. Lebovitz HE, Kreider M, Freed MI. Evaluation of liver function in type 2 diabetic patients during clinical trials: evidence that rosiglitazone does not cause hepatic dysfunction. *Diabetes Care* 2002; 25: 815–21.
220. Baba S. Pioglitazone: a review of Japanese clinical studies. *Curr Med Res Opin* 2001; 17: 166–89.
221. Ghazzi MN, Perez JE, Antonucci TK, Driscoll JH, Huang SM, Faja BW, Whitcomb RW, for the Troglitazone Study Group. Cardiac and glycemic benefits of troglitazone treatment in NIDDM. *Diabetes* 1997; 46: 433–9.
222. DeFronzo RA, Cooke CR, Andres R, Faloona GR, Davis PJ. The effect of insulin on renal handling of sodium, potassium, calcium, and phosphate in man. *J Clin Invest* 1975; 55: 845–55.
223. Clissold SP, Edwards C. Acarbose. A preliminary review of its pharmacodynamic and pharmacokinetic properties, and therapeutic potential. *Drugs* 1988; 35: 214–43.
224. Lebovitz HE, A new oral therapy for diabetes management: alpha-glucosidase inhibition with acarbose. *Clin Diabetes* 1995; 13: 99–103.
225. Krentz AJ, Ferner RE, Bailey CJ. Comparative tolerability profiles of oral antidiabetic agents. *Drug Saf* 1994; 11: 223–41.
226. Chiasson JL, Josse RG, Hunt JA, Palmason C, Rodger NW, Ross SA, Ryan EA, Tan MH, Wolever TM. The efficacy of acarbose in the treatment of patients with non-insulin-dependent diabetes mellitus. A multicenter controlled clinical trial. *Ann Intern Med* 1994; 121: 928–35.
227. Coniff RF, Shapiro JA, Robbins D, Kleinfield R, Seaton TB, Beisswenger P, McGill JB. Reduction of glycosylated hemoglobin and postprandial hyperglycemia by acarbose in patients with NIDDM. A placebo-controlled dose-comparison study. *Diabetes Care* 1995; 18: 817–24.
228. Hillebrand I, Boehme K, Frank G, Fink H, Berchtold P. The effects of the α-glucosidase inhibitor BAY g 5421 (Acarbose) on meal-stimulated elevations of circulating glucose, insulin, and triglyceride levels in man. *Res Exp Med (Berl)* 1979; 175: 81–6.
229. Bayraktar M, van Thiel DH, Adalar N. A comparison of acarbose versus metformin as an adjuvant therapy in sulfonylurea-treated NIDDM patients. *Diabetes Care* 1996; 19: 252–4.
230. Drent ML, Tollefsen AT, van Heusden FH, Hoenderdos EB, Jonker JJ, van der Veen EA. Dose-dependent efficacy of miglitol, an alpha-glucosidase inhibitor, in type 2 diabetic patients on diet alone: results of a 24-week double-blind placebo-controlled study. *Diabetes Nutr Metab* 2003; 15: 152–9.
231. Vichayanrat A, Ploybutr S, Tunlakit M, Watanakejorn P. Efficacy and safety of voglibose in comparison with acarbose in type 2 diabetic patients. *Diabetes Res Clin Pract* 2002; 55: 99–103.
232. Chiasson JL, Josse RG, Gomis R, Hanefeld M, Karasik A, Laakso M, for the STOP-NIDDM Trail Research Group. Acarbose for prevention of type 2 diabetes mellitus: the STOP-NIDDM randomised trial. *Lancet* 2002; 359: 2072–7.
233. Chiasson JL, Josse RG, Gomis R, Hanefeld M, Karasik A, Laakso M, for the STOP-NIDDM Trial Research Group. Acarbose treatment and the risk of cardiovascular disease and hypertension in patients with impaired glucose tolerance: the STOP-NIDDM trial. *JAMA* 2003; 290: 486–94.
234. Temelkova-Kurktschiev T, Koehler C, Henkel E, Leonhardt W, Fuecker K, Hanefeld M. Postchallenge plasma glucose and glycemic spikes are more strongly associated with atherosclerosis than fasting glucose or HbA1c level. *Diabetes Care* 2000; 23: 1830–4.
235. Fuhlendorff J, Rorsman P, Kofod H, Brand CL, Rolin B, MacKay P, Shymko R, Carr RD. Stimulation of insulin release by repaglinide and glibenclamide involves both common and distinct processes. *Diabetes* 1998; 47: 345–51.

236. Wolffenbuttel BH, Nijst L, Sels JP, Menheere PP, Muller PG, Kruseman AC. Effects of a new oral hypoglycaemic agent, repaglinide, on metabolic control in sulphonylurea-treated patients with NIDDM. *Eur J Clin Pharmacol* 1992; 45: 113–6.
237. Derosa G, Mugellini A, Ciccarelli L, Crescenzi G, Fogari R. Comparison of glycaemic control and cardiovascular risk profile in patients with type 2 diabetes during treatment with either repaglinide or metformin. *Diabetes Res Clin Pract* 2003; 60: 161–9.
238. Vakkilainen J, Mero N, Schweizer A, Foley JE, Taskinen MR. Effects of nateglinide and glibenclamide on postprandial lipid and glucose metabolism in type 2 diabetes. *Diabetes Metab Res Rev* 2000; 18: 484–90.
239. Marbury T, Huang WC, Strange P, Lebovitz H. Repaglinide versus glyburide: a one-year comparison trial. *Diabetes Res Clin Pract* 1999; 43: 155–66.
240. Levien TL, Baker DE, Campbell RK, White JR Jr. Nateglinide therapy for type 2 diabetes mellitus. *Ann Pharmacother* 2001; 35: 1426–34.
241. Madsbad S, Kilhovd B, Lager I, Mustajoki P, Dejgaard A, for the Scandinavian Repaglinide Group. Comparison between repaglinide and glipizide in Type 2 diabetes mellitus: a 1-year multicentre study. *Diabet Med* 2001; 18: 395–401.
242. Hollander PA, Schwartz SL, Gatlin MR, Haas SJ, Zheng H, Foley JE, Dunning BE. Importance of early insulin secretion: comparison of nateglinide and glyburide in previously diet-treated patients with type 2 diabetes. *Diabetes Care* 2001; 24: 983–8.
243. Herz M, Johns D, Reviriego J, Grossman LD, Godin C, Duran S, Hawkins F, Lochnan H, Escobar-Jimenez F, Hardin PA, Konkoy CS, Tan MH. A randomized, double-blind, placebo-controlled, clinical trial of the effects of pioglitazone on glycemic control and dyslipidemia in oral antihyperglycemic medication-naive patients with type 2 diabetes mellitus. *Clin Ther* 2003; 25: 1074–95.
244. Fonseca V, Grunberger G, Gupta S, Shen S, Foley JE. Addition of nateglinide to rosiglitazone monotherapy suppresses mealtime hyperglycemia and improves overall glycemic control. *Diabetes Care* 2003; 26: 1685–90.
245. Rosenstock J, Shen SG, Gatlin MR, Foley JE. Combination therapy with nateglinide and a thiazolidinedione improves glycemic control in type 2 diabetes. *Diabetes Care* 2002; 25: 1529–33.
246. Raskin P, Jovanovic L, Berger S, Schwartz S, Woo V, Ratner R. Repaglinide/troglitazone combination therapy: improved glycemic control in type 2 diabetes. *Diabetes Care* 2000; 23: 979–83.
247. Lebovitz HE. Stepwise and combination drug therapy for the treatment of NIDDM. *Diabetes Care* 1994; 17: 1542–4.
248. Bailey CJ. Biguanides and NIDDM. *Diabetes Care* 1992; 15: 755–72.
249. Dunn CJ, Peters DH. Metformin. A review of its pharmacological properties and therapeutic use in non-insulin-dependent diabetes mellitus. *Drugs* 1995; 49: 721–49.
250. Trischitta V, Italia S, Mazzarino S, Buscema M, Rabuazzo AM, Sangiorgio L, Squatrito S, Vigneri R. Comparison of combined therapies in treatment of secondary failure to glyburide. *Diabetes Care* 1992; 15: 539–42.
251. Cefalu WT, Schneider DJ, Carlson HE, Migdal P, Gan Lim L, Izon MP, Kapoor A, Bell-Farrow A, Terry JG, Sobel BE. Effect of combination glipizide GITS/metformin on fibrinolytic and metabolic parameters in poorly controlled type 2 diabetic subjects. *Diabetes Care* 2002; 25: 2123–8.
252. Haupt E, Knick B, Koschinsky T, Liebermeister H, Schneider J, Hirche H. Oral antidiabetic combination therapy with sulphonylureas and metformin. *Diabete Metab* 1991; 17: 224–31.
253. Garber AJ, Larsen J, Schneider SH, Piper BA, Henry D, for the Glyburide/Metformin Initial Therapy Study Group. Simultaneous glyburide/metformin therapy is superior to component monotherapy as an initial pharmacological treatment for type 2 diabetes. *Diabetes Obes Metab* 2002; 4: 201–8.
254. Blonde L, Wogen J, Kreilick C, Seymour AA. Greater reductions in A1C in type 2 diabetic patients new to therapy with glyburide/metformin tablets as compared to glyburide co-administered with metformin. *Diabetes Obes Metab* 2003; 5: 424–31.
255. Donahue SR, Turner KC, Patel S. Pharmacokinetics and pharmacodynamics of glyburide/metformin tablets (Glucovance) versus equivalent doses of glyburide and metformin in patients with type 2 diabetes. *Clin Pharmacokinet* 2002; 41: 1301–9.
256. Duckworth W, Marcelli M, Padden M, Kellick K, Duhancik T, Wilhardt M, Colgan K, Romie A. Improvements in glycemic control in Type 2 diabetes patients switched from sulfonylurea coadministered with metformin to glyburide–metformin tablets. *J Manage Care Pharm* 2002; 9: 256–62.
257. Jones TA, Sautter M, van Gaal LF, Jones NP. Addition of rosiglitazone to metformin is most effective in obese, insulin-resistant patients with type 2 diabetes. *Diabetes Obes Metab* 2003; 5: 163–70.
258. Wysowski DK, Armstrong G, Governale L. Rapid increase in the use of oral antidiabetic drugs in the United States, 1990–2001. *Diabetes Care* 2003; 26: 1852–5.
259. Koshiyama H, Shimono D, Kuwamura N, Minamikawa J, Nakamura Y. Rapid communication: inhibitory effect of pioglitazone on carotid arterial wall thickness in type 2 diabetes. *J Clin Endocrinol Metab* 2001; 86: 3452–6.
260. Minamikawa J, Tanaka S, Yamauchi M, Inoue D, Koshiyama H. Potent inhibitory effect of troglitazone on carotid arterial wall thickness in type 2 diabetes. *J Clin Endocrinol Metab* 1998; 83: 1818–20.
261. Xiang A, Peters R, Kjos S, Goico J, Ochoa C, Marroquin A, Tan S, Hodis H, Azen S, Buchanan T. Effect of troglitazone on pre-clinical carotid atherosclerosis in women with gestational diabetes. *Diabetes* 2002; 51 (suppl 2): A174.
262. Takagi T, Akasaka T, Yamamuro A, Honda Y, Hozumi T, Morioka S, Yoshida K. Troglitazone reduces neointimal tissue proliferation after coronary stent implantation in patients with non-insulin dependent diabetes mellitus: a serial intravascular ultrasound study. *J Am Coll Cardiol* 2000; 36: 1529–35.
263. Choi SH, Choi DH, Ko YK, Chang YS, Cho YL, Lim SK, Nam M-S, Lee HC, Cha BS. Preventive effects of rosiglitazone on restenosis after coronary stenting in patients with type 2 diabetes. *Diabetes* 2003; 52 (suppl 1): A19.
264. Einhorn D, Rendell M, Rosenzweig J, Egan JW, Mathisen AL, Schneider RL, for the Pioglitazone 027 Study Group. Pioglitazone hydrochloride in combination with metformin in the treatment of type 2 diabetes mellitus: a randomized, placebo-controlled study. *Clin Ther* 2002; 22: 1395–409.

265. Fonseca V, Rosenstock J, Patwardhan R, Salzman A. Effect of metformin and rosiglitazone combination therapy in patients with type 2 diabetes mellitus: a randomized controlled trial. *JAMA* 2000; 283: 1695–702.
266. Kipnes MS, Krosnick A, Rendell MS, Egan JW, Mathisen AL, Schneider RL. Pioglitazone hydrochloride in combination with sulfonylurea therapy improves glycemic control in patients with type 2 diabetes mellitus: a randomized, placebo-controlled study. *Am J Med* 2001; 111: 10–7.
267. Wolffenbuttel BH, Gomis R, Squatrito S, Jones NP, Patwardhan RN. Addition of low-dose rosiglitazone to sulphonylurea therapy improves glycaemic control in Type 2 diabetic patients. *Diabet Med* 2000; 17: 40–7.
268. Rodger NW, Chiasson JL, Josse RG, Hunt JA, Palmason C, Ross SA, Ryan EA, Tan MH, Wolever TM. Clinical experience with acarbose: results of a Canadian multicentre study. *Clin Invest Med* 1995; 18: 318–24.
269. Coniff RF, Shapiro JA, Seaton TB, Bray GA. Multicenter, placebo controlled trial comparing acarbose (BAY g 5421) with placebo, tolbutamide, and tolbutamide-plus-acarbose in non-insulin-dependent diabetes mellitus. *Am J Med* 1995; 98: 443–51.
270. Rosenstock J, Brown A, Fischer J, Jain A, Littlejohn T, Nadeau D, Sussman A, Taylor T, Krol A, Magner J. Efficacy and safety of acarbose in metformin-treated patients with type 2 diabetes. *Diabetes Care* 1998; 21: 2050–5.
271. Moses R, Slobodniuk R, Boyages S, Colagiuri S, Kidson W, Carter J, Donnelly T, Moffitt P, Hopkins H. Effect of repaglinide addition to metformin monotherapy on glycemic control in patients with type 2 diabetes. *Diabetes Care* 1999; 22: 119–24.
272. Raskin P, Klaff L, McGill J, South SA, Hollander P, Khutoryansky N, Hale PM, for the Repaglinide vs. Nateglinide Metformin Combination Study Group. Efficacy and safety of combination therapy: repaglinide plus metformin versus nateglinide plus metformin. *Diabetes Care* 2003; 26: 2063–8.
273. Yale JF, Valiquett TR, Ghazzi MN, Owens-Grillo JK, Whitcomb RW, Foyt HL. The effect of a thiazolidinedione drug, troglitazone, on glycemia in patients with type 2 diabetes mellitus poorly controlled with sulfonylurea and metformin. A multicenter, randomized, double-blind, placebo-controlled trial. *Ann Intern Med* 2001; 134: 737–45.
274. Kiayias JA, Vlachou ED, Theodosopoulou E, Lakka-Papadodima E. Rosiglitazone in combination with glimepiride plus metformin in type 2 diabetic patients. *Diabetes Care* 2002; 25: 1251–2.
275. Schwartz S, Sievers R, Strange P, Lyness WH, Hollander P, for the INS-2061 Study Team. Insulin 70/30 mix plus metformin versus triple oral therapy in the treatment of type 2 diabetes after failure of two oral drugs: efficacy, safety, and cost analysis. *Diabetes Care* 2003; 26: 2238–43.
276. Abraira C, Duckworth W, McCarren M, Emanuele N, Arca D, Reda D, Henderson W. Design of the cooperative study on glycemic control and complications in diabetes mellitus type 2 Veterans Affairs Diabetes Trial. *J Diabetes Complications* 2003; 17: 314–22.
277. Yki-Jarvinen H. Combination therapies with insulin in type 2 diabetes. *Diabetes Care* 2001; 24: 758–67.
278. Yki-Jarvinen H, Kauppila M, Kujansuu E, Lahti J, Marjanen T, Niskanen L, Rajala S, Ryysy L, Salo S, Seppala P, et al. Comparison of insulin regimens in patients with non-insulin-dependent diabetes mellitus. *N Engl J Med* 1992; 327: 1426–33.
279. Johnson JL, Wolf SL, Kabadi UM. Efficacy of insulin and sulfonylurea combination therapy in type II diabetes. A meta-analysis of the randomized placebo-controlled trials. *Arch Intern Med* 1996; 156: 259–64.
280. Landstedt-Hallin L, Adamson U, Arner P, Bolinder J, Lins PE. Comparison of bedtime NPH or preprandial regular insulin combined with glibenclamide in secondary sulfonylurea failure. *Diabetes Care* 1995; 18: 1183–6.
281. Bergenstal R, Johnson M, Whipple D, Noller D, Boyce K, Roth L, et al. Advantages of adding metformin to multiple dose insulin therapy in type 2 diabetes. *Diabetes* 1998; 7 (suppl 1): A89.
282. Shank M, Del Prato S, DeFronzo RA. Bedtime insulin/daytime glipizide. Effective therapy for sulfonylurea failures in NIDDM. *Diabetes* 1995; 44: 165–72.
283. Riddle MC. Evening insulin strategy. *Diabetes Care* 1990; 13: 676–86.
284. Groop L, Widen E. Treatment strategies for secondary sulfonylurea failure. Should we start insulin or add metformin? Is there a place for intermittent insulin therapy? *Diabete Metab* 1991; 17: 218–23.
285. Chow CC, Tsang LW, Sorenson JP, Cockram CS. Comparison of insulin with or without continuation of oral hypoglycemic agents in the treatment of secondary failure in NIDDM patients. *Diabetes Care* 1995; 18: 307–14.
286. Klein W. Sulfonylurea–metformin-combination versus sulfonylurea–insulin-combination in secondary failures of sulfonylurea monotherapy. Results of a prospective randomized study in 50 patients. *Diabetes Metab* 1991; 17: 235–40.
287. Vigneri R, Trischitta V, Italia S, Mazzarino S, Rabuazzo MA, Squatrito S. Treatment of NIDDM patients with secondary failure to glyburide: comparison of the addition of either metformin or bed-time NPH insulin to glyburide. *Diabetes Metab* 1991; 17: 232–4.
288. Groop L, Widen E, Franssila-Kallunki A, Ekstrand A, Saloranta C, Schalin C, Eriksson J. Different effects of insulin and oral antidiabetic agents on glucose and energy metabolism in type 2 (non-insulin-dependent) diabetes mellitus. *Diabetologia* 1989; 32: 599–605.
289. Schwartz S, Raskin P, Fonseca V, Graveline JF, for the Troglitazone and Exogenous Insulin Study Group. Effect of troglitazone in insulin-treated patients with type II diabetes mellitus. *N Engl J Med* 1998; 338: 861–6.
290. Buse JB, Gumbiner B, Mathias NP, Nelson DM, Faja BW, Whitcomb RW, for the Troglitazone Insulin Study Group. Troglitazone use in insulin-treated type 2 diabetic patients. *Diabetes Care* 1998; 21: 1455–61.
291. Giugliano D, Quatraro A, Consoli G, Minei A, Ceriello A, de Rosa N, D' Onofrio F. Metformin for obese, insulin-treated diabetic patients: improvement in glycaemic control and reduction of metabolic risk factors. *Eur J Clin Pharmacol* 1993; 44: 107–12.
292. Aviles-Santa L, Sinding J, Raskin P. Effects of metformin in patients with poorly controlled, insulin-treated type 2 diabetes mellitus. A randomized, double-blind, placebo-controlled trial. *Ann Intern Med* 1999; 131: 182–8.
293. Bell DSH, Mayo MS. Outcome of metformin-facilitated reinitiation of oral diabetic therapy in insulin-treated patients with non-insulin dependent diabetes mellitus. *Endocr Pract* 1997; 3: 73–6.

294. Strowig SM, Aviles-Santa ML, Raskin P. Comparison of insulin monotherapy and combination therapy with insulin and metformin or insulin and troglitazone in type 2 diabetes. *Diabetes Care* 2002; 25: 1691–8.

295. Kelley DE, Bidot P, Freedman Z, Haag B, Podlecki D, Rendell M, Schimel D, Weiss S, Taylor T, Krol A, Magner J. Efficacy and safety of acarbose in insulin-treated patients with type 2 diabetes. *Diabetes Care* 1998; 21: 2056–61.

296. de Luis DA, Aller R, Cuellar L, Terroba C, Ovalle H, Izaola O, Romero E. Effect of repaglinide addition to NPH insulin monotherapy on glycemic control in patients with type 2 diabetes. *Diabetes Care* 2001; 24: 1844–5.

51

New Drugs for the Treatment of Diabetes Mellitus

Clifford J. Bailey

Aston University, Birmingham, UK

This chapter reviews agents being considered or recently introduced for the treatment of hyperglycemia. Attention is given mainly to agents advanced in clinical development, plus selected examples of compounds that illustrate other potential therapeutic mechanisms to lower blood glucose.

Current treatment strategies for type 1 and type 2 diabetes are guidelines-lead and target-driven, based on the recognized importance of metabolic control and risk factor management [1, 2]. Reducing blood glucose serves both as a marker of metabolic control and a means of risk factor management. Improved glycemic control defers the onset and reduces the severity of chronic diabetic complications, particularly microvascular complications, and the benefits continue to accrue until euglycemia is attained [3, 4]. Existing antidiabetic drugs do not reinstate physiologically normal glucose homeostasis, and even with intensive use these drugs often fail to achieve or sustain euglycemia [5–7]. Hence the chronic complications of diabetes remain a serious burden; they are also a poignant reminder of the pressing need for new and better agents to treat hyperglycemia.

ASSESSING INTERVENTION PRIORITIES

The different pathogenic features of type 1 and type 2 diabetes dictate different therapeutic priorities. Treatment of type 1 diabetes necessitates replacement of at least some insulin or a substitute that mimics the broad spectrum of genomic and other effects of insulin to ensure vital maintenance levels of key transporters, enzymes, and metabolic pathways. Once this basal insulin requirement has been satisfied any interventions not directed at B-cells could be considered (Figure 1). For type 2 diabetes, where there is residual endogenous insulin, new agents might be targeted more selectively against underlying endocrine defects of insulin resistance and B-cell dysfunction. Interventions that directly reduce excessive glucose production or improve glucose utilization are also favored, although there is potential merit in reducing hyperglycemia by any safe means. Combinations of two or more agents that target different lesions can usefully provide additive or synergistic glucose-lowering efficacy [8, 9]. Also, potential combinations of antidiabetic drugs with agents to treat other components of the "metabolic syndrome" could provide wider management of cardiovascular risk.

A distinction exists between antihyperglycemic and hypoglycemic agents. Both reduce hyperglycemia, but the latter can reduce blood glucose below the normal range, carrying the risk of serious clinical hypoglycemia (e.g., agents that stimulate insulin secretion at subnormal glycemia) [10]. While the use of agents that can cause hypoglycemia may be necessary to achieve adequate glucose-lowering efficacy, it is prudent that new hypoglycemic drugs should not prevent or severely compromise the process of counterregulation. Since antidiabetic treatments are likely to be used long-term, issues of safety, including hypoglycemia and drug interactions, tolerability, convenient administration, and compatibility with lifestyle are crucial. Ideally, new antidiabetic agents should not aggravate known cardiovascular risk factors or features of the metabolic syndrome [11].

International Textbook of Diabetes Mellitus, Third Edition. Edited by R. A. DeFronzo, E. Ferrannini, H. Keen, and P. Zimmet.
 ISBN: 0-471-48655-8.

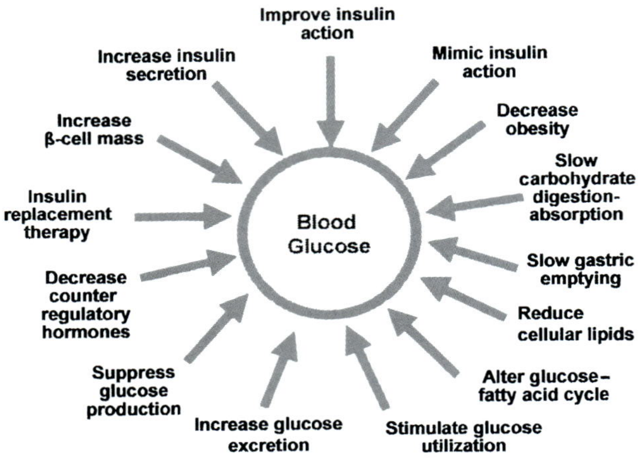

Figure 1 Potential therapeutic interventions to lower blood glucose concentrations

Table 2 Sites of action and categories of blood glucose-lowering agents considered in this chapter

Intestinal inhibitors of carbohydrate digestion and absorption
Insulin supply
Novel insulins
Insulin secretagogues
Incretin analogues
Insulin action enhancers
Insulin mimetics
Insulin potentiators
Minerals and vitamins
Inhibitors of counterregulatory hormones
Manipulators of lipid metabolism
Antiobesity agents
Stimulants of glucose utilization
Inhibitors of hepatic glucose production
Glucose elimination

PRECLINICAL AND CLINICAL STAGES OF DEVELOPMENT

Conventional stages of drug development from concept to regulatory approval are summarized in Table 1. Preclinical studies provide guidance in the selection of compounds for clinical testing, and give information on their mode of action [12]. However, blood glucose-lowering activity in animal models does not necessarily predict efficacy in clinical states, and animal studies may not reveal safety issues in long-term clinical therapy [12]. Thus, many compounds that show early promise do not proceed in pharmaceutical development, as illustrated by reference to the equivalent chapter (Chapter 38) in the second edition of this textbook published in 1997 [13]. Since then, one α-glucosidase inhibitor, two meglitinides, and two thiazolidinediones have been approved for prescription as oral antidiabetic drugs; the majority of promising compounds have not proceeded or remain in development. Fewer than 1 in 5 compounds that enter clinical development will become an approved prescription medicine, and current (year 2003) estimates suggest that, on average, the complete development life cycle of an active compound into a marketable drug is likely to take 7–10 years and cost more than US$800 million. Market analysts estimate that in the year 2000 worldwide retail sales of blood glucose-lowering drugs were over US$8 billion, of which about 63% were oral agents and 37% insulin.

Potential new antidiabetic agents and compounds with novel therapeutic mechanisms to lower blood glucose are conveniently grouped according to their main site of action or cellular target, as summarized in Table 2. It will be appreciated that some agents exert effects on several different targets.

Table 1 Preclinical and clinical stages in the development of a new drug

Preclinical stages
New chemical entity (NCE)

- Identify, extract or synthesize, chemically characterize, and patent
- Screen for biological activity *in vitro* and in animal models
- Preclinical pharmacology, mode of action, pharmacodynamics, pharmacokinetics, toxicology

Clinical stages
Investigational new drug (IND)
Permission to begin clinical studies

- Phase 1: First administration to a small number of healthy human volunteers. Dose ranging, pharmacodynamics, pharmacokinetics, drug interactions, safety
- Phase 2: First trials in small numbers of patients. Dose ranging, efficacy, further pharmacodynamics, pharmacokinetics, safety
- Phase 3: Trials, in larger numbers of patients. Multicenter trials, comparative trials with other treatments, efficacy, further pharmacodynamics, safety

New drug application (NDA)
Permission to market as a drug

- Phase 4: Use in medical practice. Further evaluation similar to phase 3, postmarketing surveillance, adverse drug reactions, use in special subgroups (e.g., elderly patients).

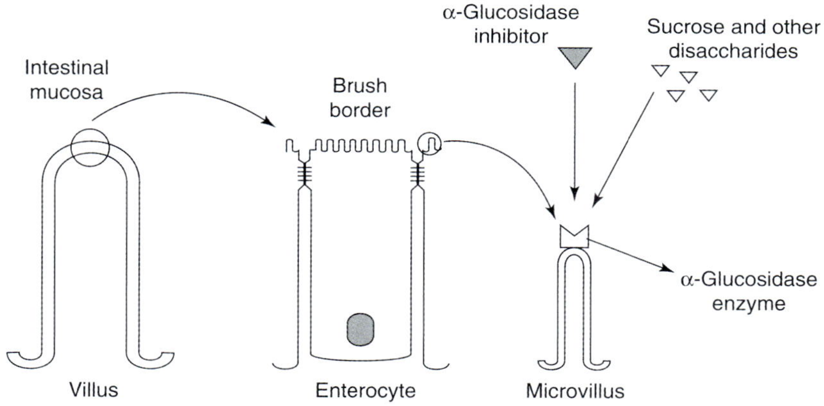

Figure 2 Mechanism of action of α-glucosidase inhibitors is by competitive inhibition of α-glucosidase enzymes in the brush-border microvilli of intestinal enterocytes

INTESTINAL INHIBITORS OF CARBOHYDRATE DIGESTION AND ABSORPTION

Excessive postprandial excursions of hyperglycemia are reported to impose an especially high risk of cardiovascular disease [14]. At the level of the alimentary tract the main approaches to reduce postprandial hyperglycemia have been alpha-glucosidase inhibitors, dietary fiber supplements, and interventions that slow the rate of gastric emptying.

α-Glucosidase Inhibitors

α-Glucosidases are brush-border oligosaccharidase and disaccharidase enzymes (e.g., maltase, glucoamylase, dextrinase, and sucrase) that cleave α-1,6 and terminal α-1,4 glucosidic bonds to release glucose [15, 16]. α-Glucosidase inhibitors such as acarbose and miglitol (see chapter 52) bind to these enzymes with high affinity and competitively inhibit access by the normal nutrient substrates (Figure 2). This slows the completion of carbohydrate digestion and consequently defers and extends the period for absorption of monosaccharides.

A new alpha-glucosidase inhibitor, voglibose, has recently been introduced in some countries (Figure 3). It is a valiolamine derivative of microbial origin, with strong affinities for α-glucosidases. Voglibose reduces the postprandial increment in glycemia similarly to acarbose and miglitol, and by delaying the appearance of glucose in the blood it can also reduce episodes of hypoglycemia during intensive insulin therapy [15, 17]. Recommendations for use of voglibose (e.g., take with carbohydrate-rich meals) and limitations of use (e.g., gastrointestinal discomfort and flatulence) are similar to acarbose and miglitol. Other alpha-glucosidase inhibitors such as castanospermine and MDL-73945 have not proceeded in clinical development [13].

α-Amylase Inhibitors

α-Amylases, present in saliva and pancreatic juice, break internal α-1,4 glucosidic bonds within starch molecules, and offer another potential site of intervention to retard carbohydrate digestion. Some α-glucosidase inhibitors (e.g. acarbose) are weak inhibitors of α-amylase activity, but attempts to specifically inhibit α-amylase activity have not given sufficiently consistent efficacy for clinical development [16].

Fiber Supplements

Many nondigestible plant polysaccharides have been tested as dietary supplements [18] and utilized in herbal

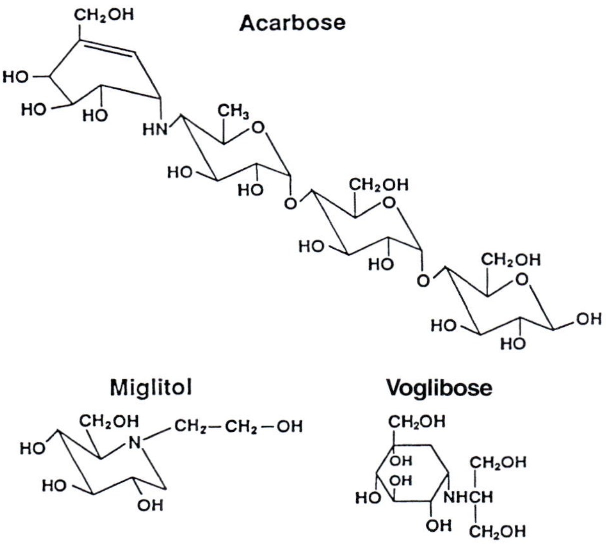

Figure 3 Structures of the α-glucosidase inhibitors acarbose, miglitol, and voglibose

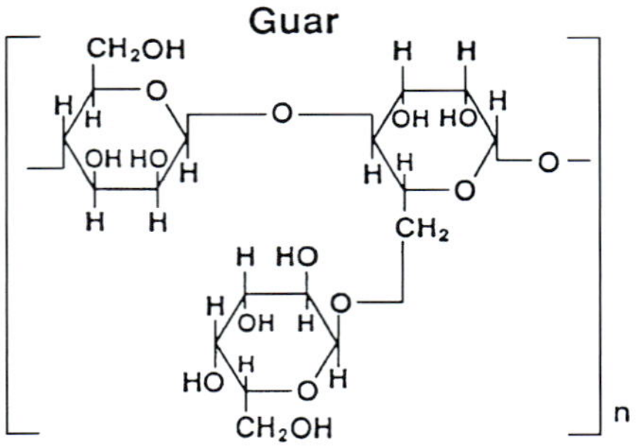

Figure 4 Structure of guar gum, a soluble galactomannan-polysaccharide fiber derived from the cluster bean *Cyamopsis tetragonolobus*

treatments for diabetes [19, 20]. They trap nutrients within the matrix of the fiber and create a diffusion barrier that reduces access by digestive enzymes and restricts contact with the intestinal epithelium [18]. Bulky viscous soluble fibers such as guar gum (Figure 4) also prolong gastric emptying and extend intestinal transit time. whereas insoluble fibers such as wheat bran can reduce transit times, depending on fiber coarseness. Supplements of soluble and insoluble fibers (Table 3) are not widely recommended because their blood glucose-lowering effects are nominal [13], especially if the patient is consuming a balanced diet that already contains sufficient fruit and vegetables [21]. Excess fiber is generally unpalatable and prone to cause abdominal discomfort and flatulence associated with fermentation in the large bowel. The potential for intestinal obstruction and impaired absorption of micronutrients and drugs has also been noted.

Other agents that include a reduced rate of gastric emptying as part of their activity profile, such as pramlintide and glucagon-like peptide 1 analogues, are considered in subsequent sections.

INSULIN SUPPLY

Other chapters in this textbook review recent developments with insulin analogues (see Chapter 56), alternative routes of insulin delivery, including inhaled and oral preparations (see Chapter 58), implantable artificial insulin delivery devices (see Chapter 59), and islet and pancreatic transplants (see Chapter 62).

Table 3 Soluble and insoluble fiber supplements

Soluble fiber	Insoluble fiber
Gums	Celluloses
Pectins	Wheat brans
Hemicelluloses	
Mucilages	

NOVEL INSULINS

Delivering exogenous insulin in a manner that mimics the physiological situation has proved a formidable challenge [22]. Insulin secretion by the pancreas into the portal vein ensures that the liver is always perfused with higher insulin concentrations than those in the periphery, and the liver also receives the full impact of rapid adjustments to the insulin concentration. An approach to enable preferential delivery of exogenous insulin to the liver has involved the construction of insulin linked to thyroxine (thyroxyl-insulin) [23]. Thyroxyl-insulin is highly bound to plasma proteins via its thyroxyl moiety, ensuring a prolonged plasma half-life and limited transport across the endothelium. In consequence, thyroxyl-insulin has relatively little metabolic influence on muscle and adipose tissue. However, in the liver where there are open sinusoids the thyroxyl-insulin has free access to hepatocytes.

A novel concept for controlling the circulating concentration of active insulin is the linkage of insulin to an organic complex that can be selectively cleaved by a catalytic aldolase antibody (38C2). The organic complex inactivates the insulin, and administration of the antibody unmasks the active insulin [24]. A so-called smart polymer approach has been considered for self-regulated insulin release in relation to the glucose concentration. For this approach insulin is interspersed between layers of a polymer that combines with glucose to create "pores" in the polymer. Raised glucose concentrations create more pores, allowing more insulin to escape.

INSULIN SECRETAGOGUES

Abnormalities of insulin secretion occur early in the pathogenesis of type 2 diabetes and severe hypoinsulinemia is a feature of advanced disease progression [25]. The onset of basal hyperglycemia is associated with a diminution and eventual loss of the acute insulin response to glucose; during further disease progression the later phase of glucose-induced insulin secretion becomes impaired. Initially, the insulin responses to other insulin secretagogues such as arginine, glucagon, sulfonylureas, gastrointestinal hormones, and β-adrenoreceptor agonists are well preserved, but these decline as B-cell failure consolidates [26]. This decline coincides with deficiencies in the synthesis and processing of proinsulin, and abnormalities in the pulsatile pattern of insulin secretion (see Chapter 8). Eventually the deterioration in B-cell function is compounded by a decline in B-cell mass in which apoptosis exceeds division and neogenesis [27].

A route map of glucose-induced insulin secretion within the islet B-cell (see Chapter 7) is illustrated in Figure 5, together with the sites of intervention by established and potential therapeutic secretagogues [28]. These can be categorized as either initiators or potentiators of insulin

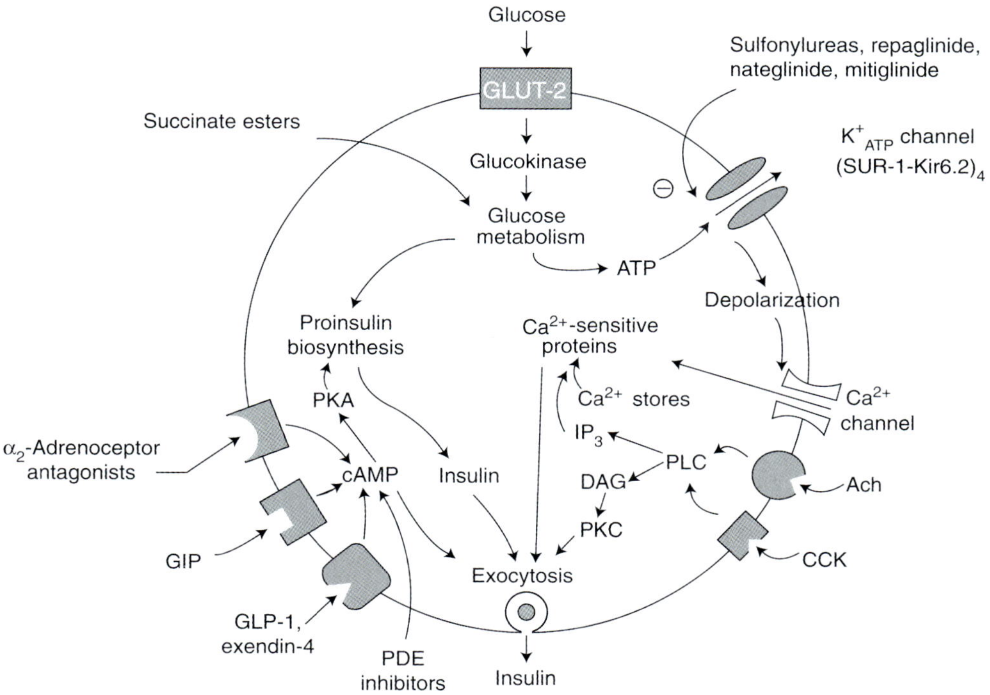

Figure 5 Route map of glucose-induced insulin secretion by an islet B-cell, showing sites at which insulin secretagogues can be targeted. Glut-2 = glucose transporter isoform 2; ATP = adenosine triphosphate; PKA = protein kinase A; IP_3 = inositol 1,4,5-trisphosphate; DAG = diacylglycerol; PKC = protein kinase C; cAMP = cyclic 3′,5′-adenosine monophosphate; K_{ATP} channel = potassium-sensitive ATP channel; SUR-1 = sulfonylurea receptor isoform 1; Kir6.2 = inwardly rectifying potassium channel 6.2; PDE = phosphodiesterase; PLC = phospholipase C; Ach = acetylcholine; CCK = cholecystokinin; GIP = gastric inhibitory polypeptide (glucose-dependent insulinotropic peptide); GLP-1 = glucagon-like peptide 1. ⊖ = inhibitory action to close K_{ATP} channels

secretion. Initiators can stimulate insulin secretion on their own, e.g. agents that close the ATP-sensitive potassium channels (K_{ATP} channels), open calcium influx channels, or contribute to energy production. Pharmacological agents that initiate insulin secretion independently of the prevailing glucose concentration carry a risk of hypoglycemia. Potentiators act predominantly to enhance the effect of glucose and other nutrient initiators, e.g. agents that increase cellular concentrations of cyclic adenosine monophosphate (cAMP). Potentiators have little insulin-releasing effect alone or at substimulatory concentrations of nutrient initiators, and therefore carry little risk of hypoglycemia.

Irrespective of the targets chosen, it would be advantageous for insulin secretagogue therapy to restore B-cell responsiveness to glucose while preserving the regulatory effects of other nutrients, ions, hormones, and neurotransmitters. It is also necessary to ensure adequate insulin biosynthesis and progression through the regulated pathway of processing and secretion. Nutrient metabolism of the B-cell to the end products of mitochondrial oxidation is required to stimulate the transcription process for the preproinsulin gene, and relevant transcription factors, such as pancreatic duodenal homeobox 1 (PDX-1), could be legitimate pharmacological targets [29, 30].

ATP-sensitive Potassium Channel Inhibitors

The K_{ATP} channels in the plasma membrane of pancreatic B-cells comprise an octameric complex of four sulfonylurea receptor 1 (SUR-1) moieties and four pore-forming Kir6.2 inwardly rectifying potassium channels. The SUR-1 moieties contain high-affinity binding sites for sulfonylureas and benzamido compounds (e.g. meglitinides) [31, 32]. Binding of ligands at these sites closes the Kir6.2 pores and prevents potassium efflux. This favors local depolarization of the plasma membrane, initiating the calcium-dependent pathway to insulin exocytosis (Figure 5). Currently available sulfonylurea and meglitinide derivatives (repaglinide and nateglinide) initiate insulin secretion via this pathway [32, 33]. The meglitinide derivative mitiglinide (KAD-1229) (Figure 4) is a prospective new insulin secretagogue that appears to bind to a site on SUR-1 to stimulate insulin secretion for a short duration [33]. SUR-1-Kir6.2 K_{ATP} channels have been identified in membranal organelles such as mitochondria within the B-cells, and in the membranes of insulin-containing β granules [34]. This raises the possibility that these sites could be pharmacological targets for sulfonylureas and benzamido compounds. Also, sulfonylureas have been shown to potentiate insulin exocytosis independently of the plasma membrane K_{ATP} channels through an interaction with protein kinase C (PKC) [35].

Certain imidazoline compounds (e.g. S22068, Figure 6) initiate insulin secretion by a mechanism that involves closure of the plasma membrane K_{ATP} channels [36]. B-cells express an imidazoline-binding site that differs from the I1 and I2 sites in other tissues, and appears to be associated with the Kir6.2 pores of the K_{ATP} channels [37]. Other imidazolines (e.g. BL11282, Figure 6) potentiate glucose-induced insulin secretion, without affecting the activity of K_{ATP} channels, possibly enhancing the exocytosis of insulin via effects on protein kinases A and C [38]. The morpholinoguanidine BTS67582 (Figure 6) stimulates insulin secretion for a short duration, at least partly by closure of K_{ATP} channels in the plasma membrane [39]. α_2-Adrenergic receptors mediate a tonic suppression of insulin secretion, and the use of α_2-adrenergic antagonists has been considered to reduce this suppression. Several such antagonists, including phentolamine, idazoxan, efaroxan, and midaglizole, which are imidazole derivatives, also showed a direct inhibitory effect on the K_{ATP} channels, but these effects have not been specific enough to customize for a therapeutic insulin secretagogue [13].

Incretins: GLP-1 and GIP

Food digestion stimulates the release of several "incretin" peptide hormones from the small intestine, which enhance insulin secretion as part of the enteroinsular axis. The two main incretins are glucagon-like peptide 1 (7-36) amide (GLP-1) and glucose-dependent insulinotropic peptide (GIP), also know as gastric inhibitory peptide (Figure 5) [40, 41]. GLP-1 and GIP bind to specific receptors in the B-cell membrane, causing activation of adenylate cyclase. This in turn raises the intracellular concentration of cAMP and protein kinase A (PKA). Cyclic AMP potentiates nutrient-initiated insulin secretion, and PKA has been implicated as a mediator of proinsulin biosynthesis and insulin exocytosis. GLP-1 also activates the phospholipase C pathway in B-cells. Meal-stimulated circulating concentrations of GLP-1 are reduced in type 2 diabetic patients, although GIP concentrations are essentially normal [42].

Much attention has recently been focused on the therapeutic potential of GLP-1. In the presence of stimulatory concentrations of glucose, GLP-1 is a potent insulin secretagogue in nondiabetic subjects, subjects with impaired glucose tolerance (IGT), and type 2 diabetic subjects [40]. In acute and chronic studies, injection or infusion of GLP-1 before or during meals has reduced postprandial hyperglycemia and improved overall glycemic contol (Figure 7) without causing clinical hypoglycemia [40, 43]. GLP-1 has also been shown to increase proinsulin

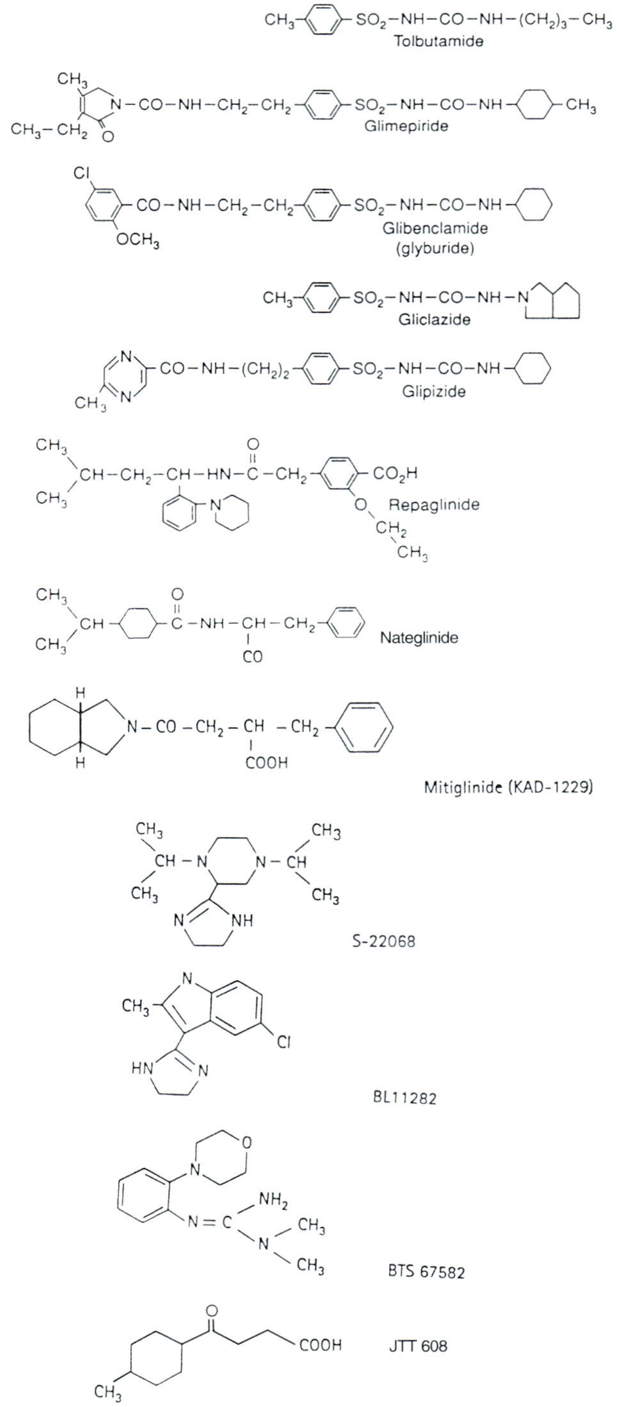

Figure 6 Insulin secretagogues that close B-cell K_{ATP} channels: structures of some sulfonylureas [tolbutamide, glimepiride, glibenclamide (glyburide), gliclazide, and glipizide] and meglitinide derivatives [repaglinide, nateglinide, and mitiglinide], and some other insulin secretagogues [S-22068, BL11282, BTS67582, and JTT608] under investigation

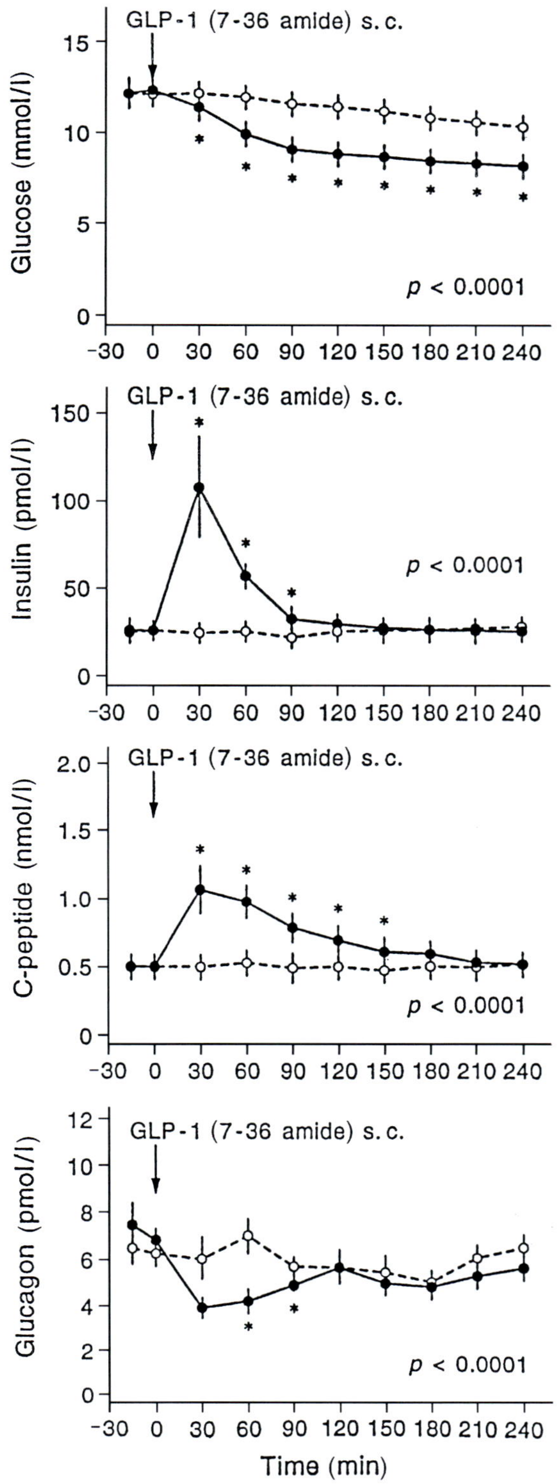

Figure 7 Effect of a single subcutaneous injection of GLP-1-(7-36 amide), 1.5 nmol/kg body weight, on plasma glucose, insulin, C-peptide, and glucagon concentrations in eight type 2 diabetic patients. Open circles – placebo; closed circles – GLP-1-(7-36 amide). Arrow shows time of injection. Values are mean with SEM. $^{*}p < 0.0001$ versus placebo. (Adapted from reference 43, with permission)

biosynthesis, involving both PKA-dependent and PKA-independent mechanisms [44]. Receptors for GLP-1 are found in various tissues including pancreatic A-cells where GLP-1 suppresses glucagon secretion, although this may be supported by the paracrine influence of increased somatostatin secretion [40]. There are GLP-1 receptors in the stomach, and GLP-1 slows gastric emptying; GLP-1 also appears to act via this effect and via direct effects in the central nervous system to exert a satiety effect. Although the slowing of gastric emptying can lead to some gastrointestinal symptoms, and there have been reports of increased heart rate and blood pressure in some studies, therapeutic doses of GLP-1 appear to be well tolerated [40]. GLP-1 has been shown to improve insulin action in some animal studies, but this has not been confirmed in clinical trials [45].

An important and therapeutically appealing feature of GLP-1 is its effect to increase growth and differentiation of B-cells [46]. GLP-1 has also been shown to increase neogenesis of B-cells, which appear to derive from cells in the exocrine pancreatic ducts [47]. These progenitor cells are sensitive to raised concentrations of GLP-1, which promotes differentiation in part by increased expression of the transcription factor PDX-1. Thus GLP-1 provides a potential means to expand the B-cell population and replace B-cells that are advanced in functional decline (Figure 8).

The main limitation to therapeutic application of GLP-1 has been its very short plasma half-life of less than 2 min after intravenous (IV) injection [about 1 h after subcutaneous (SC) injection] due mainly to rapid N-terminal degradation by the circulating enzyme dipeptidyl peptidase 4 (DPP-4) [40]. The initial breakdown product, GLP-1-(9-36) binds to the GLP-1 receptor with low affinity and may act as a competitive antagonist of the full peptide. This

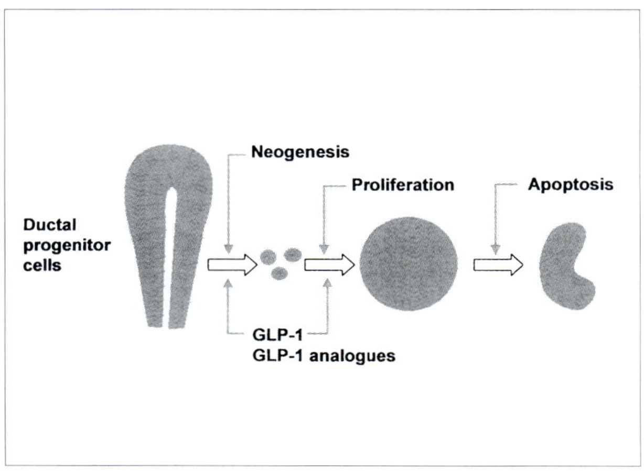

Figure 8 GLP-1-(7-36 amide) and the GLP-1 analogue, exendin-4, promote neogenesis and proliferation of pancreatic B-cells

```
                  DPP4
                   |
                   ↓
Human GLP-1       HAEGT FTSDV SSYLE GQAAK FFIAW LVKGR G       (7-37)
Human GLP-1       HAEGT FTSDV SSYLE GQAAK FFIAW LVKGR         (7-36 amide)
Exendin-4         HGEGT FTSDL SKQME EEAVR LFIEW LKNGG PSSGA PPPSG
Human GIP         YAEGT FISDY SIAMD KIHQQ DFVNW LLAQK GKKND WKHNI TQ
Human Glucagon    HSQGT FTSDY SKYLD SRRAQ DFVQW LMNT
```

Figure 9 Amino acid sequences of human glucagon-like peptide 1 (GLP-1), human GLP-1-(7-36) amide, exendin-4, human glucose-dependent insulinotropic peptide (GIP), and human glucagon. The arrow shows the site at which dipeptidyl peptidase 4 (DPP-4) cleaves GLP-1 and GIP at the Ala2 residue, and glucagon at the Ser2 residue. Exendin-4 is not cleaved by DPP-4

enzyme is specific for an Ala, Pro, or Ser residue at position 2 from the N-terminus. Hence, analogues of GLP-1 that modify the amino acid sequence to avoid this degradation have been sought. One such analogue is exendin-4 (Figure 9). Exendin-4 (AC2993) was first isolated from the venom of a North American reptile known as the Gila monster (*Heloderma suspectum*). Exendin-4 has a longer half-life than native GLP-1, but retains the same biological profile [46, 48, 49]. Recent clinical trials in type 2 diabetic patients found that SC injection or infusion of exendin-4 for up to 28 days improved the daily glucose profile, and especially reduced postprandial glucose excursions [50, 51].

Another long-acting analogue of GLP-1 is NN2211 (Liraglutide) (Arg34, Lys26-(N-ε-(γ-Glu(N-α-hexadecanoyl)))-GLP-1-(7-37)) in which GLP-1 is linked to a fatty acid [52]. This analogue binds to plasma proteins, giving a half-life of about 12 h after SC injection. During a trial in type 2 patients, NN2211 (10 ug/kg once daily SC) reduced fasting plasma glucose by 1.1 mmol/l and postprandial glycemia by 23%, the reduction being associated with an increase in postprandial insulin, a decrease in postprandial glucagon, and a delay in gastric emptying [53]. A related strategy to obviate rapid cleavage by DPP-4 has been the construction of GLP-1 linked to a drug affinity complex that conjugates to albumin *in vivo* (CJC-1131), which causes prolonged activation of the GLP-1 receptor [54]. Glycated GLP-1 analogues provide further opportunities to extend the duration of action of GLP-1 [55]. To overcome the need for parenteral delivery of GLP-1, buccal and oral formulations have been considered, including an oral preparation of D-Ala2 analogue encapsulated in poly-lactide-co-glycolide microspheres [56].

GIP stimulates insulin biosynthesis and contributes substantially to the overall incretin response [41], and its therapeutic potential has been demonstrated using the DPP4-resistant analogues such as D-Ala2 GIP and glycated GIP [57, 58]. However, GIP may tend to raise postprandial glucagon. The capacity of various gastrointestinal hormones to expand the B-cell mass, notably gastrin [59], might be an exploitable therapeutic avenue.

Dipeptidyl Peptidase 4 Inhibitors

Since endogenous and exogenous GLP-1 and GIP are rapidly inactivated at the N-terminus by circulating DPP4, inhibitors of DPP-4 have been explored to therapeutically enhance the incretin effects of these peptides [60]. Several such inhibitors (e.g. thiazolidine derivatives), administered with or without supplementary GLP-1, have shown promise as antidiabetic agents in animal models of diabetes [61–64], and have been reported to improve insulin sensitivity as well as improve B-cell function. Interestingly, the DPP-4 inhibitor NVPDPP728 reduced fasting and postprandial hyperglycemia without raising insulin concentrations, during a 4-week trial in type 2 patients [65]. DPP-4 degrades a variety of circulating peptides (e.g., PYY and NPY) including glucagon, which might contribute to the glucose-lowering effect, but it is not yet evident whether effects of DPP-4 inhibitors on other peptides could limit their use [60].

Phosphodiesterase Inhibitors

Selective suppression of phosphodiesterase (PDE) activity in islet B-cells offers a potential therapeutic approach to raise intracellular cAMP and thereby increase insulin biosynthesis and secretion. Several PDEs (PDE-1, -2, -3, -4, and -5) are expressed by pancreatic islets, and PDE-1, -3, and -5 appear to be the main types in B-cells. Isoform PDE-3B is mainly responsible for increasing glucose-induced insulin secretion, and selective inhibitors of this isoform substantially enhance insulin secretion *in vitro* [66]. Less selective inhibitors of PDEs (e.g. JTT-608, Figure 6) have increased insulin secretion and improved glycemic control in animal models of diabetes [67, 68], but the challenge is to specifically target the B-cell *in vivo* with a PDE-3B inhibitor.

Succinate Esters

Esters of succinic acid (Figure 10) stimulate proinsulin biosynthesis and insulin secretion [69]. They provide a substrate for mitochondrial energy production at the level of the Krebs cycle; hence, they can substitute for

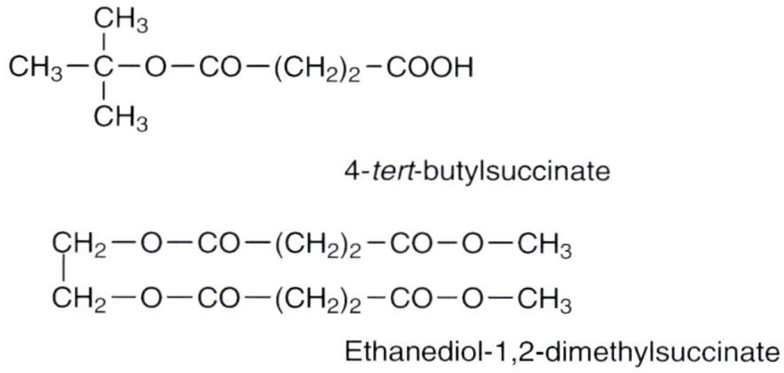

Figure 10 Examples of two succinate esters, 4-*tert*-butylsuccinate and ethanediol-1,2-dimethylsuccinate

nutrients to initiate insulin secretion and enhance submaximal stimulation of insulin secretion by glucose and other agents that close K_{ATP} channels. Succinate-induced energy production also appears to elicit transcription signals that promote proinsulin production. However, succinate esters have low enteral bioavailability, and a short duration of action and general effects as a metabolic fuel, including increased gluconeogenesis in the liver. Thus they will require specific targeting to the B-cell. Another possibility would be to target the B-cell, with an agent to stimulate succinyl-CoA synthetase [70].

OTHER INSULIN SECRETAGOGUES

α-Adrenoceptors in the B-cell membrane normally mediate a tonic suppression of insulin secretion, and in theory selective antagonism of these receptors should lift this suppression. However, potent and specific agents for pharmaceutical development have not emerged; indeed, several α-adrenoreceptor antagonists (e.g., phentolamine, idazoxan, efaroxan, and midaglizole) also bind at other sites, including K_{ATP} channels [13]. Various other types of insulin secretagogues have been considered in a pharmaceutical context, but have not proceeded in development [13]. The antibiotic erythromycin potentiates glucose-induced insulin release and might serve as a template for an antidiabetic drug (by analogy with the history of sulfonylureas from sulfonamide antibacterial drugs) [71]. The neuropeptide pituitary adenylate-cyclase-activating polypeptide (PACAP) stimulates insulin secretion in a glucose-dependent manner, might be pharmacologically exploitable [72].

INSULIN ACTION ENHANCERS

A substitute for insulin, preferably active by oral administration and able to circumvent insulin resistance, has long been sought but remains elusive. Several agents can partially substitute for insulin either by independently mimicking certain actions of insulin or by potentiating pathways of insulin action. Such agents should be helpful therapeutically to enhance insulin action in hypoinsulinemic states. Their potential therapeutic use to overcome insulin resistance is likely to depend largely on whether their site of action is distal to, or able to bypass, the rate-limiting defect(s) of the insulin action pathway. It has yet to be established that any "substitute" agents with insulin-like effects can sustain normal life indefinitely in the total absence of insulin. A route map of intracellular insulin signaling pathways is illustrated in Figure 11 showing some potential sites of therapeutic intervention.

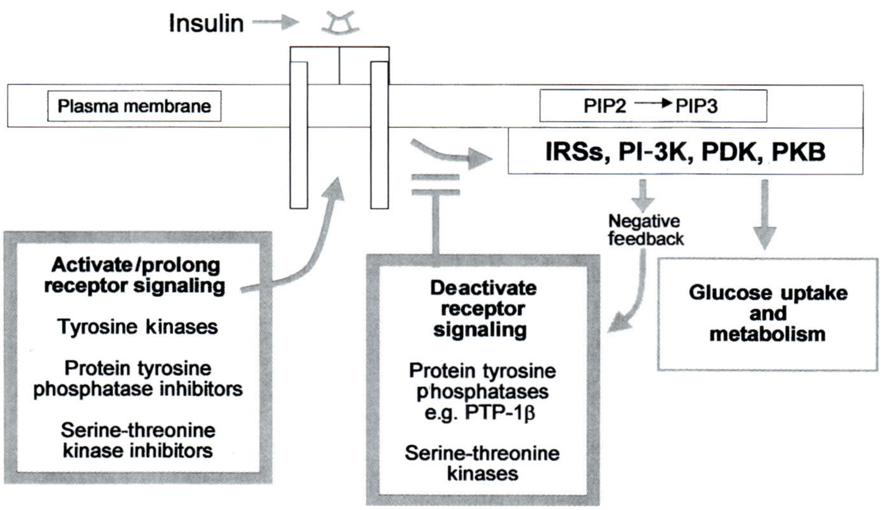

Figure 11 Intracellular pathways of insulin signaling showing some potential sites of therapeutic intervention. IRS = insulin receptor substrate; PTP-1B = protein tyrosine phosphatase 1B; PI-3K = phosphatidylinositol 3 kinase; PIP2 = phosphatidylinositol-3,4-bisphosphate; PIP3 = phosphatidylinositol-3,4, 5-trisphosphate; PDK = phosphoinositide-dependent kinase; PKB (akt) = protein kinase B; PKC = protein kinase C

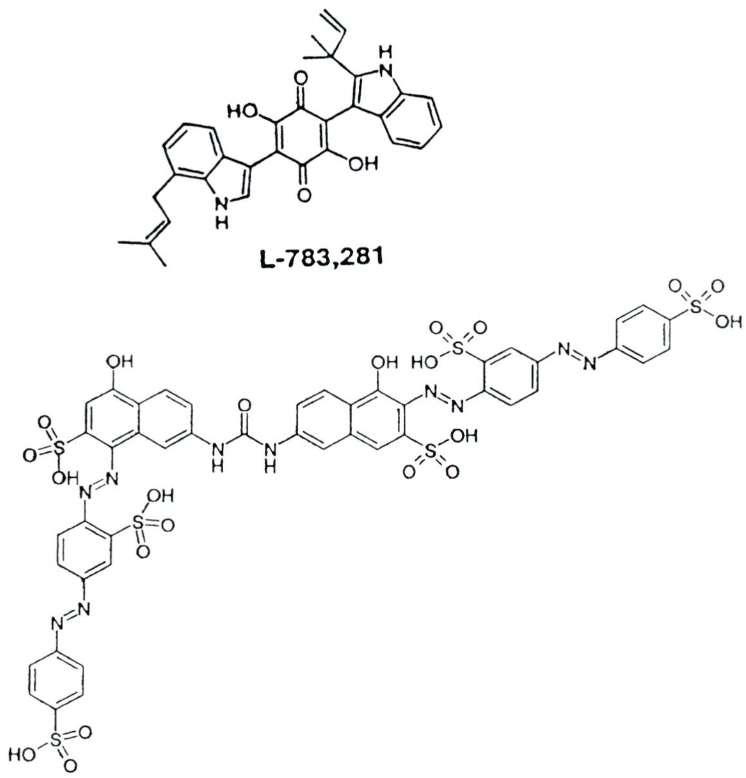

Figure 12 Structure of compounds that increase insulin action by enhancing insulin receptor signaling activity: L-783,281 and TLK16998

Insulin Receptor Activation

In principle, an agent that directly activates kinase activity of the B-subunit of the insulin receptor could elicit the full range of biological actions of insulin. The metabolite L-783,281 (Figure 12) from a *Pseudomassaria* species of fungus, which was active by oral administration, selectively and directly stimulated phosphorylation and activation of tyrosine kinase activity of the B-subunit of the insulin receptor [73, 74]. This in turn induced tyrosine phosphorylation and activation of insulin receptor substrate 1 (IRS-1), increased activity of phosphatidylinositol 3 kinase (PI-3K), and increased phosphorylation of protein kinase B (PKB, also known as akt). This resulted in a range of insulin-like effects including increased glucose uptake by adipocytes and skeletal muscle [73]. After oral administration to insulin-resistant, obese-diabetic *db*/*db* mice, L-783,281 caused acute lowering of blood glucose, which was sustained over a week of daily administration. The antihyperglycemic effect was less marked in *ob*/*ob* mice, which are more severely insulin resistant and grossly hyperinsulinemic. Although L-783,281 itself may not be suitable for clinical development, this compound appears to provide proof of concept for an orally active nonpeptide substitute for insulin.

Several mechanisms have been reported to enhance or prolong phosphorylation of the B-subunit of the insulin receptor after stimulation by insulin at the A-subunit, thereby potentiating insulin action. A nonpeptide molecule TLK16998 (Figure 12), which does not interact with the A-subunit and has no effect in the absence of insulin, increased insulin-induced phosphorylation of the insulin receptor B-subunit [74, 75]. This augmented the insulin-signaling cascade through IRS-1 and PI-3K, and increased translocation of glucose transporter isoform 4 (GLUT-4) into the plasma membrane of adipocytes. Accordingly, TLK6998 increased glucose uptake by adipocytes in response to submaximal stimulation by insulin. TLK6998 also acutely reduced the hyperglycemia in *db*/*db* mice and low-dose streptozotocin (STZ) mice after intraperitoneal injection [75].

It is recognized that administration of C-peptide along with insulin in type 1 diabetes can improve glycemic control [76]. In cultured L6 muscle cells, C-peptide increased glycogen synthesis in response to submaximal stimulation with insulin but not with a maximally effective insulin concentration [77]. At the submaximal insulin concentration, C-peptide increased insulin receptor tyrosine kinase activity, tyrosine phosphorylation of IRS-1, activity of PI-3K (but not akt in this study), and increased phosphorylation of mitogen-activated protein kinase (MAPK). Although the mechanism through which C-peptide enhances the action of a low concentration of insulin is unclear (presumably via a C-peptide receptor), it represents a possible route for therapeutic intervention.

Protein tyrosine phosphatases (PTPs), especially PTP-1B, normally dephosphorylate the insulin receptor B-subunit and terminate insulin-induced signaling. They also dephosphorylate and deactivate IRS-1 and IRS-2. Thus, mice with a homozygous PTP-1B knockout [78], and mice treated with antisense oligonucleotides against PTP-1B [79] show increased insulin sensitivity. Several selective inhibitors of PTP-1B, such as benzonaphthofurans and thiophenes, have been shown to reduce the hyperglycemia in insulin-resistant diabetic animals [80]. Vanadium salts (considered in more detail later) can inhibit PTPs including PTP-1B, and may enhance insulin action in part via this effect [81].

Negative feedback by downstream intermediates of the insulin-signaling cascades can reduce the tyroine kinase activity of the insulin receptor and IRS-1/2; for example, PI-3K and PKB (akt) appear to promote phosphorylation of serine and threonine residues on the insulin receptor B-subunit to terminate receptor signaling [82]. It is possible that certain isoforms of PKC and inhibitor factor κB kinase (IKKB) could mediate these effects; hence, selective inhibitors of these proteins could provide a means to prolong the signaling activity of the insulin receptor and IRS-1/2 to sustain insulin action [83]. Salicylates may exert beneficial effects against insulin resistance in this manner [84].

Insulin-like growth factor 1 (IGF-1) exerts weak insulin action through low-affinity binding to the insulin receptor and through cross talk between the IGF-1 receptor and postreceptor sites in the insulin-signaling cascades [85]. Accordingly, injection of IGF-1 can reduce hyperglycemia in type 1 and type 2 diabetes. The ability of IGF-1 receptor signaling to activate the insulin signaling cascade can be exploited for the treatment of rare genetic syndromes in which the number of functional insulin receptors is very severely depleted. However, since IGF-1 and analogues can exert proliferative effects these agents are not considered to be suitable for the routine treatment of diabetes. N-terminal fragments of human growth hormone (hGH) have been reported to potentiate insulin action, possibly in part by increasing insulin receptor binding, although the main effect appears to occur at a postreceptor level [86]. Stable nonpeptide analogues to mimic this effect have not been forthcoming.

Although a decreased number of insulin receptors is often a feature of insulin-resistant states it is not a rate-limiting defect for impaired insulin action in most type 2 diabetic patients. However, agents that increase the number of insulin receptors may improve insulin sensitivity. Treatment of type 2 diabetic patients with mosapride, a benzamide derivative that activates serotonin 5HT-4 receptors and hastens gastric emptying, increased the number of erythrocyte insulin receptors and their autophosphorylation, associated with improved insulin sensitivity and improved glycemic control [87].

Insulin Postreceptor Signaling

In addition to potential interventions at the level of IRS-1/2 mentioned above, several compounds have been reported to increase intracellular insulin signaling at sites distal to the insulin receptor, or prevent the effect of cytokines and other physiological signals that normally decrease expression or activity of postreceptor signaling intermediates.

PI-3K is a key enzyme in the main signaling pathway for insulin-stimulated glucose transport, and activity of this enzyme is often reduced in insulin-resistant states. PI-3K promotes phosphorylation of phosphatidylinositol 4,5-bisphosphate (PIP2) to the 1,4,5-trisphosphate (PIP3), and increased availability of precursor inositol substrate has been considered as a potential means of increasing this reaction. Administration of D-chiro-inositol (INS-1) to non-insulin-dependent animal models and to type 2 diabetic patients reduced the hyperglycemia [88]. Similarly, the 3-methoxy analogue of D-chiro-inositol (pinitol, Figure 13) improved muscle glucose uptake

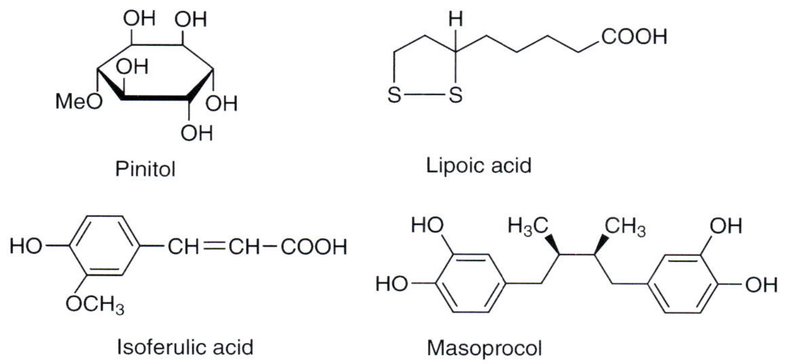

Figure 13 Structure of compounds that increase insulin action by enhancing insulin postreceptor signaling activity: pinitol, lipoic acid, isoferulic acid, and masoprocol

and reduced the hyperglycemia in hypoinsulinemic STZ-diabetic mice [89]. The therapeutic potential of boosting PI-3K-mediated PIP3 production has been further illustrated using an antisense oligonucleotide to a protein phosphatase (PTEN) that dephosphorylates PIP3. Administration of the oligonucleotide (intraperitoneally, once weekly) to *db/db* and *ob/ob* mice increased signaling downstream of PIP3, improved insulin sensitivity, and normalized glycemia [90].

The antioxidant α-lipoic acid (Figure 13) can increase insulin sensitivity and improve glycemic control in diabetic states where there is still some endogenous insulin production or exogenous insulin administration [91, 92]. This might be due in part to the action of α-lipoic acid as a cofactor for mitochondrial dehydrogenases involved in glucose metabolism. However, α-lipoic acid also enhances insulin-stimulated glucose uptake by increased tyrosine phosphorylation of IRS-1 [93], resulting in increased glucose uptake via at least two pathways: first, the PI-3K pathway that increases GLUT-4 translocation into the plasma membrane; and second, by a pathway involving MAPK that does not alter GLUT-4 translocation [94].

Several cytokines, especially those from adipose tissue (adipokines) such as tumor necrosis factor α (TNF-α) and interleukin 6 (IL-6), and adipocyte hormones such as resistin are known to promote insulin resistance. Agents designed to suppress the secretion or action of these substances to alleviate insulin resistance have not emerged, although agonists of the peroxisome proliferator-activated receptor-γ (PPAR-γ) reduce production of TNF-α and resistin (discussed below). General treatments to reduce adiposity are beyond the remit of this chapter. The adipocyte hormone leptin, which exerts centrally mediated satiety and thermogenic effects, promotes lipid oxidation apparently without inhibiting glucose metabolism [95]. Evidence from cultured muscle cells suggests that the postreceptor leptin signaling pathway may activate the postreceptor insulin pathway, but it is unclear whether this could be exploited therapeutically [96]. Another adipocyte hormone, adiponectin, has been reported to protect against insulin resistance and atherogenesis by a variety of putative processes [97, 98], making this hormone an enticing new candidate for therapeutic adaptation.

Negative effects of chronic hyperglycemia (glucotoxicity) and dyslipidemia (lipotoxicity) on postreceptor insulin-signaling pathways are known to contribute to insulin resistance, and some aspects are covered elsewhere in this chapter. However, it is noteworthy here that the detrimental effects of hyperglycemia on insulin-dependent glucose uptake appear to involve activation of certain isoforms of PKC. Thus, in theory (as mentioned earlier) isoform-specific inhibitors of PKC could reduce this cause of insulin resistance [83]. However, other isoforms of PKC can stimulate insulin-independent and/or insulin-dependent glucose uptake by muscle [99, 100]. Isoform-specific inhibitors of PKC may be useful in the treatment of micro- and macrovascular and neural complications of diabetes, but it will be crucial to ensure adequate selectivity to separate wanted and unwanted effects on glucose metabolism [99].

Increased flux of glucose through the hexosamine pathway is another route for glucotoxicity to cause insulin resistance [101]. Entry to this pathway is regulated by the enzyme glutamine:fructose-6-phosphate amidotransferase (GFAT), and this is therefore a potential therapeutic target.

Several compounds that partially mimic or improve insulin-mediated glucose metabolism have been described as possible new antidiabetic agents. The dopamine D2 receptor agonist bromocriptine improves insulin sensitivity and glycemic control in type 2 diabetes [102] but has not proceeded in development for antidiabetic use. Isoferulic acid (Figure 13) inhibits gluconeogenesis by reducing phosphoenolpyruvate carboxykinase (PEPCK) and increases muscle glucose transport by increased expression of GLUT-4 in insulinopenic rats [103]. Sibutramine, a satiety-inducing serotonin–noradrenaline reuptake inhibitor used to treat obesity, produces metabolites that increase glucose transport in muscle [104]. Angiotensin converting enzyme (ACE) inhibitors improve insulin sensitivity independently of their antihypertensive action. This effect is mediated by bradykinin, acting via kinin B2 receptors. ACE and circulating neutral endopeptidases (NEPs) normally degrade bradykinin; hence, agents that prevent the breakdown of bradykinin (for example, based on ACE and NEP inhibitors) provide an avenue to increase insulin action [105, 106].

Many extracts and purified compounds from plants improve insulin-mediated glucose metabolism [20]. Athough their mechanisms of action are often unclear, they have formed the basis of an expanding industry to find new leads for antidiabetic agents. A recent example is masoprocol (Figure 13) from creosote bush, which decreased plasma glucose and triglyceride concentrations in STZ-diabetic rats [107]. Phorbol esters and other substances have been reported to enhance the intrinsic activity of glucose transporters, but therapeutic targeting of this action has not been reported [13].

PPAR-γ Agonists

The nuclear peroxisome proliferator-activated receptor-gamma (PPAR-γ), which exists as a heterodimer with the retinoid X receptor (RXR), provides a pharmacological target to increase insulin sensitivity. Currently available thiazolidinediones (rosiglitazone and pioglitazone, Figure 14) are PPAR-γ agonists. PPAR-γ is expressed mostly by adipose tissue where it mediates adipogenesis, lipogenesis, and glucose uptake (Figure 15). In particular it promotes the development of preadipocytes into

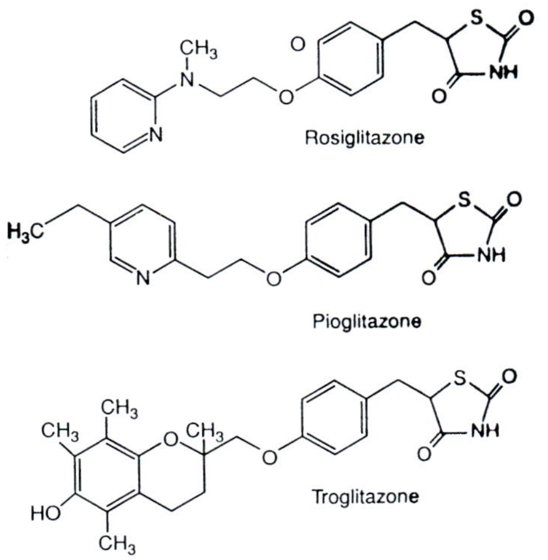

Figure 14 Structures of the PPAR-γ agonists thiazolidinediones pioglitazone, rosiglitazone, and troglitazone

new adipocytes in the subcutaneous depots. Activation of PPAR-γ induces transcription of a group of genes that are also sensitive to insulin; these include lipoprotein lipase, fatty acid transporter protein, adipocyte fatty acid binding protein (aP2), fatty acyl-CoA synthase, glycerol kinase, malic enzyme, glucokinase, and PEPCK [108]. Thiazolidinediones also induce GLUT-4 mRNA. Current wisdom attributes much of the antihyperglycemic efficacy of PPAR-γ agonists to increased adipogenesis and adipocyte lipogenesis. This decreases circulating concentrations of free fatty acids (FFAs), altering the glucose-fatty acid (Randle) cycle to favor glucose utilization by muscle [109]. Thiazolidinediones also act directly on insulin target tissues to ameliorate the lipotoxic effects of FFAs on early insulin postreceptor signaling intermediates such as IRS-1, due in part to prevention of reduced levels of fatty acid translocase (FAT/CD36) [110]. Additionally, PPAR-γ agonists reduce adipocyte production of cytokines that cause insulin resistance such as TNF-α, and the hormone resistin, and increase the production of adiponectin and activate PI-3K [16, 111, 112]. Further actions of PPAR-γ agonists to improve insulin action probably occur through the modest expression of PPAR-γ in skeletal muscle and liver, and thiazolidinediones may additionally operate via mechanisms that are independent of PPAR-γ [113, 114].

Several new PPAR-γ agonists are in development as potential antidiabetic agents (Table 4). These include both thiazolidinediones [115–122] and non-thiazolidinediones [123–126]. Although there is generally a good positive correlation between their binding affinity for PPAR-γ and their antihyperglycemic efficacy in non-insulin-dependent diabetic animals [127], there are exceptions. For example MCC-555 and NC-2100 have potent antihyperglycemic efficacy but only weak PPAR-γ agonism [118, 119]. This may be due to actions of the non-thiazolidinedione moiety of the molecule, which could have independent glucose-lowering activity or interfere with binding at the PPAR-γ-ligand binding epitope so as to alter the receptor conformation in a manner that recruits different coactivators and consequently alters the selection of genes transcribed [128, 129]. Theoretically, therefore, it should be possible to selectively modify the structure of PPAR-γ agonists, to create a preferred therapeutic profile. This might provide

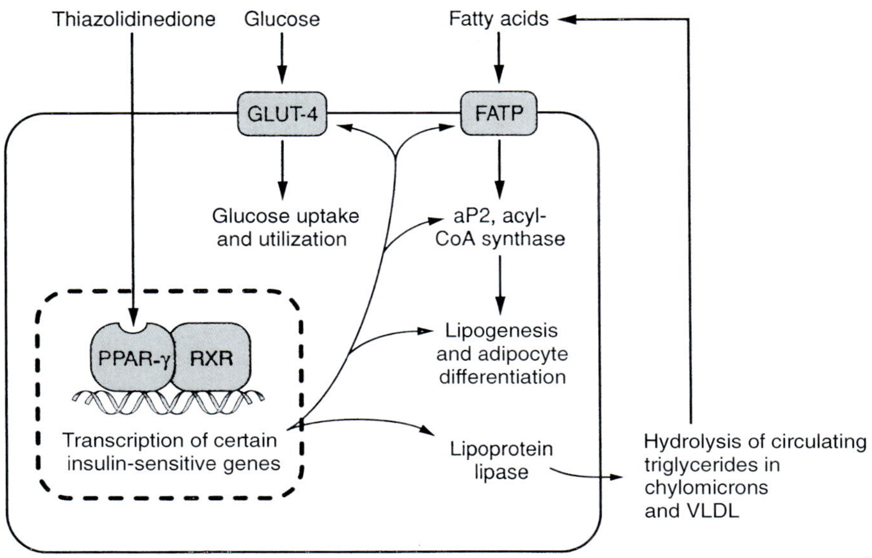

Figure 15 Cellular mechanism of action of PPAR-γ agonists on adipose tissue. PPAR-γ = peroxisome proliferator-activated receptor γ; RXR = retinoid X receptor; GLUT-4 = glucose transporter isoform 4; FATP = fatty acid transporter protein; aP2 = adipocyte fatty acid-binding protein; VLDL = very low-density lipoproteins

Table 4 Examples of thiazolidinedione and non-thiazolidinedione PPAR-γ agonists and dual PPAR-γ/α agonists under investigation as potential new oral antidiabetic agents

Thiazolidinediones	Non-thiazolidinediones
PPAR-γ agonists	
BM-13.1246 and BM-15.2054	BM-17.0744
CS-011/CI-1037*	GI-262570*†
MCC-555	GW-1929
NC-2100	
NIP-221* and NIP-223	L-764406
T-174	
TZD-300512*	
R-483	
Dual PPAR-γ/α agonists	
DRF-2189	BMS-298585
KRP-297†	AZ-242
	LY-465608
	GW-409544
	NN-622†
	JTT-501†
	CLX-0940

* May also exhibit some PPAR-α agonism.
† Believed to be discontinued in clinical development.

an opportunity to minimize side effects that appear to be associated with PPAR-γ agonism, such as fluid retention and edema. However, it will be important to exclude structures that could give rise to hepatotoxicity as seen with a previous thiazolidinedione troglitazone [130].

PPAR-γ is expressed to a small extent in many cell types including pancreatic B-cells, and there is evidence in animal models that PPAR-γ agonists can restore B-cell granulation. This raises the possiblility that PPAR-γ agonists could be selected for beneficial effects on the B-cell [131, 132]. Structure–activity relationships could be biased to enhance other effects of PPAR-γ agonists relevant to diabetes, notably to reduce chronic low-grade inflammation, markers of nephropathy, myriad vascular risk factors, and other conditions such as polycystic ovary syndrome that are associated with insulin resistance [133].

Dual PPAR-γ and PPAR-α Agonists

PPAR-α is strongly expressed by liver and muscle where it promotes the oxidation of fatty acids through increased transcription of acyl-CoA synthase and various mitochondrial enzymes of the β-oxidation pathway [108]. Fibrates are PPAR-α agonists that produce their lipid-lowering effect in this manner. Some PPAR-γ agonists are already known to exhibit low affinity binding to PPAR-α conferring substantial glucose lowering *and* lipid-lowering efficacy [111]. This has prompted the selection of potential new thiazolidinedione and non-thiazolidinedione agents with binding affinities for both PPAR-γ and PPAR-α, so-called dual PPAR-γ/α agonists [134–137] (Table 4). For optimal therapeutic efficacy it will be important that these agents have similar binding affinities for both PPAR-γ and PPAR-α to achieve a balanced glucose-lowering and lipid-lowering efficacy.

Compounds that simultaneously activate PPAR-α, -γ, and -δ (termed PPARpan agonists) have recently been described. Preliminary reports suggest that these compounds might offer better glycemic control in diabetic animal models than selective PPAR-γ agonists, and better lipid benefits than selective PPAR-α agonists [138].

Combined PPAR-γ and RXR Agonists

Activation of PPAR-γ normally requires coactivation of RXR by retinoic acid [108]. Synthetic agonists of RXR have been ascribed various effects, including reduced feeding and reduced weight gain, increased energy dissipation through increased production of mitochondrial uncoupling proteins, and possibly increased signaling through PI-3K. These effects complement those of PPAR-γ and provide justification for exploring combined PPAR-γ–RXR agonism. Indeed, coadministration of an RXR agonist with a PPAR-γ agonist can produce additive effects on glucose and lipid metabolism in muscle and counter the weight gain that often occurs with a PPAR-γ agonist alone [139–142]. However, the effects of synthetic RXR agonists may depend upon interactions with sites other than the RXR ligand-binding site on the RXR receptor, leaving the structural requirements for RXR agonists undefined.

MINERALS

Circulating concentrations of some minerals, notably magnesium, chromium, and zinc, are often reduced in diabetic patients (Table 5), and supplementation may improve glycemic control in cases of mineral deficiency [143]. Magnesium is required for phosphate transfer and kinase reactions including insulin receptor and postreceptor signaling. Hypomagnesemia is not uncommon in insulin-resistant states, and magnesium supplements have been reported to improve insulin action and B-cell function, and possibly reduce cardiovascular mortality in magnesium-deficient diabetic patients [143, 144]. Chromium deficiency is common in type 2 diabetes, especially the elderly, and trials with trivalent chromium supplements have improved glycemic control, without increasing insulin concentrations [145]. Although there is concern about over-replacement of chromium, the potential value of correcting a deficiency state is often disregarded. Adequate chromium is necessary for normal insulin sensitivity, but the site of action of chromium is unresolved. Reduced zinc concentrations in diabetes are rarely severe, and a therapeutic indication for zinc supplements is unclear [143]. High concentrations of zinc can exert various insulin-like effects *in vitro* and *in vivo*, but the mechanisms are

Table 5 Potential mineral deficiencies and supplements in diabetic patients

	Reduced levels in diabetes	Deficiency in diabetes	Cause	RDA (mg/day)	Supplementation improved glycemic control
Magnesium	Yes	About 25%*	↑excretion	350	Yes†
Zinc	Yes	Rare	↑excretion	15	Equivocal‡
Chromium	Yes	In elderly	? poor diet	<0.2	Yes§

Note: RDA = recommended daily allowance in United States. ↑ indicates "increase"; ? indicates "uncertain."
* Deficiency taken as <2 SD below normal.
† In magnesium-deficient patients.
‡ Improved glycemic control in patients with coexistent liver disease.
§ Must use trivalent form of chromium; supplementation also lowers plasma cholesterol.

unestablished [146]. Zinc can also protect against B-cell damage, and zinc supplements have been reported to improve glycemic control in diabetic patients with liver disease [147, 148].

Vanadium

Vanadium salts exert insulin-like effects on glucose metabolism *in vitro* and lower blood glucose levels in animal models of hyperinsulinemic and hypoinsulinemic animal models of diabetes [81]. Small short-term clinical studies have also provided "proof of principle" that vanadium salts can improve glycemic control in type 1 and type 2 diabetic patients; insulin requirement was reduced in type 1 patients, and there was reduced hepatic glucose output and increased peripheral glucose utilization in type 2 patients [149, 150]. One explanation is that vanadium salts prolong the signaling of insulin receptors and some postreceptor kinases by inhibition of PTPs especially PTP-1B [81]. In addition, vanadium salts can enhance glucose transport in skeletal muscle when PI-3K signaling is blocked, suggesting an effect at a more distal step in the control of glucose transport [151]. Vanadium salts also reduce appetite and slow intestinal glucose absorption [81].

Caution is noted about the cellular accumulation and potential toxicity of vanadium salts. However, a protracted cellular presence of vanadium after a short treatment period might account for the continued antidiabetic effect for weeks after treatment stopped [150], raising the possibility of an intermittent administration schedule. The highly potent effects of peroxovanadium salts, or mixtures of vanadium salts with agents such as benzylamine that give rise to pervanadates, could enable use of very small dosages of vanadium [151, 152]. Poor intestinal absorption of vanadium compounds has been addressed by organic vanadium complexes [153] (Figure 16).

Other Trace Elements

Several futher trace metals have been ascribed some insulin-like properties, including lithium, selenium, molybdenum, tungsten, mercury, and cadmium [143]. However, exploitation of these properties to treat diabetes has been overshadowed by concerns about toxicity. Anecdotal accounts of lithium use in psychiatric medicine and studies in diabetic animals suggest that lithium can modestly improve insulin sensitivity. Unfortunately, lithium also decreases insulin secretion, compromising potential use in type 2 diabetes [143]. Selenium salts reduce hyperglycemia in STZ-diabetic animals, partly through effects on enzyme expression affecting glucose metabolism in the liver [154]. Molybdate and tungstate effectively reduce hyperglycemia in models of insulin-resistant and insulinopenic diabetes [155–157]. Both of these metals beneficially alter the expression and activity of several glucoregulatory enzymes in liver, in particular to reduce gluconeogenesis and increase glycolysis.

VITAMINS

Various dietary vitamin supplements have been reported to improve glycemic control in diabetes but, to date, none has shown a sufficiently specific or potent action to warrant a pharmaceutical application. Large doses of biotin (vitamin H) have been reported to improve insulin sensitivity and improve glucose tolerance in type 2 diabetes [158]. Thiamine (vitamin B1) facilitates glucose metabolism as a cofactor in reactions of pyruvate dehydrogenase and α-ketoglutarate dehydrogenase, and could account for some of the beneficial effects of high-fiber intake in diabetic patients [159].

Bis(maltolato)oxovanadium(IV)

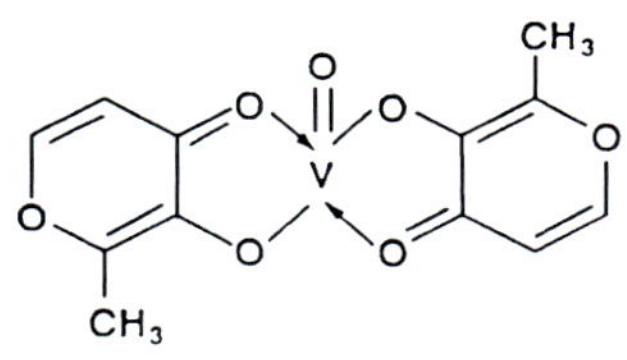

Figure 16 Structure of an organic vanadium complex (bis(maltolato)oxovanadium IV)

Mounting evidence suggests that increased activity of reactive oxygen species contribute to the development of insulin resistance and B-cell damage as well as complications associated with gluco- and lipotoxicity in diabetic states [160]. Natural antioxidant defense is impaired and concentrations of water-soluble vitamins are often reduced in diabetes [161, 162]. Nevertheless, use of antioxidant supplements, notably vitamin C (ascorbic acid), vitamin E (α-tocopherol), and β-carotene has given equivocal results with regard to glycemic control [163, 164]. Nicotinic acid (niacin), used in the treatment of dyslipidaemia, has been considered for the treatment of hyperglycemia (see lipid section below).

INHIBITORS OF COUNTERREGULATORY HORMONES

Key hormones that bring about a rise in blood glucose concentrations are glucagon, adrenaline, growth hormone, and glucocorticoids, and inappropriately raised concentrations of these hormones can occur in diabetic states. While the use of specific inhibitors against the secretion or action of these hormones has long been considered as an approach to improve glycemic control, it is essential to preserve an adequate counterregulatory response to hypoglycemia [see Chapter 64].

Glucagon Antagonists

Agents that inhibit glucagon secretion such as somatostatin analogues and the sulphonamidobenzamide MB-39890A have not been sufficiently selective for use as antidiabetic agents [13]. Some glucagon analogues that compete with native glucagon for receptor binding sites fail to elicit the normal biological effects; these peptides exerted antihyperglycemic effects, but are short-acting and not suitable for drug development [13]. Recently, nonpeptide glucagon receptor antagonists have shown more promise. Bay27-9955 is an isopropylfluorobiphenyl compound that competitively blocks the binding of native glucagon to its receptor [165]. This compound substantially reduced glucagon-stimulated hepatic glucose output in type 2 diabetes. Another nonpeptide, NNC25-2504, is a noncompetitive glucagon receptor antagonist that appears to bind to the transmembrane region of the receptor [166]. The fungal bisanthroquinone, skyrin, uncouples the glucagon receptor from its activation of adenylate cyclase, preventing glucagon-stimulated cAMP production [167].

Glucocorticoid Antagonists

Raised glucocorticoid concentrations are often implicated in the development of obesity, insulin resistance, impaired glucose tolerance, and various other features of the metabolic syndrome [168]. Chronic glucocorticoid therapy can precipitate diabetes, and a reduction of glucocorticoid concentrations improves glycemic control and ameliorates other features of the metabolic syndrome in obese diabetic animal models [169]. Reducing glucocorticoid production with agents that selectively inhibit enzymes of steroid synthesis is a potential means to achieve this, particularly to dampen early-morning spikes of glucocorticoid release. This in turn should suppress hepatic glucose output and constrain the dawn phenomenon of raised early-morning glycemia. Lowering the morning basal level of glycemia should facilitate glycemic control throughout the day [170].

Another approach to reduce the metabolic effects of glucocorticoids takes advantage of the normal cellular conversion of less active cortisone to more active cortisol. This reaction is mediated by the enzyme 11β-hydroxysteroid dehydrogenase 1 (11BHSD-1), which is strongly expressed in liver and adipose tissue [171]. Selective inhibition of 11BHSD with a benzenesulfonamide derivative, BVT2733, has been shown to improve glycemic control without increasing insulin concentrations in diabetic KKAy mice, associated with reduced hepatic expression of PEPCK and glucose-6-phosphatase [172].

Somatostatin Analogues

Somatostatin reduces intestinal motility, delays nutrient absorption, and inhibits the secretion of growth hormone and glucagon, but its therapeutic potential is restricted by a short half-life. The analogue octreotide (Figure 17) rapidly suppresses growth hormone and glucagon secretion [13, 143]. It has been considered for type 1 patients to decrease postprandial glycemia when injected subcutaneously before the meal, and to reduce daily insulin requirement. By reducing production of growth hormone and hence IGF-1, octreotide might potentially help to arrest proliferative retinopathy, and it has been suggested that it could delay the progression of advanced diabetic nephropathy. Since octreotide inhibits insulin secretion, it is not appropriate for type 2 diabetes [13].

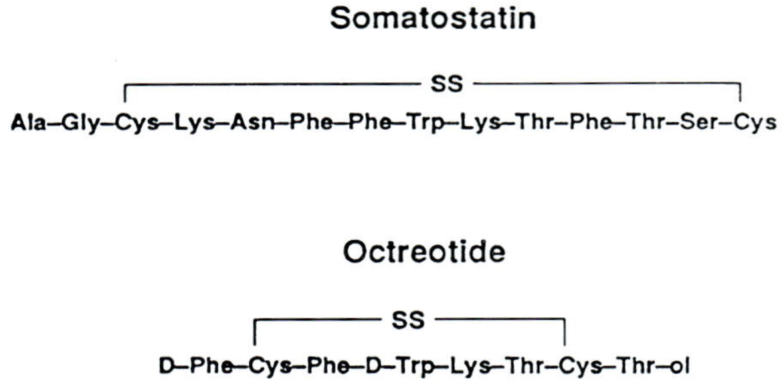

Figure 17 Amino acid sequences of somatostatin-14 and the somatostatin analogue octreotide (Sandostatin, SMS 201-995)

MANIPULATORS OF LIPID METABOLISM

Dyslipidemia occurs commonly in both type 1 and type 2 diabetes, typically including raised plasma concentrations of very low-density lipoprotein (VLDL) triglycerides and FFAs (see Chapter 55). These disturbances and associated excesses of tissue lipids contribute to the pathogenesis of type 2 diabetes [173]. Chronically raised concentrations of fatty acids impair postreceptor insulin signaling and impair B-cell function. Also, increased rates of fatty acid oxidation and re-esterification in diabetic states throw the glucose–fatty acid (Randle) cycle out of balance and contribute to impaired glucose utilization and increased gluconeogenesis. Diabetic dyslipidaemia often warrants treatment in its own right (see Chapter 55), and some of these treatments help to improve glycemic control. PPAR-γ agonists may be considered as primarily affecting lipid metabolism, and other approaches to lower blood glucose via changes in lipid metabolism have been considered.

Antilipolytic and Triglyceride-lowering Agents

Nicotinic acid (niacin) and its longer acting analogue acipimox (Figure 18) suppress lipolysis by adipose tissue and lower circulating FFAs. These agents improve glucose tolerance in type 2 diabetes but the effect is not sustained, and chronic use has not produced consistent improvements in glycemic control [13, 174]. Adenosine reduces adipocyte lipolysis partly by inhibiting cAMP formation. Adenosine agonists such as phenylisopropyladenosine (PIA) can reduce plasma FFA and improve glucose disposal [13].

PPAR-α-agonist fibric acid derivatives such as bezafibrate and gemfibrozil (Figure 19), which are routinely used for lipid lowering, can improve glycemic control but not to a clinically significant extent [175, 176]. Several novel lipid-lowering agents such as the fenfluramine analogue benfluorex and the long-chain dicarboxylic acid Medica 16 (Figure 19), increase insulin action and improve glycemic control in obese and insulin-resistant diabetic states [13, 177, 178].

Inhibitors of Fatty Acid Oxidation

Increased fatty acid oxidation in diabetic states raises the mitochondrial concentration of acetyl-CoA, which suppresses the activity of pyruvate dehydrogenase. Fatty acid oxidation also creates a more reduced NADH- to- NAD ratio and increases citrate production. NADH further suppresses pyruvate dehydrogenase, and citrate inhibits phosphofructokinase (Figure 20). The net result in muscle is a decrease in glucose oxidation, reduced glycolysis, and a decrease in glucose uptake. Raised acetyl-CoA stimulates pyruvate carboxylase, and in the liver these combined factors favor gluconeogenesis. Thus, interventions that inhibit fatty acid oxidation offer a means of increasing glucose utilization and inhibiting gluconeogenesis. A further important effect of reduced fatty acid oxidation is a decrease in ketogenesis.

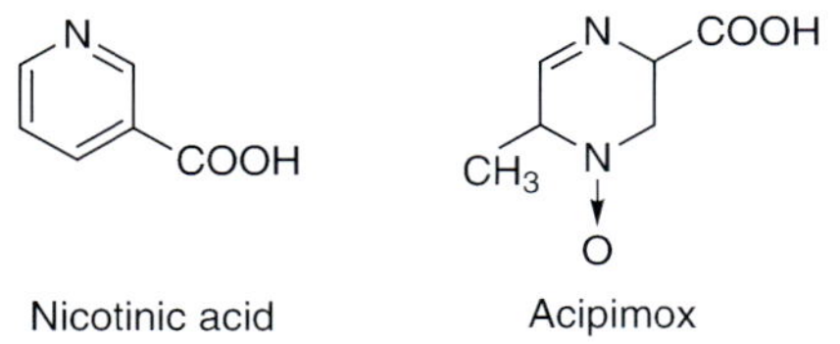

Figure 18 Structures of antilipolytic agents: nicotinic acid and acipimox

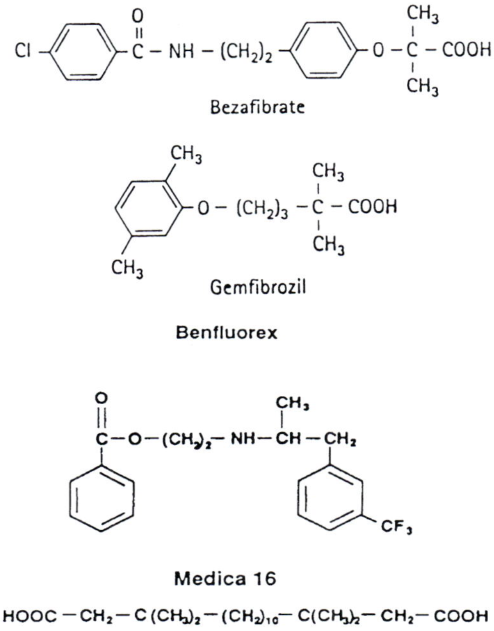

Figure 19 Structures of lipid-lowering agents: bezafibrate, gemfibrozil, benfluorex, and Medica 16

The main approach to inhibiting long-chain fatty acid oxidation has been the inhibition of carnitine palmitoyltransferase 1 (CPT-1), which is the rate-limiting enzyme for transfer of long-chain fatty acyl-CoA into the mitochondria. Such inhibitors include methyl palmoxirate and etomoxir (Figure 21); they have effective glucose-lowering effects in type 2 diabetes and have shown promise as antiketogenic agents for type 1 diabetes [13]. Other inhibitors of long-chain fatty acid oxidation have targeted intramitochondrial enzymes of the β-oxidation pathway of acyl-CoA, such as acyl-CoA dehydrogenase and thiolase. However, the effects of these inhibitors of CPT-1 and other enzymes of fatty acid oxidation have not been rapidly reversible, leaving patients vulnerable to protracted suppression of gluconeogenesis and hypoglycemia [175]. They may also have detrimental effects on lipid metabolism by cardiac muscle.

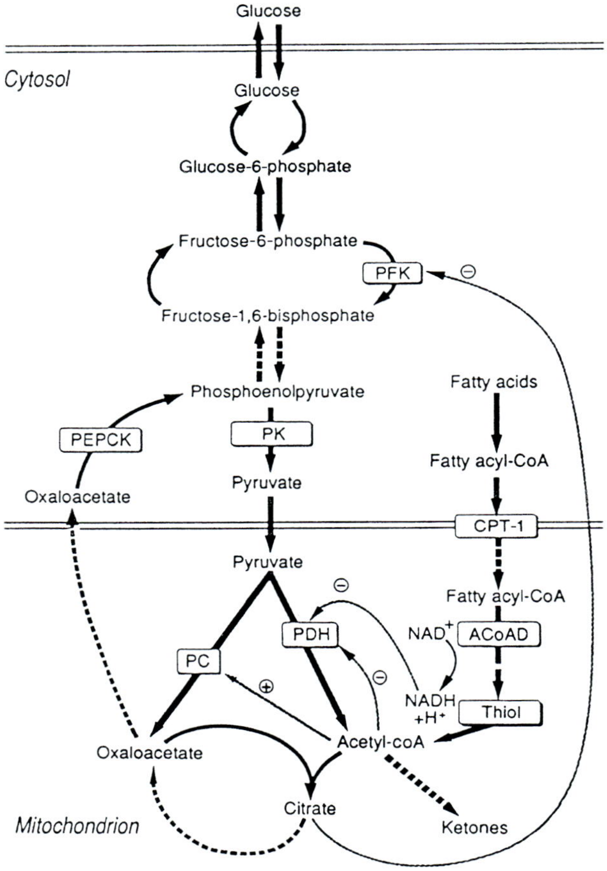

Figure 20 Pathway of long-chain fatty acid oxidation and its implications for glycolysis, glucose oxidation, and gluconeogenesis. ACoAD = acyl-CoA dehydrogenase; Thiol = thiolase; CPT1 = carnitine palmitoyl transferase 1; PDH = pyruvate dehydrogenase; PC = pyruvate carboxylase; PK = pyruvate kinase; PFK = phosphofructokinase; PEPCK = phospho-enolpyruvate carboxykinase; NAD = nicotinamide adenine dinucleotide; NADH = reduced NAD; → single-step pathway; – – → multiple-step pathway; positive (⊕) or negative (⊖) influence. Enzymes are shown in boxes

In contrast to inhibitors of fatty acid oxidation, it is possible that hyperglycemia in diabetes could be improved by agents that facilitate lipid oxidation through effects on membranal and cytosolic fatty acid transporters and binding proteins [179, 180]. Also, stimulation of lipoprotein lipase, for example with NO-1886, has been reported to increase lipid oxidation and improve insulin sensitivity [181].

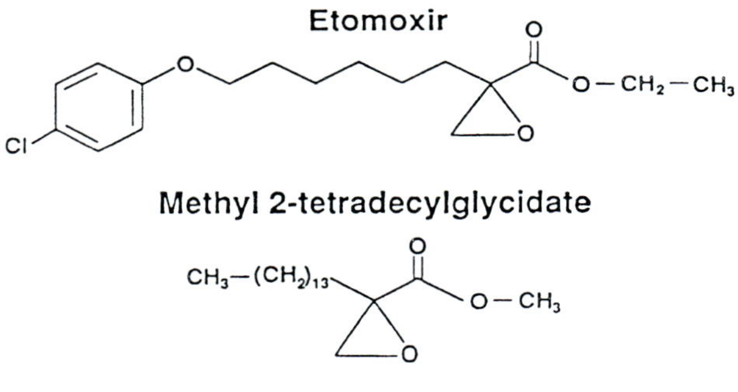

Figure 21 Structures of inhibitors of fatty acid oxidation: etomoxir and methyl palmoxirate. MeTDGA = methyl 2-tetradecylglycidate

ANTIOBESITY AGENTS

Many agents that lower blood glucose are anabolic and prone to cause weight gain, namely insulin, insulin secretagogues, and PPAR-γ agonists, and this may compromise their therapeutic efficacy. Conversely, weight reduction, especially by dieting, is well recognized to increase insulin sensitivity and improve glycemic control in overweight type 2 patients [182]. Although current antiobesity agents (orlistat and sibutramine; and in some countries, also phentermine, ephedrine, and mazindol, Figure 22) do not have a generally accepted place in most algorithms for the treatment of hyperglycemia, new safe and well tolerated antiobesity agents could provide a convenient

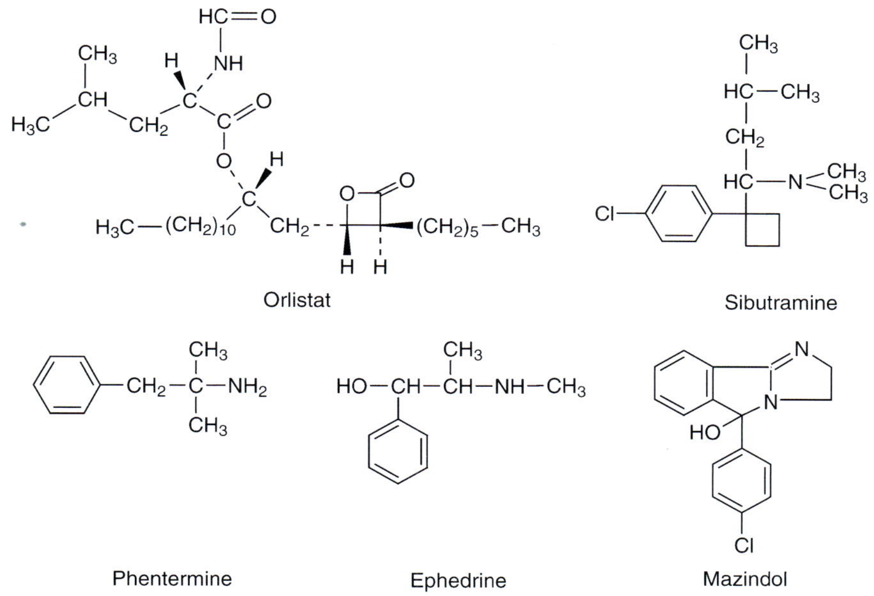

Figure 22 Structures of the antiobesity agents orlistat, sibutramine, phentermine, ephedrine, and mazindol

adjunct for lowering blood glucose in the overweight. Detailed consideration of potential future antiobesity agents, such as PYY (3-36) [183], is beyond the scope of this review, and readers are referred to an excellent recent review [184]. Several antiobesity targets receiving pharmaceutical attention are noted in Table 6, and agents with independent glucose-lowering activity are discussed herein. Several peptides involved in energy balance, such as leptin, adiponectin, and ghrelin, have recently been reported to influence glucose homeostasis, but only leptin has been tested for therapeutic use and did not show substantive weight-lowering efficacy, presumably due to leptin resistance. Etiocholanolones (Figure 23), which are metabolites of dehydroepiandrosterone (DHEA), decrease adiposity in obese diabetic animals, and have been reported to increase satiety, reduce hepatic gluconeogenesis, possibly preserve B-cell function, and increase futile cycling, but have not proceeded in development [185].

Table 6 Promising targets for development of antiobesity agents

Decrease appetite or increase satiety
Leptin sensitizers and receptor agonists,* melanin
Melanin-concentrating hormone (MCH) receptor antagonists*
Neuropeptide Y (NPY) receptor Y1 and Y5 antagonists
Cannabinoid (CB) receptor 1 antagonists*
α-Melanocyte-stimulating hormone (α-MSH) receptor agonists
Cholecystokinin (CCK) receptor agonists
Ciliary neurotrophic factor (CNTF) analogues
Melanocortin 4 (MC-4) receptor agonists
5-Hydroxytryptamine (5HT; serotonin) 2C receptor agonists
Selective centrally acting α- and β-adrenergic reuptake inhibitors
Ghrelin inhibitors and antagonists
Increase thermogenesis
Uncoupling-protein-stimulating agents
β_3-Adrenoceptor agonists
Modulators of lipids
Intestinal lipase and lipid absorption inhibitors
Inhibitors of lipogenesis

* May also increase energy expenditure.

β_3-Adrenoreceptor Agonists

β_3-Adrenoreceptors are mainly expressed in brown and white adipose tissue, and agonists of these receptors, which typically stimulate lipolysis and thermogenesis, could provide antiobesity agents. Highly selective agonists that were previously developed against rodent β_3-adrenoreceptors (e.g., the benzodioxole dicarboxylate CL316,243) were not effective in humans due to minor but crucial species differences in receptor structure. In

Etiocholanolone

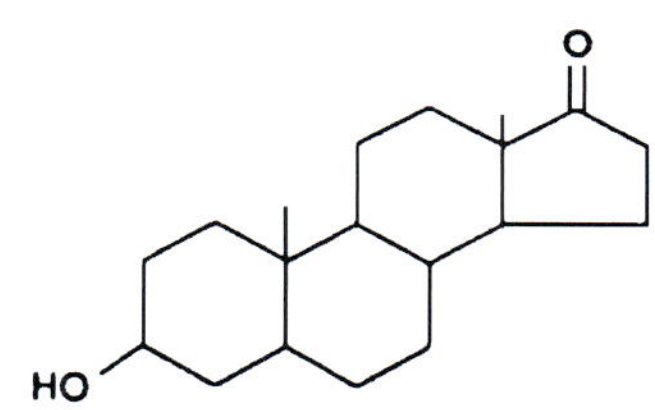

Figure 23 Structure of etiocholanolone

```
                  ┌S-S┐
Human amylin     KCNTATCATQRLANFLVHSSNNFGAILSSTNVGSNTY

                  ┌S-S┐
Pramlintide      KCNTATCATQRLANFLVHSSNNFGPILPPTNVGSNTY
```

Figure 24 Structure of amylin and the soluble amylin analogue pramlintide (three different amino acid residues are underlined)

obese diabetic rodents, one β_3-adrenoreceptor agonist (SR58611A) stimulated insulin release and reduced hyperglycemia, and another (AJ9677) reduced insulin resistance, with upregulation of GLUT-4 protein levels [186, 187].

Amylin

Islet amyloid polypeptide (IAPP or amylin) (see Chapter 12) is a peptide produced by islet B-cells and co-secreted with insulin and C-peptide. Human amylin self-aggregates intracellularly and accumulates extracellularly in the islets, and has been implicated in the pathogenesis of B-cell dysfunction in type 2 diabetes [188]. However, patients with type 1 diabetes and advanced type 2 diabetes have decreased circulating amylin levels consistent with their insulinopenia/hypoinsulinemia. Pramlintide (AC137, Figure 24), a soluble analogue of amylin that does not aggregate or accumulate in islet tissue, has been shown to improve glycemic control in insulin-treated type 1 and type 2 diabetic patients when injected subcutaneously before meals [189]. The main reduction of glycemia occurs during the postprandial period; the insulin dose can often be reduced, and chronic use is frequently associated with a modest weight loss. However, pramlintide must be injected separately to insulin, and initiation of therapy can produce mild nausea. Pramlintide acts predominantly through central pathways that are probably activated via binding to amylin receptors located in the area postrema (Figure 25). This gives rise to several therapeutic effects, particularly the suppression of glucagon secretion and a delay in gastric emptying mediated by vagal pathways. There is also a satiety effect of pramlintide that appears to contribute to the weight loss, and reduced secretion of gastric acid and pancreatic enzymes [190].

STIMULANTS OF GLUCOSE UTILIZATION

Many substances can act independently of insulin to enhance glucose metabolism and lower blood glucose. For example, vitamin K_5, certain polyamines such as spermine (Figure 26), and deoxyfrenolicin increase glucose metabolism, but mainly by the pentose phosphate pathway [13]. Oxidants such as diamide, peroxides, and phenazine methosulphate increase glucose oxidation, but they do not lend themselves to pharmaceutical development. Okadaic acid and phorbol esters can acutely initiate insulin-like effects, but subsequently impede responsiveness to insulin.

Dichloroacetate (Figure 26) and its esters stimulate pyruvate dehydrogenase activity, causing increased glucose oxidation, and reduce hepatic gluconeogenesis by interrupting the supply of substrate (e.g. lactate) and by inhibiting pyruvate carboxylase consequent to the metabolism of dichloroacetate to glyoxylate and oxalate.

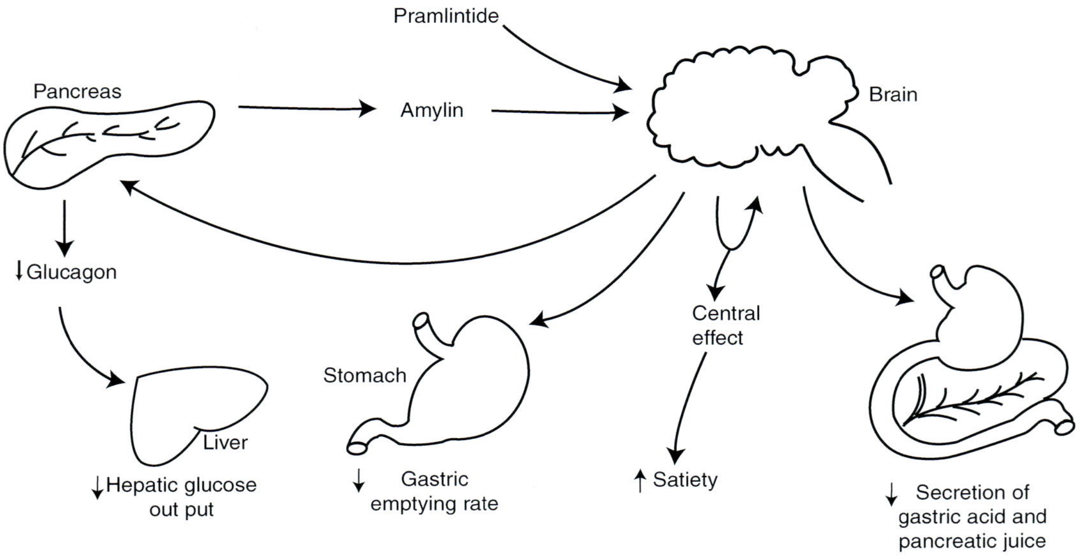

Figure 25 Main modes of actions of amylin and pramlintide to reduce hyperglycemia and reduce weight. Arrow down = inhibitory effect; arrow up = stimulatory effect

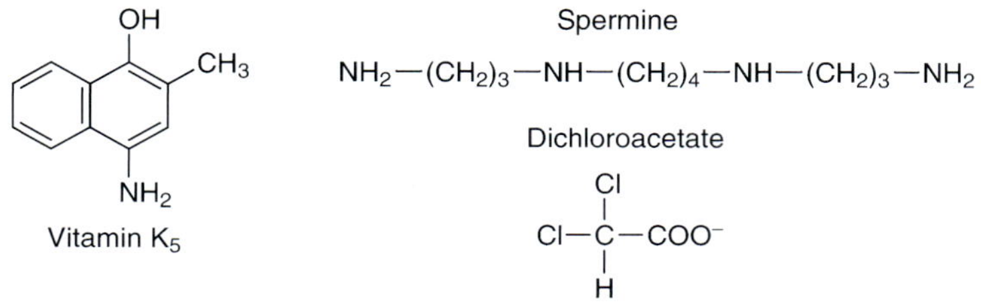

Figure 26 Structures of some agents that directly stimulate glucose utilization: vitamin K_5, spermine, and dichloroacetate

However, chronic use of dichloroacetate may adversely affect nerve function and lens structure, possibly via oxalate formation [191].

AMP-activated Protein Kinase

Adenosine monophosphate-activated protein kinase (AMPK) is an enzyme that is sensitive to the energy status of cells [192]. For example, the utilization of energy by a contracting muscle causes the concentrations of adenosine triphosphate (ATP) and creatine phosphate (CP) to become depleted, and the concentration of AMP rises. The increased concentration of AMP activates AMPK kinase, which then activates AMPK. This is partially offset by falling concentrations of CP, which inhibit AMPK. AMPK promotes the production of more energy by enhancing fatty acid oxidation and increasing glucose uptake (independently of insulin), leading to the restoration of ATP (Figure 27).

AICAR (5-aminoimidazole-4-carboxamide-1-B-D-ribofuranoside) activates AMPK, causing increases in GLUT-4 levels, glucose transport, hexokinase activity, glucose utilization, and glycogen accumulation in muscle. AICAR also inhibits fructose-1,6-bisphosphatase, reducing gluconeogenesis in liver. Accordingly, AICAR reduced the hyperglycemia in obese diabetic and insulin-resistant animals [193–196]. However, effects on circulating triglycerides and FFAs have been variable in these animals, and prolonged exposure to high concentrations of AICAR may induce apoptosis of pancreatic B-cells [197], suggesting that activation of AMPK for antidiabetic purposes may need to be tissue-selective.

INHIBITORS OF HEPATIC GLUCOSE PRODUCTION

Excess hepatic glucose output in diabetic states is mainly attributed to inadequately restrained gluconeogenesis, with a lesser contribution from increased glycogenolysis. For therapeutic purposes, agents acting to decrease gluconeogenesis and glycogenolysis will preferably cause only partial suppression; they must not be irreversible or prevent responsiveness to crucial counterregulatory hormones and neural signals in times of hypoglycemia. Several types of compounds have been described in foregoing sections of this chapter that suppress hepatic glucose output, including PPAR-γ agonists, some trace minerals, inhibitors of fatty acid oxidation, glucagon receptor antagonists, BHSD-1 inhibitors, etiocholanolones, and AMPK activators.

Among the new agents designed to specifically inhibit hepatic glucose output, attention has been focused on glycogen phosphorylase inhibitors [143, 198]. A recent addition to the list is the dihydropyridine derivative BAY R3401 (Figure 28). This acts through a metabolite to cause both allosteric inhibition of glycogen phosphorylase and dephosphorylation of glycogen phosphorylase *a* [199]. Interest has also been shown in the therapeutic potential of inhibitors of glucose-6-phosphate translocase

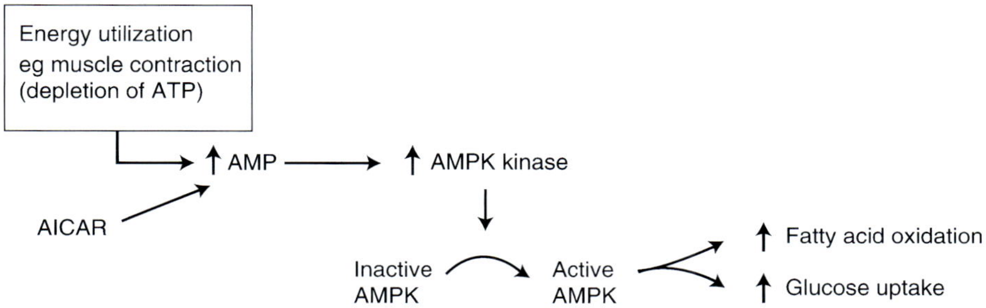

Figure 27 Activation of adenosine monophosphate-activated protein kinase (AMPK). ATP = adenosine triphosphate; AMP = adenosine monophosphate; AMPK = adenosine monophosphate-activated protein kinase; AICAR = 5-aminoimidazole-4-carboxamide-1-B-D-ribofuranoside; up arrows = increase

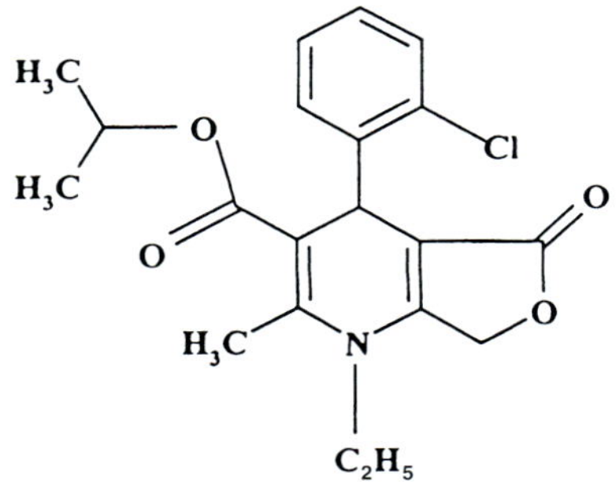

Bay R3401, glycogen phosphorylase inhibitor

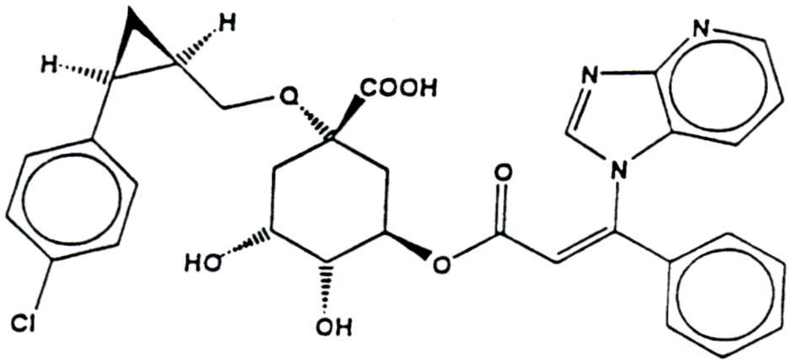

Glucose-6-phosphate translocase inhibitor

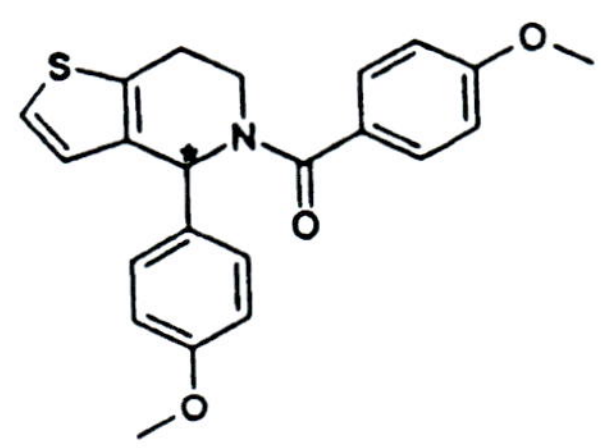

Glucose-6-phosphatase catalytic protein inhibitor

Figure 28 Structures of the glycogen phosphorylase inhibitor BAY R3401, a glucose-6-phosphate translocase inhibitor, and a glucose-6-phosphatase catalytic protein inhibitor [199–201]

and glucose-6-phosphatase catalytic protein (Figure 28) [200, 201].

INCREASED GLUCOSE ELIMINATION

Renal reabsorption of glucose is mediated by a sodium–glucose co-transporter (SGLT). If this is inhibited by phlorizin (also known as phlorhizin or phloridzin, Figure 29), the resulting glycosuria can substantially reduce hyperglycemia in diabetic animals [202]. An orally active derivative of phlorizin, T-1095 and its metabolite, inhibited renal SGLT activity and lowered blood glucose concentrations in STZ-diabetic and *db*/*db* mice, providing further evidence of the feasibility for this approach to glycemic control [203]. Development or progression of albuminuria was also decreased. However, increased glycosuria raises questions about nocturia, urinary tract infections, and pruritis.

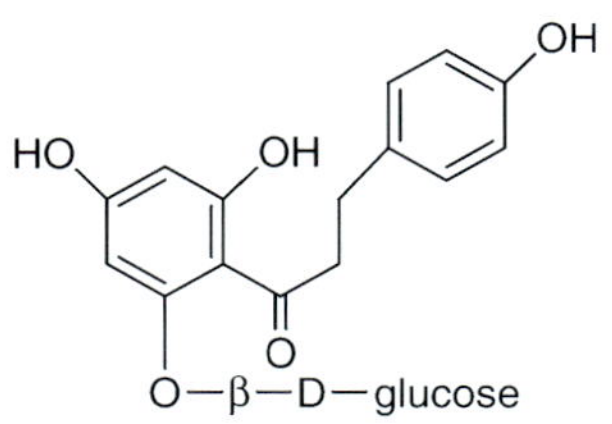

Phlorizin (phlorhizin/phloridzin)

Figure 29 Structure of phlorizin (also phlorhizin or phloridzin)

CONCLUSIONS

This chapter has reviewed many potential sites for therapeutic intervention against hyperglycemia. No single "ideal" therapy has emerged. Indeed the heterogeneous nature and multiple pathological disturbances of diabetes suggest the need for a selection of differently acting agents. Treatments that address fundamental defects may be more likely to restore normal physiological glucose homeostasis, but any safe means of treating hyperglycemia cannot be disregarded. At the present time, agents that can partially mimic or improve insulin action, and agents that reduce B-cell loss and dysfunction or promote B-cell neogenesis are creating particular interest as potential future therapies.

REFERENCES

1. European Diabetes Policy Group. A desktop guide to type 2 diabetes mellitus. *Diabet Med* 1999; 16: 716–30.
2. American Diabetes Association. Standards of medical care for patients with diabetes mellitus. *Diabetes Care* 2002; 25 (suppl 1): S33–49.
3. The Diabetes Control and Complications Trial Research Group. The absence of a glycemic threshold for the development of long-term complications: the perspective of the diabetes control and complications trial. *Diabetes* 1996; 45: 1289–98.
4. Stratton IM, Adler AI, Neil HAW, Matthews DR, Manley SE, Cull CA, Hadden D, Turner RC, Holman RR. Association of glycaemia with macrovascular and microvascular complications of type 2 diabetes (UKPDS 35): prospective observational study. *BMJ* 2000; 321: 405–12.
5. The Diabetes Control and Complications Trial Research Group. The effect of intensive treatment of diabetes on the development and progression of long-term complications in insulin-dependent diabetes mellitus. *N Engl J Med* 1993; 329: 978–86.
6. UK Prospective Diabetes Study (UKPDS) Group. Intensive blood glucose control with sulphonylureas or insulin compared with conventional treatment and risk of complications in patients with type 2 diabetes (UKPDS 33). *Lancet* 1998; 352: 837–53.
7. UKPDS Group. Effect of intensive blood glucose control with metformin on complications in overweight patients with type 2 diabetes (UKPDS 34). *Lancet* 1998; 352: 854–65.
8. Yki-Jarvinen H. Combination therapies with insulin in type 2 diabetes. *Diabetes Care* 2001; 24: 758–67.
9. Van Gaal LF, De Leeuw IH. Rationale for combining agents to control fasting and postprandial glucose. *Diabetologia* 2003; 46 (suppl 1): M44–50.
10. Bailey CJ. Hypoglycaemic, antihyperglycaemic and antidiabetic drugs. *Diabet Med* 1992; 9: 482–3.
11. Bailey CJ. Insulin resistance and antidiabetic drugs. *Biochem Pharmacol* 1999; 58: 1511–20.
12. Bailey CJ, Flatt PR. Models for testing new hypoglycemic drugs. In Bailey CJ, Flatt PR (eds), *New Antidiabetic Drugs*. London: Smith-Gordon, 1990; pp 65–82.
13. Bailey CJ. New drugs for the treatment of diabetes mellitus. In Alberti KGMM, Zimmet P, DeFronzo RA, Keen H (eds), *International Textbook of Diabetes Mellitus*, 2nd edn. Chichester, UK: Wiley, 1997; pp 865–81.
14. Bonora E, Muggeo M. Postprandial blood glucose as a risk factor for cardiovascular disease in type 2 diabetes: the epidemiological evidence. *Diabetologia* 2001; 44: 2107–14.
15. Lebovitz HE. Alpha-glucosidase inhibitors as agents in the treatment of diabetes. *Diabetes Rev* 1998; 6: 132–45.
16. Bailey CJ. New approaches to the pharmacotherapy of diabetes. In Pickup JC, Williams G (eds), *Textbook of Diabetes*, 3rd edn. Oxford: Blackwell, 2003; pp 73.1–73.21.
17. Taira M, Takasu N, Komiya I, Taira T, Tanaka H. Voglibose administration before the evening meal improves nocturnal hypoglycemia in insulin-dependent diabetic patients with intensive insulin therapy. *Metabolism* 2000; 49: 440–3.
18. Nuttall FQ. Dietary fiber in the management of diabetes. *Diabetes* 1993; 42: 503–8.
19. Day C. Hypoglycaemic compounds from plants. In Bailey CJ, Flatt PR (eds), *New Antidiabetic Drugs*. London: Smith-Gordon, 1990; pp 267–78.
20. Bailey CJ, Day C. Traditional plant medicines as treatments for diabetes. *Diabetes Care* 1989; 12: 553–64.
21. Chandalia M, Garg A, Lutjohann D, von Bergmann K, Grundy SM, Brinkley LJ. Beneficial effects of high dietary fiber intake in patients with type 2 diabetes mellitus. *N Engl J Med* 2000; 342: 1392–8.
22. Lee WL, Zinman B. From insulin to insulin analogs: progress in the treatment of type 1 diabetes. *Diabetes Rev* 1998; 6: 73–88.
23. Shojee-Moradie F, Powrie JK, Sundermann E, Spring MR, Brandenburg D, Sonksen P, Jones RH. Novel hepatoselective insulin analog: studies with a covalently linked thyroxyl-insulion complex in humans. *Diabetes Care* 2000; 23: 1124–9.
24. Worrall DS, McDunn JE, List B, Reichart D, Hevener A, Gustafson T, Barbas CF, Lerner RA, Olefsky JM. Synthesis of an organoinsulin molecule that can be activated by antibody catalysis. *Proc Natl Acad Sci USA* 2001; 98: 13514–8.
25. Kahn SE. The relative contributions of insulin resistance and beta-cell dysfunction to the pathophysiology of type 2 diabetes. *Diabetologia* 2003; 46: 3–19.
26. Porte D. B-cells in type II diabetes. *Diabetes* 1991; 40: 166–80.
27. Butler AE, Janson J, Bonner-Weir S, Ritzel R, Rizza RA, Butler PC. B-cell deficit and increased B-cell apoptosis in humans with type 2 diabetes. *Diabetes* 2003; 52: 102–10.
28. Bailey CJ. Potential new treatments for type 2 diabetes. *Trends Pharmacol Sci* 2000; 21: 259–65.
29. McKinnon CM, Docherty K. Pancreatic duodenal homeobox-1,PDX-1, a major regulator of beta cell identity and function. *Diabetologia* 2001; 44: 1203–14.
30. Melloul D, Marshak S, Cerasi E. Regulation of insulin gene transcription. *Diabetologia* 2002; 45: 309–26.
31. Ashcroft FM, Gribble FM. ATP-sensitive K+ channels and insulin secretion: their role in health and disease. *Diabetologia* 1999; 42: 903–19.
32. Dornhorst A. Insulinotropic meglitinide analogues. *Lancet* 2001; 358: 1709–16.
33. Malaisse WJ. Stimulation of insulin release by non-sulfonylurea hypoglycemic agents: the meglitinide family. *Horm Metab Res* 1995; 27: 263–6.
34. Geng X, Li L, Watkins S, Robbins PD, Drain P. The insulin secretory granule is the major site of K-ATP channels of the endocrine pancreas. *Diabetes* 2003; 52: 767–76.
35. Eliasson L, Renstrom E, Ämmälä C, Berggren P-O, Bertorello AM, Bokvist K, Chibalin A, Deeney JT, Flatt PR, Gäbel J, Gromada J, Larsson O, Lindström P, Rhodes CJ, Rorsman P. PKC-dependent stimulation of exocytosis by sulphonylureas in pancreatic B-cells. *Science* 1996; 271: 813–5.
36. Le Brigand L, Virsolvy A, Manechez D, Godfriod JJ, Guardiola-Lemaitre B, Gribble FM, et al. In vitro mechanism of action on insulin release of S-22068, a new putative antidiabetic compound. *Br J Pharmacol* 1999; 128: 1021–6.

37. Morgan NG, Chan SL. Imidazoline binding sites in the endocrine pancreas. *Curr Pharm Des* 2001; 7: 1413–31.
38. Efanov AM, Zaitsev SV, Mest HJ, Raap A, Appelskog IB, Larsson O, et al. The novel imidazoline compound BL11282 potentiates glucose-induced insulin secretion in pancreatic B-cells in the absence of modulation of K-ATP channel activity. *Diabetes* 2001; 50: 797–802.
39. Storey DA, Bailey CJ. Biphasic insulin-releasing effect of BTS67582 in rats. *J Pharm Pharmacol* 1998; 50: 1357–60.
40. Drucker DJ. Glucagon-like peptides. *Diabetes* 1998; 47: 159–69.
41. Creutzfeldt W. The entero-insular axis in type 2 diabetes. Incretins as therapeutic agents. *Exp Clin Endocrinol Diabetes* 2001; 109: 288–303.
42. Vilsboll T, Krapup T, Deacon CF, Madsbad S, Holst JJ. Reduced postprandial concentrations of intact glucagons-like peptide-1 in type 2 diabetic patients. *Diabetes* 2001; 50: 609–13.
43. Glutniak NK, Linde B, Holst JJ, Efendic S. Subcutaneous injection of the incretin hormone glucagon-like peptite-1 abolishes postprandial glycemia in NIDDM. *Diabetes Care* 1994; 17: 1039–44.
44. Skoglund G, Hussain MA, Holz GG. Glucagon-like peptide-1 stimulates insulin gene promoter activity by protein kinase a independent activation of the rat insulin 1 gene cAMP response element. *Diabetes* 2000; 48: 2270–6.
45. Vella A, Shah P, Basu R, Basu A, Holst JJ, Rizza RA. Effect of glucagon-like peptide-1 (7-36) amide on glucose effectiveness and insulin action in people with type 2 diabetes. *Diabetes* 2000; 49: 611–7.
46. Xu W, Stoffers DA, Habener JF, Bonner-Weir S. Exendin-4 stimulates both B-cell replication and neogenesis, resulting in increased B-cell mass and improved glucose tolerance in diabetic rats. *Diabetes* 1999; 48: 2270–6.
47. Hui H, Wright C, Perfetti R. Glucagon-like peptide 1 induces differentiation of islet duodenal homeobox-1-positive pancreatic ductal cells into insulin-secreting cells. *Diabetes* 2001; 50: 785–96.
48. Young AA, Gedulin BR, Bhavsar S, Bodkin N, Jodka C, Hansen B, Denaro M. Glucose-lowering and insulin sensitizing actions of exendin-4: studies in obese diabetic (*ob/ob, db/db*) mice, diabetic fatty Zucker rats, and diabetic rhesus monkeys (*Macaca mulatto*). *Diabetes* 1999; 48: 1026–34.
49. Wang Q, Brubaker PL. Glucagon-like peptide-1 treatment delays the onset of diabetes in 8-week-old *db/db* mice. *Diabetologia* 2002; 45: 1263–73.
50. Fineman MS, Bicsak T, Shen L, Taylor K, Gaines E, Varns A, Kim D, Baron A. AC2993(synthetic exendin-4) added to existing metformin and/or sulfonylurea treatment improved glycemic control in patients with type 2 diabetes during 28 days of glycemic control to patients with type 2 diabetes. *Diabetes* 2002; 52 (suppl 2). Abstract 343.
51. Taylor K, Kim D, Bicsak T, Heintz S, Varns A, Aisporna M, Fineman MS, Baron A. Continuous subcutaneous infusion of AC2993 (synthetic exendin-4) provides sustained day-long glycemic control to patients with type 2 diabetes. *Diabetes* 2002; 52 (suppl 2). Abstract 344.
52. Agerso H, Jensen LB, Elbrond B, Rolan P, Zdraavkovic M. The pharmacokinetics, pharmacodynamics, safety and tolerability of NN2211, a new long-acting GLP-1 derivative, in healthy men. *Diabetologia* 2002; 45: 195–202.
53. Juhl CB, Hollingdal M, Sturis J, Jakobsen G, Agerso H, Velduis J, Porksen N, Schmitz O. Bedtime administration of NN2211, a long-acting GLP-1 derivative, substantially reduces fasting and postprandial glycemia in type 2 diabetes. *Diabetes* 2002; 51: 424–9.
54. Kim JG, Baggio LL, Bridon DP, Castaigne JP, Robitaille MF, Jette L, Benquet C, Drucker DJ. Development and characterization of a glucagon-like peptide 1-albumin conjugate. *Diabetes* 2003; 52: 751–9.
55. Mooney MH, Abdel-Waheb YH, McKillop AM, O'Harte FP, Flatt PR. Evaluation of glycated glucagons-like peptide-1 (7-36) amide in intestinal tissue of normal and diabetic animal models. *Biochim Biophys Acta* 2002; 1569: 75–80.
56. Joseph JW, Kalitsky J, St-Pierre S, Brubakeer PL. Oral delivery of glucagon-like peptide-1 in a modified polymer preparation normalizes basal glycaemia in diabetic *db/db* mice. *Diabetologia* 2000; 43: 1319–28.
57. Hinke SA, Gelling RW, Pederson RA, Manhart S, Nian C, Demuth HU, McIntosh CHS. Dipeptidyl peptidase IV-resistant [D-Ala2] glucose-dependent insulinotropic polypeptide (GIP) improves glucose tolerance in normal and obese diabetic rats. *Diabetes* 2002; 51: 652–61.
58. O'Harte FPM, Mooney MH, Flatt PR. N-terminally modified gastric inhibitory polypeptide exhibits amino-peptidase resistance and enhanced antihyperglycemic activity. *Diabetes* 1999; 48: 758–65.
59. Rooman I, Lardon J, Bouwens L. Gastrin stimulates B-cell neogenesis and increases islet mass from transdifferentiated but not from normal exocrine pancreatic tissue. *Diabetes* 2002; 51: 686–90.
60. Holst JJ, Deacon CF. Inhibition of the activity of dipeptidyl-peptidase IV as a treatment for type 2 diabetes. *Diabetes* 1998; 47: 1663–70.
61. Pederson RA, White HA, Schlenzig D, Pauly RP, McIntosh CHS, Demuth HU. Improved glucose tolerance in Zucker fatty rats by oral administration of the dipeptidyl peptidase IV inhibitor isoleucine thiazolidide. *Diabetes* 1998; 47: 1253–8.
62. Pospisilik JA, Stafford SG, Demuth SU, Brownsey R, Parkhouse W, Finegood DT, McIntosh CHS, Pederson RA. Long-term treatment with the dipeptidyl peptidase IV inhibitor P32/98 causes sustained improvements in glucose tolerance, insulin sensitivity, hyperinsulinaemia, and B-cell glucose responsiveness in VDF (*fa/fa*) Zucker rats. *Diabetes* 2002; 51: 943–50.
63. Sudre B, Broqua P, White RB, Ashworth D, Evans DM, Haigh R, Junien JL, Aubert ML. Chronic inhibition of circulating dipeptidyl peptidase IV by FE999011 delays the occurrence of diabetes in male Zucker diabetic fatty rats. *Diabetes* 2002; 51: 1461–9.
64. Pospisilik JA, Martin J, Doty T, Ehses JA, Pamir N, Lynn FC, Piteau S, Demuth HU, McIntosh CHS, Pederson RA. Dipepidyl peptidase IV inhibitor treatment stimulates B-cell survival and islet neogenesis in streptozotocin induced diabetic rats. *Diabetes* 2003; 52: 741–50.
65. Ahren B, Simonsson E, Larsson H, Landin-Olsson M, Torgiersson H, Jansson PA, Sandqvist M, Bavenholm P, Efendic S, Eriksson JW, Dickinson S, Holmes D. Inhibition of peptidyl peptidase IV improves metabolic control over a 4-week study period in type 2 diabetes. *Diabetes Care* 2002; 25: 869–75.

66. Ahmad M, Abdel-Wahab YHA, Tate R, Flatt PR, Pyne NJ, Furman BL. Effect of type selective inhibitors on cyclic nucleotide phosphodiesterase activity and insulin secretion in the clonal insulin secreting cell line BRIN-BD11. *Br J Pharmacol* 2000; 129: 1228–34.
67. Ohta T, Furukawa N, Komuro G, Yonemori F, Wakitani K. JTT-608 restores impaired early insulin secretion in diabetic Goto-Kakizaki rats. *Br J Pharmacol* 1999; 126: 1674–80.
68. Mukai E, Ishida H, Fujimoto S, Kajikawa M, Okamoto Y, Fujita J, Hamamoto Y, Tsuura Y, Yamada Y, Furukawa N, Ohta T, Seino Y. The insulinotropic mechanism of the novel hypoglycaemic agent JTT-608: direct enhancement of Ca^{2+} efficacy and increase of Ca^{2+} influx by phosphdiesterase inhibition. *Br J Pharmacol* 2000; 129: 901–8.
69. Laghmich A, Ladriere L, Malaisse-Lagae F, Dannacher H, Bjorkling F, Malaisse W. Stimulation of biosynthetic activity by novel succinate esters in rat pancreatic islets. *Biochem Pharmacol* 1998; 55: 909–13.
70. Kowluru A. Adenine and guanine nucleotide specific succinyl-CoA synthetases in the clonal beta-cell mitochondria: implications in the beta-cell high-energy phosphate metabolism in relation to physiological insulin secretion. *Diabetologia* 2001; 44: 89–94.
71. Ueno N, Inui A, Asakawa A, Takeo F, Tani S, Komatsu Y, Itoh Z, Kasuga M. Erythromycin improves glycaemic control in patients with type II diabetes mellitus. *Diabetologia* 2000; 43: 411–5.
72. Filipsson K, Kvist-Reimer M, Ahren B. The neuropeptide pituitary adenylate cyclase-activating polypeptide and islet function. *Diabetes* 2001; 50: 1959–69.
73. Zhang B, Salituro G, Szalkowski D, Li Z, Zhang Y, Royo I, Vilella D, Diez MT, Pelaez F, Ruby C, et al. Discovery of a small molecule insulin mimetic with antidiabetic activity in mice. *Science* 1999; 284: 974–7.
74. Li M, Youngren JF, Manchem VP, Kozlowski M, Zhang BB, Maddux BA, Goldfine ID. Small molecule insulin receptor activators potentiate insulin action in insulin resistant cells. *Diabetes* 2001; 50: 2323–8.
75. Manchem VP, Goldfine ID, Kohanski RA, Cristobal CP, Lumm RT, Schow SR, Shi S, Spevak WR, Laborde E, et al. A novel small molecule that directly sensitizes the insulin receptor in vitro and in vivo. *Diabetes* 2001; 50: 824–30.
76. Wahren J, Ekberg K, Johansson J. Role of C-peptide in human physiology. *Am J Physiol* 2000; 278: E759–68.
77. Grunberger G, Quiang X, Li Z, Mathews ST, Sbrissa D, Shisheva A, Sima AAE. Molecular basis for the insulinomimetic effects of C-peptide. *Diabetologia* 2001; 44: 1247–57.
78. Elchebly M, Payette P, Michaliszyn E. Increased insulin sensitivity and obesity resistance in mice lacking the protein tyrosine phosphatase-1B gene. *Science* 1999; 283: 1544–8.
79. Gum RJ, Gaede LL, Koterski SL, Heindel M, Clampit JE, Zinker BA, Trevillyan JM, Ulrich RG, Jirousek MR, Rondinone CM. Reduction of protein tyrosine phosphatase 1B increases insulin-dependent signaling in *ob/ob* mice. *Diabetes* 2003; 52: 21–8.
80. Wrobel J, Sredy J, Moxham C, Dietrich A, Li Z, Sawicki DR, Seetaller L, Wu L, Katz A, Sullivan D, Tio C, Zhang ZY. PTP1B inhibition and antihyperglycemic activity in the *ob/ob* mouse model of novel 11-arylbenzo-[b]naphtha[2,3-d]furans and 11-arylbenzo[b]naphtha-[2,3-d]thiophenes. *J Med Chem* 1999; 42: 3199–202.
81. Tsiani E, Fantus IG. Vanadium compounds. Biological actions and potential as pharmacological agents. *Trends Endocrinol Metab* 1997; 8: 51–8.
82. Pederson TM, Kramer DL, Rondinone CM. Serine threonine phosphorylation of IRS-1 triggers its degradation; possible regulation by tyrosine phosphorylation. *Diabetes* 2001; 50: 24–31.
83. Itani S, Zhou Q, Pories WJ, et al. Involvement of protein kinase C in human skeletal muscle insulin resistance and obesity. *Diabetes* 2000; 49: 1353–8.
84. Yuan M, et al. Reversal of obesity- and diet-induced insulin resistance with salicylates or targeted disruption of IkkB. *Science* 2001; 293: 1673–7.
85. Le Roith D, Insulin-like growth factors. *N Engl J Med* 1997; 336: 633–40.
86. Ng FM. Human growth hormone fragments. In Bailey CJ, Flatt PR (eds), *New Antidiabetic Drugs*. London: Smith-Gordon, 1990; pp 197–206.
87. Ueno N, Inui A, Asakawa A, Takao F, Komatsu Y, Kotani K, Nishimura R, Kasuga M. Mosapride, a 5HT-4 receptor agonist, improves insulin sensitivity and glycaemic control in patients with type II diabetes mellitus. *Diabetologia* 2002; 45: 792–7.
88. Fleming A, Gunn R, Longo R, Sleevi M, Gregory J, Rogol A. Evaulation of D-chiro-inositol (INS-1) in combination with sulphonylureas on glycaemic control and lipids in subjects with type 2 diabetes mellitus. *Diabetes* 2001; 50 (suppl 2): A112. Abstract 448.
89. Bates SH, Jones RB, Bailey CJ. Insulin-like effect of pinitol. *Br J Pharmacol* 2000; 130: 1944–8.
90. Butler M, McKay RA, Popoff IJ, Gaarde WA, Witchell D, Murray SF, Dean NM, Bhanot S, Monia BP. Specific inhibition of PTEN expression reverses hyperglycaemia in diabetic mice. *Diabetes* 2002; 51: 1028–34.
91. Coleman MD, Eason RC, Bailey CJ. The therapeutic use of lipoic acid in diabetes: a current perspective. *Env Tox Pharmacol* 2001; 10: 167–72.
92. Eason RC, Archer HE, Akhtar S, Bailey CJ. Lipoic acid increases glucose uptake by skeletal muscles of obese-diabetic *ob/ob* mice. *Diabetes Obes Metab* 2002; 4: 29–35.
93. Yaworsky K, Somwar R, Ramial T, Tritschler HJ, Klip A. Engagement of the insulin-sensitive pathway in the stimulation of glucose transport by alpha-lipoic acid in 3T3-L1 adipocytes. *Diabetologia* 2000; 43: 294–303.
94. Konrad D, Somwar R, Sweeney G, Yaworsky K, Hayashi M, Ramlal T, Klip A. The antihyperglycemic drug a-lipoic acid stimulates glucose uptake via both GLUT4 translocation and GLUT4 activation. *Diabetes* 2001; 50: 1464–71.
95. Al-Daghri N, Bartlett WA, Jones AF, Kumar S. Role of leptin in glucose metabolism in type 2 diabetes. *Diabetes Obes Metab* 2002; 4: 147–55.
96. Bates SH, Gardiner JV, Jones RB, Bloom SR, Bailey CJ. Acute stimulation of glucose uptake by leptin in L6 muscle cells. *Horm Metab Res* 2002; 34: 111–5.
97. Yamauchi T. The fat-derived hormone adiponectin reverses insulin resistance associated with both lipoatrophy and obesity. *Nature Med* 2001; 7: 941–6.
98. Beltowski J. Adiponectin and resistin—new hormones of white adipose tissue. *Med Sci Monit* 2003; 9: RA55–61.
99. Idris I, Gray S, Donnelly R. Protein kinase C activation: isozyme specific effects on metabolism and cardiovascular complications in diabetes. *Diabetologia* 2001; 44: 659–73.

100. Houndali B, Nguyen V, Ammon HPT, Haap M, Schechinger W, Michicoa F, Rett K, Haring HU, Schleicher ED. Prolonged glucose infusion into conscious rats inhibits early steps in insulin signaling and induces translocation of GLUT4 and protein kinase C in skeletal muscle. *Diabetologia* 2002; 45: 356–68.
101. Nerlich AG, Sauer U, Kolm-Litty V, Wagner E, Kock M, Schlieicher ED. Expression of glutamine:fructose-6-phosphate amidotransferase in human tissues: evidence for high variability and distinct regulation in diabetes. *Diabetes* 1998; 47: 170–8.
102. Schwartz SL. Bromocriptine (Ergoset) improves glycemic control in type 2 diabetics on insulin. *Diabetes* 1999; 48 (suppl 1): A99. Abstract 427.
103. Liu IM, Hsu FL, Chen CF, Cheng JT. Antihyperglycemic action of isoferulic acid in streptozotocin-induced diabetic rats. *Br J Pharmacol* 2000; 129: 631–6.
104. Bailey CJ, Turner SL, Bates SH, Jones RB. Sibutramine metabolites increase glucose transport by cultured rat muscle cells. *Int J Obes* 2001; 25: 1–8.
105. Arbin V, Claperon N, Fournie-Zaluski MC, Roques BP, Peyroux J. Acute effect of the dual angiotensin-converting enzyme and neutral endopeptidase 24-11 inhibitor mixanpril on insulin sensitivity in obese Zucker rat. *Br J Pharmacol* 2001; 133: 495–502.
106. Damas J, Hallet C, Lefebvre PJ. Changes in blood glucose and plasma insulin levels induced by bradykinin in anaesthetized rats. *Br J Pharmacol* 2001; 134: 1312–8.
107. Reed MJ, Meszaros K, Entes LJ, Claypool MD, Pinkett JG, Brignetti D, Luo J, Khandwala A, Reaven GM. Effect of masoprocol on carbohydrate and lipid metabolism in a rat model of type II diabetes. *Diabetologia* 1999; 42: 102–6.
108. Desvergne B, Wahli W. Peroxisome prolfierator-activated receptors: nuclear control of metabolism. *Endocr Rev* 1999; 20: 649–88.
109. Day C. Thiazolidinediones: a new class of antidiabetic drugs. *Diabet Med* 1999; 16: 179–92.
110. Hevener AL, Reichart D, Janez A, Olefsky J. Thiazolidinedione treatment prevents free fatty acid-induced insulin resistance in male Wistar rats. *Diabetes* 2001; 50: 2316–22.
111. Bailey CJ. New pharmacologic agents for diabetes. *Curr Diabetes Rep* 2001; 1: 119–26.
112. Maeda N, Takahashi M, Funahashi T, Kihara S, Nishizawa H, Kishida K, Nagaretani H, Matsuda M, Komuro R, Ouchi N, Kuriyama H, Hotta K, Nakamura T, Shimomura I, Matsuzawa Y. PPARg ligands increase expression and plasma concentrations of adiponectin, an adipose-derived protein. *Diabetes* 2001; 50: 2094–9.
113. Brunmair B, Gras F, Neschen S, Roden M, Wagner L, Waldhausl W, Furnsinn C. Direct thiazolidinedione action on isloated rat skeletal muscle fuel handling in independent of peroxisome proliferator-activated receptor-g mediated changes in gene expression. *Diabetes* 2001; 50: 2309–15.
114. Furnsinn C, Waldhausl W. Thiazolidinediones: metabolic actions in vitro. *Diabetologia* 2002; 45: 1211–23.
115. Fursninn C, Brunmair B, Meyer M. Chronic and acute effects of thiazolidinediones BM13.1258 and BM15.2054 on rat skeletal muscle glucose metabolism. *Br J Pharmacol* 1999; 128: 1141–8.
116. Arakawa K, Ishihara T, Aoto M. Actions of novel antidiabetic thiazolidinedione T-174, in animal models of non-insulin-dependent diabetes mellitus and in cultured muscle cells. *Br J Pharmacol* 1998; 125: 429–36.
117. Araki K, Taki M, Magisawa T. Antidiabetic characterization of CS-001: a new thiazolidinedione with potent insulin-sensitising activity. *Diabetes* 2000; 49 (suppl 1): A425.
118. Upton R, Widdowson PS, Ishii S. Improved metabolic status and insulin sensitivity in obese fatty (*fa/fa*) Zucker rats and Zucker diabetic fatty (ZDF) rats treated with the thiazolidinedione MCC-555. *Br J Pharmacol* 1998; 125: 1708–14.
119. Fukiu Y, Masui S, Osada S. A new thiazolidinedione, NC-2100 which is a weak PPARg activator, exhibits potent antidiabetic effects andinduces uncoupling protein 1 in white adipose tissue of KKAy obese mice. *Diabetes* 2000; 49: 759–67.
120. Naitoh T, Nakabeppu K, Kamon J. NIP-221 is a novel and potent thiazolidinedione-based peroxisome proliferators activated receptor (PPAR) g ligand with a prolonged biological half time. *Diabetes* 2000; 49 (suppl 1): A480.
121. Sohda T, Mizuno K, Momose Y. Studies on antidiabetic agents. Novel thiazolidinedione derivatives as potent hypoglycemic and hypolipidemic agents. *J Med Chem* 1992; 35: 2617–26.
122. Yakubu-Madus FE, Stephens TW, Johnson WT. Lipid lowering explains the insulin sensitivity enhancing effects of a thiazolidinedione, 5-(4-(2-(2-phenyl-4-oxazolyl)ethoxy)benzyl)-2, 4 thiazolidinedione. *Diabetes Obes Metab* 2000; 2: 155–63.
123. Fiedorek F, Wilson GG, Frith L. Monotherapy with GI262570, a tyrosine-based non-thiazolidinedione PPARg agonist, improves metabolic control in type 2 diabetes mellitus patients. *Diabetes* 2000; 49 (suppl 1): A157.
124. Brown KK, Henke PR, Blanchard SG. A novel N-aryl tyrosine activator of peroxisome proliferator-activated receptor-g reverses the diabetic phenotype of the Zucker diabetic rat. *Diabetes* 2000; 48: 1415–24.
125. Way JM, Harrington WW, Brown KK. Comprehensive messenger ribonucleic acid profiling reveals that peroxisome proliferator activated receptor gamma activation has coordinate effects on gene expression in multiple insulin-sensitive tissues. *Endocrinology* 2001; 142: 1269–77.
126. Elbrecht A, Chen Y, Adams A. L-764406 is a partial agonist of human peroxisome proliferator-activated receptor gamma. The role of Cys313 in ligand binding. *J Biol Chem* 1999; 274: 7913–22.
127. Berger J, Bailey P, Biswas C. Thiazolidinediones produce a conformational change in peroxisome proliferators activated receptor-gamma: binding and activation correlate with antidiabetic actions in *db/db* mice. *Endocrinology* 1996; 137: 4189–95.
128. Nolte RT, Wisely GB, Westin S. Ligand binding and co-activator assembly of the peroxisome proliferators-activated receptor gamma. *Nature* 1998; 395: 137–43.
129. Camp HS, Li O, Wise SC. Differential activation of peroxisome proliferators activated receptor-g. *Diabetes* 2000; 49: 539–47.
130. Bailey CJ. The rise and fall of troglitazone. *Diabet Med* 2000; 17: 414–5.
131. Dubois M, Pattou F, Kerr-Conte J. Expression of peroxisome proliferator-activated receptor g (PPARg) in normal human pancreatic islet cells. *Diabetologia* 2000; 43: 1165–69.

132. Buckingham RE, Al-Barazanji KA, Toseland CD. Peroxisome proliferators activated receptor-g agonist, rosiglitazone, protects against nephropathy and pancreatic islet abnormalities in Zucker fatty rats. *Diabetes* 1998; 47: 1326–34.
133. Murphy GJ, Holder JC. PPAR-γ agonists: therapeutic role in diabetes, inflammation and cancer. *Trends Pharmacol Sci* 2000; 21: 469–74.
134. Shibàta T, Takeuchi S, Yokota S. Effects of peroxisome proliferator activated receptor-α and -γ agonist JTT-501, on diabetic complications in Zucker diabetic fatty rats. *Br J Pharmacol* 2000; 130: 495–514.
135. Lohray BB, Bhushan V, Rao BP. Novel euglycemic and hypolipidemic agents. *J Med Chem* 1998; 41: 619–30.
136. Murakami K, Tobe K, Ide T. A novel insulin sensitizer acts as a coligand for peroxisome proliferator-activated receptor-α (PPARα) and PPAR-γ. *Diabetes* 1998; 47: 1841–7.
137. Etgen GT, Oldham BA, Johnson WT, Broderick CL, Montrose CR, Brozinick JT, Misener EA, Bean JS, Bensch WR, Brooks DA, Shuker AJ, Rito CJ, McCarthy JR, Ardecky RJ, Tyhonas JS, Dana SI, Bilakovies JM, Paterniti JR Jr, Ogitvie KM, Liu S, Kauffman RF. A tailored therapy for the metabolic syndrome. The dual peroxisome proliferators-activated receptor-a/g agonist LY465608 ameliorates insulin resistance and diabetic hyperglycemia while improving cardiovascular risk factors in preclinical models. *Diabetes* 2002; 51: 1083–7.
138. Oliver W, Wilson J, Winegar D, Brainard T, Binz J, Banker P, Sternbach D, Lewis M. A PPARpan agonist delivers glycemic control and improved lipid profiles without weight gain and hemodilution in rodent models of type 2 DM, dyslipidemia and obesity. *Diabetes* 2003; 52 (suppl 1): A453. Abstract 1961.
139. Mukherjee R, Davies PJ, Crombie D. Sensitization of diabetic and obese mice to insulin by retinoid X receptor agonists. *Nature* 1997; 386: 407–10.
140. Emilsson V, O'Dowd J, Wang S. The effects of rexinoids and rosiglitazone on body weight and uncoupling protein isoform expression in the Zucker *fa/fa* rat. *Metabolism* 2000; 49: 1610–5.
141. Liu Y, Sennitt MV, Hislop DC. Retinoid x receptor agonists have anti-obesity effects and improve insulin sensitivity in Zucker *fa/fa* rats. *Int J Obes* 2000; 24: 997–1004.
142. Cha BS, Ciaraldi TP, Carter L. Peroxisome proliferators-activated receptor (PPAR) g and retinoid x receptor (RXR) agonists have complimentary effects on glucose and lipid metabolism in human skeletal muscle. *Diabetologia* 2001; 44: 444–52.
143. Bailey CJ. New pharmacological approaches to glycemic control. *Diabetes Rev* 1999; 7: 94–113.
144. American Diabetes Association. Magnesium supplementation in the treatment of diabetes. *Diabetes Care* 1992; 15: 1065–7.
145. Anderson RA, Cheng N, Bryden NA, Polansky MM, Cheng N, Chi J, Feng J. Elevated intakes of supplemental chromium improve glucose and insulin variables in individuals with type 2 diabetes. *Diabetes* 1997; 46: 1786–91.
146. Shisheva A, Gefel D, Shechter Y. Insulin like effects of zinc ion in vitro and in vivo. *Diabetes* 1992; 41: 982–6.
147. Ohly P, Dohle C, Abel J, Seissler J, Gleichmann H. Zinc sulphate induces metallothionein in pancreatic islets of mice and protects against diabetes induced by multiple low doses of streptozotocin. *Diabetologia* 2000; 43: 1020–30.
148. Hwang IK, Go VLW, Harris DM, Yip I, Song MK. Effects of arachidonic acid plus zinc on glucose disposal in genetically diabetic (*ob/ob*) mice. *Diabetes Obes Metab* 2002; 4: 124–31.
149. Goldfine AB, Simonson DC, Folli F, Patti ME, Kahn CR. Metabolic effects of sodium metavanadate in humans with insulin dependent and noninsulin dependent diabetes mellitus. In vivo and in vitro studies. *J Clin Endocrinol Metab* 1995; 80: 3311–20.
150. Cohn N, Halberstam M, Shlimovich M, Chang CJ, Shamoon H, Rossetti L. Oral vanadyl sulfate improves hepatic and periphertal insulin sensitivity in patients with non-insulin dependent diabetes mellitus. *J Clin Invest* 1995; 95: 2501–9.
151. Tsiani E, Bogdanovic E, Sorisky A, Nagy L, Fantus IG. Tyrosine phosphatase inhibitors, vanadate and pervanadate, stimulate glucose transport and GLUT translocation in muscle cells by a mechanism independent of phosphatidylinositol 3-kinase and protein kinase C. *Diabetes* 1998; 47: 1676–86.
152. Marti L, Abella A, Carpene C, Palacin M, Testar X, Zorzano A. Combined treatment with benylamine and low dosages of vanadate enhances glucose tolerance and reduces hyperglycemia in streptozotocin-induced diabetic rats. *Diabetes* 2001; 50: 2061–8.
153. Reul BA, Amin SS, Buchet JP, Ongemba LN, Crans DC, Brichard SM. Effects of vanadium complexes with organic ligands on glucose metabolism: a comparison study in diabetic rats. *Br J Pharmacol* 1999; 126: 467–77.
154. Becker DJ, Reul B, Ozvelikay AT, Buchet JP, Henquin JC, Brichard SM. Oral selenate improves glucose homeostasis and partly reverses abnormal expression of liver glycolytic and gluconeogenic enzymes in diabetic rats. *Diabetologia* 1996; 39: 3–11.
155. Reul BA, Becker DJ, Ongemba LM, Bailey CJ, Henquin JC, Brichard SM. Improvement of glucose homeostasis and hepatic insulin resistance in *ob/ob* mice given oral molybdate. *J Endocrinol* 1997; 155: 55–64.
156. Munoz MC, Barbera A, Dominguez J, Fernandez-Alvarez J, Gomis R, Guinovart JJ. Effects of tungstate, a new potential oral antidiabetic agent, in Zucker diabetic fatty rats. *Diabetes* 2001; 50: 131–8.
157. Barbera A, Gomis RR, Prats N, Rodriguez-Gil JE, Domingo M, Gomis R, Guinovart JJ. Tungstate is an effective antidiabetic agent in strptozotocin-induced diabetic rats: a long-term study. *Diabetologia* 2001; 44: 507–13.
158. Fernandez-Mejia C, Zendejas-Ruiz I, Revilla-Monsalve C, Islas-Andrede S. Biotin treatment increases insulin sensitivity in type 2 diabetics (T2D). *Diabetes* 2003; 52 (suppl 1): A459. Abstract 1987.
159. Bakker SJL, Hoogeveen EK, Nijpels G, Kostense PJ, Dekker JM, Gans ROB, Heine RJ. The association of dietary fibres with glucose tolerance is partly explained by concomitant intake of thiamine: the Hoorn study. *Diabetologia* 1998; 41: 1168–75.
160. Evans JL, Goldfine ID, Maddux BA, Grodsky GM. Are oxidative stress-activated signaling pathways mediators of insulin resistance and B-cell dysfunction? *Diabetes* 2003; 52: 1–8.
161. Opara EC, Abdel-Rahman E, Soliman S, Kamel WA, Souka S, Lowe JE, Abdel-Aleem S. Depletion of total antioxidant capacity in type 2 diabetes. *Metabolism* 1999; 48: 1414–7.

162. Coleman MD. Monitoring diabetic antioxidant status: a role for in vitro methaemoglobin formation. *Env Tox Pharmacol* 2001; 10: 207–13.
163. Kaneto H, Kajimoto Y, Miyagawa J, Matsuoka T, Fujitani Y, Umayahara T, Hanafusa T, Matsuzawa Y, Yamasaki Y, Hori M. Beneficial effects of antioxidants in diabetes. *Diabetes* 1999; 48: 2398–406.
164. Sargeant LA, Wareham NJ, Bingham S, Day NE, Luben RN, Oakes S, Welch A, Khaw KT. Vitamin C and hyperglycemia in the European Prospective Investigation into cancer. Norfolk (EPIC-Norfolk) study. *Diabetes Care* 2000; 23: 726–32.
165. Petersen KE, Sullivan JT. Effects of a novel glucagon receptor antagonist (Bay 27-9955) on glucagon-stimulated glucose production in humans. *Diabetologia* 2001; 44: 2018–24.
166. Knudsen LB, Brand CL, Sidelmann UG, Teston K, Ling A. NNC25-2504, apotent glucagons receptor antagonist. *Diabetologia* 2001; 44 (suppl 1): A196. Abstract 752.
167. Parker JC, McPherson RK, Andrews KM, Levy CB, Dubins JS, Chin JE, Perry PV, Bulin B, Perry DA, Inagaki T, Dekker KA, Tachikawa K, Sugie Y, Treadway JL. Effects of skyrin, a receptor-selective glucagons antagonist, in rat and human hepatocytes. *Diabetes* 2000; 49: 2079–86.
168. Bjorntorp P, Rosmond R. Obesity and cortisol. *Nutrition* 2000; 16: 924–36.
169. Reynolds RM, Walker BR. Human insulin resistance: the role of glucocorticoids. *Diabetes Obes Metab* 2003; 5: 5–12.
170. DeFronzo RA. Pharmacologic therapy for type 2 diabetes mellitus. *Ann Intern Med* 1999; 131: 281–303.
171. Stewart PM, Krozowski ZS. 11B-hydroxysteroid dehydrogenase. *Vitam Horm* 1999; 57: 249–324.
172. Alberts P, Engblom L, Edling N, Fosgren M, Klingstrom G, Larsson C, Ronquist-Nii Y, Ohman B, Abrahmsen L. Selective inhibition of 11B-hydroxysteriod dehydrogenase type 1 decreases blood glucose concentrations in hyperglycaemic mice. *Diabetologia* 2002; 45: 1528–32.
173. McGarry JD. Dysregulation of fatty acid metabolism in the etiology of type 2 diabetes. *Diabetes* 2002; 51: 7–18.
174. Saloranta C, Taskinen MR, Widen E. Metabolic consequences of sustained suppression of free fatty acids by acipimox in patients with NIDDM. *Diabetes* 1993; 42: 1559–66.
175. Foley JE. Rationale and application of fatty acid oxidation inhibition in treatment of diabetes mellitus. *Diabetes Care* 1992; 15: 773–84.
176. Vinik AJ, Colwell JA. Effects of gemfibrozil on triglyceride levels in patients with NIDDM. *Diabetes Care* 1993; 16: 37–44.
177. Hertz R, Bishara-Shieban J, Bar-Tana J. Mode of action of peroxisome proliferators as hypolipidemic drugs: suppression of apoliporotein C-III. *J Biol Chem* 1995; 270: 13470–5.
178. Atkinson LL, Kelly SE, Russell JC, Bar-Tana J, Opaschuk GD. Medica 16 inhibits hepatic acetyl-CoA carboxylase and reduced plasma triacylglycerol levels in insulin resistant JCR:LA-cp rats. *Diabetes* 2002; 51: 1548–55.
179. Fruebis J, Tsao TS, Javorschi S, Ebbets-Reed D. Proteolytic cleavage product of 30-kDa adipocyte complement-related protein increases fatty acid oxidation in muscle and causes weight loss in mice. *Proc Natl Acad Sci USA* 2001; 98: 2005–10.
180. Blaak EE, Glatz JFC, Saris WHM. Increase in skeletal muscle fatty acid binding protein (FABPC) content is directly related to weight loss and to changes in fat oxidation following a very low calorie diet. *Diabetologia* 2001; 44: 2013–7.
181. Kusunoki M, Hara T, Tsutsumi K, Nakamura T, Miyata T, Sakakibara F, Sakamoto S, Ogawa H, Nakaya Y, Storlien LH. The lipoprotein lipase activator, NO-1886, suppresses fat accumulation and insulin resistance in rats fed a high-fat diet. *Diabetologia* 2000; 43: 875–80.
182. Williams KV, Kelley DE. Metabolic consequences of weight loss on glucose metabolism and insulin action in type 2 diabetes. *Diabetes Obes Metab* 2000; 2: 121–9.
183. Batterham RL, Cohen MA, Ellis SM, Le Roux CW, Withers DJ, Frost GS, Ghatei MA, Bloom SR. Inhibition of food intake in obese subjects by peptide YY3-36. *NEJM* September 2003; 349 (10): 941–8.
184. Bray GA, Tartaglia LA. Medicinal strategies in the treatment of obesity. *Nature* 2000; 404: 672–7.
185. Pashko LL, Schwartz AG. Antihyperglycemic effect of dehydroepiandrosterone analog 16a-fluoro-5-androsten-17-one in diabetic mice. *Diabetes* 1993; 42: 1105–8.
186. Williams CA, Shih MF, Taberner PV. Sustained improvement in glucose homeostasis in lean and obese mice following chronic administration of the B3 agonist SR58611A. *Br J Pharmacol* 1999; 128: 1586–92.
187. Kato H, Ohue M, Kato K, Nomura A, Toyosawa K, Furutani Y, Kimura S, Kadawaki T. Mechanism of amelioration of insulin resistance by B3-adrenoceptor agonist AJ-9677 in the KK-Ay/Ta diabetic obese mouse model. *Diabetes* 2001; 50: 113–22.
188. Gebre-Medhim S, Olofsson C, Mulder H. Islet amyloid polypeptide in the islets of Langerhans: friend or foe? *Diabetologia* 2000; 43: 687–95.
189. Weyer C, Maggs DG, Young AA, Kolterman OG. Amylin replacement with pramlintide as an adjunct to insulin therapy in type 1 and type 2 diabetes mellitus: a physiological approach toward improved metabolic control. *Curr Pharm Res* 2001; 7: 1353–73.
190. Buse JB, Weyer C, Maggs DG. Amylin replacement with pramlintide in type 1 and type 2 diabetes: a physiological approach to overcome barriers with insulin therapy. *Clin Diabetes* 2002; 20: 137–44.
191. Stacpoole PW, Greene YJ. Dichloroacetate. *Diabetes Care* 1992; 15: 785–91.
192. Winder WW, Hardie DG. AMP-activated protein kinase, a metabolic master switch: possible roles in type 2 diabetes. *Am J Physiol* 1999; 277: E1–10.
193. Bergeron R, Previs SF, Cline GW, Perret P, Russell RR, Young LH, Shulman GI. Effect of 5-aminoimidazole-4-carboxamide-1-B-D-ribofuranoside infusion on in vivo glucose and lipid metabolism in lean and obese Zucker rats. *Diabetes* 2001; 50: 1076–82.
194. Fiedler M, Zierath JR, Selen G, Wallberg-Henriksson H, Liang Y, Sakariassen KS. 5-aminoimidazole-4-carboxyamide-1-B-D-ribofuranoside treatment ameliorates hyperglycaemia and hyperinsulinaemia but not dyslipidaemia in KKAy-CETP mice. *Diabetologia* 2001; 44: 2180–6.
195. Buhi ES, Jessen N, Schmitz O, Pedersen SB, Pedersen O, Holman GD, Lund S. Chronic treatment with 5-aminoimidazole-4-carboxamide-1-B-D-ribofuranoside increases insulin-stimulated glucose uptake and GLUT4 translocation in rat skeletal muscles in a fiber type-specific manner. *Diabetes* 2001; 50: 12–7.

196. Song XM, Fiedler M, Galuska D, Ryder JW, Fernstrom M, Chibalin AV, wallberg-Henriksson H, Zierath JR. 5-aminoimidazole-4-carboxamide ribonucleoside treatment improves glucose homeostasis in insulin resistant diabetic (*ob*/*ob*) mice. *Diabetologia* 2002; 45: 56–65.
197. Kefas BA, Heimberg H, Vaulont S, Meisse D, Hue L, Pipeleers D, Casteele M. AICA-riboside induces apoptosis of pancreatic beta cells through stimulation of AMP-activated protein kinase. *Diabetologia* 2003; 46: 250–4.
198. Treadway JL, Mendys P, Hoover DJ. Glycogen phosphorylase inhibitors for treatment of type 2 diabetes mellitus. *Expert Opin Invest Drugs* 2001; 10: 439–54.
199. Bergans N, Stalmans W, Goldmann S, Vanstapel F. Molecular mode of inhibition of glycogenolysis in rat liver by the dihydropyridine derivative BAY R3401. *Diabetes* 2000; 49: 1419–26.
200. Parker JC, VanVolkenburg A, Levy CB, Martin WH, Burk SH, Kwon Y, Giragossian C, Gant TG, Carpino PA, McPherson RK, Vestergaard P, Treadway JL. Plasma glucose levels are reduced in rats and mice treated with an inhibitor of glucose-6-phosphate translocase. *Diabetes* 1998; 47: 1630–6.
201. Westergaard N, Madsen P, Lundbeck JM, Jakobsen P, Varming A, Andersen B. Identification of two novel and potent competitive inhibitors of the glucose-6-phosphatase catalytic protein. *Diabetes Obes Metab* 2002; 4: 96–105.
202. Rossetti L. Glucose toxicity: the implications of hyperglycemia in the pathophysiology of diabetes mellitus. *Clin Invest Med* 1995; 18: 255–60.
203. Arakawa K, Ishihara T, Oku A, Nawano M, Ueta K, Kitamura K, Matsumoto M, Saito A. Improved diabetic syndrome in C57BL/KsJ-*db*/*db* mice by oral administration of the Na^+ glucose transporter inhibitor T-1095. *Br J Pharmacol* 2001; 132: 578–86.

52

Hypolipidemic Agents and Their Role in the Therapy of Diabetes Mellitus

Marja-Riitta Taskinen

University of Helsinki, Helsinki, Finland

INTRODUCTION

Patients with diabetes are at increased risk for cardiovascular disease (CVD) particularly coronary heart disease (CHD) [1, 2]. Approximately three quarters of all patients with diabetes will die of CVD and over 50% of the patients die of CHD. These comorbidities are also major causes of premature disability in people with diabetes. The prognosis of CHD is markedly worse in people with diabetes than in their nondiabetic counterparts. International Diabetes Federation (IDF) foresees a rise of epidemic proportions of type 2 diabetes that portends a rapid increase of CHD worldwide particularly among elderly subjects [3]. Today type 2 diabetes is recognized as a major risk factor for CHD. Therefore it is of paramount importance that aggressive management of CHD risk factors is initiated as early as possible to relieve the excessive burden of CVD in people with diabetes. Early screening and identification of risk factors is imperative. Conventional risk factors for CVD like hypertension, high cholesterol, and smoking are operative in people with diabetes but cannot explain the excess of CVD risk. Dyslipidemia is a major risk factor for the development of CVD in diabetes although the nature of dyslipidemia differs between type 1 and type 2 diabetes. The UK Prospective Diabetes Study (UKPDS) demonstrated that in people with type 2 diabetes, low-density lipoprotein cholesterol (LDL-C) and high-density lipoprotein cholesterol (HDL-C) were the best predictors of CHD [fatal and nonfatal myocardial infarction (MI)] among the modifiable risk factors including systolic blood pressure, smoking, and HbA_{1c} [4]. Diabetic dyslipidemia therefore represents a good target for therapeutic intervention. To date the advantages of multifactorial strategy to reduce CVD risk is convincing [5]. Overwhelming evidence also supports the benefits of lipid, modifying strategy. Recent results from the Heart Protection Study (HPS) have closed the debate whether or not LDL lowering is beneficial in people with diabetes [6]. To date the challenge is how to implement the guidelines in the clinical practice to endorse the aggressive lipid management and to achieve the target levels set by the current guidelines. Another challenge is how to tackle the lipid abnormalities of diabetic dyslipidemia beyond LDL-C to make lipid management even more successful to reduce CHD risk optimally.

DYSLIPIDEMIA IN PATIENTS WITH DIABETES

In people with diabetes the concentration of an individual lipoprotein or apoprotein can be highly variable and is totally different in the two forms of diabetes [7, 8] (Table 1). In general the lipoprotein profile is antiatherogenic in subjects with type 1 diabetes who have optimal or good glycemic control. In contrast the pattern is atherogenic in type 2 diabetes, regardless of the mode of therapy. The two forms of diabetes share the common characteristics of hyperglycemia as well as both macrovascular and microvascular complications. Likewise some abnormalities of lipoproteins and apoproteins, like glycation and oxidation linked to hyperglycemia, may be shared by both type 1 and type 2 diabetes. The presence of diabetic nephropathy also modifies lipid profiles in a similar adverse fashion in the two types of diabetes.

Lipoprotein Abnormalities in Type 1 Diabetes

Glycemic control and the regimen of insulin therapy are factors that can markedly modify lipoprotein pattern in

International Textbook of Diabetes Mellitus, Third Edition. Edited by R. A. DeFronzo, E. Ferrannini, H. Keen, and P. Zimmet.
 ISBN: 0-471-48655-8.

Table 1 Serum lipoproteins and apoproteins in treated diabetic patients

	Type 1 diabetes		Type 2 diabetes	
	Good control	Poor control	Good control	Poor control
Chylomicrons	Absent	Increased	Absent or slightly increased	Increased
VLDL	Normal or subnormal	Increased	Increased	Increased
IDL	Normal	Increased	Increased	Increased
LDL	Normal or subnormal	Normal	Normal	Increased
HDL	Normal or increased	Decreased	Decreased	Decreased
LDL size	Increased	Normal	Reduced	Reduced
Apoprotein-B	Decreased	Increased	Increased	Increased
Apoprotein-A1	Normal or increased	Decreased	Decreased	Decreased
Apoprotein-A2	Normal	Normal or decreased	Normal or decreased	Decreased
Lp(a)	Normal	Normal or increased	Normal	Normal

type 1 diabetes [8]. The hallmarks of lipid profile are normal/subnormal very low-density lipoprotein (VLDL) triglycerides, normal/subnormal LDL-C, and raised HDL-C in type 1 diabetic subjects with good glycemic control [7, 8]. Despite lack of visible abnormalities in lipoprotein concentrations, there are compositional changes and alterations in lipoprotein subclass distribution that may cause functional defects. The relevance of these alterations with respect to CHD risk is unclear. If metabolic control is poor the major lipid abnormality is the elevation of plasma triglyceride level although elevation of serum and LDL-C may also occur. Intensive insulin therapy normalizes the glycemic control, lowers VLDL and LDL, and increases HDL. In the Diabetes Control and Complication Trial (DCCT) favorable changes of serum lipid and lipoproteins were observed as a result of intensive insulin therapy [9]. Optimization of glycemic control is particularly powerful to reduce VLDL concentration.

Type 1 diabetic patients with overt albuminuria and clinical nephropathy have a broad spectrum of lipid abnormalities characterized by elevations of serum total and LDL-C, serum total and VLDL triglycerides, apo B 100, and lipoprotein (a), Lp(a). Substantial evidence shows that abnormalities of serum lipids and lipoproteins already occur in type 1 diabetic patients with microalbuminuria [10]. Suprisingly little data exists on the prevalence of lipid abnormalities in type 1 diabetic populations. The previous studies suggest that dyslipidemia in type 1 subjects is not more common than in the general population [7]. In the EURODIAB cohort, 45% of the subjects had LDL-C above 3.35 mmol/l and only 22% had LDL-C <2.6 mmol/l [11]. Thus, a high proportion of type 1 diabetic patients seem to have a LDL-C problem. The prevalence of raised triglycerides (>1.7 mmol/l) and low HDL (<0.5 mmol/l) was observed only in about 10%. Although there is limited data on lipoproteins and CHD, strong evidence indicates that cholesterol/LDL-C levels are predictors of CVD in type 1 diabetes [12, 13]. In contrast parameters associated with HDL-C are poorly related to CVD risk [14]. Finally it is important to recognize that both hypercholesterolemia and dyslipidemia may occur independently of type 1 diabetes and requests similar approach as in nondiabetic populations.

Dyslipidemia in Type 2 Diabetes

In type 2 diabetes dyslipidemia comprises a cluster of lipid aberrations that are metabolically closely linked [7, 15]. The key components are elevation of serum and VLDL triglyceride, excessive postprandial lipemia and remnant particles, small dense LDL, and lowering of HDL-C. All these abnormalities of lipid pattern have been found to be correlates of insulin resistance that plays a crucial role in the pathophysiology of diabetic dyslipidemia [15]. A much debated question has been which individual lipoprotein abnormality in diabetic dyslipidemia is most atherogenic and should be the primary target of lipid management. This debate cannot be considered fully relevant, since all components are metabolically closely linked to each others and represent together the culprit. The initiating factor seems to be overproduction of VLDL particles in the liver [15]. The most powerful atherogenic components are (1) Small dense LDL (2) Remnant particles, and (3) low concentration of HDL with its atherogenic compositional alterations. This atherogenic triad should be the target of lipid management in type 2 diabetes [15]. Obviously the malignant nature of diabetic dyslipidemia is not disclosed by the lipid measures used in the clinical practice. Small dense LDL is an integral feature of diabetic dyslipidemia and is more atherogenic than are large buoyant LDL particles. Since each LDL particle contains one molecule of apo B 100 at the same LDL-C concentration, the number of LDL particles is increased if small and dense. Thus the absolute concentration of LDL-C that is commonly normal or even subnormal can be misleading in CHD risk evaluation in people with type 2 diabetes. The implication of small dense LDL together with increased number of LDL particles is that LDL-C should be treated in type 2 diabetic people more vigorously than in nondiabetic subjects with the same LDL-C. Importantly, UKPDS

Table 2 Category of risk based on lipoprotein levels in adults with diabetes*

Risk	LDL cholesterol	HDL cholesterol†	Triglyceride
High	≥3.4 (≥130)	≤1.02 (<40)	≥4.5 (≥400)
Borderline	2.60–3.35 (100–129)	1.02–1.50 (40–59)	1.7–4.5 (150–399)
Low	≤2.6 (≤100)	≥1.50 (≥60)	≤1.7 (≤150)

Note: Data are given in millimoles per litre and in paranthesis in milligrams per deciliter.

† For women, the HDL cholesterol values should be increased by 0.26 mmol/l (by 10 mg/dl).

reported that among modifiable risk factors, LDL-C was the first and HDL-C the second variable as a predictor of CHD in Cox proportional hazards multivariate model [4].

The high prevalence of diabetic dyslipidemia has been observed in several studies in different populations. The National Health and Nutrition Examination Survey III (NHANES III) reported that 85% of patients with type 2 diabetes had LDL-C above the optimal goal of 2.6 mmol/l (>100 mg/dl), 42% had triglyceride levels >2.3 mmol/l (>200 mg/dl) and 62% had HDL-C <1.15 mmol/l (<45 mg/dl) [16]. Employing the more stringent optimal level for triglycerides <1.7 mmol/l (150 mg/dl) would increase the prevalence of subjects with elevated triglycerides. In the Botnia study from Finland, among 1130 type 2 diabetic subjects, 45% had triglyceride values > 1.7 mmol/l (>150 mg/dl), 86% had LDL-C values > 2.6 mmol/(100 mg/dl), and 16% had HDL-C values < 0.9 mmol/l (35 mg/dl), respectively [17]. Likewise in a Canadian cohorts, triglyceride values > 1.7 mmol/l were seen in 50% and values > 2.3 mmol/l in 20%; LDL-C values > 2.6 mmol/l in 77%; and HDL-C >1.15 mmol/l in 49% [17]. In these cohorts, LDL values > 3.4 mmol/l (>130 mg/dl) have been found in 45–50% of the type 2 diabetic subjects. The high incidence of lipid values above target levels has also been observed in South European and Asian populations, being a universal feature of type 2 diabetes worldwide. However, the prevalence of high LDL-C is not different from the prevalence rate in the respective nondiabetic populations. Overall the prevalence of elevated triglyceride and low HDL-C is two to three times more frequent than in the nondiabetic populations. The high incidence of dyslipidemia is a special challenge for the implementation of treatment guidelines, due to the large populations in need of intervention.

RATIONALE FOR MANAGEMENT OF DIABETIC DYSLIPIDEMIA

The National Cholesterol Education Program – Adult Treatment Panel III (NCEP-ATP III) guidelines designated diabetes as a CHD risk equivalent even in the absence of known CHD and recommended the same treatment strategy for people with diabetes as in nondiabetic individuals with established CHD [18]. This means that the goal of LDL-C is <2.6 mmol/l (<100 mg/dl). Current American Diabetes Association (ADA) guidelines also recognize LDL-C as the primary goal of therapy, the optimal LDL-C level for adults with diabetes being <2.6 mmol/l [19] (Table 2). The justification for this treatment strategy is, first, the high incidence of CVD disease in people with diabetes that relates to 10-year risk >20% of new CHD in the majority of studies [18]. Furthermore the poor early prognosis of diabetic patients with their first MI is well established in several studies [20, 21]. The higher case fatality rates signifies that a large proportion of diabetic patients with vascular events die before they reach the hospital. Thus there is a strong case for primary prevention. Likewise the excess mortality during the first year after MI in people with diabetes is well documented in several studies [22–24]. Altogether, these factors justify the designation of diabetes as a CHD risk equivalent although the actual CHD incidence may not always indicate a high risk [25, 26]. Ultimately the current LDL-C goal <2.6 mmol/l may not be low enough when one considers the recent results from the HPS, showing that lowering LDL-C from below 3.0 mmol/l to below 2.0 mmol/l (from 116 to <77 mg/dl) in people with diabetes reduced the risk of the first major vascular event by 27% [6].

ADA guidelines specify target levels for triglycerides and HDL-C [19]. Optimal HDL-C levels are >1.02 mmol/l (>40 mg/dl) and desirable triglyceride levels are <1.7 mmol/l (<150 mg/dl) (Table 2). NCEP-ATP III guidelines recommends *non-HDL-C*, defined as the difference between total and HDL-C, as a secondary target if triglycerides exceed 2.3 mmol/l (200 mg/dl) [18]. Notably non-HDL-C represents cholesterol carried on VLDL, intermediate density lipoprotein (IDL) and LDL, and triglyceride-rich lipoprotein (TRL) remnants. Since concentrations of both VLDL and IDL are elevated in diabetic dyslipidemia, this measure may be particularly practical [27, 28]. The therapeutic goal for non-HDL-C is less [<3.4 mmol/l (<130 mg/dl)]. Recent data suggest that these optimal values are appropriate for type 1 diabetic subjects also [13].

OPTIONS FOR LIPID MANAGEMENT IN PEOPLE WITH DIABETES

Lifestyle Modifications

Treatment of dyslipidemia in diabetic patients consists of a stepwise approach, with three major components [19].

The first-line therapy comprises lifestyle changes focusing at weight loss, increased physical activity, smoking cessation, and moderation of alcohol intake. These actions aim to correct metabolic risk factors linked to insulin resistance. Effective implementation of lifestyle intervention is associated with clear benefits. Weight loss is generally associated with improvements in triglyceride and HDL-C levels and also with modest lowering of LDL-C. Substantial benefits of the lipid profile are also seen with regular exercise programs aimed to improve physical fitness. ADA has given recommendations for both medical nutrition therapy (MNT) and physical activity [29, 30]. Likewise American Heart Association (AHA) has published a statement on exercise and physical activity in the prevention of CVD [31]. As most people with diabetes are overweight the nutrition therapy should emphasize reduced energy intake and aim to moderate weight loss [29]. The goal of diet therapy in people with diabetes and with dyslipidemia is to reduce the amount of saturated fat <10% of energy intake and dietary cholesterol <200 mg/dl [29, 32]. Saturated fat can be replaced with monounsaturated fat or whole grains as the principal form of carbohydrates, as well as fruits and vegetables. In addition plant stanols/sterol (2 g/day) can be used to lower plasma LDL-C, recognizing that this may lead to an increase in energy intake and weight gain if used *ad libitum*. Recent data confirmed that regular physical activity markedly reduces CVD risk and mortality in people with diabetes [33–35]. Notably even moderate physical activity such as regular walking is beneficial. Unfortunately the prescription of physical activity is an underutilized strategy. Recommendations for physical activity should be individualized and routinely prescribed. Since smoking induces insulin resistance and unfavorable lipid profile in addition to being a strong CVD risk factor the cessation of smoking is extremely important. If these actions are insufficient to improve glycemic control and lipid values the second step is to intensify glycemic control aiming to the target of HbA_{1c} <7.0%.

Management of Hyperglycemia

Although the association between glycemic control and macrovascular disease is well-established the magnitude of the association is modest [36]. Thus even optimal glycemic control may eliminate only a part of the excess CHD risk, as the power of intensive glycemic control to reduce cardiovascular events has not been convincing [37]. In UKPDS the intensive management of hyperglycemia was associated with a highly significant reduction of microvascular endpoints but there was only a 16% reduction in MI that was of borderline significance [38]. These findings support the concept that CHD is not influenced to the same extent by glycemic control as are microvascular complications. Nevertheless, observational data from UKPDS showed that there was 14% decrease of relative risk for MI per 1% decrement of HbA_{1c} [39]. Thus the observational and trial data are closely comparable. This raises the question whether the attenuated response of CVD outcomes is due to a poor efficacy of current antihyperglycemic agents to achieve good glycemic control? Whether more intense control of glycemia than achieved in UKPDS would have more impact on the prevention of CHD events remains to be confirmed in future clinical trials.

In type 2 diabetes, lipid abnormalities are present independently of the mode of treatment in cross-sectional studies [7]. There is no continuous increase of plasma triglycerides until HbA_{1c} levels exceed 8.5%, suggesting that the impact of insulin resistance on triglyceride metabolism is stronger than that of hyperglycemia *per se* [40]. In general any approach to improve glycemic control will improve lipid profile particularly reducing plasma triglyceride levels. The beneficial effects of intensified insulin therapy on lipid profiles have been shown in several studies [8]. There is also substantial evidence that metformin exerts positive effects on serum lipid profiles in type 2 diabetic patients. However, all interventions improving glucose control have only a modest effect on plasma triglyceride levels. Furthermore the optimization of glycemic control has minor or no effects on HDL and LDL-C levels. Interestingly thiazolidienediones (TZDs) raise consistently HDL-C, the change being 5–15% [41]. The response of plasma triglycerides and LDL-C is variable, depending on the compound (rosiglitazone vs pioglitazone). However, the available data suggest that TZDs have potentially beneficial actions on lipid parameters by improving insulin sensitivity. The potential clinical benefits of glitazones on vascular outcomes await results from ongoing trials.

Unfortunately optimization of glycemic control frequently fails to fully correct dyslipidemia in most type 2 diabetic patients. Nevertheless, the misconception that diabetic dyslipidemia is completely reversed if glucose control is improved is common. Therefore, efforts to improve glycemic control should not be an excuse to neglect the initiation of lipid therapy if specific targets for lipid levels are not achieved within a reasonable time (2–3 months).

LIPID MODIFYING THERAPY

Hydroxymethylglutaryl Coenzyme A Reductase Inhibitors

Hydroxymethylglutaryl coenzyme A reductase inhibitors (statins) are the most effective current tools to lower serum total and LDL-C levels. There are six available statins: atorvastatin, fluvastatin, lovastatin, pravastatin, rosuvastatin, and simvastatin. The statins act by inhibiting cholesterol synthesis in the liver. The secondary effect is the

Table 3 Effects of lipid modifying drugs on lipid profile*

Drug class	Lipid/lipoprotein effects
HMG-CoA reductase inhibitors	LDL ↓ 18–55% HDL ↑ 5–15% Tg ↓ 7–30%
Fibric acids	LDL ↓ 5–20% HDL ↑ 10–20% Tg ↓ 20–50%
Nicotinic acid	LDL ↓ 5–25% HDL ↑ 15–35% Tg ↓ 20–50%

Note: HMG-CoA = hydroxymethylglutaryl coenzyme A; Tg = triglyceride.
* Reproduced by permission of the Journal of American Medical Association (2001) 285, 2486–2497 [18].

upregulation of LDL receptor that enhances the catabolism of LDL as well as uptake of VLDL particles [42]. Thus, statins reduce not only LDL but also other apo B containing particles (VLDL and IDL). Recent studies have shown that statins do not reduce apo B production in the liver [42, 43]. In general the LDL-lowering action of statins has been the same in people with diabetes as in nondiabetic subjects averaging as much as 18–55%, depending on the dose and the efficacy of the compound (Table 3). Statins produce a substantial lowering of elevated plasma triglycerides, but the effect is only trivial in normotriglyceridemic subjects. The lowering of plasma triglycerides is proportional to LDL-C reduction and seems to be comparable at equipotent doses for LDL lowering [44]. In clinical practice the less potent statins like lovastatin and pravastatin lower plasma triglycerides to a lesser extent than do more potent statins like atorvastatin and rosuvastatin. Statins are also modestly effective to raise HDL-C usually by 5–15%. Long-term treatment in major clinical trials has confirmed that statins are well tolerated and have an excellent safety record. Importantly, statins do not have any adverse effects on the glycemic control.

Fibric Acid Derivatives

Fibrates (fibric acid derivatives) are another class of lipid-lowering drugs that is documented to be effective for the treatment of diabetic dyslipidemia. There are four fibrates available: bezafibrate, ciprofibrate, gemfibrozil, and fenofibrate. The effects of fibrates can be explained by the activation of the peroxisome proliferator-activator receptor α (PPARα), a nuclear receptor in the liver, altering transcription of genes and resulting in either stimulation or suppression of the target genes [45]. The discovery of the *PPARα* as the target of fibrate action opened a renaissance for fibrates to correct the lipoprotein abnormalities of diabetic dyslipidemia. Activation of *PPARα* by fibrates is followed by multiple effects on lipoprotein metabolism. *PPARα* activation results in downregulation of *apoC-III* gene and decrease of *apoC-III* synthesis. Fibrates also turn on the expression of *LPL* gene and genes regulating lipid oxidation. The end result is enhanced catabolism of triglyceride-rich particles, resulting in lowering of plasma fasting and postprandial triglyceride levels [43]. As a consequence of triglyceride lowering, there is a shift of LDL particle size from small dense to large buoyant subclasses. Likewise, *PPARα* activation increases plasma HDL-C by increasing *apoA-I* and *A-II* gene expression, followed by increased synthesis of these apoproteins. In addition, PPARα activators have been reported to increase expression of both ATP cassette binding protein 1 (ABCA-1) and scavenger receptor BI (SR-BI) that regulate cholesterol efflux system, accelerating reverse cholesterol transport from peripheral cells to the liver [46]. The consequence of these effects is the increase of HDL particles in plasma. In general, fibrates reduce plasma triglyceride levels by 20–50% and raise HDL-C by 10–20% (Table 3). Fibrates have a limited effect on LDL-C. Fibrates do not have any adverse effects on glycemic control.

Nicotinic Acid Derivatives

Nicotinic acid (niacin) is the most effective agent for raising HDL-C and it also substantially decreases plasma triglycerides and LDL-C [7]. Nicotinic acid inhibits free fatty acid flux from adipose tissue and secondary suppresses triglyceride synthesis and VLDL release from the liver [47]. Nicotinic acid also favorably modulates the metabolism of HDL by inhibiting HDL catabolic pathway. Therefore, nicotinic acid would be a rational choice for the treatment of diabetic dyslipidemia. However, nicotinic acid potentially worsens the glycemic control in type 2 diabetic patients and requests strict monitoring of glucose control although the effect usually is modest [7]. The Arterial Disease Multiple Intervention Trial (ADMIT) study reported that the use of niacin was safe in patients with stable well-controlled type 2 diabetes [48]. Notably, niacin has been reported to have positive action on LDL size and Lp(a), in addition to well-known effects on VLDL triglycerides, HDL-C, and LDL-C [49]. Immediate-release niacin has frequent adverse effects, i.e. flushing and hepatic toxicity, that have limited its tolerability. Consequently the use of niacin has been discouraged in diabetic patients [7]. Recently a new formulation i.e. extended-release (ER) niacin (Niaspan) has been introduced for once-daily administration. This preparation appears to be better tolerated and circumvents partly the side effects like flushing and hepatotoxicity [50]. A recent report in type 2 diabetic subjects indicates that Niaspan given alone or with a statin was efficient and well tolerated [51]. Thus ER compound may provide a potential option to target all abnormalities of diabetic dyslipidemia, but its safety profile needs to be confirmed in large-scale studies.

Combination Therapy

Acknowledging the target of LDL-C <2.6 mmol/l together with secondary target for HDL-C >1.02 and triglycerides <1.7 mmol/l or non-HDL goal < 3.4 mmol/l, it is obvious that many type 2 diabetic patients may not achieve these targets by monotherapy and there is need to reinforce the lipid-lowering therapy. Several options are available and should be considered carefully, recognizing that type 2 diabetic patients are commonly elderly, on multiple medication, and may have renal impairment. A special caution must be exercised when combining the statins with fibrate to avoid the potential for myopathy and rhabdomyolysis. Recent studies indicate that there is diversity in pharmacological interaction between statins and different fibrates [52, 53]. This difference may explain the lack of significant interaction between fenofibrate as compared to gemfibrozil with statins. The efficacy and safety of fenofibrate–atorvastatin combination has been evaluated in two small-scale studies of type 2 diabetic patients, with promising results [54, 55]. Likewise the fenofibrate–simvastatin combination was found to improve lipoprotein profile markedly more than either drugs alone in patients with combined hyperlipidemia and metabolic syndrome [56]. To minimize the risk of myopathy a once-daily fibrate (fenofibrate or bezafibrate) given in the morning together with a low-dose short-acting statin in the evening is recommended. Action to Control Cardiovascular Risk in Diabetes (ACCORD) is an ongoing large-scale intervention study that will evaluate in a factorial design the safety and efficacy of simvastatin, fenofibrate, and their combination, in type 2 diabetic patients.

An alternative option for individuals with severe hypertriglyceridemia to reduce plasma triglycerides is the use of omega-3 fatty acids that reduce plasma triglyceride levels by about 20–30% at doses of 3–5 g per day [57] but has trivial effects on HDL-C levels and may increase LDL-C. Consequently a combination with either statin or fibrate is needed to improve the whole lipoprotein profile.

The combination of statins with nicotinic acid seems to be highly effective to correct abnormalities of diabetic dyslipidemia. The safety data from recent small-scale trials are encouraging [58]. Importantly, the combination of simvastatin and niacin provided stunning clinical and angiographically measured benefits in patients with coronary artery disease (CAD) and low HDL-C [59].

If the goal of LDL-C is not achieved with a moderate dose of statins, ezetimibe as a novel cholesterol absorption inhibitor provides a promising tool for the combination therapy to lower LDL-C [60, 61]. The use of ezetimibe allows to use lower statin doses and this may improve patient compliance. Ezetimibe can also be combined with a fibrate to achieve LDL-C targets.

Overall, the combination therapies provide potential tools to achieve optimal lipid profiles in type 2 diabetic patients. However, clinical outcome studies are needed to determine the benefits and role of the different combination therapies in diabetic patients.

TRANSLATING THE TRIAL EVIDENCE INTO CLINICAL PRACTICE

Trial Evidence for Clinical Benefits by Statin Therapy

The data from the landmark secondary prevention studies [Scandinavian Simvastanin Survival Study (4S); Cholesterol and Recurrent Events (CARE); Long-Term Intervention with Pravastanin in Ischemic Disease (LIPID)] have provided strong evidence that statins reduce the risk of both CHD events and mortality by 25–35% in patients with previous CHD [62–64]. These trials have included relatively small subsets of adult type 2 diabetic subjects (altogether about 1500 patients with pre-existing CHD). The data from these trials were encouraging and strongly suggested that the diabetic subgroups had the same or even greater clinical benefits with statin treatment than did the nondiabetic CHD patients (Table 4). The Scandinavian Simvastatin Survival Trial was the first study to show that lowering LDL-C in type 2 diabetic patients decreases the risk of CHD events [65]. The reduction of the CHD events was 55% in the diabetic cohort as compared to 32% in the nondiabetic cohort. The primary endpoint of total mortality was not significant owing to a small sample size. In a post hoc analysis of 4S data, using the revised 1997 ADA criteria for diabetes the risk reduction of CHD events was 42% among diabetic patients [66]. Importantly, among the patients with impaired glucose tolerance the risk of CHD events was reduced significantly by 38%. It should be kept in mind that in the 4S study the diabetic patients had relatively high baseline cholesterol levels (between 5.5 and 8.0 mmol/l), and patients with triglycerides above 2.5 mmol/l were excluded. Hence the lipid abnormalities were not typical of diabetic dyslipidemia.

CARE trial included 586 patients with clinical diagnosis of diabetes who were randomized to receive 40 mg pravastatin or placebo for 5 years [67]. Pravastatin reduced the risks of major coronary events and revascularization procedures by 25% ($p = 0.05$) in diabetic group and 23% in nondiabetic cohort ($p < 0.001$), respectively. In LIPID study the risk reduction among diabetic patients was 19% in pravastatin group but this trend was not statistically significant [64]. In Prospective Pravastatin Poolin Project (PPP) including 1440 subjects with diabetes, the relative risk reduction of expanded end point was 26% and highly significant [68]. In CARE and LIPID the diabetic patients had moderate cholesterol levels, the LDL-C ave-raging 3.5 mmol/l (136 mg/dl) and 3.9 mmol/l (150 mg/dl), respectively. A recent combined analysis of CARE and LIPID data included 472 diabetic patients with LDL-C

<3.3 mmol/l (<125 mg/dl) [69]. The diabetic patients with low LDL-C had significantly higher subsequent CHD event rates over 5 years than did nondiabetic individuals (34 vs. 21%). In diabetic patients, pravastatin markedly decreased CHD event rates during 5.7 years follow-up, the relative risk reduction being 44% (95% CI 0.37 to 0.83, $p = 0.004$). Noteworthy, the risk reduction was significant in diabetic subgroup with low LDL-C but not in nondiabetic group. The data suggested that low HDL-C and high triglycerides have stronger effects on CHD risk in diabetic subjects with low LDL-C compared with non-diabetic subjects.

To date the HPS is the largest intervention trial involving diabetic subjects [6]. The HPS included about 6000 patients with diabetes among >20 000 participants at high risk of CVD. Patients were randomly allocated to receive either simvastatin 40 mg daily or placebo. The diabetic cohort included 5348 individuals with type 2 diabetes and 615 with type 1 diabetes, respectively. Among the diabetic participants, 1981 had previous CHD, 1070 other occlusive vascular diseases, and 2912 no history of any arterial disease. At the entry to the study the mean concentration of LDL-C averaged 3.23 mmol/l, and 40% of the subjects had LDL-C <3.0 mmol/l. The mean values for triglycerides and HDL-C were 2.38 mmol/l and 1.02 mmol/l, respectively [70]. Thus the type 2 diabetic subjects included in the HPS had a very similar lipid profile to those seen in the UKPDS study [71] and Diabetes Atherosclerosis Intervention Study (DAIS) cohort [72].

The average reduction of LDL-C in patients with diabetes allocated to simvastatin group was 1.0 mmol/l during the 5-year treatment period. The HPS also reassured the safety and tolerability of simvastatin in this broad-base population. The main results for cholesterol lowering in the diabetic patients are shown in Figure 1. In patients with diabetes first major coronary event (i.e. nonfatal MI or coronary death) and first major vascular event (i.e. major coronary event, stroke, or revascularization) were reduced in simvastatin group by 27% and 22%, which were similar to those among other high-risk participants without diabetes. Allocation to simvastatin produced a highly significant 37% proportional reduction in first MI. The proportional reduction in coronary mortality was 20% among the diabetic participants. The evidence for stroke reduction was also impressive being a significant 24% in the diabetic patients and 26% among the other participants. Noteworthy among about 3000 diabetic subjects without any history of previous vascular disease there was a highly significant 33% reduction in first major vascular events.

The proportional risk reduction among the diabetic patients appeared to be about 25%, independent of the duration of diabetes, the degree of glycemic control, body mass index (BMI), age, and sex. Additionally, the risk reduction was similar about a quarter in those diabetic subjects with LDL-C above or below 3 mmol/l or HDL- C above or below 0.9 mmol/l. The important message is that lowering LDL-C from below 3.0 mmol/l (116 mg/dl) to below 2.0 mmol/l (77 mg/dl) produced a significant reduction in proportional risk of cardiovascular events. The HPS data suggest that LDL-C lowering is beneficial at any LDL-C level for diabetic patients. Thus, the current LDL goals < 2.6 mmol/l (i.e., <100 mg/dl) may not be low enough, considering the atherogenic nature of LDL particles in people with type 2 diabetes. Three trials [Treating to New Targets (TNT); The Incremental Decrease in Endpoints through Aggressive Lipid Lowering (IDEAL); and Study on the Effectiveness of Additional Reductions in Cholesterol and Homocysteine (SEARCH)]; including substantial numbers of people with diabetes are currently

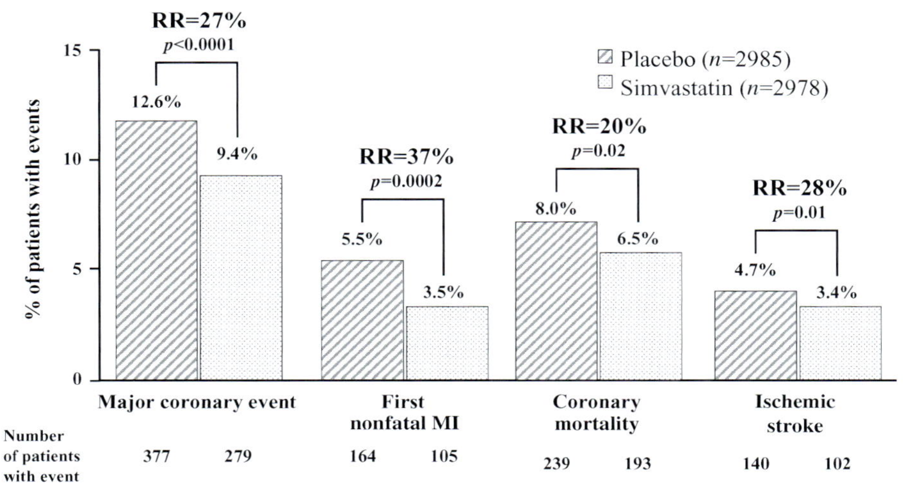

Figure 1 Impact of simvastatin in Heart Protection Study on major vascular events in people with diabetes. (Reproduced by permission of Elsevier [6])

Table 4 CHD prevention trials withs statins in diabetic subjects—subgroup analyses*

Study	Drug	N	Trial dose (mg)	LDL reduction (%)	CHD risk reduction (overall)	CHD risk reduction (diabetes)
1° Prevention						
AFCAPS/TexCAPS	Lovastatin	155	20–40	25†	−37%	−43%
HPS	Simvastatin	2912	40	29†	−24%	−26% ($p < 0.0001$)
ASCOT	Atorvastatin	2532	10	35†	−36%	−26%
2° Prevention						
CARE	Pravastatin	586	40	27	−23%	−25% ($p = 0.05$)
4S	Simvastatin	202	20–40	36	−32%	−55% ($p = 0.002$)
LIPID	Pravastatin	782	40	25†	−25%	−19%
4S Renalysis	Simvastatin	483	20–40	36	−32%	−42% ($p = 0.001$)
HPS	Simvastatin	3051	40	30	−24%	−24%
ALLHAT	Pravastatin	3638	40	10†	−9%	−11%

*Reproduced by permission of Elsevier [6, 64–67, 73–75].
†LDL reduction in the total cohort.

underway to assess the evidence for the "lower is better" hypothesis. These trials are due to be completed in 2006. Another important message from the HPS is that absolute benefits of LDL-C lowering depend chiefly on the absolute risk of CVD. The investigators estimated that in people with diabetes and without any occlusive vascular disease, 5-year statin treatment will prevent about 45 per 1000 diabetic subjects to have major vascular events and about 90 per 1000 diabetic people in those with previous vascular disease. Taken together, the HPS argues for more aggressive lipid lowering than is currently recommended in all type 2 as well as in type 1 diabetic patients.

Two other recent studies, the Antihypertensive and Lipid-Lowering Treatment to Prevent Heart Attack Trial (ALLHAT) and the Anglo-Scandinavian Cardiac Outcomes Trial (ASCOT), also included substantial number of people with type 2 diabetes (i.e. 3638 vs. 2532) [73, 74] (Table 4). In ALLHAT the average difference in LDL-C between pravastatin arm and usual care was only about 0.6 mmol/l, due to common use of nonstudy statin in the usual care group. In both nondiabetic and diabetic participants allocated to pravastatin arm there was similar but nonsignificant reduction in coronary event rates (9 vs. 11%). In ASCOT study atorvastatin, 10 mg daily, reduced the major coronary events in hypertensive people with type 2 diabetes over 3.3 years, but the relative risk reduction of the major coronary events was not significant probably due to few coronary events (38 atorvastatin vs. 46 placebo).

Thus the benefits of statin therapy in people with type 2 diabetes can no longer be questioned, also recognizing the fact that statins have additional properties that can increase their effectiveness beyond lowering LDL-C. The HPS evidence for clinical benefits in type 1 diabetes is encouraging. Today we are faced with the question should all patients with type 2 diabetes be treated with statins or not? [76] If so, this approach will have significant cost implications for diabetes care. This question may get the final answer from ongoing trials in people with type 2 diabetes, including Collaborative Atorvastatin Diabetes Study (CARDS), Atorvastatin as Prevention of Coronary Heart Disease (ASPEN), and ACCORD.

Trial Evidence for Clinical Benefits by Fibrate Therapy

The data from a subgroup analysis of diabetic subjects included in the Helsinki Heart Study, a 5-year primary prevention trial in men with a high LDL-C, were encouraging and indicated that fibrate treatment may reduce the risk of CHD events [77]. In fact the relative risk reduction was 60% in the gemfibrozil group as compared to placebo but the figure was not statistically significant. The Veterans Administration High Density Lipoprotein Intervention Trial (VA-HIT) also used gemfibrozil or placebo in a cohort of 2531 men with existing CHD [78]. The study population is unique because the subjects had both low HDL-C (mean 0.80 mmol/l vs. 31.5 mg/dl) and low LDL-C (mean 2.81 mmol/l vs. 111 mg/dl), high prevalence of diabetes (31%), obesity (39%, with BMI > 30 kg/m^2), and hyperinsulinemia (32%). In all participants, gemfibrozil treatment produced a significant 22% relative reduction in CHD events and a 31% reduction in stroke. Among diabetic subjects, gemfibrozil produced a highly significant 32% proportional risk reduction as compared to 18% in nondiabetic men [79]. The absolute risk reduction was 9.9% in the diabetes group and 3.6% in the nondiabetic group. Importantly, there was a significant 41% reduction in CHD death and 40% reduction in stroke among diabetic patients. Noteworthy, in VA-HIT the number needed to treat for diabetic cohort was lower than in CARE or LIPID [80] (Table 5). In addition there was a significant 35% reduction in major CHD events with gemfibrozil in nondiabetic subjects with high fasting insulin levels [79]. Recent results from VA-HIT show that the benefits of genfibrozil therapy were more pronounced in subjects with insulin resistance than in those without insulin resistance

Table 5 Myocardial infarction and coronary heart disease death reduction in diabetes with lipid drug therapy*

Trial	Drug	*N*	LDL-C† (mg/dl)	CHD events in DM‡ Placebo (%)	Drug (%)	Absolute RR (%)	NNT to prevent 1 event§
4S	Simvastatin	483	186 ± 26	37.5	23.5	14.0	7
CARE	Pravastatin	586	136 ± 14	20.4	17.7	2.7	37
LIPID‖	Pravastatin	782	150 ± 27	22.8	19.2	3.6	28
HPS	Simvastatin	5963	123 ± 32	12.6	3.2	3.2	31
VA-HIT	Gemfibrozil	769	108 ± 23	29.4	21.2	8.2	12

*Adapted from reference 80.
†LDL cholesterol values are mean ±SD.
‡CHD events are shown as the 5-year incidence rate of nonfatal MI or CHD death in diabetes.
§NNT = 100/Absolute RR.
‖LDL values are for the entire trial.

despite similar changes of plasma triglycerides and HDL-C by gemfibrozil [81]. Thus the VA-HIT results suggest that gemfibrozil maybe most efficacious to reduce CHD risk in subjects with the metabolic syndrome.

The DAIS was designed specifically to examine whether correcting the lipid abnormalities typically seen in type 2 diabetes will alter the course of coronary atherosclerosis [72]. The DAIS is an angiographic study in which 418 diabetic patients were randomized to receive either micronized fenofibrate or placebo. Fenofibrate treatment was associated with 40% less progression of average minimum lumen diameter and 42% less progression in percent diameter stenosis, which are the parameters of focal disease. There was 25% (NS) less progression in mean segment diameter, a measure of diffuse disease. The results of DAIS clearly demonstrated a slowing of coronary atherosclerosis, with fenofibrate treatment over 3 years in people with type 2 diabetes. DAIS was not powered to assess the effect of treatment on clinical events. However, it was encouraging to note that there were fewer fatal and nonfatal coronary endpoints in the fenofibrate than in placebo group (38 vs. 50, NS). Altogether the data from VA-HIT and DAIS emphasize treatment beyond LDL-C in patients with low LDL levels. The Fenofibrate Intervention and Event Lowering in Diabetes (FIELD) study will provide a clear answer whether fenofibrate can prevent cardiovascular events in type 2 diabetic subjects. The FIELD study includes more than 9700 type 2 diabetic patients randomly allocated to receive either micronized fenofibrate or placebo. The study will be completed in 2005.

Is Lipid-modifying Therapy Optimized in Current Clinical Practice?

The data from clinical trials argue for more aggressive lipid-lowering therapy than is currently practiced. Several recent studies have reported that diabetic patients are undertested and undertreated irrespective of whether they have or do not have clinical CAD [82–85]. In a recent survey of outpatient medical record data from 47 813 CAD patients from multiple medical practices in the United States, lipid profile testing increased from 28 to 50% between 1996 and 1998 and lipid management from 32 to 51% in people with diabetes, indicating a positive development [83]. Nevertheless the people with diabetes were 26% less likely to have a lipid profile and 17% less likely to receive a lipid-lowering drug than their nondiabetic counterparts. Furthermore the lipid management improved less rapidly in people with diabetes than is in nondiabetic, patients. In general, hypercholesterolemia and hypertension are managed with less aggressive therapy than is hyperglycemia, despite the fact that targeting lipid and hypertension management may be more likely cardioprotective than focusing on the glucose level. This is highlighted by a survey in US academic outpatient clinic where only 38% of type 2 diabetic patients with above-goal LDL-C levels (defined as <3.4 mmol/l, and <2.6 mmol/l if coronary disease was present) received any drug therapy as compared to 92% for hyperglycemia and 78% for hypertension [85]. These data probably represents the best scenario as compared to general clinical practice and emphasize the glucocentric view in the care of type 2 diabetic patients. How to improve lipid testing and ensure aggressive lipid management is the challenge of today in clinical practice.

The key question from the diabetes care perspective is how cost-effective is lipid management? *Post hoc* cost-effectiveness analysis from the 4S trial reported that simvastatin treatment reduced CVD-related hospitalization days more in diabetic patients than in nondiabetic patients and resulted in a net cost savings in direct medical cost per subject [86]. Likewise the costs per life-year gained were less in the diabetic subjects than in those without diabetes, indicating that the therapy was clearly cost-effective in diabetic patients [87]. Recently the cost-effectiveness of statin therapy for primary prevention of CHD events in type 2 diabetes was analyzed, using population estimates from NHANES III survey and results from the HPS. The estimations confirmed that statin therapy in type 2 diabetic patients with LDL-C between 2.6 and 3.39 mmol/l is affordable and costeffective relative to statin therapy for diabetic subjects with higher LDL levels [88]. A simulated health economic analysis reported that primary prevention was as cost-effective as was secondary prevention among diabetic patients [89]. These economic estimates highlight that statin therapy in diabetic patients is cost-effective and will be affordable, considering the current availability of less expensive generic compounds.

TREATMENT OF DYSLIPIDEMIAS

The top priority is to reduce LDL-C. A second priority is HDL raising and third priority is triglyceride lowering [19]. NCET-ATP III designates non-HDL lowering as a second priority [18]. A strategy to choose HDL-C over triglycerides as a second priority is scientifically justified. However, raising HDL is difficult and therefore the management of low HDL/high triglycerides goes hand in hand in clinical practice.

1. *Diabetic patients with clinical CHD, PVD, or CVD.* The current ADA guidelines advocate drug treatment at LDL-C level > 2.6 mmol/l (> 100 mg/dl) in diabetic patients with clinical CVD [19]. In post-HPS period this statement is undisputable for both type 1 and type 2 diabetic patients. Lifestyle modification should be started at the same time with pharmacological therapy. Statins are accepted to be the drug of choice.
2. *Adults with diabetes but without pre-existing CHD, PVD, and CVD, and LDL-C >3.4 mmol/l.* In diabetic patients without pre-existing CHD and LDL-C >3.4 mmol/l (>130 mg/dl) the pharmacological therapy can be instituted at the same time as lifestyle modification because effective lifestyle modification seldom reduces LDL-C more than 0.40–0.65 mmol/l (15–25 mg/dl). Statins are generally accepted as first-line treatment for these patients. A substantial number of type 2 diabetic subjects also have elevated plasma triglyceride and low HDL that remain abnormal after the statin therapy. Adding a fibrate, preferably fenofibrate or niacin is the next option to correct the lipid profile.
3. *Adults with diabetes without pre-existing CHD, DVD or CVD, and LDL-C between 2.6 and 3.4 mmol/l.* The stepwise approach starting with lifestyle modification followed by improvement of glycemic control is employed. The choice of a particular drug depends on the lipid profile achieved after 6–12 weeks of intense lifestyle modification. Figure 2 gives a proposal of drug therapy for dyslipidemia based on plasma triglyceride values in these type 2 diabetic subjects. If the major lipid abnormality is hypertriglyceridemia with triglyceride >4.5 mmol/l (>400 mg/dl), ADA suggests that strong consideration should be given to pharmacological treatment of triglycerides, the fibrates being the first choice of therapy. If HDL-C is also clearly reduced, niacin is a good option. If LDL-C is above 3.4 mmol/l in subsequent follow-up a statin or potentially exetimide should be added as a combination therapy.

In subjects with moderately elevated triglyceride levels of 2.3 mmol/l to 4.5 mmol/l the choice of therapy is dependent on the clinician's judgement. Since

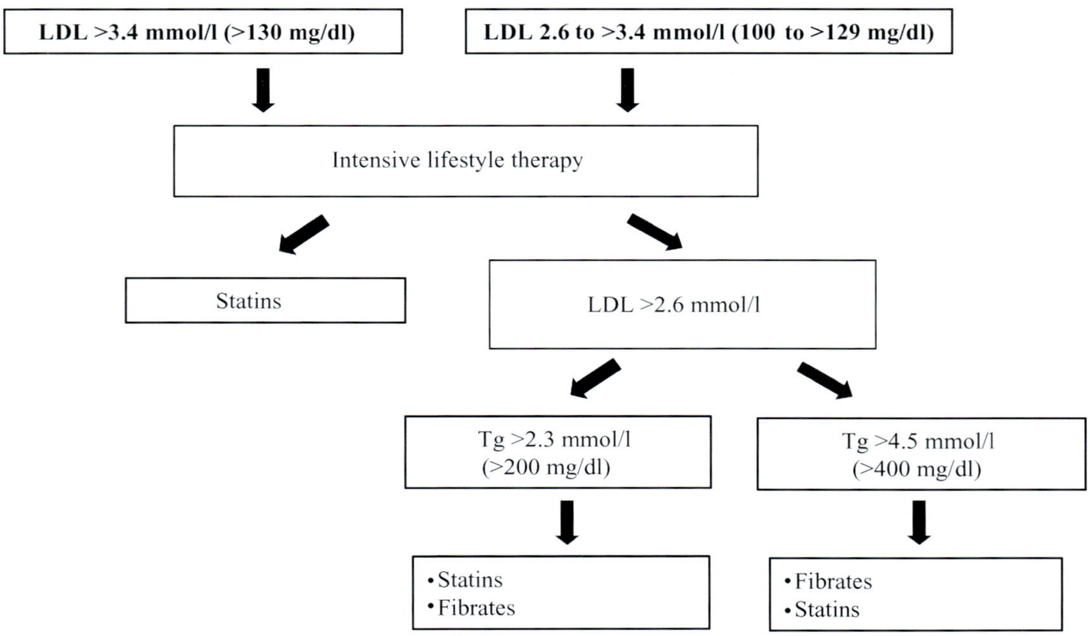

Figure 2 Management of diabetic dyslipidemia in type 2 diabetic subjects without pre-existing CHD, PVD, and CVD (Tg = triglyceride)

statins are moderately effective in lowering plasma triglycerides and raising HDL levels, a statin is a relevant first option. If elevated triglyceride and low HDL levels coexist with low LDL-C (<3.0 mmol/l) the evidence from VA-HIT and DAIS study support the use of fibrate as a first choice [72, 79].

4. *Diabetic subjects with severe hypertiglyceridemia (>11.3 mmol/l, i.e. >1000 mg/dl).* The first aim is to prevent acute pancreatitis by aggressive triglyceride lowering. The therapy includes dietary fat restriction (<10% of calories) and the initiation of fibrate. Intensive glycemic control should also be aggressively pursued. The use of omega-3 fatty acids may also be helpful [57].
5. *Adults with type 1 diabetes but without pre-existing CHD, PVD, and CVD.* Unfortunately there is a relative lack of data on lipids and CHD in type 1 diabetes. Nevertheless, type 1 diabetes is also associated with increased CHD risk, and LDL-C is a significant predictor of CHD. Therefore the treatment strategy should follow the guidelines for patients at high risk after evaluation of the global risk. In HPS the proportional risk reduction of first major vascular event was similar, although not significant, in type 1 diabetic patients as in type 2 diabetic patients [6]. In author's view type 1 diabetic patients with LDL 3.4 mmol/l should have a statin independently of HDL-C concentration.

In conclusion, the primary strategy is to achieve LDL goals but the optimum therapy should target all components of diabetic dyslipidemia.

CONCLUSIONS

Diabetic dyslipidemia represents a good target for therapeutic intervention. To date there are overwhelming data providing evidence of the ability of aggressive LDL lowering in people with diabetes to reduce the risk of CVD. There is also a good justification for a more stringent LDL target in type 2 diabetes than in nondiabetic population. In spite of the clear benefits of lipid lowering, people with diabetes are undertested and undertreated for dyslipidemia. Despite the established efficacy and good safety profile of lipid-lowering drugs there is a huge gap between guidelines and achieving the lipid targets. How to break these barriers to ensure that diabetic patients at high risk worldwide will receive the aggressive lipid management is a challenge. Strong multifaceted effort and concerted actions are needed to translate the current knowledge into routine practice worldwide. Effective intervention will be crucial to combat the wave of CVD following the epidemic of type 2 diabetes.

A multifactorial approach implies that different risk factors, also lipid factors, produce an independent reduction in relative risk and may interact in multiplicative fashion. It should be recognized that statin therapy does not wipe out the risk associated with low HDL and therefore is unlikely to reduce risk optimally. Raising HDL is a strategy gaining wide acceptance, and the complex mechanisms regulating plasma HDL are rapidly becoming elucidated. The recognition that overproduction of VLDL particles is the culprit of diabetic dyslipidemia pinpoints the regulatory steps of VLDL assembly in the liver as a primary target of therapy. Novel therapeutic strategies aimed specifically to attack the explicit components of diabetic dyslipidemia will hopefully become available in the foreseeable future and will be translated into more effective and refined treatment of all components in diabetic dyslipidemia.

REFERENCES

1. Laakso M, Lehto S. Epidemiology of macrovascular disease in diabetes. *Diabetes Rev* 1997; 5: 294–315.
2. Beckman JA, Creager MA, Libby P. Diabetes and atherosclerosis: epidemiology, pathophysiology, and management. *JAMA* 2002; 287: 2570–81.
3. Zimmet P, Shaw J, Murray S, Sicree R. The diabetes epidemic in full flight: forecasting the future. *Diabetes Voice* 2003; 48: 12–6.
4. Turner RC, Millns H, Neil HA, Stratton IM, Manley SE, Matthews DR, Holman RR. Risk factors for coronary artery disease in non-insulin dependent diabetes mellitus: United Kingdom Prospective Diabetes Study (UKPDS: 23). *BMJ* 1998; 316: 823–8.
5. Gaede P, Vedel P, Larsen N, Jensen GV, Parving HH, Pedersen O. Multifactorial intervention and cardiovascular disease in patients with type 2 diabetes. *N Engl J Med* 2003; 348: 383–93.
6. Collins R, Armitage J, Parish S, Sleigh P, Peto R, for the Heart Protection Study Collaborative Group. MRC/BHF Heart Protection Study of cholesterol-lowering with simvastatin in 5963 people with diabetes: a randomised placebo-controlled trial. *Lancet* 2003; 361: 2005–16.
7. Haffner SM. Management of dyslipidemia in adults with diabetes. *Diabetes Care* 1998; 21: 160–78.
8. Taskinen MR. Lipid disorders in diabetes. In Aldo Pinchera (ed) *Endocrinology and Metabolism. Clinical Medicine Series*, 2001; Chap 64, pp 673–84.
9. DCCT Research Group. Lipid and lipoproteins levels in patients with IDDM: Diabetes Control and Complications Trial Experience. *Diabetes Care* 1992; 15: 886–94.
10. Groop PH, Elliott T, Ekstrand A, Franssila-Kallunki A, Friedman R, Viberti GC, Taskinen MR. Multiple lipoprotein abnormalities in type I diabetic patients with renal disease. *Diabetes* 1996; 45: 974–9.
11. Idzior-Walus B, Mattock MB, Solnica B, Stevens L, Fuller JH, for the EURODIAB IDDM Complications Study Group. Factors associated with plasma lipids and lipoproteins in type 1 diabetes mellitus: the EURODIAB IDDM Complications Study. *Diabet Med* 2001; 18: 786–96.
12. Fuller JH, Stevens LK, Wang SL. Risk factors for cardiovascular mortality and morbidity: the WHO Mutinational Study of Vascular Disease in Diabetes. *Diabetologia* 2001; 44 (suppl 2): S54–64.

13. Orchard TJ, Forrest KY, Kuller LH, Becker DJ, for the Pittsburgh Epidemiology of Diabetes Complications Study. Lipid and blood pressure treatment goals for type 1 diabetes: 10-year incidence data from the Pittsburgh Epidemiology of Diabetes Complications Study. *Diabetes Care* 2001; 24: 1053–9.
14. Chaturvedi N, Fuller JH, Taskinen MR, for the EURODIAB PCS Group. Differing associations of lipid and lipoprotein disturbances with the macrovascular and microvascular complications of type 1 diabetes. *Diabetes Care* 2001; 24: 2071–77.
15. Taskinen MR. Diabetic dyslipidaemia: from basic research to clinical practice. *Diabetologia* 2003; 46: 733–49.
16. Harris MI. Health care and health status and outcomes for patients with type 2 diabetes. *Diabetes Care* 2000; 23: 754–8.
17. Report of a Round Table Discussion held during the American Diabetes Association, Philadelphia, 27 June 2001. Dyslipidaemia in type 2 diabetes: a panel discussion. *Pract Diabetes Int* 2002; 19: S1–6.
18. Expert Panel on Detection, Evaluation, and Treatment of High Blood Cholesterol in Adults. Executive Summary of The Third Report of The National Cholesterol Education Program (NCEP) Expert Panel on Detection, Evaluation, And Treatment of High Blood Cholesterol In Adults (Adult Treatment Panel III). *JAMA* 2001; 285: 2486–97.
19. Haffner SM, for the American Diabetes Association. Management of dyslipidemia in adults with diabetes. *Diabetes Care* 2003; 26 (suppl 1): S83–6.
20. Miettinen H, Lehto S, Salomaa V, Mahonen M, Niemela M, Haffner SM, Pyorala K, Tuomilehto J, for the FINMONICA Myocardial Infarction Register Study Group. Impact of diabetes on mortality after the first myocardial infarction. *Diabetes Care* 1998; 21: 69–75.
21. Kjaergaard SC, Hansen HH, Fog L, Bulow I, Christensen PD. In-hospital outcome for diabetic patients with acute myocardial infarction in the thrombolytic era. *Scand Cardiovasc J* 1999; 33: 166–70.
22. Haffner SM, Lehto S, Ronnemaa T, Pyorala K, Laakso M. Mortality from coronary heart disease in subjects with type 2 diabetes and in nondiabetic subjects with and without prior myocardial infarction. *N Engl J Med* 1998; 339: 229–34.
23. Mukamal KJ, Nesto RW, Cohen MC, Muller JE, Maclure M, Sherwood JB, Mittleman MA. Impact of diabetes on long-term survival after acute myocardial infarction: comparability of risk with prior myocardial infarction. *Diabetes Care* 2001; 24: 1422–7.
24. Malmberg K, Yusuf S, Gerstein HC, Brown J, Zhao F, Hunt D, Piegas L, Calvin J, Keltai M, Budaj A. Impact of diabetes on long-term prognosis in patients with unstable angina and non-Q-wave myocardial infarction: results of the OASIS (Organization to Assess Strategies for Ischemic Syndromes) Registry. *Circulation* 2000; 102: 1014–9.
25. Evans JM, Wang J, Morris AD. Comparison of cardiovascular risk between patients with type 2 diabetes and those who had had a myocardial infarction: cross sectional and cohort studies. *BMJ* 2002; 324: 939–42.
26. Game FL, Jones AF. Coronary heart disease risk assessment in diabetes mellitus—a comparison of PROCAM and Framingham risk assessment functions. *Diabet Med* 2001; 18: 355–9.
27. Hsia SH. Non-HDL cholesterol: into the spotlight. *Diabetes Care* 2003; 26: 240–2.
28. Lu W, Resnick HE, Jablonski KA, Jones KL, Jain AK, Howard WJ, Robbins DC, Howard BV. Non-HDL cholesterol: as a predictor of cardiovascular disease in type 2 diabetes: the strong heart study. *Diabetes Care* 2003; 26: 16–23.
29. American Diabetes Association. Evidence-based nutrition principles and recommendations for the treatment and prevention of diabetes and related complications. *Diabetes Care* 2003; 26: S51–61.
30. American Diabetes Association. Diabetes mellitus and exercise. *Diabetes Care* 2001; 24: S51–55.
31. Thompson PD, Buchner D, Pina IL, Balady GJ, Williams MA, Marcus BH, Berra K, Blair SN, Costa F, Franklin B, Fletcher GF, Gordon NF, Pate RR, Rodriguez BL, Yancey AK, Wenger NK, for the American Heart Association Council on Clinical Cardiology Subcommittee on Exercise, Rehabilitation, and Prevention., American Heart Association Council on Nutrition, Physical Activity, and Metabolism Subcommittee on Physical Activity. Exercise and physical activity in the prevention and treatment of atherosclerotic cardiovascular disease: a statement from the Council on Clinical Cardiology (Subcommittee on Exercise, Rehabilitation, and Prevention) and the Council on Nutrition, Physical Activity, and Metabolism (Subcommittee on Physical Activity). *Circulation* 2003; 107: 3109–16.
32. Hu FB, Willett WC. Optimal diets for prevention of coronary heart disease. *JAMA* 2002; 288: 2569–78.
33. Rockhill B, Willett WC, Manson JE, Leitzmann MF, Stampfer MJ, Hunter DJ, Colditz GA. Physical activity and mortality: a prospective study among women. *Am J Public Health* 2001; 91: 578–83.
34. Tanasescu M, Leitzmann MF, Rimm EB, Hu FB. Physical activity in relation to cardiovascular disease and total mortality among men with type 2 diabetes. *Circulation* 2003; 107: 2435–9.
35. Hu FB, Stampfer MJ, Solomon C, Liu S, Colditz GA, Speizer FE, Willett WC, Manson JE. Physical activity and risk for cardiovascular events in diabetic women. *Ann Intern Med* 2001; 134: 96–105.
36. Laakso M. Hyperglycemia and cardiovascular disease in type 2 diabetes. *Diabetes* 1999; 48: 937–42.
37. Laakso M. Cardiovascular disease in type 2 diabetes: challenge for treatment and prevention. *J Intern Med* 2001; 249: 225–35.
38. UK Prospective Diabetes Study (UKPDS) Group. Intensive blood-glucose control with sulphonylureas or insulin compared with conventional treatment and risk of complications in patients with type 2 diabetes (UKPDS 33). *Lancet* 1998; 352: 837–53.
39. Stratton IM, Adler AI, Neil HA, Matthews DR, Manley SE, Cull CA, Hadden D, Turner RC, Holman RR. Association of glycaemia with macrovascular and microvascular complications of type 2 diabetes (UKPDS 35): prospective observational study. *BMJ* 2000; 321: 405–12.
40. Taskinen MR. Controlling lipid levels in diabetes. *Acta Diabetol* 2002; 39 (suppl 2): S29–34.
41. Mudaliar S, Henry RR. PPAR agonists in health and disease: a pathophysiological and clinical overview. *Curr Opin Endocrinol Diabetes* 2002; 9: 285–302.
42. Forster LF, Stewart G, Bedford D, Stewart JP, Rogers E, Shepherd J, Packard CJ, Caslake MJ. Influence of atorvastatin and simvastatin on apolipoprotein B metabolism in moderate combined hyperlipidemic subjects with low

VLDL and LDL fractional clearance rates. *Atherosclerosis* 2002; 164: 129–45.

43. Watts GF, Barrett PH, Ji J, Serone AP, Chan DC, Croft KD, Loehrer F, Johnson AG. Differential regulation of lipoprotein kinetics by atorvastatin and fenofibrate in subjects with the metabolic syndrome. *Diabetes* 2003; 52: 803–11.
44. Stein EA, Lane M, Laskarzewski P. Comparison of statins in hypertriglyceridemia. *Am J Cardiol* 1998; 81: 66B–69B.
45. Fruchart JC, Duriez P, Staels B. Peroxisome proliferator-activated receptor-alpha activators regulate genes governing lipoprotein metabolism, vascular inflammation and atherosclerosis. *Curr Opin Lipidol* 1999; 10: 245–57.
46. Barbier O, Torra IP, Duguay Y, Blanquart C, Fruchart JC, Glineur C, Staels B. Pleiotropic actions of peroxisome proliferator-activated receptors in lipid metabolism and atherosclerosis. *Arterioscler Thromb Vasc Biol* 2002; 22: 717–26.
47. Kamanna VS, Kashyap ML. Mechanism of action of niacin on lipoprotein metabolism. *Curr Atheroscler Rep* 2000; 2: 36–46.
48. Elam MB, Hunninghake DB, Davis KB, Garg R, Johnson C, Egan D, Kostis JB, Sheps DS, Brinton EA. Effect of niacin on lipid and lipoprotein levels and glycemic control in patients with diabetes and peripheral arterial disease: the ADMIT study: A randomized trial. Arterial Disease Multiple Intervention Trial. *JAMA* 2000; 284: 1263–70.
49. Pan J, Lin M, Kesala RL, Van J, Charles MA. Niacin treatment of the atherogenic lipid profile and Lp(a) in diabetes. *Diabetes Obes Metab* 2002; 4: 255–61.
50. Guyton JR, Blazing MA, Hagar J, Kashyap ML, Knopp RH, McKenney JM, Nash DT, Nash SD, for the Niaspan-Gemfibrozil Study Group. Extended-release niacin vs. gemfibrozil for the treatment of low levels of high-density lipoprotein cholesterol. *Arch Intern Med* 2000; 160: 1177–84.
51. Grundy SM, Vega GL, McGovern ME, Tulloch BR, Kendall DM, Fitz-Patrick D, Ganda OP, Rosenson RS, Buse JB, Robertson DD, Sheehan JP, for the Diabetes Multicenter Research Group. Efficacy, safety, and tolerability of once-daily niacin for the treatment of dyslipidemia associated with type 2 diabetes: results of the assessment of diabetes control and evaluation of the efficacy of niaspan trial. *Arch Intern Med* 2002; 162: 1568–76.
52. Davidson MH. Combination lipid-lowering therapy in diabetes. *Curr Diabetes Rep* 2003; 3: 263–8.
53. Prueksaritanont T, Zhao JJ, Ma B, Roadcap BA, Tang C, Qiu Y, Liu L, Lin JH, Pearson PG, Baillie TA. Mechanistic studies on metabolic interactions between gemfibrozil and statins. *J Pharmacol Exp Ther* 2002; 301: 1042–51.
54. Frost RJ, Otto C, Geiss HC, Schwandt P, Parhofer KG. Effects of atorvastatin versus fenofibrate on lipoprotein profiles, low-density lipoprotein subfraction distribution, and hemorheologic parameters in type 2 diabetes mellitus with mixed hyperlipoproteinemia. *Am J Cardiol* 2001; 87: 44–8.
55. Athyros VG, Papageorgiou AA, Athyrou VV, Demitriadis DS, Kontopoulos AG. Atorvastatin and micronized fenofibrate alone and in combination in type 2 diabetes with combined hyperlipidemia. *Diabetes Care* 2002; 25: 1198–202.
56. Vega GL, Ma PT, Cater NB, Filipchuk N, Meguro S, Garcia-Garcia AB, Grundy SM. Effects of adding fenofibrate (200 mg/day) to simvastatin (10 mg/day) in patients with combined hyperlipidemia and metabolic syndrome. *Am J Cardiol* 2003; 91: 956–60.
57. Weber P, Raederstorff D, Triglyceride-lowering effect of omega-3 LC-polyunsaturated fatty acids—a review. *Nutr Metab Cardiovasc Dis* 2000; 10: 28–37.
58. Xydakis AM, Ballantyne CM. Combination therapy for combined dyslipidemia. *Am J Cardiol* 2002; 90: 21K–29K.
59. Brown BG, Zhao XQ, Chait A, Fisher LD, Cheung MC, Morse JS, Dowdy AA, Marino EK, Bolson EL, Alaupovic P, Frohlich J, Albers JJ. Simvastatin and niacin, antioxidant vitamins, or the combination for the prevention of coronary disease. *N Engl J Med* 2001; 345: 1583–92.
60. Ballantyne CM, Houri J, Notarbartolo A, Melani L, Lipka LJ, Suresh R, Sun S, LeBeaut AP, Sager PT, Veltri EP, for the Ezetimibe Study Group. Effect of ezetimibe coadministered with atorvastatin in 628 patients with primary hypercholesterolemia: a prospective, randomized, double-blind trial. *Circulation* 2003; 107: 2409–15.
61. Bruckert E, Giral P, Tellier P. Perspectives in cholesterol-lowering therapy: the role of ezetimibe, a new selective inhibitor of intestinal cholesterol absorption. *Circulation* 2003; 107: 3124–8.
62. Randomised trial of cholesterol lowering in 4444 patients with coronary heart disease: the Scandinavian Simvastatin Survival Study (4S). *Lancet* 1994; 344: 1383–9.
63. Sacks FM, Pfeffer MA, Moye LA, Rouleau JL, Rutherford JD, Cole TG, Brown L, Warnica JW, Arnold JM, Wun CC, Davis BR, Braunwald E, for the Cholesterol and Recurrent Events Trial Investigators. The effect of pravastatin on coronary events after myocardial infarction in patients with average cholesterol levels. *N Engl J Med* 1996; 335: 1001–9.
64. The Long-Term Intervention with Pravastatin in Ischaemic Disease (LIPID) Study Group. Prevention of cardiovascular events and death with pravastatin in patients with coronary heart disease and a broad range of initial cholesterol levels. *N Engl J Med* 1998; 339: 1349–57.
65. Pyorala K, Pedersen TR, Kjekshus J, Faergeman O, Olsson AG, Thorgeirsson G. Cholesterol lowering with simvastatin improves prognosis of diabetic patients with coronary heart disease. A subgroup analysis of the Scandinavian Simvastatin Survival Study (4S). *Diabetes Care* 1997; 20: 614–20.
66. Haffner SM, Alexander CM, Cook TJ, Boccuzzi SJ, Musliner TA, Pedersen TR, Kjekshus J, Pyorala K. Reduced coronary events in simvastatin-treated patients with coronary heart disease and diabetes or impaired fasting glucose levels: subgroup analyses in the Scandinavian Simvastatin Survival Study. *Arch Intern Med* 1999; 159: 2661–7.
67. Goldberg RB, Mellies MJ, Sacks FM, Moye LA, Howard BV, Howard WJ, Davis BR, Cole TG, Pfeffer MA, Braunwald E, for the Care Investigators. Cardiovascular events and their reduction with pravastatin in diabetic and glucose-intolerant myocardial infarction survivors with average cholesterol levels: subgroup analyses in the cholesterol and recurrent events (CARE) trial. *Circulation* 1998; 98: 2513–9.
68. Sacks FM, Tonkin AM, Shepherd J, Braunwald E, Cobbe S, Hawkins CM, Keech A, Packard C, Simes J, Byington R, Furberg CD. Effect of pravastatin on coronary disease events in subgroups defined by coronary risk

factors: the Prospective Pravastatin Pooling Project. *Circulation* 2000; 102: 1893–900.

69. Sacks FM, Tonkin AM, Craven T, Pfeffer MA, Shepherd J, Keech A, Furberg CD, Braunwald E. Coronary heart disease in patients with low LDL-cholesterol: benefit of pravastatin in diabetics and enhanced role for HDL-cholesterol and triglycerides as risk factors. *Circulation* 2002; 105: 1424–8.
70. Armitage J, Collins R. Need for large scale randomised evidence about lowering LDL cholesterol in people with diabetes mellitus: MRC/BHF heart protection study and other major trials. *Heart* 2000; 84: 357–60.
71. UK Prospective Diabetes Study Group. Plasma lipids and lipoproteins at diagnosis of NIDDM by age and sex. *Diabetes Care* 1997; 20: 1683–7.
72. Effect of fenofibrate on progression of coronary-artery disease in type 2 diabetes: the Diabetes Atherosclerosis Intervention Study, a randomised study. *Lancet* 2001; 357: 905–10.
73. ALLHAT Officers and Coordinators for the ALLHAT Collaborative Research Group. The Antihypertensive and Lipid-Lowering Treatment to Prevent Heart Attack Trial. Major outcomes in moderately hypercholesterolemic, hypertensive patients randomized to pravastatin vs. usual care. *JAMA* 2002; 288: 2998–3007.
74. Sever PS, Dahlof B, Poulter NR, Wedel H, Beevers G, Caulfield M, Collins R, Kjeldsen SE, Kristinsson A, McInnes GT, Mehlsen J, Nieminen M, O'Brien E, Ostergren J, ASCOT investigators. Prevention of coronary and stroke events with atorvastatin in hypertensive patients who have average or lower-than-average cholesterol concentrations, in the Anglo-Scandinavian Cardiac Outcomes Trial—Lipid Lowering Arm (ASCOT-LLA): a multicentre randomised controlled trial. *Lancet* 2003; 361: 1149–58.
75. Downs JR, Clearfield M, Weis S, Whitney E, Shapiro DR, Beere PA, Langendorfer A, Stein EA, Kruyer W, Gotto A Jr, for the AFCAPS/TexCAPS Research Group. Primary prevention of acute coronary events with Lovastanin in men and women with average cholesterol levels: results of AFCAPS/TexCAPS. *JAMA* 1998; 279: 1613–22.
76. Lindholm LH. Major benefits from cholesterol-lowering in patients with diabetes. *Lancet* 2003; 361: 2000–1.
77. Koskinen P, Manttari M, Manninen V, Huttunen JK, Heinonen OP, Frick MH. Coronary heart disease incidence in NIDDM patients in the Helsinki Heart Study. *Diabetes Care* 1992; 15: 820–5.
78. Rubins HB, Robins SJ, Collins D, Fye CL, Anderson JW, Elam MB, Faas FH, Linares E, Schaefer EJ, Schectman G, Wilt TJ, Wittes J, for the Veterans Affairs High-Density Lipoprotein Cholesterol Intervention Trial Study Group. Gemfibrozil for the secondary prevention of coronary heart disease in men with low levels of high-density lipoprotein cholesterol. *N Engl J Med* 1999; 341: 410–8.
79. Rubins HB, Robins SJ, Collins D, Nelson DB, Elam MB, Schaefer EJ, Faas FH, Anderson JW. Diabetes, plasma insulin, and cardiovascular disease: subgroup analysis from the Department of Veterans Affairs high-density lipoprotein intervention trial (VA-HIT). *Arch Intern Med* 2002; 162: 2597–604.
80. Robins SJ. Fibrates and coronary heart disease reduction in diabetes. *Curr Opin Endocrinol Diabetes* 2002; 9: 312–21.
81. Robins SJ, Rubins HB, Faas FH, Schaefer EJ, Elam MB, Anderson JW, Collins D. Insulin resistance and cardiovascular events with low HDL-C: the Veterans Affairs HDL Intervention Trial (VA-HIT). *Diabetes Care* 2003; 26: 1513–7.
82. Massing MW, Henley NS, Carter-Edwards L, Schenck AP, Simpson RJ Jr. Lipid testing among patients with diabetes who receive diabetes care from primary care physicians. *Diabetes Care* 2003; 26: 1369–73.
83. Massing MW, Foley KA, Sueta CA, Chowdhury M, Biggs DP, Alexander CM, Simpson RJ Jr. Trends in lipid management among patients with coronary artery disease: has diabetes received the attention it deserves? *Diabetes Care* 2003; 26: 991–7.
84. McFarlane SI, Jacober SJ, Winer N, Kaur J, Castro JP, Wui MA, Gliwa A, Von Gizycki H, Sowers JR. Control of cardiovascular risk factors in patients with diabetes and hypertension at urban academic medical centers. *Diabetes Care* 2002; 25: 718–23.
85. Grant RW, Cagliero E, Murphy-Sheehy P, Singer DE, Nathan DM, Meigs JB. Comparison of hyperglycemia, hypertension, and hypercholesterolemia management in patients with type 2 diabetes. *Am J Med* 2002; 112: 603–9.
86. Herman WH, Alexander CM, Cook JR, Boccuzzi SJ, Musliner TA, Pedersen TR, Kjekshus J, Pyorala K. Effect of simvastatin treatment on cardiovascular resource utilization in impaired fasting glucose and diabetes. Findings from the Scandinavian Simvastatin Survival Study. *Diabetes Care* 1999; 22: 1771–8.
87. Jonsson B, Cook JR, Pedersen TR. The cost-effectiveness of lipid lowering in patients with diabetes: results from the 4S trial. *Diabetologia* 1999; 42: 1293–301.
88. Brandle M, Davidson MB, Schriger DL, Lorber B, Herman WH. Cost effectiveness of statin therapy for the primary prevention of major coronary events in individuals with type 2 diabetes. *Diabetes Care* 2003; 26: 1796–801.
89. Grover SA, Coupal L, Zowall H, Alexander CM, Weiss TW, Gomes DR. How cost-effective is the treatment of dyslipidemia in patients with diabetes but without cardiovascular disease? *Diabetes Care* 2001; 24: 45–50.

53

Effective Insulin Therapy

Richard M. Bergenstal

International Diabetes Center, Park Nicollet Institute, Minneapolis, MN, USA

INTRODUCTION

Worldwide the incidence of diabetes is reaching epidemic proportions. In addition to focusing on ways to prevent diabetes the health care community must determine and then implement the most effective management strategies that will prevent an epidemic of *uncontrolled* diabetes. It is uncontrolled diabetes that results in devastating physical, psychological, and financial burdens [1]. Diabetes is the sixth leading cause of death in the United States. One third of individuals with diabetes are depressed during their lifetime, and treatment of diabetes and its complications and time lost from productive work costs $132 billion per year in the United States [2].

The rate of uncontrolled diabetes in the population can only be determined once there is agreement what constitutes controlled diabetes. The HbA_{1c} most often defines overall glucose control. Several leading diabetes organizations suggest different goals for the HbA_{1c} [3]. For instance, the American Diabetes Association suggests that the goal HbA_{1c} is <7%, and the American Association of Clinical Endocrinologists and the European International Diabetes Federation suggest an HbA_{1c} goal of <6.5%. Others suggest the goal should be an HbA_{1c} as close to normal as possible while avoiding serious or frequent hypoglycemia. Conflicting goals from respected organizations usually mean we do not have definitive evidence that points to one ideal HbA_{1c} value or we do not have the necessary tools that allow us to safely achieve normoglycemia, which no one would argue is ideal if it were feasible. Target ranges for self-monitored blood glucose (SMBG) values constitute an additional glycemic measure of controlled vs. uncontrolled diabetes. There is even less consensus around targets for fasting, premeal, and postmeal SMBG values. It is important for clinicians to have enough working knowledge of how SMBG values correlate with HbA_{1c} readings in order to be able to establish SMBG targets for each of his or her patients since these are the data that individuals educated in diabetes self-management principles will use on a regular basis to fine-tune their meal plan, exercise, or medications. It has been said that educated individuals with diabetes do 99% of their own management and health care professionals merely coach them and support them a few times a year [4, 5, 6, 7, 8]. We are just beginning to define appropriate premeal and postmeal glucose targets and the percentage of values needed to be in a target range in order to achieve the desired HbA_{1c} level. There are organizations suggesting premeal SMBG targets of 80–140 mg/dl (4.4–7.8 mmol/l) and postmeal (usually defined as 2 h after start of a meal, or as the peak value postmeal) SMBG targets of 140–180 mg/dl (7.8–10.0 mmol/l). Another approach to deciding on a postprandial glucose target is to teach that the glucose should not go up more that 40 mg/dl (2.2 mmol/l) after meals [9]. A very helpful clinical tip is that if the patient is able to obtain approximately 50% of their SMBG values in the predetermined target range, this will consistently result in the corresponding target HbA_{1c} value. This has been taught at the International Diabetes Center (IDC) after analyzing data from their DCCT (Diabetes Control and Complications Trial) patients and from a group of intensively treated type 2 diabetic patients. If 50% of premeal glucose values were between 70 and 140 mg/dl (3.9–7.8 mmol/l), this consistently resulted in an HbA_{1c} of 7% [10]. Brewer et al. also found that approximately 50% of SMBG values in the target range resulted in the target HbA_{1c} value in individuals with type 1 diabetes [11]. When reviewing a patient's glucose values (written logbook data or downloaded meter memory data) the clinician or educator who has a realistic expectation

International Textbook of Diabetes Mellitus, Third Edition. Edited by R. A. DeFronzo, E. Ferrannini, H. Keen, and P. Zimmet.
 ISBN: 0-471-48655-8.

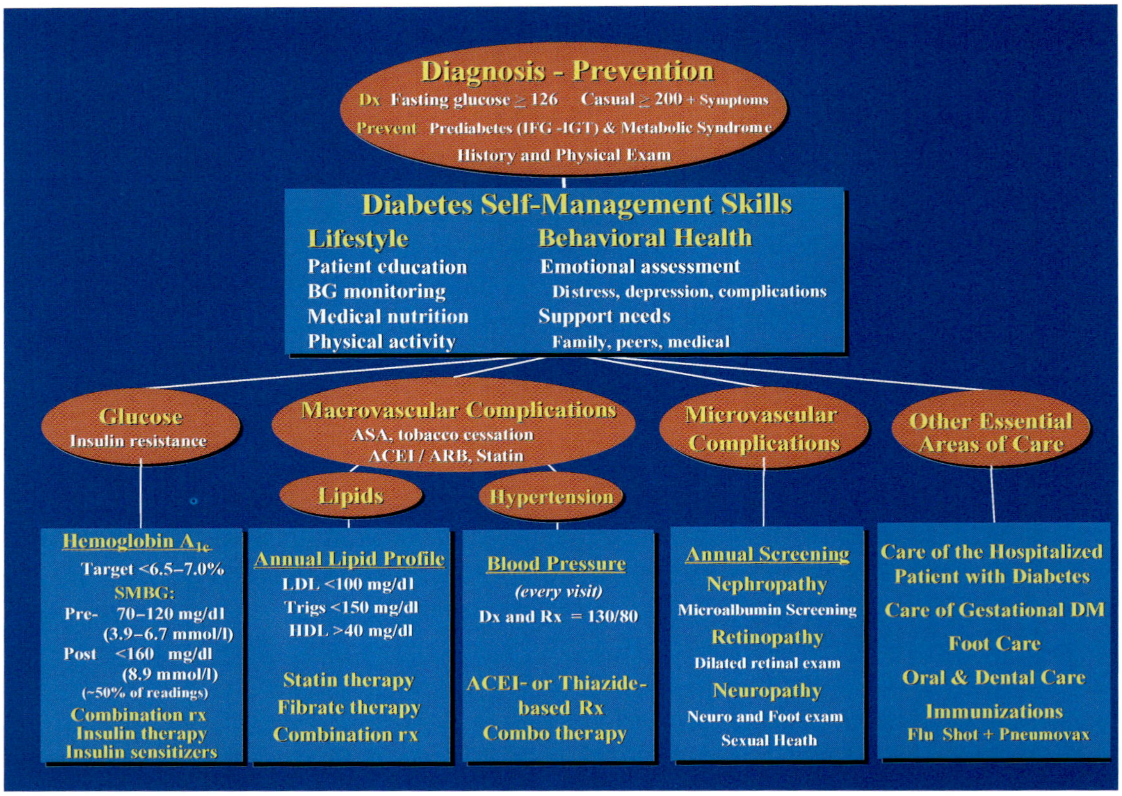

Figure 1 Priorities of care for adults with diabetes. (Reproduced by permission of the International Diabetes Center. © 2003 International Diabetes Center, Minneapolis, USA)

of the percentage to be within the target range will communicate more effectively and empathetically with his or her patients.

Control of diabetes is no longer defined only by the level of glycemic control (HbA_{1c} and SMBG values) but now has appropriately been expanded to include the psychosocial, metabolic, clinical, and therapeutic parameters as outlined in the summary of the priorities of care for adults with type 2 diabetes from the IDC (Figure 1). This figure and corresponding clinical trials [12, 13, 14] and modeling studies [15] demonstrate that effective management of diabetes utilizing a multifactorial approach, including achieving aggressive targets for glycemic, blood pressure, and lipid control as well as screening regularly for microvascular and macrovascular complications and providing education, behavioral health support, and proven preventive therapies, will reduce the complications associated with diabetes.

Studies that have evaluated how well we are achieving the accepted diabetes standards of care make it clear that more effective therapies or more uniform implementation of therapies known to be effective are definitely required. For instance, Saaddine in an article entitled "A Diabetes Report Card" reveals that 18% of patients with diabetes in the United States had an $HbA_{1c} > 9.5\%$, only 43% had an $HbA_{1c} < 7\%$, 34% had a BP > 140/90 mmHg (this number may be twice as large if the currently accepted standard for BP control of 130/80 mmHg were used), and 89% reported an LDL (low-density lipoprotein) level above the target level of 100 mg/dl [16].

Alarming is the fact that patients treated with insulin have uniformly poorer glycemic control compared to those treated with other therapies. Insulin, which is widely accepted to be the most potent glucose-lowering agent, with hypoglycemia being the only major dose-limiting factor, unlike all oral agents that have a limited maximum action, has progressively more side effects as the dose is increased. In order to establish better glycemia control it may be important to move insulin further up in the treatment algorithm of type 2 diabetes or help clinicians move their patients down the treatment algorithm to insulin therapy more quickly if they are not reaching agreed-upon glycemic targets.

Is prescribing insulin earlier or utilizing insulin more often really the answer to establishing better glycemic control in type 2 diabetes? If so, why did Saaddine's report show that overall 18% of individuals with diabetes had an $HbA_{1c} > 9.5\%$ (the value that all practitioners and quality-measurement organizations agreed represents very poor glycemic control) but 24% of those treated with insulin had an HbA_{1c} >9.5%? The most common explanation for a higher HbA_{1c} in patients on insulin is that insulin is usually started very late in the natural history of type 2 diabetes and only when the HbA_{1c} is very high. Yet, the United Kingdom Prospective Diabetes Study (UKPDS) randomized one group of newly diagnosed type 2 diabetic patients to insulin therapy, but did not achieve glucose control better than that noted in patients randomized to oral agents [17]. Also those randomized to insulin in the UKPDS saw a gradual deterioration in glycemic control that mirrored what was seen for study participants on oral agents. In addition to earlier and more frequent use of insulin in type 2 diabetes, it is essential that the practitioner, educator, parent, and/or individual with diabetes continually adjust the insulin dose or regimen in a systematic manner in order to optimize glycemic control.

How does one optimize the use of insulin therapy in order to achieve ideal glycemic control while minimizing hypoglycemia and maintaining a flexible and quality life?

Several recent reviews of insulin therapy have been published, some historical, some clinical, and others suggesting the next paradigm of insulin therapy [18–27]. Any successful implementation of insulin therapy must include consideration of the many of the following elements of type 1 and type 2 diabetes management.

In *type 1 diabetes* optimal use of insulin therapy will routinely require a well-educated patient (and family), participating actively in his or her own insulin, food, and activity adjustments, and using an advanced insulin regimen (basal–bolus). The patient must have access to a diabetes team, and have adequate finances or insurance coverage to utilize the newest insulin preparations (analogues), insulin delivery devices (pens, pumps), and glucose monitoring technology (meters, continuous glucose monitors) when required.

In *type 2 diabetes* optimal use of insulin therapy will require most of the items outlined for an individual with type 1 diabetes plus an understanding on the clinician's part of how to use insulin in someone with insulin resistance. Many real and perceived barriers to insulin initiation and intensification in type 2 diabetes must be overcome. In most of the world, up to 90% of people with diabetes are managed by primary care providers (physicians, nurse practitioners, and physician assistants). Therefore to optimize the use of insulin, on a population basis, effective patient and professional education programs and systematic evidence-based management strategies that enable primary care providers and their patients to be successful with insulin therapy must be developed and implemented [27]. Some strategies such as disease management programs and paying physicians, medical clinics, or even patients for successful performance (pay for performance) are being studied [28–30].

Optimizing insulin therapy starts with an understanding of:

- The types of insulin
- Insulin time action curves
- Rationale for selecting an insulin regimen
  - Basic insulin regimen (initial, simplified, usually one to two injections and most often basal or premixed insulin)
  - Advanced insulin regimen (intensive, multidose, flexible, functional, physiologic, or basal–bolus)

TYPES OF INSULIN

Table 1 shows the available (and in late trials) insulin preparations. They are grouped according to when they provide insulin coverage: either mealtime (bolus) insulin, or background (basal) insulin. In this table the insulins in italic are *insulin analogues*. An insulin analogue has an alteration in the amino acid sequence of human insulin, that changes the rate of insulin absorption, or some other structural change like being linked to a fatty acid chain, that alters the insulin time action curve [31].

Figure 2 demonstrates how regular insulin is modified to result in the various rapid-acting insulin analogues: insulin lispro (Humalog) [Lys(B28), Pro(B29)-insulin], insulin aspart (Novolog) [Asp(B28)-insulin], and insulin glulisine (Apidra) [Lys(B3), Glu(B29)-insulin] completing clinical trials around the world.

Figure 3 demonstrates how regular insulin is modified to result in two long-acting insulin analogues: insulin glargine (Lantus) [Gly(A21), Arg(B31), Arg(B32)-insulin] currently available in many countries around the world, and insulin detemir [Lys(B29)-*N*-ε-tetradecanoyl, des-(B30)-insulin] completing clinical trials around the world.

INSULIN TIME ACTION CURVES

Analyzing the onset of action, peak action, and the duration of action is the classic way to compare the various formulations of insulin. One must be careful to discern if a table or diagram represents the plasma insulin level achieved or the biologic (glucose-lowering) time action effect. From a clinical standpoint the most important way to compare insulin compounds is to determine from insulin/glucose clamp studies and experience in clinical practice when an insulin begins having (onset), has its greatest (peak), or ends having (duration) a clinically relevant or meaningful glucose-lowering effect. Tables listing the time action of each insulin vary considerably because some tables refer to the presence of

Table 1 Insulin action times*

Insulin	Onset of action	Peak action	Duration of clinically effective action
		Mealtime (bolus) insulin	
Rapid-acting			
Lispro (*Humalog®*)			
Aspart (*Novolog®*)	5–15 min	1–2 h	4 h
Glulisine (*Aprida®*)†			
Short-acting			
Regular (Novolin®; Humulin®)	30–45 min	2–3 h	5–8 h
Regular (U500)	Similar time action as regular insulin (U100) but concentrated five fold for individuals requiring very large doses of insulin		
		Background (basal) insulin	
Intermediate-acting			
NPH or Lente	2–4 h	4–8 h	10–16 h
Prolonged intermediate-acting			
Ultralente (Humulin® U)	3–5 h	8–12 h	16–20 h
Long-acting			
Glargine (*Lantus®*)	2 h	No peak	24 h
Insulin detemir†	Clinical trials are being completed to determine insulin detemir's time action and if it best fits a prolonged intermediate or long-acting insulin		
Background/Bolus	**Onset**	**Early peak/late peak**	**Duration of clinically effective action**
		Premixed insulin‡	
Mix 75/25 with lispro	5–15 min	1–2 h/4–8 h	10–16 h
Mix 70/30 with aspart	5–15 min	1–2 h/4–8 h	10–16 h
70/30 or 50/50 with regular	30–45 min	2–3 h/4–8 h	10–16 h

Note: *Italicized insulin* represents an insulin analogue.
* Modified with permission from *Insulin BASICS*. © 2004 International Diabetes Center, Minneapolis, USA.
† Expected to be marketed in the United States in 2004.
‡ Other premixed insulin formulations are available outside the United States.

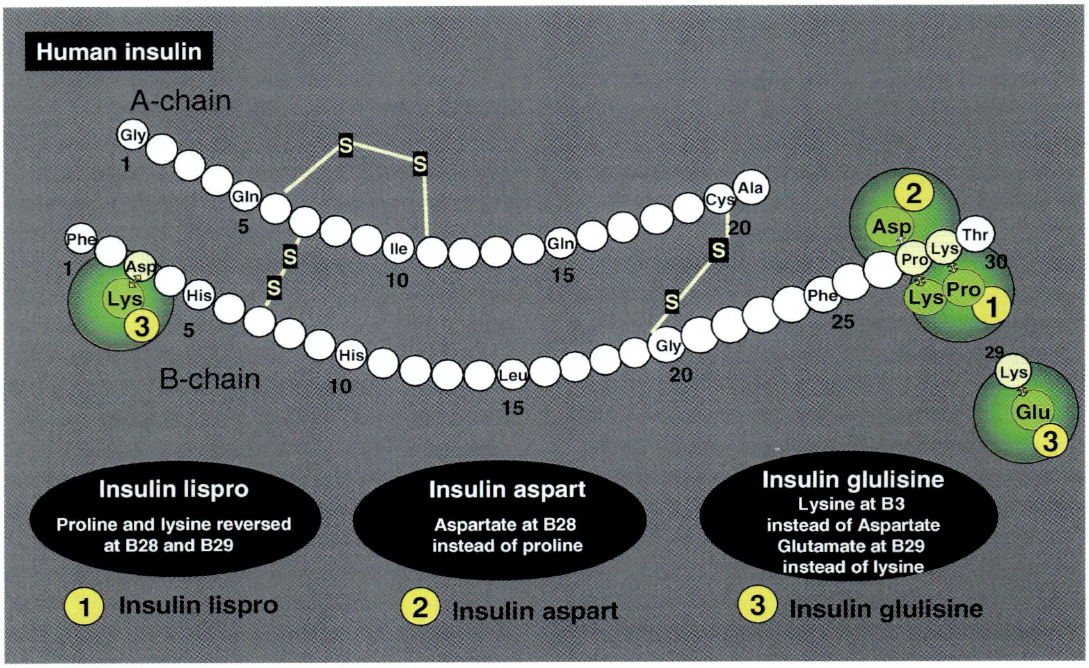

Figure 2 Rapid-acting insulin analogues: insulin lispro, insulin aspart, and insulin glulisine

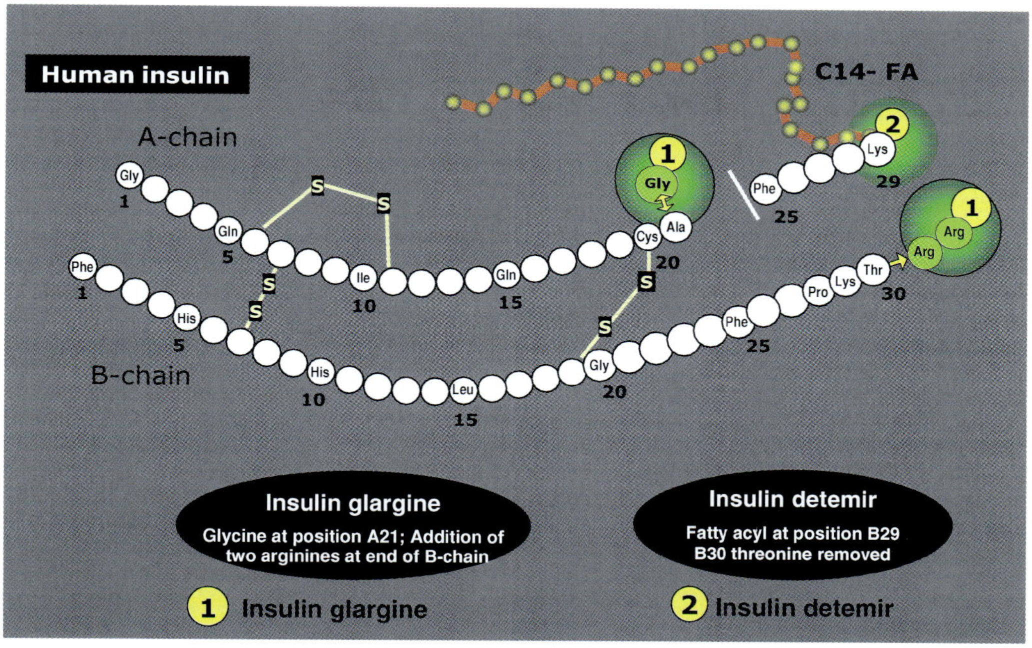

Figure 3 Long-acting insulin analogues: insulin glargine and insulin detemir

any detectable level of insulin in the plasma following an injection while others refer to any glucose-lowering effect following the injection. Perhaps the most meaningful to clinical practice is data referring to a clinically significant or clinically relevant glucose-lowering effect. Figure 4 displays glucose/insulin clamp data from a study comparing several of the insulin formulations and delivery modalities used in clinical practice today [32]. Figure 5 represents an estimate of the clinically relevant glucose-lowering time actions of the major classes of insulin in use today.

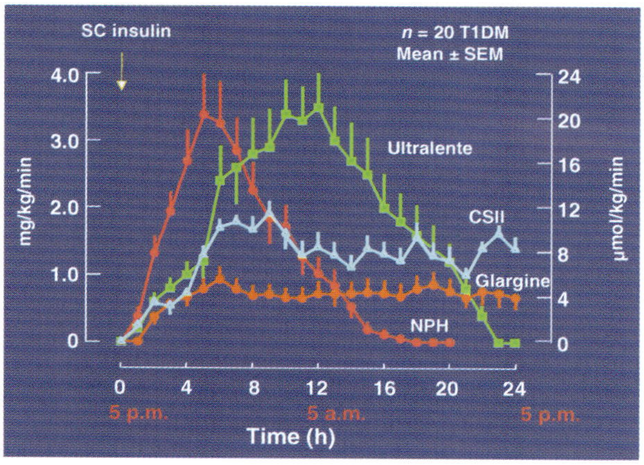

Figure 4 Pharmacodynamics of insulin in type 1 diabetes—glucose infusion rate

SELECTING THE TYPE OF INSULIN

Each group of patients has a preference for a certain insulin preparation. Practitioners need to learn some general principles about each type of insulin (rapid, short, intermediate, prolonged-intermediate, and long) to help them establish a rational approach to insulin selection and combination.

Rapid-acting Insulin

Few patients take regular or soluble insulin 30–45 min before meals as recommended in order to minimize postprandial hyperglycemia. One study demonstrated that the optimal time to take regular insulin is 58 min before a meal, which is quite impractical. Postprandial

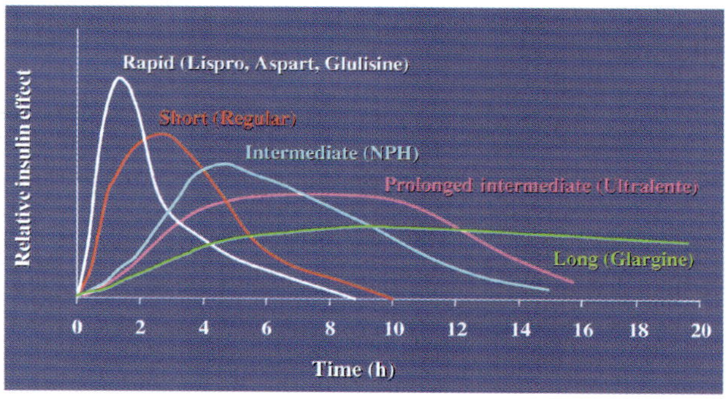

Figure 5 Insulin time action curves. (Reproduced by permission of the International Diabetes Center. © 2003 International Diabetes Center, Minneapolis, USA)

hyperglycemia can increase an HbA_{1c} level and may be linked to increased cardiovascular disease. Therefore a class of insulin that can be taken at the start of the meal and effectively target postprandial glucose control because it is absorbed rapidly from the subcutaneous tissue should be a valuable therapeutic option. When formulated for injection, regular insulin is present in solution as a hexamer. To be efficiently absorbed into the circulation the insulin hexamer must disassociate into dimers or monomers. It is the dissociation process that takes 30–60 min that determines the onset and ultimately the time action curve of regular insulin. There are two rapid-acting injectable insulins available (lispro and aspart) and a third in clinical trials (glulisine). The amino acid changes in each of the rapid-acting analogues outlined in Figure 2 results in subtle changes in the three-dimensional configuration of the insulin hexamer and an alteration in the molecular binding or association forces creating a more weakly associated or held together hexamer. Therefore, although each rapid-acting analogue still aggregates into an insulin hexamer, the analogue hexamer has a more rapid disassociation rate than does regular insulin when injected into the subcutaneous tissue. This rapid disassociation of hexamer into dimeric and monomeric insulin results in the rapid onset and peak as well as the shorter duration of action of the rapid-acting insulin analogues. The amino acid changes in all three insulin analogues have the desired and presumed beneficial result of a more rapid onset of action but are there any negative consequences of a change in structure from that of the natural human insulin molecule? To date, no adverse clinical side effects have been reported that are the result of any minimal differences these analogues may have in their antigenic or mitogenic properties compared to human insulin. The available rapid-acting insulin analogues are routinely used in pregnancy, where postprandial glycemic control is essential and often difficult to achieve with regular insulin. There have been no known adverse effects of the rapid-acting analogues on mother or baby. Compared to regular insulin the rapid-acting insulin analogues have been shown to result in better postprandial control with less hypoglycemia, particularly less nocturnal hypoglycemia. The benefit of rapid-acting insulin analogues becomes most clinically apparent when the practitioner and individual with diabetes strive for near-normal glycemia while trying to minimize hypoglycemia. Achieving an HbA_{1c} of <7% without an unacceptable amount of hypoglycemia means premeal glucose reading of approximately 120 mg/dl (6.7 mmol/l) and postmeal reading of approximately 160 mg/dl (8.9 mmol/l). A rapid-acting insulin analogue taken with a meal (preferably dose adjusted for the current glucose level and the carbohydrate content of the meal) can minimize both the postprandial glucose excursion and the potential for hypoglycemia or need for a snack between meals seen with regular insulin. Although there a few long-term trials comparing complication rates between rapid-acting analogues and regular insulin, most clinicians and patients prefer analogues for issues of ease in consistency of dosing times, better postprandial coverage, less hypoglycemia, less need for insulin between meal snacks, and a more rapid ability to correct hyperglycemia. Regular insulin, which is considerably less expensive than an insulin analogue, may be the preferred insulin if cost is the determining selection factor. In addition, in some instances patients plan to consistently snack between meals and are not willing to cover these snacks with an injection of a rapid-acting analogue and therefore may do better with broader insulin cover across the entire between-meal period that regular insulin provides. If the regular insulin is optimally adjusted to cover a meal and between-meal snacks, one must continue snacking to match the insulin or risk hypoglycemia. One can imagine this would be a formula for weight gain or at least make it difficult to lose weight as insulin doses and glycemic control are optimized.

There are a several inhaled-insulin preparations in clinical trials that utilize short-acting human regular insulin (dry powder or liquid suspension) that when delivered by pulmonary inhalation have an onset and peak action time similar to that of a rapid-acting insulin but a duration of action slightly longer than that of the currently available rapid-acting insulin analogues. There is considerable interest in inhaled-insulin technology because clinical trials have clearly shown that this mode of insulin delivery can control blood glucose levels as well as rapid- or short-acting injectable insulin preparations [33–36]. Patients are eager to try this mode of insulin delivery. Since many investigators feel that the earlier use of insulin is important for treating type 2 diabetes, it will be of great interest to see if inhaled insulin can facilitate this objective. Preliminary data from one trial showed that inhaled insulin was more effective in achieving glycemic targets than did an oral agent as first-line therapy after diet and exercise failure in subjects with type 2 diabetes [37]. Data are needed for people with type 2 diabetes to see if inhaled insulin will reduce the resistance to starting insulin on the part of both physician and patient. Studies are also needed to see if inhaled insulin results in more consistent use of what is consider the most optimal mode of insulin delivery, basal–bolus or advanced insulin management, in both type 1 and type 2 diabetes. All of these interesting clinical questions regarding the potential role of inhaled insulin must await the compounds regulatory approval that appears to be focused mainly on monitoring pulmonary function studies over an extended period of time.

Short-acting Insulin

Regular or soluble insulin that was once the fastest acting insulin available is now regarded as a short-acting insulin with a slower onset of action, later peak action, and longer duration of action than those of the rapid acting insulin analogues. Regular insulin initially was available only after extraction and purification of animal pancreases, resulting in beef, pork, or mixed beef–pork formulations. Indeed, when insulin was discovered in 1921 and became available for clinical use in 1922 regular insulin was the only formulation available. The discovery of insulin is still regarded as one of the great accomplishments in medicine. Additional medical milestones have been reached during the steady progress of purifying and refining the production process of insulin. Insulin was the first molecule produced by biosynthetic engineering, and the first molecule used for commercial development of a drug made by recombinant DNA technology. Slowly but steadily around the world, there is less access to animal insulin preparations. Regular insulin made by recombinant DNA technology is now referred to as human regular insulin because its amino acid sequence is identical to that of insulin made by the human pancreas. Human regular insulin has certainly resulted in dramatically less lipoatrophy, lipohypertrophy, and insulin allergy than previous insulin formulations. All of these side effects of injected insulin can still be found even with human insulin preparations, and patients and clinicians must be educated about how to minimize their occurrence and how to treat these side effects if they develop. There has been a debate whether human insulin results in more hypoglycemia than does animal insulin. Some investigators felt that the central nervous system recognized or responded differently to hypoglycemia induced by animal vs. human insulin. For the most part clinicians are now very comfortable using human regular insulin, which has a slightly faster onset of action and a slightly shorter duration of action than does its animal counterpart [38]. With the rapid-acting insulin analogues being considered by most clinicians more physiologic and convenient for patients the use of regular insulin is becoming relegated to situations where cost is an issue (worldwide still a very important consideration), or special circumstances such as covering snacks or in an attempt to minimize the number of insulin injections.

Intermediate-acting Insulin

The time action curve of short-acting regular insulin or a rapid-acting insulin analogue can be extended or prolonged in a variety of ways that either slow the rate of absorption from the subcutaneous tissue or slow the rate of metabolism or clearance from the circulation. If either excess zinc (lente insulin) or the protein protamine (NPH insulin, or protamine suspensions of insulin lispro or aspart) is added to short-acting regular insulin or rapid-acting insulin analogue formulations, this slows the rate of either insulin's absorption from the subcutaneous tissue into the circulation. Lente insulin has a slightly later peak action time and a longer duration of action than does NPH, but most clinicians consider then clinically interchangeable. This may be a less important distinction with the new longer acting insulins now being produced. There have been some case reports of an allergy to the protein protamine, making lente preferable when intermediate insulin was necessary. Recently some insulin manufactures have begun to discontinue the production of lente insulin.

When intermediate-acting insulin preparations were introduced there was a reduction in the frequency of multiple injections of regular insulin. Regular and NPH insulin could be mixed together in the same syringe prior to injection or could be formulated into a premixed insulin preparation. There were a few studies indicating that regular and NPH insulin when mixed together kept their separate time action curves better after injection than did a mixture of regular and lente insulin. These insulin preparations need to be taken twice daily to achieve significant insulin levels within 24 h. Evening or nighttime NPH insulin can be used to suppress hepatic glucose production overnight and normalize the fasting glucose. But NPH at night does not provide sufficient insulin to significantly cover background insulin needs far into the next day.

Prolonged-Intermediate-acting Insulin

Ultralente insulin is an extended zinc formulation of lente insulin. Ultralente has been and continues to be classified by many as long-acting insulin. Most who have used ultralente insulin extensively in clinical practice have noted that although there may be some insulin present 24 h after injection, it is not sufficient to provide adequate basal or background insulin coverage. This is particularly true of the human ultralente preparation that definitely has a shorter duration of action than does the older animal formulations of ultralente insulin. Proposed in this chapter is a new classification of ultralente insulin as a prolonged-intermediate-acting insulin as it is thought to better describe and represent ultralente's potential clinical utility. Ultralente was once a long-acting insulin if long acting is defined as the longest insulin available in practice. But if long acting is defined as usually given once a day, and having a minimal peak, it does not seem reasonable to continue classifying ultralente as long acting. Reviewing Figures 4 and 5 also makes the case for ultralente being a prolonged-intermediate-acting insulin. Ultralente insulin has an onset and peak similar to that of intermediate-acting insulin but a bit later or prolonged. Ultralente has a duration that is longer than that of intermediate (prolonged) but not as long as newer longer acting insulin preparations such as insulin glargine. Clinically it is almost always a mistake to think that ultralente insulin will consistently provide basal insulin coverage for 24 h. In most clinical practices ultralente is used either twice a day (morning and supper or in some cases morning and bedtime) or in a regimen where ultralente is given at breakfast to provide basal insulin throughout the day and evening, and NPH is given at bedtime to suppress hepatic glucose production overnight. These regimens incorporating ultralente are used less often today, with other longer acting insulin preparations available. Since insulin pump therapy has taught us that most people do not require the same basal insulin rate all day and night, there are still some situations where it is helpful to have the ability to split the basal insulin to match observed needs.

Long-acting Insulin

The only insulin available today that meets most of the characteristics of long-acting insulin is insulin glargine. One can see in Figures 4 and 5 that insulin glargine has a relatively flat insulin curve and duration close to 24 h. It is approved for use once daily, anytime of day. Initial studies and most data collected to date have been with glargine injected once daily at bedtime. But some recent studies and clinical observations from many practitioners show that there are frequently cases where control is better with once daily insulin glargine given at breakfast time. Clearly there are situations where glucose control is optimized if insulin glargine is split into two injections per day. With twice-daily injections of insulin glargine one is assured of basal coverage for 24 h without accumulation and minimal insulin peak related to the basal insulin. In most cases one starts with a single injection of insulin glargine at the time of day that is most convenient and consistent for the patient. If it appears that there is not adequate basal insulin coverage (usually determined by glucoses going up just before the next glargine injection) be sure that the problem is not lack of postprandial control that is better addressed by administering rapid-acting insulin with the meal than by splitting the insulin glargine into two injections. If postprandial glucose control is adequate but there does appear to be waning basal insulin coverage, it is appropriate to split the insulin glargine. Like every 24-h medication be it insulin of antihypertensive medications, clinical experience usually reveals that these 24-h medications all have slightly more activity over the first 12 h than over that second 12 h. Most who have had clinical experience with insulin glargine consider it a major advance in basal insulin therapy and uniformly classify it as long-acting insulin, even if on occasion it needs to be split or the clinician decides to split it in order to provide an even smoother basal profile.

Insulin glargine is created by recombinant DNA techniques, resulting in the changes in the amino acid structure of regular insulin as shown in Figure 3 and is thus called an insulin analogue. The long-acting time action curve of insulin glargine is due to the fact that insulin glargine has an isoelectric point such that in solution it has an acidic pH and when injected into the neutral pH of the subcutaneous tissue it forms microprecipitants. These microprecipitants are gradually absorbed over approximately 24 h. Insulin glargine because of its acidic pH cannot be mixed with any other insulin preparation and must be injected separately and at least a few inches away from any other insulin being injected at the same time. It is also important to note that insulin glargine is clear and not cloudy as longer acting insulins have all been to date.

The availability of long-acting basal insulin has renewed discussions and clinical trials of the most appropriate strategy for insulin initiation in both type 1 and type 2 diabetes. How early should insulin be started in type 2 diabetes and how often can insulin be initiated as a single injection of basal insulin? The clinical trials to date have shown that insulin glargine used as a basal insulin results in either less hypoglycemia for the same level of glucose control or better glucose control for the same level of hypoglycemia when compared to NPH used as a basal insulin once or twice daily. Insulin glargine is an insulin analogue and is priced higher than NPH or ultralente insulin, which may be barrier for some individuals. Studies continue on the growth-promoting effects (retinopathy studies) of insulin glargine compared to other insulin preparations. Insulin glargine like all other insulins is not approved for use in pregnancy and there is not enough data in pregnancy to make a recommendation for clinical practice at this point. Insulin glargine has been widely adopted in basal–bolus or advanced insulin regimens. Many women of childbearing age are now on an advanced insulin regimen that includes insulin glargine in order to optimize glucose control and prevent diabetes complications. Over time many of these women may become pregnant or will want to plan a pregnancy. The medical community will have to come to consensus on the safety of insulin glargine in pregnancy or be prepared to change insulin regimens for these women many of whom may have established good control for the first time. The rapid-acting insulin analogues initially faced the same dilemma but are now used regularly in pregnancy if there is an appropriate clinical indication [39].

Insulin detemir is an insulin analogue currently used in clinical trials. Attaching a fatty acyl chain at the B29 lysine amino acid of regular insulin and removing the B30 amino acid, threonine forms insulin detemir as shown in Figure 3. The insulin gets absorbed like regular insulin from the subcutaneous tissue but the fatty acyl side chain slows its metabolism and removal from the circulation, resulting in a time action curve that is longer than that of intermediate one but does not appear to be as long as insulin glargine. The initial studies appear to indicate a very consistent insulin profile that may be helpful clinically. Whether insulin detemir is eventually classified clinically as a prolonged-intermediate-acting insulin (usually requiring two injections per day and having a moderate peak) or a long-acting insulin (usually one injection per day with a minimal peak) depends on future clinical trials and clinical experience.

Premixed Insulin

Premixed insulin was developed for patient's convenience and for simplicity in ordering and dosage adjustment by the physician. Premixed insulin is available today in one of several ratios of short-acting insulin or rapid-acting insulin to intermediate-acting insulin (NPH or a protamine suspension). Some professionals consider premixed insulin a great advance because the entire day can be "covered" with just two injections. Other clinicians feel any fixed ratio of short to intermediate insulin does not allow for "fine-tuning" of each insulin component according to SMBG patterns. Some countries have only a few choices in the ratio of short to intermediate premixed insulin available (like 30/70 or 50/50) while other countries have a whole range of options in premixed insulin. Direct comparisons of premixed insulin to self-mixing and adjusting each insulin have not been done. In addition a comparison of two basic or simple insulin regimens for starting insulin in type 2 diabetes (one daily insulin glargine vs. bid premixed insulin) has not been completed.

There is enough clinical experience with premixed insulin to say that this category of insulin compounds are not appropriate for treating type 1 diabetes where frequent insulin adjustment based on pattern control and carbohydrate counting is needed to achieve optimal control in most cases. In type 2 diabetes where there appears to be great barriers to insulin initiation, the benefits of simplicity and ease of adjustment for both patient and provider may outweigh the disadvantage of the inability to fine-tune the doses. All providers and patients must learn that treating to a target HbA_{1c} of at least $<7\%$ is the goal and however insulin is started it must be advanced to more intensive or physiologic regimens if the HbA_{1c} is not at target.

Rapid-acting insulin analogues are gradually replacing regular insulin because of improved postprandial glucose control, less hypoglycemia, and more patient convenience in timing of insulin doses. For the same reasons it may be expected that premixed insulin with a rapid-acting insulin analogue (mix 75/25, mix 70/30) will replace premixed insulin with regular insulin (70/30) in most cases.

STARTING INSULIN AND SELECTING AN INSULIN REGIMEN

Type 1 Diabetes

Whether diagnosed with type 1 diabetes as a child or an adult the goal is to optimize insulin therapy to achieve near normoglycemia while minimizing significant hypoglycemia and maintaining as flexible a schedule as possible. HbA_{1c} goals may be less stringent in children with type 1 diabetes compared to adults so as to avoid severe hypoglycemia. Recent data from the Epidemiology of Diabetes Interventions and Complications (EDIC) study, which is the follow-up study to the DCCT, have shown that in type 1 diabetes there is an emerging concept of metabolic memory or imprinting [40, 41]. This implies that if glucose control is poor early in the course of diabetes the adverse effect of hyperglycemia on diabetes complications can persist for many years despite an improvement in glucose control. To date studies have been published showing a 10-year metabolic memory for the rate of development of retinopathy and nephropathy [42, 43]. One can conclude from the DCCT and EDIC studies that in type 1 diabetes it is important to establish good metabolic control as early in the course of the disease as possible and then make every effort to maintain that level of control.

There are many critical factors that need to be addressed in order to establish ideal glycemic control in type 1 diabetes. While this chapter focuses on the contribution made by optimizing insulin therapy, it is important to emphasize that most clinicians feel the best results in managing both type 1 and type 2 diabetes are obtained by ensuring a patient-centered team care approach to the disease, as outlined in Figure 6. This model involves an active involved patient, a team of educators (registered nurse (RN), registered dictitian (RD), psychologist), and a physician, all communicating effectively [44, 45]. The intersections of the overlapping circles indicate the main role of the interaction and communication between team members.

All patients with type 1 diabetes are best managed with a basal–bolus insulin regimen often referred to as intensive insulin therapy, multiple dose insulin therapy, flexible insulin therapy, or what I will call advanced insulin management. Insulin therapy in type 1 diabetes is rapidly becoming a choice between an advanced insulin regimen of insulin glargine as the basal insulin and a rapid-acting

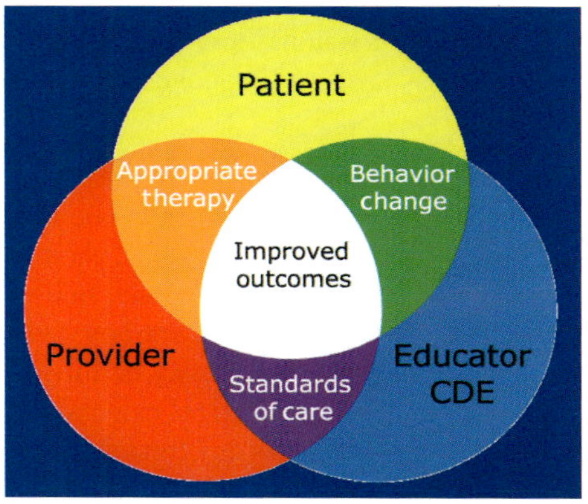

Figure 6 Patient-centered team care. (Reproduced by permission of the International Diabetes Center. © 2003 International Diabetes Center, Minneapolis, USA)

insulin analogue as the bolus insulin or the use of an external insulin pump (continuous subcutaneous insulin infusion, CSII) infusing a rapid-acting insulin analogue. (It is assumed that one can afford an insulin analogue or an insulin pump.)

General Principles of Advanced Insulin Management in Type 1 Diabetes

- Most insulin starts can be safely completed as an outpatient treatment if the patient is metabolically stable (not in diabetic ketoacidosis), has 24-h phone access to a diabetes team member, has learned SMBG and urine ketone testing, and has a glucagon emergency kit available.
- Total starting insulin dose of 0.5–0.7 units/kg; the larger amounts if ketones are present
  - 50% of the total insulin given as basal (background) insulin (insulin glargine). Start once per day in the morning or night depending on the time that is the most consistent for the patient.
  - 50% of the total insulin given as bolus (meal) insulin (rapid-acting insulin analogue) divided according to proportion of the total carbohydrates consumed at each meal.
- Management tools
  - Teach SMBG with a memory meter so that patterns can be reviewed
  - Teach how to adjust insulin for patterns of SMBG data
  - Teach carbohydrate counting
- Insulin adjustments
  - Determine an insulin-to-carbohydrate ratio (how many units of insulin are needed to cover each 15 g of carbohydrate or one carbohydrate choice)
  - Determine an insulin corrective dose schedule to correct for a high or low current glucose level (for instance one unit of insulin more (or less) for each 10–25 mg/dl (0.56–1.4 mmol/l) above (or below) glucose target
    - Using rapid-acting insulin analogue (1800/total insulin dose), determine how much one unit of supplemental insulin will lower the plasma glucose.
    - Note that recent studies by Bode, one of the international experts in insulin therapy, indicate that using 1700 in this formula may be the most accurate starting point (based on his extensive database) [46]. He emphasizes that any formula is just a starting point; further adjustments must be made based on review of food and glucose logs, looking for patterns.
  - Determine how to adjust (usually reduce insulin) for completed or anticipated exercise.

When Should a Patient with Type 1 Diabetes Consider an Insulin Pump?

- Implement a basal–bolus insulin injection regimen first and teach the principles of advanced insulin management; then the transition to a pump is straightforward and all the patient has to focus on are the pump mechanics.
- Consider a pump if maximal flexibility is needed owing to an erratic schedule
- Consider a pump if one basal rate from injected insulin glargine is not adequate
- Consider a pump if patient works shifts or frequently travels internationally
- Consider a pump if patient prefers pump boluses to multiple-daily insulin injections
- Consider a pump for optimal control during pregnancy (particularly if low glucoses overnight)
- Consider a pump if there is a need to reduce basal insulin rates for exercise

What Is the Role of Technology to Enhance Insulin Therapy in the Management of Type 1 Diabetes?

- Insulin pens make the delivery of a rapid-acting insulin analogue in a basal–bolus insulin regimen very convenient.
- Glucose meters that can be downloaded by the patient and the physician for analysis are helpful in advanced insulin management regimens.
- Continuous subcutaneous glucose monitoring for 72 h to evaluate glucose trends can be very helpful in fine-tuning insulin doses and looking for unsuspected episodes of hypoglycemia.
- Many glucose pumps now record insulin doses delivered and some pumps can receive glucose data from a glucose meter by radio frequency and integrate glucose and insulin data and even make suggestions for the next bolus dose.
- Secured e-mail messaging makes it possible for health care professionals to communicate with patients on a regular basis, if needed. This important support modality will become more widespread if there is a reimbursement system established.

Type 2 Diabetes

Controlling type 2 diabetes includes achieving an HbA_{1c} of at least <7%, a blood pressure of <130/80 mmHg, and a LDL cholesterol <100 mg/dl (5.6 mmol/l) (also with an HDL cholesterol >40 mg/dl, and triglycerides <150 mg/dl) (Figure 1). Since cardiovascular disease inflicts such a medical and financial burden on individuals with type 2 diabetes, practitioners must develop systems and expertise to manage dyslipidemia, hypertension, appropriate use of aspirin, statins, ace inhibitiors (ARBs), and smoking cessation counseling. The UKPDS epidemiological analysis revealed a significant correlation of glucose control and cardiovascular disease [47]. Many other studies have reinforced the correlation between glucose control and heart disease but none can definitively say how low the HbA_{1c} or corresponding glucose levels need to be so as to minimize the risk of cardiovascular disease. One large NIH funded trial, Action to Control Cardiovascular Risk in Diabetes (ACCORD), is studying if an HbA_{1c} less than 6% compared to more standard glycemic control will reduce the incidence of cardiovascular disease in individuals with type 2 diabetes [48]. There appears to be a continuous increase in risk of complications as glucose, blood pressure, and lipid levels increase even within the normal range of these related cardiovascular risk factors. The ACCORD trial will also evaluate the impact of achieving a systolic BP of 120 mmHg and treating dyslipidemia with both a statin and a fibrate.

Three Steps Toward Improving Overall Diabetes Management

Step 1: *Develop a personal and institutional philosophy and commitment for diabetes management*

First, develop an overall strategy or philosophy of diabetes management such as a commitment to instituting a patient-centered team care model (Figure 6), or utilizing the chronic care model developed by the Institute for Healthcare Improvement [49]. If this is an institution initiative, be sure that senior leadership is supportive of setting up the infrastructure to make the chosen model work. If patients are to work with educators toward making and sustaining healthy behavior changes, do you have diabetes educators available and are they teaching self-management skills?

Step 2: *Agree upon overall priorities and standards of care for diabetes*

Do I as a practitioner or does my clinic have an approach or policy toward screening for diabetes and strategies and team support focused on diabetes prevention in those with the insulin resistance syndrome (metabolic syndrome)? Is a plan in place to support and sustain lifestyle and behavioral changes in those diagnosed with diabetes? Finally, does each clinician, educator, and patient know the target goals for each major clinical factor in this multifactorial disease called type 2 diabetes? Figure 1 outlines the priorities and standards of care that could serve as a framework for a diabetes care plan for each practitioner or for an institution's diabetes initiative.

Step 3: *Develop a curriculum or decision path and implementation plan each priority area of care*

Once the priorities and standards of care are agreed upon it is very helpful to have a template, pathway, or algorithm for each area of focus outlined in Figure 1: a plan for self-management education, glycemic control, preventive care for macrovascular disease, lipid and BP control, screening for microvascular disease, and as detailed and standardize a plan as possible for the other important areas of care like the hospitalized patient with diabetes or managing gestational diabetes.

This chapter will deal only with the role of insulin in the glycemic control pathway. The more physicians and diabetes educators agree on the basic glycemic management pathway the more consistent they will be in their educational messages to the patient and in their practice patterns. There will always be deviations from and exceptions to any decision pathway when each patient's individual clinical needs are considered but one does not need to start from scratch with each patient. Figure 7 is an algorithm (modified from IDC diabetes management tools Staged Diabetes Management and Insulin BASICS) that is based on the two major pathophysiologic defects in type 2 diabetes insulin resistance and insulin deficiency (Figure 8). At presentation (new patient encounter or follow-up visit) any choice of therapy may be appropriate, dependent, in part, on the glucose control at that time and in the recent past [50]. If the HbA_{1c} goal is <7% and medical nutrition therapy (MNT) can lower the HbA_{1c} by 1% on average, then MNT is appropriate if the HbA_{1c} at presentation is <8%. On the other extreme of clinical presentations, if the HbA_{1c} is >11% or the fasting plasma glucose is >300 mg/dl then it is most appropriate to initiate insulin therapy. Insulin initiation at the time of extreme hyperglycemia reduces insulin resistance and enhances insulin secretion in part by correcting glucotoxicity. In some instances insulin can be stopped and oral agents can maintain good glycemic control. While most patients fear insulin injections and many physicians are slow to initiate insulin in type 2 diabetes, there is research underway evaluating the pros and cons of very early basal insulin by injection [the Outcome Reduction with Initial Glargine Intervention (ORIGIN) trial] or bolus insulin by inhalation [37] in patients with type 2 diabetes or even in individuals with prediabetes.

The most typical clinical scenario in the management of type 2 diabetes is to start one oral agent (monotherapy) while obtaining a nutrition consultation [51]. If the HbA_{1c} target is not achieved within 3 months, one proceeds to two oral agents (combination oral agent therapy). If the glucose is moderately high at presentation (HbA_{1c} >2% above target), one may consider stating two oral agents (or a fixed combination of two agents) realizing that any one oral agent will only lower the HbA_{1c} by 1–2%. If the HbA_{1c} is not at target on a combination of two oral agents, the next clinical decision is to either add a third oral agent or combine insulin with oral agents or stop the oral agents and start insulin alone. If one chooses triple oral agent therapy (which only makes sense clinically if the HbA_{1c} on two oral agents is <8% or within 1% of the target),

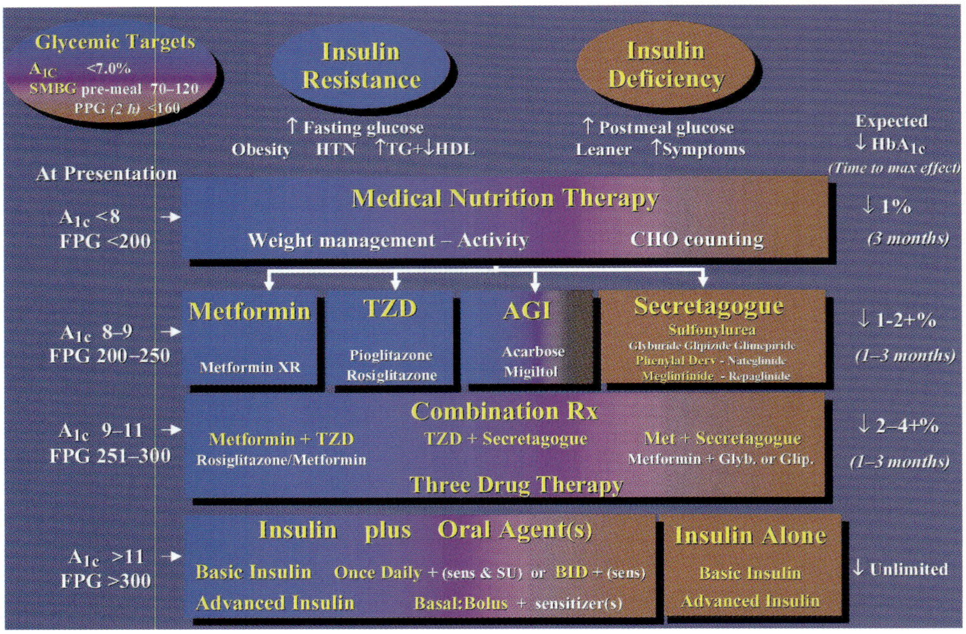

Figure 7 Treatment of type 2 diabetes. (Reproduced by permission of the International Diabetes Center. © 2003 International Diabetes Center, Minneapolis, USA)

eventually one will face the same decision in transitioning to insulin. Does one move to insulin plus oral agents or to insulin alone?

Historically, making the transition from combined oral agents to insulin (or insulin plus oral agents) has been one of the largest hurdles to overcome when trying to achieve or maintain optimal glycemic control in type 2 diabetes. There has been much discussion and speculation regarding the barriers to insulin initiation in type 2 diabetes. Barriers to insulin initiation can be classified as patient barriers, or medical provider barriers. These barriers to insulin initiation and several of the clinical and technological

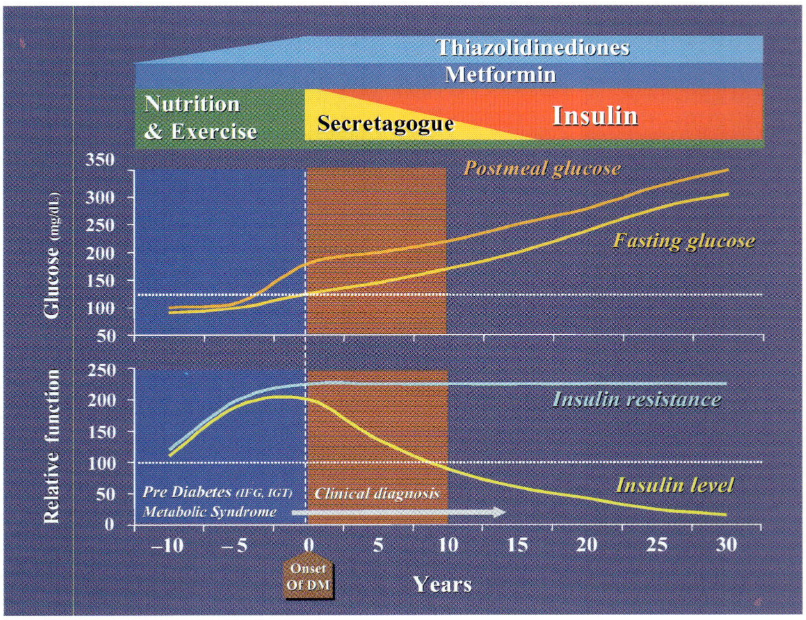

Figure 8 Natural history and treatment of type 2 diabetes. (Reproduced by permission of the International Diabetes Center. © 2003 International Diabetes Center, Minneapolis, USA)

Table 2 Barriers and solutions to insulin initiation

Barriers to insulin initiation		
Patient barriers	Provider barriers	Clinical and technology solutions*
Fear of injections	Fear of injections	Try it—there are many misconceptions: better needles, pens, watch for inhaled insulin
Fear of hypoglycemia	Fear of hypoglycemia	Lower incidence likely with insulin analogues, less frequent in type 2 diabetes mellitus, learn to recognize, watch for continuous glucose monitoring with alarms
Insulin causes weight gain	Insulin causes weight gain	More physiologic insulin delivery may minimize weight gain, do not overtreat hypoglycemia, type 2 use metformin as one agent, watch for new drugs that decrease weight or appetite and improve glucose
Insulin causes complications (like blindness/amputations)	Insulin causes or is associated with heart disease	No good evidence that exogenously administered insulin causes any complications. Watch for studies utilizing early insulin therapy, or insulin sensitizers: to see if either diminishes heart disease
Insulin means serious diabetes	Not convinced insulin needed in type 2 diabetes mellitus to reach HbA_{1c} <7%	Develop systematic approach to insulin starts and f/u • Good patient and MD education materials • Tools/kits for easy in office insulin start followed by quick referral to RN/RD education • Teach patients self-management and have systematic insulin adjustment algorithms for MD • Consider technology that suggests insulin doses
Insulin disrupts ones schedule	Insulin is hard to start and adjust–science and logistics	

* To enhance insulin use in type 2 diabetes.

solutions to help overcome these barriers are summarized in Table 2.

One key physician barrier to starting insulin is either not understanding or accepting that over time insulin will be a necessary part of the therapy for most patients with type 2 diabetes. Figure 8 depicts the natural history of type 2 diabetes, with the major therapy selections in the bar above the natural history curves. It is clear from this natural history figure that there are two main therapeutic targets in type 2 diabetes, insulin resistance, and insulin deficiency. This figure at a glance also implies that overtime exogenous insulin will play an ever more important role in glycemic control due to the steady deterioration in β-cell function over time as was nicely shown in the UKPDS. Diabetes experts feel so strongly that overcoming barriers to insulin initiation is critical to improved glycemic control and quality-of-life outcomes for patients with diabetes that focused research has begun surveying patients and providers in order to be sure that the assumptions the medical community has been making for years are indeed correct. For instance there is preliminary data available from the Diabetes Attitudes, Wishes and Needs (DAWN) study that shows health care providers should focus as much on patient attitudes and environment as on medicine when trying to improve a patient's health [52].

The trend over the last decade is toward insulin initiation in combination with oral agents [this is pictorially demonstrated in the glycemic algorithm (Figure 7) showing that insulin plus oral agents comprises some 75% of the insulin stage] [53, 54]. This trend of combined oral agents plus insulin is building in clinical use for at least three reasons.

The reasons to consider combining insulin and oral agents [54] are as follows:

- Insulin plus oral agents is perceived as an easy way to start insulin, allowing one to take only one injection of insulin per day and still achieve or maintain good glycemic control.
- Oral agents are continued with insulin for their potential benefits beyond lowering glucose levels (such as weight reduction, possible β-cell preservation, improving lipids, reducing insulin resistance associated risk factors – PAI-1, CRP, blood pressure, carotid IMT, microalbumin, etc.) [55].
- Oral agents added to any insulin regimen may help improve the level of glucose control (HbA_{1c}) one is able to achieve [56, 57, 58].

In the past when insulin was started the oral agents were stopped in type 2 diabetes. Investigators like Riddel and others started a trend of using NPH insulin at night and continuing a sulfonylurea (the only oral agent available in the United States at the time of these studies) during the day [59, 60, 61]. These studies demonstrated that the oral agent and insulin combination was as good if not better than evening insulin alone. Glycemic control was never optimized to the currently desired target levels. Many clinicians in practice (the author included) felt that the improved fasting glucose levels were a temporary phenomena and often glycemic control seemed to escape during the day. Additional NPH would often result in overnight hypoglycemia. Insulin sensitizers combined with bedtime insulin were superior to bedtime insulin alone, bedtime insulin plus sulfonylurea, or twice-daily intermediate-acting insulin. There was still a tendency for glucose levels to shoot up the day after the evening NPH injection. Insulin sensitizers added to two or more insulin injections per day showed some definite benefits such as less weight gain and better lipids, or improved glycemic control. If one uses insulin very aggressively in a basal–bolus fashion, with 1–1.2 units of insulin/kg, and supplementing insulin for carbohydrate intake (advanced insulin regimen), it is not known if insulin sensitizers added to this type of regimen would add additional glycemic benefit. Since a very small number of practitioners use truly advanced insulin regimens in type 2 diabetes in most cases it can be said that adding insulin sensitizers to an insulin regimen is likely to improve metabolic control. The insulin sensitizes may be adding additional cardiovascular protection by extraglycemic effects previously discussed.

When insulin glargine, uniformly considered long-acting and relatively peakless, became available it reenergized the waning trend of once-daily insulin (usually at night) combined with oral agents during the day. A recently published study in patients with type 2 diabetes who added either insulin glargine or NPH insulin at night to their usual oral agents during the day resulted in significantly improved fasting glucose levels, and an HbA_{1c} of $<7\%$ in over 60% of the participants [62]. Insulin glargine resulted in less hypoglycemia, particularly overnight, compared to NPH insulin. Many clinicians now feel that if the fasting glucose is significantly elevated, then starting insulin glargine and continuing oral agents is a reasonable way to start insulin and ease the patient (and provider) into more advanced insulin regimens as needed. Others feel that if the glucose is steadily going up after meals and during the day, then a basal insulin alone may not be sufficient to establish or maintain optimal glycemic control and thus would prefer to start at least two insulin injections per day (again often with an oral agent for its glycemic and extraglycemic effects).

It can be argued that every patient in whom insulin is needed should be on a basal–bolus, physiologic, or advanced insulin regimen. In type 1 diabetes using an advanced insulin regimen or an insulin pump seems necessary to optimize glycemic control, minimize hypoglycemia, and maintain a flexible schedule. In individuals with type 2 diabetes more clinical studies are needed comparing various insulin regimens with and without oral agents to make a definitive statement about the most effective approach to insulin delivery. Little data exists about the possible role of insulin pump therapy in type 2 diabetes. Since much of time in type 2 diabetes management the barrier is getting insulin started, it seems appropriate to have a strategy for getting insulin started that includes an easy or *basic insulin regimen* and then an approach to monitoring and as soon as necessary advancing insulin to a more *advanced insulin regimen*.

Basic Insulin Regimen

A basic insulin regimen may be appropriate for individuals

- With type 2 diabetes who are new to insulin
- Exhibiting barriers to insulin initiation
  - Decreased cognitive skills
  - Poor manual dexterity
  - Decreased visual acuity
  - Emotional issues—overwhelmed with insulin
- Opposed to multiple insulin injections
- Unable/willing to take a midday injection
- Having a consistent schedule/routine
  - Consistent meal times and snacks
  - Consistent carbohydrate intake
  - Less than 10–12 h between breakfast and dinner

The options for starting a basic insulin regimen include as follows:

- Daily insulin glargine with oral agents
  - Particularly effective if elevated fasting, relatively stable daytime glucose, patient desires a single injection
  - Start—0.1–0.2 units/kg glargine at bedtime or morning whichever is the more consistent injection time (package insert suggests starting 10 units/day)
  - Increase glargine every 4–7 days (by 2–5 units) until fasting glucose is approximately 120 mg/dl (6.7 mmol/l)
  - Continue oral agents (particularly helpful to have sulfonylurea + sensitizer)
- Daily split-mixed or premixed insulin
  - Particularly effective if very elevated postprandial glucose, significantly increasing daytime blood glucose, willing to pursue two injections, needs premixed pen (glargine not in a pen in the United States in 2003)
  - Start—0.3–0.5 units/kg (2/3 breakfast, 1/3 dinner)
  - Prefer rapid-acting analogue mixtures like mix 75/25 or mix 70/30
    - More flexible timing, not need snacks
  - Consider regular insulin mixture 70/30 or free mix regular + NPH
    - If cost is a major issue
    - Between meal snacks often (will not cover with insulin)
    - Eat inconsistently throughout the day ("grazers")
  - Continuing oral agents optional but usually at least an insulin sensitizer is continued

Advanced Insulin Regimen

An advanced insulin regimen (basal–bolus) is appropriate for individuals with

- Type 1 diabetes—all patients (delivered by injections or pump)
- Type 2 diabetes—all who
  - Need to optimize glucose control
  - Desire a flexible schedule
  - Need to limit the risk of hypoglycemia
  - Are willing to be educated on self-management skills, carbohydrate counting, adjusting for exercise, use of pens, pumps, and other technology
  - Have been on basic regimen and are ready to move to an advanced regimen for more flexibility or improved control

The options for starting an advanced insulin regimen are as follows:

- Basal (insulin glargine), bolus (rapid-acting insulin analogue)
  - 0.3–0.7 units/kg
  - 50% basal, 50% bolus
  - Basal—night or morning whichever is the most consistent time
  - Bolus—distribute according to usual carbohydrate intake
  - Adjust basal and bolus base doses according to glucose patterns
  - Establish insulin-to-carbohydrate ratio (see under Type 1 Diabetes)
  - Establish insulin correction factor, and correction for exercise
- Other basal insulin considerations
  - NPH is not an ideal basal insulin due to peak activity, unless taken in small doses frequently (3–4 times/day—which may not be clinically practical)
  - Multiple relatively small doses of premixed insulins of various formulations of rapid-acting to intermediate insulin, depending on size or carbohydrate content of a meal, could be used
  - Ultralente does not last 24 h, and has a quite variable time action
  - Ultralente in the morning and NPH insulin at night has been used to provide basal insulin coverage which can be adjusted to provide different basal levels at different times of day if needed (for instance, the Dawn effect)
  - Insulin detemir still in clinical trials may serve as a basal insulin taken once or twice per day (appears to have a very consistent time action profile)

Considerations When Converting From Basic to Advanced Insulin Regimen

- Transition from daily glargine to rapid-acting insulin and glargine if unable to establish or maintain HbA_{1c} in target range with basal insulin and oral agents
  - Little research has been conducted on this transition and clinical practice patterns include
    - Continue basal glargine and start rapid-acting insulin at largest meal or meal after which one has the highest postprandial glucose level. Add rapid-acting insulin progressive with meals only if needed because of postprandial hyperglycemia
    - Add rapid-acting insulin with each meal once unable to maintain HbA_{1c} in target. Add 10–20% more insulin depending on how high the HbA_{1c} is; take total insulin dose and divide it into 50% basal and 50% bolus insulin
    - Once all meals have rapid-acting insulin coverage, discontinue any insulin secretagogue and consider continuing insulin sensitizer for glycemic-lowering and non-glycemic-lowering properties
- Transition from rapid-acting or regular insulin and NPH (premixed or free mixed) to rapid-acting insulin and insulin glargine
  - The most effective transition method (derived from IDC practice incorporated into Staged Diabetes Management guidelines):
    - Take the total amount of insulin and subtract 20% (if HbA_{1c} is >9%, subtract 10% or continue entire total dose) to arrive at new total insulin
    - Divide new total insulin into 50% glargine and 50% rapid-acting insulin analogue as in starting basal–bolus regimen above

There are many insulin types available and multiple combinations that can generate endless possible insulin regimens for use in type 2 diabetes. Figure 9 narrows the options drastically in an attempt to summarize the systematic approach described here of starting with a basic insulin regimen usually combined with oral agents then eventually transitioning to an advanced basal–bolus insulin regimen. The figure does provide the option of going straight to an advanced insulin regimen if patient and physician agree. Figures 10–12 show two basic insulin therapy regimens (regular or rapid-acting insulin with intermediate insulin) and one advanced insulin therapy regimen (rapid-acting and glargine). As one progresses from short-acting regular insulin to a rapid-acting insulin analogue and from a basic insulin regimen to an advanced insulin regimen, the insulin profile more closely mimics the normal physiologic insulin profile.

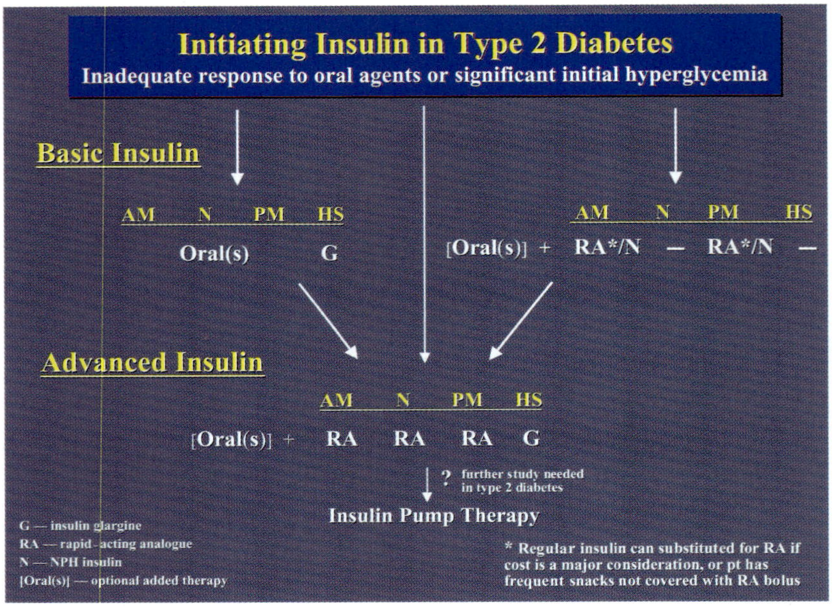

Figure 9 Summary of insulin therapy in type 2 diabetes: initiation and progression. (Reproduced by permission of the International Diabetes Center. © 2003 International Diabetes Center, Minneapolis, USA)

If a patient with type 2 diabetes on insulin has not achieved target glycemia levels, one might go through the following *checklist regarding insulin use in type 2 diabetes*:

- Is there a need to move from basic to advanced insulin regimen?
- Have more physiologic insulin analogues been used?
- Is total insulin dose close to 1–1.2 units/kg (commonly needed in type 2 diabetes)?
- Is the distribution of insulin close to 50% basal/50% bolus?
- Have you considered adding an insulin-sensitizing agent?
- Has the patient received self-management education including medical nutrition therapy?
- Has the patient been educated on how to recognize hypoglycemia?
- Is the patient using technology that might help obtain control—pens, insulin pump, memory meters, and continuous glucose monitoring to evaluate fasting, premeal, postprandial glucoses and unsuspected hypoglycemia?

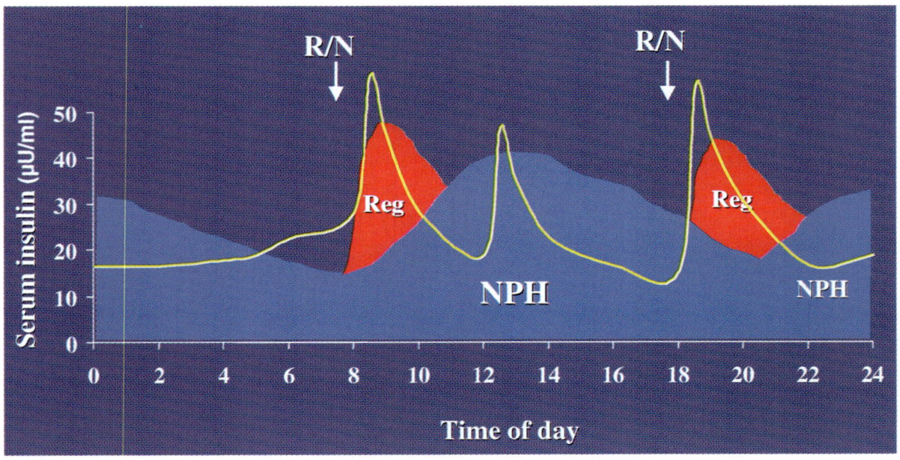

Figure 10 Basic insulin therapy: free mixed insulin (R/N) or premixed R/N (70/30). (Reproduced by permission of the International Diabetes Center. © 2003 International Diabetes Center, Minneapolis, USA)

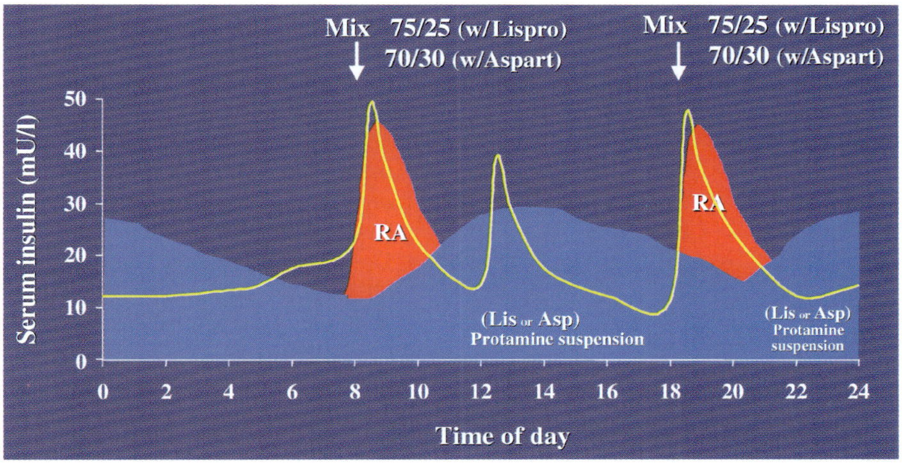

Figure 11 Basic insulin therapy: rapid-acting analogue/lispro or aspart protamine suspension. (Reproduced by permission of the International Diabetes Center. © 2003 International Diabetes Center, Minneapolis, USA)

- Has self-management education included carbohydrate counting, insulin-to-carbohydrate ratio, pattern control, insulin corrective doses for food, exercise, illness, or medications such as corticosteroids [63, 64]?
- Have depression and eating disorders been ruled out and other psychosocial support made available?

INSULIN THERAPY IN GESTATIONAL DIABETES

A good meal plan is essential in the management of gestational diabetes. In order to establish and maintain blood glucose levels as close to euglycemia as possible, insulin is often needed and recently it has been demonstrated that some women may be effectively treated with the oral agent glyburide.

A detailed discussion of the management of gestational diabetes can be found elsewhere in this textbook [65, 66, 67]. A few points on insulin therapy in gestational diabetes are worth highlighting.

If the fasting glucose on screening for gestational diabetes (using oral glucose tolerance test) is 90 mg/dl or higher, there is general agreement that insulin should be initiated. A split-mixed insulin regimen using rapid-acting insulin analogues has proven to be effective in many instances. Often the NPH is moved to nighttime and care should be taken not to induce hypoglycemia overnight since the developing fetus utilizes a fair amount of calories that are not matched by caloric intake overnight. One needs to move to as advanced an insulin regimen as is needed to achieve near normoglycemia. Particularly difficult to control can be the postbreakfast glucose levels. This requires attention to modified carbohydrate intake at

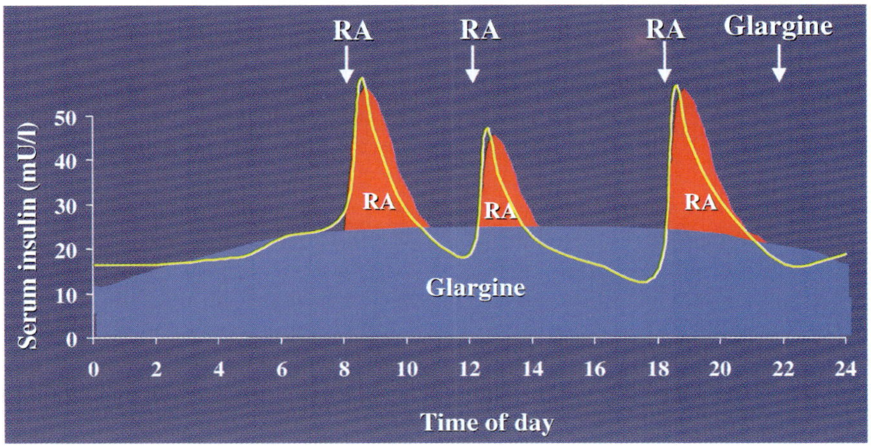

Figure 12 Advanced insulin therapy: rapid-acting analogue/glargine. (Reproduced by permission of the International Diabetes Center. © 2003 International Diabetes Center, Minneapolis, USA)

breakfast and rapid-acting insulin in whatever doses are required to normalize the 1-h postprandial glucose levels. Careful monitoring of fasting ketone levels is important and balancing insulin and caloric intake overnight to eliminate ketones is essential.

INSULIN THERAPY IN THE HOSPITALIZED PATIENT (WITH OR WITHOUT KNOWN DIABETES)

Evidence is building that optimizing glycemic control in every hospitalized patient in the critical care or intensive care unit may reduce morbidity and mortality. This usually involves using an insulin infusion and in those with diabetes making a smooth transition to insulin injection therapy. In addition, there is intriguing data that an infusion followed by a period of advanced insulin therapy can reduce morbidity and mortality in individuals with diabetes suffering from an acute myocardial infarction.

A detailed discussion of the management of the hospitalized patient with diabetes can be found elsewhere in this textbook. A few points on the use of insulin in the hospital setting are worth highlighting. Several comprehensive reviews of diabetes management in the hospital all agree that data is accumulating, indicating that the glucose goals once focused on preventing hypoglycemia in the hospital now are shifting toward avoiding hyperglycemia and in some instance trying to achieve as near normoglycemia as possible [68, 69, 70]. While clinical trials reveal advantages in striving for improved glycemic control in the hospital setting, there are few practical inpatient diabetes management tools easily implemented in the average hospital where diabetes patients account for up to 10–20% of all hospital bed days. One recent clinical trial in patients with diabetes undergoing a coronary artery bypass graft showed that the postoperative glucose levels correlated not only with infections (shown by others as well) but also with length of stay, rehospitalization rate, other morbidity and mortality [71]. In preparation for this study and in follow-up clinical translation work a series of diabetes management tools are in development by the IDC. Some of the inpatient insulin management suggestions from these materials include

- Teach all physicians treating a hospitalized patient how to write an insulin order that must include both basal and bolus insulin.
- Sliding scales can be used effectively [72] but only if they are added to a basal insulin.
- Use practical insulin infusion protocols that can be implemented by ICU staff and that take into account such factors as the rate of fall of the glucose when adjusting insulin infusion rates hourly.
- Critical to a good insulin infusion protocol is a smooth and systematic transition to insulin injections. Enough time must be allowed where the insulin infusion is continued after the insulin injections have been started.
- Basal insulin should be continued when patient is not eating (procedures, surgery)
- Use at least 4–8 capillary glucose tests per day to supplement insulin above basal insulin and then add a portion of supplemented insulin each day back to increase daily basal insulin requirements
- Do an HbA_{1c} test (if you can get results quickly) on all hospitalized patients with diabetes and all patients undergoing cardiovascular surgery
    - HbA_{1c} can help decide those who need insulin at hospital discharge
    - HbA_{1c} can pick up undiagnosed diabetes or at abnormal glucose tolerance that could affect the outcome of cardiovascular surgery
        - Fish found that of 200 patients undergoing coronary artery bypass grafting, 31% had known diabetes and 21% had undiagnosed diabetes [73]
- Set hospital-wide policy or expectation to strive for inpatient glucose control of diabetes patients similar to outpatient goals, for instance 80–140 mg/dl.

Two recent reports [74, 75] present a fascinating description of over 900 individuals who have lived with diabetes for over 50 years. They tended to have minimal complications despite what was reported as less than excellent glycemic control. They were on average fairly normal weight, had an elevated HDL cholesterol, and a very low incidence of significant renal disease. While there may be some genetic or other protective factors present in these remarkable individuals, as we care for our patients, day to day, we must assume they are all susceptible to the potentially devastating and certainly disruptive complications of diabetes and implement the most effective treatment strategies currently available. The use of a patient-centered team, with a cost-effective patient education infrastructure, consensus on targets for standards of care, and a systematic approach to treatment decisions, seems to be the prescription most likely to result in the best outcomes. Effective use of an advanced insulin regimen is a critical part of management for all individuals with type 1 diabetes. The first step in insulin therapy in type 2 diabetes is for patients and practitioners to understand that insulin will be required to achieve optimal glycemic control in most patients with type 2 diabetes. Next, one must anticipate and then overcome the barriers to insulin initiation, and then progress the insulin therapy from a basic insulin regimen to an advanced insulin regimen as needed to maintain a near-normal HbA_{1c} level [76, 77, 78]. These steps will go a long way toward preventing an epidemic of *uncontrolled* diabetes.

Acknowledgments

I would like to thank David Kendall, MD, Roger Mazze, PhD, Ellie Strock, NP, Gregg Simonson, PhD, Karol Carstensen, Katie Colon, and the rest of the International Diabetes Center clinical, education and research staff for assistance in developing and testing many of the materials and concepts presented in this chapter. Many of these materials and concepts are incorporated in Diabetes BASICS and Staged Diabetes Management, the key education and clinical management programs of the International Diabetes Center. Special thanks are due to Mary Ann Carr for her excellent work in editing and organizing the material in this chapter.

REFERENCES

1. Home P. The challenge of poorly controlled diabetes mellitus. *Diabetes Metab* April 2003; 29: 101–9.
2. American Diabetes Association. Economic costs of diabetes in the U.S. in 2002. *Diabetes Care* 2003; 26: 917–32.
3. American Diabetes Association. Standards of medical care. *Diabetes Care* 2004; 27 (suppl 1): S15–35.
4. Etzwiler DD. Chronic care: a need in search of a system. *Diabetes Educ* 1997; 23: 569–73.
5. Bodenheimer T, Lorig K, Holman H, Grumbach K. Patient self-management of chronic disease in primary care. *JAMA* 2002; 288: 2469–75.
6. Mazze RS, Etzwiler DD, Strock E, Peterson K, McClave CR, Meszaros JF, Leigh C, Owens LW, Deep LC, Peterson A, et al. Staged diabetes management: toward an integrated model of diabetes care. *Diabetes Care* 1994; 17 (suppl 1): 56–66.
7. Norris Sl, Engelgau MM, Narayan KM. Effectiveness of self-management in type 2 diabetes:systematic review of randomized controlled trials. *Diabetes Care* 2001; 24: 561–87.
8. Norris SL, Nichols PJ, Caspersen CJ, Glasgow RE, Engelgau MM, Jack L, Isham G, Snyder SR, Carande-Kulis VG, Garfield S, Briss P, McCullough D. The effectiveness of disease and case management for people with diabetes: a systematic review. *Am J Prev Med* 2002; 22 (4, suppl): 15–38.
9. Davidson J, Reader D, Rickheim P. *Blood Glucose Patterns: A Guide to Achieving Targets*. Minneapolis, MN: International Diabetes Center, Park Nicollet Institute, 2003.
10. Bergenstal R, Callahan T, Johnson M, Upham P, Hollander P, Spencer M, Castle G, Nelson J, Roth L, Etzwiler D. Management principles that most influence glycemic control: a follow-up study of former DCCT participants. *Diabetes* 1996; 45 (suppl 1): 124A.
11. Brewer KW, Chase HP, Owen S, Garg SK. Slicing the pie. Correlating HbA-values with average blood glucose values in a pie chart form. *Diabetes Care* 1998; 21 (2): 209–12.
12. Gaede P, Vedel P, Larsen N, Jensen GV, Parving HH, Pedersen O. Multifactorial intervention and cardiovascular disease in patients with type 2 diabetes. *N Engl J Med* 2003; 348 (5): 383–93.
13. Grant RW, Cagliero E, Murphy-Sheehy P, Singer DE, Nathan DM, Meigs JB. Comparison of hyperglycemia, hypertension, and hypercholesterolemia management in patients with type 2 diabetes. *Am J Med* 2002; 112 (8): 603–9.
14. Turner RC, Millns H, Neil HA, Stratton IM, Manley SE, Matthews DR, Holman RR. Risk factors for coronary artery disease in non-insulin dependent diabetes mellitus: United Kingdom Prospective Diabetes Study (UKPDS 23). *BMJ* 1998; 316: 823–8.
15. The CDC Diabetes Cost-Effectiveness Group. Cost-effectiveness of intensive glycemic control, intensified hypertension control, and serum cholesterol level reduction for type 2 diabetes. *JAMA* 2002; 287: 2542–51.
16. Saaddine JB, Engelgau MM, Beckles GL, Gregg EW, Thompson TJ, Venkat Narayan KM. A diabetes report card for the United States: quality of care in the 1990s. *Ann Intern Med* 2002; 136: 565–74.
17. UK Prospective Diabetes Study (UKPDS) Group. Intensive blood-glucose control with sulphonylureas or insulin compared with conventional treatement wand risk of complications in patients with type 2 diabetes (UKPDS 33). *Lancet* 1998; 352: 837–53.
18. DeWitt DE, Dugdale DC. Using new insulin strategies in the outpatient treatment of diabetes: clinical applications. *JAMA* 2003; 289 (17): 2265–9.
19. DeWitt DE, Hirsch IB. Outpatient insulin therapy in type 1 and type 2 diabetes mellitus: scientific review. *JAMA* 2003; 289 (17): 2254–64.
20. Greaves CJ, Brown P, Terry RT, Eiser C, Lings P, Stead JW. Converting to insulin in primary care: an exploration of the needs of practice nurses. *J Adv Nurs* 2003; 42 (5): 487–96.
21. Kazlauskaite R, Fogelfeld L. Insulin therapy in type 2 diabetes [review]. *Dis Mon* June 2003; 49 (6): 377–420.
22. McDonald K. Insulin therapy today. Focusing on the basal–bolus balance. *Adv Nurse Pract* 2003; 11 (7): 40–4.
23. Royle P, Waugh N, McAuley L, McIntyre L, Thomas S. Inhaled insulin in diabetes mellitus [review]. *Cochrane Database Syst Rev* 2003; (3): CD003890.
24. Dills DG. New aspects of insulin therapy in type 1 and type 2 diabetes. *Curr Diab Rep* 2001; 1 (2): 112–8.
25. Sasali A, Leahy JL. Insulin therapy for type 2 diabetes. *Curr Diab Rep* 2003; 3 (5): 378–85.
26. Chan JL, Abrahamson MJ. Pharmacological management of type 2 diabetes mellitus: rationale for rational use of insulin [review]. *Mayo Clin Proc* 2003; 78 (4): 459–67.
27. Bergenstal RM. Optimization of insulin therapy in patients with type 2 diabetes. *Endocr Pract* 2000; 6: 93–7.
28. Weingarten SR, Henning JM, Badamgarav E, Knight K, Hasselblad K, Gano A, Jr Offman JJ. Interventions used in disease management programs for patients with chronic illness—which ones work? Meta-analysis of published reports. *BMJ* 2002; 325: 925–32.
29. Steinberg EP. Improving the quality of care—can we practice what we preach? *N Engl J Med* 2003; 348: 2681.
30. Leatherman S, Berwick D, Iles D, et al. The business case for quality: case studies and an analysis. *Health Aff* (*Millwood*) 2003; 22 (2): 17–30.
31. Bethel MA, Feinglos MN. Insulin analogues: new therapies for type 2 diabetes mellitus [review]. *Curr Diab Rep* 2002; 2 (5): 403–8.
32. Lepore M, Pampanelli S, Fanelli C, Porcellati F, Bartocci L, DiVincenzo A, Cordoni C, Costa E, Brunetti P, Bolli G. Pharmacokinetics and pharmacodynamics of subcutaneous injection of long-acting human insulin analog glargine, NPH insulin, and ultralente human insulin and

continuous subcutaneous infusion of insulin lispro. *Diabetes* 2000; 49: 2142–8.

33. Cefalu WT. Concept, strategies, and feasibility of noninvasive insulin delivery. *Diabetes Care* 2004; 27: 239–46.
34. Heinemann L. Alternative delivery routes: inhaled insulin [review]. *Diabetes Nutr Metab* 2002; 15 (6): 417–22.
35. Cefalu WT, Skyler JS, Kourides IA, Landschulz WH, Balagtas CC, Cheng SL, Gelfan RA, Inhaled Insulin Study Group. Inhaled human insulin treatment in patients with type 2 diabetes mellitus. *Ann Intern Med* 2001; 3: 203–7.
36. Nathan DM. Inhaled insulin for type 2 diabetes: solution or distraction [editorial]. *Ann Intern Med* 2001; 134: 242–4.
37. Bergenstal RM, for the Exubera Phase III Study Group. Efficacy and safety of inhaled insulin (Exubera®) compared with rosiglitazone in type 2 diabetes patients not optimally controlled on diet and exercise: results of a 3-month, randomised, comparative trial. *Diabetologia* 2003; 46 (suppl 2): A801.
38. Richter B, Neises G. Human insulin versus animal insulin in people with diabetes mellitus [review]. *Cochrane Database Syst Rev* 2003; (3): CD003816.
39. Jovanovic L, Ilic S, Pettitt DJ, Hugo K, Gutierriez M, Bowsher RR, Bastyr EJ. The metabolic and immunologic effects of insulin lispro. *Diabetes Care* 1999; 22: 1422–7.
40. The Diabetes Control and Complications Trial/ Epidemiology of Diabetes Intervention and Complications Research Group. Retinopathy and nephropathy in patients with type 1 diabetes four years after a trial of intensive therapy. *N Engl J Med* 2000; 342: 381–9.
41. The Diabetes Control and Complications Trial/ Epidemiology of Diabetes Intervention and Complications Research Group. Effect of intensive therapy on microvascular complications of type 1 diabetes. *JAMA* 2002; 287: 2563–9.
42. The Diabetes Control and Complications Trial/ Epidemiology of Diabetes Intervention and Complications Research Group. Intensive diabetes therapy and carotid intima-media thickness in type 1 diabetes mellitus. *N Engl J Med* 2003; 348: 2294–303.
43. The Diabetes Control and Complications Trial/ Epidemiology of Diabetes Intervention and Complications Research Group. Sustained effect of intensive treatment of type 1 diabetes on development and progression of diabetic nephropathy. *JAMA* 2003; 290: 2159–67.
44. Berry LL, Seiders K, Wilder SS. Innovations in access to care: a patient-centered approach. *Ann Intern Med* 2003; 139: 568–74.
45. Heisler M, Vijan S, Anderson RM, Ubel P, Bernstein SJ, Hofer TP. Diabetes management improves when patients, doctors agree on treatment goals. *J Gen Intern Med* 2003.
46. Davidson PC, Hebblewhite HR, Bode BW, Richardson PL, Steed RD, Welch NS, Poulos E, Ybanez P. An empirical basis for modifying the "1500 rule." *Diabetes* 2002; 51 (suppl 2): A518.
47. Prospective Diabetes Study (UKPDS) Group. Association of glycaemia with macrovascular and microvascular complications of type 2 diabetes (UKPDS 35): prospective observational study. *BMJ* 2000; 321: 405–12.
48. Article available at: https://www.accordtrial.org. Accessed December 10, 2003.
49. Wagner EH, Grothhaus LC, Sandhu N, Galvin MS, McGregor M, Artz K, Coleman EA. Chronic care clinics for diabetes in primary care: a system-wide randomized trial. *Diabetes Care* 2001; 25: 695–700.
50. Inzucchi SE. Oral antihyperglycemic therapy for type 2 diabetes: scientific review. *JAMA* 2002; 287 (3): 360–72.
51. Ahmann AJ, Riddle MC. Current oral agents for type 2 diabetes. Many options, but which to choose when? *Postgrad Med* May 2002; 111 (5): 32–4, 37–40, 43–6.
52. Korytkowski M. When oral agents fail: practical barriers to starting insulin. *Int J Obes Relat Metab Disord* 2002; 26 (suppl 3): S18–24.
53. Buse J. Combining insulin and oral agents. *Am J Med* 2000; 108 (suppl 6): 23S–32S.
54. Garber AJ. Benefits of combination therapy of insulin and oral hypoglycemic agents. *Arch Intern Med* 2003; 163 (15): 1781–2.
55. Bergenstal R, Johnson M, Whipple D, Noller D, Boyce K, Roth L, Upham P, DeBold R. Advantages of adding metformin to multiple dose insulin therapy in type 2 diabetes. *Diabetes* 1998; 47 (suppl 1): A347.
56. Yki-Järvinen H, Kauppila M, Kujansuu E, Lahti J, Marjanen T, Niskanen L, Rajala S, Ryysy L, Salo S, Seppala P, et al. Comparison of insulin regimens in patients with non-insulin-dependent diabetes mellitus. *New Engl J Med* 1992; 327: 1426–33.
57. Yki-Järvinen H, Ryysy L, Nikkilä K, Tulokas T, Vanamo R, Keikkilä M. Comparison of bedtime insulin regimens in patients with type 2 diabetes mellitus: a randomized controlled trial. *Ann Inter Med* 1999; 130: 389–96.
58. Avilés-Santa L, Sinding J, Raskin P. Effects of metformin in patients with poorly controlled, insulin-treated type 2 diabetes mellitus: a randomized, double-blind, placebo-controlled trial. *Ann Intern Med* 1999; 131: 182–8.
59. Riddle M. Combining sulfonylureas and other oral agents. *Am J Med* 2000; 108 (suppl 6a): 15S–22S.
60. Pugh JA, Wagner ML, Sawyer J, Ramirez G, Tuley M, Friesderg S. Is combination sulfonylurea and insulin therapy useful in NIDDM patients? *Diabetes Care* 1992; 15: 953–8.
61. Riddle MC, Schneider J. Beginning insulin treatment of obese patients with evening 70/30 insulin plus glimepiride versus insulin alone. *Diabetes Care* 1998; 21: 1053–7.
62. Riddle MC, Rosenstock J, Gerich J. The Treat-to-Target Trial: randomized addition of glargine or human NPH insulin to oral therapy of type 2 diabetic patients. *Diabetes Care* 2003; 26: 3080–6.
63. Trence DL. Management of patients on chronic glucocorticoid therapy: an endocrine perspective. *Prim Care* 2003; 30 (3): 593–605.
64. Hoogwerf B, Danese RD. Drug selection and the management of corticosteroid-related diabetes mellitus [review]. *Rheum Dis Clin North Am* 1999; 25 (3): 489–505.
65. Jovanovic L, Pettitt D. Gestational diabetes mellitus. *JAMA* 2001; 286: 2516–8.
66. Metzger BE, Coustan DR. Summary and recommendations of the Fourth International Workshop-Conference on Gestational Diabetes Mellitus. *Diabetes Care* 1998; 21 (suppl 2): B161–7.
67. Langer O, Conway DL, Berkus MD, Xenakis EM, Gonzales O. A comparison of glyburide and insulin in women with gestational diabetes mellitus. *N Engl J Med* 2000; 343: 1134–8.
68. Trence DL, Kelly JL, Hirsch IB. The rationale and management of hyperglycemia for in-patients with cardiovascular

disease: time for change [review]. *J Clin Endocrinol Metab* 2003; 88 (6): 2430–7.

69. van den Berghe G, Wouters P, Weekers F, Verwaest C, Bruyninckx F, Schetz M, Vlasselaers D, Ferdinande P, Lauwers P, Bouillon R. Intensive insulin therapy in the critically ill patients. *N Engl J Med* 2001; 345 (19): 1359–67.
70. Mesotten D, Van den Berghe G. Clinical potential of insulin therapy in critically ill patients [review]. *Drugs* 2003; 63 (7): 625–36.
71. Buse J. Combining insulin and oral agents. *Am J Med.* 2000; 108 (suppl 6): 23S–32S.
72. Bergenstal R, Fish L, List S. The insulin sliding scale is not dead. *Arch Intern Med* 1998; 158: 298.
73. Fish LH, Weaver TW, Moore AL, Steel LG. Value of postoperative blood glucose in predicting complications and length of stay after coronary artery bypass grafting. *Am J Cardiol* 2003; 92 (1): 74–6.
74. Bain SC, Gill GV, Dyer PH, Jones AF, Murphy M, Jones KE, Smyth C, Barnett AH. Characteristics of type 1 diabetes of over 50 years duration (the Golden Years Cohort). *Diabet Med* 2003; 20 (10): 808–11.
75. Goddard L, Wong K, Bashan A, Doria A, King G. Complication-free subjects after more than 50 years of type 1 diabetes mellitus. *Diabetes* 2003; 52 (suppl 1): A796.
76. Wagner EH, Sandhu N, Newton KM, McCulloch DK, Ramsey SD, Grothaus LC. Effect of improved glycemic control on health care costs and utilization. *JAMA* 2001; 285: 182–9.
77. Hayward RH, Manning WG, Kaplan SH, Wagner EH, Greenfield S. Starting insulin therapy in patients with type 2 diabetes: effectiveness, complications, and resource utilization. *JAMA* 1997; 278: 1663–9.
78. Colwell JA. Controlling type 2 diabetes: are the benefits worth the costs? *JAMA* 1997; 278: 1700.

Index

International Textbook of Diabetes Mellitus

THIRD EDITION

Editorial Board

International Textbook of Diabetes Mellitus

THIRD EDITION

Editors-in-Chief

Ralph A. DeFronzo

The University of Texas Health Science Centre, San Antonio, TX, USA

Ele Ferrannini

Department of Internal Medicine, University of Pisa School of Medicine, Pisa, Italy

Harry Keen

Department of Diabetes Endocrinology and Metabolism, Guy's Hospital, London, UK

Paul Zimmet

International Diabetes Institute, Melbourne, Australia

VOLUME TWO

John Wiley & Sons, Ltd

Telephone (+44) 1243 779777

Email (for orders and customer service enquiries): cs-books@wiley.co.uk
Visit our Home Page on www.wileyeurope.com or www.wiley.com

Other Wiley Editorial Offices

John Wiley & Sons Inc., 111 River Street,
Hoboken, NJ 07030, USA

Jossey-Bass, 989 Market Street,
San Francisco, CA 94103-1741, USA

Wiley-VCH Verlag GmbH, Boschstr. 12,
D-69469 Weinheim, Germany

John Wiley & Sons Australia Ltd, 33 Park Road,
Milton, Queensland 4064, Australia

John Wiley & Sons (Asia) Pte Ltd, 2 Clementi Loop #02-01,
Jin Xing Distripark, Singapore 129809

John Wiley & Sons Canada Ltd, 22 Worcester Road,
Etobicoke, Ontario, Canada M9W 1L1

Wiley also publishes its books in a variety of electronic formats. Some content that appears in print may not be available in electronic books.

Library of Congress Cataloging- in-Publication Data

International textbook of diabetes mellitus / editors, Ralph A. DeFronzo
. . . [et al.]. – 3rd ed.
p. ; cm.
Includes bibliographical references and index.
ISBN 0-471-48655-8 (cloth : alk. paper)
1. Diabetes
[DNLM: 1. Diabetes Mellitus. WK 810 I60359 2004] I. DeFronzo, Ralph
A. II. Series.
RC660.I585 2004
616.4'62–dc21 2003009069

British Library Cataloguing in Publication Data

A catalogue record for this book is available from the British Library

ISBN 0-471-48655-8

Typeset in 10/12 pt Times by Techbooks, Delhi, India.
Printed and bound by Rotolito Lombarda, Milan, Italy.
This book is printed on acid-free paper responsibly manufactured from sustainable forestry in which at least two trees are planted for each one used for paper production.

About the Editors-in-Chief

Professor Ralph A. DeFronzo, MD, is a Professor of Medicine and Chief of the Diabetes Division at the University of Texas Health Science Center and the Audie L. Murphy Memorial VA Hospital in San Antonio, Texas. He also functions as the Deputy Director of the Texas Diabetes Institute. Dr DeFronzo is a graduate of Harvard Medical School and did his training in internal medicine at the Johns Hopkins Hospital. Later, he completed fellowships in endocrinology at the National Institutes of Health (NIH) and Baltimore City Hospitals and in nephrology at the Hospital of the University of Pennsylvania.

His major interests focus on the pathogenesis and treatment of type 2 diabetes mellitus, the central role of insulin resistance in the metabolic-cardiovascular cluster of disorders known collectively as the *insulin resistance syndrome*, and the etiology and treatment of diabetic nephropathy. Using the euglycemic insulin clamp technique in combination with radioisotope turnover methodology, limb catheterization, indirect calorimetry, and muscle biopsy, he has helped to define the biochemical and cellular disturbances responsible for insulin resistance in type 2 diabetes mellitus.

For his work in this area, Dr DeFronzo has received the prestigious Lilly Award from the American Diabetes Association (ADA), the Banting Lectureship from the Canadian Diabetes Association as well as many other national and international awards. He is also the recipient of the ADA's Albert Renold Award for lifetime commitment to the training of young diabetes investigators. Previously, he served on the ADA Board of Directors and as Chairman of the ADA's Medical and Scientific Oversight Committee, Research Policy Committee, Research Review Committee, and Professional Education Committee.

He is the past-editor of *Diabetes Reviews*, a co-editor of the ADA's *Physicians' Guide to Type 1 Diabetes* and the ADA's *Physicians' Guide to Type 2 Diabetes,* a co-editor of the *International Textbook of Diabetes*, and a past member of the editorial board of *Diabetologia*. With more than 400 articles published in peer-reviewed medical journals, Dr DeFronzo is a distinguished clinician, teacher, and investigator who has been an invited speaker at major national and international conferences on diabetes mellitus.

Professor Ele Ferrannini is the Professor of Internal Medicine, University of Pisa School of Medicine; Chief of the Metabolism Unit of the CNR (National Research Council) Institute of Clinical Physiology, Pisa; and Clinical Professor of Medicine, Diabetes Division, University of Texas Health Science Center at San Antonio.

From 1977 to 1978, Professor Ferrannini was a Visiting Investigator at the Karolinska Institute in Stockholm, Sweden. In 1979 he became a Post-doctoral Fellow of the Fogarty International Centre of the National Institutes of Health, Yale University School of Medicine, Connecticut, USA, in 1988 he was appointed Clinical Professor of Medicine, Diabetes Division at the University of Texas Health Science Center at San Antonio, and in 1994 he assumed his current position in Italy.

Professor Ferrannini has been involved in over 250 publications in the field of diabetes, metabolism, hypertension, obesity, and cardiovascular risk factors. He was formerly the Editor-in-Chief of *Diabetologia*, the official journal of the European Association for the Study of Diabetes (EASD) and is currently the Chairman of the European Group for the Study of Insulin Resistance.

Professor Harry Keen, CBE, MD, FRCP, qualified in 1948 at St Mary's Hospital Medical School, London, where he worked, after service in the Royal Army Medical Corps, with Sir George Pickering and Sir Stanley Peart in the Professorial Medical Unit. From 1953 to 1960 Professor Keen was Senior Clinical Assistant to Dr R.D. Lawrence and Dr W.G. Oakley in the Diabetic Department, King's College Hospital. After an International Post-doctoral Research Fellowship at NIH, Bethesda, MD, USA (1960–1961), he joined Lord Butterfield at Guy's Hospital, London, as Senior Lecturer, Reader, and from 1971, as Professor of Human Metabolism, heading the Academic Unit for Metabolic Medicine and as Consultant Physician till his retirement in 1990. He continues to work in the Department, School, and University as Professor and Consultant Physician Emeritus.

His main research and clinical interests have been in diabetes and its complications and have included basic laboratory studies, clinical research, and clinical epidemiology.

Professor Keen has published many papers, reviews, and book chapters and is editor and co-editor of various books and international peer-reviewed journals. He has received numerous honors including the Banting Memorial Lecturer of the British Diabetic Association (1984), Claude Bernard Lecturer of the European Association for the Study of Diabetes (EASD) (1987), Harold Rifkin

Distinguished Fellow of the American Diabetes Association (1979, 1987, and 1989), James Watt Lecturer of the Royal College of Physicians of Edinburgh (1988), and the Juhling Award for Diabetes Research (1995). Professor Keen was the first recipient of the United Nations/ UNESCO Hellmut Mehnert Award for the Prevention of Diabetes and its Complications (1998) and was presented with the Novartis Distinguished Service Award UK (1999). Professor Keen was awarded a CBE in 1998.

Professor Keen was appointed Director of the Diabetes and Metabolism Unit and Honorary Consultant Physician, Guy's Group of Hospitals in 1967 and was involved in research, clinical care, and undergraduate and postgraduate teaching. Following this, he was appointed Director of Medicine (1985–1990), Chairman of the British Diabetic Association (1990–1996) and has been Honorary President of the International Diabetes Federation (IDF) since 1991. Appointed Emeritus Professor of the University of London Faculty of Medicine in 1990, he continues clinical research and teaching activities at the Guy's Hospital Campus of the (now) King's College London School of Medicine, London.

Professor Paul Zimmet is currently Foundation Director of the International Diabetes Institute, a position he has held since 1985, and Professor of Diabetes at Monash University. He is also a Professor at Deakin University and is Adjunct Professor in the Graduate School of Public Health, the University of Pittsburgh. He also serves on the Australian Government's Strategic Taskforce on Diabetes. His current research interests include epidemiological, environmental, and molecular biological components in the causation of type 2 diabetes, and he has published over 500 scientific papers, chapters, and reviews in peer-reviewed journals and books.

Professor Zimmet is a member of the Editorial Board of a number of international peer-reviewed journals, and has received many awards, including the Kelly West Medal from the American Diabetes Associated, Eli Lilly Award from the IDF, and the AM Cohen Award Lecture from the EASD. In 1997, at the *16th IDF Congress* in Finland, he received the first Peter Bennett Diabetes Epidemiology Award for outstanding contributions to research on the epidemiology of diabetes. In 2002, he received the Harold Rifkin Award of the American Diabetes Association for contributions to diabetes internationally. In 1993, he was awarded the Order of Australia for distinguished services to medicine and education, particularly in the field of diabetes. In 2001, he was further honored with the Order of Australia (AO) for services to medical research of national and international significance, particularly in the field of diabetes, as a leader of investigations into social, nutritional, and lifestyle diseases, and to biotechnology development in Australia.

Contents

VOLUME ONE

VOLUME TWO

Contributors

Carl-David Agardh	Malmö University Hospital, Malmö, Sweden
Elisabet Agardh	Malmö University Hospital, Malmö, Sweden
Intekhab Ahmed	Jefferson Medical College, Thomas Jefferson University, Philadelphia, PA, USA
Bo Ahrén	Lund University, Lund, Sweden
Lloyd M. Aiello	Joslin Diabetes Center, Boston, MA, USA, and Harvard Medical School, Boston, MA, USA
J. Akwe	University of Perugia, Perugia, Italy
Abdulaziz R. Al-Harthi	University of Michigan, Ann Arbor, MI, USA
K.G.M.M. Alberti	University of Newcastle upon Tyne, Newcastle upon Tyne, UK
Marie-Christine Alessi	University Hospital Timone, Marseille, France
Stephanie A. Amiel	King's College, London, UK
James H. Anderson, Jr.	Eli Lilly and Company, Indianapolis, IN, USA
Morsi Arab	University of Alexandria, Alexandria, Egypt
Pablo Arias	University of Buenos Aires Medical School, Buenos Aires, Argentina
Arne Astrup	The Royal Veterinary and Agricultural University, Frederiksberg, Denmark
Shigeaki Baba	International Institute for Diabetes Education and Study, Kobe, Japan
Laurie L. Baggio	Banting and Best Diabetes Centre, Toronto General Hospital, University of Toronto, Toronto, Canada
Clifford J. Bailey	Aston University, Birmingham, UK
Stephen C. Bain	University of Birmingham, Birmingham, UK and Birmingham Heartlands Hospital, Birmingham, UK
Mandeep Bajaj	University of Texas Health Science Center at San Antonio, San Antonio, TX, USA
George L. Bakris	Rush Presbyterian/St. Luke's Medical Centre, Chicago, IL, USA
Alberto Barcelo	Pan American Health Organization, Washington, DC, USA
Anthony H. Barnett	University of Birmingham, Birmingham, UK, and Birmingham Heartlands Hospital, Birmingham, UK

Eugene J. Barrett	University of Virginia Health System, Charlottesville, VA, USA
M. Massi Benedetti	University of Perugia, Perugia, Italy
Richard M. Bergenstal	International Diabetes Center, Park Nicollet Institute, Minneapolis, MN, USA
Richard N. Bergman	University of Southern California, Los Angeles, CA, USA
Rudy W. Bilous	James Cook University Hospital, Middlesbrough, UK
Per Björntorp (deceased)	University of Göteborg, Göteborg, Sweden
Henry R. Black	Rush Presbyterian/St. Luke's Medical Centre, Chicago, IL, USA
Geremia B. Bolli	University of Perugia, Perugia, Italy
Riccardo C. Bonadonna	University of Verona School of Medicine, Verona, Italy
Claude Bouchard	Louisiana State University, Baton Rouge, LA, USA
Michael Brownlee	Albert Einstein College of Medicine, Bronx, NY, USA
G. Calabrese	University of Perugia, Perugia, Italy
Jerry D. Cavallerano	Joslin Diabetes Center, Boston, MA, USA
A. Cesarini	"Pretura Circondariale" of Perugia, Italy
Juliana C.N. Chan	The Chinese University of Hong Kong, Shatin, Hong Kong, China
Sudesna Chatterjee	Leicester Royal Infirmary, University Hospitals of Leicester NHS Trust, Leicester, UK
Chee W. Chia	The Johns Hopkins University School of Medicine, Baltimore, MD, USA
Jean-Louis Chiasson	Research Centre, Centre Hospitalier de l'Université de Montréal, Montréal, Canada, and Université de Montréal, Montréal, Canada
Theodore P. Ciaraldi	University of California San Diego, San Diego, CA, USA
A. Clark	Oxford Centre for Diabetes, Endocrinology and Metabolism, Oxford, UK
Deborah J. Clegg	University of Cincinnati, Cincinnati, OH, USA
Clive S. Cockram	The Chinese University of Hong Kong, Shatin, Hong Kong, China
Peter G. Colman	The Walter and Eliza Hall Institute of Medical Research, Parkville, Australia
Alberto Coppelli	University of Pisa, Pisa, Italy
Catherine Cowie	National Institutes of Health, Bethesda, MD, USA
Philip E. Cryer	Washington University School of Medicine, St. Louis, MO, USA

Michael H. Cummings Queen Alexandra Hospital, Portsmouth, UK

M.J. Davies Leicester Royal Infirmary, University Hospitals of Leicester NHS Trust, Leicester, UK

J.L. Day Ipswich Hospital, Ipswich, Suffolk, UK

Ralph A. DeFronzo University of Texas Health Science Center, San Antonio, TX, USA

Thanh L. Dinh Harvard Medical School, Boston, MA, USA

Gary Dowse Department of Health, Perth, Australia

Daniel J. Drucker Banting and Best Diabetes Centre, Toronto General Hospital, University of Toronto, Toronto, Canada

Jean-Luc Dulong Technological University of Compiègne, Compiègne, France

Michael Edmonds Kings College Hospital, London, UK

George S. Eisenbarth Barbara Davis Center for Childhood Diabetes, University of Colorado Health Sciences Center, Denver, CO, USA

Karin Ekberg Karolinska Institute, Stockholm, Sweden

Jean-Marie Ekoe Centre de Reserche CHUM, Montreal, Canada

Alison L. Every The Walter and Eliza Hall Institute of Medical Research, Parkville, Australia

Stephen R. Farmer Boston University School of Medicine, Boston, MA, USA

M. Orsini Federici University of Perugia, Perugia, Italy

Ele Ferrannini Department of Internal Medicine, University of Pisa School of Medicine, Pisa, Italy

Samuel Edwin Fineberg Indiana University School of Medicine, Indianapolis, IN, USA

Spiros Fourlanos The Walter and Eliza Hall Institute of Medical Research, Parkville, Australia

Brian M. Frier Royal Infirmary, Edinburgh, Scotland

David P. Funda The Walter and Eliza Hall Institute of Medical Research, Parkville, Australia

Henrik Galbo University of Copenhagen, Copenhagen, Denmark

Alan J. Garber Baylor College of Medicine, Houston, TX, USA

Abhimanyu Garg The University of Texas Southwestern Medical Center at Dallas, Dallas, TX, USA

W. Timothy Garvey University of Alabama at Birmingham, and the Birmingham Veterans Affairs Medical Center, Birmingham, AL, USA

Robert J. Genco State University of New York at Buffalo, Buffalo, NY, USA

G.V. Gill University of Liverpool, Liverpool, UK

Barry J. Goldstein Jefferson Medical College, Thomas Jefferson University, Philadelphia, PA, USA

Christopher S. Gray	University of Newcastle upon Tyne, Newcastle upon Tyne, UK
Rosaire P. Gray	Whittington Hospital, London, UK
Leif Groop	Lund University, Malmö, Sweden
Leonard C. Harrison	The Walter and Eliza Hall Institute of Medical Research, Parkville, Australia
Andrew T. Hattersley	Peninsula Medical School, Exeter, UK
Zhiheng He	Joslin Diabetes Center, Harvard Medical School, Boston, MA, USA
Robert R. Henry	VA San Diego Healthcare System, and University of California San Diego, San Diego, CA, USA
William H. Herman	University of Michigan, Ann Arbor, MI, USA
Rury Holman	Diabetes Trials Unit, Radcliffe Infirmary, Oxford, UK
Margo C. Honeyman	The Walter and Eliza Hall Institute of Medical Research, Parkville, Australia
Barbara V. Howard	MedStar Research Institute, Washington, DC, USA
Katrin Hücking	University of Southern California, Los Angeles, CA, USA
Giuseppina Imperatore	Centers for Disease Control and Prevention, National Center for Chronic Disease Prevention and Health Promotion, Atlanta, GA, USA
Serge Jabbour	Jefferson Medical College, Thomas Jefferson University, Philadelphia, PA, USA
Alan M. Jacobson	Joslin Diabetes Center, Harvard Medical School, Boston, MA, USA
Dimitrije Jakovljevic	National Public Health Institute, Helsinki, Finland
Kent P. Jensen	The Walter and Eliza Hall Institute of Medical Research, Parkville, Australia
Bo-Lennart Johansson	Karolinska Institute, Stockholm, Sweden
Jan Johansson	Karolinska Institute, Stockholm, Sweden
Stephen C. Jones	James Cook University Hospital, Middlesbrough, UK
Hans Jörnvall	Karolinska Institute, Stockholm, Sweden
Lois Jovanovic	Sansum Medical Research Foundation, Santa Barbara, CA, USA
Irène Juhan-Vague	University Hospital Timone, Marseille, France
Steven E. Kahn	VA Puget Sound Health Care System and University of Washington, Seattle, WA, USA
M. Ann Kelly	University of Birmingham, Birmingham, UK
George L. King	Joslin Diabetes Center, Harvard Medical School, Boston, MA, USA
Abbas E. Kitabchi	University of Tennessee Health Science Center, Memphis, TN, USA
Peter J.E.M Kitslaar	University Hospital Maastricht, Maastricht, The Netherlands, and Cardiovascular Research Institute Maastricht (CARIM), Maastricht, The Netherlands

Leslie P. Kozak	Pennington Biomedical Research Center, Baton Rouge, LA, USA
M.F. Laker	University of Newcastle upon Tyne, Newcastle upon Tyne, UK
Jonathan R.T. Lakey	University of Alberta, Edmonton, Canada
Karen S.L. Lam	The University of Hong Kong, Queen Mary Hospital, Hong Kong, China
H.E. Lebovitz	State University of New York, Brooklyn, NY, USA
Warren Lee	KK Women's and Children's Hospital, Singapore
Pierre J. Lefèbvre	University of Liège, Liège, Belgium
Cécile Legallais	Technological University of Compiègne, Compiègne, France
Eldon D. Lehmann	St Bartholomew's Hospital, London, UK, and Imperial College, London, UK
R.D.G. Leslie	St Bartholomew's Hospital, London, UK
Naomi S. Levitt	University of Cape Town, Cape Town, South Africa
N.J. Lewis-Barned	University of Newcastle Medical School, Newcastle upon Tyne, UK and North Tyneside General Hospital, Tyne and Wear, UK
Astrid M. Libman	University of Rosario Medical School, Rosario, Argentina
Julio Libman	University of Rosario Medical School, Rosario, Argentina
Robert S. Lindsay	MedStar Research Institute, Washington, DC, USA
Jaana Lindstrom	National Public Health Institute, Helsinki, Finland
Zhenqi Liu	University of Virginia Health System, Charlottesville, VA, USA
Pierre Maechler	University Medical Centre, Geneva, Switzerland
Lawrence Mandarino	University of Texas Health Science Center, San Antonio, TX, USA
J.I. Mann	University of Otago, Dunedin, New Zealand and Diabetes Service, Dunedin Hospital, Dunedin, New Zealand
Stuart I. Mannering	The Walter and Eliza Hall Institute of Medical Research, Parkville, Australia
Sally M. Marshall	The Medical School, University of Newcastle upon Tyne, Newcastle upon Tyne, UK
Nathan R. Martinez	The Walter and Eliza Hall Institute of Medical Research, Parkville, Australia
Jean Claude Mbanya	University of Yaoundé I, Yaoundé, Cameroon
Arne Melander	The NEPI Foundation, Medical Research Centre, University Hospital, Malmö, Sweden
Anoop Misra	The University of Texas Southwestern Medical Center at Dallas, Dallas, TX, USA
Braxton D. Mitchell	University of Maryland School of Medicine, Baltimore, MD, USA
Pierre Emmanuel Morange	University Hospital Timone, Marseille, France

Sunder Mudaliar VA San Diego Healthcare System, San Diego, CA, USA and University of California at San Diego, CA, USA

Dara Murphy Centers for Disease Control, Division of Diabetes, Atlanta, GA, USA

Mary Beth Murphy University of Tennessee Health Science Center, Memphis, TN, USA

Seiki Nambu Mukogawa Women's University, Nishinomiya, Japan

K.M.Venkat Narayan Centers for Disease Control and Prevention, National Center for Chronic Disease Prevention and Health Promotion, Atlanta, GA, USA

Parth Narendran The Walter and Eliza Hall Institute of Medical Research, Parkville, Australia

R.D.G. Neely Newcastle upon Tyne Hospitals NHS Trust, Newcastle upon Tyne, UK

Christopher B. Newgard Duke University Medical Center, Durham, NC, USA

Jens Høiriis Nielsen University of Copenhagen, Copenhagen, Denmark

Jane Overland Royal Prince Alfred Hospital, Camperdown, Australia, and The University of Sydney, Sydney, Australia

David R. Owens University of Wales College of Medicine, Cardiff, Wales, UK

Johanna Paronen Barbara Davis Center for Childhood Diabetes, University of Colorado Health Sciences Center, Denver, CO, USA, and University of Helsinki, Helsinki, Finland

Breay W. Paty University of Alberta, Edmonton, Canada

Ewan R. Pearson Peninsula Medical School, Exeter, UK

Louis Pérusse Laval University, Québec, Canada

John C. Pickup Guy's Hospital, London, UK

Vincent Poitout Pacific Northwest Research Institute, Seattle, WA, USA

Daniel Porte, Jr. VA Puget Sound Health Care System and University of Washington, Seattle, WA, USA

Paolo Pozzilli University Campus Bio Medico, Rome, Italy, and St Bartholomew's Hospital, London, UK

Stefano Del Prato University of Pisa, Pisa, Italy

Deepanwita Prusty Boston University School of Medicine, Boston, MA, USA

Qing Qiao University of Helsinki, Helsinki, Finland and National Public Health Institute, Helsinki, Finland

Rémi Rabasa-Lhoret Research Centre, Centre Hospitalier de l'Université de Montréal, Montréal, Canada and Université de Montréal, Montréal, Canada

Ambady Ramachandran Diabetes Research Centre, M.V. Hospital for Diabetes and WHO Collaborating Centre for Research Education and Training in Diabetes, Chennai, India

Lawrence I. Rand Joslin Diabetes Center, Boston, MA, USA, and Harvard Medical School, Boston, MA, USA

Christian Rask-Madsen	Joslin Diabetes Center, Harvard Medical School, Boston, MA, USA
Daiva Rastenyte	Kaunas Institute of Cardiology, Kaunas, Lithuania
Eric Ravussin	Pennington Biomedical Research Center, Baton Rouge, LA, USA
Gérard Reach	Hôpital Avicenne, Assistance Publique-Hôpitaux de Paris, Bobigny, France
Jane E.-B. Reusch	University of Colorado School of Medicine, Denver, CO, USA
Marian J. Rewers	University of Colorado Health Sciences Center, Denver, CO, USA
Christopher J. Rhodes	Pacific Northwest Research Institute, Seattle, WA, USA
Erik A. Richter	University of Copenhagen, Copenhagen, Denmark
Martin Ridderstråle	Lund University, Malmö, Sweden
R. Paul Robertson	Pacific Northwest Research Institute, Seattle, WA, USA
Arlan L. Rosenbloom	University of Florida College of Medicine, Gainesville, FL, USA
Kathy Rufo	Centers for Disease Control, Division of Diabetes, Atlanta, GA, USA
Giacomo Ruotolo	MedStar Research Institute, Washington, DC, USA
Sue Rutherford	University of Maryland School of Medicine, Baltimore, MD, USA
Edmond A. Ryan	University of Alberta, Edmonton, Canada
Christopher D. Saudek	The Johns Hopkins University School of Medicine, Baltimore, MD, USA
Simon A. Saunders	University Hospital Aintree, Liverpool, UK
Casper G. Schalkwijk	VU University Medical Centre, Amsterdam, The Netherlands
Nicolaas C. Schaper	University Hospital Maastricht, Maastricht, The Netherlands, and Cardiovascular Research Institute Maastricht (CARIM), Maastricht, The Netherlands
Michael W. Schwartz	Harborview Medical Center and University of Washington, Seattle, WA, USA
Randy J. Seeley	University of Cincinnati, Cincinnati, OH, USA
Palle Serup	Hagedorn Research Institute Gentofte, Denmark
Jawed Shafqat	Karolinska Institute, Stockholm, Sweden
A.M. James Shapiro	University of Alberta, Edmonton, Canada
Jonathan E. Shaw	International Diabetes Institute, Melbourne, Australia
A. Samad Shera	Diabetes Association of Pakistan and WHO Collaborating Centre, Karachi, Pakistan
Alan R. Shuldiner	University of Maryland School of Medicine, Baltimore, MD, USA
Kamran Siddiqi	University of Leeds, Leeds, UK
Richard W. Simpson	Monash University, Box Hill Hospital, Victoria, Australia

Alan J. Sinclair	University of Warwick, Coventry, UK
Jay S. Skyler	University of Miami, FL, USA
Chamukuttan Snehalatha	Diabetes Research Centre, M.V. Hospital for Diabetes and WHO Collaborating Centre for Research Education and Training in Diabetes, Chennai, India
Thomas J. Songer	University of Pittsburgh, Pittsburgh, PA, USA
Andrea K. Steck	University of Colorado Health Sciences Center, Denver, CO, USA
Coen D.A. Stehouwer	VU University Medical Centre, Amsterdam, The Netherlands
Roland Stein	Vanderbilt University Medical Center, Nashville, TN, USA
Raymond J. Steptoe	The Walter and Eliza Hall Institute of Medical Research, Parkville, Australia
Nelia P. Steyn	South African Medical Research Council, Tygerberg, Cape Town, South Africa
William V. Tamborlane	Yale University School of Medicine, New Haven, CT, USA
Kathryn C.B. Tan	The University of Hong Kong, Queen Mary Hospital, Hong Kong, China
Nauman Tarif	King Fiassel University, Riyadh, Saudi Arabia
Marja-Riitta Taskinen	University of Helsinki, Helsinki, Finland
P.K. Thomas	Institute of Neurology, London, UK
Antonio Tiengo	University of Padova, Padova, Italy
P. Tong	The Chinese University of Hong Kong, Hong Kong, China
John E. Tooke	Peninsula Medical School, Plymouth, UK
Russell P. Tracy	College of Medicine, The University of Vermont, Burlington, VT, USA
Jaakko Tuomilehto	University of Helsinki, Helsinki, Finland and National Public Health Institute, Helsinki, Finland
Guillermo E. Umpierrez	University of Tennessee Health Science Center, Memphis, TN, USA
Kristina M. Utzschneider	VA Puget Sound Health Care System and University of Washington, Seattle, WA, USA
Aristidis Veves	Harvard Medical School, Boston, MA, USA
Frank Vinicor	Centers for Disease Control, Division of Diabetes, Atlanta, GA, USA
Vijay Viswanathan	Diabetes Research Centre, MV Hospital for Diabetes and WHO Collaborating Centre for Research Education and Training in Diabetes, Chennai, India
John Wahren	Karolinska Institute, Stockholm, Sweden
Richard M. Watanabe	University of Southern California, Los Angeles, CA, USA
Stuart A. Weinzimer	Yale University School of Medicine, New Haven, CT, USA

Desmond E. Williams	Centers for Disease Control and Prevention, National Center for Chronic Disease Prevention and Health Promotion, Atlanta, GA, USA
Gareth Williams	University of Bristol, Bristol, UK
Rhys Williams	University of Leeds, Leeds, UK
Claes B. Wollheim	University Medical Centre, Geneva, Switzerland
Stephen C. Woods	University of Cincinnati, Cincinnati, OH, USA
Hannele Yki-Järvinen	Helsinki University, Helsinki, Finland
David A. York	Louisiana State University, Baton Rouge, LA, USA
John S. Yudkin	Royal Free and University College Medical School, London, UK
Paul Zimmet	International Diabetes Institute, Melbourne, Australia
Bernard Zinman	Mount Sinai Hospital, Toronto, Canada

Preface

The late and lamented David Pyke used to say that two notable things happened in 1921. First, he was born. Second, insulin was isolated. Although little has happened in diabetes since to match either event, especially the latter, our knowledge of the disease, its surrounding pathophysiology, and its roots in the basic sciences has grown stupendously. Those working with diabetes, whether in the clinics, in the laboratories, or, increasingly, in government or international health agencies, are overwhelmed by the sheer torrent of new diabetes-related information that flows daily from professional journals, from the media, and from cyberspace. In many parts of the world, the prospects for the person with diabetes have never been better. The threat of diabetic blindness has receded, kidney failure can be anticipated and its progression greatly attenuated, the spectre of gangrene and limb amputation has retreated, we have almost come to expect a successful outcome of pregnancy, and even the great atherosclerotic behemoth begins to shrink.

Nonetheless, although the devastating complications of the disease have been mollified, they are still with us and still of uncertain mechanisms. To many people with diabetes, the benefits of these advances are not available. Despite the explosion in understanding, the breathtaking technological bravura, and our well-furnished therapeutic armoury, we are actually losing the battle against diabetes and, at best, engaged in a fighting retreat. Paradoxically, this "failure" is an almost direct consequence of "success" elsewhere. The global population continues to expand, with the biggest contribution from peoples seemingly most susceptible to diabetes. A growing abundance of foods coincides with falling physical energy requirements as machines take on the hard labor. Adaptation falls far short of perfect, and obesity inexorably engulfs a growing portion of the population at an earlier age. Our much sought-after increasing longevity comes at a price, of which greater risk of diabetes is only part. In many industrialized countries, these threats to health have been recognized, often by the better educated and financially more privileged members of society, who have successfully adapted their lifestyle to maintain higher levels of physical activity and to reduce the risk of obesity and the complications which follow in its wake.

Diabetes is often represented as a prime exemplar of a maladaptive response of a genetic constitution fashioned to fit a human environment subject to intermittent famine, exotic infections, and frequent recourse to "fight and flight." This entirely plausible (but untestable) hypothesis, memorably given literary immortality by J. V. Neel with his "thrifty genotype," carried the implication that in type 2 diabetes the genetic component(s) would be likely to be found among the genomic elements concerned with adapting insulin production or insulin effects (or both) to the prevailing "nutritional climate." The clear evidence of bimodality in the distribution of glucose tolerance/intolerance in, first, the Pima Indian and then the Nauruan, Mexican American, and other high diabetes prevalence societies raised the expectation that a single gene, or at most a very small number of genes, of substantial effect would distinguish between the upper and lower modes of the distribution. To date, despite the wide application of the powerful methods of genetic analysis now available, such offending genes have not been identified and bimodality remains unexplained.

We have always been conscious of the wide front on which diabetes knowledge advances and have tried to reflect this in the breadth of subject and versatility of authorship of the *International Textbook of Diabetes Mellitus* (ITDM). At the same time, we have always tried to highlight the growing points of knowledge and, more difficult, to anticipate growth areas and to set some authoritative pointers to the future. Backing the whole enterprise, we have also attempted to present, as far as we are able to in two volumes, the firm foundation of validated knowledge on which our day-to-day clinical decisions and our broad strategies and directions of research are based. Even these laudable activities and objectives are in flux. The very process of information storage, organization, and transfer has been revolutionized by the Internet and this has affected us all. Not least, ITDM has responded to the challenge and is bringing its content to the diabetes community both in familiar hard copy and, hot from the keyboard, through the Internet (http://www.mrw.interscience.wiley.com/itdm). This will allow existing chapters to be updated as new information becomes available, and new chapters to be added, without the necessarily longer turnaround time, which has been the case with print publication. In due course it is possible that a more interactive element may also be added, allowing readers and authors a forum to comment on and discuss points of interest. We certainly welcome feedback on this latest edition of ITDM and will seriously consider readers' suggestions for future inclusions and improvements.

Harry Keen

April 2004

Introduction

INTRODUCTION TO THE THIRD EDITION

The *International Textbook of Diabetes Mellitus* (ITDM), now in its third edition, has become the most widely referenced textbook of diabetes worldwide. It is the only textbook that truly engages the expertise of clinicians, educators, and investigators from widely diverse regions of the world. It provides a comprehensive overview of the treatment of diabetes and its associated microvascular and macrovascular complications. However, it is unique in that it also addresses the specific pathogenic mechanisms, the diverse epidemiological features of diabetes and its complications, clinical presentations, diagnostic evaluation, and therapeutic approaches, that are unique to different ethnic groups and countries throughout the world.

The current edition of the *International Textbook of Diabetes Mellitus* has been extensively reorganized, with 11 major subdivisions (Epidemiology; Normal Physiology of Pancreatic Function; Normal Physiology of Insulin Action; Pathogenesis; Obesity; Management of Diabetes: Diet, Exercise, and Drugs; Management of Diabetes: Monitoring and Other Interventions; Complications: General and Microvascular; Complications: Macrovascular Disease; Management of Diabetes: Glucose and Lipid Monitoring, Specific Subgroups; and Diabetes and Public Health), each headed by a Section Editor who is an internationally recognized authority in his/her area. A number of new chapters have been added, among them:

- Development and Life Cycle of a β-Cell
- Mechanisms of Insulin Signal Transduction
- Monogenic Disorders of the β-Cell
- Is Type 2 Diabetes the Result of a "Thrifty Genotype" or a "Thrifty Phenotype"?
- The Genetics of Human Obesity
- Role of the Adipocyte in Type 2 Diabetes
- Treatment of Obesity
- The Role of the Hypothalamus in the Maintenance of Energy Balance and Peripheral Glucose Control
- Thiazolidinediones as PPAR Agonists
- Combination Therapy in Type 2 Diabetes
- Periodontal Disease and Diabetes Mellitus
- Erectile Dysfunction in Diabetes Mellitus
- The Syndrome of Insulin Resistance and Its Links to Atherosclerosis
- Endothelial Function and Dysfunction
- Cerebrovascular Disease in Diabetes Mellitus
- Prevention of Type 1 Diabetes
- Prevention of Type 2 Diabetes

In addition, several previous chapters have been combined, and all chapters (including those combined) have been revised extensively since the last edition of the Textbook seven years ago. In an attempt to introduce fresh looks and perspectives to keep the *International Textbook of Diabetes Mellitus* current, approximately one third of the authors have been replaced since the previous edition. An innovative feature of the current edition is the availability of all chapters online (http://www.mrw.interscience.wiley.com/itdm), with regular updates scheduled depending upon scientific advances and growth of knowledge in specific areas.

Ralph A. DeFronzo
Ele Ferrannini
Harry Keen
Paul Zimmet

April 2004

INTRODUCTION TO THE SECOND EDITION

It has been four years since the first edition of *International Textbook of Diabetes Mellitus* appeared. At that time we attempted to give a broader sweep to our coverage of diabetes than was customary in the available "Northern" textbooks. This was due in part to the pandemic of diabetes that was, and still is, sweeping the globe, and in part to the lack of texts dealing with diabetes in non-Europids. We felt that much could be learned by considering diabetes in relation to different ethnic groups, cultures, and geographical settings. We also attempted to cover the whole of diabetes, from the gene and cell biology to the social and economic aspects. Further background to the rationale of ITDM is given in the original introduction, which is reprinted below.

We have been encouraged by the response to the first edition: hence the present volumes. This second edition does not, however, just represent a reworking of the previous volumes. Several new chapters have been added, others replaced, and many new authors introduced. We hope that we have been able to enhance the previous edition and also remain current and relevant.

K.G.M.M. Alberti
P.Z. Zimmet
R.A. DeFronzo

INTRODUCTION TO THE FIRST EDITION

A modern textbook of diabetes should be international in scope. Not only does it draw on the knowledge and expertise of people from all over the world, but it also reminds us that no race of mankind is immune from the diabetic state. Ethnic susceptibility to diabetes varies tremendously, a variation in liability that must depend both upon the widely differing conditions in which the human species exists and upon the diversity of the genetic endowment. It is important to our understanding of the nature of diabetes mellitus and our attempts to prevent and treat it that we view the diabetic state as the outcome of the interplay of a multiplicity of causal factors, potentially varying in both the genetic and the environmental components of the mix. Although the diabetic state can itself be clearly defined—we, after all, are responsible for creating the definition—it is, nevertheless, heterogeneous in its causation and in its consequences. In investigating its mechanisms we should be prepared to find differences between, and even within, populations in the nature of the underlying susceptibility and in the factors that provoke its emergence and its pathological sequelae.

Before attempting to explain the diabetic state, we should agree upon its definition. Those who coined the term *diabetes mellitus* had little doubt: originally, it described a grave sickness characterized by dramatic symptoms—intense thirst, profuse urination, rapid wasting, inexorably proceeding through the stages of vomiting and drowsiness to coma and death. The term *diabetes* was no more than a description of these characteristic symptoms; *mellitus* was added when the sweetness of the urine indicated its high sugar content and distinguished it from the insipid, sugar-free variety.

Identification of the urinary sugar as glucose can be said to have ushered in the era of clinical chemistry. However, it was not until laboratory methods were sufficiently refined that the central importance of hyperglycemia in the diabetic state and its primacy in diabetes diagnosis were recognized. This transition from clinical to chemical diagnosis had a profound effect on the diagnostic concept of diabetes: it resulted in the addition to the same diagnostic rubric of ever-larger numbers of cases with ever-lessening degrees of symptomatology. This conceptual inflation reached its limits with the application of preemptive screening tests for diabetes to large sections of the general population. Now, the diagnosis was called upon to accommodate cases without symptoms or signs, sometimes even without glucose in the urine. The existence of a state of "pathological hyperglycemia" had become the main justification for including in the same diagnostic category a spectrum of abnormality which ranged from a totally asymptomatic transgression of an arbitrary blood glucose norm at the one extreme, to a potentially lethal metabolic catastrophe at the other. A further justification for retaining the single diagnostic term was the common liability to the ultimate development of a characteristic set of organ and tissue abnormalities—the complications of diabetes.

Population surveys for diabetes, with the new diagnostic perspectives that they generated, stemmed from the recognition of the high prevalence of unsuspected diabetes and the hope that early detection and treatment might avert its complications. Large population samples were tested, many being submitted to measurements of blood glucose concentration in response to a glucose challenge. It was difficulty with interpretation of the results of such surveys that brought the diagnostic definition of diabetes to critical review. Unexpectedly large numbers of apparently healthy people had blood glucose levels at the suspiciously high end of the range, their frequency increasing with age. At no age could a "natural" dividing line be found separating normal from diabetic glycemic responses. Depending on which set of diagnostic criteria were adopted, the estimates of diabetes frequency in a given population could vary as much as 10-fold. As a consequence, an individual diagnosed as unquestionably diabetic by one doctor could be equally emphatically reassured of normality by another. Add to this the substantial variation introduced by differences in the methods of diagnostic testing, and the reasons for the moves toward national and international standardization of the 1970s and early 1980s become clear. A measure of order was introduced in consensus meetings of a number of national diabetes organizations, principally the US National Diabetes Data Group, and soon after by the World Health Organization (WHO). They agreed upon a set of glycemic criteria for diabetes diagnosis and interposed a new category of "impaired glucose tolerance" (IGT) between clearly normal and clearly diabetic glycemic responses. Although these proposals are by no means above criticism, they have been increasingly widely applied in both clinical practice and epidemiological investigation, and provide a degree of comparability and uniformity that was previously lacking.

The international perspective is also appropriate to the classification of the diabetic state, which also has been the subject of concern and revision over the past decade. The two major types of diabetes mellitus, insulin dependent (IDDM or type 1) and non-insulin dependent

(NIDDM or type 2), are essentially defined by their clinical characteristics, although these largely correspond (in people of European origin) to underlying etiological mechanisms and, perhaps, to genetic liabilities. The frequency of IDDM or type 1 diabetes—the severe disease of classic description—is notably higher in peoples of European origin, although it has been reported almost universally in others. NIDDM also has rather different characteristics in Europeans, compared with most other ethnic groups: its prevalence is lower, it appears later in life, and it is, perhaps, less liable to lead to renal failure, possibly because of its later appearance. Malnutrition-related diabetes mellitus (MRDM) appeared in the most recent WHO classification as an independent type. Its existence as a tropical variant of diabetes, secondary to pancreatic damage and etiologically related to dietary protein deficiency or to toxic food contaminants, has been the subject of debate and investigation in recent years. More systematic investigation is needed before the size and nature of this problem can be confidently documented.

NIDDM is by far the largest problem numerically on a global scale. In the most susceptible populations, up to one person in two may expect to develop the disease. The Pima tribe of American Indians, currently topping the league tables for diabetes prevalence, has shown what appears to be an explosive increase in incidence over the course of this century. The tribe was visited in the early 1930s by Dr E.P. Joslin, the doyen of diabetes in the United States, who was interested in the reputed rarity of diabetes among its members. This dramatic transformation must have been the response to some widespread environmental change affecting a relatively inbred population carrying some underlying genetic susceptibility to the disease: a steeply rising prevalence of obesity is widely held to have been the environmental determinant; the genetic susceptibility factor has as yet eluded definition. At the present pace of genetic research and discovery, its detection can only be a matter of time. When it is found, however, will it prove to be the same as that determining susceptibility to NIDDM in other populations? On the face of it, it seems unlikely that NIDDM is a single homogeneous entity *within* populations, let alone *between* them. Its associations with age, adiposity, and clinical progression appear so diverse that a multiplicity of underlying mechanisms appears probable.

In recent years some part of this broad spectrum of NIDDM and IGT have been linked with a number of other common disorders and conditions, such as hypertension, hyperlipidemia, and hyperinsulinemia. From this has emerged the view that this form of glucose intolerance may only be part—and not an obligatory part at that—of some much more general disturbance of adaptation to the conditions of modern life. Characterized by diminished tissue sensitivity to the effects of insulin and associated with a centripetal distribution of body fat and increased liability to atherosclerosis, this so-called syndrome X currently attracts the attention of many investigators. In a continuum of interacting mechanisms that may contribute to a number of important human disorders, glucose intolerance or diabetes may have a small or even nonexistent role. Other broad classes of NIDDM may be described, without obesity, with early age of onset, and with evidence of islet autoimmunity, which highlight its probable heterogeneity.

It is the so-called complications of diabetes that today constitute the main burden for patients, their families, and the societies in which they live. Blindness due to retinopathy, such a dreaded hazard a generation ago, is now in large part a preventable disaster, provided that facilities for eye screening and timely photocoagulation are available. The long period of ill health as diabetic renal disease neared its termination in end-stage renal failure can now be reversed with modern renal substitution methods of dialysis and transplantation; there is reason to suppose that the stage of renal failure may be postponed and the number of patients entering renal failure greatly diminished, again depending upon facilities for the early recognition of those at risk and their appropriately monitored treatment. There is some evidence that people with the increased arterial disease risk of diabetes are sharing in the general diminution in coronary heart disease morbidity and mortality documented in some societies over the past 20 years. This strongly suggests that much of the aggravated risk of atherosclerotic disease in diabetes could be reduced. Even the morbid effects of that most intransigent of diabetic complications—neuropathy—can be ameliorated by the application of quite simple preventative measures. The scope of diabetes care has expanded dramatically in recent years, with the promise of longer and healthier years of life for many and (that prize so beloved of health politicians) a reduction in the enormous costs of health-care provision for diabetic complications. The remarkable advances of knowledge have firmly placed on the agenda even the prevention of diabetes itself.

It is our hope that we have been able, in this book, to cover most of this broad panorama of diabetes, from the molecular structures responsible for susceptibility, through the hormonal and biochemical mechanisms responsible for the clinical manifestations and complications of the disease, to the therapeutic agencies and their availability to ameliorate, arrest, reverse, or even prevent its damaging impact. Much remains to be discovered; we are still far short of a full understanding of the disease. Much that is known remains to be applied; it is important to translate what we know into what we do. We hope that this book will enhance the understanding of diabetes mellitus and help in applying that understanding to the better care of people with diabetes.

Harry Keen
George Alberti
Ralph DeFronzo
Paul Zimmet

Management of Diabetes: Monitoring and Other Interventions

54

Alternative Routes of Insulin Delivery

David R. Owens*, **Geremia B. Bolli**†, **and Bernard Zinman**‡

**University of Wales College of Medicine, Cardiff, Wales, UK, †University of Perugia, Perugia, Italy, and ‡Mount Sinai Hospital, Toronto, Canada*

INTRODUCTION

Identification of the pancreas as the site of the defect in diabetes mellitus by von Mehring and Minkowski in 1889 led eventually to the identification and successful extraction of insulin in 1921 by Banting and Best [1]. The availability of insulin for therapy shortly afterwards dramatically changed the lives of patients with diabetes who previously had a life expectancy of less than 2 years. In the 80 years since, major benefits have accrued. In the year 2000 alone, it is estimated that about 4.8 million years of life were gained for patients with type 1 diabetes as a result of insulin treatment, assuming a life expectancy of 1.5 years in its absence and a global prevalence of 5.1 million. Since insulin was first introduced into clinical practice there have been major developments in its production, purification, pharmaceutical formulation, and methods of delivery. However, despite these advances, microvascular and premature macrovascular complications persist as the main cause of morbidity and mortality in both type 1 and type 2 diabetes and represent a constant reminder that current therapeutic and management strategies, for the vast majority of our patients, remain woefully inadequate. Restoring near normal blood glucose levels to prevent the development and progression of the devastating complications of diabetes was strongly advocated by Joslin in the 1930s, more than 50 years before the emergence of incontrovertible evidence from both the Diabetes Control and Complication Trial and the United Kingdom Prospective Diabetes Study [2, 3]. Consequently, attempting to replicate physiological insulin secretion as a means of restoring the normal metabolic milieu and thus eliminate the risk of diabetic complications has become an essential feature of insulin treatment. The need for intensive insulin therapy regimens involving multiple daily subcutaneous injections has led to improvements in glycemic control but imposes a burden of compliance on patients. In this chapter, we describe the many attempts made to develop alternative, less invasive routes for the delivery of insulin while focusing on recent progress achieved with inhaled insulins, which may provide the first opportunity for at least partial independence from subcutaneous injections (Figure 1).

NORMAL PHYSIOLOGY—GLUCOSE HOMEOSTASIS

The plasma glucose concentration in healthy subjects is retained within a narrow range throughout the day (3.5–7.0 mmol/l) despite wide fluctuations in nutritional intake and physical exercise as well as other physiological, psychological, and iatrogenic influences. The postabsorptive (fasting) state represents a near equilibrium between the rates of endogenous glucose production and utilization. During fasting, the liver generates about 80% of the glucose entering the circulation with equal contributions from glycogenolysis and gluconeogenesis, but with increasing reliance on renal gluconeogenesis during prolonged fasting. Glucose production is under the precise control of both glucoregulatory hormones and nonhormonal mechanisms. The balance between insulin and glucagon concentration is critical in the regulation of hepatic glucose output. This is also influenced by the other glucoregulatory hormones, catecholamines, glucocorticoids, and growth hormone. In the postabsorptive state, glucose uptake occurs predominantly by the brain (~50–60%), skeletal muscle (~15–20%), and kidneys (~10–15%), and is virtually independent of basal insulin concentrations.

International Textbook of Diabetes Mellitus, Third Edition. Edited by R. A. DeFronzo, E. Ferrannini, H. Keen, and P. Zimmet.
 ISBN: 0-471-48655-8.

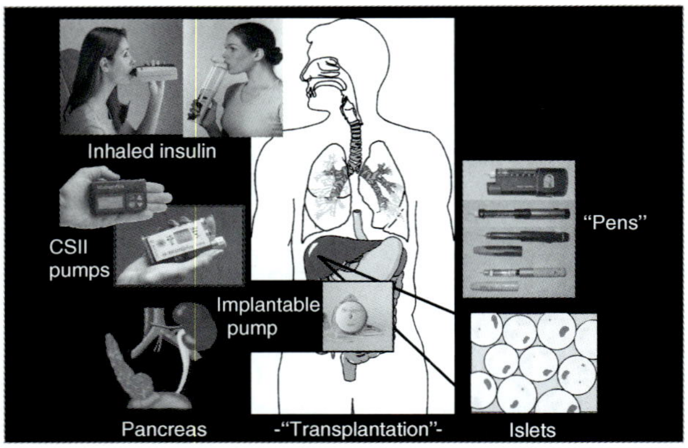

Figure 1 Routes of insulin delivery

In the postprandial state, glucose homeostasis is reliant upon the early suppression of endogenous hepatic glucose release, hepatic glucose extraction, and peripheral tissue glucose uptake. The early secretion of insulin in response to a nutrient challenge and the reciprocal inhibition of glucagon are essential in maintaining normal postprandial glucose homeostasis because of a prompt decrease in endogenous glucose production and increased hepatic glucose extraction. Approximately 80% of postprandial glucose disposal is reliant on both the direct (insulin-sensitive tissues) and indirect (limiting availability of gluconeogenic substrate) actions of insulin in promoting glucose transport. In normal subjects, the ingestion of a meal is followed by a rise in plasma glucose levels, which peaks in 30–60 min, returning to basal levels, or below, within the following 2–3 h. Plasma insulin concentrations follow a similar pattern. In persons with type 2 diabetes, the quantitative, qualitative, and temporal pattern of postprandial insulin secretion is grossly disrupted.

PERORAL (ENTERIC-GASTROINTESTINAL) ROUTE OF DELIVERY

The ability to deliver insulin orally offers convenience for patients and therefore the potential for glycemic control. Attempts, however, to develop this route of administration have met with little or no success [4]. The various epithelial surfaces of the gastrointestinal tract (GIT) are an effective barrier to the absorption of polypeptide drugs. Insulin is degraded intralumenally in the acid environment of the stomach and by digestive enzymes (trypsin and α-chymotrypsin) in the small intestine as well as being exposed to a cytosolic insulin-degrading enzyme in the gut wall. Dysmotility of the GIT associated with diabetes (gastroparesis, etc.) is another complicating factor [5] (Table 1).

Both individual and combination strategies are continuously being developed in an attempt to enhance insulin absorption sufficiently for therapeutic use. The coadministration of enzyme inhibitors and/or permeation enhancers with insulin has been extensively explored as have been methods of improving insulin's chemical stability (structural modifications, pharmaceutical formulations) and the use of muco-bioadhesive materials, liposomes, emulsions, or polymer-based delivery systems [6]. However, despite the many different strategies employed to overcome the physical and chemical barriers presented by the GIT, generally less than 1% of orally administered insulin is absorbed [7].

The concept of utilizing liposomes for drug delivery was introduced during the 1970s [8]. Incorporating insulin into liposomes has since been extensively investigated but almost exclusively in animal studies [6, 9]. Varying degrees of blood glucose lowering have been reported dependent upon such factors as lipid composition, size, surface charge, and physical state of the phospholipid bilayer employed, which help to determine the rate and site of clearance of the liposomal vesicles [10–12]. Conventional liposomes are susceptible to both enzymatic degradation and bile salt dissolution although they can be made resistant to the gastrointestinal environment by different strategies including polymerization, which allows them to be absorbed relatively intact prior to dispersion in the circulation before reaching the target cells [13, 14]. Coating the insulin with a pH-dependent acrylic-based biodegradable polymer (with or without an absorption enhancer) [15] or encapsulation into enteric coated microspheres [16] has also been tried. Microspheres in the nanosize range are absorbed intact across the intestinal epithelium before reaching in the liver where their residence time is dependent upon the degradation rate of the polymer vesicle. Oral administration of insulin encapsulated in biocompatible self-assembled "nanocubicles" appears effective in animal studies [17].

Other strategies employed to enhance absorption include modification of insulin by the covalent attachment of one or more low molecular weight amphiphilic oligomers (carriers) in order to improve both the stability against enzymatic degradation and solubility of the insulin. Absorption across the gut wall of encapsulated conjugated hexyl insulin monoconjugate 2, where the amphiphilic polymer is attached at B29 lysine, has been demonstrated in both

Table 1 *Oral-enteric* route of administration

- Advantages
  - Rapid absorption
  - Direct to liver
    - Lower systemic insulinemia
    - Restores glycogen status
    - Control hepatic glucose output
  - Enhanced compliance
- Disadvantages
  - Effect of food types
  - GIT dysmotility
  - Taste/smell

nondiabetic subjects and patients with type 1 and type 2 diabetes [18]. Nonacylated amino acids are also being utilized to facilitate the absorption of insulin. Noncovalent complexes formed between carrier molecules and insulin induce partial and reversible unfolding ('molten globule' state) of the insulin molecule. This conformational change exposes insulin's hydrophobic side chains, thereby facilitating passive diffusion across cell membranes before the complex eventually dissociates beyond the epithelial cell [19].

Another avenue being explored is transfection of the pancreas by retrograde ductal injection of a plasmid containing the human insulin coding sequence ("gut gene therapy") [20]. Other attempts include controlling insulin release by transfecting human fibroblast cell lines with fusion proteins consisting of the signal sequence for human insulin, which accumulate in the endoplasmic reticulum. Adding a synthetic ligand results in dissociation of the fusion protein aggregates, releasing insulin from the endoplasmic reticulum, employing different technologies to provide either a rapid or a slow release of insulin.

The oral route of insulin administration promises to remain a major challenge for some time to come, compounded by issues relating to dosage and timing of administration, with safety a high priority throughout.

ORAL: BUCCAL AND SUBLINGUAL ROUTES OF DELIVERY

Administering polypeptide drugs noninvasively through the mucosae of the mouth is a potentially attractive option. The oral cavity is easily accessible, has a large surface area for absorption (100–200 cm^2) with little proteolytic activity, and is highly vascularized. However, this route presents special problems for the delivery of insulin. The nonkeratinized multilayered squamous epithelium of the buccal and sublingual mucosae (~60% of oral mucosal surface area) combined with the constant flow of saliva in the mouth constitutes an effective barrier to absorption. The permeability of the keratinized mucosa of the gums, palatal mucosa, and inner lips is lower.

The use of absorption enhancers (surfactants, bile salts, chelators, alcohol, and fatty acids), alone or combined with bioadhesive delivery systems (gels, films, patches), to enhance the mucosal permeability of insulin has been extensively tested in animal studies. Reductions in blood glucose of up to 30% relative to intramuscular insulin have been reported but the studies have lacked reproducibility [21, 22].

Many other options for improving absorption have been tried including the addition of enzyme inhibitors and/or molecular modifications to increase the lipophilicity of the insulin molecule (conjugation with various polymers, acylation, methylation) and the use of prodrugs [23–25]. Further efforts have been made to develop mucoadhesive delivery systems incorporating insulin with or without enhancers into different liposomal formulations including highly deformable lipid vesicles (transfersome) that encapsulate the insulin [26, 27].

Studies in humans evaluating the buccal and sublingual routes of insulin delivery have been limited. Reductions in blood glucose have been recorded in a small number of patients with type 1 diabetes but only after multiple applications of a liquid human insulin spray [28]. In contrast to animal studies, the coadministration of an absorption enhancer (1% sodium glycocholate) had no perceived effect on blood glucose [25]. Another liquid insulin aerosol formulation has been developed that contains mixed micelles made from a combination of absorption enhancers that incorporates the insulin [29]. Limited data in patients with type 1 and type 2 diabetes suggest a more rapid and shorter lived hypoglycemic response to multiple topical (spray) applications when compared to SC human soluble insulin. Local tolerability appears acceptable, but bioavailability remains low [29, 30].

The multitude of techniques already tested illustrates the inherent difficulties associated with the oro-buccal route of insulin administration. Combined strategies seem to be the most likely route to possible future success. The safety of the various absorption enhancers used in these strategies is of paramount importance, with acute and long-term evaluation necessary prior to their clinical use in patients with diabetes.

RECTAL

Administration of insulin by the rectal route is potentially advantageous because local enzymatic degradation is avoided and most of the insulin enters the systemic circulation via the lymphatic system, circumventing the hepatic extraction of insulin that occurs by some other routes. Compared to SC injection, rectally delivered insulin acts more rapidly and is shorter lived. However, absorption of insulin from the rectum is poor and inconsistent and requires the incorporation of enhancers into suppositories or gel formulations to improve absorption. Bioavailability in humans is very low (4–10%) and appears not to be dose related.

A short-term impact on blood glucose has been reported both in normal subjects and in patients with type 1 and type 2 diabetes following single or repeated rectally applied doses [31–33]. The long-term acceptance of this route of delivery by patients seems unlikely, which, along with the relatively poor and erratic absorption and the potential for mucosal damage, mitigates against its clinical usefulness. Future options for improved absorption by this route include the concomittant use of polyunsaturated fatty acids formulated into gels or emulsions [34, 35], bioadhesive hydrogel preparations containing absorption promoters [36, 37], or suppositories containing insulin-β-cyclodextrin complexes [38]. Long-term safety and efficacy will need to be demonstrated before consideration for clinical use.

OCULAR AND INTRAVAGINAL ROUTES

The bioavailability of insulin absorbed following ocular administration is poor ($\leq$1%) and as such produces little or no effect on blood glucose in normal subjects [39]. When absorption enhancers such as saponin are present, insulin is rapidly absorbed from the conjunctival sac, [40]. The coadministration of insulin with the promoter Laureth-9 or bile salts increases overall bioavailability to between 4 and 13% [41]. Of the administered insulin most is absorbed via the nasal mucosa, which it reaches through the lacrimal duct [42]. The small volume of the conjunctival sac and consequent requirement for both higher insulin concentrations and chemical enhancers represents a major limitation of this route of administration.

Animal studies have shown that absorption of insulin across the vaginal mucosa is minimal but is increased substantially by the inclusion of absorption promoters [43, 44] or the use of bioadhesive microspheres [45]. However, severe local adverse effects and histological changes have been observed following the intravaginal application of insulin [46]. The one small pharmacokinetic study that has been carried out found highly variable absorption of insulin from the vagina according to the presence of local infection, pregnancy, or following the menopause [47]. Unsurprisingly, this latter route offers little or no real opportunities in the clinical management of the patient with insulin-requiring diabetes.

TRANSDERMAL DELIVERY

Although the skin is the largest and most accessible organ of the body with a surface area of 1–2 m^2, it is relatively impermeable to large (molecular weight >500 Da) hydrophilic polypeptides such as insulin. The impermeability of the skin is due predominately to the outermost layer of the epidermis, the stratum corneum, which consists of dead keratin filled cells in a lipid matrix [48]. The composition of the intercellular lipid layer (cholesterol, cholesteryl esters, fatty acids, ceramides) is a major determinant of the skin's permeability [49]. Attempts to optimize the transdermal drug delivery of drugs have included the breaking down or removal of the lipid barrier by a variety of chemical, electrical, or physical methods used singly or in combinations (Table 2). Iontophoresis [50–53], low frequency ultrasound (phonophoresis) [54–55], and drug carrier agents (various liposomes and lipid suspensions) [56], either with or without the pretreatment or concomittant use chemical enhancers (surfactants, solvents), are the main methodologies being explored (Figure 2).

Table 2 Strategies for enhancing absorption of insulin via the skin

- Enhancing flux by *physical* means
  - Debridement, stripping
  - Iontophoresis (direct current, alternating current)
  - Ultrasound/sonophoresis
  - Electroporation
- Enhancing flux by *chemical* means
  - Absorption enhancers
  - Vehicles
  - Modification of insulin
- Combinations

The use of cathodal iontophoresis to transfer hexameric soluble insulin across untreated skin is inefficient but can be improved by stripping off of the stratum corneum, shaving the hair, or by applying highly charged or monomeric insulin analogues following pretreatment of the skin with delipidating agents (e.g. absolute alcohol) [53]. Even so, the amount of insulin transferred is barely enough to satisfy basal insulin requirements. while some enhancement in absorption has been achieved with systems employing pulsed rather than continuous direct current, the transdermal transfer of insulin remains poor [57]. Apart from the issue of safety of the various chemical and physical pretreatment procedures being used with this approach, an assessment of the specific biophysical impact of iontophoresis [58] will be required.

The use of low frequency (20–150 kHz) ultrasound (sonophoresis) for periods up to 1.5 h results in increased transdermal transfer of insulin applied to the skin as an aqueous solution or mixed with an ultrasound coupler such as hydrogel. Several studies using this method have demonstrated reductions in blood glucose [54–56, 59]. A proposed mechanism of action of ultrasound involves the formation of aqueous pathways by disrupting the lipid matrix in the stratum corneum, a process known as cavitation. Ultrasound may also cause deactivation of skin proteolytic enzymes. The efficiency of the ultrasound

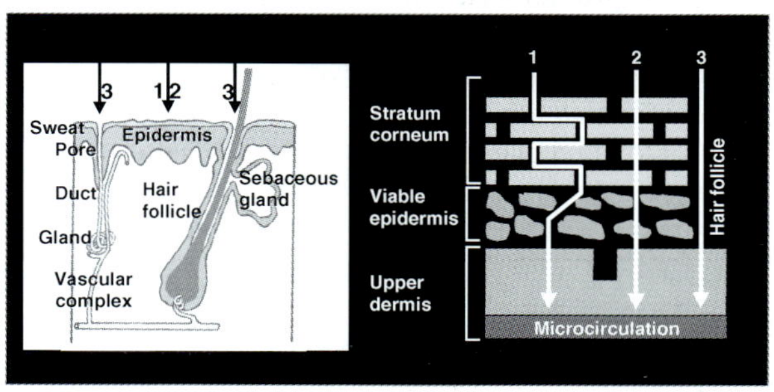

Figure 2 Dermal route of insulin delivery: paracellular (1), transcellular (2), and (3) follicular (appendages) routes of penetration

technique depends upon the energy density and length of the ultrasound pulse with no enhancement by pre-treatment of the skin [56]. It is also being proposed that iontophoresis and ultrasound may work synergistically [60]. Other physical methods of potential value include the use of microneedles or electroporation to bypass the stratum corneum, magnetophoresis, or employing a laser pulse directed at insulin in solution to generate a photomechanical wave [61].

The incorporation of insulin into highly deformable, liposome-like lipid vesicles known as transfersomes was reported to result in intercellular transdermal transfer rates of the order of 50%. However, subsequent, more recent studies have been unable to reproduce these initial results. A number of other liposomal variants are being investigated including ethosomes and niosomes produced by incorporating ethanol and nonionic surfactants respectively.

Despite the numerous strategies employed to enhance the transdermal transfer of insulin, success has been very limited. In order to provide a basal insulin supply utilizing this route of delivery, newer methods will need to be explored to include combining the different physical and/or chemical technologies available [62, 63].

INTRANASAL DELIVERY

The nasal cavity provides a relatively large epithelial surface (~150 cm^2) for the absorption of polypeptide drugs. The main respiratory area is lined with pseudostratified, ciliated columnar epithelial cells interspersed with goblet cells, which rest on a basement membrane punctuated by seromucous glands overlying a rich vascular and lymphatic subepithelium. The main barriers to absorption include the very active mucociliary clearance mechanism (flow rate 1–20 mm/min, residence half-life 10–20 min) and the presence of proteolytic enzymes (aminopeptidases) in the nasal fluid, mucosal cell, and lamina propria. Early attempts in the 1920s to explore the potential of nasal insulin delivery met with little or no success until surfactants (saponin, glycol) were added to the insulin. However, unacceptable local reactions to the absorption promotors and a requirement for large doses of insulin led researchers to discontinue their efforts. Interest resumed some 50 years later, since when a variety of physical and formulation changes (delivery devices, droplets, sprays, etc.) and chemical additives have been used in an attempt to enhance the absorption of insulin across the nasal epithelium.

An extensive variety of absorption enhancers have been tested both in normal subjects and in patients with type 1 and type 2 diabetes. These include bile salts and their derivatives [sodium deoxycholate (SDC), sodium glycocholate (SGC), sodium taurodihydrofusidate (STDHF)], surfactants [Laureth-9 spray], fatty acids and their derivatives [didecanoylphosphatidycholine (DDPC)], and cyclodextrins [dimethyl-β-cyclodextrin (DMβCD)] [64–67]. Proposed mechanisms of action of the various enhancers include opening the intercellular tight junctions, disruption of the epithelial cell membrane, and/or mucolytic activity. Histological studies in animals have revealed a variety of mucosal cell damage on exposure to absorption promoters, especially SDC and STDHF and to a lesser extent SGC, with cyclodextrins the least problematic [64, 68, 69].

Other methods used to improve insulin absorption involve inhibiting nasal proteases or retarding the removal of insulin from the nose with bioadhesive preparations [66, 67, 70]. Lipid emulsions, various liposomal particles, and nonionic surfactants such as alkylglycosides have also been used as enhancers of nasal insulin absorption.

The bioavailability of intranasal insulin varies according to the type, volume and concentration of both the enhancer and the insulin, the size, density, shape and hygroscopicity of the particles as well as the airflow characteristics and the presence of nasal pathology [66, 69, 70]. Animal studies have not necessarily been good predictors of bioavailability in humans. Compared to the IV and SC routes of administration in humans, the bioavailability of insulin delivered by the nasal route is lower, rarely exceeding 20% [65–67, 69, 71]. The coefficient of variation is also higher compared to the SC route (44 and 22% respectively) [72].

In patients with type 2 diabetes, a single application of nasal insulin produced a rapid but relatively short-lived increase in plasma insulin, which failed to adequately control prandial glucose excursions [73]. This suggested the need for either a much higher dose or repeated applications during the course of a meal [74, 75]. In patients with type 1 diabetes, serial doses of intranasal insulin at 30-min intervals from the onset of a meal were required to lower postprandial hyperglycemia [76] (Table 3). Longer term clinical studies (1–4 months) involving relatively small

Table 3 Summary of long-term clinical studies using intranasal insulin

Author	Patients	Enhancer	Duration	Efficacy	Safety
Salzman [77]	Type 1 [8]	Laureth-9 (0.25–110%)	3 m	Equivalent HbA_{1c}, "hypos"	Nasal irritation in up to 50%
Frauman [76]	Type 1 [9]	SGC (1%)/U250	4 m	Poor in 6/9; withdrawn from 3/9	Nasal irritation in 1/9
Hilsted [78]	Type 1 [31]	DDPC (2%)/U200	1 m	Withdrawn from 6/31	Minor nasal irritation
Lassman-Vague [79]	Type 1 [10]	Laureth-9 (0.25%)	1 m	Withdrawn from 4/10	Nasal irritation in 1/10

numbers of patients with type 1 diabetes demonstrated that nasal insulin given once or twice preprandially [76–78] instead of a bolus SC injection of soluble insulin resulted in either equivalent or inferior metabolic control [76–78]. In about 20% of patients it was necessary to revert to SC insulin, despite the use of high doses of the nasal insulin preparation and with increasing basal insulin supplementation, because of inferior efficacy and local (nasal) irritability. The incidence of hypoglycemic events was unaltered in patients given intranasal insulin. More recently, a lyophilized nasal insulin preparation containing sodium glycocholate given preprandially, with or without neutral protamine Hagedorn (NPH) as the basal insulin, achieved glycemic control equivalent to a regimen of twice daily NPH insulin in patients with type 2 diabetes over a 4-month period [80]. Subsequently, a gel formulation was developed and found to be equally effective to SC insulin in patients with type 1 diabetes treated over a longer period of 6 months [81]. Nasal tolerance was better with the gelified formation than the lyophilized form, but, when present, symptoms were more marked.

Although clinical experience with the different intranasal insulin formulations is limited, the findings demonstrate a need for high and repeated doses to control postprandial glycaemia because of the relatively poor bioavailability and short duration of action respectively. In addition, the occurrence of nasal irritation in up to 25% of patients and the potential for damage to the nasal mucosa and nasal-ciliary function [64, 68, 82] are points of concern, especially when viewed in the context of the need for long-term exposure. There is also little or no information on the impact of nasal pathology (common cold, allergic rhinitis, etc.) on the bioavailability of intranasal insulin. Research continues in the area of bioadhesive delivery systems using starch or chitosan based microspheres to retard nasal insulin clearance. Prodrug strategies present another possibility. In order for intranasal insulin to become a clinical and commercially viable alternative to SC insulin, major obstacles remain to be overcome to improve bioavailability, reproducibility, and time–action characteristics while ensuring local tolerance and long-term safety. At present the nasal route does not provide a viable option to subcutaneously administered insulin (Table 4).

Table 4 Intranasal delivery of insulin-limitations

Bioavailability at <10% and reproducibility (intrasubject CV ~40%) poor (influenced by insulin and excipient concentration)
Too "short-acting":
High and repeated dosing required
Nasal irritation
Toxic to nasal ciliary epithelium?
Effect of local pathology?
High failure rate
Discontinued—currently not a realistic alternative to sc injection

Table 5 Characteristics of the main absorptive surface of the lung for insulin administration*

• ~140 m^2 in adult humans	• Rich blood perfusion
• 1000-fold greater than nasal bed	• Lack of mucociliary clearance
• Bronchioles, alveolar ducts, and alveoli (300 million, >95% of total absorptive surface area)	• Painless
	• Natural
• Large surface area	• Immunotolerant
• Highly permeable membrane	

* Reference 85.

PULMONARY ROUTE

The respiratory tree, with an estimated surface area of 140 m^2, offers the greatest potential for the delivery of polypeptide drugs. The alveolar surface, which accounts for more than 95% of the absorptive area, includes an estimated 300 million alveoli lined by a very thin (0.1–0.2 μm), vesiculated and richly perfused monolayer of epithelial cells. Transport of molecules across the alveolar wall (type 1 cell) occurs by trancytosis for molecules in excess of 40 kDa and predominately by bi- or trijunctional paracellular processes for smaller molecules such as insulin (5.7 kDa) [83]. Thereafter, larger molecules proceed via the highly permeable tightjunctions of the venules and lymph vessels, with the small molecules passing mainly through the endothelial tight junctions, with cytosolic biodegradation an important determinant of bioavailability. The immunotolerant nature of the lung is of potential advantage for drug delivery [84] (Table 5).

The first attempts to deliver insulin by the pulmonary route using a variety of nebulizers took place in the 1920s shortly after insulin was first introduced [86, 87]. Modest reductions in blood glucose were achieved despite the use of doses in excess of 30-fold required by SC injection. The need for more efficient delivery systems was quickly acknowledged. However, almost 50 years elapsed before the feasibility of inhaled, aerosolized insulin was demonstrated having produced a nebulized mist containing 500 U of soluble insulin that was inhaled over a period of 5 min [88]. A relatively rapid, but variable, increase in plasma insulin concentration and consequently a fall in blood glucose was observed in both healthy subjects and adult patients with diabetes. Similar results were then achieved in children using a modified nebulizer connected to a spacer chamber at four to five times the SC dose [89]. Studies in smokers clearly demonstrated that the pulmonary absorption of insulin was enhanced threefold compared to nonsmokers [90]. Later, scintigraphic studies in nonsmoking patients with type 2 diabetes revealed that by maintaining a low rate of delivery during inspiration, about 80% of the inhaled insulin reached beyond the larynx [91]. The observed time to peak plasma insulin level averaged 40 min, but was highly variable. However, the inhaled insulin produced a more consistent decrease in blood glucose and the aerosol was well tolerated. Many studies have since confirmed the much earlier time to peak insulin concentration with inhaled insulin and the shorter duration of action compared to SC injection both in healthy subjects [92–94] and in patients with type 2 diabetes [95, 96]. In these studies, crude estimates of the bioavailability of inhaled insulin in nonsmoking subjects ranged between 7 and 25%. The intrasubject variability in absorption was comparable to that seen with SC soluble insulin [92, 97].

Many factors are known to influence the site of deposition of inhaled particles, including size or *aerodynamic diameter* (a function of the particles' geometric diameter and mass density referred to as the mass median aerodynamic diameter or MMAD), surface morphology, charge, solubility, and hygroscopicity [98]. Alveolar ('deep lung') deposition is optimal for particles with a MMAD of 1.5–2.5 μm with breath holding and 2.5–4 μm without breath holding [85]. Smaller particles (<1 μm) are mostly exhaled whereas larger particles of 5–10 and >10 μm are predominately deposited in the tracheobronchial or oropharyngeal regions respectively. The distribution of emitted particle sizes (geometric standard deviation) and the fine particle ('respirable') fraction are therefore critical determinants of the efficiency of delivery devices, along with the mass output (particle mass and number per volume).

The deposition of inhaled particles in the lung occurs by inertial impaction at bifurcations (increased by high velocity and turbulence), sedimentation (gravity), and diffusion [99]. Breathing pattern [inspiratory flow rate and inhaled ('tidal') volume] is therefore a major influence on intrapulmonary absorption [100, 101]. The presence of airflow obstruction and interstitial lung diseases [102, 103], smoking [104, 105, 106], exercise [106, 107] and patient's ability to operate inhaler devices [108] are all key factors that can influence the efficiency of inhaled insulin delivery.

Current pulmonary drug delivery systems include a variety of pressurized metered dose inhalers (pMDI), dry powder inhalers (DPI), nebulizers, and aqueous mist inhalers (AMI). The pMDI and DPI systems are associated with large degrees of inter- and intrasubject variability due to a reliance on patient technique [109] especially with the pMDI devices along with a dependence on the inspiratory flow rate [110] for effective drug delivery with the DPI delivery systems [111]. A further potential disadvantage of DPIs is powder hygroscopicity [112]. AMIs offer the advantages of nebulizers without the limited portability, excessive and wasteful consumption of the active medication.

Dispensing an insulin aerosol at the beginning of a slow and deep inspiration optimizes alveolar deposition [100, 101]. Therefore, controlling the breathing pattern, along with ensuring the delivery of a precise dose (based on mass output and particle dispersion), is critical in an attempt to achieve the desired and reproducible response.

Most of the recent clinical experience with inhaled insulin has been obtained using either a dry powder formulation in the Nektar/Exubera pulmonary inhaler (Nektar Therapeutics Inc., Aventis, Pfizer) or as liquid aerosols formulations in the AER_x® Insulin Diabetes Management System (Aradigm Corp., NovoNordisk A/S) or in the Aerosose® Inhaler (Aerogen Inc., CA, USA). Other delivery technologies include the use of modified insulin particles in the AIR™ Pulmonary Drug Delivery System (Advanced Inhalation Research Alkermes, Eli Lilly) and in the form of Technosphere™ insulin (Pharmaceutical Discovery Corporation (PDC), NY, USA).

NEKTAR/EXUBERA DELIVERY DEVICE

The Nektar/Exubera device is a DPI that uses compressed air to disperse an insulin powder formulation into a spacer reservoir ("chamber") prior to inhalation. The dry powder formulation is composed of insulin (∼60%) and excipients, principally mannitol, which stabilizes the insulin during spray drying and storage, along with glycine and sodium citrate. The insulin powder is packaged into single-dose blisters containing 1 or 3 mg (approximately 28 and 84 units) of insulin (Figure 3). For delivery, an individual blister is placed into a slot on the device and is dispersed by the inhaler into an aerosol cloud that is captured in the holding chamber. The patient then inhales the aerosol-containing particles (MMAD of ∼3 μm) at the beginning of a slow, deep breath during which air is drawn into the chamber extruding the aerosol into the pulmonary tree. The procedure is repeated if doses requiring multiple blisters are needed. Breath holding at the end of inspiration does not appear to enhance the bioavailability of the inhaled insulin. The overall system efficiency of the inhaled insulin (a product of aerosolization losses and bioavailability) has been estimated to be about 10% relative to SC insulin (18 U) (human soluble insulin and lispro insulin)

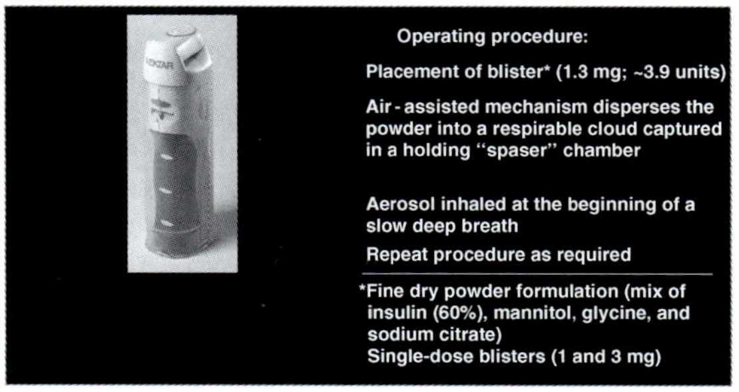

Figure 3 Nektar pulmonary inhaler for inhaled insulin (Pfizer, Nektar, Aventis)

during a glucose clamp procedure in healthy, nonsmoking subjects when observed over a 10-h postadministration period [113]. The inhaled insulin had a faster onset of action than SC human soluble insulin with a time-to-peak effect resembling the fast-acting insulin analogue, and a duration of action between 5 and 10 h—intermediate between the two insulin preparations. The two dosage formulations, 1 and 3 mg, have similar pharmacokinetic and pharmacodynamic time–action characteristics. When used at doses that comparably reduce postprandial hyperglycemia in patients with type 2 diabetes, the reproducibility of the response to the pulmonary insulin is similar to SC insulin [99]. Add-on therapy with the inhaled insulin in patients with type 2 diabetes failing on oral agents achieves an improvement in overall glycemic control with a low risk of hypoglycemia [114].

In a "proof-of-concept," open-label study, patients with type 1 diabetes were given inhaled insulin immediately before meals on a thrice-daily basis, with ultralente insulin at bedtime as the basal supplement. The control group of patients received a conventional split-mixed SC insulin regimen comprising two or mainly three daily injections of human soluble and NPH insulin at bedtime [115]. From a baseline HbA_{1c} level of 8.5% in both treatment groups at the end of a 3-month treatment period, the multiple dose inhaled insulin group achieved a HbA_{1c} level of 7.9% compared to 7.7% in the control group. The total daily insulin dose for the inhaled and SC insulin groups were approximately 60 U (60% inhaled insulin, 40% ultralente insulin) and 47 U (34% short-acting insulin, 66% NPH insulin) respectively. The estimated bioavailability of the inhaled insulin was 5–6% relative to SC insulin. The glucose profile during a test "meal" (Sustacal) was similar in the two treatment groups both at the beginning and at the end of the 3-month treatment period. The frequency and severity of hypoglycemic episodes were also similar with no changes in body weight occurring in either group. In this relatively short-term study, no significant changes in pulmonary function were observed [FEV_1, FVC, $FEF_{25-75\%}$, PEFR; lung volume (TLC, RV, VC), diffusion capacity, or resting oxygen saturation]. Patient treatment satisfaction scores favored inhaled insulin, with 82% of patients electing to continue treatment. Inhaled insulin was deemed to be more convenient and easier to use than SC insulin [116, 117]. Although the inhaled insulin therapy did not result in improvement in overall glycemic control compared to conventional treatment, the study demonstrated the feasibility of using the pulmonary route for meal-related insulin delivery.

In a longer 6 month study of patients with type 1 diabetes, inhaled insulin given preprandially with ultralente as basal insulin was again comparable to SC insulin (two to three injections daily of regular/NPH insulin) with respect to overall glycemic control (HbA_{1c}) and the number of patients achieving target blood glucose levels [118]. The risk of hypoglycemic events was lower with the inhaled insulin, with comparable rates for severe episodes in both treatment groups. An increase in insulin-binding antibodies was seen in the inhaled patient group. Coughing, although more frequent in the inhaled group, decreased over time. While there was no change in forced expiratory volume ($FEV_{1.0}$) observed, a fall in diffusing capacity (DL_{CO}) was seen in the inhaled insulin group. Further investigations are needed to explain this latter observation and further research is needed to assess its potential clinical significance.

In a 3-month controlled study, insulin-treated patients with type 2 diabetes were randomly assigned to inhaled insulin before each meal, with ultralente insulin at bedtime or remained on their original insulin regimen of two to three daily SC injections [119, 120]. A test meal (Sustacal) carried out preconversion (baseline) and after 12 weeks showed no difference in postprandial glycaemia between the two treatment regimens. A similar improvement in HbA_{1c} (~0.7%) was observed at the end of the study period in both groups and there was no difference in the frequency of hypoglycemic events during the study. Pulmonary function tests remained essentially unchanged in response to inhaled insulin. This study demonstrated the feasibility of intrapulmonary insulin delivery in patients with type 2 diabetes. In patients with type 2 diabetes who had failed to achieve adequate glycemic control on combination oral therapy, the introduction of inhaled insulin either as monotherapy or in conjunction with the existing oral agents improved glycemic control [121]. The introduction of the inhaled insulin increased the overall rate of hypoglycemia, increased weight, and insulin antibody binding was more frequent when compared to the patients who remained on their combined oral treatment. Patients on inhaled insulin did however have a greater level of overall satisfaction. The impression from continued surveillance of both type 1 and type 2 patients on inhaled insulin suggests that glycemic control and lung function tests (spirometry) remain stable for up to 2 years [122].

These studies demonstrate the feasibility of using inhaled insulin to cover meal time insulin requirements in patients with either type 1 and type 2 diabetes. However, longer term controlled clinical trials will be essential to further ensure the efficacy and safety of inhaled insulin. Therefore, comparisons should include basal bolus insulin regimens involving either constant subcutaneous insulin infusion (CSII) or combinations of long- and rapid-acting preprandial insulin analogues.

AER_x® INSULIN DIABETES MANAGEMENT SYSTEM

The AER_x Insulin Diabetes Management System (IDMS) is an aqueous mist inhaler in which single-use insulin

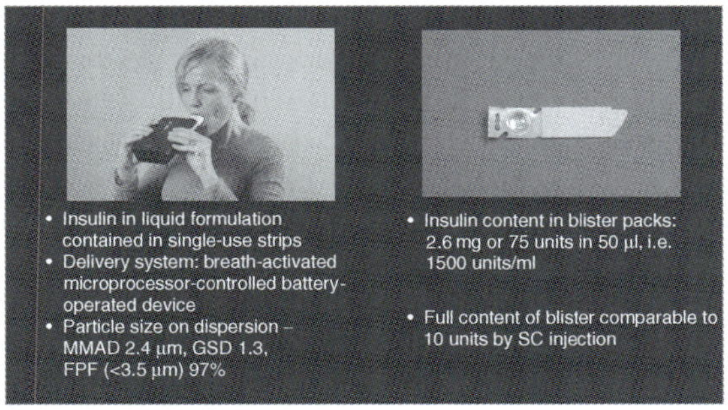

Figure 4 AER$_x$® IDMS delivery device (Aradigm/Novo Nordisk). (Reproduced by permission of Novo Nordisk)

strips are combined with a hand-held, breath-activated, microprocessor-controlled device. The insulin strips, which are disposable, contain 75 U of insulin as an aqueous solution (Figure 4). The device, which is battery operated, is designed to deliver a low-velocity fine-particle aerosol spray early during inhalation, but only when appropriate breathing conditions (inspiratory flow rate and volume) are satisfied. Scintigraphic studies have established the ability of the device to minimize patient-related variability in inhaled lung dose by controlling and thus optimizing both the inspiratory flow rate and inhaled volume [101, 123, 124]. Breath holding has been shown not be necessary to enhance the absorption of insulin using this device [125]. The inspired air is temperature controlled as it passes through the AER$_x$ device, which is also designed to monitor patient compliance by capturing dosing events.

Comparison of an early prototype of the AER$_x$ delivery system with a conventional pMDI, where both employed microprocessor-controlled actuation, revealed a predominantly central pattern (conducting airways) of distribution with the pMDI in contrast to a more homogeneous pattern (deep lung) with the AER$_x$ delivery system [123]. Lung deposition with the pMDI device was less and more variable, with a higher proportion deposited in the oropharyngeal region. This situation was largely avoided with the AER$_x$ system, which emphasizes the importance of minimizing the ballistic component associated with pMDIs. In contrast to conventional nebulizers and inhalers, where the estimated delivery of drugs to the lung is 10–20% of the loaded dose, the AER$_x$ system achieved deposition of 50% of the extruded dose, with 16–18% in the lung periphery [123, 126]. The uniform deposition throughout the deep lung was attributed to the emitted particles having a MMAD of 2 μm. Lung distribution was unaffected by posture.

Studies in healthy subjects show that insulin delivered with the AER$_x$ device is more rapidly absorbed and has a shorter time to maximum plasma insulin concentration compared to SC injection (7–20 min versus 100–120 min, respectively) [101]. The pharmacokinetics and pharmacodynamics of insulin delivered with the AER$_x$ device resemble that of rapid-acting insulin analogues when administered subcutaneously [127]. In a glucose clamp study carried out over a 10-h period, a dose–response relationship was seen for both bioavailability and metabolic effect in normal subjects [128].

Studies comparing nondiabetic smokers and nonsmokers have further demonstrated a much faster and greater degree of absorption in habitual smokers [129], with a peak serum insulin concentration threefold higher in smokers. The act of smoking immediately prior to inhalation resulted in a lower peak insulin concentration compared to that observed in the same subjects having abstained from smoking overnight. Intrasubject variability in insulin absorption associated with the AER$_x$ system appears lower (~20%) in both smokers and nonsmokers compared to SC insulin [130]. Asthmatic patients absorb less insulin, resulting in a lesser hypoglycemic effect compared to their nonasthmatic, nondiabetic counterparts [131]. Inhalation of a relatively high dose of insulin (equivalent to ~18 units SC) did not exacerbate the baseline airway hyperreactivity state of the asthmatic patients. During mild upper respiratory tract infection (nondiabetic subjects) a shorter time to peak insulin concentration with the inhaled insulin has been observed when compared to that seen after elimination of the infection, although the difference was not reflected in the glucose response [132].

A near linear dose–response relationship was seen for both pharmacokinetic (insulin profile) and pharmacodynamic (glucose infusion rate) parameters in patients with type 1 diabetes in a 10-h glucose clamp study carried out following inhalation of insulin doses in the 0.3–1.8 U/kg range via the AER$_x$ device [133]. The inspiratory flow rate was controlled within 50–70 l/min after which the patients held their breath for 10 s. For the inhaled insulin, the time to maximum plasma insulin concentration was approximately half that of SC insulin. The overall efficiency of the AER$_x$ pulmonary delivery system estimated over an initial 6-h period was 13%, based on the loaded dose. The intrasubject variability in the pharmacokinetic and pharmacodynamic parameters measured are essentially the same as SC insulin administration [134–136].

A proof-of-concept trial carried out over a 3-month period in nonsmoking patients with type 2 diabetes compared inhaled insulin delivered by the AER$_x$ device and SC human soluble insulin given preprandially with NPH insulin at bedtime in both groups [137]. The study found no difference between the groups in overall glycemic control (HbA_{1c}) although the fasting glucose was lower with the inhaled insulin despite the use of similar NPH insulin doses. Based on the bioavailability of inhaled insulin relative to SC insulin, bioeffectiveness was estimated at 16%. Although the number of hypoglycemic events was lower with inhaled insulin, the difference was not significant.

No changes in lung function tests were observed in either group. This study did not report data on the occurrence of insulin-binding antibodies. The study demonstrates that meal time inhaled insulin delivered via the AER_x system is equally safe and effective compared with SC human soluble insulin used in conjunction with NPH insulin at bedtime in patients with type 2 diabetes. Although essentially similar plasma insulin profiles have been observed in response to a single inhalation of insulin in young and elderly patients with type 2 diabetes, the glucose reduction achieved was less in the elderly [138].

Despite the technical differences between the Inhale/Exubera and AER_x pulmonary insulin delivery devices, the mean bioeffectiveness of the devices estimated in the glucose clamp studies is similar (10 and 13%, respectively) [139]. In meal challenge studies, the respective mean bioavailability is 11 and 16% and mean bioeffectiveness 13 and 17%, respectively. Advantages of the dry powder insulin formulation may include better stability at room temperature, a higher possible insulin content per puff, and reduced potential for microbial growth. However, the extrusion mechanism of the AER_x IDMS device can uniquely control the amount delivered allowing smaller dose adjustments, while also able to store the data relating to each dosing episode and therefore available for clinical review. The use of a liquid insulin formulation may also avoid problems related to the production of dry insulin powder formulations and the influence of external humidity on the dispersion of the preparation. The potential of the different pulmonary insulin formulations to induce the production of insulin antibodies and the clinical implications of such antibodies on the metabolic control and the immune system remains unknown at present [140].

AERODOSE™ INHALER

The Aerodose inhaler is a breath-activated delivery device developed by Aerogen Inc. (Sunnydale, CA, USA). The device uses a liquid insulin formulation (Humalin I™ 500 U/ml) to produce an aerosol with a mean dispersed particle size of 3.3 μm and a fine-particle (1–6 μm) ("respirable") fraction of 87% [141]. In a comparison of inhaled insulin delivered by the Aerodose inhaler and SC insulin in nondiabetic subjects, the time to peak plasma insulin concentration was shorter with the inhaler device (50 min compared to 85 min, respectively). The relative bioavailability and biopotency of the inhaled insulin, estimated over a 6-h observation period during a glucose clamp study, was 9.3 and 10.3% respectively. The inhaled insulin preparation was well tolerated and no acute changes in pulmonary function tests were seen. Aerosolization time and particle size are seen as important factors in determining the efficiency of the delivery system [142]. A study in type 2 diabetic patients confirmed the shorter time to peak insulin concentration and the earlier metabolic effect of inhaled insulin relative to SC insulin with bioavailability and biopotency over 8 h estimated at 16 and 13% respectively, relative to SC insulin [143]. Reproducibility of the inhaled and SC insulin was similar at about 20% for both absorption and action.

MODIFICATION TO INHALED PARTICLES

Advanced Inhalation Research (Alkermes/Eli Lilly)

Large, porous, insulin-containing particles (10–20 μm) of low-mass density (<0.03 gm/cm^3) have been developed by Advanced Inhalation Research (AIR) using a biodegradable polymer matrix composed of phospholipids [144–146]. The formulation, which is packaged in blisters, is easily aerosolized using a simple, breath-activated, DPI device. Although the particles are physically large, their mass mean aerodynamic diameter is within the aerodynamic window of 1–3 μm [145]. The large porous particles have a reduced tendency to aggregate (agglomeration), thereby facilitating their dispersion, and they are also less susceptible to phagocytosis in the lung [145]. In addition to short- or rapid-acting insulin-containing particles, sustained-release insulin formulations may also be incorporated into the biodegradable polymer matrix [145–147]. The results from human studies are now awaited.

Technosphere™ Insulin

Pharmaceutical Development Corp. (Elmsford, NY, USA) has developed a drug delivery system known as Technosphere™ that captures insulin or other peptides utilizing a diketopiperazine derivative [148]. The formulation self-assembles into an ordered lattice array at low pH, which dissolves at the neutral pH of the alveolar surface rapidly releasing the insulin. The formulation is designed for use with the Medtone® DPI delivery device, which is a capsule-based high-impedance inhaler using a passive powder deagglomeration mechanism.

The glucose clamp technique was used to compare inhaled Technosphere/insulin with human soluble insulin administered by the SC and IV routes in nonsmoking, nondiabetic subjects. The inhaled insulin (100 U) reached a peak plasma concentration after 13 min compared to 121 min for SC insulin (10 U) and 5 min for IV insulin (5 U) [148]. The times to maximum activity were 39, 163, and 14 min respectively and the estimated bioavailabilities of the inhaled insulin relative to SC insulin over 3 and 6 h postadministration were 26 and 16% respectively with relative biopotencies of 19 and 14% respectively. In a further dose–response study of Technosphere/insulin (25, 50, and 100 U), the peak metabolic effect occurred much earlier (47, 52, 56 min) compared with SC soluble insulin

(192 min) and the estimated relative bioavailabilities over the first 3 h were 46, 42, and 28 respectively [149]. In patients with type 2 diabetes, the intrasubject variation in peak and time to peak insulin concentration and metabolic effect with the inhaled insulin (100 U) in an euglycemic clamp study was 27, 23, and 20% respectively [150]. These observations are comparable to results obtained with SC administered soluble insulin [94].

Modification to the surface morphology of inhaled particles and/or the use of absorption promoters may result in improved absorption of insulin across the alveolar barrier [147, 151, 152]. Potential enhancers include bile salts (glycocholate) and their derivatives (dihydrofusidate), long-chain phospholipids (DPPC), surfactants, and cyclodextrins. Where attempts are made to facilitate insulin absorption, the long-term safety of such promoters will need careful evaluation [151, 153].

CLINICAL PERSPECTIVE

Ease of use and patient acceptance may greatly influence the choice of delivery system for inhaled insulin. This is especially important when considering the requirements of certain patient groups such as children, adolescents, and the elderly. For persons with significant airway obstruction and interstitial lung disease, intrapulmonary delivery of insulin is less appropriate, given the paucity of information about the influence of lung pathology on inhaled insulin absorption. In this respect, it is of interest that up to two thirds of patients with long-standing diabetes are reported to have some abnormality of lung function ("diabetic pneumopathy") [154, 155]. Special caution also needs to be exercised when inhaled insulin is used in patients who are habitual smokers, because of the very rapid and greater absorption when compared to non-smokers [89, 129, 156, 157]. Similarly, exercise may enhance the pulmonary absorption of inhaled insulin.

Current clinical experience with inhaled insulin is limited to 3-, 6-, or 12-month treatment periods, with data from longer exposure studies awaited. To date, there is little evidence of local adverse reactions other than an increase in a throat clearing type cough associated with the act of inhalation, which occurs in approximately 10% of patients, reducing with time [95]. Lung function tests (spirometry, lung volume, diffusion capacity, and oxygen saturation) show some statistically nonsignificant changes in both patients with type 1 diabetes [115] and type 2 diabetes [120, 158]. There appears to be a trend for a small but consistent fall in $FEV_{1.0}$, and more so, DL_{CO} in patients treated for periods of 6 months or more with inhaled insulin [118]. Careful appraisal of the data will be necessary before cause and effect can be established. Data from longer term controlled studies supported by limited but more specialized studies, such as lung (alveolar) lavage, are needed to better establish the safety of the different formulations of inhaled insulin. Other concerns expressed include the possibility of inducing pulmonary hypotension and pulmonary edema due to the relatively high insulin concentration achieved in the pulmonary vascular bed, especially in patients with cardiac dysfunction [159]. Insulin's proinflammatory effects may also potentially unmask airways obstruction such as asthma, again emphasizing the need for both acute and long-term surveillance [160].

The immunogenicity of inhaled insulin is another important consideration, especially as relatively high insulin-binding antibody concentrations are in evidence in patients with type 1 and type 2 diabetes treated with a dry powder insulin formulation (Nektar, Pfizer, Aventis). The potential role of excipients such as mannitol in this process needs to be elucidated. However, the impact of such insulin-binding antibodies remains to be clarified. The fate of inhaled insulin is also as yet to be described.

In clinical terms, the onset of action of inhaled insulin is comparable to the rapid-acting insulin analogues but with a slightly more prolonged effect, making it theoretically suitable for meal-related insulin supplementation. The frequency and severity of hypoglycemic events appears equivalent to that being experienced with SC human soluble insulin in patients with both type 1 and type 2 diabetes [96, 115, 119, 161].

Patients treated with inhaled insulin (Nektar-Exubera) report improved satisfaction and quality of life when compared to human insulin given by bolus SC injection [117]. However, the introduction of intrapulmonary insulin into clinical practice will depend on a satisfactory long-term efficacy profile and, more especially, safety evaluation (local tolerance and systemic incidence of hypoglycemia) and finally quality-of-life assessments and cost–benefit analyses. Having satisfied these requirements, appropriate patient education will be essential as an integral part of the introduction of inhaled insulin into clinical practice. While certain delivery devices remain fairly bulky (some more than others) considerable social stigma may persist. Translating the differences between various delivery devices into clinical benefits or not will become evident with more extensive clinical use, which will also serve in redesigning future devices for the pulmonary delivery of insulin. Insulin formulation changes are also in development, including the use of absorption enhancers, protease inhibitors, micro-nano spheres, and mucoadhesive nanoparticulate systems among others. Long-term safety relating to insulin itself and the use of excipients and absorption enhancers will remain a priority as will assessment of cost-effectiveness in this quickly evolving arena.

SUMMARY

The introduction of insulin over 80 years ago has, and will continue to, save, prolong, and improve the lives of countless millions of patients with diabetes. Since its introduction, major advances have been made in the production, purification, pharmaceutical formulation, and methods of delivery of insulin in pursuit of the ultimate goal of replicating the normal pattern of physiological secretion and thereby eliminate the adverse diabetic milieu with its associated morbidity and mortality. There is an ever-increasing acceptance of the need to achieve and sustain near normoglycemia in order to delay the onset and retard the progression of diabetic angiopathy. Physiological insulin replacement is therefore central to the optimal management of the insulin-requiring patient with diabetes. Lately, recombinant DNA technology has made it possible to design new insulins (insulin analogues) with altered characteristics in an attempt to overcome the shortcomings imposed by the SC route of administration.

Even in the first decade after its introduction, attempts were being made to deliver insulin by less invasive routes (oral, nasal, pulmonary, rectal, vaginal, etc.) as a means of avoiding life-long dependence on multiple daily SC injections. Most available orifices and exposed surfaces have since been tested, mainly in animals and mostly with limited success. Despite the academic challenge, there now appears to be little or no justification for continuing to pursue the nasal, rectal, ocular, and vaginal/uterine routes. The oral-enteric route also presents a multitude of obstacles making it an unrealistic endeavor, although new pharmaceutical formulations are providing further opportunities. There is also active research in the buccal and transdermal delivery of insulin. Currently, however, interest is centered on the intrapulmonary route as a means of providing meal-related and possibly basal insulin requirements. However, although inhaled insulin is rapidly absorbed, bioavailability is poor compared with that of SC injection (not more than 20%), and may require bulky and conspicuous devices for its delivery. With the recent development of rapid-acting insulin analogues, inhaled insulin offers little metabolic advantage, although avoidance of SC injections remains a major benefit for patients. This is well appreciated in the context of the current advocacy for four injections per day as part of intensified insulin therapy, amounting to almost 15 000 injections per decade of insulin-requiring diabetes—a sobering thought.

To date, exploring the use of alternative routes for insulin administration has been relatively unsuccessful. Although the efficiency of absorption across epithelial surfaces of the mouth, GIT, skin, and nose has increased somewhat using a wide variety of absorption enhancing techniques, bioavailability remains too low and erratic to be of any clinical value (Table 6). After being dormant for almost half a century, interest in the intrapulmonary route has been regenerated with the advent of new delivery devices and an increasing choice of dry powder or liquid aerosol formulations now being available. Improving the delivery of insulin to the "deep lung" has benefited from a greater understanding of the relevance of aerosol particle size, inspiratory flow rate, and inhaled volume. However, methods of estimating bioavailability need to be standardized so as to allow meaningful comparisons between delivery devices. Precision of dosing, dose adjustments, and reproducibility will remain key features in the viability of this approach. It is important to better delineate the functionalities of delivery devices as a means of determining overall system efficiency relative to SC insulin. Clinical studies to date suggest a possible role for inhaled insulin in the control of postprandial glucose excursions in patients

Table 6 Common strategies for promoting absorption of insulin across epithelial surfaces

Chemical	• Permeation enhancers	Surfactants Chelators Fatty acids Inclusion complexes (cyclodextrins) Bile salts
	• Enzyme inhibitors	Biodegradable polymers (particulate systems)
	• Encapsulation	Liposomes
	• Pharmaceutical formulations	Structural modification of insulin Use of bioadhesive molecules Prodrug concept Dosage forms (patches, sprays, suppositories, etc.)
Physical	• Iontophoresis • Phonophoresis (ultrasonic) • Electroporation • Microneedles, ablation	
Gene therapy	• Insufflation of "insulin coding sequence" into pancreatic duct • "Gene pill" control of protein secretion by intestinal cells	

with type 1 or type 2 diabetes. However, the need for supplementary SC basal insulin in patients with type 1 and possibly type 2 diabetes means complete avoidance of SC injections cannot be achieved at present. The availability of an intrapulmonary, long-acting insulin is much further down the road in development. Only following confirmation of its long-term safety, will inhaled insulins possibly become the first widespread non-SC route of administration. An important benefit may be for those patients with type 2 diabetes in whom insulin therapy would otherwise be delayed.

Recognizing the true cost of diabetes to both the individual patient and society has helped to stimulate the enormous effort undertaken by researchers and carers worldwide to arrive at better treatments for patients with insulin-requiring diabetes. In the near future both patients and care teams will face ever-increasing options for providing insulin. Choice must therefore be based on well-designed clinical studies and not on large volumes of mainly uncontrolled data, which may be open to misinterpretation.

The treatment of the insulin-requiring diabetic patient has come a long way since insulins were first introduced in 1922, some 80 years ago. Despite the many major achievements in insulin therapy, it is estimated that about 4 million years of life are still lost to patients with type 1 diabetes each year. This new millennium promises a revolutionary change in the delivery of insulin, which cannot come too soon for the millions of sufferers reliant on SC injections. Cautious optimism based on scientific rigor remains the only way forward.

REFERENCES

1. Banting FG, Best CH, Collip JB, Macleod JJR. The preparation of pancreatic extracts containing insulin, I: the preparation of the earlier extract. *Trans Roy Soc Can* 1922; 16 (V): 1–2.
2. Diabetes Control and Complication Trial (DCCT) Group. The effect of intensive treatment of diabetes on the development and progression of long-term complications in insulin-dependant diabetes mellitus. *N Engl J Med* 1993; 329: 977–86.
3. United Kingdom Prospective Diabetes Study Group. Intensive blood glucose control with sulphonylureas or insulin compared with conventional treatment and risk of complications in patients with type 2 diabetes (UKPDS 33). *Lancet* 1998; 352: 837–53.
4. Berger M. Oral insulin 1922–1992: the history of continuous ambition and failure. In Berger M, Gries F (eds), *Frontiers in Insulin Pharmacology*. Stuttgart: Plenum Press, 1993; pp 144–8.
5. Horowitz M. O'Donovon D, Jones KL, Feinle C, Rayner CK, Samsom M. Gastric emptying in diabetes: clinical significance and treatment. *Diabet Med* 2002; 19 (3): 177–94.
6. Damgé C. Oral insulin. In Pickup J (ed), *Biotechnology of Insulin Therapy*. Oxford: Blackwell Scientific, 1991; pp 97–112.
7. Carino GP, Mathiowitz E. Oral insulin delivery. *Adv Drug Delivery Rev* 1999; 35: 249–57.
8. Gregoriadis G. The carrier potential of liposomes in biology and medicine. *N Engl J Med* 1976; 295 (13): 704–10.
9. Patel HM, Ryman BE. Orally administered liposomally entrapped insulin. *Biochem Soc Trans* 1977; 5: 1739–41.
10. Dapergolas G, Gergoriadis G. Hypoglycemic effect of liposome-entrapped insulin administered intragastrically. *Lancet* 1976; II: 824–7.
11. Choudhari KB, Labhasetwar V, Dorle AK. Liposomes as a carrier for oral administration of insulin: effect of formulation factor. *J Microencapsul* 1994; 11: 319–25.
12. Kisel MA, Kulik LN, Tsybovsky IS, Vlasov AP, Vorob'yov MS, Kholodova EA, Zabarovskaya ZV. Liposomes with phosphatidylethanol as a carrier for oral delivery of insulin: studies in the rat. *Int J Pharm* 2001; 216: 105–14.
13. Chen H, Torchilin V, Langer R. Polymerized liposomes as potential oral vaccine carrier: stability and bioavailability. *J Control Release* 1996; 42: 263–72.
14. Langer R. Drug delivery and targeting. *Nature* 1998; 386: 410–4.
15. Gwinup G, Elias AN, Domurat ES. Insulin and C-peptide levels following oral administration of insulin in intestinal-enzyme protected capsules. *Gen Pharmacol* 1991; 22: 243–6.
16. Mathiowitz E, Jacobs JS, Jong YS, Carino GP, Chickering D, et al. Biologically erodable microspheres as potential oral drug delivery systems. *Nature* 1997; 286: 410–4.
17. Chung H, Kim J, Um JY, Kwon JC, Jeong SY. Self-assembled "nanocubicle" as a carrier for peroral delivery. *Diabetologia* 2002; 45 (3): 448–51.
18. Still JG. Development of oral insulin: progress and current status. *Diabetes Metab Res Rev* 2002; 18 (suppl 1): S29–37.
19. Milstein SJ, Leipold H, Sarubb D, Leone-Bay A, Mynek GM, Robinson JR, Kasimova M, Freire E. Partially unfolded efficiently penetrated cell membranes—implications for oral drug delivery. *J Control Release* 1998; 53: 259–67.
20. Goldfine ID, German MS, Tseng HC, Wang J, Bolaffi JL, Chen JW, Olson DC, Rothman SS. The endocrine secretion of human insulin and growth hormone by exocrine glands of the gastrointestinal tract. *Nat Biotechnol* 1997; 15: 1378–82.
21. Nagai T, Machida Y. Mucosal adhesive dosage forms. *Pharm Int* 1985; 6: 196.
22. Aungst BJ, Rogers NJ. Site dependence of absorption-promoting actions of Laureth-9, Na salicylate, Na2EDTA, and aprotinin on rectal, nasal, and buccal insulin delivery. *Pharm Res* 1988; 5 (5): 305–8.
23. YoKosuka T, Omori Y, Hirata Y, Hirai S. Nasal and sublingual administration of insulin in man. *J Jpn Diabetes Soc* 1977; 20: 146–52.
24. Hoogstraate JAJ, Wertz PW. Drug delivery via the buccal mucosa. *Pharm Sci Technol Today* 1998; 1 (7): 309–16.
25. Veuillez F, Kalia YN, Jacques Y, Deshusses J, Buri P. Factors and strategies for improving buccal absorption of peptides. *Eur J Pharm Biopharm* 2001; 51 (2): 93–109.
26. Senal S, Kremer M, Nagy K, Squier C. Delivery of bioactive peptides and proteins across the oral (buccal) mucosa. *Curr Pharm Des* 2001; 2: 175–86.
27. Yang TZ, Wang XT, Yan XY, Zhang Q. Phospholipid deformable vesicles for buccal delivery of insulin. *Chem Pharm Bull* 2002; 50 (6): 749–53.

28. Al-Walli NSD. Sublingual human insulin for hyperglycemia in type 1 diabetes. *JPMA* 1999; 49: 167–9.
29. Modi P, Mihic M, Lewin A. The evolving role of oral insulin in the treatment of diabetes usinga RapidMisttm system. *Diabetes Metab Res Rev* 2002; 18 (suppl 1): S38–42.
30. Cavello MG, Coppolino G, Romeo S, Pozzilli P. Inhaled insulin in type 1 diabetes. *Lancet* 2001; 357: 198.
31. Yamasaki Y, Shichiri M, Kawamori R, Kikuchi M, Yagi T, Arai S, Tohdo R, Hakui N, Oji N, Abe H. The effectiveness of rectal administration of insulin suppository on normal and diabetic subjects. *Diabetes Care* 1981; 4: 454–8.
32. Hildebrant R, Lius A, Lotz U, Schliack V. Effect of insulin suppositories in type 1 diabetic patients. *Exp Clin Endocrinol* 1984; 873 (2): 168–72.
33. Raz I, Bar-on H, Kidron M, Ziv E. Rectal administration of insulin. *Isr J Med Sci* 1984; 20: 173–5.
34. Barichello JM, Morishita M, Takayama K, Chiba Y, Tokiwa S, Nagai T. Enhanced rectal absorption of insulin-loaded PluronicR F-127 gels containing unsaturated fatty acids. *Int J Pharm* 1999; 183: 125–32.
35. Onuki Y, Morishita M, Takayama K, Tokiwa S, Chiba Y, Isowa K, Nagai T. In vivo effects of highly purified docosahexaenoic acid on rectal insulin absorption. *Int J Pharm* 2000; 198 (2): 147–56.
36. Yun M-O, Choi H-G, Jung J-H, Kim C-K. Development of a thermo-reversible liquid suppository with bioavailabilty enhancement. *Int J Pharm* 1999; 189: 137–45.
37. Uchida T, Sakakibara S, Toida Y, Nagareya N, Yasuda N, Matsuyama K. Rectal delivery of insulin using a bioadhesive hydrogel preparation containing lauric acid as an enhancer in rats. *Pharm Pharmacol Commun* 1999; 5 (8): 523–7.
38. Matsuda H, Arima H. Cyclodextrins in transdermal and rectal delivery. *Adv Drug Deliv Rev* 1999; 36: 81–99.
39. Bartlett JD, Turner-Henson A, Atchson JA, Woolley TW, Pillion DJ. Insulin administration to the eyes of normoglycemic human volunteers. *J Ocul Pharmacol* 1994: 10 (4): 683–91.
40. Chiou GC. Systemic delivery of insulin through eyes to lower the glucose concentration. *J Ocul Pharmacol* 1989; 5: 81–91.
41. Yamamoto A, Luo AM, Dodda-Kashi S, Lee VHL. The ocular route for systemic insulin delivery in the albino rabbit. *J Pharmacol Exp Ther* 1989; 249 (1): 489–502.
42. Yung-Chi L, Simamora P, Pinsuwan S, Yalkowsky SH. Review on the systemic delivery of insulin via the ocular route. *Int J Pharm* 2002; 233: 1–18.
43. Morimoto K, Takeeda T, Nakamoto Y, Morisaka K. Effective vaginal absorption of insulin in diabetic rats and rabbits using polyacrylic acid aqueous gel bases. *Int J Pharm* 1982; 12: 107–11.
44. Richardson JL, Illum L, Thomas NW. Vaginal absorption of insulin in the rat: effect of penetration enhancers on insulin uptake and mucosal histology. *Pharm Res* 1992; 9 (7): 878–83.
45. Richardson JL, Farraj NF, Illum L. Enhanced vaginal absorption of insulin in sheep using lysophosphatidylcholine and a bioadhesive microsphere delivery system. *Int J Pharm* 1992; 88: 319–25.
46. Rodrigues de Melo V, Valeri V. Morphological evidence for the stimulatory effect of insulin on vaginal and endometrial cells of rats. *Acta Anat* 1980; 106: 378–86.
47. Gagliardi F. Absorption of insulin by the human vagina. *Attualita di ostetricia e ginecologia* 1966; 12 (4): 599–608.
48. Cullander C, Guy RH. (D) Routes of delivery; case studies, 6: transdermal delivery of peptides and proteins. *Adv Drug Deliv Rev* 1992; 8(2–3): 291–329.
49. Foldavri M. Non-invasive administration of drugs through the skin: challenged in delivery system design. *PSTT* 2000; 3 (12): 417.
50. Stephen RL, Petelenz TJ, Jacobsen SC. Potential novel methods for insulin administration, I: iontophoresis. *Biomed Biochim Acta* 1984; 43: 553–8.
51. Sage BH Jr. Insulin iontophoresis. In Saunders LM, Hendren RW (eds), *Protein Delivery—Physical Systems*. New York: Plenum Publishing Corp., 1997; pp 319–41.
52. Siddiqui O, Shi WM, Chien YW. Transdermal iontophoretic delivery of insulin for blood glucose control in diabetic rabbits. *Proc Int Symp Control Res Bioact Mater* 1987; 14: 174.
53. Langkjaer L, Brange J, Grodsky GM, Guy RH. Iontophoresis of monomeric insulin analogues *in vitro*: effects of insulin charge and skin pretreatment. *J Control Release* 1998; 51: 47–56.
54. Tachibana K. Transdermal delivery of insulin to alloxan-diabetic rabbits by ultrasound exposure. *Pharm Res* 1992; 9 (7): 952–4.
55. Mitragotri S, Blankschtein D, Langer R. Ultrasound-mediated transdermal protein delivery. *Science* 1995; 269: 850–3.
56. Cevc G. Transfersomes, liposomes and other liquid suspensions on the skin: permeation enhancement vesicle penetration and transdermal drug delivery. *Crit Rev Ther Drug Carrier Syst* 1996; 13 (3–4); 257–388.
57. Chien YW, Banga AK. Direct current iontopheric transdermal delivery of peptide and protein drugs. *J Pharm Sci* 1989; 78 (5): 376–83.
58. Curdy C, Kalia YN, Guy RH. Non-invasive assessment of the effects of iontophoresis on human skin *in vivo*. *J Pharm Pharmacol* 2001; 53 (6): 769–77.
59. Machet L, Boucand A. Phonophoresis: efficiency, mechanisms and skin tolerance. *Int J Pharm* 2002; 243: 1–15.
60. Le L, Kost J, Mitragotri S. Combined effect of low frequency ultrasound and iotophoresis. Applications of transdermal heparin delivery. *Pharm Res* 2000; 17 (9): 151–4.
61. Barry BW. Novel mechanisms and devices to enable successful transdermal drug delivery. *Eur J Pharm Sci* 2001; 14 (2): 101–14.
62. King MJ, Badea I, Solomon J, Kumar P, Gaspar KI, Foldvari M. Transdermal delivery of insulin from a novel biphasic lipid system in diabetic rats. *Diabetes Technol Ther* 2002; 4 (4): 479–88.
63. Kost J. Ultrasound-assisted insulin delivery and noninvasive glucose sensing. *Diabetes Technol Ther* 2002; 4 (4), 489–97.
64. Hirai S, Ikenaga T, Matzuzawa T. Nasal absorption of insulin in dogs. *Diabetes* 1978; 27: 296–9.
65. Pontiroli AE, Alberetto M, Secchi A, Dossi G, Bosi I, Pozza G. Insulin given intranasally induces hypoglycemia in normal and diabetic subjects. *Br Med J* 1982; 284: 303–6.
66. Gizurarson S, Bechgaard E. Intranasal administration of insulin to humans. *Diabetes Res Clin Pract* 1991; 12: 71–84.
67. Merkus FWHM, Schipper NGM, Verhoef JC. The influence of absorption enhancers on intranasal insulin

absorption in normal and diabetic subjects. *J Control Release* 1996; 41: 69–75.
68. Duchateau GSMJE, Zuidema J, Merkus FWHM. Bile salts and intranasal drug absorption. *Int J Pharm* 1986; 31: 193–9.
69. Hinchcliffe M, Illum L. Intranasal insulin delivery and therapy. *Adv Drug Deliv Rev* 1999; 35 (2–3): 199–234.
70. Brange J, Langkjaer L. Insulin formulation and delivery. *Pharm Biotechnol* 1997; 10: 343–409.
71. Drejer K, Vaag A, Bech K, Hansen P, Sørensen AR, Mygind N. Intranasal insulin administration of insulin with phospholipid as absorption enhancer: pharmacokinetics in normal subjects. *Diabet Med* 1992; 9: 335–40.
72. Holman RR. Intranasal insulin in type 1 diabetes. In Berger M, Gries FA (eds), *Frontiers in Insulin Pharmacology*. Stuttgart: Thieme Verlag, 1993; pp 138–43.
73. Bruce DG, Chishom DJ, Storlien LH, Borkman M, Kraegen EW. Meal-time intranasal insulin delivery in type 2 diabetes. *Diabet Med* 1991; 8: 366–70.
74. Frauman AG, Jerums G, Louis WJ. Effects of intranasal insulin in non-obese type 2 diabetics. *Diabetes Res Clin Pract* 1987; 3: 197–202.
75. Coates PA, Ismail IS, Luzio SD, Griffiths I, Ollerton RL, Vølund A, Owens DR. Intranasal insulin: the effect of three dose regimens on postprandial glycemic profiles in type 2 diabetic subjects. *Diabet Med* 1995; 12: 235–9.
76. Frauman AG, Cooper ME, Parsons BJ, Jerums G, Louis WJ. Long-term use of intranasal insulin in insulin-dependant diabetic patients. *Diabetes Care* 1987; 10 (5): 573–8.
77. Salzman R, Manson JE, Griffing GT, Kimmerel R, Ruderman N, McCall A, Armstrong J, et al. Intranasal aerosolized insulin. Mixed-meal studies and long-term use in type 1 diabetes. *N Engl J Med* 1985; 312 (17): 1078–84.
78. Hilsted J, Madsbad S, Hvidberg A, Rasmussen MH, Krarup T, Ipsen H, Hansen B, Pedersen M, Djurup R, Oxenbøll B. Intranasal insulin therapy: the clinical realities. *Diabetologia* 1995; 38: 680–4.
79. Lassman-Vague V, Thiers D, Vialettes B, Vague PH. Preprandial intranasal insulin. *Lancet* 1988; 331: 367–8.
80. Lelej-Bennis D, Boillot J, Bardin C, Zirinis P, Coste A, Escudier E, Chast F, Peynegre R, Selam JL, Slama G. Efficacy and tolerance of intranasal insulin administered during 4 months in severely hyperglycemic type 2 diabetic patients with oral drug failure: a crossover study. *Diabet Med* 2001; 18: 614–8.
81. Lelej-Bennis D, Boillot J, Bardin C, Zirinis P, Coste A, Escudier E, Chast F, Peynegre R, Slama G, Selam JL. Six month administration of gelified intranasal insulin in type 1 diabetic patients under multiple injections: efficacy versus subcutaneous injections and local tolerance. *Diabetes Metab* 2001; 27 (3): 372–7.
82. Lee WA. Histological studies of insulin absorption across the nasal mucosa in the presence of sodium taurodihydrofusidate (STDHF). *Proc Int Symp Control Release Biochem Mater* 1988; 15: 77.
83. Patton JS. Mechanisms of macromolecule absorption by the lungs. *Adv Drug Deliv Rev* 1996; 19: 3–36.
84. Patton JS, Platz RM. Pulmonary delivery of peptides and proteins for systemic action. *Adv Drug Deliv Rev* 1992; 8: 179–96.
85. Byron PR. Prediction of drug residence times in regions of the human respiratory tract following aerosol inhalation. *J Pharm Sci* 1986; 75 (5): 433–9.
86. Von Heubner W, de Jongh SE, Laquer E. Uber inhalation von insulin. *Klin Wochenschr* 1924; 51: 2342–3.
87. Gansslen M. Uber inhalation von insulin. *Klin Wochenschr* 1925; 4: 71.
88. Wigley FM, Londono JH, Scott MD, Wood SH, Shipp JC, Waldman RH. Insulin across respiratory mucosae by aerosol delivery. *Diabetes* 1971; 20: 552–6.
89. Elliot RB, Edgar BW, Pilcher CC, Quested C, McMaster J. Parenteral absorption of insulin from the lung in diabetic children. *Aust Paediatr J* 1987; 23: 293–7.
90. Kohler D. Nicht radioaktives verfahren zur messung der lungenpermeabilitat: inhalation von insulin. *Atemwegs-Lungenkrankh* 1987; 13: 230–2.
91. Laube BL, Georgeopolous A, Adams GK. Preliminary study of the efficacy of insulin aerosol delivered by oral inhalation in diabetic patients. *JAMA* 1993; 269: 2106–9.
92. Galloway TA, Spradlin CT, Nelson RL, Wentworth SM, Davidson JA, Swarner JL. Factors influencing the absorption versus insulin concentration and blood glucose responses after injections of regular insulin in various insulin mixtures. *Diabetes Care* 1981; 4: 366–76.
93. Jendle JH, Karlberg BE. Intrapulmonary administration of insulin to healthy volunteers. *J Intern Med* 1996; 240 (2): 93–8.
94. Heinemann L, Traut T, Heise T. Time–action profile of inhaled insulin. *Diabet Med* 1997; 14 (1): 63–72.
95. Laube BL, Benedict GW, Dobs AS. Time to peak insulin level. Relative bioavailability, and effect of site of deposition of nebulized insulin in patients with non insulin-dependant diabetes mellitus. *J Aerosol Med* 1998; 11 (3): 153–73.
96. Gelfand RA, Schwartz SL, Horton M, Law CG, Pun EF. Pharmacological reproducibility of inhaled human insulin in patients with type 2 diabetes mellitus. *Diabetologia* 2000; 43: 773.
97. Lauritzen T, Faber OK, Binder C. Variation in ^{125}I-insulin absorption and blood glucose concentration. *Diabetologia* 1979; 17: 291–5.
98. Patton JS, Bukar J, Nagarajan S. Inhaled insulin. *Adv Drug Deliv Rev* 1999; 35: 235–47.
99. Martonen TB, Schroeter JD, Hwang D, Fleming JS, Conway JH. Human lung morphology models for particle deposition studies. *Inhal Toxicol* 2000; 12: 109–21.
100. Schultz H. Mechanisms and factors affecting intrapulmonary particle deposition: implications for efficient inhalation therapies. *Pharm Sci Technol* 1998; 1: 336–44.
101. Farr SJ, McElduff A, Mather LE, Okikawa J, Ward ME, Gonda I, Licko V, Rubsamen RM. Pulmonary insulin administration using the AER_x™ system: physiological and physiochemical factors influencing insulin effectiveness in healthy fasting subjects. *Diabetes Technol Ther* 2000; 2 (2): 185–97.
102. Wollmer P, Evander E. Biphasic pulmonary clearance of 99mTc-DPTA in smokers. *Clin Physiol* 1994; 14 (5): 547–59.
103. Bradvik I, Wollmer P, Evander E, Sloth M, Larusdottir H, Blom-Bulow B, Jonson B. One year follow-up of lung clearance of 99mTc-diethylene traimine penta-acetic acid and diseases activity in sarcodisis. *Vasc Diffuse Lung Dis* 2000; 17 (3): 281–7.
104. Jones JG, Royston D, Minty BD. Changes in alveolar–capillary barrier function in animals and humans. *Am Rev Respir Dis* 1983; 127 (5 pt 2): S51–9.

105. Minty BD, Royston D, Jones JG, Hulands GH. The effect of nicotine on pulmonary epithelial permeability in man. *Chest* 1984; 86 (1): 72–4.
106. Meignam M, Rosso J, Leveau J, Katz A, Cinotti L, Madelaine G, Galle P. Exercise increases the lung clearance of inhaled technetium-99m DPTA. *J Nucl Med* 1986; 27 (2): 274–80.
107. Schmekel B, Borgstrom L, Wollmer P. Exercise increases the rate of pulmonary absorption of inhaled terbulatie. *Chest* 1992; 1 (3): 742–5.
108. Fink JB. Metered-dose inhalers, dry powder inhalers, and transitions. *Respir Care* 2000; 456 (6): 623–35.
109. Corne J, Gillespie D, Roberts D, Younes M. Effect of inspiratory flow rate in intubated ventilated patients. *Am J Respir Crit Care Med* 1997; 156 (1): 304–8.
110. Smith KJ, Chan HK, Brown KF. Influence of flow rate on aerosol particle size distributions from pressurised and breath-actuated inhalers. *J Aerosol Med Deposit Clear Eff Lung* 1998; 11 (4): 231–45.
111. Borgstom L, Bengtsson T, Derom E, Pauwels R. Variability in lung deposition of inhaled drug, within and between asthmatic patients, with a pMDI and dry powder inhaler, Turbuhaler. *Int J Pharm* 2000; 193 (2): 227–30.
112. Maggi L, Bruni R, Conte U. Influence of the moisture on the performance of a new dry powder inhaler. *Int J Pharm* 1999; 177 (1): 83–91.
113. Heise T, Rave K, Bott S, Sha S, Willavize SA, Gruber S, Lee JD, Heinemann L. Time–action profile of an inhaled insulin preparation in comparison to insulin lispro and regular insulin. *Diabetes* 2000; 39 (suppl 1): A10.
114. Berger S, Davidson MH, Kourides I, Landshulz WH, Gelfand RA. Add-on therapy with inhaled human insulin in type 2 diabetic patients failing oral agents. Preliminary results of a multicentre trial. *Diabetologia* 1998; 41 (suppl 1): A226.
115. Skyler JS, Cefalu WT, Kourides IA, Landschulz WH, Balagtas CC, Cheng SL, Gelfand RA. Efficacy of inhaled human insulin in type 1 diabetes mellitus: a randomised proof-of-concept study. *Lancet* 2001; 357 (9253): 331–5.
116. Cappelleri JC, Kourides IA, Gerber RA, Gelfand RA. Development and factor analysis of a questionnaire to measure patient satisfaction with inhaled insulin for type 1 diabetes. *Diabetes Care* 2000; 23 (12): 1799–803.
117. Gerber RA, Kourides IA, Cappelleri JC, Gelfand RA. Treatment satisfaction with inhaled insulin in patients with type 1 diabetes. *Diabetes Care* 2001; 24 (9): 1556–9.
118. Skyler JS. Efficacy and safety of inhaled insulin (Exubera®) comparison to subcutaneous insulin therapy in an intensive insulin regimen in patienst with type 1 diabetes: results of a 6-month, randomised comparative trial. *Diabetes* 2002; 51 (suppl 2): A134.
119. Cefalu WT, Skyler JS, Kourides IA, Landschultz WH, Balagtas CC, Cheng S-L, Gelfand RA. Inhaled human insulin treatment in patients with type 2 diabetes mellitus. *Ann Intern Med* 2001; 134 (3): 203–7.
120. Cefalu WT. Inhaled insulin: a proof of concept study. *Ann Intern Med* 2001; 134 (9): 795.
121. Rosenstock J. Mealtime rapid acting inhaled insulin (Exubera®) improves glycemic control in patients with type 2 diabetes failing combination oral agents: a 3 month randomised comparative trial. *Diabetes* 2002; 51 (suppl 2): A132.
122. Cefalu WT, Balagtas CC, Landshultz WH, Gelfand RA. Sustained efficacy and pulmonary safety of inhaled insulin during 2 years of outpatient therapy. *Diabetologia* 2000; 43 (suppl 1): A47.
123. Farr SJ, Warren SJ, Lloyd P, Okikawa JK, Schuster JA, Rowe AM, Rubsamen RM, Taylor G. Comparison of *in vitro* and *in vivo* efficiencies of a novel unit-dose aerosol generator and a pressurised metered dose inhaler. *Int J Pharm* 2000; 198: 63–70.
124. Sangwan S, Agout JM, Bover LA, Otulono BA, Moristige RJ, Cipolla DC, Blanchard JD, Smalldone GC. Aersolised protein delivery in asthma; gamma analysis of regional deposition and perfusion. *J Aerosol Med* 2001; 14: 185–95.
125. Ann B, Renhardt R. *Breath Holding is not Required for Pulmonary Administration of Insulin by the AER$_x$ Insulin Diabetes Management System*. Alexandria, VA: ADA, 2002.
126. Chan H-K, Daviskas E, Eberl S, Robinson M, Bautovich G, Young I. Deposition of aqueous aerosol of technetuium-99 m diethylene triamine penta-acetic acid generated and delivered by a novel system (AER$_x$) in healthy subjects. *Eur J Nucl Med* 1999; 26 (4): 320–7.
127. McElduff A, Farr S, Ward E, Okumu F, Mather L, Gonda I, Rubsamen R, Dimarchi R, Wolff R. Comparison of the pharmacokinetics and pharmacodynamics of subcutaneous and inhaled insulin lispro in healthy fasted volunteers. *Diabetes* 1998; 47: 413.
128. Heise T, Scharling B, Bellaire S, Tusek C, Bott S. Dose–response of pulmonary insulin with the AER$_x$® insulin diabetes management system in healthy subjects. *Diabetologia* 2001; 44 (suppl 1): 812.
129. Jendle J, Himmelmann A, Mellen A, Wollmer P, Petersen AH, Dahl UL. Pharmacokinetics of pulmonary insulin in healthy smokers and non-smokers. *Diabetologia* 2001; 44 (suppl 1): 816.
130. Mellen A, Himmelmann A, Jendle J, Wollmer P. Pharmacokinetics and intra-patient variability of inhaled insulin in healthy smokers and non-smokers. *Diabetes* 2001; 50 (suppl 2): A126.
131. Henry R, Mudaliar S, Howland HI, Chu N, Kim D, An B, Reinhart R. Pulmonary delivery of insulin using the AER$_x$™ insulin diabetes management system in healthy and asthmatic subjects. *Diabetologia* 2001; 44 (suppl 1): 9.
132. McElduff A, Clauson P, Uy C, Kam P. *Pulmonary Absorption Profiles of Insulin During and After an Upper Respiratory Tract Infection in Healthy Volunteers Using the AER$_x$ Insulin Diabetes Management System. An Open Labelled Crossover Study in Healthy Volunteers*. Alexandria, VA: ADA, 2002.
133. Brunner GA, Balent B, Ellmerer M, Schnapp L, Siebenhofer A, Jendle JH, Okikawa J, Pieber TR. Dose–response relation of liquid aerosol inhaled insulin in type 1 diabetic patents. *Diabetologia* 2001; 44: 305–8.
134. Kipnes M, Otulana B, Okikawa J, Farr S, Jendle J, Thipphawong J, Schwartz S. Pharmacokinetics and pharmacodynamics of pulmonary insulin delivered via the AER$_x$® diabetes management system in type 1 diabetics, *Diabetologia* 2000; 43 (suppl 1): A201.
135. Hompesch M, Kapitza C, Scharling B, Thomsen LK, Heise T. Intrasubject variability of pulmonary insulin via the AER$_x$® insulin diabetes management system versus subcutaneous insulin, *Diabetologia* 2001; 44 (suppl 1): 813.
136. Kapitza C, Hompesch M, Thomsen LK, Heise T. *intrasubject Variability of Pulmonary Insulin via the AER$_x$*

Insulin Diabetes Management System Versus Subcutaneous Insulin. Alexandria, VA: ADA, 2002.

137. Hermansen K, Ronnemaa T, Petersen AH, Adamson U. *Intensive Treatment with Pulmonary Insulin Using the AER$_x$ Insulin Diabetes Management System. A Proof of Concept Trial in type 2 Diabetic Patients*. Alexandria, VA: ADA, 2002.
138. Henry R, Mudaliar S, Chu N, Reinhardt R. *Pharmacokinetics and Pharmacodynamics of Pulmonary Insulin in Young and Elderly type 2 Diabetic Patients Using the AER$_x$ Insulin Diabetes Management System*. Alexandria, VA: ADA, 2002.
139. Farr S, Reynolds, D, Nat A, Srinivasen S, Roach M, Jensen S, Poulsen JU. Technical development of AER$_x$ diabetes management system: essential characteristics for diabetes treatment with pulmonary insulin. In Byron PR, Dalby RN, Peart J, Farr SJ (eds), *Respiratory Drug Delivery VIII, Vol I*. Raleigh: Davies Horwood International, 2002; pp 51–9.
140. Stoever JA, Palmer JP. Inhaled insulin and insulin antibodies: a new twist to an old debate. *Diabetes Technol Ther* 2002; 4 (2): 157–61.
141. Fishman RS, Guinta D, Chambers F, Quintana R, Shapiro DA. Insulin administration via the Aerodose™ inhaler: comparison to subcutaneously injected insulin. *Diabetes* 2000; 49 (suppl 1): 38.
142. Heinemann L, Kapitza C, Heise T, Shapiro DA, Gopalakrishan V, Fishman RS. Impact of particle size and aerosolization time on the metabolic effect of an inhaled insulin aerosol. *Diabetologia* 2001; 44 (suppl 1): 10.
143. Perera AD, Kapitza C, Nosek L, Heinemann LW, Shapiro DA, Fishman TC, Heise TC. Reproducibility of inhaled and subcutaneous insulin in type 2 diabetic patients, *Diabetologia* 2001; 44 (suppl 1): 815.
144. Edwards DA, Hanes J, Caponetti G, Hrkach J, Ben-Jebria A, Eskew ML, Mintzes J, Deaver D, Lotan N, Langer R. Large porous particles for pulmonary drug delivery. *Science* 1997; 276: 1868–71.
145. Edwards DA, Ben-Jerbria A, Eskew ML, Langer R. Recent advances in pulmonary drug delivery using large, porous inhaled particles. *J Appl Physiol* 1998; 85 (2): 379–85.
146. Hrkach J, Batycky R, Chen D, Deaver D, Lloyd E, Kovalesky RA, Nice J, Schmitke J, Stapleton K, Edwards D. AIR insulin: complete diabetes therapy via inhalation of fact-acting and slow-acting dry powder aerosols. *Diabetes* 2000; 49 (suppl 1): 37.
147. Vanbever R, Ben-jebria A, Mintzes JD, Langer R, Edwards DA. Sustained release of insulin from insoluble inhaled particles. *Drug Dev Res* 1999; 48 (4): 178–85.
148. Pfutzner A, Mann A, Steiner S. Technosphere™/insulin—a new approach for effective delivery of human insulin via the pulmonary route. *Diabetes Technol Ther* 2002; 4 (5): 589–93.
149. Rave KM, Heise T, Pfutzner A, Steiner S, Heinemann L. Results of a dose–response study with a news pulmonary insulin formulation and inhaler. *Diabetes* 2000; 49 (suppl 1): 305 pp.
150. Pfutzner A, Rave K, Heise T, Steiner S, Heinemann L. Low variability in metabolic action in type 2 diabetic patients with inhaled Technosphere™/insulin. *Diabetologia* 2000; 43 (suppl 1): A202.
151. Yamamoto A, Fujita T, Muranshi S. Pulmonary absorption enhancement of peptides by absorption enhancers and protease inhibitors. *J Control Release* 1996; 41 (1–2): 57–67.
152. Heinemann L, Klappoth W, Rave K, Hompesch B, Linkeschowa R, Heise T. Intra-individual variability of the metabolic effect of inhaled insulin together with an absorption enhancer. *Diabetes Care* 2000; 23 (9) 1343–7.
153. Heinemann L, Pfutzner A, Heise T. Alternative routes of administration as an approach to improve insulin therapy: update on dermal, oral, nasal and pulmonary insulin delivery. *Curr Pharm Des* 2001; 7 (14): 1327–51.
154. Niranjan V, McBrayer DG, Ramirez LC, Raskin P, Hsai CC. glycemic control and cardiopulmonary function in patients with insulin-dependent diabetes mellitus. *Am J Med* 1997; 103 (6): 504–13.
155. Ramirez IC, Dal Nogare A, Hsia C, Arauz C, Bott C, Strowig SM, Schnurr-Brren L, Raskin P. Relationship between diabetes control and pulmonary function in insulin-dependent diabetes mellitus. *Am J Med* 1991; 91 (4): 371–6.
156. Schmekel B, Borgstrom L, Wollmer P. Difference in pulmonary absorption of inhaled terbutaine in healthy smokers and non-smokers. *Thorax* 1991; 46 (4): 225–8.
157. Wise SD, Sathirakul K, Yeo KP, Chien JY, Aftring P. Smoking increases the bioavailability of inhaled insulin, but relative insulin resistance ameliorates differences in action. *Diabetologia* 2001; 44 (suppl 1): 0048.
158. Weiss SR, Berger S, Cheng SL, Kourides I, Landshultz WH, Gelfand RA. Adjunctive therapy with inhaled human insulin in type 2 diabetic patients failing oral agents: a multicenter phase II trial. *Diabetes* 1999; 48 (suppl 1): 0048.
159. Chan NN, Baldeweg S, Tan TMM, Hurel SI, Nagaoka T, Miyakoshi H, Baker EH, Phillips BJ, Cavello MG, Coppolino G, Romeo S, Pozzilli P. Inhaled insulin in type 1 diabetes. *Lancet* 2001; 357 (9272): 1979.
160. Baker EH, Phillips BJ. Inhaled insulin in type 1 diabetes. *Lancet* 2001; 357 (9272): 1979.
161. Laube BL, Benedict W, Dobs AS. The lung as an alternative route of delivery for insulin in controlling postprandial glucose levels in patients with diabetes. *Chest* 1998: 114: 1734–9.

55

Implantable Pumps

Christopher D. Saudek and Chee W. Chia

The Johns Hopkins University School of Medicine, Baltimore, MD, USA

INTRODUCTION

Clinical approaches to insulin delivery remain crude and imperfect. While problems of purity, stability, and consistency of the insulin itself have been largely solved, particularly with the advent of recombinant DNA technology, the delivery systems remain primitive. The vast majority of people with insulin-requiring diabetes continue to take conventional insulin injections subcutaneously one to four times daily. Even as external insulin pumps become more widely used, the route of delivery remains erratic and unphysiologic.

Subcutaneous (SC) injection is imprecise, a fraction of the dose often being delivered intramuscularly [1]. And if the insulin is truly delivered subcutaneously, there are still a number of essentially uncontrollable variables [2]. The temperature of the skin, muscle contractions, and lipoatrophy each affect pharmacokinetics. Perhaps most important, subcutaneously injected insulin is absorbed into the peripheral venous circulation, instead of the hepatic portal system and liver.

Implantable insulin infusion pumps that deliver insulin into the peritoneal cavity offer the promise of being more physiologic and more acceptable to patients—more physiologic because the insulin is delivered by basal–bolus patterns into the peritoneal space where it is preferentially absorbed into the portal system [3], and more acceptable because of the freedom from insulin injections or the limitations of wearing an external insulin pump. Daily injections, perhaps more than anything else, are identified as the downside of diabetes self-care.

The development of implantable insulin pumps (IIPs), however, has been a laborious exercise in applied research, extending back for at least the past quarter century. The participants have necessarily included engineers working in collaboration with clinicians. The technical challenges of designing a safe and effective delivery system have been formidable: insulin had to be modified to survive at body temperature for months at a time; pumps had to be designed that would be reliable for years at a time, would not harm the insulin, or have excessive power requirements; microelectronics had to assure reliable, durable transcutaneous communication. A series of safety features had to be incorporated that would eliminate the chance of unintended overdelivery of insulin. And even then, designs that appeared promising on the bench were foiled at an alarming rate when used *in vivo*. Most troublesome of all is the still-vexing problem of keeping the very tip of the insulin delivery catheter open and in contact with insulin-absorbing tissue. These have not been trivial exercises in biomedical engineering.

A BRIEF HISTORY OF IIP DEVICES

The first investigational use of IIPs for the treatment of diabetes in humans dates back to the late 1970s [4, 5]. Initially, the Infusaid pump, pioneered by Buchwald and colleagues at the University of Minnesota [6], used a positive pressure exerted by a Freon® as the driving force. This original pump delivered at only one continuous rate, and to change that rate, one had to change the concentration of insulin in the reservoir. While it has frequently been mentioned that continuous insulin infusion could have specific benefit in treating type 2 diabetes [7], it is clear that variable rate delivery is necessary to treat type 1 diabetes successfully.

In the 1980s, more sophisticated pumps were introduced that could be remotely controlled and could vary

International Textbook of Diabetes Mellitus, Third Edition. Edited by R. A. DeFronzo, E. Ferrannini, H. Keen, and P. Zimmet.
 ISBN: 0-471-48655-8.

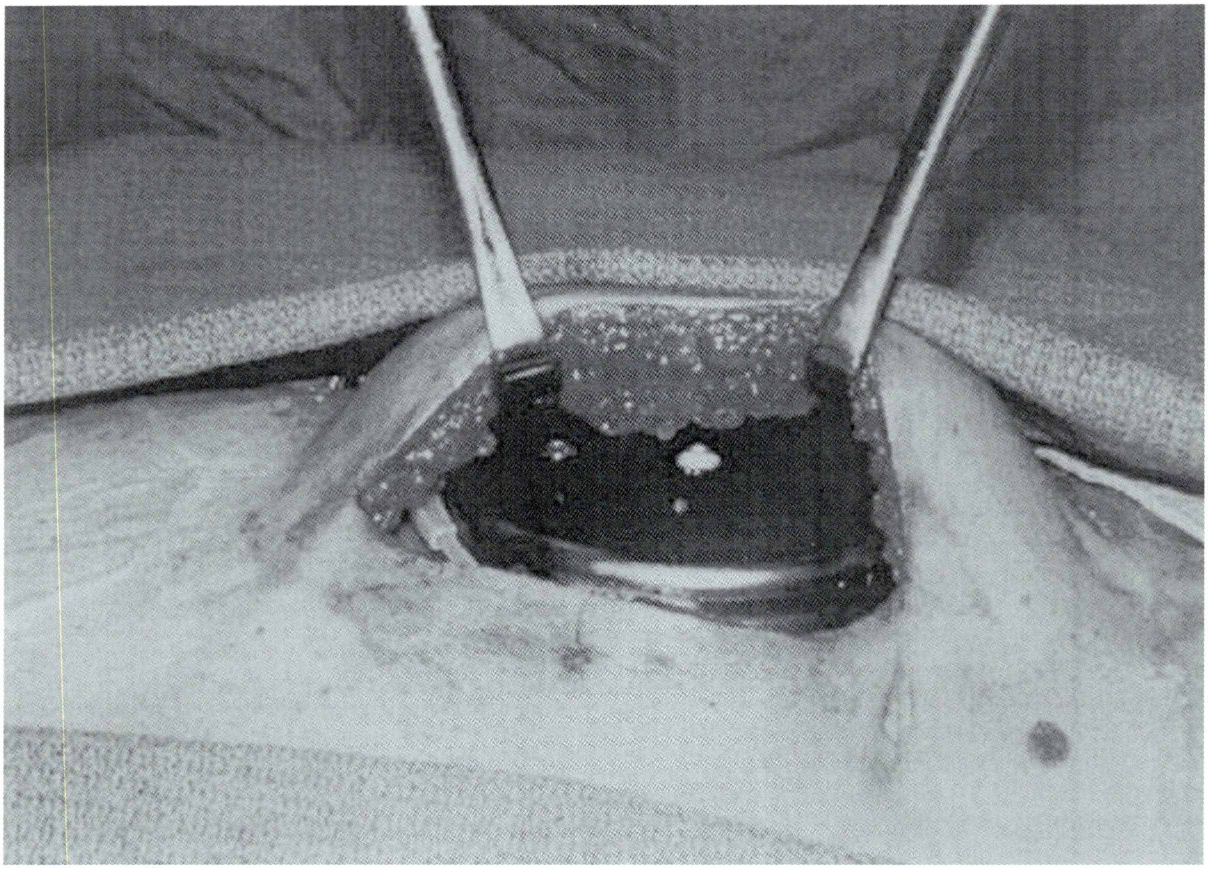

Figure 1 Medtronic MiniMed Implantable Insulin Pump

the rate of insulin delivery. Three different types of programmable insulin devices were developed:

(1) At the Johns Hopkins University Applied Physics Laboratory, the Programmable Implantable Medication System (PIMS) was designed by Fischell and coworkers [8]. License to develop and manufacture PIMS was transferred to MiniMed, Inc., and subsequent generations of the MiniMed Implantable Pump (MIP) were developed by the company that in 2000 became Medtronic MiniMed Implantable Pump, MIP (Northridge, CA, USA).
(2) Shiley Infusaid Co., no longer in existence, developed the Infusaid pump. This underwent extensive clinical trials before the project was dropped, apparently because of difficulty manufacturing a totally reliable positive-pressure pump.
(3) Siemens, Inc., developed several models of IIPs in the 1980s and 1990s before abandoning the project.

In the late 1990s, Infusaid and Siemens stopped the production of their IIPs, leaving Medtronic MiniMed MIP as the only available device.

THE ANATOMY OF IMPLANTABLE INSULIN INFUSION PUMPS

Consideration of the components that make up IIPs will provide an overview of how the current systems operate, what developmental challenges have been overcome, and what problems remain. Since the Medtronic MiniMed pump is the only device currently in widespread trials, it will be described in more detail.

The Casing

The implanted device is housed in a titanium disk of 8.1-cm diameter and 2.0-cm thickness, weighing 131 g with an empty reservoir (Figure 1). There is a central refill port on the superficial surface of the pump, which is a round cone-shaped entrance about 7 mm in diameter. It is accessed transcutaneously for refills. The insulin is delivered from an outlet port on a tangent edge of the pump, to which the catheter is attached. Also on the tangent edge of the pump are wire loops for suturing the device to the fascia.

The main determinant of overall pump size is reservoir volume, which itself determines the interval patients can go between refills. The current pump, MMT-2007C, can hold up to 15 ml of the highly concentrated insulin (400 units/ml), and the insulin preparation requires refills every three months. To make a significantly smaller implanted device, would require either even more concentrated insulin or a smaller reservoir and thus shorter refill intervals.

The Catheter

The catheter exits the pump, traverses the abdominal musculature, and delivers the insulin into the peritoneal space. It is surgically secured to the rectus muscles, with a 17-cm distal portion floating freely in the abdomen cavity. In early trials, catheters often became grossly encapsulated within the peritoneum, blocking the exit of insulin and requiring laparoscopic surgery to clean the tissue off. With the development of more flexible, more biocompatible catheters, gross encapsulation is not often seen. There remains an incidence of catheter blockage by small fibrin-containing plugs at the catheter tip, however [9, 10]. These catheter blocks, interestingly, ordinarily present gradually and intermittently, with patients noticing less responsiveness to administered insulin or short periods of unresponsiveness. If complete blockage occurs, they resume SC insulin injections until the catheters can be surgically replaced (see below).

As insulin precipitation and aggregation were noted, sideports were added to the hub of the catheter where it meets the pump. This allows a needle to be passed transcutaneously into the proximal portion of the catheter, for flushing the catheter or for drawing fluid through the pump without entering the patient. Problems with insulin aggregation within the pump, in the catheter, or catheter blocks can often be corrected with this catheter sideport.

The Pump Module

The actual pumping mechanism for delivering the insulin has required innovative engineering. Insulin is a fragile molecule, subject to physical as well as thermal and chemical damage. The pump must therefore be mechanically "gentle," but other requirements include precision, reliability, and minimal power requirement.

One suboptimal approach tried in early devices, for example, used a roller pump mechanism that was like a miniaturized tractor tread [11]. The problems were two: it required considerable electrical current to keep the pump churning, causing a short battery life; and the mechanical pressure damaged the fragile insulin molecule.

The PIMS, invented at the Johns Hopkins University Applied Physics Laboratory [8] and developed at School of Medicine, took a different approach. A tiny positive displacement pump, developed originally by the National Aeronautics and Space Administration (NASA), provides an accurate pulse with minimal power requirement and minimal trauma to the insulin. Variations on this positive displacement pump have been used in subsequent versions of the Medtronic MiniMed Implantable Pumps.

The Reservoir

Reservoirs in the current pump are not a static holding tank. Rather, one surface is a diaphragm that moves on bellows between a Freon chamber and the insulin reservoir. When the reservoir is full, the Freon chamber is collapsed, but as the reservoir empties, the Freon chamber expands. Freon serves the purpose particularly well since its maintains essentially equal pressure regardless of volume. As volume of the chamber expands, more Freon vaporizes; as volume contracts, Freon liquefies; at all points, the gas pressure exerted on the reservoir is essentially constant; just what that pressure is, depends on the type of Freon used.

The most significant difference between the MIP and the earlier Infusaid pumps is the type of Freon. In the case of the original Infusaid pump and its successors, the Freon exerts a positive pressure relative to atmosphere, a pressure that becomes the driving force of insulin delivery (4). In contrast, the MIP uses a type of Freon that exerts a pressure less than atmospheric pressure, i.e. a vacuum relative to atmosphere. This provides significant safety in the MIP, described later.

The Electronics and Power Source

In the absence of a glucose sensor (all available insulin delivery systems are "open loop," without a glucose sensor), patient-driven communication from outside the body is the key to establishing variable rate insulin delivery. The external device can of course have manyfold more energy requirement since batteries can be changed, and even failure to function is less critical than with the implanted components, since the external programmer can also be exchanged easily. But size, speed, and effectiveness of communication is most important. With the latest MIP model MMT-2007C, the external device has become smaller, quicker, and is said to be more reliable.

Remote communication systems were applied to insulin pumps in the 1980s. The reliability of such communication had been well established by the NASA space program, and since then, of course, remote control of everything from televisions to car door locks has become commonplace. Control of the implantable insulin pump requires a two-way link between the implant and the external device, and is coded to prevent other sources of radio frequency signals to interfere or cause extraneous commands to occur.

The electronics of the MIP have been redesigned several times. The object is to provide both reliability and the smallest possible energy use so as to prolong life of the implanted battery. No pump models in recent years have replaceable or rechargeable batteries, and so the entire pump must be replaced surgically when the battery runs down. The MMT-2007C devices have a battery life expectancy reputed to be about 8 years, a significant improvement from the 3-year battery life in older models. Redundant internal checks by the electronics are part of the safety profile.

The Insulin

Insulin is a highly unstable protein, subject to aggregation, precipitation, and denaturation [12, 13]. In initial design phase, the ability of insulin to remain active after months at body temperature was thought to be the main obstacle. With initial trials, however, this was not nearly so much of a problem as was insulin stability. Development of a stable insulin preparation has thus been a focus of implantable insulin pump programs since the beginning.

Early approaches to preventing insulin aggregation included use of a highly viscous solution of glycerol [14]. This was difficult to work with, even to pass through a needle for refills. A more practical solution was developed by Hoechst AG (Frankfurt, Germany), adding a surfactant material, polyethylene–polypropylene glycol (Genapol® [15]). This proved to be highly compatible in implanted pumps [16].

In addition to reservoir volume, the concentration of insulin determines the maximum refill interval. The insulin used by MIP has been U400 (400 units/ml), four times more concentrated than standard clinical insulin. We are unaware of studies indicating whether this is the maximum concentration feasible for use in implanted pumps, but it does allow a refill interval of every 3 months, which is clinically reasonable.

The insulin used, then, is called HOE 21 PH, and is a preparation of human regular insulin, stabilized by the surfactant material Genapol. One report found that lispro insulin was not useful with implanted insulin pumps [17], although it is possible that formula modifications could be made to make it so. HOE 21 PH insulin was apparently entirely stable and effective through the first 8 years or so of clinical trials, from 1986 through 1992. However that early success came to an abrupt halt.

Starting in about 1993, there was a marked increase in incidence of underdelivery. The consortium of French investigators called Evaulation dans le Diabète du Traitement par Implants Actifs (EVADIAC) Society, carefully documented the magnitude of the problem, and the fact that it reflected use of certain insulin batches, rather than pump models or duration of implantation [18]. Clinically, as with catheter blocks, it occurred gradually, and manifested as increased insulin dose requirements, sometimes to the point of doubling apparent daily dose. On refilling pumps, it was clear that the increased dose was due to underdelivery (increased volume of insulin in reservoir beyond that calculated to remain), rather than normal insulin delivery with loss of insulin potency. And unlike catheter blocks, the problem often resolved using a sodium hydroxide (NaOH) rinse of the pump.

By 1994, it was determined that there had been a change in the manufacturing procedure for insulin that significantly altered its long-term stability in implanted pumps, apparently to comply with the new regulations of *European Pharmacopoeia* [19]. Evaluation of some explanted pumps found that the new insulin formulation was causing microdeposits on one of the outlet valves, resulting in slightly impaired valve closure. The negative pressure reservoir was drawing a fraction of the stroke volume back into the reservoir.

The insulin stability problem hampered the progress of the implantable pumps for several years. During this period, a rinsing procedure using NaOH was developed to correct the backflow problems by dissolving the offending material from the valve seating [19]. Refill intervals were reduced to 30–45 days instead of the usual 90 days. A new laboratory method was developed that could test insulin stability more efficiently (without waiting months per batch), and ultimately a chromatography step was added to remove insoluble components during the manufacturing process. In 1997, the modified HOE 21 PH (now called Aventis HOE 21 PH) insulin became available, and experience showed that backflow problems were dramatically reduced [20].

Surgical Implantation

Pitt and Udelsman developed the surgical techniques in use at Johns Hopkins [21–23]. Pumps have been implanted under general anesthesia or with local anesthesia. About 45 min is required for preparation of the pump in the operating room, and the surgery itself takes a similar amount of time. The incision we have used is midline, although some surgeons prefer a transverse incision cephalad to the pump. The location of the pump in the abdomen is determined by patient preference and topography of the abdomen, but it must be either above or below the beltline, not directly under the belt. After the initial incision, a SC pocket is formed, and a small incision is made through the abdominal musculature into the abdominal cavity. The catheter is placed freely in the abdomen, the proximal portion sutured to the fascia. The pump is then placed subcutaneously and also sutured in place. Closure is accomplished and the wound heals in the usual manner. Perioperative antibiotics are started just before surgery.

Replacement of the pump and catheter or catheter alone is performed with local anesthetic. The original incision is reopened, the pump and catheter removed. Any resistance in removing the catheter tip from the abdominal cavity is noted, since that suggests an adhesion. On a sterile side table, the pump is checked for stroke volume, rinsed if necessary, and a new catheter is attached. The pump is put in place, the catheter tip inserted through the same small incision through the abdominal muscles, and the pump pocket closed separately from cutaneous closure.

It is not uncommon to have a seroma form for several weeks postoperatively. Some centers have used an abdominal wrap in the hope of reducing fluid accumulation; we have not found that useful. We do not drain the seroma unless it is so large as to threaten the integrity of the wound healing or unless we suspect infection. Antibiotics are restarted promptly if cellulitis, erythema, or fever is noted. Patients may remain hospitalized for 24 h postoperatively in the absence of complications.

Complications of surgery are unusual at our center. The most common is mild inflammation surrounding the pump, particularly when replacing a pump into the same pump pocket. The most serious complication is undoubtedly infection of the pump pocket. Frank infection (positive cultures, puss in the pocket, inflammation) is rarely if ever curable. The usual course is to require explantation followed several months later by reimplantation at a different site. The data from other centers are discussed later.

The implanted pumps are clearly visible under the skin of thinner subjects but may be well hidden in people with some degree of adiposity. They are not uncomfortable or painful and not perceived as heavy. All degrees of physical activity and athletics are routinely permissible, although we do not recommend heavy contact sports.

The incidence of local complications has varied widely from center to center, from 0 to 28% (mean 7.1%) per patient-year [24]. While postoperative seroma is common, persistent discomfort or pain at the site is not. It is most important that during long-term management of implanted pumps, the pump pocket does not become infected, though, since an established infection is virtually impossible to treat successfully without explantation. We therefore use aseptic technique in refilling the devices.

Safety Features

It is immediately apparent, in considering the safety of any approach to insulin delivery, that overdelivery of insulin is vastly more dangerous than underdelivery. Hyperglycemia and even ketoacidosis develop gradually and are readily avoidable by prompt reinstitution of conventional injections, whereas severe overdelivery could cause sudden, potentially catastrophic hypoglycemia. From the outset, therefore, designers of these devices have dealt with establishing fail-safe approaches that would prevent uncontrolled overdelivery of insulin. Put another way, all failure modes would manifest in underdelivery, not overdelivery.

The underlying mechanical safety approach of the PIMS and then the MIP has been the negative pressure reservoir. This has two major advantages. First, it allows refills to be done without any positive pressure that would push insulin into the body if the needle tip is not in the reservoir; instead, the insulin is drawn into the reservoir automatically when the needle tip is correctly placed. Second, any leaks will cause fluid to be drawn into the reservoir rather than causing insulin to be pushed out.

With patient-controlled insulin delivery, there can never be assurance that hypoglycemia will not occur, since the pump has no way of knowing when, whether, or how much of a meal is ingested. It is has always been a challenge to control postprandial hyperglycemia successfully, since insulin must be delivered at a rate 10–100 times higher postprandially than that required as a basal rate. As anyone with insulin-requiring diabetes knows, if a meal does not follow a mealtime dose of insulin, hypoglycemia can occur. Therefore, compromises had to be made that would prevent catastrophic insulin overdose while allowing adequate insulin delivery to control postprandial glycemia.

With the MIP, parameters can be programmed by the health care professional that limit both the basal and bolus insulin doses. These adjustable controls work well unless patients develop an underdelivery problem, in which case they often have to be adjusted to allow command rates that would otherwise be excessive.

While there have certainly been episodes of severe hypoglycemia, there have been no instances, in over 15 years of experience with the MIP or its predecessor, PIMS, of uncontrolled insulin delivery, or episode of catastrophic hypoglycemia.

CLINICAL USE OF IIPs

Patient Selection

Patients implanted with insulin pumps thus far are carefully selected, either in research settings or as part of specially selected centers. The devices have not been used by the general medical profession. The majority of implanted people have documented type 1 diabetes, although 59 patients in the Veterans Affairs Cooperative Study had type 2 diabetes. All patients using an implanted pump are expected to monitor their own blood glucose three to four times daily, to come in regularly for research data collection as well as routine clinical management, and they are motivated to take part in a new form of treatment. In general, patients with serious comorbidities, late-stage diabetic complications, pregnancy, and other factors, which would interfere with completion of reliable studies, have been largely excluded.

The rigorous eligibility criteria, however, should not be overemphasized. Over 100 patients have qualified at some individual centers. Subjects' age ranges at least from 14 to 75; they have a range of body weights from thin to obese; they have a wide variety of ethnic backgrounds and levels of formal education. While motivation to perform good self-care is a significant feature of the patient group, many have little formal education. It has not been our experience that management of the pump requires unusual intelligence.

There has been preliminary discussion of clinical indications for implantable insulin pump therapy [25], but much more discussion and consensus will be needed when the devices are more widely approved for clinical use.

PATIENT USE OF IIPs

Insulin is delivered in a basal–bolus pattern, i.e. at a continuous low basal rate (usually about 0.5–1 unit/h) between meals and overnight, supplemented by boluses (e.g., 2–10 units) delivered before meals. As with external pumps, the basal rates continue, recycling every 24 h, until changed by the patient. At each mealtime, the patient chooses an appropriate bolus dose, within limits established by the health care professional, places the external communicator over the pump, and presses a button on the communicator, commanding the pump to deliver the intended bolus.

Refills

Pump refills are accomplished, as noted, about every 3 months with the MIP. They are done in a medical setting, by either a carefully trained physician or a nurse. Refills by the patient are not a possibility, since the large amount of insulin put into the pump (6000 units) would be exceedingly dangerous if self-administered erroneously. After aseptic preparation of the skin, a drop of local anesthetic in the skin and a needle is placed through the skin into the pump reservoir. Old insulin is withdrawn, and the accuracy of insulin delivery by the pump can be precisely estimated by comparing the amount of insulin withdrawn with that expected to be present in the reservoir based on number of units "commanded." Underdelivery can be detected in this way. New insulin is then delivered after being drawn into a separate 50-ml syringe, and after thorough "degassing" by shaking in a relative vacuum created in the syringe. The entire refill procedure is essentially painless and ordinarily takes 10–15 min.

Management of Complications

Patients are carefully instructed to keep conventional insulin supplies available in case underdelivery occurs. If underdelivery is noted, either on the basis of unexpected amounts of insulin withdrawn at refills or because apparent dose requirement is increased, it is usually due to one of two problems—catheter block or backflow through a slightly incompetent outlet valve due to microdeposits of insulin. A rinse procedure with alkaline solution drawn through the pump (but not the catheter) corrects the backflow condition due to insulin aggregation on the pump valve, but if catheter block occurs, the catheter is surgically replaced under local anesthetic.

A low-battery condition is signaled in the MIP with an audible alarm, well before underdelivery from battery failure would occur. This is expected after 3.5 years of therapy with the older model 2000, but the latest model MMT-2007C is expected to last more than 7 years. If this longevity is correct, it would be expected that insulin and catheter issues would become rate-limiting rather than battery failure. There is no way to recharge batteries, and so battery failure requires elective replacement of the pump.

CLINICAL TRIALS OF IIP THERAPY

Initial Trials

The first clinical use of IIP therapy was by Buchwald et al. in the 1970s, using the constant-rate Infusaid pump in patients primarily with type 2 diabetes [5].

Variable rate pump trials took place in the early 1980s, with several relatively small experiences using pumps developed by the Sandia Corp. in collaboration with Schade et al. [26], and Siemens, working with Irsigler et al. [11]. While some success was achieved, the devices had short battery life, mechanical failures, and skin breakdown from the corners of the casing. Coincident with these experiences, PIMS, the predecessor of the MIP, was undergoing about 4 years of preclinical dog trial experience.

In 1986, PIMS entered clinical trials in 18 human subjects at the Johns Hopkins University and the University of California, Irvine [27]. For the first time, a variable rate pump was demonstrated to treat type 1 diabetes in reliable fashion, free of a disabling rate of device failures for an average of 3 years continuously. Glycemic control was excellent, and there were no surgical or other safety hazards. Another generation of the Siemens pump was used in 20 subjects in Europe simultaneously, with less good results [28].

Recent Clinical Trials

Table 1 lists the major clinical trials published as of September 2002, and described in more details in the text.

The MiniMed Implantable Pump Trial in Type 1 Diabetes Mellitus

The MIP trial in type 1 diabetes took place in over 26 hospitals in the United States, France, and elsewhere in Europe. Summary results have not been published, but

Table 1 Summary of major clinical studies

Study	Type of diabetes	Number of diabetic patients	Length of study (patient-years)	Type(s) of pumps
Nonrandomized trials				
MiniMed Implantable Pump Trials	Type 1	No published data available	NA	MiniMed MIP 2001
The Implantable Insulin Pump Trial Study Group [29]	Type 1	76	251	Infusaid Model 1000
Point Study II [10]	Type 1	31	51	Siemens Promedos 3
EVADIAC Registry [30, 31]	Type 1	298	NA	MiniMed MIP 2001 Infusaid Model 1000 Siemens Promedos 3
Randomized trial				
VA Cooperative Study [32]	Type 2	59	59	MiniMed MIP 2001

over 1000 pumps have been implanted, starting in 1990. The trial was not randomized or controlled. Centers were chosen largely on the basis of their ability to purchase pumps, and so the majority of implantations were in France, where the national health system agreed to purchase devices. The study was designed to collect data using the MIP in practice-based settings as well as university centers. There was a brief Food and Drug Administration (FDA)-imposed hold on new implantations in the United States in the mid-1990s, as the cause and correction of the backflow anomaly was worked out; and there was a hold of about a year as the model 2000 was replaced with model 2007 and as MiniMed, Inc. became Medtronic MiniMed. While French regulatory approval has been conditionally granted for some time now [25], in the United States, FDA approval remains pending, pending a pivotal trial.

The Infusaid Trial in Type 1 Diabetes (The Implantable Insulin Pump Trial Study Group)

The Infusaid clinical trial in type 1 diabetes began in 1989. Like the MiniMed trial, it was multicenter, carried out in Europe and the United States. And also like the MiniMed trial, it was not randomized, but was designed to expand experience with the Infusaid pump. This pump model, Infusaid Model 1000, had a positive pressure reservoire, needed refill every 4–6 weeks, and used HOE 21 PH U100 insulin (Hoechst AG, Frankfurt, Germany) [33]. Seventy-six patients with type 1 diabetes were recruited in nine centers, with duration of therapy averaged at 39.6 $\pm$10 months (range 4–58 months) for a total of 251 patient-years. The long-term outcome data showed that implantable pump therapy can maintain similar HbA_{1c} that of intensive SC therapy (mean $HbA_{1c} < 7.5\%$ during the 3 years), but with much lower incidence of hypoglycemia (33 episodes/100 patient-years for intensive SC therapy versus 4 episodes/100 patient-years for implantable pump therapy) [29].

The Siemens Implantable Pump Trial (The Point Study II Group)

For this trial, 31 patients with type 1 diabetes were enrolled in six centers in Europe [10]. Again, it was not a randomized trial. The patients were treated with implantable pump therapy for 10–30 months for a total of 51 patient-years. This pump model, Promedos 3, needed refill every 4–6 weeks and used HOE 21 PH U100 insulin (Hoechst AG, Frankfurt, Germany). The median HbA_{1c} was 7.5% (range 5.4–9.8). The rate of catheter obstruction requiring surgical intervention was noted to be very high at 25 episodes/100 patient-years, but the follow-up was short.

The EVADIAC Registry

The EVADIAC Society was founded in 1990 to provide a central registry for all patients with IIPs in France. A common protocol is used. This central registry enables exchange of information among the different centers, numbered at 15 as of 2001 [30]. From last available update in 1998, there are 1065 pumps implanted in 689 patients worldwide, and the EVADIAC group having the largest cohort, 298 patients [30, 31].

The EVADIAC group published a series of reports of a multicenter prospective study involving 224–240 type 1 diabetic patients with implantable insulin pumps in 1995 and 1996. Their results are compatible with the other trials, namely, HbA_{1c} is modestly reduced while glycemic fluctuations and hypoglycemic events are markedly reduced [9, 34, 35].

The Veterans Affairs Cooperative Study in Type 2 Diabetes

There are two crucial reasons to try implantable insulin pump therapy in type 2 diabetes [36]. First, as with type 1 diabetes, many people with type 2 diabetes are increasingly metabolically labile, indicating loss of β-cell function. Many do not, in fact, achieve good glycemic control despite multiple-dose insulin regimens. Second, there is concern that the peripheral hyperinsulinism caused by subcutaneously delivered insulin may be particularly inadvisable in people already prone to accelerated atherosclerosis. Insulin delivered into the peritoneal space not only is more rapidly absorbed than insulin delivered subcutaneously, but produces less peripheral hyperinsulinism [37], presumably because of the first-pass clearance of portally absorbed insulin by the liver.

The Veterans Affairs (VA) Cooperative Study of Implantable Insulin Pumps was therefore designed to test rigorously whether insulin delivered to people with type 2 diabetes by IIPs could control their diabetes as well as that delivered by multiple-dose insulin subcutaneously, and whether there are significant other advantages to the use of pumps in type 2 diabetes. The MIP was selected for use in the VA study. Being conceived and conducted entirely independent of corporate support, though, it was possible to accomplish the first large-scale randomized trial comparing the insulin delivery modes.

One-hundred twenty-one males with type 2 diabetes were recruited at seven VA medical centers in the United States. Fifty-nine individuals were randomized to IIP and 62 to multiple daily injection (MDI) therapy. The outcome of the study showed that, consistent with the study objective, very good glycemic control was achieved with both the implanted pumps and multiple daily doses of insulin, with HbA_{1c} at 7.34 (0.79%) (IIP) versus 7.54 (0.83%) (MDI). There was, however, significantly reduced glycemic variance in the patients treated with pumps, translating into a greatly reduced incidence of both severe and mild hypoglycemia in subjects assigned to implantable insulin pump therapy, by 87.5 and 68% respectively [32].

ENDOCRINE AND METABOLIC EFFECTS

Glycemic Control

Multiple studies have demonstrated the advantage of intraperitoneal (IP) route of insulin delivery versus SC (SC) or intravenous (IV) route in terms of more stable glycemic variance and less hypoglycemic events. Several studies were done to elucidate the underlying mechanisms of improved glycemic control.

In one report, euglycemic hyperinsulinemic glucose clamps were performed using IV versus IP form of insulin delivery. Both the IV and IP insulin delivery modes were equally effective on glucose metabolism, but the IP route can achieve similar effect at lower systemic insulin levels [38]. Selam et al. studied the effects of IP versus IV insulin in hypoglycemic clamp studies. The route of infusion significantly affected the glucose production/utilization rates in a pattern that might be expected: when insulin was delivered at rates that equalized peripheral insulinemia (i.e. more delivered IP, to account for hepatic clearance), hepatic glucose production was reduced. But when insulin was delivered at equal absolute rates, as might occur with IIP versus SC therapy, peripheral levels were lower. In this case, the lower peripheral insulin levels decreased glucose utilization, and glucose production was increased [39]. The data on IP delivery have been reviewed [3].

In type 1 diabetes, IIPs provide more physiologic free insulin profile than SC injection using continuous subcutaneous insulin infusion (CSII), with earlier higher peak and lower nighttime insulin level, consequently better postprandial glycemic profile and lower hypoglycemia [40]. Euglycemic clamp study was performed in patients with type 2 diabetes using IP or SC route on separate day, and IP route was shown to achieve more rapid and greater peak values for stimulation of glucose utilization and return quicker to basal insulin level than SC injection of regular insulin [41].

All the above studies used regular insulin for the SC route of injection. With the availability of faster acting insulin lispro, the kinetics of insulin of IIP and SC injections needed to be reevaluated. In a pilot study of 14 type 1 diabetic patients, insulin kinetics of CSII lispro was compared to that of IIP after implantation using each patient as his/her own control. Both daily blood glucose (BG) levels and preprandial BG levels were lower with IIP. Postprandial BG values tended to be lower with IIP but not statistically significant. Glucose variance and HbA_{1c} levels were lower at the end of 45 days with IIP [42].

Lipoprotein Metabolism

The effects of IIP therapy on lipid metabolism have been extensively studied but the results remain controversial. Bagdade et al. showed that after 6 months of IIP therapy in type 1 diabetes, cholesteryl ester transfer (CET) and lipoprotein lipase (LPL) activities were decreased to the normal range, with tryiglycerides, cholesterol, high-density lipoprotein 2 (HDL-2), and high-density lipoprotein 3 (HDL-3) remained unchanged at normal levels [43]. The same group also showed similar results in type 2 diabetic men after IIP therapy for 9 months where CET was normalized [44]. However, another group (Ruotolo et al.) reported an unchanged or slightly increased LPL activity, an increased hepatic lipase activity, and normalization of lipoprotein composition after 9 months of IIP therapy [45].

The VA study in type 2 diabetes showed improvement in total cholesterol level in both MDI and IIP groups, with no change in LDL, HDL, and triglycerides [46]. In another study, IIP therapy was shown to decrease chylomicron remnant levels in type 2 diabetes [47].

Hepatic Protein Synthesis

The more physiologic effect of IP insulin delivery with hepatic portal absorption of insulin seemed to normalize hepatic protein synthesis with possible positive effects on the endocrine system. Lassmann-Vague et al. showed that 3 months after switching from intensive MDI therapy to IIP treatment, sex-hormone binding globulins in both men and women decreased significantly to the normal range [48]. Hanaire-Broutin et al. showed that after 12 months of IIP therapy, growth hormone sensitivity improved with normalization of insulin-like growth factor 1 and insulin-like growth factor binding protein 3 production in type 1 diabetic patients, as compared to CSII treatment [49].

Insulin Antibodies Production

Several studies have shown that up to 40–44% of patients (responders) who were treated with IIP developed significant insulin antibodies [50, 51]. The so-called nonresponders have better metabolic control in terms of mean blood glucose and postprandial glucose [51]. Two cases of "insulin autoimmune syndrome" were reported, with one patient demonstrating a nocturnal fall in blood glucose and insulin resistance during the day [51], and another patient needed to decrease nighttime insulin requirement by 80% to avoid hypoglycemia [52]. No difference was observed overall among patients using different pump designs (PIMS, MIP, or Infusaid) or the type of insulin used (HOE 21 PH U400 versus U100) [50].

Preliminary rat studies showed that insulin aggregates due to modifications occurred during storage in the pump device may be the cause of the antigenicity [53]. IP insulin infusion was found to be more antigenic than CSII but not related to the HOE 21 PH insulin [54].

In the VA study in type 2 diabetes, no change was found in the insulin antibodies level and it tended to decrease in the IIP group compared with the MDI group [46].

ADVERSE EVENTS

Catheter Obstructions

Catheter obstruction is the major cause of surgical intervention for IIP. The rate of obstruction ranges from 7.4 to 25 events/100 patient-years at different centers [9, 10, 55], possibly, possibly because different pump manufacturers with different catheter designs were involved in these groups at different time. The causes of obstructions generally involve clots inside the catheter lumen or tissue encapsulation around the catheter tip, or both.

Several diagnostic procedures have been developed to differentiate various types of catheter malfunctions and minimize surgical interventions. A sideport to the catheter at its exit from the pump provides direct, transcutaneous access to the pump outlet and the catheter lumen. This not only allows some diagnostic maneuvers to differentiate causes of pump delivery slowdown, but also allows clearing of catheter obstructions without surgical intervention [56–58]. Further modification of the sideport catheter by Medtronic MiniMed has included the addition of three small titanium "pillows" to increase compliance of the catheter system. This change appears to further improve insulin delivery by the pump [59].

It is fair to say that the mechanisms leading to catheter obstructions are still not fully understood. There is evidence that fibrin, insulin precipitation, and tissue growth can all contribute. One study showed that patients who developed catheter obstruction seemed to have a higher capacity for macrophage activation compared to patients without obstruction [60]. Particularly as the battery life of the new pumps is prolonged, catheter blockage is likely to become more and more rate-limiting. There is a need for further investigation and development of biocompatible as well as easily replaced catheters.

Pump-Pocket Complications

The local adverse events consist of mostly pump-pocket complications. The rate of such reported complications is generally low, in the range of 2.1–8.2/100 patient-years, and varies among different centers [24, 55, 61]. There was one reported rate as high as 24/100 patient-years, but the cumulative follow-up for that center was only 58.5 patient-years [62]. The differences seemed to be correlated with the size of the center but that difference was not significant [24]. The pump-pocket complications reported to date are pump-pocket infections, local inflammatory reaction, atrophy of SC tissue, skin erosion, pump migration/exteriorization, and chronic seromas, hematomas, and local abdominal pain [9, 24, 55, 61]. There is only one reported case of small bowel obstruction caused by the peritoneal catheter [55].

Insulin Antibody Formation

Our own experience suggests that a relatively small fraction of people implanted with insulin pumps do develop high titers of anti-insulin antibody, and that these subjects are occasionally prone to prolongation of insulin action. This can cause late daytime boluses to accumulate and cause nocturnal hypoglycemia. Front-loading bolus doses given early in the day is usually effective, although the problem persisted in one of our subjects, contributing to her preference for explantation.

PATIENT SATISFACTION

In the VA Cooperative Study in type 2 diabetes and the Infusaid Pump Trial, quality of life before and after pump implantation was assessed using quality-of-life instrument developed for the DCCT (Diabetes Control and Complications Trial). The questionnaire was slightly modified for the older patient population in the type 2 diabetes group. In both studies, IIP yielded better overall quality of life and impact of disease subscale score [29, 32].

COST-BENEFIT ANALYSIS

Cost will obviously be a significant factor in the acceptance of IIP when it is available in the broader marketplace. There is only one study from over a decade ago that addresses the cost-benefit of IIP versus MDI in 10 patients with type 1 diabetes, using a randomized, prospective, 6-month, crossover design. The conclusion from that study is that IIP is more effective, equally acceptable, but much more costly than MDI [63]. However, no long-term cost–benefit analysis has ever been done.

In defense of expensive therapies, several points are worth noting. The overwhelming cost of diabetes, to the individual and to society, results from its complications, not its treatment. IIP could potentially be used early in the course of the disease as a preventive approach to avoiding devastating complications. With the longer battery life, the cost will be "amortized" across a longer time frame. And a great many other medical devices and procedures such as pancreas transplantation and renal dialysis are far more expensive, especially when applied to end-stage diabetic complications.

All this said, reasonable cost–benefit analyses are needed, as are approaches that will hold the cost of IIP down.

THE FUTURE

The relatively near-term future of implantable insulin pump therapy can be well visualized; the long-term future is always less clear. The only available device now in use is the Medtronic MiniMed MMT-2007C (Medtronic MiniMed, CA, USA). It is commercially available in France [30], but is still awaiting the results of trials that will support FDA approval in the United States. If the treatment does become generally available in the United States (after more than 16 years of largely successful research use), it would not only allow more people to benefit from a therapy that has had a high rate of patient satisfaction, but would allow further refinement of medical indications for its use, surgical and medical procedures for management of patients, and better definition of complication rates. It is fair to point out that no company has approached making a profit from IIPs despite over 25 years of corporate investment in their development. At some point, the investment will have to provide some return, which can then support further device improvements.

Scientifically, it will be of great interest to know the exact metabolic effects of insulin delivered into the peritoneal space and absorbed preferentially into the portal system. Some evidence suggests that given equal concentrations, portally and peripherally delivered insulin have the same effect [64, 65]. This observation raises some interesting possibilities to explain the apparent decrease in the rate of hypoglycemia when insulin is delivered by IIPs as discussed earlier. Many questions remain to be answered with carefully controlled metabolic studies.

It is clear that certain device improvements will continue to be made over the years, such as development of better catheters that allow the nonsurgical correction of catheter tip blockage, smaller and more flexible external communication units, and somewhat smaller implanted devices (although reservoir volume will always limit the device miniaturization). Device and insulin changes, though, are painfully slow in coming not only because even the smallest change requires careful design, preclinical and clinical testing, but because new applications must be submitted to and approved by regulatory bodies.

The question on everyone's mind when considering IIPs is whether they will become "closed loop," i.e. controlled automatically by an implanted sensor of blood glucose, and if so when. Significant breakthroughs have been made over the past few years in development of both invasive and external glucose sensors. A continuous SC glucose sensor, Medtronic MiniMed Continuous Glucose Monitoring System (CGMS), is already commercially available for interstitial glucose monitoring for up to 72 h in patients with diabetes [66], as is a GlucoWatch Biographer (by Cygnus/Sankyo Corp.). An implanted long-term IV glucose sensor system has been tested in five diabetic patients, with promising results [67, 68]. An automated closed-loop system consisting of an intravascular glucose sensor, an implanted peritoneal insulin pump, and a closed-loop algorithm downloaded on demand has been extensively tested in insulin-dependent diabetic canines, with promising results [69].

The technical barriers are formidable, though, particularly to implanting a reliable, fool-proof sensor for years at a time. The long-term goal of a fully automated, closed-loop implantable insulin pump may not be realized for years to come. Were it to happen, though, it could rightly be put in the category of a technological "cure" for diabetes, alongside such long-term goal of the biological approach as islet cell transplantation without pan-immunosuppression, or stem cell implantation.

SUMMARY

Implantable insulin pumps have developed from simple, single-rate devices through small and limited clinical trials to expanded clinical trials in which over 690 subjects have taken part [30]. They have been used to treat people with type 1 diabetes for over 14 years continuously. The complications, especially blockage of the IP catheter, are now well defined and clinically manageable. Implantable insulin pumps have a high degree of patient acceptance and enthusiasm. The therapy thus seems to be on the verge of becoming generally available. As advances are made to provide further ease of use and fewer interventions, the technology has the potential to improve the quality of life and the glycemic control of people with diabetes.

Acknowledgment

This report was supported in part by the Johns Hopkins University School of Medicine General Clinical Research Center, NIH/NCRR Grant M01 RR00052.

REFERENCES

1. Vaag A, Pedersen KD, Lauritzen M, Hildebrandt P, Beck-Nielsen H. Intramuscular versus SC injection of unmodified insulin: consequences for blood glucose control in patients with type 1 diabetes mellitus. *Diabet Med* 1990; 7 (4): 335–42.
2. Zinman B. The physiologic replacement of insulin. An elusive goal. *N Engl J Med* 1989; 321 (6): 363–70.
3. Duckworth WC, Saudek CD, Henry RR. Why intraperitoneal delivery of insulin with implantable pumps in NIDDM? *Diabetes* 1992; 41 (6): 657–61.
4. Blackshear PJ, Dorman FD, Blackshear PL Jr, Varco RL, Buchwald H. The design and initial testing of an implantable infusion pump. *Surg Gynecol Obstet* 1972; 134 (1): 51–6.
5. Blackshear PJ, Shulman GI, Roussell AM, Nathan DM, Minaker KL, Rowe JW, Robbins DC, Cohen AM. Metabolic response to three years of continuous, basal rate intravenous insulin infusion in type II diabetic patients. *J Clin Endocrinol Metab* 1985; 61 (4): 753–60.
6. Blackshear PJ, Rohde TD, Prosl F, Buchwald H. The implantable infusion pump: a new concept in drug delivery. *Med Prog Technol* 1979; 6 (4): 149–61.
7. Buchwald H, Rohde TD. It's time to reconsider the implantable insulin pump. *ASAIO J* 1994; 40 (4): 917–8.
8. Saudek CD, Fischell RE, Swindle MM. The programmable implantable medication system (PIMS): design features and pre-clinical trials. *Horm Metab Res* 1990; 22 (4): 201–6.
9. Hanaire-Broutin H, Broussolle C, Jeandidier N, Renard E, Guerci B, Haardt MJ, Lassmann-Vague V, for the Evaluation dans le Diabete du Traitement par Implants Actifs (EVADIAC) Study Group. Feasibility of intraperitoneal insulin therapy with programmable implantable pumps in IDDM. A multicenter study. *Diabetes Care* 1995; 18 (3): 388–92.
10. The Point Study II Group. Multicentre trial of a programmable implantable insulin pump in type I diabetes. *Int J Artif Organs* 1995; 18 (6): 322–5.
11. Irsigler K, Kritz H, Hagmuller G, Franetzki M, Prestele K, Thurow H, Geisen K. Long-term continuous intraperitoneal insulin infusion with an implanted remote-controlled insulin infusion device. *Diabetes* 1981; 30: 1072–5.
12. Grau U. Insulin stability. In Hepp KD, Renner R (eds) *Continuous Insulin Infusion Therapy: Experience From One Decade*. Stuttgart: Schattauer, 1985; pp 33–46.
13. Grau U. Chemical stability of insulin in a delivery system environment. *Diabetologia* 1985; 28 (7): 458–63.
14. Blackshear PJ, Rohde TD, Palmer JL, Wigness BD, Rupp WM, Buchwald H. Glycerol prevents insulin precipitation and interruption of flow in an implantable insulin infusion pump. *Diabetes Care* 1983; 6 (4): 387–92.
15. Grau U, Obermeier R, Thurow H. Stabile Insulinlosungen fur authomatische Dosiergerate. In Petersen KG, Schluter KJ, Kerp L (eds) *Neue Insuline*. Freiburg: Freiburger Graphische Betriebe, 1982; pp 411–9.
16. Grau U, Saudek CD. Stable insulin preparation for implanted insulin pumps. Laboratory and animal trials. *Diabetes* 1987; 36 (12): 1453–9.
17. Demirdjian S, Bardin C, Savin S, Zirinis P, Chast F, Slama G, Selam JL. Lispro insulin is suitable for external pumps but not for implantable pumps. *Diabetes Care* 1998; 21 (5): 867–8.
18. Boivin S, Belicar P, Melki V, for the EVADIAC Group. Assessment of *in vivo* stability of a new insulin preparation for implantable insulin pumps. A randomized multicenter prospective trial. *Diabetes Care* 1999; 22 (12): 2089–90.
19. Renard E, Bouteleau S, Jacques-Apostol D, Lauton D, Gibert-Boulet F, Costalat G, Bringer J, Jaffiol C. Insulin underdelivery from implanted pumps using peritoneal route. Determinant role of insulin pump compatibility. *Diabetes Care* 1996; 19 (8): 812–7.
20. Renard E, Souche C, Jacques-Apostol D, Lauton D, Gibert-Boulet F, Costalat G, Bringer J, Jaffiol C. Improved stability of insulin delivery from implanted pumps using a new preparation process for infused insulin. *Diabetes Care* 1999; 22 (8): 1371–2.
21. Udelsman R, Chen H, Loman K, Pitt HA, Saudek CD. Implanted programmable insulin pumps: one hundred fifty-three patient years of surgical experience. *Surgery* 1997; 122 (6): 1005–11.
22. Udelsman R, Boyne MS, Loman KE, Saudek CD. Intraperitoneal delivery of insulin via mechanical pump: surgical implications. *Langenbecks Arch Surg* 2000; 385 (6): 367–72.
23. Pitt HA, Saudek CD, Zacur HA. Long-term intraperitoneal insulin delivery. *Ann Surg* 1992; 216 (4): 483–92.
24. Belicar P, Lassmann-Vague V. Local adverse events associated with long-term treatment by implantable insulin pumps. The French EVADIAC Study Group experience. *Diabetes Care* 1998; 21 (2): 325–6.
25. Selam JL. External and implantable insulin pumps: current place in the treatment of diabetes. *Exp Clin Endocrinol Diabetes* 2001; 109 (suppl 2): S333–40.
26. Schade DS, Eaton RP, Edwards WS, Doberneck RC, Spencer WJ, Carlson GA, Bair RE, Love JT, Urenda RS, Gaona JI Jr. A remotely programmable insulin delivery system. Successful short-term implantation in man. *JAMA* 1982; 247 (13): 1848–53.
27. Saudek CD, Selam JL, Pitt HA, Waxman K, Rubio M, Jeandidier N, Turner D, Fischell RE, Charles MA. A preliminary trial of the programmable implantable medication system for insulin delivery. *N Engl J Med* 1989; 321 (9): 574–9.
28. The Point Study Group. One-year trial of a remote-controlled implantable insulin infusion system in type I diabetic patients. *Lancet* 1988; 2 (8616): 866–9.
29. Dunn FL, Nathan DM, Scavini M, Selam JL, Wingrove TG, for the Implantable Insulin Pump Trial Study Group.

Long-term therapy of IDDM with an implantable insulin pump. *Diabetes Care* 1997; 20 (1): 59–63.

30. Selam JL. External and implantable insulin pumps: current place in the treatment of diabetes. *Exp Clin Endocrin Diabetes* 2001; 109 (suppl 2): S333–40.
31. Selam JL. Implantable insulin pumps. *Lancet* 1999; 354 (9174): 178–9.
32. Saudek CD, Duckworth WC, Giobbie-Hurder A, Henderson WG, Henry RR, Kelley DE, Edelman SV, Zieve FJ, Adler RA, Anderson JW, Anderson RJ, Hamilton BP, Donner TW, Kirkman MS, Morgan NA, for the Department of Veterans Affairs Implantable Insulin Pump Study Group. Implantable insulin pump vs multiple-dose insulin for non-insulin-dependent diabetes mellitus: a randomized clinical trial. *JAMA* 1996; 276 (16): 1322–7.
33. Selam JL, Micossi P, Dunn FL, Nathan DM. Clinical trial of programmable implantable insulin pump for type I diabetes. *Diabetes Care* 1992; 15 (7): 877–85.
34. Broussolle C, Jeandidier N, Hanaire-Broutin H, for the EVADIAC Study Group. French multicentre experience of implantable insulin pumps. *Lancet* 1994; 343 (8896): 514–5.
35. Jeandidier N, Selam JL, Renard E, Guerci B, Lassman-Vague V, Rocher L, Hanaire-Broutin H, for the EVADIAC Study Group. Decreased severe hypoglycemia frequency during intraperitoneal insulin infusion using programmable implantable pumps. *Diabetes Care* 1996; 19 (7): 780.
36. Saudek CD, Duckworth WC. The Department of Veterans Affairs Implanted Insulin Pump Study. *Diabetes Care* 1992; 15 (4): 567–70.
37. Micossi P, Cristallo M, Librenti MC, Petrella G, Galimberti G, Melandri M, Monti L, Spotti D, Scavini M, Di Carlo V, Pozza G. Free-insulin profiles after intraperitoneal, intramuscular, and subcutaneous insulin administration. *Diabetes Care* 1986; 9 (6): 575–8.
38. Bouhanick B, M'Bemba J, Robert J-J, Rongier M, Slama G, Selam JL. Effects of peritoneal vs peripheral venous insulin delivery on glucose production and utilization in type 1 diabetic patients. *Diabetes Nutr Metab* 1994; 7: 213–7.
39. Selam JL, Medlej R, M'Bemba J, Chevalier A, Guyon F, Ashworth L, Slama G. Symptoms, hormones, and glucose fluxes during a gradual hypoglycaemia induced by intraperitoneal vs venous insulin infusion in type I diabetes. *Diabet Med* 1995; 12 (12): 1102–9.
40. Lassmann-Vague V, Belicar P, Alessis C, Raccah D, Vialettes B, Vague P. Insulin kinetics in type I diabetic patients treated by continuous intraperitoneal insulin infusion: influence of anti-insulin antibodies. *Diabet Med* 1996; 13 (12): 1051–5.
41. Kelley DE, Henry RR, Edelman SV, for the Veterans Affairs Implantable Insulin Pump Study Group. Acute effects of intraperitoneal versus subcutaneous insulin delivery on glucose homeostasis in patients with NIDDM. *Diabetes Care* 1996; 19 (11): 1237–42.
42. Catargi B, Meyer L, Melki V, Renard E, Jeandidier N. Comparison of blood glucose stability and HbA_{1C} between implantable insulin pumps using U400 HOE 21Ph insulin and external pumps using lispro in type 1 diabetic patients: a pilot study. *Diabetes Metab* 2002; 28 (2): 133–7.
43. Bagdade JD, Dunn FL, Eckel RH, Ritter MC. Intraperitoneal insulin therapy corrects abnormalities in cholesteryl ester transfer and lipoprotein lipase activities in insulin-dependent diabetes mellitus. *Arterioscler Thromb* 1994; 14 (12): 1933–9.
44. Bagdade JD, Kelley DE, Henry RR, Eckel RH, Ritter MC. Effects of multiple daily insulin injections and intraperitoneal insulin therapy on cholesteryl ester transfer and lipoprotein lipase activities in NIDDM. *Diabetes* 1997; 46 (3): 414–20.
45. Ruotolo G, Parlavecchia M, Taskinen MR, Galimberti G, Zoppo A, Le NA, Ragogna F, Micossi P, Pozza G. Normalization of lipoprotein composition by intraperitoneal insulin in IDDM. Role of increased hepatic lipase activity. *Diabetes Care* 1994; 17 (1): 6–12.
46. Duckworth WC, Saudek CD, Giobbie-Hurder A, Henderson WG, Henry RR, Kelley DE, Edelman SV, Zieve FJ, Adler RA, Anderson JW, Anderson RJ, Hamilton BP, Donner TW, Kirkman MS, Morgan NA. The Veterans Affairs Implantable Insulin Pump Study: effect on cardiovascular risk factors. *Diabetes Care* 1998; 21 (10): 1596–602.
47. Georgopoulos A, Saudek CD. Intraperitoneal insulin delivery decreases the levels of chylomicron remnants in patients with IDDM. *Diabetes Care* 1994; 17 (11): 1295–9.
48. Lassmann-Vague V, Raccah D, Pugeat M, Bautrant D, Belicar P, Vague P. SHBG (sex hormone binding globulin) levels in insulin dependent diabetic patients according to the route of insulin administration. *Horm Metab Res* 1994; 26 (9): 436–7.
49. Hanaire-Broutin H, Sallerin-Caute B, Poncet MF, Tauber M, Bastide R, Chale JJ, Rosenfeld R, Tauber JP. Effect of intraperitoneal insulin delivery on growth hormone binding protein, insulin-like growth factor (IGF)-I, and IGF-binding protein-3 in IDDM. *Diabetologia* 1996; 39 (12): 1498–504.
50. Olsen CL, Chan E, Turner DS, Iravani M, Nagy M, Selam JL, Wong ND, Waxman K, Charles MA. Insulin antibody responses after long-term intraperitoneal insulin administration via implantable programmable insulin delivery systems. *Diabetes Care* 1994; 17 (3): 169–76.
51. Jeandidier N, Boivin S, Sapin R, Rosart-Ortega F, Uring-Lambert B, Reville P, Pinget M. Immunogenicity of intraperitoneal insulin infusion using programmable implantable devices. *Diabetologia* 1995; 38 (5): 577–84.
52. Lassmann-Vague V, Belicar P, Raccah D, Vialettes B, Sodoyez JC, Vague P. Immunogenicity of long-term intraperitoneal insulin administration with implantable programmable pumps. Metabolic consequences. *Diabetes Care* 1995; 18 (4): 498–503.
53. Jeandidier N, Boullu S, Delatte E, Sapin R, Steibel J, Meyer P, Uhl C, Pinget M. High antigenicity of intraperitoneal insulin infusion via implantable devices: preliminary rat studies. *Horm Metab Res* 2001; 33 (1): 34–8.
54. Jeandidier N, Boullu S, Busch-Brafin MS, Chabrier G, Sapin R, Gasser F, Pinget M. Comparison of antigenicity of Hoechst 21PH insulin using either implantable intraperitoneal pump or subcutaneous external pump infusion in type 1 diabetic patients. *Diabetes Care* 2002; 25 (1): 84–8.
55. Udelsman R, Boyne MS, Loman KE, Saudek CD. Intraperitoneal delivery of insulin via mechanical pump: surgical implications. *Langenbecks Arch Surg* 2000; 385 (6): 367–72.
56. Scavini M, Reich S, Eaton RP, Charles MA, Dunn FL, for the Implantable Insulin Pump Trial Study Group. Use of an integrated sideport for diagnosis and management of decreased flow rates in a programmable implanted insulin delivery system. *Artif Organs* 1996; 20 (9): 991–6.

57. Scavini M, Hammarberg B, Dosio F, Torri M, Petrella G, Galimberti G, Vai S, Fazio F, Pozza G. A method for assessing catheter patency in implanted pumps for long-term intraperitoneal insulin delivery. *Artif Organs* 1997; 21 (5): 405–8.
58. Olsen CL, Turner DS, Iravani M, Waxman K, Selam JL, Charles MA. Diagnostic procedures for catheter malfunction in programmable implantable intraperitoneal insulin infusion devices. *Diabetes Care* 1995; 18 (1): 70–6.
59. Gin H, Melki V, Guerci B, Catargi B. Clinical evaluation of a newly designed compliant sideport catheter for an insulin implantable pump: the EVADIAC experience. *Diabetes Care* 2001; 24 (1): 175.
60. Kessler L, Tritschler S, Bohbot A, Sigrist S, Karsten V, Boivin S, Dufour P, Belcourt A, Pinget M. Macrophage activation in type 1 diabetic patients with catheter obstruction during peritoneal insulin delivery with an implantable pump. *Diabetes Care* 2001; 24 (2): 302–7.
61. Scavini M, Cristallo M, Sarmiento M, Dunn FL. Pump-pocket complications during long-term insulin delivery using an implanted programmable pump. *Diabetes Care* 1996; 19 (4): 384–5.
62. Renard E, Bringer J, Jacques-Apostol D, Lauton D, Mestre C, Costalat G, Jaffiol C. Complications of the pump pocket may represent a significant cause of incidents with implanted systems for intraperitoneal insulin delivery. *Diabetes Care* 1994; 17 (9): 1064–6.
63. Haardt MJ, Selam JL, Slama G, Bethoux JP, Dorange C, Mace B, Ramaniche ML, Bruzzo F. A cost–benefit comparison of intensive diabetes management with implantable pumps versus multiple subcutaneous injections in patients with type I diabetes. *Diabetes Care* 1994; 17 (8): 847–51.
64. Ishida T, Chap Z, Chou J, Lewis RM, Hartley CJ, Entman ML, Field JB. Effects of portal and peripheral venous insulin infusion on glucose production and utilization in depancreatized, conscious dogs. *Diabetes* 1984; 33 (10): 984–90.
65. Kryshak EJ, Butler PC, Marsh C, Miller A, Barr D, Polonsky K, Perkins JD, Rizza RA. Pattern of postprandial carbohydrate metabolism and effects of portal and peripheral insulin delivery. *Diabetes* 1990; 39 (2): 142–8.
66. Mastrototaro JJ. The MiniMed Continuous Glucose Monitoring System. *Diabetes Technol Ther* 2000; 2 (suppl 1): S19–26.
67. Renard E, Costalat G, Moran B, Shah R, Zhang Y, Villegas D, Kolopp M, Lebel R, Bringer J. First combined implantations of a long-term IV glucose sensor and an intra-peritoneal insulin pump in diabetic patients. *Diabetes* 2001; 50 (suppl 2): A3.
68. Renard E, Miller M, Stark-Weather T, Kolopp M, Costalat G, Bringer J. Accuracy of real-time blood glucose measurement by long-term sensor system allows automated insulin delivery in diabetic patients. *Diabetes* 2002; 51 (suppl 2): A126.
69. Shah R, Zhang Y, Ross P, Starkweather T, Reghabi B, Haight R, Lebel R. Automatic feedback control of plasma glucose levels in diabetic canines. *Diabetes* 2001; 50 (suppl 2): A3.

56

Artificial and Bio-artificial Pancreas Systems

Gérard Reach*, Jean-Luc Dulong†, and Cécile Legallais†

**Hôpital Avicenne, Assistance Publique-Hôpitaux de Paris, Bobigny, France, and †Technological University of Compiègne, Compiègne, France*

INTRODUCTION: DIABETES THERAPY, NAVIGATING BETWEEN TWO REEFS

The results of the Diabetes Control and Complications Trial (DCCT) indicate that although improving blood glucose control halves the rate of appearance and progression of complications (retinopathy, nephropathy, neuropathy), it also trebles the risk of severe hypoglycemia, despite intensive, but discontinuous, blood glucose monitoring [1].

The impact of hypoglycemia, the most common side effect of insulin therapy, and the one that patients with diabetes fear most, cannot be understated. Understandably, this fear of hypoglycemia is a major factor preventing patients from adopting intensified insulin therapy. This is the principal reason why normalization of HbA_{1c} is not possible in the majority of patients, despite intensified insulin therapy. Indeed, pancreas transplantation and, more recently, islet transplantation [2] represent the only treatments currently capable of consistently *normalizing* glycated hemoglobin in type 1 diabetic patients.

Furthermore, in the clinical setting, improved diabetes control can only be achieved when patients continually adjust insulin dose in response to self-monitoring of blood glucose. This is difficult to achieve for most patients. Thus the development of an artificial pancreas, a *machine* that can continuously administer insulin and be automatically controlled by concomitant blood glucose measurements, has been a long sought after goal. Together with pancreatic tissue transplantation, this has been one of the great anticipated advances for patients with diabetes.

ARTIFICIAL ORGANS

The European Society for Biomaterials defined an *artificial organ* as "a medical device that replaces, in part or in whole, the function of one of the organs of the body" [3]. It seems, therefore, that the first task in designing an artificial organ is to analyze the function of the natural organ. The function in need of replacement in the case of type 1 diabetes is the secretion of insulin by the pancreatic islet B-cells, which has four physiological characteristics: (a) it is continuous, even in the postabsorptive state, with rapid and transient peaks during meals; (b) it undergoes automatic regulation by blood glucose levels; (c) insulin is delivered into the portal blood system; (d) the endocrine pancreas is (of course) an internal organ placed within the body. The first physiological characteristic is duplicated by continuous subcutaneous insulin infusion, but none of the four characteristics can be applied to the current, discontinuous, administration of insulin via syringes or pens. An entirely different approach will be required to develop an artificial pancreas. It is important to highlight two key research objectives in improving the treatment of diabetes mellitus: (a) improving diabetes control so as to prevent the late complications of the disease without increasing the risk of severe hypoglycemia; and (b) improving patient's quality of life. In this context, it may be important that the artificial pancreas be "implantable" as this would provide the patient with a sense of a real diabetes cure. The challenge is therefore much more difficult than in the case of the artificial kidney. The new system must also of course be safe so that it adds no increased risk to a disease that can be treated by conventional insulin therapy.

International Textbook of Diabetes Mellitus, Third Edition. Edited by R. A. DeFronzo, E. Ferrannini, H. Keen, and P. Zimmet.
 ISBN: 0-471-48655-8.

A major feature of insulin secretion, which is absent with current insulin therapy, is its continuous regulation by blood glucose level. The aim of this chapter is to describe two different approaches, one electromechanical, the other bio-artificial, with the view of developing an "artificial pancreas," namely insulin delivery automatically regulated by continuous glucose sensoring.

ARTIFICIAL ELECTROMECHANICAL B-CELLS

Methods were developed 30 years ago to monitor blood glucose continuously, either by modifying standard laboratory techniques adapted to continuous flow analysis or by developing electrochemical biosensors. The glucose concentration determinations could then be processed by a computer controlling the rate insulin delivery from a pump, creating the framework of an "artificial B-cell." Interestingly, the use of the Clark oxygen electrode for the detection of glucose was proposed in the early 1970s, at the same time when the first attempts at treating type 1 diabetic patients with *continuous* intravenous insulin infusion were made [4].

With these two technological advances it was possible to develop a bedside artificial system, referred to as the "artificial pancreas." The glucose sensor had the form of a flow-through chamber containing an enzymatic glucose electrode. A double-lumen indwelling venous catheter was used to withdraw blood continuously. Venous blood was pumped to the glucose sensor chamber, which consisted of a permeable membrane designed to protect the glucose oxidase enzyme that detected the glucose. The hydrogen peroxide produced during glucose oxidation was oxidized on contact with an electrode, producing electrons. The current thus generated was transformed after calibration into an estimation of blood glucose concentration. An algorithm relating to the change in glucose over time was used to determine the amount of insulin to be delivered. This algorithm took into account not only the value of blood glucose concentration at a given time but also its rate of change; the amount of insulin to be released being higher if blood glucose concentration was increasing as compared to a stable value or a decreasing concentration. Interestingly, this resulted in an insulin delivery pattern that mimicked the biphasic insulin secretion profile of the natural B-cell. In addition, the artificial system was also able to deliver either glucose or glucagon in order to avoid hypoglycemia, a physiological characteristic performed by the liver and the A-cell of the islet of Langerhans.

These devices [5] were first used in clinical situations such as the treatment of diabetic ketoacidosis, hemodialysis, surgery, or the resection of insulinoma. They were also used to achieve normoglycemia for a short period of time after the onset of diabetes with the aim of inducing a diabetes remission (see review in reference 6). The clinical uses of the artificial pancreas were limited and it soon became a research tool. In the early 1980s it was recognized that it could be used to clamp blood glucose concentrations at a desired value, in both normal subjects and in patients with diabetes. The development of portable pumps, making continuous insulin infusion possible, and development of discontinuous blood glucose monitoring with test strips have contributed to the lack of success of bedside artificial pancreas systems in the management of acute metabolic situations (ketoacidosis, surgery, etc.). These complex and expensive devices were replaced by simple systems consisting of an intravenous insulin pump and capillary blood glucose monitoring strips, combined with simple algorithms, aimed at modifying insulin infusion in order to achieve glucose regulation during these acute circumstances.

An artificial pancreas consists of two parts: the system providing the continuous monitoring of blood glucose concentration, and the system delivering insulin. These two systems are linked by an information processing tool, using an appropriate algorithm translating glucose concentration information into an amount of physiological insulin to deliver. While this concept was developed more than 25 years ago, human clinical trials of an implantable artificial pancreas have only recently been initiated. These studies were made possible by (1) the demonstration of the safety and efficacy of wearable and implantable pumps and (2) the development of reliable glucose sensors.

Implantable Pumps

Implantable insulin infusion systems, the size of a pacemaker, are implanted under general anesthesia in the abdominal subcutaneous tissue, and a catheter delivers insulin into the peritoneal cavity. The insulin reservoir contains 2–3 months' supply of insulin and is refilled by the physician via a skin puncture. The basal rate of insulin delivery and premeal boluses can be modified by the patient using telemetry via an external programmer. There is only one implantable pump: the model 2007, Medtronic-MiniMed pump. Around 1200 implantable pumps have been used in diabetic patients worldwide [7].

In the late 1990s, the development of implantable insulin pumps was hampered by a problem of underdelivery of insulin [8], secondary to insulin aggregation and catheter occlusions. This phenomenon occurred as a result of a slight modification in the formulation resulting in insulin. In addition this problem resulted in peritoneal tissue overgrowth resulting in catheter encapsulation. Improvements in both the insulin preparation and in the catheter design resolved this problem.

The primary clinical benefit of an implantable pump appears to be a significant reduction in the frequency of severe hypoglycemia [9]. In addition, it was recently shown that switching from continuous subcutaneous insulin infusion with lispro insulin to an implantable insulin pump resulted in significantly improved metabolic control [10]. One possible metabolic advantage of infusing insulin into the peritoneal cavity may be due to more effective suppression of hepatic production and an accelerated insulin absorption. Importantly, implantable pumps delivering insulin into the peritoneal cavity may represent the most useful route of insulin delivery for closing the loop in an artificial pancreas.

Glucose Sensors

It took almost 20 years after the first publications reporting on the use of a subcutaneous enzymatic glucose sensor for a clinical continuous glucose monitoring system (CGMS) to be marketed. The "Continuous Glucose Monitoring System" developed by MiniMed-Medtronic [11], using a subcutaneous needle-type glucose sensor, is used as a "glycemic holter monitor," supplying retrospective recording of the previous 3 days. Similar systems are under development and evaluation [12]. The GlucoWatch®, developed by Cygnus [13], is based on the measurement of glucose extracted from the skin by iontophoresis. In its current configuration, it produces a value every 10 min for a 12-h period. Microdialysis-based systems are in an earlier stage of evaluation, Glucoday® being developed by Menarini [14], GlucOnline® being developed by Disetronic [15] , and the Accu-chek-Monitor® being developed by Roche [16].

In comparison to these systems that are invasive or minimally invasive, the ideal glucose monitoring system should be completely noninvasive. However, the development of these non invasive systems, largely based on change in the absorption pattern of near-infrared light [17] has been disappointing, primarily due to difficulties related to the specificity of the measurement.

The GlucoWatch® system, based on iontophoresis, can qualify as minimally invasive: its use entails a variable cutaneous reaction that generally disappears after 24 h. Implantation of the needle-type glucose sensors, as required for the MiniMed CGMS, is done by the patient. This is relatively painless and the product can also be viewed as minimally invasive. For microdialysis-based systems, implantation of the fiber is more difficult and it is unlikely the patient will be able to accomplish this on their own. Microdialysis-based systems under development use glucose oxidase (Glucoday®, Accu-chek Monitor®) or concanavaline A (GlucOnline, Disetronic). In the latter case, the presence of glucose modifies the viscosity, of the medium containing the concanavaline A pumped through the microdialysis fiber, producing a change in viscosity, which is proportional to glucose concentration. The risk of toxicity related to the use of concanavaline A has to be evaluated more carefully.

In the context of long-term implantable glucose sensors, glucose can be monitored in blood or from an alternative biological site. Monitoring glucose concentrations directly in blood would have two advantages. First, this would make the calibration step simpler, and secondly, there would be no lag time between a change in blood glucose concentration and a change in the signal generated by the sensor. Indeed, a disadvantage of using the extravascular sensor for glucose sampling is the fact that significant discrepancies between blood and interstitial glucose concentration exist [18]. Thus, the intravascular space is the ideal site for monitoring glucose concentration in a closed-loop insulin delivery system. An intravascular sensor was first shown to function for several months in dogs by Armour in the early 1990s [19], and a subsequent model was developed by Minimed-Medtronic. The system consists of the sensor implanted under general anesthesia by jugular access in the superior vena cava, and an implantable pump delivering insulin in the peritoneal cavity. This system was recently piloted in 10 diabetic patients. Remarkably, one sensor was proved to function for more than 1 year. Analysis of data obtained in the first five patients indicated that more than 95% of the measurements of glucose concentration were in the excellent or good zones (A and B) of the Clark error grid [20]. Although no significant adverse effects were observed in this first trial, the use of large vessel vascular access may represent a risk that needs further safety testing.

The development of long-term subcutaneous implantable glucose sensors was significantly advanced by the introduction of the angiogenic membrane. The system, developed by Updike, was first assessed in dogs and was shown to function for up to 3–5 months [21]. Recently, it was evaluated with promising results in 25 patients. Implantation requires a simple surgical procedure performed with local anesthesia. The system functioned well for up to 8 months [22].

Continuous glucose monitoring systems use can be classified as follows. Initially the device can be used as a simple holter glucose monitor used to help the clinician recognize hyperglycemic peaks or hypoglycemia periods so as to improve the insulin regimen of the patient. The CGMS developed by MiniMed-Medtronic is already largely used in several clinics; however, recent publications suggest that the reliability of the system may not be optimal [23]. Larger studies are underway.

The second possible use of these devices is as a hypoglycemic alarm. In addition to simple detection, a recent paper presented the principal of this being used for hypoglycemia prevention, based on risk assessment algorithm [24]. Finally, the ultimate glucose sensor would be incorporated into an artificial pancreas. The system developed by MiniMed-Medtronic utilizes the intravascular sensor and closes the loop with an implantable pump. The system functions as an artificial β-cell and was tested for a 48-h period (postabsorptive glucose). Control was excellent but postprandial glycemic regulation was not optimal.

BIO-ARTIFICIAL SYSTEMS

If type 1 diabetes mellitus is secondary to the destruction of the islet β-cells that secrete insulin, the ultimate solution would be to transplant pancreatic tissue. Indeed, these cells have the property of responding rapidly to glucose changes with a response that is proportional to the glucose concentration of the stimulating medium. The beta cell glucose sensor and the machinery responsible for insulin exocytosis from the cell have a very prompt response time (within 1 min). Moreover, the beta cells respond to other nutrients that normally stimulate insulin secretion (amino acids, free fatty acids, hormones). In addition, unlike implantable pumps, pancreatic beta cells have the potential for synthesizing insulin to restore reserves. Finally, the islet volume responsible for secretion of the daily insulin requirement (approximately 40–50 IU) is extremely small: 1 million islets of Langerhans represent a volume smaller than 1 ml. They could therefore be readily implantable.

To date, approximately 12 000 patients with type 1 diabetes mellitus have received a whole pancreatic, vascularized graft, with a success rate of approximately 70%, and a patient survival rate of 90% at 4 years. Islet transplantation has recently become a successful option primarily because of a change in the immunosuppression protocol (Edmonton protocol). Multicenter studies are underway to evaluate the feasibility of the approach in large numbers of patients (see Chapters 58 and 59).

Another way of using islet tissue is in the context of a bio-artificial pancreas. Islets would be immunoisolated in an artificial membrane, leading to that of cell immunoisolation in a *bio-artificial organ*. Indeed, a bio-artificial pancreas represents a machine at the frontier between the two disciplines of tissue transplantation and artificial organs.

A couple of approaches are possible [25]: (a) vascular devices, in which blood circulates in contact with a membrane through a semi-permeable hollow fiber so hemodialysors, with the "dialysate" compartment containing the islets being closed; or (b) a simpler system, referred to as an extravascular system, includes microencapsulated islets, a diffusion chamber, and islets placed inside a hollow fiber, which may be implanted inside the peritoneal cavity or in the subcutaneous tissue. The possible advantages of this kind of bio-artificial organ are as follows:

(1) The system works as a closed-loop insulin delivery device normalising glycemia.
(2) Islets of Langerhans can survive in an immunoisolated state, although they are neither vascularized nor innervated.
(3) The membrane is biostable.
(4) The membrane is biocompatible. If a host reaction occurs, the function of the "device" remains unaltered.
(5) The system is safe.
(6) The device can be produced on an industrial basis, which means that all its parameters, including islets and membrane characteristics, can be defined.
(7) It can be prepared in a reproducible manner and should be able to be stored.

Vascular Systems

Here the islets are placed outside a hollow fiber through which the recipient's blood circulates. This system would therefore be connected to a vascular shunt [26–30]. On the basis of the kinetic modelling of glucose and insulin transfer through the fiber [31], a system based on convective fluxes across the membrane was devised, and has yielded excellent kinetics *in vitro* [32] and *in vivo* in rats [33] and in dogs [34]. The correction of hyperglycemia in diabetic rats with this system was demonstrated over a few hours [35]. However, the system was unable to avoid blood clotting inside the fiber.

A major effort in this field was made by the group working with Chick, who used a radically opposite approach. They focused on the hemocompatibility of the system, and reported the successful graft of a vascular device in dogs over several months in the absence of any heparinization of the animals, which only received aspirin [36, 37]. Hyperglycaemia was corrected, but the authors recognize that improvements in the kinetics of insulin release by this device are still required. Recent studies showed that a device seeded with xenogeneic porcine islets implanted into pancreatectomized dogs resulted in a reduction of exogenous insulin requirement for up to 9 months [38]. This work led to FDA authorization to initiate a clinical trial. However, during one of the last preclinical transplants, the device failed, leading to the death of the animal and the program was cancelled.

A similar system was proposed by Calafiore et al., who implanted microencapsulated islets inside the wall of a dacron-based prosthesis connected to an arterial bypass. Plasma crossed the dacron meshes and perifused the islets, which were immunoprotected by the membrane of the microcapsules, and which released insulin into the bloodstream. This system was investigated in a small number of dogs [39] and in two diabetic patients [40].

It is obvious that the development of these systems is hindered by the need for vascular access and by the risk of thrombosis, anticoagulant therapy representing a formidable challenge. This may be one reason why the intravenous route for insulin delivery by implantable pumps has now been abandoned: all the systems currently implanted infuse insulin into the peritoneal space. Similarly, the successive failures of vascular access for a transplanted pancreas encouraged the above-mentioned groups to move to the extravascular concept.

Extravascular Systems

Microencapsulated Islets

Most of the studies are derived from the method initially published by Lim and Sun [41] using alginate, which is cross-linked by polylysine to form the immunoprotective membrane. *In vitro* it was possible to demonstrate that, provided the capsule size is small, microencapsulated islets do respond to glucose by increasing their insulin release [42], and that the membrane provides immunoprotection to encapsulated insulin-secreting cells against the cytotoxic effect of antibodies present in the serum of newly diagnosed diabetic patients [43]. *In vivo* experiments with microencapsulated islets have indicated that they are able to provide long-term correction of hyperglycaemia in streptozotocin-induced models of diabetes in rats and mice, in biobreeding (BB) rats and nonobese diabetic (NOD) mice [44–48]. Approximately 10 years ago, the announcement of the implantation of microencapsulated human islets in a type 1 diabetic patient was very promising, despite the fact that this patient was receiving immunosuppressive therapy for a kidney transplant [49]. This trial abolished the exogenous insulin requirement for 1 month [50], but has never been repeated. Importantly, less optimistic results have also been published ([51–54]; see review in reference 55). It is generally accepted that fibrosis around implanted microcapsules is often observed, even though the phenomenon is not universal. This reaction was supposed to increase the insulin diffusion time. The chemical nature of the membrane (in particular the respective percentages of mannuronic or glucuronic residues in the alginate used) might be a factor [56, 57], as might the fragile nature of the chemical bonding between alginate and polylysine. In contrast, the degree of purity of alginate used did not seem to be responsible of graft failure [58]. The activation of complement [59] and of macrophages to elicit interleukin 1 [60] is a subject of concern [61], since interleukin 1 is known to induce fibrosis; furthermore, it could cross the membrane and kill the islets [62]. This has led other groups to investigate other methods for micro-encapsulation, using nonsoluble biomaterials known for their biocompatibility [63–65], or using islet coated with agarose [66] or barium alginate [67]. Globally, these novel methods are based on the use of a single material that might prove to be more stable than the complex polyelectrolyte formed by alginate and polylysine. More recent results indicated that even without fibrosis around the capsule, islet necrosis occurred when alginate beads were used [68]. The fact that beads remained unattached and freely floating in the peritoneal cavity, concomitant with low oxygen supply, could explain this phenomenon.

Another point that deserves further investigation is the kinetics of insulin release by these systems *in vivo*. In all these studies, implantation of microencapsulated islets was considered to be successful when blood glucose (usually determined in a fasted state) was normalized. It should be pointed out that this can be achieved in rats by implanting a system releasing insulin without any regulation [69]. Such is not the case in diabetic humans, where a peak in insulin is necessary to normalize postprandial hyperglycemia. The only study concerning the postprandial insulin response to a glucose load in animals with peritoneal implantation of microencapsulated islet was negative [70].

Finally, another major concern is the size of the implant. It is clear that the volume of implanted material will be determined primarily by the size of the microcapsules (since the volume of a sphere is proportional to the cube of the radius). It is therefore mandatory to set up methods for reducing the size of the microcapsules, which will also facilitate diffusion of oxygen [71]. However, when this is attempted the production of inadequately encapsulated islets (empty beads, or non immunoprotected islets near the bead surface) increases [72]. It may also be necessary to design methods for recovering the microencapsulated islets, if necessary, from the cavity into which they have been implanted.

Diffusion Chambers

In the initial form of diffusion chambers (two disks of membrane separated by a ring), a severe fibrotic reaction was elicited because of the membranes themselves [73]. As a consequence, these devices were abandoned during the 1980s. More recently, however, this fibrotic reaction was used to promote neovascularization around the device. A new design has been proposed, in which the membrane consists of a microporous membrane, covered with a second membrane capable of inducing the neovascularization [74, 75]. To control the islet density and to avoid their clumping within the device, islets were first microencapsulated in alginate beads, then loaded into the planar diffusion chamber [76]. If the device was neovascularized before being loaded with islets, their survival could be increased. This could be accomplished by perfusing the device with endothelial growth factors during a month using an osmotic pump, then removing the pump and introducing the islets into the neovascularized chamber [77].

Another approach to improve the diffusion of insulin out of the chamber is to reduce the thickness of the device. An extremely thin alginate flat sheet containing allogenic islets maintained fasting euglycemia for 84 days [78]. However, these very thin devices become extremely fragile mechanically: sheet planarity could not be maintained, as observed on the explanted devices.

Macroencapsulated Islets

First proposed by Archer [79], this method was successfully applied by Altman with fragments of human insulinoma seeded into pieces of semipermeable tubes, sealed, and implanted in the peritoneal cavity of diabetic rats [80]. Less encouraging results were obtained when these fibers were implanted in pigs, since extensive fibrosis around the fibers was observed [81], as well as in rats [82]. Promising results have been published on macroencapsulated islets implanted either into the peritoneal cavity of mice or rats [83–85] or in the subcutaneous tissue of diabetic rats [86]. The implantation into the peritoneal cavity of 250 fibers containing dog islets was able to correct hyperglycemia in diabetic dogs. Plasma glucose following a meal was not normal but returned to the normal range after 2 h. Unfortunately no data on plasma insulin were reported [87].

Bio-artificial Pancreas: Unresolved Issues

As discussed, there is no doubt that islets can survive in an immunoisolated state and that some of the systems proposed, whatever their geometry (beads, chambers, fibers), were able to correct diabetes in animals, although most of the studies only demonstrated the correction of fasting blood glucose with no data on the glycemic and insulin profiles after a glucose load. Furthermore, most of them were performed in small laboratory animals, and some necrosis occurred [68, 85]. The scaling up of these systems remains a major challenge. To date, all the different device configurations failed when adapted to large animals. Even if necrosis is avoided, hypoxia causes the reduction of the functional secretory capacity of the encapsulated islets [88]. For instance within a given fiber geometry, it was shown that very low islet density was required to induce sufficient oxygenation if the system were not richly neovascularised [89, 90]. In this case, the size of a device necessary to accommodate the 500 000 islets (a therapeutic dose of islets) in man would be prohibitive. This leads to the concept of developing a *bio-artificial organoid*. It will also be necessary to demonstrate the complete safety of the system, particularly its sterility: bacterial, viral, and fungal hazards must be eliminated. Special attention will have to be paid to endogenous retrovirus in the case of porcine islet utilization. Ultimately, for the bio-artificial concept to be effective the immuno-isolation of engineered cells may be required.

CONCLUSION: ARTIFICIAL PANCREAS, AN ELUSIVE GOAL?

Research on both the artificial and the bio-artificial pancreas has spanned more than 30 years. There is no doubt that the demonstration that hyperglycaemia is the principal cause of diabetic complications, and that hypoglycemia is a major barrier in achieving normoglycemia with intensive insulin therapy, highlights the importance of developing systems in which insulin would be delivered on a regulated basis. This would also alleviate the burden on patients of having to use complex insulin treatment regimens day after day, meal after meal. In the development of an artificial pancreas, it is clear that the difficulty in developing a biocompatible glucose sensor was largely underestimated, and that the present goal of providing patients with a CGMS without giving this system the responsibility of controlling an insulin pump is a much more realistic first approach. Nevertheless, a reliable CGMS may well play a major role in the next few years as a powerful tool for facilitating the implementation of intensive insulin therapy. With respect to the bio-artificial pancreas, the major issue now is the scaling up of devices to make it possible to correct diabetes, not only in rodents, but in larger mammals, and finally in diabetic patients.

The fact that despite after 30 years of intensive research no artificial or bio-artificial pancreas has been developed as a therapeutic model should not be surprising. Thirty-two years elapsed between the discovery of the role of the pancreas in the genesis of type 1 diabetes and the first use of insulin in a diabetic dog, but within a few years enough insulin was available to treat all the diabetic patients in developed countries. It sometimes happens that for the achievement of a novel therapeutic method, research takes longer than development, and that more time is needed to move from the original concept to a prototype, than to move from the prototype to a product.

If you don't hope for the unhoped-for, you will not find it —Heraclite

REFERENCES

1. The Diabetes Control and Complications Trial Research Group. The effect of intensive treatment of diabetes on development and progression of long-term complications in insulin-dependent diabetes mellitus. *N Engl J Med* 1993; 329: 977–86.
2. Ryan EA, Lakey JR, Paty BW, Imes S, Korbutt GS, Kneteman NM, Bigam D, Rajotte RV, Shapiro AM. Successful islet transplantation: continued insulin reserve provides long-term glycemic control. *Diabetes* July 2002; 51 (7): 2148–57.
3. Williams DF. A list of terms from the European Society for Biomaterials. *Enjeux* 1986; 74: 44–5.
4. Slama G, Hautecouverture M, Assan R, Tchobroutsky G. One to five days of continuous intravenous insulin infusion on seven diabetic patients. *Diabetes* 1974; 23: 732–8.

5. Albisser AM, Leibel BS, Ewart G, Davidovac Z, Botz CK, Zingg W. An artificial endocrine pancreas. *Diabetes* 1974; 23: 389–96.
6. Albisser AM. Artificial beta cell insulin delivery systems. In Brownlee M (ed), *Diabetes Mellitus*, *Vol* V. Chichester, UK: Wiley, 1981; pp 245–72.
7. Selam JL. External and implantable pumps: current place in the treatment of diabetes. *Exp Clin Endocrinol Diabetes* 2001; 1009 (suppl 2): S333–40.
8. Renard E, Bouteleau S, Jacques-Apostol D, Lauton D, Gibert-Boulet F, Costalat G, Bringer J, Jaffiol C. Insulin underdelivery from implanted pumps using peritoneal route. Determinant role of insulin pump compatibility. *Diabetes Care* August 1996; 19 (8): 812–7.
9. Broussolle C, Jeandidier N, Hanaire Broutin H, for the Evadiac Study Group. French multicentre experience with implantable insulin pumps. *Lancet* 1994; 343: 514–5.
10. Catargi B, Meyer L, Melki V, Renard E, Jeandidier N, for the EVADIAC Study Group. Comparison of blood glucose stability and HbA1C between implantable insulin pumps using U400 HOE 21PH insulin and external pumps using lispro in type 1 diabetic patients: a pilot study. *Diabetes Metab* April 2002; 28 (2): 133–7.
11. Bode BW, Gross TM, Thornton KR, Mastrototaro JJ. Continuous glucose monitoring used to adjust diabetes therapy improves glycosylated hemoglobin: a pilot study. *Diabetes Res Clin Pract* December 1999; 46 (3): 183–90.
12. Heller A. Implanted electrochemical glucose sensors for the management of diabetes. *Annu Rev Biomed Eng* 1999; 1: 153–75.
13. Potts RO, Tamada JA, Tierney MJ. Glucose monitoring by reverse iontophoresis. *Diabetes Metab Res Rev* January–February 2002; 18 (suppl 1): S49–53.
14. Maran A, Crepaldi C, Tiengo A, Grassi G, Vitali E, Pagano G, Bistoni S, Calabrese G, Santeusanio F, Leonetti F, Ribaudo M, Di Mario U, Annuzzi G, Genovese S, Riccardi G, Previti M, Cucinotta D, Giorgino F, Bellomo A, Giorgino R, Poscia A, Varalli M. Continuous subcutaneous glucose monitoring in diabetic patients: a multicenter analysis. *Diabetes Care* February 2002; 25 (2): 347–52.
15. Beyer U, Schafer D, Thomas A, Aulich H, Haueter U, Reihl B, Ehwald R. Recording of subcutaneous glucose dynamics by a viscometric affinity sensor. *Diabetologia* April 2001; 44 (4): 416–23.
16. Jungheim K, Wientjes KJ, Heinemann L, Lodwig V, Koschinsky T, Schoonen AJ, for the Glucose Monitoring Study Group. Subcutaneous continuous glucose monitoring: feasibility of a new microdialysis-based glucose sensor system. *Diabetes Care* September 2001; 24 (9): 1696–7.
17. Koschinsky T, Heinemann L. Sensors for glucose monitoring: technical and clinical aspects. *Diabetes Metab Res Rev* March–April 2001; 17 (2): 113–23.
18. Aussedat B, Dupire-Angel M, Gifford R, Klein JC, Wilson GS, Reach G. Interstitial glucose concentration and glycemia: implications for continuous subcutaneous glucose monitoring. *Am J Physiol Endocrinol Metab* April 2000; 278 (4): E716–28.
19. Armour JC, Lucisano JY, McKean BD, Gough DA. Application of chronic intravascular blood glucose sensor in dogs. *Diabetes* December 1990; 39 (12): 1519–26.
20. Renard E, Costalat G, Bringer J. De la pompe externe à la pompe implantable: peut on fermer la boucle? *Diabetes Metab* September 2002; 28 (4, Pt 2): 19–25.
21. Updike SJ, Shults MC, Gilligan BJ, Rhodes RK. A subcutaneous glucose sensor with improved longevity, dynamic range, and stability of calibration. *Diabetes Care* February 2000; 23 (2): 208–14.
22. Edelman SV, Beatty DJ, Bouvet M, Fisher JC, Cefalu WT. Continuous glucose sensing with a long-term subcutaneous implant in patients with type 1 diabetes. *Diabetologia* 2002; 45: A26.
23. Metzger M, Leibowitz G, Wainstein J, Glaser B, Raz I. Reproducibility of glucose measurements using the glucose sensor. *Diabetes Care* 2002; 25: 1185–91.
24. Choleau C, Dokladal P, Klein JC, Ward WK, Wilson GS, Reach G. Prevention of hypoglycemia using risk assessment with a continuous glucose monitoring system. *Diabetes* November 2002; 51 (11): 3263–73.
25. Reach G. Bioartificial pancreas. *Diabet Med* 1993; 10: 105–9.
26. Chick WL, Like AA, Lauris V, Richardson PD, Panol G, Mix TW, Colton CK. A hybrid artificial pancreas. *Trans Am Soc Artif Intern Organs* 1975; 21: 8–13.
27. Tze W, Wong F, Chen L. Implantable artificial capillary unit for pancreatic islet allograft and xenograft. *Diabetologia* 1979; 16: 247–52.
28. Orsetti A, Guy C, Zouari N, Deffay F. Implantation du distributeur bio-artificiel d'insuline chez le chien utilisant des ilots d'espèce animale différente. *Compt Rend Soc Biol* 1978; 172: 144–50.
29. Sun AM, Parisius W, Healy G, Vacek I, MacMorine H. The use in diabetic rats and monkeys of artificial capillary units containing cultured islets of Langerhans (artificial endocrine pancreas). *Diabetes* 1977; 26: 1136–9.
30. Reach G, Poussier Ph, Sausse A, Assan R, Itoh M, Gerich JE. Functional evaluation of a bioartificial pancreas using isolated islets perifused with blood ultrafiltrate. *Diabetes* 1981; 30: 296–301.
31. Reach G, Jaffrin MY. Kinetic modelling as a tool for the design of a vascular bioartificial pancreas: feedback between modelling and experimental validation. *Computer Methods Programs Biomed* 1990; 32: 277–85.
32. Reach G, Jaffrin MY, Desjeux JF. A U-shaped bioartificial pancreas with rapid glucose insulin kinetics: *in vitro* evaluation and kinetic modelling. *Diabetes* 1984; 33: 752–61.
33. Reach G, Chenard PS, Darquy S, Lepeintre J, Desjeux JF, Cannon R, Jaffrin MY. Bioartificial pancreas: *in vivo* evaluation in conscious normal rats. In Nosé Y, Kjelllstrand C, Ivanovich P (eds), *Progress in Artificial Organs—1985*. Cleveland, OH: ISAO Press, 1986; pp 621–6.
34. Lepeintre J, Briandet H, Moussy F, Chicheportiche D, Darquy S, Rouchette J, Imbaud P, Duron JJ, Reach G. *Ex vivo* evaluation in normal dogs of insulin release by a bioartificial pancreas containing isolated rat islets of Langerhans. *Artif Organs* 1990; 14: 20–7.
35. Reach G, Jaffrin MY. Bioartificial pancreas as an approach to closed-loop insulin delivery. In Emsinger WD, Selam JL (eds), *Drug Delivery Systems*. Mount Kisco, NY: Futura, 1987; pp 99–102.
36. Sullivan SJ, Maki T, Borland KM, Mahoney MD, Solomon BA, Muller TE, et al. Biohybrid artificial pancreas: long-term implantation studies in diabetic, pancreatectomized dogs. *Science* 1991; 252: 718–21.
37. Monaco AP, Maki T, Ozato H, Carretta M, Sullivan SJ, Borland KM, et al. Transplantation of islet allografts and xenografts in totally pancreatectomized dogs using the hybrid artificial pancreas. *Ann Surg* 1991; 214: 339-60.
38. Maki T, Otsu I, O'Neil JJ, Dunleavy K, Mullon CJ, Solomon BA, et al. Treatment of diabetes by xenogeneic islets without immunosuppression. Use of a vascularized bioartificial pancreas. *Diabetes* 1996; 45: 342–7.

39. Calafiore R, Basta G, Falorni A, Ciabattoni P, Brotzu G, Cortesini R, et al. Intravascular transplantation of microencapsulated islets in diabetic dogs. *Transplant Proc* 1992; 24: 935–6.
40. Calafiore R. Transplantation of microencapsulated pancreatic human islets for therapy of diabetes mellitus: a preliminary report. *Am Soc Artif Intern Organs* 1992; 38: 34–7.
41. Lim F, Sun AM. Microencapsulated islets as bioartificial endocrine pancreas. *Science* 1980; 210: 908–10.
42. Chicheportiche D, Reach G. Kinetics of insulin release by microencapsulated islets: effect of the size of the microcapsule. *Diabetologia* 1988; 31: 54–7.
43. Darquy S, Reach G. Immunoisolation of pancreatic B cells by microencapsulation: an *in vitro* study. *Diabetologia* 1985; 28: 776–80.
44. O'Shea GM, Goosen MFA, Sun AM. Prolonged survival of transplanted islets of Langerhans encapsulated in a biocompatible membrane. *Biochim Biophys Acta* 1984; 804: 133–6.
45. O'Shea GM, Sun AM. Encapsulation of rat islets prolongs xenograft survival in diabetic mice. *Diabetes* 1986; 35: 943–6.
46. Fan MY, Lum ZP, Fu XW, Levesque L, Tai IT, Sun AM. Reversal of diabetes in BB rats by transplantation of encapsulated pancreatic islets. *Diabetes* 1990; 39: 519–22.
47. Lum ZP, Tait IT, Krestaw M, Norton J, Vacek I, Sun AM. Prolonged reversal of the diabetic state in NOD mice by xenografts of microencapsulated rat islets. *Diabetes* 1991; 40: 1511–6.
48. Calafiore R, Calcinaro F, Basta G, et al. A method for the massive separation of highly purified, adult porcine islets of Langerhans. *Metabolism* 1990; 39: 175–81.
49. Soon-Shiong P, Heintz RE, Merideth M, et al. Insulin independence in a type 1 diabetic patient after encapsulated islet transplantation. *Lancet* 1994; 343: 950–51.
50. Soon-Shiong P. Treatment of type I diabetes using encapsulated islets. *Adv Drug Deliv Rev* 1999; 35: 259–70.
51. Ricker AT, Stobetger SM, Halban PA, Eisenbarth GS, Bonner-Weir S. Hyperimmune response to microencapsulated xenogenic tissue in non-obese diabetic mice. In Jaworski MA, Molnar GD, Rajotte RV, Singh B (eds), *The Immunology of Diabetes Mellitus*. Amsterdam: Elsevier, 1986; pp 193–200.
52. Chicheportiche D, Darquy S, Lepeintre J, Capron F, Halban PA, Reach G. High-performance liquid chromatography analysis of circulating insulins distinguishes between endogenous insulin production (a potential pitfall with streptozotocin diabetic rats) and islet xenograft function. *Diabetologia* 1990; 33: 457–61.
53. Darquy S, Chicheportiche D, Capron F, Boitard C, Rouchette J, Reach G. Comparative study of microencapsulated rat islets implanted in different diabetic models in mice. In Federlin K, Bretzel RG, Hering BJ (eds), *Methods in Islet Transplantation Research*. Stuttgart, Germany: Georg Thieme Verlag, 1990; pp 209–13.
54. Mazaheri R, Atkison P, Stiller C, Dupré J, Vose J, O'Shea G. Transplantation of encapsulated allogeneic islets into diabetic BB/W rats. Effects of immunosuppression. *Transplantation* 1991; 51: 750–4.
55. Clayton HA, James RFL, London NJM. Islet microencapsulation: a review. *Acta Diabetol* 1994; 30: 181–9.
56. Clayton HA, London NMJ, Colloby PS, James RFL, Bell PRF. The effect of capsule composition on the viability and biocompatibility of sodium alginate/poly-L-lysine encapsulated islets. *Transplant Proc* 1992; 24: 956.
57. Wolters GHJ, Fritschy WF, de Vos P, van Schilfgaarde R. Improvement of the biocompatibility of microencapsulated pancreatic islets [abstract]. *Diabetologia* 1992; 35 (suppl 1): A190.
58. De Vos P, De Haan BJ, Wolters GH, Strubbe JH, Van Schilfgaarde R. Improved biocompatibility but limited graft survival after purification of alginate for microencapsulation of pancreatic islets. *Diabetologia* 1997; 40: 262–70.
59. Darquy S, Pueyo ME, Capron F, Reach G. Complement activation by alginate–polylysine microcapsules used for islet transplantation. *Artif Organs* 1994; 18: 898–903.
60. Pueyo ME, Darquy S, Capron F, Reach G. *In vitro* activation of human macrophages by alginate-polylysine microcapsules. *J Biomater Sci Polym Ed* 1993; 5: 197–203.
61. Siebers U, Horcher A, Bretzel RG, Federlin K, Zekorn T. Alginate-based microcapsules for immunoprotected islet transplantation. *Ann NY Acad Sci* 1997; 831: 304–12.
62. Cole DR, Waterfall M, McIntyre M, Baird JD. Microencapsulated islet grafts in the BB/E rat: a possible role for cytokines in graft failure. *Diabetologia* 1992; 35: 231–7.
63. Uludag H, De Vos P, Tresco PA. Technology of mammalian cell encapsulation. *Adv Drug Deliv Rev* 2000; 42: 29–64.
64. Gin H, Dupuy B, Baquey A, Baquey Ch, Ducassou D. Lack of responsiveness to glucose of microencapsulated islets of Langerhans after three weeks' implantation in the rat—influence of the complement. *J Microencapsul* 1990; 7: 341–6.
65. Honiger J, Darquy S, Reach G, Muscat E, Thomas M, Collier C. Preliminary report on cell encapsulation in a hydrogel made of a biocompatible material, AN69, for the development of a bioartificial pancreas. *Int J Artif Organs* 1994; 17: 46–52.
66. Tashiro H, Iwata H, Warnock GL, Ikada Y, Tsuji T. Application of agarose microcapsules to allo-islet transplantation in a canine model. *Transplant Proc* 1998; 30: 498–9.
67. Zekorn T, Siebers U, Horcher A, Schnettler R, Zimmermann U, Bretzel RG, et al. Alginate coating of islets of Langerhans: *in vitro* studies on a new method for microencapsulation for immuno-isolated transplantation. *Acta Diabetol* 1992; 29: 41–5.
68. De Vos P, Van Straaten JF, Nieuwenhuizen AG, de Groot M, Ploeg RJ, De Haan BJ, et al. Why do microencapsulated islet grafts fail in the absence of fibrotic overgrowth? *Diabetes* 1999; 48: 1381–8.
69. Brown L, Munoz C, Siemer L, Edelman E, Langer R. Controlled release of insulin from polymer matrices. Control of diabetes in rats. *Diabetes* 1986; 35: 692–7.
70. Fritschy WM, Strubbe JH, Wolters GHJ, Van Schilfgaarde R. Glucose tolerance and plasma insulin response to intravenous glucose infusion and test meal in rats with microencapsulated islets. *Diabetologia* 1991; 34: 542–54.
71. Lum ZP, Krestow M, Tai IT, Vacek I, Sun AM. Xenografts of rat islets into diabetic mice. An evaluation of new smaller capsules. *Transplantation* 1992; 53: 1180–83.
72. De Vos P, De Haan BJ, Van Schilfgaarde R. Upscaling the production of microencapsulated pancreatic islets. *Biomaterials* 1997; 18: 1085–90.
73. Theodorou NA, Vrbova H, Tyhurst M, Howell SL. Problems in the use of polycarbonate diffusion chambers for syngeneic pancreatic islet transplantation in rats. *Diabetologia* 1980; 13: 313–17.
74. Andersson A, Eizirik DL, Bremer C, Johnson RC, Pipeleers DG, Hellerstrom C. Structure and function of macroencapsulated human and rodent pancreatic islets

transplanted into nude mice. *Horm Metab Res* 1996; 28: 306–9.

75. Rafael E, Gazelius B, Wu GS, Tibell A. Longitudinal studies on the microcirculation around the TheraCyte immunoisolation device, using the laser Doppler technique. *Cell Transplant* 2000; 9: 107–13.
76. Suzuki K, Bonner-Weir S, Hollister-Lock J, Colton CK, Weir GC. Number and volume of islets transplanted in immunobarrier devices. *Cell Transplant* 1998; 7: 47–52.
77. De Vos P, Hamel AF, Tatarkiewicz K. Considerations for successful transplantation of encapsulated pancreatic islets. *Diabetologia* 2002; 45: 159–73.
78. Storrs R, Dorian R, King SR, Lakey J, Rilo H. Preclinical development of the Islet Sheet. *Ann NY Acad Sci* 2001; 944: 252–66.
79. Archer J, Kaye R, Mutter G. Control of streptozotocin diabetes in Chinese hamsters by cultured mouse islet cells without immunosuppression: a preliminary report. *J Surg Res* 1980; 28: 77–85.
80. Altman JJ, Houlbert D, Callard P, McMillan P, Solomon BA, Rosen J, et al. Long-term plasma glucose normalization in experimental diabetic rats with macroencapsulated implants of benign human insulinomas. *Diabetes* 1986; 35: 625–33.
81. Icard P, Penfornis F, Gotheil C, Boillot J, Cornec C, Barrat F, et al. Tissue reaction to implanted bioartificial pancreas in pigs. *Transplant Proc* 1990; 22: 724–6.
82. Zekorn T, Siebers U, Filip L, Mauer K, Schmitt U, Bretzel RG, et al. Bioartificial pancreas: the use of different hollow fibres as a diffusion chamber. *Transplant Proc* 1989; 21: 2748–50.
83. Lanza RP, Butler DH, Borland KM, Staruk JE, Faustman DL, Solomon BA, et al. Xenotransplantation of canine, bovine, and porcine islets in diabetic rats without immunosuppression. *Proc Natl Acad Sci USA* 1991; 88: 11100–4.
84. Kuhtreiber WM, Lanza RP, Chick WL. Secretory function of biohybrid pancreas devices containing isolated porcine islets. *ASAIO J* 1994; 40: M789–92.
85. Delaunay C, Darquy S, Honiger J, Capron F, Rouault C, Reach G. Glucose-insulin kinetics of a bioartificial pancreas made of an AN69 hydrogel hollow fiber containing porcine islets and implanted in diabetic mice. *Artif Organs* 1998; 22: 291–9.
86. Lacy PE, Hegre OD, Gerasimidi-Vazeou A, Gentile FT, Dionne KE. Maintenance of normoglycemia in diabetic mice by subcutaneous xenografts of encapsulated islets. *Science* 1991; 254: 1782–4.
87. Lanza RP, Borland KM, Lodge P, Caretta M, Sullivan S, Muller T, et al. Treatment of severely diabetic pancreatectomized dogs using a diffusion-based hybrid pancreas. *Diabetes* 1992; 41: 886–9.
88. Dionne KE, Colton CK, Yarmush ML. Effect of hypoxia on insulin secretion by isolated rat and canine islets of Langerhans. *Diabetes* 1993; 42: 12–21.
89. Dulong JL, Legallais C, Darquy S, Reach G. A novel model of solute transport in a hollow-fiber bioartificial pancreas based on a finite element method. *Biotechnol Bioeng* 2002; 78: 576–82.
90. Dulong JL, Legallais C. Contributions of a finite element model for the geometric optimization of an implantable bioartificial pancreas. *Artif Organs* 2002; 26: 583–9.

57

Pancreas Transplantation

R. Paul Robertson

Pacific Northwest Research Institute, Seattle, WA, USA

ROLE OF PANCREAS TRANSPLANTATION IN MANAGEMENT OF DIABETES

Pancreas transplantation is normally performed in tertiary care centers that have an active kidney transplant program and that are equipped to handle the complex medical and psychosocial needs of transplant patients. To answer the difficult question of which patient should be recommended for pancreas transplantation, the American Diabetes Association prepared a position statement in 2000 [1]. These recommendations were as follows:

1. Pancreas transplantation should be considered an acceptable therapeutic alternative to continued insulin therapy in diabetic patients with imminent or established end-stage renal disease who have had or plan to have a kidney transplant, because the successful addition of a pancreas does not jeopardize patient survival, may improve kidney survival, and will restore normal glycemia. Such patients also must meet the medical indications and criteria for kidney transplantation and not have excessive surgical risk for the dual transplant procedure. Medicare and other third-party payers of medical care should include coverage for pancreas transplant procedures meeting these criteria. The pancreas transplant may be done simultaneous with, or subsequent to, a kidney transplant. Pancreas graft survival is better when done simultaneously with a kidney transplant.
2. In the absence of indications for kidney transplantation, pancreas transplantation should only be considered a therapy in patients who exhibit these three criteria: 1) A history of frequent, acute, and severe metabolic complications (hypoglycemia, hyperglycemia, ketoacidosis) requiring medical attention; 2) Clinical and emotional problems with exogenous insulin therapy that are so severe as to be incapacitating; 3) Consistent failure of insulin-based management to prevent acute complications. Program guidelines for insuring an objective multidisciplinary evaluation of the patient's condition and eligibility for transplantation should be established and followed. Third-party payer coverage is appropriate only where such guidelines and procedures exist.

These carefully worded guidelines clearly indicate that pancreas transplantation should not be considered routine care for patients with type 1 diabetes. Rather, this procedure is reserved for individuals who are unable to establish control of their glucose levels and to have a reasonable quality of life by using standard intensified insulin treatment regimens using short- and long-acting insulin preparations. The availability of self-monitoring of glucose and multiple preparations of insulin, in addition to insulin pumps, have facilitated the evolution of highly sophisticated therapeutic paradigms so that greater numbers of type 1 diabetic patients are able to maintain hemoglobin A_{1c} levels that fall within the recommended range. A very small number of type 2 diabetic patients have received a pancreas transplant, but this is not normally considered to be an option for such patients.

THE TRANSPLANTATION PROCEDURE

Pancreas transplantation was first begun for the treatment of type 1 diabetes in humans in 1966 [2]. Not many procedures were performed up to 1978 because of the low rates of graft survival. Thereafter, important improvements in immunosuppressive therapy developed, most notably the use of anti-T-cell agents and cyclosporine. These new drugs, combined with new surgical techniques and the selection of healthier recipients, led to a much greater use of pancreas transplant for therapeutic intervention. By the year 2000, over 14 000 pancreas transplantations had been performed worldwide [3]. Between the years 1978 and 2000 there were many changes in surgical techniques and immunosuppressive drugs that led to progressively higher

International Textbook of Diabetes Mellitus, Third Edition. Edited by R. A. DeFronzo, E. Ferrannini, H. Keen, and P. Zimmet.
 ISBN: 0-471-48655-8.

patient and graft survival rates. Nonetheless, the operative procedure and chronic immunosuppression still carry significant acute and chronic morbidity.

Typically, an intact pancreas donated by a person who has died is placed into the pelvis of the recipient and the native pancreas is left untouched. Most grafts receive arterial blood from, and return venous blood to, iliac vessels. On occasion, hepatic portal venous drainage of the allograft is used. Uncommonly, a hemi-pancreas is donated to a sibling by a healthy, living-related donor who has undergone hemi-pancreatectomy. When a cadaveric organ is used, a small portion of the donor duodenum containing the exit of the pancreatic duct is included and oversewn onto the urinary bladder. In this manner, the exocrine drainage of the donated organ drains into the bladder and is excreted. Alternatively, enteric rather than bladder drainage is used. Currently, each is used roughly 50% of the time. Advantages of bladder drainage over enteric drainage are the use of urinary amylase to monitor for rejection of the pancreas and the avoidance of small bowel complications such as obstruction and infection. On the other hand, the advantages of enteric over bladder drainage are the avoidance of urinary bladder infection, hematuria, and reflux pancreatitis. In terms of hepatic portal venous drainage, one advantage is the avoidance of hyperinsulinemia that is caused when systemic venous drainage is used. The latter bypasses hepatic clearance of insulin, which may be as high as 80–90% in a single pass. It should also be appreciated that because of its ectopic position, it is highly unlikely that central nervous system fibers establish physiologically meaningful innervation of the transplanted organ. This is an important consideration since the central nervous system under normal physiologic conditions is considered to be an important regulator of pancreatic islet function.

Transplanted pancreases can undergo both acute and chronic rejection episodes despite the use of immunosuppressive drugs. Management involves hospitalization and intense acceleration of immunosuppression. If the pancreas is transplanted simultaneously with a kidney, detection of rejection is facilitated because an increase in serum creatinine can be easily monitored and used as a signal that both organs are at risk for undergoing a rejection episode. When a pancreas is transplanted with bladder drainage without a kidney, the less sensitive and later indices of decreasing urinary amylase, increasing serum amylase, and increasing blood glucose levels are the only available warnings of rejection. Cystoscopic transduodenal or percutaneous biopsy with ultrasound guidance is used to confirm rejection. A renewed autoimmune attack on the transplanted islet has been suggested as a possible cause of graft demise, but this is probably an unusual event, partly because the recipient receives immunosuppressive drugs that are known to suppress primary autoimmune responses effectively.

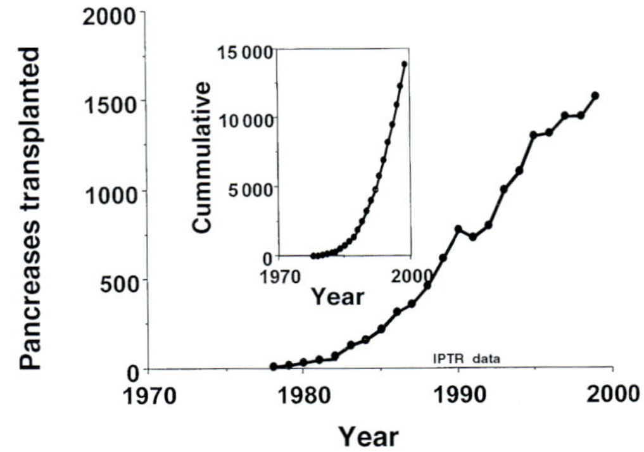

Figure 1 The frequency of pancreas transplantation worldwide according to the International Pancreas Transplant Registry. Inset illustrates the cumulative number of pancreases transplanted through the year 2000. (Reproduced by permission of Elsevier [2])

Currently, long-term maintenance of immunosuppression is provided by triple-drug therapy with either cyclosporine or tacrolimus (both calcineurin inhibitors), azathioprine or mycophenolate mofetil (both antimetabolites), and corticosteroids. Increasingly, more immunosuppressive protocols are excluding corticosteroids because of their severe adverse side effects that greatly compromise quality of life, such as metabolic bone disease and cushingnoid appearance.

The annual and cumulative pancreas transplantation event rates, as well as the success rates for patient and organ survival, have continually increased since 1978. By the year 2000 the annual number of pancreases transplanted worldwide numbered greater than 1400 with a cumulative total greater than 14 000 (Figure 1). Historically, the vast majority of pancreases are transplanted simultaneously with kidneys. However, in 1999, of 1287 pancreas transplants reported, 75% were performed simultaneously with kidneys, 18% were performed after kidney transplantation, and 7% were performed unrelated to previous or concurrent kidney transplantation [3]. The patient survival rate for simultaneous pancreas and kidney transplantation 1 year posttransplant is currently 95%. It seems likely that the 5% mortality is due more to the chronic diabetic state than the surgery itself because the vast majority of deaths do not occur in the perioperative period and are usually cardiovascular in nature. In this regard, it is important to bear in mind that the average recipient of a pancreas transplant has had diabetes mellitus for over 20 years and prior to the surgery has had serious complications including macrovascular and microvascular disease. For pancreases transplanted simultaneously with kidneys in the 1994–1997 era, the pancreas graft survival rate is currently 82% at 1 year and 78% at 3 years (Figure 2). Similar data for pancreas transplantation after a previous kidney transplantation are 71% at 1 year and 62% at 3 years. When

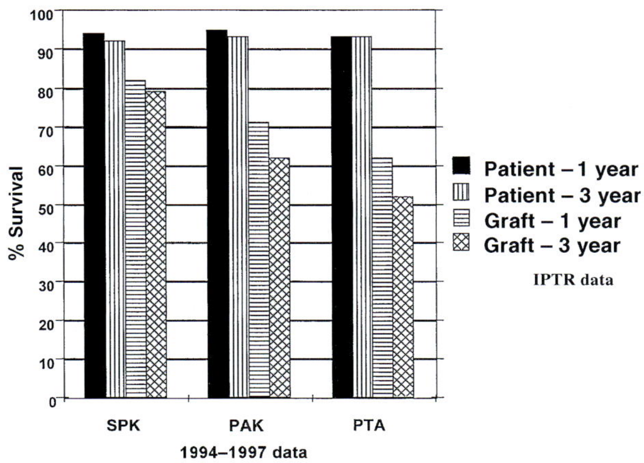

Figure 2 Patient and pancreas graft survival 1 and 3 years posttransplantation according to the International Pancreas Transplant Registry. SPK = simultaneous pancreas kidney; PAK = pancreas after kidney; PTA = pancreas transplant alone. (Reproduced by permission of Elsevier [2])

pancreases are transplanted alone, the 1-year survival rate is 62% and the 3-year survival rate is 52%. More recently, in the 1998–2000 era, 1-year pancreas survival is 82% after a simultaneous pancreas and kidney transplantation; 74% when the pancreas was transplanted after an established kidney transplant; and 76% when the pancreas was transplanted alone without kidney transplantation. When interpreting these data, it is important to remember that none of the patients were assigned to transplant categories on a randomized basis and that the data cited came from multiple worldwide transplant centers with varying degrees of experience.

Serious adverse effects often accompany the surgery required for pancreas transplantation as well as the immunosuppressive drugs used. Perioperative complications (Table 1) leading to laparotomy occur in approximately 30% of patients because of intra-abdominal infections and abscess, vascular graft thrombosis, anastomotic leakage, and duodenal stump leak. Drug-related complications include bacterial and viral infections (particularly cytomegalovirus) and malignancy (particularly skin tumors and lymphoma). Adverse metabolic side effects of the drugs include osteoporosis and insulin resistance as a consequence of using glucocorticoids and decreased renal

Table 1 Complications of pancreas transplantatation

- Intra-abdominal infection and abscess
- Vascular graft thrombosis
- Anastomotic and duodenal stump leak
- Cytomegaloviral infection
- Malignancy
- Metabolic bone disease
- Death

function as a consequence of using calcineurin inhibitors. Ironically, many of the immunosuppressive drugs, particularly the calcineurin inhibitors, have deleterious effects on pancreatic β-cell function. These include decreased β-cell insulin gene expression and insulin content as well as defective insulin secretion in response to glucose. For this reason, newer drugs are being sought that do not adversely affect β-cell function of the transplanted pancreas.

CLINICAL OUTCOMES OF SUCCESSFUL PANCREAS TRANSPLANTATION ON THE COMPLICATIONS OF DIABETES

The major metabolic defect in patients with type 1 diabetes mellitus is the total absence of insulin secretion because their β-cells have been killed by the autoimmune process that underlies this disease. Although exogenous insulin therapy has been remarkably effective in maintaining the life of such patients, it is extremely difficult, if not impossible, to maintain normal glucose levels using insulin-based therapy without excessive severe hypoglycemia. In contrast, successful pancreas transplantation is remarkably effective in restoring endogenous insulin secretion, independence from exogenous insulin therapy, normal glucose levels, and normal hemoglobin A_{1c} levels [4]. Normalization of fasting blood glucose levels has been documented to exceed 18 years (Figure 3). That not only fasting but also postprandial glucose levels are improved can be appreciated when hemoglobin A_{1c} levels in pancreas transplant recipients are compared to those observed in the Diabetes Control and Complications Trial (DCCT). Patients undergoing standard therapy in the DCCT had an average hemoglobin A_{1c} value of approximately 9% whereas those undergoing intensive insulin-based management had an average level of approximately 7% [5]. In a group of successful pancreas transplant recipients followed over 6

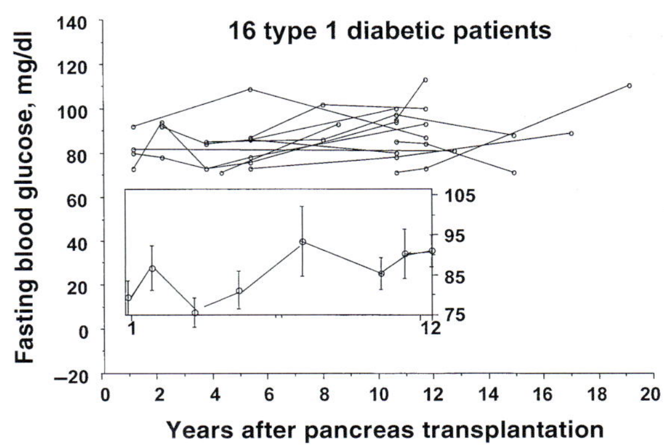

Figure 3 Fasting blood glucose levels determined longitudinally in patients with successful pancreas transplantation. Inset shows mean data for all patients 12 years posttransplantation. (Reproduced by permission of the American Diabetes Association [4])

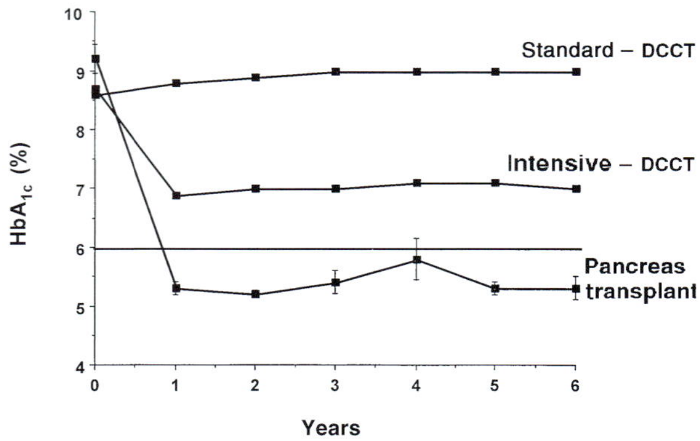

Figure 4 Comparison of hemoglobin A_{1c} levels after successful pancreas transplantation with levels observed during standard and intensive therapy in the DCCT. The solid line at 6% represents the upper limit of normal. (Copyright © 1993 Massachusetts Medical Society. All rights reserved [5, 6])

years, the average hemoglobin A_{1c} level ranged between 5 and 6% (Figure 4). These results are all the more impressive because some of the immunosuppressive drugs used compromise β-cell function and cause increased insulin resistance [7]. Concern exists that the hyperinsulinemism that is caused by systemic venous drainage of the transplanted pancreas may be harmful in terms of accelerating atherosclerosis. However, if anything, circulating lipids are under better control following pancreas transplantation [8, 9] and there have been no reports of accelerated atherosclerosis in transplant recipients. To the contrary, recent evidence suggests that successful pancreas transplant recipients have improved vascular status (see below).

Hypoglycemia was one of the major limitations to obtaining a better hemoglobin A_{1c} value in the intensive management group of the DCCT. In contrast, patients receiving a successful pancreas transplant typically do not experience hypoglycemia, because the transplanted β-cells stop secreting insulin when glucose levels fall to lower than normal values. In nondiabetic individuals, glucagon secretion from the pancreatic α-cell occurs promptly when glucose levels fall to approximately 56 mg/dl. Glucagon released from the α-cell immediately enters the hepatic portal circulation through which it travels to the liver to stimulate glycogenolysis. This promptly releases glucose into the hepatic vein and thereafter into the general circulation. Soon after the glucagon response, the adrenal medulla releases epinephrine, which also is capable of stimulating hepatic glycogenolysis. Typically, patients who have had type 1 diabetes mellitus for more than 5 years have absent glucagon responses, and after 10 years have diminished epinephrine responses, to hypoglycemia. To make matters worse, patients who are recurrently hypoglycemic do not have the usual array of physical symptoms—warmth, sweating, visual disturbances, rapid heart rate, and tremulousness—that accompany hypoglycemia. Because these warning signs are absent, patients often do not realize they are hypoglycemic until blood glucose levels drop as low as 30 mg/dl, an obviously dangerous situation because obtundation and even death may follow as values drop even lower. The loss of symptomatic responsiveness to hypoglycemia has been shown to be an example of desensitization since loosening of tight metabolic control with insulin in type 1 diabetic patients is also accompanied by a return of symptoms to subsequent hypoglycemia [10, 11].

Successful pancreas transplantation completely restores endogenous glucagon secretion to hypoglycemia (Figure 5). In experiments using hypoglycemic/hyperinsulinemic clamps, it has been demonstrated that successfully transplanted patients have virtually identical glucagon responses to those observed in non-diabetic control subjects [13]. Similar benefits are observed for epinephrine secretion (Figure 6), although this response is not completely restored. As far as the patient is concerned, the most salutary improvement is the complete return of symptom responses during hypoglycemia (Figure 7). No differences are found in symptomatology at the various glucose levels developed during a hypoglycemic clamp when comparing transplanted patients to normal controls and both groups have markedly more intense symptoms than nontransplanted type 1 diabetic patients.

Nephropathy is a major secondary complication of chronic hyperglycemia. Decreased glomerular filtration rate and mesangial thickening are commonly observed as diabetes progresses. Normal kidneys transplanted into diabetic patients who remain hyperglycemic soon undergo the same deterioration in structure and function

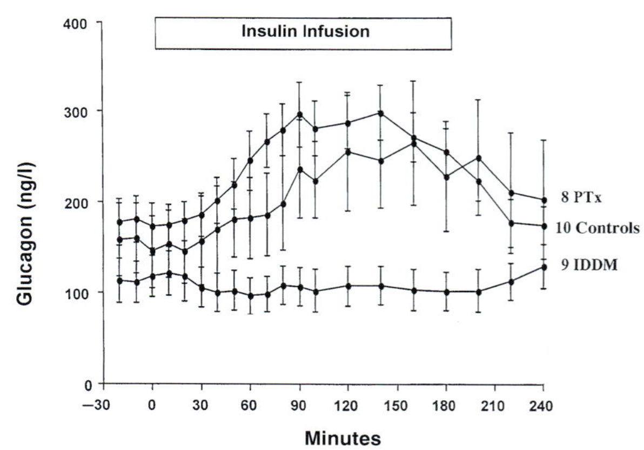

Figure 5 Comparison of glucagon responses during hypoglycemic clamps in patients with insulin-dependent diabetes mellitus (IDDM), patients with successful pancreas transplantation (PTx), and control subjects. After successful pancreas transplantation the glucagon responses are indistinguishable from those of control patients whereas responses in patients with IDDM are absent. (Reproduced by permission of the American Diabetes Association [12])

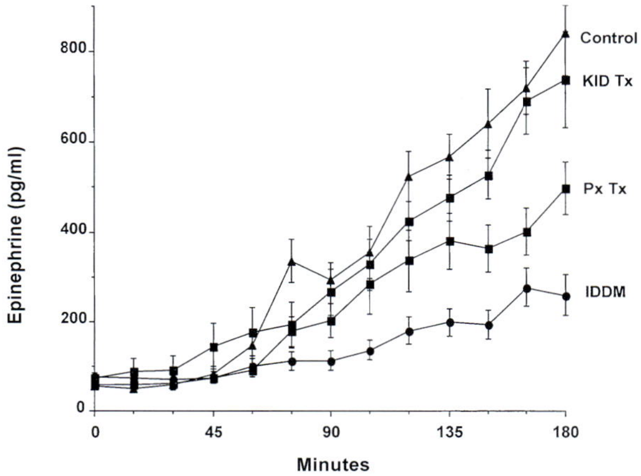

Figure 6 Epinephrine responses during hypoglycemic clamps in nondiabetic kidney transplant (KID Tx) recipients, type 1 diabetic pancreas transplant (Px Tx) recipients, untransplanted patients with type 1 diabetes mellitus, and control subjects. Epinephrine is secreted during the hypoglycemic clamp procedure in all patient groups but is significantly depressed in patients with IDDM. Pancreas transplantation in IDDM recipients partially restores the defective response. (Reproduced by permission of the American Diabetes Association [13])

experienced by native kidneys. In cases of simultaneous pancreas and kidney transplantation, transplanted kidneys fare much better because the recipients become euglycemic. Most recently, it has been appreciated that abnormal diabetic renal structure in the native kidney undergoes resolution of thickened basement membranes and mesangial accumulation after 10 years of normal glu-

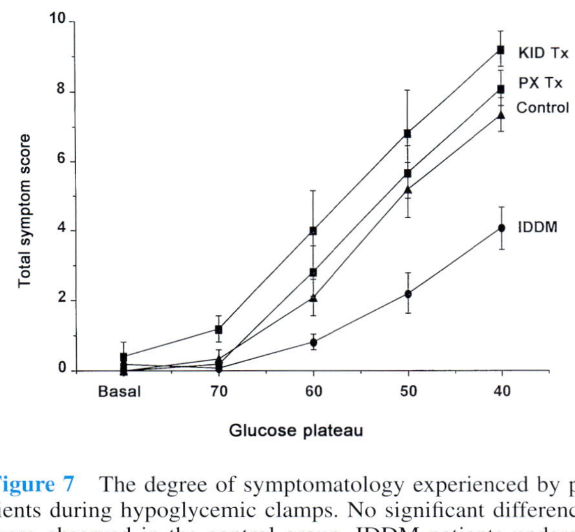

Figure 7 The degree of symptomatology experienced by patients during hypoglycemic clamps. No significant differences were observed in the control group, IDDM patients undergoing pancreas transplantation, or nondiabetic patients undergoing kidney transplantation. The nontransplanted IDDM patients had significantly less severe symptoms than the other three groups. (Reproduced by permission of the American Diabetes Association [13])

cose levels following successful pancreas transplantation [14].

Motor and sensory neuropathy greatly diminishes the quality of life in patients with chronic diabetes. Sensory neuropathy can be expressed as chronic numbness of the skin, particularly in the feet, and can also be expressed as chronic pain and exquisite sensitivity to touch. After several years of successful pancreas transplantation and return to euglycemia, indices of sensory and motor nerve function are stabilized. Recently, it has been demonstrated that parameters of nerve function, including physical examination, motor and sensory nerve conduction, and cardiorespiratory reflexes, can be stabilized for up to 10 years in successful recipients [15]. Even more impressively, the marked diminution in life expectancy that accompanies autonomic dysfunction in chronic diabetes, which approximates 50% at 5 years, is greatly improved. In one study, a group of type 1 diabetic patients with autonomic insufficiency who had successful pancreas transplantation and return to euglycemia had a 20% mortality at 5 years versus an approximate 70% mortality in failed pancreas transplant recipients [16].

The impact of successful pancreas transplantation on retinopathy has been equivocal. Several studies comparing transplanted to nontransplanted patients with chronic diabetes have indicated no significant differences in abnormal retinal changes. This generally gloomy conclusion has recently been challenged by a report indicating that less laser therapy for retinopathy was required in patients undergoing pancreas and kidney transplantation compared to those undergoing kidney transplantation alone [17].

Until recently, there was no indication that macrovascular disease in patients with diabetes might be improved by a return to euglycemia following pancreas transplantation. More recently however, three reports have appeared suggesting the opposite. Two studies involved in examination of intima media thickness of the carotid artery. In one report, thickness was significantly less in patients who had undergone pancreas and kidney transplantation compared to patients undergoing kidney transplantation alone [8]. In the second study, carotid intima media thickness 4 years after successful pancreas transplantation was no different than that found in a nondiabetic control group, but was less than that found in a pre-pancreas transplant diabetic group [9]. However, both studies were cross-sectional and did not obtain paired measures in the same patients before and after pancreas transplantation. More recently, a study of coronary artery patency indicated less narrowing over time in a group of successful pancreas transplant patients studied prospectively compared to a group of patients who failed transplantation [18].

Quality-of-life studies consistently demonstrate benefits for successful recipients of pancreas transplantation. Although this outcome is the most clinically difficult to objectively measure, it is clearly the most important indicator of success or failure. Virtually all published studies report that the quality of life after pancreas transplantation improves regardless of whether a kidney transplant is involved or not [19]. The most common question asked is whether the recipients would prefer a successfully transplanted organ and the risks of chronic immunosuppression or a return to their original diabetic state and insulin-based therapy with the hazards of hypoglycemia. Patients usually report they prefer taking immunosuppressive drugs as the price of a functioning pancreas, normal glucose levels, and decreased risk of developing secondary complications of diabetes, including hypoglycemia. An important caveat is that most diabetic patients who receive transplants have had serious difficulty avoiding extremely high and low glucose levels. Clearly, the worse the quality of life before transplantation, the more likely it is to improve after successful surgery. Very little has been published about the relative costs and benefits of pancreas transplantation versus insulin-based management.

Acknowledgment

This study was supported in part by NIH Grant RO1 DK 399994.

REFERENCES

1. American Diabetes Association Position Statement. Pancreas transplantation for patients with type 1 diabetes. *Diabetes Care* 2000; 23: S85.
2. Kelly WD, Lillehei RC, Merkel FK, Idezuki Y, Goetz FC. Allotransplantation of the pancreas and duodenum along with the kidney in diabetic nephropathy. *Surgery* 1967; 61: 827–37.
3. Gruessner AC, Sutherland DER. *Pancreas Transplant Outcomes for United States (US) Cases Reported to the United Network for Organ Sharing (UNOS) and Non-US Cases Reported to the International Pancreas Transplant Registry (IPTR) as of October, 2000*. Los Angeles: UCLA Immunogenetics Center, 2000; pp 45–71.
4. Robertson RP, Sutherland DE, Lanz KJ. Normoglycemia preserved insulin secretory reserve in diabetic patients 10–18 years after pancreas transplantation. *Diabetes* 1999; 48: 1737–40.
5. The Diabetes Control and Complications Trial Research Group. The effect of intensive treatment of diabetes on the development and progression of long-term complications in insulin-dependent diabetes mellitus. *N Engl J Med* 1993; 329: 977–86.
6. Robertson R. Pancreas and islet transplants for patients with diabetes: taking positions and making decisions. *Endocr Pract* 1998; 5: 24–8.
7. Paty BW, Harmon JS, Marsh CL, Robertson RP. Inhibitory effects of immunosuppressive drugs on insulin secretion from HIT-T15 cells and Wistar rat islets. *Transplantation* 2002; 73: 353–7.
8. Fiorina P, La Rocca E, Venturini M, Minicucci F, Fermo I, Paroni R, D'Angelo A, Sblendido M, Di Carlo V, Cristallo M, Del Maschio A, Pozza G, Secchi A. Effects of kidney–pancreas transplantation on atherosclerotic risk factors and endothelial function in patients with uremia and type 1 diabetes. *Diabetes* 2001; 50: 496–501.
9. Larsen JL, Ratanasuwan T, Burkman T, Lynch T, Erickson J, Colling C, Lane J, Mack-Shipman L, Lyden E, Loseke M, Miller S, Leone J. Carotid intima media thickness decreases after pancreas transplantation. *Transplantation* 2002; 73: 936–40.
10. Dagogo-Jack S, Rattarasarn C, Cryer PE. Reversal of hypoglycemia unawareness, but not defective glucose counterregulation, in IDDM. *Diabetes* 1994; 43: 1426–34.
11. Fanelli CG, Epifano L, Rambotti AM, Pampanelli S, Di Vincenzo A, Modarelli F, Lepore M, Annibale B, Ciofetta M, Bottini P, Porcellati F, Scionti L, Santeusanio B, Brunetti P, Bolli GB. Meticulous prevention of hypoglycemia normalizes the glycemic thresholds and magnitude of most of neuroendocrine responses to, symptoms of, and cognitive function during hypoglycemia in intensively treated patients with short-term IDDM. *Diabetes* 1993; 42: 1683–9.
12. Barrou Z, Seaquist ER Robertson RP. Pancreas transplantation in diabetic humans normalizes hepatic glucose production during hypoglycemia. *Diabetes* 1994; 43: 661–6.
13. Kendall DM, Rooney DP, Smets YF, Salazar Bolding L, Robertson RP. Pancreas transplantation restores epinephrine response and symptom recognition during hypoglycemia in patients with long-standing type I diabetes and autonomic neuropathy. *Diabetes* 1997; 46: 249–57.
14. Fioretto P, Steffes MW, Sutherland DE, Goetz FC, Mauer M. Reversal of lesions of diabetic nephropathy after pancreas transplantation. *N Engl J Med* 1998; 339: 69–75.
15. Navarro X, Sutherland DE, Kennedy WR. Long-term effects of pancreatic transplantation on diabetic neuropathy. *Ann Neurol* 1997; 42: 727–36.
16. Navarro X, Kennedy WR, Loewenson RB, Sutherland DE. Influence of pancreas transplantation on cardiorespiratory reflexes, nerve conduction, and mortality in diabetes mellitus. *Diabetes* 1990; 39: 802–6.
17. Koznarova R, Saudek F, Sosna T, Adamec M, Jedinakova T, Boucek P, Bartos V, Lanska V. Beneficial effect of pancreas and kidney transplantation on advanced diabetic retinopathy. *Cell Transplant* 2000; 9: 903–8.
18. Jukema JW, Smets YF, van der Pijl JW, Zwinderman AH, Vliegen HW, Ringers J, Reiber JH, Lemkes HH, van der Wall EE, de Fijter JW. Impact of simultaneous pancreas and kidney transplantation on progression of coronary atherosclerosis in patients with end-stage renal failure due to type 1 diabetes. *Diabetes Care* 2002; 25: 906–11.
19. Zehrer CL, Gross CR. Comparison of quality of life between pancreas/kidney and kidney transplant recipients: 1-year follow-up. *Transplant Proc* 1994; 26: 508–9.

58

Islet Transplantation

Edmond A. Ryan, Jonathan R.T. Lakey, Breay W. Paty, and A.M. James Shapiro

University of Alberta, Edmonton, Canada

INTRODUCTION

The discovery of insulin dramatically changed the outcome for patients with type 1 diabetes and the acute lethal complications of diabetes like diabetic ketoacidosis could be effectively treated. However, the improved survival allowed the development of the secondary complications of diabetes [1]. Typically the patient with type 1 diabetes develops retinopathy, nephropathy, neuropathy, or vascular disease over time. It was not until 1993 that definitive proof for the value of good glycemic control was established. The landmark Diabetes Control and Complications Trial (DCCT) study showed that the microvascular complications of diabetes could be delayed or avoided by good glycemic control, which required intensive insulin therapy [2]. Such therapy was associated with a HbA_{1c} that was 1% lower than the control group. It should be noted that the HbA_{1c} was not normalized and in the intensively treated group, remained at least 1% above the upper limit of normal. Similar evidence was provided by the United Kingdom Prospective Diabetes Study (UKPDS) in type 2 diabetes with microvascular disease, showing a significant improvement for a decline of 1% in the HbA_{1c} [3]. Thus, glycemic control is essential if the microvascular complications of diabetes are to be prevented.

Controlling glycemia with exogenous insulin remains a challenge. Given the nonphysiological subcutaneous route of insulin administration, its inherent delay in absorption, the variability of serum levels obtained, and the systemic versus portal venous delivery, it is perhaps remarkable how well the glucose levels are actually controlled. The newer insulin analogues have removed some of the variability and delay in absorption but even with intensive therapy it is difficult to achieve normoglycemia. Continuous subcutaneous insulin administration helps further but old and recent studies still did not normalize glucose values [4, 5]. Carbohydrate counting and attention to diet aids the quest for normoglycemia but is not the complete solution. The largest study using all available tools to optimize therapy was still associated with an increased risk of hypoglycemia [2]. In the DCCT, the risk for severe hypoglycemia (defined as needing third-party assistance) was increased threefold. Concern about hypoglycemia remains the limiting factor in attempts to achieve optimal glycemic control.

Many efforts have been made to generate a closed-loop system for glucose control. The first successful efforts were with the Biostator®, which involved continuous monitoring of blood glucose and then an insulin infusion using a computer-derived algorithm [6]. Although effective for a short period of time, it was impractical being bulky and plagued with flow problems from the double lumen catheter being used for sensing the glucose level. Insulin infusion pumps (especially using insulin analogues such as lispro or insulin aspart) have helped but are not closed-loop systems and require frequent glucose monitoring and rarely results in normal glycemia without severe hypoglycemia. The goal of any closed-loop system is to have reliable glucose sensing linked to appropriate insulin delivery on a continuous basis. Mechanical closed-loop systems may in the future achieve this but have been fraught with problems despite early promise. Transplantation of islets of Langerhans or of the whole pancreas can achieve a physiological closed-loop system today.

BACKGROUND HISTORY

Transplantation of pancreatic tissue was first tried in 1890 when a surgeon in England transplanted a sheep pancreas

International Textbook of Diabetes Mellitus, Third Edition. Edited by R. A. DeFronzo, E. Ferrannini, H. Keen, and P. Zimmet.
 ISBN: 0-471-48655-8.

into a boy with diabetic ketoacidosis [7]. The immune barriers, unknown at the time, were insurmountable. The modern era of transplantation began in the 1960s when the use of steroids, especially when combined with azathioprine, allowed successful renal transplantation. The steroids block several cytokines and act as inhibitors of antigen presentation, and azathioprine is an inhibitor of purine synthesis and thus impedes the generation of active T-cells. In 1972 Ballinger and Lacy proposed that it might be possible to transplant islets of Langerhans for the treatment of type 1 diabetes [8]. Cyclosporin A, a calcineurin inhibitor, which is associated with an impaired transcription in active T-cells and thus blocks interleukin 2 activation, greatly improved transplantation graft survival [9].

Many groups had been working in rodent and canine models to perfect islet isolation and maintain demonstrable β-cell insulin secretion [10, 11]. Experiments in rats and mice showed that success in transplantation of islets could be obtained in rodents [8] and the transplanted islets had a biphasic insulin secretory response to glucose [12]. Islet allotransplantation in animals was also successfully performed [13, 14] and it has been possible to isolate human islets that would function in diabetic nude mice [15, 16]. The results of these studies highlighted the need for purified islets and the importance of the site of transplantation.

Multicellular islet tissue comprises 1.5% by weight of the whole pancreas [17]. Careful digestion is necessary to achieve a purified preparation, and collagenase became the mainstay in the digestion [10]. Success with isolation from human pancreases was more problematic than in animal studies [18, 19]. Methods used for the dissociation of islets from the exocrine tissue required a combination of mechanical and enzymatic techniques.

The site of transplantation was also an issue. The pancreatic bed, because of its inaccessibility, was not a preferred option. Liver, spleen, renal subcapsule, and an omental pouch have been the primary locations tried [14, 20–22]. Work with immune privileged sites, such as the testes, has been ongoing but has not been routinely adapted [23]. A site with portal drainage has the natural advantage of mimicking the normal route of insulin delivery and is most commonly used for human islet transplantation [24]. The splenic site was associated with infarction [25] and so the liver, renal, and omental pouch have been the preferred areas for islet transplantation. All sites have disadvantages compared to the native islet bed in that oxygenation is lower [26] and the intraislet blood pressure is elevated [27]. The vascularization of the liver gives it an advantage and may help in angiogenesis of the islets while an advantage of the omental pouch or renal site is the ability to remove the islets for histologic examination. When the liver is used, an unresolved question is whether the venous drainage of the islets is into the portal sinusoids or systemic circulation. A possible drawback of the portal site is that it allows more exposure to high levels of immunosuppressive drugs and their potential toxicity as they are absorbed [28].

EARLY HUMAN STUDIES

The first human islet transplants, were performed in the 1970s [29], with insulin independence rarely reported [30]. Up to 1998, approximately 260 type 1 diabetic patients had received an islet transplant, with only 12% remaining insulin independent for more than 1 week [24]. The first two patients transplanted as part of an early cohort transplanted in Edmonton in 1989 [31] received approximately 260 000 islets at the same time as a renal transplantation. Exogenous insulin was used intravenously for 14 days with intensive glucose monitoring in order to maintain euglycemia, which may help preserve β-cell function [32]. The immunosuppression therapy included corticosteroids, azathioprine, cyclosporin A, and Minnesota antilymphocyte globulin. Both patients demonstrated positive C-peptide status posttransplant but both developed cytomegalovirus infection and lost islet mass, never having achieved insulin independence. The subsequent five patients had transplants using both fresh and cryopreserved islets so that the total islet mass given exceeded 10 000 islet equivalents/kg. One patient obtained insulin independence for 2 years [33]. One patient who was transplanted at this time had a liver transplant with partially purified islets infused. Complete portal vein thrombosis ensued necessitating an urgent repeat liver transplant [34]. One other patient attained insulin independence for a period of time but eventually all patients required insulin again. On long-term follow-up, two of these patients have continued C-peptide production, the longest being more than 9 years since her transplant. However, subsequent technical problems arose in Edmonton, particularly with the collagenase, and so purified islets could not be obtained and thus islet transplantation lapsed as an avenue for treating diabetes. Other major centers, particularly Miami/Pittsburg, St. Louis, and Milan, also reported early success [35–38] and demonstrated that the transplanted cells may survive for a prolonged time [39, 40].

PANCREAS TRANSPLANTATION

With improved immunosuppression the possibility of performing whole pancreas transplants, particularly at the time of renal transplantation, for end-stage diabetic nephropathy, became a possibility [41]. Initial efforts were associated with peritonitis from exocrine drainage of the pancreatic duct. These problems were surmounted by using bladder drainage [42] such that success rates reached over 80% for 1-year graft survival accompanied by low mortality rates [43–46]. With newer techniques of anastomosis connecting the pancreatic duct to an enteric drainage site [47], fewer problems were encountered (especially with the acidosis secondary to bicarbonate loss in the urine associated with the bladder anastomosis [48]). The 5-year graft survival is now approximately 67%. The side effects are diminishing but it remains a challenging technical surgical procedure [49–51] with some morbidity and mortality as fully reviewed in Chapter 59. The excellent glycemic control [52] can lead to reversal of diabetic renal lesions [53], stabilization or improvement in neuropathy [54, 55], vascular status [56, 57], and stabilization but not necessarily improvement of retinopathy [58, 59].

ISLET TRANSPLANTATION IN THE NEW MILLENNIUM

The unimpressive results of islet transplantation in the late 1990s, as illustrated by low rates of insulin independence [39, 60, 61], were related to the islet preparation (purity of preparations and adequate islet numbers) [62] and immunosuppression (potency and toxicity especially in terms of glucose tolerance) as has been reviewed recently by White et al. [24].

Islet Isolation

Islet mass availability remained a central issue for success. The normal pancreas has 1.0–1.7 million islets [63, 64] yet early studies showed only 250 000 islets being recovered for allotransplantation. Minimizing warm and cold ischemia time and other donor issues are important [65, 66]. The use of University of Wisconsin perfusate solution at the time of organ retrieval [67] enhanced the yield. In addition, the intraductal delivery of collagenase [18, 19, 68], particularly with improved collagenase preparations [69, 70], further enhanced the number of islets obtained. Great strides were made in characterizing the collagenase necessary for purified islet isolation, resulting in much better preparations. The current preparation (Liberase) is a blend of primarily collagenase type 1 and 2, but also has collagenase 3 and 4, clostripain, thermalysin, and proteases (trypsin, chymotrypsin, and elastase), and is associated with a low endotoxin load [70]. A major advance was the development of a metal chamber by Ricordi et al. that allowed disassociation of islets with mechanical digestion and the continuous removal and harvesting of the liberated islets [71, 72]. Purification of islets using a refrigerated COBE centrifuge and Ficoll gradient is also important while it leads to some loss of cells but the risk of intraportal hypertension with the infusion of impure preparations is substantial [34, 73]. The increased purification may also have a negative effect in that ductal elements may be important as a source for islet neogenesis [74]. Short-term culture of the islets may lead to enhanced purity without excessive loss of islets. In addition, the newer methods of islet isolation have removed all xenoproteins from the process. Final issues of islet numbers could also be overcome with the use of multiple donor pancreases. Cryopreservation may be another mechanism to save islets from low yield preparations, with a view to later pooling them with other preparations for the infusion of adequate cell numbers at one procedure [75].

Immunosuppression

More recently, tacrolimus, a more potent calcineurin inhibitor than cyclosporin A, became available [9]. Effective blockade of interleukin 2 with sirolimus, which inhibits T-cell expression and activation, and daclizumab, an antibody to interleukin 2 receptors, allows inhibition of T-cell activation and provides potent immunosuppression. Such a combination allowed the omission of steroids from the regimen, which was a major advantage in the setting of borderline islet mass by reducing β-cell toxicity. The regimen of daclizumab, tacrolimus, and sirolimus may still carry some toxicity for the β-cells and carbohydrate metabolism. Daclizumab is associated with no adverse events [76]. Sirolimus is associated with lipid abnormalities but not usually glucose intolerance [77, 78]. Tacrolimus is associated with some diabetogenicity [9, 79–81] by inhibiting insulin release [82] in a dose-dependent manner [83], a similar problem as its predecessor cyclosporin A [84, 85]. The importance of the appropriate immunosuppression regimen is demonstrated by the fact that with autotransplantation once 2500 islet equivalents/kg are provided then insulin independence can usually be achieved but three or four times this number of cells are required for insulin independence in the allotransplant environment [86]. Not surprisingly, the resurgence of autoimmune responses posttransplantation is ominous for the graft survival [87, 88].

Thus the field of islet transplantation was rejuvenated with our report of seven consecutive cases, achieving insulin independence, with islet transplantation using a steroid-free immunosuppression regimen (Edmonton Protocol) [89]. Of note was the fact that these patients were not in end-stage renal failure and thus these were islet-alone transplants. Initial 100% insulin independence sets the stage for islet transplantation to be considered as a therapy for type 1 diabetes in selected patients.

INDICATIONS

Given that immunosuppression is required posttransplant, careful consideration of the cost–benefit analysis for each patient is required. The major indications for an islet transplant at this time are (1) recurrent severe hypoglycemia, particularly if decreased awareness of hypoglycemia is present, (2) labile diabetes, and (3) progressive complications.

Subjects with diabetes who strive for good glucose control may be at increased risk for severe hypoglycemia. Typically the ready appearance of adrenergic symptoms protects the patient from neuroglycopenia but in some subjects these symptoms are lost. The situation is compounded by the fact that nearly all patients with type 1 diabetes of greater than 5 years' duration lose glucagon secretion in response to hypoglycemia [90]. Thus their immediate defense mechanisms against hypoglycemia are limited to the adrenergic response. However with recurrent mild hypoglycemia the adrenergic response becomes diminished and thus the perilous situation can arise whereby the first manifestation of hypoglycemia are neuroglycopenic symptoms. When the first symptoms of hypoglycemic are confusion, disorientation, or coma, the obvious risks of this situation are apparent in terms of driving, working (especially with small children), or living alone.

Glycemic lability is not uncommon, but it may be such that the glucose values are totally unpredictable. Patients can take the same dose of insulin, have similar meal plans and identical activity levels, but markedly different glucose levels. In addition to frustration such patterns rarely are associated with a good HA_{1c} and patients frequently have problems with severe hypoglycemia. The unpredictable response makes good glucose control impossible despite all efforts.

Finally, some patients have progressive complications despite optimization of medical therapy. Although we originally considered this group, they are now the exception, as we look at our outcomes (see below). Patients who have progression of microalbuminuria, despite being on intensive insulin therapy and an angiotensin-converting enzyme inhibitor, can be considered. If the urine protein is in excess of 1 g/day then a calcineurin-free immunosuppressant regimen is preferred, given the known nephrotoxicity of these agents. Patients who have unstable eye disease despite optimization of glucose control could also be considered; however, some patients have had retinal bleeds posttransplant and we now recommend waiting until the eyes are stable. A further group to be considered for islet transplantation is of those patients who have severe neuropathy. Since there is so little else to offer such patients, the excellent glycemic control that a transplant may provide may be of value but it is likely to take considerable time before benefits are seen. In these patients gastroparesis poses a particular difficulty in that posttransplant the glucose may be stable but maintaining adequate immunosuppression levels in the face of recurrent nausea and vomiting is difficult. Finally, we test all patients to ensure that they have C-peptide absent. More recently, we are willing to consider some people with very limited insulin reserve as evidenced by low C-peptide, who meet the above criteria. We set a weight limit of 90 kg (BMI of <30 kg/m^2) and insulin requirement of no more than 1.2 U/kg/day, as transplanting very insulin resistant patients is likely to be associated with a requirement for several pancreases with the potential added risks of donor sensitization.

Although these two major groups (decreased hypoglycemic awareness and excessive lability of glycemia) are readily identified by experienced diabetologists, characterizing them is much more difficult. There are no good objective measures of severity of hypoglycemia. Currently a month's records of glucose readings with documentation of each value < 3 mmol/l are used. The frequency of hypoglycemia, the lack of autonomic symptoms, and the number of severe reactions (requiring outside help) help guide the assessment of the severity of hypoglycemia. Lability of glycemia has also been difficult to characterize. Older studies suggested this using the mean amplitude of glycemic excursions and we have used this based on 2 days' readings of seven capillary blood glucose values per day [91]. We have found this technique of limited use and are trying to develop alternative assessment measures. Both indications are always predicated on the basis that the patient is following a diabetic meal plan carefully, is monitoring his/her glucose frequently, and has been tried on an intensive insulin therapy regimen.

EVALUATION

At the assessment visit for islet transplantation the patient should have a realistic expectation of the outcome. If the patient has frequent hypoglycemia and glycemic lability problems, then both of these are readily correctable by islet transplantation. The ability to render the patient free of the risk of progression of diabetes complications is unproven at this time, although given good glycemic control this may be expected. Patients who have active infection, a history of cancer, severe vascular disease, or active foot ulceration, who abuse alcohol or drugs, or who are younger than 18 or older than 65 years are not usually considered.

Once the patient meets the entry criteria and is willing to accept the risks of the procedure and immunosuppression, a full evaluation is required. This includes a thorough history and physical examination, the latter concentrating on diabetes complications—retinopathy, neuropathy (autonomic and peripheral), and vascular disease. Our laboratory evaluation includes details of these complications with an ophthalmology report required, 24-h urine for microalbuminuria, protein, and creatinine clearance, together with a serum creatinine, ECG, and stress MIBI scan including a lipid panel. If there is any suggestion of an abnormality either clinically or on vascular testing, coronary angiogram is performed.

In addition, the basic transplant screens are required, including blood group, complete blood count, coagulation screen, liver function tests, electrolytes, calcium, magnesium, phosphorus, checks for HIV, hepatitis, EB virus, syphilis, cytomegalovirus, and urine culture. An ultrasound of the abdomen and liver is required to ensure that no lesions are present in the liver. A hemangioma on the right side of the liver would place a patient at increased risk of bleeding during the procedure if a percutaneous approach was used. In subjects older than 40 years, mammograms are performed in women and prostate-specific antigen determinations in men. Considerable time is spent reviewing the potential complications with the patients so that each individual can make a personal assessment of the risk–benefit ratio for themselves and decide if they wish to proceed. In most other transplant settings (heart and liver) the issues are life and death but in islet transplantation this is not the case, as continuing to work with other insulin regimens is possible and thus risk–benefit issues are different.

PROCEDURE

After completion of the evaluation and once nothing untoward is found, the patient after signing an informed consent is then listed for islet transplantation. When a pancreas becomes available the patient is admitted to hospital and has a recheck coagulation screen, CBC, and chest X-ray unless performed recently. The patient is commenced on a dextrose infusion ($D_{10}W$ at 100 ml/h with KCl) and a variable insulin infusion designed to attain good glycemic control. Glucose is measured hourly and the insulin infusion rate adjusted to maintain the glucose between 6 and 10 mmol/l. Once adequate pure islets are prepared, the patient is brought to radiology and percutaneous access is established under midazolam and fentanyl sedation. After infiltration of local anesthetic a 22 mmHg gauge Cheba needle is advanced under fluoroscopic guidance into the portal vein. Others have used CT guidance or it is possible to gain access by the transjugular route or with laparoscopy [92]. A guidewire is then inserted into the main portal vein and a catheter is positioned with confirmation by venogram. Purified islets are then infused with frequent monitoring of portal pressure. If the portal pressure doubles or rises to greater than 22 mmHg, infusion is halted until it resolves and if it does not resolve, the infusion is discontinued. Initially we used a 60-ml syringe but lately have been using an intravenous bag that is prepared in the laboratory. This aids aseptic technique and may also pose less shear pressure on the islets and further provides some constant monitoring of pertal pressure during islet infusion. Once the islets are infused, the catheter is removed and the patient returns to the ward.

The glucose is monitored hourly and occasionally $D_{10}W$ is required at 50 ml/h if the glucose decreases under 4.0 mmol/l. If the glucose rises to above 10 mmol/l, subcutaneous lispro insulin is used. Typically, the plasma glucose level is normal for 16–24 h and then rises. A variable four times daily dose of insulin is used (lispro insulin premeals, neutral protamine Hagedorn at bedtime), depending on the glucose value. The following day the patient has an ultrasound, CBC, and liver function tests, and is discharged home if all results are acceptable. Immunosuppression is achieved with daclizumab 1 mg/kg every 2 weeks for 10 weeks, sirolimus with target trough levels of 12–15 μg/l for the first 3 months and then 7–10 μg/l, and tacrolimus at a target level of 3–6 μg/l. In addition, for cytomegalovirus prophylaxis patients are given ganciclovir 1000 mg t.i.d. for 3 months and trimethoprim-sulfamethoxazole or, if the white cell count is $<2.5 \times 10^9$/l, inhaled pentamidine for prevention of *Pneumocystis carinii* Pneumonia. Usually insulin requirements are halved after the first procedure and nearly all subjects need a second transplant to become insulin independent. A minority need three transplants.

OUTCOMES

Procedure Related

Details of the procedure and outcomes from our center have been published [89, 93–95]. The transplant procedure is well tolerated, with a median hospital stay of 1 day. Insertion of the needle may take more than one pass and has been associated with a 10% chance of bleeding, most of whom required blood transfusion. The gallbladder has been punctured in 2 of 17 cases and gave rise to pain but this settled with conservative management. Twenty percent of patients have moderate to severe abdominal pain but this is usually transient. About half of the patients have had a rise in the liver function tests but in all cases this has settled. The major concern is of portal vein thrombosis. This has occurred in 2 of 17 cases in both patients involving just the peripheral branch of the portal vein. In the first case a hemostat plug had been used after the transplantation and may have contributed to the problem. In the second patient the portal vein pressure rose when the final less pure layer of cells was infused. The patient was anticoagulated but then developed an expanding subcapsular and intrahepatic bleed that required surgical evacuation and partial hepatic resection. The patient made a good recovery and, although continues on insulin, is still C-peptide positive.

Glycemia

All patients became insulin independent once they received adequate islet numbers (Figure 1). A minimum of 9000 islet equivalents/kg is required. The one patient who required more than this had the peripheral portal vein thrombosis and likely lost some cells. Most patients required two transplantations to achieve insulin independence. On four occasions three procedures were required.

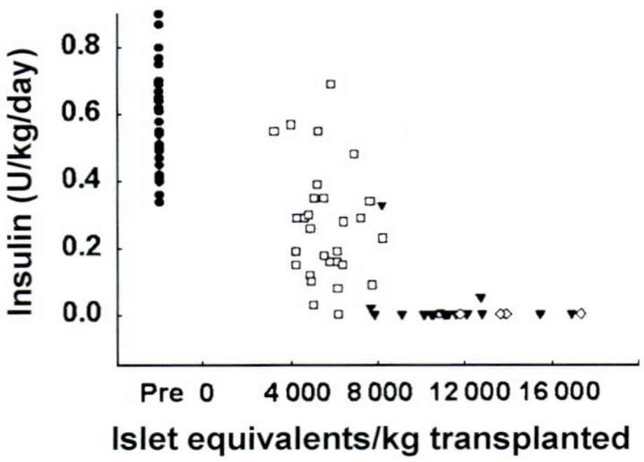

Figure 1 Number of islets infused per kilogram vs. exogenous insulin requirements (U/kg/day). Values for pretransplant (filled circles), post first transplant (open squares), post second transplant (filled inverted triangles), and after the third procedure (open diamonds) are shown. All but one patient became insulin dependent once 9000 or more islet equivalents/kg were provided (reproduced with permission, from reference 94)

On two occasions two pancreases were available at the time of isolation and both were used for a single infusion. The mean number of islet equivalents transplanted for the first infusion was $374\,283 \pm 20\,247$ and for the second transplant, $391\,647 \pm 32\,921$. As some patients had three procedures, the mean total islet mass provided was $850\,035 \pm 337\,911$. This represents a total islet mass provided of $12\,330 \pm 581$ islet equivalents/kg. Typically the insulin requirements are halved after the first transplant and most become insulin independent after the second transplant (Figure 1). On long-term follow-up the C-peptide secretion has been maintained in the majority of subjects. Of 15 patients who have reached 1 year post-transplantation, 80% were insulin independent and 4 of 6 are insulin-free at 2 years; these results are considerably better than those previously available (Figure 2). Of those patients currently back on insulin (6/17), 3 have lost C-peptide secretion, 2 of whom have had a recurrence

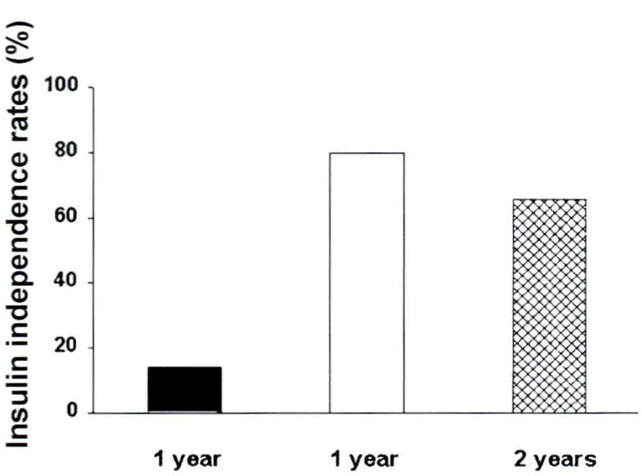

Figure 2 Insulin independence rates post islet transplantation for the Edmonton patients at 1 year ($n = 15$, open bar) and 2 years ($n = 6$, hatched bars) compared to the rates previously reported by the Islet Transplant Registry prior to the year 2000 (solid bar)

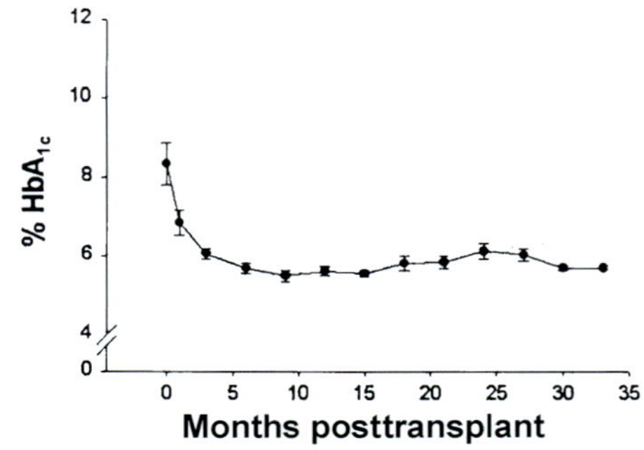

Figure 3 % HbA_{1c} (mean ± SE) pre- and posttransplant in insulin-independent subjects over time

of autoimmunity. Three have persisting C-peptide but because of imperfect glucose control they are on insulin at about half the dose of pretransplant. The HA_{1c} is normal in those subjects who are insulin independent (Figure 3). The degree of glucose control is also evident with the standard meal tolerance testing (Table 1). Of note is the finding that although insulin secretion is similar to controls, the glucose, though greatly improved, is not normal. In some patients the fasting glucose is higher than the postprandial. A minimally elevated fasting glucose (6.05 mmol/l) has also been reported in islet transplant patients with no increased hepatic glucose production [96]. The insulin reserve in our subjects is also limited as has been noted in islet autotransplantation [97]. Subjects have had an intravenous glucose tolerance test (IVGTT) and determination of the acute insulin response to glucose (AIR_g). In controls the value for the AIR_g is 56.1 ± 8.4 U/ml but in successful islet transplant patients the level at 1-month posttransplant is only 7.9 ± 1.7 U/ml (15% of control). The acute insulin response to arginine (AIR_{arg}) may be more indicative of islet mass in that the acute insulin response to arginine was 61% of that of controls. Monitoring function to predict graft loss is difficult, with no easy measure such as using the serum creatinine in post renal transplant patients. The insulin area under the curve during an IVGTT may

Table 1 Glucose and insulin responses before and after a standard mixed meal (Ensure®) in nondiabetic controls, type 1 diabetic subjects pretransplant, and in those with continued insulin independence

	Control	Pretransplant	Posttransplant
Fasting glucose, mmol/l	4.5 ± 0.1	11.5 ± 1.9	6.1 ± 0.4
90-min glucose, mmol/l	3.7 ± 0.4	19.2 ± 2.9	8.1 ± 0.8
Fasting C-peptide, nmol/l	0.56 ± 0.07	<0.1	0.92 ± 0.14
90-min C-peptide, nmol/l	1.25 ± 0.12	<0.1	1.47 ± 0.18

Note: Values are mean ± SE.

be predictive [94] as may measuring proinsulin [98] or split-proinsulin secretion [99].

Diabetes Complications

No change has been found in neuropathy, and in two patients with severe painful peripheral neuropathy there has been no improvement noted after at least 2 years of successful transplantation. One patient with necrobiosis lipoidica diabeticorum anecdotally reported that it was better [93]. Of the 17 patients who had an adequate islet mass provided, 3 have reported retinal bleeds, which required laser photocoagulation. We felt this was related to the sudden improvement in the glucose control and in all patients the eyes have stabilized [100, 101]. Two patients with elevated creatinine showed initial deterioration of the renal function but this has stabilized. Four had a worsening of their preexisting proteinuria posttransplant but this has also stabilized [94]. The two patients with the elevated creatinine have been switched to mycophenolate mofetil from tacrolimus as this is the most likely culprit [102]. No vascular deterioration has been noted although one patient who had established coronary artery disease has required an angioplasty. However, 60% of subjects have had a rise in their cholesterol, requiring statin therapy, although the triglycerides did not rise. Hyperlipidemia is well recognized as an adverse affect of sirolimus [77]. Hypertension has also been a problem with 50% of patients requiring an increase in their antihypertensive medication.

One of the major indications for the islet transplant is a problem with hypoglycemia. Typically after the first transplant the problems with the frequent occurrence of hypoglycemia are eliminated. In a subgroup we have performed a hypoglycemic clamp and measured their counterregulatory response. We have studied seven of these patients posttransplant who had stable glucose control and with the stepped hypoglycemic clamp they are still found to have a deficient glucagon and epinephrine responses although they were not having problems with clinical hypoglycemia. Interestingly this is similar to what is found in islet autotransplantation [103, 104] but different from the whole pancreas situation [105, 106] or if the intrasplenic or intraperitoneal site is used [104, 107]. In both islet and whole pancreas transplantation denervation occurs, and so this is unlikely to be the explanation although it blunts some of the insulin response [108]. Thus islet transplantation into the intrahepatic site is unique in that the glucagon response to hypoglycemia is not restored, a difference that is unexplained at this time.

Side Effects of Medications

Common side effects of sirolimus are hyperlipidemia and diarrhea [109]. As mentioned above, the majority of patients have had a rise in their cholesterol but not triglycerides. This is in contrast to the earlier use of these drugs where the combination of sirolimus and corticosteroids resulted in a rise of triglyceride in 51% of subjects and of cholesterol in 44% of subjects, which improved with a decrease in the dose of steroids and sirolimus [110]. Interestingly the combination of sirolimus and tacrolimus alone was not associated with hyperlipidemia in liver transplant patients [111] compared to when cyclosporin A was used or in our group of patients. Perhaps the background of diabetes creates the setting for hyperlipidemia. Diarrhea has been a problem in about half the patients but has usually settled down with time. Common side effects of tacrolimus are tremor, hypertension, diarrhea, and hyperglycemia [80]. Hypertension, lipid, and bowel problems were seen frequently, and tremor was only reported by 2 of 17 patients. The extent to which the tacrolimus contributed to the hyperglycemia in the 7 patients back on insulin is unknown and the mechanism of such toxicity is not defined. Certainly very high levels of tacrolimus can give decreased insulin release but we were not aiming for such levels. Finally, some patients have had acne, arthralgia, anemia, and one patient has developed arthritis. Interestingly there have been no cases of cytomegalovirus even in donor/recipient mismatches, which may be related to there being very few passenger leukocytes in the islet preparations.

SUMMARY

Islet transplantation can correct problems with glycemic lability and recurrent hypoglycemia. Given its technical ease, it is particularly suitable for those with problems with glycemic control and no other major complications. The more technically difficult whole pancreas transplant provides stable glucose control and is ideal in those undergoing simultaneous renal transplant. The islet transplant procedure has some risks both acutely (particularly bleeding, 10%, and thrombosis in the portal vein circulation, 4%) and in the long-term, the unknown but real risk of sepsis and neoplasms. For some patients with major problems with diabetes control these risks are acceptable. Whether the good glycemic control attained will prevent complications in the long-term will take years to resolve. Using the indication of progressive diabetes complications is less suitable at this time, given the problems encountered. Islet transplantation can free a patient with very difficult diabetes from the risks of frequent hypoglycemia or glycemic lability. The decision whether to proceed can only be made by an informed patient who has to cope with difficult diabetes on a daily basis.

FUTURE

Major steps have been taken in islet transplantation but more needs to be done. Currently, we are transplanting an average of 850 000 islets/patient but the insulin response to IV glucose is still less than normal and some of the islet, may have been destroyed. Whether an alternative site would help is unknown but the islets certainly respond better to hypoglycemia at sites other than the liver. Newer immunosuppression regimens may enhance survival, as may anti-inflammatory agents at the time of transplant in order to decrease the cytokine response [112, 113], which may be toxic for insulin secretion and the islets [114]. Whether tolerance can be induced is unknown but may be much more feasible with isolated islets than whole organ transplantation [115, 116]. Novel ideas for either monoclonal antibodies [117, 118] or immunosuppression [119] hold promise. Encapsulation of islets has long been sought as an alternative but to date has only had limited success [120]. Co-transplantation of islets with Sertoli cells may provide immunoprotection [121]. Simultaneous bone marrow transplantation may be another avenue to pursue [122]. However all these approaches will also have to deal with the possibility that islet autoimmunity will resurface. Finally, a major hurdle is the number of cells available. Improving isolation techniques may help increase the recovery of islets from donor organs but likely a completely new source of cells is required, such as stem cells or xenotransplantation [123, 124]. Islet transplantation has faced hurdles before and overcome them. These new challenges can be met and solved.

REFERENCES

1. Banting FG, Best CH, Collip JB, Campbell WR, Fletcher AA. Pancreatic extracts in the treatment of diabetes mellitus: preliminary report. *CMAJ* 1922; 12: 141–6.
2. The Diabetes Control and Complications Trial Research Group. The effect of intensive treatment of diabetes on the development and progression of long-term complications in insulin-dependent diabetes mellitus. *N Engl J Med* 1993; 329: 977–86.
3. The UK Prospective Diabetes Study (UKPDS) Group. Intensive blood-glucose control with sulphonylureas or insulin compared with conventional treatment and risk of complications in patients with type 2 diabetes (UKPDS 33). *Lancet* 1998; 352: 837–53.
4. Reeves ML, Seigler DE, Ryan EA, Skyler JS. Glycemic control in insulin dependent diabetes mellitus. Comparison of outpatient intensified conventional therapy with continuous subcutaneous infusion. *Am J Med* 1982; 72: 673–80.
5. Tsui E, Barnie A, Ross S, Parkes R, Zinman B. Intensive insulin therapy with insulin lispro. A randomized trial of continuous subcutaneous insulin infusion versus multiple daily insulin injection. *Diabetes Care* 2001; 24: 1722–7.
6. Ratzmann KP, Bruns W, Schulz B, Zander E. Use of the artificial B-cell (Biostator) in improving insulin therapy in unstable insulin-dependent diabetes. *Diabetes Care* 1982; 5: 11–7.
7. Williams P. Notes on diabetes treated with extract and by grafts of sheep's pancreas. *BMJ* 1894; 2: 1303–4.
8. Ballinger WF, Lacy PE. Transplantation of intact pancreatic islets in rats. *Surgery* 1972; 72: 175–86.
9. Pirsch JD, Miller J, Deierhoi MH, Vincenti F, Filo RS. A comparison of tacrolimus (FK506) and cyclosporine for immunosuppression after cadaveric renal transplantation. *Transplantation* 1997; 7: 977–83.
10. Lindall A, Steffes M, Sorensen R. Immunoassayable insulin content of subcellular fractions of rat islets. *Endocrinology* 1969; 85: 218–23.
11. Lacy PE, Walker MM, Fink CJ. Perifusion of isolated rat islets *in vitro*—participation of the microtubular system in the biphasic release of insulin. *Diabetes* 1972; 21: 987–98.
12. Brömme HJ, Hahn HJ, Blech W. Biphasic release of insulin from islets of Langerhans after their transplantation into the liver of rats. *Horm Metab Res* 1998; 20: 138–40.
13. Bowen KM, Lafferty KJ. Reversal of diabetes by allogenic islet transplantation without immunosuppression. *Aust J Exp Biol Med Sci* 1980; 58: 441–7.
14. Naji A, Silvers WK, Plotkin SA, Dafoe D, Barker CF. Successful islet transplantation in spontaneous diabetes. *Surgery* 1979; 86: 218–26.
15. Ricordi C, Scharp DW, Lacy PE. Reversal of diabetes in nude mice after transplantation of fresh and 7-day culture (24°C) human pancreatic islets. *Transplantation* 1988; 45: 994–6.
16. Gerling IC, Kotb M, Fraga D, Sabek O, Gaber AO. No correlation between *in vitro* and *in vivo* function of human islets. *Transplant Proc* 1998; 30: 587–8.
17. Hellman B. The frequency distribution of the number and volume of the islets of Langerhans in man. *Acta Soc Med Ups* 1959; 64: 432–60.
18. Rajotte RV, Warnock GL, Evans MG, Ellis D, Dawidson I. Isolation of viable islets of Langerhans from collagenase-perfused canine and human pancreata. *Transplant Proc* 1987; 19: 918–22.
19. Gray DWR, McShane P, Grant A, Morris PJ. A method for isolation of islets of Langerhans from the human pancreas. *Diabetes* 1984; 33: 1055–61.
20. Marchetti P, Scharp DW, Olack BJ, Swanson CJ, Bier D, Cobelli C, Toffolo G, Newton M, Navalesi R. Glucose metabolism, insulin sensitivity, and glucagon secretion in dogs with intraportal or intrasplenic islet autografts. *Transplant Proc* 1992; 24: 2828–9.
21. Sutton R, Gray DWR, Burnett M, McShane P, Turner RC, Morris PJ. Metabolic function of intraportal and intrasplenic islet autografts in cynomolgus monkeys. *Diabetes* 1989; 38 (suppl 1): 182–4.
22. Yasunami Y, Lacy PE, Finek EH. A new site for islet transplantation—a peritoneal–omental pouch. *Transplantation* 1983; 36: 181–2.
23. Selawry HP, Whittington K. Extended allograft survival of islets grafted into intra-abdominally placed testis. *Diabetes* 1984; 33: 405–6.
24. White SA, James RFL, Swift SM, Kimber RM, Nicholson ML. Human islet cell transplantation—future prospects. *Diabet Med* 2001; 18: 78–103.
25. White SA, London NJ, Johnson PR, Davies JE, Pollard C, Contractor HH, Hughes DP, Robertson GS, Musto PP, Dennison AR. The risks of total pancreatectomy and splenic islet autotransplantation. *Cell Transplant* 2000; 9: 19–24.
26. Carlsson P-O, Palm F, Andersson A, Liss P. Markedly decreased oxygen tension in transplanted rat pancreatic islets irrespective of the implantation site. *Diabetes* 2001; 50: 489–95.

27. Carlsson P-O, Jansson L, Andersson A, Källskog Ö. Capillary blood pressure in syngeneic rat islets transplanted under the renal capsule is similar to that of the implantation organ. *Diabetes* 1998; 47: 1586–93.
28. Shapiro AMJ, Gallant H, Hao E, Wong J, Rajotte R, Yatscoff R, et al. Portal vein immunosuppressant levels and islet graft toxicity. *Transplant Proc* 1998; 39: 641.
29. Najarian JS, Sutherland DER, Matas AJ, Steffes MW, Simmons RL, Goetz FC. Human islet transplantation: a preliminary report. *Transplant Proc* 1977; 9: 233–6.
30. Largiader F, Kolb E, Binswanger U, Illig R. Successful allotransplantation of an island of Langerhans. *Schweiz Med Wochenschr* 1979; 109: 1733–6.
31. Warnock GL, Kneteman NM, Ryan EA, Evans MG, Seelis REA, Halloran PF, Rabinovitch A, Rajotte RV. Continued function of pancreatic islets after transplantation in type 1 diabetes. *Lancet* 1989; II: 570–2.
32. The Diabetes Control and Complications Trial Research Group. Effect of intensive therapy on residual β-cell function in patients with type 1 diabetes in the Diabetes Control and Complications Trial. *Ann Intern Med* 1998; 128: 517–23.
33. Warnock GL, Kneteman NM, Ryan EA, Rabinovitch A, Rajotte RV. Long-term follow-up after transplantation of insulin-producing pancreatic islets into patients with type1 (insulin-dependent) diabetes mellitus. *Diabetologia* 1992; 35: 89–95.
34. Shapiro AMJ, Lakey JRT, Rajotte RV, Warnock GL, Friedlich MS, Jewell LD, Kneteman NM. Portal vein thrombosis after transplantation of partially purified pancreatic islets in a combined human liver/islet allograft. *Transplantation* 1995; 59: 1060–3.
35. Ricordi C, Tzakis A, Alejandro R, Zeng Y, Demetris AJ, Carroll P, Mintz DH, Starzl TE. Detection of pancreatic islet tissue following islet allotransplantation in man. *Transplantation* 1991; 52: 1079–80.
36. Tzakis AG, Ricordi C, Alejandro R, Zeng Y, Fung JJ, Todo S, Demetris AJ, Mintz DH, Starzl TE. Pancreatic islet transplantation after upper abdominal exenteration and liver replacement. *Lancet* 1990; 336: 402–5.
37. Scharp DW, Lacy PE, Santiago JV, McCullough CS, Weide LG, Boyle PJ, Falqui L, Marchetti P, Ricordi C, Gingerich RL, Jaffe AS, Cryer PE, Hanto DW, Anderson CB, Flye MW. Results of our first nine intraportal islet allografts in type 1, insulin-dependent diabetic patients. *Transplantation* 1991; 51: 76–85.
38. Socci C, Davalli AM, Vignali A, Bertuzzi F, Maffi P, Zammarchi O, et al. Evidence of *in vivo* human islet graft function despite a weak response to *in vitro* perfusion. *Transplant Proc* 1992; 24: 3056–7.
39. Alejandro R, Lehmann R, Ricordi C, Kenyon NS, Angelico MC, Burke G, et al. Long-term function (6 years) of islet allografts in type 1 diabetes. *Diabetes* 1997; 46: 1983–9.
40. Robertson RP, Lanz KJ, Sutherland DE, Kendall DM. Prevention of diabetes for up to 13 years by autoislet transplantation after pancreatectomy for chronic pancreatitis. *Diabetes* 2001; 50: 47–50.
41. Kelly WD, Lillehei RC, Merkel FK, Idezuki Y, Goetz FC. Allotransplantation of the pancreas and duodenum along with the kidney in diabetic nephropathy. *Surgery* 1967; 61: 827–37.
42. Cook K, Sollinger HW, Warner T, Kamps D, Belzer FO. Pancreaticocystostomy: an alternative method for exocrine drainage of segmental pancreatic allografts. *Transplantation* 1983; 35: 634–6.
43. Büsing M, Heimes M, Martin D, Schulz T, Dehof S, Kozuschek W. Simultaneous pancreas-/kidney transplantation—the Bochum experience. *Exp Clin Endocrinol Diabetes* 1997; 105: 92–7.
44. Sutherland DER. Pancreas transplantation as a treatment for diabetes: indications and outcome. In Bardin CW (ed) *Current Therapy in Endocrinology and Metabolism*, 6th edn. St. Louis: Mosby, 1997; pp 496–9.
45. Sutherland DE, Gruessner AC, Gruessner RWG. Pancreas transplantation: a review. *Transplant Proc* 1998; 30: 1940–3.
46. Ryan EA. Pancreas transplants: for whom? *Lancet* 1998; 351: 1072–3.
47. Kuo PC, Johnson LB, Schweitzer EJ, Bartlett ST. Simultaneous pancreas/kidney transplantation—a comparison of enteric and bladder drainage of exocrine pancreatic secretions. *Transplantation* 1997; 63: 238–43.
48. Nghiem DD, Gonwa TA, Corry RJ. Metabolic effects of urinary diversion of exocrine secretions in pancreatic transplantation. *Transplantation* 1987; 43: 70–3.
49. Humar A, Kandaswamy R, Granger D, Gruessner RW, Gruessner AC, Sutherland DER. Decreased surgical risks of pancreas transplantation in the modern era. *Ann Surg* 2000; 231: 269–75.
50. Sutherland DE, Gruessner RW, Gruessner AC. Pancreas transplantation for the treatment of diabetes mellitus. *World J Surg* 2001; 25: 487–96.
51. Sutherland DE, Gruessner RW, Dunn DL, Matas AJ, Humar A, Kandaswamy R, Mauer SM, Kennedy WR, Goetz FC, Najarian JS. Lessons learned from more than 1,000 pancreas transplants at a single institution. *Ann Surg* 2001; 233: 463–501.
52. Robertson RP, Sutherland DE, Lanz KJ. Normoglycemia and preserved insulin secretory reserve in diabetic patients 10–18 years after pancreas transplantation. *Diabetes* 1999; 48: 1737–40.
53. Fioretto P, Steffes MW, Sutherland DER, Goetz FC, Mauer M. Reversal of lesions of diabetic nephropathy after pancreas transplantation. *N Engl J Med* 1998; 339: 69–75.
54. Kennedy WR, Navarro X, Goetz FC, Sutherland DER, Najarian JS. Effects of pancreatic transplantation on diabetic neuropathy. *N Engl J Med* 1990; 322: 1031–7.
55. Martinenghi S, Comi G, Galardi G, Di Carlo V, Pozza G, Secchi A. Amelioration of nerve conduction velocity following simultaneous kidney/pancreas transplantation is due to the glycemic control provided by the pancreas. *Diabetologia* 1997; 40: 1110–2.
56. Jukema JW, Smets YFC, van der Pijl JW, Zwinderman AH, Vliegen HW, Ringers J, Reiber JH, Lemkes HHPJ, van der Wall EE, de Fijter JW. Impact of simultaneous pancreas and kidney transplantation on progression of coronary atherosclerosis in patients with end-stage renal failure due to type 1 diabetes. *Diabetes Care* 2002; 25: 906–11.
57. Fiorina P, La Rocca E, Venturini M, Minicucci F, Fermo I, Paroni R, D'Angelo A, Sblendido M, Di Carlo V, Cristallo M, Del Maschio A, Pozza G, Secchi A. Effects of kidney–pancreas transplantation on atherosclerotic risk factors and endothelial function in patients with uremia and type 1 diabetes. *Diabetes* 2001; 50: 496–501.

58. Wang Q, Klein R, Moss SE, Klein BEK, Hoyer C, Burke K, Sollinger HW. The influence of combined kidney–pancreas transplantation on the progression of diabetic retinopathy. *Ophthalmology* 1994; 101: 1071–6.
59. Königsrainer A, Miller K, Steurer W, Kieselbach G, Aichberger C, Öfner D, Margreiter R. Does pancreas transplantation influence the course of diabetic retinopathy? *Diabetologia* 1991; 34 (suppl 1): S86–8.
60. Brendel MD, Hering BJ, Schulz AO, Bretzel RG. International Islet Transplant Registry Report. *Justus-Liebig-University of Giessen,*1999; pp 1–20.
61. Benhamou PY, Oberholzer J, Toso C, Kessler L, Penfornis A, Bayle F, Thivolet C, Martin X, Ris F, Badet L, Colin C, Morel P. Human islet transplantation network for the treatment of type 1 diabetes: first data from the Swiss–French GRAGIL consortium (1999–2000). *Diabetologia* 2001; 44: 859–64.
62. Weir GC, Bonner-Weir S, Leahy JL. Islet mass and function in diabetes and transplantation. *Diabetes* 1990; 39: 401–5.
63. Korc M. Normal function of the endocrine pancreas. In Go VLW, Dimagno EP, Gardner JD, Lebenthal E, Reber HA, Scheele GA (eds). *The Pancreas*, 2nd edn. New York: Raven Press, 1993; pp 751–8.
64. Volk BW, Wellmann KF. Quantitative studies of the islets of nondiabetic patients. In Volk BW, Arquilla ER (eds) *The Diabetic Pancreas*, 2nd edn. New York: Plenum Medical Book Co.; 1985; pp 117–25.
65. Lakey JRT, Warnock GL, Rajotte RV, Suarez-Almazor ME, Ao Z, Shapiro AMJ, Kneteman NM. Variables in organ donors that affect the recovery of human islets of Langerhans. *Transplantation* 1996; 61: 1047–53.
66. Lakey JRT, Rajotte RV, Warnock GL, Kneteman NM. Human pancreas preservation prior to islet isolation. *Transplantation* 1995; 59: 689–94.
67. Kneteman NM, Warnock GL, Evans MG, Dawidson I, Rajotte RV. Islet isolation from human pancreas stored in UW solution for 6 to 26 hours. *Transplant Proc* 1990; 22: 763–4.
68. Lakey JRT, Warnock GL, Shapiro AMJ, Korbutt GS, Ao Z, Kneteman NM, Rajotte RV. Intraductal collagenase delivery into the human pancreas using syringe loading or controlled perfusion. *Cell Transplant* 1999; 8: 285–92.
69. Johnson PR, White SA, London NJ. Collagenase and human islet isolation. *Cell Transplant* 1996; 5: 437–52.
70. Linetsky E, Bottino R, Lehmann R, Alejandro R, Inverardi L, Ricordi C. Improved human islet isolation using a new enzyme blend, liberase. *Diabetes* 1997; 46: 1120–3.
71. Ricordi C, Lacy PE, Scharp DW. Automated islet isolation from human pancreas. *Diabetes* 1989; 38 (suppl 1): 140–2.
72. Ao Z, Lakey JRT, Rajotte RV, Warnock GL. Collagenase digestion of canine pancreas by gentle automated dissociation in combination with ductal perfusion optimizes mass recovery of islets. *Transplant Proc* 1992; 6: 2787.
73. Walsh TJ, Eggleston JC, Cameron JL. Portal hypertension, hepatic infarction, and liver failure complication pancreatic islet autotransplantation. *Surgery* 1982; 91: 485–7.
74. Gores PF, Sutherland DER. Pancreatic islet transplantation: is purification necessary? *Am J Surgery* 1993; 166: 538–42.
75. Warnock GL, Kneteman NM, Ryan E, Seelis REA, Rabinovitch A, Rajotte RV. Normoglycemia after transplantation of freshly isolated and cryopreserved pancreatic islets in type 1 (insulin-dependent) diabetes mellitus. *Diabetologia* 1991; 34: 55–8.
76. Eckhoff DE, McGuire B, Sellers M, Contreras J, Frenette L, Young C, Hudson S, Bynon JS. The safety and efficacy of a two-dose daclizumab (Zenapax) induction therapy in liver transplant recipients. *Transplantation* 2000; 69: 1867–72.
77. Kahan BD. Efficacy of sirolimus compared with azathioprine for reduction of acute renal allograft rejection: a randomised multicentre study. *Lancet* 2000; 356: 194–202.
78. Kneteman NM, Lakey JRT, Wagner T, Finegood D. The metabolic impact of rapamycin (Sirolimus) in chronic canine islet graft recipients. *Transplantation* 1996; 61: 1206–10.
79. Panz VR, Bonegio R, Raal FJ, Maher H, Hsu H-C, Joffe BI. Diabetogenic effect of tacrolimus in South African patients undergoing kidney transplantation. *Transplantation* 2002; 73: 587–90.
80. Gruessner RW, for the Tacrolimus Pancreas Transplant Study Group. Tacrolimus in pancreas transplantation: a multicenter analysis. *Clin Transplant* 1997; 11: 299–312.
81. Maes BD, Kuypers D, Messiaen T, Evenepoel P, Mathieu C, Coosemans W, Pirenne J, Vanrenterghem YFC. Posttransplantation diabetes mellitus in FK-506-treated renal transplant recipients: analysis of incidence and risk factors. *Transplantation* 2001; 72: 1655–61.
82. Tamura K, Fujimura T, Tsutsumi T, Nakamura K, Ogawa T, Atumaru C, Hirano Y, Ohara K, Ohtsuka K, Shimomura K, Kobayashi M. Transcriptional inhibition of insulin by FK506 and possible involvement of FK506 binding protein-12 in pancreatic β-cell. *Transplantation* 1995; 59: 1606–13.
83. Ishizuka J, Gugliuzza KK, Wassmuth Z, Hsieh J, Sato K, Tsuchiya T, Townsend CM, Fish JC, Thompson JC. Effects of FK506 and cyclosporine on dynamic insulin secretion from isolated dog pancreatic islets. *Transplantation* 1993; 56: 1486–90.
84. Cosio FG, Pesavento TE, Osei K, Henry ML, Ferguson RM. Post-transplant diabetes mellitus: increasing incidence in renal allograft recipients transplanted in recent years. *Kidney Int* 2001; 59: 732–7.
85. Nielsen JH, Mandrup-Poulsen T, Nerup J. Direct effects of cyslosporin A on human pancreatic β-cells. *Diabetes* 1986; 35: 1049–52.
86. Oberholzer J, Triponez F, Mage R, Andereggen E, Bühler L, Crétin N, Fournier B, Goumaz C, Lou J, Philippe J, Morel P. Human islet transplantation. *Transplantation* 2000; 6: 1115–23.
87. Roep BO, Stobbe I, Duinkerken G, van Rood JJ, Lernmark A, Keymeulen B, Pipeleers D, Class FHJ, de Vries RRP. Auto- and alloimmune reactivity to human islet allografts transplanted into type 1 diabetic patients. *Diabetes* 1999; 48: 484–90.
88. Jaeger C, Brendel MD, Hering BJ, Eckhard M, Bretzel RG. Progressive islet graft failure occurs significantly earlier in autoantibody-positive than in autoantibody-negative IDDM recipients of intrahepatic islet allografts. *Diabetes* 1997; 46: 1907–10.
89. Shapiro AMJ, Lakey JRT, Ryan EA, Korbutt GS, Toth EL, Warnock GL, Kneteman NM, Rajotte RV. Islet transplantation in seven patients with type 1 diabetes mellitus using a glucocorticoid-free immunosuppressive regimen. *N Engl J Med* 2000; 343: 230–8.

90. Cryer PE, Fisher JN, Shamoon H. Hypoglycemia. *Diabetes Care* 1994; 734–55.
91. Service FJ, Molnar GD, Rosevear JW, Ackerman E, Gatewood LC, Taylor WF. Mean amplitude of glycemic excursions, a measure of diabetic instability. *Diabetes* 1970; 19: 644–55.
92. Weimar B, Rauber K, Brendel MD, Bretzel RG, Rau WS. Percutaneous transhepatic catheterization of the portal vein: a combined CT- and fluoroscopy-guide technique. *Cardiovasc Intervent Radiol* 1999; 22: 342–4.
93. Ryan EA, Lakey JRT, Rajotte RV, Korbutt GS, Kin T, Imes S, Rabinovitch A, Elliott JF, Bigam D, Kneteman NM, Warnock GL, Larsen I, Shapiro AMJ. Clinical outcomes and insulin secretion after islet transplantation with the Edmonton Protocol. *Diabetes* 2001; 50: 710–9.
94. Ryan EA, Lakey JRT, Paty BW, Imes S, Korbutt GS, Kneteman NM, Bigam D, Rajotte RV, Shapiro AMJ. Successful islet transplantation. Continued insulin reserve provides long-term glycemic control. *Diabetes* 2002; 51: 2148–57.
95. Ryan EA, Lakey JRT, Shapiro AMJ. Clinical results after islet transplantation. *J Invest Med* 2001; 49 (suppl): 559–62.
96. Luzi L, Perseghin G, Brendel MD, Terruzzi I, Battezzati A, Eckhard M, Brandhorst D, Brandhorst H, Friemann S, Socci C, Di Carlo V, Sereni LP, Benedini S, Secchi A, Pozza G, Bretzel RG. Metabolic effects of restoring partial β-cell function after islet allotransplantation in type 1 diabetic patients. *Diabetes* 2001; 50: 277–82.
97. Teuscher AU, Kendall DM, Smets YFC, Leone JP, Sutherland DER, Robertson RP. Successful islet autotransplantation in humans. *Diabetes* 1998; 47: 324–30.
98. Davalli AM, Maffi P, Socci C, Sanvito F, Preshci M, Bertuzzi F, Falqui L, Di Carlo V, Pozza G, Secchi A. Insights from a successful case of intrahepatic islet transplantation into a type 1 diabetic patient. *J Clin Endocrinol Metab* 2000; 85: 3847–52.
99. White SA, Koppiker NP, Burden AC, Davies MJ, Clayton HA, Swift SM, Hales CN, Dennison AR, London NJM. Insulin deficiency and increased intact and 32/33 split proinsulin secretion following human islet autotransplantation. *Transplant Proc* 1998; 30: 627–8.
100. Lauritzen T, Frost-Larsen K, Larsen H-W, Deckert T. Effect of 1 year of near-normal blood glucose levels on retinopathy in insulin-dependent diabetics. *Lancet* 1983; i: 200–4.
101. Dahl-Jorgensen K, Brinchmann-Hansen O, Hanssen KF, Sandvik L, Aagenaes O. Rapid tightening of blood glucose control leads to transient deterioration of retinopathy in insulin dependent diabetes mellitus: the Oslo study. *BMJ* 1985; 290: 811–5.
102. de Mattos AM, Olyaei AJ, Bennett WM. Nephrotoxicity of immunosuppressive drugs: long-term consequences and challenges for the future. *Am J Kidney Dis* 2000; 35: 333–46.
103. Kendall DM, Teuscher AU, Robertson RP. Defective glucagon secretion during sustained hypoglycemia following successful islet allo- and autotransplantation in humans. *Diabetes* 1997; 46: 23–7.
104. Gupta V, Wahoff DC, Rooney DP, Poitout V, Sutherland DER, Kendall DM, Robertson RP. The defective glucagon response from transplanted intrahepatic pancreatic islets during hypoglycemia is transplantation site-determined. *Diabetes* 1997; 46: 28–33.
105. Kendall DM, Rooney DP, Smets YFC, Bolding LS, Robertson RP. Pancreas transplantation restores epinephrine response and symptom recognition during hypoglycemia in patients with long-standing type 1 diabetes and autonomic neuropathy. *Diabetes* 1997; 46: 249–57.
106. Paty BW, Lanz K, Kendall DM, Sutherland DE, Robertson RP. Restored hypoglycemic counterregulation is stable in successful pancreas transplant recipients for up to 19 years after transplantation. *Transplantation* 2001; 72: 1103–7.
107. Ansara MF, Saudek F, Newton M, Raynor AC, Cryer PE, Scharp DW. Pancreatic islet transplantation prevents defective glucose counter-regulation in diabetic dogs. *Transplant Proc* 1994; 26: 664–5.
108. Berthoud HR, Trimble ER, Siegel EG, Bereiter DA, Jeanrenaud B. Cephalic-phase insulin secretion in normal and pancreatic islet-transplanted rats. *Am J Physiol* 1980; 238: E336–40.
109. Vasquez EM. Sirolimus: a new agent for prevention of renal allograft rejection. *Am J Health Syst Pharm* 2000; 57: 437–48.
110. Groth CG, Bäckman L, Morales J-M, Calne R, Kreis H, Lang P, Touraine J-L, Claesson K, Campistol JM, Durand D, Wramner L, Brattström C, Charpentier B. Sirolimus (rapamycin)-based therapy in human renal transplantation. *Transplantation* 2002; 67: 1036–42.
111. Trotter JF, Wachs ME, Trouillot TE, Bak T, Kugelmas M, Kam I, Everson G. Dyslipidemia during sirolimus therapy in liver transplant recipients occurs with concomitant cyclosporine but not with tacrolimus. *Liver Transpl* 2001; 7: 401–8.
112. Burke GW, Alejandro R, Cirocco R, Nery J, Mintz D, Miller J. Regional cytokine changes following OKT3 induction for islet cell transplantation in humans: early increase in portal and systemic levels of interleukin-6 and tumor necrosis factors. *Transplant Proc* 1992; 24: 962–4.
113. Stevens RB, Lokeh A, Ansite JD, Field MJ, Gores PF, Sutherland DER. Role of nitric oxide in the pathogenesis of early pancreatic islet dysfunction during rat and human intraportal islet transplantation. *Transplant Proc* 1994; 26: 692.
114. Xenos ES, Farney AC, Widmer MB, Casanova D, Stevens RB, Blazar BR, Sutherland DER, Gores PF. Effect of tumor necrosis factor α and of the soluble tumor necrosis factor receptor on insulin secretion of isolated islets of Langerhans. *Transplant Proc* 1992; 24: 2863–4.
115. Mazariegos GV, Reyes G, Marino IR, Demetris AJ, Flynn B, Irish W, McMichael J, Fung JJ, Starzl TE. Weaning of immunosuppression in liver transplant recipients. *Transplantation* 1997; 63: 243–9.
116. Chatenoud L. Restoration of self-tolerance is a feasible approach to control ongoing β-cell specific autoreactivity: its relevance for treatment in established diabetes and islet transplantation. *Diabetologia* 2001; 44: 521–36.
117. Herold KC, Hagopian W, Auger JA, Poumian-Ruiz E, Taylor L, Donaldson D, Gitelman SE, Harlan DM, Xu D, Ziven RA, Bluestone JA. Anti-CD3 monoclonal antibody in new-onset type 1 diabetes mellitus. *N Engl J Med* 2002; 346: 1692–8.
118. Calne R, Moffatt SD, Friend PJ, Jamieson NV, Bradley JA, Hale G, Firth J, Bradley J, Smith KGC, Waldmann H. Campath IH allows low-dose

cyclosporine monotherapy in 31 cadaveric renal allograft recipients. *Transplantation* 1999; 68: 1613–6.

119. Rabinovitch A, Suarez-Pinzon WL, Shapiro AMJ, Rajotte RV, Power R. Combination therapy with sirolimus and interleukin-2 prevents spontaneous and recurrent autoimmune diabetes in NOD mice. *Diabetes* 2002; 51: 638–3445.

120. Soon-Shiong P, Heintz RE, Merideth N, Yao QX, Yao Z, Zheng T, Murphy M, Moloney MK, Schmehl M, Harris M, Mendez R, Sandford PA. Insulin independence in a type 1 diabetic patient after encapsulated islet transplantation. *Lancet* 1994; 343: 950–1.

121. Korbutt GS, Suarez-Pinzon WL, Power RF, Rajotte RV, Rabinovitch A. Testicular Sertoli cells exert both protective and destructive effects on syngeneic islet grafts in non-obese diabetic mice. *Diabetologia* 2000; 43: 474–80.

122. Ricordi C, Karatzas T, Nery J, Webb M, Fernandez L, Selvaggi G, Garcia R, Goldberg M, Schiff E, Olson L, Ruiz P, Esquenazi V, Miller J, Tzakis AG. Effect of timing of donor bone marrow infusions on liver allograft survival. *Transplant Proc* 1997; 29: 1186.

123. Soria B, Skoudy A, Martin F. From stem cells to β-cell: new strategies in cell therapy of diabetes mellitus. *Diabetologia* 2001; 44: 407–15.

124. Korbutt GS, Elliott JF, Ao Z, Smith DK, Warnock GL, Rajotte RV. Large scale isolation, growth, and function of porcine neonatal islet cells. *J Clin Invest* 1996; 97: 2119–29.

59

Hypoglycemia

Philip E. Cryer* **and Brian M. Frier†**

**Washington University School of Medicine, St. Louis, MO, USA, and †Royal Infirmary, Edinburgh, Scotland*

INTRODUCTION

Hypoglycemia is the limiting factor in the glycemic management of diabetes mellitus [1–3]. In the short-term it causes recurrent physical, and often psychosocial, morbidity (and occasional mortality) in most patients with type 1 diabetes mellitus (T1DM) [1–4] and many with type 2 diabetes mellitus (T2DM) [5, 6]. In the long-term it precludes maintenance of true euglycemia over a lifetime of diabetes and thus full realization of the well-established microvascular benefits and potential macrovascular benefits of strict glycemic control [4–6]. Thus, complications of diabetes—microvascular disease including diabetic retinopathy, nephropathy, and neuropathy and premature macrovascular disease—occur despite aggressive insulin therapy although at least the former occur at lower rates than during less intensive therapy [4–6].

Patients with T1DM attempting to achieve strict glycemic control suffer an untold number of episodes of asymptomatic hypoglycemia; plasma glucose concentrations may be less than 3.3 mmol/l 10% of the time [1, 3]. They suffer an average of approximately two episodes of symptomatic hypoglycemia a week and of approximately one episode of severe temporarily disabling hypoglycemia, often with seizure or coma, a year [1, 3]. Two to four percent of deaths of people with T1DM have been attributed to hypoglycemia [1, 7]. While some of those deaths are suicides, this represents an alarming iatrogenic mortality rate. Hypoglycemia is considerably less frequent in T2DM overall. However, it becomes increasingly limiting to glycemic control over time, even in T2DM [3].

Despite advances in the management of diabetes, iatrogenic hypoglycemia remains a barrier to glycemic control. Clearly, we must learn to replace insulin in a much more physiological fashion, to prevent, correct, or compensate for compromised defenses against hypoglycemia, or both if we are to achieve true glycemic control safely in people with diabetes. Nonetheless, the goals of improving glycemic control and minimizing the risk of hypoglycemia are not incompatible [8].

PHYSIOLOGY OF GLUCOSE COUNTERREGULATION

Glucose is the predominant metabolic fuel for the brain. Because the brain cannot synthesize or store glucose this fuel must be provided from the circulation. Thus, the prevention or correction of hypoglycemia is critical to survival. Effective physiological mechanisms have evolved to prevent or correct hypoglycemia. The physiology of glucose counterregulation in humans [9] involves the principles given in Table 1.

Systemic Glucose Balance

After an overnight fast, glucose is produced (by the liver and to a lesser extent by the kidneys) and utilized (largely by the brain) at a rate of approximately 12 μmol/kg/min (2.2 mg/kg/min) in adult humans [9]. Systemic glucose balance is frequently driven out of steady state with, for example, glucose appearance in the circulation increasing after ingestion of carbohydrate and glucose disappearance from the circulation increasing during physical exercise. Despite these profound changes, the blood glucose concentration normally increases only slightly after a meal and decreases little, if at all, during mild or moderate exercise. Clearly, the balance between glucose production and utilization is tightly regulated so that the blood glucose concentration is maintained within a narrow

International Textbook of Diabetes Mellitus, Third Edition. Edited by R. A. DeFronzo, E. Ferrannini, H. Keen, and P. Zimmet.
 ISBN: 0-471-48655-8.

Table 1 Principles of normal glucose counterregulation

(1) The prevention or correction of hypoglycemia is the result of both dissipation of insulin and activation of glucose counterregulatory systems
(2) Although insulin is the dominant plasma-glucose-lowering factor, there are redundant glucose counterregulatory factors
(3) There is a hierarchy among the glucoregulatory factors

range. Thus, a continuous supply of glucose to the brain is assured. Indeed, it appears that physiological defense against declining glucose levels is even more effective than defense against rising glucose levels. Hyperglycemia (diabetes mellitus) is common. With the notable exception of drug-treated diabetes, hypoglycemia is uncommon [1–3].

Glucoregulatory Factors

Insulin is the dominant blood-glucose-lowering factor. The hormone potently suppresses hepatic (and renal) glucose production; at higher circulating levels it also stimulates glucose utilization by responsive tissues, particularly skeletal muscle [9]. Thus, insulin lack causes hyperglycemia and insulin excess of sufficient magnitude causes hypoglycemia.

Theoretically, glucose counterregulatory (blood-glucose-raising) factors could include hormones, neurotransmitters, and metabolic substrates/intermediates [9]. Among the hormones, glucagon is the most potent. It is secreted from pancreatic α-cells in response to falling blood glucose levels, stimulates hepatic glucose production, and, thus, tends to raise blood glucose concentrations. The mechanisms of the glucose-raising effect of the adrenomedullary hormone, adrenaline (epinephrine), which is also secreted in response to falling blood glucose levels, are more complex. They involve both stimulation of hepatic (and renal) glucose production and limitation of glucose utilization through direct (β_2-adrenoceptor) actions on the liver (and the kidneys) and muscle respectively and through indirect actions that include particularly (α_2-adrenoceptor) limitation of insulin secretion but also (β_2, adrenoceptor) stimulation of glucagon secretion and (β_1-, β_2-, β_3-adrenoceptor) stimulation of lipolysis. While the hyperglycemic effects of glucagon and adrenaline are rapid (minutes), those of growth hormone and cortisol, which are also secreted in response to falling glucose levels, are delayed (hours). The latter hormones primarily limit glucose utilization but they also support glucose production [9–11]. A variety of other hormones are released during hypoglycemia, and are therefore potential counterregulatory factors.

Both the sympathetic and the parasympathetic nervous systems are activated by falling blood glucose levels. Noradrenaline (norepinephrine), released from sympathetic postganglionic neurones, as well as from the adrenal medullae, exerts hyperglycemic actions presumably through mechanisms similar to those of adrenaline [9]. In contrast, acetylcholine, released from parasympathetic postganglionic neurones, tends to reduce hepatic glucose production, an effect demonstrable in humans only in the absence of an increment in glucagon [12]. Some of the growing list of peptides released from autonomic neurones and the adrenal medullae might also have relevant glucoregulatory actions.

Among the metabolic substrates/intermediates, glucose itself is a potentially important glucose counterregulatory factor [9]. The phenomenon of glucose autoregulation—hepatic glucose production as an inverse function of circulating glucose levels independent of hormonal and neural glucoregulatory factors—was described in studies of animals more than 50 years ago [13]. In addition, elevated nonesterified fatty acid levels limit glucose utilization and drive glucose production [14].

Glycemic Thresholds

If glucose counterregulatory factors are involved in the prevention, as well as the correction, of hypoglycemia, they must be released in response to decrements in blood glucose within or just below the physiological range and at blood glucose levels higher than those required to produce symptoms and cognitive dysfunction. This prerequisite has been met in studies using the stepped hypoglycemic clamp technique to quantitate arterialized venous glycemic thresholds for responses to hypoglycemia [15, 16]. These plasma glucose thresholds in nondiabetic humans are summarized in Figure 1.

The earliest response to falling glucose concentrations is a decrease in insulin secretion. The threshold,

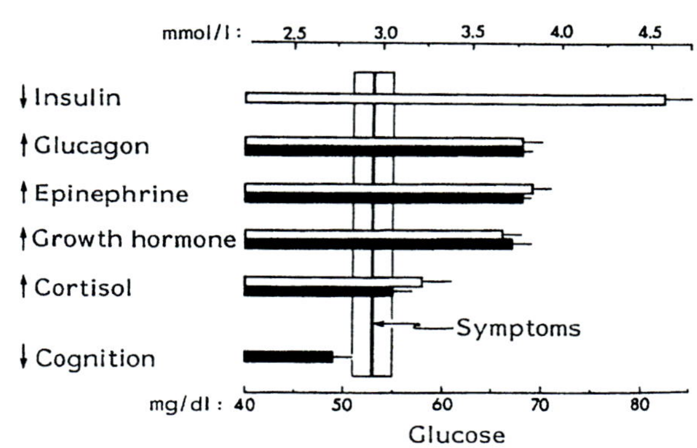

Figure 1 Mean (±SE) arterialized venous glycemic thresholds for decrements in insulin secretion, increments in glucagon, adrenaline (epinephrine), growth hormone, and cortisol secretion, symptoms and cognitive dysfunction during decrements in plasma glucose concentrations in normal humans (figure constructed from data in references 15 (open columns) and 16 (closed columns))

~4.6 mmol/l, lies within the physiological range. The thresholds for release of the counterregulatory hormones glucagon and adrenaline (~3.8 mmol/l), growth hormone (~3.7 mmol/l), and cortisol (~3.2 mmol/l, perhaps at a higher glucose level [17]) lie just below the physiological range, and are remarkably close to the plasma glucose concentration that starts to limit glucose transport into the brain [18]. The thresholds for symptoms of hypoglycemia (~3.0 mmol/l) and cognitive dysfunction (~2.7 mmol/l) are at lower plasma glucose concentrations than those for changes in glucoregulatory hormone secretion.

It is now clear that the glycemic thresholds for counterregulatory hormone release, symptoms, and cognitive dysfunction during hypoglycemia are dynamic rather than static. They shift, and can do so in a matter of hours, at least in part as a function of recent antecedent glycemia [1, 3]. This is particularly relevant to understanding the pathophysiology of glucose counterregulation in insulin-deficient diabetes (discussed later in this chapter).

Principles of Glucose Counterregulation

The principles of glucose counterregulation [9] are three (Table 1). First, the prevention or correction of hypoglycemia is the result of both dissipation of insulin and activation of glucose counterregulatory systems. It is not due solely to decreased insulin secretion. Second, although insulin is the dominant plasma-glucose-lowering factor, there are redundant glucose counterregulatory factors. In other words, there are multiple glucose-raising counterregulatory factors that collectively constitute a fail-safe system that prevents or minimizes failure of the entire system upon failure of one, or perhaps more, of its components. Third, there is a hierarchy among the glucoregulatory factors. In other words, there is a ranked series of counterregulatory factors, some more critical to the effectiveness of the fail-safe system than others, that act in concert with decrements in insulin to prevent or correct hypoglycemia.

Hierarchy of Redundant Glucoregulatory Factors

Following initial definition of the relationships between the kinetics of glucose counterregulation and activation of potentially important glucose counterregulatory systems in a model of short-term hypoglycemia [19], several studies have dissected the relative physiological importance of each of these potentially important factors. The hierarchy of the roles of the redundant glucoregulatory factors in normal glucose counterregulation is illustrated in Figure 2. This topic has been reviewed in detail elsewhere [9] and is only summarized here.

Decreased endogenous insulin secretion plays an important role in defense against falling blood glucose concentrations [21], and postabsorptive glucose concentrations are regulated primarily by variations in insulin secretion. However, the prevention or correction of hypoglycemia does not depend solely on dissipation of insulin [9, 21]. For example, despite persisting moderate hyperinsulinemia, blood glucose concentrations reach a plateau and do not fall to levels sufficient to cause neuroglycopenia [21]. Furthermore, biological recovery from hypoglycemia can occur despite approximately twofold peripheral hyperinsulinemia and in the absence of calculated portal hypoinsulinemia [21]. Clearly, additional glucose counterregulatory factors must be involved.

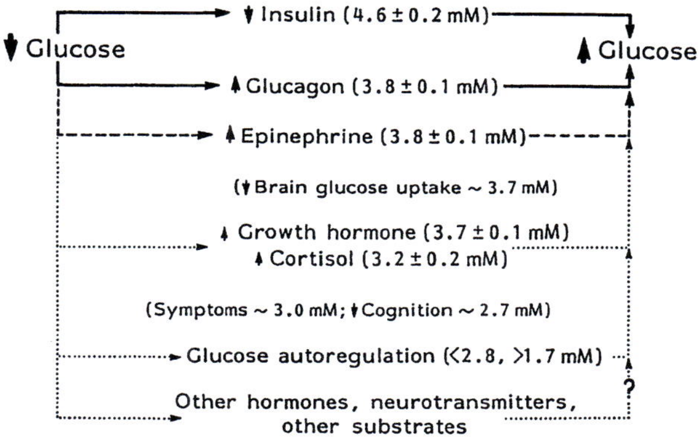

Figure 2 Hierarchy of the roles of the redundant glucoregulatory factors in normal glucose counterregulation (from reference 20, with permission)

Among the counterregulatory factors, glucagon plays a primary role. Glucose recovery from hypoglycemia is impaired, although not prevented completely, when the glucagon response is prevented [22, 23]. Similarly, selective glucagon deficiency reduces blood glucose concentrations, but does not produce hypoglycemia, in the postabsorptive state [24], the postprandial state [25, 26], after a 3-day fast [27], and, when combined with absence of decrements in insulin, during physical exercise [28, 29]. These data establish the primacy of glucagon in glucose counterregulation but they also indicate that an additional factor, or factors, plays an important role when glucagon is deficient.

Adrenaline, although demonstrably involved, is not normally critical to the correction or prevention of hypoglycemia. However, it becomes critical when glucagon is deficient. Deficient adrenaline secretion or action results in failure of recovery from hypoglycemia [22, 23] and in the development of progressive hypoglycemia in the postabsorptive state [24], the postprandial state [25, 26], after a 3-day fast [27], and during exercise [28, 29] when glucagon secretion is deficient, but not when glucagon secretion is intact.

Because hypoglycemia develops or progresses and recovery from hypoglycemia fails to occur when both glucagon and adrenaline are deficient and insulin is present, these three hormones stand high in the hierarchy of redundant glucose counterregulatory factors. Growth hormone [10] and cortisol [11], as well as glucagon [30] and adrenaline [31], are demonstrably involved in defense against prolonged hyperinsulinemia and the resultant development of hypoglycemia. However, growth hormone and cortisol are not critical to the correction of even prolonged hypoglycemia, or to the prevention of hypoglycemia after an overnight fast [32]. Thus, these hormones stand lower in the hierarchy. Glucose autoregulation may be operative, albeit only during severe hypoglycemia [33, 34]. Finally, there is evidence, discussed elsewhere [9], that factors other than insulin, glucagon, adrenaline, growth hormone, and cortisol (whether autoregulatory, neural, other hormonal or other substrate mediated) play minor roles in glucose counterregulation.

PHYSIOLOGICAL RESPONSES TO HYPOGLYCEMIA

A fall in blood glucose triggers a series of neurophysiological and neurohumoral changes within the central nervous system (CNS), which precipitate physical manifestations of hypoglycemia, some of which are perceived as subjective symptoms. The primary benefit of these responses is to activate counterregulatory mechanisms and, failing effectiveness of these, to alert the affected individual to this potential threat to the brain and so stimulate an appropriate behavioral response (ingesting food). In a person with diabetes some of these physiological changes may have pathological significance and contribute to the morbidity of severe hypoglycemia.

CNS Effects

The CNS relies on a continuous supply of glucose as its principal source of fuel and rapidly malfunctions if deprived of this substrate. Cerebral dysfunction can be demonstrated by tests of cognitive function or by neurophysiological measurements such as cortical electroencephalography (EEG) or brain evoked potentials.

Cognitive Function

Cognitive function soon becomes impaired during hypoglycemia, affecting tasks requiring selective attention, memory, rapid decision-making, analysis of visual stimuli, and hand–eye coordination [35]. Tests that require rapid responses and that are more complex and attention-demanding tend to be impaired, whereas the ability to perform simple motor and perceptual skills, such as finger tapping, forward digit span, and simple reaction time, is preserved. Many aspects of mental performance become impaired during moderate hypoglycemia when blood glucose falls below 3.0 mmol/l but considerable individual variation is evident. Tasks that involve decision-making (as in choice reaction time) are affected at higher blood glucose concentrations than simple tests (simple reaction time); accuracy is preserved at the expense of speed, and recovery of cognitive function is usually delayed for 40–90 min after normoglycemia is restored [35]. As cognitive functions are multifaceted and involve several cognitive domains, it is axiomatic that neuropsychological evaluation during hypoglycemia requires a battery of tests of cognitive ability, which preferably take little time to perform. It is difficult (if not impossible) to assess mental function at a single point in time, and this limits evaluation of the possible effect of short-term cerebral adaptation to neuroglycopenia.

Neurophysiological Changes

EEG changes occur during hypoglycemia in resting, awake subjects but are not specific, and similar changes occur with other causes of cerebral dysfunction. Alpha-wave activity is reduced and slow-wave activity (primarily theta waves) is increased as blood glucose declines, with progressive bursts of delta activity [36, 37]. The EEG changes are diffusely distributed over the cerebral cortex but regional differences occur and are more pronounced over the anterior parts of the brain, which are most sensitive to neuroglycopenia [38].

Studies of brain evoked potentials have included pattern-shift visual evoked potentials, brain stem auditory evoked potentials, and event-related brain potentials (P300, which involves decision time and uses either visual or auditory stimuli). Several studies have demonstrated abnormalities during hypoglycemia, represented principally by increased latencies of wave forms, indicating that neurophysiological transmission is delayed during neuroglycopenia. The P300 component of event-related cerebral potentials is the most sensitive index of neurophysiological dysfunction during acute hypoglycemia, while somatosensory evoked potentials are unaffected. Glycemic thresholds for the development of these neurophysiological abnormalities have been reported but vary considerably between studies [36].

Peripheral (Extra-CNS) Effects

Acute hypoglycemia is a profound stimulus to the autonomic nervous system with concurrent adrenomedullary and sympathetic and parasympathetic neural activation, with the profuse secretion of catecholamines, particularly adrenaline. These autonomic responses underlie many of the physiological changes that occur during hypoglycemia, some of which constitute overt physical manifestations and induce symptoms (Figure 3).

The principal hemodynamic effects are a transient rise in heart rate and a more sustained widening of pulse pressure (a rise in systolic blood pressure with a fall in

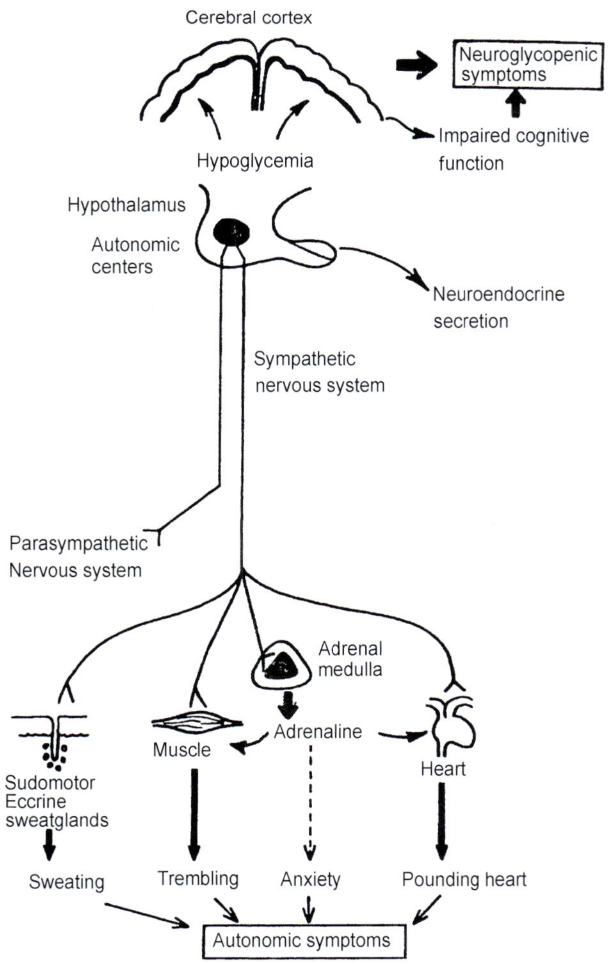

Figure 3 Diagram of the physiological autonomic, neuroglycopenic, and neuroendocrine responses to hypoglycemia (from reference 39, with permission)

diastolic blood pressure but no change in mean arterial pressure), accompanied by increased myocardial contractility and cardiac output and a fall in total peripheral vascular resistance [40]. The cardiac effects of hypoglycemia are mediated mainly via stimulation of β-adrenoceptors. Electrocardiographic changes include flattening or inversion of the T wave, which is associated with a fall in serum potassium during hypoglycemia, and lengthening of the QT interval [41].

Regional changes in blood flow occur in different vascular systems during hypoglycemia. Cerebral blood flow, measured by different techniques, increases by around 20% during marked hypoglycemia (venous blood glucose < 2.0 mmol/l) [42, 43], with the greatest rise occurring in the frontal and parietal lobes [43]. Acute hypoglycemia affects the kidney with reductions in renal plasma flow and glomerular filtration rate of about 20% [44]. Splanchnic blood flow and, more specifically, superior mesenteric arterial blood flow increase during hypoglycemia [45], while splenic blood flow is markedly reduced [46]. It is likely that hepatic blood flow increases as a consequence, which would promote the delivery of substrates to the liver for gluconeogenesis. In addition, gastric emptying is increased [47], which enhances carbohydrate delivery to the small intestine and permits faster glucose absorption. Blood flow in skeletal muscle is significantly increased [48], and is mediated by β_2-adrenoceptors. This increase in blood flow through skeletal muscle should promote the removal of lactate and alanine, which are important three-carbon precursors for hepatic gluconeogenesis. Thus the changes in regional blood flow (Table 2) appear to have potentially beneficial effects to promote metabolic recovery from hypoglycemia.

The effects on cutaneous blood flow are variable, depending upon the method of measurement and the timing related to the onset of hypoglycemia [49]. There appears to be an early rise in cutaneous blood flow (consistent with flushing and a sensation of warmth) which precedes the sweating response, and this is followed by a reduction in blood flow and pallor. The sweating response to hypoglycemia is mediated predominantly through sympathetic cholinergic stimulation [50] supplemented by the secretion of catecholamines, which stimulate β-adrenoceptors. Tremor is a cardinal feature of sympathetic stimulation and is caused primarily through β-adrenoceptor stimulation [51]. Hypoglycemia can lower core body temperature and induce hypothermia but the mechanism depends on the prevailing environmental temperature [49]. In a warm environment, body cooling occurs through heat loss by increased heat conduction from vasodilatation and sweating, while in a cold environment shivering is inhibited and the subjective sensation of cold is diminished, leading to a significant fall in body core temperature. Thus hypoglycemia disturbs thermoregulation in the cold and can provoke hypothermia. A fall in body temperature will reduce metabolic rate, and so may initially assist survival, but severe hypothermia may eventually develop.

Various hemostatic and hemorheological changes occur in response to hypoglycemia, including changes in

Table 2 Acute hypoglycemia: effects on regional blood flow with adrenoceptor mechanism for mediation (in parentheses)

Increased (vasodilatation)		Decreased (vasoconstriction)	
Heart (coronary arteries)	(β)	Kidney (renal artery)	(?)
Brain	(? β)		
Skeletal muscle	(β_2)	Spleen	(α)
Splanchnic (superior mesenteric)	(β)		
Skin (early)	(?)	Skin (late)	(?)
? Retina	(?)		

Note: "?" indicates that adrenergic receptor mediation (α or β) is unknown.

capillary blood flow, mobilization of peripheral white blood cells (with neutrophil activation), increased viscosity and fibrinolysis, platelet activation, a rise in clotting factors, and increased free radical activity. These responses are mediated primarily as a result of counterregulatory hormonal secretion, including adrenaline, cortisol, and vasopressin [52]. They may have significant pathophysiological effects on blood vessels affected by diabetic vasculopathy [41, 52].

Symptoms

The symptoms of hypoglycemia are subjective and idiosyncratic, but have a fundamental protective role by providing early warning of a fall in blood glucose [35, 53]. Some of the neuroglycopenic symptoms of hypoglycemia are considered to be the subjective impressions of impaired cognitive function, and in studies of nondiabetic subjects, the glycemic thresholds for neuroglycopenic symptoms and the onset of cognitive dysfunction usually coincide [15]. This helps to protect the individual from progressing to severe neuroglycopenia. A greater number of symptoms experienced aids the perception of hypoglycemia, but symptom profiles vary in nature and intensity between individuals; consistency is maintained over time except in diabetic patients who are exposed to varying levels of glycemic control. Individual variability of symptom profiles may be related to differences in perceptual appreciation and biological variation in the nature and intensity of the autonomic response to hypoglycemia.

The central and peripheral physiological effects of hypoglycemia determine the potential subdivision of symptoms into *neuroglycopenic*, resulting from the direct effect of glucose deprivation on the brain, and *autonomic* (*or neurogenic*), which are provoked by end-organ responses to autonomic stimulation. In addition, nonspecific symptoms such as headache and nausea are common and are difficult to allocate to either of these two groups. The classification of symptoms has undergone considerable refinement in an attempt to allocate symptoms objectively to groups based upon their etiology. One approach has applied the statistical technique of principal components (factor) analysis to historical surveys of hypoglycemia in insulin-treated diabetic populations and also by using symptom questionnaires during experimental hypoglycemia [54, 55]. This has confirmed three main groupings (or clusters) of neuroglycopenic, autonomic, and nonspecific (general malaise) symptoms. Although a wide range of symptoms is experienced, the most common symptoms have been identified in adults (Table 3) and used to construct a standardized method of measuring the symptomatic response to hypoglycemia (the Edinburgh Hypoglycemia Score) [55]. Physiological

Table 3 Common symptoms of hypoglycemia in different age groups*

Children	Young adults	Elderly
	Autonomic symptoms	
Tremor	Tremor	Tremor
Hunger	Hunger	
	Pounding heart	Pounding heart
	Sweating	Sweating
Pallor		Anxiety
	Neuroglycopenic symptoms	
Drowsiness	Drowsiness	Drowsiness
Poor concentration	Odd behavior	Poor concentration
	Confusion	Confusion
Weakness	Incoordination	Weakness
Dizziness	Speech difficulty	Dizziness
Behavioral	*Nonspecific*	*Neurological*
Tearful	Nausea	Unsteadiness
Confusion	Headache	Poor concentration
Tiredness		Double vision
Irritable		Blurred vision
Aggressive		Slurred speech

* Classified using principal components analysis [35, 53]. The symptoms in young adults are used in the Edinburgh Hypoglycemia Symptoms Score [55].

methods of symptom evaluation during experimental hypoglycemia with pharmacological blockade in nondiabetic subjects [50, 56] have produced a very similar classification. The symptoms of hypoglycemia vary with age, which has relevance to clinical practice, particularly to the education of patients and their relatives, and to the interpretation and design of clinical studies [35, 53]. Children have prominent behavioral symptoms and signs, while elderly people have neurological symptoms including visual disturbance and unsteadiness [35, 53] (Table 3), which may be misinterpreted as features of cerebrovascular disease.

External factors may modify the symptomatic response to acute hypoglycemia. These include environmental distractions, physical activity, posture, sleep, alcohol, caffeine, and some pharmacological agents such as hypnotics or nonselective β-adrenoceptor blocking drugs. Distinction should be made between symptoms ascertained in field studies, where diabetic patients record symptoms experienced during daily life, and experimental hypoglycemia induced in the supine position in the artificial setting of the laboratory. These differences may explain why neuroglycopenic and autonomic symptoms are reported with equal frequency as the principal warning symptoms experienced by diabetic patients [54], in contrast to nondiabetic subjects during controlled hypoglycemia, in whom autonomic symptoms appear to predominate [56]. In addition, the symptoms of hypoglycemia experienced by diabetic patients may become modified with time and can be influenced by strict glycemic control. This leads to the clinical phenomenon of impaired awareness of hypoglycemia.

PATHOPHYSIOLOGY OF GLUCOSE COUNTERREGULATION

Hypoglycemia is a fact of life for most patients with T1DM who attempt to achieve a reasonable degree of glycemic control [1–3]. As developed in the paragraphs that follow, iatrogenic hypoglycemia is the result of the interplay of relative or absolute therapeutic insulin excess and compromised physiological and behavioral defenses against developing hypoglycemia in T1DM [1, 3]. Although hypoglycemia is much less common early in the course of T2DM, it becomes progressively more limiting to glycemic control over time [3, 57]. Indeed, the frequencies of severe hypoglycemia are similar in patients with T2DM and T1DM matched for duration of insulin therapy [58].

Hypoglycemia in T1DM

The causes of iatrogenic hypoglycemia in T1DM are conventionally based on the premise that insulin excess, which must occur from time to time because of the imperfections of current insulin replacement regimens, is the sole determinant of risk [1, 3]. Absolute or relative insulin excess occurs when (1) insulin doses are excessive, ill-timed, or of the wrong type; (2) the intake of exogenous carbohydrate is decreased, as following a missed meal or snack or during an overnight fast; (3) endogenous glucose production is decreased as following alcohol ingestion; (4) insulin-independent glucose utilization is increased as during physical exercise; (5) sensitivity to insulin is increased as following exercise, in the middle of the night, during effective intensive therapy, or following weight loss; (6) insulin clearance is decreased as with progressive renal insufficiency. At a practical level these are the variables with which most health professionals and their patients deal as they attempt to limit the frequency of hypoglycemia while achieving the best possible glycemic control. Nonetheless, the observations of many reported studies and the extensive experience of the Diabetes Control and Complications Trial (DCCT) indicate that these conventional causal factors explain only a minority of episodes of severe iatrogenic hypoglycemia in T1DM [59]. Indeed, the most powerful predictor (relative risk = 2.5) of severe iatrogenic hypoglycemia in the DCCT experience was a history of previous severe hypoglycemia [59]. This suggests that there is something different about patients who suffer severe hypoglycemia. It is apparent that we must look beyond the conventional causes and recognized risk factors if we are to understand the pathogenesis of most episodes of severe hypoglycemia in T1DM.

Iatrogenic hypoglycemia in T1DM is more appropriately viewed as the result of the interplay of absolute or relative insulin excess and compromised glucose counterregulation [1, 3]. In other words, while insulin excess of sufficient magnitude will cause hypoglycemia despite intact counterregulatory mechanisms, the integrity of the counterregulatory mechanisms determines whether or not lesser degrees of hyperinsulinemia result in hypoglycemia.

Table 4 Syndromes of compromised glucose counterregulation in T1DM

(1) Defective glucose counterregulation
(2) Impaired awareness of hypoglycemia
(3) Elevated glycemic thresholds during intensive therapy
(4) Elevated glycemic thresholds following recent hypoglycemia
(5) Elevated glycemic thresholds during β-adrenergic blockade

Several syndromes of compromised glucose counterregulation in T1DM are now recognized (Table 4), and have been reviewed [1, 3]. These include defective glucose counterregulation [60–62], impaired awareness of hypoglycemia [63–68], elevated glycemic thresholds during effective intensive therapy [67, 69, 70], following recent antecedent hypoglycemia [71–76], or both, and, perhaps, therapy with a β-adrenoceptor antagonist [77].

Syndromes of Compromised Glucose Counterregulation in T1DM

Defective Glucose Counterregulation

As the person with T1DM becomes absolutely insulin-deficient, plasma insulin levels—which are the passive result of absorption of administered insulin—do not decrease as plasma glucose levels fall. The first defense against developing hypoglycemia is lost. The glucagon secretory response to hypoglycemia, the second defense, becomes deficient in the first few years of T1DM [78, 79]. This is a selective defect; glucagon responses to other stimuli are largely, if not entirely, intact. Therefore, it cannot be attributed to a structural abnormality of the α-cells *per se*, and must represent a signaling abnormality. The mechanism of this defect is not known, but it is tightly linked to absolute insulin deficiency [80]. The deficient glucagon response appears to be absolute; even severe hypoglycemia does not elicit a glucagon response [74]. Because glucagon is normally the primary glucose counterregulatory hormone, and a deficient glucagon response to falling plasma glucose concentrations is the rule in patients with T1DM, glucose counterregulation is altered in patients with established T1DM. Yet, it often appears to be adequate, perhaps because adrenaline compensates at least in part. A reduced adrenaline secretory response to hypoglycemia develops in most patients with T1DM [74, 79]. This, too, is selective; adrenaline secretory responses to other stimuli are intact. Therefore, the reduced adrenaline response cannot be attributed to a structural lesion of the adrenal medullae or the sympathochromaffin reflex arc that mediates all adrenaline secretory responses, and must represent a regulatory abnormality. In contrast to the reduced glucagon response, the reduced adrenaline response to a given degree of hypoglycemia represents, at least in large part, a shift to a higher glycemic threshold. Adrenaline responses can be elicited but lower blood glucose concentrations are required [74]. Thus, C-peptide negative patients have no glucagon responses to hypoglycemia and the adrenaline responses to a given degree of hypoglycemia are often reduced [1, 3, 74].

In the setting of absent glucagon responses, the development of deficient adrenaline responses is a critical event in the pathophysiology of glucose counterregulation in T1DM. Patients who have combined deficiencies of the glucagon and adrenaline responses to falling blood glucose concentrations have defective glucose counterregulation [1, 3, 60–62]. When compared with those with deficient glucagon but intact adrenaline responses, they have been shown, in prospective studies, to be at 25-fold or greater increased risk for severe iatrogenic hypoglycemia, at least during intensive therapy [60, 61], as illustrated in Figure 4.

Impaired Awareness of Hypoglycemia

Historically this has been termed hypoglycemia unawareness but there is a spectrum of impaired awareness ranging from complete unawareness to normal awareness of hypoglycemia in persons with diabetes [63–68]. Affected patients no longer have the warning, largely autonomic (neurogenic) symptoms that previously allowed them to recognize developing hypoglycemia and take appropriate

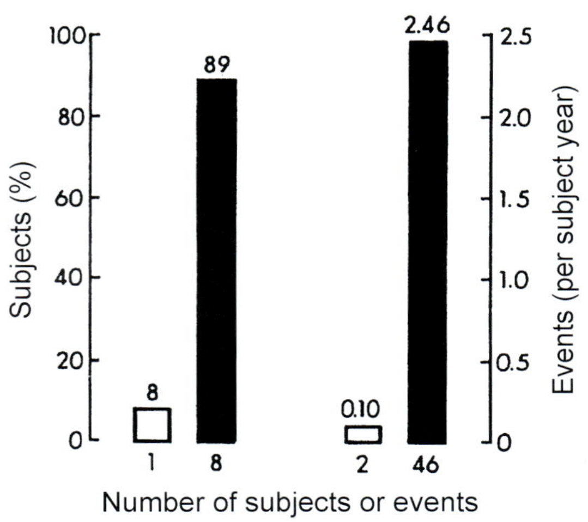

Figure 4 Proportion of patients affected (left) and frequency of severe iatrogenic hypoglycemia (right) during intensive therapy of patients with T1DM and adequate glucose counterregulation (open columns, $n = 13$) or defective glucose counterregulation (closed columns, $n = 9$) (figure constructed from data in reference 60, and reproduced with permission)

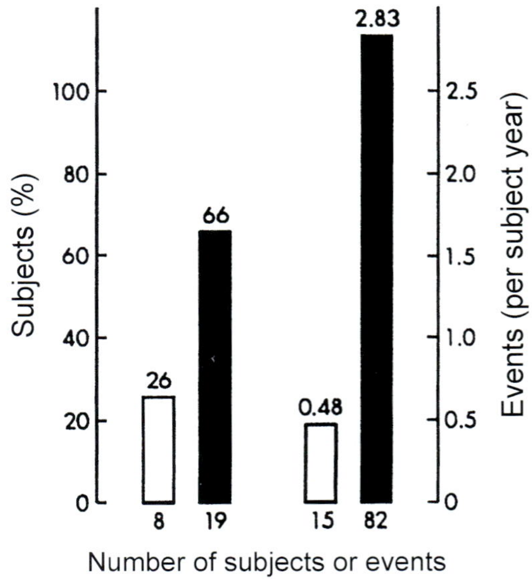

Figure 5 Proportion of patients affected (left) and frequency of severe iatrogenic hypoglycemia (right) in patients with T1DM with normal (open columns, $n = 31$) and impaired awareness of hypoglycemia (closed columns, $n = 29$) (figure constructed from data in reference 83)

action (e.g., eat) to prevent its progression to severe hypoglycemia. Thus, the initial symptoms are neuroglycopenic and the resultant cognitive dysfunction interferes with the ability for self-treatment. Attempts to define the prevalence of impaired awareness [81–83] are confounded by the dynamic nature of awareness of hypoglycemia as developed below. Lower blood glucose concentrations are required to elicit autonomic responses, including adrenaline and autonomic symptom responses, to hypoglycemia in patients with impaired awareness of hypoglycemia [66, 68]. Thus, the glycemic thresholds for these responses are elevated since a greater hypoglycemic stimulus (i.e., more profound hypoglycemia) is required to elicit them. Patients with a history of impaired awareness of hypoglycemia have been shown, in a prospective study, to have a sixfold increase in incidence of severe hypoglycemia [84], as illustrated in Figure 5. The shift in glycemic thresholds to lower blood glucose concentrations that result in reduced autonomic responses to a given level of hypoglycemia in patients with defective glucose counterregulation [1–3, 74] and with impaired awareness of hypoglycemia [1–3, 64, 65, 74, 83]—which, often cosegregate—represents, at least in large part, a functional alteration rather than the structural alteration of classical diabetic autonomic neuropathy.

Elevated Glycemic Thresholds During Intensive Therapy

The clinical impression that patients with T1DM who achieve strict glycemic control often tolerate low plasma glucose levels without symptoms provided the first clue that glycemic thresholds for autonomic and symptomatic responses to hypoglycemia are dynamic rather than static. That impression has been amply supported by objective data. During intensive therapy of T1DM lower blood glucose concentrations are required to elicit autonomic responses to, and symptoms of, hypoglycemia [69, 70]. Conversely, patients with poorly controlled T1DM [85] can experience symptoms of hypoglycemia when blood glucose falls into the normal range. The mechanism(s) of these shifts in thresholds is not known. The possibility that recent antecedent hypoglycemia causes increased blood-to-brain glucose transport at a given level of subsequent hypoglycemia has been proposed [18, 86] but challenged [87].

The large prospective experience of the DCCT [4] demonstrated that effective intensive therapy results in a threefold increase in the incidence of severe iatrogenic hypoglycemia. However, the extent to which the requirement for lower blood glucose levels to stimulate autonomic and symptomatic responses to hypoglycemia contributes to this has been debated. If lower blood glucose concentrations are not required to produce cognitive dysfunction, as suggested by some studies [88, 89], it would be reasonable to suggest that the requirement for lower glucose levels for autonomic and symptomatic responses is a major risk factor for severe hypoglycemia since neuroglycopenia might precede the onset of counterregulatory activation and autonomic symptoms. If the glycemic thresholds for cognitive dysfunction also shift, as suggested by other studies [90–92], elevated thresholds for autonomic and symptomatic responses may be less detrimental.

Elevated Glycemic Thresholds Following Recent Hypoglycemia

Recent antecedent hypoglycemia reduces autonomic and symptomatic responses to subsequent hypoglycemia in nondiabetic humans [71–73] and patients with T1DM [74–76]. For example, in nondiabetic humans, Heller and Cryer [70] found that an episode of afternoon hypoglycemia of less than 2 h reduced autonomic responses (including secretion of adrenaline and pancreatic polypeptide) and symptomatic (both autonomic and neuroglycopenic) responses to hypoglycemia the following morning. Similarly, in patients with TIDM, Dagogo-Jack et al. [74] found such an episode of afternoon hypoglycemia to reduce both autonomic responses (including secretion of adrenaline and pancreatic polypeptide) and symptomatic (both autonomic and neuroglycopenic) responses to a given degree of hypoglycemia and impair the physiological defense against hyperinsulinemia the following morning. This is a threshold shift. Autonomic and symptomatic responses can be elicited but lower plasma glucose concentrations are required. The potential clinical importance of these findings is discussed later (see under Hypoglycemia-associated Autonomic Failure).

Elevated Glycemic Thresholds During β-Adrenoceptor Blockade

By blocking β-adrenoceptor actions of adrenaline, β-adrenoceptor antagonists impair glucose recovery from experimental hypoglycemia in (glucagon-deficient) patients with T1DM [93]. This class of drugs also reduces symptoms at a given level of hypoglycemia in T1DM [77]. Since both the counterregulatory effects of adrenaline and awareness of a given level of hypoglycemia are reduced, it is reasonable to suspect that administration of a β-adrenoceptor antagonist might increase the frequency of iatrogenic hypoglycemia in patients with T1DM. However, compelling clinical support for this expectation is lacking.

Hypoglycemia-associated Autonomic Failure in T1DM

The syndromes of defective glucose counterregulation, impaired awareness of hypoglycemia, and elevated glycemic thresholds during intensive therapy (perhaps a result of recent antecedent hypoglycemia) co-segregate clinically, are associated with a high frequency of severe iatrogenic hypoglycemia, and share several pathophysiological features [94]. The latter include elevated glycemic thresholds for autonomic responses to hypoglycemia: adrenomedullary (adrenaline), parasympathetic (pancreatic polypeptide) and sympathetic (noradrenaline, autonomic symptoms) responses to a given level of hypoglycemia are reduced [74, 94]. In the setting of absent glucagon responses, reduced adrenaline responses compromise physiological defense against developing hypoglycemia. Reduced symptomatic responses compromise awareness of developing hypoglycemia and, thus, the appropriate behavioral response. This line of reasoning led one of us to propose the unifying concept of hypoglycemia-associated autonomic failure in diabetes of which these three clinical syndromes are examples [94].

The pathogenesis of hypoglycemia-associated autonomic failure is not known, need not necessarily be the same in all of these clinical syndromes of compromised glucose counterregulation, and could be multifactorial even in a given syndrome. Recent antecedent hypoglycemia may well be one pathogenetic factor. The hypothesis, illustrated in Figure 6, is that recent antecedent iatrogenic hypoglycemia is a major cause of hypoglycemia-associated autonomic failure in T1DM and that hypoglycemia-associated autonomic failure, by reducing both physiological defense against and symptoms of developing hypoglycemia, results in recurrent severe hypoglycemia, thus creating a vicious cycle [94].

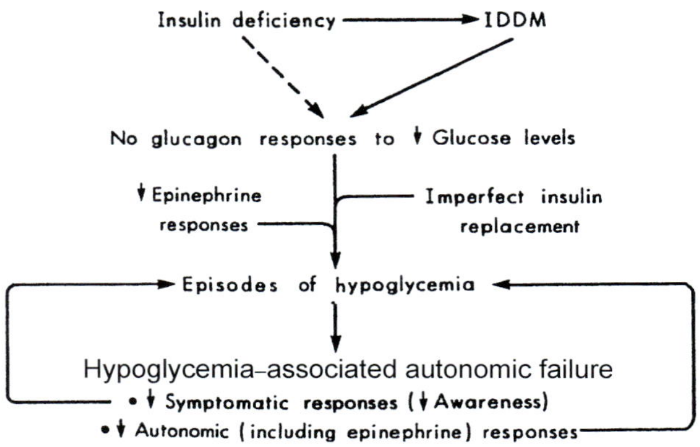

Figure 6 Schematic diagram of the concept of hypoglycemia-associated autonomic failure in T1DM (from reference 94, with permission)

There is now considerable support for the clinical impact of hypoglycemia-associated autonomic failure in diabetes. Recent antecedent hypoglycemia elevates glycemic thresholds (lower blood glucose concentrations are required) for autonomic and symptomatic responses to subsequent hypoglycemia and impairs physiological defense against hyperinsulinemia in patients with T1DM [74]. It shifts glycemic thresholds for cognitive dysfunction as well as autonomic and symptomatic responses to hypoglycemia to lower levels [91] and impairs detection of hypoglycemia in the clinical setting [92]. Finally, the phenomenon is not attributable to depletion of autonomic effectors by prior activation of the system, since preceding activation of the sympathochromaffin system (by exercise 90 min earlier) does not reduce the response of that system to subsequent hypoglycemia [95].

The most compelling support for the concept of hypoglycemia-associated autonomic failure in T1DM [74, 94] is the finding, in three independent laboratories [96–98], that as little as 2 weeks of scrupulous avoidance of hypoglycemia reverses hypoglycemia unawareness, and improves the reduced adrenaline component of defective glucose counterregulation, in most affected patients. The failure to completely reverse the reduced autonomic response may have been the result of the inability to eliminate completely hypoglycemia, a component of diabetic autonomic neuropathy [99, 100], or both.

Well-established risk factors for iatrogenic hypoglycemia in T1DM [1, 3, 8]—greater insulin deficiency; a history of severe hypoglycemia, impaired awareness of hypoglycemia, or both; and aggressive glycemic thereapy *per se* as evidenced by lower mean glycemia (hemoglobin A_{1c}), lower glycemic goals, or both—are clinical surrogates for the key pathophysiological features of hypoglycemia-associated autonomic failure. Endogenous insulin deficiency indicates that insulin levels will not decrease and predicts accurately that glucagon levels will not increase [80] as blood glucose levels fall. A history of severe hypoglycemia or of impaired awareness of hypoglycemia and lower mean glycemia imply recent antecedent iatrogenic hypoglycemia which would reduce the adrenaline and autonomic symptom responses to subsequent hypoglycemia, i.e., produce hypoglycemia-associated autonomic failure. These clinical risk factors have been confirmed along with the intriguing observation of an association of severe (but not mild) hypoglycemia with higher serum angiotensin-converting enzyme activity (and the corresponding genotype) [101].

Hypoglycemia in T2DM

Iatrogenic hypoglycemia is generally less frequent in T2DM than in T1DM. Indeed, the event rates for severe hypoglycemia are approximately 10-fold lower in T2DM even during aggressive therapy with insulin [3]. However, hypoglycemia occurs during treatment with insulin and sulfonylureas and has been reported during therapy with metformin [102]. Clinical experience, the observation that hypoglycemia becomes progressively more limiting to glycemic control over time in T2DM [57], and the finding that the rates of severe hypoglycemia are similar in patients with T2DM and those with T1DM when matched for duration of insulin therapy [58] indicate that hypoglycemia becomes a progressively more frequent clinical problem as patients approach the insulin-deficient end of the spectrum of T2DM [102]. This line of reasoning led one of us to the hypothesis that patients with advanced (i.e., insulin-deficient) T2DM have compromised glucose counterregulation analogous to that which occurs in T1DM. That hypothesis has been confirmed [103]. Glucagon responses to hypoglycemia were shown to be virtually absent in such patients, as they are in T1DM. Furthermore, glycemic thresholds for autonomic (including adrenaline) and symptomatic responses to hypoglycemia were shown to be at higher than normal plasma glucose concentrations in patients with poorly controlled T2DM, and shifted to lower plasma glucose concentrations following episodes of hypoglycemia, as they are in T1DM. Thus, patients with advanced T2DM are also at risk of developing hypoglycemia-associated autonomic failure.

The symptoms of iatrogenic hypoglycemia are similar in patients with T2DM and T1DM [58]. The conventional causes and risk factors for iatrogenic hypoglycemia in patients with T1DM, discussed earlier, also apply to patients with T2DM. Additional risk factors for sulfonylurea-induced hypoglycemia include advanced age, fasting, poor nutrition, diarrhea, intercurrent acute illnesses, alcohol ingestion, and hepatic, renal, or cardiac disease [104]. Among the sulfonylureas, the relatively long-acting drugs chlorpropamide and glibenclamide (glyburide) have been associated most often with iatrogenic hypoglycemia [104].

CLINICAL ASPECTS OF HYPOGLYCEMIA

Definition

In nondiabetic humans, hypoglycemia has been defined arbitrarily as a decline in postabsorptive venous blood glucose to below a level ranging from 2.8 to 3.3 mmol/l, although in some circumstances (such as prolonged starvation) these blood glucose concentrations may represent a normal physiological response. Asymptomatic biochemical hypoglycemia is common in patients with insulin-treated diabetes and it is impractical to define hypoglycemia as an absolute concentration of blood glucose. Glycemic thresholds for symptoms of hypoglycemia are dynamic and may alter as a consequence of exposure to hypoglycemia or hyperglycemia. However, many patients appear to tolerate relatively low blood glucose concentrations without demonstrable neuroglycopenia [69, 70], while others (particularly if their diabetes is poorly controlled) may develop florid symptoms of hypoglycemia when blood glucose falls within the normal range [85]. Reliance on symptomatic responses alone without simultaneous biochemical measurement or estimation of blood glucose may also be confused with other events affecting the CNS, such as transient cerebral ischemia.

In clinical practice, hypoglycemia is defined by the individual's ability to self-treat a low blood glucose, and is "mild" when self-treatment with oral carbohydrate suffices and "severe" when external help is required to effect recovery. Thus, severe hypoglycemia does not require the development of coma or convulsions or treatment with parenteral therapy; profound neuroglycopenia can occur without loss of consciousness and manifests as overt cognitive dysfunction. Severity is not determined by the intensity or nature of the symptomatic response.

Frequency of Severe Hypoglycemia

Mild symptomatic episodes of hypoglycemia are often quickly forgotten by the patient and can be recalled with accuracy at an interval of only 1 week [81]. Accurate estimates therefore require prospective recording. By contrast, severe hypoglycemia is a much more robust measure and a comparison of retrospective and prospective estimates has shown good congruence [81], despite occasional posthypoglycemia amnesia in some patients. The drama and disruption associated with severe hypoglycemia probably ensures that the patient is informed of the event by others and the objective accounts of witnesses such as friends and relatives are of considerable corroborative value when ascertaining the frequency of severe hypoglycemia.

Disparity between various studies in estimates of the frequency of severe hypoglycemia is principally related to differences in definition, heterogeneity of diabetic populations, quality of glycemic control, methods of ascertainment (prospective vs. retrospective), and the difficulty of determining the frequency of asymptomatic severe hypoglycemia occurring during sleep. If the above definition of severe hypoglycemia is applied, the reported incidence in unselected populations (predominantly Caucasian) of insulin-treated adult diabetic patients in Northern Europe and North America ranges from 0.2 to 1.7 episodes/patient/year [4, 81, 105–107] (Table 5), with an annual prevalence affecting between 10 and 40% of patients [4, 107, 109, 110]. In Northern European countries the estimated incidences [81, 105–107] were much higher than those recorded in North America during the DCCT [59, 110]. In the DCCT, the group with strict glycemic control had an incidence of severe hypoglycemia of 0.6 episodes/patient/year [4], which is about half the rate of other studies [105–107]. However, the participants in the DCCT were a carefully selected group of young, healthy, motivated individuals with T1DM of short duration; patients who had a preceding history of recurrent severe hypoglycemia or hypoglycemic coma without premonitory symptoms (i.e. those at high risk of severe hypoglycemia) were excluded. Estimates based on emergency treatment provided by medical and paramedical services considerably underestimate the frequency of severe hypoglycemia, as less than one third of such episodes are treated in this way [111, 112], and most are treated at home by relatives.

Table 5 Frequency of severe hypoglycemia* in adults with T1DM

	n	Episodes/ patient/year	Reference
Denmark	411	1.4	[81]
Sweden	52	1.1	[105]
Scotland	544	1.7	[106]
Netherlands	195	1.5	[107]
Denmark/England	1076	1.3	[108]
United States/Canada			
Intensive	711	0.6	[4]†
Conventional	730	0.2	

* Severe hypoglycemia = requiring external help for recovery.
† Excluded patients with a history of severe hypoglycemia or hypoglycemic coma without warning symptoms.

If the definition of severe hypoglycemia is restricted to coma requiring intravenous dextrose or glucagon therapy, the incidence is around 0.4 episodes/patient/year, with a prevalence of about 10% per annum [108], thus recording about one third of episodes that are determined using the definition of inability to self-treat. This may also partly explain the much lower frequencies of severe hypoglycemia reported in some German centers [113], where patients received an intensive education program in diabetes self-management that is considered to be beneficial in lowering the risk of severe hypoglycemia. It is difficult to estimate the frequency of hypoglycemia in children with T1DM. The above definitions cannot be used as most episodes require help from a parent and carer. There is a paucity of

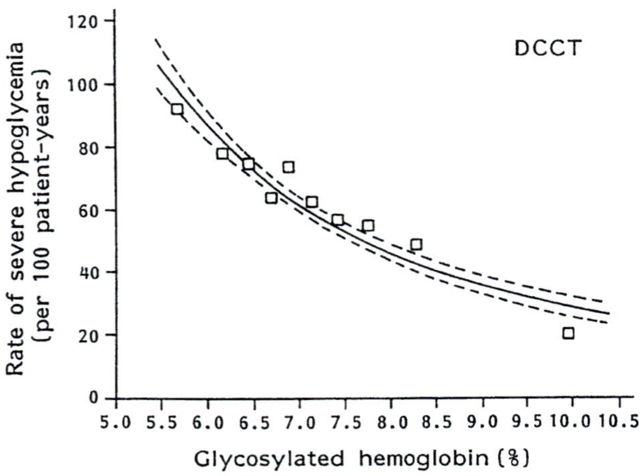

Figure 7 Inverse relationship between the frequency of severe iatrogenic hypoglycemia and overall glycemic control as assessed with glycated hemoglobin values in the DCCT (from reference 4, with permission)

accurate data on the frequency of severe hypoglycemia in insulin-treated T2DM, but this increases with duration of insulin therapy [57, 58].

Risk Factors

Various risk factors can be identified [112] and include strict glycemic control (glycated hemoglobin concentration is often close to or within the nondiabetic range), increasing age of the patient, duration of diabetes, a previous history of severe hypoglycemia [59, 110], impaired awareness of hypoglycemia [81, 83], C-peptide negativity [114], and sleep, during which normal warning symptoms either are undetectable by the patient or are diminished. In the DCCT, strict glycemic control increased the risk of severe hypoglycemia by threefold and the rate of severe hypoglycemia was inversely correlated with the mean glycated hemoglobin concentration [4, 110] (Figure 7). Three quarters of all episodes of severe hypoglycemia occurred in the intensively treated group and 55% of all episodes during sleep [59]. The risk of severe hypoglycemia may also be increased by alcohol, which blunts the normal warning symptoms of hypoglycemia and delays recovery of blood glucose by inhibiting gluconeogenesis, thus protracting its duration and severity. The risk of hypoglycemia is higher at the extremes of age and during pregnancy, with irregular lifestyle (particularly adolescents), alcoholism [112], and lower social class [114]. The relationship of many of these risk factors to the pathophysiological concept of hypoglycemia-associated autonomic failure was discussed earlier [1, 3, 8, 74, 94, 103].

Causal Factors

In the diabetic person treated with insulin, hypoglycemia usually results from a mismatch between the action of insulin, the ingestion of food, and energy expenditure. Although the principal causal factors are

(1) an excessive or inappropriate dose of insulin,
(2) inadequate or delayed ingestion of food, and
(3) sudden or sustained exercise,

the potential causes are usually multiple and seldom result from one factor in isolation. The juxtaposition of a combination of circumstances or events may precipitate isolated severe hypoglycemia, and it is often difficult to determine causation with certainty. A definitive cause can be identified only in about one third of all episodes [111, 112], and susceptibility to hypoglycemia may be increased in specific situations such as after childbirth in the insulin-treated diabetic mother or in patients with gastroparesis secondary to autonomic neuropathy. Errors of judgement in treatment (e.g. inaccurate measurement of insulin dose) and carelessness by the patient (e.g. missing a meal) are common, although the fault may sometimes rest with the physician who prescribes an unsuitable or inappropriate insulin regimen. Hypoglycemia is common in view of the problems inherent with current insulin replacement therapy in terms of insulin formulations, pharmacokinetics, and methods of delivery, which do not simulate the normal physiology of insulin secretion and action. It is also extremely difficult for patients to maintain vigilance indefinitely to prevent hypoglycemia. Recognized causal factors of hypoglycemia in diabetic patients are numerous and may operate in combination (see Table 6).

Many causes of hypoglycemia are self-limiting or remediable or can be avoided by judicious observance of the principles of diabetic self-management. However, few people taking insulin successfully avoid hypoglycemia in perpetuity, and hence the trepidation this therapeutic side effect arouses in patients and their relatives. Fear of hypoglycemia is high among patients and their relatives who equate it with the development of serious diabetic complications, such as blindness from retinopathy [81] (Figure 8), and this may influence behavior and limit enthusiasm to achieve strict glycemic control.

Nocturnal Hypoglycemia

Nocturnal glycemic control, which represents approximately one third of the patient's lifetime treatment with insulin, is remarkably uncharted territory and the vulnerability to hypoglycemia during sleep is high. The tendency of many insulin regimens to produce nocturnal hyperinsulinemia and the problem of detecting the warning symptoms of hypoglycemia during sleep combine to promote nocturnal hypoglycemia which may go undetected for long periods [2, 112]. Most episodes of nocturnal hypoglycemia are "asymptomatic" and do not wake the individuals, although the spouse or partner may be disturbed by their restless movements in bed, profuse sweating, or

Table 6 Causal factors of hypoglycemia in diabetic patients

	Problems with insulin		
Management errors	Altered pharmacokinetics	Sensitivity	Inadequate carbohydrate
Patient error	Change of insulin species	Insulin antibodies	Missed or delayed meals
Physician error	Change of formulation	Exercise	Excessive/unpremeditated exercise
Pharmacy error	Excessive dose	Weight reduction	
Drug interactions	Injection: site, size, depth	Diurnal variation	Delayed gastric emptying (autonomic neuropathy)
Factitious	Absorption: muscle exercise, massage, temperature	Diabetic pregnancy and following delivery	Malabsorption (coeliac disease, pancreatic exocrine failure)
Other related conditions	Delayed clearance: insulin antibodies, renal failure, hepatic failure	Menstrual cycle	Slimming diets (anorexia nervosa)
Endocrine failure		Acute remission following treatment of type 1 diabetes	Pregnancy: breastfeeding
Addison's disease			
Hypopituitarism		Alcohol	(*NB*: Contributory effects of change of occupation, shiftwork, travel, sport, training)
Thyroid disease			

even a convulsion. The patient who is sleeping alone is particularly vulnerable and unexplained deaths during sleep have implicated cardiac arrhythmias provoked by nocturnal hypoglycemia [115], the "dead in bed" syndrome.

Estimates of the prevalence of nocturnal hypoglycemia range from 13 to 56% in adult populations of insulin-treated patients and 25–70% of episodes are asymptomatic [116–120]. In the DCCT, 55% of all episodes of severe hypoglycemia occurred during sleep, with 43% occurring at night [59]. The clinical manifestations of recurrent nocturnal hypoglycemia are subtle and nonspecific, with complaints by the patient of poor quality of sleep, morning headaches, chronic fatigue, and vivid dreams or nightmares. Some of these features result from deep sleep being disrupted by hypoglycemia [121]. Enuresis is associated with nocturnal hypoglycemia in diabetic children. Asymptomatic nocturnal hypoglycemia can also cause hypoglycemia-associated autonomic failure [91].

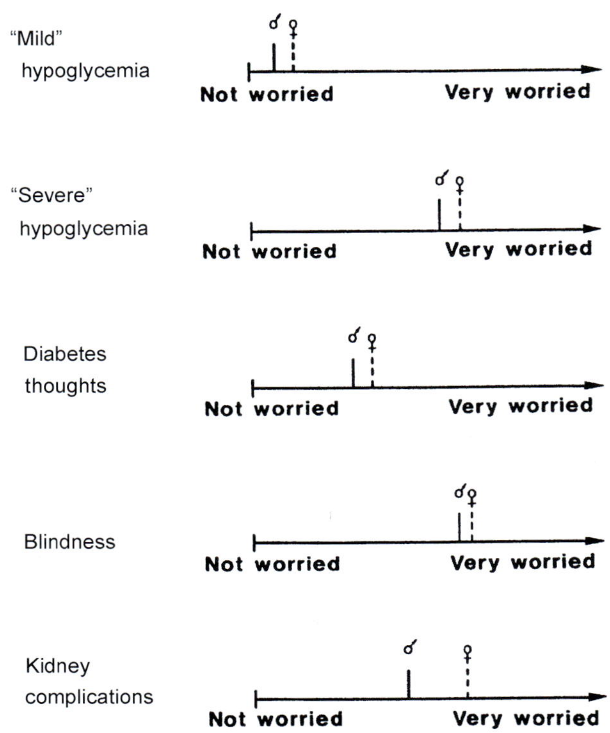

Figure 8 Degree of concern about various aspects of diabetes among 411 patients with T1DM (from reference 81, with permission)

The time of the nocturnal hypoglycemia depends on when the evening meal is taken and the time of injection of preprandial short-acting insulin before the evening meal and intermediate-acting insulin (whether before the evening meal or at bedtime). With the regimen of twice daily soluble and isophane insulins, the glucose nadir is around 0300 h [117], whereas with basal-bolus regimens, the times of maximum risk are between 2300 and 0100 h, and between 0400 and 0730 h [118]. Biochemical clues to the presence of nocturnal hypoglycemia are a glycated hemoglobin close to, or within, the nondiabetic range, low blood glucose values measured during the night, and a relatively high insulin dose (>1 unit/kg body weight). Fasting hyperglycemia (the "Somogyi effect") is not a reliable indicator of nocturnal hypoglycemia and overnight blood glucose profiles have not shown a clinically important rise in fasting glucose after hypoglycemia had occurred during the night [119, 120, 122–124]. The existence of the Somogyi effect is disputed and it does not appear to have any functional significance in T1DM. Fasting hyperglycemia may result from the nocturnal ingestion of large amounts of carbohydrate to treat hypoglycemia, or may represent the waning of insulin action and the "dawn phenomenon" [125]. Other measures to detect nocturnal hypoglycemia, including estimation of morning urinary cortisol and fasting ketonuria, are unreliable and devices that rely on physiological responses to hypoglycemia, such as sweating and skin temperature changes, have been shown to be insensitive or nonspecific [126]. The use of continuous blood glucose monitoring to detect nocturnal hypoglycemia is currently undergoing evaluation. The single most useful predictor for the risk of developing nocturnal hypoglycemia is blood glucose value at bedtime [117, 127]; a blood glucose below 6.0 mmol/l should encourage the ingestion of food. Patients who are reluctant to do any routine blood glucose monitoring should be persuaded of the value of bedtime measurements to protect themselves from the risk of asymptomatic nocturnal hypoglycemia. The development of an effective glucose sensor could transform the management of insulin-treated diabetes by reducing the risk of neuroglycopenia during sleep.

The consequences of recurrent nocturnal hypoglycemia on cerebral function are unknown. Nocturnal hypoglycemia in a group of patients with T1DM had no apparent effect on cognitive function estimated on the following morning [128, 129], but their subjective well-being was affected the following day with greater fatigue being experienced during exercise [129]. The difficulty of estimating the frequency of nocturnal hypoglycemia may underestimate the potential effect of protracted neuroglycopenia on intellectual function in the long term. Nocturnal hypoglycemia has been implicated as a cause of impaired awareness to hypoglycemia mediated by the effect of antecedent hypoglycemia [91, 130], and catecholamine responses to hypoglycemia are lower during sleep [131], indicating a general reduction in sympatho-adrenal activity.

Because most insulin regimens produce hyperinsulinemia in the early hours of the morning, they may require modification to avoid nocturnal hypoglycemia. The evening dose of intermediate-acting insulin can be administered at bedtime to prevent a nocturnal fall in blood glucose but this maneuvre may have limited success because of the unpredictable variability of insulin absorption. The use of fast-acting insulin analogues, insulin lispro and insulin aspart, before the evening meal, and the long-acting insulin analogue, insulin glargine, reduces the risk of nocturnal hypoglycemia, as does continuous subcutaneous insulin infusion [132].

Treatment of Hypoglycemia

Prevention

Hypoglycemia is a classic example of prevention being better than cure and patient education is fundamental to the avoidance of this potentially life-threatening complication of insulin therapy. Instruction on the prevention and emergency treatment of hypoglycemia should embrace the patient's relatives, friends, colleagues at work, and, if necessary, employer. Because the symptoms of hypoglycemia are idiosyncratic, early familiarization of patients with the symptom constellation peculiar to themselves is important, but because the nature and intensity of symptoms may change with time, these should be reviewed at intervals [53]. The relationships between insulin administration, timing of meals, and exercise must be explained, along with methods of self-treating hypoglycemia. Other important prophylactic measures include the choice of appropriate insulin regimens and dose schedules and the establishment of appropriate therapeutic goals by the patient's physician, tailored to the needs of the individual patient. Intensive insulin therapy is contraindicated in patients with impaired awareness of hypoglycemia and in those with a history of recurrent severe hypoglycemia, as both of these clinical problems co-segregate with defective glucose counterregulation and impaired awareness of hypoglycemia as discussed earlier. Indeed, as little as 2–3 weeks of scrupulous avoidance of hypoglycemia may reverse these problems [96–98].

Methods of Treatment

The choice of treatment is determined by the patient's ability to initiate appropriate action. Self-treatment usually involves the oral ingestion of some form of fast-acting carbohydrate, whereas more severe episodes may require interventional measures with the parenteral administration of either intravenous dextrose or intramuscular glucagon [112].

Oral carbohydrate in concentrated form should release a high load of glucose without inducing nausea. Various commercial preparations of glucose tablets are available and confectionery may be as effective. Alternatively, carbohydrate can be taken in mixed or complex form (as biscuits or sandwiches). When treating hypoglycemia a glycemic response to a glucose load occurs within 10–15 min of ingestion [133]. Glucose in liquid form may be given, provided the patient is conscious and able to swallow, but the carbohydrate content of commercial drinks is very variable. In children, a viscous gel solution ("Hypostop," Diabetic Bio-Diagnostics) applied to the buccal mucosa has been advocated; jam or honey may be as effective, but these measures should be avoided in the semiconscious individual.

Glucagon is used when the patient is unconscious or unable to take oral glucose. It acts largely by promoting hepatic glycogenolysis to release glucose. Glucagon may, therefore, be ineffective in patients who are anorectic and emaciated, or in those with protracted hypoglycemia in whom ineffective counterregulation has already occurred [134]. Hepatic stores of glycogen in these patients may be limited or already exhausted. Glucagon is also said to be contraindicated in sulfonylurea-induced hypoglycemia because it stimulates the secretion of endogenous insulin and may therefore exacerbate the hypoglycemia. Glucagon (1.0 mg) can be given subcutaneously, intramuscularly, or intravenously, with all of these routes giving a comparable glycemic response [134]. Side effects include nausea, vomiting, and headache. Glucagon can be administered at home by friends, relatives, or paramedical emergency staff as the initial treatment of the unconscious patient. After recovering consciousness the patient should be encouraged to ingest oral carbohydrate (as starch).

Intravenous glucose by injection (dextrose monohydrate) is the most effective method of treatment of the comatose patient. The usual dose of 50 ml of 50% solution provides 25 g of dextrose and had been demonstrated to induce an average rise of venous blood glucose from a nadir below 1.0 to 12.5 mmol/l within 5 min [135]. It is a safe and highly effective form of treatment but occasionally can cause localized phlebitis or venous thrombosis.

If a comatose patient does not regain consciousness after appropriate resuscitative measures, other causes of neurological impairment should be considered, such as a stroke, subarachnoid or intracerebral hemorrhage, cerebral infection, or a drug overdose. Alternatively, the patient may be postictal and remain drowsy, or have developed cerebral edema. Cerebral edema is associated with prolonged hypoglycemic coma (more than 4 h), occurs in patients who have coexisting alcohol intoxication, in parasuicide with deliberate insulin overdose, and in patients with Addison's disease or hypopituitarism [134]. This particular complication is associated with severe neurological deficit in survivors and carries a high mortality. Neuroimaging of the brain with computerized tomography or magnetic resonance imaging should be performed at an early stage to clarify the diagnosis and if cerebral edema is confirmed, treatment should be initiated with mannitol or dexamethasone. Controlled hyperventilation with high flow oxygen may be of value and convulsions should be treated with an anticonvulsant such as phenytoin.

Morbidity

The potential range of morbidity in diabetic patients exposed to hypoglycemia is shown in Table 7. Acute hypoglycemia can provoke several pathophysiological changes in diabetic patients that may underlie some of the morbidity associated with this form of metabolic stress. The profound stimulation of the sympathoadrenal system causes profuse secretion of catecholamines of a magnitude equivalent to those recorded during an acute myocardial infarction or in hemorrhagic shock. The secretion of adrenaline is accompanied by the release of hormones such as vasopressin and angiotensin II, which may also have major influences on hemodynamics and hemostasis. The increments in cardiac output and myocardial contractility, the arrhythmogenic effect of a fall in plasma potassium, the changes in regional blood flow, and effects on blood constituents and hemorheology may all potentially contribute to precipitating an acute vascular event. Myocardial ischemia and stroke during hypoglycemia have been described anecdotally in diabetic patients, particularly in those who have premature macrovascular disease. It has been postulated that the mobilization and activation of white blood cells in peripheral blood, the increase in coagulability and plasma viscosity, platelet activation and release of clotting factors and free radicals may also have a detrimental effect on established microangiopathy, causing further damage to endothelium and precipitating capillary closure, thus aggravating microvascular complications [41, 136, 137].

Table 7 Morbidity of hypoglycemia

Brain	Psychological
	Cognitive dysfunction
	Automatism
	Behavioral/personality changes
	Psychosis
	Neurological
	Coma
	Convulsions
	Focal abnormalities—motor, sensory
	Hemiplegia; transient ischemic attacks
	Ataxia; choreoathetosis
	Decortication; vegetative states
Heart	Myocardial ischemia; infarction
	Arrhythmias
Eye	Vitreous hemorrhage
	? Aggravates retinopathy
Other	Accidents (including driving)
	Hypothermia

Note: "?" indicates that effect of hypoglycemia to activate retinopathy is possible but not established.

The vital dependence of the brain on a continuous supply of glucose as its principal fuel renders it highly susceptible to acute hypoglycemia. Acute neuroglycopenia causes cognitive impairment, and progresses to drowsiness, confusion, and eventual loss of consciousness with the risk of brain damage. Antisocial or criminal activity may occur during a state of hypoglycemia-induced automatism and may necessitate medico-legal assessment of loss of reason and the level of responsibility for the actions of an individual during hypoglycemia.

Severe brain damage following hypoglycemic coma is rare, with survivors having evidence of cortical and hippocampal atrophy and secondary ventricular enlargement associated with the development of a vegetative state. These patients often have massive intellectual deficit, varying degrees of paralysis, and loss of physical independence. They probably represent the few survivors of protracted and devastating neuroglycopenia, which is usually fatal. Transient hemiplegia and cerebral ischemia are well documented and a wide range of neurological sequelae of hypoglycemia has been described [138].

Severe hypoglycemia causes focal or generalized convulsions in around 7% of all insulin-treated patients [106]. This is often misdiagnosed as idiopathic epilepsy, and as EEG changes occur with hypoglycemia and can persist for several days, investigation should be deferred for at least a week. Some patients who have experienced recurrent severe hypoglycemia have permanent EEG changes that confound clinical interpretation. Hypoglycemic convulsions *per se* have a recognized morbidity, such as joint dislocations and fractures, including wedge compression fractures of the vertebrae. Prophylactic anticonvulsants are considered to be ineffective.

Transient cognitive dysfunction during acute hypoglycemia has been studied extensively [35, 139] and has recovered fully within 1.5 days of a severe hypoglycemic coma [140]. Noncognitive effects include significant changes in mood including a state of anxious tension, unhappiness, low energy, and even irritability and anger [141], which may have clinical sequelae. One major unresolved issue is whether recurrent severe hypoglycemia can cause cumulative impairment of cognitive function as a long-term consequence of repeated exposure to neuroglycopenia. The immature brain is very vulnerable to neuroglycopenia. In young nondiabetic children with a history of neonatal hypoglycemia and in children who have developed diabetes before the age of 5 years and have been exposed to recurrent severe hypoglycemia, their subsequent intellectual development has been shown to be significantly impaired [142, 143]. There is a strong correlation between severe hypoglycemia, with or without convulsions, and a lower IQ later in childhood, and affected children have increased behavioral problems, learning difficulties, and anxiety. Evidence is accumulating that adult diabetic patients who are exposed to recurrent severe hypoglycemia over a period of years have a subtle and moderate reduction in IQ with variable forms of cognitive impairment [140, 144–148], which is not an effect of diabetes *per se* [147], in which decision processes, but not encoding mechanisms, are affected.

While the results of retrospective studies in adult diabetic patients are considered to be equivocal, prospective studies such as the DCCT [149] and the Stockholm Diabetes Intervention Study (SDIS) [105] have shown no significant deterioration in neuropsychological function over a period of up to 10 years. However, these results must be interpreted with caution, because of the atypical population of T1DM patients in the DCCT. The frequency of exposure to severe hypoglycemia was lower in patients in the DCCT [4] than in unselected populations of insulin-treated diabetic patients (Table 5). In addition, the period of study in both prospective trials may have been too short to allow the emergence of significant cognitive impairment. A neuroimaging study using magnetic resonance imaging of the brain of a small subgroup of participants of one of the cross-sectional studies [145–147] has suggested that cortical atrophy was more prevalent in those with a history of frequent exposure to severe hypoglycemia [149]. The potential problems of hypoglycemia occurring while driving, during exercise, and in relation to employment and recreational activities have been reviewed elsewhere [150].

Mortality

Where hypoglycemia has been identified as the principal cause of death in populations of insulin-treated diabetic patients, it has been estimated to cause 2–4% of all deaths [1, 7, 41, 151–154]. The postmortem diagnosis of hypoglycemia is very difficult, if not impossible, to establish with certainty, and historical and circumstantial evidence is usually necessary to identify this metabolic cause of death unless preterminal blood glucose estimates are available. A number of hypoglycemic deaths in insulin-treated diabetic patients may therefore be unrecognized and hypoglycemia may be the primary but unrecorded event in precipitating a fatal vascular events such as a stroke or a myocardial infarction. Problems with ascertainment have been highlighted by inaccurate coding of causes of death in diabetic patients [41, 154]. Death usually results from severe brain damage or secondary effects such as hypostatic pneumonia, an acute vascular event, or cardiac arrest.

Sudden death in young diabetic patients has been recognized since insulin was first introduced into clinical usage and hypoglycemia has often been implicated. Attention has been drawn again to this problem by the description of patients found "dead in bed," many of whom were sleeping alone and had a history of nocturnal hypoglycemia [115]. The actual cause of death could not be determined but hypoglycemia-induced cardiac arrhythmia and respiratory arrest have been proposed as possible mechanisms. Most of these young patients were otherwise in good health and this illustrates the unpredictable and life-threatening nature of severe hypoglycemia.

Despite its integral importance to the treatment of diabetes, insulin remains a potentially dangerous drug. A casual approach to self-management by the diabetic patient and a dismissive attitude to the risks of hypoglycemia by the physician can have a disastrous outcome. Overzealous attempts to achieve strict glycemic control run the risk of inducing frequent severe hypoglycemia, which potentially may have a more serious outcome than the prospect of vascular disease.

PREVENTION OF HYPOGLYCEMIA

Clearly, iatrogenic hypoglycemia is a problem for many patients with T1DM, and for some with T2DM. For the former, hypoglycemia is a fact of life. It cannot be prevented entirely with current insulin replacement techniques if one strives to reap the benefits of effective glycemic control [4]. However, its frequency and severity can be minimized.

Obviously, we need to learn to replace insulin in a much more physiological manner if we are to achieve euglycemia safely in the majority of patients with T1DM.

Short of that, we need to learn to prevent, correct, or compensate for compromised glucose counterregulation if we are to achieve euglycemia safely in a larger proportion of patients with IDDM. Pending these developments, we must use available techniques to their full advantage.

The principles of modern intensive therapy, coupled with prudent glycemic goals, can be used to minimize the frequency and severity of iatrogenic hypoglycemia in T1DM [8]. These principles include thorough education of the patient, since it is the individual who actually manages T1DM, and of the patient's relatives and associates in the recognition and early treatment of hypoglycemia. This includes regular self-monitoring of blood glucose, rational and flexible insulin replacement regimens, and ongoing professional support. Given these, the critical issue is the selection of appropriate glycemic goals that are tailored to the individual patient.

The degree of glycemic control achievable varies among patients with T1DM based on their motivation, intelligence, skills, and knowledge of diabetes in addition to the effect of acquired syndromes associated with recurrent severe hypoglycemia, as discussed earlier. Typically, strict glycemic control becomes more difficult over time. Glycemic goals, therefore, need to be individualized and reassessed at intervals. Episodes of biochemical or mildly symptomatic hypoglycemia are likely, and should be accepted, in a patient striving for optimal glycemic control. However, recurrent episodes of severe hypoglycemia are not acceptable as the short-term risks of physical and psychological morbidity, and the potential risk to life, are simply too great. Near-euglycemia is not a rational goal in such a patient. Since long-term benefits, at least reduction of microangiopathy, are related to overall glycemic control to generally achievable levels [4–6], glycemic control should not, and need not, be compromised completely.

Acknowledgments

Professor Cryer acknowledges the assistance of his technical staff, the research nursing staff of the Washington University General Clinical Research Center, and the secretarial assistance of Ms Karen Muehlhauser. The substantive input of his collaborators and postdoctoral fellows, most of whose names appear in the list of references, is also gratefully acknowledged. His work cited was supported, in part, by United States Public Health Service/National Institutes of Health grants R37 DK27085, M01 RR00036, P01 DK20579, and T32 DK07120 as well as the American Diabetes Association and the Juvenile Diabetes Research Foundation.

Professor Frier acknowledges the collaborative work of various colleagues including Professor Ian Deary, of the Department of Psychology, University of Edinburgh, and of several clinical research fellows, and the secretarial assistance of Ms Mhairi Weatherston. He gratefully acknowledges the support of Diabetes UK, Eli Lilly & Co. Ltd., Novo Nordisk Pharmaceuticals, and the Scottish Hospital Endowments Research Trust with research funding.

REFERENCES

1. Cryer PE. Hypoglycemia in diabetes mellitus. In Cryer PE (ed) *Hypoglycemia: Pathophysiology, Diagnosis and Treatment*. New York: Oxford University Press, 1997; pp 91–125.
2. Frier BM, Fisher BM. *Hypoglycaemia and Diabetes, Clinical and Physiological Aspects*. London: Edward Arnold, 1993.
3. Cryer PE. Hypoglycaemia: the limiting factor in the glycemic management of type I and type II diabetes. *Diabetologia* 2002; 45: 937–48.
4. The Diabetes Control and Complications Trial Research Group. The effect of intensive treatment of diabetes on the development and progression of long-term complications in insulin dependent diabetes mellitus. *N Engl J Med* 1993; 329: 977–86.
5. The United Kingdom Prospective Diabetes Study Research Group. Intensive blood-glucose control with sulfonylureas or insulin compared with conventional treatment and risk of complications in patients with type 2 diabetes (UKPDS 33). *Lancet* 1998; 352: 837–53.
6. The United Kingdom Prospective Diabetes Research Group. Effect of intensive blood-glucose control with metformin on complications in overweight patients with type 2 diabetes (UKPDS 34). *Lancet* 1998; 352: 854–65.
7. Laing SP, Swerdlow AJ, Slater SD, Botha JL, Burden AC, Waugh NR, Smith AWM, Hill RD, Bingley PJ, Patterson CC, Qiao Z, Keen H. The British Diabetic Association Cohort Study, II: cause-specific mortality in patients with insulin-treated diabetes mellitus. *Diabet Med* 1999; 16: 466–71.
8. Cryer PE, Childs BP. Negotiating the barrier of hypoglycemia in diabetes. *Diabetes Spectrum* 2002; 15: 20–7.
9. Cryer PE. The prevention and correction of hypoglycemia. In Jefferson LS, Cherrington AD (eds) *Handbook of Physiology, Section 7: The Endocrine System. Volume II: The Endocrine Pancreas and Regulation of Metabolism*. New York: Oxford University Press, 2001; pp 1057–92.
10. De Feo P, Perriello G, Torlone E, Ventura MM, Santeusanio F, Brunetti P, Gerich JE, Bolli GB. Demonstration of a role for growth hormone in glucose counterregulation. *Am J Physiol* 1989; 256: E835–43.
11. De Feo P, Perriello G, Torlone E, Ventura MM, Fanelli C, Santeusanio F, Brunetti P, Gerich JE, Bolli GB. Contribution of cortisol to glucose counterregulation in humans. *Am J Physiol* 1989; 257: E35–42.
12. Boyle PJ, Liggett SB, Shah SD, Cryer PE. Direct muscarinic cholinergic inhibition of hepatic glucose production in humans. *J Clin Invest* 1988; 82: 445–9.
13. Soskin S, Essex H, Herrick J, Mann F. The mechanism of regulation of the blood sugar by the liver. *Am J Physiol* 1938; 124: 558–67.
14. Fanelli C, De Feo P, Porcellati F, Perriello G, Torlone E, Santeusanio F, Brunetti P, Bolli GB. Adrenergic mechanisms contribute to hypoglycemic glucose counterregulation in man largely by accelerating lipolysis. *J Clin Invest* 1992; 89: 2005–13.

15. Schwartz NS, Clutter WE, Shah SD, Cryer PE. Glycemic thresholds for activation of glucose counterregulatory systems are higher than the threshold for symptoms. *J Clin Invest* 1987; 79: 777–81.
16. Mitrakou A, Ryan C, Veneman T, Mokan M, Jenssen T, Kiss I, Durant J, Cryer P, Gerich J. Hierarchy of glycemic thresholds for counterregulatory hormone secretion, symptoms and cerebral dysfunction. *Am J Physiol* 1991; 260: E67–74.
17. Mitrakou A, Mokan M, Ryan C, Veneman T, Cryer P, Gerich J. Influence of plasma glucose rate of decrease on hierarchy of responses to hypoglycemia. *J Clin Endocrinol Metab* 1993; 76: 462–5.
18. Boyle PJ, Nagy R, O'Connor AM, Kempers SF, Yeo RA, Qualls C. Adaptation in brain glucose uptake following recurrent hypoglycemia. *Proc Natl Acad Sci USA* 1994; 91: 9352–6.
19. Garber AJ, Cryer PE, Santiago JV, Haymond MW, Pagliara AS, Kipnis DM. The role of adrenergic mechanisms in the substrate and hormonal response to insulin induced hypoglycemia in man. *J Clin Invest* 1976; 58: 7–15.
20. Cryer PE. Glucose counterregulation: the prevention and correction of hypoglycemia in humans. *Am J Physiol* 1993; 264: E149–55.
21. Heller SR, Cryer PE. Hypoinsulinemia is not critical to glucose recovery from hypoglycemia in humans. *Am J Physiol* 1991; 261: E41–8.
22. Gerich J, Davis J, Lorenzi M, Rizza R, Bohannon N, Karam J, Lewis S, Kaplan S, Schultz T, Cryer P. Hormonal mechanisms of recovery from insulin induced hypoglycemia in man. *Am J Physiol* 1979; 236: E380–5.
23. Rizza RA, Cryer PE, Gerich JE. Role of glucagon, epinephrine and growth hormone in human glucose counterregulation: effects of somatostatin and adrenergic blockade on plasma glucose recovery and glucose flux rates following insulin-induced hypoglycemia. *J Clin Invest* 1979; 64: 62–71.
24. Rosen SG, Clutter WE, Berk MA, Shah SD, Cryer PE. Epinephrine supports the postabsorptive plasma glucose concentration, and prevents hypoglycemia, when glucagon secretion is deficient in man. *J Clin Invest* 1984; 73: 405–11.
25. Tse TF, Clutter WE, Shah SD, Miller JP, Cryer PE. Neuroendocrine responses to glucose ingestion in man: specificity, temporal relationships and quantitative aspects. *J Clin Invest* 1983; 72: 270–7.
26. Tse TF, Clutter WE, Shah SD, Cryer PE. The mechanisms of postprandial glucose counterregulation in man: physiologic roles of glucagon and epinephrine vis-à-vis insulin in the prevention of hypoglycemia late after glucose ingestion. *J Clin Invest* 1983; 72: 278–86.
27. Boyle PJ, Shah SD, Cryer PE. Insulin, glucagon and catecholamines in the prevention of hypoglycemia during fasting in humans. *Am J Physiol* 1989; 256: E651–61.
28. Hirsch IB, Marker JC, Smith LJ, Spina RJ, Parvin CA, Holloszy JO, Cryer PE. Insulin and glucagon in the prevention of hypoglycemia during exercise in humans. *Am J Physiol* 1991; 260: E695–704.
29. Marker JC, Hirsch IB, Smith LJ, Parvin CA, Holloszy JO, Cryer PE. Catecholamines in the prevention of hypoglycemia during exercise in humans. *Am J Physiol* 1992; 260: E705–12.
30. De Feo P, Perriello G, Torlone E, Fanelli C, Ventura MM, Santeusanio F, Brunetti P, Gerich JE, Bolli GB. Evidence against important catecholamine compensation for absent glucagon counterregulation. *Am J Physiol* 1991; 260: E203–12.
31. De Feo P, Perriello G, Torlone E, Fanelli C, Ventura MM, Santeusanio F, Brunetti P, Gerich JE, Bolli GB. Contribution of adrenergic mechanisms to glucose counterregulation in humans. *Am J Physiol* 1991; 261: E725–36.
32. Boyle PJ, Cryer PE. Growth hormone, cortisol, or both are involved in defense against, but are not critical to recovery from, prolonged hypoglycemia in humans. *Am J Physiol* 1991; 260: E395–402.
33. Bolli GB, De Feo P, Perriello G, De Cosmo S, Ventura M, Campbell P, Brunetti P, Gerich JE. Role of hepatic autoregulation in defense against hypoglycemia in humans. *J Clin Invest* 1985; 75: 1623–31.
34. Hansen I, Firth R, Haymond M, Cryer P, Rizza R. The role of autoregulation of hepatic glucose production in man: response to a physiologic decrement in plasma glucose. *Diabetes* 1986; 35: 186–91.
35. Deary IJ. Symptoms of hypoglycaemia and effects on mental performance and emotions. In Frier BM, Fisher BM (eds) *Hypoglycaemia in Clinical Diabetes*. Chichester: Wiley, 1999; pp 29–54.
36. Bendtson I. Neurophysiological changes of hypoglycaemia. In Frier BM, Fisher BM (eds) *Hypoglycaemia and Diabetes, Clinical and Physiological Aspects*. London: Edward Arnold, 1993; pp 72–9.
37. Tallroth G, Lindgren M, Stenberg G, Rosen I, Agardh C-D. Neurophysiological changes during insulin-induced hypoglycaemia and in the recovery period following glucose infusion in Type I (insulin-dependent) diabetes mellitus and in normal man. *Diabetologia* 1990; 33: 319–23.
38. Bjorgaas M, Sand T, Vik T, Jorde R. Quantitative EEG during controlled hypoglycaemia in diabetic and nondiabetic children. *Diabet Med* 1998; 15: 30–7.
39. Hepburn DA, Frier BM. Hypoglycaemia and diabetes. In Lawson DH (ed) *Current Medicine 4*. Edinburgh: Churchill Livingstone/Royal College of Physicians of Edinburgh, 1994; pp 97–120.
40. Fisher BM, Frier BM. Haemodynamic responses and functional changes in major organs. In Frier BM, Fisher BM (eds) *Hypoglycaemia and Diabetes, Clinical and Physiological Aspects*. London: Edward Arnold, 1993; pp 144–55.
41. Fisher BM, Heller SR. Mortality, cardiovascular morbidity and possible effects of hypoglycaemia on diabetic complications. In Frier BM, Fisher BM (eds) *Hypoglycaemia in Clinical Diabetes*. Chichester: Wiley, 1999; pp 167–86.
42. Neil HAW, Gale EAM, Hamilton SJC, Lopez-Espinoza I, Kaura R, McCarthy ST. Cerebral blood flow increases during insulin-induced hypoglycaemia in Type I (insulin-dependent) diabetic patients and control subjects. *Diabetologia* 1987; 30: 305–9.
43. Tallroth G, Ryding E, Agardh C-D. Regional cerebral blood flow in normal man during insulin-induced hypoglycemia and in the recovery period following glucose infusion. *Metabolism* 1992; 41: 717–21.
44. Patrick AW, Hepburn DA, Craig KJ, Thomson I, Swainson CP, Frier BM. The effects of acute insulin-induced hypoglycaemia on renal function in normal human subjects. *Diabet Med* 1989; 6: 703–8.
45. Braatvedt GD, Flynn MD, Stanners A, Halliwell M, Corrall RJM. Splanchnic blood flow in man: evidence

for mediation via a beta-adrenergic mechanism. *Clin Sci* 1993; 84: 201–7.

46. Fisher BM, Gillen G, Hepburn DA, Dargie HJ, Barnett E, Frier BM. Splenic responses to acute insulin-induced hypoglycaemia in humans. *Clin Sci* 1990; 78: 469–74.
47. Schvarcz E, Palmer M, Aman J, Berne C. Hypoglycemia increases the gastric emptying rate in healthy subjects. *Diabetes Care* 1995; 18: 674–6.
48. Allwood MJ, Hensel H, Papenberg J. Muscle and skin blood flow in the human forearm during insulin hypoglycaemia. *J Physiol* 1959; 147: 269–73.
49. Maggs DG, Scott AR, Macdonald IA. Thermoregulatory responses to hyperinsulinemic hypoglycemia and euglycemia in humans. *Am J Physiol* 1994; 267: R1266–72.
50. Corrall RJM, Frier BM, Davidson NMcD, Hopkins WM, French EB. Cholinergic manifestations of the acute autonomic reaction to hypoglycaemia in man. *Clin Sci* 1983; 64: 49–53.
51. Heller SR, Macdonald IA, Herbert M, Tattersall RB. Influence of sympathetic nervous system on hypoglycaemic warning symptoms. *Lancet* 1987; ii: 359–63.
52. Fisher BM, Frier BM. Peripheral blood, hemostasis and hemorheology. In Frier BM, Fisher BM (eds) *Hypoglycaemia and Diabetes, Clinical and Physiological Aspects*. London: Edward Arnold, 1993; pp 156–64.
53. McAulay V, Deary IJ, Frier BM. Symptoms of hypoglycaemia in people with diabetes. *Diabet Med* 2001; 18: 690–705.
54. Hepburn DA, Deary IJ, Frier BM. Classification of symptoms of hypoglycaemia in insulin-treated diabetic patients using factor analysis: relationship to hypoglycaemia unawareness. *Diabet Med* 1992; 9: 70–5.
55. Deary IJ, Hepburn DA, MacLeod KM, Frier BM. Partitioning the symptoms of hypoglycaemia using multisample confirmatory factor analysis. *Diabetologia* 1993; 36: 771–7.
56. Towler DA, Havlin CE, Craft S, Cryer PE. Mechanism of awareness of hypoglycemia: perception of neurogenic (predominantly cholinergic) rather than neuroglycopenic symptoms. *Diabetes* 1993; 42: 1791–8.
57. The United Kingdom Prospective Diabetes Study Research Group. A 6-year, randomized, controlled trial comparing sulfonylurea, insulin and metformin therapy in patients with newly diagnosed type 2 diabetes that could not be controlled with diet therapy. *Ann Intern Med* 1998; 128: 165–75.
58. Hepburn DA, MacLeod KM, Pell ACH, Scougal IJ, Frier BM. Frequency and symptoms of hypoglycaemia experienced by patients with type 2 diabetes treated with insulin. *Diabet Med* 1993; 10: 231–7.
59. The Diabetes Control and Complications Trial Research Group. Epidemiology of severe hypoglycemia in the Diabetes Control and Complications Trial. *Am J Med* 1991; 90: 450–9.
60. White NH, Skor DA, Cryer PE, Levandoski L, Bier DM, Santiago JV. Identification of type I diabetic patients at increased risk for hypoglycemia during intensive therapy. *N Engl J Med* 1983; 308: 485–91.
61. Bolli GB, De Feo P, De Cosmo S, Perriello G, Ventura MM, Massi Benedetti M, Santeusanio F, Gerich JE, Brunetti P. A reliable and reproducible test for adequate glucose counterregulation in type I diabetes mellitus. *Diabetes* 1984; 33: 732–7.
62. Clausen-Sjbom N, Adamson U, Lins PE. The prevalence of impaired glucose counterregulation during an insulin infusion test in insulin-treated patients prone to severe hypoglycaemia. *Diabetologia* 1989; 32: 818–25.
63. Heller SR, Herbert M, Macdonald IA, Tattersall RB. Influence of sympathetic nervous system on hypoglycaemic warning symptoms. *Lancet* 1987; ii: 359–63.
64. Hepburn DA, Patrick AW, Eadington DW, Ewing DJ, Frier BM. Unawareness of hypoglycaemia in insulin-treated diabetic patients: prevalence and relationship to autonomic neuropathy. *Diabet Med* 1990; 7: 711–7.
65. Ryder REJ, Owens DR, Hayes TM, Ghatei M, Bloom SR. Unawareness of hypoglycaemia and inadequate glucose counterregulation: no causal relationship with diabetic autonomic neuropathy. *Br Med J* 1990; 301: 783–7.
66. Grimaldi A, Bosquet F, Davidoff P, Digy JP, Sachon C, Landau C, Thervet F, Zoghbi F, Legrand JC. Unawareness of hypoglycaemia by insulin-dependent diabetics. *Horm Metab Res* 1990; 22: 90–5.
67. Clarke WL, Gonder-Frederick LA, Richards FE, Cryer PE: Multifactorial origin of hypoglycemic symptom awareness in insulin dependent diabetes mellitus. *Diabetes* 1991; 40: 680–5.
68. Hepburn DA, Patrick AW, Brash HM, Thomson I, Frier BM. Hypoglycaemia unawareness in type I diabetes: a lower plasma glucose is required to stimulate sympathoadrenal activation. *Diabet Med* 1991; 8: 934–45.
69. Amiel SA, Tamborlane WV, Simonson DC, Sherwin RS. Defective glucose counterregulation after strict control of insulin-dependent diabetes mellitus. *N Engl J Med* 1987; 316: 1376–83.
70. Amiel SA, Sherwin RS, Simonson DC, Tamborlane WV. Effect of intensive insulin therapy on glycemic thresholds for counterregulatory hormone release. *Diabetes* 1988; 37: 901–7.
71. Heller SR, Cryer PE. Reduced neuroendocrine and symptomatic responses to subsequent hypoglycemia after one episode of hypoglycemia in nondiabetic humans. *Diabetes* 1991; 40: 223–6.
72. Davis M, Shamoon H. Counterregulatory adaptation to recurrent hypoglycemia in normal humans. *J Clin Endocrinol Metab* 1991; 73: 995–1001.
73. Widom B, Simonson DC. Intermittent hypoglycemia impairs glucose counterregulation. *Diabetes* 1992; 41: 1597–602.
74. Dagogo-Jack SE, Craft S, Cryer PE. Hypoglycemia-associated autonomic failure in insulin dependent diabetes mellitus. *J Clin Invest* 1993; 91: 819–28.
75. Davis MR, Mellman M, Shamoon H. Further defects in counterregulatory responses induced by recurrent hypoglycemia in type I diabetes. *Diabetes* 1992; 41: 1335–40.
76. Lingenfelser T, Renn W, Sommerwerck U, Jung MF, Buettner UW, Zaiser-Kaschel H, Kaschel R, Eggstein M, Jakober B. Compromised hormonal counterregulation, symptom awareness, and neurophysiological function after recurrent short-term episodes of insulin-induced hypoglycemia in IDDM patients. *Diabetes* 1993; 42: 610–8.
77. Hirsch IB, Boyle PJ, Craft S, Cryer PE. Higher glycemic thresholds for symptoms during β-adrenergic blockade in IDDM. *Diabetes* 1991; 40: 1177–86.
78. Gerich J, Langlois M, Noacco C, Karam J, Forsham P. Lack of glucagon response to hypoglycemia in diabetes: evidence for an intrinsic pancreatic alpha-cell defect. *Science* 1973; 182: 171–3.
79. Bolli G, De Feo P, Compagnucci P, Cartechini MG, Angeletti G, Santeusanio F, Brunetti P, Gerich JE. Abnormal glucose counterregulation in insulin-dependent

diabetes mellitus: interaction of anti-insulin antibodies and impaired glucagon and epinephrine secretion. *Diabetes* 1983; 32: 134–41.
80. Fukuda M, Tanaka A, Tahara Y, Ikegami H, Yamamoto Y, Kumahara Y, Shima K. Correlation between minimal secretory capacity of pancreatic α-cells and stability of diabetic control. *Diabetes* 1988; 37: 81–8.
81. Pramming S, Thorsteinsson B, Bendtson I, Binder C. Symptomatic hypoglycemia in 411 type I diabetic patients. *Diabet Med* 1991; 8: 217–22.
82. Gerich JE, Mokan MT, Korytkowski M, Mitrakou A. Hypoglycemia unawareness. *Endocr Rev* 1991; 12: 356–71.
83. Frier BM, Fisher BM. Impaired hypoglycaemia awareness. In Frier BM, Fisher BM (eds) *Hypoglycaemia in Clinical Diabetes*. Chichester: Wiley, 1999; pp 111–46.
84. Gold AE, MacLeod KM, Frier BM. Frequency of severe hypoglycemia in patients with type I diabetes with impaired awareness of hypoglycemia. *Diabetes Care* 1994; 17: 697–703.
85. Boyle PJ, Schwartz NS, Shah SD, Clutter WE, Cryer PE. Plasma glucose concentrations at the onset of hypoglycemic symptoms in patients with poorly controlled diabetes and in nondiabetics. *N Engl J Med* 1988; 318: 1487–92.
86. Boyle PJ, Kempers SF, O'Connor AM, Nagy RJ. Brain glucose uptake and unawareness of hypoglycemia in patients with insulin dependent diabetes mellitus. *N Engl J Med* 1995: 333: 1726–31.
87. Segel SA, Fanelli CG, Dence CS, Markham J, Videen TO, Paramore DS, Powers WJ, Cryer PE. Blood-to-brain glucose transport, cerebral glucose metabolism and cerebral blood flow are not increased following hypoglycemia. *Diabetes* 2001; 50: 1911–7.
88. Amiel SA, Pottinger RC, Archibald HR, Chusney G, Cunnah DTF, Prior PF, Gale EAM. Effect of antecedent glucose control on cerebral function during hypoglycemia. *Diabetes Care* 1991; 14: 109–18.
89. Widom B, Simonson D. Glycemic control and neuropsychologic function during hypoglycemia in patients with insulin dependent diabetes mellitus. *Ann Intern Med* 1990; 112: 904–12.
90. Hvidberg A, Fanelli CG, Hershey TG, Terkamp C, Craft S, Cryer PE. Impact of recent antecedent hypoglycemia on hypoglycemic cognitive dysfunction in nondiabetic humans. *Diabetes* 1996; 45: 1030–6.
91. Fanelli CG, Paramore DS, Hershey T, Terkamp C, Ovalle F, Craft S, Cryer PE. Impact of nocturnal hypoglycemia on hypoglycemic cognitive dysfunction in type 1 diabetes. *Diabetes* 1998; 47: 1920–7.
92. Ovalle F, Fanelli CG, Paramore DS, Craft S, Cryer PE. Brief twice weekly episodes of hypoglycemia reduce detection of clinical hypoglycemia in type 1 diabetes mellitus. *Diabetes* 1998; 14: 1472–9.
93. Popp DA, Tse TF, Shah SD, Clutter WE, Cryer PE. Oral propranolol and metoprolol both impair glucose recovery from insulin induced hypoglycemia in insulin dependent diabetes mellitus. *Diabetes Care* 1984; 7: 243–7.
94. Cryer PE. Iatrogenic hypoglycemia as a cause of hypoglycemia-associated autonomic failure in IDDM: a vicious cycle. *Diabetes* 1992; 41: 255–60.
95. Rattarasarn C, Dagogo-Jack SE, Zachwieja JJ, Cryer PE. Hypoglycemia-associated autonomic failure in IDDM is specific for the stimulus of hypoglycemia and is not attributable to prior autonomic activation *per se*. *Diabetes* 1994; 43: 809–18.
96. Fanelli C, Pampanelli S, Epifano L, Rambotti AM, Di Vincenzo A, Modarelli F, Ciofetta M, Lepore M, Annibale B, Torlone E, Perriello G, De Feo P, Santeusanio F, Brunetti P, Bolli GB. Long-term recovery from unawareness, deficient counterregulation and lack of cognitive dysfunction during hypoglycaemia, following institution of rational, intensive therapy in IDDM. *Diabetologia* 1994; 37: 1265–76.
97. Cranston I, Lomas J, Maran A, Macdonald I, Amiel S. Restoration of hypoglycaemia awareness in patients with long-duration insulin-dependent diabetes. *Lancet* 1994; 344: 283–7.
98. Dagogo-Jack SE, Rattarasarn C, Cryer PE. Reversal of hypoglycemia unawareness, but not defective glucose counterregulation, IDDM. *Diabetes* 1994; 43: 1426–34.
99. Bottini P, Boschetti E, Pampanelli S, Ciofetta M, Del Sindaco P, Scionti L, Brunetti P, Bolli GB. Contribution of autonomic neuropathy to reduced plasma adrenaline responses to hypoglycemia in IDDM. *Diabetes* 1997; 46: 814–23.
100. Meyer C, Grobmann R, Mitrakou A, Mahler R, Veneman T, Gerich J, Reinhard G. Effects of autonomic neuropathy on counterregulation and awareness of hypoglycaemia in type 1 diabetic patients. *Diabetes Care* 1998; 21: 1960–6.
101. Pedersen-Bjergaard U, Agerholm-Larsen B, Pramming S, Hougaard P, Thorsteinsson B. Activity of angiotensin converting enzyme and risk of severe hypoglycaemia in type 1 diabetes mellitus. *Lancet* 2001; 357: 1248–53.
102. The United Kingdom Prospective Diabetes Study Research Group. Overview of 6 years of therapy of type II diabetes: a progressive disease. *Diabetes* 1995; 44: 1249–58.
103. Segel SA, Paramore DS, Cryer PE. Hypoglycemia-associated autonomic failure in advanced type 2 diabetes. *Diabetes* 2002; 51: 724–33.
104. McAulay V, Frier BM. Hypoglycaemia. In Sinclair AJ, Finucane P (eds) *Diabetes in Old Age*, 2nd edn., Chichester: Wiley, 2001; pp 133–52.
105. Reichard P, Pihl M, Rosenqvist U, Sule J. Complications in IDDM are caused by elevated blood glucose level: the Stockholm Diabetes Intervention Study (SDIS) at 10-year follow up. *Diabetologia* 1996; 39: 1483–8.
106. MacLeod KM, Hepburn DA, Frier BM. Frequency and morbidity of severe hypoglycaemia in insulin-treated diabetic patients. *Diabet Med* 1993; 10: 238–45.
107. Ter Braak EWMT, Appleman AMMF, Van de Laak MF, Stolk RP, Van Haeften TW, Erkelens DW. Clinical characteristics of type 1 diabetic patients with and without severe hypoglycemia. *Diabetes Care* 2000; 23: 1467–71.
108. Pramming S, Pederson-Bjergaard U, Heller SR, Wallace T, Rasmussen AK, Jorgensen HV, Matthews Dr, Thorsteinsson B. Severe hypoglycaemia in unselected patients with type 1 diabetes: a cross-sectional multicentre survey [abstract]. *Diabetologia* 2000; 43 (suppl 1): A194.
109. The EURODIAB IDDM Complications Study Group. Microvascular and acute complications in IDDM patients: the EURODIAB IDDM complications study. *Diabetologia* 1994; 37: 278–85.
110. The Diabetes Control and Complications Trial Research Group. Hypoglycaemia in the Diabetes Control and Complications Trial. *Diabetes* 1997; 46: 271–86.
111. Moses RG, Hubert PA, Lewis-Driver DJ. Severe hypoglycaemia. A one-year prospective survey in Wollongong. *Med J Aust* 1985; 142: 294–6.
112. Tattersall RB. Frequency, causes and treatment of hypoglycaemia. In Frier BM, Fisher BM (eds) *Hypoglycaemia*

in Clinical Diabetes, Chichester: Wiley, 1999; pp 55–87.
113. Bott S, Bott U, Berger M, Mühlhauser I. Intensified insulin therapy and the risk of severe hypoglycaemia. *Diabetologia* 1997; 40: 926–32.
114. Mühlhauser I, Overmann H, Bender R, Bott U, Berger M. Risk factors of severe hypoglycaemia in adult patients with type 1 diabetes—a prospective population based study. *Diabetologia* 1998; 41: 1274–82.
115. Tattersall RB, Gill GV. Unexplained deaths of type 1 diabetic patients. *Diabet Med* 1991; 8: 49–58.
116. Gale EAM, Tattersall RB. Unrecognised nocturnal hypoglycemia in insulin-treated diabetics. *Lancet* 1979; i: 1049–52.
117. Pramming S, Thorsteinsson B, Bendtson I, Ronn B, Binder C. Nocturnal hypoglycaemia in patients receiving conventional treatment with insulin. *Br Med J* 1985; 291: 376–9.
118. Vervoort G, Goldschmidt HMG, van Doorn LG. Nocturnal blood glucose profiles in patients with type 1 diabetes mellitus on multiple (>4) daily insulin injection regimens. *Diabet Med* 1996; 13: 794–9.
119. Stephenson JM, Schernthaner G. Dawn phenomenon and Somogyi effect in IDDM. *Diabetes Care* 1989; 12: 245–51.
120. Lerman IG, Wolfsdorf JI. Relationship of nocturnal hypoglycemia to daytime glycemia in IDDM. *Diabetes Care* 1988; 11: 636–42.
121. Bendtson I, Gade J, Thomsen CE, Rosenfalck A, Wildschiödtz G. Sleep disturbances in IDDM patients with nocturnal hypoglycemia. *Sleep* 1992; 15: 74–81.
122. Havlin CE, Cryer PE. Nocturnal hypoglycemia does not commonly result in major morning hyperglycemia in patients with diabetes mellitus. *Diabetes Care* 1987; 10: 141–7.
123. Tordjman KM, Havlin CE, Levandoski LA, White NH, Santiago JV, Cryer PE: Failure of nocturnal hypoglycemia to cause fasting hyperglycemia in patients with insulin dependent diabetes mellitus. *N Engl J Med* 1987; 317: 1552–9.
124. Hirsch IB, Smith LB, Havlin CE, Shah SD, Clutter WE, Cryer PE. Failure of nocturnal hypoglycemia to cause daytime hyperglycemia in patients with insulin dependent diabetes mellitus. *Diabetes Care* 1990; 13: 133–42.
125. Cryer PE. Morning hyperglycemia in insulin dependent diabetes mellitus: insulin lack versus the dawn and Somogyi phenomena. In Mazzaferri EL (ed) *Advances in Endocrinology and Metabolism, Volume 1*. Chicago: Year Book Medical Publishers, 1990; pp 231–43.
126. Clarke WL, Carter MR, Moll M, Cox DJ, Gonder-Frederick LA, Cryer PE. Metabolic and cutaneous events associated with hypoglycemia detected by SleepSentry. *Diabetes Care* 1988; 11: 630–5.
127. Schiffrin A, Suissa S. Predicting nocturnal hypoglycemia in patients with type 1 diabetes mellitus with continuous subcutaneous insulin infusion. *Am J Med* 1987; 82: 1127–32.
128. Bendtson I, Gade J, Theilgaard A, Binder C. Cognitive function in type 1 (insulin-dependent) diabetic patients after nocturnal hypoglycaemia. *Diabetologia* 1992; 35: 898–903.
129. King P, Kong M-F, Parkin H, Macdonald IA, Tattersall RB. Well-being, cerebral function, and physical fatigue after nocturnal hypoglycemia in IDDM. *Diabetes Care* 1998; 21: 341–5.
130. Veneman T, Mitrakou A, Mokan M, Cryer P, Gerich J. Induction of hypoglycemia unawareness by asymptomatic nocturnal hypoglycemia. *Diabetes* 1993; 42: 1233–7.
131. Jones TW, Porter P, Sherwin RS, Davis EA, O'Leary P, Frazer F, Byrne G, Sticks S, Tamborlane WV. Decreased epinephrine responses to hypoglycemia during sleep. *N Engl J Med* 1998; 338: 1657–62.
132. Kanc K, Janssen MMJ, Keulen ETP, Jacobs MAJM, Popp-Snijders C, Snoek FJ, Heine RJ. Substitution of night-time continuous subcutaneous insulin in a multiple injection regimen improved counterregulatory hormonal; responses and warning symptoms of hypoglycaemia in IDDM. *Diabetologia* 1998; 41: 322–9.
133. Brodows RG, Williams C, Amatruda JM. Treatment of insulin reactions in diabetics. *J Am Med Assoc* 1984; 252: 3378–81.
134. MacCuish AC. Treatment of hypoglycaemia. In Frier BM, Fisher BM (eds) *Hypoglycaemia and Diabetes, Clinical and Physiological Aspects*. London: Edward Arnold, 1993; pp 212–21.
135. Collier A, Steedman DJ, Patrick AW, Nimmo GR, Matthews DM, MacIntyre CCA, Little K, Clarke BF. Comparison of intravenous glucagon and dextrose in treatment of severe hypoglycemia in an accident and emergency department. *Diabetes Care* 1987; 10: 712–5.
136. Frier BM, Hilsted J. Does hypoglycaemia aggravate the complications of diabetes? *Lancet* 1985; ii: 1175–7.
137. Fisher BM, Frier BM. Effect on vascular disease. In Frier BM, Fisher BM (eds) *Hypoglycaemia and Diabetes, Clinical and Physiological Aspects*. London: Edward Arnold, 1993; pp 355–61.
138. Lins P-E, Adamson U. Neurological manifestations of hypoglycaemia. In Frier BM, Fisher BM (eds) *Hypoglycaemia and Diabetes, Clinical and Physiological Aspects*. London: Edward Arnold, 1993; pp 347–54.
139. Richardson JTE. Cognitive function in diabetes mellitus. *Neurosci Biobehav Revs* 1990; 14: 385–8.
140. Strachan MWJ, Deary IJ, Ewing FME, Frier BM. Recovery of cognitive function and mood after severe hypoglycemia in adults with insulin-treated diabetes. *Diabetes Care* 2000; 23: 305–12.
141. Gold AE, Deary IJ, Frier BM. Hypoglycaemia and non-cognitive aspects of psychological function in insulin-dependent (type 1) diabetes mellitus (IDDM). *Diabet Med* 1997; 14: 111–8.
142. Soltesz G. Hypoglycaemia in the diabetic child. *Bailliere's Clin Endocrinol Metab* 1993; 7 (3): 741–55.
143. Swift PGF. Hypoglycaemia in children with diabetes. In Frier BM, Fisher BM (eds) *Hypoglycaemia in Clinical Diabetes*. Chichester: Wiley, 1999; pp 211–42.
144. Wredling R, Levander S, Adamson U, Lins P-E. Permanent neuropsychological impairment after recurrent episodes of severe hypoglycaemia in man. *Diabetologia* 1990; 33: 152–7.
145. Langan SJ, Deary IJ, Hepburn DA, Frier BM. Cumulative cognitive impairment following recurrent severe hypoglycaemia in adult patients with insulin-treated diabetes mellitus. *Diabetologia* 1991; 34: 337–44.
146. Deary IJ, Langan SJ, Graham KS, Hepburn DA, Frier BM. Recurrent severe hypoglycemia, intelligence, and speed of information processing. *Intelligence* 1992; 16: 337–59.
147. Deary IJ, Crawford JR, Hepburn DA, Langan SJ, Blackmore LM, Frier BM. Severe hypoglycemia and

intelligence in adult patients with insulin-treated diabetes. *Diabetes* 1993; 42: 341–4.

148. Lincoln NB, Faleiro RM, Kelly C, Kirk BA, Jeffcoate WJ. Effect of long-term glycemic control on cognitive function. *Diabetes Care* 1996; 19: 656–8.
149. The Diabetes Control and Complications Trial Research Group. Effects of intensive diabetes therapy on neuropsychological function in adults in the Diabetes Control and Complications Trial. *Ann Intern Med* 1996; 124: 379–88.
150. Frier BM. Living with hypoglycaemia. In Frier BM, Fisher BM (eds). *Hypoglycaemia in Clinical Diabetes*. Chichester: Wiley, 1999; pp 261–90.
151. Deckert T, Poulsen JE, Larsen M. Prognosis of diabetics with diabetes before the age of thirty-one, 1: survival, cause of deaths and complications. *Diabetologia* 1978; 14: 363–70.
152. Connell FA, Louden JM. Diabetes mortality in persons under 45 years of age. *Am J Pub Health* 1983; 73: 1174–7.
153. Borch-Johnsen K, Nissen H, Hendriksen E, Kreiner S, Salling N, Deckert T, Nerup J. The natural history of insulin-dependent diabetes mellitus in Denmark: long term survival with and without late diabetic complications. *Diabet Med* 1987; 4: 201–10.
154. Tattersall RB, Gale EAM. Mortality. In Frier BM, Fisher BM (eds) *Hypoglycaemia and Diabetes, Clinical and Physiological Aspects*. London: Edward Arnold, 1993; pp 190–8.

60

Diabetic Ketoacidosis and Hyperglycemic Hyperosmolar State

Abbas E. Kitabchi, Guillermo E. Umpierrez, and Mary Beth Murphy

University of Tennessee Health Science Center, Memphis, TN, USA

INTRODUCTION

Diabetic ketoacidosis (DKA) and hyperglycemic hyperosmolar state (HHS) are two of the most serious acute metabolic emergencies in type 1 and type 2 diabetes. In spite of advances in our understanding of the underlying mechanisms that lead to the development of hyperglycemic crises, DKA continues to be an important cause of morbidity and mortality among patients with diabetes. DKA is reported to be responsible for more than 100 000 hospital admissions per year in the United States [1], and recent epidemiological data indicate that the admission rate for DKA may be on the rise [2].

In this chapter, we review recent advances on the epidemiology, diagnosis, and pathogenesis of DKA and HHS, and provide recommendations for their therapy based on the recent American Diabetes Association (ADA) guidelines for management of hyperglycemic crises [3].

DIABETIC KETOACIDOSIS

Definition and Classification

Diabetic ketoacidosis consists of three distinct components: hyperglycemia, acidemia, and ketonemia. Each of these components may be caused by a variety of conditions, which are depicted in [3] Figure 1. According to the recent ADA guidelines, DKA is now classified as mild, moderate, or severe based primarily on the blood pH, bicarbonate, ketones, and alteration of sensorium [3, 5] (Table 1). This table also provides the criteria for the diagnosis of HHS.

Epidemiology

The annual incidence for DKA on population-based studies is reported to be between 4.6 and 8 per thousand patients with diabetes. However, these figures are from reports of the 1980 census [6, 7]. The most recent epidemiological study suggests that the hospitalization rates are about 4–9% on all patients admitted with the diagnosis of diabetes [1]. In one study that included 172 796 admissions to a county teaching hospital from 1981 to 1989, DKA accounted for 28.7% of all patients admitted with a primary diagnosis of diabetes and 6.2% of patients with a secondary diagnosis of diabetes [8]. The mortality rate in the same study was 2.7 and 9.3% for patients with DKA admitted with a primary or secondary diagnosis of diabetes, respectively. These studies are in agreement with the recent national discharge survey showing a mortality rate of 2–5% for DKA [1, 2].

Precipitating Factors

Although the most common precipitating factor for the development of DKA is infection [1, 6, 7, 9], some centers with patients in a lower socioeconomic class have noted that the most common precipitating factor is inadequate insulin or omitted insulin [10–12]. Table 2 summarizes the results of various studies on precipitating factors for DKA [5, 6, 8, 13–17]. Although infection was considered to be the major precipitating event in most series, omission or inadequate dose of insulin accounts for approximately 30% of the precipitating factors in DKA. Urinary tract infection and pneumonia are the most common infections noted as precipitating factors for DKA [5, 9, 18, 19]. About

International Textbook of Diabetes Mellitus, Third Edition. Edited by R. A. DeFronzo, E. Ferrannini, H. Keen, and P. Zimmet.
 ISBN: 0-471-48655-8.

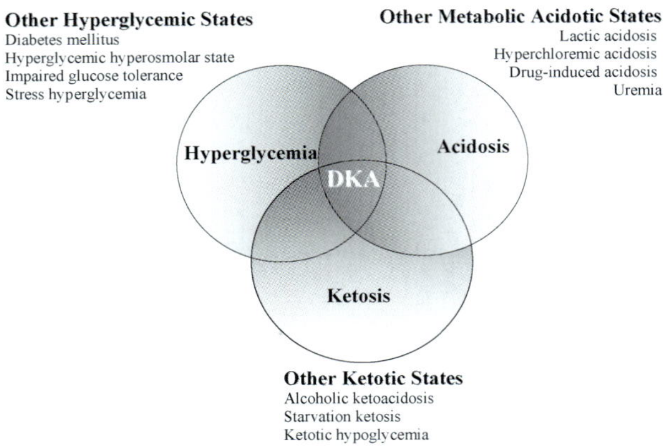

Figure 1 Triad of DKA consists of hyperglycemia, acidosis, and ketosis; and other conditions associated with each of the above components of DKA. (Reproduced by permission of WB Saunders Company/LWW [3])

20% of DKA admissions may be due to undiagnosed diabetes brought about by various conditions including drug and alcohol abuse, cerebrovascular accident, pancreatitis, myocardial infarction, thyroid disorder, and pulmonary embolism [8, 17].

In contrast to popular belief, DKA is more common in adults than in children [20]. In community-based studies, 45% of patients with DKA were older than 44 years and 26% older than 60 years [6, 7]. During the past decade, an increasing number of ketoacidosis cases have been reported in adult African Americans [21, 22, 23] and in other minority ethnic groups [24]. Many of these adult patients with DKA have type 2 diabetes, since the majority of them are obese, have a strong family history of diabetes, and have signs of insulin resistance, measurable insulin secretion, and a low prevalence of autoimmune markers of β-cell destruction [10, 23, 25]. A large number of these patients, after a few months of aggressive insulin therapy, achieve near-normoglycemic remission and can be controlled with diet, or diet and oral hypoglycemic agents [22, 23, 25]. Thus, DKA can no longer be considered a pathognomonic of type 1 diabetes mellitus [5].

Malfunction of continuous subcutaneous insulin infusion (CSII) devices or insulin pumps may lead to DKA, particularly if the problem is not identified early [26]. The overall incidence of DKA during CSII is higher than with conventional insulin injections as shown in the Diabetes Control and Complications Trial (DCCT) study [27], and is more likely to occur during the first few weeks to months of CSII therapy [28]. Most of these cases are caused by inadvertent interruption of insulin delivery or infection [29, 30]. The development of severe hyperglycemia or ketoacidosis can be reduced by increased physician and patient awareness and by the use of frequent home glucose monitoring [28, 31].

Pathogenesis

DKA is the result of an absolute deficiency or ineffective concentration of circulating insulin with concomitant stimulation of counterregulatory hormones, which results in an abnormal metabolism of carbohydrate, protein, and fat as well as disturbances of fluid and electrolyte balances [3, 8, 32]. The temporal relationship of counterregulatory hormones (glucagon, cortisol, catecholamines, growth hormone) to the genesis of metabolic decompensation in DKA is the subject of debate. Data on the role of these hormones are based on the results of studies on acute insulin withdrawal in patients with type 1 diabetes [33–36]. Insulin withdrawal in patients with type 1 leads to complex changes in the circulating concentration of stress hormones [8] (Figure 2), which lead to the activation of protein-kinase-induced stimulation of hormone-sensitive lipase in adipose tissue (37–39). The increased activity of tissue lipase causes breakdown of triglycerides to glycerol and free fatty acids (FFAs). The increased availability of glycerol is utilized as a substrate for gluconeogenesis in the liver and kidney, whereas the massive release of FFAs serves as the main precursor of ketoacids in the liver

Table 1 Diagnostic criteria for DKA and HHS*

	Diagnostic criteria and classification			
	DKA			
	Mild	Moderate	Severe	HHS
Plasma glucose (mg/dl)	>250	>250	>250	>600
Arterial pH	7.25 to 7.30	7.00 to <7.24	<7.00	>7.30
Serum bicarbonate (mEq/l)	15 to 18	10 to <15	<10	>15
Urine ketone†	Positive	Positive	Positive	Small
Serum ketone†	Positive	Positive	Positive	Small
Effective serum osmolality (mOsm/kg)‡	Variable	Variable	Variable	>320
Alteration in sensorium or mental obtundation	Alert	Alert/drowsy	Stupor/coma	Stupor/coma

*(Reproduced by permission of the American Diabetes Association [4]).
† Nitroprusside reaction method.
‡ Calculation: Effective serum osmolality = 2[measured Na (mEq/l)] + glucose (mg/dl)/18.

Table 2 Precipitating factors (% of all cases) for DKA

Study location (Time period)	Ref. no.	Number of episodes	Infections (%)	Concomitant cardiovascular disease (%)	Inadequate insulin rx (%)	New onset (%)	Other (%)	Unknown cause (%)
Frankfurt, Germany	[13]	472	19	6	38	+	+	+
Birmingham, UK (1968–1972)	[14]	258	28	3	23	+	+	+
Erfurt, Germany (1970–1971)	[15]	133	35	4	21	+	+	+
Basel, Switzerland (1968–1978)	[16]	163	56	5	31	+	+	+
Rhode Island, USA (1975–1979)	[6]	152	43	—	26	+	+	+
Memphis, TN, USA (1974–1985)	[8]	202	38	—	28	22	10	4
Atlanta, GA, USA (1993–1994)	[17]	144	28	—	41	17	10	4

Note: + denotes that complete data on these items were not given as total numbers did not reach 100%.
(Reproduced by permission of the American Diabetes Association).

[37, 39, 40]. Increased production of FFAs plays a pivotal role in ketogenesis in DKA [5, 8, 41], by (1) suppressing glycolytic pathway through inhibiting the rate-limiting enzymes of glycolysis (hexokinase, phosphofructokinase, and pyruvate kinase) as well as pyruvate dehydrogenase; (2) increasing production of fatty acyl-CoA, which (a) inhibits the rate-limiting enzyme citrate synthetase, the first step in the TCA (tricarboxylic acid; Krebs) cycle, and (b) stimulates hyperlipidemia through conversion to triacylglycerol; and (c) increases β-oxidation of FFAs, leading to increased ketogenesis.

Carbohydrate Metabolism

As a result of increased counterregulatory hormones, particularly glucagon, and catecholamines, in combination with reduction of insulin, five major pathways of carbohydrate metabolism are affected in DKA:

(1) glycogen synthesis is decreased secondary to reduction in glycogen synthase as a result of insulin deficiency (33);
(2) glycogenolysis is accelerated [32, 42] as a result of stimulation of glycogen phosphorylase through

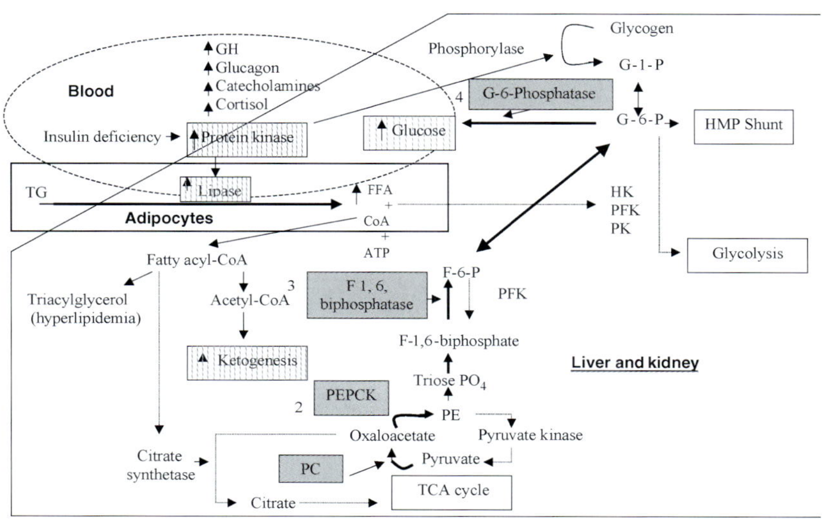

Figure 2 Proposed biochemical pathways in diabetic ketoacidosis, which leads to increased lipolysis, glycogenolysis, ketogenesis, and decreased glycolysis. Lipolysis mainly occurs in adipose tissue. Other events occur mainly in the liver (with the exception of gluconeogenesis which may occur in the kidney). Darker arrows indicate stimulated pathways, and lighter arrows indicate inhibited pathways in DKA. G-1-P = glucose-1-phosphate; G-6-P = glucose-6-phosphate; HK = hexokinase; PFK = phosphofructokinase; PK = pyrvate kinase; HMP = hexomono-phosphate shunt; PEP = phosphoenolpyruvate; PEPCK = phosphoenolpyruvate carboxykinase; FFA = FFAs; GH, growth hormone; ATP = adenosinetriphosphate; TCA = tricarboxylic acid; TG = triglycerides; CoA = coezyme A; CPT-1 = carnitine palmitoyl transferase 1. Gray boxes depict the rate-limiting enzymes in gluconeogenic pathway. Striped boxes depict processes or substrates which are increased in DKA (modified from reference 5)

catecholamines' β-receptor stimulation and cyclic-AMP; glycogen is then broken down to glucose-1-phosphate;

(3) inhibition of glycolysis, as result of FFA-induced inhibition of rate-limiting glycolytic enzymes (see above);
(4) decreased glucose utilization by peripheral tissues as a result of insulin deficiency;
(5) stimulation of gluconeogenesis by activation of four rate-limiting enzymes: (a) pyruvate carboxylase, (b) (c) fructose-1,6-bisphosphatase, and (d) glucose-6-phosphatase [42, 43].

Additionally, increased levels of alanine (in the liver) and glutamine (from the kidney), as a result of increased proteolysis [44, 45]; lactate, as a result of decreased glucose oxidation [33, 44]; and glycerol from increased lipolysis serve as substrates for gluconeogenesis [33]. The hepatic glucose production in DKA may be as much as 500 g/day [46]. Although gluconeogenesis occurs mainly in the liver, the kidneys also contribute to this process in patients with DKA [47]. Increased glucagon/insulin ratio also (a) inhibits the level of fructose-2,6-biphosphate, leading to a stimulation of fructose-1,6-biphosphatase, (b) stimulation of phosphoenolpyruvate carboxykinase, and (c) stimulation of glucose-6-phosphatase. Thus, the initial counterregulatory hormone response to acute insulin withdrawal appears to be primarily a combination of increased glucagon and catecholamines and decreased free insulin [5]. The combination of the above five pathways leads to hyperglycemia in DKA.

Fat and Ketone Body Metabolism

With decreased availability of insulin, the major antilipolytic hormone, and increased counterregulatory hormones such as catecholamines, glucagon, cortisol, and growth hormone, there is an accelerated breakdown of triglycerides to glycerol and FFAs through activation of hormone-sensitive lipase [37–39, 48]. Glycerol, which serves as a carbon skeleton for gluconeogenesis and accelerated production of FFAs, leads to its further β-oxidation to ketone bodies. This process is predominantly stimulated by glucagon [32, 49]. FFAs are also converted to triacylglycerol, which may lead to increased very low density lipoprotein production and hyperlipidemia. In DKA, the combination of increased glucagon and low insulin levels decreases liver malonyl-CoA because of a reduction in hepatic carnitine. Reduced malonyl-CoA will permit activation of the rate-limiting enzyme of ketogenesis, carnitine palmitoyltransferase 1 (CPT-1), which allows transesterification of fatty acyl carnitine and oxidation of FFAs to ketone bodies [39, 41, 45, 49]. CPT-1 is necessary to move FFAs into the mitochondria [41, 49, 50]. Thus, ketone body production is accelerated as a result of increased fatty acyl-CoA and CPT-1 activity. In addition, metabolism and clearance of these bodies are decreased in DKA [51–53].

Although some studies have suggested that the increased level of glucagon or the ratio of glucagon to insulin is the major stimulator of ketogenesis [41, 49, 50, 54], the role of a physiologic dose of glucagon in ketogenesis is not certain [55]. In addition, some studies have suggested that a synergistic effect of certain counterregulatory hormones, in the absence of insulin, may stimulate ketogenesis [5, 56]. These biochemical pathways are depicted in Figure 2 [8].

Protein and Amino Acid Metabolism

Negative nitrogen balance is the hallmark of DKA, which was described in the original work of Atchley et al. [57], Butler et al. [58], and Nabarro et al. [59]. These pioneers demonstrated that insulin deficiency results in a loss of 9–12 g of nitrogen per day, with slow recovery after insulin therapy. Furthermore, it was shown that during insulin withdrawal, the levels of gluconeogenic amino acids (glutamine, alanine, threonine, serine, glutamate, and glycine) were decreased but levels of ketogenic amino acids (such as leucine, valine, and isoleucine) were increased during DKA [60, 61]. It has been suggested that both increased proteolysis and decreased protein synthesis are responsible for these observations, but the detailed mechanism for these steps is not clearly elucidated. However, increased levels of glucagon and cortisol appear to play major synergistic roles [62–64].

Water and Electrolyte Metabolism

Table 3 illustrates electrolyte and water deficits in DKA as well as in HHS [54, 65]. The severe derangement of water and electrolytes in DKA and HHS is the result of insulin deficiency, hyperglycemia, and hyperketonemia. Hyperglycemia leads to glycosuria and osmotic diuresis when the renal threshold of glucose (~200 mg/dl) is exceeded. The osmotic effects of glucosuria result in impairment of NaCl and H_2O reabsorption in the proximal

Table 3 Typical total body deficits of water and electrolytes in DKA and HHS*

	DKA	HHS
Total water (l)	6	9
Water (ml/kg)†	100	100–200
Na^+ (mEq/kg)	7–10	5–13
Cl^- (mEq/kg)	3–5	5–15
K^+ (mEq/kg)	3–5	4–6
PO_4 (mmol/kg)	5–7	3–7
Mg^{2+} (mEq/kg)	1–2	1–2
Ca^{2+} (mEq/kg)	1–2	1–2

* Data from references 54 and 65.
† Per kg of body weight.

tubule and loop of Henle, resulting in loss of water, sodium, potassium, as well as other electrolytes [57, 66]. In addition, insulin deficiency *per se* may also contribute to renal losses of water, sodium, potassium, and ammonium salts because insulin stimulates salt and water reabsorption in the proximal and distal nephron [66–68]. However, in DKA, the osmotic effects of urinary ketoanion excretion are half that of glucose excretion, which makes the loss of water much less in DKA than in HHS [68]. Therefore, in DKA, the net loss of minerals such as potassium, sodium, calcium, magnesium, chloride, and phosphate can be replaced adequately by the use of sodium, potassium, or chloride, but other minerals require days to be replenished. During the development of DKA, intracellular dehydration also occurs as hyperglycemia and water loss lead to increased plasma tonicity, leading to a shift of water out of cells. This shift of water is also associated with a shift of potassium out of cells into the extracellular space. Potassium shifts are further enhanced by the presence of acidosis and the breakdown of intracellular protein secondary to insulin deficiency [69]. Furthermore, entry of potassium into cells is impaired in the presence of insulinopenia. Marked renal potassium losses occur as a result of osmotic diuresis and ketonuria. Progressive volume depletion leads to decreased glomerular filtration rate and greater retention of glucose and ketoanions in the plasma [32]. During treatment of DKA with insulin, hydrogen ions are consumed as ketoanion metabolism is facilitated. This process contributes to regeneration of bicarbonate, correction of metabolic acidosis, and a decrease in plasma anion gap. The urinary loss of ketoanions, as sodium and potassium salts, therefore represents the loss of potential bicarbonate [70], which is gradually recovered within a few days or weeks.

Pathophysiologic Basis of Clinical Presentation

In DKA, an absolute insulin deficiency coupled with a concomitant elevation of counterregulatory hormones leads to a series of events, which is initiated by the stimulation of hormone-sensitive lipase. This leads to an increased production of excess FFAs that, upon presentation to the liver, inhibits glycolysis and also stimulates conversion to triacylglycerol and hyperlipidemia (in certain cases) [5, 42]. β-Oxidation of FFAs also results in increased ketogenesis, which is followed by ketonemia and ketonuria. Ketonuria consumes positively charged cations such as Na^+, K^+, and NH_4^+. Hydrogen ions are then titrated by bicarbonate, resulting in acidosis.

Of the three ketone bodies, β-hydroxybutyrate, acetoacetate, and acetone, the former two are the stronger acids, and the level of β-hydroxybutyrate is about three times greater than that of acetoacetate [8]. During therapy of DKA, because of a higher oxidation rate of acetoacetate to β-hydroxybutyrate, there is a greater amount of conversion of acetoacetate to β-hydroxybutyrate. Acetoacetate and acetone are the only two ketones that react with nitroprusside. Thus the use of nitroprusside test for follow-up of DKA may be misleading [5, 8]. As stated earlier, the hyperglycemia of DKA is the result of increased gluconeogenesis (both in the liver and in the kidney), glycogenolysis (through activation of phosphorylase), and decreased glucose utilization by muscle and fat tissues. Hyperglycemia results in glycosuria, osmotic diuresis, and loss of water, glucose, and electrolytes. Thus, patients in DKA feel thirsty and hungry and are dehydrated. Severely malnourished and dehydrated patients with DKA may have further deterioration of their kidney functions, resulting in a greater anion gap, higher ketonemia, lower ketonuria, and less hyperchloremic acidosis [71]. Figure 3 provides a synopsis of these events in both DKA and HHS [8].

Diagnostic Procedures

History and Physical Examination

The clinical evaluation of patients with DKA consists of a prompt and careful medical history and physical examination with attention to all body systems [3–5, 8, 18]. Of particular importance is the assessment of precipitating events and the state of hydration, which delineates the priorities for therapeutic options and laboratory procedures. Development of signs and symptoms are rapid with polyuria, polydipsia, and weight loss. Acidosis stimulates the medullary respiratory center, thereby resulting in deep Kussmaul respirations. Acetone, a volatile ketoacid, is noted by its characteristic fruity odor on the patient's breath. Dehydration and osmotic diuresis result in dry mucous membranes, orthostasis, tachycardia, and loss of skin turgor. In DKA, unless there is an increase in serum osmolality above 300 mOsm/kg, there is very little change in mentation. However, approximately one third of DKA patients may present in a hyperosmolar state in which case their mental state may be correlated to the level of serum osmolality [72].

Abdominal pain, sometimes mimicking an acute abdomen, is reported in 40–75% of cases of DKA [73, 74]. The etiology of the abdominal pain in most patients could not be identified by clinical and radiological studies, but the pain spontaneously resolves after resolution of ketoacidosis. The presence of abdominal pain in patients with DKA correlates with the severity of metabolic acidosis, but not with the initial blood glucose level or severity of dehydration. In a prospective study of 200 patients with hyperglycemic crises, abdominal pain was present in 86% of patients with serum bicarbonate ≤ 5 mmol/l, in 66% of patients with serum bicarbonate levels 5 to <10 mmol/l, in 36% of patients with bicarbonate levels 10 to <15 mmol/l, and in 13% of patients with bicarbonate levels 15–18 mmol/l [74]. Patients with DKA and

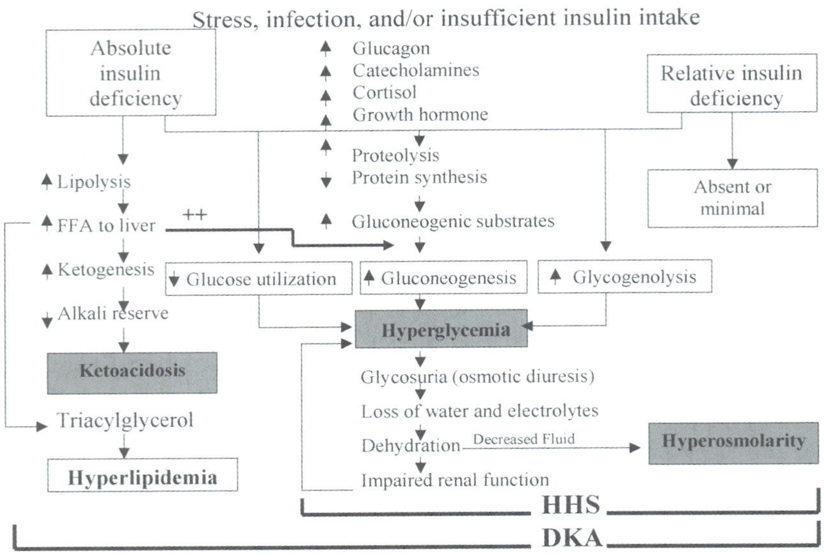

Figure 3 Pathogenesis of DKA and HHS (adopted from reference 8)

abdominal pain had a more frequent history of alcohol and cocaine abuse than those without abdominal pain. In that study, none of the 11 patients with HHS presented with abdominal pain despite an admission mean blood glucose level greater than 1000 mg/dl and a mean serum osmolality greater than 350 mOsm/kg.

In spite of infection, which occurs in a considerable number of patients, the presence of fever is rare, as patients may present with hypothermia due to either vasodilatation of the skin or low fuel substrate levels.

Laboratory Evaluation

The type of laboratory assessments for DKA will be determined largely by the history, physical examination, and precipitating event(s). The initial laboratory evaluation should include determination of arterial blood gases, blood glucose, blood urinary nitrogen (BUN), serum electrolytes, creatinine, ketones, osmolality, and urinalysis as well as a complete blood count with differential and bacterial culture for various tissues, as indicated. While waiting for the laboratory tests, an initial blood glucose test by finger stick as well as a dipstick urinalysis for glucose, ketone, nitrite, and leukocyte esterase can give the clinician an insight into the severity and precipitating factors leading to metabolic decompensation.

Because of the rather restrictive criteria for the diagnosis of DKA in the past, the recent ADA guidelines have provided three classification levels of DKA to outline different approaches to therapy, depending on the degree of ketoacidosis (Table 1).

The plasma anion gap, which is not a criterion for diagnosis, is calculated by subtracting the major measured anions (chloride and bicarbonate) from the major measured cation (sodium). The normal anion gap has been historically reported to be 12 ± 2 mEq/l [3, 17]. Most laboratories, however, currently measure sodium and chloride concentrations using ion-specific electrodes, which measure plasma chloride concentration 2–6 mEq/l higher than with prior methods [75]. Thus, the normal anion gap using the current methodology is between 7 and 9 mEq/l, and an anion gap $>$ 10–12 mEq/l indicates the presence of increased anion gap acidosis [4]. Although most subjects with DKA present with a high anion gap acidosis, some patients present with mixed acid–base disorders. It has been reported that 46% of patients admitted with DKA had predominant anion gap acidosis, 43% had mixed anion gap acidosis and hyperchloremic metabolic acidosis, and 11% had hyperchloremic metabolic acidosis [71]. During treatment, a transient hyperchloremic nonanion gap metabolic acidosis has been reported in the majority of patients [76, 77].

Effective osmolality can be calculated by the following formula: 2[measured Na^+ (mEq/l)] + glucose (mg/dl)/18. BUN, in general, is not used for calculation of effective osmolality but may be used for calculation of total osmolality. The sodium concentration in DKA is not adjusted to the glucose concentration for calculation of osmolality. However, the sodium concentration should be adjusted by glucose concentration for clinical treatment decisions when assessing actual serum sodium concentration.

Laboratory Pitfalls

Clinical assessment of ketonuria and ketonemia has traditionally been done by the use of the nitroprusside tablet or Ketostix, which only reacts with acetoacetate and acetone. Thus the most prevalent ketone body, beta-hydroxybutyrate, is not measured. Furthermore, during therapy, β-hydroxybutyrate is converted to acetoacetate, which if used as an indication of DKA recovery, will be misleading. The recent availability of self-glucose monitoring systems, which also contain a mechanism for measurement of β-hydroxybutyrate by finger stick, is a marked improvement in the management of patients with DKA [78, 79].

Leukocytosis, which is a hallmark of DKA, may not be indicative of an infectious process, particularly when total white blood cell counts are below 25 000 [18, 80]. The reason for this elevation has not been established. The majority of white cells in leukocystosis are granulocytes with no detectable eosinophil counts (as a result of hypercortisolism). Leukocystosis (total white blood cell counts > 25 000) requires further assessment for an underlying infection. The admission serum sodium is usually low because of the osmotic flux of water from the intracellular to the extracellular space in the presence of hyperglycemia. An increase in serum sodium concentration in the presence of hyperglycemia indicates a rather profound degree of water loss. To assess the severity of sodium and water deficit, serum sodium may be corrected by adding 1.6 mg/dl to the measured serum sodium for each 100 mg/dl of glucose above 100 mg/dl [32]. Extreme hypertriglyceridemia, which may be present during the DKA due to impaired lipoprotein lipase activity, may cause lipemic serum with spurious lowering of serum sodium (pseudohyponatremia) [82]. Abnormally low glucose may be seen in severe hypertriglyceridemia [81]; this however needs to be reassessed by high centrifugal forces so as to separate the plasma from the lipid layer. Serum potassium may also be high as a result of cellular dehydration and shift of potassium from the cell to the extracellular space [83]. Hyperkalemia may also be partially due to the breakdown of intracellular protein secondary to insulin deficiency. Serum creatinine in DKA may be artificially elevated in the presence of excess ketone bodies if a colorimetric assay is used for this measurement as ketone bodies interfere with this assay [84].

Other laboratory abnormalities in patients with DKA include hyperamylasemia, which has been reported in 21–79% of cases [85, 86]. There is little correlation between the presence, degree, or isoenzyme type of hyperamylasemia and the presence of gastrointestinal symptoms, triglyceride concentration, or pancreatic imaging studies [85, 87]. The cause of hyperamylasemia in DKA is postulated to be multifactorial; the most important causes include the existence of salivary amylase, reduced renal clearance of amylase, and increased leakage from acinar cell secondary to neural and metabolic disturbances. Nonspecific serum lipase elevation has also been noted in 29–41% of patients with DKA in the absence of clinical or radiological evidence of acute pancreatitis [88]. Recent studies have shown decreased serum leptin in obese and thin patients with DKA as well as obese hyperglycemic patients. These levels normalize after correction of hyperglycemia [89]. Furthermore, recent studies on proinflammatory factors in hyperglycemic crises demonstrate significant increases in TNF α, IL-1, IL-6, and IL-8 [90]. These increased cytokines are also associated with *de novo* emergence of growth factor in activated T-lymphocytes for insulin, IGF-1 and IL-2 [91].

HYPERGLYCEMIC HYPEROSMOLAR STATE

Definition

Hyperglycemic hyperosmolar syndrome (HHS) was first described by Dreschfed [92] over a century ago, but this condition received little attention until 1957, when Sament and Schwartz [93] reported their experience of a diabetic syndrome characterized by marked stupor without ketosis (diabetic hyperosmolar syndrome). HHS is one of the most serious acute complications of diabetes and represents an important cause of morbidity among patients with diabetes. Hyperglycemia in HHS is usually more severe than in DKA (see Table 1). The hyperglycemia is associated with normal bicarbonate and a normal pH. Ketosis by nitroprusside method is usually negative, but may be mildly positive. Altered sensorium (lethargy, stupor, coma) correlates better with hyperosmolality than with patient's age or severity of acid–base disturbance. Several reports have shown that the mean total serum osmolality in patients who presented in coma is greater than 340 mmol/kg, and that levels are higher than in noncomatose patients [8, 21, 65, 72, 94]. Hence, the term *hyperosmolar nonketotic coma* does not accurately depict the nature of the disease state, since not all patients are comatose or free of ketones [95]. Therefore, a more apt description for this syndrome is hyperglycemic hyperosmolar state (HHS) as defined by the ADA guideline [3].

Epidemiology

Although epidemiological reports on HHS are sparse, data collected from 1979 to 1981 by an NIH data group suggest an incidence of 10 cases per 100 000 of the general population (1). This is about one sixth that of DKA. More recently, the incidence of HHS in two different teaching institutions in the United States was 0.05% of all diabetes-related admissions [8, 21]. Mortality attributed to HHS is considerably higher than with DKA, with recent mortality rates of 5–35%, most likely depending on the underlying illness or co-morbidities [1, 7, 8, 96].

Precipitating and Predisposing Factors

In general, subjects with HHS have a longer history of symptoms of hyperglycemia and patients present to the emergency room with an altered mental status [65]. The typical patient with HHS has undiagnosed type 2 diabetes, is between 55 and 70 years old, and frequently is a nursing home resident or someone who has delayed seeking medical attention [95].

Infection is the major precipitating factor occurring in 30–60% of patients, with urinary tract infections and pneumonia being the most common infections [65, 94]. HHS is the initial manifestation of diabetes in 7–17% of patients [21, 65]. Other precipitating causes of HHS include an acute illness, such as cerebrovascular accident or myocardial infarction, that provokes the release of counterregulatory hormones and/or compromises access to water. Certain medications that cause DKA may also precipitate the development of HHS, including glucocorticoid, thiazide diuretics, dilantin, and β-blockers [97, 98] (Table 4).

Table 4 Predisposing or precipitating factors for HHS*

Acute illness
Acute infection (32–60%)
Pneumonia
Urinary tract infection
Sepsis
Cerebral vascular accident
Myocardial infarction
Acute pancreatitis
Acute pulmonary edema
Intestinal obstruction
Dialysis, peritoneal
Mesenteric thrombosis
Renal failure
Heat stroke
Hypothermia
Subdural hematoma
Severe burns
Endocrine
Acromegaly
Thyrotoxicosis
Cushing's syndrome
Drugs/therapy
β-Adrenergic blockers
Calcium channel blockers
Chlorpromazine
Cimetidine
Diazoxide
Diuretics
Encainide
Ethacrynic acid
Immunosuppressive agents
L-Asparaginase
Loxapine
Phenytoin
Propranolol
Steroids
Total parenteral nutrition
Previously undiagnosed diabetes

*(Reproduced by permission of the American Diabetes Association [65]).

Pathogenesis

The underlying pathogenic mechanism for HHS is a reduction in the net effective concentration of circulating insulin and a concomitant elevation of counterregulatory or stress hormones such as glucagon, catecholamines, cortisol, and growth hormone in association with severe dehydration [8, 32, 65, 95]. DKA and HHS represent opposite ends of the spectrum of hyperglycemia with and without ketosis respectively. However, mixed mild ketotic hyperosmolar conditions may exist [8, 21, 72, 95, 99]. In one report approximately one third of DKA patients were also hyperosmolar [72].

Several mechanisms have been proposed to explain the absence or minimal presence of ketosis in patients with HHS. Key differences between DKA and HHS include (1) higher levels of endogenous insulin reserve in HHS (i.e., adequate insulin concentration to prevent lipolysis but inadequate to inhibit hepatic glucose production and/or stimulate glucose use), (2) lower levels of counterregulatory hormones and FFAs in HHS, and (3) inhibition of lipolysis by the hyperosmolar state, thereby decreasing ketogenesis [45, 100–102]. Early studies suggested that the level of FFAs, cortisol, and growth hormone were lower in HHS than in DKA [45]. However, a subsequent study by Chupin et al. [101] comparing 12 cases of HHS and 22 cases of DKA confirmed a higher level of growth hormone, but revealed no significant difference in either FFAs or cortisol in the two groups. Although earlier studies were not able to demonstrate differences in pancreatic insulin secretion between patients with HHS and DKA, it is important to note that prior to 1980, the measurement of insulin was not specific and could not separate proinsulin from insulin and a standardized C-peptide assay was not used. More recent studies [101] have demonstrated a higher level of C-peptide in HHS than in DKA (Table 5). Similar results were observed recently in lean African American patients with DKA as compared to obese DKA and obese nonketotic hyperglycemia state [10, 25] (Table 6). Therefore, the most likely reason for the lack of ketoacidosis in HHS appears to be a higher level of pancreatic reserve (as determined by C-peptide) than in DKA. This is due to the fact that the antilipolytic effect of insulin is about one tenth of that of glucose utilization [103, 104]. Another potential mechanism for the lack of ketosis in HHS involves the effect of hyperosmolality on inhibiting lipolysis, insulin secretion, and glucose uptake [105].

A major cause of HHS in older patients may be related to their inability to recognize the need for water [106], and therefore, hyperglycemia results in accelerated dehydration. Hepatic glucose production in HHS is higher than that in DKA and may be as high as 1 kg/day [46]. Equally important is the glomerular filtration rate, which may be decreased with increasing age, exacerbating the

Table 5 Admission biochemical data in patients with HHS or DKA[†*]

	Mean ± SEM	
Parameters measured	HHS ($n = 12$)	DKA ($n = 22$)
Glucose (mg/dl)	930 ± 83	616 ± 36
Na^+ (mEq/l)	149 ± 3.2	134 ± 1.0
K^+ (mEq/l)	3.9 ± 0.2	4.5 ± 0.13
BUN (mg/dl)	61 ± 11	32 ± 3
Creatinine (mg/dl)	1.4 ± 0.1	1.1 ± 0.1
pH	7.3 ± 0.03	7.12 ± 0.04
Bicarbonate (mEq/l)	18 ± 1.1	9.4 ± 1.4
3-β-Hydroxybutyrate (mM)	1.0 ± 0.2	9.1 ± 0.85
Total osmolality[†]	380 ± 5.7	323 ± 2.5
IRI (nM)[‡]	0.08 ± 0.01	0.07 ± 0.01
C-peptide (nM)	1.14 ± 0.1	0.21 ± 0.03
FFA (nM)	1.5 ± 0.19	1.6 ± 0.16
Human growth hormone (ng/ml)	1.9 ± 0.2	6.1 ± 1.2
Cortisol (ng/ml)	570 ± 49	500 ± 61
IRI (nM)[§]	0.27 ± 0.05	0.09 ± 0.01
C-peptide (nM)[§]	1.75 ± 0.23	0.25 ± 0.05

* Data are from reference 98.
† According to the formula: 2(Na + K) + urea (mM) + glucose (mM).
‡ IRI = immunoreactive insulin.
§ Values following IV administration of tolbutamide.

level of hyperglycemia, decreasing intravascular space, and leading to tachycardia and hypotension. Studies in a group of comatose and noncomatose patients with DKA showed that those who were comatose had higher serum BUN, lower blood pressure, and high serum osmolality than noncomatose patients, but no significant differences were noted in blood pH, ketone bodies, serum cortisol, or glucagons [99].

Diagnosis

As shown in Table 1, the diagnosis of HHS is characterized by a higher level of glucose levels, absence of metabolic acidosis, minimal or negative ketosis, and higher serum osmolality [4]. These patients are obtunded more often than DKA patients. Furthermore, biochemical data on admission suggest slightly higher sodium, BUN, creatinine, osmolality, and possibly higher serum lactate levels than in DKA (Table 5).

Pathophysiologic Basis of Clinical Presentation

In the pathogenesis of HHS, there is a relative (rather than absolute) deficiency of insulin and greater dehydration, as shown in Figure 3 and Table 5, than in DKA. The major differences between these two hyperglycemic emergencies are the absence of severe ketosis and acidosis, and greater losses of fluids and electrolytes in HHS than in DKA. However, approximately 50% of HHS patients still have an increased anion gap secondary to mild acidosis or increased lactate [95].

Differential Diagnosis

Patients may present with metabolic conditions resembling DKA or HHS, which emphasizes the need for laboratory and physical evaluation to assess the metabolic causes of various acidosis and coma. Patients with alcoholic ketoacidosis (AKA), with an initial concentration of insulin or counterregulatory hormones similar to those of subjects with DKA, have a normal or low blood glucose concentration, equal or slightly lower total ketone bodies, but higher β-hydroxybutyrate to acetoacetate and lactate to pyruvate ratios compared to patients with AKA [77, 107]. The absence of hyperglycemia in AKA results from the combination of prolonged starvation with glycogen depletion [107] and impaired gluconeogenesis due to decreased nicotinamide adenosine dinucleotide (NAD), a cofactor critical for the utilization of gluconeogenic precursors [108]. In the liver, as alcohol is metabolized to acetaldehyde by the enzyme alcohol dehydrogenase,

Table 6 Clinical characteristics and pancreatic C-peptide of DKA and hyperglycemia subjects vs. controls*

	Lean DKA	Obese DKA	Obese hyperglycemia	Obese control
n	54	77	51	25
Age (years)	36 ± 2	40 ± 2	46 ± 2	38 ± 2
Sex (M/F)	34/20	49/28	34/17	9/16
New-onset diabetes (% of total)	15 (28)	64 (83)	40 (78)	—
BMI (kg/m^2)	22 ± 1	37 ± 1	37 ± 1	30 ± 2
Glucose (mmol/1)	36 ± 2	36 ± 2	37 ± 2	5 ± 1
Venous pH	7.18 ± 0.02	7.24 ± 0.01	7.4 ± 0.01	—
Bicarbonate (mEq/l)	12 ± 1	14 ± 1	22 ± 1	24 ± 2
HbA_{1c} (%)	13.0 ± 0.4	13.5 ± 0.4	12.4 ± 0.4	5.4 ± 0.1
Basal C-peptide (ng/ml)	0.5 ± 0.1[†]	1.5 ± 0.1	1.8 ± 0.1	1.9 ± 0.1
Stimulated C-peptide[‡]	0.6 ± 0.1[†]	2.5 ± 0.1	3.5 ± 0.3[†]	4.2 ± 0.3
Acute C-peptide response[‡]	0.2 ± 0.13[†]	1.0 ± 0.1	1.7 ± 0.2[†]	2.3 ± 0.2

Note: Data are means ± SEM.
* From reference 25.
† $P < 0.01$ vs. obese DKA.
‡ In response to IV glucagon stimulation.

NAD is reduced to nicotinamide adenine dinucleotide (NADH) [109]. The increase in NADH/NAD ratio alters the cellular redox state and results in impaired gluconeogenesis and a shift in the β-hydroxybutyrate/acetoacetate equilibrium reaction toward β-hydroxybutyrate formation [108, 110].

Patients with a low intake of food (less than 500 k/cal/day) may present with mild ketoacidosis (starvation ketosis) [111]. However, a healthy subject is able to adapt to prolonged fasting by increasing the clearance of ketone bodies in peripheral tissues and by enhancing the kidneys' ability to excrete ammonium to compensate for the increased ketoacid production [112]. Patients with starvation ketosis rarely present with serum bicarbonate concentration less than 18, and do not exhibit hyperglycemia [111].

DKA must also be distinguished from other causes of high anion gap acidosis, including lactic acidosis, chronic renal failure as well as ingestion of drugs such as salicylate, methanol, and ethylene glycol. These conditions have been reviewed elsewhere [5, 113, 114] and the laboratory findings are presented in Table 7.

TREATMENT OF HYPERGLYCEMIC CRISES

Because DKA and HHS have essentially the same underlying pathogenesis consisting of insufficient insulin and loss of fluid and electrolytes, the major therapeutic goals include (1) improvement of organ perfusion by increasing circulatory volume, (2) gradual reduction of osmolality, (3) gradual correction of serum glucose, (4) clearance of both serum and urine of ketones, and (5) normalization of electrolytes levels. As stated in many previous reviews [3, 5, 17, 18, 25, 32, 59, 96, 114, 116, 117], careful and frequent monitoring of these patients every 30–60 min for the first 4 h and subsequently every hour is the most important aspect of management of patients with hyperglycemic crises. Figures 4 and 5 summarize the algorithm for the treatment of DKA and HHS [3].

Hydration and Fluid Therapy

As reported by previous investigators, hydration in hyperglycemia crises alone has been shown to increase extra cellular volume [118], lower serum glucose, decrease hyperosmolality, reduce circulating levels of counterregulatory hormones [72, 119], and improve insulin resistance [120]. Because of severe loss of intravascular volume and electrolytes in both DKA and HHS, the initial fluid therapy should be one liter of isotonic saline, which will expand extracellular fluid and restore renal perfusion [118]. The rate of isotonic solution should be given at 15–20 ml/kg/h. The tonicity and volume of subsequent sodium chloride solutions should be determined by the state of hydration and by the corrected serum sodium value (Figures 4 and 5). In general, 0.45% sodium chloride solution after the initial normal saline will expand intracellular and interstitial space volume and normalize the contracted volume within a few hours, and should continue until blood glucose reaches 250 mg/dl in DKA or 300 mg/dl in HHS [5]. At this time, the hydrating fluid should be changed to 5–10% glucose-containing saline with a concomitant reduction of insulin to 0.05–0.1 units/kg/h. Plasma glucose levels should remain ~200 mg/dl until bicarbonate and pH reach normal levels in DKA and serum osmolality and mental status in patients with HHS is normalized. There is some evidence that the use of 10% dextrose solutions may enhance clearance of ketone bodies faster than 5% glucose [117].

Insulin Therapy

Low-dose insulin therapy, which was reported as early as 1923 [121], and subsequently in the 1970s [122, 123], is the method of choice for both DKA and HHS. Randomized control trials have indicated that low-dose insulin therapy is preferable to high-dose insulin administration with lower incidence of hyperglycemia and hypokalemia [124] and is effective by any route with [125] and without [126] the use of albumin in the infusion system. The efficacy of low-dose therapy in children was also demonstrated in prospective randomized trials [127, 128]. Since DKA is now classified as mild, moderate, and severe, the method of therapeutic approach may be different for each. Thus with careful monitoring, most patients with mild to moderate DKA can be managed by IM or SC insulin injections on an hourly or 2-hourly basis in general wards as long as (1) there is an available quick turnaround method of laboratory assessment for glucose and electrolytes and (2) there is a knowledgeable team of health care providers on site. Severe DKA as well as HHS patients should be admitted to an intensive care unit (ICU) setting such as a stepdown unit or ICU facility where frequent monitoring and emergency care are available. This is due to the fact that there are no data on the comparative efficacy of such parameters on outcome, morbidity, or recovery time of severe cases of DKA or HHS in a general ward setting versus an ICU. Availability of a glucose meter with the capability of measuring glucose and β-hydroxybutyrate by finger stick has made the follow-up of patients with DKA, even in a general ward, quite feasible, and should be utilized in place of the nitroprusside test for assessment of β-hydroxybutyrate level.

As shown in Figures 4 and 5, the IV insulin protocol requires an initial bolus of regular insulin of 0.15 unit/kg body weight, followed by a continuous infusion of regular insulin at a dose of 0.1 unit/kg/h (5–10 units/h). This will result in a fairly predictable decrease in plasma glucose concentration at a rate of 65–125 mg/h [8, 54]. When

Table 7 Laboratory evaluation of metabolic causes of acidosis and coma*

	Starvation or high fat intake	DKA	Lactic acidosis	Uremic acidosis	Alcoholic ketosis (starvation)	Salicylate Intoxication	Methanol or ethylene glycol intoxication	Hyperosmolar coma	Hypoglycemic coma	Rhabdomyolysis
pH	Normal			Mild		†		Normal	Normal	Mild may be
Plasma glucose	Normal		Normal	Normal	Normal	Normal	Normal	>500 mg/dl	<30 mg/dl	Normal
Glycosuria	Negative	++	Negative	Negative	Negative	Negative‡	Negative	++	Negative	Negative
Total plasma ketones§	Slight		Normal	Normal	Slight to moderate	Normal	Normal	Normal or slight	Normal or slight	Normal
Anion gap	Slight			Slight				Normal	Normal or slight	
Osmolality	Normal		Normal		Normal	Normal		>330 mOsm/kg	Normal	Normal or slight
Uric acid	Mild (starvation)		Normal	Normal		Normal	Normal	Normal	Normal	
Miscellaneous		May give false-positive for ethylene glycol‖	Serum lactate >7 mmol/l	BUN >200 mg/dl		Serum salicylate positive	Serum levels positive			Myoglobinuria, hemoglobinuria

Note: +, positive.
* From reference 5.
† Acetest and Ketostix measure acetoacetic acid only, thus, misleading low values may be obtained because the majority of "ketone bodies" are β-hydroxybutyrate.
‡ Respiratory alkalosis/metabolic acidosis.
§ May get false-positive or false-negative urinary glucose caused by the presence of salicylate or its metabolites.
‖ From reference 113. All other data are from reference 115.
(Reproduced by permission of the American Diabetes Association).

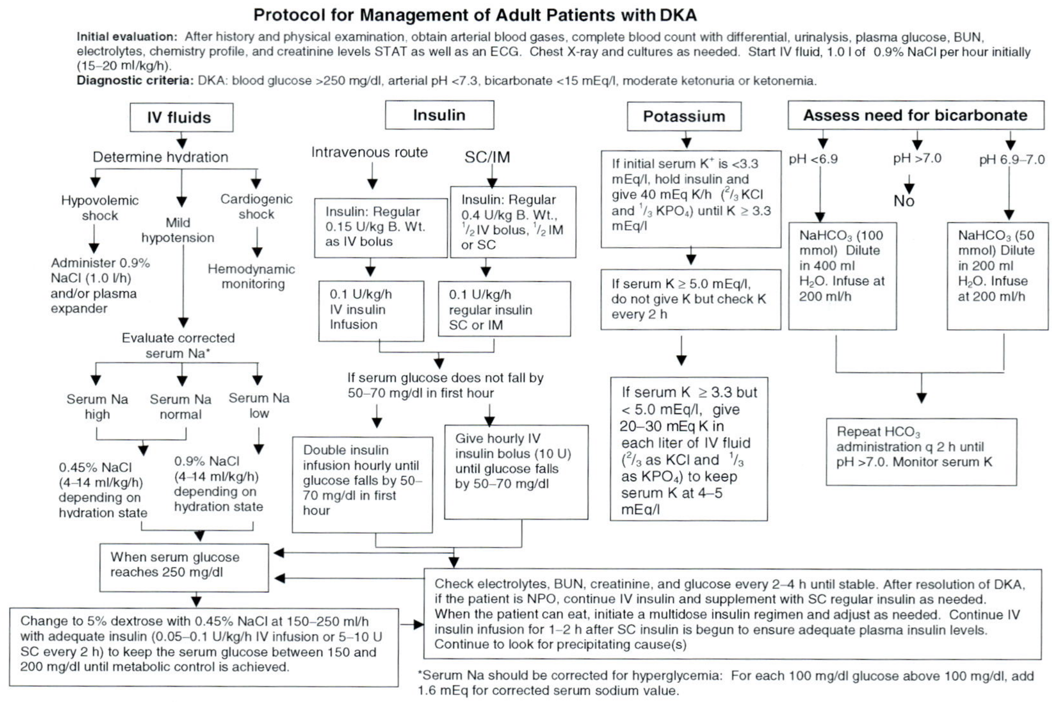

Figure 4 ADA guidelines for management of DKA in adults. (Reproduced by permission of the American Diabetes Association [4])

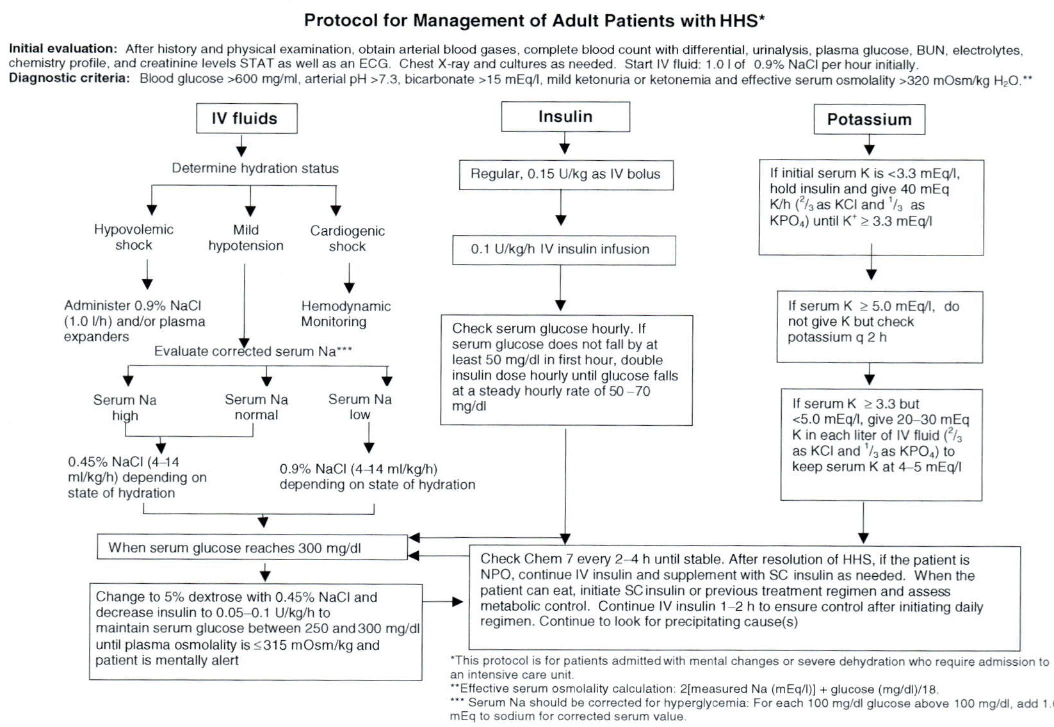

Figure 5 ADA guidelines for management of HHS in adults. (Reproduced by permission of the American Diabetes Association [4])

plasma glucose levels reach 250 mg/dl in DKA or 300 mg/dl in HHS, the insulin infusion rate is reduced to 0.05 unit/kg/h (3–5 units/h), and dextrose (5–10%) should be added to IV fluids. Thereafter, the rate of insulin administration may need to be adjusted to maintain the above glucose values until ketoacidosis or mental obtundation and hyperosmolality are resolved. During therapy, capillary blood glucose should be determined every 1–2 h at the bedside using a glucose oxidase reagent strip; and blood should be drawn every 2–4 h for serum electrolytes, glucose, blood urea nitrogen, creatinine, magnesium, phosphorus, and venous pH. A conscious patient with mild DKA could be treated with SC or IM insulin in a general hospital ward. In such patients, the administration of regular insulin every 1–2 h by the SC or IM route has been shown to be as effective in lowering blood glucose and ketone bodies concentration as giving the entire insulin dose by IV infusion without addition of albumin [125, 126]. However, low-dose IM or SC insulin alone does not seem to clear serum ketones as quickly as the same dose of IV insulin [125, 126, 129]. Such patients should receive the recommended initial "priming" dose of regular insulin of 0.4 unit/kg body weight, given half as an IV bolus and half as an SC or IM injection (Figures 4 and 5). Blood insulin levels using IM and SC route may take 1–2 h before reaching postprandial physiologic levels (70–100 microunits/ml), whereas IV insulin reaches supraphysiologic insulin level in a few minutes [124, 129]. The combined use of IV and SC (or IM) insulin is an acceptable therapeutic approach in a non-ICU setting [124, 126].

Recent prospective randomized studies comparing the use of rapid-acting insulin (lispro) SC route versus IV infusion in the ICU, in mild to moderate DKA patients, has been reported to be as effective as a standard IV low-dose regular insulin protocol [130]. In this preliminary study, the mean time of insulin treatment to correct hyperglycemia and ketoacidosis was similar between SC lispro and IV infusion of regular insulin. Further studies are needed to demonstrate the efficacy and safety of this procedure in general medical wards.

Potassium

The deficit of potassium in both DKA and HHS is the most profound and serious electrolyte imbalance. In spite of a low total body potassium concentration, the admission serum potassium may be normal or elevated [32, 83]. Although fluid therapy and insulin correct hypokalemia, replacement of potassium at the beginning of therapy is of utmost importance. Potassium supplementation should start before the initiation of the insulin therapy, particularly in those patients whose potassium on admission is below 3.3 mEq/l [131]. In patients whose initial potassium level is <3.3 mEq/l, insulin administration should be withheld until the serum potassium level is demonstrated to be ≥3.3 mEq/l in adult patients. Such patients should receive potassium chloride at 20–40 mEq/l in the first hour, and thereafter, 20–30 mEq/l is needed to maintain plasma potassium levels between 4 and 5 mEq/l. We recommend electrocardiogram monitoring in patients who present with hypokalemia or in patients with any abnormal cardiac rhythms other than sinus tachycardia. Elevations in serum chloride, i.e. hyperchloremic acidosis, may be prevented by replacing part of the chloride ion by a solution of potassium phosphate at a ratio of 1:3 as a supplemented potassium solution. If hyperkalemia develops during potassium replacement (>5.0 mEq/l), potassium infusion should withheld and levels should be checked every 2 h until it is normal.

Bicarbonate

Most current reviews [5, 18, 114, 116, 117, 132], including the recent ADA guidelines (4), do not recommend the routine use of alkali therapy in DKA because bicarbonate levels tend to correct with insulin therapy. Insulin administration inhibits ongoing lipolysis and ketoacid production and promotes ketoanion metabolism. Because protons are consumed during ketoanion metabolism, bicarbonate is regenerated, leading to partial correction of metabolic acidosis. The use of bicarbonate in HHS is not recommended, as patients exhibit normal serum bicarbonate, unless there is a condition of mixed hyperosmolar ketoacidosis.

The use of bicarbonate in DKA, however, is recommended for conditions where either severe bicarbonate deficiency (below 5 mM) or severe acidemia (pH less than 6.9) is present. Even the use of bicarbonate in DKA at this level of acidosis is controversial [133] because of the potential deleterious effects of bicarbonate including paradoxical CSF acidosis, rebound alkalosis, hypokalemia [5, 8], and increased lactate production [133–135] as well as local irritation with bicarbonate administration [117]. The theoretical advantage of bicarbonate therapy may be due to its salutary effect on advanced acidosis and improvement of the negative ionotropic effect on the heart and peripheral vasodilatation [136]. There are, however, no prospective randomized studies to demonstrate a beneficial or deleterious effect of bicarbonate therapy on cardiac function and the various parameters of severe DKA. Several prospective and retrospective studies have demonstrated conflicting results regarding the use of biocarbonate therapy in DKA. Two studies have shown increases in blood pH when bicarbonate therapy was compared to saline infusion [134, 135, 137, 138]. Another study showed no changes in blood pH when biocarbonate therapy was used [139]. None of the above studies, however, have enough power to detect significant differences between two treatment regimens, and therefore further studies with larger number of patients are necessary to settle this issue [133]. Furthermore, there are no large studies to demonstrate the efficacy of bicarbonate therapy in patients with DKA and pH less than 6.9. In the absence of such data, the ADA guidelines recommend that patients with pH lower than 6.9 should receive two ampules of bicarbonate (100 mmol) as an isotonic solution (in 400 ml of water) at the rate of 50 mmol/h with 15 mEq of potassium [4]. For follow-up of acidosis, we recommend measuring venous rather than arterial pH every 2 h, realizing that venous pH is approximately 0.03 lower than the arterial pH.

Phosphate

Patients with DKA and HHS present with decreased phosphate and (2,3-diphosphoglycerate) (2,3-DPG) levels, which shifts the O_2 dissociation curve to the left, resulting in hypoxemia [140]. Hypophosphatemia is a result of both insulin deficiency and osmotic diuresis in spite of normal or increased level of serum phosphate on admission [141]. This is possibly due to an extracellular shift that may exist, similar to the shift seen with potassium. However, during insulin therapy this rapid shift of phosphate into the cell results in lower levels of intravascular phosphate. Although severe hypophosphatemia is rare, some patients with phosphorus concentration <1 mg/dl may be at risk of muscle cramps and cardiorespiratory compromise and may benefit from the use of phosphate [141].

In two randomized prospective protocols, in both children and adults, the use of phosphate therapy failed to show any benefit on various metabolic parameters [41, 42]. Excessive administration of phosphorus can lead to hypocalcemia and soft tissue calcifications [142, 143]. Therefore, if phosphate replacement is needed, 20–30 mEq/l potassium phosphate can be added to replacement fluids and given over several hours. In such patients, because of the risk of hypocalcemia, serum calcium and phosphate levels must be monitored during phosphate infusion [144, 145].

MANAGEMENT OF PATIENTS IN POSTHYPERGLYCEMIC CRISIS

Because low-dose insulin will maintain a physiologic level of insulin (40–100 microunits/ml) [124, 127], sudden disruption or cessation of insulin, particularly when the IV route is used, will result in an immediate drop in serum insulin concentration culminating in a relapse of DKA or HHS. It is therefore recommended that when hyperglycemia is reduced to a desirable level (but patients are not eating), insulin may be changed from the IV to the SC or IM route with an overlap of the IV insulin infusion of 1–2 h. Once the patient is able to tolerate food intake, rapid-acting insulin should be given before each meal in combination with intermediate or long-acting insulin. The patients should also receive adequate education for management of their diabetes and dietary education.

Figures 4 and 5 illustrate step-by-step guidelines for management of patients with DKA and HHS approved by the ADA. It is important to point out, however, that no set of guidelines can replace individualized management of the patient in DKA or HHS.

Complications of Therapy

The most common complications of DKA are hypoglycemia and hypokalemia. The use of low-dose insulin has reduced these problems considerably [5, 124]. The use of dextrose-containing solutions when blood glucose reaches 250 mg/dl in DKA and a simultaneous reduction in the rate of insulin delivery should further reduce the incidence of hypoglycemia. Similarly, the addition of potassium to the hydrating solution and frequent monitoring of serum potassium during the early phases of DKA and HHS therapy should reduce the incidence of hypokalemia.

Relapse of DKA is also noted after sudden interruption of IV insulin therapy, or in patients without concomitant use of SC or IM insulin or lack of frequent monitoring. Another complication of the treatment of DKA is the development of nonanion gap hyperchloremic metabolic acidosis [70, 71]. This acidosis has no adverse clinical effects and is gradually corrected over the subsequent 24–48 h by enhanced renal acid excretion. The hyperchloremia can be prevented with reduction of the chloride load by judicious use of hydration solutions [76, 146].

Cerebral edema is a rare but serious complication of DKA, occurring in approximately 1% of episodes of diabetic ketoacidosis in children [147–149], and is associated with a mortality rate of 40–90% [149]. Cerebral edema is rarely reported in adult patients with DKA. Clinically, cerebral edema is characterized by decreasing level of consciousness and headache, followed by seizures, sphincter incontinence, pupillary changes, papilledema, bradycardia, and respiratory arrest. Although no single factor has been identified that can be used to predict the development of cerebral edema [148, 149], it has been hypothesized that cerebral edema in DKA results from a rapid shift in extracellular and intracellular fluids, resulting in changes in osmolality [150–152]. Recent data also suggest that cerebral edema in children may also be related to brain ischemia [151]. In children with diabetic ketoacidosis, both hypocapnia (which causes cerebral vasoconstriction) and extreme dehydration are associated with increased risk for cerebral edema. Prevention might include a gradual decrease in serum glucose and maintenance of serum glucose between 250 and 300 mg/dl until the patient's serum osmolality is normalized and mental status is improved. Treatment of cerebral edema should include transfer to ICU and use of mannitol and mechanical ventilation.

Adult respiratory disease syndrome (ARDS) has been reported as a complication of DKA [153]. It has been proposed that hypoxemia can reduce the oncotic pressure, resulting in reduction of lung compliance since patients with DKA have a widened alveolar arteriolar oxygen gradient and thus could be more vulnerable to pulmonary edema [3, 5, 118]. Patients with an increased AaO_2 gradient or those who have pulmonary rales on physical examination may be at an increased risk for development of this syndrome [3]. Monitoring of PaO_2 with pulse oximetry and monitoring of AaO_2 gradient may assist in the management of such patients. Because crystalloid solutions may be a precipitating factor, we advise that such patients should receive lower rate of IV fluids.

As DKA and HHS are both associated with a hypercoagulable state, thromboembolic conditions may occur in which case the use of an anticoagulant such as low-molecular-weight heparin may be of benefit [18, 117].

PREVENTION OF HYPERGLYCEMIC CRISES

One of the major precipitating factors in both DKA and HHS is inadequate insulin dosing or omission of insulin injection. The frequency of hospitalizations for DKA has been reduced following diabetes education programs, improved follow-up care, and access to medical advice [13, 79, 154, 155]. Outpatient management is more cost-effective and can minimize missed days of school and work for patients with diabetes and their family members [154]. Important aspects of preventive care in HHS include frequent monitoring and adequate hydration as well as prevention and early treatment of hyperglycemia [5, 65, 67, 95]. Furthermore, recent studies in DKA patients suggest that frequent endocrine clinic visits on a quarterly rather than on an annual basis reduces DKA events significantly as compared to an annual visit [154].

Recent studies in both surgical wards as well as general wards have clearly demonstrated that the mortality rate is greatly increased in those patients with hyperglycemia with or without a previous history of diabetes [156, 157]. Therefore, it is important to note that frequent monitoring of inhospital patients, and nursing home residents, is an important mechanism to diagnose and treat diabetes and to reduce mortality.

FUTURE PROSPECTS

Areas of future investigations include the following:

(1) The mechanism for low or absent ketones in HHS versus DKA
(2) Left ventricular cardiac status of patients in severe DKA
(3) Use of bicarbonate in severe DKA
(4) C-peptide responses in various hyperglycemic states, with specific emphasis on the role of glucotoxicity and lipotoxicity in these conditions [158]
(5) Resource utilization for the management of patients with mild, moderate, and severe DKA and HHS in various inpatient settings (ICU versus stepdown units versus general wards).

REFERENCES

1. Harris MI, Hamman RF (eds). *Diabetes in America (National Diabetes Group)*. Washington, DC: US Department of Health and Human Sciences, 1985; pp XII-1–16.
2. Centers for Disease Control. *Division of Diabetes Translations: Diabetes Surveillance, 1991*. Washington, DC: US Government Printing Office, 1992; pp 635–1150.
3. American Diabetes Association. Hyperglycemic crises in patients with diabetes mellitus. *Diabetes Care* 2001; 25 (1): 5100–8.
4. Kitabchi AE, Wall BM. Diabetic ketoacidosis. *Med Clin North Am* 1995; 79: 9–37.
5. Kitabchi AE, Umpierrez GE, Murphy MB, Barrett EJ, Kreisburg RA, Malone JI, Wall BM. Management of hyperglycemic crises in patients with diabetes. *Diabetes Care* 2001; 24: 131–53.
6. Faich GA, Fishbein HA, Ellis SE. The epidemiology of diabetic acidosis: a population-based study. *Am J Epidemiol* 1983; 117: 551–8.
7. Johnson DD, Palumbo PJ, Chu CP. Diabetic ketoacidosis in a community-based population. *Mayo Clin Proc* 1980; 55: 83–8.
8. Kitabchi AE, Fisher JN, Murphy MB, Rumbak MJ. Diabetic ketoacidosis and the hyperglycemic hyperosmolar nonketotic state. In Kahn CR, Weir GC (eds) *Joslin's Diabetes Mellitus*, 13th edn. Philadelphia: Lea & Febiger, 1994; pp 738–70.
9. Ellemann K, Soerensen JN, Pedersen L, Edsberg B, Anderson OO. Epidemiology and treatment of diabetic ketoacidosis in a community population. *Diabetes Care* 1984; 7: 528–32.
10. Umpierrez GE, Casals MM, Gebhart SP, Mixon PS, Clark WS, Phillips LS. Diabetic ketoacidosis in obese African-Americans. *Diabetes* 1995; 44: 790–5.
11. Musey VC, Lee JK, Crawford R, Klatka MA, McAdams D, Phillips LS. Diabetes in urban African-Americans, I: cessation of insulin therapy is the major precipitating cause of diabetic ketoacidosis. *Diabetes Care* 1995; 18: 483–9.
12. Polonsky WH, Anderson BJ, Lohrer PA, et al. Insulin omission in women with IDDM. *Diabetes Care* 1994; 17: 1178–85.
13. Petzold R, Trabert C, Walter A, Schoffling K. Etiology and prognosis of diabetic coma: a retrospective study. *Verh Dtsch Ges Inn Med* 1971; 77: 637–40.
14. Soler NG, Bennett MA, FitzGerald MG, Malins JM. Intensive care in the management of diabetic ketoacidosis. *Lancet* 1973; 1: 951–4.
15. Panzram G. Epidemiology of diabetic coma. *Schweiz Med Wochenschr* 1973; 103: 203–8.
16. Berger W, Keller U, Vorster D. Mortality from diabetic coma at the Basle Cantonal Hospital during 2 consecutive observation periods 1968–1973 and 1973–1978, using conventional insulin therapy and treatment with low dose insulin. *Schweiz Med Wochenschr* 1979; 109: 1820–4.
17. Umpierrez GE, Khajavi M, Kitabchi AE. Review: diabetic ketoacidosis and hyperglycemic hyperosmolar nonketotic syndrome. *Am J Med Sci* 1996; 311: 225–33.

18. Lebovitz HE. Diabetic ketoacidosis. *Lancet* 1995; 345: 767–72.
19. EURODIAB IDDM Complications Study. Microvascular and acute complications in IDDM patients. *Diabetologia* 1994; 37: 278–85.
20. Graves EJ, Gillium BS. Detailed diagnosis and procedures: National Discharge Survey, 1995. National Center for Health Statistics. *Vital Health Stat* 1997; 13: 133.
21. Umpierrez GE, Kelly JP, Navarrete JE, Casals MM, Kitabchi AE. Hyperglycemic crises in urban blacks. *Arch Intern Med* 1997; 157: 669–75.
22. McFarlane SI, Chaiken RL, Hirsch S, Harrington P, Lebovits HE, Banerji MA. Near-normoglycaemic remission in African-Americans with type 2 diabetes mellitus is associated with recovery of beta cell function. *Diabet Med* 2001; 18: 10–6.
23. Banerji MA, Chaiken RL, Huey H, Tuomi T, Norin AJ, Mackey IR, Rowley MJ, Zimmet PZ, Lebovitz HE. GAD antibody negative NIDDM in adult black subjects with diabetic ketoacidosis and increased frequency of human leukocyte antigen DR3 and DR4. Flatbush diabetes. *Diabetes* 1994; 43: 741–5.
24. Balasubramanyam A, Zern JW, Hyman DJ, Pavlik V. New profiles of diabetic ketoacodosis: type 1 vs type 2 diabetes and the effect of ethnicity. *Arch Intern Med* 1999; 159: 2317–22.
25. Umpierrez GE, Woo W, Hagopian WA, Issacs SD, Palmer JP, Gaur LK, Nepom GT, Clark WS, Mixon PS, Kitabchi AE. Immunogenetic analysis suggests different pathogenesis for obese and lean African-Americans with diabetic ketoacidosis. *Diabetes Care* 1999; 22: 1517–23.
26. Teutsch SM, Herman WH, Dwyer DM, Lane JM. Mortality among diabetic patients using continuous subcutaneous insulin-infusion pumps. *N Engl J Med* 1984; 310: 361–8.
27. The DCCT Study Group. Implementation of treatment protocols in the Diabetes Control and Complications Trial. *Diabetes Care* 1995; 18: 361–76.
28. Bending JJ, Pickup JC, Keen H. Frequency of diabetic ketoacidosis and hypoglycemic coma during treatment with continuous subcutaneous insulin infusion. Audit of medical care. *Am J Med* 1985; 79: 685–91.
29. Siperstein MD. Diabetic ketoacidosis and hyperosmolar coma. *Endocrinol Metab Clin North Am* 1992; 21: 415–32.
30. Kitabchi AE, Fisher JN, Burghen GA, Tsiu W, Huber T. Problems associated with continuous insulin infusion. *Horm Metab Res Suppl* 1982; 12: 271–6.
31. Delaney MF, Zisman A, Kettyle WM. Diabetic ketoacidosis and hyperglycemic hyperosmolar nonketotic syndrome. *Endocrinol Metab Clin North Am* 2000; 29: 683–705.
32. DeFronzo RA, Matzuda M, Barret E. Diabetic ketoacidosis: a combined metabolic–nephrologic approach to therapy. *Diabetes Rev* 1994; 2: 209–38.
33. Miles JM, Rizza RA, Haymond MW, Gerich JE. Effects of acute insulin deficiency on glucose and ketone body turnover in man: evidence for the primacy of overproduction of glucose and ketone bodies in the genesis of diabetic ketoacidosis. *Diabetes* 1980; 29: 926–30.
34. Owen, OE, Block BS, Patel M, Boden G, McDonough M, Kreulen T, Shuman CR, Richard GA Jr. Human splanchnic metabolism during diabetic ketoacidosis. *Metabolism* 1977; 26: 381–98.
35. Miles JM, Haymond MW, Nissen SL, Gerich JE. Effects of free fatty acid availability, glucagons excess, and insulin deficiency on ketone body production in postabsorptive man. *J Clin Invest* 1983; 71: 1554–61.
36. Schade DS, Eaton RP. The temporal relationship between endogenously secreted stress hormones and metabolic decompensation in diabetic man. *J Clin Endocrinol Metab* 1980; 50: 131–6.
37. Jensen MD, Caruso M, Heiling V, Miles JM. Insulin regulation of lipolysis in nondiabetic and IDDM subjects. *Diabetes* 1989; 38: 1595–601.
38. Arner P, Kriegholm E, Engfeldt P, Bolinder J. Adrenergic regulation in lipolysis *in situ* at rest and during exercise. *J Clin Invest* 1990; 85: 893–8.
39. Nurjhan N, Consoli A, Gerich J. Increased lipolysis and its consequences on gluconeogenesis in non-insulin-dependent diabetes mellitus. *J Clin Invest* 1992; 89: 169–75.
40. Exton JH. Mechanisms of hormonal regulation of hepatic glucose metabolism. *Diabetes Metab Rev* 1987; 3: 163–83.
41. McGarry JD, Woeltje KF, Kuwajima M, Foster DW. Regulation of ketogenesis and the renaissance of carnitine palmitoyltransferase. *Diabetes Metab Rev* 1989; 5: 271–84.
42. van de Werve G, Jeanrenaud B. Liver glycogen metabolism: an overview. *Diabetes Metab Rev* 1987; 3: 47–78.
43. Pilkis SJ, el-Maghrabi MR, Claus TH. Fructose-2,6-bisphosphate in control of hepatic gluconeogenesis: from metabolites to molecular genetics. *Diabetes Care* 1990; 13: 582–99.
44. Foster DW, McGarry JD. The metabolic derangements and treatment of diabetic ketoacidosis. *N Engl J Med* 1983; 309: 159–69.
45. Gerich JE, Lorenzi M, Bier DM, Tsalikian E, Schneider V, Karan JH, Forsham PH. Effects of physiologic levels of glucagon and growth hormone on human carbohydrate and lipid metabolism. Studies involving administration of exogenous hormone during suppression of endogenous hormone secretion with somatostatin. *J Clin Invest* 1976; 57: 875–84.
46. Luzi L, Barrett EJ, Groop LC, Ferrannini E, DeFronzo RA. Metabolic effects of low-dose insulin therapy on glucose metabolism in diabetic ketoacidosis. *Diabetes* 1988; 37: 1470–7.
47. Meyer C, Stumvoll M, Nadkarni V, Dostou J, Mitrakou A, Gerich J. Abnormal renal and hepatic glucose metabolism in type 2 diabetes mellitus. *J Clin Invest* 1998; 102: 619–24.
48. McGarry JD. Lilly Lecture 1978. New perspectives in the regulation of ketogenesis. *Diabetes* 1979; 28: 517–23.
49. McGarry JD, Foster DW. Regulation of hepatic fatty acid oxidation and ketone body production. *Annu Rev Biochem* 1980; 49: 395–420.
50. Cook GA, King MT, Veech RL. Ketogenesis and malonyl coenzyme: a content of isolated rat hepatocytes. *J Biol Chem* 1978; 253: 2529–31.
51. Reichard GA Jr, Skutches CL, Hoeldtke RD, Owen OE. Acetone metabolism in humans during diabetic ketoacidosis. *Diabetes* 1986; 35: 668–74.
52. Ruderman NB, Goodman MN. Inhibition of muscle acetoacetate utilization during diabetic ketoacidosis. *Am J Physiol* 1974; 226: 136–43.

53. Nosadini R, Avogaro A, Doria A, Fioretto P, Trevisan R, Morocutti A. Ketone body metabolism: a physiological and clinical overview. *Diabetes Metab Rev* 1989; 5: 299–319.
54. Kreisberg RA. Diabetic ketoacidosis: an update. *Crit Care Clin* 1987; 3: 817–34.
55. Beylot M, Picard S, Chambrier C, Vidal H, Laville M, Cohen R, Cotisson A, Mornax R. Effect of physiological concentrations of insulin and glucagon on the relationship between nonesterified fatty acids availability and ketone body production in humans. *Metabolism* 1991; 40: 1138–46.
56. Shamoon H, Hendler R, Sherwin RS. Synergistic interactions among antiinsulin hormones in the pathogenesis of stress hyperglycemia in humans. *J Clin Endocrinol Metab* 1981; 52: 1235–41.
57. Atchley DW, Loebre DWR, Richards DW, Benedict EM, Driscoll ME. A detailed study of electrolyte balances following the withdrawal and reestablishment of insulin therapy. *J Clin Invest* 1933; 12: 297–326.
58. Butler AM, Talbot NB, Burnett CH. Metabolic studies in diabetic coma. *Trans Assoc Am Physicians* 1947; 60: 102–9.
59. Nabarro JDN, Spence AG, Stowers JM. Metabolic studies in severe diabetic ketosis. *Q J Med* 1952; 21: 222–4.
60. Felig P, Marliss E, Ohman JL, Cahill CF Jr. Plasma amino acid levels in diabetic ketoacidosis. *Diabetes* 1970; 19: 727–8.
61. Blackshear PJ, Alberti K. Sequential amino acid measurements during experimental diabetic ketoacidosis. *Am J Physiol* 1975; 228: 205–11.
62. Genuth SM, Castro J. Effect of oral alanine on blood β-hydroxybutyrate and plasma glucose, insulin, FFAs, and growth hormone in normal and diabetic subjects. *Metabolism* 1974; 23: 375–86.
63. Gerich JE, Lorenzi M, Bier DM, Schneider V, Tsalikian E, Karam JH, Forsham PH. Prevention of human diabetic ketoacidosis by somatostatin: evidence for an essential role of glucagon. *N Engl J Med* 1975; 292: 985–9.
64. May RC, Kelly RA, Mitch WE. Metabolic acidosis stimulates protein degradation in rat muscle by a glucocorticoid-dependent mechanism. *J Clin Invest* 1986; 77: 614–62.
65. Ennis ED, Stahl EJVB, Kreisberg RA. The hyperosmolar hyperglycemic syndrome. *Diabetes Rev* 1994; 2: 115–26.
66. DeFronzo RA, Cooke CR, Andres R, Faloona GR, Davis PJ. The effect of insulin on renal handling of sodium, potassium, calcium and phosphate in man. *J Clin Invest* 1975; 55: 845–55.
67. Wachtel TJ, Silliman RA, Lamberton P. Predisposing factors for the diabetic hyperosmolar state. *Arch Intern Med* 1987, 147: 499–501.
68. DeFronzo RA, Goldberg M, Agus ZS. The effects of glucose and insulin on renal electrolyte transport. *J Clin Invest* 1976; 58: 83–90.
69. DeFronzo RA, Felig P, Ferrannini E, Wahren J. Effect of graded doses of insulin on splanchnic and peripheral potassium metabolism in man. *Am J Physiol* 1980; 238: E421–7.
70. Halperin ML, Cheema-Dhadli S. Renal and hepatic aspects of ketoacidosis: a quantitative analysis based on energy turnover. *Diabetes Metab Rev* 1989; 5: 321–36.
71. Adrogue HJ, Wilson H, Boyd AE III, Sukiw N, Eknoyan G. Plasma acid–base patterns in diabetic ketoacidosis. *N Engl J Med* 1982; 307: 1603–10.
72. Kitabchi AE, Fisher JN. Insulin therapy of diabetic ketoacidosis: physiologic versus pharmacologic doses of insulin and their routes of administration. In Brownlee M (ed) *Handbook of Diabetes Mellitus*. New York: Garland Press, 1981; pp 95–149.
73. Campbell IW, Duncan LJ, Innes JA, MacCuish AC, Munro JF. Abdominal pain in diabetic metabolic decompensation. Clinical significance. *JAMA* 1975; 233: 166–8.
74. Umpierrez G, Freire AX. Abdominal pain in patients with hyperglycemic crises. *J Crit Care* 2002; 17: 63–7.
75. Winter SD, Pearson JR, Gabow PA, Schultz AL, Lepoff RB. The fall of the serum anion gap. *Arch Intern Med* 1990; 150: 311–3.
76. Adrogue HJ, Eknoyan G, Suki WK. Diabetic ketoacidosis: role of the kidney in the acid–base homeostasis reevaluated. *Kidney Int* 1984; 25: 591–8.
77. Umpierrez G, DiGirolamo M, Tuvlin JA, Issacs SD, Bhoola SM, Kokko JP. Differences in metabolic and hormonal milieu in diabetic- and alcohol-induced ketoacidosis. *J Crit Care* 2000; 15: 52–9.
78. Byrne HA, Tieszen KL, Hollis S, Dornan TL, New JP. Evaluation of an electrochemical sensor for measuring blood ketones. *Diabetes Care* 2000; 23: 500–3.
79. Laffel L. Sick-day management in type 1 diabetes. *Endocrinol Metab Clin North Am* 2000; 29: 707–23.
80. Slovis CM, Mork VG, Slovis RJ, Bain RP. Diabetic ketoacidosis and infection: leukocyte count and differential as early predictors of serious infection. *Am J Emerg Med* 1987: 5: 1–5.
81. Rumbak MJ, Hughes TA, Kitabchi AE. Pseudonormoglycemia in diabetic ketoacidosis with elevated triglycerides. *Am J Emerg Med* 1991; 9: 61–3.
82. Kaminska ES, Pourmotabbed G. Spurious laboratory values in diabetic ketoacidosis and hyperlipidemia. *Am J Emerg Med* 1993; 11: 77–80.
83. Adrogue HJ, Lederer ED, Suki WN, Eknoyan G. Determinants of plasma potassium levels in diabetic ketoacidosis. *Medicine (Baltimore)* 1986; 65: 163–72.
84. Gerard SK, Khayam Bashi H. Characterization of creatinine error in ketotic patients. A prospective comparison of alkaline picrate methods with an enzymatic method. *Am J Clin Pathol* 1985; 84: 659–64.
85. Vinicor F, Lehrner LM, Karn RC, Merritt AD. Hyperamylasemia in diabetic ketoacidosis: sources and significance. *Ann Intern Med* 1979; 91: 200–4.
86. Vantyghem MC, Haye S, Balduyck M, Hober C, Degand PM, LeFebvre J. Changes in serum amylase, lipase and leukocyte elastase during diabetic ketoacidosis and poorly controlled diabetes. *Acta Diabetol* 1999; 36: 39–44.
87. Yadav D, Nair S, Norkus EP, Pitchumoni CS. Nonspecific hyperamylasemia and hyperlipasemia in diabtic ketoacidosis: incidence and correlation with biochemical abnormalities. *Am J Gastroenterol* 2000; 95: 3123–8.
88. Nair S, Yadav D, Pitchumoni CS. Association of diabetic ketoacidosis and acute pancreatitis: observations in 100 consecutive episodes of DKA. *Am J Gastroenterol* 2000; 95: 2795–800.
89. Kitabchi AE, Umpierrez GE. Changes in serum leptin in lean and obese subjects with acute hyperglycemia crises. *J Clin Endo Metab* 2003; 88 (6): 2593–6.
90. Umpierrez G, Culbreath B, Crisler J, Stentz F, Kitabchi AE. Cytokine response in patients with diabetic ketoacidosis. *J Invest Med* 2002; 50: 141A [Abstract 742].

91. Stentz F, Umpierrez G, Cuvero R, Kitabchi A. *In situ* activation of T-lymphocytes in patients with diabetic ketoacidosis. *Diabetes* 2003; 52 (suppl): A295.
92. Dreschfeld J. The Bradshawe Lecture on diabetic coma. *Br Med J* 1886; 2: 358–63.
93. Sament S, Schwartz MB. Severe diabetic stupor without ketosis. *S Afr Med J* 1957; 31: 893–4.
94. Wachtel TJ, Tetu-Mouradjian LM, Goldman DL, Ellis SE, O'Sullivan PS. Hyperosomolarity and acidosis in diabetes mellitus: a three year experience in Rhode Island. *J Gen Intern Med* 1991; 6: 495–502.
95. Wachtel TJ. The diabetic hyperosmolar state. *Clin Geriatr Med* 1990; 6: 797–806.
96. Wachtel TJ, Silliman RA, Lamberton P. Prognostic factors in the diabetic hyperosmolar state. *J Am Geriatr Soc* 1987; 35: 737–41.
97. Cruz-Caudillo JC, Sabatini S. Diabetic hyperosmolar syndrome. *Nephron* 1995; 69: 201–10.
98. Lorber D. Nonketotic hypertonicity in diabetes mellitus. *Med Clin North Am* 1995; 79: 39–52.
99. Morris LR, Kitabchi AE. Efficacy of low-dose insulin therapy for severely obtunded patients in diabetic ketoacidosis. *Diabetes Care* 1980; 3: 53–6.
100. Rosenthal NR, Barrett EJ. An assessment of insulin action in hyperosmolar hyperglycemic nonketotic diabetic patients. *J Clin Endocrinol Metab* 1985; 60: 607–10.
101. Chupin M, Charbonnel B, Chupin F. C-peptide blood levels in ketoacidosis and in hyperosmolar nonketotic diabetic coma. *Acta Diabetol Lat* 1981; 18: 123–8.
102. Gerich JE, Martin MM, Recant L. Clinical and metabolic characteristics of hyperosmolar nonketotic coma. *Diabetes* 1971; 20: 228–38.
103. Yu SS, Kitabchi AE. Biological activity of proinsulin and related polypeptides in the fat tissue. *J Biol Chem* 1973; 248: 3753–61.
104. Schade DS, Eaton RP. Dose response to insulin in man: differential effects on glucose and ketone body regulation. *J Clin Endocrinol Metab* 1977; 44: 1038–53.
105. Bratusch-Marrain PR, DeFronzo RA. Impairment of insulin-mediated glucose metabolism by hyperosmolality in man. *Diabetes* 1983; 32: 1028–34.
106. Phillips PA, Rolls BJ, Ledingham JG, Forsling ML, Morton JJ, Crowe MJ, Wollner L. Reduced thirst after water deprivation in healthy elderly men. *N Engl J Med* 1984; 311: 753–9.
107. Kreisberg RA. Acid–base and electrolyte disturbances in the alcoholic. *Probl Crit Care* 1987; 1: 66–72.
108. Krebs HA, Freedland RA, Hems R, Stubbs M. Inhibition of hepatic gluconeogenesis by ethanol. *Biochem J* 1969; 112: 117–24.
109. Ehrig T, Bosron WF, Li TK. Alcohol and aldehyde dehydrogenase. *Alcohol* 1990; 25: 105–16.
110. Cusi K, Consoli A. Alcoholic ketoacidosis and lactic acidosis. *Diabetes Rev* 1994; 2: 195–208.
111. Cahill GF Jr. Ketosis. *Kidney Int* 1981; 20: 416–25.
112. Cahill GF Jr. Starvation in man. *N Engl J Med* 1970; 282: 668–75.
113. Bjellerup P, Kaliner A, Kollind M. GLC determination of serum–ethylene glycol interferences in ketotic patients. *J Toxicol Clin Toxicol* 1994; 32: 85–7.
114. Carroll P, Matz R. Uncontrolled diabetes mellitus in adults: experience in treating diabetic ketoacidosis and hyperosmolar coma with low-dose insulin and uniform treatment regimen. *Diabetes Care* 1983; 6: 579–85.
115. Morris LE, Kitabchi AE. Coma in the diabetic. In Schnatz JD (ed) *Diabetes Mellitus: Problems in Management*. Menlo Park, CA: Addison-Wesley, 1982; pp 234–51.
116. Ennis ED, Stahl EJ, Kreisberg RA. Diabetic ketoacidosis. In Porte D. Jr, Sherwin RS (eds) *Diabetes Mellitus: Theory and Practice*. Amsterdam: Elsevier, 1997; pp 827–44.
117. Marshall SM, Walker M, Alberti KGMM. Diabetic ketoacidosis and hyperglycaemic nonketotic coma. In Alberti KGMM, Zimmet P, DeFronzo RA (eds) *International Textbook of Diabetes Mellitus.* New York: Wiley, 1997; pp 1215–29.
118. Hillman K. Fluid resuscitation in diabetic emergencies—a reappraisal. *Intensive Care Med* 1987; 13: 4–8.
119. Waldhausl W, Kleinberger G, Korn A, Dudczak R, Bratusch-Marrain P, Nowotny P. Severe hyperglycemia effects of rehydration on endocrine derangements and blood glucose concentration. *Diabetes* 1979; 28: 557–84.
120. Bratusch-Marrain PR, Komajati M, Waldhausal W. The effect of hyperosmolarity on glucose metabolism. *Pract Cardiol* 1985; 11: 153–63.
121. Foster NB. The treatment of diabetic coma with insulin. *Am J Med Sci* 1923; 166: 699–709.
122. Alberti KG, Hockaday TD, Turner RC. Small doses of intramuscular insulin in the treatment of diabetic "coma." *Lancet* 1973; 2: 515–22.
123. Genuth SM. Constant intravenous insulin infusion in diabetic ketoacidosis. *JAMA* 1973; 223: 1348–51.
124. Kitabchi AE, Ayyagari V, Guerra SM. The efficacy of low-dose versus conventional therapy of insulin for treatment of diabetic ketoacidosis. *Ann Intern Med* 1976; 84: 633–8.
125. Fisher JN, Shahshahani MN, Kitabchi AE. Diabetic ketoacidosis: low-dose insulin therapy by various routes. *N Engl J Med* 1977; 297: 238–41.
126. Sacks HS, Shahshahani MN, Kitabchi AE, Fisher JN, Young RT. Similar responsiveness of diabetic ketoacidosis to low-dose insulin by intramuscular injection and albumin-free infusion. *Ann Intern Med* 1979; 90: 36–42.
127. Burghen GA, Etteldorf JN, Fisher JN, Kitabchi AE. Comparison of high-dose and low-dose insulin by continuous intravenous infusion in the treatment of diabetic ketoacidosis in children. *Diabetes Care* 1980; 3: 15–20.
128. Edwards GA, Kohaut EC, Wehring B, Hill LL. Effectiveness of low-dose continuous intravenous insulin infusion in diabetic ketoacidosis: a prospective comparative study. *J Pediatr* 1977; 91: 701–5.
129. Kitabchi AE, Young RT, Sacks HS, Morris L. Diabetic ketoacidosis: reappraisal of therapeutic approach. *Annu Rev Med* 1979; 30: 339–57.
130. Latif K, Umpierrez GE, Stoever J, Kitabchi AE. Subcutaneous lispro insulin in the treatment of diabetic ketoacidosis. *Diabetes* 2002; 51 (suppl 2): A427.
131. Abramson E, Arky R. Diabetic acidosis with initial hypokalemia. Therapeutic implications. *JAMA* 1966; 196: 401–3.
132. Barnes HV, Cohen RD, Kitabchi AE, Murphy MB. When is biocarbonate appropriate in treating metabolic acidosis including diabetic ketoacidosis? In Gitnick G, Barnes HV, Duffy TP, et al. (eds) *Debates in Medicine.* Chicago: Yearbook Medical Publishers, 1990; pp 200–33.
133. Latif K, Freire A, Kitabchi AE, Umpierrez GE, Qureshi N. The use of alkali therapy in severe diabetic ketoacidosis (DKA). *Diabetes Care* 2002; 25: 2113–4.
134. Gamba G, Oseguera J, Castrejon M, Gomez-Perez FJ. Bicarbonate therapy in severe diabetic ketoacidosis: a

double blind, randomized, placebo controlled trial. *Rev Invest Clin* 1991; 43: 234–8.
135. Hale PJ, Crase J, Nattrass M. Metabolic effects of bicarbonate in the treatment of diabetic ketoacidosis. *Br Med J (Clin Res Ed)* 1984; 289: 1035–8.
136. Wildenthal K, Mierzwiak DS, Myers RW, Mitchell JH. Effect of acute lactic acidosis on left ventricular performance. *Am J Physiol* 1986; 214: 1252–9.
137. Lever E, Jaspan JB. Sodium bicarbonate therapy in severe diabetic ketoacidosis. *Am J Med* 1983; 75: 263–8.
138. Green SM, Rothrock SG, Ho JD, Gallant RD, Borger R, Thomas TL, Zimmerman GJ. Failure of adjunctive bicarbonate to improve outcome in severe pediatric diabetic ketoacidosis. *Ann Emerg Med* 1998; 31: 41–8.
139. Morris LR, Murphy MB, Kitabchi AE. Bicarbonate therapy in severe diabetic ketoacidosis. *Ann Intern Med* 1986; 105: 836–40.
140. Gibby OM, Veale KE, Hayes TM, Jones JG, Wardrop CA. Oxygen availability from the blood and the effect of phosphate replacement on erythrocyte 2,3-diphosphoglycerate and haemoglobin-oxygen affinity in diabetic ketoacidosis. *Diabetologia* 1978; 15: 381–5.
141. Kreisberg RA. Phosphorus deficiency and hypophosphatemia. *Hosp Pract* 1977; 12: 121–8.
142. Fisher JN, Kitabchi AE. A randomized study of phosphate therapy in the treatment of diabetic ketoacidosis. *J Clin Endocrinol Metab* 1983; 57: 177–80.
143. Zipf WB, Bacon GE, Spencer ML, Kelch RP, Hopwood NJ, Hawker CD. Hypocalcemia, hypomagnesemia, and transient hypoparathyroidism during therapy with potassium phosphate in diabetic ketoacidosis. *Diabetes Care* 1979; 2: 265–8.
144. White NH. Diabetic ketoacidosis in children. *Endocrinol Metab Clin North Am* 2000; 29: 657–82.
145. Wilson HK, Keuer SP, Lea AS, Boyd AE III, Eknoyan G. Phosphate therapy in diabetic ketoacidosis. *Arch Intern Med* 1982; 142: 517–20.
146. Kitabchi AE, Murphy MB, Matteri R, Spencer J. Contributing factors in the development of hyperchloremic metabolic acidosis during the treatment of diabetic ketoacidosis. *Diabetes* 1991; 40: 42A. Abstract 167.
147. Bello FA, Sotos JF. Cerebral oedema in diabetic ketoacidosis in children. *Lancet* 1990; 336: 64.
148. Duck SC, Wyatt DT. Factors associated with brain herniation in the treatment of diabetic ketoacidosis. *J Pediatr* 1988; 113 (1, pt 1): 10–4.
149. Rosenbloom AL. Intracerebral crises during treatment of diabetic ketoacidosis. *Diabetes Care* 1990; 13: 22–33.
150. Silver SM, Clark EC, Schroeder BM, Sterns RH. Pathogenesis of cerebral edema after treatment of diabetic ketoacidosis. *Kidney Int* 1997; 51: 1237–44.
151. Glaser N, Barnett P, McCaslin I, Nelson D, Trainor J, Louie J, Kaufman F, Quayle K, Roback M, Malley R, Kupperman N. for the Pediatric Emergency Medicine Collaborative Research Committee of the American Academy of Pediatrics. Risk factors for cerebral edema in children with diabetic ketoacidosis. *N Engl J Med* 2001; 344: 264–9.
152. Arieff AI, Kleeman CR. Cerebral edema in diabetic comas, II: Effects of hyperosmolality, hyperglycemia and insulin in diabetic rabbits. *J Clin Endocrinol Metab* 1974; 38: 1057–67.
153. Carroll P, Matz R. Adult respiratory distress syndrome complicating severely uncontrolled diabetes mellitus: report of nine cases and a review of the literature. *Diabetes Care* 1982; 5: 574–80.
154. Vanelli M, Chiari G, Ghizzoni L, Costi G, Giacalone T, Chiarelli F. Effectiveness of a prevention program for diabetic ketoacidosis in children. *Diabetes Care* 1999; 22: 7–9.
155. Laffel LM, Brackett J, Ho J, Anderson BJ. Changing the process of diabetes care improves metabolic outcomes and reduces hospitalizations. *Qual Manag Health Care* 1998; 6: 53–62.
156. van den Berghe G, Wouters P, Weekers F, Verwaest C, Bruyninckx F, Schetz M, Vlasselaers D, Ferdiande P, Lauwers P, Bouillon R. Intensive insulin therapy in the critically ill patients. *N Engl J Med* 2001; 345: 1359–67.
157. Umpierrez GE, Isaacs SD, Bazargan N, You X, Thaler YM, Kitabchi AE. Hyperglycemia: an independent marker of in-hospital mortality in patients with undiagnosed diabetes. *J Clin Endocrinol Metab* 2002; 87: 978–82.
158. Poitout V, Robertson RP. Secondary β-cell in type 2 diabetes: a convergence of glucotoxity and lipotoxicity. *Endocrinology* 2002; 143: 339–42.

61

Complications of Insulin Therapy

Samuel Edwin Fineberg* and James H. Anderson, Jr.†

*Indiana University School of Medicine, Indianapolis, IN, USA, and †Eli Lilly and Company, Indianapolis, IN, USA

INTRODUCTION

Insulin Purification and Structure

The use of highly purified animal insulins, semisynthetic, and recombinant DNA human insulins has resulted in a dramatic reduction in the immunological complications of insulin therapy [1]. Even in countries that for economic reasons continue to use purified beef insulin, anti-insulin-antibody-related problems are seldom seen [2]. However, anti-insulin antibodies are detectable by solid-phase assays in the majority of nondiabetic individuals, and insulin immunity demonstrable by radioimmunoassay (RIA) can arise spontaneously in normal individuals associated with insulin injection, viral infections, inflammatory states, and the use of various drugs [3]. Further, anti-insulin antibodies commonly precede the appearance of type 1 diabetes, especially in children [4]. Insulin when used as a therapeutic agent cannot be administered in a physiological manner and must be modified to alter activity profiles and delivered in a nonpulsitile fashion via nonphysiological routes. Insulin manufacturers have introduced various insulin analogues in an attempt to overcome the shortcomings of unmodified injected insulins. Alternative route insulin delivery via mucosal (respiratory or gastrointestinal tract) dermal or serosal surfaces (peritoneum) is under active exploration in order to enhance the convenience of insulin delivery and possibly provide for access to portal venous drainage [5]. Modification of manufacturing techniques, the development of insulin analogues, and differences in delivery mode may induce immune tolerance or enhance immunological responses through presentation of new epitopes, stimulation of natural immunity via B1 lymphocytes, presence of manufacturing by-products, or unanticipated delivery-related factors [6].

Prior to the 1970s insulin preparations were produced by repeated recrystallization of pancreatic insulin extracts. These insulins contained non-insulin peptides and insulin degradation products [7]. Patients treated with these conventionally purified insulins sustained an up to 30% incidence of allergic phenomena related to insulin antibodies and had antibodies to glucagon as well as other pancreatic peptides [8, 9]. It has also been proposed that antigen complexes containing both insulin and glucagon may contribute to insulin's immunogenicity [10]. After the application of gel and ion-exchange chromatography, the proinsulin content of animal insulins decreased from 3000 ppm to less than 3 ppm [11–13]. Non-insulin pancreatic peptides are present in virtually undetectable concentrations in currently available highly purified porcine or bovine insulins [13]. Reversed-phase high-performance liquid chromatography has been added to the purification steps in semisynthetic and biosynthetic human insulins [14, 15]. Semisynthetic human insulin is converted from porcine insulin by substitution of alanine (B30) by threonine [14]. Biosynthetic human insulin is enzymatically derived from either an intact human proinsulin gene inserted in a nonpathogenic strain of *Escherichia coli* or alternatively from foreshortened synthetic proinsulin produced from genes inserted in yeast [15, 16]. Residual bacterial or yeast proteins are undetectable in these insulins and have not produced detectable antibody responses [17].

There are three commercially available insulin analogues (see Table 1). Two are similar in their rapid subcutaneous absorption and short duration profiles because of decreased affinity for hexamer formation, insulin lispro (B28 lys, B29 pro) and insulin aspart (B28 asp). Insulin glargine has a diarginyl moiety, added to B30 and glycine substituted at A21 for stability [18, 19]. At physiological

International Textbook of Diabetes Mellitus, Third Edition. Edited by R. A. DeFronzo, E. Ferrannini, H. Keen, and P. Zimmet.
 ISBN: 0-471-48655-8.

Table 1 Sequence differences among insulins

	A chain				B chain		
	8	9	10	21	28	29	30
Unmodified insulins							
Human	Thr	Ser	Ile	Asn	Pro	Lys	Thr
Pork	Thr	Ser	Ile	Asn	Pro	Lys	Ala
Beef	Ala	Ser	Val	Asn	Pro	Lys	Ala
Human analogues							
Lispro	Thr	Ser	Ile	Asn	Lys	Pro	Thr
Aspart	Thr	Ser	Ile	Asn	Asp	Lys	Thr
Glargine	Thr	Ser	Ile	Gly	Pro	Lys	Thr(+Arg − Arg)
Detemir	Thr	Ser	Ile	Asn	Pro	Lys	Thr
						C14 fatty acid	

pH, insulin glargine precipitates, resulting in its delayed systemic absorption. The immunology of these preparations is discussed below. In addition, intermediate duration insulin, insulin detemir, is under clinical investigation and achieves prolongation of activity by attachment of a C14 fatty acid to B29, which in turn leads to albumin binding after absorption [20].

Regardless of modifications in the insulin molecule, hypoglycemia and other nonimmunological complications due to the intrinsic activity of insulin as well as those attributable to faulty timing or injection techniques are likely to be seen until true closed-loop feedback therapies or transplantation of β-cells can be perfected and made widely available.

This chapter reviews insulin immunology and the immunological and nonimmunological complications of insulin therapy (see Table 2).

IMMUNOLOGICAL COMPLICATIONS OF THERAPY

Insulin Immunology

Insulin allergic reactions were seen in the first insulin preparations used for therapy of diabetes mellitus. The earliest report of human insulin's ability to incite antibody responses in normal individuals was associated with the use of cadaveric human insulin extracts in insulin shock therapy [17]. Subcutaneous human insulin administration with biosynthetic insulins has now been shown to incite antibody responses in nondiabetic individuals as well as in diabetic individuals treated via subcutaneous, respiratory, and peritoneal routes. Insulin autoimmunity has been demonstrated in the Hirata syndrome associated with thiourea therapy in hyperthyroidism, other drug therapies, collagen vascular diseases, and various viral illnesses [21–24]. Insulin autoimmunity is common prior to the development of type 1 diabetes and very low levels of autoantibodies may be detectable by Enzyme-linked immunosorbent assay (ELISA) in normal individuals that may be directed against epitopes differing from those detectable by liquid-phase RIA [25]. Studies in transgenic mice suggest that the low levels of antibodies seen with ELISA may be a reflection of natural immunity, whereas most of the insulin antibody response in nondiabetic individuals is under active T-cell suppression stimulated by circulating levels of endogenous insulin [25]. The antibody responses after injection therapy and in insulin autoimmunity that are detectable by RIA seem to bypass these suppressive mechanisms and

Table 2 Complications of insulin therapy

Nonimmunological	
Hypoglycemia	Injection site infection
Lipohypertrophy	Insulin edema
Pseudoallergy	Diabetic ketoacidosis associated with continuous subcutaneous insulin infusion
Immunological	
Insulin allergy	Localized: immediate, biphasic, delayed, localized Arthus reaction
Injection site lipoatrophy	Systemic: anaphylaxis, serum sickness, angioedema, hematological, gastrointestinal, dermatological
Antibody-related hypoglycemia	Protamine allergy
Insulin resistance	Zinc allergy
Immune complex related disorders antibody transfer	Maternal–Fetal insulin and antibody transfer

Table 3 Potential immunogens in pharmaceutical insulins

Pancreas-derived insulin	Biosynthetic insulin
Insulin	Insulin
Proinsulin	Proinsulin
Noninsulin pancreatic peptides	Yeast or *E. coli* peptides
Protamine	Protamine
Zinc	Zinc
Insulin covalent dimers	Insulin covalent dimmers
Insulin storage products	Insulin storage products
Preservatives	Preservatives
Plasticizers (cap materials)	Plasticizers (cap materials)

may reflect activation of sequestered B1 lymphocytes [25].

The Immunology of Pharmaceutical Insulins

Complications attributable to circulating antibodies and cellular immunity have not been totally averted, even with the *de novo* treatment of patients with human insulin. Over 80 naturally occurring species of insulin (including a small number of human insulin structural variants) have been described. More than 1000 structural variants of insulin have been produced. Biologically effective insulins share little variation in receptor-binding motifs but they may vary in portions of the molecule responsible for immunogenicity and hexamer- and dimer-forming attributes [15]. All insulins must be pharmaceutically modified to assure storage stability and these modifications can also alter absorption. Thus, the production of commercial insulin formulations increases the potential for antigens and haptens that might evoke insulin antibody responses. A list of potential immunogens found in insulin formulations can be found in Table 3.

Amino acids critical in receptor binding include A1–3, A5, A19, and A21 and B6, B12, B16, B22, and B23 [18, 24] (see Table 4). The receptor-binding and immunogenic portions of the molecule are not coincident. B6 probably plays a critical role in preserving the structure of the receptor-binding groove. The hexamer- and dimer-forming faces of the insulin molecule are on the backside of the insulin monomer, opposite to the receptor groove. Only B10, a weakly immunogenic site, is on the hexamer face.

With regard to the immunogenic portions of the insulin molecule, the A loop region of the insulin monomer, A8–10, is in an outer portion of the monomer and is closely adjacent to B3. B30 is in a mobile portion of the B chain that must swing out of the way to permit insulin receptor binding. In studies performed in transgenic mice it has been demonstrated that alterations in the amino acid structure of the A loop region (A8–10) are immunodominant and result in significant immunogenicity with the most likelihood of producing high affinity, structure-specific immune responses [26]. Alterations at B10 and B30 have weak effects upon immunogenicity while the terminal end of the B chain is important in efficient dimer formation. Alterations in the order or structure of the 28th and/or 29th amino acids or omission of the terminal 5 amino acids of the B chain result in insulins that resist crystal formation. Therefore one could predict that insulin analogues that affect the amino acid structure of the insulin molecule in areas outside the A loop structure would be relatively weak immunogens. This has been confirmed for insulin lispro, insulin aspart, and insulin glargine [27–29]. A comparison of the structures of the various human insulins with animal source insulin is shown in Table 1 and factors affecting the immunogenicity of insulin are summarized in Table 5.

Table 4 Relationship of insulin structure to its bioactivity and immunogenicity

Receptor binding	A1–3, A5, A19, A21 and B6, B12, B22, B23
Immunogenicity	A8–10, B10, and B30

Table 5 Factors affecting the development of insulin antibodies

Insulin-related	
Purity	Formulation
Molecular structure	Excipients
Storage conditions	Dimer and oxidation products
Patient-related	
Age	Endogenous insulin
HLA type	Delivery route and pattern

Animal insulins are more immunogenic than human insulins [11–13, 30]. Even the most highly purified beef insulin exceeds pork and human insulins in inciting circulating antibodies and in the incidence of insulin injection site lipoatrophy and local allergy. Insulin antibody levels have been shown to be increased in individuals who are positive for HLA-DR4 and -DR7, whereas lower levels were seen in those individuals positive for HLA-B8, -DR3, and C4 QA0 [31]. There may be a link in immune responsiveness to genes for IgG heavy chains. There also seems to be an age relationship and relationship to levels of circulating insulin in the development of insulin antibodies, with younger type 1 patient being more prone to develop an immune response to porcine and human insulins than do older patients with type 2 diabetes [32]. Older individuals have been found to be less responsive to immunogens than do younger individuals and insulin antibodies preceding the onset of type 1 diabetes are much more common in individuals below the age of 20 [33]. Patients previously treated with conventional insulin preparations not only had antibodies to insulin and non-insulin peptides, but also had high levels of antibodies directed against the animal proinsulins [30]. However, clinical trials with human biosynthetic proinsulin have demonstrated that human proinsulin is quite a weak immunogen as is glargine (diarginyl attached to B30) [29, 34]. Adverse storage conditions accelerate the formation of covalent insulin dimers. It has been suggested that a substantial portion of the immunogenicity may be linked to insulin covalent dimers that form over time in insulins [35, 36]. Dimer-directed antibodies can be demonstrated in a high proportion of conventional insulin-treated individuals. Insulin suspension formulations have been shown to be significantly more antigenic than soluble preparations when injected subcutaneously, although lente and protamine insulins are equivalent [12]. There is also some evidence that if soluble insulin is delivered by continuous subcutaneous infusion, this route may contribute to increased immunogenicity [37]. Intravenous insulin therapy with recrystallized insulin has also been shown to evoke antibody responses in the past [38]. Intraportal insulin delivery using highly concentrated human insulin delivered intraperitoneally results in enhanced antibody formation [39, 40]. While a portion of the enhanced immunogenicity of intraperitoneal insulin is due to degradation products, injection of the same insulin into subcutaneous sites produces less antibody response. In addition, preliminary reports regarding inhaled insulin also suggest that insulin delivered via this route is also immunogenic [6]. There is no question that a significant number of individuals treated with protamine insulins develop detectable anti-protamine antibodies [41, 42]. Combined insulin allergy with protamine allergy has also been reported, which required desensitization to insulin and protamine. However, protamine antibodies become a problem only rarely during the rapid reversal of heparin anticoagulation [43]. The presence of such antibodies does not predict protamine-related anaphylaxis [43]. Zinc present in various concentrations in insulin formulations may also precipitate local or systemic immune reactions [44]. Also, it is possible that insulin oxidation products as well as plasticizers in cap material, preservatives, or diluents may contribute to insulin immunogenicity or to injection site reactions.

Altered Pharmacokinetics and Antibody-induced Hypoglycemia

Most large-scale analyses of anti-insulin antibody levels usually seen in clinical practice have not shown consistent effects on insulin pharmacokinetics and insulin dose requirements, whereas some analyses do confirm an effect of moderate or high levels of antibodies on increasing insulin dose per day [45, 46]. When patients have been transferred from conventional bovine to highly purified insulins, dose requirements may decrease by up to 14% [45]. Careful monitoring of glucose levels is advisable during the transfer of patients from conventional to highly purified porcine or human insulins or when switching between various formulations of human insulin or human insulin analogues. In a study of the relationship of circulating antibodies, it has been shown that treatment with moderate doses of insulin (20–40 U/day) results in a predominant IgG-1 and IgG-2 response whereas high doses of 90–135 U/day were associated with increased levels of IgG-4 [47]. High levels of insulin antibodies result in inhibition of cellular binding of insulin, which may be demonstrated *in vitro*, or may act as a carrier protein, resulting in clearance by the reticuloendothelial system. In addition to insulin resistance, antibody binding of insulin may interfere or delay the onset of insulin action following a premeal dosage [48]. Such effects have been reported when radiotracer insulin binding in an RIA is $>10\%$. The presence of insulin antibodies also interferes with the detection of insulin by immunoassay [49]. Therefore in insulin-treated individuals, it is advisable to measure free insulin levels after bedside precipitation of antibody-bound insulin by polyethylene glycol [50]. Anti-insulin antibodies may also serve as an insulin buffer as first suggested by Dixon [51]. The reported benefits of such binding are a decreased incidence of diabetic ketoacidosis and prolonged insulin activity [51]. However, detrimental effects of the release of antibody-bound insulin include unpredictable hypoglycemia, delayed recovery from hypoglycemia, a disturbed time action profile, and possibly metabolic instability [52]. Insulin-antibody-mediated hypoglycemia has been reported in the insulin autoimmune syndrome, most commonly seen in women who are being treated with thioureas for hyperthyroidism [53]. Insulin-antibody-related hypoglycemia has also been reported in insulin-treated patients and in patients whose antibodies arise spontaneously.

Transplacental Transfer of Insulin Antibodies

Maternal insulin crosses the placenta associated with anti-insulin antibodies. Increased insulin levels seen in infants of diabetic mothers are associated with such transfer and such insulin is present in immune complexes in the infant [54]. However, the persistence of antibodies well into postnatal life may be the harbinger of type 1 diabetes [55]. It has been proposed that transferred antibodies might increase the need for fetal insulin secretion and might lead to postnatal complications such as postpartum hyperglycemia secondary to antibody binding or hypoglycemia secondary to β-cell hypertrophy [56]. Macrosomia may be related to fetal serum insulin levels independent of glucose levels. Whether other fetal complications of pregnancy in diabetes, such as an increased frequency of spontaneous abortions or perinatal deaths, are related to transplacental insulin transfer has been suggested but not been confirmed.

Insulin Allergy, Pseudoallergic Reactions, and Injection Site Infection

Allergic reactions to insulin therapy that were once seen in up to 55% of patients now occur in 2–3% of individuals

Table 6 Mechanisms of insulin antibody-mediated allergic complications

Mechanism	Effect
IgE → mast cell discharge	Local immediate and anaphylaxis
IgG → compliment fixation	Arthus reaction, serum sickness
Lymphocyte mediated	Delayed hypersensitivity (tuberculin-like)

[57]. Positive skin tests with purified pork insulin have been detected in 40% of otherwise asymptomatic insulin-treated patients [58]. Most commonly, allergic reactions are localized to insulin injection sites and occur within the first 1–4 weeks of therapy. Injection site pseudoallergic reactions can be confused with allergic reactions because of intradermal injections of insulin. These reactions are associated with marked pain at the injection site and occur rapidly after injection [59]. Sites become reddened within an hour and later become violet in color. Purulent reactions associated with intradermal injections are characterized by perivascular cuffing with a mononuclear infiltrate. Such reactions may take several days to resolve. In patients treated *de novo* with purified porcine, beef/pork, or human insulins, the incidence of local allergy was found to be 3.9, 12, and 2.4% respectively [57].

Mechanisms leading to allergic reactions to insulin are shown in Table 6. Localized skin reactions to insulin are usually mild and may occur within minutes to 4 h after injection. These symptoms tend to remit spontaneously over a period of 3–4 weeks as therapy is continued [60, 61]. Antihistamines, such as diphenylhydramine, are useful in blocking wheal-and-flare reactions and may be used to ease patients" symptoms. Less commonly an IgE-mediated biphasic reaction may occur with an immediate reaction within 1 h, followed by a deep indurated, often painful lesion that lasts over 24 h. Late-phase, lymphocyte-mediated reactions can occur in isolation without an immediate reaction. Rarely, an Arthus-type reaction can be seen with histological evidence of ischemic cellular damage at the injection site [60, 61]. Histamine blockers are ineffective in modifying late-phase or tuberculin-like reactions. In some individuals, severe local reactions persist longer than 14–30 days. Proper injection technique should be emphasized and observed. Patients should then switch to human insulin if they are not already on this therapy. The human insulin analogues, insulin lispro and insulin aspart, have proven useful in treatment of insulin allergic reactions [62, 63].

If switching insulins is ineffective, then intradermal testing should be carried out to ascertain the least reactive insulin. As mentioned above, testing with even highly purified, low immunogenicity pork insulin produces positive skin tests in a significant proportion of asymptomatic insulin-treated individuals. During intradermal testing, reactivity to zinc sulfate should also be assessed along with a comparison of protamine and protamine-free insulins. Testing consists of the intradermal injection of 0.02 ml at 1:1 dilutions of U100 insulin, human, porcine, and bovine insulins in phenol-saline diluent; 0.02 ml of a 700 μg/ml solution of zinc sulfate; 0.02 ml of histamine phosphate (0.1 mg/ml), and diluent alone. Histamine phosphate serves as a positive control and the saline serves as a negative control. Reactions should be observed at 20 min, 6 h, and 24 h. Positive wheal-and-flare reactions should exceed the phenol saline control by 5 mm, 20 min after injection. Induration should exceed 1 cm. Patients should then be treated with the least reactive insulin. Zinc sulfate reactivity indicates the possible usefulness of protamine insulins that are low in zinc content. If the above measures are not successful, then the following should be considered: (1) divide dosage and deliver into multiple sites, (2) use soluble insulin delivered by constant subcutaneous insulin infusion (CSII), (3) add dexamethasone to each unit of insulin delivered (1 or 2 mg of dexamethasone/1000 unit vial), and (4) add systemic antihistamines [64, 65]. In addition, two relatively untested approaches have been suggested: cimetidine 300 mg t.i.d. or oral insulin plus aspirin in individuals unresponsive to dermal desensitization [66, 67].

Systemic Allergy

Systemic allergy has been seen in less than 0.01% in patients treated with highly purified porcine and human insulins [65, 68]. Most commonly systemic allergy is characterized by cutaneous reactions such as urticaria, generalized rash, pruritis, or paresthesias. Cardiorespiratory reactions include angioedema palpitations, pallor, and circulatory collapse. Gastrointestinal manifestations have also been reported and include nausea, vomiting, cramps, and diarrhea. Hematological complications such as hemolytic anemia have also been reported [69].

Anaphylaxis due to insulin must be differentiated from anaphylaxis due to protamine hypersensitivity [70]. In only one case has anaphylaxis occurred in an individual who had interrupted treatment with protamine insulin. Most instances of protamine anaphylaxis have occurred during rapid reversal of heparin anticoagulation [71]. Reported mild protamine allergic reactions include flushing, urticaria, and angioedema often accompanied by transient hypotension. However, more prolonged hypotension, cardiac arrest, and respiratory obstruction have also been reported. In addition, transient hematological disorders have been seen. Anaphylaxis from either insulin or protamine is treated with life support measures, epinephrine by injection, and possibly steroids in an intensive care setting [72, 73].

Discontinuation of insulin is usually not advisable because of the possibility of future anamnestic reactions but could be considered in individuals who might be diet or oral hypoglycemic agent responsive. Desensitization with purified porcine and human insulins is successful in over 94% of individuals [64]. A thorough discussion of the problems surrounding drug challenge and desensitization protocols is included in an article by Greenberger [73]. The mechanism of benefit from desensitization is unknown.

Skin Testing

Prior to desensitization, one should perform skin testing to determine the least reactive insulin. Begin with intradermal injections of 0.02 ml of neutral regular human insulin containing 0.001 units and proceeding to 0.01 and 0.1 units. If positive wheal-and-flare reactions are observed, test with porcine insulin in the same matter and then if positive, proceed to insulin lispro or insulin aspart. A positive test results in a wheal-and-flare reaction 5 mm greater than negative control. If initial testing is negative, then proceed to test with 1 unit of insulin and if this is also negative, proceed to treat the patient with this insulin. If skin testing is positive, one should proceed to formal desensitization.

Desensitization

Desensitization should be carried out in a hospital setting, with a syringe of 1:1000 epinephrine, life support equipment, and an intravenous line in place. It is not advisable to mask reactions with prior administration of steroids or antihistamines. In medically stable patients in whom therapy ceased less than 24 h prior to desensitization, administer one third of the last dose of the same type of therapeutic insulin subcutaneously and increase the dosage by 5 units every 12 h. If reactions occur, reduce to the previous dosage, otherwise begin therapy with intermediate duration insulins when satisfactory metabolic control is achieved [74].

If reactions occur even with the reduction of dosage, if patients are medically unstable, or the last insulin therapy was less than 24 h prior to desensitization, proceed to a rapid desensitization protocol [73]. Using sterile saline, one should make a 1:1 dilution of U100 insulin and then serial 1:10 dilutions of the least reactive soluble U100 insulin down to 0.005 U/ml (50, 5, 0.5, 0.05, and 0.005 U/ml). Then every 20 min beginning with 0.05 U/ml, administer increasing doses of insulin subcutaneously, proceeding from 0.02 to 0.04 and 0.08 cm^3 for each dilution. The absolute amounts of insulin injected would be from 0.001 to 4 units in 12 steps until a wheal-and-flare reaction is observed. If such a reaction or induration >1 cm is observed with 0.02 ml of the 0.05 U/ml solution, one should begin desensitization with 0.005 U/ml. Reduce the injectate by two dilution steps if higher concentrations produce a reaction. When patients tolerate the highest desensitization steps, double the dose every 4 h until metabolic stability is achieved. Patients should then be treated for 48–72 h with injections of short-acting insulin at least every 6 h prior to switching to intermediate or long-action insulins. Rarely desensitization is not successful in a metabolically unstable individual. Then use of steroid therapy or delivery of soluble insulin by CSII may become necessary. An infrequent accompaniment of desensitization is the initiation of insulin resistance [75].

Insulin-Antibody-mediated Resistance

Insulin-antibody-mediated insulin resistance has been previously estimated to occur in less than 0.1% of patients. Occasionally, antibody-mediated insulin resistance can lead to diabetic ketoacidosis [76]. Rare reports of antibody-mediated insulin resistance have been seen with human and pork insulins, although most individuals have had exposure to animal source insulins in the past [76–79]. Such resistance has been defined as an insulin requirement of >2.5 U/kg in adults and >1.5 U/kg in children. The vast majority of individuals requiring high doses of insulin have insufficient antibody binding to account for increased insulin requirements (>15 units/l) [78]. Insulin antibody binding is usually determined in liquid-phase assays in which antibodies are titered against fixed amounts of radiotracer insulin and varying amounts of nonlabeled beef, pork, and human insulins. Unlike the cross-reactivity that is usually seen with antibody levels in nonresistant patients, it is not uncommon to observe preferential binding of a heterologous population of antibodies for one species over all others. Predisposing factors for insulin resistance include a history of atopy, interrupted insulin therapy (especially with beef-containing insulins), and desensitization for systemic allergy [79]. In assessing patients for resistance, one should determine whether insulin therapy can be replaced with diet and/or oral hypoglycemic agents. Intercurrent illness, neoplasia, drugs, factitious insulin dosage, and other known causes of insulin resistance should be actively sought [80]. Patients on beef-containing insulins should be switched to highly purified porcine or human insulin or human insulin analogues, which are effective in the reduction of dose requirements in over 40% of individuals [81]. Sulfated beef insulin (which is no longer available) was proven to be effective in reduction of antibody-mediated resistance in the past [78]. If these measures prove to be ineffective, the institution of 40–80 mg of prednisone a day in a tapering manner over 4–6 weeks should be begun. Steroids have proven to be effective in about 50% of individuals. Steroid therapy must be approached with caution since in responsive individuals it is not unusual to observe dramatic falls in insulin requirements with subsequent hypoglycemia. Plasmaphoresis has also been used to reduce the antibody load in immunological insulin resistance [82]. If all of the above fail, the use of U500 porcine or human regular insulin administered two to three times per day, which in this concentrated form has delayed absorption characteristics, may prove effective in glycemic control and reduction of dose [83]. While antibody-mediated resistance in most patients spontaneously remits, patients have been seen whose resistance persisted for >5 years.

Injection Site Lipoatrophy

In contrast to reports of up to 55% incidence of insulin injection site lipoatrophy with older preparations of bovine insulins, *de novo* treatment with highly purified bovine insulin resulted in a 9% incidence [11]. There are only scattered reports of lipoatrophy with highly purified porcine or human insulins [84]. These hollowed out areas are characterized by local loss of fat cells and are largely noninflammatory in histological appearance. Lipoatrophy occurs more often in individuals with dermal reactions to insulin and a predilection for young children has been reported. While lesions usually are limited to injection sites, they may also occur distally. In a study of 14 patients with lipoatrophy, Reeves demonstrated that lipoatrophic lesions occurred in individuals with high levels of circulating anti-insulin antibodies [85]. The edges of these lesions were characterized by deposition of immunologic proteins within dermal vessels, most commonly IgM and C3 or fibrin. Reaccumulation of fat cells occurs over 90% of the time when highly purified porcine or human insulins (including short-acting insulin analogues) are repeatedly injected into the affected areas [86, 87]. Once such areas are filled out, occasional injection of insulin is required to maintain normal appearance (see Figure 1). If reaccumulation of fat does not occur, injection of dexamethasone 4 μg/unit added to the insulin injection has been found to be effective in restoration of fat [88].

Immune-Complex-related Disorders in Diabetes—Possible Relationship Between Anti-insulin Antibodies and Diabetic Complications

Microangiopathy in diabetes has a similar histological appearance to lesions in immune complex disorders [89]. Elevated levels of immune complexes have been reported in individuals with advanced microvascular complications. However, there is little evidence to support the idea that insulin antibodies are contained in increased amounts within these complexes. Significant correlations have been found between soluble immune complexes, insulin dosage, and evidence of small and large vessel damage. [90]. *In vitro*, evidence has been presented that beef insulin–anti-insulin immune complexes are significantly more potent activators of procoagulant activity than does pork or human insulin [91]. Thus it is possible, but unproven, that high levels of anti-insulin antibodies may indirectly relate to diabetic vasculopathy.

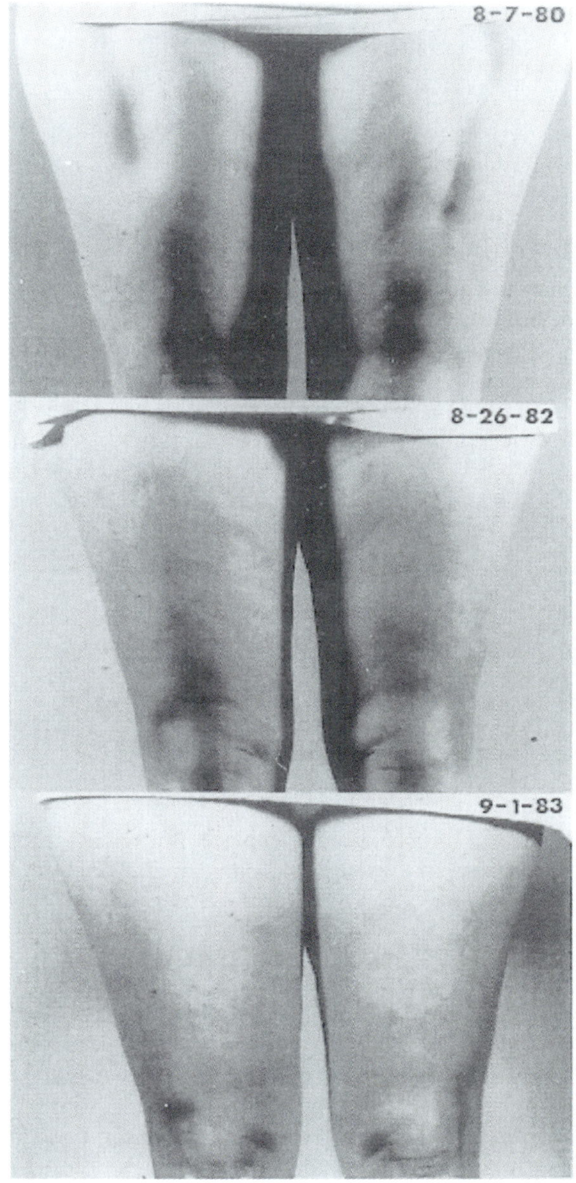

Figure 1 Injection site lipoatrophy (top panel) secondary to injection of beef-containing insulin. Repeated injections of highly purified soluble porcine insulin resulted in reaccumulation of lost fat (middle and lower panels). Photographs were obtained through the courtesy of J.A. Galloway, MD, Lilly Research Laboratories

NONIMMUNOLOGICAL COMPLICATIONS OF INSULIN THERAPY

Injection Site Lipohypertrophy

Hypertrophy of subcutaneous fat at sites of repeated insulin injections continues to be a common nonimmunological complication of therapy [92]. Also, hypertrophy of omental fat has been reported to be a cause of catheter

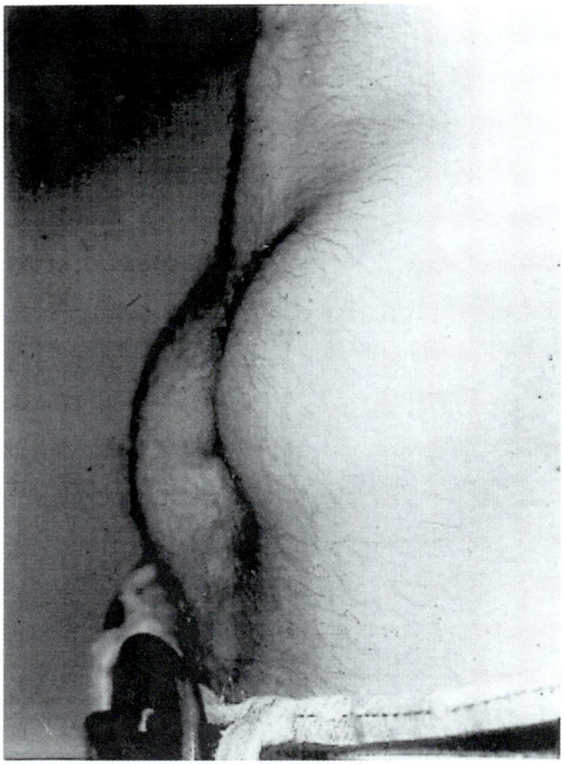

Figure 2 Injection site lipohypertrophy resulting from repeated injections into the same areas. The photograph was obtained through the courtesy of J.A. Galloway, MD, Lilly Research Laboratories

occlusion during the course of intraperitoneal delivery of concentrated insulin by implantable insulin pumps [93]. Such examples of fat cell hypertrophy are likely to result from the natural mitogenic activity of insulin. Pathologically, such fatty tumors are fibrous and have decreased vascularity. Patients often continue to select these injection sites owing to their relative anesthesia. Absorption from hypertrophic sites has been shown to be significantly impaired in studies by Young and coworkers, utilizing clearance of ^{125}I-insulin in 12 insulin-dependent patients [94]. If avoidance of affected sites does not result in regression and removal is desirable, liposuction is advised [95] (see Figure 2).

Insulin Edema

Edema associated with insulin therapy is an unusual and usually self-limited disorder. This is infrequently reported in the current literature but should be suspected when the institution of insulin therapy is associated with a sudden weight gain over short periods of time [96]. Although Leifer first reported insulin edema in 1928, the incidence of this condition is unknown [97]. However, 3.5% of 491 patients in a series from Africa developed edema associated with malnutrition and insulin-induced hypoglycemia [98]. This complication of therapy has been most often reported after the initiation of insulin, following a large change in dosage, or following treatment for diabetic ketoacidosis. Perhaps the most dramatic reported results of sodium retention secondary to insulin therapy is congestive cardiac failure or ascites in individuals for whom a cardiac or renal etiology could not be demonstrated [99, 100]. Saudek and coworkers studied fluid retention in five individuals with poorly controlled diabetes and one with diabetic ketoacidosis during optimization of insulin [101]. Sodium retention did not correlate with decreases in glycemia or ketonemia and was felt to be attributable in the past to a fall in glucagon levels. Others have proposed that persistent elevation of aldosterone or antidiuretic hormone during refeeding might play a role in the mechanisms of edema [102].

Wheatley and Edwards have demonstrated that there was an increased transcapillary albumin escape in three subjects whose edema followed the institution of excessive insulin [103]. Therapy consists of reduction in dosage. Diuretic therapy is usually not advisable. Oral epinephrine has been used successfully in a patient with recurrent edema secondary to treatment of poorly controlled diabetes. The mechanism may be correction of hyperaldosteronism [104].

Insulin-induced Hypoglycemia and Hypoglycemic Unawareness

Hypoglycemia secondary to insulin therapy is the expected outcome of a mismatch between nutrients, insulin levels, insulin action, and glucose counterregulatory mechanisms. It is apparent that the risk factors for severe hypoglycemic events include a previous history of severe hypoglycemia and is inversely related to HbA_{1c} levels [105]. Additionally, the duration of insulin therapy may also be related [106]. Although attempts have been made to predict which individuals would be especially prone to develop hypoglycemia, by use of insulin infusion studies, the magnitude of counterregulatory responses does not predict susceptibility of all individuals. Hypoglycemic unawareness is likely to be the result of repeated episodes of hypoglycemia [107]. Thus, intensified insulin therapy merits careful glycemic monitoring, proper patient selection, and heightened precautions regarding hypoglycemic episodes. A complete discussion of hypoglycemia is present in Chapter 60.

REFERENCES

1. Fineberg SE. Insulin allergy and insulin resistance. In Leibovitz HE (ed) *Therapy for Diabetes Mellitus and Related Diseases.* Alexandia, VA: American Diabetes Association, 1995; pp 178–84.

2. Goswami R, Jaleal A, Kochupillai NP. Insulin antibody response to bovine insulin therapy, functional significance among insulin requiring young diabetics in India. *Diabetes Res Clin Pract* 2000; 49 (suppl): 7–15.
3. Fineberg SE, Biegel AA, Durr KL, Hufferd S, Fineberg NS, Anderson JH. Presence of insulin autoantibodies as a regular autoantibodies as a regular feature of nondiabetic repertoire of immunity. *Diabetes* 1991; 40: 1187–93.
4. Yu L, Cuthbertson DD, Maclaren N, Jackson R, Palmer JP, et al. Expression of GAD 65 and islet cell antibody (ICA 512) autoantibodies among cytoplasmic ICA + relatives is associated with eligibility for the diabetes prevention trial-type 1. *Diabetes* 2001; 50: 1735–40.
5. Owens DR. New horizons—alternative routes for insulin delivery. *Nat Rev* 2002; 1: 520–30.
6. Stoever JA, Palmer JP. Inhaled insulin and insulin antibodies: a new twist to an old debate. *Diapers Technol Ther* 2002; 4: 157–61.
7. Mirsky IA, Kawamura K. Heterogenicity of crystalline insulin. *Endocrinology* 1966; 78: 1115–9.
8. Fitz-Patrick D, Patel YC. Antibodies to insulin, pancreatic polypeptide, glucagon and somatostatin in insulin-treated diabetics. *J Clin Endocrinol Metab* 1981; 52: 948–52.
9. Bloom SR, Barnes AJ, Adiran TE, Polak JM. Autoimmunity in diabetes induced by hormonal contaminants of insulin. *Lancet* 1979; 1: 14–7.
10. Root-Bernstein TS, Dobbelstein C. Insulin binds to glucagon a complex that is hyperantigenic and inducing antibodies having an idiotype–antiidiotype relationship. *Autoimmunity* 2001; 33: 153–69.
11. Wilson RM, Douglas CA, Tattersall RB, Reeves WG. Immunogenicity of highly purified bovine insulin: a comparison with conventional, bovine and highly purified human insulins. *Diabetologia* 1985; 28: 667–70.
12. Fineberg SE, Galloway JA, Fineberg NS, Goldman J. Effects of species of origin, purification levels and formulation on insulin immunogenicity. *Diabetes* 1983; 32: 592–9.
13. Heding LG, Marshall MO, Persson B, Dahlquist G, Thalme B, Lindgren F, Akerbloom HK, Rivla A, Knip M, Ludvigsson I, Stenhammar L, Stromberg L, Sovik O, Belevre H, Weiring K, Vidnes I, Kjaergard II, Bro P, Kaad PH. Immunogenicity of monocomponent human and porcine insulin in newly diagnosed type I (insulin-dependent) diabetic children. *Diabetologia* 1984; 27: 96–8.
14. Markussen J, Damgaard U, Pingel M, Snel L, Sorensen A, Sorensen E. Human insulin (NOVO): chemistry and characteristics. *Diabetes Care* 1983; 6 (suppl 1): 4–8.24.
15. Frank BH, Pettee JM, Zimmerman RE, Burck PJ. The production of human proinsulin and its transformation to human insulin and C-peptide. In Rich DH, Gross R (eds) *Peptides, Synthesis–Structure–Function*, Proceedings of the Seventh American Peptide Symposium. Rockford, IL: Pierce Cheurreal Co., 1981; pp 729–38.
16. Thim L, Han sen MT, Norris K, Hoegh I, Boel E, Forstom J, Ammerer G, Filil NP. Secretion and processing of insulin precursors in yeast. *Proc Natl Acad Sci USA* 1986; 83: 6766–70.
17. Fineberg SE, Galloway JA, Fineberg NS, Rathbun MJ, Hufferd S. Immunogenicity of recombinant DNA human insulin. *Diabetologia* 1983; 25: 465–9.
18. Vano Z, Fawcett J, Duckworth WC. Recombinant DNA technology in the treatment of diabetes: insulin analogues. *Endocr Rev* 2001; 22: 706–17.
19. Bolli GB, Di Marchi RD, Park BD, Pramming S, Kovisto VA. Insulin analogues and their potential use in the management of diabetes mellitus. *Diabetologia* 1999; 42: 1151–67.
20. Dea MK, Hamilton-Wessler M, Ader M, Moore D, Shaffer L, Loftager M, Volund A, Bergman RN. Albumin binding of acetylated insulin (NN304) does not deter action to stimulate glucose uptake. *Diabetes* 2002; 51: 762–9.
21. Uchigata Y, Tokunaga K, Nepom G, Bannai M, Shoji D, et al. Differential immunogenetic determinants of polyclonal insulin autoimmune syndrome (Hirata's disease) and monoclonal insulin autoimmune disease. *Diabetes* 1995; 44: 1227–32.
22. Lidar M, Rachman R, Half E, Ravid M. Insulin autoimmune syndrome after therapy with imipenem. *Diabetes Care* 1999; 22: 524–5.
23. Shah P, Mares D, Fineberg E, Pescovitz M, Jindal R, Mahoney S, Lumeng L. Insulin autoimmune syndrome as a cause of spontaneous hypoglycemia in alcoholic cirrhosis. *Gastroenterology* 1995; 109: 1673–6.
24. Kahn CR, Rosenthal AS, Immunological reactions to insulin: insulin allergy, insulin resistance and the insulin autoimmune syndrome. *Diabetes Care* 1979; 2: 283–95.
25. Thomas JW. Antigen-specific responses in autoimmunity and tolerance. *Immunol Res* 2001; 23 (2/3): 235–44.
26. Ottesen JL, Nilsson P, Weilguny D, et al. The potential immunogenicity of human insulin and insulin analogues evaluated in a transgenic mouse model. *Diabetologia* 1994; 37: 1178–85.
27. Fineberg NS, Fineberg SE, Anderson JH, Birkett M, Gibson RG, Hufferd S. Effects of insulin lispro (Lys (B28), Pro (B29) human insulin)in IDDM and NIDDM previously treated with insulin. *Diabetes* 1996; 45: 1750–4.
28. Lindholm A, Jensen LB, Home P, Raskin P, Boehn BO, Rastam J. Immune responses to insulin aspart and biphasic insulin aspart in people with type 1 and type 2 diabetes. *Diabetes Care* 2002; 25: 876–82.
29. Yki-Jarvinen H, Dressler A, Ziemen M. Less nocturnal hypoglycemia and better post diner glucose control with bedtime insulin glargine compared with bedtime NPH insulin during combination therapy in type 2 diabetes. *Diabetes Care* 2000; 23: 1130–6.
30. Klaff LJ, Vinik AI, Berelowitz M, Jackson WPU. Circulating antibodies in diabetes treated with conventional and purified insulins. *S Afr Med J* 1979; 54: 149–53.
31. Reeves WG, Barr D, Douglas CA, Gelsthorpe K, Hanning I, Skene A, Wells L, Wilson RM, Tattersall RB. Factors governing the human immune response to injected insulin. *Diabetologia* 1984; 26: 266–71.
32. Fineberg NS, Fineberg SE, Galloway J. Does age at initiation of insulin therapy determine who will develop an immune response? *Diabetes* 1992; 41 (suppl 1): 191A.
33. Graham J, Hagopian WA, Kockam I, Li LS, Sanjeevi CB, et al. Genetic effects on age-dependent onset and islet cell autoantibody markers in type 1 diabetes. *Diabetes* 2002; 51: 1346–55.
34. Fineberg SE, Rathbun MJ, Hufferd S, Fineberg NS, Spradlin CT, Galloway JA, Frank BH. Immunologic aspects of human proinsulin therapy. *Diabetes* 1988; 37: 276–80.
35. Robbins DC, Mead PM. Free covalent aggregates of therapeutic insulins in the blood of insulin-dependent diabetics. *Diabetes* 1987; 36: 147–51.

36. Robbins DC, Cooper SM, Fineberg E, Mead PM. Antibodies to covalent aggregates of insulin in blood of insulin-using diabetic patients. *Diabetes* 1987; 36: 838–41.
37. Dahl-Jorgensen K, Torjensen P, Hanssen KF, Sandvik L, Aagenaes O. Increase in insulin antibodies during continuous subcutaneous insulin infusion and multiple-injection therapy in contrast to conventional treatment. *Diabetes* 1987; 36: 1–5.
38. Deckert T, Anderson OO, Grundahl E, Kerp L. Isoimmunization of man by recrystallized human insulin. *Diabetologia* 1972; 8: 358–1.
39. Georges LP, O'Brian JT, Davidson PC, Thornton KR, Fineberg SE, Fineberg NS and the MiniMed investigators. Intraperitoneal delivery of U400 insulin is immunogenic. *Diabetes* 1993; 42: 183A.
40. Jeandidier N, Boullu S, Busch-Brafin M, Chabrier G, et al. Comparison of Hoechst 21 PH insulin using either implantable intraperitoneal pump or subcutaneous external pump infusion in type 1 diabetic patients. *Diabetes Care* 2002; 25: 84–8.
41. Kim R. Anaphylaxis masquerading as an insulin allergy. *Del Med J* 1993; 65: 17–23.
42. Bollinger ME, Hanilton RG, Wood TA. Protamine Allergyas a complication of insulin hypersensitivity: a case report. *J Allergy Clin Immunol* 1999; 104 (pt 1): 462–5.
43. Weiler JM, Gellhaus MA, Carter JG, Meng RL, Benson PM, Hottel RA, Schillig KB, Vegh AB, Clarke WR. A prospective study of the risk of an immediate adverse reaction to protamine sulfate during cardiopulmonary bypass surgery. *J Allergy Clin Immunol* 1990; 85: 713–9.
44. Bruni B, Campana M, Gamba S, Grassi G, Blatto A. A generalized allergic reaction to zinc in insulin preparation. *Diabetes Care* 1985; 8: 201.
45. Walford S, Allison SP, Reeves WG. The effect of insulin antibodies on insulin dose and diabetic control. *Diabetologia* 1982; 22: 106–10.
46. Haumont D, Dorchy H, Toussaint D, Despontin M. Exogenous insulin needs. Relationship with duration of diabetes, C-peptidemia, insulin antibodies and retinopathy. *Helv Paediatr Acta* 1982; 37: 143–50.
47. Siddiqui MA, Wangnoo SK. Selective IgG subclass antibody response to insulin in diabetic patients receiving animal insulin replacement therapy. *Int Arch Allergy Appl Immunol* 1989; 89: 49–53.
48. Peters A, Klose O, Keck F, Kerner W. The influence of insulin antibodies on the pharmacokinetics of NPH insulin in patients with type 1 diabetes treated with human insulin. *Diabet Med* 1995; 12: 925–30.
49. Hayford JT, Thompson RG. Free and total insulin integrated concentrations in insulin dependent diabetes. *Metabolism* 1982; 31: 387–97.
50. Rudkowski R, Antony G. The effect of immediate polyethylene glycol precipitation on free insulin measurements in diabetic patients with insulin antibodies. *Diabetes* 1986; 35: 253–7.
51. Dixon K, Exon PD, Hughes HR. Insulin antibodies in the etiology of labile diabetes. *Lancet* 1972; 1: 343–7.
52. Bolli GB, Dimitriadis GD, Pehling GB, Baker BA, Haymond MW, Cryer PE, Gerich JE. Abnormal glucose counterregulation after subcutaneous insulin in insulin-dependent diabetes mellitus. *N Engl J Med* 1984; 310: 1706–11.
53. Hirata Y, Tominaga M, Ito JI, Noguchi A. Spontaneous hypoglycemia with insulin autoimmunity in Graves' disease. *Ann Int Med* 1974; 81: 214–21.
54. Heding LG, Persson B, Stangenberg M. B cell function in newborn infants of diabetic mothers. *Diabetologia* 1980; 19: 427–32.
55. Hamalainen AM, Ronkainen MS, Akerblom HK, Knip M. Postnatal elimination of transplacentally acquired disease-associated antibodies in infants born to families with type 1 diabetes. The Finnish TIGIGR Study: trial to reduce IDDM in the genetically at risk. *J Clin Endocrinol Metab* 2000; 85: 4249–53.
56. Menon RK, Cohen RM, Sperling MA, Cutfield WS, Mimouni F, Khoury JC. Transplacental passage of insulin in pregnant women with insulin-dependent diabetes mellitus. Its role in fetal macrosomia. *N Engl J Med* 1990; 323: 309–15.
57. Galloway JA, Fireman P, Fineberg SE. Complications of insulin therapy: a brief review of four years experience with human insulin (rDNA). In Church J (ed) *Diabetes Mellitus Achievements and Skepticism* (Royal Society of Medicine International Congress and Symposium Series, Vol 77). Oxford: Oxford University Press, 1984; pp 55–64.
58. Grammer LC. Part C: Immunological reaction to high molecular weight therapeutic agents. *Patterson's Allergic Diseases*. Philadelphia, PA: Lippencott, Williams & Wilkins, 2002; pp 360–85.
59. Pietri A, Raskin P. Cutaneous complications of chronic continuous subcutaneous insulin infusion therapy. *Diabetes Care* 1981; 4: 624–6.
60. deShazo RD, Mather P, Grant W, Carrington D, Frentz JM, Lueg M, Lauritano AA, Falholt K. Evaluation of patients with local reactions to insulin with skin tests and *in vitro* techniques. *Diabetes Care* 1987; 10: 330–6.
61. deShazo RD, Boehm TM, Kumar D, Galloway JA, Dvorak HF. Dermal hypersensitivity, reactions to insulin: correlations of three patterns to their histopathology. *J Allergy Clin Immunol* 1982; 69: 229–37.
62. Abraham M, Al-Sharif BA, Saavedra GA, Khardori R. Lispro in the treatment of insulin allergy. *Diabetes Care* 1999; 22: 1916–17.
63. Airaghi L, Lorini M, Tedeschi A. The insulin analog aspart. A safe alternative in insulin allergy. *Diabetes Care* 2000; 24: 2000.
64. Galloway JA. Chemistry and clinical use of insulin in diabetes mellitus. In Galloway JA, Potvin JH, Suman CR (eds) *Diabetes Mellitus*. Indianapolis, IN: Eli Lilly Co., 1988; pp 105–37.
65. Granic M, Renar IP, Metelko Z, Skrabalo Z. Insulin allergy. *Diabetes Care* 1986; 9: 99–100.
66. Chideckel EW, Mullin CJ, Michael BE. Cimetidine in insulin allergy. *Diabetes Care* 1981; 4: 503–4.
67. Holdaway IM, Wilson JD. Cutaneous allergy responsive to oral desensitization and aspirin. *Br Med J Clin Res* 1984; 289A: 1565–6.
68. Hannauer L, Batson JM. Anaphylactic shock following insulin injection. *Diabetes* 1961; 10: 105–9.
69. Yamreudeewong W, Cavell RM, Hennan NE. Possible hemolytic anemia associated with human insulin therapy. *Drug Intelligence Clin Pharm Ann Pharmacother* 1990; 24: 887.
70. Weiler JM, Freiman P, Sharath MD, Metzger WJ, Smith JM, Richerson HB, Ballas ZK, Halveson PC, Shulan DJ, Matsuo S, Wilson RL. Serious adverse reactions to

protamine sulfate: are alternatives needed? *J Allergy Clin Immunol* 1985; 297–303.
71. Weiler JM, Gellhaus MA, Carter JG, Meng RL, Benson PM, et al. A Prospective study of the risk of an immediate adverse reaction to protamine sulfate during cardiopulmonary bypass surgery. *J Allergy Clin Immunol* 1990; 85: 713–9.
72. Soto-Aguillar MC, deShazo RD, Waning NP. Anaphylaxis. *Postgrad Med* 1987; 82: 154–70.
73. Greenberger P. Drug challenge and desensitisation protocols. *Immunol Allergy Clin North Am* 1998; 18: 759–72.
74. Mattson JR, Patterson R, Roberts M. Insulin therapy in patients with systemic insulin allergy. *Arch Int Med* 1975; 135: 818–21.
75. Witters LE, Ottman JL, Weir GC, Raymond LW, Lowell FC. Insulin antibodies in the pathogenesis of insulin allergy and persistence. *Am J Med* 1977; 63: 703–9.
76. Nasri F, Dib SA, Sa JR, Russo EM, Viera JP, Chacra AR. Diabetic ketoacidosis induced by immunologic insulin resistance. *Rev Assoc Med Bras* 1995; 41: 37–42.
77. Ganz MA, Unterman T, Roberts M, et al. Resistance and allergy to recombinant human insulins. *J Allergy Clin Immunol* 1990; 86: 45–52.
78. Davidson JK, Fineberg SE, DeMeyts P, Fineberg NS, Galloway JA. Immunological and metabolic responses of patients with a history of antibody-induced beef insulin resistance to treatment with beef, pork, human and sulfated beef insulin. *Diabetes Care* 1992; 15: 702–4.
79. Davidson JK, DeBra DW. Immunological insulin resistance. *Diabetes* 1978; 27: 307–18.
80. Tobe HK, Uchigata Y, Nakazomo M, Yasuda K, Terauchi Y, Iwamoto Y, Nakazono M, Iyuamoto Y, Akanuma Y, Kimura S, Kadowaki T. Antibody mediated insulin resistance treated by cessation of insulin administration. *Invest Med* 2000; 39: 143–5.
81. Lahtela JT, Knip M, Antonin J, Salmi J. Severe antibody mediated human insulin resistance: successful treatment with the insulin analog lispro. A case report. *Diabetes Care* 1997; 20: 71–3.
82. Micic D, Birkic S, Kendereski A, Popovic V, Zoric S, Nicolic JA, Ingrutinovic L, Ivanoska D, Manojlovic D, Micic J. Immunological resistance to human biosynthetic insulin—effects of immunosuppression and plasmaphoresis. *Diabetes Res Clin Pract* 1993; 19: 83–9.
83. Nathan DM, Axelrod L, Flier JS, Carr DB. U-500 insulin in the treatment of antibody-mediated insulin resistance. *Ann Int Med* 1981; 94: 653–6.
84. Page MD, Bodansky JH. Human insulin and lipoatrophy. *Diabet Med* 1992; 9: 779.
85. Reeves WG, Allen BR, Tattersall RB. Insulin-induced lipoatrophy: evidence for an immune pathogenesis. *Br Med J* 1980; 1: 1500–3.
86. Czyzyk A, Rogala H, Laweki J. Controlled study comparing treatment with monocomponent and conventional insulin in patients with lipoatrophy. *Acta Diabetol Lat* 1989; 26: 17–26.
87. Valenta LJ, Elias AN. Insulin induced lipodystrophy in diabetic patients resolved by treatment with human insulin. *Ann Int Med* 1985; 102: 790–1.
88. Kumar O, Miller L, Mehtalia S. Use of dexamethasone in treatment of insulin lipodystrophy. *Diabetes* 1977; 26: 296–9.
89. Blumenthal HT, Hirata Y, Owens CT, Beris AW. A histo- and immunological analysis of diabetes in the human and rabbit. In Sipperstein Wowell AR, Myer K (eds) *Small Blood Vessel Involvement in Diabetes Mellitus*. Washington, DC: American Institute of Biological Sciences, 1964; pp 279–87.
90. Iavicoli M, DiMario U, Pazzili P, Canalese J, Ventriglia L, Galfo C, Andreani D. Impaired phagocytic function and increased immune complexes in diabetes with severe microangiopathy. *Diabetes* 1982; 30: 7–11.
91. Uchman B, Bang NU, Rathbun MJ, Fineberg NS, Davidson JK, Fineberg SE. Effect of insulin immune complexes in human blood monocyte and endothelial cell procoagulant activity. *J Lab Clin Med* 1988; 112: 652–9.
92. Galloway JA, Peck FB Jr, Fineberg SE, Spradlin CT, Marsden JH, Allemends D, Ingulli-Fattio J. The US "new patient" and "transfer" studies. *Diabetes Care* 1982; 5 (suppl 2): 135–9.
93. Pitt HA, Saudek CD, Zacur HA. Long term intraperitoneal insulin delivery. *Ann Surg* 1992; 216: 483–91.
94. Young RJ, Hannan WT, Frier BM, Steel J, Duncan LJP. Diabetic lipohypertrophy delays insulin absorption. *Diabetes Care* 1984; 7: 479–80.
95. Bodansky HJ, Browning FS. Treatment of insulin lipohypertrophy with liposuction. *Diabet Med* 1992; 9: 395–6.
96. Hirshberg B, Nuiszkat M, Marom T, Shalit M. Natural course of insulin edema. *J Endocrinol Invest* 2000; 187–8.
97. Leifer A. Case of insulin edema. *JAMA* 1928; 90: 610–1.
98. Shaper AG. The insulin-oedema syndrome in African diabetic subjects. *Trans R Soc Trop Med Hyg* 1966; 60: 519–25.
99. Sheehan JP, Sisam DA, Schumacher OP. Insulin-induced cardiac failure. *Am J Med* 1985; 79: 147–8.
100. Bronstein HD, Kantrowitz PA, Schaffner F. Marked enlargement of the liver and transient ascites with treatment of diabetic acidosis. *N Engl J Med* 1959; 261: 1314–8.
101. Saudek CD, Boulter PR, Knopp RH, Arky RA. Sodium retention accompanying insulin treatment of diabetes mellitus. *Diabetes* 1974; 23: 240–6.
102. Spark RF, Arky RA, Boulter PR, Saudek CD, O'Brian JT. Adolsterone and glucagon in the natriuresis of fasting. *N Engl J Med* 1975; 292: 1335–40.
103. Wheatley T, Edwards OM. Insulin oedema and its clinical significance: metabolic studies in three cases. *Diabet Med* 1985; 2: 400–4.
104. Hopkins DFC, Carton SJ, Williams G. Effective treatment of insulin-induced edema using eprinephrine. *Diabetes Care* 1993; 16: 1026–8.
105. The Diabetes Control and Complications Trial (DCCT) Research Group. Epidemiology of severe hypoglycemia in the Diabetes Control and Complications Trial. *Am J Med* 1991; 90: 450–9.
106. MacLeod KM, Hepburn DA, Frier BM. Frequency and morbidity of severe hypoglycemia in insulin-treated diabetic patients. *Diabet Med* 1993; 10: 238–45.
107. Lingenfelser T, Renn W, Sommerwerk U, Jung MF, Buettner UW, Zaiser-Kaschel H, Kaschel R, Eggstein M, Jakober B. Compromised normal counterregulation, symptom awareness, and neurophysiological function after recurrent short-term episodes of insulin-induced hypoglycemia in IDDM patients. *Diabetes* 1993; 42: 610–8.

Complications: General and Microvascular

62

Pathogenesis of Diabetic Microvascular Complications

Zhiheng He, Christian Rask-Madsen, and George L. King

Joslin Diabetes Center, Harvard Medical School, Boston, MA, USA

GENERAL INTRODUCTION

Vascular and neuropathic complications are the major cause of mortality and morbidity of diabetes. Several clinical studies including the Diabetes Control and Complications Trial (DCCT) and the United Kingdom Prospective Diabetes Study (UKPDS) have shown that the severity of these complications are directly associated with hyperglycemia, regardless of the different pathogenesis of type 1 or 2 diabetes [1–3]. The cardiovascular complications, of diabetes could be classified into three categories including cardiomyopathy, macrovascular complications, and microvascular complications. Diabetic cardiomyopathy constitutes pathological and functional changes intrinsic to cardiomyocytes in diabetic states that are independent of coronary artery diseases [4]. Such changes include ventricular diastolic dysfunctions, interstitial fibrosis, and gradual loss of cardiomyocytes and contractility [4]. Macrovascular complications mainly involve coronary artery diseases, atherosclerosis, and peripheral vasculopathy [5]. Microvascular complications consist of pathological changes in the microvasculature that mainly affect the functions of retina, kidney, and neurovascular perfusion and might also contribute to reduced myocardium vascularization and wound healing. The development and progression of diabetic vascular complications are clearly associated with the severity and duration of hyperglycemia as established by the DCCT and UKPD studies as well as numerous other clinical observations. Tight glycemic control is by far the most effective approach in the prevention of diabetic vascular complications. However, current therapeutic regimen has not yet provided satisfactory glycemic control to a level that can prevent the onset of these complications. Recent progress in the mechanistic study on diabetic vasculopathy is gradually advancing our understanding of these formidable complications in cellular and molecular level. Findings from these studies provide rational for the design of novel interventions. Several theories have been proposed to explain the mechanisms underlying diabetes-induced vasculopathy. Such theories include (1) enhanced vascular oxidative stress and generation of reactive oxygen species (ROS); (2) flux through polyol pathway; (3) formation of advanced glycation end-products (AGEs); (4) formation of glycoxidation products through increased flux through hexosamine pathway; (5) activation of diacylglycerol (DAG)-protein kinase C (PKC); (6) inflammation; and (7) expression and action of vascular mediators. Derangement of any of these mechanisms has been shown to result in vascular pathology and their inhibition can partially normalize diabetes-induced damages. Furthermore, these theories also share extensive cross-interaction that form a complicated network.

PATHOLOGICAL AND FUNCTIONAL CHANGES IN VASCULAR TISSUES IN DIABETIC STATES

Hyperglycemia and diabetes-associated metabolic derangements cause many pathological and functional changes in vasculature that even present before clinical onset of diabetic vasculopathy. These changes are characterized by the thickening of vascular basement membrane,

International Textbook of Diabetes Mellitus, Third Edition. Edited by R. A. DeFronzo, E. Ferrannini, H. Keen, and P. Zimmet.
 ISBN: 0-471-48655-8.

cellular growth and death, and changes in blood flow and vessel permeability [6]. Basement membrane thickening is a common pathological change observed in many of the complications including retinopathy, nephropathy, neuropathy, and cardiomyopathy and is the most prominent structure change observed by electron microscopy. The thickening of basement membrane is a direct consequence of the expression and deposition of extracellular matrix (ECM) proteins in the vasculature. Such proteins include collagen type I, III, IV, and VI, fibronectin, and laminin. The increased expression of ECM components is well documented in the vessels from retina, kidney, and neurovascular tissues from diabetic subjects [7] and even from vascular cells cultured under hyperglycemic conditions [8]. Vascular cell growth or death is both cell-type-dependent and tissue-specific in diabetic states. Premature retinal pericyte death is the earliest and a specific change observed in diabetic retinopathy [9]. In contrast to pericyte loss, retinal endothelial cells generally undergo proliferation in diabetes to form cell clusters at the sites of pericyte loss, also known as microaneurysm, and is a hallmark change of diabetic retinopathy [9]. Further, endothelial proliferation might also contribute substantially to the pathological angiogenesis in proliferative diabetic retinopathy (PDR) [9]. The endothelial growth and angiogenesis seem to be tissue-specific, since reduced angiogenesis is observed in cutaneous wounding in diabetic rodents and patients, which results in the impaired wound healing [10–12]. In conjunction with these structural changes, gene expression for vascular tone mediators such as endothelin 1 (ET-1) and prostacyclins is also regulated to induce hemodynamic abnormalities in diabetes.

Although vascular complications in diabetes share certain common structural and functional changes, characteristic manifestations are found in the vasculopathy in a tissue-specific manner as discussed below in brief.

Retinopathy

Key features of diabetic retinopathy are loss of capillary pericytes, formation of microaneurysms, thickening of basement membrane, increased vessel permeability, vascular occlusion, and ischemia-induced neovascularization. In later stages, hemorrhage and tractional retinal detachment occur that eventually lead to vision loss [9, 13]. Poor glycemic control is the most important risk factor associated with retinopathy in both type 1 and type 2 diabetes, supported by several landmark clinical trials [1–3, 14]. Severity and duration of hyperglycemia are directly linked to the pathological changes and cause vascular dysfunctions such as retinal angiogenesis and vascular permeability [15–17]. Loss of pericytes is probably one of the earliest specific findings in diabetic retinopathy and the sites of pericytes loss are often associated with microaneurysms formation and vascular obstruction [9]. The subsequent retinal hypoxia will therefore increase the expression of angiogenic factors such as vascular endothelial growth factor (VEGF) and placenta growth factor (PLGF) that in turn promote neovascularization [9]. The importance of VEGF in the pathogenesis of diabetic retinopathy is underlined by the close association between ocular and retinal VEGF concentration and the severity of proliferative diabetic retinopathy [18, 19]. In addition to VEGF, retinal platelet-derived growth factor (PDGF) is receiving increasing attention. Mice that are genetically deficient for PDGF-BB develop vascular abnormalities including pericyte loss and microaneurysm [20, 21] that are similar to those of diabetic retinopathy. A recent study using genetic approach to disrupt the retention of PDGF-BB within the pericellular space also suggests the essential roles of PDGF in pericytes survival [22]. However, PDGF-BB expression was found increased rather than decreased in the retina from streptozotocin-(STZ)-induced diabetic rats [23], and pericytes cultured in media containing high glucose also showed an induction of PDGF-BB expression [23]. This discreet finding might suggest that the induction of PDGF-BB gene expression is likely a consequence of hyperglycemia-mediated downregulation of PDGF signaling cascade, the activation of which is required for pericyte survival.

Nephropathy

Diabetes mellitus is the leading cause of end-stage renal disease (ERSD) worldwide [24, 25]. Diabetic nephropathy is characterized by early hemodynamic changes, glomerular hyperfiltration, mesangial expansion, glomerular hypertrophy, and thickening of glomerular basement membrane that ultimately progress to glomerulosclerosis and renal insufficiency. Diabetic nephropathy is the malignant sequelae of chronic hyperglycemia, as supported by multiple evidence showing that accumulation of AGE, enhanced oxidative stress, activation of PKC, and altered expression and action of growth factors and vasoactive mediators are all observed in the glomerular tissues from diabetic subjects [26]. Furthermore, suppression of AGE formation and action [26], oxidative stress [27], and PKC activation [28, 29] respectively are all protective against the development of diabetic nephropathy, both in animal model of experimental diabetes and in diabetic patients [26]. Multiple growth factors such as the profibrotic factors transforming growth factor $\beta 1$ (TGF-$\beta 1$) and connective tissue growth factor (CTGF) are all increased in the kidney tissues from diabetic subjects and are suggested to play important roles in the accumulation of ECM proteins and the induction of mesangial expansion [26]. The upregulation of gene expression for TGF-β and CTGF have been shown to be the downstream events following the accumulation of AGE, increased oxidative stress, and the activation of PKC as discussed in the next section. In addition, the activation of vasoactive mediators such as ET-1 and angiotensin pathways is reported to increase in diabetic glomerular tissues [26] and their inhibition is clearly documented to be protective against diabetic nephropathy [26].

Neuropathy

Peripheral polyneuropathy is the most common form of diabetic neuropathy with distal symmetrical sensory loss or sensorimotor dysfunctions that often affect distal lower limbs [30]. Several pathological changes, including the loss of nerve fibers, paranodal or segmental demyelination, axonal thickening, and endoneurinal capillary narrowing, have been reported [31]. The precise pathogenesis of diabetic neuropathy is still not fully understood. However, clinical observation and studies using animal models of experimental diabetes suggest that hyperglycemia and other metabolic derangement might directly induce damages to neurons and nerve parenchyma [6]. In parallel, reduced neurovascular blood flow might also cause ischemic–neuronal damages [6]. Multiple abnormalities in diabetic states, including the activation of PKC, enhanced oxidative stress, formation of AGE in neuronal tissues, and altered expression of neurotrophic factors such as nerve growth factor (NGF) and insulin-like growth factors 1 (IGF-1), have all been reported to be important determinants for the pathogenesis of diabetic neuropathy [30, 32]. Furthermore, vascular etiology in diabetic neuropathies is supported by multiple abnormalities in the neurovasculature, including the deposition of AGE in the perineuronal vascular wall, basement thickening, endothelial cell swelling and the loss of pericytes, reduced endothelial nitric oxide activity and capillary occlusion [30], and degeneration of blood vessels supplying neuronal tissues [33]. All these changes eventually contribute to hyperglycemia-induced decreases in neurovascular blood flow and the subsequent hypoxia–ischemic damage [34]. Gene transfer of VEGF in experimental diabetic animal models has been reported to restore blood flow in neuronal tissues and rectify the conductivity of the nerves that were impaired in diabetic states [33], providing supportive evidence for the involvement of vascular component in the pathogenesis of diabetic neuropathy.

Impaired Wound Healing

Patients with diabetes and diabetic animals are often associated with impaired cutaneous wound healing [10, 35–37]. This is partly due to dermal circulation insufficiency derived from diabetic microangiopathy. In accordance with this hypothesis, several abnormalities have been reported, such as the presence of morphologically abnormal blood vessels near wound edge [11], reduced dermal angiogenesis in response to wounding, and loss of local vascular tone [12]. The importance of microvascular dysfunction in impaired wound healing is also supported by evidence showing that restoring blood supply using VEGF gene transfer enhances wound healing in diabetic animals [38]. In addition, recombinant PDGF-BB, which is a potent angiogenic factor [39], is effective in promoting chronic ulcer healing in diabetic patients in several clinical trials [40–42]. Multiple cellular abnormalities associated with diabetic microvascular dysfunctions, such as increased oxidative stress, activation of PKC, and increased AGE, are all observed in the wound site in diabetes, and suppression of their action has been reported to restore a physiological wound healing [37].

CELLULAR AND BIOCHEMICAL MECHANISMS CONTRIBUTING TO DIABETIC VASCULAR COMPLICATIONS

Over the past two decades, several mechanisms have been proposed to explain the pathogenesis of diabetic vascular complications. Although it is tempting to speculate a mechanistic frame that accommodates the diverse aspects of diabetic complications, the pathogenesis of vasculopathy is complicated beyond the simplified explanation by a unified mechanism. Seven mechanisms have been suggested to contribute to the development of diabetic vascular complications as shown in Figure 1. Instead of working alone, they share extensive cross talks and cause the multiple complications in a coordinated manner.

The understanding of these mechanisms is of particular importance in the development of pharmacological interventions treating diabetic vascular complications. By far, glycemic control is still the best therapeutic approach to prevent these vascular complications. However, strict euglycemic control is difficult to achieve and is likely to be associated with hypoglycemia. Intermittent high glucose derived from alternative fluctuation between hyper- and hypoglycemia is believed to have a much more pronounced effect on the generation of free radical and oxidative stress mediated through a PKC-dependent pathway [43]. In addition, once hyperglycemia occurred, the detrimental effects persisted for a prolonged period of time even if the risk factor was corrected via mechanisms that are not fully understood [44, 45]. Because of these side effects, interventional approaches to prevent or treat complications in the presence of hyperglycemia are urgently needed. Based on the mechanisms discussed below, several rational targets have been chosen and agents developed that show promising results in treating the vascular complications.

Oxidative-Stress-induced Vascular Pathology in Diabetes

Physiologically, tissue concentration of ROS is regulated by the balanced action of pro-oxidative and antioxidative

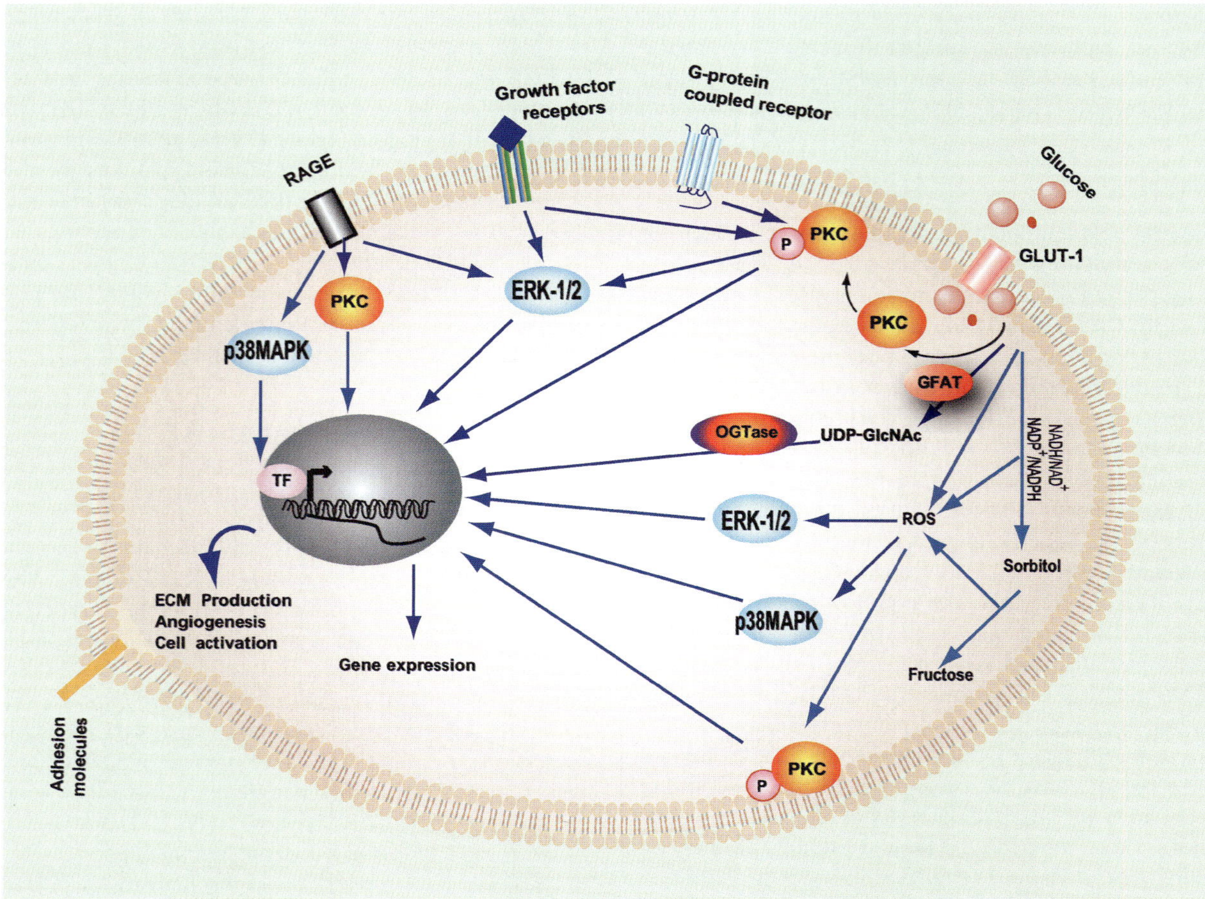

Figure 1 Schematic illustration of the proposed mechanisms underlying hyperglycemia-induced vascular complications. Formation of the reactive oxygen species (ROS), accumulation of advanced glycation end products (AGE), increased flux through the polyol and hexosamine pathways, activation of the intracellular signaling cascades such as the diacylglycerol (DAG)-protein kinase C (PKC) pathway, as well as the expression and actions of the multiple hormones, growth factors, and cytokines are all suggested to be induced by hyperglycemia in diabetes and contributes to the pathogenesis of diabetic microvascular complications. These pathways also share extensive interaction in this process. TF = transcriptional factors

mechanisms as illustrated in Figure 2. Nicotinamide adenine dinucleotide phosphate [NAD(P)H] oxidases and xanthine oxidases actively catalyze the formation of superoxide particles ($O_2^{\cdot -}$) from oxygen and can be further converted to hydrogen peroxide by superoxide dismutase (SOD). Mitochondria also contribute to the formation of ROS via the enhanced flux through the mitochondrial electron transport chain complexes. To maintain the redox homeostasis and prevent the overproduction of ROS such as $O_2^{\cdot -}$ and H_2O_2, catalase and glutathione peroxidase will further convert H_2O_2 to H_2O (Figure 2). In pathological conditions, such as diabetes mellitus, this balance cannot be maintained and will lead to the accumulation of ROS and increase oxidative stress [46]. A great deal of clinical observations have shown that both type 1 and type 2 diabetes are always accompanied by parallel induction of oxidative stress, likely to be induced by metabolic abnormalities such as hyperglycemia, dyslipidemia, and the accumulation of metabolic byproducts [27, 47, 48]. Elevated circulating levels of isoprostants, lipid peroxides, and 8-epiprostaglandin $F_{2\alpha}$ (8-epi-PGF$_{2\alpha}$), all surrogate markers for oxidative stress, are strongly associated with diabetes in patients [27, 49]. This is sometimes accompanied by the reduction of antioxidants such as reduced glutathione [50], vitamin C [51], and vitamin E [52]. However, others reported the lack of decreases of these antioxidants in diabetes [53, 54]. In the Framingham Heart Study, oxidative stress was suggested to have a close link with diabetes and might be a significant risk factor for cardiovascular diseases [49]. Serum level of ROS is also suggested to correlate with the severity of diabetic retinopathy [55]. Similar to that observed in diabetic patients, animals with experimental diabetes or even vascular cells cultured in media containing diabetic level of glucose have increased production of ROS and oxidative stress [27, 56].

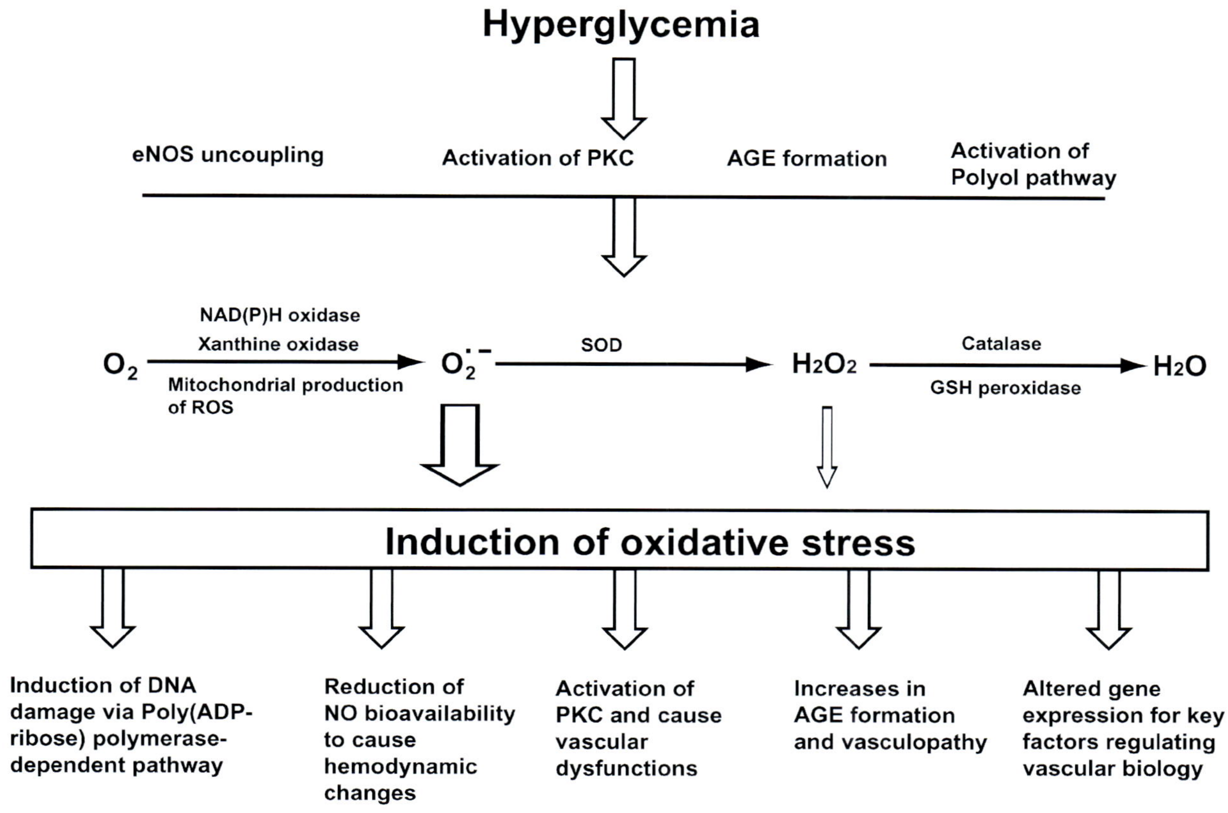

Figure 2 The roles of hyperglycemia-induced accumulation of ROS and oxidative stress in diabetic vascular complications. In diabetic states, hyperglycemia regulates the multiple steps of the production and clearance of ROS and is in favor of ROS accumulation. Such events include the production of superoxide from endothelial nitric oxide synthase (eNOS) uncoupling, activation of PKC, AGE formation, and increased flux through polyol pathway. In addition to the increased activity of NAD(P)H oxidase, mitochondrial production of ROS is also increased and results in the overproduction of superoxide $O_2^{\cdot -}$, which is the major form of ROS that causes vascular oxidative stress. This in turn, contributes to diabetic vascular complications as illustrated

Hyperglycemia can induce oxidative stress via several mechanisms [48, 56–61]. Accumulation of AGE in diabetes and AGE–receptor for AGE (RAGE) interaction have been shown to cause vascular oxidative stress. This action is probably mediated through the activation of NAD(P)H oxidase since mice null for gp91^{phox}, a crucial component of NAD(P)H oxidase, failed to generate tissue factors in response to AGE [62] whereas angiotensin II infusion resulted in the production of ROS via the induction of NAD(P)H oxidase activity [63]. Enhanced vascular oxidative stress is also found to be downstream of PKC activation. In cultured vascular cells including endothelial cells and vascular smooth muscle cells, hyperglycemia-induced generation of ROS and oxidative stress is through PKC-dependent activation of NAD(P)H oxidase [64]. One of the major sources of ROS formation in diabetes is through the marked increase flux through the mitochondrial respiratory chain [56]. Increased activity of glycolysis and tricarboxylic acid cycle in response to hyperglycemia produces abundant reducing protons that dramatically upregulate the proton gradient and in turn, increase the generation of superoxides. Increases in mitochondrial manganese superoxide dismutase (MnSOD) or uncoupling protein 1 (UCP-1) prevent hyperglycemia-induced production of ROS through the reduction of proton gradient [61, 65], providing supportive evidence for the role of increased activity of mitochondrial respiratory chain. Animal studies using mice overexpressing Cu^{2+}/Zn^{2+}-SOD showed reduced pathological changes in diabetic nephropathy, including albuminuria and glomerular hypertrophy [66]. Given the major role for SOD in the clearance of superoxide anion, it is likely that these actions are mediated by reducing ROS formation and oxidative stress. In addition, activation of aldose reductase in diabetic states will decrease cellular NADPH and alter the cellular redox balance to further induce tissue oxidative stress [6]. Uncoupling of endothelial nitric oxide synthase (eNOS) has been reported to contribute to the generation of superoxide due to either substrate [67] or cofactor deficiency [68, 69]. This mechanism might partly responsible for hyperglycemia-induced ROS generation [70].

Formation of ROS and increased oxidative stress might contribute to the multiple vascular damages in diabetes, such as endothelial dysfunctions, changes in vascular permeability, induction of leukocyte adhesion, cell-type-dependent apoptosis, abnormality in vascular cell cycle regulation, and altered vasomotor tone [6, 56] (Figure 2). These effects are regulated through the induction of cellular DNA damage [71, 72] that might be partly mediated through the activation of poly(ADP-ribose) polymerase [73]. Accumulation of ROS is known to impair vasodilation by uncoupling eNOS activity. Although it has been clearly shown that increases of oxidative stress can be achieved by increased AGE–RAGE actions and activation of PKC, oxidative stress can also activate multiple pathways including AGE–RAGE, PKC, and aldose reductase pathways to induce vascular cell damage in diabetic states [61]. Endothelial cell culture experiments showed that the suppression of mitochondrial superoxide formation could inhibit hyperglycemia-induced AGE formation, activation of PKC, and sorbitol formation [61], and therefore suggest a profound network of interactions between mechanisms utilized by hyperglycemia to mediate its adverse effects.

The contribution of oxidative stress to the development of diabetic vascular complications is supported by a great deal of studies showing the beneficial effects of antioxidants. Applications of antioxidants such as vitamin C, *d*-α-tocopherol (vitamin E), and lipoic acid in animal models of diabetes can prevent part of the vascular pathological changes. Effects on retinopathy [74, 75], neuropathy [76, 77], and nephropathy [78] have all been reported. However, clinical assessment of antioxidants in the prevention of diabetic vascular complications has yielded inconclusive results. Some of the trials involving small number of patients showed beneficial effects of antioxidants. For example, oral treatment with raxofelast, an antioxidant, improves endothelial functions in patients with type 2 diabetes and downregulate plasma 8-epi-$PGF_{2\alpha}$, a surrogate marker for oxidative stress [79]. Combined application of vitamin C and E reduces urinary albumin excretion rate [80]. Vitamin E at a dose of 1000 IU/day or higher normalizes hemodynamic changes in the retinas as well as renal functions in these patients [81]. However, large-scale clinical studies, for example, the Heart Outcome Prevention Evaluation (HOPE) study, have suggested that antioxidant treatment failed to show beneficial effects in the cardiovascular outcome in more than 1800 patients receiving vitamin E at a dose of 400 IU daily [82]. In the MICRO-HOPE study that involves 3654 diabetic patients, similar dose of vitamin E also yielded negative results in preventing cardiovascular outcome and diabetic nephropathy [83]. These results suggested that increased oxidative stress might provide supportive effects rather than being a major pathway leading to diabetic vasculopathy. It should also be noted that vitamin E at high dose (1800 IU daily) could suppress the activation of DAG-PKC [84] and rectify retinal abnormalities as reported [81] and thus is antioxidant-independent. Nevertheless, enhanced oxidative stress might provide supportive effects in the development of vascular complications, and antioxidants might require the additional therapeutic regimens to achieve satisfactory effects.

Activation of Aldose Reductase (Polyol) Pathway in Diabetes

Accumulation of metabolic products of aldose reductase (polyol) pathway has been clearly documented in vascular tissues in both diabetic patients and animals. It is thus postulated to play a role in the pathogenesis of diabetic vascular complications [85]. When challenged with hyperglycemia, intracellular aldose reductase reduces glucose to sorbitol by the utilization of NADPH. Sorbitol is in turn oxidized to fructose by another enzyme sorbitol dehydrogenase [6, 56] (Figure 3). Activation of polyol pathway has been suggested to cause vascular damages in several ways, including the osmotic damage induced by the accumulation of sorbitol [85]; overconsumption of NADPH reduces nitric oxide in vasculature [86], and increased $NADH/NAD^+$ ratio might also increase oxidative stress and reduce Na^+–K^+-ATPase activity [56]. Although inhibitors of aldose reductase have been shown to prevent some pathological changes in animal model of diabetic retinopathy [87, 88], nephropathy [89], and neuropathy [90, 91], these results are not conclusive, since long-term application of aldose reductase inhibitor failed to alter diabetic retinopathy and nephropathy in diabetic canine [92]. Further, clinical trials using aldose reductase inhibitors

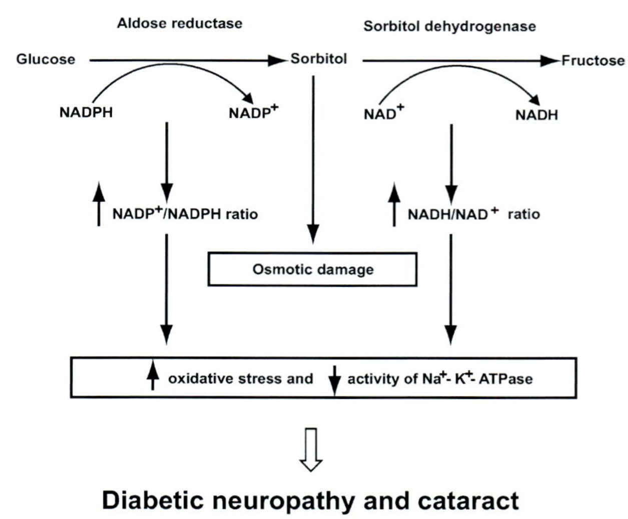

Figure 3 Increased flux through polyol pathway in diabetes and the development of vascular complications. It has been shown in cell culture and animal studies that flux through the polyol pathway is increased when challenged with hyperglycemia that lead to osmotic damage, induction of oxidative stress, and reduced activity of the Na^+–K^+-ATPase. These changes are suggested to contribute to the development of vascular pathologies in diabetes

yielded largely negative outcomes in diabetic retinopathy and nephropathy in patients. Application of Sorbinil failed to confer prevention against the development of diabetic retinopathy in the Sorbinil retinopathy trial [93]. However, Zenarestat, a potent aldose reductase inhibitor, is shown to suppress sorbitol, in biopsies of contralateral sural nerves, by more than 80%, and improves nerve conduction velocity (NCV) and nerve morphology in diabetic peripheral polyneuropathy (DPN) [94].

Formation of Advanced Glycation End Products

Hyperglycemia in diabetic states can induce irreversible glycation of both intracellular and extracellular proteins that results in AGEs, the formation of which plays important roles in aging process and the development of diabetic vascular complications [95–97] (Figure 4). The glycation process that leads to AGE formation occurs both intracellularly and extracellularly with different kinetics. Cytoplasmic proteins are the primary targets of intracellular glycation and form AGE at a rate much faster than that of extracellular glycation [98], although they have a much shorter lifespan as compared to that of extracellular AGEs [97]. AGEs are formed by the irreversible covalent modification and cross-linking of glucose and its derivatives such as glyoxal [99], methylglyoxal, and 3-deoxyglucosone [100]. Amongst all the modified proteins, carboxy(methyl)lysine (CML), pentosidine, and pyralline are the major AGEs found in diabetes.

A role for AGEs in the pathogenesis of diabetic vasculopathy is well supported by many experimental and clinical observations. High level of AGE deposition is detected in the glomerular tissues in diabetic rats that eventually develop renal insufficiency [101–104]. AGE is found in the serum [105] or glomeruli [106] of patients with diabetes and therefore has been proposed as a biomarker to predict the development or progression of renal insufficiency in these patients. The accumulation of AGE is also localized to retinal tissues from diabetic animals [107, 108] and might cause pericyte loss [109]. Infusion of AGE into animals results in pathological changes similar to those induced by hyperglycemia, such as vascular leakage and reduced nitric-oxide-mediated vasodilation [110, 111]. Inhibition of AGE formation using pharmacological inhibitors such as aminoguanidine can prevent some of the pathological changes observed in nephropathy [112, 113] and retinopathy [114] in animal model of diabetes. Excessive formation of AGE is postulated to

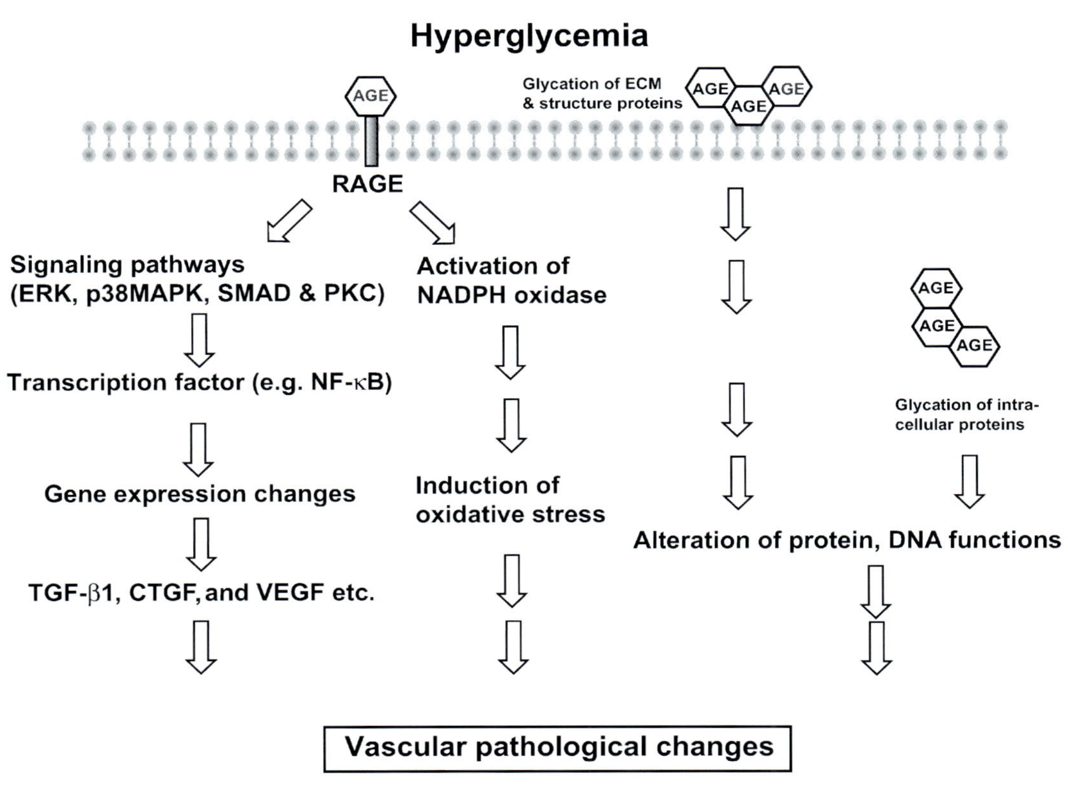

Figure 4 Role of AGE accumulation in diabetic vascular complications. Hyperglycemia induces the glycation of multiple extracellular and intracellular proteins known collectively as AGE. The glycation modification of proteins not only alter the function of structure proteins, but also activate intracellular signaling pathways through receptor for AGE (RAGE) that contributes to the development of diabetic vascular complications

induce cellular damage via several mechanisms including the modification of extracellular structure proteins such as collagen type I and IV and laminin [115, 116] and the subsequent alteration of their functions, which in turn not only change the integrity of the ECM, but also disrupt cell and ECM interaction [117]. It has been shown that adhesion of endothelial cells to glycated laminin and type IV collagen was impaired and might have profound functional impacts on the proliferation and migration of endothelial cells [117]. AGE modification of ECM protein might also decrease the plasticity of blood vessels and change vascular tone [56]. In addition, the glycated ECM proteins might have higher reactivity toward glomerular basement membrane in diabetic nephropathy [101].

Through the direct interaction with cellular proteins, AGE might also induce the activation of intracellular signaling pathways to alter vascular cell biology (Figure 4). Over the years, several cell surface binding proteins for AGEs have been identified and are known as AGE receptors that include many independent components such as receptor for AGE (RAGE), scavenger receptor class A (ScR-A), AGE-R1 (OST-48), AGE-R2 (80 K-H), and AGE-R3 (Galectin-3) [118–123]. These receptors possess diverse biological functions in the mediation of AGE endocytosis, degradation, and clearance as well as the activation of intracellular signaling pathways. A novel splice variant of RAGE has been identified in vascular endothelial cells and pericytes and its activation in diabetic states might also induce vascular damages [124]. Some of these receptors are expressed in vascular cells including endothelial cells, pericytes, vascular smooth muscle cells, mesangial cells, monocytes/macrophages, and lymphocytes that are all involved in the development of diabetic vascular complications [107, 123]. AGE-R1 has been reported to process AGE endocytosis and degradation, the downregulation of which might cause the accumulation of AGEs [123]. This observation is further supported by evidence showing that nonobese diabetic (NOD) mice have reduced gene expression for AGE-R1 and AGE-R1-mediated processing of AGE [123, 125]. Consistent with this finding, expression of AGE-R1 was found to be decreased in monocytes from patients with type 1 diabetes [123]. On the contrary, the expression of AGE-R3 in glomeruli from diabetic rats is increased, although the significance of this upregulation is not clear [126]. In addition, many studies provided supporting evidence that AGE receptors are involved in the development of diabetic vascular complications. A small-scale analysis of kidney tissues from patients with diabetes and healthy control donors revealed the upregulation of RAGE protein and mRNA level in glomeruli from diabetic patients versus their healthy controls [104]. As the best characterized receptors for AGE, RAGE is found to have ligand-mediated cellular signaling event and actions [110, 127] instead of being a mediator for endocytosis and degradation of AGEs [128]. To explore the role of RAGE in diabetic vascular complications, Yamamoto and colleagues specifically overexpressed *RAGE* gene in mouse vascular cells using *flk-1* promoter and crossed the RAGE transgenic to mice with type 1 diabetes [129]. The descendents showed exacerbated diabetic nephropathy manifested by nephromegaly, mesangial expansion, albuminuria, glomerular-hypertrophy, -sclerosis, and decreased renal functions. All these changes can be prevented by the inhibition of AGE [129]. Results from this study provide clear evidence that enhanced action of AGE–RAGE contributes to the development of diabetic nephropathy. Of all the AGE receptors, AGE-R2 is the only one that is known to be phosphorylated following AGE stimulation [97, 130] although this phosphorylation has not been associated with the activation of intracellular signaling pathway yet. RAGE, on the other hand, can activate intracellular signal transduction pathways by AGE. Such signaling cascades include RAS-MEK/Erk-1/2 pathway and stress kinase pathway that eventually lead to the activation of nuclear transcription factor κB (NF-κB) [131–133]. Activation of RAGE also led to the activation of proinflammatory programs in vascular tissues [134] and was recently shown to induce the activation of p38 mitogen-activated protein kinase (MAPK) cascades and SMAD pathway independent of TGF-β1 [135]. AGE-mediated vascular cell damage acts through the induced expression of multiple cytokines and growth factors in the target cells, among which interleukin 1 (IL-1), tumor necrosis factor α (TNF-α), insulin-like growth factor 1 (IGF-1), fibroblast growth factor (FGF), TGF-β1, CTGF, PDGF, and VEGF are all known to regulate inflammation and vascular biology and might contribute to the development of diabetic vascular complications [56]. Another mechanism for AGE to induce vascular damage in diabetic states is believed to mediate through the induction of vascular oxidative stress. AGE–RAGE interaction might activate NADPH oxidase, generate ROS such as H_2O_2 [62], and further interfere with vasodilation by uncoupling eNOS activity.

Several approaches have been developed to disrupt the formation of AGEs, including chemical inhibitors that interrupt AGE-mediated cross-linking such as aminoguanidine [136] and OPB-9195 [113], cross-linker breakers that breakdown the cross-linked proteins including *N*-phenylthiazolium bromide [137] and ALT-711 [138, 139], neutralizing antibodies against glycated proteins [140], antisera against receptor for AGEs [110], soluble recombinant RAGE (sR-RAGE) that block AGE–RAGE interaction [127, 141], and lysozyme-linked matrix that capture AGEs [142]. However, most of these strategies are still being tested in animal models except for aminoguanidine, which is being evaluated in a phase I clinical trial for its effect on advanced glycation modification of hemoglobin in human subjects [6, 97, 143].

Activation of Hexosamine Pathway

Hexosamine biosynthesis pathway has been proposed to be an autoregulatory sensing mechanism for cells to regulate glucose uptake and utilization [144]. Instead of being metabolized to fructose-1,6-biphosphate in the glycolysis pathway, fructose-6phosphate is converted to glucosamine-6-phosphate, catalyzed by glutamine: fructose-6-phosphate aminotransferase (GFAT) (Figure 5) The activation of hexosamine pathway ultimately results in the formation of uridine-diphosphate-*N*-acetylglucosamine (UDP-GlcNAC) and the O-linked glycoproteins. UDP-GlcNAC serves as a donor of *N*-acetylglucosamine (GlcNAC) to induce O-linked glycosylation of downstream proteins at the serine and threonine residues (Figure 5). When challenged with hyperglycemia in diabetes, hexosamine pathway is activated to shunt the excess metabolites from the overburdened glycolysis pathway. However, it might also cause vascular damages [56] and insulin resistance [145, 146], probably through the inhibitory effects of glucosamine on insulin-induced PI-3K/Akt activation [147]. In addition to shunting from the overwhelmed glycolysis pathway, hexosamine pathway can also be activated in vasculature by the activation of PKC [148] and the increased oxidative stress [149], both of which are activated in diabetic states (see other section in this chapter). Furthermore, GFAT expression might also be regulated by angiotensin II

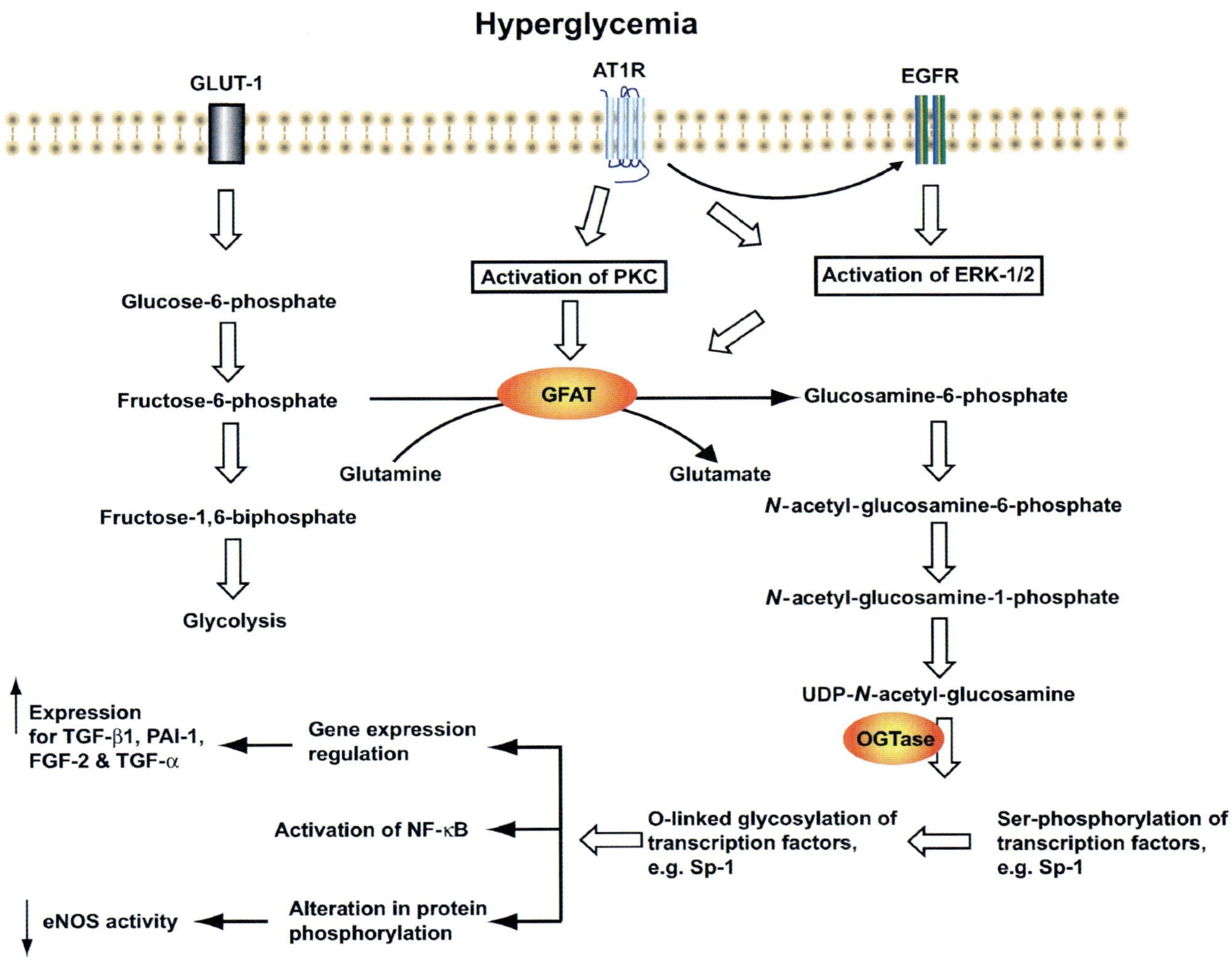

Figure 5 Activation of the hexosamine pathway in response to hyperglycemia and its role in diabetic vascular complications. Increased action of the key enzymes in the hexosamine pathway including glutamine: fructose-6-phosphate aminotransferase GFAT and O-GlcNAC transferase OGTase induces the flux through the hexosamine pathway that can result in the O-linked glycosylation of many proteins. Increased glycolysis induces the induction of flux through the hexosamine pathway. There is also cell culture study suggested the increased transcription of GFAT in response to AT-1R activation that requires the transactivation of epidermal growth factor receptor (EGFR). The increased hexosamine pathway activity is modification can prevent the serine phosphorylation of multiple key enzymes and transcriptional factors that alter vascular hemodynamic and gene expression. These changes have been suggested to play a role in the development of diabetic vascular complications

signaling pathway that is also involved in the development of diabetic vascular complications [150].

Hexosamine pathway is activated in the vasculature in diabetic states. In biopsies from diabetic patients or rats, mRNA and protein levels of GFAT, the rate-limiting enzyme catalyzing this pathway, as well as the enzyme O-GlcNAC transferase (OGTase) that catalyzes the O-linked glycosylation, are all upregulated in vascular smooth muscle cells [151, 152]. These activations have been recapitulated in vascular cells (endothelial cells and vascular smooth muscle cells) cultured in media containing high levels of D-glucose that mimic hyperglycemia [149, 152–154]. Activation of the hexosamine pathway results in the aberrant overexpression of growth factors in the vascular cells, including the profibrotic factor plasminogen activator inhibitor 1 (PAI-1), TGF-β1, FGF-2, and TGF-α [149, 155–157], the action of which regulates vascular remodeling and pathologies in diabetes (see later sections). Investigation into the mechanisms underlying this regulation reveal that this is mediated mainly through the O-linked glycosylation of the serine and threonine residues of key nuclear transcriptional factors. The glycosylation of these residues competes for the phosphorylation modification and therefore might alter their biological activities. This process might be mediated through a PKC-β1 and -δ isoform-dependent pathway, demonstrated at least in cultured mesangial cells [157]. Hyperglycemia induces the gene expression for TGF-α and PAI-1 in cultured vascular smooth muscle cells [155, 158] and mesangial cells [159]. Anatomic analysis of the TGF-α gene promoter region revealed a glucose responsive motif that contains three binding sites for Sp1 [155]. Sp1 belongs to the family of transcription factors that interact with RNA polymerase II to regulate the transcription of multiple target genes [160]. Both the serine and threonine residues on Sp1 determine the transcription activities of this protein with a suppressed activity in its phosphorylated form and enhanced activity in glycosylated states [161, 162]. Consistent with these observations, glucosamine, a metabolite of the hexosamine pathway, can also upregulate the expression of many growth factors such as TGF-β1 and PAI-1 in a pattern similar to that induced by hyperglycemia [163]. Therefore, hexosamine-mediated Sp1 activation might be a potential link leading to hyperglycemia-induced gene expression that contributes to vascular complications. This hypothesis is supported by observations made by Du and colleagues. They showed that the activation of hexosamine pathway flux by hyperglycemia induces O-linked glycosylated form of Sp1 accompanied by a reciprocal reduction of its serine and threonine phosphorylation [149] and therefore establish the link between hyperglycemia-induced O-link glycosylation on the regulation of gene expression (Figure 5).

In addition to Sp1, other nuclear or cytosolic proteins might also undergo O-linked glycosylation due to activation of hexosamine pathway. One such example is eNOS. Activation of eNOS requires the phosphorylation of serine 1177 (Ser1177), which is believed to be the target site of PKB/Akt that is downstream of PI-3K [164, 165]. In endothelial cells cultured in media containing high glucose, O-linked glycosylation of Ser1177 competitively suppresses its phosphorylation and downregulates eNOS activity [65, 166], the action of which contributes to hemodynamic changes observed in diabetes. Similar scenario has also been observed in vascular tissues from diabetic animals [65].

Extensive cross talks exist between the activation of hexosamine pathway, PKC activation, and AGE and ROS accumulation. Activation of PKC as well as enhanced oxidative stress in diabetic states are all known to increase flux through the hexosamine pathway by upregulating the activity of the rate-limiting enzyme GFAT [167]. AGE accumulation, which is known to induce oxidative stress and the activation of PKC (see other sections in this chapter), might also induce hexosamine pathway activation indirectly. The detrimental effect of hexosamine pathway activation might also be due to activation of PKCs [168] that are known to play key roles in the development of diabetic complications (see later section in this chapter).

All these evidences clearly support a role for hexosamine pathway in regulation of vascular biology and, furthermore, their chronic activation might contribute to the development of diabetic vascular complications.

Activation of Protein Kinase C

Altered activities of the multiple intracellular signaling cascades have been documented in the vascular tissues in diabetes, amongst which activation of DAG-PKC has been suggested to be a key component by which hyperglycemia mediates its adverse effects [6, 95, 169]. Protein kinase C is a family of structurally and functionally related serine/threonine kinases that consists of at least 12 members, with 9 of them that can be activated by DAG [170]. Activation of PKC in vascular cells exposed to diabetic states can be achieved through multiple routes including the action of cell surface receptors, intermediates from metabolic pathways, oxidative stress, and AGE–RAGE activation [6, 56] (Figure 6). The conformational changes in the process of PKC activation is not fully understood, but has been reported to involve the phosphorylation of key residues in the activation loop of PKC, thus leading to the exposure of their substrate-binding domain and translocation to the active pool [171]. Multiple PKC isoforms are expressed in cardiovascular systems and display tissue specificity. In addition, PKC activity has been shown to increase in response to hyperglycemic exposure and has been attributable to specific isoforms [5]. In diabetic states, accumulation of glyceraldehyde-3-phosphate due to the increased flux through glycolysis pathway can

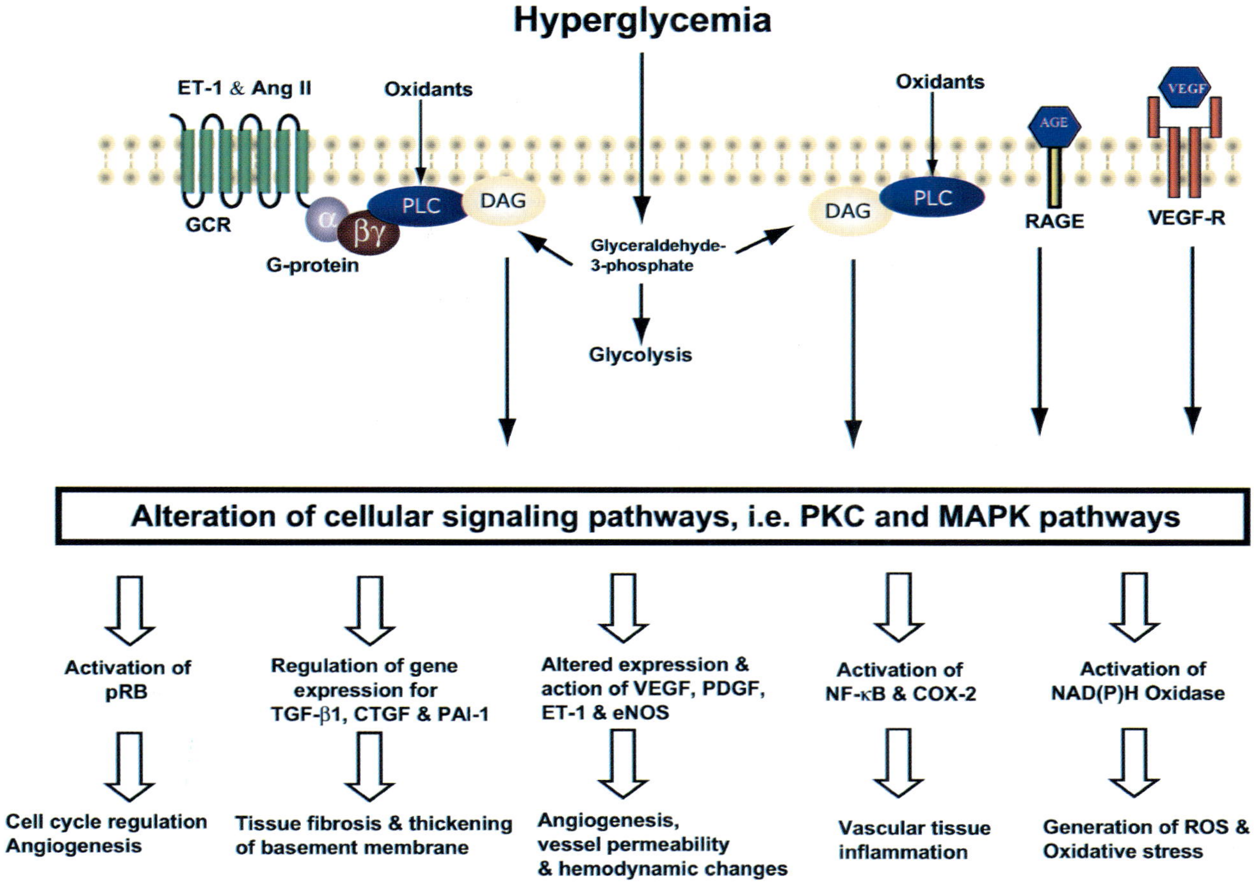

Figure 6 Activation of intracellular signaling cascades by hyperglycemia lead to multiple vascular pathological changes in diabetes. Hyperglycemia could activate intracellular signaling pathways via several mechanisms independently, including actions of cell surface receptors, formation of AGE, oxidative stress, and intermediates of the glycolysis pathways. The activation of these intracellular signaling molecules, especially the PKC-β and -δ isoforms, have been shown to regulate vascular cell growth and apoptosis, gene expression, vascular permeability, hemodynamic changes, oxidative stress, and inflammation. Clinical trials are ongoing evaluating selective inhibition of PKC-β in the treatment of diabetic retinopathy and neuropathy

result in the *de novo* synthesis of DAG, which in turn can activate different isoforms of PKC [6, 172–174] (Figure 6). Diabetes is often associated with derangement of metabolisms such as dyslipidemia. Increased circulating free fatty acid (FFA) in diabetes has been shown to activate PKC in vascular cells [64, 175]. Aberrant expression of growth factors and cytokine also contribute to the activation of vascular PKC in diabetes and this action is clearly associated with pathological changes in diabetic vascular complications. VEGF is one of the most potent growth factors regulating angiogenesis [176]. Activation of PKC has been documented in culture vascular cells stimulated by VEGF through the activation of phospholipase C-γ [177] and mediates *in vitro* angiogenesis such as endothelial cell proliferation and migration [177, 178] as well as the pathological angiogenesis in retina *in vitro* [178]. Formation of AGE and interaction with their cell surface receptors in diabetes are also believed to contribute to the activation of PKC [179]. In addition, enhanced oxidative stress in the vasculature in diabetes can also lead to the activation of PKC [61, 180].

Activation of PKC, especially the β isoform, both in cultured vascular cells and in diabetic animals causes multiple pathological changes in the vasculature. Retinal blood flow abnormality [173, 181], increased vascular permeability [182–184], and synthesis of ECM proteins [28, 185] are all reported to be caused by PKC-β activation. The structural and hemodynamic effects of PKC activation are probably mediated through the inhibition of nitric oxide production and the alteration of gene expression for vasoactive and growth factors. PKC has been shown to inhibit both the mRNA expression and activation of eNOS [186–188]. Its activation can also increase the expression of vasomotor mediator ET-1 [23], VEGF [189] as well as profibrotic factor TGF-β1 [28] and CTGF [190]. It has been reported that PKC can be activated by VEGF [177] and can mediate its effect on vessel leakage [191] and retinal angiogenesis as well, especially the β and δ isoforms of PKC [178]. Further, PKC induces the expression of adhesion molecules such as platelet/endothelial cell adhesion molecule (PECAM) and intracellular adhesion molecule (ICAM) and regulates cellular growth and apoptosis—all these have a role in diabetic vasculopathy [6]. PKC activation by hyperglycemia might also downregulate gap-junction of the vascular cells to increase their permeability [192]. In addition, suppression of PKC-β isoform increases retinal blood flow reduced by STZ-induced diabetic rats [193], whereas the inhibition of DAG kinase results in the accumulation of DAG that in turn activates PKC and decreases retinal blood flow, mimicking diabetic retinopathy [193].

Activation of PKC in vascular tissues share extensive cross talks with the involvement of other mechanisms in diabetic vascular complications (Figure 6). Hyperglycemia-induced PKC activity is suggested to cause inflammatory responses including the upregulation of cyclooxygenase-2 (*COX-2*) gene expression [194], activation of NF-κB probably by enhancing the action of TNF-α [195], and the induction of a spectrum of gene expression in favor of tissue fibrosis [28, 190]. Activation of PKC can be achieved by stimulations from growth factors and cytokines that are involved in diabetic vascular complications. For example, activation of PKC, especially the β and δ isoforms, are essential for VEGF-induced vascular permeability as well as angiogenic response [178, 191]. Both PKC-β1 and -δ isoforms are suggested to play a role in *PAI-1* gene expression induced by the activation of hexosamine pathway [157]. PKC also lies downstream of AGE–RAGE interaction and its activation is required for RAGE-induced vascular inflammatory responses and the formation of ROS [122]. However, the activation of PKC can also lead to the generation of ROS and increase vascular oxidative stress [6, 56]. This action is probably mediated through PKC-induced expression of $p22^{phox}$, a key component of NAD(P)H oxidases [194].

Given the central role of PKC activation in the development of diabetic vascular complications as discussed above, targeting PKC has been proposed to be an effective approach in the prevention or reversal of vasculopathy. Indeed, large number of experimental data, either from cell culture studies, animal model of diabetes, or in clinical trials provide supportive evidence [6, 56]. Many approaches have been used, including the amelioration of PKC gene expression by antisense techniques and suppression of PKC translocation by synthetic peptides or PKC activity by chemical inhibitors [170]. Amongst these approaches, a PKC-β-selective inhibitor LY333531 has shown by far the most promising effects in the prevention of diabetic vascular complications. Oral treatment with this inhibitor normalizes retinal blood flow, leukocyte entrapment, leakage, and pathological angiogenesis in retinopathy [181, 193, 196–198]. It can also prevent renal changes in diabetic nephropathy such as nephromegaly, mesangial expansion, and renal dysfunctions [28, 29, 181, 199] and restore neurovascular blood flow and nerve conduction velocity (NCV) [200–202]. In clinical studies, oral application of LY333531 normalized the reduced endothelium-dependent vasodilation in healthy subjects with acute hyperglycemia by glucose infusion [203]. LY333531 is being evaluated in phase II/III clinical trials in the treatment of diabetic retinopathy and neuropathy [198, 204]. Oral treatment with LY333531 is effective in the restoration of certain physiological markers that are abnormal in patients with diabetic retinopathy although conclusive results are not yet available [198]. In addition to retinopathy, preliminary results suggested that LY333531 is able to improve clinical symptoms of diabetic neuropathy in a multicenter clinical trial [204]. Because of the isoform-specific effects of PKC activation in vascular biology, many attempts have been made to develop PKC isoform selective inhibitors or activators with a hope to specifically regulate those that are involved in diabetic vasculopathy. However, these attempts have yielded little satisfactory results due to the poor selectivity of the inhibitors [170]. Since the activation of PKCs require their translocation to the active pools that is determined by the interaction between a peptide sequence in their regulatory domain and a cellular protein receptor for activated C kinase (RACK), several synthetic peptides corresponding to this sequence have been shown to confer isoform selective PKC activation or inhibition [205]. These peptide PKC-isoform selective activators or inhibitors have not been tested in animal model of diabetic vasculopathy to date. PKC activation has tissue-selectivity with tissue-dependent isoform specificity and therefore, tissue-selective manipulation of PKC isoforms should also be considered.

Role of Inflammation in Diabetic Vascular Complications

Inflammation is observed in both type 1 and type 2 diabetes and associated with endothelial dysfunction that contributes to the development of diabetic cardiovascular complications [206–208]. Increased inflammation and diabetes have been associated in clinical observations although this correlation is not sufficient to identify inflammation as a causal factor for diabetic vascular complications. In EURODIAB prospective complications study, diabetic patients have increased plasma level of inflammation markers such as C-reactive protein, IL-6, and TNF-α that are associated with endothelial dysfunction [207]. Proinflammatory TNF-α has been suggested to play a role in proliferative diabetic retinopathy [209, 210]. Through its cell surface receptor, TNF-α induces the activation of NF-κB, the action of which upregulates inflammatory gene expression, including cell adhesion molecules ICAM-1 and TNF-α. Activation of

NF-κB has been documented in the vascular tissues in diabetic rats [211]. Cyclooxygenase-2 is responsible for the production of prostanoids that regulate inflammatory responses and vascular tone in response to stimulations, for example, the presence of tissue inflammation or injury [212]. Hyperglycemia induces the gene expression for COX-2 in cultured vascular endothelial cells via a PKC-dependent pathway [194]. In addition, increased production of prostanoids has been reported in the glomeruli tissues from diabetic rodents [28] or glomeruli mesangial cells cultured in media containing high glucose [213]. All these evidences suggest a role for inflammation in the pathogenesis of diabetic vascular complications.

Several mechanisms have been proposed to explain the induction of vascular inflammation, including activation of PKC [28, 194, 213], AGE–RAGE action [122], and ROS formation [194]. Suppression of RAGE and the inhibition of oxidative stress have been clearly shown to reduce vascular inflammation, improve endothelial function [122, 214], and prevent hyperglycemia-induced vascular complications [6, 56]. One of such model is the impaired wound healing in diabetic subjects. Chronic inflammation has been associated with chronic wounds whereas inhibition of RAGE using sR-RAGE can suppress the inflammation and results in effective wound healing in diabetic animals [37].

Anti-inflammatory intervention has been shown to be beneficial in the treatment of diabetic retinopathy. Nonsteroidal anti-inflammatory agents could reduce leukocyte adhesion and prevent diabetic retinopathy in rodents [211]. Such agents, including the salicylate and aspirin, could inhibit the activity of both COX-2 and NF-κB although the later requires a much higher dose [215]. However, use of anti-inflammatory agents in the treatment of diabetic vascular complications has not yet shown beneficial effects. In the Early Treatment Diabetic Retinopathy Study (ETDRS), daily use of 650 mg anti-inflammatory agent aspirin failed to prevent the development of diabetic retinopathy [216] and cardiovascular mortality [217].

Altered Expression and Actions of Hormones, Growth factors, Cytokines, and Vasomotor mediators

Maintenance of vascular homeostasis is governed by the coordinated actions of multiple extra- and intracellular mediators that determine the status of the vascular cells (endothelial cells, pericytes, and vascular smooth muscle cells). These factors consist of hormones, growth factors, cytokines, signaling molecules, and transcriptional factors that form a complicated network [218]. Altered expression and actions of these factors have been reported in diabetic vascular complications.

Vascular Endothelial Growth Factor

VEGF family of growth factors are highly specific for endothelial cells and mediate their proangiogenic actions through cell surface receptors Flt-1 and Flk-1 [176, 218, 219]. VEGF has been suggested to be a key factor in the pathological changes in diabetic retinopathy. Increased concentration of VEGF has been reported in the ocular fluids [18] as well as retina tissues [19, 220] from diabetic patients. Level of VEGF concentration is associated with the severity of proliferative diabetic retinopathy [18, 19], probably through the induction of retinal inflammation, leukocyte entrapment [221], vascular leakage, and neovascularization [13]. Overexpression of VEGF and its receptors are also observed in the kidney tissues from diabetic patients [222] and rats [223, 224]. Neutralizing the actions of VEGF has been reported to improve renal function in diabetic rats [224, 225], suggestive of the detrimental role of VEGF in nephropathy. However, whether blocking VEGF's action will be beneficial to the nephropathy in diabetic patients awaits further investigation. Reduced nerve blood flow, hypoxia, and ischemia in diabetic neuropathy have led to the hypothesis that VEGF gene transfer might improve circulation insufficiency and furthermore, nerve functions. This hypothesis has been substantiated in diabetic animals [33]. The expression and actions of VEGF are decreased in the myocardium from both diabetic patients and rats suffering from ischemic heart disease (IHD), in contrast to the enhanced expression in IHD patients without diabetes [226]. Mice null for cardiac-specific VEGF have reduced coronary microvessels, reduced contractility, and impaired responses to β-adrenergic stimulations [227], similar to certain manifestations observed in diabetic patients [228]. Although the significance of this differential expression in the impaired cardiac angiogenesis needs further investigation, a great deal of studies have shown that *in situ* delivery of VEGF can restore myocardium perfusion and improve cardiac function, both in experimental animal model of IHD [15] and in clinical trials [229, 230], providing evidence that VEGF insufficiency might cause microvascular complications that further affect macrovasculopathy in diabetic states. Antiangiogenic therapy by targeting VEGF system has been evaluated in clinical trials on prevention of cancer metastasis; its application in treating diabetic microvascular complications [231], however, awaits further clinical trials.

Platelet-derived Growth Factor

PDGFs are also potent proangiogenic factors that regulate vascular cell proliferation, apoptosis, and migration, although less specific for endothelial cells than are VEGFs [232]. PDGF, especially PDGF-BB, is of particular importance in the recruitment of supportive mural cells (pericytes and vascular smooth muscles cells) to the blood vessels [233]. The mural cells stabilize the newly formed blood vessels, without which blood vessels will degenerate [21, 22]. Mice null for *PDGF-B* gene developed abnormalities in vasculatures in multiple tissues including myocardium, renal, and retinas [20, 21]. Some of the phenotypes such as pericytes loss, microaneurysm, and acellular capillaries resemble the pathology of diabetic retinopathy [20–22]. Long-term absence of PDGF-BB action on pericytes is recently shown to induce glomerulosclerosis and proteinuria [22], both of which are observed in diabetic nephropathy. However, mRNA expression for PDGF-BB is increased instead of decreased in the retinal tissues from diabetic rats [23]. It is not clear whether this upregulation of gene expression is due to the impairment of PDGF-BB-mediated intracellular signaling pathway, and an affirmative role for PDGF-BB in diabetic vasculopathy will require further investigation.

Transforming Growth Factor β1

One of the most prominent pathological changes in vasculature in diabetes is the thickening of basement membrane that has been suggested to be induced by TGF-β1-mediated accumulation of ECM proteins, and tissue fibrosis. Through its cell surface receptor, TGF-β1 activates intracellular SMAD pathways and induce the expression of ECM proteins and inhibit the degradation of proteases that lead to the overexpression and deposition of ECM proteins. In addition, TGF-β1 is also known to induce cell cycle arrest, apoptosis, angiogenesis, and cell mass growth [234] that is cell-type-dependent and contributes to glomerular hypertrophy. Increased expression of TGF-β1 has been reported in kidney tissues from diabetic patients [235–237] or animals [238, 239]. This induction of expression is probably mediated through the activation of PKC [28], increased oxidative stress [56], AGE–RAGE interaction [240], increased flux through polyol pathway [241], and hexosamine pathway [163]. Ablation of TGF-β1 and its actions have been clearly shown to prevent the gene expression for ECM proteins and structural and functional changes in kidneys in diabetic states [242–244]. However, TGF-β is involved in the regulation of a wide array of vital physiological processes including inflammation, cell proliferation, and angiogenesis. Mice null for TGF-β1 died shortly after birth because of multiple organ failure [245, 246]. Therefore, targeting to downstream effectors mediating only the profibrotic effects of TGF-β1 might be able to avoid the unwanted side effects. Connective tissue growth factor is such a mediator that will be discussed in the following section.

Connective Tissue Growth Factor

CTGF belongs to the CCN (CTGF, cyr 61/cef 10, nov) family of proteins and is a potent profibrotic factor [247]. Increased gene expression for CTGF has been reported in the kidneys from diabetic subjects [247–250] or in mesangial cells cultured in media containing high level of glucose [248, 249] and suggested to play key roles in the development of glomerulosclerosis. The induction of CTGF expression in diabetic states may be the result of hyperglycemia [249], AGE–RAGE action [251–253], and activation of PKC [248, 254], TGF-β1 [249, 254], or VEGF [255]. CTGF stimulation has been reported to arrest the cell cycle of mesangial cells at G1 phase to induce mesangial expansion and mesangial hypertrophy [256]. In addition, CTGF is a potent profibrotic factor that induces the gene expression for ECM components that characterize the glomerulosclerosis observed in diabetic nephropathy [249]. All these effects are downstream of TGF-β1, since blockade of CTGF action using either antisense approach or a neutralizing antibody effectively abolishes TGF-β1-mediated proliferation of cultured fibroblasts as well as the gene expression for collagens [257]. Although the identity of the receptor for CTGF is still elusive, CTGF has been reported to stimulate MAPK signal cascade probably via integrin-mediated pathway [250] or through the receptor for bone morphogenetic protein (BMP) and TGF-β1 [258]. A recent study using enzyme-linked immunosorbent assay (ELISA) approach suggested that urinary secretion of CTGF was significantly increased in diabetic patients with nephropathy and has been suggested to be a potential predictor of diabetic nephropathy [259]. Although CTGF might be a promising target to block diabetic glomerulosclerosis without altering the vital functions of TGF-β1, an effective CTGF antagonist is currently unavailable.

Renin–Angiotensin System

Angiotensin II is a potent vasoconstrictor that has been implicated in many of the deleterious effects of hyperglycemia on vasculature, likely due to the increased tissue sensitivity to angiotensin II [260]. Angiotensin II might have both blood-pressure-dependent or -independent effects. In addition to its role in the induction of hypertension [260], angiotensin II can directly act through its cell surface AT1 receptor and regulate tissue remodeling, fibrosis, cell hypertrophy, and apoptosis [261], presumably through the induction of gene expression for growth factors such as TGF-β1 [262], PAI-1 [263], and VEGF [264, 265] that contribute substantially to the pathogenesis of diabetic vascular complications. In addition to its direct effects on vasculatures, angiotensin II is also know to down-regulate cellular sensitivity to insulin through the interaction of insulin receptor substrate 1 (IRS-1) [266] and therefore may also likely antagonize insulin's action on vasculatures. Suppression of angiotensin II production or action, either by angiotensin converting enzyme (ACE) inhibitors or AT1 receptor antagonists, have been shown to be beneficial in preventing diabetic retinopathy [265, 267], nephropathy [268–274], and neuropathy [275] and substantially reduce mortality and morbidity in a growing number of clinical studies [276]. It has been clearly shown that these effects are achieved via both anti-hypertension-dependent and -independent mechanisms since the protective effects are also observed in normotensive patients. Targeting RAS system is by far the most effective supporting strategy in lowering morbidity and mortality in diabetes.

Endothelin 1

Endothelin family of peptides is the most potent vasoconstrictors amongst which ET-1 is the predominant form. Through the cell surface ET_A receptor, ET-1 acts on vascular smooth muscle cells to induce vasoconstriction. ET-1-mediated vasoconstriction has been suggested to induce endoneurial hypoxia and ischemia, and furthermore, neuropathy [277]. In the kidney, ET-1 not only causes vasoconstriction, but also enhances glomerular proliferation and the production of ECM proteins that characterize diabetic nephropathy [277]. Increased expression and action of ET-1 have been reported in the retinas of diabetic animals and associated with reduced blood flow in diabetic retinopathy [278, 279]. The altered expression is presumably through the activation of PKC by hyperglycemia as well as other factors such as PDGF-BB [23, 279]. Although controversy remains with regards to the expression changes of ET-1 in diabetic states [277], the beneficial effects of ET-1 antagonists in the prevention of vascular complications clearly provide supportive evidence. Blockade of ET_A, but not ET_B, restored the impaired endoneuronal blood flow as well as nerve conduction [280, 281]. Several ET_A antagonists rectify renal pathological changes and dysfunctions in diabetic states [282, 283]. ET_A-selective antagonists BQ-123 [278] or Bosentan [284] can normalize retinal blood flow changes in diabetic rats. This effect can also be reproduced by the reduction of retinal ET-1 levels achieved by endothelin converting-enzyme inhibitor (CEI) phosporamindon [284]. However, no clinical data is available to assess the effects of ET-1 antagonism on the development of diabetic vascular complications in human subjects.

Cross-talk Between Growth Factors, Cytokines, Hormones, and Vasoactive Mediators

In diabetic states, changes in the expression of these growth factors and cytokines occurred simultaneously, suggesting a coordinated working pattern. VEGF expression and its effect on angiogenesis are affected by the action of angiotensin II in many tissues [285–288], although the mechanisms underlying this regulation is not clear. ACEI can reverse the progression of diabetic retinopathy, probably not only via the regulation of blood pressure, but also by inhibiting the overexpression of angiogenic factors such as VEGF in the retina tissue [287, 289, 290]. Growth factors, when added together, might display a synergistic working pattern. For example, simultaneous application of PDGF and FGF-2 showed a strong angiogenic effect that is not the sum of these two factors [233]. In addition, effects of some factors might require the presence of others. TGF-β1 does not directly regulate endothelial cells to differentiate into vessel-tubule-like structure, but rather through the increased expression and action of other growth factors such as VEGF.

RATIONAL DESIGN OF MECHANISM-BASED THERAPEUTIC STRATEGIES IN THE TREATMENT OF DIABETIC VASCULAR COMPLICATIONS

The understanding of the multiple mechanisms mentioned above has provided potential targets for the rational design of therapeutic approaches in the prevention and treatment of vascular complications, in addition to tight glycemic control. Such strategies include antioxidants [27, 83]; various inhibitors of AGE–RAGE action [136] and signaling molecules such as DAG-PKC activation [5]; aldose reductase [93]; anti-inflammatory agents [217]; activation of transketolase-regulated pentose phosphate pathway by benfotiamine, therefore shunting the flux from the glycolysis pathway [291, 292]; and antagonists of growth factors, cytokines, or vasoactive mediators [260, 277]. However, most clinical trials of these approaches are not yet conclusive except for the ACE inhibitors, which clearly show beneficial effects [260]. The discrepancy between animal study and clinical observations might reflect the complexity of diabetic vascular complications in human patients that cannot be mimicked in animal models. Furthermore, utilization of only one approach might not be effective, given the extensive cross-talk between these mechanisms and the activation of alternative pathways. Therefore, it might be necessary to use several of these inhibitors simultaneously to achieve optimal effects.

REFERENCES

1. The Diabetes Control and Complications Trial Research Group. The effect of intensive treatment of diabetes on the development and progression of long-term complications in insulin-dependent diabetes mellitus. *N Engl J Med* 1993; 329: 977–86.
2. The UK Prospective Diabetes Study (UKPDS) Group. Intensive blood-glucose control with sulphonylureas or insulin compared with conventional treatment and risk of complications in patients with type 2 diabetes (UKPDS 33). *Lancet* 1998; 352: 837–53.

3. Ohkubo Y, Kishikawa H, Araki E, Miyata T, Isami S, Motoyoshi S, Kojima Y, Furuyoshi N, Shichiri M. Intensive insulin therapy prevents the progression of diabetic microvascular complications in Japanese patients with non-insulin-dependent diabetes mellitus: a randomized prospective 6-year study. *Diabetes Res Clin Pract* 1995; 28: 103–17.
4. Spector KS. Diabetic cardiomyopathy. *Clin Cardiol* 1998; 21: 885–7.
5. Way KJ, Katai N, King GL. Protein kinase C and the development of diabetic vascular complications. *Diabet Med* 2001; 18: 945–59.
6. Sheetz MJ, King GL. Molecular understanding of hyperglycemia's adverse effects for diabetic complications. *JAMA* 2002; 288: 2579–88.
7. Williamson JR, Kilo C. Capillary basement membranes in diabetes. *Diabetes* 1983; 32 (suppl 2): 96–100.
8. Haneda M, Kikkawa R, Horide N, Togawa M, Koya D, Kajiwara N, Ooshima A, Shigeta Y. Glucose enhances type IV collagen production in cultured rat glomerular mesangial cells. *Diabetologia* 1991; 34: 198–200.
9. Cai J, Boulton M. The pathogenesis of diabetic retinopathy: old concepts and new questions. *Eye* 2002; 16: 242–60.
10. Greenhalgh DG, Sprugel KH, Murray MJ, Ross R. PDGF and FGF stimulate wound healing in the genetically diabetic mouse. *Am J Pathol* 1990; 136: 1235–46.
11. Ferguson MW, Herrick SE, Spencer MJ, Shaw JE, Boulton AJ, Sloan P. The histology of diabetic foot ulcers. *Diabet Med* 1996; 13: S30–3.
12. Galeano M, Torre V, Deodato B, Campo GM, Colonna M, Sturiale A, Squadrito F, Cavallari V, Cucinotta D, Buemi M, Altavilla D. Raxofelast, a hydrophilic vitamin E-like antioxidant, stimulates wound healing in genetically diabetic mice. *Surgery* 2001; 129: 467–77.
13. Ferris FL III, Davis MD, Aiello LM. Treatment of diabetic retinopathy. *N Engl J Med* 1999; 341: 667–78.
14. The Diabetes Control and Complications Trial Research Group. Progression of retinopathy with intensive versus conventional treatment in the Diabetes Control and Complications Trial. *Ophthalmology* 1995; 102: 647–61.
15. Engerman RL. Pathogenesis of diabetic retinopathy. *Diabetes* 1989; 38: 1203–6.
16. Robison WG Jr, McCaleb ML, Feld LG, Michaelis OE, Laver N, Mercandetti M, Robinson WG Jr. Degenerated intramural pericytes ('ghost cells') in the retinal capillaries of diabetic rats. *Curr Eye Res* 1991; 10: 339–50.
17. Mizutani M, Kern TS, Lorenzi M. Accelerated death of retinal microvascular cells in human and experimental diabetic retinopathy. *J Clin Invest* 1996; 97: 2883–90.
18. Aiello LP, Avery RL, Arrigg PG, Keyt BA, Jampel HD, Shah ST, Pasquale LR, Thieme H, Iwamoto MA, Park JE, Nguyen HV, Aiello LM, Ferrara N, King GL. Vascular endothelial growth factor in ocular fluid of patients with diabetic retinopathy and other retinal disorders. *N Engl J Med* 1994; 331: 1480–7.
19. Boulton M, Foreman D, Williams G, McLeod D. VEGF localisation in diabetic retinopathy. *Br J Ophthalmol* 1998; 82: 561–8.
20. Leveen P, Pekny M, Gebre-Medhin S, Swolin B, Larsson E, Betsholtz C. Mice deficient for PDGF B show renal, cardiovascular, and hematological abnormalities. *Genes Dev* 1994; 8: 1875–87.
21. Lindahl P, Johansson BR, Leveen P, Betsholtz C. Pericyte loss and microaneurysm formation in PDGF-B-deficient mice. *Science* 1997; 277: 242–5.
22. Lindblom P, Gerhardt H, Liebner S, Abramsson A, Enge M, Hellstrom M, Backstrom G, Fredriksson S, Landegren U, Nystrom HC, Bergstrom G, Dejana E, Ostman A, Lindahl P, Betsholtz C. Endothelial PDGF-B retention is required for proper investment of pericytes in the microvessel wall. *Genes Dev* 2003; 17: 1835–40.
23. Yokota T, Ma RC, Park JY, Isshiki K, Sotiropoulos KB, Rauniyar RK, Bornfeldt KE, King GL. Role of protein kinase C on the expression of platelet-derived growth factor and endothelin-1 in the retina of diabetic rats and cultured retinal capillary pericytes. *Diabetes* 2003; 52: 838–45.
24. Friedman EA. Renal syndromes in diabetes. *Endocrinol Metab Clin North Am* 1996; 25: 293–324.
25. Ritz E, Orth SR. Nephropathy in patients with type 2 diabetes mellitus. *N Engl J Med* 1999; 341: 1127–33.
26. Cooper ME. Pathogenesis, prevention, and treatment of diabetic nephropathy. *Lancet* 1998; 352: 213–9.
27. Kuroki T, Isshiki K, King GL. Oxidative stress: the lead or supporting actor in the pathogenesis of diabetic complications. *J Am Soc Nephrol* 2003; 14 (suppl 3): S216–20.
28. Koya D, Jirousek MR, Lin YW, Ishii H, Kuboki K, King GL. Characterization of protein kinase C beta isoform activation on the gene expression of transforming growth factor-beta, extracellular matrix components, and prostanoids in the glomeruli of diabetic rats. *J Clin Invest* 1997; 100: 115–26.
29. Koya D, Haneda M, Nakagawa H, Isshiki K, Sato H, Maeda S, Sugimoto T, Yasuda H, Kashiwagi A, Ways DK, King GL, Kikkawa R. Amelioration of accelerated diabetic mesangial expansion by treatment with a PKC beta inhibitor in diabetic *db/db* mice, a rodent model for type 2 diabetes. *FASEB J* 2000; 14: 439–47.
30. Harati Y. Diabetes and the nervous system. *Endocrinol Metab Clin North Am* 1996; 25: 325–59.
31. Malik RA, Tesfaye S, Thompson SD, Veves A, Sharma AK, Boulton AJ, Ward JD. Endoneurial localisation of microvascular damage in human diabetic neuropathy. *Diabetologia* 1993; 36: 454–9.
32. Sugimoto K, Murakawa Y, Sima AA. Diabetic neuropathy—a continuing enigma. *Diabetes Metab Res Rev* 2000; 16: 408–33.
33. Schratzberger P, Walter DH, Rittig K, Bahlmann FH, Pola R, Curry C, Silver M, Krainin JG, Weinberg DH, Ropper AH, Isner JM. Reversal of experimental diabetic neuropathy by VEGF gene transfer. *J Clin Invest* 2001; 107: 1083–92.
34. Cameron NE, Eaton SE, Cotter MA, Tesfaye S. Vascular factors and metabolic interactions in the pathogenesis of diabetic neuropathy. *Diabetologia* 2001; 44: 1973–88.
35. Goodson WH III, Hunt TK. Wound healing and the diabetic patient. *Surg Gynecol Obstet* 1979; 149: 600–8.
36. King L. Impaired wound healing in patients with diabetes. *Nurs Stand* 2001; 15: 39–45.
37. Goova MT, Li J, Kislinger T, Qu W, Lu Y, Bucciarelli LG, Nowygrod S, Wolf BM, Caliste X, Yan SF, Stern DM, Schmidt AM. Blockade of receptor for advanced glycation end-products restores effective wound healing in diabetic mice. *Am J Pathol* 2001; 159: 513–25.
38. Galeano M, Deodato B, Altavilla D, Cucinotta D, Arsic N, Marini H, Torre V, Giacca M, Squadrito F, Adeno-associated viral vector-mediated human vascular endothelial growth factor gene transfer stimulates

angiogenesis and wound healing in the genetically diabetic mouse. *Diabetologia* 2003; 46: 546–55.
39. Bornfeldt KE, Raines EW, Graves LM, Skinner MP, Krebs EG, Ross R. Platelet-derived growth factor. Distinct signal transduction pathways associated with migration versus proliferation. *Ann NY Acad Sci* 1995; 766: 416–30.
40. Steed DL, for the Diabetic Ulcer Study Group Clinical evaluation of recombinant human platelet-derived growth factor for the treatment of lower extremity diabetic ulcers. *J Vasc Surg* 1995; 21: 71–81.
41. Wieman TJ, Smiell JM, Su Y. Efficacy and safety of a topical gel formulation of recombinant human platelet-derived growth factor-BB (becaplermin) in patients with chronic neuropathic diabetic ulcers. A phase III randomized placebo-controlled double-blind study. *Diabetes Care* 1998; 21: 822–7.
42. Wieman TJ, for the Becaplermin Gel Studies Group. Clinical efficacy of becaplermin (rhPDGF-BB) gel. *Am J Surg* 1998; 176: 74S–79S.
43. Quagliaro L, Piconi L, Assaloni R, Martinelli L, Motz E, Ceriello A. Intermittent high glucose enhances apoptosis related to oxidative stress in human umbilical vein endothelial cells: the role of protein kinase C and NAD(P)H-oxidase activation. *Diabetes* 2003; 52: 2795–804.
44. Kannel WB, McGee DL, for the The Framingham Study. Diabetes and cardiovascular disease. *JAMA* 1979; 241: 2035–8.
45. Uusitupa MI, Niskanen LK, Siitonen O, Voutilainen E, Pyorala K. 5-year incidence of atherosclerotic vascular disease in relation to general risk factors, insulin level, and abnormalities in lipoprotein composition in non-insulin-dependent diabetic and nondiabetic subjects. *Circulation* 1990; 82: 27–36.
46. Halliwell B. Antioxidant characterization. Methodology and mechanism. *Biochem Pharmacol* 1995; 49: 1341–8.
47. Giugliano D, Ceriello A, Paolisso G. Oxidative stress and diabetic vascular complications. *Diabetes Care* 1996; 19: 257–67.
48. Evans JL, Goldfine ID, Maddux BA, Grodsky GM. Oxidative stress and stress-activated signaling pathways: a unifying hypothesis of type 2 diabetes. *Endocr Rev* 2002; 23: 599–622.
49. Keaney JF Jr, Larson MG, Vasan RS, Wilson PW, Lipinska I, Corey D, Massaro JM, Sutherland P, Vita JA, Benjamin EJ. Obesity and systemic oxidative stress: clinical correlates of oxidative stress in the Framingham Study. *Arterioscler Thromb Vasc Biol* 2003; 23: 434–9.
50. Jain SK, McVie R. Effect of glycemic control, race (white versus black), and duration of diabetes on reduced glutathione content in erythrocytes of diabetic patients. *Metabolism* 1994; 43: 306–9.
51. Jennings PE, Chirico S, Jones AF, Lunec J, Barnett AH. Vitamin C metabolites and microangiopathy in diabetes mellitus. *Diabetes Res* 1987; 6: 151–4.
52. Karpen CW, Cataland S, O'Dorisio TM, Panganamala RV. Production of 12-hydroxyeicosatetraenoic acid and vitamin E status in platelets from type I human diabetic subjects. *Diabetes* 1985; 34: 526–31.
53. Will JC, Ford ES, Bowman BA. Serum vitamin C concentrations and diabetes: findings from the Third National Health and Nutrition Examination Survey, 1988–1994. *Am J Clin Nutr* 1999; 70: 49–52.
54. Campoy C, Baena RM, Blanca E, Lopez-Sabater C, Fernandez-Garcia JM, Miranda MT, Molina-Font JA, Bayes R. Effects of metabolic control on vitamin E nutritional status in children with type 1 diabetes mellitus. *Clin Nutr* 2003; 22: 81–6.
55. Augustin AJ, Dick HB, Koch F, Schmidt-Erfurth U. Correlation of blood-glucose control with oxidative metabolites in plasma and vitreous body of diabetic patients. *Eur J Ophthalmol* 2002; 12: 94–101.
56. Brownlee M. Biochemistry and molecular cell biology of diabetic complications. *Nature* 2001; 414: 813–20.
57. Oberley LW. Free radicals and diabetes. *Free Radic Biol Med* 1988; 5: 113–24.
58. Sakurai T, Tsuchiya S. Superoxide production from nonenzymatically glycated protein. *FEBS Lett* 1988; 236: 406–10.
59. Baynes JW. Role of oxidative stress in development of complications in diabetes. *Diabetes* 1991; 40: 405–12.
60. Van Dam PS, Van Asbeck BS, Erkelens DW, Marx JJ, Gispen WH, Bravenboer B. The role of oxidative stress in neuropathy and other diabetic complications. *Diabetes Metab Rev* 1995; 11: 181–92.
61. Nishikawa T, Edelstein D, Du XL, Yamagishi S, Matsumura T, Kaneda Y, Yorek MA, Beebe D, Oates PJ, Hammes HP, Giardino I, Brownlee M. Normalizing mitochondrial superoxide production blocks three pathways of hyperglycaemic damage. *Nature* 2000; 404: 787–90.
62. Wautier MP, Chappey O, Corda S, Stern DM, Schmidt AM, Wautier JL. Activation of NADPH oxidase by AGE links oxidant stress to altered gene expression via RAGE. *Am J Physiol Endocrinol Metab* 2001; 280: E685–94.
63. Mollnau H, Wendt M, Szocs K, Lassegue B, Schulz E, Oelze M, Li H, Bodenschatz M, August M, Kleschyov AL, Tsilimingas N, Walter U, Forstermann U, Meinertz T, Griendling K, Munzel T. Effects of angiotensin II infusion on the expression and function of NAD(P)H oxidase and components of nitric oxide/cGMP signaling. *Circ Res* 2002; 90: E58–65.
64. Inoguchi T, Li P, Umeda F, Yu HY, Kakimoto M, Imamura M, Aoki T, Etoh T, Hashimoto T, Naruse M, Sano H, Utsumi H, Nawata H. High glucose level and free fatty acid stimulate reactive oxygen species production through protein kinase C dependent activation of NAD(P)H oxidase in cultured vascular cells. *Diabetes* 2000; 49: 1939–45.
65. Du XL, Edelstein D, Dimmeler S, Ju Q, Sui C, Brownlee M. Hyperglycemia inhibits endothelial nitric oxide synthase activity by posttranslational modification at the Akt site. *J Clin Invest* 2001; 108: 1341–8.
66. Craven PA, Melhem MF, Phillips SL, DeRubertis FR. Overexpression of $Cu2^+/Zn2^+$ superoxide dismutase protects against early diabetic glomerular injury in transgenic mice. *Diabetes* 2001; 50: 2114–25.
67. Xia Y, Dawson VL, Dawson TM, Snyder SH, Zweier JL. Nitric oxide synthase generates superoxide and nitric oxide in arginine-depleted cells leading to peroxynitrite-mediated cellular injury. *Proc Natl Acad Sci USA* 1996; 93: 6770–4.
68. Cosentino F, Katusic ZS. Tetrahydrobiopterin and dysfunction of endothelial nitric oxide synthase in coronary arteries. *Circulation* 1995; 91: 139–44.
69. Cosentino F, Patton S, d'Uscio LV, Werner ER, Werner-Felmayer G, Moreau P, Malinski T, Luscher TF. Tetrahydrobiopterin alters superoxide and nitric oxide release in prehypertensive rats. *J Clin Invest* 1998; 101: 1530–7.

70. Cosentino F, Hishikawa K, Katusic ZS, Luscher TF. High glucose increases nitric oxide synthase expression and superoxide anion generation in human aortic endothelial cells. *Circulation* 1997; 96: 25–8.
71. Dandona P, Thusu K, Cook S, Snyder B, Makowski J, Armstrong D, Nicotera T. Oxidative damage to DNA in diabetes mellitus. *Lancet* 1996; 347: 444–5.
72. Suzuki S, Hinokio Y, Komatu K, Ohtomo M, Onoda M, Hirai S, Hirai M, Hirai A, Chiba M, Kasuga S, Akai H, Toyota T. Oxidative damage to mitochondrial DNA and its relationship to diabetic complications. *Diabetes Res Clin Pract* 1999; 45: 161–8.
73. Garcia Soriano F, Virag L, Jagtap P, Szabo E, Mabley JG, Liaudet L, Marton A, Hoyt DG, Murthy KG, Salzman AL, Southan GJ, Szabo C. Diabetic endothelial dysfunction: the role of poly(ADP-ribose) polymerase activation. *Nat Med* 2001; 7: 108–13.
74. Kowluru RA, Tang J, Kern TS. Abnormalities of retinal metabolism in diabetes and experimental galactosemia, VII: Effect of long-term administration of antioxidants on the development of retinopathy. *Diabetes* 2001; 50: 1938–42.
75. Kowluru RA, Koppolu P. Diabetes-induced activation of caspase-3 in retina: effect of antioxidant therapy. *Free Radic Res* 2002; 36: 993–9.
76. Cameron NE, Cotter MA, Archibald V, Dines KC, Maxfield EK, Anti-oxidant and pro-oxidant effects on nerve conduction velocity, endoneurial blood flow and oxygen tension in non-diabetic and streptozotocin-diabetic rats. *Diabetologia* 1994; 37: 449–59.
77. Nagamatsu M, Nickander KK, Schmelzer JD, Raya A, Wittrock DA, Tritschler H, Low PA. Lipoic acid improves nerve blood flow, reduces oxidative stress, and improves distal nerve conduction in experimental diabetic neuropathy. *Diabetes Care* 1995; 18: 1160–7.
78. Lal MA, Korner A, Matsuo Y, Zelenin S, Cheng SX, Jaremko G, DiBona GF, Eklof AC, Aperia A. Combined antioxidant and COMT inhibitor treatment reverses renal abnormalities in diabetic rats. *Diabetes* 2000; 49: 1381–9.
79. Chowienczyk PJ, Brett SE, Gopaul NK, Meeking D, Marchetti M, Russell-Jones DL, Anggard EE, Ritter JM. Oral treatment with an antioxidant (raxofelast) reduces oxidative stress and improves endothelial function in men with type II diabetes. *Diabetologia* 2000; 43: 974–7.
80. Gaede P, Poulsen HE, Parving HH, Pedersen O. Double-blind, randomised study of the effect of combined treatment with vitamin C and E on albuminuria in Type 2 diabetic patients. *Diabet Med* 2001; 18: 756–60.
81. Bursell SE, Clermont AC, Aiello LP, Aiello LM, Schlossman DK, Feener EP, Laffel L, King GL, High-dose vitamin E supplementation normalizes retinal blood flow and creatinine clearance in patients with type 1 diabetes. *Diabetes Care* 1999; 22: 1245–51.
82. Yusuf S, Dagenais G, Pogue J, Bosch J, Sleight P. (The Heart Outcomes Prevention Evaluation Study Investigators). Vitamin E supplementation and cardiovascular events in high-risk patients. *N Engl J Med* 2000; 342: 154–60.
83. Lonn E, Yusuf S, Hoogwerf B, Pogue J, Yi Q, Zinman B, Bosch J, Dagenais G, Mann JF, Gerstein HC. Effects of vitamin E on cardiovascular and microvascular outcomes in high-risk patients with diabetes: results of the HOPE study and MICRO-HOPE substudy. *Diabetes Care* 2002; 25: 1919–27.
84. Kunisaki M, Bursell SE, Clermont AC, Ishii H, Ballas LM, Jirousek MR, Umeda F, Nawata H, King GL. Vitamin E prevents diabetes-induced abnormal retinal blood flow via the diacylglycerol-protein kinase C pathway. *Am J Physiol* 1995; 269: E239–46.
85. Gabbay KH. Hyperglycemia, polyol metabolism, and complications of diabetes mellitus. *Annu Rev Med* 1975; 26: 521–36.
86. Tesfamariam B. Free radicals in diabetic endothelial cell dysfunction. *Free Radic Biol Med* 1994; 16: 383–91.
87. Robison WG Jr, Nagata M, Laver N, Hohman TC, Kinoshita JH. Diabetic-like retinopathy in rats prevented with an aldose reductase inhibitor. *Invest Ophthalmol Vis Sci* 1989; 30: 2285–92.
88. Kador PF, Akagi Y, Takahashi Y, Ikebe H, Wyman M, Kinoshita JH. Prevention of retinal vessel changes associated with diabetic retinopathy in galactose-fed dogs by aldose reductase inhibitors. *Arch Ophthalmol* 1990; 108: 1301–9.
89. Mauer SM, Steffes MW, Azar S, Brown DM. Effects of sorbinil on glomerular structure and function in long-term-diabetic rats. *Diabetes* 1989; 38: 839–46.
90. Yue DK, Hanwell MA, Satchell PM, Turtle JR. The effect of aldose reductase inhibition on motor nerve conduction velocity in diabetic rats. *Diabetes* 1982; 31: 789–94.
91. Cameron NE, Leonard MB, Ross IS, Whiting PH. The effects of sorbinil on peripheral nerve conduction velocity, polyol concentrations and morphology in the streptozotocin-diabetic rat. *Diabetologia* 1986; 29: 168–74.
92. Engerman RL, Kern TS, Larson ME. Nerve conduction and aldose reductase inhibition during 5 years of diabetes or galactosaemia in dogs. *Diabetologia* 1994; 37: 141–4.
93. Sorbinil Retinopathy Trial Research Group. A randomized trial of sorbinil, an aldose reductase inhibitor, in diabetic retinopathy. *Arch Ophthalmol* 1990; 108: 1234–44.
94. Greene DA, Arezzo JC, Brown MB, for the Zenarestat Study Group. Effect of aldose reductase inhibition on nerve conduction and morphometry in diabetic neuropathy. *Neurology* 1999; 53: 580–91.
95. King GL, Brownlee M. The cellular and molecular mechanisms of diabetic complications. *Endocrinol Metab Clin North Am* 1996; 25: 255–70.
96. Brownlee M, Cerami A, Vlassara H. Advanced glycosylation end products in tissue and the biochemical basis of diabetic complications. *N Engl J Med* 1988; 318: 1315–21.
97. Vlassara H, Palace MR. Diabetes and advanced glycation endproducts. *J Intern Med* 2002; 251: 87–101.
98. Giardino I, Edelstein D, Brownlee M. Nonenzymatic glycosylation in vitro and in bovine endothelial cells alters basic fibroblast growth factor activity. A model for intracellular glycosylation in diabetes. *J Clin Invest* 1994; 94: 110–7.
99. Wells-Knecht KJ, Zyzak DV, Litchfield JE, Thorpe SR, Baynes JW. Mechanism of autoxidative glycosylation: identification of glyoxal and arabinose as intermediates in the autoxidative modification of proteins by glucose. *Biochemistry* 1995; 34: 3702–9.
100. Thornalley PJ. The glyoxalase system: new developments towards functional characterization of a metabolic pathway fundamental to biological life. *Biochem J* 1990; 269: 1–11.
101. Gugliucci A, Bendayan M. Reaction of advanced glycation endproducts with renal tissue from normal and streptozotocin-induced diabetic rats: an ultrastructural

study using colloidal gold cytochemistry. *J Histochem Cytochem* 1995; 43: 591–600.
102. Makino H, Shikata K, Hironaka K, Kushiro M, Yamasaki Y, Sugimoto H, Ota Z, Araki N, Horiuchi S. Ultrastructure of nonenzymatically glycated mesangial matrix in diabetic nephropathy. *Kidney Int* 1995; 48: 517–26.
103. Horie K, Miyata T, Maeda K, Miyata S, Sugiyama S, Sakai H, van Ypersole de Strihou C, Monnier VM, Witztum JL, Kurokawa K. Immunohistochemical colocalization of glycoxidation products and lipid peroxidation products in diabetic renal glomerular lesions. Implication for glycoxidative stress in the pathogenesis of diabetic nephropathy. *J Clin Invest* 1997; 100: 2995–3004.
104. Tanji N, Markowitz GS, Fu C, Kislinger T, Taguchi A, Pischetsrieder M, Stern D, Schmidt AM, D'Agati VD. Expression of advanced glycation end products and their cellular receptor RAGE in diabetic nephropathy and nondiabetic renal disease. *J Am Soc Nephrol* 2000; 11: 1656–66.
105. Berg TJ, Bangstad HJ, Torjesen PA, Osterby R, Bucala R, Hanssen KF. Advanced glycation end products in serum predict changes in the kidney morphology of patients with insulin-dependent diabetes mellitus. *Metabolism* 1997; 46: 661–5.
106. Suzuki D, Miyata T, Saotome N, Horie K, Inagi R, Yasuda Y, Uchida K, Izuhara Y, Yagame M, Sakai H, Kurokawa K. Immunohistochemical evidence for an increased oxidative stress and carbonyl modification of proteins in diabetic glomerular lesions. *J Am Soc Nephrol* 1999; 10: 822–32.
107. Stitt AW, Li YM, Gardiner TA, Bucala R, Archer DB, Vlassara H. Advanced glycation end products (AGEs) co-localize with AGE receptors in the retinal vasculature of diabetic and of AGE-infused rats. *Am J Pathol* 1997; 150: 523–31.
108. Hammes HP, Wellensiek B, Kloting I, Sickel E, Bretzel RG, Brownlee M. The relationship of glycaemic level to advanced glycation end-product (AGE) accumulation and retinal pathology in the spontaneous diabetic hamster. *Diabetologia* 1998; 41: 165–70.
109. Yamagishi S, Hsu CC, Taniguchi M, Harada S, Yamamoto Y, Ohsawa K, Kobayashi K, Yamamoto H. Receptor-mediated toxicity to pericytes of advanced glycosylation end products: a possible mechanism of pericyte loss in diabetic microangiopathy. *Biochem Biophys Res Commun* 1995; 213: 681–7.
110. Wautier JL, Zoukourian C, Chappey O, Wautier MP, Guillausseau PJ, Cao R, Hori O, Stern D, Schmidt AM. Receptor-mediated endothelial cell dysfunction in diabetic vasculopathy. Soluble receptor for advanced glycation end products blocks hyperpermeability in diabetic rats. *J Clin Invest* 1996; 97: 238–43.
111. Vlassara H, Fuh H, Makita Z, Krungkrai S, Cerami A, Bucala R. Exogenous advanced glycosylation end products induce complex vascular dysfunction in normal animals: a model for diabetic and aging complications. *Proc Natl Acad Sci USA* 1992; 89: 12043–7.
112. Soulis-Liparota T, Cooper M, Papazoglou D, Clarke B, Jerums G. Retardation by aminoguanidine of development of albuminuria, mesangial expansion, and tissue fluorescence in streptozocin-induced diabetic rat. *Diabetes* 1991; 40: 1328–34.
113. Nakamura S, Makita Z, Ishikawa S, Yasumura K, Fujii W, Yanagisawa K, Kawata T, Koike T. Progression of nephropathy in spontaneous diabetic rats is prevented by OPB-9195, a novel inhibitor of advanced glycation. *Diabetes* 1997; 46: 895–9.
114. Hammes HP, Martin S, Federlin K, Geisen K, Brownlee M. Aminoguanidine treatment inhibits the development of experimental diabetic retinopathy. *Proc Natl Acad Sci USA* 1991; 88: 11555–8.
115. Tanaka S, Avigad G, Brodsky B, Eikenberry EF. Glycation induces expansion of the molecular packing of collagen. *J Mol Biol* 1988; 203: 495–505.
116. Tsilibary EC, Charonis AS, Reger LA, Wohlhueter RM, Furcht LT. The effect of nonenzymatic glucosylation on the binding of the main noncollagenous NC1 domain to type IV collagen. *J Biol Chem* 1988; 263: 4302–8.
117. Haitoglou CS, Tsilibary EC, Brownlee M, Charonis AS. Altered cellular interactions between endothelial cells and nonenzymatically glucosylated laminin/type IV collagen. *J Biol Chem* 1992; 267: 12404–7.
118. Li YM, Mitsuhashi T, Wojciechowicz D, Shimizu N, Li J, Stitt A, He C, Banerjee D, Vlassara H. Molecular identity and cellular distribution of advanced glycation end-product receptors: relationship of p60 to OST-48 and p90 to 80K-H membrane proteins. *Proc Natl Acad Sci USA* 1996; 93: 11047–52.
119. Smedsrod B, Melkko J, Araki N, Sano H, Horiuchi S. Advanced glycation end products are eliminated by scavenger-receptor-mediated endocytosis in hepatic sinusoidal Kupffer and endothelial cells. *Biochem J* 1997; 322 (pt 2): 567–73.
120. Vlassara H, Li YM, Imani F, Wojciechowicz D, Yang Z, Liu FT, Cerami A. Identification of galectin-3 as a high-affinity binding protein for advanced glycation end products (AGE): a new member of the AGE-receptor complex. *Mol Med* 1995; 1: 634–46.
121. Neeper M, Schmidt AM, Brett J, Yan SD, Wang F, Pan YC, Elliston K, Stern D, Shaw A. Cloning and expression of a cell surface receptor for advanced glycosylation end products of proteins. *J Biol Chem* 1992; 267: 14998–5004.
122. Schmidt AM, Stern DM. RAGE: a new target for the prevention and treatment of the vascular and inflammatory complications of diabetes. *Trends Endocrinol Metab* 2000; 11: 368–75.
123. Vlassara H. The AGE-receptor in the pathogenesis of diabetic complications. *Diabetes Metab Res Rev* 2001; 17: 436–43.
124. Yonekura H, Yamamoto Y, Sakurai S, Petrova RG, Abedin MJ, Li H, Yasui K, Takeuchi M, Makita Z, Takasawa S, Okamoto H, Watanabe T, Yamamoto H. Novel splice variants of the receptor for advanced glycation end-products expressed in human vascular endothelial cells and pericytes, and their putative roles in diabetes-induced vascular injury. *Biochem J* 2003; 370: 1097–109.
125. He CJ, Zheng F, Stitt A, Striker L, Hattori M, Vlassara H. Differential expression of renal AGE-receptor genes in NOD mice: possible role in nonobese diabetic renal disease. *Kidney Int* 2000; 58: 1931–40.
126. Pugliese G, Pricci F, Leto G, Amadio L, Iacobini C, Romeo G, Lenti L, Sale P, Gradini R, Liu FT, Di Mario U. The diabetic milieu modulates the advanced glycation end product-receptor complex in the mesangium by inducing or upregulating galectin-3 expression. *Diabetes* 2000; 49: 1249–57.
127. Park L, Raman KG, Lee KJ, Lu Y, Ferran LJ Jr, Chow WS, Stern D, Schmidt AM. Suppression of accelerated

diabetic atherosclerosis by the soluble receptor for advanced glycation endproducts. *Nat Med* 1998; 4: 1025–31.

128. Mackic JB, Stins M, McComb JG, Calero M, Ghiso J, Kim KS, Yan SD, Stern D, Schmidt AM, Frangione B, Zlokovic BV. Human blood–brain barrier receptors for Alzheimer's amyloid-beta 1-40. Asymmetrical binding, endocytosis, and transcytosis at the apical side of brain microvascular endothelial cell monolayer. *J Clin Invest* 1998; 102: 734–43.
129. Yamamoto Y, Kato I, Doi T, Yonekura H, Ohashi S, Takeuchi M, Watanabe T, Yamagishi S, Sakurai S, Takasawa S, Okamoto H, Yamamoto H. Development and prevention of advanced diabetic nephropathy in RAGE-overexpressing mice. *J Clin Invest* 2001; 108: 261–8.
130. Stitt AW, He C, Vlassara H. Characterization of the advanced glycation end-product receptor complex in human vascular endothelial cells. *Biochem Biophys Res Commun* 1999; 256: 549–56.
131. Yan SD, Schmidt AM, Anderson GM, Zhang J, Brett J, Zou YS, Pinsky D, Stern D. Enhanced cellular oxidant stress by the interaction of advanced glycation end products with their receptors/binding proteins. *J Biol Chem* 1994; 269: 9889–97.
132. Lander HM, Tauras JM, Ogiste JS, Hori O, Moss RA, Schmidt AM. Activation of the receptor for advanced glycation end products triggers a p21(ras)-dependent mitogen-activated protein kinase pathway regulated by oxidant stress. *J Biol Chem* 1997; 272: 17810–4.
133. Huttunen HJ, Fages C, Rauvala H. Receptor for advanced glycation end products (RAGE)-mediated neurite outgrowth and activation of NF-kappaB require the cytoplasmic domain of the receptor but different downstream signaling pathways. *J Biol Chem* 1999; 274: 19919–24.
134. Hofmann MA, Drury S, Fu C, Qu W, Taguchi A, Lu Y, Avila C, Kambham N, Bierhaus A, Nawroth P, Neurath MF, Slattery T, Beach D, McClary J, Nagashima M, Morser J, Stern D, Schmidt AM. RAGE mediates a novel proinflammatory axis: a central cell surface receptor for S100/calgranulin polypeptides. *Cell* 1999; 97: 889–901.
135. Li JH, Huang XR, Zhu HJ, Oldfield M, Cooper M, Truong LD, Johnson RJ, Lan HY. Advanced glycation end products activate Smad signaling via TGF-beta-dependent and -independent mechanisms: implications for diabetic renal and vascular disease. *FASEB J* April 22, 2003. Available at: http://www.fasebj.org. doi: 10.1096/fj.02-1117fje.
136. Brownlee M, Vlassara H, Kooney A, Ulrich P, Cerami A. Aminoguanidine prevents diabetes-induced arterial wall protein cross-linking. *Science* 1986; 232: 1629–32.
137. Vasan S, Zhang X, Kapurniotu A, Bernhagen J, Teichberg S, Basgen J, Wagle D, Shih D, Terlecky I, Bucala R, Cerami A, Egan J, Ulrich P. An agent cleaving glucose-derived protein crosslinks in vitro and in vivo. *Nature* 1996; 382: 275–8.
138. Wolffenbuttel BH, Boulanger CM, Crijns FR, Huijberts MS, Poitevin P, Swennen GN, Vasan S, Egan JJ, Ulrich P, Cerami A, Levy BI. Breakers of advanced glycation end products restore large artery properties in experimental diabetes. *Proc Natl Acad Sci USA* 1998; 95: 4630–4.
139. Kass DA, Shapiro EP, Kawaguchi M, Capriotti AR, Scuteri A, deGroof RC, Lakatta EG. Improved arterial compliance by a novel advanced glycation end-product crosslink breaker. *Circulation* 2001; 104: 1464–70.
140. Clements RS Jr, Robison WG Jr, Cohen MP. Anti-glycated albumin therapy ameliorates early retinal microvascular pathology in *db/db* mice. *J Diabetes Complications* 1998; 12: 28–33.
141. Bonnardel-Phu E, Wautier JL, Schmidt AM, Avila C, Vicaut E. Acute modulation of albumin microvascular leakage by advanced glycation end products in microcirculation of diabetic rats in vivo. *Diabetes* 1999; 48: 2052–8.
142. Zheng F, Cai W, Mitsuhashi T, Vlassara H. Lysozyme enhances renal excretion of advanced glycation endproducts in vivo and suppresses adverse age-mediated cellular effects in vitro: a potential AGE sequestration therapy for diabetic nephropathy? *Mol Med* 2001; 7: 737–47.
143. Freedman BI, Wuerth JP, Cartwright K, Bain RP, Dippe S, Hershon K, Mooradian AD, Spinowitz BS. Design and baseline characteristics for the aminoguanidine Clinical Trial in Overt Type 2 Diabetic Nephropathy (ACTION II). *Control Clin Trials* 1999; 20: 493–510.
144. McClain DA, Crook ED. Hexosamines and insulin resistance. *Diabetes* 1996; 45: 1003–9.
145. Rossetti L, Hawkins M, Chen W, Gindi J, Barzilai N. In vivo glucosamine infusion induces insulin resistance in normoglycemic but not in hyperglycemic conscious rats. *J Clin Invest* 1995; 96: 132–40.
146. Baron AD, Zhu JS, Zhu JH, Weldon H, Maianu L, Garvey WT. Glucosamine induces insulin resistance in vivo by affecting GLUT 4 translocation in skeletal muscle. Implications for glucose toxicity. *J Clin Invest* 1995; 96: 2792–801.
147. Singh L, Gennerette D, Simmons S, Crook E. Glucose-induced insulin resistance of phosphatidylinositol 3′-OH kinase and AKT/PKB is mediated by the hexosamine biosynthesis pathway. *J Diabetes Complications* 2001; 15: 88–96.
148. Fujii N, Kaji T, Yamamoto C, Fujiwara Y, Koizumi F. Phorbol 12-myristate 13-acetate stimulates the release of glycosaminoglycans from cultured vascular endothelial cells: possible involvement of protein kinase C activation. *Thromb Res* 1996; 82: 379–87.
149. Du X, Edelstein D, Rossetti L, Fantus I, Goldberg H, Ziyadeh F, Wu J, Brownlee M. Hyperglycemia-induced mitochondrial superoxide overproduction activates the hexosamine pathway and induces plasminogen activator inhibitor-1 expression by increasing Sp1 glycosylation. *Proc Natl Acad Sci USA* 2000; 97: 12222–6.
150. James L, Ingram A, Ly H, Thai K, Cai L, Scholey J. Angiotensin II activates the GFAT promoter in mesangial cells. *Am J Physiol Renal Physiol* 2001; 281: F151–62.
151. Nerlich AG, Sauer U, Kolm-Litty V, Wagner E, Koch M, Schleicher ED. Expression of glutamine:fructose-6-phosphate amidotransferase in human tissues: evidence for high variability and distinct regulation in diabetes. *Diabetes* 1998; 47: 170–8.
152. Akimoto Y, Kreppel LK, Hirano H, Hart GW. Hyperglycemia and the O-GlcNAc transferase in rat aortic smooth muscle cells: elevated expression and altered patterns of O-GlcNAcylation. *Arch Biochem Biophys* 2001; 389: 166–75.
153. Wu G, Haynes TE, Yan W, Meininger CJ. Presence of glutamine:fructose-6-phosphate amidotransferase for glucosamine-6-phosphate synthesis in endothelial cells: effects of hyperglycaemia and glutamine. *Diabetologia* 2001; 44: 196–202.

154. Tannock LR, Little PJ, Wight TN, Chait A. Arterial smooth muscle cell proteoglycans synthesized in the presence of glucosamine demonstrate reduced binding to LDL. *J Lipid Res* 2002; 43: 149–57.
155. McClain DA, Paterson AJ, Roos MD, Wei X, Kudlow JE. Glucose and glucosamine regulate growth factor gene expression in vascular smooth muscle cells. *Proc Natl Acad Sci USA* 1992; 89: 8150–4.
156. Daniels MC, McClain DA, Crook ED. Transcriptional regulation of transforming growth factor beta1 by glucose: investigation into the role of the hexosamine biosynthesis pathway. *Am J Med Sci* 2000; 319: 138–42.
157. Goldberg HJ, Whiteside CI, Fantus IG. The hexosamine pathway regulates the plasminogen activator inhibitor-1 gene promoter and Sp1 transcriptional activation through protein kinase C-beta I and -delta. *J Biol Chem* 2002; 277: 33833–41.
158. Chen YQ, Su M, Walia RR, Hao Q, Covington JW, Vaughan DE. Sp1 sites mediate activation of the plasminogen activator inhibitor-1 promoter by glucose in vascular smooth muscle cells. *J Biol Chem* 1998; 273: 8225–31.
159. James LR, Fantus IG, Goldberg H, Ly H, Scholey JW. Overexpression of GFAT activates PAI-1 promoter in mesangial cells. *Am J Physiol Renal Physiol* 2000; 279: F718–27.
160. Black AR, Black JD, Azizkhan-Clifford J. Sp1 and kruppel-like factor family of transcription factors in cell growth regulation and cancer. *J Cell Physiol* 2001; 188: 143–60.
161. Kadonaga JT, Courey AJ, Ladika J, Tjian R. Distinct regions of Sp1 modulate DNA binding and transcriptional activation. *Science* 1988; 242: 1566–70.
162. Haltiwanger RS, Grove K, Philipsberg GA. Modulation of O-linked *N*-acetylglucosamine levels on nuclear and cytoplasmic proteins in vivo using the peptide O-GlcNAc-beta-*N*-acetylglucosaminidase inhibitor O-(2-acetamido-2-deoxy-D-glucopyranosylidene)amino-*N*-phenylcarbamate. *J Biol Chem* 1998; 273: 3611–7.
163. Goldberg HJ, Scholey J, Fantus IG. Glucosamine activates the plasminogen activator inhibitor 1 gene promoter through Sp1 DNA binding sites in glomerular mesangial cells. *Diabetes* 2000; 49: 863–71.
164. Fulton D, Gratton JP, McCabe TJ, Fontana J, Fujio Y, Walsh K, Franke TF, Papapetropoulos A, Sessa WC. Regulation of endothelium-derived nitric oxide production by the protein kinase Akt. *Nature* 1999; 399: 597–601.
165. Dimmeler S, Fleming I, Fisslthaler B, Hermann C, Busse R, Zeiher AM. Activation of nitric oxide synthase in endothelial cells by Akt-dependent phosphorylation. *Nature* 1999; 399: 601–5.
166. Federici M, Menghini R, Mauriello A, Hribal ML, Ferrelli F, Lauro D, Sbraccia P, Spagnoli LG, Sesti G, Lauro R. Insulin-dependent activation of endothelial nitric oxide synthase is impaired by O-linked glycosylation modification of signaling proteins in human coronary endothelial cells. *Circulation* 2002; 106: 466–72.
167. James LR, Ingram A, Ly H, Thai K, Cai L, Scholey JW. Angiotensin II activates the GFAT promoter in mesangial cells. *Am J Physiol Renal Physiol* 2001; 281: F151–62.
168. Schleicher ED, Weigert C. Role of the hexosamine biosynthetic pathway in diabetic nephropathy. *Kidney Int* 2000; 77 (suppl): S13–8.
169. Ishii H, Koya D, King GL. Protein kinase C activation and its role in the development of vascular complications in diabetes mellitus. *J Mol Med* 1998; 76: 21–31.
170. Way KJ, Chou E, King GL. Identification of PKC-isoform-specific biological actions using pharmacological approaches. *Trends Pharmacol Sci* 2000; 21: 181–7.
171. Newton AC. Regulation of the ABC kinases by phosphorylation: protein kinase C as a paradigm. *Biochem J* 2003; 370: 361–71.
172. Inoguchi T, Battan R, Handler E, Sportsman JR, Heath W, King GL. Preferential elevation of protein kinase C isoform beta II and diacylglycerol levels in the aorta and heart of diabetic rats: differential reversibility to glycemic control by islet cell transplantation. *Proc Natl Acad Sci USA* 1992; 89: 11059–63.
173. Shiba T, Inoguchi T, Sportsman JR, Heath WF, Bursell S, King GL. Correlation of diacylglycerol level and protein kinase C activity in rat retina to retinal circulation. *Am J Physiol* 1993; 265: E783–93.
174. Xia P, Inoguchi T, Kern TS, Engerman RL, Oates PJ, King GL. Characterization of the mechanism for the chronic activation of diacylglycerol-protein kinase C pathway in diabetes and hypergalactosemia. *Diabetes* 1994; 43: 1122–9.
175. Yu HY, Inoguchi T, Kakimoto M, Nakashima N, Imamura M, Hashimoto T, Umeda F, Nawata H. Saturated non-esterified fatty acids stimulate de novo diacylglycerol synthesis and protein kinase c activity in cultured aortic smooth muscle cells. *Diabetologia* 2001; 44: 614–20.
176. Ferrara N, Gerber HP, LeCouter J. The biology of VEGF and its receptors. *Nat Med* 2003; 9: 669–76.
177. Xia P, Aiello LP, Ishii H, Jiang ZY, Park DJ, Robinson GS, Takagi H, Newsome WP, Jirousek MR, King GL. Characterization of vascular endothelial growth factor's effect on the activation of protein kinase C, its isoforms, and endothelial cell growth. *J Clin Invest* 1996; 98: 2018–26.
178. Suzuma K, Takahara N, Suzuma I, Isshiki K, Ueki K, Leitges M, Aiello LP, King GL. Characterization of protein kinase C beta isoform's action on retinoblastoma protein phosphorylation, vascular endothelial growth factor-induced endothelial cell proliferation, and retinal neovascularization. *Proc Natl Acad Sci USA* 2002; 99: 721–6.
179. Kim YS, Kim BC, Song CY, Hong HK, Moon KC, Lee HS. Advanced glycosylation end products stimulate collagen mRNA synthesis in mesangial cells mediated by protein kinase C and transforming growth factor-beta. *J Lab Clin Med* 2001; 138: 59–68.
180. Taher MM, Garcia JG, Natarajan V. Hydroperoxide-induced diacylglycerol formation and protein kinase C activation in vascular endothelial cells. *Arch Biochem Biophys* 1993; 303: 260–6.
181. Ishii H, Jirousek MR, Koya D, Takagi C, Xia P, Clermont A, Bursell SE, Kern TS, Ballas LM, Heath WF, Stramm LE, Feener EP, King GL. Amelioration of vascular dysfunctions in diabetic rats by an oral PKC beta inhibitor. *Science* 1996; 272: 728–31.
182. Lynch JJ, Ferro TJ, Blumenstock FA, Brockenauer AM, Malik AB. Increased endothelial albumin permeability mediated by protein kinase C activation. *J Clin Invest* 1990; 85: 1991–8.
183. Oliver JA. Adenylate cyclase and protein kinase C mediate opposite actions on endothelial junctions. *J Cell Physiol* 1990; 145: 536–42.

184. Stasek JE Jr, Patterson CE, Garcia JG. Protein kinase C phosphorylates caldesmon77 and vimentin and enhances albumin permeability across cultured bovine pulmonary artery endothelial cell monolayers. *J Cell Physiol* 1992; 153: 62–75.
185. Studer RK, Craven PA, DeRubertis FR. Role for protein kinase C in the mediation of increased fibronectin accumulation by mesangial cells grown in high-glucose medium. *Diabetes* 1993; 42: 118–26.
186. Craven PA, Studer RK, DeRubertis FR. Impaired nitric oxide-dependent cyclic guanosine monophosphate generation in glomeruli from diabetic rats. Evidence for protein kinase C-mediated suppression of the cholinergic response. *J Clin Invest* 1994; 93: 311–20.
187. Ganz MB, Seftel A. Glucose-induced changes in protein kinase C and nitric oxide are prevented by vitamin E. *Am J Physiol Endocrinol Metab* 2000; 278: E146–52.
188. Kuboki K, Jiang ZY, Takahara N, Ha SW, Igarashi M, Yamauchi T, Feener EP, Herbert TP, Rhodes CJ, King GL. Regulation of endothelial constitutive nitric oxide synthase gene expression in endothelial cells and in vivo: a specific vascular action of insulin. *Circulation* 2000; 101: 676–81.
189. Williams B, Gallacher B, Patel H, Orme C. Glucose-induced protein kinase C activation regulates vascular permeability factor mRNA expression and peptide production by human vascular smooth muscle cells in vitro. *Diabetes* 1997; 46: 1497–503.
190. Way KJ, Isshiki K, Suzuma K, Yokota T, Zvagelsky D, Schoen FJ, Sandusky GE, Pechous PA, Vlahos CJ, Wakasaki H, King GL. Expression of connective tissue growth factor is increased in injured myocardium associated with protein kinase C beta2 activation and diabetes. *Diabetes* 2002; 51: 2709–18.
191. Aiello LP, Bursell SE, Clermont A, Duh E, Ishii H, Takagi C, Mori F, Ciulla TA, Ways K, Jirousek M, Smith LE, King GL. Vascular endothelial growth factor-induced retinal permeability is mediated by protein kinase C in vivo and suppressed by an orally effective beta-isoform-selective inhibitor. *Diabetes* 1997; 46: 1473–80.
192. Kuroki T, Inoguchi T, Umeda F, Ueda F, Nawata H. High glucose induces alteration of gap junction permeability and phosphorylation of connexin-43 in cultured aortic smooth muscle cells. *Diabetes* 1998; 47: 931–6.
193. Bursell SE, Takagi C, Clermont AC, Takagi H, Mori F, Ishii H, King GL. Specific retinal diacylglycerol and protein kinase C beta isoform modulation mimics abnormal retinal hemodynamics in diabetic rats. *Invest Ophthalmol Vis Sci* 1997; 38: 2711–20.
194. Cosentino F, Eto M, De Paolis P, van der Loo B, Bachschmid M, Ullrich V, Kouroedov A, Delli Gatti C, Joch H, Volpe M, Luscher TF. High glucose causes upregulation of cyclooxygenase-2 and alters prostanoid profile in human endothelial cells: role of protein kinase C and reactive oxygen species. *Circulation* 2003; 107: 1017–23.
195. Yerneni KK, Bai W, Khan BV, Medford RM, Natarajan R. Hyperglycemia-induced activation of nuclear transcription factor kappaB in vascular smooth muscle cells. *Diabetes* 1999; 48: 855–64.
196. Danis RP, Bingaman DP, Jirousek M, Yang Y. Inhibition of intraocular neovascularization caused by retinal ischemia in pigs by PKCbeta inhibition with LY333531. *Invest Ophthalmol Vis Sci* 1998; 39: 171–9.
197. Nonaka A, Kiryu J, Tsujikawa A, Yamashiro K, Miyamoto K, Nishiwaki H, Honda Y, Ogura Y. PKC-beta inhibitor (LY333531) attenuates leukocyte entrapment in retinal microcirculation of diabetic rats. *Invest Ophthalmol Vis Sci* 2000; 41: 2702–6.
198. Aiello LP. The potential role of PKC beta in diabetic retinopathy and macular edema. *Surv Ophthalmol* 2002; 47 (suppl 2): S263–9.
199. Kelly DJ, Zhang Y, Hepper C, Gow RM, Jaworski K, Kemp BE, Wilkinson-Berka JL, Gilbert RE. Protein kinase C beta inhibition attenuates the progression of experimental diabetic nephropathy in the presence of continued hypertension. *Diabetes* 2003; 52: 512–8.
200. Nakamura J, Kato K, Hamada Y, Nakayama M, Chaya S, Nakashima E, Naruse K, Kasuya Y, Mizubayashi R, Miwa K, Yasuda Y, Kamiya H, Ienaga K, Sakakibara F, Koh N, Hotta N. A protein kinase C beta-selective inhibitor ameliorates neural dysfunction in streptozotocin-induced diabetic rats. *Diabetes* 1999; 48: 2090–5.
201. Cotter MA, Jack AM, Cameron NE. Effects of the protein kinase C beta inhibitor LY333531 on neural and vascular function in rats with streptozotocin-induced diabetes. *Clin Sci (Lond)* 2002; 103: 311–21.
202. Cameron NE, Cotter MA. Effects of protein kinase C beta inhibition on neurovascular dysfunction in diabetic rats: interaction with oxidative stress and essential fatty acid dysmetabolism. *Diabetes Metab Res Rev* 2002; 18: 315–23.
203. Beckman JA, Goldfine AB, Gordon MB, Garrett LA, Creager MA. Inhibition of protein kinase Cbeta prevents impaired endothelium-dependent vasodilation caused by hyperglycemia in humans. *Circ Res* 2002; 90: 107–11.
204. Bastyr E III, Price K, Skljarevski V, Lledo A, Vignati L. Ruboxistaurin (RBX) mesylate treatment in patients with diabetic peripheral neuropathy (DPN) improves clinical global impression (CGI) and correlates with change in patient symptoms and signs. *Diabetes* 2003; 52: A191.
205. Schechtman D, Mochly-Rosen D. Isozyme-specific inhibitors and activators of protein kinase C. *Methods Enzymol* 2002; 345: 470–89.
206. Dandona P. Endothelium, inflammation, and diabetes. *Curr Diab Rep* 2002; 2: 311–5.
207. Schram MT, Chaturvedi N, Schalkwijk C, Giorgino F, Ebeling P, Fuller JH, Stehouwer CD. Vascular risk factors and markers of endothelial function as determinants of inflammatory markers in type 1 diabetes: the EURODIAB Prospective Complications Study. *Diabetes Care* 2003; 26: 2165–73.
208. Theuma P, Fonseca VA. Inflammation and emerging risk factors in diabetes mellitus and atherosclerosis. *Curr Diab Rep* 2003; 3: 248–54.
209. Limb GA, Chignell AH, Green W, LeRoy F, Dumonde DC. Distribution of TNF alpha and its reactive vascular adhesion molecules in fibrovascular membranes of proliferative diabetic retinopathy. *Br J Ophthalmol* 1996; 80: 168–73.
210. Limb GA, Soomro H, Janikoun S, Hollifield RD, Shilling J. Evidence for control of tumour necrosis factor-alpha (TNF-alpha) activity by TNF receptors in patients with proliferative diabetic retinopathy. *Clin Exp Immunol* 1999; 115: 409–14.
211. Joussen AM, Poulaki V, Mitsiades N, Kirchhof B, Koizumi K, Dohmen S, Adamis AP. Nonsteroidal anti-inflammatory drugs prevent early diabetic retinopathy via TNF-alpha suppression. *FASEB J* 2002; 16: 438–40.

212. Pairet M, Engelhardt G. Distinct isoforms (COX-1 and COX-2) of cyclooxygenase: possible physiological and therapeutic implications. *Fundam Clin Pharmacol* 1996; 10: 1–17.
213. Williams B, Schrier RW. Glucose-induced protein kinase C activity regulates arachidonic acid release and eicosanoid production by cultured glomerular mesangial cells. *J Clin Invest* 1993; 92: 2889–96.
214. Zhang L, Zalewski A, Liu Y, Mazurek T, Cowan S, Martin JL, Hofmann SM, Vlassara H, Shi Y. Diabetes-induced oxidative stress and low-grade inflammation in porcine coronary arteries. *Circulation* 2003; 108: 472–8.
215. Yuan M, Konstantopoulos N, Lee J, Hansen L, Li ZW, Karin M, Shoelson SE. Reversal of obesity- and diet-induced insulin resistance with salicylates or targeted disruption of Ikkbeta. *Science* 2001; 293: 1673–7.
216. The Early Treatment Diabetes Control and Complications Trial Research Group. Effects of aspirin treatment on diabetic retinopathy. ETDRS report number 8. Early Treatment Diabetic Retinopathy Study Research Group. *Ophthalmology* 1991; 98: 757–65.
217. The Early Treatment Diabetic Retinopathy Study Investigators. Aspirin effects on mortality and morbidity in patients with diabetes mellitus. Early Treatment Diabetic Retinopathy Study Report 14. *JAMA* 1992; 268: 1292–300.
218. Yancopoulos GD, Davis S, Gale NW, Rudge JS, Wiegand SJ, Holash J. Vascular-specific growth factors and blood vessel formation. *Nature* 2000; 407: 242–8.
219. Neufeld G, Cohen T, Gengrinovitch S, Poltorak Z. Vascular endothelial growth factor (VEGF) and its receptors. *FASEB J* 1999; 13: 9–22.
220. Hammes HP, Lin J, Bretzel RG, Brownlee M, Breier G. Upregulation of the vascular endothelial growth factor/vascular endothelial growth factor receptor system in experimental background diabetic retinopathy of the rat. *Diabetes* 1998; 47: 401–6.
221. Ishida S, Usui T, Yamashiro K, Kaji Y, Amano S, Ogura Y, Hida T, Oguchi Y, Ambati J, Miller JW, Gragoudas ES, Ng YS, D'Amore PA, Shima DT, Adamis AP. VEGF164-mediated inflammation is required for pathological, but not physiological, ischemia-induced retinal neovascularization. *J Exp Med* 2003; 198: 483–9.
222. Bortoloso E, Del Prete D, Gambaro G, Dalla Vestra M, Sailer A, Baggio B, Antonucci F, Fioretto P, Anglani F. Vascular endothelial growth factor (VEGF) and VEGF receptors in diabetic nephropathy: expression studies in biopsies of type 2 diabetic patients. *Ren Fail* 2001; 23: 483–93.
223. Cooper ME, Vranes D, Youssef S, Stacker SA, Cox AJ, Rizkalla B, Casley DJ, Bach LA, Kelly DJ, Gilbert RE. Increased renal expression of vascular endothelial growth factor (VEGF) and its receptor VEGFR-2 in experimental diabetes. *Diabetes* 1999; 48: 2229–39.
224. Tsuchida K, Makita Z, Yamagishi S, Atsumi T, Miyoshi H, Obara S, Ishida M, Ishikawa S, Yasumura K, Koike T. Suppression of transforming growth factor beta and vascular endothelial growth factor in diabetic nephropathy in rats by a novel advanced glycation end product inhibitor, OPB-9195. *Diabetologia* 1999; 42: 579–88.
225. de Vriese AS, Tilton RG, Elger M, Stephan CC, Kriz W, Lameire NH. Antibodies against vascular endothelial growth factor improve early renal dysfunction in experimental diabetes. *J Am Soc Nephrol* 2001; 12: 993–1000.
226. Chou E, Suzuma I, Way KJ, Opland D, Clermont AC, Naruse K, Suzuma K, Bowling NL, Vlahos CJ, Aiello LP, King GL. Decreased cardiac expression of vascular endothelial growth factor and its receptors in insulin-resistant and diabetic States: a possible explanation for impaired collateral formation in cardiac tissue. *Circulation* 2002; 105: 373–9.
227. Giordano FJ, Gerber HP, Williams SP, VanBruggen N, Bunting S, Ruiz-Lozano P, Gu Y, Nath AK, Huang Y, Hickey R, Dalton N, Peterson KL, Ross J Jr, Chien KR, Ferrara N. A cardiac myocyte vascular endothelial growth factor paracrine pathway is required to maintain cardiac function. *Proc Natl Acad Sci USA* 2001; 98: 5780–5.
228. Yarom R, Zirkin H, Stammler G, Rose AG. Human coronary microvessels in diabetes and ischaemia. Morphometric study of autopsy material. *J Pathol* 1992; 166: 265–70.
229. Hedman M, Hartikainen J, Syvanne M, Stjernvall J, Hedman A, Kivela A, Vanninen E, Mussalo H, Kauppila E, Simula S, Narvanen O, Rantala A, Peuhkurinen K, Nieminen MS, Laakso M, Yla-Herttuala S. Safety and feasibility of catheter-based local intracoronary vascular endothelial growth factor gene transfer in the prevention of postangioplasty and in-stent restenosis and in the treatment of chronic myocardial ischemia: phase II results of the Kuopio Angiogenesis Trial (KAT). *Circulation* 2003; 107: 2677–83.
230. Henry TD, Annex BH, McKendall GR, Azrin MA, Lopez JJ, Giordano FJ, Shah PK, Willerson JT, Benza RL, Berman DS, Gibson CM, Bajamonde A, Rundle AC, Fine J, McCluskey ER. The VIVA trial: Vascular endothelial growth factor in Ischemia for Vascular Angiogenesis. *Circulation* 2003; 107: 1359–65.
231. Ferrara N, Alitalo K. Clinical applications of angiogenic growth factors and their inhibitors. *Nat Med* 1999; 5: 1359–64.
232. Heldin CH, Ostman A, Ronnstrand L. Signal transduction via platelet-derived growth factor receptors. *Biochim Biophys Acta* 1998; 1378: F79–113.
233. Cao R, Brakenhielm E, Pawliuk R, Wariaro D, Post MJ, Wahlberg E, Leboulch P, Cao Y. Angiogenic synergism, vascular stability and improvement of hind-limb ischemia by a combination of PDGF-BB and FGF-2. *Nat Med* 2003; 9: 604–13.
234. Lang F, Klingel K, Wagner CA, Stegen C, Warntges S, Friedrich B, Lanzendorfer M, Melzig J, Moschen I, Steuer S, Waldegger S, Sauter M, Paulmichl M, Gerke V, Risler T, Gamba G, Capasso G, Kandolf R, Hebert SC, Massry SG, Broer S. Deranged transcriptional regulation of cell-volume-sensitive kinase hSGK in diabetic nephropathy. *Proc Natl Acad Sci USA* 2000; 97: 8157–62.
235. Yamamoto T, Nakamura T, Noble NA, Ruoslahti E, Border WA. Expression of transforming growth factor beta is elevated in human and experimental diabetic nephropathy. *Proc Natl Acad Sci USA* 1993; 90: 1814–8.
236. Border WA, Yamamoto T, Noble NA. Transforming growth factor beta in diabetic nephropathy. *Diabetes Metab Rev* 1996; 12: 309–39.
237. Sharma K, Ziyadeh FN, Alzahabi B, McGowan TA, Kapoor S, Kurnik BR, Kurnik PB, Weisberg LS. Increased renal production of transforming growth factor-beta1 in patients with type II diabetes. *Diabetes* 1997; 46: 854–9.
238. Pankewycz OG, Guan JX, Bolton WK, Gomez A, Benedict JF. Renal TGF-beta regulation in spontaneously

diabetic NOD mice with correlations in mesangial cells. *Kidney Int* 1994; 46: 748–58.

239. Park IS, Kiyomoto H, Abboud SL, Abboud HE. Expression of transforming growth factor-beta and type IV collagen in early streptozotocin-induced diabetes. *Diabetes* 1997; 46: 473–80.
240. Throckmorton DC, Brogden AP, Min B, Rasmussen H, Kashgarian M. PDGF and TGF-beta mediate collagen production by mesangial cells exposed to advanced glycosylation end products. *Kidney Int* 1995; 48: 111–7.
241. Wong TY, Phillips AO, Witowski J, Topley N. Glucose-mediated induction of TGF-beta 1 and MCP-1 in mesothelial cells in vitro is osmolality and polyol pathway dependent. *Kidney Int* 2003; 63: 1404–16.
242. Sharma K, Jin Y, Guo J, Ziyadeh FN. Neutralization of TGF-beta by anti-TGF-beta antibody attenuates kidney hypertrophy and the enhanced extracellular matrix gene expression in STZ-induced diabetic mice. *Diabetes* 1996; 45: 522–30.
243. Ziyadeh FN, Hoffman BB, Han DC, Iglesias-De La Cruz MC, Hong SW, Isono M, Chen S, McGowan TA, Sharma K. Long-term prevention of renal insufficiency, excess matrix gene expression, and glomerular mesangial matrix expansion by treatment with monoclonal antitransforming growth factor-beta antibody in db/db diabetic mice. *Proc Natl Acad Sci USA* 2000; 97: 8015–20.
244. Han DC, Hoffman BB, Hong SW, Guo J, Ziyadeh FN. Therapy with antisense TGF-beta1 oligodeoxynucleotides reduces kidney weight and matrix mRNAs in diabetic mice. *Am J Physiol Renal Physiol* 2000; 278: F628–34.
245. Shull MM, Ormsby I, Kier AB, Pawlowski S, Diebold RJ, Yin M, Allen R, Sidman C, Proetzel G, Calvin D, et al. Targeted disruption of the mouse transforming growth factor-beta 1 gene results in multifocal inflammatory disease. *Nature* 1992; 359: 693–9.
246. Kulkarni AB, Huh CG, Becker D, Geiser A, Lyght M, Flanders KC, Roberts AB, Sporn MB, Ward JM, Karlsson S. Transforming growth factor beta 1 null mutation in mice causes excessive inflammatory response and early death. *Proc Natl Acad Sci USA* 1993; 90: 770–4.
247. Gupta S, Clarkson MR, Duggan J, Brady HR. Connective tissue growth factor: potential role in glomerulosclerosis and tubulointerstitial fibrosis. *Kidney Int* 2000; 58: 1389–99.
248. Murphy M, Godson C, Cannon S, Kato S, Mackenzie HS, Martin F, Brady HR. Suppression subtractive hybridization identifies high glucose levels as a stimulus for expression of connective tissue growth factor and other genes in human mesangial cells. *J Biol Chem* 1999; 274: 5830–4.
249. Riser BL, Denichilo M, Cortes P, Baker C, Grondin JM, Yee J, Narins RG. Regulation of connective tissue growth factor activity in cultured rat mesangial cells and its expression in experimental diabetic glomerulosclerosis. *J Am Soc Nephrol* 2000; 11: 25–38.
250. Weston BS, Wahab NA, Mason RM. CTGF mediates TGF-beta-induced fibronectin matrix deposition by upregulating active alpha5beta1 integrin in human mesangial cells. *J Am Soc Nephrol* 2003; 14: 601–10.
251. Twigg SM, Cao Z, MCLennan SV, Burns WC, Brammar G, Forbes JM, Cooper ME. Renal. connective tissue growth factor induction in experimental diabetes is prevented by aminoguanidine. *Endocrinology* 2002; 143: 4907–15.
252. Candido R, Forbes JM, Thomas MC, Thallas V, Dean RG, Burns WC, Tikellis C, Ritchie RH, Twigg SM, Cooper ME, Burrell LM. A breaker of advanced glycation end products attenuates diabetes-induced myocardial structural changes. *Circ Res* 2003; 92: 785–92.
253. Forbes JM, Cooper ME, Oldfield MD, Thomas MC. Role of advanced glycation end products in diabetic nephropathy. *J Am Soc Nephrol* 2003; 14: S254–8.
254. Chen Y, Blom IE, Sa S, Goldschmeding R, Abraham DJ, Leask A. CTGF expression in mesangial cells: involvement of SMADs, MAP kinase, and PKC. *Kidney Int* 2002; 62: 1149–59.
255. Suzuma K, Naruse K, Suzuma I, Takahara N, Ueki K, Aiello LP, King GL. Vascular endothelial growth factor induces expression of connective tissue growth factor via KDR, Flt1, and phosphatidylinositol 3-kinase-akt-dependent pathways in retinal vascular cells. *J Biol Chem* 2000; 275: 40725–31.
256. Abdel-Wahab N, Weston BS, Roberts T, Mason RM. Connective tissue growth factor and regulation of the mesangial cell cycle: role in cellular hypertrophy. *J Am Soc Nephrol* 2002; 13: 2437–45.
257. Duncan MR, Frazier KS, Abramson S, Williams S, Klapper H, Huang X, Grotendorst GR. Connective tissue growth factor mediates transforming growth factor beta-induced collagen synthesis: down-regulation by cAMP. *FASEB J* 1999; 13: 1774–86.
258. Abreu JG, Ketpura NI, Reversade B, De Robertis EM. Connective-tissue growth factor (CTGF) modulates cell signalling by BMP and TGF-beta. *Nat Cell Biol* 2002; 4: 599–604.
259. Riser BL, Cortes P, DeNichilo M, Deshmukh PV, Chahal PS, Mohammed AK, Yee J, Kahkonen D. Urinary CCN2 (CTGF) as a possible predictor of diabetic nephropathy: preliminary report. *Kidney Int* 2003; 64: 451–8.
260. Feener EP. The renin-angiotensin system in diabetic cardiovascular complications. In Johnston MT, Veves A (eds), *Diabetes and Cardiovascular Disease*. Totowa, NJ: Humana press; 2001.
261. Ardaillou R. Angiotensin II receptors. *J Am Soc Nephrol* 1999; 10 (suppl 11): S30–9.
262. Kagami S, Border WA, Miller DE, Noble NA. Angiotensin II stimulates extracellular matrix protein synthesis through induction of transforming growth factor-beta expression in rat glomerular mesangial cells. *J Clin Invest* 1994; 93: 2431–7.
263. Chen HC, Bouchie JL, Perez AS, Clermont AC, Izumo S, Hampe J, Feener EP. Role of the angiotensin AT(1) receptor in rat aortic and cardiac PAI-1 gene expression. *Arterioscler Thromb Vasc Biol* 2000; 20: 2297–302.
264. Pupilli C, Lasagni L, Romagnani P, Bellini F, Mannelli M, Misciglia N, Mavilia C, Vellei U, Villari D, Serio M. Angiotensin II stimulates the synthesis and secretion of vascular permeability factor/vascular endothelial growth factor in human mesangial cells. *J Am Soc Nephrol* 1999; 10: 245–55.
265. Hogeboom van Buggenum IM, Polak BC, Reichert-Thoen JW, de Vries-Knoppert WA, van Hinsbergh VW, Tangelder GJ. Angiotensin converting enzyme inhibiting therapy is associated with lower vitreous vascular endothelial growth factor concentrations in patients with proliferative diabetic retinopathy. *Diabetologia* 2002; 45: 203–9.
266. Folli F, Kahn CR, Hansen H, Bouchie JL, Feener EP. Angiotensin II inhibits insulin signaling in aortic smooth

muscle cells at multiple levels. A potential role for serine phosphorylation in insulin/angiotensin II crosstalk. *J Clin Invest* 1997; 100: 2158–69.

267. Chaturvedi N, Sjolie AK, Stephenson JM, Abrahamian H, Keipes M, Castellarin A, Rogulja-Pepeonik Z, Fuller JH, for the The EUCLID Study Group. Effect of lisinopril on progression of retinopathy in normotensive people with type 1 diabetes. EURODIAB controlled trial of lisinopril in insulin-dependent diabetes mellitus. *Lancet* 1998; 351: 28–31.
268. Lewis EJ, Hunsicker LG, Bain RP, Rohde RD, for the The Collaborative Study Group. The effect of angiotensin-converting-enzyme inhibition on diabetic nephropathy. *N Engl J Med* 1993; 329: 1456–62.
269. Laffel LM, McGill JB, Gans DJ, for the North American Microalbuminuria Study Group. The beneficial effect of angiotensin-converting enzyme inhibition with captopril on diabetic nephropathy in normotensive IDDM patients with microalbuminuria. *Am J Med* 1995; 99: 497–504.
270. The Microalbuminuria Captopril Study Group. Captopril reduces the risk of nephropathy in IDDM patients with microalbuminuria. *Diabetologia* 1996; 39: 587–93.
271. The EUCLID Study Group. Randomised placebo-controlled trial of lisinopril in normotensive patients with insulin-dependent diabetes and normoalbuminuria or microalbuminuria. *Lancet* 1997; 349: 1787–92.
272. Ravid M, Brosh D, Levi Z, Bar-Dayan Y, Ravid D, Rachmani R. Use of enalapril to attenuate decline in renal function in normotensive, normoalbuminuric patients with type 2 diabetes mellitus. A randomized, controlled trial. *Ann Intern Med* 1998; 128: 982–8.
273. Mathiesen ER, Hommel E, Hansen HP, Smidt UM, Parving HH. Randomised controlled trial of long term efficacy of captopril on preservation of kidney function in normotensive patients with insulin dependent diabetes and microalbuminuria. *BMJ* 1999; 319: 24–5.
274. Heart Outcome Prevention Evaluation Study Investigators. Effects of ramipril on cardiovascular and microvascular outcomes in people with diabetes mellitus: results of the HOPE study and MICRO-HOPE substudy. *Lancet* 2000; 355: 253–9.
275. Malik RA, Williamson S, Abbott C, Carrington AL, Iqbal J, Schady W, Boulton AJ. Effect of angiotensin-converting-enzyme (ACE) inhibitor trandolapril on human diabetic neuropathy: randomised double-blind controlled trial. *Lancet* 1998; 352: 1978–81.
276. The UKPDS Group. Tight blood pressure control and risk of macrovascular and microvascular complications in type 2 diabetes: UKPDS 38. *BMJ* 1998; 317: 703–13.
277. Hopfner RL, Gopalakrishnan V. Endothelin: emerging role in diabetic vascular complications. *Diabetologia* 1999; 42: 1383–94.
278. Takagi C, Bursell SE, Lin YW, Takagi H, Duh E, Jiang Z, Clermont AC, King GL. Regulation of retinal hemodynamics in diabetic rats by increased expression and action of endothelin-1. *Invest Ophthalmol Vis Sci* 1996; 37: 2504–18.
279. Park JY, Takahara N, Gabriele A, Chou E, Naruse K, Suzuma K, Yamauchi T, Ha SW, Meier M, Rhodes CJ, King GL. Induction of endothelin-1 expression by glucose: an effect of protein kinase C activation. *Diabetes* 2000; 49: 1239–48.
280. Cameron NE, Dines KC, Cotter MA. The potential contribution of endothelin-1 to neurovascular abnormalities in streptozotocin-diabetic rats. *Diabetologia* 1994; 37: 1209–15.
281. Cameron NE, Cotter MA. Effects of a nonpeptide endothelin-1 ETA antagonist on neurovascular function in diabetic rats: interaction with the renin-angiotensin system. *J Pharmacol Exp Ther* 1996; 278: 1262–8.
282. Nakamura T, Ebihara I, Fukui M, Tomino Y, Koide H. Effect of a specific endothelin receptor A antagonist on mRNA levels for extracellular matrix components and growth factors in diabetic glomeruli. *Diabetes* 1995; 44: 895–9.
283. Hocher B, Lun A, Priem F, Neumayer HH, Raschack M. Renal endothelin system in diabetes: comparison of angiotensin-converting enzyme inhibition and endothelin-A antagonism. *J Cardiovasc Pharmacol* 1998; 31 (suppl 1): S492–5.
284. Deng D, Evans T, Mukherjee K, Downey D, Chakrabarti S. Diabetes-induced vascular dysfunction in the retina: role of endothelins. *Diabetologia* 1999; 42: 1228–34.
285. Chua CC, Hamdy RC, Chua BH. Upregulation of vascular endothelial growth factor by angiotensin II in rat heart endothelial cells. *Biochim Biophys Acta* 1998; 1401: 187–94.
286. Otani A, Takagi H, Suzuma K, Honda Y. Angiotensin II potentiates vascular endothelial growth factor-induced angiogenic activity in retinal microcapillary endothelial cells. *Circ Res* 1998; 82: 619–28.
287. Otani A, Takagi H, Oh H, Suzuma K, Matsumura M, Ikeda E, Honda Y. Angiotensin II-stimulated vascular endothelial growth factor expression in bovine retinal pericytes. *Invest Ophthalmol Vis Sci* 2000; 41: 1192–9.
288. Fujiyama S, Matsubara H, Nozawa Y, Maruyama K, Mori Y, Tsutsumi Y, Masaki H, Uchiyama Y, Koyama Y, Nose A, Iba O, Tateishi E, Ogata N, Jyo N, Higashiyama S, Iwasaka T. Angiotensin AT(1) and AT(2) receptors differentially regulate angiopoietin-2 and vascular endothelial growth factor expression and angiogenesis by modulating heparin binding-epidermal growth factor (EGF)-mediated EGF receptor transactivation. *Circ Res* 2001; 88: 22–9.
289. Gilbert RE, Kelly DJ, Cox AJ, Wilkinson-Berka JL, Rumble JR, Osicka T, Panagiotopoulos S, Lee V, Hendrich EC, Jerums G, Cooper ME. Angiotensin converting enzyme inhibition reduces retinal overexpression of vascular endothelial growth factor and hyperpermeability in experimental diabetes. *Diabetologia* 2000; 43: 1360–7.
290. Morisaki N, Watanabe S, Fukuda K, Saito Y. Angiogenic interaction between retinal endothelial cells and pericytes from normal and diabetic rabbits, and phenotypic changes of diabetic cells. *Cell Mol Biol* 1999; 45: 67–77.
291. Stracke H, Lindemann A, Federlin K. A benfotiamine-vitamin B combination in treatment of diabetic polyneuropathy. *Exp Clin Endocrinol Diabetes* 1996; 104: 311–6.
292. Hammes HP, Du X, Edelstein D, Taguchi T, Matsumura T, Ju Q, Lin J, Bierhaus A, Nawroth P, Hannak D, Neumaier M, Bergfeld R, Giardino I, Brownlee M. Benfotiamine blocks three major pathways of hyperglycemic damage and prevents experimental diabetic retinopathy. *Nat Med* 2003; 9: 294–9.

63

The Role of Glycemia in Diabetic Complications

Stephanie A. Amiel

King's College, London, UK

Several biochemical features are linked to diabetes, of which the most obvious are hyperglycemia and inadequate insulin action. Risk of chronic complications varies among the different types of diabetes, but the nature of those complications is shared: microvascular disease causing renal and retinal and some neurological damage, and macrovascular disease causing premature stroke, myocardial infarction, and peripheral vascular disease. It is logical to implicate glycemia *per se* as a causative agent in the etiopathogenesis of the diabetic complications; this chapter examines the evidence.

GLYCEMIC CONTROL AND MICROVASCULAR COMPLICATIONS

Epidemiological Evidence

The connection between worse glycemic control and higher prevalence of microvascular complications was first made in the early 1950s. Marble described greater frequency of nephropathy and retinopathy in more poorly controlled diabetes in 1951 [1], and Johnsson, writing in 1960 [2], unfavorably compared the data from 107 patients managed in Sweden on a "free diet" in whom 93.4% had vascular complications at 10 years' duration [3], with those from 34 patients managed in the United States on a more strict regimen, of whom 30 were free of nephropathy and 20% of more than minimal retinopathy after a mean duration of over 26 years [4]. Thereafter, one of the most quoted studies linking glycemic control to risk of microvascular complications of diabetes is a clinical observational study from Pirart [5]. Pirart classified his patients' glycemic control on the basis of urinary glucose level and documented the presence of retinopathy, neuropathy, and nephropathy. He made two very important observations: one that diabetic complications increase in prevalence with diabetes duration, and second, that there is a strong association of diabetic complications with glycemic control. He described the negligible prevalence of microvascular complications in those patients he considered well controlled, intermediate prevalence in the moderately controlled, and highest prevalence in the patients he defined as poorly controlled, with functional loss (renal failure, blindness) only making an appearance in the latter group. His data on retinopathy are reproduced in Figure 1. Until the advent of the prospective intervention trials (see below), these data were the most robust to defend the hypothesis that glycemic control was important in the pathogenesis of at least the microvascular complications of diabetes, and to support discussions with patients that they should strive for better diabetic control than that which controlled acute symptoms alone.

More recent population studies continue to provide evidence for a link between glycemic control and risk of microvascular complications. The diabetic condition is defined according to measurements of plasma glucose and its surrogates, and the redefining of appropriate glucose levels in 1997–1998 was based in part on the glycemic levels defining risk of the diabetes-specific microvascular complication of diabetic retinopathy in population studies. Plasma glucose in the fasting state and 2 h after a 75-g oral glucose load in standardized oral glucose tolerance tests has been plotted against prevalence of diabetic microvascular complications in three large epidemiological surveys. In three very different populations—the Pima Indians [6], Egyptians [7], and Americans (aged

International Textbook of Diabetes Mellitus, Third Edition. Edited by R. A. DeFronzo, E. Ferrannini, H. Keen, and P. Zimmet.
 ISBN: 0-471-48655-8.

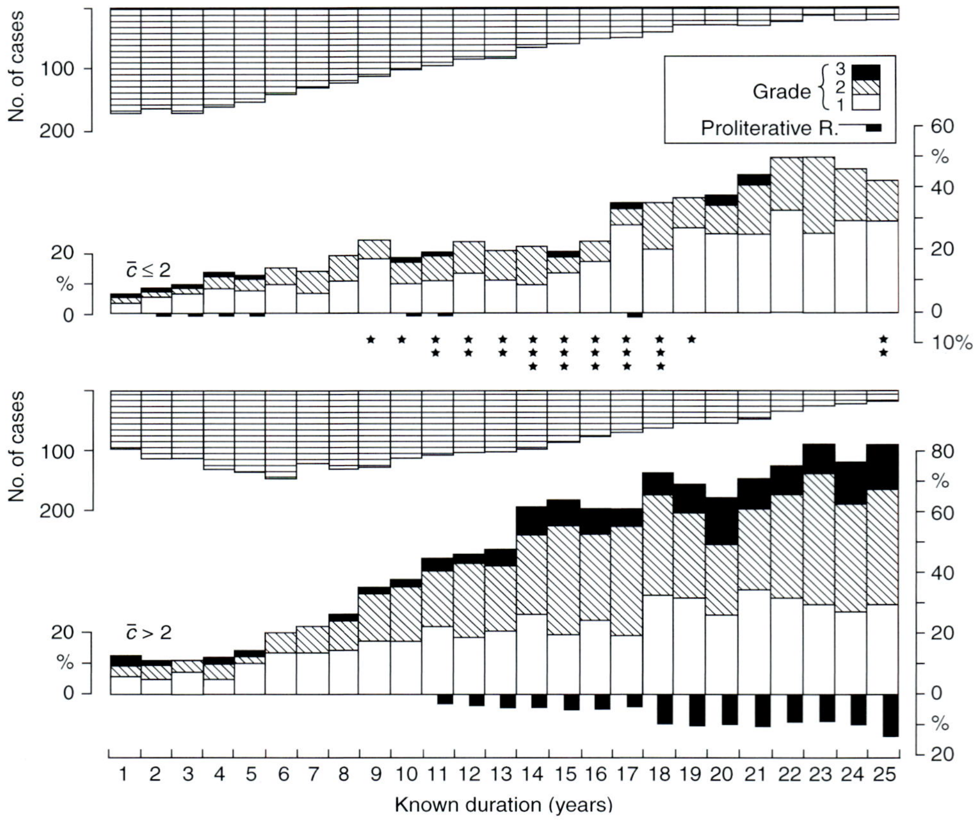

Figure 1 Association between worsening glycemic control and retinopathy. The bars show the extent of all retinopathy increasing over time (x axis) and to a greater degree as control is worse (best controlled, top panel; least well controlled, bottom panel). Significant visual loss (solid bars below line) occurs almost exclusively in the worst controlled. (From reference 5)

40–74 years) [8], diabetic retinopathy begins to occur in populations where the 2-h venous plasma glucose is around 11.0 mmol/l or more (Figure 2) (Table 1). Equivalent fasting levels were 7.0 and glycated hemoglobin 6%, with similar values for nephropathy, although these data are a little less clear-cut, perhaps because of the less specific measurement used to assess its presence (proteinuria). These definitions imply that microvascular disease does not occur in abnormalities of glucose tolerance short of diabetes. This is in contrast to macrovascular disease, discussed below. The association between the different measures of plasma glucose concentration and retinopathy is very robust, but again does not confirm causality.

Although the most recent epidemiological data increasingly recognize the role of other factors such as hypertension and hyperlipidemia in the etiopathogenesis of microvascular complications, they continue to support the role for an independent effect of hyperglycemia. In the large, long-term multinational WHO survey, fasting plasma glucose was associated with retinopathy [9], had an independent association with albuminuria in type 1 and type 2 diabetes [10], and was also an independent predictor of renal failure in type 2 diabetes [11].

Table 1 Epidemiological associations between glycemia and retinopathy

	FPG (mmol/l)	2-h PG (mmol/l)
NHANES III [7]	6.7	10.8
Egyptians [6]	7.2	11.5
Pima [8]	6.8	11.1

Note. FPG = fasting plasma glucose; PG = post-glucose.

The major criticism that can be leveled against all the above studies is that the plasma glucose concentrations may be a co-incident marker of some other causal agent for microvascular complications. Perhaps those diabetic patients that experience complications have a more complicated disease that is both prone to complications and has more difficult glycemic control. It needs intervention studies, where the effect of different glycemic control strategies on the evolution of complications is examined, to determine a causal—and modifiable—link.

Intervention Studies

One of the earliest studies that suggested that the risk of microvascular complications might be altered by treatment strategy in presumed type 1 diabetes was a

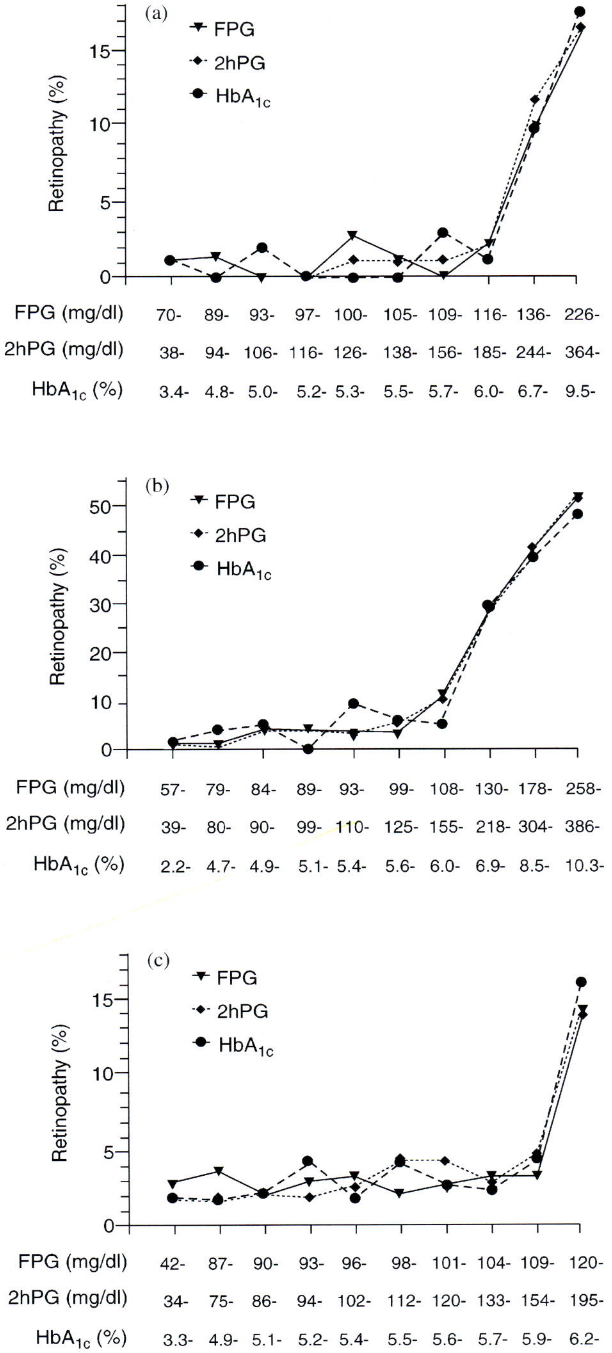

Figure 2 Plots of data from three epidemiological surveys, showing prevalence of diabetic retinopathy against measurements of glycemic control. The x axes show the lower limit of each decile group. In each panel, the triangles and dashed lines refer to fasting plasma glucose (FPG); the diamonds and dotted lines refer to 2-h post-glucose (2hPG) load plasma glucose; and the solid circles and solid lines are the NbA_{1c} data. The top panel shows data from Pima Indians [6], the middle panel from Egyptians [7], and the lower panel from Americans [8]. The data indicate the precise and reproducible relationship between glucose control and retinopathy. (Reproduced from reference 8)

retrospective analysis of the evolution of complications in two cohorts of diabetic patients, diagnosed before the age of 40 years, one treated with strict diet and premeal injections of soluble insulin intended to achieve aglycosuria between 1922 and 1935; the other treated with a more flexible diet and the newly available intermediate-acting insulins between 1935 and 1945. Despite a shorter follow-up, the latter group developed strikingly more retinopathy [2]. In view of what was to follow, it is worth noting that the prevalence of hypoglycemia was higher in the earlier group.

Type 1 Diabetes

Since then there have been a series of studies performed in the more robust prospective controlled way. In the late 1970s and early 1980s, a series of small studies was done, examining intensified insulin therapy in type 1 diabetes in a randomized controlled trial setting. This was the time of the development of insulin pump therapy (continuous subcutaneous insulin therapy, or CSII), developed as a new, more physiological way to deliver exogenous insulin [12, 13]. Table 2 shows the sample size and summarizes the main points about these studies [14–28]. The Kroc study, one of the largest of these early trials, was designed as a feasibility study for a larger trial. It was funded by the Kroc Foundation (started by the family that own McDonald's) and set out to determine whether it was feasible to reduce parameters of glycemic control in a multicenter study of type 1 diabetes. It was not designed to address issues of efficacy of therapy in reducing complications; nevertheless it did demonstrate stabilization of retinal status and reduction in urine albumin excretion rate (albeit after only a single baseline measurement) with CSII, while both features tended to progress in the conventionally treated arm.

Of note, these studies continued despite early failure to improve or frank deterioration in retinal status within the first few months of instituting intensified therapy. Accelerated progression of retinopathy with the institution of tight control was seen in some of the studies, primarily the appearance of cotton wool spots [20, 26]. The investigators and patients bravely continued to show the resolution of these changes and some evidence for slowing of progression of the retinopathy with intensive therapy and continued better control [21, 27, 28]. Worsening of retinopathy with the institution of good glycemic control has since been seen elsewhere [29]. It has been attributed to the removal of hyperglycemia-driven hyperperfusion, and it shows stabilization and then improvement in retinal or nephropathy status after about 2 years [30].

A meta-analysis of many of these early trials convincingly demonstrated the ability of strict glycemic control to reduce the risk of retinopathy and slow progression of nephropathy, but did comment on the increased risk of

Table 2 Early intervention studies and microvascular disease

Study	Type 1 patients	*n*	Duration	Mode of intensive Rx and treatment allocation	Effects seen in intensively treated group	
					Retinopathy	Nephropathy
Steno 1 [14]	Background retinopathy	30	2 years	CSII RCT	Initial deterioration in more patients, then stable with fewer deteriorated at 2 years	Elevated GFR reduced in CSII Urine albumin excretion stable
Steno 2 [15]	Microalbuminuria	36	2 years	CSII RCT	—	Reduced annual increase in albumin excretion. No patient developed proteinuria (vs. 5 in conventional group, who had highest albuminuria at baseline)
Steno follow-up [16]			8 and 5 years			Continued reduction in rate of decline of GFR 3 deaths with DKA in CSII five cardiovascular events in 3 patients in conventional group
Oxford [17]	Background retinopathy	74	2 years	MDI, with home monitoring RCT	6 patients developed new vessels (vs. 2 in control group)	Renal and nerve function better preserved
Aarhus [18, 19]	Normal albumin excretion and minimal or no retinopathy	24	1 year 5 year	CSII	No difference No statistically significant effect	Reduced GFR GFR had fallen in both
Oslo [20, 21]	Minimal or no retinopathy No proteinuria	45	2 years	MDI or CSII RCT	Early deterioration, mostly regressing by 1 year and no increase in microaneurysm count in intensive groups only	Reduced GFR but no change in albumin excretion
			7 years		Lower HbA_{1c} and fall during treatment reduced risk	
Stockholm [22, 23]	Nonproliferative retinopathy	102		MDI or CSII RCT	Lower prevalence of serious retinopathy	No subnormal GFR in intensive arm and less fall in nerve conduction velocity
		91	10 years		Lower prevalence of serious retinopathy	Lower prevalence of nephropathy and neuropathy
Dallas [24, 25]	Background retinopathy with 3 patients then put on CSII having proliferative	54	31 months	Patient preference	Significantly less progression	
Kroc collaborative [26–28]	Mild to moderate retinopathy 11 proteinuria, 39 normo- and 20 microalbuminuric	70 47	8 months 2 years	CSII RCT	Worsened with CSII Worsened with conventional	Albumin excretion rates fell in microalbuminuric group with CSII

Note. GFR = glomerular filtration rate; DKA = diabetic ketoacidosis; MDI = multiple daily injection therapy; RCT = randomized controlled trial; Rx = therapy.

diabetic ketoacidosis with insulin pump therapy and more severe hypoglycemia in intensified treatment in general [31]. The case for type 1 diabetes however was considered finally proven with the publication of the results of the US National Institutes of Health funded Diabetes Control and Complications Trial (DCCT) [32]. This large multicenter prospective randomized controlled trial of intensified vs. conventional insulin therapy for type 1 patients was based on the Kroc study, which had originally been designed as its feasibility arm. The DCCT did not enrol patients with advanced complications but did recruit two cohorts: one of recent-onset (up to 5 years' duration) type 1 diabetes with no evidence of microvascular complications; the other had diabetes for 5–15 years and had very early retinopathy. Some had microalbuminuria. This enabled the investigators to examine the effect of intensified therapy on both primary prevention and rate of progression of microvascular complications. In both groups the intervention consisted of frequent home blood glucose monitoring, multiple daily insulin injections and a treatment adjusted to achieve home blood glucose monitoring results of 3.9–6.7 mmol/l premeals, less than 10 mmol/l after meals, and, as a late innovation, more than 3.5 mmol/l at 3 a.m. The goal was an HbA_{1c} <6.05%. In the event, the mean HbA_{1c} achieved by intensive therapy over the whole study was about 7%. The equivalent figure in the conventionally treated patients was 8.9%.

The DCCT was powered on the basis of the ability to prevent progression of retinopathy, which was defined as at least a three-step progression of retinal disease assessed by seven-field stereoscopic fundal photography. Risk reduction for primary prevention of new retinopathy in the short-duration patients was 76%, with a risk reduction of 54% for secondary prevention (see Figures 3 and 4). There were similarly significant risk reductions in development and progression of nephropathy, assessed by albumin and protein excretion, and neuropathy. The risk reduction continued as HbA_{1c} fell (Figure 5). There were no deleterious effects on cardiovascular risk factors but no significant effect on macrovascular events, which was thought to be because the patients were all of relatively short duration and the event rate was low. Based on the microvascular data, the study was terminated early, after 9 rather than the planned 10 years [32].

At the close of the DCCT, patients in the conventionally treated group were offered intensified therapy and all were transferred back to their own physicians. Within 4 years,

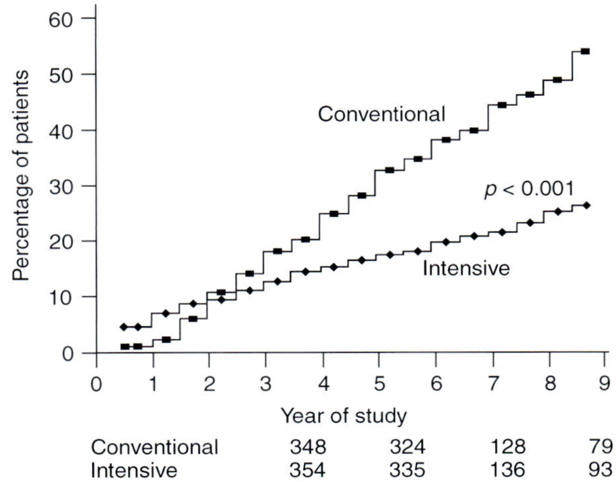

Figure 4 Cumulative incidence of a sustained change in secondary prevention cohort of type 1 diabetic patients in the DCCT. The numbers of patients in each group are shown under the *x* axis. (© 1993 Massachusetts Medical Society)

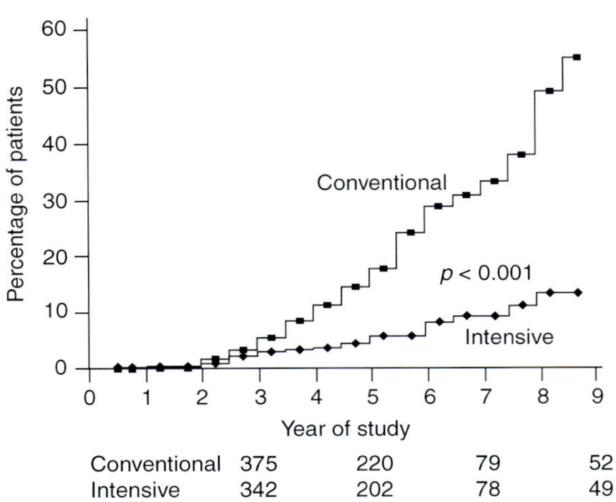

Figure 3 Cumulative incidence of a sustained change in primary prevention cohort of type 1 diabetic patients in the DCCT. The numbers of patients in each group are shown under the *x* axis. (© 1993 Massachusetts Medical Society)

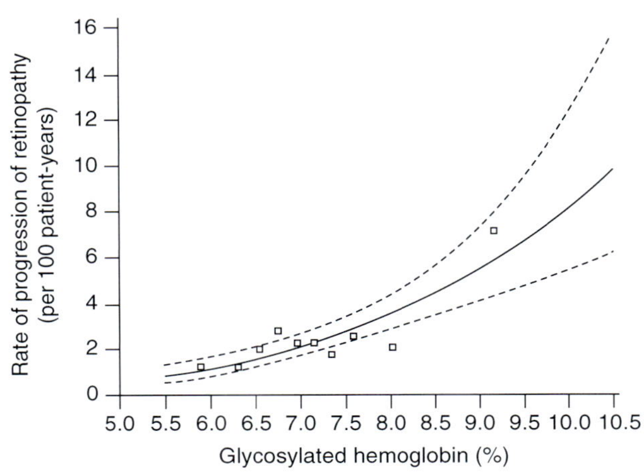

Figure 5 Risk of sustained progression of retinopathy by glycemic control in the DCCT. Squares denote crude rates within deciles of mean HbA_{1c}; the solid line is a regression line estimated as a function of the log of the mean HbA_{1c}, with 95% confidence intervals (dashed lines). (© 1993 Massachusetts Medical Society)

the gap in HbA_{1c} result had closed, with some improvement in the original conventional treatment group and some loss in the former intensively treated group of the tight control they had sustained while involved with the trial and the trialists. The development of clinically significant and sight-threatening retinopathy has remained slower and the proportion of patients with an increase in urinary albumin excretion has remained less in the former intensive treatment group, both at 4 years [33] and at over 6 years [34].

Intensive diabetes therapy is not without cost. In all the studies mentioned above there has been an increase in severe hypoglycemia rates with intensified diabetes therapies and weight gain. In the DCCT, the increase in risk of severe hypoglycemia was threefold, and although the absolute numbers of such hypoglycemic episodes were reduced during the course of the study, the difference between the intensively and conventionally treated patients remained the same [35]. There do not appear to have been any neurological or psychological problems associated with this increased risk although one of three deaths in the DCCT was of someone not enrolled in the trial, who died in a road traffic accident, associated with hypoglycemia in the driver. Most importantly, there have been several more recent reports of techniques of delivering improved glycemic control with intensified insulin therapy without increasing severe hypoglycemia since the DCCT [36–39].

Type 2 Diabetes

The equivalent trial to the DCCT for patients with type 2 diabetes is considered to be the United Kingdom Prospective Diabetes Study (UKPDS) [40]. The design of this trial was more complex, as it also sought to address issues around treatment modality (especially the benefit of insulin vs. oral agents) and also looked at the effects of an intensified therapy program for hypertension.

In contrast to the DCCT, the UKPDS trial ran for longer than originally planned. Nearly 4000 people with newly diagnosed type 2 diabetes from 15 centers in the United Kingdom were randomized to intensive or conventional diabetes therapy, if 3 months' lifestyle therapy failed to restore fasting plasma glucose to less than 6 mmol/l. The therapies used reflect the era in which the trial began. Thus intensified therapy was targeted solely at a fasting blood glucose concentration of less than 6 mmol/l and comprised oral hypoglycemic agents or single injections of intermediate-acting insulin. Although the patients were newly diagnosed, the rate of complications at trial entry (50% if cardiovascular complications are included) suggests a prolonged phase of diabetes prior to diagnosis.

Many important observations were made in the course of this trial, which will be explored in more detail elsewhere in this textbook. Most notable however was the progressive nature of the hyperglycemia of type 2 diabetes, as in all groups, measures of glycemic control deteriorated over time. Associated with this was the observation that polypharmacy was inevitable in the long-term control of both glucose and blood pressure in type 2 patients. Of most relevance to our argument here however were the observations of the effect of intensified glycemic management on the progression of complications. Assessed by HbA_{1c}, the difference in control over the course of the trial between the intensively and conventionally managed groups was not large—7% vs. 7.9%. Nevertheless, there was a significant and important effect of glycemic control, particularly on miscrovascular complications. Risk of microvascular events, defined as retinopathy requiring photocoagulation, vitreous hemorrhage, or fatal or nonfatal renal failure, was 25% less in the intensively treated patients, with a 12% reduction in the occurrence of any diabetes-related endpoint and a 10% reduction in diabetes-related deaths. The major effect was seen in the reduction of need for photocoagulation. The evolution of microalbuminuria was reduced over 9 years in the intensively treated cohort, while beneficial effects on the appearance of abnormalities of vibration perception was seen after 15 years. From the patients' perspective these data have been translated into risk associated with any given improvement in HbA_{1c}. Thus it was calculated that for every 1% increase in HbA_{1c}, the risk of any diabetes-related endpoint is increased by 21%, with a similar increase in risk for a diabetes-related death. For microvascular complications, this increase in risk is 37% [40].

UKPDS produced no convincing evidence for preferring one modality of treatment over another, although there was a trend for chlorpropamide to perform less well than the other sulfonylureas used, and in an obese subgroup, metformin conveyed survival advantage for equivalent levels of glycemic control [41].

Severe hypoglycemia was slightly less of a problem in UKPDS, as would be expected of newly diagnosed type 2 patients with residual insulin secretion, but the same relationship between risk of hypoglycemia and intensified therapy was seen, and hypoglycemia rates were highest with insulin therapy, despite the fact that this was allocated randomly.

The patients of UKPDS were newly diagnosed, and the use of insulin was less intensive than might be considered today. There are other albeit much smaller trials that have sought to examine whether even more intensified regimens in type 2 diabetes might yield additional benefit in type 2 diabetes. The Kumamoto study ramdomised 110 Japanese type 2 diabetic patients with less than 15 years' duration to a multiple daily insulin injection regimen aimed at establishing an HbA_{1c} $<6.5\%$ or to once or twice daily intermediate-acting insulins only. Half the patients had no retinopathy at enrolment, and the other 55 had background retinopathy [42]. At eight years, the multiple daily insulin injection regimen group had less progression of retinopathy and an improvement rather than a deterioration in nerve conduction velocity, compared to the less intensively managed group. The Veteran's Affairs Cooperative Study on Glycemic Control and Complications in type 2 diabetes is looking at a similar group of 153 men with established (<15 years') disease, using a stepped management plan of background insulin; background insulin plus sulfonylurea therapy; twice daily insulin; and more than twice daily insulin [43]. Having proven feasibility, a larger trial is now ongoing to determine efficacy of such strict control [44].

NEUROLOGICAL COMPLICATIONS AND GLYCEMIC CONTROL

Peripheral neuropathy is less well studied as an endpoint in the trials of glycemic control in diabetes—perhaps in part because of the difficulty in assessing it. There is no easy universal measure of peripheral nerve function in diabetes equivalent to the assessment of retinal status or the measurement of albumin excretion, proteinuria, or glomerular filtration rate. There is often a major discrepancy between the symptoms of diabetic neuropathy and the detectable signs, and even specifics such as nerve conduction may not match the clinical picture and may be influenced by ambient glucose at the time of assessment. In general, where neurological factors have been assessed, they have paralleled the findings for retinopathy and nephropathy; in the Oxford [17] and Stockholm [22, 23] studies and in the DCCT [32], for example, intensified therapy was clearly associated with reduced progression of neuropathy.

The existence of a central (brain) neuropathy in diabetes remains controversial. Preliminary studies that attempted to measure cortical function in diabetes were dogged by problems such as failure to account for comorbidities such as depression. There are some studies that find evidence for limited impairment of cortical function in diabetes [45]. Some studies have found an association between some impairment in aspects of cortical function with other diabetic complications, implying a central effect of chronic hyperglycemia [46, 47]. This observation has been supported more recently in a study suggesting that cognitive function may decline over time in type 1 diabetes in association with occurrence of other complications, such as proliferative retinopathy and hypertension [48]. On the other hand, there have been concerns that recurrent hypoglycemia, experienced during pharmacological treatment of diabetes, may cause central neurological impairment. However, in two recent cross-sectional studies, severe hypoglycemia was not found to be associated with either worse performance of cognitive function tests or increased abnormalities on magnetic resonance brain imaging. In contrast, some evidence for impaired function and structural abnormalities was found in patients with retinopathy, where the retinopathy itself was not enough to impair vision [45, 49]. The long-term studies of cognitive function in the trials of intensive insulin therapy have also not found a problem attributable to hypoglycemia. The data show no worsening of cortical function in those who have undergone the intensive treatment arms, despite obviously higher rates of exposure to severe hypoglycemia [23, 50]. However, this may not be the case in children where there is some evidence that recurrent severe hypoglycemia in children may later be associated with poorer performance on cortical function testing [51].

Recent data suggest that some impairment of psychomotor skills in type 2 diabetic patients is also associated with worse glycemic control, as reflected by HbA_{1c} [52]. In type 2 diabetes, new concerns are being raised by epidemiological evidence linking insulin resistance to dementia [53–55]. There are no data to suggest whether this effect is related to the hyperglycemia itself or other aspects of insulin resistance [56].

MACROVASCULAR COMPLICATIONS AND GLYCEMIC CONTROL

Epidemiological Studies

Macrovascular disease is the major cause of premature mortality in diabetes. In the WHO multinational study, cardiovascular disease accounted for 44% deaths in type 1 and 52% in type 2 diabetic populations [57, 58]. Possibly the highest rates are recorded from the United States [59], but rates of 44% are reported from Italy [60] and 35% in Japan [61]. Macrovascular disease is commonly thought to be a particular problem for people with type 2 diabetes; the early studies from Framingham showed that people with type 2 diabetes have a two- to threefold increased incidence of atheromatous disease [62] and data from the United Kingdom suggest that the incidence of macrovascular disease is twice that of microvascular disease in type 2 diabetic patients [63]. However, as suggested by the WHO multinational study, there is also a significantly increased risk of cardiovascular death in type 1 diabetic patients, confirmed in a UK study in which type 1 diabetes was diagnosed on the basis of age <30 at diagnosis and insulin treatment was started early in the course of the disease [64].

The data linking glycemia to macrovascular disease are more complex than those conclusively showing its relationship with microvascular complications. This may be in part because macrovascular disease is not specific to diabetes, although occurring more frequently, more aggressively, and earlier in diabetic than nondiabetic peers [65]. Furthermore, hyperglycemia is only one of several important vascular risk factors that tend to be abnormal especially in insulin resistance syndromes and type 2 diabetes, including obesity, hypertension, and dyslipidemia. In the Whitehall study, a survey of 18 403 male civil servants aged between 40 and 64 years, the 10-year mortality rate from coronary heart disease and stroke was increased in the men with glucose intolerance and diabetes [66], while within the glucose intolerant and diabetic group, the main predictor of cardiovascular death was baseline blood pressure [67].

Recent epidemiological data suggest that if there is a link between glycemia and macrovascular disease it may be occurring at glucose levels lower than those associated with microvascular damage. Thus, the risk for cardiovascular disease is already increased in people with impaired glucose tolerance. This finding is not new. In the Bedford study conducted in the 1970s, cardiovascular mortality was higher in people with impaired glucose tolerance and highest in those with diabetes diagnosed by oral glucose tolerance testing [68]. In three more recent studies that included nondiabetic European men, there was increased risk of cardiovascular death in those at the top end of the range of both fasting and 2-h post-glucose load plasma glucose levels [69]. In the DECODE study, an analysis of data from 17 European studies where large populations had undergone glucose tolerance testing, the risk of cardiovascular disease was primarily predicted by 2-h post-glucose load [70]. Similar data are available from a study of five Finnish cohorts [71] and have also been described in the Japanese and Chinese [72–74].

An association between cardiovascular risk and impaired glucose tolerance does not confirm that it is the minor elevation in blood glucose that is causally responsible as people with impaired glucose tolerance have other features of the metabolic syndrome. Undoubtedly, other risk factors are involved in the proneness of diabetic subjects to macrovascular disease [75] and the risk of cardiovascular disease in impaired glucose tolerance is not due to progression to diabetes [76]. Nevertheless, several studies have shown an independent effect of blood glucose [77–81]. As described above, the current diagnostic criteria for diabetes come primarily from epidemiological studies linking the microvascular complication of retinopathy with indicators of glycemic control; similar data plotted for macrovascular risk are likely to reproduce these curves but shifted markedly to the left. If the cardiovascular disease is causally related to usual glycemic control, then very minor elevations above normal may be responsible. As with microvascular disease, the proof of causality depends on appropriate prospective trials in which the outcomes of differing degrees of glycemic control are compared.

Intervention Trials

Type 1 Diabetes

DCCT: The impressive effect of intensified therapy on microvascular disease in the DCCT was not replicated on macrovascular disease. However, risk factors for cardiovascular disease did improve with intensified therapy and the trial was not powered to look at cardiovascular outcomes [32]. The type 1 patients, all within 15 years' diagnosis at enrolment, had a low rate of cardiovascular events as one might anticipate. A beneficial effect on atheromatous disease has become more apparent in the follow-up studies of the DCCT patients (EDIC). A subgroup of patients underwent serial ultrasonic measurement of intima-medial arterial wall thickness, a measure of atherosclerosis generally accepted as a surrogate marker of macrovascular disease. At the end of the DCCT itself, this measure was not different from controls but 6 years later it had increased in both diabetic cohorts. However, the increase was significantly less in those subjects who had undertaken intensified therapy in the DCCT—good evidence for the role of hyperglycemia *per se* on the evolution of macrovascular disease in type 1 diabetes [82]. A meta-analysis of all appropriate trial data in type 1 confirms the benefits of glycemic control on macrovascular disease [83].

Type 2 Diabetes

The data for type 2 diabetes are less certain. One of the earliest prospective studies of intensified diabetes control, the University Group Diabetes Program or UGDP, was designed to test whether type 2 patients would do better on insulin [84]. In addition to comparing insulin therapy with diet and with oral hypoglycemic agents, UGDP compared two insulin regimens against placebo—in one the insulin dose was fixed according to body weight, and in the other doses were adjusted according to blood glucose readings taken during fasting and 1 h after meals. "Poor control" assessed on the basis of three monthly glucose profiles and an annual oral glucose tolerance test was reported to occur in only 14.6% of the variable insulin regimen group, compared to 33.7% of the standardized insulin group and 44.6% of those not on insulin. However, there was no effect on mortality by insulin regimen; indeed, the only reported difference was between the standard insulin group and the controls in terms of the proportion of people who developed an elevated creatinine. At the same time, there was reported an increase in cardiovascular mortality in a separate group on tolbutamide [85], as well as increased mortality with phenformin [86]. The former has been dismissed as a statistical quirk [87] and doubts about the safety of sulfonylureas were not upheld by the data in UKPDS (see below). In the later Veteran's Affairs Cooperative Study, despite a 2% difference in HbA_{1c} between groups, there was no significant impact on cardiovascular events. This trial was however short (27 months) [88].

In UKPDS, intensive therapy was associated with a reduced myocardial infarction rate but this did not achieve statistical significance [40]. This was disappointing, but also not conclusive, as the p value achieved was 0.056

[40]. The overall event rate was not high. There was no impact of intensive therapy on stroke in this study. Likewise, although cardiovascular event rate was more than 50% lower in the 8-year follow-up of the Kumamoto study, this too did not achieve statistical significance [42].

Further analysis of the UKPDS data has however suggested that hyperglycemia has an independent effect on macrovascular disease. A 14% risk reduction for myocardial infarction was observed for every 1% reduction in HbA_{1c}, which was highly significant [89]. Adler et al. examined risk factors for peripheral vascular disease in the UKPDS cohorts and found a 28% increased risk of peripheral vascular disease for every 1% rise in HbA_{1c} [90]. There was no such association for stroke [91].

There are data to suggest that strict glycemic control *after* a cardiovascular event can reduce mortality. In the DIGAMI study, intensive insulin therapy at the time of the initial event and for at least 3 months thereafter was associated with reduced mortality, although the relative influence of the acute vs. the continued insulin management is still under investigation. The data from DIGAMI cannot separate out the effect of insulin therapy *per se* from that of lower glycemic levels however [92].

The above data have led some to suggest that glycemic control is of less importance in complication prevention in type 2 patients than in type 1, and can be ignored while attention is focused upon blood pressure control. This is clearly not true, if only because of the importance of glycemic control on microvascular complications in both disease groups. However, in terms of macrovascular disease, the importance of glycemic control remains uncertain in the type 2 population, although it is hard to understand why the effect that is proven in type 1 would not operate in type 2. Several arguments have been raised to explain the failure of prospective studies to demonstrate macrovascular effect in type 2 diabetes. One would suggest that other elements of the insulin resistance syndrome may be overriding any effect of glucose control alone. Another is based on the observations of high cardiovascular risk in people with impaired glucose tolerance and would suggest that in studies to date, intensive therapies have not been intensive enough and that to reduce the risk of cardiovascular disease in type 2 diabetes, glucose levels and HbA_{1c} need to be reduced to nondiabetic levels, which has not been achieved. Further randomized controlled trials of intensive control in type 2 diabetes are probably unethical, because of the proven worth of the therapy on microvascular disease but it might be permissible and instructive to examine the effects of treating to normoglycemic targets (assuming these can be achieved) in type 2 patients in whom other risk factors, such as lipids and blood pressure, have been managed optimally and as discussed above, trials are in progress to ascertain the potential of near normalization of glycemic levels to influence macrovascular prognosis [44].

MEAN GLYCEMIA, FASTING, OR POSTPRANDIAL—WHAT MATTERS MOST?

The failure to demonstrate conclusively a direct relationship between glycemic control as judged by fasting blood glucose and HbA_{1c} and risk of macrovascular disease and the convincing demonstrations of the impact of impaired glucose tolerance on macrovascular disease have led to suggestions that nonfasting blood glucose concentrations may be an independent risk factor for large vessel damage. There are undoubtedly good data to link the 2-h post-glucose load blood glucose concentration (i.e. the 2-h value of an oral glucose tolerance test) to cardiovascular risk. The DECODE study calculated hazard ratios for death from myocardial infarction in people with impaired glucose tolerance. The data from this study also suggested that, within diabetes, the highest risk of macrovascualr disease was in those defined on the basis of their 2-h post-glucose load plasma glucose being 11.1 mmol/l or more. The rates were nearly 75% higher in people with diabetic fasting plasma glucose in both men and women but were also increased by two to three times in people with a 2-h post-glucose load value of greater than 11.1 [70]. In the Rancho Bernardo study too, isolated postchallenge hyperglycemia was a major risk factor for cardiovascular disease [93].

More controversial in interpretation are the data relating macrovascular risk to impaired glucose tolerance. Several studies demonstrate increased vascular risk in people with impaired glucose tolerance and are quoted to support the hypothesis that high non-fasting glucose concentrations confer specific risk for macrovascular disease [70, 72–74]. In contrast, a recent paper from the American Third National Health and Nutrition Examination Survey failed to find an association between isolated postchallenge hyperglycemia and cardiovascular risk [94]. While fasting glucose predicts cardiovascular risk only once it is in the diabetic range (>7 mmol/l) [95], several authors suggest that it is the postchallenge glucose load that mostly predicts cardiovascular risk [71]. Nevertheless, once again this does not confirm causality.

The 2-h blood glucose concentration is not the same as the postprandial glucose concentration in daily life. There are some data that have examined the latter. In the German Diabetes Intervention Study, 1-h postbreakfast blood glucose estimation (not fasting glucose) was an independent predictor of all-cause mortality [96], and Bonora quotes similar data from the Verona Diabetes Complications Study [97]. It is possible that type 2 patients for a given HbA_{1c} experience more significant post prandial hyperglycaemic excursions than do type 1 patients with the equivalent HbA_{1c}, and that this may explain their increased risk of cardiovascular disease at given HbA_{1c} concentrations. Nevertheless, HbA_{1c} does correlate well with both values [98]. More important, although there are some epidemiological data to link postmeal blood glucose concentrations with cardiovascular risk, there are no data to suggest that targeting treatment specifically toward controlling postprandial glucose will have any impact. Until we have such data, it is difficult to defend the additional expense and stress of routine post prandial glucose monitoring in patients with type 2 diabetes using oral agents [99].

There are few studies examining the effect of treating impaired glucose tolerance and those that do exist are mainly powered to examine the rate of progression to diabetes [74, 100–102]. There is evidence that this is independent of cardiovascular risk [76]. The only data available are old and negative. For example, hypoglycemic agents and diet advice did not alter mortality in the Whitehall survey [67].

GLYCEMIC CONTROL IN PERSPECTIVE

There is no doubt that factors other than glycemic control influence the development of diabetic complications. Genetic factors play a role; parents of type 1 diabetic patients with microalbuminuria themselves have high prevalence of hypertension [103] and other cardiovascular risk [104]. There is evidence that specific genotypes may influence progression of microvascular complications in some settings; for example, the DD genotype of the ACE (angiotensin-converting enzyme) gene is reported to predispose to faster progression of diabetic nephropathy and may interact with other genes in this regard [105]. Even in these settings however, hyperglycemia has additional and important effect; in one study of nephropathy in diabetic patients with parental hypertension and high sodium/potassium countertransport (another association with high risk of nephropathy), poor glycemic control increased the odds ratio of developing nephropathy in those with parental hypertension from 3.7 to 4.5 and for those with high sodium/potassium countertransport to 7.7 [106], and in another, hypertension had impact on the development of nephropathy only in the setting of hyperglycemia [107].

There is clear evidence that managing nonglycemic risk factors for vascular damage is essential if risk of chronic complications is to be minimized in diabetic populations. The Heart Protection Study showed benefits of cholesterol-lowering agents against cardiovascular disease in type 2 diabetes[108]; the use of ACE inhibitors has been shown to reduce premature mortality [109]. There may still be some questions about the magnitude of the benefit to be obtained from glucose lowering alone on macrovascular disease in patients with type 2 diabetes and it is clear that a multifactorial approach is required. Nevertheless, the data for the importance of glycemic control itself on microvascular complications in both type 1 and type 2 diabetes and for macrovascular disease in type 1 are irrefutable. Glycemic control clearly plays a major, direct role in the pathogenesis of the vascular complications of diabetes, and the evidence for achieving benefit by controlling glycemia is now unequivocal.

REFERENCES

1. Keiding NR, Root HF, Marble A. *JAMA* 1952; 150: 964.
2. Johnsson SL. Retinopathy and nephropathy in diabetes mellitus: comparison of the effect of two forms of treatment. *Diabetes* 1960; 9: 1–8.
3. Englesson G. *Studies in Diabetes Mellitus*. Thesis report, University of Lund, 1954.
4. Sherrill JW. Diabetic retinitis: the relationship between retinal degenerative changes and the degree of diabetic control. *Scripps Metab Clin* 1951; 2: 1.
5. Pirart J. Diabetes mellitus and its degenerative complications. A prospective study of 4400 patients observed between 1947 and 1973. *Diabet Metab* 1977; 3: 97–107.
6. McCance DR, Hanson RL, Charles MA, Jacobssen LTH, Pettitt DJ, Bennett PH, et al. Comparison of tests for glycated haemoglobin and fasting and two hour plasma glucose concentrations as diagnostic methods for diabetes. *BMJ* 1994; 308: 1323–8.
7. Engelgau MM, Thompson TJ, Herman WH, Boyle JP, Aubert RE, Kenny SJ, et al. Comparison of fasting and 2 hour blood glucose and HbA1c levels for diagnosing diabetes: diagnostic criteria and performance revisited. *Diabetes Care* 1997; 20: 785–91.
8. The Expert Committee on the Diagnosis and Classification of Diabetes Mellitus. Report of the Expert Committee on the Diagnosis and Classification of Diabetes Mellitus. *Diabetes Care* 1997; 20: 1183–91058.
9. Keen H, Lee ET, Russell D, Miki E, Bennett PH, Lu M. The appearance of retinopathy and progression to proliferative retinopathy: the WHO Multinational Study of Vascular Disease in Diabetes. *Diabetologia*. September 2001; 44 (suppl 2): S22–30.
10. Bennett PH, Lee ET, Lu M, Keen H, Fuller JH. Increased urinary albumin excretion and its associations in the WHO Multinational Study of Vascular Disease in Diabetes. *Diabetologia*. September 2001; 44 (suppl 2): S37–45.
11. Colhoun HM, Lee ET, Bennett PH, Lu M, Keen H, Wang SL, Stevens LK, Fuller JH. Risk factors for renal failure: the WHO Multinational Study of Vascular Disease in Diabetes. *Diabetologia*. 2001; 44 (suppl 2): S46–53.
12. Pickup JC, Keen H, Parsons JA, Alberti KG. Continuous subcutaneous insulin infusion: an approach to achieving normoglycaemia. *Br Med J* 1978; 1: 204–7.
13. Tamborlane WV, Sherwin RS, Genel M, Felig P. Reduction to normal of plasma glucose in juvenile diabetes by subcutaneous administration of insulin with a portable infusion pump. *N Engl J Med* 1979; 300: 573–8.
14. Lauritzen T, Frost-Larsen K, Larsen HW, Deckert T. Two years experience with continuous subcutaneous insulin infusion in relation to retinopathy and neuropathy. *Diabetes* 1985; 34 (suppl 3): 74–9.
15. Feldt-Rasmussen B, Mathiesen ER, Deckert T. Effect of two years of strict metabolic control on progression of incipient nephropathy in insulin dependent diabetes. *Lancet* 1986; 2: 1300–4.

16. Feldt-Rasmussen B, Mathiesen ER, Jensen T, Lauritzen T, Deckert T. Effect of improved metabolic control on loss of kidney function in type 1 (insulin-dependent) diabetic patients: an update of the Steno studies. *Diabetologia* 1991; 34: 164–70.
17. Holman RR, Dornan TL, Mayon-White V, Howard-Williams J, Orde-Peckar C, Jenkins L, Steemson J, Rolfe R, Smith B, Barbour D, McPherson K, Poon P, Rizza C, Mann JI, Knight AH, Bron AJ, Turner RC. Prevention of deterioration of renal and sensory-nerve function by more intensive management of insulin-dependent diabetic patients. A two-year randomised prospective study. *Lancet* 1983; 1 (8318): 204–8.
18. Beck-Nielsen H, Richelsen B, Morgensen CE, Olsen T, Ehlers N, Nielsen CB, Charles P. Effect of insulin pump treatment for one year on renal function and retinal morphology in patients with IDDM. *Diabetes Care* 1985; 8: 585–9.
19. Beck-Neilsen H, Olesen T, Morgensen CE, Richelsen B, Olsen HW, Ehlers N, Charles P, Sorensen NS. Effect of near normoglycemia for 5 years on progression of early diabetic retinopathy and renal involvement. *Diabetes Res* 1990; 15: 185–90.
20. Dahl-Jorgensen K, Brinchmann-Hansen O, Hanssen KF, Ganes T, Kierulf P, Smeland E, Sandvik L, Aagenaes O. Effect of near normoglycaemia for two years on progression of early diabetic retinopathy, nephropathy, and neuropathy: the Oslo study. *Br Med J (Clin Res Ed)* 1986; 293: 1195–9.
21. Brinchmann-Hansen O, Dahl-Jorgensen K, Sandvik L, Hanssen KF. Blood glucose concentrations and progression of diabetic retinopathy: the seven year results of the Oslo study. *BMJ* 1992; 304: 19–22.
22. Reichard P, Nilsson BY, Rosenqvist U. The effect of long term intensified treatment on the development of microvascular complications of diabetes mellitus. *N Engl J Med* 1993; 329: 304–9.
23. Reichard P, Pihl M, Rosneqvist U, Sule J. Complications in IDDM are caused by elevated blood glucose level: the Stockholm Diabetes Intervention Study at 10 year follow up. *Diabetologia* 1996; 39: 1438–88.
24. Rosenstock J, Friberg T, Raskin P. Effect of glycemic control on microvascular complications in patients with type I diabetes mellitus. *Am J Med* 1986; 81: 1012–8.
25. Friberg TR, Rosenstock J, Sanborn G, Vaghefi A, Raskin P. The effect of long-term near normal glycemic control on mild diabetic retinopathy. *Ophthalmology* 1985; 92: 1051–8.
26. Kroc Collaborative Study Group. Blood glucose control and the evolution of diabetic retinopathy and albuminuria. A preliminary multicenter trial. *N Engl J Med* 1984; 311: 365–72.
27. Kroc Collaborative Study Group. Diabetic retinopathy after two years of intensified insulin treatment. Follow up of the Kroc Collaborative Study. *JAMA* 1988; 260: 37–41.
28. Bending JJ, Viberti GC, Bilous RW, Keen H. Eight month correction of hyperglycaemia in insulin dependent diabetes mellitus is associated with a significant and sustained reduction of urinary albumin excretion rates in patients with microalbuminuria. *Diabetes* 1985; 34 (suppl 3): 69–73.
29. Hendricsson M, Janzon L, Groop L. Progression of retinopathy after change in treatment from oral antihyperglycemic agents to insulin in patients with NIDDM. *Diabetes Care* 1995; 18: 1571–6.
30. Dahl-Jorgensen K, Brinchmann-Hansen O, Hanssen KF, Sandvik L, Aagenaes O Rapid tightening of blood glucose control leads to transient deterioration of retinopathy in insulin dependent diabetes mellitus: the Oslo study. *Br Med J (Clin Res Ed)* March 1985; 16; 290: 811–5.
31. Wang PH, Lau J, Chalmers TC, Meta-analysis of effects of intensive blood glucose control on late complications of type 1 diabetes. *Lancet* 1993; 341: 1306–9.
32. Diabetes Control and Complications Research Group. The effect of intensive treatment of diabetes on the development and progression of long-term complications in insulin dependent diabetes mellitus. *N Engl J Med* 1993; 329: 977–86.
33. Diabetes Control and Complications Trial/Epidemiology of Diabetes Interventions and Complications Research Group. Retinopathy and nephropathy in patients with type 1 diabetes four years after a trial of intensive therapy. *N Engl J Med* 2000; 342: 381–92.
34. Writing Team for the Diabetes Control and Complications Trial/Epidemiology of Diabetes Interventions and Complications Research Group. Effect of intensive therapy on microvascular complications of type 1 diabetes mellitus. *JAMA* 2002; 287: 2563–9.
35. Diabetes Research and Complications Trial Research Group. Hypoglycemia in the Diabetes Control and Complications Trial. *Diabetes* 1997; 46: 271–86.
36. Muhlhauser J, Jorgens V, Berger M, Graninger W, Gurtler W, Hornke L, Kunz A, Schernthaner G, Scholz V, Voss HE. Bicentric evaluation of a teaching and training programme for Type 1 (insulin dependent) diabetic patients. Improvement of metabolic control and other measures of diabetes care for up to 22 months. *Diabetologia* 1983; 25: 470–6.
37. Muhlhauser I, Bruckner I, Berger M, Cheta D, Jorgens V, Ionescu-Tirgoviste C, Scholtz V, Mincu I. Evaluation of an intensified insulin treatment and teaching programme as routine management of type 1 (insulin dependent) diabetes: the Bucharest-Dusseldorf Study. *Diabetologia* 1997; 40: 926–32.
38. Pieber TR, Brunner GA, Schnedl WJ, Schattenberg S, Kaufamn P, Krehs GI. Evaluation of a structured outpatient group education program for intensive insulin therapy. *Diabetes Care* 1995; 18: 625–30.
39. DAFNE Study Group. Training in flexible, intensive insulin management to enable dietary freedom in people with Type 1 diabetes: dose adjustment for normal eating (DAFNE) randomised controlled trial. *Br Med J* 2002; 325: 746.
40. UK Prospective Diabetes Study (URPDS) Group. Intensive blood glucose control with sulphonylureas or insulin compared with conventional therapy and risk of complications in patients with Type 2 diabetes mellitus (UKPDS 33). *Lancet* 1998; 352: 837–53.
41. UKPDS Group. Effect of intensive blood glucose control with metformin on complications in overweight patients with type 2 diabetes (UKPDS 34). *Lancet* 1998; 352: 854–65.
42. Shichiri M, Kishikawa H, Ohkubo Y, Wake N. Long term results of the Kumamoto study on optimal diabetes control in Type 2 patients. *Diabetes Care* 200; 23 (suppl 2): B21–9.
43. Emanuele N, Klein R, Abrairta C, Colwell J, Comstock J, Henderson WG, Levin S, Nuttall F, Sawin C, Silbert C,

Less HS, Johnson-Nagel N. Evaluations of retinopathy in the VA Cooperative Study on Glycemic control and Complications in Type II Diabetes (VA CSDM): a feasibility study. *Diabetes Care* 1996; 19: 1375–81.
44. Abraira C, Duckworth W, McCarren M, Emanuele N, Arca D, Reda D, Henderson W. Design of the cooperative study on glycemic control and complications in diabetes mellitus Type 2: Veterans Affairs Diabetes Trial. *J Diabet Complications* 2003; 17: 314–22.
45. Kramer L, Fasching P, Madl C, Schneider B, Damjancic P, Waldhausl W, Irsigler K, Grimm G. Previous episodes of hypoglycaemic coma are not associated with permanent cognitive brain dysfunction in IDDM patients on intensive insulin treatment. *Diabetes* 1998; 47: 1909–114.
46. Ryan CM, Williams TM, Finegold DN, Orchard TJ. Cognitive dysfunction in adults with type 1 (insulin dependent) diabetes mellitus of long duration: effects of recurrent hypoglycaemia and other chronic complications. *Diabetologia* 1993; 36: 329–34.
47. Ryan CM, Williams TM, Orchard TJ, Finegold DN. Psychomotor slowing is associated with distal symmetrical polyneuropathy in adults with diabetes mellitus. *Diabetes* 1992; 41: 107–13.
48. Ryan CM, Geckle MO, Orchard TJ. Cognitive efficiency declines over time in adults with Type 1 diabetes: effects of micro- and macro-vascular complications. *Diabetologia* 2003; 46: 940–8.
49. Ferguson SC, Blane A, Perros P, McCrimmon RJ, Best JJ, Wardlaw J, Deary IK, Frier BM. Cognitive ability and brain structure in Type 1 diabetes: relation to microangiopathy and preceding severe hypoglycaemia. *Diabetes* 2003; 52: 149–56.
50. Austin EJ, Deary IJ. Effects of repeated hypoglycaemia on cognitive function: a psychometrically validated reanalysis of the Diabetes Control and Complications Trial data. *Diabetes Care* 1999; 22: 1273–77.
51. Hershey T, Bhagava N, Sadler M, White NH, Craft S. Conventional vs intensive therapy in children with Type 1 diabetes: effects on memory and motor speed. *Diabetes Care* 1999; 22: 1318–24.
52. Ryan CM, Geckle MO. Circumscribed cognitive dysfunction in middle aged adults with type 2 diabetes, *Diabetes Care* 2000; 23: 1486–93.
53. Ott A, et al. Diabetes mellitus and the risk of dementia: the Rotterdam Study. *Neurology* 1999; 53: 1937–42.
54. Stolk RP, et al. Insulin and cognitive function in an elderly population: the Rotterdam Study. *Diabetes Care* 1997; 20: 792–5.
55. Kuusisto J, et al. Association between features of the insulin resistance syndrome and Alzheimer's disease independently of apolipoprotein E4 phenotype: cross-sectional population based study. *BMJ* 1997; 315: 1045–9.
56. Razay J, Wilcock GK. Hyperinsulinaemia and Alzheimer's disease. *Age Aging* 1994; 23: 396–9.
57. Morrish NJ, Wang SL, Stevens LK, Fuller JH, Keen H. Mortality and causes of death in the WHO Multinational Study of Vascular Disease in Diabetes. *Diabetologia* 2001; 44 (suppl 2): S14–21.
58. Lee ET, Keen H, Bennett PH, Fuller JH, Lu M. Follow-up of the WHO Multinational Study of Vascular Disease in Diabetes: general description and morbidity. *Diabetologia* 2001; 44 (suppl 2): S3–13.
59. Gu K, Cowie CC, Harris MI. Mortality in adults with and without diabetes in a national cohort of the US population. *Diabetes Care* 1998; 21: 1138–45.
60. Brun E, Nelson RG, Bennett PH, Imperatore G, Zoppini G, Verlato G, Muggeo M. Diabetes duration and cause specific mortality in the Verona Diabetes Study. *Diabetes Care* 2000; 23: 1119–23.
61. Sasaki A, Uehara M, Horiuchi N, Hasegawa K, Shimizu T. A 15 year follow up study of patients with non-insulin dependent diabetes mellitus (NISSM) in Osaka, Japan. Long term prognosis and cause of death. *Diabetes Res Clin Pract* 1996; 34: 47–55.
62. Garcia MJ, McNamara PM, Gordon T, Kannell WB. Morbidity and mortality in diabetics in the Framingham population: sixteen year follow up. *Diabetes* 1974; 23: 105–11.
63. Panzram G. Mortality and survival in type 2 (non-insulin dependent) diabetes mellitus. *Diabetologia* 1987; 30: 123–31.
64. Laing SO, Swerdlow AJ, Slater SD, Botha JL, Burden ACM, Waught NR, Smith AW, Hill RD, Bingley PJ, Patterson CC, Qiao Z, Keen H. The British Diabetic Association Cohort Study II: cause specific mortality in patients with insulin treated diabetes mellitus. *Diabet Med* 1999; 16: 446–7.
65. De Marco R, Locatelli F, Zoppini G, Verlato G, Bonora E, Muggeo M. Cause-specific mortality in Type 2 diabetes. *Diabetes Care* 1999; 22: 756–61.
66. Fuller JH, Shipley MJ, Rose G, Jarrett RJ, Keen H. Mortality from coronary heart disease and stroke in relation to degree of glycaemia: the Whitehall study. *Br Med J (Clin Res Ed)* 1983; 287: 867–70.
67. Jarrett RJ, Keen H, McCartney P. The Whitehall Study: ten year follow-up report on men with impaired glucose tolerance with reference to worsening to diabetes and predictors of death. *Diabet Med* 1984; 1: 279–83.
68. Jarrett RJ, McCartney P, Keen H. The Bedford survey: ten year mortality rates in newly diagnosed diabetics and normoglycaemic controls and risk factors for coronary heart disease in borderline diabetics. *Diabetologia* 1982; 22: 79–84.
69. Balkau B, Shipley M, Jarrett RJ, Pyorala K, Pyorala M, Forhan A, Eschwege E. High blood glucose concentration is a risk factor for mortality in middle-aged nondiabetic men. 20-year follow-up in the Whitehall Study, the Paris Prospective Study, and the Helsinki Policemen Study. *Diabetes Care* 1998; 21: 360–7.
70. DECODE Study Group. Glucose tolerance and mortality: comparison of WHO and American Diabetes Diagnostic Criteria. *Lancet* 1999; 617–21.
71. Qiao Q, Pyorala K, Pyorala M, Nissinen A, Lindstrom J, Tilvis R, Tuomilehto J. Two hour glucose is a better risk predictor for incident coronary heart disease and cardiovascular mortality than fasting glucose. *Eur Heart J* 2002; 23: 1267–75.
72. Tominaga M, Eguchi H, Manaka H, Igarashi K, Kato T, Sekikawa A. Impaired glucose tolerance in a risk factor for cardiovascular disease but not impaired fasting glucose: the Funagata Study. *Diabetes Care* 1999; 22: 920–4.
73. Fujishma M, Kiohara Y, Kato I, Ohmura T, Iwatmoto H, Nakayama K, Ohmori S, Yoshitake T. Diabetes and cardiovascular disease in a prospective in population survey in Japan: the Hisayama Study. *Diabetes* 1996; 45 (suppl): S14–6.
74. Pan XR, Hu YH, Li GW, Liu PA, Bennett PH, Howard BV. Impaired glucose tolerance and its relationship to

ECG indicated coronary heart disease and risk factors among Chinese: Da Qing IGT and Diabetes Study. *Diabetes Care* 1993; 16: 150–6.
75. Turner RC, Mills H, Neil HAW, Stratton IM, Manely SA, Matthews DR, Holman RR, for the United Kingdom Prospective Diabetes Study Group. Risk factors for coronary artery disease in non-insulin dependent diabetes mellitus: United Kingdom Prospective Diabetes Study (UKPDS 23). *Br Med J* 1998; 316: 823–8.
76. Qiao Q, Jousiahti P, Eriksson J, Tuomilehto J. Predictive properties of impaired glucose tolerance for cardiovascular disease are not explained by the development of overt diabetes during follow up. *Diabetes Care* 2003; 26: 2910–4.
77. Butler WJ, Ostrander LD, Carman WJ, Lamphiear DE. Mortality form coronary heart disease in the Tecumseh study. Long term effect of diabetes mellitus, glucose tolerance and other risk factors. *Am J Epidemiol* 1985; 121: 541–7.
78. Gall MA, Borch-Johnsen K, Hougaard P, Nielsen FS, Parving HH. Albuminuria and poor glycaemic control predict mortality in NIDDM. *Diabetes* 1985; 44: 1303–9.
79. Kuusisto J, Mykkanen L, Pyorala K, Laakso M. NIDDM and its metabolic control predict coronary heart disease in elderly subjects. *Diabetes* 1994; 43: 960–7.
80. Lehto S, Ronnemaa T, Haffner SM, Pyorala K, Kallio V, Laakso M. Dyslipidemia and hyperglycemia predict coronary heart disease in middle aged patients with NIDDM. *Diabetes* 1997; 48: 1354–9.
81. Walters DP, Gatling W, Houston AC, Mullee AA, Julious SA, Hill RD. Mortality in diabetic subjects: an eleven year follow up of a community based population. *Diabet Med* 1994; 11: 968–73.
82. Nathan DM, Lachin J, Cleary P, Orchard T, Brillon DJ, Backlund JY, O'Leary DH, Genuth S. The Diabetes Control and Complications Trial/Epidemiology of Diabetes Interventions and Complications Research Group Intensive diabetes therapy and carotid intima-media thickness in type 1 diabetes mellitus. *N Engl J Med* June 5, 2003; 348: 2294–303.
83. Diem P, Steffes MW, Egger M, and the Cochrane Collaborative Review Group. Macrovascular disease in Type 1 diabetes mellitus: effects of intensified insulin treatment. *Diabetes* 2001; 50 (suppl 2): A151.
84. University Group Diabetes Program. Effects of hypoglycaemic agents on vascular complications in patients with adult-onset diabetes. Evaluation of Insulin therapy, final report. *Diabetes* 1982; 31 (suppl 5): 1–26.
85. University Group Diabetes Program. A study of the effects of hypoglycaemic agents on vascular complications in patients with adult onset diabetes, 2: Mortality results. *Diabetes* 1970; 19 (suppl 2): 785–830.
86. University Group Diabetes Program. Effect of hypoglycaemic agents on vascular complications in patients with adult onset diabetes, 4: a preliminary report on phenformin results. *JAMA* 1971; 217: 777–84.
87. Blume JD. Likelihood methods for measuring evidence. *Stat Med* 2002; 21: 2563–99.
88. Abraira C, Colwell JA, Nuttall FQ, et al. Cardiovascular Events and correlates in the Veterans Affairs Diabetes Feasibility Trial. Veterans Affairs Cooperative Study on glycemic control and complications in type 2 diabetes (VA CSDM). *Arch Intern Med* 1997; 157: 181–8.
89. Stratton IM, Adler AI, Neil HA, Atthews DR, Manely SE, Cull CA, Hadden D, Turner RC, Holman RR. Association of glycaemia with macrovascular and microvascular complications of type 2 diabetes (UKPDS 35): prospective observational study. *Br Med J* 2000; 321: 405–12.
90. Adler AI, Stevens RJ, Neil A, Stratton IM, Boulton AJ, Holman RR. UKPDS 59 hypoergycaemia and other potentially modifiable risk factors for peripheral vascular disease in type 2 diabetes. *Diabetes care* 2002; 25: 894–9.
91. Kothari V, Stevens RJ, Adler AI, Stratton IM, Manley SE, Neil HA, Holman RR. UKPDS 60: risk of stroke in type 2 diabetes estimated by the UK Prospective Diabetes Study risk engine. *Stroke* 2002; 33: 1776–81.
92. Malmerberg K. Prospective randomised study of intensive insulin treatment on long term survival after acute myocardial infarction in patients with diabetes mellitus. DIAGAM (Diabetes Mellitus, Insulin Glucose Infusion in Acute Myocardial Infarction Study Group). *Br Med J* 1997; 314: 1512–5.
93. Bennett Connor E, Ferrara A. Isolated post challenge hyperglycemia and the risk of fatal cardiovascular disease in older women and men. *Diabetes Care* 1998; 21: 1236–9.
94. Resnick HE, Harris MI, Brock DB, Harris TB. American Diabetes Association diabetes diagnostic criteria, advancing age and cardiovascular disease risk profiles: results from the Third National Health and Nutrition Examination Survey. *Diabetes Care* 2000; 23: 176–80.
95. Unwin N, Shaw J, Zimmet P, Alberti KG. Impaired glucose tolerance and impaired fasting glycemia: the current status on definition and intervention. *Diabet Med* 2002; 19: 708–23.
96. Hanefeld M, Fischer S, Julius U, et al. Risk factors for myocardial infarction and death in newly detected NIDDM: the Diabetes Intervention Study. 11 year follow up. *Diabetologia* 1996; 39: 1577–83.
97. Bonora E. Post prandial peaks as a risk factor for cardiovascular disease: epidemiological perspectives. *Int J Clin Pract* 2002; (suppl 129): 5–11.
98. Bonora E, Calcaterra F, Lombardi S, et al. Plasma glucose levels throughout the day and HbA1c interrelationships in type 2 diabetes. Implication for treatment and monitoring of metabolic control. *Diabetes Care* 2001; 24: 2023–9.
99. Franciosi M, Pellegrini F, De Berardis G, Belfiglio M, Cavaloere D, Di Nardo B, Greenfield S, Kaplan SH, Sacco M, Tognoni G, Valentini M, Nicolucci A, QuED Study Group. The impact of self monitoring on metabolic control and quality of life in type 2 diabetic patients. An urgent need for better educational strategies. *Diabetes Care* 2001; 24: 1870–7.
100. Chiasson JL, Josse RG, Gomis R, et al., for the STOP-NIDDM Trial Research Group. Acarbose for prevention of type 2 diabetes mellitus: the STOP-NIDDM trial. *Lancet* 2002; 359: 2072–7.
101. Tuomilehto J, Lindstrom J, Eriksson JG, Valle TT, Hamalainen H, Ilanne-Parikka P, Keinanen-Kiukaanniemi S, Laakso M, Louheranta A, Rastas M, Saliminen V, Uusitupa M, for the Finnish Diabetes Prevention Study Group. *N Engl J Med* 2001; 344: 1343–50.
102. Hernan WH, Brandle M, Zhang P, Williamson DF, Matulik MJ, Ratner RE, Lachin JM, Engelgau MM, for the Diabetes Prevention Program Research Group. Costs associated with the primary prevention of type 2 diabetes mellitus in the diabetes prevention program. *Diabetes Care* 2003; 26: 36–47.

103. Viberti GC, Keen H, Wiseman MJ. Raised arterial pressure in proteinuric insulin dependent diabetics. *Br Med J* 1987; 295: 515–7.

104. De Cosmo S, Bacci S, Piras GP, Cignarelli M, Placentino G, Margaglione M, Colaizzo D, DiMinno G, Giogino R, Liuzzi A, Viberti GC. High prevalence of risk factors for cardiovascular disease in parents of IDDM patients with albuminuria. *Diabetologia* 1997; 40: 1191–6.

105. De Cosmo S, Miscio G, Zucaro L, Maraglione AM, Argiolas A, Thomas S, Piras G, Trevisan R, Perin PC, Bacci S, Frittitta L, Pizzuti A, Tassi V, Di Monno G, Viberti G, Trischitta V. The role of PC-1 and ACE genes in diabetic nephropathy in Type 1 diabetic patients. Evidence for polygenic control of kidney disease progression. *Nephrol Dial Transplant* 2002; 17: 1402–7.

106. Krowleski AS, Canessa M, Warram JH, Laffel LMB. Christlieb AR, Knowler WC, Rand LI. Predisposition to hypertension and susceptibility to renal disease in insulin dependent diabetes mellitus. *N Engl J Med* 1988; 318: 140–5.

107. Derby L, Warram JH, Laffel MB, Krowleski AS. Elevated blood pressure predicts the development of persistent proteinuria in the presence of poor glycaemic control in patients with Type 1 diabetes. *Diabete Metab* 1989; 15: 320–6.

108. Heart Protection Study Collaborative Group. The MRC/BHF Heart Protection Study of cholesterol lowering with simvastatin in 20,536 high risk individuals: a randomised controlled trial. *Lancet* 2002; 360: 7–22.

109. Heart Outcomes Prevention Evaluation Study Investigators. Effects of ramipril on cardiovascular and microvascular outcomes in people with diabetes mellitus: results of the HOPE study and MICRO-HOPE substudy. *Lancet* 2000; 355: 253–9.

64

The Microcirculation in Diabetes Mellitus

John E. Tooke

Peninsula Medical School, Plymouth, UK

INTRODUCTION

Structural change to the microcirculation is widespread in diabetes mellitus irrespective of the organ studied, and it is generally accepted that the so-called late-specific complications of diabetes have their basis in failure of microvascular function. For the most part, clinical manifestations of microvascular failure in diabetes represent the end stage of a protracted process that begins, at least it is currently believed in insulin-dependent disease, with the development of raised glucose levels. Former theories based on basement membrane changes suggesting prediabetic changes have been discounted, although endothelial dysfunction may antedate the appearance of non-insulin-dependent diabetes. The picture the clinician sees of such late microvascular failure is colored by secondary phenomena such as bleeding from neovascularization in the retina or thrombosis of a damaged vessel supplying a nerve, dramatic events that draw attention away from the clinically silent impairment of microvascular function that accrues with increasing disease duration. Even the appearance of the first retinal microaneurysm, dismissively termed *background retinopathy*, is in pathophysiological terms a late stage of microvascular damage.

Our limited understanding of the preclinical phase of microangiopathy owes much to the relative paucity of techniques for studying human microvascular function; study of the human condition is important, for no animal model precisely mirrors human diabetic complications. Lack of technology has arguably contributed to the wealth of studies purporting to reveal a pathogenetic role for myriad biochemical and cellular abnormalities that accompany the diabetic state, regardless of whether the abnormalities are specific for diabetes or conform to criteria that fit the clinical and epidemiological characteristics of a prime-moving mechanism [1] (Table 1).

Similar confusion has surrounded the interpretation of microvascular structural change in diabetes [2]. Capillary basement membrane thickening is observed in many vascular beds including the retina, kidney, skin, and muscle. Nevertheless, changes in a particular bed (e.g. muscle) do not correlate well with the presence or absence of clinical microangiopathy in another tissue (e.g. the retina) [3]. Furthermore, at first sight it is difficult to associate thickening of the capillary wall with an increase in microvascular permeability, another general characteristic of the diabetic microcirculation, although a more thorough analysis (see below) suggests such a combination of features is explicable.

A far more profitable line of enquiry has been the unraveling of the biochemical sequelae that stem from hyperglycemia that could have an impact on microvascular function, including the genesis of products of advanced glycation, activation of the Diacyl glycerol–PKC pathway, and increased flux through the sorbitol pathway, which are dealt with in detail in other parts of this book. Further insight has been gained from study of endothelial function in diabetes, and this cell type is arguably the best placed to account for the ubiquity of the angiopathic process in diabetes. Nonetheless, all relevant biochemical and endothelial mechanisms must manifest themselves as disturbances of microvascular function, and the capacity to measure the key determinants of microvascular function in normal humans has made it possible to test unifying functional hypotheses as well as enlighten the pursuit of candidate cellular and molecular mechanisms [4]. Accordingly this chapter is concerned with microvascular function and its breakdown, predominantly in human diabetes. Although patients with both insulin-dependent type 1 diabetes mellitus (T1DM) and non-insulin-dependent type 2 diabetes mellitus (T2DM) develop microangiopathy, differences are evident in the epidemiology of the various

International Textbook of Diabetes Mellitus, Third Edition. Edited by R. A. DeFronzo, E. Ferrannini, H. Keen, and P. Zimmet.
 ISBN: 0-471-48655-8.

Table 1 Characteristics of a prime-moving mechanism involved in the pathogenesis of microangiopathy in patients with insulin-dependent diabetes

- Operative from day one of diabetes
- Linked in some way to blood glucose levels
- Responsive to improvements in blood glucose levels
- Aggravated or accelerated with passage through puberty
- More marked in patients at high risk of microangiopathy
- Less marked in patients with a long disease duration, who avoid complications
- Aggravated by hypertension

complications between these two major types of the disease and recent work points to modified pathophysiological mechanisms in T2DM [5]. For this reason the abnormalities of microvascular function are considered separately in the two main forms of the disease, as well as in the rarer monogenic causes of the condition.

ABNORMALITIES OF MICROVASCULAR FUNCTION IN T1DM

Normal Function

The microcirculation involves the arterioles and those vessels distal to them yet before the veins. An often forgotten yet important component is the peripheral lymphatic system including the prenodal collector, precollector, and terminal lymphatics, about which virtually nothing is known in diabetes. The principal functions of the microcirculation concern the transport and distribution of nutrients, water, and waste products between blood and tissue fluid, thereby subserving tissue metabolism, growth, defense, and repair, yet at the same time maintaining tissue fluid economy. Local and extrinsic mechanisms combine to regulate peripheral vascular resistance in response to the potentially conflicting demands of maintaining total peripheral resistance, and therefore central arterial blood pressure, yet meeting local tissue flow requirements. Different microvascular beds possess varying capacities to override central extrinsic mechanisms and maintain flow in the face of falling perfusion pressure, a phenomenon known as *autoregulation*.

Thus, it can be seen that any analysis of microvascular function in diabetes must consider microvascular flow and pressure, and their regulation including autoregulatory capacity, as well as vessel wall permeability.

Microvascular Blood Flow

Although the diabetic state is normally associated with ischemic events, measures of blood flow in relevant organs under resting conditions early in the disease process paradoxically suggest an increase in microvascular perfusion [6]. In support of this broad contention are observations suggesting that under these circumstances cardiac output is slightly increased [7].

Renal plasma flow appears to be elevated in a manner dependent on metabolic control in early T1DM [8], and estimates of retinal microvascular flow from fluoroscein transit time [9] and laser Doppler velocimetry [10] suggest an increase before the emergence of clinically obvious structural damage. The situation in the limbs is complicated by the dual nature of skin blood flow, the majority of acral blood flow under normal thermal conditions occurring through arteriovenous shunts rather than through the nutritive capillary bed. Total blood flow to the extremities is increased, particularly during poor diabetic control [11], although the distribution of blood flow under these circumstances favors the arteriovenous shunts [12]. As passage through puberty results in an accelerated rate of development of microangiopathy, it is interesting to note that postpubertal diabetic children exhibit increased peripheral capillary flow compared to prepubertal children [13]. Furthermore, whereas healthy children acquire an increased capacity to vasoconstrict the skin microcirculation under certain physiological circumstances with passage through puberty, acquisition of such responses is impaired in T1DM [14]. Although there is little doubt that the increase in microvascular blood flow in early T1DM is related to glycemic control, short-term intra-arterial infusion of glucose in the upper limb in healthy subjects (a technique that arguably avoids the activation of systemic mechanisms) fails to result in an increase in either muscle or skin blood flow in the infused arm [15]. This may, however, imply that relevant local mechanisms take several hours to be induced, rather than a lack of mechanisms that depend upon local glucose toxicity.

It should be emphasized that the early microvascular hyperemia alluded to above is under resting conditions. When the microcirculation is challenged by, for example, a period of arterial occlusion, local heat, or tissue injury, a limited hyperemic response is typically seen in diabetes [16]. It is much easier to demonstrate such phenomena in skin than in muscle. Measurements of superficial skin microvascular blood flow using laser Doppler fluximetry show a reduction in maximum hyperemia irrespective of site or stimulus, which is more marked in patients with a long duration of disease or evidence of microangiopathy [17]. Furthermore, patients with microalbuminuria who are at high risk of microangiopathic complications possess reduced microvascular hyperemic capacity compared to patients with similar disease duration and levels of glycemic control who have avoided this problem [18]. Specific techniques for visualizing nutritive capillary flow confirm that skin capillary hyperemia is reduced in terms of both the peak value obtained and the time taken to reach peak flow [19]. Although both these measures appear to be related to blood glucose control early in the disease process, normalization of glucose tolerance by pancreas transplantation fails to correct deficient microvascular hyperemia fully in patients with complications and a long disease duration [20], soon after transplantation, although longer term studies suggest at least partial restitution [21]. Retinal blood flow begins to fall as a prelude (and probable stimulus) to proliferative change [22], and a decline in renal blood flow signals deteriorating renal function in patients with nephropathy [23]. It is likely that this represents a reduction in the total number of perfused capillaries, rather than a reduction in average flow velocity throughout an entire microvascular bed; indeed, it has been suggested that flow through remaining individual vessels may well be increased [24].

At first sight the reduction in microvascular hyperemic responses appears to contradict the observed increase in resting flow. Such observations are compatible, however, if it is appreciated that it is the physiological circumstance that dictates the level of flow required. Under resting conditions organ flow should be the minimum required to sustain tissue health; in contrast, following injury for example, it is physiologically appropriate for skin blood flow to increase perhaps 30-fold. The limitation of maximum hyperemia observed in the skin has been correlated with the degree of basement membrane thickness [25].

Impaired autoregulatory function in insulin-dependent diabetes has been demonstrated in the retina, kidney, and skin [6]. In the retina, autoregulatory capacity is more impaired during poor glycemic control [26]. The impairment of autoregulation of skin blood flow is related to the degree of arteriolar hyalinosis that may be seen on tissue biopsy [27].

Microvascular Pressure

Although it is often assumed that increased organ blood flow implies increased microvascular pressure, such is not inevitably the case: a reduction in both pre- and post-capillary resistance may increase flow yet mean capillary pressure remains constant. Nevertheless, studies of animal models of diabetes suggest glomerular capillary pressure is increased [28], and indirect assessment of filtration pressure in young patients with T1DM suggests a similar abnormality [29]. Direct measurement of human capillary pressure is possible in the nailfold, and increased values have been demonstrated in insulin-dependent patients compared to age- and sex-matched control subjects [30]. Pressure is higher in those subjects with poor glycemic control and is responsive to improvement in control at least in subjects with minimal complications and short to moderate disease duration. Pressure is high within the first year of T1DM and, in keeping with the criteria for a prime-moving mechanism, is particularly high in those subjects at high risk of microangiopathy, yet indistinguishable from normal in patients who have survived a long duration of T1DM without significant complications [31]. Although there are as yet no systematic studies of capillary pressure in hypertensive insulin-dependent diabetic patients, it is known that capillary pressure is elevated in nondiabetic patients with essential hypertension [32], and can be lowered by hypotensive therapy. Allied to an inability to autoregulate capillary pressure in the face of an increase in arterial perfusion pressure (personal observations), it is likely that capillary pressure values in normotensive subjects at rest underestimate the disturbance occurring in hypertensive subjects during normal physiological activity. Given that both pregnancy and exposure to the combined oral contraceptive pill may accelerate microangiopathy, it is interesting to note that both circumstances are associated with increased capillary pressure [33, 34].

Microvascular Permeability

Although it is generally believed that microvascular permeability is increased in T1DM, an increased flux of solute or solvent across the capillary wall can be a function of many factors other than the leakiness of this barrier. These include intra- and extravascular hydrostatic and colloid osmotic pressures, microvascular blood flow, and the surface area available for exchange. Accurate assessment of capillary wall permeability in human diabetes is difficult, as many of these other key variables can only be assumed.

In early T1DM there is an increase in the capillary filtration coefficient (CFC), and the transcapillary escape rate (TER) of albumin [35], which is related to blood glucose control. Both abnormalities could simply reflect the observed increase in capillary hydrostatic pressure [30]. Recently however, more sophisticated plethysmographic techniques have been applied to the estimation of CFC, which minimize any impact of differences in hydrostatic pressure in diabetic and control groups, and an increased flux of water is still observed [36].

The passage of most small solutes is largely diffusive and in the case of very freely diffusible molecules flow-limited. Tracer clearance studies suggest that capillary diffusion capacity is increased in long duration T1DM (despite a tendency for maximum blood flow to be reduced) [37], whereas no early increase that can be related to blood glucose control is observed [35].

Access to capillary filtrate (urine) has facilitated further investigation of the nature of the increased permeability observed in T1DM, at least as far as the glomerulus is concerned [38]. Increased albumin flux appears to be a function both of increased pressure and reduced charge barrier; with advancing disease both molecular size and charge selectivity are lost.

The Hemodynamic Hypothesis

The array of functional microvascular abnormalities alluded to above has been marshaled to devise a

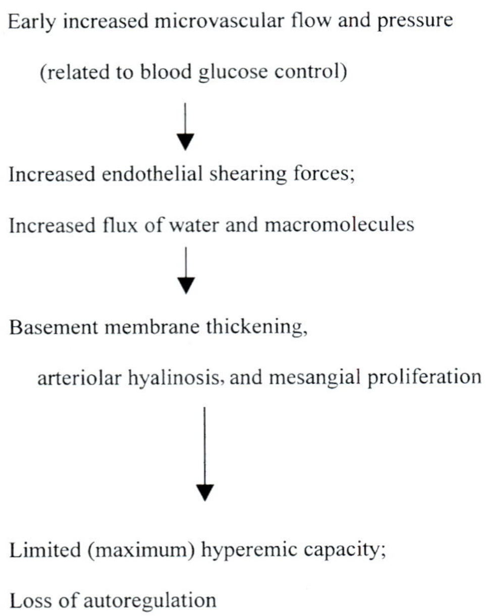

Figure 1 The hemodynamic hypothesis of the pathogenesis of diabetic microangiopathy in insulin-dependent diabetes

hemodynamic hypothesis of pathogenesis of diabetic microangiopathy [6, 24, 39] (Figure 1). The hypothesis states that early in T1DM, increased microvascular flow and pressure occurs in a manner that is dependent on blood glucose control. Increased pressure, through increased shearing forces, induces an "injury" response by the microvascular endothelium, resulting in manufacture of perivascular matrix proteins and structural remodeling of the microcirculation. In addition, the increased pressure contributes to the increased water and macromolecular flux observed. As capillary basement membranes thicken and arterioles become more hyalinosed, vasodilatory capacity becomes limited, resulting in a reduction in (maximal) perfusion and a limited autoregulatory potential. Anecdotal clinical evidence exists in support of the central tenet of the hypothesis that increased capillary pressure is the fundamental stimulus: both renal artery [40] and carotid artery [41] stenosis protect against the development of microangiopathy in the organ supplied. Furthermore, conditions associated with high intraocular pressure (which will tend to offset raised capillary pressure), such as glaucoma, are associated with lesser degrees of microangiopathy [42].

The association between elevated pressure and basement membrane thickening is supported by the fact that capillary basement membrane is increased in area in the distal extremity [43] (where hydrostatic pressure is highest in the upright posture) and in other conditions in which hydrostatic pressure is increased (e.g. congestive cardiac failure) [44].

MICROVASCULAR FUNCTION IN T2DM

As is observed in T1DM, cutaneous microvascular overperfusion has been described in T2DM, particularly during poor glycemic control, with the majority of increased blood flow occurring through arteriovenous shunts [45]. Increased renal plasma flow has also been described in newly diagnosed T2DM [46]; retinal blood flow measured by the technique of laser Doppler velocimetry is also raised and can be reduced by an insulin-induced fall in blood glucose concentration [47].

More striking, however, than the blood-glucose-related increases in perfusion observed under resting conditions soon after diagnosis of diabetes, is the profound reduction in microvascular vasodilatation observed under conditions designed to stress the microcirculation. In the skin microcirculation there is a reduction in the maximal hyperemic response to local heat that is present at diagnosis of T2DM [48]. Although it is well accepted that T2DM may be present for many years before the diagnosis is made, the derangement in hyperemic response observed equates to that seen after a median duration of T1DM of 18 years. Reductions in the cutaneous reactive hyperemia that follows release of arterial occlusion have also been documented [49]. In muscle tissue, reduction in total muscle blood flow after exercise has been described [50], which has more recently been attributed to impaired endothelium-dependent vasodilatation secondary to elevated plasma glucose [51]. To what extent this reflects a defect in capillary recruitment in T2DM (and insulin resistance), which may also underlie defects in postprandial, insulin-mediated glucose disposal in such tissue, remains a point of contention [52, 53].

In contrast to the clear elevation in skin capillary pressure observed in T1DM, skin nailfold capillary pressure does not appear to be elevated in normotensive T2DM patients [54]. However, pressure is elevated in non-insulin-dependent patients with raised blood pressure and falls with hypotensive treatment [55]. Studies of microvascular permeability in T2DM are characterized by inconsistency: retinal vitreous fluorophotometry reveals no evidence of increased retinal permeability in T2DM patients without retinopathy [56]; similarly no increase in forearm CFC was observed in a group of normotensive T2DM patients who were relatively free of microvascular complications [57] despite the fact that the technique employed was capable of revealing abnormalities in young, well-controlled insulin-dependent patients who showed no diabetic complications [36]. However, an increase in sodium fluorescein flux in the skin has been observed [58], as has an increase in the permeability/surface area product of the small lipophilic molecule pentetic acid in the tissues of the forearm [59]. An increased flux of radiolabeled albumin in the tissues of the forearm seems at first to be inconsistent with the normal fluid permeability alluded to above, as the majority of macromolecular transfer occurs by the process of solvent drag. However, the increased albumin retention in forearm tissue was most marked in hypertensive T2DM patients and seemed to relate to a decrease in lymphatic washout in a number of subjects. Other workers have demonstrated that the transcapillary flux of albumin assessed by the TER following intravenous injection is not increased in normotensive T2DM patients with no clinical evidence of microangiopathy [60]. In contrast, in the kidney, increased permeability to both fluid and macromolecules is demonstrable at an early stage in T2DM [61]; although some studies have observed an early increase in glomerular filtration as is found in T1DM [62], which reduces with improved glycemic control [63], others have found glomerular filtration to be normal [62, 63].

The Hemodynamic Hypothesis and T2DM

Just how sustainable is the hemodynamic hypothesis of diabetic microangiopathy, given the normal skin capillary pressure and fluid filtration coefficients observed in (normotensive) T2DM? It seems intuitively unlikely that a similar array of microvascular complications in the two types of diabetes could have different pathogenetic origins. The key to this puzzle may lie in the differences in prevalence of arterial hypertension in T2DM compared to T1DM: prevalence rates are in the region of 30–40% in T2DM [64], whereas in T1DM, in the absence of nephropathy, prevalence of hypertension is comparable with that of the nondiabetic population [65]. Sustained high blood pressure relies upon an increase in peripheral resistance that may be associated with the insulin-resistant state that predates the emergence of non-insulin-dependent diabetes. It is possible to construct a modification of the hemodynamic hypothesis for T2DM (Figure 2) that asserts that insulin resistance is associated with a modification of arteriolar resistance as well as raising blood pressure by other mechanisms; when glucose tolerance breaks down, the resultant precapillary vasodilatation does not result in the same increase in capillary pressure and fluid filtration as in T1DM patients at rest because of the protective increase in proximal resistance (which also contributes to the excessive prevalence of hypertension). However, the autoregulation of capillary pressure is disturbed, allowing for breakthrough capillary hypertension, particularly in the presence of arterial hypertension, which commonly coexists; such an interdependence between microangiopathy and arterial hypertension in T2DM is exemplified by several epidemiological studies [66, 67], and has been further emphasized by the protective effect of blood pressure control on the development of microangiopathy in the United Kingdom Prospective Diabetes Study [68].

In support of this modified hypothesis, increased peripheral microvascular resistance is demonstrable in nondiabetic populations with minor degrees of impaired glucose tolerance [69] and in other patient groups with insulin resistance but normal glucose tolerance [70].

MICROVASCULAR FUNCTION IN MONOGENIC FORMS OF DIABETES

In recent years the genetic origins of maturity-onset diabetes of the young (MODY) have largely been elucidated. Mutations of the genes for glucokinase, and the transcription factors HNF-1α and -4γ, and insulin promoter factor account for the majority of cases of MODY. In United Kingdom the *HNF-1* gene accounts for about three quarters of MODY [71]. Despite its name, implying similarities with T2DM (once commonly termed maturity-onset diabetes), in contrast to T2DM the principal problem in MODY appears to be a pancreatic β-cell secretory defect rather than insulin resistance. One might therefore anticipate that the microvascular physiological changes observed in MODY mirror those observed in T1DM (in which β-cell failure is the proximal cause) rather than T2DM. In keeping with this hypothesis, a disease-duration-related decline in maximum microvascular hyperemia is observed in MODY secondary to HNF-1, very similar to that observed in T1DM [72]. The blood glucose excursion observed in MODY secondary to glucokinase gene polymorphisms is modest, reflecting the role of glucokinase as the β-cell glucose sensor, defects in which alter the glucose set point. It is thus not surprising that patients with glucokinase MODY remain relatively free of microangiopathic complications. In contrast, hyperglycemia is more marked in MODY secondary to other genetic defects with consequent greater expression of microangiopathy.

THE CELLULAR AND BIOCHEMICAL BASIS OF MICROVASCULAR MALFUNCTION IN DIABETES MELLITUS

The definition of the pattern of functional breakdown of the microcirculation in diabetes points to several pivotal processes, the elucidation of the biochemical and cellular basis of which are major research issues. Detailed consideration of these processes are the subject of Chapter 76 in this book but the molecular determinants of certain pathophysiological features described above deserve special mention here. These include (a) the link between hyperglycemia and reduced precapillary resistance; (b) the link between insulin resistance and increased peripheral vascular resistance; (c) the transduction of increased microvascular pressure into the formation of extravascular matrix proteins; and (d) the physicochemical basis of increased permeability in diabetes.

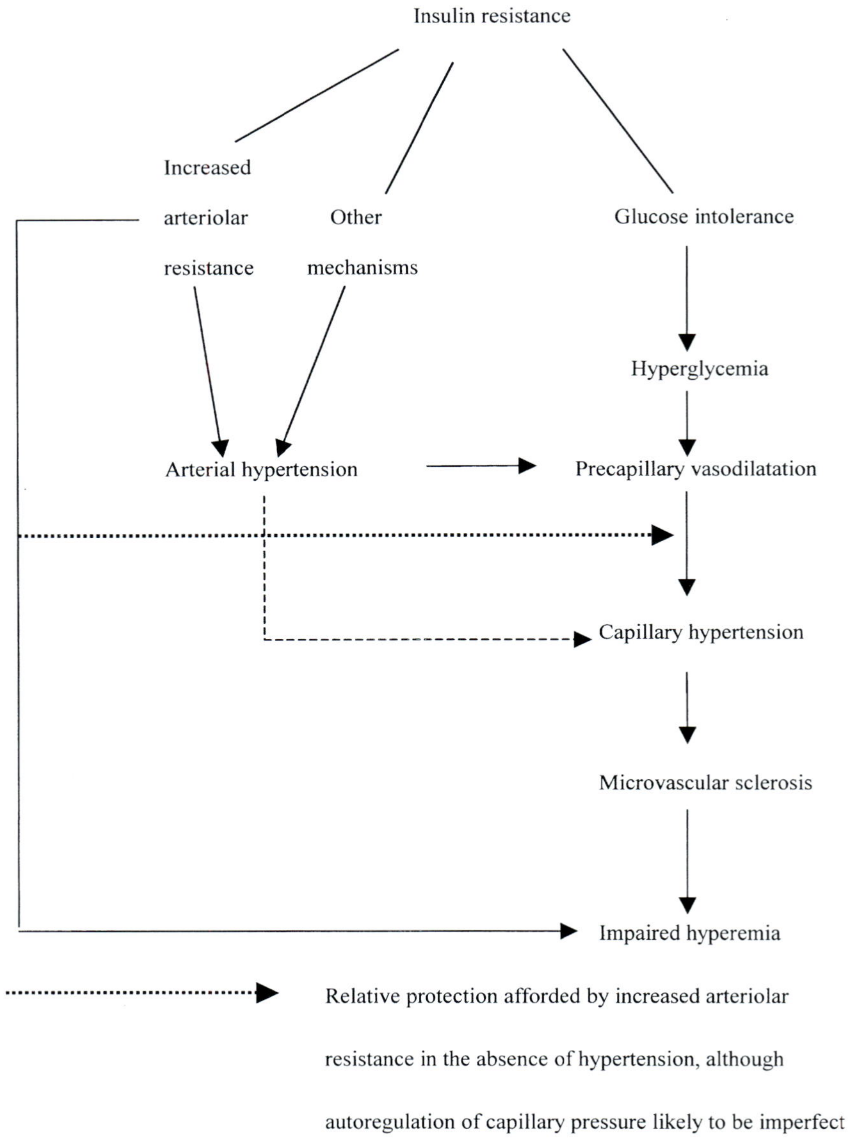

Figure 2 Hemodynamic factors in the pathogenesis of diabetic microangiopathy in non-insulin-dependent diabetes

Hyperglycemia and Reduced Precapillary Resistance

Precapillary vascular tonus represents the integrated influence of a great many factors, including extrinsic neural and humoral influences, intrinsic myogenic tone, and the function of, and response to, products derived from the vascular endothelium. Many if not all of these factors may be modified by the diabetic state, and different factors may be of greater importance in particular microvascular beds. Thus, sympathetic neuropathy, which in subtle form may be an early feature of T1DM, may account in part for the high blood flow observed in the skin, although it cannot be an adequate explanation for retinal hyperperfusion as this tissue is not under significant neurogenic vascular control.

Reduced precapillary resistance could be due to either an increase in circulating levels of vasodilator mediators or a reduction in vasoconstrictors, or a disturbance of both with a net balance in favour of vasodilation in the early part of the disease process. Insulin is one such vasodilatory hormone [73] that may be present in excess in both T1DM and T2DM, although its direct influence may be offset by the activation of the sympathetic nervous system [74].

In T1DM patients without complications atrial natriuretic peptide (ANP) levels are elevated [75], and it has been demonstrated that infusion of physiological quantities into the brachial artery of healthy humans results in an increase in forearm blood flow [76], although to date no such studies have been performed in early T1DM. Indeed in long-term T1DM patients the forearm vasodilator response to intra-arterial ANP infusion appears to be impaired [77].

Bradykinin and histamine are also potential candidates, although their levels in early T1DM are not currently known. An accumulation of either lactate or ketone bodies, metabolic products of insulin deficiency, to levels seen during poor diabetic control may induce an increase in renal plasma flow [78]. More compeling, however, is the central role played by that more obvious product of relative insulin deficiency, namely hyperglycemia. Although many animal studies suggest that hyperglycemia may induce vasodilatation and an increase in permeability through an action on the endothelium, little such evidence exists in humans; indeed stimulated endothelium-dependent vasodilatation appears to be unchanged in short-term T1DM patients, and there is some indirect evidence suggesting that their basal nitric oxide production is decreased [79]. This latter observation argues against the attractive hypothesis that blood rheological changes, including increased red cell aggregability and impaired deformability that are present from early in T1DM in a manner dependent on blood glucose control, create shear stresses on the endothelium, resulting in an abundance of vasodilator products [1]. The evidence in favor of an increased production of vasodilator prostaglandins is confused [80, 81].

What then are the mechanisms by which hyperglycemia can influence endothelial and/or vascular smooth muscle function? *In vivo* animal studies suggest that hyperglycemia leads to an intracellular accumulation of sorbitol and fructose with a secondary reduction in myoinositol uptake and decreased Na–K-ATPase activity [82], the latter having complex effects on cellular growth, differentiation, and smooth muscle contraction. A further result of increased flux through the sorbitol pathway is an increased NADH/NAD ratio that facilitates diacylglycerol production. The latter compound activates protein kinase C that may result in arteriolar vasodilatation either directly [83] or through increased endothelial production of nitric oxide. As far as early human T1DM is concerned much of the above remains a hypothesis, but a plausible one that is amenable to investigation. Finally, vasodilatation may represent a failure of vascular smooth muscle response to vasoconstrictor mediators. Recent evidence suggests that agonist receptor expression may be diminished in aortic smooth muscle in a hyperglycemic environment [84], although no such data exist for microvascular resistance vessels.

The Transduction of Increased Microvascular Pressure

The vascular endothelium responds to the physical forces that play upon its surface by the production of mediators that modulate vascular tone, as well as by the excitation of intracellular machinery that results in the increased production of extravascular matrix proteins and cytokines that modify vascular smooth muscle structure.

In particular, the synthesis of both nitric oxide and prostacyclin is known to be dependent upon the prevailing shear rate and pulsatility of blood flow [85]. In a rat model of diabetes, the mesangial stretching that results from increased glomerular pressure has been shown to correlate with increased mRNA expression of a number of mesangial proteins [86]. In human mesangial cells, stretch activates p38 MAP kinase, which induces TGF-β1 and fibronectin via a PKC-dependent mechanism [87].

Insulin Resistance and Increased Peripheral Vascular Resistance

The link between insulin resistance and increased peripheral vascular resistance is central to an understanding of the microvascular pathology of T2DM. Elucidation of the precise nature of the link is clouded by the lack of certainty regarding the association between hyperinsulinemia and hypertension, for the latter abnormality will have effects on microvascular structure independent of any underlying common metabolic basis. Nonetheless, it is known that Na^+–K^+-ATPase activity is insulin-sensitive [88], and a resulting increase in intracellular Na^+ concentrations would be expected to increase intracellular Ca^+ concentrations (the effector mechanism of increased vascular tone), which could be further increased by insulin effects on Ca^+-ATPase. Insulin resistance has also been linked to elevated Na/Li countertransport [89], which is known to be abnormal in essential hypertension. In recent years considerable evidence has been accumulated showing that endothelium-dependent vasodilatory mechanisms might be impaired not only in nondiabetic subjects with one or more features of the insulin resistance syndrome, but also in subjects at risk of developing T2DM without such features, raising the possibility that endothelial dysfunction may be a common antecedent.

Finally, theories suggesting that insulin resistance may stem, in some instances, from impaired intrauterine nutrition resulting in reduced vascularity of peripheral tissues would imply that increased peripheral vascular resistance might have an anatomical basis [90]. Although altered muscle morphology and capillary density may play a role [91], skin capillary density appears to be normal [92] in insulin-resistant subjects in the absence of hypertension, despite a reduction in cutaneous vasodilatory reserve.

The Physicochemical Basis of Permeability Change

At the present time it is only possible to speculate about the physicochemical changes that account for the increases in permeability observed: water and large molecules, the passage of which is largely convective, pass predominantly through interendothelial cell junctions that are filled with a basement-membrane-like glycocalyx. The interendothelial junction also involves a complex array of adhesion molecules, the expression of which may be altered under hyperglycemic conditions [93]. Furthermore, actin filaments within the cell are tethered to parts of the complex; filament tension (which may be modified by nitric oxide bioavailability and/or oxidative stress) will influence the integrity of the interendothelial junction. The biochemical milieu of diabetes may not only alter interendothelial cell junction integrity but may also result in alteration of the charge barrier as well as the tertiary structure of basement membrane due to cross-linking. Even though the path length may be increased because of basement membrane thickening, steric hindrance and charge repulsion are arguably less, and these are important determinants of permeability.

In the glomerulus the determinants of permeability to albumin are even more complex, reflecting the multicomponent nature of the barrier. The components comprise (i) an endothelial layer with substantial spaces (fenestrae) between cells filled with filamentous material; (ii) a glomerular endothelial surface covered with a glycocalyx comprising a charged glycoprotein framework onto which are adsorbed certain plasma proteins; (iii) the basement membrane separating the endothelium from the epithelium layer, which is thickened and less compressible in the presence of diabetes, probably reflecting glycation cross-linking; and (iv) the epithelial foot processes separated by highly specialized structures, the slit diaphragms, the molecular architecture of which is beginning to be appreciated and may be disrupted by diabetes.

CONCLUSIONS

Disturbance of microvascular function precedes the development of clinically relevant diabetic microangiopathy. Plausible candidate cellular and molecular mechanisms responsible for such microangiopathy must be able to account for the pathophysiological changes observed.

Although the pattern of microvascular pathophysiology is common to all forms of diabetes, important distinctions in microvascular behavior are also observed between the two major forms of the condition. In the case of T2DM, evidence exists that microvascular functional derangement occurs prior to the development of hyperglycemia, associated with the insulin resistance that commonly antedates this form of diabetes. Capillary hypertension is an important mediator of adverse microvascular change, aggravated by coexistent arterial hypertension. Until the molecular mechanisms responsible for microvascular decompensation are better defined, protecting the diabetic capillary bed from pressure excess through judicious use of hypotensive therapy in appropriate patient groups remains an important disease-modifying strategy in addition to strategies aimed at achieving optional glycemic control.

REFERENCES

1. Tooke JE. Microvascular hemodynamics in diabetes. *Eye* 1993; 7: 227–9.
2. Dornan TL, Tattersall RB. Blind alleys in diabetes research: muscle capillary basement membrane thickening—marker of microvascular complications or false prophet? *Diabet Med* 1986; 3: 413–8.
3. Klein RF, Feingold KR, Morgan C, Stern WH, Siperstein MD. Relationship of muscle capillary basement membrane thickness and diabetic retinopathy. *Diabetes Care* 1987; 10: 195–9.
4. Tooke JE. Microvascular physiology and its clinical relevance with special reference to diabetes. *Q J Med* 1992; 304: 567–73.
5. Jaap A, Tooke JE. The pathophysiology of microvascular disease in non-insulin-dependent diabetes. *Clin Sci* 1995; 89: 3–12.
6. Tooke JE. Microvascular hemodynamics in diabetes mellitus. *Clin Sci* 1986; 70: 119–25.
7. Thuesen L, Christiansen JS, Mogensen CE, Henningsen P. Cardiac hyperfunction in insulin-dependent diabetic patients developing microvascular complications. *Diabetes* 1988; 37: 851–6.
8. Christiansen JS, Gammelgaard J, Tronier B, Svendsen PA, Parving H-H. Kidney function and size in diabetics, before and during initial insulin treatment. *Kidney Int* 1982; 21: 683–8.
9. Kohner EM, Hamilton AM, Saunders SJ, Sutcliffe BA, Bulpitt CJ. The retinal blood flow in diabetes. *Diabetologia* 1975; 11: 27–33.
10. Grunwald JE, Riva CE, Baine J, Brucker AJ. Total retinal volumetric blood flow rate in diabetic patients with poor glycemic control. *Invest Ophthalmol Vis Sci* 1992; 33: 356–63.
11. Gundersen HJG. Peripheral blood flow and metabolic control in juvenile diabetes. *Diabetologia* 1974; 10: 225–31.
12. Tymms DJ, Tooke JE. The effect of continuous subcutaneous insulin infusion (CSII) on microvascular blood flow in diabetes mellitus. *Int J Microcirc Clin Exp* 1988; 7: 347–56.
13. Shore AC, Price KJ, Mawson DM, Tripp JH, Tooke JE. Nailfold capillary blood flow velocity in prepubertal and late pubertal diabetic children. In *Proceedings of the Fifth World Congress for Microcirculation*, Louisville, USA, September 1991 (abstract 604).
14. Shore AC, Price KJ, Sandeman DD, Mawson DM, Tripp JH, Tooke JE. Posturally induced vasoconstriction in children and adolescents with diabetes mellitus. *Arch Dis Child* 1994; 70: 22–6.
15. Houben AJHM. *Early (Micro)Circulatory Hemodynamic Changes in Type 1 Diabetes Mellitus*, MD Thesis. Maastricht, The Netherlands: University of Maastricht, 1993; Chap 9.
16. Rayman G, Williams SA, Spencer PD, Smaje LH, Wise PH, Tooke JE. Impaired microvascular hyperemic response to minor skin trauma in type I diabetes. *Br Med J* 1986, 292: 1295–8.
17. Walmsley D, Wales JK, Wiles PG. Reduced hyperemia following skin trauma: evidence for an impaired microvascular response to injury in the diabetic foot. *Diabetologia* 1989; 32: 736–9.

18. Shore AC, Donohoe M, Jaap AJ, Tooke JE. The effect of increasing doses of an angiotensin converting enzyme inhibitor on capillary pressure levels in patients with insulin-dependent-diabetes mellitus and microalbuminuria. *Diabet Med* 1993; 10 (suppl 1): S5.
19. Ostergren J, Fagrell B, Karlander SG. Skin capillary blood flow dynamics in patients with diabetes mellitus [abstract]. *Int J Microcirc Clin Exp* 1982; 1: 300.
20. Jörneskog G, Tyden G, Bolinder J, Fagrell B. Skin microvascular reactivity in fingers of diabetic patients after combined kidney and pancreas transplantation. *Diabetologia* 1991; 34 (suppl 1): SS135–7.
21. Cheung ATW, Perez RV, Chen PCY. Improvements in diabetic microangiopathy after successful simultaneous pancreas–kidney transplantation. *Transplantation* 1999; 68: 927–32.
22. Bresnick GH, de Venecia G, Myers EL, Harris JA, Davis MD. Retinal ischaemia in diabetic retinopathy. *Arch Ophthalmol* 1975; 93: 1300–10.
23. Mogensen CF, Christensen CK, Vittinghus E. The stages in diabetic renal disease. *Diabetes* 1983; 32 (suppl 2): 64–78.
24. Zatz R, Brenner BM. Pathogenesis of diabetic microangiopathy: the hemodynamic view. *Am J Med* 1986; 80: 443–53.
25. Rayman GA. *Microvascular Hemodynamics of the Foot Skin in Diabetes Mellitus*, MD Thesis. University of London: England, 1991.
26. Patel V, Rassam SMB, Chen HC, Kohner EM. Oxygen reactivity in diabetes mellitus: the effect of hypertension and hyperglycemia. *Clin Sci* 1994; 86: 689–95.
27. Kastrup J, Norgaard T, Parving H-H, Henriksen O, Lassen NA. Impaired autoregulation of blood flow in subcutaneous tissue of long-term type 1 (insulindependent) diabetic patients with microangiopathy: an index of arteriolar dysfunction. *Diabetologia* 1985; 28: 711–7.
28. Hostetter TH, Troy JL, Brenner BM. Glomerular hemodynamics in experimental diabetes mellitus. *Kidney Int* 1981; 19: 410–5.
29. Paulsen EP, Pauly FL, Croft BY, Teates CD. Simultaneous measurement of glomerular filtration rate and effective renal plasma flow reveals increased glomerular capillary pressure among teenage diabetic subjects. *Contrib Nephrol* 1990; 79: 52–7.
30. Sandeman DD, Shore AC, Tooke JE. Relation of skin capillary pressure in patients with insulin-dependent diabetes mellitus to complications and metabolic control. *N Engl J Med* 1992; 327: 760–4.
31. Shore AC, Jaap AJ, Tooke JE. Capillary pressure in insulin dependent diabetic patients of long disease duration with and without microangiopathy. *Diabet Med* 1992; 9 (suppl 2): S11.
32. Williams SA, Boolell M, MacGregor GA, Smaje LH, Wassermann S, Tooke JE. Capillary hypertension and abnormal pressure dynamics in patients with essential hypertension. *Clin Sci* 1990; 79: 5–8.
33. Tooke JE, Tindall H, Hancock KW. Capillary pressure during pregnancy [abstract]. *Microvasc Res* 1982; 24: 238.
34. Tooke JE, Tindall H, McNicol GP. The influence of a combined oral contraceptive pill and menstrual cycle phase on digital microvascular hemodynamics. *Clin Sci* 1981; 61: 91–5.
35. Parving H-H, Noer I, Deckert T, Evrin PE, Nielsen SL, Lyngsoe J, Mogensen CE, Rorth M, Svendsen PA, Trap-Jensen J, Lassen NA. The effect of metabolic regulation on microvascular permeability to small and large molecules in short-term juvenile diabetics. *Diabetologia* 1976; 12: 161–6.
36. Jaap AJ, Shore AC, Gartside IB, Gamble J, Tooke JE. Increased microvascular fluid permeability in young type 1 (insulin-dependent) diabetic patients. *Diabetologia* 1993; 36: 648–52.
37. Trap-Jensen J, Lassen NA. Increased capillary diffusion capacity for small ions in skeletal muscle in longterm diabetics. *Scand J Clin Lab Invest* 1968; 21: 116–22.
38. Tooke JE. Methodologies used in the study of the microcirculation in diabetes mellitus. *Diabetes Metab Rev* 1993; 9 (1): 57–70.
39. Parving H-H, Viberti GC, Keen H, Christiansen JS, Lassen NA. Hemodynamic factors in the genesis of diabetic microangiopathy. *Metabolism* 1983; 32: 943–9.
40. Berkman J, Rifkin H. Unilateral nodular diabetic glomerulosclerosis (Kimmelstiel–Wilson). Report of a case. *Metab Clin Exp* 1973; 22: 715–22.
41. Behrendt T, Duane TD. Unilateral complications in diabetic retinopathy. *Trans Am Acad Ophthalmol Otol* 1970; 74: 28–32.
42. Becker B. Diabetes and glaucoma. In Kimura SJ, Caygill WM (eds), *Vascular Complications of Diabetes Mellitus with Special Emphasis on Microangiopathy of the Eye*. St Louis: Mosby, 1967; pp 657–63.
43. Vracko R. Skeletal muscle capillaries in diabetics. *Circulation* 1970; 41: 271–83.
44. Fahr GE, Ershler I. Studies of factors concerned in edema formation: hydrostatic pressure in capillaries during edema formation in right heart failure. *Ann Intern Med* 1941; 15: 798–810.
45. Tooke JE. Capillary pressure in non-insulin-dependent diabetes. *Int Angiol* 1983; 2: 167–71.
46. Ishida K, Ishibashi F, Takashina S. Comparison of renal hemodynamics in early non-insulin-dependent and insulin-dependent diabetes mellitus. *J Diabet Complications* 1991; 5: 143–5.
47. Grunwald JE, Riva CE, Martin DB, Quint AR, Epstein PA. Effect of an insulin-induced decrease in blood glucose on the human diabetic retinal circulation. *Ophthalmology* 1987; 94: 1614–20.
48. Sandeman DD, Pym CA, Green EM, Seamark C, Shore AC, Tooke JE. Microvascular vasodilatation in feet of newly diagnosed non-insulin-dependent diabetic patients. *BMJ* 1991; 302: 1122–3.
49. Tur E, Yosipovitch G, Bar-On Y. Skin reactive hyperemia in diabetic patients. A study by laser Doppler flowmetry. *Diabetes Care* 1991; 14: 958–62.
50. Menon RK, Grace AA, Burgoyne W, Fonseca VA, James IM, Dandona P. Muscle blood flow in diabetes mellitus. Evidence of abnormality after exercise. *Diabetes Care* 1992; 15: 693–5.
51. Kingwell BA, Formosa M, Muhlmann M, Bradley SJ, McConell GK. Type 2 Diabetic individuals have impaired leg blood flow responses to exercise. *Diabetes Care* 2003; 26: 899–904.
52. Baron AD, Steinberg HO, et al. *Insulin-mediated* skeletal muscle vasodilation contributes to both insulin sensitivity and responsiveness in lean humans. *J Clin Invest* 1995; 96: 786–92.
53. Yki-Jarvinen H, Utriainen T. Insulin-induced vasodilation: physiology or pharmacology? *Diabetologia* April1998; 41 (4): 369–79.
54. Shore AC, Sandeman DD, Jaap AJ, Sampson KJ, Tooke JE. Is capillary pressure elevated in patients with

non-insulin-dependent diabetes [abstract]. *Int J Microcirc Clin Exp* 1992; 11 (suppl 1): S210–358.

55. Fegan PG, MacLeod KM, Tooke JE, Shore AC. N-3 NEFA: vascular implications. *J Hypertens* 2003; 5: 1111–7.
56. Yoshida A, Kojima M, Ogasawara H, Ishiko S. Oscillatory potentials and permeability of the blood–retinal barrier in non-insulin-dependent diabetes mellitus without retinopathy. *Ophthalmology* 1991; 98: 1266–71.
57. Jaap AJ, Shore AC, Gamble J, Gartside IB, Tooke JE. Capillary filtration coefficient in type 2 (non-insulin-dependent) diabetes. *J Diabet Complications* 1994; 8: 111–6.
58. Bollinger A, Frey J, Jäger K, Furrer J, Seglias J, Siegenthaler W. Patterns of diffusion through skin capillaries in patients with long-term diabetes. *New Engl J Med* 1982; 307: 1305–10.
59. Katz MA, McCuskey P, Begg JL, Johnson PC, Gaines JA. Relationship between microvascular function and capillary structure in diabetic and non-diabetic human skin. *Diabetes* 1989; 38: 1245–50.
60. O'Hare JA, Ferriss JB, Twomey B, O'Sullivan DJ. Poor metabolic control, hypertension and microangiopathy independently increase the transcapillary escape rate of albumin in diabetes. *Diabetologia* 1983; 25: 260–3.
61. Vora JP, Dolben J, Dean JD, et al. Renal hemodynamics in newly presenting non-insulin-dependent diabetes mellitus. *Kidney Int* 1992; 41: 829–35.
62. Ishida K, Ishibashi F, Takashina S. Comparison of renal hemodynamics in early non-insulin-dependent and insulin-dependent diabetes mellitus. *J Diabet Complications* 1991; 5: 143–5.
63. Schmitz A, Christensen T, Taagehoej Jensen F. Glomerular filtration rate and kidney volume in normoalbuminuric non-insulin-dependent diabetics. Lack of glomerular hyperfiltration and renal hypertrophy in uncomplicated T2DM. *Scand J Clin Lab Invest* 1989; 49: 103–8.
64. The United Kingdom Prospective Diabetes Study Group. United Kingdom Prospective Diabetes Study III. Prevalence of hypertension and hypotensive therapy in patients with new diagnosed diabetes. *Hypertension* 1985; 7 (suppl 2): 8–13.
65. Norgaard K, Feldt-Rasmussen B, Borch-Johnsen K, Saelan H, Deckert T. Prevalence of hypertension in type 1 (insulin-dependent) diabetes mellitus. *Diabetologia* 1990; 33: 407–10.
66. Knowler WC, Bennett PH, Ballintine EJ. Increased incidence of retinopathy in diabetics with elevated blood pressure: a six-year follow-up study in Pima Indians. *N Engl J Med* 1980; 302: 645–50.
67. Gall M-A, Rossing P, Skott P, et al. Prevalence of micro- and macroalbuminuria, arterial hypertension, retinopathy and large vessel disease in European type 2 (non-insulin-dependent) diabetic patients. *Diabetologia* 1991; 34: 655–61.
68. Holman R, Turner R, et al. Efficacy of atenolol and captopril in reducing risk of macrovascular and microvascular complications in type 2 diabetes: UKPDS 39. *BMJ* 1998; 317: 713–20.
69. Jaap AJ, Hammersley MS, Shore AC, Tooke JE. Reduced microvascular hyperemia in subjects at risk of developing type 2 (non-insulin-dependent) diabetes mellitus. *Diabetologia* 1994; 37: 214–6.
70. Tooke JE, Goh K. Vascular function in Type 2 diabetes mellitus and pre-diabetes: the case for intrinsic endotheliopathy. *Diabet Med* 1999; 16: 710–5.
71. Frayling T, Bulman MP, Ellard S, Appleton M, Dronsfield MJ, Mackie ADR, et al. Mutations in the hepatocyte nuclear factor 1 alpha gene are a common cause of maturity-onset diabetes of the young in the UK. *Diabetes* 1997; 46: 720–5.
72. Lee BC, Appleton M, Shore AC, Tooke JE, Hattersley AT. Impaired maximum microvascular hyperemia in patients with MODY 3 (hepatocyte nuclear factor-1α (gene mutations). *Diabet Med* 1999; 16: 1–5.
73. Tooke JE, Lins PE, Ostergren J, Adamson U, Fagrell B. The effects of intravenous insulin infusion on skin microcirculatory flow in type 1 diabetes. *Int J Microcirc Clin Exp* 1985; 69: 69–83.
74. Anderson EA, Hoffman RP, Balon TW, Sinkley CA, Mark AL. Hyperinsulinemia produces both sympathetic neural activation and vasodilation in normal humans. *J Clin Invest* 1991; 87: 2246–52.
75. Trevisan R, Fioretto P, Semplicini A, Opocher G, Mantero F, Rocco S, et al. Role of insulin and atrial natriuretic peptide in sodium retention in insulin-treated T1DM patients during isotonic volume expansion. *Diabetes* 1990; 39: 289–98.
76. Bolli P, Muller FB, Linder L, Raine AEG, Resink TJ, Erne P, et al. The vasodilator potency of atrial natriuretic peptide in man. *Circulation* 1987; 75: 221–8.
77. Smits P, Hersbach F, Jansen T, Lutterman J, Thien T. Impaired vasodilator response to atrial natriuretic factor in insulin-dependent (type 1) diabetes mellitus. *Diabetes* 1993; 42: 1454–61.
78. Trevisan R, Nosadini R, Fioretto P, Velussi M, Avogaro A, Duner E, et al. Metabolic control of kidney hemodynamics in normal and insulin-dependent diabetic subjects. Effects of acetoacetic, lactic and acetic acids. *Diabetes* 1987; 36: 1073–81.
79. Calver A, Collier J, Vallance P. Inhibition and stimulation of nitric oxide synthesis in the human forearm arterial bed of patients with insulin-dependent diabetes. *J Clin Invest* 1992; 90: 2548–54.
80. Jeremy JY, Mikhailidis DP, Dandona P. Simulating the diabetic environment modifies *in vitro* prostacyclin synthesis. *Diabetes* 1983; 32: 217–21.
81. Harrison HE, Reece AH, Johnson M. Decreased vascular prostacyclin in experimental diabetes. *Life Sci* 1978; 23: 351–6.
82. Williamson JR, Kilo C, Tilton RG. Mechanisms of glucose- and diabetes-induced vascular dysfunction. In Ruderman N, Williamson JR, Brownlee M (eds), *Hyperglycemia, Diabetes, and Vascular Disease*. New York: Oxford University Press, 1992; pp 107–32.
83. Wolf BA, Williamson JR, Easom RA, Chang K, Sherman WR, Turk J. Diacylglycerol accumulation and microvascular abnormalities induced by elevated glucose levels. *J Clin Invest* 1991; 87: 31–8.
84. Williams B, Tsai P, Schrier RW. Glucose-induced downregulation of angiotensin II and arginine vasopressin receptors in cultured rat aortic vascular smooth muscle cells. *J Clin Invest* 1992; 90: 1992–9.
85. Rubanyi GM, Romero JC, Vanhoutte PM. Flowinduced release of endothelium-derived relaxing factor. *Am J Physiol* 1986; 250: H1145–9.
86. Riser BL, Cortes P, Zhao X, et al. Intraglomerular pressure and mesangial stretching stimulate extracellular matrix formation in the rat. *J Clin Invest* 1993; 90: 1932–43.

87. Gruden G, Zonca S, Hayward A, Thomas S, Maestrini S, Gnudi L. Mechanical stretch-induced fibronectin and transforming growth factor-β1 production in human mesangial cells 1s p38 mitogen-activated protein kinase-dependent. *Diabetes* 2000; 49: 655–61.
88. Smith U. Insulin resistance in hypertension. In Moller AE (ed), *Insulin Resistance*. Chichester, UK: Wiley, 1993; pp 327–54.
89. Dovia A, Fioretto P, Avogaro A, Carraro A, Morocutti A, Trevisan R, et al. Insulin resistance is associated with high sodium-lithium countertransport in essential hypertension. *Am J Physiol* 1991; 261: E684–91.
90. Barker DJP, Hales CN, Fall CHD, Osmond C, Phipps K, Clark PMS. Type 2 (non-insulin-dependent) diabetes mellitus, hypertension and hyperlipidaemia (syndrome X): relation to reduced fetal growth. *Diabetologia* 1993; 36: 62–7.
91. Ganrot PO. Insulin resistance syndrome: possible key role of blood flow in resting muscle. *Diabetologia* 1993; 36: 876–9.
92. Katz MA, McCuskey P, Beggs JL, Johnson PC, Gaines JA. Relationship between microvascular function and capillary structure in diabetic and nondiabetic human skin. *Diabetes* 1989; 38: 1245–50.
93. Baumgartner-Parzer SM, Wagner L, et al. Modulation by high glucose of adhesion molecule expression in cultured endothelial cells. *Diabetologia* 1995; 38: 1367–70.

65

Diabetic Retinopathy

Elisabet Agardh and Carl-David Agardh

Malmö University Hospital, Malmö, Sweden

The term *diabetic retinopathy* refers to all vascular changes in the retina occurring in diabetes. The lesions may vary from occasional hemorrhages and microaneurysms, to multiple hemorrhages and microaneurysms, prominent retinal thickening and exudates along blood vessels and in the macular region, new vessels, fibrosis, and retinal detachment. The severe vascular lesions result in visual impairment and blindness due to an accumulation of extracellular fluid, lipids, and lipoproteins from leaking vessels in the macular region (Figure 1) and/or to hemorrhages and retinal detachment as a result of growth of abnormal vessels (Figure 2). Diabetic retinopathy has been shown to be the cause of visual impairment and blindness in 86% of type 1 diabetic patients and in 33% of type 2 diabetic patients [1]. In the 1980s, the annual incidence of blindness due to diabetes was estimated to be 2 per 100 000 population in southern Germany [2], and 3.3 per 100 000 in Wisconsin, USA [3]. Diabetic retinopathy has been reported to be the most common cause of blindness among people in working age in western Europe and the incidence does not seem to decline [4].

Although the visible manifestations of diabetic retinopathy are vascular lesions, it cannot be regarded solely as a microvascular abnormality [5]. Neurons and glial cells comprise more than 95% of the retinal tissue. Visual information is perceived by photoreceptors, modulated and transmitted by chains of neurons, bipolar, horizontal, amacrine and ganglion cells, and finally, by the optic nerve to the brain. Numerous glial cells, Mueller cells and astroglia, support the neurons and the retinal blood vessels. These elements play a role in the regulation of extracellular ion concentrations and neurotransmitters. In addition, they are probably of importance for the preservation of the inner blood retinal barrier by securing the tight junctions between endothelial cells. Apart form the inner blood retinal barrier, there is also an outer barrier between the choroid and the photoreceptors, which is maintained by the retinal pigment epithelium.

The tone in the vasculature is maintained by smooth muscle cells in the retinal arterial vessels and by pericytes in the capillaries, arterioles, and venules. Like the brain, the retina is dependent on a continuous vascular supply unaffected by changes in the systemic arterial blood pressure. Hence, retinal circulation is maintained by autoregulation in response to systemic and local metabolic demands. Normally, this autoregulation responds to the partial pressure of carbon dioxide and oxygen. Diabetes results in an imbalance between retinal metabolism and vascular supply and subsequently, in vascular damage.

NATURAL COURSE OF DIABETIC RETINOPATHY

The major sight-threatening manifestations of diabetic retinopathy, macular edema, and proliferative retinopathy are the end manifestations of increased vascular permeability and vascular occlusion.

The retinal capillary wall consists of endothelial cells connected with tight junctions, intramural pericytes, and a basement membrane. Early in the course of diabetic retinopathy, intramural pericytes are lost and the basement membrane is thickened, resulting in the formation of acellular (nonperfused) capillaries and microaneurysms [6–8]. Impaired contractility of the vessels due to pericyte loss leads to a weakening of the vessel walls, and subsequently, harmed tight junctions between the endothelial cells [9]. Saccular outpouchings and focal endothelial cell proliferation result in formation of microaneurysms. Vascular

International Textbook of Diabetes Mellitus, Third Edition. Edited by R. A. DeFronzo, E. Ferrannini, H. Keen, and P. Zimmet.
 ISBN: 0-471-48655-8.

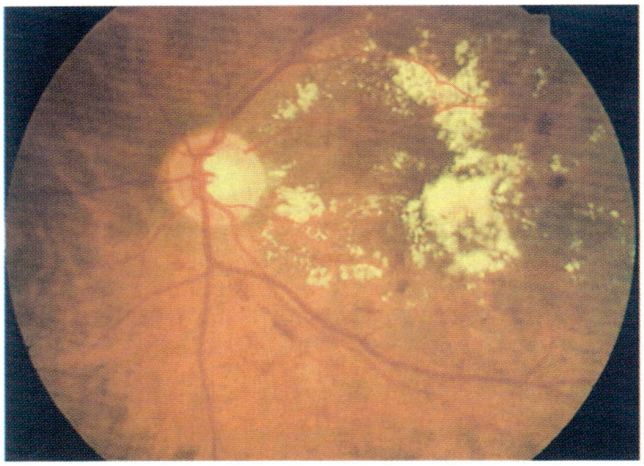

Figure 1 Extensive accumulation of hard exudates in the macular region. Fundus photograph

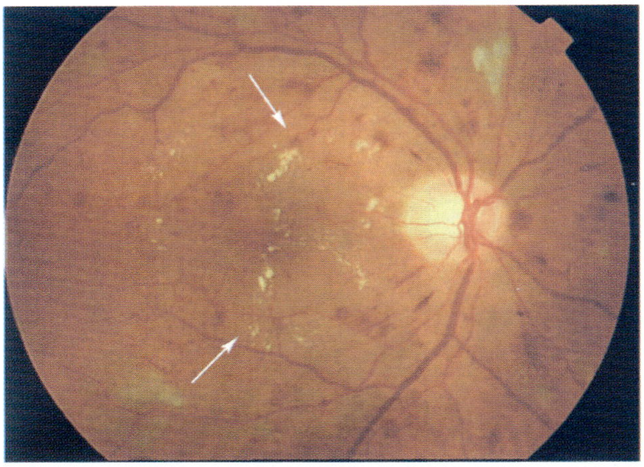

Figure 3 Rings of hard exudates from focal sources of leakage. Fundus photograph

occlusion, caused by thickened basement membranes, platelet aggregation, leucocyte activation [10], and/or migration of glial cells through the vessel walls [11], results in nonperfusion and hypoxia. Subsequent autoregulation of the blood flow leads to dilation of the arterioles and an increased hydrostatic pressure in the capillaries and venules [12]. The pressure lays an extra burden on the already weakened vessel walls, which can no longer maintain the inner blood retinal barrier. The vascular permeability increases, which results in retinal hemorrhages and an extracellular accumulation of fluid, lipids, and lipoproteins. Microaneurysms and dilated segments of retinal capillaries and arterioles are the main sources of leakage [13]. The leakage from microaneurysms and subsequent retinal thickening is focal, often surrounded by rings of hard exudates (Figure 3), representing deposits of lipids and/or lipoproteins in the outer retinal layers or even beneath the retina. A generalized breakdown of the inner blood retinal barrier results in a diffusely dilated capillary bed and adjacent thickening of the retina. In those eyes, hard exudates are usually absent (Figure 4) suggesting that the inner blood retinal barrier can be sufficient for retaining large lipoprotein molecules within the vascular bed. Accumulation of fluid in the deeper layers of the retina often appears as cysts (Figure 5). Apart from a resilient inner retinal barrier, there is also evidence for a breakdown of the outer barrier function, i.e. the pigment epithelium [9].

Occlusion of capillaries results in areas of nonperfusion, and in subsequent, dilation of preexisting capillaries or formation of new intraretinal vessels, i.e. intraretinal microvascular abnormalities (IRMA) (Figure 6). These vessels can often be found adjacent to cotton-wool spots, which are signs of impaired axonal transport, probably secondary to hypoxia in the nerve fiber layer. Areas of nonperfusion stimulate the growth of new vessels, which

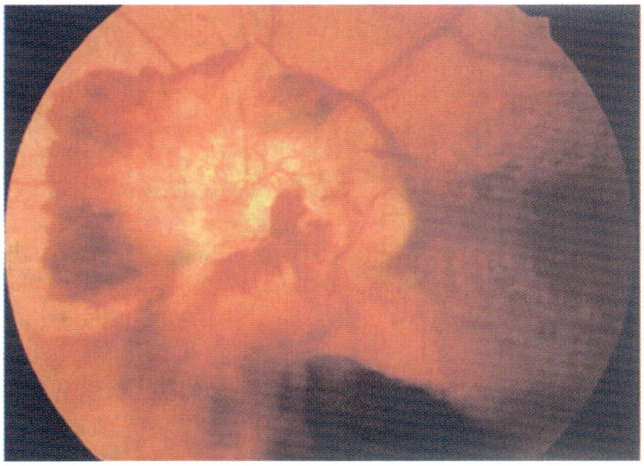

Figure 2 Preretinal and vitreous hemorrhage from new vessels on the optic disc. Fundus photograph

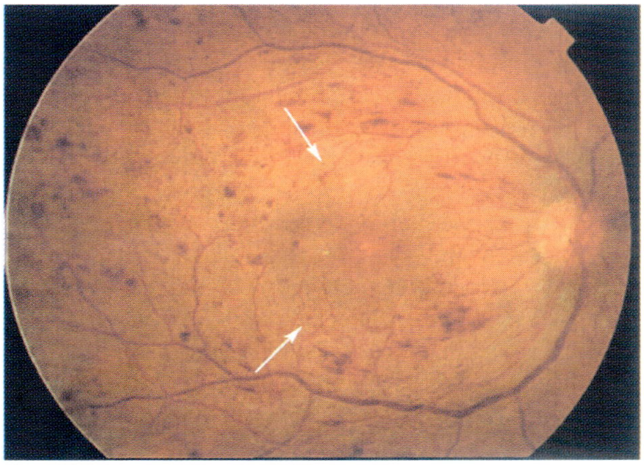

Figure 4 Diffuse leakage from dilated vessels and accumulation of fluid in deep layers of the retina. Fundus photograph

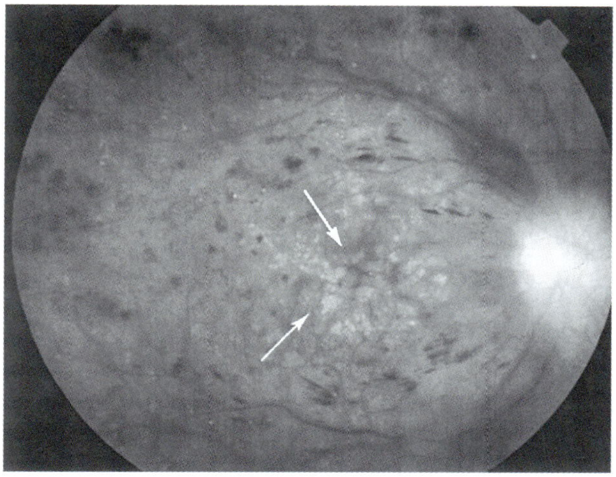

Figure 5 Deep leakage and cyst formation in Figure 4. Fluorescein angiogram

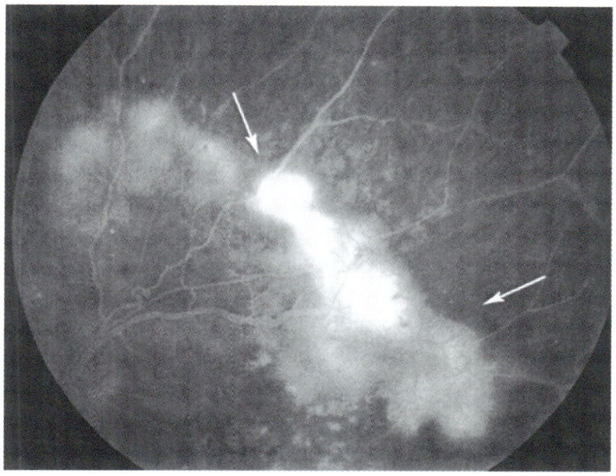

Figure 7 Leaking new vessels bordering nonperfused retina in the upper right part of the figure. Fluorescein angiogram

often occur in the margin between perfused and nonperfused areas (Figure 7). Formation of new vessels activates glial cells, which appear to loosen the tight junctions of the endothelial cells [14]. The new vessels initially grow on the surface of the retina or on the optic disc forming networks, but may later extend and in conjunction with fibrous tissue adhere to the posterior vitreous membrane, break through and grow further into the posterior vitreous cortex. Since the new vessels are fragile, adhesion to the vitreous membrane frequently results in preretinal (Figure 8) and/or vitreous (Figure 2) hemorrhages in case of a partial or complete posterior vitreous detachment due to vitreous contraction and shrinkage of the posterior surface [15]. As the shrinkage of posterior vitreous membrane becomes more prominent, the attached fibrovascular complexes are pulled forward, increasing the traction on the retina (Figure 9), which may result in localized areas of retinal detachment. If the fibrovascular tissue is extensive, it may cause a complete retinal detachment.

New vessels can also appear on the iris. They start as small tufts at the pupillary margin or in the anterior chamber angle. Initially, they are asymptomatic but as they grow they may occlude the chamber angle, resulting in neovascular glaucoma, a painful condition which results in blindness and may necessitate enucleation [16].

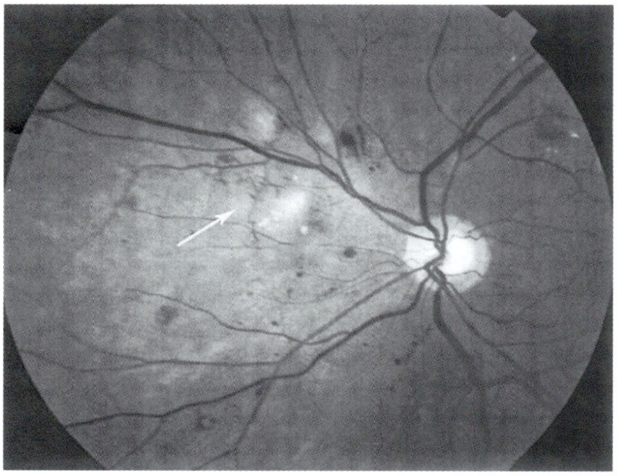

Figure 6 Intraretinal microvascular abnormalities nasal to the optic disc adjacent to cotton-wool spots. Fundus photograph (red-free illumination)

Diabetic Retinopathy and Pregnancy

Deterioration of diabetic retinopathy during pregnancy is not uncommon [17, 18]. Retinopathy, already present before pregnancy, may worsen during the second trimester, remain stable during the third, but improve postpartum.

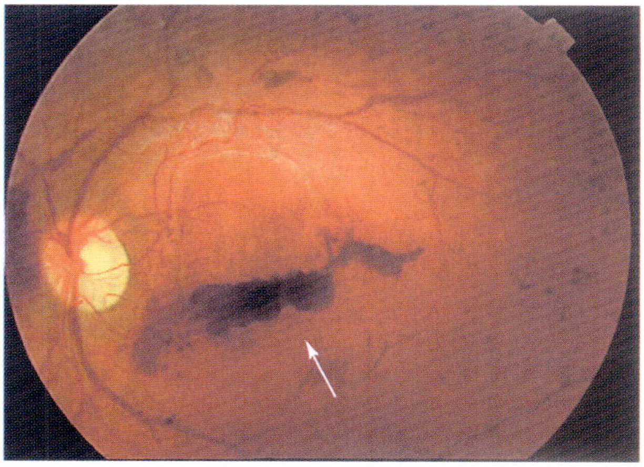

Figure 8 Preretinal hemorrhage from new vessels along the upper temporal vessel arc. Fundus photograph

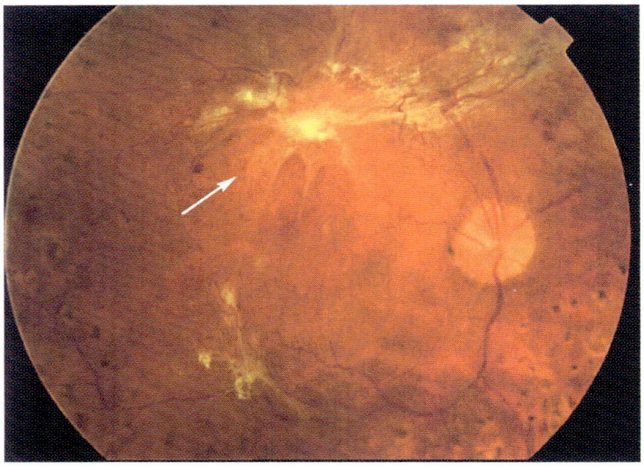

Figure 9 Fibrovascular complexes and macular traction. Fundus photograph

If the preexisting retinopathy is more pronounced, proliferative changes may occur and result in severe visual impairment. In addition, transient edema in the macular region may develop and although the edema resolves postpartum in most cases, it may persist and cause irreversible visual loss.

PATHOGENESIS

The molecular pathophysiology of diabetic retinopathy is still not fully understood. Recent advances in biomedical and genetic research have, however, substantially expanded our understanding of the underlying processes.

At the cellular level, possible factors that initiate and promote the vascular disease are hyperglycemia, the polyol pathway, nonenzymatic glycation, oxidative stress, activation of protein kinase C (PKC), and different growth and vasoactive hormones.

Several changes also take place in the retinal vasculature, which cause change of retinal blood flow, including an increase in retinal blood flow and heterogeneity of its distribution. These microvascular abnormalities can lead to areas of nonperfusion and ischemia. The retina responds to this hypoxia by increased production of vascular endothelial growth factor (VEGF), which promotes neovascularization [19].

Polyol Pathway

Aldose reductase is the first enzyme in the polyol pathway. During normal glucose concentrations the metabolism in this pathway is very slow, but is activated at the levels of hyperglycemia seen in diabetes, which results in enzymatic conversion to sorbitol, with a concomitant decrease in NADPH. Sorbitol is further oxidized to fructose by the enzyme sorbitol dehydrogenase, with NAD^+ being reduced to NADH. Increased flux through the sorbitol pathway increases osmotic pressure, decreases myoinositol concentrations, and in combination with glycolysis, alters the intracellular redox balance. Studies of inhibition of the polyol pathway *in vivo* have given conflicting results in diabetic animal models regarding inhibition of retinopathy, and since several clinical studies in humans have given negative results, the relevance of this mechanism in humans is questioned [20].

Nonenzymatic Glycation

Long-term exposure of hyperglycemia results in nonenzymatic conjunction of glucose of extracellular matrix proteins, which leads to advanced glycated end products (AGEs). AGE formation may cause pathologic changes by altering protein function in target tissues directly, signal transduction pathways involving ligands on extracellular matrix, and the gene expression through interactions with AGE-specific cellular receptors. AGE will also increase the generation of reactive oxygen species (ROS), which are capable of damaging biological macromolecules, such as DNA and carbohydrates and of causing membrane damage through lipid peroxidation [21].

Oxidative Stress

Oxidative stress is defined as an increase in the steady-state levels of ROS. Sources of ROS in diabetes include autoxidation of glucose, AGE-formation and binding of AGE to AGE receptors, increased flux through the polyol pathway, and stimulation of eicosanoid metabolism. Several endogenous enzyme-scavenging systems protect cells and tissues from ROS, like superoxide dismutases, catalase, and gluthathione peroxidase. Increased ROS could cause cellular dysfunction and induce mutations in mitochondrial DNA, and may impair endothelium-dependent vasodilation through inactivation of NO. Both altered gene expression of scavenging enzymes and overexpression of the cell death protease gene have been suggested to increase apoptosis of retinal capillary cells in diabetic retinopathy [10].

Protein Kinase C

Protein kinase C has important roles in intracellular signal transduction for hormones and cytokines. Increased activation of the diacylglycerol–PKC signal transduction pathway has been identified in vascular tissues from diabetic animals, and in vascular cells, like retinal endothelial cells, exposed to high glucose. In the retina of diabetic rats, the PKCβ isoforms exhibit the greatest increase. PKC activation regulates a number of vascular functions, such as vascular permeability, contractility, cellular proliferation, membrane synthesis, and signal transduction mechanisms for hormones and growth factors. A novel isoform specific inhibitor of PKC, Ly333531, has shown selectivity for PKCβ. In animal experiments, orally administered Ly333531 decreased the retinal mean circulation time. In diabetic rats, intravitreal injection of Ly333531 decreased retinal PKC activation, reduced retinal mean circulation time, and increased retinal blood flow to levels that were comparable to that of control group. In other studies, Ly333531 treatment of diabetic rats showed a normalization of the diabetes-induced reductions in activity of both Na^+–K^+-ATPase and Ca^+-ATPase in the retina and confirmed the involvement of PKCβ in VEGF-mediated retinal vessel permeability in rats [22]. The results from ongoing clinical studies in diabetic patients assessing potential benefits of Ly333531-interventional therapy for the progression of macular edema and retinal neovascularization associated with diabetic retinopathy will be presented in future.

Retinal Blood Flow

There is a fluctuation of retinal blood flow in diabetic patients, with a decrease in blood flow at the early stage of retinopathy and a progressive increase in blood flow in more advanced stages of retinopathy [23]. The retinal vasculature is dependent on local mechanisms for regulation of an appropriate blood flow. The most important endothelium-derived relaxing factors are NO, endothelium-derived hyperpolarizing factor, and prostacyclin. These relaxing factors are balanced by contracting factors like endothelin-1 and different cyclooxygenase products. Local glucose levels regulate these factors, and hyperglycemia leads to a decrease in relaxing and an increase in constricting factors leading to a change in retinal blood flow and heterogenity of distribution of retinal blood flow resulting in retinal ischemia [10, 24]. Other factors contribute to the development of retinal ischemia, like an increase in the synthesis of basement membrane components in the retina, which may contribute to the closure of capillaries. PKC stimulates endothelial cells, leukocytes, and platelets to produce platelet-activating factor (PAF), which stimulates PAF receptors on platelets, activating these platelets, which in turn contribute to thrombus formation. Also, activated leukocytes, which adhere more tightly to the endothelial cells, may contribute. Damage to the retinal vascular bed can lead to progressive retinal hypoxia. Chronic hypoxia induces the expression of several angiogenic factors, which results in retinal neovascularization and proliferative retinopathy. Retinal neovascularization has been observed to occur close to nonperfused areas, which supports that angiogenic factors are released from hypoxic tissues [10].

Growth Factors and Vasoactive Hormones

Diabetes induces abnormalities in the expression and actions of several growth factors that regulate retinal vasculature and are involved in the development and progression of diabetic retinopathy, like VEGF, pigment epithelium-derived factor (PEDF), and insulin-like growth factor 1 (IGF-1).

Increased levels of VEGF have been shown in the vitreous and retina of diabetic patients. This increase is probably hypoxia-induced, and VEGF protein and mRNA have been demonstrated in the ischemic retina adjacent to areas of neovascularization, both in animals and humans. VEGF also appears to play a role in the development of nonproliferative diabetic retinopathy, and is likely to initiate the increased permeability associated with the retinal vasculature in diabetes [10].

PEDF has a wide variety of functions, among them a regulator of development of retinal vasculature and inhibitor of retinal and choroidal neovascularization in a number of animal models. PEDF is downregulated by hypoxia and in eyes with proliferative retinopathy, which suggests that PEDF acts as a negative regulator of angiogenesis [10].

IGF-1 has been shown to induce endothelial cell proliferation, migration, and basement membrane degradation *in vitro*. These results have been confirmed in experimental animals, and increased levels of IGF-1 have been found in the vitreous of patients with proliferative retinopathy, indicating a localized effect of IGF-1 in the development of neovascularization [10]. Ongoing studies in diabetic patients using the somatostatin analogue octreotide will hopefully show whether growth hormone and IGF-1 play any important role in the development of retinopathy in humans.

CLASSIFICATION OF DIABETIC RETINOPATHY

Classification of diabetic retinopathy serves two main purposes. The first is to set cutoff limits for different stages of retinopathy, which can be useful in clinical research and trials. The second is to identify stages that present an immediate threat to visual acuity or that may confer a high risk for progression to those stages. Since visual impairment can be prevented by proper and timely treatment, it is particularly important for clinicians in everyday practice to recognize sight-threatening retinopathy.

In clinical trials, different scales have been developed over the years [25–27]. The scales have been used in randomized clinical trials, in which one eye of each patient was assigned to laser treatment and the other to deferral of treatment. The modified Airlie House classification identified eight levels ranging from absence of retinopathy to severe vitreous hemorrhage. The study design allowed observation of the natural course of retinopathy in the initially untreated eye, and in 1991 the Early Treatment

Table 1 Summary of the Early Treatment Diabetic Retinopathy Study final retinopathy severity scale*

Level	Severity	Definition
10	DR absent	
14–15	DR questionable	
20	Very mild NPDR	Microaneurysms only
35	Mild NPDR	Microneurysms and hemorrhages, soft exudates, and/or venous loops
43	Moderate NPDR	Microaneurysms and hemorrhages moderate in four fields, or severe in one field, or IRMA
47	Moderately severe NPDR	Two out of three level 43 characteristics and/or one of the following: microaneurysms and hemorrhages severe in two to three fields, IRMA present in four to five fields, or venous beading present in one field
53	Severe NPDR	Microaneurysms and hemorrhages severe in four to five fields, or IRMA moderate in one field, or venous beading definite in two to three fields
61	Mild PDR	Fibrous proliferations on the optic disc or elsewhere, or visible NVE
65	Moderate PDR	NVE $\geq 1/2$ disc area, or visible NVD, or vitreous or preretinal hemorrhage and NVE $< 1/2$ disc area
71–75	High-risk PDR	NVD $\geq 1/4$–$1/3$ disc area, or NVD $< 1/4$ disc area and vitreous or preretinal hemorrhage, or NVE $\geq 1/2$ disc area and vitreous or preretinal hemorrhage, or vitreous or preretinal hemorrhage obscuring ≥ 1 disc area
81–85	Advanced PDR	Fundus partially obscured by vitreous hemorrhage and/or retinal detachment
90	Cannot grade	

Note: DR = diabetic retinopathy; NPDR = nonproliferative diabetic retinopathy; PDR = proliferative retinopathy; IRMA = intraretinal microvascular abnormalities; NVD = new vessels on or within one disc diameter from the optic disc margin; NVE = new vessels elsewhere, i.e., outside one optic disc diameter from the optic disc margin.

* From reference 28.

Diabetic Retinopathy Study (ETDRS) came up with a "final retinopathy severity scale" for individual eyes [28]. Based on stereophotographs of seven defined fields, this scale divided diabetic retinopathy into 13 levels ranging from absence of retinopathy to severe vitreous hemorrhage and retinal detachment (Table 1). Since the progression rates were quite similar across baseline levels, the scale was shown to be useful for assessing change in retinopathy, at least for shorter follow-up periods, i.e. 1–3 years [28]. However, this scale is too complicated in daily practice, and to that end, a variety of simplified scales are in use all over the world. A simplified globally accepted scale would be of great value for doctors as well as for patients worldwide and facilitate the communication between general practitioners and diabetologists on one hand and ophthalmologists on the other. In 2002, the American Academy of Ophthalmology organized a workshop with ophthalmologists and endocrinologists from all over the world. This Global Diabetic Retinopathy Project Group agreed upon a simplified retinopathy scale, which characterizes five stages of diabetic retinopathy [29], corresponding to levels 10–15, 20, 35–47, 53, and $\geq$61, respectively, in the ETDRS severity scale (Table 1).

In clinical practice, it is also of importance to identify sight-threatening stages that confer a high risk for impaired visual acuity as well as those which may predict severe progression within 1–2 years, i.e., diabetic macular edema, severe nonproliferative retinopathy, and proliferative retinopathy. It is important that patients with sight-threatening retinopathy are referred to specialists in ophthalmology for proper and timely treatment.

Diabetic Macular Edema

Diabetic macular edema constitutes a severe threat to visual function, particularly in the elderly, and visual acuity impairment secondary to macular edema can rarely be restored, [30, 31]. The edema is the result of an abnormal collection of extracellular fluid in the retina due to deficient barriers in the central part of the eye. In clinical practice, thickening of the retina and hard exudates within about two disc diameters from the fovea is usually regarded as macular edema. In its prospective study of laser therapy, the ETDRS Group had a more restrict definition of macular edema, i.e., thickening of the retina within one disc diameter of the center of the macula or definite hard exudates in this region [30]. It was found, however, that visual acuity was good and did not change significantly during the 3-year follow-up period in some of those eyes, i.e. those with limited areas of retinal thickening or hard exudates away from the center of the macula. Thus a new term was created, *clinically significant macular edema* (CSME), which was defined as retinal thickening that involves or threatens the center of the macula (Figure 10), more specifically

(1) thickening of the retina at or within 500 μm of the center of the fovea;
(2) hard exudates at or within 500 μm of the center of the fovea associated with a thickening of the adjacent retina;
(3) one or more zones of thickening of the retina of at least one disc area, any part of which is within one optic disc diameter of the center of the fovea.

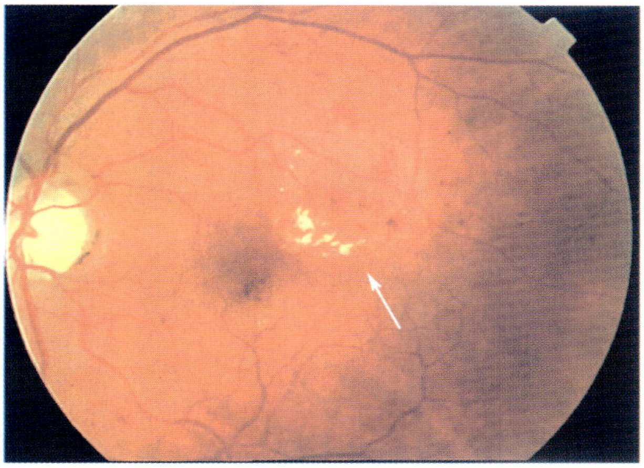

Figure 10 Clinically significant macular edema with hard exudates within 500 μm from the center of the macula in combination with a thickening of the retina. Fundus photograph

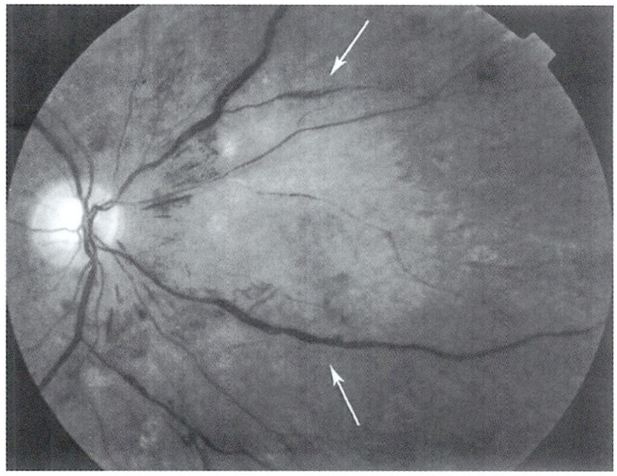

Figure 12 Venous beading. Fundus photograph (red-free illumination)

The Global Diabetic Retinopathy Project Group agreed upon three severity levels for macular edema, defined as hard exudates and/or leakage in the posterior pole, depending on the proximity to the center of the macula [29].

Severe Nonproliferative Retinopathy

Although severe nonproliferative retinopathy *per se* does not threaten visual acuity, it is important to recognize this stage because of the risk for progression to proliferative retinopathy [28]. Factors that have been identified as the most important in predicting rapid progression are

- severe intraretinal hemorrhages (in four quadrants) (Figure 11)
- venous beading (in two quadrants) (Figure 12)
- IRMA (in one quadrant) (Figure 6).

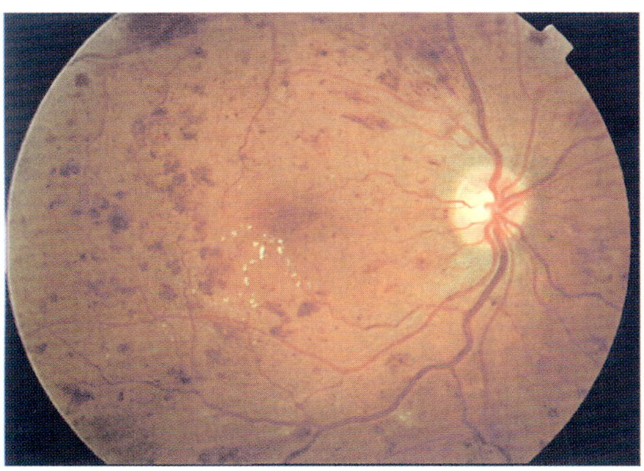

Figure 11 Severe hemorrhages. Fundus photograph

At those stages, the 1-year progression rate to proliferative retinopathy is 32%, the 3- and 5-year progression rates are 58 and 68%, respectively. Progression to severe proliferative retinopathy occurs in 14, 38, and 53%, respectively [32].

Proliferative Retinopathy

Proliferative retinopathy is asymptomatic at its early stages, but as the vessels grow and attach to the posterior capsule of the vitreous, the risk for visual acuity impact increases [33–35]. The growth rate of new vessels varies considerably. Neovascularizations may remain stable for years and even undergo spontaneous regression, whereas in some cases progression is rapid and confers a high risk for subsequent severe visual loss. Eyes with new vessels of about one-fourth disc area on or within one disc diameter from the optic disc and eyes with new vessels and preretinal or vitreous hemorrhages are at high risk [36]. More specifically, the term *high-risk proliferative diabetic retinopathy* refers to

(1) new vessels on or within one disc diameter from the optic disc covering an area of more than one fourth to one third of the optic disc area (Figure 13);
(2) new vessels on or within one disc diameter from the optic disc associated with vitreous or preretinal hemorrhage (Figure 8);
(3) new vessels separated from the optic disc by one or more disc diameters and greater than half disc area in size associated with vitreous or preretinal hemorrhage.

In those eyes, the 1-year cumulative rate of severe visual loss, defined as visual acuity less than 5/200, was

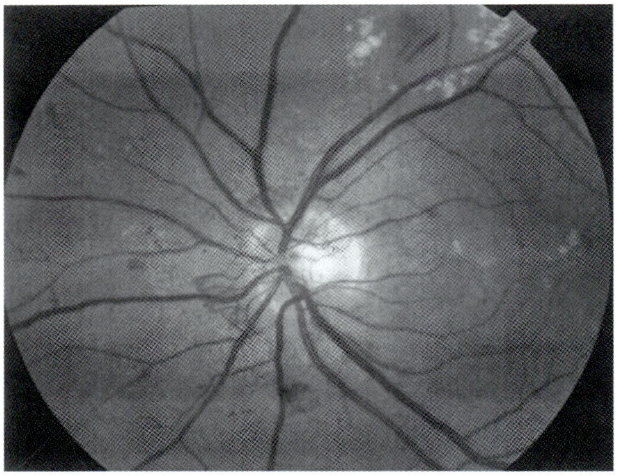

Figure 13 New vessels on the optic disc. Fundus photograph (red-free illumination)

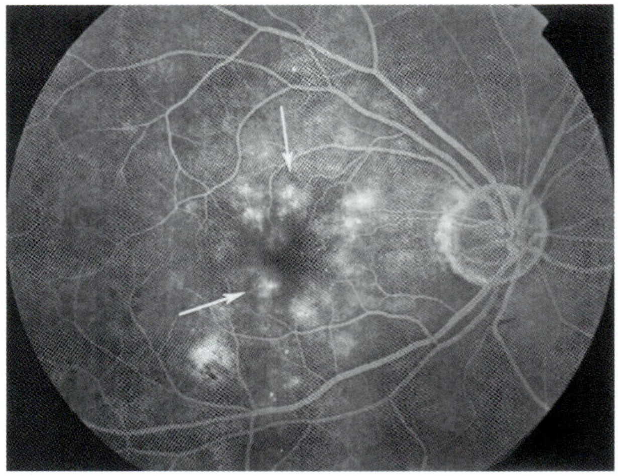

Figure 14 Focal leakage from microaneurysms. Flourescein angiogram

about 10%, and the 3- and 5-year rates about 35 and 50%, respectively [36]. Corresponding figures for proliferative retinopathy without high-risk characteristics were close to 0, 5, and 25%, respectively.

DIAGNOSTIC TOOLS

Clinical Examination and Photography

In addition to clinical examination through dilated pupils using a slit lamp and a magnifying lens or by direct ophthalmoscopy, photography tends to play an increasingly important role not only for diagnosis but also for documentation of the retinal lesions. In the Wisconsin Study [37], the eight-level classification scale was based on stereo fundus color photographs of seven 30° fields, but it was shown that for four retinopathy levels, the agreement of interpretation between seven and two to four fields was good, 91%. By using wider angles of 45–60°, improved coverage allows identification also of more peripherally located lesions, e.g. new vessels.

Stereopsis is necessary for any evaluation of thickening of the retina. If stereo fundus photography or slit lamp examination with the use of a magnifying lens is not possible to perform, patients with microaneurysms and/or hard exudates within two disc diameters from the center of the macula should be referred to an ophthalmologist.

Color photographs can be replaced by digital retinal imaging [38–42], which fully developed will facilitate transmission of retinal images to ophthalmologists or specific reading centers for interpretation [43, 44]. In the future, the present manual interpretation might even be replaced by automatic detection of retinopathy lesions [45, 46].

Fluorescein Angiography

The retinal vasculature can be further visualized by fluorescein angiography [47]. Intravenously injected sodium fluorescein bound to albumin diffuses freely through the choriocapillaris but not, under normal conditions, through the pigment epithelium or tight junctions between the endothelial cells. Fluorescein angiography is of particular importance for a qualitative assessment of diabetic macular edema. Focal spots of leakage (Figure 14) and areas of diffuse edema (Figure 15) can be identified, as well as the extension of the avascular zone (Figure 16). In addition, the fluorescein angiogram can be useful in mapping areas of nonperfusion (Figure 17) and in distinguishing between the nonleaking IRMA and leaking neovascularizations.

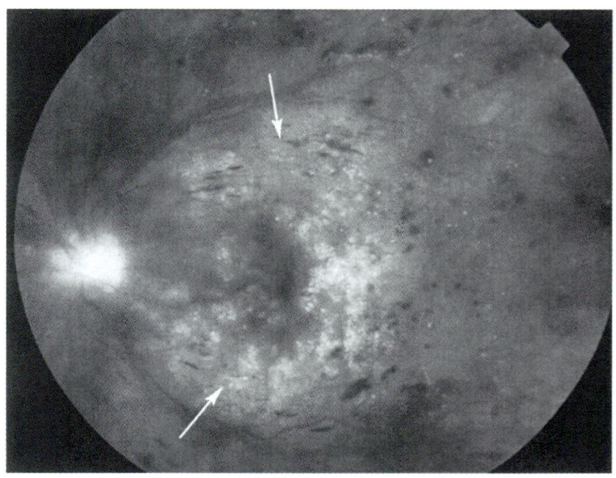

Figure 15 Diffuse leakage from dilated vessels. Fluorescein angiogram

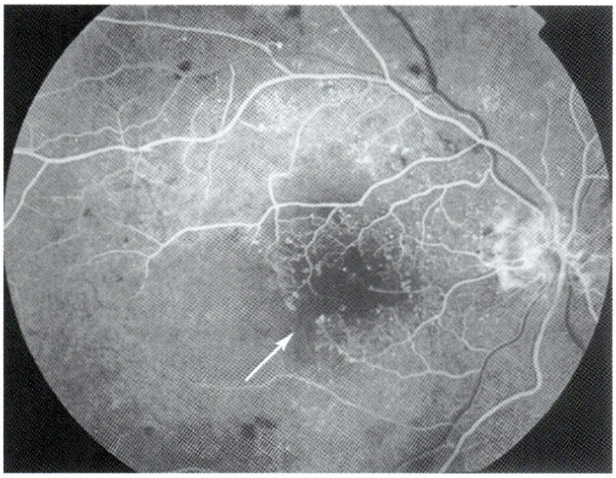

Figure 16 Increased extension of the foveal avascular zone. Fluorescein angiogram

Ultrasonography

Ultrasound has important implications in patients with ocular media opacities and diabetic vitreoretinopathy, i.e. when cataract, vitreous hemorrhages, or other media opacities hinders a thorough retinal examination [48, 49]. In such cases, contact B-scan ultrasonography (Figure 18) makes it possible to detect posterior vitreous detachment, fibrovascular membranes, and areas of focal or widespread retinal detachment.

Optical Coherence Tomography

Optical coherence tomography (OCT) is a laser-based noninvasive technique, which utilizes reflections of infrared light waves from different structures in the eye in

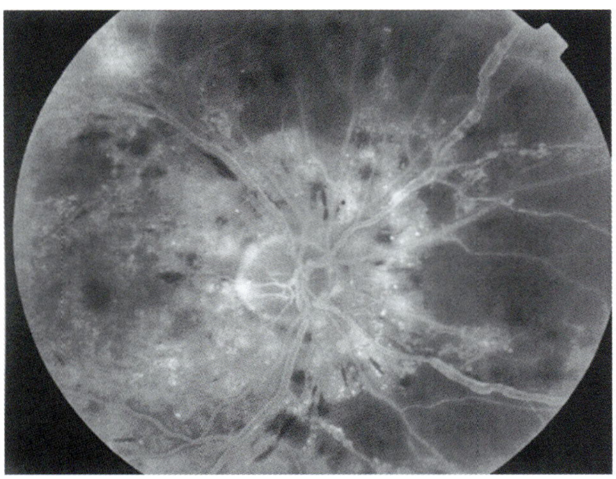

Figure 17 Extended areas of nonperfusion nasal to the optic disc. Fluorescein angiogram

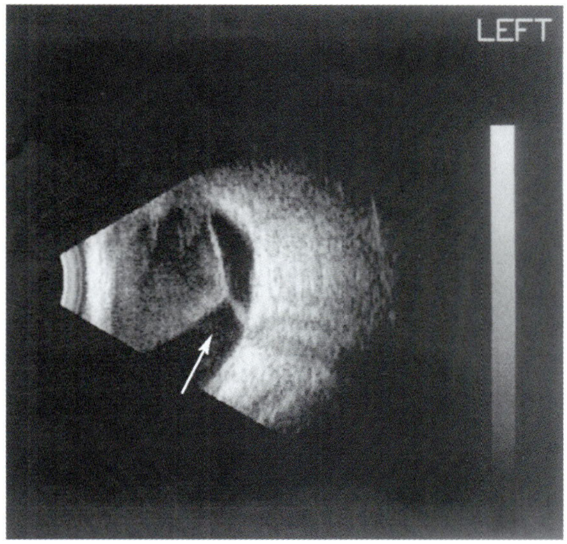

Figure 18 Vitreous hemorrhage and detachment. One cord is still attached but the underlying retina has not detached. B-scan ultrasonography

a manner similar to ultrasonography. It produces cross-sectional images of the retina in two dimensions. With a resolution of 10 μm, optical coherence tomography is an important new diagnostic tool for noninvasive high-resolution imaging of the retina and adjacent ocular tissues. The technique can visualize patterns of structural changes in macula edema [50–52] (Figures 19 and 20) and appears to be of particular value in revealing taut posterior hyaloid membranes and vitreomacular traction (Figure 20) [53]. In addition, it has been suggested as a valuable and reliable tool for monitoring retinal thickness [54–58].

PREVALENCE OF DIABETIC RETINOPATHY

The Wisconsin Epidemiologic Study of Diabetic Retinopathy [59] is the widest and most prolonged population-based ophthalmologic survey of people with diabetes. The study described the prevalence and incidence of diabetic retinopathy in two groups of individuals. One group had an age at onset of diabetes before 30 years and was on insulin, in this book chapter referred to as type 1 diabetes, and the other with an age at onset at or after 30 years, referred to as type 2 diabetes. In the latter group, those with and without insulin treatment were described separately. In individuals with type 1 diabetes, the overall prevalence of any diabetic retinopathy was 71%, of CSME 14%, and of proliferative retinopathy 23%. Corresponding frequencies for those with type 2 diabetes taking insulin were 70, 11, and 14%, respectively, and for those not taking insulin 39, 4, and 2%, respectively [59]. Higher prevalence was associated with longer duration of diabetes in all groups [60] (Figure 21). In persons with type 1

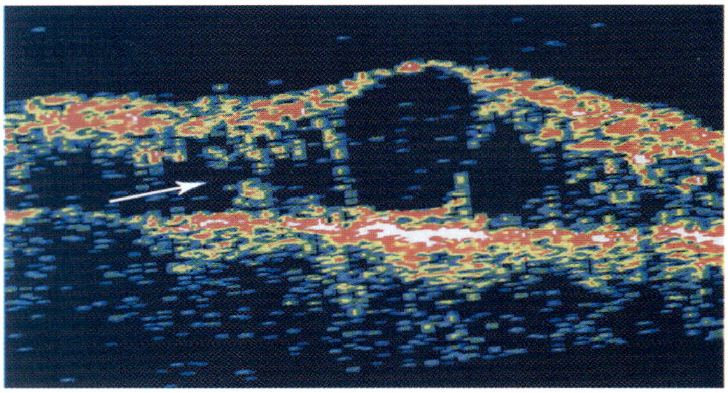

Figure 19 Cystic macular edema. A transsection of the retina visualized by optical coherence tomography

diabetes and less than 5 years of duration, the prevalence of retinopathy was about 10%, whereas it ranged from 25 to 40% in individuals with type 2 diabetes, probably due to delayed diagnosis of diabetes in this patient group. With increased duration of diabetes, the prevalence of retinopathy became more frequent, reaching nearly 100% in type 1 diabetes, 85% in patients with type 2 diabetes taking insulin, and 65% in those not taking insulin. The prevalence of macular edema (Figure 22) and proliferative retinopathy (Figure 23) also varied considerably with duration of diabetes. In the type 1 diabetes group, the rate of macular edema ranged from 0 to 20% between 2 and 35 years of diabetes, and proliferative retinopathy from 0 to 60%. Corresponding figures in the type 2 diabetes group taking insulin were 5–35% for macular edema and less than 5–30% for proliferative retinopathy. In the type 2 diabetes group not taking insulin, the prevalence of both macular edema and proliferative retinopathy reached maximum after 22 years of diabetes duration, 15 and 10%, respectively, followed by declining rates, probably due to decreasing numbers of survivors by time in this patient group.

Thus, the prevalence of diabetic retinopathy is highly correlated to the duration of diabetes. In type 1 diabetes, the rate is initially low but follows a steep curve and affects almost 100% after 25 years of diabetes. In type 2 diabetes, retinopathy is much more prevalent after only a few years of known diabetes and eventually affects the majority but not all patients. The prevalence of macular edema over time is quite similar in type 1 and type 2 diabetes, whereas the increase of proliferative retinopathy over time is considerably more pronounced in people with type 1 diabetes, particularly when compared to those not taking insulin.

MEDICAL RISK FACTORS AND SYSTEMIC TREATMENT

Blood Glucose Control

In 1982, the National Institute of Diabetes, Digestive and Kidney Diseases initiated and designed a trial to assess whether intensive treatment regimen aimed at achieving blood glucose values as close to the nondiabetic range as

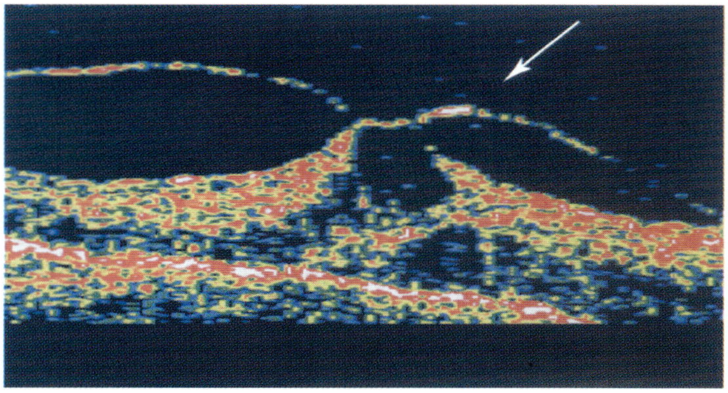

Figure 20 Vitreomacular traction from a taut posterior hyaloid membane. A transsection of the retina visualized by optical coherence tomography

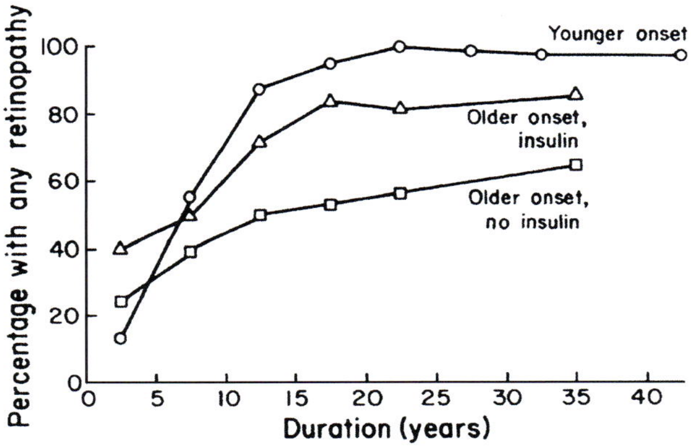

Figure 21 Percentage of persons with diabetic retinopathy by duration of diabetes in each of the three age-at-diagnosis groups. The number of persons in each duration interval in each group was at least 70, with the following exceptions: younger-onset group, 30–34 year interval, 43; younger-onset group, 35 or more years interval, 44; noninsulin-taking group, 20–24 year interval, 41; noninsulin-taking group, 25 or more year interval, 15 (from reference 60, reproduced by permission)

possible would affect the onset and progression of early retinopathy in type 1 diabetic patients compared to conventional treatment. The Diabetes Control and Complications Trial (DCCT) was started in 1983 and included 726 patients with no retinopathy and a urine albumin excretion rate of less than 40 mg/day in a primary prevention group and 715 patients with mild to moderate retinopathy (≤47/47 on the ETDRS scale) and an albumin excretion rate of 40–199 mg/day in a secondary prevention group. The primary and secondary prevention cohorts were randomized to either intensive diabetes treatment with three to four injections of insulin or insulin pump treatment and four self-monitored blood glucose tests daily, or conventional treatment with one to two injections of insulin and either urine glucose testing several times daily, or later in the study, self blood glucose testing once a day [61].

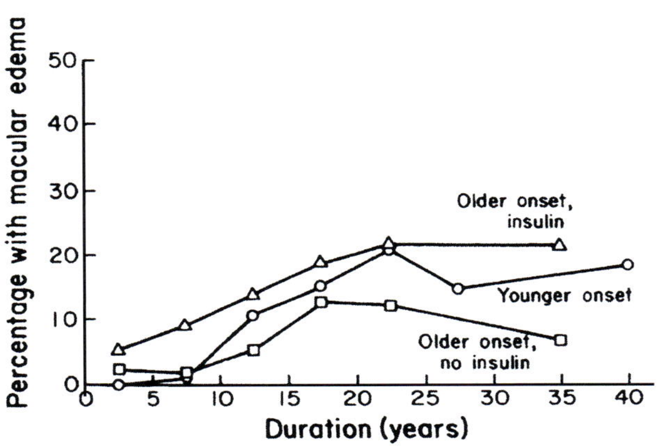

Figure 22 Percentage of persons with macular edema by duration of diabetes in each of the three age-at-diagnosis groups (from reference 60, reproduced by permission)

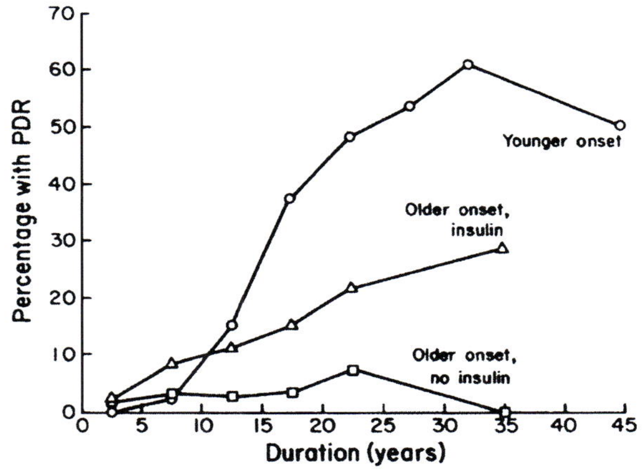

Figure 23 Percentage of persons with proliferative retinopathy by duration of diabetes in each of the three age-at-diagnosis groups (from reference 60, reproduced by permission)

The DCCT ended in 1993 after a mean follow-up of 6.5 years. Patients on intensive treatment achieved a substantially better metabolic control and maintained a median HbA_{1c} of 7.3% compared with 9.1% with conventional treatment. Intensified treatment reduced the progression of retinopathy, measured as a three-step increase on the ETDRS scale, by 76% in the primary prevention cohort and by 54% in the secondary intervention cohort, progression to severe nonproliferative diabetic retinopathy by 47%, and necessity of laser treatment by 56% [62]. Further analysis of the DCCT data has demonstrated a strong exponential relationship between the risk of retinopathy and the mean HbA_{1c} measured on a regular basis throughout the study, which was similar in the two groups, strongly supporting that lowering of blood glucose resulted in the decreased risk for retinopathy. The shorter the duration of type 1 diabetes at entry of the study, the greater were the benefits of intensive therapy. In each treatment group, the mean HbA_{1c} was the dominant predictor for progression of retinopathy, and the risk reduction was similar in the two groups, e.g. a 10% lower HbA_{1c}, i.e., from 8.0 to 7.2%, was associated with 43–45% reduced risk in both groups. No glycemic threshold was seen above the nondiabetic range, below which the risk of retinopathy was eliminated. Taken together, these results show the importance of both the duration and the glucose exposure for the development of retinopathy in type 1 diabetes [63]. Although DCCT indicated that tight control of blood glucose levels had a salutary effect on the development and progression of diabetic retinopathy in many patients, a subpopulation of diabetic subjects in the study did not benefit from tight control of blood glucose during the study period and in no case did tight control halt or reverse progression of diabetic retinopathy during the initial three-year study period. There was also evidence for that the severity of diabetic retinopathy was influenced by familial, possibly genetic factors [64], which may explain why some patients with good metabolic control developed retinopathy, while a subgroup with poor metabolic control did not [65].

At the closure of the DCCT Study in 1993, a total of 1375 of the DCCT subjects (95%) participated in an open follow-up study, the Epidemiology of Diabetes Interventions and Complications (EDIC) Research Group, to assess whether the benefits achieved during the DCCT persisted after a four-year period. All patients were offered intensified therapy and all patients were referred to their own physicians. Retinopathy was evaluated on the basis of centrally graded fundus photographs. Although the degree of metabolic control between the conventional-therapy and intensive-therapy groups were quite similar during the four-year follow-up period, $HbA1_{1c}$ 8.2% versus 7.9%, the proportion of patients who had worsening retinopathy, including proliferative retinopathy, macular edema, and need for laser treatment, was lower in the former intensive-treated group with an odds reduction of 72–87%. Even after 7 years of EDIC follow-up, the cumulative incidence of further three-step progression on the ETDRS scale from the level at the end of the DCCT was still less in the former intensive-treatment group [66]. These results indicate that hyperglycemia has long-term chronic effects on the underlying pathophysiology, and that the reduced risk of progression of retinopathy resulting from intensified therapy in patients with type 1 diabetes persists for at least four years despite increasing hyperglycemia. They also indicate that intensified therapy shall be implemented as early as possible.

The influence of metabolic control on the development and progression of retinopathy has also been investigated in type 2 diabetic patients. The United Kingdom Prospective Diabetes Study (UKPDS) enrolled 3867 newly diagnosed type 2 diabetic patients aged 48–60 years, who were randomized either to intensified treatment with sulfonylureas or insulin, or to diet alone. Endpoints for retinopathy included visual acuity <6/60 in one eye, a two-step worsening of diabetic retinopathy on the ETDRS scale, a three-line worsening of visual acuity, and an aggregate endpoint including vitreous hemorrhage, laser treatment, and cataract extraction. During a 12-year study period ending in 1998, a 0.9 percentage difference in HbA_{1c} was maintained between the groups. The improved metabolic control in the intensive-treated group was associated with a reduced risk of retinopathy worsening by 21%, laser treatment by 29%, and cataract extraction by 24%, while no differences were seen for vitreous hemorrhage and blindness in one eye [67].

Hypertension

Hypertension is a common feature in diabetic patients, and an association between hypertension and the presence and severity of diabetic retinopathy has been suggested from cross-sectional studies [68].

In the Wisconsin Study, the prevalence of hypertension in type 1 diabetic patients, defined by ongoing antihypertensive treatment or a mean blood pressure ≥160/95 mmHg (or ≥140/90 mmHg in those under 25 years) at baseline, was 17.3% and the 10-year incidence was 25.9% [69]. Hypertension is even more common in type 2 diabetic patients, and in the UKPDS, 38% of newly diagnosed patients had hypertension with a blood pressure ≥160/90 mmHg (or ≥150/85 mmHg in those on antihypertensive treatment).

In the Wisconsin epidemiologic study of diabetic retinopathy in type 1 diabetes, systolic blood pressure at baseline was related to progression to proliferative retinopathy, and diastolic blood pressure to progression of retinopathy, progression to proliferative retinopathy, and incidence of macular edema. Hypertension at baseline was associated with a 91% increase in the risk of having proliferative retinopathy develop and a 40% increased risk of having macular edema develop during the 14-year follow-up period [70]. Similar results have been found in type 2 diabetic patients. In the UKPDS, development of retinopathy was strongly associated with baseline glycemia, glycemic exposure over 6 years, and systolic blood pressure, while there was no correlation of retinopathy progression with systolic blood pressure [71]. Each 10 mmHg decrease in updated mean systolic blood pressure was associated with reductions in risk for microvascular complications (retinopathy requiring photocoagulation, vitreous hemorrhage, and fatal or nonfatal renal failure) of 10–16%, and no threshold of risk was observed [72]. In other studies, patients with hypertension have been more likely to develop diabetic retinopathy, and more severe levels of retinopathy and to have a more rapid progression of retinopathy compared to diabetic patients without hypertension [73, 74].

Most studies have shown an association between blood pressure and retinopathy. A causal relationship between hypertension and diabetic retinopathy was strongly suggested by the results from the UKPDS, in which patients were randomized to one tight and one less-tight blood pressure treatment group. The mean blood pressure in the intensive group was 144/82 mmHg compared with 154/87 mmHg in the less-tight control group. The patients were followed for a median of 8.5 years. A 37% reduction in diabetic microvascular endpoints was found, mainly due to a reduction in need for laser treatment. In the group with tight blood pressure control, there was a 34% reduction in the risk of progression of retinopathy and a 47% reduction in moderate visual acuity loss. These effects were seen independent of the degree of glycemic control. Atenolol (a β-blocker) and captopril (an ACE-inhibitor) were equally effective in reducing the risk of developing retinal microvascular complications [75].

In the Appropriate Blood Pressure Control in Diabetes (ABCD) Trial, type 2 diabetic patients with hypertension (diastolic blood pressure ≥90 mmHg) were randomized to treatment with the calcium-channel blocker nisoldipine or the ACE-inhibitor enalapril. The mean blood pressure achieved was 132/78 mmHg in the intensive group and 138/86 mmHg in the group with moderate treatment. During the 5-year follow-up period no difference between the groups was seen regarding progression of diabetic retinopathy and there was no difference in effect between nisoldipine and enalapril [76].

The EURODIAB Controlled Trial of Lisinopril in Insulin Dependent Diabetes Mellitus (EUCLID) Study investigated the effect of lisinopril on retinopathy in mainly normotensive type 1 diabetic patients. After 2 years ACE inhibition was found to be associated with a reduction in progression of retinopathy by at least one EURODIAB level. However, the placebo group had higher mean glycosylated hemoglobin than did the treated group [77]. In both the ABCD trial and the EUCLID Study, diabetic retinopathy was not the primary endpoint and the results of ongoing studies are awaited.

Taken together, the results from different studies are conflicting, but hypertension appears to be a risk factor for development and progression of diabetic retinopathy and should be controlled. So far, no specific type of antihypertensive medication has been shown to be superior in its effects.

Regardless of diabetes, patients with hypertension alone, especially systolic hypertension, may also develop retinopathy with macro- and microaneurysms, flame hemorrhages, cotton-wool spots, macular exudates, and optic disc edema [78].

Diabetic Nephropathy

The association between nephropathy and retinopathy was described in the 1954 [79], and seems to start already at the level of microalbuminuria. In a prospective study of 211 type 1 diabetic patients, the prevalence of proliferative diabetic retinopathy increased from 7% at onset of microalbuminuria to 29% 4 years after the onset of microalbuminuria compared to 3 and 8%, respectively, in patients without microalbuminuria [80]. When nephropathy progresses, proteinuria develops and has been shown to predict proliferative retinopathy [81], and 80% of patients with persistent proteinuria have proliferative diabetic retinopathy compared to 25% of those without proteinuria [82]. When nephropathy progresses to end-stage renal disease, almost all type 1 diabetic patients and two thirds of type 2 diabetic patients on dialysis have retinopathy, usually proliferative retinopathy [83]. Diabetic retinopathy is found in 85–99% of patients with type 1 diabetes and persistent proteinuria but only in 47–63% of patients with type 2 diabetes, suggesting that about 30% of proteinuria in type 2 diabetes has other causes than diabetic nephropathy [84]. Interestingly, about one third of diabetic patients with proliferative retinopathy have no signs of diabetic nephropathy, suggesting different pathogenic mechanisms [85].

Elevated Serum Lipids and Lipoproteins

The effects of serum lipids and lipoproteins on the development and progression of diabetic retinopathy have been studied mainly in cross-sectional studies. In type 1 diabetes, an association was found between more severe retinopathy and total cholesterol and high-density lipoprotein cholesterol, but not with the level of triglycerides [86]. In other cross-sectional studies, total cholesterol levels were associated with the severity of hard exudates [87], and the incidence of macular edema in type 1 diabetic patients, but not in type 2 diabetic patients [88]. Lipid modulation using statins may have an effect on microvascular outcomes, but there are no conclusive results so far. It is hoped that ongoing studies will give the answer.

Smoking

Smoking is a risk factor for progression of albuminuria and nephropathy in both type 1 and type 2 diabetes, but the effects of smoking on diabetic retinopathy are less clear. In a review on the subject, Muhlhauser concluded that the association between smoking and retinopathy remains less consistent than the association between smoking and nephropathy [89].

PHOTOCOAGULATION AND VITREO-RETINAL SURGERY

Current treatment guidelines for diabetic retinopathy are based mainly on three large prospective controlled and randomized clinical trials: The Diabetic Retinopathy Study (DRS) 1971–1978, The ETDRS 1980–1989, and the Diabetic Vitrectomy Study 1976–1983. The results of these studies are still applicable, although lasers and vitreo-retinal surgical techniques have improved considerably since then. The xenon arc lamp is no longer used for photocoagulation, modern solid-state lasers like the frequency-doubled neodymium:yttrium–aluminum garnet (Nd:YAG:green) or diode lasers will probably gradually replace the argon lasers, and instrumentation and vitreo-retinal surgical techniques have certainly been refined since the first pars-plana vitrectomy in the 1970s [90].

Photocoagulation

Photocoagulation results in the absorption of highly directional laser light by melanin in the retinal pigment epithelium and the choroid. The outcome is a conversion of light energy to heat generating an increased chorioretinal temperature [91]. Rapidly, within milliseconds, heat conduction spreads thermal energy to the overlaying transparent retina, the contiguous retinal pigment epithelium, and the choroid.

The mechanisms of the action of photocoagulation are not clear. The absorption of light in the pigment epithelium may cause a release of chemical substances, which in turn may affect the retinal vessels. It has been shown that laser treatment causes endothelial cell proliferation in the capillaries and venules of the inner retina [92, 93]. The laser burns result in loss of photoreceptors and hence a reduced thickness of the retina. This may in turn improve oxygen diffusion and decrease oxygen consumption resulting in a narrowing of dilated vessels [94]. The beneficial effect of photocoagulation would thus be improved oxygenation, a normalization of the vessel diameter and secondary, a decreased hydrostatic pressure [95]. It has also been found that panretinal photocoagulation reduces the amount of VEGF in the vitreous [19], and thereby, one of the most important drives for new vessel growth.

Photocoagulation for Macular Edema

The ETDRS demonstrated that laser photocoagulation reduced the risk of moderate and severe visual loss by about 50% for eyes with CSME but gain of visual acuity was uncommon [30, 31]. Photocoagulation, spot size 50–200 μm, was applied directly to focal fluorescein leaks of microaneurysms (Figure 24) and/or in a grid-like pattern to areas of thickened retina of diffuse fluorescein leakage (Figure 25) [96]. The ETDRS showed that photocoagulation for macular edema halts the progression of visual loss but that it rarely restores visual acuity.

The beneficial effects of laser treatment may be counteracted by damage to the retina and result in scarring

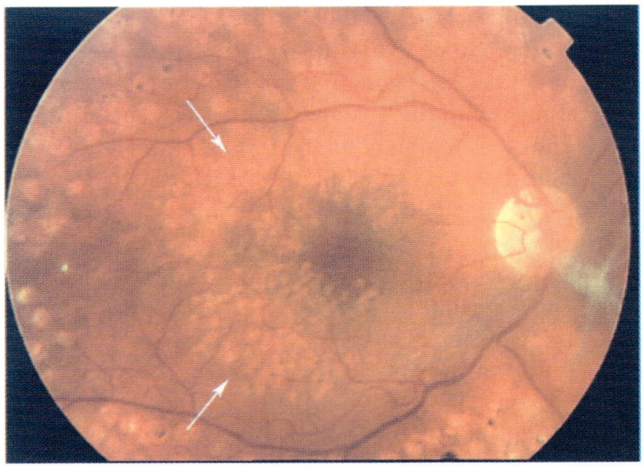

Figure 25 Laser scars above, temporal, and below the center of the macula after a grid laser treatment. Fundus photograph

caused by direct thermal injury and/or by thermal damage adjacent to treatment areas. Atrophic creep of the pigment epithelium (Figure 26), fibrosis, and neovascularization membranes [97–105] have all been described in conjunction with argon laser photocoagulation for diabetic macular edema. In order to limit retinal damage, subthreshold laser photocoagulation for CSME has been suggested. This approach aims at causing undetectable retinal burns at treatment time. Pilot studies indicate that subthreshold treatment can be successful [106–108] but so far, there are no prospective randomized clinical trials to confirm the results.

Intravitreal Injection of Steroids

In patients with diffuse macular edema resistant to photocoagulation, intravitreal steroid injections might be beneficial for improvement of visual acuity [109, 110]. However,

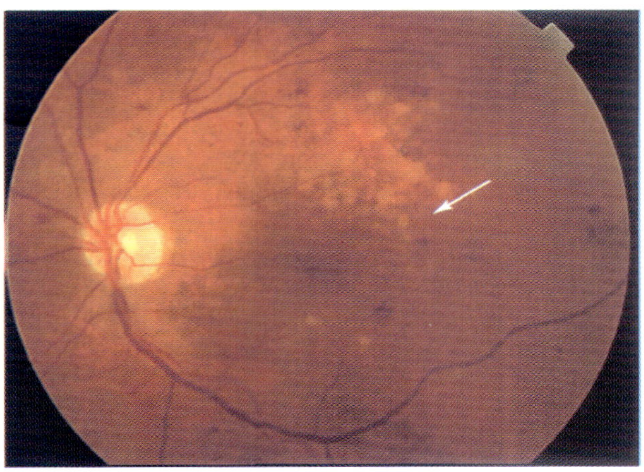

Figure 24 Laser scars above and temporal to the center of the macula after a focal laser treatment. Fundus photograph

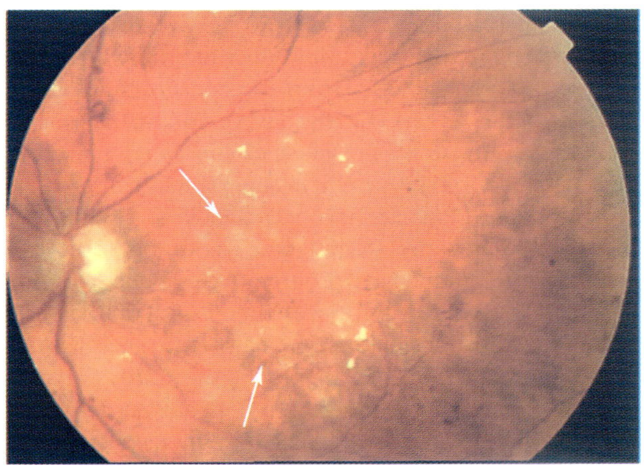

Figure 26 Atrophic laser scars as a result of creeping. Fundus photograph

results from prospective randomized trials are necessary before this treatment can be recommended.

Photocoagulation for Proliferative Diabetic Retinopathy

The DRS showed that panretinal photocoagulation reduced the rate of severe visual loss by at least 50% in patients with proliferative retinopathy and high-risk characteristics [36, 111]. Panretinal photocoagulation is generally given in two or three sessions. A total of 1200–2000 laser burns of 500 μm is usually required, and should be applied in a scattered pattern separated from each other by one burn width (Figure 27). The treatment should extend from just outside the retinal vascular arcades to or, if possible, beyond the equator in the periphery (Figure 28).

In the DRS, two types of light sources were used: a xenon arc lamp and an argon laser. The beneficial effect on visual outcome was similar for the two techniques but an adverse effect on the peripheral visual fields was more common among those in the xenon-treatment group who had a modest loss of visual field in 25% and a more severe loss in an additional 25%. Only 5% had a moderate visual loss in the argon-treatment group. The patients also noted that both treatments resulted in a prolonged dark adaptation. Since the xenon arc lamp was replaced by other light sources, side effects nowadays are considerably less common and pronounced.

Panretinal photocoagulation may worsen a preexisting macular edema [31, 112]. In case of a macular edema, focal and/or grid treatment should take place before or at the beginning of the treatment sessions [31]. Panretinal photocoagulation may also be considered for patients with severe nonproliferative retinopathy. It was shown that with this treatment approach, visual acuity could be stabilized in type 2 diabetic patients [31].

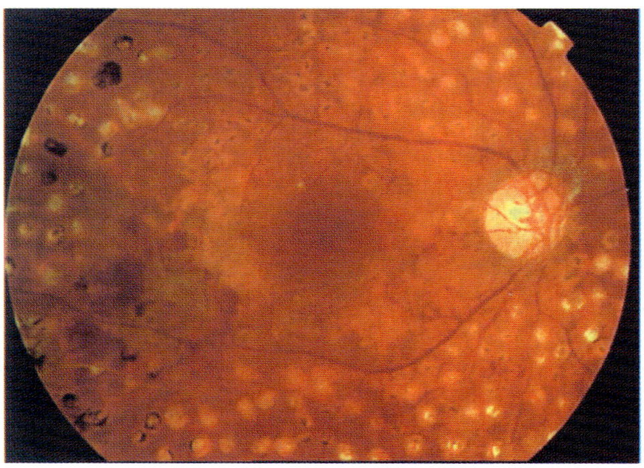

Figure 27 Laser scars after a panretinal photocoagulation

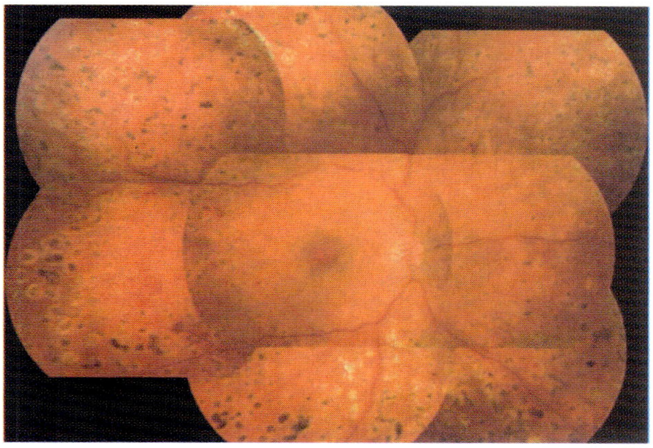

Figure 28 Panretinal photocoagulation from the vessel arcades to the periphery. Fundus photograph mosaic

Vitrectomy for Macular Edema

It is still not known whether the vitreous has a pathogenic role in the development of diabetic macular edema, but it has been suggested that an attached taut and condensed posterior hyaloid may aggravate and sustain diffuse diabetic macular edema [113]. Posterior vitreous detachment is less common in older diabetic patients with than without macular edema [114] and spontaneous resolution of edema occurs more frequently in eyes with a vitreomacular separation than in those without [115].

Visual acuity can be preserved or improved by surgical release of vitreomacular traction in nondiabetic eyes with no or incomplete posterior vitreous detachment [116]. In accordance, it has been suggested that vitrectomy and stripping of the posterior hyaloid might be beneficial in eyes with diffuse macular edema and an attached thickened and taut posterior hyaloid (Figure 20) [113, 117–119]. However, randomized prospective trials are necessary before vitrectomy can be established as a treatment for diffuse macular edema.

Vitrectomy for Proliferative Retinopathy

Panretinal photocoagulation reduces the risk for severe visual loss substantially, but in some patients new vessels and fibrovascular complexes may continue to grow despite appropriate photocoagulation, and there are still people with diabetes who for various reasons have not been offered or who actively have avoided laser treatment. In eyes with vitreous hemorrhage or tractional retinal detachment, there is a chance for visual recovery or stabilization if the opacities in the vitreous are removed and if the traction from the fibrovascular proliferations can be eliminated [120]. A randomized clinical trial [121] demonstrated that overall, 25% had a visual acuity of 20/40 or better 2 years after early vitrectomy for severe vitreous hemorrhage from proliferative retinopathy compared to 15% after deferral.

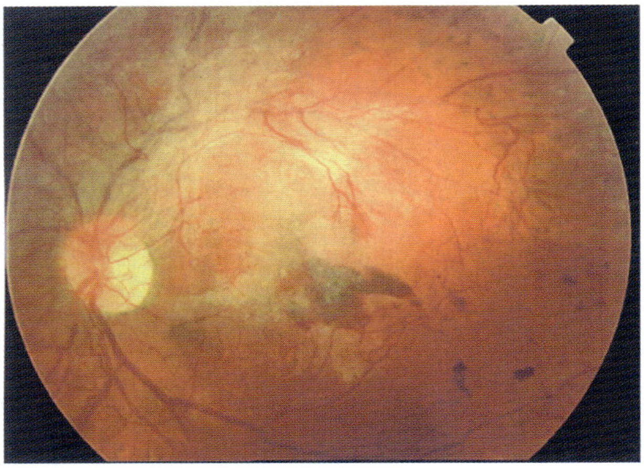

Figure 29 Fibrovascular proliferations involving the macula before vitrectomy. Fundus photograph

In type 1 diabetic patients with less than 20 years of diabetes duration, the difference was even greater, 35% versus <5%, and after 4 years of follow-up, visual acuity was 20/40 or better in 50% in the early vitrectomy group compared to 10% in the deferral group. Early vitrectomy for advanced active neovascularizations resulted in a 4-year rate of visual acuity greater than or equal to 20/40 in 44% compared to 28% for the conventionally treated group [122]. Since the 1980s, both instrumentation and surgical techniques have improved and broadened indications for vitrectomy [120]. Thus, vitreo-retinal surgery should be considered in case of severe vitreous hemorrhage showing no sign of spontaneous clearing, extensive subhyaloidal macular hemorrhage, progressive fibrovascular proliferations, tractional detachment which threatens to involve the macula (Figures 29 and 30), or traction associated with retinal tears. Side effects like recurrent vitreous hemorrhages, retinal detachment, and rubeosis iridis may occur [120].

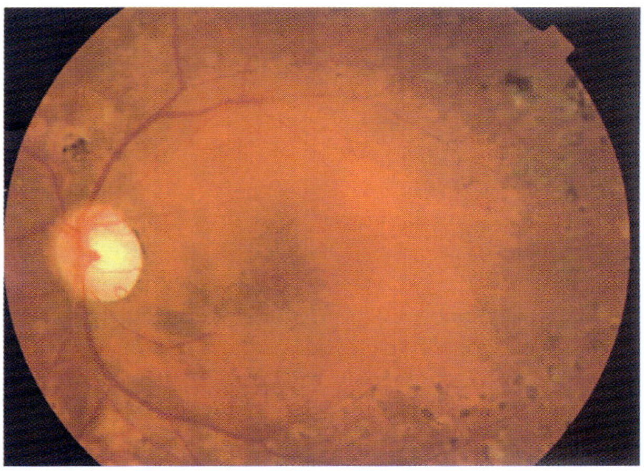

Figure 30 Photograph of the same patient as in Figure 29 after vitrectomy. Fundus photograph

SCREENING

Severe vascular changes may well be present without symptoms and visual outcome is dependent on timely photocoagulation, which ideally should be performed before visual function is affected. To that end, regular retinal examinations are important and should be available to all diabetic patients, also in the absence of retinopathy, and they are cost-effective [4, 123]. The most reliable screening test is mydriatic retinal photography [124]. Several reports from the Nordic countries in Europe have demonstrated low figures of visual impairment and blindness in regions where screening programs for early detection of sight-threatening diabetic retinopathy have been implemented successfully [123]. For patients without retinopathy, most screening protocols recommend retinal examinations with 1–2 year intervals starting at puberty in type 1 and at diagnosis of diabetes in type 2 diabetes since the duration of diabetes is most uncertain in the latter group. Recently, even 3-year intervals have been suggested for type 2 diabetic patients [125]. For patients with retinopathy, examination intervals should be individualized depending not only on the degree of retinopathy but also on medical risk factors.

REFERENCES

1. Klein R, Klein BE, Moss SE. Visual impairment in diabetes. *Ophthalmology* 1984; 91: 1–9.
2. Trautner C, Haastert B, Giani G, Berger M. Incidence of blindness in southern Germany between 1990 and 1998. *Diabetologia* 2001; 44: 147–50.
3. Moss SE, Klein R, Klein BE. The incidence of vision loss in a diabetic population. *Ophthalmology* 1988; 95: 1340–8.
4. Porta M, Bandello F. Diabetic retinopathy. A clinical update. *Diabetologia* 2002; 45: 1617–34.
5. Gardner TW, Antonetti DA, Barber AJ, LaNoue KF, Levison SW, and The Penn State Retina Research Group. Diabetic retinopathy: more than meets the eye. *Surv Ophthalmol* 2002; 47 (suppl): 253–62.
6. Engerman RL. Pathogenesis of diabetic retinopathy. *Diabetes* 1989; 38: 1203–6.
7. Engerman RL, Kern TS. Retinopathy in animal models of diabetes. *Diabetes Metab Rev* 1995; 11: 109–20.
8. Garner A. Histopathology of diabetic retinopathy in man. *Eye* 1993; 7: 250–3.
9. Antcliff RJ, Marshall J. The pathogenesis of edema in diabetic maculopathy. *Semin Ophthalmol* 1999; 14: 223–32.
10. Cai J, Boulton M. The pathogenesis of diabetic retinopathy: old concepts and new questions. *Eye* 2002; 16: 242–60.
11. Bek T. Glial cell involvement in vascular occlusion of diabetic retinopathy. *Acta Ophthalmol Scand* 1997; 75: 239–43.

12. Kristinsson JK, Gottfredsdottir MS, Stefansson E. Retinal vessel dilatation and elongation precedes diabetic macular oedema. *Br J Ophthalmol* 1997; 81: 274–8.
13. Bresnick GH. Diabetic maculopathy. A critical review highlighting diffuse macular edema. *Ophthalmology* 1983; 90: 1301–17.
14. Ohira A, de Juan E Jr. Characterization of glial involvement in proliferative diabetic retinopathy. *Ophthalmologica* 1990; 201: 187–95.
15. Davis MD. Vitreous contraction in proliferative diabetic retinopathy. *Arch Ophthalmol* 1965; 74: 741–51.
16. Gartner S, Henkind P. Neovascularization of the iris (rubeosis iridis) [review]. *Surv Ophthalmol* 1978; 22: 291–312.
17. Best RM, Chakravarthy U. Diabetic retinopathy in pregnancy. *Br J Ophthalmol* 1997; 81: 249–51.
18. Soubrane G, Coscas G. Influence of pregnancy on the evolution of diabetic retinopathy. *Int Ophthalmol Clin* 1998; 38: 187–94.
19. Aiello LP, Avery RL, Arrigg PG, Keyt BA, Jampel HD, Shah ST, Pasquale LR, Thieme H, Iwamoto MA, Park JE, Nguyen HV, Aiello LM, Ferrara N, King GL. Vascular endothelial growth factor in ocular fluid of patients with diabetic retinopathy and other retinal disorders. *N Engl J Med* 1994; 331: 1480–7.
20. Sorbinil Retinopathy Trial Research Group. A randomised trial of sorbinil, an aldose reductase inhibitor, in diabetic retinopathy. *Arch Ophthalmol* 1990; 108: 1234–44.
21. Brownlee M. Biochemistry and molecular cell biology of diabetic complications. *Nature* 2001; 414: 813–20.
22. Way KJ, Katai N, King GL. Protein kinase C and the development of diabetic vascular complications. *Diabet Med* 2001; 18: 945–59.
23. Clermont AC, Aiello LP, Mori F, Aiello LM, Bursell SE. Vascular endothelial growth factor and severity of nonproliferative diabetic retinopathy mediate retinal hemodynamics in vivo: a potential role for vascular endothelial growth factor in the progression of nonproliferative retinopathy. *Am J Ophthalmol* 1997; 124: 433–46.
24. Alder VA, Su EN, Yu DY, Cringle S, Yu PY. Overview of studies on metabolic and vascular regulatory changes in early diabetic retinopathy. *Aust N Z J Ophthalmol* 1998; 26: 141–8.
25. Davis MD, Norton EWD, Myers FL. The Airlie House classification of diabetic retinopathy. In Goldberg MF, Fine SL (eds), *Symposium on the Treatment of Diabetic Retinopathy*. Washington, DC, 1969; pp 7–22. USPHS Publication No. 1890.
26. Diabetic Retinopathy Study Research Group. A modification of the Airlie House classification of diabetic retinopathy. DRS Report Number 7. *Invest Ophthalmol Vis Sci* 1981; 21: 210–26.
27. Early Treatment Diabetic Retinopathy Study Research Group. Grading diabetic retinopathy from stereoscopic color fundus photographs: an extension of the modified Airlie House classification. ETDRS Report Number 10. *Ophthalmology* 1991; 98 (suppl): 786–806.
28. Early Treatment Diabetic Retinopathy Study Research Group. Fundus photographic risk factors for progression of diabetic retinopathy. ETRDS Report Number 12. *Ophthalmology* 1991; 98: 823–33.
29. Wilkinson CP, Ferris FL III, Klein RE, Lee PP, Agardh CD, Davis M, Dills D, Kampik A, Pararajasegaram R, Verdaguer JT. International clinical diabetic retinopathy and diabetic macular edema disease severity scales. *Ophthalmology* 2003; 110: 1677–82.
30. Early Treatment Diabetic Retinopathy Study Research Group. Photocoagulation for diabetic macular edema. ETDRS Report Number 1. *Arch Ophthalmol* 1985; 103: 1796–806.
31. Early Treatment Diabetic Retinopathy Study Research Group. Early photocoagulation for diabetic retinopathy: ETDRS Report Number 9. *Ophthalmology* 1991; 98: 766–85.
32. Davis MD, Fisher MR, Gangnon RE, Barton F, Aiello LM, Chew EY, Ferris FL III, Knatterud GL. Risk factors for high-risk proliferative diabetic retinopathy and severe visual loss. Early Treatment Diabetic Retinopathy Study (ETDRS) Report Number 18. *Invest Ophthalmol Vis Sci* 1998; 39: 233–52.
33. Beetham WP. Visual prognosis of proliferating diabetic retinopathy. *Br Ophthalmol J* 1963; 47: 611–9.
34. Spencer R, McMeel JW, Franks EP. Visual outcome in moderate and severe proliferative diabetic retinopathy. *Arch Ophthalmol* 1981; 99: 1551–4.
35. Diabetic Retinopathy Vitrectomy Study Research Group. Two-year course of visual acuity in severe proliferative diabetic retinopathy with conventional treatment. DRVS Report Number 1. *Ophthalmology* 1985; 92: 492–502.
36. Diabetic Retinopathy Study Research Group. Photocoagulation treatment of proliferative diabetic retinopathy. Clinical application of Diabetic Retinopathy Study (DRS) findings. DRS Report Number 8. *Ophthalmology* 1981; 88: 583–600.
37. Moss SE, Meuer SM, Klein R, Hubbard LD, Brothers RJ, Klein BE. Are seven standard photographic fields necessary for classification of diabetic retinopathy? *Invest Ophthalmol Vis Sci* 1989; 30: 823–8.
38. Bursell SE, Cavallerano JD, Cavallerano AA, et al. Stereo nonmydriatic digital-video color retinal imaging compared with Early Treatment Diabetic Retinopathy Study seven standard field 35-mm stereo color photos for determining level of diabetic retinopathy. *Ophthalmology* 2001; 108: 572–85.
39. Tennant MT, Greve MD, Rudnisky CJ, Hillson TR, Hinz BJ. Identification of diabetic retinopathy by sterescopic digital imaging via teleophthalmology: a comparison to slide film. *Can J Ophthalmol* 2001; 36: 187–96.
40. Gomez-Ulla F, Fernandez MI, Gonzalez F, Rey P, Rodriguez M, Rodriguez-Cid MJ, Casanueva FF, Tome MA, Garcia-Tobio J, Gude F. Digital retinal images and teleophthalmology for detecting and grading diabetic retinopathy. *Diabetes Care* 2002; 25: 1384–9.
41. Fransen SR, Leonard-Martin TC, Feuer WJ, Hildebrand PL, and the Inoveon Health Research Group. Clinical evaluation of patients with diabetic retinopathy: accuracy of the Inoveon Diabetic Retinopathy-3DT system. *Ophthalmology* 2002; 109: 595–601.
42. Lin DY, Blumenkranz MS, Brothers RJ, Grosvenor DM. The sensitivity and specificity of single-field nonmydriatic monochromatic digital fundus photography with remote image interpretation for diabetic retinopathy screening: a comparison with ophthalmoscopy and standardized mydriatic color photography. *Am J Ophthalmol* 2002; 134: 204–13.
43. Lamminen H, Ruohonen K. Fundus imaging and the telemedical management of diabetes. *J Telemed Telecare* 2002; 8: 255–8.
44. Liesenfeldt B, Kohner E, Piehlmeier W, Kluthe S, Aldington S, Porta M, Bek T, Obermaier M, Mayer H,

Mann G, Holle R, Hepp KD. A telemedical approach to the screening of diabetic retinopathy: digital fundus photography. *Diabetes Care* 2000; 23: 345–8.

45. Teng T, Lefley M, Claremont D. Progress towards automated diabetic ocular screening: a review of image analysis and intelligent systems for diabetic retinopathy. *Med Biol Eng Comput* 2002; 40: 2–13.
46. Larsen M, Godt J, Larsen N, Lund-Andersen H, Sjolie AK, Agardh E, Kalm H, Grunkin M, Owens DR. Automated detection of fundus photographic red lesions in diabetic retinopathy. *Invest Ophthalmol Vis Sci* 2003; 44: 761–6.
47. Cunha-Vaz JG. Studies on the pathophysiology of diabetic retinopathy. The blood–retinal barrier in diabetes. *Diabetes* 1983; 32 (suppl 2): 20–7.
48. McLeod D, Restori M. Ultrasonic examination in severe diabetic eye disease. *Br J Ophthalmol* 1979; 63: 533–8.
49. Jalkh AE, Avila MP, El-Markabi H, Trempe CL, Schepens CL. Immersion A- and B-scan ultrasonography. Its use in preoperative evaluation of diabetic vitreous hemorrhage. *Arch Ophthalmol* 1984; 102: 686–90.
50. Baumal CR. Clinical applications of optical coherence tomography. *Curr Opin Ophthalmol* 1999; 10: 182–8.
51. Otani T, Kishi S, Maruyama Y. Patterns of diabetic macular edema with optical coherence tomography. *Am J Ophthalmol* 1999; 127: 688–93.
52. Imai M, Iijima H, Hanada N. Optical coherence tomography of tractional macular elevations in eyes with proliferative diabetic retinopathy. *Am J Ophthalmol* 2001; 132: 458–61.
53. Kaiser PK, Riemann CD, Sears JE, Lewis H. Macular traction detachment and diabetic macular edema associated with posterior hyaloidal traction. *Am J Ophthalmol* 2001; 131: 44–9.
54. Hee MR, Puliafito CA, Duker JS, Reichel E, Coker JG, Wilkins JR, Schuman JS, Swanson EA, Fujimoto JG. Topography of diabetic macular edema with optical coherence tomography. *Ophthalmology* 1998; 105: 360–70.
55. Rivellese M, George A, Sulkes D, Reichel E, Puliafito C. Optical coherence tomography after laser photocoagulation for clinically significant macular edema. *Ophthalmic Surg Lasers* 2000; 31: 192–7.
56. Massin P, Vicaut E, Haouchine B, Erginay A, Paques M, Gaudric A. Reproducibility of retinal mapping using optical coherence tomography. *Arch Ophthalmol* 2001; 119: 1135–42.
57. Sanchez-Tocino H, Alvarez-Vidal A, Maldonado MJ, Moreno-Montanes J, Garcia-Layana A. Retinal thickness study with optical coherence tomography in patients with diabetes. *Invest Ophthalmol Vis Sci* 2002; 43: 1588–94.
58. Goebel W, Kretzchmar-Gross T. Retinal thickness in diabetic retinopathy: a study using optical coherence tomography (OCT). *Retina* 2002; 22: 759–67.
59. Klein R, Klein BE, Moss SE. The Wisconsin epidemiological study of diabetic retinopathy: a review. *Diabetes Metab Rev* 1989; 5: 559–70.
60. Klein R, Davis MD, Moss SE, Klein BEK, DeMets DL. The Wisconsin epidemiologic study of diabetic retinopathy: a comparison of retinopathy in younger and older onset diabetic persons. In Vranic M, Hollenberg C, Steiner G (eds), *Comparison of Type I and II Diabetes*. New York: Plenum, 1985; pp 321–5.
61. The Diabetes Control and Complications Trial (DCCT) Research Group. Design and methodological considerations for the feasibility phase. *Diabetes* 1986; 35: 530–45.
62. The DCCT Research Group. The effect of intensive treatment of diabetes on the development and progression of long-term complications in insulin-dependent diabetes mellitus. *N Engl J Med* 1993; 329: 977–86.
63. The Writing team for the Diabetes Control and Complications Trial/Epidemiology of Diabetes Interventions and Complications Research Group. Effect of intensive theraphy on the microvascular complications of type 1 diabetes mellitus. *JAMA* 2002; 287: 2563–9.
64. The DCCT Research Group. Clustering of long-term complications in families in the diabetes control and complications trial. *Diabetes* 1997; 46: 1829–39.
65. Zhang LY, Krzentowski G, Albert A, Lefebvre PJ. Risk of developing retinopathy in diabetes control and complications trial type 1 diabetic patients with good or poor metabolic control. *Diabetes Care* 2001; 24: 1275–9.
66. The Diabetes Control and Complications Trial/ Epidemiology of Diabetes Interventions and Complications Research Group. Retinopathy and nephropathy in patients with type 1 diabetes four years after a trial of intensive therapy. *N Engl J Med* 2000; 342: 381–9.
67. The UKPDS Group. Intensive blood-glucose control with sulphonylureas or insulin compared with conventional treatment and risk of complications in patients with type 2 diabetes (UKPDS 33). *Lancet* 1998; 352: 837–53.
68. Klein R, Klein BEK. Blood pressure control and diabetic retinopathy. *Br J Ophthalmol* 2002; 86: 365–7.
69. Klein R, Klein BE, Lee KE, Cruickshanks KJ, Moss SE. The incidence of hypertension in insulin-dependent diabetes. *Arch Intern Med* 1996; 156: 622–7.
70. Klein R, Klein BEK, Moss SE, Cruickshanks KJ. The Wisconsin epidemiologic study of diabetic retinopathy, XVII: The 14-year incidence and progression of diabetic retinopathy and associated risk factors in type 1 diabetes. *Ophthalmology* 1998; 105: 1801–15.
71. Stratton IM, Kohner EM, Aldington SJ, Turner RC, Holman RR, Manley SE, Matthews DR, for the UK Prospective Diabetes Study Group. UKPDS 50: Risk factors for incidence and progression of retinopathy in type II diabetes over 6 years from diagnosis. *Diabetologia* 2001; 44: 156–63.
72. Adler AI, Stratton IM, Neil HA, Yudkin JS, Matthews DR, Cull CA, Wright AD, Turner RC, Holman RR. Association of systolic blood pressure with macrovascular and microvascular complications of type 2 diabetes (UKPDS 36): prospective observational study. *BMJ* 2000; 321: 412–19.
73. Marshall G, Garg SK, Jackson WE, Holmes DL, Chase HP. Factors influencing the onset and progression of diabetic retinopathy in subjects with insulin-dependent diabetes mellitus. *Ophthalmology* 1993; 100: 1133–9.
74. Agardh E, Tallroth G, Bauer B, Cavallin-Sjöberg U, Agardh CD. Retinopathy and nephropathy in insulin-dependent diabetics: an inconsistent relationship? *Diabet Med* 1987; 4: 248–50.
75. The UKPDS Group. Tight blood pressure control and risk of macrovascular and microvascular complications in type 2 diabetes (UKPDS 38). *BMJ* 1998; 317: 703–13.
76. Estacio RO, Jeffers BW, Gifford N, Schrier RW. Effect of blood pressure control on diabetic microvascular complications in patients with hypertension and type 2 diabetes. *Diabetes Care* 2000; 23 (suppl 2): B54–64.
77. Chaturverdi N, Sjolie AK, Stephenson JM, Abrahamian H, Keipes M, Castellarin A, Rogulja-Pepeonik Z, Fuller J, and the EUCLID Study Group. Effect of lisinopril on

progression of retinopathy in normotensive people with type 1 diabetes. *Lancet* 1998; 351: 28–31.

78. Yu T, Mitchell P, Berry G, Li W, Wang JJ. Retinopathy in older persons without diabetes and its relationship to hypertension. *Arch Ophthalmol* 1998; 116: 83–9.
79. Root HF, Pote WH, Frehner H. Triopathy of diabetes: a consequence of neuropathy, retinopathy and nephropathy. *Arch Intern Med* 1954; 94: 931–41.
80. Mathiesen ER, Ronn B, Storm B, Foght H, Deckert T. The natural course of microalbuminuria in insulin-dependent diabetes: a 10-year prospective study. *Diabet Med* 1995; 12: 482–7.
81. Klein R, Moss SE, Klein BE. Is gross proteinuria a risk factor for the incidence of proliferative diabetic retinoparhy? *Ophthalmology* 1993; 100: 1140–6.
82. Krolewski AS, Warram JH, Rand LI, Christlieb AR, Busick EJ, Kahn CR. Risk of proliferative diabetic retinopathy in juvenile-onset type I diabetes: a 40-yr follow-up study. *Diabetes Care* 1986; 9: 443–52.
83. Watanabe Y, Yuzawa Y, Mizumuto D, Tamai H, Itoh Y, Kumons S, Yamazaki C. Long-term follow-up study of 268 diabetic patients undergoing haemodialysis, with special attention to visual acuity an heterogeneity. *Nephrol Dial Transplant* 1993; 8: 725–34.
84. Parving HH, Gall MA, Skott P, Jorgensen HE, Lokkegaard H, Jorgensen F, Nielsen B, Larsen S. Prevalence and causes of albuminuria in non-insulin-dependent diabetic patients. *Kidney Int* 1992; 41: 758–62.
85. Agardh CD, Agardh E, Torffvit O. The association between retinopathy, nephropathy, cardiovascular disease and long-turn metabolic control in type 1 diabetes: a 5 year follow-up study of 442 adult patients in routine care. *Diabetes Res Clin Pract* 1997; 35: 113–21.
86. Larsson LI, Alm A, Lithner F, Dahlén G, Bergström R. The association of hyperlipidemia with retinopathy in diabetic patients aged 15–50 yeras in the county of Umeå. *Acta Ophthalmol Scand* 1999; 77: 585–91.
87. Klein BE, Moss SE, Klein R, Surawicz TS. The Wisconsin epidemiologic study of diabetic retinopathy, XIII: Relationship of serum cholesterol to retinopathy and hard exudate. *Ophthalmology* 1991; 98: 1261–5.
88. El-Asrar AM, Al-Rubeaan KA, Al-Amro SA, Kangave D, Moharram OA. Risk factors for diabetic retinopathy among Saudi diabetics. *Int Ophthalmol* 1998; 22: 155–61.
89. Muhlhauser I. Cigarette smoking and diabetes: an update. *Diabet Med* 1994; 11: 336–43.
90. Machemer R, Buettner H, Norton EW, Parel JM. Vitrectomy: a pars plana approach. *Trans Am Acad Ophthalmol Otolaryngol* 1971; 75: 813–20.
91. Mainster MA. Decresing retinal photocoagulation damage: principles and techniques. *Semin Ophthalmol* 1999; 14: 200–9.
92. Marshall J, Clover G, Rothery S. Some new findings on retinal irradiation by krypton and argon lasers. *Doc Ophthalmol Proc Ser* 1984; 36: 21–37.
93. Clover GM. The effects of argon and krypton photocoagulation on the retina: implications for the inner and outer blood retinal barriers. In Gitter KA, Schatz H, Yannuzzi LA, McDonald HR (eds), *Laser Photocoagulation of Retinal Disease*. San Fransisco: Pacific Medical Press, 1988; pp 11–7.
94. Gottfredsdottir MS, Stefansson E, Jonasson F, Gislason I. Retinal vasoconstriction after laser treatment for diabetic macular edema. *Am J Ophthalmol* 1993; 115: 64–7.
95. Stefànsson E. The therapeutic effects of retinal laser treatment and vitrectomy. A theory based on oxygen and vascular physiology. *Acta Ophthalmol Scand* 2001; 79: 435–40.
96. Early Treatment Diabetic Retinopathy Study Research Group. Treatment techniques and clinical guidelines for photocoagulation of diabetic macular edema. ETDRS Report Number 2. *Ophthalmology* 1987; 94: 761–74.
97. Lewen RM. Subretinal neovascularization complicating laser photocoagulation of diabetic maculopathy. *Ophthalmic Surg* 1988; 19: 734–7.
98. Varley MP, Frank E, Purnell EW. Subretinal neovasularization after focal argon laser for diabetic macular edema. *Ophthalmology* 1988; 95: 567–73.
99. Lewis H, Schachat AP, Haimann MH, et al. Choroidal neovascularization after laser photocoagulation for diabetic macular edema. *Ophthalmology* 1990; 97: 503–10.
100. Schatz H, Madeira D, McDonald HR, Johnson RN. Progressive enlargement of laser scars following grid laser photocoagulation for diffuse diabetic macular edema. *Arch Ophthalmol* 1991; 109: 1549–51.
101. Guyer DR, D'Amico DJ, Smith CW. Subretinal fibrosis after laser photocoagulation for diabetic macular edema. *Am J Ophthalmol* 1992; 113: 652–6.
102. Han DP, Mieler WF, Burton TC. Submacular fibrosis after photocoagulation for diabetic macular edema. *Am J Ophthalmol* 1992; 113: 513–21.
103. Rutledge BK, Wallow IH, Poulsen GL. Sub-pigment epithelial membranes after photocoagulation for diabetic macular edema. *Arch Ophthalmol* 1993; 111: 608–13.
104. Fong DS, Segal PP, Myers F, Ferris FL, Hubbard LD, Davis MD. Subretinal fibrosis in diabetic macular edema. ETDRS Report Number 23. *Arch Ophthalmol* 1997; 115: 873–7.
105. Lovestam-Adrian M, Agardh E. Photocoagulation of macular oedema—complications and visual outcome. *Acta Ophthalmol Scand* 2000; 78: 667–71.
106. Akduman L, Olk RJ. Subthreshold (invisible) modified grid diode laser photocoagulation in diffuse diabetic macular edema (DDME). *Ophthalmic Surg Lasers* 1999; 30: 706–14.
107. Moorman CM, Hamilton AM. Clinical applications of the MicroPulse diode laser. *Eye* 1999; 13: 145–50.
108. Roider J. Laser treatment of retinal diseases by subthreshold laser effects. *Semin Ophthalmol* 1999; 14: 19–26.
109. Martidis A, Duker JS, Greenberg PB, Rogers AH, Puliafito CA, Reichel E, Baumal C. Intravitreal triamcinolone for refractory diabetic macular edema. *Ophthalmology* 2002; 109: 920–7.
110. Jonas JB, Kreissig I, Sofker A, Degenring RF. Intravitreal injection of triamcinolone for diffuse diabetic macular edema. *Arch Ophthalmol* 2003; 121: 57–61.
111. Diabetic Retinopathy Study Research Group. Photocoagulation treatment of proliferative diabetic retinopathy: the second report of Diabetic Retinopathy Study (DRS) findings. *Ophthalmology* 1978; 85: 82–106.
112. Ferris FL III, Podgor MJ, Davis MD. Macular edema in diabetic retinopathy study patients. DRS Report Number 12. *Ophthalmology* 1987; 94: 754–60.
113. Pendergast SD. Vitrectomy for diabetic macular edema associated with a taut premacular posterior hyaloid. *Curr Opin Ophthalmol* 1998; 9: 71–5.
114. Nasrallah FP, Jalkh AE, Van Coppenolle F, Kado M, Trempe CL, McMeel JW, Schepens CL. The role of

the vitreous in diabetic macular edema. *Ophthalmology* 1988; 95: 1335–9.

115. Hikichi T, Fujio N, Akiba J, Azuma Y, Takahashi M, Yoshida A. Association between the short-term natural history of diabetic macular edema and the vitreomacular relationship in type II diabetes mellitus. *Ophthalmology* 1997; 104: 473–8.
116. McDonald HR, Johnson RN, Schatz H. Surgical results in the vitreomacular traction syndrome. *Ophthalmology* 1994; 101: 1397–402.
117. Lewis H, Abrams GW, Blumenkranz MS, Campo RV. Vitrectomy for diabetic macular traction and edema associated with posterior hyaloidal traction. *Ophthalmology* 1992; 99: 753–9.
118. Harbour JW, Smiddy WE, Flynn HW Jr, Rubsamen PE. Vitrectomy for diabetic macular edema associated with a thickened and taut posterior hyaloid membrane. *Am J Ophthalmol* 1996; 121: 405–13.
119. Pendergast SD, Hassan TS, Williams GA, Cox MS, Margherio RR, Ferrone PJ, Garretson BR, Trese MT. Vitrectomy for diffuse diabetic macular edema associated with a taut premacular posterior hyaloid. *Am J Ophthalmol* 2000; 130: 178–86.
120. Smiddy WE, Flynn HW. Vitrectomy in the management of diabetic retinopathy. *Surv Ophthalmol* 1999; 43: 491–507.
121. Diabetic Retinopathy Vitrectomy Study Research Group. Early vitrectomy for severe vitreous hemorrhage in diabetic retinopathy. Four-year results of a randomized trial. DRVS Report Number 5. *Arch Ophthalmol* 1990; 108: 958–64.
122. Diabetic Retinopathy Vitrectomy Study Research Group. Early vitrectomy for severe proliferative diabetic retinopathy in eyes with useful vision. Results of a randomized trial. DRVS Report Number 3. *Ophthalmology* 1988; 95: 1307–20.
123. Stefànsson E, Bek T, Porta M, Larsen N, Kristinsson JK, Agardh E. Screening and prevention of diabetic blindness. *Acta Ophthalmol Scand* 2000; 78: 374–85.
124. Hutchinson A, McIntosh A, Peters J, O'Keeffe C, Khunti K, Baker R, Booth A. Effectiveness of screening and monitoring tests for diabetic retinopathy. *Diabet Med* 2000; 17: 495–506.
125. Younis N, Broadbent DM, Vora JP, Harding SP, and the Liverpool Diabetic Eye Study. Incidence of sight-threatening retinopathy in patients with type 2 diabetes in the Liverpool Diabetic Eye Study: a cohort study. *Lancet* 2003; 361: 195–200.

66

Nonretinal Ocular Complications of Diabetes Mellitus

Lawrence I. Rand*†, Jerry D. Cavallerano*, and Lloyd M. Aiello*†

**Joslin Diabetes Center, Boston, MA, USA, and †Harvard Medical School, Boston, MA, USA*

Diabetic eye disease is not limited to diabetic retinopathy: all structures of the eye are susceptible to the deleterious effects of diabetes. Some of these effects are of minor consequence, and may go unnoticed by both the patient and the doctor. Other effects, while not sight-threatening, result in uncomfortable vision or other symptoms interfering with normal visual function. Still other effects, while common in diabetes, must be fully evaluated to rule out potentially life-threatening underlying causes other than diabetes. Nevertheless, careful examination and treatment and appropriate patient counseling and education can generally mitigate effects of nonretinal ocular complications of diabetes. This chapter reviews common nonretinal ocular complications of diabetes mellitus.

OPHTHALMOPLEGIA

Mononeuropathy of the third, fourth, or sixth cranial nerves is an uncommon but dramatic complication of diabetes, afflicting 0.4–0.97% of persons with diabetes [1, 2]. Presentation of such neuropathy, however, is of serious concern to the patient, because the presenting symptom is frequently frank diplopia, sometimes accompanied by eye pain. The mononeuropathies also present a serious clinical challenge for the examiner, as a misdiagnosis may result in an overlooked cranial neoplasm or aneurysm. On the other hand, complete neurological evaluation may prove time-consuming, costly, and sometimes uncomfortable for the patient.

In the diabetic mononeuropathies, the third nerve (oculomotor) is most commonly affected, followed by the sixth (abducens) cranial nerve [3, 4]. Less frequently the fourth nerve (trochlear) or seventh (facial) nerve may be involved alone or in combination with one of the other nerves. The presenting complaint is usually diplopia and may be associated with ipsilateral headache or eye pain, which can precede the onset of diplopia. The combination of third, sixth, and fourth nerve palsies is rarely of diabetic origin (Table 1).

Third nerve palsies usually result in a ptosis of the eyelid on the affected side. The eye is directed down and out, and supraorbital pain may precede or be associated with the palsy. A common clinical impression is that in diabetic third nerve palsies the pupil is generally spared, although pupillary evaluation may be compromised either by the diabetic condition itself or by previous scatter (panretinal) laser photocoagulation [6–10]. In a prospective study of 26 patients with a diabetes-related third nerve palsy, however, internal ophthalmoplegia occurred in 38% of the cases, although the anisocoria was 1 mm or less in most patients and no patients had a fully dilated, unreactive pupil [11]. Patients with sixth nerve palsies usually have the affected eye turned inward toward the nose. Movement of the eye laterally past the midline is restricted or absent. The sixth nerve has a long intracranial course and multiple causes may be responsible for sixth nerve palsies, necessitating careful neurologic evaluation, particularly if bilateral. Weakness of the fourth nerve results in a combination of vertical and lateral diplopia, and the patient may present with a head tilt or a complaint of tilting images. Fourth nerve palsies are comparatively rare.

Complete recovery of function usually occurs in 1–9 months. Recurrence may develop, but aberrant regeneration of the nerve is not seen. Particularly important in

International Textbook of Diabetes Mellitus, Third Edition. Edited by R. A. DeFronzo, E. Ferrannini, H. Keen, and P. Zimmet.
 ISBN: 0-471-48655-8.

Table 1 Nonretinal ocular complications of diabetes mellitus*

Structure	Symptoms	Comment
III (Oculomotor)	1. Complete or partial ptosis 2. Horizontal and vertical diplopia 3. Affected eye "down and out" 4. Possible supraorbital pain 5. Pupillary sparing (80% of cases) 6. Decreased sursumduction and adduction	1. Examination to rule out other causes 2. Consultation with internist or diabetologist 3. Neurologic referral 4. Patient education 5. Follow-up 6 weeks or as indicated
IV (Trochlear)	1. Vertical diplopia with associated esotropia 2. Vertical deviation increases in downward gaze or when head is tilted to side of affected muscle 3. Vertical deviation decreases with abduction of the affected eye 4. Esotropia increases with downward gaze	
VI (Abducens)	1. Lateral or horizontal diplopia 2. Esotropia of the affected eye 3. Decreased abduction 4. Possible head turn in the direction of the affected eye	
Cornea		
Decreased sensitivity	1. None	1. Artificial tears
Recurrent erosion	2. Eye pain	2. Patient education
Poor re-epithelialization	3. Blurred vision	3. Careful contact lens-patient selection
Abrasion		
Ulceration		
Iris		
Iris neovascularization (Rubeosis iridis)	1. None	1. Referral for possible panretinal photocoagulation
Ectropion uveae	2. Eye pain	2. Management of glaucoma
Neovascular glaucoma		
Lens		
Diabetic cataract	1. None	1. Optimal refractive correction
Premature cataract	2. Blurred vision	2. Surgical referral for cataract extraction and intraocular lens implant
Refractive fluctuations	3. Fluctuating vision	3. Control of blood glucose level

*Modified from reference 5.

third nerve palsies of diabetic origin is the frequent sparing of the pupillary fibers, which may help distinguish these third nerve palsies from those due to intracranial aneurysms and tumors, which affect the pupil in 80–90% of the cases. In situations where all third nerve function is absent with the exception of the pupil, an aneurysm is highly improbable. In partial third nerve palsy pupillary sparing is not as reassuring. Ocular palsies in a diabetic patient should prompt a thorough medical and neurological evaluation, as 42% of such palsies seen in diabetic patients in one series were of nondiabetic origin [12]. Other diagnoses include myasthenia gravis, Graves' disease, herpes zoster, demyelinating disease, idiopathic orbital myositis and other orbital inflammatory disease, primary and metastatic brain tumor, prolactinoma, and hypoglycemia [13].

In a retrospective case-control study of 100 patients with ischemic cranial nerve palsies in association with diabetes, aspirin use was not associated with a reduced rate of ischemic third, fourth, sixth, and seventh nerve palsies [14]. Treatment of ophthalmoplegia is symptomatic to relieve diplopia, and usually consists of temporary occlusion of one eye, together with a mild analgesic if needed. Severe pain is not characteristic, and so the need for strong analgesics should arouse suspicion that an intracranial aneurysm may be present. Diabetic nerve palsies are usually self-limited, with resolution occurring in a few weeks to up to 6–9 months later. Nerve palsies that have not begun to resolve after approximately 6 months are most probably not of diabetic origin.

CORNEA

Diabetes affects the cornea in a variety of fashions. The cornea of a person with diabetes may injure more easily and heal more slowly and less completely than the cornea of a person who does not have diabetes. One significant factor is reduced corneal sensitivity related to diabetes, compared with age-matched nondiabetic individuals [15]. This reduction was symmetrical in each patient, and the thresholds increased with the duration of diabetes, although diabetic patients did not exhibit more clinically significant corneal disease than nondiabetic patients did. Furthermore, in a separate study, impairment of corneal sensitivity was found to correlate significantly with duration of diabetes in experiments conducted on diabetic dogs [16].

Corneal nerve alterations in diabetic rats have been demonstrated in the basal lamina of Schwann cells, as well as occasional axonal degenerations [17]. Such alterations are probably implicated in the development of neurotrophic corneal ulcerations with diabetes [18]. Histological studies of the endothelial cells of the diabetic cornea show morphological abnormalities resulting in a less stable and more vulnerable cell layer [19]. Minute folds in Descemet's membrane probably represent an alteration in the tissue fluid level of the cornea (1). The corneal epithelium and its basement membrane have also been implicated in corneal disease associated with diabetes. As the human corneal epithelium contains significant levels of both sorbitol and fructose, it is likely that the sorbitol pathway operates in this tissue [20]. Poor adhesion of epithelial cells to its basement membrane is probably the result of osmotic changes within the cornea.

Such corneal changes pose numerous clinical problems. The patient with diabetes may be a poor candidate for contact lenses, as discomfort from a poorly fitting or damaged lens may be absent because of reduced corneal sensitivity, although a prospective, controlled study comparing soft contact lens wear in 40 patients with diabetes to 40 nondiabetic control subjects suggests that current generation daily wear soft contact lenses resulted in no appreciable clinical risk for persons with diabetes [21]. Corneal abrasions or minor erosions, which may be detected early in an otherwise healthy cornea, may develop into significant ulcerations. Corneal erosions may also be more likely to become recurrent because of slow or poor wound healing. Minor infections, which might otherwise be of little or no consequence, may become sight-threatening in the presence of diabetes. Daily wear soft contact lenses are probably the best alternative for the diabetic patient. Extended wear lenses should be avoided. Compulsive adherence to lens hygiene regimens is essential.

Another complication of compromised corneal integrity relates to the treatment for diabetic retinopathy. In order to perform a thorough ocular evaluation of the anterior segment or of the retina of the eye, a contact lens for examining purposes is frequently necessary. The mechanical action of the lens, although cushioned by a solution, may be enough to damage the cornea. Furthermore, similar types of contact lenses are required for laser treatments, and the mechanical action of the lens, in conjunction with the length of time that the lens must be placed on the eye, may result in an iatrogenic corneal abrasion; this potential complication also applies to vitrectomy surgery. Nonhealing or delayed healing corneal abrasions are not uncommon following vitrectomy. Recurrent erosion (that is, reopening of epithelial defects without new trauma) is also more common in patients with diabetes.

The tendency for corneal abrasion may necessitate the use of tear replacement drops, collagen or silicon punctual plug occlusion, or punctual cauterization to retain tear volume, particularly in dry environments. In a study of 95 patients with type 2 diabetes and 58 nondiabetic controls, corneal sensation, total tear secretion, and reflex tear secretion were all reduced in the diabetic subjects [22] and the loss of corneal sensation was correlated with the level of diabetic retinopathy. In the Beaver Dam Eye Study, diabetes was independently and significantly associated with dry eye syndrome [23].

Keratorefractive surgery has become an increasingly accepted method to correct myopia, astigmatism, or hyperopia. Laser *in situ* keratomileusis (LASIK) is a popular and generally well-tolerated procedure. Studies have shown, however, that patients undergoing LASIK may develop dry eye and compromised tear function, especially in the first postoperative month [24]. Additionally, reduced corneal sensitivity following LASIK has been documented, with disruption of ocular surface tear dynamics [25]. A retrospective study of 30 eyes from patients with diabetes and 150 age- and gender-matched control eyes showed that over a 6-month follow-up period, patients with diabetes undergoing LASIK had a significantly higher risk of developing postoperative corneal epithelial complications and had poorer final refractive results [26]. The diabetic eyes had an overall complication rate of 47% compared with a 6.9% complication rate in the control group. Consequently, persons with diabetes should be counseled on these potential complications and the added risk that may be posed by diabetes.

In summary, patients with diabetes should be alerted to the potential side effects of contact lenses, and follow-up evaluations need to be frequent and thorough. The necessity for safety glasses and goggles should be emphasized for appropriate work and sport environments. For ocular examination and treatment, a soft contact lens may be used between the cornea and the examining or treating lens, particularly if the patient has had a corneal abrasion in the past. Although evolving procedures may have fewer side effects and complications, keratorefractive surgery for persons with diabetes should be undertaken only after careful consideration of risks and benefits of the procedure.

GLAUCOMA

Primary open angle glaucoma is reported to be more common among individuals with diabetes (4.0%) than it is among those without it (1.8%); in addition, diabetes has been found to be more common among glaucoma patients (4–18%) than in the general population (2%) [27]. In the Wisconsin Epidemilogic Study of Diabetic Retinopathy, the self-reported incidence of glaucoma was 3.7% in persons diagnosed prior to age 30 years, 6.9% in persons diagnosed at age 30 years or older and not using insulin, and 11.8% in persons diagnosed at age 30 years or older and taking insulin [28]. In this cohort of patients (2366 with diabetes and 381 nondiabetic subjects as control), diabetic persons had a higher mean intraocular pressure than did the control group [29]. The Beaver Dam Eye Study, a population-based study of age-related eye disease in 4926 persons, found 4.2% of persons with diabetes to have definite glaucoma, compared with 2.0% in the nondiabetic group [30]. The Blue Mountains Eye Study, which enrolled 3654 persons near Sydney, Australia, found a 5.5% prevalence of glaucoma in diabetic persons compared with 2.8% in nondiabetic persons [31]. The study concluded that there is a "significant and consistent association between diabetes and glaucoma." Similarly, among the 4178 persons participating in the Rotterdam Study, there was a strong association between elevated intraocular pressure and high-tension glaucoma and newly diagnosed diabetes mellitus and elevated blood glucose levels [32].

Why glaucoma may be more common in diabetes is not well understood, as the pathogenesis of primary open angle glaucoma remains unclear. Glaucoma or elevated intraocular pressure has been proposed as protecting an eye from developing severe diabetic retinopathy, based on studies of patients with diabetes and unilateral glaucoma. As the intra-ocular pressure is the main component of tissue pressure in the eye, and retinal venous pressure usually just barely exceeds intra-ocular pressure, it would not be surprising if alterations in the regulation of intraocular pressure and its relationship with vascular resistance could play a major part in the pathogenesis of diabetic retinopathy.

Treatment of open angle glaucoma in diabetic individuals is influenced by the patient's general medical condition. Caution must be exercised with the use of topical β-blockers in possibly masking hypoglycemic symptoms or affecting frequently occurring cardiovascular disease. Acetazolamide or other carbonic anhydrase inhibitors may be used if needed, but as these medications can cause a metabolic acidosis, more frequent electrolyte monitoring should be done. The presence of renal disease may influence how these and other pressure-lowering drugs may be used, and close cooperation between the internist and eye doctor is important. The recent addition of new antiglaucoma medications, including topical carbonic anhydrase inhibitors, selective topical β-blockers, and different classes of topical agents, has aided in managing glaucoma. Among these, prostaglandin analogues have been rarely associated with macular edema in pseudophakic patients [33]; consequently, prostaglandin analogues should be used with caution in pseudophakic persons with diabetes who are more susceptible to this complication [34]. Laser trabeculoplasty has either eliminated or reduced the need for topical glaucoma agents in some cases.

Narrow angle glaucoma or acute angle closure glaucoma is comparatively rare. Narrow angle glaucoma does not seem to be more common in persons with diabetes than in the general population, but recent investigations suggest that the shallower the anterior chamber of the eye, the more likely a person is to have an abnormal response to an oral glucose tolerance test [35]. The postulated mechanism for this association is the autonomic dysfunction within the anterior segment of the eye, resulting in a hypersensitivity to both sympathetic and parasympathetic autonomic mediators, with the iris–lens diaphragm moving forward, resulting in shallowing of the filtration angle and possible closing of the angle.

In acute angle closure glaucoma, the outflow angle in the anterior chamber of the eye formed by the iris plane and the posterior corneal surface becomes closed, blocking outflow to the outflow channels of the trabecular meshwork. The result is a dramatic and rapid rise in intraocular pressure with ocular pain, decreased vision, colored halos around lights, and frequently nausea and vomiting. Angle closure glaucoma should be considered as part of the differential diagnosis for a diabetic patient presenting with nausea and vomiting.

Angle closure glaucoma is considered to be a medical emergency. Treatment consists of attempting to break the angle closure medically with miotic drops and to lower the pressure with either systemic or topical medications. A surgical peripheral iridectomy or laser iridotomy may restore the normal aqueous outflow in the eye if the angle closure is broken. As pupil dilation can trigger an angle closure attack, care needs to be exercised before any pupil is dilated.

Another type of glaucoma that is common in diabetic individuals is neovascular glaucoma, in which a proliferation of new blood vessels on the iris (NVI) extends into the filtration angle of the anterior chamber. This fibrovascular proliferation interferes with normal aqueous outflow, resulting in neovascular glaucoma. NVI is related to the vascular proliferation on the retina of the eye, and is probably the result of growth factors such as vascular endothelial growth factor being produced by an ischemic retina and circulating forward to the anterior segment to stimulate neovascularization [36–39].

NVI usually is first seen around the pupillary margin, although the vessels can grow initially in or near the filtration angle. Evaluation with a slit-lamp biomicroscope is necessary to observe and evaluate these vessels. The development of neovascular glaucoma in one eye is strongly correlated to the development of the same condition in the patient's other eye. Prognosis for the eye is usually guarded if neovascular glaucoma is present [1].

Treatment with either scatter (panretinal) laser photocoagulation or cryotherapy has been shown to be beneficial in the management of NVI [39–41]. Neovascular glaucoma also can be treated by goniophotocoagulation if the surgeon is unable to dilate the pupil, or if cloudy media or vitreous hemorrhage prevents visualization of the fundus [42]. In this procedure, discrete laser applications are applied directly to the new vessels as they arborize in the angle, resulting in angle synechiae. Frequently, a combination of panretinal photocoagulation and goniophotocoagulation is used to treat neovascular glaucoma. Adjunct medical therapy may include topical agents to lower intraocular pressure. Cycloplegic agents and topical steroid drops may reduce local ocular inflammation and relieve some of the associated pain. YAG contact laser ablation of the ciliary body may control high pressures when medical therapy fails. Conventional filtration surgery has had poor results but other surgical and laser techniques such as Molteno valves and trans-scleral laser have greatly improved results [43]. It is not unusual to save eyes with this previously uniformly blinding condition.

DIABETES AND CATARACT

Opacification of the crystalline lens or cataract is another important ocular manifestation of diabetes [44]. Traditionally, three types of cataract have been noted in diabetes [1]: these are the "snowflake" or metabolic cataract, the senile cataract, and the cataracta complicata or secondary cataract.

Snowflake cataracts are seen primarily in young diabetic patients with uncontrolled diabetes [1]; the name is derived from the snowflake or flocculent appearance, which starts in the subcapsular regions of the lens. The cataract may progress rapidly, and total opacification of the lens resulting in a mature cataract can occasionally occur over a period of a few days. The cataract may be unilateral or bilateral, and institution of adequate diabetic control has been reported to stop or to reverse these lens opacities when they are discovered in their incipient stages [45–48].

Development of a metabolic cataract occurs in most animal models of diabetes. Investigation of this cataract led to the discovery of the sorbitol pathway [49, 50], an alternative route for glucose metabolism requiring the enzyme aldose reductase and in which sorbitol, a sugar alcohol, is the by-product. Inhibition of sorbitol production by use of an aldose reductase inhibitor prevents the development of cataract in these diabetic experimental animals and in galactosemia as well. The possible role of sugar alcohol accumulation as an underlying factor in other diabetic complications, including neuropathy and possibly retinopathy, has received much attention. Aldose reductase inhibitors have been shown to slow reduction in nerve conduction velocities in persons with diabetes, but the effect of aldose reductase inhibitors on retinopathy or cataract in humans has not been proven [51].

Cataracta complicata, or cataracts associated with other ocular disease such as iridocyclitis chorioretinitis, high myopia or retinal detachment, were seen in 6% of a large group of diabetic patients examined by Waite and Beetham, a figure not significantly different from that seen in the nondiabetic group [1].

Senile cataract is the most common form of cataract seen in diabetes, and cannot be distinguished from the senile cataract of nondiabetic individuals. With diabetic patients, however, the senile changes of nuclear sclerosis and cortical and subcapsular opacification develop at an earlier age than in nondiabetic patients (in 59% of older-onset diabetic individuals at 30–54 years of age, compared with 12% of age-matched nondiabetic individuals) [44, 52]. The cataracts also may progress to a vision-impairing level more rapidly, necessitating cataract extraction. In the United Kingdom Prospective Diabetes Study patients in the intensive control of blood glucose group had a 24% reduction in need for cataract surgery compared with the conventional control group [53].

The indications for cataract extraction are, in general, similar for those with diabetes and those without, but the retinopathy status of the patient should influence the surgical procedure performed and the timing of surgery [54]. Modern cataract surgery with posterior chamber intraocular lens implant is generally successful. There is debate concerning rate of complications and risk of progression of retinopathy depending on surgical technique (e.g., extracapsular cataract extraction, phacoemulsfication, one-stitch or no-stitch procedures), and intraocular surgery is a risk factor for progression of diabetic retinopathy [55–61]. In the Early Treatment Diabetic Retinopathy Study results of cataract surgery were better than previously published reports [62]. Patients with severe nonproliferative diabetic retinopathy or worse before lens surgery had poorer visual outcomes, although 55% of these patients had vision improvement after 1 year; the main causes of poor visual results following cataract surgery were diabetic macular edema and/or proliferative diabetic retinopathy. Increased severity of retinopathy and poorer visual acuity prior to surgery were risk factors for less favorable results, and cataract surgery was associated with a borderline statistically significant increased risk of progression of diabetic retinopathy; no such increased risk of new-onset diabetic macular edema was noted [62]; nevertheless, anecdotal reports from experienced ophthalmologists suggest that there may be an increased risk of macular edema.

Delay of cataract surgery until functional vision is impaired is probably the best course when significant retinopathy is present. Presurgical laser treatment for macular edema and proliferative diabetic retinopathy and close attention to pre-surgical retinal status, including presence of epiretinal membranes, can reduce the risk of postoperative complications. Close retinal follow-up with laser treatment is indicated. Use of topical nonsteroidal anti-inflammatory agents postoperatively may limit postoperative macular edema. The incidence of rubeosis iridis and neovascular glaucoma in these eyes following cataract extraction is reported to be significant [63].

In summary, cataracts develop at an earlier age and progress faster in patients with diabetes; high-risk proliferative diabetic retinopathy and clinically significant macular edema should be treated before cataract surgery when possible; and cataract surgery and laser treatment (if indicated) should be considered before cataract prevents adequate view of the retina. Phacoemulcification is safe in persons with diabetes and may be preferable to extracapsular cataract extraction. Both acrylic and polymethylmethacrylate intraocular lenses are safe for intraocular lens implants for persons with diabetes, although the use of silicon lenses has generally been avoided in diabetic patients. Nevertheless, if there is minimal retinopathy, the risk of using silicon lenses is small if it is unlikely that vitrectomy surgery or silicon oil tamponade will be necessary in the future.

REFRACTIVE ERRORS

Diabetic individuals have the same range of refractive errors as does the general population [1, 64]. The effects of blood glucose level on refractive error, however, have been well documented and investigators now have a better understanding of the relationship of refractive changes to the effects of the sorbitol pathway [49, 50, 64, 65]. Hyperglycemia is usually recognized as resulting in a myopic shift, and Waite and Beetham [1] measured shifts of up to 10 diopters, although hyperopic shifts have been documented [66, 67]. A lowering of blood glucose level is similarly recognized as causing a reduction in myopia and an increase in hyperopia. The mechanism remains open to debate, but it is suggested that in a hyperglycemic state, glucose enters the intracellular spaces of the lens, resulting in lens swelling and an associated increase in myopia [65].

Sudden refractive shifts are frequently the presenting sign for a person with new diabetes. Patients who could see clearly at distance, either with or without their glasses, may complain that their distance vision is now blurred. On the other hand, those who required reading glasses or who were experiencing difficulty with near work may now find they can read more easily without their glasses, misinterpreting the change as "an improvement" in their eyes. Patients with uncontrolled or poorly controlled blood glucose levels should be encouraged to postpone spectacle purchase until their blood glucose levels have stabilized; this stabilization may take 4–6 weeks to occur, although the effects of a rise in blood glucose on refractive state are generally recognized as being more sudden. Any coexisting physical condition that affects blood glucose level, such as infection, cold, or even stress, should be considered a reason not to prescribe glasses if a patient recognizes recent or sudden changes in vision.

The Early Treatment Diabetic Retinopathy Study demonstrated that diabetes and duration of diabetes are independent risk factors for reduced amplitude of accommodation. A transient reduction in accommodation amplitude was also measured following scatter (panretinal) laser photocoagulation [68].

MISCELLANEOUS OCULAR EFFECTS

There are other nonretinal effects of diabetes that, while not frequently reported by patients, may have an impact on their vision or visual function. Because of autonomic nervous system abnormalities, pupil size is frequently smaller in a diabetic person than in an age-matched and sex-matched individual without diabetes. Pupil size has been shown to be related to duration of diabetes and metabolic control and that there is a smaller pupil size and a loss of spontaneous fluctuation of pupil diameter with increased duration or poor diabetes control [6–9, 69–71]. These abnormalities, once believed to be related to stiffness of iris tissues, are probably related to autonomic neuropathy predominantly affecting the sympathetic innervation to the iris dilator muscle, with the parasympathetic innervation to the iris sphincter muscle being relatively spared. Laser injury to the long ciliary nerves as they course anteriorly on the inner surface of the retina can, similarly, result in pupillary abnormalities and reduced amplitude of accommodation [10]. Reduction in accommodative ability can also occur, especially in the young, newly diagnosed diabetic individual [72].

CONCLUSION

Diabetic eye disease is not restricted to diabetic retinopathy alone. Early diagnosis and treatment of diabetes mellitus, identification of ocular abnormalities, and patient education can mitigate many of these effects. As with all aspects of diabetes care, interaction with the patient and other health care providers is necessary to assist patients properly in managing their diabetic condition.

REFERENCES

1. Waite JH, Beetham WP. The visual mechanism in diabetes mellitus: a comparative study of 2002 diabetics and 457 non-diabetics for control. *N Engl J Med* 1935; 212: 367–79, 429–43.
2. Watanabe K, Hagura R, Akanuma Y, Takasu T, Kajinuma H, Kuzuya N, Irie M. Characteristics of cranial nerve palsies in diabetic patients. *Diabetes Res Clin Pract* 1990; 10 (1): 19–27.
3. Rucker CW. The causes of paralysis of the third, fourth and sixth cranial nerves. *Am J Ophthalmol* 1966; 61 (5): 1293–8.

4. Rucker CW. Paralysis of the thrid, fourth, and sixth cranial nerves. *Am J Ophthalmol* 1958; 46: 787–94.
5. Aiello LM, Aiello LP, Cavallerano JD. Ocular complications of diabetes mellitus. *Joslin's Diabetes Mellitus*, 14th edn. Philadelphia: Lea & Febiger (in press).
6. Hreidarsson AB. Pupil size in insulin-dependent diabetes. Relationship to duration, metabolic control, and long-term manifestations. *Diabetes* 1982; 31 (5, pt 1): 442–8.
7. Hreidarsson AB. Pupil motility in long-term diabetes. *Diabetologia* 1979; 17 (3): 145–50.
8. Smith SE, Smith SA, Brown PM, Fox C, Sonksen PH. Pupillary signs in diabetic autonomic neuropathy. *Br Med J* September 30, 1978; 2 (6142): 924–7.
9. Clapp CA. Diabetic iridopathy. *Am J Ophthalmol* 1945; 28: 617–23.
10. Rogell GD. Internal ophthalmoplegia after argon laser panretinal photocoagulation. *Arch Ophthalmol* 1979; 97 (5): 904–5.
11. Jacobson DM. Pupil involvement in patients with diabetes-associated oculomotor nerve palsy. *Arch Ophthalmol* 1998; 116 (6): 723–7.
12. Zorrilla E, Kozak GP. Ophthalmoplegia in diabetes mellitus. *Ann Intern Med* 1967; 67 (5): 968–76.
13. Sergott RC, Glaser JS, Berger LJ. Simultaneous, bilateral diabetic ophthalmoplegia. Report of two cases and discussion of differential diagnosis. *Ophthalmology* 1984; 91 (1): 18–22.
14. Johnson LN, Stetson SW, Krohel GB, Cipollo CL, Madsen RW. Aspirin use and the prevention of acute ischemic cranial nerve palsy. *Am J Ophthalmol* 2000; 129 (3): 367–71.
15. Schwartz DE. Corneal sensitivity in diabetics. *Arch Ophthalmol* 1974; 91 (3): 174–8.
16. MacRae SM, Engerman RL, Hatchell DL, Hyndiuk RA. Corneal sensitivity and control of diabetes. *Cornea* 1982; 1: 223–6.
17. Ishida N, Rao GN, del Cerro M, Aquavella JV. Corneal nerve alterations in diabetes mellitus. *Arch Ophthalmol* 1984; 102 (9): 1380–4.
18. Hyndiuk RA, Kazarian EL, Schultz RO, Seideman S. Neurotrophic corneal ulcers in diabetes mellitus. *Arch Ophthalmol* 1977; 95 (12): 2193–6.
19. Schultz RO, Matsuda M, Yee RW, Edelhauser HF, Schultz KJ. Corneal endothelial changes in type I and type II diabetes mellitus. *Am J Ophthalmol* October 15, 1984; 98 (4): 401–10.
20. Foulks GN, Thoft RA, Perry HD, Tolentino FI. Factors related to corneal epithelial complications after closed vitrectomy in diabetics. *Arch Ophthalmol* 1979; 97 (6): 1076–8.
21. O'Donnell C, Efron N, Boulton AJ. A prospective study of contact lens wear in diabetes mellitus. *Ophthalmic Physiol Opt* 2001; 21 (2): 127–38.
22. Saito J, Enoki M, Hara M, Morishige N, Chikama T, Nishida T. Correlation of corneal sensation, but not of basal or reflex tear secretion, with the stage of diabetic retinopathy. *Cornea* 2003; 22 (1): 15–8.
23. Moss SE, Klein R, Klein BE. Prevalence of and risk factors for dry eye syndrome. *Arch Ophthalmol* 2000; 118 (9): 1264–8.
24. Toda I, Asano-Kato N, Komai-Hori Y, Tsubota K. Dry eye after laser *in situ* keratomileusis. *Am J Ophthalmol* 2001; 132 (1): 1–7.
25. Battat L, Macri A, Dursun D, Pflugfelder SC. Effects of laser *in situ* keratomileusis on tear production, clearance, and the ocular surface. *Ophthalmology* 2001; 108 (7): 1230–5.
26. Fraunfelder FW, Rich LF. Laser-assisted *in situ* keratomileusis complications in diabetes mellitus. *Cornea* 2002; 21 (3): 246–8.
27. Armstrong JR, Daily RK, Dobson HL, Gerard LJ. The incidence of glaucoma in diabetes mellitus: a comparison with the incidence in the general population. *Am J Ophthalmol* 1960; 50: 55–63.
28. Klein BE, Klein R, Moss SE. Incidence of self-reported glaucoma in people with diabetes mellitus. *Br J Ophthalmol* 1997; 81 (9): 743–7.
29. Klein BE, Klein R, Moss SE. Intraocular pressure in diabetic persons. *Ophthalmology* 1984; 91 (11): 1356–60.
30. Klein BE, Klein R, Jensen SC. Open-angle glaucoma and older-onset diabetes: the Beaver Dam Eye Study. *Ophthalmology* 1994; 101 (7): 1173–7.
31. Mitchell P, Smith W, Chey T, Healey PR. Open-angle glaucoma and diabetes: the Blue Mountains Eye Study, Australia. *Ophthalmology* 1997; 104 (4): 712–8.
32. Dielemans I, de Jong PT, Stolk R, Vingerling JR, Grobbee DE, Hofman A. Primary open-angle glaucoma, intraocular pressure, and diabetes mellitus in the general elderly population: the Rotterdam Study. *Ophthalmology* 1996; 103 (8): 1271–5.
33. Warwar RE, Bullock JD, Ballal D. Cystoid macular edema and anterior uveitis associated with latanoprost use. Experience and incidence in a retrospective review of 94 patients. *Ophthalmology* 1998; 105 (2): 263–8.
34. Moroi SE, Gottfredsdottir MS, Schteingart MT, Elner SG, Lee CM, Schertzer RM, Abrams GW, Johnson MW. Cystoid macular edema associated with latanoprost therapy in a case series of patients with glaucoma and ocular hypertension. *Ophthalmology* 1999; 106 (5): 1024–9.
35. Mapstone R, Clark CV. Prevalence of diabetes in glaucoma. *Br Med J (Clin Res Ed)* July 13, 1985; 291 (6488): 93–5.
36. Aiello LP, Avery RL, Arrigg PG, Keyt BA, Jampel HD, Shah ST, Pasquale LR, Thieme H, Iwamoto MA, Park JE. Vascular endothelial growth factor in ocular fluid of patients with diabetic retinopathy and other retinal disorders. *N Engl J Med* December 1, 1994; 331 (22): 1480–7.
37. Fernandez-Vigo J, Castro J, Macarro A. Diabetic iris neovascularization. Natural history and treatment. *Acta Ophthalmol Scand* 1997; 75 (1): 89–93.
38. Bandello F, Brancato R, Lattanzio R, Galdini M, Falcomata B. Relation between iridopathy and retinopathy in diabetes. *Br J Ophthalmol* 1994; 78 (7): 542–5.
39. Hamanaka T, Akabane N, Yajima T, Takahashi T, Tanabe A. Retinal ischemia and angle neovascularization in proliferative diabetic retinopathy. *Am J Ophthalmol* 2001; 132 (5): 648–58.
40. Wand M, Dueker DK, Aiello LM, Grant WM. Effects of panretinal photocoagulation on rubeosis iridis, angle neovascularization, and neovascular glaucoma. *Am J Ophthalmol* 1978; 86 (3): 332–9.
41. Pavan PR, Folk JC, Weingeist TA, Hermsen VM, Watzke RC, Montague PR. Diabetic rubeosis and panretinal photocoagulation. *Arch Ophthalmol* 1983; 101 (6): 882–4.
42. Simmons RJ, Dueker DK, Kimbrough RL, Aiello LM. Goniophotocoagulation for neovascular glaucoma. *Trans Am Acad Ophthalmol Otolaryngol* 1977; 83 (1): 80–9.
43. Mermoud A, Salmon JF, Alexander P, Straker C, Murray AD. Molteno tube implantation for neovascular glaucoma. Long-term results and factors influencing the outcome. *Ophthalmology* 1993; 100 (6): 897–902.

44. Klein BE, Klein R, Moss SE. Prevalence of cataracts in a population-based study of persons with diabetes mellitus. *Ophthalmology* 1985; 92 (9): 1191–6.
45. Epstein DL. Reversible unilateral lens opacities in a diabetic patient. *Arch Ophthalmol* 1976; 94 (3): 461–3.
46. Brown CA, Burman D. Transient cataracts in a diabetic child with hyperosmolar coma. *Br J Ophthalmol* 1973; 57 (6): 429–33.
47. Dickey JB, Daily MJ. Transient posterior subcapsular lens opacities in diabetes mellitus. *Am J Ophthalmol* 2-15-1993; 115 (2): 234–8.
48. Gelvin JB, Thonn VA. The formation and reversal of acute cataracts in diabetes mellitus. *J Am Optom Assoc* 1993; 64 (7): 471–4.
49. Kinoshita JH, Merola LO, Satoh K, Dikmak E. Osmotic changes caused by the accumulation of dulcitol in the lenses of rats fed with galactose. *Nature* 1962; 194: 1085–7.
50. Gabbay KH. The sorbitol pathway and the complications of diabetes. *N Engl J Med* April 19, 1973; 288 (16): 831–6.
51. The Sorbinil Retinopathy Trial Research Group. The Sorbinil Retinopathy Trial: neuropathy results. *Neurology* 1993; 43 (6): 1141–9.
52. Klein BE, Klein R, Wang Q, Moss SE. Older-onset diabetes and lens opacities: the Beaver Dam Eye Study. *Ophthalmic Epidemiol* 1995; 2 (1): 49–55.
53. The UK Prospective Diabetes Study (UKPDS) Group. Intensive blood-glucose control with sulphonylureas or insulin compared with conventional treatment and risk of complications in patients with type 2 diabetes (UKPDS 33). *Lancet* September 12, 1998; 352 (9131): 837–53.
54. Pollack A, Leiba H, Bukelman A, Abrahami S, Oliver M. The course of diabetic retinopathy following cataract surgery in eyes previously treated by laser photocoagulation. *Br J Ophthalmol* 1992; 76 (4): 228–31.
55. Klein BE, Klein R, Moss SE. Incidence of cataract surgery in the Wisconsin Epidemiologic Study of Diabetic Retinopathy. *Am J Ophthalmol* 1995; 119 (3): 295–300.
56. Zaczek A, Olivestedt G, Zetterstrom C. Visual outcome after phacoemulsification and IOL implantation in diabetic patients. *Br J Ophthalmol* 1999; 83 (9): 1036–41.
57. Kato S, Fukada Y, Hori S, Tanaka Y, Oshika T. Influence of phacoemulsification and intraocular lens implantation on the course of diabetic retinopathy. *J Cataract Refract Surg* 1999; 25 (6): 788–93.
58. Mittra RA, Borrillo JL, Dev S, Mieler WF, Koenig SB. Retinopathy progression and visual outcomes after phacoemulsification in patients with diabetes mellitus. *Arch Ophthalmol* 2000; 118 (7): 912–7.
59. Raskauskas PA, Walker JP, Wing GL, Fletcher DC, Elsner AE. Small incision cataract surgery and placement of posterior chamber intraocular lenses in patients with diabetic retinopathy. *Ophthalmic Surg Lasers* 1999; 30 (1): 6–11.
60. Sadiq SA, Sleep T, Amoaku WM. The visual results and changes in retinopathy in diabetic patients following cataract surgery. *Eur J Ophthalmol* 1999; 9 (1): 14–20.
61. Hykin PG, Gregson RM, Stevens JD, Hamilton PA. Extracapsular cataract extraction in proliferative diabetic retinopathy. *Ophthalmology* 1993; 100 (3): 394–9.
62. Chew EY, Benson WE, Remaley NA, Lindley AA, Burton TC, Csaky K, Williams GA, Ferris FL III. Results after lens extraction in patients with diabetic retinopathy: Early Treatment Diabetic Retinopathy Study Report Number 25. *Arch Ophthalmol* 1999; 117 (12): 1600–6.
63. Aiello LM, Wand M, Liang G. Neovascular glaucoma and vitreous hemorrhage following cataract surgery in patients with diabetes mellitus. *Ophthalmology* 1983; 90 (7): 814–20.
64. Duke-Elder WS. Changes in refraction in diabetes mellitus. *Br J Ophthalmol* 1925; 9: 167–87.
65. Gwinup G, Villarreal A. Relationship of serum glucose concentration to changes in refraction. *Diabetes* 1976; 25 (1): 29–31.
66. Fledelius HC. Refractive change in diabetes mellitus around onset or when poorly controlled. A clinical study. *Acta Ophthalmol* (Copenh) 1987; 65 (1): 53–7.
67. Saito Y, Ohmi G, Kinoshita S, Nakamura Y, Ogawa K, Harino S, Okada M. Transient hyperopia with lens swelling at initial therapy in diabetes. *Br J Ophthalmol* 1993; 77 (3): 145–8.
68. Braun CI, Benson WE, Remaley NA, Chew EY, Ferris FL III. Accommodative amplitudes in the Early Treatment Diabetic Retinopathy Study. *Retina* 1995; 15 (4): 275–81.
69. Cahill M, Eustace P, de Jesus V. Pupillary autonomic denervation with increasing duration of diabetes mellitus. *Br J Ophthalmol* 2001; 85 (10): 1225–30.
70. Bitsios P, Prettyman R, Szabadi E. Changes in autonomic function with age: a study of pupillary kinetics in healthy young and old people. *Age ageing* 1996; 25 (6): 432–8.
71. Rogell GD. Internal ophthalmoplegia after argon laser panretinal photocoagulation. *Arch Ophthalmol* 1979; 97 (5): 904–5.
72. Marmor MF. Transient accommodative paralysis and hyperopia in diabetes. *Arch Ophthalmol* 1973; 89 (5): 419–21.

67

Preserving Vision

Lloyd M. Aiello*† and Jerry D. Cavallerano*

**Joslin Diabetes Center, Boston, MA, USA, and †Harvard Medical School, Boston, MA, USA*

Vision preservation provides a more suitable topic for discussion than vision impairment for persons with diabetes. Multicentered clinical trials conducted in the Untied States, the United Kingdom, and Europe over the past 30 years have provided the scientific basis for management of diabetic eye disease, with the expectation that the risk of severe vision loss from diabetic retinopathy can be virtually eliminated. Similarly, the risk of moderate visual loss, legal blindness, and other loss of vision can be reduced substantially. Nevertheless, diabetes remains a significant cause of vision loss and blindness worldwide. This chapter reviews the epidemiology of vision loss in diabetes and methods to preserve vision for persons with diabetes.

EPIDEMIOLOGY OF VISUAL LOSS

The World Health Organization identifies diabetic retinopathy as the leading cause of preventable blindness and visual disability in adults in economically developed societies. Approximately 120 million people worldwide have diabetes, and it is estimated that after 15 years' duration of diabetes, 2% of people become blind and 10% develop severe visual disability [1]. In the Cost of Diabetes in Europe – Type II (CODE-2) study, which enrolled over 7000 patients with type 2 diabetes in eight European countries, the prevalence of diabetic retinopathy was 20%, with 6.5% requiring laser treatment for sight-threatening eye disease within the past 6 months [2]. In a population-based study in Germany, diabetes was the second leading cause of blindness (vision <1/50), with an incidence of 2.01/100 000, and the leading cause of preventable vision loss [3].

In the EURODIAB IDDM Complications Study, a clinic-based study that enrolled 3250 patients with insulin-dependent (type 1) diabetes from 31 European countries, vision loss was a common complication [4]. Visual acuity (VA) was graded as a decimal of the Snellen fraction, and was considered *good* if VA was greater than or equal to 1.0 (20/20 or 6/6), *reduced* if VA measured less than or equal to 0.3 (20/60) in at least one eye, and *poor* if VA measured less than or equal to 0.3 in the better eye. Severe visual impairment was defined as best corrected VA less than or equal to 0.1 (20/200 or 6/60) in the better eye. Visual acuity was measured in 3024 patients. Severe visual impairment was present in 69 (2.3%) patients. Good VA was measured in 2109 (69.7%) patients, reduced VA was measured in 804 (26.6%) patients, and poor VA was measured in 42 (1.4%) patients.

In the Wisconsin Epidemiologic Study of Diabetic Retinopathy (WESDER), visual impairment (defined as visual acuity of 20/40 or worse in the better eye), and blindness (defined as visual acuity of 20/200 or worse in the better eye), and moderate visual loss (defined as a doubling of the visual angle) were measured in a sample ($n = 880$) of younger onset (diagnosed prior to age 30 years) patients who were also taking insulin [5]. Over a course of 14 years, the cumulative incidence of visual impairment was 12.7%, the cumulative incidence of moderate visual loss was 14.2%, and the cumulative incidence of blindness was 2.4%.

In a cross-sectional study chart review of 1047 patients with diabetes mellitus in a group model health maintenance organization, 687 of these patients had VA measurements [6]. Best acuity of 20/200 or worse (legal blindness) in the better eye was present in 10 patients (1.5%); acuity between 20/40 and 20/200 in the better eye was present

International Textbook of Diabetes Mellitus, Third Edition. Edited by R. A. DeFronzo, E. Ferrannini, H. Keen, and P. Zimmet.
 ISBN: 0-471-48655-8.

in 46 patients (6.7%); and acuity better than 20/40 was present in 631 patients (91.8%). Best acuity of 20/200 or worse in the worse eye was present in 56 patients (8.2%); acuity between 20/40 and 20/200 in the better eye was present in 107 patients (16.6%); and acuity better than 20/40 was present in 524 patients (76.3%).

In an effort to assess the extent of visual impairment among persons with diabetes, the Behavioral Risk Factor Surveillance System (BRFSS) survey interviewed 3391 adults with diabetes to measure their subjective assessment of visual functioning [7]. The BRFSS is a continuous, random-digit-dialed telephone survey of state population-based samples of the civilian noninsitutionalized adult population aged 18 years and older and conducted in all 50 states and the District of Columbia in the United States. In the survey, the prevalence of self-rated visual impairment was 24.8%. The prevalence was similar for persons with (1) type 1 diabetes (25.2%), (2) type 2 diabetes who were using insulin (29.2%), and (3) type 2 diabetes who were not using insulin (22.7%) [8]. Prevalence did increase with age, ranging from 18.6% for those aged 18–44 years, to 24.7% for those aged 45–64 years, to 28.0% for those aged 65 years.

VISION PRESERVATION

Visual loss in diabetes generally results from diabetic macular edema, nonresolving vitreous hemorrhage, and/or traction retinal detachment resulting from fibrovascular proliferation. Proper treatment, however, can significantly reduce the risk of severe vision loss (best corrected vision of 5/200 or worse), moderate vision loss (a doubling of the visual angle; e.g., 20/20 reduced to 20/40), and legal blindness (best corrected vision of 20/200 in the better seeing eye). In the Early Treatment Diabetic Retinopathy Study (ETDRS), a multicentered clinical trial that enrolled 3711 patients at 22 clinical centers in the United States and Puerto Rico, scatter (panretinal) laser photocoagulation reduced the 5-year rate of severe visual loss for eyes assigned to early photocoagulation to 2.6% [9, 10] (Figure 1). Focal laser photocoagulation reduced the risk of moderate vision loss from clinically significant diabetic

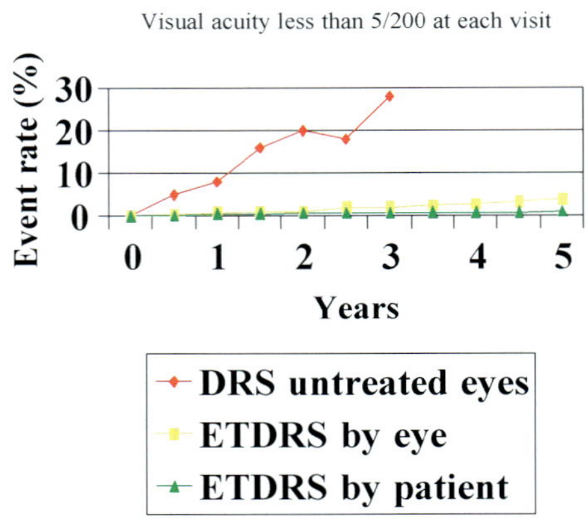

Figure 1 Laser photocoagulation according to Early Treatment Diabetic Retinopathy Study (ETDRS) protocol significantly reduces the risk of severe vision loss compared to eyes in the Diabetic Retinopathy Study that received no laser photocoagulation

macular edema by 50% or more [11–14]. Furthermore, vitrectomy surgery was performed in 208 of the 3711 patients enrolled in the ETDRS. Vitrectomy was effective in restoring or preserving vision for eyes that had either vitreous hemorrhage or retinal detachment with or without vitreous hemorrhage. Before vitrectomy, VA was 5/200 or worse in 66.7% of the eyes and better than 20/100 in 6.2% of the eyes. One year after vitrectomy, VA was 20/100 or better in 47.6% of eyes, including 24.0% with VA of 20/40 or better [15].

The Diabetes Control and Complications Trial (DCCT), a multicentered clinical trial that enrolled 1441 patients with type 1 diabetes nationwide in the United States, investigated whether intensive glycemic control, compared to conventional control, reduced the risk of onset (primary prevention cohort) or progression (secondary intervention cohort) of diabetic retinopathy [16–19]. In the primary prevention group, intensive control reduced the risk of onset of retinopathy by 27%, and a three-step progression of retinopathy by 78%. In the secondary intervention group, intensive control resulted in a 54% reduction in three-step progression of retinopathy, 47% reduction in progression to severe nonproliferative diabetic retinopathy and

Table 1 Summary of associated risk factors for vision loss

Condition/factor	Comment
Poor glycemic control	The DCCT and the UKPDS demonstrated that for type 1 and type 2 DM respectively, intensive blood glucose control reduced the risk of onset of DR and progression of DR
Renal disease	Renal disease associated with DM can lead to uncontrolled hypertension, exacerbating diabetic retinopathy and resulting in hypertensive retinal changes
Hypertension	Hypertension can be an independent risk factor for progression of DR, and can result in hypertensive retinal changes
Anemia	Associated with progression of DR in ETDRS
Dyslipidemia	Associated with increased hard exudates and macular edema in the WESDR and ETDRS

Note: DCCT = Diabetes Control and Complications Trial; DM = diabetes mellitus; DR = diabetic retinopathy; ETDRS = Early Treatment Diabetic Retinopathy Study; UKPDS = United Kingdom Prospective Diabetes Study; WESDR = Wisconsin Epidemilogic Study of Diabetic Retinopathy.

Table 2 Recommended eye examination schedule*

Type of DM	Recommended initial eye examination	Routine follow-up
Type 1 DM	Within 3–5 years after diagnosis of diabetes, once a person is age 10 years or older	Yearly
Type 2 DM	At time of diagnosis	Yearly
Pregnancy with preexisting DM	Prior to pregnancy for counseling	• Early in first trimester • Each trimester or more frequently as indicated • 6 weeks *postpartum*

*Abnormal findings will dictate more frequent follow-up examinations.

proliferative diabetic retinopathy, a 23% reduction in developing diabetic macular edema, and a 56% reduction in the need for laser photocoagulation [16–19]. These benefits of intensive control persisted, and 4 years after the conclusion of the DCCT, the intensive control group compared with the conventional control group showed a 75% risk reduction in progression of retinopathy, a 69% risk reduction in progression to severe levels of nonproliferative diabetic retinopathy and proliferative diabetic retinopathy, a 58% risk reduction in developing diabetic macular edema, and a 52% risk reduction in need for laser photocoagulation [20, 21].

The United Kingdom Prospective Diabetes Study (UKPDS) investigated whether intensive glycemic control, compared to conventional control, reduced the risk of onset (primary prevention cohort) or progression (secondary intervention cohort) of diabetic retinopathy in 4209 patients with newly diagnosed type 2 diabetes. Intensive blood glucose control resulted in a 17% reduction in a two-step progression of retinopathy, 23% reduction in vitreous hemorrhage, 16% reduction in legal blindness, 29% reduction in need for laser photocoagulation, and 24% reduction in need for cataract surgery [22]. Based on the findings of the DCCT and the UKPDS, the recommendation is that persons with diabetes initiate intensive control of blood glucose levels as early as possible, and maintain intensive blood glucose control for as long as possible, with the expectation that better glycemic control will reduce the risk of onset and progression of diabetic retinopathy and vision loss.

Systemic factors associated with diabetes are also associated with progression of diabetic retinopathy to sight-threatening stages. In addition to striving for optimal glycemic control, it is recommended that associated risk factors such as hypertension, renal disease, dyslipidemia, and anemia be monitored and treated aggressively in order to reduce the risk of visual loss [20, 23–29] (Tables 1 and 2).

CONCLUSION

Diabetes is a significant cause of preventable visual loss worldwide. Human vision can be preserved by applying the results of clinical trials that spanned the last 30 years of the twentieth century [28, 30–32]. Specifically, the goal to preserve human vision can be achieved by identifying persons who have diabetes; striving for intensive glycemic control as demonstrated in the DCCT and the UKPDS; striving to control coexisting medical conditions such as hypertension, anemia, renal disease, and dyslipidemia; examining for level of diabetic retinopathy at least annually; performing laser photocoagulation for diabetic macular edema and proliferative diabetic retinopathy as demonstrated in the ETDRS; and performing vitrectomy surgery to prevent visual loss or recover vision. Applying this evidence-based care can result in significant preservation of human vision until a cure for the complications of diabetes and diabetes itself can be achieved.

REFERENCES

1. World Health Organization. Diabetes Mellitus. Report No. 138. 2002.
2. Williams R, Van Gaal L, Lucioni C. Assessing the impact of complications on the costs of type II diabetes. *Diabetologia* 2002; 45 (7): S13–7.
3. Krumpaszky HG, Ludtke R, Mickler A, Klauss V, Selbmann HK. Blindness incidence in Germany: a population-based study from Wurttemberg-Hohenzollern. *Ophthalmologica* 1999; 213 (3): 176–82.
4. Sjolie AK, Stephenson J, Aldington S, Kohner E, Janka H, Stevens L Fuller J. Retinopathy and vision loss in insulin-dependent diabetes in Europe: the EURODIAB IDDM Complications Study. *Ophthalmology* 1997; 104 (2): 252–60.
5. Moss SE, Klein R, Klein BE. The 14-year incidence of visual loss in a diabetic population. *Ophthalmology* 1998; 105 (6): 998–1003.
6. Fong DS, Sharza M, Chen W, Paschal JF, Ariyasu RG, Lee PP. Vision loss among diabetics in a group model health maintenance organization (HMO). *Am J Ophthalmol* 2002; 133 (2): 236–41.
7. Kini MM, Leibowitz HM, Colton T, Nickerson RJ, Ganley J, Dawber TR. Prevalence of senile cataract, diabetic retinopathy, senile macular degeneration, and open-angle glaucoma in the Framingham Eye Study. *Am J Ophthalmol* 1978; 85 (1): 28–34.
8. Saaddine JB, Narayan KM, Engelgau MM, Aubert RE, Klein R, Beckles GL. Prevalence of self-rated visual impairment among adults with diabetes. *Am J Public Health* 1999; 89 (8): 1200–5.

9. The Early Treatment Diabetic Retinopathy Study Research Group. Early photocoagulation for diabetic retinopathy: Early Treatment Diabetic Retinopathy Study Report No. 9. *Ophthalmology* 1991; 98 (5, suppl): 766–85.
10. The Early Treatment Diabetic Retinopathy Study Research Group. Techniques for scatter and local photocoagulation treatment of diabetic retinopathy: Early Treatment Diabetic Retinopathy Study Report No. 3. *Int Ophthalmol Clin* 1987; 27 (4): 254–64.
11. The Early Treatment Diabetic Retinopathy Study Research Group. Photocoagulation for diabetic macular edema: Early Treatment Diabetic Retinopathy Study Report No. 1. *Arch Ophthalmol* 1985; 103 (12): 1796–806.
12. Photocoagulation treatment of proliferative diabetic retinopathy: the second report of diabetic retinopathy study findings. *Ophthalmology* 1978; 85 (1): 82–106.
13. The Early Treatment Diabetic Retinopathy Study Research Group. Photocoagulation for diabetic macular edema: Early Treatment Diabetic Retinopathy Study Report No. 4. *Int Ophthalmol Clin* 1987; 27 (4): 265–72.
14. The Early Treatment Diabetic Retinopathy Study Research Group. Case reports to accompany Early Treatment Diabetic Retinopathy Study Reports 3 and 4. *Int Ophthalmol Clin* 1987; 27 (4): 273–333.
15. Flynn HW Jr, Chew EY, Simons BD, Barton FB, Remaley NA, Ferris FL III, for the Early Treatment Diabetic Retinopathy Study Research Group. Pars plana vitrectomy in the Early Treatment Diabetic Retinopathy Study: Early Treatment Diabetic Retinopathy Study Research Group Report No. 17. *Ophthalmology* 1992; 99 (9): 1351–7.
16. The relationship of glycemic exposure (HbA_{1c}) to the risk of development and progression of retinopathy in the Diabetes Control and Complications Trial. *Diabetes* 1995; 44 (8): 968–83.
17. The Diabetes Control and Complications Trial Research Group. Progression of retinopathy with intensive versus conventional treatment in the Diabetes Control and Complications Trial. *Ophthalmology* 1995; 102 (4): 647–61.
18. The Diabetes Control and Complications Trial Research Group. The effect of intensive treatment of diabetes on the development and progression of long-term complications in insulin-dependent diabetes mellitus. *N Engl J Med* September 30, 1993; 329 (14): 977–86.
19. The Diabetes Control and Complications Trial. The effect of intensive diabetes treatment on the progression of diabetic retinopathy in insulin-dependent diabetes mellitus. *Arch Ophthalmol* 1995; 113 (1): 36–51.
20. The Diabetes Control and Complications Trial/Epidemiology of Diabetes Interventions and Complications Research Group. Retinopathy and nephropathy in patients with type 1 diabetes four years after a trial of intensive therapy. *N Engl J Med* October 2, 2000; 342 (6): 381–9.
21. Epidemiology of Diabetes Interventions and Complications (EDIC). Design, implementation, and preliminary results of a long-term follow-up of the Diabetes Control and Complications Trial Cohort. *Diabetes Care* 1999; 22 (1): 99–111.
22. UK Prospective Diabetes Study (UKPDS) Group. Intensive blood-glucose control with sulphonylureas or insulin compared with conventional treatment and risk of complications in patients with type 2 diabetes (UKPDS 33). Lancet December 9, 1998; 352 (9131): 837–53.
23. Aiello LP, Cahill MT, Wong JS. Systemic considerations in the management of diabetic retinopathy. *Am J Ophthalmol* 2001; 132: 760–6.
24. Davis MD, Fisher MR, Gangnon RE, Barton F, Aiello LM, Chew EY, Ferris FL III, Knatterud GL. Risk factors for high-risk proliferative diabetic retinopathy and severe visual loss: Early Treatment Diabetic Retinopathy Study Report No. 18. *Invest Ophthalmol Vis Sci* 1998; 39 (2): 233–52.
25. Turner RC. The UK Prospective Diabetes Study: a review. *Diabetes Care* 1998; 21 (suppl 3): C35–8.
26. Chew EY, Klein ML, Ferris FL III, Remaley NA, Murphy RP, Chantry K, Hoogwerf BJ, Miller D. Association of elevated serum lipid levels with retinal hard exudate in diabetic retinopathy: Early Treatment Diabetic Retinopathy Study Report No. 22. *Arch Ophthalmol* 1996; 114 (9): 1079–84.
27. Fong DS, Ferris FL III, Davis MD, Chew EY, for the Early Treatment Diabetic Retinopathy Study Research Group. Causes of severe visual loss in the early treatment diabetic retinopathy study: Early Treatment Diabetic Retinopathy Study Report No. 24. *Am J Ophthalmol* 1999; 127 (2): 137–41.
28. Aiello LP, Gardner TW, King GL, Blankenship G, Cavallerano JD, Ferris FL III, Klein R. Diabetic retinopathy. *Diabetes Care* 1998; 21 (1): 143–56.
29. The UK Prospective Diabetes Study Group. Tight blood pressure control and risk of macrovascular and microvascular complications in type 2 diabetes: UKPDS 38. BMJ December 9, 1998; 317 (7160): 703–13.
30. Aiello LM. *Am J Ophthalmol* (in press).
31. Aiello LM, Cavallerano J, Cavallerano A, Bursell S. The Joslin Vision Network (JVN): innovative telemedicine care for diabetes. *Ophthalmol Clin N Am* 2000; 13: 213–24.
32. Bursell SE, Cavallerano JD, Cavallerano AA, Clermont AC, Birkmire-Peters D, Aiello LP, Aiello LM. Stereo nonmydriatic digital-video color retinal imaging compared with early treatment diabetic retinopathy study seven standard field 35-mm stereo color photos for determining level of diabetic retinopathy. *Ophthalmology* 2001; 108 (3): 572–85.

68

Diabetic Nephropathy

Stephen C. Jones*, Sally M. Marshall†, and Rudy W. Bilous*

James Cook University Hospital, Middlesbrough, UK, and †The Medical School, University of Newcastle upon Tyne, Newcastle upon Tyne, UK

INTRODUCTION

The first description of proteinuria in a person with diabetes was given by Cotunnius in 1764, who described the separation of a clot when a sample of urine was heated. Authors from the nineteenth century onward had begun to describe microscopic pathological changes in the kidneys of people with diabetes. Indeed, in 1877 Armanni and Epstein described the first microscopic lesion specific to diabetes as swelling of renal tubular cells. It was not until 1936 when Kimmelstiel and Wilson reported specific glomerular histopathology in proteinuric patients with diabetes that a diabetes specific glomerulopathy was accepted. Further reports in the 1940s described a clinical syndrome that was associated with intercapillary glomerulosclerosis, though it was recognized from postmortem studies that not all patients with proteinuria had typical glomerular changes. In 1951, the term "diabetic nephropathy" was suggested to describe a clinical syndrome of proteinuria, hypertension, and falling GFR, based upon a cohort of 62 patients.

Boiling urine and observing clot formation as a test for proteinuria was replaced by quantitative tests and test strips. The latter remain the mainstay for the detection of proteinuria in clinical practice today. In the 1960s, a threshold for proteinuria of 0.5–1 g/24 h was proposed as the level of proteinuria that defines "overt or clinical nephropathy." This level of protein excretion equates to a protein concentration in the urine that is roughly the same as the lower limit of detection of standard test strips.

Further developments of more specific and sensitive assays, particularly for albumin, led to the realization that patients developing nephropathy gradually passed increasing amounts of protein in their urine, which were not detected by routine tests including standard test strips. This level of urinary protein excretion that exceeds the upper limit of normal but is too low to be detected by standard strip tests has been termed incipient nephropathy or microalbuminuria. Albumin is the main protein excreted in diabetic nephropathy. It has become the convention to classify the stage of diabetic nephropathy upon the basis of precise urinary albumin concentrations or particularly for research-purposes-timed urinary albumin excretion rates (UAER). In this chapter the terms clinical nephropathy and microalbuminuria will be used to describe the clinical syndromes. The term diabetic kidney disease will be used when both stages are combined and the term diabetic glomerulopathy will be used to describe the typical histological changes.

DEFINITIONS AND DIAGNOSIS

The diagnosis of clinical nephropathy is based upon the detection of proteinuria using dipstick urinalysis. Such tests are based largely on the detection of albumin and are positive at a concentration of >300 mg/l (Table 1). Concentrations of urine albumin above normal but below 300 mg/l are termed microalbuminuria and can only be detected by sensitive immunoassays specifc for albumin. A number of factors such as intercurrent illness and diabetic ketoacidosis, in addition to diabetic kidney disease, can temporarily increase UAER. As a result a number of positive tests, usually at least two over a period of several months, are required to confirm the diagnosis of microalbuminuria or clinical nephropathy (Figure 1). It has been assumed until recently that microalbuminuria which is detected consistently over 6 or more months persists; however, it does appear that microalbuminuria

International Textbook of Diabetes Mellitus, Third Edition. Edited by R. A. DeFronzo, E. Ferrannini, H. Keen, and P. Zimmet.
 ISBN: 0-471-48655-8.

Table 1 Definitions of stages of diabetic kidney disease

	Normoalbuminuria	Microalbuminuria	Clinical nephropathy
Urinary albumin concentration (UAC)	<20 mg/l	20–300 mg/l	>300 mg/l (>30 mg/dl)
Timed overnight collection	<20 μg/min	20–199 μg/min	≥200 μg/min (dipstick-positive if >300 μg/min)
24-h collection	<30 mg/24 h	30–299 mg/24 h	≥300 mg/24 h
Albumin:creatinine ratio (ACR)			
Men	<2.5 mg/mmol	2.5–20 mg/mmol	>2 mg/mmol
	<25 mg/g	25–300 mg/g	>300 mg/g
Women	<3 mg/mmol	3–30 mg/mmol	>30 mg/mmol
	<30 mg/g	30–300 mg/g	>300 mg/g

Note: False positive results with concentrated urine, biological variation related to posture/diurnal variation, exercise, intercurrent illness, urinary infection, and nondiabetic kidney disease. False negative results with dilute urine or diuresis.

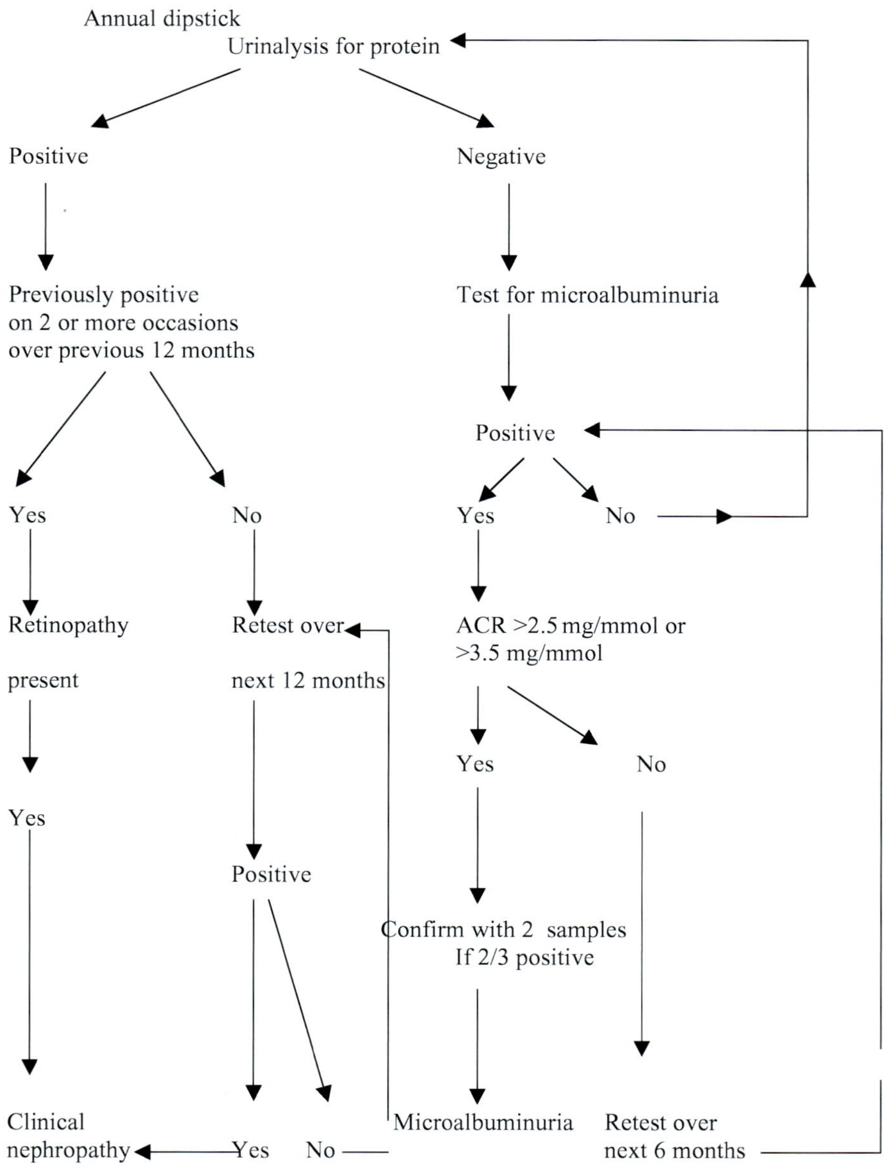

Figure 1 Flowchart for diagnosis of incipient and clinical nephropathy. Sterile urine assumed throughout. Exclude urinary tract infection when proteinuria is first detected

may be detected for many years before reverting to normal in a proportion of people [1].

Exclusion of Nondiabetic Kidney Disease

It is important to exclude nondiabetic kidney disease that might require specific therapy as clearly people with diabetes are not precluded from having any other renal condition. In clinical practice, a diagnosis of diabetic nephropathy can be made without resorting to renal biopsy when the typical features of the clinical syndrome are present; these include a duration of diabetes for at least 10 years, hypertension, and the presence of diabetic retinopathy (Figure 1). In type 1 diabetes when the onset is clearly defined clinical diagnosis is usually straight forward. In type 2 diabetes the clinical diagnosis may be more complicated as diabetes may have been present for a number of years before being recognized.

It is difficult to be certain of the precise prevalence of nondiabetic kidney disease, which has been described in different series as occurring in 8–22% of patients. These figures are very likely to be strongly affected by selection bias and overestimate the incidence of nondiabetic kidney disease as most patients with typical clinical features of diabetic nephropathy will not undergo renal biopsy. Those with atypical features are much more likely to undergo this procedure. The investigation of patients with hematuria is controversial. If red cell casts are detected on microscopy then further investigation, including biopsy, should be considered, although such casts have been noted in 4% cases of biopsy-proven diabetic glomerulopathy. If there are no casts then one large series of 136 patients with type 1 and type 2 diabetes suggested that the presence of hematuria (detected in 66% of patients) was of little help in distinguishing between diabetic and nondiabetic kidney disease.

If there is any doubt then renal biopsy should be considered (Table 2). The risks of the procedure when undertaken by a skilled practitioner (under ultrasound guidance) are small and the benefits, if treatable nondiabetic kidney disease is detected, may be large.

PATHOLOGY

Macroscopic Changes

Kidney enlargement has been recognized as a feature of newly diagnosed type 1 diabetes for a number of years.

Table 2 Features that suggest nondiabetic kidney disease

Rapid deterioration in renal function
Sudden development of nephrotic syndrome
Heavy hematuria/red cell casts
Absence of diabetic retinopathy
Short duration of type 1 diabetes
Clinical or laboratory evidence of nondiabetic systemic disease
Blood pressure higher than expected for degree of proteinuria

Experimental and *in vitro* studies suggest that expansion occurs as a result of tubular hypertrophy and hyperplasia [2, 3], probably as a compensatory response to increased glucose and fluid filtration and the need for active reabsorption in uncontrolled diabetes [4].

As urinary tract infection is relatively common in women with diabetes, renal scaring may occur. Papillary necrosis is a feature of long-standing diabetes and can occur as a result of hyperosmolar coma. Atheromatous renal artery stenosis is also well described in type 2 diabetes; however, functional stenosis is relatively rare.

Microscopic Appearances

Light Microscopy

The glomerulus Glomerular enlargement is an early feature of both human and experimental diabetes. In the rat, this occurs as the result of increases in capillary length and diameter. As basement membrane width is unchanged there must be a significant increase in matrix material production [4, 5].

In humans, enlargement is also present in patients with established nephropathy, particularly in type 2 diabetes. By using plastic embedded tissue, mean glomerular volumes of around (4 and 6) $\times 10^6$ μm^3 have been reported in type 1 and type 2 diabetes respectively, compared to a normal nondiabetic range of $(1-2.3) \times 10^6$ μm^3 [6].

The reasons why glomerular enlargement occurs in humans are unclear. In early diabetes, altered glomerular, hemodynamics, and hyperfiltration may be the major factors, while in established nephropathy a compensatory response to glomerular capillary closure and global glomerulosclerosis may predominate. Morphometric analysis of glomeruli from type 2 patients suggests that the proportion of patients who showed marked glomerular enlargement had a different structural response to diabetes, perhaps because of preexisting essential hypertension, which would tend to ameliorate diabetes-induced increases in glomerular capillary pressure [6].

The hallmark of diabetic glomerulopathy is diffuse mesangial expansion, which is associated with nodule formation in a minority of patients. Most patients with long-standing diabetes show an increase in *para*-aminosalicylic acid- (PAS-) positive matrix material, although these changes are much more prominent in those with clinical nephropathy. Initially, this material is central to the tuft but later it expands and effectively obliterates the capillaries, eventually leading to global glomerulosclerosis [5].

Nodules are more or less pathognomonic for diabetes and were the first specific glomerular pathological abnormality to be described. They comprise acellular, eosinophilic, and lamellated structures, usually located at the tuft periphery. Their pathogenesis is unclear but they may represent obliterated capillary microaneurysms or may result from focal mesangiolysis at the junction of the glomerular basement membrane (GBM) with the mesangium. This would lead to endothelial cell detachment and subsequent ballooning into the capillary, quickly followed by matrix deposition [5].

These characteristic features are not as universal in type 2 patients with microalbuminuria [7]; a proportion of patients have appearances more suggestive of glomerular ischemia or tubulointerstitial disease. However, type 2 patients with clinical nephropathy and significant retinopathy have glomerular changes similar to those of patients with type 1 diabetes [8].

Capsular drops of PAS-positive matrix material lying between the matrix membrane and parietal epithelium of Bowman's capsule are commonly seen but their significance is unclear.

In end-stage renal disease, glomeruli appear as sclerosed hyalinized structures and a percentage are actually reabsorbed. This global sclerosis appears to be due to a combination of mesangial expansion and ischemia secondary to afferent arteriolar hyalinosis [9].

Tubulointerstitium The first renal pathological abnormality to be described in diabetes was the presence of glycogen-rich granules in proximal tubular cells—the Armanni–Ebstein lesion. These changes are entirely preventable by glycemic correction and abolition of glycosuria.

Tubulointerstitial expansion contributes to whole kidney enlargement in early diabetes. It is also a feature of established nephropathy and is found in a significant number of microalbuminuric type 2 patients. It is not clear whether these changes are a response to glomerulosclerosis and subsequent tubular atrophy, or to a more fundamental mechanism leading to progressive renal failure [6]. As with glomerular enlargement, the causes are almost certainly different in early diabetes compared to established nephropathy. Acute changes in the juxta glomerular apparatus are seen within hours of development of diabetes in the rat. More subtle, long-term abnormalities in this structure have also been described in microalbuminuric type 1 patients and may reflect increased activity of tubuloglomerular feedback mechanisms and an upregulation of the renin–angiotensin system [10, 11].

Afferent and efferent arteriolar hyalinosis is a characteristic feature of diabetes and is more prominent in those with microalbuminuria [12].

Immunofluorescence Microscopy

Nonspecific linear staining for IgG (mainly IgG4) and albumin is found in the GBM, tubular basement membrane (TBM), and Bowman's capsule. Incubation in conditions of a low pH removes the staining implying strong ionic binding. There is no direct correlation with severity of glomerulopathy or nephropathy and pathophysiological significance is unclear [5].

Immunohistochemical analysis shows an increase in not only (mainly) type 4 collagen, but also type 6 collagen, tenascin, laminin and fibronectin in the mesangium, GBM, and TBM. The proportion differs however, with α-3 and α-4 chains of type 4 collagen predominating in thickened GBM of patients with rapidly developing glomerulopathy, and a reduced density of type 6 collagen in the subendothelial regions of the GBM and mesangium. These changes are undoubtedly due to an imbalance between the production and degradation of matrix proteins with perhaps differences in emphasis in different parts of the nephron and at different stages in nephropathy development [5].

Electron Microscopy

Glomerulus Structure of GBM is normal at the onset of type 1 diabetes, but GBM thickening up to three times the normal range of 270–359 nm is an almost universal feature in patients with a duration of >10 years (Figure 2). This thickening is more marked in those with microalbuminuria and clinical nephropathy. There is an accumulation of type IV collagen with a net reduction in heparan sulfate proteoglycan. This combination disrupts both normal GBM structure as well as its electrostatic charge properties, resulting in abnormal permselectivity to circulating proteins [5].

The expanded mesangium occurs as a result of excess matrix accumulation. In normal human, the ratio of cellular to matrix components is about 1:1, with a mean fractional volume of mesangium between 14 and 20% in the glomerular tuft [13]. In patients with nephropathy, the proportion of matrix increases and the mesangium may comprise over 40% of total tuft volume. This accumulation disrupts the microfibrillar structure of the mesangium, altering its porosity to proteins, and weakening attachments to the endothelium and GBM, perhaps predisposing to nodule formation [5]. Nodules comprise matrix of similar composition to the mesangial areas, but with a prominent accumulation of microfibrils.

Some patients with advanced nephropathy have thin irregular segments of GBM lined by an abnormal looking endothelium. These could represent new capillary growth analogous to the situation in the retina or possibly microaneurysms. Their significance is uncertain but they might lead to microscopic hematuria (occasionally seen in diabetes) as it occurs in nondiabetic patients with thin basement membrane disease, or it might even represent a highly porous "shunt pathway" contributing to total proteinuria [5, 14].

Tubulointerstitium The structure and constitution of the TBM is largely similar to GBM but it is almost twice as wide. In diabetes, TBM increases to about two to three

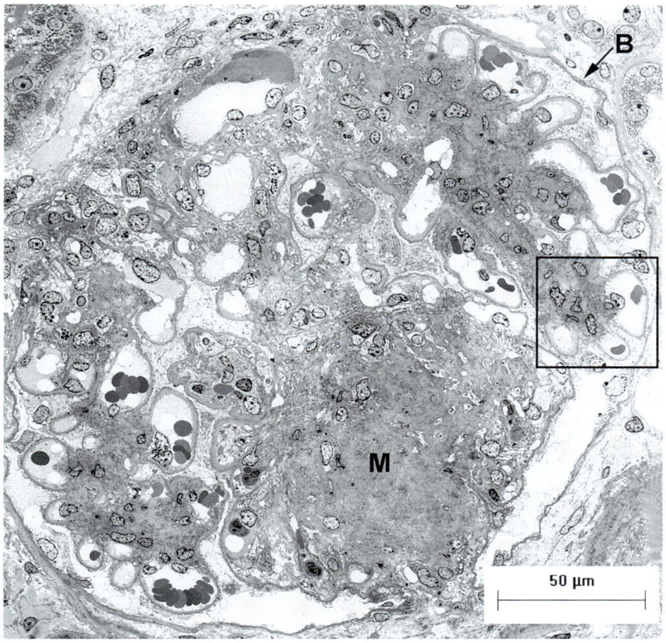

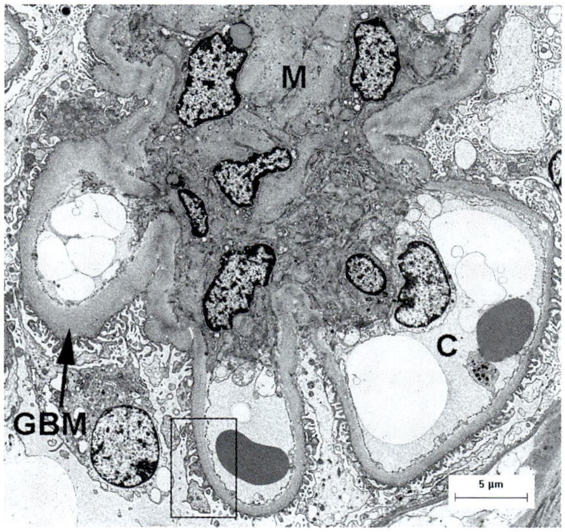

Figure 2 Electron micrograph of a glomerulus from a patient with clinical nephropathy. Low-powered view indicating typical changes of diabetic glomerulopathy including diffuse mesangial expansion and associated with nodule formation (M). High-powered view demonstrating glomerular basement membrane (GBM) thickening

times normal width and often appears split [15]. This could lead to macromolecular penetration of the interstitial space leading to an activation of cytokines, setting in train pathways that ultimately lead to fibrosis.

Early tubulointerstitial expansion is largely a result of an increase in cellular components [16], with fibrosis and collagen accumulation occurring much later in established nephropathy.

EPIDEMIOLOGY AND NATURAL HISTORY

Studies of the prevalence and incidence of diabetic kidney disease have reported widely differing results. This is because the prevalence of diabetic kidney disease is strongly influenced by factors such as population selection (hospital- or primary-care-based patients), and ethnicity as well as technical factors related to the number and type of tests that are undertaken and the diagnostic levels that are chosen. Although the stages of diabetic kidney disease for type 1 and type 2 diabetes will be described separately according to UAER, it is important to bear in mind that proteinuria is a continuous variable, and any diagnostic cutoff points are somewhat arbitary.

Type 1 Diabetes

At the Time of Diagnosis

A number of abnormalities have been described in relation to kidney function at the time of diagnosis of type 1 diabetes. These include a raised glomerular filtration rate (GFR) [17], increased UAER [18, 19], and increased renal size. Shortly after commencement of insulin treatment, UAER returns to normal levels in most patients [20–22]. However, in around one third of patients GFR remains high [17, 23]. The significance of this hyperfiltration has been debated. It has been suggested that it is associated with a later progression to nephropathy [24]; however, this has not been universally confirmed [25, 26].

Microalbuminuria

In those patients who are destined never to develop diabetic nephropathy, UAER remains, for the most part, in the normal range. However, this can change temporarily during times of poor glycemic control, after an episode of diabetic ketoacidosis, during acute intercurrent illnesses, or after vigorous exercise and high-protein meals. At these times UAER may increase to the microalbuminuric or even the proteinuric range, but usually returns promptly to normal values. This "natural variation" is one of the reasons why several abnormal measurements, over a period of time, are required before the diagnosis of microalbuminuria, and indeed clinical nephropathy, can be established (Figure 1).

This variability may also contribute to the wide variation in the reported prevalence of microalbuminuria in patients with type 1 diabetes (Table 3), although other factors relating to the population under investigation and

Table 3 Reported prevalence of microalbuminuria in type 1 and 2 diabetic populations with a sample size > 200 individuals

Study	Number	Age (years)	Definition	Type of sample	Prevalence (%)
Type 1					
Hospital/clinics					
Denmark	982	>18	>30 mg/day	24-h collection	22
United States (Pittsburgh)	627	15–54	>20 μg/min	4-h collection	22
EURODIAB	3250	15–60	>20 μg/min	24-h collection	21
United Kingdom (Newcastle)	416	14–87	>30 μg/min	Timed overnight	7
Population-based					
Norway	351	18–32	>15 μg/min	Timed O/N × 2	12.5
United States (Wisconsin)	706	8–71	>30 mg/l	Spot urine	21
Type 2					
Newly diagnosed					
United Kingdom (UKPDS)	5097	Mean 52.1	>50 mg/l	Spot urine	6.5
Denmark	1267	Median 65.3	ACR >2 mg/mmol	Spot urine	34
Hospital/clinic					
United Kingdom (Newcastle)	524	19–86	>30 μg/min	Timed overnight	10
United Kingdom (Belfast)	216	Mean 63.9	>25 mg/l	Spot urine	22
Denmark	549	<76	>31 mg/day	? 24 h urine	27
Population-based					
Pacific Islanders	228	>20	>30 mg/l	Spot urine	42
United Kingdom (Poole)	329	?	>30 μg/min	Timed O/N	11
Denmark	204	60–74	>15 μg/min	Timed O/N	25
New Zealand (Europid)	297	20–80	>30 mg/day	24-h collection	22
United States (Pima)	830	15–87	>30 mg/g ACR (3.5 mg/mmol)	Spot urine	25

Note: O/N = overnight.

the chosen diagnostic levels are also important. The reported prevalence of microalbuminuria in hospital-based patients from the United Kingdom and United States is around 20%, although in a European population based study the prevalence was lower at around 12% and this is likely to be closer to the true value in unselected Europid patients.

In patients who are destined to develop end-stage renal failure (ESRF) UAER rises progressively, with microalbuminuria developing within 10 years of the diagnosis of diabetes. It has been thought that UAER remained within the normal range for several years after diagnosis [21, 22, 27]. Recently, however, microalbuminuria has been detected in up to 19% of patients with a relatively short duration (1–5 years) [28, 29].

Duration of diabetes remains, however, closely related to the prevalence of microalbuminuria in type 1 diabetes, reaching 40–50% after 30 years [30, 31]. The annual incidence of microalbuminuria in patients with an initially normal UAER has been estimated to be around 2% [32–34], although there is some evidence that with good glycemic control this can be reduced [35]. This might explain why the prevalence of microalbuminuria in more recently described cohorts is somewhat lower [28, 36].

A number of clinical and biochemical parameters influence the progression from normoalbuminuria to microalbuminuria. Perhaps, not surprisingly, the strongest factor is the baseline UAER, with those in the "high normal" range most likely to progress to microalbuminuria [32]. Indeed it has been suggested that the upper limit of "normal" UAER should be 10 μg/min rather than the conventional 20 μg/min. The latter figure of 20 μg/min was adopted somewhat arbitrarily at a consensus meeting and remains in use today. There may be a period of intermittent microalbuminuria before persistent microalbuminuria is established. This presumably reflects the high day-to-day variation in UAER of up to 40–50% [37]. Other factors that have consistently been associated with the development of microalbuminuria are poor glycemic control, increased blood pressure, and the presence of retinopathy. There is a much less consistent association with smoking and plasma lipid abnormalities.

Blood pressure is particularly important in the rate of progression from microalbuminuria to clinical nephropathy, patients with a mean arterial pressure >94 mmHg being more likely to progress [38]. In those who do progress, the rate of change of albumin excretion is very variable from individual to individual, but is on average 20% per annum [39], so that it takes 10–15 years for UAER to reach clinical nephropathy levels. As the cutoff between microalbuminuria and proteinuria is reached, patients pass through a phase of intermittent proteinuria, before it becomes persistent [40]. Thereafter, protein excretion rises continuously, occasionally into the nephrotic range, with the main determinant being systemic blood pressure [41].

Clinical Nephropathy

Diabetic kidney disease has always been regarded as a disease of inevitable progression from one stage to another. Indeed the early initial studies suggested that approximately 80% of microalbuminuric type 1 diabetic patients would develop clinical nephropathy proteinuria [42–44]. However, more recent studies suggest that in approximately 30% of microalbuminuric patients, albumin excretion reverts to normal, 50% remain microalbuminuric, and 20% progress to proteinuria over a 5–9-year period [22, 38, 45, 46]. However, while it is now clear that not all microalbuminuric patients progress to clinical nephropathy their risk remains much higher than patients whose UAER remains within normal range.

Epidemiological studies suggest that those who develop microalbuminuria after a short duration of diabetes have a more aggressive disease and are more likely to progress to clinical nephropathy [47]. Such patients have been termed "fast trackers" while those with microalbuminuria and duration of diabetes >15 years are less likely to progress and appear to have relatively well-preserved renal function [48]. However, with general improvements, particularly in glycemic and blood pressure control, it is likely that this pattern is altering—the whole disease process being slowed and the natural history delayed. Thus microalbuminuria and proteinuria may now develop after longer durations of diabetes. Recent evidence appears to confirm this with the description of a long-duration cohort of patients in whom diabetic kidney disease continued to progress despite a duration of diabetes for more than 30 years [49].

In historical series, the cumulative incidence of clinical nephropathy after 25-year duration of type 1 diabetes was approximately 41% in those diagnosed from 1933 to 1942 and 25% in patients diagnosed from 1953 to 1962 [50, 51]. In some more recent series, after 15–29 years of duration of diabetes, the cumulative incidence of clinical nephropathy was similar at 26% in 1986 data [52] with a further fall to 14–17% in some cohorts reported in the 1990s [28, 36, 52, 53]. However, in other populations, no change in the incidence of proteinuria by year of diagnosis has been observed [54, 55].

The prevalence of clinical nephropathy also varies considerably between hospital-based patients and population-based studies for similar reasons as for the reported variation in microalbuminuria, i.e. selection criteria, methodology used to define UAER, and ethnicity. The range is from 6 to 27% in type 1 diabetes (Table 4).

End-Stage Renal Disease

In type 1 diabetes GFR can start to decline with increasing UAER in the microalbuminuric range. The rate of fall varies considerably from person to person but is relatively constant within each individual. Historically, the average rate of fall is 10–12 ml/min/year, so that it would take 8–10 years from the onset of proteinuria to end-stage renal disease (ESRD) [56–58]. Blood pressure is the most important determinant of the rate of fall of GFR [57, 59] and with the advent of intensive blood pressure management regimes, the rate of fall is now around 4 ml/min/year. As renal function deteriorates, fluid overload and pulmonary edema may occur even in the absence

Table 4 Reported prevalence of clinical nephropathy in type 1 and 2 diabetes with a sample size >200 individuals

Study	Number	Age	Definition	Type of sample	Prevalence (%)
Type 1 and 2					
World Health Organization study	6695	35–54	Positive acid test	Spot urine	25
Type 1					
Hospital					
EURODIAB	3250	15–60	>200 μg/min	24-h collection	9
United States (Pittsburgh)	627	15–45	>200 μg/min	4-h collection	27
United Kingdom (Newcastle)	416	14–87	>150 μg/min	Timed O/N	6
United States (Boston)	292	20–40	>300 mg/l	Spot urine	18 (20 years dd)
Denmark	1475	20–50	>300 mg/day	24-h collection	21 (20–25 years dd)
Population-based					
United Kingdom (Poole)	202	10–85	>300 mg/l	Timed O/N	6
Type 2					
Hospital					
United Kingdom (Newcastle)	524	19–86	>150 μg/min	Timed O/N	6
Denmark	549	<76	>300 mg/day	24-h collection	14
Newly diagnosed					
UKPDS	5097	Mean 52	>300 mg/l	Spot	1
Population based					
United Kingdom (Poole)	640	20–85	>300 mg/l	Timed O/N	7
United States (Wisconsin)	1292	35–85	>300 mg/l	Spot	16
United States (Hispanic)	317	Mean 54	>300 mg/l	Spot	17
United States (Pima)	830	15–87	>300 mg/g ACR	Spot	21
New Zealand (Europid)	297	20–80	>300 mg/day	24-h urine	5
Pacific Islanders	228	>20	>300 mg/l	Spot	33

Note: O/N = overnight; dd = diabetes duration.

of hypoalbuminemia, partly because of associated poor left ventricular function due to cardiovascular disease.

Type 2 Diabetes

Recent data suggest that the course of the development of nephropathy in type 2 diabetes is in general very similar to that seen in type 1 diabetes, although there are some differences. Longitudinal studies in the Pima Indians, including data obtained during normal and impaired glucose tolerance, have been particularly informative.

At the Time of Diagnosis

Diabetes may have been present for many years before a clinical diagnosis is made. As a result, therefore, UAER at the time of diagnosis of type 2 diabetes may be normal or high [60–63]. As blood glucose is controlled, albumin excretion returns to the normal range in many patients [63–65]. However, in 10–48% of the patients microalbuminuria is persistent, presumably reflecting the long period of diabetes prior to diagnosis and underlying irreversible renal structural damage [63, 64, 66]. Some studies have suggested that blood glucose and glycated hemoglobin levels at diagnosis of diabetes are higher in those in whom microalbuminuria persists [64].

Microalbuminuria

In cross-sectional studies in established diabetes, the prevalence of microalbuminuria varies considerably between 10 and 42%, depending upon population selection and ethnicity [67–72] (Table 3). Higher prevalences are reported in UK Asians [68], Pima Indians [72], African Americans, Native Americans [73], and in Maori and Pacific Islanders [70] compared to White Europid patients who seem, in relative terms, to be protected from this complication. Perhaps because of the uncertainties associated with estimating the precise onset of diabetes the relationship of prevalence of microalbuminuria to duration of type 2 diabetes is not as strong as in type 1 diabetes. Longitudinal studies suggest that the rate of progression from normal albumin excretion to microalbuminuria is 2–4% per annum, at least as high, if not higher than in type 1 diabetes [72, 74–77]. Factors most consistently associated with progression include baseline albumin excretion, glycated hemoglobin, systemic blood pressure, and serum cholesterol [74, 76, 78].

Clinical Nephropathy

There is less information on progression from microalbuminuria to proteinuria in type 2 diabetes. In White Europid populations, approximately one third of microalbuminuric type 2 diabetic patients develop clinical nephropathy within 5 years [79, 80]. After 20-year duration of type 2 diabetes, the cumulative incidence of clinical nephropathy is 27%, similar to that observed in type 1 diabetes [81] (Table 4). In the Pima Indians, more than 50% develop proteinuria within 20 years [78]. In contrast to the decline in the cumulative incidence of clinical nephropathy in type 1 diabetes with onset in the 1970s and 1980s in some populations, the incidence in Pima Indians has doubled in the last 40 years [82], despite improvements in glucose and blood pressure control. This suggests a rapidly changing environmental or behavioral effect.

Because of the high prevalence of systemic hypertension in newly diagnosed and established type 2 diabetes, the relationship of hypertension to microalbuminuria and proteinuria is more complex than that in type 1 diabetes. However, most people with microalbuminuria or proteinuria have concomitant systemic hypertension and blood pressure rises further as albuminuria increases.

End-Stage Renal Disease

The progression to ESRF is broadly similar in type 1 and 2 diabetes. GFR remains stable or occasionally high with the onset of microalbuminuria, and begins to decline only when clinical nephropathy has developed [78, 83, 84].

In patients with established clinical nephropathy, the rate of decline of GFR is similar to that seen in type 1 diabetes, at 10–12 ml/min/year [45, 81] although there is some suggestion that it may be greater in non-Caucasian subjects [85]. In England, the age-standardized acceptance ratios for renal replacement therapy are reported as 4.2 and 3.7 times higher in African Caribbean and Indo-Asian compared to White Europid diabetic patients [86]. This is in agreement with data from studies based in other countries [87–89].

The number of diabetic patients requiring renal replacement therapy continues to increase rapidly worldwide, although wide variation in the absolute incidence rates remains. In 2000, the highest reported annual incidence was in the United States (145 diabetic patients per million population), with Japan and Taiwan reporting rates of just less than 100 per million (Table 5) [90]. The highest rate reported in the European Union was in Germany at 63 per million population. In most countries, diabetes is now the single commonest cause of ESRD.

Despite limitations in these epidemiological data, it is clear that the increase is not entirely due to increasing numbers of patients with type 2 diabetes. Reasons for this include a greater willingness to treat ESRD in elderly patients and a progressively declining premature cardiovascular mortality in this high-risk population. However, there also appears to be a greater than expected increase in numbers reaching ESRD, particularly in non-Europid populations, despite improvements in glucose and blood pressure control [82]. Reasons for this might be reduced a renoprotective effect of inhibition of the renin–angiotensin

Table 5 Annual incidence of patients with end-stage renal failure commencing renal replacement therapy and proportion of those with diabetes*

Country	All patients incidence of ESRD per million population	Proportion of patients with diabetes
Austria	90	33
Brunei	210	45
Bulgaria	78	9.4
Canada	143	32
Finland	94	31
Germany	175	36
Japan	252	37
Philippines	27	23.4
Russia	15	3.6
United States	326	43.5

*Data from reference 90.

system in Indo-Asian patients [85] and also reduced nephron endowment due to relative fetal growth retardation [91]. However, the rapid rate of increase also suggests environmental factors [82]. A distinct form of obesity-related glomerulopathy has been reported and it may be that population increases in body weight are influencing the development of ESRD in type 2 diabetes [92].

Overall, the development and course of nephropathy in Europid patients with type 2 diabetes is remarkably similar to those with type 1, the differences seen probably relating to delayed diagnosis and to the older age and consequently more marked concomitant cardiovascular disease. In non-Europid populations, the prevalence of diabetic kidney disease is higher and progression to ESRD may be faster.

STRUCTURAL–FUNCTIONAL CORRELATES

The relatively slow progressive nature of renal functional loss in diabetic nephropathy and the fact that only a minority of patients develop the condition has led to studies of renal structure to see if this can provide clues as to the pathogenesis and evolution of the condition.

Renal Structure and GFR

Glomerular capillary filtration surface area is the major structural factor determining GFR. Cross-sectional studies in type 1 patients show that mesangial volume was inversely, and glomerular volume positively correlated to the surface area of the peripheral GBM and GFR. Moreover, in more advanced nephropathy the number of globally sclerosed glomeruli was negatively correlated to GFR. As the number of glomeruli per kidney ranges from 0.3 to 1.4×10^6 in normal human being, the structural determinants of GFR become

(1) capillary filtration surface area, which is dependent upon glomerular volume and the degree of mesangial expansion.
(2) number of functioning glomeruli, which is dependent upon the original number at diagnosis minus those lost to global sclerosis.

Glomerular volumes are known to be large at diagnosis of diabetes and can be normalized by insulin therapy in diabetic animals. There is continuing controversy over whether glomerular enlargement is itself a risk factor for later nephropathy development in humans. Studies on isolated glomeruli demonstrate that volume can change dramatically with alterations in perfusion pressure, and it is recognized that average volume varies throughout the renal cortex, with larger glomeruli in the juxta medullary region. Finally, the method of processing tissue can affect the estimate of glomerular size with generally larger values for plastic embedded tissue, and the measurement technique can also produce estimates that are subject to varying degrees of unquantifiable bias. Thus associative studies between glomerular volume changes and GFR are sometimes difficult to interpret.

Notwithstanding these caveats the consistent glomerular enlargement seen in early diabetes is noteworthy and almost certainly reflects an increase in intraglomerular pressure and hyperfiltration. Intriguing data on the effects of mechanical stretch on mesangial cells provide a plausible link between glomerular enlargement and subsequent development of glomerulopathy [93].

In more advanced clinical nephropathy glomerular enlargement may be an adaptive response to an expanding mesangium and glomerulosclerosis [5]. In these circumstances, such enlargement would tend to preserve GFR. Interestingly, some type 2 patients with clinical nephropathy have much larger glomeruli than do type 1 patients with a similar GFR [6]. As many type 2 patients have hypertension prior to developing nephropathy (in direct distinction to type 1), it is possible that intraglomerular pressures may be lower than in those individuals with hypertension as a result of glomerulopathy. (It is known that nondiabetic patients with essential hypertension have normal intraglomerular capillary pressure.) Thus any mechanical effect on the mesangium would be reduced with perhaps less matrix production, less stiffening of the glomerulus, and thus permitting a greater adaptive enlargement to loss of filtration surface.

Interstitial volume changes have also been related to GFR both in cross-sectional and follow-up biopsy studies, although the correlations are generally weaker than for mesangial volume [5]. In type 2 patients, interstitial changes can be more prominent than in those with type 1 diabetes. In a proportion of type 2 patients such changes are the dominant lesion (see above). In advanced nephropathy interstitial lesions are closely related to GFR, even though they are not closely related to mesangial expansion. Thus changes in these two structures may have different impacts on nephropathy progression at different stages in its evolution, and may also lead to differences between type 1 and type 2 diabetes.

Renal Structure and Albumin Excretion Rate

Initial increases in albumin excretion rate (AER) in diabetes are probably related to subtle changes in the composition and structure of the GBM that are difficult to visualize. It is likely that reduction or dilution of heparan sulfate proteoglycan associated positive electrostatic charge leads to slight increases in AER into the microalbuminuric range. By using cuprolinic blue staining, a dispersal and loss of anionic charge sites has been demonstrated in the GBM of diabetic patients with microalbuminuria [5].

As AER increases into the clinically nephropathic range, the development of a shunt pathway results in a decline in size selectivity of the GBM to circulating macromolecules [14]. The structural counterpart of this shunt is not clear. It could be a general leakiness of the peripheral GBM as a result of disruption of the collagen lattice due to matrix accumulation. It may also result from new vessel growth or thin GBM development. It could even originate from the mesangio-urinary interface, which is increased in established glomerulopathy, particularly in type 1 patients.

Cross-sectional studies in both types of diabetes reveal positive correlations between GBM width and AER [6]. Moreover, in a longitudinal study of type 1 patients change in GBM width was correlated with change in AER over 2–3 years, and baseline GBM width was predictive of AER at follow-up 6 years later.

More detailed ultrastructural study has shown that changes in epithelial foot process width also relate to AER. This is thought to be an adaptive response in an attempt to narrow and shorten the filtration slit between adjacent foot processes. More recently, a reduction in podocyte number has been found by some in both type 1 and 2 diabetic patients with clinical nephropathy, although these findings have not been confirmed in microalbuminuric type 1 patients [94]. There are major methodological problems involved in estimating podocyte number in human beings, and changes in podocyte number and function are currently the subject of intense research. Their role in nephropathy will undoubtedly become clearer in the future.

Cross-sectional studies in large cohorts of type 1 patients continue to show a degree of overlap in glomerulopathy between those with normal AER, microalbuminuria, and clinical nephropathy. While the latter group almost always have well-established mesangial lesions, some patients with apparently normal function in terms of AER can have quite advanced glomerulopathy. Microalbuminuric patients generally have increased mesangial volumes, particularly if they are hypertensive. These results have prompted a vigorous debate on the importance of glomerular lesions for nephropathy development and progression. One school of thought suggests that the lesions are the inevitable result of diabetes itself and not important. The opposing view is that as some patients with microalbuminuria regress to normal and do not appear to progress, and that renal failure must inevitably be the result of nephron loss, then structural progression must be paramount [95]. It is likely that some pathological change such as GBM thickening and minor increases in mesangial matrix may be a consequence of prolonged exposure to hyperglycemia. It is the degree of change that must characterize those individuals who will progress to renal failure. Preliminary results suggesting that those with normal AER and glomerulopathy are more likely to progress to clinical nephropathy imply that lesions may precede functional changes. The results of prospective studies are eagerly awaited [96]. As renal biopsy remains for the most part an experimental procedure in routine diabetes care, however, measurement of AER remains the most important clinical assessment of progression.

Tubulointerstitial changes also correlate with AER and may be an important consequence of increased protein trafficking in patients with advanced nephropathy [16].

PATHOPHYSIOLOGY

Hyperglycemia

The specificity of the glomerular pathological lesions for diabetes was established 50 years ago, and the association between poor glycemic control and an increased frequency of complications has been known for over 30 years. Deeper explorations of the relationship between glycemia and nephropathy have been aided by the development of tests that estimate average glucose control over a period of time, such as glycated hemoglobin (HbA_{1c}, 8–12 weeks) or fructosamine (2 weeks). However, it is important to realize that these tests tell us little about the moment to moment variation in glycemia and there is now a growing body of evidence linking postprandial peaks of blood glucose to risk of development of complications. Many patients with a satisfactory HbA_{1c} were found to have long day-time periods of relative hypo- and hyperglycemia, when studied over 3 days using an implantable glucose sensor. Also related to this problem is the of duration of diabetes, which is itself closely related to the risk of nephropathy development. Thus it is crucial to allow for these factors when interpreting cross-sectional or longitudinal studies in diabetic patients.

Much of our current understanding has come from trials of improved vs. standard glycemic control. In the DCCT (Diabetes Control and Complications Trial) a cohort of

726 patients without retinopathy (the primary prevention cohort) within 5 years of onset of type 1 diabetes was randomized to intensive vs. conventional glycemic control [35]. The conventionally treated group had a significantly increased risk of developing microalbuminuria compared to those on intensive therapy. A similar relationship was seen in the UKPDS (United Kingdom Prospective Diabetes Study) of intensive vs. standard control in nearly 4000 newly diagnosed type 2 patients [97]. It is important to note, however, that the development of microalbuminuria is not completely abolished even in intensively treated patients. For example, 15% of intensively treated patients in the DCCT developed microalbuminuria over 9 years suggesting that inherited susceptibility (see below) and/or postprandial glucose peaks referred to above also play important roles in the development of this condition.

Numerous cross-sectional as well as prospective studies in both types of diabetes and in all ethnic populations have confirmed the relationship between hyperglycemia and nephropathy. The more important question is how hyperglycemia causes nephropathy. It is highly likely that at any one time there is an interaction between different mechanisms and that different factors are operating at different stages in nephropathy evolution.

Glycation

Glucose is able to react spontaneously with proteins, lipids, and nucleic acids to form stable but potentially reversible compounds [98]. Structural proteins such as collagen, which have a slow turnover, undergo a slow transformation to form chemically irreversible advanced glycation end products or AGEs. These compounds can also be formed as a result of oxidative processes. Specific receptors for AGE have now been found to be present in many tissues that are prone to diabetic complications, such as the retina, peripheral nerve, and blood vessels. In the kidney, AGE binding sites have been described in cultured mesangial cells and proximal tubular epithelium.

AGE molecules could promote the development of nephropathy in three ways.

(1) Glycation of structural proteins such as collagen increases disulfide cross-linking. Such changes are likely to affect matrix assembly and permeability to macromolecules and may also impair degradation and turnover.
(2) Receptor binding has been shown to activate a range of cytokines implicated in the etiology of diabetic kidney disease, including transforming growth factor β (TGF-β), interleukin 1, tumor necrosis factor, and vascular endothelial growth factor (VEGF). Circulating AGE molecules can also bind to other cytokines such as SPARC, vascular cell adhesion molecule 1 (VCAM-1), and Platelet-derived growth factor (PDGF), as well as directly increasing oxidized LDL cholesterol.
(3) AGE molecules blunt the effect of endogenous nitric oxide inhibiting its vasodilatory and antiproliferative actions.

Injection of AGEs into nondiabetic mice leads to a glomerulopathy with some similarities to diabetes. Moreover plasma AGE levels are increased in diabetic patients with nephropathy and renal impairment. Because AGEs are so highly reactive via both receptor- and nonreceptor-mediated mechanisms, it is hard to distinguish between potentially protective clearance pathways and pathologically damaging reactions. The development of AGE cross-link inhibitors such as aminoguanidine has provided a tool to explore these possibilities [98]. However, concerns have been raised with regards to the toxicity of these compounds and the promising results observed in animal models of diabetic kidney disease have not been replicated in humans.

Polyol Pathway

The enzyme aldose reductase, which is present throughout the kidney, catalyzes the conversion of D-glucose to a metabolically inert alcohol, sorbitol. This enzyme is upregulated by increases in circulating glucose thus leading to an accumulation of sorbitol in tissues exposed to prolonged hyperglycemia [99]. The physiological role of aldose reductase in the kidney is unclear but it is probably important in maintaining medullary cell osmolality. In human and experimental diabetes, sorbitol concentrations are increased in many tissues, particularly the lens and peripheral nerve. The metabolism of sorbitol consumes NADPH, leading to reduced myoinositol levels and to an altered REDOX balance, which some have linked to the development of microvascular complications.

Much of the evidence for the role of this pathway in diabetic nephropathy has come from the use of aldose reductase inhibitor drugs, which can prevent the early abnormalities of a raised GFR and increased tissue permeability to proteins in experimental animals. The data in humans are less clear-cut [100].

Protein Kinase Cβ

High-glucose concentrations have been shown to increase intracellular production of protein kinase C (PKC) in many tissues, but specifically the retina and glomerulus. This increase is probably mediated via excessive activation of the glycolytic pathway leading to enhanced diacylglycerol (DAG) production. PKC can induce extracellular matrix production, cell growth, and angiogenesis as well as increasing vascular permeability and cell contractility, all of which have been described at various stages of animal and human diabetic nephropathy [101].

PKC comprise a family of kinases that act as intracellular signal transduction systems for cytokines and hormones. They are classified according to structure and at least 11 have been described. PKC-β isoforms appear to be those consistently activated by diabetes and they are sensitive to both DAG and calcium. Potential mechanisms by which PKC-β activation could mediate some of the functional changes of diabetes include the following:

(1) Enhancement of arachidonic acid production with consequent prostaglandin E2 and prostacyclin release.
(2) Inhibition of Na^+–K^+-ATPase with consequent effects on contractility, growth, and differentiation.
(3) Increased expression of mRNA for TGF-β leading to excess extracellular matrix production.
(4) Increased capillary permeability to macromolecules possibly related to an overexpression of VEGF.

The development of a specific PKC-β isoform inhibitor has shown that many of the functional and structural features of experimental diabetes in the rat can be ameliorated or prevented. This agent is currently undergoing phase 2 studies in human beings.

Oxidative Stress

The implication of oxidative stress in the development of diabetic complications is long-standing [102]. There are many *in vitro* data linking hyperglycemia to the generation of reactive oxygen species in a range of tissues, including endothelial and mesangial cells. However, it is not entirely clear whether these reactions are independent or a result of other pathways such as AGE production or PKC-β activation. *In vitro* antioxidant therapies block most of the responses to reactive oxygen species but trials in intact animals and human beings are largely negative or inconclusive. Better markers of oxidative stress *in vivo*, and more specific therapies are needed to explore this potential causative mechanism.

Nuclear Factor κB

This transcription factor is widely expressed and can activate many genes encoding a range of proteins and cytokines implicated in nephropathy. High glucose, AGEs, and PKC can all activate it, and inhibition in nondiabetic models of renal fibrosis confers nephro-protection. Its potential role in diabetic nephropathy requires further study [102].

Hexosamine Pathway

Hexokinase converts glucose to glucose-6-phosphate, which subsequently converts to fructose-6-phosphate by glycolysis. Glutamine:fructose-6-phosphate amidotransferase (GFAT) activation produces glucosamine-6-phosphate, using glutamine as an amino donor. Overexpression of this enzyme by glucose leads to PKC activation and TGF-β expression. GFAT blockade is possible using azaserine and its impact on diabetic nephropathy is currently being explored [102].

A number of potential therapies that could block glucose-mediated kidney damage have been developed. AGE cross-link inhibitors such as aminoguanidine have been available for some time. However, the relatively few clinical trials in patients with diabetic kidney disease have not reproduced the positive results that have been observed in animal studies. This may reflect species differences, or the different stages at which therapy has been attempted. In animal studies treatment has been given from the onset of diabetes, whereas in humans therapy has been attempted in patients with diabetic kidney disease in whom structural lesions are established and are likely to be difficult to reverse. In addition, as there are many routes by which glucose can exert damaging effects on the kidney, it is possible that blocking a single pathway will be ineffective. The role of newer agents such as PKC-β inhibitors have yet to be defined in clinical trials.

Growth Factors

Whole kidney enlargement in early diabetes and matrix overproduction in glomerulosclerosis imply a possible role of growth factors in the pathophysiology of nephropathy [103]. Growth factor is a generic term that includes a variety of compounds that can induce cellular proliferation or differentiation. These can range from hypothalamic or pituitary hormones, such as growth hormone, to substances that have paracrine or autocrine actions, such as TGF-β. Many of these growth factors are interrelated and activation of one family will have stimulatory effects on another. Most of our current understanding of the role of these factors is based upon *in vitro* cell culture or experimental diabetes in rodents. The development of specific antagonists opens therapeutic avenues in human beings that are as yet unexplored.

Growth Hormone and Insulin-like Growth Factor

Historically, an association between growth hormone (GH) and diabetes was first demonstrated in 1937 by Young, who found that administration of anterior pituitary extracts induced diabetes in dogs [103]. The later development of GH assays led to the discovery of increased levels in many diabetic patients, and the observation of regression of retinopathy in a diabetic woman who developed postpartum hypopituitarism (Sheehan's syndrome) suggested a role of GH in microvascular complications.

It is now realized that GH mediates its effects by inducing local tissue production of insulin-like growth factor 1 (IGF-1) and IGF-2 by interacting with specific growth hormone receptors. These receptors have intracellular, transmembrane, and extracellular components. After GH binding, there is posttranslational cleavage of the extracellular component, which is lost to the circulation where it can be detected as GH binding protein. IGF-1 and -2 are circulating hormones in their own right and as such have their own specific receptors. The IGF-1 and insulin receptors have a high degree of homology and the intracellular consequences of hormone receptor binding are also similar. The IGF-2 receptor is quite different and linked to lysosymal enzyme activation [103].

There are six well characterized high-affinity binding proteins for IGF-1 and -2. These prolong circulatory half-life and can directly stimulate or inhibit local tissue action.

mRNA expression for all the components of this complex system is found in normal kidney tissues, although each constituent has a specific localization in the nephron. Cell culture studies have shown that IGF-1 can stimulate matrix production from mesangial cells and reduce metalloproteinase 2 activity, a protein that plays an important role in matrix breakdown.

In human beings the low-insulin levels associated with poorly controlled diabetes result in deceased hepatic IGF-1 production. In a classical endocrine feedback loop this results in stimulation of the anterior pituitary somatotrophs to release GH. This in turn is thought to lead to stimulation of local IGF-1 and -2 production in the kidney and other tissues.

In rodents there is a direct link between renal production of IGF-1 and the early kidney enlargement in both streptozotocin-induced and spontaneous diabetes. GH-deficient diabetic rats have an ameliorated kidney and glomerular enlargement supporting a role of GH in initiating these changes. While IGF-1 receptor activation occurs in both early and sustained diabetes, the IGF-2 system appears to be activated only in the first few days. The impact of diabetes on the IGF binding proteins is highly complex and there are inconsistencies between animal models. However, a striking redistribution of IGF binding protein 1 from medulla to cortex has been thought to accentuate IGF-1 actions, perhaps leading to the tubular cell hypertrophy and hyperplasia observed in early experimental diabetes in the rat [103]. In experimental models of diabetes, GH anatagonists such as octreotide have been shown to ameliorate renal changes. However short term studies in patients with established renal disease have produced disappointing results.

Transforming Growth Factor β

After GH and IGF-1, the evidence linking TGF-β to nephropathy is the strongest [103, 104]. There are three mammalian isoforms (TGF-β1, -β2 and -β3) and these belong to a larger family of related compounds including activins, inhibins, and bone morphometric proteins.

TGF-β1 remains the best characterized of the family and the most studied in diabetes. This nuclear transcription factor acts via intracellular signaling, following binding and interaction with specific type 1 and type 2 receptors on the cell membrane. mRNA for the TGF-β isoforms and their receptors has been identified in all glomerular cell types and in the proximal tubule.

In vivo, glomerular, endothelial, and mesangial cells produce extracellular matrix in response to TGF-β. Moreover, the action of collagenases is inhibited and metalloproteinase inhibitors stimulated. High-glucose levels induce both mRNA expression and TGF-β release from cultured mesangial, glomerular epithelial, and proximal tubular cells probably via PKC-β stimulation of the TGF-β1 promoter gene. Other mechanisms for glucose-stimulated TGF-β release involve upregulation of the glucose transporter GLUT1 by TGF-β, thus increasing glucose uptake and further enhancing TGF-β production, or direct stimulation of production by glucosamine, thrombospondin, and connective tissue growth factor, which are all induced by high glucose [102, 103].

In intact animals an increase in TGF-β mRNA can be detected within 24 h of diabetes onset and this is sustained for up to 40-week duration. These changes can be attenuated by insulin treatment. Absolute concentrations of TGF-β isoforms and their receptors are not consistently elevated, however. In the glomerulus, TGF-β1 levels are low whereas TGF-β2 and the type 2 receptor are increased. The upregulation of this receptor could lead to increased activation of the system, however, as its initial binding to TGF-β is a crucial first step.

In humans TGF-β production is upregulated in kidney tissue from patients with nephropathy. There is an increase in immunostaining for all three isoforms as well as enhanced expression of mRNA in human diabetic glomeruli. Studies in 14 type 2 patients undergoing cardiac catheterization found a positive gradient of TGF-β concentration between the renal artery and vein implying net production by the kidney. The gradient was negative in 11 nondiabetic controls implying renal extraction in these patients. Urinary levels of TGF-β were also higher in the diabetic patients, supporting the conclusion that there was a net overproduction of this growth factor.

Vascular Endothelial Growth Factor

There are at least five different isoforms of VEGF and at least two high-affinity receptors [103, 105]. It is a glycoprotein with two main effects of angiogenesis and increased vascular permeability. It is highly expressed in vascular tumors and appears crucial for embryonic development as its absence in knockout mice is lethal. In the normal kidney VEGF may function to maintain the integrity of glomerular endothelium.

Specific VEGF binding has been noted in glomerular epithelial cells as well as the tubules and collecting ducts. In tissue culture, hypoxia and angiotensin II have been shown to stimulate VEGF production from mesangial and other glomerular and tubular cells. High glucose can stimulate VEGF from smooth muscle cells and this action is probably PKC-β mediated. Numerous other growth factors and cytokines have been shown to increase VEGF production in a variety of nonrenal tissues.

Glomerular endothelial and epithelial cells from diabetic rats were found to have increased expression of VEGF and its type 2 receptor and their respective mRNAs at 3 and 32 weeks of diabetes. Interestingly, as for TGF-β, the time course was different with VEGF increased at both time points and its receptor only at 3 weeks. There are relatively few data linking VEGF to diabetic or other nephropathies in humans. However, a recent study has demonstrated that circulating VEGF levels are increased in patients with type 2 diabetes and nephropathy [106]. Strong VEGF expression has been found in nonsclerosed glomeruli from diabetic patients but much less expression is observed in severely sclerosed glomeruli.

Epidermal Growth Factor

Kidney is one of the main sites of epidermal growth factor (EGF) synthesis and several different cell types exhibit its receptors. *In vitro* studies have shown EGF to stimulate proliferation of proximal tubular cells and this is enhanced by angiotensin II. EGF infusion can increase urine flow rates in normal animals. Urinary excretion of EGF is increased in early experimental diabetes and there is a parallel increase in mRNA expression over the same time period. After 2–3 weeks, urinary levels are normal suggesting that any involvement of EGF in diabetic changes is likely to be acute and perhaps confined to tubular hypertrophy and hyperplasia [103].

Angiotensin II

Angiotensin II (AII) has both vasoactive (see later) as well as growth-promoting properties [107]. AII is an octa-peptide hormone produced from its precursor angiotensin I by the action of converting enzyme ACE (angiotensin-converting enzyme). This reaction can be activated both systemically and locally.

AII has two known receptors in human beings AT1 and AT2. The AT1 is a seven transmembrane domain receptor linked to intracellular Gq proteins. The AT2 receptor has 34% homology and also has seven transmembrane domains but is linked to Giα2 and Giαα3 protein.

The distribution of the receptors is quite distinct but widespread throughout the kidney (Table 6).

Until recently it was thought that the AT2 receptor was not expressed in the adult human kidney, but it is now estimated to account for up to 10% of AII receptors.

Many of the profibrotic properties and excess matrix production observed with AII are dependent upon other growth factor release and can be blocked using specific antibodies (e.g. TGF-β) [108] or inhibitors (e.g. PKC-β) [101].

In diabetic animals and human beings circulating levels of renin and AII are low. However, circulating prorenin is increased in many type 1 patients and elevated levels are predictive of the later development of microalbuminuria and retinopathy. The functional significance of this observation is unclear. Short periods of poor glycemic control can induce renin release, however, with measurable increases in blood pressure and renal vascular resistance.

Table 6 Distribution throughout the kidney and functional effects of AT1 and AT2 receptors

Localization	Function: AT1	Function: AT2
Mesangium	Contraction, increased matrix, increased TGF-β	? Inhibits cell growth
Endothelium	Stimulates PAI-1	Production RANTES
Podocytes	? contraction	
Juxta glomerular cells	Inhibits renin release	
Macula densa	Increased sodium transport	
Proximal tubule	Cell hypertrophy increased and TGF-β increased sodium/water transport	Inhibits cell growth, increases apoptosis, and decreases sodium absorption
Medullary thick ascending limb	Increased sodium transport	
Distal tubule	Increased bicarbonate transport	
Collecting ducts	Increased bicarbonate transport	
Vascular smooth muscle	Vasoconstriction	
Vasa rectae	Vasoconstriction	
Afferent glomerular arteriole		Vasodilatation
Efferent glomerular arteriole	Vasoconstriction	
Interstitium	Increased matrix	Decreased cell growth, increased apoptosis, and increased matrix

Note: Here "?" stands for probably.

These responses appear to be reversible by the AT1 receptor blocker Losartan. Similarly, low-renin levels have also been found in type 2 patients. This paradox of low-circulating levels but evidence of increased tissue activation is reminiscent of that seen with other growth factors and strongly suggests either intrarenal upregulation or increased sensitivity to AII [107].

AII concentrations are high in both the glomerular ultrafiltrate and the lumen of the proximal tubule in diabetic animals, implying increased local production. However, the only evidence so far for altered local RAS activity in the diabetic kidney is the observation of a redistribution of ACE from the tubular cells to the glomerulus.

The number of AT1 receptors is reduced in rats with diabetes of up to 12-week duration. In addition mRNA for the AT1 receptor is markedly reduced in renal biopsy material from type 2 patients. These findings could result from downregulation secondary to local overproduction of AII. There are data, however, suggesting that hyperglycemia *per se* can reduce AT1 receptor number but at the same time augment AII responsiveness, at least in vascular smooth muscle cells. No conclusive data exist on the effect of diabetes on AT2 receptor expression, although downregulation has been reported in some diabetic animals.

The importance of AII-mediated effects in the pathophysiology of nephropathy remains speculative, but the clinical effectiveness of agents that block the RAS infer a significant role that needs further clarification [103].

Platelet-derived Growth Factor

PDGF expression is up regulated in the diabetic rat glomerulus and its production appears necessary for the secretion and activation of TGF-β in cultured human mesangial and proximal tubular cells [103]. PDGF receptors are expressed by mesangial, endothelial, and vascular smooth muscle cells in response to high ambient glucose levels. Urinary levels of PDGF are increased in diabetic patients with microalbuminuria and clinical nephropathy compared to those with a normal AER.

Connective Tissue Growth Factor

Connective tissue growth factor (CTGF) is a cysteine-rich peptide secreted by several glomerular tissues, including mesangial and endothelial cells. Synthesis is stimulated by mechanical stretch and hyperglycemia *in vitro* and it is thought to be a mediator of some of the effects of TGF-β such as cell proliferation and collagen production [102]. Recent studies have demonstrated an overexpression of CTGF mRNA in glomeruli from microalbuminuric type 1 patients [109].

Vasoactive Hormones and Cytokines

Prostaglandins

Increased urinary levels of vasodilatory and vasoconstricting prostaglandins have been found in acutely diabetic rats, and can be prevented by insulin treatment [110]. There are species differences in the type of prostaglandin produced with PGE_2 more prominent in the rat and prostacyclin in human. However, after 1 month of experimental diabetes there are no detectable differences in prostaglandin production from the kidney. Thromboxane stimulates fibronectin production from cultured mesangial cells and inhibitors of its synthesis reduce both albuminuria and mesangial matrix expression. Cyclooxygenase inhibitors reduce vasodilatory prostaglandin synthesis and have been shown by some to blunt the initial rise in GFR seen in acutely diabetic rats.

It is likely that the balance between vasodilatory and vasoconstricting prostaglandins is important in determining glomerular capillary pressure. There is also evidence linking them to TGF-β bioactivity. The results of studies exploring the impact of PG inhibitors such as indomethacin on human nephropathy have been contradictory, probably because of confounding factors such as diabetes duration, prevalent glycemia at the time of study, and variable intravascular volume status at the time of the investigations.

Angiotensin II and Other Vasoconstictors

Angiotensin II directly increases glomerular capillary pressure by virtue of its vasoconstricting action on the efferent arteriole and is therefore implicated in the development of hyperfiltration (see later) [107]. This mechanism would also result in an increased tension in the glomerular capillary wall with consequent release of growth factors such as TGF-β. AII blockade reduces filtration fraction (and by implication, intracapillary pressure) in acutely diabetic rats.

Other vasoconstrictors such as endothelins have also been implicated [111]. Increased circulating levels were found in type 2 patients compared to the nondiabetic population, and in those with, compared to those without, retinopathy. Endothelin blockade reduces hyperfiltration and proteinuria in diabetic rats, as well as decreases mRNA levels for growth factors and matrix proteins. Finally, abnormal catecholamine sensitivity has also been found in experimental diabetes.

Atrial Natriuretic Peptide

Atrial natriuretic peptide (ANP) levels have been found to be increased in diabetic animals and human beings probably as a consequence of changes in circulating volumes secondary to hyperglycemia [112]. Circulating ANP levels have been correlated to GFR in type 1 patients. Blockade reduces hyperfiltration in rats but low-dose infusion has no impact on GFR in normal man. Recent data suggest that ANP responses may be abnormal in microalbuminuric type 1 patients but it is not clear whether these abnormalities are a potential cause or effect of early nephropathy.

Kinins

Bradykinin stimulates nitric oxide production and causes glomerular efferent arteriolar vasodilatation leading to a reduction in GFR in the diabetic rat. ACE inhibitor drugs also block kininase and thus increase bradykinin levels. There is some evidence of an effect of a potential kinins in the diabetic kidney [107]. Evidence of a role in human diabetes is inconclusive, however, but many studies of ACE inhibitors vs. AT1 receptor blockers (which have no effect on kinins) show marginally greater but statistically insignificant reductions in AER with the former agents.

Endothelial function Glomerular capillary endothelium actively regulates vascular tone, permeability to macrophages and macromolecules, the composition of subendothelial matrix and the proliferation of smooth muscle cells, as well as maintaining the balance between coagulation and fibrinolysis. It performs these functions directly by the production of matrix proteins, and indirectly via mediators such as nitric oxide, prostanoids, endothelins, AII, von Willebrand factor (vWF), tissue type plasminogen activator (tPA) and plasminogen activator inhibitor 1 (PAI-1), and other cytokines and adhesion molecules [113].

Alterations in the endothelium could result in changes in some or all of these functions, many of which have been implicated in the pathogenesis of diabetic complications. Changes may occur in one or more endothelial function at different sites in the body and at different stages in the evolution of vascular complications. It is not possible to measure endothelial function directly in humans. Most research has relied upon techniques measuring vascular permeability (of which the presence of microalbuminuria is most relevant to the kidney), measures of endothelium-dependent vasodilatation (the NO synthase pathway), and circulating levels of endothelially derived compounds such as vWF.

NO is a direct dilator of vascular smooth muscle and is produced in endothelial cells from its precursor L-arginine by NO synthase. This reaction is enhanced by a wide range of compounds including bradykinin, prostanoids, insulin, and AII.

Inhibition of NO synthase reduces hyperfiltration in the rat probably via reduction in neuronally mediated enzyme activity. Other workers, however, have found increased endothelial NO synthase activity in the diabetic kidney [102].

In human beings, abnormalities of NO production have been described in patients with both type 1 and type 2 diabetes, and seem more marked in those with microalbuminuria. Both sensitivity and production are impaired, at least in type 2 patients. There are several potential mechanisms that might result in these observations:

(1) Abnormal number or function of acetyl choline receptors.
(2) Imbalance between vasoconstrictor (endothelins, thromboxane) and vasodilator production from the endothelium.
(3) "Quenching" of NO function from circulating AGE, free oxygen radicals, and oxidized low-density lipoproteins.

Circulating vWf is increased in diabetic patients, and baseline levels are correlated to a subsequent increase in AER in microalbuminuric type 2 patients [114]. Moreover in this study new cardiovascular events occurred only in those patients with a baseline vWf above the median. A close relationship between retinopathy, microalbuminuria, and circulating vWf was found in the EURODIAB Study in type 1 diabetes. However, those microalbuminuric patients without retinopathy had no relationship between AER and circulating vWf [115]. In type 2 patients, a positive correlation was found between vWf levels and AER in those with typical diabetic glomerulopathy, but no relationship in those patients with less typical lesions. Again the majority of the former group had coexistent retinopathy.

Although the link between endothelial dysfunction and nephropathy offers an attractive hypothesis linking cardiovascular disease and increased AER, there is little evidence supporting a causative role in microvascular complications. vWf levels are normal in normoalbuminuric patients, even in those with early retinopathy but there are some data linking an increase in vWf to the development of microalbuminuria 3 years later. Thus endothelial dysfunction does not seem to be an inevitability of diabetes alone but is a possible factor in the progression of micro- and perhaps more likely macrovascular complications.

Renal Hemodynamics

A potential link between the elevated GFR seen in diabetic patients and subsequent development of nephropathy was suggested over 40 years ago and was given added impetus by the finding of glomerulopathy only in the nonstenosed kidney from a patient with unilateral renal artery stenosis [116]. Since then studies in diabetic animals, that were known to increase GFR (such as unilateral or 5/6 total nephrectomy, high protein diet or experimental renal artery stenosis), resulted in more severe glomerulopathy and increased AER compared to intact controls [117]. Moreover, micropuncture studies demonstrated an increased single-nephron GFR in the diabetic rat and the key hemodynamic change related to subsequent pathological damage was an elevated glomerular intracapillary pressure. In diabetic animals, this pressure was increased due to relatively greater vasodilatation of the afferent compared to the efferent arteriole. Therapeutic interventions that directly reduce glomerular capillary pressure, such as dietary protein restriction, glycemic control with insulin, and ACE inhibitors, ameliorated subsequent glomerulosclerosis and increases in AER. These findings led to the proposal that elevated GFR and consequent increases in glomerular capillary pressure initiated diabetic glomerulopathy—the hyperfiltration hypothesis.

Not all studies support this hypothesis. Severely hyperglycemic animals develop glomerulopathy with normal GFR and capillary pressures [118]. Spontaneously hypertensive rats with diabetes have demonstrable glomerular capillary hypertension but similar AER and glomerulopathy to their normotensive controls after 6 months. Finally, in a rat model of left sided 2/3 nephrectomy plus either right nephrectomy or ureteral diversion, glomerular hypertrophy did not occur in the diverted kidneys despite persistent hyperfiltration [119].

There are some confounding factors in interpreting these results. Nephrectomy and experimental renal artery stenosis both lead to compensatory hypertrophy, presumably mediated by growth factors that may directly influence mesangial matrix production and glomerular pathology. Diabetic animals are also hyperphagic and protein intake is high if they are fed *ad libitum*. The mechanisms leading to hyperfiltration and which could subsequently give rise to glomerulopathy are many. Perhaps the most intriguing relates to mechanical alterations in the mesangium and glomerular capillary, secondary to raised intraglomerular capillary pressure, and these will be dealt with separately (see section Mechanical Factors below).

Around 20–40% of diabetic patients have hyperfiltration at diagnosis but this number is highly dependent upon GFR methodology and the population under study. Although it is not possible to measure glomerular capillary pressure directly in humans, the filtration fraction is a reasonable proxy and is usually increased in hyperfiltering type 1 patients. Latterly more complex mathematical models have been developed to derive estimates of capillary pressure. These have shown increased glomerular capillary pressure in type 2 patients with microalbuminuria (53 vs. 43 mmHg, $p < 0.001$), although their normoalbuminuric controls also had higher than normal pressures (<35 mmHg) [120].

Despite this evidence, no consistent association between hyperfiltration and subsequent nephropathy development in diabetic patients has been found. One of the difficulties is that often only single GFR estimates have been made at baseline and follow-up; the follow-up periods have varied from 4 to 20 years; and, crucially, the definition of hyperfiltration is highly methodological and population dependent, with different GFR levels being used by different workers. Studies in both type 1 and type 2 patients suggest that GFR decline may be more rapid in those with higher baseline values, although remaining within the normal range, but no excess in numbers developing microalbuminuria. Such a phenomenon may represent a regression to the mean. Because hyperfiltration may be a response to altered cytokine or growth factor secretion and function, current research has concentrated more on the underlying mechanisms rather than the elevated GFR alone.

Mechanical Factors

The association of glomerular enlargement and hyperfiltration in early diabetes has led to an exploration of the mechanical processes that lead to cytokine release and matrix accumulation. The following two potential mechanisms may operate:

(1) Shear stress induced by increased blood flow has been shown to induce growth factor release from endothelium.
(2) Stretching glomerular capillaries and mesangial cells as a result of increased pressure.

The elastic properties of the glomerulus have been recognized for many years and have been explored using isolated microperfused glomeruli [121]. As the intracapillary pressure is increased to levels seen in diabetes, glomerular volume increases by 30%. The elasticity of the glomerulus permits this maximum volume to be reached within 3–4 s of the pressure being applied. Because of the specialized microstructure of the mesangial–basement membrane junction, such changes in tension within the capillary wall will be transmitted to the mesangium. Moreover, the central location of the mesangium within the tuft lobules probably amplifies the effect. As most of the capacity for enlargement resides within the capillaries, it has been estimated that maximum mesangial contraction could reduce glomerular volume by less than 5%. Studies of whole, microprofused glomeruli as well as mesangial cell cultures exposed to stretching have revealed a consistent production and release of profibrotic cytokines such as TGF-β1, VEGF, and connective tissue growth factor and their receptors. These responses are magnified in the presence of high glucose [122].

The signaling mechanism for these cytokines involves kinases such as ERK as well as PKC and mitogen-activated protein kinase [123] and their activation, resulting in a realignment of actin within mesangial cells.

It is suggested that early loss of autoregulation of intraglomerular pressure induced by diabetes results in the transmission of higher mean pressures. This leads to wide minute to minute oscillations, which may induce volume changes up to 18-fold larger than those encountered in normal conditions (7.3% vs. 0.4% distension) [122]. The evidence for glomerular enlargement as a cause *per se* of glomerulopathy is reviewed later.

Fetal Origins Hypothesis

Malnutrition or placental insufficiency in early pregnancy tends to result in small infants of low-birth weight. In mid-pregnancy the result will be a short and thin low birth weight baby associated with a small placenta, whereas later in pregnancy the result will be a thin infant of normal length. An association between geographical variations in cardiovascular mortality and neonatal mortality has led to the idea that intrauterine nutrition may predispose to later development of diabetes, hypertension, and cardiovascular disease. This hypothesis has prompted vigorous debate and is not consistently supported by observational data in humans [124].

As far as the kidney is concerned, a link has been made between low birth weight and glomerular number. Rats whose dams were exposed to low-protein diets in pregnancy had fewer glomeruli than did normally fed control animals. Naturally occurring low birth weight animals, however, had numbers of glomeruli similar to those of their normal birth weight littermates [124].

Human neonates with intrauterine growth retardation or with low birth weight and who subsequently died postpartum had 30% fewer glomeruli than did normal birth weight infants [124]. These observations have lent support to a hypothesis that links low birth weight to a reduction in glomeruli, which could perhaps be more vulnerable to hyperglycemia, thus placing such an individual at high risk of nephropathy if they should develop diabetes.

This hypothesis is difficult to prove because of the difficulty of obtaining an unbiased estimate of glomerular number in living intact person. Postmortem studies using whole kidneys have failed to show fewer glomeruli in diabetic vs. nondiabetic individuals, neither was found any relationship with recorded birth weight in these series [125].

It is likely that severely growth retarded infants will have fewer glomeruli but the significance of this in relation to diabetic nephropathy is uncertain.

Genetic Factors

Nephropathy affects only a minority of diabetic patients and epidemiological studies of the incidence of clinical nephropathy suggest that the number of individuals developing the condition after 20-year duration declines. This suggests that there is a subgroup at high risk of developing nephropathy. Moreover nephropathy is more common in certain ethnic peoples such as Indo-Asians; African, Hispanic, and Native Americans; Aboriginals in Australia and Maori in New Zealand; and Pacific Islanders. These observations point to nonmetabolic, perhaps inherited factors.

Familial clustering has been noted in three major studies in type 1 diabetes, each showing a significant concordance for nephropathy in diabetic siblings of index cases with the condition. One of these reports concluded that the observed association was consistent with a major gene effect [126, 127]. In addition, the DCCT found a strong association for nephropathy between mothers with diabetes and their diabetic offspring [128]. Type 2 families are harder to study because of a greater mortality in this generally older population. However, nephropathy is more common in diabetic Pima Indians if both parents have nephropathy (46%) than if one (23%) or none (14%) have the condition. Preliminary results in Europid patients support this association [129].

There is also a link between a parental history of cardiovascular mortality and nephropathy in their type 1 diabetic offspring. Approximately twice as many parents of 61 type 1 diabetic patients with nephropathy died of cardiovascular disease than did parents of 61 age- and duration-matched normoalbuminuric controls (40% vs. 22%) [130]. Studies in both type 1 and 2 diabetes have found increased insulin resistance and/or hypertension in first degree, nondiabetic relatives. These findings provide a possible explanation of the increased cardiovascular disease in patients with nephropathy.

Several methods have been used to explore the genetic basis for these observations.

Association Studies

Case control analysis compares diabetic patients with nephropathy to those without. A candidate gene is then examined in the two groups and any differences in frequency noted.

This type of analysis is time consuming and theoretically inefficient [129]. It is also subject to error, the most common being too few numbers of cases and controls. Because the number of genes involved in nephropathy is unknown, it is not possible to be precise with regard to sample size but at least 200 patients in each group are probably needed to exclude a type 2 statistical error.

However, using this method many candidate genes have been examined, particularly polymorphisms in those linked to the renin–angiotensin system.

A polymorphism at intron 16 of the ACE gene has been described which accounts for over 50% of the variation in circulating ACE levels. Homozygous individuals for the insertion polymorphism (II) have lower levels than heterozygotes (ID) who, in turn, have lower levels than homozygous people with a deletion genotype (DD). In nondiabetic populations, DD individuals are more prone

Table 7 Candidate genes studied in diabetic nephropathy

Renin/angiotensin system	Vasoactive factors	Matrix proteins	Lipids	Metabolic/hormonal growth factors
ACE	Kallikrein	HSPG core protein	Lipoprotein lipase	Insulin
AII receptor	Bradykinin receptor	Type IV collagen	ApoE	Aldose reductase
Angiotensinogen	No synthase	α Adducin	Cholesterol ester transfer	Sorbitol dehydrogenase
Renin	ANP		ApoA1	Methylenetetra hydrofolate reductase
	PAI-1			β_3-Adrenergic receptor
	Platelet glycoprotein IIIa			TGF-β
	Paraoxonase			
Immunological				
HLA				
Interleukin 1				

Note: ACE = angiotensin I converting enzyme; AII = angiotensin II; NO = nitric oxide; ANP = atrial natriuretic peptide; PAI = plasminogen activator inhibitor; HSPG = heparan sulfate proteoglycan; Apo = apolipoprotein; TGF-β = transforming growth factor β.

to ischemic heart disease. Numerous studies in patients with both type 1 and 2 diabetes and nephropathy have been reported with variable results [129]. There are some data suggesting that homozygous II patients with nephropathy have a slower rate of decline of GFR and a greater response in terms of reduction of AER when treated with ACE inhibitor drugs (51.3 vs. 14.8 vs. 7.7% in II, ID, and DD respectively) [131]. Thus it is possible that although the polymorphism is unlikely to predispose to nephropathy development, it may have a major role in its rate of progression and/or response to treatment; a so-called additive response.

Other polymorphisms of the angiotensinogen and AII type 1 receptor gene have been linked to nephropathy by some, but not confirmed by others.

Many other candidate gene polymorphisms have been examined and are listed in Table 7. Of these, those in the aldose reductase, apolipoprotein E and heparan sulfate core protein genes have shown the most consistent associations.

Family Studies

These studies use families with sibling pairs who have diabetes but are either concordant or discordant for nephropathy. Discordant sibpair analysis needs many fewer families to detect an effect [126]. However, these families are difficult to identify partly because of the uncertainty of knowing that the apparently discordant sibling will always be free from nephropathy and partly because of the increased mortality in patients with nephropathy and their parents.

Preliminary results in concordant pairs have shown linkage to chromosomes 12 and 20 in a small study in Europid families, and to chromosomes 3, 7, 9, and 20 in the Pima Indians. In this latter study the strongest association was on chromosome 7, which has three known genes with the potential for involvement in nephropathy: aldose reductase, nitric oxide synthase, and the T-cell receptor B chain. Sixty-six discordant type 1 diabetic sib pairs demonstrated linkage of nephropathy to an area of the long arm of chromosome 3, which contains the AII type 1 receptor genes [129].

Another form of linkage examines the transmission of genes from heterozygous parents to their affected offspring and is termed transmission disequilibrium analysis. Using this method positive associations have been established between nephropathy and the apolipoprotein E and endothelial nitric oxide genes.

An important confounder in all of these studies lies in the phenotypic definition of nephropathy. Nearly all have used AER. However type 1 patients with normal AER can have significant glomerular pathology and a significant number with microalbuminuria spontaneously revert to normal [95]. Confining study to patients with clinical nephropathy is safer but is problematic in type 2 diabetes because of the heterogeneity in glomerulopathy and a significant percentage of nondiabetic causes of proteinuria. A robust definition of nephropathy phenotype must be included in any study exploring genetic causes.

Several multicenter and multinational family cohorts have now been established to explore this rapidly moving area of diabetic nephropathy research.

Hypertension

It is now recognized that systemic blood pressure is higher in those type 1 patients who go on to develop microalbuminuria compared to those who have a persistently normal AER [132]. Some studies have also shown an association between parental hypertension and nephropathy in their type 1 diabetic offspring.

There is also an association between prediabetic blood pressure and later nephropathy in the Pima Indians and in type 2 diabetic Japanese patients [133].

The demonstration of an inherited defect in red blood cell membrane sodium transport in patients with essential hypertension prompted several studies in patients with diabetic nephropathy [134, 135]. These workers found increased sodium-stimulated lithium efflux from previously lithium-loaded red blood cells (so-called sodium/lithium countertransport) in type 1 patients with nephropathy, compared to age- and duration-matched controls, as well as patients with nondiabetic renal impairment. Careful analysis of this phenomenon has shown that the increased sodium/lithium exchange in diabetic nephropathy is probably due to a more generalized abnormality in cell membrane function influenced by the metabolic milieu, rather than an inherited defect alone [136]. Red cell sodium/lithium countertransport has no known physiological function in human beings. However abnormalities of another cell membrane transporter, the sodium/hydrogen exchanger, have also been described in diabetic nephropathy. So far, at least five subtypes of sodium/hydrogen exchanger (NHE) have been described, the isoform NHE-1 being the most widely studied.

The sodium/hydrogen antiporter is involved in the maintenance of intracellular pH, cell volume control, stimulus/release coupling, and cell proliferation. In addition, its activity can be modulated by many cytokines, growth factors, and protein kinases including PKC, all of which have been implicated in nephropathy development. Increased sodium/hydrogen antiporter activity has been found in both circulating white cells and cultured fibroblasts from patients with nephropathy. In this latter study, intracellular pH was lower in cells from type 1 patients with nephropathy. Cultured fibroblasts from patients with nephropathy have also shown increases in DNA synthesis and extracellular matrix production, both of which could be mediated by changes in sodium/hydrogen transport [137].

The overactivity of the sodium/hydrogen antiporter is probably a result of increased function of individual sites, as the density of NHE-1 exchangers was no different in immortalized lymphoblasts from patients with, compared to matched controls without, nephropathy.

Biochemical Changes in the Basement Membrane

A major component of the charge selective property of GBM resides in noncollagenous components, notably glycosaminoglycans and sialoglycoproteins. The former account for >90% and the principal molecule is heparan sulfate. Together with sialic acid, these compounds are responsible for maintaining the integrity of the charge selective properties of the filtration barrier.

The heparan sulfate content of GBM is reduced in patients with nephropathy, as are siliac acid residues. These reductions are thought to be secondary to impaired production and have been proposed as an important cause of albuminuria and subsequent renal impairment [138]. However, hyperglycemia-induced changes in charge selectivity cannot fully explain why only a minority of diabetic patients develop nephropathy and it is possible that the observed reductions in proteoglycan are secondary rather than primary phenomena. They may well contribute to increases in AER as glomerulopathy progresses.

Other Potential Factors

Hyperlipidemia

Data from models of renal insufficiency in obese diabetic animals suggest a role for circulating plasma lipoproteins in progressive renal injury [139]. In addition, cultured mesangial cells possess LDL cholesterol receptors and binding initiates a proliferative response.

Patients with established nephropathy have abnormally raised total and LDL cholesterol, total and VLDL triglyceride and apolipoprotein B, and reduced HDL (particularly HDL2) cholesterol. These abnormalities are present in microalbuminuric patients and almost certainly contribute to the observed increase in cardiovascular disease. Higher serum cholesterol levels were associated with progressive loss of GFR in a cohort of 301 type 1 patients with nephropathy, with an approximately twofold greater decline in the uppermost (mean serum cholesterol 7.3 mmol/l) compared to the lowermost (4.2 mmol/l) quintile. A plasma cholesterol >5.25 mmol/l was linked with a greater than 20-fold odds ratio for progression to microalbuminuria in 574 normoalbuminuric Israeli type 2 diabetic patients [133]. HDL and LDL cholesterol were also associated but with smaller odds ratios. Weaker but similar associations have been found in the Pima Indians, but they were only apparent after 10 years of diabetes duration. In European populations, serum triglyceride has been linked to increases in AER in the UKPDS and in Holland, and to nephropathy development in the update of the WHO Multinational Study of Vascular Disease in Diabetes [140].

Protein Intake

Animal models show a convincing association between dietary protein intake and nephropathy progression in experimental diabetes. In type 1 diabetes, the EURODIAB cross-sectional survey of 3250 patients found that dietary protein intake amounting to >20% total energy was linked to the presence of microalbuminuria. Patients with levels <20% were more likely to have an AER <20 μg/min. This effect was more marked in those with hypertension [141]. The HOORN Study of 680 Europid individuals found an increasing risk of microalbuminuria for every 0.1 g/kg body weight/day increase in dietary protein intake [133].

The effects of increased dietary protein ingestion have been studied in both normal and diabetic patients. Usually there is an increase in GFR and RPF, possibly mediated by prostaglandins, glucagon, or ketoacids. These effects are not seen with protein from vegetable rather than animal sources [142].

Smoking

Reported smoking rates are higher in both type 1 and 2 diabetic patients with nephropathy [143]. However, no conclusive or consistent data links smoking with subsequent nephropathy development. There are no data on the impact of stopping smoking on AER or GFR.

Hydrocarbons

As with other renal diseases occupational exposure to hydrocarbons has been found to be associated with nephropathy development in at least one study.

Obesity

There are some data linking body mass index (BMI) and subsequent development of nephropathy in type 2 diabetes. Many but not all cross-sectional studies in type 1 diabetes have also found that BMI is increased in patients with diabetic kidney disease. It is difficult to dissociate the effects of obesity from hypertension and hyperlipidemia [133]. A description of an obesity-related glomerulopathy may explain the association, particularly in type 2 diabetes [92].

DIABETIC KIDNEY DISEASE AND CARDIOVASCULAR DISEASE

At all stages, patients with diabetic kidney disease are at increased risk of cardiovascular disease compared to those with normal albumin excretion. In type 1 diabetes, the relative risk of premature cardiovascular disease is 1.2-fold in microalbuminuric patients [54, 144] and at least 10-fold in those with clinical nephropathy [145, 146]. In type 2 diabetes, risk is increased two-to threefold in microalbuminuria [147] and nine fold in proteinuria [148]. It is noteworthy that, as with renal risk, the increase in cardiovascular risk is apparent at levels of albuminuria below that conventionally considered to lie within the microalbuminuric range [149]. Recent data from the Heart Outcomes Prevention Evaluation (HOPE) Study confirms the increased cardiovascular risk in type 2 diabetic patients with even minimally elevated serum creatinine [150]. Patients with ESRD who enter renal replacement programs have a particularly poor prognosis. In type 2 diabetic patients beginning hemodialysis, mortality is around 50% at 3 years largely as a result of vascular disease [151].

Although microalbuminuric and proteinuric patients have an excess of conventional cardiovascular risk factors (higher glucose, more marked dyslipidemia with higher triglycerides, lower HDL-cholesterol and smaller dense LDL-cholesterol, higher blood pressure, excess smoking, higher fibrinogen, and more marked insulin resistance), these do not fully account for the increased cardiovascular risk. There is growing evidence of a familial effect, not just for nephropathy [152–154] but also for cardiovascular risk factors and disease. First degree relatives of both type 1 and type 2 diabetic patients with microalbuminuria or proteinuria are more likely to have hypertension, dyslipidemias, and cardiovascular disease than relatives of diabetic patients with normal albumin excretion [130, 155–158]. This suggests that the genetic susceptibility that influences the development of nephropathy also affects the cardiovascular system. Suggested mechanisms linking renal and vascular disease include endothelial dysfunction, abnormalities of the renin–angiotensin system, and widespread vascular basement membrane defects.

In assessing cardiovascular risk in diabetic patients it has been suggested that the presence of microalbuminuria or proteinuria should be taken into account. Omission of such information is likely to underestimate risk significantly [159]. However most of the currently used cardiovascular risk calculators do not take this into account.

TREATMENT

The Role of Glycemic Control

Primary Prevention of Microalbuminuria

The maintenance of good glycemic control, in both type 1 and type 2 diabetes, has been shown to reduce the cumulative incidence of microalbuminuria [160–162]. The landmark study in type 1 diabetes was the DCCT in which patients with (primary prevention) or without (secondary prevention) diabetic retinopathy were randomized to receive either intensive insulin therapy or routine care. Follow-up was for an average of 6.5 years. Intensively treated patients received three or more injections a day or used and insulin pump, performed four or more capillary blood glucose tests a day, and were reviewed every month with telephone contact between visits. Those receiving routine care were reviewed every 3 months, usually took two injections of insulin a day, and had more variable levels of blood glucose monitoring. At the end of the study there was a difference in HbA_{1c} of nearly 2% in the intensively treated group (7.2%) compared to the conventionally treated patients (9.1%). This difference in glucose control resulted in a 34% (95% CI 2–56%, $p < 0.04$) risk reduction for the development of microalbuminuria in the primary-prevention cohort and a 43% (95% CI 21–58%, $p < 0.001$) reduction in the secondary-prevention cohort.

Some authors have suggested that there is a “glycemic threshold” in type 1 diabetes below which microalbuminuria does not occur [163]. Although this is disputed, the relationship between glycemic control and microvascular complications in type 1 diabetes appears to be curvilinear with the risk of developing microalbuminuria rising markedly as HbA_{1c}increases above 7.5–8 (DCCT standardized) [163, 164].

In type 2 diabetes the UKPDS is the largest trial to have investigated the effect of improving glycemic control on the primary prevention of microalbuminuria. In this study 3041 newly diagnosed, mainly White Europid patients were randomized to either conventional treatment, with a target fasting plasma glucose <15 mmol/l or intensive treatment with insulin of oral hypoglycaemic therapies, with a target fasting plasma glucose of <6 mmol/l. The median follow-up in this study was for 10 years with the intensively treated group reaching a median HbA_{1c} of 7.0% compared to 7.9% in the conventionally treated group. At 9 years there was a relative risk reduction of 24% (99% CI 9–38%, $p < 0.001$) for the development of microalbumiuria in the intensively treated group, with 19.2% of the intensively treated group progressing compared to 25.2% in the conventionally treated group.

In the UKPDS there was a linear reduction in risk as HbA_{1c} is reduced to 7% and even below, with no evidence of a glycemic threshold for the development of microvascular complications [165]. A threshold for intervention to improve glycemic control is therefore recommended at an HbA_{1c} value of 8%. Ideally HbA_{1c} should be reduced to and maintained at 7% or less.

Secondary Prevention of the Development of "Overt" Diabetic Nephropathy

Observational studies have shown that the rate of progression from microalbuminuria to dipstick-positive proteinuria is associated with poor glycemic control. A recent observational study in people with type 1 diabetes has suggested that progression can be reduced if HbA_{1c} is maintained below 8.5% [166]. However, randomized controlled trials (RCTs) have failed to demonstrate that improved glycemic control can reduce the rate of progression, possibly because of small numbers of patients and a type 2 statistical error, and relatively short periods of follow up [167]. Nevertheless, an intervention threshold for HbA_{1c} of 8% and a goal of 7% has been recommended in microalbuminuric patients with type 1 and type 2 diabetes in order to prevent the progression of other microvascular complications such as retinopathy.

Reducing the Rate of Decline of Renal Function

There is no convincing evidence from RCTs to suggest that good glycemic control can slow progression of diabetic nephropathy once renal function starts to decline, although these studies were probably underpowered. However, in an observational study of 158 people with type 1 diabetes followed up for a median of 8 years, good glycemic control (HbA_{1c} <8%) was associated with a slower rate of decline in renal function [168]. Good glycemic control is clearly also important in reducing the rate of progression of other microvascular complications.

In type 2 diabetes the UKPDS showed that there was a significant reduction in the number of patients in the intensive versus the conventionally treated group in whom serum creatinine doubled from baseline. However the numbers were very small in both groups (7 vs. 10) and although the relative risk reduction reached statistical significance the fact that the 99% confidence interval was wide (0.07–0.91) means that the finding should be interpreted with some caution [97].

Effective Early Treatment with Antihypertensive Agents

Primary Prevention of Microalbuminuria

In normotensive, normoalbuminuric patients with type 1 diabetes there is no convincing evidence that antihypertensive treatment prevents or delays the onset of microalbuminuria. The EUCLID study suggested that ACE inhibition may reduce the rate of change of UAER within the normoalbuminuric range, [169]. However the numbers of patients developing microalbuminuria in this study was not significantly. Normoalbuminuric, normotensive patients with type 1 diabetes are therefore not routinely treated with antihypertensive agents.

In patients with type 1, diabetes blood pressure rises as UAER enters the microalbuminuric range and continues to rise thereafter [170]. The presence of either hypertension or microalbuminuria should prompt screening for the other. Both require treatment in their own right to prevent progression to more advanced forms of diabetic nephropathy. Details of the therapeutic strategies are described in the section below relating to secondary prevention.

In contrast in type 2 diabetes, hypertension commonly precedes microalbuminuria. In the UKPDS, hypertension was present in 38% of the cohort at diagnosis but only 21% of these individuals had a raised UAER [162]. Treatment with β-blockers or angiotensin converting enzyme inhibitors (ACEIs) was equally effective in reducing the development of microalbuminuria in type 2 diabetes. There does not appear to be a "blood pressure threshold" below which there is no risk of developing microvascular complications and below which there is no benefit of reducing blood pressure further [171].

Secondary Prevention of the Development of "Overt" Diabetic Nephropathy

Treatment with antihypertensive agents, particularly those which modulate the renin–angiotensin axis, are of proven benefit in reducing the rate of progression from microalbuminuria to proteinuria. In patients with type 1 diabetes there appears to be an advantage in using ACEIs, even if blood pressure is within the "normal" range [172]. A recent meta-analysis of "normotensive" patients has confirmed the efficacy of ACE inhibitors with an average 75% reduction in UAER after 1 year treatment [173]. Interestingly, the effects of ACE inhibition were most marked in subjects with a higher UAER at baseline and the impact appeared to decline over time.

In type 2 diabetes there are less data relating to ACE inhibitors. Three studies in which a total of 248 patients with microalbuminuria and a blood pressure of less than 140/90 mmHg were randomized to receive an ACE inhibitor or placebo have been published. Although UAER was stabilized in ACE inhibitor treated patients, compared to a 9–20% annual increase in those treated with placebo, it may not be possible to extend the results to all patients with type 2 diabetes. This is because the subjects were relatively young (aged <50 years) and slim (mean BMI was <25).

A low-sodium diet (less then 50 mmol/day) increases the efficacy of ACEIs and should be recommended [174] when therapy is commenced. In addition to preventing progression of microalbuminuria, ACEIs appear to have a beneficial effect on cardiovascular mortality and morbidity in diabetic patients with a raised UAER [175].

The largest study reported to date in microalbuminuric patients with type 2 diabetes compared two doses of the AII receptor blocker (AIIRB) irbesartan (150 or 300 mg) to placebo in 590 patients [176]. After 2 years, significantly fewer subjects treated with 300 mg of irbesartan developed clinical nephropathy. The relative risk reduction of 0.32 observed in this study was similar to that observed in the meta-analysis of the effect of ACE inhibitors in patients with type 1 diabetes of 0.38 [173]. It is possible to speculate therefore that as both agents have a similar effect on UAER, then blockade of the renin–angiotensin system by any means would be clinically effective. Although there have been several studies in which ACE inhibitors have been compared directly with AIIRBs none were long term or had end-points, such as the development of clinical nephropathy.

One short-term study compared the effect of the ACE inhibitor lisinopril with the AIIRB candesartan. Both agents appeared equally effective in reducing both blood pressure and UAER [177]. Interestingly, an additional effect on both blood pressure and UAER was observed if both agents were used in combination. In a review of short-term studies there appears to be a consistent extra benefit on reduction of UAER in patients with microalbuminuria and those with clinical nephropathy when dual blockade of the renin–angiotensin has been attempted [178]. Long-term trials are awaited, however, and if combination therapy is contemplated, careful monitoring of serum chemistry is recommended.

Treatment with either ACEIs or AIIRBs should therefore be commenced once microalbuminuria is detected. Blood pressure should ideally be maintained at or below 130/80 mmHg, particularly in younger subjects [179, 180]. This requires intensive effort on the part of the patient and physician, usually requiring multiple antihypertensive agents. While drugs that block the renin–angiotensin system (RAS) are recommended as first line treatment, combination therapy with β-blockers, calcium channel blockers, diuretics, and α-blockers and possibly a combination of renin–angiotensin blocking agents is often required.

Reducing the Rate of Decline in Renal Function

Antihypertensive agents, especially those that modulate the renin–angiotensin axis, are of proven benefit in reducing the rate of decline in GFR in diabetic patients with established clinical nephropathy [181–183]. In type 1 diabetes the ACE inhibitor captopril (50 mg twice daily) has been shown to reduce the numbers doubling baseline serum creatinine over 4 years [184]. The effect was significant only in those whose baseline creatinine was greater than 133 μmol/l (1.5 mg/dl) at baseline and in whom a 68% reduction in the risk of serum creatinine doubling was observed. It has been suggested that ACEIs exert a specific renal protective effect with their blood pressure lowering action and appear to be more effective in reducing UAER than other agents. However this added reduction in albuminuria has not always been associated with a different impact in the rate of decline of GFR [185].

In type 2 diabetes there have been two large studies in which 3228 patients with advanced clinical nephropathy were enrolled; these studies have investigated the effect of AIIRBs on renal outcome [186, 187]. Both irbesartan and losartan reduced proteinuria by around one third, compared to near stabilization in those treated with conventional regimes that excluded ACE inhibitors. This reduction in UAER was associated with a significant reduction in the numbers of patients in whom serum creatinine doubled between 25 and 33%. The blood pressure achieved in both studies was almost identical in both treatment groups. These findings suggest that reducing UAER as well as blood pressure has an important role in reducing the rate of decline in renal function. However the effect of RAS blockade with AIIRBs in type 2 diabetes on the doubling of serum creatinine was relatively modest, roughly 50% of that observed when ACE inhibition was used in type 1 diabetes. This may be explained in part by the heterogeneity of renal pathology seen in type 2 diabetes and the fact that the patients with type 2 diabetes had more advanced nephropathy with greater levels of UAER and lower derived GFRs.

Treatment with ACE inhibitors or AIIRBs is recommended in all diabetic patients with clinical nephropathy even if blood pressure is not elevated. Ideally most patients should have started such therapy at the microalbuminuric stage. An initial blood pressure target of 130/80 mmHg has been recommended in patients with proteinuria. Once renal function starts to decline and protein excretion reaches 1 g in 24 h even more stringent blood pressure targets of less than 125/75 mmHg have been suggested [179]. Meeting such targets in patients with declining renal function invariably requires combination therapy, often including a loop diuretic. The latter are particularly important should the patient develop peripheral edema or the nephrotic syndrome.

Blood pressure targets for all people with diabetes usually reflect consensus opinion and are aimed at reducing both cardiovascular events and renal failure. Such targets must balance aspiration against what can be achieved in practice. An intervention threshold for hypertension in normoalbuminuric patients, initially with nonpharmacological measures, is recommended if blood pressure exceeds 140/90 mmHg. If antihypertensive agents are required the Antihypertensive and Lipid-Lowering Treatment to Prevent Heart Attack Trial (ALLHAT) Study demonstrated that treatment with an ACEI diuretic or calcium channel blockers are all similar in their ability to reduce cardiovascular events [188]. Angiotensin II receptor blockers and β-blockers may be equally effective. Ideally blood pressure should be maintained at or below 140/80 mmHg in all people with diabetes [180]. More than one agent may be required, for example in the UKPDS blood pressure study 29% of patients in the intensively treated arm required three or more agents to achieve a mean blood pressure of 142/82 mmHg, well short of the targets described above [162]. The optimal combination of antihypertensive agents in hypertensive patients with diabetes is yet to be defined and should be tailored to the individual.

Dietary Protein Restriction

There does not appear to be role for dietary protein restriction until the stage of overt nephropathy has been reached and possibly renal function (GFR) has begun to decline. Even at this stage the role of protein restriction is controversial; however, there does appears to be a benefit of a modest reduction in dietary protein intake. The general consensus is to restrict protein intake to approximately that of the adult recommended dietary allowance of 1.07 g/kg/day in patients with clinical nephropathy, approximately 10% of daily calories, with a further reduction to 0.8 g/kg/day once GFR begins to fall [142].

Other Measures

Smoking Cessation

There is some evidence to suggest that smoking can hasten the progression of microalbuminuria to proteinuria [189]. In addition as patients with diabetic nephropathy are at increased risk of premature death from cardiovascular disease smoking should be strongly discouraged.

Monitoring Renal Function

Once proteinuria is established, the aim of treatment is to holt or at least reduce the rate of decline in renal function. Historically, the rate of decline of GFR has been in the order of 10 ml/min/year. This rate of decline can be modified by aggressive antihypertensive therapy as described above and can be monitored clinically by plotting the reciprocal serum creatinine against time. Such a plot enables the clinician to determine the impact of intervention, detect sudden changes in renal function that might require additional investigation and specific treatments, and to estimate when individual patients are likely to require renal replacement therapy.

Management of Cardiovascular Risk Factors and Cardiovascular Disease

Patients with diabetic nephropathy are at particularly high risk of cardiovascular disease and premature death. As such they need to be screened carefully for other cardiovascular risk factors which, if detected, should be treated aggressively. Treatments such as cholesterol lowering therapies, antihypertensive regimes, particularly with ACEIs, and smoking cessation may have the twin benefits of reducing the risk of cardiovascular events and preventing progression of diabetic nephropathy. In the Steno 2 study such a multifactorial approach was adopted. In this study patients with type 2 diabetes and microalbuminuria were aggressively treated to target, with regards to hyperglycemia, hypertension, dyslipidemia as well as with aspirin. As a result of this combined approach cardiovascular events were reduced by nearly 50% in the intensively treated group [190]. In addition the rate of progression to clinical nephropathy was also significantly lower. As a result of this study treatment with aspirin should be considered in all patients with diabetic kidney disease.

Multidisciplinary Approach

As diabetic kidney disease progresses treatment becomes increasingly complicated and involves multiple therapies, lifestyle modifications, and a large number of health care professionals. The latter is likely to include all members of the diabetes team, ophthalmologists, cardiologists, and nephrologists. An important task for the diabetologist is the coordination of these services to ensure that treatment of one part of the condition does not occur at the expense of other elements. The treatment of diabetic kidney disease is summarized in Table 8.

Table 8 Summary of the management of diabetic nephropathy

	Stage of diabetic nephropathy		
	Normal UAER	Microalbuminuria	Proteinuria
Key features	UAER normal Blood pressure may be raised (type 2 diabetes)	UAER raised BP increased CV risk increased	UAER raised BP increased GFR declines CV risk increased Other complications of diabetes likely
Main aim	Primary prevention	Prevent progression	Prevent decline in renal function
Glycemic control	Intervention threshold: HbA_{1c} >8% Ideal: <7%	Intervention threshold: HbA_{1c} >8% Ideal: <7%	Prevent nonrenal complications
Antihypertensive therapy	Intervention threshold: 140/90 mmHg Ideal: 130/80 mmHg ACEI first line	Intervention threshold: 140/90 mmHg Ideal: 130/80 mmHg ACEI or AIIRB first line	Intervention threshold: 140/90 mmHg 125/75 mmHg if protein excretion ≥1 g/24 h ACEI or AIIRB first line
Lifestyle modification	Carbohydrate restriction Smoking cessation Modest salt intake	Carbohydrate restriction Smoking cessation Modest salt intake	Carbohydrate restriction Smoking cessation Modest salt intake Protein restriction Low-fat diet
Agencies involved	Diabetes team*	Diabetes team* Possibly: Ophthalmologist Cardiologist	Diabetes team* Nephrologist Probably: Ophthalmologist Cardiologist Possibly: Vascular surgeon Radiologist
Additional aims		Reduce CV risk	Reduce CV risk

Note: UAER = urinary albumin excretion rate; CV risk = cardiovascular risk; ACEI = angiotensin converting enzyme inhibitor; AIIRB = angiotensin type 2 receptor blocker.
* Diabetes team includes, physician, diabetes specialist nurse, dietitian, retinal screener, and podiatrist.

END-STAGE RENAL DISEASE

General Management

Management of end-stage diabetic nephropathy is extremely difficult, primarily because of concomitant cardiovascular disease. In type 2 diabetes metformin should be withdrawn when serum creatinine >150 μmol/l, because of the potential risk of lactic acidosis, and in type 2 diabetes short-acting sulfonylureas used. As glomerular filtration declines, the doses of sulfonylureas and insulin, which are for the most part excreted by the kidney, commonly need to be substantially reduced.

Referral to nephrology is generally recommended when serum creatinine exceeds 200 μmol/l, although it should be considered earlier if control of blood pressure, electrolyte, or fluid balance is difficult. In addition, using creatinine alone in individuals with low muscle mass (such as elderly patients) will significantly over estimate residual kidney function and referral in such patients may need to occur at substantially lower levels. Early referral allows optimization of management of all aspects of renal disease and preparation, both psychological and physical, for renal replacement therapy. In addition to optimization of fluid balance and blood pressure, particular attention should be directed at the correction of anemia, which may be required relatively early in diabetic kidney disease because of a specific deficiency of erythropoietin activity [191]. In addition, left ventricular hypertrophy is more common in diabetic compared to nondiabetic patients with ESRD and is exacerbated by anemia. In the uremic diabetic patient, serum parathyroid hormone levels and bone turnover are generally low. Treatment with calcium-containing phosphate binders and Vitamin D may be necessary.

Preparation for Renal Replacement Therapy

The prognosis for patients who require emergency renal replacement therapy (RRT) is less good than those who begin therapy in a planned fashion. Diabetic patients commonly require dialysis at a lower serum creatinine than nondiabetic individuals because of their poor tolerance of fluid overload, presumably because of cardiovascular disease and diabetic cardiomyopathy [192]. In most countries diabetes is no longer a contraindication for consideration for renal replacement therapy. Older patients (>60 years) have a worse prognosis because of cardiovascular disease, so are generally offered dialysis rather than transplantation. In younger patients, renal transplantation, sometimes combined with pancreatic transplantation, is the treatment of choice.

Transplantation

Full cardiovascular investigation is now recommended before acceptance for transplantation because of the early death from CAD shortly after transplantation [193].

No randomized-controlled trials have been performed, but observational data have suggested that survival after transplantation is better than with dialysis. Preparation for transplantation is as in the nondiabetic individual, apart from the intensive cardiovascular assessment and management of other aspects of diabetes. Transplantation should be performed if at all possible before dialysis is needed. Simultaneous renal–pancreatic transplantation is the method of choice [194], as 10-year survival following combined renal–pancreas transplant is significantly better than after a kidney alone [195]. For isolated renal transplantation, outlook is better after living-related donor transplant than cadaveric transplantation [196]. With thorough pretransplantation work-up and newer immunosuppressive drugs [197], patient survival at 1 (approximately 100%), 3 (>90%), and 5 years (82%) is now almost as good as in nondiabetic kidney disease [198–200].

Histological changes of diabetic glomerulosclerosis develop in the transplanted kidney if good glucose control is not achieved posttransplantation. After 2 years, thickening of the GBM can be seen, with mesangial expansion after 4–5 years. There are reports of recurrent end-stage disease in transplanted kidneys.

Hemodialysis

Hemodialysis poses special problems for the diabetic patient. Vascular access may be technically more difficult because of arteriosclerosis and medial calcification. Arteriovenous fistulas fail prematurely: about 67% remain functional at 1 year compared to 83% in nondiabetic patients [201]. Synthetic grafts may have better survival. Distal ischemic pain or digital necrosis may occur, requiring amputation or closure of the fistula.

It may be difficult to achieve satisfactory and stable metabolic control. Dialysate containing 5–8 mmol/l glucose will prevent hypoglycaemia. Insulin requirements may be very variable. Rapid progression of retinopathy may rarely occur on chronic hemodialysis. Despite hypertension predialysis, hypotension during dialysis sessions may make it impossible to remove enough fluid in order to achieve the optimal "dry weight."

Peritoneal Dialysis

Peritoneal dialysis in theory offers specific benefits to the diabetic person. Vascular access is not required and blood pressure and fluid volume control is more stable. Intraperitoneal insulin may be administered, usually as four doses divided between the dialysis bags. Insulin requirements are usually much higher than the previous subcutaneous dose. However, high rates of peritonitis have limited its use.

Survival of Type 2 Diabetic Patients on Renal Replacement Therapy

Although the survival of type 2 diabetic patients receiving renal replacement therapy has improved somewhat, it remains extremely poor. Approximately 25% of patients die within 1 year of commencing dialysis, 50% within 3 years, and 75% within 5 years [200, 202, 203]. Cardiovascular disease is the commonest cause of death. It remains contentious whether survival is better on hemodialysis than CAPD.

Pregnancy and Nephropathy

Evidence is accruing that the prognosis for mother and child is worse in the presence of microalbuminuria and proteinuria. Preexisting microalbuminuria and proteinuria are strong predictors of preeclampsia [204, 205]. Microalbuminuria developing during pregnancy also indicates a higher risk of preeclampsia [206]. Treatment with ACE inhibitors for at least 6 months before pregnancy and tight glycemic control for at least 3 months prior seems to reduce risk [207] but administration of aspirin has no effect [205].

Perinatal/neonatal mortality, congenital malformations, and cesarean section rate are all higher in women with nephropathy [208]. However, a meta-analysis and other studies have concluded that with good care, fetal survival rates of 95% are achievable [209, 210]. Also, although there may be a decline in renal function during pregnancy, there is debate as to whether this is a temporary phenomenon or a permanent phenomenon [209, 211, 212]. There is some concern that withdrawal of ACE inhibition because of the risks of fetal malformation might accelerate the decline in renal function.

The fetus of mothers with diabetic kidney disease is at increased risk in the short and long term. In two small longitudinal studies of infants born to mothers with diabetic nephropathy, birth weight was lower than in infants of diabetic women without nephropathy [213, 214]. Premature delivery and respiratory distress syndrome were commoner. Three years postpartum, more children had body weight <50th centile and linguistic development was later and infections more common in children from women with nephropathy.

In light of the above, women with diabetes and any evidence of nephropathy, should plan pregnancy and contraception be continued until glucose and blood pressure management has been optimized. The mother should be counseled about the risks, ACE inhibitors must be withdrawn, and blood pressure control optimized using other agents, methyldopa and calcium channel blocking agents being preferred.

REFERENCES

1. Perkins BA, Ficociello LH, Silva KH, Finkelstein DM, Warram JH, Krolewski AS. Regression of microalbuminuria in type 1 diabetes. *N Engl J Med* 2003; 348 (23): 2285–93.
2. Seyer- Hansen K, Gundersen HJG. Renal hypertrophy in experimental diabetes. A morphometric study. *Diabetologia* 1982; 18: 501–5.
3. Jones SC, Saunders HJ, Pollock CA. High glucose increases growth and collagen synthesis in cultured human tubulointerstitial cells. *Diabet Med* 1999; 16 (11): 932–8.
4. Wolf G, Ziyadeh FN. Molecular mechanisms of diabetic renal hypertrophy. *Kidney Int* 1999; 56 (2): 393–405.
5. Bilous RW. The pathology of diabetic nephropathy. In Alberti KG, Zimmet P, de Fronzo RA (eds), *International Textbook of Diabetes Mellitus*, 2nd edn. Chichester: Wiley, 1997; pp 1349–62.
6. White KE, Bilous RW. Type 2 diabetic patients with nephropathy show structural–functional relationships that are similar to type 1 disease. *J Am Soc Nephrol* 2000; 11 (9): 1667–73.
7. Fioretto P, Mauer M, Brocco E, Velussi M, Frigato F, Muollo B, Sambataro M, Abaterusso C, Baggio B, Crepaldi G, Nosadini R. Patterns of renal injury in NIDDM patients with microalbuminuria. *Diabetologia* 1996; 39 (12): 1569–76.
8. Olsen S, Mogensen CE. How often is NIDDM complicated with non-diabetic renal disease? An analysis of renal biopsies and the literature. *Diabetologia* 1996; 39 (12): 1638–45.
9. Harris RD, Steffes MW, Bilous RW, Sutherland DE, Mauer SM. Global glomerular sclerosis and glomerular arteriolar hyalinosis in insulin dependent diabetes. *Kidney Int* 1991; 40 (1): 107–14.
10. Gulmann C, Osterby R, Bangstad HJ, Long-term studies of the juxtaglomerular apparatus in young microalbuminuric type 1 diabetic patients. *APMIS* 2001; 109 (11): 767–73.
11. Gulmann C, Osterby R, Bangstad HJ, Rudberg S. The juxtaglomerular apparatus in young type-1 diabetic patients with microalbuminuria. Effect of antihypertensive treatment. *Virchows Archiv* 2001; 438 (6): 618–23.
12. Olsen S. Light microscopy of diabetic glomerulopathy: The classic lesions. In Mogensen CE (ed), *TheKidney and Hypertension in Diabetes Mellitus*, 5th edn. Boston: Kluwer, 2001; pp 201–10.
13. Steffes MW, Bilous RW, Sutherland DE, Mauer SM. Cell and matrix components of the glomerular mesangium in type I diabetes. *Diabetes* 1992; 41 (6): 679–84.
14. Tomlanovich S, Deen WM, Jones HW III, Schwartz HC, Myers BD. Functional nature of glomerular injury in progressive diabetic glomerulopathy. *Diabetes* 1987; 36 (5): 556–65.
15. Ziyadeh FN, Goldfarb S. The renal tubulointerstitium in diabetes mellitus. *Kidney Int* 1991; 39 (3): 464–75.
16. Lane PH, Steffes MW, Fioretto P, Mauer SM. Renal interstitial expansion in insulin-dependent diabetes mellitus. *Kidney Int* 1993; 43 (3): 661–7.
17. Sandahl CJ, Gammelgaard J, Tronier B, Svendsen PA, Parving HH. Kidney function and size in diabetics before and during intial insulin treatment. *Kidney Int* 1982; 21: 683–8.
18. Mogensen CE, Andersen MJ. Increased kidney size and glomerular filtration rate in untreated juvenile diabetes: normalization by insulin-treatment. *Diabetologia* 1975; 11 (3): 221–4.
19. Parving HH, Noer I, Deckert T, Evrin PE, Nielsen SL, Lyngsoe J, et al. The effect of metabolic regulation on microvascular permeability to small and large molecules in short-term juvenile diabetics. *Diabetologia* 1976; 12 (2): 161–6.
20. Mogensen CE. Urinary albumin excretion in early and long-term juvenile diabetes. *Scand J Clin Lab Invest* 1971; 28 (2): 183–93.
21. Lind B, Jensen T, Feldt-Rasmussen B, Deckert T. Normal urinary albumin excretion in recently diagnosed type 1 diabetic patients. *Diabet Med* 1989; 6 (8): 682–4.
22. The Diabetes Control and Complications (DCCT) Research Group. Effect of intensive therapy on the development and progression of diabetic nephropathy in the Diabetes Control and Complications Trial. *Kidney Int* 1995; 47 (6): 1703–20.
23. Brochner-Mortensen J, Ditzel J. Glomerular filtration rate and extracellular fluid volume in insulin-dependent patients with diabetes mellitus. *Kidney Int* 1982; 21 (5): 696–8.
24. Dahlquist G, Stattin EL, Rudberg S. Urinary albumin excretion rate and glomerular filtration rate in the prediction of diabetic nephropathy: a long-term follow-up study of childhood onset type-1 diabetic patients. *Nephrol Dial Transplant* 2001; 16 (7): 1382–6.
25. Lervang HH, Jensen S, Brochner-Mortensen J, Ditzel J. Early glomerular hyperfiltration and the development of late nephropathy in type 1 (insulin-dependent) diabetes mellitus. *Diabetologia* 1988; 31 (10): 723–9.
26. Yip JW, Jones SL, Wiseman MJ, Hill C, Viberti G. Glomerular hyperfiltration in the prediction of nephropathy in IDDM: a 10-year follow-up study. *Diabetes* 1996; 45 (12): 1729–33.
27. Microalbuminuria Collaborative Study Group. Microalbuminuria in type I diabetic patients. Prevalence and clinical characteristics. *Diabetes Care* 1992; 15 (4): 495–501.
28. Microvascular and acute complications in IDDM patients: the EURODIAB IDDM Complications Study. *Diabetologia* 1994; 37 (3): 278–85.
29. Warram JH, Gearin G, Laffel L, Krolewski AS. Effect of duration of type I diabetes on the prevalence of stages of diabetic nephropathy defined by urinary albumin/creatinine ratio. *J Am Soc Nephrol* 1996; 7 (6): 930–7.
30. Mackin P, Macleod JM, New JP, Marshall SM. Renal function in long-duration type I diabetes. *Diabetes Care* 1996; 19 (3): 249–51.
31. Orchard TJ, Dorman JS, Maser RE, Becker DJ, Drash AL, Ellis D, et al. Prevalence of complications in IDDM by sex and duration. Pittsburgh Epidemiology of Diabetes Complications Study II. *Diabetes* 1990; 39 (9): 1116–24.
32. Mathiesen ER, Ronn B, Jensen T, Storm B, Deckert T. Relationship between blood pressure and urinary albumin excretion in development of microalbuminuria. *Diabetes* 1990; 39 (2): 245–9.
33. The Microalbuminuria Collaborative Study Group. Predictors of the development of microalbuminuria in patients with Type 1 diabetes mellitus: a seven-year prospective study. *Diabet Med* 1999; 16 (11): 918–25.

34. Chaturvedi N, Bandinelli S, Mangili R, Penno G, Rottiers RE, Fuller JH. Microalbuminuria in type 1 diabetes: Rates, risk factors and glycemic threshold. *Kidney Int* 2001; 60 (1): 219–27.
35. The Diabetes Control and Complications Trial Research Group. The effect of intensive treatment of diabetes on the development and progression of long-term complications in insulin-dependent diabetes mellitus. *N Engl J Med* 1993; 329 (14): 977–86.
36. Harvey JN, Rizvi K, Craney L, Messenger J, Shah R, Meadows PA, Population-based survey and analysis of trends in the prevalence of diabetic nephropathy in Type 1 diabetes. *Diabet Med* 2001; 18 (12): 998–1002.
37. Feldt-Rasmussen B, Mathiesen E. Variability of urinary albumin excretion in incipient diabetic nephropathy. *Diabet Nephropathy* 1984; 3: 101–3.
38. Microalbuminuria Collaborative Study Group, United Kingdom. Intensive therapy and progression to clinical albuminuria in patients with insulin dependent diabetes mellitus and microalbuminuria. *BMJ* 1995; 311 (7011): 973–7.
39. Christensen CK, Mogensen CE. The course of incipient diabetic nephropathy: studies of albumin excretion and blood pressure. *Diabet Med* 1985; 2 (2): 97–102.
40. Bending JJ, Viberti GC, Watkins PJ, Keen H. Intermittent clinical proteinuria and renal function in diabetes: evolution and the effect of glycaemic control. *Br Med J (Clin Res Ed)* 1986; 292 (6513): 83–6.
41. Hasslacher C, Stech W, Wahl P, Ritz E. Blood pressure and metabolic control as risk factors for nephropathy in type 1 (insulin-dependent) diabetes. *Diabetologia* 1985; 28 (1): 6–11.
42. Mogensen CE, Christensen CK. Predicting diabetic nephropathy in insulin-dependent patients. *N Engl J Med* 1984; 311 (2): 89–93.
43. Viberti GC, Hill RD, Jarrett RJ, Argyropoulos A, Mahmud U, Keen H. Microalbuminuria as a predictor of clinical nephropathy in insulin-dependent diabetes mellitus. *Lancet* 1982; 1 (8287): 1430–2.
44. Parving HH, Oxenboll B, Svendsen PA, Christiansen JS, Andersen AR. Early detection of patients at risk of developing diabetic nephropathy. A longitudinal study of urinary albumin excretion. *Acta Endocrinol (Copenh)* 1982; 100 (4): 550–5.
45. Myers BD, Nelson RG, Tan M, Beck GJ, Bennett PH, Knowler WC, et al. Progression of overt nephropathy in non-insulin-dependent diabetes. *Kidney Int* 1995; 47 (6): 1781–9.
46. Almdal T, Norgaard K, Feldt-Rasmussen B, Deckert T. The predictive value of microalbuminuria in IDDM. A five-year follow-up study. *Diabetes Care* 1994; 17 (2): 120–5.
47. Krolewski AS. Clinical features and epidemiology of diabetic nephropathy. In Pickup J, Williams G (eds), *Textbook of Diabetes*, 2nd edn: Cambridge, MA: Blakewell Science, 1997; pp 53.1–13.
48. Forsblom CM, Groop PH, Ekstrand A, Groop LC. Predictive value of microalbuminuria in patients with insulin-dependent diabetes of long duration. *BMJ* 1992; 305 (6861): 1051–3.
49. Arun CS, Stoddart J, Mackin P, MacLeod JM, New JP, Marshall SM. Significance of microalbuminuria in long-duration type 1 diabetes. *Diabetes Care* 2003; 26 (7): 2144–9.
50. Kofoed-Enevoldsen A, Borch-Johnsen K, Kreiner S, Nerup J, Deckert T. Declining incidence of persistent proteinuria in type I (insulin-dependent) diabetic patients in Denmark. *Diabetes* 1987; 36 (2): 205–9.
51. Krolewski AS, Warram JH, Christlieb AR, Busick EJ, Kahn CR. The changing natural history of nephropathy in type I diabetes. *Am J Med* 1985; 78 (5): 785–94.
52. Parving HH, Hommel E, Mathiesen E, Skott P, Edsberg B, Bahnsen M, et al. Prevalence of microalbuminuria, arterial hypertension, retinopathy and neuropathy in patients with insulin dependent diabetes. *Br Med J (Clin Res Ed)* 1988; 296 (6616): 156–60.
53. Bojestig M, Arnqvist HJ, Hermansson G, Karlberg BE, Ludvigsson J. Declining incidence of nephropathy in insulin-dependent diabetes mellitus. *N Engl J Med* 1994; 330 (1): 15–8.
54. Rossing P, Hougaard P, Borch-Johnsen K, Parving HH. Predictors of mortality in insulin dependent diabetes: 10 year observational follow up study. *BMJ* 1996; 313 (7060): 779–84.
55. Klein R, Klein BE, Moss SE, Cruickshanks KJ, Brazy PC. The 10-year incidence of renal insufficiency in people with type 1 diabetes. *Diabetes Care* 1999; 22 (5): 743–51.
56. Watkins PJ, Blainey JD, Brewer DB, Fitzgerald MG, Malins JM, O'Sullivan DJ, et al. The natural history of diabetic renal disease. A follow-up study of a series of renal biopsies. *Q J Med* 1972; 41 (164): 437–56.
57. Mogensen CE, Long-term antihypertensive treatment inhibiting progression of diabetic nephropathy. *Br Med J (Clin Res Ed)* 1982; 285 (6343): 685–8.
58. Parving HH, Andersen AR, Smidt UM, Svendsen PA. Early aggressive antihypertensive treatment reduces rate of decline in kidney function in diabetic nephropathy. *Lancet* 1983; 1 (8335): 1175–9.
59. Hasslacher C, Ritz E, Terpstra J, Gallasch G, Kunowski G, Rall C. Natural history of nephropathy in type I diabetes. Relationship to metabolic control and blood pressure. *Hypertension* 1985; 7 (6, pt 2): II74–8.
60. UK Prospective Diabetes Study (UKPDS). Urinary albumin excretion over 3 years in diet-treated type 2, (non-insulin-dependent) diabetic patients, and association with hypertension, hyperglycaemia and hypertriglyceridaemia. *Diabetologia* 1993; 36 (10): 1021–9.
61. Standl E, Stiegler H. Microalbuminuria in a random cohort of recently diagnosed type 2 (non-insulin-dependent) diabetic patients living in the greater Munich area. *Diabetologia* 1993; 36 (10): 1017–20.
62. Uusitupa M, Siitonen O, Penttila I, Aro A, Pyorala K. Proteinuria in newly diagnosed type II diabetic patients. *Diabetes Care* 1987; 10 (2): 191–4.
63. Schmitz A, Hansen HH, Christensen T. Kidney function in newly diagnosed type 2 (non-insulin-dependent) diabetic patients, before and during treatment. *Diabetologia* 1989; 32 (7): 434–9.
64. Patrick AW, Leslie PJ, Clarke BF, Frier BM. The natural history and associations of microalbuminuria in type 2 diabetes during the first year after diagnosis. *Diabet Med* 1990; 7 (10): 902–8.
65. Vasquez B, Flock EV, Savage PJ, Nagulesparan M, Bennion LJ, Baird HR, et al. Sustained reduction of proteinuria in type 2 (non-insulin-dependent) diabetes following diet-induced reduction of hyperglycaemia. *Diabetologia* 1984; 26 (2): 127–33.
66. Martin P, Hampton KK, Walton C, Tindall H, Davies JA. Microproteinuria in type 2 diabetes mellitus from diagnosis. *Diabet Med* 1990; 7 (4): 315–8.

67. Marshall SM, Alberti KG. Comparison of the prevalence and associated features of abnormal albumin excretion in insulin-dependent and non-insulin-dependent diabetes. *Q J Med* 1989; 70 (261): 61–71.
68. Allawi J, Rao PV, Gilbert R, Scott G, Jarrett RJ, Keen H, et al. Microalbuminuria in non-insulin-dependent diabetes: its prevalence in Indian compared with Europid patients. *Br Med J (Clin Res Ed)* 1988; 296 (6620): 462–4.
69. Gall MA, Rossing P, Skott P, Damsbo P, Vaag A, Bech K, et al. Prevalence of micro- and macroalbuminuria, arterial hypertension, retinopathy and large vessel disease in European type 2 (non-insulin-dependent) diabetic patients. *Diabetologia* 1991; 34 (9): 655–61.
70. Collins VR, Dowse GK, Finch CF, Zimmet PZ, Linnane AW. Prevalence and risk factors for micro- and macroalbuminuria in diabetic subjects and entire population of Nauru. *Diabetes* 1989; 38 (12): 1602–10.
71. Damsgaard EM, Mogensen CE. Microalbuminuria in elderly hyperglycaemic patients and controls. *Diabet Med* 1986; 3 (5): 430–5.
72. Nelson RG, Knowler WC, Pettitt DJ, Hanson RL, Bennett PH. Incidence and determinants of elevated urinary albumin excretion in Pima Indians with NIDDM. *Diabetes Care* 1995; 18 (2): 182–7.
73. Dasmahapatra A, Bale A, Raghuwanshi MP, Reddi A, Byrne W, Suarez S, et al. Incipient and overt diabetic nephropathy in African Americans with NIDDM. *Diabetes Care* 1994; 17 (4): 297–304.
74. Gall MA, Hougaard P, Borch-Johnsen K, Parving HH. Risk factors for development of incipient and overt diabetic nephropathy in patients with non-insulin dependent diabetes mellitus: prospective, observational study. *BMJ* 1997; 314 (7083): 783–8.
75. John L, Rao PS, Kanagasabapathy AS. Rate of progression of albuminuria in type II diabetes. Five-year prospective study from south India. *Diabetes Care* 1994; 17 (8): 888–90.
76. Ravid M, Brosh D, Ravid-Safran D, Levy Z, Rachmani R. Main risk factors for nephropathy in type 2 diabetes mellitus are plasma cholesterol levels, mean blood pressure, and hyperglycemia. *Arch Intern Med* 1998; 158 (9): 998–1004.
77. Forsblom CM, Groop PH, Ekstrand A, Totterman KJ, Sane T, Saloranta C, et al. Predictors of progression from normoalbuminuria to microalbuminuria in NIDDM. *Diabetes Care* 1998; 21 (11): 1 932–8.
78. Nelson RG, Meyer TW, Myers BD, Bennett PH. Course of renal disease in Pima Indians with non-insulin-dependent diabetes mellitus. *Kidney Int Suppl* 1997; 63: S45–8.
79. Schmitz A, Vaeth M, Mogensen CE. Systolic blood pressure relates to the rate of progression of albuminuria in NIDDM. *Diabetologia* 1994; 37 (12): 1251–8.
80. Ravid M, Savin H, Jutrin I, Bental T, Katz B, Lishner M, Long-term stabilizing effect of angiotensin-converting enzyme inhibition on plasma creatinine and on proteinuria in normotensive type II diabetic patients. *Ann Intern Med* 1993; 118 (8): 577–81.
81. Hasslacher C, Ritz E, Wahl P, Michael C. Similar risks of nephropathy in patients with type I or type II diabetes mellitus. *Nephrol Dial Transplant* 1989; 4 (10): 859–63.
82. Nelson RG, Morgenstern H, Bennett PH. An epidemic of proteinuria in Pima Indians with type 2 diabetes mellitus. *Kidney Int* 1998; 54 (6): 2081–8.
83. Vedel P, Obel J, Nielsen FS, Bang LE, Svendsen TL, Pedersen OB, et al. Glomerular hyperfiltration in microalbuminuric NIDDM patients. *Diabetologia* 1996; 39 (12): 1584–9.
84. Lee KU, Park JY, Hwang IR, Hong SK, Kim GS, Moon DH, et al. Glomerular hyperfiltration in Koreans with non-insulin-dependent diabetes mellitus. *Am J Kidney Dis* 1995; 26 (5): 722–6.
85. Earle KK, Porter KA, Ostberg J, Yudkin JS. Variation in the progression of diabetic nephropathy according to racial origin. *Nephrol Dial Transplant* 2001; 16 (2): 286–90.
86. Roderick PJ, Jones I, Raleigh VS, McGeown M, Mallick N. Population need for renal replacement therapy in Thames regions: ethnic dimension. *BMJ* 1994; 309 (6962): 1111–4.
87. Cowie CC, Port FK, Wolfe RA, Savage PJ, Moll PP, Hawthorne VM. Disparities in incidence of diabetic end-stage renal disease according to race and type of diabetes. *N Engl J Med* 1989; 321 (16): 1074–9.
88. Tell GS, Hylander B, Craven TE, Burkart J. Racial differences in the incidence of end-stage renal disease. *Ethn Health* 1996; 1 (1): 21–31.
89. Hebert LA, Kusek JW, Greene T, Agodoa LY, Jones CA, Levey AS, et al. Effects of blood pressure control on progressive renal disease in blacks and whites. Modification of Diet in Renal Disease Study Group. *Hypertension* 1997; 30 (3, pt 1): 428–35.
90. US Renal Data System Annual Data Report 2003.; Bethesda, MD, 2003.
91. Hinchliffe SA, Lynch MR, Sargent PH, Howard CV, Van Velzen D. The effect of intrauterine growth retardation on the development of renal nephrons. *Br J Obstet Gynaecol* 1992; 99 (4): 296–301.
92. Kambham N, Markowitz GS, Valeri AM, Lin J, D'Agati VD, Obesity-related glomerulopathy: an emerging epidemic . *Kidney Int* 2001; 59 (4): 1498–509.
93. Gruden G, Thomas S, Burt D, Zhou W, Chusney G, Gnudi L, et al. Interaction of angiotensin II and mechanical stretch on vascular endothelial growth factor production by human mesangial cells. *J Am Soc Nephrol* 1999; 55 (6): 2526–7.
94. White KE, Bilous RW, Marshall SM, El Nahas M, Remuzzi G, Piras G, et al. Podocyte number in normotensive type 1 diabetic patients with albuminuria. *Diabetes* 2002; 51 (10): 3083–9.
95. Caramori ML, Fioretto P, Mauer M. The need for early predictors of diabetic nephropathy risk: is albumin excretion rate sufficient? *Diabetes* 2000; 49 (9): 1399–408.
96. Mauer M, Drummond K. The early natural history of nephropathy in type 1 diabetes: I. Study design and baseline characteristics of the study participants. *Diabetes* 2002; 51 (5): 1572–9.
97. UK Prospective Diabetes Study (UKPDS) Group. Intensive blood-glucose control with sulphonylureas or insulin compared with conventional treatment and risk of complications in patients with type 2 diabetes (UKPDS 33). *Lancet* 1998; 352: 837–53.
98. Singh R, Barden A, Mori T, Beilin L. Advanced glycation end-products: A review. *Diabetologia* 2001; 44 (2): 129–46.
99. Dunlop M. Aldose reductase and the role of the polyol pathway in diabetic nephropathy. *Kidney Int* Suppl 2000; 77: S3–12.

100. Oates PJ, Mylari BL. Aldose reductase inhibitors: Therapeutic implications for diabetic complications. *Expert Opin Invest Drugs* 1999; 8 (12): 2095–2119.
101. Idris I, Gray S, Donnelly R. Protein kinase C activation: isozyme-specific effects on metabolism and cardiovascular complications in diabetes. *Diabetologia* 2001; 44 (6): 659–73.
102. Cooper ME. Interaction of metabolic and haemodynamic factors in mediating experimental diabetic nephropathy. *Diabetologia* 2001; 44 (11): 1957–72.
103. Flyvbjerg A. Putative pathophysiological role of growth factors and cytokines in experimental diabetic kidney disease. *Diabetologia* 2000; 43 (10): 1205–23.
104. Sharma K, Ziyadeh FN. Hyperglycemia and diabetic kidney disease. The case for transforming growth factor-beta as a key mediator. *Diabetes* 1995; 44 (10): 1139–46.
105. Duh E, Aiello LP. Vascular endothelial growth factor and diabetes: the agonist versus antagonist paradox. *Diabetes* 1999; 48 (10): 1899–906.
106. Shimada K, Baba TNS, Onozaki A, Yamada D, Midorikawa S, Sato W, et al. Plasma vascular endothelial growth factor in Japanese type 2 diabetic patients with and without nephropathy. *J Diabetes Complications* 2002; 16: 386–90.
107. Burns KD. Angiotensin II and its receptors in the diabetic kidney. *Am J Kidney Dis* 2000; 36 (3): 449–67.
108. Chen S, Cohen MP, Ziyadeh FN, Amadori-glycated albumin in diabetic nephropathy: Pathophysiologic connections. *Kidney Int Suppl* 2000; 77: S40–4.
109. Adler SG, Kang SW, Feld S, Cha DR, Barba L, Striker L, et al. Glomerular mRNAs in human type 1 diabetes: biochemical evidence for microalbuminuria as a manifestation of diabetic nephropathy. *Kidney Int* 2001; 60 (6): 2330–6.
110. de Rubertis FR, Craven PA. Eicosanoids in the pathogenesis of the functional and structural alterations of the kidney in diabetes. *Am J Kid Dis* 1993; 22: 727–35.
111. Hopfner RL, Gopalakrishnan V. Endothelin: emerging role in diabetic vascular complications. *Diabetologia* 1999; 42(12): 1383–94.
112. Zietse R, Weimar W, Schalekamp MA. Atrial naturetic peptide in diabetic nephropathy. *Kidney Int* 1997; 51: S33–41.
113. Stehouwer CDA, Lambert JR, Donker AJM, van Hinsbergh VWM. Endothelial dysfunction and the pathogenesis of diabetic angiopathy. *Cardiovasc Res* 1997; 34: 55–68.
114. Bilous R. Blood pressure control in type 2 diabetes—what does the United Kingdom Prospective Diabetes Study (UKPDS) tell us? *Nephrology Dial Transplant* 1999; 14 (11): 2562–4.
115. Karamanos B, Porta M, Songini M, Metelko Z, Kerenyi Z, Tamas G, et al. Different risk factors of microangiopathy in patients with type I diabetes mellitus of short versus long duration. The EURODIAB IDDM Complications Study. *Diabetologia* 2000; 43 (3): 348–55.
116. Berkman J, Rifkin H. Unilateral nodular diabetic glomerulosclerosis (Kimmelstiel-Wilson): Report of a case. *Metabolism* 1973; 22: 715–22.
117. Anderson S, Komers R. Pathogenesis of diabetic glomerulopathy: The role of glomerular haemodynamic factors. In Mogensen CE (ed), *The Kidney and Hypertension in Diabetes Medllitus*, 5th edn. Boston: Kluwer, 2000.
118. Bank N, Close R, Aynedjian HS, Nguyen D, Sablay LB. Evidence against increased glomerular pressure initiating diabetic nephropathy. *Kidney Int* 1987; 31: 898–905.
119. Bilous RW, Marshall SM. Clinical aspects of nephropathy. In Alberti KG, Zimmet P (eds), *International Textbook of Diabetes Mellitus*, 2nd edn. Chichester: Wiley, 1997; pp 1364–1411.
120. Imanishi M, Yoshioka K, Konishi Y, Okumura M, Okada N, Sato T, et al. Glomerular hypertension as one cause of albuminuria in type II diabetic patients. *Diabetologia* 1999; 42 (8): 999–1005.
121. Riser BL, Cortes P, Zhao X, Bernstein J, Dumler F, Narins RG. Intraglomerular pressure and mesangial stretching stimulate extracellular matrix formation in the rat. *J Clin Invest* 1992; 90 (5): 1932–43.
122. Riser BL, Cortes P. Pressure induced and metabolic alterations in the glomerulus: Role in cytokine activity and progressive sclerosis. In Mogensen CE (ed), *The Kidney in Hypertension and Diabetes*, 5th edn. Boston: Kluwer, 2000; pp 1–11.
123. Tomlinson DR, Mitogen-activated protein kinases as glucose transducers for diabetic complications. *Diabetologia* 1999; 42 (11): 1271–81.
124. Jones S, Nyengaard JR. Birth, Barker and Brenner, the concept of low birthweight and renal disease. In Mogensen CE, (ed), *The Kidney in Hypertension and Diabetes*, 5th edn. Boston: Kluwer, 2000; pp 129–139.
125. Nyengaard JR, Bendtsen TF, Mogensen CE. Low birth weight—is it associated with few and small glomeruli in normal subjects and NIDDM patients? *Diabetologia* 1996; 39 (12): 1634–7.
126. Quinn M, Angelico MC, Warram JH, Krolewski AS. Familial factors determine the development of diabetic nephropathy in patients with IDDM. *Diabetologia* 1996; 39 (8): 940–5.
127. Fava S, Hattersley AT. The role of genetic susceptibility in diabetic nephropathy: evidence from family studies. *Nephrol Dial Transplant* 2002; 17 (9): 1543–6.
128. The Diabetes Control and Complications Trial Research Group. Clustering of long-term complications in families with diabetes in the diabetes control and complications trial. *Diabetes* 1997; 46 (11): 1829–39.
129. Chowdhury TA, Dyer PH, Kumar S, Barnett AH, Bain SC. Genetic determinants of diabetic nephropathy. *Clin Sci (Lond)* 1999; 96 (3): 221–30.
130. Earle K, Walker J, Hill C, Viberti G. Familial clustering of cardiovascular disease in patients with insulin-dependent diabetes and nephropathy. *N Engl J Med* 1992; 326 (10): 673–7.
131. Penno G, Chaturvedi N, Talmud PJ, Cotroneo P, Manto A, Nannipieri M, et al. Effect of angiotensin-converting enzyme (ACE) gene polymorphism on progression of renal disease and the influence of ACE inhibition in IDDM patients: findings from the EUCLID Randomized Controlled Trial. EURODIAB Controlled Trial of Lisinopril in IDDM. *Diabetes* 1998; 47 (9): 1507–11.
132. Microalbuminuria Collaborative Study Group, United Kingdom. Risk factors for development of microalbuminuria in insulin dependent diabetic patients: A cohort study. *BMJ* 1993; 306 (6887): 1235–9.
133. Bilous RW. Risk factors for the progression of renal disease in Type 2 diabetes. In Ritz E, Rychlik I (eds), *Nephropathy in Type 2 Diabetes*. Oxford: Oxford University Press; 1999; pp 89–110.
134. Krolewski AS, Canessa M, Warram JH, Laffel LM, Christlieb AR, Knowler WC, et al. Predisposition to

hypertension and susceptibility to renal disease in insulin-dependent diabetes mellitus. *N Engl J Med* 1988; 318 (3): 140–5.
135. Mangili R, Bending JJ, Scott G, Li LK, Gupta A, Viberti G. Increased sodium-lithium countertransport activity in red cells of patients with insulin-dependent diabetes and nephropathy. *N Engl J Med* 1988; 318 (3): 146–50.
136. Rutherford PA, Thomas TH, Wilkinson R. Erythrocyte sodium-lithium countertransport: clinically useful, pathophysiologically instructive or just phenomenology? *Clin Sci (Lond)* 1992; 82 (4): 341–52.
137. Trevisan R, Yip J, Sarika L, Li LK, Viberti G. Enhanced collagen synthesis in cultured skin fibroblasts from insulin-dependent diabetic patients with nephropathy. *J Am Soc Nephrol* 1997; 8 (7): 1133–9.
138. Deckert T, Feldt-Rasmussen B, Borch-Johnsen K, Jensen T, Kofoed-Enevoldsen A. Albuminuria reflects widespread vascular damage. The Steno hypothesis. *Diabetologia* 1989; 32 (4): 219–26.
139. Keane WF. Lipids and the kidney. *Kidney Int* 1994; 46 (3): 910–20.
140. Bennett PH, Lee ET, Lu M, Keen H, Fuller JH. Increased urinary albumin excretion and its associations in the WHO Multinational Study of Vascular Disease in Diabetes. *Diabetologia* 2001; 44 (suppl 2): S37–45.
141. Toeller M, Buyken A, Heitkamp G, Bramswig S, Mann J, Milne R, Gries FA, Keen H. Protein intake and urinary albumin excretion rates in the EURODIAB IDDM Complications Study. *Diabetologia* October 1997; 40 (10): 1219–26.
142. Walker J. Non-glycaemic intervention in diabetic nephropathy: the role of dietary protein intake. In Mogensen CE (ed), *The Kidney and Hypertension in Diabetes Mellitus*, 5 edn. Boston: Kluwer, 2000.
143. Orth SR. Smoking and the kidney. *J Am Soc Nephrol* 2002; 13 (6): 1663–72.
144. Deckert T, Yokoyama H, Mathiesen E, Ronn B, Jensen T, Feldt-Rasmussen B, et al. Cohort study of predictive value of urinary albumin excretion for atherosclerotic vascular disease in patients with insulin dependent diabetes. *BMJ* 1996; 312 (7035): 871–4.
145. Borch-Johnsen K, Kreiner S. Proteinuria: Value as predictor of cardiovascular mortality in insulin-dependent diabetes mellitus. *BMJ* 1989; 294: 1651–54.
146. Tuomilehto J, Borch-Johnsen K, Molarius A, Forsen T, Rastenyte D, Sarti C, et al. Incidence of cardiovascular disease in Type 1 (insulin-dependent) diabetic subjects with and without diabetic nephropathy in Finland. *Diabetologia* 1998; 41 (7): 784–90.
147. Dinneen SF, Gerstein HC. The association of microalbuminuria and mortality in non-insulin-dependent diabetes mellitus. A systematic overview of the literature. *Arch Intern Med* 1997; 157 (13): 1413–8.
148. Fuller JH, Stevens LK, Wang SL. Risk factors for cardiovascular mortality and morbidity: the WHO Mutinational Study of Vascular Disease in Diabetes. *Diabetologia* 2001; 44 (suppl 2): S54–64.
149. MacLeod JM, Lutale J, Marshall SM. Albumin excretion and vascular deaths in NIDDM. *Diabetologia* 1995; 38 (5): 610–6.
150. Mann JF, Gerstein HC, Pogue J, Bosch J, Yusuf S. Renal insufficiency as a predictor of cardiovascular outcomes and the impact of ramipril: the HOPE randomized trial. *Ann Intern Med* 2001; 134 (8): 629–36.
151. Koch M, Kutkuhn B, Grabensee B, Ritz E. Apolipoprotein A, fibrinogen, age and history of stroke are predictors of death in dialysed diabetic patients: a prospective study in 412 subjects. *Nephrol Dial Transplant* 1997; 12: 2603–11.
152. Seaquist ER, Goetz FC, Rich S, Barbosa J. Familial clustering of diabetic kidney disease. Evidence for genetic susceptibility to diabetic nephropathy. *N Engl J Med* 1989; 320 (18): 1161–5.
153. Pettitt DJ, Saad MF, Bennett PH, Nelson RG, Knowler WC. Familial predisposition to renal disease in two generations of Pima Indians with type 2 (non-insulin-dependent) diabetes mellitus. *Diabetologia* 1990; 33 (7): 438–43.
154. Freedman BI, Tuttle AB, Spray BJ. Familial predisposition to nephropathy in African-Americans with non-insulin-dependent diabetes mellitus. *Am J Kidney Dis* 1995; 25 (5): 710–3.
155. De Cosmo S, Bacci S, Piras GP, Cignarelli M, Placentino G, Margaglione M, et al. High prevalence of risk factors for cardiovascular disease in parents of IDDM patients with albuminuria. *Diabetologia* 1997; 40 (10): 1191–6.
156. Fogarty DG, Rich SS, Hanna L, Warram JH, Krolewski AS. Urinary albumin excretion in families with type 2 diabetes is heritable and genetically correlated to blood pressure. *Kidney Int* 2000; 57 (1): 250–7.
157. Canani LH, Gerchman F, Gross JL. Increased familial history of arterial hypertension, coronary heart disease, and renal disease in Brazilian type 2 diabetic patients with diabetic nephropathy. *Diabetes Care* 1998; 21 (9): 1545–50.
158. Tarnow L, Rossing P, Nielsen FS, Fagerudd JA, Poirier O, Parving HH. Cardiovascular morbidity and early mortality cluster in parents of type 1 diabetic patients with diabetic nephropathy. *Diabetes Care* 2000; 23 (1): 30–3.
159. Yudkin JS, Chaturvedi N. Developing risk stratification charts for diabetic and nondiabetic subjects. *Diabet Med* 1999; 16 (3): 219–27.
160. The Diabetes Control and Complications Trial Research Group. The effect of intensive treatment of diabetes on the development and progression of long-term complications in insulin-dependent diabetes mellitus. *N Eng J Med* 1993; 329 (14): 977–86.
161. The Diabetes Control and Complications (DCCT) Research Group. Effect of intensive therapy on the development and progression of diabetic nephropathy in the Diabetes Control and Complications Trial. *Kidney Int* 1995; 47 (6): 1703–20.
162. UK Prospective Diabetes Study Group. Tight blood pressure control and risk of macrovascular and microvascular complications in type 2 diabetes: UKPDS 38. *BMJ* 1998; 317 (7160): 703–13.
163. Krolewski AS, Laffel LM, Krolewski M, Quinn M, Warram JH. Glycosylated hemoglobin and the risk of microalbuminuria in patients with insulin-dependent diabetes mellitus. *N Eng J Med* 1995; 332 (19): 1251–5.
164. The Diabetes Control and Complications Trial Research Group. The absence of a glycemic threshold for the development of long-term complications: the perspective of the Diabetes Control and Complications Trial. *Diabetes* 1996; 45 (10): 1289–98.
165. Stratton IM, Adler AI, Neil HA, Matthews DR, Manley SE, Cull CA, et al. Association of glycaemia with macrovascular and microvascular complications of type 2

diabetes (UKPDS 35): prospective observational study. *BMJ* 2000; 12: (321): 405–12.

166. Warram JH, Scott LJ, Hanna LS, Wantman M, Cohen SE, Laffel LM, et al. Progression of microalbuminuria to proteinuria in type 1 diabetes: nonlinear relationship with hyperglycemia. *Diabetes* 2000; 49: 94–100.

167. Microalbuminuria Collaborative Study Group, United Kingdom. Intensive therapy and progression to clinical albuminuria in patients with insulin dependent diabetes mellitus and microalbuminuria. *BMJ* 1995; 311: 973–7.

168. Mulec H, Blohme G, Grande B, Bjorck S. The effect of metabolic control on rate of decline in renal function in insulin-dependent diabetes mellitus with overt diabetic nephropathy. *Nephrology Dial Transplant* 1998; 13 (3): 651–5.

169. The EUCLID Study Group. Randomised placebo-controlled trail of lisinopril in normotensive patients with insulin-dependent diabetes and normoalbuminuria or microalbuminuria. *Lancet* 1997; 349: 1787–92.

170. Hansen WH, Poulsen PL, Ebbehoj E. Blood pressure elevation in diabetes: The results from 24-h ambulatory blood pressure recordings. In Mogensen CE (ed), *The Kidney and Hypertension in Diabetes Mellitus*, 5 edn. Boston: Kluwer, 2000; pp 339–62.

171. Adler AI, Stratton IM, Neil HA, Yudkin JS, Matthews DR, Cull CA, et al. Association of systolic blood pressure with macrovascular and microvascular complications of type 2 diabetes (UKPDS 36): prospective observational study. *BMJ* 2000; 12 (321): 412–9.

172. Viberti G, Mogensen CE, Groop LC, Pauls JF. Effect of captopril on progression to clinical proteinuria in patients with insulin-dependent diabetes mellitus and microalbuminuria. European Microalbuminuria Captopril Study Group. *Jama* 1994; 271 (4): 275–9.

173. The ACE Inhibitors in Diabetic Nephropathy Trialist Group. Should all patients with type 1 diabetes mellitus and microalbuminuria receive angiotensin-converting enzyme inhibitors? A meta-analysis of individual patient data. *Ann Intern Med* 2001; 134 (5): 370–9.

174. Heeg JE, de Jong PE, vanderHem GK, de Zeeuw D. Efficacy and variability of the antiproteinuric effect of ACE inhibition by lisinopril. *Kidney Int* 1989; 36: 272–9.

175. Heart Outcomes Prevention Evaluation Study Investigators. Effects of ramipril on cardiovascular and microvascular outcomes in people with diabetes mellitus: results of the HOPE study and MICRO-HOPE substudy. *Lancet* 2000; 355 (9200): 253–9.

176. Parving HH, Lehnert H, Brochner-Mortensen J, Gomis R, Andersen S, Arner P, et al. The effect of irbesartan on the development of diabetic nephropathy in patients with type 2 diabetes. *N Eng J Med* 2001; 345 (12): 870–8.

177. Mogensen CE, Neldam S, Tikkanen I, Oren S, Viskoper R, Watts RW, et al. Randomised controlled trial of dual blockade of renin-angiotensin system in patients with hypertension, microalbuminuria, and non-insulin dependent diabetes: the candesartan and lisinopril microalbuminuria (CALM) study. *BMJ* 2000; 321: 1440–4.

178. Noris M, Remuzzi G. ACE inhibitors ans AT1 receptor anatgonists: is two better than one? *Kidney Int* 2002; 61 (4): 1462–8.

179. Joint national committee on prevention, evaluation and treatment of high blood pressure, the national high blood pressure education program coordinating committee. The sixth report of the joint national committee on prevention, detection, evaluation and treatment of high blood pressure. *Arch Internal Med* 1997; 157: 2413–46.

180. American Diabetes Association. Clinical practice recommendations 2001. *Diabetes Care* 2001; 24 (S1): S3.

181. Lewis EJ, Hunsicker LG, Bain RP, Rohde RD, for the Collaborative Study Group. The effect of angiotensin-converting-enzyme inhibition on diabetic nephropathy. *N Eng J Med* 1993; 329 (20): 1456–62.

182. Lewis EJ, Hunsicker LG, Clarke WR, Berl T, Pohl MA, Lewis JB, et al. Renoprotective effect of the angiotensin-receptor antagonist irbesartan in patients with nephropathy due to type 2 diabetes. *N Eng J Med* 2001; 345 (12): 851–60.

183. Brenner BM, Cooper ME, de Zeeuw D, Keane WF, Mitch WE, Parving HH, et al. Effects of losartan on renal and cardiovascular outcomes in patients with type 2 diabetes and nephropathy. *N Eng J Med* 2001; 345 (12): 861–9.

184. Lewis EJ, Hunsicker LG, Bain RP, Rohde RD. The effect of angiotensin-converting-enzyme inhibition on diabetic nephropathy. The Collaborative Study Group. *N Engl J Med* 1993; 329 (20): 1456–62.

185. Tarnow L, Rossing P, Jensen C, Hansen BV, Parving HH. Long-term renoprotective effect of nisoldipine and lisinopril in type 1 diabetic patients with diabetic nephropathy. *Diabetes Care* 2000; 23 (12): 1725–30.

186. Lewis EJ, Hunsicker LG, Clarke WR, Berl T, Pohl MA, Lewis JB, et al. Renoprotective effect of the angiotensin-receptor antagonist irbesartan in patients with nephropathy due to type 2 diabetes. *N Engl J Med* 2001; 345 (12): 851–60.

187. Brenner BM, Cooper ME, de Zeeuw D, Keane WF, Mitch WE, Parving HH, et al. Effects of losartan on renal and cardiovascular outcomes in patients with type 2 diabetes and nephropathy. *N Engl J Med* 2001; 345 (12): 861–9.

188. Major outcomes in high-risk hypertensive patients randomized to angiotensin-converting enzyme inhibitor or calcium channel blocker vs diuretic: The Antihypertensive and Lipid-Lowering Treatment to Prevent Heart Attack Trial (ALLHAT). *JAMA* 2002; 288 (23): 2981–97.

189. Sawicki P, Didjugeit U, Mulhauser I, Bender R, Heinemann L, Berger M. Smoking is associated with progression of diabetic nephropathy. *Diabetes Care* 1994; 1994: 126–31.

190. Gaede P, Vedel P, Larsen N, Jensen GV, Parving HH, Pedersen O. Multifactorial intervention and cardiovascular disease in patients with type 2 diabetes. *N Engl J Med* 1993; 348 (5): 383–93.

191. Bilous R. Anaemia—a diabetologist's dilemma? *Acta Diabetologica* 2002; 39 (suppl 1): S15–9.

192. Ritz E, Koch M, Fliser D, Schwenger V. How can we improve prognosis in diabetic patients with end-stage renal disease? *Diabetes Care* 1999; 22 (suppl 2): B80–3.

193. Manske CL, Wang Y, Rector T, Wilson RF, White KW. Coronary revascularisation in insulin-dependent diabetic patients with chronic renal failure. *Lancet* 1992; 340: 998–1002.

194. Califiore R. Perspectives in pancreatic and islet cell transplantation for the therapy of IDDM. *Diabetes Care* 1999; 20: 889–96.

195. Tyden G, Bolinder J, Solders G, Brattstrom C, Tibell A, Groth CG. Improved survival in patients with insulin-dependent diabetes mellitus and end-stage diabetic nephropathy 10 years after combined pancreas and kidney transplantation. *Transplantation* 1999; 67 (5): 645–8.

196. Krakauer H, Grauman JS, McMullan MR, Creede CC. The recent U.S. experience in the treatment of end-stage renal disease by dialysis and transplantation. *N Engl J Med* 1983; 308 (26): 1558–63.
197. Stratta RJ. Simultaneous use of tacrolimus and mycophenolate mofetil in combined pancreas-kidney transplant recipients: a multi-center report. The FK/MMF Multi-Center Study Group. *Transplant Proc* 1997; 29 (1–2): 654–5.
198. Sutherland DE, Pirenne J. Current status of pancreas transplantation for treatment of type I diabetes mellitus. *Acta Gastroenterol Belg* 1997; 60 (4): 294–7.
199. Sutherland DE. Pancreas transplantation as a treatment for diabetes: Indications and outcome. *Curr Ther Endocrinol Metab* 1997; 6: 496–9.
200. Biesenbach G, Hubmann R, Grafinger P, Stuby U, Eichbauer-Sturm G, Janko O. 5-year overall survival rates of uremic type 1 and type 2 diabetic patients in comparison with age-matched nondiabetic patients with end-stage renal disease from a single dialysis center from 1991 to 1997. *Diabetes Care* 2000; 23 (12): 1860–2.
201. Martin LC, Lewin NW, Smith DW. Hamodialysis access site morbidity. *Proc Clin Dialysis Transpl Forum* 10: 277–82.
202. US Renal Data System 1998 Annual Data Report. *Am J Kidney Dis* 1998; 32: 69–80.
203. Brunner FP, Selwood NH. Profile of patients on RRT in Europe and death rates due to major causes of death groups. The EDTA Registration Committee. *Kidney Int Suppl* 1992; 38: S4–15.
204. Ekbom P, Damm P, Nogaard K, Clausen P, Feldt-Rasmussen U, Feldt-Rasmussen B, et al. Urinary albumin excretion and 24-hour blood pressure as predictors of pre-eclampsia in Type I diabetes. *Diabetologia* 2000; 43 (7): 927–31.
205. Sibai BM. Risk factors, pregnancy complications, and prevention of hypertensive disorders in women with pregravid diabetes mellitus. *J Matern Fetal Med* 2000; 9 (1): 62–5.
206. Schroder W, Heyl W, Hill-Grasshoff B, Rath W. Clinical value of detecting microalbuminuria as a risk factor for pregnancy-induced hypertension in insulin-treated diabetic pregnancies. *Eur J Obstet Gynecol Reprod Biol* 2000; 91 (2): 155–8.
207. Bar J, Chen R, Schoenfeld A, Orvieto R, Yahav J, Ben-Rafael Z, et al. Pregnancy outcome in patients with insulin dependent diabetes mellitus and diabetic nephropathy treated with ACE inhibitors before pregnancy. *J Pediatr Endocrinol Metab* 1999; 12 (5): 659–65.
208. Dunne FP, Chowdhury TA, Hartland A, Smith T, Brydon PA, McConkey C, et al. Pregnancy outcome in women with insulin-dependent diabetes mellitus complicated by nephropathy. *Q J Med* 1999; 92 (8): 451–4.
209. Reece EA, Leguizamon G, Homko C. Pregnancy performance and outcomes associated with diabetic nephropathy. *Am J Perinatol* 1998; 15 (7): 413–21.
210. Gordon M, Landon MB, Samuels P, Hissrich S, Gabbe SG. Perinatal outcome and long-term follow-up associated with modern management of diabetic nephropathy. *Obstet Gynecol* 1996; 87 (3): 401–9.
211. Kaaja R, Sjoberg L, Hellsted T, Immonen I, Sane T, Teramo K, Long-term effects of pregnancy on diabetic complications. *Diabet Med* 1996; 13 (2): 165–9.
212. Purdy LP, Hantsch CE, Molitch ME, Metzger BE, Phelps RL, Dooley SL, et al. Effect of pregnancy on renal function in patients with moderate-to-severe diabetic renal insufficiency. *Diabetes Care* 1996; 19 (10): 1067–74.
213. Biesenbach G, Grafinger P, Zazgornik J, Helmut, Stoger. Perinatal complications and three-year follow up of infants of diabetic mothers with diabetic nephropathy stage IV. *Ren Fail* 2000; 22 (5): 573–80.
214. Kimmerle R, Zass RP, Cupisti S, Somville T, Bender R, Pawlowski B, et al. Pregnancies in women with diabetic nephropathy: long-term outcome for mother and child. *Diabetologia* 1995; 38 (2): 227–35.

69

The Pathology of Diabetic Neuropathy

P. K. Thomas

Institute of Neurology, London, UK

INTRODUCTION

The considerable variety of disturbances of peripheral nerve function observed clinically in patients with diabetes mellitus indicates that a corresponding diversity is to be expected in the underlying pathological alterations. These will be considered under the headings of changes in nerve fibers and their parent nerve cell bodies and changes in supporting tissues, i.e. the neural vasculature and connective tissues. The literature on this topic is extensive and this review must therefore be selective. An attempt will be made to relate the pathological changes to the clinical syndromes.

A number of different classifications for the diabetic neuropathies have been proposed. Broadly speaking they can be classified into rapidly reversible phenomena and more persistent manifestations [1]. The former consist of sensory symptoms that are most prominent in the lower limbs ("hyperglycemic neuropathy"), reduced nerve conduction velocity [2], and an abnormal tolerance to ischemic conduction failure [3]. All three phenomena occur in patients with poorly controlled diabetes and are rapidly corrected by the establishment of euglycemia. Nothing is known about any underlying pathological changes. Their rapid reversibility suggests that they are more likely to depend upon metabolic changes rather than structural alterations. Similar phenomena are observed in streptozotocin-induced diabetes in rats where they are unaccompanied by nerve fiber loss or demyelination [4].

The more persistent manifestations of diabetic neuropathy can be subdivided into focal and multifocal neuropathies on the one hand, and symmetric polyneuropathies on the other. Mixed forms are quite frequently encountered. Focal and multifocal neuropathies include isolated cranial nerve lesions, most commonly the nerves to the extra-ocular muscles and the facial nerves, thoraco-abdominal neuropathy, focal limb nerve lesions, and diabetic amyotrophy (proximal lower limb motor neuropathy). The polyneuropathies include diabetic sensory or sensorimotor polyneuropathy, within which acute painful diabetic neuropathy [5] represents a distinct syndrome, and autonomic neuropathy.

The peripheral nerves are more susceptible to compression in patients with diabetes, accounting for the increased frequency of entrapment neuropathies and nerve lesions secondary to external pressure [6]. It is also likely that chronic inflammatory demyelinating polyneuropathy (CIDP) is more frequent in diabetic subjects [7, 8].

PERIKARYAL AND NERVE FIBER CHANGES

Anterior Horn Cells and Sensory and Autonomic Ganglia

Few systematic observations have been made on abnormalities affecting the anterior horn and intermediolateral cell neurons in the spinal cord, or on the neurons of the dorsal root and autonomic ganglia. Earlier reports have described loss of anterior horn cells [9], but these are difficult to assess as adequate clinical details are not available. Severe loss of lumbar anterior horn cells was described in a patient by Greenbaum et al. [10]; it was a somewhat atypical case which showed extensive lower limb wasting and weakness. Some loss of dorsal root ganglion cells may occur [10] but severe loss, as was found in another atypical case reported by Bosanquet and Henson [11], involving an acute sensory neuropathy, is unusual, raising the possibility of an alternative basis. Vacuolation of dorsal root and autonomic ganglion cells has been reported [10, 12]. Abnormal enlargement of sympathetic ganglion

International Textbook of Diabetes Mellitus, Third Edition. Edited by R. A. DeFronzo, E. Ferrannini, H. Keen, and P. Zimmet.
 ISBN: 0-471-48655-8.

cells that contain periodic acid-schiff (PAS)-positive material has been noted [12, 13], together with swelling and degenerative changes in dendritic processes of postganglionic neurons [13]. But the distinctive feature appears to be the neuroaxonal dystrophy of the distal preterminal axons and synapses consisting of disorganized neurofilaments aggregates, mitochondria, dense bodies, lucent proteinaceous materials, and tubulovesicular elements. The change is particularly prominent in the superior mesenteric and celiac ganglia [14].

In an autopsy study on five cases of severe autonomic neuropathy, Duchen et al. [15] described conspicuous inflammatory infiltrates in autonomic ganglia. Such infiltrates were also observed in or around bundles of unmyelinated nerve fibers in the walls of viscera. Smith [16] described inflammatory infiltrates in the ganglia of the myenteric plexuses of the esophagus. Such infiltrates are not a universal finding in cases of autonomic neuropathy.

Nerve Fiber Changes

Nerve Fiber Loss

It is clearly established that in distal symmetric sensory or sensorimotor neuropathy there is loss of both myelinated (Figure 1) and unmyelinated axons [17–22]. This is distally accentuated [10–13, 15–18] but it may also involve the spinal roots [18], particularly the dorsal roots [23]. The distal accentuation could have two possible explanations. In an autopsy study of two patients with an "essentially symmetrical" distal sensorimotor neuropathy, Sugimura and Dyck [23] found multifocal areas of fiber loss in proximal nerves that had summated distally to give rise to diffuse loss. These nerve fiber lesions were thought to have a vascular basis, which seems likely, as was the interpretation of fiber loss in focal areas, found by Johnson et al. [24]. These patients were elderly. The other explanation for distally accentuated fiber loss is a distal axonopathy of "dying-back" type, as was found in younger patients with sensory polyneuropathy of pseudosyringomyelic type by Said et al. [20]. It may well represent the salient pathological change in the sensory polyneuropathy.

Dyck et al. [21] reported that in sural nerve biopsies from patients with diabetic neuropathy, fiber loss is multifocal, which was again interpreted as indicating an ischemic causation [25]. Nevertheless, an identical pattern of loss is observable in patients with hereditary motor and sensory neuropathy [26], a condition in which a vascular basis can be discounted. The explanation for such focality of fiber loss in distal nerves is uncertain. It is possible that there is a segregation of fibers in nerve trunks in relation to their distribution in the periphery. Loss of fibers in a length-related neuropathy could therefore appear to be multifocal at proximal levels.

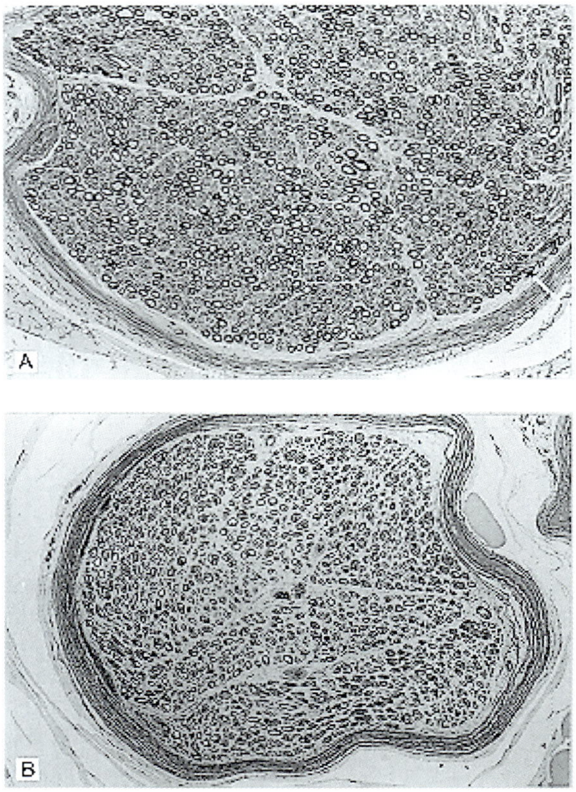

Figure 1 Transverse sections through sural nerve biopsy specimens from a control subject (A) and a patient with diabetic sensory polyneuropathy (B). The latter shows a severe depletion of myelinated nerve fibers. Semi-thin sections of plastic-embedded specimen. Thionin and acridine orange stain (both $\times 110$)

The question of possible selectivity of fiber loss in relation to fiber size has been investigated but is not yet resolved. Some initial studies suggested that loss of unmyelinated axons was a feature in early cases, but these were based on identification using silver stains. Brown et al. [27] reported two cases of painful sensory neuropathy wherein morphometric studies on sural nerve biopsies suggested predominant involvement of small myelinated and unmyelinated axons. A less clear-cut conclusion was reached by Said et al. [20] in a series of patients with pseudosyringomyelic diabetic neuropathy. Dyck et al. [21], in a large series of nerve biopsies, failed to find clear evidence of selective loss and considered that cases with evidence of greater loss of small or large fibers represented either end of a spectrum in which fibers of all diameters are lost. Llewelyn et al. [28] obtained a similar result but pointed out that regenerative activity, giving rise to clusters of small myelinated axons, would mask a selective small fiber neuropathy.

Evidence of acute axonal degeneration of Wallerian type may be found at times, for example in acute painful diabetic neuropathy [5]. Degenerative changes short of axonal breakdown may be detectable by electron microscopy, including the presence of dense filamentous arrays, glycogenosomes, and paranodal axon–Schwann cell networks indicative of the scavenging of degenerate material from axons by the adaxonal Schwann cell [29].

In patients with autonomic neuropathy, including patients with gastric atony [30, 31], fiber loss has been observed in the vagus nerve. Fiber loss has also been recorded from the greater splanchnic nerve [32] and the myenteric plexuses of the intestine [33] and esophagus [16]. Another study [34] failed to detect abnormalities both in the vagus nerve and in the myenteric plexus, although only light microscopy was employed. Degenerative axonal changes have been noted in the bladder wall [35] and in the corpora cavernosa of impotent diabetic males [36]. A reduction in the innervation of arterioles in the sural nerve was documented by Grover-Johnson and her colleagues [37]. Budzilovich [38] reported neuromatous lesions consisting of bundles of axons and associated Schwann cells related to the communicating rami from spinal nerves as well as to perivascular nerves in the spinal subarachnoid space, suggesting aberrant reinnervation.

Loss of nerve fibers in the spinal cord may be evident in the lumbosacral region and in the posterior columns, particularly in the gracile fasciculi [10, 39]. This has been attributed to loss of dorsal root ganglion cells. It is not yet established whether the fiber loss in the gracile fasciculi is more prominent rostrally. If so, it would suggest the existence of a central–peripheral distal axonopathy of dying-back type.

The pathological changes in focal peripheral nerve lesions are discussed later.

Axonal Atrophy

This is a feature of some neuropathies. Its occurrence in diabetic neuropathy is disputed. It can be assessed by measuring the relationship between myelin thickness and axon diameter, for example, by the *g* ratio (axon diameter/total fiber diameter), which is reduced in the presence of atrophy. The occurrence of axonal atrophy in diabetic neuropathy has been claimed by Malik et al. [40], but was not detected by Sugimura and Dyck [41] or Llewelyn et al. [28]. Malik et al. suggested a possible relationship between the occurrence of atrophy and painful neuropathy.

Regeneration

Axonal regeneration is vigorous in the earlier stages of diabetic neuropathy, giving rise to clusters of myelinated and unmyelinated axon sprouts as may be seen in transverse sections of the affected nerves (Figure 2), or detected in teased fiber preparations by the presence of uniformly short internodes for the diameter of the fiber [42]. The proportion of regenerating fibers increases with worsening of

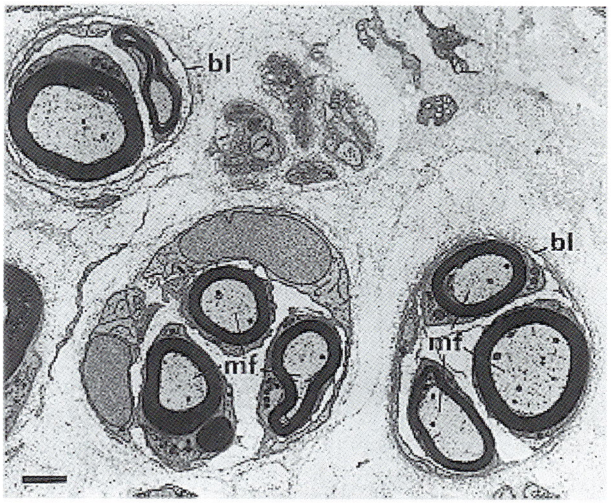

Figure 2 Electron micrograph of transverse section through a sural nerve biopsy specimen from a patient with a chronic distal diabetic sensory polyneuropathy, showing three regenerative clusters containing several myelinated nerve fibers (mf). Each cluster is surrounded by a circular basal lamina (bl) that represents the persisting basal lamina that had surrounded the original fibers before they degenerated (bar = 2 μm)

neuropathy [28]. Regenerative activity later fails so that in severe cases distal nerves may be almost totally devoid of nerve fibers [17].

Brown et al. [27] attempted to relate the occurrence of pain with the presence of regenerative activity in small nerve fibers with the proposal that the pain arose as a consequence of the generation of ectopic impulses in regenerating axon sprouts. This view was supported by Llewelyn et al. [43]. However, in a later study, Llewelyn et al. [28] found little correlation between the occurrence of pain and evidence of regenerative activity both in myelinated and in unmyelinated axons. This explanation for pain therefore appears to be unconvincing.

Demyelination and Remyelination

Apart from axonal degeneration, the other major pathological abnormality displayed by nerve fibers is demyelination. This may be restricted to the region of nodes of Ranvier (paranodal demyelination) or affect whole internodal segments (segmental demyelination). Recovery is by remyelination, either by extension from the adjacent Schwann cells if restricted paranodal demyelination has occurred, or by the migration of proliferated Schwann cells to produce new intercalated internodes. With repeated demyelination and remyelination, supernumerary Schwann cells may remain around the remyelinated fibers to give rise to a concentric or "onion bulb" arrangement of proliferated cells, sometimes referred to as hypertrophic neuropathy.

Both segmental and paranodal demyelination are features of diabetic neuropathy [17, 19, 20, 44–46]. As a general phenomenon, demyelination may be primary or secondary. If primary, it implies abnormality of the myelin sheath itself or the ability of the Schwann cell to maintain it. Secondary demyelination is the consequence of axonal pathology, such as atrophy. Behse et al. [45] found little correlation between the occurrence of axonal loss and demyelination, and therefore concluded that the demyelination was primary, due to an independent effect of the diabetic state on Schwann cell function. A similar conclusion was reached by Yagihashi and Matsunaga [46]. Said et al. [20], from teased fiber studies, found evidence of both primary and secondary demyelination, the latter occurring in fibers that showed distal axonal degeneration. Dyck et al. [47] found that in untreated diabetic subjects without symptoms of neuropathy, demyelination and remyelination were the predominant changes; in treated cases with symptomatic neuropathy, there was a combination of axonal loss and demyelination; in long-standing treated cases, axonal degeneration predominated.

Minor hypertrophic changes are not infrequently seen in nerve biopsies from patients with diabetic neuropathy. The finding of prominent hypertrophic changes in a patient with diabetes suggests the superimposition of another disorder, such as CIDP, hereditary demyelinating neuropathy, or paraproteinemic neuropathy. There is some evidence that CIDP occurs with increased frequency in diabetic patients [7, 8], raising the possibility that it can be triggered as a secondary immune event as seems likely at times in patients with hereditary motor and sensory neuropathy [48].

Sima et al. [49] have described abnormalities in the attachment of the terminal myelin helix at the nodes of Ranvier ("axoglial dysjunction") that could precede the occurrence of paranodal demyelination. The importance of this phenomenon in the evolution of the changes of diabetic neuropathy is still uncertain. The occurrence of axoglial dysjunction was related to expansion of the paranodal axon secondary to an influx of sodium ions and water consequent upon a failure of the axolemmal sodium pump.

The best studied instance of focal neuropathy in pathological terms is the third cranial nerve palsy. In a case reported by Dreyfus et al. [50] a focal lesion was found, situated centrally in the nerve. This presumably explains the characteristic sparing of pupillary function in this condition as the pupillomotor fibers are located peripherally in the nerve trunk. In the case documented by Dreyfus et al. [50] there was interruption of axons but in a later case reported by Asbury et al. [51] the lesion, which was again situated centrally in the nerve, was primarily demyelinating in nature. This type of pathological change presumably underlies the usual rapid improvement that is observed clinically, recovery being associated with remyelination. The generally good prognosis in diabetic amyotrophy [52] suggests that a demyelinating pathology figures in this disorder, although the frequent electromyographic demonstration of denervation indicates that axonal interruption also occurs. In the case investigated by Raff et al. [53], the morphological techniques employed did not permit the authors to establish whether demyelination was present.

Entrapment neuropathies and neuropathies related to external compression are the result of mechanical displacement of myelin [54, 55]. Axonal interruption occurs in more severe instances. No information is available as yet as to whether the appearances differ in compression lesions in diabetic subjects or why there is increased susceptibility to compression in diabetes.

CHANGES IN SUPPORTING TISSUES

Connective Tissue Changes

Nerve fascicles are surrounded by a lamellated cellular sheath, the perineurium, which provides a diffusion barrier around the intrafascicular compartment. The perineurial cells are flattened and are closely associated with each other at their lateral margins by tight junctions. These junctions provide the morphological expression of the perineurial diffusion barrier. The cells are covered both on the internal and external aspects by basal lamina and are separated by layers of collagenous connective tissue. The fascicles are bound together by collagenous epineurial connective tissue. Within the fascicles is collagenous endoneurial connective tissue that shows condensations around the nerve fibers and blood vessels. Individual nerve fibers are ensheathed by a continuous basal laminal tube.

If axonal degeneration occurs, under normal circumstances, following removal of axonal and myelin debris, the basal laminal tubes that had surrounded the nerve fibers collapse and assume a corrugated appearance as seen in transverse sections through the nerve (Figure 3). Schwann cell proliferation occurs within the tubes to produce "bands of Büngner." With regeneration, the Schwann cells associated with regenerating axons become invested with new basal lamina and the original basal laminal tube disappears. In diabetic neuropathy, if axonal degeneration occurs, the basal laminal tubes frequently fail to collapse and remain circular as seen in transverse section [56] (Figure 4). They become filled with dense collagen. In addition, if axonal regeneration occurs, the basal laminae tend to persist for an abnormal length of time. Such appearances are pathognomonic of diabetic neuropathy and are the only really unequivocal feature that identifies that a neuropathy is due to diabetes. They suggest that the basal laminae are both abnormally rigid and abnormally resistant to proteolytic degradation. It is possible that the dense collagen that appears within the basal laminal tubes could impede axonal regeneration.

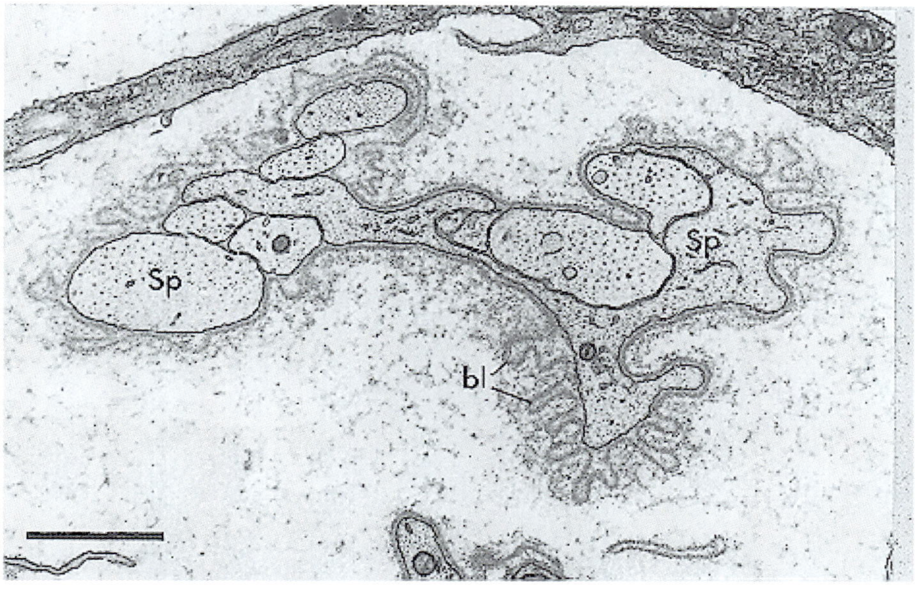

Figure 3 Electron micrograph through a group of Schwann cell processes (Sp) following degeneration of a myelinated nerve fiber in the sural nerve of a patient with chronic inflammatory demyelinating polyneuropathy. The processes are surrounded by a collapsed convoluted basal lamina (bl) (bar = 1 μm) (from reference 56, with permission)

Thickening of the basal laminae of the perineurial cells is also a feature of diabetic neuropathy [57, 58]. The widened basal laminae may display electron-lucent areas, giving them a "moth-eaten" appearance. This thickening is not specific to diabetes; it also occurs with aging. Perineurial calcification may be prominent in diabetic neuropathy [58–60] (Figure 5), mainly localized to the outer laminae. The deposits are composed of hydroxyapatite [61]. In the presence of diabetic nephropathy, the calcification may be related to a high calcium–phosphorus ion product [61]. The functional significance of these perineurial changes is uncertain.

Recent work by Bradley et al. [62] showed extensive endoneurial collagen deposition to be predominantly type I and III.

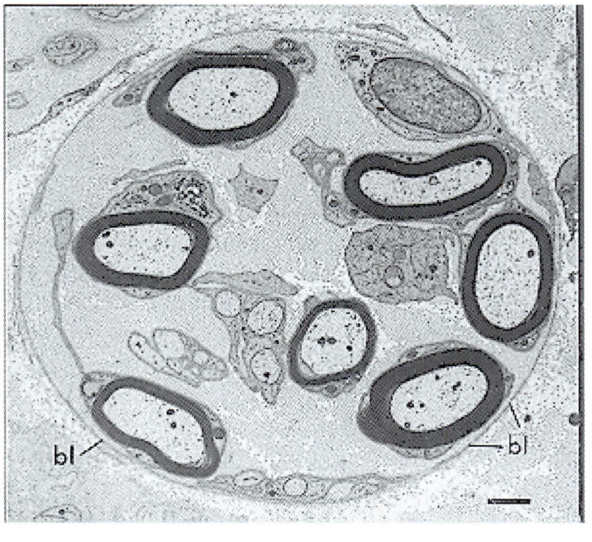

Figure 4 Electron micrograph of a regenerative cluster in the sural nerve from a patient with diabetic sensory polyneuropathy. The original Schwann cell basal lamina (bl) is still intact and is circular (bar = 1 μm) (from reference 56, with permission)

Vascular Changes

Peripheral nerves have a rich blood supply. Nutrient arteries and veins reach the nerve trunks from neighboring blood vessels and enter a longitudinal anastomotic network in the epineurium. From this, vessels penetrate the perineurium to join a longitudinal capillary network in the endoneurium. The capillaries in the epineurium are fenestrated whereas those in the intrafascicular compartment are not. The endothelial cells of the endoneurial capillaries are linked by tight junctions, a reflection of the existence of the blood–nerve barrier.

Abnormalities of the endoneurial microvessels are consistently found in diabetic neuropathy. Fagerberg [63] initially reported thickening and hyalinization of the walls of these vessels by PAS-positive material. This was subsequently shown to represent reduplication of the basal lamina surrounding the endothelial cells [31, 45, 64–66] (Figure 6). This change is not specific for diabetic neuropathy. It is common in chronic neuropathies, but statistically is greater in diabetes [66]. In comparison with type I hereditary motor and sensory neuropathy, the individual reduplicated basal laminae tend to be thicker and more

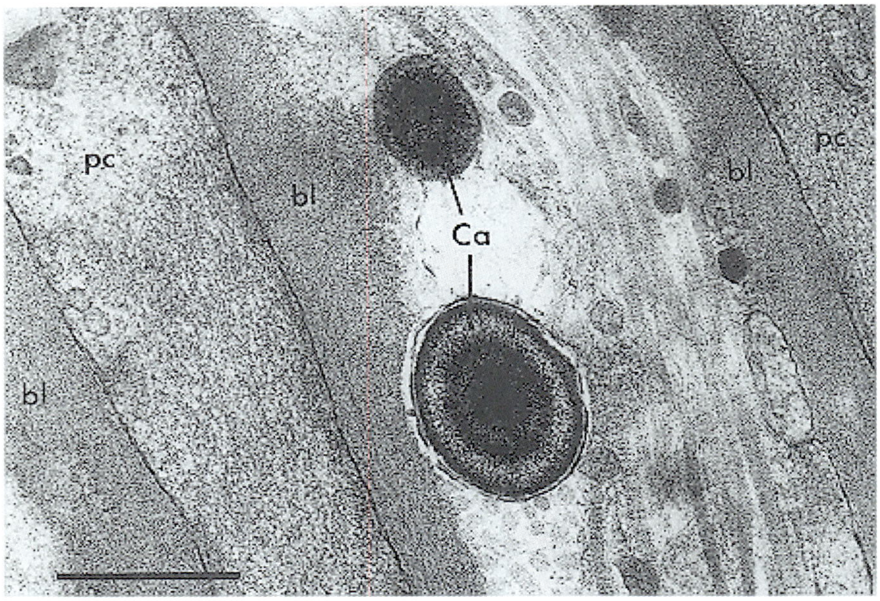

Figure 5 Electron micrograph through perineurium in the sural nerve of a patient with diabetic sensory polyneuropathy. The basal lamina (bl) around the perineurial cells (pc) is thickened and deposits of calcium (Ca) are visible in the interlamellar space (bar = 0.5 μm)

continuous in diabetic neuropathy [68]. This may explain the abnormal persistence of Schwann cell basal laminae during nerve fiber degeneration [58]. Both may be related to abnormal glycation of basement membrane collagen. The reason for the reduplication of the pericapillary basal laminae is uncertain. A further feature of diabetic and other chronic neuropathies is endothelial cell hyperplasia [67–70]. It is possible that division of these cells leads to repeated shedding of the surrounding basal lamina. These

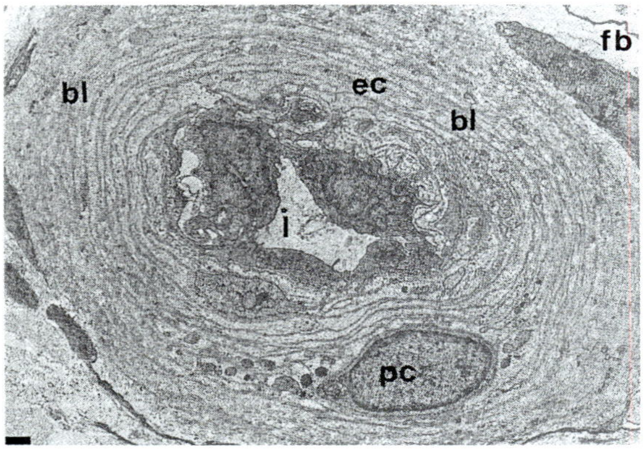

Figure 6 Electron micrograph of transverse section through an endoneurial capillary from a patient with a chronic distal diabetic sensory polyneuropathy showing multiple layers of reduplicated basal lamina (bl) surrounding the endothelial cells (ec); pc, pericyte; fb, fibroblast; l, capillary lumen (bar = 1 μm) (from reference 67, with permission)

changes in endoneurial microvessels are correlated with the severity of the neuropathy [70]. This does not necessarily imply a causal connection as both may reflect the adequacy or otherwise of diabetic control. Dyck et al. [71] found that the number of "closed" capillaries was increased in diabetic neuropathy and that this was also correlated with the severity of neuropathy. An increased incidence of closed capillaries has not been found in other studies of diabetic neuropathy [67, 70].

Increased quantities of albumin and serum proteins are present in the endoneurium in patients with diabetes, with and without neuropathy [72], and increased permeation of glycated albumin across the blood–nerve barrier is demonstrable [73]. The explanation for this is uncertain. Fenestrated endoneurial capillaries have not been detected.

The intima of the epineurial arterioles has been shown to be thickened in diabetic neuropathy but this is not correlated with the severity of the neuropathy [74]. Timperley et al. [69] reported occlusion of vessels by accumulations of fibrin and platelets in nerve biopsies from patients with diabetic neuropathy. Some but not all of these patients were acutely ill with disseminated intravascular coagulation. Such appearances have not been noted by others.

A recent finding of some interest is that in a proportion of patients with diabetic amyotrophy with accompanying sensory loss, biopsy of the intermediate cutaneous nerve of the thigh has shown evidence of vasculitis, and also intrafascicular inflammatory changes [75–77]. An inflammatory infiltrate related to a vessel is evident in the obturator nerve of the autopsied case reported by Raff et al. [53].

There is a correlation between diabetes and Mönckeberg's medial sclerosis [78], and also a positive correlation with neuropathy and, to a lesser extent, with proliferative retinopathy and proteinuria [79]. This is a specific complication of diabetes: it is not related merely to age or to duration of diabetes. It has been suggested that this form of vascular pathology is related to sympathetic denervation of arterial smooth muscle. It begins distally in the lower limbs and later develops distally in the upper limbs.

REFERENCES

1. Thomas PK, Tomlinson DR. Diabetic and hypoglycemic neuropathy. In Dyck PJ, Thomas PK, Griffin JW, Low PA, Poduslo JF (eds), *Peripheral Neuropathy*, 3rd edn. Philadelphia: Saunders, 1993; pp 1219–50.
2. Gregersen G. Diabetic neuropathy: influence of age, sex, metabolic control and duration of diabetes on motor conduction velocity. *Neurology* 1967; 17: 972–80.
3. Steiness IB. Vibratory perception in diabetics during arrested blood flow to the limb. *Acta Med Scand* 1959; 163: 195–205.
4. Sharma AK, Thomas PK. Animal models: pathology and pathophysiology. In Dyck PJ, Thomas PK, Asbury AK, Porte D, Winegrad AI (eds), *Diabetic Neuropathy*. Philadelphia: Saunders, 1987; pp 237–52.
5. Archer AG, Watkins PJ, Thomas PK, Sharma AK, Payan J. The natural history of acute painful neuropathy in diabetes mellitus. *J Neurol Neurosurg Psychiatry* 1983; 46: 491–9.
6. Mulder DW, Lambert EH, Bastron JA, Sprague RG. The neuropathies associated with diabetes mellitus: a clinical and electromyographic study of 103 unselected diabetic patients. *Neurology* 1961; 11: 275–84.
7. Cornblath DR, Drachman DB, Griffin JW. Demyelinating motor neuropathy in patients with diabetic polyneuropathy. *Ann Neurol* 1987; 22: 126–31.
8. Stewart JD, Mckelvey R, Duncan L, Carpenter S, Karpati G. Chronic inflammatory demyelinating polyneuropathy (CIDP) in diabetics. *J Neurol Sci* 1996; 142: 59–64.
9. Alderman JE. Anterior neuropathy in diabetes. *J Mt Sinai Hosp* 1938; 5: 396–402.
10. Greenbaum D, Richardson PC, Salmon MV, Urich H. Pathological observations on six cases of diabetic neuropathy. *Brain* 1964; 87: 201–14.
11. Bosanquet FD, Henson RA. Sensory neuropathy in diabetes mellitus. *Folia Psychiatr Neurol Neurochirur Neerl* 1957; 60: 107–17.
12. Appenzeller O, Richardson EP Jr. The sympathetic chain in patients with diabetic and alcoholic neuropathy. *Neurology* 1966; 16: 1203–9.
13. Hensley GT, Soergel KH. Neuropathologic findings in diabetic diarrhea. *Arch Pathol* 1968; 85: 341–8.
14. Schmidt RE. The neuropathology of human sympathetic autonomic ganglia. *Microsc Res Tech* 1996; 35: 107–21.
15. Duchen LW, Anjorin A, Watkins PJ, Mackay JD. Pathology of autonomic neuropathy in diabetes. *Ann Intern Med* 1980; 92: 301–3.
16. Smith B. Neuropathology of the esophagus in diabetes mellitus. *J Neurol Neurosurg Psychiatry* 1974; 37: 1151–4.
17. Thomas PK, Lacelles RG. The pathology of diabetic neuropathy. *Q J Med* 1966; 35: 489–97.
18. Olsson Y, Säve-Södebergh K, Sourander P, Angevall L. A pathoanatomical study of the central and peripheral nervous system in diabetes of early onset and long duration. *Pathol Eur* 1968; 3: 62–9.
19. Chopra JS, Hurwitz LJ, Montgomery DAD. The pathogenesis of sural nerve changes in diabetes mellitus. *Brain* 1969; 92: 391–6.
20. Said G, Slama G, Selva J. Progressive centripetal degeneration of axons in small fiber type diabetic polyneuropathy. A clinical and pathological study. *Brain* 1983; 106: 791–807.
21. Dyck PJ, Lais A, Karnes JL, O'Brien P, Rizza R. Fiber loss is primary and multifocal in sural nerves in diabetic polyneuropathy. *Ann Neurol* 1986; 19: 425–39.
22. Veves A, Malik RA, Lye RH, Masson EA, Sharma AK, Schady W, Boulton AJM. The relationship between sural nerve morphometric findings and measures of peripheral nerve function in mild diabetic neuropathy. *Diabet Med* 1991; 8: 917–21.
23. Sugimura K, Dyck PJ. Multifocal fiber loss in proximal sciatic nerve in symmetric distal diabetic neuropathy. *J Neurol Sci* 1982; 53: 501–9.
24. Johnson PC, Doll SC, Cromey DW. Pathogenesis of diabetic neuropathy. *Ann Neurol* 1986; 19: 450–7.
25. Dyck PJ, Karnes JL, O'Brien P, Okazaki H, Lais A, Engelstad J. The spatial distribution of fiber loss in diabetic polyneuropathy suggests ischemia. *Ann Neurol* 1986; 19: 440–9.
26. Llewelyn JG, Thomas PK, Gilbey SG, Watkins PJ, Muddle JR. Pattern of myelinated fiber loss in the sural nerve in neuropathy related to type 1 (insulin-dependent) diabetes. *Diabetologia* 1988; 31: 162–7.
27. Brown MJ, Martin JR, Asbury AK. Painful diabetic neuropathy. A morphometric study. *Arch Neurol* 1976; 33: 164–71.
28. Llewelyn JG, Gilbey SG, Thomas PK, King RHM, Muddle JR, Watkins PJ. Sural nerve morphometry in diabetic autonomic and painful sensory neuropathy. *Brain* 1991; 114: 867–92.
29. Spencer PS, Thomas PK. Ultrastructural studies of the dying-back process, II: the sequestration and removal by Schwann cells and oligodendrocytes of organelles from normal and diseased axons. *J Neurocytol* 1974; 3: 763–83.
30. Kristensson K, Nordborg C, Olsson Y, Sourander P. Changes in the vagus nerve in diabetes mellitus. *Acta Pathol Microbiol Scand A* 1971; 79: 684–5.
31. Guy RJC, Dawson JL, Garrett JR. Diabetic gastroparesis from autonomic neuropathy: surgical considerations and changes in vagus morphology. *J Neurol Neurosurg Psychiatry* 1984; 47: 686–91.
32. Low PA, Walsh JC, Huang CY, McLeod JG. The sympathetic nervous system in diabetic neuropathy—a clinical and pathological study. *Brain* 1975; 98: 357–62.
33. Frančois R, Mouriquand C. Diarrhée incoercible et fatale chez une jeune diabétique: études de plexus myentériques. *Sem Hop Paris* 1958; 34: 1526–31.
34. Yoshida MM, Schuffler MD, Sumi SM. There are no morphological abnormalities in the gastric wall or abdominal vagus in patients with diabetic gastroparesis. *Gastroenterology* 1988; 94: 907–11.
35. Faerman I, Glocer L, Celener D, Jadzinsky MN, Fox D, Maler M, Alverez E. Autonomic nervous system and diabetes: histological and histochemical study of the autonomic nerve fibers of the urinary bladder in diabetic patients. *Diabetes* 1973; 22: 225–37.

36. Faerman I, Glocer L, Fox D, Jadzinsky MN, Rapaport M. Impotence and diabetes: histological studies of the autonomic nervous fibers of the corpora cavernosa in impotent diabetic males. *Diabetes* 1974; 23: 971–6.
37. Grover-Johnson NM, Baumann FG, Imparato AM, Kim GE, Thomas PK. Altered pattern of innervation of epineurial vessels in the lower limb of patients with diabetes mellitus. *Diabetologia* 1981; 20: 31–8.
38. Budzilovich GN. Peripheral sympathetic nervous system in diabetes mellitus. In *Proceedings of the 6th International Congress of Neuropathology*. Paris: Masson et Cie, 1970; p 275.
39. Dolman CL. The morbid anatomy of diabetic neuropathy. *Neurology* 1963; 13: 135–42.
40. Malik RA, Newrick PG, Sharma AK, Tomlinson DR, Ward JD. Pathogenesis of human diabetic neuropathy. In Ward JD, Goto Y (eds), *Diabetic Neuropathy*. Chichester, UK: Wiley, 1990; pp 219–33.
41. Sugimura K, Dyck PJ. Sural nerve myelin thickness and axis cylinder caliber in human diabetes. *Neurology* 1981; 31: 1087–91.
42. Sima AAF, Bril V, Nathaniel V, McEwen TAJ, Brown MB, Lattimer SA, Greene DA. Regeneration and repair of myelinated fibers in sural nerve biopsies from patients with diabetic neuropathy treated with sorbinil, an investigational aldose reductase inhibitor. *N Engl J Med* 1988; 319: 548–55.
43. Llewelyn JG, Thomas PK, Fonseca V, King RHM, Dandona P. Acute painful diabetic neuropathy precipitated by strict glycaemic control. *Acta Neuropathol (Berl)* 1986; 72: 157–63.
44. Chopra JS, Fannin T. Pathology of diabetic neuropathy. *J Pathol* 1971; 104: 175–83.
45. Behse F, Buchthal F, Carlsen F. Nerve biopsy and conduction studies in diabetic neuropathy. *J Neurol Neurosurg Psychiatry* 1977; 40: 1072–82.
46. Yagihashi S, Matsunaga M. Ultrastructural pathology of peripheral nerves in patients with diabetic neuropathy. *Tohoku J Exp Med* 1979; 129: 358–66.
47. Dyck PJ, Sherman WR, Hallcher LM. Human diabetic endoneurial sorbitol, fructose, and myo-inositol related to sural nerve morphometry. *Ann Neurol* 1980; 8: 590–97.
48. Dyck PJ, Low PA, Bartelson JD, Daube J, Swanson CJ. Prednisone responsive hereditary motor and sensory neuropathy. *Mayo Clin Proc* 1982; 57: 239–45.
49. Sima AAF, Nathaniel V, Bril V, McEwen TAJ, Greene DA. Histopathological heterogeneity of neuropathy in insulin-dependent and non-insulin-dependent diabetes and demonstration of axoglial dysjunction in human diabetic neuropathy. *J Clin Invest* 1988; 81: 349–64.
50. Dreyfus PM, Hakim S, Adams RD. Diabetic ophthalmoplegia. Report of a case with postmortem study and comments of vascular supply of human oculomotor nerve. *Arch Neurol Psychiatr* 1957; 77: 337–43.
51. Asbury AK, Aldredge H, Herschberg R, Fisher CM. Oculomotor palsy in diabetes mellitus: a clinico-pathological study. *Brain* 1970; 93: 555–66.
52. Watkins PJ. The natural history of the diabetic neuropathies. *Q J Med* 1990; 77: 1209–18.
53. Raff M, Sangalang V, Asbury AK. Ischemic mononeuropathy multiplex associated with diabetes mellitus. *Arch Neurol* 1968; 18: 487–95.
54. Ochoa J. Nerve fiber pathology in acute and chronic compression. In Omer GE, Spinner M (eds), *Management of Peripheral Nerve Problems*. Philadelphia: Saunders, 1980; pp 487–98.
55. Neary D, Eames RA. The pathology of ulnar compression in man. *Neuropathol Appl Neurobiol* 1975; 1: 69–76.
56. King RHM, Llewelyn JG, Thomas PK, Gilbey SG, Watkins PJ. Diabetic neuropathy: abnormalities of the Schwann cell and perineurial basal laminae. Implications for diabetic vasculopathy. *Neuropathol Appl Neurobiol* 1989; 15: 339–55.
57. Johnson PC, Brendel K, Meezan E. Human diabetic perineurial basement membrane thickening. *Lab Invest* 1981; 44: 265–74.
58. King RHM, Llewelyn JG, Thomas PK, Gilbey SG, Watkins PJ. Perineurial calcification. *Neuropathol Appl Neurobiol* 1988; 14: 105–23.
59. Paetau A, Haltia M. Calcification of the perineurium. *Acta Neuropathol (Berl)* 1976; 36: 185–97.
60. Vanlis JM, Jennekens FGI, Veldman H. Calcium deposits in the perineurium and their relation to lipid accumulation. *J Neurol Sci* 1979; 43: 367–73.
61. Kalimo H, Mäki J, Paetau A, Haltia M. Microanalysis of perineurial calcification in diabetic nephropathy. *Muscle Nerve* 1981; 4: 228–34.
62. Bradley JL, King RHM, Muddle JR, Thomas PK. The extracellular matrix of peripheral nerve in diabetic polyneuropathy. *Acta Neuropathol (Berl)* 2000; 99: 450–7.
63. Fagerberg SE. Diabetic neuropathy: a clinical and histological study on the significance of vascular affections. *Acta Med Scand* 1959; 164 (suppl 345): 1–7.
64. Bischoff A. Die Ultrastruktur peripherer Nerven bei der diabetische Neuropathie. *Verh Dtsch Inn Med* 1967; 72: 1138–41.
65. Vital C, Vallat JM, Leblanc MF, Coquet M. Les neuropathies périphériques du diabète sucre: étude ultrastructurale des 12 cas biopsiés. *J Neurol Sci* 1973; 18: 381–6.
66. Vital C, Leblanc M, Vallat JM. Étude ultrastructurale du nerf périphérique chez 16 diabétiques sans neuropathie clinique. Comparaison avec 16 neuropathies diabétiques et 16 neuropathies non diabétiques. *Acta Neuropathol (Berl)* 1974; 30: 63–72.
67. Bradley J, Thomas PK, King RHM, Llewelyn JG, Muddle JR, Watkins PJ. Morphometry of endoneurial capillaries in diabetic sensory and autonomic neuropathy. *Diabetologia* 1990; 33: 611–18.
68. Powell HC, Rosoff J, Myers RR. Microangiopathy in human diabetic neuropathy. *Acta Neuropathol* 1985; 68: 295–305.
69. Timperley WR, Ward JD, Preston FE, Duckworth T, O'Malley BC. Clinical and histological studies in diabetic neuropathy. A reassessment of vascular factors in relation to intravascular coagulation. *Diabetologia* 1976; 12: 237–43.
70. Malik RA, Newrick PG, Sharma AK, Jennings A, Ah-See AK, Mayhew TM, Jakubowski J, Boulton AJ, Ward JD. Microangiopathy in human diabetic neuropathy: relationship between capillary abnormalities and the severity of neuropathy. *Diabetologia* 1989; 32: 92–102.
71. Dyck PJ, Hansen S, Karnes J, O'Brien P, Yasuda H, Windebank A, Zimmerman B. Capillary number and percentage closed in human diabetic sural nerve. *Proc Natl Acad Sci USA* 1985; 82: 2513–17.
72. Poduslo JF, Curran GL, Dyck PJ. Increase in albumin, IgG, and IgM blood–nerve barrier indices in human diabetic neuropathy. *Proc Natl Acad Sci USA* 1988; 85: 4879–83.

73. Poduslo JF, Curran GL. Increased permeability across the blood–nerve barrier of albumin glycated *in vitro* and *in vivo* from patients with diabetic polyneuropathy. *Proc Natl Acad Sci USA* 1992; 89: 2218–22.
74. Korthals JK, Gieron MA, Dyck PJ. Intima of epineurial arterioles is increased in diabetic polyneuropathy. *Neurology* 1988; 38: 1582–6.
75. Said G, Goulon-Goeau C, Lacroix C, Moulonguet A. Proximal diabetic neuropathy—clinical aspects and morphological findings in biopsy specimens of the intermediate cutaneous nerve of the thigh. *Ann Neurol* 1994; 35: 559–69.
76. Llewelyn JG, Thomas PK, King RHM. Epineural microvasculitis in proximal diabetic neuropathy. *J Neurol* 1998; 245: 159–65.
77. Dyck PJB, Norell JE, Dyck PJ. Microvasculitis and ischemia in diabetic lumbosacral radiculoplexus neuropathy. *Neurology* 1999; 53: 2113–21.
78. Bowen BD, Koenig EC, Viele A. A study of the lower extremities in diabetes as compared with non-diabetic states from the standpoint of X-ray findings, with particular reference to the relationship of arteriosclerosis and diabetes. *Bull Buffalo Gen Hosp* 1924; 2: 35–42.
79. Edmonds ME, Morrison N, Laws JW, Watkins PJ. Medial calcification and diabetic neuropathy. *Br Med J* 1982; 284: 928–35.

70

Autonomic Neuropathy

Michael Edmonds

Kings College Hospital, London, UK

INTRODUCTION

Autonomic neuropathy is an important complication of diabetes, resulting in increased patient morbidity and mortality. Cardiovascular autonomic neuropathy represents a serious complication and leads to an approximately five-fold risk of mortality. Autonomic dysfunction is common although symptomatic autonomic neuropathy is rare. However, when present, it can involve many systems including cardiovascular, gastrointestinal, genitourinary, and respiratory systems. Autonomic neuropathy results in hemodynamic and structural changes in the arterial system.

This chapter will be divided into the following parts:

- Epidemiology
- Etiology
- Pathology
- Cardiovascular autonomic neuropathy
- Circulatory changes in neuropathy (peripheral vascular system and cerebrovascular system)
- Gastrointestinal autonomic neuropathy
- Genitourinary autonomic neuropathy
- Respiratory autonomic neuropathy
- Abnormal patterns of sweating
- Abnormalities in eyes and pupils
- Abnormal responses to hypoglycemia
- Clinical associations of autonomic neuropathy
- Erythropoetin depletion in autonomic neuropathy
- Natural history and mortality
- Management

EPIDEMIOLOGY

Symptomatic autonomic neuropathy is an occasional but devastating complication of diabetes mellitus, especially type 1. Although the full-blown clinical syndrome is not common, abnormal cardiovascular tests are found in at least 16% of the diabetic population, although others describe up to 40% [1]. Sweating abnormalities have been described in as many as 84% of diabetic patients and abnormalities of pupillary function in about 14%. A recent prospective study has shown the prevalence of autonomic neuropathy in the EURODIAB IDDM Complications Study to be 36% [2]. The prevalence of symptomatic autonomic neuropathy (other than impotence) has not been established but is uncommon. A survey suggested that it was present in 12% of type 1 patients and 0.5% of patients with type 2 diabetes [3].

A distinct syndrome exists in young insulin-dependent diabetic subjects in their twenties and thirties, often women, who develop symptomatic autonomic neuropathy often associated with Charcot joints and foot ulceration, and associated with grossly abnormal autonomic function tests, serious loss of thermal sensation, and increased peripheral blood flow. They demonstrate medial calcification of the arteries of the feet despite their youth, yet do not experience numbness of their feet, retaining normal light touch, and near-normal vibration perception. The clinical manifestations are almost solely due to small nerve fiber damage. This striking syndrome is not rare, is highly destructive, and is clearly different from the commoner problem of numb, ulcerated feet [4].

ETIOLOGY

The cause of autonomic neuropathy is not fully understood. Major metabolic changes develop in nerves of diabetic patients; their impact on the neural circulation causes reduced blood flow and hypoxia, which could be important factors in the development of neuropathy [5]. However, it is probable that diabetic autonomic neuropathy may have

International Textbook of Diabetes Mellitus, Third Edition. Edited by R. A. DeFronzo, E. Ferrannini, H. Keen, and P. Zimmet.
 ISBN: 0-471-48655-8.

multiple causative mechanisms leading to the differing presentations of autonomic injury in diabetes [6].

Immunological mechanisms might underlie symptomatic autonomic neuropathy. An association of severe autonomic deficit with iritis was initially described [7]. Autoantibodies to autonomic nervous tissue structures, including vagus nerve, cervical ganglion, and adrenal medulla, is a feature of patients with symptomatic diabetic autonomic neuropathy [8]. Furthermore, such antibodies have been shown to persist, and in studies 2 years apart, there is a high degree of concordance of both positive and negative results [9].

Autoantibodies against sympathetic and parasympathetic nervous tissues are relatively specific for type 1 diabetes. Autoantiobodies against sympathetic nervous tissue in cardiac autonomic denervation have been described in type 1 diabetes mellitus [10]. However, in type 2 diabetes mellitus autoantibodies against autonomic nervous tissues showed no association with cardiac autonomic dysfunction [11]. Thus, it has not been established whether these autoantibodies cause, contribute to, or simply reflect nervous tissue damage.

PATHOLOGY

In an autopsy study of patients with symptoms of autonomic neuropathy, Duchen and colleagues found infiltration of lymphocytes, macrophages, and plasma cells in and about autonomic nerve bundles and ganglia [12].

Further studies in diabetic rodents and human sympathetic ganglia at autopsy have demonstrated axonal and dendritic pathology in sympathetic ganglia in the absence of significant neuron loss as the neuropathologic hallmark of diabetic autonomic neuropathy [6].

A recurring theme in sympathetic ganglia, as well as in the postganglionic autonomic innervation of various end organs, is the involvement of distal portions of axons and nerve terminals by degenerative or dystrophic changes. There is a marked enlargement of distal preterminal axons and synapses, and this is the most notable alteration in sympathetic ganglia in diabetic patients [13].

CARDIOVASCULAR AUTONOMIC NEUROPATHY

Cardiovascular autonomic neuropathy will be discussed in three parts:

(1) Cardiac denervation
(2) Blood pressure (BP) abnormalities
(3) Cardiovascular autonomic function tests

Cardiac Denervation

Resting Tachycardia and Diminished Heart Rate Variability

Resting tachycardia is an early sign of autonomic neuropathy. Tachycardia increases the risk of atherosclerosis [14], and distensibility of the vascular wall is reduced by tachycardia [15].

Depression of heart rate variability (HRV) has been observed in autonomic neuropathy, heart transplantation, congestive heart failure, myocardial infarction (myocardial ischemia), and other cardiac and noncardiac diseases. However, it is important to realize that clinical implication of HRV analysis has been clearly recognized in only two clinical conditions [16]:

(1) as a predictor of risk of arrhythmic events or sudden cardiac death after acute myocardial ischemia, and
(2) as a clinical marker of evolving diabetic neuropathy.

The demonstration of loss of HRV during deep breathing indicates the presence of vagal denervation of the heart, which becomes increasingly common with the lengthening duration of diabetes. In population studies, decreased HRV has had predictive value for mortality among healthy adults. It is a well-established risk factor for arrhythmic events and mortality among post-myocardial-infarction patients but has only moderate sensitivity and specificity [17]. It is thought that decreased parasympathetic innervation exposes the heart to unopposed stimulation by sympathetic nerves [18]. Reduced HRV is associated with increased progression of coronary atherosclerosis [19].

Sympathetic and Parasympathetic Abnormalities

Cardiac denervation involves both parasympathetic and sympathetic fibers. Resting tachycardia due to parasympathetic damage may represent one of the earlier signs. Sympathetic denervation was thought to develop after parasympathetic changes had occurred, but newer techniques suggest that sympathetic changes might occur very early in the course of diabetes. The progress of diabetic cardiac parasympathetic dysfunction as reflected by loss of HRV may parallel the impairment of sympathetic function as measured by of the uptake of radiolabeled analogues of norepinephrine, by the sympathetic nerve terminals of the heart [20].

Quantitative scintigraphic assessment of the cardiac sympathetic innervation of the heart is possible with either 123I-metaiodobenzylguanidine (MIBG) and single-photon-emission computed tomography (SPECT) or [11C]-hydroxyephedrine (HED) and positron emission tomography (PET).

Deficits of left ventricular [123I]-MIBG and [11C]-HED retention have been identified in diabetic subjects without abnormalities on cardiovascular reflex testing, indicating an increased sensitivity to detect cardiac autonomic neuropathy.

Several studies have shown an early sympathetic involvement before evidence of vagal neuropathy. The finding of a higher than expected prevalence of MIBG regional abnormalities in patients without signs or symptoms of autonomic neuropathy suggests that cardiac autonomic nerve damage occurs earlier than previously thought in diabetic patients whose cardiovascular tests are still completely normal [21].

Deficits begin distally in the left ventricle and may extend proximally. Since this abnormality occurs in the inferior segment, an inferior-to-anterior count ratio, an index of regional MIBG uptake, may be suitable for the evaluation of this condition [22]. The clinical significance and subsequent fate of these small regional defects is unknown [23]. However, impaired myocardial MIBG uptake correlates with altered left ventricle diastolic filling and myocardial electrophysiological deficits and is predictive of sudden death.

Thus 123I-MIBG myocardial scintigraphy is a useful diagnostic tool both in the early detection and evaluation of the progression of myocardial sympathetic nerve dysfunction in patients with diabetes mellitus [24].

Left Ventricular Dysfunction

There is evidence of left ventricular dysfunction, in particular, diastolic dysfunction, in patients with autonomic neuropathy [25]. Left ventricular diastolic dysfunction may be detected early in type-1 diabetic patients. Parasympathetic impairment and nocturnal elevations in BP could be the link between autonomic neuropathy and diastolic ventricular dysfunction [26]. Diastolic function is usually impaired first, followed by systolic dysfunction [27].

Decreased Myocardial Reserve

Diabetic autonomic neuropathy is also associated with an impaired vasodilator response of coronary resistance vessels to increased sympathetic stimulation, which is related to the degree of sympathetic neuropathy [28]. There was a significant correlation between BP response to dipyridamole and myocardial perfusion reserve index. Type 1 diabetic patients with autonomic neuropathy have a decreased myocardial perfusion reserve capacity when challenged with a vasodilatator. The underlying mechanism may be defective myocardial sympathetic vasodilatation, a lack of ability to maintain BP during vasodilatation, or both [29]. The heart rate BP and cardiac output responses to exercise are significantly impaired in diabetic neuropathic patients [30].

Silent Myocardial Ischemia

Asymptomatic coronary artery disease and myocardial infarctions are common in diabetic subjects. It is assumed that autonomic neuropathy is responsible for painless myocardial ischemia and silent acute myocardial infarction—but this is not proven.

Indeed, the available clinical and epidemiological data suggest that the increased incidence of asymptomatic myocardial infarctions and coronary artery disease in diabetic patients mainly reflects accelerated coronary atherosclerosis and the proportion of silent disease relative to symptomatic disease or episodes is not increased in diabetes. In spite of the theoretical background, there is no convincing clinical or epidemiological evidence that diabetic autonomic neuropathy plays a major part in the lack of ischemic pain. This is not surprising because the mechanisms of silent myocardial ischemia are complex and controversial even without diabetes [31].

Although the association between autonomic neuropathy and silent myocardial ischemia is controversial, data indicate that event-free survival among diabetic patients with silent myocardial ischemia is predicted by the presence of autonomic neuropathy. During a 4.5-year follow-up of diabetic patients with autonomic neuropathy accompanied by silent myocardial ischemia, a serious cardiovascular event was recorded in 50% [32].

On a practical basis, autonomic neuropathy is independently associated with asymptomatic coronary artery disease. Thus patients may experience equivalents of angina, such as breathlessness or fatigue. Silent myocardial ischemia should be suspected in patients presenting with acute left ventricular failure, collapse, vomiting, and ketoacidosis.

Autonomic Neuropathy and Coronary Heart Disease Risk

Recent studies have shown an association between autonomic neuropathy and increased coronary heart disease risk [33]. The EURODIAB IDDM Complications Study group [2] has recently shown the strong relationship between autonomic neuropathy and the presence of cardiovascular disease risk factors, including cigarette smoking, total cholesterol/high-density lipoprotein (HDL)-cholesterol ratio, fasting triglyceride, diastolic BP, and low HDL-cholesterol, as well as confirming significant correlations between autonomic neuropathy and age, duration of diabetes, and HbA_{1c}.

Indeed cardiovascular autonomic neuropathy may be a component of the metabolic syndrome. Autonomic neuropathy 5 years after diagnosis of type 2 diabetes is associated with an unfavourable metabolic risk profile, and parasympathetic neuropathy in type 2 diabetic patients is associated with features of the insulin resistance syndrome [34]. However, in a further study, autonomic neuropathy was associated with BP levels, but not with dyslipidemia, smoking, or obesity [35].

Nevertheless, a high insulin level seems to have a predictive role in the development of parasympathetic autonomic neuropathy, irrespective of obesity and glycemia [36]. Insulin resistance may be associated with altered balance between parasympathetic and sympathetic pathways [37] and there may be a link between hepatic parasympathetic denervation and insulin resistance [38]. Alternatively, insulinemia as a feature of metabolic syndrome may alter autonomic tone [39].

Cardiovascular autonomic neuropathy is associated with platelet activation in type 1 diabetes mellitus. The high platelet activation may reflect an increased prothrombotic state in diabetic cardiovascular autonomic dysfunction [40]. Furthermore, cardiovascular autonomic neuropathy is related to increased plasminogen activator inhibitor [41]. In women with type 1 diabetes there is a correlation between increased aortic stiffness and parasympathetic dysfunction. Increased arterial stiffness may be of importance in the increased susceptibility to cardiovascular complications in diabetic women [42]. Sympathetic denervation of arteries leads to medial smooth muscle degeneration and calcification [43].

Blood Pressure Abnormalities

These include loss of circadian rhythm, postural hypotension, and postprandial hypotension.

Loss of Circadian Rhythm

Patients with autonomic neuropathy have disturbed circadian rhythms of BP [44]. They lose the normal diurnal/nocturnal BP variation in which nighttime BP is overall lower than that during the daytime, suggesting that there is a relative sympathetic overdrive due to predominantly parasympathetic impairment of cardiovascular innervation.

This occurs in both normotensive and hypertensive type 2 patients with asymptomatic autonomic neuropathy. Nocturnal BP in patients with diabetic autonomic neuropathy is higher than in nondiabetic subjects. Monitoring BP over 24 h confirms this flattening in nocturnal BP reduction at night and shows increased BP values [45]. This may cause cardiac hypertrophy and is postulated as one possible cause of their increased mortality [46].

Postural Hypotension

Presentation Maintenance of BP on standing depends on afferent impulses from baroreceptors (namely in the carotid sinus and aortic arch) and on efferent sympathetic impulses to the heart and blood vessels. *Postural hypotension*, that is a fall in systolic pressure of more 30 mmHg on standing, occurs in diabetic subjects with advanced neuropathy, although symptoms are infrequent. Disabling hypotension when systolic pressure falls below 70 mmHg on standing is rare.

Blood flow studies show that the reduction in foot blood flow on standing observed in normal subjects is diminished in diabetic patients with postural hypotension, although significant vasoconstriction still occurs [47]. Another important mechanism is the failure of the splanchnic bed to vasoconstrict on standing. However, this was no worse than in diabetic patients without hypotension so that the importance of this mechanism in diabetic autonomic neuropathy remains uncertain [48].

Failure of cardiac acceleration and reduced cardiac output both contribute to the problems. Noradrenaline levels are generally reduced in diabetic patients with postural hypotension. An excess of noradrenaline is found in some patients with hypotension because of reduced intravascular volume rather than autonomic neuropathy. Failure of renin responses on standing, though probably not responsible for acute postural hypotension, may or may not be present. Anemia may also contribute to postural hypotension, as treatment with erythropoetin has been shown to improve the anemia and postural hypotension (see below).

Insulin is known to have cardiovascular effects [49]. It causes a reduction in plasma volume, an increase of peripheral blood flow from vasodilatation and an increase in heart rate. In patients with autonomic neuropathy, insulin may cause or exacerbate postural hypotension to the point of fainting whether it is given intravenously or subcutaneously, and occasionally a blackout may occur from hypotension and this may be confused with hypoglycemia. These effects of insulin are likely to be due to the insulin itself and not to changes in blood glucose concentration.

Both hypotension and its symptoms fluctuate spontaneously to a remarkable degree and may persist for many years without necessarily deteriorating [50]. This explanation in our patients is unclear although insulin itself may partly be responsible for exacerbating the condition and fluid retention may improve it.

Management Few patients develop symptoms sufficiently severe to need treatment. When they do, it is first essential to stop any drugs that exacerbate hypotension, notably diuretics, tranquilizers, and antidepressants. Simple treatment should always be tried and include raising the head of the bed and wearing full-length elastic stockings, but the benefits are slight. Mild symptoms may respond to raising the head of the bed about 10 cm, which helps to maintain postural vascular tone.

Measures that increase plasma volume are the most effective, although edema is a troublesome side effect that renders the treatment unacceptable. A high salt uptake or fludrocortisone sometimes in high doses up to 0.4 mg daily can be effective. It acts by increasing peripheral vascular tone and extracellular fluid and blood volume.

The use of an orally active adrenergic agonist midodrine can help. It has an exclusively peripheral pressor effect on arterial and venous capacitance of vessels. Intranasal administration of an antidiuretic agent such as desmopressin (DDAVP) can, by reducing noctural diuresis, improve symptomatic postural hypotension. Erythropoietin administered subcutaneously to anaemic autonomic neuropathy patients has been described [51].

Many other treatments have been suggested. Their effectiveness is inconsistent. Some regimes are hazardous and supine hypertension is a common sequel, and these treatments include β-blockers with partial agonist activity, such as pindolol, and the use of ergotamine, caffeine, nonsteroidal anti-inflammatory drugs, clonidine, and metoclopramide.

Postprandial Hypotension

In diabetic patients with autonomic neuropathy, postprandial hypotension may also occur. Observations on insulin-dependent diabetic patients established that while food causes a large increase in mesenteric blood flow, the latter does not coincide with an exacerbation of their hypotension [52]. In a small number of patients, octreotide is of value in the treatment of postural hypotension in diabetic autonomic neuropathy.

Cardiovascular Autonomic Function Tests

Bedside cardiovascular tests have been developed that indicate the presence or absence of autonomic neuropathy (Table 1). Their use to exclude the condition is at least as important as its confirmation; the tests are extremely sensitive and as many as one fifth of all diabetic patients have one or more abnormalities, while only rarely suffering from symptomatic autonomic neuropathy. When symptoms such as diarrhea or gastroparesis occur, autonomic tests must be abnormal, and other conditions excluded, before they can be attributed to diabetic autonomic neuropathy.

Table 1 Normal values for autonomic function*

Test	Normal	Abnormal
Heart rate variation on deep breathing (beats/min)	>15	<10
Heart rate increase on standing, at 15 s (beats/min)	>15	<12
Heart rate increase on standing, 30:15 ratio	>1.04	<1.00
Valsalva ratio	>1.21	<1.20
Postural systolic pressure fall at 2 min (mmHg)	<10	>30

Note. These tests decline with age. The figures given here generally apply in those less than 60 years old.
* From reference 53.

The tests fall into four groups:

- Simple noninvasive cardiovascular reflex tests
- Spectral analysis of heart rate variation
- Measurement of baroreflex sensitivity
- Measurement of QT interval

Simple Noninvasive Cardiovascular Reflex Tests

Beat to beat variation of heart rate has been used to assess dysfunction of the vagal nerve for many years. The most commonly used battery of noninvasive tests includes heart rate response to deep breathing, heart rate response to standing and Valsalva maneuver, and BP fall on standing. A further test was designed to evaluate BP changes during sustained handgrip.

These tests form the core of diagnosis of cardiac autonomic neuropathy. They are validated, reliable, and reproducible. They correlate with each other with tests of peripheral somatic nerve function. Computerized systems are available to make the performance of the tests easier and to improve the analysis of results during tests on the changes of heart rate. The computer program measures the length of individual RR intervals with immediate display of the results.

A recent study has provided age-specific and sex-specific reference values for a wide range of different autonomic function measures in an elderly population [54].

Spectral Analysis of Heart Rate Variability

The development of power-spectrum analysis has facilitated the diagnosis of autonomic neuropathy. HRV can be assessed in the time domain (by statistical analysis of RR intervals) and in the frequency domain (by spectral analysis of a series of successive RR intervals). Electrocardiogram (ECG) recordings are made for at least 5 min to allow spectral analysis to be carried out. However, the optimum duration of the tracing is 10 min. Where there are slow fluctuations in heart rate, a prolonged 24-h recording is necessary [55].

In the time domain, the simplest parameter is the standard deviation of RR intervals, whereas the most commonly used indices are the mean calculated from the differences of consecutive RR intervals and the number of RR intervals recorded over a period where the difference of consecutive RR intervals exceeds 50 ms. HRV can also be measured in the frequency domain. Plotting the length of the RR interval against time produces a periodic curve that can be broken down in to different wave components. These are characterized by their frequency (range) and amplitude representing a given power. Three frequency components are usually measured:

- A high frequency (HF) component that is a reflection of respiratory sinus arrhythmia and is an index of vagal activity;

- A low frequency (LF) component reflecting vasomotor activity and is dependent on both sympathetic and vagal tone;
- A very low frequency (VLF) band representing the influence of the peripheral vasomotor and renin–angiotensin system [56].

Diabetic autonomic neuropathy is associated with a reduction of HRV. Both the LF and HF components diminish before the onset of clinical neuropathy. This suggests similar damage to both sympathetic and parasympathetic pathways of the heart. HRV in long-term diabetic patients using 24-h ambulatory recordings is abnormal and reproducible over a 12-month interval with very little variation in all HRV parameters, especially in parameters of parasympathetic activity [57].

Twenty-four-hour assessments of heart, including spectral analysis, compare favorably with conventional tests [58]. In a study that performed four cardiovascular tests of autonomic function (deep breathing, lying to standing, Valsalva maneuver, and postural hypotension) and simultaneous 24-h recordings of BP and ECG, the significant correlation of day–night pattern of BP and sympathovagal activity to standard cardiovascular reflex tests, supported the usefulness of 24-h BP monitoring and spectral analysis of HRV in diabetic neuropathy [59].

In conclusion, spectral analysis of HRV appears a convenient method to assess various degrees of diabetic autonomic dysfunction; it appears easy to perform, while giving results similar to traditional methods, with greater sensibility [60].

Measurement of Baroreflex Sensitivity

The arterial baroreflex maintains the stability of BP. Changes in BP lead to stimulation of the baroreceptors, which activates cardiac vagal fibers and sympathetic outflow to the heart and the peripheral blood vessels. Vagal tone is maintained by reflex mechanisms that are activated by continuous input from baroreceptors. Thus baroreflex sensitivity can be measured from the reflex heart rate response to changes in BP. A change in BP can be induced pharmacologically, or the spontaneous fluctuations of BP in steady state conditions may be used [46].

Thus, short noninvasive recording of the BP and RR interval signals are taken in the supine patient, i.e. under conditions suitable for routine outpatient evaluation. The baroreflex sensitivity is determined by the regression analysis of changes induced in the length of RR interval by spontaneous fluctuations in BP.

Baroreflex sensitivity is impaired in diabetes and is helpful in the early detection of cardiac autonomic neuropathy [61]. After myocardial infarction the analysis of baroreflex sensitivity has a significant prognostic value independent of left ventricular ejection fraction and ventricular arrhythmias, and it significantly adds to the prognostic value of HRV.

In conclusion, these estimates of baroreceptor-HR function may provide a powerful tool for assessing cardiovascular autonomic neuropathy at any stage, including the early stage, which is not detected by the conventional tests [62].

Measurement of the QT Interval

The length of the QT interval is influenced by autonomic nervous tone. A long QT interval may reflect imbalance between right and left heart sympathetic nerve activity. Electric instability reflected by abnormally long QT intervals increases the risk of severe abnormal rhythms and sudden death. This was first described with the long QT syndrome. A prolonged QT interval due to autonomic neuropathy can be seen in a proportion of patients with type 1 diabetes. The length of the QT interval is dependent on heart rate. Therefore a corrected QT interval must be obtained by dividing the QT length measured in seconds with the square root of the length of RR interval. Corrected QT (QTc) values above 440 ms are considered abnormal.

In the EURODIAB IDDM Complications Study, 16% had prolonged corrected QT interval. Studies have shown that QTc prolongation is associated with major degrees of autonomic neuropathy [63]. In a cohort-based prospective study QTc prolongation was predictive of increased mortality in type 1 diabetic patients [64].

The usefulness of the QTc interval is under debate. A meta-analysis concluded that QTc prolongation is a specific albeit insensitive indicator of autonomic failure [65]. Other data suggest that in type 1 diabetic patients, QT abnormalities can occur independently of autonomic dysfunction or myocardial ischemia and may be related to the processes that increase urinary albumin leakage [66]. Experimental hypoglycemia in adults with type 1 diabetes causes an abnormal ECG, with increases in QT interval [67].

The significance of the QTc in type 2 diabetes is not clear. QT dispersion may be more important than the measurement QT interval length [68]. QT dispersion is the difference between the longest and shortest QT intervals recorded by the 12-lead ECG. Increasing QT dispersion reflects electrical instability of the left ventricular musculature. Increase of QT dispersion is a major determinant of risk of mortality in type 2 diabetes, but this may be related more to structural factors and local ischemia than to autonomic neuropathy [69].

CIRCULATORY CHANGES IN NEUROPATHY

Peripheral Arterial System

Sympathetic denervation of the peripheral arterial system may occur quite early in the evolution of neuropathy and has major effects on blood flow and vascular responses and causes structural changes in the arterial wall [49].

Blood Flow and Vascular Responses

Sympathetic denervation causes loss of vasoconstrictor tone and peripheral vasodilatation, associated with opening of arteriovenous shunts. Skin blood flow increases substantially and this can occur in the absence of other clinical evidence of neuropathy. These blood flow changes explain some of the clinical features of the neuropathic foot, notably the excessively warm skin, bounding pulses, and marked venous distension. The venous po_2 is increased because of arteriovenous shunting. Capillary pressure is increased and may contribute to neuropathic edema, which can occasionally be severe and sometimes reversed by administration of ephedrine. However, nutritive capillary blood flow is not compromised by shunting and has been shown directly by television microscopy to be normal or even increased [70].

Blood flow responses to various stimulai are also abnormal. Sympathetic stimulation by coughing or standing normally induces peripheral vasoconstriction. Neuropathic patients show blunting of these responses. Maximal vasodilatation in response to heating is reduced. Although this defect is partly attributable to the effects of hyperglycemia on the microvasculature, failure of nitric oxide dependent smooth muscle vasodilatation in neuropathy has been described in diabetic foot patients [71].

Increased blood flow in the neuropathic foot may sometimes be related to the presence of pain, and a reduction of blood flow can be associated with diminution of pain in these cases. Bone blood flow is also elevated in these patients and this is thought to contribute to the osteopenia that predisposes to the development of Charcot joints in diabetic patients.

Structural Changes

Vascular sympathetic denervation can lead to degeneration of the smooth muscle of arteries, leading to medial arterial calcification and stiffening of the arteries (Figure 1). This calcification may assume the histological characteristics of bone.

Unilateral lumbar sympathectomy in humans, both in diabetic and nondiabetic patients, has been shown to result in medial wall calcification on the ipsilateral side [72]. Unilateral sympathectomy in animals leads to excess deposition of cholesterol on the operated side, and the occurrence of cholesterol sclerosis in the rabbit's aorta was accelerated by removal of the celiac ganglion [73]. Furthermore, in animal models, denervation of smooth muscle leads to striking pathological changes, including atrophy of muscle fibers with foci of degeneration [74], and arterial calcification is initiated within senescent atrophic smooth muscle [75].

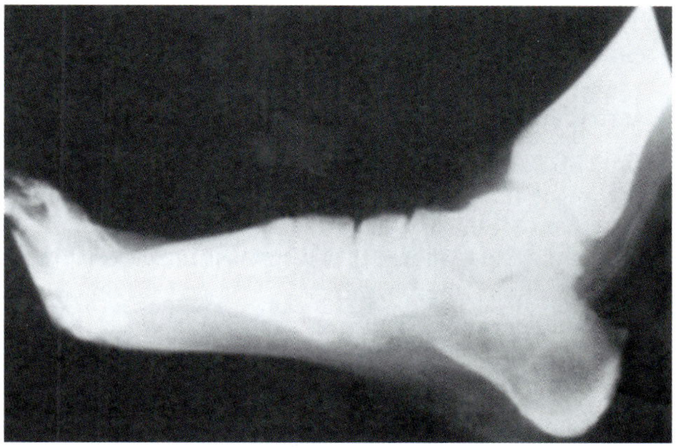

Figure 1 Medial arterial calcification

Medial arterial calcification in the Pima Indians is significantly associated with an increased prevalence of cardiovascular mortality [76]. Medial calcification may be an important factor in the development of peripheral vascular disease, which in diabetes shows a prediliection for the distal arteries below the knee and is unexplained. Chantelau reported an association of below knee atherosclerosis to medial arterial calcification [77].

Thus, a peripheral autonomic neuropathy by causing sympathetic denervation can lead to calcification and stiffening of the arteries. This can predispose to loss of arterial elasticity and abnormal flow, which results in injury to the endothelium and predisposes to atherosclerosis. The influence of peripheral autonomic neuropathy in predisposing to stiffening of the peripheral arteries may provide an explanation for the distal distribution of the atheroscerosis.

Cerebrovascular System

Impaired cerebrovascular reactivity and autoregulation has been reported in patients with diabetes mellitus. However, the contribution of cardiovascular diabetic autonomic neuropathy is not known. A recent study indicates that patients with cardiovascular autonomic neuropathy and orthostatic hypotension show instability in cerebral blood flow upon standing [78].

Cardiovascular autonomic neuropathy is associated with atherosclerosis and narrowing of the carotid artery [79]. In type 2 diabetic patients autonomic neuropathy predicts the development of stroke in patients with non-insulin-dependent diabetes mellitus [80].

GASTROINTESTINAL AUTONOMIC NEUROPATHY

Oesophageal Problems

Abnormal oesophageal motility has been described but no symptoms have been attributed to this functional abnormality. Thus autonomic damage to the upper gastrointestinal tract is often asymptomatic.

Gastroparesis

Presentation

Gastric emptying can be normal, accelerated, or retarded in patients with diabetes [81, 82]. Gastric stasis is a feature of autonomic neuropathy [83, 84], which sometimes, though rather surprisingly not always, causes vomiting. Although radionuclide studies to measure gastric emptying indicate delay in 30–50% of outpatients with long-standing type 1 [85] or type 2 diabetes [86], symptomatic gastroparesis is a rare diabetic complication. The vomiting may be due to vagal denervation of the stomach. Studies have demonstrated the loss of myelinated and unmyelinated fibers in the vagus nerve.

However, there is also evidence of smooth muscle degeneration, characterized by subtotal smooth muscle cell atrophy in the muscularis propria, associated with transformed smooth muscle cells undergoing a form of necrobiosis, appearing as highly distinctive, homogeneous, round eosinophilic bodies. Since vagal degeneration does not normally cause gut smooth muscle degeneration, these changes might represent an independent gastromyopathic process as the cause of gastroparesis [87].

Investigation

The diagnosis is difficult to establish and three approaches are needed. First, other obstructive causes should be excluded by endoscopic and barium studies; second, the presence of gastric stasis must be established with videography to detect decreased or absent peristalsis; and third, the presence of abnormal autonomic function should be demonstrated. Most patients with this complication suffer from other symptoms of autonomic neuropathy.

Gastric stasis must be confirmed by radioisotopic studies, using anterior and posterior cameras to exclude artifacts from stomach movements during the test. Liquids, solids, and indigestible solids, are emptied by the stomach at different rates and by different mechanisms. Radioisotope studies in diabetic patients with autonomic neuropathy have variously shown normal solid emptying, impairment of the usual differentiation between solid and liquid emptying, abnormal liquid emptying, and abnormal solid and liquid emptying. Abnormal liquid emptying probably represents advanced disease.

Management

Glycemic control should be optimized as hyperglycemia per se can delay gastric emptying. Dopamine antagonists (metoclopramide and domperidone) enhance gastric tone and emptying. They may accelerate gastric emptying in diabetic autonomic neuropathy. Intravenous erythromycin (3 mg/kg every 8 h) causes a substantial acceleration of gastric emptying. Oral administration is less effective in alleviating symptoms. The very rare cases of intractable vomiting from gastroparesis may require more invasive treatment. Vomiting should be sufficiently severe to cause recurrent hospital admissions over a considerable period of time, since occasionally it may remit spontaneously even after an interval of as long as 2 years [88].

The introduction of percutaneous endosocopic jejunostomy or gastrostomy may benefit patients in the short term. This may alleviate the problem until a natural remission of vomiting occurs even after protracted periods of time. Sometimes a more definitive procedure is required and a two-thirds gastrectomy with Roux-en-Y loop anastomosed 60 mm from the gastric stump has proved to be successful [89].

The long-term outlook for patients who have symptomatic gastroparesis and who have generally suffered multiple diabetic complications is poor [90]. However, patients with abnormal gastric emptying tests but not necessarily symptoms have a better prognosis [91].

Diabetic Diarrhea

Presentation

Diarrhea is a very disagreeable symptom of autonomic neuropathy. Borborygmi and discomfort precede attacks of watery diarrhea without pain or bleeding and usually without malabsorption. Fecal incontinence is common, especially at night, when exacerbations seem to be worse. Symptoms last from a few hours to a few days and then remit, with normal bowel action or even constipation (sometimes induced by treatment in between attacks). Constipation is not otherwise a particular problem experienced by diabetic patients with neuropathy.

Intermittent attacks of diabetic diarrhea tend to persist over many years and rarely remit completely. Very few patients suffer almost continuous diarrhea for which no other cause is discovered and they are very difficult to treat. The underlying cause of diabetic diarrhea is not established. Gut denervation probably alters gut motility. And bacterial overgrowth has been demonstrated in these cases. Yet many mechanisms are responsible and have not been well studied. Thus gastroparesis might result in maldigestion of disaccharides and result in malabsorption of bile acids that may in turn cause diarrhea. Neuromuscular dysfunction might exist causing a shortened transit time. The possibility of a secretory diarrhea also exists, while the idea that intestinal permeability might be altered has not been studied.

Investigation

Full investigation of diarrhea in a diabetic patient is crucial in order not to overlook easily treatable causes such as celiac disease that may be increased in type 1 patients, pancreatic malabsorption, or other rarer causes. Autonomic function tests should be abnormal otherwise autonomic diarrhea is very unlikely and normal tests virtually exclude this as a cause. Nevertheless, the presence of abnormal autonomic function is not alone sufficient to lead to a diagnosis of diabetic diarhoea and may thus be very deceptive. The diagnosis is most likely to be correct in long-standing type 1 patients with other autonomic symptoms such as gustatory sweating and postural hypotension.

Treatment

Tetracycline offers effective treatment in approximately half the patients and is given in one or two doses of 250 mg at the onset of the attack, which is abruptly aborted. If this fails, a range of the antidiarrhea remedies could be tried, notably codeine phosphate, lomotil, or loperamide. Clonidine reduces propulsive contractions and restores sympathetic tone, and octreotide may be useful in intractable diarrhea [84].

Various methods have been used to treat fecal incontinence, ranging from relaxation and biofeedback techniques to surgical reconstruction of the anal sphincter. They are only partially successful. Control of associated diarrhea often helps.

Gall Bladder

Enlargement of the gall bladder, probably due to poor contraction, may be a feature of diabetes related to autonomic neuropathy. Studies by ultrasonography have not confirmed the enlargement of the gall bladder, but do suggest impaired muscular contraction. There are no known clinical effects from this.

GENITOURINARY AUTONOMIC NEUROPATHY

Bladder Dysfunction

Presentation

Autonomic neuropathy affecting the sacral nerves causes bladder dysfunction [92]. Bladder function tests are commonly abnormal in neuropathic diabetic patients, but symptoms from neurogenic bladder in diabetes are relatively rare, usually occurring in diabetic patients who already have advanced complications. Most men with neurogenic bladder are also impotent.

Impairment of bladder function is chiefly the result of neurogenic detrusor muscle abnormality, while pudendal innervation of perineal and periurethral striated muscle is usually unaffected in diabetic neuropathy. Afferent damage results in impaired sensation of bladder filling and leads to detrusor areflexia. Thus the bladder pressure during cystometrography fails to increase as the bladder is filled. In advanced cases, bladder emptying is reduced because of impaired detrusor activity and possibly failure of the internal sphincter to open adequately. Measurements of urine flow show that the peak flow rate is reduced and that duration of flow is increased.

There are no symptoms in the early stages but later patients experience hesitancy during micturition, develop the need to strain, a feeble stream, and a tendency to dribble. Micturition is sometimes in short, interrupted spurts, which result from straining. Patients may be aware of lengthening intervals between micturition and also experience a sensation of inadequate bladder emptying. Gradually residual urine volume increases and in severe cases gross bladder retention occurs with abdominal swelling and sometimes overflow incontinence as well. Bladder capacity may exceed 1 l.

Investigation

Diagnosis of neurogenic bladder is usually possible especially in those patients with clinical evidence of severe neuropathy. It is however important to exclude bladder neck obstruction and especially prostatic obstruction in men. Ultrasound examination before and after emptying should be performed and cystoscopy is usually needed. Rarely diabetic neurogenic bladder causes hydroureter and hydronephrosis. Occasionally more sophisticated bladder function tests are needed. These include cystograms, cystometrography, and urine flow rate measurements.

Treatment

The principles of treatment are to compensate for a deficient bladder sensation and thus prevent the development of a high residual urine volume. For those diabetic patients who have symptoms of cystopathy, education is important and may suffice. In particular the patient should be told to void every 3 h during the daytime. Manual suprapubic pressure can increase the efficiency of bladder emptying. With more severe symptoms more active measures are needed. An α-1 adrenoceptor blocker may help by reducing urethral resistance. Self-catherization three times daily is now the recommended treatment for patients with chronic retention. Recurrent urinary tract infections are often troublesome in those patients and protracted courses of antibiotics changing monthly may be needed to prevent this problem.

Impotence

Presentation

Autonomic neuropathy is the main etiological factor in diabetic impotence [93]. It is due to erectile failure resulting from damage to both parasympathetic and sympathetic innervation of the corpora cavernosa. Vasoactive intestinal peptidergic (VIPergic) nerves are also important in the vasodilatation of erection, and the concentration of VIP is low in the penile corpora in diabetic patients with autonomic neuropathy. Failure to achieve erection may also be the result of a concomitant sensory deficit in the dorsal nerve of the penis. The onset of neuropathic impotence is usually gradual, progressing slowly over months, but complete erectile failure is usually present within 2 years of the onset of symptoms. This history contrasts with psychogenic impotence, which begins suddenly and in which nocturnal erections are present. Impotence may be due to vascular occlusions of the branches of internal pudendal artery. Furthermore in rare cases erectile failure may be caused by Leriche syndrome.

The diagnosis of neuropathic impotence is diabetes is difficult. The use of intracavernosal injections of prostaglandin E1 is to some extent helpful in distinguishing neurogenic from vasculogenic impotence—it causes an erection in the former and fails to do so in the latter. This is helpful both in terms of diagnosis and in giving guidance in the choice of treatment. For centers with particular interest, other techniques are available. Thus, it is possible to record nocturnal penile tumescence and rigidity during sleep. The absence of tumescence and rigidity over three successive nights is a strong indication of an organic cause of impotence. Vasculogenic impotence can be confirmed by a measurement of penile BP and by comparing it with the brachial systolic pressure thereby achieving a penile–brachial index. When the ratio of penile to brachial pressure is 0.75 or less the diagnosis of penile vascular disease can be considered. Autonomic function tests give some guidance regarding the presence of autonomic neuropathy but they do not establish conclusively in an individual that it is the cause of impotence. A neuropathic cause can be more exactly defined by electophysiological testing of reflex sexual pathways. Conduction velocity is reduced in the dorsal nerve of the penis in diabetic impotent patients and latency of the bulbocavernosus reflex is prolonged.

Treatment

Stop medications causing impotence Medications associated with erectile dysfunction should be stopped, if possible. These include antihypertensive drugs, diuretics, vasodilators, β-blockers, angiotensin converting enzyme (ACE) inhibitors, calcium channel blockers, and antidepressants, both tricyclics and monoaminoxidase inhibitors.

Counselling If the history reveals a psychological component, then the patient and his partner may be helped by appropriate discussion and advice. Counselling is always needed, especially if the impotence is psychogenic in origin. Neuropathic impotence is, however, permanent and there is no cure. This needs to be understood to eliminate suspicion and mistrust. Proper explanation often suffices and many seek no further treatment. Androgen treatment is contraindicated unless there is evidence of its deficiency, because it merely serves to increase libido without restoring potency.

Oral pharmacological agents The introduction of sildenafil (Viagra) has revolutionized the treatment of erectile dysfunction [94]. Sildenafil produces a natural erectile response to sexual stimulation by enhancing the relaxant effect of nitric oxide on the corpora cavernosa. Nitric oxide is the pivotal neurotransmitter involved in the relaxation of the corpus cavernosal smooth muscle. It acts through a second messenger system involving guanylate cyclase. This enzyme converts guanosine triphosphate (GTP) into intracellular cyclic guanosine monophosphate (cGMP), a potent second messenger for smooth muscle relaxation. Detumescence is caused by sympathetic vasoconstrictor activity and the enzyme breakdown of cGMP by phosphodiesterase type 5 (PDE5), which exists principally in the corpora cavernosa [95].

Sildenafil is a selective inhibitor of GMP-specific PDE5 and therefore enhances the normal vasodilatory erectile mechanisms. The therapeutic window is up to 4 h after administration of the single dose. Recommended dose is 50 mg taken approximately 60 min before sexual activity. It should be taken no more than once daily. The dose may be increased to 100 mg or reduced to 25 mg depending on its effect.

Sildenafil has peripheral vasodilatory properties and this results in modest decreases in BP in some patients, which is consistent with its known effects on the nitric oxide cGMP pathway. Sildenafil is contraindicated in patients using nitrates, such as glyceryl trinitrate, or nitric oxide donors, such as sodium nitroprusside. It is contraindicated in patients with significant cardiac disease [96].

Other phosphodiesterase inhibitor drugs available include tadalafil and vardenafil. For patients taking tadalafil, the duration of the therapeutic window of effectiveness is at least 24 h in 80% of men. It has a rapid tissue distribution but a half-life of 17.5 h. These characteristics potentially reduce the need for planning associated with most other treatments for erectile dysfunction, but like other PDE5 inhibitors it is contraindicated in those taking nitrates.

Vacuum devices Erection can be induced by application of a partial vacuum to the penis after venous occlusion. This is applied with a specially designed reusable condom with a vacuum pump attached [97]. It is noninvasive, but the apparatus is cumbersome and relatively expensive. A vacuum is applied to the penis for a few minutes, causing tumescence and rigidity that are sustained using a constricting ring at the base of the penis but trabecular smooth muscle relaxation does not occur. By this mechanism, blood is simply trapped in both the intracorporal and extracorporal compartments of the penis. Many different devices are now manufactured. They all have three common components: a vacuum chamber, a pump, and a constriction band that is applied to the base of the penis once an erection is achieved.

Vasoactive therapy This includes intracavernosal and intraurethral drug therapy and is useful in diabetic neuropathy where there is a normal hemodynamic mechanism but lack of a control system that initiates the erectile response. High local concentrations of smooth muscle relaxant drugs act on both the trabecular muscle and the arteriolar vasculature.

When the arterial supply is severely compromised, pharmacologically induced arterial dilatation is ineffective because it cannot facilitate sufficient inflow to engorge the lacunar spaces and thereby operate the veno-occlusive mechanism.

Intracavernosal therapy Direct injection of a vasodilator into the corpus cavernosum is a satisfactory treatment. Papaverine is a powerful direct smooth muscle relaxant that acts on both the trabecular muscle of the erectile tissue and the vascular tone, inducing an erection that last for several hours. When vasoactive drugs were introduced, papaverine was initially the most widely used agent for intracorporal self-injection. If papaverine alone fails, then combination therapy with phentolamine and papaverine may be beneficial. Phentolamine acts directly on the α-adrenoceptors of the vascular smooth muscle and potentiates the effects of papaverine. Prostaglandin E1 (as alprostadil or caverject) is the best available agent.

Recently alprostadil has become the drug of choice for intracavernous pharmacotherapy. Prostaglandin E1 plays a natural role as a neurotransmitter in the natural erectile mechanism and alprostadil is at least as effective in treating erectile dysfunction as combination therapy with papaverine and phentolamine and has fewer side effects. The effective dose ranges from 5 mcg to 20 mcg.

Patients need instruction; with alprostadil the recommended starting dose is 1.25 mcg for patients with neurogenic impotence. The skin is drawn taut and the needle and syringe held at right angles. The injection is given near to the base of the penis on either side and avoiding any visible veins. Injection sites should be varied.

After starting with a small dose the patient should titrate this upwards under medical supervision until a satisfactory erection lasting not more than 1 h is achieved. The chief hazard is from a sustained erection (i.e. lasting more than 4 h), which can lead to permanent damage if it is not treated promptly. Patients must be given written instructions; if vigorous exercise fails to reduce the erection, they should receive emergency treatment consisting of aspiration of blood and phenylephrine injection, which leads to prompt detumescence. Failure to achieve detumescence after 6–8 h can cause irreversible ischemic damage to the corpora cavernosa with subsequent fibrotic damage and permanent loss of erectile function. Other long-term problems are sepsis and penile fibrosis, but these occur infrequently. Papaverine, phentolamine, and alprostadil have a low rate of leakage into the systemic circulation.

Many patients with erectile dysfunction will be given a trial injection of vasoactive agents to establish the possible origin of the problem and to test the efficacy of the drug as potential therapy.

Intraurethral therapy Alprostadil has been developed for insertion into the urethra as a pellet through a specific polypropylene applicator. Once delivered the pellet dissolves into the urethral mucosa and from there it enters the corpora. In a comparative study of intracavernosal and intraurethral application of alprostadil, the intracavernosal administration was shown to be more effective though there was a slightly higher incidence of local side effects than with the intraurethral route of administration [98]. It would seem that while the intraurethral route of administraton is associated with a lower overall success rate, the improved side effect profile and acceptability to patients makes it a preferred option for some patients [78].

Surgical treatment Surgical treatment of erectile dysfunction is usually reserved for patients in whom more conservative therapy has failed or for whom conservative therapy is contraindicated. Most of these patients will have significant arterial or venous disease. Surgically implantable penile prostheses are classified as either semi-rigid or inflatable.

The simplest technique is the insertion of a malleable silastic rod that is often effective especially when ejaculation is retained. Semi-rigid rod devices were the first prostheses designed to restore erectile function and are used extensively. More elaborate inflatable prostheses can be inserted but the apparatus is more complex, prone to failure, and very expensive.

Although the incidence of postoperative complications has decreased markedly, mechanical malfunction can still occur with any of the penile prosthetic devices. Another potential complication is infection [99].

In conclusion, sildenafil has been a major advance. Prescribed as an oral agent, it can be administered comfortably and its use relieves patients from the use of cumbersome vacuum devices, as well as the discomfort and risks associated with self-injections.

RESPIRATORY RESPONSES AND ARRESTS

Sudden respiratory arrests have been described in diabetes with autonomic neuropathy. Autonomic neuropathy may be responsible for spontaneous respiratory arrest and unexplained sudden death. In most of these episodes there was some interference with respiration either by anesthesia, drugs, or bronchopneumonia. These episodes are transient and while temporary ventilation may be needed, recovery to normal health is expected. Anesthetists need to be forewarned of this possibility when symptomatic autonomic neuropathy patients require even minor surgery.

These observations have led to further investigation of the respiratory system of diabetic patients with autonomic neuropathy and this falls into three parts.

1. The control of ventilation in response to hypoxia with hypocapnia
2. The pattern of respiration during sleep
3. The bronchal reactivity to chemical and physical agents

The integrity of the ventilatory responses in autonomic neuropathy has been studied by measuring responses to hypoxia and hypercapnia in diabetic patients with and without neuropathy. The majority of studies have found a defective response to hypoxia in autonomic neuropathy [100]. The results regarding responses to hypercapnia are conflicting, as both normal ventilatory and reduced responses have been detected. Thus the true importance of abnormal ventilatory responses as a cause of respiratory arrest has yet to be established.

Sleep apnea has been reported in type 1 diabetes, occasionally in association with autonomic neuropathy [101]. Heart rate responses to apneic episodes may be abnormal. Uncertainty still exists however, and in the study of Catterall et al. [102] there was no evidence for sleep apnea in diabetic patients with autonomic neuropathy. However, recently a large group of diabetic patients have been studied and 26% of patients suffering from autonomic neuropathy had obstructive sleep apnes and none of the patients without autonomic neuropathy showed any breathing abnormalities [103].

The third area of study has assessed the integrity of respiratory reflexes, which affect bronchomotor tone. Airway tone is mainly under vagal control and is reduced in diabetic patients with autonomic neuropathy with diminished bronchodilatation in response to anticholinergic agents. Diabetic patients with autonomic neuropathy also show decreased bronchoconstriction during inhalation of cold air and even more strikingly a diminished or even absent cough reflex in response to an inhaled irritant such as citric acid [104].

These deficits are due to neuropathic denervation and not due to any intrinsic abnormality in bronchial smooth muscle that responds normally to direct stimulation by inhaled histamine. The perception of respiratory sensations in diabetic patients has also been measured in patients breathing through a tube manifold apparatus with resistance to airflow that was randomly varied. Diminished perception or respiratory resistance loads occurred in diabetic patients with neuropathy, and this may render the patient prone to subclinical episodes of respiratory illness. Respiratory arrests in diabetic patients with autonomic neuropathy continue to be reported. It is difficult to know whether they are responsible for the sudden unexplained deaths reported in diabetic autonomic neuropathy.

SWEATING ABNORMALITIES

Peripheral

The sweat gland is an important structure with a complex peptidergic as well cholinergic innervation. Neuropeptide immunoreactivity especially of vasoactive intestinal polypeptide is low in diabetic sudomotor nerves [105]. Measurement of sweating in the periphery is one of the few quantitative methods for assessing cholinergic nerve function.

There are various methods for studying sweat responses. The thermoregulatory sweat test involves whole body heating, and sweating is detected by the application of alizarin red powder. This method assesses peripheral sympathetic function, both pre- and postganglionic). The quantitative sudomotor axon reflex test (QSART) stimulates sweating by iontophoresis of acetylcholine and assesses postganglionic sympathetic function by the axon reflex. Direct stimulation of sweat glands either by iontophoresis of pilocarpine and counting sweat droplets on a silastic imprint or by acetylcholine injection and counting iodine starch sweat spots assesses postganglionic sweat gland denervation. The *sympathetic skin response* (SSR) is a potential generated by a change in the electrical resistance of the skin, caused by activity of the sweat glands innervated by sympathetic sudomotor fibers. The potential difference between electrode plates placed on opposite surfaces of the foot is measured [106].

Studies of sympathetic peripheral neuropathy suggest that QSART can evaluate early diabetic neuropathy more precisely than can SSR [107]. More important than differences in sensitivity is the specificity of QSART, which evaluates the postganglionic axon (instead of polysynaptic pathways in SSR) and provides quantitative data on the severity and pattern of autonomic deficit. Peripheral sympathetic adrenergic and cholinergic fibers simultaneously undergo early alterations in diabetic patients, even when there is no clinical neuropathy [108]. There is a close relationship between sudomotor and vagal cardiac neuropathy. This may reflect a C-fiber directed selectivity of the pathological process in autonomic diabetic neuropathy [109].

The commonest sweating abnormality in diabetic neuropathy is in the feet, in the classical stocking distribution. Loss of sweating causes dryness of the feet and cracked skin, which might serve as a portal of entry for infection as a part of the pathogenesis of diabetic foot problems.

Patients with diabetic neuropathy typically have decreased sweating in the feet but excessive sweating in the upper body. Redistribution of sudomotor responses is an early sign of sympathetic dysfunction with decreased sweating in the feet and increased sweating in the upper body [110].

Gustatory Sweating

Gustatory sweating is a highly characteristic and not uncommon symptom of diabetic autonomic neuropathy. Sweating begins soon after starting to chew tasty food, especially cheese. It starts on the forehead, and spreads to involve the face, scalp, and neck, and sometimes the shoulders and upper part of the chest, compelling patients to keep a towel at the dinner table. Distribution of the sweating is in the territory of the superior cervical ganglion. It may be of sudden onset; its cause is unknown, although aberrant nerve regeneration has been suggested. It is occasionally sufficiently severe to need treatment. Gustatory sweating, once established, generally persists over many years although there can be remarkable and unexplained remission after renal transplantation.

Gustatory sweating is occasionally sufficiently severe to need treatment. Anticholinergic drugs are highly effective although side effects may limit their use. Poldine methylsulphate is the best agent, and propantheline bromide can also be used. They are given half an hour before meals, but may also be effective if given before single meals at social occasions. Recently the use of glycopyrrolate cream has been described made from glycopyrrolate powder and made into a cream, using a standing cream base called cetamacrogol normally at 0.5% but 1 or 2% may be more effective. The cream is applied on alternate days to the areas affected by sweating, avoiding contact with the mouth, nose, and eyes. The area must not be washed for 4 h after application. The only contraindication known is narrow angle glaucoma that might be exacerbated if the eye is accidentally contaminated.

Some neuropathic patients complain of drenching night sweats requiring a change of clothes and bed clothes, and not precipitated by hypoglycemia. This symptom is unexplained and rare.

ABNORMALITIES IN PUPIL

The pupil receives a substantial sympathetic and parasympathetic innervation and has been extensively studied as a visible mirror of autonomic denervation [111]. In diabetic neuropathy, various abnormalities have been reported. These include a decrease in pupil size, greater than expected for age; slowness to redilate after constricting to light; and a diminished light reflex amplitude. Hippus, i.e. the natural oscillatory movement of the pupil, is reduced in patients with neuropathy [112]. Finally, there is evidence of denervation hypersensitivity in the exaggerated response to directly acting sympathomimetic agents. Most of these observations require sophisticated apparatus with which to measure them, and they have not generally been adapted for bedside tests.

ABNORMAL RESPONSES TO HYPOGLYCEMIA

Hypoglycemia is a powerful stimulus of autonomic function, causing sweating, tremor, tachycardia, and an increase of pulse pressure, with a notable rise of systolic BP. There are also major circulatory and endocrine changes in response to hypoglycemia. Glucagon, adrenaline, noradrenaline, pancreatic polypeptide, somatostatin, adrenocorticotropic harmone (ACTH), growth hormone, and corticosteroids all increase in response to hypoglycemia. The presence of autonomic neuropathy prevents the stimulated increase of pancreatic polypeptide and possibly of somatostatin, while responses of the remaining hormones are unaffected beyond the diminished responses that occur anyway in long-term type 1 diabetes regardless of the presence of neuropathy, notably for glucagon and adrenaline. Noradrenaline release is of course reduced in patients with autonomic neuropathy but responses to hypoglycemia are unaffected. Glucose recovery following hypoglycemia may be impaired in type 1 diabetes, especially following repeated episodes, but this deficit is not related to the presence of autonomic neuropathy.

Loss of warning of hypoglycemia has often in the past been attributed to autonomic neuropathy, but it is now established that the phenomenon occurs chiefly in those subjected to repeated hypoglycemia and can be reversed [113].

Studies in type 1 patients of more than 15 years, with and without loss of warnings of hypoglycemia, showed equal proportions of autonomic damage in the two groups. Furthermore, patients with established autonomic neuropathy have similar autonomic and neuroglycopenic symptoms to those without autonomic neuropathy [114, 115]. The Diabetes Control and Complications Trial (DCCT) study also showed a lack of relationship between loss of warning in those with tight control and the presence of autonomic neuropathy [116]. In long-standing diabetes with duration over 20 years, autonomic neuropathy results in an irreversible loss of adrenaline response to hypoglycemia and impairment of autonomic symptoms [117].

The concept, however, that diminished autonomic symptoms and counterregulatory changes may occur as a result of reduced central nervous system responses to hypoglycemia has gained substantial support, but these changes are independent of the presence or absence of autonomic neuropathy itself.

The use of β-blocking drugs can, however, cause abrupt loss of warning of hypoglycemia in delayed metabolic recovery. This occurs infrequently, perhaps in as few as 1 in 50 patients on β-blockers. Yet, when it occurs it is dramatic and potentially dangerous and patients should always be warned of this hazard.

CLINICAL ASSOCIATIONS OF AUTONOMIC NEUROPATHY

Nephropathy

There is increasing evidence of a link between autonomic neuropathy and nephropathy. There is an association of 24-h cardiac parasympathetic activity and degree of nephropathy and the urinary albumin in IDDM patients [118]. The urinary albumin excretion rate (UAER) is independently related to subclinical autonomic neuropathy in type 2 diabetes [119]. The remarkable covariation of degree of neuropathy and nephropathy has suggested a common pathogenetic mechanism. Furthermore, the reduced 24-hr vagal activity, even in the early stages of nephropathy, could be an important risk factor for cardiac death in insulin-dependent diabetic patients.

Retinopathy

In a study of risk factors for early onset proliferative retinopathy in insulin-dependent diabetes, a striking relationship with cardiovascular autonomic neuropathy was found [120]. In a further study of IDDM patients with proteinuria, abnormal cardiac autonomic neuropathy was notably demonstrated in patients suffering from proliferative retinopathy [121]. Cardiac autonomic neuropathy is thus significantly associated with the presence of retinopathy; an impairment of autonomic peripheral blood flow control might be a contributing factor in the formation of microvascular lesions [122].

ERYTHROPOIETIN DEPLETION IN AUTONOMIC NEUROPATHY

Renal erythropoietin production is stimulated chiefly by the presence of anaemia and hypoxia. However, sympathetic innervation of the kidney appears to have a modulating influence, and renal denervation leads to a reduction of stimulated erythropoiesis due to a decreased reduction of erythropoietin. Studies of human autonomic neuropathy with postural hypotension, including some patients with diabetes, have demonstrated erythropoietin depletion. Diabetic autonomic neuropathy may cause both anemia and diminished erythropoietin production in patients without renal impairment [123]. Certainly, an erythropoietin-deficient anemia is recognized in type 1 diabetic patients with early nephropathy and symptomatic autonomic neuropathy. Diabetic patients with autonomic neuropathy have inappropriately low erythropoietin levels for the severity of their anemia but they can mount an appropriate erythropoietin response to moderate hypoxia [124]. The mechanism underlying the erythropoietin-deficient anaemia present in some diabetic patients remains unclear. Administration of erythropoietin may improve symptomatic postural hypotension.

NATURAL HISTORY AND MORTALITY

Autonomic function tests have been used to detect early changes in the natural history and abnormalities can be detected in children. Studies in diabetic children have shown that heart rate variation analysis can detect early subclinical alterations of the autonomic nervous system in asymptomatic patients with IDDM, which seem to consist mainly of a parasympathetic impairment. Autonomic dysfunction is associated with both the duration and an inadequate metabolic control of the disease [125]. Neurological abnormalities were also demonstrable in a small proportion of diabetic children, who were younger than the rest of the population at the time of onset of their disease [126].

Autonomic function declines with age but in diabetes it deteriorates, on average, faster than in normal subjects. Thus HRV, which normally decreases at approximately one beat per minute per 3 years, declines three times faster in diabetic patients although there is substantial variation. Most patients who develop abnormal autonomic function do not become symptomatic.

Established symptoms of autonomic neuropathy, including diarrhea, vomiting from gastroparesis, and postural hypotension, run a very protracted though intermitting course and rarely become disabling even over the 10–15 years during which these patients have been seen. Postural hypotension fluctuates substantially with corresponding variation in intensity of symptoms. Type 2 diabetic patients with abnormal autonomic function tests have increased mortality, and those combined with postural hypotension have higher mortality than those without [127]. Gustatory sweating also tends to persist without remission although many patients describe disappearance of this symptom after renal transplantation.

Mortality of asymptomatic patients with autonomic dysfunction may be increased but the prognosis is generally good with 90% of patients (all under 50 years old) still alive 10 years later [128]. In contrast the outcome for those with symptomatic autonomic neuropathy is not as good, although even in this group 73% were still alive after a decade. Ewing and Clark described a poorer prognosis although patient selection was different [129]. The patients were older and some had renal damage. Those with postural hypotension appeared to have the highest mortality perhaps because of a premature development of left ventricular hypertrophy. Most deaths of these patients were from renal failure or myocardial infarction.

Autonomic neuropathy is clearly associated with increased mortality, and this may be explained by associations with complications (e.g., nephropathy) and increased cardiovascular risk factors (e.g., hypertension) [130]. In a study that investigated the incidence rate and potential predictors for cardiovascular autonomic neuropathy in a cohort of childhood-onset type 1 diabetic patients (subjects from the Epidemiology of Diabetes Complications Study), beyond age and poor glycemic control, nephropathy was a significant risk factor for cardiac autonomic neuropathy and this association may explain some of the increased mortality. As a key finding, autonomic neuropathy was related to the presence of cardiovascular disease ($P < 0.0001$) [131].

In addition to increased mortality, autonomic neuropathy may also be responsible for spontaneous respiratory arrest and unexplained sudden death [132]. Possible causes and mechanisms of sudden death include silent myocardial ischemia/infarction, ventricular arrhythmias, prolongation of the QT interval, impaired respiratory reflexes to hypoxia, and sleep apnea syndrome.

MANAGEMENT

Near normoglycemia is now generally accepted as the primary approach to the prevention of diabetic neuropathy but is not achievable in most patients. The natural history of neuropathy is governed by the degree of glycemic control. The deleterious effect of long-term poor glycemic control on the development and progression of autonomic neuropathy is now accepted, in the light of evidence from prospective large scale studies, including the DCCT and the UK Prospective Diabetes Study.

In diabetic subjects with early cardiovascular denervation, institution of good glycemic control may prevent the development of further myocardial, sympathetic, and enhanced cardiac risk [23]. A target-driven, long-term, intensified intervention aimed at multiple risk factors in patients with type 2 diabetes and microalbuminuria reduced the risk of cardiovascular and microvascular events by about 50%, including a significant reduction in autonomic neuropathy [133].

As to specific treatment of the neuropathy, clinical experience with aldose reductase inhibitors has been disappointing. Treatment of autonomic neuropathy with α-lipoic acid has been promising. This is a powerful, free-radical scavenger that improves nerve blood flow, reduces nerve oxygen, and lipid peroxidation and oxidative stress. Improvement of cardiac autonomic function as assessed by HRV was demonstrated in the DEKAN study [134]. A recent study has shown that quinapril significantly increases parasympathetic activity in patients with autonomic neuropathy 3 months after treatment initiation and sustains this effect until the 6th month [135].

CONCLUSION

This chapter has focused on autonomic denervation in diabetic patients. Autonomic neuropathy as defined by abnormal autonomic tests is common, but symptoms are rare. However, when present they can be devastating. The unfavorable connection between autonomic neuropathy and cardiovascular disease is notable and illustrates how the autonomic nervous system interacts between diabetes and vascular disease.

REFERENCES

1. Neil HAW. The epidemiology of diabetic autonomic neuropathy. In Banister R, Matthias CJ (eds), *Autonomic Failure* Oxford: Oxford Medical Publications, 1992; pp 682–97.
2. Kempler P, Tesfaye S, Chaturvedi N, Stevens LK, Webb DJ, Eaton S, Kerenyi Z, Tamas G, Ward JD, Fuller JH. Autonomic neuropathy is associated with increased cardiovascular risk factors: the EURODIAB IDDM Complications Study Group. *Diabet Med* November 2002; 19 (11): 900–9.
3. Niel HA, Thompson AV, John S, McCarthy ST, Mann JI. Diabetic autonomic neuropathy: the prevalence of impaired heart rate variability in a geographically defined population. *Diabet Med* January–February 1988; 6 (1): 20–4.
4. Winkler AS, Ejskjaer N, Edmonds M, Watkins PJ. Dissociated sensory loss in diabetic autonomic neuropathy. *Diabet Med* June 2000; 17 (6): 457–62.
5. Stevens MJ. Nitric oxide as a potential bridge between metabolic and vascular hypothesis of diabetic neuropathy. *Diabet Med* 1995; (12): 292–5.
6. Schmidt RE. Neuropathology and pathogenesis of diabetic autonomic neuropathy. *Int Rev Neurobiol* 2002; 50: 257–92.
7. Guy RJC, Richards F, Edmonds ME, Watkins PJ. Diabetic autonomic neuropathy and iritis: an association suggesting an immunological cause. *Br Med J* 1984; 789: 343–5.
8. Ejskjaer NT, Zanone MM, Peakman M. Autoimmunity in diabetic autonomic neuropathy: does the immune system get on your nerves? [Review]. *Diabet Med* September 1998; 15 (9): 723–9.
9. Cachia MJ, Peakman M, Zanone M, Watkins PJ, Vergani D. Reproducibility and persistence of neural and adrenal autoantibodies in diabetic autonomic neuropathy. *Diabet Med* June 1997; 14 (6): 461–5.
10. Schsnell O, Muhr D, Dresel S, Tatsch K, Ziegler AG, Haslbeck M, Standl E. Autoantibodies against sympathetic ganglia and evidence of cardiac sympathetic dysinnervation in newly diagnosed and long-term IDDM patients. *Diabetologia* August 1996; 39 (8): 970–5.
11. Schnell O, Schwarz A, Muhr-Becker D, Standl E. Autoantibodies against autonomic nervous tissues in type 2 diabetes mellitus: no association with cardiac autonomic dysfunction. *Exp Clin Endocrinol Diabetes* 2000; 108 (3): 181–6.
12. Duchen LW, Anjorin A, Watkins PJ, MacKay JD. Pathology of autonomic neuropathy in diabetes mellitus. *Ann Intern Med* 1980; 92: 301–3.
13. Schroer JA, Plurad SB, Schmidt RE. Fine structure of presynaptic axonal terminals in sympathetic autonomic

ganglia of aging and diabetic human subjects. *Synapse* 1992; 12: 1–13.
14. Beer PA, Glagor S, Zariu CK. Retarding effect of lowered heartrate on coronary atheroscerosis. *Science* 1984; 226: 180–2.
15. Mangoni AA, Mircoli L, Giannattasio C, Ferrari AU, Mancia G. Heartrate-dependence of arterial distensibilty in vivo. *J Hypertens* 1996; 14: 802–97.
16. Stys A, Stys T. Current clinical applications of heart rate variability. *Clin Cardiol* 1998; 21 (10): 719–24.
17. Stein PK, Kleiger RE. Insights from the study of heart rate variability. *Annu Rev Med* 1999; 50: 249–61.
18. Gorman JM, Sloan RP. Heart rate variability in depressive and anxiety disorders. *Am Heart J* October 2000; 140 (4 suppl): 77–83.
19. Uikuri HV, Jokinen V, Syvanne M, Nieminen MS, Airaksinen KE, Ikaheimo MJ, Koistinen JM, Kauma H, Kesaniemi AY, Majahalme S, Niemela KO, Frick MH. Heart rate variability and progression of coronary atherosclerosis. *Arterioscler Thromb Vasc Biol* August 1999; 19 (8): 1979–85.
20. Stevens MJ. New imaging techniques for cardiovascular autonomic neuropathy: a window on the heart. *Diabetes Technol Ther* Spring 2001; 3 (1): 9–22.
21. Giordano A, Calcagni ML, Verrillo A, Pellegrinotti M, Frontoni S, Spallone V, Gambardella S. Assessment of sympathetic innervation of the heart in diabetes mellitus using 123I-MIBG. *Diabetes Nutr Metab Clin Exp* December 2000; 13 (6): 350–5.
22. Hattori N, Tamaki N, Hayashi T, Masuda I, Kudoh T, Tateno M, Tadamura E, Yonekura Y, Nakao K, Konishi J. Regional abnormality of iodine-123-MIBG in diabetic hearts. *J Nucl Med* December 1996; 37 (12): 1985–90.
23. Stevens MJ, Raffel DM, Allman KC, Schwaiger M, Wieland DM. Regression and progression of cardiac sympathetic dysinnervation complicating diabetes: an assessment by C-11 hydroxyephedrine and positron emission tomography. *Metab* 1999; 48 (1): 92–101.
24. Nagamachi S, Jinnouchi S, Nakahara H, Flores LG II, Ohnishi T, Hoshi H, Futami S, Watanabe K, Nakatsuru K, Toshimori T, Matsukura S. 123I-MIBG myocardial scintigraphy in diabetic patients: relationship to autonomic neuropathy. *Nucl Med Commun* July 1996; 17 (7): 621–32.
25. Willenheimer RB, Erhardt LR, Nilsson H, Lilja B, Juul-Moller S, Sundkvist G. Parasympathetic neuropathy associated with left ventricular diastolic dysfunction in patients with insulin-dependent diabetes mellitus. *Scand Cardiovasc J* 1998; 32 (1): 17–22.
26. Monteagudo PT, Moises VA, Kohlmann O Jr, Ribeiro AB, Lima VC, Zanella MT, for the Department of Medicine, Escola Paulista de Medicina, UNIFESP, Sao Paulo, Brazil. Influence of autonomic neuropathy upon left ventricular dysfunction in insulin-dependent diabetic patients. *Clin Cardiol* May 2000; 23 (5): 371–5.
27. Irace L, Iarussi D, Guadagno I, Tedesco MA, Perna B, Ratti G, Spadaro P, Rogliani G, Armentano V, Iacono A. Left ventricular performance and autonomic dysfunction in patients with long-term insulin-dependent diabetes mellitus. *Acta Diabetol* December 1996; 33 (4): 269–73.
28. Di Carli MF, Bianco-Batlles D, Landa ME, Kazmers A, Groehn H, Muzik O, Grunberger G. Effects of autonomic neuropathy on coronary blood flow in patients with diabetes mellitus. *Circulation* 1999; 100 (8): 813–9.
29. Taskiran M, Fritz-Hansen T, Rasmussen V, Larsson HB, Hilsted J. Decreased myocardial perfusion reserve in diabetic autonomic neuropathy. *J Diabetes* November 2002; 51 (11): 3306–10.
30. Roy TM, Peterson HR, Snider HL, Cyrus J, Broadstone VL, Fell RD, Rothchild AH, Samols E, Pfeifer MA. Autonomic influence on cardiovascular performance in diabetic subjects. *Am J Med* October 1989; 87 (4): 382–8.
31. Airaksinen KE. Silent coronary artery disease in diabetes—a feature of autonomic neuropathy or accelerated atherosclerosis? *Diabetologia* February 2001; 44 (2): 259–66.
32. Valensi P, Sachs RN, Harfouche B, Lormeau B, Paries J, Cosson E, Paycha F, Leutenegger M, Attali JR. Predictive value of cardiac autonomic neuropathy in diabetic patients with or without silent myocardial ischemia. *Diabetes Care* February 2001; 24 (2): 339–43.
33. Ziegler D. Cadiovascular autonomic neuropathy: clinical manifestations and measurement. *Diabetes Rev* 1999; 7: 342–57.
34. Gottsater A, Ahmed M, Fernlund P, Sundkvist G. Autonomic neuropathy in type 2 diabetic patients is associated with hyperinsulinaemia and hypertriglyceridaemia. *Diabet Med* January 1999; 16 (1): 49–54.
35. Spallone V, Maiello MR, Cicconetti E, Menzinger G. Autonomic neuropathy and cardiovascular risk factors in insulin-dependent and non insulin-dependent diabetes. *Diabet Res Clin Pract* January 1997; 34 (3): 169–79.
36. Toyry JP, Niskanen LK, Mantysaari MJ, Lansimies EA. Uusitupa myocardial ischemia occurrence, predictors, and clinical significance of autonomic neuropathy in NIDDM. Ten-year follow-up from the diagnosis. *Diabetes* March 1996; 45 (3): 308–15.
37. Lindmark S, Wiklund U, Bjerle P, Eriksson JW. Does the autonomic nervous system play a role in the development of insulin resistance? A study on heartrate variabilty in first-degree relatives of type 2 diabetes patients, and control subjects. *Diabet Med* 2003; 20: 399–405.
38. Takayama S, Legare DJ, Lautt WW, Dose-related atropine-induced insulin resistance: comparing intraportal vs. intravenous administration. *Proc West Pharmacol Soc* 2000; 43: 33–4.
39. Van De Borne P, Hausberg M, Hoffman RP, Mark AL, Anderson EA. Hyperinsulinaemia produces cardiac vagal withdrawal and nonuniform sympathetic activation in normal subjects. *Am J Physiol* January 1999; 276 (1, pt 2): R178–83.
40. Rauch U, Ziegler D, Piolot R, Schwippert B, Benthake H, Schultheiss HP, Tschoepe D. Platelet activation in diabetic cardiovascular autonomic neuropathy. *Diabet Med* October 1999; 16 (10): 848–52.
41. Zelag B, Wroblewski M, Castenfors J, Henricsson M, Berntorp K, Fernlund P, Sundkvist G. Obesity, microalbuminuria, hyperinsulinemia, and increased plasminogen activator inhibitor 1 activity associated with parasympathetic neuropathy in type 2 diabetes. *Diabetes Care* November 1999; 22 (11): 1907–8.
42. Ahlgren AR, Sundkvist G, Wollmer P, Sonesson B, Lanne T. Increased aortic stiffness in women with type 1 diabetes mellitus is associated with diabetes duration and autonomic nerve function. *Diabet Med* April 1999; 16 (4): 291–7.
43. Edmonds ME, Morrison N, Laws JW, Watkins PJ. Medial aterial calcification & diabetic neuropathy. *Br Med J* 1982; 284: 928–30.

44. Spallone V, Menzinger G, Ziegler D. Diabetic autonomic neuropathy cardiovascular system. In Gries R, Cameron N, Low P, Ziegler D (eds), Textbook of Diabetic Neuropathy. Stuttgart: Georg Thieme verlag, 2003; pp 225–40.
45. Ikeda T, Matsubara T, Sato Y, Sakamoto N. Circadian blood pressure variation in diabetic patients with autonomic neuropathy. *J Hypertens* May 1993; 11 (5): 581–7.
46. Jermendy G, Ferenczi J, Hernandez E, Farkas K, Nadas J. Day-night blood pressure variation in normotensive and hypertensive NIDDM patients with asymptomatic autonomic neuropathy. *Diabetes Res Clin Pract* October 1996; 34 (2): 107–14.
47. Flyn ME, et al. Direct measurement of capillary blood flow in the diabetic neuropathic foot. *Diabetologia* 1988; 31: 652–6.
48. Watkins PJ, Edmonds ME. Diabetic autonomic failure. In *Autonomic Failure,* 4th edn. Oxford: OUP, 1999; pp 378–86.
49. Yki-Jarvinen H, Utriainent T. Insulin-induced vasodilatation: physiology or pharmacology? *Diabetologia* 1998; 41: 369–79.
50. Sampson MJ, et al. Progression of diabetic autonomic neuropathy over a decade in insulin dependent diabetics. *Q J Med* 1990; 75: 635–46.
51. Winkler AS, Landau S, Watkins PJ. Erythropoietin treatment of postural hypotension in anemic type 1 diabetic patients with autonomic neuropathy: a case study of four patients. *Diabetes Care* June 2001; 24 (6): 1121–3.
52. Purewal TS, Watkins PJ, Postural-hypotension in diabetic autonomic neuropathy: a review. *Diabet Med* 1995; 12: 192–200.
53. Ewing DJ. Analysis of heartrate variablity and other non-invasive tests with special reference to diabetes mellitus. In Bannister R, Matthias CJ (eds), *Autonomic Failure*. Oxford: Oxford Medical Publications, 1992; pp 312–33.
54. Gerritsen J, TenVoorde BJ, Dekker JM, Kingma R, Kostense PJ, Bouter LM, Heethaar RM. Measures of cardiovascular autonomic nervous function: agreement, reproducibility, and reference values in middle age and elderly subjects. *Diabetologia* March 2003; 46 (3): 330–8.
55. Kempler P. Clinical features, diagnosis and therapy of autonomic neuropathy in neuropathies. Budapest, Hungary: Springer Scientific, 2002; pp 79–141.
56. Stein P, Kleiger R. Insights from the study of heart rate variability. *Annu Rev Med* 1999; 50: 249–61.
57. Burger AJ, Charlamb M, Weinrauch LA, D'Elia JA. Short- and long-term reproducibility of heart rate; variability in patients with long-standing type 1 diabetes mellitus. *Am J Cardiol* 1997; 80 (9): 1198–202.
58. Takase B, Kitamura H, Noritake M, Nagase T, Kurita A, Ohsuzu F, Matsuoka T. Assessment of diabetic autonomic neuropathy using twenty-four-hour spectral analysis of heart rate variability: a comparison with the findings of the Ewing battery *Japanese Heart J* 2002; 43 (2): 127–35.
59. Spallone V, Bernardi L, Maiello MR, Cicconetti E, Ricordi L, Fratino P, Menzinger G. Twenty-four-hour pattern of blood pressure and spectral analysis of heart rate variability in diabetic patients with various degrees of autonomic neuropathy. Comparison to standard cardiovascular tests. *Clin Sci* 1996; 91 (suppl): 105–7.
60. Pagani M. Heart rate variability and autonomic diabetic neuropathy. Diabetes, Nutri Metab—Clin Exp 2000: 13 (6); 341–6.
61. Frattola A, Parati G, Gamba P, Paleari F, Mauri G, Di Rienzo M, Castiglioni P, Mancia G. Time and frequency domain estimates of spontaneous baroreflex sensitivity provide early detection of autonomic dysfunction in diabetes mellitus. *Diabetologia* December 1997; 40 (12): 1470–5.
62. Ziegler D, Laude D, Akila F, Elghozi JL. Time- and frequency-domain estimation of early diabetic cardiovascular autonomic neuropathy. *Clin Auton Res* December 2001; 11 (6): 369–76.
63. Tentolouris N, Katsilambros N, Papazachos G, Papadogiannis D, Linos A, Stamboulis E, Papageorgiou K. Corrected QT interval in relation to the severity of diabetic autonomic neuropathy. *Euro J Clin Invest* 1997; 27 (12): 1049–54.
64. Veglio M, Sivieri R, Chinaglia A, Scaglione L, Cavallo-Perin P. QT interval prolongation and mortality in type 1 diabetic patients: a 5-year cohort prospective study. Neuropathy Study Group of the Italian Society of the Study of Diabetes, Piemonte Affiliate. *Diabetes Care* September 2000; 23 (9): 1381–3.
65. Whitsel EA, Boyko EJ, Siscovick DS. Reassessing the role of QTc in the diagnosis of autonomic failure among patients with diabetes: a meta-analysis. *Diabetes Care* 2000; 23 (2): 241–7.
66. Earle KA, Mishra B, Morocutti A, Barnes D, Chambers J, Viberti GC. QT dispersion in microalbuminuric type 1 diabetic patients without myocardial ischemia. *J Diabetes Complications* 2000; 14 (5): 277–80.
67. Heller SR. Abnormalities of the electrocardiogram during hypoglycaemia: the cause of the dead in bed syndrome? *Int J Clin Pract Suppl* July 2002; 129: 27–32.
68. Kumhar MR, Agarwal TD, Singh VB, Kochar DK, Chadda VS. Cardiacautonomic neuropathy and its correlation with QTc dispersion in type 2 diabetes. *Indian Heart J* July 2000; 52 (4): 421–6.
69. Sawicki PT, Kiwitt S, Bender R, Berger M. The value of QT interval dispersion for identification of total mortality risk in non-insulin-dependent diabetes mellitus. *J Intern Med* January 1998; 243 (1): 49–56.
70. Watkins PJ, Edmonds ME. Diabetic autonomic failure. In *Autonomic Failure*, 4th edn. Oxford: OUP, 1999; pp 378–86.
71. Pitei DL, Watkins PJ, Edmonds ME. NO-Dependent smooth muscle vasodilatation is reduced in the NIDDM patients with peripheral sensory neuropathy. *Diabet Med* 1997; 14: 284–90.
72. Goebel F-D, Fuessl HS. Monckeberg's sclerosis after sympathetic denervation in diabetic and non diabetic subjects. *Diabetologia* 1983; 24: 347–50.
73. Harrison CV. The effect of sympathectomy on the development of experimental arterial disease. *J Pathol* 1938; 616: 353–60.
74. Kerper HA, Collier WD. Pathological changes in arteries following partial denervation. *Proc Soc Exp Biol Med* 1926; 24: 493–4.
75. Morgan AJ. Mineralised deposits in the thoracic aorta of aged rats: ultrastructural and electron probe x-ray microanalysis study. *Ext Gerontol* 1980; 15: 563–73.
76. Everhart JE, Pettitt DJ, Knowler WC, Rose FA, Bennett PH. Medial arterial calcification and its association with mortality and complications of diabetes. *Diabetologia* 1988; 31: 16–33.
77. Chantelau E, Lee KM, Jungblut R. Association of below knee athrosclerosis to medial arterial calcification in

diabetes mellitus. *Diabetes Res Clin Pract* 1995; 29: 169–72.

78. Mankovsky BN, Piolot R, Mankovsky OL, Ziegler D. Impairment of cerebral autoregulation in diabetic patients with cardiovascular autonomic neuropathy and orthostatic hypotension. *Diabet Med* February 2003; 20 (2): 119–26.
79. Gottsater A, Ryden-Ahlgren A, Szelag B, Hedblad D, Persson J, Berglund G, et al. Cardiovascular autonomic neuropathy associated with charotid atherosclerosis in Type 2 diabetic patients. *Diabet Med* 2003; 20: 495–9.
80. Toyry JP, Niskanen LK, Lansimies EA, Partanen KP. Uusitupa myocardial ischemia. Autonomic neuropathy predicts the development of stroke in patients with non-insulin-dependent diabetes mellitus. *Stroke* 1996. 27 (8): 1316–8.
81. Horowitz M, Wishart JM, Jones KL, Hubbard GS. Gastric emptying in diabetes: an overview. *Diabet Med* 1996; 13 (suppl): 16–22.
82. Kong MFFSC, MacDonald IA, Tattersal RB. Gastric emptying in diabetes. *Diabet Med* 1996; 13: 112–9.
83. Stacher G. Gastric stasis is a feature of autonomic neuropathy. Diabetes mellitus and the stomach. [Review]. *Diabetologia* September 2001; 44 (9): 1080–93.
84. Stacher G, Lenglinger J, Bergmann H, Schneider C, Brannath W, Festa A, Meghdadi S, Stacher-Janotta G. Impaired gastric emptying and altered intragastric meal distribution in diabetes mellitus related to autonomic neuropathy? *Dig Dis Sci* June 2003; 48 (6): 1027–34.
85. Ziegler D, Schadewaldt P, Pour Mirza A, Piolot R, Schommartz B, Reinhardt M, Vosberg H, Brosicke H, Gries FA. [13C] octanoic acid breath test for non-invasive assessment of gastric emptying in diabetic patients: validation and relationship to gastric symptoms and cardiovascular autonomic function. *Diabetologia* June 1996; 39 (7): 823–30.
86. O'Donovan D, Samson M, Feinle C, Jones KL, Horowitz M. Gasrointestinal tract. In Gries R, Cameron N, Low P, Ziegler D (eds), *Textbook of Diabetic Neuropathy*. Stuttgart, Georg Thieme verlag, Germany: 2003; pp 246–62.
87. Watkins PJ. The enigma of autonomic failure in diabetes. *J R Coll Phys Lond* 1998; 32: 360–5.
88. Dowling CJ, Kumar S, Boulton AJM, Edmonds ME, Fielding ME, Jenkins DJ, et al. Severe gastro-perisis diabeticorum in a young patient with insulin dependent diabetes. *Br Med J* 1985; 310: 308–11.
89. Ejskjaer N, Bradley JL, Buxton-Thomas MS, Edmonds ME, Howard ER, Purewal T, et al. Novel surgical treatment and gastric pathology in diabetic gastroperisis. *Diabet Med* 1999; 16: 488–95.
90. Watkins PJ, Buxton-Thomas MS, Howard ER, Long-term outcome after gastrectomy for intractable diabetic gastroparesis. *Diabet Med* January 2003; 20 (1): 58–63.
91. Kong MF, Horowitz M, Jones KL, Wishart JM, Harding PE. Natural history of diabetic gastroparesis patients with abnormal. *Diabetes Care* March 1999: 22 (3): 503–7.
92. Stief CG, Ziegler D. Urogenital system. In Gries R, Cameron N, Low P, Ziegler D (eds), *Textbook of Diabetic Neuropathy*. Stuttgart, Georg Thieme verlag, Germany: 2003; pp 262–74.
93. Carson C, Holmes S, Kirby RS. *Erectile Dysfunction*. Oxford: Health Press, 2002.
94. Goldstein I, Lue TF, Padma-Nathan H, et al. Oral sildenafil in the treatment of erectile dysfunction. *N Engl J Med* 1998; 338: 1397–404.
95. Rendell M, Ragfer J, Wicker PA. Sidenafil for treatment of ED in men with diabetes. *JAMA* 1999; 281: 421–6.
96. Jackson G, Betteridge J, Dean J, et al. A systematic approach to ED in the cardiovascular patient: a consensus statement. *Int J Clin Pract* 1999; 53: 445–51.
97. Bosshardt RJ, Farwerk R, Sikora R, et al. Objective measurement of the effectiveness, therapeutic success and dynamic mechanisms of vacuam device. *Br J Urol* 1995; 75: 786–91.
98. Linet OI, Ogring FG. Efficacy and safety of intracavernosal Alprostadil in men with erectile dysfunction. *N Engl J Med* 1996; 334: 873–7.
99. Carson CC. Diagnosis, treatment and prevention of penile prosthesis infection. *Int J Impot Res* October 2003; 15 (suppl 5): S139–46.
100. Scionti L, Bottini P. Respiratory tract. In Gries R, Cameron N, Low P, Ziegler D (ed), *Textbook of Diabetic Neuropathy*. Stuttgart, Georg Thieme verlag, Germany: 2003; pp 242–5.
101. Rees PJ, Prior JG, Cochrane GM, Clark TJ. Sleep apnoea in diabetic patients with autonomic neuropathy. *J R Soc Med* 1981; 74: 192–5.
102. Catterall JR, Calverley PM, Ewing DJ, Shapiro CM, Clarke BF, Douglas NJ. Breathing, sleep and diabetic autonomic neuropathy. *Diabetes* 1984; 33: 1025–7.
103. Ficker JH, Dertinger SH, Siegfried W, Konig HJ, Pentz M, Sailer D, Katalinic A, Hahn EG. Obstructive sleep apnoea and diabetes mellitus: the role of cardiovascular autonomic neuropathy. *Eur Respir J* January 1998; 11 (1): 14–9.
104. Vianna LG, Gilbey SG, Barnes NC, Guy RJ, Gray BJ. Cough threshold to citric acid in diabetic patients with and without autonomic neuropathy. *Thorax* July 1988; 43 (7): 569–71.
105. Levy DM, Karanth SS, Springall DR, Polak JM. Depletion of cutaneous nerves and neuropeptides in diabetes mellitus: an immunopsytochemical study. *Diabetologia* 1989; 32: 427–33.
106. Nazhel B, Yetkin I, Irkec C, Kocer B. Sympathetic skin response in diabetic neuropathy. *Auton Neurosci* September 2001; 92 (1/2): 72–5.
107. Shimada H, Kihara M, Kosaka S, Ikeda H, Kawabata K, Tsutada T, Miki T. Comparison of SSR and QSART in early diabetic neuropathy—the value of length-dependent pattern in QSART. *Auton Neurosci* 2001; 92 (1–2): 72–5.
108. Cacciatori V, Dellera A, Bellavere F, Bongiovanni LG, Teatini F, Gemma ML, Muggeo M. Comparative assessment of peripheral sympathetic function by postural vasoconstriction arteriolar reflex and sympathetic skin response in NIDDM patients. *Am J Med* April 1997; 102 (4): 365–70.
109. Spitzer A, Lang E, Birklein F, Claus D. Cardiac autonomic involvement and peripheral nerve function in patients with diabetic neuropathy. *Neundorfer Funct Neurol* May 1997; 12 (3/4): 115–22.
110. Hoeldtke RD, Bryner KD, Horvath GG, Phares RW, Broy LF, Hobbs GR. Redistribution of sudomotor responses is an early sign of sympathetic dysfunction in type 1 diabetes. *Diabetes* February 2001; 50 (2): 436–43.
111. Smith SA, Smith SE. Pupil function: tests and disorders. In Matthias CJ, Bannister R (eds), *Autonomic Failure*. Oxford: Oxford Medical Publications, 1999; pp 245–53.

112. Hreidarsson AB. The pupil of the eye in diabetes mellitus, an indicator of autonomic nervous dysfunction. *Dan Med Bull* 1992; 39: 400–8.
113. Cranston, et al. Restoration of hypoglycaemia unawareness in patients with long-duration insulin-dependent diabetes *Lancet* 1994; 344: 283–7.
114. Hepburn DA, et al. Unawareness of hypoglycaemia in insulin trated diabetic patients: prevalence and relationship to autonomic neuropathy. *Diabet Med* 1990; 7: 711–7.
115. Frier BM. *Hypoglycaemia unwareness in hypoglycaemia and diabetes*. London: Edward Arnold, 1993; pp 291–3.
116. The effect of intensive treatment of diabetes on the development and progression of long-term complications in insulin-dependent diabetes mellitus. The Diabetes Control and Complications Trial Research Group. *N Engl J Med* September 1993; 30; 329 (14): 977–86.
117. Bottini P, Boschetti E, Pampanelli S, Ciofetta M, Del Sindaco P, Scionti L, Brunetti P, Bolli GB. Contribution of autonomic neuropathy to reduced plasma adrenaline responses to hypoglycaemia in IDDM: evidence for a nonselective defect. *Diabetes* May 1997; 46 (5): 814–23.
118. Molgaard H, Christensen PD, Sorensen KE, Christensen CK, Mogensen CE. Association of 24-h cardiac parasympathetic activity and degree of nephropathy in IDDM patients. *Diabetes* July 1992; 41 (7): 812–7.
119. Wirta OR, Pasternack AI, Mustonen JT, Laippala PJ, Reinikainen PM. Urinary albumin excretion rate (UAER) is independently related to subclinical autonomic neuropathy in type 2 diabetes. *J Intern Med* April 1999; 245 (4): 329–35.
120. Krolewski AS, Barzilay J, Warram JH, Martin BC, Pfeifer M, Rand LI. Risk of early onset proliferative retinopathy in IDDM is closely related to cardiovascular autonomic neuropathy. *Diabetes* 1992; 41: 430–7.
121. Zander E, Seidlein I, Herfurth S, Heinfe P, Chlup R, Badendick K, et al. Increased prevalence of proliferative retinopathy and cardiovascular autonomic dysfunction in IDDM patients with protein urea. *Exp Clin Endcrinol* 1992; 99: 102–7.
122. Valensi P, Huard JP, Giroux C, Attali JR. Factors involved in cardiac autonomic neuropathy in diabetic patients. *J Diabetes Complications* May 1997; 11 (3): 180–7.
123. Winkler AS, Marsden J, Chaudhuri KR, Hambley H, Watkins PJ. Erythropoietin depletion and anaemia in diabetes mellitus. *Diabet Med* October 1999; 16 (10): 813–9.
124. Bosman DR, Osborne CA, Marsden JT, Macdougall IC, Gardner WN, Watkins PJ. Erythropoietin response to hypoxia in patients with diabetic autonomic neuropathy and non-diabetic chronic renal failure. *Diabet Med* January 2002; 19 (1): 65–9.
125. Chessa M, Butera G, Lanza GA, Bossone E, Delogu A, De Rosa G, Marietti G, Rosti L, Carminati M. Role of heart rate variability in the early diagnosis of diabetic autonomic neuropathy in children. *Herz* December 2002; 27 (8): 785–90.
126. Karavanaki K, Baum JD. Prevalence of microvascular and neurologic abnormalities in a population of diabetic children. *J Pediatr Endocrinol Metab* 1999; 12 (3): 411–22.
127. Chen HS, Hwu CM, Kuo BI, Chiang SC, Kwok CF, Lee SH, Lee YS, Weih MJ, Hsiao LC, Lin SH, Ho LT. Abnormal cardiovascular reflex tests are predictors of mortality in Type 2 diabetes mellitus. *Diabet Med* April 2001; 18 (4): 268–73.
128. O'Brien IA, McFadden JP, Corrall RJ. The influence of autonomic neuropathy on mortality in insulin-dependent diabetes. *Q J Med* June 1991; 79 (290): 495–502.
129. Ewing DJ, Clarke BF. Autonomic neuropathy: its diagonosis and prognosis. In Watkins PJ (ed), *Clinics in Endocrinology & Metabalism*. London: Saunders, 1986; pp 855–88.
130. Orchard TJ, Lloyd CE, Maser RE, Kuller LH. Why does diabetic autonomic neuropathy predict IDDM mortality? An analysis from the Pittsburgh Epidemiology of Diabetes Complications Study. *Diabetes Res Clin Pract* 1996; 34 (suppl): S165–71.
131. Stella P, Ellis D, Maser RE, Orchard TJ. Cardiovascular autonomic neuropathy (expiration and inspiration ratio) in type 1 diabetes. Incidence and predictors. *J Diabetes Complications* January 2000; 14 (1): 1–6.
132. Rathmann W, Ziegler D, Jahnke M, Haastert B, Gries FA. Mortality in diabetic patients with cardiovascular autonomic neuropathy. *Diabet Med* November 1993; 10 (9): 820–4.
133. Gaede P, Vedel P, Larsen N, Jensen GV, Parving HH, Pedersen O. Multifactorial intervention and cardiovascular disease in patients with type 2 diabetes. *N Engl J Med* January 2003; 348 (5): 383–93.
134. Ziegler D, Schatz H, Conrad F, Gries FA, Ulrich H, Reichel G. Effects of treatment with the antioxidant alpha-lipoic acid on cardiac autonomic neuropathy in NIDDM patients. A 4-month randomized controlled multicenter trial (DEKAN Study). Deutsche Kardiale Autonome Neuropathie. *Diabetes Care* March 1997; 20 (3): 369–73.
135. Kontopoulos AG, Athyros VG, Didangelos TP, Papageorgiou AA, Avramidis MJ, Mayroudi MC, Karamitsos DT. Effect of chronic quinapril administration on heart rate variability in patients with diabetic autonomic neuropathy. *Diabetes Care* 1997; 20 (3): 355–61.

This chapter is based in part on a chapter of the same title which was published in an earlier edition of the *International Textbook of Diabetes Mellitus*, by P J Watkins and M E Edmonds.

71

Connective Tissue Disorders in Diabetes

Arlan L. Rosenbloom

University of Florida College of Medicine, Gainesville, FL, USA

Connective tissue disorders in diabetes encompass the major long-term complications, which can be attributed to alteration in the quantity and quality of structural macromolecules of the extracellular matrix [1]. These alterations affect vascular basement membrane in the retina, kidney, heart, and skeletal muscle; muscle fiber basement membrane (e.g. with cardiomyopathy) [2]; nervous system basement membrane; lens capsule and crystallin; and trophoblastic basement membrane of the placenta in both gestational diabetes and overt diabetic pregnancies [3]. Other sections of this volume treat the connective tissue abnormalities in the major chronic complications and their biochemical basis. This chapter reviews the abnormalities of interstitial connective tissue involving skeleton, joints, skin, and periarticular tissues that have been considered to be associated with diabetes, including osteopenia in children and adults; hyperostosis; osteoarthritis; rheumatoid arthritis; osteolysis; scleroderma diabeticorum; Dupuytren disease; stiff hand syndrome of Lundbaek [4]; carpal tunnel syndrome; flexor tenosynovitis; adhesive capsulitis of the shoulder and shoulder–hand syndrome; and limited joint mobility (LJM) [5]. Despite an extensive literature defining the characteristic features of the six distinct conditions resulting in limitation of hand-joint mobility, it is often not appreciated that these are different entities, although they may coexist [6–10]. Among these conditions affecting hand-joint mobility, LJM is unique in that it can occur in children and adolescents, in whom it was originally described, does not occur in the nondiabetic young population, and is an important risk marker for other complications [5, 11–13].

SKELETON

Osteopenia

Decreased bone mineral content (BMC) has long been recognized in type 1 diabetes mellitus (T1DM) and type 2 diabetes mellitus (T2DM), although there is far greater inconsistency regarding this finding in T2DM [14]. There is also uncertainty about the clinical significance of the osteopenia, i.e. whether there is an increased risk of skeletal fracture. The first population-based study, comprising 1000 persons with diabetes, failed to reveal an increased risk of fracture [15]. In T2DM, increased weight appears to be associated with increased bone density, as is true in those without diabetes, and it has long been recognized that this heavier group comprised a larger proportion of T2DM patients than the group with bone loss [16]; this admixture of patients might explain the difficulty in demonstrating a population risk [14].

Direct comparisons among various studies of bone integrity in diabetes are difficult. Various techniques have been used to demonstrate reduced bone mass, including conventional radiographs, computerized tomography, single and dual photon absorption densitometry, radiographic measurement of cortical width (radiogrammetry), resonance frequency of the ulna, total body neutron activation analysis, X-ray microdensitometry, and since the mid-1990s, dual energy X-ray absorptiometry (DEXA). Controls in a number of reports are from previous studies or the literature, rather than concurrent and analyzed simultaneously. Finally, there are wide differences in age groups studied, as well as in diabetes types, and distinction is not always made between T1DM and T2DM in a particular study, or between insulin use and other treatment.

International Textbook of Diabetes Mellitus, Third Edition. Edited by R. A. DeFronzo, E. Ferrannini, H. Keen, and P. Zimmet.
 ISBN: 0-471-48655-8.

Type 1 Diabetes

Early studies preceding the availability of contemporary bone mineral density (BMD) measurement techniques described osteopenia in T1DM from X-ray films [17, 18]. Table 1 summarizes bone density studies by photon absorptiometry, radiogrammetry, and more recently, DEXA in T1DM patients. The single photon absorption (SPA) technique detects a transmission of radiation from a ^{125}I-crystal through the bones, usually of the forearm. An analyzer determines bone width and mineral content, expressing bone density as grams of calcium per square centimeter of bone width [19, 21]. Dual photon absorptiometry measures radiation transmission of two separate photon energies from a ^{153}GD source through bone and soft tissue. This permits study of the axial skeleton and determination of fat mass. DEXA uses the more rapid, reliable, and consistent binocular X-ray transmission instead of photon emission. Hand radiogrammetry involves the measurement of cortical bone thickness and percentage cortical area at the midshaft of the second metacarpal bone on the left hand [20].

The original SPA studies by Levin et al. [19] included 35 T1DM patients of whom over half had osteopenia defined as greater than 10% bone mineral loss; there was no sex difference nor any difference in mean duration between those with more than 10% loss and those with less than 10% loss. Using the same technique in a much larger population of 190 patients aged 6–26 years compared with a control population matched for age and sex, Rosenbloom et al. [21] found that 48% of girls and 29% of boys had more than 10% loss in bone density, and that this was much more severe in Whites than in Blacks. Abnormalities were associated with the early stages of diabetes, particularly in the White females. When the groups were divided into those with duration of diabetes less than 5 years and those with duration greater than 5 years, most of the abnormality was seen in the first 5 years among White females. After 5 years, there was no sex difference in mean percentage bone mass change. In this study the predominance of abnormality in White female youngsters with diabetes is similar to the sex-specific and race-specific adult risk for bone loss.

The initial study of cortical thickness in 107 patients described a 3:1 male preponderance of abnormality defined as cortical thickness less than the 5th percentile of published controls, and in this study there was no effect of diabetes duration [20]. Later study in 45 patients found less abnormality but no information was provided on sex differences [25]. The impression that these abnormalities were due to a failure to gain adequate endosteal bone rather than a loss of bone was derived from studies of Wiske et al. [27], showing decreased cortical area with normal subperiosteal diameter among 78 patients aged 8–25 years. In the same group, radial midshaft determination by SPA correlated with the metacarpal cortical area. These authors also found a negative correlation between bone mass and duration of diabetes, in contrast to the studies describing either no effect of duration [20], improved bone mass with longer duration [19, 21], or a plateau after 3–5 years [20, 26]. Findings similar to those of Santiago et al. [20] have been reported by Hough [29] among 206 patients aged 7–20 years, also using radiogrammetry; values less than 2 SD below the mean for reference standards were found in 31% of males and 12% of females. There was no relationship to duration of diabetes.

Using the technique of dual photon absorptiometry of the axial skeleton along with radiogrammetry of the metacarpal and single photon absorptiometry of the distal radius, Auwerx et al. [31] found that adults with uncomplicated long-standing T1DM had decreased mean bone mass of the peripheral skeleton. Only women had reduction of spinal BMC with decreased vertebral cortical thickness. In children studied by computed tomography, cortical bone density of the spine was reported as slightly but significantly decreased [35]; however, when the BMD is adjusted for body weight differences between those with diabetes and age/sex/race-matched controls, these differences disappear [36]. This reflects the normal correlation between spinal bone mineral and weight-bearing load.

Since 1994, almost all studies have used DEXA for determining BMC or BMD. In comparable size and age adult populations with T1DM, BMD has been reported to be normal [37] or <2 SD from normal [38], in both studies correlating with duration and control measures. Other studies in adults with T1DM (see Table 1) generally indicate modest reduction in BMD, either independently, or related to renal function, diabetes control, oral contraceptive use, duration of diabetes, or menopausal status. In both children and adults, reduced BMD has been reported soon after diagnosis [57, 58], as in the initial studies with the less sophisticated SPA technique [19, 21].

The above findings are all from cross-sectional studies. In an 11-year follow-up of 7 adult patients with well-controlled T1DM and absence of long-term complications, an annual decrease in BMC of 0.5% was estimated. This was not considered clinically significant [60]. In a study of 62 adult patients with T1DM before and after 7 years of intensive therapy, 69% had osteopenia or osteoporosis in at least one site, and there was no correlation with HbA_{1c}. Over the period of the study, however, HbA_{1c} improved and BMD stabilized [61]. A 12.5-year longitudinal study indicated that bone loss was at the expected rate in patients with T1DM, with maintenance of the early deficit [62].

The bone mineral loss in young patients with insulin deficiency diabetes appears to be unrelated to the etiology of the diabetes. In a unique morphometric study, ribs and vertebrae were examined in postmortem specimens from 8 children and young adults (1.5–24 years)

Table 1 Bone density in type 1 diabetes mellitus

Reference	Method	Population		Findings
		No.	Ages (years)	
[19]	SPA	35	9–57	54% with BM loss > 10%, no sex difference
[20]	RG	107	4.5–18	41% males, 13% females with CT < 5th percentile
[21]	SPA	196	6–26	29% males, 48% females with BM loss > 10% only during first 5 years
[22]	SPA	86 129	7–25 26–70	10% BM loss for group, with 2× loss (14%) in young vs. old (7%)
[23]	SPA	51	Mean 12	14.5% females, 11.7% males with BM loss
[24]	SPA	34	7–18	1.7% BM loss attributed to delayed bone age
[25]	RG	45	7–18	16% with CT > 2 SD below mean for age
[26]	SPA	58	23–64	9.6% BM loss
[27]	SPA/RG	78	8–25	Decreased BM, CT
[28]	SPA/RG	69	8–24	Mean BM SD 0.86; mean 3-year follow-up no change
[29]	RG	206	7–20	85% below mean for age/sex: 22% below 2 SD—M 31%/F 12%
[30]	SPA	29	2.6–18	Mean BM 12.8%
[31]	SPA/DPA/RG/	31	41 ± 16	Distal radial BM density and spinal cortical decrease in females
[32]	SPA	53	17–74	No differences from normal
[33]	RG	87	[Children]	9.5% with BM < 10% control mean
[34]	SPA	66	9–18.5	11% females, 12% males <2 SD
[35]	CAT	48	5–20	Vertebral cortical density decrease
[36]	DPA	56	5–18	No vertebral abnormality when adjusted for weight
[37]	DEXA	94	18–62	Lumbar BMD normal, correlates with HbA_{1c}, age, duration
[38]	DEXA	90	18–54	BMD < 2 SD in 34% correlating with duration, control, chronic complications
[39]	DEXA	94	20–56	19% with osteoporosis (lumbar spine, femoral neck, Ward triangle)
[40]	DPA	41	[Adults]	Mean 10% decrease BMD femoral neck, 12% distal limb
[41]	CAT	21	7–18	19% decrrease trabecular, 9% total, 5% cortical BMD, correlated with HbA_{1c}
[42]	DEXA	24 females	43–69	Whole-body BM less than that of controls; no difference in whole-body or lumbar BMD; femoral neck and trochanter decreased BMD
[43]	DEXA	36 males	[Adults]	BMD (cortical and cancellous) reduction only with decreased renal function
[44]	DEXA	55	Mean 10.4	No correlation BMD with HbA_{1c}, duration
[45]	DEXA	99 females	Median 42	BMD not different from controls, + association with BMI, height, oral contraceptive use
[46]	DEXA	31 females	42 ± 9	BMD reduced at femoral neck
[47]	DEXA	78	18–39	Reduced BMD correlates with duration, albuminuria, insulin dose
[48]	DEXA	54	39 ± 9	Reduced BMD compared to controls
[49]	DEXA	42 males	58 ± 27	Neuropathy independent risk factor for BMD loss
[50]	DEXA	23	12.5 ± 3.7	No abnormality first years of diabetes; BMD highly correlated with height
[51]	DEXA	26	7–14	Decreased lumbar BMD not related to HbA_{1c} or duration
[52]	DEXA	30	11–16	Lumbar BMD decreased, no effect of disease duration or HbA_{1c}
[53]	DEXA	56	52–72	BMD reduced—all developed diabetes >30 years of age
[54]	DEXA	31 22	40 ± 7 (premenopause) 65 ± 9 (postmenopause)	Only postmenopausal decrease in BMD
[55]	DEXA	45	5–19	Decreased lumbar/forearm BMD, mainly during puberty, related to HbA_{1c}, duration
[56]	DEXA	88	30 ± 9	Lumbar BMD but not femoral neck decreased, not independently related to albuminuria, retinopathy
[57]	DEXA	23	9.5 ± 2.2	Decreased lumbar BMD with mean duration < 6 months
[58]	DEXA	32	20–39	Decreased BMD at onset
[59]	DEXA	27	13 ± 1.7	BMD decreased related to HbA_{1c}

Note: SPA = single photon absorptiometry; DPA = dual photon absorptiometry; BM = bone mineral; BMD = bone mineral density; RG = radiogrammetry; CT = cortical thickness; CAT = computerized axial tomography; DEXA = dual energy X-ray absorptiometry.

dying with diabetes—2 with T1DM, 4 secondary to cystic fibrosis, and 2 associated with thalassemia major. There were no differences related to the etiology of the diabetes; cancellous bone and epiphyseal activity of the ribs were approximately half normal, while there were no changes in the vertebrae [63].

A specific mechanism for bone mineral loss in T1DM remains elusive. In the reported studies where diabetes control has been examined, findings are mixed. While several studies of adults with T1DM show correlation of BMC or BMD with control [37, 38, 47], others do not [26, 43, 61]. Similarly, in children several studies show such a correlation [22, 41, 55, 59], while more do not [14, 21, 25, 29, 35, 36, 44, 51, 52]. Similar disparities are seen when considering insulin dose and C-peptide levels, age, and duration of diabetes.

A wide variety of metabolic findings has been reported in association with osteopenia in T1DM, including hypercalciuria and hyperphosphaturia [64, 65], increased serum concentrations of alkaline phosphatase [25, 26, 29, 37, 65], decreased levels of 1,25-dihydroxyvitamin D_3 [25, 30], and 25-hydroxyvitamin D_3 [25], decreased parathormone (PTH) [65], decreased osteocalcin indicative of decreased bone formation [30, 37, 66, 67], and increased urinary deoxypyridineum cross-links as an indicator of increased bone resorption [68]. An early study described a strong correlation between bone mineral loss and fasting blood glucose concentration, glucosuria, and insulin requirement, suggesting that calcium loss was directly related to hyperglycemia and glucosuria, because urinary excretion of calcium and phosphorus correlated with these manifestations [22]. A later study [29], however, was unable to demonstrate any great difference between osteopenic and non-osteopenic patients in terms of calcium or phosphate excretion, when these subjects were matched for age, size, and diabetes control. Rosenbloom et al. [21] found no correlation of bone mineral loss with serum concentrations of calcium, magnesium, or alkaline phosphatase. There does not appear to be a correlation between osteopenia and 24-h calciuria [51]. Hyperphosphaturia and hypercalciuria in T1DM may reflect poor diabetes control [64, 65].

D-metabolite levels were normal in the study of Auwerx et al. [31] and did not correlate with BMC. In the study of Olmos et al. [37], serum alkaline phosphatase, serum tartrate resistant acid phosphatase, and urinary hydroxyproline were higher and serum osteocalcin lower in those with diabetes, but there was no relationship between these bone remodeling markers and BMD. Leon et al. [33] described normal calcium, phosphorus, alkaline phosphatase, magnesium, PTH, hydroxyproline, and osteocalcin in 87 children with T1DM, which did not correlate with bone mass deficit. Hough [29] did calcium loading studies that demonstrated intense intestinal hyperabsorption of calcium, absorptive hypercalciuria, and phosphaturia, which, together with hypomagnesemia, hypophosphatasemia, and decreased circulating PTH, may form the basis of bone mass loss. Calcitonin levels in serum have been found to be elevated in children with diabetes and osteopenia with, however, a normal reserve demonstrated by calcium stimulation. This increased calcitonin activity may have reflected increased bone reabsorption [69].

Decreased osteocalcin has been related to the presence of retinopathy in adults with T1DM [70, 71]. A controlled study at the onset of T1DM and 15 days after metabolic improvement in 31 children found serum osteocalcin and PTH levels markedly lower than those in control children, but no difference from control subjects after metabolic stabilization [72]. PTH secretion in response to EDTA infusion is diminished in patients with poorly controlled diabetes [73]. Among 23 recently diagnosed prepubertal children found to have decreased lumbar spine BMD, bone turnover was increased as determined by increased serum concentrations of carboxy-terminal propeptide of type 1 collagen (PICP) and the carboxy-terminal cross-linked telopeptide of type 1 collagen (ICTP) [57]. In a 2-year follow-up study of 54 patients with long-standing T1DM, serum alkaline phosphatase and osteocalcin were higher than in controls while pyridinoline and deoxypyridinoline were normal and did not correlate with BMD, leading to the conclusion that osteopenia was associated with normal bone turnover, uninfluenced by duration or degree of metabolic control [48].

The growth hormone (GH)/insulin-like growth factor (IGF)/IGF-binding protein (IGFBP) axis components are critical in bone formation, development, and turnover. Twenty-seven adults with T1DM had reduced levels of GH-dependent IGF-1, IGFBP-3, and IGFBP-5, and elevated concentrations of IGFBP-1 (indicative of diminished insulin concentration/effect) [74]. BMD of the hip correlated negatively with IGFBP-1 and -4, but positively with IGFBP-5, as did bone markers indicating bone loss (ICTP) and increased bone turnover (PTH, osteocalcin).

Some of the variability in BMD effects of diabetes might be attributable to genetic background. Homogeneity for one vitamin D receptor gene polymorphism was associated with a lower mean BMD at the lumbar spine and femoral neck in Brazilian T1DM adults, but this was a relatively small influence [47]. Collagen type 1 genotypes have been examined in postmenopausal British women with T1DM because the type 1 alpha 1 gene has been shown to be associated with low bone mass in British women. This genotype was a predictor of bone mass at the femoral neck only [46].

The mechanism for the influence of diabetes on bone formation has been suggested by an examination of the effect of advanced glycation end products on type 1 collagen, the predominant matrix protein of bone. *In vitro* studies have indicated that glycated collagen has reduced ability to promote differentiation of preosteoblasts to mature osteoblasts [75].

Type 2 Diabetes

The original report of 101 T2DM patients studied by SPA noted greater than 10% bone mass loss in 60% of subjects. Particularly noteworthy was that 80% of patients receiving oral hypoglycemic agents had osteopenia, compared with a not significantly different 57% for those on diet therapy alone, but highly significantly different from the 44% abnormal who were receiving insulin [19]. In this study, in contrast to T1DM patients in whom density improved with duration of diabetes, T2DM patients showed no influence of diabetes duration on bone loss. Because of the presence of this finding at onset, its lack of relationship to control measures and to duration of diabetes, and experimental evidence to suggest defective osteon formation, constitutional rather than metabolic factors were proposed as causative [19].

Quite different findings come from a study of 138 Belgian patients who had only a 20% rate of bone loss exceeding 10%. Most striking in this study was the presence of increased bone density in twice this proportion, with the greatest densities in those receiving oral hypoglycemic agents, who were also the heaviest patients [16]. Japanese investigators used microdensitometry of hand radiographs to examine 168 T2DM patients and found bone mass clearly diminished in 26% and severely decreased in 12%. They noted that the cortical bone width and volume in diabetes are relatively well preserved, whereas the mineral content is decreased, which differs from typical osteoporosis. They suggest that the preservation of volume may explain why there is no increased risk of fracture with this type of osteopenia. Levels of 25-hydroxyvitamin D_3 and 1,25-dihydroxyvitamin D_3 were not different among control subjects and those with T2DM with or without osteopenia [76]. Similarly, among 79 older women with T2DM examined by SPA, BMD loss with age was about half that of those without diabetes [77]. Others have reported no diminution in BMD in patients with T2DM [32, 53, 54, 78–80], or increased BMD even after adjustment for BMI [81–83], especially in women, associated with increased osteoclast activity [84, 85]. A contributor to increased BMD in patients with T2DM has been noted in patients with T2DM who are taking HMG-CoA reductase inhibitors [86].

Fracture Risk

As noted above, the initial population-based study of fracture risk with diabetes failed to show an association among 986 patients with both T1DM and T2DM [15]. A review of studies before 1990 by Bouillon [87] indicated an increased risk of 1.2–4.6-fold. An early brief report from Israel examined 2000 patients aged 55–84 years, of whom 340 had fracture of the proximal femur. There appeared to be slightly increased representation of those with diabetes among the fracture patients (22%) than among the population as a whole (13%) [88]. A Danish case control study involving patients with both T1DM and T2DM found no increased rates of hip or forearm fractures compared to the general population [89]. In contrast, another Scandinavian study found hip fractures to be significantly increased in females, but not in males, with T1DM and T2DM [90]. Quite different findings emerged from a study in Netherlands of women with T2DM who had lower frequency of fractures over the previous 5 years than did women without diabetes; there were no differences among men [82]. A study of risk factors for ankle and foot fractures among 9704 women over 65 years of age provided a contrasting observation that diabetes conferred a relative risk of 2.9, and that this risk was unrelated to bone mass [91]. A more recent study adds to this contrasting picture; in a population of 9654 women aged 65 or older, of whom 657 had diabetes onset after 40 years of age, at least one nonvertebral fracture was experienced by 2624 women during nearly 10 years of follow-up, and 388 had at least one vertebral fracture during approximately 4 years of follow-up. Diabetes conferred substantial increased fracture risks of ~2–2.5-fold for various sites, controlling for age, BMI, BMD, and other factors associated with fractures [92]. Thus, if diabetes confers an added risk for fracture, it would not be on the basis of osteopenia, but the result of complications such as neuropathy, muscle wasting, retinopathy, and renal disease.

Hyperostosis

Increased BMD in T2DM in a number of studies may be related to the association of this disease with diffuse idiopathic skeletal hyperostosis (DISH), which may involve the spine as hyperostotic spondylosis (HS), the skull as hyperostosis frontalis interna, the pelvis as osteitis condensans ilii, the pelvic or other ligaments, or as large bony spurs at the heel or elbow [93, 94]. There may be mild stiffness on arising in the morning, but spinal mobility is preserved and symptoms are usually absent. Heel and elbow pain can occur from calcaneal and olecranon spurs in about one third of affected patients and dysphagia has been described in 16% of those with hyperostosis of the spine.

While 2–4% of the general population may have hyperostotic changes, these changes are present in ~25% of the diabetes population. Pima Indians, with the world's highest prevalence of diabetes, also have a high prevalence of vertebral ankylosing hyperostosis, comparable to their diabetes rate of 50% [95]. Of those hyperostotic

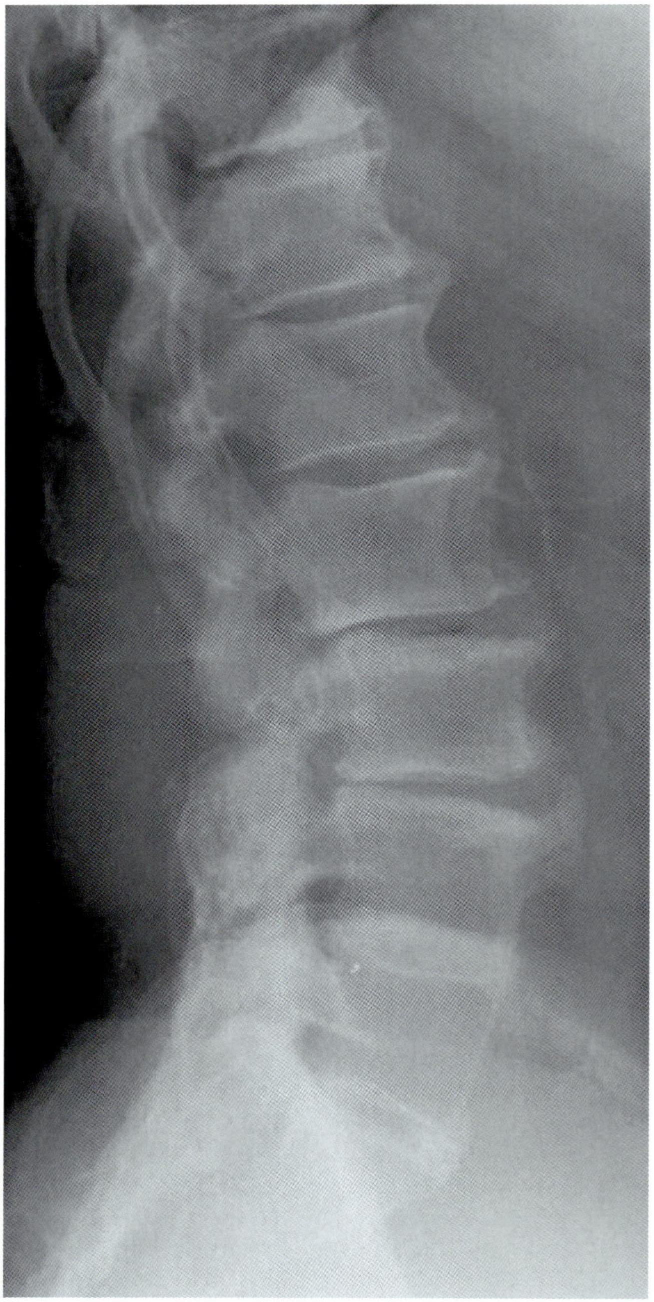

Figure 1 Radiographs of lumbosacral spine showing flowing osteophytes and soft tissue ligamentous ossification indicative of diffuse idiopathic skeletal hyperostosis

patients with spine changes, 83% are male and 30% are obese. One half of all patients with hyperostosis will have manifest diabetes or impaired glucose tolerance. Obesity and diabetes appear to operate independently in the determination of this condition. Radiography reveals preservation of the disc spaces with hyperostosis seen as a line of calcification in the right anterolateral portion of the spine, typically in the thoracic region. Radiolucency is seen between the deposited bone and the cortex of the underlying vertebral body (Figure 1). The principal differential diagnosis of HS is from ankylosing spondylitis, which occurs in a younger population and produces more serious problems, with morning stiffness and incapacitating loss of spinal movement. Radiographic differences are straightforward [94].

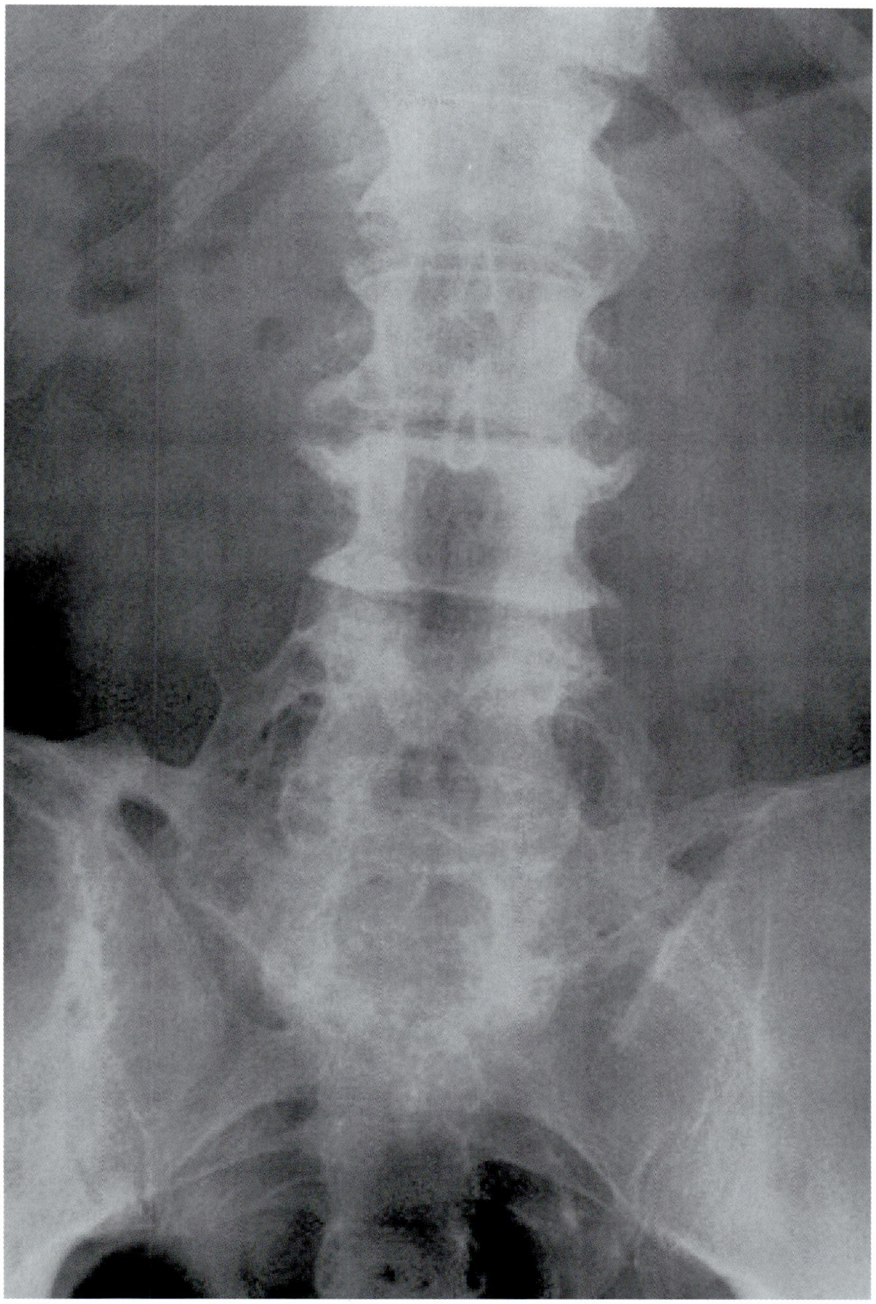

Figure 1 *Continued*

Not surprisingly, the total hip BMD of 35 post-menopausal patients with DISH-related T2DM was greater than that of T2DM controls and nondiabetic controls without DISH [96]. The etiology of hyperostosis in diabetes is not clear. It would be attractive to invoke growth hormone hypersecretion, in view of the similarity to acromegalic lesions, but growth hormone metabolism has been described as normal [94].

JOINTS

Osteoarthritis

Osteoarthritis and diabetes would be expected to be associated in T2DM through the common pathogenic factor of obesity. Additionally, there are a number of processes that have been described *in vitro* or with experimental diabetes, such as loss of glycosaminoglycans from

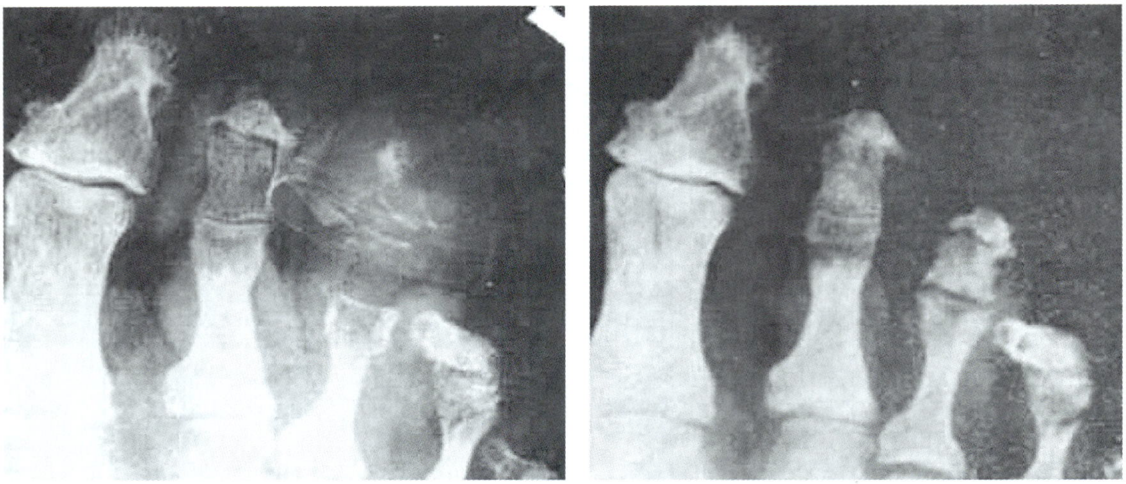

Figure 2 Severe osteolysis (diabetic osteopathy) of third toe and less severe of second toe (a) with reversal and disappearance of all inflammatory signs 1 year later (b) (reproduced with permission from reference 102)

arti-cular cartilage, which may be pertinent to the pathogenesis [97]. Nonetheless, it has not been possible to establish an increased risk for osteoarthritis conferred by diabetes. Neither overt diabetes nor that detected by glucose tolerance testing was associated with osteoarthritis in a study of 632 men and 882 women aged 52–95 years [98]. Among 809 patients undergoing knee or hip joint replacement for osteoarthritis, T2DM was more often associated with bilateral changes, but not with generalized osteoarthritis; without an explanation for this finding, the authors considered that bilaterality might be a chance finding [99]. Similarly, diabetes had no influence on the emergence of osteoarthritis of the hand in elderly patients from Israel [100].

Osteolysis

Osteolysis (also known as diabetic osteopathy) of the forefoot is seen as a localized or generalized osteoporosis of the distal metatarsus and proximal phalanges. Pain is variable and there may be erythema over the joint, inevitably leading to a suspicion of cellulitis or osteomyelitis. The juxta-articular erosions may resemble those of rheumatoid arthritis and gout. The etiology of this lesion is unknown, and perfect reconstruction usually occurs spontaneously [94, 101] (Figure 2).

Rheumatoid Arthritis

The genetic interrelationship between T1DM and rheumatoid arthritis has been studied in informative families by HLA haplotype analysis, suggesting co-inheritance [103]. Insulin resistance has been noted to be a feature of rheumatoid arthritis, together with other features of the metabolic syndrome [104, 105]. The decreased insulin sensitivity has been quantitatively documented, correlating with C-reactive protein elevation and with dyslipidemia [106].

SKIN AND PERIARTICULAR TISSUE

Scleredema Diabeticorum

Fifty-four cases of scleredema diabeticorum associated with long-standing diabetes were summarized by Jelinek [107]. This condition occurs with a male preponderance (4:1) in middle-aged adults who have a long-standing history of poorly controlled diabetes and are obese. Ischemic heart disease, hypertension, and retinopathy are common. There is thickening of the skin with a predilection for the posterior and lateral aspects of the neck and upper back, with induration extending to the face and anterior and posterior trunk and potentially involving most of the body. The condition has been described in Whites, Orientals, and Blacks. Prospective studies indicate that it may be more common than the number of reported cases suggests. For example, 17 patients have been seen over a 15-year period in one clinic and it is noteworthy that 16 of them had T2DM. In a prospective study of 484 outpatients with diabetes, scleredema was seen in 2.5%. Angina pectoris was the only complication occurring more frequently in those with scleredema than in the diabetic patients without this complication [108].

Hyperplasia of collagen is seen on histological examination, and one study has shown accumulation of glycogen in unmyelinated nerve fibers [109].

Scleroderma-like conditions occur with diabetes, which should not be confused with scleredema diabeticorum, such as generalized scleroderma changes, digital sclerosis, and joint contracture in the 21-year-old Japanese woman with maturity-onset diabetes of the young [110]. We have seen a similar patient, a young man with T1DM who had generalized scleroderma-like changes, digital sclerosis, and contractures of the fingers.

Dupuytren Disease

Dupuytren disease (DD) refers to subcutaneous fibrosis of the palmar aponeurotic space of the hands. In those without diabetes the process is sex-linked with a 6:1 male predominance, and occurs only in people of European origin. There has been disagreement about whether DD is more prevalent in persons with diabetes, but this question has been resolved by the recognition of milder expression in patients with diabetes. Not only does careful examination reveal that the true incidence approaches 40%, but, as with cardiovascular risk, the presence of diabetes abolishes the sex difference. However, women with diabetes tend to have knuckle pads, nodules, and skin tethering without contraction. DD is also more radial in the hands of those with diabetes than in those without diabetes, affecting the third and fourth digits predominantly instead of the fourth and fifth. Characteristic lesions may precede the development of diabetes and are present in 16% of newly diagnosed older patients [111]. A study from Finland found that the prevalence of DD was similar in T1DM and T2DM, ~14%, but tended to occur at a younger age in T1DM; no information was provided for the frequency in the nondiabetic population. There was also no sex difference, and in T2DM, DD was an indicator of macroalbuminuria independent of time variables [112].

DD lesions causing sufficient contracture to be removed by surgery were found to contain higher contents of water, collagen, and chondroitin sulfate, as well as increased proportions of soluble collagen and of reducible cross-links, indicating synthesis of new collagen. The lesions also showed increased amounts of type III collagen and increased hydroxylation and glycation of reducible cross-links, characteristics of granulation, and scar tissues [113]. Recent evidence places DD in the category of autoimmune T-cell-mediated disorders, which are relatively common with diabetes [114].

Peyronie disease, involving the penis, and Ledderhose disease, affecting the plantar aponeurosis, are so rarely seen as to be difficult to relate to diabetes, although the impression is that they are more frequent with diabetes and have a similar pathogenesis to DD [94].

Stiff Hand Syndrome

This "severe and sometimes incapacitating form of vascular disease of the hands" was described by Lundbaek in 1957, in 5 patients with long-standing T1DM [4]. The problem typically began with complaints of tingling or burning sensations in the hand, with increasing symptoms and pain aggravated by movement, leading in 2 patients to invalidism. The subcutaneous tissue of the fingers and palms was stiff and hard, and in 2 patients there were marked nail changes. There was no muscle atrophy. Radiographic study revealed calcification of the arteries of the hand in all five cases. Skin biopsy showed very few elastic fibers, but no other changes. Further reports of this dramatic condition are lacking, although the term has been erroneously applied to the markedly different limited joint mobility that occurs in young patients and is without pain or paresthesias, is nondisabling, and lacks the dramatic skin changes and radiologic findings [115].

Carpal Tunnel Syndrome

Compression of the median nerve within the carpal tunnel at the wrist is the most common entrapment neuropathy, resulting in paresthesia of the thumb, index finger, and little finger, with pain that is often worse at night. Diabetes is the most common associated disorder, accounting for 5–16% of cases [93].

In persons with diabetes, carpal tunnel syndrome (CTS) may not be simply due to nerve compression but a manifestation of diabetic neuropathy with decreased conduction velocity of both median and ulnar nerves with, in addition to typical thenar muscle atrophy, atrophy of the intrinsic and hypothenar muscles. The contractures involve the metacarpophalangeal (MCP) and proximal interphalangeal (PIP) joints of all fingers equally. The 23 patients with 'diabetic hand syndrome' described by Jung et al. [116] included 6 who were not taking insulin. The average age of the 23 patients was 43 years and diabetes duration 17 years. These authors were impressed with the bilateral and symmetrical involvement of all distal and PIP and MCP joints and the involvement of the ulnar nerves. This indicated a neuropathic etiology as opposed to an entrapment origin of this condition in their patients. As with the "stiff hand syndrome" of Lundbaek [4], the term "diabetic hand syndrome" coined by Jung et al. [116] has been misapplied to the very different limited joint mobility of childhood diabetes [117].

A literature review of 64 articles on CTS confirmed diabetes or a family history of diabetes as a primary risk factor, along with menopausal age, obesity, lack of fitness, smoking, alcohol intake, and osteoarthritis of the carpal–metacarpal joint of the thumb [118].

Flexor Tenosynovitis

Flexor tenosynovitis (FTS), also known as "trigger finger" or stenosing tenovaginitis, can be congenital or hereditary in children, almost exclusively involving the thumb. In adults, it is estimated that one third of multiple palmar FTS is due to diabetes, although the prevalence in those with diabetes is not known [93]. There is marked female predominance, predilection for the right hand, and preferential involvement of the thumb, middle, and ring fingers. Fibrous tissue proliferates in the tendon sheath, particularly where the tendon is constricted in its passage through a fibrous ring or pulley or over a bony prominence, with swelling distal to this constriction and pain with movement of the enlarged segment through the narrowed ring. Palpable or audible crepitus may be present with movement; locking in flexion or extension occurs with impaction of the nodule proximal or distal to the thickened segment of tendon sheath [94].

Adhesive Capsulitis of the Shoulder and Shoulder–Hand Syndrome

Thickening of the joint capsule and its adherence to the head of the humerus results in marked reduction in the volume of the glenohumeral joint. In some cases this periarthritis may precede, accompany, or follow diffuse swelling, coldness, erythema, tenderness, and hyperhydrosis of the hand. Subsequently, swelling and vasomotor instability resolve, with the development of trophic skin changes and contractures. After weeks or months, the tenderness, swelling, and vasomotor dysfunction completely resolve, with residual atrophic or dystrophic changes, finger contractures and, occasionally, frozen shoulder with atrophy of the shoulder girdle muscles. Osteoporosis of the bones of the hand and shoulder is seen. In addition to shoulder–hand syndrome, this has been referred to as reflex sympathetic dystrophy, causalgia, post-traumatic osteoporosis, and Sudeck atrophy [93].

The above description of classic adhesive capsulitis and shoulder–hand syndrome appears to differ considerably from what is often seen with diabetes. In one large study, 11% of 800 patients with diabetes had frozen shoulder compared with 2.3% of 600 controls without diabetes [119]. Among 15 patients with frozen shoulder identified by the criteria of pain for more than 3 months with over 50% loss of range of motion, in the absence of such causes as trauma or myocardial infarction, minimal functional disability was noted, with the principal pain being relatively mild discomfort around the shoulder joint.

Prevalence of frozen shoulder was 45% among 29 individuals with finger-joint stiffness, aged 23–65 years, with a duration of diabetes of 14–48 years. Ten of these people had DD and 10 flexor tenosynovitis, in both situations considered not sufficient to account for the finger-joint limitation. Only 7% of subjects of similar age and diabetes duration without finger-joint limitation had frozen shoulder. In 10 out of the 13 with LJM and 1 out of the 2 controls, the frozen shoulder was bilateral, an uncommon circumstance in the spontaneous disease (5%). On radiographic examination, one patient was found to have periarticular calcification and no joint abnormalities were noted. Suspicion that finger contractures in these patients are attributable to more than the syndrome of LJM as described in young patients [5] arises from the findings of digital or radial artery calcification in 50% of those with finger-joint contraction, compared with 14% of controls, and of a fourfold increase in peripheral neuropathy in those with joint contracture. This study demonstrated important clinical, radiological, and natural history differences from the isolated (not associated with diabetes) lesion, which would be expected in view of the histological findings in this condition (those of DD), in contrast to the inflammatory reaction (the synovial cell proliferation, collagen degeneration, and infiltration by inflammatory cells) seen in the isolated syndrome [120].

Another study of 49 T1DM and 60 T2DM patients, compared with 75 controls, found comparable frequencies of finger-joint contracture (50%) in both types of diabetes as opposed to 20% of controls; the contractures were all mild in the last group. Shoulder capsulitis was seen in 20% of T1DM patients, 18.3% of T2DM patients, and 5.3% of controls, applying criteria that were similar to, but somewhat less stringent than, those in the previous study. In this study, no correlation was observed between shoulder and finger-joint limitation [121]. In contrast to the study of Fisher et al. [120], who eliminated half their original patient population on the basis of their joint contractures being obviously due to DD, osteoarthritis, or flexor tenosynovitis, Pal et al. [121] made no attempt to distinguish the causes of the finger-joint limitation.

Swedish investigators identified a subset of 60 diabetic patients with painful shoulder from a rehabilitative referral population. Their patients had difficulties in activities of daily living: in 25% working capacity was affected and 42% also had restricted hip-joint mobility. In contrast to the series of Fisher et al. [37], this group had a rate of recovery comparable to that of the nondiabetic population, with 35% of the shoulders regaining normal mobility, 48% having clinical limitation, and 17% having functional limitation over a median observation time of 29 months. T1DM was associated with worse prognosis. Nearly two thirds of the group had associated hand syndromes [122]. Among 291 patients with T1DM at a mean age of 33 years, and 134 with T2DM at a mean age of 61 years, the prevalence of shoulder capsulitis was 10.3% in the former and 22.4% in the latter. Its presence was associated with age in both groups but with duration of diabetes only in T1DM. In both, the shoulder capsulitis was associated with greatly increased presence of autonomic neuropathy [123].

Limited Joint Mobility

The initial observation of striking limitation of extension and flexion of the interphalangeal, MCP, and wrist joints, in association with short stature, thick, tight, waxy skin, delayed sexual maturation, and early microvascular complications, in 3 older teenagers with long-standing diabetes

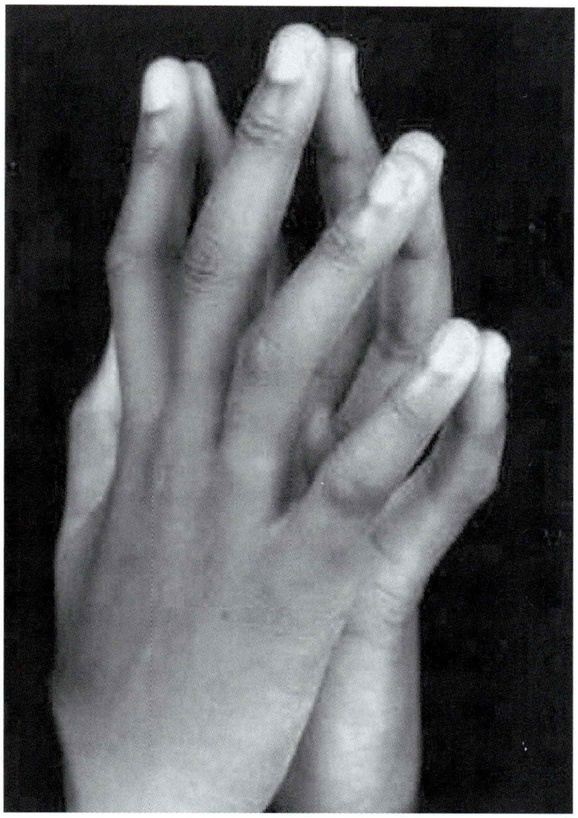

Figure 3 Inability to approximate the palmar surfaces of the fingers in a 14-year-old girl with diabetes for 7 years

[124], was followed by the description of milder manifestations in 28% of 229 campers with diabetes aged 7–18 years [125] (Figure 3). Subsequent studies from Japan [126], Italy [127], Ireland [128], England [129–132], Scotland [133], Mexico [134], Ethiopia [135], Hungary [136], Canada [137], France [138], Cuba [139], Greece [140], Croatia [141], Australia [142], Finland [143], Germany [144], Russia [145], Israel [146], and from various populations in the United States [12, 13, 147–154] have reported prevalences of 9–63% among T1DM patients, depending on the age of the population and the duration of diabetes, as well as the examination techniques; these studies are summarized in Table 2. A comparison of the findings in 1998 to those done by the same examiners using the same techniques 20 years earlier found a greater than fourfold reduction in frequency of LJM together with a decrease in the proportion having more advanced changes, attributed to improved blood glucose control measures [155]. A lower frequency than generally noted earlier has also recently been reported from England [156].

Several reports have described LJM from a broad geographical range in T2DM also, summarized in Table 3: frequencies range from 25 to 76%, except for a single study which involved only patients not taking insulin [157].

There is no influence of sex or race on prevalence. In control pediatric populations, stiffness of the little fingers only was usually found in fewer than 4% (Table 2), whereas older populations may have as much as 25% involvement, probably related to occupation and aging (Table 3). A significant independent contribution of cigarette smoking to both LJM and DD has been described in Scottish adults with T1DM and T2DM. Controls without diabetes who smoked had substantial frequencies of these hand changes, and smoking more than doubled the risk for LJM and DD in those with diabetes [133, 162]. LJM did not correlate with smoking status in Finnish patients with T2DM [165].

Changes begin in the MCP and PIP joints of the little finger and extend medially; the distal interphalangeal joint may also be involved. Changes are also seen in the metatarsophalangeal joints [142, 164] and larger joints, most commonly wrist and elbow but also ankles and cervical and thoracolumbar spine [166]. The limitation is painless, unresponsive to physical therapy, and nondisabling. Unrecognized cervical spine involvement can complicate endotracheal intubation [167, 168], although the existence of this problem has been challenged [169]. Involvement of the foot can contribute to abnormal foot pressures and damage [164, 170, 171].

Examination and Classification

The original method for demonstrating milder LJM was to have the patient place the hands on a flat surface palm down with the fingers fanned; the examiner would then determine contact with the plane surface by viewing at table level. Normally, the entire palmar surface of the fingers makes contact [166]. A simpler method is to have the patient attempt to approximate the palmar surfaces of the interphalangeal joints with the fingers fanned (Figure 1). Whether either of these approximations is possible or not, the examiner extends the proximal and distal interphalangeal and MCP joints. In addition to finding these limited to less than 180° and 60° respectively, the examiner may find resistance to the permitted movement [11, 166]. Studies that depend on the simple demonstration of inability to approximate the proximal surfaces of the fingers [156, 164] are difficult to compare to those in which the complete examination is pursued [139, 165]. A comparison of "the prayer sign" to range of motion measurements in 50 adults with T1DM and 44 controls concluded that there was sufficient correlation to justify the use of the simple test as a clinical indicator for LJM [171]. Thickening of the tissues surrounding the limited joints and inability to tent the skin may also be noted, particularly over the dorsa of the fingers and hand. The examiner also attempts to extend the wrist maximally to

Table 2 Population-based studies of LJM in T1DM

Reference	Age group (years)	T1DM patients		Controls		% Location
		No.	% LJM	No.	% LJM	
[125]	7–18	229	28	201	1	Florida
[21]	6–26	196	40	124	0	Florida
[126]	3–18	68	30	92	1	Japan
[11]	1–28	309	30	—	—	Florida
[127]	?	210	9	—	—	Italy
[128]	5–57	115	36	90	3	Belfast
[147]	3–22	100	32	—	—	Boston
[129]	2–16	112	42	50	21	Nottingham
[148]	5–24	137	19	52	0	New Jersey
[134]	15–32	34	41	34	3	Mexico City
[149]	7–23	204	21	90	1	Florida
[130]	?	215	46	—	—	London
[150]	?	104	19	—	—	California
[151]	6–27	311	36	—	—	Florida
[152]	3–24	95	40	39	3	New York
[135]	14–62	110	44	300	2	Ethiopia
[131]	6–39	254	15	110	4	Bath
[12]	11–83	238	55	45	4	Boston
[136]	5–18	55	44	—	—	Hungary
[153]	7–25	375	33	—	—	California
[121]	18–82	49	49	75	20	Newcastle
[154]	3–30	211	19	239	0	Florida
[132]	8–17	70	31	51	12	Surrey
[133]	18–81	266	37	150	23	Edinburgh
[137]	35 ± 2 (SD)	58	31	25	0	Toronto
[13]	14–?	357	26	—	—	Colorado
[139]	9–23	183	63	—	—	Cuba
[144]	1–32	322	31	200	2	Germany
[143]	7–21	174	30	—	—	Finland
[145]	6–22	108	44	—	—	Russia
[146]	9–30	35	43	—	—	Israel
[140]	12 ± 4	148	28	648	7.5	Greece
[141]	2–20	100	36	100	0	Croatia
[142]	11–20	302	26	51	14	Australia
[155]	7–18	312	7	—	—	Florida
[156]	4–17	129	9	144	2	Bristol

Table 3 Population-based studies of LJM in T2DM

Reference	Age group (years)	T2DM patients		Controls		Location
		No.	% LJM	No.	% LJM	
[130]	?	241	34	—	—	London
[157]	?	80	45	47	15	Montreal
[135]	28–79	190	25	300	2	Ethiopia
[158]	?	165	4	—	—	Italy
[12]	?	41	76	45	9	Boston
[159]	mean 55	168	47	100	26 M/9 F	Scotland
[121]	34–85	60	52	75	20	Newcastle
[160]	54 ± 12 (SD)	256	19	56	2	Nigeria
[161]	40–65	262	34	—	—	Sheffield
[137]	54 ± 2 (SD)	42	38	20	0	Toronto
[162]	36–84	200	31	170	25	Edinburgh
[146]	41–76	83	37	—	—	Israel
[163]	?	170	54	?	7	Taiwan
[164]	58 ± 6	216	20	216	5	Sri Lanka
[165]	38–84	139	60	—	—	Finland

at least 70° and the elbow to at least 180°. The ankle should flex maximally to at least 100°, the cervical spine lateral flexion should permit ear-to-shoulder juxtaposition, and thoracolumbar spine lateral flexion should be at least 35° in young people [11].

This examination will reveal obvious LJM but, as noted, the clinical sensation of joint limitation without absolute reduction in maximum extension is quite subjective. Buithieu et al. [154] compared MCP and wrist maximal extension in 239 controls and 211 T1DM patients aged 9–30 years using a goniometer, and found a significant proportion of those without clinical LJM to have MCP and wrist limitation, defined as less than 2 SD of the control mean. The 172 subjects without apparent LJM included 25% with MCP limitation and 13% with wrist limitation. Similar findings have been reported from France [138]. Thus, earlier detection of LJM may be possible through objective measurement. This is also likely for the associated changes in the lower extremity [172].

The staging of LJM has been useful in describing relationships of other findings to LJM and for patient follow-up. *No limitation* includes equivocal or unilateral findings, including failure to approximate the palmar surfaces to tabletop or in the prayer position, but with normal range of passive motion. *Mild limitation* indicates involvement of one or two PIP joints, one large joint, or only the MCP joints bilaterally. *Moderate limitation* refers to involvement of three or more PIP joints or one finger joint and one large joint bilaterally. *Severe limitation* refers to obvious hand deformity at rest or associated cervical spine involvement [11].

In describing 11 patients with severe LJM at the time that this problem was first being recognized, Benedetti and Noacco [173] used the term "juvenile diabetic cheiroarthropathy," based on the Greek word for hand. Because LJM may involve more than hand joints, the term "cheiroarthropathy" is not adequate, leading to such incongruous statements as, "Cheiroarthropathy ... may also affect the large joints" [174]. Referring to this condition as "the scleroderma-like syndrome" [175] is not appropriate because only the more severely affected individuals will have "digital sclerosis" [166].

Natural History

Cross-sectional studies demonstrate that duration of diabetes is the most important variable in the appearance of LJM. When Rosenbloom et al. [176] were able to determine the time of development of joint changes in 76 patients, however, they found that age attained was much more important than duration of diabetes in the development of LJM. The interval between detection of mild LJM and progression to moderate or severe changes varies from 3 months to 4 years, with a mean of 2 years. After this period, progression (if any) is very slow. Most do not progress beyond mild changes.

In one study, there was no correlation between loss of BMC by photon absorptiometry and the presence or absence of LJM, which is to be expected in view of the different timing of these findings in the course of T1DM [21]. One half of young patients affected with more than 5 years' duration of diabetes had moderate or severe limitation, defined as at least three interphalangeal joints or one finger joint and one large joint bilaterally. Approximately one third of the affected group had severe limitation, i.e. involvement of all the fingers and often of the cervical spine as well [176]. In adult populations, about two thirds of patients affected had at least two fingers involved [128, 130].

A relationship between LJM and diabetes control as measured by HbA_{1c} levels or clinical criteria has not been demonstrable in the cross-sectional studies involving controls without LJM who are of comparable age and diabetes duration [5, 125]. Nonetheless, hepatomegaly and proteinuria in many of the initial patients who were severely affected by LJM and had associated thick, tight, waxy skin, suggested that LJM was the result of poor control [124, 166, 173]. Higher mean HbA_{1c} levels over a period of years were noted in those with severe LJM but not in those with mild changes, compared to those without LJM in one study, but the subjects without LJM or with mild changes had significantly shorter diabetes duration, a serious confound [13]. LJM was associated with both longer duration of diabetes and greater average HbA_{1c} in the previous year in a Cuban population [139]. The only controlled study of metabolic regulation from the onset of diabetes until the occurrence of LJM, in order to avoid the numerous biases of cross-sectional study, described a strong association of long-term control and the appearance of LJM. For every 1% increase in average HbA_{1c} from onset, there was an approximately 46% increase in the risk of LJM; the odds ratio for $HbA_{1c} > 8\%$ was 2.55, and for $HbA_{1c} > 12\%$ the odds ratio was 4.54 [177]. As noted above, the greater than fourfold decrease in prevalence of LJM and in severity in those affected between 1976–1978 and 1998 can only be explained by the improvement in control measures [155] (Figures 4 and 5).

Effects on Growth

It has long been recognized that chronic poor diabetes control is associated with poor growth, delayed maturation, and reduced adult height [179]. The original patients described with severe LJM had growth failure [125, 173]. The subsequent population study demonstrated that more severe changes of LJM were associated with growth limitation, but that milder LJM was not [166]. A later study of individuals with more than 3 years' duration of diabetes, with onset before adolescence (thus permitting sufficient time for growth failure to occur), was more informative

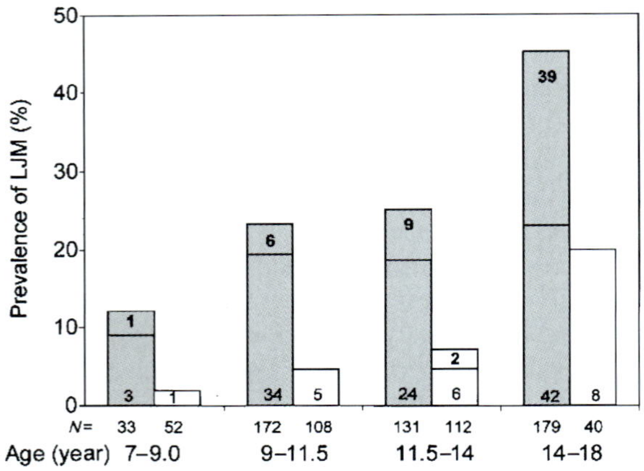

Figure 4 Frequency of LJM by age group in children with diabetes in 1976–1978 (solid bars) and 1998 (open bars). Number of subjects in each age group is shown beneath the bar. The line dividing the bar separates the proportion with moderate to severe LJM (upper) and mild LJM (lower); numbers of subjects affected are shown within the bar [178]. (Reproduced by permission of Mosby)

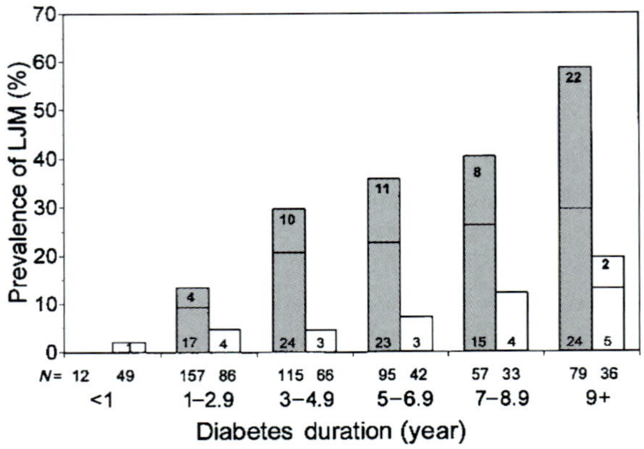

Figure 5 Frequency of LJM by duration of diabetes in children examined in 1976–1978 (solid bars) and 1998 (open bars). Number of subjects in each diabetes duration group is shown beneath the bar. The line dividing the bar separates the proportion with moderate to severe LJM (upper) and mild LJM (lower); numbers of subjects affected are shown within the bar [178]. (Reproduced by permission of Mosby)

than previous cross-sectional studies; 142 such patients were assessed, including 31 with mild LJM and 43 with more severe changes. Of subjects without LJM, 68% were below the 50th percentile for height rather than the expected 50%, and most of this discrepancy was below the 25th percentile (38% vs. expected 25%). Mild LJM resulted in four times the excess below the 25th percentile (72%), and moderate to severe limitation was not associated with significantly smaller stature (77% below the 25th percentile). The small proportion above the 75th percentile was similar for those without LJM (12%), and with mild or more severe LJM (both 10%) [176]. As with the marked reduction in frequency of LJM, the associated impairment in growth and the modest growth impairment in those without LJM virtually disappeared in the ~20 years following the initial study; 175 children with greater than 2 years duration before puberty and overall duration greater than 3 years, corresponding to the criteria of the earlier study, were examined; without LJM, only 22% in 1998 versus 37% in 1982 were <25th percentile for height and with LJM, only 33% in 1998 were <25th percentile compared to 77% in 1982 [178].

Differential Diagnosis

The differential diagnosis from other joint problems should be straightforward [5]. Nevertheless, since the original description, numerous reports have referred to the various conditions listed in Table 4 as LJM, or have

Table 4 Differential diagnosis of joint syndromes involving the hand in diabetes

Condition	Usual fingers involved	Pain/paresthesia	Muscle	Frequency	Other distinctive features
LJM	Begins 5th, extends radially	No	Normal	>50% of T1DM after 5 years and puberty	Not disabling; associated with thick, tight, waxy skin
Dupuytren disease	3rd, 4th	No	Normal	Up to 40% over age 40, 16% at diagnosis	Milder expression common in women; may precede diabetes
Flexor tenosynovitis	1st, 3rd, 4th	Yes	Normal	1/3 associated with diabetes	Marked female predominance; locking, disability
Carpal tunnel (diabetic hand)	All	Yes	Intrinsic, palmar atrophy	5–16% due to diabetes	Ulnar as well as median nerve involvement in diabetes
Stiff hand	All	Yes	Normal	Rare: T1DM >20 years	Disability; calcified vessels; hard palmar skin, soft dorsal
Shoulder–hand (reflex dystrophy)	All	Yes	Atrophy	Shoulder limitation in 10–20% of older T1DM, T2DM; reflex dystrophy unusual	Most bilateral; often associated with other hand syndromes

considered several of these conditions to be varying manifestations of the same process, using the terms for the distinctive diagnostic conditions interchangeably, in particular referring to LJM as diabetic hand syndrome or stiff hand syndrome [115, 117, 146]. LJM is easily distinguishable from DD, the only other condition involving the hand that is not associated with pain, by the absence of palmar fascial thickening and nodules, and by the finger distribution. DD is not seen in young patients; in older patients, DD and LJM may be seen together [122, 130, 159, 161, 162]. All the other conditions are associated with pain and other characteristic findings, as noted in Table 4. Rheumatoid arthritis is rarely associated with diabetes, and patients with LJM do not meet the pain or inflammatory criteria for rheumatoid arthritis [5, 103].

There have been several examples of diagnostic confusion in this area. The finding that LJM could precede the development of diabetes by 3 years in a teenage patient has suggested an important constitutional component [10]. The patient described developed stiffness in the MCP and PIP joints and wrists more or less simultaneously, had thickening and contraction of flexor tendons in the palm, and progressive disability, indicative of precocious FTS [180, 181]. Robertson et al. [182] described a patient in her late 20s who also had characteristic features of flexor tenosynovitis but was reported as "juvenile diabetic cheiroarthropathy." Three patients reported as having LJM appeared to have the diabetic hand syndrome, with additional features of shoulder–hand syndrome in one and flexor tenosynovitis in another [183, 184].

The superimposition of other hand syndromes on LJM as patients age is not surprising, especially with prolonged duration [185, 186]. The presence of pain or paresthesia, neurologic findings, disability, finger locking, swelling, muscle atrophy, palmar skin or fascia thickening, or absence of greater involvement of the ring and little fingers could be indicators of additional problems. One would expect people with LJM to be at greater risk for other connective tissue proliferative problems and neuropathy. As noted above, generalized scleroderma can rarely be associated with diabetes, but should provide no diagnostic confusion [187]. In older patients, osteoarthritis and occupation-related limitation should be easily distingued by history and physical examination.

Neuropathy

Kennedy et al. [188] noted prolonged nerve conduction velocity for the ulnar and median nerves in older patients with LJM, compared with those without LJM and comparable durations of diabetes. Also noted was decreased vibratory sense in both upper and lower extremities in the presence of LJM. Starkman et al. [12] found that LJM was associated with a 4.3-fold relative risk of clinical neuropathy in T1DM. More recently, Ficicioglu et al. [189] found reduced nerve conduction velocities in those with LJM, affecting the peroneal and sural nerves; symptomatic neuropathy was present in those with severe LJM.

Cardiac Function

Cardiac response to dynamic exercise in a group of otherwise healthy adolescents with T1DM was compared with a nondiabetic control group by postexercise echocardiography. Abnormalities were found in the diabetic group in indicators of systolic function indicating subclinical cardiomyopathy. Twelve of the 25 patients had LJM. Five of the patients and 1 of the 26 controls had flat interventricular septal motion; all 5 T1DM patients with this abnormality had LJM [190].

Pulmonary Changes

Decreased elastic recoil at low lung volumes was initially described in 11 young men with T1DM who also had decreased pulmonary capacity [191]. The association of limited pulmonary capacity with LJM was first noted by Barta in a single patient [192]. A study of 12 adolescents and young adults with severe LJM who were matched for age, sex, height, and duration of T1DM to 11 without LJM, found that LJM subjects had significantly less total lung capacity, thoracic gas volume, residual volume, forced vital capacity, and forced expiratory volume (1 s). What could not be ascertained was whether these individuals had limited pulmonary compliance, decreased mobility of the chest wall, or both [193]. A subsequent report noted that 19% of T1DM patients had vital capacities more than 2 SD below those normal for age, but this was not associated with LJM [153]. In contrast, Madacsy et al. [136] found that 24 patients with LJM had a significant decrease in total lung capacity, airway resistance, and peak expiratory flow, compared with 26 without LJM. Among 51 Cuban patients with T1DM of whom 31 had LJM, no differences in diabetes duration, stature, or metabolic control were present between those with and those without LJM; however, those with LJM had highly significant reductions in vital capacity, forced expiratory volume, and mean maximal expiratory flow [194].

Fibrous Disease of the Breast

Twelve women with breast lumps were identified from among 88 with T1DM, aged 20–40 years, and 11 of these 12 were found to have LJM. The duration of their diabetes ranged from 8 to 30 years, and all but 1 had retinopathy [195]. While this might be a significant association, no data were provided about the prevalence of LJM in the rest of the population. The prevalence of breast lumps in this study (14%) is similar to that in nondiabetic populations.

Skin Changes

Thick, tight, waxy skin, most prominent over the dorsum of the hands and the forearms, was noted in the initial patients and in about one third of those with LJM described subsequently; this change was apparent only in those with moderate to severe LJM [11, 125]. Seibold [148] found abnormal tenting of the skin to be more frequent than LJM, but that LJM was present only in those who had skin changes (47 out of 137, of whom 26 had LJM). Similarly, in a study of 375 patients aged 7–25 years, skin changes were present in 34% of those without LJM, in 70% of those with mild LJM (involving only the fifth PIP joint) and in 100% of those with more severe limitation [153].

Ultrasound studies of 92 T1DM patients aged 20–38 years, with a wide range of disease durations, demonstrated that those with LJM had thicker skin than those without LJM, who in turn had thicker skin than those without diabetes [196]. Skin thickness assessed by ultrasound measurement was also noted to correlate with LJM in 80 children and adolescents [197].

Biopsy studies have shown thickening of the dermis and epidermis with accumulation of collagen and loss of skin appendages compared with control biopsies [125, 150] (Figure 6). The pathological features have been more carefully defined by Hanna et al. [198]. They found clinical evidence of skin thickening in 22% of T1DM patients and 4% of controls. Full-thickness skin biopsy specimens from the forearm were analyzed in 9 patients with T1DM and thick skin, 4 patients with T1DM and clinically normal skin, 4 patients with progressive systemic sclerosis, and 4 normal control subjects. They defined distinct differences from sclerodermatous and normal individuals: the T1DM patients with thick skin showed active fibroblasts and extensive collagen polymerization in the rough endoplasmic reticulum. Unlike scleroderma, in which there is bimodality of collagen fiber sizes, the thick skin of diabetes demonstrated predominance of large fibers, a finding that was also present in those with diabetes who did not have thick skin. Thus, the fibrosis in these two conditions appears basically different. Biochemical studies are discussed below.

Hyaluronan is an ubiquitously distributed glycosaminoglycan in connective tissue, seen in all layers of normal skin but especially in the papillary dermis and basement membrane zones. This distribution did not differ from normal in the skin of patients with T1DM who had no or mild LJM, but in the skin of those with severe LJM there was weak hyaluronan staining of the papillary dermis and the basement membrane zone was almost devoid of hyaluronan. This was associated with epidermal thickening. The hyaluronan abnormality was considered to cause disturbances in skin function that would result in stiffness and poor wound healing [199].

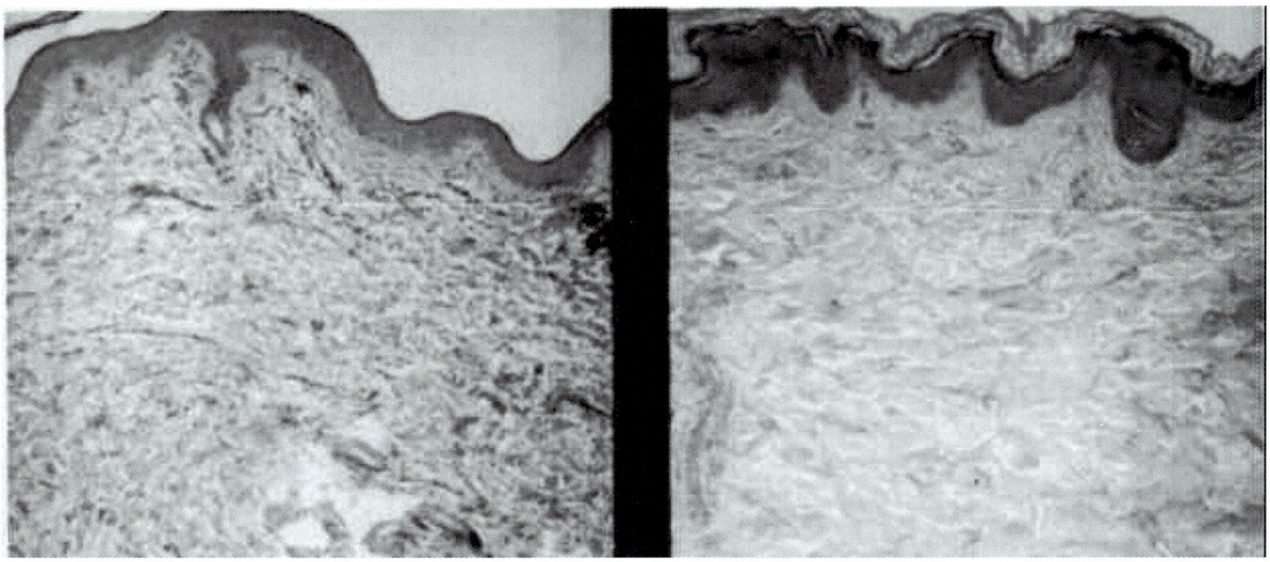

Figure 6 Biopsies of skin from the dorsal wrist crease of a normal 16-year-old female on the left and a 16-year-old with type 1 diabetes for 9 years with severe LJM on the right (patient 3 in Table 2 of reference 125). The biopsy from the girl with diabetes shows thickened dermis and epidermis, loss of skin appendages, loss of elastic fibers, and accumulation of collagen (Reproduced by permission of Mosby).

Association with Microvascular Disease

The initial 7 patients with severe LJM involving fingers and large joints included 5 with clinically apparent retinopathy or proteinuria before the age of 18 years [125]. In a unique longitudinal study of a clinic cohort in which the onset of LJM and of microvascular complications could be documented, who had diabetes duration of more than 4.5 years (the shortest duration at which microvascular complications were noted), 82 of 169 patients had LJM, of whom 41 also had microvascular complications, in contrast to only 10 of the 87 patients without LJM. Severity of LJM correlated directly with the frequency and severity of the microvascular disease. Actuarial analysis indicated an 83% risk for microvascular complications after 16 years of diabetes if joint limitation was present, but only a 25% risk in the absence of LJM. The differences between the LJM and non-LJM groups could not be accounted for by differences in patients' ages or durations of diabetes. The 4.5-fold greater likelihood of microvascular disease in the group with LJM in this population indicated that LJM identified a group exceptionally at risk for the development of early complications [11] (Figure 7).

Benedetti and Noacco [127] reported that 8 of their 19 patients with LJM had clinical retinopathy, and this was exclusively in the group over 21 years of age (range 21–48 years) among whom only 1 individual did not have retinopathy. No data were provided on a case control population. Among adult Irish patients with T1DM, retinopathy was present in 52.4% with LJM compared with only 12.3% without. Those with LJM and retinopathy had much longer durations of diabetes than those with LJM and no retinopathy. To assess whether the presence of LJM was a risk factor for the development of retinopathy, independent of duration of diabetes, two subgroups of 20 patients each, with and without LJM, were matched for duration. Retinopathy was much more common in the group with LJM (85% vs. 40%), with a highly significant difference in the prevalence of proliferative retinopathy—70% in patients with LJM compared with 15% in patients with normal joint mobility [128].

A similar attempt was made to correct for duration of diabetes in a young population of 311 subjects aged 6–27 years undergoing fluorescein angiography to determine the prevalence of early retinopathy. The relationship between LJM and retinopathy was highly significant ($P < 0.0001$), and this was not due to the effect of duration on both complications: the interaction of LJM, retinopathy, and duration was insignificant. The presence of LJM was predictive of associated retinopathy at the level of clinical recognition (more than 10 microaneurysms); 43% of those with LJM and more than 4 years' disease duration had retinopathy compared with 15% of a matched duration group without LJM [151]. Among the 45% of 110 Ethiopian patients with T1DM who had LJM, retinopathy was found to be twice as frequent as in those without LJM [135].

Among 150 Joslin Clinic patients under 40 years old, of whom 75 had LJM, the relative risk of retinopathy conferred by the presence of LJM was 3.7, and of preproliferative and proliferative retinopathy, 4.2 [12]. Two thirds of young patients with LJM reported from Hungary had preclinical retinopathy as opposed to one third of those without LJM [136].

The largest survey reported, involving 375 persons aged 7–25 years, noted positive correlations between skin involvement, severity of joint limitation, and diabetic

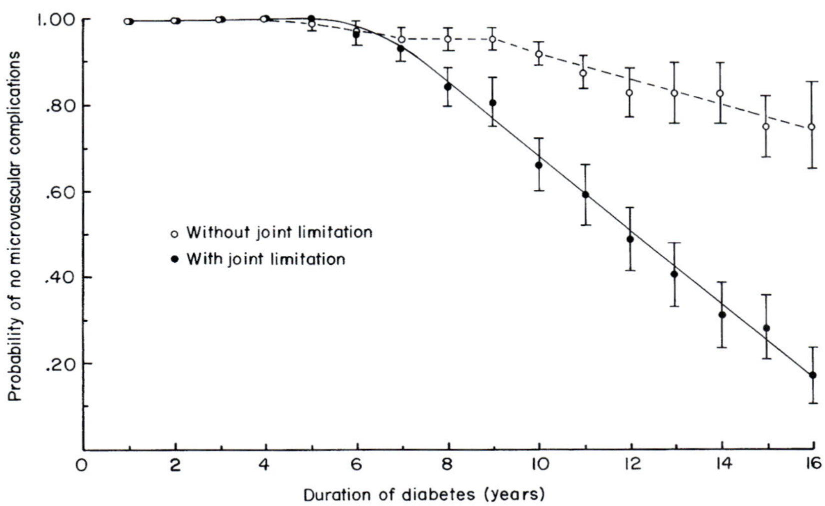

Figure 7 Actuarial analysis of risk for development of microvascular complications with and without LJM, based on a longitudinal study of 169 patients with diabetes duration ≥4.5 years followed from before the development of LJM or microvascular disease [11]. (Reproduced by permission of the Massachusetts Medical Society)

retinopathy, although the latter was evaluated only through the undilated pupil [153]. Another large study, of 357 subjects, noted significant association of LJM with retinopathy and proteinuria [13]. In a controlled study of 63 Spanish T1DM patients aged 18–57 years, in which correction was made for age and duration of diabetes, LJM was significantly associated with microalbuminuria and retinopathy [200]. Among 335 T1DM patients from Germany aged 14–40 years, 34% had LJM, which was significantly associated with higher albumin excretion rates and hypertension in men and women; LJM was also an independent predictor of retinopathy only in men, and of macrovascular disease (increased intima-media thickness of the carotids and atherosclerotic plaques) only in women [201]. In a study of 12 adolescent patients with proteinuria or hypertension and LJM, the increase in the mesangial matrix and basement membrane thickening on renal biopsy correlated with the severity of LJM [202].

Significant correlations between LJM and microvascular disease have been reported with T2DM, but these correlations have been less impressive than in T1DM. This difference is particularly apparent in studies that involve both T1DM and T2DM [130, 135, 137, 157]. The most recent study, involving 139 patients with T2DM with a mean age of 61 years (SD 12 years), however, suggests a substantial relationship. Subjects with LJM had a threefold risk for coronary heart disease and a fourfold risk for cerebrovascular disease when the confounding effects of age, duration of diabetes, and diabetes control were controlled. There was also a ninefold increased risk for proliferative retinopathy and a threefold increased risk for nephropathy, controlling for duration of diabetes, but these correlations disappeared when diabetes control was included in the model [203].

Biochemical Studies

Increased accumulation of dermal collagen that is relatively insoluble and resistant to enzymatic digestion has been recognized as a characteristic of connective tissue aging in both T1DM and T2DM [204]. Two out of 3 youngsters with multiple LJM and skin changes had decreased acid solubility of skin collagen, suggesting increased cross-linkage; however, the 3 patients taken together did not have a significantly greater resistance of their collagen to digestion than did 7 nondiabetic controls, and no comparison was made to T1DM without LJM [205]. In a subsequent study, skin biopsies from the lateral thigh of 23 patients with T1DM yielded 8 with less than 2.5% collagen extractable in 0.5 mol/l acetic acid. Compared with the 15 with more than 2.5% acid-soluble collagen, there was no difference in age or mean duration of diabetes. However, the rates of retinopathy (50% vs. 0%), LJM (63% vs. 20%), skin changes (63% vs. 20%), HbA_{1c} values greater than 12% (63% vs. 27%), and decreased vital capacity (57% vs. 0%) were all significantly different [206].

Skin collagen glycation is increased with diabetes but this does not correlate with LJM [188, 204, 205] or microvascular complications [206]. This glycation correlates with HbA_{1c} level, and reflects the ketoamine link, an early step in the nonenzymatic browning [Maillard] reaction that leads to stable end products (advanced glycation end products, AGEs). These AGEs are fluorescent and thought to be responsible for increased cross-linking of collagen. Monnier et al. [206] demonstrated that skin collagen fluorescence increased linearly with age, but that 95% of 41 T1DM patients had abnormal increases for age and that their fluorescence of skin collagen correlated with the presence of retinopathy, nephropathy, and LJM. In a comparison of Maillard reaction products and collagen-linked fluorescence in skin collagen from 39 T1DM and 52 controls, a modest increase (33%) was seen over the age span from 20 to 85 years in the controls. In those with diabetes, there was a threefold increase in collagen fluorescence, which correlated strongly with HbA_{1c}, but not with age, and twofold increases in the Maillard products [207]. These same investigators further demonstrated association of these findings with retinopathy and nephropathy, but not with LJM [208]. AGE serum concentrations have been found to be increased in young patients with T1DM, correlating significantly with HbA_{1c}, and to decrease with improved control, consistent with the early appearance of LJM and its correlation with long-term control [177, 209]. Most impressive has been the demonstration in the Diabetes Control and Complications Trial (DCCT) that indicators of skin collagen glycation, glycoxidation, and cross-linking, which correlated strongly with complications in the secondary intervention cohort, were markedly reduced in both cohorts undergoing intensive treatment compared to conventional treatment [210].

The accumulation of AGEs of the Maillard reaction, with increased cross-linking, dehydration, and condensation of collagen, is quite distinct from the more hydrated and soluble collagen with increased reducible cross-links in the thickened tissue of DD and shoulder capsulitis associated with diabetes [113, 114]. Thus, the suggestion that hypertrophied polyol pathway activity resulting in increased hydration of connective tissue, as in the connective tissue in DD, might also be associated with LJM appears unlikely [211]. Indeed, aldose reductase inhibition has been ineffective in reducing LJM [212].

Constitutional vs. Metabolic Considerations

The intuitive attribution of LJM and associated skin changes to metabolic control along with the other long-term complications of diabetes has received extensive experimental support since publication of the DCCT results [213]. The definitive demonstration of the importance of long-term diabetes control in the emergence of LJM [177] and the marked decrease in prevalence of this complication with improved control measures over the past 20 years [155] have indicated that the findings of the DCCT can be extended to the specific complication of LJM.

Although no differences in HLA distribution between those with and without LJM have been described [144, 176, 188], and there is no difference in frequency of organ-specific autoimmunity [176], a genetic component had been suggested by the observation of LJM in nondiabetic relatives of T1DM patients [129, 214]. Traisman et al. [214] found a greater frequency of LJM among 106 nondiabetic siblings (9.4%) than among 310 probands (8.4%). In the oldest age group (15–18 years), however, 9% of siblings but 17% of patients had LJM. Data are not provided on duration of diabetes. The overall percentage for this patient population is lower than any other reported in that era, except for that of the Italian investigators who used a handprint method for determining LJM, which might only pick up the more severe contractures [127]; Brice et al. [129] found 42% of 112 T1DM patients aged 2–12 years to have LJM, with 78% of those with duration of diabetes of more than 7 years being affected; this is three to four times the prevalence reported by others for this largely preadolescent age group. This diagnostic exuberance may explain their finding among 214 nondiabetic first-degree relatives, that 35% of the relatives of children with LJM were similarly affected as were 13% of relatives of those children without LJM.

Rosenbloom and colleagues [149] examined 204 T1DM patients aged 7–23 years and 336 of their firt-degree relatives. They also examined simplex and multiplex pedigrees with T1DM and normal controls. Only 1 of the non-diabetes-related normal controls had LJM; 3% of 225 nondiabetic parents were affected compared with 21% of the probands. Of the 108 nondiabetic siblings, only 1 had LJM. Three parents had adult-onset diabetes and had LJM. Of the nondiabetic relatives with joint limitation, none was related to a proband with LJM and all tested were negative for islet cell antibodies. Among 11 T1DM multiplex families with at least 1 member having joint limitation, the concordance rate for LJM was no greater than expected for age and duration of diabetes. Thus, the evidence for LJM being a metabolic consequence of diabetes included the absence of limitation among nondiabetic first-degree relatives of probands, including of probands with LJM, and that concordance for joint involvement was not increased in first-degree relatives with T1DM.

Further evidence for a metabolic explanation for LJM in T1DM comes from its description in non-HLA-associated, nonautoimmune T1DM, in 2 siblings with the syndrome of diabetes insipidus, diabetes mellitus, and optic atrophy [215], as well as in 2 siblings with diabetes from infancy due to pancreatic hypoplasia [216].

As with other complications, the suggestion of a genetic component comes from the difficulty in identifying close correlation with control over the short term and the inability to recognize exceptional control in those individuals who do not develop LJM. The case previously noted in which purported LJM appeared years before clinical diabetes was clearly an erroneous classification of the joint problem [10, 180]. However, LJM has been noted in a teenage sibling of a patient with T1DM who had mild impaired glucose tolerance, and 2 adolescents have been found to have LJM at the time of diagnosis of their diabetes [166, 176]. The latter circumstance does not preclude primary metabolic pathogenesis, as a substantial degree of hyperglycemia can be present for an extended time, particularly in an older child, before clinical symptoms appear.

Tissue culture studies provide the opportunity to examine genetically determined donor characteristics generations of cells removed from the donor metabolic milieu. The viability of cultured fibroblasts from 2 patients with severe LJM and growth failure was found to be completely normal for age, indicating that there is not an inherent cellular defect in growth in these youngsters [217]. Seibold et al. [148] studied 5 older patients with T1DM and 3 with T2DM, all of whom had "digital sclerosis.' They found that dermal fibroblasts from these subjects produced less collagen and had less DNA replication but normal collagenase activity. However, there were only 3 controls, and they were substantially younger than the patients, a factor that would significantly alter the DNA replication and collagen synthesis results. Furthermore, there were no comparisons with age-matched people with diabetes who did not have digital sclerosis, because the purpose of this study was to demonstrate differences *in vitro* from systemic sclerosis, which these authors accomplished. Systemic sclerosis is associated with increased collagen synthesis by fibroblasts in culture. The finding of decreased collagen production from cultured dermal fibroblasts from patients with diabetes is consistent with the decrease in collagen production *in vivo* by streptozotocin-induced diabetic rats [218]. These animals had specific decrease in collagen production in their bone and cartilage but normal non-collagen protein production. In contrast to the suggestion of a genetic component from the studies of Seibold et al. [148], these studies in nongenetic diabetes, using fresh tissue, indicate a metabolic etiology.

The essential (apparently) metabolic derangement for the development of LJM and associated skin findings as well as other complications of diabetes that occur despite the type of diabetes (T1DM, T2DM, secondary) must require a constitutional predisposition, which is not specific. Monnier and colleagues [219] proposed a means by which this constitutional factor may be expressed. They noted that the age-related collagen-linked fluorescence in skin biopsies from long-standing T1DM reflecting AGEs was, as previously noted, greatly increased compared with controls. The rate of browning was not significantly different from normal in those without retinopathy but was 2.5 times greater in the presence of retinopathy. These findings suggested that there was a mechanism controlling the browning rate of collagen in those individuals who did not develop retinopathy.

An alternative metabolic pathway for ketoamine products could provide such a mechanism [220]. The oxidation of earlier glycation products to form relatively inert carboxymethyllysine rather than AGEs would reduce the ill effects of protein glycation. Differences in response to this process could explain different susceptibility to the development of complications.

CONCLUSION

The abnormalities in bone, joints, skin, and periarticular tissue described in this chapter cannot be attributed to a single pathogenic mechanism. As osteopenia is seen early in the course of diabetes and does not appear to worsen with duration, a basic metabolic abnormality concomitant with the development of hyperglycemia and unlikely to be related to other complications is probable. Vascular insufficiency associated with vessel calcification can explain the stiff hand syndrome, and neuropathy the carpal tunnel syndrome as it appears in diabetes, where it is referred to as the diabetic hand syndrome. The lesions attributable to connective tissue proliferation, involving palmar fascia (DD), the periarticular tissue (adhesive capsulitis of the shoulder, LJM), the tendon sheaths (flexor tenosynovitis), and the skin, may have the most relevance to the long-term disabling or fatal complications of diabetes in which connective tissue of basement membranes is abnormal.

Although the lesions of diabetes complications are frequently compared to those of aging, the skin and periarticular lesions (and perhaps the osteopenia) of diabetes either are unique or differ substantially from comparable lesions in nondiabetic individuals. This is also true for the complications of the retina, the heart, the kidneys, and the peripheral nerves. LJM is of particular interest because of its early onset, the associated skin, and lung changes, the established relationship to microvascular disease, and the dramatic reduction in its frequency in T1DM during an era of improved ability to control glycemia.

REFERENCES

1. Brownlee M. Glycation products and the pathogenesis of diabetic complications. *Diabetes Care* 1992; 15: 1835–43.
2. Regan TJ, Lyons MM, Ahmed SS, Levinson GE, Oldewurtel HA, Ahmed MR, Haider B. Evidence for cardiomyopathy in familial diabetes mellitus. *J Clin Invest* 1977; 60: 885–9.
3. Luishner JRA, Tevaarwerk GJM, Clarson CL, Harding PGR, Chance GW, Haust MD. Analysis of the collagens of diabetic placental villi. *Cell Mol Biol* 1986; 32: 27–35.
4. Lundbaek K. Stiff hands in long-term diabetes. *Acta Med Scand* 1957; 158: 447–51.
5. Rosenbloom AL, Silverstein JH. Connective tissue and joint disease in diabetes mellitus. *Endocrinol Metab Clin North Am* 1996; 25: 473–83.
6. Kim RP. The musculoskeletal complications of diabetes. *Curr Diabetes Rep* 2002; 2: 49–52.
7. Eaton RP, Sibbitt WL, Shah VO, Dorin RI, Zager PG, Bicknell JM. A commentary on 10 years of aldose reductase inhibition for limited joint mobility in diabetes. *J Diabetes Complications* 1998; 12: 34–8.
8. Cropley TG. The diagnostic challenge of diabetic hands. *Arch Dermatol* 1993; 129: 40–1.
9. Verrotti A, Chiarelli F, Morgese G. Limited joint mobility in children with type 1 diabetes mellitus. A critical review. *J Pediatr Endocrinol Metab* 1996; 9: 3–8.
10. Sherry DD, Rothstein RRL, Petty RE. Joint contractures preceding insulin-dependent diabetes mellitus. *Arthritis Rheum* 1982; 25: 1362–4.
11. Rosenbloom AL, Silverstein JH, Lezotte DC, Richardson K, McCallum M. Limited joint mobility in childhood diabetes indicates increased risk for microvascular disease. *N Engl J Med* 1981; 305: 191–4.
12. Starkman HS, Gleason RE, Rand LI, Miller DE, Soeldner JS. Limited joint mobility (LJM) of the hand in patients with diabetes mellitus: relation to chronic complications. *Ann Rheum Dis* 1986; 45: 130–5.
13. Garg SK, Chase HP, Marshall G, Jackson WE, Holmes D, Hoops S, Harris S. Limited joint mobility in subjects with insulin dependent diabetes mellitus: relationship with eye and kidney complications. *Arch Dis Child* 1992; 67: 96–9.
14. Hough FS. Alterations of bone and mineral metabolism in diabetes mellitus, Part I: An overview. *S Afr Med J* 1987; 72: 116–9.
15. Heath H, Melton LJ, Chic GP. Diabetes mellitus and risk of skeletal fracture. *N Engl J Med* 1980; 303: 567–70.
16. DeLeeuw I, Abs R. Bone mass and bone density in maturity-type diabetes measured by the ^{125}I photon-absorption technique. *Diabetes* 1977; 26: 1130–5.
17. Albright N, Reifenstein EC. Bone development in diabetic children: a roentgen study. *Am J Med Sci* 1948; 174: 313–9.
18. Berney PW. Osteoporosis and diabetes mellitus. *J Iowa Med Soc* 1952; 42: 10–2.
19. Levin ME, Boisseau VC, Avioli LV. Effects of diabetes mellitus on bone mass in juvenile and adult-onset diabetes. *N Engl J Med* 1976; 294: 241–5.
20. Santiago JV, McAlister WH, Ratzan SK, Bussman Y, Haymond MW, Shackelford G, Weldon VY. Decreased cortical thickness and osteopenia in children with diabetes mellitus. *J Clin Endocrinol Metab* 1977; 45: 845–8.
21. Rosenbloom AL, Lezotte DC, Weber FT, Gudat J, Heller DR, Weber ML, Klein S, Kennedy BB. Diminution of bone mass in childhood diabetes. *Diabetes* 1977; 26: 1052–5.
22. McNair P, Madsbad S, Christiansen C, Faber OK, Transbol I, Binder C. Osteopenia in insulin-treated diabetes mellitus. Its relation to age at onset, sex and duration of disease. *Diabetologia* 1978; 15: 87–90.
23. Shore RM, Chesney RW, Mazess RB, Rose PG, Bergman GJ. Osteopenla in juvenile diabetes. *Calcif Tissue Int* 1981; 33: 455–457.

24. Nielsen CT, Ibsen KK, Christiansen JS, Pieterson B, Uhrenholdt A. Diabetes mellitus, skeletal age and bone mineral content in children [abstract]. *Acta Endocrinol* 1978; 219 (suppl): 58.
25. Frazer TE, White NH, Hough S, Santiago JV, McGee BR, Bryce G, Mallon J, Avioli LV. Alterations in circulating vitamin D metabolites in the young insulin-dependent diabetic. *J Clin Endocrinol Metab* 1981; 53: 1154–9.
26. McNair P, Christiansen MS, Madsbad S, Christiansen C, Transbol I. Hypoparathyroidism in diabetes mellitus. *Acta Endocrinol* 1981; 96: 81–6.
27. Wiske PS, Wentworth SM, Norton JA, Epstein S, Johnston C. Evaluation of bone mass and growth in young diabetics. *Metabolism* 1982; 31: 848–54.
28. Hui SL, Epstein S, Johnston CC. A prospective study of bone mass in patients with type I diabetes. *J Clin Endocrinol Metab* 1985; 60: 74–80.
29. Hough FS. Alterations of bone and mineral metabolism in diabetes mellitus, Part II: Clinical studies in 206 patients with type I diabetes mellitus. *S Afr Med J* 1987; 72: 120–6.
30. Saggese G, Bertelloni S, Baroncelli GI, Federico G, Calisti L, Fusaro C. Bane demineralization and impaired mineral metabolism in insulin-dependent diabetes mellitus. *Helv Paediatr Acta* 1988; 43: 405–14.
31. Auwerx J, Dequeker J, Bouillon R, Geusens P, Nijs J. Mineral metabolism and bone mass at peripheral and axial skeleton in diabetes mellitus. *Diabetes* 1988; 37: 8–12.
32. Giacca A, Fassina A, Caviezel E, Cattaneo AG, Caldirola G, Pozza G. Bane mineral density in diabetes mellitus. *Bone* 1988; 9: 29–36.
33. Leon M, Larroderaa L, Lledo G, Hawkins F. Study of bone loss in diabetes mellitus type 1. *Diabetes Res Clin Pract* 1989; 6: 237–42.
34. Weber G, Beccaria L, deAngelis M, Mora S, Galli L, Cazzuffi MA, Turbo S, Frisone F, Guarneri ME, Chiumelo G. Bone mass in young patients with type I diabetes. *Bone Miner* 1990; 8: 23–30.
35. Roe TF, Mora S, Costin G, Kaufman F, Carlson ME, Gilsanz V. Vertebral bone density in insulin-dependent diabetic children. *Metabolism* 1991; 40: 967–71.
36. Ponder SW, McCormick DP, Fawcett HD, Tran AD, Ogelsby GW, Brouhard BH, Travis LB. Bone mineral density of the lumbar vertebrae in children and adolescents with insulin-dependent diabetes mellitus. *J Pediatr* 1992; 120: 541–5.
37. Olmos JM, Perez-Castrillón JL, Garcia MT, Garrido JC, Amado JA, Gonzalez-Macias J. Bone densitometry and biochemical bone remodeling markers in type 2 diabetes mellitus. *Bone Miner* 1994; 26: 1–8.
38. Kayath MJ, Dib SA, Vieiaa JG. Prevalence and magnitude of osteopenia associated with insulin-dependent diabetes mellitus. *J Diabetes Complications* 1994; 8: 97–104.
39. Munoz-Torres M, Jodar E, Escobar-Jimenez F, Lópezt-Ibarra PJ, Luna 1D. Bone mineral density measured by dual X-ray absorptiometry in Spanish patients with insulin-dependent diabetes mellitus. *Calcif Tissue Int* 1996; 58: 316–9.
40. Forst T, Pfutzner A, Kann P, Schehler B, Lobmann R, Schafer H, Andreas J, Bockisch A, Beyer J. Peripheral osteopenia in adult patients with insulin-dependent diabetes mellitus. *Diabet Med* 1995; 12: 874–9.
41. Lettgen B, Hauffa B, Mohlmann C, Jeken C, Reiners C. Bone mineral density in children and adolescents with juvenile diabetes: selective measurement of bone mineral density of trabecular and cortical bone using peripheral quantitative computer tomography. *Horm Res* 1995; 43: 173–5.
42. Compston JE, Smith EM, Matthews C, Schofield P. Whole body composition and regional bone mass in women with insulin-dependent diabetes mellitus. *Clin Endocrinol* 1994; 41: 289–93.
43. Clauson P, Feldt-Rasmussen B, Jacobsen P, Rossing K, Parving HH, Nielsen PK, Feldt-Rasmussen U, Olgaard K. Microalbuminuria as an early indicator of osteopenia in male insulin-dependent diabetic patients. *Diabet Med* 1997; 14: 1038–43.
44. Pascual J, Argente J, Lopez MB, Munoz M, Martinez G, Vazquez MA, Jodar E, Perez-Cano R, Hawkins F. Bone mineral density in children and adolescents with diabetes mellitus type 1 of recent onset. *Calcif Tissue Int* 1998; 62: 31–5.
45. Lunt H, Florkowski CM, Cundy T, Kendall D, Brown LJ, Elliot JR, Wells JE, Turner JG. A population based study of bone mineral density in women with long-standing type 1 (insulin-dependent) diabetes. *Diabetes Res Clin Pract* 1998; 40: 31–8.
46. Hampson G, Evans C, Petitt RJ, Evans WD, Woodhead SJ, Peters JR, Ralston SH. Bone mineral density, college in type 1 alpha 1 genotypes and bone turnover in premenopausal women with diabetes mellitus. *Diabetologia* 1998; 41: 1314–20.
47. Hauache OM, Lazaretti-Castro M, Andreoni S, Gimeno SG, Brandao C, Ramalho AC, Kasamatsu TS, Kunii I, Hayashi LF, Dib SA, Vieira JG. Vitamin D receptor gene polymorphism: correlation with bone mineral density in a Brazilian population with insulin-dependent diabetes mellitus. *Osteoporos Int* 1998; 8: 204–10.
48. Miazgowski T, Czekalski S. A two-year follow-up study of bone mineral density and markers of bone turnover in patients with long-standing insulin-dependent diabetes mellitus. *Osteoporos Int* 1998; 8: 399–403.
49. Rix M, Andreassen H, Eskildsen P. Impact of peripheral neuropathy on bone density in patients with type 1 diabetes. *Diabetes Care* 1999; 22: 827–31.
50. De Schepper J, Smitz J, Rosseneu S, Bollen P, Louis O. Lumbar spine bone mineral density in diabetic children with recent onset. *Horm Res* 1998; 50: 193–6.
51. Gunczler P, Lanes R, Paz-Martinez V, Martins R, Esaa S, Colmenares V, Weisinger JR. Decreased lumbar spine bone mass and low bone turnover in children and adolescents with insulin-dependent diabetes mellitus followed longitudinally. *J Pediatr Endocrinol Metab* 1998; 11: 413–9.
52. Ersoy B, Goksen D, Darcan S, Mavi E, Ozturk C. Evaluation of bone mineral density in children with diabetes mellitus. *Indian J Peditr* 1999; 66: 375–9.
53. Tuominen JT, Impivaara O, Puukka P, Ronnema T. Bone mineral density in patients with type 1 and type 2 diabetes. *Diabetes Care* 2000; 23: 564–5.
54. Christensen JO, Svendsen OL. Bone mineral in pre- and postmenopausal women with insulin-dependent and non-insulin-dependent diabetes mellitus. *Osteoporos Int* 1999; 10: 307–11.
55. Vina Simon E, Bueno Lozano G, Armada Maresca MI, et al. Bone mineral density in juvenile onset diabetes mellitus. *An Esp Pediatr* 2000; 52: 507–15.
56. Rozadilla A, Nolla JM, Montana E, Fiter J, Gomez-Vaquero C, Soler J, Roig-Escofet D. Bone mineral density in patients with type 1 diabetes mellitus. *Joint Bone Spine* 2000; 67: 215–8.

57. Gunczler P, Lanes R, Paoli M, Martinis R, Villaroel O, Weisinger JR. Decreased bone mineral density and bone formation markers shortly after diagnosis of clinical type 1 diabetes mellitus. *J Pediatr Endocrinol Metab* 2001; 14: 525–8.
58. López-Ibarra PJ, Escobar-Jiménez F, Pardo MD, et al. Bone mineral density at time of clinical diagnosis of adult-onset type 1 diabetes mellitus. *Endocr Pract* 2001; 7: 346–51.
59. Valerio G, Del Puente A, Esposito-Del Puente A, Buono P, Mozzillo E, Franzese A. The lumbar bone mineral density is affected by long-term for metabolic control in adolescents with type 1 diabetes mellitus. *Horm Res* 2002; 58: 266–72.
60. Mathiassen B, Nielsen S, Ditzel J, Rodbro P, Long-term bone loss in insulin-dependent diabetes mellitus. *J Int Med* 1990; 227: 325–7.
61. Campos-Pastor MM, López-Ibarra PJ, Escobar-Jíménez F, Serrano Pardo MD, García-Cervigón AG. Intensive insulin therapy and bone mineral density in type 1 diabetes mellitus: a prospective study. *Osteoporos Int* 2000; 11: 455–9.
62. Krakauer JC, McKenna MJ, Buderer NF, Rao DS, Whitehouse FW, Parfitt AM. Bone loss and bone turnover in diabetes. *Diabetes* 1995; 44: 775–82.
63. Soejima D, Landing BH. Osteoporosis in juvenile-onset diabetes mellitus: morphometric and comparative studies. *Pediatr Pathol* 1986; 6: 289–99.
64. Malone JI, Lowitt S, Duncan JA, Shah S, Vargas A, Root A. Hypercalciuria, hyperphosphaturia, and growth retardation in children with diabetes mellitus. *Pediatrics* 1986; 78: 298–304.
65. Thalassinos NC, Hadjiyauni P, Tzanela M, Akvizaki C, Philokiprou D. Calcium metabolism in diabetes mellitus; effect of improved blood glucose control. *Diabet Med* 1993; 10: 341–4.
66. Pedrazzoni M, Ciotti G, Pioli G, Gimsole G, Davo BL, Paturrmmen E, Passers M. Osteocalcin levels in diabetic subjects. *Calcif Tissue Int* 1989; 45: 331–6.
67. Rico H, Hernandez ER, Calibrates JA, Gomez-Cmtresame F. Suggestion of a deficient osteoblsstic function in diabetes mellitus: the possible cause of osteopenia in diabetics. *Calcif Tissue Int* 1989; 45: 71–3.
68. Bjorgaas M, Haug E, Johnsen ID. The urinary excretion of deoxypyridinium cross-links is higher in diabetic than in nondiabefic adolescents. *Calcif Tissue Int* 1999; 65: 121–4.
69. Saggese G, Bertelloni S, Baroncelli GI, Ghirri P. Calcitonin secretion in children with insulin-dependent diabetes mellitus. *Eur J Pediatr* 1991; 150: 464–7.
70. Pietschmann P, Schernthaner G, Wolosmzuk W. Seman ostemalcin levels in diabetes mellitus: analysis of the type of diabetes and microvascular complications. *Diabetologia* 1988; 31: 892–5.
71. Pasaoglu H, Kumandas S, Kelestimur F. Serum osteocalcin levels in type 1 diabetes mellitus. *Turk J Pediatr* 1995; 37: 323–9.
72. Guarneri MP, Weber G, Gallia P, Chiumello G. Effect of insulin treatment on osteocalcin levels in diabetic children and adolescents. *J Endocrinol Invest* 1993; 16: 505–9.
73. Paula FJ, Lanna CM, Shuhama T, Foss MC. Effect of metabolic control on parathyroid hormone secretion in diabetic patients. *Braz J Med Biol Res* 2001; 34: 1139–45.
74. Jehle PM, Jehle DR, Mohan S, Bohm BO. Serum levels of insulin like growth factor system components and relationship to bone metabolism in type 1 and type 2 diabetes mellitus patients. *J Endocrinol* 1998; 159: 297–306.
75. Katayama Y, Celic S, Nagat N, Martin TJ, Findlay DM. Nonenzymatic glycation of type I collagen modifies interaction with UMR 201–108 preosteoblastic cells. *Bone* 1997; 21: 237–42.
76. Ishide H, Seino Y, Matsukura S, Ikeda M, Yawata M, Yamashita G, Ishizuka S, Imura H. Diabetic osteopenia and circulating levels of vitamin D metabolites in type 2 (non-insulin-dependent) diabetes. *Metabolism* 1985; 34: 797–801.
77. Johnston CC, Hui SL, Longcope C. Bone mass and sex steroid concentrations in postmenopausal Caucasian diabetics. *Metabolism* 1985; 34: 544–50.
78. Weinstock RS, Goland RS, Shane E, Clemens TL, Lindsay R, Bilezikian JP. Bone mineral density in women with type II diabetes mellitus. *J Bone Miner Res* 1989; 4: 97–101.
79. Hafner SM, Bauer RL. The association of obesity and glucose and insulin concentrations with bone density in premenopausal and postmenopausal women. *Metabolism* 1993; 42: 735–9.
80. Wakasugi M, Wakao R, Tawata M, Gan N, Koizumi K, Onaya T. Bone mineral density measured by dual energy x-ray absorptiometry in patients with non-insulin-dependent diabetes mellitus. *Bone* 1989; 14: 29–33.
81. Bauer DC, Browner WS, Canter JA, Orwell ES, Scott JC, Black DM, Tao JL, Cunmtings SR, for the Study of Osteoporosic Fractures Research Group. Factors associated with eppendicular bone mass in older women. *Ann Intern Med* 1993; 118: 657–65.
82. Van Daele P, Stolk RP, Burger H, et al. Bone density in non-insulin-dependent diabetes mellitus. The Rotterdam Study. *Ann Intern Med* 1995; 122: 409–14.
83. Sahin G, Bagis S, Cimen OB, Ozisik S, Guler H, Erdogan C. Lumbar and femoral bone mineral density in type 2 Turkish diabetic patients. *Acta Med* 2001; 44: 141–3.
84. Barrett-Connor E, Holbrook TL. Sex differences in osteoporosis in older adults with non-insulin-dependent diabetes mellitus. *JAMA* 1992; 268: 3333–7.
85. Miedany YM, el Gaafary S, el Baddinie MA. Osteoporosis in older adults with non-insulin-dependent diabetes mellitus: is it sex related? *Clin Exp Rheumatol* 1999; 36: 35–8.
86. Chung YS, Lee MD, Lee SK, Kim HM, Fitzpatrick LA, HMG-CoA reductase inhibitors increase BMD in type 2 diabetes mellitus patients. *J Clin Endocrinol Metab* 2000; 85: 1137–42.
87. Bouillon R. Diabetic bone disease. *Calcif Tissue Int* 1991; 49: 155–60.
88. Menczel 1, Makin M, Robin G. Prevalence of diabetes mellitus in Jerusalem: its association with osteoporosis. *Isr J Med Sci* 1972; 88: 918–9.
89. Melchior TM, Sorensen H, Torp-Pedersen C. Hip and distal arm fracture rates in peri- and postmenapausal insulin-treated diabetic femalses. *J Intern Med* 1994; 236: 203–8.
90. Forsón L, Meyer HE, Midlhjell K, Edna TH. Diahetes mellitus and the incidence of hip fracture: results from the Nord-Trondelag Health Survey. *Diabetologia* 1999; 42: 920–5.
91. Schwartz AV, Sellmeyer DE, Ensrud KE, Cauley JA, Tabor KA, Schreiner PJ, Jamal SA, Black DM, Cummings SR. Older women with diabetes have an

increased risk of fracture: a prospective study. *J Clin Endocrinol Metab* 2001; 86: 32–8

92. Seeley DG, Kelsey J, Jergas M, Nevitt MC, for the Study of Osteoporotic Fractures Research Group. Predictors of ankle and foot fractures in older women. *J Bone Miner Res* 1996; 11: 1347–55.
93. Bland JH, Frymoyer JW, Newberg AH. Rheumatic syndromes in endocrine disease. *Semin Arthritis Rheum* 1979; 9: 23–65.
94. Crisp AJ, Heathcote JG. Connective tissue abnormalities in diabetes mellitus. *J R Coll Physicians Lond* 1984; 18: 132–41.
95. Spagnola AM, Bennett PH, Ternsald PI. Vertebral ankylosing hyperostosis (Forestier's disease) and HLA antigens in pima indiam. *Arthritis Rheum* 1978; 21: 467–72.
96. Sahin G, Polat G, Bagis S, Milcan A, Erdogan C. Study of axial bone mineral density in postmenopausal women with diffuse idiopathic skeletal hyperostosis related to type 2 diabetes mellitus. *J Womens Health* 2002; 11: 801–4.
97. Mobasheri A, Vannuci SJ, Bondy CA, Carter SD, Innes JF, Arteaga MF, Trujillo E, Ferraz I, Shakibaei M, Martin-Vasallo P. Glucose transport and metabolism in chondrocytes: a key to understanding chondrogenesis, skeletal development and cartilage degradation in osteoarthritis. *Histol Histopathol* 2002; 17: 1239–67.
98. Frey MI, Barrett-Connor E, Sledge PA, Schneider DL, Weissman MH. The effect of noninsulin-dependent diabetes mellitus on the prevalence of clinical osteoarthritis. A population based study. *J Rheumatol* 1996; 23: 716–22.
99. Sturmer T, Brenner H, Brenner RE, Gunther KP. Non-insulin-dependent diabetes mellitus (NIDDM) and patterns of osteoarthritis the Ulm osteoarthritis study. *Scand J Rheumatol* 2001; 30: 169–71.
100. Caspi D, Flusser G, Farber I, Ribak J, Leibovitz A, Habot B, Yaron M, Segal R. Clinical, radiologic, demographic, and occupational aspects of hand osteoarthritis in the elderly. *Semin Arthritis Rheum* 2001; 30: 321–31.
101. Pastan RS, Cohen AS. The rheumatologic manifestations of diabetes mellitus. *Med Clin North Am* 1978; 62: 829–39.
102. Marble A, Krall LP, Bradley RF, Christlieb AR, Soeldner JS (eds), *Joslin's Diabetes Mellitus*, 12 th edn. Philadelphia: Lea & Febiger, 1985; p 846.
103. Dessein PH, Joffe BI, Stanwix A, Botha AS, Moomal Z. The acute phase response does not fully predict the presence of insulin resistance and dyslipidemia in inflammatory arthritis. *J Rheumatol* 2002; 29: 462–6.
104. Svenson KLG, Pollare T, Lithell H, Hallgren R. Impaired glucose handling in active rheumatoid arthritis: relationship to peripheral insulin resistance. *Metabolism* 1998; 37: 125–30.
105. Torfs CP, King M-C, Huey B, Malmgren J, Grumet FC. Genetic interrelationship between insulin-dependent diabetes mellitus, the autoimmune thyroid diseases, and rheumatoid arthritis. *Am J Hum Genet* 1986; 38: 170–87.
106. Dessein PH, Stanwix A, Joffe BI. Cardiovascular risk in rheumatoid arthritis versus osteoarthritis: acute phase response related decreased insulin sensitivity and high-density lipoprotein cholesterol as well as clustering of metabolic syndrome features in rheumatoid arthritis. *Arthritis Res* 2002; 4: R5.
107. Jelinek JE. Collagen disorders in which diabetes and cutaneous features coexist. In Jelinek JE (ed), *The Skin in Diabetes*. Philadelphia: Lea & Febiger, 1986; pp 155–73.
108. Cole GW, Headley J, Skowsky R. Scleredema diabeticorum: a common and distinct cutaneous manifestation of diabetes mellitus. *Diabetes Care* 1983; 6: 189–92.
109. Van De Staak WJBM, Bergers AMG. Ultrastructural abnormalities in the skin nerves of a patient with scleroderma adultorum (Buschke) and diabetes mellitus. *Dermatologia* 1975; 151: 223–7.
110. Iwasaki T, Kohama T, Houjou S, et al. Diabetic scleredema and scleroderma-like changes in a patient with maturity onset type diabetes of young people. *Dermatology* 1994; 188: 228–31.
111. Noble J, Heathcote JG, Cohn H. Diabetes mellitus in the aetiology of Dupuytren's disease (DD). *J Bone Joint Surg Br* 1984; 66: 322–5.
112. Arkkila PE, Kantola IM, Viikari JS. Dupuytren's disease: association with chronic diabetic complications. *J Rheumatol* 1997; 24: 153–9.
113. Bazin S, LeLous M, Duance VC, Sims TJ, Bailey AJ, Gabbiani G, D'Andiran G, Pizzolato G, Browski A, Nicoletis C, Delaunay A. Biochemistry and histology of the connective tissue of Dupuytren's disease lesions. *Eur J Clin Invest* 1980; 10: 9–16.
114. Baird KS, Crossan JF, Alwan WH, Wojciak B. T cell-mediated response in Dupuytren's disease. *Lancet* 1993; 341: 1622–3.
115. Sugrue D, McEvoy M, Dempsey J, Fitzgerald G, Drury MI. Diabetic stiff hand syndrome. *Ir J Med Sci* 1983; 152: 152–6.
116. Jung Y, Hohmann TC, Gerneth JA, Novak J, Wasserman RC, D'Andrea BJ, Newton RH, Danowski TS. Diabetic hand syndrome. *Metabolism* 1971; 20: 1008–14.
117. Ceruso M, Lauri G, Bufalini C, Bartolozzi G, Bernardini S, Cinti S, Morroni M, Matucci-Cerinic M. Diabetic hand syndrome. *J Hand Surg* 1988; 13A: 765–70.
118. Falkiner S, Myers S. When exactly can carpal tunnel syndrome be considered work-related? *Aust N Z J Surg* 2002; 72: 204–9.
119. Bridgeman JF. Periarthritis of the shoulder and diabetes mellitus. *Ann Rheum Dis* 1972; 312: 69–71.
120. Fisher L, Kurtz A, Shipley M. Association between cheiroarthropathy and frozen shoulder in patients with insulin-dependent diabetes mellitus. *Br J Rheumatol* 1986; 25: 1141–6.
121. Pal B, Andersen J, Dick WR, Griffiths ID. Limitation of joint mobility and shoulder capsulitis in insulin- and non-insulin-dependent diabetes mellitus. *Br J Rheumatol* 1986; 25: 147–51.
122. Morén-Hybbinette I, Moritz U, Schersten B. The clinical picture of the painful diabetic shoulder—natural history, social consequences and analysis of concomitant hand syndrome. *Acta Med Scand* 1987; 221: 73–82.
123. Arkkila PE, Kantola IM, Viikari JS, Ronnemaa T. Shoulder capsulitis in type I and II diabetic patients: association with diabetic complications and related diseases. *Ann Rheum Dis* 1996; 55: 907–14.
124. Rosenbloom AL, Frias JL. Diabetes, short stature and joint stiffness—a new syndrome. *Clin Res* 1974; 22: 92A.
125. Grgic A, Rosenbloom AL, Weber FT, Giordano B. Joint contracture in childhood diabetes. *N Engl J Med* 1975; 292: 372.

126. Isshiki G, Osasa Y, Fujiwara Y, Izumi K, Kuno S, Okuno G. Joint contractures in childhood diabetes. In Mimura G, Kitagawa T, Hibi I (eds), *Childhood Diabetes in Asia*. Tokyo: Medical Journal Sha, 1979; pp 226–30.
127. Benedetti A, Noacco C. Hand changes in childhood onset diabetes. *Pediatr Adolesc Endocr* 1981; 9: 149–55.
128. Kennedy L, Beacom R, Archer DB, Carson DJ, Campbell SL, Johnston PB, Maguire CJ. Limited joint mobility in type I diabetes mellitus. *Postgrad Med J* 1982; 58: 481–4.
129. Brice JEH, Johnston DI, Noronha JL. Limited finger joint mobility in diabetes. *Arch Dis Child* 1982; 157: 879–80.
130. Lawson PM, Maneschi F, Kohner EM. The relationship of hand abnormalities to diabetes and diabetic retinopathy. *Diabetes Care* 1983; 6: 140–3.
131. Campbell RR, Hawkins SJ, Maddison PJ, Reckless JPD. Limited joint mobility in diabetes mellitus. *Ann Rheum Dis* 1985; 44: 93–7.
132. Clarke CF, Piesowicz AT, Spathis GS. Limited joint mobility in children and adolescents with insulin dependent diabetes mellitus. *Ann Rheum Dis* 1990; 49: 236–7.
133. Eadington DW, Patrick AW, Collier A, Frier BM. Limited joint mobility, Dupuytren's contracture, and retinopathy in type 1 diabetes: association with cigarette smoking. *Diabet Med* 1989; 6: 152–7.
134. Garza-Elizondo MA, Diaz-Jouanen E, Franco-Casique JJ, Alarcon-Segovia D. Joint contractures and scleroderma-like skin changes in the hands of insulin-dependent juvenile diabetics. *J Rheumatol* 1983; 10: 797–800.
135. Mengistu M, Abdulkadir J. Limited finger joint mobility in insulin-dependent and non-insulin-dependent Ethiopian diabetics. *Diabet Med* 1985; 2: 387–9.
136. Madacsy L, Peja M, Korompay K, Biro B. Limited joint mobility in diabetic children: a risk factor of diabetic complications? *Acta Paediatr Hung* 1986; 27: 91–6.
137. Gertner E, Sukenik S, Gladman DD, Hanna W, Lee P, Bombardier C, Hanna AK. HLA antigens and nailfold capillary microscopy studies in patients with insulin dependent and non-insulin dependent diabetes mellitus and limited joint mobility. *J Rheumatol* 1990; 17: 1375–9.
138. Tubiana-Rufi N, Prieur AM, Bourden R, Pridlet P, Czernichow P. Détection précoce limitation de la mobilité articulaire chez l'enfantet l'adolescent diabetiques. *Diabète Métab* 1991; 17: 504–11.
139. Vera M, Rosales C, Alvarez MC, Guell R. Limitacion de los movimientos articulares (LMA) en diabeticos insulino dependientes. Consideraciones y hallazgos clinicos. *Av Diabetol* 1990; 3: 135–40.
140. Kakourou T, Dacou-Voutetakis C, Kavadias G, Bakoula C, Aroni K. Limited joint mobility and lipodystrophy in children and adolescents with insulin-dependent diabetes mellitus. *Pediatr Dermatol* 1994; 11: 310–4.
141. Vukovic J, Dumic M, Radica A, Filipovic-Grcic B, Jovanovic V. Risk factors for expression and progression of limited joint mobility in insulin-dependent childhood diabetes. *Acta Diabetol* 1996; 33: 15–8.
142. Duffin AC, Donaghue KC, Potter M, McInnes A, Chan AK, King J, Howard NJ, Silink M. Limited joint mobility in hands and feet of adolescents with type 1 diabetes mellitus. *Diabet Med* 1999; 16: 125–30.
143. Veijola R, Knip M, Risteli L, Risteli J, Kaar ML, Puuka R, Ilonen J. Clinical characteristics and circulating collagen and laminin metabolites in insulin-dependent diabetic children with joint and skin manifestations. *Pediatr Res* 1993; 33: 501–5.
144. Reimer-Veit M, Burger W, Kroll M, Oberdisse U, Hovener G, Enders I, Weber B. Prevalence and development of limited joint mobility in type 1 diabetic children and adolescents. *Pediatr Adolesc Endocr* 1988; 111–21.
145. Lebedev NB, Kuraeva TL. Limited mobility of the joints: a complication of diabetes mellitus in children and adolescents. *Probl Endokrinol (Mosk)* 1994; 40: 4–7.
146. Sukenik S, Weitzman S, Buskila D, Eyal A, Gross J, Horwitz J. Limited joint mobility and other rheumatological manifestations in diabetic patients. *Diabete Metab* 1987; 13: 187–92.
147. Starkman H, Brink S. Limited joint mobility of the hand in type I diabetes mellitus. *Diabetes Care* 1982; 5: 534–6.
148. Seibold J. Digital sclerosis in children with insulin dependent diabetes mellitus. *Arthritis Rheum* 1982; 25: 1357–61.
149. Rosenbloom AL, Silverstein JH, Riley WJ, Maclaren NK. Limited joint mobility in childhood diabetes: family studies. *Diabetes Care* 1983; 6: 370–3.
150. Buckingham BA, Uitto J, Sandborg C, Keens T, Roe T, Costin G, Kaufman F, Bernstein B, Landing B, Castellano A. Scleroderma-like changes in insulin-dependent diabetes mellitus: clinical and biochemical studies. *Diabetes Care* 1984; 7: 163–9.
151. Rosenbloom AL, Malone JI, Yucha J, Van Cader TC. Limited joint mobility and diabetic retinopathy demonstrated by fluorescein angiography. *Eur J Pediatr* 1984; 141: 163–4.
152. Costello PB, Tambar PK, Green FA. The prevalence and possible prognostic importance of arthropathy in childhood diabetes. *J Rheumatol* 1984; 11: 62–5.
153. Buckingham B, Perejda AJ, Sandborg C, Kershnar AK, Uitto J. Skin, joint, and pulmonary changes in type I diabetes mellitus. *Am J Dis Child* 1986; 140: 420–3.
154. Buithieu M, Rosenbloom AL, Conlon M, Thomas JL. Joint mobility and control in IDDM patients. *Diabetes* 1988; 37: 129A.
155. Infante JR, Rosenbloom AL, Silverstein JH, Garzarella L, Pollock BH. Changes in frequency and severity of limited joint mobility in children with type 1 diabetes mellitus between 1976–78 and 1998. *J Pediatr* 2001; 138: 33–7.
156. Karavanaki K, Baum JD. Prevalence of microvascular and neurologic abnormalities in a population of diabetic children. *J Pediatr Endocrinol Metab* 1999; 12: 411–22.
157. Fitzcharles MA, Duby S, Waddell RW, Banks E, Karsh J. Limitation of joint mobility (cheiro-arthropathy) in adult non-insulin-dependent diabetic patients. *Ann Rheum Dis* 1984; 43: 251–7.
158. Rossi P, Fossaluzza V. Diabetic cheiroarthropathy in adult non-insulin-dependent diabetes. *Ann Rheum Dis* 1985; 44: 141–2.
159. Larkin JG, Frier BM. Limited joint mobility and Dupuytren's contracture in diabetic, hypertensive, and normal populations. *Br Med J* 1986; 292: 1494.
160. Akanji AO, Bella AF, Osotimehin BO. Cheiroarthropathy and long-term diabetic complications in Nigerians. *Ann Rheum Dis* 1990; 49: 28–30.
161. Jennings AM, Milner PC, Ward JD. Hand abnormalities are associated with the complications of diabetes in type 2 diabetes. *Diabet Med* 1989; 6: 43–7.
162. Eadington DW, Patrick AW, Frier BM. Association between connective tissue changes and smoking habit in type 2 diabetes and in non-diabetic humans. *Diabetes Res Clin Pract* 1991; 11: 121–6.

163. Lu YC, Wang PW, Liu RT, Tung SC, Chien WY, Hung SL, Chen M. Limited joint mobility of the hand: prevalence and relation to chronic complications in nine insulin-dependent diabetes mellitus patients. *J Formos Med Assoc* 1993; 92: 139–43.
164. Fernando DJF, Vernidharan J. Limited joint mobility in Sri Lankan patients with non-insulin-dependent diabetes. *Br J Rheumatol* 1997; 36: 374–6.
165. Arkkila PET, Kantola IM, Viikari JSA. Limited joint mobility in non-insulin-dependent diabetic (NIDDM) patients: correlation to control of diabetes, atherosclerotic vascular disease, and other diabetic complications. *J Diabetes Complications* 1997; 11: 208–17.
166. Grgic A, Rosenbloom AL, Weber FT, Giordano B, Malone JI, Shuster JJ. Joint contracture—common manifestation of childhood diabetes mellitus. *J Pediatr* 1976; 8: 584–8.
167. Salzarulo HH, Taylor LA. Diabetic "stiff joint syndrome" as a cause of difficult endotracheal intubation. *Anesthesiology* 1986; 64: 366–8.
168. Vani V, Kamath SK, Naik LD. The palm print as a sensitive indicator of difficult laryngoscopy in diabetics: a comparison with other airway evaluation indices. *J Postgrad Med* 2000; 46: 75–9.
169. Warner ME, Contreras MG, Warner MA, Schroeder DR, Munn SR, Maxson PM. Diabetes mellitus and difficult laryngoscopy in renal and pancreatic transplant patients. *Anesth Analg* 1998; 86: 516–9.
170. Fernando DJS, Masson EA, Veves A, Boulton AJM. Relationship of limited joint mobility to abnormal foot pressures and diabetic foot ulceration. *Diabetes Care* 1991; 14: 8–11.
171. Sauseng S, Kastenbauer T, Irsigler K. Limited joint mobility in selected hand and foot joints in patients with type 1 diabetes mellitus: a methodology comparison. *Diabetes Nutr Metab* 2002; 15: 1–6.
172. Tinley P, Tatanto M. Clinical and dynamic range of motion techniques in subjects with and without diabetes mellitus. *J Am Podiatr Med Assoc* 2002; 92: 136–42.
173. Benedetti A, Noacco C. Juvenile diabetic cheiroarthropathy. *Acta Diabet Lat* 1976; 13: 54–66.
174. Aljahian M, Lee K-C, Toth E. Limited joint mobility in diabetes: diabetic cheiroarthropathy may be a clue to more serious complications [online]. *Postgrad Med* 1999; 105: 1–5.
175. Brik R, Berant M, Vardi P. The scleroderma-like syndrome of insulin-dependent diabetes mellitus. *Diabetes Metab Rev* 1991; 7: 121–8.
176. Rosenbloom AL, Silverstein JH, Lezotte DC, Riley WJ, Maclaren NK. Limited joint mobility in diabetes mellitus in childhood: natural history and relationship to growth impairment. *J Pediatr* 1982; 101: 874–8.
177. Silverstein JH, Gordon G, Pollock BH, Rosenbloom AL. Long-term glycemic control influences the onset of limited joint mobility in type 1 diabetes. *J Pediatr* 1998; 132: 944–7.
178. Infante R, Rosenbloom AL, Silverstein JH, Garzarella L, Pollock BH. Limited joint mobility (LJM) and stature in childhood type 1 diabetes mellitus (DM1): improved methods of control are making a difference. In *Proc Endocr Soc 81st Ann Mtg*, San Diego, CA, 1999.
179. Penfold J, Chase HP, Marshall G, Walravens CF, Walravens PA, Garg SK. The final adult height and its relationship to blood glucose control and microvascular complications in IDDM. *Diabet Med* 1995; 12: 129–33.
180. Rosenbloom AL. Joint contractures preceding insulin-dependent diabetes mellitus. *Arthritis Rheum* 1983; 26: 931.
181. Sieratzki JS, Charnley G, Morgan MH, Witherow PJ. Case of the month: an 8-year-old girl with clumsiness, grip weakness, and hypoplasia of the right hand. *Eur J Pediatr* 1997; 156: 579–80
182. Robertson JR, Earnshaw PM, Campbell IW. Tenolysis in juvenile diabetic cheiroarthropathy. *Br Med J* 1979; 2: 971–2.
183. Eaton RP, Sibbett WL, Harsh A. The effect of an aldose reductase inhibiting agent on limited joint mobility in diabetic patients. *JAMA* 1985; 253: 1437–40.
184. Rosenbloom AL. Sorbinil and limited joint mobility in diabetes. *JAMA* 1985; 254: 1453–4.
185. Gamstedt A, Holm-Glad J, Ohlson CG, Sundstrom M. Hand abnormalities are strongly associated with the duration of diabetes mellitus. *J Intern Med* 1993; 234: 189–93.
186. Chammas M, Bousquet P, Renard E, Poirer JL, Jaffiol C, Allieu Y. Dupuytren's disease, carpal tunnels syndrome, trigger finger, and diabetes mellitus. *J Hand Surg* 1995; 20: 109–14.
187. Polak M, Le Luyer B, Rybojab M, Czernichow P. Case report: insulin-dependent diabetes mellitus in childhood associated with scleroderma. *Diabetes Metab* 1996; 22: 192–6.
188. Kennedy L, Richie C, Lyons TJ, Beacom R. Limited joint mobility in diabetes—some clinical and biochemical aspects. In Serrano-Rios M, Lefèbvre PJ (eds), *Diabetes 1985*. Amsterdam: Elsevier, 1986; pp 767–70.
189. Ficicioglu C, Kiziltan M, Aydin A, Basio P. Relation between limited joint mobility and peripheral nerve function in diabetic children. *Turk J Pediatr* 1996; 38: 431–7.
190. Baum VC, Levitsky LL, Englander RM. Abnormal cardiac function after exercise in insulin-dependent diabetic children and adolescents. *Diabetes Care* 1987; 10: 319–23.
191. Schuyler MR, Niewoehner E, Inkley SR, Kohn R. Abnormal lung elasticity in juvenile diabetes mellitus. *Am Rev Respir Dis* 1976; 113: 37–41.
192. Barta L. Flexion contractures in a diabetic child (Rosenbloom syndrome). *Eur J Pediatr* 1980; 135: 101–2.
193. Schnapf BM, Banks R, Silverstein JH, Rosenbloom AL, Chesrown S, Loughlin G. Pulmonary function in insulin dependent diabetes mellitus with limited joint mobility. *Am Rev Respir Dis* 1984; 130: 930–2.
194. Vera M, Suffos R, Carriles M, Guell R, Picasso N, Alvarez MC, A study of the respiratory function in insulin-dependent diabetic patients with and without limited joint mobility (LJM). *Acta Diabetol Lat* 1998; 27: 113–7.
195. Soler NG, Khardori R. Fibrous disease of the breast, thyroiditis, and cheiroarthropathy in type I diabetes mellitus. *Lancet* 1984; i: 193–5.
196. Collier A, Matthews DM, Kellett HA, Clarke BF, Hunter JA. Change in skin thickness associated with cheiroarthropathy in insulin dependent diabetes mellitus. *Br Med J* 1986; 292: 936.
197. Lieberman LS, Rosenbloom AL. Changes in growth and body composition related to control in children with diabetes. In Borms J, Hauspie R, Sand A, Susanne C, Hebbelink M (eds), *Human Growth and Development*. New York: Plenum, 1984; pp 619–25.

198. Hanna W, Friesen D, Bombardier C, Gladman D, Hanna A. Pathologic features of diabetic thick skin. *J Am Acad Dermatol* 1987; 16: 546–53.
199. Bertheim U, Engstrom-Laurent A, Hofer P-A, Hallgren P, Asplund J, Hellstrom S. Loss of hyaluronan in the basement membrane zone of the skin correlates to the degree of stiff hands in diabetic patients. *Acta Derm Venereol* 2002; 82: 329–34.
200. Montana E, Rozadilla A, Nolla JM, Gomez N, Escofet DR, Soler J. Microalbuminuria is associated with limited joint mobility in type 1 diabetes mellitus. *Ann Rheum Dis* 1995; 54: 582–6.
201. Frost D, Beischer W. Limited joint mobility in type 1 diabetic patients. Associations with microangiopathy and subclinical macroangiopathy are different in men and women. *Diabetes Care* 2001; 24: 95–9.
202. Silverstein JH, Fennell R, Donnelly W, Banks R, Stratton R, Spillar R, Rosenbloom AL. Correlates of biopsy-studied nephropathy in young patients with insulin-dependent diabetes mellitus. *J Pediatr* 1985; 106: 196–201.
203. Arkkila PE, Kantola IM, Viikari JS. Limited joint mobility in non-insulin-dependent diabetic (NIDDM) patients: correlation to control of diabetes, atherosclerotic vascular disease, and other diabetic complications. *J Diabetes Complications* 1997; 11: 208–17.
204. Kohn RR, Schnider SL. Glucosylation of human collagen. *Diabetes* 1982; 31 (suppl 3): 47–51.
205. Perejda A, Buckingham B, Uitto J, Kaufman F, Sandborg C, Kershnar A. Correlation of increased collagen cross-linking with diabetic complications. *Diabetes* 1985; 34 (suppl 1): 105A.
206. Monnier VM, Vishwanath V, Frank KE, Elmets CA, Dauchot P, Kohn RR. Relation between complications of type 1 diabetes mellitus and collagen-linked fluorescence. *N Engl J Med* 1986; 314: 403–8.
207. Dyer G, Dunn JA. Thorpe SR, Bailie KE, Lyons TJ, McCance DR, Baynes JW. Accumulation of Maillard reaction products in skin collagen in diabetes and aging. *J Clin Invest* 1993; 91: 2463–9.
208. McCance DR, Dyer G, Dunn JA, Bailie KE, Thorpe SR, Baynes JW, Lyons TJ. Maillard reaction products and their relation to complications in insulin-dependent diabetes mellitus. *J Clin Invest* 1993; 91: 2470–8.
209. Chiarelli F, de Martino M, Mezzetti A, Catino M, Morgese G, Cuccurullo F, Verrotti A. Advanced glycation and products in children and adolescents with diabetes: relation to glycemic control and early microvascular complications. *J Pediatr* 1999; 134: 486–91.
210. Monnier VM, Bautista O, Kenny D, Sell DR, Fogarty J, Dahms W, Cleary PA, Lachin J, Genuth S, for the DCCT Skin Collagen Ancillary Study Group. Skin collagen glycation, glycoxidation, and cross-linking are lower in subjects with long-term intensive versus conventional therapy of type 1 diabetes.relevance of glycated collagen products versus HbA1c as markers of diabetic complications. *Diabetes* 1999; 48: 870–80.
211. Eaton RP. Aldose reductase inhibition and the diabetic syndrome of limited joint mobility: implications for altered collagen hydration. *Metabolism* 1986; 35 (suppl 1): 119–21.
212. Rosenbloom AL, Buithieu M, Jellife KA, Atchison RD, Truglia JA. Effect of an aldose reductase inhibiting agent on limited joint mobility in insulin dependent diabetes mellitus. *Diabetes Care* 1992; 15: 588–9.
213. The Diabetes Control and Complications Trial (DCCT): the effect of intensive treatment of diabetes on the development and progression of long-term complications in insulin-dependent diabetes mellitus. *N Engl J Med* 1993; 329: 977–86.
214. Traisman H, Traisman ES, Marr TJ, Wise J. Joint contractures in patients with juvenile diabetes and their siblings. *Diabetes Care* 1978; 1: 360–1.
215. Fitzgerald GA, Greally JF, Drury MI. The syndrome of diabetes insipidus, diabetes mellitus and optic atrophy (DIDMOA) with diabetic cheiroarthropathy. *Postgrad Med J* 1978; 54: 815–7.
216. Winter WE, Maclaren NK, Riley WR, Toskes PP, Andres J, Rosenbloom A. Congenital pancreatic hypoplasia: a syndrome of exocrine and endocrine pancreatic insufficiency. *J Pediatr* 1986; 109: 465–8.
217. Rosenbloom AL, Rosebloom EK. Insulin-dependent childhood diabetes: normal viability of cultured fibroblasts. *Diabetes* 1978; 27: 338–41.
218. Spanheimer RG, Umpierrez GE, Stumpf V. Decreased collagen production in diabetic rats. *Diabetes* 1988; 37: 371–6.
219. Monnier VM, Elmets CA, Frank KE, Vishwanath V. Yamashita T. Age-related normalization of the browning rate of collagen in diabetic subjects without retinopathy. *J Clin Invest* 1986; 78: 832–5.
220. Kennedy L, Lyons TJ. Non-enzymatic glycosylation. *Br Med Bull* 1989; 445: 174–90.

72

Periodontal Disease and Diabetes Mellitus

Robert J. Genco

State University of New York at Buffalo, Buffalo, NY, USA

Periodontal disease has been recognized in the past decade as the sixth complication of diabetes mellitus [1]. This is based on strong evidence showing that both type 1 and type 2 diabetic patients have more severe periodontal disease than do individuals without diabetes. In fact, signs and symptoms of periodontal disease may be among the first manifestations of diabetes. Furthermore, there is evidence that diabetic patients who have periodontal disease suffer from poor glycemic control, as evidenced by increased levels of glycated hemoglobin, and that treatment of periodontal disease in diabetic patients often results in improvement of metabolic control, as evidenced by a reduction in glycated hemoglobin. Therefore, an understanding of the relationship between diabetes and periodontal disease is essential to the management of the diabetic patient.

OVERVIEW OF PERIODONTAL DISEASE

There are two main types of periodontal disease: gingivitis, in which the gingiva surrounding the teeth is reddened, inflamed, and bleeds easily; and periodontitis, in which the infection and inflammation surrounding the teeth has proceeded to destroy the ligamentous attachment of the teeth as well as the alveolar bone surrounding the teeth. The ultimate result of periodontal disease is loss of the teeth by exfoliation.

Periodontal diseases are caused by infections with oral organisms that form biofilms around the teeth. These biofilms are constantly forming and maturing, difficult to remove and highly resistant to antibiotics and other antimicrobial agents. The main pathologic changes in periodontal disease are thought to occur as a result of the body's response to infection with these microbial pathogens.

Periodontitis is often an asymptomatic or silent infection that goes undetected by both the patient and the physician. Even an oral examination may reveal nothing more than gingival redness, spacing between the teeth, and occasional bleeding of the gingiva. Periodontal disease is highly prevalent, estimated to affect 35% of the adult population of the United States. Severe forms of the disease are age related and affect 1–30% of the population from the second decade to the seventh and eighth decade of life [2].

In view of the high prevalence of periodontal disease in the general population and its strong association with diabetes mellitus, it is incumbent upon the physician to be alert to any signs or symptoms of periodontal disease in the diabetic patient. These signs and symptoms include gingival redness, swelling, periodontal pockets, halitosis, painful periodontal abscesses, with looseness and loss of teeth in severe cases.

PATHOGENESIS OF PERIODONTAL DISEASE

Periodontal disease is a complex interplay between specific pathogenic organisms, host response to these microorganisms, and environmental risk factors [3]. There are approximately 15 bacterial species implicated in periodontal pathogenesis. These include *Actinobacillus actinomycetemcomitans*, *Porphyromonas gingivalis*, *Prevotella intermedia*, *Bacteroides forsythus*, and *Treponema denticola* [4]. Viruses such as Epstein-Barr virus type 1 (EBV-1) and human cytomegalovirus (HCMV) may also play a role in the development of periodontal disease by altering local host responses [5].

The host immune response to these microbial insults determines the course of disease. For example, polymorphonuclear leukocyte function is especially instrumental in the pathogenesis of periodontal disease [6].

International Textbook of Diabetes Mellitus, Third Edition. Edited by R. A. DeFronzo, E. Ferrannini, H. Keen, and P. Zimmet.
 ISBN: 0-471-48655-8.

Patients who suffer from abnormalities or reduction in polymorphonuclear leukocyte function suffer from more severe periodontal disease. This condition may be relevant to some diabetic patients who have reduced polymorphonuclear leukocyte function. Proinflammatory mediators triggered by periodontal organisms, such as prostaglandin E_2 (PGE_2), interleukin 1 (IL-1), tumor necrosis factor α (TNF-α), and the matrix metalloproteinases are thought to play a major role in the destruction of the collagenous fibers of the gingiva and periodontal ligament, as well as being responsible, in part, for pathologic alveolar bone resorption.

Environmental factors, most notably smoking, influence a patient's susceptibility to periodontal disease. For example, cigarette smoking has been established as a significant independent risk factor for periodontal disease. Even moderate smokers have nearly a fourfold relative risk of developing severe periodontitis when compared with nonsmokers [7, 8].

THE RELATIONSHIP BETWEEN DIABETES MELLITUS AND PERIODONTAL DISEASE

Periodontal disease is more prevalent in diabetic patients. In fact, periodontal disease and diabetes mellitus have a mutually detrimental effect. It is reasonable to expect that since diabetic patients are well known to have increased vulnerability to infection, diabetic patients will also have an increased risk of developing periodontal infections. Many epidemiologic studies have confirmed the strength of this association. For example, the prevalence of periodontal disease among individuals with type 1 diabetes is about 10 times higher than that in a nondiabetic control population. There is a juvenile form of periodontitis found in people with type 1 diabetes, which resembles localized juvenile periodontitis, an unrelated entity, which is particularly subtle and patients are rarely aware that they have the condition [9].

A fairly definitive series of studies of type 2 diabetes has been carried out in Pima Indians, a population with the world's highest reported prevalence of type 2 diabetes. In these studies, the age of onset, severity, and prevalence of periodontal disease are all adversely affected by type 2 diabetes [10, 11]. In fact, individuals with diabetes are up to four times as likely to develop periodontal disease as their nondiabetic counterparts [12]. Poorly controlled diabetes increases the risk of experiencing progressive periodontal bone loss more than diabetes that is under good glycemic control [13]. Periodontal disease is also more severe in patients with diabetes mellitus if they also suffer from other complications such as retinopathy [14].

It is clear from these studies that good control of diabetes will reduce the likelihood of patients developing periodontal disease. It is also clear that diabetic patients who practice good oral hygiene will be less likely to develop periodontal disease. The approach to managing periodontal disease in diabetic patients is recognition of the relationship and proper prevention and management of both conditions.

DECREASED GLYCEMIC CONTROL IN PERIODONTAL PATIENTS

The relationship between diabetes and periodontal disease is a two-way relationship [15]. The diabetic patient with active periodontal disease has been shown to have decreased glycemic control over time. It has been reported that when periodontal infections are treated in diabetic patients, the patient's glycemic control is improved. For example, severe periodontitis has been found to be strongly associated with poor glycemic control, defined as glycated hemoglobin of 9% or more [16]. Patients treated to resolve periodontal infections show significant reductions, up to 10% from pretreatment values, in their HbA_{1c} levels [17].

These studies provide compelling evidence of the close link between periodontal disease and diabetes mellitus, and the paramount importance of maintaining good periodontal health in the diabetic patient.

RELATIONSHIP OF PERIODONTAL DISEASE TO DIABETIC COMPLICATIONS

Related findings further emphasize the important role of periodontal health in diabetic patients. It has long been known that individuals with diabetes are at heightened risk for cardiovascular disease. Recently, it has been demonstrated that periodontal disease appears to be an independent risk factor for heart disease. Several longitudinal epidemiologic studies show that patients with severe periodontal disease are at increased risk of developing atherosclerosis, myocardial infarction, and stroke over time. For example, the odds ratio for developing fatal coronary heart disease in patients with periodontal disease is 1.9 [18], and for developing stroke is 2.2 [19]. This connection between cardiovascular disease, stroke, diabetes, and periodontal disease is of great concern as it implies that the diabetic patient with periodontal disease has a very high likelihood of developing cardiovascular disease. This concern is confirmed by a study of Pima Indians, showing that death from cardiovascular disease is approximately five times greater in diabetic patients with periodontal disease than in patients who have little or no periodontal disease [20].

MECHANISMS LINKING DIABETES AND PERIODONTAL INFECTIONS

The infectious complications of diabetes, including periodontal disease, likely result in most part from the adverse effects of hyperglycemia. These cause increased susceptibility to infection, impaired wound healing capabilities, and vascular injury. The molecular mechanisms underlying these pathologic manifestations, which, in turn, affect infections such as periodontal disease, can be associated with (1) sorbitol–myoinositol osmolarity changes; (2) oxidative–redox stress; (3) nonenzymatic glycation reactions (advanced glycation endproducts – AGEs); and (4) activation of the protein kinase C–diacylglycerol pathway.

AGE-related processes have been associated with periodontal disease [21, 22]. The primary effects of these AGE-related processes are effects on collagen metabolism, altered immune responses, and compromised vascular integrity. The presence of AGEs decreases collagen solubility and prevents normal collagen turnover. This effect on collagen metabolism, in turn, contributes to both impaired wound healing and loss of vascular integrity. Insulin treatment of hyperglycemic patients has been found to return collagen turnover rates to nearly normal [23].

In addition, AGEs bind monocytes and macrophages, leading to a hyperreactive immune state. This state results in an increase in production of proinflammatory cytokines such as TNF-α and IL-1. This reaction is likely triggered in the periodontium by bacterial products such as lipopolysaccharide (LPS), increasing the local production of these tissue-destructive cytokines, which, in turn, lead to enhanced chronic destructive periodontal disease. It is possible that the chronic inflammatory state that AGEs promote also has the systemic effect of encouraging atheroma formation and vascular disease [24]. Finally, AGEs contribute to vascular injury by decreasing vascular integrity with increasing oxidative stresses in diabetic tissues. The exaggerated, destructive response of the periodontal tissues in diabetic patients to infection may also result in part from AGE-related microvascular injury.

SIGNS AND SYMPTOMS OF PERIODONTAL DISEASE THAT CAN BE DETERMINED BY QUESTIONING THE PATIENT, AND AN ORAL EXAMINATION

It is important to ask patients with diabetes several key questions about their oral health. Table 1 lists eight questions that should be asked routinely. The next step in assessing a patient's oral status is through an oral examination. The physician should look for signs and symptoms that may indicate the presence of periodontitis. These signs may include red or swollen gingiva; the presence of copious amounts of dental plaque or stain and tartar; gingiva that is pulled away from the teeth; teeth that are loose or have recently developed spaces; and halitosis. In severe cases of periodontal disease, the patient may have one or more painful periodontal abscesses and have teeth that are noticeably loosened.

Table 1 Key questions for your diabetic patients

(1) Do your gums bleed?
(2) Do your gums feel swollen or tender?
(3) Do you have or have you had any abscesses or swellings on your gums?
(4) Are your teeth loose, or have spaces developed between the teeth?
(5) Do you have persistent bad breath?
(6) Do you smoke?
(7) Have you ever been told that you have periodontal disease?
(8) If you have had periodontal disease in the past, have you had periodontal treatment?

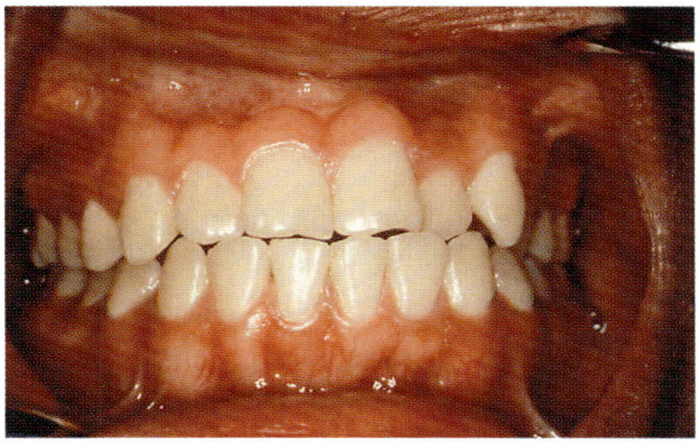

Figure 1 Healthy periodontium with pink, firm gingiva; no evidence of swelling; spaces between the teeth are filled with gingiva

Healthy gingiva is firm and pink, and fits snugly against the tooth (Figure 1). In the presence of bacterial plaque, the gingiva becomes inflamed and appears red and swollen (Figure 2). The gingiva may appear to have pulled away from the tooth (Figure 3). It may be helpful to compare adjacent areas within the patient's mouth to detect the presence of inflammation.

Dental plaque, a white or yellowish deposit, is found on most teeth. However, if the plaque is calcified, it is often darkly stained. This usually suggests the presence of calculus at or below the gumline, which is often associated with periodontal infection. Most patients experience gingival bleeding when they brush or floss their

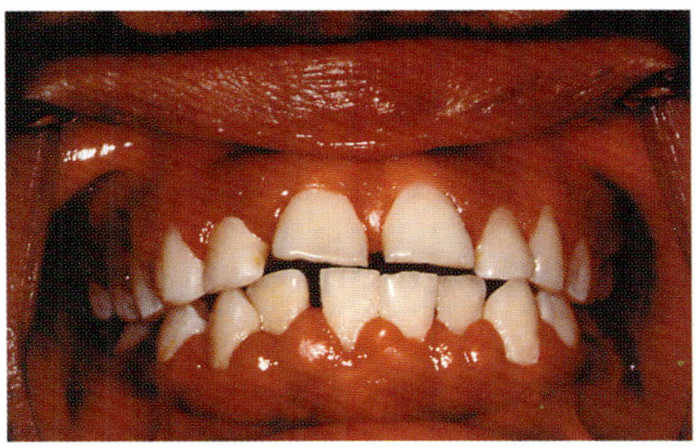

Figure 2 Gingivitis with enlarged gingiva, particularly between the teeth; red, glistening surface; bleeds easily

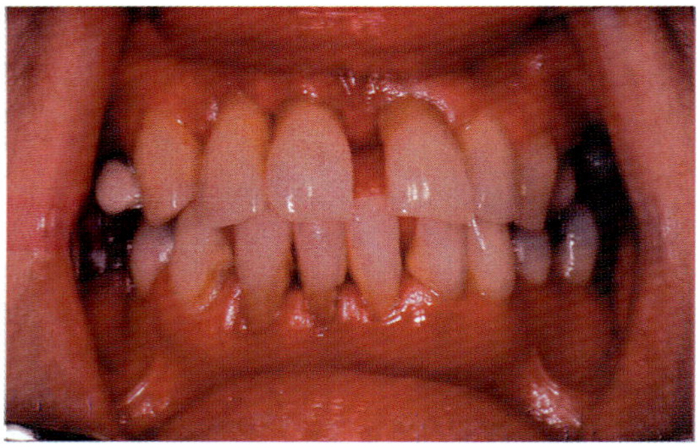

Figure 3 Recession with exposed root surfaces; often this area is yellow since it represents the portion of the tooth not covered by the enamel of the crown

teeth; however, persistent gingival bleeding is abnormal and usually a sign of the presence of disease. In addition, spontaneous gingival bleeding, or "blood on the pillow," is often a sign of periodontal disease.

Loose teeth often occur when periodontal disease has destroyed half or more of the alveolar bone, and hence is indicative of late-stage periodontal disease. Loose teeth often migrate in the jaw, resulting in the development of spaces between the teeth (Figure 4). These newly developed spaces can indicate the presence of periodontal disease.

Oral malodor, or halitosis, often accompanies periodontitis. Such malodor results from volatile sulfur compounds released by oral bacteria. However, malodor associated with gastrointestinal or respiratory abnormalities or food should be distinguished from periodontal-associated malodor.

Noticeable swelling or abscesses of the gingiva, often accompanied by an abscess or fistula through which suppurative exudate can be seen, accompanies late forms of periodontal disease (Figure 5). The patient may complain of pain on biting or throbbing and radiating pain.

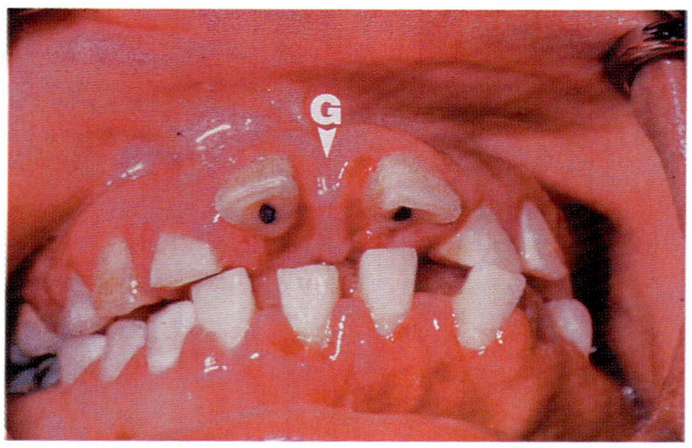

Figure 4 Represents spacing of the teeth seen in periodontitis where the teeth have loosened and migrated out of position. Inflamed gingiva around the upper front teeth and fistula on the gingiva around the lower front teeth

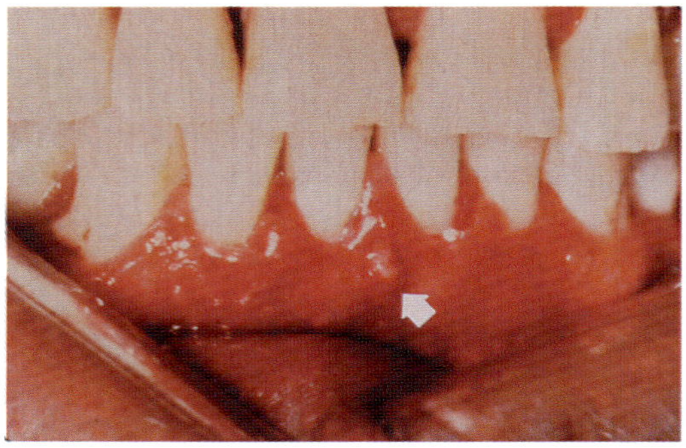

Figure 5 Gingival abscess. Often the abscess will rupture, leaving a fistula with suppuration. Again, a sign of advanced periodontal disease

These are often signs of very severe, untreated periodontal disease.

A positive intraoral examination finding, or a "yes" answer to any of the questions in Table 1, indicates that the patient either has periodontal disease or is at risk for developing periodontal disease. Such a patient should be referred to a periodontist.

OTHER ORAL FINDINGS

A number of oral conditions, besides periodontal disease, have been linked to diabetes. However, none of these correlations are as strong as the link between periodontal disease and diabetes. Increased dental caries, xerostomia, candidiasis, lichen planus, and burning mouth have been found in individuals with diabetes, but there is conflicting data regarding the relative prevalence of most of these conditions in patients with diabetes. Some studies show increased caries in people with diabetes, apparently caused by increased salivary glucose concentrations. Other studies suggest a low caries rate among their nondiabetic counterparts, presumably because of the carbohydrate-restricted diet followed by many diabetic patients.

Xerostomia, or dry mouth, is the only nonperiodontal oral condition that has been consistently found to be increased in patients with diabetes. Although autonomic neuropathy may be a cause, in part, of decreased salivation, it appears that diabetic xerostomia is most often a side effect of the patient's medications. Over 200 commonly used drugs including some antihistamines, antihypertensives, and antidepressants have xerostomic effects. Many diabetic patients take such drugs to treat complications of diabetes or for unrelated disorders and may, therefore, develop xerostomia [24]. A decrease in salivary flow can, in turn, promote caries, candidiasis, or burning mouth syndrome. Patients with xerostomia require special dental attention to prevent and treat the effects of reduced salivary flow. In some cases, it may be necessary for the

Table 2 Dental therapy of the diabetic patient

Patients known to have periodontal disease

(1) Patients with a prior diagnosis of periodontitis
(2) Patients currently under the care of a periodontist or dentist for periodontal treatment
(3) Patients who report periodontal symptoms when questioned (e.g., abscesses)
(4) Patients with signs of periodontitis on intraoral examination
(5) Patients who have been told they have "pockets"

All patients in this category who are not already under the care of a periodontist should be referred to one. In either case, the physician and periodontist should be in contact to ensure the patient receives optimal care.

High-risk patients with no obvious sign of periodontal disease

(1) Patients who smoke
(2) Patients with poor glycemic control

All diabetic smokers are to be considered at high risk for developing periodontal disease. Smokers frequently do not exhibit the usual signs of periodontitis. They tend to have deceivingly pink, fibrotic gingiva and little or no gingival bleeding.

Patients with poor glycemic control are more likely to develop periodontitis than do well-controlled patients. The severity of periodontal disease is also greater in poorly controlled patients with diabetes.

Patients in this category should be referred for a dental examination. The dentist should be made aware of the patient's diabetes and should perform a baseline periodontal examination. Referral to a periodontist is recommended if periodontal disease is diagnosed.

The low-risk patient

(1) Patients with well-controlled diabetes
(2) Nonsmoking patients
(3) Patients with no positive findings on intraoral examination or questioning

Such patients are at low risk for developing periodontal disease. Careful follow-up by the patient's physician and dentist may be all that is required as long as the patient maintains low-risk status.

physician to replace xerostomic medication with one less likely to cause dry mouth, or to recommend use of a saliva substitute.

REFERRAL RECOMMENDATIONS

Physicians should be alert to the diabetic patient's periodontal status and risk profile. Oral examinations should be performed regularly to ensure that any change in the patient's periodontal health is not overlooked. A referral system is recommended to ensure that the patient receives appropriate follow-up care (Table 2).

MANAGEMENT OF DENTAL DISEASE IN PATIENTS WITH DIABETES MELLITUS

Patients with poorly controlled diabetes should receive mainly emergency dental care. The dentist should refer patients with suspected poorly controlled diabetes to a physician, and only when the patient's glycemic control has been evaluated and managed, should advanced dental treatment proceed. Generally speaking, well-controlled diabetic patients require no changes in the normal dental treatment plan. However, the treating dentist should work with the physician to ensure that an acceptable level of glycemic control has been obtained.

Hypoglycemia is a serious complication likely to occur in well-controlled diabetic patients under stress. Diabetic patients should be asked to bring their blood glucose meter to dental appointments and the blood glucose should be tested before treatment is begun. If the blood glucose level is found to be low, the patient may be given a small amount of carbohydrate by mouth to help prevent hypoglycemia. In addition, the blood glucose meter is useful in monitoring a patient's recovery from hypoglycemia and in differentiating between hypoglycemia and hyperglycemia, especially in symptomatic patients who take insulin.

Patients should be reminded to eat normal meals and take their medications as prescribed while undergoing dental treatment. It may be advantageous to schedule dental treatment appointments in the morning when the endogenous steroid levels are high and the patient's tolerance for stressful dental procedures is optimal. Dental appointments should be scheduled before or after insulin peaks to prevent hypoglycemia.

It is important that the dentist use local anesthetics with the amount of vasocontrictor agents required to achieve adequate pain control, again to reduce stress. Antibiotics are not needed if the patient is undergoing routine dental treatment. If the patient presents with an infection, especially if the patient's glycemic control is suboptimal, antibiotic use can be considered. In fact, there is some evidence that antibiotic use as an adjunct to periodontal therapy is useful in managing periodontal infections in most diabetic patients [17].

Patients with poor metabolic control may respond poorly to dental implant placement because of their impaired wound healing. However, there is clinical evidence suggesting that dental implants can be used as tooth replacements in diabetic patients who are under reasonable metabolic control [24].

CONCLUSIONS

Periodontal disease is more severe and has an earlier onset in diabetic patients. However, periodontal disease will be better managed in diabetic patients who are well-controlled metabolically. Furthermore, intense monitoring of prevention as well as early treatment are often necessary for those suffering with diabetes to prevent the ravaging effects of periodontal disease. Recent evidence supports the role of periodontal infections in worsening of glycemic control in diabetic patients. A series of studies have been reported showing that aggressive periodontal therapy, especially using adjunctive systemic and local antibiotics, is effective in treating periodontal disease in diabetic patients. Aggressive management of periodontal infections often results in reduced glycated hemoglobin.

REFERENCES

1. Loe H. Periodontal disease. The sixth complication of diabetes mellitus. *Diabetes Care* 1993; 16 (suppl 1): 329–34.
2. Albandar JM, Brunelle JA, Kingman A. Destructive periodontal disease in adults 30 years of age and older in the United States, 1988–1994. *J Periodontol* 1999; 70: 13–29.
3. Research, Science, and Therapy Committee of the American Academy of Periodontology. The pathogenesis of periodontal diseases. *J Periodontol* 1999; 70: 457–70.
4. Tanner A, Stillman N. Oral and dental infections with anaerobic bacteria: Clinical features, predominant pathogens, and treatment. *Clin Infect Dis* 1993; 16 (suppl 4): S304–9.
5. Contreras A, Umeda M, Chen C, Bakker I, Morrison JL, Slots J. Relationship between herpes viruses and adult periodontitis and periodontopathic bacteria. *J Periodontol* 1999; 70: 478–84.
6. Genco RJ, Van Dyke TE, Levine MJ, Nelson RD, Wilson ME. 1985 Kreshover Lecture. Molecular factors influencing neutrophil defects in periodontal disease. *J Dent Res* 1986; 65: 1379–91.
7. Johnson GK. Tobacco use and the periodontal patient. *J Periodontol* 1999; 70: 1419–27.
8. Grossi SG, Zambon JJ, Ho AW, Koch G, Dunford RG, Machtei EE, Norderyd OM, Genco RJ. Assessment of risk for periodontal disease, I: risk indicators for attachment loss. *J Periodontol* 1994; 65: 260–7.
9. Cianciola LJ, Park BH, Bruck E, Mosovich L, Genco RJ. Prevalence of periodontal disease in insulin-dependent diabetes mellitus (juvenile diabetes). *J Am Dent Assoc* 1982; 104: 653–60.
10. Shlossman M, Knowler WC, Pettitt DJ, Genco RJ. Type 2 diabetes mellitus and periodontal disease. *J Am Dent Assoc* 1990; 121: 532–6.
11. Emrich LJ, Shlossman M, Genco RJ. Periodontal disease in non-insulin-dependent diabetes mellitus. *J Periodontol* 1991; 62: 123–30.
12. Taylor GW, Burt BA, Becker MP, Genco RJ, Shlossman M, Knowler WC, Pettitt DJ. Non-insulin dependent diabetes mellitus and alveolar bone loss progression over 2 years. *J Periodontol* 1998; 69: 76–83.
13. Oliver RC, Tervonen T. Diabetes—a risk factor for periodontal disease in adults? *J Periodontol* 1994; 65 (suppl 5): 530–8.
14. Glavind L, Lund B, Loe H. The relationship between periodontal state and diabetes duration, insulin dosage and retinal changes. *J Periodontol* 1968; 39: 341–7.
15. Grossi S, Genco RJ. Periodontal disease and diabetes mellitus: a two-way relationship. *Ann Periodontol* 1998; 3 (1): 51–61.
16. Taylor Gw, Burt BA, Becker MP. Severe periodontitis and risk for poor glycemic control in patients with non-insulin-dependent diabetes mellitus. *J Periodontol* 1996; 67 (suppl 10): 1085–93.
17. Grossi SG, Skrepcinski FB, DeCaro T, et al. Treatment of periodontal disease in diabetics reduces glycated hemoglobin. *J Periodontol* 1997; 68: 713–9.
18. Beck J, Garcia R, Heiss G, Vokonas P, Offenbacher S. Periodontal disease and cardiovascular disease. *J Periodontol* 1996; 67: (suppl 10): 1123–37.
19. Wu T, Trevisan M, Genco RJ, Dorn JP, Falkner KL, Sempos CT. Periodontal disease and risk of cerebrovascular disease: The First National Health and Nutrition Examinations Survey and its follow-up study. *Arch Intern Med* 2000; 160: 2749–55.
20. Saremi A, Nelson RG, Hanson RL, Tulloch-Reid M, Shlossman M, Genco RJ, Knowler WC. Effect of periodontal disease on mortality in Type 2 diabetes. *Diabetes* 2003; 52 (suppl 1): 978 (abstract 228).
21. Research, Science, and Therapy Committee of the American Academy of Periodontology. Diabetes and periodontal disease. *J Periodontol* 1999; 70: 935–49.
22. Schmidt AM, Weidman E, Lalla E, Yan SD, Hori O, Cao R, Brett JG, Lamster IB. Advanced glycation endproducts (AGEs) induce oxidant stress in the gingiva. A potential mechanism underlying accelerated periodontal disease associated with diabetes. *J Periodontal Res* 1996; 31: 508–15.
23. Golub LM, Schneir M, Ramamurthy N. Enhanced collagenase activity in diabetic rat gingiva: in vitro and in vivo evidence. *J Dent Res* 1978; 57: 520–5.
24. Mealey B. Diabetes mellitus. In Rose LF, Genco RJ, Mealey BL, Cohen DW (eds), *Periodontal Medicine*. Lewiston, NY: BC Decker, 1999; pp 121–50.

73

The Diabetic Foot

Thanh L. Dinh and Aristidis Veves

Harvard Medical School, Boston, MA, USA

INTRODUCTION

Diabetic foot complications are common manifestations with potentially devastating consequences. Foot pathology encountered in the clinical setting ranges from benign skin and nail changes to the more severe and debilitating ulcerations and infections. Despite adequate therapy, these more serious ulcerations and infections may progress to extensive hospitalizations, lower extremity amputations, and premature death.

Foot pathology remains the leading diabetic complication requiring hospitalization [1]. As the incidence of diabetes in the general population is expected to rise, the prevalence of diabetic foot complications will follow. The resulting cost to society can be measured in direct costs attributed to treatment, as well as indirect costs in lost productivity. However the costs are measured, diabetic foot problems represent a major public health challenge of growing proportions.

Over the last decade, considerable strides have been gained in identifying the risk factors and causal pathways leading to diabetic foot problems. Major risk factors for the development of diabetic foot ulcers include peripheral neuropathy, peripheral vascular disease, and high foot pressures. These, along with other predisposing elements in the formation of diabetic foot complications, will be discussed in greater detail later in the chapter. With a greater understanding of the pathogenesis of diabetic foot complications, preventative strategies aimed at limb salvage have been met with greater success.

EPIDEMIOLOGY

Discussions of diabetic foot complications focus on two major problems, foot ulcers and lower extremity amputations. Combined, these two entities represent substantial utilization of medical efforts and healthcare resources, in addition to contributing to significant morbidity and mortality in the patient with diabetes.

Foot ulcers result from a number of etiologic factors, and are characterized by an underlying inability to heal in a timely fashion. These etiologic factors arise from pathophysiologic changes in the diabetic state, anatomic deformities in the diabetic foot, and environmental influences. Annually, 2% of all diabetic patients will develop a foot ulcer [2], while 15% will ulcerate over a lifetime [2, 3]. The prevalence of diabetic foot ulcers has been reported to range from 5.3 to 10.5% [2, 4–6]. This wide variation in range has been attributed to the lack of awareness and appropriate preventative care on the part of both patient and provider. Furthermore, this wide variation may be due to the fact that most studies select only diabetic patients at risk for diabetic foot complications for inclusion in evaluation of ulcer formation.

The cost of diabetic foot complications vary considerably, depending on the outcome and extent of intervention required. The majority of the costs are attributed to inpatient expenditures [7]. Cost for an entire ulcer episode not requiring surgery averages close to $7000, while those ulcers that ultimately required amputation exceeds $44 000 [8].

The link between diabetic foot ulcers and lower extremity amputations is indisputable, given the fact that foot ulcers precede 85% of amputations [9, 10]. Alarmingly, 15% of all foot ulcers will ultimately require amputation, representing the major risk factor for amputation [2]. Other risk factors for amputation include increased duration of diabetes, poor glycemic control, peripheral neuropathy, peripheral vascular disease, history of foot ulcers, previous amputations, retinopathy, and nephropathy [11–16].

International Textbook of Diabetes Mellitus, Third Edition. Edited by R. A. DeFronzo, E. Ferrannini, H. Keen, and P. Zimmet.
 ISBN: 0-471-48655-8.

In the United States, approximately one half of all amputations are performed on patients with diabetes [17]. Amputation rates have also been shown to vary with both gender and ethnicity. Being male, African American, or Hispanic has been associated with greater risk for amputation [18, 19]. The reasons for this appear to be due to lack of access to education and routine preventative care. When programs designed to prevent and promote awareness of diabetic foot complications were instituted in high-risk populations, the rate of amputations was decreased by nearly 50% [20, 21].

Lower extremity amputations in the diabetic population is estimated at 60 000 cases annually with an estimated expense of $30 000–60 000 per case [22]. More disturbingly, the incidence of lower extremity amputations continues to escalate despite greater awareness levels and promotion of preventative care. Since 1990, the rate of lower extremity amputation in patients with diabetes increased by a staggering 26%.

As evidenced by the statistics, diabetic foot complications can be an overwhelming burden to patients, their families, and health care professionals. The total cost of diabetic foot complications in the United States has been estimated to approach 4 billion annually, as extrapolated from the costs of ulcer care and amputations [23]. Continued efforts to identify high-risk patients, ensure adequate availability of preventative care, and prompt treatment remain the best means of reducing the destructive consequences of amputations and death.

DIABETIC FOOT ULCERATION

The Pathway to Foot Ulceration

The risk factors for diabetic foot ulceration can be categorized into three distinct groups: pathophysiologic, anatomic deformities, and environmental influences. Pathophysiologic changes at the biomolecular level lead to peripheral sensory neuropathy, peripheral vascular disease, and a compromised immune system with alteration in wound-healing capabilities. Motor neuropathy and Charcot neuroarthropathy are the major contributors to foot deformity. Finally, external factors in the form of acute or chronic trauma often precipitates the initiation of ulceration.

It is important to note that most of these risk factors do not act independently to produce foot ulceration. Instead, a combination of these risk factors triggers a pathway leading to ulceration. The causal pathway to foot ulceration can consist of a number of component causes such as peripheral neuropathy, foot trauma, foot deformity, lower limb ischemia, foot edema, and callus formation. However, a critical triad of neuropathy, minor foot trauma, and foot deformity was found in greater than 63% of foot ulcers in one study [24].

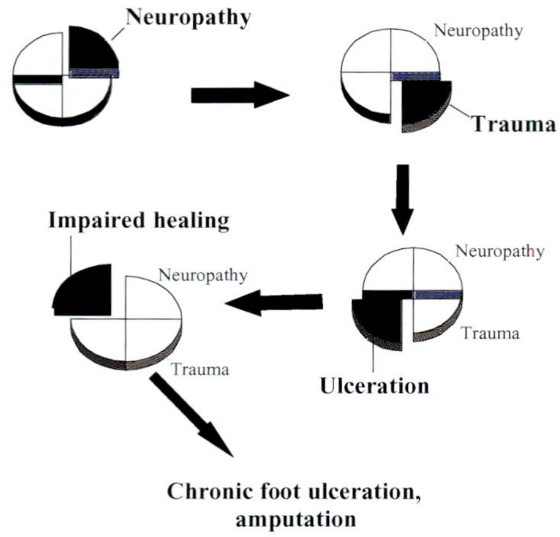

Figure 1 The pathway to foot ulceration. Sensory neuropathy, associated with pain insensitivity is the first component of the pathway. However, the development of ulceration also requires the existence of trauma, usually related to the plantar tissue stress and injury that results from the development of high foot pressures during walking. The presence of the third component, impaired wound healing due to reduced blood flow in the ulcer area and aberrant expression of growth factors and cytokines, prevents the wound closure and leads to the development of chronic ulceration an, in some cases, amputation. (modified from reference 10)

As shown in Figure 1, in the vast majority of diabetic foot ulceration, the first major component is the development of sensory neuropathy that causes pain insensitivity [10]. The next component is the development of trauma, usually related to the high foot pressures that develop under the foot during walking. The third major component is the impaired wound healing, related to reduced blood supply at the wound area and abnormal expression of growth factors and other cytokines that are involved in the healing process. It is usually the combination of these three major components that leads to the development of chronic ulceration and, in a substantial number of cases, amputation of the lower extremity.

Peripheral Sensory Neuropathy

Reported in approximately 30–50% of all diabetic patients, peripheral sensory neuropathy has been found to be the most common and sensitive predictor for foot ulceration in the diabetic patient [25, 26]. In a study that specifically studied casual pathways of diabetic foot ulceration, the presence of neuropathy was reported in 78% of cases [24].

The presence of peripheral sensory neuropathy initiates a series of events that eventually results in foot ulceration. With an inability to detect the pain signals that warn of impending tissue trauma, the insensate foot is exposed to increased pressures that hasten tissue damage, leading to ulceration. The propagation of this vicious cycle, of increased forces coupled with impaired protective sensation, causes the ulcer to worsen.

Autonomic and Motor Neuropathy

Autonomic neuropathy is a common finding in patients with long-standing diabetes. In the lower extremity, autonomic neuropathy can cause arteriovenous shunting, resulting in a vasodilatory condition in the small arteries [27]. The resultant distension of the foot veins is not diminished even with foot elevation. Consequently, a neuropathic edema recalcitrant to diuretic therapy is observed. In addition to swelling, the neuropathic foot is also noted to be warm as a result of arteriovenous shunting [28]. Abnormalities in autonomic neuropathy are also responsible for the decreased activity of the sweat glands of the feet. These changes in the diabetic foot can result in skin that is prone to dryness and fissuring, predisposing the patient to the risk of infection [29].

Motor neuropathy in the foot causes weakness and wasting of the small intrinsic muscles, classically termed the "intrinsic minus" foot (Figure 2). This leads to muscular imbalance with a characteristic clawing of the toes and plantar flexion of the metatarsal heads. The prominences at the plantar metatarsal head level and the digital level serve as areas of focal pressures with possible irritation from footwear. Coupled with sensory neuropathy, these prominences are susceptible to increased forces with subsequent ulceration.

Peak Plantar Pressures

Diabetic ulcers can occur on any part of the foot, but are clinically observed most frequently on the plantar surfaces. The predilection of diabetic foot ulcers to the plantar surfaces is related to the trauma that develops in these areas because of the increased peak plantar pressures during walking [30].

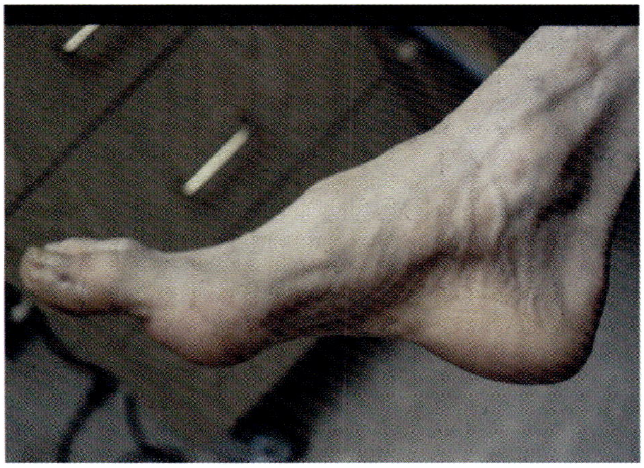

Figure 2 Changes related to motor neuropathy (minor foot). There is extensive wasting of the intrinsic muscles of the foot that results in clawing of the toes and prominence of the metatarsal heads

Under normal conditions, the foot has the ability to distribute high forces that are applied on the plantar surface and therefore avoid the development of high foot pressures. This ability is greatly impaired in diabetes and is mainly related to the foot changes that are related to motor neuropathy (and were described above) and to the restriction of joint mobility (see below). As a result of this, the pressures under certain areas of the diabetic foot can be considerably high and lead to tissue injury even after walking short distances. In the presence of sensory neuropathy, the patient is unaware of initial warning signs of this injury, such as pain, and continues to walk until tissue integrity is compromised and foot ulceration occurs.

Numerous studies have shown that foot pressures are high in diabetic neuropathic patients [31–34]. The high pressures tend to aggregate in the forefoot area or sites with bony prominence in the case of patients with Charcot neuroarthropathy. Usually, most ulcers develop under these areas of high foot pressures but the development of ulceration in other foot areas can also occur.

The development of high foot pressures starts in the early stages of diabetic neuropathy, even in the subclinical phase of the disease. One of the first steps is the transfer of high peak pressures from the heel area to the forefoot area, in the absence of any clinically detectable neuropathy [33]. As neuropathy worsens and the clawing of the toes develops, there is further transfer of peak pressures from the toes to the forefoot area. In cases of severe neuropathy, the forefoot pressures are so high that the ratio between forefoot to rear foot pressures is increased and can be used as an alternative of foot pressure measurement in identifying the at-risk patient for foot ulceration [35].

There is ample evidence, either from cross-sectional or prospective clinical studies, that high foot pressures can predict foot ulceration [31, 32, 36, 37]. However, foot pressure measurements are characterized by a relatively low sensitivity and are not recommended as a screening tool [30]. However, as they also have a satisfactory specificity, they can be employed in selected cases of at-risk patients to guide for the provision of proper footwear that reduces high pressures and therefore, decreases the risk of foot ulceration [38].

Limited Joint Mobility

Restriction of joint mobility is well documented in diabetes and is related mainly to collagen glycosylation that results in thickening of the periarticular structures such as tendons, ligaments, and joint capsules [39, 40]. At the foot level, the subtalar and metatarsophalangeal joints are most commonly involved. The involvement of the subtalar joint seems critical as it impairs the ability of the foot to adapt to the ground surface and absorb the shock that develops when the heel makes contact with the ground during walking. As a result of this, high foot pressures develop, mainly in the forefoot area and are believed to further contribute to the development of foot ulceration [34, 41–43]. Interestingly, limited joint mobility appears to vary with racial differences, with patients of Caucasian background having significantly less joint mobility compared to Black patients [44].

Collagen glycosylation is also implicated in decreasing the resiliency of the Achilles tendon in diabetic patients. Decreased motion of the Achilles tendon creates an equinus deformity with a subsequent shift of plantar forces to the forefoot region that sets the stage for foot ulcers in the metatarsal region [45]. Surgical lengthening of the Achilles tendon has been found to effectively distribute plantar pressures more uniformly, decreasing the peak forces at the metatarsal region [46].

Peripheral Vascular Disease

Macrocirculation Peripheral vascular disease in not uncommon in diabetic foot ulceration and can be present in 30% of this population [24]. Ischemia in itself is not only a risk factor for development of a foot ulcer, but it also complicates and slows wound healing, as a result of insufficient blood flow. Peripheral vascular disease in the diabetes is characterized by impairment at both the microcirculation and macrocirculation level. Macrocirculatory disease in the diabetic patient is identical to the atherosclerotic changes found in nondiabetic patients and is discussed in greater detail elsewhere in this book. Microcirculatory disease, on the other hand, is unique to the diabetic patient.

Microcirculation Changes in the microcirculation of the diabetic foot contribute significantly to the impaired wound healing. While there are no occlusive lesions in the diabetic microcirculation, structural changes do exist, most notably, thickening of the basement membrane. However, this does not result in narrowing of the capillary lumen [47]. Instead, these changes decrease the elastic properties of the capillary vessel walls and therefore limit vasodilatation capacity. The basement membrane thickening may also act as a barrier to the normal exchange of nutrients and cellular migration, decreasing the ability of the diabetic foot to fight infection [48].

Despite these structural changes, it is currently understood that the most important changes in the microcirculation are functional. More specifically, over the last decade, it has been realized that these changes are related mainly to the dysfunction of the endothelial cells and vascular smooth muscle cells of the arterioles, and the impairment of the nerve–axon reflex.

The endothelium, one-cell-layer in thickness, forms the luminal surface of all blood vessels. Normally, the endothelium synthesizes and releases substances such as nitric oxide, endothelin, and prostaglandins that are vital for regulating vasoconstriction and vasodilation and therefore in maintaining vascular tone and regulating blood flow [49]. The main action of the vasomodulators is directed to the vascular smooth muscle cells that are adjacent to the endothelial cells. It should also be emphasized that, in contrast to large vessels, no atherosclerotic changes, such as monocyte migration or foam cell formation are observed in the microcirculation. In addition, endothelial cells are involved in the angiogenesis, an important factor of the wound-healing process.

Recent work over the last decade has shown that both the endothelium-dependent vasodilation and the independent one (that reflects the function of the vascular smooth muscle cell function) are impaired not only in diabetes but in the prediabetic stage as well [50] (Figure 3). Furthermore, even in healthy subjects the microcirculation vasodilatory capacity at the foot level is reduced when compared to the forearm level. Thus, the additional reduction in vasodilation that is caused by diabetes can be critical for the skin and other foot tissues, as it restricts the maximal blood flow to levels that cannot sustain

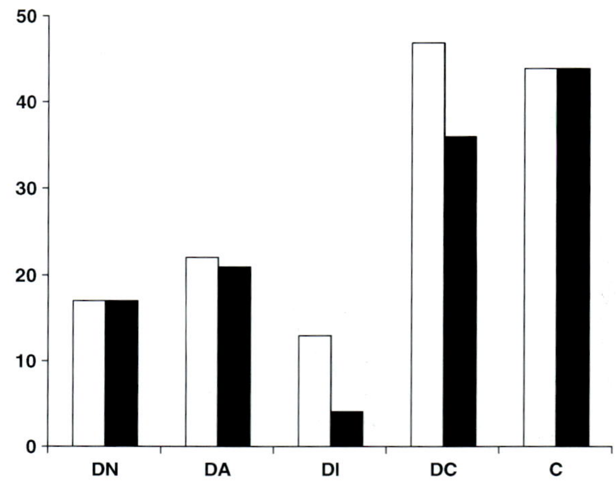

Figure 3 The vasodilatory response to the iontophoresis of acetylcholine (empty bars) and sodium nitroprusside (SNP, black bars) at the foot level. The response to acetylcholine (endothelium-dependent vasodilation) was equally reduced in the diabetic neuropathic patients with a history of foot ulceration (DN group), the patients with both neuropathy and peripheral vascular disease (DI), and the patients with Charcot neuroarthropathy (DA) when compared to non-neuropathic diabetic patients (D) and healthy controls (C), $p < 0.0001$. The response to SNP (endothelium-independent vasodilation) was more pronounced in the DI group, and also reduced in the DN and DA groups compared to D and C groups, $p < 0.0001$. These results indicate that both the endothelial cells and vascular smooth muscle cells of the skin microcirculation are impaired in the neuropathic diabetic foot (from reference 50)

normal wound healing [51]. Studies in our unit have shown that the endothelium-dependent vasodilation is equally impaired in diabetic neuropathic patients without large-vessel disease and adequate arterial blood flow, and in patients with obstructive arterial disease requiring bypass operation. The endothelium-dependent vasodilation was also impaired in both groups but was more pronounced in the patients with large vessel disease [52, 53].

Another important factor that affects the neuropathic foot microcirculation is the impairment of the nerve axon reflex. Under normal conditions, stimulation of the C-nociceptive fibers leads to retrograde stimulation of adjacent fibers that secrete a number of vasomodulators, such as substance P, CGRP, and histamine, and produce vasodilation (also known as Lewis triple-flare response) (Figure 4). This response is equal to one third of the maximal vasodilatory capacity and is responsible for the hyperemia that is observed in areas that are close to injury.

As it would be expected, the nerve–axon-reflex-related vasodilation is almost absent in diabetic naturopathic patients. This response remains absent even after successful bypass surgery to the pedal arteries that establishes satisfactory blood flow in the large vessels of the foot [54]. This is probably the main reason that hyperemia, a major sign of inflammation, is absent in diabetic patients with infection of the foot. Thus, even the presence of neuropathy alone can lead to impaired blood flow under conditions of stress [55–57].

At the molecular level, the reduction of endothelium-dependent vasodilation seems to be related to the reduced expression of endothelial nitric oxide synthase (eNOS) by

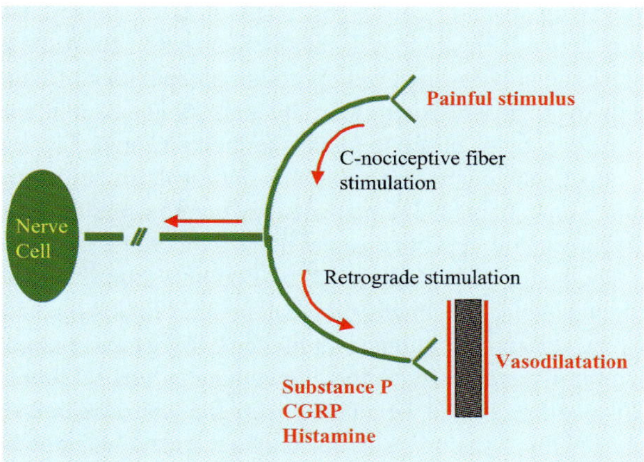

Figure 4 The nerve–axon reflex. Stimulation of the C-nociceptive fibers causes retrograde stimulation of adjacent fibers that release active vasodilators such as histamine, substance P, and calcitonin gene-related peptide (CGRP). The final result is hyperemia during injury or inflammation. Because of the presence of peripheral neuropathy, this response (also known in physiology as Lewis triple-flare response) is absent in diabetic patients

the endothelial cells of the microvasculature that is located in the skin of neuropathic foot [50]. Whether this reduction is also related to the development of neuropathy is not clear. However, the expression of eNOS by endothelial cells at the forearm level is not affected by diabetes. Other mechanisms that contribute to the observed functional changes include reduced poly (ADP-ribose) polymerase (PARP) activity and increased nitrotyrosine formation [53].

Despite the lack of complete understanding of the involved mechanisms, the main understanding from work that was conducted over the last decade is that the microcirculation of diabetic neuropathic foot fails to maximally vasodilate under conditions of stress. Thus, even in the absence of any peripheral disease and in the presence of good blood blow in the large vessels, the skin blood flow is impaired when injury occurs, and this is one of the major factors that are related to impaired wound healing. Therefore the neuropathic diabetic foot should be considered functionally ischemic regardless of the presence or absence of vascular disease. In addition, lack of hyperemia should not be interpreted as lack of inflammation or infection.

Impaired Wound Healing

As shown in Figure 1, impaired wound healing is a major factor that contributes to the development of chronic foot ulceration and amputation. Initially it was thought that failure to heal a diabetic ulcer was related to continuous walking on the injured foot, mainly because of the pain insensitivity, and the existence of peripheral arterial disease. However, it is currently realized that two other major factors contribute to this impairment, namely the functional changes in the microcirculation and changes in cellular activity, and the expression of the various growth factors and cytokines that are normally involved in tissue repair and wound healing.

The normal wound-healing process entails a complex interplay between connective tissue formation, cellular activity, and growth-factor activation. All three of these physiologic processes are altered in the diabetic state and contribute to the poor healing of diabetic foot ulcers. Collagen, the most abundant protein in connective tissue, is an integral component of dermis, bones, tendons, and ligaments. Collagen synthesis and degradation in wound repair are complex processes that continue at the wound site long after the injury. The resulting scar tissue following wound repair never fully regains the tensile strength of the original intact skin. Instead, scar collagen retains only 70–80% tensile strength of the original collagen [58]. The balance between collagen synthesis and degradation in wound repair is tenuous, and disease states such as diabetes can shift the balance to one side, disrupting the wound-healing process.

The normal inflammatory stage of wound repair involves an orchestrated interaction of resident cells such as epithelial cells, fibroblasts, dendritic cells, and endothelial cells with biochemical activity [58]. In addition to these resident cells, platelets, neutrophils, T-cells, natural killer cells, and macrophages are recruited to the wound site. These cells migrate to the injury site to mediate the inflammation, coagulation, and angiogenesis processes occurring in the wound-healing process.

Growth factors influence the wound-healing process through inhibitory or stimulatory effect on the local wound environment. Growth factors such as-platelet-derived growth factor (PDGF), basic fibroblast growth factor (bFGF), and vascular endothelial growth factor (VEGF) have all been found in wound fluid. These growth factors are known to be integral in the chemotaxis, migration, stimulation, and proliferation of cells and matrix substances necessary for wound healing. Therefore, the altered secretion or absence of these growth factors in diabetic foot ulcers can potentially impair wound healing. Recent investigation of the role these growth factors play in wound healing appears to support this hypothesis [59].

In diabetes, there are major abnormalities in all the above mechanisms. Thus, collagen synthesis markedly decreased, at both the collagen peptide production level as well as the posttranslational modification of collagen degradation [39]. In addition, hyperglycemia can potentially mitigate the cellular activity in the inflammatory process. More specifically, the morphological characteristics of macrophages are transformed in such a manner that impairs their function [60]. Furthermore, inhibition of skin keratinocyte proliferation in the presence of increased cellular differentiation leads to an imbalance in keratinocyte production, an essential step in the wound-healing process [61]. Finally, the expression of various growth factors, such as PDGF and VEGF is reduced, while the expression of matrix metalloproteinases (MMPs) is increased. The upgraded expression of the MMPs results in increased proteolytic activity and inactivation of the growth factors that are necessary for proper wound healing.

The final result of the above changes is that diabetic ulcers are "stuck" in the inflammatory phase of the wound-healing process. Under normal circumstances, during this phase that lasts only 2–3 days, the wound is cleaned by any bacteria and is covered by an eschar that is devoid of any tensile strength. The inflammatory phase is followed by the proliferative phase that is characterized by angiogenesis, expression of numerous growth factors, cell migration, collagen production, and results in complete wound closure. It is currently believed that aberrant expression of growth factors and cytokines is the main reason that the diabetic foot ulcers fail to progress to the proliferative phase and remain in a chronic inflammatory state. Further understanding of this process will help in the development of new treatments in the future [62, 63].

Additional Risk Factors

Other risk factors for the development of diabetic foot ulcers include long duration of diabetes, prior foot ulcer, and prior amputation. Duration of diabetes of greater than 20 years has been found to increase the risk of ulceration sixfold when compared to patients with a history of diabetes of less than 9 years [64]. A number of studies have demonstrated that a prior history of ulceration or amputation significantly increases the likelihood of a subsequent ulcer [5, 65].

Clinical Examination and Screening Techniques to Identify the Patient At Risk of Foot Ulceration

Prevention remains the best means of averting the potentially devastating results of diabetic foot complications. It has been estimated that up to 80% of diabetic foot ulcers are preventable [66]. To that end, screening for risk factors by way of clinical examination of the diabetic foot has been recommended on a routine basis [67]. Routine examination of the "at-risk" diabetic foot should include clinical inspection, neurologic examination, and vascular assessment.

Clinical evaluation of the diabetic foot should begin with a history of previous ulceration or amputation. A past history of ulceration or amputation increases the risk for future ulceration, infection, and amputation. It has been demonstrated that 60% of diabetic patients with a history of a foot ulcer will develop another ulcer within a year following wound healing [68]. This is due to three distinct factors. First, the risk factors that were necessary to cause the previous ulceration remain present. Second, the skin over the previous ulcer site may be weakened and therefore, more prone to subsequent breakdown. Finally, areas of previous amputation may demonstrate deformity and biomechanical imbalances that create areas of high pressure allowing for resultant ulcerations.

The history of symptoms of neuropathy should also be elicited. More specifically, the patient should be asked for the existence of numbness in his feet or legs and painful symptoms such as described elsewhere in this textbook. However, it should be emphasized that the absence of neuropathic symptoms is not equated to the absence of neuropathy and that a large number of patients develop neuropathic ulceration without having ever noticed any symptoms.

Clinical examination usually starts with the inspection for foot deformities and limitation of joint mobility. Both of these entities increase foot pressures that lead to ulceration. Osseous prominences can be observed secondary to Charcot neuroarthropathy, motor neuropathy, and common foot deformities such as hallux abductovalgus and hammertoes, not confined to the diabetic foot. In addition, the examiner should look for callus formation and areas of erythema due to irritation from shoewear. In the past, the presence of calluses was speculated to be a protective mechanism with debridement of these lesions not recommended. However, it is now well known that calluses are actually focal areas of increased pressure and can serve as sites of potential ulceration [69]. Any areas of erythema secondary to shoewear irritation should be protected with padding or appropriate accommodative shoewear dispensed to alleviate the pressure.

The next step in screening should involve neurologic testing for identification of the foot with loss of protective sensation. The perception of pain, touch, and vibration can be easily tested using simple standard equipment such as a pin prick, cotton wool, and a tuning fork. The main feature the clinician should look for is a sensory level below which all the above modalities are reduced. The examination should be completed by testing the ability of the patient to feel a 5.07 Semmes–Weinstein monofilament (SWM) at the great toe or the metatarsal heads (Figure 5). Inability to feel the 5.07 SWM and/or the presence of a sensory level can identify 99% of all diabetic patients who are at risk of foot ulceration [70, 71]. As both these techniques are simple, not time-consuming, and do not require any expensive equipment, they should be performed at least once a year in all diabetic patients. Patients with abnormality in any of these two tests should be considered at risk of ulceration and should be provided preventive care as described below in this chapter [66, 71, 72].

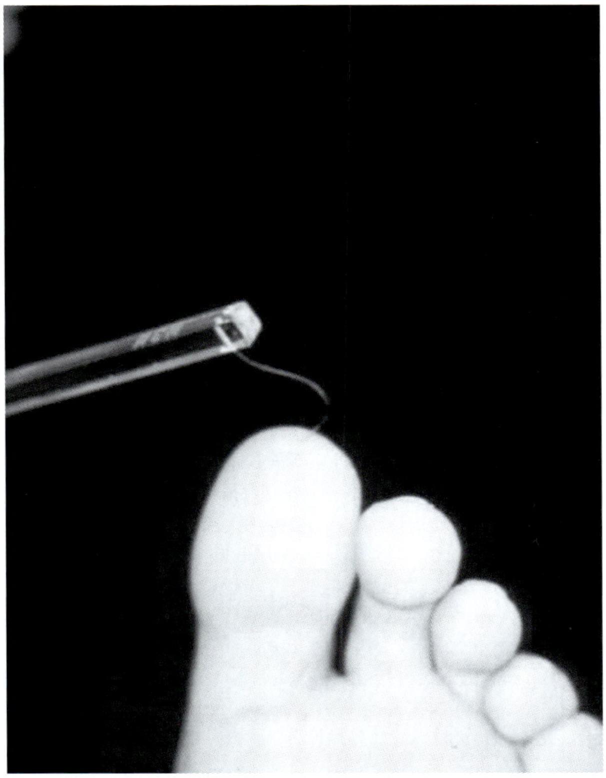

Figure 5 The 5.07 Semmes–Weinstein monofilament. The filaments is flexed when 10 gr of pressure is applied on the skin. Failure to feel a 5.07 SWM strongly indicates that the patient is at risk of developing foot ulceration

High vibration pressure threshold (VPT) is another effective technique to identify patients at risk of ulceration. Vibration pressure threshold is commonly measured with a hand-held biothesiometer device that applies voltage in the range of 0–50 V. The test is performed by placing the vibrating stylus on the pulp of the great toe or the malleolus. Failure to detect a value of 25 V is considered indicative of a foot at risk for ulceration [25]. When compared to SWF, the sensitivity of VPT approaches only 79%, and as it requires more sophisticated equipment it cannot be recommended as the technique of choice [70, 71].

The final part of the examination should involve the vascular assessment. Peripheral vascular disease is the cause in roughly 25% of foot ulcers and can contribute to the nonhealing of foot ulcers [73]. Vascular assessment includes a brief history for the existence of claudication and the palpation of all lower extremity pulses. The absence of palpable foot pulses or the existence of a nonhealing ulceration should prompt noninvasive vascular examination along with consultation with a vascular surgeon. Vascular intervention in the diabetic foot is discussed in further detail elsewhere in this book.

Classification of Diabetic Foot Ulcers

There have been numerous classification schemes proposed for describing diabetic foot ulcers. The most commonly used and most often referred to is the Wagner system [74]. The Wagner system classifies diabetic foot ulcers into five distinct grades on the basis of anatomical location, depth, and presence of ischemia. Wagner grade 0 describes a preulcerative or postulcerative lesion. There is no break in skin, but risk factors such as calluses and foot deformities are present. Wagner grade 1 ulcerations are superficial, full thickness ulcers with penetration past the epidermis. Grade 1 lesions are indicative of the presence of peripheral sensory neuropathy along with at least one other risk factor for ulceration. Continued weight bearing on grade 1 ulcerations will cause deepening of foot ulcers past the dermis with involvement of deeper structures such as tendons, ligaments, joint capsules, and neurovascular structures. Ulcers to this depth are considered Wagner grade 2 lesions. Grade 2 lesions do not probe to bone and osteomyelitis is not present. Wagner grade 3 ulcerations are characterized by the presence of deep infection with bone involvement. Abscess formations or osteomyelitis is commonly present in these deep ulcerations. Wagner grade 4 ulcers present with partial gangrene of the foot. Grade 4 ulcers demonstrate extensive vascular insufficiency, sepsis, and tissue necrosis that will necessitate aggressive management by a limb salvage team in order to limit tissue loss and possible amputation. Grade 5 ulcers are characterized by extensive necrosis and gangrene, which is usually best addressed with primary amputation.

The Wagner classification system for diabetic foot ulcers has withstood the test of time because of its simplicity, ease of use, and universal ability to be communicated amongst various medical personnel. However, criticisms of the Wagner classification system include its failure to gauge the degree of ischemia in grades 1 through 3 and its inability to address the combination of infection and ischemia. Additionally, it does not provide predictions on healing and outcomes. In response, other classification systems have been proposed to address these deficiencies.

Other classification systems proposed include one described by Brodsky and Lavery that aims to be more inclusive of all types of neuropathic foot lesions in addition to providing predictors of outcomes and response to therapy [75]. The San Antonio wound classification system mirrors the Wagner classification, but instead incorporates the presence or absence of infection and/or ischemia within each grade [76]. This classification scheme has the added benefit of predicting outcomes, with results deteriorating with increasing stage and grade. While these newer classifications are more inclusive, the comprehensiveness makes them difficult to remember and use in the clinical setting.

As a result of the lack of a universally accepted classification system, the American Diabetes Association has formed a working committee to propose a new system. Although the final report is not ready as yet, the consensus is that the new system will be based on the Wagner classification allowing for some alterations, such as using infection as a separate parameter.

TREATMENT PRINCIPLES OF FOOT ULCERATION

Treatment of diabetic foot ulcers varies greatly depending on the severity of the ulceration as well as the presence of ischemia. However, the cornerstones of treatment for full thickness ulcers should consist of adequate debridement, off-loading of pressure, treatment of infection, and local wound care. In addition to these basic tenets of ulcer treatment, greater understanding of the pathophysiology of wound healing has led to advanced wound care products demonstrating promise in accelerating wound healing.

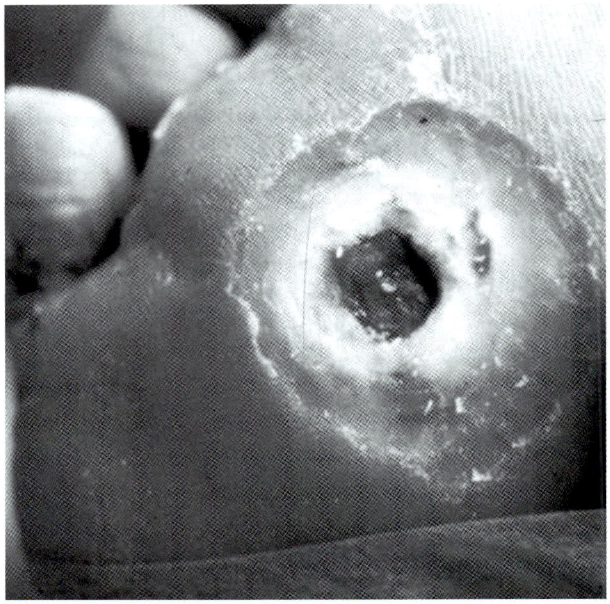

Figure 6 A grade 2 ulcer after surgical debridement. Adequate debridement is achieved when all exuberant callous tissue and necrotic tissue have been removed and a clean granular base is revealed

Debridement

The goal of wound debridement is the complete removal of all necrotic, dysvascular, and nonviable tissue in order to achieve a red, granular wound bed. Sharp surgical debridement using sharp instruments such as a scalpel blade is considered the treatment of choice [77] (Figure 6). Using this technique all nonviable tissue can be removed until a healthy bleeding ulcer bed is produced with saucerization of the wound edges. This procedure can be performed in the office setting except the rare cases when extensive debridement is required or sensation to the foot intact and the use of the operating room may be required. In addition, in the event that ischemia is suspected, aggressive debridement should be delayed until vascular examination and revascularization is achieved.

Other debridement techniques are also available but none has gained universal acceptance. *Autolytic debridement* refers the body's own mechanism of removing devitalized tissue. This process is primarily undertaken by macrophages, which release proteolytic enzymes to degrade nonviable tissue [78]. However, this method requires adequate arterial perfusion as well as wound hydration and can be slow and tedious. Enzymatic debridement involves the use of topical agents with the ability to degrade necrotic tissue via proteolytic enzymes. These agents are typically applied to a wound under an occlusive dressing. Indications for use are limited and generally indicated to slowly soften large eschars or debride decubitus ulcerations in sensate limbs. Drawbacks to this form of debridement include the lengthy process and considerable expense of these agents [79]. Finally, mechanical debridement gently loosens and removes slough from the wound bed. The simplest form of this technique is the commonly applied wet-to-dry saline gauze. Upon removable of this dressing, the dried gauze will be slightly adhered to the wound bed, thereby removing the very superficial tissue. While this is an inexpensive and relatively easy technique, it can remove both viable and nonviable tissue and cause pain in the sensate foot.

Pressure Off-loading

Reduction of pressures is essential in the healing of plantar foot ulcers. As discussed previously, ulcerations occur in high pressure areas of the insensate foot. There are a number of methods employed for the reduction of foot pressures, with varying success rates. The most popular methods include total contact casting, half shoes, short leg walkers, and felted foam dressings.

Total contact casting has been considered the most effective means of off-loading diabetic foot ulcers as measured by wound-healing rate [80]. Described by Paul Brand, total contact casting involves the use of a well-molded minimally padded plaster cast to distribute pressures evenly to the entire limb. It allows for patient mobility during treatment and has been found to help control edema linked to impairment of healing [81]. The main advantage and likely effectiveness of total contact casting however, is the forced patient compliance due to the inability to remove the apparatus. Disadvantages include the considerable skill and time required for application, the possibility of secondary skin lesions due to cast irritation, and the inability to assess the wound daily.

Because of the considerable disadvantages associated with the total contact cast, few clinicians use it as the technique of choice in regular clinical practice. Instead, commercially available off-the-shelf devices such as the half-shoe and short leg walker are more commonly used. Both these devices are relatively inexpensive, easy to use, and readily accepted by the patient. However, pressure reduction is significantly less compared to total contact casting, and patient compliance cannot be assured because of the removable nature of the devices [82].

Felted foam dressings are accommodative off-loading devices fashioned from a felt-foam pad with an aperture corresponding to the ulceration for customized pressure relief. The pad is generally attached by tape or rubber cement directly to the patients skin, preventing migration of the pad and ensuring a degree of patient compliance (Figure 7). Wound care and wound assessment can be performed through the aperture portion. The felted foam is often used in conjunction with a surgical shoe or half-shoe and must be changed every 10–14 days to ensure integrity of the dressing. Felted foam dressings in combination with a surgical shoe or half-shoe were found to be more effective in pressure reduction when compared to a short leg walker or a half-shoe alone [83].

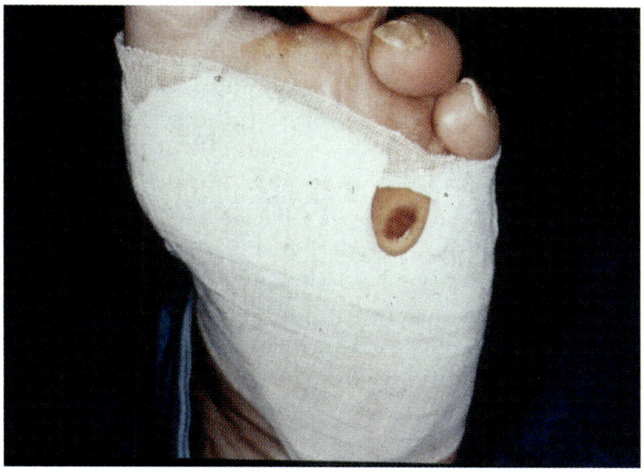

Figure 7 The felted foam dressing is an effective pressure off-loading modality for patients with Wagner 1 and 2 foot ulcers. The felted foam can stay in place for 1 week while wound care and wound assessment can be performed through the aperture portion

Treatment of Infection

A diabetic foot ulcer serves as a portal of entry for bacteria with subsequent infection. Diagnosis of infection is primarily based on clinical appearance, relying on clinical signs such as erythema, edema, pain, tenderness, and warmth. The severity of the infection can range from a superficial cellulitis to a deep abscess or necrotizing fasciitis with systemic toxicity. Care must be taken to diagnose and treat infections sufficiently, as mild cellulitis can rapidly progress to a limb-threatening infection if left untreated.

The diagnosis and course of treatment can be facilitated with diagnostic tools such as cultures, radiographs, and more advanced imaging techniques. When clinical infection of an ulcer is suspected, cultures of the wound will aid in directing subsequent antibiotic therapy. It should be noted that clinically uninfected ulcers should not be cultured, as the organisms recovered will only consist of colonizing flora. Empirical antibiotic therapy should be started, with revision of therapy following culture results.

Radiographic imaging of the infected foot can demonstrate increased density and thickening of the subcutaneous fat along with blurring of the usually visible fat planes [84, 90]. Presence of osseous changes such as periosteal reaction, cortical bone destruction, and focal osteopenia may suggest a diagnosis of osteomyelitis. However, these changes only become evident after osteomyelitis has been present for 10–14 days and require up to 50%

bone loss before becoming recognizable [85]. Advanced imaging techniques such as magnetic resonance imaging and computed tomography may aid in the accurate diagnosis of osteomyelitis, as well as demonstrate abscess formations.

Treatment of infection involves debridement of all necrotic tissue and drainage of purulent collections along with antibiotic therapy. Antibiotic selection should take into account the likely causative organisms while bearing in mind the potential toxicity of the agents. In the diabetic foot, the bacteria most likely responsible for non-limb-threatening infections are staphylococcus and streptococci, while limb-threatening infections are generally the consequence of a polymicrobial infection [86].

Empiric antibiotic selection should be based on the suspected bacterial pathogens along with modifications to address anticipated resistant pathogens that may have been selected during prior hospitalizations. Antibiotic selection should minimize toxicity and be cost-effective. Broad-spectrum antimicrobial therapy should be begun empirically with reassessment following the results of culture and sensitivities. Treatment regimens should then be simplified on the basis of the culture data. The main antibiotic regimens for initial empiric therapy that are employed in our unit is shown in Table 1 [88].

The duration of antimicrobial therapy for severe soft-tissue infections of the foot is based on response to the antibiotics and wound care. Two weeks of therapy is the usual guideline, however, recalcitrant infections may require longer courses. Even if the ulcer has not fully healed, antibiotics can be discontinued when evidence of infection has resolved. Continuation of antibiotics beyond this duration has not demonstrated any effect on wound healing [87, 89].

Wound Care

The effective use of dressings is essential to ensure the optimal management of diabetic foot ulcers. In recent years, the concept of a clean, moist wound-healing environment has been widely accepted. Benefits to this approach include prevention of tissue dehydration and cell death, acceleration of angiogenesis, and facilitating the interaction of growth factors with the target cells [90]. In addition, patients have reported less discomfort with moist wound dressings. The notion that a moist wound environment increases the risk of developing an infection appears to be unfounded. There are a multitude of wound care products available on the market that promote moist wound healing; however, wet-to-dry-normal saline gauze remains the standard of care.

Advanced Wound Care Products

Advanced wound care products have been developed in response to an improved understanding of the impaired wound healing integral in the diabetic foot ulcer. Pathophysiologic defects such as decreased growth factors production and cellular inactivity have led to the development of products that address these deficiencies. Products in this category include recombinant PDGF and biological skin substitutes.

Recombinant human-platelet-derived growth factor BB (rhPDGF-BB) (becaplermin) is the only growth factor to date approved by the US Food and Drug Administration for the treatment of diabetic foot ulcers. PDGF-B is a potent mitogen and chemotactic agent for connective tissue and stromal cells and may act to increase the wound vascularization by stimulating endothelial cell proliferation, movement, and tube formation. Levels of PDGF have been shown to be lower in chronic wounds [91]. Administered

Table 1 Selected antibiotic regimens for initial empiric therapy of foot infections in patients with diabetes mellitus*

Infection	Antimicrobial regimen†
Non-limb-threatening	Cephalexin 500 mg p.o. q6h
	Clindamycin 300 mg p.o. q8h
	Amoxicillin-clavulanate (875/125 mg) 1 q12h
	Dicloxacillin 500 mg p.o. q6h
	Levofloxacin 500–750 mg p.o. qd
Limb-threatening	Ceftriaxone‡ 1 g IV daily plus clindamycin 450–600 mg IV q8h
	Ciprofloxacin 400 mg IV q12h plus clindamycin 450–600 mg IV q8h
	Ampicillin/sulbactam 3 g IV q6h
	Ticarcillin/clavulanate 3.1 g IV q4–6h
	Piperacillin/tazobactam 3.375 g IV q4h or 4.5 g IV q6h
	Fluoroquinolone§ IV plus metronidazole 500 mg IV q6h
Life-threatening	Imipenem cilastatin 500 mg IV q6h
	Piperacillin/tazobactam 4.5 g IV q6h plus gentamicin‖ 1.5 mg/kg IV q8h
	Vancomycin 1 g IV q12h plus gentamicin plus metronidazole

* From reference 87.
† Doses for patients with normal renal function.
‡ An alternative is cefotaxime 2 g IV q8h.
§ Fluoroquinolone with increased activity against gram positive cocci, e.g. levofloxacin 500–750 mg IV qd.
‖ Can be given as single daily dose 5.1 mg/kg/day.

in a gel formulation concurrent with a standard wound care, becaplermin gel increased both the incidence of complete wound closure and decreased the time to achieve complete wound healing [92].

Biological skin substitutes, also known as living skin equivalents (LSE), are commercially offered in both autograft and allergenic form. The allergenic LSEs are produced from neonatal fibroblasts and keratinocytes using tissue-engineering technology. Available for epidermal, dermal, and composite (epidermal and dermal) wounds, LSEs offer distinct advantages over traditional skin grafting as their use is noninvasive, does not require anesthesia, can be performed in an outpatient setting, and avoids potential-donor-site complications such as infection and scarring [93]. Furthermore, more rapid wound coverage of chronic diabetic foot ulcers with the use of LSEs can provide both social and economic advantages by reducing the number of office visits and hospital stays, and preventing serious wound complications that often lead to amputation.

Two LSEs are currently approved for use in diabetic foot ulcers, the Dermagraft (Advanced Tissue Sciences Inc., La Jolla, CA, USA) and Apligraf (Organogenesis, Inc., Canton, MA, USA, distributed by Novartis Pharmaceutical Corp., East Hanover, NJ, USA). Dermagraft consists of neonatal dermal fibroblasts cultured *in vitro* onto a bioabsorbable polyglactin mesh, producing a living, metabolically active tissue containing the normal dermal matrix proteins and cytokines. Dermagraft has been shown to incorporate quickly into the wound with good vascularization and with no adverse side effects [94, 95]. In a prospective randomized multicenter study, Dermagraft-treated ulcers were associated with more complete and rapid healing with the added benefit of a reduction in the ulcer recurrence rate compared to conventional therapy [96].

Apligraf is considered a composite graft, containing both epidermal and dermal components. The outer layer consists of allergenic human keratinocytes constructed with an inner dermal layer consisting of human fibroblasts on type 1 collagen dispersed in a protein matrix. While Apligraf histologically resembles human skin, it does not contain structures such as blood vessels, hair follicles, or sweat glands. Interestingly, Apligraf acts like human skin, producing all the cytokines and growth factors produced by normal skin during the wound-healing process [97]. In diabetic foot ulcers, Apligraf was shown to significantly increase the wound-healing rate as well as decrease the median time to complete wound closure [98, 99]. Ulcer recurrence rate was similar in both Apligraf-treated ulcers and standard treatment groups [99].

While the precise mechanism of action of Dermagraft and Apligraf is not completely understood, it is believed that improved wound healing is due to filling of the wound with extracellular matrix proteins and with the subsequent induction and expression of growth factors and cytokines necessary for wound healing. Additionally, the matrix components may further facilitate the recruitment of cells to the wound, improving wound repair.

Algorithms for Ulcer Treatment and the Appropriate Use of Advanced Wound Care Products

Although advanced wound care products can increase the rate of complete wound healing, they carry the disadvantage of being very expensive, to the extent that their use is prohibited in some societies with limited resources. However, even in prosperous societies their use is not recommended in all patients as they carry a heavy economic cost. The current consensus is that they should be employed only in cases that are likely to fail standard care. The identification of such patients is therefore very important as it can help individual patients heal their ulcers while at the same time do not impose a disadvantageous economical burden to the society.

Observing the changes in wound area over a 4-week period while intensive standard care is administered is the best method currently available to identify the patients who do not respond to standard care and are more likely to benefit by advanced wound care products (Figure 8).

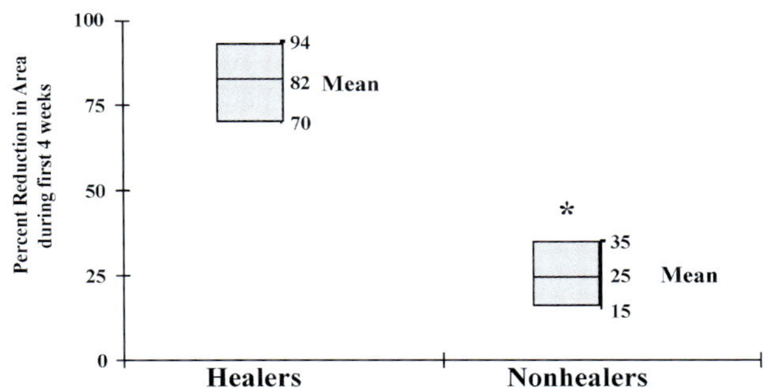

Figure 8 Mean percent ulcer area reduction during the first 4 weeks of a prospective study that followed up a large number of patients for a 12-week period. Patients who completely healed their ulcer during the 12-week period of the study are characterized as *healers* and those who failed to heal their ulcer as *nonhealers*. The ulcer area was measured by multiplying the length by the width of the ulcer. During the first 4 weeks of the study, the healers had a mean percent ulcer area reduction of 82% (95% CI 70–94) significantly higher to that of the nonhealers who had a 25% reduction (95% CI 15–35, $p < 0.001$). The midpoint between the percentage area reduction from baseline at 4 weeks in patients healed vs. those not healed at 12 weeks was 53%. Subjects with an ulcer area reduction above the 4-week median had a 12-week healing rate of 58%, while those below had a healing rate of only 9% ($p < 0.01$). Thus, patients who fail to reduce their ulcer area to half over a 4-week period should be considered as to be unlikely to heal, and the use of advanced wound care products may be justifiable. * indicates $p < 0.01$. (from reference 100)

The wound area is calculated by measuring the maximal width and length of the ulcer. Patients who fail to reduce the wound area by 50% during this period are unlikely to achieve complete wound closure in the next few months and should be selected for additional advanced treatment [100]. Patients who exceed the 50% reduction should continue to receive standard care; in the event, ulcer area reduction slows to less than 50% in subsequent visits should a change in wound care be considered.

Treatment by Ulcer Severity

Treatment of the diabetic foot ulcer should be individually tailored according to the size, depth, location, and presence/absence of infection or ischemia. Location of the ulcer will give clues as to the etiology of the wound, whether it is due to shoe pressure or an osseous prominence. Size and depth plays a key role in determining the length of time required for wound healing. The presence of infection should be addressed with appropriate antibiotic therapy or surgical incision and drainage when required. Ischemic ulcers demand revascularization techniques in order for wound healing to proceed.

The treatment of ulcers based on grade, as delineated by the Wagner classification, will be presented here. It is important to note that as a general rule, Wagner grades 0 and 1 ulcers and the vast majority of grade 2 ulcers are largely managed on an outpatient basis, while patients with Wagner Grades 3,4, and 5 ulcers may require hospitalization. Table 2 describes the management of specific Wagner-classified foot ulcers based on treatment rendered and medical personnel involved.

Wagner Grade 0

As mentioned earlier, all patients identified as being at risk of developing foot ulceration should be classified as grade 0. The management of the grade 0 foot ulcers consists primarily of patient education and regular foot care in an effort to prevent the development of foot ulceration. Regarding education, the patients should be informed of the risks associated with the neuropathic foot along with the early signs and symptoms of infection. In addition, the need of regular foot care by a specialist and the avoidance of self-care should be emphasized. Finally the daily inspection of the foot by the patient or a member of his close environment should be arranged. Literature with simple and easily understood guidelines is available worldwide by various sources, and all patients should have access to this information.

Regular visits for podiatric care should be part of the patients health care management. Clinical inspection of the feet should be performed with evaluation of vascular perfusion to the foot. Hyperkeratotic lesions such as corns and calluses should be debrided at these visits. Shoe and sock modifications may be necessary to accommodate and pad any foot deformities. Extra-depth diabetic shoes and custom-molded inserts both serve to protect osseous prominences and also effectively reduce plantar foot pressures [101]. High foot pressures can also be alleviated with the use of padded hosiery [102].

Wagner Grade 1

Grade 1 ulceration is defined as one that has penetrated beyond the epidermis. The presence of sensory neuropathy and at least one other risk factor is assured. The ulcer should be evaluated for size, depth, location, and any signs of infection. The presence of drainage, as well as the type of drainage should be noted.

The hallmark of treatment in these ulcers is debridement of all nonviable tissue, local wound care, off-loading of pressures, and antibiotic therapy if warranted. Sharp debridement of the ulcer should be performed as previously discussed in this chapter. Following debridement, the foot must be off-loaded to eliminate all pressure from the site of ulceration to promote epithelialization. The authors commonly use the felted foam dressing for off-loading. This method is easy to perform, relatively inexpensive, and

Table 2 Principles of treatment and medical personnel involved in diabetic foot ulcers based on the Wagner classification

	Principles of treatment	Provider involved
Wagner grade 0	Patient education, outpatient routine preventative foot care, and protective shoewear	diabetes educator, podiatrist, pedorthotist
Wagner grade 1	Outpatient ulcer care with debridement and off-loading	podiatrist
Wagner grade 2	Outpatient ulcer care with debridement, off-loading, and wound care. Treatment of infection as warranted	podiatrist
Wagner grade 3	Outpatient/inpatient ulcer care consisting of bedside or surgical debridement with off-loading and wound care. Treatment of infection as necessary	podiatrist, surgeon, infectious disease specialist
Wagner grade 4	Inpatient care consisting of surgical debridement and antibiotic therapy. Revascularization may be required with possible amputation	podiatrist, vascular surgeon, Infectious disease, orthopedic surgeon
Wagner grade 5	Inpatient care consisting of revascularization if possible and probable amputation	vascular surgeon, orthopedic surgeon, rehabilitation therapy

reproducible. Wound care can be performed through the window of the felted foam dressing.

Ulcerations that recur may warrant surgical correction of any underlying structural deformity. Surgical procedures such as digital arthroplasties, metatarsal osteotomies, metatarsal head resections, and midfoot and hindfoot exostectomies have all proved useful in the prevention of recurrent ulcerations [103–107].

Wagner Grade 2

Grade 2 ulcer is a full thickness ulcer that penetrates beyond the dermis with involvement of deeper structures such as tendons, ligaments, or joint capsules. The management of such ulcers is usually based on an outpatient basis although hospitalization can be considered in deep wounds that expose tendons, and complications such as peripheral vascular disease and infection are suspected.

Outpatient care for the full thickness ulcer that has a noninfected granulating basis is similar to the grade 1 ulceration described above. Broad-spectrum antibiotics may be added in case infection is suspected and dressing changes may be performed more often in cases of heavy exudates. Advanced wound care products may be considered for patients who are not exhibiting a satisfactory progress using the criteria previously described.

Involvement of deep structures to the base of the ulcer should be managed with aggressive debridement, complete bed rest, empiric use of broad-spectrum antibiotics, and occasionally hospitalization [108]. The foot may require surgical debridement in order to remove all necrotic and nonviable tissue that may impede granulation tissue. Debridement should be carried out until there is evidence of healthy, red, granulation tissue to the base. Additionally, all sinus tracts should be explored and drained. Intraoperative deep cultures should be taken for identification of the pathogen responsible for infection.

In the event that vascular insufficiency is suspected, incision and drainage of the infected foot should not be delayed. Adequate drainage of the infected foot is paramount to limb salvage. Delaying of surgical drainage may lead to further tissue loss as well as potential limb loss [109]. Instead, vascular consultation should be initiated as soon as possible, even if it occurs after surgical drainage.

Wagner Grade 3

Grade 3 ulcerations are characterized by the presence of deep infection with bone involvement and abscess collections. Grade 3 ulcers are usually the result of grade 2 ulcers that fail to respond, aggressive bacterial infections, or puncture wounds resulting in direct inoculation of bone. Because of the depth of these ulcers and the presence of purulent collections and bone infection, patients with these ulcers require hospitalization with adequate drainage of all infection and debridement of all infected bone. Prolonged antibiotic therapy may be required.

Adequate drainage of infection is key in managing grade 3 ulcerations. All sinus tracts must be explored and all necrotic and nonviable tissue debrided. In cases of severe infection, open amputations of digits or rays may be required to prevent the spread of infection. Once the infection has cleared and granulation of the wound bed observed, thought can be given to coverage of the wound. In instances where soft-tissue coverage is adequate, delayed primary closure can be undertaken. However, more often than not in these extensive wounds, significant soft-tissue defects may be present, requiring osseous remodeling in addition to tissue flaps or skin grafts to provide wound coverage [110]. No single technique can be applied universally. Instead, a flexible approach will maximize limb salvage.

Wagner Grade 4

Grade 4 ulcerations demonstrate partial foot gangrene. These ulcers are usually complicated by ischemia, osteomyelitis, and sepsis. A team approach is required in order to minimize the extent of tissue loss and prevent amputation. Consultations with vascular surgeons, podiatrists, infectious disease specialists, and plastic surgeons are essential for limb salvage. The primary goal in the management of these ulcers is to limit the extent of tissue loss.

Gangrenous changes can result from minor trauma in the face of severe arterial insufficiency or when overwhelming infection results in occlusion of digital arterial branches [10, 111]. Initial treatment of gangrene secondary to severe arterial insufficiency should begin with vascular assessment followed by revascularization when possible [109]. In severe infections resulting in local ischemia, aggressive drainage along with appropriate antibiotic therapy should be instituted to limit tissue loss.

Wagner Grade 5

Grade 5 ulcerations demonstrate extensive necrosis of the entire foot as a direct result of arterial insufficiency. Primary amputation is the only treatment for extensive gangrene. However, vascular assessment and revascularization should always be attempted to allow for amputation at the most distal level of the foot.

CHARCOT NEUROARTHROPATHY

Charcot neuroarthropathy is a noninfectious progression of joint destruction characterized by pathologic fractures and joint dislocations. Described initially in 1868 by J.M. Charcot [112], it described joint destruction accompanying common diseases that manifested peripheral neuropathy such as leprosy, tertiary syphilis, chronic alcoholism and spina bifida [113]. However, diabetes mellitus is currently the primary cause of Charcot neuroarthropathy.

Etiology

The exact etiology of Charcot neuroarthropathy remains unclear. There are two leading theories: the neurotraumatic (German) theory, and the neurovascular (French) theory. The neurotraumatic theory proposed that repeated microtrauma on neuropathic joints results in the eventual joint destruction [114]. Thus, repetitive minor stresses on insensate joints produce intracapsular effusions, ligamentous laxity, and joint instability. With continued use of the foot, degeneration of the joints continues, often resulting in severe joint dislocation and deformity.

In contrast, the neurovascular theory suggested that the main factor is the autonomic-neuropathy-related hyperemia that causes excessive bone resorption and leads to weakening of the bone [115]. The hyperemic bone resorption thus allows for increased risk of pathologic fractures with joint dislocation and destruction evident in Charcot joints. This theory corresponds to the clinical observation that Charcot neuroarthropathy occurs most commonly in patients with palpable pedal pulses [116]. Further support to this hypothesis is provided by studies in our unit that have shown that the nonspecific hyperemic response to skin heating is increased in patients with neuroarthropathy when compared to diabetic patient with equally severe neuropathy [50]. The current consensus is that the process of Charcot neuroarthropathy is secondary to a combination of both the neurovascular and neurotraumatic theories.

Clinical Findings

Regardless of the exact etiology, the Charcot foot usually presents as a warm, nonpainful, swelling of the foot. Usually there is no evidence of an open wound and an infectious process can be excluded based on lack of a portal of entry. Occasionally, patients may describe a precedent history of minor trauma; however, this is frequently so trivial that the patient is unable to recall the incident. Trauma in the form of foot surgery can also be another precipitating factor. The Charcot neuroarthropathy can occur in either the ipsilateral or contralateral limb following foot surgery. This phenomenon can be attributed to the likely alteration in weight-bearing forces in joints of the foot, triggering the Charcot joint changes.

Initial evaluation of Charcot neuroarthropathy requires a thorough clinical and radiographic examination of the foot. Clinical examination reveals a warm, edematous foot with evidence of crepitus with joint range of motion. Most commonly, pain is absent or significantly less than expected from the clinical presentation. Radiographic findings demonstrate osseous debris and fragmentation with mild to frank joint subluxation. The most common site affected in the foot is the tarsometatarsal joint [117]. The extent of fragmentation and joint destruction is variable and most often related to the particular joints affected and the degree of ambulation prior to diagnosis. Advanced imaging techniques such as CT scans and MRIs are rarely necessary to make the diagnosis of Charcot joint and instead may be more useful in preoperative surgical planning in certain cases.

There are three identifiable clinical phases of Charcot neuroarthropathy: acute, coalescence, and remodeling. The acute phase is characterized by clinical findings of edema, erythema, localized warmth, and joint crepitus with range of motion examination. The coalescence phase begins when skin temperature normalizes and joint crepitus diminishes. With a period of duration lasting from months to years, the remodeling phase is characterized by joint stabilization and remodeling.

Resolution of Charcot neuroarthropathy can result in a deformed foot with obvious boney prominences susceptible to ulceration [113] (Figure 9). If diagnosed early and sufficient immobilization is rendered, the possibility of joint collapse with resulting osseous prominences may be mitigated. However, in instances of misdiagnosis or inadequate immobilization, a "rocker-bottom" type foot can result, with gross deformities of the involved joint and prominent areas to the plantar aspect of the foot. These prominent areas are prone to increased pressure and ulceration. Ulcerations secondary to Charcot deformities should be evaluated surgically, as discussed in the treatment section below.

Treatment

The treatment of choice for acute Charcot foot is complete immobilization and nonweight bearing. Immobilization can be achieved with casts, splints, or braces and nonweight bearing aided with the use of crutches, walkers, or wheelchairs. Failure to adequately nonweight bear the foot may result in further fragmentation of bone with progression of the joint deformity, resulting in a nonplantigrade foot. The ultimate goal of immobilization therapy is to allow for the foot to coalesce in a shape that will allow for eventual ambulation.

Immobilization and nonweight bearing should continue until the acute phase of Charcot has ended and the coalescence phase commenced. The duration of immobilization varies from 8 to 32 weeks [118, 119]. The decision to begin weight bearing may be best made by clinical parameters such as foot temperature (should be the same with the contralateral limb) and resolution of erythema and edema, rather than an arbitrary time period. Serial radiographs may also aid in the decision-making process. Evidence of osseous consolidation, union of fractures, and

(a)

(b)

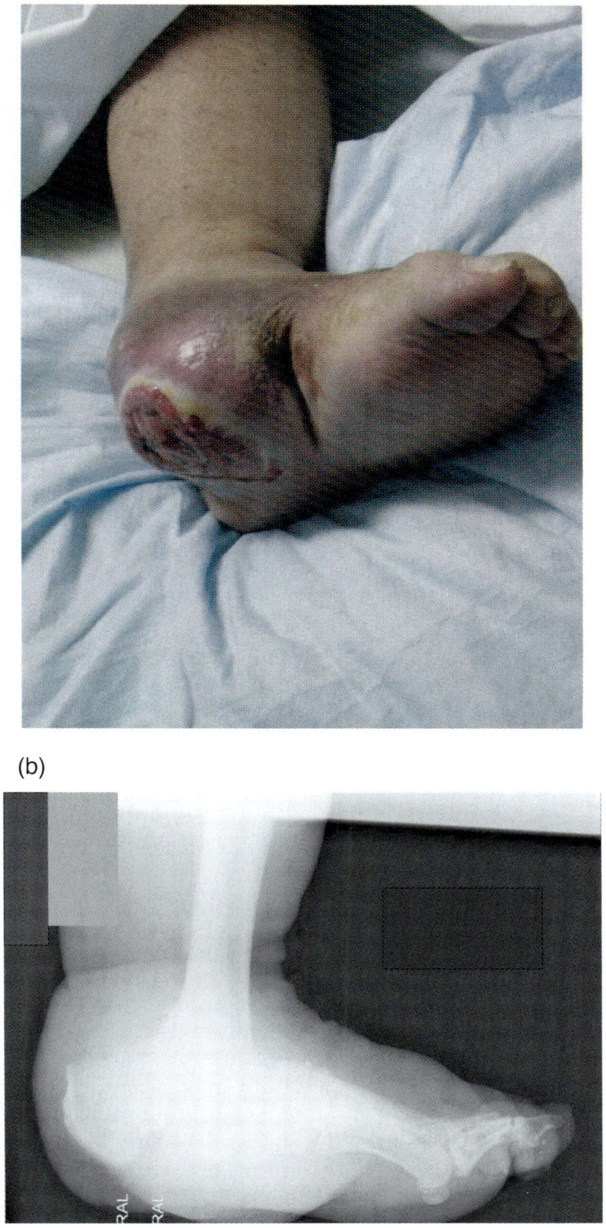

Figure 9 (a) Midfoot Charcot neuroarthropathy in a diabetic patient with severe peripheral neuropathy. Severe foot deformity has resulted in an area where high pressures have been applied during walking leading to extensive ulceration. (b) X-ray from the same patient shows extensive destruction of the midfoot joints

reduction in soft-tissue edema are radiographic clues that coalescence has begun.

Once weight bearing is deemed safe, return to ambulation should be performed in a gradual manner. Typically, weight bearing is begun allowing only 15–20 lb of weight on the affected limb, with 10-lb increments added on a weekly basis. Should symptoms of the acute phase such as edema, erythema, and warmth appear, immobilization and nonweight bearing should be resumed until resolution of these symptoms occur. As weight bearing progresses, the patient is eventually allowed to fully ambulate short distances without the use of assistive devices.

In recent years, increased attention has been given to surgical reconstruction of the severely deformed Charcot foot. In cases where immobilization and nonweight bearing have failed to prevent extensive joint dislocation, a rocker-bottom type foot with osseous prominences can be the end result. This type of foot is not amenable to ambulation and is highly susceptible to ulceration. Therefore, arthrodesis of the involved joints may provide a stable platform for ambulation in addition to preventing future ulcerations. However, patients undergoing joint fusions will require extended periods of immobilization and nonweight bearing postoperatively, and therefore should be screened carefully.

REFERENCES

1. Gibbons G, Eliopolos G. Infection of the diabetic foot. In Kozak G, Hoar CJ, Rowbotham J, Wheelock F, Gibbons G, Campbell D (eds), *Management of Diabetic Foot Problems*. Philadelphia: Saunders, 1984; pp 97–102.
2. Ramsey SD, Newton K, Blough D, McCulloch DK, Sandhu N, Reiber GE, Wagner EH. Incidence, outcomes, and cost of foot ulcers in patients with diabetes. *Diabetes Care* 1999; 22: 382–7.
3. Palumbo PJ, Melton LJ. Peripheral vascular disease and diabetes. In Harris MI, Hamman RF (eds), *Diabetes in America*. Washington, DC: US Government Printing Office, 1985; pp XV, 1–21.
4. Borssen B, Bergenheim T, Lithner F. The epidemiology of foot lesions in diabetic patients aged 15–50 years. *Diabet Med* 1999; 7: 438–44.
5. Kumar S, Asche HA, Fernando DJS. The prevalence of foot ulceration and its correlates in type 2 diabetic patients: a population-based study. *Diabet Med* 1994; 11: 480–4.
6. Moss SE, Klein R, Klein BEK. The prevalence and incidence of lower extremity amputation in a diabetic population. *Arch Intern Med* 1992; 152: 610–6.
7. Harrington C, Zagari MJ, Corea J, Klitenic J. A cost analysis of diabetic lower extremity ulcers. *Diabetes Care* 2000; 23: 1333–8.
8. Apelqvist J, Ragnarson-Tennvall G, Persson U, Larson J. Diabetic foot ulcers in a multi-disciplinary setting: an economic analysis of primary healing and healing with amputation. *J Intern Med* 1994; 235: 463–71.
9. Reiber GE, Boyko E, Smith DG. Lower extremity ulcers and amputations in individuals with diabetes. In Boyko EJ, Reiber GE, Bennett PH (eds), *Diabetes in America*. Washington, DC: US Government Printing Office, 1995; pp 409–27.
10. Pecoraro RE, Reiber GE, Burgess EM. Pathways to diabetic limb amputation: basis for prevention. *Diabetes Care* 1990; 13: 513–21.

11. Reiber GE, Pecorraro RE, Koepsell TD. Risk factors for amputation in patients with diabetes mellitus: a case-control study. *Ann Int Med* 1992; 117: 97–105.
12. Lehto S, Pyorala K, Ronnemaa T, Laakso M. Risk factors predicting lower extremity amputations in patients with NIDDM. *Diabetes Care* 1996; 19: 607–12.
13. Nelson RG, Gohdes DM, Everhart JE, Hartner JA, Zwemer DJ, Dettitt DJ, Knowler WC. Lower extremity amputations in NIDDM: 12 yr follow-up study in Pima Indians. *Diabetes Care* 1988; 11: 8–16.
14. Sitonen OI, Niskanen LK, Laakso M, Sittonen J, Pyoral K. Lower-extremity amputations in diabetic and nondiabetic patients. *Diabetes Care* 1988; 16: 16–20.
15. Resnick HE, Valsania P, Phillips CL. Diabetes mellitus and nontraumatic lower extremity amputation in black and white Americans: the National Health and Nutrition Examination Survey epidemiologic follow-up study, 1971–1992. *Arch Intern Med* 1999; 159: 2470–5.
16. Wrobel JS, Mayfield JA, Reiber GE. Geographic variation of lower-extremity major amputation in individuals with and without diabetes in the Medicare population. *Diabetes Care* 2001; 24: 1–5.
17. Most RS, Sinnock P. The epidemiology of lower extremity amputations in diabetic individuals. *Diabetes Care* 1983; 6: 87–91.
18. Flegal KM, Ezzati TM, Harris M, Haynes SG, Juarez RZ, Knowler WI, Perez-Stable EJ, Stern MP. Prevalence of diabetes in Mexican Americans, Cubans and Puerto Ricans from the Hispanic Health and Nutrition Examination Survey, 1982–1984. *Diabetes Care* 1991; 14: 628–38.
19. Roseman JM. Diabetes in black Americans. In *Diabetes in America*. Washington, DC: US Government Printing Office, 1985.
20. Edmonds ME, Blundell MP, Morris ME, Thomas EM, Cotton LT, Watkins PJ. Improved survival of the diabetic foot: the role of a specialized foot clinic. *J Med* 1986; 60: 763–71.
21. Lippmann HI. Must loss of a limb be a consequence of diabetes mellitus? *Diabetes Care* 1979; 2: 432–6.
22. Reiber GE. Diabetic foot care: guidelines and financial implications. *Diabetes Care* 1992; 15: 29–31.
23. Bakker K, Rauwerda JA, Schaper NC. *Diabetes Metab Res Rev* 2000; 16 (suppl 1): S1.
24. Reiber GE, Vileikyte L, Boyko EJ, Del Aguila M, Smith DG, Lavery LA, Boulton AJM. Causal pathways for incident lower-extremity ulcers in patients with diabetes from two settings. *Diabetes Care* 1999; 22: 157–62.
25. Young MJ, Breddy JL, Veves A, Boulton AJM. The prediction of diabetic neuropathic foot ulceration using vibration perception thresholds: a prospective study. *Diabetes Care* 1994; 17: 557–60.
26. Adler AI, Boyko EJ, Ahroni JH, Stensel V, Forsberg RC, Smith DG. Risk factors for diabetic peripheral sensory neuropathy. Results of the Seattle prospective diabetic foot study. *Diabetes Care* 1997; 96: 223–8.
27. Ward JD, Simms JM, Knight G, Boulton AJM, Sandler DA. Venous distension in the diabetic neuropathic foot. *J R Soc Med* 1983; 76: 1011–4.
28. Boulton AJM, Scarpello JHB, Ward JD. Venous oxygenation in the diabetic neuropathic foot: evidence of arteriovenous shunting? *Diabetologia* 1982; 22: 6–8.
29. Tegner R. The effect of skin temperature on vibratory sensitivity in polyneuropathy. *J Neurol Neurosurg Psychiatry* 1985; 48: 176–8.
30. Boulton AJ, Hardisty CA, Betts RP, Franks CI, Worth RC, Ward JC, Duckworth T. Dynamic foot pressure and other studies as diagnostic and management aids in diabetic neuropathy. *Diabetes Care* 1983; 1: 26–33.
31. Stokes IA, Furis IB, Hutton WC. The neuropathic ulcer and loads on the foot in diabetic patients. *Acta Orthop Scand* 1975; 46: 839–47.
32. Ctercteko G, Dhanendran M, Hutton WC, et al. Vertical forces acting on the feet of diabetic patients with neuropathic ulceration. *Br J Surg* 1981; 68: 608–14.
33. Veves A, Fernando DK, Walewski P, Boulton AJ. A study of plantar pressures in a diabetic clinic population. *Foot* 1991; 2: 89–92.
34. Fernando DJ, Masson EA, Veves A, Boulton AJ. Relationship of limited joint mobility to abnormal foot pressures and diabetic foot ulceration. *Diabetes Care* 1991; 14 (1): 8–11.
35. Caselli A, Pham HT, Giurini JM, Armstrong DG, Veves A. The forefoot/rearfoot plantar pressure ratio is increased in severe diabetic neuropathy and can predict foot ulceration. *Diabetes Care* 2002; 25: 1066–71.
36. Veves A, Murray HJ, Young MJ, et al. The risk of foot ulceration in diabetic patients with high foot pressure: a prospective study. *Diabetologia* 1992; 35: 660–3.
37. Kelly PJ, Coventry MB. Neurotrophic ulcers of the feet: review of 47 cases. *JAMA* 1958; 168: 388–90.
38. Sarnow MR, Veves A, Giurini JM, et al. In-shoe foot pressure measurements in diabetic patients with at-risk feet and in healthy subjects. *Diabetes Care* 1994; 17: 1002–6.
39. Crisp AJ, Heathcote JG. Connective tissue abnormalities in diabetes mellitus. *J R Coll Phys* 1984; 18: 132–41.
40. Vlassara H, Brownlee M, Cerami A. Nonenzymatic glycosylation: rose in the pathogenesis of diabetic complications. *Clin Chem* 1986; 32: B37–41.
41. Delbridge L, Perry P, Marr S, Arnold N, Yue DK, Turtle JR, Reeve TS. Limited joint mobility in the diabetic foot: relationship to neuropathic ulceration. *Diabet Med* 1988; 5: 333–7.
42. Mueller MJ, Diamond JE, Delitto A, Sinacore DR. Insensitivity, limited joint mobility, and plantar ulcers in patients with diabetes mellitus. *Phys Ther* 1989; 69: 453–62.
43. Birke JA, Franks BD, Foto JG. First ray joint limitation, pressure, and ulceration of the first metatarsal head in diabetes mellitus. *Foot Ankle* 1995; 16: 277–84.
44. Veves A, Sarnow MR, Giurini JM, Rosenblum BI, Lyons TE, Chrzan JS, Habershaw GM. Differences in joint mobility and foot pressures between black and white diabetic patients. *Diabet Med* 1995; 12: 585–9.
45. Grant WP, Sullivan R, Soenshine DE, et al. Electron microscopic investigation of the effects of diabetes mellitus on the Achilles tendon. *J Foot Ankle Surg* 1997; 36: 272–8.
46. Armstrong DG, Stacpoole-Shea S, Nguyen HC, Harkless LB. Lengthening of the Achilles tendon in diabetic patients who are at high risk for ulceration of the foot. *J Bone Joint Surg* 1999; 81A: 535–8.
47. Parving HH, Viberti GC, Keen H, Christiansen JS, Lassen NA. Hemodynamic factors in the genesis of diabetic microangiopathy. *Metabolism* 1983; 32: 943–9.
48. Rayman G, Williams SA, Spencer PD, et al. Impaired microvascular hyperaemic response to minor skin trauma in type I diabetes. *BMJ* 1986; 292: 1295–8.

49. Vane JR, Anggard EE, Botting RM. Regulatory functions of the vascular endothelium. *N Engl J Med* 1990; 323: 27–36.
50. Veves A, Akbari CM, Primavera J, et al. Endothelial dysfunction and the expression of endothelial nitric oxide synthetase in diabetic neuropathy, vascular disease, and foot ulceration. *Diabetes* 1998; 47: 457–63.
51. Arora S, Smakowski P, Frykberg RG, Freeman R, LoGerfo FW, Veves A. Differences in foot and forearm skin microcirculation in diabetic patients with and without neuropathy. *Diabetes Care* 1998; 21: 1339–44.
52. Caballero AE, Arora S, Saouaf R, Lim SC, Smakowski P, Park JY, King GL, LoGerfo FW, Horton ES, Veves A. Microvascular and macrovascular reactivity is reduced in subjects at risk for type 2 diabetes. *Diabetes* 1999; 48: 1856–62.
53. Szabo C, Zanchi A, Komjati K, Pacher P, Krolewski AS, Quist WC, LoGerfo FW, Horton ES, Veves A. Poly(ADP-ribose) polymerase is activated in subjects at risk of developing type 2 diabetes and is associated with impaired vascular reactivity. *Circulation* 2002; 106: 2680–6.
54. Arora S, Pomposelli F, LoGerfo FW, Veves A. Cutaneous microcirculation in the neuropathic diabetic foot improves significantly but not completely after successful lower extremity revascularization. *J Vasc Surg* 2002; 35: 501–5.
55. Caselli A, Rich J, Hanane T, Uccioli L, Veves A. Role of C-nociceptive fibers in the nerve axon reflex-related vasodilation in diabetes. *Neurology* 2003; 60: 297–300.
56. Hamdy O, Abou-Elenin K, LoGerfo FW, Horton ES, Veves A. Contribution of nerve–axon reflex-related vasodilation to the total skin vasodilation in diabetic patients with and without neuropathy. *Diabetes Care* 2001; 24: 344–9.
57. Parkhouse N, LeQueen PM. Impaired neurogenic vascular response in patients with diabetes and neuropathic foot lesions. *N Engl J Med* 1988; 318: 1306–9.
58. Schilling JA. Wound healing. *Physiol Rev* 1968; 48: 374–423.
59. Cooper DM, Yu EZ, Hennesey P, et al. Determination of endogenous cytokines in chronic wounds. *Ann Surg* 1994; 219: 688–92.
60. Zykova SN, Jenssen TG, Berdal M, et al. Altered cytokine and nitric oxide secretion in vitro by macrophages from diabetic type II-like *db/db* mice. *Diabetes* 2000; 40: 1451–8.
61. Spravchikov N, Sizyakov G, Gartsbein M, et al. Glucose effects on skin keratinocytes. *Diabetes* 2001; 50: 1627–35.
62. Jude EB, Boulton AJ, Ferguson MW, Appleton I. The role of nitric oxide synthase isoforms and arginase in the pathogenesis of diabetic foot ulcers: possible modulatory effects by transforming growth factor beta 1. *Diabetologia* 1999; 42: 748–57.
63. Loots MA, Lamme EN, Zeegelaar J, Mekkes JR, Bos JD, Middelkoop E. Differences in cellular infiltrate and extracellular matrix of chronic diabetic and venous ulcers versus acute wounds. *J Invest Dermatol* 1998; 111: 850–7.
64. Rith-Najarian SJ, Stolusky T, Gohdes DM. Identifying diabetic patients at high risk for lower-extremity amputation in a primary health care setting. *Diabetes Care* 1992; 22: 1036–42.
65. Boyko E, Ahroni JH, Stensel V, et al. A prospective study of risk factors for diabetic foot ulcer: the Seattle Diabetic Foot Study. *Diabetes Care* 1999; 22: 1036–42.
66. Mayfield JA, Reiber GE, Sanders LJ, et al. Preventative foot care in people with diabetes. *Diabetes Care* 1998; 21: 2161–77.
67. Boulton AJM, Gries FA, Jervell J. Guidelines for the diagnosis and outpatient management of diabetic periperal neuropathy. *Diabet Med* 1998; 15: 508–14.
68. Helm PA, Walker SC, Pulliam GF. Recurrence of neuropathic ulcerations following healing in a total contact cast. *Arch Phys Med Rehabil* 1991; 72: 967–70.
69. Young MJ, Cavanagh PR, Thomas G, Johnson MM, Murray H, Boulton AJM. The effect of callus removal on dynamic plantar pressures in diabetic patients. *Diabet Med* 1992; 9: 55–7.
70. Kumar S, Fernando DJ, Veves A, Knowles EA, Young MJ, Boulton AJ. Semmes-Weinstein monofilaments: a simple, effective and inexpensive screening device for identifying diabetic patients at risk of foot ulceration. *Diabetes Res Clin Pract* 1991; 13: 63–7.
71. Pham H, Armstrong DG, Harvey C, Harkless LB, Giurini JM, Veves A. Screening techniques to identify people at high risk for diabetic foot ulceration. *Diabetes Care* 2000; 23: 606–11.
72. McNeely MJ, Boyko E, Ahroni JH. The independent contributions of diabetic neuropathy and vasculopathy in foot ulceration: how great are the risks? *Diabetes Care* 1995; 18: 216–9.
73. Thompson FJ, Veves A, Ashe H, et al. A team approach to diabetic foot care-the Manchester experience. *Foot* 1991; 1: 75–82.
74. Wagner FW. The dysvascular foot: a system for diagnosis and treatment. *Foot Ankle* 1981; 2: 64–122.
75. Lavery LA, Armstrong DG, Harkless LB. Classification of diabetic foot wounds. *J Foot Ankle Surg* 1996; 36: 528–31.
76. Armstrong DG, Lavery L, Harkless LB. Validation of a diabetic wound classification system. *Diabet Med* 1998; 21: 855–9.
77. Steed DL, Donohoe D, Wbster MW, Lindsley L, for the Diabetic Ulcer Study Group. Effect of extensive debridement and treatment on the healing of diabetic foot ulcers. *J Am Coll Surg* 1996; 183: 61–4.
78. Clark RAF. Mechanisms of cutaneous wound repair. In Fitzpatrick TB, Austen KF, Wolff K, Eisen Az, Freedberg IM (eds), *Dermatology in General Medicine*. New York: McGraw-Hill, 1993.
79. Bale S. A guide to wound debridement. *J Wound Care* 1997; 6: 179–82.
80. Armstrong DG, Nguyen HC, Lavery LA, et al. Offloading the diabetic foot wound: a randomized clinical trial. *Diabetes Care* 2001; 24: 1019–22.
81. Mueller MJ, Diamond JE, Sinacore DR, et al. Total contact casting in treatment of diabetic plantar ulcers. *Diabetes Care* 1989; 12: 364–87.
82. Lavery LA, Vela SA, Lavery DC, et al. Reducting dynamic foot pressures in high-risk diabetics with foot ulcerations: a comparison of treatments. *Diabetes Care* 1996; 19: 818–21.
83. Birke JA, Fred B, Krieger LA, Sliman K. The effectiveness of an accommodative dressing in off loading pressure over areas of previous metatarsal head ulceration. *Wounds* 2003; 15: 33–9.
84. Cheung Y, Hochman M, Brophy DP. Radiographic changes in the diabetic foot. In Veves A, Giurini JM,

Logerfo FW (eds), *The Diabetic Foot*. Totawa, NJ: Humana Press, 2002; pp 179–205.

85. Bonakdar-Pour A, Gaines VD. The radiology of osteomyelitis. *Orthop Clin North Am* 1983; 14: 21–37.
86. Lipsky BA, Pecoraro RE, Wheat LJ. The diabetic foot: soft tissue and bone infection. *Infect Dis Clin North Am* 1990; 4: 409–32.
87. Jones EW, Edwards R, Finch R, Jaffcoate WJ. A microbiologic study of diabetic foot lesions. *Diabet Med* 1984; 2: 213–5.
88. Karchmer AW. Microbiology and treatment of diabetic foot infections. In Veves A, Giurini JM, LoGerfo FW (eds), *The Diabetic Foot. Medical and Surgical Management*. Totawa, NJ: Humana Press, 2002; pp 207–20.
89. Lipsky BA, Pecoraro RE, Larson SA, Hanley ME, Ahroni JH. Outpatient management of uncomplicated lower-extremity infections in diabetic patients. *Arch Intern Med* 1990; 150: 790–7.
90. Field FK, Kerstein MD. Overview of wound healing in a moist environment. *Am J Surg* 1994; 167 (1A): 2S–6S.
91. Cooper DM, Yu EZ, Hennesey P, et al. Determination of endogenous cytokines in chronic wounds. *Ann Surg* 1994; 219: 688–92.
92. Wieman TJ, Smiell JM, Su Y. Efficacy and safety of a topical gel formulation of recombinant human platelet-derived growth factor-BB (Becaplermin) in patients with chronic neuropathic diabetic ulcers. *Diabetes Care* 1998; 21: 822–7.
93. Muhart M, McFalls S, Kirsner RS, et al. Behavior of tissue-engineered skin. *Arch Dermatol* 1999; 135: 913–8.
94. Hansbrough JF, Dore C, Hansbrough WB. Clinical trials of a living dermal tissue replacement placed beneath meshed, split-thickness skin grafts on excised burn wounds. *J Burn Care Rehabil* 1992; 13: 519–29.
95. Cooper ML, Hansbrough JF, Spielvogel RL, et al. In vivo optimization of a living dermal substitute employing cultured human fibroblasts on a biodegradable polyglycolic acid or polyglactin mesh. *Biomaterials* 1991; 12: 243–8.
96. Gentzkow GD, Iwasaki SD, Hershon KS, et al. Use of Dermagraft, a cultured human dermis, to treat diabetic foot ulcers. *Diabetes Care* 1996; 19: 350–4.
97. Eaglstein WH, Iriondo M, Laszio K. A composite skin substitute (Graftskin) for surgical wounds: a clinical experience. *Dermat Surg* 1995; 21: 839, 834.
98. Brem H, Balledux J, Bloom T, Kerstein M, Hollier L. Healing of diabetic foot ulcers and pressure ulcers with human skin equivalent. *Arch Surg* 2000; 135: 627–34.
99. Veves A, Falanga V, Armstrong DG, Sabolinski ML. Graftskin, a human skin equivalent, is effective in the management of noninfected neuropathic diabetic foot ulcers. *Diabetes Care* 2001; 24: 290–5.
100. Sheehan P, Jones P, Caselli A, Giurini JM, Veves A. Percent change in wound area of diabetic foot ulcers over a 4-week period is a robust predictor of complete healing in a 12-week prospective trial. *Diabetes Care* 2003; 26: 1879–82.
101. Chanteleau E, Kushner T, Spraul M. How effective is cushioned therapeutic footwear in protecting diabetic feet. *Diabet Med* 1990; 7: 355–9.
102. Veves A, Masson EA, Fernando DJS, Boulton AIM. Studies of experimental padded hosiery to reduce foot pressures in diabetic neuropathy. *Diabetes Care* 1989; 12: 653–5.
103. Gudas CJ. Prophylactic surgery in the diabetic foot. *Clin Podiatr Med Surg* 1987; 4: 445–58.
104. Tillo TH, Giurini JM, Habershaw GM, Chrzan JS, Rowbotham JL. Review of metatarsal osteotomies for the treatment of neuropathic ulcerations. *J Am Podiatr Med Assoc* 1990; 80: 211–7.
105. Giurini JM, Basile P, Chrzan JS, Habershaw GM, Rosenblum BI. Panmetatarsal head resection: a viable alternative to the transmetatarsal amputation. *J Am Podiatr Med Assoc* 1993; 83: 101–7.
106. Giurini JM, Rosenblum BI. The role of foot surgery in patients with diabetes. *Clin Podiatr Med Surg* 1995; 12: 119–27.
107. Rosenblum BI, Giurini JM, Chrzan JS, Habershaw GM. Preventing loss of the great toe with the hallux interphalangeal joint arthroplasty. *J Foot Ankle Surg* 1994; 33: 557–60.
108. Gibbons GW. The diabetic foot: amputations and drainage of infection. *J Vasc Surg* 1987; 5: 791–3.
109. Taylor LM, Porter JM. The clinical course of diabetic patients who require emergent foot surgery because of infection or ischemia. *J Vasc Surg* 1987; 6: 454–9.
110. Attinger CE. Use of soft tissue techniques for the salvage of the diabetic foot. In Kominsky SJ (ed), *Medical and Surgical Management of the Diabetic Foot* Boston: Mosby-Year Book, Inc, 1994; pp 323–36.
111. Edmonds M, Foster A, Oreenhill M, et al. Acute septic vasculitis not diabetic micro antiopathy leads to digital necrosis in the neuropathic foot. *Diabet Med* 1992; 9 (suppl): P85.
112. Charcot JM. Sur quelques arthropathies qui paraissent dependre d'une lesion du cerveau ou de la moelle epiniere. *Arch Physiol Norm Pathol* 1868; 1: 161–78.
113. Sanders LJ, Frykberg RG. Diabetic neuropathic osteoarthropathy: Charcot Foot. In Frykberg RG (ed), *The High Risk Foot in Diabetes Mellitus* New York: Churchill Livingstone, 1991; pp 297–338.
114. Delano PJ. The pathogenesis of Charcot's joint. *Am J Rheumatol* 1946; (56) 2: 189–200.
115. Edmonds ME, Roberts VC, Watkins PJ. Blood flow in the diabetic neuropathic foot. *Diabetologia* 1982; 22: 9–15.
116. Edelman SV, Kosofsky Em, Paul RA, et al. Neuro-osteoarthropathy (Charcot's joint) in diabetes mellitus following revascularization surgery: three case reports and a review of the literature. *Arch Intern Med* 1987; 147: 1504–8.
117. Sinha S, Munichoodappa C, Kozak GP. Neuroarthropathy (Charcot joints) in diabetes mellitus: clinical study of 101 cases. *Medicine* 1972; 52: 191–210.
118. Giurini JM, Chrzan JS, Gibbons GW, Habershaw GH. Charcot's disease in diabetic patients. *Postgrad Med* 1991; 89: 163–9.
119. Frykberg RG. Charcot changes in the diabetic foot. In Veves A, Giurini JM, LoGerfo FW (eds), *The Diabetic Foot.* Totawa, NJ: Humana Press, 2002; pp 221–46.

74

Erectile Dysfunction in Diabetes Mellitus

Michael H. Cummings

Queen Alexandra Hospital, Portsmouth, UK

In keeping with many other areas of diabetes care, there have been considerable advances in our understanding of the prevalence, pathogenesis, and management of erectile dysfunction (ED). It is now recognized that ED is perhaps the most common complication in diabetic men. There is also a greater understanding of the biochemical pathways that lead to vasodilation and smooth muscle relaxation within the penile muscle, facilitating tumescence. Abnormalities of these biochemical pathways have been identified in diabetic men with ED and have led to the development of a number of successful therapeutic options to treat the condition. In particular, the development of oral phosphodiesterase type 5 inhibitors (PDE5I) has revolutionized management not only because of ease of treatment but also because the publicity around their launch has led to a wider understanding and more open discussion of the subject by patients and health care professionals. Prior to the launch of this class of drugs, ED was considered a taboo subject and both diabetic patients and their health care professionals were embarrassed to talk about the problem [1].

Previously, our understanding of ED in diabetic men has been hampered by studies that predominantly focused upon the general population with this condition. The knowledge that diabetes is the single most common cause of ED has led to a barrage of diabetes-specific studies being undertaken, and this evidence forms the basis of this chapter examining epidemiology, pathophysiology, and clinical management.

EPIDEMIOLOGY

Despite the variation in populations studied and differing methodologies used to define ED, the overall prevalence of this condition is universally consistent, lying between 30 and 50% [1–7] and is far higher than in nondiabetic men where this figure does not exceed 20% [8]. In these studies, there has been little attempt to segregate findings in type 1 and type 2 diabetic subjects; however, one study reported a similar prevalence of ED in both forms of diabetes [9]. Up to 40% of patients with ED may have underlying diabetes [10] and the incidence of new cases of diabetes has been shown to be 11–12% [11, 12], justifying the screening for diabetes in all previously undiagnosed patients presenting with ED.

Figure 1 demonstrates the exponential rise in ED with age and that the prevalence is always higher in the diabetic male compared with that in the nondiabetic population. The likelihood of ED in a 35-year-old male is equivalent to that of a 60-year-old nondiabetic male.

McCulloch et al. [4] showed that in diabetic men with ED, the most significant associations with its development were age ($p < 0.001$), treatment with oral hypoglycemic agents or insulin ($p < 0.001$), retinopathy ($p < 0.001$), symptomatic peripheral as well as symptomatic autonomic neuropathy ($p < 0.001$ and $p < 0.005$, respectively). There was also a weaker association with duration of diabetes, poor glycemic control, ischemic heart disease, and nephropathy. This cohort was re-examined 5 years later at which stage only 9% had regained potency [13], reflecting the progressive and nonreversible nature of the condition, supporting the concept that the etiology is primarily organic in most cases.

In practical terms when attempting to forecast the likelihood of ED in diabetic men presenting for routine review, the probabilities are less than 5% in a 20-year-old male with no diabetic complications, 40–80% in a 40-year-old male with diabetic complications, rising to 80–100% in a 65-year-old male with diabetic complications.

International Textbook of Diabetes Mellitus, Third Edition. Edited by R. A. DeFronzo, E. Ferrannini, H. Keen, and P. Zimmet.
 ISBN: 0-471-48655-8.

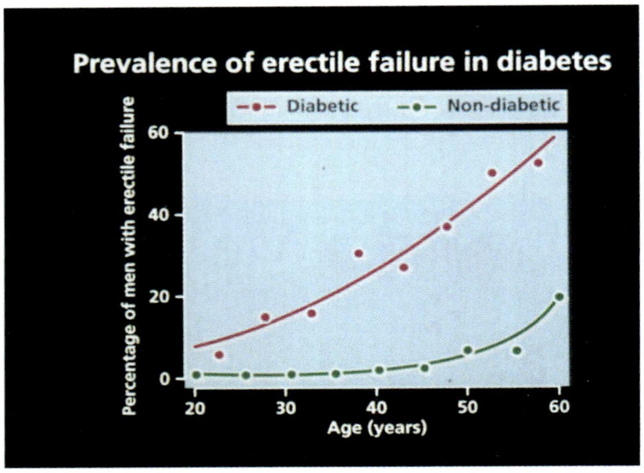

Figure 1 The prevalence of erectile dysfunction in diabetic and nondiabetic men

PATHOPHYSIOLOGY

Table 1 shows the factors that may contribute to the development of ED in the diabetic male. The most influential factors are considered to be local changes within the corpus cavernosum and aberrant neurovascular supply to this organ.

Changes Within the Corpus Cavernosum

It is now recognized from studies of diabetic animal and human corpus cavernosum that there are abnormalities in the availability or effectiveness of several key chemical mediators involved in smooth muscle relaxation and constriction (Table 2).

Nitric oxide (NO) is released either directly from the parasympathetic nerve terminal (PNT) or from the local vascular endothelium, following stimulation by PNT-released acetylcholine (ACh) and is integral, via its messenger cyclic guanosine monophosphate (GMP), in reducing intracellular calcium concentrations and facilitating smooth muscle relaxation. It has been demonstrated in diabetic men with ED that there is an impairment in both parasympathetic nerve and endothelium-dependent mechanisms that mediate smooth muscle relaxation [14–16]. ACh administration was associated with a lesser degree of muscle relaxation in corpus cavernosum from diabetic men with ED, and the degree of impairment was associated with the duration of diabetes [14]. Experimental studies in Wistar rats have provided a mechanism linking chronic dysglycemia and ED. When glycated hemoglobin was added to isolated corpus cavernosum from this animal model, ACh-mediated relaxation of this smooth muscle was impaired [17]. Moreover, this effect of glycated hemoglobin was mimicked by the addition of pyrogallol (a donor of superoxide anions) and partially reversed by the addition of L-arginine (the precursor of NO) [18]. In summary, these studies support the concept that dysglycemia impairs NO-induced smooth muscle relaxation and vasodilation in the diabetic male with ED.

Table 1 Factors that may be associated with the development of erectile dysfunction in diabetic men

Functional and structural changes within the corpus cavernosum
Neurological factors (changes within the parasympathetic nervous system)
Vascular factors (atherosclerosis and endothelial dysfunction)
Endocrine factors
Iatrogenic factors (drug use)
Psychological factors and psychiatric disorders
Primary penile abnormalities (for example, Peyronie's disease)
Venous leaks
Infections (balanitis)

Table 2 Biochemical mediators of smooth muscle relaxation and constriction within the corpus cavernosum that may be affected in diabetic men with erectile dysfunction

Relaxant	Contractile
Neuronal release	
Nitric oxide	Noradrenaline
Acetylcholine	
Vasoactive intestinal polypeptide	
Local release	
Nitric oxide	Endothelin 1
Vasodilator prostanoids	Vasoconstrictor prostanoids
Adenosine triphosphate	

The PNT within the corpus cavernosum also releases another smooth muscle relaxant, vasoactive intestinal polypeptide (VIP), capable of reducing intracellular calcium via its messenger, cyclic adenosine monophosphate (AMP). It has been shown that VIP immunoreactivity is reduced in penile tissue of streptozotocin-induced diabetic rats [19] and of diabetic men with ED [15]. It is possible that vasoactive prostanoids synthesized and released by the corpus cavernosum may also affect smooth muscle relaxation in the diabetic rat corpus cavernosum although addition of indomethacin, a cyclooxygenase inhibitor, had no effect upon the glycated-hemoglobin-mediated impaired cavernosal muscle response to ACh in rats [17].

Noradrenaline, the principal mediator of smooth muscle contraction within the penis, appears to be less abundant in the corpus cavernosum of diabetic men with ED [16] although the responsiveness of smooth muscle to noradrenaline seems to be unaffected [15]. Endothelin-1-induced smooth muscle contraction also appears unaltered in corporal smooth muscle strips of diabetic men with ED [20].

Structural abnormalities of penile tissue from diabetic men with ED and rats have also been identified. These include fibrosis of the penile arteries, corpus cavernosum, and reduced amounts of cavernous nerve fibres of unmyelinated axons with collagen, factors that will impair smooth muscle relaxation and vasodilation. Altered gene expression (downregulated mRNA transcript) [21] and increased apoptosis [22] have been noted in penile tissue from diabetic men with ED and rats respectively.

Neurological Factors

Neuropathy has been linked to the development of ED in approximately 80% of diabetic men [23], particularly under the age of 60 [24], and the principal abnormality appears to be within the parasympathetic nervous system, responsible for achieving tumescence. This is evident from clinical, observational [4, 13], and physiological studies. Abnormalities in deep-breathing tests [25], thermal sensation [26], and urinary flow rates [27] that are linked to the integrity of the parasympathetic nervous system are all impaired in diabetic males with ED. By contrast, there appears to be no impairment of the sympathetic nervous system [25]. Perhaps surprisingly, despite the clinical link between ED and a symptomatic sensory neuropathy [4], physiological studies undertaken using several different tools have largely shown no difference in sensory innervation between diabetic men with ED and potent males [27–29].

At the cellular level, neurological changes in diabetic men with ED may be due to hyperglycemia-induced activation of protein kinase C, aldose reductase pathways, and nonenzymatic glycation that provokes oxidative stress [30].

Vascular Factors

The penis is a highly vascular organ and diabetes may be associated with diffuse atherosclerosis or isolated disease of the external iliac artery [31] both of which may contribute to the development of ED. Observational studies have linked the presence of ED with complications in other microvascular and macrovascular beds of men with diabetes [4, 13]. Diabetic neuropathy is integrally linked to impaired microvascular blood supply. Abnormalities of vascular function, in particular NO-mediated vasodilation have been described earlier (see section Changes Within the Corpus Cavernosum). Up to 95% of diabetic men with ED show impaired penile blood flow [32] that has been suggested to be more likely as an etiological factor in type 1 compared with type 2 diabetic men with ED [33].

Endocrine Factors

It is well recognized that hypogonadism, hyperprolactinemia, thyrotoxicosis, or hypothyroidism or growth hormone deficiency can be associated with the development of ED. The majority of studies have shown no difference in the circulating levels of these hormones in the diabetic population with and without ED compared with the general population, whether examining random measurements or during dynamic testing [34–38]. While mean concentrations of thyroid stimulating hormone (TSH), thyroxine, and triiodothyronine do not differ in the diabetic and nondiabetic populations who are either potent or have ED, it is recognized that thyroid abnormalities are more commonly observed in diabetes [39].

Drugs

Recent therapeutic advances and large-scale studies in diabetic patients, examining the impact of these drugs on disease progression or symptom relief has resulted in an exponential escalation in the use of polypharmacy regimens in the diabetic individual. Many of these drugs may be associated with the development of ED, and it is not surprising, therefore, that iatrogenic causes of ED may be on the increase. For many drugs (for example, antihypertensive agents) the mechanism responsible for the development of ED is clear; for many other drugs the etiological process is obscure. Although ED is more common in patients on oral hypoglycemic agents or insulin [4], this is more likely to be due to disease duration and hyperglycemia rather than the treatment *per se*.

Table 3 highlights drugs that may be commonly used in treating diabetes and are associated with the development of ED and also drugs used in the general population that commonly precipitate ED.

Psychological Factors

There has been a diverse reporting of the prevalence of psychological or psychiatric disease in diabetic men with ED, ranging between 9 and 39% [11, 33, 40, 41]. Moreover, it is not possible to categorically implicate these factors as the primary etiological precipitant of ED. It is generally held that organic disease predominates although performance anxiety [42] and other psychological factors that are common in patients with ED (particularly those with other vascular complications) may perpetuate the problem. Libido, the degree of coital, masturbatory, and sleep-related erections, and frequency of sexual satisfaction and coital activity is also reduced in diabetic men [43].

Other Factors

The association between chronic hyperglycemia and ED, and the mechanisms that may be implicated in dysglycemia-induced ED have been discussed. It is also recognized that acute deterioration in glycemic control may result in temporary ED in hitherto potent diabetic males although the mechanism is less clearly understood. Painful balanitis is more commonly observed in diabetic males, particularly those with poor glycemic control. Autonomic dysfunction has been suggested as being

Table 3 Drugs associated with the development of erectile dysfunction in diabetic men

Drugs commonly prescribed in the management of diabetes
Cardiovascular protective drugs
Thiazide diuretics and spironolactone
β-blockers
Angiotensin converting enzyme inhibitors
Calcium channel blockers and other antihypertensive agents
Digoxin
Drugs for symptomatic relief of painful peripheral neuritis
Tricyclic antidepressant agents
Carbamazepine
Gabapentin
Nonsteroidal anti-inflammatory agents
Lipid-lowering agents
HMG-CoA reductase inhibitors (statin therapy)
Fibrates
Drugs of a general nature commonly associated with development of erectile dysfunction
Alcohol
Anticonvulsant agents
Antiarrhythmic agents
Antipsychotic agents
Antidepressant agents
Anabolic steroids
Allopurinol
Acetazolamide
Baclofen
Bromocriptine
Cimetidine
Ketoconazole
Metoclopramide
Oestogen
Opiates

causative in penile venous leaks, observed in two thirds of diabetic males with vascular ED [44]. Structural abnormalities of the penis that may cause ED, for example Peyronie's disease, are no more frequently observed in the diabetic individual compared with the general population.

MANAGEMENT

The clinical assessment and management of ED in the diabetic male is broadly similar to that of the ED in non-diabetic men, but a few areas are worthy of particular mention. In addition more modern therapeutic approaches are discussed, with emphasis on their effectiveness in the diabetic male.

Clinical Assessment

History and Examination

The presence of other microvascular or macrovascular complications may give a clue to the underlying etiology of ED in a given patient. Conversely, it is extremely important to assess for previously unrecognized cardiovascular disease in diabetic men with ED, given the strong associations between this triad and the very high prevalence of cardiovascular disease. Not only may ED precipitate vascular events in some susceptible diabetic men but also it is likely to influence treatment choice.

Jackson et al. [45] have provided helpful guidelines in assessing the "cardiovascular" patient in relation to considering treatment of ED. When considering whether patients are fit from the cardiovascular perspective to engage in sexual activity, it has been shown this activity is no more strenuous on the heart than a number of other natural daily activities, such as walking at normal pace on the flat for 20 min, lifting and carrying objects (weighing 9–20 kg), gardening, and golf. Jackson et al. broadly classified patients with ED into three groups. The low-risk group comprised diabetic patients with controlled hypertension and less than two other cardiovascular risk factors or mild stable angina (including those postsuccessful revascularization), whose ED could be safely managed in the primary care setting. In the intermediate group [myocardial infarction (MI) or cerebrovascular accident within the previous 6 weeks, patients with New York Heart Association Class I or II heart failure or moderate stable angina] diabetic patients received specialized evaluation (for example, exercise test, echocardiogram), which placed them in the high- or low-risk grouping. In the high-risk group [diabetic patients with unstable or refractory angina, uncontrolled hypertension (systolic BP > 180 mmHg), patients with New York Heart Association Class III or IV heart failure or recent MI (within 14 days)] patients were referred for specialist cardiac evaluation with the recommendation that ED treatment be deferred until their cardiac condition was stabilized and/or specialist evaluation completed.

Investigations

Table 4 shows the investigative tools available in clinical practice to assess the etiology of ED in the diabetic male. There is considerable variation worldwide, surrounding the extent of routine investigation that should be

Table 4 Investigations of erectile dysfunction in diabetic men

Measurements to assess glycemic control (glycated hemoglobin, fructosamine)
Hormone measurements (testosterone axis, prolactin, thyroid function tests, growth hormone, IGF-1)
Prostatic specific antigen measurement
Penile doppler studies
Responsiveness to a standard intracavernosal injection ("papaverine test")
Physiological tests of the autonomic nervous system
Detailed psychosexual assessment
Nocturnal penile rigidity
Invasive radiological procedures (cavernosography and arteriography)

undertaken and this remains controversial. In our own practice, we restrict investigations to hormonal blood tests although it is recognized that the yield of hitherto unrecognized endocrine abnormalities is low. We avoid extensive investigation unless indicated on a clinical basis, since in our experience this rarely influences individual management plans.

Treatment Options

General Considerations

While chronic hyperglycemia is integrally linked to the development of ED, there is no evidence that supports restoration of or enhanced erectile performance if glycemic control is improved. However, ED developing concomitantly with the onset of acute deterioration in glycemic control has a more positive outcome if good glucose control can be re-established. Testosterone should be considered only in diabetic patients with proven hypogonadism. Although diabetic men with ED are commonly taking drugs associated with the development of ED, it is our experience that restoration of potency is usually successful in only those patients where there has been a temporal relationship between the commencement of a drug (within 2 weeks) and the development of ED. Moreover, even if implicated in the etiology, there is often compelling clinical grounds to continue with the drug. The majority of patients will need to consider the therapeutic options summarized in Table 5.

Oral Treatment

The biggest single advance in the treatment of diabetic ED has been the development of oral phosphodiesterase type 5 inhibitors (PDE5I). PDE5 is the isoenzyme responsible for the breakdown of cyclic GMP, the final chemical messenger promoting smooth muscle relaxation within the penis. Thus PDE5I facilitate erections through prolonging the availability of cyclic GMP within the corpus cavernosum. Currently, there are three commercial forms of PDE5I available: sildenafil [46], tadalafil [47], and vardenafil [48]. Their effectiveness is in part determined by the severity of ED, the underlying etiology, the clinical characteristics of the diabetic male being treated, and the tool used to evaluate response. These factors make it difficult to reliably interpret any clinical differences in effectiveness between these three agents. Broadly speaking, however, most clinicians agree that their effectiveness is similar (between three and four out of five patients will respond), a response rate that is less than that of the general population with ED. Sildenafil use in diabetes has the advantage of greater clinical experience and a larger research base confirming its efficacy and safety. In particular there has been no evidence of increased cardiovascular events in patients using the drug [49]. The use of sildenafil and other PDE5I in patients taking nitrates, however, is absolutely contraindicated because of the increased risk of cardiovascular events. Vardenafil has a similar chemical structure to sildenadil and their pharmacokinetic and side effect profiles are similar. Tadalafil has a longer duration of action (half-life 17.5 h) compared with sildenafil and vardenafil (half-life < 4 h) and appears to have less interaction with fatty food and alcohol [47]. PDE5I are well tolerated with very few patients stopping treatment because of unacceptable side effects. Reported side effects are often transitory and usually relate to effects on other PDE isoenzymes. They include dyspepsia, vomiting, facial flushing, headaches, and visual disturbances. PDE5I have been demonstrated to be a cost-effective approach in the management of ED [50].

Sublingual apomorphine is a dopamine receptor agonist that has been shown to stimulate the central nervous system (probably hypothalamic and limbic neural pathways) producing an arousal response [51]. There are no diabetes-specific studies evaluating its effectiveness, but examination of diabetic subpopulations in larger studies [52] and our own clinical experience suggests that it is less effective than PDE5I. Unlike PDE5I, concomitant nitrate use is considered as a relative rather than absolute contraindication. Side effects include nausea, headaches, dizziness, and drowsiness although these are experienced much less at the doses used for treating ED (2–3 mg) compared with the higher doses prescribed for treating parkinsonism. There are no published studies that have examined the combination of PDE5I and apomorphine. Oral yohimbine, an indole alkaloid, has been previously used to treat ED but is less effective than other currently available licensed preparations. It is thought to act through blockade of central α-2 adrenergic activity and has been more effective in treating psychological ED [53] than organic disease but its use has now virtually ceased since the development of PDE5I.

Table 5 Options used in clinical practice for treating erectile dysfunction in diabetic men

Therapy	Comment
Oral therapy	Phosphodiesterase type 5 inhibitors (sildenafil, tadalafil, vardenafil) Sublingual apomorphine Yohimbine
Intracavernosal therapy	Prostaglandin E1 (alprostadil), thymoxamine, papaverine, phentolamine
Transurethral therapy	Alprostadil ("MUSE")
Vacuum tumescence devices	Manual or battery operated
Psychosexual therapy	Most commonly sensate focusing
Testosterone	Reserved for proven hypogonadism
Penile implants	Usually reserved for men who fail to respond to less invasive measures
Corrective surgery	Peyronie's disease, phimosis, trauma, venous leaks

Intracavernosal Injections

In the early 1980s, intracavernosal injections with papaverine [54] and phentolamine [55] were reported as being effective in the treatment of ED. There is a high incidence of priapism and other side effects with both drugs and neither have been licensed for this specific indication. Their use has been superseded by a licensed intracavernosal preparation (prostaglandin E1, alprostadil), which can be self-administered directly into the corpus cavernosum (Figure 2). It is the most potent available treatment for ED (approximately 9 out of 10 injections in the general population resulted in successful erections) and has a lower incidence of priapism [57] compared with previous intracavernosal preparations. The occurrence of priapism (erections lasting greater than 6 h) should be considered a medical emergency, and treatment options to facilitate detumescence include leg exercise, locally applied icepacks, aspiration of blood from the corpus cavernosum, or intracavernosal injection of α-adrenergic drugs such as phenylephrine [56]. Corrective surgery is rarely required. Other side effects include local pain and tingling, bruising,

(a)

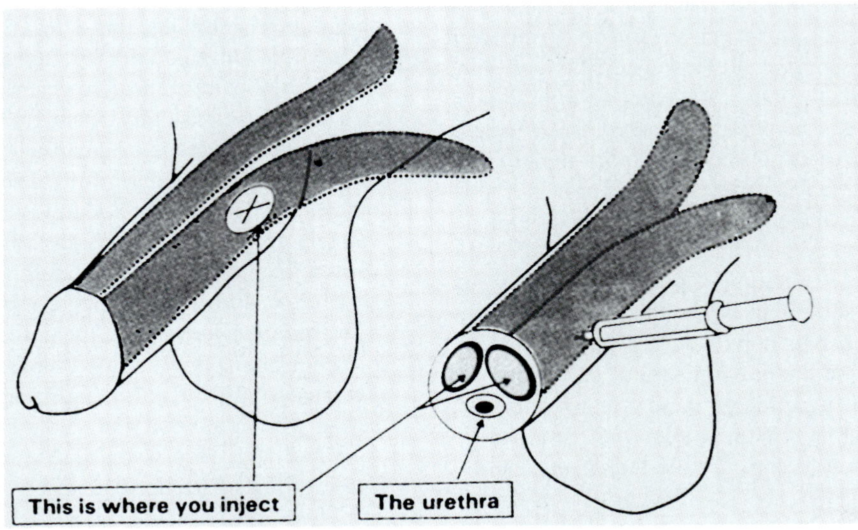

(b)

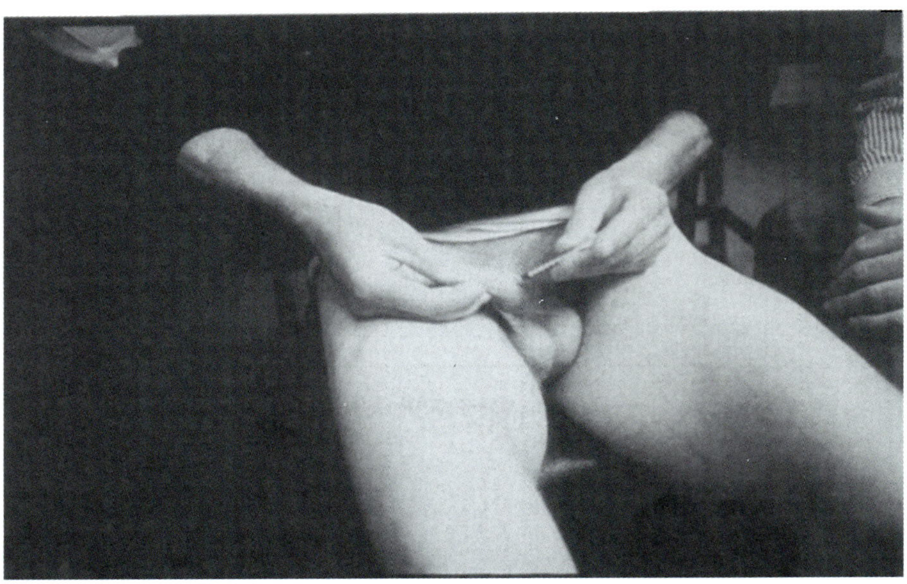

Figure 2 The technique of self-administration of intracavernosal therapy. (From reference 56, p. 82)

fibrosis, scarring, and occasional infection that may limit its use. Recently, one of the largest studies of diabetic men with ED has showed that intracavernosal alprostadil was at least as effective in diabetic men compared with the non-diabetic population and no differences in responses were observed between type 1 and type 2 diabetic patients [58].

Transurethral Alprostadil

The application of alprostadil in the form of a pellet (MUSE) into the urethra has been associated with a 65.9% success rate in achieving erections suitable for sexual intercourse, in the general population [59]. Although there are no major prospective diabetes-specific reports of its use, the above study examined a subgroup of diabetic men with ED and reported similar success rates. Penile pain was reported in one third of patients taking this form of alprostadil and other side effects more commonly reported as compared with placebo were minor urethral trauma and dizziness, although priapism was not reported.

Vacuum Devices

Vacuum devices provide a safe alternative strategy to pharmacological approaches (Figure 3). A cylinder with a constriction rubber band at its base is placed over the penis. A manual- or battery pump is operated to create a vacuum in the cylinder leading to tumescence. The rubber band is slipped on to the base of the penis and can be left in place for up to 30 min. Side effects are rare and include bruising, ejaculatory failure, and penile discomfort. They require a moderate degree of manual dexterity and are usually suitable only for diabetic men in stable relationships. Their success in diabetic patients has not been well reported. One of the largest diabetes-specific studies examined just 19 patients [60]. Eleven patients continued to use the device over 6 months with reports of enhanced sexual satisfaction, partners' sexual satisfaction, and patients' self-esteem with a low incidence of pain and ejaculatory failure.

Psychosexual Counseling

Clearly, this is the treatment of choice for diabetic men with an overt psychological or psychiatric etiology to their ED. It may also provide an additional approach to patients receiving physical treatment, given the performance anxiety seen in many diabetic men with organic ED. There are many different psychological therapies available. One of the most well known forms is sensate focusing employing the Masters and Johnson technique [61]. It requires staged exercises broadly divided into three phases—nongenital, genital, and vaginal containment.

Surgery

Penile prostheses may be considered in diabetic patients who have failed to respond to less invasive measures. There are various complexities of prostheses that range from simple malleable devices that produce a permanent semirigid erection to more complex inflatable devices that are associated with an implanted reservoir system enabling tumescence or detumescence as required (Figure 4). Mechanical failure is relatively common, particularly with the inflatable devices. Also extrusion of the prosthesis, pain, and bruising may occur, but in centers with good

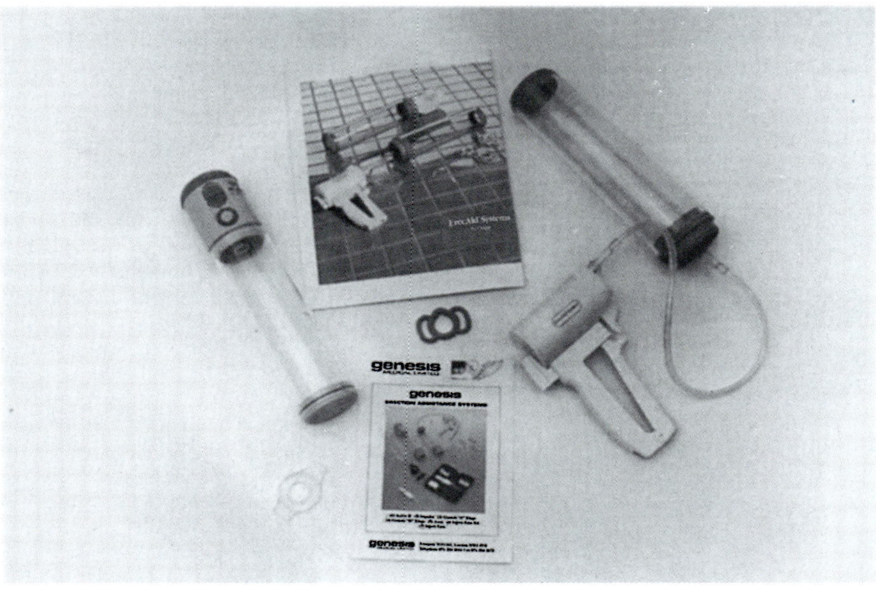

Figure 3 Vacuum tumescence devices. (From reference 56, p. 86)

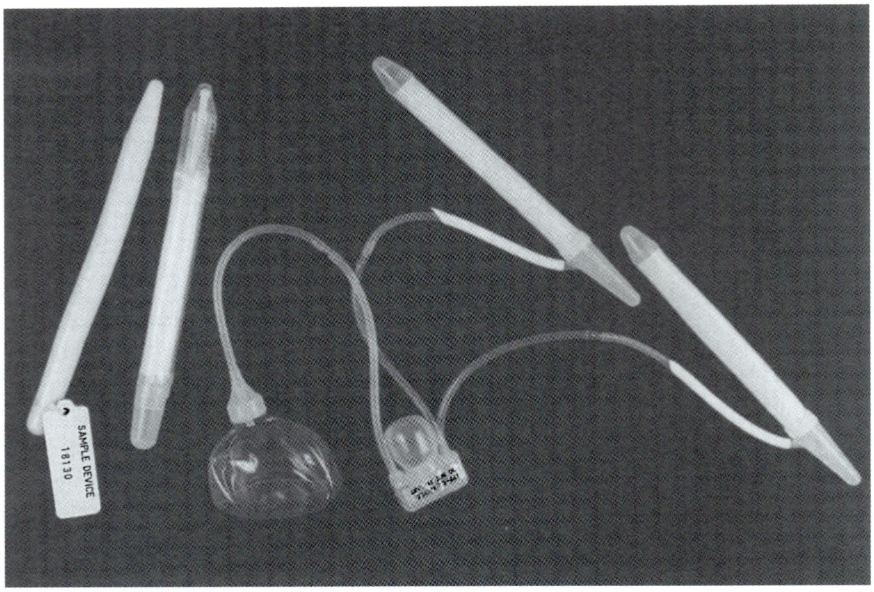

Figure 4 Penile prostheses. (From reference 56, p. 90)

experience of inserting these devices, these complications are rare [62].

Corrective surgery may be considered in patients with primary penile abnormalities such as Peyronie's disease, and venous ligation may be undertaken in diabetic patients with established venous leaks. In diabetic patients with impaired penile blood flow, microvascular surgical techniques have proved disappointing and are rarely performed.

Future Treatment Options

Topical agents either as monotherapy (nitrates) or combination therapy (for example, aminophylline, isosorbide dinitrates, and co-dergocrine [63]) applied to the penis continue to be explored as do other oral agents such as L-arginine. The effectiveness of other intracavernosal agents, for example VIP is also being evaluated. Although controversial, gene therapy through introduction of vectors that promote the synthesis of NO synthase (responsible for the production of NO) have been shown to be effective in promoting erections in diabetic rats [64].

CONCLUSIONS

In the 1980s it was common for diabetic patients with ED to suffer in silence. Both patients and health care professionals avoided discussing the subject, and treatment options were not known about, services to provide treatment were scanty, and successful therapeutic treatments were mainly unlicensed and poorly tolerated. Today, many health care professionals involved in diabetes care adopt a holistic approach and can successfully treat ED within their own service, without the need for referral to specialist services. The previous, common approach of ushering diabetic patients with ED out of the consultation room with no treatment other than being told "not to worry, it will get better with time" should no longer be employed.

REFERENCES

1. Cummings MH, Meeking D, Warburton F, Alexander WD. The diabetic male's perception of erectile dysfunction. *Pract Diabetes Int* 1997; 14 (4): 100–2.
2. UCSF-Fresno Family Practice Residency Program, California 93702, USA. Barriers to recognition of erectile dysfunction among diabetic Mexican–American men 1998. *J Am Board Fam Pract* 1998; 11 (4): 327–30.
3. Alonso Sandoica E, Sanchez Sanchez MD, Benito Fernandez, Giron M, Palancar de LaTorre JL, Tejero Cabello I, Jara Rascon J. Impotence in diabetic patients: detection of prevalence and social-health implications. *Aten Primaria* 1997; 20 (8): 435–9.
4. McCulloch DK, Campbell IW, Wu FC, Prescott RJ, Clarke BF. The prevalence of diabetic impotence. *Diabetologia* 1980; 18 (4): 279–83.
5. Rubin A, Babbott D. Impotence and diabetes mellitus. *JAMA* 1958; 168: 498–500.
6. Kolodny RC, Kahn CB, Goldstein HH, Barnett DM. Sexual dysfunction in diabetic men. *Diabetes* 1974; 23: 306–9.
7. Faerman I, Vilar O, Rivarola MA, Rosner JM, Jadzinsky MN, Fox D, Perez Loret A, Bernstein-Hahn L, Saraceni D. Impotence and diabetes. Studies of androgenic function in diabetic impotent males. *Diabetes* 1972; 21: 23–30.
8. Kinsey AC, Pomeroy WB, Martin CE. Age and sexual outlet. In Kinsey AC, Porneroy WB, Martin CE (eds). *Sexual Behaviour in the Human Male*. Philadelphia: Saunders, 1948; pp 218–62.

9. Pointel JP, Got I, Ziegler O, Jan P, Kolopp M, Drouin P, Debry G. Impotence in the diabetic. *J Mal Vasc* 1989; 14 (2): 133–7.
10. Zonszein J. Diagnosis and management of endocrine disorders of erectile dysfunction. *Urol Clin North Am* 1995; 22: 789–802.
11. Maatman TJ, Montague DK, Martin LM. Erectile dysfunction in men with diabetes mellitus. *Urology* 1987; 29 (6): 589–92.
12. Deutsch S, Sherman L. Previously unrecognized diabetes mellitus in sexually impotent men. *JAMA* 1980; 244 (21): 2430–2.
13. McCulloch DK, Young RJ, Prescott RJ, Campbell IW, Clarke BF. The natural history of impotence in diabetic men. *Diabetologia* 1984; 26 (6): 437–40.
14. Saenz de Tejada I, Goldstein I, Azadzoi K, Krane RJ, Cohen RA. Impaired neurogenic and endothelium-mediated relaxation of penile smooth muscle from diabetic men with impotence. *N Engl J Med* 1989; 320 (16): 1025–30.
15. Kim SC, Ahn SY, Park SH, Lee MY, Uhm DY. A comparison of the relaxation responses of isolated cavernosal smooth muscles by endothelium-independent and endothelium-dependent vasodilators in diabetic men with impotence. *J Korean Med Sci* 1995; 10 (1): 1–6.
16. Lincoln J, Crowe R, Blacklay PF, Pryor JP, Lumley JS, Burnstock G. Changes in the VIPergic, cholinergic and adrenergic innervation of human penile tissue in diabetic and non-diabetic impotent males. *J Urol* 1987; 137 (5): 1053–9.
17. Cartledge JJ, Eardley I, Morrison JF. Impairment of corpus cavernosal smooth muscle relaxation by glycosylated human haemoglobin. *BJU Int* 2000; 85 (6): 735–41.
18. Ari G, Vardi Y, Finbeg JPM. Nitric oxide and penile erection in streptozotocin-diabetic rats. *Clin Sci* 1999; 96: 365–71.
19. Crowe R, Lincoln J, Blacklay PF, Pryor JP, Lumley JS, Burnstock G. Vasoactive intestinal polypeptide-like immunoreactive nerves in diabetic penis. A comparison between streptozotocin-treated rats and man. *Diabetes* 1983; 32 (11): 1075–7.
20. Christ GJ, Lerner SE, Kim DC, Melman A. Endothelin-1 as a putative modulator of erectile dysfunction, I: Characteristics of contraction of isolated corporal tissue strips. *J Urol* 1995; 153 (6): 1998–2003.
21. Autieri MV, Melman A, Christ GJ. Identification of a down-regulated mRNA transcript in corpus cavernosum from diabetic patients with erectile dysfunction. *Int J Impot Res* 1996; 8 (2): 69–73.
22. Alici B, Gumustas MK, Ozkara H, Akkus E, Demirel G, Yencilek F, Hattat H. Apoptosis in the erectile tissues of diabetic and healthy rats. *BJU Int* 2000; 85 (3): 326–9.
23. Ellenberg M. Inmpotence in diabetes: the neurological factor. *Ann Intern Med* 1971; 75: 213–9.
24. Yamaguchi Y, Kumamoto Y. Etiological analysis of male diabetic erectile dysfunction with particular emphasis on findings of vascular and neurological examinations. *Nippon Hinyokika Gakkai Zasshi* 1994; 85: 1474–83.
25. Quadri R, Veglio M, Flecchia D, Tonda L, De Lorenzo F, Chiandussi L, Fonzo D. Autonomic neuropathy and sexual impotence in diabetic patients: analysis of cardiovascular reflexes. *Andrologia* 1989; 21: 346–52.
26. Fowler CJ, Ali Z, Kirby RS, Pryor JP. The value of testing for unmyelinated fibre, sensory neuropathy in diabetic impotence. *Br J Urol* 1988; 61: 63–7
27. Buvat J, Lemaire A, Buvat-herbaut M, Guieu JD, Bailleul JP, Fossati P. Comparative investigations in 26 impotent and 26 non-impotent diabetic patients. *J Urol* 1985; 133: 34–8.
28. Bird SJ, Hanno PM. Bulbocavernous reflex studies and autonomic testing in the diagnosis of erectile dysfunction. *J Neurol Sci* 1998; 154: 8–13.
29. Ho KH, Ong BK, Chong PN, Teo WL. The bulbocavernous reflex in the assessment of neurogenic impotence in diabetic and non-diabetic men. *Ann Acad Singapore* 1996; 25: 558–61.
30. Vinik AI, Park TS, Stansberry KB, Pittenger GL. Diabetic neuropathies. *Diabetologia* 2000; 43: 957–73.
31. Goldwasser B, Carson CC, Braun SD, McCann RL. Impotence due to the pelvic steal syndrome: treatment by transilluminal angioplasty. *J Urol* 1985; 133: 860–1.
32. Jevtich MJ, Edson M, Jarman WD, Herrera HH. Vascular factors in erectile failure amongst diabetics. *Urology* 1982; 19: 163–8.
33. Lehman TP, Jacobs JA. Etiology of diabetic impotence. *J Urol* 1983; 129: 291–4.
34. Zeidler A, Gelfand R, Tamagna E, Marrs R, Chopp R, Kletzky O. Pituitary gonadal function in diabetic male patients with and without impotence. *Andrologia* 1982; 14 (1): 62–8.
35. Daubresse JC, Meunier JC, Wilmotte J, Luyckx AS, Lefebvre PJ. Pituitary-testicular axis in diabetic men with and without sexual impotence. *Diabete Metab* 1978; 4 (4): 233–7.
36. Ando S, Rubens R, Rottiers R. Androgen plasma levels in male diabetics. *J Endocrinol Invest* 1984; 7 (1): 21–4.
37. Levitt NS, Vinik AI, Sive AA, Klaff LJ, Phillips C. Synthetic luteinizing hormone-releasing hormone in impotent male diabetics. *S Afr Med J* 1980; 57 (17): 701–4.
38. Maneschi F, White MC, Porta M, Kohner EM. 24 hour studies of prolactin and growth hormone levels in diabetic impotence. *Horm Res* 1981; 14 (2): 79–86.
39. Smithson MJ. Screening for thyroid dysfunction in a community population of diabetic patients. *Diabet Med* 1998; 15 (2): 148–50.
40. El-Bayoumi M, el-Sebini O, Mostafa M. Impotence in diabetics: organic versus psychogenic factors. *Urology* 1984; 24 (5): 459–63.
41. Melman A, Tiefer L, Pedersen R. Evaluation of first 406 patients in urology department based centre for male sexual dysfunction. *Urology* 1988; 32 (1): 6–10.
42. Morse WI, Morse JM. Erectile impotence precipitated by organic factors and perpetuated by performance anxiety. *Can Med Assoc J* 1982; 127: 599–601.
43. Schiavi RC, Stimmel BB, Mandeli J, Rayfield EJ. Diabetes mellitus and male sexual function: a controlled study. *Diabetologia* 1993; 36: 745–51.
44. Colakoglu Z, Kutluay E, Ertekin C, Altay B, Killi R, Alkis A. Autonomic nerve involvement and venous leakage in diabetic men with impotence. *BJU Int* 1999; 83 (4): 453–6.
45. Jackson G, Betterdige J, Dean J, Hall R, Holdright D, Holmes S, Kirby M, Riley A, Sever P. A systematic approach to erectile dysfunction in the cardiovascular patient: a consensus statement. *Int J Clin Pract* 1999; 53: 445–51.
46. Rendell MS, Rajfer J, Wicker PA, Smith MD. Sildenafil for treatment of erectile dysfunction in men with diabetes: a randomised control trial. *JAMA* 1999; 281: 424–6.

47. Saenz de Tejada I, Anglin G, Knight JR, Emmick J. Effects of tadalafil on erectile dysfunction in men with diabetes. *Diabetes Care* 2002; 25 (12): 2159–64.
48. Goldstein I, Young JM, Fischer J. Vardenafil, a new highly selective PDE-5 inhibitor, improves erectile function in patients with diabetes mellitus. *Diabetes* 2001; 50 (suppl 2): 114.
49. Morales A, Gingell C, Collins M. Clinical safety of oral sildenafil citrate (viagra) in the treatment of erectile dysfunction. *Int J Impot Res* 1998; 10: 69–74.
50. Ashton-Key M, Sadler M, Walmsley B, Holmes S, Randall S, Cummings MH. UK department of health guidance on prescribing for impotence following the introduction of sildenafil: potential to contain costs in the average health authority district. *Pharmacoeconomics* 2002; 20 (12): 839–46.
51. Melis M, Argiolas A, Gessa G. Apomorphine induced penile erection and yawning: site of action in brain. *Brain Res* 1987; 415: 98–105.
52. Stief C, Padley RJ, Perdok RJ, Sleep DJ, Cross-study review of the clinical efficacy of apomorphine SL 2 and 3 mg: pooled data from three placebo-controlled, fixed-dose crossover studies. *Eur Urol* 2002; 1: 12–20.
53. Reid K, Morales A, Harris C, Surridge DHC, Condra M, Owen J, Fenemore J. Double-blind trial of yohimbine in treatment of psychogenic impotence. *Lancet* 1987; 1: 421–3.
54. Virag R. Intracavernous injection of papaverine for erectile failure. *Lancet* 1982; 2: 938.
55. Brindley GS. Cavernosal alpha blockade: a new technique for investigating and treating erectile impotence. *Br J Psychiatry* 1983; 143: 332–7.
56. Alexander WD, Cummings M. Erectile dysfunction and its treatment. In Shaw KM (ed), *Diabetic Complications*. Chichester, UK: Wiley, 1996; pp 67–100.
57. Linet OI, Ogrinc FG. Efficacy and safety of intracavernosal alprostadil in men with erectile dysfunction. *N Engl J Med* 1996; 334: 873–7.
58. Heaton JP, Lording D, Liu SN, Litonjua AD, Guangwei L, Kim SC, Kim JJ, Zhi-Zhai S, Israr D, Niagi D, Rajatanaven R, Suyons S, Berad F, Casey R, Brock G, Belanger A. Intracavernosal alprostadil is effective for the treatment of erectile dysfunction in diabetic men. *Int J Impot Res* 2001; 13: 317–21.
59. Padma-Nathan H, Hellstrom W, Kaiser FE. Treatment of men with erectile dysfunction with transurethral alprostadil. *N Engl J Med* 1997; 336: 1–7.
60. Bodansky HJ. Treatment of male erectile dysfunction using the active vacuum assist device. *Diabet Med* 1994; 11 (4): 410–2.
61. Masters WH, Johnson VE. *Human Sexual Inadequacy*. London: Churchill, 1970.
62. Montague DK. Treatment of erectile dysfunction. *J Urol* 1993; 150 (6): 1833.
63. Gomaa A, Shalaby M, Osman M. Topical treatment of erectile dysfunction: randomised double blind placebo controlled trial of cream containing aminophylline, isosorbide dinitrate and co-dergocrine mesylate. *BMJ* 1996; 312: 1512–5.
64. Bivalacqua TJ, Usta MF, Champion HC, Adams D, Namara DB, Abdel-Mageed AB, Kadowitz PJ, Hellstrom WJ. Gene transfer of endothelial nitric oxide synthase partially restores nitric oxide synthesis and erectile function in streptozotocin diabetic rats. *J Urol* 2003; 169 (5): 1911–7.

Complications: Macrovascular Disease

75

Epidemiology of Macrovascular Disease and Hypertension in Diabetes Mellitus

Jaakko Tuomilehto*†, Daiva Rastenyte‡, Qing Qiao*†, and Dimitrije Jakovljevic*

**National Public Health Institute, Helsinki, Finland, †Department of Public Health, University of Helsinki, Helsinki, Finland, and ‡Kaunas Institute of Cardiology, Kaunas, Lithuania*

INTRODUCTION

Diabetic patients suffer from cardiovascular disease (CVD) and the majority of both type 1 diabetes mellitus (T1DM) and type 2 diabetes mellitus (T2DM) patients die from CVD. Epidemiological studies of CVD in diabetes are important for the estimation of the magnitude and the nature of the problem, for the identification of the risk factors for CVD in diabetic subjects, and for the development of preventive measures. Risk factor studies in the diabetic population are complicated because of very close interrelations between diabetes, hypertension, and other macrovascular diseases. For instance, diabetes and hypertension, which commonly coexist, are both known to increase the risk of coronary heart disease (CHD) and stroke. It is extremely difficult to find out their independent effects even with modern and sophisticated statistical methods. It has been proposed that diabetes and macrovascular disease may both have common genetic or environmental antecedents. This "common soil" hypothesis for diabetes and macrovascular diseases has received more support from the numerous epidemiologic studies during the last few years [1]. The major forms of CVD, i.e. CHD, stroke and peripheral vascular disease (PVD), share both an atherosclerotic background and several common risk factors.

HYPERTENSION

Prevalence and Incidence

It has been known for decades that the prevalence of hypertension in diabetic individuals appears to be approximately twice as high as in nondiabetic people in the same population [2–4]. It is more frequent in men than in women before the fifth decade and more frequent in women thereafter [5]. The prevalence of coexisting diabetes and hypertension is higher in Blacks compared with Whites; both conditions are more common among the lower socioeconomic groups [6–8].

The prevalence of hypertension among young T1DM patients is dramatically increased. Data from the Joslin clinic showed that 15.5% of males with diabetes aged 18–24 years had hypertension compared with only 1.7% in the general population—excess risk of 13.8% [9]. A much lower prevalence of hypertension was found in females in the same age group: 2.4% vs. 0.8%, respectively. Others have also reported a significant increase in blood pressure (BP) in T1DM males but not in T1DM females [10]. In the general population BP levels are higher in men than in women until the age of 45–50 years, and this may also be reflected in young diabetic subjects. Nevertheless, other studies suggest that significant increases in BP in T1DM patients are seen in both sexes [11].

Epidemiological evidence is unequivocal and uniform, showing that patients with T2DM have a higher prevalence of hypertension than do nondiabetic subjects at any age, in both sexes and regardless of BP levels in the background population [12]. The problem for the interpretation of the available epidemiological data is that in many studies control for degree of obesity was not done or remained unclear. The increased prevalence of hypertension in the diabetic population (especially T2DM) may to some extent be due to improved screening since diabetic patients

International Textbook of Diabetes Mellitus, Third Edition. Edited by R. A. DeFronzo, E. Ferrannini, H. Keen, and P. Zimmet.
 ISBN: 0-471-48655-8.

use more health services, and due to the lower thresholds for treatment of high BP in diabetic patients [13].

The definition for hypertension has changed over the years, and also varies to some extent between countries. The most recent criteria of the World Health Organization/International Society of Hypertension (WHO/ISH) were issued in 1999 [14]. In general, the WHO and the ISH define hypertension as an office BP exceeding 140 and/or 90 mmHg (Korotkoff I–V), and borderline hypertension as being below these limits but above 130 systolic and/or 85 mmHg diastolic. Established hypertension is diagnosed when readings consistently exceed 140/90 mmHg over several weeks, or when the pressure is very high (diastolic pressure >110 mmHg), or when there are clinical signs of tissue organ damage due to long-standing hypertension. However, it is clear from numerous epidemiological studies that these thresholds are too high in diabetic subjects because of their additional risk of both macrovascular and microvascular diseases. Therefore, the WHO/ISH recommendation is to consider diabetes as an indication (comparable to the presence of multiple other risk factors) to consider a lower BP level to initiate medical action. Various other expert bodies have also suggested alternative, generally lower, target levels. A consensus would be to aim for a BP of less than 130–140 mmHg systolic and under 85 mmHg diastolic. There are, however, dangers in extrapolating from epidemiological data to make treatment recommendations. Interventional advice should depend on evidence, and thus far for cardiovascular endpoints there is no evidence that a BP of <140/80 mmHg is an appropriate target.

There are a few studies that have shown that in T2DM the increase in BP is, at last in part, independent of body weight [12, 15, 16]. While T1DM patients are usually normotensive until overt renal disease develops, the prevalence of hypertension increases markedly in T2DM before the proteinuric state [17, 18]. About one fourth of T2DM patients are already hypertensive at the time of diagnosis of diabetes [3, 17, 19].

Proteinuria/Microalbuminuria and BP

Microalbuminuria is in most cases the first sign of the diabetic renal disease in both T1DM and T2DM patients. The prevalence of microalbuminuria among diabetic patients is 15–20% [20–22] and it is higher in T1DM than T2DM patients. On the other hand, more or less severe signs of diabetic renal disease may be found in as many as 41% of both T1DM and T2DM patients once the duration of diabetes is long enough [22]. It is possible that high BP in diabetic patients with either microalbuminuria or nephropathy is genetically determined, but the susceptibility genes have not been identified yet. There is little question that BP is higher, even within the normal range, in T1DM patients with microalbuminuria compared with normoalbuminuric patients [23]. However, whether BP rises before or after the development of microalbuminuria has been debated. Mathiesen et al. [24] found no difference in BP between those who did and those who did not develop persistent microalbuminuria until microalbuminuria had been present at least 3 years, indicating that BP elevation is secondary to the initiation of diabetic nephropathy. Raal et al. [25] found no difference in BP at baseline between individuals who remained normoalbuminuric and those who later progressed to diabetic renal disease. Nevertheless, the development of microalbuminuria was accompanied by a parallel rise in diastolic BP, indicating that BP elevation and the initial stage of diabetic renal disease are concurrent events. Kimball et al. [23] also suggested that the alterations in cardiovascular and renal function may occur in parallel in adolescents with T1DM. However, some studies suggested that BP may rise before the detection of microalbuminuria and may even serve as a predictor of its development [26–28]. Results from the EURODIAB T1DM Complications Study [29] also suggest that raised albumin excretion is a response to, and not necessarily a cause of, mildly raised BP.

The pathogenetic relationship between elevated BP and renal disease in T2DM is more difficult to establish than in T1DM. Often the time of onset of T2DM cannot be precisely defined, and some 40–50% of T2DM patients receive antihypertensive treatment at the time of diagnosis [30]. It has been shown that elevated BP is an independent predictor of T2DM and glucose intolerance [4]. However, BP starts to increase steeply when persistent proteinuria develops in T2DM patients [31], and evidence exists that BP may start to rise before the development of microalbuminuria not only in T2DM patients but also in T1DM patients [27, 31]. It is possible that in many hypertensive patients with T2DM, diabetes itself is not causally related to elevated BP, since even in nondiabetic populations of the same age hypertension is very common.

Hyperinsulinemia/Insulin Resistance and BP

Numerous conditions associated with insulin resistance and/or hyperinsulinemia are frequently accompanied by hypertension. This conclusion applies not only to obesity [32, 33], impaired glucose tolerance (IGT) [34], or T2DM [35], but also to T1DM [36] when insulin sensitivity is impaired [37]. It has been suggested that hyperinsulinemia, which occurs with insulin resistance, increases BP primarily through an increase of sodium retention, stimulation of sympathetic nervous activity, or both [38]. However, epidemiological and clinical data linking hyperinsulinemia to hypertension are inconsistent. There is support for the insulin–BP association in some Caucasoid populations [34, 39], case-control studies [40–42], or cross-sectional studies [43, 44], but a number of studies in ethnic groups including Europids [45–47], Micronesians, Polynesians, and Melanesians [48], Pima Indians [49, 50], African Americans [49], Asian Indian, Creole, and Chinese Mauritians [51] do not support the hypothesis. Interestingly, these latter populations have substantially higher circulating insulin concentrations than do, for instance, Europid populations, and yet, their BP levels are not higher or may be even somewhat lower. In addition, insulin resistance has not always been demonstrated in patients with essential hypertension. In the study by Pollare et al. [42] approximately 50% of the hypertensive individuals were able to dispose of glucose at a rate that was within the range of normotensive subjects. On the other hand, not all subjects with hyperinsulinemia are insulin resistant. Patients with severe hyperinsulinemia due to an islet cell tumor, for example, display neither hypertension nor hyperglycemia [52]. Likewise, the supraphysiologic dose of insulin administered to patients with T1DM is not always associated with hypertension [53]. One study indicated a correlation between insulin and BP only in subjects with a positive family history of hypertension or diabetes and suggested a possible genetic influence on insulin resistance [54]. A role of a familial component in insulin resistance syndrome is also suggested by studies showing that young adult normotensive offspring of hypertensive parents are more insulin resistant than offspring of normotensive parents [55]. Doria et al. [56] suggested that insulin resistance occurs only in those hypertensive subjects with high erythrocyte sodium–lithium countertransport.

Inconsistency in association between insulin and hypertension can be in part explained by the hemodynamic effects of insulin. There is a strong evidence that acute physiological increments in plasma insulin concentrations (euglycemic clamp) stimulate the sympathetic noradrenergic activity, which is offset by its vasodilator action on skeletal muscle blood flow [57]. The acute vasodilatory effect of insulin may be through alteration of intracellular calcium handling. Saito et al. [58] found that insulin attenuated angiotensin II stimulated increases in cytosolic free calcium by decreasing the pool of inositol triphosphate (IP_3) releasable calcium, an effect blocked by inhibition of nitric oxide generation. More recent studies show an important effect of insulin on the vascular production of endothelin 1 [59].

The opposing hemodynamic effects of insulin help explain why acute physiologic hyperinsulinemia does not elevate BP in normal human beings [60]. Baron et al. [61] hypothesize that insulin resistance and hyperinsulinemia are markers of the hypertensive process in the muscle and not contributors to elevated BP. A sympathetic overactivity could also lead to insulin resistance and a compensatory increase in plasma insulin levels [62, 63]. The recent line of research related to insulin has been targeted to endothelial dysfunction [64]. Hyperinsulinemia (or insulin resistance) seems to abrogate endothelium-dependent vasodilation in large arteries. One of the proposed mechanisms includes oxidative stress caused by hyperinsulinemia.

Attenuation in the balance between insulin's depressor and pressor effects could influence BP regulation. Insulin-mediated stimulation of skeletal muscle blood flow is reduced in obese subjects [65] and T2DM patients [66]. However, several clinical studies have failed to show any effect of acute physiologic hyperinsulinemia on BP in obese, insulin-resistant hypertensive patients [67–69]. Thus it is probable that hyperinsulinemia is not directly causing hypertension, but may serve as an indicator of a common antecedent (either genetic or environmental) of T2DM and hypertension. In studies of Mexican Americans a number of factors including typical CVD risk factors such as high total cholesterol, BP, fasting glucose, body mass index (BMI), triglycerides, and low high-density lipoprotein (HDL) cholesterol predicted the development of T2DM, but their effect was virtually removed after adjusting for fasting insulin [70]. This study strongly suggested that prediabetic individuals who are insulin resistant are at a higher risk of developing CVD than do insulin-sensitive prediabetic individuals, pointing out the importance of hyperinsulinemia in targeting prevention [71].

Hyperglycemia and BP

Hyperglycemia is the distinguishing feature of diabetes. The joint data from Finnish and Dutch cohorts of the Seven Countries Study with 30 years of follow-up showed that in men with T2DM or IGT, BP levels and the prevalence of hypertension were higher than in normoglycemic men. Interestingly, these differences in BP had already been seen 20–30 years earlier. An elevation in BP preceded abnormal glucose tolerance but not hyperinsulinemia. BMI levels of men with hyperinsulinemia had been shown to be higher 20–30 years earlier, but BP levels had not. Thus, it was proposed that glucose intolerance is a stronger correlate of hypertension than is hyperinsulinemia [72].

The hypothesis of oxidative stress through which high glucose levels may play a role in cardiovascular complications has been increasingly discussed [73, 74]. The endothelium has been shown to release a substance that induces smooth muscle relaxation by increasing the production of cyclic guanosine monophosphate. This factor is called endothelium-derived relaxing factor, and nitric oxide is believed to be one of such factors [75]. Vessels of healthy people are continuously dilated by nitric oxide released from endothelial cells. Exposure to elevated concentrations of glucose *in vitro* causes selective impairment of endothelium-dependent relaxation [76]. Oxidative stress induced by hyperglycemia is implicated as a source of altered endothelially mediated relaxation in diabetes. It was shown in experimental studies that oxygen-derived free radicals inactivate endothelium-derived releasing factors [77] and selectively attenuate endothelium-dependent relaxation [78]. One possible source of oxygen-derived free radicals in diabetes is autoxidation of glucose [79]. Glucose can autoxidize, generating free radicals, hydrogen peroxide, and reactive ketoaldehydes. These last compounds may largely participate in the formation of glycated proteins, which are themselves a source of oxygen-derived free radicals [80, 81]. The possibility that oxygen-derived free radicals play a role in the pathogenesis of vascular complications of diabetes is suggested by studies that have shown that antioxidants such as vitamin E, superoxide dismutase, catalase, glutathione, and ascorbic acid are all decreased in tissues and blood of diabetic patients [82, 83]. Also elevated levels of products of oxygen-derived free radicals have been reported in diabetic patients [84, 85]. In a study by Ceriello et al. [86], the plasma concentration of O_2^- was elevated in patients with T1DM, but showed a trend to normalization after strict metabolic control. There was a strong correlation between plasma glucose concentrations and O_2^- concentrations in both normal subjects and diabetic patients over a wide range of glucose concentrations. An acute antihypertensive effect of antioxidant agents, such as vitamin C, thiopronine, and glutathione, has been reported in hypertensive subjects, regardless of whether they are diabetic patients [86]. During the postprandial state, not only hyperglycemia occurs, but also hyperlipidemia. More recently, it was confirmed that both postprandial hypertriglyceridemia and hyperglycemia have independent and cumulative deleterious effect on endothelial function and suggested that oxidative stress is the common mediator through which they exert such effect [87].

Diurnal Blood Pressure Variability

BP and heart rate are principally under the control of the autonomic nervous system. It has been proposed that loss of the normal day–night difference in BP may be a sign of early autonomic dysfunction in diabetic patients. In normotensive T1DM and T2DM patients during sleep there is loss of the nocturnal dip of BP seen in normal subjects, and diabetic patients also have increased BP variability [88–90]. These may be contributing factors to the development of hypertension and the accelerated cardiovascular damage seen in diabetes [88]. In addition, left ventricular mass is increased [91–94], asymptomatic cerebrovascular damage is more advanced [95], and history of stroke is more frequent [96] in nondiabetic hypertensive nondippers as compared with dippers. Thus, for any given level of daytime BP, a persistent pressure overload could speed the progression of hypertensive organ damage and thereby result in a higher incidence of cardiovascular events. Since cardiovascular risk in hypertension is somewhat lower in nondiabetic women than in men, the detrimental effect of persistently high BP levels over 24 h would become particularly evident in diabetic women, thus raising their risk to the level occurring in men [97]. A study on determinants of ambulatory 24-h BP in T1DM patients has shown that the mean male–female difference in 24-h diastolic BP was 5.6 mmHg less in diabetic patients than in healthy individuals after adjusting for all other variables [98]. These findings are in concert with the reported loss in diabetic women of the relative female protection against cardiovascular and cerebrovascular diseases [99, 100].

Atherosclerosis

Diabetic subjects show more widespread and more severe coronary atherosclerosis. Data supporting this opinion emerge equally from postmortem [101–103] and from clinical and epidemiological studies [104]. Five Town Study [105] found more extensive atherosclerosis in the coronary arteries and abdominal aortae of diabetic subjects than in the groups which represented "standardized average" atherosclerosis in the background population. In addition, there was a tendency for an increased severity of atherosclerosis when both diabetes and hypertension had been present in life. Another WHO study on the prevalence of large vessel disease among diabetic population in 14 European centers suggested the following [106]:

(1) The prevalence of large vessel disease varies considerably between different centers, the highest being in Eastern Europe. This corresponds to the prevalence of CVD in the general population.
(2) The prevalence of all large vessel disease is at least the same in diabetic women as in diabetic men. The overrepresentation of women seems particularly great in centers where the overall prevalence of atherosclerotic diseases is high.
(3) The female overrepresentation is due to CHD while the prevalence of PVD is higher in men than in women in most centers.

The first statement is in agreement with the observations from the International Atherosclerosis Project [107]. This was a population-based pathological study that noted that the severity of coronary atherosclerosis in diabetic patients varied in parallel with the general severity in the population from which they were sampled, with the effect of diabetes superimposed. There was no good evidence of a positive association between duration of diabetes and degree of coronary atherosclerosis.

At least two studies were designed to evaluate the severity of coronary artery disease specifically in juvenile-onset T1DM. One was an autopsy study, in which coronary pathology of nine young patients with T1DM was compared with a group of nine age-matched individuals without diabetes [107, 108]. None of the individuals in either group had a clinical history of angina pectoris. Six of the nine diabetic patients had a >75% reduction in luminal diameter, while none of the nondiabetic subjects had this degree of narrowing. Another study examined clinical and angiographic findings in 32 patients with T1DM and 31 nondiabetic patients, matched for age and symptoms [109]. In comparison with nondiabetic individuals, patients with T1DM were significantly more likely to have severe (>70%) narrowings, to have them in all three major coronary arteries (47% vs. 6%), and to have them in distal segments. Severe narrowings of multiple vessels were significantly more common in men than in women and in individuals who also had hypercholesterolemia.

In the only population-based autopsy study, autopsies were evaluated in 83 diabetic and 159 nondiabetic Japanese American men from the Honolulu Heart Program [103]. Diabetic men had an excess of coronary atherosclerosis and of acute, healing, or fibrotic myocardial lesions; the latter but not the former association was independent of major CHD risk factors. This suggests that the atherosclerotic process is mediated by BP, cholesterol, and smoking, while in men with diabetes one or more modes of action besides atherosclerosis also seem to account for the excess of heart disease.

Results from other autopsy studies have shown that diabetic patients have a higher incidence of two- and three-vessel disease, and a lower incidence of single-vessel disease, compared with patients without diabetes. In a report by Natali et al., the incidence of multivessel disease was as high as 36% in individuals with diabetes compared with 17% in nondiabetic individuals ($p < 0.0001$) [110]. Retrospective analyses of patients undergoing elective percutaneous transluminal coronary angioplasty (PTCA) support these data. Stein and coworkers analyzed results from 1133 diabetic and 9300 nondiabetic patients undergoing PTCA and showed that the patients with diabetes had a higher rate of multivessel disease than did those without diabetes [111]. The Thrombolysis and Angioplasty in Myocardial Infarction Trial involved 148 diabetic patients and 923 nondiabetic patients [112]. Patients with diabetes had a significantly higher incidence of multivessel disease (66%) than did the patients without diabetes (46%, $p = 0.0001$). In addition, the number of diseased vessels per patient was greater among patients with diabetes compared with those without diabetes.

The effect of diabetes on cerebral and peripheral circulation has been studied extensively during the last decades. Chan et al. [113], using noninvasive methods, compared the prevalence of carotid artery stenoses (50% reduction or more) in 286 volunteer T2DM subjects and 135 controls of similar age (mean 61 and 60 years, respectively); 7% of the diabetic subjects and 1% of controls had severe stenoses. Pujia et al. [114] examined carotid arteries of 54 T2DM subjects and 54 sex- and age-matched control subjects using echo-Doppler examination. The prevalence of carotid atherosclerosis was 46% in T2DM subjects and 18% in control subjects. Yamasaki et al. [115] assessed the carotid arteries in 105 patients with T1DM (age 4–25 years, duration of diabetes 0.5–17 years), 529 patients with T2DM (age 31–86 years, duration of diabetes 0.5–49 years), and 104 nondiabetic healthy subjects using ultrasound high-resolution B-mode imaging. The intimal plus medial thickness (IMT) values of the arterial wall for T1DM patients aged 10–25 years were significantly greater than those in age-matched nondiabetic subjects. T2DM patients showed IMT values equivalent to those in normal adults over 20 years old. A cross-sectional study on the relation of carotid artery stiffness indices with glucose intolerance and serum insulin concentrations found that persons with T2DM or borderline glucose intolerance had stiffer arteries than did their counterparts with normal glucose tolerance [116]. According to the recently published results of the Insulin Resistance Atherosclerosis Study, diabetes was significantly associated with increased atherosclerosis in the internal carotid artery as determined by IMT [117]. Several studies reported a higher degree of early atherosclerosis in newly detected type 2 diabetic patients than in nondiabetic subjects [118, 119]. This suggests that hyperglycemia together with clustering of risk factors, particularly dyslipidemia, may cause intimal–medial thickening already in the early phases of diabetes.

Kingsbury [120] studied 338 male nondiabetic subjects referred to a surgical clinic specializing in PVD. Arteriography was performed in each subject and the degree of irregularity classified into three grades of severity. Both fasting and 2-h blood glucose levels were related to the degree of irregularity, independent of age. The mean ages of men in the "moderate" and "extensive" categories of PVD were 59 and 61 years respectively. Thus, nondiabetic men at increased risk of T2DM (because of relative glucose intolerance) seem to have more extensive PVD. In the Schwabing Study [121], more than 600 T1DM and T2DM patients were prospectively followed for low-extremity arterial disease, e.g. PVD by ultrasonic Doppler measurements. Both at the 5-year and 9-year follow-up, the incidence of mostly asymptomatic was consistently and significantly associated with baseline BP and the dyslipidemic complex of high-serum triglycerides/low-HDL cholesterol, but not with total cholesterol or weight. The association with HbA_1, plasma C-peptide, and daily insulin dose (in insulin-treated T2DM) was weaker and at 9-year follow-up only significant in univariate analysis. Of diabetic patients dying from cardiovascular causes within 5-year observation, 67% had PVD (mostly asymptomatic) at baseline compared with 15% in those who survived.

Mozes et al. [122] compared the histomorphologic appearance of atherosclerosis in amputated legs of diabetic (10 type 2, 4 unclassified) and nondiabetic patients ($n = 14$). In diabetic patients occlusive disease in amputated legs was more severe in arteries above the ankle than in nondiabetic patients while no difference was found in this series in arteries of the ankle and foot. Also medial calcification in the arteries tended to be more prominent in diabetic patients than in nondiabetic patients [122]. Jude and collaborators [123] performed the first study that compared angiographic findings between diabetic and nondiabetic patients with PVD. This study showed that in a group of patients referred for angiography of the lower extremity, diabetic patients have worse angiographic findings, more amputations (41.4% vs. 11.5%), and higher mortality than do nondiabetic patients [123].

Many other studies confirm an association between diabetes and increased prevalence of PVD. Individuals with diabetes have 2–4-fold increase in the rates of PVD [124], more often have femoral bruits and absent pedal pulses [125], and have rates of abnormal ankle–brachial indices ranging from 11.9% to 16% [126, 127]. The duration and severity of diabetes correlate with incidence and extent of PVD [123]. Patients with diabetes have a greater risk of intermittent claudication, gangrene (10-fold), and amputations (15–20-fold) [128, 129]. In the Framingham cohort, the presence of diabetes increased the risk of claudication by 3.5-fold in men and 8.6-fold in women [130]. Overall, diabetes causes most nontraumatic lower extremity amputations in the United States [131]. The relative risk estimate for lower extremity amputation in patients with diabetes was 12.7 compared with that of nondiabetic patients in Medicare population and as high as 23.5 for diabetic persons aged 65–74 years. Inconsistency exists regarding the question of whether PVD is more commonly symptomatic or asymptomatic among patients with diabetes [129, 132].

CORONARY HEART DISEASE

Prevalence and Incidence

There are geographical differences in the prevalence of CHD among cohorts of diabetic patients, and in the incidence of CHD in the general population [133]. Although CHD is a relatively rare cause of death in the first 30 years of T1DM, it is much more common in later years, accounting for up to 30% of deaths in those with T1DM for more than 40 years. A study of 370 male employees with T1DM of a US company showed that death rates in diabetic subjects were more than double than in healthy controls during a 10-year period [134]. Mortality ratios were highest under the age 45, mainly because of increased risk of CHD. Researchers at the Joslin clinic reported that after 20–40 years duration of diabetes 33% of patients aged 45–59 years had either symptomatic or asymptomatic CHD [135]. This is likely to be an underestimate however, as only survivors were included in the study population. Four occupational/population-based studies from the United States found an increased risk of incident heart disease (fatal and nonfatal combined) among diabetic persons [104, 136–138]. National survey data from the United States on adults with T2DM have shown a prevalence of fatal and nonfatal CHD events of around 4% for those aged 18–44 years and 20% for those older than 65 years [139]. These rates are 2–20 times higher than corresponding ones for similar-aged people without T2DM, the rate-ratios being highest among younger patients with T2DM. Uusitupa et al. [140] have also found that age-standardized prevalence of acute myocardial infarction (AMI) among newly diagnosed T2DM men (17%) and women (18%) was significantly higher than among nondiabetic ones (10% and 4%, respectively). Also the incidence of first myocardial infarction (MI) was significantly higher among diabetic compared with nondiabetic persons (for men 27% vs. 19%; for women 12% vs. 2%) during the 10-year follow-up. Age-standardized cardiovascular mortality was substantially higher in diabetic men (15%) and women (17%) than in nondiabetic men (5%) and women (2%).

In one population-based study, the 7-year incidence of first MI or death for patients with diabetes was 20% but was only 3.5% for nondiabetic patients [141]. History of MI increased the rate of recurrent MI or cardiovascular death for both groups (18.8% in nondiabetic persons and 45% in those with diabetes). Thus, patients with diabetes but without previous MI carry the same level of risk for subsequent acute coronary events as nondiabetic patients with previous MI. This study and other findings were considered when the US National Cholesterol Education Program Adult Treatment Panel III proposed that more intense interventions should be considered for diabetic than nondiabetic subjects to prevent CHD [142].

Many studies have shown a considerable 2–8-fold excess in CVD mortality in insulin-treated diabetic subjects compared with the general population [143–147]. Cardiovascular mortality has been estimated to be 2.5-fold higher in T2DM men and 2.9-fold higher in T2DM women compared with nondiabetic subjects. Those treated with oral hypoglycemic agents had higher rates of cardiovascular mortality than did those treated with diet alone, indicating that the severity of diabetes contributes to the risk of cardiovascular mortality [148, 149].

Recent extensive evidence confirms the excess risk of cardiovascular mortality in diabetic patients. Data from the intensive blood-glucose treatment arm of the United Kingdom Prospective Diabetes Study (UKPDS) examined the reasons for death in patients with newly diagnosed type 2 diabetes over a 10-year follow-up period. The UKPDS showed that 8.4% of type 2 diabetic patients died of either fatal MI or sudden death, whereas mortality associated with other disease was relatively very low [150]. Data from an age- and sex-matched group in the Framingham Study show that for nondiabetic individuals the equivalent mortality rate over 10 years is only 4% [151].

Women in general have a lower unadjusted risk of CHD than do men. In many studies, rates of CVD in women with diabetes equal or exceed those in men [152–154], although not all studies have demonstrated this relationship [155, 156]. More research is also needed to determine whether this is true for both T1DM and T2DM. The Wisconsin population-based study reported similar risk ratio in both T2DM men (2.4) and women (2.2) vs. nondiabetic persons. Nevertheless, in T1DM women the risk ratio (13.5) was significantly higher than that in T1DM men (9.1) [157]. The reason for the accelerated atherogenesis among diabetic women is not completely understood, but it may relate to hyperglycemia itself since this phenomenon is seen both in young-onset T1DM patients [158] and in older T2DM patients [104]. It may also relate, at least in part, to more severe lipid and lipoprotein abnormalities, particularly elevated levels of triglycerides and reduced levels of HDL, among diabetic women [159, 160]. A recent study [161] suggests greater impairment of endothelial function associated with T2DM in women than in men. The role of hyperinsulinemia and insulin resistance is important in understanding the link between female gender and risk of CVD in diabetic patients. Insulin resistance is associated with lower estrogen and higher androgen levels. Premenopausal women with insulin resistance or diabetes do not benefit from the protective effects of menstruation experienced by women without these conditions [162]. In addition, the magnitude of increased risk of reinfarction and fatality rate following an acute MI among diabetic patients compared with nondiabetic patients was greater in women than in men [163]. Several studies have noted that CVD mortality in diabetic patients was related to age at the onset of diabetes or to duration of diabetes [145–147, 164]. In the Diabetes Epidemiology Research International Study of young-onset T1DM patients, cardiovascular deaths were relatively few during a follow-up of 8–15 years, although significantly increased as compared with the rates in the background population [165].

Excess mortality, CVD mortality in particular, extends beyond the limits of diabetes to IGT. Studies in the United Kingdom, in Bedford [166] and in Whitehall, London [167], have all consistently shown increased mortality at the upper end of the blood glucose distribution before T2DM is manifest. This is in agreement with the findings of Uusitupa et al. [168] who showed that a considerable number of T2DM patients had already suffered an MI before the time of diagnosis of their diabetes. Similar findings were also observed in the Pacific Island populations where CHD is much less common than in Europid populations [169].

Mortality and Case-Fatality in AMI

There are wide differences in the age-adjusted incidence of fatal CHD in T2DM patients between populations: the highest rates were in Framingham [170] where they were 4% per year for men, but the rates were only 1% per year in the Chicago Heart [171] and MRFIT [172] studies. In Europe, the CHD incidence varied from 2.6% per year in Finland [173] and 2.2% in the Schwabing cohort [174], to 1 to 1.4% per year in the United Kingdom [175] and in another study in Finland [140] and 0.4% per year in the Paris Prospective study in France [176]. Prospective studies from Japan have reported very low mortality from CHD in both T2DM and T1DM [165, 177], corresponding to the general rates in Japan. Also in Pima Indians who have the highest prevalence of T2DM in the world, mortality from CHD is not a particularly high [178]. Nevertheless, the most recent information on total and CVD mortality among the Native Americans in the Strong Heart Study has revealed that currently American Indian populations have higher CVD mortality rates than in other ethnic groups in the United States [153].

A number of studies have demonstrated that diabetes mellitus negatively influences the survival after MI, including increased rates of reinfarction, congestive heart failure, and death [112, 179–187]. The largest population-based study of the impact of diabetes on mortality after the first MI was the FINMONICA Study [185]. The 1-year case-fatality rate for first MI (including prehospitalization mortality) was 45% in diabetic men and 39% in diabetic women. These case-fatality rates were significantly higher than rates in nondiabetic male and female subjects (38 and 25%, respectively). Furthermore, diabetic patients were more likely than nondiabetic patients to die from sudden cardiac death before reaching hospital. In unstable angina pectoris or non-Q-wave MI, the presence of diabetes increases the risk of inhospital MI, complications of MI, and mortality [186]. In the OASIS Registry, a six-nation study of unstable angina and non-Q-wave MI, diabetes independently increased the risk of death by 57% [187]. In the SHOCK Trial of revascularization for MI complicated by cardiogenic shock, the relative risk of death for patients with diabetes was 1.36 compared with that of nondiabetic patients [188].

There also seems to be a differential gender-related effect regarding the type of diabetes on case-fatality in AMI. Data from the GISSI-2 Study have shown that in men, both T1DM and T2DM were associated with moderately higher mortality rate after MI compared with nondiabetic men [183]. In women, diabetes was a strong risk factor for death following an MI. In the Framingham Study [163], which included a much higher proportion of women than men taking insulin (27% vs. 15%), the relative risk of fatal CHD was higher for women than men. In men, the presence of diabetes may lead to an overall decreased survival rate independent from the type of diabetes, whereas in women, T1DM is uniquely associated with major alterations in cardiovascular function that have a strong impact on mortality after MI.

Reviewed by Jacoby and Nesto [189], the reasons for the increased case-fatality in AMI in diabetic patients still remain debated. Some of the studies suggested that a higher prevalence of other risk factors (hypertension, hyperlipidemia, extensive coronary artery disease, and advanced age) or higher degree of left ventricular damage after infarction may explain the higher mortality rate in diabetic patients. Conversely, other studies [190] indicate that the detrimental effect of diabetes on survival is most evident in patients whose baseline risk factor profile would indicate a relatively low risk of death after MI, thus suggesting that pathophysiologic derangements accompanying diabetes that apparently do not affect the clinical status of the patients may play a subtle but critical role as they reduce survival after MI. A study from the community-based AMI register in Finland demonstrated that there were no differences in cardiac enzyme or ECG findings between diabetic and nondiabetic patients who had their first AMI [184]. Thus, there was no evidence that the size of AMI is larger in diabetic than nondiabetic subjects. It is known that AMI is often associated with an acute hyperglycemia. This may be particularly aggravated in diabetic AMI patients leading to various metabolic and cardiac problems during the first 1–2 weeks after AMI. The DIGAMI Study suggests benefit from glucose lowering post-AMI [191], and so this problem might be reversible. The current evidence has also revealed that diabetic patients without previous MI have as high a risk of developing MI as nondiabetic patients with previous MI [141], although these findings have not been supported by all more recent, larger, studies [192, 193]. It is possible that this effect is more pronounced in women than in men; thus studies comprising only men may not have reconfirmed this initial finding from a study where both sexes were included.

Risk Factors for CHD in Diabetic Patients

Several studies have examined risk factors for CHD in T2DM patients, whereas little population-based prospective data are available on the risk and determinants of CHD in T1DM. The traditional risk factors, such as cigarette smoking, serum cholesterol, or BP, play an important role in the development of CHD in diabetic patients [172], but they explain only a part of the excess risk of ischemic heart lesions in diabetes [194–196]. The greater the number of coronary risk factors, the higher the susceptibility to CHD whether diabetic or not [140, 166, 172, 173]. Hyperglycemia was found to be predictive of CHD death for T2DM in several studies [140, 173, 175, 194, 195]. The recently published results from the Nurses' Health Study indicated duration of T2DM as an important factor associated with increased risk of death from all causes and fatal CHD [164]. Compared with those in nondiabetic persons, the multivariate relative risks of fatal CHD across categories of diabetes duration (5, 6–10, 11–15, 16–25, >25 years) were 2.75, 3.63, 5.51, 6.38, and 11.9 ($p < 0.001$ for trend), respectively. The combination of prior CHD and a long duration of clinical diabetes (i.e., >15 years) was associated with a 30-fold (95% CI 20.7–43.5) increased risk of fatal CHD [164]. These results need to be confirmed by other studies.

Serum cholesterol level has been found to be particularly important in predicting cardiovascular mortality [196]. In men with and without diabetes, CHD death rates increased markedly with increasing cholesterol levels. At every level of serum cholesterol, however, the CHD death rate was several times higher for diabetic than nondiabetic men, and the increase in absolute CHD mortality rate with higher serum cholesterol level tended to be disproportionately greater for diabetic men than for nondiabetic men [172].

The lipid profiles predictive of cardiovascular death were assessed in the Paris Prospective Study [197]. The relationship between baseline triglyceride levels alone was clear: individuals with the lowest baseline triglyceride levels had the lowest risk of death from CHD during 15 years of follow-up. Conversely, individuals with CHD had the highest triglyceride levels [197]. Also previous cross-sectional findings from the WHO Multinational Study suggested that triglycerides were a stronger predictor of CHD and PVD in several countries than was total cholesterol [198]. Adults with diabetes do not have total cholesterol or low-density lipoprotein (LDL) cholesterol concentrations that are significantly increased compared with the general population [199]. However, significantly more patients with diabetes have low HDL-C levels and elevated triglyceride levels compared with individuals without diabetes. Thus, lipid abnormalities, although not necessarily hypercholesterolemia, contribute to the prediction of CHD [140, 173, 174, 197]. Elevated levels of triglyceride-rich lipoproteins lower HDL levels by promoting exchanges of cholesterol from HDL to very low density lipoprotein (VLDL) via cholesteryl ester transfer protein [200]. Diabetic persons with CHD more commonly have the combination of elevated triglycerides and low HDL than elevated total and LDL cholesterol levels [201].

Risk factors for CHD related to increased triglyceride concentrations include an increase in postprandial accumulation of remnant lipoproteins, which form highly atherogenic particles [202, 203]. Erkelens [204] has recently summarized available data on the altered composition of lipoproteins and lipids, so-called diabetic dyslipidemia, in patients with T2DM. Thus, diabetic dyslipidemia is characterized by (1) elevated levels of triglyceride; (2) normal levels of total cholesterol and LDL-C; (3) reduced levels of HDL-C; (4) elevated levels of apolipoprotein B; (5) a preponderance of small, dense LDL particles; and (6) increased levels of cholesterol-rich VLDL [204].

Central fat distribution appears to be one of the prominent indicators of CHD risk in the Paris, Gothenburg, and Framingham studies [197, 205, 206]. Also, android fat distribution independently of BMI contributes to the development of T2DM. This is particularly striking in women, as demonstrated in the Gothenburg Study [207]. Also in studies from Iowa [208] and Mauritius [209] the risk of developing diabetes increased with BMI as well as with the waist-to-hip ratio; the highest risk was observed for the highest combined tertiles. Björntorp [210] has suggested that the intra-abdominal tissue, particularly the portion drained by the portal circulation, has an exceedingly sensitive lipomobilization capacity. This results in high portal free fatty acid concentrations, which in turn generate through hepatic regulation hyperinsulinemia, hyperglycemia, and T2DM. This is associated with a cluster of metabolic abnormalities defined as the insulin resistance syndrome. To explain what makes fat accumulate intra-abdominally rather than subcutaneously, Björntorp suggested a number of possibilities that involve, besides genetic predisposition, endocrine perturbations, which could, for example, affect glucocorticoid and androgen levels. These perturbations can occur as a consequence of certain modern lifestyle factors such as stress, smoking, alcohol consumption, lack of physical activity, and the excessive intake of saturated fat.

Since the first suggestions of the insulin–atheroma relationship in the 1960s [211, 212] there have been many clinical, experimental, and epidemiological studies addressing this question. Insulin may directly promote atherosclerosis [213]. Although insulin correlates with a number of cardiovascular risk factors, such as BMI, body fat distribution, serum triglycerides, and HDL cholesterol, epidemiological studies of the insulin–CHD relationship have provided inconsistent findings, both cross-sectionally and longitudinally. Moreover, populations that are clearly hyperinsulinemic such as Pima Indians, Naurans, Polynesians, etc., do not have a particularly high mortality from CHD [178, 214–217]. Data from the Multiple Risk Factor Intervention Trial [218] demonstrated that insulin appears to contribute to cardiovascular risk in persons with apolipoprotein E 3/2 phenotype but does not explain the increased risk seen in these subjects. The authors suggested that this new finding, if confirmed, may throw further light on the role of insulin in atherosclerosis.

Long-term hyperglycemia may explain a large proportion of excessive cardiovascular mortality among T2DM patients not explained by classical coronary risk factors [140]. In addition, it was recently hypothesized that increased plasma and tissue glucose levels may be one important source of the increased oxidative stress seen in diabetic patients, which through various metabolic mechanisms could predispose to atheroma [73].

Albumin excretion rate has also been shown to be significantly associated with CHD morbidity after taking into account the confounding effects of raised BP and other coronary risk factors [219–221]. Also Nielsen et al. [222] has noted that the prevalence of CVD increases with increasing albumin excretion in T2DM. It was shown that the simultaneous occurrence of hyperinsulinemia and microalbuminuria is a strong predictor of CHD events in elderly nondiabetic people [223]. Several earlier studies performed among T1DM patients also observed a substantial increase in mortality from, and incidence of, CHD in those with nephropathy compared with T1DM patients without nephropathy [224, 225]. In the Finnish cohort of childhood-onset T1DM patients the risk of CHD was high, about 3–4% after 20–33 years of follow-up when the patients were aged 19–49 years [158]. The risk of CHD was 10-fold in those who had developed nephropathy compared with those without nephropathy, and increased with increasing duration of nephropathy.

Prothrombotic and fibrinolytic factors act in concert to maintain hemostasis. Plasminogen activator inhibitor 1 (PAI-1), an enzyme needed to lyse a thrombus once formed, is synthesised in endothelial cells, vascular smooth muscle cells, adipose tissue, and the liver. Insulin resistance is associated with a shift toward the prothrombotic state and highly correlated with an increased risk of MI [226]. In an analysis of the Framingham population, levels of PAI-1 were measured in men and women with normal glucose tolerance, and those with IGT or previously undiagnosed diabetes [227]. In the latter two groups, levels of PAI-1 were consistently twofold higher than in the group with normal glucose tolerance. This finding suggests that these persons have a reduced ability to eliminate clots once they have formed.

The ARIC Study examined the association of traditional and nontraditional risk factors with incidence of CHD in adults with diabetes [228]. After adjustment for hypertension, smoking, total cholesterol level, and low HDL cholesterol level, levels of albumin, fibrinogen, and von Willebrand factor, factor VII activity, and leukocyte count were predictors of CHD among persons with diabetes. The authors suggested that these associations may reflect the underlying inflammatory reaction or microvascular injury related to atherosclerosis and a tendency toward thrombosis or common antecedents for both diabetes and coronary heart disease [228]. C-reactive protein has been shown to have predictive value in nondiabetic populations [229] but has not been well studied in persons with diabetes.

Similarly to hypertension, it has been suggested that an activation of the renin–angiotensin system might play a role in the pathogenesis of CHD [230]. Both T1DM and T2DM patients with abnormal albumin excretion have increased plasma angiotensin-I-converting enzyme (ACE) concentration [231]. Several studies have demonstrated that an insertion (I)/deletion (D) polymorphism of the ACE gene is strongly associated with the level of circulating ACE and may increase the risk of MI and severe CHD in nondiabetic subjects and T2DM patients [232]. Ruiz et al. studied 132 patients with T2DM with either MI or severe coronary stenosis verified by angiography, and 184 T2DM patients with no history of CHD. They found a significant 1.8-fold increase in risk of MI or severe coronary stenosis in subjects with the DD genotype. Tarnow et al. [233] performed a similar study in T1DM. They found no difference in genotype or allele frequency (D/I) between T1DM patients with and without nephropathy, although the prevalence of CHD was more than twice as high in patients with diabetic nephropathy as compared to patients with normoalbuminuria. Nevertheless, the plasma ACE concentration was elevated in patients with nephropathy.

STROKE AND CEREBROVASCULAR DISEASES

Incidence and Mortality

Cerebrovascular diseases, also known in the literature as a stroke, apoplexy, and/or cerebrovascular accident, are a major cause of disability and mortality. They require considerable health care resources, particularly in an aging population.

Diabetes mellitus magnifies the risk of cerebrovascular morbidity and mortality [162, 234–241] (Table 1). Cerebrovascular disease is the predominant long-term cause of morbidity and mortality in patients with both T1DM and T2DM. Several large population studies have shown an increase in the prevalence of stroke in the diabetic population. The Framingham Study was one of the earliest to demonstrate an increased morbidity and mortality from cerebrovascular disease in patients with diabetes. Similar conclusions have been drawn from most, although not all, subsequent studies of patients with T2DM [235–240]. In a prospective study from Finland with a follow-up of 15 years, diabetes was the strongest single factor for stroke in a multivariate analysis (relative risk for men 3.4 and for women 4.9) [241]. Diabetes is a prominent risk factor for ischemic but not hemorrhagic stroke [241, 256, 257]. However, the recent joint report from the Honolulu Heart Program and the Framingham Study suggested that an increased risk of hemorrhagic stroke might also exist in T2DM [237].

Ischemic cerebrovascular disease accounts for about 80% of all strokes [258], but the female-to-male mortality ratio differs for stroke subtypes by ethnicity and age [259]. Diabetes mellitus is a definite independent risk factor for atherosclerosis and atherothrombotic brain infarction [240, 247, 260, 261]. In the Framingham Study the incidence of atherothrombotic cerebral infarction for both sexes aged 45–74 years was greater by a factor of 2.5–3.5 in diabetic men that in nondiabetic subjects. Among the diabetic cohort, ischemic cerebral infarction comprised 88% of stroke events, 8% were subarachnoid or intracerebral hemorrhages and the rest of the strokes were of unknown type. Diabetes mellitus may also cause microatheroma in small vessels, such as lenticulostriate arteries, leading to lacunar stroke, one of the most common subtype of ischemic stroke. Lacunar stroke is a unique subtype and requires specific clinical and radiological features for diagnosis. The presence of diabetes mellitus was associated only with symptomatic cerebral infarcts but not with silent infarcts [262], which are five times as prevalent as symptomatic brain infarcts in the general population [263].

Table 1 Relative risk of stroke in the diabetic population

	Relative risk in diabetic patient
USA, 1970 [242]	Hospitalized patients ×1.4 aged 45–69 years
Seal Beach and Chicago, USA, 1972 [243]	×1.7 males; ×2.8 females
Jerusalem, Israel, 1973 [244]	Hospitalized patients ×6 in 5th decade; ×3 in 6th decade; ×2 after age 60
Chicago, USA, 1974 [245]	×1.3 in elderly patients receiving financial assistance
Hawaii, USA, 1980 [246]	×2.0
Tilsburg, The Netherlands, 1982 [247]	Hospitalized patients ×2.2
Framingham, USA, 1983 [248]	Males ×4 in 5th and 6th decade; ×1 in 7th decade; females ×1 in 5th decade; ×4 in 6th decade; ×3 in 7th decade
Rochester, USA, 1983 [249]	×1.4 in population with median age of 75 years
Monroe Co., USA, 1983 [250]	Hospitalized patients ×3.3
USA, 1987 [251]	×4 45–64-year-olds; ×2.5 65–74-year-olds
Sweden, 1987 [252]	×6 males; ×13 females
USA, NHANES, 1990 [239]	×2.5 males; ×2.5 females; 35–74-year-olds
Framingham, USA, 1991 [236]	×1.4 males; ×1.7 females; 55–84-year-olds
MRFIT, USA, 1993 [253]	×3.8 in males
Oslo, Norway, 1995 [254]	×7.9 males; 40–49-year-olds
Sweden, 1995 [255]	×4.4 males; ×5.1 females; 35–74-year-olds
MRFIT, USA, 1998 [238]	×1.8 males; ×2.1 females
USA, 2002 [237]	population-based study ×2.1 in Hawaii and ×3.6 in Framingham; only men age-adjusted for thromboembolic stroke; ×4.9 for hemorrhagic strokes in Framingham

A negative correlation has been reported between diabetes, especially T1DM, and aneurysmal subarachnoidal hemorrhage (SAH) [256]. While diabetes is one of the major risk factors for stroke in general, patients with aneurysmal SAH have a lower or equal prevalence of diabetes mellitus than does the general population. In particular, T1DM is rarely present prior to aneurysmal rupture [256]. However, there are also opposite opinions, since two studies claim that diabetes is closely associated with SAH and stroke [264, 265]. Stroke patients with diabetes, or with hyperglycemia in the acute stage of stroke, have a higher mortality rate, worse neurologic outcome, and more severe disability than did those without [260–269]. The presence of diabetes, however, did not influence the outcome of parenchymatous hemorrhage or SAH [264, 270]. There is insufficient information on the association of diabetes mellitus and radiologically confirmed SAH [271]. In a recent study, there was no difference in the presence of diabetes among SAH patients and controls [272]. New data from Finland (J. Tuomilehto, personal communication, 2003) are of a particular interest since Finland has one of the highest incidences of SAH [273]. During 1990–1998, 5630 first stroke events were registered in a community-based stroke register [274]. The subtype of the stroke was ischemic in 81%, hemorrhagic in 12%, and subarachnoid hemorrhage in 7% of the cases. The percentage of CT, MRI, angiography, or autopsy was 98%. The number of patients with diabetes was 1148 (20%). Of these, 19% were on insulin therapy and 81% were on diet alone or oral drug therapy. SAH was less common in patients with diabetes (1.0%) than patients without diabetes (8.2%, $p < 0.00001$).

There is much less information concerning the risk of stroke in T1DM. Deckert et al. [144] studying a group of patients who had had T1DM for more than 40 years, reported a 10% cumulative incidence of stroke and 7% mortality from stroke. The World Health Organization Multinational Study of vascular disease in diabetes has indicated an overall raised cerebrovascular mortality in patients with T1DM, but with considerable variation between countries [275].

T1DM patients generally are much younger than T2DM patients, and stroke is known as a disease of elderly people, two thirds of all stroke cases in the population occurring in people aged 65 years or older. Thus, future studies are needed to show what the true risk of stroke in T1DM patients will be once they have reached the age when stroke is common. The data from the large nationwide cohort of Finnish childhood-onset T1DM patients showed that by the age of 50 years, and after 20–40 years duration of diabetes, the risk of stroke was equally high as that of acute CHD [158]. Also, the risk of stroke was equally common in both sexes. Previously, many T1DM patients who also had other risk factors for stroke (e.g., hypertension, smoking, dyslipidemia) had a high probability of dying relatively young from diabetic renal diseases or CHD, and so the number of T1DM patients surviving until "stroke risk age" (older than 65 years) has thus far been small. It is likely that improved treatment for hypertension and better blood glucose control will change this situation markedly, and stroke will become an important late complication of T1DM in the future.

Risk Factors for Stroke in Diabetic Patients

Diabetes mellitus is a well-established risk factor for small-artery occlusive disease affecting the distal extremities, kidneys, retinas, peripheral and cranial nerves, and other tissues. However, its role in cerebral small-vessel disease is less well characterized. Epidemiological studies have demonstrated an independent contribution of diabetes to the risk of stroke.

In a Finnish study [276], fasting and 2-h glucose, a HbA_{1c} duration of diabetes, and atrial fibrillation were the baseline variables predicting both fatal and nonfatal stroke events in T2DM patients during a 3.5-year follow-up. The association between duration of diabetes and risk of stroke was reported by these authors and also by other prospective studies from Finland [158, 241]. This study showed that the risk factors for stroke were the same for diabetic and nondiabetic subjects, except smoking, which was not significant in diabetic women (probably because few diabetic women smoked in Finland). Others have not found a significant relationship between ischemic stroke and diabetes duration, fasting glucose level, and serum HDL-cholesterol [277]. The Pima Indian Study did not find any relation between duration of T2DM and the risk of fatal stroke [278]. Results from the Honolulu Heart Program indicated that the serum glucose level at baseline was an independent risk factor for all cerebrovascular accidents and for thromboembolic strokes [237]. In a study from Oslo, nonfasting serum glucose was a risk factor for stroke mortality only in men with BMI above the median value, and only in univariate but not in multivariate analysis [254].

Several studies have provided sufficient evidence to indicate that hypertension and diabetes mellitus have direct effect on the occurrence of moderate to severe atherosclerotic stenosis of extracranial and intracranial arteries [279, 280]. Furthermore some clinical series have suggested that patients with single lacunes may represent an entity different from those with multiple lacunes in that only the latter group have an increased frequency of arterial hypertension and diabetes mellitus [281, 282]. However, in comparison with nonhemorrhagic lacunar stroke, patients with hemorrhagic lacunar stroke are less likely to have diabetes mellitus [283].

Blood pressure is a well-known risk factor for stroke in both types of diabetes [275], and the UKPDS trial suggested that controlling blood pressure in patients with

T2DM reduced the stroke risk although not the risk of AMI [284]. Diabetic subjects have higher systolic BP than does the general population, particularly females [5, 11, 240, 241, 285]. It is suggested that diabetes may enhance the risk of stroke even in the absence of increased BP. In the nondiabetic population, there is a 40% increase in stroke risk and a 25% increase in CHD risk with an elevation of 6 mmHg in excess of 75 mmHg diastolic BP. Diabetes increases the risk of both conditions by a factor of 2 or 3, and in diabetic subjects hypertension augments these risks [286]. Tuomilehto et al. [241] did not find evidence for an interaction between BMI, diabetes, and BP in a prospective study of stroke in a random population sample. There were neither additive nor multiplicative effects between diabetes and other CVD risk factors. Thus, it is unlikely that the risk of stroke associated with diabetes would be restricted to a particular subgroup, such as obese or hypertensive subjects. Moreover, it is possible that a part of the increased risk of stroke seen in hypertensive subjects is related to abnormalities of glucose metabolism, which are a common correlate of hypertension, particularly in the elderly [241, 287, 288].

It has been noted that the relative significance of risk factors for stroke varies with age and sex [289]. Hypertension, BP, smoking, hematocrit, and left-ventricular hypertrophy are strongly associated with stroke in patients younger than 65 years. Diabetes seems to be a stronger risk factor for stroke in females than in males [255, 290]. Diabetes adversely affects cerebrovascular arterial circulation, akin to its effects in the coronary and lower extremity vasculature. Patients with diabetes have more severe extracranial atherosclerosis [291].

Besides being a risk factor for stroke, it has been shown that diabetes in the aftermath of the stroke event increases regional brain damage due to acute vascular insufficiency [292, 293] and may have deleterious effects in both the short- and long-term prognosis of stroke [266–269, 294]. It was shown that hyperglycemia directly increases regional brain damage due to acute vascular insufficiency [292]. Some studies have claimed, however, that neither a history of diabetes nor the glucose levels on admission are related to the outcome in an acute stroke event [295–300]. A number of studies have investigated whether diabetes has influence on the volume of damaged brain tissue in patients with stroke, as newer imaging methods have made the comparisons of stroke size possible. Most studies using computed tomography [267, 268, 300] and autopsy [301] have not found differences in the size of cerebral infarction between patients with and without diabetes mellitus.

There are at least three possible explanations for the worsening of stroke damage in the presence of hyperglycemia [302]. First, under the hypoxic conditions caused by a stroke, glucose is anaerobically metabolized to lactic acid, and the resultant cerebral intracellular and extracellular acidosis causes damage to neurones, glial, and vascular tissue. The effects of glycemia may also differ at different anatomical sites. In the center of an infarct, excess glucose will worsen damage, whereas in the surrounding ischemic area, an increase in glucose level may lessen damage. Secondly, under hyperglycemic and hypoxic conditions the extracellular concentration of amino acids is increased because of excessive release combined with failure of energy-dependent re-uptake that would normally result in detoxification of glutamate and aspartate. A third theory is that with ischemia and hyperglycemia, together with neuronal hyperstimulation, intracellular calcium concentration increases, which may cause neuronal damage.

Excessive alcohol intake may increase the risk for stroke among patients with diabetes [303, 304]. In addition, the Gothenburg population cohort study of mostly T2DM showed that alcohol combined with diabetes are important risk factors for cerebral infarction [252].

The increased incidence of and mortality from stroke in patients with T1DM is strongly related to the development of diabetic nephropathy [158, 305]. The presence of nephropathy increases the stroke risk up to 10-fold compared with T1DM patients without nephropathy, and the stroke risk increases with increasing duration of nephropathy [158]. When proteinuria develops, not only is there an increase in systolic and diastolic BP but also an increase in von Willebrand factor, fibrinogen, platelet adhesiveness and number, and stimulated levels of tissue plasminogen activator and plasminogen activator inhibitor [305, 306]. No evidence associates background diabetic retinopathy or proliferative retinopathy with an increased prevalence of stroke in T1DM [307]. Only one study has shown an increase in the relative risk of nonembolic ischemic stroke in diabetic subjects with retinopathy (4.0; 95% CI 1.0–14.5) after adjustment for age, sex, smoking, use of insulin, average systolic BP, and average random glucose [308]. However, that study was unable to distinguish T1DM and T2DM subjects and duration of diabetes was not taken into account.

ASYMPTOMATIC HYPERGLYCEMIA AND CVD RISK

It has been known for quite some time that individuals with overt diabetes have an increased risk for CVD, but the fact that subjects with asymptomatic diabetes or hyperglycemia are also at high risk for the development of CVD has been recognized only recently. Earlier studies such as the International Collaborative Group [309] in 1979 did not show consistent evidence for a threshold or graded association between asymptomatic hyperglycemia and CHD. In 1985, Epstein [310] reviewed 13 cohort studies that had studied postchallenge glucose and CHD. Five of them demonstrated a direct association between postchallenge glucose and CHD that remained significant in multivariate analysis. In two studies the direct association was no longer persistent after adjusting for other risk factors or no multivariate analysis was done, and the remaining six showed no association even before consideration of other risk factors.

Over the past decades, the prevalence of diabetes has increased markedly worldwide. Only around 1980, the National Diabetes Data Group (NDDG) [311] and WHO [312, 313] formulated criteria for diagnosing diabetes based on glucose levels 2-h after a 75-g oral glucose load. The near-universal adoption of these diagnostic criteria has created order out of the confusion in the diagnostic criteria for diabetes and stimulated the interest in studying outcomes related to different categories of hyperglycemia. Now, after about two decades from the adoption of standard criteria for diabetes and glucose intolerance, epidemiological evidence has been accumulated showing that asymptomatic diabetes, as well as hyperglycemia in the nondiabetic range was associated with the increased risk of CVD. Coutinho et al. recently made a metaregression analysis of the data published between 1966 and 1996 from 20 studies comprising 95 783 individuals (94% male) followed on average for 12.4 years, and demonstrated that the progressive relationship between glucose levels and CVD risk extends below the diabetic threshold [314]. In data from the 23-year follow-up of the Paris Prospective Study of 7018 men, aged 44–55 years at baseline, Balkau et al. found that the relationship of fasting and 2-h postload glucose with mortality from all-causes and CHD were curvilinear, and that the increased risks already became apparent at the upper levels of the nondiabetic glucose distribution [315]. Results from a 22-year follow-up of nondiabetic Norwegian men (aged 40–59 years) showed a multivariate adjusted relative risk of 1.4 (95% CI 1.0–1.8) for CVD mortality in men with fasting whole blood glucose >4.7 mmol/l compared with <4.7 mmol/l [316]. An increased risk of developing CHD associated with the highest quartile of normal fasting glucose distribution was also observed in Australian nondiabetic women, but not in men [317].

Increasing evidence has been accumulated on the importance of hyperglycemia after an oral glucose challenge as an independent risk factor for CVD. In the Chicago Heart Study of 11,554 White men and 666 Black men aged 35–64 years, asymptomatic hyperglycemia (>11.1 mmol/l) 1 h after a 50-g glucose load showed increased CVD mortality in both White and Black men [318]. The 23-year follow-up of the Honolulu Heart Program among 8006 Japanese American middle-aged men also suggested an increasing risk gradient between 1-h postload glucose and CHD [319]. In the Hisayama Study, the multivariate adjusted relative risk for the incidence of CHD and stroke in Japanese aged 40–79 years was 1.9 (95% CI 1.2–3.2) for subjects with IGT compared with those who had a normal glucose tolerance [320].

In the late 1990s, a new surge of interest to study the relationship between asymptomatic hyperglycemia and the risk of CVD developed following the 1997 revision of diagnostic criteria for diabetes and milder degrees of hyperglycemia by the American Diabetes Association. In the Funagata diabetes study of a Japanese cohort aged 40 years or over, IGT but not impaired fasting glycemia (IFG) was associated with increased CVD mortality [321]. In the Hoorn study in the Netherlands in subjects with no prior history of diabetes, 2-h postload glucose proved to be a better risk predictor of CVD mortality than does fasting glucose or HbA_{1c} [322]. Pooled longitudinal data from Mauritius, Fiji, and Nauru showed that isolated postchallenge hyperglycemia (>11.1 mmol/l) with a nondiabetic fasting plasma glucose (<7.0 mmol/l) doubled the CVD mortality risk [323]. Similar results were also observed in older Californian women [324]. A recent analysis of the data from US Second National Health and Nutrition Survey, including 3092 adults aged 30–74 years, revealed that subjects with IGT and undiagnosed diabetes defined by isolated postload hyperglycemia had 40% higher CVD mortality rates compared with those with a normal glucose tolerance [325]. Thus, there is no doubt that the risk of CVD starts to increase much before the development of fasting hyperglycemia. A 20-year follow-up of 117,629 women aged 30–55 years in the Nurses' Health Study in the United States revealed that the risk of incident nonfatal MI and stroke started to increase 15 years before a clinical diagnosis of diabetes [326]. The multivariate adjusted relative risk for MI or stroke was 2.4, 3.2, and 3.6, respectively, for female nurses 15 years, 10–14.9 years, and <10 years before the onset of diabetes, in comparison with those who remained nondiabetic throughout the study.

The most convincing evidence of increased CVD risk related to asymptomatic hyperglycemia was provided by the DECODE (Diabetes Epidemiology: Collaborative Analysis of Diagnostic Criteria in Europe) Study. In this study, data from 10 prospective European cohort studies including 15,388 men and 7,126 women aged 30–89 years were collaboratively analyzed [327, 328]. Multivariate Cox proportional hazard analyses showed that the risk for death from all-cause, CVD, CHD, and stroke significantly increased in subjects with asymptomatic diabetes defined according to either the fasting plasma glucose >7.0 mmol/l or the 2-h postload plasma glucose >11.1 mmol/l. People with IGT also had an increased risk of death compared with those whose glucose tolerance was normal, but subjects with IFG did not have increased risk of death [327, 328] (Table 2). Furthermore, the DECODE Study revealed that elevated 2-h glucose was a better predictor of mortality from all-cause, CVD, and CHD than did elevated fasting glucose alone [327, 328]. A high 2-h glucose concentration was found to be associated with an increased risk of death, independent of

Table 2 Multivariate adjusted hazard ratios for deaths from cardiovascular diseases (CVD), coronary heart diseases (CHD), stroke, and all-cause according to the fasting and the 2-h glucose criteria: the DECODE Study

	Plasma (whole blood) glucose categories (mmol/l), subjects not known as diabetic				
	Fasting glucose criteria*		2-h glucose criteria†		
	IFG 6.1–6.9 (5.6–6.0)	Diabetes ≥7.0 (6.1)	IGT 7.8–11.0 (6.7–9.9)	Diabetes ≥11.1 (10.0)	Known diabetes†
CVD	1.09 (0.90–1.30)	1.48 (1.15–1.91)	1.34 (1.14–1.57)	1.55 (1.20–2.01)	1.96 (1.62–2.37)
CHD	1.07 (0.83–1.39)	1.43 (1.02–2.02)	1.28 (1.02–1.59)	1.64 (1.18–2.28)	1.94 (1.51–2.50)
Stroke	1.04 (0.70–1.56)	1.92 (1.16–3.17)	1.26 (0.88–1.79)	1.74 (1.01–2.99)	1.72 (1.11–2.66)
All-cause	1.11 (1.00–1.23)	1.65 (1.43–1.91)	1.40 (1.27–1.54)	1.92 (1.66–2.22)	1.81 (1.60–2.05)

Note: Data are given as hazards ratios (95% confidence intervals), adjusted for age, center, total cholesterol, body mass index, systolic blood pressure, smoking, and sex.
* Using fasting plasma (whole blood) glucose <6.1 (5.6) mmol/l as reference group.
† Using 2-h postload plasma (whole blood) glucose <7.8 (6.7) mmol/l as reference group.

the level of fasting blood glucose, whereas mortality associated with the fasting glucose concentration depended on the simultaneous level of 2-h glucose [327] (Table 3). Addition of 2-h glucose to a model based on fasting glucose improved the prediction (all p values <0.05, except for stroke). Conversely, fasting glucose did not add any further information once the 2-h glucose concentration was in the model (all p values >0.10) [327]. The largest absolute number of excess deaths was observed in subjects with IGT, especially those with IGT but normal fasting glucose, reflecting the fact that this category is the most prevalent abnormality in glucose regulation [327, 328].

The observations from the DECODE Study on mortality related to 2-h glucose versus fasting glucose have also been extended to the prediction of the risk of serious incident CHD events (CHD death and nonfatal MI) based on five Finnish DECODE Study cohorts [329]. These results confirmed that in subjects without a prior history of diabetes the association of 2-h glucose with CHD incidence is graded and independent, and that 2-h glucose is superior to fasting glucose in assessing the risk of future CHD events (Figure 1). Thus, the DECODE Study unequivocally confirmed that asymptomatic postchallenge hyperglycemia independently increases cardiovascular morbidity and mortality and is a better predictor of the events than fasting hyperglycemia.

Whether postchallenge hyperglycemia is a true risk factor for CHD or merely a reflection of a high-risk phenotype remains to be determined [330]. Postchallenge plasma glucose concentrations are more strongly correlated with a variety of risk factors than are those of fasting plasma glucose in nondiabetic subjects, including central obesity, low-grade inflammation, and endothelial dysfunction [331]. It also remains unclear as to whether postchallenge hyperglycemia and postprandial hyperglycemia are similar or distinct characteristics. One study has suggested that mild-to-moderate mealtime hyperglycemia is an independent risk factor for increased IMT [332]. In a cohort at risk for diabetes, postchallenge glucose and glycemic excursions were found to be more strongly associated with carotid IMT than fasting glucose or HbA_{1c} level [333]. More recently, Ceriello et al. has shown an independent and cumulative deleterious effect of postprandial hypertriglyceridemia and hyperglycemia on endothelial function and suggested that oxidative stress is the common mediator through which they exert such effects [87].

Table 3 Adjusted hazards ratios for death from cardiovascular diseases (CVD), coronary heart diseases (CHD), stroke, and all-cause with both the fasting and the 2-h glucose classes in the same model: The DECODE Study

	Plasma (whole blood) glucose categories (mmol/l), subjects not known as diabetic						
	Fasting glucose criteria*			2-h glucose criteria†			
	IFG 6.1–6.9 (5.6–6.0)	Diabetes ≥7.0 (6.1)	χ^2 (p value)‡	IGT 7.8–11.0 (6.7–9.9)	Diabetes ≥11.1 (10.0)	χ^2 (p value)§	Known diabetes*
CVD	1.01 (0.84–1.22)	1.20 (0.88–1.64)	1.34 (>0.10)	1.32 (1.12–1.56)	1.40 (1.02–1.92)	12.09 (<0.005)	1.96 (1.62–2.37)
CHD	1.01 (0.77–1.31)	1.09 (0.71–1.67)	0.15 (>0.10)	1.27 (1.01–1.58)	1.56 (1.03–2.36)	6.81 (<0.05)	1.94 (1.51–2.50)
Stroke	1.00 (0.66–1.51)	1.64 (0.88–3.07)	2.35 (>0.10)	1.21 (0.84–1.74)	1.29 (0.66–2.54)	1.23 (>0.10)	1.73 (1.12–2.68)
All-cause	1.03 (0.93–1.14)	1.21 (1.01–1.44)	4.32 (>0.10)	1.37 (1.25–1.51)	1.73 (1.45–2.06)	61.35 (<0.001)	1.82 (1.60–2.06)

Note: Data are given as hazards ratios (95% confidence intervals), adjusted for age, sex, center, total cholesterol, body mass index, systolic blood pressure, and smoking.
* Using fasting plasma (whole blood) glucose <6.1 (5.6) mmol/l as reference group.
† Using 2-h postload plasma (whole blood) glucose <7.8 (6.7) mmol/l as reference group.
‡ Compared with the models in Table 1, with only the 2-h glucose criteria, 2 df.
§ Compared with the models in Table 1, with only the fasting glucose criteria, 2 df.

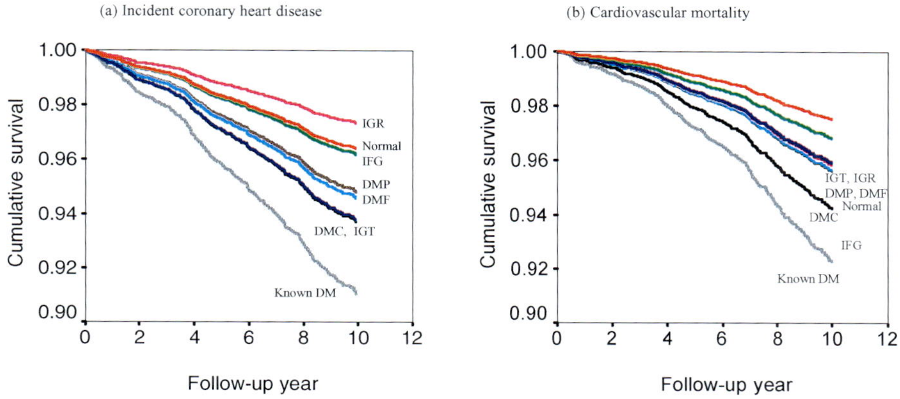

Figure 1 Cumulative survival curves for incidence of coronary heart disease (a) and for cardiovascular mortality (b) according to the glucose categories defined by both fasting and 2-h plasma glucose criteria. The cumulative survival are estimated from Cox proportional hazards models and adjusted for age, cohorts, sex, body mass index, blood pressure, serum cholesterol, and smoking. Normal = fasting plasma glucose <6.1 mmol/l and 2-h plasma glucose <7.8 mmol/l; IFG = impaired fasting glycaemia only; IGT = impaired glucose tolerance only; IGR = impaired glucose regulation (IFG and IGT); DMF = undiagnosed diabetes by fasting glucose criteria alone (fasting plasma glucose ≥7.0 mmol/l and 2-h plasma glucose <11.1 mmol/l); DMP = undiagnosed diabetes by 2-h postload glucose criteria alone (2-h plasma glucose ≥11.1 mmol/l and fasting plasma glucose <7.0 mmol/l); DMC = undiagnosed diabetes by both fasting and 2-h glucose criteria combined (fasting plasma glucose ≥7.0 mmol/l and 2-h plasma glucose ≥11.1 mmol/l); known DM = previously diagnosed diabetes

These findings may be important especially in the elderly population because postchallenge glucose levels increase to a much greater extent with advancing age than fasting glucose [324, 334]. In the DECODE population, the prevalence of isolated postload hyperglycemia, i.e. 2-h plasma glucose ≥11.1 mmol/l and fasting plasma glucose <7.0 mmol/l, was 0.7% in people 49 years or younger and 4.6% in those older than 70 years. In contrast, the prevalence of isolated fasting hyperglycemia, i.e. 2-h plasma glucose <11.1 mmol/l and fasting plasma glucose ≥7.0 mmol/l, in these two age groups was 1.3 and 2.3%, respectively [335]. Fasting glucose levels in this aspect can be compared with diastolic blood pressure that beyond middle age does not rise with aging, whereas systolic blood pressure does and also is a stronger predictor of cardiovascular events [336]. With conclusive evidence, the guidelines for the treatment of hypertension have been modified to emphasize the importance of systolic blood pressure [14]. These recommendations are, however, more firmly based on intervention studies, and not only on epidemiological evidence. The need for similar reassessment regarding postchallenge or postprandial versus fasting glucose, and for evaluating possible benefit of treatments focused on postprandial hyperglycemia, is required, especially in the elderly population.

REFERENCES

1. Stern MP. Diabetes and cardiovascular disease. The "common soil" hypothesis. *Diabetes* 1995; 44: 369–74.
2. Klein BE, Klein R, Moss SE. Blood pressure in a population of diabetic persons diagnosed after 30 years of age. *Am J Public Health* 1984; 74: 336–9.
3. Teuscher A, Egger M, Herman JB. Diabetes and hypertension. Blood pressure in clinical diabetic patients and a control population. *Arch Intern Med* 1989; 149: 1942–5.
4. Salomaa VV, Strandberg TE, Vanhanen H, Naukkarinen V, Sarna S, Miettinen TA. Glucose tolerance and blood pressure: long term follow up in middle aged men. *BMJ* 1991; 302: 493–6.
5. Aromaa A, Reunanen A, Pyorala K. Hypertension and mortality in diabetic and non-diabetic Finnish men. *J Hypertens* 1984; 2 (suppl): S205–7.
6. Sowers JR, Levy J, Zemel MB. Hypertension and diabetes. *Med Clin North Am* 1988; 72: 1399–414.
7. Sowers JR. Insulin resistance and hypertension. *Mol Cell Endocrinol* 1990; 72: C87–9.
8. Harris MI. Noninsulin-dependent diabetes mellitus in black and white Americans. *Diabetes Metab Rev* 1990; 6: 71–90.
9. Krolewski AS, Warram JH, Cupples A, Gorman CK, Szabo AJ, Christlieb AR. Hypertension, orthostatic hypotension and the microvascular complications of diabetes. *J Chronic Dis* 1985; 38: 319–26.
10. Tarn AC, Drury PL. Blood pressure in children, adolescents and young adults with type 1 (insulin-dependent) diabetes. *Diabetologia* 1986; 29: 275–81.
11. Cruickshank KJ, Orchard TJ, Becker DJ. The cardiovascular risk profile of adolescents with insulin-dependent diabetes mellitus. *Diabetes Care* 1985; 8: 118–24.
12. Tuomilehto J, Zimmet P, Taylor R, Bennett P, Kankaanpaa J, Wolf E. A cross-sectional ecological analysis of blood pressure and its determinants in eleven Pacific populations. *J Am Coll Nutr* 1989; 8: 151–65.
13. Cooper R, Cutler J, Desvigne-Nickens P, Fortmann SP, Friedman L, Havlik R, Hogelin G, Marler J, McGovern P, Morosco G, Mosca L, Pearson T, Stamler J, Stryer D, Thom T. Trends and disparities in coronary heart disease, stroke, and other cardiovascular diseases in the United States: findings of the national conference on cardiovascular disease prevention. *Circulation* 2000; 102: 3137–47.

14. 1999 World Health Organization–International Society of Hypertension Guidelines for the Management of Hypertension. Guidelines Subcommittee. *J Hypertens* 1999; 17: 151–83.
15. Jarrett RJ, Keen H, McCartney M, Fuller JH, Hamilton PJ, Reid DD, Rose G. Glucose tolerance and blood pressure in two population samples: their relation to diabetes mellitus and hypertension. *Int J Epidemiol* 1978; 7: 15–24.
16. Barrett-Connor E, Criqui MH, Klauber MR, Holdbrook M. Diabetes and hypertension in a community of older adults. *Am J Epidemiol* 1981; 113: 276–84.
17. Schnack C, Scheithauer W, Gisinger C, Winkler J, Schernthaner G. Prevalence of microalbuminuria in maturity onset primarily non-insulin-requiring diabetes mellitus: effect of disease duration, glycemic control, and mean systemic blood pressure. *J Diabet Complications* 1987; 1: 132–6.
18. Hasslacher C, Ritz E, Tschope W, Gallasch G, Mann JF. Hypertension in diabetes mellitus. *Kidney Int Suppl* 1988; 25: S133–7.
19. Ritz E, Hasslacher C, Tschope W, Koch M, Mann JF. Hypertension in diabetes mellitus. *Contrib Nephrol* 1987; 54: 77–85.
20. Parving HH, Hommel E, Mathiesen E, Skott P, Edsberg B, Bahnsen M, Lauritzen M, Hougaard P, Lauritzen E. Prevalence of microalbuminuria, arterial hypertension, retinopathy and neuropathy in patients with insulin dependent diabetes. *BMJ* 1988; 296: 156–60.
21. Gall MA, Rossing P, Skott P, Damsbo P, Vaag A, Bech K, Dejgaard A, Lauritzen M, Lauritzen E, Hougaard P, Beck-Nielsen H, Parving HH. Prevalence of micro- and macroalbuminuria, arterial hypertension, retinopathy and large vessel disease in European type 2 (non-insulin-dependent) diabetic patients. *Diabetologia* 1991; 34: 655–61.
22. Tarnow L, Rossing P, Gall MA, Nielsen FS, Parving HH. Prevalence of arterial hypertension in diabetic patients before and after the JNC-V. *Diabetes Care* 1994; 17: 1247–51.
23. Kimball TR, Daniels SR, Khoury PR, Magnotti RA, Turner AM, Dolan LM. Cardiovascular status in young patients with insulin-dependent diabetes mellitus. *Circulation* 1994; 90: 357–61.
24. Mathiesen ER, Ronn B, Jensen T, Storm B, Deckert T. Relationship between blood pressure and urinary albumin excretion in development of microalbuminuria. *Diabetes* 1990; 39: 245–9.
25. Raal FJ, Kalk WJ, Taylor DR, Osler CE, Panz VR. The relationship between the development and progression of microalbuminuria and arterial blood pressure in type 1 (insulin-dependent) diabetes mellitus. *Diabetes Res Clin Pract* 1992; 16: 221–7.
26. Microalbuminuria Collaborative Study Group, United Kingdom. Risk factors for development of microalbuminuria in insulin dependent diabetic patients: a cohort study. *BMJ* 1993; 306: 1235–9.
27. Coonrod BA, Ellis D, Becker DJ, Bunker CH, Kelsey SF, Lloyd CE, Drash AL, Kuller LH, Orchard TJ. Predictors of microalbuminuria in individuals with IDDM: Pittsburgh Epidemiology of Diabetes Complications Study. *Diabetes Care* 1993; 16: 1376–83.
28. Virdis R, Vanelli M, Street M, Zampolli M, De Fanti A, Cantoni S, et al. Blood pressure tracking in adolescents with insulin-dependent diabetes mellitus. *J Hum Hypertens* 1994; 8: 313–7.
29. Stephenson JM, Fuller JH, Viberti GC, Sjolie AK, Navalesi R. Blood pressure, retinopathy and urinary albumin excretion in IDDM: the EURODIAB IDDM Complications Study. *Diabetologia* 1995; 38: 599–603.
30. The United Kingdom Prospective Diabetes Study Group. Relative efficacy of randomly allocated diet, sulphonylurea, insulin, or metformin in patients with newly diagnosed non-insulin dependent diabetes followed for three years: UKPDS 13. *BMJ* 1995; 310: 83–8.
31. Baba T, Neugebauer S, Watanabe T. Diabetic nephropathy. Its relationship to hypertension and means of pharmacological intervention. *Drugs* 1997; 54: 197–234.
32. Christlieb AR, Krolewski AS, Warram JH, Soeldner JS. Is insulin the link between hypertension and obesity? *Hypertension* 1985; 7: II54–7.
33. Landsberg L. Diet, obesity and hypertension: an hypothesis involving insulin, the sympathetic nervous system, and adaptive thermogenesis. *Q J Med* 1986; 61: 1081–90.
34. Modan M, Halkin H, Almog S, Lusky A, Eshkol A, Shefi M, Shitrit A, Fuchs Z. Hyperinsulinemia: a link between hypertension obesity and glucose intolerance. *J Clin Invest* 1985; 75: 809–17.
35. Harris M. *Summary*. Washington, DC: National Institutes of Health, 1995. NIH Publication 95–1468.
36. Krolewski AS, Canessa M, Warram JH, Laffel LM, Christlieb AR, Knowler WC, et al. Predisposition to hypertension and susceptibility to renal disease in insulin-dependent diabetes mellitus. *N Engl J Med* 1988; 318: 140–5.
37. Yki-Jarvinen H, Koivisto VA. Natural course of insulin resistance in type I diabetes. *N Engl J Med* 1986; 315: 224–30.
38. Ferrannini E, Natali A. Essential hypertension, metabolic disorders, and insulin resistance. *Am Heart J* 1991; 121: 1274–82.
39. Ferrannini E, Haffner SM, Stern MP, Mitchell BD, Natali A, Hazuda HP, Patterson JK. High blood pressure and insulin resistance: influence of ethnic background. *Eur J Clin Invest* 1991; 21: 280–7.
40. Ferrannini E, Buzzigoli G, Bonadonna R, Giorico MA, Oleggini M, Graziadei L, Pedrinelli R, Brandi L, Bevilacqua S. Insulin resistance in essential hypertension. *N Engl J Med* 1987; 317: 350–7.
41. Falkner B, Hulman S, Tannenbaum J, Kushner H. Insulin resistance and blood pressure in young black men. *Hypertension* 1990; 16: 706–11.
42. Pollare T, Lithell H, Berne C. Insulin resistance is a characteristic feature of primary hypertension independent of obesity. *Metabolism* 1990; 39: 167–74.
43. Ohmori S, Kiyohara Y, Kato I, Ohmura T, Iwamoto H, Nakayama K, et al. Hyperinsulinaemia and blood pressure in a general Japanese population: the Hisayama Study. *J Hypertens* 1994; 12: 1191–7.
44. Boyko EJ, Leonetti DL, Bergstrom RW, Newell-Morris L, Fujimoto WY. Visceral adiposity, fasting plasma insulin, and blood pressure in Japanese-Americans. *Diabetes Care* 1995; 18: 174–81.
45. Cambien F, Warnet JM, Eschwege E, Jacqueson A, Richard JL, Rosselin G. Body mass, blood pressure, glucose, and lipids. Does plasma insulin explain their relationships? *Arteriosclerosis* 1987; 7: 197–202.
46. Asch S, Wingard DL, Barrett-Connor EL. Are insulin and hypertension independently related? *Ann Epidemiol* 1991; 1: 231–44.

47. Muller DC, Elahi D, Pratley RE, Tobin JD, Andres R. An epidemiological test of the hyperinsulinemia–hypertension hypothesis. *J Clin Endocrinol Metab* 1993; 76: 544–8.
48. Collins VR, Dowse GK, Finch CF, Zimmet PZ. An inconsistent relationship between insulin and blood pressure in three Pacific island populations. *J Clin Epidemiol* 1990; 43: 1369–78.
49. Saad MF, Lillioja S, Nyomba BL, Castillo C, Ferraro R, De Gregorio M, Ravussin E, Knowler WC, Bennett PH, Howard BV, Bogardus C. Racial differences in the relation between blood pressure and insulin resistance. *N Engl J Med* 1991; 324: 733–9.
50. Saad MF, Knowler WC, Pettitt DJ, Nelson RG, Mott DM, Bennett PH. Insulin and hypertension. Relationship to obesity and glucose intolerance in Pima Indians. *Diabetes* 1990; 39: 1430–5.
51. Zimmet PZ, Collins VR, Dowse GK, Alberti KG, Tuomilehto J, Knight LT, Gareeboo H, Chitson P, Fareed D, for the Mauritius Noncommunicable Disease Study Group. Is hyperinsulinaemia a central characteristic of a chronic cardiovascular risk factor clustering syndrome? Mixed findings in Asian Indian, Creole and Chinese Mauritians. *Diabet Med* 1994; 11: 388–96.
52. O'Brien T, Young WF Jr, Palumbo PJ, O'Brien PC, Service FJ. Hypertension and dyslipidemia in patients with insulinoma. *Mayo Clin Proc* 1993; 68: 141–6.
53. Pyorala K, Laakso M, Uusitupa M. Diabetes and atherosclerosis: an epidemiologic view. *Diabetes Metab Rev* 1987; 3: 463–524.
54. Weisser B, Grune S, Spuhler T, Kistler T, Vetter W. Plasma insulin is correlated with blood pressure only in subjects with a family history of hypertension or diabetes mellitus: results from 11,001 participants in the Heureka Study. *J Hypertens Suppl* 1993; 11 (suppl 5): S308–9.
55. Beatty OL, Harper R, Sheridan B, Atkinson AB, Bell PM. Insulin resistance in offspring of hypertensive parents. *BMJ* 1993; 307: 92–6.
56. Doria A, Fioretto P, Avogaro A, Carraro A, Morocutti A, Trevisan R, Frigato F, Crepaldi G, Viberti G, Nosadini R. Insulin resistance is associated with high sodium–lithium countertransport in essential hypertension. *Am J Physiol* 1991; 261: E684–91.
57. Anderson EA, Hoffman RP, Balon TW, Sinkey CA, Mark AL. Hyperinsulinemia produces both sympathetic neural activation and vasodilation in normal humans. *J Clin Invest* 1991; 87: 2246–52.
58. Saito F, Hori MT, Fittingoff M, Hino T, Tuck ML. Insulin attenuates agonist-mediated calcium mobilization in cultured rat vascular smooth muscle cells. *J Clin Invest* 1993; 92: 1161–7.
59. Eringa EC, Stehouwer CD, Merlijn T, Westerhof N, Sipkema P. Physiological concentrations of insulin induce endothelin-mediated vasoconstriction during inhibition of NOS or PI3-kinase in skeletal muscle arterioles. *Cardiovasc Res* 2002; 56: 464–71.
60. Anderson EA, Mark AL. The vasodilator action of insulin. Implications for the insulin hypothesis of hypertension. *Hypertension* 1993; 21: 136–41.
61. Baron AD, Brechtel-Hook G, Johnson A, Hardin D. Skeletal muscle blood flow. A possible link between insulin resistance and blood pressure. *Hypertension* 1993; 21: 129–35.
62. Jamerson KA, Julius S, Gudbrandsson T, Andersson O, Brant DO. Reflex sympathetic activation induces acute insulin resistance in the human forearm. *Hypertension* 1993; 21: 618–23.
63. Julius S. Corcoran Lecture. Sympathetic hyperactivity and coronary risk in hypertension. *Hypertension* 1993; 21: 886–93.
64. Arcaro G, Cretti A, Balzano S, Lechi A, Muggeo M, Bonora E, Bonadonna RC. Insulin causes endothelial dysfunction in humans: sites and mechanisms. *Circulation* 2002; 105: 576–82.
65. Laakso M, Edelman SV, Brechtel G, Baron AD. Decreased effect of insulin to stimulate skeletal muscle blood flow in obese man. A novel mechanism for insulin resistance. *J Clin Invest* 1990; 85: 1844–52.
66. Laakso M, Edelman SV, Brechtel G, Baron AD. Impaired insulin-mediated skeletal muscle blood flow in patients with NIDDM. *Diabetes* 1992; 41: 1076–83.
67. O'Hare JA, Minaker KL, Meneilly GS, Rowe JW, Pallotta JA, Young JB. Effect of insulin on plasma norepinephrine and 3,4-dihydroxyphenylalanine in obese men. *Metabolism* 1989; 38: 322–9.
68. Rocchini AP. Insulin resistance and blood pressure regulation in obese and nonobese subjects [Special lecture]. *Hypertension* 1991; 17: 837–42.
69. Anderson EA, Balon TW, Hoffman RP, Sinkey CA, Mark AL. Insulin increases sympathetic activity but not blood pressure in borderline hypertensive humans. *Hypertension* 1992; 19: 621–7.
70. Haffner SM, Stern MP, Hazuda HP, Mitchell BD, Patterson JK. Cardiovascular risk factors in confirmed prediabetic individuals. Does the clock for coronary heart disease start ticking before the onset of clinical diabetes? *JAMA* 1990; 263: 2893–8.
71. Haffner SM, Mykkanen L, Festa A, Burke JP, Stern MP. Insulin-resistant prediabetic subjects have more atherogenic risk factors than insulin-sensitive prediabetic subjects: implications for preventing coronary heart disease during the prediabetic state. *Circulation* 2000; 101: 975–80.
72. Feskens EJ, Tuomilehto J, Stengard JH, Pekkanen J, Nissinen A, Kromhout D. Hypertension and overweight associated with hyperinsulinemia and glucose tolerance: a longitudinal study of the Finnish and Dutch cohorts of the Seven Countries Study. *Diabetologia* 1995; 38: 839–47.
73. Giugliano D, Ceriello A, Paolisso G. Diabetes mellitus, hypertension, and cardiovascular disease: which role for oxidative stress? *Metabolism* 1995; 44: 363–8.
74. Ceriello A. The post-prandial state and cardiovascular disease: relevance to diabetes mellitus. *Diabetes Metab Res Rev* 2000; 16: 125–32.
75. Palmer RM, Ferrige AG, Moncada S. Nitric oxide release accounts for the biological activity of endothelium-derived relaxing factor. *Nature* 1987; 327: 524–6.
76. Tesfamariam B, Brown ML, Deykin D, Cohen RA. Elevated glucose promotes generation of endothelium-derived vasoconstrictor prostanoids in rabbit aorta. *J Clin Invest* 1990; 85: 929–32.
77. Gryglewski RJ, Palmer RM, Moncada S. Superoxide anion is involved in the breakdown of endothelium-derived vascular relaxing factor. *Nature* 1986; 320: 454–6.
78. Rubanyi GM, Vanhoutte PM. Oxygen-derived free radicals, endothelium, and responsiveness of vascular smooth muscle. *Am J Physiol* 1986; 250: H815–21.
79. Hunt JV, Dean RT, Wolff SP. Hydroxyl radical production and autoxidative glycosylation. Glucose autoxidation

as the cause of protein damage in the experimental glycation model of diabetes mellitus and ageing. *Biochem J* 1988; 256: 205–12.
80. Gillery P, Monboisse JC, Maquart FX, Borel JP. Glycation of proteins as a source of superoxide. *Diabete Metab* 1988; 14: 25–30.
81. Sakurai T, Tsuchiya S. Superoxide production from nonenzymatically glycated protein. *FEBS Lett* 1988; 236: 406–10.
82. Wohaieb SA, Godin DV. Alterations in free radical tissue-defense mechanisms in streptozocin-induced diabetes in rat. Effects of insulin treatment. *Diabetes* 1987; 36: 1014–8.
83. Wolff SP, Dean RT. Glucose autoxidation and protein modification. The potential role of "autoxidative glycosylation" in diabetes. *Biochem J* 1987; 245: 243–50.
84. Collier A, Wilson R, Bradley H, Thomson JA, Small M. Free radical activity in type 2 diabetes. *Diabet Med* 1990; 7: 27–30.
85. Ceriello A, Giugliano D, Quatraro A, Dello Russo P, Lefebvre PJ. Metabolic control may influence the increased superoxide generation in diabetic serum. *Diabet Med* 1991; 8: 540–2.
86. Ceriello A, Quatraro A, Caretta F, Varano R, Giugliano D. Evidence for a possible role of oxygen free radicals in the abnormal functional arterial vasomotion in insulin dependent diabetes. *Diabete Metab* 1990; 16: 318–22.
87. Ceriello A, Taboga C, Tonutti L, Quagliaro L, Piconi L, Bais B, Da Ros R, Motz E. Evidence for an independent and cumulative effect of postprandial hypertriglyceridemia and hyperglycemia on endothelial dysfunction and oxidative stress generation: effects of short- and long-term simvastatin treatment. *Circulation* 2002; 106: 1211–8.
88. Hassan MO, al Shafie OT, Johnston WJ. Loss of the nocturnal dip and increased variability of blood pressure in normotensive patients with noninsulin-dependent diabetes mellitus. *Clin Physiol* 1993; 13: 519–23.
89. Gilbert R, Phillips P, Clarke C, Jerums G. Day–night blood pressure variation in normotensive, normoalbuminuric type I diabetic subjects. Dippers and non-dippers. *Diabetes Care* 1994; 17: 824–7.
90. McKinlay S, Foster C, Clark A, Clark S, Kemp F, Denver E, et al. Increased blood pressure variability during 24 h blood pressure monitoring as an early sign of autonomic dysfunction in non-insulin-dependent diabetics. *J Hum Hypertens* 1994; 8: 887–90.
91. Verdecchia P, Schillaci G, Boldrini F, Guerrieri M, Porcellati C. Sex, cardiac hypertrophy and diurnal blood pressure variations in essential hypertension. *J Hypertens* 1992; 10: 683–92.
92. Palatini P, Penzo M, Racioppa A, Zugno E, Guzzardi G, Anaclerio M, Pessina AC. Clinical relevance of nighttime blood pressure and of daytime blood pressure variability. *Arch Intern Med* 1992; 152: 1855–60.
93. Rizzoni D, Muiesan ML, Montani G, Zulli R, Calebich S, Agabiti-Rosei E. Relationship between initial cardiovascular structural changes and daytime and nighttime blood pressure monitoring. *Am J Hypertens* 1992; 5: 180–6.
94. Cardillo C, De Felice F, Campia U, Folli G. Psychophysiological reactivity and cardiac end-organ changes in white coat hypertension. *Hypertension* 1993; 21: 836–44.
95. Shimada K, Kawamoto A, Matsubayashi K, Nishinaga M, Kimura S, Ozawa T. Diurnal blood pressure variations and silent cerebrovascular damage in elderly patients with hypertension. *J Hypertens* 1992; 10: 875–8.
96. O'Brien E, Sheridan J, O'Malley K. Dippers and non-dippers. *Lancet* 1988; 2: 397.
97. Verdecchia P, Porcellati C, Schillaci G, Borgioni C, Ciucci A, Battistelli M, Guerrieri M, Gatteschi C, Zampi I, Santucci A, Santucci C, Reboldi G. Ambulatory blood pressure. An independent predictor of prognosis in essential hypertension. *Hypertension* 1994; 24: 793–801.
98. Hansen KW, Poulsen PL, Christiansen JS, Mogensen CE. Determinants of 24-h blood pressure in IDDM patients. *Diabetes Care* 1995; 18: 529–35.
99. Bell DS. Stroke in the diabetic patient. *Diabetes Care* 1994; 17: 213–9.
100. Pyorala K. Diabetes and heart disease. In Mogensen C, Standl E (eds), *Prevention and Treatment of Diabetic Late Complications*. New York: Walter de Grutyer, 1989; pp 151–68.
101. van Hoeven KH, Factor SM. A comparison of the pathological spectrum of hypertensive, diabetic, and hypertensive-diabetic heart disease. *Circulation* 1990; 82: 848–55.
102. Yarom R, Zirkin H, Stammler G, Rose AG. Human coronary microvessels in diabetes and ischaemia. Morphometric study of autopsy material. *J Pathol* 1992; 166: 265–70.
103. Burchfiel CM, Reed DM, Marcus EB, Strong JP, Hayashi T. Association of diabetes mellitus with coronary atherosclerosis and myocardial lesions. An autopsy study from the Honolulu Heart Program. *Am J Epidemiol* 1993; 137: 1328–40.
104. Wingard DL, Barrett-Connor E. Heart disease and diabetes. In Harris MI, Cowie CC, Stern MP, Boyko EJ, Reiber GE, Bennett PH (eds), *Diabetes in America*, 2nd edn. Washington, DC: US Government Printing Office, 1995; pp 429–48.
105. Zdanov VS, Vihert AM. Atherosclerosis and diabetes mellitus. *Bull World Health Organ* 1976; 53: 547–53.
106. The Diabetes Drafting Group. Prevalence of small vessel and large vessel disease in diabetic patients from 14 centers. The World Health Organisation Multinational Study of Vascular Disease in Diabetics. *Diabetologia* 1985; 28 (suppl): 615–40.
107. Robertson WB, Strong JP. Atherosclerosis in persons with hypertension and diabetes mellitus. *Lab Invest* 1968; 18: 538–51.
108. Crall FV Jr, Roberts WC. The extramural and intramural coronary arteries in juvenile diabetes mellitus: analysis of nine necropsy patients aged 19 to 38 years with onset of diabetes before age 15 years. *Am J Med* 1978; 64: 221–30.
109. Valsania P, Zarich SW, Kowalchuk GJ, Kosinski E, Warram JH, Krolewski AS. Severity of coronary artery disease in young patients with insulin-dependent diabetes mellitus. *Am Heart J* 1991; 122: 695–700.
110. Natali A, Vichi S, Landi P, Severi S, L'Abbate A, Ferrannini E. Coronary atherosclerosis in Type II diabetes: angiographic findings and clinical outcome. *Diabetologia* 2000; 43: 632–41.
111. Stein B, Weintraub WS, Gebhart SP, Cohen-Bernstein CL, Grosswald R, Liberman HA, Douglas JS Jr, Morris DC, King SB 3rd. Influence of diabetes mellitus on early and late outcome after percutaneous transluminal coronary angioplasty. *Circulation* 1995; 91: 979–89.

112. Granger CB, Califf RM, Young S, Candela R, Samaha J, Worley S, Kereiakes DJ, Topol EJ, for The Thrombolysis and Angioplasty in Myocardial Infarction (TAMI) Study Group. Outcome of patients with diabetes mellitus and acute myocardial infarction treated with thrombolytic agents. *J Am Coll Cardiol* 1993; 21: 920–5.
113. Chan A, Beach KW, Martin DC, Strandness DE Jr. Carotid artery disease in NIDDM diabetes. *Diabetes Care* 1983; 6: 562–9.
114. Pujia A, Gnasso A, Irace C, Colonna A, Mattioli PL. Common carotid arterial wall thickness in NIDDM subjects. *Diabetes Care* 1994; 17: 1330–6.
115. Yamasaki Y, Kawamori R, Matsushima H, Nishizawa H, Kodama M, Kajimoto Y, et al. Atherosclerosis in carotid artery of young IDDM patients monitored by ultrasound high-resolution B-mode imaging. *Diabetes* 1994; 43: 634–9.
116. Salomaa V, Riley W, Kark JD, Nardo C, Folsom AR. Non-insulin-dependent diabetes mellitus and fasting glucose and insulin concentrations are associated with arterial stiffness indexes: the Atherosclerosis Risk in Communities (ARIC) Study. *Circulation* 1995; 91: 1432–43.
117. Haffner SM, Agostino RD Jr, Saad MF, O'Leary DH, Savage PJ, Rewers M, Selby J, Bergman RN, Mykkanen L. Carotid artery atherosclerosis in type-2 diabetic and non-diabetic subjects with and without symptomatic coronary artery disease (The Insulin Resistance Atherosclerosis Study). *Am J Cardiol* 2000; 85: 1395–400.
118. Temelkova-Kurktschiev TS, Koehler C, Leonhardt W, Schaper F, Henkel E, Siegert G, Hanefeld M. Increased intimal-medial thickness in newly detected type 2 diabetes: risk factors. *Diabetes Care* 1999; 22: 333–8.
119. Frost D, Frohlich B, Beischer W. Subclinical arteriosclerosis in patients with newly diagnosed type 2 diabetes mellitus. Demonstration by high-resolution ultrasound measurements of intima–media thickness of the common carotid and femoral arteries. *Dtsch Med Wochenschr* 2000; 125: 648–54.
120. Kingsbury KJ. The relation between glucose tolerance and atherosclerotic vascular disease. *Lancet* 1966; 2: 1374–9.
121. Janka HU, Standl E, Mehnert H. Peripheral vascular disease in diabetes mellitus and its relation to cardiovascular risk factors: screening with the doppler ultrasonic technique. *Diabetes Care* 1980; 3: 207–13.
122. Mozes G, Keresztury G, Kadar A, Magyar J, Sipos B, Dzsinich S, Gloviczki P. Atherosclerosis in amputated legs of patients with and without diabetes mellitus. *Int Angiol* 1998; 17: 282–6.
123. Jude EB, Oyibo SO, Chalmers N, Boulton AJ. Peripheral arterial disease in diabetic and non-diabetic patients: a comparison of severity and outcome. *Diabetes Care* 2001; 24: 1433–7.
124. Newman AB, Siscovick DS, Manolio TA, Polak J, Fried LP, Borhani NO, Wolfson SK, for the Cardiovascular Heart Study (CHS) Collaborative Research Group. Ankle–arm index as a marker of atherosclerosis in the Cardiovascular Health Study. *Circulation* 1993; 88: 837–45.
125. Abbott RD, Brand FN, Kannel WB. Epidemiology of some peripheral arterial findings in diabetic men and women: experiences from the Framingham Study. *Am J Med* 1990; 88: 376–81.
126. Meijer WT, Hoes AW, Rutgers D, Bots ML, Hofman A, Grobbee DE. Peripheral arterial disease in the elderly: the Rotterdam Study. *Arterioscler Thromb Vasc Biol* 1998; 18: 185–92.
127. Hiatt WR, Hoag S, Hamman RF. Effect of diagnostic criteria on the prevalence of peripheral arterial disease: the San Luis Valley Diabetes Study. *Circulation* 1995; 91: 1472–9.
128. Most RS, Sinnock P. The epidemiology of lower extremity amputations in diabetic individuals. *Diabetes Care* 1983; 6: 87–91.
129. Uusitupa MI, Niskanen LK, Siitonen O, Voutilainen E, Pyorala K. 5-year incidence of atherosclerotic vascular disease in relation to general risk factors, insulin level, and abnormalities in lipoprotein composition in non-insulin-dependent diabetic and non-diabetic subjects. *Circulation* 1990; 82: 27–36.
130. Kannel WB, McGee DL. Update on some epidemiologic features of intermittent claudication: the Framingham Study. *J Am Geriatr Soc* 1985; 33: 13–8.
131. Reiber GE, Boyko EJ, Smith DG. Lower extremity foot ulcers and amputations in diabetes. In Harris MI, Cowie CC, Stern MP, Boyko EJ, Reiber GE, Bennett PH (eds), *Diabetes in America*, 2nd edn. Washington, DC: US Government Printing Office, 1995; pp 409–28.
132. Mackaay AJ, Beks PJ, Dur AH, Bischoff M, Scholma J, Heine RJ, Rauwerda JA. The distribution of peripheral vascular disease in a Dutch Caucasian population: comparison of type II diabetic and non-diabetic subjects. *Eur J Vasc Endovasc Surg* 1995; 9: 170–5.
133. Fuller JH, Stevens LK, Wang SL. Risk factors for cardiovascular mortality and morbidity: the WHO Mutinational Study of Vascular Disease in Diabetes. *Diabetologia* 2001; 44 (suppl 2): S54–64.
134. Pell S, D'Alonzo CA. Factors associated with long-term survival of diabetics. *JAMA* 1970; 214: 1833–40.
135. Nesto RW, Phillips RT, Kett KG, Hill T, Perper E, Young E, Leland OS Jr. Angina and exertional myocardial ischemia in diabetic and non-diabetic patients: assessment by exercise thallium scintigraphy. *Ann Intern Med* 1988; 108: 170–5.
136. Wilson PW, Cupples LA, Kannel WB. Is hyperglycemia associated with cardiovascular disease? The Framingham Study. *Am Heart J* 1991; 121: 586–90.
137. Laws A, Marcus EB, Grove JS, Curb JD. Lipids and lipoproteins as risk factors for coronary heart disease in men with abnormal glucose tolerance: the Honolulu Heart Program. *J Intern Med* 1993; 234: 471–8.
138. Manson JE, Colditz GA, Stampfer MJ, Willett WC, Krolewski AS, Rosner B, Arky RA, Speizer FE, Hennekens CH. A prospective study of maturity-onset diabetes mellitus and risk of coronary heart disease and stroke in women. *Arch Intern Med* 1991; 151: 1141–7.
139. Wingard DL, Barrett-Connor EL, Ferrara A. Is insulin really a heart disease risk factor? *Diabetes Care* 1995; 18: 1299–304.
140. Uusitupa MI, Niskanen LK, Siitonen O, Voutilainen E, Pyorala K. Ten-year cardiovascular mortality in relation to risk factors and abnormalities in lipoprotein composition in type 2 (non-insulin-dependent) diabetic and non-diabetic subjects. *Diabetologia* 1993; 36: 1175–84.
141. Haffner SM, Lehto S, Ronnemaa T, Pyorala K, Laakso M. Mortality from coronary heart disease in subjects with type 2 diabetes and in non-diabetic subjects with and

without prior myocardial infarction. *N Engl J Med* 1998; 339: 229–34.

142. Expert Panel on Detection E, and Treatment of High Blood Cholesterol in Adults. Executive Summary of the Third Report of the National Cholesterol Education Program (NCEP) Expert Panel on Detection, Evaluation, and Treatment of High Blood Cholesterol in Adults (Adult Treatment Panel III). *JAMA* 2001; 285: 2486–97.
143. Deckert T, Poulsen JE, Larsen M. Prognosis of diabetics with diabetes onset before the age of thirty-one, I: survival, causes of death, and complications. *Diabetologia* 1978; 14: 363–70.
144. Deckert T, Poulsen JE, Larsen M. Prognosis of diabetics with diabetes onset before the age of thirty-one, II: factors influencing the prognosis. *Diabetologia* 1978; 14: 371–7.
145. Krolewski AS, Czyzyk A, Janeczko D, Kopczynski J. Mortality from cardiovascular diseases among diabetics. *Diabetologia* 1977; 13: 345–50.
146. Shenfield GM, Elton RA, Bhalla IP, Duncan LJ. Diabetic mortality in Edinburgh. *Diabete Metab* 1979; 5: 149–58.
147. Green A, Hougaard P. Epidemiological studies of diabetes mellitus in Denmark, 5: mortality and causes of death among insulin-treated diabetic patients. *Diabetologia* 1984; 26: 190–4.
148. Reunanen A. Mortality in type 2 diabetes. *Ann Clin Res* 1983; 15: 26–8.
149. Stengard JH, Tuomilehto J, Pekkanen J, Kivinen P, Kaarsalo E, Nissinen A, Karvonen MJ. Diabetes mellitus, impaired glucose tolerance and mortality among elderly men: the Finnish Cohorts of the Seven Countries Study. *Diabetologia* 1992; 35: 760–5.
150. The UK Prospective Diabetes Study (UKPDS) Group. Intensive blood-glucose control with sulphonylureas or insulin compared with conventional treatment and risk of complications in patients with type 2 diabetes (UKPDS 33). *Lancet* 1998; 352: 837–53.
151. Nesto R. CHD: a major burden in type 2 diabetes. *Acta Diabetol* 2001; 38: S3–8.
152. Rewers M, Shetterly SM, Baxter J, Marshall JA, Hamman RF. Prevalence of coronary heart disease in subjects with normal and impaired glucose tolerance and non-insulin-dependent diabetes mellitus in a biethnic Colorado population: the San Luis Valley Diabetes Study. *Am J Epidemiol* 1992; 135: 1321–30.
153. Howard BV, Cowan LD, Go O, Welty TK, Robbins DC, Lee ET. Adverse effects of diabetes on multiple cardiovascular disease risk factors in women: the Strong Heart Study. *Diabetes Care* 1998; 21: 1258–65.
154. Barrett-Connor EL, Cohn BA, Wingard DL, Edelstein SL. Why is diabetes mellitus a stronger risk factor for fatal ischemic heart disease in women than in men? The Rancho Bernardo Study. *JAMA* 1991; 265: 627–31.
155. Kleinman JC, Donahue RP, Harris MI, Finucane FF, Madans JH, Brock DB. Mortality among diabetics in a national sample. *Am J Epidemiol* 1988; 128: 389–401.
156. Head J, Fuller JH. International variations in mortality among diabetic patients: the WHO Multinational Study of Vascular Disease in Diabetics. *Diabetologia* 1990; 33: 477–81.
157. Moss SE, Klein R, Klein BE. Cause-specific mortality in a population-based study of diabetes. *Am J Public Health* 1991; 81: 1158–62.
158. Tuomilehto J, Borch-Johnsen K, Molarius A, Forsen T, Rastenyte D, Sarti C, Reunanen A. Incidence of cardiovascular disease in Type 1 (insulin-dependent) diabetic subjects with and without diabetic nephropathy in Finland. *Diabetologia* 1998; 41: 784–90.
159. Walden CE, Knopp RH, Wahl PW, Beach KW, Strandness E Jr. Sex differences in the effect of diabetes mellitus on lipoprotein triglyceride and cholesterol concentrations. *N Engl J Med* 1984; 311: 953–9.
160. Siegel RD, Cupples A, Schaefer EJ, Wilson PW. Lipoproteins, apolipoproteins, and low-density lipoprotein size among diabetics in the Framingham Offspring Study. *Metabolism* 1996; 45: 1267–72.
161. Steinberg HO, Paradisi G, Cronin J, Crowde K, Hempfling A, Hook G, Baron AD. Type II diabetes abrogates sex differences in endothelial function in premenopausal women. *Circulation* 2000; 101: 2040–6.
162. Resnick HE, Shorr RI, Kuller L, Franse L, Harris TB. Prevalence and clinical implications of American Diabetes Association-defined diabetes and other categories of glucose dysregulation in older adults: the health, aging and body composition study. *J Clin Epidemiol* 2001; 54: 869–76.
163. Abbott RD, Donahue RP, Kannel WB, Wilson PW. The impact of diabetes on survival following myocardial infarction in men vs women: the Framingham Study. *JAMA* 1988; 260: 3456–60.
164. Hu FB, Stampfer MJ, Solomon CG, Liu S, Willett WC, Speizer FE, Nathan DM, Manson JE. The impact of diabetes mellitus on mortality from all causes and coronary heart disease in women: 20 years of follow-up. *Arch Intern Med* 2001; 161: 1717–23.
165. Sex differences in the mortality associated with insulin-dependent diabetes mellitus in four countries: the Diabetes Epidemiology Research International (DERI) Study. *Am J Epidemiol* 1991; 133: 577–84.
166. Jarrett RJ, McCartney P, Keen H. The Bedford survey: ten year mortality rates in newly diagnosed diabetics, borderline diabetics and normoglycaemic controls and risk indices for coronary heart disease in borderline diabetics. *Diabetologia* 1982; 22: 79–84.
167. Fuller JH, Shipley MJ, Rose G, Jarrett RJ, Keen H. Mortality from coronary heart disease and stroke in relation to degree of glycaemia: the Whitehall Study. *BMJ* 1983; 287: 867–70.
168. Uusitupa M, Siitonen O, Aro A, Pyorala K. Prevalence of coronary heart disease, left ventricular failure and hypertension in middle-aged, newly diagnosed type 2 (non-insulin-dependent) diabetic subjects. *Diabetologia* 1985; 28: 22–7.
169. Li N, Tuomilehto J, Dowse G, Virtala E, Zimmet P. Prevalence of coronary heart disease indicated by electrocardiogram abnormalities and risk factors in developing countries. *J Clin Epidemiol* 1994; 47: 599–611.
170. Kannel WB, McGee DL. Diabetes and cardiovascular risk factors: the Framingham Study. *Circulation* 1979; 59: 8–13.
171. Pan WH, Cedres LB, Liu K, Dyer A, Schoenberger JA, Shekelle RB, Stamler R, Smith D, Collette P, Stamler J. Relationship of clinical diabetes and asymptomatic hyperglycemia to risk of coronary heart disease mortality in men and women. *Am J Epidemiol* 1986; 123: 504–16.
172. Stamler J, Vaccaro O, Neaton JD, Wentworth D. Diabetes, other risk factors, and 12-yr cardiovascular mortality for men screened in the Multiple Risk Factor Intervention Trial. *Diabetes Care* 1993; 16: 434–44.
173. Laakso M, Lehto S, Penttila I, Pyorala K. Lipids and lipoproteins predicting coronary heart disease mortality

and morbidity in patients with non-insulin-dependent diabetes. *Circulation* 1993; 88: 1421–30.

174. Janka HU, Ziegler AG, Standl E, Mehnert H. Daily insulin dose as a predictor of macrovascular disease in insulin treated non-insulin-dependent diabetics. *Diabete Metab* 1987; 13: 359–64.
175. Jarrett RJ, Shipley MJ. Type 2 (non-insulin-dependent) diabetes mellitus and cardiovascular disease—putative association via common antecedents: further evidence from the Whitehall Study. *Diabetologia* 1988; 31: 737–40.
176. Fontbonne A, Charles MA, Thibult N, Richard JL, Claude JR, Warnet JM, Rosselin GE, Eschwege E. Hyperinsulinaemia as a predictor of coronary heart disease mortality in a healthy population: the Paris Prospective Study, 15-year follow-up. *Diabetologia* 1991; 34: 356–61.
177. Sasaki A, Horiuchi N, Hasegawa K, Uehara M. Mortality and causes of death in type 2 diabetic patients. A long-term follow-up study in Osaka District, Japan. *Diabetes Res Clin Pract* 1989; 7: 33–40.
178. Nelson RG, Sievers ML, Knowler WC, Swinburn BA, Pettitt DJ, Saad MF, Liebow IM, Howard BV, Bennett PH. Low incidence of fatal coronary heart disease in Pima Indians despite high prevalence of non-insulin-dependent diabetes. *Circulation* 1990; 81: 987–95.
179. Sprafka JM, Burke GL, Folsom AR, McGovern PG, Hahn LP. Trends in prevalence of diabetes mellitus in patients with myocardial infarction and effect of diabetes on survival: the Minnesota Heart Survey. *Diabetes Care* 1991; 14: 537–43.
180. Cooper RS, Pacold IV, Ford ES. Age-related differences in case-fatality rates among diabetic patients with myocardial infarction. Findings from National Hospital Discharge Survey, 1979–1987. *Diabetes Care* 1991; 14: 903–8.
181. Barbash GI, White HD, Modan M, Van de Werf F, for the Investigators of the International Tissue Plasminogen Activator/Streptokinase Mortality Trial. Significance of diabetes mellitus in patients with acute myocardial infarction receiving thrombolytic therapy. *J Am Coll Cardiol* 1993; 22: 707–13.
182. Karlson BW, Herlitz J, Hjalmarson A. Prognosis of acute myocardial infarction in diabetic and non-diabetic patients. *Diabet Med* 1993; 10: 449–54.
183. Zuanetti G, Latini R, Maggioni AP, Santoro L, Franzosi MG. Influence of diabetes on mortality in acute myocardial infarction: data from the GISSI-2 study. *J Am Coll Cardiol* 1993; 22: 1788–94.
184. Lehto S, Pyorala K, Miettinen H, Ronnemaa T, Palomaki P, Tuomilehto J, Laakso M. Myocardial infarct size and mortality in patients with non-insulin-dependent diabetes mellitus. *J Intern Med* 1994; 236: 291–7.
185. Miettinen H, Lehto S, Salomaa V, Mahonen M, Niemela M, Haffner SM, Pyorala K, Tuomilehto J, for The FINMONICA Myocardial Infarction Register Study Group. Impact of diabetes on mortality after the first myocardial infarction. *Diabetes Care* 1998; 21: 69–75.
186. Kjaergaard SC, Hansen HH, Fog L, Bulow I, Christensen PD. In-hospital outcome for diabetic patients with acute myocardial infarction in the thrombolytic era. *Scand Cardiovasc J* 1999; 33: 166–70.
187. Malmberg K, Yusuf S, Gerstein HC, Brown J, Zhao F, Hunt D, Piegas L, Calvin J, Keltai M, Budaj A. Impact of diabetes on long-term prognosis in patients with unstable angina and non-Q-wave myocardial infarction: results of the OASIS (Organization to Assess Strategies for Ischemic Syndromes) Registry. *Circulation* 2000; 102: 1014–9.
188. Shindler DM, Palmeri ST, Antonelli TA, Sleeper LA, Boland J, Cocke TP, Hochman JS. Diabetes mellitus in cardiogenic shock complicating acute myocardial infarction: a report from the SHOCK Trial Registry. Should we emergently revascularize occluded coronaries for cardiogenic shock? *J Am Coll Cardiol* 2000; 36: 1097–103.
189. Jacoby RM, Nesto RW. Acute myocardial infarction in the diabetic patient: pathophysiology, clinical course and prognosis. *J Am Coll Cardiol* 1992; 20: 736–44.
190. Singer DE, Moulton AW, Nathan DM. Diabetic myocardial infarction. Interaction of diabetes with other preinfarction risk factors. *Diabetes* 1989; 38: 350–7.
191. Malmberg K, Ryden L. Myocardial infarction in patients with diabetes mellitus. *Eur Heart J* 1988; 9: 259–64.
192. Hu FB, Stampfer MJ, Solomon CG, Liu S, Willett WC, Speizer FE, Nathan DM, Manson JE. The impact of diabetes mellitus on mortality from all causes and coronary heart disease in women: 20 years of follow-up. *Arch Intern Med* 2001; 161: 1717–23.
193. Cho E, Rimm EB, Stampfer MJ, Willett WC, Hu FB. The impact of diabetes mellitus and prior myocardial infarction on mortality from all causes and from coronary heart disease in men. *J Am Coll Cardiol* 2002; 40: 954–60.
194. Wingard DL, Barrett-Connor E, Criqui MH, Suarez L. Clustering of heart disease risk factors in diabetic compared to non-diabetic adults. *Am J Epidemiol* 1983; 117: 19–26.
195. Abu-Lebdeh HS, Hodge DO, Nguyen TT. Predictors of macrovascular disease in patients with type 2 diabetes mellitus. *Mayo Clin Proc* 2001; 76: 707–12.
196. Syvanne M, Pajunen P, Kahri J, Lahdenpera S, Ehnholm C, Nieminen MS, Taskinen MR. Determinants of the severity and extent of coronary artery disease in patients with type-2 diabetes and in non-diabetic subjects. *Coron Artery Dis* 2001; 12: 99–106.
197. Fontbonne A, Thibult N, Eschwege E, Ducimetiere P. Body fat distribution and coronary heart disease mortality in subjects with impaired glucose tolerance or diabetes mellitus: the Paris Prospective Study, 15-year follow-up. *Diabetologia* 1992; 35: 464–8.
198. West KM, Ahuja MM, Bennett PH, Czyzyk A, De Acosta OM, Fuller JH, Grab B, Grabauskas V, Jarrett RJ, Kosaka K, Keen H, Krolewski AS, Miki E, Schliack V, Teuscher A, Watkins PJ, Stober JA. The role of circulating glucose and triglyceride concentrations and their interactions with other "risk factors" as determinants of arterial disease in nine diabetic population samples from the WHO multinational study. *Diabetes Care* 1983; 6: 361–9.
199. Garg A, Grundy SM. Management of dyslipidemia in NIDDM. *Diabetes Care* 1990; 13: 153–69.
200. Sniderman AD, Scantlebury T, Cianflone K. Hypertriglyceridemic hyperapob: the unappreciated atherogenic dyslipoproteinemia in type 2 diabetes mellitus. *Ann Intern Med* 2001; 135: 447–59.
201. Rubins HB, Robins SJ, Collins D, Iranmanesh A, Wilt TJ, Mann D, Mayo-Smith M, Faas FH, Elam MB, Rutan GH, Anderson JW, Kashyap ML, Schectman G, for the Department of Veterans Affairs HDL Intervention Trial Study Group. Distribution of lipids in 8,500 men with coronary artery disease. *Am J Cardiol* 1995; 75: 1196–201.

202. Karpe F, Taskinen MR, Nieminen MS, Frick MH, Kesaniemi YA, Pasternack A, Hamsten A, Syvanne M. Remnant-like lipoprotein particle cholesterol concentration and progression of coronary and vein-graft atherosclerosis in response to gemfibrozil treatment. *Atherosclerosis* 2001; 157: 181–7.
203. Karpe F, Boquist S, Tang R, Bond GM, de Faire U, Hamsten A. Remnant lipoproteins are related to intima–media thickness of the carotid artery independently of LDL cholesterol and plasma triglycerides. *J Lipid Res* 2001; 42: 17–21.
204. Erkelens DW. Insulin resistance syndrome and type 2 diabetes mellitus. *Am J Cardiol* 2001; 88: 38J–42J.
205. Kannel WB, Cupples LA, Ramaswami R, Stokes J III, Kreger BE, Higgins M. Regional obesity and risk of cardiovascular disease: the Framingham Study. *J Clin Epidemiol* 1991; 44: 183–90.
206. Larsson B, Bengtsson C, Bjorntorp P, Lapidus L, Sjostrom L, Svardsudd K, Tibblin G, Wedel H, Welin L, Wilhelmsen L. Is abdominal body fat distribution a major explanation for the sex difference in the incidence of myocardial infarction? The study of men born in 1913 and the study of women, Goteborg, Sweden. *Am J Epidemiol* 1992; 135: 266–73.
207. Ohlson LO, Larsson B, Svardsudd K, Welin L, Eriksson H, Wilhelmsen L, Bjorntorp P, Tibblin G. The influence of body fat distribution on the incidence of diabetes mellitus. 13.5 years of follow-up of the participants in the study of men born in 1913. *Diabetes* 1985; 34: 1055–8.
208. Kaye SA, Folsom AR, Sprafka JM, Prineas RJ, Wallace RB. Increased incidence of diabetes mellitus in relation to abdominal adiposity in older women. *J Clin Epidemiol* 1991; 44: 329–34.
209. Dowse GK, Zimmet PZ, Gareeboo H, George K, Alberti MM, Tuomilehto J, Finch CF, Chitson P, Tulsidas H. Abdominal obesity and physical inactivity as risk factors for NIDDM and impaired glucose tolerance in Indian, Creole, and Chinese Mauritians. *Diabetes Care* 1991; 14: 271–82.
210. Björntorp P. "Portal" adipose tissue as a generator of risk factors for cardiovascular disease and diabetes. *Arteriosclerosis* 1990; 10: 493–6.
211. Nikkila EA, Miettinen TA, Vesenne MR, Pelkonen R. Plasma-insulin in coronary heart-disease: response to oral and intravenous glucose and to tolbutamide. *Lancet* 1965; 2: 508–11.
212. Stout RW, Vallance-Owen J. Insulin and atheroma. *Lancet* 1969; 1: 1078–80.
213. Stout RW. Insulin and atheroma. 20-yr perspective. *Diabetes Care* 1990; 13: 631–54.
214. Collins VR, Dowse GK, Zimmet PZ, Tuomilehto J, Alberti KG, Gareeboo H, Nan L. Serum insulin and ECG abnormalities suggesting coronary heart disease in the populations of Mauritius and Nauru: cross-sectional and longitudinal associations. *J Clin Epidemiol* 1993; 46: 1373–93.
215. Tuomilehto J, Zimmet P, Kankaanpaa J, Wolf E, Hunt D, King H, Ram P. Prevalence of ischaemic ECG abnormalities according to the diabetes status in the population of Fiji and their associations with other risk factors. *Diabetes Res Clin Pract* 1988; 5: 205–17.
216. Sicree RA, Tuomilehto J, Zimmet P, King H, Ram P, Hunt D, Coventry J. Electrocardiographic abnormalities amongst Melanesian and Indian men of Fiji: prevalence and associated factors. *Int J Cardiol* 1988; 19: 27–38.
217. Jackson L, Whitehouse S, Zimmet P, Sloman G. Electrocardiographic findings in a partly urbanised Polynesian population: the Funafuti Survey. *N Z Med J* 1980; 91: 210–2.
218. Orchard TJ, Eichner J, Kuller LH, Becker DJ, McCallum LM, Grandits GA. Insulin as a predictor of coronary heart disease: interaction with apolipoprotein E phenotype. A report from the Multiple Risk Factor Intervention Trial. *Ann Epidemiol* 1994; 4: 40–5.
219. Mattock MB, Keen H, Viberti GC, el-Gohari MR, Murrells TJ, Scott GS, Wing JR, Jackson PG. Coronary heart disease and urinary albumin excretion rate in type 2 (non-insulin-dependent) diabetic patients. *Diabetologia* 1988; 31: 82–7.
220. Neil A, Hawkins M, Potok M, Thorogood M, Cohen D, Mann J. A prospective population-based study of microalbuminuria as a predictor of mortality in NIDDM. *Diabetes Care* 1993; 16: 996–1003.
221. Bennett PH, Lee ET, Lu M, Keen H, Fuller JH. Increased urinary albumin excretion and its associations in the WHO Multinational Study of Vascular Disease in Diabetes. *Diabetologia* 2001; 44 (suppl 2): S37–45.
222. Nielsen FS, Voldsgaard AI, Gall MA, Rossing P, Hommel E, Andersen P, Dyerberg J, Parving HH. Apolipoprotein(a) and cardiovascular disease in type 2 (non-insulin-dependent) diabetic patients with and without diabetic nephropathy. *Diabetologia* 1993; 36: 438–44.
223. Kuusisto J, Mykkanen L, Pyorala K, Laakso M. Hyperinsulinemic microalbuminuria. A new risk indicator for coronary heart disease. *Circulation* 1995; 91: 831–7.
224. Krolewski AS, Kosinski EJ, Warram JH, Leland OS, Busick EJ, Asmal AC, Rand LI, Christlieb AR, Bradley RF, Kahn CR. Magnitude and determinants of coronary artery disease in juvenile-onset, insulin-dependent diabetes mellitus. *Am J Cardiol* 1987; 59: 750–5.
225. Jensen T, Borch-Johnsen K, Kofoed-Enevoldsen A, Deckert T. Coronary heart disease in young type 1 (insulin-dependent) diabetic patients with and without diabetic nephropathy: incidence and risk factors. *Diabetologia* 1987; 30: 144–8.
226. Juhan-Vague I, Alessi MC, Morange PE. Hypofibrinolysis and increased PAI-1 are linked to atherothrombosis via insulin resistance and obesity. *Ann Med* 2000; 32 (suppl 1): 78–84.
227. Meigs JB, Mittleman MA, Nathan DM, Tofler GH, Singer DE, Murphy-Sheehy PM, Lipinska I, D'Agostino RB, Wilson PW. Hyperinsulinemia, hyperglycemia, and impaired hemostasis: the Framingham Offspring Study. *JAMA* 2000; 283: 221–8.
228. Saito I, Folsom AR, Brancati FL, Duncan BB, Chambless LE, McGovern PG. Nontraditional risk factors for coronary heart disease incidence among persons with diabetes: the Atherosclerosis Risk in Communities (ARIC) Study. *Ann Intern Med* 2000; 133: 81–91.
229. Ridker PM, Stampfer MJ, Rifai N. Novel risk factors for systemic atherosclerosis: a comparison of C-reactive protein, fibrinogen, homocysteine, lipoprotein(a), and standard cholesterol screening as predictors of peripheral arterial disease. *JAMA* 2001; 285: 2481–5.
230. Cambien F, Poirier O, Lecerf L, Evans A, Cambou JP, Arveiler D, Luc G, Bard JM, Bara L, Ricard S, Tiret L, Amoyel P, Alhenc-Gelas F, Soubrier F. Deletion polymorphism in the gene for angiotensin-converting enzyme

is a potent risk factor for myocardial infarction. *Nature* 1992; 359: 641–4.

231. Hallab M, Berrut G, Bouhanick B, Bled F, Suraniti S, Girault A, Fressinaud P, Marre M. Increase of activity of angiotensin-converting enzyme in insulin-dependent diabetic patients with permanent microalbuminuria. *Arch Mal Coeur Vaiss* 1992; 85: 1185–8.
232. Ruiz J, Blanche H, Cohen N, Velho G, Cambien F, Cohen D, Passa P, Froguel P. Insertion/deletion polymorphism of the angiotensin-converting enzyme gene is strongly associated with coronary heart disease in non-insulin-dependent diabetes mellitus. *Proc Natl Acad Sci USA* 1994; 91: 3662–5.
233. Tarnow L, Cambien F, Rossing P, Nielsen FS, Hansen BV, Lecerf L, Poirier O, Danilov S, Boelskifte S, Borch-Johnsen K. Insertion/deletion polymorphism in the angiotensin-I-converting enzyme gene is associated with coronary heart disease in IDDM patients with diabetic nephropathy. *Diabetologia* 1995; 38: 798–803.
234. Lehto S, Ronnemaa T, Pyorala K, Laakso M. Predictors of stroke in middle-aged patients with non-insulin-dependent diabetes. *Stroke* 1996; 27: 63–8.
235. Garcia MJ, McNamara PM, Gordon T, Kannel WB. Morbidity and mortality in diabetics in the Framingham population. Sixteen year follow-up study. *Diabetes* 1974; 23: 105–11.
236. Wolf PA, D'Agostino RB, Belanger AJ, Kannel WB. Probability of stroke: a risk profile from the Framingham Study. *Stroke* 1991; 22: 312–8.
237. Rodriguez BL, D'Agostino R, Abbott RD, Kagan A, Burchfiel CM, Yano K, Ross GW, Silbershatz H, Higgins MW, Popper J, Wolf PA, Curb JD. Risk of hospitalized stroke in men enrolled in the Honolulu Heart Program and the Framingham Study: a comparison of incidence and risk factor effects. *Stroke* 2002; 33: 230–6.
238. Yusuf HR, Giles WH, Croft JB, Anda RF, Casper ML. Impact of multiple risk factor profiles on determining cardiovascular disease risk. *Prev Med* 1998; 27: 1–9.
239. Kittner SJ, White LR, Losonczy KG, Wolf PA, Hebel JR. Black–white differences in stroke incidence in a national sample. The contribution of hypertension and diabetes mellitus. *JAMA* 1990; 264: 1267–70.
240. Barrett-Connor E, Khaw KT. Diabetes mellitus: an independent risk factor for stroke? *Am J Epidemiol* 1988; 128: 116–23.
241. Tuomilehto J, Rastenyte D, Jousilahti P, Sarti C, Vartiainen E. Diabetes mellitus as a risk factor for death from stroke. Prospective study of the middle-aged Finnish population. *Stroke* 1996; 27: 210–5.
242. Kuller L, Anderson H, Peterson D, Cassel J, Spiers P, Curry H, Paegel B, Saslaw M, Winkelstein W Jr, Lilienfeld A, Seltser R. Nationwide cerebrovascular disease morbidity study. *Stroke* 1970; 1: 86–99.
243. Report of the Joint Committee for Stroke Facilities, I: epidemiology for stroke facilities planning. *Stroke* 1972; 3: 359–71.
244. Lavy S, Melamed E, Cahane E, Carmon A. Hypertension and diabetes as risk factors in stroke patients. *Stroke* 1973; 4: 751–9.
245. Ostfeld AM, Shekelle RB, Klawans H, Tufo HM. Epidemiology of stroke in an elderly welfare population. *Am J Public Health* 1974; 64: 450–8.
246. Kagan A, Popper JS, Rhoads GG. Factors related to stroke incidence in Hawaii Japanese men: the Honolulu Heart Study. *Stroke* 1980; 11: 14–21.
247. Herman B, Leyten AC, van Luijk JH, Frenken CW, Op de Coul AA, Schulte BP. Epidemiology of stroke in Tilburg, the Netherlands. The population-based stroke incidence register, 2: incidence, initial clinical picture and medical care, and three-week case fatality. *Stroke* 1982; 13: 629–34.
248. Wolf PA, Kannel WB, Verter J. Current status of risk factors for stroke. *Neurol Clin* 1983; 1: 317–43.
249. Roehmholdt ME, Palumbo PJ, Whisnant JP, Elveback LR. Transient ischemic attack and stroke in a community-based diabetic cohort. *Mayo Clin Proc* 1983; 58: 56–8.
250. Barker W, Feldt KS, Feibel JH. Community surveillance of stroke in persons under 70 years old: contribution of uncontrolled hypertension. *Am J Public Health* 1983; 73: 260–265.
251. Hadden WC, Harris MI. Prevalence of diagnosed diabetes, undiagnosed diabetes, and impaired glucose tolerance in adults 20–74 years of age. *Vital Health Stat* 1987 11: 1–55.
252. Lindegard B, Hillbom M. Associations between brain infarction, diabetes and alcoholism: observations from the Gothenburg population cohort study. *Acta Neurol Scand* 1987; 75: 195–200.
253. Neaton JD, Wentworth DN, Cutler J, Stamler J, Kuller L, for the Multiple Risk Factor Intervention Trial Research Group. Risk factors for death from different types of stroke. *Ann Epidemiol* 1993; 3: 493–9.
254. Haheim LL, Holme I, Hjermann I, Leren P. Nonfasting serum glucose and the risk of fatal stroke in diabetic and non-diabetic subjects: 18-year follow-up of the Oslo Study. *Stroke* 1995; 26: 774–7.
255. Stegmayr B, Asplund K. Diabetes as a risk factor for stroke. A population perspective. *Diabetologia* 1995; 38: 1061–8.
256. Adams HP Jr, Putman SF, Kassell NF, Torner JC. Prevalence of diabetes mellitus among patients with subarachnoid hemorrhage. *Arch Neurol* 1984; 41: 1033–5.
257. Qureshi AI, Suarez JI, Parekh PD, Sung G, Geocadin R, Bhardwaj A, Tamargo RJ, Ulatowski JA. Risk factors for multiple intracranial aneurysms. *Neurosurgery* 1998; 43: 22–7.
258. Mohr JP, Caplan LR, Melski JW, Goldstein RJ, Duncan GW, Kistler JP, Pessin MS, Bleich HL. The Harvard Cooperative Stroke Registry: a prospective registry. *Neurology* 1978; 28: 754–62.
259. Ayala C, Croft JB, Greenlund KJ, Keenan NL, Donehoo RS, Malarcher AM, Mensah GA. Sex differences in US mortality rates for stroke and stroke subtypes by race/ethnicity and age, 1995–1998. *Stroke* 2002; 33: 1197–201.
260. Abbott RD, Donahue RP, MacMahon SW, Reed DM, Yano K. Diabetes and the risk of stroke: the Honolulu Heart Program. *JAMA* 1987; 257: 949–52.
261. Burchfiel CM, Curb JD, Rodriguez BL, Abbott RD, Chiu D, Yano K. Glucose intolerance and 22- year stroke incidence: the Honolulu Heart Program. *Stroke* 1994; 25: 951–7.
262. Longstreth WT Jr, Dulberg C, Manolio TA, Lewis MR, Beauchamp NJ Jr, O'Leary D, Carr J, Furberg CD. Incidence, manifestations, and predictors of brain infarcts defined by serial cranial magnetic resonance imaging in the elderly: the Cardiovascular Health Study. *Stroke* 2002; 33: 2376–82.

263. Vermeer SE, Koudstaal PJ, Oudkerk M, Hofman A, Breteler MM. Prevalence and risk factors of silent brain infarcts in the population-based Rotterdam Scan Study. *Stroke* 2002; 33: 21–5.
264. Simpson RK Jr, Contant CF, Fischer DK, Cech DA, Robertson CS, Narayan RK. The influence of diabetes mellitus on outcome from subarachnoid hemorrhage. *Diabetes Res* 1991; 16: 165–9.
265. Hu HH, Chu FL, Chiang BN, Lan CF, Sheng WY, Lo YK, Wong WJ, Luk YO. Prevalence of stroke in Taiwan. *Stroke* 1989; 20: 858–63.
266. Oppenheimer SM, Hoffbrand BI, Oswald GA, Yudkin JS. Diabetes mellitus and early mortality from stroke. *BMJ* 1985; 291: 1014–5.
267. Kushner M, Nencini P, Reivich M, Rango M, Jamieson D, Fazekas F, Zimmerman R, Chawluk J, Alavi A, Alves W. Relation of hyperglycemia early in ischemic brain infarction to cerebral anatomy, metabolism, and clinical outcome. *Ann Neurol* 1990; 28: 129–35.
268. Kiers L, Davis SM, Larkins R, Hopper J, Tress B, Rossiter SC, Carlin J, Ratnaike S. Stroke topography and outcome in relation to hyperglycemia and diabetes. *J Neurol Neurosurg Psychiatry* 1992; 55: 263–70.
269. Toni D, Sacchetti ML, Argentino C, Gentile M, Cavalletti C, Frontoni M, Fieschi C. Does hyperglycemia play a role on the outcome of acute ischaemic stroke patients? *J Neurol* 1992; 239: 382–6.
270. Tuhrim S, Dambrosia JM, Price TR, Mohr JP, Wolf PA, Hier DB, Kase CS. Intracerebral hemorrhage: external validation and extension of a model for prediction of 30-day survival. *Ann Neurol* 1991; 29: 658–63.
271. Lukovits TG, Mazzone TM, Gorelick TM. Diabetes mellitus and cerebrovascular disease. *Neuroepidemiology* 1999; 18: 1–14.
272. Kissela BM, Sauerbeck L, Woo D, Khoury J, Carrozzella J, Pancioli A, Jauch E, Moomaw CJ, Shukla R, Gebel J, Fontaine R, Broderick J. Subarachnoid hemorrhage: a preventable disease with a heritable component. *Stroke* 2002; 33: 1321–6.
273. Sarti C, Tuomilehto J, Salomaa V, Sivenius J, Kaarsalo E, Narva EV, Salmi K, Torppa J. Epidemiology of subarachnoid hemorrhage in Finland from 1983 to 1985. *Stroke* 1991; 22: 848–53.
274. Tuomilehto J, Rastenyte D, Sivenius J, Sarti C, Immonen-Raiha P, Kaarsalo E, Kuulasmaa K, Narva EV, Salomaa V, Salmi K, Torppa J. Ten- year trends in stroke incidence and mortality in the FINMONICA Stroke Study. *Stroke* 1996; 27: 825–32.
275. Fuller JH, Stevens LK, Wang SL. International variations in cardiovascular mortality associated with diabetes mellitus: the WHO Multinational Study of Vascular Disease in Diabetes. *Ann Med* 1996; 28: 319–22.
276. Kuusisto J, Mykkanen L, Pyorala K, Laakso M. Non-insulin-dependent diabetes and its metabolic control are important predictors of stroke in elderly subjects. *Stroke* 1994; 25: 1157–64.
277. Kim JS, Sunwoo IN. Risk factors of ischemic brain stroke in Korean diabetic patients—a retrospective study. *Yonsei Med J* 1989; 30: 288–93.
278. Sievers ML, Nelson RG, Knowler WC, Bennett PH. Impact of NIDDM on mortality and causes of death in Pima Indians. *Diabetes Care* 1992; 15: 1541–9.
279. Longstreth WT Jr, Bernick C, Manolio TA, Bryan N, Jungreis CA, Price TR. Lacunar infarcts defined by magnetic resonance imaging of 3660 elderly people: the Cardiovascular Health Study. *Arch Neurol* 1998; 55: 1217–25.
280. Arboix A, Padilla I, Massons J, Garcia-Eroles L, Comes E, Targa C. Clinical study of 222 patients with pure motor stroke. *J Neurol Neurosurg Psychiatry* 2001; 71: 239–42.
281. Boiten J, Lodder J, Kessels F. Two clinically distinct lacunar infarct entities? A hypothesis. *Stroke* 1993; 24: 652–6.
282. Mast H, Thompson JL, Lee SH, Mohr JP, Sacco RL. Hypertension and diabetes mellitus as determinants of multiple lacunar infarcts. *Stroke* 1995; 26: 30–3.
283. Arboix A, Garcia-Eroles L, Massons J, Oliveres M, Targa C. Hemorrhagic lacunar stroke. *Cerebrovasc Dis* 2000; 10: 229–34.
284. The UK Prospective Diabetes Study Group. Tight blood pressure control and risk of macrovascular and microvascular complications in type 2 diabetes: UKPDS 38. *BMJ* 1998; 317: 703–13.
285. Sprafka JM, Bender AP, Jagger HG. Prevalence of hypertension and associated risk factors among diabetic individuals: the Three-City Study.. *Diabetes Care* 1988; 11: 17–22.
286. Yudkin JS. Factors influencing threshold and choice of treatment for hypertension in NIDDM. Cardiovascular factors. *Diabetes Care* 1991; 14 (suppl 4): 27–32.
287. Reaven PD, Barrett-Connor EL, Browner DK. Abnormal glucose tolerance and hypertension. *Diabetes Care* 1990; 13: 119–25.
288. Haffner SM, Valdez R, Morales PA, Mitchell BD, Hazuda HP, Stern MP. Greater effect of glycemia on incidence of hypertension in women than in men. *Diabetes Care* 1992; 15: 1277–84.
289. Chukwuma C Sr, Tuomilehto J. Diabetes and the risk of stroke. *J Diabetes Complications* 1993; 7: 250–62.
290. Sacco RL, Wolf PA, Gorelick PB. Risk factors and their management for stroke prevention: outlook for 1999 and beyond. *Neurology* 1999; 53: (7): S15–24.
291. Fabris F, Zanocchi M, Bo M, Fonte G, Fiandra U, Poli L. Risk factors for atherosclerosis and aging. *Int Angiol* 1994; 13: 52–8.
292. de Falco FA, Sepe Visconti O, Fucci G, Caruso G. Correlation between hyperglycemia and cerebral infarct size in patients with stroke. A clinical and X-ray computed tomography study in 104 patients. *Schweiz Arch Neurol Psychiatr* 1993; 144: 233–9.
293. Vannucci SJ, Willing LB, Goto S, Alkayed NJ, Brucklacher RM, Wood TL, Towfighi J, Hurn PD, Simpson IA. Experimental stroke in the female diabetic, *db/db*, mouse. *J Cereb Blood Flow Metab* 2001; 21: 52–60.
294. Asplund K, Hagg E, Helmers C, Lithner F, Strand T, Wester PO. The natural history of stroke in diabetic patients. *Acta Med Scand* 1980; 207: 417–24.
295. Power MJ, Fullerton KJ, Stout RW. Blood glucose and prognosis of acute stroke. *Age Ageing* 1988; 17: 164–70.
296. Woo E, Ma JT, Robinson JD, Yu YL. Hyperglycemia is a stress response in acute stroke. *Stroke* 1988; 19: 1359–64.
297. Woo J, Lam CW, Kay R, Wong AH, Teoh R, Nicholls MG. The influence of hyperglycemia and diabetes mellitus on immediate and 3-month morbidity and mortality after acute stroke. *Arch Neurol* 1990; 47: 1174–7.
298. Matchar DB, Divine GW, Heyman A, Feussner JR. The influence of hyperglycemia on outcome of cerebral infarction. *Ann Intern Med* 1992; 117: 449–56.

299. Gray CS, French JM, Bates D, Cartlidge NE, Venables GS, James OF. Increasing age, diabetes mellitus and recovery from stroke. *Postgrad Med J* 1989; 65: 720–4.
300. Murros K, Fogelholm R, Kettunen S, Vuorela AL, Valve J. Blood glucose, glycosylated haemoglobin, and outcome of ischemic brain infarction. *J Neurol Sci* 1992; 111: 59–64.
301. Cambon H, Derouesne C, Yelnik A, Duyckaerts C, Hauw JJ. Effect of diabetes mellitus and blood glucose on the size of cerebral infarction and causes of death. Neuropathological study of 77 cases of infarction in the sylvian artery area. *Rev Neurol* 1991; 147: 727–34.
302. McCall AL. The impact of diabetes on the CNS. *Diabetes* 1992; 41: 557–70.
303. Wannamethee SG, Shaper AG, Perry IJ, Alberti KG. Alcohol consumption and the incidence of type II diabetes. *J Epidemiol Community Health* 2002; 56: 542–8.
304. Cucchiara BL, Kasner SE. Atherosclerotic risk factors in patients with ischemic cerebrovascular disease. *Curr Treat Options Neurol* 2002; 4: 445–53.
305. Ibrahim HA, Vora JP. Diabetic nephropathy. *Baillieres Best Pract Res Clin Endocrinol Metab* 1999; 13: 239–64.
306. Keane WF. Metabolic pathogenesis of cardiorenal disease. *Am J Kidney Dis* 2001; 38: 1372–5.
307. Klein R, Sharrett AR, Klein BE, Moss SE, Folsom AR, Wong TY, Brancati FL, Hubbard LD, Couper D, ARIC Group. The association of atherosclerosis, vascular risk factors, and retinopathy in adults with diabetes: the Atherosclerosis-Risk in-Communities Study. *Ophthalmology* 2002; 109: 1225–34.
308. Petitti DB, Bhatt H. Retinopathy as a risk factor for nonembolic stroke in diabetic subjects. *Stroke* 1995; 26: 593–6.
309. Asymptomatic hyperglycemia and coronary heart disease. A series of papers by the International Collaborative Group, based on studies in fifteen populations. *J Chronic Dis* 1979; 32: 681–837.
310. Epstein FH. Hyperglycaemia as a risk factor for coronary heart disease. *Monogr Atheroscler* 1985; 13: 92–7.
311. The National Diabetes Data Group. Classification and diagnosis of diabetes mellitus and other categories of glucose intolerance. *Diabetes* 1979; 28: 1039–57.
312. WHO Expert Committee. WHO Expert Committee on Diabetes Mellitus: second report. *World Health Organ Tech Rep Ser* 1980; 646: 1–80.
313. Diabetes mellitus. Report of a WHO Study Group. *World Health Organ Tech Rep Ser* 1985; 727: 1–113.
314. Coutinho M, Gerstein HC, Wang Y, Yusuf S. The relationship between glucose and incident cardiovascular events. A metaregression analysis of published data from 20 studies of 95,783 individuals followed for 12.4 years. *Diabetes Care* 1999; 22: 233–40.
315. Balkau B, Bertrais S, Ducimetiere P, Eschwege E. Is there a glycemic threshold for mortality risk? *Diabetes Care* 1999; 22: 696–9.
316. Bjornholt JV, Erikssen G, Aaser E, Sandvik L, Nitter-Hauge S, Jervell J, Erikssen J, Thaulow E. Fasting blood glucose: an underestimated risk factor for cardiovascular death. Results from a 22-year follow-up of healthy non-diabetic men. *Diabetes Care* 1999; 22: 45–9.
317. Simons LA, Friedlander Y, McCallum J, Simons J. Fasting plasma glucose in non-diabetic elderly women predicts increased all-causes mortality and coronary heart disease risk. *Aust N Z J Med* 2000; 30: 41–7.
318. Lowe LP, Liu K, Greenland P, Metzger BE, Dyer AR, Stamler J. Diabetes, asymptomatic hyperglycemia, and 22-year mortality in black and white men. The Chicago Heart Association Detection Project in Industry Study. *Diabetes Care* 1997; 20: 163–9.
319. Rodriguez BL, Lau N, Burchfiel CM, Abbott RD, Sharp DS, Yano K, Curb JD. Glucose intolerance and 23-year risk of coronary heart disease and total mortality: the Honolulu Heart Program. *Diabetes Care* 1999; 22: 1262–5.
320. Fujishima M, Kiyohara Y, Kato I, Ohmura T, Iwamoto H, Nakayama K, Ohmori S, Yoshitake T. Diabetes and Cardiovascular Disease in a Prospective Population Survey in Japan. The Hisayama Study. *Diabetes* 1996; 45 (suppl): S14–6.
321. Tominaga M, Eguchi H, Manaka H, Igarashi K, Kato T, Sekikawa A. Impaired glucose tolerance is a risk factor for cardiovascular disease, but not impaired fasting glucose: the Funagata Diabetes Study. *Diabetes Care* 1999; 22: 920–4.
322. de Vegt F, Dekker JM, Ruhe HG, Stehouwer CD, Nijpels G, Bouter LM, Heine RJ. Hyperglycaemia is associated with all-cause and cardiovascular mortality in the Hoorn population: the Hoorn Study. *Diabetologia* 1999; 42: 926–31.
323. Shaw JE, Boyko EJ, Courten de M, Zimmet PZ. Impact of new diagnostic criteria for diabetes on different populations. *Diabetes Care* 1999; 22: 762–6.
324. Barrett-Connor E, Ferrara A. Isolated postchallenge hyperglycemia and the risk of fatal cardiovascular disease in older women and men: the Rancho Bernardo Study. *Diabetes Care* 1998; 21: 1236–9.
325. Saydah SH, Miret M, Sung J, Varas C, Gause D, Brancati FL. Postchallenge hyperglycemia and mortality in a national sample of US adults. *Diabetes Care* 2001; 24: 1397–402.
326. Hu FB, Stampfer MJ, Haffner SM, Solomon CG, Willett WC, Manson JE. Elevated risk of cardiovascular disease prior to clinical diagnosis of type 2 Diabetes. *Diabetes Care* 2002; 25: 1129–34.
327. The DECODE Study Group. Glucose tolerance and cardiovascular mortality: comparison of fasting and 2- hour diagnostic criteria. *Arch Intern Med* 2001; 161: 397–405.
328. The DECODE Study Group. Glucose tolerance and mortality: comparison of WHO and American Diabetes Association diagnostic criteria. *Lancet* 1999; 354: 617–21.
329. Qiao Q, Pyorala K, Pyorala M, Nissinen A, Lindstrom J, Tilvis R, Tuomilehto J. Two-hour glucose is a better risk predictor for incident coronary heart disease and cardiovascular mortality than fasting glucose. *Eur Heart J* 2002; 23: 1267–75.
330. Heine RJ, Dekker JM. Beyond postprandial hyperglycemia: metabolic factors associated with cardiovascular disease. *Diabetologia* 2002; 45: 461–75.
331. Yudkin JS. Post-load hyperglycemia—an inappropriate therapeutic target. *Lancet* 2002; 359: 166–7.
332. Hanefeld M, Koehler C, Schaper F, Fuecker K, Henkel E, Temelkova-Kurktschiev T. Postprandial plasma glucose is an independent risk factor for increased carotid intima–media thickness in non-diabetic individuals. *Atherosclerosis* 1999; 144: 229–35.
333. Temelkova-Kurktschiev TS, Koehler C, Henkel E, Leonhardt W, Fuecker K, Hanefeld M. Postchallenge

plasma glucose and glycemic spikes are more strongly associated with atherosclerosis than fasting glucose or HbA_{1c} level. *Diabetes Care* 2000; 23: 1830–4.

334. Resnick HE, Harris MI, Brock DB, Harris TB. American diabetes association diabetes diagnostic criteria, advancing age, and cardiovascular disease risk profiles. Results from the Third National Health and Nutrition Examination Survey. *Diabetes Care* 2000; 23: 176–80.

335. The DECODE Study Group. Age- and sex-specific prevalences of diabetes and impaired glucose regulation in 13 European cohorts. *Diabetes Care* 2003; 26: 61–9.

336. Zimmet P. Epidemiology of diabetes and its macrovascular manifestations in Pacific populations: the medical effects of social progress. *Diabetes Care* 1979; 2: 144–53.

76

Effect of Intensive Glycemic Control on Macrovascular Events in Patients with Diabetes Mellitus

Abdulaziz R. Al-Harthi and William H. Herman

University of Michigan, Ann Arbor, MI, USA

Diabetes mellitus is associated with an increased risk of cardiovascular disease. In general, the relative risk of cardiovascular disease is two- to fourfold higher in people with diabetes than in those without diabetes [1]. In one study, the incidence of myocardial infarction was as high in diabetic adults without previous myocardial infarction as it was in nondiabetic adults with previous myocardial infarction [2]. In people with diabetes, cardiovascular disease appears earlier in life, affects women almost as often as men, and is more often fatal [3]. After an acute myocardial infarction, people with diabetes have an increased risk of re-infarction, congestive heart failure, and death [4]. When people with diabetes develop a cerebrovascular accident (CVA), they are at increased risk of recurrent CVA, CVA-related dementia, and death [5–7]. Similarly, when peripheral vascular disease occurs in people with diabetes, it is more likely to be symptomatic and associated with complications [8]. In general, approximately 65% of people with diabetes die from cardiovascular disease. Although cardiovascular mortality has declined in recent decades in individuals without diabetes, it has declined more slowly in men with diabetes and has increased in women with diabetes [3].

The increased prevalence of conventional risk factors for cardiovascular disease (hypertension, dyslipidemia, and in young persons with diabetes, cigarette smoking) contributes in part to the increased risk of cardiovascular disease in people with diabetes. Yet not all of the risk can be explained on the basis of these risk factors [9]. Other risk factors associated with diabetes may also contribute. These include insulin resistance, tissue glycation, oxidative stress, chronic inflammation, endothelial dysfunction, thrombosis, and renal disease [10]. Although hyperglycemia has been associated with cardiovascular disease in cross-sectional and observational studies, the impact of aggressive blood glucose control on cardiovascular disease in diabetes is less clear.

HYPERGLYCEMIA AND MACROVASCULAR DISEASE IN THE GENERAL POPULATION

An association between glucose and cardiovascular disease exists at levels below those used to define diabetes. The Norfolk cohort of the European Prospective Investigation of Cancer and Nutrition (EPIC-Norfolk) demonstrated that hemoglobin A_{1c} (HbA_{1c}) was continuously related to all-cause, cardiovascular, and ischemic heart disease mortality through the whole population distribution. A 1% increase in HbA_{1c} was associated with a 28% ($p < 0.002$) increase in risk of death in men independent of age, blood pressure, serum cholesterol, body mass index, and cigarette smoking. This effect remained [relative risk (RR) 1.46, $p = 0.05$ adjusted for age and risk factors] after men with known diabetes, $HbA_{1c} \geq 7\%$, or history of myocardial infarction or stroke were excluded. The lowest rates of cardiovascular mortality occurred in men with HbA_{1c} concentrations $< 5\%$, and 82% of the population excess mortality risk associated with HbA_{1c} occurred in men

International Textbook of Diabetes Mellitus, Third Edition. Edited by R. A. DeFronzo, E. Ferrannini, H. Keen, and P. Zimmet.
 ISBN: 0-471-48655-8.

with HbA_{1c} concentrations of 5–6.9% [11]. A recent meta-analysis of 20 studies including nearly 96 000 nondiabetic individuals showed that cardiovascular events increased by one-third as the fasting glucose level increased from 4.2 to 6.1 mmol/l and by nearly two-thirds when the 2-h glucose level was ≥7.8 mmol/l [12]. Many of the studies included in the meta-analysis showed a significant association between glucose levels and cardiovascular disease even after adjustment for other cardiovascular risk factors (age, weight, blood pressure, lipids, smoking, and insulin levels). Thus, there is a graded relationship between glucose levels and cardiovascular risk. While it might appear that glucose is a continuous cardiovascular risk factor, like blood pressure or serum cholesterol, it is not yet clear that glucose is an independent risk factor rather than merely a risk marker [13,14]. The best proof of cause would be to demonstrate that in randomized controlled clinical trials, lower glucose levels reduce risk.

GLYCEMIC CONTROL AND MACROVASCULAR DISEASE IN TYPE 1 DIABETES

A number of clinical trials have reported the impact of intensive glycemic control on cardiovascular outcomes and survival in type 1 diabetes. Unfortunately, none of the trials was designed to assess the impact of therapy on macrovascular disease, and the youth of the subjects and the relative shortness of follow-up made the detection of treatment-related differences in macrovascular events unlikely. For this reason, most analyses have reported surrogate endpoints. A cross-sectional analysis of the Stockholm Diabetes Intervention Study (SDIS) demonstrated an association between HbA_{1c}, stiffness of the carotid wall, and endothelial dysfunction in type 1 diabetic subjects [15]. In contrast, the Epidemiology of Diabetes Interventions and Complications (EDIC) study [16], a large multicenter observational follow-up of the Diabetes Control and Complications Trial (DCCT) cohort [17], demonstrated that prior intensive therapy and HbA_{1c} levels measured during the DCCT or at the time of the ultrasound, about 18 months after the end of the DCCT, were not associated with carotid intima-media wall thickness. Conventional cardiovascular risk factors, including older age, hypertension, high low-density lipoprotein (LDL) cholesterol levels, and smoking, and duration of diabetes were significantly associated with carotid intima-media wall thickness. In addition, there was no significant difference in the mean intima-media wall thickness between the EDIC subjects and age- and sex-matched control subjects, except for internal carotid intima-media thickness among men.

Recently, Lawson and colleagues critically reviewed the randomized, controlled, clinical trials to estimate the impact of intensive insulin therapy on the risk of developing cardiovascular, cerebrovascular, and peripheral vascular disease events and macrovascular death in type 1 diabetes [18]. The initial search identified 30 studies, but only 6 studies met all inclusion criteria. These studies are described in Table 1. Intensive insulin therapy significantly reduced the total number of first major macrovascular events (OR = 0.55, 95% CI 0.35–0.88, $p = 0.015$) (Figure 1). In 3 of the studies, subjects had more than one type of event (e.g. cardiovascular, cerebrovascular, peripheral vascular, and macrovascular death). When events within the same class (for example, angina and myocardial infarction) were counted only once, the results became nonsignificant. Although there was a trend toward a decrease in the number of subjects having one or more macrovascular events with intensive insulin therapy, the difference between intensive insulin therapy and conventional therapy was not statistically significant (OR = 0.72, 95% CI 0.44–1.17, $p = 0.22$).

Prospective observational studies have suggested an association between hyperglycemia and mortality in type 1 diabetes. In the Wisconsin Epidemiologic Study of Diabetic Retinopathy (WESDR), after a median follow-up of 10 years, the hazard ratio for mortality from ischemic heart disease in younger-onset (<30 years of age) insulin-treated diabetic subjects for a 1-percentage-point change in glycosylated hemoglobin was 1.18 (95% CI 1.00–1.40) [24]. Glycosylated hemoglobin was also significantly associated with all-cause mortality in younger-onset insulin-treated subjects ($p < 0.005$). Ten-year survival in the first quartile of glycosylated hemoglobin was 96.3% compared to 93.0% in the fourth quartile. After correcting for age and sex, the hazard ratio of dying for the fourth relative to the first quartile was 1.9 (95% CI not reported).

To the extent that intensive insulin therapy prevents the development and delays the progression of diabetic nephropathy [17], and to the extent that diabetic kidney disease is associated with excess mortality in type 1 diabetes [25], intensive therapy might be associated with improved survival. Indeed, a computer simulation model developed by the DCCT Research Group to assess the long-term benefits and costs of intensive therapy suggested that intensive therapy might be associated with a 5.1-year increase in survival compared to conventional therapy [26]. This intriguing hypothesis must, however, be tested empirically. In the meta-analysis by Lawson and colleagues, rates of macrovascular mortality were not different between intensive insulin therapy and conventional therapy (OR = 0.91, 95% CI 0.31–2.65, $p = 0.93$).

In summary, studies of surrogate markers have yielded conflicting results as to the impact of glycemic control on atherosclerosis in type 1 diabetes. Although observational studies have suggested an association, a meta-analysis of prospective randomized controlled clinical trials demonstrated that intensive insulin therapy significantly decreased the total number of macrovascular events but

Table 1 Effect of intensive glycemic control on macrovascular events in type 1 diabetes*

Study [reference]	Number of participants	Age at entry (years)	Duration of type 1 diabetes (years)	Study duration (years)	ΔHbA_{1c} (%)	Number of first MVD events		Number of patients with ≥1 MVD event		Number of deaths attributed to MVD	
						IIT	CT	IIT	CT	IIT	CT
Holman et al. [19]	74	42 ± 12	18.6 ± 6.1	2	0.9	0	3	0	3	0	1
Steno 1 [20]	34	34 ± 7	19.0 ± 3.0	8	0.5	1	0	1	0	0	0
Steno 2 [20]	36	18 – 50	5 – 26	5	0.9	0	2	0	2	0	1
Oslo Norway [21]	45	26 ± 5	12.8 ± 3.6	7	1.2	0	0	0	0	0	0
Stockholm [22]	102	31 ± 8	17.0 ± 5.0	8	1.4	3	5	3	3	2	2
DCCT [23]	Primary: 726 Secondary: 715	27 ± 8 27 ± 7	2.6 ± 1.4 8.8 ± 3.8	7	1.9	23	40	22	30	2	1
Common OR (95% CI)						0.55 (0.350–0.88)		0.72 (0.44–1.17)		0.91 (0.31–2.65)	

Note. Data for age at entry and diabetes duration are means ± SD or ranges. Study duration includes intervention and follow-up. MVD: macrovascular disease; IIT: intensive insulin therapy; CT: conventional therapy.

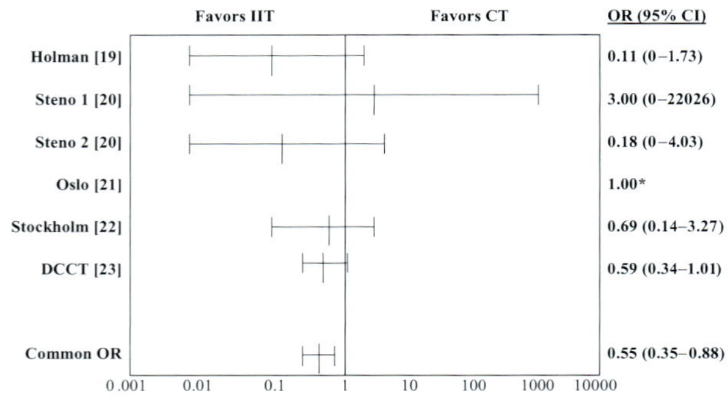

Figure 1 Effect of intensive glycemic control on number of macrovascular events in type 1 diabetes. IIT: intensive insulin therapy; CT: conventional therapy. *Accurate determination of CI not possible due to zero-event rate in both groups. (Copyright © 1999, American Diabetes Association from Diabetes Care, Vol 22, Suppl. 2, 1999; B35–B39. Reprinted with permission from the American Diabetes Association) [18]

had no significant effect on the number of subjects with type 1 diabetes developing macrovascular disease and had no impact on mortality. Given the proven beneficial effects of intensive glycemic control on microvascular complications, future trials of intensive therapy are not likely to be conducted in patients with type 1 diabetes. Thus, the relationship between glycemia and macrovascular disease in type 1 diabetes may never be more definitely answered.

GLYCEMIC CONTROL AND MACROVASCULAR DISEASE IN TYPE 2 DIABETES

Table 2 summarizes the major trials of glycemic control in type 2 diabetes and the impact of improved glycemic control on cardiovascular disease.

The University Group Diabetes Program (UGDP) reported no benefit of variable insulin therapy relative to placebo therapy on cardiovascular outcomes [29, 30]. Because of inadequate randomization, poor patient compliance, and the lack of both self-monitoring of blood glucose and HbA_{1c} measurements to objectively assess glycemic control, the results from this study are difficult to interpret.

The Veterans Administration Cooperative Study on Glycemic Control and Complications in Type 2 Diabetes (VACSDM) reported a higher rate of cardiovascular events in the intensively treated group but the difference was not statistically significant (32% in the intensive therapy vs. 21% in the conventional therapy group, $p < 0.10$) [31–33].

The Kumamoto study involved 110 nonobese type 2 diabetic patients. There were only four (7.2%) cardiovascular events in the intensive therapy group versus seven (12.7%) in the conventional therapy group. This difference in this relatively small population was not statistically significant [34].

The United Kingdom Prospective Diabetes Study (UKPDS) involved 3867 subjects with newly diagnosed type 2 diabetes mellitus. It demonstrated a 16% reduction in myocardial infarctions in the intensive therapy group compared to the conventional therapy group after 10 years of follow-up [35]. The effect was of borderline statistical significance (95% CI 0–29, $p = 0.052$). In a UKPDS substudy, 342 obese patients treated with metformin were compared to 411 diet-controlled obese patients and 951 obese patients treated with insulin or sulfonlyurea [36]. Compared to diet therapy, metformin resulted in a 39% reduction in the incidence of myocardial infarction ($p = 0.010$), a 30% reduction in all cardiovascular events ($p = 0.020$), and a 42% reduction in diabetes-related death ($p = 0.017$) (Figure 2). Both metformin and insulin/sulfonylurea treated groups achieved comparable levels of glycemic control, but metformin resulted in a 32% reduction in any diabetes-related endpoints ($p = 0.003$), a 41% reduction in the incidence of stroke ($p = 0.032$), and a 36% decrease in all-cause mortality ($p = 0.021$). The epidemiological analysis of glucose and diabetes-related complications in the UKPDS showed that a 1% difference in HbA_{1c} was associated with a significant difference in the risk of myocardial infarction, heart failure, stroke, and amputation [39] (Figure 3 and Table 3).

In the Diabetes Mellitus Insulin Glucose Infusion in Acute Myocardial Infarction (DIGAMI) study, 620 patients with diabetes and acute myocardial infarction were randomized to treatment with insulin-glucose infusion followed by a minimum of 3 months of multiple daily injections of insulin or to conventional therapy [37, 38]. The inhospital mortality was 9.1% in the insulin-glucose infusion group versus11.1% in the control group (p value = not significant). However, the mortality rate at 3 months, 1 year, and 3 years was significantly lower in insulin-glucose infusion group with relative risk reductions of 52, 30, and 25% respectively. At the end of follow-up (mean 3.4 years), the difference in cardiovascular mortality between the two groups was still significant (RRR 28%, 95% CI 8–45, $p = 0.011$).

The meta-analysis of the five clinical trials discussed above showed that intensive glycemic control compared to conventional therapy reduced the rate of nonfatal myocardial infarction and coronary death (15/1000 person-years versus 18/1000 person-years) [27]. However, this reduction in incidence was not statistically significant (RR = 0.87, 95% CI 0.74–1.01; person-years needed to treat 419, CI 197–∞).

A number of ongoing clinical trials may provide more definitive answers as to the impact of intensive glycemic control on cardiovascular outcomes in persons with type 2 diabetes. In the Veterans Administration Diabetes Trial (VADT), 1700 older patients with type 2 diabetes who have failed diet, exercise, and maximum dose of one or more oral antidiabetic agents will be treated with either metformin (obese patients) or glimepiride (nonobese patients) in combination with rosiglitazone and with insulin

Table 2 Effect of intensive glycemic control on macrovascular events in type 2 diabetes*

Study [reference]	Number of participants	Mean age (years)	Duration of type 2 diabetes (years)	Study History of CAD (%)	Intensive therapy	Conventional therapy	Follow-up (years)	ΔHbA_{1c} (%)	Cardiovascular events (%)		
									IT	CT	p
UGDP [29, 30]	619	53	≤1	4	Variable insulin	Placebo	13	NA	21	20	NS
VACSDM [31–33]	153	60	8	19	Ins/glipizide	Insulin	2	2.1	32	21	NS
Kumamoto [34]	110	50	9	0	MDI[c]	Twice daily insulin	8	2.2	7	13	NS
UKPDS [35, 36]											
Main arm	3867	53	≤1	0	Insulin/SU	Diet/SU/insulin	10	0.9	21	23	NS
Obese arm	1704	53	≤1	0	Insulin/SU (951 patients)	Diet (411 patients)	11	0.6	22	26	NS
					Metformin (342 patients)	Diet (411 patients)	11	0.6	17	26	<0.02
DIGAMI [37, 38]	620	68	NA	100	Insulin-glucose infusion and MDI for ≥3 months	Usual ICU care	3	0.3	33	44	0.011
Common OR (95% CI)										0.91 (0.78–1.05)	

Note. CAD: coronary artery disease; Ins: insulin; MDI: multiple daily injection; SU: sulfonylurea; IT: intensive therapy; CT: conventional therapy; NA: not available; NS: not significant; Cardiovascular events defined as: fatal and nonfatal MI in UGDP; fatal and nonfatal MI, angina, CHF, CABG, PTCA, TIA, CVA, and PVD, in VACSDM; MI, angina, CVA, and intermittent claudication in Kumamoto study; MI, CVA, and PVD in UKPDS; and cardiovascular mortality in DIGAMI.

*(Reprinted from American Journal of Medicine, 111, 633–542, © 2001 with permission from Excerpta Medica Inc. [27, 28]).

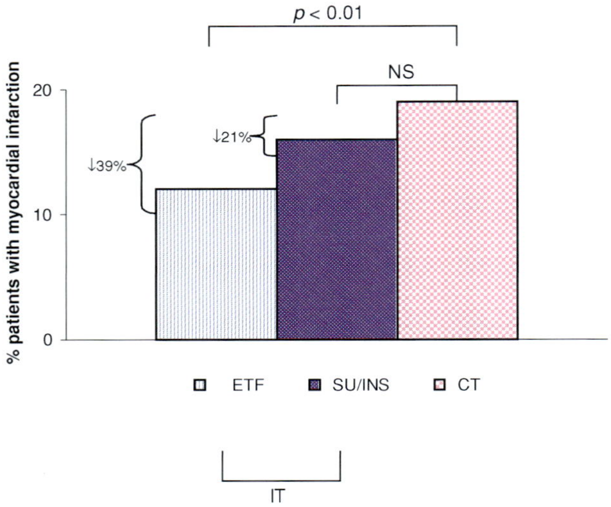

Figure 2 Effect of intensive glycemic control on the incidence of myocardial infarction in obese patients with type 2 diabetes in the UKPDS. Despite the comparable glycemic control between the sulfonylurea/insulin and metformin arms, only metformin led to a significant 39% reduction in myocardial infarction ($p < 0.01$) [36]. NS: not significant; CT: conventional therapy (diet); IT: intensive therapy (metformin, sulfonylurea, insulin). (With permission from the BMJ Publishing Group)

as needed [40]. Both the intensive therapy and the conventional therapy arms will be treated with the same agents but with different intensities. The target HbA_{1c} will be 6.5% in the intensive arm and 8.5% in the conventional arm. Multiple daily insulin injections and insulin glargine will be used in the intensive therapy arm versus Neutral Protamine Hagedorn (NPH) insulin in the conventional therapy arm. Cardiovascular risk factors will be treated aggressively in both arms. The primary outcome is timely to major cardiovascular events (myocardial infarction, stroke, heart failure, amputation, cardiovascular intervention, and cardiovascular death). Secondary outcomes will include angina,

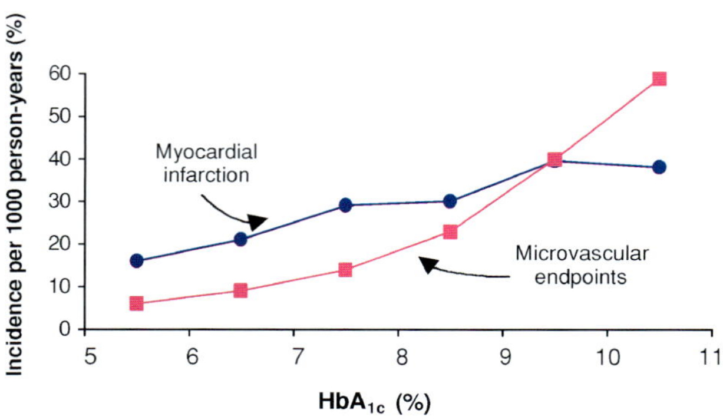

Figure 3 Incidence of myocardial infarction and microvascular complications in relation to HbA_{1c} in the UKPDS [39]. (Reprinted with permission from Elsevier, The Lancet, Vol 352, 1998, 854–865)

Table 3 Epidemiological data on influence of 1% change in HbA_{1c} on risk of macrovascular complications in the UKPDS*

Complication	Decrease in risk per 1% HbA_{1c} reduction	*p* value
Myocardial infarction	14%	<0.0001
Heart failure	16%	0.021
Amputation or death from peripheral vascular disease	43%	<0.0001
Stroke	12%	0.035

*(With permission from the BMJ Publishing Group [39]).

transient ischemic attack, intermittent claudication, critical limb ischemia, and total mortality.

The Action to Control Cardiovascular Risk in Diabetes (ACCORD) is a multicenter 3 × 2 factorial randomized clinical trial designed to determine the impact of intensive control of glycemia, blood pressure, and lipids and insulin resistance lowering therapy on major cardiovascular events in type 2 diabetic subjects (www.clinicaltrials.gov). A total of 5000 patients will be randomized to one of three glycemic treatment strategies on one axis and two lipid and blood pressure control strategies on the other axis. Glycemic control strategies include (1) conventional glycemic control with non-insulin resistance lowering drugs (sulfonylureas or meglitinides ± insulin) with a target HbA_{1c} of 7–8%; (2) intensive glycemic control with non-insulin resistance lowering drugs with a target HbA_{1c} of 6–6.5%; or (3) intensive glycemic control with insulin resistance lowering drugs (biguanides or thiazolidinediones with or without α-glucosidase inhibitors and insulin) with a target HbA_{1c} of 6–6.5%. Subjects will also be randomized to either conventional blood pressure and lipid control treatment strategies (with target systolic BP < 130 mmHg and LDL cholesterol < 3.4 mmol/l, or < 2.6 mmol/l in persons with clinical cardiovascular disease) or intensive blood pressure and lipid control treatment strategies (with target systolic BP < 120 mmHg, and LDL cholesterol < 2.6 mmol/l, or < 1.9 mmol/l in persons with clinical cardiovascular disease). The primary outcome will be major cardiovascular disease event rates defined as myocardial infarction, stroke, or death attributed to cardiovascular disease. Secondary outcomes will include total mortality, myocardial infarction, stroke, heart failure, amputation, retinopathy, albuminuria, renal function, peripheral neuropathy, quality of life, and cost-effectiveness.

The Bypass Angioplasty Revascularization Investigation in Type 2 Diabetes (BARI 2D) is a multicenter 2 × 2 factorial randomized clinical trial designed to determine the best therapy for established cardiovascular disease in patients with type 2 diabetes (www.clinicaltrials.gov). The effect of initial elective coronary revascularization with aggressive medical therapy is compared with aggressive medical therapy alone. Whether the strategy of glucose control affects the prognosis of these patients will also be determined. Approximately 2600 patients will be randomized to (1) surgical or balloon revascularization plus best medical therapy for cardiac disease, plus insulin-sensitizing drugs (metformin or rosiglitazone); (2) surgical or balloon revascularization plus best medical therapy for cardiac disease, plus insulin-providing drugs (insulin or sulfonylureas); (3) best medical therapy for cardiac disease, plus insulin-sensitizing drugs; or (4) best medical therapy for cardiac disease, plus insulin-providing drugs. Cardiovascular disease risk factors will be treated aggressively in all participants. The target HbA_{1c} will be 7.5%. The primary outcome will be all-cause mortality. Secondary outcomes will include cardiac mortality, myocardial infarction, angina, and quality of life.

In summary, the weight of evidence from recent large clinical trials demonstrates no adverse effect and indeed support a small beneficial effect of intensive glycemic control on macrovascular complications in patients with type 2 diabetes. In obese patients with newly diagnosed type 2 diabetes, metformin therapy appears superior to sulfonylureas or insulin. The relative benefits of other specific therapeutic classes will require further study.

CONCLUSIONS

In the nondiabetic population, higher levels of glucose and HbA_{1c} are associated with an increased risk of cardiovascular disease. In patients with diabetes, cardiovascular disease is common and represents the major cause of morbidity and mortality. These data suggest that glucose may be a continuous cardiovascular risk factor, similar to blood pressure and serum cholesterol. While there is strong evidence that intensive glycemic control reduces the risk of microvascular complications in patients with diabetes, its impact on cardiovascular disease is less clear. Meta-analyses of trials in both type 1 and type 2 diabetes have generally failed to demonstrate a statistically significant impact of intensive glycemic control on cardiovascular events. Unfortunately, none of the trials included in the meta-analyses was designed to assess the impact of treatment on cardiovascular disease. It is possible that if the differences in HbA_{1c} levels between treatment groups had been greater, the trials had been larger, and the follow-up had been longer, the trials might have demonstrated cardiovascular benefit. It is also possible that they might not have demonstrated cardiovascular benefit. Although hyperglycemia is clearly associated with cardiovascular disease, hyperglycemia itself may not cause cardiovascular disease. The association between hyperglycemia and features of the metabolic syndrome, including abdominal obesity, insulin resistance, hypertension, hypertriglyceridemia, and low high-density lipoprotein cholesterol, suggest many alternative causal pathways.

What should we conclude? Intensive glycemic control reduces the risk of microvascular and neuropathic complications in both type 1 and type 2 diabetes. There is no evidence that intensive glycemic control causes adverse cardiovascular outcomes or reduced quality of life. Accordingly, intensive glycemic control should be the standard of care for patients with type 1 and type 2 diabetes who are likely to benefit from it: those without advanced complications of diabetes, major comorbidities, or reduced life expectancies. For people likely to have limited benefit or increased risk with intensive treatment, it may be more appropriate to negotiate less intensive goals for glycemic management that reflect the persons self-determined goals of care and willingness to make lifestyle modifications.

REFERENCES

1. Feskens EJ, Kromhout D. Glucose tolerance and the risk of cardiovascular disease: the Zutphen Study. *J Clin Epidemiol* 1992; 45: 1327–34.
2. Haffner S, Lehto S, Ronnemaa T, et al. Mortality from coronary artery disease in subjects with type 2 diabetes and in nondiabetic subjects with and without prior myocardial infarction. *N Engl J Med* 1998; 339: 229–34.
3. Gu K, Cowie C, Harris M. Diabetes and decline in heart disease mortality in US adults. *JAMA* 1999; 281: 1291–7.
4. Malmberg K, Yusuf S, Gerstein HC, Brown J, Zhao F, Hunt D, Piegas L, Calvin J, Keltai M, Budaj A. Impact of diabetes on long-term prognosis in patients with unstable angina and non-Q-wave myocardial infarction: results of the OASIS (Organization to Assess Strategies for Ischemic Syndromes) Registry. *Circulation* 2000; 102: 1014–9.
5. Hankey GJ, Jamrozik K, Broadhurst RJ, Forbes S, Burvill PW, Anderson CS, Stewart-Wynne EG. Long-term risk of first recurrent stroke in the Perth Community Stroke Study. *Stroke* 1998; 29: 2491–500.
6. Luchsinger JA, Tang MX, Stern Y, Shea S, Mayeux R. Diabetes mellitus and risk of Alzheimer's disease and dementia with stroke in a multiethnic cohort. *Am J Epidemiol* 2001; 154: 635–41.
7. Tuomilehto J, Rastenyte D, Jousilahti P, Sarti C, Vartiainen E. Diabetes mellitus as a risk factor for death from stroke. *Stroke* 1996; 27: 210–5.
8. Jude EB, Oyibo SO, Chalmers N, Boulton AJ. Peripheral arterial disease in diabetic and nondiabetic patients. *Diabetes Care* 2001; 24: 1433–7.
9. Geiss LS, Herman WH, Smith PJ. Mortality in non-insulin-dependent diabetes. In National Diabetes Data Group (ed) *Diabetes in America*, 2nd edn. Bethesda, MD: National Institutes of Health, 1995; pp 233–57. DHHS publication no (NIH) 95-1468.
10. Beckman J, Creager M, Libby P. Diabetes and atherosclerosis. *JAMA* 2002; 287: 2570–81.
11. Khaw KT, Wareham N, Luben R, Bingham S, Oakes S, Welch A, Day N. Glycated hemoglobin, diabetes, and mortality in men in Norfolk cohort of European Prospective Investigation of Cancer and Nutrition (EPIC-Norfolk). *BMJ* 2001; 322: 1–6.
12. Coutinho M, Gerstein HC, Wang Y, Yusuf S. The relationship between glucose and incident cardiovascular events. *Diabetes Care* 1999; 22: 233–40.

13. Gerstein HC. The plasma glucose level—a continuous risk factor for vascular disease in both diabetic and nondiabetic people. *Adv Exp Med Biol* 2001; 498: 35–9.
14. Gerstein HC. Dysglycemia: a cardiovascular risk factor. *Diabetes Res Clin Pract* 1998; 40 (suppl): S9–14.
15. Jensen-Urstad KJ, Reichard PG, Rosfors JS, Lindblad LEL, Jensen-Urstad MT. Early atherosclerosis is retarded by improved long-term blood glucose control in patients with IDDM. *Diabetes* 1996; 45: 1253–8.
16. Epidemiology of Diabetes Interventions and Complications (EDIC) Research Group. Effect of intensive diabetes treatment on carotid artery wall thickness in the Epidemiology of Diabetes Interventions and Complications. *Diabetes* 1999; 48: 383–90.
17. The Diabetes Control and Complications Trial (DCCT) Research Group. The effect of intensive treatment of diabetes on the development and progression of long-term complications in insulin-dependent diabetes mellitus. *N Engl J Med* 1993; 329: 977–86.
18. Lawson ML, Tsui E, Gerstein HC, Zinman B. Effect of intensive therapy on early macrovascular disease in young individuals with type 1 diabetes—a systematic review and meta-analysis. *Diabetes Care* 1999; 22: B35–9.
19. Holman RR, Dornan TL, Mayon-White V, Howard-Williams J, Orde-Peckar C, Jenkins L, Steemson J, Rolfe R, Smith B, Barbour D, McPherson K, Poon P, Rizza C, Mann JI, Knight AH, Bron AJ, Turner RC. Prevention of deterioration of renal and sensory-nerve function by more intensive management of insulin-dependent diabetic patients: a two-year randomized prospective study. *Lancet* 1983; 204–8.
20. Feldt-Radmussen B, Mathiesen ER, Jensen T, Lauritzen T, Deckert T. Effect of improved metabolic control on loss of kidney function in type 1 (insulin-dependent) diabetic patients: an update of the Steno studies. *Diabetologia* 1991; 34: 164–70.
21. Brinchmann-Hansen O, Dahl-Jorgensen K, Sankvik L, Hanssen KF. Blood glucose concentrations and progression of diabetic retinopathy: the seven year results of the Oslo study. *BMJ* 1992; 304: 19–22.
22. Reichard P, Pihl M. Mortality and treatment side-effects during long-term intensified conventional insulin treatment in the Stockholm Diabetes Intervention Study. *Diabetes* 1994; 43: 313–7.
23. The DCCT Research Group. Effects of intensive diabetes management on macrovascular events and risk factors in the Diabetes Control and Complications Trial. *Am J Cardiol* 1995; 75: 894–903.
24. Klein R. Hyperglycemia and microvascular and macrovascular disease in diabetes. *Diabetes Care* 1995; 18: 258–68.
25. Dorman JS, Laporte RE, Kuller LH, et al. The Pittsburgh insulin-dependent diabetes mellitus (IDDM) morbidity and mortality study: mortality results. *Diabetes* 1984; 33: 271–6.
26. The DCCT Research Group. Lifetime benefits and costs of intensive therapy as practiced in the Diabetes Control and Complications Trial. *JAMA* 1996; 276: 1409–15.
27. Huang ES, Meigs JB, Singer DE. The effect of interventions to prevent cardiovascular disease in patients with type 2 diabetes mellitus. *Am J Med* 2001; 111: 633–42.
28. Cusi K. Cardiovascular risk management in type 2 diabetes. *Endocrinologist* 2001; 11: 474–90.
29. University Group Diabetes Program. Effects of hypoglycemic agents on vascular complications in patients with adult-onset diabetes, VIII: evaluation of insulin therapy. Final report. *Diabetes* 1982; 31: 1–81.
30. Feinglos MN, Bethel MA. Therapy of type 2 diabetes, cardiovascular death, and the UGDP. *Am Heart J* 1999; 138: S346–52.
31. Abraira C, Colwell JA, Nuttall FQ, Sawin CT, Nagel NJ, Comstock JP, Emanuele NV, Levin SR, Henderson W, Lee HS. Veterans Affairs Cooperative Study on Glycemic Control and Complications in Type II Diabetes (VACSDM). Results of the feasibility trial. Veterans Affairs Cooperative Study in Type II Diabetes. *Diabetes Care* 1995; 18: 1113–23.
32. Abraira C, Colwell J, Nuttall F, Sawin CT, Henderson W, Comstock JP, Emanuele NV, Levin SR, Pacold I, Lee HS. Cardiovascular events and correlates in the Veterans Affairs Diabetes Feasibility Trial. Veterans Affairs Cooperative Study on Glycemic Control and Complications in Type II Diabetes. *Arch Intern Med* 1997; 157: 181–8.
33. Abraira C, Henderson WG, Colwell JA, Nuttall FQ, Comstock JP, Emanuele NV, Levin SR, Sawin CT, Silbert CK. Response to intensive therapy steps and to glipizide dose in combination with insulin in type 2 diabetes. VA Feasibility Study on Glycemic Control and Complications (VACSDM). *Diabetes Care* 1998; 21: 574–9.
34. Shichiri M, Kishikawa H, Ohkubo Y, Wake N. Long-term results of the Kumamoto study on optimal diabetes control in type 2 diabetic patients. *Diabetes Care* 2000; 23 (suppl 2): B21–9.
35. The UK Prospective Diabetes Study (UKPDS) Group. Intensive blood-glucose control with sulfonylureas or insulin compared with conventional treatment and risk of complications in patients with type 2 diabetes (UKPDS 33). *Lancet* 1998; 352: 837–53.
36. The UKPDS Group. Effect of intensive blood-glucose control with metformin on complications in overweight patients with type 2 diabetes (UKPDS 34). *Lancet* 1998; 352: 854–65.
37. Malmberg K, Ryden L, Efendic S, Herlitz J, Nicol P, Waldenstrom A, Wedel H, Welin L. Randomized trial of insulin-glucose infusion followed by subcutaneous insulin treatment in diabetic patients with acute myocardial infarction (DIGAMI study): effects on mortality at 1 year. *J Am Coll Cardiol* 1995; 26: 57–65.
38. Malmberg K, for the Diabetes Mellitus, Insulin Glucose Infusion in Acute Myocardial Infarction (DIGAMI) Study Group. Prospective randomized study of intensive insulin treatment on long term survival after myocardial infarction in patients with diabetes mellitus. *BMJ* 1997; 314: 1512–5.
39. The UKPDS Group. Association of glycemia with macrovascular and microvascular complications of type 2 diabetes (UKPDS 35). *BMJ* 2000; 321: 405–12.
40. Duckworth WC, McCarren M, Abraira C. Glucose control and cardiovascular complications: the VA Diabetes Trial. *Diabetes Care* 2001; 24: 942–5.

77

The Syndrome of Insulin Resistance and Its Links to Atherosclerosis

Riccardo C. Bonadonna

University of Verona School of Medicine, Verona, Italy

WHY A SYNDROME?

Insulin resistance is a common feature in obesity and in type 2 diabetes mellitus [1, 2]. More recently, insulin resistance has also been associated with other cardiovascular risk factors, such as dyslipidemia [high triglycerides/low high-density lipoprotein (HDL) cholesterol] [3, 4] and hypertension [5]. These and other observations have led to postulate the existence of the so-called insulin resistance syndrome, or dysmetabolic syndrome X, or metabolic syndrome, or plurimetabolic syndrome, in which obesity, central fat distribution, altered glucose tolerance, dyslipidemia, and hypertension cluster together to a variable extent presumably because of the common pathogenetic denominator represented by insulin resistance [6]. The primary relevance of such a syndrome to human disease is in its possible involvement in the etiology and/or pathophysiology of atherosclerosis [7].

There exist several definitions of this syndrome, but in this chapter I refer to only two of them: the one proposed by the WHO Consultation Group [8] (Table 1) and the one recently put forward by the NCEP/ATP III Panel [9] (Table 2). Only for conventional reasons, I will use the term *dysmetabolic syndrome X* (DSX) throughout this chapter, without attributing to this denomination and/or to the definition of DSX by the NCEP/ATP III Panel any right of primacy over other denominations and definitions. Nevertheless, even without dwelling on all the fine details and pros/cons that differentiate the WHO and the NCEP definitions, two remarks are in order:

(1) the WHO definition needs an assessment of insulin sensitivity in all individuals with normal glucose regulation

(2) the NCEP/ATP III definition highlights a clinical cluster of risk factors and infers insulin resistance.

The WHO definition rests on pathophysiological grounds, whereas the NCEP/ATP III definition is based on purely clinical elements and lends itself to a much more widespread application, but it does not assess the putative main component, i.e. insulin resistance. The efforts devoted to the identification and the elucidation of the DSX should first raise the question: is there a need for it? The relevant point is that classical risk factors of cardiovascular disease (age, gender, family history of cardiovascular disease, cholesterol, glucose, blood pressure, and left ventricular hypertrophy) do not explain all, and perhaps not even the majority, of vascular atherosclerosis [10]. Thus, some important pieces of the puzzle are missing, and the DSX may be one of them.

It could be argued that little is gained by defining the DSX through a cluster of clinical parameters that are already known to be cardiovascular risk factors on their own. However, there is a distinct advantage in unifying some modifiable classical (diabetes and blood pressure) and nonclassical (central obesity, dyslipidemia) risk factors in a single pathophysiological scheme, which could be defined as *insulin-resistance-associated (or -mediated) atherosclerosis*. As a corollary, all other modifiable risk factors, first and foremost low-density lipoprotein (LDL) cholesterol, could be covered under the umbrella of *insulin-resistance-independent atherosclerosis*. A different pathological, diagnostic, prognostic, and therapeutic profile might be associated to either domain, lending clinical, as well as biological, relevance to this diagnostic exercise.

International Textbook of Diabetes Mellitus, Third Edition. Edited by R. A. DeFronzo, E. Ferrannini, H. Keen, and P. Zimmet.
 ISBN: 0-471-48655-8.

Table 1 The metabolic syndrome*

Presence of
(1) Impaired glucose regulation or diabetes mellitus; or
(2) Insulin resistance (assessed by the euglycemic insulin clamp)
Plus
Two or more of the following:
(1) Impaired glucose regulation or diabetes mellitus
(2) Insulin resistance (assessed by the euglycemic insulin clamp)
(3) Hypertension (≥140/90 mmHg)
(4) Hypertriglyceridemia (≥150 mg/dl) and or low HDL cholesterol (<35 mg/dl in males, <39 mg/dl in females)
(5) Central adiposity (waist-to-hip ratio >0.9 in males, >0.85 in females) and/or BMI >30kg/m^2
(6) Microalbuminuria (UAER[†] ≥20 μg/min or albumin/creatinine ratio ≥20 mg/g)

*WHO Consultation Group; reference 8.
[†]UAER = urinary albumin excretion rate.

The second potential advantage might be that through the use of a correct definition and assessment of the DSX, one could widen significantly our present skills to predict and, hence, prevent cardiovascular disease.

In this chapter, I review the available evidence linking the DSX to atherogenesis and clinical atherosclerosis, trying to illuminate the present relevance of this syndrome in the etiology and pathophysiology of atherosclerosis.

THE EVIDENCE FOR A SYNDROME

The trend of several modifiable traits to aggregate in the same individuals in proportions greater than predicted by chance alone has been appreciated for longer than a decade and is the seminal observation that has led to the recognition of the DSX (Tables 1 and 2).

Each of the entities listed in Tables 1 and 2, including atherosclerosis *per se* [11], have been found to be associated with insulin resistance in many human studies. Genetic manipulations in the experimental animal leading to insulin resistance have also prompted the onset of a syndrome resembling human DSX, thereby proving the concept that insulin resistance/hyperinsulinemia underlies DSX [12].

Table 2 Clinical identification of the metabolic syndrome*

Presence of three or more among	
(1) Abdominal obesity (waist circumference)	
(a) Men	>102 cm
(b) Women	>88 cm
(2) Triglycerides	≥150 mg/dl
(3) HDL cholesterol	
(a) Men	<40 mg/dl
(b) Women	<50 mg/dl
(4) Blood pressure	≥130/≥85 mmHg
(5) Fasting glucose	≥110 mg/dl

*The National Cholesterol Education Program (NCEP) Expert Panel on Detection, Evaluation, and Treatment of High Blood Cholesterol in Adults; reference 9.

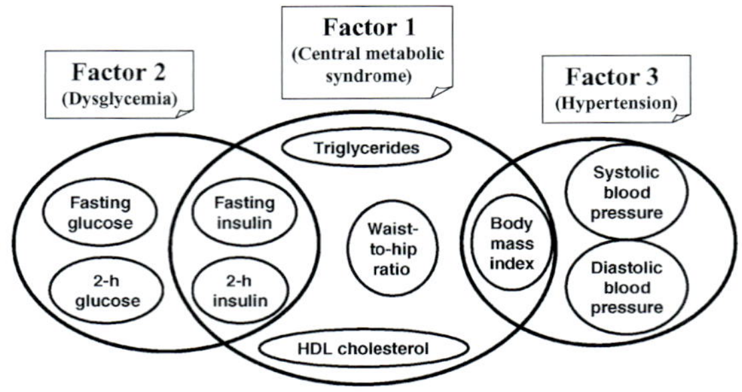

Figure 1 Factor analysis (principal components) of the main variables of the DSX in the Framingham Offspring Study (redrawn with permission from reference 13)

Perhaps the most elegant tool to demonstrate in humans that the existence of such cluster(s) is not a biased observer-dependent phenomenon is the application of factor analysis to data drawn from population-based studies. Factor analysis is a statistical technique that explores the possibility, if any, to identify a limited number of unknown and unmeasured factors underlying and explaining most of the variance of a larger number of continuous variables.

For example, in the Framingham Offspring Study, this "neutral" statistical tool extracted three factors (Figure 1), possibly identifiable as pathophysiological domains, which underlay the biological parameters most commonly included in the DSX: a *central metabolic syndrome*, a *hypertensive syndrome*, and a *dysglycemic syndrome* [13]. Importantly, some biological parameters were included in more than one factor, thereby bridging the three factors to form a communicating, albeit articulated, system. Indeed, insulin was included in both the dysglycemic and central metabolic syndromes, and adiposity, as reflected by body mass index (BMI), was included in both the central metabolic and hypertensive syndromes. These results have been replicated to a greater or a lesser extent also in other studies [14, 15], some of which also have reported data compatible with ethnic-specific patterns of factor extraction [16–19].

Studies conducted in twins have shown that factors extracted through factor analysis of the variables composing the DSX are heritable to a variable extent, with the dysglycemic syndrome possibly being the one most sensitive to inheritable (genetic) influences [20].

Finally, a genome-wide scan has been carried out in 27 extended Mexican American families in quest of genetic determinants of three factors extracted from insulin-resistance related phenotypes. Evidence for linkage to two regions on chromosome 6 was found for a BMI-leptin-insulin factor, and to one region on chromosome 7 for a triglyceride/HDL-cholesterol factor [21]. Note that these two factors are encompassed by the central metabolic syndrome in the Framingham Offspring Study [13].

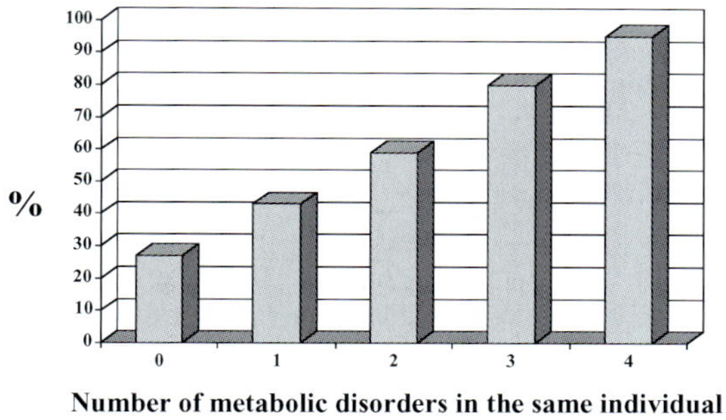

Figure 2 Prevalence of insulin resistance in the subjects of the Bruneck Study with no abnormalities or one or more abnormalities among glucose intolerance (diabetes or impaired glucose tolerance), hypertension, dyslipidemia (low HDL- cholesterol and/or high triglycerides), and hyperuricemia (drawn with permission from data in reference 23)

LINKS BETWEEN THE SYNDROME AND ATHEROSCLEROSIS

Clustering of cardiovascular risk factors obviously brings about an enhanced prevalence of atherosclerosis in the patients affected by the DSX [22]. Conversely, the richer is the cluster of cardiovascular risk factors, the more severe is the degree of insulin resistance (and *vice versa*) (Figure 2), [23]. This undisputable fact, however, is a reason for controversy. Indeed, one can envision quite different scenarios.

At one end of the spectrum, a common antecedent [24], or a "common soil" [25], is the reason for the concomitant presence of insulin resistance and cardiovascular risk factors in the same individual, with more or less involvement of insulin resistance in the pathogenesis of atherosclerosis.

At the other end of the spectrum, insulin resistance directly favors atherosclerosis on the one hand, and the appearance of disturbances in glucose, lipoprotein, and blood pressure homeostasis, on the other, the latter then adding their own contribution to atherosclerosis. Between these two extremes, there are several intermediate possibilities.

At the simplest level, justification for the relevance of insulin resistance in atherogenesis can be sought by investigating the statistical independence of the link between insulin resistance and atherosclerosis. This evidence can be looked for in either cross-sectional or longitudinal studies.

In the Bruneck Study, a population-based study conducted in northern Italy, hyperinsulinemia, as an indicator of insulin resistance, is independently associated with carotid atherosclerosis, as assessed by ultrasound scans [26], and with coronary heart disease [27]. It is worth noting that this relationship is neither linear nor coherent, because it actually shows increased atherosclerotic risk in the lowest quintile of insulin distribution, thereby shaping a J- or U-like function connecting hyperinsulinemia to atherosclerosis (Figure 3).

The Insulin Resistance Atherosclerosis Study Investigators have reported that insulin resistance, as assessed by the intravenous glucose tolerance test, was independently associated with carotid atherosclerosis, but this was so in Caucasians and in Hispanics, not in African Americans [28].

As to longitudinal studies, a recent meta-analysis has reassessed the role of insulin concentration as an independent risk factor of cardiovascular disease [29]. A doubling of the typical average fasting insulin value is associated with an 18% increase in the risk of experiencing a

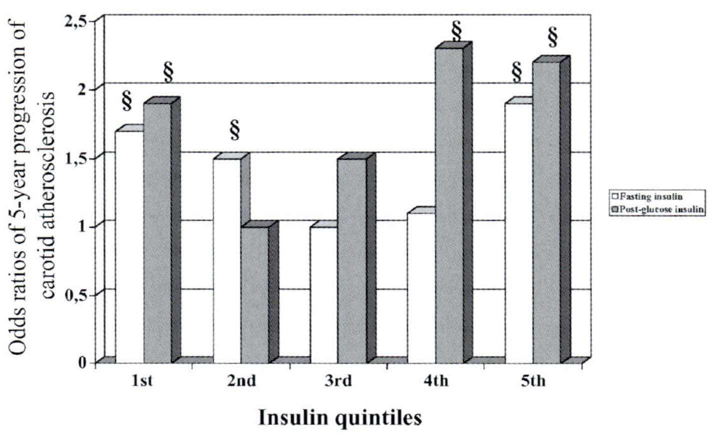

Figure 3 Odds ratio of progression of carotid atherosclerosis over 5 years in the Bruneck Study according to increasing quintiles of fasting (empty bars) and post-glucose (2 h after ingestion of a standard oral glucose load; shaded bars) insulin concentrations. The multivariate model is adjusted for gender, age, vascular status at baseline, BMI, glucose tolerance, smoking, physical activity level, socioeconomic status, alcohol consumption, hypertension, triglycerides, apoproteins A1 and B, and fibrinogen (drawn with permission from data of reference 26). §$p < 0.05$ or less vs. the reference (odds ratio = 1) quintile

cardiovascular event over the following 10 years. This increase in risk was much more evident when insulin was measured with recent, specific assays, than with older radioimmunoassays, which show significant cross-reactivity with proinsulin and other fragments of the proinsulin molecule. If one takes fasting insulin as a surrogate marker of insulin resistance, these data seem to invest the latter with a sort of definitive designation as an important precursor of atherosclerosis. In the Bruneck Study, a J-shaped pattern linking insulin and carotid atherosclerosis was also observed in the prospective data [26].

In some reports, proinsulin has shown a statistically better relationship with prevalent atherosclerosis [30, 31] and with incident cardiovascular disease [32] than insulin itself. This finding may be due to one or more of several factors. First, since proinsulin clearance is significantly lower than that of insulin, proinsulin may serve as a better integrated index of β-cell secretion. Therefore, were insulin resistance and/or insulin itself causally related to atherosclerosis, proinsulin would be more robust than insulin in reflecting such a relationship. Furthermore, in some studies proinsulin has shown a biological activity of its own in stimulating plasminogen activator inhibitor 1 (PAI-1) gene expression in endothelial cells [33, 34], thereby possibly favoring thrombosis.

Finally, in patients with type 2 diabetes, insulin resistance, as assessed by a mathematical model based on fasting insulin concentration, is a predictor of cardiovascular events over a 5-year follow-up independently of classical risk factors, duration of disease, and HbA_{1c} [35].

The factors extracted by factor analysis applied to the parameters of the DSX have also been reported to predict cardiovascular disease. In elderly nondiabetic Finnish men, an insulin-resistance factor formed by total and central adiposity, triglycerides, fasting glucose, and insulin was an independent predictor of clinical events due to coronary heart disease [36]. A similar finding was reported in two other surveys conducted in Finnish men, one in nondiabetic and the other in diabetic individuals [37, 38]. Oddly, this finding was not replicated in Finnish women [36], perhaps pointing to gender-related differences.

However, this evidence should be considered less cogent, at least on statistical grounds, than that obtained with the use of insulin resistance in comparison with the classical cardiovascular risk factors. This is because "factors" embody the variance of the raw variables from which they were extracted, and hence a good deal of their predictive power. This, in turn, may well be rooted in the predictive power of dyslipidemia, blood presssure, and alterations in glucose homeostasis, not in the biological phenomenon of insulin resistance.

Moreover, since a great number of studies have used hyperinsulinemia, or other indexes derived from it, as a proxy for insulin resistance [13–27, 29, 35–38], epidemiologic evidence cannot solve the dilemma whether insulin resistance or compensatory hyperinsulinemia determines the potentially lethal association between DSX and atherosclerosis.

Furthermore, even in the situation where insulin resistance had been actually measured, at the epidemiological level it might be unjustified to interpret a statistically independent power of insulin resistance to predict atherosclerosis as a definite proof that insulin resistance bears a causal relationship to atherosclerosis more than hyperinsulinemia does.

INSULIN ACTION ON THE VESSEL WALL

Pathophysiological studies may shed some light on the role of insulin resistance and/or hyperinsulinemia in atherogenesis, although they are not devoid of ambiguities.

As a first confounder, hyperinsulinemia/insulin resistance, as currently assessed in humans, essentially reflects insulin sensitivity for glucose metabolism [39], but a direct pathophysiologic link between insulin-mediated whole body glucose utilization, which is primarily determined by glucose uptake in skeletal muscle [2], and atherogenesis can hardly be sustained. Thus, even the gold standard assessment of insulin sensitivity, namely the glucose clamp technique, is an index of some unidentified, although related, biological phenomenon, which is involved in atherogenesis.

The most obvious candidates to account for such a relationship are some nonclassical effects of insulin, which are potentially endowed with some bearing on atherogenesis.

A second confounder is that insulin sensitivity/resistance in any given individual has a strong familiar/genetic component [40], but it is also heavily influenced by environmental and acquired factors, such as diet, physical exercise, and drugs [41].

The major genes responsible for insulin sensitivity have not yet been identified [40], but their relationship to a polygenic trait such as atherosclerosis [42] is likely to be complex.

The experimental evidence *in vivo* in humans generally shows that the acute physiological effects of hyperinsulinemia on lipids [43], blood pressure [44], endothelial [45, 46] and platelet [47, 48] functions appear to be antiatherogenic. More specifically, acute experimental hyperinsulinemia in humans causes a fall in very low density lipoprotein (VLDL) triglycerides, which are potential precursors of atherogenic lipoproteins [43]. In many studies, acute hyperinsulinemia has been shown to reduce arterial blood pressure in healthy individuals [44]. Finally, insulin causes vasodilation of resistance vessels via an endothelium- and nitric oxide (NO)-dependent

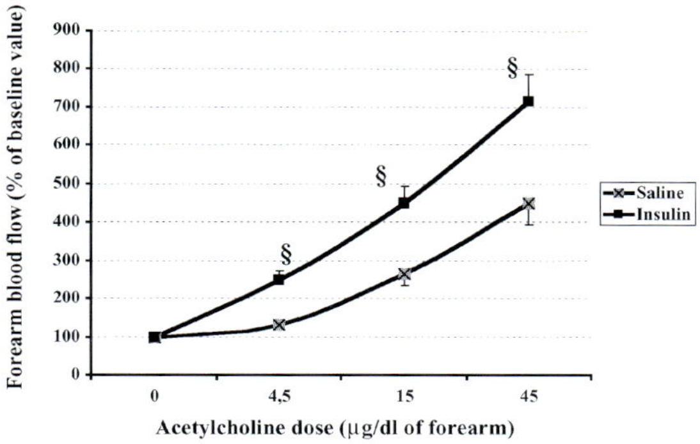

Figure 4 Local insulin infusion amplifies acetylcholine-induced (endothelium-dependent) vasodilation in the forearm vascular bed of healthy subjects (redrawn with permission from reference 40) §$p < 0.05$ or less insulin vs. saline

mechanism and amplifies vasodilation induced by endothelium- and NO-dependent agents in resistance arterioles [45, 46] (Figure 4). During acute hyperinsulinemia, there also is a fall in platelet sensitivity to aggregant agents and again this effect is, at least partially, mediated by NO [47, 48].

Lipids, and in particular free fatty acids, seem to be able to counteract insulin's effects on endothelium-dependent vasodilation and lead, therefore, to endothelial dysfunction [49]. These data raise the possibility that insulin resistance of fat cells and metabolism may be an inducer of endothelial dysfunction, a critical event in atherogenesis [50]. Endothelium is a crossroad cell, and endothelial dysfunction, activation, and damage are obligate steps in atherosclerosis [42]. Importantly, in all states of insulin resistance thus far investigated, endothelial dysfunction is also present [50], suggesting that vascular endothelium may be particularly vulnerable to insulin resistance *per se* or to some other factor regularly associated with insulin resistance.

Hyperinsulinemia also causes an activation of the noradrenergic arm of the sympathetic nervous system (SNS) [51]. This also occurs in the classic insulin-resistant state—obesity. Twenty-four hour profiles of heart rate variability and blood pressure have shown that during postprandial phases the low frequency domain of heart rate variability, reflecting primarily cardiac effects of SNS, prevails over the high frequency domain, reflecting vagal action, in obese individuals. This alteration is related to hyperinsulinemia, not to body fatness, and is reversed by weight loss [52]. A further possible consequence of insulin-induced activation of the SNS is prolongation of the QT interval, which occurs within 30 min of sustained physiological hyperinsulinemia [53]. Prolongation of the ECG QT interval reflects abnormalities in cardiomyocyte repolarization and predisposes to sudden death owing to fatal arrythmias [54].

To this picture, recent data have added new dimensions. Quinones-Galvan et al. have reported that hyperinsulinemia *in vivo* in humans diminishes the circulating levels of vitamin E, an important antioxidant, and causes an increased susceptibility of LDL to oxidation [55]. Arcaro and colleagues in turn have reported that mild physiological hyperinsulinemia in humans causes a complete abrogation of endothelium-dependent vasodilation in large conduit arteries, an effect that appears to be mediated by increased oxidant stress [56] (Figure 5). These data are in apparent contrast with insulin's amplifying effects on endothelium-dependent vasodilation observed in other studies [45, 46]. However, it should be noted that the latter findings were obtained in resistance vessels, whereas the detrimental effects of insulin described in reference 56 have been documented in conduit arteries, the ones that are susceptible to develop plaques. These data indeed highlight that there is significant heterogeneity of endothelial function *in vivo*, depending on the type of vessel and on the vascular bed.

Thus, physiological hyperinsulinemia may cause an imbalance between prooxidant and antioxidant systems with ensuing damage to lipoproteins and endothelium in conduit arteries, the ones that are susceptible to atherosclerosis.

Cardillo et al. have demonstrated elegantly that hyperinsulinemia stimulates not only the nitrergic but also the endothelinergic system in the human forearm vascular bed, which mainly reflects resistance arterioles [57]. Endothelin 1 is the most powerful vasoconstrictor known to date, and is an effective stimulator of smooth muscle cell proliferation. Evidence shows that it is upregulated in several instances of both animal and human atherosclerosis [58]. Thus, it is believed to play an important role in disease

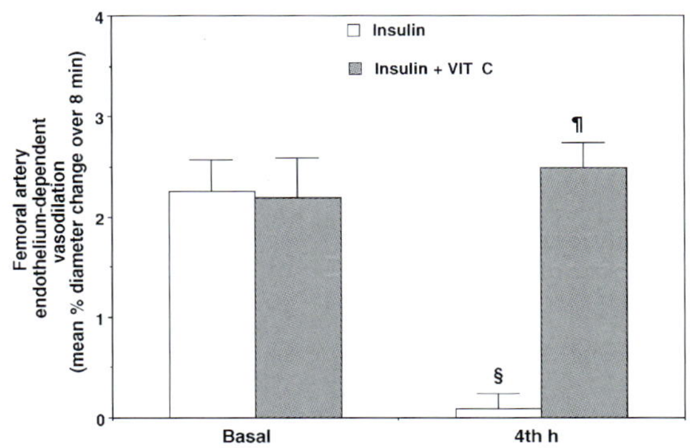

Figure 5 Modest (≈110 pmol/l) systemic hyperinsulinemia abrogates flow-mediated (endothelium-dependent) vasodilation in the common femoral artery of healthy subjects (empty bars). This effect of insulin is prevented by infusion of vitamin C, an antioxidant (shaded bars.) §$p < 0.01$ insulin vs. basal; ¶$p < 0.01$ insulin + VITC vs. insulin (redrawn with permission from reference 51)

progression, although some cautionary remarks have been offered recently [59].

Also the positive effect of insulin on circulating VLDL triglycerides has been questioned on the grounds that insulin simultaneously causes a fall in circulating free fatty acids and amino acids, which are important substrates for the assembly of VLDL by the liver. When this is not the case, as in insulin-resistant states, then the promoting effect of insulin on VLDL secretion by the liver would be unveiled [60].

In summary, *in vivo* studies show that insulin activates the SNS, the nitrergic, the endothelinergic, and the oxidant stress systems, in sites, with time courses and to extents which may greatly vary within the cardiovascular system and between individuals. A likely example of these potential ambiguities is offered by the effects of insulin on lipids, which may differ according to whether individuals are insulin resistant or not. In the former case, hyperinsulinemia may promote increased secretion of VLDL triglycerides in a metabolic stage, which would favor the formation of atherogenic lipoproteins.

INSULIN ACTION AND ATHEROGENESIS: THE MOLECULAR LEVEL

In the last decade, a number of studies have elucidated, at least in part, the molecular basis of insulin action in the vascular wall.

Insulin action in both endothelium and vascular smooth muscle cells (VSMCs) is mediated by the insulin receptor, which phosphorylates tyrosine residues of several downstream signaling proteins. The two most relevant ones in the vascular wall may be insulin receptor substrate 1 (IRS-1) and Shc. The former leads to activation of phosphatidylinositol 3 kinase (PI3K) and several downstream PI3K-dependent pathways. The latter eventually results into the activation of mitogen-activated protein kinases (MAPKs) and several pathways controlled by them [61].

In particular, insulin, through an IRS-1/PI3K/Akt-dependent pathway, enhances endothelial constitutive NO synthase (ecNOS) expression and activity, resulting in increased NO generation [62–64]. This pathway is also involved in acceleration of glucose transport/phosphorylation and glycogen synthesis in skeletal muscle [61]. Thus, impairments in this pathway may lead to insulin resistance of glucose metabolism in skeletal muscle and to an NO-deficient state in the vessel wall, with endothelial dysfunction as just one of the prominent signs of this process. Furthermore, NO is a powerful vasodilator and inhibits platelet aggregation [65]. Further effects of NO include inhibition of the expression of adhesion molecules, which favor monocyte migration within the vascular wall [66].

Recent experiments have demonstrated that insulin, through the IRS-1/PI3K/Akt-dependent pathway and stimulation of ecNOS, causes decreased expression and activation of matrix metalloproteinases (MMPs) 2 and 9 and opposite effects on tissue inhibitor of metalloproteinases (TIMPs) [67]. These MMPs and their main inhibitor TIMP play a major role in regulating the rate at which vascular extracellular matrix is degraded and, through it, the process of vascular remodeling [68].

Also the antiapoptotic effect of insulin may be of potential relevance, although it has been studied more in detail in β-cells [69]. This effect is also mediated through an IRS/PI3K/Akt-dependent pathway and may also be involved in vascular remodeling [70].

Thus the IRS-1/PI3K/Akt pathway plays a relevant role in preserving vascular integrity. Insulin resistance of this pathway is to be considered detrimental to vascular health. As the first committed molecule in transmitting insulin signal through this specific pathway, IRS-1 may play a critical role. The activity of IRS-1 is modulated positively by tyrosine phosphorylation [e.g., through insulin receptor and insulin-like growth factor (IGF-1) receptor] and negatively by serine phosphorylation [e.g., as a consequence of cell exposure to tumor necrosis factor α (TNF-α and to hyperglycemia] [71, 72]. Therefore, the phosphorylation status of IRS-1 may be of paramount importance to insulin action in the vascular wall.

Earlier *in vitro* and *in vivo* evidence supported the concept that hyperinsulinemia can promote atherogenesis essentially by virtue of its growth-factor-like action [73]. Insulin is a proliferant agent on its own [72], but, perhaps more importantly, it greatly amplifies the proliferative responses to several growth factors, in particular angiotensin II and platelet-derived growth factor (PDGF) [74, 75]. These effects of insulin are mediated primarily through Shc/MAPK-dependent pathways [74]. Downstream to MAPK activation is also insulin-induced increased transcription of the endothelin receptor A (ET-A) receptor [76], whose ligand is endothelin 1, a powerful vasoconstrictor with a strong proliferant effect on VSMC. Finally, insulin-mediated increased production of PAI-1, the main negative regulator of fibrinolysis, via increased transcription of PAI-1 gene, seems to be activated through a MAPK-dependent pathway [77].

Thus, an imbalance between IRS-1/PI3K-mediated processes, which are impaired in insulin resistance, and Shc/MAPK-mediated processes, which may retain insulin sensitivity even in insulin resistant states and would be overstimulated by compensatory hyperinsulinemia, may turn out to be a good molecular paradigm to explain the links between insulin resistance/hyperinsulinemia and atherosclerosis (Figure 6).

Indeed, in humans insulin resistance of the PI3K pathway exists in association with normal sensitivity of MAPK

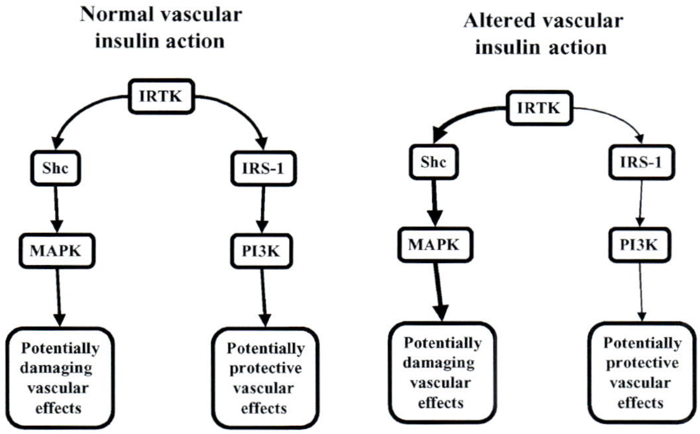

Figure 6 A current popular paradigm to explain the links between the binomial insulin resistance/hyperinsulinemia and atherosclerosis. In the vessel of a normal individual (left), there is a balanced stimulation of both Shc/MAPK- and IRS-1/PI3K-dependent pathways. In the vessel of an individual with insulin resistance (right), there is overstimulation (shown as thicker arrows) of Shc/MAPK-dependent pathways, due to compensatory hyperinsulinemia, and understimulation (shown as thinner arrows) of IRS-1/PI3K-dependent pathways, due to insulin resistance

[78] at least in skeletal muscle (Figure 7). It is unknown whether the same applies to vascular cells.

Blockade of PI3K in endothelial cells does not affect MAPK-mediated signaling, amplifies insulin-induced prenylation and activation of Rho proteins, and leads to increased expression of vascular cell adhesion molecule 1 (VCAM-1) and E-selectin, as well as increased rolling of monocytes on endothelium [79].

These and other recent data open new potential avenues to insulin action. VCAM-1 and E-selectin gene transcription is typically increased by the transcription factor named nuclear factor κB (NF-κB) [80], and raise the possibility of a possible interaction between insulin action and this important inflammatory pathway. Recent evidence suggests that NF-κB may be an important crossroad between inflammation and metabolic insulin resistance.

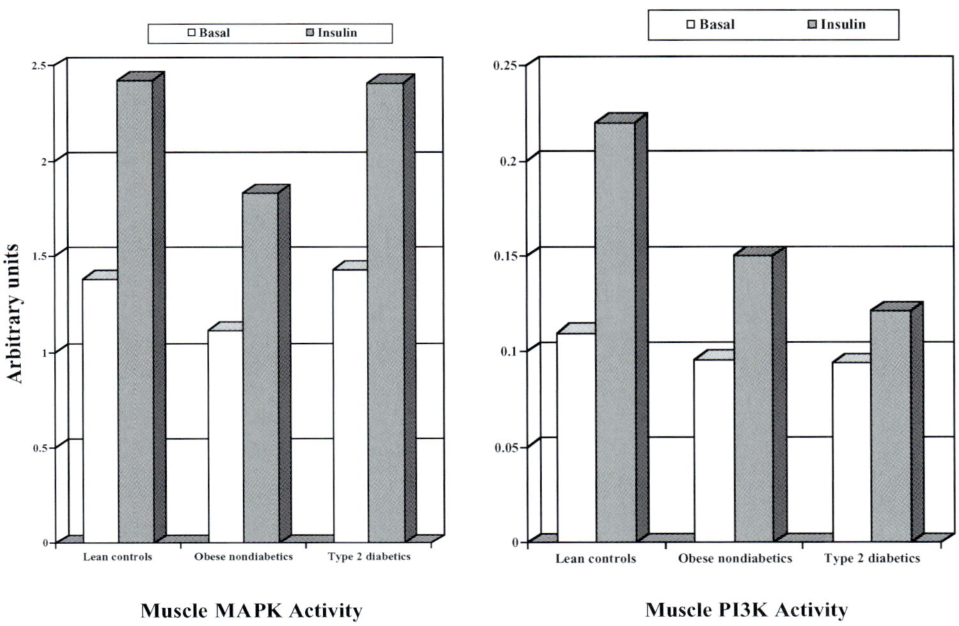

Figure 7 Effects of systemic hyperinsulinemia (shaded bars) on MAPK activity (left panel) and on IRS-1-associated PI3K activity (right panel) in skeletal muscle of lean controls, obese nondiabetic subjects, and patients with type 2 diabetes mellitus. It can be seen that in both insulin-resistant states (obesity and diabetes) there is normal insulin sensitivity of MAPK, and insulin resistance of PI3K, as postulated in the paradigm of Figure 6 (drawn with permission from data of reference 72)

Indeed, lipid-induced insulin resistance might be attributable to activation of NF-κB via some isoforms of protein kinase C (PKC) and/or ceramide [81], which in skeletal muscle would be responsible for inducing insulin resistance for glucose metabolism [82]. The intermediate molecular event is thought to be activation of I-κB kinase, which neutralizes I-κB, the inhibitor of NF-κB. I-κB kinase can also modulate negatively IRS-1 through serine phosphorylation and lead to metabolic/vascular insulin resistance [83].

However, as a more generalized phenomenon, activation of the NF-κB system may be a critical step in causing a subinflammatory state in the vascular wall and in promoting atherogenesis [42]. Thus, I-κB kinase/NF-κB activation may be a common mechanism involved in the etiology of at least some varieties of metabolic insulin resistance and in bridging insulin resistance and atherogenesis (Figure 8).

Since in humans modest hyperinsulinemia may cause increased oxidant stress in conduit arteries [56] and NF-κB typically is activated by superoxide anion [80], it may be envisioned that both insulin resistance and compensatory hyperinsulinemia are associated with, or are a direct cause of, NF-κB activation.

This likely relationship between insulin resistance and the NF-κB system is made more plausible by the presence of increased levels of acute reactant phase proteins in insulin resistance, especially C-reactive protein (CRP), a finding particularly evident in obesity and correlated to adiposity [84]. These proteins are to be considered the footprints of an upregulation of the innate immune system. Activation of the innate immune system leads to activation of NF-κB, and all its downstream effectors.

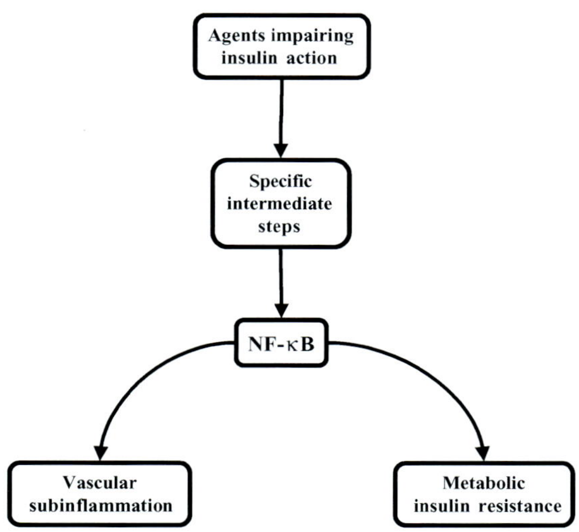

Figure 8 The system of transcription factor NF-κB as a common mediator of metabolic insulin resistance and vascular subinflammatory injury. See text for details

These mechanisms have been considered to offer an evolutionary advantage in terms of response to infections, yet at the expense of susceptibility to the consequences of low-grade inflammation, including glucose intolerance and atherosclerosis [85].

Indeed, in the Bruneck Study, a variant of the Toll-4-like receptor gene, a receptor which has a paramount role in raising innate immunity responses through downstream activation of NF-κB, is associated with reduced CRP and adhesion molecule levels, increased susceptibility to infections, and decreased risk of both prevalent and incident atherosclerosis [86]. To close the circle, most recent evidence shows that application of factor analysis in male Europeans yields an insulin resistance factor, formed by insulin, proinsulin, triglycerides, and BMI, and a low-grade inflammation factor, formed by fibrinogen, CRP, and interleukin 6 (IL-6), which are significantly related to each other, even independently of obesity, and are both strong indicators of previous myocardial infarction [87].

ATHEROGENESIS, INSULIN RESISTANCE, AND HYPERINSULINEMIA

The current view of atherogenesis recognizes several phases [42, 88, 89]. The first of them is the process(es) that leads to lesion initiation [88]. At least three different, not mutually exclusive, mechanisms can be hypothesized. The first one requires the presence of circulating atherogenic lipoproteins, which, after being trapped within the vessel wall, induce a biological process with striking resemblance to a chronic inflammatory reaction [42, 88, 89]. The second one is represented by endothelial activation, triggered by stimuli which are independent of lipids and hemostatic factors, which in turn leads to monocyte migration within the vessel wall and the induction of an inflammatory-like process [88]. The third one postulates an initial layer of fibrin/platelets on the endothelium, which again leads to transendothelial migration of monocytes and an inflammatory-like process [88]. All of these mechanisms (e.g., levels and composition of atherogenic lipoproteins) are most likely to be influenced by genetic determinants [42, 88], which may turn out to display significant interaction with the degree of insulin resistance (Figure 9).

In this phase, insulin action on the metabolism of nonclassical atherogenic lipoproteins, such as triglyceride-rich remnants and small dense LDL [90, 91], may be critical. Indeed, in insulin-resistant states, especially in obesity, lipoprotein lipase activity is increased in the fasting state and does not respond to insulin in the postprandial phase. This leads to an increase in substrate supply for the hepatic triglyceride lipase pathway, which in turn favors a decrease in HDL and a shift of LDL toward a small

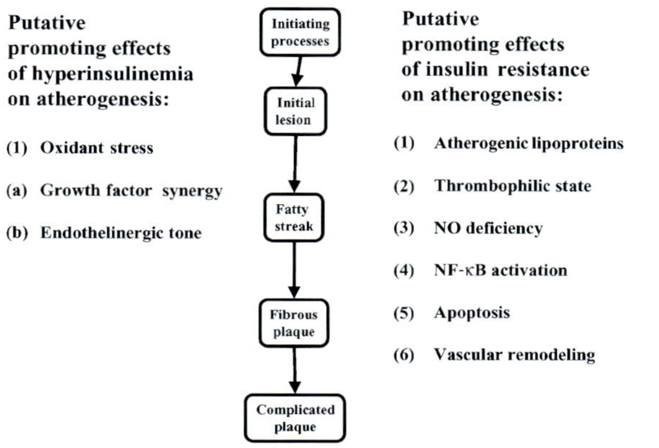

Figure 9 Recognized phases of plaque formation, with lists of some main biological events, due to either hyperinsulinemia or insulin resistance, which could promote atherogenesis. See text for details

dense phenotype. These LDL particles are more readily oxidized, when trapped within the vessel wall [42]. Furthermore, as already mentioned, acute hyperinsulinemia can increase LDL susceptibility to oxidation [55].

There exists a large body of literature showing that insulin can regulate ecNOS in vascular cells [62–64]. Endothelial dysfunction and activation might be related to a NO-deficient state, secondary to the loss of insulin action on ecNOS.

Layering of fibrin/platelets on endothelium may be facilitated by the decrement in insulin effects on platelets of insulin-resistant individuals [50, 92], again mediated by a loss of insulin action on ecNOS. To this, the compensatory increased secretion of beta-cell products, i.e. insulin and proinsulin, further stimulates PAI-1 expression and secretion, which impairs fibrinolysis [77]. It is noteworthy that insulin-induced activation of PAI-1 synthesis occurs primarily at the PAI-1 gene promoter level, through a peculiar cascade which sequentially involves PI3K, PKC, and MAPK [77]. Thus, the general paradigm that sees a separation, and an opposition, between PI3K- and MAPK-mediated actions does not apply to this case.

The subsequent phases of plaque formation are characterized by the unambiguous presence of lesions that are the result of the atherogenetic process. Current classifications list the initial lesion, the fatty streak, the intermediate lesion, the fibrous plaque, and the complex (calcified) plaque [42, 88, 89]. The last one is most likely to undergo rupture, with local thrombosis and ensuing clinical event [42, 89]. All of these diverse lesions share, as a common feature, the presence of lipid deposits and the cell reactions associated with them [42, 89].

An important pathogenetic step in the lesion progression is the modification of the lipoproteins that are trapped in the vessel wall [42, 89]. The best known modification is oxidation of LDL, which is a multistage process. The lesion progression also depends on the liability of the arterial wall to build an active chronic inflammatory response to different stimuli. This susceptibility is believed to have strong genetic determinants, some of which may have already been identified [42, 86]. Necessary steps include monocyte adhesion, migration, and transformation into macrophages, as well as proliferation and migration of smooth muscle cells. A variety of adhesion molecules, such as P- and E-selectin, intercellular adhesion molecule 1, VCAM-1, platelet endothelial cell adhesion molecule 1, etc.; chemokines, such as IL-1β, IL-6, TNF-α, monocyte chemoattractant protein 1, etc.; and growth factors, such as angiotensin II, PDGF, IGF-1, fibroblast growth factors, transfoming growth factors, etc., are involved in this process [42].

The condition of hyperinsulinemia/insulin resistance presumably leads to seed the arterial wall with more readily oxidizable lipoproteins, but it may also be linked to a condition of increased oxidant stress, both directly and through its complex relationships with some other systems (e.g., the angiotensinergic and the kininergic system) that regulate the balance between NO synthesis and reactive radical generation, such as superoxide anion and others [93–98]. To this, the decreased HDL-cholesterol levels usually seen in insulin-resistant states may add the loss of the protective effect of HDL against LDL oxidation, primarily mediated by paraoxonase [99, 100].

Furthermore, the recognition of ecNOS as an effector of insulin action [62–64] raises the possibility that insulin resistance plays a role in modulating the degree of the chronic inflammatory reaction involved in atherogenesis through the loss of the anti-inflammatory effects exerted by low NO concentrations [66]. Indeed, in obese subjects the capability of insulin to stimulate endothelium- and NO-dependent vasodilation in resistance vessels is typically lost, featuring an elegant example of insulin resistance of the vascular NO synthetic pathway [46] (Figure 10).

Notably, this state of vascular insulin resistance is present in obesity-related insulin resistance, but not in essential hypertension [44], which is a salient component of the DSX. This is one clue that there exists significant heterogeneity in metabolic-/vascular-insulin-resistant phenotypes. There is also some sparse evidence that the acute antagonistic effects of insulin toward the angiotensinergic system are typically lost in insulin-resistant states, whereas (see below) the chronic synergistic effects of insulin with angiotensin II may be preserved.

Finally, smooth muscle cell proliferation might be a sensitive target of compensatory hyperinsulinemia [101]. Insulin is a proliferant agent on its own, but, perhaps more importantly, it greatly amplifies the proliferative responses to several growth factors, with special regard to angiotensin II and PDGF, and stimulates endothelin

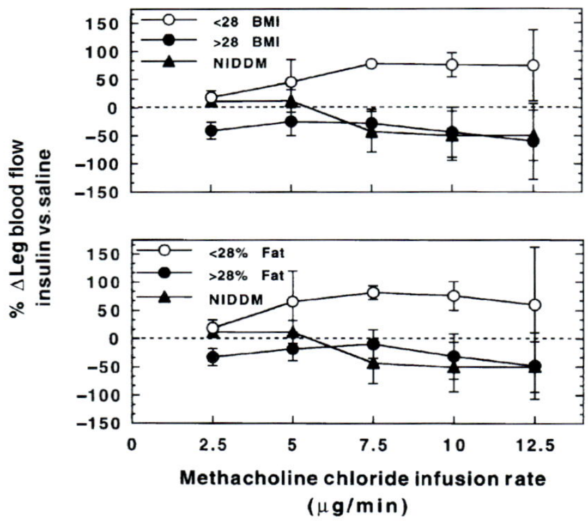

Figure 10 Insulin amplifying effects on metacholine-induced (endothelium-dependent) vasodilation of the leg vascular bed in lean controls (BMI < 28 kg/m^2 or % body fat < 28), in obese nondiabetic subjects (BMI > 28 kg/m^2 or % body fat > 28), and in patients with type 2 diabetes (NIDDM). It can be seen that in both insulin-resistant states (obesity and diabetes) insulin causes no amplification of methacholine-induced vasodilation, thereby featuring a pattern of vascular insulin resistance (from reference 41 with permission)

expression [102]. These effects of insulin are mediated primarily through MAPK-dependent pathways.

However, NO deficiency due to insulin resistance should also cause a decrease in TIMP and increase in MMP-2 and -9, thereby accelerating the processes of extracellular matrix (ECM) reabsorption [67]. This in turn through integrin-mediated signaling may favor smooth muscle cell migration and proliferation [68]. The entire process leads to profound disturbances in vascular remodeling.

The final events of plaque rupture and thrombosis are influenced by the activation of the MMP system, especially at the shoulder of a vulnerable plaque, as well as by the balance between vasoconstrictors and vasodilators and the balance between thrombohemostatic factors and antagonists [42, 89]. Compensatory hyperinsulinemia due to metabolic insulin resistance, if acting on a vascular-insulin-sensitive PI3K, may shift the balance between MMP and TIMP, thereby leading to critical activation of MMP in vulnerable sites [67, 68].

Once the plaque has undergone rupture, loss of anticoagulant and vasodilatory endothelial properties, increased levels of coagulation factors, reduced fibrinolytic activity, and increased platelet reactivity may be predictors of a poor outcome [42]. Insulin resistance of the PI3K pathway in the vessel wall leads to reduced NO generation [62–64] with subsequent reduced vasodilation and increased vasoconstriction [46]. Insulin also stimulates the endothelinergic system *in vivo* [57]. Both fibrinogen and PAI-1 increase in insulin-resistant states, primarily as a consequence of compensatory hyperinsulinemia [77]. Insulin-induced inhibition of platelet aggregation, in turn, is lost in insulin resistance and may be considered a cofactor of platelet hyperactivity [92].

Thus, the prevalence of vasoconstrictive action, the thrombophilic state, and the impairment in fibrinolysis commonly due to insulin resistance/hyperinsulinemia may well be involved in facilitating and/or triggering and/or sustaining the thrombotic episodes that usually underlie the clinical events.

REVISITING THE MAIN HYPOTHESES

Revisiting Hyperinsulinemia/Insulin Resistance as a Primary Step in Atherogenesis

Primacy of hyperinsulinemia/insulin resistance is deemed possible on the basis of some key facts:

(1) Even in healthy, lean individuals there are a substantial number of individuals who display a degree of insulin (in)sensitivity similar to that observed in many individuals affected by the classic insulin-resistant states such as obesity.
(2) These individuals display some features of the DSX.
(3) These features contribute to the relationship between hyperinsulinemia and coronary heart disease at the epidemiological level.

In these individuals, who have been classified as metabolically obese normal-weight subjects [103], the impairment in insulin action is due to a reduction in IRS1/PI3K-dependent pathways, with the concomitant fall in ecNOS function, increase in MMP/TIMP ratio, and alterations in vascular remodeling. Concomitantly, compensatory hyperinsulinemia may overstimulate the Shc/MAPK-dependent pathways in the vessel wall, with increased endothelinergic tone and proliferation of VSMC. These two phenomena may lead to atheroma. Mice with partial knockout of IRS-1 gene may be considered a reasonable model of this condition. They indeed develop alterations in blood pressure regulation and endothelial dysfunction, typical intermediate phenotypes of cardiovascular disease [12]. Their susceptibility to atherosclerosis is still unknown.

A possible counterpart in humans may be offered by individuals with the Arg972 polymorphism in the IRS-1 gene. The frequency of this variant is approximately twice as high in patients with type 2 diabetes as in the general population and is associated with a reduction in β-cell function [104]. However, in nondiabetic individuals the presence of this polymorphism conveys a much higher risk of cardiovascular events, which is particularly evident in obese and diabetic patients, but is still detectable in nonobese nondiabetic individuals [105].

Thus, IRS-1 and its state of phosphorylation/activity are likely to provide a molecular basis to a primitive role of insulin resistance in atherogenesis.

Revisiting the Common Antecedent or "Common Soil" Hypothesis

The paradigmatic examples of this condition may be the phenotypes that are thought to result from "thrifty gene(s)" [106] or from very early, particularly *in utero*, undernutrition ("thrifty phenotype") [107] or from various combinations of these two possibilities in westernized societies. In the former case, the interaction between a "thrifty" genotype, selected by evolution to ensure survival during famines, and westernized, affluent societies is cause of disease. In the latter case, undernutrition in critical, very early stages of life causes a "resetting" of metabolism, which results in maladaptive responses when the individual is exposed to a westernized environment later in life.

Both of these hypotheses converge in predicting the onset of, and/or the interaction with, obesity at some point in life. From (central) obesity one can start to outline some biological events linked to insulin resistance, which can promote plaque formation and growth. There cannot be an increase in body weight without a higher than needed food intake. This increase in food intake, especially if rich in lipids, leads to widespread intracellular deposition of lipids, and triggers lipotoxicity [108]. Lipotoxicity leads to insulin resistance of the IRS-1/PI3K pathway, with apparently preserved sensitivity of the Shc/MAPK-dependent pathway. Concomitantly, the obese individual activates a complex response with the dual aim of decreasing body weight (leptin and other adipocytokines), and overcoming insulin resistance (hyperinsulinemia) [108–111]. The common second messenger(s) of some of these effects may be sphingomyosins, especially ceramide and lactosyl ceramide [112, 113]. These may cause peripheral insulin resistance in muscle, vascular insulin resistance of the IRS-1/PI3K pathway, increased anion superoxide preduction. There are data that also involve some isoforms of PKC (θ and ε) as downstream effectors of sphingomyosins. However, in humans, diacylglycerol, but not total ceramide, is increased in skeletal muscle following prolonged lipid infusion. These changes are associated with activation of PKC-βII and -δ, but not PKC-θ and -ε. NF-κB is eventually activated, through stimulation of I-κB kinase that neutralizes I-κBα, the inhibitor of NF-κB [114]. I-κB kinase is believed to be able to phosphorylate serine residues of IRS-1 [83], thereby reducing transmission of insulin signal to PI3K-dependent pathways. Thus, I-κB kinase/NF-κB may be the molecular crossroad that causes insulin resistance in skeletal muscle and vascular dysfunction, with the latter eventually resulting in plaque formation.

Restenosis, Insulin Resistance, and Hyperinsulinemia

About 25 years ago percutaneous revascularization was introduced successfully in the therapy of advanced atherosclerotic lesions [115], both in the coronary circulation [116] and in other peripheral territories [115]. Quite soon it was realized that in many patients, after successful discharge, symptoms would reappear after a variable period of time, and that those who would suffer from this problem within 6 months, would be most likely to have developed restenosis of the same diseased segment of vessel.

From the pathological viewpoint, it is known that this is a model of acute fibrointimal proliferation with negative remodeling of the vascular wall [42]. Indeed, a number of studies have shown that hyperinsulinemia is a powerful risk indicator of restenosis especially after balloon angioplasty [117, 118]. It is conceivable that, in this process, insulin concentrations are a marker of the loss PI3K sensitivity to insulin itself, and hence, it represents an indicator of vessel vulnerability. Furthermore, treatment with a PPAR-γ agonist, such as troglitazone, seems to prevent restenosis [119]. Although PPAR-γ ligands exert a variety of effects, including an antiinflammatory action and, for troglitazone, a direct antioxidant effect [120], it is tempting to attribute at least part of this alleged preventive effect on restenosis to the improvement in insulin sensitivity, possibly at the level of the vascular wall.

CONCLUSIONS

Since it impacts on a tightly controlled homeostatic variable such as glucose, insulin resistance is never present without a complicated and articulated homeostatic response, of which hyperinsulinemia is only the most evident component. The profile of this response may vary greatly according to variable effects of genes and environment. Furthermore, all the interactions of the insulin-resistant phenotype we have described occur with other phenotypes, such as obesity, hypertension, diabetes, and dyslipidemia, each of which has long been known to be a complex phenotype on its own.

Finally, on top of this pyramid sits the atherosclerotic plaque, with its potential to become a complicated lesion. This ascending hierarchy is also a hierarchy of complexity.

Better understanding of these processes will be rooted necessarily in novel technologies, but also in innovative thinking tools. Sophisticated improvements in factor analysis, neural networks, and applications of chaos theory may be the heralds of this new era [121].

Acknowledgments

This work was supported in part by University of Verona Medical School Grants (60%) to R.C. Bonadonna. I am deeply indebted to many colleagues and friends, who over the years have shared with me their reflections and in-depth insights on the topic of this chapter. They are too many to be quoted, and I apologize to them for not doing so, but special thanks are due to Enzo Bonora and Stefano Del Prato. I thank John Yudkin for critically reading the manuscript and for offering many helpful suggestions.

REFERENCES

1. Bonadonna R, Groop L, Kraemer N, Ferrannini E, Del Prato S, DeFronzo RA. Obesity and insulin resistance in man: a dose–response study. *Metabolism* 1990; 39: 452–8.
2. Bonadonna RC, Del Prato S, Bonora E, Saccomani MP, Gulli G, Natali A, Frascerra S, Pecori N, Ferrannini E, Bier D, Cobelli C, DeFronzo RA. Roles of glucose transport and glucose phosphorylation in muscle insulin resistance of type 2 (non-insulin-dependent) diabetes mellitus. *Diabetes* 1996; 45: 915–25.
3. McKane WR, Stevens AB, Woods R, Andrews WJ, Henry RW, Bell PM. The assessment of hepatic and peripheral insulin sensitivity in hypertriglyceridemia. *Metabolism* 1990; 39: 1240–5.
4. Karhapaa P, Malkki M, Laakso M. Isolated low HDL cholesterol. An insulin-resistant state Diabetes 1994; 43 (3): 411–7.
5. Ferrannini E, Buzzigoli G, Bonadonna R, Giorico MA, Oleggini M, Graziadei L, Pedrinelli R, Brandi L, Bevilacqua S. Insulin resistance in essential hypertension: sites and mechanisms. *N Engl J Med* 1987; 317: 350–7.
6. Reaven GM. The role of insulin resistance and hyperinsulinemia in coronary heart disease. *Metabolism* 1992; 41 (5, suppl 1): 16–9.
7. Reaven GM. Banting lecture 1988. Role of insulin resistance in human disease. *Diabetes* 1988; 37: 1595–607.
8. WHO Consultation Group. Definition, diagnosis and classification of diabetes mellitus and its complications. Report of a WHO consultation. Part 1: diagnosis and classification of diabetes mellitus. Geneva: WHO, 1999. WHO/NCD/NCS/99.2.
9. Executive Summary of the Third Report of the National Cholesterol Education Program (NCEP) Expert Panel on Detection, Evaluation, and Treatment of High Blood Cholesterol in Adults (Adult Treatment Panel III). *JAMA* 2001; 285: 2486–97.
10. Natali A, Vichi S, Landi P, Severi S, L'Abbate A, Ferrannini E. Coronary atherosclerosis in type 2 diabetes: angiographic findings and clinical outcome. *Diabetologia* 2000; 43: 632–41.
11. Laakso M, Sarlund H, Salonen R, Suhonen M, Pyorala K, Salonen JT, Karhapaa P. Asymptomatic atherosclerosis and insulin resistance. *Arterioscler Thromb* 1991; 11: 1068–76.
12. Abe H, Yamada N, Kamata K, Kuwaki T, Shimada M, Osuga J, Shionoiri F, Yahagi N, Kadowaki T, Tamemoto H, Ishibashi S, Yazaki Y, Makuuchi M. Hypertension, hypertriglyceridemia, and impaired endothelium-dependent vascular relaxation in mice lacking insulin receptor substrate-1. *J Clin Invest* 1998; 101: 1784–8.
13. Meigs JB, D'Agostino RB Sr, Wilson PW, Cupples LA, Nathan DM, Singer DE. Risk variable clustering in the insulin resistance syndrome: the Framingham Offspring Study. *Diabetes* 1997; 46: 1594–600.
14. Gray RS, Fabsitz RR, Cowan LD, Lee ET, Howard BV, Savage PJ. Risk factor clustering in the insulin resistance syndrome: the Strong Heart Study. *Am J Epidemiol* 1998; 148: 869–78.
15. Chen W, Srinivasan SR, Elkasabany A, Berenson GS. Cardiovascular risk factors clustering features of insulin resistance syndrome (syndrome X) in a biracial (Black–White) population of children, adolescents, and young adults: the Bogalusa Heart Study. *Am J Epidemiol* 1999; 150: 667–74.
16. Chen CH, Lin KC, Tsai ST, Chou P. Different association of hypertension and insulin-related metabolic syndrome between men and women in 8437 nondiabetic Chinese. *Am J Hypertens* 2000; 13: 846–53.
17. Snehalatha C, Sivasankari S, Satyavani K, Vijay V, Ramachandran A. Insulin resistance alone does not explain the clustering of cardiovascular risk factors in southern India. *Diabet Med* 2000; 17: 152–7.
18. Shmulewitz D, Auerbach SB, Lehner T, Blundell ML, Winick JD, Youngman LD, Skilling V, Heath SC, Ott J, Stoffel M, Breslow JL, Friedman JM. Epidemiology and factor analysis of obesity, type II diabetes, hypertension, and dyslipidemia (syndrome X) on the Island of Kosrae, Federated States of Micronesia. *Hum Hered* 2001; 51: 8–19.
19. Hodge AM, Boyko EJ, de Courten M, Zimmet PZ, Chitson P, Tuomilehto J, Alberti KG. Leptin and other components of the metabolic syndrome in Mauritius—a factor analysis. *Int J Obes Relat Metab Disord* 2001; 25: 126–31.
20. Edwards KL, Newman B, Mayer E, Selby JV, Krauss RM, Austin MA. Heritability of factors of the insulin resistance syndrome in women twins. *Genet Epidemiol* 1997; 14: 241–53.
21. Arya R, Blangero J, Williams K, Almasy L, Dyer TD, Leach RJ, O'Connell P, Stern MP, Duggirala R. Factors of insulin resistance syndrome-related phenotypes are linked to genetic locations on chromosomes 6 and 7 in nondiabetic Mexican-Americans. *Diabetes* 2002; 51: 841–7.
22. Grundy SM. Obesity, metabolic syndrome, and coronary atherosclerosis. *Circulation* 2002; 105: 2696–8.
23. Bonora E, Kiechl S, Willeit J, Oberhollenzer F, Egger G, Targher G, Alberiche M, Bonadonna RC, Muggeo M. Prevalence of insulin resistance in metabolic disorders. The Bruneck Study. *Diabetes* 1998; 47: 1643–9.
24. Yudkin JS. Abnormalities of coagulation and fibrinolysis in insulin resistance. Evidence for a common antecedent? *Diabetes Care* 1999; 22 (suppl 3): C25–30.
25. Stern MP. Diabetes and cardiovascular disease. The "common soil" hypothesis. *Diabetes* 1995; 44: 369–74.
26. Bonora E, Willeit J, Kiechl S, Oberhollenzer F, Egger G, Bonadonna R, Muggeo M. Relationship between insulin and carotid atherosclerosis in the general population. The Bruneck Study. *Stroke* 1997; 28: 1147–52.
27. Bonora E, Willeit J, Kiechl S, Oberhollenzer F, Egger G, Bonadonna R, Muggeo M. U-shaped and J-shaped relationships between serum insulin and coronary heart disease in the general population: the Bruneck Study. *Diabetes Care* 1998; 21: 221–30.

28. Howard G, O'Leary DH, Zaccaro D, Haffner S, Rewers M, Hamman R, Selby JV, Saad MF, Savage P, Bergman R, for the The Insulin Resistance Atherosclerosis Study (IRAS) Investigators. Insulin sensitivity and atherosclerosis. *Circulation* 1996; 93: 1809–17.
29. Ruige JB, Assendelft WJ, Dekker JM, Kostense PJ, Heine RJ, Bouter LM. Insulin and risk of cardiovascular disease: a meta-analysis. *Circulation* 1998; 97: 996–1001.
30. Boquist S, Ruotolo G, Tang R, Bjorkegren J, Bond MG, de Faire U, Karpe F, Hamsten A. Alimentary lipemia, postprandial triglyceride-rich lipoproteins, and common carotid intima-media thickness in healthy, middle-aged men. *Circulation* 1999; 100: 723–8.
31. Bokemark L, Wikstrand J, Wedel H, Fagerberg B. Insulin, insulin propeptides and intima-media thickness in the carotid artery in 58-year-old clinically healthy men: the Atherosclerosis and Insulin Resistance (AIR) Study. *Diabet Med* 2002; 19: 144–51.
32. Yudkin JS, May M, Elwood P, Yarnell JWG, Greenwood R, Davey Smith G. Concentrations of proinsulin like molecules predict coronary heart disease risk independently of insulin: prospective data from the Caerphilly study. *Diabetologia* 2002; 45: 327–36.
33. Schneider DJ, Nordt TK, Sobel BE. Stimulation by proinsulin of expression of plasminogen activator inhibitor type-I in endothelial cells. *Diabetes* 1992; 41: 890–5.
34. Nordt TK, Sawa H, Fujii S, Bode C, Sobel BE. Augmentation of arterial endothelial cell expression of the plasminogen activator inhibitor type-1 (PAI-1) gene by proinsulin and insulin *in vivo*. *J Mol Cell Cardiol* 1998; 30: 1535–43.
35. Bonora E, Formentini G, Calcaterra F, Lombardi S, Marini F, Zenari L, Saggiani F, Poli M, Perbellini S, Raffaelli A, Cacciatori V, Santi L, Targher G, Bonadonna R, Muggeo M. HOMA—estimated insulin resistance is an independent predictor of cardiovascular disease in type 2 diabetic subjects: prospective data from the Verona Diabetes Complications Study. *Diabetes Care* 2002; 25: 1135–41.
36. Lempiainen P, Mykkanen L, Pyorala K, Laakso M, Kuusisto J. Insulin resistance syndrome predicts coronary heart disease events in elderly nondiabetic men. *Circulation* 1999; 100: 123–8.
37. Pyorala M, Miettinen H, Halonen P, Laakso M, Pyorala K. Insulin resistance syndrome predicts the risk of coronary heart disease and stroke in healthy middle-aged men: the 22-year follow-up results of the Helsinki Policemen Study. *Arterioscler Thromb Vasc Biol* 2000; 20: 538–44.
38. Kuusisto J, Lempiainen P, Mykkanen L, Laakso M. Insulin resistance syndrome predicts coronary heart disease events in elderly type 2 diabetic men. *Diabetes Care* 2001; 24: 1629–33.
39. DeFronzo RA, Tobin JD, Andres R. Glucose clamp technique: a method for quantifying insulin secretion and resistance. *Am J Physiol* 1979; 237: E214–23.
40. Stern MP. Strategies and prospects for finding insulin resistance genes. *J Clin Invest* 2000; 106: 323–7.
41. American Diabetes Association. Consensus Development Conference on Insulin Resistance. *Diabetes Care* 1998; 21: 310–4.
42. Lusis AJ. Atherosclerosis. *Nature* 2000; 407: 233–41.
43. Lewis GF, Steiner G. Acute effects of insulin in the control of VLDL production in humans. Implications for the insulin-resistant state. *Diabetes Care* 1996; 19: 390–3.
44. Baron AD, Brechtel-Hook G, Johnson A, Hardin D. Skeletal muscle blood flow. A possible link between insulin resistance and blood pressure. *Hypertension* 1993; 21: 129–35.
45. Taddei S, Virdis A, Mattei P, Natali A, Ferrannini E, Salvetti A. Effect of insulin on acetylcholine-induced vasodilation in normotensive subjects and patients with essential hypertension. *Circulation* 1995; 92: 2911–8.
46. Steinberg HO, Chaker H, Leaming R, Johnson A, Brechtel G, Baron AD. Obesity/insulin resistance is associated with endothelial dysfunction. Implications for the syndrome of insulin resistance. *J Clin Invest* 1996; 97: 2601–10.
47. Trovati M, Anfossi G, Cavalot F, Massucco P, Mularoni E, Emanuelli G. Insulin directly reduces platelet sensitivity to aggregating agents. Studies *in vitro* and *in vivo*. *Diabetes* 1988; 37: 780–6.
48. Trovati M, Anfossi G, Massucco P, Mattiello L, Costamagna C, Piretto V, Mularoni E, Cavalot F, Bosia A, Ghigo D. Insulin stimulates nitric oxide synthesis in human platelets and, through nitric oxide, increases platelet concentrations of both guanosine-3′,5′-cyclic monophosphate and adenosine-3′,5′-cyclic monophosphate. *Diabetes* 1997; 46: 742–9.
49. Steinberg HO, Baron AD. Vascular function, insulin resistance and fatty acids. *Diabetologia* 2002; 45: 623–34.
50. De Caterina R. Endothelial dysfunctions: common denominators in vascular disease. *Curr Opin Clin Nutr Metab Care* 2000; 3: 453–67.
51. Sartori C, Scherrer U. Insulin, nitric oxide and the sympathetic nervous system: at the crossroads of metabolic and cardiovascular regulation. *J Hypertens* 1999; 17: 1517–25.
52. Emdin M, Gastaldelli A, Muscelli E, Macerata A, Natali A, Camastra S, Ferrannini E. Hyperinsulinemia and autonomic nervous system dysfunction in obesity: effects of weight loss. *Circulation* 2001; 103: 513–9.
53. Gastaldelli A, Emdin M, Conforti F, Camastra S, Ferrannini E. Insulin prolongs the QTc interval in humans. *Am J Physiol* 2000; 279: R2022–5.
54. Khan IA. Clinical and therapeutic aspects of congenital and acquired long QT syndrome. *Am J Med* 2002; 112: 58–66.
55. Quinones-Galvan A, Sironi AM, Baldi S, Galetta F, Garbin U, Fratta-Pasini A, Cominacini L, Ferrannini E. Evidence that acute insulin administration enhances LDL cholesterol susceptibility to oxidation in healthy humans. *Arterioscler Thromb Vasc Biol* 1999; 19: 2928–32.
56. Arcaro G, Cretti A, Balzano S, Lechi A, Muggeo M, Bonora E, Bonadonna RC. Insulin causes endothelial dysfunction in humans. Sites and mechanisms. *Circulation* 2002; 105: 576–82.
57. Cardillo C, Nambi SS, Kilcoyne CM, Choucair WK, Katz A, Quon MJ, Panza JA. Insulin stimulates both endothelin and nitric oxide activity in the human forearm. *Circulation* 1999; 100: 820–5.
58. Luft FC. Proinflammatory effects of angiotensin II and endothelin: targets for progression of cardiovascular and renal diseases. *Curr Opin Nephrol Hypertens* 2002; 11: 59–66.
59. Dashwood MR, Tsui JC. Endothelin-1 and atherosclerosis: potential complications associated with endothelin-receptor blockade. *Atherosclerosis* 2002; 160: 297–304.

60. Reaven GM. Insulin resistance, compensatory hyperinsulinemia, and coronary heart disease: syndrome X revisited. In Jefferson LS, Cherrington AD (eds) *The Endocrine Pancreas and Regulation of Metabolism*. Oxford: Oxford University Press, 2001; pp 1169–97. Goodman HM (sect ed.) *Handbook of Physiology, Sect 7: The Endocrine System*; Vol II.
61. Saltiel AR, Kahn CR. Insulin signalling and the regulation of glucose and lipid metabolism. *Nature* 2001; 414 (6865): 799–806.
62. Kuboki K, Jiang ZY, Takahara N, Ha SW, Igarashi M, Yamauchi T, Feener EP, Herbert TP, Rhodes CJ, King GL. Regulation of endothelial constitutive nitric oxide synthase gene expression in endothelial cells and *in vivo*: a specific vascular action of insulin. *Circulation* 2000; 101: 676–81.
63. Zeng G, Nystrom FH, Ravichandran LV, Cong LN, Kirby M, Mostowski H, Quon MJ. Roles for insulin receptor, PI3-kinase, and Akt in insulin-signaling pathways related to production of nitric oxide in human vascular endothelial cells. *Circulation* 2000; 101: 1539–45.
64. Montagnani M, Chen H, Barr VA, Quon MJ. Insulin-stimulated activation of eNOS is independent of Ca^{2+} but requires phosphorylation by Akt at Ser (1179). *J Biol Chem* 2001; 276: 30392–8.
65. Radomski MW, Salas E. Nitric oxide—biological mediator, modulator and factor of injury: its role in the pathogenesis of atherosclerosis. *Atherosclerosis* 1995; 118 (suppl): S69–80.
66. De Caterina R, Libby P, Peng HB, Thannickal VJ, Rajavashisth TB, Gimbrone MA Jr, Shin WS, Liao JK. Nitric oxide decreases cytokine-induced endothelial activation. Nitric oxide selectively reduces endothelial expression of adhesion molecules and proinflammatory cytokines. *J Clin Invest* 1995; 96: 60–8.
67. Federici M, Menghini R, Mauriello A, Hribal ML, Ferrelli F, Lauro D, Sbraccia P, Spagnoli LG, Sesti G, Lauro R. Insulin-dependent activation of eNOS is impaired by O-linked-glycosylation modification of signaling proteins in human coronary endothelial cells. *Circulation* 2002; 106: 466–72.
68. Galis ZS, Khatri JJ. Matrix metalloproteinases in vascular remodeling and atherogenesis. The good, the bad, and the ugly. *Circ Res* 2002; 90: 251–62.
69. Accili D. A kinase in the life of the beta cell. *J Clin Invest* 2001; 108: 1575–6.
70. Walsh K, Smith RC, KimH-S. Vascular cell apoptosis in remodeling, restenosis, and plaque rupture. *Circ Res* 2000; 87: 184–8.
71. Mothe I, Van Obberghen E. Phopshorylation of insulin receptor substrate 1 multiple serine residues 612, 662, and 731 modulates insulin action. *J Biol Chem* 1996; 271: 11222–7.
72. Kanety H, Feinstein R, Papa MZ, Hemi R, Karasik A. Tumor necrosis factor-alpha induced phosphorylation of insulin receptor substrate-1 (IRS-1). Possible mechanisms for suppression of insulin-stimulated tyrosine phosphorylation of IRS-1. *J Biol Chem* 1995; 270: 23780–4.
73. Stout RW. Insulin as a mitogenic factor: role in the pathogenesis of cardiovascular disease. *Am J Med* 1991; 90 (2A): 62S–5S.
74. Hsueh WA, Law RE. Insulin signaling in the arterial wall. *Am J Cardiol* 1999; 84 (1A): 21J–4J.
75. Nickenig G, Bohm M. Interaction between insulin and AT1 receptor. Relevance for hypertension and arteriosclerosis. *Basic Res Cardiol* 1998; 93 (suppl 2): 135–9.
76. Hopfner RL, Hasnadka RV, McNeill JR, Wilson TW, Gopalakrishnan V. Differential regulation of endothelin-1 action by insulin and vanadate in vascular smooth muscle. *J Cardiovasc Pharmacol* 1998; 31 (suppl 1): S196–8.
77. Banfi C, Eriksson P, Giandomenico G, Mussoni L, Sironi L, Hamsten A, Tremoli E. Transcriptional regulation of plasminogen activator inhibitor type 1 gene by insulin: insights into the signaling pathway. *Diabetes* 2001; 50: 1522–30.
78. Cusi K, Maezono K, Osman A, Pendergrass M, Patti ME, Pratipanawatr T, DeFronzo RA, Kahn CR, Mandarino LJ. Insulin resistance differentially affects the PI 3-kinase- and MAP kinase-mediated signaling in human muscle. *J Clin Invest* 2000; 105: 311–20.
79. Montagnani M, Golovchenko I, Kim I, Koh GY, Goalstone ML, Mundhekar AN, Johansen M, Kucik DF, Quon MJ, Draznin B. Inhibition of phosphatidylinositol 3-kinase enhances mitogenic actions of insulin in endothelial cells. *J Biol Chem* 2002; 277: 1794–9.
80. Barnes PJ, karin M. Nuclear factor-κB—a pivotal transcription factor in chronic inflammatory diseases. *N Engl J Med* 1997; 336: 1066–71.
81. Shulman GI. Cellular mechanisms of insulin resistance. *J Clin Invest* 2000; 106: 171–6.
82. Kim JK, KimY-J, Fillmore JJ, Chen Y, Moore I, Lee J, Yuan M, Zhi Wei Li, Karin M, Perret P, Shoelson SE, Shulman GI. Prevention of fat-induced insulin resistance by salicylate. *J Clin Invest* 2001; 108: 437–46.
83. Gao Z, Hwang D, Bataille F, Lefevre M, York D, Quon MJ, Ye J. Serine phosphorylation of insulin receptor substrate 1 by inhibitor kappa B kinase complex. *J Biol Chem* 2002; 277: 48115–21.
84. Yudkin JS, Stehouwer CDA, Emeis JJ, Coppack SW. C-reactive protein in healthy subjects: associations with obesity, insulin resistance, and endothelial dysfunction. A potential role for cytokine originating from adipose tissue? *Arterioscler Thromb Vasc Biol* 1999; 19: 972–8.
85. Pickup JC, Crook MA. Is type II diabetes mellitus a disease of the innate immune system? *Diabetologia* 1998; 41: 1241–8.
86. Kiechl S, Lorenz E, Reindl M, Wiedermann CJ, Oberhollenzer F, Bonora E, Willeit J, Schwartz DA. Toll-like receptor 4 polymorphisms and atherogenesis in humans. *N Engl J Med* 2002; 347: 185–92.
87. Yudkin JS, Juhan-Vague I, Hawe E, Humphries SE, Di Minno G, Mergaglione M, Tremoli E, Kooistra T, Morange PE, Lundman P, Mohamed-Ali V, Hamsten A. On behalf of the HIFMECH Study Group. The insulin resistance syndrome and inflammatory markers in relation to myocardial infarction in North and South Europe (HIFMECH Study). In press.
88. Stary HC, Chandler AB, Glagov S, Guyton JR, Insull W Jr, Rosenfeld ME, Schaffer SA, Schwartz CJ, Wagner WD, Wissler RW. A definition of initial, fatty streak, and intermediate lesions of atherosclerosis. A report from the Committee on Vascular Lesions of the Council on Arteriosclerosis, American Heart Association. *Circulation* 1994; 89: 2462–78.
89. Berliner JA, Navab M, Fogelman AM, Frank JS, Demer LL, Edwards PA, Watson AD, Lusis AJ. Atherosclerosis:

basic mechanisms. Oxidation, inflammation, and genetics. *Circulation* 1995; 91: 2488–96.

90. Rapp JH, Lespine A, Hamilton RL, Colyvas N, Chaumeton AH, Tweedie-Hardman J, Kotite L, Kunitake ST, Havel RJ, Kane JP. Triglyceride-rich lipoproteins isolated by selected-affinity anti-apolipoprotein B immunosorption from human atherosclerotic plaque. *Arterioscler Thromb* 1994; 14: 1767–74.
91. Coresh J, Kwiterovich PO Jr, Smith HH, Bachorik PS. Association of plasma triglyceride concentration and LDL particle diameter, density, and chemical composition with premature coronary artery disease in men and women. *J Lipid Res* 1993; 34: 1687–97.
92. Trovati M, Mularoni EM, Burzacca S, Ponziani MC, Massucco P, Mattiello L, Piretto V, Cavalot F, Anfossi G. Impaired insulin-induced platelet antiaggregating effect in obesity and in obese NIDDM patients. *Diabetes* 1995; 44: 1318–22.
93. Dzau VJ. Cell biology and genetics of angiotensin in cardiovascular disease. *J Hypertens* 1994; 12 (suppl): S3–10.
94. Rajagopalan S, Kurz S, Munzel T, Tarpey M, Freeman BA, Griendling KK, Harrison DG. Angiotensin II-mediated hypertension in the rat increases vascular superoxide production via membrane NADH/NADPH oxidase activation. Contribution to alterations of vasomotor tone. *J Clin Invest* 1996; 97: 1916–23.
95. Busse R, Fleming I. Molecular responses of endothelial tissue to kinins. *Diabetes* 1996; 45 (suppl 1): S8–13.
96. Yagi S, Takata S, Kiyokawa H, Yamamoto M, Noto Y, Ikeda T, Hattori N. Effects of insulin on vasoconstrictive responses to norepinephrine and angiotensin II in rabbit femoral artery and vein. *Diabetes* 1988; 37: 1064–7.
97. Folli F, Kahn CR, Hansen H, Bouchie JL, Feener EP. Angiotensin II inhibits insulin signaling in aortic smooth muscle cells at multiple levels. A potential role for serine phosphorylation in insulin/angiotensin II crosstalk. *J Clin Invest* 1997; 100: 2158–69.
98. Ritchie RH, Marsh JD, Lancaster WD, Diglio CA, Schiebinger RJ. Bradykinin blocks angiotensin II-induced hypertrophy in the presence of endothelial cells. *Hypertension* 1998; 31: 39–44.
99. Parthasarathy S, Barnett J, Fong LG. High-density lipoprotein inhibits the oxidative modification of low-density lipoprotein. *Biochim Biophys Acta* 1990; 1044: 275–83.
100. Navab M, Imes SS, Hama SY, Hough GP, Ross LA, Bork RW, Valente AJ, Berliner JA, Drinkwater DC, Laks H, Fogelman AM. Monocyte transmigration induced by modification of low density lipoprotein in cocultures of human aortic wall cells is due to induction of monocyte chemotactic protein 1 synthesis and is abolished by high density lipoprotein. *J Clin Invest* 1991; 88: 2039–46.
101. Cavalot F, Russo I, Mattiello L, Anfossi G, Massucco P, Mularoni E, Hahn AW, Trovati M. Influence of protamine on adhesion, chemotaxis and proliferation of human vascular smooth muscle cells. *Diabetologia* 1997; 40: 67–75.
102. Trovati M, Anfossi G. Influence of insulin and of insulin resistance on platelet and vascular smooth muscle cell function. *J Diabetes Complications* 2002; 16: 35–40.
103. Ruderman N, Chishiolm D, Pi-Sunyer X, Schneider S. The metabolically obese, normal-weight individuals revisited. *Diabetes* 1998; 47: 699–713.
104. Marchetti P, Lupi R, Federici M, Marselli L, Masini M, Boggi U, Del Guerra S, Patane G, Piro S, Anello M, Bergamini E, Purrello F, Lauro R, Mosca F, Sesti G, Del Prato S. Insulin secretory function is impaired in isolated human islets carrying the Gly(972)–> Arg IRS-1 polymorphism. *Diabetes* 2002; 51: 1419–24.
105. Baroni MG, D'Andrea MP, Montali A, Pannitteri G, Barilla F, Campagna F, Mazzei E, Lovari S, Seccareccia F, Campa PP, Ricci G, Pozzilli P, Urbinati G, Arca M. A common mutation of the insulin receptor substrate-1 gene is a risk factor for coronary artery disease. *Arterioscler Thromb Vasc Biol* 1999; 19: 2975–80.
106. Neel JV. The "thrifty genotype" in 1998. *Nutr Rev* 1999; 57: S2–9.
107. Petry CJ, Ozanne SE, Hales CN. Programming of intermediary metabolism. *Mol Cell Endocrinol* 2001; 185: 81–91.
108. Unger RH. Lipotoxic diseases. *Annu Rev Med* 2002; 53: 319–36.
109. Havel PJ. Control of energy homeostasis and insulin action by adipocyte hormones: leptin, acylation stimulating protein, and adiponectin. *Curr Opin Lipidol* 2002; 13: 51–9.
110. Moller DE. Potential role of TNF-α in the pathogenesis of insulin resistance and type 2 diabetes. *Trends Endocrinol Metab* 2000; 11: 212–7.
111. Cummings DE, Weigle DS, Frayo RS, Breen PA, Ma MK, Dellinger EP, Purnell JQ. Plasma ghrelin levels after diet-induced weight loss or gastric bypass surgery. *N Engl J Med* 2002; 346: 1623–30.
112. Levade T, Augé N, Veldman RJ, Cuvillier O, Negre-Salvayre A, Salvayre R. Sphingolipid mediators in cardiovascular cell biology and pathology. *Circul Res* 2001; 89: 957–68.
113. Kolesnick R. The therapeutic potential of modulating the ceramide/sphingomyelin pathway. *J Clin Invest* 2002; 110: 3–8.
114. Itani SI, Ruderman NB, Schmieder F, Boden G. Lipid-induced insulin resistance in human muscle is associated with changes in diacylglycerol, protein kinase C, and I-κB-α. *Diabetes* 2002; 51: 2005–11.
115. Gruntzig A, Kuhlmann U, Vetter W, Lutolf U, Meier B, Siegenthaler W. Treatment of renovascular hypertension with percutaneous transluminal dilatation of a renal-artery stenosis. *Lancet* 1978; 1: 801–2.
116. Gruntzig AR, Senning A, Siegenthaler WE. Nonoperative dilatation of coronary-artery stenosis: percutaneous transluminal coronary angioplasty. *N Engl J Med* 1979; 301: 61–8.
117. Nishimoto Y, Miyazaki Y, Toki Y, Murakami R, Shinoda M, Fukushima A, Kanayama H. Enhanced secretion of insulin plays a role in the development of atherosclerosis and restenosis of coronary arteries: elective percutaneous transluminal coronary angioplasty in patients with effort angina. *J Am Coll Cardiol* 1998; 32: 1624–9.
118. Osanai H, Kanayama H, Miyazaki Y, Fukushima A, Shinoda M, Ito T. Usefulness of enhanced insulin secretion during an oral glucose tolerance test as a predictor of restenosis after direct percutaneous transluminal coronary angioplasty during acute myocardial infarction in patients without diabetes mellitus. *Am J Cardiol* 1998; 81: 698–701.

119. Takagi T, Akasaka T, Yamamuro A, Honda Y, Hozumi T, Morioka S, Yoshida K. Troglitazone reduces neointimal tissue proliferation after coronary stent implantation in patients with non-insulin dependent diabetes mellitus: a serial intravascular ultrasound study. *J Am Coll Cardiol* 2000; 36: 1529–35.
120. Ghanim H, Garg R, Aljada A, Mohanty P, Kumbkarni Y, Assian E, Hamouda W, Dandona P. Suppression of nuclear factor-kappaB and stimulation of inhibitor kappaB by troglitazone: evidence for an anti-inflammatory effect and a potential antiatherosclerotic effect in the obese. *J Clin Endocrinol Metab* 2001; 86: 1306–12.
121. Lisboa PJ. A review of evidence of health benefit from artificial neural networks in medical intervention. *Neural Netw* 2002; 15: 11–39.

78

Metabolic Stress and Atherosclerosis

Jane E.-B. Reusch* **and Michael Brownlee†**

**University of Colorado School of Medicine, Denver, CO, USA, and*
†Albert Einstein College of Medicine, Bronx, NY, USA

INTRODUCTION

Diabetes is associated with accelerated atherosclerotic macrovascular disease affecting arteries that supply the heart, brain, and lower extremities. As a consequence, patients with diabetes have a much higher risk of myocardial infarction (MI), stroke, and limb amputation. The excess risk associated with diabetes remains even after adjustment for traditional coronary heart disease risk factors such as smoking, hypertension, and hypercholesterolemia [1–3]. Type 2 diabetic patients without a previous myocardial infarction have as high a risk of MI over 7 years as nondiabetic patients with a previous MI [4]. The mechanisms by which diabetes confers this increased risk are much less clear than those responsible for diabetic microvascular disease, but associational studies suggest that the metabolic derangements caused by insulin resistance (IR) are involved. The continuum of cardiovascular disease (CVD) risk with increasing glucose levels has also been identified in patients with type 1 diabetes, and in subjects without clinically overt diabetes but with varying degrees of glucose tolerance [5, 6]. High glucose levels in individuals with acute MI or stroke without previous known diabetes can be used to identify high-risk patients. A recent trial indicates that 66% of individuals (without prior known diabetes) presenting with an acute MI have either diabetes mellitus (31%) or impaired glucose tolerance (35%) [7]. Thus high glucose worsens prognosis and is very common in persons with acute MI and stroke. These observations are consistent with a causal role for hyperglycemia, but are equally consistent with a causal role for insulin resistance, with hyperglycemia simply being a marker of IR. In patients spanning the spectrum of glucose tolerance from normal to impaired glucose tolerance to frank diabetes, IR positively correlates with the degree of atherosclerosis [8].

Prospective studies have demonstrated that hyperglycemia contributes significantly to the microvascular complications of diabetes including retinopathy, neuropathy, and nephropathy, but they have not conclusively demonstrated that hyperglycemia causes macrovascular disease. The DCCT (Diabetes Control and Complications Trial), which was not powered to examine cardiovascular end points, showed a trend toward decreased cardiovascular events that did not reach statistical significance ($P = 0.06$) [9]. The largest prospective trial examining glycemic control in type 2 diabetic patients, the UKPDS (UK Prospective Diabetes Study), did not find improved cardiovascular outcomes in the intensive control group. This cohort did see improvements in microvascular disease and so the intervention was effective for microvascular disease [10]. To date, we do not have interventional data to demonstrate that glycemic control improves cardiovascular outcomes. In contrast, there are positive correlations between glycemic control and cardiovascular events in epidemiological studies [11]. Epidemiological studies of large cohorts from northern Finland indicate a direct correlation between glycosylated hemoglobin and coronary heart disease in type 2 diabetic patients [12, 13]. In the UKPDS, there was also a correlation of hemoglobin A_{1c} with cardiovascular events, but this relationship was only apparent at the lower levels of hemoglobin A_{1c}. These data suggest that despite important effects of hyperglycemia on the vessel wall, normalization of blood glucose alone has modest impact on diabetes-induced acceleration of CVDs. Rather, it appears that the aggregate of metabolic

International Textbook of Diabetes Mellitus, Third Edition. Edited by R. A. DeFronzo, E. Ferrannini, H. Keen, and P. Zimmet.
 ISBN: 0-471-48655-8.

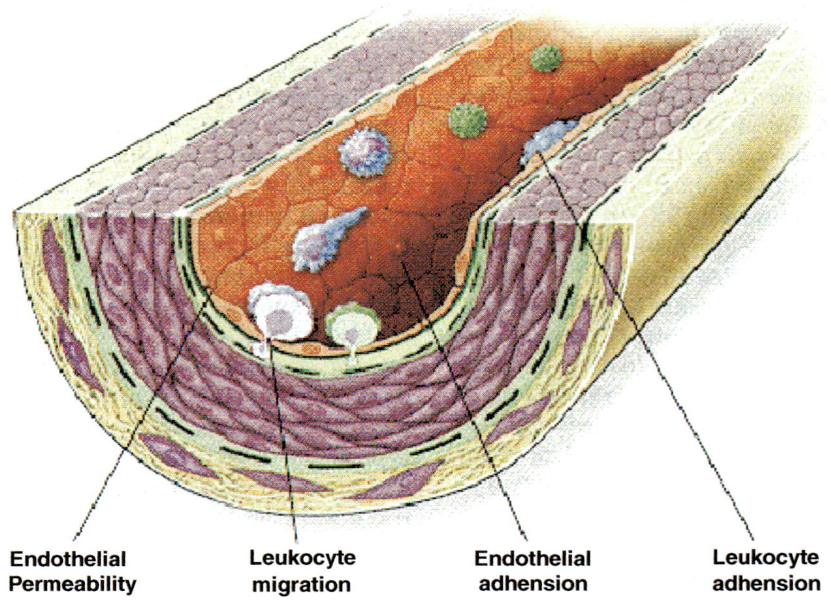

Figure 1 Diagrammatic representation of the vessel wall: The endothelial lining of the vessel wall is vasodilatory, anti-inflammatory, antioxidant, and antiproliferative. Under circumstances of chronic metabolic stress (glucose and FFA) the endothelium is injured and loses these antiatherogenic properties

alterations resulting from IR (including hyperglycemia, increased free fatty acid (FFA) flux, hypertension, lipoprotein abnormalities, and a prothrombotic state—collectively termed the metabolic syndrome) lead to progressive macrovascular disease [14, 15]. Alternatively it could result from an effect of a common antecedent (e.g. low-grade inflammation) from adipocyte-derived cytokines [16]. Preliminary data suggest that increased FFA flux into arterial endothelial cells (due to IR) may be a central element in this process (M.B. and coworkers, unpublished data).

The case-fatality rate following MI is substantially higher in patients with diabetes [1, 3, 4]. Hyperglycemia itself appears to play a major role in CVD mortality, patients with the highest levels of fasting blood glucose having a CVD mortality rate nearly five times higher than that in patients with lower levels [17]. This may reflect differences in the response to plaque rupture and chronic vascular inflammation, rather than to differences in atherosclerosis. The DIGAMI (Diabetes Mellitus, Insulin Glucose Infusion in Acute Myocardial Infarction) trial [18] demonstrated that in subjects with either known diabetes or newly diagnosed diabetes, intensive treatment with insulin improves short-term and long-term mortality. Thus, acute hyperglycemia appears to play a major role in the response to acute ischemic cardiac events.

In this chapter, the mechanisms by which the metabolic stress of hyperglycemia and increased FFA flux may damage arterial vascular cells are reviewed, and a unified model for diabetes-induced accelerated atherosclerosis is presented.

The pathogenesis of atherosclerosis in nondiabetic patients has been extensively described in recent reviews (Figure 1), and begins with endothelial dysfunction [19]. Under normal circumstances, the endothelial cell layer serves to protect the arterial intima and media against circulating cells and factors such as glucose, FFAs, and lipoproteins. The endothelial cell layer also provides an anticoagulant and fibrinolytic surface by producing tissue plasminogen activator and prostacyclin, which counter the effects of procoagulant factors such as fibrinogen and plasminogen activator inhibitor (PAI-1). In addition, endothelial-cell-derived nitric oxide (NO) leads to vasodilation, and opposes the activity of vasoconstrictors such as angiotensin II and endothelin 1. NO also limits smooth muscle cell (SMC) migration and proliferation. Finally, healthy endothelium has minimal binding sites for platelets and inflammatory cells and only selective permeability. In the diabetic environment, evidence suggests that IR increases metabolic stress, leading to an overproduction of reactive oxygen species (ROS) that increases inflammation and undermines the protective mechanisms of the endothelium. This loss of normal endothelial function promotes the development of atherosclerosis.

The endothelial cell is the pivot point of normal vascular function as it has vasodilatory, anti-inflammatory, and antiproliferative functions. The metabolic environment in type 1 and type 2 diabetes, and to a lesser extent in the pre-diabetic state, is characterized by hyperglycemia, increased levels of FFA, and modified lipoproteins. Unfortunately, the endothelial cell is exquisitely sensitive to changes in glucose, FFAs, and lipoproteins. The impact of hyperglycemia on endothelial function (*in vivo* and *in vitro*) has been extensively studied by a number of groups. Changes in endothelial function observed *in vitro* with exposure to high glucose include increased generation of intracellular ROS, which leads to accumulation of intracellular advanced glycation end products (AGEs) increased flux through the polyol and glucosamine pathways, and stimulation of the proinflammatory transcription factor NF-κB [20]. In addition, hyperglycemia leads to accumulation of DAG, which activates protein kinase C (PKC). Together, these changes interfere with endothelial cell NO generation, increase expression of adhesion molecules that attract and activate platelets and white blood cells, and inactivate prostacyclin synthase [21, 22] (M.B. and coworkers, unpublished data). *In vivo*, acute infusion of either glucose or FFA decreases flow-mediated and acetylcholine-mediated vasodilation, a measure of NO-mediated endothelial function [23, 24]. In addition to interference with vasodilation, loss of NO may release the chronic restraint by NO on SMC activation (proliferation and migration). Hyperglycemia also stimulates PAI-1 production [25].

Both IR and hyperglycemia have been implicated in the pathogenesis of diabetic dyslipidemia. The role of IR has been reviewed recently [14, 15]. Indeed, with significant vascular endothelial dysfunction, the entire context at the vessel wall could be expected to switch. The combined loss of NO and attraction of platelets and inflammatory cells, which release platelet-derived growth factor (PDGF) and other growth promoting cytokines, leads to increased SMC migration and proliferation, while loss of prostacyclin synthase activity and increased PAI-1 would significantly increase thrombus formation after endothelial injury [26–30]. All of these effects potentially contribute to the development of atherosclerotic plaques and thrombus formation after plaque rupture. The potent effects of hyperglycemia *per se* on the endothelium make it somewhat surprising that glucose lowering does not have a more profound impact on clinical cardiovascular outcomes. This disconnection suggests that the other dysmetabolic factors are even more potent agents of vascular injury.

The effects of elevated levels of FFAs on the vasculature have been studied less extensively but are also proposed as an etiologic factor in diabetic vasculopathy. Similar to glucose, acute infusion of FFA leads to endothelial dysfunction [19, 31] and to accumulation of DAG and ceramide, which interfere with regulation of NO synthase (NOS). Additionally, fibrinolysis may be impaired by an FFA-induced increase in the level of PAI-1 [32]. In type 2 diabetic patients, the augmentation of PAI-1 levels

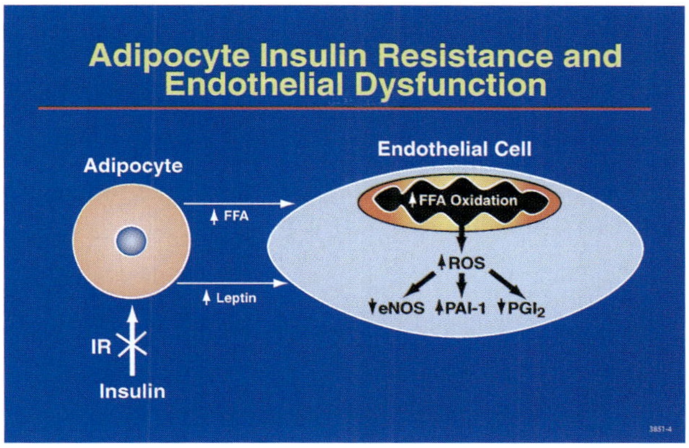

Figure 2 Schematic mechanism by which increased FFA flux may mediate the injurious effects of IR on arterial endothelial cells. PGI_2 = prostacyclin

may be exacerbated by hyperinsulinemia [33]. Similar to glucose, FFA infusion will decrease endothelial function acutely as will the FFA flux that occurs postprandially [34] *In vitro*, increased FFA rapidly leads to accumulation of intracellular ROS and activation of NFkB, which in turn increases expression of endothelial adhesion molecules. FFA-induced ROS also inhibit prostacylin synthase, activate PKC, increase intracellular AGE formation, and stimulate the polyol pathway and the hexosamine pathway (M.B. and coworkers, unpublished data). Since IR may result in increased FFA release from visceral fat, this may be the mechanism by which impaired glucose tolerance confers the same increased CVD risk as frank diabetes, rather than hyperglycemia (Figure 2).

Diabetic dyslipidemia occurs primarily in patients with type 2 diabetes or in those with the metabolic syndrome and is characterized by elevated triglycerides, small dense low-density lipoprotein (LDL) particles, and low high-density lipoprotein (HDL) concentrations. The finding that LDL cholesterol levels are not higher in patients with diabetes than in the general population [35] is offset by a number of other factors. The number of LDL particles in patients with diabetic dyslipidemia is usually increased because of abnormal composition of these particles, termed small dense LDL or B pattern [36]. Small dense LDL particles are oxidized more easily and interact with hepatic LDL receptors less effectively and are more readily taken up by scavenger LDL receptors located in the vasculature, which may explain why small dense LDL is more atherogenic [37]. The atherogenic interaction of small dense LDL particles may also be potentiated by elevated levels of postprandial lipoproteins [38] and decreased HDL, which occur by a variety of mechanisms [39]. The impact of lipids upon diabetic vascular disease is addressed in detail in other chapters of this textbook and is mentioned here because of clinical evidence that they represent modifiable cardiovascular risk factors that are known to affect outcomes. The remainder of this chapter discusses changes in vascular cellular function secondary to hyperglycemia, although recent work demonstrates that increased FFA flux causes increased mitochondrial generation of ROS and activates the same pathways in arterial endothelial cells as does hyperglycemia (M.B. and coworkers, unpublished data).

MECHANISMS OF METABOLITE-INDUCED DAMAGE

How does macrovascular pathology result from hyperglycemia and increased FFA? Four major hypotheses about how hyperglycemia and FFA cause diabetic complications have generated a large amount of data, as well as several clinical trials based on specific inhibitors of these mechanisms. The four hypotheses are increased polyol pathway flux, increased AGE formation, activation of PKC isoforms, and increased hexosamine pathway flux. These injurious pathways modified by hyperglycemia and FFA are considered primarily in terms of microvascular disease. It is becoming clear that these same destructive cellular responses are relevant for macrovascular disease because these pathways are dramatically dysregulated in the vascular endothelium. Until quite recently, there was no unifying hypothesis linking these four mechanisms together.

Increased Polyol Pathway Flux

Aldose reductase (alditol:NAD(P)$^+$ 1-oxidoreductase, EC 1.1.1.21) is the first enzyme in the polyol pathway. Aldose reductase has a low affinity (high K_m) for glucose, and at the normal glucose concentrations found in nondiabetic patients, metabolism of glucose by this pathway constitutes a very small percentage of total glucose utilization. However, in a hyperglycemic environment, increased intracellular glucose results in increased enzymatic conversion to the polyalcohol sorbitol, with concomitant decreases in NADPH. In the polyol pathway, sorbitol is oxidized to fructose by the enzyme sorbitol dehydrogenase, with NAD$^+$ reduced to NADH. Flux through this pathway during hyperglycemia varies from 33% of total glucose utilization in the rabbit lens to 11% in human erythrocytes. Thus, the contribution of this pathway to diabetic complications may be very much species-, site-, and tissue-dependent.

A number of mechanisms have been proposed to explain the potential detrimental effects of hyperglycemia-induced increases in polyol pathway flux. These include sorbitol-induced osmotic stress, decreased Na$^+$/K$^+$-ATPase activity, increased cytosolic NADH/NAD$^+$, and decreased cytosolic NADPH. Sorbitol does not diffuse easily across cell membranes, and it was originally suggested that this resulted in osmotic damage to microvascular cells. However, sorbitol concentrations measured in diabetic vessels and nerves are far too low to cause osmotic damage.

Another early suggestion was that increased flux through the polyol pathway decreased Na$^+$/K$^+$-ATPase activity. Although this was originally thought to be mediated by polyol-pathway-linked decreases in phosphatidylinositol synthesis, it has recently been shown to result from activation of PKC (see below). Hyperglycemia-induced activation of PKC increases cytosolic phospholipase A_2 activity, which increases the production of two inhibitors of Na$^+$/K$^+$-ATPase, arachidonate, and prostaglandin E_2 [40].

More recently, it has been proposed that oxidation of sorbitol by NAD$^+$ increases the cytosolic ratio of NADH/NAD$^+$, thereby inhibiting activity of the enzyme glyceraldehyde-3-phosphate dehydrogenase (GAPDH), and increasing concentrations of triose phosphate [41]. Elevated triose phosphate concentrations could increase formation of both methylglyoxal, a precursor of AGEs, and DAG (via α-glycerol-3-phosphate), thus activating PKC (discussed in subsequent sections). Although hyperglycemia does increase the NADH/NAD$^+$ ratio in endothelial cells, this reflects a marked decrease in the absolute concentration of NAD$^+$ due to consumption by activated poly(ADP-ribose) polymerase, rather than reduction of NAD$^+$ to NADH [42]. The source of hyperglycemia-induced ROS is discussed later in this review.

It has also been proposed that reduction of glucose to sorbitol by NADPH consumes the cofactor NADPH. Since NADPH is required for regenerating reduced glutathione (GSH), this could induce or exacerbate intracellular oxidative stress. Less reduced GSH has in fact been found in the lens of transgenic mice that overexpress aldose reductase, and this is the most likely mechanism by which increased flux through the polyol pathway has deleterious consequences [43]. This conclusion is further supported by recent experiments with aldose reductase deficient homozygous knockout mice, showing that in contrast to wild-type mice, diabetes neither decreases sciatic nerve GSH content nor reduces motor nerve conduction velocity (S.K. Chung, personal communication).

In vivo studies of polyol pathway inhibition have yielded inconsistent results. In a 5-year study in dogs, aldose reductase inhibition prevented diabetic neuropathy, but failed to prevent retinopathy or capillary basement membrane thickening in the retina, kidney, or muscle [44]. Several negative clinical trials have questioned the relevance of this mechanism in humans [45]. However, the positive effect of aldose reductase inhibition on diabetic neuropathy has been confirmed in humans in a rigorous multidose, placebo controlled trial with the potent aldose reductase inhibitor zenarestat [46].

Increased Intracellular AGE Formation

AGEs are found in increased amounts in diabetic retinal vessels [47], renal glomeruli [48], and arterial wall [49], where they can cause damage by mechanisms described later in this section. These AGEs were originally thought to arise from nonenzymatic reactions between extracellular proteins and glucose. However, the rate of AGE formation from glucose is orders of magnitude slower than the rate of AGE formation from glucose-derived dicarbonyl precursors generated intracellularly, and it now seems likely that intracellular hyperglycemia is the primary initiating event in the formation of both intracellular and extracellular AGEs [50]. AGEs can arise from intracellular autoxidation of glucose to glyoxal [51], decomposition of the Amadori product to 3-deoxyglucosone (perhaps accelerated by an amadoriase), and fragmentation of glyceraldehyde-3-phosphate and dihydroxyacetonephosphate to methylglyoxal [52]. These reactive intracellular dicarbonyls react with amino groups of intracellular and extracellular proteins to form AGEs. Methylglyoxal and glyoxal are detoxified by the glyoxalase system [52]. All three AGE precursors are also substrates for other reductases [53].

The potential importance of AGEs in the pathogenesis of diabetic complications is suggested by the observation in animal models that two structurally unrelated AGE inhibitors partially prevented various functional and structural manifestations of diabetic microvascular disease in retina, kidney, and nerve [54–56].

Intracellular production of AGE precursors damages target cells by three general mechanisms. First, intracellular proteins modified by AGEs have altered function. Second, extracellular matrix components modified by AGE precursors interact abnormally with other matrix components and with matrix receptors (integrins) on cells. Third, plasma proteins modified by AGE precursors bind to AGE receptors on endothelial cells, mesangial cells, and macrophages, inducing receptor-mediated ROS production. This AGE-receptor ligation activates the pleiotrophic transcription factor NF-κB, causing pathologic changes in gene expression.

In endothelial cells exposed to high glucose, intracellular AGE formation occurs within 1 week. Basic fibroblast growth factor is one of the major AGE-modified proteins in endothelial cells [57]. Proteins involved in macromolecular endocytosis are also modified by AGEs, since the increase in endocytosis induced by hyperglycemia is prevented by overexpression of the methylglyoxal-detoxifying enzyme glyoxalase I [58]. Glyoxalase-I overexpression also completely prevents the hyperglycemia-induced increase in Muller cell expression of angiopoietin-2 (T. Matsumura and coworkers, unpublished data), a factor that has been implicated in both pericyte loss and capillary regression [59].

AGE formation alters the functional properties of several important matrix molecules. On type I collagen, intermolecular cross-linking by AGEs induces an expansion of the molecular packing [60]. These AGE-induced cross-links alter the function of intact vessels. For example, AGEs decrease elasticity in large vessels from diabetic rats, even after vascular tone is abolished, and increase fluid filtration across the carotid artery [61]. AGE formation on type IV collagen from basement membrane inhibits lateral association of these molecules into a normal network-like structure by interfering with binding of the noncollagenous NC1 domain to the helix-rich domain [62]. AGE formation on laminin causes decreased polymer self-assembly, decreased binding to type IV collagen, and decreased binding of heparan sulfate proteoglycan [63].

AGE formation on extracellular matrix not only interferes with matrix–matrix interactions, it interferes with matrix–cell interactions as well. For example, AGE modification of type IV collagen's cell-binding domains decreases endothelial cell adhesion [64], and AGE modification of a six-amino acid growth-promoting sequence in the A chain of the laminin molecule markedly reduces neurite outgrowth [65].

Multiple cell-associated binding proteins for AGEs have been identified, including OST-48, 80K-H, galectin-3, the macrophage scavenger receptor type II, and RAGE (receptor for AGE) [30, 66–68]. Certain of these are more likely to contribute to clearance of AGEs, whereas others may underlie sustained cellular perturbations mediated by AGE-ligand binding. In cell culture systems, the receptors identified to date appear to mediate long-term effects of AGEs on key cellular targets of diabetic complications such as macrophages, glomerular mesangial cells, and vascular endothelial cells, although not all these receptors bind AGE-modified proteins having levels of AGEs found in diabetes. These effects include expression of cytokines and growth factors by macrophages and mesangial cells (IL-1, IGF-1, TNF-α, TGF-β, M-CSF, GM-CSF, and PDGF), and expression of procoagulatory/proinflammatory molecules by endothelial cells (thrombomodulin, tissue factor, and vascular cell adhesion molecule 1 [49, 69–73]. In addition, endothelial AGE receptor binding appears to mediate in part the hyperpermeability induced by diabetes, probably through the induction of vascular endothelial growth factor [74].

Consistent with this concept, blockade of one such receptor, RAGE, a member of the immunoglobulin superfamily with three immunoglobulin-like regions on a single polypeptide chain, suppressed macrovascular disease in an atherosclerosis-prone type 1 diabetic mouse model in a glucose- and lipoprotein-independent fashion [75]. RAGE has been shown to mediate signal transduction via generation of ROS, which activates both NF-κB and p21 ras [76, 77]. AGE signaling is blocked in cells by expression of RAGE antisense cDNA [78] or anti-RAGE ribozyme [79].

Activation of PKC

PKC comprises a family of at least 11 isoforms, 9 of which are activated by the lipid second messenger DAG. Intracellular hyperglycemia increases DAG content in cultured microvascular cells and in the retina and renal glomeruli of diabetic animals. Intracellular hyperglycemia appears to increase DAG content primarily by increasing its *de novo* synthesis from the glycolytic intermediate dihydroxyacetonephosphate *via* reduction to glycerol-3-phosphate and stepwise acylation [29]. Increased *de novo* synthesis of DAG activates PKC both in cultured vascular cells and in retina and glomeruli of diabetic animals [29, 80, 81]. Increased DAG primarily activates the β and δ isoforms of PKC, but increases in other isoforms have also been found, such as PKC-α and -ε isoforms in the retina [29] and PKC-α and -β in the glomerulus [82] of diabetic rats. Hyperglycemia may also activate PKC isoforms indirectly through both AGE-receptor ligation [83] and increased polyol pathway activity [84] presumably by increasing ROS.

In early experimental diabetes, activation of PKC-β isoforms has been shown to mediate retinal and renal blood flow abnormalities [84] perhaps by depressing NO production and/or increasing endothelin 1 activity. Abnormal activation of PKC has been implicated in the decreased glomerular production of NO induced by experimental diabetes [85], and in the decreased SMC NO production induced by hyperglycemia [86]. PKC activation also inhibits insulin-stimulated expression of endothelial NO synthase (eNOS) mRNA in cultured endothelial cells. Hyperglycemia increases endothelin 1-stimulated mitogen-activated protein kinase activity in glomerular mesangial cells by activating PKC isoforms [87]. The increased endothelial cell permeability induced by high glucose in cultured cells is mediated by activation of PKC-α, however [88]. Activation of PKC by elevated glucose also induces expression of the permeability-enhancing factor VEGF (vascular endothelial growth factor) in SMCs [89].

In addition to affecting hyperglycemia-induced abnormalities of blood flow and permeability, activation of PKC contributes to increased microvascular matrix protein accumulation by inducing expression of transforming growth factor β_1 (TGF-β_1), fibronectin, and α1(IV) collagen in both cultured mesangial cells [90] and in glomeruli of diabetic rats [80]. This effect appears to be mediated through PKC's inhibition of NO production [91, 92]. Hyperglycemia-induced activation of PKC has also been implicated in the overexpression of the fibrinolytic inhibitor PAI-1 [93], and in the activation of the pleiotrophic transcription factor NFκB in cultured endothelial cells and vascular SMCs [94]. PKC activation also regulates and activates various membrane-associated NAD(P)H-dependent oxidases.

Treatment with a β-isoform-specific PKC inhibitor significantly reduced PKC activity in the retina and renal glomeruli of diabetic animals. Concomitantly, treatment significantly reduced diabetes-induced increases in retinal mean circulation time, normalized increases in glomerular filtration rate, and partially corrected urinary albumin excretion [95]. Treatment of a type 2 diabetic mouse model (*db/db*) with a β-isoform-specific PKC inhibitor ameliorated accelerated glomerular mesangial expansion [95]. These inhibitors also decrease postangioplasty restentosis in the Zucker diabetic rat model [96].

Increased Hexosamine Pathway Flux

Shunting of excess intracellular glucose into the hexosamine pathway may also cause several manifestations of diabetic complications [97, 98]. In this pathway, fructose-6-phosphate is diverted from glycolysis to provide substrates for reactions that require uridine diphosphate-*N*-acetylglucosamine (UDP-GlcNAc), such as proteoglycan synthesis and the formation of O-linked glycoproteins (O-GlcNacylation). Inhibition of the rate-limiting enzyme in the conversion of glucose to glucosamine, glutamine:fructose-6-phosphate amidotransferase (GFAT), blocks hyperglycemia-induced increases in the transcription of TGF-α [97], TGF-β_1, and PAI-1 [25, 97]. This pathway has also been shown to play an important role in hyperglycemia-induced and fat-induced IR [98–101].

The mechanism by which increased flux through the hexosamine pathway mediates hyperglycemia-induced increases in gene transcription has not been clear, but the observation that Sp1 sites regulate hyperglycemia-induced activation of the PAI-1 promoter in vascular SMCs [99] suggested that covalent modification of Sp1 by *N*-acetylglucosamine might explain the link between hexosamine pathway activation and hyperglycemia-induced changes in PAI-1 gene transcription. Glucosamine itself was subsequently shown to activate the PAI-1 promoter through Sp1 sites in glomerular mesangial cells [102]. The glycosylated form of Sp1 appears to be more transcriptionally active than the deglycosylated form of the protein [103]. A fourfold increase in Sp1 O-GlcNacylation caused by inhibition of the enzyme O-GlcNac-β-*N*-acetylglucosaminidase resulted in a reciprocal 30% decrease in its level of serine/threonine phosphorylation, supporting the concept that O-GlcNacylation and phosphorylation compete to modify the same sites on this protein [104].

Recently, hyperglycemia was shown to induce a 2.4-fold increase in hexosamine pathway activity in aortic endothelial cells, resulting in a 1.7-fold increase in Sp1 O-linked GlcNAc and a 70–80% decrease in Sp1 O-linked phosphothreonine and phosphoserine [25]. Concomitantly, hyperglycemia increased expression from an

85-bp truncated PAI-1 promoter luciferase reporter containing two Sp1 sites by 3.8-fold, but failed to increase expression when the two Sp1 sites were mutated [25].

GlcNAc modification of Sp1 may regulate other glucose-responsive genes in addition to PAI-1. Since virtually every RNA polymerase II transcription factor examined has been found to be O-GlcNacylated [105] it is possible that reciprocal modification by O-GlcNacylation and phosphorylation of transcription factors other than Sp1 may function as a more generalized mechanism for regulating glucose-responsive gene transcription.

In addition to transcription factors, many other nuclear and cytoplasmic proteins are dynamically modified by O-GlcNAc moieties, and may exhibit reciprocal modification by phosphorylation in a manner analogous to Sp1 [105]. One example relevant to diabetic complications is the inhibition of eNOS activity by hyperglycemia-induced O-GlcNacylation at the Akt site of the eNOS protein [106]. Another example may be various PKC isoforms, which are activated by glucosamine without membrane translocation [102]. Thus, activation of the hexosamine pathway by hyperglycemia may result in many changes in both gene expression and in protein function that together contribute to the pathogenesis of diabetic complications.

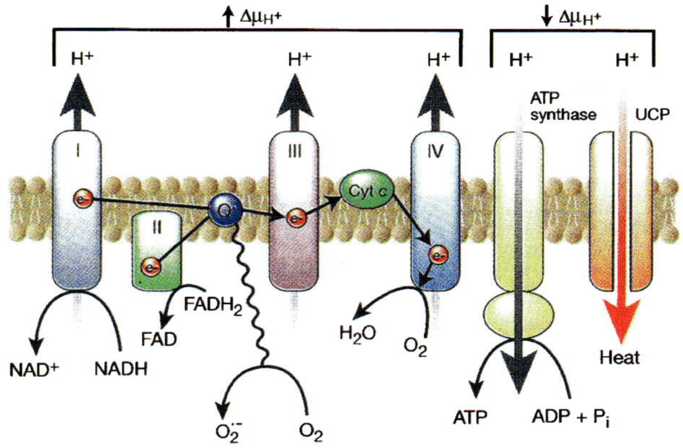

Figure 3 Production of superoxide by the mitochondrial electron transport chain. Increased hyperglycemia or FFA derived electron donors from the TCA cycle (NADH and $FADH_2$) generate a high mitochondrial membrane potential ($\Delta\mu H^+$) by pumping protons across the mitochondrial inner membrane. This inhibits electron transport at complex III, increasing the half-life of free-radical intermediates of coenzyme Q, which reduces O_2 to superoxide. Coenzyme Q is ubiquinone, which becomes the ubisemiquinone radical upon addition of an unpaired electron; O_2.− is superoxide. (Reprinted with permission from Nature, 2001; 414:813 © 2001 Macmillan Magazines Limited). [20]

DIFFERENT PATHOGENIC MECHANISMS REFLECT A SINGLE HYPERGLYCEMIA-INDUCED PROCESS

Although specific inhibitors of aldose reductase activity, AGE formation, PKC activation, and the hexosamine pathway each ameliorate various diabetes-induced abnormalities in cell culture and animal models, there has been no apparent common element linking the four mechanisms of hyperglycemia-induced damage discussed in the preceding section [43, 44, 54–56, 84, 85, 107]. This issue has now been resolved by the recent discovery that each of the four different pathogenic mechanisms reflects a single hyperglycemia-induced process: overproduction of superoxide by the mitochondrial electron transport chain [25, 107]. A large literature had established that diabetes and hyperglycemia increase oxidative stress [108], but neither the underlying mechanism nor the consequences on other pathways of hyperglycemic damage were known.

To understand how hyperglycemia increases ROS production inside cultured aortic endothelial cells [99], a brief overview of glucose metabolism is helpful. Intracellular glucose oxidation begins with glycolysis in the cytoplasm, which generates NADH and pyruvate. Cytoplasmic NADH can donate reducing equivalents to the mitochondrial electron transport chain via two shuttle systems, or it can reduce pyruvate to lactate, which exits the cell to provide substrate for hepatic gluconeogenesis. Pyruvate can also be transported into the mitochondria, where it is oxidized by the tricarboxylic acid (TCA) cycle to produce CO_2, H_2O, four molecules of NADH, and one molecule of $FADH_2$. Mitochondrial NADH and $FADH_2$ provide energy for ATP production via oxidative phosphorylation by the electron transport chain [100, 109].

Electron flow through the mitochondrial electron transport chain (Figure 3) is carried out by four inner-membrane-associated enzyme complexes, plus cytochrome *c* and the mobile carrier ubiquinone (for review see reference 20]. NADH derived from both cytosolic glucose oxidation and mitochondrial TCA cycle activity donates electrons to NADH:ubiquinone oxidoreductase (complex I). Complex I ultimately transfers its electrons to ubiquinone. Ubiquinone can also be reduced by electrons donated from several $FADH_2$-containing dehydrogenases, including succinate:ubiquinone oxidoreductase (complex II) and glycerol-3-phosphate dehydrogenase. Electrons from reduced ubiquinone are then transferred to ubiquinol:cytochrome *c* oxidoreductase (complex III) by the ubisemiquinone radical-generating Q cycle. Electron transport then proceeds through cytochrome *c*, cytochrome *c* oxidase (complex IV), and finally, molecular oxygen.

Electron transfer through complexes I, III, and IV generates a proton gradient that drives ATP synthase (complex V). When the electrochemical potential difference generated by this proton gradient is high, the life of superoxide-generating electron transport intermediates such as ubisemiquinone is prolonged (Figure 3). There appears to be a threshold value above which superoxide production is markedly increased [109]. Hyperglycemia was found to increase the proton electrochemical gradient generated by the mitochondrial electron transport chain above this threshold [106], because of overproduction of electron donors by the TCA cycle. This, in turn, caused a dramatic increase in the production of superoxide by endothelial cells. Overexpression of manganese superoxide dismutase (MnSOD), the mitochondrial form of this enzyme, abolished the ROS signal [110], and overexpression of uncoupling protein 1 (UCP-1) collapsed the proton electrochemcial gradient and prevented hyperglycemia-induced overproduction of ROS [107]. Inhibition of hyperglycemia-induced mitochondrial superoxide overproduction by MnSOD or UCP-1 completely prevented increased polyol pathway flux in endothelial cells. Sorbitol accumulation, a measure of polyol pathway flux, increased 2.6-fold when incubation medium glucose concentration was switched from 5 to 30 mM. No increase occurred with 30 mM glucose when the rise in mitochondrial superoxide production was prevented [107]. Since hyperglycemia-induced mitochondrial superoxide overproduction induces a 66% decrease in GAPDH activity [25], the effect of hyperglycemia on polyol pathway flux may reflect the accumulation of glycolytic metabolites, including glucose, upstream of GAPDH (Figure 4). Although the direct inhibition of GAPDH by reactive oxygen species has been well described *in vitro*, the inhibition of GAPDH by hyperglycemia-induced reactive oxygen species *in vivo* actually reflects activation of poly(ADP-ribose) polymerase and depletion of NAD^+ [15], rather

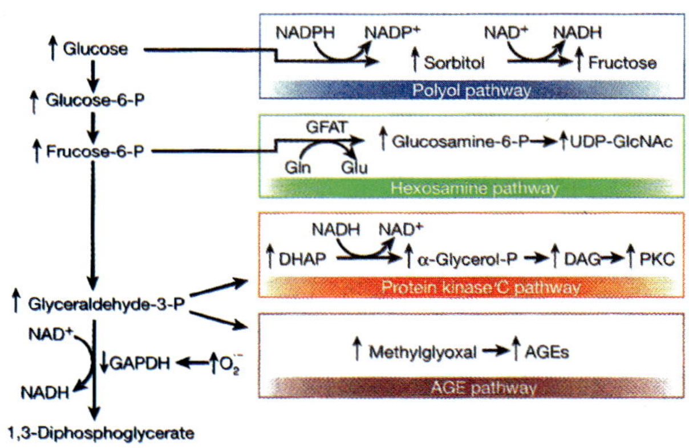

Figure 4 Potential mechanism by which excess metabolite-induced mitochondrial superoxide overproduction activates four pathways of hyperglycemic damage. Excess superoxide partially inhibits the glycolytic GAPDH, thereby diverting upstream metabolites from glycolysis into pathways of glucose overutilization. This results in increased flux of DHAP (dihydroxyacetonephosphate) to DAG, an activator of PKC, and of triose phosphates to methylglyoxal, the major intracellular AGE precursor. Increased flux of fructose-6-phosphate to UDP-GlcNAc increases modification of proteins by O-linked GlcNAc, and increased glucose flux through the polyol pathway consumes NADPH and depletes GSH. (Reprinted with permission from Nature, 2001; 414:813 © 2001 Macmillan Magazines Limited). [20]

than direct oxidative inactivation of the enzyme (M.B. and coworkers, unpublished data).

Inhibition of hyperglycemia-induced mitochondrial superoxide overproduction by MnSOD or UCP-1 also prevented increased intracellular AGE formation in endothelial cells. Methylglyoxal-derived AGE, the primary intracellular AGE induced by hyperglycemia [58], increased nearly two-fold when incubation medium glucose concentration was switched from 5 to 30 mM. No increase occurred with 30 mM glucose when the rise in mitochondrial superoxide production was prevented [107]. Since methylglyoxal is formed by fragmentation of triose phosphates, the effect of hyperglycemia on intracellular AGE formation also likely reflects increased triose phosphate levels because of inhibition of GAPDH by mitochondrial overproduction of ROS [25] (Figure 4). This hypothesis is supported by the observation that GAPDH antisense oligonucleotides caused identical intracellular AGE increases in the absence of hyperglycemia (M.B. and coworkers, unpublished data).

Inhibition of hyperglycemia-induced mitochondrial superoxide overproduction by MnSOD or UCP-1 also prevented increased PKC activation in endothelial cells. PKC activity in the membrane increased 1.8-fold when incubation medium glucose concentration was switched from 5 to 30 mM. No increase occurred with 30 mM glucose when the rise in mitochondrial superoxide production was prevented [107]. Since hyperglycemia activates PKC by increasing the *de novo* synthesis of diacylglycerol [54], the effect of hyperglycemia on PKC activation also likely reflects increased dihydroxyacetonephosphate levels because of inhibition of GAPDH by ROS [25] (Figure 4). This hypothesis is supported by the observation that GAPDH antisense oligonucleotides also caused activation of PKC in the presence of physiologic glucose concentrations (M.B. and coworkers, unpublished data).

Inhibition of hyperglycemia-induced mitochondrial superoxide overproduction by MnSOD or UCP-1 also prevented increased hexosamine pathway activity in endothelial cells. Hexosamine pathway activity, measured as UDP-GlcNAc accumulation, increased 2.5-fold when incubation medium glucose concentration was switched from 5 to 30 mM. No increase occurred with 30 mM glucose when the rise in mitochondrial superoxide production was prevented. Since hyperglycemia increases hexosamine pathway flux by providing more fructose-6-phosphate for the rate-limiting enzyme of the pathway, GFAT, the effect of hyperglycemia on hexosamine pathway flux likely reflects increased fructose-6-phosphate levels also because of inhibition of GAPDH by ROS [25] (Figure 4). This hypothesis is supported by the observation that GAPDH antisense oligonucleotides also caused identical increases in hexosamine pathway flux in the absence of hyperglycemia (M.B. and coworkers, unpublished data). Hyperglycemia-induced activation of the redox-sensitive pleiotrophic transcription factor NF-κB was also prevented by inhibition of mitochondrial superoxide overproduction [107].

Overexpression of UCP-1 or MnSOD corrects a variety of hyperglycemia-induced phenotypes in target cells of diabetic complications. In cultured glomerular mesangial cells, overexpression of MnSOD suppresses the increase in collagen synthesis induced by high glucose [111]. In dorsal root ganglion neurons from both wild-type and MnSOD +/− mice, overexpression of MnSOD decreases hyperglycemia-induced programmed cell death, and in embryonic rat dorsal root ganglion neurons, overexpression of UCP-1 inhibits cleavage of programmed cell death effector caspases (J.W. Russell, personal communication). In aortic endothelial cells, overexpression of either UCP-1 or MnSOD completely blocks hyperglycemia-induced monocyte adhesion (J.L. Nadler and C.C. Hedrick, personal communication), and prevents hyperglycemia-induced inhibition of the antiatherogenic enzyme prostacyclin synthase. Overexpression of either MnSOD or UCP-1 also prevents inhibition of eNOS activity by hyperglycemia [106]. In platelets, chemical uncouplers and superoxide dismutase mimetics both prevent potentiation by hyperglycemia of collagen-induced platelet activation and aggregation [112].

In streptozotocin (STZ) diabetic transgenic mice overexpressing human cytoplasmic Cu^{2+}/Zn^{2+} superoxide dismutase, albuminuria, glomerular hypertrophy and glomerular content of TGF-β and collagen α1(IV) were all attenuated compared to wild-type littermates after 4 months of diabetes. The wild-type STZ-diabetic mice developed modest increases in fractional mesangial volume after 8 months of diabetes, and this change was also suppressed in the SOD transgenic diabetic mice [111]. Overexpression of the human SOD1 transgene in *db/db* diabetic mice similarly attenuated the extensive expansion of the glomerular mesangial matrix that was otherwise evident by age 5 months in the nontransgenic *db/db* littermates (F.R. DeRubertis, P.A. Craven, M.F. Melhem, H. Liachenko, and S.L. Phillips, unpublished observations).

Recently, another important downstream target of chronic glycemia-mediated increases in intracellular ROS has been identified the transcription factor CREB (cAMP response element binding protein) [111, 113, 114]. CREB plays a pivotal role in vascular SMC function. CREB restrains SMC proliferation and migration [115, 118] decreases expression of the growth factor receptors for PDGF-α and endothelin 1, and decreases expression of the proinflammatory cytokine IL-6 (interleukin 6) [115]. Exposure of SMC and endothelial cells to glucose concentrations that elevate intracellular ROS, leads to decreased CREB content and function. In the case of the SMC, the increased proliferative and migratory response of SMC to mitogens (i.e. PDGF) induced by ROS or high glucose can be restored by overexpression of constitutively active CREB [113, 114]. Thus loss of this important nuclear protein in diabetes may contribute to macrovascular complications by increasing SMC activation. Insulin-resistant and insulin-deficient diabetic rodents all have loss of intravascular CREB content [113]. In the insulin-resistant *ob/ob* mouse, CREB protein content can be restored by treatment with PPAR-γ (peroxisome proliferator-activated receptor γ) agonists. PPAR-γ agonists also increase SMC CREB content *in vitro* (J.E.B.R., D. Klemm, and P. Watson, unpublished data). Recent studies have demonstrated accumulation of intravascular ROS and markers of increased oxidant stress in the vessel wall of NOD mice. Loss of vascular CREB and enhanced expression of the PDGFR-α is also observed in this model. These abnormalities are reversed by treatment with an SOD mimetic (K. Haskins, S. Flores, P.A. Watson, and J.E.B.R., unpublished data). These observations support a major role for mitochondrial ROS generation as a contributor to CREB downregulation and diabetic macrovascular disease (Figure 5). In related studies, loss of CREB and CREB-dependent gene expression is also observed in the nervous system in diabetes. In STZ animals CREB expression is decreased in the sural nerve and the hippocampus [116]. CREB downregulation is associated with decreased expression of the CREB-dependent survival factor bcl-2. Glycemia-mediated interference with neuronal CREB and bcl-2 expression can be restored by treatment of the neurons *in vitro* with a SOD mimetic [116]. In the nervous system CREB is well accepted as playing an essential role in survival and neuronal plasticity [117]. Loss of CREB in other neurodegenerative diseases such as Alzheimer's is also likely secondary to ROS and may

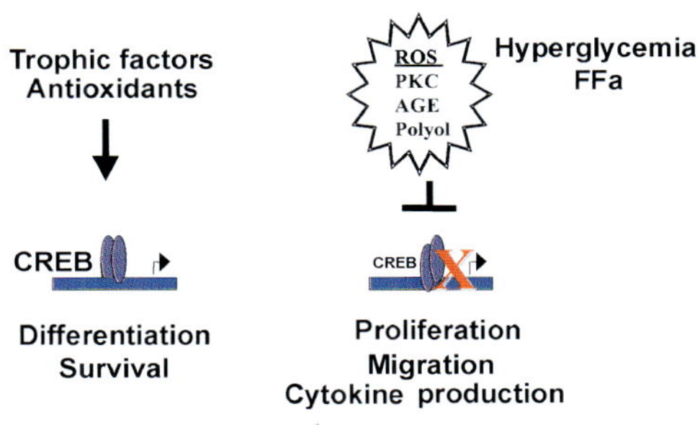

Figure 5 CREB impact on vascular smooth muscle proliferative capacity: CREB is critical for vascular SMC differentiation. It is also important for differentiation and survival of adipocytes, neurons, and cardiac myocytes. This transcription factor restrains SMC proliferation and migration. In the setting of chronic metabolic stress (such as animal models of diabetes and IR) CREB content and function is lost in the vasculature. This is secondary to generation of ROS and activation of the AGEs, PKC, and the polyol intracellular signaling pathways. The result of loss of CREB function in SMC, adipocytes, and the nervous system is dedifferentiation and decreased survival. This phenomenon can be reversed by antioxidants

provide a pathogenetic link between these two disorders. Similar loss of CREB content has been observed in diabetic myocardium. Myocardial CREB content is increased by treatment with PPAR-γ agonists (P. A. Watson, C. Brurant, and J.E.B.R., unpublished data). Changes in the function of this key transcriptional regulator may represent a pivotal consequence of glycemia-mediated dysfunction in numerous target tissues. The effects of FFA on CREB expression and function are currently under investigation.

FUTURE DIRECTIONS

The paradigm discussed in this chapter suggests that interrupting the overproduction of superoxide by the mitochondrial electron transport chain would normalize polyol pathway flux, AGE formation, PKC activation, hexosamine pathway flux, NF-κB activation, prostacylin synthase activity, and CREB function. It may be difficult to accomplish this using conventional antioxidants, however, since these agents scavenge ROS in a stoichiometric manner. Thus, although long-term administration of a multi-anti-oxidant diet inhibited the development of early diabetic retinopathy in rats [118], and vitamin C improved endothelium-dependent vasodilation in diabetic patients, low-dose vitamin E failed to alter the risk of cardiovascular and renal disease in patients with diabetes [119, 120]. Novel, small molecular weight compounds that act as superoxide dismutase/catalase mimetics have the theoretical advantage of scavenging ROS continuously by acting as catalysts with efficiencies approaching those of the native enzymes [121]. These and other agents discovered using high throughput chemical and biological methods may have unique clinical efficacy in preventing the development and progression of diabetic macrovascular disease.

Acknowledgments

This work was supported by grants from NIH, Veterans Affairs, JDRFI, and ADA. Owing to space limitations, a comprehensive list of reference citations could not be included. We apologize to those colleagues whose work is not specifically referenced, and gratefully acknowledge their contributions to the field.

REFERENCES

1. Stone PH, Muller JE, Hartwell T, York BJ, Rutherford JD, Parker CB, Turi ZG, Strauss HW, Willerson JT, Robertson T, Braun Wald E, Jaffe A, for The MILIS Study Group. The effect of diabetes mellitus on prognosis and serial left ventricular function after acute MI: contribution of both coronary disease and diastolic left ventricular dysfunction to the adverse prognosis. *J Am Coll Cardiol* 1989; 14: 49–57.
2. Smith JW, Marcus FI, Serokman R. Prognosis of patients with diabetes mellitus after acute MI. *Am J Cardiol* 1984; 54: 718–21.
3. Stamler J, Vaccaro O, Neaton JD, Wentworth D. Diabetes, other risk factors, and 12-yr cardiovascular mortality for men screened in the Multiple Risk Factor Intervention Trial. *Diabetes Care* 1993; 16: 434–44.
4. Haffner SM, Lehto S, Ronnemaa T, Pyorala K, Laakso M. Mortality from coronary heart disease in subjects with type 2 diabetes and in nondiabetic subjects with and without prior MI. *N Engl J Med* 1998; 339: 229–34.
5. Capes SE, Hunt D, Malmberg K, Gerstein HC. Stress hyperglycaemia and increased risk of death after MI in patients with and without diabetes: a systematic overview. *Lancet* 2000; 355: 773–8.
6. Wingard DL, Barrett-Connor EL, Scheidt-Nave C, McPhillips JB. Prevalence of cardiovascular and renal complications in older adults with normal or impaired glucose tolerance or NIDDM. A population-based study. *Diabetes Care* 1993; 16: 1022–5.
7. Norhammar A, Tenerz A, Nilsson G, Hamsten A, Efendic S, Ryden L, Malmberg K. Glucose metabolism in patients with acute MI and no previous diagnosis of diabetes mellitus: a prospective study. *Lancet* 2002; 359: 2140–4.
8. Howard G, O'Leary DH, Zaccaro D, Haffner S, Rewers M, Hamman R, Selby JV, Saad MF, Savage P, Bergman R, for The Insulin Resistance Atherosclerosis Study (IRAS) Investigators. Insulin sensitivity and atherosclerosis. *Circulation* 1996; 93: 1809–17.
9. The Diabetes Control and Complications Trial Research Group. The effect of intensive treatment of diabetes on the development and progression of long-term complications in insulin-dependent diabetes mellitus. *N Engl J Med* 1993; 329: 977–86.
10. UK Prospective Diabetes Study (UKPDS) Group. Intensive blood-glucose control with sulphonylureas or insulin compared with conventional treatment and risk of complications in patients with type 2 diabetes (UKPDS 33). *Lancet* 1998; 352: 837–53.
11. Haffner SM. Epidemiological studies on the effects of hyperglycemia and improvement of glycemic control on macrovascular events in type 2 diabetes. *Diabetes Care* 1999; 22 (suppl 3): C54–6.
12. Kuusisto J, Mykkanen L, Pyorala K, Laakso M. NIDDM and its metabolic control predict coronary heart disease in elderly subjects. *Diabetes* 1994; 43: 960–7.
13. Laakso M. Glycemic control and the risk for coronary heart disease in patients with non-insulin-dependent diabetes mellitus. The Finnish studies. *Ann Intern Med* 1996; 124: 127–30.
14. Ginsberg HN. Insulin resistance and cardiovascular disease. *J Clin Invest* 2000; 106: 453–8.
15. Hsueh WA, Law RE. Cardiovascular risk continuum: implications of IR and diabetes. *Am J Med* 1998; 105: 4S–14S.
16. Yudkin JS, Stehouwer CD, Emeis JJ, Coppack SW. C-reactive protein in healthy subjects: associations with obesity, IR, and endothelial dysfunction. A potential role for cytokines originating from adipose tissue? *Arterioscler Thromb Vasc Biol* 1999; 19: 972–8.
17. Wei M, Gaskill SP, Haffner SM, Stern MP. Effects of diabetes and level of glycemia on all-cause and cardiovascular mortality. The San Antonio Heart Study. *Diabetes Care* 1998; 21: 1167–72.

18. Malmberg K for the DIGAMI (Diabetes Mellitus, Insulin Glucose Infusion in Acute Myocardial Infarction) Study Group. Prospective randomised study of intensive insulin treatment on long term survival after acute MI in patients with diabetes mellitus. *BMJ* 1997; 314: 1512–5.
19. Lusis AJ. Atherosclerosis. *Nature* 2000; 407: 233–41.
20. Brownlee M. Biochemistry and molecular cell biology of diabetic complications. *Nature* 2001; 414: 813–20.
21. Eckel RH, Wassef M, Chait A, Sobel B, Barrett E, King G, Lopes-Virella M, Reusch J, Ruderman N, Steiner G, Vlassara H. Prevention Conference VI: diabetes and Cardiovascular Disease. Writing Group II: pathogenesis of atherosclerosis in diabetes. *Circulation* 2002; 105: e138–43.
22. Zou MH, Shi C, Cohen RA. High glucose via peroxynitrite causes tyrosine nitration and inactivation of prostacyclin synthase that is associated with thromboxane/prostaglandin H(2) receptor-mediated apoptosis and adhesion molecule expression in cultured human aortic endothelial cells. *Diabetes* 2002; 51: 198–203.
23. Steinberg HO, Tarshoby M, Monestel R, Hook G, Cronin J, Johnson A, Bayazeed B, Baron AD. Elevated circulating FFA levels impair endothelium-dependent vasodilation. *J Clin Invest* 1997; 100: 1230–9.
24. Beckman JA, Goldfine AB, Gordon MB, Creager MA. Ascorbate restores endothelium-dependent vasodilation impaired by acute hyperglycemia in humans. *Circulation* 2001; 103: 1618–23.
25. Du XL, Edelstein D, Rossetti L, Fantus IG, Goldberg H, Ziyadeh F, Wu J, Brownlee M. Hyperglycemia-induced mitochondrial superoxide overproduction activates the hexosamine pathway and induces PAI-1 expression by increasing Sp1 glycosylation. *Proc Natl Acad Sci USA* 2000; 97: 12222–6.
26. Taher MM, Garcia JG, Natarajan V. Hydroperoxide-induced diacylglycerol formation and PKC activation in vascular endothelial cells. *Arch Biochem Biophys* 1993; 303: 260–6.
27. Natarajan V, Scribner WM, Taher MM. 4-Hydroxynonenal, a metabolite of lipid peroxidation, activates phospholipase D in vascular endothelial cells. *Free Radic Biol Med* 1993; 15: 365–75.
28. Kawano Y, Rincon J, Soler A, Ryder JW, Nolte LA, Zierath JR, Wallberg-Henriksson H. Changes in glucose transport and PKC beta(2) in rat skeletal muscle induced by hyperglycaemia. *Diabetologia* 1999; 42: 1071–9.
29. Koya D, King GL. PKC activation and the development of diabetic complications. *Diabetes* 1998; 47: 859–66.
30. Vlassara H, Fuh H, Donnelly T, Cybulsky M. Advanced glycation endproducts promote adhesion molecule (VCAM-1, ICAM-1) expression and atheroma formation in normal rabbits. *Mol Med* 1995; 1: 447–56.
31. Itani SI, Ruderman NB, Schmieder F, Boden G. Lipid-induced IR in human muscle is associated with changes in diacylglycerol, PKC, and IkappaB-alpha. *Diabetes* 2002; 51: 2005–11.
32. Toft I, Bonaa KH, Ingebretsen OC, Nordoy A, Jenssen T. Fibrinolytic function after dietary supplementation with omega3 polyunsaturated fatty acids. *Arterioscler Thromb Vasc Biol* 1997; 17: 814–9.
33. Schneider DJ, Sobel BE. Synergistic augmentation of expression of PAI type-1 induced by insulin, very-low-density lipoproteins, and fatty acids. *Coron Artery Dis* 1996; 7: 813–7.
34. Ceriello A, Taboga C, Tonutti L, Quagliaro L, Piconi L, Bais B, Da Ros R, Motz E. Evidence for an independent and cumulative effect of postprandial hypertriglyceridemia and hyperglycemia on endothelial dysfunction and oxidative stress generation: effects of short- and long-term simvastatin treatment. *Circulation* 2002; 106: 1211–8.
35. Siegel RD, Cupples A, Schaefer EJ, Wilson PW. Lipoproteins, apolipoproteins, and low-density lipoprotein size among diabetics in the Framingham offspring study. *Metabolism* 1996; 45: 1267–72.
36. Haffner SM, Mykkanen L, Stern MP, Paidi M, Howard BV. Greater effect of diabetes on LDL size in women than in men. *Diabetes Care* 1994; 17: 1164–71.
37. Gardner CD, Fortmann SP, Krauss RM. Association of small low-density lipoprotein particles with the incidence of coronary artery disease in men and women. *JAMA* 1996; 276: 875–81.
38. Karpe F. Postprandial lipoprotein metabolism and atherosclerosis. *J Intern Med* 1999; 246: 341–55.
39. Goldberg IJ. Clinical review 124. Diabetic dyslipidemia: causes and consequences. *J Clin Endocrinol Metab* 2001; 86: 965–71.
40. Xia P, Kramer RM, King GL. Identification of the mechanism for the inhibition of Na^+, K^+-adenosine triphosphatase by hyperglycemia involving activation of PKC and cytosolic phospholipase A2. *J Clin Invest* 1995; 96: 733–40.
41. Williamson JR, Chang K, Frangos M, Hasan KS, Ido Y, Kawamura T, Nyengaard JR, van den Enden M, Kilo C, Tilton RG. Hyperglycemic pseudohypoxia and diabetic complications. *Diabetes* 1993; 42: 801–13.
42. Garcia Soriano F, Virag L, Jagtap P, Szabo E, Mabley JG, Liaudet L, Marton A, Hoyt DG, Murthy KG, Salzman AL, Southan GJ, Szabo C. Diabetic endothelial dysfunction: the role of poly(ADP-ribose) polymerase activation. *Nat Med* 2001; 7: 108–13.
43. Lee AY, Chung SS. Contributions of polyol pathway to oxidative stress in diabetic cataract. *FASEB J* 1999; 13: 23–30.
44. Engerman RL, Kern TS, Larson ME. Nerve conduction and aldose reductase inhibition during 5 years of diabetes or galactosaemia in dogs. *Diabetologia* 1994; 37: 141–4.
45. Sorbinil Retinopathy Trial Research Group. A randomized trial of sorbinil, an aldose reductase inhibitor, in diabetic retinopathy. *Arch Ophthalmol* 1990; 108: 1234–44.
46. Greene DA, Arezzo JC, Brown MB. Effect of aldose reductase inhibition on nerve conduction and morphometry in diabetic neuropathy. Zenarestat Study Group. *Neurology* 1999; 53: 580–91.
47. Stitt AW, Li YM, Gardiner TA, Bucala R, Archer DB, Vlassara H. Advanced glycation end products (AGEs) co-localize with AGE receptors in the retinal vasculature of diabetic and of AGE-infused rats. *Am J Pathol* 1997; 150: 523–31.
48. Horie K, Miyata T, Maeda K, Miyata S, Sugiyama S, Sakai H, van Ypersole de Strihou C, Monnier VM, Witztum JL, Kurokawa K. Immunohistochemical colocalization of glycoxidation products and lipid peroxidation products in diabetic renal glomerular lesions. Implication for glycoxidative stress in the pathogenesis of diabetic nephropathy. *J Clin Invest* 1997; 100: 2995–3004.
49. Schmidt AM, Hori O, Chen JX, Li JF, Crandall J, Zhang J, Cao R, Yan SD, Brett J, Stern D. Advanced glycation endproducts interacting with their endothelial receptor induce expression of vascular cell adhesion molecule-1 (VCAM-1) in cultured human endothelial cells and in mice. A potential mechanism for the accelerated

vasculopathy of diabetes. *J Clin Invest* 1995; 96: 1395–403.

50. Degenhardt TP, Alderson NL, Arrington DD, Beattie RJ, Basgen JM, Steffes MW, Thorpe SR, Baynes JW. Pyridoxamine inhibits early renal disease and dyslipidemia in the streptozotocin-diabetic rat. *Kidney Int* 2002; 61: 939–50.
51. Wells-Knecht KJ, Zyzak DV, Litchfield JE, Thorpe SR, Baynes JW. Mechanism of autoxidative glycosylation: identification of glyoxal and arabinose as intermediates in the autoxidative modification of proteins by glucose. *Biochemistry* 1995; 34: 3702–9.
52. Thornalley PJ. The glyoxalase system: new developments towards functional characterization of a metabolic pathway fundamental to biological life. *Biochem J* 1990; 269: 1–11.
53. Suzuki K, Koh YH, Mizuno H, Hamaoka R, Taniguchi N. Overexpression of aldehyde reductase protects PC12 cells from the cytotoxicity of methylglyoxal or 3-deoxyglucosone. *J Biochem (Tokyo)* 1998; 123: 353–7.
54. Soulis-Liparota T, Cooper M, Papazoglou D, Clarke B, Jerums G. Retardation by aminoguanidine of development of albuminuria, mesangial expansion, and tissue fluorescence in streptozocin-induced diabetic rat. *Diabetes* 1991; 40: 1328–34.
55. Nakamura S, Makita Z, Ishikawa S, Yasumura K, Fujii W, Yanagisawa K, Kawata T, Koike T. Progression of nephropathy in spontaneous diabetic rats is prevented by OPB-9195, a novel inhibitor of advanced glycation. *Diabetes* 1997; 46: 895–9.
56. Hammes HP, Martin S, Federlin K, Geisen K, Brownlee M. Aminoguanidine treatment inhibits the development of experimental diabetic retinopathy. *Proc Natl Acad Sci USA* 1991; 88: 11555–8.
57. Giardino I, Edelstein D, Brownlee M. Nonenzymatic glycosylation *in vitro* and in bovine endothelial cells alters basic fibroblast growth factor activity. A model for intracellular glycosylation in diabetes. *J Clin Invest* 1994; 94: 110–7.
58. Shinohara M, Thornalley PJ, Giardino I, Beisswenger P, Thorpe SR, Onorato J, Brownlee M. Overexpression of glyoxalase-I in bovine endothelial cells inhibits intracellular AGE formation and prevents hyperglycemia-induced increases in macromolecular endocytosis. *J Clin Invest* 1998; 101: 1142–7.
59. Maisonpierre PC, Suri C, Jones PF, Bartunkova S, Wiegand SJ, Radziejewski C, Compton D, McClain J, Aldrich TH, Papadopoulos N, Daly TJ, Davis S, Sato TN, Yancopoulos GD. Angiopoietin-2, a natural antagonist for Tie2 that disrupts *in vivo* angiogenesis. *Science* 1997; 277: 55–60.
60. Tanaka S, Avigad G, Brodsky B, Eikenberry EF. Glycation induces expansion of the molecular packing of collagen. *J Mol Biol* 1988; 203: 495–505.
61. Huijberts MS, Wolffenbuttel BH, Boudier HA, Crijns FR, Kruseman AC, Poitevin P, Levy BI. Aminoguanidine treatment increases elasticity and decreases fluid filtration of large arteries from diabetic rats. *J Clin Invest* 1993; 92: 1407–11.
62. Charonis AS, Tsilbary EC. Structural and functional changes of laminin and type IV collagen after nonenzymatic glycation. *Diabetes* 1992; 41 (suppl 2): 49–51.
63. Charonis AS, Reger LA, Dege JE, Kouzi-Koliakos K, Furcht LT, Wohlhueter RM, Tsilibary EC. Laminin alterations after *in vitro* nonenzymatic glycosylation. *Diabetes* 1990; 39: 807–14.
64. Haitoglou CS, Tsilibary EC, Brownlee M, Charonis AS. Altered cellular interactions between endothelial cells and nonenzymatically glucosylated laminin/type IV collagen. *J Biol Chem* 1992; 267: 12404–7.
65. Federoff HJ, Lawrence D, Brownlee M. Nonenzymatic glycosylation of laminin and the laminin peptide CIKVAVS inhibits neurite outgrowth. *Diabetes* 1993; 42: 509–13.
66. Smedsrod B, Melkko J, Araki N, Sano H, Horiuchi S. Advanced glycation end products are eliminated by scavenger-receptor-mediated endocytosis in hepatic sinusoidal Kupffer and endothelial cells. *Biochem J* 1997; 322 (pt 2): 567–73.
67. Neeper M, Schmidt AM, Brett J, Yan SD, Wang F, Pan YC, Elliston K, Stern D, Shaw A. Cloning and expression of a cell surface receptor for advanced glycosylation end products of proteins. *J Biol Chem* 1992; 267: 14998–5004.
68. Li YM, Mitsuhashi T, Wojciechowicz D, Shimizu N, Li J, Stitt A, He C, Banerjee D, Vlassara H. Molecular identity and cellular distribution of AGE receptors: relationship of p60 to OST-48 and p90 to 80K-H membrane proteins. *Proc Natl Acad Sci USA* 1996; 93: 11047–52.
69. Abordo EA, Westwood ME, Thornalley PJ. Synthesis and secretion of macrophage colony stimulating factor by mature human monocytes and human monocytic THP-1 cells induced by human serum albumin derivatives modified with methylglyoxal and glucose-derived AGEs. *Immunol Lett* 1996; 53: 7–13.
70. Doi T, Vlassara H, Kirstein M, Yamada Y, Striker GE, Striker LJ. Receptor-specific increase in extracellular matrix production in mouse mesangial cells by advanced glycosylation end products is mediated via platelet-derived growth factor. *Proc Natl Acad Sci USA* 1992; 89: 2873–7.
71. Kirstein M, Aston C, Hintz R, Vlassara H. Receptor-specific induction of insulin-like growth factor I in human monocytes by advanced glycosylation end product-modified proteins. *J Clin Invest* 1992; 90: 439–46.
72. Skolnik EY, Yang Z, Makita Z, Radoff S, Kirstein M, Vlassara H. Human and rat mesangial cell receptors for glucose-modified proteins: potential role in kidney tissue remodelling and diabetic nephropathy. *J Exp Med* 1991; 174: 931–9.
73. Vlassara H, Brownlee M, Manogue KR, Dinarello CA, Pasagian A. Cachectin/TNF and IL-1 induced by glucose-modified proteins: role in normal tissue remodeling. *Science* 1988; 240: 1546–8.
74. Lu M, Kuroki M, Amano S, Tolentino M, Keough K, Kim I, Bucala R, Adamis AP. Advanced glycation end products increase retinal vascular endothelial growth factor expression. *J Clin Invest* 1998; 101: 1219–24.
75. Park L, Raman KG, Lee KJ, Lu Y, Ferran LJ Jr, Chow WS, Stern D, Schmidt AM. Suppression of accelerated diabetic atherosclerosis by the soluble receptor for AGEs. *Nat Med* 1998; 4: 1025–31.
76. Lander HM, Tauras JM, Ogiste JS, Hori O, Moss RA, Schmidt AM. Activation of the receptor for advanced glycation end products triggers a p21(ras)-dependent mitogen-activated protein kinase pathway regulated by oxidant stress. *J Biol Chem* 1997; 272: 17810–4.
77. Yan SD, Schmidt AM, Anderson GM, Zhang J, Brett J, Zou YS, Pinsky D, Stern D. Enhanced cellular oxidant stress by the interaction of advanced glycation end products with their receptors/binding proteins. *J Biol Chem* 1994; 269: 9889–97.

78. Yamagishi S, Fujimori H, Yonekura H, Yamamoto Y, Yamamoto H. Advanced glycation endproducts inhibit prostacyclin production and induce PAI-1 in human microvascular endothelial cells. *Diabetologia* 1998; 41: 1435–41.
79. Tsuji H, Iehara N, Masegi T, Imura M, Ohkawa J, Arai H, Ishii K, Kita T, Doi T. Ribozyme targeting of receptor for advanced glycation end products in mouse mesangial cells. *Biochem Biophys Res Commun* 1998; 245: 583–8.
80. Koya D, Jirousek MR, Lin YW, Ishii H, Kuboki K, King GL. Characterization of PKC beta isoform activation on the gene expression of transforming growth factor-beta, extracellular matrix components, and prostanoids in the glomeruli of diabetic rats. *J Clin Invest* 1997; 100: 115–26.
81. Xia P, Inoguchi T, Kern TS, Engerman RL, Oates PJ, King GL. Characterization of the mechanism for the chronic activation of diacylglycerol-PKC pathway in diabetes and hypergalactosemia. *Diabetes* 1994; 43: 1122–9.
82. Portilla D, Dai G, Peters JM, Gonzalez FJ, Crew MD, Proia AD. Etomoxir-induced PPARalpha-modulated enzymes protect during acute renal failure. *Am J Physiol Renal Physiol* 2000; 278: F667–75.
83. Keogh RJ, Dunlop ME, Larkins RG. Effect of inhibition of aldose reductase on glucose flux, diacylglycerol formation, PKC, and phospholipase A2 activation. *Metabolism* 1997; 46: 41–7.
84. Ishii H, Jirousek MR, Koya D, Takagi C, Xia P, Clermont A, Bursell SE, Kern TS, Ballas LM, Heath WF, Stramm LE, Feener EP, King GL. Amelioration of vascular dysfunctions in diabetic rats by an oral PKC beta inhibitor. *Science* 1996; 272: 728–31.
85. Craven PA, Studer RK, DeRubertis FR. Impaired NO-dependent cyclic guanosine monophosphate generation in glomeruli from diabetic rats. Evidence for PKC-mediated suppression of the cholinergic response. *J Clin Invest* 1994; 93: 311–20.
86. Ganz MB, Seftel A. Glucose-induced changes in PKC and NO are prevented by vitamin E. Am J Physiol Endocrinol *Metab* 2000; 278: E146–52.
87. Glogowski EA, Tsiani E, Zhou X, Fantus IG, Whiteside C. High glucose alters the response of mesangial cell PKC isoforms to endothelin 1. *Kidney Int* 1999; 55: 486–99.
88. Hempel A, Maasch C, Heintze U, Lindschau C, Dietz R, Luft FC, Haller H. High glucose concentrations increase endothelial cell permeability via activation of PKC alpha. *Circ Res* 1997; 81: 363–71.
89. Williams SB, Goldfine AB, Timimi FK, Ting HH, Roddy MA, Simonson DC, Creager MA. Acute hyperglycemia attenuates endothelium-dependent vasodilation in humans *in vivo*. *Circulation* 1998; 97: 1695–701.
90. Studer RK, Craven PA, DeRubertis FR. Role for PKC in the mediation of increased fibronectin accumulation by mesangial cells grown in high-glucose medium. *Diabetes* 1993; 42: 118–26.
91. Craven PA, Studer RK, Felder J, Phillips S, DeRubertis FR. Nitric oxide inhibition of transforming growth factor-beta and collagen synthesis in mesangial cells. *Diabetes* 1997; 46: 671–81.
92. Phillips SL, DeRubertis FR, Craven PA. Regulation of the laminin C1 promoter in cultured mesangial cells. *Diabetes* 1999; 48: 2083–9.
93. Feener EP, Xia P, Inoguchi T, Shiba T, Kunisaki M, King GL. Role of PKC in glucose- and angiotensin II-induced PAI expression. *Contrib Nephrol* 1996; 118: 180–7.
94. Yerneni KK, Bai W, Khan BV, Medford RM, Natarajan R. Hyperglycemia-induced activation of nuclear transcription factor kappaB in vascular SMCs. *Diabetes* 1999; 48: 855–64.
95. Koya D, Haneda M, Nakagawa H, Isshiki K, Sato H, Maeda S, Sugimoto T, Yasuda H, Kashiwagi A, Ways DK, King GL, Kikkawa R. Amelioration of accelerated diabetic mesangial expansion by treatment with a PKC beta inhibitor in diabetic *db/db* mice, a rodent model for type 2 diabetes. *FASEB J* 2000; 14: 439–47.
96. Jiang ZY, Lin YW, Clemont A, Feener EP, Hein KD, Igarashi M, Yamauchi T, White MF, King GL. Characterization of selective resistance to insulin signaling in the vasculature of obese Zucker (*fa/fa*) rats. *J Clin Invest* 1999; 104: 447–57.
97. Kolm-Litty V, Sauer U, Nerlich A, Lehmann R, Schleicher ED. High glucose-induced transforming growth factor beta1 production is mediated by the hexosamine pathway in porcine glomerular mesangial cells. *J Clin Invest* 1998; 101: 160–9.
98. Marshall S, Bacote V, Traxinger RR. Discovery of a metabolic pathway mediating glucose-induced desensitization of the glucose transport system. Role of hexosamine biosynthesis in the induction of IR. *J Biol Chem* 1991; 266: 4706–12.
99. Chen YQ, Su M, Walia RR, Hao Q, Covington JW, Vaughan DE. Sp1 sites mediate activation of the PAI-1 promoter by glucose in vascular SMCs. *J Biol Chem* 1998; 273: 8225–31.
100. Goldberg HJ, Scholey J, Fantus IG. Glucosamine activates the PAI 1 gene promoter through Sp1 DNA binding sites in glomerular mesangial cells. *Diabetes* 2000; 49: 863–71.
101. Hawkins M, Barzilai N, Liu R, Hu M, Chen W, Rossetti L. Role of the glucosamine pathway in fat-induced IR. *J Clin Invest* 1997; 99: 2173–82.
102. Goldberg HJ, Whiteside CI, Fantus IG. The hexosamine pathway regulates the plasminogen activator inhibitor-1 gene promoter and Sp1 transcriptional activation through PKC-beta I and -delta. *J Biol Chem* 2002; 277: 33833–41.
103. Kadonaga JT, Courey AJ, Ladika J, Tjian R. Distinct regions of Sp1 modulate DNA binding and transcriptional activation. *Science* 1988; 242: 1566–70.
104. Haltiwanger RS, Grove K, Philipsberg GA. Modulation of O-linked *N*-acetylglucosamine levels on nuclear and cytoplasmic proteins *in vivo* using the peptide *O*-GlcNAc-beta-*N*-acetylglucosaminidase inhibitor *O*-(2-acetamido-2-deoxy-D-glucopyranosylidene)amino-*N*-phenylcarbamate. *J Biol Chem* 1998; 273: 3611–7.
105. Jackson SP, Tjian R. O-Glycosylation of eukaryotic transcription factors: implications for mechanisms of transcriptional regulation. *Cell* 1988; 55: 125–33.
106. Du XL, Edelstein D, Dimmeler S, Ju Q, Sui C, Brownlee M. Hyperglycemia inhibits endothelial NO synthase activity by posttranslational modification at the Akt site. *J Clin Invest* 2001; 108: 1341–8.
107. Nishikawa T, Edelstein D, Du XL, Yamagishi S, Matsumura T, Kaneda Y, Yorek MA, Beebe D, Oates PJ, Hammes HP, Giardino I, Brownlee M. Normalizing mitochondrial superoxide production blocks three pathways of hyperglycaemic damage. *Nature* 2000; 404: 787–90.
108. Giugliano D, Ceriello A, Paolisso G. Oxidative stress and diabetic vascular complications. *Diabetes Care* 1996; 19: 257–67.

109. Korshunov SS, Skulachev VP, Starkov AA. High protonic potential actuates a mechanism of production of reactive oxygen species in mitochondria. *FEBS Lett* 1997; 416: 15–8.
110. Craven PA, Phillips SL, Melhem MF, Liachenko J, DeRubertis FR. Overexpression of manganese superoxide dismutase suppresses increases in collagen accumulation induced by culture of mesangial cells in high-media glucose. *Metabolism* 50: 1043–8.
111. Craven PA, Melhem MF, Phillips SL, DeRubertis FR. Overexpression of Cu^{2+}/Zn^{2+} superoxide dismutase protects against early diabetic glomerular injury in transgenic mice. *Diabetes* 2001; 50: 2114–25.
112. Yamagishi SI, Edelstein D, Du XL, Brownlee M. Hyperglycemia potentiates collagen-induced platelet activation through mitochondrial superoxide overproduction. *Diabetes* 2001; 50: 1491–4.
113. Watson PA, Nesterova A, Burant CF, Klemm DJ, Reusch JE. Diabetes-related changes in cAMP response element-binding protein content enhance smooth muscle cell proliferation and migration. *J Biol Chem* 2001; 276: 46142–50.
114. Watson PA, Vinson C, Nesterova A, Reusch JE. Content and activity of cAMP response element-binding protein regulate platelet-derived growth factor receptor-alpha content in vascular smooth muscles. *Endocrinology* 2002; 143: 2922–9.
115. Klemm DJ, Watson PA, Frid MG, Dempsey EC, Schaack J, Colton LA, Nesterova A, Stenmark KR, Reusch JE. cAMP response element-binding protein content is a molecular determinant of smooth muscle cell proliferation and migration. *J Biol Chem* 2001; 276: 46132–41.
116. Pugazhenthi S, Reusch JEB. *J Neurochem* 2003; 84: 982–96.
117. Finkbeiner S. CREB couples neurotrophin signals to survival messages. *Neuron* 2000; 25: 11–4.
118. Kowluru RA, Tang J, Kern TS. Abnormalities of retinal metabolism in diabetes and experimental galactosemia, VII: effect of long-term administration of antioxidants on the development of retinopathy. *Diabetes* 2001; 50: 1938–42.
119. Ting HH, Timimi FK, Boles KS, Creager SJ, Ganz P, Creager MA. Vitamin C improves endothelium-dependent vasodilation in patients with non-insulin-dependent diabetes mellitus. *J Clin Invest* 1996; 97: 22–8.
120. Heart Outcomes Prevention Evaluation Study Investigators. Effects of ramipril on cardiovascular and microvascular outcomes in people with diabetes mellitus results of the HOPE study and MICRO-HOPE substudy. *Lancet* 2000; 355: 253–9.
121. Salvemini D, Wang ZQ, Zweier JL, Samouilov A, Macarthur H, Misko TP, Currie MG, Cuzzocrea S, Sikorski JA, Riley DP. A nonpeptidyl mimic of superoxide dismutase with therapeutic activity in rats. *Science* 1999; 286: 304–6.

79

Endothelial Function and Dysfunction

Coen D.A. Stehouwer and Casper G. Schalkwijk

VU University Medical Centre, Amsterdam, The Netherlands

INTRODUCTION

Micro- and macroangiopathy cause most of the excess morbidity and mortality in diabetes mellitus. Retinal and renal microangiopathy cause diabetic retinopathy and nephropathy, and microangiopathy of the vasa nervorum contributes to diabetic neuropathy. Macroangiopathy in diabetes consists mainly of an accelerated form of atherosclerosis and affects all clinically important sites, i.e., the coronary, the carotid, and the peripheral arteries [1–3].

Diabetic patients with the most severe hyperglycemia have the highest risk of microangiopathy. Hyperglycemia, however, is a necessary but not a sufficient cause of clinically important microangiopathy. Hypertension is an additional major cause, and smoking, hypercholesterolemia, diabetic dyslipidemia (i.e., low high-density lipoprotein (HDL) cholesterol and high triglycerides), obesity, and hyperhomocysteinemia may also contribute. Risk of macroangiopathy, as in nondiabetic individuals, is related to general risk factors for atherothrombosis, such as age, smoking, hypertension, hypercholesterolemia, dyslipidemia, obesity, and hyperhomocysteinemia. Risk factors for micro- and macroangiopathy thus show much overlap except that risk of macroangiopathy does not appear to be strongly related to hyperglycemia, although this is controversial [1–9]. Hypertension, dyslipidemia, and obesity are seen more often in patients with type 2 than in those with type 1 diabetes. In addition, the latter three risk factors occur together more commonly than expected by chance and are thus said to *cluster* in the metabolic (or insulin resistance) syndrome, which further consists of insulin resistance, hyperinsulinemia, and impaired fibrinolysis.

In both types of diabetes, risk of macroangiopathy is strongly determined by the presence of nephropathy, even in its early stages (microalbuminuria), which identifies a group of patients at very high risk of developing severe complications, i.e., proliferative retinopathy, renal insufficiency, severe neuropathy, and cardiovascular disease. On the other hand, a substantial fraction of diabetic patients, perhaps 50%, will never develop this cluster of severe complications, i.e., they appear “protected.”

Dysfunction of the vascular endothelium is thought to play a key role in the pathogenesis of micro- and macroangiopathy in diabetes. This chapter will review how endothelial dysfunction relates to the pattern of disease occurrence described above and what current biochemical mechanisms have been proposed as an explanation for the development of endothelial dysfunction in diabetes.

WHAT IS ENDOTHELIAL DYSFUNCTION AND HOW CAN IT BE MEASURED IN HUMANS?

The endothelium is an important locus of control of vascular and thus organ functions [10–32]. It actively regulates vascular tone and permeability, the balance between coagulation and fibrinolysis, the composition of the subendothelial matrix, the adhesion and extravasation of leukocytes, inflammatory activity in the vessel wall, and the functioning of vascular smooth muscle cells. It also affects (and can be affected by) the functions of other cell types, such as platelets, leukocytes, retinal pericytes, renal mesangial cells, and large artery macrophages. To carry out its functions, the endothelium produces components of the extracellular matrix and a variety of regulatory mediators, such as nitric oxide, prostanoids, endothelin, angiotensin II, tissue-type plasminogen activator (tPA) and plasminogen activator inhibitor 1 (PAI-1), von Willebrand factor (vWF), adhesion molecules, and cytokines.

International Textbook of Diabetes Mellitus, Third Edition. Edited by R. A. DeFronzo, E. Ferrannini, H. Keen, and P. Zimmet.
 ISBN: 0-471-48655-8.

Normal functions of the endothelium include the following:

(1) It actively decreases vascular tone.
(2) It limits leukocyte adhesion and thus inflammatory activity in the vessel wall.
(3) It maintains vascular permeability to nutrients, hormones, other macromolecules, and leukocytes within narrow bounds.
(4) It inhibits platelet adhesion and aggregation by producing prostacyclin, nitric oxide, and ectonucleotidases.
(5) It limits activation of the coagulation cascade by the thrombomodulin–protein C, heparan sulfate–antithrombin and tissue factor – tissue factor pathway inhibitor interactions.
(6) It regulates fibrinolysis by producing tPA and its inhibitor, PAI-1.

Nitric oxide is a particularly important endothelium-derived mediator, because of its vasodilator, antiplatelet, antiproliferative, permeability-decreasing, and anti-inflammatory properties. Nitric oxide inhibits leukocyte adhesion and rolling as well as cytokine-induced expression of vascular cell adhesion molecule 1 (VCAM-1) and monocyte chemotactic protein 1, effects that are at least in part attributable to inhibition of the transcription factor NF-κB through increased expression of its inhibitor, IκB.

The endothelium can adapt to temporal and local requirements. Thus, for example, the increase in venular endothelial permeability observed in local inflammation is an adaptive and useful response. However, injury to the endothelium can cause endothelial dysfunction. Dysfunction of the endothelium can be considered present when its properties, either in the basal state or after stimulation, have changed in a way that is inappropriate with regard to the preservation of organ function. For example, basement membrane synthesis may be altered, resulting in changes in cell–matrix interactions, which can contribute to arterial stiffening and increased microvascular permeability; vascular tone and permeability may increase, which contributes to increased blood pressure and atherogenesis; and the endothelium may lose its antithrombotic and profibrinolytic properties and may instead acquire prothrombotic and antifibrinolytic properties. Such alterations (*endothelial dysfunctions*) do not necessarily occur simultaneously. Furthermore, they may differ according to the nature of the injury and may depend on the intrinsic properties of the endothelium (e.g., venous versus arterial versus microvascular endothelium). Endothelial *activation* designates one specific set of dysfunctions characterized by (usually inflammatory-cytokine-induced) increased interactions with blood leukocytes, in which adhesion molecules (such as E-selectin and VCAM-1) and chemoattractants (such as monocyte chemotactic protein 1 and interleukin-8) are essential.

Endothelial dysfunctions are thought to play important roles not only in the initiation of atherosclerosis, but also in its progression and clinical sequelae. Endothelial dysfunctions, notably endothelial activation, can be conceptualized as a transducer of atherogenic risk factors. In this view, risk factors such as oxidatively modified low-density lipoprotein (LDL) cholesterol, smoking, and diabetes initiate atherosclerosis through endothelial activation, whereas the protective effect of HDL is mediated by its ability to decrease LDL oxidation. Atherosclerosis is often especially severe at arterial branching points, biturcations, and convexities. This predilection is explained by the fact that blood flow there is nonlaminar or even turbulent and shear stress low or oscillatory, and that these conditions increase endothelial activation, effects that are enhanced by high blood pressure. Experimental models of hypercholesterolemia, hypertension, and diabetes also have in common that endothelial nitric oxide availability is decreased, whether through decreased production or through increased degradation. For example, high LDL cholesterol increases the production of reactive oxygen species and thus nitric oxide scavenging, but also increases the interaction between nitric oxide synthase and caveolin 1, which decreases nitric oxide production. Another important example is angiotensin II, which increases activity of vascular NAD(P)H oxidases, superoxide production, and nitric oxide scavenging, and thus decreases nitric oxide availability. These processes will increase endothelial activation.

Endothelial function cannot be measured directly in humans. Estimates of different types of endothelial dysfunction may be obtained indirectly by measuring endothelium-dependent vasodilation, plasma levels of endothelium-derived regulatory proteins, and, possibly, microalbuminuria (Table 1). Some other vascular properties, such as arterial stiffness, are probably in part endothelium-dependent, but it is not known to what extent [21, 31, 32]. Are the measurements listed in Table 1 valid estimates of endothelial dysfunction? On the one hand, many cross-sectional studies have shown impaired endothelium-dependent vasodilation and high levels of endothelium-derived regulatory proteins in patients with diseases that involve injury to the endothelium, such as atherothrombosis, preeclampsia, and vasculitis, as well as in individuals with risk factors for atherothrombosis. Moreover, prospective studies have shown that individuals with impaired endothelium-dependent vasodilation, high levels of endothelium-derived regulatory proteins, or microalbuminuria (regardless of the presence of diabetes) have an adverse cardiovascular prognosis. On the other hand, the interpretation of the tests listed in Table 1 is not as straightforward as one would wish. First, tests intended to estimate nitric oxide mediated endothelium-dependent

Table 1 Proposed estimates of endothelial dysfunction in humans

Measurement	Interpretation of altered endothelial function
Impaired endothelium-dependent vasodilation	Decreased production of vasodilators such as nitric oxide and/or increased production of vasoconstrictors
Increased transcapillary escape rate of intravenously injected radiolabeled albumin	Increased permeability to macromolecules
Microalbuminuria	
Endothelin*	Increased production of vasoconstrictors
von Willebrand factor*	Increased prothrombotic and procoagulant activity
sThrombomodulin*	Decreased anticoagulant activity
Tissue-type plasminogen activator*	Decreased profibrinolytic activity
Plasminogen activator inhibitor 1*	
sE-selectin*	Increased adhesion of and permeability to leukocytes; inflammatory activation
sVCAM 1*	
sICAM 1*	
Cellular fibronectin*	Altered extracellular matrix synthesis
Type IV collagen fragments*	

Note: s = soluble; VCAM = vascular cell adhesion molecule; ICAM = intercellular adhesion molecule.
* Increased plasma or serum level.

vasodilation in part measure effects of other endothelial vasodilators such as prostacyclin and endothelium-derived hyperpolarizing factor, and in part may be confounded by impaired vascular smooth muscle function. Second, the concept that high plasma levels of endothelium-derived mediators reflect endothelial dysfunction in clinically relevant arteries (such as the coronary and carotid) requires (1) that other cell types are not an important source; (2) that synthesis is more important than clearance, unless the latter is endothelium-dependent; and (3) that endothelial function in the microvasculature parallels that in large arteries, because microvascular endothelium, with its very large surface area and synthetic capacity, is the most important determinant of plasma levels of endothelium-derived mediators. Information on the validity of these assumptions is as yet scarce. In some cases, the assumptions are clearly invalid. For example, PAI-1 can be produced not only by endothelial cells, but also by hepatocytes, adipocytes, and vascular smooth muscle cells. Third, it is likely that the transcapillary escape rate of albumin is determined not only by the endothelium, but also by the biochemical and biophysical properties of the extracellular matrix and by hemodynamic forces. Finally, it is unlikely that the presence of microalbuminuria always and exclusively reflects a generalized increase of endothelial permeability; it may be wholly or partly a local renal hemodynamic phenomenon in at least some cases. Thus, the estimates that exist for assessing endothelial function *in vivo* in humans are reasonable but not perfect.

ENDOTHELIAL DYSFUNCTION IN DIABETES: GENERAL REMARKS

The literature on endothelial function in diabetes is large and complex [33–43], in part because endothelial function can be measured in many ways and in many vascular beds (see above). In addition, investigators have studied endothelial function in diabetes to answer several distinct questions, namely,

(1) Is the occurrence of microalbuminuria accompanied by severe endothelial dysfunction, and, if so, can this explain why microalbuminuria is accompanied by an increased risk of other microangiopathic complications and of atherothrombotic disease?
(2) Is hyperglycemia a sufficient cause of at least some types of endothelial dysfunction and is diabetes therefore usually a state of endothelial dysfunction?
(3) What is the significance of the finding that insulin resistance (regardless of the presence of diabetes) is associated with endothelial dysfunction?
(4) What are the mechanisms that cause diabetes-associated endothelial dysfunction?

The importance of these questions lies in the expected consequences of persistent endothelial dysfunction, which include

(1) increased blood pressure through increased peripheral arteriolar resistance, impaired renal function, and increased large arterial stiffness;
(2) increased susceptibility to microangiopathy through both hemodynamic (increased microvascular pressure and permeability) and other mechanisms, such as inflammation; and
(3) increased susceptibility to atherothrombosis through increases in blood pressure, vascular permeability, leukocyte adhesion and inflammation, and procoagulant and antifibrinolytic changes.

These concepts have a firm experimental basis but have as yet not been rigorously tested in humans, for two reasons. First, such testing can be difficult because there is no established method of measurement (e.g., for large artery endothelial permeability) or because the outcome (e.g., myocardial infarction) is many years away. Second, specific interventions to improve endothelial function are not available. Statins, angiotensin-converting-enzyme (ACE) inhibitors, angiotensin receptor blockers, estrogen, L-arginine, antioxidants, and folic acid have all been shown to improve endothelial function, but these compounds have many other effects, and so it has not been possible to determine to what extent such improvement of endothelial function explains clinical effects (e.g., ACE-inhibitor-induced decrease of blood pressure or statin-induced reduction of risk of myocardial infarction).

GENERALIZED ENDOTHELIAL DYSFUNCTION, CHRONIC, LOW-GRADE INFLAMMATION, MICROALBUMINURIA, AND ATHEROTHROMBOSIS

In both type 1 and type 2 diabetes, patients with advanced nephropathy (macroalbuminuria) have a greatly increased risk of severe retinopathy, neuropathy, and atherothrombotic disease. This pattern can be observed even in early nephropathy, i.e. microalbuminuria, which has raised the question of what common mechanisms may be at work [1, 2, 33]. Because (micro)albuminuria is often associated with classic risk factors for microangiopathy and atherothrombosis, notably poor glycemic control, hypertension, obesity, dyslipidemia, and smoking, an obvious possibility is that such risk factors cause both (micro)albuminuria and atherothrombosis and thus explain their association. Many studies have investigated this and have concluded that common risk factors explain at most a small part of the association between (micro)albuminuria and atherothrombosis [44, 45]. Other mechanisms must therefore be at work, which may include severe, generalized endothelial dysfunction and chronic, low-grade inflammation.

Indeed, in both types of diabetes, micro- and macroalbuminuria are accompanied by a variety of markers of endothelial dysfunction [33]. Prospective studies using markers such as plasma vWF have shown that high vWF concentrations are associated with an increased risk of developing microalbuminuria, with increased progression of microalbuminuria, with the occurrence of diabetic retinopathy and neuropathy, and with an increased risk of cardiovascular events and death. Endothelial dysfunction in type 1 and 2 diabetes complicated by micro- or macroalbuminuria is generalized, in that it affects many aspects of endothelial function and occurs both in the kidney and elsewhere. Such data, together with more limited data showing that microalbuminuria is also associated with endothelial dysfunction in the absence of diabetes, have led to the concept that microalbuminuria itself is a marker of generalized renal and extrarenal endothelial dysfunction. Endothelial dysfunction is a central feature of the pathogenesis of atherothrombosis and could thus explain the latter's association with (micro)albuminuria. It is less clear how endothelial dysfunction might cause (micro)albuminuria. Theoretically, endothelial dysfunction could contribute to the pathogenesis of albuminuria both directly, by causing increased glomerular pressure and the synthesis of a leaky glomerular basement membrane, and indirectly, by influencing glomerular mesangial and epithelial cell function in a paracrine fashion (e.g., through inflammatory mechanisms). Importantly, the molecular pathways by which endothelial dysfunction causes (micro)albuminuria have yet to be worked out.

Chronic, low-grade inflammation [as assessed from markers such as plasma C-reactive protein (CRP) concentration] is another candidate to explain the association between (micro)albuminuria and extrarenal complications [46–48]. Indeed, regardless of the presence of diabetes, chronic, low-grade inflammation is associated with the occurrence and progression of (micro)albuminuria [47], and with risk of atherothrombotic disease [10]. In addition, chronic, low-grade inflammation can be both the cause and consequence of endothelial dysfunction, and the two appear tightly linked [46–48]. Nevertheless, recent data indicate that the association between (micro)albuminuria and atherothrombotic disease cannot be explained entirely by markers of endothelial dysfunction and chronic inflammation [47, 48]. One (likely) possibility is that such markers do not fully capture the processes they are meant to reflect; but an alternative or additional explanation is that there are other pathways that link (micro)albuminuria to extrarenal complications, such as autonomic neuropathy [49, 50] or prothrombotic mechanisms (Figure 1).

It must be noted that diabetes is associated with activation of the coagulation cascade [1]. Hyperglycemia, nonenzymatic glycation, and oxidative stress increase tissue factor activity and factor VII activity, decrease antithrombin activity, and impair heparan sulfate synthesis. Initially, anticoagulant defenses such as the response to activated protein C and the secretion of tissue factor

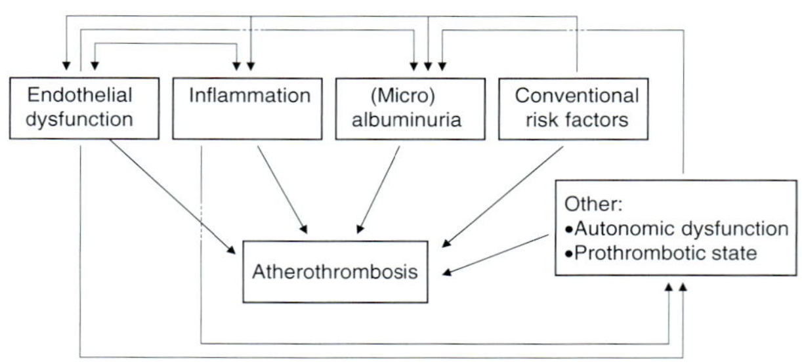

Figure 1 Postulated pathways linking conventional risk factors, endothelial dysfunction, inflammatory activity, (micro)albuminuria, and atherothrombosis in diabetes

pathway inhibitor may be enhanced. In patients with micro- and macroalbuminuria, i.e., in those with severe endothelial dysfunction, activation of the coagulation cascade increases further and endothelial anticoagulant defenses may be overwhelmed. In addition, patients with the metabolic syndrome have high PAI-1 levels and thus impaired fibrinolysis. In these patients, PAI-1 probably originates mainly from adipocytes and possibly from other cell types such as endothelial cells and hepatocytes, in response to several diabetes-associated stimuli, such as increased levels of glucose, insulin, proinsulin, very low density lipoprotein (VLDL), tumor necrosis factor α (TNF-α), and transforming growth factor β (TGF-β). Thrombin and fibrin thus generated may further increase endothelial activation. Importantly, increased coagulation and impaired fibrinolysis may increase thrombus formation and persistence after plaque rupture, and in part explain the poor prognosis of diabetic patients after myocardial infarction.

AT WHAT STAGE OF DIABETES DOES ENDOTHELIAL DYSFUNCTION BECOME MANIFEST?

Type 1 Diabetes

In type 1 diabetes, patients who have had the condition for more than 5–10 years and who have normal urinary albumin excretion, as compared to nondiabetic individuals, are characterized by subtle increases in blood pressure and large artery stiffness and by autonomic dysfunction, and some or perhaps most have impaired endothelial function and increased low-grade inflammation. All these abnormalities are worse in the microalbuminuric stage [33, 46, 51–53]. It is not clear how they interact nor whether impaired endothelial function is a common antecedent or a consequence, but these data illustrate that cardiovascular function, including endothelial function, does become impaired before the onset of microalbuminuria, at least when the latter is defined as ≥30 mg/24 h. The possibility remains, however, that patients with "normal" urinary albumin excretion who show such cardiovascular abnormalities are those in whom urinary albumin excretion is in fact increased albeit within the normal range as conventionally defined, i.e., the (arbitrary) cutoff of 30 mg/24 h may be too high. This has a parallel in type 2 diabetes and in nondiabetic individuals, in whom *any* increase in microalbuminuria appears associated with increased risk of atherothrombosis [44, 45].

Endothelial dysfunction thus occurs before microalbuminuria sets in. However, is endothelial dysfunction a feature of type 1 diabetes *per se* and is moderate hyperglycemia sufficient to impair endothelial function? On the one hand, plasma vWF levels are not increased in patients with early, uncomplicated, and reasonably well-regulated type 1 diabetes, suggesting normal endothelial function. On the other hand, it has been argued that nitric oxide mediated endothelium-dependent vasodilation is impaired in short-term uncomplicated diabetes and that hyperglycemia, in the absence of other factors, acutely impairs endothelium-dependent vasodilation in nondiabetic individuals [33, 54, 55]. Several findings are however in conflict with these concepts [56–61]. First, studies that carefully stratified patients according to the presence or absence of a normal urinary albumin excretion rate have concluded that, in reasonably well-controlled type 1 diabetes, endothelium-dependent and -independent vasodilation of resistance and conduit arteries are neither impaired nor enhanced [56–58]. Second, early uncomplicated type 1 diabetes is accompanied by dilation, not constriction, of small and large blood vessels, and an increase in microvascular blood flow, both in humans and in animal models [1, 58]. Microvascular dilation may cause capillary hypertension, and, according to the so-called hemodynamic hypothesis of the pathogenesis of microangiopathy, capillary hypertension will, in time, damage the microvascular endothelium and thus set the stage for more advanced stages of microangiopathy, such as microalbuminuria. It is at this stage that a general impairment of endothelial function, including impaired endothelium-dependent vasodilation, can usually be clearly observed, although endothelial function may sometimes be normal even among microalbuminuric individuals [62]. Notably, the mediators responsible for the vasodilation typical of early type 1 diabetes remain to be identified, and it is not known whether the endothelium is involved. Taken together, these data suggest that impaired endothelium-dependent vasodilation may occur early in a subset of type 1 diabetic patients, apparently dependent on other, environmental or genetic, factors [63]. In other words, the diabetic state predisposes to the development of endothelial dysfunction, but in and of itself is not a sufficient cause. Other factors, genetic or environmental, are likely to play a role in determining who among type 1 diabetic patients goes on to develop aggressive angiopathy and who does not.

Type 2 Diabetes

Endothelial dysfunction (e.g., impaired endothelium-dependent vasodilation and increased plasma concentrations of markers of endothelial function) is common in early and otherwise uncomplicated type 2 diabetes. For example, vWF and soluble VCAM-1 levels are increased and have been found to be associated with an increased risk of cardiovascular mortality and with an increased risk of development and progression of microalbuminuria [30, 33, 47, 48]. Impairment of endothelial function may be especially severe among diabetic women [64].

It is not clear to what extent this endothelial dysfunction is caused by hyperglycemia. Type 2 diabetes typically occurs in the context of a cluster of cardiovascular risk factors, notably obesity, hypertension, high triglyceride levels, low HDL cholesterol levels, abnormal LDL composition, hyperinsulinemia, insulin resistance, and chronic low-grade inflammation, all of which may impair endothelial function. Endothelial dysfunction in type 2 diabetes appears to be independent of that induced by hypertension and obesity [64, 65], but the role of the other variables (versus hyperglycemia) remains to be established [48, 66]. An important contender is increased inflammatory activity. Endothelial dysfunction, inflammation, and urinary albumin excretion in type 2 diabetes are progressive and closely interrelated [48]. Nevertheless, as in type 1 diabetes, microalbuminuria in type 2 diabetes can occur in the absence of severe endothelial dysfunction [62, 67], and then has a relatively good prognosis [68].

ENDOTHELIAL DYSFUNCTION, INSULIN RESISTANCE, AND THE METABOLIC (INSULIN RESISTANCE) SYNDROME

Insulin resistance usually precedes the development of type 2 diabetes and is often accompanied by a cluster of other risk factors (see above). The mechanisms underlying this clustering are still unclear, but all elements of the cluster share two important pathophysiological features, namely insulin resistance and endothelial dysfunction. A widely accepted theory states that insulin resistance is the primary abnormality that gives rise to type 2 diabetes, hypertension, and dyslipidemia, and that endothelial dysfunction merely represents the impact of hyperglycemia and other features of the metabolic syndrome. An alternative concept is that endothelial dysfunction is at the heart of the metabolic syndrome. According to this concept, the endothelial dysfunction in large arteries, which is an early and prominent event in atherothrombotic disease, is parallelled by endothelial dysfunction in resistance vessels and metabolically important capillary beds, which contributes to the development of the metabolic syndrome [69].

How can endothelial dysfunction impair insulin-induced glucose disposal? First, insulin is a vasoactive hormone. Insulin increases muscle blood flow in a time- and concentration-dependent fashion through a mechanism that involves binding to the insulin receptor on the endothelial cell membrane and that can be abolished by inhibiting nitric oxide synthase. Nevertheless, insulin-induced increases in glucose uptake and total blood flow have different concentration–effect curves as well as time kinetics. Therefore, it is unlikely that a simple insulin-induced increase in total blood flow *per se* can increase glucose disposal [34]. Second, however, in a process termed *capillary recruitment*, insulin can redirect blood flow in skeletal muscle from nonnutritive capillaries (those that are not coupled to muscle cells) to nutritive capillaries (those that are) and thus increase glucose disposal even without increasing total blood flow [70, 71]. In this way, physical integrity and normal function of the arteriolar and capillary endothelium are prerequisites for normal metabolic insulin action. Indeed, insulin's vasodilator actions have been shown to be impaired in classic insulin-resistant states, notably type 2 diabetes, obesity, and hypertension, and to be decreased by mediators closely associated with insulin resistance, namely TNF-α and free fatty acids [72–75]. Taken together, these data suggest that endothelial dysfunction and impaired capillary recruitment can cause insulin resistance with respect to glucose disposal both when the microvascular endothelium is otherwise healthy but cannot react properly to insulin (endothelial insulin resistance) and when the microvascular endothelium is injured through other mechanisms, such as age-related capillary drop-out ("rarefaction", i.e., reduced capillary density per volume of tissue). Specifically, decreased capillary density and impaired capillary recruitment may decrease insulin-mediated glucose disposal by increasing the diffusion distance of glucose and insulin to glucose-metabolizing tissues; by impairing transendothelial insulin transport, if this should be surface-area-dependent; and by impairing recruitment of previously underperfused muscle tissue.

Decreased capillary density and impaired capillary recruitment may in part explain why insulin resistance is associated with hypertension [76–78], as capillaries can contribute to control of peripheral vascular resistance by virtue of their narrow caliber and relative nondistensibility; by rarefaction (modeling indicates that for ~40% rarefaction, there is a ~20% increase in peripheral vascular resistance); and through active deformations, i.e. contractility [79]. In turn, the association of decreased capillary density and impaired recruitment with low birth weight [80, 81] and increasing age may help explain the propensity of such individuals both to insulin resistance and hypertension.

Decreased capillary density and impaired capillary recruitment may also play a role in the development of atherogenic changes in lipoprotein concentrations, through impaired action of endothelium-bound lipoprotein lipase (LPL). LPL is the rate-limiting enzyme for triglyceride utilization and its physiological site of action is the capillary endothelial surface. Studies in transgenic mice and in individuals with mutations in the *LPL* gene suggest that LPL dysfunction leads to increased plasma triglycerides and reduced plasma HDL cholesterol. A reduced capillary endothelial surface area may in turn result in reduced access of triglyceride-rich lipoprotein particles to LPL. Such a mechanism could explain why the dyslipidemia of the metabolic syndrome is confined to triglycerides and HDL cholesterol [34].

The molecular pathways through which insulin increases nitric oxide synthesis, endothelium-dependent

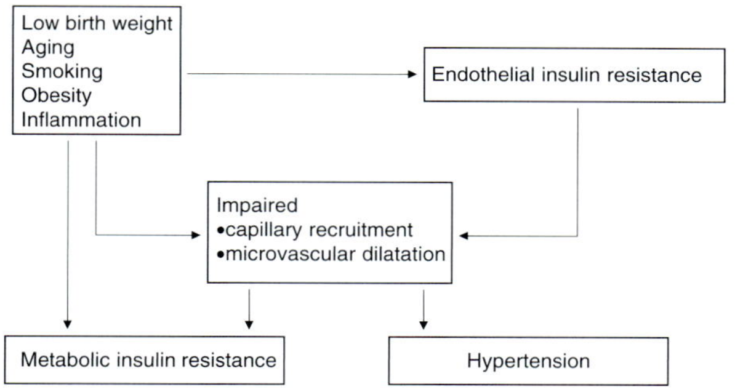

Figure 2 Postulated pathways linking cardiovascular risk factors, insulin resistance, and microvascular function

vasodilation, and capillary recruitment have not yet been fully elucidated, nor how TNF-α, free fatty acids, and perhaps hyperinsulinemia itself [82, 83] impair these actions of insulin. First, insulin can act on insulin receptors on endothelial cells to produce nitric oxide but also endothelin 1, a potent vasoconstrictor. Endothelial insulin resistance can thus be conceptualized as a shift in the balance between vasodilators and vasoconstrictors produced by insulin, with vasodilation as the normal response and impaired vasodilation or even net vasoconstriction as abnormal responses. Second, although insulin's endothelial actions have been shown to occur in cell culture and in isolated vessels, this does not exclude that, *in vivo*, insulin may act at insulin receptors on vascular smooth cells to cause vasodilation and (or) on skeletal muscle to activate glucose metabolism to produce a metabolite (e.g., adenosine) that then acts on local endothelial and (or) smooth muscle cells. Third, regardless of the presence of diabetes, chronic, low-grade inflammation is closely associated with, and may link, endothelial dysfunction and metabolic insulin resistance [84–89]. These postulated pathways are summarized in Figure 2.

MOLECULAR CELL BIOLOGY OF ENDOTHELIAL DYSFUNCTION IN DIABETES

General Remarks

Endothelial dysfunction in diabetes originates from three main sources [1, 3, 34, 90–98].

First, hyperglycemia and its immediate biochemical sequelae *directly* alter endothelial function. Glucose transport into endothelial and vascular smooth muscle cells occurs by facilitated diffusion and is thus insulin-independent. Glucose transport is autoregulated by glucose in smooth muscle cells, but not in endothelial cells, in which an increase in blood glucose concentration will thus increase the intracellular accumulation of glucose and its metabolites. Thus, endothelial cells exposed to high glucose *in vitro* increase the production of extracellular matrix components, such as collagen and fibronectin, and of procoagulant proteins, such as vWF and tissue factor, and show decreased proliferation, migration, and fibrinolytic potential, and increased programmed cell death (apoptosis). Second, high glucose influences endothelial cell functioning *indirectly* by the synthesis of growth factors (e.g., TGF-β and vascular endothelial growth factor (VEGF)), cytokines (e.g., TNF-α), and vasoactive agents in other cells. Third, the components of the metabolic syndrome can affect endothelial function.

Hyperglycemia and Its Immediate Biochemical Sequelae

An increase in intracellular glucose will lead to an increase in the flux of glucose to sorbitol via the polyol pathway, an increase in glucosamine-6-phosphate via the hexosamine pathway, and the activation of protein kinase C (PKC) via *de novo* synthesis of diacylglycerol (DAG). In addition, glucose and glucose-derived dicarbonyl compounds react nonenzymatically with the basic amino acids, lysine and arginine, in proteins to form advanced glycation end products (AGEs) both extra- and intracellularly. Figure 3 shows how, intracellularly, these four biochemical mechanisms may all be the consequence of hyperglycemia-induced overproduction of reactive oxygen species in mitochondria [90, 96].

The Sorbitol Pathway

In most cells, excess glucose can be metabolized to sorbitol and fructose by aldose reductase and sorbitol dehydrogenase, which is accompanied by increased oxidation of NADPH to $NADP^+$ and increased reduction of NAD^+ to NADH. This pathway may impair endothelial function through three mechanisms. First, increased sorbitol accumulation will increase osmotic stress. Sorbitol accumulation decreases other osmolytes such as *myo*-inositol and taurine, which in turn can impair DAG formation and PKC activation, and exacerbate oxidative stress and disrupt calcium homeostasis, respectively. However, the relatively low expression of aldose reductase in endothelial cells may not be sufficient to cause significant sorbitol accumulation.

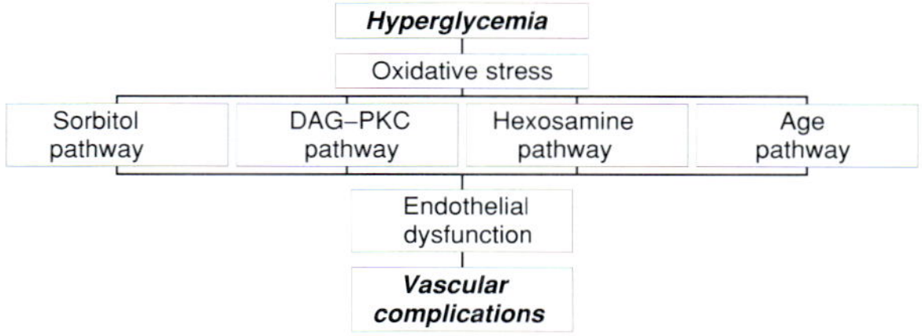

Figure 3 Four biochemical pathways through which hyperglycemia can cause endothelial dysfunction and vascular complications

Second, the increase in the cytosolic NADH/NAD$^+$ ratio results in a redox imbalance that resembles that which occurs in tissue hypoxia and therefore is termed *hyperglycemic pseudohypoxia*. It is caused not only by oxidation of sorbitol but especially by increased glycolysis, i.e., the oxidation of glyceraldehyde-3-phosphate to 1,3-diphosphoglycerate by glyceraldehyde-3-phosphate dehydrogenase (GAPDH). Consequences include inhibition of GAPDH, increased *de novo* synthesis of DAG, and activation of PKC. The effect of hyperglycemia on DAG and PKC may thus be cell- and tissue-specific, because, in cells with high levels of aldose reductase, *myo*-inositol depletion may decrease rather than increase PKC activity. Third, the redox imbalance favors the accumulation of triose phosphates, which increases the formation of methylglyoxal and AGEs, and enhances oxidative stress, which can be exacerbated by NADPH-deficiency-induced depletion of reduced glutathione [1].

The full impact of the sorbitol pathway in vascular dysfunction is not completely understood and the role of inhibition of aldose reductase in the prevention and treatment of diabetic complications remains unclear. Aldose reductase activity in endothelial cells is low and it thus appears unlikely that the improved nerve conduction in diabetic neuropathy observed with aldose reductase inhibitors or *myo*-inositol supplementation is related to improved endothelial function [1].

The DAG–PKC Pathway

The cellular pathogenic consequences of hyperglycemia-induced activation of PKC are multiple and include dysregulation of vascular permeability directly or indirectly (the latter through the induction of VEGF in smooth muscle cells); dysregulation of blood flow by decreasing endothelial nitric oxide synthase activity, and (or) increasing endothelin 1 synthesis; basement membrane thickening through TGF-β-mediated increased synthesis of type IV collagen and fibronectin; impaired fibrinolysis through increased expression of PAI-1; and increased oxidative stress by the regulation of several NADPH oxidases.

Hyperglycemia-induced activation of PKC occurs through increased levels of the PKC activator DAG, which, in cells with a low aldose reductase activity such as endothelial cells, is synthesized *de novo* from the glycolytic intermediates dihydroxyacetone phosphate and glyceraldehyde-3-phosphate. Interestingly, vitamin E can inhibit PKC-β activity, indicating a link between oxidative stress and PKC activation.

The PKC family consists of at least 11 isoforms. In vascular cells, the PKC-βII isoform appears preferentially activated. In diabetic animals, an oral PKC-β inhibitor prevented diabetes-induced abnormalities in mRNA expression of TGF-β1, type IV collagen, and fibronectin; ameliorated increases in glomerular filtration rate and accelerated glomerular mesangial expansion; and partly corrected urinary albumin excretion. Studies to evaluate the importance of the DAG–PKC pathway in humans are underway [1].

The Hexosamine Pathway

The vascular effects of the hexosamine pathway, in which fructose-6-phosphate is converted to glucosamine-6-phosphate by the enzyme glutamine : fructose-6-phosphate amidotransferase, are just beginning to be understood but may be profound. In aortic endothelial cells, hyperglycemia was shown to increase levels of hexosamine-6-phosphate and subsequently *N*-acetylglucosamine (GlcNAc). This, by the addition of GlcNAc to serine and threonine residues, increased O-linked glycosylation of the transcription factor SP-1, which decreased SP-1 phosphorylation and increased SP-1 activity, which in turn can increase transcription of PAI-1 and TGF-β1 [96]. Other proteins, such as PKC and endothelial cell nitric oxide synthase can be modified in a similar way. For example, such a modification of the Akt site of endothelial cell nitric oxide synthase has been shown to decrease enzyme activity [97].

Nonenzymatic Glycation

Nonenzymatic glycation of proteins is the condensation reaction of the carbonyl group of sugar aldehydes with the N-terminus of free amino acids of proteins and initially leads to a Schiff base, which then undergoes rearrangement to early glycation Amadori-adducts such as fructosamine. Amadori-adducts are relatively stable and only a small fraction undergoes rearrangements to irreversible AGEs. AGEs are a mixture of different moieties. When oxidation is involved in their formation, so-called glycoxidation products such as pentosidine and N^{ε}-(carboxymethyl)lysine result. Initially, AGEs were thought to form only on long-lived extracellular molecules, because of the slow rate of reaction of glucose with proteins. However, intracellular and short-lived molecules have now also been shown to be targets for AGE formation through reactions with other sugars such as glucose-6-phosphate and glyceraldehyde-3-phosphate, which form AGEs at a much faster rate than glucose. In addition, the highly reactive dicarbonyl compounds methylglyoxal, glyoxal, and 3-deoxyglucosone, which are formed from the degradation of glycolytic intermediates, are believed to contribute importantly to the formation of AGEs *in vivo*. This so-called carbonyl stress has been implicated in the accelerated vascular damage in both diabetes and uremia. In endothelial cells, methylglyoxal is probably the main AGE-forming compound and can be degraded to D-lactate by the glyoxylase system [91, 92].

The introduction of AGEs in the extracellular matrix can interfere with endothelial function in several ways. AGE-modified type I and IV collagen inhibit normal matrix formation and cross-linking, and decrease arterial elasticity; AGE-modified matrix stimulates interactions with mononuclear cells and macromolecules such as LDL; and AGEs may act as oxidants. For example, AGEs can quench nitric oxide. In addition, AGE-modified plasma proteins can bind to AGE receptors, including the receptor for AGE (RAGE), the macrophage scavenger receptor A, galectin-3, AGE-R1/*p60*, and AGE-R2/*p90*, on different cell types including endothelial cells [98]. Ligation of RAGE has been shown to mediate signal transduction via a receptor-mediated induction of reactive oxygen species and activation of the transcription factors NF-κB and $p21^{ras}$. In endothelial cells, the expression of the thrombomodulin, tissue factor, and VCAM-1 genes is adversely affected; in macrophages and mesangial cells, there is an increased expression of cytokines and growth factors such as interleukin 1, TNF-α, and TGF-β. In animal models, blockade of RAGE inhibited the development of macrovascular disease and diabetic nephropathy [98].

Many aspects of diabetic complications are thus potentially related to the effect of Amadori-adducts [99] and AGEs. Clinical trials with aminoguanidine, an AGE formation inhibitor that had shown promise in animal experiments, have unfortunately been halted because of unforeseen side effects, but trials with other AGE formation inhibitors and with AGE cross-link breakers are underway or are being planned.

Hyperglycemia-induced Oxidative Stress as a Common Activator of the Polyol, DAG-PKC, Hexosamine, and AGE Formation Pathways

Recent evidence [90] suggests that hyperglycemia-induced mitochrondrial overproduction of superoxide anion radicals plays a key role in the activation of the above pathways (Figures 3 and 4). The principal mitochondrial substrate is pyruvate, which is derived from aerobic glycolysis. In endothelial cells, glucose phosphorylation determines the rate of glycolysis and of pyruvate generation. Thus, when blood glucose concentration is high, glycolysis and pyruvate generation in endothelial cells will increase. Pyruvate carbons enter the Krebs cycle in the mitochondrial matrix, in which substrates are oxidized with the formation of CO_2 and the reduction of NAD^+ and FADH to NADH and $FADH_2$, respectively. NADH derived from both cytosolic glucose oxidation and the Krebs cycle provides electrons to complex I of the respiratory chain, while $FADH_2$ derived from the Krebs cycle donates electrons to complex II. The electron flow along the respiratory chain drives the extrusion of protons from the mitochondrial matrix, which establishes a steep electrochemical gradient across the inner mitochondrial membrane (inside negative). ATP synthase in the mitochondrial membrane catalyzes the condensation of ADP with inorganic phosphate to yield ATP. The generation of this high-energy bond is powered by the diffusion of protons back into the matrix through ATP synthase. Finally, ATP is transferred to the cytosol in exchange for ADP by the adenine nucleotide translocator. Because of the high membrane potential, electron transport is imperfect and mitochondria are the principal source of superoxide production. However, normally only 0.1% of total oxygen consumption leaks to reactive oxygen species. Hyperglycemia causes a marked increase in superoxide production by increasing the membrane potential as a result of an overproduction of electron donors by the Krebs cycle (Figure 5). Since

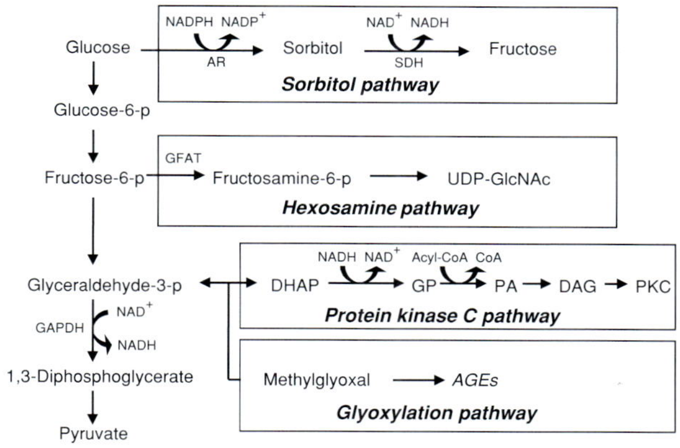

Figure 4 Potential mechanisms by which hyperglycemia and its immediate biochemical sequelae can induce hyperglycemic damage. AR = aldose reductase; SDH = sorbitol dehydrogenase; P = phosphate; GFAT = glutamine:fructose-6-phosphate amidotransferase; GlcNAc = *N*-acetylglucosamine; DHAP = dihydroxyacetone phosphate; GP = glycerol-3-phosphate; PA = phosphatidic acid; DAG = 1,2-diacylglycerol; PKC= protein kinase C [90]

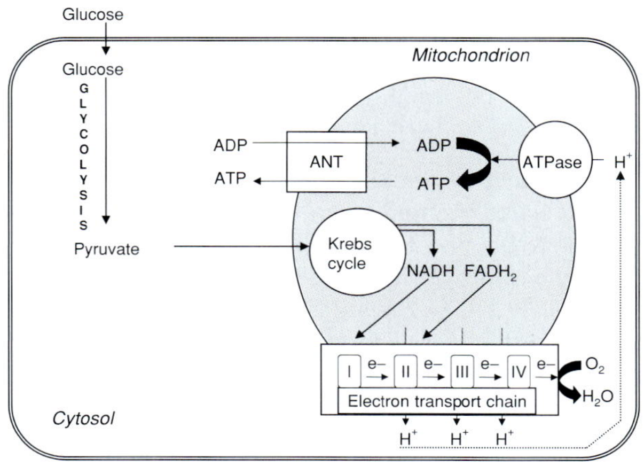

Figure 5 Overview of how glucose metabolism leads to energy (ATP) production. ADP = adenosine diphosphate; ATP = adenosine triphosphate; ANT = adenine nucleotide translocator

inhibition of hyperglycemia-induced reactive oxygen species production in cultured bovine endothelial cells prevented the hyperglycemia-associated activation of the pathways of damage described above, oxidative stress may be the initial event in endothelial cell dysfunction [90, 97].

Oxidative Stress as a Final Common Pathway of Hyperglycemia-induced Vascular Dysfunction

Hyperglycemic pseudohypoxia, glucose autooxidation, and AGE formation increase oxidative stress. In addition, hyperglycemia impairs endothelial free-radical scavenging by reducing the activity of the pentose phosphate pathway and thus decreasing the availability of NADPH to the glutathione redox cycle [92].

Reactive oxygen species can affect many signaling pathways, such as G-proteins, protein kinases, ion channels, and transcription factors, and may modify endothelial function by a variety of mechanisms. These include direct effects on the endothelium such as peroxidation of membrane lipids, activation of NF-κB, interference with the availability of nitric oxide, and increased matrix metalloproteinase activity [100] (which is involved in monocyte invasion and smooth muscle cell migration); and indirect effects such as increasing the oxidation of LDL and the activation of platelets and monocytes. On the other hand, endothelial cells can respond to high glucose levels by increasing the expression of antioxidant enzymes such as superoxide dismutase, catalase, and glutathione peroxidase.

It is not known whether oxidative stress causes endothelial dysfunction in human diabetes. It has been difficult to assess the presence of increased oxidative stress *in vivo*, mainly because of questionable specificity and reproducibility of the methods used. In short-term experiments, high doses of vitamin C can improve some aspects of endothelial dysfunction in diabetes [1]. On the other hand, randomized clinical trials have failed to show a decrease in macrovascular disease. The reasons for this discrepancy are unclear.

Growth Factors and Cytokines: TGF-β, VEGF, and TNF-α

There is solid evidence that TGF-β (with other growth factors such as insulin-like growth factor 1 and epidermal growth factor) plays a major role in diabetic nephropathy [101], while VEGF is important in severe retinopathy [102]. TNF-α may cause insulin resistance and impair endothelial function in large arteries and also in the microcirculation, suggesting that it may be important both in atherothrombosis and in microangiopathy.

Transforming Growth Factor β

TGF-β mediates glomerular capillary basement thickening and mesangial matrix expansion. Its role in the thickening of capillary basement membranes elsewhere (e.g., in the retina) is less well established. TGF-β has three isoforms. TGF-β1 is secreted by different cell types as an inactive dimer consisting of a latency-associated peptide and the mature TGF-β1, and is activated by serine proteases such as plasmin. TGF-β1 is increased through hyperglycemia-induced PKC activation (which involves the transcription factors c-fos and c-jun, and the AP-1 binding site in the promoter region of the *TGF-β1* gene); through Amadori-albumin and AGEs; through stretch and angiotensin II; and through cytokine activation of endothelial cells, which also increases plasmin-induced activation of the latent form. Three TGF-β receptors are involved in signal transduction. TGF-β1 stimulates the production of matrix components such as type I and IV collagen, fibronectin, laminin, and proteoglycans in cultured glomerular mesangial cells and epithelial cells; is involved in the regulation of glomerular endothelial, epithelial, and mesangial proliferation; and also has potent anti-inflammatory effects on vascular cells, downregulating cytokine-induced expression of E-selectin, VCAM-1, and monocyte chemotactic protein 1 [101].

Vascular Endothelial Growth Factor

VEGF is a potent and apparently endothelium-specific mitogenic cytokine, whose expression can be induced by hypoxia through hypoxia-inducible factor 1, but also by insulin-like growth factor 1 and TGF-β1. VEGF binds to several receptors, of which VEGF receptors 1 and 2, also known as fms-like tyrosine kinase and fetal liver kinase 1, have been best characterized. Hypoxia stimulates the expression of these receptors, ligation of which induces the proliferation and migration of vascular endothelial cells leading to angiogenesis, neovascularization, and increased vascular permeability. Several studies have shown increased vitreous VEGF levels in patients with proliferative diabetic retinopathy, and antagonists of VEGF and its receptors have been shown to reduce retinopathy in animal models. The role of increased or decreased VEGF in other diabetic complications is the subject of much ongoing research [102].

Tumor Necrosis Factor α and Inflammation

TNF-α is an inflammatory cytokine produced by neutrophils, macrophages, and, importantly, adipocytes. TNF-α can induce other powerful cytokines such as interleukin-6, which in turn regulates the expression of CRP. These mediators alone or in combination can impair endothelial function and contribute to atherothrombosis. In addition, TNF-α can induce insulin resistance, which may at least in part explain why insulin resistance, endothelial dysfunction, and atherothrombosis are so closely related (see above). Finally, recent studies have shown that

TNF-α and inflammation in general can contribute to the pathogenesis of diabetic nephropathy.

Vascular cells are both a target for cytokines and a source. The spectrum of endothelial cell responses elicited by cytokines is varied. Briefly, inflammatory cytokines increase vascular permeability; alter vasoregulatory responses; increase leukocyte adhesion to endothelium; and facilitate thrombus formation by inducing procoagulant activity, by inhibiting anticoagulant pathways and by impairing fibrinolysis via stimulation of PAI-1. Activation of the transcription factor NF-κB is crucial in cytokine regulation of gene expression in endothelial cells [14, 15]. NF-κB consists of a family of transcription factors that serve as important regulators of the inflammatory response and vascular cell function. NF-κB is activated not only by TNF-α and interleukin 1, but also by hyperglycemia, AGEs, angiotensin II, oxidized lipids, and insulin. Examples of NF-κB-regulated genes include VCAM-1, E-selectin, ICAM-1, interleukins 1, 6, and 8, tissue factor, PAI-1, and inducible nitric oxide synthase. On the other hand, NF-κB protects against apoptosis and activates the antioxidant enzyme, superoxide dismutase. Taken together, these data suggest that the NF-κB pathway is an important contributor to the pathogenesis of vascular disease in diabetes mellitus.

The Metabolic Syndrome: Insulin Resistance, Insulin, Insulin Precursor Molecules, Hypertension, Dyslipidemia, and Obesity

Insulin Resistance

How metabolic and endothelial insulin resistance occur and why they are closely related is not fully understood (see above). Endothelial insulin resistance, whether primary or secondary (Figure 2), can be regarded as a form of endothelial dysfunction and conceivably contributes to both atherothrombosis and microangiopathy. Both TNF-α and free fatty acids can cause metabolic and endothelial insulin resistance. TNF-α may induce endothelial insulin resistance through its ability to impair intracellular signaling by inhibition of insulin-stimulated autophosphorylation and phosphorylation of insulin receptor substrate 1. How nonesterified fatty acids impair insulin's endothelial actions is not clear.

Insulin

Both type 1 and type 2 diabetes are usually accompanied by chronic hyperinsulinemia. Whether insulin has atherogenic effects is controversial, mainly because it is not clear whether effects such as increased vascular permeability to macromolecules and increased vascular smooth muscle cell proliferation occur at physiological concentrations. In addition, insulin can increase nitric oxide synthesis and may have anti-inflammatory and antiatherogenic effects [103]. Taken together, these data raise the possibility that insulin may have adverse effects when insulin signaling in vascular cells is abnormal.

Insulin Precursor Molecules

Type 2 diabetes is characterized by high levels of molecules that arise as a by-product of insulin synthesis and secretion, notably intact proinsulin, proinsulin split products, and C-peptide. In contrast, levels of these peptides are abnormally low in type 1 diabetes. The vascular effects of these peptides have not been extensively investigated. Insulin precursors may increase plasma levels of PAI-1. C-peptide may affect vascular tone and permeability, although the molecular basis for these effects has not been fully elucidated.

Hypertension

Hypertension is a major determinant of microangiopathy and atherothrombosis in diabetes. Hypertension causes endothelial activation and impaired nitric oxide availability (see above); whether the latter then contributes to increased blood pressure is not clear. Experimental data indicate that decreased nitric oxide availability in the kidney may contribute to vasoconstriction and decreased glomerular filtration; impaired tubuloglomerular feedback; decreased medullary blood flow and impaired pressure natriuresis; and progressive proteinuria. Salt sensitivity of blood pressure may denote an inability to increase nitric oxide availability in response to increased blood pressure [104].

Impaired endothelial function in secondary hypertension is usually reversible upon reduction of blood pressure; in contrast, some patients with essential hypertension do not normalize endothelial function with blood pressure lowering [20, 104]. Data on this issue in diabetes are scarce.

Dyslipidemia

The general effects of LDL cholesterol have been discussed above. These may be enhanced in type 2 diabetes, which is associated with increased small dense LDL particles. In addition, type 2 diabetes, especially when glycemic control is poor, is characterized by increased postprandial triglyceride-rich lipoproteins (chylomicrons and VLDL particles), which can enhance oxidative stress and impair endothelial function both directly and indirectly (by increasing the production of small dense LDL particles and by reducing HDL [105–107]). These changes contribute to atherothrombosis and may also play a role in nephropathy, as such dyslipidemia can damage glomerular podocytes and mesangial cells [108]. Dyslipidemia has been associated with increases in urinary albumin excretion in both type 1 and type 2 diabetes [109, 110].

Obesity

Obesity, especially visceral obesity, is associated with increased risk of atherothrombosis and microangiopathy. These effects may be mediated through the associations of obesity with hypertension, dyslipidemia, and insulin resistance, and also through mediators directly secreted by adipocytes, such as TNF-α, leptin, and PAI-1. For example, obesity-associated proteinuria may be related to hyperfiltration, increased renal venous pressure, glomerular hypertrophy, and increased matrix production through increased synthesis of vasoactive and fibrogenic mediators, such as angiotensin II, insulin, leptin, and TGF-β1 [111].

SUMMARY

(1) The endothelium is an important locus of control of vascular functions.
(2) Reasonable but not perfect methods exist for assessing endothelial function *in vivo* in humans.
(3) Endothelial dysfunction in diabetes complicated by micro- or macroalbuminuria is generalized, in that it affects many aspects of endothelial function. The close linkage between microalbuminuria and endothelial dysfunction in diabetes is an attractive explanation for the fact that microalbuminuria is a risk marker for atherothrombosis.
(4) In type 1 diabetes, endothelial dysfunction precedes and may cause diabetic microangiopathy, but it is not clear whether endothelial dysfunction is a feature of the diabetic state *per se*.
(5) In type 2 diabetes, endothelial function is impaired from the onset of the disease and is strongly related to adverse outcomes. It is not clear whether impaired endothelial function is caused by hyperglycemia or by other factors.
(6) Impaired endothelial function is closely associated with and may contribute to insulin resistance regardless of the presence of diabetes.
(7) Endothelial dysfunction in diabetes originates from three main sources.
    (a) Hyperglycemia and its immediate biochemical sequelae *directly* alter endothelial function.
    (b) Hyperglycemia influences endothelial cell functioning *indirectly* by the synthesis of growth factors, cytokines, and vasoactive agents in other cells.
    (c) The components of the metabolic syndrome can impair endothelial function.

REFERENCES

1. Tooke JE (ed). *Diabetic Angiopathy*. London: Arnold, 1999.
2. Mogensen CE (ed). *The Kidney and Hypertension in Diabetes Mellitus*, 5th edn. Boston: Kluwer, 2000.
3. Stehouwer CDA, Yudkin JS (eds). Diabetic angiopathy. *Semin Vasc Med* 2002; 2: 1–228.
4. Hoogeveen EK, Kostense PJ, Eysink PED, Polak BCP, Beks PJ, Jakobs C, Dekker JM, Nijpels G, Heine RJ, Bouter LM, Stehouwer CDA. Hyperhomocysteinemia is associated with the presence of retinopathy in type 2 diabetes mellitus. The Hoorn Study. *Arch Intern Med* 2000; 160: 2984–90.
5. Jager A, Kostense PJ, Nijpels G, Dekker JM, Heine RJ, Bouter LM, Donker AJM, Stehouwer CDA. Serum homocysteine levels are associated with the development of (micro)albuminuria. The Hoorn Study. *Arterioscler Thromb Vasc Biol* 2001; 21: 74–81.
6. Stehouwer CDA, Gall MA, Hougaard P, Jakobs C, Parving HH. Plasma homocysteine concentration predicts mortality in non-insulin-dependent diabetic patients with and without albuminuria. *Kidney Int* 1999; 55: 308–14.
7. Hoogeveen EK, Kostense PJ, Jakobs C, Dekker JM, Nijpels G, Heine RJ, Bouter LM, Stehouwer CDA. Hyperhomocysteinemia increases risk of death, especially in type 2 diabetes: 5-year follow-up of the Hoorn Study. *Circulation* 2000; 101: 1506–11.
8. The Epidemiology of Diabetes Intervention and Complications (EDIC) Research Group. Effect of intensive diabetes treatment on carotid artery wall thickness in the epidemiology of diabetes interventions and complications. *Diabetes* 1999; 48: 383–90.
9. Laakso M. Hyperglycemia and cardiovascular disease in type 2 diabetes. *Diabetes* 1999; 48: 937–42.
10. Ross R. Atherosclerosis—an inflammatory disease. *N Engl J Med* 1999; 340: 115–26.
11. Cines DB, Pollak E, Buck CA, Loscalzo J, Zimmerman GA, McEver RP, Pober JS, Wick TM, Konkle BA, Schwartz BS, Barnathan ES, McCrae KR, Hug BA, Schmidt AM, Stern DM. Endothelial cells in the physiology and in the pathophysiology of vascular disorders. *Blood* 1998; 91: 3527–61.
12. De Caterina R. Endothelial dysfunctions: common denominators in vascular disease. *Curr Opin Lipidol* 2000; 11: 9–23.
13. Kinlay S, Libby P, Ganz P. Endothelial dysfunction and coronary artery disease. *Curr Opin Lipidol* 2001; 12: 383–9.
14. de Martin R, Hoeth M, Hofer-Warbinek R, Schmid JA. The transcription factor NF-κB and the regulation of vascular cell function. *Arterioscler Thromb Vasc Biol* 2000; 20: e83–8.
15. Tedgui A, Mallat Z. Anti-inflammatory mechanisms in the vascular wall. *Circ Res* 2001; 88: 877–87.
16. Resnick N, Yahav H, Schubert S, Wolfovitz E, Shay A. Signaling pathways in vascular endothelium activated by shear stress: relevance to atherosclerosis. *Curr Opin Lipidol* 2000; 11: 167–77.
17. John S, Schmieder RE. Impaired endothelial function in arterial hypertension and hypercholesterolemia: potential mechanisms and differences. *J Hypertens* 2000; 18: 363–74.
18. Ishani A, Raij L. Hypertension, nitric oxide and end-organ damage. *Curr Opin Nephrol Hypertens* 1999; 8: 237–41.
19. Berry C, Brosnan MJ, Fennell J, Hamilton CA, Dominiczak AF. Oxidative stress and vascular damage in hypertension. *Curr Opin Nephrol Hypertens* 2001; 10: 247–55.

20. Sowers JR. Hypertension, angiotensin II, and oxidative stress. *N Engl J Med* 2002; 346: 1999–2001.
21. McVeigh GE, Hamilton PK, Morgan DR. Evaluation of mechanical arterial properties: clinical, experimental and therapeutic aspects. *Clin Sci* 2002; 102: 51–67.
22. Celermajer DS. Endothelial dysfunction: does it matter? Is it reversible? *J Am Coll Cardiol* 1997; 30: 325–33.
23. Vanhoutte PM. How to assess endothelial function in human blood vessels. *J Hypertens* 1999; 17: 1047–58.
24. Stehouwer CDA. Is measurement of endothelial dysfunction clinically useful? *Eur J Clin Invest* 1999; 29: 459–61.
25. Cannon RO. Cardiovascular benefit of cholesterol-lowering therapy: does improved endothelial vasodilator function matter? *Circulation* 2000; 102: 820–2.
26. Vita JA, Keaney JF. Hormone replacement therapy and endothelial function. *Arterioscler Thromb Vasc Biol* 2001; 21: 1867–9.
27. Munford RS. Statins and the acute-phase response. *N Engl J Med* 2001; 344: 2016–8.
28. Schächinger V, Britten MB, Zeiher AM. Prognostic impact of coronary vasodilator dysfunction on adverse long-term outcome of coronary heart disease. *Circulation* 2000; 101: 1899–906.
29. Jager A, van Hinsbergh VWM, Kostense PJ, Emeis JJ, Yudkin JS, Nijpels G, Dekker JM, Heine RJ, Bouter LM, Stehouwer CDA. Von Willebrand factor, C-reactive protein and 5-year mortality in diabetic and nondiabetic subjects: the Hoorn Study. *Arterioscler Thromb Vasc Biol* 1999; 19: 3071–8.
30. Jager A, van Hinsbergh VWM, Kostense PJ, Emeis JJ, Nijpels G, Dekker JM, Heine RJ, Bouter LM, Stehouwer CDA. Increased levels of soluble vascular cell adhesion molecule 1 are associated with risk of cardiovascular mortality in type 2 diabetes. *Diabetes* 2000; 49: 485–91.
31. Kinlay S, Creager MA, Fukumoto M, Hikita H, Fang JC, Selwyn AP, Ganz P. Endothelium-derived nitric oxide regulates arterial elasticity in human arteries *in vivo*. *Hypertension* 2001; 38: 1049–53.
32. Silacci P, Desgeorges A, Mazzolai L, Chambaz C, Hayoz D. Flow pulsatility is a critical determinant of oxidative stress in endothelial cells. *Hypertension* 2001; 38: 1162–6.
33. Stehouwer CDA, Lambert J, Donker AJM, van Hinsbergh VWM. Endothelial dysfunction and the pathogenesis of diabetic angiopathy. *Cardiovasc Res* 1997; 34: 55–68.
34. Stehouwer CDA, Serné EH, Gans ROB. Endothelial function in diabetes. In Walker M, Butler P, Rizza RA (eds) *The Diabetes Annual*, 13th edn. Amsterdam: Elsevier Science, 2000; pp 77–95.
35. Goligorsky MS, Chen J, Brodsky S. Endothelial cell dysfunction leading to diabetic nephropathy. *Hypertension* 2001; 37 (pt 2): 744–8.
36. Flyvbjerg A. Putative pathophysiological role of growth factors and cytokines in experimental diabetic kidney disease. *Diabetologia* 2000; 43: 1205–23.
37. Cooper ME. Interaction of metabolic and hemodynamic factors in mediating experimental diabetic nephropathy. *Diabetologia* 2001; 44: 1957–72.
38. Jandeleit-Dahm K, Cooper ME. Hypertension and diabetes. *Curr Opin Nephrol Hypertens* 2002; 11: 221–8.
39. Boeri D, Maiello M, Lorenzi M. Increased prevalence of microthromboses in retinal capillaries of diabetic individuals. *Diabetes* 2001; 50: 1432–9.
40. Lorenzi M, Cerhardinger C. Early cellular and molecular changes induced by diabetes in the retina. *Diabetologia* 2001; 44: 791–804.
41. Cameron NE, Eaton SEM, Cotter MA, Tesfaye S. Vascular factors and metabolic interactions in the pathogenesis of diabetic neuropathy. *Diabetologia* 2001; 44: 1973–88.
42. Beckman JA, Creager MA, Libby P. Diabetes and atherosclerosis. Epidemiology, pathophysiology, and management. *JAMA* 2002; 287: 2570–81.
43. James RW. Diabetes and other coronary heart disease equivalents. *Curr Opin Lipidol* 2001; 12: 425–31.
44. Jager A, Kostense PJ, Ruhé HG, Heine RJ, Nijpels G, Dekker JM, Bouter LM, Stehouwer CDA. Microalbuminuria and peripheral arterial disease are independent predictors of cardiovascular and all-cause mortality, especially among hypertensive subjects. Five-year follow-up of the Hoorn Study. *Arterioscler Thromb Vasc Biol* 1999; 19: 617–24.
45. Gerstein HC, Mann JFE, Yi Q, Zinman B, Dinneen SF, Hoogwerf B, Hallé JP, Young J, Rashkwo A, Joyce C, Nawaz S, Yusuf S, for the HOPE Study Investigators. Albuminuria and risk of cardiovascular events, death, and heart failure in diabetic and nondiabetic individuals. *JAMA* 2001; 286: 421–6.
46. Schalkwijk CG, Poland DCW, van Dijk W, Kok A, Emeis JJ, Dräger AM, Doni A, van Hinsbergh VWM, Stehouwer CDA. Plasma concentration of C-reactive protein is increased in type I diabetic patients without clinical macroangiopathy and correlates with markers of endothelial dysfunction: evidence for chronic inflammation. *Diabetologia* 1999; 42: 351–7.
47. Jager A, van Hinsbergh VWM, Kostense PJ, Emeis JJ, Nijpels G, Dekker JM, Heine RJ, Bouter LM, Stehouwer CDA. C-reactive protein and soluble vascular cell adhesion molecule-1 are associated with elevated urinary albumin excretion but do not explain its link with cardiovascular risk. *Arterioscler Thromb Vasc Biol* 2002; 22: 593–8.
48. Stehouwer CDA, Gall MA, Twisk JWR, Knudsen E, Emeis JJ, Parving HH. Increased urinary albumin excretion, endothelial dysfunction, and chronic low-grade inflammation in type 2 diabetes. Progressive, interrelated, and independently associated with risk of death. *Diabetes* 2002; 51: 1157–65.
49. Smulders YM, Jager A, Gerritsen J, Dekker JM, Nijpels G, Heine RJ, Bouter LM, Stehouwer CDA. Cardiovascular autonomic function is associated with (micro-)albuminuria in elderly Caucasian subjects with impaired glucose tolerance or type 2 diabetes: the Hoorn Study. *Diabetes Care* 2000; 23: 1369–74.
50. Gerritsen J, Dekker JM, TenVoorde BJ, Kostense PJ, Heine RJ, Bouter LM, Heethaar RM, Stehouwer CDA. Impaired autonomic function is associated with increased mortality, especially in subjects with diabetes, hypertension, or a history of cardiovascular disease. *Diabetes Care* 2001; 24: 1793–8.
51. van Ittersum FJ, Spek JJ, Praet IJA, Lambert J, IJzerman RG, Fischer HRA, Nikkels RE, Van Bortel LMAB, Donker AJM, Stehouwer CDA. Ambulatory blood pressures and autonomic nervous function in normoalbuminuric type I diabetic patients. *Nephrol Dial Transplant* 1998; 13: 326–32.
52. Schalkwijk CG, Smulders RA, Lambert J, Donker AJM, Stehouwer CDA. ACE-inhibition modulates some endothelial functions in healthy subjects and in normotensive type 1 diabetic patients. *Eur J Clin Invest* 2000; 30: 853–60.
53. Vervoort G, Lutterman JA, Smits P, Berden JHM, Wetzels JF. Transcapillary escape rate of albumin is increased and

related to hemodynamic changes in normo-albuminuric type 1 diabetic patients. *J Hypertens* 1999; 17: 1911–6.
54. Dogra G, Rich L, Stanton K, Watts GF. Endothelium-dependent and -independent vasodilation studied at normoglycemia in type I diabetes mellitus with and without microalbuminuria. *Diabetologia* 2001; 44: 593–601.
55. Giugliano D, Marfella R, Coppola L, Verazzo G, Acampora R, Giunta R, Nappo F, Lucarelli C, D'Onofrio F. Vascular effects of acute hyperglycemia in humans are reversed by L-arginine: evidence for reduced availability of nitric oxide during hyperglycemia. *Circulation* 1997; 95: 1783–90.
56. Chan NN, Vallance P, Colhoun HM. Nitric oxide and vascular responses in type 1 diabetes. *Diabetologia* 2000; 43: 137–47.
57. Huvers FC, de Leeuw PW, Houben AHJM, de Haan CHA, Hamulyak K, Schouten H, Wolffenbuttel BHR, Schaper NC. Endothelium-dependent vasodilation, plasma markers of endothelial function, and adrenergic vasoconstrictor responses in type 1 diabetes under near-normoglycemic conditions. *Diabetes* 1999; 48: 1300–7.
58. Vervoort G, Wetzels JF, Lutterman JA, van Doorn LG, Berden JHM, Smits P. Elevated skeletal muscle blood flow in uncomplicated type 1 diabetes mellitus. Role of nitric oxide and sympathetic tone. *Hypertension* 1999; 34: 1080–5.
59. O'Byrne S, Forte P, Roberts LJ, Morrow JD, Johnston A, Änggard E, Leslie RDG, Benjamin N. Nitric oxide synthesis and isoprostane production in subjects with type 1 diabetes and normal urinary albumin excretion. *Diabetes* 2000; 49: 857–62.
60. Chiarelli F, Cipollone F, Romano F, Tumini S, Costantini F, di Ricco L, Pomilio M, Pierdomenico SD, Marini M, Cuccurullo F, Mezzetti A. Increased circulating nitric oxide in young patients with type 1 diabetes and persistent microalbuminuria. *Diabetes* 2000; 49: 1258–63.
61. Pieper GM. Enhanced, unaltered and impaired nitric oxide-mediated endothelium-dependent relaxation in experimental diabetes mellitus: importance of disease duration. *Diabetologia* 1999; 42: 204–13.
62. Stehouwer CDA, Yudkin JS, Fioretto P, Nosadini R. How heterogeneous is microalbuminuria? The case for "benign" and "malignant" microalbuminuria. *Nephrol Dial Transplant* 1998; 13: 2751–4.
63. Miller JA, Thai K, Scholey JW. Angiotensin II type 1 receptor gene polymorphism and the response to hyperglycemia in early type 1 diabetes. *Diabetes* 2000; 49: 1585–9.
64. Steinberg HO, Paradisi G, Cronin J, Crowde K, Hempfling A, Hook G, Baron AD. Type II diabetes abrogates sex differences in endothelial function in premenopausal women. *Circulation* 2000; 101: 2040–6.
65. Hogikyan RV, Galecki AT, Pitt B, Halter JB, Greene DA, Supiano MA. Specific impairment of endothelium-dependent vasodilation in subjects with type 2 diabetes independent of obesity. *J Clin Endocrinol Metab* 1998; 83: 1946–52.
66. Bagg W, Ferri C, Desideri G, Gamble G, Ockelford P, Braatvedt G. The influences of obesity and glycemic control on endothelial activation in patients with type 2 diabetes. *J Clin Endocrinol Metab* 2001; 86: 5491–7.
67. Fioretto P, Stehouwer CDA, Mauer M, Chiesura-Corona M, Brocco E, Carraro A, Bortoloso E, van Hinsbergh VWM, Crepaldi G, Nosadini R. Heterogeneous nature of microalbuminuria in non-insulin-dependent diabetes: studies of endothelial function and renal structure. *Diabetologia* 1998; 41: 233–6.
68. Jager A, van Hinsbergh VWM, Kostense PJ, Nijpels G, Emeis JJ, Dekker JM, Heine RJ, Bouter LM, Stehouwer CDA. Prognostic implications of retinopathy and a high plasma von Willebrand factor concentration in type 2 diabetic subjects with microalbuminuria. *Nephrol Dial Transplant* 2001; 16: 529–36.
69. Pinkney JH, Stehouwer CDA, Coppack SW, Yudkin JS. Endothelial dysfunction: cause of the insulin resistance syndrome. *Diabetes* 1997; 46 (suppl 2): S9–13.
70. Coggins M, Lindner J, Rattigan S, Jahn L, Fasy E, Kaul S, Barrett E. Physiologic hyperinsulinemia enhances human skeletal muscle perfusion by capillary recruitment. *Diabetes* 2001; 50: 2682–90.
71. Serné EH, IJzerman RG, Gans ROB, Nijveldt R, de Vries G, Evertz R, Donker AJM, Stehouwer CDA. Direct evidence for insulin-induced capillary recruitment in skin of healthy subjects during physiological hyperinsulinemia. *Diabetes* 2002; 51: 1515–22.
72. Youd JM, Rattigan S, Clark MG. Acute impairment of insulin-mediated capillary recruitment and glucose uptake in rat skeletal muscle *in vivo* by TNF-α. *Diabetes* 2000; 49: 1904–9.
73. Steinberg HO, Paradisi G, Hook G, Crowder K, Cronin J, Baron AD. Free fatty acid elevation impairs insulin-mediated vasodilation and nitric oxide production. *Diabetes* 2000; 49: 1231–8.
74. Steinberg HO, Baron AD. Vascular function, insulin resistance and fatty acids. *Diabetologia* 2002; 45: 623–34.
75. Clerk LH, Rattigan S, Clark MG. Lipid infusion impairs physiologic insulin-mediated capillary recruitment and muscle glucose uptake *in vivo*. *Diabetes* 2002; 51: 1138–45.
76. Serné EH, Stehouwer CDA, ter Maaten JC, ter Wee PM, Rauwerda JA, Donker AJM, Gans ROB. Microvascular function relates to insulin sensitivity and blood pressure in normal subjects. *Circulation* 1999; 99: 896–902.
77. Serné EH, Gans ROB, ter Maaten JC, ter Wee PM, Donker AJM, Stehouwer CDA. Capillary recruitment is impaired in essential hypertension and relates to insulin's metabolic and vascular actions. *Cardiovasc Res* 2001; 49: 161–8.
78. Serné EH, Gans ROB, ter Maaten JC, Tangelder GJ, Donker AJM, Stehouwer CDA. Impaired skin capillary recruitment in essential hypertension is caused by both functional and structural capillary rarefaction. *Hypertension* 2001; 38: 238–42.
79. Levy BI, Ambrosio G, Pries AR, Struijker Boudier HAJ. Microcirculation in hypertension. A new target for treatment? *Circulation* 2001; 104: 735–40.
80. Serné EH, Stehouwer CDA, ter Maaten JC, ter Wee PM, Donker AJM, Gans ROB. Birth weight relates to blood pressure and microvascular function in normal subjects. *J Hypertens* 2000; 18: 1421–7.
81. IJzerman RG, Voordouw JJ, Weissenbruch MM, Delemarre-van der Waal HA, Stehouwer CDA. The association between birth weight and capillary recruitment is independent of blood pressure and insulin sensitivity: a study in prepubertal children. *J Hypertens* 2002; 20: 1957–63.
82. Eringa EC, Stehouwer CDA, Merlijn T, Westerhof N, Sipkema P. Physiological concentrations of insulin induce endothelin-mediated vasoconstriction during

inhibition of NOS or PI3-kinase in skeletal muscle arterioles. *Cardiovasc Res* 2002; 56: 464–71.
83. Arcaro G, Cretti A, Balzano S, Lechi A, Muggeo M, Bonora E, Bonadonna RC. Insulin causes endothelial dysfunction in humans. Sites and mechanisms. *Circulation* 2002; 105: 576–82.
84. Fernández-Real JM, Ricart W. Insulin resistance and inflammation in an evolutionary perspective: the contribution of cytokine genotype/phenotype to thriftiness. *Diabetologia* 1999; 42: 1367–74.
85. Yudkin JS, Stehouwer CDA, Emeis JJ, Coppack SW. C-reactive protein in healthy subjects: associations with obesity, insulin resistance and endothelial dysfunction. A potential role for cytokines originating from adipose tissue? *Arterioscler Thromb Vasc Biol* 1999; 19: 972–8.
86. Hak AE, Pols HAP, Stehouwer CDA, Meijer J, Kiliaan AJ, Hofman A, Breteler MMB, Witteman JCM. Markers of inflammation and cellular adhesion molecules in relation to insulin resistance in nondiabetic elderly. The Rotterdam Study. *J Clin Endocrinol Metab* 2001; 86: 4398–405.
87. Weyer C, Yudkin JS, Stehouwer CDA, Schalkwijk CG, Pratley RE, Tataranni PA. Humoral markers of inflammation and endothelial dysfunction in relation to adiposity and *in vivo* insulin action in Pima Indians. *Atherosclerosis* 2002; 161: 233–42.
88. Perticone F, Ceravolo R, Candigliota M, Ventura G, Iacopino S, Sinopoli F, Mattioli PL. Obesity and body fat distribution induce endothelial dysfunction by oxidative stress. *Diabetes* 2001; 50: 159–65.
89. Festa A, D'Agostino R, Tracy RP, Haffner SM. Elevated levels of acute-phase proteins and plasminogen activator inhibitor-1 predict the development of type 2 diabetes. The Insulin Resistance Atherosclerosis Study. *Diabetes* 2002; 51: 1131–7.
90. Brownlee M. Biochemistry and molecular cell biology of diabetic complications. *Nature* 2001; 414: 813–20.
91. Singh R, Barden A, Mori T, Beilin L. Advanced glycation end-products: a review. *Diabetologia* 2001; 44: 129–46.
92. Baynes JW, Thorpe SR. Role of oxidative stress in diabetic complications. *Diabetes* 1999; 48: 1–9.
93. Spitaler MM, Graier WF. Vascular targets of redox signaling in diabetes mellitus. *Diabetologia* 2002; 45: 476–94.
94. Saltiel AR, Kahn CR. Insulin signaling and the regulation of glucose and lipid metabolism. *Nature* 2001; 414: 799–806.
95. Ginsberg HN. Insulin resistance and cardiovascular disease. *J Clin Invest* 2000; 106: 453–8.
96. Du XL, Edelstein D, Dimmeler S, Ju Q, Sui C, Brownlee M. Hyperglycemia inhibits endothelial nitric oxide synthase activity by posttranslational modification at the Akt site. *J Clin Invest* 2001; 108: 1341–8.
97. Du XL, Edelstein D, Rossetti L, Fantus IG, Goldberg H, Ziyadeh F, Wu J, Brownlee M. Hyperglycemia-induced mitochondrial superoxide overproduction activates the hexosamine pathway and induces plasminogen activator inhibitor-1 expression by increasing Sp1 glycosylation. *Proc Natl Acad Sci USA* 2000; 97: 12222–6.
98. Stern DM, Yan SD, Yan SF, Schmidt AM. Receptor for advanced glycation endproducts (RAGE) and the complications of diabetes. *Ageing Res Rev* 2002; 1: 1–15.
99. Schalkwijk CG, Ligtvoet N, Twaalfhoven H, Jager A, Blaauwgeers HGT, Schlingemann RO, Tarnow L, Parving HH, Stehouwer CDA, van Hinsbergh VWM. Amadori-albumin in type 1 diabetic patients: correlation with markers of endothelial function, association with diabetic nephropathy and localization in retinal capillaries. *Diabetes* 1999; 48: 2446–53.
100. Uemura S, Matsushita H, Li W, Glassford AJ, Asagami T, Lee KH, Harrison DG, Tsao PS. Diabetes mellitus enhances vascular matrix metalloproteinase activity. *Circ Res* 2001; 88: 1291–8.
101. Chen S, Hong SW, Iglesias-de la Cruz MC, Isono M, Casaretto A, Ziyadeh FN. The key role of the transforming growth factor-beta system in the pathogenesis of diabetic nephropathy. *Ren Fail* 2002; 23: 471–81.
102. Duh E, Aiello LP. Vascular endothelial growth factor and diabetes. *Diabetes* 1999; 48: 1899–906.
103. Dandona P, Aljada A, Mohanty P. The anti-inflammatory and potential anti-atherogenic effect of insulin: a new paradigm. *Diabetologia* 2002; 45: 924–30.
104. Leclercq B, Jaimes EA, Raij L. Nitric oxide synthase and hypertension. *Curr Opin Nephrol Hypertens* 2002; 11: 185–9.
105. Evans M, Khan N, Rees A. Diabetic dyslipidemia and coronary heart disease: new perspectives. *Curr Opin Lipidol* 1999; 10: 387–91.
106. Hayden JM, Reaven PD. Cardiovascular risk factors in diabetes mellitus type 2: a potential role for novel cardiovascular risk factors. *Curr Opin Lipidol* 2000; 11: 519–28.
107. Nappo F, Esposito K, Cioffi M, Giugliano G, Molinari AM, Paolisso G, Marfella R, Giugliano D. Postprandial endothelial activation in healthy subjects and in type 2 diabetic patients: role of fat and carbohydrate meals. *J Am Coll Cardiol* 2002; 39: 1145–50.
108. Sahadevan M, Kasiske BL. Hyperlipidemia in kidney disease: causes and consequences. *Curr Opin Nephrol Hypertens* 2002; 11: 323–9.
109. Chaturvedi N, Bandinelli S, Mangili R, Penno G, Rottiers RE, Fuller JH, on behalf of the EURODIAB Prospective Complications Study Group. Microalbuminuria in type 1 diabetes: rates, risk factors and glycemic threshold. *Kidney Int* 2001; 60: 219–27.
110. Smulders YM, Rakic M, Stehouwer CDA, Weijers RNM, Slaats EH, Silberbusch J. Determinants of progression of microalbuminuria in patients with non-insulin-dependent diabetes mellitus. *Diabetes Care* 1997; 20: 999–1005.
111. Adelman RD. Obesity and renal disease. *Curr Opin Nephrol Hypertens* 2002; 11: 331–5.

80

Hemostatic Abnormalities in Diabetes

Irène Juhan-Vague, Pierre Emmanuel Morange, and Marie-Christine Alessi

University Hospital Timone, Marseille, France

INTRODUCTION

Insulin- and non-insulin-dependent diabetes, obesity, and insulin resistance represent risk factors for cardiovascular mortality. Diabetic patients present accelerated atherosclerosis and 80% of diabetic patients die from thrombotic complications. It has been proposed that the dysregulation of hemostasis they present, which leads to a prothrombotic state, is involved in the accelerated atherothrombotic process.

In this chapter, after a brief survey of the hemostasis system, we review the changes of cells involved in thrombosis, the changes of coagulation and fibrinolysis, and the possible mechanisms responsible.

THE HEMOSTATIC SYSTEM

Hemostasis is the physiological process that aims to limit blood loss at the level of the vascular lesion. The rupture of the monolayer of endothelial cells exposes subendothelial structures to the blood components, leading to adhesion and activation of platelets at the site of injury, and simultaneously, the exposure of tissue factor induces a local activation of coagulation, which leads to fibrin formation. The thrombus is constituted of aggregated platelets and fibrin, stops bleeding, and allows cicatrization to take place. The fibrinolytic process, which is involved as soon as fibrin is formed, allows the destruction of the thrombus and the repermeation of the vessel. Hemostasis is a very powerful localized phenomenon with local autoamplification, but which is downregulated by several inhibitory pathways that limit the extension of the thrombus.

Any changes in the equilibrium between activators and inhibitors lead to a hemorragic or thrombotic disorder. The latter not only influences the development of intravascular occlusive thrombus, but also plays a part in vessel wall remodeling.

The Role of Platelets

Platelet adhesion to the sites of vessel damage is triggered by subendothelial components, such as collagen, microfibrils, and von Willebrand factor (vWF), and involves the platelet cell surface glycoprotein GPIb. Adhering platelets become activated, which leads to a conformational change on the surface of specific receptors, the so-called GPIIbIIIa receptors. Fibrinogen binds to these receptors and facilitates the platelet aggregation phenomenon. Adhering platelets change their shape and either release the contents of intracellular granules, including serotonin and ADP, which promotes further platelet aggregation, or produces other agents, like thromboxane A2 (TXA2), which further reinforces platelet aggregation. Activated platelets also release substances that have mitogenic and chemotactic properties like platelet-derived growth factor (PDGF) and transforming growth factor β (TGF-β), as well as an antiheparin substance (PF4). Several molecular mechanisms are involved in this platelet aggregation process, and also with the production of inositol triphosphate and diaglycerol, calcium mobilization, and protein kinase C activation and the further activation of calmodulin-dependent intracellular reactions. The activation of platelets also leads to a change in the phospholipid membrane, exposing negative charges at the outer surface. This facilitates coagulation by concentrating vitamin K-dependent coagulation factors on the cell surface.

International Textbook of Diabetes Mellitus, Third Edition. Edited by R. A. DeFronzo, E. Ferrannini, H. Keen, and P. Zimmet.
 ISBN: 0-471-48655-8.

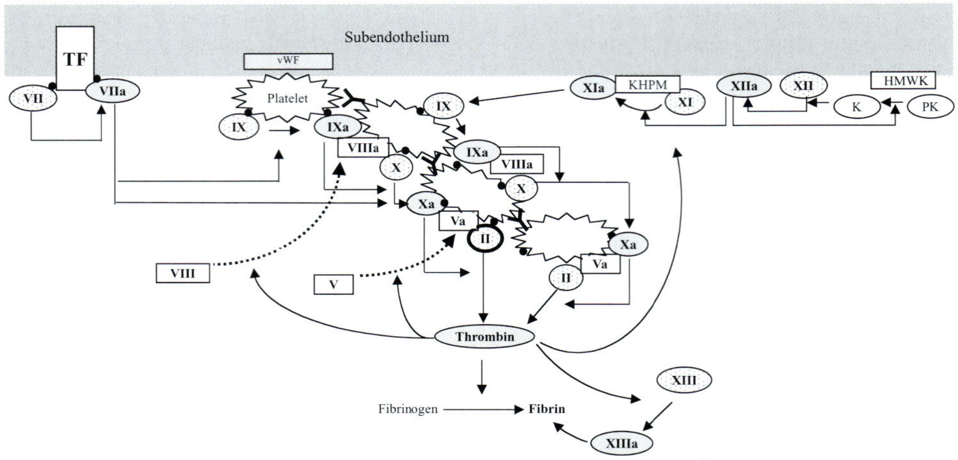

Figure 1 The coagulation system with cascade of enzymatic reactions that take place at the surface of activated platelets. TF = tissue factor; a = activated; PK = prekallicrein; K = kallicrein; HMWK = high-molecular-weight kininogen; VWF = von Willebrand factor

The Role of Coagulation

The coagulation pathway is initiated by tissue factor (TF), which is a membrane protein constitutively present in the adventitia of the vessel wall.

The coagulation factors are produced by the liver, and can be classified as inactive proenzymes (factor (F) II, VII, IX, X, XI, VII, XIII, and prekallikrein), cofactors (FV and VIII, protein S), inhibitors of serine proteases such as antithrombin, protein C, or TFPI (tissue factor pathway inhibitor), or substrate such as fibrinogen. FII, VII, IX, X, Proteins C and S are vitamin K-dependent proteins.

The cascade of enzymatic reaction (Figure 1) takes place on the surface of activated platelets. Exposition of TF to the blood allows activation of FVII (VIIa), which initiates the exogenous pathway of coagulation. The complex TF/VIIa activates FIX or FX. Activated FIX reinforces the activation of FX. FXa transforms prothrombin (FII) intro thrombin (IIa). Thrombin transforms fibrinogen into fibrin and activates FXIII, which covalently link the D domains of two adjacent fibrin molecules; this effect results in the stabilization of the clot. As soon as some molecules of thrombin are generated, they amplify their own production by activating cofactors V and VIII, and FXI, which are fixed on platelets. FXIa reinforces the production of thrombin by the activation of FIX (endogenous pathway) and recruits new platelets for the platelet aggregates.

Coagulation is regulated by three systems of inhibition (Figure 2):

(1) Antithrombin, fixed to heparan sulfate on the surface of endothelial cells, which inhibits thrombin, FXa,

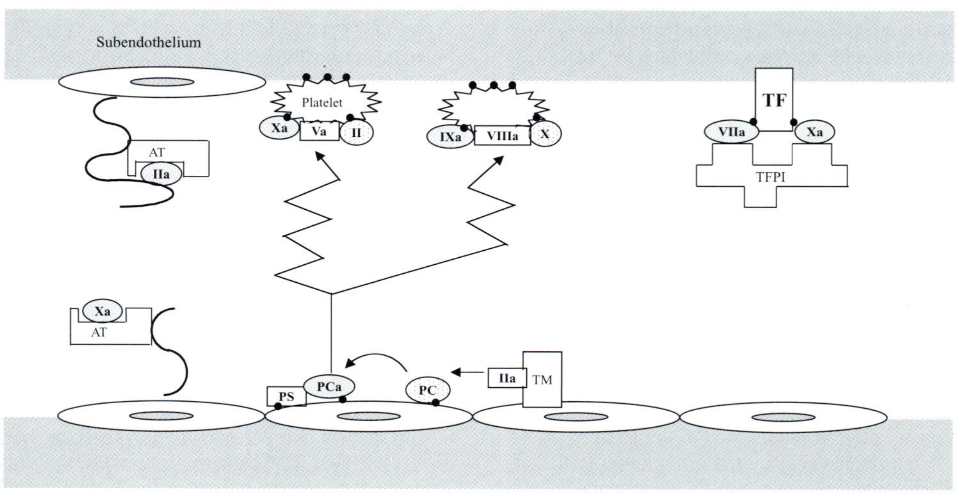

Figure 2 Inhibition of the coagulation system. AT = antithrombin; TFPI = tissue factor pathway inhibitor; PC = Protein C; PS = Protein S; TM = thrombomodulin

IXa, XIa, and XIIa when they diffuse from the platelet aggregates, and which forms irreversible complexes with these enzymes.

(2) Activated protein C (PCa) with its cofactor protein S (PS) produces its anticoagulant effect by proteolysis of FVa and FVIIIa. The common mutation Arg506Gln described in FV as FV Leiden transfers to the muted FV, a resistance to PCa inactivation. PC is activated by the thrombin/thrombomodulin complex: thrombomodulin (TM) situated at the endothelial cell surface binds thrombin and transforms it into an activator of PC.

(3) The pathway of TF is regulated by the TFPI attached to glycosaminoglycans on the surface of the endothelial cells. TFPI linked to FXa inhibits the VIIa and TF activity.

The Role of Fibrinolysis

Fibrinolysis is a proteolytic system in which plasmin is the main enzyme (Figure 3). Plasmin is formed from its inactive precursor plasminogen by the action of tissue plasminogen activator (tPA) or urokinase plasminogen activator (uPA). Its principal substrate is fibrin, which is degraded into soluble fragments containing a specific antigenic motif, the D dimer. The system is controlled by inhibitors α_2-antiplasmin (α_2AP), which inhibits plasmin, and plasminogen activator inhibitor 1 (PAI-1), which inhibits tPA and uPA and which is considered to be the predominant inhibitor of fibrinolysis. Intravascular fibrinolysis mainly involves tPA as an activator: In the absence of fibrin, tPA, which is regularly released from endothelial cells, is rapidly complexed to PAI-1 and is eliminated by the liver. Fibrin represents a surface for the binding of tPA and plasminogen, involving specific fibrin receptors, and facilitates the plasminogen activation into plasmin. tPA bound to fibrin is protected from PAI-1 inhibition. The plasmin released from the clot is rapidly inhibited by α_2AP.

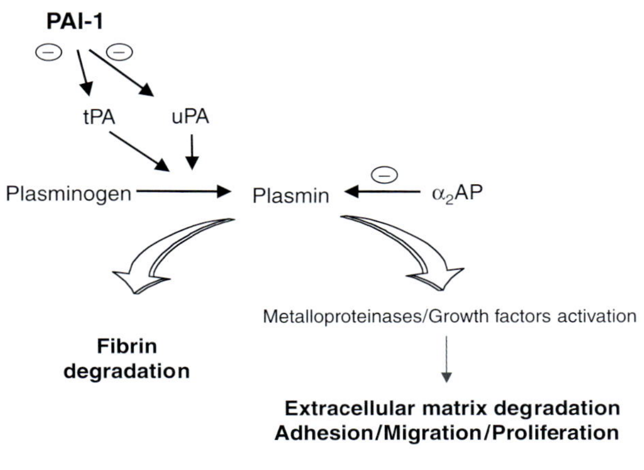

Figure 3 The Fibrinolytic System. PAI-1 = plasminogen activator inhibitor-1; tPA = tissue-type plasminogen activator; uPA = urokinase plasminogen activator; α_2AP = α_2-antiplasmin

The Role of Endothelial Cells

The endothelium is pivotal in the control of hemostasis and thrombosis because it is the primary source of many of the major hemostatic regulatory molecules. It acts at every step in the hemostasis process. Healthy endothelial cells, unlike extravascular cells, are anticoagulant and antithrombotic. This is due to the regulated secretion of antiplatelet agents, including prostacyclin and nitric oxide. The surface of the endothelium is additionally the site for the inactivation of thrombin by antithrombin, and its conversion to a coagulation inhibitor by interaction with TM. Endothelial cells are also the source of TFPI, which counteracts the initiation of coagulation and tPA, the primary activator of fibrinolysis. In disease states, many of these endothelial cell properties are changed into a procoagulant and prothrombotic phenotype, resulting in the expression of inducible tissue factor and the release of PAI-1 and vWF.

The Contribution of Leukocytes

Inflammation and immune activation have been associated with thrombosis in a number of settings. Several mechanisms have been proposed including the exhibiting of TF expression by activated monocytes and the transfer of TF-positive particles by leukocytes to platelet thrombi, making them capable of triggering and propagating thrombus growth. The adherence of activated platelets to polymorphonuclear may be a key event in the sequence of thrombus formation. In addition, leukocytes produce cytokines, which are able to stimulate the synthesis of hemostatic parameters. Fibrinogen, for example, is an acute phase protein synthesized by the liver in response to circulating interleukin-6 (IL-6). Autoantibodies could also directly or indirectly alter the hemostasis.

The Extravascular Role of Hemostasis

Many of the hemostasis components perform extravascular functions. These findings are probably relevant to the evolutionary change of molecule functions. Thrombin is able to activate all the cellular types with the exception of red blood cells. The cellular responses are mainly due to the activation of cellular receptors belonging to the protease-activated receptors (PARS), which are seven-domain transmembrane receptors coupled to G-proteins [1]. *In vitro* thrombin transfers a procoagulant and proinflammatory phenotype to the endothelial cells and exerts mitogenic and chemotactic effects on inflammatory cells such as lymphocytes and macrophages. Therefore thrombin is a factor in thrombotic complication, and also, by its effects on vascular cells, in the progression of atherosclerosis itself. Atherosclerotic plaques contain TF, expressed by macrophages and smooth muscle cells, or brought by microparticles derived from apoptotic cells, and the presence of active thrombin has been demonstrated in the neo intima. TF is considered not only a cofactor of coagulation but also a cellular receptor. The fixation of its ligand FVIIa induces signals and the expression of at least 24 different genes [2]. Extravascular fibrinolysis also takes place in tissues. Plasminogen binds to lysine-rich protein on the cell surface and is activated by uPA bound to its receptor (uPAR). Generated plasmin participates in the degradation of the extracellular matrix directly or by activating metalloproteinases (MMP) and in the activation and release of growth factors. The system is controlled by PAI-1, and by MMP inhibitors (TIMP). PAI-1 could participate directly in the control of cellular adhesion independently of its anti-uPA effect. It binds to vitronectin (RGD site) and inhibits the binding of vitronectin to its specific receptor $\alpha v\beta 3$ and to the uPAR. Therefore these properties of extravascular fibrinolysis influence the adhesion, migration, and proliferation process of vascular cells, which affect the vessel wall remodeling [3]. These properties clearly indicate that the hemostatic process has a role to play in thrombosis, and also, when amplified, in tissue remodeling, similar to that observed during atherosclerosis. [4]

DYSREGULATION OF HEMOSTASIS IN DIABETES

It is widely reported in the literature that diabetic and insulin-resistant patients present a prothrombotic state.

Qualitative and quantitative changes of cells involved in thrombosis and of coagulation and fibrinolysis proteins have been demonstrated. Disturbances of the hemostatic system may favor the development of vascular damage and the final occlusion event in the progress of coronary heart disease, by promoting thrombosis at the site of an acutely ruptured atherosclerotic plaque. Changes in the hemostatic system may have several aspects that are often encountered simultaneously:

- activation of endothelial cells and leukocytes, which presents a prothrombotic phenotype
- hyperactivity of platelets
- hypercoagulability with increased formation of the multipotent thrombin
- high levels of fibrinogen, which promotes platelet aggregation and induces rheological changes and the formation of a rich fibrin clot
- decreased fibrinolytic activity due to an increased plasma level of PAI-1,which leads to decreased removal of fibrin deposits and changes in the components of the blood vessel.

The mechanisms that induce a prothrombotic state in diabetic or nondiabetic obese patients are multifactorial. Hyperglycemia, inflammation, and insulin-resistance are the main contributors, and the importance of proinflammatory cytokines is at present emphasized.

Hyperglycemia per se plays an important role [5]. It can lead to the modification of macromolecules by forming advanced glycation end products (AGE) [6]. By binding surface receptors such as RAGE (receptor for AGE), these AGE-modified proteins can induce cell activation via the pleiotropic transcription factor NF-κB. They augment the production of proinflammatory cytokines and other inflammatory pathways in vascular endothelial cells and monocytes/macrophages. This results in the appearance of cell surface adhesion molecules, such as vWF, and a decrease production of NO. Besides hyperglycemia, the diabetic state also promotes an oxidative stress mediated by reactive oxygen species [7].

The glycation of proteins also induces functional changes. The new properties of glycated fibrin or of glycated platelet glycoproteins have been specifically analyzed in the literature.

Inflammation: In clinical studies both atherosclerosis and diabetes are associated with elevated plasma levels of C reactive protein (CRP), IL-6, and increased circulating adhesion molecules. A prolonged cytokine-mediated acute phase reaction may be part of a wide-ranging innate immune response, which through the action of cytokines on the hepatocytes, monocytes/macrophages, endothelial cells, and adipose tissue contributes to the biochemical and clinical features of the metabolic syndrome [8, 9] and to the development of atherothrombotic lesions [10]. Tumor necrosis factor α (TNF-α) is overexpressed in the adipose tissue of obese insulin-resistant patients, and the adipose tissue is an important source of IL-6 [11]. Furthermore, inflammation may contribute to the genesis of insulin resistance [12–14] and this may be a common precursor of atherosclerosis, cardiovascular disease, and diabetes.

Insulin resistance with obesity also plays an important role in hemostatic changes, principally by increasing plasma PAI-1 levels and PAI-1 expression in tissues such as adipose tissue, liver, or vessel wall [15–21]. The mechanisms leading to PAI-1 overproduction have been extensively studied recently, and the intervention of TNF-α as a connecting cytokine is recognized. Hyperinsulinemia and insulin resistance in the context of the inflammatory state associated with it are also slightly accompanied by elevated fibrinogen, vWF, and FVIII levels [16, 21] as well as increased platelet aggregation and shortened platelet survival *in vivo*.

In vitro studies have demonstrated that insulin and free fatty acid affect platelet functions or endothelial cells or the hepatocyte synthesis of hemostatic factors. These results could attribute a direct role to the hyperinsulinemia presented by prediabetic obese and type 2 diabetic patients. The long-lasting influence of these metabolic disturbances during the prediabetic state may have therefore progressive consequences on the atherothrombotic process.

We are now going to review the changes in the hemostatic system in diabetes.

DIABETES AND CELLS INVOLVED IN THE THROMBOTIC PROCESS

Endothelial Hemostatic Dysfunction

Diabetes induces a dysfunction in endothelial cells, which is considered an important factor in the atherothrombosis development. Endothelial cell activation is only partly dependent on hyperglycemia. In type 2 diabetic patients, obesity and specially abdominal obesity and not hyperglycemia is the most important and the only independent predictor of endothelial cell activation [22]. Indeed, an improved glycemic control with the administration of insulin and sulfonylureas in type 2 diabetic patients treated for 16 weeks did not influence the markers of endothelial cell activation [23]. However, in poorly controlled non-insulin-dependent diabetic patients, sE-selectin levels are increased and significantly fall to normal levels after an intensive insulin treatment [24]. An endothelial activation correlated with visceral body fat in obese women, possibly through inappropriate secretion of cytokines, and was ameliorated by weight loss [25].

The plasma concentration of vWF is also increased in diabetes, and specially in microalbuminuric patients [26, 27]. vWF is weakly [16] or not at all [28] related to the metabolic factors involved in the insulin-resistance syndrome, but as fibrinogen, it is a marker of the acute phase reaction. vWF levels are positively correlated with fibrinogen or CRP levels [29].

Monocyte/Macrophage Dysfunction

Monocytes/macrophages from diabetic patients express more TF than monocytes from normal subjects [30, 31]. This overexpression of TF is directly related to the cytokines production and to glycated proteins [32]. Hyperglycemia and oxidative stress, by inducing the appearance of cell surface adhesion molecules, increase the adherence of monocytes and the production of monocyte chemoattractant proteins and other mechanisms that activate and perpetuate chronic low-grade inflammation [33].

The Hyperactivity of Platelets

The hyperfunction of platelets from diabetic patients has been well recognized a long time ago (see review in reference 34). The platelets are bigger and this has been reported to be secondary to the increased ploidy of megakaryocytes [35]. *In vitro* platelets from diabetic patients present the ability to aggregate, with a hypersensitivity to stimulating agents. The platelet surface presents increased expression of the adhesive protein P selectin, increased in GPIb-IX, and GPIIb-IIIa receptors, increased fibrinogen binding, and accentuated TXA2 synthesis. Several changes occur in intraplatelet signaling pathways, with intensified calcium mobilization [36]. Once activated, the platelets from diabetic patients present a higher capacity for producing procoagulant microvesicules [37]. The secretion of platelet alpha-granule contents in blood (thromboxane B2 and PF4) is evidence of platelet hyperactivity *in vivo*. There is also evidence for activation of circulating platelets *in vivo* [38] with a reduced survival time, due to the accelerated sequestration in the circulation.

Generally, these platelet abnormalities were described in subjects with both insulin- and non-insulin-dependent-diabetes mellitus, early in the course of the disease and may precede the development of vascular disease [39]. The platelet hyperactivity has been directly related to hyperglycemia. The hyperglycation of platelet membrane proteins leads to decreased membrane fluidity [39]. Oral hypoglycemic agents have a beneficial effect on platelet function, which is associated with the improvement in glycemic control [40]. The acute administration of insulin has been shown to directly reduce platelet reactivity [41] via the platelet insulin receptor. Insulin resistance could also be implicated. *In vitro* insulin inhibits the platelet interaction with collagen and reduces aggregation to several agonists of platelets from normal subjects but not from obese insulin-resistant patients [42]. Interestingly, it was recently demonstrated that leptin, an adipose tissue synthesized protein, which is increased in the plasma of the obese subjects, induces platelet aggregation via leptin receptors on platelet membrane [43].

No specific trial on antiplatelet therapy has been conducted for diabetes and the results available concern subgroup analyses [40]. In the Physician Health Study, the Early Treatment Retinopathy Study, and in the Hypertension Optimal Treatment Study, it was shown that aspirin was even more beneficial in diabetic patients than in high-risk nondiabetic subjects [40].

Recently published recommendations of the American Diabetes Association [44], based on meta-analysis of all primary and secondary prevention trials with use of aspirin, support the view that aspirin therapy (recommended dose: 81–325 mg/day) should be prescribed as a secondary prevention strategy in males and females with diabetes, with evidence of a large vessel disease, as a primary prevention strategy, in high-risk males and females with type 1 and 2 diabetes. Persons at high risk include diabetic individuals over the age of 30 years with a familial history of cardiovascular disease, dyslipidemia, smoking, hypertension, obesity, micro- or macroalbuminuria, poor physical activity and sedentary life style, and elevated HbA_{1c}

(chronic hyperglycemia). More than 50% of patients with type 2 diabetes belong to this category [40].

Other therapeutic agents such as ticlopidine or clopidogrel have been used in diabetic patients. No differences between diabetic and nondiabetic patients have been recorded as regards the antiplatelet effects. In the acute situation, the response of diabetic patients to anti-GPIIbIIIa is no different from that of nondiabetic subjects [45].

DIABETES AND HYPERCOAGULABILITY

The overexpression of TF in monocytes/macrophages and endothelial cells, the increased procoagulant activity of platelets, and plasma hypercoagulability, evidenced by shorter clotting times [46], explain why diabetic patients are prone to arterial thrombotic events. Plasma markers of activation of coagulation, such as thrombin–antithrombin complex, fibrinopeptide A (released when fibrinogen is converted to fibrin by thrombin), prothrombin activation fragments, and D dimers, are also increased in diabetes. The severity of diabetic micro- and macroangiopathies correlated with the progression of the titer of activation markers, which were stronger determinants of the presence of diabetic vascular complications than other clinical variables including the degree of glycemia in stable, relatively well-controlled patients with type 2 diabetes [47].

The increased concentration of fibrinogen is the most consistently described plasma abnormality. It is now considered that the fibrinogen level is determined by overall adiposity rather than insulin resistance [48]. It is related to glycemic control and to obesity *per se* and weakly related to abdominal obesity [49] and insulin levels [16, 29, 50]. IL-6 is thought to be at the basis of this abnormality. IL-6 is produced by adipose tissue [11] and will directly stimulate the hepatic synthesis of fibrinogen. IL-6 could therefore represent a link between obesity and the fibrinogen level in plasma. Fibrinogen synthesis is partly controlled by genetic polymorphisms in the β-chain gene. Interestingly, Ceriello et al. [51] have shown that 3 months of insulin treatment decreases fibrinogen levels only in carriers of the a2 alleles, the latter having the highest level before treatment. These results indicate a possible relationship between genotypes and glycemic control in determining the plasma fibrinogen concentration in diabetic patients.

The plasma levels of several other clotting factors are elevated in diabetes [26]: FVIII, FVII, FXI, FXII, kallikrein, etc. The concentrations of soluble TM [52] and TFPI, which are released from the endothelial cell membrane, are also increased. Several studies have documented reversal of numerous disturbances in the plasma coagulation cascade induced by the correction of hyperglycemia [51, 53–55] or by loosing weight [29, 56].

Diabetes is associated not only with a quantitative modification of hemostatic proteins but also with qualitative alterations. The glycation of protein modifies their activity. This has been shown for fibrinogen for which the resulting fibrin is composed of small diameter fibers [57]. Such fibrin is markedly resistant to degradation by plasmin [58].

Some polymorphisms described on hemostatic parameters such as mutations on FV (FV Leiden) increase the risk of developing venous thrombosis but not arterial thrombosis. In diabetes as well as in smokers or in patients with hypertension, this mutation might be considered as a risk factor for arterial thrombosis [59].

Mutation in the FXIII gene Val34Leu has been shown to be protective against myocardial infarction [60]. This effect was also observed in diabetic patients [61].

DIABETES AND HYPOFIBRINOLYSIS

It is now well established that hypofibrinolysis due to elevated plasma PAI-1 levels is a core feature of the insulin-resistance syndrome. PAI-1 levels are elevated in obese insulin-resistant patients as well as in non-insulin-dependent diabetic patients and are in the normal range in type 1 diabetic patients [62, 63]. Plasma PAI-1 levels have been shown for a long time to be associated with the parameters of the insulin-resistance syndrome [64]. They correlate with body mass index, visceral fat (which characterizes android obesity), blood pressure, and plasma levels of insulin or proinsulin, triglycerides, small dense low-density lipoprotein particles, and free fatty acids, and are inversely related to HDL cholesterol [15, 65–72], whereas no correlation is observed to measures of glycemic control [62].

The modulation of insulin resistance by hypocaloric diet coupled with losing weight [73], physical training, change in dietary composition, or the use of oral antidiabetic drugs such as metformin [74] induces a decrease in PAI-1 levels, which correlate with the decrease in weight and in plasma metabolic parameters. It was recently shown that the use of thiazolinediones such as troglitazone is associated with a decrease in plasma PAI-1 levels in persons with type 2 diabetes [75]. Although insulin added *in vitro* to hepatocytes induces an increase in PAI-1 synthesis [76], and hyperinsulinemia is associated with elevated plasma PAI-1 levels [15], an acute administration of insulin does not modify plasma PAI-1 concentration [77, 78] or decrease it [55].

One uncertainty about PAI-1 synthesis in insulin resistance is its cell origin. Undoubtedly many cells/tissues are able to synthesize PAI-1, but since PAI-1 gene expression is inducible rather than constitutive, one of the foremost problems is to recognize the inducer that is involved in insulin resistance. One approach was to propose that metabolic disturbances observed during this syndrome—excess of insulin, triglycerides, free fatty acid, angiotensin II—directly affect PAI-1 synthesis. Indeed, most cell culture experiments confirm these hypotheses:

insulin [76, 79, 80], glucocorticoids [79], very low-density lipoprotein [81], free fatty acid [82], glucose [83], and angiotensin II [84] increase the PAI-1 production by cells in culture. And despite the fact that clinical observations do not always support such a direct effect, interesting concepts have emerged.

Among the other potential inducers of PAI-1 synthesis the proinflammatory cytokines TNF-α [85, 86] appears of particular relevance in the context of insulin resistance. Indeed, it has deleterious effects on both glucose homeostasis and β-cell function, and can disrupt insulin signaling pathways in both pancreatic β-cells and liver and adipose tissue [12]. In mice the adipose tissue was shown to contain a high amount of PAI-1, and the inactivation of both TNF-α receptors resulted in a significantly reduced adipose tissue PAI-1 expression and plasma PAI-1 levels [85, 86].

We have described [18], as have others [87–89], PAI-1 synthesis by human adipose tissue. We have shown a decrease of PAI-1 expression in adipose tissue by weight loss [90] and a variability of PAI-1 expression, depending on fat territory. Visceral fat produces more PAI-1 than subcutaneous or femoral fat [18, 88–90]. The main PAI-1-producing cells have been identified as stroma cells [91], some of them being of monocyte or smooth muscle cell origin. Thus the adipose tissue could represent a PAI-1 reservoir. However these results do not exclude the contribution of other tissues. Indeed, the liver is also a good candidate since some groups have observed a strong relationship between plasma PAI-1 and liver steatosis levels [92, 93]. The PAI-1 antigen content in human adipose tissue was found to correlate highly with those of TNF-α receptors and TGF-β, but not to that of TNF-α or IL-6, which were both strongly correlated to each other [94, 95]. These results from mice and human studies suggest that the TNF-α pathway could be a common link between elevated PAI-1 and insulin resistance. On the other hand, the levels of TGF-β, one of the strongest inducers of PAI-1 synthesis *in vitro*, are also associated with those of PAI-1 within human adipose tissue and could be involved in the regulation of PAI-1 in insulin resistance.

What are the consequences of PAI-1 overexpression in insulin resistance?

The high expression of PAI-1 in insulin resistance raises questions on the causality of this phenomenon. As PAI-1 is involved in tissue remodeling, it can be suggested that the elevated expression of PAI-1 observed in obesity is involved in adipose tissue development. The modulation of the PAI-1 gene in mice fed with high-fat diet induces change in weight gain: PAI-1 knockout mice gain weight faster [96] whereas PAI-1 transgenic mice with an overexpression of PAI-1 gain less weight [97]. On the same line, plasminogen knockout mice fed a high-fat diet gained less weight [98]. And *in vitro* experiments support the fact that the hypofibrinolysis induced by the excess of PAI-1 [97] or the absence of plasminogen [98] leads to a decrease of preadipocyte differentiation with consequences for the adipose growth. Thus, the PAI-1 overexpression in insulin resistance could control the fat mass mainly by reducing adiposity. This needs further investigation in more physiological models and in humans.

Despite this suspected protective effect on obesity, an excess of PAI-1 could increase the rate of atherosclerosis and diabetes. Indeed, high plasma PAI-1 levels have been considered a risk factor for coronary heart disease [99–102]. PAI-1 has been shown to be predictive of events in univariate analysis. However the predictability disappeared after adjustment for BMI, triglycerides, HDL cholesterol, and markers of insulin resistance [102]. Sobel [19] and Pandolfi [103] have provided evidence that type 2 diabetes is associated with an increased PAI-1 expression in the arterial wall. This increased PAI-1 concentration in the vessel wall, as well as the increased plasma PAI-1 level, could participate in the accelerated vasculopathy of these patients. Very interestingly, it was recently demonstrated in a large cohort of healthy nondiabetic subjects, that patients who develop an incident diabetes within 5 years presented higher levels of fibrinogen, CRP, and PAI-1 at baseline than nonconverters [14]. PAI-1 predicted type 2 diabetes independently of insulin resistance and other known risk factors for diabetes.

In this line, treatment with an angiotensin-converting enzyme (ACE) inhibitor has been shown to decrease not only PAI-1 levels [104] and the rate of cardiovascular events [105] but also the incidence of type 2 diabetes [106]. Therefore PAI-1 could play a part in the development of cardiovascular diseases, and in type 2 diabetes. Both these properties indicate that PAI-1 represents an ideal target for therapeutic intervention that aims to decrease the risk of both cardiovascular disease and type 2 diabetes.

CONCLUSION

A procoagulant state has been described in diabetes mellitus. Intensive glycemic control with insulin is effective in reducing the impact of this procoagulant state by favorably affecting platelet, coagulation, and fibrinolysis dysfunction. Decreased fibrinolytic activity due to elevated PAI-1 levels may be favorably affected by weight loss, exercise, low calorie diet, or by insulin sensitizer agents or ACE inhibitor therapy. Insulin has a variable effect on plasma PAI-1 levels. Recognition of and therapy for a procoagulant state in diabetes mellitus is likely to result in a decrease in the atherothrombotic events that characterize the later stages of diabetes.

REFERENCES

1. Coughlin SR. Thrombin signalling and protease-activated receptors. *Nature* 2000; 407: 258–64.

2. Camerer E, Gjernes E, Wiiger M, Pringle S, Prydz H. Binding of factor VIIa to tissue factor on keratinocytes induces gene expression. *J Biol Chem* 2000; 275: 6580–5.
3. Chapman HA. Plasminogen activators, integrins and the coordinated regulation of cell adhesion and migration. *Curr Opin Cell Biol* 1997; 9: 714–24.
4. Carmeliet P. Clotting factors build blood vessels. *Science* 2001; 293: 1602–4.
5. Brownlee M. Biochemistry and molecular cell biology of diabetic complications. *Nature* 2001; 414: 813–20.
6. Schmidt AM, Yan SD, Wautier JL, Stern D. Activation of receptor for advanced glycation end products: a mechanism for chronic vascular dysfunction in diabetic vasculopathy and atherosclerosis. *Circ Res* 1999; 84: 489–97.
7. Baynes JW, Thorpe SR. Role of oxidative stress in diabetic complications: a new perspective on an old paradigm. *Diabetes* 1999; 48: 1–9.
8. Pickup JC, Crook MA. Is type II diabetes mellitus a disease of the innate immune system? *Diabetologia* 1998; 41: 1241–8.
9. Yudkin JS, Stehouwer CDA, Emeis JJ, Coppack SW. C-reactive protein in healthy subjects: association with obesity, insulin resistance, and endothelial dysfunction. *Arterioscler Thromb Vasc Biol* 1999; 19: 972–8.
10. Libby P, Ridker PM, Maseri A. Inflammation and atherosclerosis. *Circulation* 2002; 105: 1135–43.
11. Mohamed-Ali V, Goodrick S, Rawesh A, Miles JM, Katz D, Yudkin JS, Coppack SW. Human subcutaneous adipose tissue secretes interleukin-6 but not tumour necrosis factor-α *in vivo*. *J Clin Endocrinol Metab* 1997; 82: 4196–200.
12. Hotamisligil GS, Peraldi P. Budavari A, Ellis R, White MF, Spiegelman BM. IRS-1-mediated inhibition of insulin receptor tyrosine kinase activity in TNF-α- and obesity-induced insulin resistance. *Science* 1996; 271: 665–8.
13. Pradhan AD, Manson JE, Rifai N, Buring JE, Ridker PM. C-reactive protein, interleukin 6 and risk of developing type 2 diabetes mellitus. *JAMA* 2001; 286: 327–34.
14. Festa A, D'Agostino R, Tracy RP, Haffner SM. Elevated levels of acute-phase proteins and plasminogen activator inhibitor-1 predict the development of type 2 diabetes. The Insulin Resistance Atherosclerosis Study. *Diabetes* 2002; 51: 1131–7.
15. Juhan-Vague I, Alessi MC, Vague P. Increased plasma plasminogen activator inhibitor-1 levels. A possible link between insulin resistance and atherothrombosis. *Diabetologia* 1991; 34: 457–62.
16. Juhan-Vague I, Thompson SG, Jespersen J. Involvement of the hemostatic system in the insulin resistance syndrome. A study of 1,500 patients with angina pectoris. *Arterioscler Thromb* 1993; 13: 1865–73.
17. Samad F, Loskutoff DJ. Tissue distribution and regulation of plasminogen activator inhibitor-1 in obese mice. *Mol Med* 1996; 2: 568–82.
18. Alessi MC, Peiretti F, Morange P, Henry M, Nalbone G, Juhan-Vague I. Production of plasminogen activator inhibitor-1 by human adipose tissue: possible link between visceral fat accumulation and vascular disease. *Diabetes* 1997; 46: 860–7.
19. Sobel BE, Woodcock-Mitchell J, Schneider DJ, Holt RE, Marutsuka K, Gold H. Increased plasminogen activator inhibitor type 1 in coronary artery atherectomy specimens from type 2 diabetic compared with nondiabetic patients: a potential factor predisposing to thrombosis and its persistence. *Circulation* 1998; 97: 2213–21.
20. Juhan-Vague I, Alessi MC. Regulation of fibrinolysis in the development of athero-thrombosis: role of adipose tissue. *Thromb Haemost* 1999; 82: 832–6.
21. Meigs JB, Mittleman MA, Nathan D, Tofler GH, Singer DE, Murphy-Sheehy PM, Lipinska I, D'Agostino RB, Wilson PW. Hyperinsulinemia, hyperglycemia and impaired hemostasis. The Framingham Offspring Study. *JAMA* 2000; 283: 221–8.
22. Bagg W, Ferri C, Desideri G, Gamble G, Ockelford P, Braatvedt GD. The influences of obesity and glycemic control on endothelial activation in patients with type 2 diabetes. *J Clin Endocrinol Metab* 2001; 86: 5491–3.
23. Yudkin JS, Panahloo A, Stehouwer C, Emeis JJ, Bulmer K, Mohamed-Ali V, Denver AE. The influence of improved glycemic control with insulin and sulphonylureas on acute phase and endothelial markers in type II diabetic subjects. *Diabetologia* 2000; 43: 1099–106.
24. Albertini JP, Valensi P, Lormeau B, Aurousseau MH, Ferriere F, Attali JR, Gattegno L. Elevated concentrations of soluble E-selectin and vascular cell adhesion molecule-1 in NIDDM. Effect of intensive insulin treatment. *Diabetes Care* 1998; 21: 1008–13.
25. Ziccardi P, Nappo F, Giugliano G, Esposito K, Marfella R, Cioffi M, D'Andrea F, Molinari AM, Giugliano D. Reduction of inflammatory cytokine concentrations and improvement of endothelial functions in obese women after weight loss over one year. *Circulation* 2002; 105: 9075–6.
26. Collier A, Rumley A, Rumley AG, Paterson JR, Leach JP, Lowe GD, Small M. Free radical activity and hemostatic factors in NIDDM patients with and without microalbuminuria. *Diabetes* 1992; 41: 909–13.
27. Kario K, Matsuo T, Kobayashi H, Matsuo M, Sakada T, Miyata T. Activation of tissue factor-induced coagulation and endothelial cell dysfunction in non insulin dependent diabetic patients with microalbuminuria. *Arterioscler Thromb Vasc Biol* 1995; 1114–20.
28. Nilsson TK, Boman K, Bjerle P, Hallmans G, Hellsten G. von Willebrand factor and fibrinolytic variables are differently affected in the insulin resistance syndrome. *J Intern Med* 1994; 235: 419–23.
29. Juhan-Vague I, Alessi MC, Joly P, Thirion X, Vague P, Declerck PJ, Serradimigni A, Collen D. Plasma plasminogen activator inhibitor-1 in angina pectoris. Influence of plasma insulin and acute-phase response. *Arteriosclerosis* 1989; 9: 362–7.
30. Vambergue A, Rugeri L, Gaveriaux V, Devos P, Martin A, Fermon C, Fontaine P, Jude B. Factor VII, tissue factor pathway inhibitor, and monocyte tissue factor in diabetes mellitus: influence of type of diabetes, obesity index, and age. *Thromb Res* 2001; 101: 367–75.
31. Ichikawa K, Yoshinari M, Iwase M, Wakisaka M, Doi Y, Iino K, Yamamoto M, Fujishima M. Advanced glycosylation end products induced tissue factor expression in human monocyte-like U937 cells and increased tissue factor expression in monocytes from diabetic patients. *Atherosclerosis* 1998; 136: 281–7.
32. Khechai F, Ollivier V, Bridey F, Amar M, Hakim J, de Prost D. Effect of advanced glycation end product-modified albumin on tissue factor expression by monocytes. Role of oxidant stress and protein tyrosine kinase activation. *Arterioscler Thromb Vasc Biol* 1997; 17: 2885–90.
33. Morigi M, Angioletti S, Imberti B, Donadelli R, Micheletti G, Figliuzzi M, Remuzzi A, Zoja C, Remuzzi G. Leukocyte–endothelial interaction is augmented by

high glucose concentrations and hyperglycemia in a NF-κB-dependent fashion. *J Clin Invest* 1998; 101: 1905–15.

34. Vinik AI, Erbas T, Park TS, Nolan R, Pittenger GL. Platelet dysfunction in type 2 diabetes. *Diabetes Care* 2001; 24: 1476–85.
35. Brown AS, Hong Y, Belder A, Beacon H, Beeso J, Sherwood R, Edmonds M, Martin JF, Erusalimsky JD. Megakaryocyte ploidy and platelet changes in human diabetes and atherosclerosis. *Arterioscler Thromb Vasc Biol* 1997; 17: 802–7.
36. Srivastava K, Dash D. Changes in membrane microenvironment and signal transduction in platelets from NIDDM patients—a pilot study. *Clin Chim Acta* 2002; 317: 213–20.
37. Omoto S, Nomura S, Shouzu A, Hayakawa T, Shimizu H, Miyake Y, Yonemoto T, Nishikawa M, Fukuhara S, Inada M. Significance of platelet-derived microparticles and activated platelets in diabetic nephropathy. *Nephron* 1999; 81: 271–7.
38. Fukuda K, Ozaki Y, Satoh K, Kume S, Tawata M, Onaya T, Sakurada K, Seto M, Sasaki Y. Phosphorylation of myosin light chain in resting platelets from NIDDM patients is enhanced—correlation with spontaneous aggregation. *Diabetes* 1997; 46: 488–93.
39. Winocour PD, Bryszewska M, Watala C, Rand ML, Epand RM, Kinlough-Rathbone RL, Packham MA, Mustard JF. Reduced membrane fluidity in platelets from diabetic patients. *Diabetes* 1990; 39: 241–4.
40. Colwell JA. Treatment for the procoagulant state in type 2 diabetes. *Endocrinol Metab Clin North Am* 2001; 30: 1011–30.
41. Juhan I, Buonocore M, Jouve R, Vague Ph, Moulin JP, Vialettes B. Abnormalities of erythrocyte deformability and platelet aggregation in insulin-dependent diabetics corrected by insulin *in vivo* and *in vitro*. *Lancet* 1982; 1: 535–7.
42. Westerbacka J, Yki-Jarvinen H, Turpeinen A, Rissanen A, Vehkavaara S, Syrjala M, Lassila R. Inhibition of platelet–collagen interaction: an in vivo action of insulin abolished by insulin resistance in obesity. *Arterioscler Thromb Vasc Biol* 2002; 22: 167–72.
43. Konstantinides S, Schafer K, Koschnick S, Loskutoff DJ. Leptin-dependent platelet aggregation and arterial thrombosis suggests a mechanism for atherothrombotic disease in obesity. *J Clin Invest* 2001; 108: 1533–40.
44. American Diabetes Association. Clinical practice. Recommendation 2000. Aspirin therapy in diabetes. *Diabetes Care* 2000; 23 (suppl 1): 561–70.
45. Steinhubl SR, Kottke-Marchant K, Moliterno DJ, Rosenthal ML, Godfrey NK, Coller BS, Topol EJ, Lincoff AM. Attainment and maintenance of platelet inhibition through standard dosing of abciximab in diabetic and nondiabetic patients undergoing percutaneous coronary intervention. *Circulation* 1999; 100: 1977–82.
46. Aoki I, Shimoyama K, Aoki N, Homori M, Yanagisawa A, Nakahara K, Kawai Y, Kitamura SI, Ishikawa K. Platelet-dependent thrombin generation in patients with diabetes mellitus: effects of glycemic control on coagulability in diabetes. *J Am Coll Cardiol* 1996; 27: 560–6.
47. Yamada T, Sato A, Nishimori T, Mitsuhashi T, Terao A, Sagai H, Komatsu M, Aizawa T, Hashizume K. Importance of hypercoagulability over hyperglycemia for vascular complication in type 2 diabetes. *Diabetes* 2000; 49: 23–31.
48. Juhan-Vague I, Morange PE, Renucci JF, Alessi MC. Fibrinogen, obesity and insulin resistance. *Blood Coagul Fibrinolysis* 1999; 10 (suppl 1): 25–8.
49. Krobot K, Hense HW, Cremer P, Eberle E, Keil U. Determinants of plasma fibrinogen: relation to body weight, waist-to-hip ratio, smoking, alcohol, age, and sex. Results from the second MONICA Augsburg Survey 1989–1990. *Arterioscler Thromb* 1992; 12: 780–8.
50. Landin K, Stigendal L, Eriksson E, Krotkiewski M, Risberg B, Tengborn L, Smith U. Abdominal obesity is associated with an impaired fibrinolytic activity and elevated plasminogen activator inhibitor-1. *Metabolism* 1990; 39: 1044–8.
51. Ceriello A, Mercuri F, Fabbro D, Giacomello R, Stel G, Taboga C, Tonutti L, Motz E, Damante G. Effect of intensive glycemic control on fibrinogen plasma concentrations in patients with Type II diabetes mellitus. Relation with beta-fibrinogen genotype. *Diabetologia* 1998; 41: 1270–3.
52. Reverter JL, Reverter JC, Tassies D, Rius F, Monteagudo J, Rubies-Prat J, Escolar G, Ordinas A, Sanmarti A. Thrombomodulin and induced tissue factor expression on monocytes as markers of diabetic microangiopathy: a prospective study on hemostasis and lipoproteins in insulin-dependent diabetes mellitus. *Am J Hematol* 1997; 56 (2): 93–9.
53. Osende JI, Badimon JJ, Fuster V, Herson P, Rabito P, Vidhun R, Zaman A, Rodriguez OJ, Lev EI, Rauch U, Heflt G, Fallon JT, Crandall JP. Blood thrombogenicity in type 2 diabetes mellitus patients is associated with glycemic control. *J Am Coll Cardiol* 2001; 38: 1307–12.
54. Standeven KF, Ariëns RAS, Whitaker P, Ashcroft AE, Weisel JW, Grant PJ. The effect of dimethylbiguanide on thrombin activity, FXIII activation, fibrin polymerization and fibrin clot formation. *Diabetes* 2002; 51: 189–97.
55. Aljada A, Ghanim H, Mohanty P, Kapur N, Dandona P. Insulin inhibits the pro-inflammatory transcription factor early growth response gene 1 (Eg2-1) expression in mononuclear cells and reduces plasma tissue factor and plasminogen activator inhibitor 1 concentrations. *J Clin Endocrinol Metab* 2002; 87: 1419–22.
56. Folsom AR, Qamhieh HT, Wing RR, Jeffery RW, Stinson VL, Kuller LH, Wu KK. Impact of weight loss on plasminogen activator inhibitor (PAI-1), factor VII, and other hemostatic factors in moderately overweight adults. *Arterioscler Thromb* 1993; 13: 162–9.
57. Carr ME, Alving BM. Effect of fibrin structure on plasmin-mediated dissolution digestion of plasma clots. *Blood Coagul Fibrinolysis* 1995; 6: 567–73.
58. Mirshahi M, Soria J, Soria C, Bertrand O, Mirshahi M, Basdevant A. Glycosylation of human fibrinogen and fibrin *in vitro*; its consequences on the properties of fibrin(ogen). *Thromb Res* 1987; 48: 279–89.
59. Doggen CJ, Cats VM, Bertina RM, Rosendaal FR. Interaction of coagulation defects and cardiovascular risk factors: increased risk of myocardial infarction associated with factor V Leiden or prothrombin 20210A. *Circulation* 1998; 24 (97): 1037–41.
60. Kohler HP, Stickland MH, Ossei-Gerning N, Carter A, Mikkola H, Grant PJ. Association of a common polymorphism in the factor XIII gene with myocardial infarction. *Thromb Haemost* 1998; 79: 8–13.
61. Franco RF, Pazin-Filho A, Tavella MH, Simoes MV, Marin-Neto JA, Zago MA. Factor XIII Val34 Leu and the risk of myocardial infarction. *Haematologica* 2000; 85: 67–71.

62. Auwerx J, Bouillon R, Collen D, Geboers J. Tissue-type plasminogen activator antigen and plasminogen activator inhibitor in diabetes mellitus. *Arteriosclerosis* 1988; 8: 68–72.
63. Juhan-Vague I, Roul C, Alessi MC, Ardissone JP, Heim M, Vague P. Increased plasminogen activator inhibitor activity in non-insulin dependent diabetic patients-relationship with plasma insulin. *Thromb Haemost* 1989; 61: 370–3.
64. Vague Ph, Juhan-Vague I, Aillaud MF, Badier C, Viard R, Alessi MC, Collen D. Correlation between blood fibrinolytic activity, PA-inhibitor level, plasma insulin level and relative body weight in normal and obese subjects. *Metabolism* 1986; 35: 250–3.
65. Potter van Loon BJ, Kluft C, Radder JK, Blankenstein MA, Meinders AE. The cardiovascular risk factor plasminogen activator inhibitor type 1 is related to insulin resistance. *Metabolism* 1993; 42: 945–9.
66. Henry M, Tregouët DA, Alessi MC, Aillaud MF, Visvikis S, Siest G, Tiret L, Juhan-Vague I. Metabolic determinants are much more important than genetic polymorphisms in determining the PAI-1 activity and antigen plasma concentrations: a family study with part of the Stanislas cohort. *Arterioscler. Thromb. Vasc. Biol.* 1998; 18: 84–91.
67. Gray RP, Panahloo A, Mohamed-Ali V, Patterson DL, Yudkin JS. Proinsulin-like molecules and plasminogen activator inhibitor type 1 (PAI-1) activity in diabetic and nondiabetic subjects with and without myocardial infarction. *Atherosclerosis* 1997; 130: 171–8.
68. Nordt T, Sawa H, Fujii S, Sobel BE. Induction of plasminogen activator inhibitor type-1 (PAI-1) by proinsulin and insulin *in vivo*. *Circulation* 1995; 91: 764–70.
69. Haffner S, Mykkänen L, Stern MP, Valdez RA, Heisserman JA, Bowsher RR. Relationship of proinsulin and insulin to cardiovascular risk factors in nondiabetic subjects. *Diabetes* 1993; 42: 1297–302.
70. Shimomura I, Funahashi T, Takahashi M, Maeda K, Kotani K, Nakamura T, Yamashita S, Miura M, Fukuda Y, Takemura K, Tokunaga K, Matsuzawa Y. Enhanced expression of PAI-1 in visceral fat: possible contributor to vascular disease in obesity. *Nat Med* 1996; 2: 800–3.
71. Cigolini M, Targher G, Bergamo Andreis IA, Tonoli M, Agostino G, De Sandre G. Visceral fat accumulation and its relation to plasma hemostatic factors in healthy men. *Arterioscler Thromb Vasc Biol* 1996; 16: 368–74.
72. Festa A, D'Agostino R, Mykkänen L, Tracy R, Howard BV, Haffner SM. Low-density lipoprotein particle size is inversely related to plasminogen activator inhibitor-1 levels. The Insulin Resistance Atherosclerosis Study. *Arterioscler Thromb Vasc Biol* 1999; 19: 605–10.
73. Janand-Delenne B, Chagnaud C, Raccah D, Alessi MC, Juhan-Vague I, Vague P. Visceral fat as a main determinant of plasminogen activator inhibitor 1 level in women. *Int J Obes Relat Metab Disord* 1998; 22: 312–7.
74. Nagi DK, Yudkin JS. Effects of metformin on insulin resistance, risk factors for cardiovascular disease, and plasminogen activator inhibitor in NIDDM subjects: a study of two ethnic groups. *Diabetes Care* 1993; 16: 621–9.
75. Kruszynska YT, Yu JG, Olefsky JM, Sobel BE. Effects of troglitazone on blood concentrations of plasminogen activator inhibitor 1 in patients with type 2 diabetes and in lean and obese normal subjects. *Diabetes* 2000; 49: 633–9.
76. Alessi MC, Juhan-Vague I, Kooistra T, Declerck PJ, Collen D. Insulin stimulates the synthesis of plasminogen activator inhibitor 1 by the human hepatocellular cell line Hep G2. *Thromb Haemost* 1988; 60: 491–4.
77. Grant PJ, Stickland MH, Wiles PG, Davies JA, Wales JK, Prentice CRM. Hormonal control of hemostasis during hypoglycemia in diabetes mellitus. *Thromb Haemost* 1987; 57: 341–4.
78. Panahloo A, Mohamed-Ali V, Andres C, Denver AE, Yudkin JS. Effect of insulin versus sulfonylurea therapy on cardiovascular risk factors and fibrinolysis in type 2 diabetes. *Metabolism* 1998; 47: 637–43.
79. Morange PE, Aubert J, Peiretti F, Vague P, Lijnen HR, Verdier M, Negrel R, Juhan-Vague I, Alessi MC. Glucocorticoids and insulin promote plasminogen activator inhibitor 1 production by human adipose tissue. *Diabetes* 1999; 48: 890–5.
80. Vulin AI, Stanley FM. A forkhead/winged helix-related transcription factor mediates insulin-increased plasminogen activator inhibitor-1 gene transcription. *J Biol Chem* 2002; 277: 20169–76.
81. Stiko-Rahm A, Wiman B, Hamsten A, Nilsson J. Secretion of plasminogen activator inhibitor-1 from cultured human umbilical vein endothelial cells is induced by very low density lipoprotein. *Arteriosclerosis* 1990; 10: 1067–73.
82. Nilsson L, Banfi C, Diczfalusy U, Tremoli E, Hamsten A, Eriksson P. Unsaturated fatty acids increase plasminogen activator inhibitor-1 expression in endothelial cells. *Arterioscler Thromb Vasc Biol* 1998; 18: 1679–85.
83. Nordt TK, Klassen KJ, Schneider DJ, Sobel BE. Augmentation of synthesis of plasminogen activator inhibitor type-1 in arterial endothelial cells by glucose and its implications for local fibrinolysis. *Arterioscler Thromb* 1993; 13: 1822–8.
84. Vaughan D. Angiotensin and vascular fibrinolytic balance. *Am J Hypertens* 2002; 15: 3S–8S.
85. Samad F, Yamamoto K, Pandey M, Loskutoff DJ. Elevated expression of transforming growth factor-beta in adipose tissue from obese mice. *Mol Med* 1997; 3: 37–48.
86. Samad F, Uysal T, Wiesbrock S, Pandey M, Hotamisligil S, Loskutoff J. Tumor necrosis factor α is a key component in the obesity-linked elevation of plasminogen activator inhibitor 1. *Proc Natl Acad Sci USA* 1999; 96: 6902–7.
87. Eriksson P, Reynisdottir S, Lönnqvist F, Stemme V, Hamsten A, Arner P. Adipose tissue secretion of plasminogen activator inhibitor-1 in non obese and obese individuals. *Diabetologia* 1998; 41: 65–71.
88. Cigolini M, Tonoli M, Borgato L, Frigotto L, Manzato F, Zeminian S, Cardinale C, Camin M, Chiaramonte E, De Sandre G, Lunardi C. Expression of plasminogen activator inhibitor-1 in human adipose tissue: a role for TNF-α? *Atherosclerosis* 1999; 143: 81–90.
89. Gottschling-Zeller H, Birgel M, Rohrig K, Hauner H. Effect of tumor necrosis factor alpha and transforming growth factor beta 1 on plasminogen activator inhibitor-1 secretion from subcutaneous and omental human fat cells in suspension culture. *Metabolism* 2000; 49: 666–71.
90. Mavri A, Alessi MC, Bastelica D, Geel-Georgelin O, Fina F, Sentocnik JT, Stegnar M, Juhan-Vague I. Subcutaneous abdominal, but not femoral fat expression of plasminogen activator inhibitor-1 (PAI-1) is related to plasma PAI-1 levels and insulin resistance and decreases after weight loss. *Diabetologia* 2001; 44: 2025–31.
91. Bastelica D, Morange PE, Berthet B, Borghi H, Lacroix O, Grino M. Juhan-Vague I, Alessi MC. Stromal cells are the main PAI-1 producing cells in human fat. Evidence of

differences between visceral and subcutaneous deposits. *Arterioscler Thromb Vasc Biol* 2002; 22: 173–8.

92. Cigolini M, Targher G, Agostino G, Tonoli M, Muggeo M, De Sandre G. Liver steatosis and its relation to plasma hemostatic factors in apparently healthy men—role of the metabolic syndrome. *Thromb Haemost* 1996; 76: 69–73.
93. Bruckert E, Ankri A, Giral P, Turpin G. Relationship between plasma plasminogen activator inhibitor 1 and hepatic enzyme concentrations in hyperlipidemie patients. *Thromb Haemost* 1994; 72: 434–7.
94. Alessi MC, Bastelica D, Morange PE, Berthet B, Leduc I, Verdier M, Geel O, Juhan-Vague I. Plasminogen activator inhibitor-1, transforming growth factor β1 and body mass index are closely associated in human adipose tissue during morbid obesity. *Diabetes* 2000; 49: 1374–80.
95. Bastelica D, Mavri A, Verdier M, Bergoin M, Berthet B, Juhan-Vague I, Alessi MC. Relationships between fibrinolytic and inflammatory parameters in human adipose tissue: strong contribution of TNFalpha receptors to PAI-1 levels. *Thromb Haemost* 2002; 88: 481–7.
96. Morange PE, Lijnen HR, Alessi MC, Kopp F, Collen D, Juhan-Vague I. Influence of PAI-1 on adipose tissue growth and metabolic parameters in a murine model of diet-induced obesity. *Arterioscler Thromb Vasc Biol* 2000; 20: 1150–4.
97. Lijnen HR, Maquoi E, Morange P, Voros G, Van Hoef B, Kopp F, Collen D, Juhan-Vague I, Alessi MC. Nutritionally induced obesity is attenuated in transgenic mice overexpressing plasminogen activator inhibitor-1. *Arterioscler Thromb Vasc Biol* January 1, 2003; 23 (1): 78–84.
98. Hoover-Plow J, Ellis J, Yuen L. *In vivo* plasminogen deficiency reduces fat accumulation. *Thromb Haemost* 2002; 87: 1011–9.
99. Hamsten A, de Faire U, Walldius G, Dahlen G, Szamosi A, Landou C, Blombäck M, Wiman B. Plasminogen activator inhibitor in plasma: risk factor for recurrent myocardial infarction. *Lancet* 1987; II: 3–9.
100. Cesari M, Rossi GP. Plasminogen activator inhibitor type 1 in ischemic cardiomyopathy. *Arterioscler Thromb Vasc Biol* 1999; 19: 1378–86.
101. Haffner SM, D'Agostino R, Mykkänen L, Hales CN, Savage PJ, Bergman RN, O'Leary D, Rewers M, Selby J, Tracy R, Saad MF. Proinsulin and insulin concentrations in relation to carotid wall thickness: Insulin Resistance Atherosclerosis Study. *Stroke* 1998; 29: 1498–503.
102. Juhan-Vague I, Pyke SDM, Alessi MC, Jespersen J, Haverkate F, Thompson SG. Fibrinolytic factors and the risk of myocardial infarction or sudden death in patients with angina pectoris. *Circulation* 1996; 94: 2057–63.
103. Pandolfi A, Cetrullo D, Polishuck R, Alberta MM, Calafiore A, Pellegrini G, Vitacolonna E, Capani F, Consoli A. Plasminogen activator inhibitor type 1 is increased in the arterial wall of type II diabetic subjects. *Arterioscler Thromb Vasc Biol* 2001; 21: 1378–82.
104. Vaughan DE, Rouleau J-L, Ridker PM, Arnold JMO, Menapace FJ, Pfeffer MA. Effects of ramipril on plasma fibrinolytic balance in patients with acute anterior myocardial infarction. *Circulation* 1997; 96: 442–7.
105. The Heart Outcomes Prevention Evaluation Study Investigators. Effects of an angiotensin-converting-enzyme inhibitor, ramipril on cardiovascular events in high-risk patients. *N Engl J Med* 2000; 342: 145–53.
106. Hansson L, Lindholm LH, Niskanen L, Lanke J, Hedner T, Niklason A, Luomanmäki K, Dahlöf B, de Faire U, Mörlin C, Karlberg BE, Wester PO, Björck J-E. Effect of angiotensin-converting-enzyme inhibition compared with conventional therapy on cardiovascular morbidity and mortality in hypertension: the Captopril Prevention Project (CAPPP) randomised trial. *Lancet* 1999; 353: 611–6.

81

Atherogenesis and Coronary Heart Disease

Russell P. Tracy

College of Medicine, The University of Vermont, Burlington, VT, USA

INTRODUCTION

Diabetes, and the cluster of pathophysiological changes called the metabolic syndrome, is strongly associated with cardiovascular disease (CVD) in general, and coronary heart disease (CHD) in particular. CVD is the largest single cause of death in those with diabetes, and the association of diabetes with CVD is so strong that the recent report of the third Adult Treatment Panel (ATP III) of the National Cholesterol Education Panel recommended that the presence of diabetes be considered equivalent in risk to the presence of clinical CVD in global risk assessment [1].

In the United States, death from CHD is up to threefold higher in diabetic men and up to sevenfold higher in diabetic women, when compared to persons without diabetes [2]. The CHD population attributable risk due to diabetes is of the order of 10%, again somewhat higher in women than in men [2]. There is excess CHD risk associated with both type 1 and type 2 diabetes, in men and in women, and in older persons as well as younger.

This chapter, using a predominantly epidemiological perspective, attempts to describe some of the known pathophysiological relationships between diabetes and heart disease, and in so doing provides support for the "common soil" hypothesis, which suggests that there are similar underlying causes of both diabetes (at least type 2 diabetes) and atherosclerotic heart disease [3]. In particular, the chapter emphasizes recent work in the areas of hemostasis and inflammation.

AN OVERVIEW OF ATHEROSCLEROSIS

The molecular details of the atherosclerotic process have been the target of intense research over the past 30 years or more. A picture has emerged that has great complexity at the cellular and molecular levels and includes lipid abnormalities, oxidative damage, immune activation, vessel wall and blood inflammation, calcification, and thrombosis. This process has been summarized by Libby and Ross in recent publications [4, 5], and is graphically shown in Figure 1.

A number of changes occur in diabetes that have atherosclerotic implications. The general prevalences of potentially atherogenic changes in type 1 and type 2 diabetes are shown in Tables 1 and 2. The general changes in lipoprotein profile are well known and have been used to argue for a large fraction of the increased risk of CHD seen in diabetes [2]. Recently, new linkages have been made with alterations in lipoprotein particle size, and in other areas as well, such as impaired fibrinolytic potential and low-level, chronic inflammation (microinflammation).

Table 3 offers a brief discussion of some potential mechanistic pathways through which these changes might be associated with CHD. Some of these are speculative, although all are supported by some degree of biochemical or animal data. In aggregate they describe a set of pathological changes that affect atherosclerotic initiation and progression throughout the natural history of the disease. The remainder of the chapter predominantly addresses type 2 diabetes and macrovascular disease; the implications for diabetic microvascular disease are less clear, and the connection of microvascular disease to clinical atherosclerotic CVD is not well understood at all.

ATHEROSCLEROSIS, THROMBOSIS, AND INFLAMMATION: A COMPLEX INTERPLAY

Atherosclerotic CHD commonly manifests itself clinically via a thrombotic event, so-called atherothrombosis.

International Textbook of Diabetes Mellitus, Third Edition. Edited by R. A. DeFronzo, E. Ferrannini, H. Keen, and P. Zimmet.
 ISBN: 0-471-48655-8.

(a)

(b)

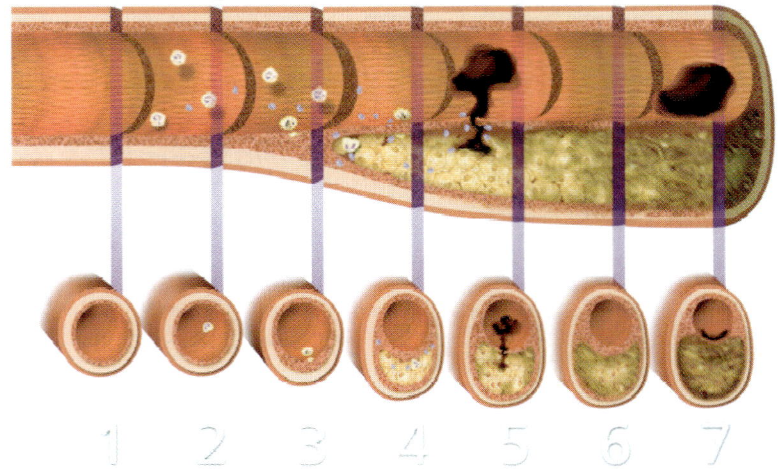

Figure 1 Initiation, progression, and complication of human coronary atherosclerotic plaque. (a) Longitudinal section of artery depicting "timeline" of human atherogenesis from normal artery [1] to atheroma that caused clinical manifestations by thrombosis or stenosis [5–7]. (b) Cross sections of artery during various stages of atheroma evolution. (1) Normal artery. Note that in human arteries, the intimal layer is much better developed than in most other species. The intima of human arteries contains resident smooth muscle cells often as early as first year of life. (2) Lesion initiation occurs when endothelial cells, activated by risk factors such as hyperlipoproteinemia, express adhesion and chemoattractant molecules that recruit inflammatory leukocytes such as monocytes and T lymphocytes. Extracellular lipid begins to accumulate in intima at this stage. (3) Evolution to fibrofatty stage. Monocytes recruited to artery wall become macrophages and express scavenger receptors that bind modified lipoproteins. Macrophages become lipid-laden foam cells by engulfing modified lipoproteins. Leukocytes and resident vascular wall cells can secrete inflammatory cytokines and growth factors that amplify leukocyte recruitment and cause smooth muscle cell migration and proliferation. (4) As lesion progresses, inflammatory mediators cause expression of tissue factor, a potent procoagulant, and of matrix-degrading proteinases that weaken fibrous cap of plaque. (5) If fibrous cap ruptures at point of weakening, coagulation factors in blood can gain access to thrombogenic, tissue-factor-containing lipid core, causing thrombosis on nonocclusive atherosclerotic plaque. If balance between prothrombotic and fibrinolytic mechanisms prevailing at that particular region and at that particular time is unfavorable, occlusive thrombus causing acute coronary syndromes may result. (6) When thrombus resorbs, products associated with thrombosis such as thrombin and mediators released from degranulating platelets, including platelet-derived growth factor and transforming growth factor-β, can cause healing response, leading to increased collagen accumulation and smooth muscle cell growth. In this manner, the fibrofatty lesion can evolve into advanced fibrous and often calcified plaque, one that may cause significant stenosis, and produce symptoms of stable angina pectoris. (7) In some cases, occlusive thrombi arise not from fracture of fibrous cap but from superficial erosion of endothelial layer. Resulting mural thrombus, again dependent on local prothrombotic and fibrinolytic balance, can cause acute myocardial infarction. Superficial erosions often complicate advanced and stenotic lesions, as shown here. However, superficial erosions do not necessarily occur after fibrous cap rupture, as depicted in this idealized diagram. (Reproduced by permission of the American Heart Association [4])

Table 1 Prevalence of potentially atherogenic changes in type 1 and type 2 diabetes

	Type 1		
Factor	Normal renal function	Impaired renal function	Type 2
Hypertension	0	+++	++
Hypercholesterolemia	0/+	+++	+
Hypertriglyceridemia	0/+	+++	+++
Remnant particles	?	+++	++
Decreased high-density lipoprotein cholesterol	0/+	+++	++
Decreased low-density lipoprotein particle size	+	?	+++
Obesity	0	0	+++
Hyperinsulinemia	+	++	++
Immune complexes	++	?	0
Impaired fibrinolysis	+	?	+++
Microinflammation	++	+++	+++

Source: Modified from reference 2, copyright © 1996 by Oxford University Press, Inc. Used by permission of Oxford University Press, Inc. Additional information from references 8–10.
0, +, ++, +++ = degrees of increased prevalence compared to nondiabetic subjects. ? = unknown.

Table 2 Alterations in plasma lipoproteins in patients with type 1 and type 2 diabetes

Lipoprotein	Alteration
Low-density lipoproteins	Increased plasma level Glycation Modification in the arterial wall to enhance uptake by macrophage Triglyceride enrichment Decreased particle size
High-density lipoproteins	Decreased plasma level Glycation Triglyceride enrichment
Very low density lipoproteins	Increased plasma level Impaired degradation leading to remnant accumulation Altered composition → endothelial toxicity; increased lipid uptake by macrophage
Chylomicra	Impaired degradation leading to remnant accumulation
Remnants	Increased levels in some type 2 diabetic subjects

Source: Modified from reference 2, copyright © 1996 by Oxford University Press, Inc. Used by permission of Oxford University Press, Inc. Additional information from references 8–10.
0, +, ++, +++ = degrees of increased prevalence compared to nondiabetic subjects.

This has been clearly understood only since the early 1970s, and the work of DeWood and colleagues [6]. The process of hemostasis, which includes the formation of a blood clot, might be considered as composed of coagulation, limited and controlled by anticoagulation; and the counterbalancing process of fibrinolysis, limited and controlled by antifibrinolysis. Examples of factors include *coagulation*: prothrombin, factor V, fibrinogen; *anticoagulation*: protein C, protein S; *fibrinolysis*: plasminogen, tissue-type plasminogen activator (tPA); *antifibrinolysis*: plasminogen activator inhibitor 1 (PAI-1), α_2-antiplasmin.

Since it has been known for a long time that changes in coagulation factor levels are associated with risk of venous clotting or bleeding (e.g., lack of factor VIII or factor IX leading to bleeding in hemophilia A or B, or deficiency in the anticoagulant protein C leading to deep vein thrombosis), researchers pursued the importance of differences in coagulation factor levels to atherothrombotic risk. Meade, Miller, and colleagues pioneered this work in the Northwick Park Heart Study, and demonstrated the clear importance of fibrinogen as a CVD risk factor [7]. They also made early observations concerning factor VIII (which were later substantiated) and factor VII (which have not been substantiated), as well as preliminary findings about the complementary process of fibrinolysis.

As this work was confirmed and extended by others [11–13], it became clear that fibrinogen, factor VIII, and several other plasma proteins were risk factors, at least in part because they reflected low-level chronic inflammation associated with atherosclerosis. That is, the coagulation factors that were elevated in the presence of clinical CVD and whose levels in otherwise healthy people predicted the occurrence of future CVD, were all in the class of liver proteins known as acute phase reactants. These proteins respond to inflammatory stimulation via the hepatic effects of the proinflammatory cytokine interleukin-6 (IL-6). In fact, even an anticoagulant protein such as protein C, which is a very weak acute phase protein, was shown to be weakly, but positively, associated with CVD (i.e., contrary to initial hypotheses higher levels, not lower levels, were found in those with CVD), suggesting that it was not so much the process of clotting that was related to CVD but the process of inflammation [14].

It was, and remains, less clear that these factors also reflect risk because higher levels are associated with a hypercoagulable state. For example, there are several plausible

Table 3 Some potential mechanistic pathways associated with pathophysiological changes seen in diabetes

Change	Pathway
Hypertension	Turbulent flow; arterial wall alterations
Hypercholesterolemia	Increased opportunity for oxidative modification; uptake by macrophage
Hypertriglyceridemia	Increased VLDL → increased surface for coagulation
Remnant particles	Increased uptake of lipids by macrophage
Decreased HDL	Impaired cholesterol metabolism
Decreased LDL particle size	Increased uptake by macrophage
Obesity	Increased cytokine production
Hyperinsulinemia	Reflection of peripheral insulin resistance
Immune complexes	Vascular wall pathology; renal pathology
Impaired fibrinolysis	Thrombosis; plaque formation
Microinflammation	Increased insulin resistance; increased lipid oxidation and uptake; immune system activation; CRP and/or cytokine-induced damage to vascular endothelium

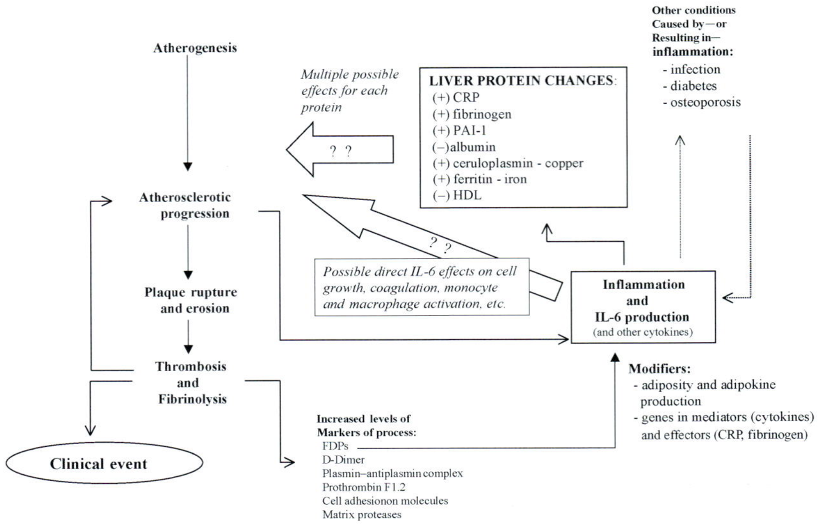

Figure 2 The complex interplay of atherothrombotic disease with plasma markers of CVD risk: a positive feedback pathway. Inflammation and the proinflammatory cytokines, e.g., IL-6, are increased by a variety of mechanisms in atherothrombosis. For example, atherothrombosis results in the production of FDPs, which in turn cause the elaboration of IL-6 by monocytes [16]. In addition, other causes of inflammation feed into this system, such as chronic infections and diabetes. This process is also modified by an individual's capacity for inflammatory response; recent data suggest that an important modifying factor is adiposity, especially visceral adiposity [17]. A wide variety of genetic influences are easily conceived. Increased IL-6 itself may aggravate the atherothrombotic process, since it can act as a potent growth regulator, cause monocytes and other cells to express procoagulant tissue factor, activate the immune system thereby exacerbating lipid uptake by foam cells, among other potential mechanisms. The plasma proteins affected by IL-6, such as CRP, fibrinogen, and others, may also directly participate in the atherothrombotic process to make it worse. Here "??" indicates uncertainty about multiple possible mechanisms. (Reproduced by permission of Schattauer)

mechanisms by which higher levels of fibrinogen might cause an increased propensity for blood clots, including increased platelet cross-linking, increased fibrin clot formation, and increased blood viscosity [15]. However, it remains unproven whether any of these mechanisms are actually at play *in situ*. Having said this, given all the available data, it seems most likely that while a number of these factors reflect the underlying atherosclerotic process, they may well also participate in that process, making it proceed at a faster rate. This "positive feedback" is illustrated in Figure 2.

Meade and colleagues were also the first to suggest that deficiencies in fibrinolysis, the process that limits clot production and ultimately removes clots from the circulation, might also be predictive of future atherothrombosis [18]. Others went on to show that levels of the major plasma antifibrinolysis protein, PAI-1, were elevated in those with CVD and did offer some risk prediction, a finding not always confirmed [19–22]. Juhan-Vague and colleagues have speculated that the degree of predictive power may be a function of the adjustment done for other variables [22]. This is of particular note in a discussion of type 2 diabetes, since PAI-1 levels are associated with levels of insulin, and there is some evidence that insulin and proinsulin are capable of directly stimulating endothelial and/or liver cells to produce PAI-1 [23, 24]. PAI-1 is also known to be a weak acute phase reactant [25]. Finally, adipocytes are also capable of PAI-1 synthesis and secretion, a fact that helps explain the known association of PAI-1 levels with measurements such as waist circumference and BMI (body mass index: weight [kg]/height [m]^2) [26]. To determine any underlying relationships among this set of correlated variables, we performed a factor analysis including metabolic, inflammation, and hemostasis factors [27]. PAI-1 did not associate with coagulation factors, fibrinolytic factors, or inflammation factors, but rather with insulin and/or body composition, supporting the notion that PAI-1 reflects both hyperinsulinemia/insulin resistance and adiposity, but not inflammation.

As we have noted above for coagulation factors, the question remains whether PAI-1 simply reflects these underlying associations or contributes to the disease process. Also as before, the most likely answer is that both views are correct.

INFLAMMATION MARKERS AND CVD RISK

Much recent research has implicated inflammation in atherosclerosis and CVD. This use of the word *inflammation* does not denote the full form of the condition with the classical four cardinal signs of warmth, redness, swelling, and pain. Rather it implies a "microinflammation," where a person with this condition might be characterized by

Table 4 Inflammation markers shown to be associated with atherosclerosis and CVD*

Marker	Reference	Description
Fibrinogen	[18]	APR; substrate for thrombin—becomes fibrin
Factor VIII	[28]	APR; clotting cofactor
CRP	[29]	APR; assists complement; activates monocytes
Ceruloplasmin	[30]	APR; transports copper
Albumin	[31]	(−) APR; binds many substances; produces COP
PAI-1	[20]	Weak APR; fibrinolytic inhibitor
IL-6	[32]	Major proinflammatory cytokine
SAA	[33]	APR; function not known

Note. APR = acute phase reactant; COP = colloid osmotic pressure; SAA = serum amyloid A.
*Additional information from references 28–31 and 33.

being in the upper part of the normal distribution for inflammation status, but not exhibiting the signs and symptoms of overt, clinical inflammation. Population-based research has played a key role in characterizing the relationship of inflammation to CVD, and recently it has become clear that inflammation is connected to the metabolic syndrome in a complex and important manner.

A number of markers of inflammation, many of which are in the category of so-called acute phase reactants, have been shown to be associated with CVD. Table 4 lists a number of these markers. Some are known acute phase reactants; others are not. Most are produced in the liver in response to IL-6. These markers have many different functions, yet have a similarity in that they all are moderately to strongly associated with the presence of CVD (in all cases clinical CVD; in some cases subclinical CVD as defined by techniques such as carotid artery ultrasonography).

While inflammation is usually estimated in human studies by a simple measurement of a plasma acute phase protein such as c-reactive protein (CRP) or fibrinogen, the term *inflammation* includes a wide variety of activities related to the response to environmental challenge, such as coagulation and fibrinolysis [34]; complement activation [35]; endothelial cell, neutrophil, and monocyte activation [36]; antioxidation [37]; immune response [38]; and others. In addition, these inflammation responses are modified by genetic architecture (e.g., variances in the IL-6 gene [39, 40]), other environmental factors (e.g., diet and smoking [41, 42]), and the volume of inflammation-mediating tissue (e.g., visceral fat [17]). Therefore it is clear that the relationship of inflammation to atherosclerosis should be expected to be (and is) complex and the full story will emerge only after much additional research.

In addition, several inflammatory markers have been shown to be predictive of future CVD events. In a number of cases, this independent predictive ability is similar among the different markers. For example, in the MONICA Augsburg cohort, ceruloplasmin had similar risk prediction to CRP [43]; in the Cardiovascular Health Study cohort, fibrinogen, factor VIII, and CRP each independently predicted future CVD events [44]; and in the Iowa 65+ Rural Health Study, both CRP and IL-6 predicted future fatal CVD events [32]. While the risk prediction is similar this does not, however, mean that these markers are identical, since there are differences in the strength of association and each marker may participate in the CVD process in a different way. In one of the few side-by-side comparisons, Ridker and colleagues have concluded that CRP offered the greatest benefit from the standpoint of risk prediction [45]. However, a recent meta-analysis observed no real difference between CRP and fibrinogen in risk prediction [46].

INFLAMMATION MARKERS, THE METABOLIC SYNDROME, AND DIABETES

In general, markers of inflammation are associated with diabetes status and the metabolic syndrome [27]. These associations take a number of forms. For example, CRP values increase with the number of components of the metabolic syndrome present [8]. Also, fibrinogen levels are correlated with albumin excretion, even in those without demonstrable impaired glucose tolerance (N. Jenny, manuscript in preparation). While these are strong relationships, factor analysis suggests that inflammation represents a distinct underlying pathophysiological pathway [27].

It has been proposed that inflammation may be an important independent component of the metabolic syndrome [8]. While many of the metabolic correlates of the various inflammation markers are the same, there are some differences. Whether these differences represent true physiological variations or reflect different populations under study, different analytical techniques, or different analytical precision is unclear.

For the purposes of discussing the correlates of inflammation, Table 5 lists the known associated variables for CRP [8, 27, 41, 42, 49]. Key among these correlates are adiposity, insulin sensitivity status, and coagulation activity. Yudkin has suggested that adipose tissue is a key producer of inflammatory cytokines (so-called adipokines), and that a prominent member of this group, IL-6, may be the major pathophysiological mediator of

Table 5 Known correlates of CRP

Correlate	Reference	Comment
Sex	[42]	(+) Women > men
Race	[42]	(+) Black > Hispanic/White
Age	[42]	(+) Increases with age
Adiposity	[42, 47]	(+++) Strongly associated with BMI, waist, and others
Glucose status	[8]	(++) Associated with diabetes
Insulin sensitivity	[8]	(++) Negatively associated with FSIGTT
Smoking status	[41, 42]	(+) Smoking and pack-years of smoking
Coagulation status	[42, 48]	(++) Associated with "ambient coag status"
IMT	[42]	(+/−) Weak association with wall thickness
Hypertension	[42]	(+/−) Weak association with blood pressure
CAC	[42]	(+/−) Weak association with calcification

Note. FSIGTT = frequently sampled intravenous glucose tolerance test; IMT = ultrasound intimal medial wall thickness of the carotid artery; CAC = coronary artery calcification; "ambient coag status" = random measurement of fibrin degradation products or plasmin–antiplasmin complex formation.

diabetes and the metabolic syndrome [47]. In this model, the metabolic syndrome is a contributor to increased inflammation through the visceral obesity component: increased visceral fat leads to increased proinflammatory response to a variety of stimulants, resulting in a chronic upregulation of IL-6 production.

Clearly, IL-6 is a potent endocrine mediator of many critical functions, and has been associated with activities ranging from T helper cell differentiation [50] to heart rate variability [51]. We have demonstrated in a murine model of atherosclerosis that weekly injections of small amounts of IL-6 will result in a two- to fivefold increase in atherosclerotic burden, supporting a direct role for IL-6 in CVD [52]. As discussed by Desprès and colleagues [53], the key adipose depot appears to be the viscera. Visceral adiposity—as a result of poor diet, lack of exercise, genetics, and other predisposing variables—may be a critical component of not only the metabolic syndrome but atherosclerotic CVD as well [17, 49, 53, 54]. This provides an important link between inflammation and obesity, especially abdominal obesity.

Although adiposity is strongly related to the other components of the metabolic syndrome, the link of CRP with insulin status is at least partially independent of adiposity, and strongly related to insulin sensitivity [27]. A possible link exists through the key proinflammatory cytokine, and also an adipokine, tumor necrosis factor α (TNF-α). While TNF-α has many functions, as a so-called first-wave cytokine TNF-α influences IL-6 production [55]. While the true role(s) of circulating TNF-α in humans remains unclear, it has been shown to affect insulin sensitivity negatively in tissue culture and in animal models [56, 57]; in addition, plasma levels are elevated in the metabolic syndrome, and associated with insulin resistance in humans [58]. TNF-α influences IL-6 levels, which in turn influence CRP; together these data suggest a possible mechanistic link between CRP and insulin sensitivity.

CRP is also associated with coagulation activity status, as estimated by markers such as D-dimer (a fibrin degradation product (FDP) that reflects first the formation of fibrin and then fibrinolysis) and plasmin–antiplasmin complex (PAP; a marker reflecting plasmin formation rate, itself depending on the stimulation of fibrin formation, as well as the levels of tPA and PAI-1) [27, 42, 48]. Increases in coagulation status in the metabolic syndrome and diabetes have been well documented [59, 60]. The exact mechanism for the association of CRP with coagulation status is not clear; however the work of Fuller and colleagues suggests a possible pathway [16]. Monocytes appear capable of binding FDPs and subsequently producing IL-6, which goes to the liver and affects the wide range of proteins known to be in the acute phase response. This has been proposed to be the mechanism by which fibrinogen consumption is replaced, and may be an important mechanism connecting coagulation and inflammation. This may have far reaching implications both in the general biology we have been discussing and in areas such as drug development, where the coagulation–inflammation connection in sepsis, as described by Esmon [34], has been recently exploited [61].

INFLAMMATION, CVD, AND CHRONIC DISEASES OF OLD AGE

Throughout this chapter a hypothesis of "positive feedback" has been proffered (illustrated in Figure 2), which suggests that we enter a downward spiral with respect to vascular disease (and possibly other diseases of old age), the slope of which is strongly affected by our genetic architecture and our environment [62]. Such a "positive feedback" pathway would raise an important question: why would our response to the process of atherosclerosis actually make the disease worse rather than better? Several hypotheses are emerging that involve evolutionary biology and the risks and benefits of various protective systems. The concept of a "thrifty gene" was first offered by Neel in 1962 to help explain the presence of diabetes in many populations [63]. He suggested that while there was an advantage to a genetic architecture that could make use of every calorie in the diet for either energy or storage when calories were scarce, this actually became a disadvantage when food became abundant, i.e., in modern times. This thrifty genotype predisposed toward insulin resistance, the metabolic syndrome, and, ultimately, diabetes when the environment included modern diets rich in calories, fats, and short-chain sugars. There is also a complementary "thrifty phenotype" hypothesis, offered by Hales and Barker, that proffers poor maternal and fetal nutrition in place of an evolved genotype as a cause for developing a "thrifty metabolism" [64]. In this hypothesis poor nutrition in early life (as estimated by birth weight) causes permanent changes in glucose metabolism, which when coupled with overnutrition as an adult, results in insulin resistance.

Recently, Fernández-Real and Ricart have expanded this view in two ways [65]. First, they have added to the general scheme what we now know about inflammation and its relationship to the metabolic syndrome and diabetes; second, through inflammation, they connect metabolic dysregulation, diabetes, and atherosclerotic CVD. In their view, just as there was a selective advantage to having a genetic framework that was as efficient as possible with respect to extracting calories from the diet, there was a selective advantage to having an immune response and an inflammatory response that were as efficient as possible at protecting us from infection, trauma, and the various other insults we have experience over evolution. And, just as there is now a disadvantage to the "thrifty" metabolic genetic makeup because of the abundance and nature of modern foodstuffs, and the longer human life span, there is also a disadvantage to an aggressive inflammatory response under these same conditions.

Through inflammation (and the damage caused by an aggressive "defense") one can expand these theories to include many (all?) of the chronic diseases of old age. Disorders in this category include, but are not limited to, CHD; other CVDs such as heart failure and sudden cardiac death that have, at least in part, atherosclerotic origins; peripheral atherosclerotic disease; the metabolic syndrome; type 2 diabetes; osteoporosis; dementia; and frailty. There may be an inflammatory component even in the case of some cancers. Recent work has demonstrated for each of these an inflammatory component, and has suggested that any chronic proinflammatory stimulation will exacerbate the condition. Indeed, recent work has shown that inflammatory markers are able to predict noncardiovascular mortality as well as that from CVD [32].

Among the many implications of these theories, two stand out. First, it seems likely that anything that increases chronic low-level proinflammation will increase the likelihood of these disorders occurring sooner rather than later. In fact, each of them can act as such a stimulant, possibly helping to explain, for example, why heart disease occurs so frequently in diabetic patients: the increasing low-level inflammation associated with increasing severity of the metabolic syndrome and diabetes accelerates the atherosclerosis, and *vice versa*. This might be considered an expanded version of the "positive feedback" model we have been discussing. Conversely, anything that decreases chronic low-level inflammation may have benefits in a number of areas. As a possible example, aspirin has been suggested as useful in Alzheimer's disease [66] and cancer [67], in addition to heart disease (both in diabetic [68] and nondiabetic [69] patients); in fact, aspirin may ultimately prove to be beneficial for the prevention or delay of insulin resistance and type 2 diabetes itself [70].

Second, the interruption of these chronic disease processes may be difficult since a large fraction of the pathophysiology is coincident with our natural homeostatic physiology. As an example, a blood clot is the proximal event in many acute coronary syndromes. Our evolved response to a ruptured atherosclerotic plaque in a coronary artery is the same as our response to a ruptured blood vessel due to a traumatic wound; we did not evolve a different response. The capability of modifying the system to provide for two separate responses is currently out of our reach, and would require manipulation of our normal physiological responses, a delicate operation indeed.

MEDICATIONS AND INFLAMMATION

Having said that it will be difficult to interrupt the normal physiology that is coincident with the pathophysiology of these chronic diseases, we do have evidence that some existing medications can play an important role. One of the first reports of the use of CRP as an inflammation marker was in the Physicians' Health Study (PHS) [71]. In this study, higher CRP values at baseline were strongly and independently associated with increased risk of incident myocardial infarction in otherwise healthy, middle-aged men. PHS was also a placebo-controlled, randomized, double-blind clinical trial of aspirin for the prevention of myocardial infarction. The investigators noted that the majority of the benefit of aspirin was in those with higher CRP values, suggesting that even the low dose of aspirin used in this study may have had an anti-inflammatory effect. Since that time, Ridker and colleagues have demonstrated in several studies a similar effect of statins, i.e., statins appear to be at least partially anti-inflammatory. For example, the AFCAPS/TexCAPS study demonstrated that statin therapy was useful not only in those with higher cholesterol levels, but also in those with lower levels; secondary analyses suggested that this benefit in those with lower lipid levels was restricted to those who also had higher CRP values [72].

These studies, and others, raise the possibility that a number of very effective drugs in the area of vascular disease may have anti-inflammatory effects in addition to effects based on their primary targets. These drugs may also have effects across a number of the chronic diseases we have been discussing. Possible multiple applications of aspirin are noted above, and statins are being explored in diabetes [73], dementia [74], cancer [75], and osteoporosis [76].

THE ROLE OF GENETICS

A comprehensive review of the known and possible roles of genetics in atherosclerotic disease in particular and inflammation in general is beyond the scope of this chapter. It is also doomed to obsolescence before this book can come to print, given the speed with which genetic information is being generated. There are many genes involved in inflammation and atherosclerosis, and many variances in these genes [77]. It remains unclear whether any of these variances are important in the processes we discussed, but it seems the likelihood is high that at least some are.

There is a variety of ways investigators are studying genes for contribution to these diseases. The first dichotomy involves family studies vs. population-based studies of unrelated individuals. While family studies are powerful from the standpoint of interpretation, they are limited in the observable variation. Population studies are by their very nature rich in variation, but this limits their power for detecting associations. Initial studies using variances (usually single nucleotide polymorphisms or SNPs) in "candidate genes" have revealed some associations of genotypes with vascular and/or inflammatory outcomes, but these associations have generally been relatively modest in strength, especially in population-based studies, and often irreproducible in multiple studies. Many investigators believe at this point that continued work in the candidate gene mode will not reveal important population-based genetic contributions, and other methods are needed. An emerging variation of this approach is to study not single candidate genes, but a modest number of genes, whose products are known to act in a pathway.

A second approach has emerged that uses "SNP maps" or "genome scans" [78]. In this method, the entire genome (or large sections) is genotyped at various positions for SNPs, and these data are used in association studies of endpoints such as myocardial infarction. The SNPs need not have any functional significance, but rather represent regions of the chromosome through the inheritance process summarized in the term *linkage disequilibrium*. The greater the number of SNPs, the smaller the region that is represented. SNP maps have been used in a number of populations, and some consistent findings are emerging [79, 80]. However, to date, the density of the mapping (i.e., the number of SNPs per unit length of DNA) has not been high enough to provide much resolution, and the statistical validity of some of the analytical approaches has been questioned [81]. A variant of this approach is to focus on "functional SNPs," that is SNPs in genes; this can be even further restricted by limiting the SNPs to those in the known coding or regulatory sections of genes.

While the Human Genome Project has given us a beginning, most of the variation among different people is currently unknown. A number of epidemiological projects are underway that will help provide this information. However, even if we were to know all the variation, we are uncertain how to organize it. For example, if we were to produce SNP maps of much greater density than those used today (e.g., 10–20 000 SNP/genome compared to several hundred), it is not clear how to use these data in the most meaningful way. A number of investigators have suggested that reducing the variance by focusing on haplotypes may provide the method, although the estimated number of haplotypes is still a very large number, and a comprehensive "haplotype map" is still several years away [82].

Whatever the molecular genetic method, much of the variation in the human genome will need to be interpreted in the context of interaction. For example, a given variance in a gene related to cardiac function might not be important in younger people, but may become important in older people, when the heart no longer functions optimally. This would constitute Gene × Age interaction. This is the emerging picture with the so-called channelopathies or disorders in ion channels, which are in part based on structural differences due to genetic variance. These variances are "transparent" to proper function in the young, healthy heart, but may be critical in the older, failing heart [83, 84]. Even brief consideration of this point reveals many possible environments that may be important to consider. For example, there are several known variances in coagulation factor genes related to venous thrombosis, including FV_{Leiden} (in the factor V gene) and 20210A (in the prothrombin gene); the susceptibility to venous thrombosis increases dramatically when other risk factors are present [85]. In addition to the environment, other genes may play a role in the expression of a particular genotypic variance, the so-called Gene × Gene interactions. Having knowledge about both types of interactions will be critical if we are to fully understand the role of common genetic variances in chronic diseases such as CVD and diabetes.

CONCLUSIONS

There appear to be two major pathways by which atherosclerosis progresses: excess lipids in blood, which end up in the subendothelium and as part of atherosclerotic plaque, and inflammatory forces, including innate immune response and T lymphocyte mediated cytokine production in the vascular wall. Much recent research has demonstrated the association of chronic low-level inflammation (microinflammation) with both diabetes and CVD. It appears that microinflammation is not only a result of these diseases but also exhibits "positive feedback," causing the disease process to accelerate. This downward spiral has a slope that is modified by genetic architecture and environmental variables, and may prove difficult to interrupt or modify effectively, since the pathways involved represent not only pathophysiology but also normal homeostatic physiology. Having said that, we currently have some medications that do seem to work to modify this process, such as aspirin and statins. The role of the environment is important, and this research emphasizes the need for more effective public health efforts in education and behavior modification, as well as economic and political approaches to arrest the burgeoning global epidemic of obesity.

We already know that if the lipid burden is decreased, atherosclerosis will decrease. If we can understand the microinflammatory pathways in enough detail, and learn how to modify these activities, we may be able to decrease atherosclerosis through this mechanism as well. By attacking both major arms we may finally be able to limit this chronic progressive disease, and possibly the other chronic diseases of old age as well.

REFERENCES

1. Grundy SM. Approach to lipoprotein management in 2001 National Cholesterol Guidelines. *Am J Cardiol* 2002; 90: 11i–21i.
2. Manson J, Spelsberg A. Risk modification in the diabetic patient. In Manson JE, Ridker P, Gaziano J, Hennekens C (eds) *Prevention of Myocardial Infarction.* New York: Oxford University Press, 1996; pp 241–73.
3. Stern MP. Diabetes and cardiovascular disease. The "common soil" hypothesis. *Diabetes* 1995; 44: 369–74.
4. Libby P. Current concepts of the pathogenesis of the acute coronary syndromes. *Circulation* 2001; 104: 365–72.
5. Ross R. Atherosclerosis—an inflammatory disease. *N Engl J Med* 1999; 340: 115–26.
6. DeWood M, Spores J, Notske R, Mouser L, Burroughs R, Goldens M, Lang H. Prevalence of total coronary occlusion during the early hours of transmural myocardial infarction. *N Engl J Med* 1980; 303: 897–902.
7. Meade T, Chakrabarti R, Haines A, North W, Stirling Y, Thompson S. Haemostatic function and cardiovascular death: early results of a prospective study. *Lancet* 1980; i: 1050–4.
8. Festa A, D'Agostino R, Jr., Howard G, Mykkänen L, Tracy RP, Haffner SM. Chronic subclinical inflammation as part of the insulin resistance syndrome: the Insulin Resistance Atherosclerosis Study (IRAS). *Circulation* 2000; 102: 42–7.
9. Festa A, D'Agostino R Jr, Mykkanen L, Tracy RP, Hales CN, Howard BV, Haffner SM. LDL particle size in relation to insulin, proinsulin, and insulin sensitivity: the Insulin Resistance Atherosclerosis Study [In Process Citation]. *Diabetes Care* 1999; 22: 1688–93.
10. Juhan-Vague I, Alessi MC, Vague P. Thrombogenic and fibrinolytic factors and cardiovascular risk in non-insulin-dependent diabetes mellitus. *Ann Med* 1996; 28: 371–80.
11. Wilhelmsen L, Svardsudd K, Korsan-Bengtsen K, Larsson B, Welin L, Tibblin G. Fibrinogen as a risk factor for stroke and myocardial infarction. *N Engl J Med* 1984; 311: 501–5.
12. Stone M, Thorp J. Plasma fibrinogen—a major coronary risk factor. *J R Coll Gen Pract* 1985; 35: 565–9.
13. Kannel W, Wolf P, Castelli W, D'Agostino R. Fibrinogen and risk of cardiovascular disease: the Framingham study. *JAMA* 1987; 258: 1183–6.
14. Folsom AR, Wu KK, Rosamond WD, Sharrett AR, Chambless LE. Prospective study of hemostatic factors and incidence of coronary heart disease: the Atherosclerosis Risk in Communities (ARIC) Study. *Circulation* 1997; 96: 1102–8.
15. Tracy R, Bovill E. Hemostasis and risk of ischemic disease: epidemiologic evidence with emphasis on the elderly. In Califf R, Mark D, Wagner G (eds) *Acute Coronary Care in the Thrombolytic Era*, 2nd edn. St. Louis, MO: Mosby-Year Book, Inc, 1995; pp 27–43.
16. Ritchie DG, Levy BA, Adams MA, Fuller GM. Regulation of fibrinogen synthesis by plasmin-derived fragments of fibrinogen and fibrin: an indirect feedback pathway. *Proc Natl Acad Sci USA* 1982; 79: 1530–4.
17. Tracy RP. Is visceral adiposity the "enemy within"? *Arterioscler Thromb Vasc Biol* 2001; 21: 881–3.
18. Meade T, Brozovic M, Chakrabarti R, Haines A, Imeson J, Mellows S, Miller G, North W, Stirling Y, Thompson S. Haemostatic function and ischaemic heart disease: principal results of the Northwick Park Heart Study. *Lancet* 1986; ii: 533–7.
19. Hamsten A, Wiman B, de Faire U, Blomback M. Increased plasma levels of a rapid inhibitor of tissue plasminogen activator in young survivors of myocardial infarction. *N Engl J Med* 1985; 313: 1557–63.
20. Hamsten A, de Faire U, Walldius G, Dahlen G, Szamosi A, Landou C, Blomback M, Wiman B. Plasminogen activator inhibitor in plasma: risk factor for recurrent myocardial infarction. *Lancet* 1987; ii: 3–9.
21. Iacoviello L, Burzotta F, Di Castelnuovo A, Zito F, Marchioli R, Donati MB. The 4G/5G polymorphism of PAI-1 promoter gene and the risk of myocardial infarction: a meta-analysis [letter]. *Thromb Haemost* 1998; 80: 1029–30.
22. Juhan-Vague I, Alessi M, Morange P. PAI-1, obesity, and insulin resistance. In Reaven G, Laws A (eds) *Insulin Resistance: The Metabolic Syndrome X.* Totowa: Humana Press, 1999; pp 317–32.
23. Alessi M, Juhan-Vague I, Kooistra T, Declerck P, Collen D. Insulin stimulates the synthesis of plasminogen activator inhibitor 1 by the human hepatocellular cell line HepG2. *Thromb Haemost* 1988; 60: 491–4.
24. Schneider DJ, Absher PM, Ricci MA. Dependence of augmentation of arterial endothelial cell expression of plasminogen activator inhibitor type 1 by insulin on soluble factors released from vascular smooth muscle cells. *Circulation* 1997; 96: 2868–76.
25. Kluft C, Verheijen J, Jie A, Rijken D, Preston F, Sue-Ling H, Jespersen J, Aasen A. The post-operative fibrinolytic shutdown: a rapidly reverting acute phase pattern for the fast acting inhibitor of tissue-type plasminogen activator after trauma. *Scand J Clin Lab Invest* 1985; 45: 605–10.

26. Loskutoff DJ, Samad F. The adipocyte and hemostatic balance in obesity: studies of PAI-1. *Arterioscler Thromb Vasc Biol* 1998; 18: 1–6.
27. Sakkinen PA, Wahl P, Cushman M, Lewis MR, Tracy RP. Clustering of procoagulation, inflammation, and fibrinolysis variables with metabolic factors in insulin resistance syndrome. *Am J Epidemiol* 2000; 152: 897–907.
28. Meade T, Ruddock V, Stirling Y, Chakrabarti R, Miller G. Fibrinolytic activity, clotting factors, and long-term incidence of ischaemic heart disease in the Northwick Park Heart Study. *Lancet* 1993; 342: 1076–9.
29. Kuller L, Tracy R, Shaten J, Meilahn E, for the MRFIT Research Group. Relationship of C-reactive protein and coronary heart disease in the MRFIT nested case-control study. *Am J Epidemiol* 1996; 144: 537–47.
30. Reunanen A, Knekt P, Aaran RK. Serum ceruloplasmin level and the risk of myocardial infarction and stroke. *Am J Epidemiol* 1992; 136: 1082–90.
31. Phillips A, Shaper A, Whincup P. Association between serum albumin and mortality from cardiovascular disease, cancer, and other causes. *Lancet* 1989; i: 1434–6.
32. Harris TB, Ferrucci L, Tracy RP, Corti MC, Wacholder S, Ettinger WH Jr, Heimovitz H, Cohen HJ, Wallace R. Associations of elevated interleukin-6 and C-reactive protein levels with mortality in the elderly. *Am J Med.* 1999; 106: 506–12.
33. Liuzzo G, Biasucci L, Gallimore J, Grillo R, Rebuzzi A, Pepys M, Maseri A. The prognostic value of C-reactive protein and serum amyloid A protein in severe unstable angina. *N Engl J Med* 1994; 331: 417–24.
34. Esmon C, Taylor F, Snow T. Inflammation and coagulation: linked processes potentially regulated through a common pathway mediated by protein C. *Thromb Haemost* 1991; 66: 160–5.
35. Lagrand WK, Visser CA, Hermens WT, Niessen HW, Verheugt FW, Wolbink GJ, Hack CE. C-reactive protein as a cardiovascular risk factor: more than an epiphenomenon? *Circulation* 1999; 100: 96–102.
36. Ross R. Inflammation, growth regulatory molecules and atherosclerosis. *J Cell Biochem* 1992; 16A (suppl): 1–30.
37. Berliner J, Navab M, Fogelman A, Frank J, Demer L, Edwards P, Watson A, Lusis A. Atherosclerosis: basic mechanisms. Oxidation, inflammation, and genetics. *Circulation* 1995; 91: 2488–96.
38. Hansson GK. Immune mechanisms in atherosclerosis. *Arterioscler Thromb Vasc Biol* 2001; 21: 1876–90.
39. Fishman D, Faulds G, Jeffery R, Mohamed-Ali V, Yudkin JS, Humphries S, Woo P. The effect of novel polymorphisms in the interleukin-6 (IL-6) gene on IL-6 transcription and plasma IL-6 levels, and an association with systemic-onset juvenile chronic arthritis. *J Clin Invest* 1998; 102: 1369–76.
40. Jenny NS, Tracy RP, Ogg MS, Luong le A, Kuller LH, Arnold AM, Sharrett AR, Humphries SE. In the elderly, interleukin-6 plasma levels and the $-174G \rightarrow C$ polymorphism are associated with the development of cardiovascular disease. *Arterioscler Thromb Vasc Biol* 2002; 22: 2066–71.
41. Mendall MA, Patel P, Ballam L, Strachan D, Northfield TC. C reactive protein and its relation to cardiovascular risk factors: a population based cross sectional study. *BMJ* 1996; 312: 1061–5.
42. Tracy R, Macy E, Bovill E, Cushman M, Psaty B, Cornell E, Kuller L. Lifetime smoking exposure affects the association of C-reactive protein with cardiovascular disease risk factors and subclinical disease in healthy elderly subjects. *Arterioscler Thromb Vasc Biol* 1997; 17: 2167–76.
43. Koenig W, Sund M, Frohlich M, Fischer HG, Lowel H, Doring A, Hutchinson WL, Pepys MB. C-Reactive protein, a sensitive marker of inflammation, predicts future risk of coronary heart disease in initially healthy middle-aged men: results from the MONICA (Monitoring Trends and Determinants in Cardiovascular Disease) Augsburg Cohort Study, 1984 to 1992. *Circulation* 1999; 99: 237–42.
44. Tracy RP, Arnold AM, Ettinger W, Fried L, Meilahn E, Savage P. The relationship of fibrinogen and factors VII and VIII to incident cardiovascular disease and death in the elderly: results from the Cardiovascular Health Study. *Arterioscler Thromb Vasc Biol* 1999; 19: 1776–83.
45. Ridker PM, Stampfer MJ, Rifai N. Novel risk factors for systemic atherosclerosis: a comparison of C-reactive protein, fibrinogen, homocysteine, lipoprotein(a), and standard cholesterol screening as predictors of peripheral arterial disease. *JAMA* 2001; 285: 2481–5.
46. Danesh J, Collins R, Appleby P, Peto R. Association of fibrinogen, C-reactive protein, albumin, or leukocyte count with coronary heart disease: meta-analyses of prospective studies. *JAMA* 1998; 279: 1477–82.
47. Yudkin JS, Kumari M, Humphries SE, Mohamed-Ali V. Inflammation, obesity, stress and coronary heart disease: is interleukin-6 the link? *Atherosclerosis* 2000; 148: 209–14.
48. Sakkinen PA, Cushman M, Psaty BM, Rodriguez B, Boineau R, Kuller LH, Tracy RP. Relationship of plasmin generation to cardiovascular disease risk factors in elderly men and women. *Arterioscler Thromb Vasc Biol* 1999; 19: 499–504.
49. Yudkin JS, Stehouwer CD, Emeis JJ, Coppack SW. C-reactive protein in healthy subjects: associations with obesity, insulin resistance, and endothelial dysfunction: a potential role for cytokines originating from adipose tissue? *Arterioscler Thromb Vasc Biol* 1999; 19: 972–8.
50. Rincon M, Anguita J, Nakamura T, Fikrig E, Flavell RA. Interleukin (IL)-6 directs the differentiation of IL-4 producing $CD4^+$ T cells. *J Exp Med* 1997; 185: 461–9.
51. Aronson D, Mittleman MA, Burger AJ. Interleukin-6 levels are inversely correlated with heart rate variability in patients with decompensated heart failure. *J Cardiovasc Electrophysiol* 2001; 12: 294–300.
52. Huber SA, Sakkinen P, Conze D, Hardin N, Tracy R. Interleukin-6 exacerbates early atherosclerosis in mice. *Arterioscler Thromb Vasc Biol* 1999; 19: 2364–7.
53. Lemieux I, Pascot A, Prud'homme D, Almeras N, Bogaty P, Nadeau A, Bergeron J, Desprès JP. Elevated C-reactive protein: another component of the atherothrombotic profile of abdominal obesity. *Arterioscler Thromb Vasc Biol* 2001; 21: 961–7.
54. Montague CT, O'Rahilly S. The perils of portliness: causes and consequences of visceral adiposity. *Diabetes* 2000; 49: 883–8.
55. Aggawal B, Puri R (eds). *Human Cytokines: Their Role in Disease and Therapy* Cambridge, MA: Blackwell Science, 1995.
56. Qi C, Pekala PH. Tumor necrosis factor-alpha-induced insulin resistance in adipocytes. *Proc Soc Exp Biol Med* 2000; 223: 128–35.
57. Hotamisligil GS. The role of TNFalpha and TNF receptors in obesity and insulin resistance. *J Intern Med* 1999; 245: 621–5.

58. Nilsson J, Jovinge S, Niemann A, Reneland R, Lithell H. Relation between plasma tumor necrosis factor-alpha and insulin sensitivity in elderly men with non-insulin-dependent diabetes mellitus. *Arterioscler Thromb Vasc Biol* 1998; 18: 1199–202.
59. Fuller J, Keen H, Jarrett R, Omer T, Meade T, Chakrabarti R, North W, Stirling Y. Haemostatic variables associated with diabetes and its complications. *BMJ* 1979; 2: 964–6.
60. Yudkin JS. Abnormalities of coagulation and fibrinolysis in insulin resistance. Evidence for a common antecedent? *Diabetes Care.* 1999; 22 (suppl 3): C25–30.
61. Ely EW, Bernard GR, Vincent JL. Activated protein C for severe sepsis. *N Engl J Med* 2002; 347: 1035–6.
62. Tracy RP. Inflammation in cardiovascular disease: cart, horse or both—revisited. *Arterioscler Thromb Vasc Biol* 2002; 22: 1514–5.
63. Neel JV, Weder AB, Julius S. Type II diabetes, essential hypertension, and obesity as "syndromes of impaired genetic homeostasis": the "thrifty genotype" hypothesis enters the 21st century. *Perspect Biol Med* 1998; 42: 44–74.
64. Hales CN, Barker DJ. The thrifty phenotype hypothesis. *Br Med Bull* 2001; 60: 5–20.
65. Fernández-Real JM, Ricart W. Insulin resistance and inflammation in an evolutionary perspective: the contribution of cytokine genotype/phenotype to thriftiness. *Diabetologia* 1999; 42: 1367–74.
66. Broe GA, Grayson DA, Creasey HM, Waite LM, Casey BJ, Bennett HP, Brooks WS, Halliday GM. Anti-inflammatory drugs protect against Alzheimer disease at low doses. *Arch Neurol* 2000; 57: 1586–91.
67. Bosetti C, Gallus S, La Vecchia C. Aspirin and cancer risk: an update to 2001. *Eur J Cancer Prev* 2002; 11: 535–42.
68. Krein SL, Vijan S, Pogach LM, Hogan MM, Kerr EA. Aspirin use and counseling about aspirin among patients with diabetes. *Diabetes Care* 2002; 25: 965–70.
69. Hayden M, Pignone M, Phillips C, Mulrow C. Aspirin for the primary prevention of cardiovascular events: a summary of the evidence for the U.S. Preventive Services Task Force. *Ann Intern Med* 2002; 136: 161–72.
70. Hundal RS, Petersen KF, Mayerson AB, Randhawa PS, Inzucchi S, Shoelson SE, Shulman GI. Mechanism by which high-dose aspirin improves glucose metabolism in type 2 diabetes. *J Clin Invest* 2002; 109: 1321–6.
71. Ridker P, Cushman M, Stampfer M, Tracy R, Hennekens C. Inflammation, aspirin, and the risk of cardiovascular disease in apparently healthy men. *N Engl J Med* 1997; 336: 973–9.
72. Ridker PM, Rifai N, Clearfield M, Downs Jr, Weis SE, Miles JS, Gotto AM Jr. Measurement of C-reactive protein for the targeting of statin therapy in the primary prevention of acute coronary events. *N Engl J Med* 2001; 344: 1959–65.
73. Paniagua JA, Lopez-Miranda J, Escribano A, Berral FJ, Marin C, Bravo D, Paz-Rojas E, Gomez P, Barcos M, Moreno JA, Perez-Jimenez F. Cerivastatin improves insulin sensitivity and insulin secretion in early-state obese type 2 diabetes. *Diabetes* 2002; 51: 2596–603.
74. Bollen EL, Gaw A, Buckley BM. Statin therapy and the prevention of dementia. *Arch Neurol* 2001; 58: 1023–4.
75. Wong WW, Dimitroulakos J, Minden MD, Penn LZ. HMG-CoA reductase inhibitors and the malignant cell: the statin family of drugs as triggers of tumor-specific apoptosis. *Leukemia* 2002; 16: 508–19.
76. Pasco JA, Kotowicz MA, Henry MJ, Sanders KM, Nicholson GC. Statin use, bone mineral density, and fracture risk: Geelong Osteoporosis Study. *Arch Intern Med* 2002; 162: 537–40.
77. Tang Z, Tracy RP. Candidate genes and confirmed genetic polymorphisms associated with cardiovascular diseases: a tabular assessment. *J Thromb Thrombolysis* 2001; 11: 49–81.
78. Altshuler D, Pollara VJ, Cowles CR, Van Etten WJ, Baldwin J, Linton L, Lander ES. An SNP map of the human genome generated by reduced representation shotgun sequencing. *Nature* 2000; 407: 513–6.
79. Mahtani MM, Widen E, Lehto M, Thomas J, McCarthy M, Brayer J, Bryant B, Chan G, Daly M, Forsblom C, Kanninen T, Kirby A, Kruglyak L, Munnelly K, Parkkonen M, Reeve-Daly MP, Weaver A, Brettin T, Duyk G, Lander ES, Groop LC. Mapping of a gene for type 2 diabetes associated with an insulin secretion defect by a genome scan in Finnish families. *Nat Genet* 1996; 14: 90–4.
80. Meigs JB, Panhuysen CI, Myers RH, Wilson PW, Cupples LA. A genome-wide scan for loci linked to plasma levels of glucose and HbA(1c) in a community-based sample of Caucasian pedigrees: the Framingham Offspring Study. *Diabetes* 2002; 51: 833–40.
81. Lander ES, Schork NJ. Genetic dissection of complex traits. *Science* 1994; 265: 2037–48. [published erratum appears in *Science* October 21, 1994; 266 (5184): 353].
82. Gabriel SB, Schaffner SF, Nguyen H, Moore JM, Roy J, Blumenstiel B, Higgins J, DeFelice M, Lochner A, Faggart M, Liu-Cordero SN, Rotimi C, Adeyemo A, Cooper R, Ward R, Lander ES, Daly MJ, Altshuler D. The structure of haplotype blocks in the human genome. *Science* 2002; 296: 2225–9.
83. Priori S, Barhanin J, Hauer R, Haverkamp W, Jongsma H, Kleber A, McKenna W, Roden D, Rudy Y, Schwartz K, Schwartz P, Towbin J, Wilde A. Genetic and molecular basis of cardiac arrythmias: impact on clinical management, parts I and II. *Circulation* 1999; 99: 518–28.
84. Priori S, Barhanin J, Hauer R, Haverkamp W, Jongsma H, Kleber A, McKenna W, Roden D, Rudy Y, Schwartz K, Schwartz P, Towbin J, Wilde A. Genetic and molecular basis of cardiac arrhythmias: impact on clinical management, part III. *Circulation* 1999; 99: 674–81.
85. Bertina RM, Rosendaal FR. Venous thrombosis—the interaction of genes and environment. *N Engl J Med* 1998; 338: 1840–1.

82

Clinical Features and Treatment of Coronary Heart Disease in Diabetes

Rosaire P. Gray* **and John S. Yudkin†**

**Whittington Hospital, London, UK, and †Royal Free and University College Medical School, London, UK*

Coronary heart disease (CHD) is the leading cause of mortality and is responsible for significant morbidity in diabetic subjects. Approximately 50% of deaths in diabetic subjects are due to CHD [1]. Many large randomized trials have evaluated primary and secondary prevention therapies; however, until recently, most trials have not randomized large numbers of diabetic subjects and therefore much of the evidence is based on subgroup analysis and extrapolation from nondiabetic populations. In addition, there is evidence that diabetic subjects have not shared the fall in cardiovascular mortality seen in the general population [2–4].

MORTALITY FROM CHD IN DIABETES

Most deaths in non-insulin-dependent diabetic patients are due to cardiovascular disease, and in particular CHD. Overall, the age-adjusted, cause-specific mortality from cardiovascular disease is 2–5 times higher in diabetic subjects than in comparable nondiabetic controls [5–11] and 12 times higher in men with both diabetes and CHD [11]. The relative risk of death from cardiovascular disease is higher in women, although their absolute risk is lower [12, 13]. The prevalence of diabetes is high in South East Asians and Afro-Caribbeans compared to the general population [14]. While both have an increased cardiovascular mortality, this is predominantly due to CHD in South East Asians and cerebrovascular disease in Afro-Caribbeans [15]. These ethnic differences are reflected in the risk factor profiles of the two groups, with insulin resistance in South East Asians and a favorable atherogenic profile coupled with a high prevalence of hypertension in Afro-Carribbeans. Cardiovascular mortality is also increased in insulin-dependent diabetic subjects compared to nondiabetic subjects [16–19], and approximately 35% of subjects with insulin-dependent diabetes mellitus (IDDM) die from cardiovascular causes. Subjects with impaired glucose tolerance also have an increased risk of cardiovascular disease [20–22]. As shown in Figure 1 diabetic subjects with angiographically proven coronary artery disease show consistently poorer survival compared with nondiabetic subjects. A recent study in Finland found that patients with non-insulin-dependent diabetes mellitus (NIDDM) without established cardiovascular disease have as high a risk of cardiovascular events and death as nondiabetic patients who have had a myocardial infarction (MI) [24] and the risk remained after adjustment for age, sex, and cardiovascular risk factors.

PATHOLOGY OF CHD IN DIABETES

The atherosclerotic lesion in diabetes mellitus is histologically similar to that in nondiabetic populations but appears to be more extensive and severe. In general, autopsy studies indicate that diabetic subjects have more extensive coronary artery lesions than nondiabetic subjects [25]. The results of angiographic studies are conflicting, with some studies showing an increased prevalence of either left main stem disease or three-vessel disease [26–29], while others have failed to show any association between the presence of diabetes and the severity of coronary artery disease [30]. However, most of these studies are retrospective and take no account of referral patterns. There is also evidence that coronary artery disease progresses more rapidly in

International Textbook of Diabetes Mellitus, Third Edition. Edited by R. A. DeFronzo, E. Ferrannini, H. Keen, and P. Zimmet.
 ISBN: 0-471-48655-8.

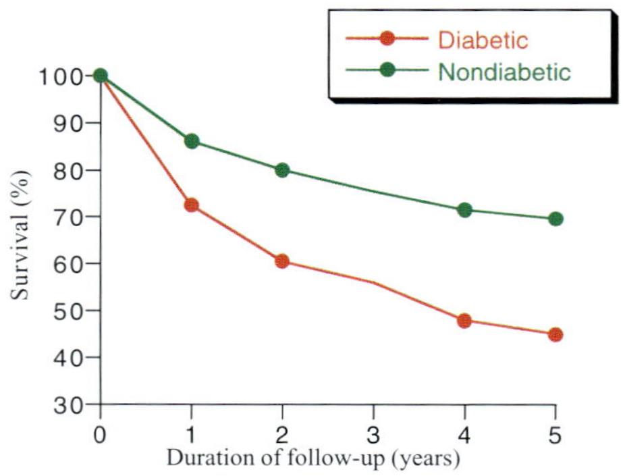

Figure 1 Survival rates for diabetic and nondiabetic subjects aged 65 years or more, with angiographically proven coronary artery disease [23]. (Reprinted from American Journal of Cardiology 81, 7–11, © 1998 with premission from Excerpta Medica Inc)

diabetic subjects [31]. Figure 2 shows typical angiographic features of coronary disease in a young woman with diabetes.

RISK FACTORS FOR CHD IN DIABETES

Data from population studies indicate that the major risk factors for cardiovascular disease, smoking, hypertension, and hyperlipidemia apply in diabetic as well as in nondiabetic subjects [32, 33]. The risk of CHD that they confer is enhanced by the presence of diabetes as shown by the additive effects on mortality of diabetes combined with hypertension or hypercholesterolemia (Figure 3). Table 1 shows 16-year CHD mortality in the Multiple Risk Factor Intervention Trial (MRFIT) in Black and White diabetic men by levels of baseline cardiovascular risk factors. Table 2 shows data from the United Kingdom Prospective Diabetes Study (UKPDS), confirming that increased low-density lipoprotein (LDL) cholesterol concentration, reduced high-density lipoprotein (HDL) cholesterol concentration, hyperglycemia, blood pressure, and smoking are all important risk factors for CHD in diabetes.

The lipid abnormalities of patients with type 2 diabetes include increased triglycerides, low HDL cholesterol, and a predominance of small dense LDL particles that are more atherogenic than LDL particles in nondiabetic subjects [34, 35]. Total cholesterol concentrations are generally similar to those in nondiabetic subjects. The composition of HDL particles is also different from nondiabetic subjects with lower concentrations of the larger, more antiatherogenic particles [36].

There is clustering of cardiovascular risk factors in diabetic subjects; however, the adjusted excess risk is still higher in diabetic subjects, suggesting that diabetes is an independent risk factor for cardiovascular disease [37, 38]. Studies have shown that between 75 and 90% of the excess risk of CHD in diabetic subjects remains after adjusting for levels of all other known risk factors [6, 7].

Microalbuminuria is an independent risk factor for CHD in diabetic subjects and is associated with a doubling of cardiovascular risk [39]. There is evidence that reducing albumin excretion rate reduces the risk of nephropathy but to date there is insufficient evidence to determine whether cardiovascular morbidity or mortality is reduced.

The increase in CHD mortality in diabetic subjects is sometimes considered synonymous with an increased risk of atherosclerosis. Clearly, the atherosclerotic plaque is necessary for the development of CHD, but it is not sufficient, and superimposed inflammation and thrombosis on an inflamed or eroded surface are important contributors to acute coronary syndromes, including unstable angina and MI. Diabetes is recognized as a hypercoagulable state [40]. Increased platelet aggregation, reduced fibrinolytic capacity, increased concentrations of hemostatic proteins, and endothelial dysfunction have been described and may promote thrombosis at the site of plaque rupture [41]. Increased levels of fibrinogen, plasminogen activator inhibitor 1 (PAI-1), and tissue-type plasminogen activator (tPA) have been linked to the increased risk of MI in diabetic subjects [36]. Other factors that contribute to a prothrombotic state in diabetic subjects include increased von Willebrand factor antigen and decreased antithrombin III levels.

CLINICAL MANIFESTATIONS OF CHD IN DIABETES

The main clinical manifestations of CHD are similar to that in nondiabetic subjects:

(1) stable angina
(2) unstable angina
(3) myocardial infarction
(4) heart failure
(5) sudden death

Angina

Exertional angina is a common symptom of CHD in diabetic patients. The investigation of diabetic subjects with stable angina in general parallels that in nondiabetic subjects. The indications for exercise testing, thallium imaging, coronary angiography, and echocardiography are similar and the results have similar implications [42]. Conventional therapy for angina with nitrates, β-blockers, calcium-channel blockers, K^+-channel openers, and aspirin have similar indications in diabetic and nondiabetic subjects [43]. Risk factors such as smoking, elevated cholesterol, and hypertension should be treated aggressively as described for secondary prevention after MI. Table 3 shows the interventions recommended in the United Kingdom National Service Framework for Coronary Heart Disease for people with diagnosed CHD [44].

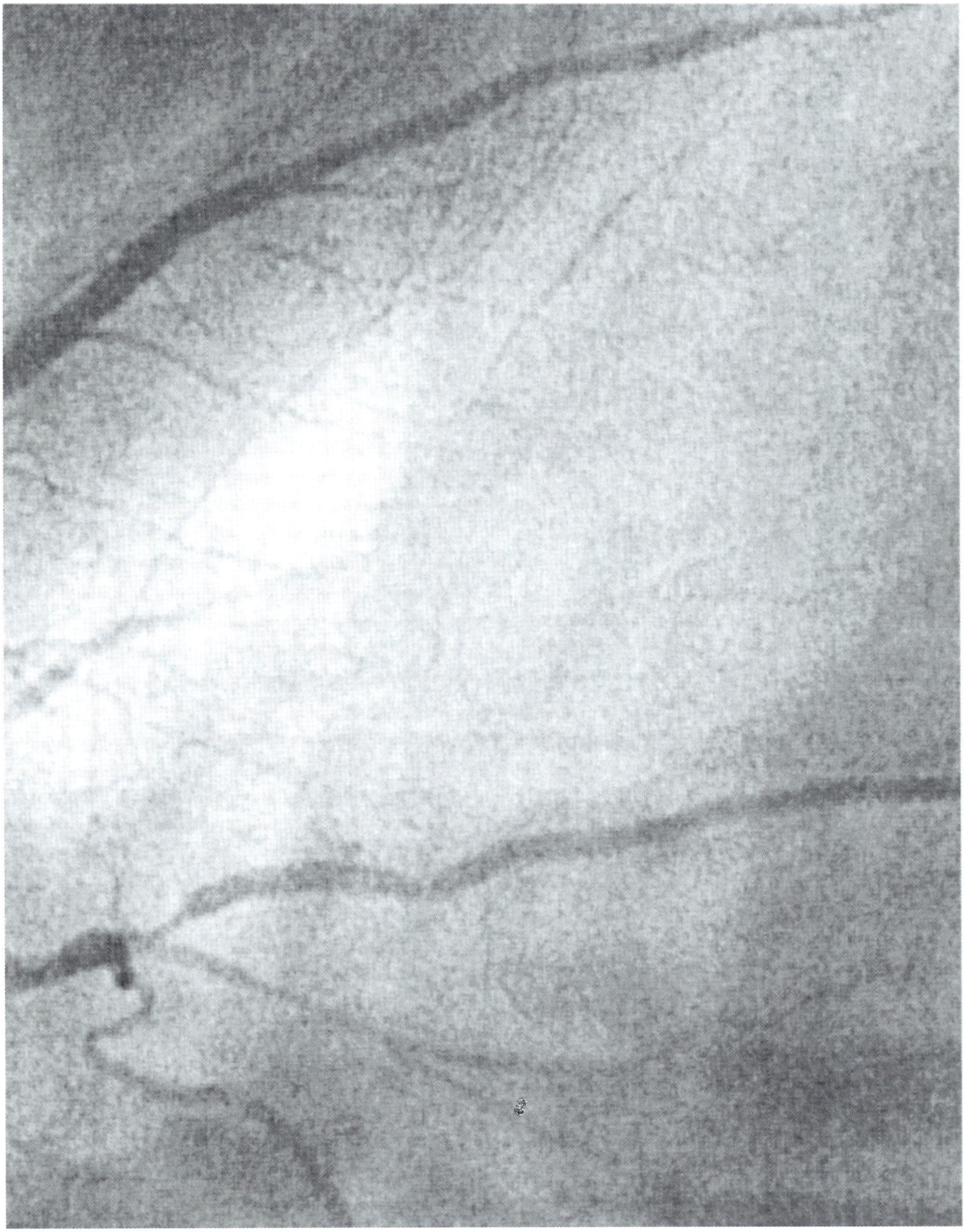

(a)

Figure 2 Coronary angiogram in a young woman with diabetes presenting with angina. (a) Right anterior oblique view of left coronary artery, showing tight proximal stenoses in proximal left anterior descending and circumflex arteries. (b) Left anterior oblique view of right coronary artery, showing patchy disease in the main vessel with significant stenosis in large right ventricular branch

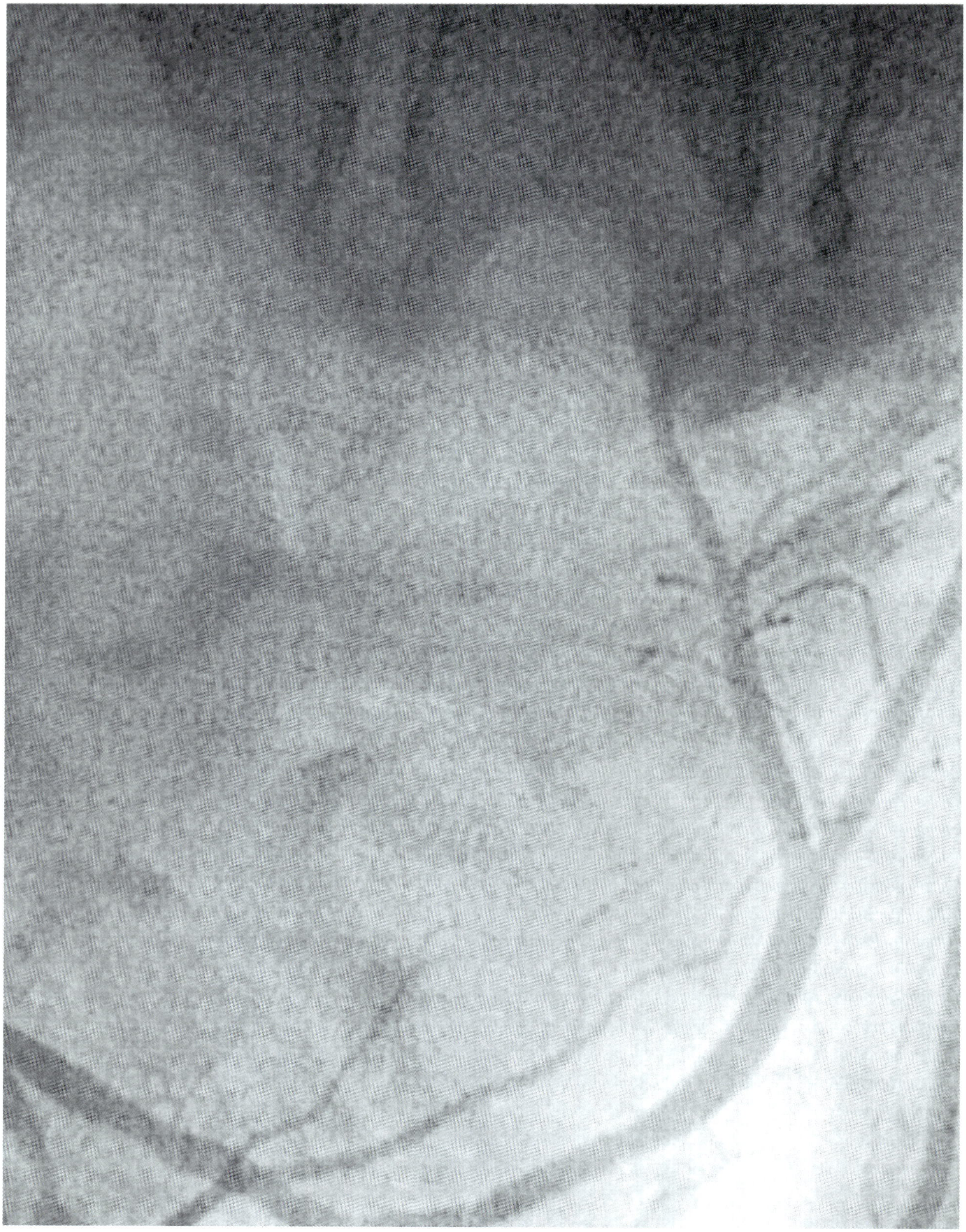

(b)

Figure 2 Continued

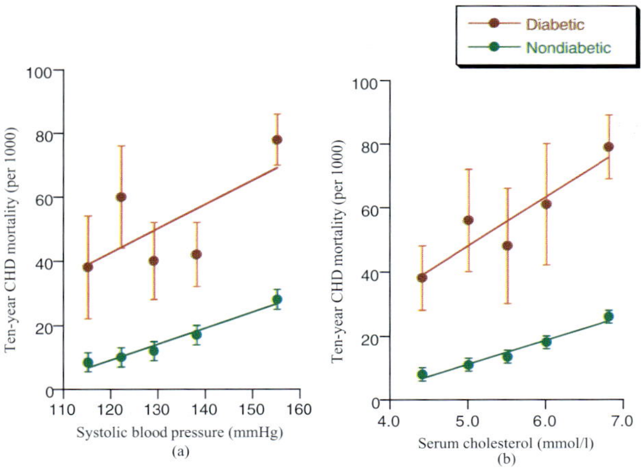

Figure 3 Effects of systolic blood pressure (a) and serum cholesterol (b) on 10-year mortality from CHD in 342 815 nondiabetic and 5163 diabetic subjects aged 35–57 years without prior MI. (data adapted from Vaccaro, the Multiple Risk Factor Intervention Trial. The 26th Annual Meeting of the European Diabetes Epidemiology Group, Lund, 1991)

More aggressive targets for modification of cardiovascular risk factors have been produced by the American Diabetes Association (ADA) for subjects with diabetes irrespective of the presence of established CHD and are summarized in Table 4 [45–49]. Coronary revascularization procedures are discussed below.

Silent Ischemia

Asymptomatic myocardial ischemia and infarction occur more frequently in diabetic patients. The reported prevalence of silent myocardial ischemia ranges from 10 to 20% in diabetic populations compared to 1 to 4% in nondiabetic populations [50–59]. One study showed no difference in the prevalence of silent ischemia between diabetic and nondiabetic subjects; however, this may reflect baseline differences between the groups [60]. The definition of silent myocardial ischemia used in these studies varies; some authors include patients without clinical symptoms but resting ECG evidence of previous infarction or ischemia, others include patients with atypical clinical symptoms and others restrict the definition to asymptomatic patients with positive functional tests or angiographically documented coronary artery disease.

Numerous explanations have been proposed for the lack of ischemic pain in patients with diabetes, including different patterns of pain sensitivity, or the presence of autonomic neuropathy leading to sensory denervation. As yet there is little convincing evidence linking these, which is hardly surprising as the mechanisms of silent ischemia are complex and controversial even in nondiabetic subjects. It has recently been suggested that silent myocardial ischemia in diabetic subjects reflects accelerated coronary atherosclerosis and that the proportion of silent disease relative to symptomatic disease is not increased in diabetes [61].

In nondiabetic subjects the presence of silent ischemia predicts adverse clinical outcome and poor survival [62–64] with a threefold increase in cardiac death [62]. There is little prognostic information in diabetic subjects, although data from the CASS registry showed that diabetic subjects with CHD and silent ischemia had a worse prognosis than nondiabetic subjects [65].

Various screening methods for silent myocardial ischemia are available, including 24–48-h Holter monitoring, exercise ECG, thallium myocardial scintigraphy with exercise testing and/or dipyridamole injection, and stress echocardiography. Evaluation of these techniques indicates that Holter monitoring is poorly sensitive, exercise ECG is fairly specific and sensitive, and thallium

Table 1 Sixteen-year CHD mortality in the MRFIT*

	White men ($n = 3997$)		Black men ($n = 610$)	
Baseline risk factor	No. of deaths	Relative Risk	No. of deaths	Relative Risk
Serum cholesterol (mmol/l)				
<6.2 (240 mg/dl)	402	1.0	45	1.0
≥6.2 (240 mg/dl)	162	1.35†	23	1.45
Systolic blood pressure (mmHg)				
<140	243	1.0	31	1.0
≥140	321	1.89†	37	1.77‡
Diastolic blood pressure (mmHg)				
<90	318	1.0	33	1.0
≥90	246	1.58†	35	1.59
Smoking status				
Nonsmoker	341	1.0	37	1.0
Smoker	223	1.49†	31	1.26

Note: RR = relative risk.
* Reproduced by permission of Oxford University Press [32].
† $p < 0.001$.
‡ $p < 0.05$.

Table 2 Cox model estimated hazard ratios (95% confidence intervals) for coronary artery disease in the UKPDS*

Dependent variable	Coronary artery disease ($n=335$)	Fatal or nonfatal MI ($n=233$)	Fatal MI ($n=103$)
LDL cholesterol (mmol/l)			
<3.02	1	1	1
≥3.02–<3.89	1.41 (1.05–1.90)	1.41 (1.00–2.00)	1.15 (0.67–1.97)
≥3.89	2.26 (1.70–3.00)	2.11 (1.50–2.95)	2.32 (1.41–3.81)
HDL cholesterol (mmol/l)			
<0.95	1	1	1
≥0.95–<1.15	0.90 (0.71–1.15)	0.94 (0.70–1.26)	1.16 (0.73–1.84)
≥1.15	0.55 (0.41–0.73)	0.65 (0.47–0.91)	0.84 (0.51–1.39)
Hemoglobin A_{1c}(%)			
<6.2	1	1	1
≥6.2–<7.5	1.47 (1.12–1.95)	1.26 (0.91–1.75)	0.98 (0.58–1.65)
≥7.5	1.52 (1.15–2.01)	1.42 (1.03–1.98)	1.72 (1.06–2.77)
Systolic blood pressure (mmHg)			
<125	1	1	1
≥125–>142	1.52 (1.12–2.06)	1.45 (1.01–2.08)	1.22 (0.66–2.24)
≥142	1.82 (1.34–2.47)	1.73 (1.22–2.54)	2.36 (1.33–4.18)
Smoking			
Never smoked	1	1	1
Ex-smoker	1.03 (0.77–1.37)	1.08 (0.75–1.54)	0.65 (0.39–1.09)
Current smoker	1.41 (10.6–1.88)	1.58 (1.11–2.25)	1.03 (0.62–1.70)

Note: n = no. of patients.
* Reproduced by permission of the British Medical Journal [33].

scintigraphy and stress echocardiography are useful but more expensive alternatives in patients who are not suitable for exercise ECG [66, 67].

Routine screening for silent ischemia in diabetic subjects is a debatable strategy. The benefits of appropriate treatment are not yet proven in diabetic subjects and there is no consensus concerning screening methods and interpretation of findings. Subjects with NIDDM between age 37 and 57 with less than two cardiovascular risk factors have an age-adjusted annual cardiovascular mortality of 0.3–0.6%, whereas in those with two or more risk factors this increases to 1.2–5.4% [38, 68]. Recent studies support screening of high-risk patients with diabetes [58, 69, 70]. However, further studies are needed to define treatment modalities for those with positive screening tests. The ongoing BARI 20 trial will examine the benefit of early revascularization in diabetic subjects with evidence of cardiac ischemia, irrespective of symptomatology. The high prevalence of silent ischemia in type 2 diabetic patients emphasizes the importance of aggressive primary and secondary prevention strategies in these patients.

CHD is the main cause of death among diabetic patients following renal transplantation. It has been advocated that the coronary angiography should be undertaken in those aged >45 years, and younger patients who smoke or have abnormal resting ECGs. Revascularization in these patients has been shown to reduce the risks of subsequent MI [71].

Unstable Angina

Unstable angina is characterized by a deteriorating pattern of myocardial ischemia, with angina at rest or on minimal exertion, which may be prolonged and is poorly responsive to nitrates. These symptoms may be associated with ECG abnormalities or elevation of sensitive biochemical markers of minimal myocardial injury, such as troponin [72], both of which indicate a worse prognosis. Non-Q wave

Table 3 Interventions recommended in the National Service Framework for Coronary Heart Disease for people with diagnosed CHD*

- Advice about how to stop smoking, including advice on the use of nicotine replacement
- Information about modifiable risk factors and personalised advice about how they can be reduced
- Advice and treatment to maintain blood pressure <140/85 mmHg
- Low-dose aspirin
- Statin therapy and dietary advice to either reduce total serum cholesterol below 5.0 mmol/l (or LDL cholesterol below 3.0 mmol/l) or by 20–25% (or LDL cholesterol by 30%), whichever results in the lowest level
- ACE inhibitors for people with left ventricular dysfunction
- β-Blockers for people who have had an MI
- Warfarin or aspirin for people over 60 years of age who have atrial fibrillation

* Reference 44.

Table 4 Goals for risk factor management in patients with diabetes (ADA recommendations)

Risk factor	Goal of therapy
Cigarette smoking	Complete cessation [45]
Blood pressure	<130/80 mmHg [46]
LDL cholesterol	<100 mg/dl [47]
Prothrombotic state	Low-dose aspirin therapy [48]
Glucose	Hemoglobin A_{1c} < 7% [46]
Physical inactivity	Exercise prescription [49]

MI presents in a similar way and is differentiated by its association with a substantial rise (greater than twofold) in cardiac enzymes. The term acute coronary syndrome (ACS) has been introduced to encompass these two groups as distinct from acute MI with ST segment elevation. In common with acute MI, ACS is initiated by rupture or erosion of an atheromatous plaque, platelet aggregation, and superimposed thrombus formation. ACS is associated with a high incidence of recurrent adverse events, and registry data show that even in treated patients the risk of death or MI is approximately 10% and repeat or refractory angina occurs in a further 20% [72, 73]. The risks are higher in diabetic subjects with a 2-year relative risk of death or MI of 1.84 and 1.44 respectively [74]. A recent meta-analysis on more than 24 000 patients with ACS taking part in 4 major trials showed that the mortality rate was 5.5% in the 5400 diabetic subjects compared to 3.3% in nondiabetic subjects [75]. Specific evaluation of treatment strategies for diabetic subjects is required. In the interim, aggressive management of these patients is indicated.

The British Cardiac Society, European Cardiac Society, and the joint American College of Cardiology/American Heart Association Task Force on Practice Guidelines [76–78] have published guidelines for management of unstable angina/ACSs in the general population and these should be followed in diabetic subjects. The aim of acute treatment is to prevent further thrombosis and ischemia using antiplatelet therapy (aspirin, clopidrogel, and glycoprotein IIb/IIIa receptor blockers), antithrombotic therapy (unfractionated or low-molecular-weight heparin), and coronary revascularization in selected patients. These three modalities of treatment have all been shown to reduce the rate of adverse cardiac events in unstable angina [79–85] but there are no specific studies in diabetic subjects. Because of ease of administration, predictable pharmokinetics, and cost, low-molecular-weight heparin is now favored over unfractionated heparin by most units. Substudy analysis of a large randomized trial in ACSs has shown that the addition of clopidrogel to aspirin over 3–12 months reduces the risk of fatal or nonfatal MI or stroke by 20% in diabetic patients [83] but there are some concerns about the increased risk of bleeding with this combination. The use of glycoprotein IIb/IIIa inhibitors has been shown to reduce mortality in ACS [85] and has been endorsed by the National Institute for Clinical Excellence (NICE) in the United Kingdom [84] and the ACC/AHA guidelines [86]. The benefit is greatest in high-risk patients undergoing percutaneous coronary intervention (PCI). Diabetic subjects have also been shown to benefit [87–89]. Risk stratification is important; clopidrogel should be added to aspirin in all patients and glycoprotein IIb/IIIa inhibitors in high-risk patients with ECG changes or raised troponin and those undergoing PCI.

Myocardial Infarction

The symptoms of MI in diabetes are usually classical, with chest pain being the dominant feature. However, painless MI is more common in diabetic than nondiabetic subjects [52] and the diabetic patient may present atypically with malaise, sweating (which may be confused with hypoglycemia), dyspnea, or syncope.

Both immediate and long-term mortality from MI are increased in diabetic subjects and this is still true in the thrombolytic era [4, 90–93] (Figure 4). This increased mortality is largely due to an increased risk of heart failure and cardiogenic shock. The increased risk is not related to increased infarct size in diabetic subjects [94–96] and persists after correction for other adverse risk factors during the acute event [97, 98]. Recent evidence from the DIGAMI study showed that mortality was predicted by age, previous heart failure, and severity of the glycometabolic state on admission but not by hypertension or previous MI [99]. Impaired infarction-induced remodeling aggravated by metabolic decompensation has been implicated in as a cause of the increased risk of heart failure after MI in diabetic subjects [100]. Patients with stress hyperglycemia in the absence of diabetes also have increased mortality and increased risk of heart failure and cardiogenic shock [101].

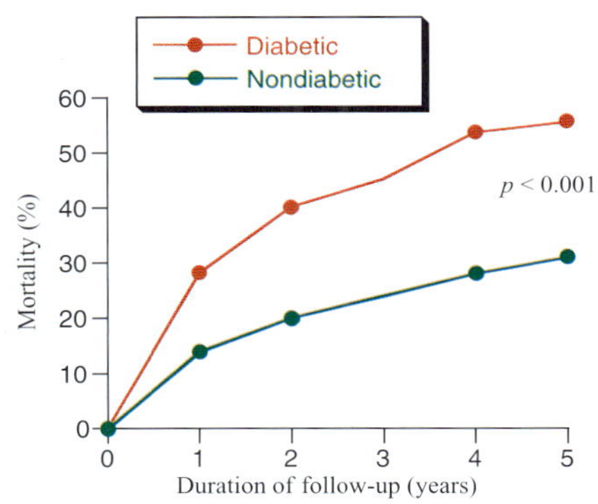

Figure 4 Five-year mortality among diabetic and nondiabetic patients during follow-up after MI [90]

Diagnosis of MI in the Diabetic Subject

The diagnostic criteria for MI are the same as in nondiabetic patients. As chest pain may be less frequent than in nondiabetic subjects, a high index of suspicion is required in diabetic subjects presenting with unexplained dyspnea, syncope, sweating, or malaise. Until recently the diagnosis of MI was based on the WHO criteria of a combination of two of three criteria of chest pain, ECG changes (ST segment elevation of 2 mm in contiguous leads, new Q waves), and a rise in cardiac enzymes [aspartate transaminase (AST)/creatine kinase (CK)/CK-MB isoenzyme] to at least twice the upper limit of the reference range. The Joint European Society of Cardiology and American College of Cardiology Committee have now revised this definition recommending the use of troponin I or T in the diagnosis of MI [102]. Troponin is highly sensitive and specific for myocardial damage, and the introduction of these new diagnostic criteria is likely to result in an increased diagnosis of MI. The impact of this remains to be determined.

Management of Acute MI in the Diabetic Subject

The principles of management of acute MI are similar to that in the nondiabetic population [103].

Thrombolytic therapy The advent of thrombolytic therapy has had a major impact in terms of reducing mortality from acute MI. Subgroup analyses of large intervention trials show that in terms of proportionate benefit the reduction in 35-day mortality with thrombolysis is similar in diabetic and nondiabetic patients [104] (Figure 5). However, given the excess in absolute 35-day mortality of diabetic patients, the absolute benefit in terms of number of lives saved per treatment is greater in diabetic patients [105], and likely to outweigh any risk of eye damage even in patients with severe retinopathy. There are only rare reports of intraocular bleeding in patients with proliferative retinopathy, which must be set against the fact that for every 1000 diabetic patients treated with thrombolytic therapy, 37 lives are saved at 35 days [106].

There is some evidence from angiographic and enzyme-release studies that the coronary artery thrombus of the diabetic patient is more resistant to thrombolytic therapy than that of nondiabetic patients [107, 108]. However, in the GUSTO study, the 90-min patency rate was similar in diabetic and nondiabetic subjects [109]. There is no evidence that complications from thrombolytic therapy such as hemorrhage are more common in diabetic subjects [109, 110]. Data from the overviews of thrombolytic therapy suggest there is little difference in benefit of different agents in the general population [104, 111] and numbers are insufficient to make such comparisons in diabetic subpopulations. Whether newer thrombolytic agents or combinations of thrombolytic agents with glycoprotein IIb/IIIa receptor blockers will be more effective remains to be seen.

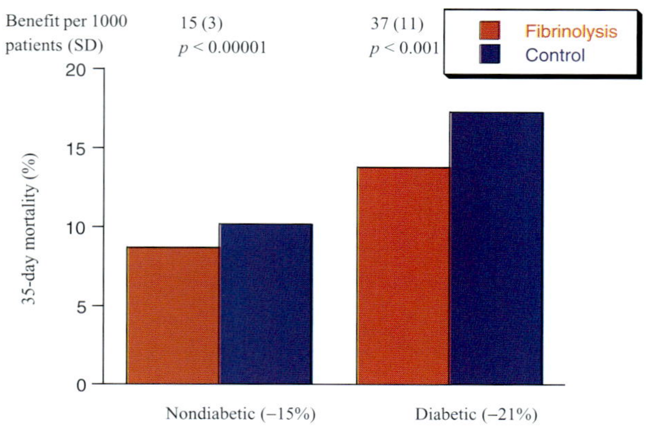

Figure 5 The benefits of thrombolytic therapy on 35-day mortality in diabetic and nondiabetic subjects [104]. (Reproduced by permission of Elsevier)

Primary coronary angioplasty Subgroup analysis has shown that primary coronary angioplasty has a similar success rate in diabetic and nondiabetic patients with acute MI and may be more effective than thrombolytic therapy [112–114]. Primary angioplasty should be considered depending on local expertise and availability and especially if thrombolytic therapy is contraindicated.

Aspirin The use of aspirin in diabetic patients has been debated. Subgroup analysis of diabetic subjects in the ISIS-2 study found a significant interaction implying that they did not benefit from aspirin [115]. However, caution must be exercised in interpreting data from multiple subgroups and other investigations of aspirin use show similar benefits in diabetic and nondiabetic subjects with reduction in nonfatal reinfarction, nonfatal stroke, and cardiovascular mortality [116]. It is estimated that 38 ± 12 vascular events per 1000 diabetic patients would be prevented if they were treated with aspirin as a secondary prevention strategy [116]. Therefore, 150–300 mg aspirin should be initiated in diabetic patients with acute MI and continued long-term.

β-Blockers The use of β-blockers has been shown to reduce reinfarction and coronary mortality in diabetic subjects [99, 117] and should be prescribed unless contraindicated. The risks of masking warning symptoms of hypoglycemia and disturbing glycemic control have been over emphasized and are largely avoided with the use of selective β-blockers.

Angiotensin-converting enzyme inhibitors Numerous studies demonstrate benefit of angiotensin-converting enzyme (ACE) inhibitors in reducing mortality, heart failure,

Table 5 Protocol for insulin-glucose infusions to achieve tight glycemic control in acute MI*

Infusion mixture	
Add 80 units soluble insulin to 500 ml 5% dextrose	
Infuse initially at 30 ml/h	
Measure blood every 1–2 h	
Titrate infusion rate	
Blood glucose (mmol/l)	*Adjustment*
>15	Give 8 units soluble insulin as IV bolus
11–14.9	Increase infusion rate by 3 ml/h
7–10.9	Maintain current rate
4–6.9	Decrease infusion rate by 6 ml/h
<4	Stop infusion until glucose >7 mmol/l Give 20 ml 30% glucose IV if symptomatic hypoglycemia Restart infusion with rate decrease by 6 ml/h

and reinfarction following MI in subjects with evidence of left ventricular dysfunction [118–120]. The benefits occur early and are greatest in those at high risk [121]. Given the high morbidity and mortality from heart failure and reinfarction in diabetic subjects with MI, it is expected that these agents will be of equal or perhaps even greater benefit in diabetic subjects. In the GISSI-III study, early institution of lisinopril was followed by a reduction in mortality in diabetic but not in nondiabetic subjects [122], and in the TRACE study, trandolapril reduced the risk of progression to severe heart failure in diabetic but not in nondiabetic subjects [123]. Other studies of ACE inhibitors in heart failure suggest the benefit is similar in diabetic patients and nondiabetic subjects [124, 125].

Glycemic control Hyperglycemia after MI is associated with a poor short- and long-term prognosis but it is unclear whether this represents cause or effect. A prospective randomized study of intensive insulin treatment on long-term survival after MI in diabetic subjects demonstrates that tight metabolic control improves the outcome. Insulin-glucose infusion for at least 24 h (Table 5) to achieve good glycemic control (blood glucose 7–10 mmol/l), followed by multidose insulin treatment for at least 3 months, was shown to improve short- and long-term survival with an absolute reduction in mortality after a mean of 3.4 years of 11% [126, 127] (Figure 6). It is not clear which element of the treatment or whether the withdrawal of other treatment such as sulfonylureas led to this improvement in survival, and a further study is in progress to clarify this. However, this should not delay implementation of insulin therapy to diabetic patients with MI.

Secondary Prevention following MI

Risk stratification As diabetic patients are at particularly high risk following MI, it is therefore important to identify those patients who may benefit from further investigations and/or treatment to improve outcome. Few prognostic studies have been carried out specifically in diabetic subjects and most guidelines are based on data from studies in the general population of patients with MI. The ideal time to undertake assessment has not been clearly established. Exercise tolerance testing is used principally to identify patients with reversible ischemia who may benefit from revascularization [128–130] and should be performed in all patients unless they are judged unable to undertake the test. Patients unable to undertake an exercise test, those with early positive tests, and those with continued angina should be referred for coronary angiography. Because of the high incidence of heart failure following MI in diabetic subjects, echocardiography should be performed in all patients even if there are no clinical signs of heart failure. Radionuclide studies have been shown to be of value in distinguishing areas of ischemia from infarction in patients who have received thrombolytic therapy

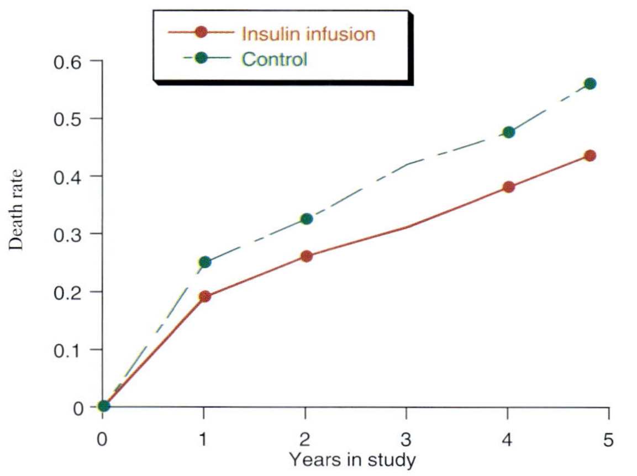

Figure 6 Long-term actuarial mortality curves after acute MI in diabetic patients treated conventionally or with insulin-glucose infusion to achieve tight glycemic control [127]. Absolute risk reduction was 11%; relative risk 0.72 (0.55–0.92), $p < 0.05$. (Reproduced by permission of the British Medical Journal)

[131] and are also useful in detecting silent ischemia in diabetic patients.

Management of risk factors A number of publications now exist to guide secondary prevention post-MI [44, 103, 132–134]. These are summarized below with particular reference to the diabetic patient.

Lifestyle modification Changes in lifestyle can have a significant effect on the secondary prevention of CHD following acute MI. Diabetic subject should be advised to stop smoking, reduce dietary intake of saturated fat and increase consumption of fruit and vegetables, reduce weight, avoid excess alcohol consumption, increase physical activity, and reduce weight if obese.

Hypertension Hypertension is a major risk factor for subsequent cardiovascular events in patients post-MI [135]. There are no large clinical trials of antihypertensive treatment in patients with MI; however, epidemiological data support the treatment of hypertension post-MI to reduce the risk of subsequent cardiac events [136, 137]. Furthermore, in the diabetic subgroup of the HOPE study, ramipril therapy reduced cardiovascular mortality and more that 50% of the subjects had previous coronary artery disease [138]. The benefits of intensive blood-pressure lowering was also seen in the subset of patients in the Hypertension Optimal Treatment (HOT) study with prior MI and preexisting CHD [139]. The Joint British Guidelines on prevention of CHD in clinical practice [132] recommend a target blood pressure of <140/85 mmHg in patients with CHD or patients with diabetes and the ADA guidelines [46] recommend a target of <130/80 mmHg in all diabetic subjects. The target blood pressure in diabetic and nondiabetic patients following MI has not been established.

Hyperlipidemia Serum cholesterol and LDL cholesterol are major risk factors for recurrent cardiac events following MI [140]. There is now evidence from large randomized controlled trials in patients with CHD that lowering serum cholesterol with HMG-CoA reductase inhibitors (statins) reduces both cardiovascular mortality and subsequent cardiovascular events even in patients with average cholesterol levels (<6.2 mmol/l) [141–143]. Subgroup analysis of the Scandanavian Simvastatin Study (4S) and the Cholesterol and Recurrent Events (CARE) Study showed that diabetic patients had a similar or even greater benefit as compared to nondiabetic patients [144, 145]. Subgroup analysis of the Long Term Intervention with Pravastatin in Ischaemic Disease (LIPID) study showed a trend toward a reduction in recurrent coronary events in diabetic subjects [142]. In the Heart Protection Study (HPS), treatment with simvastatin reduced the rates of MI, stroke, and revascularization by about a quarter for a wide range of high-risk patients and this effect was also seen in the diabetic subgroup with and without previous CHD [146]. Low HDL cholesterol is also an important cardiovascular risk factor in diabetes. In the VA-HIT study, gemfibrozil treatment reduced coronary events in men with known CHD and diabetes and low HDL [147] and should be initiated for secondary prevention in diabetic subjects with HDL cholesterol <1.0 mmol/l. The Diabetes Atherosclerosis Intervention Study (DAIS) has shown that treatment with micronized fenofibrate corrects lipid abnormalities and reduces the progression of angiographic coronary disease in type 2 diabetic subjects even in asymptomatic subjects [148].

Lipid-lowering therapy is therefore indicated in all diabetic subjects with CHD. Statins lower both LDL and VLDL and increase HDL concentrations, making this class of agent acceptable first-line therapy. In subjects with primary hypertriglyceridemia without a significant elevation in total or LDL cholesterol, a fibric acid derivative such as bezafibrate is more appropriate. Neither niacin nor bile acid sequestrants are ideal agents because of the potential adverse effects on insulin sensitivity by the former and a worsening of hypertriglyceridemia by the latter. In subjects with mixed hyperlipidemia combination therapy may be necessary. However, higher doses of statins may be moderately effective at lowering triglycerides and reduce the need for combination therapy. Optimal LDL cholesterol levels for diabetic subjects are <100 mg/dl (2.6 mmol/l), optimal HDL cholesterol levels are >45 mg/dl (>1.15 mmol/l), and desirable triglyceride levels are <150 mg/dl (<1.7 mmol/l) [47].

Revascularization in Diabetic Subjects

Recommendations for revascularization in the general population are available for stable angina and ACSs [78, 149] and should also be applied to diabetic subjects with suitable anatomy for revascularization. Indications for surgical revascularization include three-vessel disease, left main stem stenosis, two-vessel disease including proximal left anterior descending artery, and two-vessel disease with left ventricular dysfunction. Patients with diabetes have increased mortality and morbidity following revascularization. The increased risk in diabetic patients appears at least in part to be due to a number of confounding factors, including female sex, more severe and diffuse disease, impaired left ventricular function, and renal impairment [150].

Diabetes is associated with an increased early mortality and morbidity after coronary artery bypass grafting (CABG) [23, 150, 151] and long-term survival is also reduced [150, 152–154]. Heart failure is an important cause of late mortality [153, 155]. In spite of the higher mortality, available data suggest that CABG is superior to medical treatment in diabetic subjects [152] (Figure 7). As in nondiabetic subjects the use of internal mammary

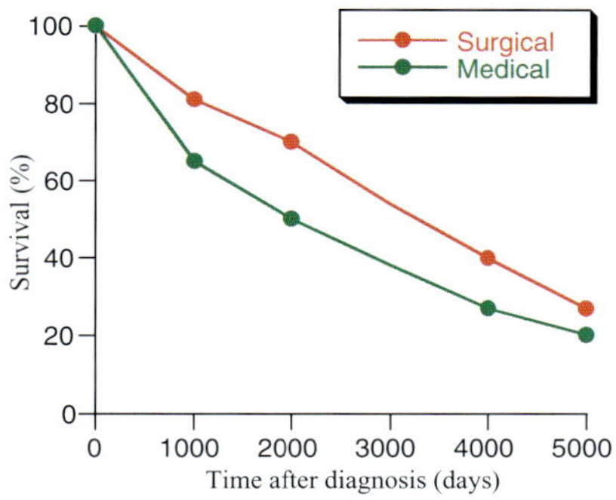

Figure 7 Survival rates for diabetic patients aged 65 years or more, with angiographically proven coronary artery disease treated either surgically (bypass grafting) or medically [152]. (Reprinted from American Journal of Cardiology 74, 334–339, © 1994 with premission from Excerpta Medica Inc)

artery grafting is associated with an improved outcome in diabetic subjects [156, 157]. The use of radial arteries is increasing [158], in the hope that they will maintain greater late patency than saphenous veins, and is feasible in diabetic patients [159]. Recent retrospective data suggest that off-pump bypass is associated with a reduced stroke risk in diabetic patients especially in high-risk groups [160] but prospective studies are needed.

Diabetic patients also benefit symptomatically from percutaneous transluminal coronary angioplasty (PTCA). Procedural success rates are similar to that in the nondiabetic population [161, 162] but mortality [162, 163] and restenosis rates are higher than in the nondiabetic population [164, 165]. Stents have been shown to improve the outcome after PTCA [166–168] in nondiabetic populations and should be employed where feasible. However, diabetes remains a risk factor for restenosis following stenting [164, 169–171]. Factors associated with the worse outcome in diabetic patients include incomplete revascularization [156, 172], insulin treatment [173], and sulfonylurea therapy [156, 174]. In one study improved glycemic control was associated with a reduced restenosis rate [175]. Platelet glycoprotein IIb/IIIa receptor antagonists have also been shown to reduce mortality after PTCA with or without stenting in diabetic subjects [88, 89, 176–179]. The value of drug-eluting stents and brachytherapy to reduce restenosis rates remain to be evaluated in the diabetic population.

Recently, concern has been raised regarding PTCA for multivessel disease in diabetic patients. Diabetic subjects with multivessel disease had a significantly reduced 7-year survival rate with PTCA than with CABG using internal mammary arteries (55.7% vs. 76.4%) in the BARI study [180] (Figure 8). A higher rate of infarction and a greater need for additional revascularization procedures were observed, probably because of early restenosis and late progression of CHD [161]. The benefit of CABG appears to be at least in part due to a reduced mortality from subsequent MI in diabetic subjects [181]. Other trials have also shown an advantage for CABG in diabetic subjects [156, 172, 173, 182, 183]. Most of these trials were conducted prior to the routine use of stents and glycoprotein IIa/IIIb inhibitors. However, even with stenting the outcome of diabetic patients with multivessel disease is worse than with CABG [184]. Further studies in diabetic patients are required to address these issues. Until results of such studies are available, CABG with the use of internal mammary arteries is recommended for diabetic patients with multivessel disease suitable for revascularization.

Heart Failure

The prevalence of heart failure is high in diabetes mellitus and much of this is related to CHD. In the Framingham study, diabetic males had a twofold and diabetic females a fivefold excess of congestive cardiac failure when compared to nondiabetic subjects, and this excess risk was still evident after excluding other risk factors and prevalent disease [5].

While ischemic heart disease is the commonest cause of heart failure in diabetic subjects, heart failure and asymptomatic abnormalities of left ventricular function have also been demonstrated in diabetic patients in the absence of CHD [185, 186]. These abnormalities correlate to a large degree with duration of diabetes and the extent of microvascular complications and this has led to the suggestion that a specific diabetic cardiomyopathy exists. The earliest manifestation of this is evidence of abnormal diastolic relaxation on Doppler flow patterns as shown in Figure 9.

The pathogenesis of diabetic cardiomyopathy remains uncertain. Small vessel disease, interstitial fibrosis, microvascular changes, hypertension, and metabolic derangements have all been implicated [187]. Abnormalities

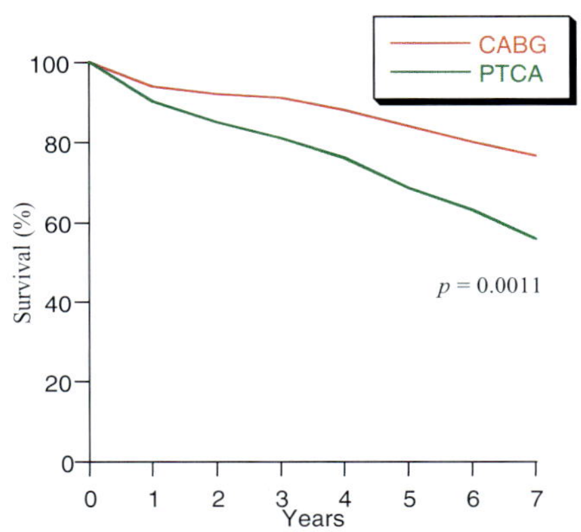

Figure 8 Kaplan–Meier estimates of survival for diabetic patients with multivessel disease randomized to CABG or PTCA in the BARI study [180]. (Reprinted from Journal of American College of Cardiology 26, 57–65, © 1995 with premission from American College of Cardiology Foundation)

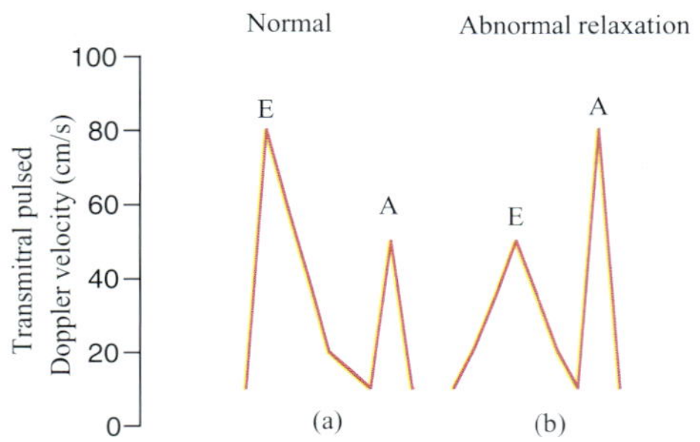

Figure 9 Schematic patterns of mitral inflow velocity as recorded by pulsed-wave Doppler technique. E, peak velocity in early diastole; A, peak velocity at atrial contraction. The normal pattern (a) shows high velocity in early diastole, minimal inflow during mid-diastole, and high velocity at end of diastole due to atrial contraction; the E/A ratio is >1.0. In a diabetic subject with abnormal relaxation (b), early diastolic filling is reduced and there is increased dependence on atrial contraction, with an E/A ratio < 1.0. Similar diastolic abnormalities are seen in CHD and left ventricular hypertrophy

of left ventricular function have been described in the absence of hypertension but it is likely that superimposed hypertension may accelerate the development of myocardial fibrosis and scarring [188]. Fisher et al. demonstrated microangiopathic changes in diabetic patients with abnormal cardiac function but without evidence of coronary artery disease [189]. Subclinical diastolic dysfunction in diabetic patients with microalbuminuria has been described [190], providing further support for the role of microangiopathy. At a cellular level defects in calcium homeostasis have been identified. Peak systolic Ca^{2+} transients in cardiac myocytes are reduced, the decay phase of the Ca^{2+} transients is slowed [191], and both Ca^{2+} uptake and sarcoplasmic reticulum Ca^{2+}-ATPase mRNA levels are reduced [192]. Increased free fatty acid production in diabetes may have deleterious effects on cardiac function as it will increase myocardial oxygen consumption and may enhance the accumulation of toxic metabolites [193].

There are no specific trials addressing therapy of heart failure in diabetic patients. Therefore investigation and management should follow guidelines for heart failure in the general population [194–197]. These guidelines stress the importance of echocardiography in confirming left ventricular systolic dysfunction in heart failure (Figure 10). Recent evidence suggests that natriuretic peptides and in particular brain natriuretic peptide are useful "rule out" tests for heart failure because of high negative predictive values, and in the future these are likely to prove useful in selecting patients with shortness of breath for echocardiography [193]. It is important to remember that diabetic subjects may present with heart failure as the sole manifestation of CHD. Recent evidence suggests that diabetes and CHD may interact to accelerate the progression of myocardial dysfunction [198]. Evaluation of

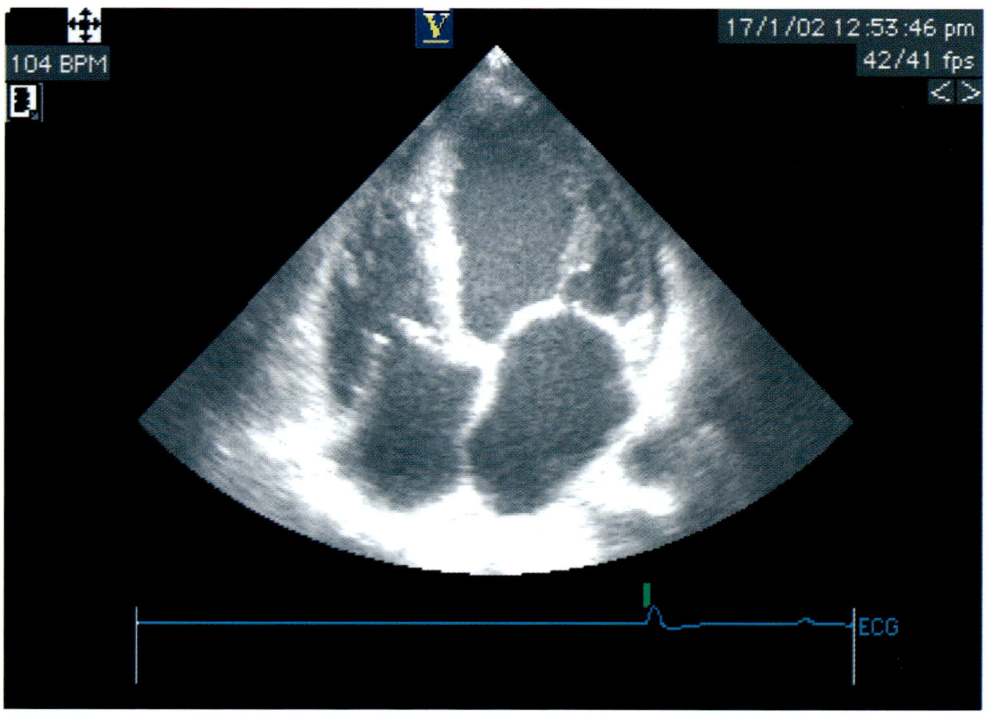

Figure 10 Two-dimensional echocardiogram (apical four-chamber view) showing dilated left ventricle in a diabetic patient presenting with dyspnea on exertion

the potential for revascularization in diabetic subjects with heart failure is therefore important, as is aggressive management of risk factors for CHD.

As in other groups, diuretics and ACE inhibitors form the mainstay of treatment. ACE inhibitors have been shown to improve the outcome for patients with heart failure and diabetic patients with left ventricular dysfunction share these benefits [199]. Large randomized trials have shown conclusively that the addition of β-blockers to standard therapy with diuretics and ACE inhibitors substantially reduces mortality and morbidity in all grade of symptomatic heart failure [200–203]. Diabetic patients were not excluded from these trials and given the high risk in diabetic patients with heart disease they are more likely, in absolute terms, to benefit from treatment. The role of AT_1 receptor antagonists in heart failure remains unclear. The ELITE II study showed that mortality was similar in patients treated with captopril and lorsartan [204]. More recently, the addition of valsartan to ACE inhibitor therapy in patients with heart failure showed no benefit in terms of survival (ValHEFT), although there was a reduction in hospital admission rates with the combination [205]. At present AT_1 receptor antagonists are recommended in patients intolerant of ACE inhibitors. Spironolactone has shown benefit in terms of mortality and morbidity in patients with severe heart failure (New York Heart Association (NYHA) grade III and IV) and should be instituted in the diabetic patient [206]. Careful monitoring of serum potassium concentrations especially in those with renal impairment is important. Heart transplantation should be considered in young patients with severe heart failure as 3-year survival, rejection rates, and development of post-transplantation coronary artery disease are similar in diabetic and nondiabetic subjects [207]. Nephropathy in diabetic patients may result in fluid retention, hypertension, and increased symptoms of pulmonary congestion that may be difficult to treat because of the lack of response to diuretic therapy and worsening renal function and may necessitate dialysis.

Sudden Cardiac Death

Sudden cardiac death, frequently defined as death occurring within 1 h of onset of symptoms, is a recognized presentation of CHD. It is often presumed to be arrhythmic in nature, although most of these deaths are not witnessed and outcome from resuscitation is poor [208]. The traditional risk factors for CHD are also predictive of sudden cardiac death [209] but long-term risk factors that predispose specifically to sudden death have not yet been identified. Diabetes is associated with sudden death in both univariate and multivariate analyses [209–211]. It has been suggested that autonomic neuropathy or microvascular disease affecting the conducting system increases the propensity for sudden death in diabetes but direct evidence for this is lacking. To date, there is limited evidence that primary [212, 213] and secondary prevention [214] strategies reduce the risk of sudden death in the general population but given the high risk of CHD in diabetic subjects, aggressive risk factor reduction is indicated.

PRIMARY PREVENTION OF CHD IN DIABETES

Treatment of Hypertension

Hypertension is very common in type 2 diabetic subjects with a prevalence of 40–60% over the age range of 45–75 years [215] and doubles the already elevated risk of future cardiac events [38, 216]. In the UKPDS [217] tight control of blood pressure (average blood pressure $<$144/82 mmHg) was associated with a significant 36% reduction in the combined risk of macrovascular disease, including MI, stroke, sudden death, and peripheral vascular disease. The 21% reduction in the risk of MI alone was not significant, but is similar to the risk reduction reported in the general population [218]. This evidence, together with that from other studies [139, 219, 220], led the British Hypertension Society to set an optimal target of $<$140/85 mmHg for diabetic subjects [221]. The National Service Framework for Diabetes [222] and the Scottish Intercollegiate Guidelines Network (SIGN) clinical guideline on the management of diabetes [223] have set similar targets for tight blood pressure control in diabetic subjects. The sixth Joint National Commission (JNC VI) guidelines [224] singled out diabetes as a high-risk state and recommended a target of $<$135/85 mmHg. The ADA goes further and recommends a goal of $<$130/80 mmHg [46].

The choice of antihypertensive agent in patients with diabetes is still debated. Thiazides, β-blockers, ACE inhibitors, and calcium-channel blockers are all effective in lowering blood pressure and reducing the risk of cardiovascular events. The relative benefits of treatment with different agents and differences between treatment intensities in nondiabetic subjects have recently been reviewed [225, 226] but as yet there are no firm recommendations for the use of one class of medication over another. In diabetic subjects, ACE inhibitors are recommended as first-line therapy in patients with microalbuminuria because of their additional benefits on renal function. The UKPDS showed no advantage of captopril over atenolol in reducing the risk of macro- and microvascular complications [227], suggesting that it is the blood pressure reduction *per se* that is important. However, in a substudy analysis of the Captopril Prevention Project, captopril was associated with a greater reduction in cardiovascular mortality than conventional therapy with diuretics and/or β-blockers [228]. More recently, the addition of angiotensin II receptor antagonists to conventional antihypertensive therapy

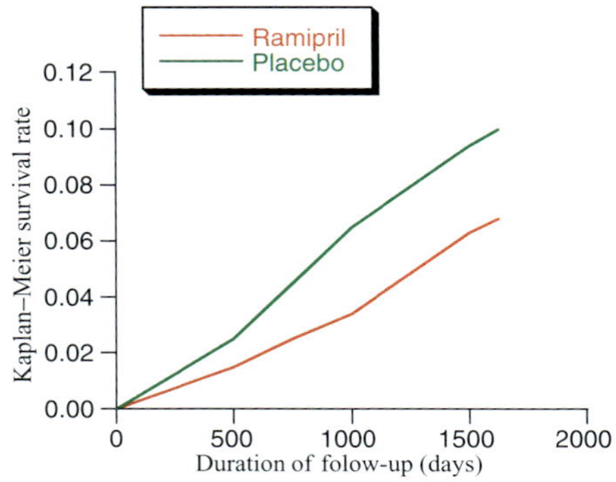

Figure 11 Kaplan–Meier survival curve for cardiovascular death in diabetic participants in the HOPE study [138]. (Reproduced by permission of Elsevier)

have been shown to delay the progression of renal disease in diabetic subjects [229–231]. In the LIFE study, lorsartan was superior to atenolol in reduced cardiovascular morbidity and mortality in diabetic patients with hypertension and LVH [232], and hospitalization for heart failure was significantly reduced in the losartan-treated group in the RENAAL study [231] (16.7–11.9%, $p = 0.005$). However, in choosing drug therapy for the diabetic patient with hypertension, it is important to remember that subgroup analysis must be interpreted with caution.

ACE Inhibitors

The recently published HOPE study showed that ramipril treatment in diabetic subjects over age 55, and with at least one other cardiovascular risk factor, reduced cardiovascular death by 37%, MI by 22%, and stroke by 33% and the effects were still significant after adjusting for the reduction in office blood pressure [138]. It is should be noted, however, that this study was unique in that the active drug and placebo were taken at night and a substudy with ambulatory blood pressure monitoring showed that 24-h blood pressure was lower by 10/6 mmHg in the ramipril treatment group, mainly because of substantially lower overnight blood pressure [233]. Figure 11 shows the Kaplan–Meier survival curve for cardiovascular death over 4.5 years of follow-up in diabetic subjects in the HOPE study ($p<0.001$). Ramipril therapy should be considered for diabetic subjects aged >55, who either smoke or have total cholesterol >5.2 mmol/l, HDL cholesterol <0.9 mmol/l, hypertension, or microalbuminuria. The soon-to-be-reported ALLHAT study is comparing different antihypertensive strategies in 48 000 subjects, of whom one third have diabetes, and will contribute substantially to the debate as to whether specific classes of antihypertensive drugs provide particular benefit in CHD risk reduction in diabetic patients.

Treatment of hyperlipidemia

Total cholesterol and LDL cholesterol are important risk factors for CHD in diabetic subjects [33, 38]. In the UKPDS, for each increment of 1 mmol/l of LDL cholesteral there was a 1.57-fold increased risk of CHD. This equates to a 36% risk reduction for a decrement of 1 mmol/l, which is similar to the reduction achieved with pravastatin in men with hypercholesterolemia [234]. To date, there are no primary prevention trials of lipid-lowering therapy specifically in type 2 diabetic subjects without CHD. However, in the diabetic subgroup of the HPS, significant reductions in coronary and other cardiovascular events were observed with simvastatin therapy irrespective of the pretreatment cholesterol or triglyceride levels [146]. Ongoing studies such as CARDS (Collaborative AtoRvastatin Diabetes Study) and LDS (Lipids in Diabetes Study) will provide further information in diabetic subjects. In the interim, because of the high mortality for diabetic subjects with first MI, aggressive treatment of dyslipidemia is indicated and the guidelines for secondary prevention discussed above should be applied.

Triglycerides are an independent marker of increased cardiovascular disease in type 2 diabetes [235]. The evidence that lowering triglycerides is beneficial in primary prevention remains unclear. The ongoing Fenofibrate Intervention and Event Lowering in Diabetes (FIELD) study is addressing whether lowering serum triglycerides will reduce CHD events in 8000 diabetic subjects with and without CHD. ω-3 Fatty acids are also effective in lowering serum triglycerides and may be beneficial in diabetic subjects.

Glycemic Control

In the UKPDS, increasing glycaemia results in an increased cardiovascular mortality [33]. Each 1% reduction in glycated HbA_{1c} was associated with a 21% reduction in the risk of diabetes-related death and a 14% reduction in MI over 10 years [236] in subjects with NIDDM. The Diabetes Control and Complications Trial (DCCT) provided clear evidence that intensive management of IDDM delays the onset and progression of microvascular complications [237] but the reduction in macrovascular events in the intensive treatment group did not reach statistical significance [238]. In a substudy of the UKPDS, patients allocated intensive blood glucose control with metformin had a greater benefit in terms of reduction in all-cause mortality, any diabetes-related end point, and stroke compared to those on sulfonylureas or insulin [239]. Therefore metformin should be considered as the first-line oral hypoglycemic agent in overweight patients with type 2 diabetes.

Recently there have been concerns that sulfonylurea therapy may have an adverse effect on diabetic patients with CHD. Sulfonylureas act by inhibiting K_{ATP} channels that are not only present in the pancreas but also in the heart and vascular smooth muscle. Experimentally they have been shown to prevent cardiac preconditioning and thus may contribute to increased cardiac mortality in diabetic subjects [240, 241]. The UKPDS found no adverse cardiovascular effects from sulfonylureas; however, few patients had preexisting CHD and only 2% had had an MI prior to recruitment to the study [242].

Smoking Cessation

Smoking is an independent risk factor in patients with diabetes [33, 38] and the prevalence of smoking is significantly higher among them [243]. Effective approaches to smoking cessation include behavioral intervention and pharmacotherapy, in particular nicotine replacement therapy and sustained-release bupropion. These should be provided for all diabetic patients who smoke.

Aspirin Therapy

The role of aspirin in primary prevention remains uncertain and the benefit must be balanced against the risk of bleeding. In the HOT study low-dose aspirin further reduced cardiovascular risk in well-controlled hypertensive patients with diabetes [139], and in the US Physicians' Health Study a reduction in MI from 10.1% to 4% was observed in diabetic men on aspirin therapy [244]. There are good overviews in nondiabetic subjects, suggesting that all subjects with 10-year cardiovascular risk >20% should be on aspirin. Therefore, low-dose aspirin therapy (up to 325 mg daily) is recommended for primary prevention in diabetic subjects [48, 223].

No randomized trials have been conducted to determine the effects of weight reduction, increasing physical activity, lowering plasma insulin, fibrinogen or plasminogen activator inhibitor concentrations on the incidence or mortality from cardiovascular disease and so the role of these risk factors in decisions about therapy remain to be determined.

REFERENCES

1. Morrish NJ, Stevens LK, Head J, Fuller JH, Jarrett RJ, Keen H. A prospective study of mortality among middle-aged diabetic patients (the London Cohort of the WHO Multinational Study of Vascular Disease in Diabetics), I: causes and death rates. *Diabetologia* 1990; 33: 538–41.
2. Gu K, Cowie CC, Harris MI. Diabetes and decline in heart disease mortality in US adults. *JAMA* 1999; 281: 1291–7.
3. Stephenson J, Swerdlow AJ, Devis T, Fuller JH. Recent trends in diabetic mortality in England and Wales. *Diabet Med* 1992; 9: 417–21.
4. Löwel H, Koenig W, Engel S, Hörmann A, Keil U. The impact of diabetes on survival after myocardial infarction? Can it be modified by drug treatment? Results of a population-based myocardial infarction register follow-up study. *Diabetologia* 2000; 43: 218–26.
5. Kannel WB, McGee DL. Diabetes and glucose tolerance as risk factors for cardiovascular disease: the Framingham Study. *Diabetes Care* 1979; 2: 120–6.
6. Fuller JH, Shipley MJ, Rose G, Jarrett RJ, Keen H. Coronary heart disease risk and impaired glucose tolerance. The Whitehall Study. *Lancet* 1980; 28: 1373–6.
7. Rosengren A, Welin L, Tsipogianni A, Wilhelmsen L. Impact of cardiovascular risk factors on coronary heart disease and mortality among middle aged diabetic men: a general population study. *BMJ* 1989; 299: 1127–31.
8. Schernthaner G. Cardiovascular mortality and morbidity in type-2 diabetes mellitus. *Diabetes Res Clin Pract* 1996; 31 (suppl): S3–13.
9. Kanthers SD, Banga JD, Stolk RP, Algra A. Incidence and determinants of mortality and cardiovascular events in diabetes mellitus. *Vasc Med* 1999; 4: 67–75.
10. Hu FB, Stampfer MJ, Solomon CG, et al. The impact of diabetes on mortality from all causes and coronary heart disease in women: 20 years of follow-up. *Arch Intern Med* 2001; 161: 1717–23.
11. Lotufo PA, Gaziano JM, Chae CU, et al. Diabetes and all-cause coronary heart disease mortality among US male physicians. *Arch Intern Med* 2001; 161: 242–7.
12. Howard BV, Cowan LD, GO O, Welty TK, Robbins DC, Lee ET. Adverse effects of diabetes on multiple cardiovascular risk factors in women: the Strong Heart Study. *Diabetes Care* 1998; 21: 1258–65.
13. Lee WL, Cheung AM, Cape D, Zinman B. Impact of diabetes on coronary artery disease in women and men: a meta-analysis of prospective studies. *Diabetes Care* 2000; 23: 962–8.
14. McKeigue PM, Shah B, Marmot MG. Relation of central obesity and insulin resistance with high diabetes prevalence and cardiovascular risk in South Asians. *Lancet* 1991; 337: 382–6.
15. Chaturvedi N, Fuller JH. Ethnic differences in mortality from cardiovascular disease in the UK: do they persist in patients with diabetes? *J Epidemiol Community Health* 1996; 50: 137–9.
16. Barrett-Connor E, Orchard TJ. Insulin dependent diabetes mellitus and ischaemic heart disease. *Diabetes Care* 1985; 8 (suppl 1): 65–70.
17. Borch-Johnsen K, Kreiner S. Proteinuria: value as a predictor of cardiovascular mortality in insulin dependent diabetes mellitus. *BMJ* 1987; 294: 1651–4.
18. Jensen T, Borch-Johnsen K, Kofoed-Enevoldsen A, Deckert T. Coronary artery disease in young Type 1 (insulin dependent) diabetic patients with and without diabetic nephropathy: incidence and risk factors. *Diabetologia* 1987; 30: 144–8.
19. Manske CL, Wilson RF, Wang Y, Thomas W. Prevalence of, and risk factors for, angiographically determined coronary artery disease in Type 1 diabetic patients with nephropathy. *Arch Intern Med* 1992; 152: 2450–5.
20. Fuller JH, McCartney P, Jarrett RJ, et al. Hyperglycemia and coronary heart disease: the Whitehall study. *J Chronic Dis* 1979; 32: 721–8.
21. Barrett-Connor E, Wingard DL, Criqui MH, Suarez L. Is borderline fasting hyperglycemia a risk factor for cardiovascular death? *J Chronic Dis* 1984; 37: 773–9.
22. Mykkänen L, Laasko M, Pyörälä K. Asymptomatic hyperglycemia and atherosclerotic vascular disease in the elderly. *Diabetes Care* 1992; 15: 1020–30.

23. Cohen Y, Raz I, Merin G, Mozes B, for the Israeli Coronary Artery Bypass (ISCAB) Study Consortium. Comparison of factors associated with 30-day mortality after coronary artery bypass grafting in patients with versus without diabetes mellitus. *Am J Cardiol* 1998; 81: 7–11.
24. Haffner SM, Lehto S, Ronnemaa T, Pyörälä K, Laasko M. Mortality from coronary heart disease in subjects with type-2 diabetes and in nondiabetic subjects with and without myocardial infarction. *N Engl J Med* 1998; 339: 229–43.
25. Burchfiel CM, Reed DM, Marcus EB, Strong JP, Hayashi T. Association of diabetes mellitus with coronary atherosclerosis and myocardial lesions: an autopsy study from the Honolulu Heart Program. *Am J Epidemiol* 1993; 137: 1328–40.
26. Hubbard BL, Gibbons RJ, Lapeyre AC III, Zinsmeister AR, Clements IP. Identification of severe coronary artery disease using simple clinical parameters. *Arch Intern Med* 1992; 152: 309–12.
27. Kanojia A, Kasliwal R, Seth A, Bhandari S, Kler TS, Bhatia ML. Clinical and coronary arteriographic features and outcome of recent onset unstable angina. *Int J Cardiol* 1993; 39: 173–80.
28. Valsania P, Zarich SW, Kowalchuk GJ, Kosinski E, Warram JH, Krolewski AS. Severity of coronary artery disease in young patients with insulin dependent diabetes. *Am Heart J* 1991; 122: 695–700.
29. Caracciolo EA, Chaitman BR, Forman SA, et al, for the ACIP Investigators. Diabetics with coronary disease have a prevalence of asymptomatic ischemia during exercise treadmill testing and ambulatory ischemia monitoring similar to that of nondiabetic patients: and ACIP database study. *Circulation* 1996; 93: 2097–105.
30. Bhan A, Das B, Wasir HS, Kaul U, Venugopal P. Profile of coronary artery disease in diabetic patients undergoing coronary artery bypass grafting. *Int J Cardiol* 1991; 31: 155–9.
31. Alderman EL, Corley SD, Fisher LD, et al. Five-year angiographic follow-up of factors associated with progression of coronary artery disease in the Coronary Artery Surgery Study (CASS). *J Am Coll Cardiol* 1993; 22: 1141–54.
32. Vaccaro O, Stamler J, Neaton JD, for the Multiple Risk factor Intervention Trial Research Group. Sixteen-year coronary mortality in black and white men with diabetes screened for the Multiple Risk factor Intervention Trial (MRFIT). *Int J Epidemiol* 1998; 27: 636–41.
33. Turner RC, Millns H, Neil HAW, et al, for the United Kingdom Prospective Diabetes Study Group. Risk factors for coronary artery disease in non-insulin dependent diabetes mellitus: United Kingdom Prospective Diabetes Study Group (UKPDS 23). *BMJ* 1998; 316: 823–828.
34. Laasko M, Lehto S, Pentillä I, et al. Lipids and lipoproteins predicting coronary heart disease mortality and morbidity in patients with non-insulin dependent diabetes. *Circulation* 1993; 88: 1421–30.
35. Stewart MW, Laker MF, Dyer RG, et al. Lipoprotein compositional abnormalities and insulin resistance in type II diabetic patients with mild hyperlipidemia. *Atheroscler Thromb* 1993; 13: 1046–52.
36. Frohlich J, Steiner G. Dyslipidaemia and coagulation defects of insulin resistance. *Int J Clin Pract Suppl* 2000; 113: 14–22.
37. Fitzgerald AP, Jarrett RJ. Are conventional risk factors for mortality relevant in Type 2 diabetes? *Diabet Med* 1991; 8: 475–80.
38. Stamler J, Vaccaro O, Neaton JD, Wentworth D, for the Multiple Risk Factor Intervention Trial Research Group. Diabetes, other risk factors and 12-year cardiovascular mortality for men screened in the multiple risk factor intervention trial. *Diabetes Care* 1993; 16: 434–44.
39. Dineen SF, Gerstein HC. The association of microalbuminuria and mortality in non-insulin-dependent diabetes. A systemic overview of the literature. *Arch Intern Med* 1997; 157: 1413–8.
40. Carr ME. Diabetes mellitus: a hypercoagulable state. *J Diabetes Complications* 2001; 15: 44–54.
41. Aronson D, Rayfield EJ, Chesebro JH. Mechanisms determining course and outcome of diabetic patients who have had acute myocardial infarction. *Ann Intern Med* 1997; 126: 296–306.
42. Williams SV, Fihn SD, Gibbons RJ, for the American College of Cardiology; American Heart Association; American College of Physicians—American Society of Internal Medicine. Guidelines for the management of patients with chronic stable angina: diagnosis and risk stratification. *Ann Intern Med* 2001; 135: 530–47.
43. Fihn SD, Williams SV, Daley J, Gibbons RJ, for the American College of Cardiology; American Heart Association; American College of Physicians—American Society of Internal Medicine. Guidelines for the management of patients with chronic stable angina: treatment. *Ann Intern Med* 2001; 135: 616–32.
44. Department of Health. National Service Framework for Coronary Heart Disease. Available at: http://www.doh.gov.uk/-nsf/.
45. American Diabetes Association. Smoking and diabetes: Clinical Practice Guideline 2001. *Diabetes Care* 2001; 24 (suppl 1): S44–7.
46. American Diabetes Association. Standards of medical care for patients with diabetes mellitus: Clinical Practice Recommendations 2001. *Diabetes Care* 2001; 24 (suppl 1) S33–43.
47. American Diabetes Association. Management of dyslipidaemia in adults with diabetes: Clinical Practice Recommendations 2001. *Diabetes Care* 2001; 24 (suppl 1) S58–61.
48. American Diabetes Association. Aspirin therapy in diabetes: Clinical Practice Recommendations 2001. *Diabetes Care* 2001; 24 (suppl 1) S62–3.
49. American Diabetes Association. Diabetes mellitus and exercise: Clinical Practice Recommendations 2001. *Diabetes Care* 2001; 24 (suppl 1) S51–5.
50. Fazzani PF, Prati PL, Rovelli F, et al. Epidemiology of silent myocardial ischemia in middle-aged men (the ECCIS project). *Am J Cardiol* 1993; 72: 1383–8.
51. Koistinen MJ. Prevalence of asymptomatic myocardial ischemia in diabetic subjects. *BMJ* 1990; 301: 92–5.
52. Scheidt-Nave C, Barrett-Connor E, Wingard DL. Resting electrocardiographic abnormalities suggestive of asymptomatic ischaemic heart disease associated with non-insulin dependent diabetes mellitus in a defined population. *Circulation* 1990; 81: 899–906.
53. Langer A, Freeman DR, Josse RG, Steiner G, Armstrong PW. Detection of silent myocardial ischemia in diabetes mellitus. *Am J Cardiol* 1991; 67: 1073–8.
54. Naka M, Hiramatsu K, Aizawa T, et al. Silent myocardial ischemia in patients with non-insulin-dependent diabetes as judged by treadmill exercise testing and coronary angiography. *Am Heart J* 1992; 123: 46–53.
55. Valensi P, Sachs RN, Lormeau B, et al. Silent myocardial ischemia and left ventricular hypertrophy in

diabetic patients. *Diabetes Metab* 1997; 23: 409–16.
56. Milan Study on Atherosclerosis and Diabetes (MiSAD) Group. Prevalence of unrecognized silent myocardial ischemia and its association with atherosclerotic risk factors in non insulin-dependent diabetes mellitus. *Am J Cardiol* 1997; 79: 134–9.
57. May O, Arildsen H, Damsgaard EM, Mickley H. Prevalence and prediction of silent ischemia in diabetes mellitus: a population-based study. *Cardiovasc Res* 1997; 34: 241–7.
58. Janand-Delenne B, Bory M, Savin B, Vague P, Habib G, Lassmann-Vague V. Silent myocardial ischemia in patients with diabetes. *Diabetes Care* 1999; 22: 1396–1400.
59. Ditchburn CJ, Hall JA, de Belder M, Davies A, Kelly W, Bilous R. Silent myocardial ischemia in patients with proved coronary artery disease: a comparison of diabetic and nondiabetic patients. *Postgrad Med J* 2001; 77: 395–8.
60. Caracciolo EA, Chaitman BR, Forman SA, et al, for the ACIP Investigators. Diabetics with coronary disease have a prevalence of asymptomatic ischemia during exercise treadmill testing and ambulatory monitoring similar to that of nondiabetic patients: an ACIP database study. *Circulation* 1996; 93: 2097–105.
61. Airaksinen KEJ. Silent coronary disease in diabetes—a feature of autonomic neuropathy or accelerated atherosclerosis? *Diabetologia* 2001; 44 (2): 259–66.
62. Weiner DA, Ryan TJ, McCabe CH, et al. Significance of silent myocardial ischemia during exercise testing in patients with coronary artery disease. *Am J Cardiol* 1987; 59: 725–9.
63. Deedwania PC, Carbagal EV. Silent ischemia during daily life is an independent predictor of mortality in stable angina. *Circulation* 1990; 81: 748–56.
64. Thaulow E, Erikssen J. Prognostic implications of asymptomatic cardiac ischemia. *Cardiology* 1994; 85: 11–5.
65. Weiner DA, Ryan TJ, Parsons L, et al. Significance of silent myocardial ischemia during exercise testing in patients with diabetes mellitus: a report from the Coronary Artery Surgery Study (CASS) Registry. *Am J Cardiol* 1991; 68: 729–34.
66. Palliole V, Ruiz J, Juliard JM Leblanc H, Gourgon R, Passa P. Detection of coronary artery disease in diabetic patients. *Diabetologia* 1995; 38: 726–31.
67. Penforis A, Zimmermann C, Boumal D, et al. Use of dobutamine stress echocardiography in detecting silent myocardial ischemia in asymptomatic diabetic patients: a comparison with thallium scintigraphy and exercise testing. *Diabet Med* 2001; 18: 900–5.
68. Nathan DM, Meigs J, Singer DE. The epidemiology of cardiovascular disease in type-2 diabetes mellitus: how sweet it is or . . . is it? *Lancet* 1997; 350: 4–9.
69. Vanzetto G, Benhamou PY, Halmi S, et al. Prediction of cardiovascular events in clinically selected high-risk NIDDM patients. *Diabetes Care* 1999; 22: 19–26.
70. Passa P, Drouin P, Issa-Sayegh M, et al. Coronaires et diabète. *Diabete Metab* 1995; 21: 446–51.
71. Manske CL, Wang Y, Rector T, et al. Coronary revascularization in insulin-dependent diabetic patients with renal failure. *Lancet* 1992; 340: 998–1002.
72. Collinson J, Flather MD, Fox KA, et al. Clinical outcomes, risk stratification and practice patterns of unstable angina and myocardial infarction without ST elevation: Prospective Registry of Acute Ischemic Syndromes (PRAIS-UK). *Eur Heart J* 2000; 21: 1450–7.
73. Yusuf S, Flather M, Pogue J, et al, for the OASIS (Organization to Assess Strategies for Ischemic Syndromes) Registry Investigators. Variations between countries in invasive cardiac procedures and outcomes in patients with suspected unstable angina or myocardial infarction without ST elevation. *Lancet* 1998; 352: 507–14.
74. Malmberg K, Yusuf S, Gerstein HC, et al. for the OASIS Registry Investigators. Impact of diabetes on long-term prognosis in patients with unstable angina and non-Q-wave myocardial infarction. Results of the OASIS (Organisation to assess Strategies for Ischemic Syndromes) Registry. *Circulation* 2000; 102: 1014–22.
75. *51st Annual Scientific Session of the American College of Cardiology*, Atlanta, GA, March 2002.
76. British Cardiac Society Guidelines and Medical Practice Committee and Royal College of Physicians Clinical Effectiveness and Evaluation Unit. Guideline for the management of patients with acute coronary syndromes without persistent ECG ST segment elevation. *Heart* 2001; 85: 133–42.
77. Bertrand ME, Simoons M, Fox KAA, et al. Management of acute coronary syndromes without persistent ST segment elevation. *Eur Heart J* 2002; 21: 1406–32.
78. Braunwald E, Antman EM, Beasley JW, et al. ACC/AHA guidelines for the management of patients with unstable angina and non-ST-segment elevation myocardial infarction. A report of the American College of Cardiology/American Heart Association Task Force on Practice Guidelines (Committee on the Management of Patients with Unstable Angina). *J Am Coll Cardiol* 2000; 36: 970–1062.
79. Theroux P, Oiumet H, Mccans J, et al. Aspirin, heparin or both to treat acute unstable angina. *N Engl J Med* 1988; 319: 1105–11.
80. The RISC Group. Risk of myocardial infarction and death during treatment with low dose aspirin and intravenous heparin in men with unstable coronary artery disease. *Lancet* 1990; 336: 827–30.
81. The Fragmin during Instability in Coronary Artery Disease (FRISC) Study Group. Low-molecular weight heparin during instability in coronary artery disease. *Lancet* 1996; 347: 561–8.
82. Eikelboom JW, Anand SS, Malmberg K, Weitz JI, Ginsberg JS, Jusuf S. Unfractionated heparin and low-molecular-weight heparin in acute coronary syndromes without ST elevation: a meta-analysis. *Lancet* 2000; 355: 1936–42.
83. Yusuf S, Zhao F, Mehta Sr, Chrolavicius S, Tognoni G, Fox KK, for the Clopidrogel in Unstable angina to Prevent Recurrent Events Trial Investigators. Effects of clopidrogel in addition to aspirin in patients with acute coronary syndromes without ST-segment elevation. *N Engl J Med* 2001; 345: 494–502.
84. National Institute for Clinical Excellence (NICE). Guidelines on the use of glycoprotein IIb/IIIa inhibitors for the treatment of acute coronary syndromes. Technology Appraisal Guidance No. 12, 2001. Available at: http://www.nice.org.-uk.
85. Boersma E, Harrington RA, Moliterno DJ, et al. Platelet glycoprotein IIb/IIIa inhibitors in acute coronary syndromes: a metanalysis of all major randomized trials. *Lancet* 2002; 359: 189–198.
86. Braunwald E, Antman EM, Beasley JW, et al. ACC/AHA 2002 Guideline update for the management of Patients with Unstable Angina and Non-ST-Segment

Elevation Myocardial infarction, 2002. Available at: http://www.acc.org/clinical/guidelines/unstable/incorporated/index.htm.

87. Kleiman NS, Lincoff AM, Kereiakes DJ, et al. Diabetes mellitus, glycoprotein IIb/IIIa blockade, and heparin: evidence for a complex interaction in a multicentre trial. EPILOG Investigators. *Circulation* 1998; 97: 1912–20.
88. Morso SP, Lincoff AM, Ellis SG, et al. Optimising the percutaneous intervention outcomes for patients with diabetes mellitus: results of the EPISTENT (evaluation of platelet IIb/IIIa inhibitor for stenting trial) diabetic substudy. *Circulation* 1999; 100: 2477–84.
89. Bhatt DL, Morso SP, Lincoff AM, et al. Abciximab reduces mortality in diabetic following percutaneous coronary intervention. *J Am Coll Cardiol* 2000; 35: 922–8.
90. Herlitz J, Malmberg K, Karlson BW, Rydén L, Hjalmarson Å. Mortality and morbidity during a five-year follow-up of diabetics with myocardial infarction. *Acta Med Scand* 1988; 224: 31–8.
91. Orlander PR, Goff DC, Morrisey M, et al. The relation of diabetes to the severity of acute myocardial infarction and post-myocardial infarction survival in Mexican-Americans and non-Hispanic whites: the Corpus Christi Heart Project. *Diabetes* 1994; 43: 897–902.
92. Melchior T, Rask-Madsen C, Torp-Pedersen C, Hildebrandt P, Kober L, Jensen G. The impact of heart failure on prognosis of diabetic and nondiabetic patients with myocardial infarction: a 15-year follow-up study. *Eur J Heart Fail* 2001; 3: 83–90.
93. Mukamel KJ, Nesto RW, Cohen MC, et al. Impact of diabetes on long-term survival after myocardial infarction: comparability of risk with prior myocardial infarction. *Diabetes Care* 2001; 24: 1422–27.
94. Gray RP, Yudkin JS, Patterson DLH. Plasminogen activator inhibitor—a risk factor for myocardial infarction in diabetic subjects. *Br Heart J* 1993; 69: 228–32.
95. Jaffe AS, Spadaro JJ, Schechtman K, Roberts R, Geltman EM, Sobel BE. Increased congestive heart failure after myocardial infarction of modest extent in patients with diabetes mellitus. *Am Heart J* 1984; 108: 31–7.
96. Yudkin JS, Oswald GA. Determinants of hospital admission and case fatality in diabetic patients with myocardial infarction. *Diabetes Care* 1988; 11: 351–8.
97. Smith JW, Marcus FI, Serokman R, with the Multicentre Postinfarction Research Group. Prognosis of patients with diabetes mellitus after acute myocardial infarction. *Am J Cardiol* 1984; 54: 718–21.
98. Stone PH, Muller JE, Hartwell T, et al. The effect of diabetes mellitus on prognosis and serial left ventricular function after acute myocardial infarction: contribution of both coronary disease and diastolic left ventricular dysfunction to the adverse prognosis. *J Am Coll Cardiol* 1989; 14: 49–57.
99. Malmberg K, Norhammar A, Wedel H, Rydén L. Glycometabolic state at admission: important risk marker of mortality in conventionally treated patients with diabetes mellitus and acute myocardial infarction. *Circulation* 1999; 99: 2626–32.
100. Standl E, Schnell O. A new look at the heart in diabetes mellitus: from ailing to failing. *Diabetologia* 2000; 43: 1455–69.
101. Capes SE, Hunt D, Malmberg K, Gerstein HC. Stress hyperglycemia and increased risk of vascular death after myocardial infarction inpatients with and without diabetes: a systemic review. *Lancet* 2000; 355: 773–8.
102. The Joint European Society of Cardiology/American College of Cardiology Committee. Myocardial infarction redefined—a consensus statement of the Joint European Society of Cardiology/American College of Cardiology. *Eur Heart J* 2000; 21: 1502–13.
103. Ryan TJ, Antman EM, Brooks NH, et al. ACC/AHA guidelines for the management of patients with acute myocardial infarction: 1999 update. A report of the American College of Cardiology/American Heart Association Task Force on Practice Guidelines (Committee on Management of Acute Myocardial Infarction), 1999. Available at http://www.acc.org.
104. Fibrinolytic Therapy Trialists (FTT) Collaborative Group. Indications for fibrinolytic therapy in suspected acute myocardial infarction: collaborative overview of early mortality and major morbidity results from all randomized trials of more than 1000 patients. *Lancet* 1994; 343: 311–22.
105. Ward H, Yudkin JS. Thrombolysis in patients with diabetes. *BMJ* 1995; 310: 3–4.
106. Yudkin JS. Managing the diabetic patient with acute myocardial infarction. *Diabet Med* 1998; 15: 276–81.
107. Fava S, Azzopardi J, Agius Muscat H, Fenech FF. Factors that influence outcome in diabetic subjects with myocardial infarction. *Diabetes Care* 1993; 16: 1615–8.
108. Gray RP, Yudkin JS, Patterson DL. Enzymatic evidence of impaired reperfusion in diabetic patients after thrombolytic therapy for acute myocardial infarction: a role for plasminogen activator inhibitor? *Br Heart J* 1993; 70: 530–6.
109. Mahaffey KW, Granger CB, Toth CA, et al, for the GUSTO-1 Investigators. Diabetic retinopathy should not be a contraindication to thrombolytic therapy for acute myocardial infarction: review of ocular haemorrhage incidence and locations in the GUSTO-1 trial. *J Am Coll Cardiol* 1997; 30: 1606–10.
110. Barbash GI, White HD, Modan M, Van de Werf F, for the Investigators of the International Tissue Plasminogen Activator/Streptokinase Mortality Trial. Significance of diabetes mellitus in patients with acute myocardial infarction receiving thrombolytic therapy. *J Am Coll Cardiol* 1993; 22: 707–13.
111. Collins R, Peto R, Baigent C, Sleight P. Aspirin, heparin, and fibrinolytic therapy in suspected acute myocardial infarction. *N Engl J Med* 1997; 336: 847–60.
112. Thomas K, Ottervanger JP, de Boer MJ, Suryapranata H, Hoorntje JC, Zijlstra F. Primary angioplasty compared with thrombolysis in acute myocardial infarction in diabetic subjects. *Diabetes Care* 1999; 22: 647–9.
113. Hasdai D, Granger CB, Srivatsa SS, et al. Diabetes mellitus and outcome after primary angioplasty for acute myocardial infarction: lessons from the GUSTO-IIb angioplasty substudy. Global use of strategies to open occluded arteries in acute coronary syndromes. *J Am Coll Cardiol* 2000; 35: 1502–12.
114. Waldecker B, Steen-Müller MK, Waas W, et al. Type 2 diabetes and acute myocardial infarction. *Diabetes Care* 1999; 22: 1832–8.
115. ISIS-2 (Second International Study of Infarct Survival Collaborative Group). Randomized trial of intravenous streptokinase, oral aspirin, both or neither among 17,185 cases of suspected acute myocardial infarction: ISIS-2. *Lancet* 1988; ii; 349–60.
116. Antiplatelet Trialists' Collaboration. Collaborative overview of randomized trials of antiplatelet therapy, I: prevention of death, myocardial infarction, and stroke by

prolonged antiplatelet therapy in various categories of patients. *BMJ* 1994; 308: 81–106.
117. Malmberg K, Herlitz J, Hjalmarson Å, Rydén L. Effects of metaprolol on mortality and late infarction in diabetics with suspected acute myocardial infarction: retrospective data from two large studies. *Eur Heart J* 1989; 10: 423–8.
118. Ball SG, on behalf of the AIRE Study Group. Effect of ramipril on mortality and morbidity of survivors of acute myocardial infraction with clinical evidence of heart failure: the acute infarction ramipril efficacy (AIRE) study. *Lancet* 1993; 342: 821–8.
119. Pleffer MA, Braunwald E, Moyé LA, et al, on behalf of the SAVE Investigators. Effect of captopril on mortality and morbidity in patients with left ventricular dysfunction after myocardial infarction; results of the survival and left ventricular enlargement trial. *N Engl J Med* 1992; 327: 669–77.
120. Kober L, Torp-Pedersen C, Carlsen JE, et al, for the Trandolapril Cardiac Evaluation (TRACE) Study Group. A clinical trial of the angiotensin-converting enzyme inhibitor trandolapril in patients with left ventricular dysfunction after myocardial infarction. *N Engl J Med* 1995; 333: 1670–6.
121. Garg R, Yusuf S. Overview of randomized trials of angiotensin-converting enzyme inhibitors on mortality and morbidity in patients with heart failure. Collaborative Group on ACE inhibitor trials. *JAMA* 1995; 273: 1450–6.
122. Zuanetti G, Latini R, Maggioni A, Franzoni M, Santoro L, Tognioni G. Effect of the ACE-inhibitor lisinopril on mortality in diabetic patients with acute myocardial infarction: data from the GISSI-3 study. *Circulation* 1997; 96: 4239–45.
123. Gustafsson I, Torp-Pedersen C, Kober L, Gustafsson F, Hildebrandt P, for the TRACE Study Group. Effect of the angiotensin-converting enzyme inhibitor trandolapril on mortality and morbidity in diabetic patients with left ventricular dysfunction after acute myocardial infarction. *J Am Coll Cardiol* 1999; 34: 83–9.
124. Moye L, Pfeffer M, Wun C, et al. Uniformity of captopril benefit in the SAVE study: subgroup analysis. *Eur Heart J* 1994; 15 (suppl B): 2–8.
125. The SOLVD Investigators. Effect of enalapril on survival in patients with reduced left ventricular ejection fractions and congestive heart failure. *N Engl J Med* 1991; 325: 293–302.
126. Malmberg K, Rydén L, Efendic S, et al. Randomized trial of insulin-glucose infusion followed by subcutaneous insulin treatment in diabetic patients with acute myocardial infarction (DIGAMI study): effect on mortality at 1 year. *J Am Coll Cardiol* 1995; 26: 57–65.
127. Malmberg K, for the DIGAMI (Diabetes Mellitus, Insulin Glucose Infusion in Acute Myocardial Infarction) Study Group. Prospective randomized study of intensive insulin treatment on longterm survival after acute myocardial infarction in patients with diabetes mellitus. *BMJ* 1997; 314: 1512–5.
128. Theroux P, Waters D, Halphen C, Debaisieux JC, Mizgala HF. Prognostic value of exercise testing soon after myocardial infarction. *N Engl J Med* 1979; 301: 341–50.
129. Davidson DM, Debusk RF. Prognostic value of a single exercise test 3 weeks after uncomplicated acute myocardial infarction. *Circulation* 1980; 61: 236–42.
130. Villella A, Maggioni AP, Villella M, et al, for the Gruppo Italiano per lo Studio della Sopravvivenza Nell'Infarto. Prognostic significance of maximal exercise testing after myocardial infarction treated with thrombolytic agents: the GISSI-2 data-base. *Lancet* 1995; 346: 523–9.
131. Basu S, Senior R, Dore C, Lahiri A. Value of thallium-201 imaging in detecting adverse cardiac events after myocardial infarction and thrombolysis: a follow-up of 100 consecutive patients. *BMJ* 1996; 313: 844–8.
132. Wood D, Durrington P, Poulter N, McInnes G, Rees A, Wray R, on behalf of the British Cardiac Society, British Hyperlipidemia Association, British Hypertension Society and British Diabetic Association. Joint British Recommendations on prevention of coronary heart disease in clinical practice. *Heart* 1999; 80 (suppl 2): S12–29.
133. Scottish Intercollegiate Guidelines Network. *Secondary Prevention of Coronary Heart Disease Following Myocardial Infarction: A National Clinical Guideline*. Edinburgh: SIGN, 2000. SIGN publication number 41. Available at: http://www.sign.ac.uk.
134. National Institute for Clinical Excellence (NICE). Prophylaxis for patients who have experienced a myocardial infarction; drug treatment, cardiac rehabilitation and dietary manipulation, 2001. Available at: http://www.nice.org.uk.
135. Kannel WB. Hypertension and the risk of cardiovascular disease. In Laragh JH, Brenner BM (eds). *Hypertension: Pathophysiology, Diagnosis and Management*. New York: Raven Press, 1990; pp 101–17.
136. Connolly DC, Elveback LR, Oxman HA. Coronary heart disease in residents of Rochester, Minnesota, 1950–1975, III: Effect of hypertension and its treatment on survival of patients with coronary artery disease. *Mayo Clin Proc* 1983; 58: 249–54.
137. Langford HG, Stamler J, Wessertheil-Smoller S, Prineas RJ. All cause mortality in the Hypertension Detection and Follow-up Program: findings for the whole cohort and for persons with less severe hypertension, with and without other traits related to risk of mortality. *Prog Cardiovasc Dis* 1986; 29: 29–54.
138. Heart Outcomes Prevention Evaluation Study Investigators. Effects of ramipril on cardiovascular and microvascular outcomes in people with diabetes mellitus: results of the HOPE study and MICRO-HOPE substudy. *Lancet* 2000; 355: 253–9.
139. Hansson L, Zanchetti A, Carruthers SG, et al, for the HOT Study Group. Effects of intensive blood-pressure lowering and low-dose aspirin in patients with hypertension: principal results of the Hypertension Optimal Treatment (HOT) randomized trial. *Lancet* 1998; 351: 1755–62.
140. Pekkanen J, Linn S, Heiss G, et al. Ten-year mortality from cardiovascular disease in relation to cholesterol level in men with and without pre-existing cardiovascular disease. *N Engl J Med* 1990; 322: 1700–7.
141. Scandinavian Simvastatin Survival Study Group. Randomized controlled trial of cholesterol lowering in 4444 patients with coronary heart disease: the Scandinavian Simvastatin Survival Study (4S). *Lancet* 1994; 344: 1383–9.
142. The Long-Term Intervention with Pravastatin in Ischaemic Disease (LIPID) Study Group. Prevention of cardiovascular events and death with pravastatin in patients with coronary heart disease and a broad range of initial cholesterol levels. *N Engl J Med* 1998; 339: 1349–57.
143. Sacks FM, Pfeffer MA, Moye LA, et al, for the Cholesterol and Recurrent Events Trial Investigators. The effect of pravastatin on coronary events after myocardial infarction in patients with average cholesterol levels. *N Engl J Med* 1996; 335: 1001–9.

144. Pyörälä K, Pedersen TR, Kjekshus J. The effect of cholesterol lowering with simvastatin on coronary artery disease in diabetic patients with coronary heart disease. *Diabetes* 1995; 44 (suppl): 35A.
145. Goldberg RB, Mellies MJ, Sacks FM, et al. Cardiovascular events and their reduction with pravastatin in diabetic and glucose-intolerant myocardial infarction survivors with average cholesterol levels; subgroup analysis in the cholesterol and recurrent events (CARE) trial. *Circulation* 1998; 98: 2513–9.
146. MRC/BHF Heart Protection Study of cholesterol lowering with simvastatin in 20536 high-risk individuals: a randomized placebo-controlled trial. *Lancet* 2002; 360; 7–22.
147. Rubins HB, Robins SJ, Collins D, et al, for the Veterans Affairs High-Density Lipoprotein Cholesterol Intervention Trial Study Group. Gemfibrozil for the secondary prevention of coronary heart disease in men with low levels of high-density lipoprotein cholesterol. *N Engl J Med* 1999; 34: 410–8.
148. The Diabetes Atherosclerosis Intervention Study Group. Effect of fenofibrate on progression of coronary-artery disease in type 2 diabetes: the Diabetes Atherosclerosis Intervention Study, a randomized study. *Lancet* 2001; 357: 905–10.
149. Scottish Intercollegiate Guidelines Network (SIGN). *Coronary Revascularization in the Management of Stable Angina Pectoris: A National Clinical Guideline*. Edinburg: SIGN, 1998. SIGN publication number 32. Available at: http://www.sign.ac.uk.
150. Thourani VH, Weintraub WS, Stein B, et al. Influence of diabetes mellitus on early and late outcome after coronary artery bypass grafting. *Ann Thorac Surg* 1999; 67: 1045–52.
151. Herlitz J, Wognsen GB, Emanuelsson H, et al. Mortality and morbidity in diabetic and nondiabetic patients during a 2-year period after coronary artery bypass grafting. *Diabetes Care* 1996; 19: 698–703.
152. Barzilay JI, Kronmal RA, Bittner V, Eaker E, Evans C, Foster ED. Coronary artery disease and coronary artery bypass grafting in diabetic patients aged > 65 years: report from the Coronary Artery Surgery Study (CASS) Registry. *Am J Cardiol* 1994; 74: 334–9.
153. Herlitz J, Wognsen GB, Karlson BW, et al. Mortality, mode of death and risk factors for death during 5 years after coronary artery bypass grafting among patients with and without a history of diabetes mellitus. *Coron Artery Dis* 2000; 11: 339–46.
154. Barsness GW, Peterson ED, Ohman EM, et al. Relationship between diabetes mellitus and long-term survival after coronary bypass and angioplasty. *Circulation* 1997; 96: 2551–66.
155. Halon DA, Merdler A, Flugelman MY, et al. Late-onset heart failure as a mechanism for adverse long-term outcome in diabetic patients undergoing revascularization (a 13 year report from the Lady Davis Carmel medical Centre Registry). *Am J Cardiol* 2000; 85: 1420–6.
156. O'Keefe JH, Blackstone EH, Sergeant P, McCallister BD. The optimal mode of coronary revascularization for diabetics. A risk-adjusted long-term study comparing coronary angioplasty and coronary artery bypass surgery. *Eur Heart J* 1998; 19: 1601–3.
157. Hirotani T, Kameda T, Kumamoto T, Shirota S, Yamano M. Effects of coronary artery bypass grafting using internal mammary arteries for diabetic patients. *J Am Coll Cardiol* 1999; 34: 532–8.
158. Tatoulis J, Royse AG, Buxton BF, et al. The radial artery in coronary surgery: a 5-year experience—clinical and angiography results. *Ann Thorac Surg* 2002; 73: 143–7.
159. Reddy VS, Parikh SM, Drinkwater DC Jr, et al. Morbidity after procurement of radial arteries in diabetic patients and the elderly undergoing coronary revascularization. *Ann Thorac Surg* 2002; 73: 803–7.
160. Abraham R, Karamanoukian HL, Jajkowski MR, et al. Does avoidance of cardiopulmonary bypass decrease the incidence of stroke in diabetics undergoing coronary surgery? *Heart Surg Forum* 2001; 4: 135–40.
161. Stein B, Weintraub WS, Gebhart SP, et al. Influence of diabetes mellitus on early and late outcome after percutaneous transluminal coronary angioplasty. *Circulation* 1995; 91: 979–89.
162. Kip KE, Faxon DP, Detre KM, Yeh W, Kelsey SF, Currier JW, for the The National, Heart, Lung and Blood Institute Percutaneous Transluminal Coronary Angioplasty Registry. Coronary angioplasty in diabetic patients. *Circulation* 1996; 94; 1804–6.
163. Kurbaan AS, Bowker TJ, Isley CD, Sigwart U, Rickards AF, on behalf of the CABRI (Coronary Angioplasty versus Bypass Revascularization Investigation) Investigators. Differences in mortality of the CABRI diabetic and nondiabetic populations and its relation to coronary artery disease and the revascularization mode. *Am J Cardiol* 2001; 87; 947–50.
164. Mercado N, Boersma E, Wijns W, et al. Clinical and quantitative coronary angiographic predictors of coronary restenosis: a comparative analysis from the balloon to-stent era. *J Am Coll Cardiol* 2001; 38: 645–52.
165. Johansen O, Abdelnoor M, Brekke M, Seljeflot I, Hostmark AT, Arnesen H. Predictors of restenosis after coronary angioplasty. A study on demographic and metabolic variables. *Scand Cardiovsac J* 2001; 35: 86–91.
166. Serruys PW, de Jaegere P, Kiemeneij F, et al, for the Benestent Study Group. A comparison of balloon-expansable-stent implantation with balloon angioplasty in patients with coronary artery disease. *N Engl J Med* 1994; 25: 489–95.
167. Fischman DL, Leon MB, Baim DS, et al, for the Stent Restenosis Study Investigators. A randomized comparison of coronary-stent placement and balloon angioplasty in the treatment of coronary artery disease. *N Engl J Med* 1994; 25: 496–501.
168. Serruys PW, van Hout B, Bonnier H, et al. Randomized comparison of implantation of heparin-coated stents with balloon angioplasty in selected patients with coronary artery disease (Benestent II). *Lancet* 1998; 352: 673–81.
169. Huynh T, Eisenberg MJ, Deligonul U, et al. Coronary stenting in diabetic patients: results from ROSETTA registry. *Am Heart J* 2001; 142: 960–4.
170. Carrozza JP Jr, Kuntz RE, Fishman RF, Baim DS. Restenosis after arterial injury caused by coronary stenting in patients with diabetes mellitus. *Ann Intern Med* 1993; 118: 344–9.
171. Elezi S, Kastrati A Pache J, et al. Diabetes mellitus and the clinical and angiographic outcome after coronary artery stent placement. *J Am Coll Cardiol* 1998; 32: 1866–73.
172. Gum PA, O'Keefe JH Jr, Borkon AM, et al. Bypass surgery versus coronary angioplasty for revascularization of treated diabetic patients. *Circulation* 1997; 96 (9, suppl): II7–10.
173. Weintraub WS, Stein B, Kosinki A, et al. Outcome of coronary bypass surgery versus coronary angioplasty in

diabetic subjects with multi-vessel disease. *J Am Coll Cardiol* 1998; 31: 10–9.
174. Garratt KN, Brady PA, Hassinger NL, Grill DE, Terzie A, Holmes DR Jr. Sulfonylurea drugs increase early mortality in patients with diabetes mellitus after direct angioplasty for acute myocardial infarction. *J Am Coll Cardiol* 1999; 33: 119–24.
175. Asakura Y, Suzuki M, Nonogi H, et al. Restenosis after percutaneous transluminal coronary angioplasty in patients with non-insulin-dependent diabetes mellitus (NIDDM). *J Cardiovasc Risk* 1998; 5: 331–4.
176. The EPIC Investigation. Use of monoclonal antibody directed against the platelet glycoprotein IIb/IIIa receptor in high-risk coronary angioplasty. *N Engl J Med* 1994; 330: 956–61.
177. The EPILOG Investigators. Platelet glycoprotein IIb/IIIa receptor blockade and low-dose heparin during percutaneous coronary revascularization. *N Engl J Med* 1997; 336: 1689–96.
178. IMPACT-II. Randomized placebo-controlled trial of the effect of eptifibatide on complications of percutaneous coronary intervention: Integrilin to Minimise Platelet Aggregation and Coronary Thrombosis-II. *Lancet* 1997; 349: 1422–8.
179. The CAPTURE Study. Randomized placebo-controlled trial of abciximab before and during coronary intervention in refractory unstable angina. *Lancet* 1997; 349: 1429–35.
180. The Bypass Angioplasty Investigators Study Group. Seven-year outcomes in the Bypass Angioplasty Revascularization Investigation (BARI) by treatment and diabetic status. *J Am Coll Cardiol* 2000; 35: 1122–9.
181. Detre KM, Lombardero MS, Brooks MM, et al. The effect of previous coronary-artery bypass surgery on the prognosis of patients with diabetes who have acute myocardial infarction. Bypass Angioplasty Revascularization Investigation Investigators. *N Engl J Med* 2000; 342: 989–97.
182. King SB III, Kosinski A, Guyton RA, Lembo NJ, Weintraub WS, for the Emory Angioplasty Versus Surgery Trial (EAST) Investigators. Eight year mortality in the Emory Angioplasty versus Surgery Trial (EAST). *J Am Coll Cardiol* 2000; 35: 1116–21.
183. Niles NW, McGrath PD, Malenka D, et al, for the Northern New England Cardiovascular Disease Study Group. Survival of patients with diabetes and multivessel coronary artery disease after surgical or percutaneous coronary revascularization: results of a large regional prospective study. *J Am Coll Cardiol* 2001; 37: 1008–15.
184. Abizaid A, Costa MA, Centemero M, et al, for the Arterial Revascularization Therapy Study Group. Clinical and economic impact of diabetes mellitus on percutaneous and surgical treatment of multivessel coronary disease patients: insights from the Arterial Revascularization Therapy Study (ARTS) trial. *Circulation* 2001; 104: 533–8.
185. Paillole C, Dahan M, Paycha F, Cohen A, Passa P, Gourgon R. Prevalence and significance of left ventricular filling abnormalities determined by Doppler echocardiography in young type 1 (insulin dependent) diabetic patients. *Am J Cardiol* 1990; 64: 1010–6.
186. Uusitupa M, Mustonen J, Laakso M, et al. Impairment of diastolic function in middle-aged Type 1 (insulin dependent) and Type 2 (non insulin dependent) diabetic patients free of cardiovascular disease. *Diabetologia* 1988; 31: 783–9.
187. Zarich SW, Nesto RW. Diabetic cardiomyopathy. *Am Heart J* 1989; 118: 1000–12.
188. Factor SM, Minese T, Sonnenblick EM. Clinical and morphological features of human hypertensive diabetic cardiomyopathy. *Am Heart J* 1980; 79: 446–58.
189. Fisher BM, Gillen G, Lindop GBM, Dargie HJ, Frier BM. Cardiac function and coronary arteriography in asymptomatic type-1 (insulin dependent) diabetic patients: Evidence for a specific diabetic heart disease. *Diabetologia* 1986; 29: 706–12.
190. Watschinger B, Brunner C, Wagner A, et al. Left ventricular diastolic impairment in type 1 diabetic patients with microalbuminuria. *Nephron* 1993; 63: 145–51.
191. Lagadic-Gossmann D, Buckler KJ, Le-Prigent K, Feuvray D. Altered Ca^{2+} handling in ventricular myocytes from diabetic rats. *Am J Physiol* 1996; 270: H1529–37.
192. Kim HW, Ch YS, Lee HR, Park SY, Kim YH. Diabetic alterations in cardiac sarcoplasmic reticulum Ca^{2+}-ATPase and phospholamban protein expression. *Life Sci.* 2001; 70: 367–79.
193. Rodrigues B, Cam MC, McNeill JH. Metabolic disturbances in diabetic cardiomyopathy. *Mol Cell Biol Biochem* 1998; 180: 53–7.
194. Remme JE, Swedberg K, for the Task Force for the Diagnosis and Treatment of Chronic Heart Failure, European Cardiac Society. Guidelines for the diagnosis and treatment of heart failure. *Eur Heart J* 2001; 22: 1527–60.
195. Scottish Intercollegiate Guidelines Network. *Diagnosis and Treatment of Heart Failure due to Left Ventricular Systolic Dysfunction: A National Clinical Guideline*. Edinburg: SIGN, 1999. SIGN publication number 35. Available at: http://www.sign.ac.uk.
196. Hunt SA, Baker DW, Chin MH, et al. ACC/AHA guidelines for the evaluation and management of chronic heart failure in the adult: executive summary. *J Heart Lung Transplant* 2002; 21: 189–203.
197. Lavine SJ, Gellman SD. Treatment of heart failure in patients with diabetes mellitus. *Drugs* 2002; 62: 285–307.
198. Dries DL, Sweitzer NK, Drazner MH, Stevenson LW, Gersh BJ. Prognostic impact of diabetes mellitus in patients with heart failure according to the etiology of left ventricular systolic dysfunction. *J Am Coll Cardiol* 2001; 38: 421–8.
199. Shindler DM, Kostis JB, Yusuf S, et al. Diabetes mellitus, a predictor of morbidity and mortality in the studies of left ventricular dysfunction (SOLVD) trials and registry. *Am J Cardiol* 1996; 77: 1017–20.
200. MERIT-HF Study Group. Effect of metaprolol CR/XL in chronic heart failure: Metaprolol CR/XL Randomized Intervention Trial in Congestive Heart Failure (MERIT-HF). *Lancet* 1999; 353: 2001–7.
201. CIBIS II Investigators. The Cardiac Insufficiency Bisoprolol Study II (CIBIS II): a randomized trial. *Lancet* 1999; 353: 9–13.
202. Australia/New Zealand Heart Failure Research Collaborative Group. Randomized, placebo-controlled trial of carvedilol in patients with congestive heart failure due to ischemic heart disease. *Lancet* 1997; 349: 375–80.
203. Packer M, Coats AJS, Fowler MB, et al, for the Carvedilol Prospective Randomized Cumulative Study Group. Effect of carvedilol on survival in severe heart failure. *N Engl J Med* 2001; 344; 1651–8.
204. Pitt B, Poole-Wilson P, Segal R, et al. Effect of losartan compared with captopril on mortality in patients with symptomatic heart failure: randomise trial—the

Lorsartan Heart Failure Survival Study (ELITE II). *Lancet* 2000; 355: 1582–7.
205. Cohn JN, Tognini G, for the Valsartan Heart Failure Trial Investigators. A randomized trial of the angiotensin receptor blocker valsartan in chronic heart failure (Val-HEFT). *N Engl J Med* 2001; 345: 1667–75.
206. Pitt B, Zannad F, Remme WJ, et al, for the Randomized Aldactone Evaluation Study Investigators. The effect of spironolactone on morbidity and mortality in patients with severe heart failure. *N Engl J Med* 1999; 341: 709–17.
207. Munoz E, Lonquist JL, Radovancevic B, et al. Long-term results in diabetic patients undergoing heart transplantation. *J Heart Lung Transplant* 1992; 11: 943–9.
208. Vreede-Swagemakers J, Gorgels A, Dubois-Arbouw W, et al. Out-of-hospital cardiac arrest in the 1990's: a population-based study in the Maastricht area on incidence, characteristics and survival. *J Am Coll Cardiol* 1997; 30: 1500–5.
209. Jouven X, Desnos M, Guerot C, Ducimetière P. Predicting sudden death in the population: the Paris Prospective Study 1. *Circulation* 1999; 99: 1978–83.
210. Balkau B, Jouven X, Ducimetière P, et al. Diabetes as a risk factor for sudden death. *Lancet* 1999; 354: 1968–70.
211. Curb JD, Rodriguez BL, Burchfiel CM, Abbot RD, Chiu D, Yano K. Sudden death, impaired glucose tolerance and diabetes in Japanese American men. *Circulation* 1995; 91: 2591–5.
212. Siscovick DS, Raghunathan TE, King I, et al. Dietary intake and cell membrane levels of long-chain n-3 polyunsaturated fatty acids and the risk of primary cardiac arrest. *JAMA* 1995; 274: 1363–7.
213. Kannel WB. Update on the role of cigarette smoking in coronary artery disease. *Am Heart J* 1981; 101: 319–28.
214. Hämäläinen H, Luurila OJ, Kallio V, Knuts LR, Arstila M, Hakkila J. Long term reduction in sudden deaths after a multifactorial intervention programme in patients with myocardial infarction: 10 year results of a controlled investigation. *Eur Heart J* 1989; 10: 55–62.
215. Adler AI, Stratton IM, Neil HA, et al, for the United Kingdom Prospective Diabetes Study Group. Association of systolic blood pressure with macrovascular and microvascular complications of type-2 diabetes (UKDPS 36). *BMJ* 2000; 321: 412–9.
216. The Hypertension in Diabetes Study Group: Hypertension in Diabetes Study II (HDS). Increased risk of cardiovascular complications in hypertensive type 2 diabetic patients. *J Hypertens* 1993; 11: 319–25.
217. United Kingdom Prospective Diabetes Study Group. Tight blood pressure control and risk of macrovascular and microvascular complications in type-2 diabetes. UKPDS 38. *BMJ* 1998; 317: 703–13.
218. Collins R, MacMahon. Blood pressure, antihypertensive drug treatment and the risks of stroke and of coronary heart disease. *Br Med Bull* 1994; 50: 272–98.
219. Dahlöf B, Lindholm LH, Hansson L, Scherstén B, Ekbom T, Wester P-O. Morbidity and mortality in the Swedish Trial in Old Patients with Hypertension (STOP-hypertension). *Lancet* 1991; 338, 1281–5.
220. SHEP Cooperative Research Group. Prevention of stroke by antihypertensive drug treatment in older persons with isolated systolic hypertension. Final results of the Systolic Hypertension in the Elderly Program (SHEP). *JAMA* 1991; 265: 3255–64.
221. Ramsay LE, Williams B, Johnstone DG, et al. Guidelines for the management of hypertension: report of the third working party of the British Hypertension Society. *J Hum Hypertension* 1999; 13: 569–92.
222. Department of Health. National Service Framework for Diabetes. Available at: http://www.doh.gov.uk/nsf/diabetes.
223. Scottish Intercollegiate Guidelines Network (SIGN). *Management of Diabetes: A National Clinical Guideline*. Edinburgh: SIGN, 2001. SIGN publication number 55. Available at: http://www.sign.ac.uk.
224. US Government Printing Office. *The Sixth Report of the Joint National Committee on Detection, Evaluation, and Treatment of High Blood Pressure*. Washington, DC: US Government Printing Office, November 1997. NIH publication no 98–4080.
225. Blood Pressure Lowering Treatment Trialists' Collaboration. Effects of ACE inhibitors, calcium antagonists, and other blood-pressure-lowering drugs: results of prospectively designed overviews of randomized trials. *Lancet* 2000; 356; 1955–64.
226. Porter P, Psaty BM, Alderman MH, et al. Health outcomes associated with calcium antagonists compared with other first-line antihypertensive therapies: a meta-analysis of randomized controlled trials. *Lancet* 2000; 356: 1949–54.
227. UK Prospective Diabetes Study Group: Efficacy of atenolol and captopril in reducing risk of macrovascular and microvascular compliactions in type 2 diabetes: UKPDS 39. *BMJ* 1998; 317: 713–20.
228. Niskanen L, Hedner T, Hansson L, Lanke J, Niklason A, for the CAPPP Study Group. Reduced cardiovascular morbidity and mortality in hypertensive diabetic patients on first-line therapy with an ACE inhibitor compared with a diuretic/β-blocker-based treatment regimen. *Diabetes Care* 2001; 24: 2091–6.
229. Brenner BM, Cooper ME, de Zeeuw D, et al, for the RENAAL Study Investigators. Effects of lorsartan on renal and cardiovascular outcomes in patients with type 2 diabetes and neuropathy. *N Engl J Med* 2001; 345: 861–9.
230. Parving HH, Lehnert H, Brochner-Mortensen J, Gomis R, Andersen S, Arner P, for the Irbesartan in Patients with Diabetes and Microalbuminuria Study Group. The effect of irbesartan on the development of diabetic nephropathy in patients with type 2 diabetes. *N Engl J Med* 2001; 345: 870–8.
231. Lewis EJ, Hunsicker LG, Clarke WR, et al, for the Collaborative Study Group. Renoprotective effect of the angiotensin-receptor antagonist irbesartan in patients with nephropathy due to type 2 diabetes. *N Engl J Med* 2001; 345: 851–60.
232. Lindholm LH, Ibsen H, Dahlof B, et al, for the LIFE Study Group. Cardiovascular morbidity and mortality in patients with diabetes in the Lorsartan Intervention For Endpoint reduction in hypertension study (LIFE): a randomized trial against atenolol. *Lancet* 2002; 359: 1004–10.
233. Yusuf S, Sleight P, Pogue J, Bosch J, Davies R, Dagenais G, for the Heart Outcomes Prevention Evaluation Study Investigators. Effects of an angiotensin-converting-enzyme inhibitor, ramipril, on death from cardiovascular causes, myocardial infarction, and stroke in high-risk patients. *N Engl J Med* 2000; 342: 145–53.
234. Shepherd J, Cobbe SM, Ford I, et al, for the West of Scotland Coronary Prevention Study Group. Prevention of coronary heart disease with pravastatin in men

with hypercholesterolaemia. *N Engl J Med* 1995; 333: 1301–7.

235. Fontbonne A, Eschwege E, Cambien F, et al. Hypertriglyceridaemia as a risk factor of coronary artery disease mortality in subjects with impaired glucose tolerance or diabetes. Results from the 11 year-follow-up of the Paris prospective Study. *Diabetologia* 1989; 32: 300–4.
236. Stratton IM, Adler AI, Neil HA, et al, on behalf of the United Kingdom Prospective Diabetes Study Group. Association of glycaemia with macrovascular and microvascular complications of type-2 diabetes (UKPDS 35). *BMJ* 2000; 321: 405–12.
237. The Diabetes Control and Complications Trial Research Group. The effect of intensive treatment of diabetes on the development and progression of long-term complications in insulin-dependent diabetes mellitus. *N Engl J Med* 1993; 329: 977–86.
238. The Diabetes Control and Complications Trial Research Group. Effect of intensive diabetes management on macrovascular events and risk factors in the diabetes control and complication trial. *Am J Cardiol* 1995; 75: 894–903.
239. UK Prospective Diabetes Study Group. Effect of intensive blood-glucose control with metformin on complications in overweight patients with type 2 diabetes (UKPDS 34). *Lancet* 1998; 352: 854–65.
240. Engler RL, Yellon DM. Sulphonylurea K_{ATP} blockade in type 2 diabetes and preconditioning in cardiovascular disease. Time for reconsideration. *Circulation* 1996; 94: 2297–301.
241. Cleveland JC, Meldrum DR, Cain BS, Banarjee A, Harken AH. Oral sulphonylurea hypoglycemic agents prevent ischaemic preconditioning in human myocardium. *Circulation* 1997; 96: 29–32.
242. UK Prospective Diabetes Study (UKPDS) Group. Intensive blood-glucose control with sulphonylureas or insulin compared with conventional treatment and risk of complications in patients with type 2 diabetes (UKPDS 33). *Lancet* 1998; 352: 837–53.
243. Dierkx RI, van de Hoek W, Hoekstra JB, et al. Smoking and diabetes mellitus. *Neth J Med* 1996; 48: 150–62.
244. Steering Committee of the Physicians' Health Study Research Group. Final report on the aspirin component of the ongoing Physicians' Health Study. *N Engl J Med* 1989; 321: 129–35.

83

Arterial Hypertension in Diabetes: Etiology and Treatment

George L. Bakris*, Nauman Tarif†, and Henry R. Black*

Rush Presbyterian/St. Luke's Medical Centre, Chicago, IL, USA, and †King Fiassel University, Riyadh, Saudi Arabia

INCIDENCE AND PREVALENCE OF HYPERTENSION IN DIABETES

The most recent data indicate that about 12% of Americans have both diabetes and hypertension [1–3]. The prevalence of diabetes has been steadily increasing around the world over the past decade, primarily accounted for by increases in type 2, rather than type 1, diabetes (Figure 1). With the significant reduction in CV deaths that has occurred over the past few decades, people are living longer [5]. This observation coupled with the increasing prevalence of type 2 diabetes has resulted in an increasing number of people with diabetes who require renal replacement therapy, i.e. dialysis (Figure 2). This is evidenced by trends in the United States Renal Data Service (USRD) over the past two decades, where the percentage of people requiring dialysis secondary to treatment for diabetes has increased from 27% in 1982 to almost 50% in 2000 [6]. Similar trends are also evident in other countries [7].

Much of the increased prevalence of type 2 diabetes as well as hypertension is likely related to the global rise in obesity [8–10]. The influence of obesity on the development of hypertension is exemplified by a study of 2437 newly diagnosed individuals with type 2 diabetes, who demonstrated an earlier onset of hypertension (early onset: 18–44 years; late onset: >44 years of age) strongly associated with the presence of higher body mass index (BMI; 39 kg/m^2 vs. 33 kg/m^2), female sex, and diastolic hypertension [11]. Weight loss is well known to reduce both the risk of new-onset type 2 diabetes and the level of blood pressure [12–14].

The prevalence of hypertension is twofold higher among those with diabetes as compared to those without diabetes [15, 16]. Yet, the incidence of CV (CV) events is sixfold higher in those with diabetes and accounts for more than half of the deaths of people with diabetes receiving end-stage renal disease (ESRD) within the first year of starting dialysis [17–20]. This increase in macrovascular and microvascular complications including retinopathy, need for dialysis and associated CV mortality in those with diabetes could be reduced by lowering blood pressure to within the current recommended goal of <130/80 mmHg [4, 21].

The prevalence of hypertension is higher in those with type 2 compared to type 1 diabetes [22]. This higher prevalence of hypertension in type 2 diabetes was noted as early as 1967 when Pell and D'Alonzo reported a 50% higher prevalence than in matched nondiabetic controls [16]. Ritz and coworkers also showed a prevalence of hypertension of 70% among his cohort of people with type 2 diabetes with normoalbuminuria [23]. Similarly Fuller in 1094 patients with type 1 diabetes and 2642 with type 2 diabetes evaluated for WHO Multinational Study of Vascular Disease in Diabetes reported a prevalence of hypertension of 41.9% in those with type 1 diabetes and of 46.8% in those with type 2 diabetes [24]. It should be noted that isolated or predominantly systolic hypertension, an independent risk factor for CV death, is more common in type 2 diabetes compared to those without diabetes, with as many as two thirds of the individuals with type 2 diabetes having systolic hypertension in one series [25–27].

International Textbook of Diabetes Mellitus, Third Edition. Edited by R. A. DeFronzo, E. Ferrannini, H. Keen, and P. Zimmet.
 ISBN: 0-471-48655-8.

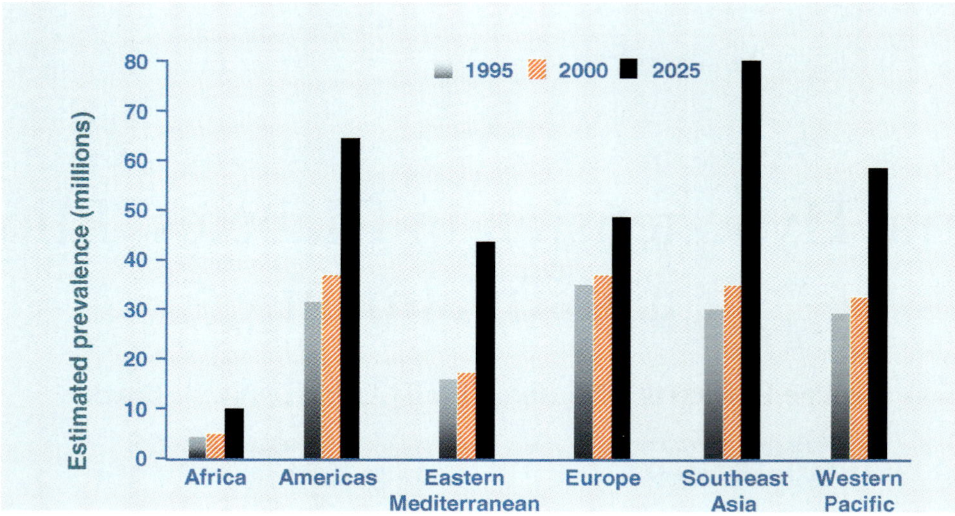

Figure 1 Current and projected prevalence rates for diabetes worldwide. (© Copyright World Health Organization (WHO) [1])

ALBUMINURIA AND HYPERTENSION

Microalbuminuria (MA), i.e. <300 mg albumin/day, is a well-known indicator of vascular dysfunction and an independent CV risk factor associated with a higher prevalence of hypertension in type 2 diabetes [28–32]. Studies by Clausen and colleagues in normotensive, nondiabetic individuals noted that those with MA had a markedly blunted vasodilatory response to nitroglycerine as well as following prolonged ischemia compared to those with albumin excretion in the normal range [30]. This coupled with earlier studies strongly suggests that MA is an indicator of vascular dysfunction, defined as reduced vasodilation in response to stimuli such as nitroprusside [33, 34].

Diabetic patients with MA have an abnormal circadian variation in blood pressure as exemplified by the absence of nocturnal dipping of blood pressure, while normoalbuminuric hypertensive diabetic patients have a normal diurnal variation [35–39]. MA hypertensive type 2 diabetic patients fail to "dip" at night to levels of systolic blood pressure below 120 mmHg [40]. Even in type 2 diabetic patients with a normal circadian blood pressure pattern, those with MA had significantly higher 24-h mean arterial pressures (MAPs), though still in the normal range. Although unusual, MA and the loss of nocturnal dipping of blood pressure also occurs in type 1 diabetic patients [39,41,42]. In these patients, MA is associated with higher nocturnal blood pressure and signs of autonomic dysfunction, such as increased heart rate variability and pupillary dilation [41].

In children with type 1 diabetes, the relationship between glycemic control and development of MA and

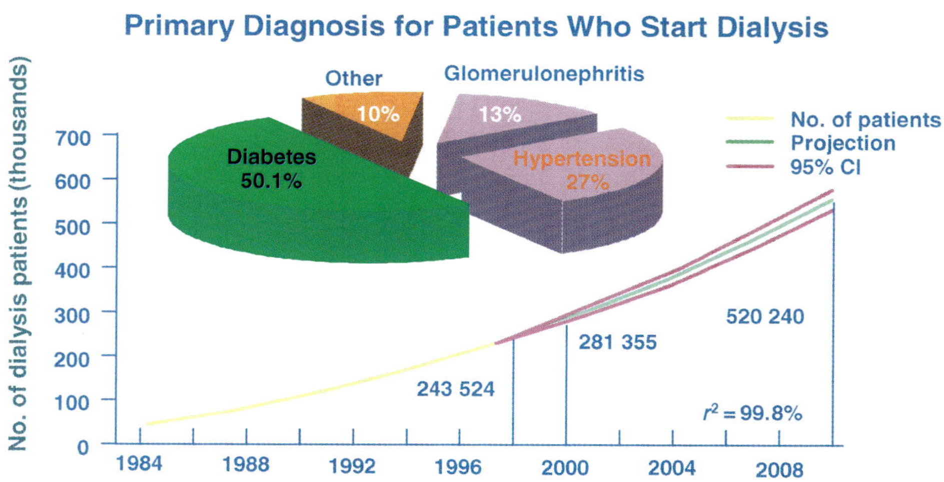

Figure 2 Diabetes: the most common cause of ESRD. (Reprinted from American Journal of Kidney Diseases, 39 (Suppl. 1), S1-S231, © 2002 with permission from National Kidney Foundation [4])

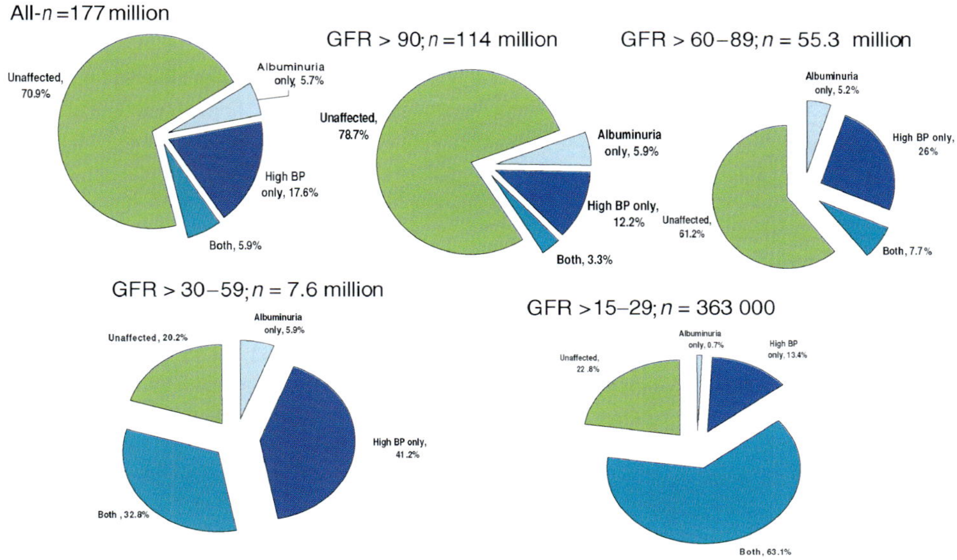

Figure 3 Prevalence of albuminuria and high blood pressure (%), NHANES III. (Reprinted from American Journal of Kidney Diseases, 39 (Suppl. 1), S1–S231, © 2002 with permission from National Kidney Foundation [4])

hypertension is clear. In one study, 12.9% of 494 patients developed MA after a median follow-up of 5 years. Poor glycemic control was the main determinant for those who developed MA and hypertension (BP > 140/90 mmHg) and MA occurred before significant elevations in blood pressure were noted [43]. This supports data from other studies in both type 1 and type 2 diabetic individuals [such as the Diabetes Control and Complications Trial (DCCT), the VA trial, and the United Kingdom Prospective Diabetes Study (UKPDS)] that intensive glycemic control can prevent increases in blood pressure and development of MA [44–46].

The prevalence of albuminuria (≥300 mg/day) associated with the presence of hypertension, and magnitude of renal insufficiency, is shown in Figure 3. Using the Joint National Committee (JNC V) definition of hypertension (BP > 140/90 mmHg), the Steno diabetes group noted that the prevalence of hypertension among 1506 people, with either type 1 or type 2 diabetes, was lowest in those with normoalbuminuria, i.e. <30 mg albumin/day, and highest in those with macroalbuminuria [22]. Other studies showed that those with the highest level of albumin excretion are at the highest risk not only for renal disease progression but also for coronary artery disease events and stroke [21, 47–50] (Figure 4).

PATHOGENESIS

Any discussion regarding pathogenetic factors that contribute to the development of hypertension in diabetes is complicated by the fact that hypertension and diabetes are both frequently associated with obesity, which may be an important etiologic factor for both of these powerful CV risk factors [52]. In National Health and Nutrition Examination Survey III (NHANES III), for example, the prevalence of hypertension is approximately 50% and type 2 diabetes occurs in more than 10% among those with BMI of >30 kg/m^2 [2].

Numerous studies demonstrate that subjects with essential hypertension, even when they do not have clinical

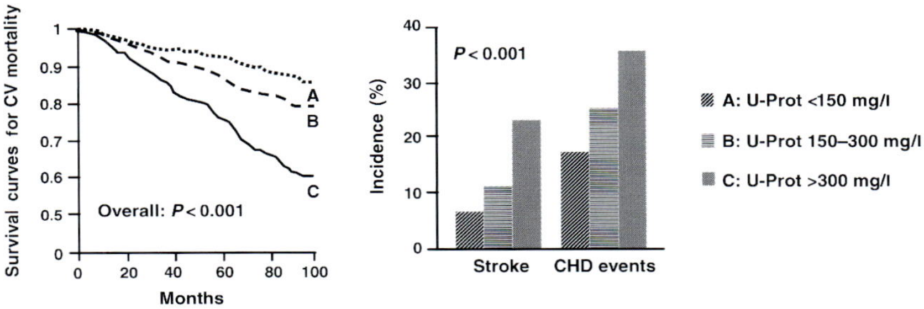

Figure 4 Proteinuria predicts stroke and coronary heart disease events in type 2 diabetes. U-Port = urinary protein concentration; CHD = Coronary heart disease. (Adapted by permission of the American Heart Association [51])

diabetes, have more insulin resistance and impaired glucose tolerance, and have a higher risk for developing type 2 diabetes than do normotensive individuals [53–58]. In the San Antonio Heart Study, where almost 9% of the 1093 normotensive individuals developed hypertension, those who became hypertensive had both higher fasting insulin levels and levels of insulin secretion 30 min after an oral glucose tolerance test [59]. Each of the factors that contribute is discussed separately.

Genetic Factors

There is clear epidemiological evidence to support a genetic predisposition for development of diabetes and hypertension in specific ethnic groups such as Native American Indians and African Americans [60–71]. An attempt to isolate the genes responsible for development of hypertension, however, has not been very fruitful. While genes specific for rare disorders associated with hypertension have been identified, the polygenic associations to truly alter the level of blood pressure have not been fully characterized [72].

Genes associated with components of the renin–angiotensin–aldosterone system (RAAS) have been linked to a predisposition for development of hypertension and modification of CV and renal risk [73, 74]. Studies such as those of Fagerudd et al. noted that parents of 73 people with type 2 diabetes with nephropathy were more likely to have essential hypertension than those of the control group without evidence of nephropathy [75]. These investigators also reported that CV morbidity and mortality was higher in the parents of those with type 2 diabetes and that fathers of diabetic patients homozygous for the I-allele [II] of the ACE-ID polymorphism had fewer myocardial infarctions [76]. Additionally, Earle and Viberti showed family clustering of coronary heart disease in parents of type 1 diabetic patients with nephropathy [77].

Another *RAAS* gene extensively studied is the angiotensinogen gene (*AGT*). Jeunemaitre et al. found a higher frequency of *AGT* gene variation at M235T location in hypertensive individuals than in normotensive controls [78]. It is, however, unclear whether the *AGT* gene M235T variant is responsible for development of hypertension or whether other additional variants may also impart the risk. Moreover, studies by other investigators cast doubt on the contribution of this allele to the genesis of hypertension. For example, Bengtsson et al. did not find that the *AGT* gene conferred any increased risk for nephropathy or hypertension [79].

The angiotensin-converting enzyme gene (*ACE*) located on chromosome 17 has also been extensively studied. The presence of deletion homozygosity (DD) of this gene has emerged as a risk factor for the development of hypertension and nephropathy in people with type 2 diabetes [80–82]. This gene also has implications for the choice of therapy. Two separate investigators have demonstrated that the presence of the DD allele was associated with greater antiproteinuric response to ACE inhibitors in people with type 2 diabetes [83–85].

Other genes have been associated with the development of hypertension late in the course of type 2 diabetes and are likely more prevalent in people with type 2 diabetes who have developed nephropathy [86]. One such gene is the G825T allele of the β-3 chain of G-protein [87]. A higher frequency of the T allele was found in people with type 2 diabetes on dialysis compared to the nondiabetic individuals on dialysis [88].

Alterations in genes that modulate β-receptors have been described in people with hypertension prone to develop diabetes. Specifically, mutations in β_3-adrenergic receptor gene are more prevalent in people with abdominal obesity, higher insulin levels, and higher blood pressure [89]. Additionally, those who either have a β_1-adrenergic receptor gene homozygous for Arg389 allele or are homozygous carriers of the Arg16 allele of β_2-adrenergic receptors have a higher likelihood of being hypertensive and having the dysmetabolic syndrome [60, 90].

It is clear from these studies that hypertension in the person with diabetes is a polygenic disorder. Moreover, those who develop sequelae of diabetes, such as nephropathy, do not necessarily have hypertension. Thus, gene interactions occur and may account for some of the differences seen in the natural history of diabetes on renal and CV outcomes [91]. The dissociation between hypertension and type 2 diabetes has been clearly characterized in certain Native American tribes of the United States, such as Pima Indians, Zuni Indians, and Alaskan natives, in which diabetic renal disease was not associated with hypertension [91–93]. Various investigators evaluated insulin levels, and presence of insulin resistance with the prevalence of hypertension in normotensive and nondiabetic Pima Indians, Whites, and African Americans [94]. Pima Indians had higher fasting plasma insulin levels than did Whites or Blacks, but the concentrations did not correlate with the presence of hypertension.

The aforementioned data on various genetic markers and their varied contribution to CV and renal risk clearly indicate that we need more studies to dissect out how these genes interact with environmental factors such as diet, lifestyle, and birth environment that leads to decreased nephron number to increase risk. One such example would include the interaction of certain ACE genotypes with the intrauterine environment (the Barker hypothesis) leading to a smaller birth weight and lower than normal numbers of nephrons. As a result of fewer nephrons, it has been noted that there is an increasing propensity to develop renal insufficiency and hypertension [95]. Thus, as of this writing there is no clear distinction between the importance of susceptibility genes and the interaction of such genes with specific environmental factors such as nephron number.

Ion Transport Homeostasis

Substantial evidence from animal and human investigation supports an association between the presence of hypertension and changes in intracellular pH and cellular electrolyte composition. The key cellular changes are the increase in the intracellular sodium and calcium and the decrease in magnesium [96–110]. These changes in the cellular milieu are linked to altered function of certain membrane ion transporters such as the Na^+/H^+ antiporter, Na/K-ATPase, Mg^{2+}/Na^+ exchanger, Ca^{2+}/H^+ exchanger, Ca^{2+}-ATPase, and others [111–119]. Evidence for genetic linkage of these transporters comes from the studies of parents of people with type 2 diabetes [77, 120]. Mead et al. measured the Na^+/Li^+ flux rate and kinetics in nondiabetic first-degree relatives of people with diabetic nephropathy and the relatives of people with type 2 diabetes but no nephropathy [121]. They found a 60% higher rate in the nondiabetic relatives of those with nephropathy and only a 20% higher rate in the relatives of those with diabetes but no nephropathy. This suggests that familial clustering of the Na^+/Li^+ countertransporter occurs in those with a higher likelihood of developing nephropathy, a hypothesis supported by data from other studies [122, 123].

Elevated Na^+/H^+ antiporter activity has been associated with diabetic nephropathy and hypertension in both type 1 and type 2 diabetic patients [104, 107, 124–126]. However, elevations of Na^+/H^+ antiporter activity may also be due to hyperglycemia or renal failure [110]. This antiporter is affected by several factors including insulin and sodium delivery to the tubule and is a key regulator of sodium homeostasis in those with diabetes or obese individuals with the dysmetabolic syndrome [127]. Na^+/H^+ antiporter activity was assessed in skin fibroblasts from 17 sibling pairs with type 2 diabetes and compared with 12 normal controls [107]. A strong familial concordance in V_{max}, intracellular pH, and buffering capacity of the Na^+/H^+ antiporter was noted in those with type 2 diabetes. They also noted that the Na^+/H^+ antiporter activity was greater in the subjects with higher albumin excretion rate than in the normoalbuminuric patients, thus confirming the association of this cellular phenotype with renal disease in diabetes. Blood pressure was not significantly different between probands and siblings, suggesting that the blood pressure in type 2 diabetes is not under the influence of this antiporter, unlike that of those with essential hypertension.

Alterations in the cellular calcium handling have also been postulated to be the key link that explains the co-existence between hypertension and insulin resistance [109, 111, 112, 128]. Insulin increases Ca^{2+}-ATPase activity after fasting in normal subjects and in the renal cortex of a rat model of type 2 diabetes [129, 130]. However, this stimulatory effect of both insulin and atrial natriuretic peptide on Ca^{2+}-ATPase pumps is attenuated over time. These data prompted the still unconfirmed concept that hormonal tolerance of the Ca^{2+}-ATPase pump in most people with type 2 diabetes contributes to the genesis of hypertension [129, 131].

Increases in intracellular calcium have been noted in offspring of people with either type 1 or type 2 diabetes who also have hypertension [132–136]. This increase in Ca^{2+} concentration is due to the reduction in plasma membrane calcium ATPase activity, modulation of Na^+/Ca^{2+} exchange, and increased Ca^{2+} flux across the plasma membrane.

SYMPATHETIC NERVOUS SYSTEM DYSFUNCTION

People with diabetes are known to have increased sympathetic tone. Moreover, there is a strong association between increased adrenergic activity and insulin levels [137, 138]. Increased sympathetic activity along with increased insulin levels contributes to increased sodium reabsorption by the proximal tubule, resulting in volume expansion and increased blood pressure [139–141]. The Steno diabetes group noted that most people with type 2 diabetes are volume expanded compared to those who are not diabetic [40].

Recent studies in animals demonstrated that the hormone leptin results in increased sympathetic outflow to the kidneys and to the hind limb vasculature, an effect similar to the sympathetic activity seen in obese hypertensive individuals [142, 143]. The role of leptin in renal diseases including diabetes has been recently reviewed and evaluated by several investigators who all noted high serum leptin levels in type 2 diabetic subjects [144–147]. Leptin, therefore, may be a factor in the genesis of hypertension in those with diabetes by increasing the sympathetic activity.

The etiologic role of leptin in essential or obesity-related hypertension is controversial and may be secondary to that of the RAAS. Nakata and colleagues observed that inhibition of the RAAS with losartan, when injected intracerebroventricularly, abolished sympathetically induced increases in blood pressure in the rat [148]. Other studies by Muntzel and colleagues demonstrate that hyperinsulinemia increases local angiotensin II levels in the brain, which modulate the increase in the sympathetic activity that results in hypertension [149]. To date, however, leptin has not been shown to be an independent factor responsible for increases in blood pressure in humans.

RENIN–ANGIOTENSIN–ALDOSTERONE SYSTEM

The contribution of the RAAS to the genesis of essential hypertension is beyond the scope of this chapter and has been recently reviewed by Burns [150]. The association of the RAAS with diabetic hypertension may be related to the fact that hyperglycemia is a stimulus for the intrarenal production of angiotensin II in both the proximal tubule and the glomerulus [151]. This local increase in RAAS is associated with enhanced sodium and water retention by the proximal tubule, leading to volume expansion and a decrease in the production of renin and angiotensin II, both of which have been observed in diabetes [152, 153]. However, angiotensin receptors are unregulated and have a greater affinity for the angiotensin II that is produced [154]. Moreover, non-ACE pathways also modulate activity of this system, and hence, could account for greater vasoconstriction and subsequent increase in blood pressure [155, 156].

NITRIC OXIDE

Endothelial dysfunction, defined as altered responsiveness to nitric oxide (NO) maintenance of vascular tone regulation, is perhaps one of the earliest cellular abnormalities noted in persons with diabetes. In the diabetic milieu of hyperglycemia, hyperinsulinemia, hypertension, and lipid abnormalities, there is an increased generation of advanced glycosylation end products (AGEs) [157–160]. It is likely that these factors lead to advancing atherosclerosis, a consequence and not the cause of endothelial dysfunction. MA is one of the earliest clinical manifestations of this vascular injury [161–163].

NO is a vasodilator produced by the endothelial cells and modulates the vascular tone in response to various stimuli. Loss or decreased production of NO is associated with the development of hypertension in both experimental animals and humans. In addition, NO has an important intrarenal regulatory function of modulating autoregulation and inhibiting renal tubular Na^+ reabsorption through inhibition of the Na/K-ATPase [164, 165].

Brands and Fitzgerald recently hypothesized that NO at the early stages of diabetes produces hyperfiltration and natriuresis leading to the activation of RAAS as a compensatory response [166]. The overall development of hypertension in these people depended on the state of the endothelium and the release of the homeostatic mechanisms controlled by NO.

NO can be inactivated by oxygen free radicals. Evidence to support this hypothesis comes from a study by Maejima et al. who examined the role of free radicals in NO regulation in 129 diabetic subjects and 76 normal controls [167]. The groups were found to have similar basal levels of NO_2; however, the levels of NO_3 were significantly higher in the diabetic subjects. This further correlated with the presence of higher lipid peroxides and microvascular abnormalities in that group. Further evidence comes from a study using human coronary endothelial cells incubated in a hyperglycemic, insulinopenic, hyperglucagonemic milieu. This resulted in decreased production of NO compared to controls [168].

In addition to these studies, there is an enormous literature concerning NO generation and quenching in patients with diabetes, the role of AGEs, and many other cytokines that affect processes of atherosclerosis that cannot be covered in this book; however, the reader is referred to some reviews and original studies [160, 169–172].

TREATMENT TRIALS IN HYPERTENSION

At the time the diagnosis of type 2 diabetes is made, more than 40% of people have an elevated arterial pressure (>140/90 mmHg), along with the presence of microvascular complications [173]. In the UKPDS, the prevalence of hypertension was around 40%. Hypertension itself is a major risk factor for the occurrence of CV events, including coronary heart disease and stroke as well as associated mortality, and in the presence of diabetes this risk is more than doubled [174]. This is supported by many epidemiological studies including the Multiple Risk Factor Intervention Trial (MRFIT) where 5625 diabetic men were found to have a higher risk of CV death at all levels of blood pressure even extending into the normotensive range after a mean follow-up of 12 years [175]. Moreover, two recent meta-analyses document that lowering of blood pressure in all people regardless of agents reduces the risk of CV events [176, 177].

In prospectively randomized intervention trials, treatment of the diabetic cohort is generally associated with greater risk reduction for CV events compared to the general population. This is exemplified by a *post hoc* analysis of the 583 participants with type 2 diabetes in the Systolic Hypertension in Elderly People (SHEP) trial, which showed a decrease in major CV events by 34% in those who received a thiazide diuretic compared to placebo at 5 years [178, 179]. Additionally, in the Systolic Hypertension in Europe [Syst-Eur] trial, a *post hoc* analysis of the 492 participants with type 2 diabetes randomized to a dihydropyridine calcium-channel blocker (DHP-CCB) showed a reduction in CV mortality, all CV events, and stroke by 70%, 62%, and 69%, vs. 16%, 25%, and 36%, respectively, in nondiabetic subjects [180]. These trials, taken together with other prospective trials, indicate that a *post hoc* analysis of a diabetic cohort in any given trial demonstrates greater risk reduction for CV events, renal disease progression, and stroke compared to the nondiabetic participants in any given trial [181–183].

A cost-effectiveness analysis of intensive therapies in people with diabetes from the SHEP trial, using a model analysis, showed that intensive treatment of hypertension was more cost saving than was intensive glycemic control [172]. Similar results were seen in the cost-effectiveness

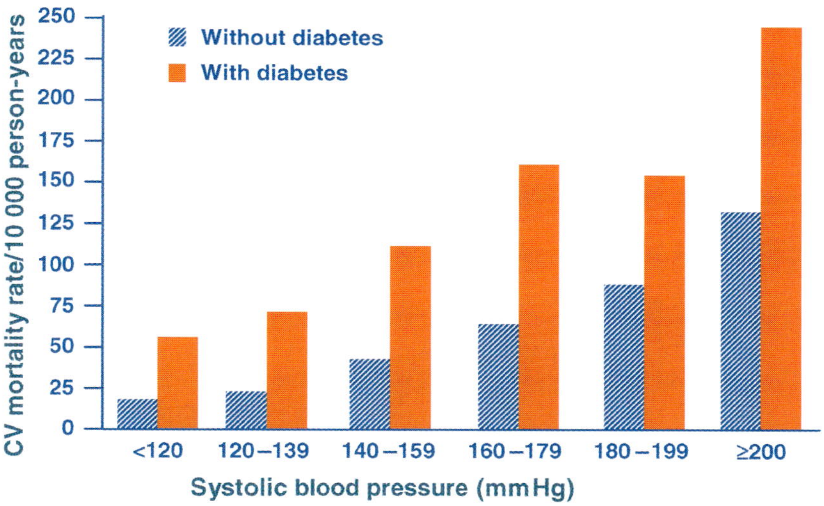

Figure 5 Association of systolic blood pressure and CV death in type 2 diabetes. (Reprinted with permission from Elsevier Science (The Lancet, Vol 356, 2000, 1955–64 [175])

analyses of UKPDS. [184, 185]. Moreover, separate analyses using data from the Captopril Trial in type 1 diabetes as well as JNC VI recommended blood pressure goals showed the same cost-saving benefits and reduced morbidity with intensive control [186, 187].

GOAL BLOOD PRESSURE

In people with diabetes a blood pressure goal of <130/85 mmHg was put forth by JNC VI and WHO reports prior to the year 2000 [188, 189]. This recommendation was based on the results of only a few *post hoc* analyses of trials and observational studies, which showed that lower blood pressure at around such levels was associated with lower CV mortality (Figure 5). Since 1999, other groups from around the world have lowered the goal to <130/80 mmHg in light of evidence from recently completed trials that reflect the greater predominance *systolic hypertension* in those with type 2 diabetes and the result of lower diastolic pressures being associated with better outcomes [4, 190–192] (Table 1). However, a close look at the data of achieved blood pressures observed in randomized trials of advanced renal disease and CV outcomes makes it apparent that <140/80 mmHg is the most defensible blood pressure goal (Figure 6). One must remember that the subgroups with the best outcomes at the lowest pressures in all these trials are those with the least amount of disease burden.

While the goal blood pressure for those with type 2 diabetes is now recommended at <130/80 mmHg, a 10-year CV incidence study of more than 500 people with type 1 diabetes by Orchard and colleagues suggests that the goal blood pressure be <120/80 mmHg to maximally reduce CV risk [193]. Thus, age and preexisting vascular disease may have a bearing on the needed blood pressure goal. This is further exemplified by the results of the MICRO-HOPE study of 3577 type 2 diabetic participants [194]. Results from this trial also suggest that blood pressure lowering to levels around 120/80 mmHg was associated with a decrease in CV events by 22% and in microvascular complications including retinopathy and nephropathy, defined as progression to MA, by 16%. It should be noted that while most of these participants were "normotensive" by usual standards (BP <140/90 mmHg) the intervention group as a whole achieved mean blood pressures around 134/82 mmHg.

The argument of lower blood pressure goals comes from over two decades of data of large, long-term studies.

Table 1 Goal blood pressure and first line (initial) *therapy* in patients with kidney disease or diabetes to reduce CV risk

Group	Goal blood pressure (mmHg)	Initial therapy
American Diabetes Association (2002) [191]	<130/80	ACE inhibitor/ARB
National Kidney Foundation-CKD (2002) [4]	<130/80	ACE inhibitor/ARB
Canadian HTN Society (2001) [192]	<130/80	ACE inhibitor/ARB
National Kidney Foundation (2000) [21]	<130/80	ACE inhibitor
British HTN Society (2000) [190]	<140/80	ACE inhibitor
WHO/ISH (1999) [189]	<130/85	ACE inhibitor
JNC VI (1997) [188]	<130/85	ACE inhibitor

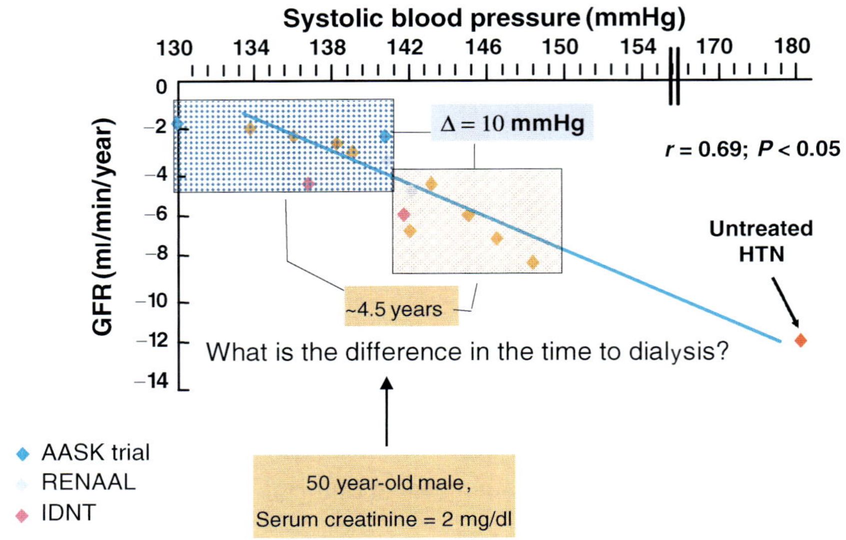

Figure 6 Summary of studies on nephropathy progression. (Reprinted from American Journal of Kidney Diseases, 36: 646–661, © 2000 with permission from National Kidney Foundation [21])

In a 12-year follow-up of 5163 diabetic men in the MRFIT, a linear relationship between coronary mortality and decreasing blood pressure was noted [175] (Figure 5). Compared with the nondiabetic individuals the risk was significantly higher in diabetic men with all grades of systolic blood pressure even at normotensive levels. Many studies in people with type 2 diabetes, using ambulatory blood pressure monitoring, showed the presence of higher microvascular complications at higher MAP levels, an observation that was true even in the prehypertensive range, independent of glycemic control [42, 195, 196]. In the UKPDS of people with type 2 diabetes tight control of blood pressure over a period of 9 years was able to decrease the microvascular and macrovascular complications (24% decrease in diabetes related endpoints, 32% in death related to diabetes, 44% in strokes, and 37% decrease in microvascular endpoints) [197]. Moreover, a *post hoc* observational analysis showed a strong relationship between the level of systolic blood pressure reduction and risk of myocardial infarction [198] (Figure 7).

The benefit of lower blood pressure goal is also true for CV events as shown in a *post hoc* analysis of the diabetic cohort in the Hypertension Outcome Treatment (HOT) trial [181]. The HOT study showed safety of decreasing the blood pressure to lower levels as 120/70 mmHg without any adverse events, although the study as a whole did not show major differences in outcome between the three randomized blood pressure groups. Differences were, however, noted in the subgroup of diabetic people ($n = 1501$) in which patients with target diastolic blood pressure lower

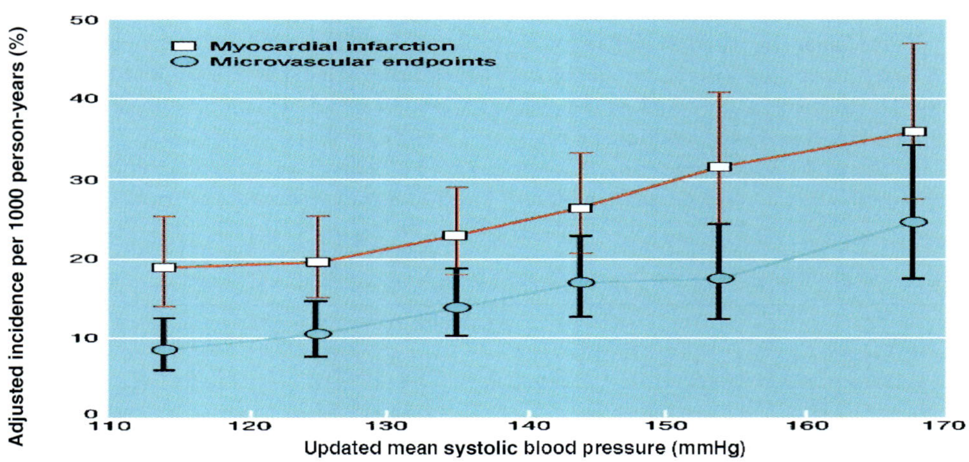

Figure 7 Systolic blood pressure with macrovascular and microvascular complications of type 2 diabetes (UKPDS 36). (BMJ 1998; 317: 703–13, with permission from the BMJ Publishing Group [197])

than 80 mmHg had a 51% reduction in major CV events and 30% reduction in stroke.

The first trial to assess the effect of blood pressure level on renal disease progression in a predominantly non-diabetic cohort (<10% with diabetes) was the Modification of Diet in Renal Disease (MDRD) [199]. While the primary results failed to support the concept that a lower level of blood pressure slowed progression of nondiabetic kidney disease, a *post hoc* analysis demonstrated that at the lowest levels of baseline glomerular filtration rate (GFR) or the highest levels of albuminuria, the lower blood pressure goal slowed disease progression [200]. More recent reports in both diabetic and nondiabetic cohorts strongly support the conclusion that the higher the level of baseline albuminuria, the greater the risk reduction from lower levels of blood pressure [201, 202].

A follow-up of the Collaborative Study Group Captopril Trial assessed the level of blood pressure reduction in the cohort of people with type 1 diabetes with nephropathy. One hundred twenty-nine of the original 307 people concluding the study were enrolled in the follow-up trial [203]. People were grouped by MAP of <92 or 100–107 mmHg, corresponding to a diastolic blood pressure of <80 and <90 mmHg respectively. At the end of 2 years, those who received the ACE inhibitor had a lower MAP and significant declines in macroalbuminuria, with 57% manifesting reductions in macroalbuminuria into the microalbuminuric or normal range. Declines in GFR, however, between groups were not significantly different, although one explanation for this was a short, i.e. <3-year, follow-up in people with relatively normal GFR values.

Earlier data from small studies suggested an increase in CV events, a J-curve phenomenon, when diastolic blood pressure has been decreased to levels well below 60 mmHg [204]. While no definitive evidence supports this observation of a "J-curve phenomenon" in the absence of preexisting symptomatic coronary disease, a blunted CV benefit–risk ratio has been noted at diastolic levels below 60 mmHg [205]. A *post hoc* analysis of a trial on isolated systolic hypertension documented a failure to reduce risk of CV events when diastolic blood pressure was lowered to <65 mmHg compared to people with levels above this pressure [206]. However, in the HOT trial no significant adverse events were noted even at blood pressure as low as 120/70 mmHg. This was also true in the Appropriate Blood Pressure Control in Diabetes (ABCD) trial of type 2 diabetic patients [201]. Thus, older people with systolic hypertension, especially with coronary disease, should not have their diastolic pressure lowered to levels below 60 mmHg.

Albuminuria as a Guide to Blood Pressure Goal

Baseline level of albuminuria strongly correlates with both adverse CV and renal outcomes [47, 207–212] (Figures 4 and 8). There is a direct correlation between the level of baseline albuminuria and level of renal dysfunction present in a given individual [214]. Therefore, those with greater than a gram of macroalbuminuria will have far lower GFRs than those with MA (<300 mg albumin/day). Data from every renal outcome trial of participants with diabetes and baseline MA (>300 mg albumin/day) demonstrate a benefit from lower levels of blood pressure and use of ACE inhibitors or ARBs (angiotensin receptor blockers) over DHP-CCBs; those with MA show no difference in outcome (Table 2). Moreover, the higher the level of baseline albuminuria, the greater the renal protection provided by lower blood pressure goals [21, 202, 215, 216]. Yet, beyond the benefits of blood pressure reduction, there may be specific benefits for agents that reduce albuminuria. A review of all trials with primary renal

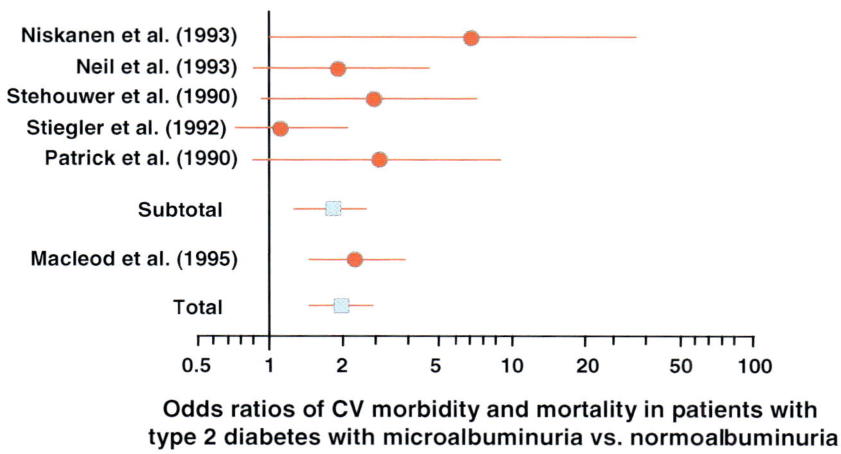

Figure 8 Association of MA and CV morbidity and mortality in type 2 diabetes. (Reproduced by permission of the Journal of the American Medical Association [213])

Table 2 Outcome differences in kidney disease progression comparing ACE inhibitors or ARBs to CCBs

	Baseline GFR	Baseline albuminuria
Captopril Trial [223]	68	<300 and >300 mg/day
Tarnow [263]	*85**	*<300 mg/day*
Guasch et al. [267]	*<60*	>300 mg/day
Bakris et al. [266]	*59*	*>300 mg/day*
Bakris [265]	*62*	*>300 mg/day*
IDNT [233]	*<70*	*>300 mg/day*
RENAAL [232]	<70	>300 mg/day
ABCD [259]	*84**	*<300 mg/day*

*Indicates no difference in outcome between ACE inhibitor and DHP-CCB. Note these are people with early diabetic nephropathy, stage 1, and MA. Studies in italic indicate comparators to DHP-CCBs.

outcomes over the past decade consistently demonstrates that a 30–35% reduction in albuminuria predicts a greater risk reduction for development of ESRD, death, or doubling of creatinine compared to blood pressure reduction without a change in albuminuria (Table 3).

Pharmacological Therapy

In the majority of individuals with diabetes, reduction of blood pressure to goal is not possible with monotherapy, and so multiple medications are needed. A summary of the number of antihypertensive medications needed to achieve blood pressure goals in clinical trials, which randomized to different blood pressure goals and which included participants with diabetes, indicates that a mean of 3.2 different medications are required to achieve the lower blood pressure targets recommended by various guideline committees [21, 217] (Figure 9). Since multiple factors are involved in the pathogenesis of hypertension in those with diabetes, failure of monotherapy to effectively achieve blood pressure target levels is not a surprise.

All national and international recommendations, including the JNC VI, WHO, and American Diabetes Association, provide an evidence-based rationale for selecting antihypertensive medications. A consensus approach for achieving blood pressure goals has been put forward by the National Kidney Foundation Hypertension and Diabetes Executive Committees Working Group for people with diabetes with and without nephropathy [20, 188, 191]. A proposed paradigm to achieve blood pressure goal and reduce CV and renal disease progression is summarized in Figure 10.

The rationale for this paradigm comes from all the clinical trial evidence demonstrating that antihypertensive medications that block the RAAS play a significant role in modulating outcomes in diabetic renal disease [177, 183, 218–220] although the evidence is less clear for coronary heart disease. Evidence for reduction of risk associated with ischemic heart disease is exemplified by results from the Captopril Prevention Project (CAPP), where captopril use in diabetic hypertensive subpopulation resulted in 66% lower incidence of myocardial infarction; any cardiac event was reduced by 33% and total mortality reduced by 46% compared to those on conventional therapy with diuretic or β-blocker [221]. In the Heart Outcomes Prevention Evaluation (HOPE) trial of people at high risk for CV disease treated with ramipril vs. placebo, 3577 diabetic people had a 25% reduction in cardiac endpoints [183]. Furthermore, a 24% decrease in incidence of MA also occurred. However patients in the HOPE and MICRO-HOPE studies may well have had lower nocturnal blood pressure, detected by ambulatory monitoring, as a result of the agent being administered at bedtime [222]. These trials need to be taken together with several other CV trials, recently summarized in a meta-analysis, which demonstrate that it is the level of blood pressure reduction that is important [177]. It is possible that in high-risk individuals, ACE inhibitors may have an edge over other agents for reducing CV events except for stroke [176], although large head-to-head comparisons such as those being made in the ALLHAT (Antihypertensive and Lipid-Lowering Treatment to Prevent Heart Attack Trial) will be necessary to make such conclusions. In people with nephropathy from type 1 diabetes, beneficial effects of slowing the decline of renal function are clearly established with ACE inhibitors [223–225]. In type 2 diabetic individuals other antihypertensive agents that also inhibit the RAAS, i.e., ARBs, may have similar efficacy to ACE inhibitors [226–228]. This is the basis for initial therapy being blockade of the RAAS. Achieving blood pressure goal, however, will require additional medications and is necessary to reduce CV and renal risk in type 2 diabetic individuals [21, 176, 177].

Data on the use of ARBs for CV or renal outcomes are sparse compared to that on ACE inhibitors. A comparison of the influence of ARBs to that of ACE inhibitors on CV outcomes has been performed only with losartan in heart failure with no trials in renal disease. The ELITE-I (Evaluation of Losartan in the Elderly I) trial compared the ARB losartan with captopril in people with congestive heart failure and found that losartan treatment was associated with lower mortality and was better tolerated [229]. However, the results of the ELITE-II trial, which was of longer duration than the ELITE-I, showed no greater reduction in mortality with losartan compared to captopril, although the side-effect profile in those who received losartan was

Table 3 Clinical trials and renal outcomes based on proteinuria reduction

Increased time to dialysis (*30–35% proteinuria reduction*)	No change in time to dialysis (*No proteinuria reduction*)
• Captopril Trial [222] • AASK Trial [202] • RENAAL [231] • IDNT [232]	• DHP-CCB arm–IDNT [232] • DHP–CCB arm–AASK [202]

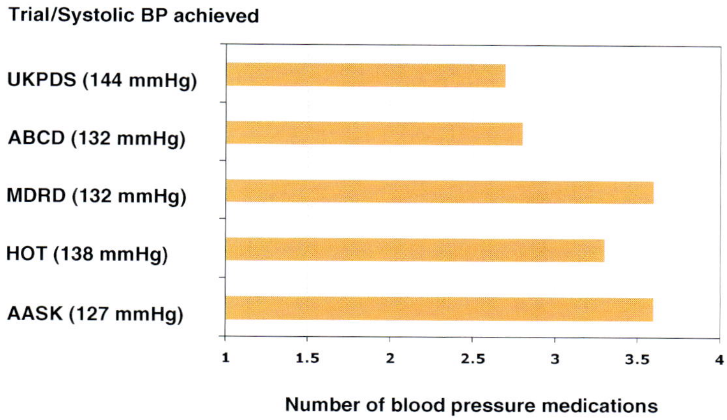

Figure 9 Average number of antihypertensive agents needed per patient to achieve target systolic blood pressure goals. (Reprinted from American Journal of Kidney Diseases, 39 (Suppl. 1), S1–S231, © 2002 with permission from National Kidney Foundation [4])

better [230]. Recent trials of ARBs with renal and CV outcomes confirm the efficacy of these agents in lowering blood pressure and reversing the adverse effects of hypertension on CV and renal function in diabetic people [226, 228, 231–233].

The recently concluded Losartan Intervention for Endpoint (LIFE) trial, a noninferiority trial that compares initial treatment with a β-blocker to that losartan with, demonstrated an unadjusted risk reduction in CV outcomes of 26% and 40% in the diabetic cohort treated with losartan and that treated with atenolol respectively [231]. In diabetic nephropathy the two seminal trials are the RENAAL and IDNT [232, 233]. In both these trials, a significant risk reduction in doubling of serum creatinine, ESRD, and death was noted in the groups randomized to the ARB. Moreover, in the longer term follow-up of the RENAAL study, a significant reduction in ESRD incidence was also seen [232]. Thus, in patients with macroalbuminuria and established nephropathy from type 2 diabetes, an ARB has clearly been shown to reduce progression over conventional therapy or the DHP-CCB, amlodipine. The common predictor of outcome in these trials was reduction in macroalbuminuria by at least 30% at similar levels of blood pressure control. An effect on MA was also seen in trials of nondiabetic renal disease with ACE inhibitors [234]. Of note, in RENAAL study there was a 32% reduction in first hospitalizations for congestive heart failure [232].

Lastly, in all ARB trials, side-effect profiles were more favorable for the ARB (Table 4). The frequency of cough is similar to that placebo with, and hyperkalemia is significantly less with ARB use than with ACE inhibitors

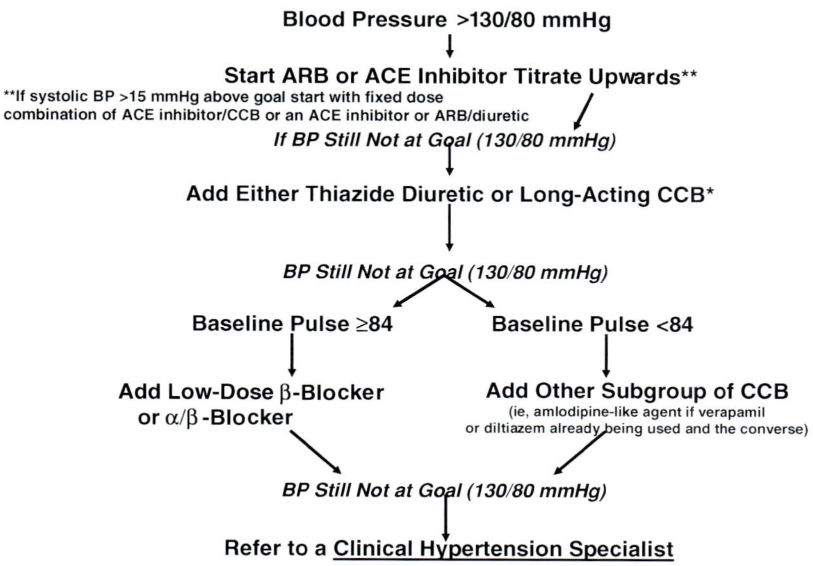

Figure 10 Algorithm for achieving target blood pressure goals in those with diabetes. (Reprinted from American Journal of Kidney Diseases, 39 (Suppl. 1), S1–S231, © 2002 with permission from National Kidney Foundation [4])

Table 4 Positive outcome trials of morbidity and mortality in renal and CV outcomes with ARBs

Trial	Diagnosis	Number of patients and medications	Other antihypertensives	BP achieved	Results	Side effects
LIFE [172]	Essential hypertension	Losartan: 4650 (DM 586); Atenolol: 4588 (DM 609)	≥2 (44%)	140/90 (49%)	Stroke = 24.9%; CVS = 13%; albuminuria	Better profile than β-blocker; K^+ = stable (↑K^+ not mentioned)
RENAAL [220]	Type 2 diabetes (24 h proteinuria > 500 mg; serum creatinine = 114–264 μmol/l)	Losartan: 751; Placebo: 762	3 medications > 75%; DHP–CCB = 61%	140/74	Primary endpoint = 16%; 1st hospitalization for CHF = 32%; decline in CrCl = 15.2%	↑K^+ causing discontinuation of ARB = 1.1%; risk profile favorable for losartan
IDNT 221	Type 2 diabetes (24 h proteinuria > 900 mg; serum creatinine = 88–264 μmol/l)	Irbesartan: 579; Amlodipine: 567; Placebo: 569	Mean = 3 medications	140/70	Primary endpoint = 33%; proteinuria = 33%	↑K^+ causing discontinuation of ARB = 1.9%; risk profile favorable for irbesartan

Note. DM = diabetes mellitus; CHF = congestive heart failure.

(1.1–1.9% compared with 10%) [229, 230, 235]. The reasons for lower incidence of hyperkalemia with ARBs over ACE inhibitors relates to the reduced inhibition of aldosterone in those with renal insufficiency, although the mechanism for this relative lack of effect is unclear [235].

An additional advantage of agents that block the RAAS is increased sensitization to insulin as glycemic control may be easier [183, 231]. In two separate large-scale trials, HOPE and LIFE, agents, which blocked the RAAS, produced a marked reduction in risk for new-onset diabetes. Given these data, it is recommended by all major guidelines that ACE inhibitors or alternatively ARBs be used as first line agents for those with nephropathy or diabetes.

It is known that multiple antihypertensive agents will usually be needed to achieve blood pressure goals in those with diabetes. Medication adherence in people with diabetes is critical to ensure optimal CV and renal risk reduction. A recent analysis of the NHANES III database revealed that only 11% of people with diabetes and hypertension achieve the JNC VI recommended goal of <130/85 mmHg [236]. A much higher percentage of blood pressure reduction to goal is possible if a focused approach is used with an eye on the target blood pressure. One hypertension clinic in the United States, achieved this goal in more than half the people with diabetes and hypertension [237]. Moreover, in a recently completed multicenter randomized trial (SHIELD), more than 200 people with type 2 diabetes were randomized to either initial therapy with a fixed-dose combination or monotherapy with the dose of both agents titrated upwards and subsequent addition of a diuretic to the monotherapy group [238]. At the end of 8 weeks more than 2.5 times as many people achieved the blood pressure goal of <130/85 mmHg compared to monotherapy. Moreover, at 12 weeks the number of people achieving goal blood pressure was still twofold higher in the fixed-dose combination group even with the addition of a diuretic for monotherapy patients. Thus, given that all antihypertensive agents reduce systolic blood pressure by a maximum of 12–15 mmHg, patients whose systolic blood pressure is more than 15 mmHg above goal should consider a fixed-dose combination as initial therapy to help achieve blood pressure goal [21]. To aid in this effort a number of fixed-dose antihypertensive combinations are available around the world (Table 5).

Given this information, it is suggested by the algorithm (Figure 10) that a diuretic or CCB be added to the RAAS blocker to potentiate the blood pressure lowering effect if blood pressure goal is not met within the first 2 months of therapy initiation [21, 239–242]. Fixed-dose combination of RAAS blockers and either thiazide diuretics or CCBs are available and should be considered first-line under specific circumstances (Table 5).

Data do exist to suggest that ACE inhibitors do not totally block the action of the RAAS [243]. Thus, the question of combining an ARB with ACE inhibitors has been tested to evaluate almost total blockade of the RAAS. In experiments in diabetic and hypertensive animal models, combinations of ARB and ACE inhibitors were more effective in nephroprotection than either agent alone [244–246]. Plasma angiotensin II levels were similarly reduced with the ACE inhibitors and combination therapy whereas the kidney tissue angiotensin II levels were more decreased with the combination therapy. This may reflect less binding and increased internalization of the angiotensin II in the presence of AT1 receptor blocker [247]. Where low doses of these drugs are combined, while most studies show a benefit, in the one well-designed and appropriately dosed human study of 13 people using a combination of lisinopril with losartan for 1 month, there was no further reduction of blood pressure and macroalbuminuria [248]. Thus, to date, clinical evidence does not exist, indicating that addition of an ARB to appropriately dosed ACE inhibitor is additive in effects on albuminuria independently of blood pressure reduction.

People with diabetes have a tendency to be volume expanded, since insulin increases sodium reabsorption at the proximal tubule. Thus, in these people a diuretic is a good second choice for achieving blood pressure goals. Similar beneficial CV effects were seen with the use of diuretics compared to β-blocker in SHEP trial of diabetic, hypertensive people, despite unfavorable metabolic profile [178, 249]. Nephropathy, however, is quite common with declining renal function and in these people thiazide diuretics may not be as helpful as addition of a loop diuretic.

Calcium-Channel Blockers

After use of RAAS blockers combined with diuretics, CCBs clearly have a role to help achieve BP goals. There are two subclasses of CCBs: DHP-CCB (amlodipine, felodipine, and nifedipine) and non-dihydropyridine [non-DHP-CCB] (verapamil and diltiazem). Studies have shown that differences exist among these subclasses of CCBs [250–253]. DHP-CCBs, regardless of half-life, are not beneficial in slowing nephropathy of either diabetic or nondiabetic etiologies, when MA is present, compared to agents that block the RAAS [202, 233]. However, non-DHPCCBs demonstrate preservation of renal morphology in animal models and blunting of the rise in macroalbuminuria as well as slowing of progression of nephropathy in long-term follow-up studies in humans [254–256]. The reasons for these differences relate to the different effects of these subclasses on renal autoregulation (Figure 11).

Three separate analyses of CCB effects on the kidney, including two separate meta-analyses, show clear differences between the subgroups. One meta-analysis

Table 5 Combination drugs for hypertension

β–Adrenergic blockers and diuretics
Atenolol (50 or 100 mg)/chlorthalidone (25 mg)
Bisoprolol fumarate (2.5, 5, or 10 mg)/hydrochlorothiazide (6.25 mg)
Metoprolol tartrate (50 or 100 mg)/hydrochlorothiazide (25 or 50 mg)
Nadolol (40 or 80 mg)/bendroflumethiazide (5 mg)
Propranolol hydrochloride (40 or 80 mg)/hydrochlorothiazide (25 mg)
Propranolol hydrochloride (extended release) (80, 120, or 160 mg)/hydrochlorothiazide (50 mg)
Timolol maleate (10 mg)/hydrochlorothiazide (25 mg)
ACE inhibitors and diuretics
Benazepril hydrochloride (5, 10, or 20 mg)/hydrochlorothiazide (6.25, 12.5, or 25 mg)
Captopril (25 or 50 mg)/hydrochlorothiazide (15 or 25 mg)
Enalapril maleate (5 or 10 mg)/hydrochlorothiazide (12.5 or 25 mg)
Lisinopril (10 or 20 mg)/hydrochlorothiazide (12.5 or 25 mg)
Angiotensin II receptor antagonists and diuretics
Losartan potassium (50 mg)/hydrochlorothiazide (12.5 mg)
Irbesartan (300 mg)/hydrochlorothiazide (12.5 mg)
Valsartan (160 mg)/hydrochlorothiazide (12.5 mg)
Telmesartan (80 mg)/hydrochlorothiazide (12.5 mg)
Calcium antagonists and ACE inhibitors
Amlodipine besylate (2.5 or 5 mg)/benazepril hydrochloride (10 or 20 mg)
Verapamil hydrochloride (extended release) (180 or 240 mg)/trandolapril (1, 2, or 4 mg)
Felodipine (5 mg)/enalapril maleate (5 mg)
Other combinations
Triamterene (37.5, 50, or 75 mg)/hydrochlorothiazide (25 or 50 mg)
Spironolactone (25 or 50 mg)/hydrochlorothiazide (25 or 50 mg)
Amiloride hydrochloride (5 mg)/hydrochlorothiazide (50 mg)
Guanethidine monosulfate (10 mg)/hydrochlorothiazide (25 mg)
Hydralazine hydrochloride (25, 50, or 100 mg)/hydrochlorothiazide (25 or 50 mg)
Methyldopa (250 or 500 mg)/hydrochlorothiazide (15, 25, 30, or 50 mg)
Reserpine, (0.125 mg)/hydrochlorothiazide (25 or 50 mg)
Reserpine (0.10 mg)/hydralazine hydrochloride (25 mg)/hydrochlorothiazide (15 mg)
Clonidine hydrochloride (0.1, 0.2, or 0.3 mg)/chlorthalidone (15 mg)
Methyldopa (250 mg)/chlorothiazide (150 or 250 mg)
Reserpine (0.125 or 0.25 mg)/chlorthalidone (25 or 50 mg)
Reserpine (0.125 or 0.25 mg)/chlorothiazide (250 or 500 mg)
Prazosin hydrochloride (1, 2, or 5 mg)/polythiazide (0.5 mg)

of diabetic and non diabetic renal disease found that ACE inhibitors and non-DHP-CCBs reduced MA and had an associated improvement on declines in renal function (0.18 ml/min/month) whereas DHP-CCBs failed to preserve renal function [250, 257, 258]. Smith et al. in a randomized crossover study compared the effects of extended-release diltiazem and extended-release nifedipine and found a threefold reduction in MA in the diltiazem group with no change in the DHP-CCB group [256]. This change was related to altered glomerular membrane permeability. Thus, not all subclasses of CCBs are protective in those with nephropathy from diabetes. It should further be noted that DHP-CCBs have not been shown to reduce risk unless used with an ACE inhibitor or ARB. This is exemplified by results of two renal outcome trials. African-American Study of Kidney Disease (AASK) in non-diabetic renal disease and Irbesartan Diabetic Nephropathy Trial (IDNT) in diabetic renal disease [202, 233]. Use of a DHP-CCB failed to reduce renal disease progression in the AASK and IDNT, where GFR was less than 60 ml/min at baseline.

There may also be subclass differences in regard to CV disease. While a controversy about the safety of DHP-CCBs appeared several years ago, subsequent outcome trials have failed to demonstrate any harm with regard to CV events. In fact, a benefit on stroke reduction was consistent and significant [176, 177]. Thus, DHP-CCBs reduce CV events in people without nephropathy, macroalbuminuria, or heart failure. In the ABCD study, where the mean GFR was approximately 85 ml/min and MA was present, the DHP-CCBs failed to reduce risk of CV events compared with ACE inhibitors, although their impact on kidney function was not different from that of ACE inhibitors [259, 260]. Moreover, DHP-CCBs failed to show a reduction in morbidity and mortality when used in people with cardiomyopathy and mild to moderate heart failure [261, 262].

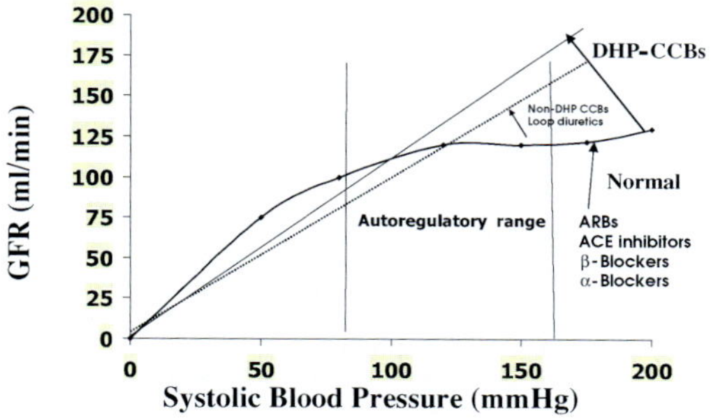

Figure 11 Effects of drug classes on renal autoregulation

Note. The normal ability of the kidney to maintain GFR and renal blood flow over a range of blood pressures is noted as "normal". Use of DHPCCBs transforms this sigmoidal curve into a linear line and loop diuretics and non-DHPCCBs (verapamil, diltiazem) have an intermediate effect. Therefore, when DHPCCBs are used blood pressure needs to be reduced well beyond the recommended level of 130 or <140 by British guidelines in diabetes to obtain any type of renal benefit. (Modified by permission of Kluwer [4, 250])

To date, none of the DHP-CCBs has been shown to reduce ischemic events in randomized secondary prevention trials of survivors of acute myocardial infarction when used in the absence of an ACE inhibitor or a β-blocker [261, 263]. Consistent with a benefit of DHP-CCBs on CV events, the Syst-Eur trial in elderly people with hypertension and absence of nephropathy as well as macroalbuminuria, demonstrated a significant risk reduction in CV events but primarily stroke reduction. Note, however, that even in the trials demonstrating risk reduction of CV events, like HOT and Syst-Eur, at least half of the participants in both groups were also receiving either an ACE inhibitor or a β-blocker along with the DHP-CCB. The results of the ALLHAT trial ($N = 42\,000$), however, will answer the issue of DHP-CCBs on CV risk reduction.

A place for DHP-CCBs in treatment of hypertension does exist in people with diabetes because of their potent antihypertensive effects and their apparent benefit on slowing progression in very early diabetic renal disease [259, 264]. However, these agents cannot be recommended as the first line medications except in elderly people with diabetes and no evidence of nephropathy or MA [265]. Non-DHP-CCBs have been shown in small, long-term follow-up studies to slow nephropathy progression and reduce CV risk; hence they are recommended by the American Diabetes Association as alternatives to ACE inhibitors and ARBs, when these agents are not tolerated [191, 266–268]. Thus, CCBs should be thought of as very useful agents to lower blood pressure, with DHP-CCBs being very useful in the presence of other agents that reduce CV risk, while non-DHP-CCBs have been shown to reduce mortality from CV events in clinical trials and work well in the absence of ACE inhibitors or ARBs.

β-Blockers

In the algorithm shown in Figure 10, β-blockers are used not only because they reduce CV risk but also because in advanced renal disease they slow progression of nephropathy. This was shown in a subanalysis of diabetic people in the SHEP trial, where atenolol and chlorthalidone, a diuretic, were both able to decrease the risk of stroke, either ischemic or hemorrhagic, when blood pressure was decreased to a target of <160 mmHg [178]. Similarly in the UKPDS, strict control of blood pressure with atenolol was as effective as captopril in decreasing the blood pressure and reducing macro- and microvascular complications [269].

β-Blockers are cardioprotective, with long-term β-blocker therapy being associated with improved long-term survival in people with non-insulin-dependent diabetes mellitus and coronary artery disease [270–272]. Despite this, their use has been limited to only 40–50% in diabetic patients after myocardial infarction. This reluctance is due to the notion that use of β-blockers may mask the symptoms of hypoglycemia and have adverse metabolic side effects. This has been most commonly seen in type 1 diabetes, but has not been a prominent problem in clinical trials, nor has been borne out from literature reviews of studies in participants with type 2 diabetes who received selective β_1-adrenoreceptor blockers [269, 273]. The hypoglycaemic effect is related to blockade of β_2 receptors, which increase hepatic glucose production and decrease peripheral utilization in the tissues, thus having a protective effect in hypoglycemic states [270]. Additionally, β-blockers are known to worsen insulin resistance and glucose control in people with type 2 diabetes, which is another reason why they are not used as much in this disease [197, 274]. Two agents with α,β-blocking properties are suggested for adjunct use to achieve BP goals in diabetes. The two agents representing this subclass are carvedilol, a multiple-action antihypertensive drug with nonselective β-adrenoreceptor and selective α-adrenoreceptor blocking activity [275]; and labetalol, which has a β-blocking potency that is 50% lower than that of carvedilol.

In a comparison between an α,β-blocker carvedilol and β-blocker atenolol, both effectively decreased blood pressure and left ventricular mass in people with diabetes and hypertension [276]. The metabolic effects, however, were different; fasting plasma glucose and insulin levels decreased during carvedilol treatment and increased during atenolol treatment, indicating different effects on insulin sensitivity. Carvedilol also produced more favorable lipid profile with a decrease in triglycerides and increase in the high-density lipoprotein cholesterol concentrations. Carvedilol, but not atenolol, significantly reduced levels

Table 6 Pharmacologic properties of commonly used antihypertensive agents

Drug	Dosage (mg/day)	Doses/day	Mechanisms of action	Special considerations
Diuretics				
Thiazides and related drugs	12.5–25	1	Decreased body sodium and extracellular fluid volume, also vasodilation	More effective antihypertensive agents than loop diuretics, unless serum creatinine is ≥2.0 ml/min or creatinine clearance ≥50 ml/min
Hydrochlorothiazide				
Loop diuretics				
Furosemide	20–320	2	Inhibit 2Cl Na pump ascending loop of Henle	Effective even in patients with advanced renal or congestive heart failure
Bumetanide	0.5–5	2		
Ethacrynic acid	25–100	2		
Torasemide	5–20	1		
Fixed-dose diuretics (potassium sparing)				
HCTZ/amiloride			Increase K^+ reabsorption	Weak diuretics
HCTZ/triampterene				
Spironolactone	25–100	2–3	Aldosterone antagonist	May cause hyperkalemia in with serum creatinine >2.5 mg/dl, particularly when combined with ACE inhibitors, K^+ supplements, or NSAIDS
Triamterene	50–100	2		
Adrenergic inhibitors				
β-Blockers				
Cardioselective				
Atenolol	25–100	1	Inhibit β_1 receptors, decrease CO; increase SVR, decrease plasma renin activity (PRA); inhibit β_1 and β_2 receptors	In higher doses, will also inhibit β_2 receptors; more likely to cause metabolic side effects, e.g. increased insulin resistance and triglycerides
Metoprolol	50–200	1–2		
Noncardioselective				
Nadolol	20–240	1		
Propranolol	40–240	1–2		
Timolol	20–40	2		
With intrinsic sympathomimetic activity (ISA)				
Acebutolol	200–1200	2	Partial agonist activity on β-adrenergic receptors	No clear advantage expect for less bradycardia and metabolic side effects than other β-blockers
Pindolol	10–60	2		
Antiadrenergic agents				
Centrally acting				
α-Methyldopa	250–1500	2	Stimulate α_2-adrenergic receptors in the brainstem, resulting in inhibition of efferent sympathetic activity; decrease SVR	Sudden withdrawal may result in hypertensive crisis.
Clonidine	0.1–0.6	2		
Clonidine TTS	0.1–0.3	Once/week		
Guanfacine	1–3	1		

Peripherally acting				
Guanethidine	10–100	1	Inhibit norepinephrine release from sympathetic nerve terminals; decrease SVR	Frequently cause orthostatic hypotension and sexual dysfunction
Reserpine	0.05–0.25	1	Depletion of norepinephrine	Causes frequent neurologic symptoms α_1-receptor blockers
Doxazosin	2–16	1	Inhibit α_1-adrenergic receptors; decrease SVR; CO same or increases	First-dose effect; postural hypotension; useful for prostatic hypertrophy
Prazosin	2–20	1–2		
Terazosin	1–20	1		
α,β-blockers				
Labertolol	200–800	2–3	Blocksα- and β-aderenergic receptors (7 : 1β : α blockade)	Same as β-blockers
Carvediol	3.75–25	2	Blocks α and β-aderenergic receptors (3 : 1 β : α blockade)	Same as β-blockers
ACE inhibitors				
Benazepril	10–40	1–2	Block convertion of angiotensin I to angiotensin II; decrease aldosterone; may increase bradykinin and vasodilatory prostaglandins; decrease SVR; no change in CO	When added to diuretics may cause hypotension; may cause hyperkalemia in patients with renal failure, those with hypoaldosteronism, those receiving K-sparing diuretics or NSAIDS; can cause acute renal failure in patients with bilateral renal artery stenosis, renal artery stenosis of a solitary kidney, creatinine >3 mg/dl, or severe congestive heart failure
Captopril	12.5–100	2–3		
Cilazapril	2.5–5	1–2		
Enalapril	2.5–40	1–2		
Fosinopril	10–40	1		
Lisinopril	5–40	1		
Perindopril	1–16	1–2		
Quinapril	5–80	1–2		
Ramipril	1.25–20	1		
Spirapril	12.5–50	1–2		
Trandolapril	1–4	1		
Calcium antagonists				
Diltiazem	90–360	3–4	Blocks entry of calcium into smooth muscle cells resulting in vasodilation; decrease SVR; blunt increases in exercise heart rate	May cause heart block, particularly when combined with β-blocker
Diltiazem CD	180–360	1		
Verapamil	80–480	2–3		
Verapamil SR	120–480	1–2		
Verapamil-Covera HS	180–240	1 (at bedtime)		
Dihydropiridines				
Amlodipine	2.5–10	1	Same as diltiazem and verapamil; do not blunt increase exercise heart rate	More potent vasodilators than diltiazem and verapamil, may cause dizziness, headache, tachycardia, flushing, edema
Felodipine	5–20	1		
Isradipine	2.5–10	2		
Nicardipine	60–120	3		
Nifedipine	30–120	3		
Nifedipine (GITS)	30–120	1		
Nisoldipine	10–10	1–2		
Direct vasodilators				
Hydralazine	50–200	2–4	Direct relaxation of smooth muscle cells, causing arteriolar vasodilation secondary to opening K^+ channels	Limited efficacy if given alone due to fluid retention and reflex vasodilation; should be combined with a diuretic and a β-blocker to prevent edema and tachycardia
Minoxidil	2.5–80	1		

of oxidants, supporting its antioxidant effect [275]. Thus, carvedilol distinguishes itself as the agent that inhibits the sympathetic nervous system without aggravating metabolic control.

Carvedilol has been used in many trials of people with heart failure. In a recent trial (COPERNICUS), participants with heart failure randomized to carvedilol in comparison to placebo improved CV mortality by 35% [277]. Similarly in comparison to metoprolol, carvedilol significantly increased left ventricular ejection fraction [275]. Thus diabetic people may benefit from these additional actions of carvedilol. No such data are available for labetalol.

Other Antihypertensive Medications

α-Blockers alone increase the incidence of congestive heart failure (ALLHAT) and have no effect on MA, a marker of vascular dysfunction [278]. Thus, α-blockers alone or as a second line medication are not recommended in diabetic, hypertensive people; however their use in males with benign prostate hypertrophy should be a consideration for add-on medication. Direct vasodilators such as hydralazine and minoxidil, which work through opening of specific potassium channels, may be needed in unusual circumstances but may be avoided through the use of two different low-dosed CCBs, a non-DHP and a DHP-CCB [279]. Specifically, low doses of diltiazem and nifedipine have been shown to have synergistic reductions in blood pressure without increases in edema or other side effects. The mechanisms of action and precautions of antihypertensive medications have been outlined in Table 6.

CONCLUSION

This information taken together clearly mandates that blood pressure reduction occur and be maintained to levels below 130/80 mmHg in order to maximally reduce both CV and renal risk. A "cocktail" of antihypertensive agents anchored on an ACE inhibitor or, if not tolerated, an ARB with a diuretic should be the cornerstone of therapy. Other agents such as CCBs and β-blockers will be needed in many cases to achieve this level of blood pressure. Achievement of this level of blood pressure along with other interventions such as glucose and lipid management will help reduce the risk of CV and renal events.

REFERENCES

1. WHO Web site for diabetes: www.who.int/ncd/dia/databases2.htm#t2, 2002.
2. Sundquist J, Winkleby MA, Pudaric S. CV disease risk factors among older black, Mexican-American, and white women and men: an analysis of NHANES III, 1988–1994. Third National Health and Nutrition Examination Survey. *J Am Geriatr Soc* 2001; 49: 109–16.
3. King H, Aubert RE, Herman WH. Global burden of diabetes, 1995–2025: prevalence, numerical estimates, and projections. *Diabetes Care* 1998; 21: 1414–31.
4. Anonymous. Clinical Practice Guidelines for Chronic Kidney Disease: Evaluation, Classification and Stratification. *Am J Kidney Dis* 2002; 39 (suppl 1): S1–231.
5. Zimmet P, Alberti KG, Shaw J. Global and societal implications of the diabetes epidemic. *Nature* 2001; 414: 782–7.
6. Cooper L. USRDS. 2001 Annual Data Report. *Nephrol News Issues* 2001; 15: 31, 34–5, 38.
7. van Dijk PC, Jager KJ, de Charro F, Collart F, Cornet R, Dekker FW, Gronhagen-Riska C, Kramer R, Leivestad T, Simpson K, Briggs JD. Renal replacement therapy in Europe: the results of a collaborative effort by the ERA-EDTA registry and six national or regional registries. *Nephrol Dial Transplant* 2001; 16: 1120–9.
8. Haffner SM. Epidemiology of type 2 diabetes: risk factors. *Diabetes Care* 1998; 21 (suppl 3): C3–6.
9. Rahman Al-Nuaim A. Effect of overweight and obesity on glucose intolerance and dyslipidemia in Saudi Arabia, epidemiological study. *Diabetes Res Clin Pract* 1997; 36: 181–91.
10. Ramachandran A, Snehalatha C, Viswanathan V, Viswanathan M, Haffner SM. Risk of noninsulin dependent diabetes mellitus conferred by obesity and central adiposity in different ethnic groups: a comparative analysis between Asian Indians, Mexican Americans and Whites. *Diabetes Res Clin Pract* 1997; 36: 121–5.
11. Hillier TA, Pedula KL. Characteristics of an adult population with newly diagnosed type 2 diabetes: the relation of obesity and age of onset. *Diabetes Care* 2001; 24: 1522–7.
12. Sjostrom CD, Peltonen M, Sjostrom L. Blood pressure and pulse pressure during long-term weight loss in the obese: the swedish obese subjects (sos) intervention study. *Obes Res* 2001; 9: 188–95.
13. Mooradian AD. Obesity: a rational target for managing diabetes mellitus. *Growth Horm IGF Res* 2001; 11 (suppl A): S79–83.
14. Su HY, Sheu WH, Chin HM, Jeng CY, Chen YD, Reaven GM. Effect of weight loss on blood pressure and insulin resistance in normotensive and hypertensive obese individuals. *Am J Hypertens* 1995; 8: 1067–71.
15. Teuscher A, Egger M, Herman JB. Diabetes and hypertension. Blood pressure in clinical diabetic patients and a control population. *Arch Intern Med* 1989; 149: 1942–5.
16. Pell S, D'Alonzo CA. Some aspects of hypertension in diabetes mellitus. *JAMA* 1967; 202: 104–10.
17. United States Renal Data System (USRDS). Causes of death. *Am J Kidney Dis* 1997; 30: S107–17.
18. United State Renal Data System (USRDS). Patient mortality and survival. *Am J Kidney Dis* 1997; 30: S86–106.
19. Baigent C, Burbury K, Wheeler D. Premature CV disease in chronic renal failure. *Lancet* 2000; 356: 147–52.
20. Collins AJ, Li S, Ma JZ, Herzog C. CV disease in end-stage renal disease patients. *Am J Kidney Dis* 2001; 38: S26–9.
21. Bakris GL, Williams M, Dworkin L, Elliott WJ, Epstein M, Toto R, et al, for the National Kidney Foundation Hypertension and Diabetes Executive Committees Working Group. Preserving renal function in adults with

hypertension and diabetes: a consensus approach. *Am J Kidney Dis* 2000; 36: 646–61.
22. Tarnow L, Rossing P, Gall MA, Nielsen FS, Parving HH. Prevalence of arterial hypertension in diabetic patients before and after the JNC-V. *Diabetes Care* 1994; 17: 1247–51.
23. Sowers JR, Epstein M. Diabetes mellitus and associated hypertension, vascular disease and nephropathy. An update. *Hypertension* 1995; 26: 869–79.
24. Fuller JH. Hypertension and diabetes: epidemiologic aspects as a guide to management. *J Cardiovasc Pharmacol* 1993; 21 (suppl 2): S63–6.
25. Mykkanen L, Haffner SM, Kuusisto J, Pyorala K, Laakso M. MA precedes the development of NIDDM. *Diabetes* 1994; 43: 552–7.
26. Borovkov NN, Sidorova NV. 24-hour arterial hypertension profile and heart rhythm variability in patients with arterial hypertension and NIDDM. *Klin Med (Mosk)* 2002; 80: 19–21.
27. Coulston AM. Diabetes mellitus in 2002. *Nutr Today* 2002; 37: 163–6.
28. Garg JP, Bakris GL. MA: marker of vascular dysfunction, risk factor for CV disease. *Vasc Med* 2002; 7: 35–43.
29. Jensen JS, Feldt-Rasmussen B, Borch-Johnsen K, Clausen P, Appleyard M, Jensen G. MA and its relation to CV disease and risk factors. A population-based study of 1254 hypertensive individuals [see comments]. *J Hum Hypertens* 1997; 11: 727–32.
30. Clausen P, Jensen JS, Jensen G, Borch-Johnsen K, Feldt-Rasmussen B. Elevated urinary albumin excretion is associated with impaired arterial dilatory capacity in clinically healthy subjects. *Circulation* 2001; 103: 1869–74.
31. Ismail N, Becker B, Strzelczyk P, Ritz E. Renal disease and hypertension in non-insulin-dependent diabetes mellitus. *Kidney Int* 1999; 55: 1–28.
32. Jensen JS, Feldt-Rasmussen B, Strandgaard S, Schroll M, Borch-Johnsen K. Arterial hypertension, MA, and risk of ischemic heart disease. *Hypertension* 2000; 35: 898–903.
33. Deckert T, Kofoed-Enevoldsen A, Norgaard K, Borch-Johnsen K, Feldt-Rasmussen B, Jensen T. MA: Implications for micro- and macrovascular disease. *Diabetes Care* 1992; 15: 1181–91.
34. Feldt-Rasmussen B. MA, endothelial dysfunction and CV risk. *Diabetes Metab* 2000; 26 (suppl 4): 64–6.
35. Cohen CN, Albanesi FMF, Goncalves M, Gomes M. Ambulatory blood pressure monitoring and MA in normotensive subjects with insulin-dependent diabetes mellitus [In Process Citation]. *Arq Bras Cardiol* 2000; 75: 200–4.
36. Cuspidi C, Macca G, Sampieri L, Fusi V, Severgnini B, Michev I, et al. Target organ damage and non-dipping pattern defined by two sessions of ambulatory blood pressure monitoring in recently diagnosed essential hypertensive patients. *J Hypertens* 2001; 19: 1539–45.
37. Pickering TG. Cardiorenal protection in diabetes. *Heart Dis* 2000; 2: S18–22.
38. Redon J. Ambulatory blood pressure and the kidney. *Blood Press Monit* 1998; 3: 157–61.
39. Lurbe E, Redon J, Kesani A, Pascual JM, Tacons J, Alvarez V, et al. Increase in nocturnal blood pressure and progression to MA in type 1 diabetes. *N Engl J Med* 2002; 347: 797–805.
40. Nielsen FS, Hansen HP, Jacobsen P, Rossing P, Smidt UM, Christensen NJ, et al. Increased sympathetic activity during sleep and nocturnal hypertension in type 2 diabetic patients with diabetic nephropathy. *Diabet Med* 1999; 16: 555–62.
41. Lafferty AR, Werther GA, Clarke CF. Ambulatory blood pressure, MA, and autonomic neuropathy in adolescents with type 1 diabetes. *Diabetes Care* 2000; 23: 533–8.
42. Voros P, Lengyel Z, Nagy V, Nemeth C, Rosivall L, Kammerer L. Diurnal blood pressure variation and albuminuria in normotensive patients with insulin-dependent diabetes mellitus. *Nephrol Dial Transplant* 1998; 13: 2257–60.
43. Schultz CJ, Neil HA, Dalton RN, Konopelska BT, Dunger DB, for the Oxford Regional Prospective Study Group. Blood pressure does not rise before the onset of MA in children followed from diagnosis of type 1 diabetes. *Diabetes Care* 2001; 24: 555–60.
44. Levin SR, Coburn JW, Abraira C, Henderson WG, Colwell JA, Emanuele NV, et al, for the Veterans Affairs Cooperative Study on Glycemic Control and Complications in type 2 Diabetes Feasibility Trial Investigators Effect of intensive glycemic control on MA in type 2 diabetes [In Process Citation]. *Diabetes Care* 2000; 23: 1478–85.
45. UK Prospective Diabetes Study (UKPDS) Group. Effect of intensive blood-glucose control with metformin on complications in overweight patients with type 2 diabetes (UKPDS 34). *Lancet* 1998; 352: 854–65.
46. The Diabetes Control and Complications (DCCT) Research Group. Effect of intensive therapy on the development and progression of diabetic nephropathy in the Diabetes Control and Complications Trial. *Kidney Int* 1995; 47: 1703–20.
47. Keane WF, Eknoyan G. Proteinuria, albuminuria, risk, assessment, detection, elimination (PARADE): a position paper of the National Kidney Foundation. *Am J Kidney Dis* 1999; 33: 1004–10.
48. Ruggenenti P, Perna A, Mosconi L, Pisoni R, Remuzzi G, for the Gruppo Italiano di Studi Epidemiologici in Nefrologia (GISEN). Urinary protein excretion rate is the best independent predictor of ESRF in non-diabetic proteinuric chronic nephropathies. *Kidney Int* 1998; 53: 1209–16.
49. Damsgaard EM, Froland A, Jorgensen OD, Mogensen CE. Eight to nine year mortality in known non-insulin dependent diabetics and controls. *Kidney Int* 1992; 41: 731–5.
50. Borch-Johnsen K, Feldt-Rasmussen B, Strandgaard S, Schroll M, Jensen JS. Urinary albumin excretion. An independent predictor of ischemic heart disease. *Arterioscler Thromb Vasc Biol* 1999; 19: 1992–7.
51. Miettinen AH, Haffner SM, Lehto S, Ronnemaa T, Pyorala K, Laakso M. Proteinuria predicts stroke and other atherosclerotic vascular disease events in nondiabetic and non-insulin-dependent diabetic subjects. *Stroke* 1996; 27 (11): 2033–9.
52. *Obesity: Preventing and Managing the Global Epidemic*. Report of a World Health Organization Consultation on Obesity. Geneva: WHO, 1998.
53. DeFronzo RA, Ferrannini E. Insulin resistance. A multifaceted syndrome responsible for NIDDM, obesity, hypertension, dyslipidemia, and atherosclerotic CV disease. *Diabetes Care* 1991; 14: 173–94.
54. Singer P, Godicke W, Voigt S, Hajdu I, Weiss M. Postprandial hyperinsulinemia in patients with mild essential hypertension. *Hypertension* 1985; 7: 182–6.

55. Shen DC, Shieh SM, Fuh MM, Wu DA, Chen YD, Reaven GM. Resistance to insulin-stimulated-glucose uptake in patients with hypertension. *J Clin Endocrinol Metab* 1988; 66: 580–3.
56. Ferrannini E, Buzzigoli G, Bonadonna R, Giorico MA, Oleggini M, Graziadei L, et al. Insulin resistance in essential hypertension. *N Engl J Med* 1987; 317: 350–7.
57. Julius S, Jamerson K, Mejia A, Krause L, Schork N, Jones K. The association of borderline hypertension with target organ changes and higher coronary risk. Tecumseh Blood Pressure study. *JAMA* 1990; 264: 354–8.
58. Sowers JR, Epstein M. Diabetes mellitus and associated hypertension, vascular disease, and nephropathy. An update. *Hypertension* 1995; 26: 869–79.
59. Haffner SM, Miettinen H, Gaskill SP, Stern MP. Metabolic precursors of hypertension. The San Antonio Heart Study. *Arch Intern Med* 1996; 156: 1994–2001.
60. Bengtsson K, Orho-Melander M, Melander O, Lindblad U, Ranstam J, Rastam L, et al. Beta(2)-adrenergic receptor gene variation and hypertension in subjects with type 2 diabetes. *Hypertension* 2001; 37: 1303–8.
61. Chaves FJ, Pascual JM, Rovira E, Armengod ME, Redon J. Angiotensin II AT1 receptor gene polymorphism and MA in essential hypertension. *Am J Hypertens* 2001; 14: 364–70.
62. Dudley CR, Keavney B, Stratton IM, Turner RC, Ratcliffe PJ. U.K. Prospective Diabetes Study, XV: relationship of renin–angiotensin system gene polymorphisms with MA in NIDDM. *Kidney Int* 1995; 48: 1907–11.
63. Fisher ND, Hurwitz S, Jeunemaitre X, Hopkins PN, Hollenberg NK, Williams GH. Familial aggregation of low-renin hypertension. *Hypertension* 2002; 39: 914–8.
64. Fradin S, Goulet-Salmon B, Chantepie M, Grandhomme F, Morello R, Jauzac P, et al. Relationship between polymorphisms in the renin–angiotensin system and nephropathy in type 2 diabetic patients. *Diabetes Metab* 2002; 28: 27–32.
65. Freedam BI, Yu H, Spray BJ, Rich SS, Rothschild CB, Bowden DW. Genetic linkage analysis of growth factor loci and end-stage renal disease in African Americans. *Kidney Int* 1997; 51: 819–25.
66. Kato N, Sugiyama T, Morita H, Kurihara H, Sato T, Yamori Y, et al. Association analysis of beta(2)-adrenergic receptor polymorphisms with hypertension in Japanese. *Hypertension* 2001; 37: 286–92.
67. Lesage S, Velho G, Vionnet N, Chatelain N, Demenais F, Passa P, et al. Genetic studies of the renin–angiotensin system in arterial hypertension associated with non-insulin-dependent diabetes mellitus. *J Hypertens* 1997; 15: 601–6.
68. Marre M, Jeunemaitre X, Gallois Y, Rodier M, Chatellier G, Sert C, et al, for the Genetique de la Nephropathie Diabetique (GENEDIAB) Study Group. Contribution of genetic polymorphism in the renin–angiotensin system to the development of renal complications in insulin-dependent diabetes. *J Clin Invest* 1997; 99: 1585–95.
69. Meigs JB, Ordovas JM, Cupples LA, Singer DE, Nathan DM, Schaefer EJ, et al. Apolipoprotein E isoform polymorphisms are not associated with insulin resistance: the Framingham Offspring Study. *Diabetes Care* 2000; 23: 69–74.
70. Price DA, Crook ED. Kidney disease in African Americans: genetic considerations. *J Natl Med Assoc* 2002; 94: 16S–27S.
71. Thomas GN, Tomlinson B, Chan JC, Sanderson JE, Cockram CS, Critchley JA. Renin–angiotensin system gene polymorphisms, blood pressure, dyslipidemia, and diabetes in Hong Kong Chinese: a significant association of tne ACE insertion/deletion polymorphism with type 2 diabetes. *Diabetes Care* 2001; 24: 356–61.
72. Lifton RP, Dluhy RG, Powers M, Ulick S, Lalouel JM. The molecular basis of glucocorticoid-remediable aldosteronism, a Mendelian cause of human hypertension. *Trans Assoc Am Physicians* 1992; 105: 64–71.
73. Remuzzi G, Schieppati A, Ruggenenti P. Clinical practice. Nephropathy in patients with type 2 diabetes. *N Engl J Med* 2002; 346: 1145–51.
74. Yoshida H, Kon V, Ichikawa I. Polymorphisms of the renin–angiotensin system genes in progressive renal diseases. *Kidney Int* 1996; 50: 732–44.
75. Fagerudd JA, Tarnow L, Jacobsen P, Stenman S, Nielsen FS, Pettersson-Fernholm KJ, et al. Predisposition to essential hypertension and development of diabetic nephropathy in IDDM patients. *Diabetes* 1998; 47: 439–44.
76. Tarnow L, Rossing P, Nielsen FS, Fagerudd JA, Poirier O, Parving HH. CV morbidity and early mortality cluster in parents of type 1 diabetic patients with diabetic nephropathy. *Diabetes Care* 2000; 23: 30–3.
77. Earle K, Viberti GC. Familial, hemodynamic and metabolic factors in the predisposition to diabetic kidney disease. *Kidney Int* 1994; 45: 434–7.
78. Jeunemaitre X, Soubrier F, Kotelevtsev YV, Lifton RP, Williams CS, Charru A, et al. Molecular basis of human hypertension: role of angiotensinogen. *Cell* 1992; 71: 169–80.
79. Bengtsson K, Orho-Melander M, Lindblad U, Melander O, Bog-Hansen E, Ranstam J, et al. Polymorphism in the angiotensin converting enzyme but not in the angiotensinogen gene is associated with hypertension and type 2 diabetes: the Skaraborg Hypertension and diabetes project. *J Hypertens* 1999; 17: 1569–75.
80. Wong TY, Szeto CC, Chow KM, Chan JC, Li PK. Contribution of gene polymorphisms in the renin–angiotensin system to macroangiopathy in patients with diabetic nephropathy. *Am J Kidney Dis* 2001; 38: 9–17.
81. Hadjadj S, Belloum R, Bouhanick B, Gallois Y, Guilloteau G, Chatellier G, et al. Prognostic value of angiotensin-I converting enzyme I/D polymorphism for nephropathy in type 1 diabetes mellitus: a prospective study. *J Am Soc Nephrol* 2001; 12: 541–9.
82. Sagnella GA, Rothwell MJ, Onipinla AK, Wicks PD, Cook DG, Cappuccio FP. A population study of ethnic variations in the angiotensin-converting enzyme I/D polymorphism: relationships with gender, hypertension and impaired glucose metabolism. *J Hypertens* 1999; 17: 657–64.
83. Ha SK, Yong LS, Su PH, Ho SJ, Jung KS, Hun KD, et al. ACE DD genotype is more susceptible than ACE II and ID genotypes to the antiproteinuric effect of ACE inhibitors in patients with proteinuric non-insulin-dependent diabetes mellitus. *Nephrol Dial Transplant* 2000; 15: 1617–23.
84. Tarnow L, Parving HH, Jacobsen P, Rossing P, Lecerf L, Poirier O, et al. The significance of deletion polymorphism in the ACE gene for progression of diabetic

nephropathies treated with ACE inhibitors. *Ugeskr Laeger* 1998; 160: 4886–9.
85. Kuznetsova T, Staessen JA, Wang JG, Gasowski J, Nikitin Y, Ryabikov A, et al. Antihypertensive treatment modulates the association between the D/I ACE gene polymorphism and left ventricular hypertrophy: a meta-analysis. *J Hum Hypertens* 2000; 14: 447–54.
86. Bluthner M, Schmidt S, Siffert W, Knigge H, Nawroth P, Ritz E. Increased frequency of G-protein beta 3-subunit 825 T allele in dialyzed patients with type 2 diabetes. *Kidney Int* 1999; 55: 1247–50.
87. Fogarty DG, Zychma MJ, Scott LJ, Warram JH, Krolewski AS. The C825T polymorphism in the human G-protein beta3 subunit gene is not associated with diabetic nephropathy in type 1 diabetes mellitus. *Diabetologia* 1998; 41: 1304–8.
88. Siffert W. G protein beta3 subunit 825T allele, hypertension, obesity, and diabetic nephropathy [In Process Citation]. *Nephrol Dial Transplant* 2000; 15: 1298–306.
89. Nannipieri M, Manganiello M, Pezzatini A, De Bellis A, Seghieri G, Ferrannini E. Polymorphisms in the hANP (human atrial natriuretic peptide) gene, albuminuria, and hypertension. *Hypertension* 2001; 37: 1416–22.
90. Widen E, Lehto M, Kanninen T, Walston J, Shuldiner AR, Groop LC. Association of a polymorphism in the beta 3-adrenergic-receptor gene with features of the insulin resistance syndrome in Finns. *N Engl J Med* 1995; 333: 348–51.
91. Broussard BA, Valway SE, Kaufman S, Beaver S, Gohdes D. Clinical hypertension and its interaction with diabetes among American Indians and Alaska Natives. Estimated rates from ambulatory care data. *Diabetes Care* 1993; 16: 292–6.
92. Dowse GK, Collins VR, Alberti KG, Zimmet PZ, Tuomilehto J, Chitson P, et al, for the Mauritius Noncommunicable Disease Study Group. Insulin and blood pressure levels are not independently related in Mauritians of Asian Indian, Creole or Chinese origin. *J Hypertens* 1993; 11: 297–307.
93. Charles MA, Pettitt DJ, Hanson RL, Bennett PH, Saad MF, Liu QZ, et al. Familial and metabolic factors related to blood pressure in Pima Indian children. *Am J Epidemiol* 1994; 140: 123–31.
94. Saad MF, Lillioja S, Nyomba BL, Castillo C, Ferraro R, De Gregorio M, et al. Racial differences in the relation between blood pressure and insulin resistance. *N Engl J Med* 1991; 324: 733–9.
95. Hoy WE, Rees M, Kile E, Mathews JD, Wang Z. A new dimension to the Barker hypothesis: low birthweight and susceptibility to renal disease. *Kidney Int.* 1999; 56: 1072–7.
96. Kelly DJ, Skinner SL, Gilbert RE, Cox AJ, Cooper ME, Wilkinson-Berka JL. Effects of endothelin or angiotensin II receptor blockade on diabetes in the transgenic (mRen-2)27 rat. *Kidney Int.* 2000; 57: 1882–94.
97. Clausen T, Everts ME. Regulation of the Na,K-pump in skeletal muscle. *Kidney Int* 1989; 35: 1–13.
98. Davidson JS, Opie LH, Keding B. Sodium–potassium cotransport activity as genetic marker in essential hypertension. *Br Med J (Clin Res Ed)* 1982; 284: 539–41.
99. Boon NA, Harper C, Aronson JK, Grahame-Smith DG. Cation transport functions *in vitro* in patients with untreated essential hypertension: a comparison of erythrocytes and leucocytes. *Clin Sci (Lond)* 1985; 68: 511–5.
100. Postnov YV, Orlov SN. Ion transport across plasma membrane in primary hypertension. *Physiol Rev.* 1985; 65: 904–45.
101. Canessa M, Spalvins A, Adragna N, Falkner B. Red cell sodium countertransport and cotransport in normotensive and hypertensive blacks. *Hypertension* 1984; 6: 344–51.
102. Garay RP, Dagher G, Pernollet MG, Devynck MA, Meyer P. Inherited defect in a Na^+,K-co-transport system in erythrocytes from essential hypertensive patients. *Nature* 1980; 284: 281–3.
103. Hilton PJ. Cellular sodium transport in essential hypertension. *N Engl J Med* 1986; 314: 222–9.
104. Tepel M, Bauer S, Husseini S, Raffelsiefer A, Zidek W. Increased cytosolic free sodium concentrations in platelets from type 2 (non-insulin-dependent) diabetic patients is associated with hypertension. *J Endocrinol* 1993; 138: 565–72.
105. Ng LL, Davies JE, Siczkowski M, Sweeney FP, Quinn PA, Krolewski B, et al. Abnormal Na^+/H^+ antiporter phenotype and turnover of immortalized lymphoblasts from type 1 diabetic patients with nephropathy. *J Clin Invest* 1994; 93: 2750–7.
106. Delva P, Pastori C, Provoli E, Degan M, Arosio E, Montesi G, et al. Erythrocyte Na^+–H^+ exchange activity in essential hypertensive and obese patients: role of excess body weight. *J Hypertens* 1993; 11: 823–30.
107. Herman WH, Prior DE, Yassine MD, Weder AB. Nephropathy in NIDDM is associated with cellular markers for hypertension. *Diabetes Care* 1993; 16: 815–8.
108. Mimura M, Makino H, Kanatsuka A, Asai T, Yoshida S. Reduction of erythrocyte (Na^+–K^+)ATPase activity in type 2 (non-insulin-dependent) diabetic patients with MA. *Horm. Metab Res.* 1994; 26: 33–8.
109. Picado MJ, de la SA, Aguilera MT, Coca A, Urbanomarquez A. Increased activity of the Mg^{2+}/Na^+ exchanger in red blood cells from essential hypertensive patients. *Hypertension* 1994; 23: 987–91.
110. Resnick LM, Barbagallo M, Gupta RK, Laragh JH. Ionic basis of hypertension in diabetes mellitus. Role of hyperglycemia. *Am J Hypertens* 1993; 6: 413–7.
111. Draznin B. Cytosolic calcium and insulin resistance. *Am J Kidney Dis* 1993; 21: 32–8.
112. Papageorgiou P, Morgan KG. Intracellular free Ca^{2+} is elevated in hypertrophic aortic muscle from hypertensive rats. *Am J Physiol* 1991; 260: H507–15.
113. Mazzanti L, Rabini RA, Faloia E, Fumelli P, Bertoli E, De Pirro R. Altered cellular Ca^{2+} and Na^+ transport in diabetes mellitus. *Diabetes* 1990; 39: 850–4.
114. Sahai A, Ganguly PK. Lack of response of (Ca^{2+}+ Mg^{2+}) ATPase to atrial natriuretic peptide in basolateral membranes from kidney cortex of chronic diabetic rats. *Biochem Biophys Res Commun* 1990; 169: 537–44.
115. Ferrannini E, Taddei S, Santoro D, Natali A, Boni C, Del Chiaro D, et al. Independent stimulation of glucose metabolism and Na^+–K^+ exchange by insulin in the human forearm. *Am J Physiol* 1988; 255: E953–8.
116. Schmouder RL, Weder AB. Platelet sodium–proton exchange is increased in essential hypertension. *J Hypertens* 1989; 7: 325–30.
117. Canessa M, Adragna N, Solomon HS, Connolly TM, Tosteson DC. Increased sodium–lithium countertransport in red cells of patients with essential hypertension. *N Engl J Med* 1980; 302: 772–6.

118. Mangili R, Bending JJ, Scott G, Li LK, Gupta A, Viberti G. Increased sodium–lithium countertransport activity in red cells of patients with insulin-dependent diabetes and nephropathy. *N Engl J Med* 1988; 318: 146–50.
119. Williams RR, Hunt SC, Kuida H, Smith JB, Ash KO. Sodium–lithium countertransport in erythrocytes of hypertension prone families in Utah. *Am J Epidemiol* 1983; 118: 338–44.
120. Walker JD, Tariq T, Viberti G. Sodium–lithium countertransport activity in red cells of patients with insulin dependent diabetes and nephropathy and their parents. *BMJ* 1990; 301: 635–8.
121. Mead PA, Wilkinson R, Thomas TH. Na/Li countertransport abnormalities in type 1 diabetes with and without nephropathy are familial. *Diabetes Care* 2001; 24: 527–32.
122. Pinkney JH, Foyle WJ, Denver AE, Mohamed-Ali V, McKinlay S, Yudkin JS. The relationship of urinary albumin excretion rate to ambulatory blood pressure and erythrocyte sodium–lithium countertransport in NIDDM. *Diabetologia* 1995; 38: 356–62.
123. Rutherford PA, Thomas TH, Taylor R, Wilkinson R. Nephropathy and changes in sodium–lithium countertransport kinetics in type 2 (non-insulin-dependent) diabetes mellitus. *J Hum Hypertens* 1994; 8: 29–35.
124. Trevisan R, Fioretto P, Barbosa J, Mauer M. Insulin-dependent diabetic sibling pairs are concordant for sodium–hydrogen antiport activity. *Kidney Int* 1999; 55: 2383–9.
125. Trevisan R, Cipollina MR, Duner E, Trevisan M, Nosadini R. Abnormal Na^+/H^+ antiport activity in cultured fibroblasts from NIDDM patients with hypertension and MA. *Diabetologia* 1996; 39: 717–24.
126. Noel J, Pouyssegur J. Hormonal regulation, pharmacology, and membrane sorting of vertebrate Na^+/H^+ exchanger isoforms. *Am J Physiol* 1995; 268: C283–96.
127. Hall JE, Louis K. Dahl Memorial Lecture. Renal and CV mechanisms of hypertension in obesity. *Hypertension* 1994; 23: 381–94.
128. Tschope D, Rosen P, Gries FA. Increase in the cytosolic concentration of calcium in platelets of diabetics type II. *Thromb Res* 1991; 62: 421–8.
129. Draznin B, Sussman KE, Eckel RH, Kao M, Yost T, Sherman NA. Possible role of cytosolic free calcium concentrations in mediating insulin resistance of obesity and hyperinsulinemia. *J Clin Invest* 1988; 82: 1848–52.
130. Levy J, Grunberger G, Karl I, Gavin JR III. Effects of food restriction and insulin treatment on ($Ca^{2+} + Mg^{2+}$)-ATPase response to insulin in kidney basolateral membranes of noninsulin-dependent diabetic rats. *Metabolism* 1990; 39: 25–33.
131. Schaefer W, Priessen J, Mannhold R, Gries AF. Ca^{2+}–Mg^{2+}-ATPase activity of human red blood cells in healthy and diabetic volunteers. *Klin Wochenschr* 1987; 65: 17–21.
132. Ohno Y, Suzuki H, Yamakawa H, Nakamura M, Otsuka K, Saruta T. Impaired insulin sensitivity in young, lean normotensive offspring of essential hypertensives: possible role of disturbed calcium metabolism. *J Hypertens* 1993; 11: 421–6.
133. Resnick LM, Gupta RK, Bhargava KK, Gruenspan H, Alderman MH, Laragh JH. Cellular ions in hypertension, diabetes, and obesity. A nuclear magnetic resonance spectroscopic study. *Hypertension* 1991; 17: 951–7.
134. Rocchini AP. The relationship of sodium sensitivity to insulin resistance. *Am J Med Sci* 1994; 307 (suppl 1): S75–80.
135. Sharma AM, Ruland K, Spies KP, Distler A. Salt sensitivity in young normotensive subjects is associated with a hyperinsulinemic response to oral glucose. *J Hypertens* 1991; 9: 329–35.
136. Zhu Z, Tepel M, Neusser M, Mehring N, Zidek W. Concentration-dependent effects of insulin on Ca^{2+} influx in vascular smooth muscle cells of normotensive and spontaneously hypertensive rats. *Clin Sci (Lond)* 1993; 85: 425–9.
137. Hollister AS, Inagami T. Atrial natriuretic factor and hypertension. A review and metaanalysis. *Am J Hypertens* 1991; 4: 850–65.
138. Scherrer U, Sartori C. Insulin as a vascular and sympathoexcitatory hormone: implications for blood pressure regulation, insulin sensitivity, and CV morbidity. *Circulation* 1997; 96: 4104–13.
139. Sechi LA. Mechanisms of insulin resistance in rat models of hypertension and their relationships with salt sensitivity. *J Hypertens* 1999; 17: 1229–37.
140. Reaven GM, Hoffman BB. A role for insulin in the aetiology and course of hypertension? *Lancet* 1987; 2: 435–7.
141. Reaven GM. The kidney: an unwilling accomplice in syndrome X. *Am J Kidney Dis* 1997; 30: 928–31.
142. Rumantir MS, Vaz M, Jennings GL, Collier G, Kaye DM, Seals DR, et al. Neural mechanisms in human obesity-related hypertension. *J Hypertens* 1999; 17: 1125–33.
143. Haynes WG, Sivitz WI, Morgan DA, Walsh SA, Mark AL. Sympathetic and cardiorenal actions of leptin. *Hypertension* 1997; 30: 619–23.
144. Wolf G, Chen S, Han DC, Ziyadeh FN. Leptin and renal disease. *Am J Kidney Dis* 2002; 39: 1–11.
145. Villarreal D, Reams G, Freeman RH. Effects of renal denervation on the sodium excretory actions of leptin in hypertensive rats. *Kidney Int* 2000; 58: 989–94.
146. Widjaja A, Stratton IM, Horn R, Holman RR, Turner R, Brabant G. UKPDS 20: plasma leptin, obesity, and plasma insulin in type 2 diabetic subjects. *J Clin. Endocrinol. Metab* 1997; 82: 654–7.
147. Fruehwald-Schultes B, Kern W, Beyer J, Forst T, Pfutzner A, Peters A. Elevated serum leptin concentrations in type 2 diabetic patients with MA and macroalbuminuria. *Metabolism* 1999; 48: 1290–3.
148. Nakata T, Takeda K, Hatta T, Kiyama M, Moriguchi J, Miki S, et al. Blockade of angiotensin II receptors inhibits the increase in blood pressure induced by insulin. *J Cardiovasc Pharmacol* 1998; 31: 248–52.
149. Muntzel MS. Insulin-mediated sympathoexcitation in obesity and type 2 diabetes. *Nephrol Dial Transplant* 1999; 14: 2282–5.
150. Burns KD. Angiotensin II and its receptors in the diabetic kidney. *Am J Kidney Dis* 2000; 36: 449–67.
151. Navar LG, Lewis L, Hymel A, Braam B, Mitchell KD. Tubular fluid concentrations and kidney contents of angiotensins I and II in anesthetized rats. *J Am Soc Nephrol* 1994; 5: 1153–8.
152. Quan A, Baum M. Endogenous angiotensin II modulates rat proximal tubule transport with acute changes in extracellular volume. *Am J Physiol* 1998; 275: F74–8.
153. De'Oliveira JM, Price DA, Fisher ND, Allan DR, McKnight JA, Williams GH, et al. Autonomy of the renin system in type II diabetes mellitus: dietary sodium and

renal hemodynamic responses to ACE inhibition. *Kidney Int* 1997; 52: 771–7.
154. Siragy HM. AT(1) and AT(2) receptors in the kidney: role in disease and treatment. *Am J Kidney Dis* 2000; 36: S4–9.
155. Bonnet F, Candido R, Carey RM, Casley D, Russo LM, Osicka TM, et al. Renal expression of angiotensin receptors in long-term diabetes and the effects of angiotensin type 1 receptor blockade. *J Hypertens* 2002; 20: 1615–24.
156. Hollenberg NK. AT(1)-receptor blockade and the kidney: importance of non-ACE pathways in health and disease. *J Hum Hypertens* 2002; 16 (suppl 3): S59–63.
157. Abiko A, Eto M, Makino I, Araki N, Horiuchi S. Increased levels of advanced glycosylation end products in the kidney and liver from spontaneously diabetic Chinese hamsters determined by immunochemical assay. *Metabolism* 2000; 49: 567–73.
158. Chibber R, Ben Mahmud BM, Coppini D, Christ E, Kohner EM. Activity of the glycosylating enzyme, core 2 GlcNAc (beta1,6) transferase, is higher in polymorphonuclear leukocytes from diabetic patients compared with age-matched control subjects: relevance to capillary occlusion in diabetic retinopathy. *Diabetes* 2000; 49: 1724–30.
159. Cohen MP, Sharma K, Jin Y, Hud E, Wu VY, Tomaszewski J, et al. Prevention of diabetic nephropathy in *db/db* mice with glycated albumin antagonists. A novel treatment strategy. *J Clin Invest* 1995; 95: 2338–45.
160. Forbes JM, Soulis T, Thallas V, Panagiotopoulos S, Long DM, Vasan S, et al. Renoprotective effects of a novel inhibitor of advanced glycation. *Diabetologia* 2001; 44: 108–14.
161. Chiarelli F, Cipollone F, Romano F, Tumini S, Costantini F, di Ricco L, et al. Increased circulating nitric oxide in young patients with type 1 diabetes and persistent MA: relation to glomerular hyperfiltration. *Diabetes* 2000; 49: 1258–63.
162. Mykkanen L, Zaccaro DJ, Wagenknecht LE, Robbins DC, Gabriel M, Haffner SM. MA is associated with insulin resistance in nondiabetic subjects: the insulin resistance atherosclerosis study. *Diabetes* 1998; 47: 793–800.
163. Mangrum A, Bakris GL. Predictors of renal and CV mortality in patients with non- insulin-dependent diabetes: a brief overview of MA and insulin resistance. *J Diabetes Complications* 1997; 11: 352–7.
164. Pallone TL, Mattson DL. Role of nitric oxide in regulation of the renal medulla in normal and hypertensive kidneys. *Curr Opin Nephrol Hypertens* 2002; 11: 93–8.
165. Kone BC, Higham S. Nitric oxide inhibits transcription of the Na^+–K^+-ATPase alpha1-subunit gene in an MTAL cell line. *Am J Physiol* 1999; 276: F614–21.
166. Brands MW, Fitzgerald SM. Blood pressure control early in diabetes: a balance between angiotensin II and nitric oxide. *Clin Exp Pharmacol Physiol* 2002; 29: 127–31.
167. Maejima K, Nakano S, Himeno M, Tsuda S, Makiishi H, Ito T, et al. Increased basal levels of plasma nitric oxide in type 2 diabetic subjects. Relationship to microvascular complications. *J Diabetes Complications* 2001; 15: 135–43.
168. Ding Y, Vaziri ND, Coulson R, Kamanna VS, Roh DD. Effects of simulated hyperglycemia, insulin, and glucagon on endothelial nitric oxide synthase expression. *Am J Physiol Endocrinol. Metab* 2000; 279: E11–7.
169. Goligorsky MS, Chen J, Brodsky S. Workshop: endothelial cell dysfunction leading to diabetic nephropathy. Focus on nitric oxide. *Hypertension* 2001; 37: 744–8.
170. Erley CM, Heyne N, Friedrich B, Schmidt T, Strobel U, Wehrmann M, et al. Differential renal response to Nomega-nitro-L-arginine methyl ester and L-arginine in rats with hypertensive or diabetic nephropathy. *J Cardiovasc Pharmacol* 2002; 40: 780–8.
171. Gewaltig MT, Kojda G. Vasoprotection by nitric oxide: mechanisms and therapeutic potential. *Cardiovasc Res* 2002; 55: 250–60.
172. Henningsson R, Salehi A, Lundquist I. Role of nitric oxide synthase isoforms in glucose-stimulated insulin release. *Am J Physiol Cell Physiol* 2002; 283: C296–304.
173. Turner RC. The U.K. Prospective Diabetes Study. A review. *Diabetes Care* 1998; 21 (suppl 3): C35–8.
174. Wong ND, Cupples LA, Ostfeld AM, Levy D, Kannel WB. Risk factors for long-term coronary prognosis after initial myocardial infarction: the Framingham Study. *Am J Epidemiol* 1989; 130: 469–80.
175. Stamler J, Vaccaro O, Neaton JD, Wentworth D. Diabetes, other risk factors, and 12-yr CV mortality for men screened in the Multiple Risk Factor Intervention Trial. *Diabetes Care* 1993; 16: 434–44.
176. Neal B, Macmahon S, Chapman N, for the Blood Pressure Lowering Treatment Trialists' Collaboration. Effects of ACE inhibitors, calcium antagonists, and other blood-pressure-lowering drugs: results of prospectively designed overviews of randomized trials. *Lancet* 2000; 356: 1955–64.
177. Staessen JA, Wang JG, Thijs L. Cardiovascular protection and blood pressure reduction: a meta-analysis. *Lancet* 2001; 358: 1305–15.
178. Curb JD, Pressel SL, Cutler JA, Savage PJ, Applegate WB, Black H, et al, for the Systolic Hypertension in the Elderly Program Cooperative Research Group. Effect of diuretic-based antihypertensive treatment on CV disease risk in older diabetic patients with isolated systolic hypertension. *JAMA* 1996; 276: 1886–92.
179. Celis H, Fagard RH, Staessen JA, Thijs L. Risk and benefit of treatment of isolated systolic hypertension in the elderly: evidence from the Systolic Hypertension in Europe Trial. *Curr. Opin. Cardiol* 2001; 16: 342–8.
180. Gasowski J, Birkenhager WH, Staessen JA, de Leeuw PW. Benefit of antihypertensive treatment in the diabetic patients enrolled in the Systolic Hypertension in Europe (Syst-Eur) trial. *Cardiovasc Drugs Ther* 2000; 14: 49–53.
181. Hansson L, Zanchetti A, Carruthers SG, Dahlof B, Elmfeldt D, Julius S, et al, for the HOT Study Group. Effects of intensive blood-pressure lowering and low-dose aspirin in patients with hypertension: principal results of the Hypertension Optimal Treatment (HOT) randomized trial. *Lancet* 1998; 351: 1755–62.
182. Kjeldsen SE, Dahlof B, Devereux RB, Julius S, Aurup P, Edelman J, et al. Effects of Losartan on CV morbidity and mortality in patients with isolated systolic hypertension and left ventricular hypertrophy: a Losartan Intervention for Endpoint Reduction (LIFE) Substudy. *JAMA* 2002; 288: 1491–8.
183. Yusuf S, Sleight P, Pogue J, Bosch J, Davies R, Dagenais G, for the Heart Outcomes Prevention Evaluation Study Investigators. Effects of an angiotensin-converting-enzyme inhibitor, ramipril, on CV events in high-risk patients. *N Engl J Med* 2000; 342: 145–53.
184. UKPDS Group. Cost effectiveness analysis of improved blood pressure control in hypertensive patients with type 2 diabetes: UKPDS 40. *BMJ* 1998; 317: 720–6.

185. Cost-effectiveness of intensive glycemic control, intensified hypertension control, and serum cholesterol level reduction for type 2 diabetes. *JAMA* 2002; 287: 2542–51.
186. Elliott WJ, Weir DR, Black HR, for the Joint National Committee on Prevention, Detection, Evaluation, and Treatment of High Blood Pressure. Cost-effectiveness of the lower treatment goal (of JNC VI) for diabetic hypertensive patients. *Arch Intern Med* 2000; 160: 1277–83.
187. Rodby RA, Firth LM, Lewis EJ, for the Collaborative Study Group. An economic analysis of captopril in the treatment of diabetic nephropathy. *Diabetes Care* 1996; 19: 1051–61.
188. The sixth report of the Joint National Committee on prevention, detection, evaluation, and treatment of high blood pressure. *Arch Intern Med* 1997; 157: 2413–46.
189. 1999 World Health Organization–International Society of Hypertension Guidelines for the management of Hypertension. Guidelines Subcommittee. *J Hypertens* 1999; 17: 151–83.
190. Ramsey L, Williams B, Johnston G, MacGregor G, Poston L, Potter J, Poulter N, Russell G. Guidelines for management of hypertension: report of the third working party of the British Hypertension Society. *J Human Hypertension* 1999; 13: 569–92.
191. American Diabetes Association. Clinical Practice Recommendations 2002. *Diabetes Care* 2002; 25 (suppl 1): S1–147.
192. McAlister FA, Campbell NR, Zarnke K, Levine M, Graham ID. The management of hypertension in Canada: a review of current guidelines, their shortcomings and implications for the future. *CMAJ* 2001; 164: 517–22.
193. Orchard TJ, Forrest KY, Kuller LH, Becker DJ. Lipid and blood pressure treatment goals for type 1 diabetes: 10-year incidence data from the Pittsburgh Epidemiology of Diabetes Complications Study. *Diabetes Care* 2001; 24: 1053–9.
194. The Heart Outcomes Prevention Evaluation Study Investigators. Effects of ramipril on CV and microvascular outcomes in people with diabetes mellitus: results of the HOPE study and MICRO-HOPE substudy [see comments]. *Lancet* 2000; 355: 253–9.
195. Stephenson JM, Fuller JH, Viberti GC, Sjolie AK, Navalesi R. Blood pressure, retinopathy and urinary albumin excretion in IDDM: the EURODIAB IDDM Complications Study. *Diabetologia* 1995; 38: 599–603.
196. Vasan RS, Larson MG, Leip EP, Evans JC, O'Donnell CJ, Kannel WB, et al. Impact of high-normal blood pressure on the risk of CV disease. *N Engl J Med* 2001; 345: 1291–7.
197. UKPDS Group. Tight blood pressure control and risk of macrovascular and microvascular complications in type 2 diabetes: UKPDS 38. *BMJ* 1998; 317: 703–13.
198. Adler AI, Stratton IM, Neil HA, Yudkin JS, Matthews DR, Cull CA, et al. Association of systolic blood pressure with macrovascular and microvascular complications of type 2 diabetes (UKPDS 36): prospective observational study. *BMJ* 2000; 321: 412–9.
199. Klahr S, Levey AS, Beck GJ, Caggiula AW, Hunsicker L, Kusek JW, et al, for the Modification of Diet in Renal Disease Study Group. The effects of dietary protein restriction and blood-pressure control on the progression of chronic renal disease. *N Engl J Med* 1994; 330: 877–84.
200. Hebert LA, Kusek JW, Greene T, Agodoa LY, Jones CA, Levey AS, et al, for the Modification of Diet in Renal Disease Study Group. Effects of blood pressure control on progressive renal disease in blacks and whites. *Hypertension* 1997; 30: 428–35.
201. Schrier RW, Estacio RO, Esler A, Mehler P. Effects of aggressive blood pressure control in normotensive type 2 diabetic patients on albuminuria, retinopathy and strokes. *Kidney Int* 2002; 61: 1086–97.
202. Agodoa LY, Appel L, Bakris GL, Beck G, Bourgoignie J, Briggs JP, et al. Effect of ramipril vs amlodipine on renal outcomes in hypertensive nephrosclerosis: a randomized controlled trial. *JAMA* 2001; 285: 2719–28.
203. Lewis JB, Berl T, Bain RP, Rohde RD, Lewis EJ, for the Collaborative Study Group. Effect of intensive blood pressure control on the course of type 1 diabetic nephropathy. *Am J Kidney Dis* 1999; 34: 809–17.
204. Bulpitt CJ, Palmer AJ, Fletcher AE, Beevers DG, Coles EC, Ledingham JG, et al. Optimal blood pressure control in treated hypertensive patients. Report from the Department of Health Hypertension Care Computing Project (DHCCP). *Circulation* 1994; 90: 225–33.
205. Kaplan NM. What is goal blood pressure for the treatment of hypertension? *Arch Intern Med* 2001; 161: 1480–2.
206. Voko Z, Bots ML, Hofman A, Koudstaal PJ, Witteman JC, Breteler MM. J-shaped relation between blood pressure and stroke in treated hypertensives. *Hypertension* 1999; 34: 1181–5.
207. Cziraky MJ, Mehra IV, Wilson MD, Bakris GL. Current issues in treating the hypertensive patient with diabetes: focus on diabetic nephropathy. *Ann. Pharmacother* 1996; 30: 791–801.
208. Deckert T, Feldt-Rasmussen B, Borch-Johnsen K, Jensen T, Kofoed-Enevoldsen A, Mathiesen ER. Natural history of diabetic complications: early detection and progression. *Diabet Med* 1991; 8 (special issue): S33–7.
209. Jerums G, Panagiotopoulos S, Tsalamandris C, Allen TJ, Gilbert RE, Comper WD. Why is proteinuria such an important risk factor for progression in clinical trials? *Kidney Int* 1997; 63 (suppl): S87–92.
210. Haffner SM, Mitchell BD, Pugh JA, Stern MP, Kozlowski MK, Hazuda HP, et al. Proteinuria in Mexican Americans and non-Hispanic whites with NIDDM. *Diabetes Care* 1989; 12: 530–36.
211. Gerstein HC, Mann JF, Yi Q, Zinman B, Dinneen SF, Hoogwerf B, et al. Albuminuria and risk of CV events, death, and heart failure in diabetic and nondiabetic individuals. *JAMA* 2001; 286: 421–6.
212. Gerstein HC, Mann JF, Pogue J, Dinneen SF, Halle JP, Hoogwerf B, et al, for the HOPE Study Investigators. Prevalence and determinants of MA in high-risk diabetic and nondiabetic patients in the Heart Outcomes Prevention Evaluation Study. *Diabetes Care* 2000; 23 (suppl 2): B35–9.
213. Dinneen SF, Gerstein HC. The association of microalbuminuria and mortality in non-insulin dependent diabetes mellitus. A systematic overview of the literature. *Arch Intern Med* 1997; 157: 1413–8.
214. Ruggenenti P, Perna A, Benini R, Bertani T, Zoccali C, Maggiore Q, et al, for the Investigators of the GISEN Group. In chronic nephropathies prolonged ACE inhibition can induce remission: dynamics of time-dependent changes in GFR. *J Am Soc Nephrol* 1999; 10: 997–1006.
215. Peterson JC, Adler S, Burkart JM, Greene T, Hebert LA, Hunsicker LG, et al. Blood pressure control, proteinuria, and the progression of renal disease. The Modification of Diet in Renal Disease Study. *Ann Intern Med* 1995; 123: 754–62.

216. Ruggenenti P, Perna A, Gherardi G, Benini R, Remuzzi G. Chronic proteinuric nephropathies: outcomes and response to treatment in a prospective cohort of 352 patients with different patterns of renal injury. *Am J Kidney Dis* 2000; 35: 1155–65.
217. Bakris GL. Maximizing cardiorenal benefit in the management of hypertension: achieve blood pressure goals. *J Clin Hypertens* (Greenwich) 1999; 1: 141–7.
218. Neal B, Macmahon S. The World Health Organization–International Society of Hypertension Blood Pressure Lowering Treatment Trialists' Collaboration: prospective collaborative overviews of major randomized trials of blood pressure-lowering treatments. *Curr Hypertens Rep* 1999; 1: 346–56.
219. Cohn JN, Tognoni G. A randomized trial of the angiotensin-receptor blocker valsartan in chronic heart failure. *N Engl J Med* 2001; 345: 1667–75.
220. The SOLVD Investigators. Effect of enalapril on mortality and the development of heart failure in asymptomatic patients with reduced left ventricular ejection fractions. *N Engl J Med* 1992; 327: 685–91.
221. Hansson L, Lindholm LH, Niskanen L, Lanke J, Hedner T, Niklason A, et al. Effect of angiotensin-converting-enzyme inhibition comparred with conventional therapyon CV morbidity and mortality in hypertension: the Captopril Prevention Project (CAPPP) randomized trial. *Lancet* 1999; 353: 611–6.
222. Svensson P, de Faire U, Sleight P, Yusuf S, Ostergren J. Comparative effects of ramipril on ambulatory and office blood pressures: a HOPE Substudy. *Hypertension* 2001; 38: E28–32.
223. Lewis EJ, Hunsicker LG, Bain RP, Rohde RD, for the Collaborative Study Group. The effect of angiotensin-converting-enzyme inhibition on diabetic nephropathy. *N Engl J Med* 1993; 329: 1456–62.
224. Parving HH, Andersen AR, Smidt UM, Svendsen PA. Early aggressive antihypertensive treatment reduces rate of decline in kidney function in diabetic nephropathy. *Lancet* 1983; 1: 1175–9.
225. Bakris GL, Slataper R, Vicknair N, Sadler R. ACE inhibitor mediated reductions in renal size and MA in normotensive, diabetic subjects. *J Diabetes Complications* 1994; 8: 2–6.
226. Garg J, Bakris GL. Angiotensin converting enzyme inhibitors or Angiotensin receptor blockers in nephropathy from type 2 diabetes. *Curr Hypertens Rep* 2002; 4: 185–90.
227. Lacourciere Y, Belanger A, Godin C, Halle JP, Ross S, Wright N, et al. Long-term comparison of losartan and enalapril on kidney function in hypertensive type 2 diabetics with early nephropathy. *Kidney Int* 2000; 58: 762–9.
228. Sica DA, Bakris GL. Type 2 diabetes: RENAAL and IDNT—the emergence of new treatment options. *J Clin Hypertens* (Greenwich) 2002; 4: 52–7.
229. Pitt B, Segal R, Martinez FA, Meurers G, Cowley AJ, Thomas I, et al. Randomised trial of losartan versus captopril in patients over 65 with heart failure (Evaluation of Losartan in the Elderly Study, ELITE). *Lancet* 1997; 349: 747–52.
230. Pitt B, Poole-Wilson PA, Segal R, Martinez FA, Dickstein K, Camm AJ, et al. Effect of losartan compared with captopril on mortality in patients with symptomatic heart failure: randomized trial—the Losartan Heart Failure Survival Study ELITE II. *Lancet* 2000; 355: 1582–7.
231. Dahlof B, Devereux RB, Kjeldsen SE, Julius S, Beevers G, Faire U, et al. CV morbidity and mortality in the Losartan Intervention for Endpoint reduction in hypertension study (LIFE): a randomized trial against atenolol. *Lancet* 2002; 359: 995–1003.
232. Brenner BM, Cooper ME, De Zeeuw D, Keane WF, Mitch WE, Parving HH, et al. Effects of losartan on renal and CV outcomes in patients with type 2 diabetes and nephropathy. *N Engl J Med* 2001; 345: 861–9.
233. Lewis EJ, Hunsicker LG, Clarke WR, Berl T, Pohl MA, Lewis JB, et al. Renoprotective effect of the angiotensin-receptor antagonist irbesartan in patients with nephropathy due to type 2 diabetes. *N Engl J Med* 2001; 345: 851–60.
234. Jafar TH, Schmid CH, Landa M, Giatras I, Toto R, Remuzzi G, et al. Angiotensin-converting enzyme inhibitors and progression of nondiabetic renal disease. A meta-analysis of patient-level data. *Ann Intern Med* 2001; 135: 73–87.
235. Bakris GL, Siomos M, Richardson D, Janssen I, Bolton WK, Hebert L, et al, for the VAL-K Study Group. ACE inhibition or angiotensin receptor blockade: impact on potassium in renal failure. *Kidney Int* 2000; 58: 2084–92.
236. Coresh J, Wei GL, McQuillan G, Brancati FL, Levey AS, Jones C, et al. Prevalence of high blood pressure and elevated serum creatinine level in the United States: findings from the third National Health and Nutrition Examination Survey (1988–1994). *Arch Intern Med* 2001; 161: 1207–16.
237. Singer GM, Izhar M, Black HR. Goal-oriented hypertension management: translating clinical trials to practice. *Hypertension* 2002; 40: 464–9.
238. Bakris G, Weir M, for the SHIELD Trial Investigators. Achieving goal blood pressure in patients with type 2 diabetes: conventional versus fixed-dose combination approaches. *J Clin Hypertens (Greenwich)* 2003; 5: 201–10.
239. Bakris GL. The role of combination antihypertensive therapy and the progression of renal disease hypertension: looking toward the next millennium. *Am J Hypertens* 1998; 11: 158S–62S.
240. Bakris GL. A practical approach to achieving recommended blood pressure goals in diabetic patients. *Arch Intern Med* 2001; 161: 2661–7.
241. Christensen CK, Pedersen MM, Mogensen CE. Combining antihypertensive agents in early diabetic nephropathy. *J Diabet Complications* 1990; 4: 88–90.
242. Fernandez R, Puig JG, Rodriguez-Perez JC, Garrido J, Redon J. Effect of two antihypertensive combinations on metabolic control in type-2 diabetic hypertensive patients with albuminuria: a randomized, double-blind study. *J Hum Hypertens* 2001; 15: 849–56.
243. Hollenberg NK. AT(1)-receptor blockade and the kidney: importance of non-ACE pathways in health and disease. *J Hum Hypertens* 2002; 16 (suppl 3): S59–63.
244. Komine N, Khang S, Wead LM, Blantz RC, Gabbai FB. Effect of combining an ACE inhibitor and an angiotensin II receptor blocker on plasma and kidney tissue angiotensin II levels. *Am J Kidney Dis* 2002; 39: 159–64.
245. Wilkinson-Berka JL, Gibbs NJ, Cooper ME, Skinner SL, Kelly DJ. Renoprotective and anti-hypertensive effects of combined valsartan and perindopril in progressive diabetic nephropathy in the transgenic (mRen-2)27 rat. *Nephrol Dial Transplant* 2001; 16: 1343–9.
246. Bidani AK, Griffin KA, Bakris G, Picken MM. Lack of evidence of blood pressure-independent protection by

renin–angiotensin system blockade after renal ablation. *Kidney Int* 2000; 57: 1651–61.
247. Zou LX, Hymel A, Imig JD, Navar LG. Renal accumulation of circulating angiotensin II in angiotensin II-infused rats. *Hypertension* 1996; 27: 658–62.
248. Agarwal R. Add-on angiotensin receptor blockade with maximized ACE inhibition. *Kidney Int* 2001; 59: 2282–9.
249. Savage PJ, Pressel SL, Curb JD, Schron EB, Applegate WB, Black HR, et al, for the SHEP Cooperative Research Group. Influence of long-term, low-dose, diuretic-based, antihypertensive therapy on glucose, lipid, uric acid, and potassium levels in older men and women with isolated systolic hypertension: the Systolic Hypertension in the Elderly Program. *Arch Intern Med* 1998; 158: 741–51.
250. Koshy S, Bakris GL. Therapeutic approaches to achieve desired blood pressure goals: focus on calcium channel blockers. *Cardiovasc Drugs Ther* 2000; 14: 295–301.
251. Tarif N, Bakris GL. Preservation of renal function: the spectrum of effects by calcium-channel blockers. *Nephrol Dial Transplant* 1997; 12: 2244–50.
252. Griffin KA, Picken M, Bakris GL, Bidani AK. Comparative effects of selective T- and L-type calcium channel blockers in the remnant kidney model. *Hypertension* 2001; 37: 1268–72.
253. Griffin KA, Picken MM, Bakris GL, Bidani AK. Class differences in the effects of calcium channel blockers in the rat remnant kidney model. *Kidney Int* 1999; 55: 1849–60.
254. Brown SA, Walton CL, Crawford P, Bakris GL. Long-term effects of antihypertensive regimens on renal hemodynamics and proteinuria. *Kidney Int* 1993; 43: 1210–8.
255. Gaber L, Walton C, Brown S, Bakris G. Effects of different antihypertensive treatments on morphologic progression of diabetic nephropathy in uninephrectomized dogs. *Kidney Int* 1994; 46: 161–9.
256. Smith AC, Toto R, Bakris GL. Differential effects of calcium channel blockers on size selectivity of proteinuria in diabetic glomerulopathy. *Kidney Int* 1998; 54: 889–96.
257. Maki DD, MA JZ, Louis TA, Kasiske BL. Long-term effects of antihypertensive agents on proteinuria and renal function. *Arch Intern Med* 1995; 155: 1073–80.
258. Kloke HJ, Branten AJ, Huysmans FT, Wetzels JF. Antihypertensive treatment of patients with proteinuric renal diseases: risks or benefits of calcium channel blockers? *Kidney Int* 1998; 53: 1559–73.
259. Estacio RO, Jeffers BW, Gifford N, Schrier RW. Effect of blood pressure control on diabetic microvascular complications in patients with hypertension and type 2 diabetes. *Diabetes Care* 2000; 23 (suppl 2): B54–64.
260. Estacio RO, Jeffers BW, Hiatt WR, Biggerstaff SL, Gifford N, Schrier RW. The effect of nisoldipine as compared with enalapril on CV outcomes in patients with non-insulin-dependent diabetes and hypertension. *N Engl J Med* 1998; 338: 645–52.
261. Packer M, O'Connor CM, Ghali JK, Pressler ML, Carson PE, Belkin RN, et al, for the Prospective Randomized Amlodipine Survival Evaluation Study Group. Effect of amlodipine on morbidity and mortality in severe chronic heart failure *N Engl J Med* 1996; 335: 1107–14.
262. Cohn JN, Ziesche S, Smith R, Anand I, Dunkman WB, Loeb H, et al, for the Vasodilator-Heart Failure Trial (V-HeFT) Study Group. Effect of the calcium antagonist felodipine as supplementary vasodilator therapy in patients with chronic heart failure treated with enalapril: V-HeFT III. *Circulation* 1997; 96: 856–63.
263. Tatti P, Pahor M, Byington RP, Di mauro P, Guarisco R, Strollo G, et al. Outcome results of the Fosinopril Versus Amlodipine CV Events Randomized Trial (FACET) in patients with hypertension and NIDDM. *Diabetes Care* 1998; 21: 597–603.
264. Tarnow L, Rossing P, Jensen C, Hansen BV, Parving HH. Long-term renoprotective effect of nisoldipine and lisinopril in type 1 diabetic patients with diabetic nephropathy. *Diabetes Care* 2000; 23: 1725–30.
265. Voyaki SM, Staessen JA, Thijs L, Wang JG, Efstratopoulos AD, Birkenhager WH, et al, for the Systolic Hypertension in Europe (Syst-Eur) Trial Investigators. Follow-up of renal function in treated and untreated older patients with isolated systolic hypertension. *J Hypertens* 2001; 19: 511–9.
266. Bakris GL, Mangrum A, Copley JB, Vicknair N, Sadler R. Effect of calcium channel or beta-blockade on the progression of diabetic nephropathy in African Americans. *Hypertension* 1997; 29: 744–50.
267. Bakris GL, Copley JB, Vicknair N, Sadler R, Leurgans S. Calcium channel blockers versus other antihypertensive therapies on progression of NIDDM associated nephropathy. *Kidney Int* 1996; 50: 1641–50.
268. Guasch A, Parham M, Zayas CF, Campbell O, Nzerue C, Macon E. Contrasting effects of calcium channel blockade versus converting enzyme inhibition on proteinuria in African Americans with non-insulin-dependent diabetes mellitus and nephropathy. *J Am Soc Nephrol* 1997; 8: 793–8.
269. UKPDS Group. Efficacy of atenolol and captopril in reducing risk of macrovascular and microvascular complications in type 2 diabetes: UKPDS 39. *BMJ* 1998; 317: 713–20.
270. Jonas M, Reicher-Reiss H, Boyko V, Shotan A, Mandelzweig L, Goldbourt U, et al, for the Bezafibrate Infarction Prevention (BIP) Study Group. Usefulness of beta-blocker therapy in patients with non-insulin-dependent diabetes mellitus and coronary artery disease. *Am J Cardiol* 1996; 77: 1273–7.
271. Landray MJ, Toescu V, Kendall MJ. The cardioprotective role of beta-blockers in patients with diabetes mellitus. *J Clin Pharm Ther* 2002; 27: 233–42.
272. Jacob S, Rett K, Henriksen EJ. Antihypertensive therapy and insulin sensitivity: do we have to redefine the role of beta-blocking agents? *Am J Hypertens* 1998; 11: 1258–65.
273. Sawicki PT, Siebenhofer A. Betablocker treatment in diabetes mellitus. *J Intern Med* 2001; 250: 11–7.
274. Sowers JR, Bakris GL. Antihypertensive therapy and the risk of type 2 diabetes mellitus [editorial; comment]. *N Engl J Med* 2000; 342: 969–70.
275. Metra M, Giubbini R, Nodari S, Boldi E, Modena MG, Dei CL. Differential effects of beta-blockers in patients with heart failure: a prospective, randomized, double-blind comparison of the long-term effects of metoprolol versus carvedilol. *Circulation* 2000; 102: 546–51.
276. Giugliano D, Acampora R, Marfella R, De Rosa N, Ziccardi P, Ragone R, et al. Metabolic and CV effects of carvedilol and atenolol in non-insulin-dependent diabetes

mellitus and hypertension. A randomized, controlled trial. *Ann Intern Med* 1997; 126: 955–9.

277. Packer M, Coats AJ, Fowler MB, Katus HA, Krum H, Mohacsi P, et al. Effect of carvedilol on survival in severe chronic heart failure. *N Engl J Med* 2001; 344: 1651–8.

278. ALLHAT Collaborative Research Group. Major CV events in hypertensive patients randomized to doxazosin vs chlorthalidone: the antihypertensive and lipid-lowering treatment to prevent heart attack trial (ALLHAT). *JAMA* 2000; 283: 1967–75.

279. Saseen JJ, Carter BL, Brown TE, Elliott WJ, Black HR. Comparison of nifedipine alone and with diltiazem or verapamil in hypertension. *Hypertension* 1996; 28: 109–14.

84

Cerebrovascular Disease in Diabetes Mellitus

Christopher S. Gray

University of Newcastle upon Tyne, Newcastle upon Tyne, UK

INTRODUCTION

The diagnostic label of cerebrovascular disease encompasses a spectrum of disorders ranging from reversible neurological symptoms and signs due to transient ischemic attacks (TIAs) to fixed neurological deficits resulting from an established stroke consequent upon cerebral infarction or primary intracerebral hemorrhage. In addition, there is increasing recognition that cerebrovascular disease is not only a major cause of cognitive impairment through what is conventionally termed vascular dementia but also contributes to Alzheimer's dementia through a mixed vascular and Alzheimer's type pathology. Against this diversity in presentation, the economic and health care burden of cerebrovascular disease has been well described but is often ignored. It is estimated that in North America and the United Kingdom cerebrovascular disease is the third major cause of death, the major cause of severe disability in the community, and the single most expensive medical disorder, consuming up to 6% of the total clinical budget [1]. Worldwide, the age-adjusted incidence of stroke ranges between 246 (US), 260 (UK), and 486 (Russia) per 100 000 population aged 45–74 years. Stroke is, however, primarily a disorder of older people, with the peak incidence occurring in those aged 75 years or older [2, 3]. Against this background of high cost and social burden, the major risk factors for stroke have been well defined and the management of modifiable risk factors is now detailed not only in specialty guidelines but also in National Service Frameworks (UK). Despite the increased use of such guideline-based interventions it is likely that the incidence of stroke will continue to rise, not only as a result of the demographic shift in our population toward the extreme of old age but also as a result of the changing prevalence of existing risk factors in this aging population [4].

Both type 1 (insulin-dependent) and type 2 (non-insulin-dependent) diabetes mellitus are important risk factors for cerebrovascular disease conferring a two- to threefold increased risk of first ever and recurrent stroke [5, 6]. For older people the prevalent form of diabetes is type 2, occurring in up to 7% of individuals. Glucose tolerance declines with age and it is estimated that an additional 7.7–14.8% of older adults >65 years will have unrecognized type 2 diabetes according to 1997 American Diabetes Association and 1985 World Health Organisation criteria respectively [7]. Thus, the prevalence of diabetes in an elderly Caucasian population may be as high as 20%, with even higher rates in other ethnic groups such as Blacks, Hispanics, Pima Indians, Scandinavians, and Japanese Americans. Accepting that most strokes occur in older people, it follows that the majority of diabetic stroke patients will have type 2 diabetes or varying degrees of hyperglycemia with impaired glucose tolerance. However, the relationship between diabetes, hyperglycemia, and stroke extends beyond a causal one, with accumulating evidence for an association with stroke severity, recovery, and long-term prognosis.

DIABETES MELLITUS, IMPAIRED GLUCOSE TOLERANCE, AND ACUTE STROKE

Although both type 1 and type 2 diabetes are important risk factors for stroke, this link is primarily for cerebral infarction, there being no proven association with primary intracerebral hemorrhage [8, 9]. In addition to diabetes, there is accumulating evidence that impaired glucose tolerance, asymptomatic nonfasting hyperglycemia, and hyperinsulinemia are also associated with increased stroke risk. Since 1966 there have been at least 22 cohort studies

International Textbook of Diabetes Mellitus, Third Edition. Edited by R. A. DeFronzo, E. Ferrannini, H. Keen, and P. Zimmet.
 ISBN: 0-471-48655-8.

that have sought to examine the relationship between fasting, postprandial, and casual glucose levels upon risk of incident cardiovascular disease. A meta-analysis of these studies has demonstrated not only a progressive relationship between glucose levels and overall cardiovascular risk but also that this risk extends below the diabetic and impaired glucose tolerance thresholds and into "normal" range [10].

In any given acute stroke population it is generally accepted that the prevalence of previously recognized diabetes may be as high as 20%. In addition, a further 6–42% are likely to have previously unrecognized diabetes (as defined by a raised HbA_{1c} and no previous history of diabetes) [11]. There are obvious limitations to studies describing the prevalence of diabetes in acute stroke, including variations in the populations studied, the diagnostic criteria for diabetes employed, and the use of indirect measures such as a raised HbA_{1c} or fructosamine. Notwithstanding these issues, the totality of the evidence suggests that diabetes and impaired glucose tolerance are both underdiagnosed prestroke and underrecognized following the acute event.

In the immediate aftermath of acute stroke, hyperglycemia (with or without a history of diabetes) is an extremely prevalent finding. There is now accumulating evidence that poststroke hyperglycemia has important prognostic implications and thus the clinical relevance of this finding extends beyond merely the discovery of an established risk factor.

DIABETES, HYPERGLYCEMIA, AND STROKE PATHOLOGY

While many diabetic patients have associated stroke risk factors such as hypertension and coronary artery disease, diabetes remains an independent risk factor for atherothrombotic cerebral infarction at all ages [12]. Cerebral infarction is responsible for over 80% of all first ever strokes and primary intracerebral hemorrhage for up to 15%. It is important to recognize that early 30-day mortality from cerebral infarction is as low as 10% compared with up to 50% for cerebral hemorrhage [13]. Thus the majority of stroke patients are likely to survive their first event not only with varying degrees of disability but also with a continuing risk of stroke recurrence and thereby cumulative disability.

Within the group of patients with ischemic stroke, differing pathophysiological mechanisms will have been causal. Approximately 29–44% will be due to thrombosis *in situ*, 20–25% due to cardio embolism, 13–21% due to small artery disease (lacunar stroke), and 15–17% will be due to mixed or undetermined etiologies [14]. Lacunar strokes are clinical syndromes arising as a result of a small deep infarct in the territory of a single deep perforating artery, the so-called *lacune*. Diabetes increases the risk of lacunar infarction, especially in the distribution of the posterior (vertebrobasilar) circulation [9]. The majority of lacunes occur in clinically silent areas however, and are detected only on CT (computed tomography) radiological imaging. Such silent strokes may be of relevance in diabetic patients who present with cognitive decline, as discussed later. Lacunes occurring at strategic areas within the brain where ascending and descending motor and sensory pathways are grouped close together may present with quite devastating clinical syndromes in relation to the actual volume of brain affected.

It is probable that diabetes and hyperglycemia increase the risk of atherothrombotic stroke through a number of mechanisms, direct and indirect. Ultrasonographic studies of the carotid arteries have shown that there is increased thickening of the vascular intima and medial complex throughout life. These atherosclerotic changes are accelerated in patients with diabetes in addition to those with impaired glucose tolerance. Furthermore, the process is considerably accelerated in patients with type 2 diabetes. Whilst prevalent in diabetic patients, it is important to recognize that significant carotid stenosis (>50% occlusion) is also a frequent finding in the general population, especially in older people, with the prevalence rising dramatically from less than 1% in individuals 60 years or younger to 10% in those 80 years or older [15].

The finding of significant carotid stenosis is a marker for increased risk of stroke although important differences in risk exist between so-called asymptomatic (no previous TIA or stroke in the distribution of an affected artery) and symptomatic stenosis (previous TIA or stroke in the distribution of an affected artery). The estimated annual probability of stroke in an elderly male population is on average <1%. In the absence of any previous symptomatic TIA or stroke the estimated annual risk of stroke in the distribution of a stenotic carotid artery (>70% stenosis) is approximately 2–3%. Such increased risk is low when compared to symptomatic carotid stenosis (previous ipsilateral stroke or TIA) where, even with best medical therapy, the estimated 3-year risk of ischemic stroke (disabling or fatal) in the distribution of a stenosis >70% is 11% [16–18]. For the diabetic patient who is found to have a carotid bruit on clinical examination, there can be little doubt that while this is a marker for increased risk of all vascular events (cardiovascular and cerebrovascular), in the absence of previous symptoms in the distribution of the affected artery, the absolute risk of stroke is relatively low.

Beyond the carotid arteries and within the cerebral circulation, diabetes appears to predispose to intracranial atheroma of large, medium sized, and smaller vessels [8]. Arteries and arterioles demonstrate characteristic changes of atheroma, whereas in the small intraparenchymal vessels there may be microatheroma, basement membrane thickening, and lipid transformation of the vessel wall, leading to partial or complete occlusion. In addition, there may be endothelial proliferation within the small intraparenchymal cerebral arteries, veins, and meningeal veins. These changes have previously been referred to as a diabetic encephalopathy or diabetic angiopathy [19]. A detailed understanding of these neuropathological changes explains how diabetic patients have a greater predisposition to small vessel lacunar stroke disease in addition to an increased risk of larger vessel atherothrombotic occlusive vascular disease.

There are several potential mechanisms through which glucose may exert a pathological effect upon the cerebral and systemic circulation. It is probable that glucose itself is causally related to the development of atherosclerosis, perhaps through increased oxidative stress, enhanced leukocyte–endothelial interaction, and widespread glycation of body proteins including lipoproteins, apolipoproteins, and clotting factors. Furthermore, repeated oxidative stress over time leads to the formation of so-called advanced glycation end products (AGEs), which can induce excessive cross-linking of collagen and other extracellular matrix proteins in the vessel wall. These changes may lead to increased accumulation of low-density lipoprotein particles and an enhanced effect upon atherogenesis through endothelial cell dysfunction [20].

DIABETES, HYPERGLYCEMIA, AND RISK OF STROKE

Diabetes is a major risk factor for all cardiovascular disease conferring a twofold increased risk upon an individual. Furthermore, this increase in risk also extends to patients with hypertension who already have a high absolute risk of cardiovascular disease [5, 21]. Although most intervention studies have demonstrated that improved glucose control in both type 1 and type 2 diabetes can delay the development and progression of retinopathy, nephropathy, and neuropathy, it is important to recognize that patients with type 2 diabetes are more likely to develop macrovascular complications (20% within 9 years of diagnosis) compared with microvascular complications (9% within 9 years). Furthermore, macrovascular complications account for 59% of deaths in such patients [22–24].

Although intensive treatment of type 2 diabetes can be shown to result in better maintenance of euglycemia, the clinical benefits of such a strategy are largely confined to preventing microvascular complications. The United Kingdom Prospective Diabetes Study (UKPDS) sought to determine by means of a randomized controlled trial the effect of intensive blood glucose control with either sulfonylureas or insulin compared with conventional care upon the risk of both microvascular and macrovascular complications [25]. In this study intensive treatment was associated with a significant (11%) reduction in HbA_{1c}, which was maintained throughout 10 years of follow-up. Despite this improvement in glucose control, there was no reduction in rate of stroke, with 5.6% of patients in the intensive treatment group and 5.2% in the conventional treatment group experiencing a fatal or nonfatal stroke. Intensive treatment was, however, associated with a nonsignificant reduction in myocardial infarction (Figure 1). Within the intensive treatment group there was a nonsignificant trend ($p = 0.07$) toward an increase in stroke risk with glibenclamide treatment (7.3% experienced stroke) compared with chlorpropamide (5.3%) or insulin (4.6%) treatment.

Accepting that intensive treatment of type 2 diabetes with either a sulphonylurea or insulin does not reduce stroke risk, is there a role for metformin? Evidence from UKPDS suggests that while treatment with insulin, glibenclamide, or chlorpropamide can achieve similar degrees of glycemic control, there is the attendant risk of weight gain. For overweight subjects, treatment with metformin can achieve equivalent levels of glycemic control without affecting weight or increasing risk of hypoglycemia [26]. Long-term follow-up of overweight UKPDS subjects randomized to diet alone versus intensive treatment with sulphonylurea, insulin, or metformin actually demonstrated additional clinical benefits with metformin therapy [27]. Compared with dietary management alone, metformin treatment reduced not only the risk of all cause mortality by 36% but also the combined risk of myocardial infarction, sudden death, angina, peripheral vascular disease, and stroke by 30%. When compared with sulphonylurea or insulin, metformin was associated with significantly greater reductions in any diabetes-related end point, all-cause mortality, and stroke. Although there is the suggestion from UKPDS 34 that the addition of metformin to sulphonylurea therapy may actually increase mortality, it is likely that the need for such treatment identifies those patients at greatest risk of diabetes-related death for whom a poor prognosis is already conferred (older, poorly controlled, and of average weight).

HYPERTENSION, DIABETES, AND RISK OF STROKE

Hypertension remains the single most important and potentially reversible risk factor for stroke. Observational studies have demonstrated that usual blood pressure levels (systolic and diastolic) are directly and continuously associated with risk of both cerebral infarction and cerebral hemorrhage in patients with or without a previous history of hypertension [28, 29]. There is a similar linear relationship between systolic and diastolic blood pressures and risk of recurrent stroke among survivors of recurrent TIA or stroke [30]. Treatment of blood pressure (mean

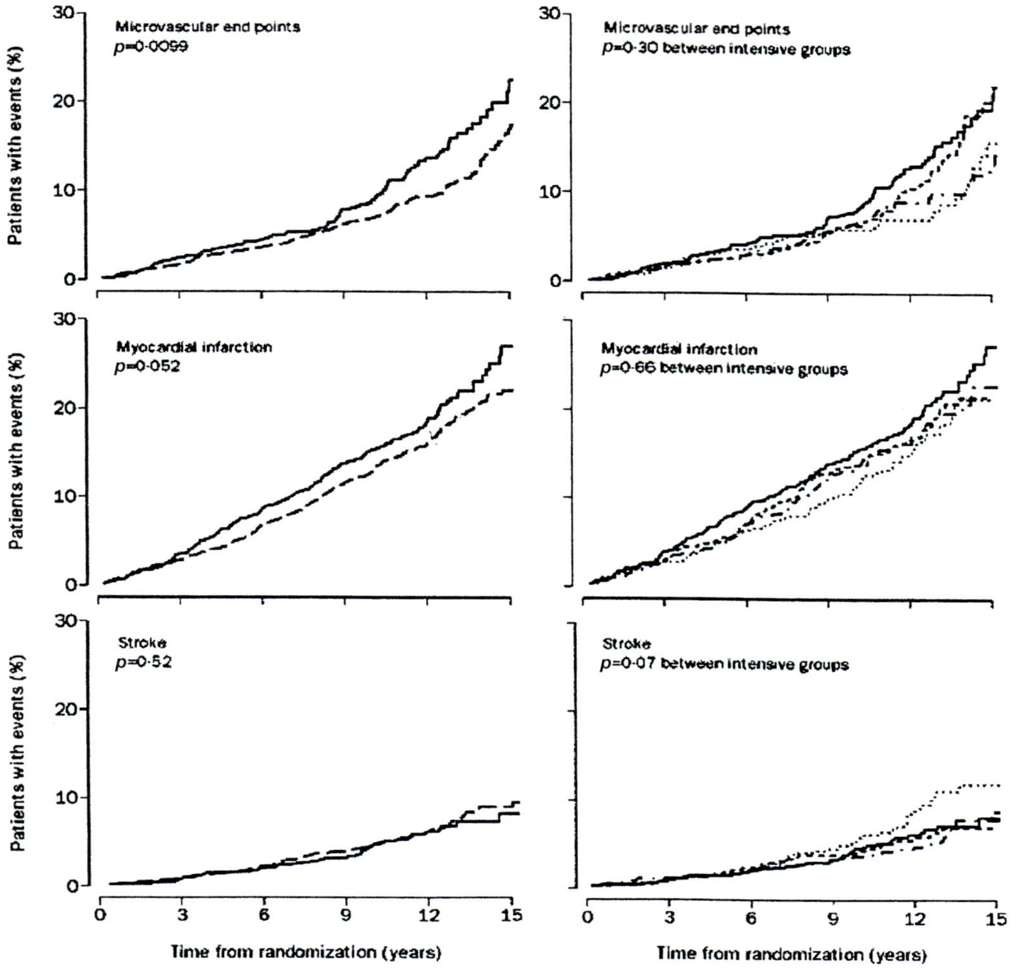

Figure 1 Kaplan–Meier plots of aggregate end points: microvascular disease, myocardial infarction, and stroke for intensive and conventional treatment and by individual intensive therapy in UKPDS 33. (Reprinted with permission from Elsevier Science (The Lancet, 1998, 352; 837–853) [25])

reduction in diastolic pressure 5–6 mmHg) in hypertensive patients without preexisting cerebrovascular disease has been shown to reduce the risk of stroke by approximately one third, with no large differences being apparent between the main drug classes [31]. While it is accepted that blood pressure is a major determinant of stroke risk, the majority of diabetic patients have multiple risk factors for whom choice of antihypertensive therapy may be influenced not only by efficacy but also comorbidity and tolerability. Accepting that tight control of glucose may not directly influence risk of stroke, how should blood pressure be managed?

Embedded within the UKPDS was a randomized controlled trial to determine whether tight control of blood pressure (<150/85 mmHg) could reduce morbidity and mortality in patients with type 2 diabetes [32]. Hypertensive diabetic patients already on treatment (blood pressure ≥150 mmHg systolic and/or ≥85 mmHg diastolic) or previously untreated (≥160 and/or ≥90 mmHg) were randomized to intensive treatment based upon an angiotensin-converting enzyme inhibitor (captopril) or β-blocker (atenolol), aiming for a target blood pressure <150/85 mmHg, or to less tight control (target <180/105 mmHg) using a treatment regimen avoiding angiotensin-converting enzyme inhibitors or β-blockers. Almost one third (29%) of patients in the tight control group required three or more agents to control their blood pressure compared with only 11% in the control group. This intensive treatment was associated with significantly greater lowering in blood pressure; mean blood pressure over 9 years of follow-up was 144/82 mmHg in the intensive group compared with 154/87 mmHg in the less intensive group. There was no significant difference in control of blood glucose between the two groups (mean HbA_{1c} 7.2% respectively). After a median follow-up period of 8.4 years, intensive treatment of blood pressure in patients with type 2 diabetes was associated with a significant 24% relative reduction in risk of

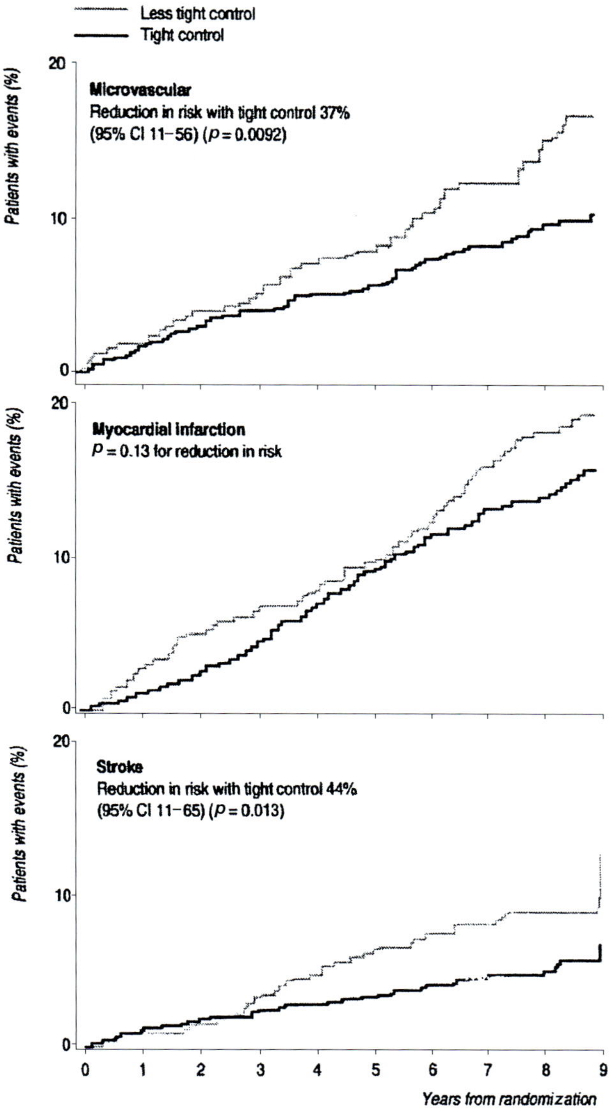

Figure 2 The effect of tight blood pressure control upon risk of microvascular end points, fatal or nonfatal myocardial infarction or sudden death and fatal or nonfatal strokes. Kaplan–Meier plots comparing proportion of patients experiencing events with tight control of blood pressure with those experiencing events less tight control (UKPDS 38). (With permission from the BMJ Publishing Group). [32]

developing any end point related to diabetes. Although there was no significant reduction in risk of myocardial infarction, there was a highly significant 44% relative reduction in risk of stroke (fatal and nonfatal) (Figure 2). These benefits are similar to those demonstrated in the SHEP and STOP trials of treating hypertension in older people [33, 34].

Therefore, for type 2 diabetic patients, tight control of glycemia may not be associated with a reduction in risk of stroke unless simultaneous intensive management of blood pressure is also instituted. The UKPDS 38 also demonstrated that intensive blood pressure treatment would likely require multiple antihypertensive agents based around a β-blocker or angiotensin-converting enzyme inhibitor, with the lowest risk of diabetes-related complications being in those with systolic blood pressure less than 120 mmHg [35].

Accepting that the early identification and treatment of high blood pressure is of critical importance in reducing stroke risk, there is accumulating evidence that for diabetic and other high-risk vascular patients the benefits of antihypertensive therapy may extend beyond a simple blood pressure lowering effect and also address attendant cardiovascular risk.

Two large randomized controlled trials have demonstrated that the angiotensin-converting enzyme inhibitor class of drugs is of value in preventing first ever and recurrent stroke in both diabetic and other high-risk vascular patients [36, 37]. In the HOPE study, 9297 high-risk vascular patients aged 55 years or older, including 3577 (38%) with diabetes (plus one additional risk factor), were randomized to receive up to 10 mg of the angiotensin-converting enzyme inhibitor ramipril or placebo on a double blind basis. Treatment with ramipril was associated with only modest reductions in office (although likely larger reductions in 24-h ambulatory) systolic/diastolic blood pressures when compared with the placebo group (3.8/2.8 mmHg). However the relative risk of any stroke or fatal stroke was reduced by 32 and 61% respectively. The beneficial effects of ramipril therapy were observed regardless of baseline blood pressure and across all baseline conditions, including those with diabetes [38]. These results are consistent with the findings from the UKPDS where the benefits seen with reductions in blood pressure were larger than those predicted from epidemiological data—perhaps suggesting improvements in 24-h blood pressure profiles [39] or perhaps some vasculoprotective effect from both angiotensin-converting enzyme inhibitors and β-blockers [35].

The PROGRESS trial, which recruited 6105 hypertensive and nonhypertensive patients with a previous history of stroke or TIA (13% with a previous history of diabetes), also found that an angiotensin-converting enzyme inhibitor (perindopril) based blood pressure lowering regimen could reduce the risk of stroke. In this study benefit was maximal in patients who received both perindopril and the diuretic indapimide (where blood pressure lowering was on average 12/5 mmHg) compared with patients who received only monotherapy with perindopril (mean blood pressure lowering 5/3 mmHg). Combination therapy reduced stroke risk (relative) by 43% compared with single therapy, which reduced risk by a nonsignificant 5%, providing further evidence for the benefits of intensive management of blood pressure in diabetic and other high-risk patients [36].

Thus, when managing blood pressure in diabetic patients it is important to recognize that it is probably the intensity of blood pressure treatment that confers benefit rather than the choice of initial antihypertensive agent. The HOT study (a trial to determine optimum diastolic blood pressure) demonstrated not only that the incidence of cardiovascular events (including stroke) was approximately twice as great in hypertensive diabetic subjects, but also that their intensive treatment to lower diastolic blood pressure to <80 mmHg was associated with a 30% reduction in risk of stroke when compared with only modest blood pressure reductions to <90 mmHg [40]. The benefits observed in this trial were achieved with a calcium-channel blocker based regimen although in many trial patients this was combined with an angiotensin-converting enzyme inhibitor or β-blocker.

Beyond the choice of treatment, how low should blood pressure actually be reduced? The management goal for systolic blood pressure in patients with diabetes was set to below 130 mmHg in the 1999 WHO/International Society of Hypertension guidelines [41]. Accumulating evidence suggests that for diabetic and other high-risk patients, intensive treatment to even lower levels, with an angiotensin-converting enzyme inhibitor and perhaps also with other agents, will substantially reduce their risk of first ever or recurrent stroke irrespective of baseline blood pressure.

In the immediate aftermath of acute stroke, blood pressure invariably rises in association with the acute systemic stress response. It remains unclear as to what extent this response contributes to further ischemic cerebral damage or whether in some patients it may protect against further damage. For many patients blood pressure falls spontaneously over the first 1–2 weeks following stroke as the acute stress response dissipates. In the PROGRESS and HOPE trials treatment with an angiotensin-converting enzyme inhibitor was initiated beyond 2–4 weeks poststroke when clinical stability had been achieved. Consequently, the optimum timing (or indeed benefit) of routine antihypertensive treatment immediately following acute stroke is not clear and in the absence of progressing neurological signs or accelerated hypertension it would seem prudent to wait until the patient is neurologically and clinically stable before initiating antihypertensive therapy [42].

DYSLIPIDEMIA, DIABETES, AND STROKE

It is generally accepted that dyslipidemia is an important risk factor for coronary heart disease across a large number of at-risk patient populations. This risk extends not just to patients with raised levels of cholesterol but in the presence of additional cardiovascular risk factors may extend to so-called normal or lower levels. The relationship between cholesterol and cardiovascular disease appears to be qualitatively similar in diabetic and nondiabetic individuals although for a given level of cholesterol the absolute risk is higher in diabetic patients.

Epidemiological evidence linking stroke risk to dyslipidemia has been inconsistent with a recent meta-analysis, concluding that there is no clear evidence of such an association [29]. Much of this evidence is constrained by a failure to distinguish between ischemic and hemorrhagic stroke, and epidemiological evidence of an association does not, of course, prove cause and effect. Studies in both Western and Asian populations have demonstrated a positive association between total cholesterol levels and risk of ischemic stroke; however, this positive association may be offset by a negative association between cholesterol levels and risk of hemorrhagic stroke [43, 44]. Consequently, concern has long existed that a simple extrapolation from this evidence to routine treatment may confer risk upon patients. Despite effective lowering of cholesterol levels, early trials using diet, fibrates (clofibrate, gemfibrozil), niacin, colestipol, and surgery had no effect on reducing the rate of stroke. Although patients with diabetes are at much greater risk of both cardiovascular and cerebrovascular disease, there has until recently been no specific trial to determine the effects of lipid-lowering agents on vascular risk in diabetic patients with no previous history of cardiovascular disease.

In contrast, early trials of cholesterol-lowering interventions demonstrated a reduction in coronary heart disease although not to the magnitude that might have been predicted from extrapolations from the epidemiological data. More recently, trials with the HMG-CoA reductase inhibitor class of drugs (statins) have demonstrated not only more marked lowering of cholesterol (total and low density lipoprotein, cholesterol) and triglyceride, but also small increases in high-density lipoprotein concentrations. These larger reductions in cholesterol were associated with much greater reductions in coronary heart disease.

Evidence for the benefits of reducing cholesterol among patients with diabetes and coronary heart disease comes mainly from *post hoc* analyses of the large secondary prevention trials where the beneficial reductions in coronary heart disease were similar in diabetic and nondiabetic patients [45, 46].

It is important to remember that the majority of diabetic patients at risk of stroke are older type 2 diabetic patients for whom the predominant lipid abnormality is hypertriglyceridemia (and reduced high-density lipoprotein cholesterol). In comparison with the evidence linking dyslipdiaemia to coronary heart disease, it is only recently that evidence has emerged demonstrating that treatment with statins can reduce stroke risk. A meta-analysis of the randomized controlled trials of statin therapy demonstrated that in patients with preexisting coronary artery disease, statin therapy when used to lower cholesterol could significantly reduce the risk of stroke by around 30% [47]. In addition, contrary to what the epidemiological data had suggested, this benefit was not offset by any increased risk of hemorrhagic stroke. These benefits are conferred in patients with high or only moderately elevated cholesterol levels. When used in patients for primary prevention, despite impressive reductions in coronary heart disease, the beneficial effects of statins on stroke risk in a number of studies appeared to be much less [48]. This apparent lack of stroke-risk benefit may reflect the lower overall rate of stroke in the primary prevention populations studied.

The benefits of cholesterol-lowering therapy in diabetic and other patients at high risk of coronary heart disease were recently studied in the United Kingdom Medical Research Council/British Heart Foundation coordinate Heart Protection Study [49]. In this large clinical trial, 20 536 patients aged 40–80 years in whom there was uncertainty of benefit for lipid lowering (diabetic patients, patients aged 70 years or older, those with noncoronary vascular disease, and those with average to below average cholesterol levels) were randomized to high-dose simvastatin (40 mg/day) or placebo and followed for an average of 5 years. This study demonstrated substantial reductions in major vascular events across all patient groups irrespective of their initial cholesterol concentrations. Furthermore, the benefits of statin therapy were additional to other cerebro- and cardioprotective treatments, including antihypertensive therapies, aspirin, β-blockers, and angiotensin-converting enzyme inhibitors. For cerebrovascular disease there was an overall 25% reduction in incidence of first ever stroke (4.3% vs. 5.7%), which extended across all patient groups. This benefit was primarily due to a reduction in ischemic stroke, there being no increase in hemorrhagic stroke. Simvastatin therapy also significantly reduced the risk of TIAs (2.0% vs. 2.4%). For diabetic patients (and indeed other patient groups) these benefits were realized irrespective of whether there was a previous history of coronary heart disease.

Therefore treatment with a statin (simvastatin in the Heart Protection Study) should be a routine part of primary and secondary stroke prevention, as well as coronary heart disease prevention in diabetic subjects, regardless of cholesterol level. This evidence particularly applies to older (>70 years) patients with type 2 diabetes who are at greatest absolute risk of stroke.

STROKE, DIABETES, AND VASCULAR DEMENTIA

Vascular dementia is a general diagnostic label that implies a degree of intellectual impairment arising owing to organic brain disease resulting from cerebrovascular disease. There are numerous diagnostic criteria for vascular dementia but in general it is accepted that the term should only be applied when there is evidence of dementia, cerebrovascular disease, and a temporal link between these two features. Overall, vascular dementia accounts for 10–30% of all dementia cases, with the estimated prevalence poststroke being around 10–16% [50].

Dementia following stroke may arise as a result of a single strategically located infarct or as a result of multiple infarcts—traditionally termed multi-infarct dementia. In addition, a proportion of patients may have diffuse small-vessel disease that manifests as dementia. These patients may have characteristic radiological features of symmetrically decreased density of periventricular and subcortical white matter on computerized tomography. The presence and extent of these lesions correlates with the degree of cognitive impairment [51].

Accepting that diabetes is a major risk factor for stroke, it follows that diabetes will be an important risk factor for post stroke dementia. Of interest is that in patients with vascular dementia, the prevalence of diabetes is higher than expected. Furthermore, there is some evidence from community studies that diabetes is associated with a twofold increased risk of not only vascular dementia but also Alzheimer's dementia. In addition, the risk of dementia may be greatest in those treated with insulin [52]. The increased risk of vascular dementia in diabetes can in part be explained by both silent and manifest stroke; however, the relationship with Alzheimer's dementia is not entirely clear. For some diabetic patients it is possible that a critical silent stroke has uncovered early and previously asymptomatic Alzheimer's dementia. For others it is possible that a specific pathological process is taking place. There is evidence to suggest that vascular risk factors may increase the risk of Alzheimer's dementia *per se* although epidemiological studies suggest that vascular risk factors alone cannot solely account for this increased risk [53]. Beyond a direct vascular etiology it is possible that neurodegeneration may also occur as a result of a number of potential mechanisms including neuronal insulin receptor resistance and impaired cerebral glucose metabolism. Interestingly, nonenzymatic glycation of proteins (so-called AGEs), which as previously discussed may be implicated in the development of long-term complications of diabetes, has been found in the plaques and tangles of Alzheimer's brains. Accumulation of these AGEs may be mediated through β-amyloid, which is important in the development of Alzheimer's pathology [54, 55].

On the basis of current evidence it seems probable that cognitive decline and dementia are linked to diabetes through processes that extend beyond simply manifest and silent stroke. There is evolving evidence for an overlap between the pathophysiological changes leading to complications of diabetes and degenerative brain disease due to Alzheimer's pathology. Unfortunately there is as yet no evidence that intensive control of diabetes can prevent vascular dementia.

DIABETES, POSTSTROKE HYPERGLYCEMIA, AND RECOVERY FROM STROKE

Beyond increasing the risk of first ever or recurrent stroke, diabetes is also associated with a poor prognosis, increasing both mortality and dependency. Such an association also extends to the finding of hyperglycemia in the immediate aftermath of stroke. This post stroke hyperglycemia may reflect the metabolic stress of the acute event, so-called stress hyperglycemia, and/or impaired glucose metabolism (impaired glucose tolerance or diabetes) previously manifest or otherwise. Most recently, admission hyperglycemia >6.0 mmol/l has been shown to be present in up to 68% of acute stroke patients [56]. This association between post stroke hyperglycemia and poor outcome from stroke has now been demonstrated in a number of clinical studies and overall it is estimated to be associated with a two- to sixfold increased risk of death. In contrast with early reports that hyperglycemia and a poor prognosis was confined to patients with the largest strokes, studies now demonstrate this risk extending across all clinical subtypes of stroke [57].

Post stroke hyperglycemia may occur as a result of a number of different mechanisms, which may independently or in combination influence subsequent outcome. In the past, post stroke hyperglycemia was thought to be largely due to an acute stress response occurring in association with elevations in plasma cortisol, glucagon, catacholamines, and often a leukocytosis [42]. Although these acute physiological responses may be contributory, accumulating clinical data suggests that much of this response is associated with impaired glucose metabolism, with the prevalence of previously unrecognized diabetes or impaired glucose tolerance preceding stroke as high as 42%. On the basis of the acute stroke patient's admission plasma glucose and HbA_{1c} status it is possible to determine whether or not stress is a major component of their hyperglycemia (Table 1).

While associations between post stroke hyperglycemia and outcome exist both in the presence and absence of impaired glucose tolerance or diabetes, the finding of both stress hyperglycemia and impaired glucose metabolism is likely to be associated with the worst prognosis [58]. Demonstrating an association between hyperglycemia and stroke outcome does not prove a cause and effect relationship however, although the totality of the clinical evidence tends to support a direct relationship.

THE PATHOPHYSIOLOGY OF STROKE AND HYPERGLYCEMIA

The brain is an obligatory aerobe deriving all of its energy from the metabolism of oxygen and glucose. Cerebral metabolism is therefore critically dependent upon blood flow. Following acute stroke due to either cerebral infarction or hemorrhage, blood flow to the affected area of the brain falls and within seconds a sequence of events occurs at a cellular level, leading eventually to irreversible cell death within the infarct core (Figure 3). This sequence of events has been termed the ischemic cascade and is thought to begin when cerebral blood flow falls to below 10–15 ml/100 g/min. It seems probable that within the core of the affected area these changes do not occur uniformly and cell death advances irregularly in both time and space. Around this central core is an area in which blood flow is reduced and cellular metabolism is impaired but not irreversibly so. This zone of potentially viable cells, the ischemic penumbra, is the target for acute stroke treatments to potentially minimize further cell death [59, 60].

Following focal cerebral ischaemia there is a local increase in glycolysis and a rapid decline in tissue glucose levels. Consequently, glucose metabolism at the center of the ischemic area decreases whereas at the periphery glucose metabolism is enhanced. With prolonged hypoxia, cellular metabolism fails and cerebral lactate levels increase rapidly. Associated with this, the supply of high-energy phosphates to the membrane ion pump decreases, resulting in pump failure, efflux of potassium, and influx of sodium and calcium ions along with water-producing cytotoxic edema. Calcium ions activate enzymatic lipolysis of the cell membrane releasing free fatty acids, which facilitate production of toxic free radicals, inflammatory responses, and prostaglandins. Consequent upon these changes there is membrane depolarization and irreversible cellular damage. This cell damage further enhances ischaemia through the release and impaired

Table 1 Admission glycemic status and stress hyperglycemia in acute stroke*

	Admission plasma glucose	Admission glycosylated hemoglobin (HbA_{1c})
Stress hyperglycemia	↑	→
Impaired glucose Tolerance/diabetes with stress hyperglycemia	↑	↑
Impaired glucose tolerance/diabetes without stress hyperglycemia	→	↑
Normal glucose tolerance without stress hyperglycemia	→	→

Note. → within normal laboratory range; ↑ above normal laboratory range.
* Adapted from reference 58.

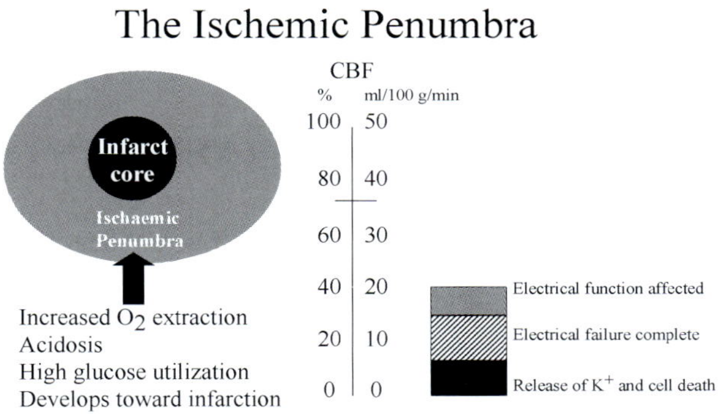

Figure 3 Schematic representation of cerebral blood flow and the ischemic penumbra

re-uptake of neurotransmitters. Toxic levels of these neurotransmitters, which include excitatory amino acids (aspartate and glutamate), are thought to further potentiate the ischemic cascade. Cerebral edema may worsen hypoxia through a direct effect upon small blood vessels in addition to increasing the oxygen diffusion distance. Disruption to the blood–brain barrier at the periphery of the penumbra results in secondary vasogenic edema, thus further potentiating ischemic damage (Figure 4).

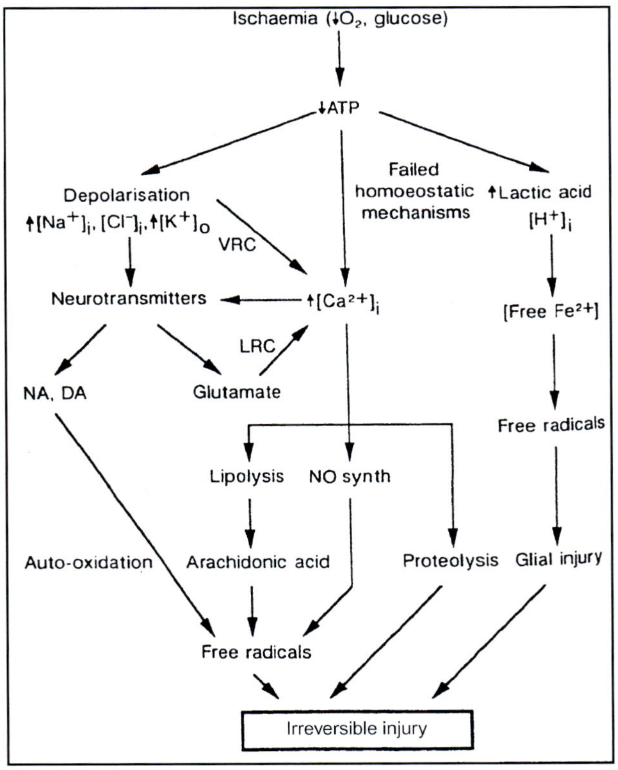

Figure 4 Potential mechanisms of ischemic brain damage. (Reprinted with permission from Elsevier Science (The Lancet, 1992, 339; 534) [60])

The French physician Claude Bernard first described a link between hyperglycemia and brain injury in 1887. By artificially inducing a lesion in the floor of the fourth ventricle of an experimental rabbit, Bernard demonstrated transient hyperglycemia and glycosuria. While Bernard originally postulated that this focal brain lesion had rendered the rabbit diabetic, this was the first recorded evidence for stress hyperglycemia in response to focal brain injury [61].

Hyperglycemia at the onset of cerebral ischaemia is thought to increase infarction by enhancing intracellular and extracellular acidosis. It seems probable that the extent of the metabolic changes, and thereby the ensuing cerebral damage, is dependent upon the degree of hyperglycemia. Clinical neuroradiological studies also suggest that hyperglycemia at the time of stroke may increase the permeability of ischemic capillary endothelium in the absence of overt vessel rupture, thus contributing to hemorrhagic transformation of an infarct. These changes further enhance ischemic damage through energy depletion and lactate accumulation. Hyperglycemia at the time of stroke has also been shown to cause more cerebral edema and slower recovery [57].

While many of the postulated effects of hyperglycemia are at a cellular level, it is possible that it also has a direct effect upon the cerebral vasculature, with evidence for impaired reperfusion after both global and focal experimental ischaemia in the presence of hyperglycemia. Hyperglycemia may also directly influence vascular tone and enhance formation of vasoconstrictive prostaglandins such as thromboxane A2 [62]. Although the experimental evidence linking hyperglycemia to enhanced cerebral damage again does not prove cause and effect, there is a suggestion that insulin may be able to reverse these changes, with evidence for a neuroprotective effect in both global and focal models of cerebral ischaemia [57, 63].

In summary, there is now very good evidence from animal models of stroke and clinical neuroradiological studies for a causative relationship between hyperglycemia and enhanced cerebral damage and the potential for an insulin treatment effect.

MANAGEMENT OF DIABETES AND HYPERGLYCEMIA FOLLOWING STROKE

While there is accumulating evidence for a link between hyperglycemia, diabetes, and enhanced ischemic cerebral damage, such an association has never been confirmed by any clinical trial. Similarly, any potential insulin treatment effect has not been examined in appropriate clinical trials.

In contrast, clinical trials in patients with acute myocardial infarction and diabetes/hyperglycemia have shown that treatment of acute myocardial infarction with a glucose/potassium/insulin based regimen reduces in-hospital mortality by 28% [64]. There is some evidence that such treatment may also confer survival benefits even in the absence of initial hyperglycemia [65].

In the DIGAMI study patients presenting with acute myocardial infarction and admission plasma glucose >11 mmol/l (with or without a past history of diabetes) were randomized to a glucose/potassium/insulin infusion for ≥24 h and then subcutaneous insulin four times daily for ≥3 months. Overall, treatment conferred a significant 29% relative reduction in mortality up to 12 months after the acute event. Maximum benefit was observed in those patients with a low cardiovascular risk profile and no previous insulin treatment, for whom there was a 52% reduction in 12-month mortality rate [66]. Such a prolonged insulin treatment regimen in acute stroke patients is not feasible in routine practice, where the complexity of clinical stroke care combined with the practical difficulties in maintaining hydration and nutrition potentially makes routine treatment with insulin beyond 24 h both illogical and unsafe. Furthermore, while the majority of acute stroke patients may present with hyperglycemia, this is usually mild and less than 11 mmol/l in most cases [67]. The management of diabetes and hyperglycemia following stroke is further complicated by the fact that up to one third of all stroke patients have swallowing difficulties in the immediate aftermath of the acute event. These difficulties resolve in two thirds of cases during the first week. Nutritional support and supplementation in acute stroke patients is often fraught with practical and ethical difficulties, thus creating a challenge for tight glycemic control in the first few days. Where persisting difficulties exist or may be envisaged, semipermanent nutritional support through a percutaneous gastrostomy feeding tube provides the basis for instituting a stable euglycemic treatment regimen.

As already discussed, the relationship between glucose and stroke risk is continuous, extending down to so-called normal values. It is probable that any association between glucose and stroke outcome also extends across a range of glucose levels, and like blood pressure, no precise threshold exists above which risk is suddenly conferred. Furthermore, the metabolic and rheological changes that occur in association with hyperglycemia are likely to evolve and persist beyond the first 24 h, thus extending the potential therapeutic time window for insulin treatment and/or glucose modulation. For clinicians caring for stroke patients it is accepted that up to 40% deteriorate neurologically following admission to hospital [68]. This neurological deterioration may reflect natural progression of the initial stroke but may also be due to enhanced ischemic damage through changes in physiological variables such as glucose, temperature, and blood pressure. Although there is similar evidence to that for glucose linking these variables to stroke outcome, it is probable that they are inexorably linked and treatment of one will have effects upon the other [69].

DIABETES, HYPERGLYCEMIA, AND ACUTE STROKE TREATMENT

There is still no safe, simple, and effective medical therapy for the majority of acute stroke patients. Even in the absence of a simple medical treatment, increased recognition of the benefits of organized and coordinate stroke care (reduced mortality, dependency, and need for institutional care) has led to the wide-scale introduction of specialist stroke services [70]. In addition, clinical trial evidence demonstrating the efficacy of recombinant tissue plasminogen activator as an acute stroke treatment for a small proportion of patients with cerebral infarction has led to the introduction of specialist acute stroke units. The rationale behind thrombolytic therapy in acute stroke is that lysis of an acute thrombus will result in early restoration of cerebral blood flow, which in turn should be followed by removal of lactate, restoration of intracellular and extracellular pH, and salvage of the ischemic penumbra with reduced tissue damage. Thrombolysis with tissue plasminogen activator if administered within 3 h of symptom onset in CT-proven cerebral infarction can reduce disability 3 months after the acute event and improve the chance of a complete recovery. This benefit is offset, however, by an increased risk of fatal and nonfatal intracranial hemorrhage within the first 7–10 days of treatment [71]. The problem with thrombolysis therapy for acute stroke is in identifying which patients will benefit maximally and in whom increased risk may be conferred. Factors such as increasing age, stroke severity, hypertension, and baseline CT appearances of extensive infarction have been shown to increase the risk of complications. There is also evidence that hyperglycemia (≥11.2 mmol/l) may increase the risk of intracranial hemorrhage fivefold following routine thrombolysis. Furthermore, clinical outcome following thrombolysis is worse in hyperglycemic patients despite successful restoration of blood flow [72].

In the absence of a simple medical therapy an essential component of acute stroke unit care is the intensive monitoring of physiological variables (hydration, glucose, temperature, blood pressure, oxygen saturation) and their early correction. It remains to be determined, however, whether such intervention does actually improve patient outcomes. Although clinical trial evidence to support the routine management of hyperglycemia is currently lacking, it is probable that hyperglycemia can actually influence the safety and efficacy of other stroke interventions. In patients for whom thrombolysis is contemplated it would seem prudent to attempt to correct hyperglycemia although the therapeutic time window for thrombolytic therapy is so short that effective glycemic control may actually follow rather than precede such treatment.

How should hyperglycemia and diabetes be managed in the aftermath of acute stroke? Thresholds for the routine management of hyperglycemia vary across centers and between clinicians although the evidence does suggest that no true threshold exists above which risk is suddenly conferred. Treatment with a variable insulin dose glucose/potassium/insulin infusion regimen has been shown to be associated with a physiological lowering of plasma glucose, mimicking the "normal" hyperglycemic response to stroke, with no adverse effect upon patient outcome [67]. Although it is feasible to routinely deliver such treatment to acute stroke patients in the first 24 h, the clinical efficacy of such an intervention remains unproven and results of an ongoing randomized controlled clinical trial to evaluate glucose/potassium/insulin-maintained euglycemia are awaited [73].

REFERENCES

1. Isarol PA, Forbes JF. The cost of stroke to the National Health Service in Scotland. *Cerebrovasc Dis* 1992; 1: 47–50.
2. Bamford J, Sandercock P, Dennis M, Warlow C, Jones L, McPherson K, Vessey M, Fowler G, Molyneux A, Hughes T. A prospective study of acute cerebrovascular disease in the community; the Oxfordshire Community Stroke Project. Methodology, demography and incident cases of first ever stroke. *J Neurol Neurosurg Psychiatr* 1988; 51: 1373–80.
3. Broderick JP, Philips SJ, Whisnant JP, O'Fallon WM, Bergstrahl EJ. Incidence rates of stroke in the eighties. The end of a decline in stroke. *Stroke* 1989; 20: 577–82.
4. Brown RD, Whisnant JP, Sicks JD, O'Fallon WM, Wiebers DO. Stroke incidence, prevalence and survival: secular trends in Rochester Minnesota, through 1989. *Stroke* 1996; 27: 373–80.
5. Kannel WB, McGee DL. Diabetes and cerebrovascular disease. The Framingham Study. *JAMA* 1979; 241: 2035–8.
6. Fuller JH, Shipley MJ, Rose G, Jarret RJ, Keen M. Mortality from coronary heart disease and stroke in relation to degree of glycemia: The Whitehall Study. *BMJ* 1983; 287: 867–70.
7. Wahl PW, Savage PJ, Psaty BM, Orchard TJ, Robbins JA, Tracy RP. Diabetes in older adults: comparison of 1997 American Diabetes Association classification of diabetes mellitus with 1985 WHO classification. *Lancet* 1998; 352: 1012–5.
8. Alex M, Baron EK, Goldenberg S, Blumenthal HT. An autopsy study of cerebrovascular accident in diabetes mellitus. *Circulation* 1962; 25: 663–73.
9. Peress NS, Kane WC, Aronson SM. Central nervous system findings in a tenth decade autopsy population. *Prog Brain Res* 1972; 40: 473–83.
10. Coutinho M, Wang Y, Gerstein HC, Yusuf S. The relationship between glucose and incident cardiovascular events. *Diabetes Care* 1999; 22: 233–40.
11. Scott JF, Gray CS, O'Connell JE, Alberti KGMM. Glucose insulin therapy in acute stroke: why delay further? *Q J Med* 1998; 91: 511–5.
12. Wolf PA, Kannel WB, Verter J. Current status of risk factors for stroke. *Neurol Clin* 1983; 1: 330–1.
13. Bamford J, Sandercock P, Dennis M, Burn J, Warlow C. Classification and natural history of clinically identifiable subtypes of cerebral infarction. *Lancet* 1991; 337: 1521–6.
14. Adams HP, Bendixen B, Kapelle J, Biller J, Lore BB, Gordon DL, Marsh EE. Classification of subtypes of acute ischemic stroke. *Stroke* 1993; 24: 35–41.
15. Carolei A, Marini C. Surgical and medical therapy in asymptomatic carotid lesions. In Fieschi C, Fisher M. (eds) *Prevention of Ischemic Stroke* London: Dunitz M Ltd, 2000.
16. Norris JW, Zhu CZ, Bornstein NM, Chambers BR. Vascular risks of asymptomatic carotid stenosis. *Stroke* 1991; 22: 1485–90.
17. European Carotid Surgery Trialists' Collaborative Group. Randomized trial of endarterectomy for recently symptomatic carotid stenosis: final results of the MRC European Carotid Surgery Trial (ECST). *Lancet* 1998; 351: 1379–87.
18. European Carotid Surgery Trialists' Collaborative Group. MRC European Carotid surgery Trial: interim results for symptomatic patients with severe (70–99%) or with mild (0–29%) carotid stenosis. *Lancet* 1991; 337: 1235–43.
19. Reske-Nielsen E, Lundback K, Rafaelsen OJ. Pathologic changes in the central and peripheral neurons system of young long term diabetics, I: diabetic encephalopathy. *Diabetologia* 1965; 1; 233–41.
20. Laakso M. Hyperglycemia and cardiovascular disease in type 2 diabetes. *Diabetes* 1999; 48: 937–42.
21. Stamler J, Vaccaro O, Neaton JD, Wentworth D. Diabetes, other risk factors and 12 year cardiovascular mortality for men screened in Multiple Risk Factor Intervention Trial. *Diabetes Care* 1993; 16: 434–44.
22. Reichard P, Berglund B, Britz A, Cars I, Nilsson BY, Rosenqvist U. Intensified conventional insulin treatment retards the microvascular complications of insulin dependant diabetes mellitus (IDDM): the Stockholm Diabetes International Study (SDIS) after 5 years. *J Intern Med* 1991; 230: 101–8.
23. Ohkubo Y, Kishikawa H, Araki E, et al. Intensive insulin therapy prevents the progression of diabetic microvascular complications in Japanese patients with non-insulin dependant diabetes mellitus: a randomized prospective study. *Diabetes Res Clin Pract* 1995; 28: 103–17.
24. UK Prospective Diabetes Study (UKPDS) Group UK Prospective Diabetes Study 17, a nine year update of a randomized controlled trial on the effect of improved metabolic control on complications in non insulin dependent diabetes mellitus. *Ann Intern Med* 1996; 124: 136–45.
25. UKPDS Group Intensive blood-glucose control with sulfonylureas or insulin compared with conventional treatment and risk of complications in patients with type 2 diabetes (UKPDS 33). *Lancet* 1998; 352: 837–53.
26. UKPDS Group. UK Prospective Diabetes Study 13: relative efficacy of randomly allocated diet, sulphonylurea, insulin, or metformin in patients with newly diagnosed non-insulin dependent diabetes followed for three years. *BMJ* 1995; 310: 83–8.
27. UKPDS Group Effect of intensive blood-glucose control with metformin in overweight patients with type 2 diabetes (UKPDS 34). *Lancet* 1998; 352: 854–65.
28. Eastern Stroke and Coronary Heart Disease Collaborative Research Group. Blood pressure, cholesterol and stroke in eastern Asia. *Lancet* 1998; 352: 1801–7.
29. Prospective Studies Collaboration 1995. Cholesterol, diastolic blood pressure and stroke. 13000 strokes in 450,000

people in 45 prospective cohorts. *Lancet* 1995; 346: 1647–53.
30. Rodgers A, MacMahon S, Gamble G, Slattery J, Sandercock P, Warlow C on behalf of the United Kingdom. Transient Ischemic Attack Collaborative Group. Blood pressure and risk of stroke in patients with cerebrovascular disease. *BMJ* 1996; 313: 147.
31. Blood Pressure Lowering Treatment Trialist's Collaboration. Effects of ACE inhibitors, calcium antagonists and other blood pressure lowering drugs: results of prospectively designed overviews of randomized trials. *Lancet* 2000; 356: 1955–64.
32. UKPDS Group. Tight blood pressure control and risk of macrovascular and microvascular complications in type 2 diabetes: UKPDS 38. *BMJ* 1998; 317: 703–13.
33. SHEP Co-operative Research Group. Prevention of stroke by hypertensive drug therapy in older persons with isolated systolic hypertension: final results of the systolic hypertension in the elderly programme. *JAMA* 1991; 265: 3255–64.
34. Dahlof B, Lindholm LH, Hansson L, Schersten B, Ekbom T, West Po. Morbidity and mortality in the Swedish trial in old patients with hypertension (STOP-Hypertension). *Lancet* 1991; 338: 1281–5.
35. Adler A, Stratton IM, Neil HAW, Yudkin JS, Matthews DR, Cull CA, Wright AD, Turner RC, Holman RR. Association of systolic blood pressure with macrovascular and microvascular complications of type-2 diabetes (UKPDS 36): prospective observational study. *BMJ* 2000; 321: 412–9.
36. PROGRESS Collaborative Group. Randomized trial of a perindopril-based blood pressure-lowering regimen among 6105 individuals with previous stroke or transient ischemic attack. *Lancet* 2001; 358: 1033–41.
37. The Heart Outcomes Prevention Evaluation Study Investigators Effects of an angiotensin converting enzyme inhibitor, ramipril, on cardiovascular events in high-risk patients. *N Engl J Med* 2000; 342: 145–53.
38. Bosch J, Yusuf S, Pogue J, Sleight P, Lonn E, Rangoonwala B, Davies R, Ostergren J, Probstfield J. Use of ramipril in preventing stroke: double blind randomized trial. *BMJ* 2002; 324: 699–702.
39. Svensson P, de Faire U, Sleight P, Yusuf S, Ostergren J. Comparative effects of ramipril on ambulatory and office blood pressures: a HOPE Substudy. Hypertension. December 1 2001: 38 (6): E28–32.
40. Hansson L, Zanchetti A, Carruthers SG, Dahlof B, Elmfeldt D, Julius S, Menard J, Rahn KH, Wedel H, Westerling S. Effects of intensive blood pressure lowering and low dose aspirin in patients with hypertension: principal results of the Hypertension Optimal treatment (HOT) randomized trial. *Lancet* 1998; 351: 1755–62.
41. Guidelines Sub-Committee. 1999 World Health Organisation—International Society of Hypertension guidelines for the management of hypertension. *J Hypertens* 1999; 17: 151–83.
42. O'Connell JE, Gray CS. Treating hypertension after stroke [Editorial]. *BMJ* 1994; 308: 1523–4.
43. Yano K, Reed DM, MacLean CJ. Serum cholesterol and hemorrhagic stroke in the Honolulu Heart Program. *Stroke* 1989; 20: 1460–5.
44. Iso H, Jacobs DR Jr, Wentworth D, Neaton JD, Cohen JD, for the MRFIT Research Group. Serum cholesterol levels and six year mortality from stroke in 350,977 men screened for the Multiple Risk Factor Intervention Trial. *N Eng J Med* 1989; 320: 904–10.
45. Isles C (ed). Consensus conference on lipid lowering to prevent vascular events. In *Proceedings of the Royal College of Physicians of Edinburgh*, Vol 29, No 2, suppl 5. Edinburgh: Metro Press, 1999; pp 10–5.
46. American Diabetes Association Management of dyslipidemia in adults with diabetes. *Diabetes Care* 2001; 24 (suppl 1): 58–61.
47. Bucher HC, Griffith LE, Guyatt GH. Effect of HMGcoA reductase inhibitors on stroke. A meta-analysis of randomized controlled trials. *Ann Intern Med* 1998; 128: 89–95.
48. Hess DC, Demchuk AM, Brass LM, Yatsu FM, HMG-CoA reductase inhibitors (statins). A promising approach to stroke prevention. *Neurology* 2000; 54: 790–6.
49. MRC/BHF Heart Protection Study of cholesterol lowering with simvastatin in 20 536 high-risk individuals: a randomized placebo controlled trial. *Lancet* 2002; 360: 7–22.
50. Barba R, Martinez-Espinosa S, Rodriguez-Garcia E, Podal M, Vivancos J, Del Ser T. Post stroke dementia: clinical features and risk factors. *Stroke* 2000; 31 (7): 1494–501.
51. Hachinski VC, Potter P, Merskey H. Leukoariosis—an ancient term for an old problem? *Can J Neurol Sci* 1986; 13: 533–4.
52. Ott A, Stolk RP, van Harskamp F, Pols HAP, Hofman A, Breteler MMB. Diabetes mellitus and the risk of dementia. The Rotterdam Study. *Neurology* 1999; 53: 1937–42.
53. Lovenstone S. Diabetes and dementia. *Neurology* 1999; 53: 1907–9.
54. Munch G, Schinzel R, Loske C, et al. Alzheimer's disease—synergistic effects of glucose deficits, oxidative stress and advanced glycation end products. *J Neural Transm* 1998; 105: 439–61.
55. Thomas T, Thomas G, McLendon C, Sutton T, Mullan M. β Amyloid-mediated vasoactivity and vascular endothelial damage. *Nature* 1996; 380: 168–71.
56. Scott JF, Robinson G, O'Connell JE, Alberti KGMM, Gray CS. Prevalence of admission hyperglycemia across clinical sub types of acute stroke. *Lancet* 1999; 353: 376–7.
57. Gray CS, O'Connell JE, Lloyd H. Diabetes hyperglycemia and recovery from stroke. *Geriatr Gerontol Int* 2001; 1: 2–7.
58. Gray CS, Taylor R, French JM, Alberti KGMM, Bates TD. The prognostic value of stress hyperglycemia and previously unrecognized diabetes following acute stroke. *Diabet Med* 1987; 4: 237–40.
59. Pulsinelli WA, Kraig RP, Plum F. Hyperglycemia, cerebral acidosis and ischemic brain damage. In Plum F, Pulsinelli WA (eds) *Cerebrovascular Diseases 14th Princeton Conference*. New York: Raven Press, 1985; pp 201–10.
60. Pulsinelli WA. Pathophysiology of acute stroke. *Lancet* 1992; 339: 533–6.
61. Bernard C. Leçons sur le Diabète. Paris: J-B Bailliere, 1887.
62. Kent TA, Soukup VM, Fabian RH. Heterogeneity affecting outcome from acute stroke therapy. Making reperfusion worse. *Stroke* 2001; 32: 2318–27.
63. Capes SE, Hunt D, Malmberg K, Pathak P, Gerstein HC. Stress hyperglycemia and prognosis of stroke in nondiabetic and diabetic patients. A systematic overview. *Stroke* 2001; 32: 2426–32.
64. Fath-Ordoubadi F, Beatt KJ. Glucose-insulin–potassium therapy for treatment of acute myocardial infarction: an overview of randomized placebo controlled trials. *Circulation* 1997; 96: 1152–6.
65. Diaz R, Paolasso EA, Piegas LS, Tajer CD, Moreno MG, Corvalan R, Isea JE, Romero G. Metabolic modulation of

acute myocardial infarction. The ECLA Glucose-Insulin-Potassium Pilot Trial. *Circulation* 1998; 98: 2227–34.
66. Malmberg K, Ryden L, Efendic S, Herlitz J, Nicol P, Waldenstrom A, Wedel H, Welin L Randomized trial of insulin glucose infusion followed by subcutaneous insulin treatment in diabetic patients with acute myocardial infarction (DIGAMI study): effects on mortality at one year. *JACC* 1995; 26: 57–65.
67. Scott JF, Robinson G, O'Connell JE, Alberti KGMM, Gray CS. Glucose Potassium Insulin (GKI) infusion in the treatment of acute stroke patients with mild to moderate hyperglycemia. (The GIST Trial). *Stroke* 1999; 30: 793–9.
68. Toni D, Fiorelli M, Gentile M, Bastianello S, Sacchetti ML, Argentino C, Pozzilli C. Fieschi C. Progressing neurological deficit secondary to acute ischemic stroke. A study on predictability, pathogenesis and prognosis. *Arch Neurol* 1995; 52: 670–5.
69. Scott JF, Robinson G, French JM, O'Connell JE, Alberti KGMM, Gray CS. Blood pressure response to glucose potassium insulin therapy in patients with acute stroke with mild to moderate hyperglycemia. *J Neurol Neurosurg Psychiatry* 2001; 70: 401–4.
70. UK Stroke Trialists Collaboration. Collaborative systematic review of the randomized trials of organised in patient (stroke unit) care after stroke. *BMJ* 1997; 314: 1151–60.
71. Wardlaw J, Yamaguchi T, Del Zoppo G. Thrombolysis for acute ischemic stroke. *The Cochrane Library,* Issue 2. Oxford Update Software, 2002.
72. Els T, Klisch J, Orszagh M, et al. Hyperglycemia in patients with focal cerebral ischaemia after intravenous thrombolysis: influence on clinical outcome and infarct size. *Cerebrovasc Dis* 2002; 13: 89–94.
73. Gray CS, Alberti KGMM, Scott J, O'Connell JE, French J, Hildreth A, Lloyd H. The United Kingdom Glucose Insulin in Stroke Trial (GIST UK). *Stroke* 2000; 31 (suppl 46): 382.

85

Peripheral Vascular Disease in Diabetes

Nicolaas C. Schaper*† and Peter J.E.M Kitslaar*†

*University Hospital Maastricht, Maastricht, The Netherlands, and †Cardiovascular Research Institute Maastricht (CARIM), Maastricht, The Netherlands

INTRODUCTION

Peripheral arterial disease (PAD) is a common finding in patients with diabetes mellitus. In many patients the disease has no or few symptoms and runs a relatively benign course. However, in others it leads to gangrene or impaired healing of a neuro-ischemic foot ulcer, with amputation as a final result. Moreover, PAD can be seen as a sign of severe generalized atherosclerosis, which should be treated aggressively. Peripheral arterial disease of the lower extremities, here abbreviated as PAD, is defined as signs, symptoms, or abnormal noninvasive tests in one or both legs attributable to obstructive atherosclerotic disease [1]. Critical limb ischemia (CLI) was recently defined as chronic ischemic rest pain, ulceration, or gangrene attributable to objectively proven arterial occlusive disease [1]. The term critical limb ischemia implies chronicity. In contrast, acute limb ischemia is a sudden event, usually due to an embolus or thombosis in preexistent PAD. In this chapter we discuss basic and clinical aspects of PAD in diabetic patients, with the patient in a diabetic clinic as a starting point. In the treatment of these patients a close cooperation between diabetologist and vascular surgeon is needed. Therefore, background information is given on several surgical procedures. For further details the reader is referred to surgical textbooks on (peripheral) vascular disease [2, 3].

PREVALENCE AND PROGNOSIS

Several population studies have shown that diabetes is a strong risk factor for PAD [4]. Population studies suggest that diabetic patients are three times more likely to develop PAD than the general population [5, 6]. In both nondiabetic and diabetic subjects the prevalence of PAD increases markedly with age. In the general population, PAD is a rare disease under the age of 50 years [7]. However, in one study of type 1 diabetic patients with a mean age of 28 years, signs of (asymptomatic) PAD had already developed in 12% of the patients after 6 years of follow-up [8]. Prevalence data in the elderly population depends, of course, to a large extent on the age of the subjects studied. In several studies in subjects aged >50 years, an ankle–brachial index (ABI) <0.9 was found in approximately 20% of the diabetic patients [9–11]. In the United Kingdom Prospective Diabetes Study (UKPDS), PAD was rare at the time of the diagnosis of type 2 diabetes, but after 6 years of follow-up at least one indicator of PAD had developed in 11% of the patients [12] (see Figure 1). It can be safely concluded, based on these population studies, that PAD is a highly prevalent disorder, in particular in the elderly diabetic patient. Unfortunately, the awareness of physicians that these patients have PAD is low, resulting in inadequate prevention of lower extremity amputations and inadequate treatment of the grossly elevated cardiovascular risk [13, 14].

Several epidemiological studies have found that in the general population only a minority of patients with PAD, defined as an ABI<0.9, report intermittent claudication [1, 7, 13]. This low proportion of patients might be explained by the fact that many elderly patients do not walk far enough to experience symptoms of intermittent claudication. Moreover, in diabetic patients with PAD classical intermittent claudication seems to be reported even less frequently, perhaps because of concomitant neuropathy. These neuro-ischemic patients more frequently report a poor lower extremity function with atypical pain [15]. In the UKPDS symptoms of claudication were reported in

International Textbook of Diabetes Mellitus, Third Edition. Edited by R. A. DeFronzo, E. Ferrannini, H. Keen, and P. Zimmet.
 ISBN: 0-471-48655-8.

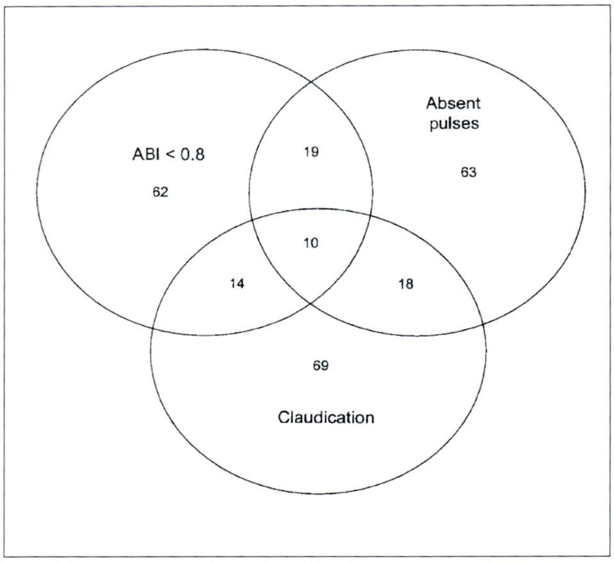

Figure 1 Results of the individual measures for PAD in 2398 individuals in the UKPDS [12]. (Copyright © 2002 American Diabetes Association. From Diabetes Care, Vol 25, 2002; 894–899. Reprinted with permission from *The American Diabetes Association*)

only 23% of the patients with an ABI <0.8 (see Figure 1), indicating that for each patient with claudication there are three patients with silent PAD [12].

The Fate of the Leg

In nondiabetic patients, PAD is a surprisingly benign disease with respect to the legs; the risk of limb loss is overshadowed by the risk of concomitant cardiovascular morbidity and mortality [16, 17]. Only a minority of nondiabetic patients with intermittent claudication will need a surgical or endovascular procedure and approximately 2% of the claudicators will ever need a major amputation [1]. However, in the case of CLI the risk of limb loss is much higher and most patients will need a revascularization procedure to save the leg [1]. In diabetic patients the atherosclerotic changes in PAD seem to be more extensive and also more aggressive, resulting in a faster progression of disease [1, 9, 18, 19]. In one prospective study in diabetic patients, vascular laboratory results worsened after 2-year follow-up in 74% of the patients with initial abnormal measurements [20]. In another study diabetic patients with claudication had a 35% risk of sudden ischemia and a 21% risk of major amputation [21]. In diabetic patients with critical limb ischemia the risk of limb-loss is markedly increased, gangrene being reported to develop in 40% of such patients [1]. This more aggressive course and the coexistent generalized atherosclerosis probably contribute to the longer in-hospital-stay and greater use of resources by diabetic patients with PAD [22]. In diabetic subjects aged 65–74 years and participating in the American Medicare system, the relative risk for lower extremity amputation was 23.5 times the risk in nondiabetic individuals [4]. Approximately 40–60% of all lower extremity amputations are performed in diabetic patients and 85% of these amputations are preceded by a foot ulcer [14]. These foot ulcers are usually caused by a combination of factors, such as loss of protective sensation, increased biomechanical stress, inadequate footwear, PAD, and/or edema [23–25]. The major reasons for a lower extremity amputation are PAD and/or a deep infection [14, 26, 27].

The Fate of the Patient

PAD is closely associated with occlusive disease in other arterial territories and is a strong predictor of future cardiovascular morbidity and mortality [1]. Mortality is increased in patients with PAD in parallel to the severity of the disease [28]. Patients with asymptomatic PAD, defined as either abnormal pedal pulses or abnormal ankle pressure, already have an increased risk for cardiovacular disease [28, 29]. In claudicant patients mortality rate is further increased, with the worst outcome in patients with critical limb ischemia. The presence of diabetes further worsens this poor cardiovascular prognosis [1, 30–32]. In one study approximately 20% of the patients with intermittent claudication and diabetes had died after 2 years [33]. The poorest outcome is observed in the diabetic patient who has had a major amputation. In a prospective Swedish study, 50% of such patients had undergone a second amputation (both minor and major) and 73% had died after 5 years [34].

PATHOGENESIS OF PAD IN DIABETES

Histologically there seems to be no major difference in the atherosclerotic lesions of the legs between diabetic and nondiabetic patients [35]. However, PAD in diabetes does have certain typical characteristics, which can be viewed as a sign of premature aging of the vascular tree (see Table 1) [24]. In nondiabetic patients the prevalence of peripheral arterial disease increases with age, but younger (<50 years) patients more frequently have aortoiliac disease, while in the elderly patients it tends to be localized more distally in the legs [1, 36]. The same pattern is seen in diabetic patients. The proximal vessels are relatively spared, with less involvement of the aorta and iliac

Table 1 Characteristics of PAD in diabetes

- More common
- Affects younger individuals
- No sex difference
- Faster progress
- Multisegmental
- More distal (aortailiac arteries less frequently involved)

arteries, and with relatively more extensive disease in the deep femoral artery and the arteries below the knee [18, 19, 37, 38]. Involvement of the deep femoral artery can impair the formation of collaterals in case of occlusions in the superficial femoral artery. Despite the more extensive crural disease, the arteries of the foot are relatively spared in many patients, rendering these distal segments suitable for bypass surgery [39]. Why atherosclerosis preferably affects the lower legs of diabetic patients has received relative little attention and is at present difficult to explain.

Risk Factors

As in the general population, older age, smoking, hypertension, and probably cholesterol are important risk factors for PAD in patients with diabetes [1, 24]. Although clinically PAD and coronary heart disease (CHD) are clearly associated, some studies suggest that the risk factors for obstructive atherosclerotic disease in these two different vascular beds might not be identical and/or might have a different impact [40]. Hyperglycemia seems to be a stronger risk factor for PAD than for CHD in both type 1 and type 2 diabetic patients [8, 12]. In the UKPDS each 1% increment in HbA_{1c} was associated with a 28% increase in the risk for PAD [12]. Smoking was also a stronger risk factor for PAD than for CHD in a general population [41]. Both hyperglycemia and smoking can result in the formation of advanced glycation end products and in enhanced oxidative stress within the vessel wall, suggesting that these processes might play a central role in the development or progression of PAD [42, 43]. The role of lipids in the pathogenesis of PAD is less clear. Although hypercholesterolemia was a risk factor for PAD in several epidemiological studies, not all have consistently shown a relationship between total cholesterol or LDL cholesterol and PAD [44, 45]. The same pattern is seen in intervention studies in which (LDL) cholesterol was pharmacologically lowered, with results being both negative and positive [1, 44, 46]. However, several studies suggest that in diabetic (and nondiabetic) subjects, PAD is associated with an atherogenic dyslipidemia, which is characterized by elevated triglycerides, low levels of HDL cholesterol, and increased number of small dense LDL particles [1, 11, 12, 44, 45]. In addition, lipoprotein (a) [Lp(a)] was associated with PAD in two cross-sectional studies in both diabetic and nondiabetic subjects [47, 48].

Apart from the classic risk factors, several novel risk factors have been identified for the development of PAD and atherosclerosis in other vascular beds. Hyperhomocysteinemia is associated with premature PAD [1, 49] and in one study elevated plasma homocysteine levels were associated with a more rapid progression of PAD [49]. In diabetic patients plasma homocysteine levels are closely linked to kidney function [50], and hyperhomocysteinemia could help explain why patients with diabetic nephropathy more frequently have PAD and why the disease runs a more severe course in these patients [32, 51]. Several studies have shown that circulating inflammatory mediators can predict CHD [52]. The same pattern, with elevated levels of acute phase proteins, cytokines, and white blood cell count, has been observed in patients with PAD [40].

Impaired Remodelling and Collateral Formation

Until now most research has been focused on the development of atherosclerosis in the legs of diabetic patients. Why PAD runs such an aggressive course in diabetic patients remains largely unexplained. Reduction in flow and perfusion pressure in the affected leg results from a gradual reduction in lumen diameter due to growth of the atherosclerotic plaque, with sudden episodes of deterioration caused by superimposed thrombosis [1, 17]. During the growth of the atherosclerotic plaque, the atherosclerotic vessel also undergoes a remodeling process of compensatory enlargement to preserve the original diameter [52]. In one study diabetic patients with coronary artery atherosclerosis had less compensatory coronary enlargement compared to nondiabetic patients [53]. Impaired outward remodeling might be due to nonenzymatic glycation of the extracellular matrix of the vessel wall, which renders it more resistant to degradation [24]. In addition, diabetic polyneuropathy could also affect vascular remodeling in the large arteries of the leg, which are relatively richly innervated [54]. Polyneuropathy is associated with media calcification in the arteries of the leg and the foot, which could be related to enhanced synthesis of calcium-binding proteins by the denervated smooth muscle cells [55–57]. Media calcification does not impair blood flow, but could impair the compensatory outward expansion of the vessel wall [58–60] (see Figure 2). In addition, prospective studies have shown that these calcifications are associated with a marked increase in cardiovascular mortality [61].

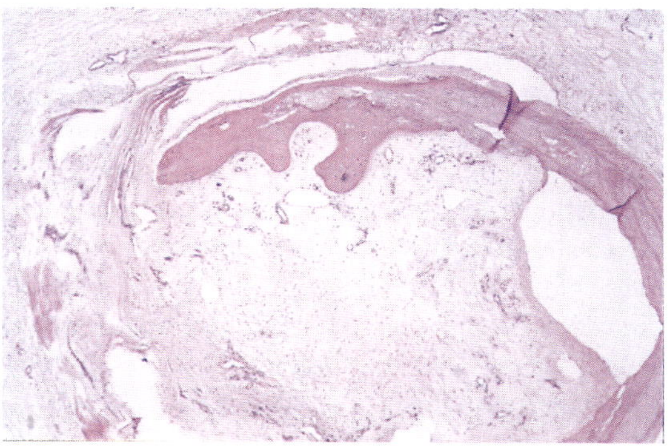

Figure 2 Cross section of atherosclerotic tibial artery, showing calcification and ossification in the media. Slide supplied by M. E. Edmonds, Diabetic Department, Kings College Hospital, London

Outward remodeling is also important during the development of a collateral network. Animal studies suggest that in the legs these collaterals are preformed and, in case of a severe reduction in blood flow, grow in diameter to restore peripheral blood flow in a process called arteriogenesis [62]. However, as recently shown in the coronary circulation, the formation of these collateral vessels seems to be impaired in diabetic patients with ischemic heart disease [63]. The same observation was made in diabetic animals with peripheral ischemia [64]. It is likely that in diabetic patients several mechanisms contribute to the impaired arteriogenesis during ischemia, such as endothelial dysfunction, diminished cellular responses to several growth factors or cytokines, and impaired degradation of the extracellular matrix [24, 65, 66]. Preliminary results suggest that treatment with growth factors such as vascular endothelial growth factor or fibroblast growth factor can improve peripheral circulation in patients with critical limb ischemia [67, 68]. The same observation was made in diabetic animals with peripheral ischemia, suggesting that chronic hyperglycemia does not preclude a favorable response to such therapy [64].

ABNORMAL MICROCIRCULATION AND PAD

The primary defect in PAD is obstructive atherosclerosis in the macrocirculation. In parallel with the reduction in flow and pressure, several compensatory mechanisms are probably activated in the microcirculation. But once critical ischemia has developed the microcirculation finally fails, resulting in rest pain and/or skin ulceration [1]. Although diabetic microangiopathy is presently not seen as a primary factor in the development of tissue ischemia, several abnormalities can be observed in the skin microcirculation of diabetic patients, which could render the skin more susceptible to a reduction in perfusion pressure [23]. The maximal vasodilator capacity of the skin microcirculation is greatly reduced in patients with type 2 diabetes [69]. To a lesser extent this abnormality was also observed in type 1 diabetic patients with (incipient) nephropathy [70]. Diabetic neuropathy, in both type 1 and 2 diabetic patients, results in increased shunt blood flow and an impaired inflammatory response to various (noxious) stimuli [71]. In type 2 diabetic patients, but not in type 1 patients, this increased shunt flow is associated with a reduction in skin capillary blood flow, which might further jeopardize the skin in case of ischemia [72, 73]. These microcirculatory abnormalities probably explain why severe skin ischemia can develop more easily in diabetic patients when perfusion pressure drops [74]. Because of sensory neuropathy, a patient with severe ischemia may have no rest pain, and because of autonomic neuropathy, subcutaneous shunt blood flow is increased, resulting in a relatively warm skin, thereby falsely reassuring the clinician.

DIAGNOSIS, INVESTIGATION, AND MANAGEMENT

Three distinct types of problems are frequently encountered in the diabetic clinic: the asymptomatic patient without foot pulses; the patient with intermittent claudication; and the patient with foot ulceration and/or other signs of critical limb ischemia. Each of these problems will be discussed separately, as management of these patients differs. In general terms management is similar to that in the nondiabetic patient with PAD, but the macrovascular disease must be seen in the context of the diabetes and its multiple effects on the lower extremity.

The Asymptomatic Diabetic Patient with Signs of PAD

Yearly palpation of foot pulses is advised in many national and international guidelines [23]. But what are the consequences of absent pulses in an asymptomatic patient? One of the two pedal pulses can be congenitally absent in a minority of subjects [1]. Although reproducibility and interobserver agreement are clearly not optimal, absent foot pulses do predict the presence of PAD and identify patients at high risk for foot ulceration or lower extremity amputation [12, 75–77]. Moreover, absent foot pulses are associated with an increased risk for cardiovascular disease [78]. On the other hand, the presence of foot pulses does not exclude PAD; for instance, claudication can be observed in patients with palpable pulses (see Figure 1).

When pulses are absent, three important additional items need to be addressed:

(1) Additional signs of PAD and assessment of its severity
(2) The risk for foot ulceration
(3) The increased cardiovascular risk

Assessment of the Severity of PAD

Apart from palpation of pulses clinical examination is not particularly helpful in assessing the severity of PAD, in the absence of rest pain or tissue loss [75]. Blanching of the feet on elevation, with a red-purple discoloration on dependency, in the absence of infection, suggests severe ischemia [1]. In our experience, a purple-reddish color of the (fore)foot during dependency is associated with a systolic toe pressure <30 mmHg in diabetic patients. Because of neuropathy the color and the temperature of the skin are usually unreliable. A temperature difference between the two legs can be helpful, but unfortunately both legs are usually affected by PAD [76]. Finally, the auscultation of a femoral bruit has also been shown to predict the presence of PAD [76]. To document objectively the presence of PAD and to estimate the severity of the vascular occlusions, noninvasive vascular tests, such as ABI, toe pressure, and transcutaneous pressure of oxygen ($tcpO_2$) can be used.

Ankle pressure and toe pressures The systolic arterial blood pressures at the ankle can be measured with a hand-held Doppler probe. The patient is placed in the supine position. A cuff, usually the same as used for the brachial pressure and connected to a sphygmomanometer, is applied to the lower calf just above the ankle. The Doppler probe is positioned over the dorsalis pedis or posterior tibial artery and the cuff is rapidly inflated to a pressure sufficient to arrest blood flow. Subsequently, the cuff is deflated slowly and the cuff pressure at which pulsatile flow returns is determined. The higher pressure of the two arteries is used to calculate the ABI, by dividing this ankle pressure by the Doppler pressure measured in the brachial artery [79]. The same principles are used in the measurement of systolic pressures in the toe arteries. A small cuff (2 cm) is recommended and blood flow is determined in the hallux by techniques as photoplethysmography or Laser Doppler fluxmetry [79]. An ABI <0.9 confirms hemodynamically significant occlusive disease between the heart and the ankle, which in most cases lies distal to the renal arteries. Moreover, the ABI can give a rough estimate of the severity of the occlusive disease in nondiabetic subjects [1]. The index is decreased to 0.5–0.9 in asymptomatic patients or in patients with claudication and most of these patients will have single segment occlusions [1, 17, 80]. Values below 0.5 indicate severe multisegment disease and in (nondiabetic) patients with rest pain the absolute ankle pressure is usually $\leq$40 mmHg [1, 80]. Measurement of ankle pressure is an easy procedure to perform. Unfortunately this technique has some severe limitations in the diabetic patient. Because of media calcification the arteries of the lower leg may be less compressible and incompressible arteries have been observed in up to 30% of diabetic patients [79]. An ABI ≥ 1.15 suggests that the ankle pressure is falsely elevated [79]. In one study the ABI failed to identify diabetic patients who were at risk for foot ulceration [81], and several studies have shown that the ABI or the absolute ankle pressure is a poor predictor of outcome in diabetic patients with PAD and/or a foot ulcer [82–84]. The toe pressure is normally approximately 10 mmHg less than the ankle pressure [1]. For screening purposes a toe systolic blood pressure index of >0.60 can be interpreted as normal [80]. Toe pressures can predict outcome in diabetic patients with foot ulcers and primary healing of a foot ulcer occurred in most patients with a toe pressure $\geq$ 30 mmHg [1, 82, 84, 85]. Unfortunately, this measurement also has limitations. Toe arteries can be affected by media calcification, although to a lesser extent than the arteries in the lower leg, resulting in falsely elevated values [79]. In addition, falsely low values can be obtained if the skin temperature of the toe is too low and in these cases the foot must be warmed prior to the investigation.

$tcpO_2$ The $tcpO_2$ can be measured with a heated oxygen-sensitive probe, which is placed on the dorsum of the foot. After an equilibration period of at least 15–20 min the skin oxygen tension can be determined, reflecting local microcirculatory blood flow [79]. In healthy subjects a wide range of values can be observed, but normal values are usually >60 mmHg. Several studies have shown that $tcpO_2$ values can identify patients at risk for foot ulceration and can predict healing or amputation in patients with a foot ulcer [1, 12, 26, 81, 83, 84]. As described elsewhere, an oxygen tension of $\leq$30 mmHg suggests ischemia, but a range of $\pm$10 mmHg must be allowed [1]. Therefore, in case of a $tcpO_2 > 40$ mmHg severe tissue ischemia is unlikely and in case of a $tcpO_2 < 20$ mmHg severe ischemia is likely [1]. However, it should be noted that various systemic factors (such as hypoxia) or local factors (such as edema and inflammation) can affect the measurement, resulting in falsely low values [79].

Conclusions Despite its limitations, palpation of foot pulses is the first step in identifying the asymptomatic patient with PAD. In the case of absent pulses or auscultation of a femoral bruit it has been recommended to always determine the ABI [80]. However, although an ABI <0.9 confirms PAD, a normal value does not exclude this diagnosis. Therefore, we tend to rely solely on clinical examination in the asymptomatic patient. When in doubt, the vessels can be more easily identified with the Doppler probe and if a normal bi- or triphasic acoustic signal is heard over these palpable vessels, PAD is less likely [23]. Measurement of toe pressures and $tcpO_2$ can be used further to exclude PAD and/or to determine the degree of ischemia.

Reduction of Other Risk Factors for Foot Ulceration

Once PAD is documented, other risk factors for foot ulceration must also be determined and should be treated accordingly. As described in the International Consensus on the Diabetic Foot, this examination should include evaluation of the skin, bone/joints, neurological status, and footwear [14]. The majority of patients with PAD usually have loss of protective sensation. Detection of these neuro-ischemic patients, with subsequent education, regular chiropody, and prescription of adequate footwear, are essential to prevent foot ulceration [23]. As in the pure neuropathic patient, also in the neuro-ischemic patient, trauma due to inadequate footwear is usually the penultimate event leading to ulceration and subsequent progressive gangrene [23].

Reduction of the Increased Cardiovascular Risk

As discussed earlier, the outcome in subjects with moderate PAD is determined mainly by the poor cardiovascular outcome and aggressive treatment of cardiovascular risk

Table 2 Effects of tobacco on progression of PAD

- Promotes progression of PAD
  - from asymptomatic to claudication
  - from claudication to CLI
- Increases failure rates of revascularization procedures
- Increases cardiovascular morbidity and mortality

factors is clearly indicated. First of all the patient should be advised to abstain completely from tobacco use (see Table 2). It is advisable to offer pharmacological (nicotine patches and/or bupropion) or behavioral interventions to assist the patient in the difficult task of coping with the nicotine addiction [17, 86]. Antiplatelet therapy should be prescribed to all patients, given its beneficial effect on cardiovascular disease in patients with PAD [87]. In case of contraindications for aspirin, clopidogrel can be offered as a substitute [88]. Other measures include life-style modification with a regular exercise program, treatment of elevated blood pressure, and prescription of lipid-lowering medication. Treatment of PAD patients with a statin reduces the risk of major vascular events, as shown in the Heart Protection Study [89]. The results of this latter study suggest that lowering of the LDL-cholesterol concentration is beneficial in these high-risk patients, irrespective of the initial cholesterol concentration [89]. In case of a low HDL-cholesterol level also, a fibrate should be considered [90]. In addition, niacin can effectively raise HDL cholesterol without any negative effects on glucose control in diabetic patients with PAD [91]. PAD is sometimes seen as a contraindication to β-adrenergic blockers, but in a meta-analysis of randomized controlled trials it was concluded that β-blockers are not contraindicated in the treatment of hypertension in patients with moderate PAD [92]. However, in patients with critical limb ischemia we are more circumspect in prescribing these drugs, given the potential negative effects on skin microcirculation. Intensive blood glucose control in the UKPDS did not reduce the risk of macrovascular disease, including PAD [12]. However, the interaction of hyperglycemia with other risk factors for foot ulceration and/or amputation suggests that patients with PAD will benefit from intensive glucose control.

The Diabetic Patient with Claudication

In subjects with intermittent claudication, the following items need to be addressed (in addition to those discussed above):

(1) Are the complaints related to PAD?
(2) The anatomical location and hemodynamic significance of the occlusive lesion(s)
(3) Exercise training
(4) Indication for and risks of a revascularization procedure

Diagnosis

Intermittent claudication is characterized by leg pain sufficient to cause the patient to stop walking, which is relieved within minutes by rest, and is caused by PAD [1]. An additional characteristic is that the pain is reproducibly caused by a given degree of exercise and the walking distance should be documented. In most patients the diagnosis can be made on the basis of history, clinical examination, and ankle or toe pressure [1, 17]. It is recommended that the ABI should be determined in all new patients with claudication to confirm and assess the severity of PAD [1]. As discussed above, in diabetic patients it is advisable also to measure toe pressures. In patients with an atypical history a treadmill exercise test is a very sensitive technique to detect or to exclude the presence of PAD [1]. The patient walks at a standard speed and inclination on a treadmill until claudication pain is experienced or a time limit is reached [1]. The ABI is measured before and after the exercise, and a drop in ABI is indicative of PAD. The drop in perfusion pressure is caused by exercise-induced vasodilatation and the reduction in downstream vascular resistance will magnify the pressure gradient across a stenotic arterial lesion, resulting in lower poststenotic perfusion pressures [1]. Once the presence and the severity of claudication are documented, the combination of history and clinical examination can correctly predict the segmental location of the occlusive lesion(s) in the majority of patients with moderate to severe PAD [93].

Segmental pressure measurements, Doppler waveform analysis, and pulse volume recording Noninvasive vascular assessment with techniques such as segmental pressure measurements, Doppler waveform analysis, pulse volume recording, and Duplex scanning can be helpful to determine the need and feasibility of some form of intervention [1]. These techniques can localize and assess the hemodynamic significance of an occlusive lesion. With segmental pressure measurements, Doppler systolic pressures are determined proximal to the ankle. A drop in pressure of 30 mmHg or more between two segments predicts hemodynamically significant occlusive disease [17]. However, these more proximal measurements can also be affected by calcification. These problems are not encountered with two other techniques. Differences in magnitude and contour of the Doppler waveform between two measurement points can identify an occlusive lesion [1]. The same principle is used with pulse volume recordings, when the relative changes with each cardiac cycle are measured in the thigh, calf, ankle, and forefoot [79].

Duplex scanning The disadvantage of the aforementioned techniques is that they do not give information about the length or number of lesions. With Duplex scanning, information is obtained about both anatomy and hemodynamic significance of an occlusive lesion, by the combined use of echography and Doppler analysis to measure blood flow velocity. Duplex scanning detects and localizes hemodynamically significant lesions in the aortofemoral segment as effectively as angiography [94, 95]. Moreover, with this technique crural and pedal occlusive lesions can also be detected [96]. However, the measurement is time-consuming, dependent on the skills of the technician and relatively expensive. Therefore, Duplex scanning is usually reserved for a specific segment selected by prior clinical examination and/or simpler noninvasive tests, in particular if a catheter-based intervention is considered [97].

Angiography Angiography should be performed once the decision has been made to proceed to a revascularization procedure or in case of a nonhealing ulcer. Usually this will be full angiography, with visualization from the infrarenal aorta to the toes using digital subtraction angiography [1]. Adequate visualization of the foot circulation is essential to identify potential sites for a distal bypass. Although with modern contrast agents the risk of nephrotoxicity is low, the patient should be adequately hydrated prior to and after the procedure. If the patient is using metformin and has renal impairment, metformin should be withheld for 48 h prior to the procedure and restarted after measurement of the serum creatinine level [98]. Angiography might be replaced in the future by magnetic resonance angiography [99].

Treatment of Intermittent Claudication

In addition to treating the increased cardiovascular risk and abstinence from smoking, an exercise program should be prescribed. Patients are instructed to walk until mild pain develops, to rest until the pain abates, and subsequently to resume walking. Such exercise, three times a week for 30–60 min, can markedly improve walking distance and physical functioning [1]. Similar results have been reported in diabetic patients [100]. The best results have been obtained with a walking training program conducted for ≥3 months, and indeed in the study quoted, walking distance in diabetic patients was still improving after 6 months of training [100]. This training should preferably be given in a supervised environment and as part of a multidisciplinary treatment [1]. Prior to the training, patients should be evaluated for loss of protective sensation, foot deformities, and/or other signs of increased biomechanical stress (such as callus), and footwear should be adapted, if necessary.

Several drugs have a statistically significant effect on walking distance in patients with claudication. However, as the clinical benefit is small these drugs are not used routinely [1, 17]. Given the relative benign course of the disease and the effectiveness of a walking training program, a revascularization procedure is rarely indicated. Such a procedure should be considered in patients in whom exercise treatment has failed and who have severe disabling claudication [1]. Subsequently, the choice is between percutaneous transluminal angioplasty (PTA) and a surgical procedure. Generally, surgery has better long-term results but the risks are also higher and in most patients a PTA will be the procedure of choice [101]. The results of an aortoiliac PTA can be further improved by the use of stents [1]. However as discussed elsewhere, stenting is advised only in selected cases such as iliac artery occlusion or when results of a PTA are inadequate [1]. The indications for more distal stenting are at present very limited. The patency of a PTA depends on the type of the lesion (stenosis or occlusion), the length, the location, and the distal run-off. The best results are obtained in single short stenoses above the inguinal ligament with good outflow into the lower leg (≥2 patent calf arteries) [102–104]. For both aortoiliac and femoropopliteal lesions a morphological stratification has been proposed, which guides the clinician in the choice between PTA and surgery [1].

Several studies suggest that diabetes mellitus is associated with a poorer long-term outcome of a PTA, which is not unexpected given the more extensive disease and the poorer run-off in these patients [102, 103, 105]. Although studies specifically addressing the effect of PTA in diabetic patients with claudication are scarce, acceptable results have been reported with 5-year iliac patency-rates of 70% and femoral patency-rates of 50–60% [102, 103, 106]. Much poorer results are obtained in diabetic patients with critical limb ischemia and in many patients a surgical procedure is necessary to save the leg, as discussed in the next section.

Diabetic Foot Ulceration and Critical Limb Ischemia

Diabetic foot ulcers are usually caused by multiple factors, with the combination of PAD and neuropathy playing a causal role in approximately 30–40% of these ulcers [25]. Only a minority of patients have classical ischemic rest pain [107]. In the majority of these neuro-ischemic ulcers ill-fitting shoes are the direct cause [23, 108]. It should be noted that poorly fitting shoes can result in gangrene of one or more toes in neuropathic feet with adequate perfusion. Also, a toe infection in these neuropathic feet can mimic PAD, as gangrene of a toe can be caused by septic thrombosis of the digital arteries.

Diagnosis

On clinical examination patients frequently have a painless, indolent ulcer on the margins of the foot or on the toes, but in our experience they may occur in any location [23]. The first step is to determine if the foot ulcer is caused predominantly by PAD and if skin perfusion is sufficient to guarantee healing. In addition, infection should be ruled out. Because of autosympathectomy, the skin can be relatively warm in diabetic patients with CLI. Although palpable pulses render severe PAD unlikely, several authors have reported that in diabetic patients ankle pulses can be present despite severe ischemia (based on angiography) [109, 110]. Given these caveats, noninvasive measurements are indicated in all ulcer patients with signs of PAD and in patients in whom a foot operation is considered. These measurements should also be performed if the foot ulcer shows no tendency to heal in 2–3 weeks despite optimal treatment. Probably the combination of ABI, toe pressure, and $tcpO_2$ is the optimal initial procedure to evaluate the degree of ischemia [111]. Angiography should also be performed in patients with a nonhealing foot ulcer after 6 weeks of optimal treatment, irrespective of the results of the aforementioned measurements, given the moderate accuracy of these tests [79]. Although clear guidelines have been published, a substantial number of patients with PAD do not receive an adequate vascular evaluation prior to amputation or are referred for vascular intervention only once extensive tissue loss has occurred [14, 23, 112]. Revacularisation should be considered in all patients with an ankle pressure <55 mmHg, a toe pressure <30 mmHg, and/or $tcpO_2 < 20(-30)$ mmHg [1, 23, 79].

Infection

The combination of a deep foot infection and neuroischemia is a medical emergency, given its poor prognosis. In one study a forefoot or lower extremity amputation was performed in 76% of diabetic patients with an infected ischemic ulcer [27]. Infection of one of the muscle compartments of the foot can result in tissue edema with a rise in compartmental pressure and subsequent microvascular occlusion. This foot compartment syndrome, with its vicious cycle of infection, edema, and microvascular failure, can result in extensive tissue necrosis [113]. Moreover, ischemia will impair the penetration of antibiotics into the foot [114]. For these reasons aggressive treatment of the infection is needed in patients with deep foot infections, with high-dose broad-spectrum antibiotics given intravenously. In every patient the need for surgery, comprising extensive debridement, decompression of the infected compartment, and/or a minor amputation, should be evaluated. If indicated, these procedures should be performed as soon as possible (<24 h) [23]. Once infection is controlled, which usually takes 4–5 days, bypass surgery can be performed. With this approach excellent long-term results have been obtained [115].

Revascularization

General aspects Once a neuro-ischemic ulcer is optimally off-loaded, infection is ruled out or adequately treated, and blood glucose levels are adequately controlled, healing is mainly determined by skin perfusion. If healing is deemed unlikely, based on clinical evaluation and noninvasive measurements, the first choice is between revascularization and lower extremity amputation. Critical limb ischemia in a patient with a nonfunctional leg should be treated with an amputation at such a level that further problems are extremely unlikely [116]. Based on the preoperative evaluation the expected risk/benefit ratio must be determined. Most patients have (silent) ischemic heart disease or cerebrovascular disease. In comparison to distal bypass surgery, the surgical risks are greater in proximal surgery, necessitating more extensive preoperative evaluation of cardiopulmonary risk factors. Patients with CLI usually have multilevel disease, which can be classified as supra- and infrainguinal disease, depending on the location of the obstructive lesions.

Suprainguinal disease Although most diabetic patients have primarily infrainguinal disease, hemodynamically significant proximal lesions should be treated before the more distal ones are corrected. Aortoiliac PTA, with or without stenting, can be sufficient to improve blood flow into the leg in some patients with relatively mild distal disease. In other diabetic patients excellent results can be obtained by the combination of iliac PTA and distal bypass surgery [117]. For more severe unilateral iliac obstructions the femoro–femoral crossover bypass is a valuable surgical treatment [1]. The aorto(bi)femoral bypass, performed with a prosthetic graft, is the traditional treatment for aortoiliac disease and has excellent long-term patency rates [1, 17]. An axillo(bi)femoral bypass is an alternative procedure, with less surgical risks but lower patency rates [1]. Diabetes does not seem to have major adverse effects on the outcome of these proximal procedures and, if necessary, an infrainguinal procedure can be performed successfully in a second stage [118].

Infrainguinal disease Infrainguinal lesions are divided in femoropopliteal and more distal (below the trifurcation) disease. Infrainguinal PTA is at present feasible in less than 50% of diabetic patients and has poor long-term results [102, 105, 106, 119, 120]. However, the complication rate is low and acceptable short-term patency rates have been reported in diabetic patients: 65–85% at 1 year after femoropopliteal PTA and in one study 32% at 1 year after crural PTA [105, 106, 120]. The temporary improvement of skin perfusion can be sufficient to promote healing of a chronic ulcer and to avoid amputation in a patient with a relatively short life expectancy [119]. Moreover, once the ulcer is healed lower perfusion pressures are necessary to maintain skin integrity.

Given its superior results and relatively low complication rate, peripheral bypass surgery will be the first choice in many diabetic patients with CLI (see Figure 3). The

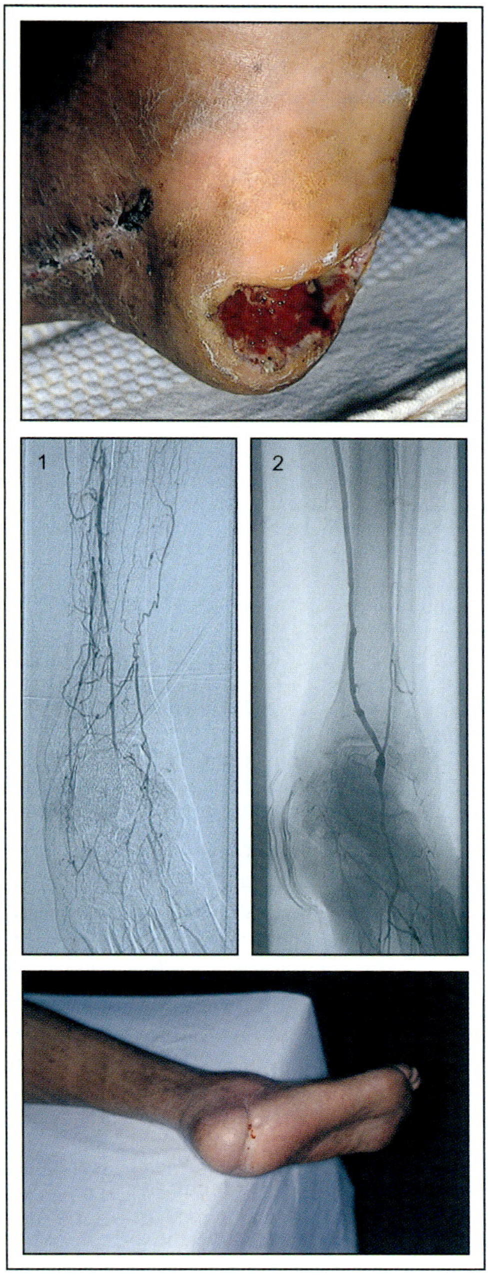

Figure 3 A deep, infected, ulcer at the calcaneal region. Angiography showed multiple crural lesions and a popliteal-pedal bypass was performed, resulting in healing of the ulcer. (Reproduced by permission of Dr. N.C. Schaper)

basic principle of this type of surgery are that any artery can be used for the proximal anastomosis, provided inflow is uncompromised. The graft should bypass the major obstructive lesions and for the distal anastomoses an artery relatively free of occlusive disease, providing the best outflow into the arteries of the foot, should be selected [1]. The bypass graft should preferably be constructed with autogenous vein(s), although acceptable results have been obtained with prosthetic grafts that do not cross the knee [1, 17]. An adequate ipsilateral saphenous vein is preferred in a below-knee bypass, but other good quality veins can be used [1]. If possible the contralateral saphenous vein should be spared, as a substantial number of patients will require a bypass on the contralateral leg in the future [121]. The crural and pedal arteries are common outflow sites of the graft in diabetic patients, given the characteristic anatomic pattern of PAD. Long-term results of these distal procedures in diabetic patients are good, with 5-year secondary patency rates of $\geq$70% and limb salvage rates of 75–85% [1, 122, 123]. In addition, such distal procedures in diabetic patients are more cost-effective than primary amputation [124]. After bypass surgery, patients should participate in a Duplex-scan surveillance program to preserve long-term patency of the graft and to reduce the number of major amputations [125]. Antiplatelet therapy should be started preoperatively and continued after an endovascular or surgical procedure [1].

Diabetes does not seem to have an important negative effect on the long-term patency rate and the limb salvage rate of bypass surgery [122, 123]. However, in one study diabetes did have a marked negative effect on long-term functional status and health-related quality of life after lower extremity revacularization [126]. This poorer outcome compared to that in nondiabetic subjects was probably caused by the more extensive comorbidity in the diabetic patients, highlighting the need for a multidisciplinary approach to improve the poor outcome of these patients.

CONCLUSIONS

PAD is a sign of generalized atherosclerosis, and in diabetic patients measures should be taken to reduce the increased cardiovascular risk, including life-style modification, complete tobacco abstinence, and pharmacological treatment. This latter treatment should include a lipid-lowering drug and antiplatelet therapy. If present, hypertension should be treated aggressively. The patient should be evaluated for the presence of other risk factors for foot ulceration and adequate footwear should be prescribed. In case of intermittent claudication a supervised walking program should be initiated.

Noninvasive tests, such as measurement of ABI, toe pressure, and tcpO_2 can be helpful to quantify the severity of the PAD. Because of calcification the ABI in diabetic patients is frequently unreliable and a combination of the above three is the best procedure in the case of a suspected (neuro-)ischemic foot ulcer. In all patients with critical limb ischemia a revascularization procedure should be considered and excellent long-term results have been obtained in diabetic patients. The combination of ischemia and infection is frequently a medical emergency and the patient should be evaluated immediately. If indicated, debridement and decompression surgery should be performed as soon as possible. The evaluation and treatment of diabetic patients with (suspected) PAD is clearly a multidisciplinary effort, which involves amongst others physicians, surgeons, chiropodists, and diabetic nurses [14]. With such an approach and with a policy of aggressive revascularization, major reductions in the number of lower leg amputations are possible [127].

REFERENCES

1. Management of peripheral arterial disease (PAD). TransAtlantic Inter-Society Consensus (TASC). Eur J Vasc Endovasc Surg 2000; 19 (suppl A): Si–xxviii, S1–250.
2. Rutherford RB. *Vascular Surgery*, 4th edn. Philadelphia: Saunders, 1995.
3. Eastcott HHG. *Arterial Surgery*, 3rd edn. New York: Churchill-Livingstone, 1992.
4. Beckman JA, Creager MA, Libby P. Diabetes and atherosclerosis: epidemiology, pathophysiology, and management. *J Am Med Assoc* 2002; 287: 2570–81.
5. Newman AB, Siscovick DS, Manolio TA, Polak J, Fried LP, Borhani NO, Wolfson SK. Ankle–arm index as a marker of atherosclerosis in the Cardiovascular Health Study. Cardiovascular Heart Study (CHS) Collaborative Research Group. *Circulation* 1993; 88: 837–45.
6. Garcia MJ, McNamara PM, Gordon T, Kannel WB. Morbidity and mortality in diabetics in the Framingham population. Sixteen year follow-up study. *Diabetes* 1974; 23: 105–11.
7. Meijer WT, Hoes AW, Rutgers D, Bots ML, Hofman A, Grobbee DE. Peripheral arterial disease in the elderly: The Rotterdam Study. *Arterioscler Thromb Vasc Biol* 1998; 18: 185–92.
8. Forrest KY, Becker DJ, Kuller LH, Wolfson SK, Orchard TJ. Are predictors of coronary heart disease and lower-extremity arterial disease in type 1 diabetes the same? A prospective study. *Atherosclerosis* 2000; 148: 159–69.
9. Beach KW, Bedford GR, Bergelin RO, Martin DC, Vandenberghe N, Zaccardi M, Strandness DE Jr. Progression of lower-extremity arterial occlusive disease in type II diabetes mellitus. *Diabetes Care* 1988; 11: 464–72.
10. Beks PJ, Mackaay AJ, de Neeling JN, de Vries H, Bouter LM, Heine RJ. Peripheral arterial disease in relation to glycaemic level in an elderly Caucasian population: the Hoorn study. *Diabetologia* 1995; 38: 86–96.
11. MacGregor AS, Price JF, Hau CM, Lee AJ, Carson MN, Fowkes FG. Role of systolic blood pressure and plasma triglycerides in diabetic peripheral arterial disease. The Edinburgh Artery Study. *Diabetes Care* 1999; 22: 453–8.
12. Adler AI, Stevens RJ, Neil A, Stratton IM, Boulton AJ, Holman RR. UKPDS 59: hyperglycemia and other potentially modifiable risk factors for peripheral vascular disease in type 2 diabetes. *Diabetes Care* 2002; 25: 894–9.
13. Hirsch AT, Criqui MH, Treat-Jacobson D, Regensteiner JG, Creager MA, Olin JW, Krook SH, Hunninghake DB, Comerota AJ, Walsh ME, McDermott MM, Hiatt WR. Peripheral arterial disease detection, awareness, and treatment in primary care. *JAMA* 2001; 286: 1317–24.
14. Apelqvist J, Larsson J. What is the most effective way to reduce incidence of amputation in the diabetic foot? *Diabetes Metab Res Rev* 2000; 16 (suppl 1): S75–83.
15. Dolan NC, Liu K, Criqui MH, Greenland P, Guralnik JM, Chan C, Schneider JR, Mandapat AL, Martin G, McDermott MM. Peripheral artery disease, diabetes, and reduced lower extremity functioning. *Diabetes Care* 2002; 25: 113–20.
16. Hooi JD, Stoffers HE, Knottnerus JA, van Ree JW. The prognosis of non-critical limb ischaemia: a systematic review of population-based evidence. *Br J Gen Pract* 1999; 49: 49–55.
17. Ouriel K. Peripheral arterial disease. *Lancet* 2001; 358: 1257–64.
18. Osmundson PJ, O'Fallon WM, Zimmerman BR, Kazmier FJ, Langworthy AL, Palumbo PJ. Course of peripheral occlusive arterial disease in diabetes. Vascular laboratory assessment. *Diabetes Care* 1990; 13: 143–52.
19. Jude EB, Oyibo SO, Chalmers N, Boulton AJ. Peripheral arterial disease in diabetic and nondiabetic patients: a comparison of severity and outcome. *Diabetes Care* 2001; 24: 1433–7.
20. Bendick PJ, Glover JL, Kuebler TW, Dilley RS. Progression of atherosclerosis in diabetics. *Surgery* 1983; 93: 834–8.
21. McDaniel MD, Cronenwett JL. Basic data related to the natural history of intermittent claudication. *Ann Vasc Surg* 1989; 3: 273–7.
22. Currie CJ, Morgan CL, Peters JR. The epidemiology and cost of inpatient care for peripheral vascular disease, infection, neuropathy, and ulceration in diabetes. *Diabetes Care* 1998; 21: 42–8.
23. Apelqvist J, Bakker K, van Houtum WH, Nabuurs-Franssen MH, Schaper NC. *International Consensus on the Diabetic Foot*. Maastricht: International Working Group on the Diabetic Foot, 1999.
24. Schaper NC, Nabuurs-Franssen MH, Huijberts MS. Peripheral vascular disease and type 2 diabetes mellitus. *Diabetes Metab Res Rev* 2000; 16 (suppl 1): S11–5.
25. Reiber GE, Vileikyte L, Boyko EJ, del Aguila M, Smith DG, Lavery LA, Boulton AJ. Causal pathways for incident lower-extremity ulcers in patients with diabetes from two settings. *Diabetes Care* 1999; 22: 157–62.
26. Reiber GE, Pecoraro RE, Koepsell TD. Risk factors for amputation in patients with diabetes mellitus. A case-control study. *Ann Intern Med* 1992; 117: 97–105.
27. Armstrong DG, Lavery LA, Harkless LB. Validation of a diabetic wound classification system. The contribution of depth, infection, and ischemia to risk of amputation. *Diabetes Care* 1998; 21: 855–9.
28. Criqui MH, Langer RD, Fronek A, Feigelson HS, Klauber MR, McCann TJ, Browner D. Mortality over a period of 10 years in patients with peripheral arterial disease. *N Engl J Med* 1992; 326: 381–6.
29. Hooi JD, Stoffers HE, Kester AD, van RJ, Knottnerus JA. Peripheral arterial occlusive disease: prognostic value of signs, symptoms, and the ankle-brachial pressure index. *Med Decis Making* 2002; 22: 99–107.
30. Brand FN, Abbott RD, Kannel WB. Diabetes, intermittent claudication, and risk of cardiovascular events. The Framingham Study. *Diabetes* 1989; 38: 504–9.
31. Boyko EJ, Ahroni JH, Smith DG, Davignon D. Increased mortality associated with diabetic foot ulcer. *Diabet Med* 1996; 13: 967–72.
32. Cheng SW, Ting AC, Lau H, Wong J. Survival in patients with chronic lower extremity ischemia: a risk factor analysis. *Ann Vasc Surg* 2000; 14: 158–65.
33. Coffman JD. Intermittent claudication: not so benign. *Am Heart J* 1986; 112: 1127–8.

34. Apelqvist J, Larsson J, Agardh CD. Long-term prognosis for diabetic patients with foot ulcers. *J Intern Med* 1993; 233: 485–91.
35. Clausell N, Kalil P, Biolo A, Molossi S, Azevedo M. Increased expression of tumor necrosis factor-alpha in diabetic macrovasculopathy. *Cardiovasc Pathol* 1999; 8: 145–51.
36. Hansen ME, Valentine RJ, McIntire DD, Myers SI, Chervu A, Clagett GP. Age-related differences in the distribution of peripheral atherosclerosis: when is atherosclerosis truly premature? *Surgery* 1995; 118: 834–9.
37. Conrad MC. Large and small artery occlusion in diabetics and nondiabetics with severe vascular disease. *Circulation* 1967; 36: 83–91.
38. Faglia E, Favales F, Quarantiello A, Calia P, Clelia P, Brambilla G, Rampoldi A, Morabito A. Angiographic evaluation of peripheral arterial occlusive disease and its role as a prognostic determinant for major amputation in diabetic subjects with foot ulcers. *Diabetes Care* 1998; 21: 625–30.
39. LoGerfo FW, Coffman JD. Current concepts. Vascular and microvascular disease of the foot in diabetes. Implications for foot care. *N Engl J Med* 1984; 311: 1615–9.
40. Schaper NC, Nabuurs-Franssen MH. The diabetic foot: pathogenesis and clinical evaluation. *Seminars in Vascular Medicine* 2002; 2: 221–8.
41. Price JF, Mowbray PI, Lee AJ, Rumley A, Lowe GD, Fowkes FG. Relationship between smoking and cardiovascular risk factors in the development of peripheral arterial disease and coronary artery disease: Edinburgh Artery Study. *Eur Heart J* 1999; 20: 344–53.
42. Cerami C, Founds H, Nicholl I, Mitsuhashi T, Giordano D, Vanpatten S, Lee A, Al-Abed Y, Vlassara H, Bucala R, Cerami A. Tobacco smoke is a source of toxic reactive glycation products. *Proc Natl Acad Sci USA* 1997; 94: 13915–20.
43. Baynes JW, Thorpe SR. Role of oxidative stress in diabetic complications: a new perspective on an old paradigm. *Diabetes* 1999; 48: 1–9.
44. Vigna GB, Fellin R. Dyslipidemia in peripheral vascular disease. *Curr Opin Lipidol* 1996; 7: 254–9.
45. O'Neal DN, Lewicki J, Ansari MZ, Matthews PG, Best JD. Lipid levels and peripheral vascular disease in diabetic and nondiabetic subjects. *Atherosclerosis* 1998; 136: 1–8.
46. Pedersen TR, Kjekshus J, Pyorala K, Olsson AG, Cook TJ, Musliner TA, Tobert JA, Haghfelt T. Effect of simvastatin on ischemic signs and symptoms in the Scandinavian Simvastatin Survival Study (4S). *Am J Cardiol* 1998; 81: 333–5.
47. Valentine RJ, Grayburn PA, Vega GL, Grundy SM. Lp(a) lipoprotein is an independent, discriminating risk factor for premature peripheral atherosclerosis among white men. *Arch Intern Med* 1994; 154: 801–6.
48. Wollesen F, Dahlen G, Berglund L, Berne C. Peripheral atherosclerosis and serum lipoprotein(a) in diabetes. *Diabetes Care* 1999; 22: 93–8.
49. Taylor LM Jr, DeFrang RD, Harris EJ Jr, Porter JM. The association of elevated plasma homocyst(e)ine with progression of symptomatic peripheral arterial disease. *J Vasc Surg* 1991; 13: 128–36.
50. Smulders YM, Rakic M, Slaats EH, Treskes M, Sijbrands EJ, Odekerken DA, Stehouwer CD, Silberbusch J. Fasting and post-methionine homocysteine levels in NIDDM. Determinants and correlations with retinopathy, albuminuria, and cardiovascular disease. *Diabetes Care* 1999; 22: 125–32.
51. Olson JC, Erbey JR, Forrest KY, Williams K, Becker DJ, Orchard TJ. Glycemia (or, in women, estimated glucose disposal rate) predict lower extremity arterial disease events in type 1 diabetes. *Metabolism* 2002; 51: 248–54.
52. Ross R. Atherosclerosis—an inflammatory disease. *N Engl J Med* 1999; 340: 115–26.
53. Vavuranakis M, Stefanadis C, Toutouzas K, Pitsavos C, Spanos V, Toutouzas P. Impaired compensatory coronary artery enlargement in atherosclerosis contributes to the development of coronary artery stenosis in diabetic patients. An in vivo intravascular ultrasound study. *Eur Heart J* 1997; 18: 1090–4.
54. Daemen MJ, De Mey JG. Regional heterogeneity of arterial structural changes. *Hypertension* 1995; 25: 464–73.
55. Edmonds ME, Morrison N, Laws JW, Watkins PJ. Medial arterial calcification and diabetic neuropathy. *Br Med J* 1982; 284: 928–30.
56. Shanahan CM, Cary NR, Salisbury JR, Proudfoot D, Weissberg PL, Edmonds ME. Medial localization of mineralization-regulating proteins in association with Monckeberg's sclerosis: evidence for smooth muscle cell-mediated vascular calcification. *Circulation* 1999; 100: 2168–76.
57. Edmonds ME. Medial arterial calcification and diabetes mellitus. *Z Kardiol* 2000; 89: 101–4.
58. Neubauer B, Gundersen HJ. Calcifications, narrowing and rugosities of the leg arteries in diabetic patients. *Acta Radiol Diagn* 1983; 24: 401–13.
59. Gilbey SG, Walters H, Edmonds ME, Archer AG, Watkins PJ, Parsons V, Grenfell A. Vascular calcification, autonomic neuropathy, and peripheral blood flow in patients with diabetic nephropathy. *Diabet Med* 1989; 6: 37–42.
60. Chantelau E, Ma XY, Herrnberger S, Dohmen C, Trappe P, Baba T. Effect of medial arterial calcification on O2 supply to exercising diabetic feet. *Diabetes* 1990; 39: 938–41.
61. Lehto S, Niskanen L, Suhonen M, Ronnemaa T, Laakso M. Medial artery calcification. A neglected harbinger of cardiovascular complications in non-insulin-dependent diabetes mellitus. *Arterioscler Thromb Vasc Biol* 1996; 16: 978–83.
62. Schaper W, Buschmann I. Arteriogenesis, the good and bad of it. *Cardiovasc Res* 1999; 43: 835–7.
63. Abaci A, Oguzhan A, Kahraman S, Eryol NK, Unal S, Arinc H, Ergin A. Effect of diabetes mellitus on formation of coronary collateral vessels. *Circulation* 1999; 99: 2239–42.
64. Rivard A, Silver M, Chen D, Kearney M, Magner M, Annex B, Peters K, Isner JM. Rescue of diabetes-related impairment of angiogenesis by intramuscular gene therapy with adeno-VEGF. *Am J Pathol* 1999; 154: 355–63.
65. Waltenberger J. Impaired collateral vessel development in diabetes: potential cellular mechanisms and therapeutic implications. *Cardiovasc Res* 2001; 49: 554–60.
66. Loots MAM, Kenter SB, Au AL, Van Galen WJM, Middelkoop E, Bos JD, Mekkes JR. Fibroblast derived from chronic diabetic ulcers differ in their response to stimulation with AGF, IGF-1, bFGF and PDGF-AB compared to controls. *Eur J Cell Biol* 2002; 81: 153–60.
67. Isner JM, Asahara T. Angiogenesis and vasculogenesis as therapeutic strategies for postnatal neovascularization. *J Clin Invest* 1999; 103: 1231–6.

68. Lederman RJ, Mendelsohn FO, Anderson RD, Saucedo JF, Tenaglia AN, Hermiller JB, Hillegass WB, Rocha-Singh K, Moon TE, Whitehouse MJ, Annex BH. Therapeutic angiogenesis with recombinant fibroblast growth factor-2 for intermittent claudication (the TRAFFIC study): a randomized trial. *Lancet* 2002; 359: 2053–8.
69. Jaap AJ, Hammersley MS, Shore AC, Tooke JE. Reduced microvascular hyperaemia in subjects at risk of developing type 2 (non-insulin-dependent) diabetes mellitus. *Diabetologia* 1994; 37: 214–6.
70. Houben AJ, Nieuwenhuijzen Kruseman AC, Bouhouch E, Slaaf DW, Schaper NC. Peripheral macro- and microcirculation in short-term insulin-dependent diabetes mellitus: the role of prostaglandins in early hemodynamic changes. *Eur J Clin Invest* 1993; 23: 662–7.
71. Flynn MD, Tooke JE. Diabetic neuropathy and the microcirculation. *Diabet Med* 1995; 12: 298–301.
72. Nabuurs-Franssen MH, Houben AJ, Tooke JE, Schaper NC. The effect of polyneuropathy of the foot microcirculation in type 2 diabetes. *Diabetologia* 2002; 45: 1164–71.
73. Netten PM, Wollersheim H, Thien T, Lutterman JA. Skin microcirculation of the foot in diabetic neuropathy. *Clin Sci* (Lond) 1996; 91: 559–65.
74. Jorneskog G, Brismar K, Fagrell B. Skin capillary circulation is more impaired in the toes of diabetic than nondiabetic patients with peripheral vascular disease. *Diabet Med* 1995; 12: 36–41.
75. de Heus-van Putten MA, Schaper NC, Bakker K. The clinical examination of the diabetic foot in daily practise. *Diabet Med* 1996; 13: S55–7.
76. McGee SR, Boyko EJ. Physical examination and chronic lower-extremity ischemia: a critical review. *Arch Intern Med* 1998; 158: 1357–64.
77. Pham H, Armstrong DG, Harvey C, Harkless LB, Giurini JM, Veves A. Screening techniques to identify people at high risk for diabetic foot ulceration: a prospective multicenter trial. *Diabetes Care* 2000; 23: 606–11.
78. Stoffers HE, Kester AD, Kaiser V, Rinkens PE, Knottnerus JA. Diagnostic value of signs and symptoms associated with peripheral arterial occlusive disease seen in general practice: a multivariable approach. *Med Decis Making* 1997; 17: 61–70.
79. Takolander R, Rauwerda JA. The use of noninvasive vascular assessment in diabetic patients with foot lesions. *Diabet Med* 1996; 13: S39–42.
80. Orchard TJ, Strandness DE Jr. Assessment of peripheral vascular disease in diabetes. Report and recommendations of an international workshop sponsored by the American Diabetes Association and the American Heart Association, September 18–20, 1992 New Orleans, Louisiana. *Circulation* 1993; 88: 819–28.
81. McNeely MJ, Boyko EJ, Ahroni JH, Stensel VL, Reiber GE, Smith DG, Pecoraro RF. The independent contributions of diabetic neuropathy and vasculopathy in foot ulceration. How great are the risks? *Diabetes Care* 1995; 18: 216–9.
82. Apelqvist J, Castenfors J, Larsson J, Stenstrom A, Agardh CD. Prognostic value of systolic ankle and toe blood pressure levels in outcome of diabetic foot ulcer. *Diabetes Care* 1989; 12: 373–8.
83. Pecoraro RE, Ahroni JH, Boyko EJ, Stensel VL. Chronology and determinants of tissue repair in diabetic lower-extremity ulcers. *Diabetes* 1991; 40: 1305–13.
84. Kalani M, Brismar K, Fagrell B, Ostergren J, Jorneskog G. Transcutaneous oxygen tension and toe blood pressure as predictors for outcome of diabetic foot ulcers. *Diabetes Care* 1999; 22: 147–51.
85. Holstein P. The distal blood pressure predicts healing of amputations on the feet. *Acta Orthop Scand* 1984; 55: 227–33.
86. Hirsch AT, Treat-Jacobson D, Lando HA, Hatsukami DK. The role of tobacco cessation, antiplatelet and lipid-lowering therapies in the treatment of peripheral arterial disease. *Vasc Med* 1997; 2: 243–51.
87. Collaborative meta-analysis of randomized trials of antiplatelet therapy for prevention of death, myocardial infarction, and stroke in high risk patients. *Br Med J* 2002; 324: 71–86.
88. CAPRIE Steering Committee. A randomized, blinded, trial of clopidogrel versus aspirin in patients at risk of ischaemic events (CAPRIE). *Lancet* 1996; 348: 1329–39.
89. Heart Protection Study Collaborative Group. MRC/BHF Heart Protection Study of cholesterol lowering with simvastatin in 20,536 high-risk individuals: a randomized placebo-controlled trial. *Lancet* 2002; 360: 7–22.
90. Rubins HB, Robins SJ, Collins D, Fye CL, Anderson JW, Elam MB, Faas FH, Linares E, Schaefer EJ, Schectman G, Wilt TJ, Wittes J. Gemfibrozil for the secondary prevention of coronary heart disease in men with low levels of high-density lipoprotein cholesterol. Veterans Affairs High-Density Lipoprotein Cholesterol Intervention Trial Study Group. *N Engl J Med* 1999; 341: 410–8.
91. Elam MB, Hunninghake DB, Davis KB, Garg R, Johnson C, Egan D, Kostis JB, Sheps DS, Brinton EA. Effect of niacin on lipid and lipoprotein levels and glycemic control in patients with diabetes and peripheral arterial disease: the ADMIT study: a randomized trial. Arterial Disease Multiple Intervention Trial. *J Am Med Assoc* 2000; 284: 1263–70.
92. Radack K, Deck C. Beta-adrenergic blocker therapy does not worsen intermittent claudication in subjects with peripheral arterial disease. A meta-analysis of randomized controlled trials. *Arch Intern Med* 1991; 151: 1769–76.
93. Baker WH, String ST, Hayes AC, Turner D. Diagnosis of peripheral occlusive disease: comparison of clinical evaluation and noninvasive laboratory. *Arch Surg* 1978; 113: 1308–10.
94. Legemate DA, Teeuwen C, Hoeneveld H, Ackerstaff RG, Eikelboom BC. The potential of duplex scanning to replace aortoiliac and femoro-popliteal angiography. *Eur J Vasc Surg* 1989; 3: 49–54.
95. Taylor LM Jr, Yeager RA, Moneta GL, McConnell DB, Porter JM. The incidence of perioperative myocardial infarction in general vascular surgery. *J Vasc Surg* 1992; 15: 52–61.
96. Karacagil S, Lofberg AM, Granbo A, Lorelius LE, Bergqvist D. Value of duplex scanning in evaluation of crural and foot arteries in limbs with severe lower limb ischaemia—a prospective comparison with angiography. *Eur J Vasc Endovasc Surg* 1996; 12: 300–3.
97. Elsman BH, Legemate DA, van der Heyden FW, de Vos H, Mali WP, Eikelboom BC. The use of color-coded duplex scanning in the selection of patients with lower extremity arterial disease for percutaneous transluminal angioplasty: a prospective study. *Cardiovasc Intervent Radiol* 1996; 19: 313–6.
98. Nawaz S, Cleveland T, Gaines PA, Chan P. Clinical risk associated with contrast angiography in metformin treated patients: a clinical review. *Clin Radiol* 1998; 53: 342–4.

99. Ho KY, Leiner T, de Haan MW, Kessels AG, Kitslaar PJ, van Engelshoven JM. Peripheral vascular tree stenoses: evaluation with moving-bed infusion-tracking MR angiography. *Radiology* 1998; 206: 683–92.
100. Ubels FL, Links TP, Sluiter WJ, Reitsma WD, Smit AJ. Walking training for intermittent claudication in diabetes. *Diabetes Care* 1999; 22: 198–201.
101. Hunink MG, Wong JB, Donaldson MC, Meyerovitz MF, de Vries J, Harrington DP. Revascularization for femoropopliteal disease. A decision and cost-effectiveness analysis. *J Am Med Assoc* 1995; 274: 165–71.
102. Capek P, McLean GK, Berkowitz HD. Femoropopliteal angioplasty. Factors influencing long-term success. *Circulation* 1991; 83: I70–80.
103. Johnston KW. Femoral and popliteal arteries: reanalysis of results of balloon angioplasty. *Radiology* 1992; 183: 767–71.
104. Matsi PJ, Manninen HI, Vanninen RL, Suhonen MT, Oksala I, Laakso M, Hakkarainen T, Soimakallio S. Femoropopliteal angioplasty in patients with claudication: primary and secondary patency in 140 limbs with 1–3-year follow-up. *Radiology* 1994; 191: 727–33.
105. Davies AH, Cole SE, Magee TR, Scott DJ, Baird RN, Horrocks M. The effect of diabetes mellitus on the outcome of angioplasty for lower limb ischaemia. *Diabet Med* 1992; 9: 480–1.
106. Stokes KR, Strunk HM, Campbell DR, Gibbons GW, Wheeler HG, Clouse ME. Five-year results of iliac and femoropopliteal angioplasty in diabetic patients. *Radiology* 1990; 174: 977–82.
107. Estes JM, Pomposelli FB Jr. Lower extremity arterial reconstruction in patients with diabetes mellitus. *Diabet Med* 1996; 13: S43–7.
108. Apelqvist J, Larsson J, Agardh CD. The influence of external precipitating factors and peripheral neuropathy on the development and outcome of diabetic foot ulcers. *J Diabet Complications* 1990; 4: 21–5.
109. Andros G, Harris RW, Dulawa LB, Oblath RW, Salles-Cunha SX. The need for arteriography in diabetic patients with gangrene and palpable foot pulses. *Arch Surg* 1984; 119: 1260–3.
110. Rivers SP, Scher L, Veith FJ. Indications for distal arterial reconstruction in the presence of palpable pedal pulses. *J Vasc Surg* 1990; 12: 552–7.
111. Ubbink DT, Tulevski II, den Hartog D, Koelemay MJ, Legemate DA, Jacobs MJ. The value of noninvasive techniques for the assessment of critical limb ischaemia. *Eur J Vasc Endovasc Surg* 1997; 13: 296–300.
112. Van Houtem W, Bakker K, Rauwerda JA, Heine RJ. Vascular assessment before lower extrimity amputation. *Diabet Foot* 2001; 4: 185–93.
113. Rauwerda JA. Foot debridement: anatomic knowledge is mandatory. *Diabetes Metab Res Rev* 2000; 16 (suppl 1): S23–6.
114. Raymakers JT, Houben AJ, van der Heyden JJ, Tordoir JH, Kitslaar PJ, Schaper NC. The effect of diabetes and severe ischaemia on the penetration of ceftazidime into tissues of the limb. *Diabet Med* 2001; 18: 229–34.
115. Tannenbaum GA, Pomposelli FB Jr, Marcaccio EJ, Gibbons GW, Campbell DR, Freeman DV, Miller A, LoGerfo FW. Safety of vein bypass grafting to the dorsal pedal artery in diabetic patients with foot infections. *J Vasc Surg* 1992; 15: 982–90.
116. Lepantalo M, Biancari F, Tukiainen E. Never amputate without consultation of a vascular surgeon. *Diabetes Metab Res Rev* 2000; 16 (suppl 1): S27–32.
117. Spence LD, Hartnell GG, Reinking G, Gibbons G, Pomposelli F, Clouse ME. Diabetic versus nondiabetic limb-threatening ischemia: outcome of percutaneous iliac intervention. *Am J Roentgenol* 1999; 172: 1335–41.
118. Faries PL, LoGerfo FW, Hook SC, Pulling MC, Akbari CM, Campbell DR, Pomposelli FB Jr. The impact of diabetes on arterial reconstructions for multilevel arterial occlusive disease. *Am J Surg* 2001; 181: 251–5.
119. Faglia E, Favales F, Quarantiello A, Calia P, Brambilla G, Rampoldi A, Morabito A. Feasibility and effectiveness of peripheral percutaneous transluminal balloon angioplasty in diabetic subjects with foot ulcers. *Diabetes Care* 1996; 19: 1261–4.
120. Danielsson G, Albrechtsson U, Norgren L, Danielsson P, Ribbe E, Thorne J, Zdanowski Z. Percutaneous transluminal angioplasty of crural arteries: diabetes and other factors influencing outcome. *Eur J Vasc Endovasc Surg* 2001; 21: 432–6.
121. Tarry WC, Walsh DB, Birkmeyer NJ, Fillinger MF, Zwolak RM, Cronenwett JL. Fate of the contralateral leg after infrainguinal bypass. *J Vasc Surg* 1998; 27: 1039–48.
122. Akbari CM, Pomposelli FB Jr, Gibbons GW, Campbell DR, Pulling MC, Mydlarz D, LoGerfo FW. Lower extremity revascularization in diabetes: late observations. *Arch Surg* 2000; 135: 452–6.
123. Panneton JM, Gloviczki P, Bower TC, Rhodes JM, Canton LG, Toomey BJ. Pedal bypass for limb salvage: impact of diabetes on long-term outcome. *Ann Vasc Surg* 2000; 14: 640–7.
124. Panayiotopoulos YP, Tyrrell MR, Arnold FJ, Korzon-Burakowska A, Amiel SA, Taylor PR. Results and cost analysis of distal [crural/pedal] arterial revascularization for limb salvage in diabetic and nondiabetic patients. *Diabet Med* 1997; 14: 214–20.
125. Visser K, Idu MM, Buth J, Engel GL, Hunink MG. Duplex scan surveillance during the first year after infrainguinal autologous vein bypass grafting surgery: costs and clinical outcomes compared with other surveillance programs. *J Vasc Surg* 2001; 33: 123–30.
126. Holtzman J, Caldwell M, Walvatne C, Kane R. Long-term functional status and quality of life after lower extremity revascularization. *J Vasc Surg* 1999; 29: 395–402.
127. Holstein P, Ellitsgaard N, Olsen BB, Ellitsgaard V. Decreasing incidence of major amputations in people with diabetes. *Diabetologia* 2000; 43: 844–7.

Management of Diabetes: Glucose and Lipid Monitoring, Specific Subgroups

86

Diabetes Mellitus in Children and Adolescents

Stuart A. Weinzimer and William V. Tamborlane

Yale University School of Medicine, New Haven, CT, USA

INTRODUCTION

Diabetes mellitus is a heterogeneous group of disorders characterized by impaired metabolism of glucose and other energy-yielding fuels, as well as the late development of vascular and neuropathic complications. Diabetes can be divided into at least three subclasses involving distinct pathogenic mechanisms: type 1 or insulin-dependent diabetes mellitus (T1DM); type 2, or non-insulin-dependent diabetes mellitus (T2DM); and secondary diabetes linked to another identifiable condition or syndrome. It is important to recognize that not all children with diabetes have T1DM: the prevalence of T2DM is increasing dramatically, especially in obese adolescents of African American, Native American, and Hispanic origin. Regardless of the cause, the disease is associated with insulin deficiency, which in T1DM is usually total, and in T2DM partial or relative when viewed in the context of coexisting insulin resistance. Lack of insulin plays a primary role in the metabolic derangements linked to diabetes, and hyperglycemia, in turn, plays a key role in the complications of the disease.

T1DM in childhood and adolescence presents special challenges to pediatric health care providers. The combination of severe insulin deficiency and the physical and psychosocial changes that accompany normal growth and development make day-to-day management of pediatric patients especially difficult. Moreover, the results of the Diabetes Control and Complications Trial (DCCT) have raised the bar considerably higher with respect to goals of treatment, since intensive treatment significantly reduced the risk of progression of retinopathy and the development of microalbuminuria. Current recommendations mandate that youth with T1DM should aim to achieve glycemic control as close to normal as possible and as early in the course of the disease as possible, while still allowing normal childhood and adolescent psychosocial development. Remarkably, a much greater proportion of young patients are meeting strict standards of care than ever imagined possible only a few years ago, although such intensive care typically requires a specialized pediatric health care team consisting of physicians, nurse practitioners, dietitians, and mental health specialists.

EPIDEMIOLOGY

Diabetes is the second most common chronic disease in childhood, occurring in 1 of every 1500 children by the age of 5 and 1 in 350 by age 18 [1] in the United States. There are two peaks in age of presentation, the first at ages 5–7 and second in early puberty. One third of people with diabetes do not present until adulthood. Diabetes affects boys and girls equally.

T1DM is primarily a disease of Caucasians of Northern European, especially Scandinavian, background. The highest incidence rates of diabetes worldwide are found in Finland, Sweden, and Denmark, where about 30 new cases per 100 000 population are diagnosed annually. For comparison, the annual incidence rate of diabetes in the United States is about 12–15 per 100 000 population, whereas Africa is about 5 per 100 000 per year and East Asia less than 2 per 100 000 per year [2]. There are striking geographical differences related to diabetes incidence: countries located at a greater distance from the equator and with lower mean annual temperatures have greater incidence

International Textbook of Diabetes Mellitus, Third Edition. Edited by R. A. DeFronzo, E. Ferrannini, H. Keen, and P. Zimmet.
 ISBN: 0-471-48655-8.

rates for diabetes, although whether this finding may be related to genetic differences in populations or exposure to certain infectious agents is unclear. Migrant studies show increased rates of diabetes in populations moving from areas of lower diabetes incidence to those with higher diabetes incidence [3]. However, because general trends of migration are from poor, tropical, developing countries to more affluent, temperate countries in the Western world, confounding influences such as diet and lifestyle make implication of certain geographical areas or environmental exposures problematic.

CLINICAL PRESENTATION IN CHILDHOOD

Classically, children with T1DM present with a triad of polyuria, polydipsia, and polyphagia. However, there is great variation within the spectrum and severity of presentation, and a wide differential diagnosis can exist. Furthermore, the fact that the initial presentation of T1DM is often triggered by an intercurrent illness can also confound the diagnosis. In children with T1DM, polyuria and compensatory polydipsia result once the renal threshold for glucose has been exceeded (at serum glucose concentrations of about 180 mg/dl), and glucosuria occurs. Hyperglycemia and resultant hyperosmolarity state induce an osmotic diuresis, leading to the polyuria, polydipsia, and enuresis. On presentation, these symptoms have often been present for several weeks. This is all the more true in babies and active adolescents, in whom it is difficult for parents to note the symptoms of excessive urination. Progressive insulin deficiency leads to weight loss, fatigue, and general malaise, as protein and fat stores are lost. As counterregulatory hormones increase and ketosis worsens, symptoms of acute illness develop, including nausea, anorexia, abdominal pain, and vomiting. At this point the acute worsening of dehydration and acidosis may produce symptoms of lethargy, confusion, stupor, even coma, and the respiratory compensation for the metabolic acidosis produces hyperpnea, the deep sighing "Kussmaul" respirations. Table 1 summarizes the typical symptoms present at diagnosis.

Table 1 Symptoms of T1DM

Polyuria
Polydipsia
Polyphagia
Weight loss
Recurrence of enuresis in previously trained child
Candidal vaginitis
Lethargy
Blurred vision
Abdominal pain*
Vomiting*
Difficulty breathing*
Alteration in mental status*

*Indicative of DKA.

Table 2 Physical findings in T1DM

Dehydration
Dry mucous membranes
Decreased skin turgor*
Delayed capillary refill*
Tachycardia*
Hypotension*
Vulvovaginitis
Fruity odor to breath*
Kussmaul respirations*
Ileus, guarding*
Depressed level of consciousness*

*Indicative of DKA.

The physical examination should focus on the state of hydration and include careful evaluation of heart rate and blood pressure, description of mucous membranes, capillary refill, pulses, and warmth of extremities. A rough estimation of degree of dehydration (~5, 10, or 15%) may be made in order to calculate the fluid deficit and facilitate rehydration therapy, with the understanding that such estimates are only fairly accurate at best. A careful examination and written documentation of the neurological status is also critical, to serve as a baseline in case of deterioration in neurological status later in therapy. General physical examination should include respiratory and abdominal examinations, as well as a search for an intercurrent illness that may have served as the "trigger." Evaluation of the thyroid for goiter and skin for hyperpigmentation allows for the diagnosis of potential comorbidities such as thyroiditis or Addison's disease. Girls should be evaluated for the presence of candidal vulvovaginitis, and both boys and girls should have documentation of height, weight, and sexual maturity rating. The discovery of a "fruity" odor to the breath is characteristic of diabetic ketoacidosis, but significant ketosis may be present even in the absence of this finding. Table 2 summarizes common findings at diagnosis of T1DM.

Appropriate laboratory studies begin with the measurement of serum blood glucose. As mentioned earlier, random "casual" blood glucose levels are indicated in the setting of a child with symptoms suggestive of diabetes. In the symptomatic child, blood glucose should be checked promptly; children should *not* be instructed to have a fasting blood glucose level measured the next day. In the obviously well-appearing child, minimal laboratory testing is required: electrolytes, blood urea nitrogen (BUN), and creatinine, along with a formal urinalysis for glucose and ketones, may suffice. In children with clinical evidence of more severe dehydration and/or other organ system signs, the evaluation should be expanded to include blood count with differential, venous, or arterial blood gas, and in the setting of fever or shock, blood culture. Other studies depend on the clinical scenario and should be individualized.

A careful history, physical examination, and laboratory investigation should allow the diagnosis of diabetes

Table 3 Differential diagnoses in T1DM and tests to consider

Clinical findings	Differential diagnosis	Tests/interpretation
Polyuria, nocturia, enuresis	Urinary tract infection (UTI), benign nocturnal enuresis	Urinalysis will demonstrate glycosuria +/− ketonuria characteristic of diabetes, instead of pyuria and other markers of UTI
Polydipsia	Psychogenic polydipsia, diabetes insipidus	Urinalysis will demonstrate glycosuria +/− ketonuria in diabetes, instead of low specific gravity (alone)
Weight loss	Anorexia nervosa, gastrointestinal or chronic disease	Careful history should reveal behaviors and ideations characteristic of anorexia nervosa; plasma glucose diagnostic of diabetes
Vomiting	Gastroenteritis, toxic ingestion, other metabolic disorders	Serum glucose and electrolytes in vomiting child will reveal diabetes; electrolyte disturbances and acidosis without hyperglycemia suggests other metabolic disorders, requiring more directed testing
Abdominal pain	Gastroenteritis, appendicitis, other intra-abdominal process	Careful history and physical examination should elicit typical symptoms of diabetes and exclude surgical abdomen; measurement of serum glucose and urinalysis will differentiate diabetes
Hyperpnea	Pneumonia, asthma, anxiety	Kussmaul respirations (deep sighing breaths) suggest metabolic acidosis, whereas tachypnea suggests a primary respiratory disorder; no rales or wheezes; serum glucose and electrolytes characteristic of diabetes and metabolic acidosis
Hyperglycemia	Medication- or stress-induced hyperglycemia	May be mistaken for diabetes, although careful history will not demonstrate characteristic prodromal weight loss or urinary symptoms
Glycosuria	Benign renal glycosuria	May be mistaken for diabetes. Measurement of serum glucose will differentiate diabetes from renal glycosuria

mellitus to be deduced in a rapid, efficient manner. The presence of polyuria, polydipsia, and weight loss in a child should be considered T1DM until proven otherwise. The primary differential for T1DM in children is urinary tract infection, due to the symptoms of excessive or frequent urination. If the symptoms of polydipsia and polyuria predominate, diabetes insipidus should be considered. However, formal urinalysis can easily differentiate the two conditions, as the urine of diabetes mellitus contains glucose, ketones, and osmotically active electrolytes, while the urine of diabetes insipidus is bland and dilute. If the presentation includes dehydration and vomiting, gastroenteritis should be considered, as should streptococcal pharyngitis and pneumonia. Pneumonia or asthmatic exacerbation may also be suggested in the setting of metabolic acidosis and abnormal breathing. In children presenting with fever, vomiting, and abdominal pain, appendicitis or other acute abdominal events may also be possibilities, a situation made more confusing by the fact that children in diabetic ketoacidosis (DKA) often have leukocytosis. Other conditions in the differential diagnosis of T1DM include toxic ingestion, pelvic inflammatory disease in a sexually active adolescent, and in any age, sepsis. Patients with persistent hyperglycemia may also present with various forms of fungal infections. Infants and toddlers may have thrush and/or diaper candidiasis, and adolescents may present with genital yeast infections. Patients and parents are often unaware that these symptoms are in any way related to diabetes. Thus, a careful genitourinary examination is necessary on admission. In a prepubertal child, the presence of candidiasis should always trigger blood glucose testing by the primary care physician. It should also be stressed that the diagnosis of diabetes requires measurement of blood glucose; the finding of glycosuria alone is not sufficient. Renal glycosuria, a benign condition in which the threshold for urinary excretion of glucose occurs even at normal blood glucose concentrations, may occasionally masquerade as diabetes in the child in whom routine urinalysis is performed in the absence of true symptoms of diabetes. Table 3 summarizes the differential diagnostic considerations in T1DM.

TREATMENT OF NEW-ONSET T1DM

The goals of management of the child with new-onset T1DM are twofold: metabolic stabilization of the child and education of the family to care for the child after the stabilization has been completed. Treatment of the newly diagnosed child with T1DM depends upon the acuity of the illness at presentation: the ambulatory well-appearing child without severe dehydration may be handled quite differently than the acutely ill, dehydrated patient with vomiting. It is still general practice to admit the newly diagnosed diabetic child to the hospital, because the frequent monitoring and intense teaching that are required cannot often be accomplished in the ambulatory setting by an untrained family still recovering from the shock of the diagnosis. Small pilot projects have, however, demonstrated that outpatient management of the new-onset diabetic patient may be accomplished in some situations [4]. The development of diabetes in the sibling of a known patient may be managed in an ambulatory setting, if the child is not acutely ill and the family well-trained in diabetes management. Management of the acutely ill child in DKA will be discussed separately.

Newly diagnosed patients may use a traditional "split-mixed" regimen, in which combinations of shorter and longer acting insulins are given together as two injections daily, with breakfast and dinner, typically using regular insulin as the shorter acting insulin and NPH (neutral protamine Hagedorn) or Lente as the longer acting insulin. The total dose is divided into 2/3 NPH/Lente and 1/3 regular.

However, the traditional "short-acting" regular insulin has now been supplanted by new insulin analogues with a more rapid activity profile. Lispro (Lilly) and Aspart (Novo Nordisk) insulins are produced by the substitution of amino acids in the C-terminal region of the B-chain (the reversal of proline at position 28 and lysine at position 29 to Lys28-Pro29 for Lispro, and a substitution of aspartic acid for Pro28 for Aspart). This bioengineering renders the insulin molecules less likely to aggregate into hexamers in the subcutaneous tissue after injection, and thus allows more rapid absorption into the bloodstream. The advantages of Lispro or Aspart to regular insulin include more rapid onset and shorter duration of activity, so that insulin is available immediately to cover meal-related glucose excursions and is not persistent after the complete absorption of the meal. Clinical trials of Lispro and Aspart have demonstrated improvements in postprandial hyperglycemia and lower rates of hypoglycemia compared to regular insulin [5]. Because of these improvements, Lispro and Aspart have essentially replaced regular insulin as the short-acting insulin of choice for most patients with diabetes, and most of our new-onset diabetic children are initiated on a two-shot regimen of Lispro or Aspart mixed with NPH or Lente, in a 1/3–2/3 ratio.

The NPH and Lente type insulins can now also be replaced by another new long-acting insulin analogue, insulin glargine. Glargine (Aventis) insulin is a new analogue of human insulin with C-terminal elongation of the β-chain by two arginine residues and replacement of asparagine in position A21 by glycine. This molecule is soluble in the acidic solution in which it is packaged but relatively insoluble in the physiologic pH of the extracellular fluid. Consequently, microprecipitates of glargine insulin are formed following subcutaneous injection, which markedly delays its absorption into the systemic circulation. Pharmacokinetic and pharmacodynamic studies have demonstrated that the insulin analogue has a very flat and prolonged time-action profile [6]. Results of preliminary studies of the efficacy and safety of glargine in children and adolescents with diabetes showed modestly lower fasting blood glucose levels and reduced risk of nocturnal hypoglycemia with glargine compared to human NPH insulin, although no differences in HbA_{1c} were noted [7, 8]. Additional studies and more clinical experience need to be accumulated regarding use of this analogue in youth with type 1 diabetes. Because glargine cannot be mixed with other insulins, it has to be given by separate injection, which might affect its acceptability by some youngsters. A list of available insulin preparations is shown in Table 4.

The rationale for using two rather than three or more injections at onset of diabetes is that with aggressive control of blood levels, most children enter a "honeymoon" or partial remission period after a few weeks of therapy. This remission period is a result of increased insulin

Table 4 Pharmacodynamic properties of common insulin formulations

Category	Onset (h)	Peak (h)	Duration (h)
Rapid-acting			
Insulin Lispro	0.25–0.5	0.5–1	3–4
Insulin Aspart	0.25–0.5	0.5–1	3–5
Short-acting			
Regular	0.5–1	2–4	4–8
Intermediate-acting			
NPH	2–4	4–10	12–18
Lente	3–4	6–12	12–18
Long-acting			
Ultralente	4–6	6–12	18–24
Insulin glargine	2–4	n/a	24+
Premixed			
70/30 (70% NPH/30% Regular)	0.5–1	2–8	12–18
50/50 (50% NPH/50% Regular)	0.5–1	2–6	12–18
Mix 25 (75% NPH/25% Lispro)	0.25–0.5	1–2	12–18
Novolog Mix (70% NPH/30% Aspart)	0.25–0.5	1–2	12–18

secretion by residual β-cells and improved insulin sensitivity with normalization of blood glucose levels [9]. To achieve these effects, patients are started on a total daily dose of at least 1 U/kg body weight/day. Even more important, each component of the insulin regimen is adjusted on the basis of finger stick blood glucose levels measured at least four times a day. The goal is to obtain premeal blood glucose values within the normal range and is achieved via daily telephone contact with the family for at least the first 3 weeks of treatment. The DCCT data indicate that strict control of diabetes also serves to prolong the period of residual β-cell function in patients with T1DM [10].

Infants and young toddlers may require modifications to the standard initial therapy, because of greater insulin sensitivity, smaller carbohydrate content of meals, and unpredictability of eating. Total daily insulin doses may be reduced to 0.5–0.7 U/kg/day and titrated as necessary. For picky eaters the rapid-acting insulin may be administered *after* the meal, to minimize hypoglycemia due to missed meals. Infants may require only NPH/Lente and not short-acting meal-related insulin. At the present time the safety and effectiveness of glargine in infants and toddlers has not been studied.

Prior to discharge, an assessment of the family's overall level of coping and functioning should be made. Special situations, such as blended families or alternate/additional caretakers in the home, should be worked out before hospital discharge. Families typically experience shock and grief at the child's diagnosis, but consideration should be made for referrals for psychosocial counseling if grief, anxiety, or depression appears to be excessive or interferes with diabetes education.

DIABETIC KETOACIDOSIS

Diabetic ketoacidosis is a life-threatening, preventable complication of diabetes mellitus characterized by inadequate insulin action, hyperglycemia, dehydration, electrolyte loss, metabolic acidosis, and ketosis. It is associated with a significant mortality rate and is the most frequent cause of death in children with T1DM. Children whose diabetes has not yet been diagnosed may present with DKA, and so the diagnosis must be considered in any child with confusion or coma of undetermined etiology. In children whose diabetes has already been diagnosed, DKA can usually be prevented by patient and family education, frequent monitoring of blood glucose and urinary ketones during intercurrent illness, adequate oral hydration, and supplemental insulin ("sick day rules").

Diabetic ketoacidosis is defined as a condition in which blood glucose concentration is greater than 200 mg/dl, together with ketonemia/ketonuria and pH <7.3. The primary abnormality is insulin deficiency, which leads to hyperglycemia because of both decreased glucose utilization and increased gluconeogenesis. As glucose levels exceed the renal threshold of 180 mg/dl, an osmotic diuresis occurs, resulting in the loss of extracellular water and electrolytes and worsening of the hyperglycemia. Insulin deficiency also leads to accelerated lipolysis with subsequent conversion of free fatty acids to β-hydroxybutyric acid and acetoacetic acid. This results in a metabolic acidosis. Acetone is also formed and gives a fruity odor to the patient's breath, but it does not contribute to the acidosis. Potassium, primarily an intracellular ion, is transported out of the cell into the plasma in exchange for hydrogen and is lost in the urine. Thus, virtually all patients with DKA develop a "total body" deficiency of potassium, regardless of their serum potassium level. Phosphate, another predominantly intracellular ion, is handled similarly. Deficiency of 2,3-diphosphoglycerate, a phosphate-containing glycolytic intermediate in red blood cells that facilitates release of oxygen from hemoglobin, may contribute to the development of lactic acidosis complicating the ketoacidosis. Although insulin deficiency is the principal abnormality, elevations in the counterregulatory hormones (glucagon, cortisol, catecholamines, and growth hormone) and reduction in circulating free insulin-like growth factor 1 contribute to accelerated gluconeogenesis and lipolysis [11].

Diabetic ketoacidosis is not difficult to recognize in a child with known diabetes who is dehydrated, hyperventilating, and obtunded. In the child whose diabetes has not yet been diagnosed, however, it may be confused with Reye syndrome, toxic ingestion (especially salicylate or alcohol), and central nervous system (CNS) infection or trauma. Persistent vomiting may suggest gastroenteritis, or with abdominal pain, acute appendicitis or other intra-abdominal process. The diagnosis of diabetes (if not already established) is suggested by a history of polyuria, polydipsia, polyphagia, nocturia, or enuresis in a previously toilet-trained child. Weakness and unexplained weight loss may also be presenting features. When the diagnosis of DKA is suspected, an attempt should be made to identify precipitating causes (e.g., infection, stress, or noncompliance). In a child with known diabetes, it is important to review briefly the recent blood glucose history and to ascertain not only the usual insulin dosage but also the quantity and timing of the most recent injection.

The physical examination should focus initially on the adequacy of the airway, breathing, and an assessment of the circulatory status (pulse, blood pressure, peripheral perfusion), degree of dehydration (including weight if possible), and mental status. Deep, rapid respirations (Kussmaul breathing) and a fruity odor to the breath are classic signs but are not present in every patient. A careful search should be made for a source of infection that may have precipitated the episode of DKA. Bedside determination of the blood glucose with a glucose monitoring device and evaluation of the urine for glucose and ketones should be performed as quickly as possible, and treatment should be initiated without waiting for the results of the laboratory assessment to become available.

The laboratory evaluation of patients suspected to have DKA includes determination of the blood glucose, plasma or urinary ketones, serum electrolyte concentration, BUN, creatinine, osmolarity, and a baseline calcium and phosphorus. A baseline blood gas measurement should also be made to determine the pH and P_{CO_2}. While venous blood gas measurements may suffice in milder episodes of DKA, an arterial blood gas measurement should be obtained in patients suspected to have incomplete respiratory compensation and/or those expected to require bicarbonate therapy (see below). If hypertriglyceridemia is present, the serum sodium concentration may be artifactually lowered. Similarly, the serum sodium will be reduced by approximately 1.6 mEq/l for each 100 mg/dl rise in glucose because of the reequilibration of the intra- and extracellular compartments at a higher osmolarity [12]. In the presence of ketones (and lactate), a large anion gap acidosis will be present. The degree of elevation of the BUN and creatinine, as well as the hematocrit, may indicate the extent of dehydration (and the possibility of renal damage). The initial serum potassium may be low, normal, or high, depending on the degree of acidosis and the quantitative urinary losses.

The acute management of DKA is directed at correction of the dehydration, electrolyte deficits, hyperglycemia, and acidosis (Table 5). Initial fluid therapy is aimed at rapid stabilization of the circulation to correct impending shock, but as in other forms of hypertonic dehydration, too rapid fluid administration must be avoided. Fluid replacement in excess of 4 $l/m^2/24$ h has been associated with the development of potentially fatal cerebral edema in DKA. For this reason, an initial fluid bolus is usually advised to expand the vascular compartment and improve peripheral circulation, but once the patient has been stabilized, subsequent rehydration is accomplished with caution. Typically, one aims to correct the fluid defect gradually, over 36–48 h. Gradual correction is particularly important in children at an increased risk of developing cerebral edema. This includes children with altered mental status, history of symptoms >48 h, pH <7.0, glucose >1000 mg/dl, corrected sodium >155 mEq/l, extreme hyperosmolarity (>375 mOsm/l), or age <3 years. A corrected sodium level that fails to rise with treatment may signify excessive free water accumulation and an increased risk of cerebral edema. Therefore, rehydration fluids should contain at least 115–135 mEq/l sodium chloride to ensure a gradual decline in serum osmolarity and minimize the risk of cerebral edema [13, 14]. Early potassium replacement is also important, to correct the potassium depletion that occurs because of both the severe initial intracellular losses and the subsequent potassium shift from the extracellular to the intracellular compartment (that occurs when treatment with insulin is initiated and the acidosis is corrected). Potassium is administered only after urine output is ensured to prevent hyperkalemia in the setting of unrecognized renal impairment. Potassium is usually given at a dose of 20–40 mEq/l of fluid, either as potassium chloride, or combinations of potassium chloride with potassium phosphate (which has the additional advantage of replacing the phosphate deficit). Electrocardiographic monitoring facilitates early recognition of either hyperkalemia (peaked T waves) or hypokalemia (flat or inverted T waves) and the development of potentially dangerous cardiac arrhythmias. Serum calcium should be monitored if phosphate is given, since phosphate administration may precipitate hypocalcemia.

Insulin therapy should be initiated immediately after the patient has been stabilized with an initial fluid bolus, typically at a dose of 0.1 U/kg/h. As with fluid replacement,

Table 5 Guidelines for management of DKA

Insulin	0.1 U/kg/h as continuous intravenous infusion is typical. For very young or severely acidotic, hyperosmolar patients, 0.05 U/kg/h may be initiated to prevent rapid changes during metabolic stabilization. In hyperglycemic, hyperosmolar, nonketotic coma (which is rarely seen in children except in some adolescents with type 2 diabetes), insulin may be withheld during the first several hours
Fluids	10–20 ml/kg 0.9% saline bolus to restore intravascular volume. Repeat as needed to treat shock. Base subsequent fluid administration upon estimated degree of dehydration, and plan to replace deficit evenly over 48 h
Sodium	Na^+ deficit at presentation generally resolves with administration of isotonic fluids during resuscitation phase. Measured $[Na^+]$ typically underestimates true Na^+ levels due to effects of hyperglycemia. Calculation and assessment of true $[Na^+]$ over time may decrease risk of cerebral edema
Potassium	K^+ deficit at presentation requires aggressive therapy. Replacement depends on serum $[K^+]$ at presentation; 20–40 mEq (1/2 as KCl and 1/2 as K^+ phosphate) added to each liter of rehydration fluid is typical
Glucose	Added to rehydration fluids once the blood glucose level falls <300 mg/dl. Goal generally is to reduce blood glucose 50–100 mg/dl/h, although recent evidence suggests that rapid fall in blood glucose may not increase risk of cerebral edema
Bicarbonate	Considered in extreme acidosis only—bicarbonate use may increase risk of cerebral edema
Clinical monitoring	Assess vital signs, neurological status, state of hydration, and fluid intake and output at least hourly
Laboratory monitoring	Measure blood glucose hourly, electrolytes, and pH at least q2h until stable. Follow BUN, creatinine, calcium, and phosphate if abnormal at presentation

the aim of therapy is gradual correction: reduction of the blood glucose by 50–100 mg/dl/h. Usually, the glucose falls significantly with initial rehydration alone. Dextrose is added to the intravenous solution when the serum glucose level falls below 300 mg/dl, and is titrated to provide a continued gradual decline in blood glucose to target levels. This is easily accomplished with the simultaneous use of two intravenous solutions, which differ only in the dextrose concentration. Usually the lowering of the blood glucose concentration precedes the decrease in ketones. Thus, in the situation of continued acidosis with a glucose less than 300 mg/dl, it is important not to decrease the insulin infusion rate, but rather to add glucose. Determination of serum ketones, though helpful diagnostically, is not an accurate guide to clinical improvement, as only acetoacetate is measured by the usual method and not β-hydroxybutyrate, which predominates early (but not later) in the course of untreated DKA. Newer home glucose meters that also measure serum β-hydroxybutyrate levels by fingerstick samples, however, may be useful in monitoring clinical improvement in DKA [15].

Bicarbonate therapy for the acidosis of DKA remains controversial. Frequently, dramatic clinical improvement results simply from initial expansion of extracellular fluid volume, reestablishment of adequate peripheral perfusion, and insulin administration. An elevation in blood pH following bicarbonate administration may be attended by worsening acidosis in the CNS, since carbon dioxide (but not bicarbonate) diffuses across the blood–brain barrier. Furthermore, the organic acids in DKA, in contrast to metabolic acidosis from other causes, are metabolized to bicarbonate. Thus, administration of "additional" bicarbonate may result in a late alkalosis. Bicarbonate may have a place in the treatment of DKA but only in the more severe degrees of acidosis (pH <7.10, which may be associated with myocardial depression) and in the setting of inadequate respiratory compensation. Use of bicarbonate in otherwise uncomplicated DKA has recently been demonstrated to prolong therapy, and may in fact be associated with an increased risk of cerebral edema [16]. If bicarbonate is given, the dosage is calculated to bring the pH only to around 7.20, paying attention to the sodium administered concomitantly; slow infusion is preferable to bolus injection.

Acute cerebral edema is a rare, potentially catastrophic complication of DKA that occurs without warning within the first 24 h of treatment, and which may be fatal. This is to be distinguished from the asymptomatic brain swelling detectable on CT scan that may occur in some children with DKA. Although a number of causes of acute cerebral edema have been suggested from uncontrolled, retrospective studies, the etiology in many cases is not known. Proposed contributing factors to the development of cerebral edema include excessive rates of fluid administration greater than 4 $l/m^2/24$ h [17], decline in plasma sodium and/or plasma osmolality during the course of treatment [13, 18], and use of sodium bicarbonate [16]. However, until the precise mechanisms underlying the development and progression are elucidated, these contributing factors cannot be considered to be causative. Therefore, careful monitoring of neurological status, fluid input/output, and corrected sodium and effective osmolality is essential for early recognition of cerebral edema. Treatment of cerebral edema is aimed at lowering intracranial pressure: intravenous mannitol (an osmotic diuretic), intubation/hyperventilation, and, if needed, ventriculostomy.

It is clear that therapy requires frequent modifications based on an individual patient's response. This can only be accomplished with a carefully maintained flow sheet that includes such items as vital signs, neurological status, intake and output volumes, weight, insulin dosage administered, and measurement of blood glucose, urinary ketones, serum electrolytes (with calculation of corrected serum sodium and effective serum osmolality), calcium, phosphorus, BUN, and creatinine (plus blood gases as necessary). Measurements are performed hourly at first and less frequently as the patient's condition stabilizes.

MEDICAL THERAPY OF THE CHILD WITH T1DM

General Principles

Optimal management of the child with diabetes requires an integrated approach, taking into account the overall level of functioning of the child and family, the nutritional and lifestyle patterns specific to that child, and attention to the overall developmental stages of childhood and adolescence. There is no one appropriate insulin regimen or meal plan. The overriding principle should be that the diabetes care plan should fit wherever possible into the surrounding home and school environments, and that the primary childhood tasks of education, socialization, growth, and maturity continue unhindered by the extra responsibilities that diabetes care entails. This potentially daunting task requires a multidisciplinary team, consisting of physicians, nurses, dietitians, and mental health professionals, all trained and experienced in the nuances of diabetes care. Children with diabetes should be seen by the team at frequent intervals for assessment of glycemic control; growth and development; evaluation for related disorders and complications; education, trouble shooting, and problem solving; and screening for adjustment problems that may affect diabetes and/or the overall health of the child.

The rationale for this intensive approach to diabetes care comes from the DCCT, a national multicenter study designed to test the hypothesis that "intensive" diabetes management would be associated with fewer long-term complications of diabetes than "standard" therapy. At the time of the DCCT, standard diabetes therapy consisted of two injections of insulin daily, infrequent home testing of the blood glucose, and basic nutritional and exercise counseling. Intensive management entailed at least three to four injections of insulin daily or use of continuous subcutaneous insulin infusion via programmable portable pumps ("pump therapy"), frequent self-monitoring of the blood glucose (SMBG) through home glucose meter use, and frequent contact with the diabetes care team to adjust insulin dosages and the nutritional and exercise programs. In the DCCT study, intensive treatment in adults was associated with improvement in glycemic control (HbA_{1c} 7.1% vs. 9.0% in the standard group) and dramatically reduced incidence and progression of microvascular complications. Development and progression of retinopathy was reduced 70%, while nephropathy was reduced 35%, and neuropathy was reduced 60% [19]. Significantly, there was an almost linear relationship between the HbA_{1c} and the risk of complications. There was no real threshold effect: the risk decreased with each improvement in the HbA_{1c} but remained elevated for any HbA_{1c} greater than normal. However, intensive control was also associated with a threefold increase in severe hypoglycemia and twofold increase in overweight (as defined by body mass index [BMI] $\geq$ 27.8 kg/m^2 for men or 27.3 kg/m^2 for women).

The DCCT also demonstrated that intensive control was possible in adolescents. Intensively treated adolescents achieved a mean HbA_{1c} of 8.1%, vs. 9.8% in the standard group [20]. Intensive control in adolescents was associated with a 60% reduction in risk of retinopathy and 35% reduction in risk of nephropathy. As in adults, adolescents undergoing intensification of therapy were at threefold risk of severe hypoglycemia and twofold risk of overweight (also as determined by BMI). It is worthwhile to note, however, that the benefits of intensive control persisted even after the conclusion of the trial. In a 4-year follow-up study of adolescents participating in the DCCT, despite equivalent HbA_{1c} levels, subjects who had been intensively controlled during the DCCT period continued to have a 74–78% reduction in risk of worsening retinopathy and 48–85% reduction in risk of nephropathy [21].

It is recognized that intensive treatment places extra burdens on patients and families and that practical considerations such as acceptability of and compliance to the treatment regimens must be balanced appropriately in order to obtain all of these aims of therapy. Nevertheless, recent data suggest that an intensive approach to diabetes education and aggressive self-management by patients and families may reduce rather than increase the adverse psychosocial effects of this chronic illness [22].

Insulin Regimens

During the "honeymoon" phase, insulin requirements rapidly decrease. Commonly, the doses of rapid-acting insulin are sharply reduced or discontinued during this time; many children are well managed with two injections of intermediate-acting insulin and some may not even require an evening injection. A major reason why the two daily injection regimen is effective during the honeymoon phase is that endogenous insulin secretion provides much of the overnight basal insulin requirements, leading to normal fasting blood glucose values. Conversely, increased and more labile prebreakfast glucose levels often herald the loss of the relatively small amount of residual endogenous insulin secretion that is required for overnight glucose control. When residual β-cell function wanes, problems with the two-injection regimen become apparent. One problem is that the peak of the predinner intermediate-acting insulin may coincide with the time of minimal insulin requirements (i.e., midnight to 4 a.m.). Subsequently, insulin levels fall off when basal requirements are increasing (i.e., 4 to 8 a.m.). Increasing the predinner dose of intermediate-acting insulin to lower fasting glucose values often leads to hypoglycemia in the middle of the night without correcting hyperglycemia before breakfast. Another problem with the conventional two-injection regimen is high predinner glucose levels, despite normal or low prelunch and mid-afternoon values. This is due, in part, to eating an afternoon snack when the effects of the prebreakfast dose of intermediate-acting insulin are waning.

One way to deal with these problems without increasing the number of injections is to add Ultralente insulin to the prebreakfast and presupper mixtures of Lispro/Aspart and NPH/Lente. The added Ultralente helps to extend the basal coverage of the NPH/Lente and reduce predinner and prebreakfast highs. However, when strict control cannot be achieved with two daily injections, we do not hesitate to switch to a regimen involving three or more daily injections, in which the predinner NPH/Lente is given at bedtime instead (the Lispro/Aspart is still given at dinner). Alternately, the NPH/Lente dose itself may be split, so that 25–50% is given with dinner and the remainder at bedtime. In youngsters who go to bed early, the third shot may be given at the parents' bedtime (i.e., 10 to 11 p.m.). For patients with elevated predinner glucose levels, a prelunch- or a preafternoon-snack dose of Lispro/Aspart or regular can be added. Such extra doses of insulin can be facilitated by the use of insulin pens, which are small, light, and easy to use.

Alternatively, the NPH or Lente may be replaced with insulin glargine, the basal–bolus approach. In this method, a one-time dose of glargine provides the background insulin coverage or "basal" insulin requirements, and meal-related insulin requirements are covered with rapid-acting insulin "bolus" doses, which may easily be administered with an insulin pen. Multiple daily injection regimens with glargine in children have been associated with lower rates of nocturnal hypoglycemia as compared to regimens with NPH [7, 8]. Such regimens have become increasingly popular, but the inability to "fine-tune" basal insulin over the course of the day and the difficulty of administering four to five insulin injections daily may account for the recent finding that adolescents randomized to insulin pumps had greater improvement in HbA_{1c} and satisfaction with their regimen compared to those randomized to basal/bolus multiple injection therapy with glargine [23].

Over the past few years, there has been a rediscovery of the effectiveness of insulin pump therapy in the management of young patients with diabetes. Indeed, we are much more likely to turn to this method of insulin replacement rather than more frequent injections in patients who are coming out of their honeymoon phase of diabetes. The pumps are battery-powered and about the size of a beeper. The pump employs a reservoir (syringe) to hold the insulin and the infusion set, which consists of tubing with a small plastic catheter at the end. The insertion site can be the abdomen or hip area, except in the young child in whom there may not be sufficient subcutaneous tissue in the abdomen. Our patients are encouraged to change their catheters every 2–3 days. Initially used with regular insulin, insulin pumps are most often used with the rapid-acting insulin analogues, which are associated with improved meal coverage and less hypoglycemia [24, 25].

With insulin pump treatment, small amounts of rapid-acting insulin are infused as a basal rate and larger bolus doses are given at each meal or snack. The basal rate can be programmed to change every half hour; varying the basal rate can be particularly helpful in regulating overnight blood glucose levels, since it can be lowered for the early part of the night to prevent hypoglycemia and increased in the hours before dawn to keep glucose from rising. However, younger children may need a higher basal rate during the earlier part of the night, perhaps because of earlier nocturnal peaks of growth hormone in this age group. Bolus doses are given before meals on the basis of glucose level, carbohydrate content of the meal, and anticipated exercise after the meal. Pump therapy also enhances flexibility in children with variable exercise and meal routines, and employing a temporary basal rate for the evening following vigorous physical activity is a simple means of preventing exercise-related nocturnal hypoglycemia. Most children and parents are encouraged to use carbohydrate counting (see below) as a means to adjust premeal bolus doses.

When used correctly, insulin pump therapy has been shown to improve glycemic control in children, reduce severe hypoglycemia, and improve quality of life [26]. This is especially true for infants and toddlers, in whom we recently demonstrated durable improvements in HbA_{1c} and risk of hypoglycemia for over 2 years of treatment [27]. In this group, in whom unpredictable eating and activity patterns make multiple daily injection regimens problematic, part of the usual premeal bolus can be given prior to the meal and the rest given at the end of the meal, depending on the actual amount of carbohydrate intake. However, children using insulin pumps and their families must be reminded that, because only rapid-acting insulin is used in the pump, discontinuation of the insulin infusion for more than 4 h at a time may lead to significant ketoacidosis and preventable hospitalization [28, 29].

Self-Monitoring

It should be readily apparent from the discussion of intensive insulin therapy that the safety and success of any insulin regimen is dependent upon frequent monitoring of blood glucose. Intensive diabetes control would have been impossible without the development of inexpensive, accurate, easy-to-use home glucose meters. There are many brands of glucose meters that are commercially available, most of which have similar reliability and accuracy to within about 5–10% of laboratory measurements. Current models utilize a peroxidase system that generates a small electric current, which is then converted to a numerical value based on calibration standards. Current meters are fast (results in 5 s) and require very small volumes of blood (0.1 μl). The smaller blood volume requirement has allowed alternate site lancing (forearm, thigh, calf), which may minimize discomfort and improve adherence to self-monitoring regimens. Alternate site testing has been associated with a time lag under conditions of rapidly changing blood glucose, so that it should be used for routine testing instead of after meals or exercise [30].

Children with diabetes should routinely test the blood glucose four times daily (premeal and prebedtime) and record the results in a log for later review by the family and diabetes care team. A target range is established, typically 80–120 mg/dl at breakfast and 80–150 mg/dl at other times of day, but may be altered based on the age of the child and the ability of the family. Ideally, 80% of the blood glucose values should fall within the target range. Information gained from frequent testing is used to titrate insulin dosages according to need. For example, a regular pattern of prebreakfast hyperglycemia should prompt the family to increase the bedtime long-acting insulin dose incrementally over several days until the majority of prebreakfast readings fall within the target range, while frequent hypoglycemia during school may suggest reducing the morning rapid- or intermediate-acting insulin. Additionally, supplemental insulin doses may be given when blood glucose values outside the target range are discovered, according to a predetermined formula. For example, a younger child with a premeal blood glucose outside the goal range may be given an extra 0.5–1.0 U of rapid-acting insulin analogue to reduce the blood glucose by 100 mg/dl in addition to the usual insulin dose at that mealtime, while an adolescent may use 2–3 U to "correct" the glucose by 100 mg/dl.

Supplemental blood glucose testing should be performed after correction doses are given, before exercise or during intercurrent illness.

Even when performed correctly, four (or even six) blood tests daily gives only a limited glimpse into the wide fluctuations in blood glucose that occur during a 24-h period in children with diabetes. Consequently, the recent introduction of continuous glucose monitoring systems has the potential to be the most important advance in assessing diabetes control in the past 20 years. There are presently two US FDA-approved devices for continuous glucose monitoring, the Continuous Glucose Monitoring System (CGMS, Medtronic MiniMed) and GlucoWatch Biographer (GWB, Cygnus). The CGMS employs an electrode that is inserted into the subcutaneous space and connected to a belt-worn pager-like monitor. Glucose in the interstitial fluid is oxidized by the electrode, and the resultant electric signal is relayed to the monitor by a cable, stored, and using a calibration against four capillary glucose levels obtained by routine SMBG, downloaded after a wear period of up to 72 h. The currently available CGMS is like a Holter device, in that the data are unavailable to the user, and the data are obtained retrospectively. The GWB utilizes reverse iontophoresis, in which a small current is applied to the skin by two hydrogel pads on the underside of the watch. Positively charged ions migrate to the anode, and the glucose present in the interstitial fluid that is pulled across the skin surface along with the ion flow is measured in 20-min cycles. After calibrating to one SMBG value, glucose values are available to the wearer by an LCD display every 10 min, for up to 13 h, before the pads require replacement.

In intensively treated children and adolescents with type 1 diabetes, preliminary results in a relatively small number of children suggest that continuous glucose monitoring will provide a wealth of data regarding postprandial glycemic excursions and asymptomatic nocturnal hypoglycemia that were unavailable from capillary blood glucose measurements [31]. Small outcome studies in children with both the CGMS [32, 33] and GWB [34] have demonstrated improvements in glycemic control and reduction in hypoglycemic episodes. Because the error of these current devices may exceed 20% [35, 36], frequent SMBG is still required for making treatment decisions. Nevertheless, we anticipate that these technological breakthroughs will have a great impact on diabetes management over the next few years, as accuracy and performance of these systems improve. Continuous monitoring is likely to be particularly useful in reducing postprandial hyperglycemia, reducing hypoglycemia (particularly at night), and programming overnight basal rates in pump-treated patients. Ultimately, continuous glucose sensors may be employed as part of a closed-loop system, in which sensor data drive an insulin pump, thus creating an artificial β-cell.

Medical Nutrition Therapy

Proper nutritional management is critical to the short- and long-term health of children with diabetes. Generally, terms such as "diet" should be avoided in favor of "meal plan," both for the negative connotation associated with the former and for the simple fact that nutritional requirements for normal growth and development are the same in diabetic and nondiabetic children. However, adherence to meal plans and accurate assessment of carbohydrate are important for optimal glycemic control.

The American Diabetes Association has adopted formal recommendations regarding general nutritional principles in diabetes, taking into account the short-term goals of blood glucose stabilization and the long-term goals of prevention/amelioration of macrovascular and microvascular complications of diabetes [37]. The currently favored model of nutritional therapy is carbohydrate counting, based on the conceptual model of matching carbohydrate "doses" to insulin doses [38]. As the carbohydrate content of foods has the greatest impact on blood glucose, the amount of carbohydrates ingested per meal or snack should be accurately assessed. Protein and fat intake, while important in the larger context of a healthy meal plan, are not counted to simplify the procedure. Recent changes in food labeling requirements have simplified the process, as most foods are clearly labeled with both the amount of carbohydrate grams per serving and the serving size. Foods less easily quantified may be weighed or estimated.

Two popular approaches to regulating carbohydrate intake are (1) consistent carbohydrate servings per meal/snack and (2) insulin-to-carbohydrate ratios. In the former, a standard amount of carbohydrates are eaten per meal or snack (e.g., 45 g for breakfast, lunch, and dinner, and 30 g each for mid-afternoon and bedtime snack). In this way, the insulin dose may be kept reasonably constant. In the latter, more flexible approach, there is no set intake. Rather, the child or parent decides upon the meal content, the carbohydrates are counted, and an insulin dose is calculated on the spot, based on a ratio of the number of insulin units per grams of carbohydrate. In younger children typical insulin-to-carbohydrate ratio is 1 U:15 g, while an older child may require 1:10 and an insulin-resistant adolescent 1:5–7. Actual insulin-to-carbohydrate ratios vary from child to child, and may even vary in the same child from meal to meal or during periods of exercise.

Long-term goals of nutritional management of diabetes include maintenance of nutrient intake balance of about 50% carbohydrate, 20% protein, and 30% fat (of which no more than 10% should be saturated). Most important, growth and weight gain should be monitored, and regular follow-up with a dietitian trained in diabetes management should be encouraged to individualize a meal plan for each child on the basis of his/her needs and food preferences.

Exercise

Establishment and maintenance of an active lifestyle should be a goal for all children, but is especially important for children with diabetes. Exercise and increased physical fitness are associated with improved insulin sensitivity and glucose utilization, the clinical correlates of which are lower insulin requirements in general, and frequently, less pronounced blood glucose excursions after meals. Improvements in physical fitness are also frequently associated with greater self-esteem and motivation to participate in diabetes care.

However, the effects of exercise must be carefully considered in the context of the entire diabetes care plan, as episodic exercise may predispose to acute hypoglycemia, if the insulin dose is not reduced or extra carbohydrates added proactively. Furthermore, intense physical activity in the setting of insulin deficiency (chronically poor diabetes control or recent omission of insulin) may provoke metabolic decompensation and DKA. Children participating in school sports or other programs should be counseled to monitor blood glucose before, during, as well as after exercise, as the hypoglycemic effects of exercise may be delayed and/or prolonged over the next 12–18 h. We frequently recommend reduction of dinner/bedtime NPH and for pump users decreases in basal rates, to account for these exercise effects.

Hypoglycemia

Severe hypoglycemia is a common problem in patients striving for strict glycemic control with intensive treatment regimens. In the DCCT, the risk of severe hypoglycemia was threefold higher in intensively treated than in conventionally treated patients, and being an adolescent was an independent risk factor for a severe hypoglycemic event [20]. The majority of severe hypoglycemic events occur overnight, partly because of sleep-induced defects in counterregulatory hormone responses to hypoglycemia [39].

Monitoring glucose is critical in order to detect asymptomatic hypoglycemia, especially in the young child with diabetes. The older child is usually aware of symptoms such as weakness, shakiness, hunger, or headache and is encouraged to treat these symptoms as soon as they occur. The older child who can accurately recognize symptoms is taught to immediately treat with 15 g of carbohydrate (e.g., three to four glucose tablets, 4 oz of juice or 15 g of a glucose gel) without waiting to check a glucose level. Each episode should be assessed in order to make proper adjustments if a cause can be identified. Every family should have a glucagon emergency kit at home in order to treat severe hypoglycemia.

Sick Days

Children with intercurrent illnesses, such as infections or vomiting, should be closely monitored for elevations in blood glucose levels and ketonuria. On sick days blood glucose levels should be checked every 2 h, and the urine should be checked for ketones with every void. Supplemental doses of short-acting insulin (0.1–0.3 U/k) should be given every 2–4 h for elevations in glucose and/or ketones. Even in the absence of hyperglycemia, the presence of ketones indicates insulin deficiency and, therefore, the need for supplemental insulin. Adequate fluid intake is essential to prevent dehydration and hasten the excretion of ketones. Fluids such as flat soda, clear soups, popsicles, and gelatin water are recommended to provide some electrolyte and carbohydrate replacement. In the child tolerating oral rehydration, a fluid "dose" of 1 oz/year of age/h serves as a rough guideline, the sugar content of which depends on the serum glucose. For blood glucose values $>$200 mg/dl, sugar-free fluids should be given; between 100 and 200 mg/dl, a mixture of sugar-free and sugar-containing fluids; and for blood sugar $<$100 mg/dl, all sugar-containing fluids. If emesis precludes normal oral intake, the intermediate- or long-acting insulin should be discontinued, and small, frequent doses of short- or rapid-acting insulin only should be given. Once the ketones have cleared and the child is tolerating an oral diet, the family may resume the normal routine. If vomiting is persistent and ketones remain moderate or large after several supplemental insulin doses, arrangements should be made for parenteral hydration and evaluation in the emergency department.

Outpatient Care

The importance of frequent follow-up by the diabetes health care team cannot be overemphasized. Children and adolescents with T1DM should be routinely cared for by a diabetes center that uses a multidisciplinary team knowledgeable about and experienced in the management of young patients. This team should ideally consist of pediatric diabetologists, diabetes nurse specialists, nutritionists, and social workers or psychologists.

Regular follow-up visits on a 2- to 3-monthly basis are recommended for most patients. The main purpose of these visits is to ensure that the patient is achieving primary treatment goals. Routine outpatient visits provide an opportunity to review glucose monitoring, to adjust the treatment regimen, and to assess child and family adjustment. At each visit, the blood glucose logbooks should be reviewed and appropriate dosage or schedule changes should be instituted as needed. Follow-up advice and support are given by the nutritionist, diabetes nurse specialist, and psychologist or social worker.

A detailed interim history should include questions relating to general health, energy, fatigue, polyuria or nocturia, intercurrent illnesses, hypoglycemic episodes, and the presence of the corresponding symptoms such as pain, bloating, or diarrhea. It is important to remember the comorbidities of other autoimmune disorders that occur with an increased frequency in children with T1DM: thyroiditis, adrenal insufficiency, and celiac disease. The child should be weighed and measured at each visit, and pulse and blood pressure also documented. Physical examination of the child should focus not only on the general organ systems, but also on examination of the skin and insulin injection/pump insertion sites for signs of lipohypertrophy or pigmentary changes, palpation of the thyroid and determination of the sexual development stage. In older children or those with longer diabetes duration, examination should include the feet. A deceleration in growth, delay in sexual development, or finding of goiter may herald hypothyroidism. The astute clinician should also consider that frequent, unexplained hypoglycemia or reduction in insulin requirements in the absence of exercise or activity may be a subtle indicator of hypothyroidism or adrenal insufficiency. Similarly, while the history of frequent, foul-smelling, greasy stools are more obvious indicators of celiac disease, the presence of abdominal pain, poor weight gain, and unexplained hypoglycemia may be the first and only signs. Indeed, many patients are asymptomatic and diagnosed by screening for celiac-related autoantibodies, tissue transglutaminase IgA. There are currently no formal recommendations for screening for thyroid/adrenal autoimmunity and celiac disease for pediatric patients with T1DM. However, since the prevalence of thyroid autoantibodies in children with diabetes may be as high as 21% [40], and of celiac disease in children with T1DM about 4% [41], we routinely screen with T4, thyroid-stimulating hormone, and tissue tranglutaminase IgA every 1–2 years.

Measurement of glycosylated hemoglobin (HbA_{1c}) provides the gold standard by which to judge the adequacy of the insulin regimen. A variety of methods are available for assaying glycosylated hemoglobin. A simple method that can be performed in the office in 6 min (Bayer DCA 2000) offers the opportunity to make immediate changes in the insulin regimen, while the patient is being seen. The goal of treatment is to achieve HbA_{1c} levels as close to normal as possible. Based on DCCT results, our general goal of therapy is to try to keep all patients under 8.0%. HbA_{1c} levels are determined at least every 3 months. The conversion of the HbA_{1c} to the mean blood glucose level may be estimated by the formula

$$\text{glu}_{\text{mean}}(\text{mg/dl}) = \text{HbA}_{1c}(\%) \times 30 - 60$$

In children with decreased red cell survival time, however, as occurs in sickle cell disease or spherocytosis, the HbA_{1c} may be artificially low, as the time available for glycosylation is decreased. In these children, HbA_{1c} measurements are not useful, and measurement of other glycosylated proteins, such as albumin, should be considered for analysis of long-term control. Discrepancies between the logs and the HbA_{1c} may suggest improper testing technique, or more seriously, falsifying the data. In the case of the latter, deeper questioning into the family dynamics and psychosocial functioning of the child are warranted.

Monitoring of the diabetic child for complications is an important function of the clinic visit, as many early complications do respond to prompt intervention. Urinary albumin excretion may be measured in a spot sample by comparison to urinary creatinine. Urinary albumin/creatinine ratio should be <30 mg albumin/g creatinine. Elevated spot samples should be confirmed by collections of first morning void or a timed overnight period to eliminate the confounding variable of benign orthostatic proteinuria. If the first morning void or timed overnight collection demonstrates microalbuminuria (>30 mg albumin/g creatinine or >30 mg albumin excretion/24 h), treatment with angiotensin-converting enzyme inhibitor (ACE-I) therapy or referral to pediatric nephrologist may be indicated. All diabetic children with hypertension, regardless of albumin excretion status, should be considered candidates for ACE-I therapy. While there are no specific guidelines for diabetic children, current recommendations for nondiabetic children are that blood pressures above the 90th percentile for age warrant lifestyle intervention and those above the 95th percentile merit the use of pharmacological agents [42].

Other screening studies for complications of diabetes include measurement of serum lipid concentrations and referral for dilated retinal examination, both of which should be performed on a yearly basis in all pubertal children with diabetes, or even in prepubertal children with diabetes duration of at least 5 years. The current standards put forth by the American Diabetes Association for adults [43], maintaining serum low-density lipoprotein concentrations below 100 mg/dl and serum triglycerides below 150 mg/dl, are less rigorous from those put forth by the American Academy of Pediatrics for nondiabetic children and youth [44]. There are no published recommendations specifically for diabetic children. Treatment for dyslipidemia should include intensification of diabetes control and dietary interventions. There are little data on the efficacy and safety of specific lipid-lowering therapeutic agents in the pediatric population.

T2DM IN CHILDREN

Within the last 10 years, there has been a striking increase in the incidence and prevalence of T2DM in children and adolescents, which has reached near epidemic proportions [45]. Noted first in African American, Latino-American, and Native American populations, it is now recognized to occur in greater frequency in all ethnic groups. It is estimated now that as many as 15–33% of children newly diagnosed with diabetes in the United States have T2DM [46]. Similar increases have been documented worldwide.

This alarming increase in pediatric T2DM is almost certainly causally related to the simultaneous increasing prevalence of obesity in the pediatric population. Impaired glucose tolerance has been demonstrated in up to 25% of obese children [47]. The pathogenesis of T2DM in children, as in adults, is a combination of underlying insulin resistance with superimposed β-cell defect in insulin secretion, causing a relative insulin deficiency. Peak age at presentation of pediatric T2DM is mid-late puberty, which corresponds to the puberty-associated increase in insulin resistance. Girls appear to be affected more frequently than boys, which may also be related to the relatively gender-related differences in the insulin resistance of puberty [48], although measurements of insulin response to glucose in pubertal adolescents also demonstrate a gender-related pancreatic β-cell component [49].

The clinical presentation of T2DM in children ranges from asymptomatic glycosuria and hyperglycemia documented on routine testing for school or camp, to life-threatening dehydration. The typical symptoms of polyuria, polydipsia, and weight loss are typically absent. The most reliable historical feature is the strong family history of diabetes, usually in at least one parent or sibling. The physical examination may demonstrate acanthosis nigricans, a hyperpigmented, hypertrophic skin lesion, typically found along the posterior neck folds or axilla, a reliable indicator of insulin resistance in children. T2DM in children may also frequently occur in the setting of the metabolic syndrome, which also includes (besides abnormal glucose tolerance) obesity, hypertension, dyslipidemia (low high-density-lipoprotein cholesterol and high triglycerides), and in girls, ovarian hyperandrogenism.

Treatment of T2DM in childhood is much more challenging than T1DM, as the cornerstone of therapy is lifestyle modification. However, pediatric T2DM disproportionately affects segments of the population with fewer resources, both at the family and community levels. The goals of treatment are weight loss and normalization of glucose, blood pressure, and lipids. These are best accomplished through a combination of education, medical nutrition therapy, exercise, and pharmacotherapy. Behavior change is critical to the management of T2DM in children, in order to retrain the whole family unit on food choices and approach to physical activity.

Until last year the only hypoglycemic agent for which there was any pediatric data or experience was insulin. The biguanide metformin has shown clinical efficacy in the treatment of T2DM in children, and is now considered the first-line therapy, along with diet and exercise therapy [50]. Metformin is believed to improve insulin resistance by reducing hepatic glucose production. Metformin also has an anorexic effect that promotes weight loss, and improves lipid profiles as well, but is contraindicated in patients with any renal impairment and should be discontinued before radiological or surgical procedures.

Other oral hypoglycemic agents have had relatively little use in pediatric T2DM. The other major class of insulin sensitizer, thiazolidinediones, improves insulin resistance through effects on peripheral muscle and adipose tissue, but has not been adequately studied in children to date. Sulfonylureas and other insulin secretagogues do not target insulin resistance and may actually worsen insulin resistance by promoting weight gain. Glucosidase inhibitors such as acarbose are associated with gastrointestinal side effects that are usually unacceptable to youth.

We currently recommend an intense lifestyle modification program with weight loss and exercise, in conjunction with metformin, as first-line therapy. Metformin may be initiated at 500 mg b.i.d. and increased to 2000–2500 mg daily as needed. Thiazolidinediones may be added in older adolescents or young adults with severe insulin resistance. If this regimen is insufficient to reduce the HbA_{1c} to 6.5% or lower, we will not hesitate to add insulin, either as a bedtime injection of Lente or glargine, or a combination rapid/intermediate-acting insulin, such as Humalog Mix 25 (Lilly) or Novolog Mix 70/30 (Novo Nordisk), with breakfast and dinner. As important as treating the diabetes is treating the comorbid hypertension and dyslipidemia with a combination of ACE-Is, bile acid binding resins, and statins. Our children with T2DM also meet regularly with dietitians and social workers or psychologists to reinforce desired behaviors and identify individual or family factors that may complicate adherence.

REFERENCES

1. Sperling MA. Diabetes mellitus. In Sperling MA (ed), *Pediatric Endocrinology*. Philadelphia: Saunders, 2002; pp 323–66.
2. Karvonen M, Vilik-Kajander M, Moltchanova E, Libman I, LaPorte R, Tuomilehto J. Incidence of childhood type 1 diabetes worldwide. *Diabetes Care* 2000; 23: 1516–26.
3. Drash A. Diabetes mellitus in the child: classification, diagnosis, epidemiology, and etiology. In Lifshitz F (ed), *Pediatric Endocrinology*. New York: Marcel Dekker, 1990; pp 663–80.
4. Chase HP, Crews KR, Garg S, Crews MJ, Cruickshanks KJ, Klingensmith G, Gay E, Hamman RF. Outpatient management vs. in-hospital management of children with new-onset diabetes. *Clin Pediatr* 1992; 31: 450–6.
5. Vajo Z, Fawcett J, Duckworth WC. Recombinant DNA technology in the treatment of diabetes: insulin analogs. *Endocr Rev* 2001; 22: 706–17.
6. Lepore M, Pampanelli S, Fanelli C, Porcellati F, Bartocci L, Di Vincenzo A, Cordoni C, Costa E, Brunetti P, Bolli GB. Pharmacokinetics and pharmacodynamics of subcutaneous injection of long-acting human insulin analog

glargine, NPH insulin, and ultralente human insulin and continuous subcutaneous infusion of insulin lispro. *Diabetes* 2000; 49: 2142–8.
7. Schober E, Schoenle E, Van Dyk J, Wernicke-Panten K, and the Pediatric Study Group of Insulin Glargine. Comparative trial between insulin glargine and NPH insulin in children and adolescents with type 1 diabetes mellitus. *J Pediatr Endocrinol Metab* 2002; 15: 369–76.
8. Murphy NP, Keane SM, Ong KK. Randomized cross-over trial of insulin glargine plus lispro or NPH insulin plus regular human insulin in adolescents with type 1 diabetes on intensive insulin regimens. *Diabetes Care* 2003; 26: 799–804.
9. Yki-Jarvinen H, Koivisto VA. Natural course of insulin resistance in type 1 diabetes. *N Engl J Med* 1986; 315: 224–30.
10. The DCCT Research Group. The effect of intensive diabetes treatment in the DCCT on residual insulin secretion in IDDM. *Ann Int Med* 1998; 128: 517–23.
11. Attia N, Caprio S, Jones TW, Heptulla R, Holcombe J, Silver D, Sherwin RS, Tamborlane WV. Changes in free insulin-like growth factor-1 and leptin concentrations during acute metabolic decompensation in insulin withdrawn patients with type 1 diabetes. *J Clin Endocrinol Metab* 1999; 84: 2324–8.
12. Katz MA. Hyperglycemia-induced hyponatremia. *N Engl J Med* 1973; 289: 843–4.
13. Harris GD, Fiordalisi I, Harris WL, Mosovich LL, Finberg L. Minimizing the risk of brain herniation during treatment of diabetic ketoacidemia: a retrospective and prospective study. *J Pediatr* 1990; 117: 22–31.
14. Harris GD, Fiordalisi I. Physiologic management of diabetic ketoacidemia: a 5-year prospective pediatric experience in 231 episodes. *Arch Pediatr Adolesc Med* 1994; 148: 1046–52.
15. Ham MR, Okada P, White PC. Bedside ketone determination in diabetic children with hyperglycemia and ketosis in the acute care setting. *Pediatr Diabetes* (in press).
16. Glaser N, Barnett P, McCaslin I, Nelson D, Trainor J, Louie J, Kaufman F, Quayle K, Roback M, Malley R, Kuppermann N. Risk factors for cerebral edema in children with diabetic ketoacidosis. *N Engl J Med* 201; 344: 264–9.
17. Duck SC, Wyatt DT. Factors associated with brain herniation in the treatment of diabetic ketoacidosis. *J Pediatr* 1988; 113: 10–4.
18. Bello FA, Sotos JF. Cerebral edema in diabetic ketoacidosis in children. *Lancet* 1990; 336: 64.
19. The Diabetes Control and Complications Trial Research Group. The effect of intensive treatment of diabetes on the development and progression of long-term complications in insulin-dependent diabetes mellitus. *N Engl J Med* 1993; 329: 977–86.
20. The Diabetes Control and Complications Trial Research Group. Effect of intensive diabetes treatment on the development and progression of long-term complications in adolescents with insulin-dependent diabetes mellitus: Diabetes Control and Complications Trial. *J Pediatr* 1994; 125: 177–88.
21. White NH, Cleary PA, Dahms W, Goldstein D, Malone J, Tamborlane WV; Diabetes Control and Complications Trial (DCCT)/Epidemiology of Diabetes Interventions and Complications (EDIC) Research Group. Beneficial effects of intensive therapy of diabetes during adolescence: outcomes after the conclusion of the Diabetes Control and Complications Trial (DCCT). *J Pediatr* 2001; 139: 804–12.
22. Grey M, Boland EA, Davidson M, Li J, Tamborlane WV. Coping skills training for youth on intensive therapy has long lasting effects on metabolic control and quality of life? *J Pediatr* 2000; 137: 107–14.
23. Boland EA, Weinzimer SA, Steffen AT, Tamborlane WV. Randomized, prospective trial of CSII vs. MDI with glargine in children: a preliminary report. *Diabetes* 2003; 52 (suppl 2): A45.
24. Zinman B, Tildesley H, Chiasson JL, Tsui E, Strack T. Insulin lispro in CSII: results of a double-blind crossover study. *Diabetes* 1997; 46: 440–3.
25. Bode BW, Strange P. Efficacy, safety, and pump compatibility of insulin aspart used in continuous subcutaneous insulin infusion therapy in patients with type 1 diabetes. *Diabetes Care* 2001; 24: 69–72.
26. Boland EA, Grey M, Fredrickson L, Tamborlane WV. CSII: a "new" way to achieve strict metabolic control, decrease severe hypoglycemia and enhance coping in adolescents with type I diabetes. *Diabetes Care* 1999; 22: 1779–894.
27. Weinzimer SA, Ahern JH, Boland EA, Steffen AT, Tamborlane WV. Continuous subcutaneous insulin infusion is safe and effective in infants and toddlers. *Diabetes* 2003; 52 (suppl 2): A402.
28. Attia N, Jones TW, Holcombe J, Tamborlane WV. Comparison of human regular and lispro insulins after interruption of continuous subcutaneous insulin infusion and in the treatment of acutely decompensated IDDM. *Diabetes Care* 1998; 21: 817–21.
29. Celona-Jacobs N, Weinzimer SA, Rearson MA, Hartz D, Katz LEL, Murphy K. Insulin pump therapy in children: a cautionary tale. *Diabetes* 2001; 50 (suppl 2): A67.
30. Bina DM, Anderson RL, Johnson ML, Bergenstal RM, Kendall DM. Clinical impact of prandial state, exercise, and site preparation on the equivalence of alternative-site blood glucose testing. *Diabetes Care* 2003; 26: 981–5.
31. Boland EA, DeLucia M, Brandt C, Grey MJ, Tamborlane WV. Limitations of conventional methods of self blood glucose monitoring: lessons learned from three days of continuous glucose monitoring in pediatric patients with type I diabetes. *Diabetes Care* 2001; 24: 1858–62.
32. Chase HP, Kim LM, Owen SL, MacKenzie TA, Klingensmith GJ, Murtfeldt R, Garg SK. Continuous subcutaneous monitoring in children with type 1 diabetes. *Pediatrics* 2001; 107: 222–6.
33. Kaufman FR, Gibson LC, Halvorson M, Carpenter S, Fisher LK, Pitukcheewanont P. A pilot study of the continuous glucose monitoring system: clinical decisions and glycemic control after its use in pediatric type 1 diabetic subjects. *Diabetes Care* 2001; 24: 2030–4.
34. Chase HP, Roberts MD, Wightman C, Klingensmith G, Garg SK, Van Wyhe M, Desai S, Harper W, Lopatin M, Bartkowiak M, Tamada J, Eastman RC. Use of the GlucoWatch biographer in children with type 1 diabetes. *Pediatrics* 2003; 111: 790–4.
35. The Diabetes Research in Children Network (DirecNet) Study Group. The accuracy of the CGMS™ in children with type 1 diabetes: results of the Diabetes Research in Children Network (DirecNet) accuracy study. *Diabetes Technol Ther* 2003; 5: 781–9.
36. The Diabetes Research in Children Network (DirecNet) Study Group. The accuracy of the GlucoWatch® G2™

Biographer in children with type 1 diabetes: results of the Diabetes Research in Children Network (DirecNet) accuracy study. *Diabetes Technol Ther* 2003; 5: 791–800.

37. American Diabetes Association Task Force for Writing Nutrition Principles and Recommendations for the Management of Diabetes and Related Complications. American Diabetes Association position statement: evidence-based nutrition principles and recommendations for the treatment and prevention of diabetes and related complications. *J Amer Diet Assoc* 2002; 102: 109–18.
38. Gregory RP, Davis DL. Use of carbohydrate counting for meal planning in type 1 diabetes. *Diabetes Educ* 1994; 20: 406.
39. Jones TW, Porter P, David EA, O'Leary P, Frazer F, Byrne G, Stick S, Tamborlane WV. Suppressed epinephrine responses during sleep: a contributing factor to the risk of nocturnal hypoglycemia in insulin-dependent diabetes. *N Engl J Med* 1999; 338: 1657–62.
40. Kordonouri O, Klinghammer A, Lang EB, Gruters-Kieslich A, Grabert M, Holl RW. Thyroid autoimmunity in children and adolescents with type 1 diabetes. *Diabetes Care* 2002; 25: 1346–50.
41. Freemark M, Levitsky LL. Screening for celiac disease in children with type 1 diabetes: two views of the controversy. *Diabetes Care* 2003; 26: 1932–9.
42. Update on the 1987 task force report on high blood pressure in children and adolescents: a working group report for the national high blood pressure education program. *Pediatrics* 1996; 98: 649–57.
43. American Diabetes Association. Management of dyslipidemia in adults with diabetes. *Diabetes Care* 2003; 26: S83–6.
44. American Academy of Pediatrics. Cholesterol in childhood. *Pediatrics* 1998; 101: 141–7.
45. Rosenbloom AL, Joe JR, Young RS, Winter WE. The emerging epidemic of type 2 diabetes mellitus in youth. *Diabetes Care* 1999; 22: 345–54.
46. Pinhas-Hamiel O, Dolan LM, Daniels SR, Standiford D, Khoury PR, Zeitler P. Increased incidence of non-insulin-dependent diabetes mellitus among adolescents. *J Pediatr* 1996; 37: 97–102.
47. Sinha R, Fisch G, Teague B, Tamborlane WV, Banyas B, Allen K, Savoye M, Rieger V, Taksali S, Barbetta G, Sherwin RS, Caprio S. Prevalence of impaired glucose tolerance among children and adolescents with marked obesity. *N Engl J Med* 2002; 346: 802–10.
48. Travers SH, Jeffers BW, Bloch CA, Hill JO, Eckel RH. Gender and Tanner stage differences in body composition and insulin sensitivity in early pubertal children. *J Clin Endocrinol Metab* 1995; 80: 172–8.
49. Guzzaloni G, Grugni G, Mazzilli G, Moro D, Morabito F. Comparison between beta-cell function and insulin resistance indexes in prepubertal and pubertal obese children. *Metabolism* 2002; 51: 1011–6.
50. Jones KL, Arslanian S, Peterokova VA, Park JS, Tomlinson MJ. Effect of metformin in pediatric patients with type 2 diabetes: a randomized controlled trial. *Diabetes Care* 2002; 25: 89–94.

87

Difficult Diabetes

Simon A. Saunders* **and Gareth Williams†**

**University Hospital Aintree, Liverpool, UK, and †University of Bristol, Bristol, UK*

Diabetes influences many aspects of a patients' life and carries with it numerous potentially life-threatening complications; consequently the long-term management of diabetes continues to be a challenge for the patients, their family, and the diabetes care team. In this sense much diabetes care is arguably "difficult."

Here, we will focus on problems in achieving good glycemic control and the practical difficulties in managing many such patients. These issues overlap to some extent with the psychological and behavioral aspects discussed in Chapter 67.

Good glycemic control is one of the central tenets of diabetes care and its benefits are now well known [1], to physicians and increasingly to patients. All clinical practitioners will encounter occasional patients who fall far short of accepted targets for glycemic control. Some present with recurrent hypoglycemia others with persistent hyperglycemia (often with repeatedly high insulin dosages and recurrent episodes of diabetic ketoacidosis), and a few with a combined picture that swings between hypo- and hyperglycemia. Historically, some of these cases have been given the snappy but unhelpful label of "brittle" diabetes. Each of these patterns of glycemic instability can be caused by "organic" conditions (e.g. coexistent endocrine disease), but their origins are often psychosocial and due to poor self-management and/or deliberate interference with treatment.

We shall discuss each of these presentations in turn, ending with a review of whether brittle diabetes can usefully be regarded as a true disease entity. This chapter relates mostly to insulin-treated and especially type 1 disease patients, but many aspects also apply to type 2 patients requiring oral hypoglycemic drugs.

RECURRENT HYPOGLYCEMIA

Hypoglycemia, the commonest and perhaps the major side effect of insulin treatment, is covered in detail in Chapter 60. The restoration of blood glucose depends critically on the "counterregulatory" response—increased secretion of hormones whose metabolic action opposes those of insulin—and on other responses, notably hunger and increased splanchnic blood flow (Figure 1).

Susceptibility to hypoglycemia, and poor recovery from it, is enhanced by deficiencies in one or more of the normal neuroendocrine responses. This can occur with chronic endocrine deficiencies: Addison's disease, growth hormone (GH) deficiency, and also hypothyroidism (thyroid hormones also oppose insulin action). Other counterregulatory failures can develop in type 1 diabetes [2]. In particular, glucagon secretion in response to hypoglycemia (even profound) declines after approximately 3–5 years of disease [3]. This is not wholesale failure of the α-cells *per se* as glucagon responses to other stimuli remain intact and suggests that a selective signaling deficiency exists. Initially, affected subjects can still mount a counterregulatory response mainly mediated by epinephrine, but this can also become blunted in some cases. Those with this "combined" counterregulatory defect are at great risk of severe hypoglycemia and often show impaired awareness of hypoglycemic symptoms as well (see Chapter 60). The cause is unknown but may represent failure of the central nervous system (CNS) and/or peripheral sensors of hypoglycemia.

Episodes of recurrent hypoglycemia may therefore be due to counter-regulatory failure; however, other pathological processes or drug use may also be responsible (Box 1).

International Textbook of Diabetes Mellitus, Third Edition. Edited by R. A. DeFronzo, E. Ferrannini, H. Keen, and P. Zimmet.

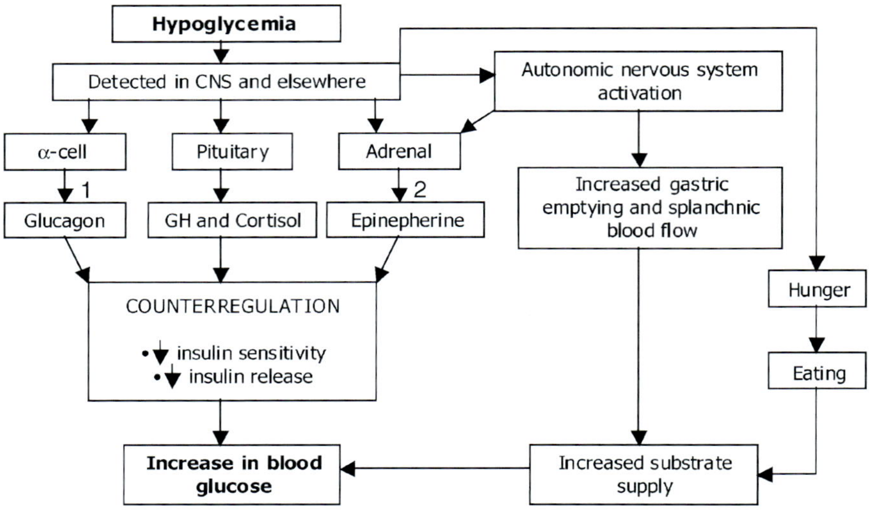

Figure 1 Showing normal physiological response to hypoglycemia (1 and 2 become impaired in type 1 diabetes)

Clinical Endocrine Diseases Causing Recurrent Hypoglycemia

Other autoimmune endocrinopathies are more common in type 1 diabetic patients than in the general population, particularly Addison's disease and hypothyroidism [4, 5]. Many patients with type 1 diabetes have circulating antibodies to the adrenal cortex while *postmortem* studies show evidence of cell-mediated autoimmune damage to the adrenal cortex [6]. Hypothyroidism coexists with type 1 diabetes, with a prevalence estimated at between 7 and 24%, depending on race, age, and geographical distribution [4, 7, 8] and affects women more frequently than men [9].

Pituitary disturbances appear to be no more common than in the general population, but GH deficiency can predispose to hypoglycemia. Patients with type 1 diabetes who suffer recurrent hypoglycemic attacks must always be investigated for coexistent endocrine disease, notably adrenal insufficiency and hypothyroidism; it is not clear whether it is cost-effective to screen for hypothyroidism or other endocrinopathies in the absence of clinical suspicion [10]. Adrenal failure classically presents with frequent hypoglycemia (persisting despite reduction in insulin dosage) and weight loss; other features such as hyperpigmentation may not be obvious, and postural hypotension (a late feature anyway) may be wrongly attributed to autonomic neuropathy. These patients respond well to steroid replacement, resuming their premorbid levels of insulin therapy and glycemic control [11, 12] (Box 2).

The onset of hypothyroidism may cause a tendency toward hypoglycemia and decreasing insulin requirements,

Box 1 Organic [genuine] causes of recurrent hypoglycemia

Genuine causes
- Endocrine disease
  - Addisons
  - Hypothyroidism
  - Pituitary failure
- Drugs
- Gut and pancreatic disorders
- Hypoglycemia unawareness

Box 2 Case History

Case history
- 29-year-old male with type 1 diabetes, 11 years duration.
- Detailed history revealed previous stability of diabetes, on 44 units of human insulin per day (3 × 10 units short-acting, 1 × 14 units long-acting injection) with an HbA_{1c} of 7.4%, 9 months earlier. He had no other medical problems.
- Five emergency room attendances over 2 months, with symptomatic hypoglycemia. The last two attendances requiring prolonged treatment before correction with intravenous glucose.
- During the last 4 months he had lost 7 kg of weight despite continuing his normal diet, and no change in bowel habit. Hypoglycemia was first noticed after exercise, something that had not occurred previously. Insulin requirements decreased over this period; hypoglycemia was occurring with increasing frequency and at rest.
- On admission he was taking 26 units of insulin, his HbA_{1c} was 6.6%. He denied overuse of insulin or other drug use.
- He was mildly hypotensive on presentation with a blood pressure of 96/68 mmHg, urea was 11.0 mmol/l, plasma sodium 128 mmol/l, and potassium 5.1 mmol/l. Adrenal insufficiency was suspected and confirmed by a short synacthen test. Baseline cortisol was 104 nmol/l and 30-min value was 360 nmol/l. Plasma adrenocorticotropic hormone (ACTH) levels were elevated 114 ng/l [Normal range (NR) 10–80 ng/l].
- Adrenal steroid replacement was started (hydrocortisone 20 mg o.d. and 10 mg o.d.). Within 36 h his insulin requirement had increased to 36 units daily. He was discharged once stable, at follow up 6 weeks later he reported no further episodes of hypoglycemia, his weight had increased by 3 kg, and his insulin requirement was 42 units daily.

Box 3 Some drugs that cause hypoglycemia

Powerful effects
- Insulin
- Sulfonylureas
- Alcohol
- Quinine
- Pentamidine
- Salicylates

Mild and occasional effects
- Antibiotics
  - Ketoconazole, chloramphenicol, sulphonamides, methicillin, and oxytetracycline
- Cardiovascular
- β-blockers, ACE-inhibitors, and lidocaine
- Psychological
  - Monoamine oxidase inhibitors, tryptophan, haloperidol, chlorpromazine, lithium, imipramine, and doxepin
- Rheumatological
  - Cochicine, azapropazone, phenylbutazone, indomethacin, and penicillamine
- Other
  - Ranitidine, cimetidine, bezafibrate, and clofibrate

but only rarely causes severe recurrent hypoglycemia [9, 13].

Drugs

Many drugs can induce hypoglycemia under various conditions. Sometimes, these can exacerbate or even cause glycemic instability; a complete drug history must always be taken from patients who suffer frequent hypoglycemic events. Occasionally they may be used to induce factitious hypoglycemia (see Table 2) (Box 3).

Gut and Pancreatic Disorders

Vomiting from any cause can lead to variable hypoglycemia in insulin-treated patients. Autonomic diabetic gastropathy (gastroparesis) is usually associated with severe autonomic neuropathy [14], although acute and reversible gastric dilatation can accompany hyperglycemia and occasionally diabetes ketoacidosis (DKA). Gastroparesis impairs emptying of the stomach, which may be severe, leading to dilatation of the stomach and vomiting. Gastric dysmotility can affect between 20 and 50% of the diabetic population (depending on how it is defined), most frequently those with poor control [15]. Although mild and even symptomless in some, in others it can cause severe glycemic instability, dominated by recurrent hypoglycemia, due to erratic food absorption. Investigation, diagnosis, and treatment are discussed in Chapter 84. Malabsorption, whether due to gut diseases such as celiac disease or pancreatic disease, can result in decreased insulin requirements and hypoglycemic attacks. Celiac disease is more prevalent in type 1 diabetes than in the general population [16, 17] and often goes undetected; this diagnosis must be considered in a diabetic patient with weight loss and decreasing insulin requirements, and some physicians have advocated screening for this disease in the diabetic population with anti-gliadin and (better) anti-endomyseal antibodies [18–20]. Pancreatic exocrine disease such as chronic pancreatitis, which results in malabsorption of fat and carbohydrate, can disturb diabetic control with unpredictable episodes of hypoglycemia. Pancreatic destruction (e.g. pancreatectomy or severe pancreatitis) can also lead to severe hypoglycemia because of impaired glucagon secretion and counterregulatory failure as described above.

Hypoglycemia Unawareness

The neuroendocrine counterregulatory responses and symptoms initiated by hypoglycemia usually occur at particular glucose concentrations. In the "hierarchy" of responses first, at a glucose concentration of ~3.2 mmol/l sweating, trembling, weakness, visual disturbances, and hunger occur. These are then followed by such symptoms as tiredness, drowsiness, and confusion at ~3.0 mmol/l and cognitive dysfunction supervenes at ~2.8 mmol/l and may progress to coma if the hypoglycemia is not treated. These values may show some intraindividual variability if glycemic control is poor. Early symptoms are classified as "autonomic", while the later features are viewed as "neuroglycopenic".

The inability to recognize the symptoms of hypoglycemia—so called hypoglycemia unawareness, is a major risk factor for developing severe and recurrent hypoglycemia. Hypoglycemia unawareness becomes increasingly common with lengthening duration of insulin-treated diabetes [21], affecting up to 50% after 25 years [22]. The underlying mechanisms are not known and are likely to be multifactorial; altered glycemic threshold of core glucose sensors (including specified neurons in the hypothalamus and hindbrain) has been invoked, although peripheral glucose sensors (e.g. in the liver and portal vein) could also be involved. Peripheral autonomic neuropathy is associated with hypoglycemia unawareness [23] and it was suggested that diminished secretion of epinephrine in response to hypoglycemia could play a role [24] by preventing the generation of autonomic symptoms or reducing their intensity. However, the relationship of epinephrine to hypoglycemic symptoms is uncertain, and most diabetic patients with autonomic neuropathy have normal physiological responses and experience typical autonomic symptoms during induced hypoglycemia. Moreover, the prevalence of autonomic neuropathy is similar in patients with type 1 diabetes whether or not they have impaired awareness of hypoglycemia [21, 25, 26]. It has been shown convincingly that a single episode of hypoglycemia (even relatively mild) can diminish symptomatic and neuroendocrine responses to a subsequent hypoglycemic episode for at least 24 h [27, 28], and this may help to set up a vicious circle of recurrent hypoglycemia that leads to hypoglycemia unawareness.

Thus, numerous factors can influence the perception of hypoglycemic symptoms, and in turn this unawareness can contribute to an increasing frequency of hypoglycemia. Interestingly, some insulin-treated diabetic patients who have poor control may experience symptoms of hypoglycemia when glucose falls but still remains within the *hyper*glycemic range [29]. This is further evidence that thresholds for responses to altered glucose levels can be modified by current diabetic control, and is a reminder that the patients' complaints of "hypoglycemia" may need to be documented carefully before changing their insulin therapy.

PERSISTENT HYPERGLYCEMIA

Hyperglycemia is almost a natural state for most patients with insulin-dependent diabetes, and current practice centers on minimizing this. Recurrent hyperglycemia and its more serious counterpart, DKA, often reflect chronic poor control, but serious disruption to lifestyle and recurrent hospital admissions occur in only a small minority.

It is important to consider physiological or pathological causes in a patient presenting with recurrent episodes of hyperglycemia/DKA or apparent insulin resistance; such causes are seen in Box 4.

Obesity and Sedentary Lifestyle

Impairment of insulin sensitivity can occur in the obese and/or sedentary patient, particularly in skeletal muscle. Glucose removal form the peripheral circulation may also be decreased. Obesity may be induced by excessive insulin administration, as hyperinsulinemia inhibits lipolysis and favors triglyceride deposition in fat that remains relatively insulin sensitive. This may lead to spiraling weight gain and increasing insulin doses, similar to that seen in type 2 diabetes.

Box 4 Organic and psychosocial [genuine and apparent] causes of insulin resistance in type 1 diabetes

Organic [genuine] causes
- Obesity and sedentary lifestyle
- Age
- Chronic infections, e.g. tuberculosis
- Endocrinopathies: Excessive counterregulatory hormones
  - Hyperthyroidism
  - Acromegaly
  - Cushing's Syndrome
  - Pheochromocytoma
- Drugs
  - Glucocorticoids
  - B-agonists
- Overinsulinization
- Defects in insulin pharmacokinetics or action (all rare)
  - Antibody-mediated insulin resistance
  - Accelerated insulin degradation
  - Insulin-receptor-associated problems

Psychosocial [apparent] causes
- Psychiatric and psychological causes
- Deliberate omission or underusing insulin
- Failure to manage or understand own diabetes

Age

Age itself is not a cause of glycemic instability, although instability is seen more frequently in certain age groups. However, changes in physiological processes, attitudes toward diabetes, and the occurrence of further medical problems are influenced by age, and as a result age may be a factor in glycemic instability.

Puberty

Glycemic control may be very variable around the time of puberty [30], a variety of reasons have been suggested for this. Growth and sex hormone levels change during development and although the influence of GH is more clearly defined, the effects of the sex hormones upon diabetes are less well characterized.

GH secretion increases during puberty, contributing to a relative insulin-resistant state. Children with type 1 diabetes, particularly those who are poorly controlled, generally have higher GH levels than their nondiabetic counterparts. This is due to a relative deficiency of insulin-like growth factor 1 (IGF-1) secondary to insulin deficiency and this results in a failure of feedback control in inhibiting GH secretion. Puberty frequently features marked glycaemia with increased insulin requirements (1.5–2.0 units/kg/day) and girls appear more affected than boys although the cause for this is not known.

Disturbances of the menstrual cycle are seen in poorly controlled diabetes, but the improvement of glycemic control does not lead to the resumption of regular menses [31]. Therefore, it seems likely that the sex hormones have a very limited role in the development of poor control. Poor control at this time is likely to be secondary to a complex interplay between social factors, behavioral attitudes, self image, and preconceptions about diabetes as a chronic disease that frequently manifest themselves around the time of puberty [32, 33].

Old Age

Although poor glycemic control is often a feature of adolescence, it can occur in the older age groups [34]. Mixed glycemic control is the commonest presentation, although recurrent hypoglycemia and recurrent ketoacidosis also occur. The etiology is again not clear; the elderly are more likely to have concomitant diseases, some of which may be undiagnosed [35] and these may affect glycemic stability. They may also be on multiple medications some of which can cause hypoglycemia and thus influence diabetic control. A further exploration of this topic can be seen in the chapter on this topic.

Infections

Intercurrent infection can cause hyperglycemia, and as a result an increased insulin requirement; the patient should adequately manage this by applying sick-day rules. However, on occasion, the infection may be serious enough and the patient ill enough to warrant hospital admission. Chronic infections may occasionally cause insulin resistance; this was seen in the 1950s with pulmonary tuberculosis, but it may also be a feature of occult infections such as abscesses, or infections in the diabetic foot.

ENDOCRINE DISEASES

Hyperthyroidism

Metabolic control in a diabetic subject can deteriorate rapidly when hyperthyroidism supervenes [13] and increasing doses of insulin may be required to control worsening hyperglycemia, and DKA may be precipitated [36]. A history of progressive weight loss and finding resting tachycardia should raise suspicion. Effective treatment with imidazoles, surgery, or radioiodine should stabilize diabetic control.

Acromegaly

Acromegaly can cause increasing insulin requirements and hyperglycemia, particularly in the fasting state, but is a very rare cause of persistent hyperglycemia. As already mentioned, pubertal adolescents, particularly those already poorly controlled, show more frequent and greater pulses of GH over 24-h than do nondiabetic controls [37–39]; although this is due to dysregulation of GH secretion because of decreased bioavailability of IGF-1 in diabetes, clinical features of acromegaly (often with much higher and sustained GH levels) are not seen. An overall improvement in control tends to return the GH levels toward normality.

Cushing's Syndrome

There is no evidence supporting a higher prevalence rate of Cushing's syndrome in patients with type 1 diabetes than in the general population. Predictably, the rate of diabetes is higher in patients with Cushing's disease than those without Cushing's, but this is usually in the form of type 2 diabetes, affecting about 25% of patients. Clinically, the development of Cushing's syndrome may be obvious, with persisting hyperglycemia despite rising insulin dosages and weight gain.

Pheochromocytoma

Pheochromocytoma may occur spontaneously in a patient with diabetes; the prevalence rate for such an occurrence is not known. Worsening of glycemic control associated with persistent or paroxysmal hypertension is a feature of this problem. It is usually amenable to initial medical therapy before definitive surgical intervention; glycemic control should stabilize, and in patients where the pheochromocytoma was causing the hyperglycemia, the "diabetes" may also resolve [40–42].

Drugs

Administration of either glucocorticoids or β-agonists may result in a transient rise in blood glucose; rarely will persistent hyperglycemia be a problem. In patients who require long-term and/or high-dose glucocorticoid therapy, adjustment of insulin doses should stabilize glycemic control.

Overinsulinization

Hyperinsulinemia causes fat deposition and consequently increasing insulin resistance; it may also cause frequent, overt, or occult hypoglycemia. It has previously been argued that, in the 1970s, up to two thirds of children were overtreated with insulin [43]. Some of these features were noted in reports of patients with idiopathic "brittle" diabetes. To what degree overinsulinization contributes to this problem is something that remains unknown.

ABNORMAL INSULIN PHARMACOKINETICS

Antibody-mediated Insulin Resistance

In the era of more impure insulin, particularly bovine, this effect was more commonly seen [44]. The insulin antibodies are capable of binding circulating insulin and reducing its free concentration; subsequently the antibody–insulin complex is removed by the reticuloendothelial system. As a result, the insulin requirements were high, sometimes more than 200 units/day and occasionally several thousand units/day. Insulin resistance has been purported to exacerbate hyperglycemia in patients with type 1 diabetes [45]. Insulin resistance is a rather arbitrary term with no specific definition. Generally, most lean type 1 diabetes patients will require 30–60 units of insulin per day, or between 0.5 and 1.2 units/kg/day. Artificial levels to define insulin resistance have been used previously, for example, >200 units of insulin per day or greater than 1.5–2.0 units/kg/day. Certainly insulin requirements in these ranges are extremely rare and would usually indicate an underlying problem. Since highly purified insulin, particularly human, has become more frequently used, this problem has largely disappeared from the western world.

Accelerated Insulin Degradation

In the 1980s considerable interest was raised by the suggestion that defects in insulin absorption and clearance could cause high insulin requirements and/or poor glycemic control. The defects were supposed either to occur in the subcutaneous tissue (the so called subcutaneous insulin resistance syndrome) or to affect circulating insulin. All the defects described are now recognized as extremely rare; in retrospect, it seems likely that deliberate interference by the patient with investigation or treatment (see below) could explain at least some of the abnormal results. Schade and Duckworth, who in well constructed trials, found no evidence of defects in either subcutaneous insulin absorption or the glucose-lowering potency of insulin in any of 30 patients referred for investigation into subcutaneous insulin resistance syndrome [46]. These subjects had persistent hyperglycemia (with or without glycemic instability), were prone to ketoacidosis, and required high doses of subcutaneous insulin, but apparently responded well to conventional intravenous doses of insulin. These routes were thought to have bypassed the barrier to insulin absorption [47–49]. Suggested mechanisms included enzymatic degradation [46], but most were not proven [41–47]. The subcutaneous insulin resistance syndrome was put forward as an explanation for the observed problems with glycemic control and recurrent ketosis in some patients. However, the evidence to support this is minimal, and it is likely that if this syndrome does exist, then it is extremely rare. There is sufficient evidence supporting deliberate interference by this group of patients; the dramatic responses noted when treated with different methods of insulin administration, such as the intravenous route, may be explained by improved insulin compliance and closer observation of administration. In three patients who appeared to exhibit massive insulin resistance to insulin administered by all methods [50–52] the explanation may well be accelerated clearance of insulin from the circulation. This obviously points past the proposed subcutaneous "barrier" to a systemic abnormality. All three cases had inappropriately low plasma levels of circulating insulin during high rates of intravenous insulin administration (up to 20 000 units/day). Where the excessive clearance of insulin occurs is not known, but it could include the liver or vascular endothelium, which are known to take up insulin.

Insulin Receptor Defects

Although rare, numerous mutations affecting the insulin receptor have been identified (see Chapter 13). Some of these cause insulin resistance with hyperglycemia and recurrent ketoacidosis; additional phenotypic features identify some syndromes clinically. Antibodies can develop against the insulin receptor in certain autoimmune diseases [e.g. systemic lupus erythematosus (SLE)] and can lead to insulin resistance. A variety of abnormalities of insulin receptors have been described in the adipose tissue of patients with idiopathic "brittle" diabetes, who as a group were resistant to insulin [53, 54]. It is possible, however, that these defects may simply be the result of preceding poor glycemic control and/or high insulin doses.

Psychiatric and Psychological Problems

Such problems have increasingly being recognized in patients with problematic control, particularly those previously labeled as "brittle". Eating disorders can cause severe problems with glycemic control; it is estimated that eating disorders may affect up to 10% of young women with type 1 diabetes [55]—substantially more common than nondiabetic women [56]. Bulimia nervosa (with food bingeing and purging) is the commonest eating disorder seen. The bingeing can lead to episodes of hyperglycemia, which may be countered by increased doses of insulin that result in obesity. The further disturbance of body image continues to drive the vicious circle and leads to poor diabetic control. Episodes of bulimia followed by purging and/or vomiting can lead to a mixed picture of unpredictable episodes of hyper- and hypoglycemia. Deliberate underdosing of insulin is another common and neglected problem. These patients are often prescribed large doses of insulin but reports have demonstrated that the full dose is not often taken, something which may be more widespread than previously known, one US survey showing that this may occur in up to 9% of women with type 1 diabetes [57–59]. Similarly, insulin omission was the conclusion drawn on a group of patients investigated for severe insulin resistance. These patients often had doses of approaching 2000 units/day; no evidence was found of impaired absorption or the action of insulin injected at normal doses under very controlled circumstances [60, 61]. The motivation for such behavior is not entirely clear. Certainly in young women, who make up the vast majority of this group, insulin omission is a convenient way to control body weight [58, 59, 62–64]. This method of weight control may well be a manifestation of disturbed body image similar to that of anorexia nervosa. Other patients may use the omission of insulin to induce ketosis as a way of escaping intolerable situations in their life; single parents, family problems, and physical and sexual abuse appear more common in these patients. Insulin omission may also be performed to avoid hypoglycemia, in those with a fear of developing such symptoms; others prefer to run chronically hyperglycemic. Finally, others may simply not understand or carry out instructions regarding insulin administration, and evidence of communication or comprehension problems have been found in a highly selected population [60, 61].

One distinct case demonstrates the effect of environmental and emotional stress on behavior and the resulting diabetic consequences. In the 1950s Peck and Peck reported on a single case featuring multiple admissions for DKA. The number of admissions increased progressively until the patient was removed from her drunken and abusive parents to a new home and regular employment [65]. More recent reports from the United Kingdom and United States confirm that psychosocial disruption is seen more frequently in the "brittle" groups than in control groups [46, 66, 67].

INVESTIGATING GLYCEMIC INSTABILITY

When faced with a patient who has severe and recurrent glycemic instability, whether predominantly hypoglycemia, hyperglycemia, or both, it is useful to have an ordered scheme of investigation. Given the problems associated with managing such patients, it is better all round if the same health care professionals are responsible for the care and investigations at each visit so as to avoid further potential areas for confusion. A schematic protocol for investigating such patients is given in Figure 2; this is useful for all types of glycemic instability. Most of the investigations can be performed in an outpatient investigation unit or in a day case investigation unit, and if the underlying problem is not determined at this stage, then admission to hospital for more detailed tests and supervision is appropriate.

Problems such as obesity, infection, and drug-induced as well as obvious endocrine causes may be elicited by careful history and examination. Given that the patients' understanding of diabetes is crucial to the management of the disease, it is useful to determine skills and knowledge at this stage, as well as reviewing injection technique before proceeding on to more detailed investigations. Since coexistent endocrine disease may have major affects on diabetic control, a full workup in this regard is worthwhile.

Although, in general, the investigation of glycemic instability as described in Figure 2 can be used for any type

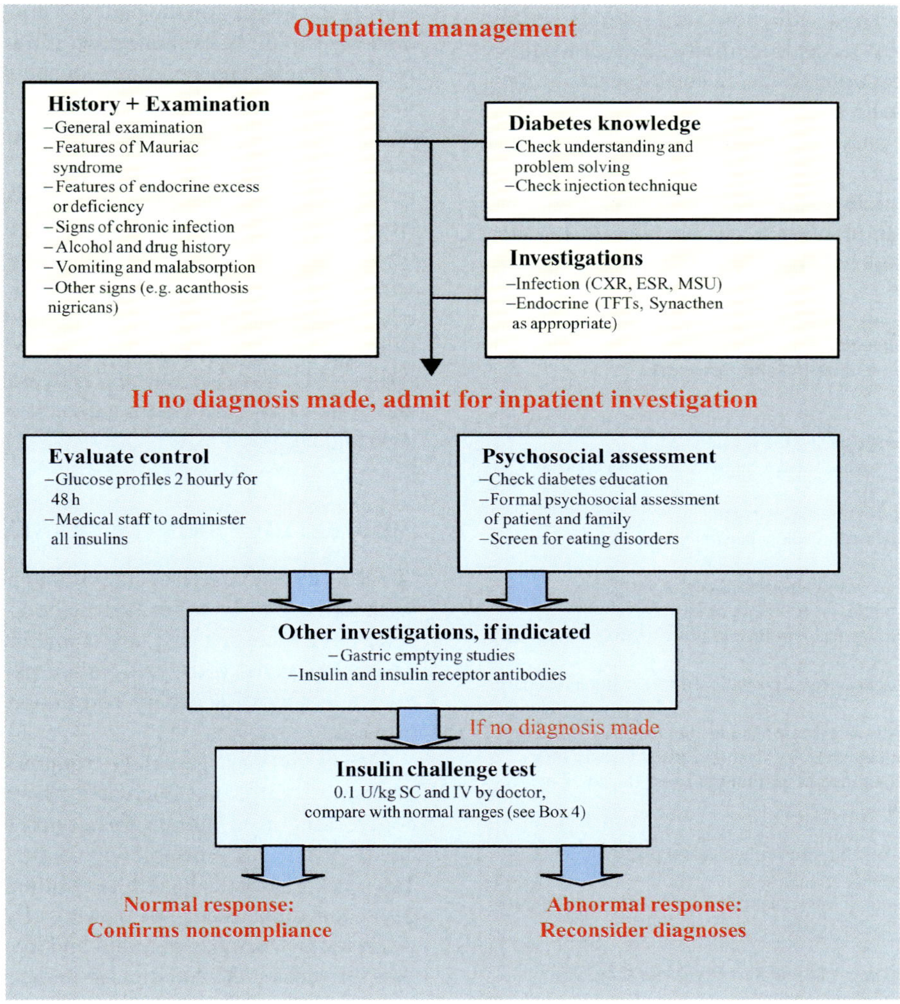

Figure 2 Scheme for investigation of glycemic instability. CXR = chest x-ray; ESR = erythrocyte sedimentation rate; MSU = midstream urine culture; TFTs = thyroid function tests; SC = subcutaneous; IV = intravenous

of instability, specific areas may need to be explored for predominant hypo- and hyperglycemia states.

Predominant Hypoglycemia

Here, a thorough alcohol history and examination for endocrine disease will identify most causes. This is the most fruitful line of investigation and most problems are amenable to treatment. Remaining cases that have not had a cause identified at this point are likely to be factitious. It is noteworthy to point out that some patients may "overtreat" themselves, resulting in recurrent hypoglycemia. The impetus for such behavior may well be based in a strong fear of developing the complications of diabetes. Admission to hospital is recommended so the patient may be closely supervised and conditions controlled to rule out excessive use of insulin, adherence to a suitable diet, and exclusion of eating disorders.

Predominant Hyperglycemia

Endocrine disease and infection (also, rarely insulin antibody and insulin receptor antibody disease) would be responsible for most organic causes and these can be identified by the outlined investigations. If no organic cause is identified, then possibly nonorganic insulin resistance should be considered. Useful in this regard is the insulin challenge test; rises in plasma insulin concentration and corresponding falls in plasma glucose should be seen, following an insulin challenge (Box 5). It is likely that patients being investigated at this stage will have nonorganic disease; consequently, they may be skilled at manipulating circumstances, family members, and health care professionals. It is then essential that the tests are performed in very controlled conditions. This should be explained firmly but sympathetically to the patient and the patient's family.

Box 5 Insulin challenge test for detection of subcutaneous or intravenous insulin resistance

Before the test
- No long-acting insulin during the previous 24 h
- Intravenous insulin and saline overnight to maintain control
- Fast patient overnight

Subcutaneous (SC) insulin resistance test
- 9 a.m.: Discontinue insulin, allow plasma glucose to rise to 12–15 mmol/l
- Inject 0.1 U/kg short-acting insulin subcutaneously
- Insulin from new bottle, given by physician
- Take blood samples for free insulin and glucose every 30 min for 4 h
- Physician to be present and observe patient during entire procedure

After SC test
- If blood glucose falls as expected (no insulin resistance) end test.
- If proceeding to intravenous (IV) test (because SC resistance demonstrated), continue IV insulin until next day to maintain control

IV test
- The next day, stop insulin infusion and allow plasma glucose to rise to 12–15 mmol/l
- Inject 0.1 U/kg insulin intravenously as a *bolus* and take blood for insulin and glucose as before

Expected results
- Subcutaneous: Maximum fall in plasma glucose should be >5.3 mmol/l (no SC resistance)
- Intravenous: Maximum fall in plasma glucose should be >3.4 mmol/l (no IV resistance)

MANAGEMENT OF POOR GLYCEMIC CONTROL

Any diagnosis reached should be discussed at length with the patient and if appropriate, the patients' family. Those with reduced awareness of hypoglycemia due to overzealous insulin administration may benefit from relaxing control and allowing blood glucose levels to rise [68]. Such patients, who may have obsessive–compulsive traits, will require convincing that their overall risk of developing the complications of diabetes will not be greatly increased. During the admission the patient's ability to manage their diabetes should be evaluated and if misconceptions or errors are found, appropriate reeducation made. It may be useful to draw up guidelines for future management goals and subsequent follow-up with the patient, allowing clear intentions to be seen by both sides. If the patient is diagnosed with noncompliance then the situation will require careful handling. Psychological therapy may be beneficial; obviously this depends on a great deal of patient cooperation and the attitude and approach of the treating physician. In the mid 1980s psychological therapy was found to help a number of patients shown to be noncompliant [46, 60, 61]; however, success is by no means guaranteed and these cases may absorb a great deal of psychologist's time and energy.

"IDIOPATHIC" BRITTLE DIABETES

"Brittle" diabetes, a term supposedly coined in the 1930s to describe poorly controlled diabetic patients [69], has been used inconsistently and sometimes pejoratively to describe patients with type 1 diabetes who struggle with glycemic control and defy conventional attempts to improve it.

The term was generally supposed to characterize glycemic control that fluctuated between hyper- and hypoglycemia, even though this seems to be the least frequent pattern of unstable glycemic control. In 1977, Tattersall pragmatically defined brittle diabetes as insulin-dependent diabetes in patients whose lives were constantly disrupted by episodes of hypo- and hyperglycemia, whatever the cause [70]. Attempts to refine this definition have included adding that failure to achieve glycemic control with an optimized insulin regime (continuous subcutaneous insulin infusion) was a hallmark of "brittle" patients

Table 1 Characteristics of patients with brittle diabetes and presentation type

Recurrent ketoacidosis	Recurrent hypoglycemia
>50% of all brittle patients	10–15% of brittle patients
Commonly young females	Roughly equal female : male ratio
Usually high insulin doses	Age variable
Psychosocial problems possible	Psychosocial problems possible
Omission of insulin noted	Factitious hypoglycemia common common
	Overuse of insulin

[66] and characterizing the degree of life disruption seen in these patients [67, 71].

Although it was initially thought that patients with brittle diabetes would fluctuate between hyper- and hypoglycemic states, it appears that this situation is relatively uncommon. Currently, the patient with "brittle" disease will tend to present with either predominantly hypoglycemic or hyperglycemic/recurrent DKA symptoms. A small minority will present with a pattern of mixed glycemic instability. Such examples may be seen in work from the United Kingdom [67, 72]. Why this polarization should occur is not known, but the social setting in which the problems initiated or indeed the ability of the patients to tolerate the symptoms may be influential. There are slight differences in the characteristics of the groups who present with recurrent ketoacidosis compared to hypoglycemic instability (Table 1).

Clinical Features of Brittle Diabetes: A Time Syndrome?

Most reports have originated in the United Kingdom or United States [60, 66, 67, 72, 73] with relatively few elsewhere. Even in the United Kingdom and United States the estimated prevalence of brittle diabetes is considerably less than 1% [73]. It is predominantly seen in young women (particularly in series from the United Kingdom) who mostly display moderate obesity and high insulin requirements. Such common characteristics (as in Table 2)

Table 2 The commonest features seen in idiopathic brittle diabetes

- Predominantly young women
- Life disruption with poor glycemic control and recurrent hospital admissions
- Onset of brittleness around puberty
- Major problems at home, work, or school common
- Mild to moderate obesity
- Unresponsive to CSII and other intensive insulin regimes
- Chronic oligo/amenorrhea
- [Deliberate?] interference with treatment may be common (and concealed)

Note. "?" means possibly or potentially.

could point to a discrete syndrome with an underlying cause; however, these features may be a result of referral patterns to units known to be interested in such cases, because other reports have suggested a more diverse picture, including wider age ranges and a more equal sex distribution [72, 74].

Most of the literature on brittle diabetes suggests that females predominate especially among those attending with recurrent DKA [66, 67, 71]. In the general diabetic population, glycosylated hemoglobin levels tend to be higher in females, and there is some evidence that females do not cope as well as males with diabetes [75–79]. Young female diabetic patients are more commonly seen as inpatients and have higher bed occupancy rates than do age-matched males. They also seem more susceptible to injection-site infections and appear less well controlled despite intensive type insulin regimes. As already mentioned, this patient group suffers from more eating disorders as well [80–82]. These numerous cultural and social pressures may make women, and in particular young women, struggle to cope with diabetes, which may also occur in other chronic diseases [83–85] such as asthma and Addison's disease.

Since brittle diabetes occurs most frequently in young women and there appears to be a correlation between the onset of "brittleness" and the age of menarche, accordingly, it has been suggested that endocrine or emotional changes at this time may be influential. As detailed earlier, GH may aggravate insulin resistance and hyperglycemia around the time of puberty [30], but this does not explain the higher prevalence in females; instead, the problems with body image in this group may play a role, e.g. underusing or omission of insulin to induce weight loss [58, 63, 64]. Those who naturally tend to obesity or those who suffer weight gain through overinsulinization may be particularly at risk. Anorexia, bulimia, and subclinical eating disorders all appear more prevalent in this group [62, 86] and may be major contributors to the problem of brittleness in these patients [66, 67, 87]. It is likely that chronically poor glycemic control, possibly combined with periods of under- and overinsulinisation, may itself worsen metabolic state in some cases. Hyperinsulinemia may tend to result in receptor downregulation, while chronic hyperglycemia can impair insulin action to some degree. However, the abnormalities are relatively minor and possibly less important than underdosing or omitting insulin and other noncompliant behaviors.

Many of these patients apparently take high doses of insulin, often in the region of >2.0 units/kg/day, but this apparent insulin resistance is spurious, as they show normal insulinemic and glycemic responses to conventional insulin administered subcutaneously or intravenously given under close supervision. Similarly, implantable insulin pumps [88–90] are effective at normal insulin dosages, presumably because they avoid the manipulation of insulin administration by the patient. The impression of insulin resistance is very likely to be created by the physician, who increases insulin doses to control persistent hyperglycemia, while the patient continues to use insufficient insulin to maintain good control. Reasons for the patient's behavior are discussed above.

Psychosocial and sometimes overt psychiatric conditions are a feature in many cases of brittle diabetes, but may not be apparent without a detailed search. These problems are likely to contribute to the development of, and indeed the maintenance of glycemic instability in a considerable proportion of these patients and require careful management.

If glycemic control continues to be unstable despite continued attempts to optimize control, it should be remembered that the patient may be interfering with the treatment so as to ensure persistence of the "brittle" state; indeed, this is suspected to be the main if not the only cause of brittleness in two thirds of some outpatients [72, 91]. Much inventiveness and dedication may be required on the part of the patient to avoid detection. Insulin injections should be witnessed and blood glucose monitoring checked. A search of the patient's possessions, although morally questionable, is often useful as it may reveal, concealed insulin or high-sugar supplements, which may be used to manipulate blood glucose levels by the patient. Patients do not frequently admit that they have been manipulating their own treatment, and it is often difficult to confront them, even though it is clear to all involved that this is what is happening (Table 3). It is likely that an underlying psychological/psychiatric issue exists in such cases and that this is clearly not an intentional behavior designed by the patient to frustrate the managing physician. Some patients may admit to such behavior many years after the brittleness has resolved. The reasons for such behavior are not always clear, but as in nonorganic hypo- and hyperglycemia it may involve manipulation of weight and therefore control of body image, or refuge-seeking behavior [59, 71].

Many "organic" mechanisms have been suggested as the underlying cause of "brittle" diabetes, but the evidence supporting them is poor. An exaggerated hormonal response to stress (both chronically and acutely) mediated via the counterregulatory hormones was held responsible [92]. For some years numerous reports focused on the relationship between diabetic instability and emotional or social "stressors" [93], and it was believed that emotional stress could disturb metabolic control [94] (although it was never explained how such stress could cause both hyper- and hypoglycemia). No convincing evidence has emerged for an exaggerated neuroendocrine and metabolic response to stress in "brittle" diabetic patients. Standardized mental stress in patients with type 1 diabetes, in an experimental setting, does not appear to elevate blood glucose or ketone levels despite detectable rises in plasma cortisol and epinephrine [95]. Overall, therefore, it seems that stress may change behavior, leading to manipulation of insulin therapy, rather than directly cause metabolic decompensation. The debate continues regarding the role of stress in influencing metabolic control [96, 97], but general opinion is agreed that psychological stress has a limited effect, at best, on metabolic control in type 1 diabetes.

Medical Management

It has been suggested that the management of brittle diabetes should be "primarily an exercise in the organisation and delivery of medical care" [98]. Certainly only experienced and specialist staff should be involved and the different members of the diabetes care team should work closely together with an agreed plan of approach. Some argue that the ability to contact a senior doctor at any time via telephone, by the patient or indeed the patient's family, can help to avert sometimes-lengthy hospital admissions.

Table 3 Examples of deliberate manipulation of treatment in type 1 diabetes patients with "brittle" diabetes

Technique of manipulation	Method of detection
Insulin manipulation	
Faked injections (through skin fold into swab)	Radiolabeled insulin found in swab, not in injection site
Air drawn up, not insulin	Syringe check before injection
Extra injections given	Concealed insulin and syringes found
Sabotage of pump devices	
Batteries removed or inverted	In all cases routine checks at random times revealed the method of sabotage
Infusion cannulae punctured	
Cannulae pulled out or disconnected	
Insulin in reservoir diluted	
Disinformation about diabetes control	
Faking hypoglycemic symptoms	Recheck blood glucose, in venous sample if necessary
Fingertips dipped in glucose drinks prior to blood glucose test	
Fabrication of home blood glucose data	Compare machine memory values with recorded values

Note. Most evaded detection initially despite close supervision.

Table 4 Methods used in the treatment of brittle diabetes

Method of treatment	Reference
Intramuscular insulin injection/infusion	[99]
Intravenous insulin infusion	[100–102]
Intraperitoneal insulin injection/infusion	[103–105]
Implantable insulin pump*	[88, 90, 106–108]
Pancreatic transplant*	[109]
Subcutaneous insulin + aprotonin	[47]
Subcutaneous insulin + vasodilators	[110]
Hemodialysis	[111]
Plasmapheresis	[112]
Insulin-like growth factor 1 (IGF-1)	[113]
Octreotide	[114]
Danazol	[115]
Counseling and support*	[116, 117]
Psychoanalysis*	[118]

* Indicates methods of proven benefit.

The patient should also never be viewed in isolation; social and family dynamics must always be considered in the overall care strategy.

Over the years, numerous methods have been employed in managing patients with brittle diabetes (see Table 4). Most were developed when the underlying cause of brittle diabetes was attributed to either severe insulin resistance or defects in subcutaneous insulin absorption. Their rationale is therefore dubious and it is best to regard these of historical interest only.

Implanted pumps that infuse insulin intraperitoneally [88–90] (e.g., Infusaid type pumps) have been successful in patients unresponsive to intensified subcutaneous insulin regimes, including CSII [99, 103–105]. Risks include cannula obstruction and infection (sometimes life-threatening); some pumps are also amenable to patient interference and manipulation [88, 90, 106–108]. Use is also limited by expense and the implantation procedure [100–102]. Pumps pose potential problems in patients subject to self-destructive behavior and manipulation but can maintain reasonably stable metabolic control and allow complementary approaches such as a psychological intervention to be started [119].

Psychological Methods

Psychological approaches would seem attractive for these predominantly behavioral problems; unfortunately success may be limited. In a few cases counseling, support, and education have been shown to be useful, sometimes dramatically so [116, 117, 120]. Such counseling may be done alone or in small groups, which may include the patient's family/carers. A small study of "brittle" diabetic children who had repeated hospital attendances, showed that psychotherapy [118] given to half of the group led to a reduction in HbA_{1c}, and slightly fewer diabetes-related hospital admissions, although the overall hospital admission rate remained the same.

Natural History of Brittle Diabetes

There are few long-term follow-up data on "brittle" diabetes. The dearth of patients aged over 30 years suggests that either they die, or the problem resolves. Four longitudinal studies have been performed. In 1988, Williams and Pickup reported on 13 "brittle" females followed up for 3–6 years. There was one death and some persisting problems but generally most patients showed an improvement in their "brittle" behavior [121]. Gill and Alberti reported a further study of 20 female patients with recurrent DKA in 1991; the mean follow-up duration was 8 years. Two patients had died, 2 were worse, and 2 the same; the 14 remaining patients had either improved or the "brittle" disease had resolved. Diabetic complications had arisen in six patients [91]. Another report in that year by Tattersall and colleagues on a group of 25 "brittle" diabetic patients followed up for 12 years compared them to matched controls. Again most patients improved and there was no increase in deaths or complications in the "brittle" group. A strong temporal relationship between life stresses and brittleness was noted by the authors [72]. The inclusion criteria for brittle diabetes in this study was not as stringent as in the two previous studies, and this may explain the relatively large number of patients managed in one center.

The final study published in 1993 with a 10-year follow-up reported on the combined cohorts of the first two studies referred to above. Only 26 of the original 33 patients could be traced. Of the 26 identified, 5 had died and of the surviving 21 only 2 patients were still considered to be "brittle". When compared with a matched stable group of type 1 patients, the "brittle" group had more microvascular complications, poorer quality of life, and more psychosocial problems. Among the patients who became pregnant, the "brittle" group had more miscarriages, fetal malformations, and deaths. These figures were much worse than matched nonbrittle controls [71].

Overall, brittle diabetes has a tendency to resolve or improve with time, and this resolution appears to be related to positive life events such as moving away from unhappy home circumstances, getting married, or becoming pregnant. There is a notable excess of deaths in people who exhibit "brittle" behavior, and there is a serious threat of long-term diabetic complications in those who do survive.

SUMMARY AND CONCLUSIONS

Metabolic instability in a patient with diabetes can be of great concern. Poor control increases the risks of long-term microvascular complications, and the short-term consequences of severe metabolic instability are potentially fatal.

Every patient who presents with metabolic instability deserves careful evaluation to try to understand the underlying cause. In many cases, especially those traditionally labeled as brittle diabetes much effort and skill may be required to tease out the noncompliant behaviors that are responsible, and to identify and manage their root causes. This process often requires the full cooperation of the whole diabetes care team and the patient's family.

REFERENCES

1. The Diabetes Control and Complications Trial Research Group. The effect of intensive treatment of diabetes on the development and progression of long-term complications in insulin-dependent diabetes mellitus. *N Engl J Med* 1993; 329 (14): 977–86.
2. Sjobom NC, Adamson U, Lin PE. The prevalence of impaired glucose counter-regulation during an insulin-infusion test in insulin-treated diabetic patients prone to severe hypoglycaemia. *Diabetologia* 1989; 32 (11): 818–25.
3. Gerich JE, Langlois M, Noacco C, Karam JH, Forsham PH. Lack of glucagon response to hypoglycaemia in diabetes: evidence for an intrinsic pancreatic alpha cell defect. *Science* 1973; 182 (108): 171–3.
4. Lindberg B, Ericsson UB, Ljung R, Ivarsson SA. High prevalence of thyroid autoantibodies at diagnosis of insulin-dependent diabetes mellitus in Swedish children. *J Lab Clin Med* 1997; 130 (6): 585–9.
5. Gharib H, Gastineau CF. Coexisting Addison's disease and diabetes mellitus: report of 24 cases with review of literature. *Mayo Clin Proc* 1969; 44 (4): 217–27.
6. Brown FM, Smith AM, Longway S, Rabinowe SL. Adrenal medullitis in type I diabetes. *J Clin Endocrinol Metab* 1990; 71 (6): 1491–5.
7. Park YS, Kim TW, Kim WB, Cho BY. Increased prevalence of autoimmune thyroid disease in patients with type 1 diabetes. *Korean J Intern Med* 2000; 15 (3): 202–10.
8. Mouradian M, Abourizk N. Diabetes mellitus and thyroid disease. *Diabetes Care* 1983; 6 (5): 512–20.
9. Gerstein HC. Incidence of postpartum thyroid dysfunction in patients with type I diabetes mellitus. *Ann Intern Med* 1993; 118 (6): 419–23.
10. Feely J, Isles TE. Screening for thyroid dysfunction in diabetics. *BMJ* 1979; 1 (6179): 1678.
11. Hardy KJ, Burge MR, Boyle PJ, Scarpello JH. A treatable cause of recurrent severe hypoglycaemia. *Diabetes Care* 1994; 17 (7): 722–4.
12. Armstrong L, Bell PM. Addison's disease presenting as reduced insulin requirement in insulin dependent diabetes. *BMJ* 1996; 312 (7046): 1601–2.
13. Cooppan R, Kozak GP. Hyperthyroidism and diabetes mellitus. An analysis of 70 patients. *Arch Intern Med* 1980; 140 (3): 370–3.
14. Enck P, Frieling T. Pathophysiology of diabetic gastroparesis. *Diabetes* 1997; 46 (suppl 2): S77–81.
15. Feldman M, Schiller LR. Disorders of gastrointestinal motility associated with diabetes mellitus. *Ann Intern Med* 1983; 98 (3): 378–84.
16. Page SR, Lloyd CA, Hill PG, Peacock I, Holmes GK. The prevalence of coeliac disease in adult diabetes mellitus. *QJM* 1994; 87 (10): 631–7.
17. Cacciari E, Salardi S, Volta U, Biasco G, Partesotti S, Mantovani A, Cicognani A, Tonioli S, Tassoni P, Pirazzoli P. Prevalence and characteristics of coeliac disease in type 1 diabetes mellitus. *Acta Paediatr Scand* 1987; 76 (4): 671–2.
18. Holmes GK. Screening for coeliac disease in type 1 diabetes. *Arch Dis Child* 2002; 87 (6): 495–8.
19. Schober E, Rami B, Granditsch G, Crone J. Coeliac disease in children and adolescents with type 1 diabetes mellitus: to screen or not, to treat or not? *Horm Res* 2002; 57 (suppl 1): 97–100.
20. Holmes GK. Coeliac disease and Type 1 diabetes mellitus—the case for screening. *Diabet Med* 2001; 18 (3): 169–77.
21. Hepburn DA, Patrick AW, Eadington DW, Ewing DJ, Frier BM. Unawareness of hypoglycaemia in insulin-treated diabetic patients: prevalence and relationship to autonomic neuropathy. *Diabet Med* 1990; 7 (8): 711–7.
22. Pramming S, Thorsteinsson B, Bendtson I, Binder C. Symptomatic hypoglycaemia in 411 type 1 diabetic patients. *Diabet Med* 1991; 8 (3): 217–22.
23. Hoeldtke RD, Boden G. Epinephrine secretion, hypoglycaemia unawareness, and diabetic autonomic neuropathy. *Ann Intern Med* 1994; 120 (6): 512–7.
24. Hepburn DA, MacLeod KM, Frier BM. Physiological, symptomatic and hormonal responses to acute hypoglycaemia in type 1 diabetic patients with autonomic neuropathy. *Diabet Med* 1993; 10 (10): 940–9.
25. Hilsted J, Richter E, Madsbad S, Tronier B, Christensen NJ, Hildebrandt P, Damkjaer M, Galbo H. Metabolic and cardiovascular responses to epinephrine in diabetic autonomic neuropathy. *N Engl J Med* 1987; 317 (7): 421–6.
26. Hilsted J, Madsbad S, Krarup T, Sestoft L, Christensen NJ, Tronier B, Galbo H. Hormonal, metabolic, and cardiovascular responses to hypoglycemia in diabetic autonomic neuropathy. *Diabetes* 1981; 30 (8): 626–33.
27. George E, Harris N, Bedford C, Macdonald IA, Hardisty CA, Heller SR. Prolonged but partial impairment of the hypoglycaemic physiological response following short-term hypoglycaemia in normal subjects. *Diabetologia* 1995; 38 (10): 1183–90.
28. Davis SN, Shavers C, Mosqueda-Garcia R, Costa F. Effects of differing antecedent hypoglycemia on subsequent counterregulation in normal humans. *Diabetes* 1997; 46 (8): 1328–35.
29. Boyle PJ, Schwartz NS, Shah SD, Clutter WE, Cryer PE. Plasma glucose concentrations at the onset of hypoglycemic symptoms in patients with poorly controlled diabetes and in nondiabetics. *N Engl J Med* 1988; 318 (23): 1487–92.
30. Amiel SA, Sherwin RS, Simonson DC, Lauritano AA, Tamborlane WV. Impaired insulin action in puberty. A contributing factor to poor glycemic control in adolescents with diabetes. *N Engl J Med* 1986; 315 (4): 215–9.
31. O'Hare JA, Eichold BH II, Vignati L. Hypogonadotropic secondary amenorrhea in diabetes: effects of central opiate blockade and improved metabolic control. *Am J Med* 1987; 83 (6): 1080–4.
32. Peyrot M, McMurry JF. Jr. Psychosocial factors in diabetes control: adjustment of insulin-treated adults. *Psychosom Med* 1985; 47 (6): 542–57.
33. Dumont RH, Jacobson AM, Cole C, Hauser ST, Wolfsdorf JI, Willett JB, Milley JE, Wertlieb D. Psychosocial predictors of acute complications of diabetes in youth. *Diabet Med* 1995; 12 (7): 612–8.
34. Benbow SJ, Walsh A, Gill GV. Brittle diabetes in the elderly. *J R Soc Med* 2001; 94 (11): 578–80.
35. Jolobe OM, Khin N. Brittle diabetes in the elderly. *J R Soc Med* 2002; 95 (1): 58.

36. Sola E, Morillas C, Garzon S, Gomez-Balaguer M, Hernandez-Mijares A. Association between diabetic ketoacidosis and thyrotoxicosis. *Acta Diabetol* 2002; 39 (4): 235–7.
37. Rother KI, Levitsky LL. Diabetes mellitus during adolescence. *Endocrinol Metab Clin North Am* 1993; 22 (3): 553–72.
38. Batch JA, Werther GA. Changes in growth hormone concentrations during puberty in adolescents with insulin dependent diabetes. *Clin Endocrinol (Oxf)* 1992; 36 (4): 411–6.
39. Press M, Caprio S, Tamborlane WV, Bhushan R, Thorner M, Vale W, Rivier J, Sherwin RS. Pituitary response to growth hormone-releasing hormone in IDDM. Abnormal responses to insulin and hyperglycemia. *Diabetes* 1992; 41 (1): 17–21.
40. Zanin L, Rossi G, Poletti A, Piotto A, Chiesura-Corona M, Pessina AC. Necrosis of a pheochromocytoma associated with spontaneous remission of diabetes and hypertension. *Clin Endocrinol (Oxf)* 1993; 39 (5): 613–7.
41. Stenstrom G, Sjostrom L, Smith U. Diabetes mellitus in pheochromocytoma. Fasting blood glucose levels before and after surgery in 60 patients with pheochromocytoma. *Acta Endocrinol (Copenh)* 1984; 106 (4): 511–5.
42. Isles CG, Johnson JK. Pheochromocytoma and diabetes mellitus: further evidence that alpha 2 receptors inhibit insulin release in man. *Clin Endocrinol (Oxf)* 1983; 18 (1): 37–41.
43. Rosenbloom AL, Giordano BP. Chronic overtreatment with insulin in children and adolescents. *Am J Dis Child* 1977; 131 (8): 881–5.
44. Witters LA, Ohman JL, Weir GC, Raymond LW, Lowell FC. Insulin antibodies in the pathogenesis of insulin allergy and resistance. *Am J Med* 1977; 63 (5): 703–9.
45. Greenbaum CJ, Insulin resistance in type 1 diabetes. *Diabetes Metab Res Rev* 2002; 18 (3): 192–200.
46. Schade DS, Duckworth WC. In search of the subcutaneous-insulin-resistance syndrome. *N Engl J Med* 1986; 315 (3): 147–53.
47. Freidenberg GR, White N, Cataland S, O'Dorisio TM, Sotos JF, Santiago JV. Diabetes responsive to intravenous but not subcutaneous insulin: effectiveness of aprotinin. *N Engl J Med* 1981; 305 (7): 363–8.
48. Home PD, Massi-Benedetti M, Gill GV, Capaldo B, Shepherd GA, Alberti KG. Impaired subcutaneous absorption of insulin in 'brittle' diabetics. *Acta Endocrinol* 1982; 101 (3): 414–20.
49. Pickup JC, Home PD, Bilous RW, Keen H, Alberti KG. Management of severely brittle diabetes by continuous subcutaneous and intramuscular insulin infusions: evidence for a defect in subcutaneous insulin absorption. *BMJ (Clin Res Ed)* 1981; 282 (6261): 347–50.
50. Blazar BR, Whitley CB, Kitabchi AE, Tsai MY, Santiago J, White N, Stentz FB, Brown DM. In vivo chloroquine-induced inhibition of insulin degradation in a diabetic patient with severe insulin resistance. *Diabetes* 1984; 33 (12): 1133–7.
51. McElduff A, Eastman CJ, Haynes SP, Bowen KM. Apparent insulin resistance due to abnormal enzymatic insulin degradation: a new mechanism for insulin resistance. *Aust NZJ Med* 1980; 10 (1): 56–61.
52. Williams G, Pickup JC, Keen H. Massive insulin resistance apparently due to rapid clearance of circulating insulin. *Am J Med* 1987; 82 (6): 1247–52.
53. Taylor SI. Receptor defects in patients with extreme insulin resistance. *Diabetes Metab Rev* 1985; 1 (1/2): 171–202.
54. Taylor R, Husband DJ, Marshall SM, Tunbridge WM, Alberti KG. Adipocyte insulin binding and insulin sensitivity in 'brittle' diabetes. *Diabetologia* 1984; 27 (4): 441–6.
55. Verrotti A, Catino M, De Luca FA, Morgese G, Chiarelli F. Eating disorders in adolescents with type 1 diabetes mellitus. *Acta Diabetol* 1999; 36 (1/2): 21–5.
56. Jones JM, Lawson ML, Daneman D, Olmsted MP, Rodin G. Eating disorders in adolescent females with and without type 1 diabetes: cross sectional study. *BMJ* 2000; 320 (7249): 1563–6.
57. Takii M, et al. Differences between bulimia nervosa and binge-eating disorder in females with type 1 diabetes: the important role of insulin omission. *J Psychosom Res* 1999; 47 (3): 221–31.
58. Polonsky WH, Anderson BJ, Lohrer PA, Aponte JE, Jacobson AM, Cole CF. Insulin omission in women with IDDM. *Diabetes Care* 1994; 17 (10): 1178–85.
59. Biggs MM, Basco MR, Patterson G, Raskin P. Insulin withholding for weight control in women with diabetes. *Diabetes Care* 1994; 17 (10): 1186–9.
60. Schade DS, Eaton RP, Drumm DA, Duckworth WC. A clinical algorithm to determine the etiology of brittle diabetes. *Diabetes Care* 1985; 8 (1): 5–11.
61. Schade DS, Drumm DA, Duckworth WC, Eaton RP. The etiology of incapacitating, brittle diabetes. *Diabetes Care* 1985; 8 (1): 12–20.
62. Neumark-Sztainer D, et al. Weight control practices and disordered eating behaviors among adolescent females and males with type 1 diabetes: associations with sociodemographics, weight concerns, familial factors, and metabolic outcomes. *Diabetes Care* 2002; 25 (8): 1289–96.
63. Rodin GM, Craven J, Littlefield C, Goldbloom D, Daneman D. Insulin misuse through omission or reduction of dose. *Psychosomatics* 1989; 30 (4): 465–6.
64. Rodin G, Craven J, Littlefield C, Murray M, Daneman D. Eating disorders and intentional insulin undertreatment in adolescent females with diabetes. *Psychosomatics* 1991; 32 (2): 171–6.
65. Peck FB, Peck FB. Tautologous diabetic coma—a behavior syndrome. Multiple unnecessary episodes of diabetic coma. *Diabetes* 1956; 5: 44–46.
66. Pickup J, Williams G, Johns P, Keen H. Clinical features of brittle diabetic patients unresponsive to optimized subcutaneous insulin therapy (continuous subcutaneous insulin infusion). *Diabetes Care* 1983; 6 (3): 279–84.
67. Gill GV. The spectrum of brittle diabetes. *J R Soc Med.* 1992; 85 (5): 259–61.
68. Cranston I, Lomas J, Maran A, Macdonald I, Amiel SA. Restoration of hypoglycaemia awareness in patients with long-duration insulin-dependent diabetes. *Lancet* 1994; 344 (8918): 283–7.
69. Tattersall RB. Brittle diabetes revisited: the Third Arnold Bloom Memorial Lecture. *Diabet Med* 1997; 14 (2): 99–110.
70. Tattersall R. Brittle diabetes. *Clin Endocrinol Metab* 1977; 6 (2): 403–19.
71. Kent LA, Gill GV, Williams G. Mortality and outcome of patients with brittle diabetes and recurrent ketoacidosis. *Lancet* 1994; 344 (8925): 778–91.
72. Tattersall R, Gregory R, Selby C, Kerr D, Heller S. Course of brittle diabetes: 12 year follow up. *BMJ* 1991; 302 (6787): 1240–3.

73. Gill GV, Lucas S, Kent LA. Prevalence and characteristics of brittle diabetes in Britain. *QJM* 1996; 89 (11): 839–43.
74. Griffith DN, Yudkin JS. Brittle diabetes in the elderly. *Diabet Med* 1989; 6 (5): 440–3.
75. Gill G, Walford S. The fragile female diabetic. *Diabet Med* 1986; 3 (3): 284.
76. Gill G. Poor glycaemic control in female type 1 adolescents—the "fragile *female diabetic" revisited? Diabet Med* 2002; 19 (8): 699–700; author reply 700–1.
77. Child DF, Williams CP. Lack of relation between glycosylated hemoglobin concentrations and number of daily insulin injections. *BMJ (Clin Res Ed)* 1985; 291 (6502): 1126.
78. Jones RB, Johnston DI, Allison SP, Peacock I, Hosking DJ, Tattersall RB. Hemoglobin A1c concentrations in men and women with diabetes. *BMJ (Clin Res Ed)* 1984; 289 (6455): 1381.
79. Stickland MH, Paton RC, Wales JK. Hemoglobin A1c concentrations in men and women with diabetes. *BMJ (Clin Res Ed)* 1984; 289 (6447): 733.
80. Williams DR. Hospital admissions of diabetic patients: information from hospital activity analysis. *Diabet Med* 1985; 2 (1): 27–32.
81. Hardy KJ, Jones KE, Gill GV. Deterioration in blood glucose control in females with diabetes changed to a basal-bolus regimen using a pen-injector. *Diabet Med* 1991; 8 (1): 69–71.
82. Steel JM, Young RJ, Lloyd GG, Macintyre CC. Abnormal eating attitudes in young insulin-dependent diabetics. *Br J Psychiatry* 1989; 155: 515–21.
83. Barnes PJ, Chung KF. Difficult asthma. *BMJ* 1989; 299 (6701): 695–8.
84. Barnes PJ, Woolcock AJ. Difficult asthma. *Eur Respir J* 1998; 12 (5): 1209–18.
85. Gill GV, Williams G. Brittle Addison's disease: a new variation on a familiar theme. *Postgrad Med J* 2000; 76 (893): 166–7.
86. Meltzer LJ, Johnson SB, Prine JM, Banks RA, Desrosiers PM, Silverstein JH. Disordered eating, body mass, and glycemic control in adolescents with type 1 diabetes. *Diabetes Care* 2001; 24 (4): 678–82.
87. Gill G, Walford S, Alberti KG. Brittle Diabetes-all in the mind? *Diabetologia* 1984; 267: 279A.
88. Campbell IW, Kritz H, Najemnik C, Hagmueller G, Irsigler K. Treatment of type I diabetic with subcutaneous insulin resistance by a totally implantable insulin infusion device ("Infusaid"). *Diabetes Res* 1984; 1 (2): 83–8.
89. Pozza G, Spotti D, Micossi P, Cristallo M, Melandri M, Piatti PM, Monti LD, Pontiroli AE. Long-term continuous intraperitoneal insulin treatment in brittle diabetes. *BMJ (Clin Res Ed)* 1983; 286 (6361): 255–6.
90. Wood DF, Goodchild K, Guillou P, Thomas DJ, Johnston DG. Management of "brittle" diabetes with a preprogrammable implanted insulin pump delivering intraperitoneal insulin. *BMJ* 1990; 301 (6761): 1143–4.
91. Gill GV, Alberti KG. Outcome of brittle diabetes. *BMJ* 1991; 303 (6797): 285–6.
92. Bradley C. Life events and the control of diabetes mellitus. *J Psychosom Res* 1979; 23 (2): 159–62.
93. Rosen H, Lidz T. Emotional factors in the precipitation of recurrent diabetic acidosis. *Psychosom Med* 1949; 11: 211–15.
94. Hinkle LE, Wolf S. Importance of life stress in course and management of diabetes mellitus. *JAMA* 1952; 148: 513–20.
95. Kemmer FW, Bisping R, Steingruber HJ, Baar H, Hardtmann F, Schlaghecke R, Berger M. Psychological stress and metabolic control in patients with type I diabetes mellitus. *N Engl J Med* 1986; 314 (17): 1078–84.
96. Williams G, Pickup J, Keen H. Psychological factors and metabolic control: time for reappraisal? *Diabet Med* 1988; 5 (3): 211–5.
97. Helz JW, Templeton B. Evidence of the role of psychosocial factors in diabetes mellitus: a review. *Am J Psychiatry* 1990; 147 (10): 1275–82.
98. Gale EA. Basic principles in the mangement of unstable diabetic control. In Pickup J (ed) *Brittle Diabetes*. Oxford: Blackwell, 1985; pp 183–99.
99. Brossard JH, Havrankova J, Rioux D, Bertrand S, D'Amour P. Long-term use of intramuscular insulin therapy in a type I diabetic patient with subcutaneous insulin resistance. *Diabet Med* 1993; 10 (2): 174–6.
100. Bayliss J. Brittle diabetes: long-term control with a portable, continuous, intravenous insulin infusion system. *BMJ (Clin Res Ed)* 1981; 283 (6301): 1207–9.
101. Williams G, Pickup JC, Keen H. Continuous intravenous insulin infusion in the management of brittle diabetes: etiologic and therapeutic implications. *Diabetes Care* 1985; 8 (1): 21–7.
102. Husband DJ, Marshall SM, Walford S, Hanning I, Wright PD, Alberti KG. Continuous intraperitoneal insulin infusion in the management of severely brittle diabetes—a metabolic and clinical comparison with intravenous infusion. *Diabet Med* 1984; 1 (2): 99–104.
103. Fonseca VA, Menon RK, O'Brien PM, Fernando ON, Stephen R, Dandona P. Diabetic pregnancy managed with intraperitoneal insulin. *Diabet Med* 1987; 4 (1): 74–6.
104. Schade DS, Eaton RP, Warhol RM, Gregory JA, Doberneck RC. Subcutaneous peritoneal access device for type I diabetic patients nonresponsive to subcutaneous insulin. *Diabetes* 1982; 31 (5, pt 1): 470–3.
105. Stephen RL, Kablitz C, Maxwell JG, Nelson E, Hanover BK, Jacobsen SC. Long-term intraperitoneal insulin administration by multiple injections. *Diabetologia* 1984; 27: 334A–5A.
106. Peacey SR, Burr WA. Management of a case of insulin resistance with an implantable programmable intraperitoneal insulin pump. *Diabet Med* 1992; 9 (suppl 1): 52A.
107. Jeandidier N, et al. Successful pregnancy in severe diabetes. *Lancet* 1992; 339 (8806): 1428.
108. Gill GV, Husband DJ, Wright PD, Sharpe G, Taylor R, Walford S, Marshall SM, Alberti KG. The management of severe brittle diabetes with "Infusaid" implantable pumps. *Diabetes Res* 1986; 3 (3): 135–7.
109. du Toit DF, et al. Pancreatic transplantation in a patient with severe insulin resistance. A case report. *S Afr Med J* 1988; 73 (12): 723–5.
110. Williams G, Pickup JC, Collins AC, Keen H. Prostaglandin E1 accelerates subcutaneous insulin absorption in insulin-dependent diabetic patients. *Diabet Med* 1984; 1 (2): 109–13.
111. Sheldon J, Hollis PR, Trafford JA, Cook JG. Diabetic ketoacidosis due to insulin resistance treated by haemodialysis. *Diabet Med* 1985; 2 (1): 59–60.
112. Antony G, Berdoukas VA, Charlton B, Cooper SG, Gurtunca N, Kelly WH. Plasmapheresis in intractable insulin-resistant diabetes. *Lancet* 1983; 2 (8359): 1148–9.
113. Usala AL, Madigan T, Burguera B, Sinha MK, Caro JF, Cunningham P, Powell JG, Butter PC. Brief report: treatment of insulin-resistant diabetic ketoacidosis with

insulin-like growth factor I in an adolescent with insulin-dependent diabetes. *N Engl J Med* 1992; 327 (12): 853–7.
114. Bello F, Falko JM, O'Dorisio TM, Osei K. The use of continuous subcutaneous octreotide infusion in brittle type 1 diabetic patients. *Diabet Med* 1991; 8 (4): 385–7.
115. Davis SN, Stephenson P. Improvement of recurrent diabetic ketoacidosis due to danazol. *Pract Diabet* 1988; 5: 251.
116. Henderson G. The psychosocial treatment of recurrent diabetic ketoacidosis: an interdisciplinary team approach. *Diabetes Educ* 1991; 17 (2): 119–23.
117. Gill G, Robinson M, Marrow J. Hypoglycaemic brittle diabetes successfully managed by social worker intervention. *Diabet Med* 1989; 6 (5): 448–50.
118. Moran G, Fonagy P, Kurtz A, Bolton A, Brook C. A controlled study of psychoanalytic treatment of brittle diabetes. *J Am Acad Child Adolesc Psychiatry* 1991; 30 (6): 925–35.
119. DeVries JH, Eskes SA, Snoek FJ, Pouwer F, Van Ballegooie E, Spijker AJ, Kostense PJ, Seubert M, Heine RJ. Continuous intraperitoneal insulin infusion in patients with 'brittle' diabetes: favourable effects on glycaemic control and hospital stay. *Diabet Med* 2002; 19 (6): 496–501.
120. Snoek FJ, Skinner TC. Psychological counselling in problematic diabetes: does it help? *Diabet Med* 2002; 19 (4): 265–73.
121. Williams G, Pickup JC. The natural history of brittle diabetes. *Diabetes Res* 1988; 7 (1): 13–8.

88

Diabetes Mellitus, Pregnancy, and Gestational Diabetes

Lois Jovanovic

Sansum Medical Research Foundation, Santa Barbara, CA, USA

TYPE 1 DIABETES MELLITUS AND PREGNANCY

Since the discovery of insulin in 1921, the woman who has been diagnosed with type 1 diabetes mellitus has had improvement in the outcome of her pregnancies. Prior to the advent of insulin, few women with type 1 diabetes survived to the childbearing years. At the Joslin Clinic, during the early years of insulin therapy, Dr Priscilla White devoted her career to children and women with diabetes of juvenile onset. By 1949, she reported [1, 2] 439 pregnancies; however, there was a 25% incidence of spontaneous abortions, 18% fetal loss rate (of these losses 80% were due to stillbirths), and 57% were neonatal deaths. In addition, 80% of the live born infants were macrosomic and metabolically unstable. Dr White concluded early on that "good treatment of diabetes" [2] clearly improved the outcome of pregnancies complicated by diabetes.

In the 1950s, other American centers confirmed Dr White's impression that pregnancy outcome was optimized when attention was paid to "good treatment" [3]. In these reports [4–7] the perinatal deaths ranged from 14 to 30%. Long et al. [8] were the first to state categorically that "excellent diabetic control was needed to carry the pregnancy safely to term."

Meanwhile, the Europeans were also noting that improved glycemic control resulted in improved outcome of pregnancies complicated by diabetes. Oakley and Peel in London [9, 10], Drury in Dublin [11], and Pedersen in Copenhagen [12] all developed treatment plans to improve outcome of pregnancies complicated by diabetes. These investigators reported that they could minimize their perinatal loss rates to 11–13%, by the end of the 1960s, with liberal use of hospitalization to maintain glycemia; Pedersen's work became the foundation for many of the treatment protocols today [12–15]. The importance of good diabetic control derived from a partnership between the obstetrician and internist led to his conclusion that there is a threefold higher fetal/neonatal loss rate when care is given only for a short period. In 1965, he reported an amazingly low rate of 6.9% in 176 pregnancies in patients who had continuous care throughout pregnancy. In addition he coined his quartet of "prognostic bad signs of pregnancy" that identified the highest risk pregnancies: (1) diabetic ketoacidosis, (2) preeclampsia, (3) pyelonephritis, and (4) neglect of prenatal care [16]. In 130 pregnancies with only one of the prognostic bad signs there was a 31% loss rate [17, 18]. The Pedersen hypothesis that related maternal glucose levels to fetal well-being was astutely formulated in 1977 [12] in his classic textbook on diabetes and pregnancy. He wrote in this revered tome,

> The key to many problems is the fact that fetal homeostasis has been disturbed and reset due to maternal hyperglycemia and the ensuing fetal hyperinsulinemia. One consequence is the finding that as a group the infants are at the same time heavy for dates and premature for dates.

In the late 1960s and early 1970s it became clear [19–21] that the higher the mean maternal glucose, the higher the risk for fetal/neonatal loss. The Karlsson and Kjellmer article [21] became the foundation upon which the next level of glycemic control was attempted. Their "normoglycemic" group had only a 3.8% fetal/neonatal loss rate. The next goal was to bring the mortality rate down to that seen in the general population. The initial attempts to completely normalize the 24-h glucose profile

International Textbook of Diabetes Mellitus, Third Edition. Edited by R. A. DeFronzo, E. Ferrannini, H. Keen, and P. Zimmet.
 ISBN: 0-471-48655-8.

were all in hospitalized patients [22–26]. When self blood glucose monitoring became available for outpatient surveillance of glucose control [27], normalization programs could be continued and the use of hospitalizations then could be minimized. By the 1980s, all the metabolic problems of the infant of the diabetic mother were eliminated with normalization of maternal glucose [28–30].

Congenital malformations in the infant of the diabetic mother emerged as the major cause of perinatal loss [31–34]. It was then realized that to minimize the losses due to congenital anomalies, programs to normalize maternal blood glucose needed to begin before conception because organogenesis is complete by the eighth gestational week.

Although today, treatment strategies all adopt the concepts of normoglycemia for the type 1 (insulin-dependent) diabetic woman, the success rate in achieving and maintaining normoglycemia has not been uniform in all centers [35–38]. This review includes one program that has proven over the last 15 years to improve the outcome of pregnancies complicated by diabetes and to equal the outcome of pregnancies seen in the normal population [39]. This study has been validated by the subsequent reports that clearly show that the original report of 1990 remains true [40–42].

PREPREGNANCY PLANNING

The normoglycemia program should ideally begin whenever pregnancy is contemplated by the diabetic woman. The program should include a complete physical and laboratory workup, with attention to pregnancy-related risk factors of (1) eye status, (2) kidney status, and (3) cardiovascular status. Although evidence of disease in any of these organ systems is not an absolute contraindication to pregnancy, there is an increased risk of complications for both mother and child (independent of glucose) if any pathology is present [43]. The glucose-related treatment program needs time. Until the woman's blood glucose levels are ideal to insure the best possible start of a pregnancy, adequate birth control must be prescribed. Most reports indicate that low dose oral contraceptives are safe and effective for the type 1 (insulin-dependent) diabetic woman [44].

The literature suggests [31–36, 38, 45–47] that a glycosylated hemoglobin level that is within 4 SDs above the mean of a nondiabetic population minimizes the risk of spontaneous abortion and congenital malformations. Diabetic women as a group have a spontaneous-abortion rate similar to that of the general population; however, when the preconception blood glucose is elevated, the risk of spontaneous abortion rises. It has been shown that diabetic women with poor glycemic control in the periconception period and early in pregnancy have increased spontaneous-abortion rate. In addition, women with excellent diabetes control actually have a lower spontaneous-abortion rate than does the general population [36]. Several investigators have shown a correlation between an increase in spontaneous-abortion rate with increasing values of first-trimester glycosylated hemoglobin [35–37]. The glycosylated hemoglobin is only a rough measure of glycemic control and reflects the mean blood glucose values only in the preceding 4–8 weeks. Albumin, however, also is glycosylated when exposed to glucose and because it has a higher turnover rate than does the glycosylated hemoglobin, albumin measurements reflect the mean blood glucose values in the preceding 2–4 weeks. Using this assay, Miodovnik and coworkers [48] showed that women who later had spontaneous abortions had significantly elevated glycosylated hemoglobin levels at about 8 weeks of gestation, but no elevation of either glycosylated albumin or glycosylated total protein. They therefore concluded that spontaneous abortion was related to poor glycemic control around the time of conception rather than control immediately before the abortion occurred. In general, diabetic women with good glycemic control before conception have a spontaneous-abortion rate approximately equal to that of the general population, thus emphasizing the role for preconception counseling.

Congenital malformations can be divided into three categories: (1) malformations incompatible with life, (2) major malformations, and (3) minor malformations. Major malformations, defined as those that significantly affect the health of the child or require surgical correction, have been reported in 4–11% of infants of diabetic mothers compared with only 1.2–2.1% of infants of nondiabetic women [34, 38, 46, 47]. Retrospective and prospective studies have shown that poor glycemic control in the early weeks of gestation was correlated with an increase in malformations [34–48]. The cause of these diabetes-related malformations is still unclear. A number of studies have been carried out in different animal models, with the aim of discovering mechanisms that may be operative in human diabetic pregnancy. Many of these studies implicate glucose as the major teratogen. The human studies, however, do not clearly implicate glucose as the sole teratogen. Organogenesis is completed by the sixth week after conception [49], and thus the critical period for malformation is almost over at the time pregnancy becomes clinically apparent. The fact that organogenesis is completed before most women recognize that they are pregnant adds further merit to the need for preconceptional counseling in diabetic women. Although the literature strongly supports the relationship between hyperglycemia and increased prevalence of malformations, the controversial Diabetes in Early Pregnancy (DIEP) Study failed to confirm the claim that glycemic control is related to congenital malformation [50]. There is an alternative way of interpreting the data in this study, however. If only the severely handicapping malformations, the lethal malformations, and the malformations classically attributed to diabetes are considered, and the nonspecific pathologic characteristics that may or may not be caused by hyperglycemia are ignored, it can be seen that almost 80% of the malformations reported in the DIEP Study occurred beyond 3 SDs above the normal mean glycosylated hemoglobin. In addition, over 50% of the mothers who gave birth to malformed infants had peri-conception glycosylated hemoglobin levels beyond 6 SDs above the mean [51]. Also, poorer glycemic control could explain the higher malformation rate of 9% seen in the late-entry group if one assumes that before coming for care these diabetic women were in poorer control than did the early-entry group. Thus all the articles cited earlier, even the DIEP Study, suggest that poor glycemic control explains some, if not all, diabetes-associated malformations. This includes the metabolic abnormalities associated with low insulin levels.

PROTOCOLS TO ACHIEVE NORMOGLYCEMIA IN THE PREPREGNANT DIABETIC WOMAN

In the moderately active nonpregnant woman, the insulin requirement is about 0.6 units/kg/day [52]. We affectionately call this 24-h need the "Big I." The "Big I" is equal to the total 24-h insulin requirement and comprises the basal dosage (the insulin requirement necessary to maintain normoglycemia when the woman is not eating) and the meal-related insulin dosage. For a 60-kg woman, the 24-h insulin requirement is 36 units/day. Our standing orders are shown in Table 1. These orders are an example of the methods to calculate doses of insulin for insulin-sensitive women with a stable body weight. The initially calculated dose is evaluated by eight blood glucose determinations a day (before and after the meal, before bedtime, and at 3:00 a.m.).

These orders allow for the adjustment of each of the injections daily. The percent change for the sliding scales is 3% of the total insulin requirement. The initial calculations divide "Big I" into 4/9 I as neutral protamine Hagedorn (NPH) before breakfast, 2/9 I as regular insulin (or the fast-acting insulin analogue, lispro or aspart, now that the literature is emerging that these analogues are safe; see discussion below and references 53 and 54) before breakfast, 1/6 I as regular insulin (or the fast-acting insulin analogue, lispro or aspart) before dinner, and 1/6 I as NPH before bedtime. Timings of the injections and the meals are key if regular insulin is used. If the regular insulin is injected too close to a meal plan with a high carbohydrate content, the blood sugars swing from high to low. A lag time of 30–45 min between injection and a breakfast of 30% or less of carbohydrate, complete with a mid-morning snack, produces normoglycemia. The use of fast-acting insulin analogues completely eliminates this timing problem. Note that the sliding scale stops at 140 mg/dl. We have not increased our sliding scales to give higher doses of regular insulin above 140 mg/dl, for large doses of regular or fast-acting insulin analogues may produce severe hypoglycemia. It is gentler to take insulin in two separate doses spaced several hours apart than try to "conquer hyperglycemia" by a large dose of insulin. We suggest that a woman who has a high glucose level before the meal take enough insulin to normalize her blood glucose and wait to eat until her blood glucose is less than 120 mg/dl. If her blood glucose level is not low enough to eat 2 h after the injection, then she may supplement the dose of insulin with 2–4 units of extra insulin and continue to wait for the insulin to lower her blood glucose to less than 120 mg/dl. If a woman cannot wait until her blood glucose is less than 120 mg/dl, then she may eat the protein and fat portions of her meal plan and save the carbohydrates and use them as dessert to extend the waiting period as long as possible. The lunchtime dose of insulin suggested in Table 1 is intended to be a "touch up" and would only be necessary if the blood glucose is high before lunch. Once the doses of breakfast NPH and regular (or fast-acting) insulin that normalize the blood glucose are achieved, there may not be a need for a lunchtime "touch up" dose of regular or fast-acting insulin, although others prefer to have the women take a daily dose of regular (or fast-acting) insulin before lunch to allow for flexibility of the meal plan's composition. Each dose of insulin will be changed as outlined in the established orders shown in Table 1. A special note needs to be made about adjusting the NPH at bedtime. This NPH dose at bedtime requires three blood glucose checks before it can be safely adjusted. The NPH dose before bedtime is designed to "fix the fasting" or "conquer" the wake-up blood glucose for the following morning. Other forces come into play, however, which may make the interpretation of a high fasting blood glucose difficult. There are six ways to end up with a high fasting blood glucose level:

(1) One can go to bed with a high glucose level because of a persisting high level at dinner, and the level will remain elevated all night long. The cause is not enough regular (or fast-acting) insulin at dinner or too much food at dinner.
(2) One can go to bed with a normal blood glucose level, but have a bedtime snack, which then produces the high wake-up glucose level. This can be avoided by having a smaller bedtime snack.
(3) One can go to bed with a normal blood glucose level, but "drift up" throughout the night because the bedtime NPH dose was not sufficient to prevent this rise.
(4) One can go to bed with a normal blood glucose level, become hypoglycemic in the middle of the night, and wake up with a high level because of a nice

Table 1 Prepregnancy (nonpregnant) routine NPH plus regular or fast-acting insulin orders

Nurse will calculate and administer the starting dose of insulin as outlined below:

"Big I" = Total daily insulin = 0.6 × weight kg/24 h = ______

Divide so that 4/9 of "Big I" is NPH given before breakfast
1/6 of "Big I" is NPH given before bedtime
2/9 of "Big I" is regular or fast-acting insulin given before breakfast
1/6 of "Big I" is regular or fast-acting insulin given before dinner
Amount of regular or fast-acting insulin is titrated based on the blood glucose (BG)

Prebreakfast: NPH = 4/9 "Big I" = ______

Check predinner BG to adjust for the next day morning NPH dose
If the predinner BG < 70, then decrease the morning NPH by 2 units
If the predinner BG = 71–120, then no change in the morning NPH
If the predinner BG > 121, then increase the morning NPH by 2 units

Regular or fast-acting (lispro or aspart) = 2/9 "Big I" adjusted based on BG

BG <70 = ______ = (2/9 "Big I" dose) − 3% "Big I"
71–100 = ______ = 2/9 "Big I" dose
101–140 = ______ = (2/9 "Big I" dose) + 3% "Big I"
>141 = ______ = (2/9 "Big I") + 6% "Big I"

Check the BG 1 h after the start of breakfast to adjust for the next day prebreakfast dose
If the BG 1 h after the meal is <110, then decrease the next day prebreakfast regular or fast-acting insulin by 2 units
If the BG 1 h after the meal is 111–150, then no change in the next day prebreakfast regular fast-acting insulin doses
If the BG 1 h after the meal is >151, then increase the next day prebreakfast regular or fast-acting insulin by 2 units

Prelunch: Regular or fast-acting insulin (lispro or aspart) is given based on the BG
BG <120 = no insulin
121–140 = ______ = 1/18 "Big I"
141–180 = ______ = 1/18 "Big I" + 2 units
>181 = ______ = 1/18 "Big I" + 4 units

Predinner: Regular or fast-acting insulin (aspart or lispro) dose is 1/6 "Big I" adjusted based on the BG
BG <70 = ______ = (1/6 "Big I") – 3% of "Big I"
71–100 = ______ = 1/6 "Big I"
101–140 = ______ = (1/6 "Big I") + 3% of "Big I"
>141 = ______ = (1/6 "Big I") + 6% of "Big I"

Check the BG 1 h after the start of dinner to adjust for the next day predinner dose
If the BG 1 h after dinner is <110, then decrease the next day predinner insulin by 2 units
If the BG 1 h after dinner is 111–150, then no change in the next day predinner insulin
If the BG 1 h after dinner is >151, then increase the next day insulin by 2 units

Bedtime NPH: Give 1/6 of "Big I"______

Test 3 a.m. BG
Check prebreakfast, HS (hour of sleep), and initially the 3 a.m. BG to adjust the HS insulin
If the prebreakfast BG is <70, then decrease the bedtime NPH by 2 units
If the prebreakfast BG is 71–120, then no change in the bedtime NPH
If the prebreakfast BG is >121, then increase the bedtime NPH by 2 units
If the HS, 3 a.m., and prebreakfast BG are >121, decrease the bedtime NPH by 2 units
If the HS and 3 a.m. BG are 70–120 but the prebreakfast BG is >121, then increase the bedtime NPH by 2 units

counterregulatory response to the low sugar. The cause is too much bedtime NPH or an inadequate bedtime snack.

(5) One can go to bed with a high glucose level, but still have a hypoglycemic reaction in the middle of the night, mount a counterregulatory response, and wake up with a high glucose level. The cause is not enough regular or fast-acting insulin at dinner (or too much dinner) and too much bedtime NPH.

(6) One can have a normal bedtime level and stay normal until after 3 a.m., when the blood glucose rises with increasing insulin needs (the Dawn phenomenon). More bedtime insulin is needed. Thus, the adjustment of the bedtime dose of NPH requires all three readings: bedtime, 3 a.m., and wake-up blood glucose.

If the wake-up blood glucose is low (less than 70 mg/dl) then the bedtime NPH dose should be decreased by 2 units.

If the wake-up blood glucose is high and if the previous night's bedtime and 3 a.m. levels were also high, then the NPH should be increased at bedtime by 2 units. If the 3 a.m. glucose is low, no matter what the bedtime or the wake-up blood glucose was, the bedtime dose of NPH needs to be cut back. Here, the physician would need to write separate orders to indicate if the quantity of food at dinner or for the bedtime snack should be adjusted. These established orders would also increase the NPH dose before bedtime if the wake-up blood glucose is high but the bedtime and 3 a.m. blood glucose levels are normal, because there is room for a little more bedtime NPH insulin to "conquer" the fasting.

One additional order that can speed the normalization process is to prescribe regular insulin at 3 a.m. After all, if the blood glucose is high at 3 a.m., it definitely will be high at 7:30 a.m. Therefore, a convenient and worthwhile addition to these orders is a sliding scale for regular insulin at 3 a.m., which is the same at the lunchtime "touch-up":

BG $<120 = 0$

$121–140 = 1/18$ "Big I"

$141–180 = 1/18$ "Big I" $+ 2$ units

$>181 = 1/18$ "Big I" $+ 4$ units

Compliance with this 3 a.m. regular insulin injection is excellent because the frustration associated with a high wake-up blood glucose is easily resolved when the woman can make decisions at night to assure that the fasting blood glucose will be normal. If a woman is able to check her 3 a.m. blood glucose only three or four times a week, when the majority of the week's fasting blood glucose levels are normal, the glycosylated hemoglobin level improves in parallel. As suggested by other authors, adding a bedtime dose of regular insulin along with a bedtime snack does not produce consistent results. We also feel that a bedtime "touch up" of regular or fast-acting insulin is dangerous. Between 11 p.m. and 3 a.m., patients are exquisitely sensitive to regular or fast-acting insulin. It is better to leave a high bedtime glucose level untreated, but wake the patient at 3 a.m. and give the extra insulin if the blood glucose is still elevated because the blood glucose will rise spontaneously from 3 a.m. onward [52].

MEDICAL NUTRITIONAL THERAPY FOR DIABETES AND PREGNANCY

This protocol for standing insulin orders was designed to go hand in hand with a 40% carbohydrate diet. The reason a 40% carbohydrate diet (20% protein and 40% fat) is prescribed is that the calculation for the relationship between regular insulin and grams of carbohydrate in the meal plan is very easy. A 60-kg woman requires 30 kcal/kg/day or 1800 cal of which 40% is carbohydrate [or 180 g of carbohydrate calculated by taking 40% of (1800 divided by 4 kcal/g carbohydrate)]. One unit of regular or fast-acting insulin will cover approximately 10 g of carbohydrate at lunch and dinner (however it takes approximately 1.5 units of regular or fast-acting insulin to cover 10 g of carbohydrate at breakfast) and thus matching the insulin dose to the meal plan is facilitated [52].

FIRST-TRIMESTER INSULIN REQUIREMENTS AND THEREAFTER

Once the woman's blood glucose levels have been documented to be in the target ranges associated with a lower risk of complications, more frequent interaction between the patient and the health care team is necessary. When the target glycosylated hemoglobin (within 4 SDs above the mean of a normal population [51]) is achieved, it is safe to attempt to conceive. It is helpful to use a basal body temperature thermometer to allow the couple to optimize the chances of conception. After ovulation occurs, as indicated by a persistent rise of basal body temperature, the team "pretends" the woman is pregnant and helps with daily insulin adjustments. Once the woman has missed her period by 1 day and her temperature remains elevated, then an early pregnancy test is ordered. If the pregnancy test is positive then the pregnancy insulin orders are undertaken (Table 2).

The first-trimester insulin doses are recalculated to be 0.7 units/kg/24 h. The target blood glucose levels are lower in pregnancy and thus the standing orders (Table 2) are designed to achieve and maintain these lower glucose levels: fasting and preprandial glucose levels, 60–90 mg/dl; and 1 h after meals, <120 mg/dl. These target glucose levels have been associated with decreased risk of macrosomia [27–29, 55]. There is a smooth rise of insulin requirement throughout pregnancy [28] and thus by the second trimester the insulin requirement is 0.8 unit/kg/day, by the third trimester it is 0.9 units/kg/day, and by term it is 1.0 unit/kg/day.

As is the case with the prepregnancy insulin orders, these insulin orders during pregnancy are also designed to "match" a calculated diet that is calculated as 30 kcal/kg/day for a normal weight (80–120% ideal body weight) woman and is divided into 40% carbohydrate, 40% fat, and 20% protein. This diet is then subdivided into three meals and frequent small snacks (Table 3). When women are overweight, fewer calories are needed per present pregnant weight: 24 cal/kg/day for a woman 120–150% over ideal body weight and 12 cal/kg/day for woman greater than 150% over ideal body weight [56]. The rationale for the 30-kcal/kg/day diet is that it has been shown that this caloric intake will result in 22–28 lb weight gain for the entire pregnancy.

Table 2 Pregnancy (nonpregnant) routine NPH plus regular or fast-acting insulin orders

Nurse will calculate and administer the starting dose of insulin as outlined below:

"*Big I*" = Total daily insulin = Weeks 5–12 = 0.6 × weight kg/24 h = ______
12–24 = 0.6 × weight kg/24 h = ______
24–28 = 0.6 × weight kg/24 h = ______
28–36 = 0.6 × weight kg/24 h = ______
36–40 = 0.6 × weight kg/24 h = ______

Divide "Big I" such that 4/9 of "Big I" is NPH given before breakfast
1/6 of "Big I" is NPH given before bedtime
2/9 of "Big I" is regular or fast-acting insulin given before breakfast
1/6 of "Big I" is regular or fast-acting insulin given before dinner
Amount of regular or fast-acting insulin is titrated based on the blood glucose (BG)

Prebreakfast: NPH = 4/9 "Big I" = ______
Check predinner BG to adjust for the next day morning NPH dose
If the predinner BG < 60, then decrease the morning NPH by 2 units
If the predinner BG = 61–90, then no change in the morning NPH
If the predinner BG > 91, then increase the morning NPH by 2 units

Regular or fast-acting (lispro or aspart) = 2/9 "Big I" adjusted based on BG

BG <60 = ______ = (2/9 "Big I" dose) − 3% "Big I"
61–90 = ______ = 2/9 "Big I" dose
91–120 = ______ = (2/9 "Big I" dose) + 3% "Big I"
>121 = ______ = (2/9 "Big I") + 6% "Big I"

Check the BG 1 h after the start of breakfast to adjust for the next day prebreakfast dose
If the BG 1 h after the meal is <90, then decrease the next day prebreakfast regular or fast-acting insulin by 2 units
If the BG 1 h after the meal is 91–120, then no change in the next day prebreakfast regular or fast-acting insulin dose
If the BG 1 h after the meal is >121, then in the next day prebreakfast regular or fast-acting insulin by 2 units

Prelunch: Regular or fast-acting insulin (lispro or aspart) is given based on the BG
BG <90 = no insulin
91–120 = ______ = 3% "Big I"
121–140 = ______ = 6% "Big I" + 2 units
>141 = ______ = 9% "Big I" + 4 units

Predinner: Regular or fast-acting insulin (aspart or lispro) dose is 1/6 "Big I" adjusted based on the BG
BG <60 = ______ = (1/6 "Big I") − 3% of "Big I"
61–90 = ______ = 1/6 "Big I"
91–120 = ______ = (1/6 "Big I") + 3% of "Big I"
>121 = ______ = (1/6 "Big I") + 6% of "Big I"
Check the BG 1 h after the start of dinner to adjust for the next day predinner dose
If the BG 1 h after dinner is <90, then decrease the next day predinner insulin by 2 units
If the BG 1 h after dinner is 91–120, then no change in the next day predinner insulin
If the BG 1 h after dinner is >121, then increase the next day insulin by 2 units

Bedtime NPH: Give 1/6 of "Big I"______

Test 3 a.m. BG
Check prebreakfast, HS (hour of sleep), and initially the 3 a.m. BG to adjust the HS insulin
If the prebreakfast BG is <60, then decrease the bedtime NPH by 2 units
If the prebreakfast BG is 61–90, then no change in the bedtime NPH
If the prebreakfast BG is >121, then increase the bedtime NPH by 2 units
If the HS, 3 a.m., and prebreakfast BG are >121, decrease the bedtime NPH by 2 units
If the HS and 3 a.m. BG are 70–120 but the prebreakfast BG is >121, then increase the bedtime NPH by 2 units

For a type 1 diabetic woman on an insulin pump, the basal infusion rate is calculated as one half of the total daily dose (based on weight and gestational week as above) but the meal-related insulin dose is calculated as insulin to carbohydrate ratio (1 unit/10 g of carbohydrate at lunch and dinner and 1.5 units/10 g of carbohydrate at breakfast) [57–66] (Table 4). Only carbohydrate need be equated with units of regular or fast-acting insulin. Overlapping insulin covers the glucose that is slowly converted from protein. Patients need only to count grams of carbohydrate in order to deviate from the very rigid distribution of calories shown in Table 3.

Table 3 The "euglycemic diet" for gestational diabetic women: calorie distribution to maintain normoglycemia and diet calculation for women 80–120% of ideal body weight*

Time	Meal	Fraction (kcal/24 h)	% of daily carbohydrate allowed
8:00 a.m.	Breakfast	2/18	10
10:30 a.m.	Snack	1/18	5
12:00 p.m.	Lunch	5/18	30
3:00 p.m.	Snack	2/18	10
5:00 p.m.	Dinner	5/18	30
8:00 p.m.	Snack	2/18	5
11:00 p.m.	Snack	1/18	10

* For women less than 80% of their ideal body weight, calculate as 40 kcal/kg/day; for women 120–150% above ideal body weight, calculate as 18 kcal/kg/day; and for women greater than 150% above ideal body weight, calculate as 12 k cal/kg/day. (adapted from reference 52, Table 29)

CLINIC VISITS

The frequency of clinic visits is determined by the degree of glycemic control attained by patients on an outpatient basis. Those in good control may be seen in clinic weekly, while those in less than optimal control may need to be admitted to the hospital. Since normoglycemia throughout pregnancy is the therapeutic goal, there are strict standards set for defining good diabetic control. All the following criteria must be met, or control is classified as suboptimal: fasting blood glucose, 55–65 mg/dl (60–75 mg/dl plasma); mean/24-h, 80–87 mg/dl (90–100 mg/dl plasma); 1-h postprandial, <120 mg/dl (<140 mg/dl plasma); and glycosylated hemoglobin within laboratory normal range for pregnancy. These glucose targets are the normal glucose concentrations seen in pregnancy [27]. Management of the pregnant diabetic woman becomes a process of constant surveillance as term approaches. In the past, the greater incidence of sudden intrauterine death in pregnant diabetic women often prompted elective termination after 34–38 weeks of gestation. In view of the fact that 80% of preterm infants have some form of morbidity, the current aim is to delay delivery, when possible, at least until pulmonary maturity has been attained and documented. This can usually be done as long as maternal health and normoglycemia are maintained, fetal stability documented by antepartum fetal surveillance, and the patient reports no sudden decrease in fetal movement.

Table 4 Basal insulin pump program*

Period	Basal requirement	Rationale
Hourly infusion rate		
12:00–4:00 a.m.	50% less basal ($B/24 \times 0.5$)	Maternal cortisol at nadir
4:00–10:00 a.m.	50% more basal ($B/24 \times 1.5$)	Maternal cortisol at peak
10:00–12:00 a.m.	Basal (B/24)	

Note: To refine basal settings, have the patient perform self blood glucose monitoring at the end of each period to determine whether adjustments are needed. For instance, at the 4:00 a.m. test, blood glucose should be 60–90 mg/dl. If blood glucose is out of this range, dial up or down insulin in increments of 0.10 units/h. (Consider using 0.1 units/kg as NPH insulin at bedtime to prevent diabetic ketoacidosis secondary to needle slippage. Then decrease the overnight basal from 4:00 a.m. to 10:00 a.m. by 0.02 units/kg/h.)

* Using human regular, insulin lispro, or insulin aspart, whereas basal (B) equals one half of total daily insulin dose (I) or $B = (1/2)I$ or an hourly rate of B/24.

The insulin requirement may drop during the last 4 weeks of the pregnancy. As the fetus grows the glucose shunted to the fetus accelerates and the overnight insulin requirement falls if the bedtime snack is not sufficient to sustain the fetal needs. As the overnight insulin requirement falls, the daytime insulin requirement may continue to rise and thus the daily needs may not change, only the distribution. The daytime needs will change if the woman finds that her ability to eat a substantial meal is impaired by her enlarging uterus. Rapidly falling insulin requirements not explained by these two phenomena are ominous, however, and concern for the well-being of the fetus should initiate immediate testing and a decision about immediate delivery.

Timing of the final admission for intensive daily fetal surveillance and delivery depends on the quality of glucose control throughout the pregnancy. Delivery decisions are also preferably based on accurate dating information gathered throughout pregnancy. Patients being considered for induction should have fetal pulmonary maturity confirmed by amniotic fluid testing when possible, particularly when glucose control has been suboptimal, or dates are unsure. A trend toward decreasing maternal insulin requirements must be followed up by daily antepartum fetal surveillance if these tests are not already in progress.

LABOR AND DELIVERY

Maintenance of normoglycemia continues to dominate patient management during labor and delivery, to assure the best possible outcome of pregnancy [67]. The night before labor the usual doses of NPH insulin is given. Then, on the day of induction no subcutaneous insulin should be given. Insulin requirements are relatively high before active labor begins, with no need for glucose infusion. When active labor (3 contractions/10 min lasting 60 s each) is established, insulin requirements decrease to 0 and the glucose infusion rate needs to be increased to 2.55 mg/kg/min to maintain normoglycemia during active labor. Guided by hourly blood glucose determinations, glucose and insulin administration are regulated to maintain normoglycemia (80–100 mg/dl) throughout labor.

ELECTIVE CESAREAN SECTION

The following guidelines should be followed for a scheduled elective cesarean section [52]:

(1) give usual bedtime NPH insulin the night before surgery;

(2) give same NPH (bedtime) dose the morning of surgery; and every 8 h before delayed surgery;
(3) monitor fingerstick blood glucose hourly before surgery, and throughout surgery using two-tone visual-read strips or a reflectance meter. Keep blood glucose level at 80–100 mg/dl;
(4) manage intravenous infusions and insulin as in spontaneous labor. If the blood glucose level is greater than 120 mg/dl, an alternative protocol for lowering the glucose level is to start a constant infusion of insulin at a rate of 0.05 units/kg/h and increase the rate of infusion of insulin until the glucose level is stabilized at a blood glucose level near 10 mg/dl. If additional fluid is needed, give as normal saline.

POSTPARTUM MANAGEMENT

Bear in mind that insulin requirements may drop precipitously in the immediate postpartum, and remain much lower for 48–96 h. Any suspected postpartum infections should be cultured, and aggressively treated. In addition, pregestational diabetic women should have a repeat ophthalmologic examination regardless of the degree of retinopathy during the pregnancy. Those woman who did have evidence of retinopathy by their examinations performed every trimester need special attention at this moment, although retinopathy that has developed during pregnancy tends to regress in the postpartum state [68], and advice as to the follow-up plans for the best eye care. Postpartum care should be routine with a calculated diet based on 25 cal/kg/day of 20% protein, 40% carbohydrate, and 40% fat if not breastfeeding. Diet should be calculated on the basis of postpartum weight, and should be divided into antepartum meal and snack proportions. pregestational diabetic women's total daily insulin should be calculated on the basis of postpartum body weight: 0.6 unit/kg/day if not breastfeeding. NPH and regular or fast-acting insulins are divided in the same proportions and doses as antepartum insulin. The blood glucose level is checked five times a day (fasting, 1-h postmeals, and 1-h before dinner).

INSULIN AND DIET FOR NURSING MOTHERS

The caloric requirement for a nursing mother is approximately 27 kcal/kg/24 h. These calories should be divided as usual; however, the feeding routine of each infant will directly impact on the mother's feeding schedule [69]. Specifically, if baby consumes a majority of its calories at bedtime or in the middle of the night, then the mother must also consume her calories then. Thus, many women need only a few units of NPH insulin before bedtime and some can stop the bedtime NPH insulin dose entirely. The daytime insulin requirement remains approximately the same (5/6 of the daily dose at 0.6 × weight in kg) with the morning NPH and regular or fast-acting insulin still 2/3 of the daily dose, dinner regular or fast-acting insulin 1/6 of the daily dose, and the bedtime NPH insulin omitted (which would have been 1/6 of the daily doses).

GESTATIONAL DIABETES MELLITUS

Gestational diabetes mellitus (GDM) is defined as carbohydrate intolerance of varying degrees of severity recognized with onset of or during pregnancy [70, 71], regardless of whether insulin is used for treatment or the condition persists after the pregnancy. This diagnosis does not apply to pregnant women with previously diagnosed diabetes. Gestational diabetes has been well recognized for decades [72], but the potential significance of the condition as well as criteria for screening and diagnosis remain controversial. Until such time as universal multinational screening and diagnostic criteria are adopted, we are left with several sets of criteria that are in current use around the globe, and these criteria remain in a state of flux. In addition, once the diagnosis is made, there is controversy as to the optimal monitoring and treatment strategy. It is apparent that even mild degrees of hyperglycemia may result in fetal developmental defects [61].

EPIDEMIOLOGY

Gestational diabetes is a common obstetrical complication afflicting 1–14% of the pregnant population or approximately 135 000 women per year in the United States [73]. Insulin resistance occurs to some degree in all normal pregnancies [74], but those women who are unable to compensate develop GDM. Women at greatest risk of developing GDM are those who are obese, over 25 years of age, have a previous history of abnormal glucose metabolism or poor obstetric outcome, have first-degree relatives with diabetes, or are members of certain ethnic groups with very high prevalence rates of diabetes. Fetal macrosomia, defined as an oversized baby with a birth weight that is either >90th percentile for gestational age and sex or ≥2 SDs above the normal mean weight [74], may affect up to 40% of the offspring of pregnancies complicated by GDM in those series in which only preprandial glucose was measured or no care was given [75]. One study observed macrosomia in 17.9% of the offspring of pregnancies complicated by gestational diabetes despite treatment compared with 5.6% of control subjects [76]. The other neonatal complications result from the macrosomia. The greatest danger of macrosomia lies in its association with increased risk of birth injuries and asphyxia [77, 78]. Birth trauma is a direct result of the large size of the fetus [79]. Accrual of fat that is deposited differentially in the trunk with preponderance in the shoulder girdle causes dystocia (impedance of delivery of the infant because the shoulder locks onto the pubic bone after the head has passed through the birth canal, resulting in injury of the cephalic vessels and nerves). The risk of shoulder dystocia is increased by as much as 30-fold in pregnancies complicated by diabetes when the infants weigh more than 4500 g [80]. When the obstetrician delivers the infant early to stop the accelerated growth and thus to deliver a smaller baby, complications related to prematurity, such as hyperbilirubinemia, erythremia, hypocalcemia, and respiratory distress [81], may result. Ever after birth, the infant of a woman with gestational diabetes is still at higher risk of developing obesity, impaired glucose tolerance, or diabetes at an early age [82–84]. This appears to be the result of the hyperglycemic intrauterine environment superimposed on a genetic predisposition to diabetes [85, 86].

The maternal complications of GDM include pregnancy-associated hypertension, higher rates of preeclampsia, and urinary tract infections [87]. Although these complications of mother and infant are associated with gestational diabetes, to date there is no evidence showing that prevention and rigorous treatment of gestational diabetes result in minimizing these complications. Given the current recommended standards of care [88, 89], it is unlikely that such studies could ethically be done today. The risk of subsequent gestational diabetes occurring after one pregnancy complicated by gestational diabetes is reported to be 60–90%, depending on the woman's first-trimester weight in the subsequent pregnancies [90]. In addition, after a pregnancy complicated by gestational diabetes, the mother has an increased risk of developing type 2 diabetes. In one study, by 7–10 years postpartum, 30% of women had developed diabetes or impaired glucose tolerance.

OPTIMAL SCREENING AND DIAGNOSTIC STRATEGIES

Table 5 shows the most commonly recommended screening and diagnostic criteria for GDM. Most of the world uses some modification of the criteria of the World Health Organization (WHO) [71], which are based on a glucose load of 75 g. The same test load and the same criteria for diagnosis of diabetes and impaired glucose tolerance are used in nonpregnant adults, with the recommendation that even the diagnosis of gestational impaired glucose tolerance should alert the physician to the high-risk nature of the pregnancy, and that gestational impaired glucose tolerance should be treated in the same way as gestational diabetes [71]. These criteria, therefore, make the diagnosis of gestational diabetes at the lowest glucose concentrations. Several studies have shown that the WHO criteria [91–93] identify more adverse outcomes than do other criteria.

Table 5 Criteria for the diagnosis of gestational diabetes mellitus

Time	NDDG*	ADA†	WHO‡	IGT‡	Diabetes
Fasting	105	95	95	—	140
1-h	190	180	180	—	—
2-h	165	155	155	140	200
3-h	145	140	—	—	—

Note: Glucose load for oral glucose tolerance test – NDDG, 100 g; ADA, 100 g; WHO, 75 g; IGT, 75 g; Diabetes, 75 g. Values in this table are in mg/dl.

* NDDG = National Diabetes Data Group. Two or more concentrations as high as or higher than those shown make the diagnosis of gestational diabetes [92].

† ADA = American Diabetes Association. May be done as primary test or only if screening glucose 1 h after a 50-g oral glucose load ≥140 mg/dl. Two or more concentrations as high as or higher than those shown make the diagnosis of gestational diabetes [70].

‡ WHO = World Health Organization; IGT = Impaired glucose tolerance. See reference 71.

The WHO, however, has no recommendation for routine screening of diabetes during pregnancy.

In the United States and a few centers scattered around the world the criteria endorsed by the National Diabetes Data Group [92] and the American Diabetes Association [70] are in general use. At the Fourth International Workshop-Conference on Gestational Diabetes Mellitus, sponsored by the American Diabetes Association, the glucose concentrations considered diagnostic of gestational diabetes were lowered [70]. This change was made more than a decade after these criteria were originally proposed. During the intervening years, data were generated, suggesting that lower degrees of glucose intolerance were associated with increased risk of adverse perinatal outcome [70]. Gestational diabetes is now diagnosed as two or more numbers above a fasting plasma glucose of 95 mg/dl, a 1-h post 100-g oral glucose load of 180 mg/dl, a 2-h post glucose load of 155 mg/dl, and a 3-h post glucose load of 140 mg/dl. However, the recommendation to test all pregnant women was removed. Therefore women who appear to be at low risk by lacking all the risk factors for GDM will no longer be screened. This includes women who are members of ethnic groups with a low prevalence of GDM, who have no known diabetes in first-degree relatives, are below 25 years of age, were of normal weight before pregnancy, and have no history of abnormal glucose metabolism and no history of a poor obstetric outcome [70]. While still recommending the use of a 100-g glucose load for diagnosis, criteria for glucose concentrations following a 75-g load were endorsed as an alternative.

The confusion of having different recommendations for screening and diagnosis of gestational diabetes, along with periodic changes in the recommendations, has made it difficult for the physician to know what is best for his or her patients. To date, the attempt to relate glucose thresholds to pregnancy outcome has been sparse; thus the guidelines by necessity have been somewhat arbitrary. New data should provide a basis for the development of international agreements on the best criteria for diagnosing GDM and the best protocol for identifying women at risk. The recommendation of the Fourth International Workshop-Conference on Gestational Diabetes allows some women to go untested during pregnancy [70]. In an identified low-risk group, the risk of gestational diabetes is less than 2%.

IMPORTANCE OF BLOOD GLUCOSE MONITORING FOR GESTATIONAL DIABETIC WOMEN

There are three articles in the literature that suggest that the risk of macrosomia rises as the postprandial glucose increases [75, 94, 95]. Therefore, although therapy begins with diet, insulin therapy should be initiated when peak postprandial response exceeds this target [51].

Women with gestational diabetes have been known to deliver very large newborns despite only modest elevations of glucose as determined by whole blood capillary glucose [96]. Continuous glucose monitoring system (CGMS) use has enabled the detection of previously missed postprandial blood glucose peaks in gestational diabetes [97]. We used CGMS in 10 gestational diabetic women and discovered that, on average, the women spent 1.8 h/day with glucose concentrations greater than or equal to 120 mg/dl. CGMS in these women revealed high postprandial blood glucose levels that were previously unrecognized by intermittent fingerstick evaluation [97]. Further research using CGMS in gestational diabetes may finally put to rest the controversy as to the role of maternal hyperglycemia in the etiology of neonatal macrosomia.

DIETS DESIGNED TO MINIMIZE POSTPRANDIAL GLYCEMIA FOR GESTATIONAL DIABETIC WOMEN

Diabetic fetopathy that is a result of maternal postprandial hyperglycemia can be minimized when the peak postprandial response is blunted [96, 98]. The peak postprandial response is best blunted when the meal plan restricts carbohydrates [99]. The optimal dietary prescription would be a diet that provides the caloric and nutrient needs to sustain pregnancy but does not cause postprandial hyperglycemia. To date, there are no randomized controlled trials specifically focused on the development of an optimal diet for the gestational diabetic woman. Because there was no consensus as to the ideal diet for a woman with gestational diabetes, the American Diabetes Association recommendations for nonpregnant persons were adopted. The American Diabetes Association's diet for non-pregnant persons suggested that meal plans could have up to 60% carbohydrate composition. Instituting this high-carbohydrate diet for gestational diabetes results in necessitating insulin therapy in greater than 50% of women [56]. The logical step would be to restrict carbohydrates even at the expense of prescribing a hypocaloric diet. The National Academy of Science concluded that healthy, obese pregnant women need to gain no more than 15 lb when a woman is greater than 150% of her ideal body weight. In addition, the subsequent infant birth weight was optimized if the maternal weight gain was minimized to less than 3 kg or if no weight was gained [100]. In their report no dietary recommendations were made to either obese or lean diabetic pregnant women. Intrauterine growth retardation is associated with subsequent diabetes in populations with a high prevalence of malnutrition [101, 102]. Magee et al. [103] reported the only randomized trial that studied the impact of a calorie-restricted diet in gestational diabetic women. They compared a 2400-kcal/day diet with a 1200-kcal/day diet. The two groups, after more than 6 weeks of assigned diet, differed significantly in mean glucose levels and ketonemia developed in the calorie-restricted group after 1 week on the 1200-kcal/day diet. They went on to study a 33% restricted diet and showed that this mildly restricted diet did not cause ketonemia and did result in normal birth weight infants [104]. The role of ketones in pregnancies complicated by diabetes has also remained controversial [105, 106]. Ketonuria develops in 10–20% of normal pregnancies after an overnight fast and may in fact protect the fetus from starvation. In addition there may be a difference between the ketonuria produced from starvation and the ketonemia produced from diabetes that is out of control. The study by Rizza et al. [107] and the DIEP Study Group [108] related the neonatal complications to maternal ketones only in those mothers with ketonemia from hyperglycemia, not from starvation [105]. It is hoped that the National Institutes of Health funded multinational, muticenter randomized clinical trial of hyperglycemia and adverse pregnancy outcome will report the definitive diagnostic and treatment goals for glycemia [109]. Until there is a definitive study, however, we have used a minimally restricted carbohydrate diet to treat gestational diabetes and have shown that this diet does not result in excessive weight gain and has normalized the birth weight in Santa Barbara County [98]. This diet consists of 30 kcal/kg/day for normal weight women, 24 kcal/kg/day for overweight women, and 12 kcal/kg/day for morbidity obese women with less than 40% of the calories composed of carbohydrates. (The diet shown in Table 3 is also applied to the gestational diabetic woman.) To date, there are no data on long-term follow-up of these infants.

INSULIN TREATMENT FOR GESTATIONAL DIABETIC WOMEN

When dietary strategies fail to achieve the glucose goals for the gestational diabetic woman, insulin therapy needs to be initiated. There is only one report in the United States in which glyburide was used during pregnancies complicated by gestational diabetes [110]. Until there is a multicenter clinical trial with more data, both the American College of Obstetrics and Gynecology [87] and the American Diabetes Association do not recommend the use of oral hypoglycemic agents during pregnancy [70]. The type of insulin chosen should be based on the specific glucose abnormalities. The frequency of monitoring and the criteria for initiation of insulin are also controversial. Some authors' reports show that insulin does decrease the macrosomia rate [98, 111] but does not decrease the cesarean section rate. Apparently, obstetricians believe that women who require insulin therapy are at higher risk for difficulties during delivery, and that therefore the criteria for cesarean section are liberalized. Others have shown that decreased macrosomia rates do decrease the cesarean section rate if the indications for cesarean section are not changed for the insulin-requiring gestational diabetic woman [98].

Once the decision to initiate insulin has been made, the type and insulin administration schedule should be prescribed to lower the fasting (and premeal) and postprandial glucose levels. Here the initial doses of insulin can be administered as per the orders in Table 2.

The fast-acting insulin analogues, lispro and aspart, have been shown to be safe and efficacious in the treatment of gestational diabetic women [107, 108]. The rapid absorption of these insulin analogues allows for a faster peak insulin concentration than that seen with regular human insulin [112]. This effect more closely mimics the physiologic first-phase insulin release and results in lower postprandial glucose concentrations. In a study designed to assess the safety and efficacy of insulin lispro for the treatment of gestational diabetes, Jovanovic et al. [53, 54, 113] studied 42 gestational diabetic women randomized to treatment with either NPH and regular insulin or NPH and insulin lispro. After 6 weeks of therapy, the lispro group had significantly lower postprandial glucose levels without an increase in hypoglycemic events. In addition, no increase in lispro-specific or insulin-specific antibodies was demonstrated in the lispro group. Recently, insulin aspart has also been shown to be safe and efficacious for the treatment of gestational diabetic women [54]. The studies of the safety and efficacy of insulin analogues for the treatment of type 1 and type 2 diabetic women are still in progress. As new insulin analogues (fast-acting and long-acting analogues, such as glargine and detemir) come into the marketplace, they must be individually tested for safety and efficacy in pregnancy. It is hoped that there will be many treatment options to optimize the care of the insulin-requiring gestational diabetic woman.

CONCLUSION

Pregnancy is a time when metabolic changes are carefully regulated to provide optimum substrate to both mother and fetus. Subtle perturbations in metabolism can have implications not only for the index pregnancy but also for future generations. The goal of management during the past century has focused on the delivery of a live born infant. The challenge for the twenty-first century is to develop management strategies that establish a maternal/fetal environment that does not place the mother, infant, or subsequent generations at risk for abnormal metabolic homeostasis with the associated risks of obesity, hypertension, and diabetes mellitus. It is hoped that there will be resolution of the controversy over the best methods and optimal cut points for screening and initiation of treatment. Since 1977 and the inception of the programs described in this review, "tight glycemic control" achieved by "intensive conventional therapy" (including patient selfmonitoring of blood glucose) has become an integral part of various treatment plans for diabetes mellitus. In obstetrics, corroboration of the benefits of tight glycemic control can be seen at the conclusion of each diabetic pregnancy. There is now a wealth of literature and experience to justify intensive approach toward achieving normoglycemia through obstetric supervision. When normoglycemia is achieved and maintain throughout pregnancies complicated by type 1, type 2, or gestational diabetes mellitus, the outcome is a normal healthy infant. Now it is our challenge to create a cost-effective means to spread these techniques worldwide and thus ensure that all women in their childbearing years can have access to an intensive care program.

REFERENCES

1. White P. Pregnancy complicating diabetes. *JAMA* 1945; 128: 181–2.
2. White P. Pregnancy complicating diabetes. *Am J Med* 1949; 7: 609–16.
3. White P, Gillespie L, Sexton L. Use of female sex hormone therapy in pregnant diabetic patients. *Am J Med* 1956; 71: 57–69.
4. Hurwitz D, Hignao N. Diabetes and pregnancy. *N Engl J Med* 1952; 247: 305–9.
5. Eastman NJ. Diabetes mellitus and pregnancy. *Obstet Gynecol Surv* 1946; 1: 3–31.
6. Reis RA, deCosta EJ, Allweiss MD. The management of the pregnant diabetic woman and her newborn infant. *Am J Obstet Gynecol* 1950; 60: 1023–39.
7. Jones WL. Diabetes in pregnancy. *Am J Obstet Gynecol* 1953; 66: 322–34.
8. Long NW, Hartmann WL, Futcher PH, Eastman NJ. Diabetes mellitus and pregnancy. *Obstet Gynecol* 1954; 3: 160–8.
9. Oakley WG. The evolution of the management of diabetic pregnancy. *Postgrad Med J* 1969; 45: 802–5.
10. Peel J. A historical review of diabetes and pregnancy. *J Obstet Gynaecol Br Commonw* 1972; 79: 385–95.
11. Drury MI, Greene AT, Stronge JM. Pregnancy complicated by clinical diabetes mellitus: a study of 600 pregnancies. *Obstet Gynecol* 1977; 49: 519–22.

12. Pedersen J. *The Pregnant Diabetic and Her Newborn: Problems and Management*. Baltimore: Williams & Wilkins, 1977.
13. Pedersen J. Course of diabetes during pregnancy. *Acta Endocrinol* 1952; 9: 342–64.
14. Pedersen J. Fetal morality in diabetics in relation to management during the latter part of pregnancy. *Acta Endocrinol* 1954; 15: 282–94.
15. Pedersen J, Brandstrup E. Fetal mortality in pregnant diabetics: strict control of diabetes with conservative obstetric management. *Lancet* 1956; i: 607–12.
16. Pedersen J, Molsted-Pedersen L. Prognosis of the outcome of pregnancies in diabetics: a new classification. *Acta Endocrinol* 1965; 50: 70–8.
17. Pedersen J, Molsted-Pedersen L, Andersen B. Assessors of fetal perinatal mortality in diabetic pregnancy. *Diabetes* 1974; 23: 302–5.
18. Pedersen J. Weight and length at birth of infants of diabetic mothers. *Acta Endocrinol* 1954; 16: 330–42.
19. Harley JMG, Montgomery DAD. Management of pregnancy complicated by diabetes. *Br Med J* 1965; 1: 14–8.
20. Delany JJ, Ptacek J. Three decades of experience with diabetic pregnancies. *Am J Obstet Gynecol* 1970; 106: 550–6.
21. Karlsson K, Kjellmer I. The outcome of diabetic pregnancies in relation to the mother's blood sugar level. *Am J Obstet Gynecol* 1972; 112: 213–20.
22. Persson B, Lunell N, Carlstrom K, Furhjelm M. Urinary oestriol excretion in strictly controlled diabetic pregnancies. *Acta Obstet Gynecol Scand* 1970; 49: 379–84.
23. Persson B. Treatment of diabetic pregnancy. *Isr J Med Sci* 1975; 11: 609–18.
24. Brudenell M, Beard R. Diabetes in pregnancy. *Clin Endocrinol Metab* 1972; 1: 673–95.
25. Brudenell M. Care of the clinical diabetic woman in pregnancy and labor. In Sutherland HW, Stowers JM (eds) *Diabetes and Pregnancy* New York: Chruchill Livingstone, 1975; pp 221–9.
26. Gabbe SG, Mestman JJ, Freeman RK, Goeblesmann UT, Lowensohn RI, Nochimson D, Cetrulo C, Quilligan EJ. Management and outcome of pregnancy in diabetes mellitus: classes B to R. *Am J Obstet Gynecol* 1977; 129: 723–31.
27. Jovanovic L, Peterson C, Saxena B, Sawood MY, Saudek C. Feasibility of maintaining normal glucose profiles in insulin-dependent pregnant diabetic women. *Am J Med* 1980; 68: 105–12.
28. Jovanovic L, Druzin M, Peterson CM. Effect of euglycemia on the outcome of pregnancy in insulin-dependent diabetic women as compared with normal control subjects. *Am J Med* 1981; 71: 921–7.
29. Jovanovic L, Peterson CM. Optimal insulin delivery for pregnant diabetic patients. *Diabetes Care* 1982; 5 (suppl 1): 24–31.
30. Jovanovic L, Peterson C, Reed G, Metzger B, Mills J, Knopp R, Aarons J. The National Institute of Child Health and Human Development—Diabetes in Early Pregnancy Study: maternal postprandial glucose levels and infant birth weight. *Am J Obstet Gynecol* 1991; 164: 103–11.
31. Fuhrmann K, Reiher H, Semmler K, Fischer F, Fisher M, Glockner E. Prevention of congenital malformations in infants of insulin-dependent diabetic mothers. *Diabetes Care* 1983; 6: 219–23.
32. Goldman JA, Dickerd D, Feldberg D. Pregnancy outcome in patients with insulin-dependent diabetes mellitus with pre-conceptual diabetic control: a comparative study. *Am J Obstet Gynecol* 1986; 155: 193–7.
33. Damm P, Molsted-Pedersen L. Significant decrease in congenital malformations in newborn infants of an unselected population of diabetic women. *Am J Obstet Gynecol* 1989; 161: 1163–7.
34. Kitzmiller JL, Gavin LA, Gin GD, Jovanovic L, Main EK, Zigrang WD. Preconception care of diabetes: glycemic control prevents congenital anomalies. *JAMA* 1991; 265: 731–6.
35. Miodovnik M, Skillman C, Holroyde JC, Butler JB, Wendel JS, Siddiqi TA. Elevated maternal glycohemoglobin in early pregnancy and spontaneous abortion among insulin-dependent diabetic women. *Am J Obstet Gynecol* 1985; 153: 439–42.
36. Mills JL, Simpson JL, Driscoll SG, Jovanovic L, Van Allen M, Aarons JH, Metzger B, Bieber FR, Knopp RH, Holmes L, Peterson CM, Withiam-Wilson M, Brown ZP, Ober C, Harley E, Macpherson TA, Duckles A, Mueller-Geubach E. The National Institute of Child Health and Human Development—Diabetes in Early Pregnancy Study: incidence of spontaneous abortion among normal women and insulin-dependent diabetic women whose pregnancies were identified within 21 days of conception. *N Engl J Med* 1988; 319: 1617–23.
37. Cousins L. The California Diabetes and Pregnancy Program: a statewide collaborative program for the preconception and prenatal care of diabetic women. *Clin Obstet Gynecol* 1991; 5: 443–60.
38. Rosenn B, Miodovnik M, Combs CA, Khoury J, Siddiqi TA. Pre-conception management of insulin-dependent diabetes: improvement of pregnancy outcome. *Obstet Gynecol* 1991; 77: 846–9.
39. Jovanovic L, Peterson CM. Moment in history: turning point in the management of pregnancies complicated by diabetes, normoglycemia with self blood glucose monitoring of diet and insulin dosing. *Trans Am Soc Artif Intern Organs* 1990; 36: 799–804.
40. Jovanovic L, Bevier W, Peterson CM. The Santa Barbara County Health Care Services Program: birth weight change concomitant with screening for and treatment of glucose-intolerance of pregnancy. A potential cost-effective intervention. *Am J Perinatol* 1997; 14: 221–8.
41. Jovanovic L, Metzger BE, Knopp RH, Conley MR, Park E, Lee YJ, Simpson JL, Holms L, Aarons JH, Mills JL, and The NICHD—Diabetes in Early Pregnancy Study Group. The Diabetes in Early Pregnancy Study: β-hydroxybutyrate levels in type 1 diabetic pregnancy compared with normal pregnancy. *Diabetes Care* 1998; 21: 1978–84.
42. Jovanovic L, Mills Jl, Knopp RH, Metzger BE, Park E, Aarons JH, Holmes LB, Simpson JL, Brown Z, Conley MR, and the National Institute of Child Health and Human Development—Diabetes in Early Pregnancy Study Group. Declining insulin requirement in the late first trimester of diabetic pregnancy. *Diabetes Care* 2001; 24: 1130–36.
43. Combs CA, Wheeler B, Gunderson E, Gavin L, Kitzmiller JL. Significance of microproteinuria in the first trimester of pregnancies complicated by diabetes. *Diabetes* 1990; 39: 36A.

44. Jovanovic L, Peterson CM. Diabetes and Pregancy, Part I: a preconception and prenatal plan. *Med Aspects Hum Sex* 1992; 26: 54–65.
45. Dicker D, Feldberg D, Samuel N, Yeshaya A, Karp M, Goldman JA. Spontaneous abortion in patients with insulin-dependent diabetes mellitus: the effect of preconceptional diabetic control. *Am J Obstet Gynecol* 1988; 158: 1161–4.
46. Steel JM, Johnstone FD, Hepburn DA, Smith A. Can prepregnancy care of diabetic women reduce the risk of abnormal babies? *Br Med J* 1990; 301: 1070–4.
47. Fuhrmann K, Reiher H, Semmler K, Glockner E. The effect of intensified conventional insulin therapy before and during pregnancy on the malformation rate in offspring of diabetic mothers. *Exp Clin Endocrinol* 1984; 83: 173–7.
48. Miodovnik M, Mimouni F, Tsang RC. Glycemic control and spontaneous abortion in insulin-dependent diabetic women. *Obstet Gynecol* 1986; 68: 366–9.
49. Mill JL, Baker L, Goldman AS. Malformations in infants of diabetic mothers occur before the seventh gestational week: implications for treatment. *Diabetes* 1979; 28: 292–3.
50. Mills JL, Knopp RH, Simpson JL, Jovanovic L, and the DIEP Study Group. Lack of relation of increased malformation rates in infants of diabetic mother to glycemic control during organogenesis. *N Engl J Med* 1988; 319: 1617–23.
51. Jovanovic L. Summary and comment on expanded care in obstetrics for the 1980's: preconception and early post conception counseling. *Diabetes Spectrum* 1990; 3: 179–80.
52. Jovanovic L (ed). *Medical Management of Pregnancy Complicated by Diabetes*. Alexandria, VA: American Diabetes Association, 2000.
53. Jovanovic L, Ilic S, Pettitt DJ, Hugo K, Gutierrez M, Bowsher RR, Bastyr EJ III. The metabolic and immunologic effects of insulin lispro. *Diabetes Care* 1999; 22: 1422–7.
54. Pettitt DJ, Ospina P, Kolaczynski JW, Jovanovic L. Comparison of an insulin analog, insulin aspart, and regular human insulin with no insulin in gestational diabetes mellitus. *Diabetes Care* 2003; 26: 183–6.
55. Langer O. Prevention of macrosomia. *Clin Obstet Gynecol* 1991; 5: 333–48.
56. Jovanovic L, Peterson CM. Dietary manipulation as a primary treatment strategy for pregnancies complicated by diabetes. *Am Coll Nutr* 1990; 9: 320–5.
57. Potter JM, Beckless JP, Cullen DR. Subcutaneous insulin infusion control of blood glucose concentration in diabetics in third trimester of pregnancy. *Br Med J* 1980; 26: 1099–101.
58. Kitzmiller JL, Younger MD, Hare JW, Phillippe M, Vignati L, Fargnoli B, Grause A. Continuous subcutaneous insulin therapy during early pregnancy. *Obstet Gynecol* 1985; 66: 606–11.
59. Coustan DR, Reece A, Sherwin RS, Rudolf MC, Bates SE, Sockin SM, Holford T, Tamborlane WV. A randomized clinical trial of the insulin pump versus intensive conventional therapy in diabetic pregnancies. *JAMA* 1986; 255: 631–5.
60. Carta O, Meriggi E, Trossarelli GF, Catella G, Molin VD, Menato G, Gagliardi L, Massobrio M, Vitelli A. Continuous subcutaneous insulin infusion versus intensive conventional insulin therapy in type 1 and type 2 diabetic pregnancy. *Diabetes Metab* 1986;12: 121–9.
61. Mancuso S, Caruso A, Lanzone A, Bianchi V, Massidda M, Codipetro F, Fulghesu. Continuous subcutaneous insulin infusion in pregnant diabetic women. *Acta Endocrinol* 1986 77: (suppl 277); 112–6.
62. Leveno KJ, Fortunato SJ, Raskin P, Williams ML, Whalley PJ. Continuous subcutaneous insulin infusion during pregnancy. *Diabetes Res Clin Pract* 1988; 257–68.
63. Caruso A, Lanzone V, Massidda M, Castelli MP, Fulghesu AM. Continuous subcutaneous insulin infusion in pregnant diabetic patients. *Prenatal Diagnosis* 1987; 7: 41–50.
64. Simmons D, Thompson CF, Conroy C, Scott DJ. Use of insulin pumps in pregnancies complicated by type 2 diabetes and gestational diabetes in a multiethnic community. *Diabetes Care* 2002; 24: 2078–82.
65. Jensen BM, Kuhl C, Petersen LM, Saurbrey N, Pedersen JF. Preconceptional treatment with insulin infusion pumps in insulin-dependent diabetic women with particular reference to prevention of congenital malformations. *Acta Endocrinol* 1986; 77 (suppl 2): 81–5.
66. Gabbe SG, Holing E, Temple P, Brown ZA. Benefits, risks, costs, and patient satisfaction associated with insulin pump therapy for the pregnancy complicated by type 1 diabetes mellitus. *Am J Obstet Gynecol* 2000; 182: 1283–91.
67. Jovanovic L, Peterson CM. Insulin and glucose requirements during the first stage of labor in insulin-dependent diabetic women. *Am J Med* 1983; 75: 607–12.
68. Chew EY, Mills JL, Metzger BE, Remaley NA, Jovanovic L, Knopp RH, Conley M, Rand L, Simpson JL, Holms LB, Aarons JH, and The NICHD-DIEP. Metabolic control and progression of retinopathy. *Diabetes Care* 1995; 18: 631–7.
69. Jovanovic L, Peterson CM. Maternal milk and plasma glucose and insulin levels: studies in normal and diabetic subjects. *J Am Coll Nutr* 1989; 8: 125–31.
70. Metzger BE, Coustan DR. Summary and recommendations of the Fourth International Workshop-Conference on Gestational Diabetes Mellitus. *Diabetes Care* 1998; 21: B161–7.
71. World Health Organization (WHO) Study Group. Prevention of diabetes mellitus. WHO Technical Report Series No. 844. Geneva: WHO, 1994.
72. Freinkel N, Josimovich J. Conference planning committee: American Diabetes Association Workshop-Conference on Gestational Diabetes. Summary and recommendations. *Diabetes Care* 1980; 3: 499–501.
73. Coustan DR, Gestational diabetes. In Harris MI, Cowie CC, Stern MP, Boyko EJ, Reiber GE, Bennett PH (eds), *Diabetes in America*, 2nd edn. Washington, DC: National Institutes of Health, 1995; chap 35, pp 703–17. NIH Publication No. 95–1468.
74. Xiang AH, Peters RK, Trigo E, Kjos SL, Lee WP, Buchanan TA. Multiple metabolic defects during late pregnancy in women at high risk for type 2 diabetes. *Diabetes* 1999; 48: 848–54.
75. De Veciana M, Major CA, Morgna MA, et al. Postprandial versus preprandial blood glucose monitoring in women with gestational diabetes mellitus requiring insulin therapy. *N Engl J Med* 1995; 333: 1237–41.
76. Hod M, Rabinerson D, Peled Y. Gestational diabetes mellitus: is it a clinical entity? *Diabetes Rev* 1995; 3: 603–13.

77. Persson B, Hanson U. Neonatal morbidities in gestational diabetes mellitus. *Diabetes Care* 1998; 21 (suppl 2): B79–84.
78. Gonen R, Bader D, Ajami M. Effects of a policy of elective cesarean delivery in cases of suspected fetal macrosomia on the incidence of brachial plexus injury and the rate of cesarean delivery. *Am J Obstet Gynecol* 2000; 183 (5): 1296–300.
79. Zamorski MA, Biggs WS. Management of suspected fetal macrosomia. *Am Fam Phys* 2001; 63 (2): 302–6.
80. Pettitt DJ, Baird HR, Aleck KA, Bennett PH, Knowler WC. Excessive obesity in offspring of Pima Indian women with diabetes during pregnancy. *N Engl J Med* 1983; 308: 242–5.
81. Silverman BL, Rizzo T, Green OC, Cho NH, Winter RJ, Ogata ES, Richards GE, Metzger BE. Long-term prospective evaluation of offspring of diabetic mothers. *Diabetes* 1991; 40 (suppl 2): 121–5.
82. Pettitt DJ, Aleck KA, Baird HR, Carraher MJ, Bennett PH, Knowler WC. Congenital susceptibility to NIDDM: role of intrauterine environment. *Diabetes* 1988; 37: 622–8.
83. Silverman BL, Metzger BE, Cho NH, Loeb CA. Impaired glucose tolerance in adolescent offspring of diabetic mothers. Relationship to fetal hyperinsulinism. *Diabetes Care* 1995; 18: 611–7.
84. Dabelea D, Hanson RL, Lindsay RS, Pettitt DJ, Imperatore G, Gabir MM, Roumain J, Bennett PH, Knowler WC. Intrauterine exposure to diabetes conveys risks for type 2 diabetes and obesity: a study of discordant sibships. *Diabetes* 2000; 49: 2208–11.
85. Kjos SL, Henry OA, Montoro M, Buchanan TA, Mestman JH. Insulin-requiring diabetes in pregnancy: a randomized trial of active induction of labor and expectant management. *Am J Obstet Gynecol* 1993; 169: 611–5.
86. American Diabetes Association. Gestational diabetes mellitus (Position Statement). *Diabetes Care* 2001; 24 (suppl 1): S77–9.
87. American College of Obstetricians and Gynecologists. *Diabetes and Pregnancy*. Washington, DC: American College of Obstetricians and Gynecologists, 1994; pp 1–8. Technical Bulletin No. 200.
88. Lupo VR, Stys SJ. Recurrence of gestational diabetes in subsequent pregnancies. In Weiss PAM, Coustan DR (eds) *Gestational Diabetes*. Vienna: Springer-Verlag, 1988; pp 123–6.
89. Amadin RA, Famuyiwa OO, Adelusi BO. Glycemic response to 75 gms and 100 gms glucose load during pregnancy in Nigerian women. *Diabetol Croatica* 1989; 18: 159–61.
90. Pettitt DJ, Bennett PH, Hanson RL, Narayan KMV, Knowler WC. Comparison of World Health Organization and National Diabetes Data Group procedures to detect abnormalities of glucose tolerance during pregnancy. *Diabetes Care* 1994; 17: 1264–8.
91. Deerochanawong C, Putiyanun C, Wongsuryrat M, Serirat S, Junayon P. Comparison of national diabetes data group and world health organization criteria for detecting gestational diabetes mellitus. *Diabetologia* 1996; 39: 1070–3.
92. National Diabetes Data Group. Classification and diagnosis of diabetes mellitus and other categories of glucose intolerance. *Diabetes* 1979; 28: 1039–57.
93. Carpenter MW, Coustan DR. Criteria for screening tests for gestational diabetes. *Am J Obstet Gynecol* 1982; 144: 768–73.
94. Combs CA, Gunderson E, Kitzmiller JL, Gavin LA, Main EK. Relationship of fetal macrosomia to maternal postprandial glucose control during pregnancy. *Diabetes Care* 1992; 15: 1251–7.
95. Jovanovic L, Peterson CM, Reed GF, et al. Maternal postprandial glucose levels and infant birth weight: the diabetes in early pregnancy study. *Am J Obstet Gynecol* 1991; 164: 103–11.
96. Bevier WC, Fischer R, Jovanovic L. Treatment of women with an abnormal glucose challenge test (but a normal oral glucose tolerance test) decreases the prevalence of macrosomia. *Am J Perinatol* 1999; 16: 269–75.
97. Jovanovic L. The role of continuous glucose monitoring in gestational diabetes mellitus. *Diabetes Technol Ther* 2000; 2 (suppl 1): 67–71.
98. Jovanovic L, Bevier W, Peterson CM. The Santa Barbara County Health Care Services Program: birthweight change concomitant with screening for and treatment of glucose-intolerance of pregnancy. A potential cost-effective intervention. *Am J Perinatal* 1997; 14: 221–8.
99. Peterson CM, Jovanovic L. Percentage of carbohydrate and glycemia response to breakfast, lunch and dinner in women with gestational diabetes. *Diabetes* 1991; 40 (suppl 2): 172–4.
100. King J, Allen L. *Nutrition During Pregnancy*. Washington, DC: National Academy Press, 1990.
101. Ericksson UJ, SwenneI. Diabetes in pregnancy: fetal macrosomia, hyperinsulinism, and islet hyperplasia in offspring of diabetic rates subjected to temporary protein-energy malnutrition in early life. *Pediat Res* 1993; 34: 791–5.
102. Barker DJP, Bull AR, Osmond C, Simmonds SJ. Fetal and placental size and risk of hypertension in adult life. *BMJ* 1990; 301: 259–62.
103. Magee MS, Knopp RH, Benedetti TJ. Metabolic effects of 1,200-kcal diet in obese pregnant women with gestaiona fiabets. *Diabetes* 1990; 39: 234–40.
104. Knopp RH, Magee M, Raisys V. Hypocaloric diets and ketogenesis in the management of obese gestational diabetic women. *J Am Coll Nutr* 1991; 10: 649–67.
105. Jovanovic L. Sweet success but an acid aftertaste? *N Engl J Med* 1991; 325: 959–60.
106. Churchill JA, Berendes HW, Nemore J. Neuropsychological deficients in children of diabetic mothers. *Am J Obstet Gynecol* 1969; 105: 257–68.
107. Rizza T, Metzger BE, Urns WJ, Burns K. Correlations between antepartum maternal metabolism and intelligence of offspring. *N Engl J Med* 1991; 325: 911–6.
108. Jovanovic L, Metzger B, Knopp RH. Beta-hydroxybutyrate levels in type 1 diabetic pregnancy compared with normal pregnancy. *Diabetes Care* 1998; 21: 1–5.
109. Metzger B, for the Hyperglycemia and Adverse Pregnancy Outcome (HAPO) Group. Study design of the Hypoglycemia and Adverse Pregnancy Outcome (HAPO) Protocol. *Int J Gynaecol Obstet* 2002; 78: 69–77.
110. Langer O, Conway DL, Berkus MD, Xenakis EM, Gonzales O. A comparison of glyburide and insulin in women with gestational diabetes mellitus. *N Engl J Med* 2000; 343: 1134–8.

111. Naylor CD, Sermer M, Chen E, Sykora K. Cesarean delivery in relation to birth weight and gestational glucose tolerance: pathophysiology or practice style? *JAMA* 1996; 275: 1165–70.
112. Balsells M, Corcoy R, Mauricio D, Morales J, Garcia-Patterson A, Carreras G, Puig-Domingo M, de Leiva A. Insulin antibody response to a short course of human insulin therapy in women with gestational diabetes. *Diabetes Care* 1997; 20: 1172–5.
113. Anderson JH Jr, Brunelle RL, Koivisto VA, Pfutzner A, Trautmann ME, Vignati L, DiMarchi R. Reduction of postprandial hyperglycemia and frequency of hypoglycemia in IDDM patients on insulin-analog treatment. *Diabetes* 1997; 46: 265–70.

89

Aging and Diabetes Mellitus

Alan J. Sinclair

University of Warwick, Coventry, UK

INTRODUCTION

Diabetes care systems for older people require an integrated approach between general practitioners, hospital specialists, and other members of the health care team. This should be multidimensional, with an emphasis on prevention of diabetes and its complications, early intervention for vascular disease, and assessment of disability due to limb problems, eye disease, and stroke.

Variations in clinical practice are common in most health care systems, resulting in inequalities of care. For older people with diabetes, this may be manifest as lack of access to services, inadequate specialist provision, poorer clinical outcomes, and patient and family dissatisfaction. The development of clinical guidelines that are responsive to the needs of older people with diabetes may be an important step to minimize deficits in care from country to country, worldwide.

Type 2 diabetes mellitus is a common disabling chronic medical disorder that has a tremendous health, social, and economic burden [1], and has a high prevalence across Europe of 10–30% of subjects older than 65 years [2]. Acute care hospitalizations account for about 60% of the total expenditure on this special group [3], and compared with nondiabetic counterparts, the relative risk for admission to hospital is 5.0. At any one time, about 1 in 12 district hospital beds are occupied by older people who have diabetes and their length of stay is doubled, compared with nondiabetic inpatients [4]. The introduction of insulin to their regimen results in expenditure quadrupling, presumably because of the additional resources required in both hospital and community settings to monitor and support the use of insulin [5].

One therapeutic approach to the management of type 2 diabetes in aging subjects is to concentrate on strategies designed to limit and ameliorate both defective insulin secretion and insulin resistance. The term *metabolic syndrome* now embraces this view that type 2 diabetes represents a cluster of cardiovascular risk factors which represent a significant vascular threat [6]. In older subjects, the added effects of aging and renal impairment increase the impact of this syndrome, while some of the features may be present up to 10 years before the onset of overt hyperglycemia, thus increasing the cardiovascular risk before the onset of diabetes [7]. When you also consider that up to 50% of the variability in insulin action in insulin-resistant states may be associated with lifestyle differences—obesity, physical activity levels, and cigarette smoking [8]—you realize that environmental, preventative, and health promotional strategies are of vital importance in limiting the impact of this epidemic.

Management of diabetes in older people can be relatively straightforward especially when patients have no other comorbidities and when vascular complications are absent. In many cases, however, special issues arise which increase the complexity of management and lead to difficult clinical decision making. It is thus not surprising that the present state of diabetes care for older patients varies throughout Europe and North America. Although geriatric diabetes is developing as a subspeciality interest in the United Kingdom, there is little evidence of its presence in other national diabetes care systems and virtually no specific provision for those who are housebound or in institutional care. Diabetes in older subjects is characterized by a series of factors that highlight deficiencies in care and tend to increase the complexity of management (Table 1); however, there is emerging evidence that diabetes care for the elderly may be improving [9, 10].

International Textbook of Diabetes Mellitus, Third Edition. Edited by R. A. DeFronzo, E. Ferrannini, H. Keen, and P. Zimmet.
 ISBN: 0-471-48655-8.

Table 1 Defining characteristics of older subjects with diabetes

- Common comorbidities of diabetes
- Age-related impairment of functional ability
- Increased vulnerability to hypoglycemia
- Age-specific complications
- Increased mortality from acute metabolic decompensation
- Poor medical follow-up by primary-care physicians, diabetic specialists, and geriatricians
- Need to involve spouses and informal carers in management

AGING AND GLUCOSE TOLERANCE

An age-related impairment in glucose tolerance was originally observed in 1921 by Spence [11], which has been confirmed by recent studies, indicating that glucose intolerance begins in the third decade, or even earlier in the obese population, and continues throughout adulthood [12]. The extent of the rise is estimated to be 0.33–0.72 mmol/l (5.9–13.0 mg/dl) per decade in 1-h and 2-h post-glucose load samples. Women exhibit a more pronounced rise [about 0.55 mmol/l (9.9 mg/dl) higher than in men]. The Third National Health and Nutrition Examination Survey (NHANES III) of 19 000 adult US residents conducted between 1988 and 1994 found a rise in impaired glucose tolerance of 11.9% in those aged 40–49 years to 20.7% in those aged 60–74 [13]. Prevalence rates of diabetes rose with advancing age but reached a plateau at age 60–74 years.

Mechanisms of Age-related Glucose Intolerance

The impairment is multifactorial and is characterized by alterations in glucose-induced insulin release (more apparent in response to an oral load rather than an intravenous one) and resistance to insulin-mediated glucose disposal. This latter defect may be the most important in aged subjects [14], with the principal site of defect implicated to be skeletal muscle [12]. Since insulin receptor number or binding are not usually affected by age, the impairment is due primarily to a so-called postreceptor defect. Table 2 is a list of those factors that may contribute to the glucose intolerance. Metabolic alterations in elderly subjects with and without diabetes have been studied in detail by Meneilly and coworkers [15] using glucose-clamp techniques. In contrast to younger subjects, fasting hepatic glucose production is normal in both lean and obese elderly subjects. However, although insulin resistance is minimal, lean elderly subjects have a profound impairment in pancreatic insulin secretion. In obese elderly subjects, in contrast, insulin secretory ability is maintained but there is a marked resistance to insulin-mediated glucose disposal. The ability of insulin to enhance blood flow was also markedly reduced in obese older insulin-resistant subjects: insulin-mediated vasodilation is thought to account for about 30% of normal glucose disposal. Recently it has been demonstrated that in healthy elderly subjects, glucose effectiveness (the ability of glucose to stimulate its own uptake in the absence of insulin) is impaired but is normal during hypoglycemia [16]. This is an important finding since under fasting conditions, this mechanism accounts for 70% of glucose uptake (primarily in the central nervous system), and after a meal, 50% of glucose uptake occurs via this process primarily involving skeletal muscle. This is a potential new site for therapeutic action since in younger patients, exercise, anabolic steroids, and a reduction in free fatty acids may increase glucose effectiveness [17].

Table 2 Glucose intolerance in old age: contributory factors

Impaired glucose disposal and utilization
↓ Insulin-mediated uptake into skeletal muscle
↓ Insulin-mediated vasodilatation in muscle
↓ Non-insulin-mediated glucose uptake
Impaired glucose-induced insulin secretion
Other factors
Obesity
Physical inactivity
Reduced dietary carbohydrate
Diabetogenic drugs (thiazides, glucocorticoids)

EPIDEMIOLOGY

It is projected that by 2010, the number of diabetic individuals in the world will reach the number of 221 million, compared with 151 million in 2000. This increase in prevalence will be attributed to several important risk factors such as advancing age of the population, greater numbers of people from ethnic minority backgrounds adopting a "transitional" lifestyle, greater levels of overweight and obesity, and more sedentary lifestyles. From an epidemiological perspective, aging is an important factor: in the United States, the number of people with diabetes (75 years and older) doubled between 1980 and 1987 [2]. The rise in prevalence of diabetes begins in early adulthood: for example, in Pima Indians aged 25–34 years are 10 times more likely to have diabetes than those aged 15–24 years, and in Americans aged 45–55 years, diabetes is four times more common than in those aged 20–44 years. Peak prevalence rates in Pima Indians are noted at age 40 years for men and 50 years for women and declines in men after the age of 65 years and after 55 years in women. In other populations, peak rates are generally found in the sixth decade and subsequently Figure 1 shows the prevalence rates of diabetes in both sexes in different age groups taken from the NHANES III Study in the United States [13].

Most developed countries have a prevalence rate of about 17% in White elderly subjects and 25% in non-White subjects. Racial differences in prevalence rates of diabetes are also apparent in older people. In NHANES III, for subjects 75 years and older, the rates for non-Hispanic

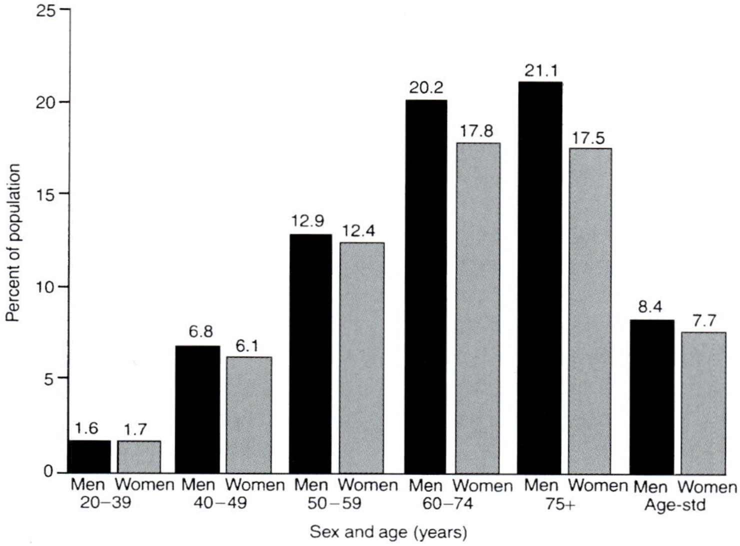

Figure 1 Prevalence of diabetes in men and women in the US population aged ≥20 years, based on NHANES III. Diabetes includes previously diagnosed and undiagnosed diabetic patients, defined by fasting plasma glucose ≥126 mg/dl. Age-std = age-standardized. (Reproduced with permission from reference 13)

Whites, non-Hispanic Blacks, and Mexican Americans were 17.5, 22.4, and 29.7% (compared with the corresponding rates in younger subjects of 17.3, 28.6, and 29.3% in those aged 60–74 years) [13]. The prevalence of White British elderly is only around 9% although the prevalence in non-White British elderly is about 25% [18, 19] and the prevalence in British care homes is 25% [20]. The prevalence of previously diagnosed diabetes in the United Kingdom has increased over the last few decades and this may be due to increased ascertainment combined with a true increase in prevalence.

MODES OF PRESENTATION

Presentation of diabetes in older people is often varied and may be insidious, which ultimately delays diagnosis [1] (Table 3). Many cases are detected by noting hyperglycemia during hospital admissions for other comorbidities or acute illnesses. Even when hyperglycemia has been recognized in hospital about half the subjects receive no further evaluation for diabetes or treatment [21]. Some patients do not have the classic features of either diabetic ketoacidosis or hyperosmolar nonketotic coma but present with a "mixed" disturbance of hyperglycemia (blood glucose levels 15–25 mM; arterial blood pH of 7.2 or 7.3, not particularly acidotic), and without marked dehydration or change in level of consciousness.

Recognition of the symptom profile of hyperglycemia in older subjects can be helpful in making an early diagnosis but perusal of the items listed in Table 3 demonstrate the atypical presentation and diverse effects of this metabolic disorder.

BURDEN OF DIABETES MELLITUS

Older patients with diabetes appear to burden the hospital care system two to three times more than the general population [5] and use primary care services two to three times more than nondiabetic controls [22]. This latter primary care study from Denmark indicated that insulin-treated patients accounted for more than half of the service provision, mainly because of chronic vascular disease, with a correspondingly high number of hospital clinic visits. The

Table 3 Varying presentation of diabetes in older people

Asymptomatic (coincidental finding)	
Classical osmotic symptoms	
Metabolic disturbances	Diabetic ketoacidosis Hyperosmolar non-ketotic coma "Mixed" metabolic disturbance
Spectrum of vague symptoms	Depressed mood Apathy Mental confusion
Development of "geriatric" syndromes	Falls or poor mobility: muscle weakness, poor vision, cognitive impairment Urinary incontinence Unexplained weight loss Memory disorder or cognitive impairment
Slow recovery from specific illnesses or increased vulnerability	Impaired recovery from stroke Repeated infections Poor wound healing

average number of bed-days occupied per person-year was 6.8 for males and 8.2 for females, whereas the figure for insulin-treated type 2 diabetic patients was 23.9, which was considerably higher than for insulin-treated patients with type 1 diabetes (15.2) [5]. Similar bed-occupancy rates for patients with known diabetes have been reported by others [23].

Several studies have attempted to estimate the prevalence of diabetes mellitus in elderly hospital in patients. In a study from Edinburgh Royal Infirmary, elderly patients with diabetes (65 years and older) accounted for 60% of the bed occupancy, giving a mean hospital prevalence of 4.6% [24]. A Cardiff-based study of three district general hospitals found a hospital prevalence (pooled data) of 8.4%, with a mean age of 65 years [4].

Diabetes in older subjects is associated with considerable morbidity, mainly because of the long-term complications of diabetes. A population-based study from Oxford [25] measured the incidence of complications over a median period of 6 years in 188 patients 60 years and older by using a structured questionnaire and clinical examination. Incidence rates of ischemic heart disease, stroke, and peripheral vascular disease (PVD) were 56, 22, and 146 per 1000 person-years, which were comparable to rates found in the Framingham study [26] but slightly higher as the Oxford study involved an older age group. Retinopathy occurred at a rate of 60 and cataract at 29 per 1000 person-years, while proteinuria (albumin concentration > 300 mg/l) was at 19 per 1000 person-years. Incidence rates appeared to be unrelated to sex or duration of diabetes but stroke and PVD rose significantly with age.

In Southern England, a study of 1077 diabetic subjects revealed an overall prevalence of diabetic neuropathy to be 16.3% (compared with 2.9% in nondiabetic controls) with similar values in both insulin-dependent diabetic and non-insulin-dependent diabetic patients, with three quarters of patients reporting symptoms [27]. In this study, duration of diabetes and metabolic control were significant predictors of neuropathy. The prevalence of neuropathy increased with age in all groups, with one in four type 2 diabetic patients 80 years and older being affected.

A community survey from Nottingham, England [28], of 98 elderly diabetic patients (mean age 73 years) registered with two inner-city general practices, used several measures such as stroke with residual disability, visual impairment, or previous amputation to document the impact of diabetes on older patients. Disability of any nature was present in four out of five patients. Cataract was the commonest cause of disability associated with visual impairment.

In the Welsh Community Diabetes Study of patients (and controls) 65 years and older living in three separate districts of Wales [29], one in three subjects with diabetes had been hospitalized in the previous 12 months (compared with one in six nondiabetic controls), and diabetic subjects had significantly increased levels of both physical and cognitive disability. One in four diabetic subjects required assistance with personal care and based on SF-36 health status data, older people with diabetes had significantly lower levels of well-being in the majority of domains examined.

The prevalence of some diabetic complications has been reported to increase with advancing age. In a cross-sectional study of non-insulin-dependent diabetic patients aged 53–80 years [30], the prevalence of retinopathy, peripheral neuropathy, and hypertension were evaluated at different ages. Logistic regression demonstrated a significant increase in the prevalence of retinopathy with aging, independent of the effects of metabolic control, duration of disease, and other risk variables. Age was also related to the prevalence of peripheral neuropathy, hypertension, and impotence. The independent contribution of age *per se* to retinopathy was not seen in a study by Ballard et al. [31] in Minnesota, USA, who found a positive relationship with persistent proteinuria only, or in a study by Knuiman et al. [32], who studied both type 1 and type 2 diabetic patients and found independent associations of age with renal impairment, macrovascular complications, and sensory neuropathy only.

Diabetic Retinopathy and Visual Loss

In Avon, UK, the third leading cause of blindness and partial sight registration is diabetic retinopathy [33]. Blind registrations for diabetic subjects in Nottingham, UK, are eight times higher that the subjects not known to have diabetes [28], with 16% of the elderly diabetic subjects having blind or partial sight registrations. The majority of older patients with diabetes will have diabetic retinopathy of some description although about one in twenty show no evidence of retinal damage even after 15 years [34].

In the Welsh Community Diabetes Study [35], impaired distance visual acuity was screened for in an elderly population of both diabetic and nondiabetic subjects. Visual acuity was impaired in 40% of diabetic subjects (compared with 31% controls) and diabetes was found to be associated with an increased risk of visual impairment (OR 1.50 [1.09–2.05]). Factors that were significantly associated with visual loss in diabetic subjects included advanced age, female sex, history of foot ulceration, duration of diabetes, and treatment with insulin. Reduced visual acuity was significantly associated with poorer health status (quality of life) measured by the SF-36 questionnaire.

The underlying problem in diabetic retinopathy is capillary occlusion; this may cause retinal hypoxia and increased vascular permeability, with new vessel formation secondary to vascular endothelial growth factor production. However, other capillaries become dilated, which causes microaneurysms if focal, or leakage from the capillaries if generalized. It is this capillary leakage that causes exudative and edematous maculopathies, which are the main forms of sight-threatening retinopathy in the older subject with type 2 diabetes.

The Diabetes Control and Complications Trial (DCCT) in type 1 diabetes and the United Kingdom Prospective Diabetes Study (UKPDS) in type 2 diabetes has demonstrated convincingly that tight control of hyperglycemia leads to a reduction in retinopathy [36]. Unfortunately, there are no specific intervention studies in elderly type 2 diabetic subjects. The UKPDS demonstrated a 25% risk reduction in retinopathy when tight control was present (HbA_{1c} <7.0% [37]). Duration of disease is also associated with increased risk of retinopathy. Achieving a target systolic blood pressure of <140 mmHg in the UKPDS, a 37% reduced rate of progression of retinopathy was demonstrated [38] providing support for the additional benefits of blood pressure control. Diabetic retinopathy is already present at diagnosis in 23.8% of subjects of all ages in the UKPDS.

Without laser intervention in proliferative diabetic retinopathy, the risk of severe visual loss is 50–70% at 2 and 5 years [39]. Laser photocoagulation can preserve vision in edematous (reduces risk of visual deterioration by 50% [40]) and exudative maculopathies if visual acuity is 6/9 or better [41], and it has been calculated that screening and treating diabetic retinopathy would prevent 56% of blind registrations due to this condition. Cataract is the most common cause of deteriorating vision in the elderly population and has been shown to be more common in diabetic subjects, even at the time of diagnosis, and its presence suggests increased future mortality [19].

Age-related macular degeneration is common in diabetic patients and its prevalence increases with age. It is an important cause of central vision loss [34]. Risk factors include atherosclerosis, diastolic blood pressure > 95 mmHg, antihypertensive medication, and elevated serum cholesterol.

Screening for retinopathy in the elderly is particularly important as deteriorating vision may not be regarded as a significant event by the subject who expects "age-related" changes. Retinopathy may be the presenting feature of diabetes in older people, and screening using digital fundus photography is being developed as a screening tool. If photography is not available, subjects need measurements of visual acuity and dilated fundoscopy by experienced observers each year, although in the absence of poor metabolic control and/or hypertension, some ophthalmologists may accept an interval of 2–3 years; this is probably worth doing anyway opportunistically, as even photography misses 11% of retinopathy. Although exudative maculopathy is easy to spot in the dilated eye (exudates around or within 1 disc's diameter of the macula), macular edema is practically impossible to distinguish from a normal eye by ophthalmoscopy, hence the importance of measuring the corrected visual acuity. Indications for referral to an ophthalmologist are virtually identical to younger counterparts but the threshold for referral may vary.

Diabetic Foot Syndrome

Amputation of a limb remains an important and expensive health problem in the diabetic population, with the elderly being particularly affected [42]. A recent study from the Netherlands [43] identified increasing age and a higher level of amputation as important factors leading to increases in both the period of hospitalization and the associated costs (estimated to be over £10 000 per hospitalization, with a mean inpatient stay of 42 days).

The 3-year survival following lower extremity amputation is about 50% [44], and in about 70% of cases, amputation is precipitated by foot ulceration [45]. The principal antecedents include peripheral vascular disease, sensorimotor and autonomic neuropathy, limited joint mobility (which impairs the ability of older people to inspect their feet), and high foot pressures [42].

The majority of the elderly diabetic population is at increased risk of developing foot ulcers. Factors that have been identified as increasing the likelihood of foot ulceration are shown in Table 4. Peripheral sensorimotor neuropathy is the primary cause or contributory factor in the vast majority of cases. This may cause common symptoms of numbness, lancinating and burning pain, 'pins and needles,' and hyperesthesia (which is typically worse at night), and evidence of high foot pressures leading to gait disturbances, falls, and other foot injuries. The presence of visual loss increases the consequences of this situation [46]. A trivial foot injury in a patient with severe neuropathy can eventually lead to the development of a Charcot joint; the majority of cases have had diabetes for at least 10 years and most are elderly.

Treatment of painful neuropathy in older patients is often difficult but may improve in pain of recent onset by improved metabolic control. Pain associated with loss of sensation and of greater than 6 months duration requires specific therapy. Patients with localized pain may respond to a topical cream called capsaicin (0.075%), which works by depleting the neurotransmitter, substance P. Alternative treatments include transcutaneous nerve stimulation or acupuncture. Drug therapies include tricyclic antidepressants (TCADs) and antiepileptics such as carbamazepine,

Table 4 Risk factors for foot ulceration in the elderly

- Peripheral sensorimotor neuropathy
- Automatic neuropathy
- Peripheral vascular disease
- Limited joint mobility
- Foot pressure abnormalities, including deformity
- Previous foot problems
- Visual loss
- History of alcohol abuse

although these are given "off-license" by some physicians. Lower doses are recommended initially for older patients but in the presence of cardiac disease, e.g. arrhythmias, TCADs are not advised, and with carbamazepine, a history of cardiac, renal, or hepatic disease may not allow its use. Gabapentin has recently been licensed for the treatment of painful neuropathy, and a recent review of five randomized clinical trials examining the effects of gabapentin in managing the pain of diabetic neuropathy found that the drug relieved the symptoms of allodynia, burning pain, shooting pain, and hyperaesthesia [47], at a dosage of 1800–3600 mg/day with reasonably good tolerance.

Both the micro- and macrocirculations are disturbed in diabetic limbs. Some of these abnormalities may be reversible or ameliorated by improved glycemic control [48]. Chronic change in peripheral blood vessels is usually manifested by atherosclerosis, with the pattern of PVD tending to involve vessels below the knee more often in diabetic than in nondiabetic individuals. Risk factors for PVD include smoking, hypertension, and dyslipidmia, with prevalence increasing with both advancing age and duration of diabetes. Symptoms include intermittent claudication and/or rest pain, with lower limb ulceration or gangrene being important clinical outcomes. Radiological investigation may show medial arterial calcification and this may be associated with both diabetic peripheral somatosensory and autonomic neuropathy. Objective assessment of limb blood flow by Doppler ultrasound can be affected by extensive medial calcification, giving rise to a misleadingly high ankle-pressure index. An appropriate and early referral for vascular assessment is mandatory in elderly patients with PVD who may benefit from arterial reconstruction or angioplasty. This is best organized through joint protocols developed by the diabetes specialist and the vascular surgeon [49]. A reasonable life-expectancy is considered important by surgeons since concomitant cardiac and cerebrovascular disease may account for death in 50% cases within 5 years [50].

Interventions designed to prevent diabetic foot disease and amputations in patients with diabetes should be directed to the prevention of peripheral neuropathy and PVD including the prevention, early detection, and treatment of foot lesions. Several studies using staff and patient education and a multidisciplinary approach to foot care have demonstrated a reduction in diabetes-related amputations. In proximal arterial reconstruction, the 5-year patency averages 70% and in those patients with high comorbidity levels, graft patency may exceed life-expectancy; for distal reconstruction surgery, 5-year limb salvage rates approach 85% [50].

For many elderly patients having great difficulty in performing the most routine foot care [51], often as a result of poor vision and reduced mobility, it becomes very important that strategies are designed which enable both spouses and other carers to have a role in prevention and treatment of foot lesions. Educational material needs to be concise and repeated regularly and video presentations may also be helpful.

Erectile Dysfunction

Erectile dysfunction (ED) due to diabetes in older adults is age related, and occurs earlier and more commonly than in the general population [52], and may be associated with cardiovascular disease. At least three important studies indicate the importance of ED in older people which is often neglected and may be an obvious reason for a diminished quality of life or depressive illness [53, 54]. After the age of 60 years, 55–95% of diabetic men are affected, while the corresponding figure for nondiabetic counterparts is 50%. The etiology of ED, defined as the inability to attain and maintain an erection satisfactory for sexual intercourse, is a complex problem involving several mechanisms. Vasculopathy, autonomic neuropathy, hormonal dysregulation, endothelial dysfunction, and psychogenic factors have all been implicated. Drug-related causes may be a particular problem in older patients, with thiazide diuretics, cimetidine, β-blockers and spironolactone especially being implicated. An alcohol history must be looked for. ED is evaluated initially by carrying out an interview with the patient and sexual partner where appropriate. A comprehensive history, full medical examination, blood testing for diabetes control, and lipids, testosterone, and thyroid function tests are necessary. Other more sophisticated tests are available through diabetes ED clinics in most large centers and may involve testing for prolactin, other gonadotrophins, and for nocturnal penile tumescence. For many older patients, extensive testing is often avoided. As treatment is available for some patients, e.g. oral sildenafil (achieved erections in 67% of elderly men in one study [52], where available), vacuum tumescence device, misaprostil urethral suppositories, or self-injection therapy with intracorporeal injection of vasoactive drugs (e.g. prostaglandin E1), ED should always be enquired about. Although intracavernous therapy is relatively successful, up to 50% of men discontinue eventually because of pain, loss of effect, or lack of interest [55]. Apomorphine is currently being evaluated in the treatment of ED, and surgery (penile prostheses, revascularization) is another option but requires expert evaluation beforehand.

Metabolic Comas

Diabetic ketoacidosis (DKA) and hyperglycemic hyperosmolar nonketotic (HONK) comas also occur in older subjects with diabetes; HONK comas are predominant in subjects aged over 50 years. Compared with the young, older subjects with hyperglycemic comas have a higher mortality, have a higher length of stay in hospital following admission, are less likely to have had diabetes diagnosed previously, are more likely to have renal impairment, and require a greater amount of insulin as treatment [56].

In an early study from Birmingham, UK, 22% of admissions with DKA were in subjects 60 years and older [57]; in contrast, 82 out of 610 admissions (13.4%) with hyperglycemic coma of all ages in Melbourne were due to HONK comas [58].

It appears that in hyperglycemic comas most subjects with type 2 diabetes have just enough residual insulin secretion to suppress lipolysis and ketogenesis, thus avoiding DKA, and develop a HONK coma instead. The tendency to hyperosmolarity in HONK comas may be worsened in elderly people, who may not appreciate thirst well, may have difficulty drinking enough to compensate for their osmotic diuresis, and may also be on diuretics. It also appears that hyperosmolarity not only worsens insulin resistance but may also inhibit lipolysis.

Death may be due to the metabolic disturbance and to acute illnesses such as pneumonia and myocardial infarction. The cause of the hyperglycemia may be infection, infarction, inadequate hypoglycemic treatment, or inappropriate drug treatment. Often a particular cause cannot be identified; for instance, there was no apparent cause in 354 out of 929 admissions with DKA in Birmingham [57], but in a study of HONK, 55% of cases were precipitated by infection [59]. Residents of care homes are also at increased risk of HONK coma associated with appreciable mortality [60]. Thiazide diuretics and steroids are known to increase blood glucose levels and may precipitate DKA; thiazide diuretics and frusemide may be particularly likely to precipitate HONK coma.

Treatment of Hyperglycemic Comas

The history and examination should pay special attention to previous diabetic symptoms and treatment, any precipitating infection, infarction, or medication, evidence of heart failure, and the degree of dehydration. Initial investigations are as for younger patients but it is essential to measure arterial blood gases. Attention to pressure areas is essential and monitoring of renal function paramount in an older patient.

Each major hospital unit will have an agreed fluid and insulin and potassium replacement protocol to use in these cases. Intravenous fluid replacement at a rate of 500 ml/h over the initial 4 h, reducing to 250 ml/h afterwards, should take place. The patient needs more rapid infusion if he or she is shocked, and here a central line is invaluable to monitor quick infusions, particularly in the presence of cardiac failure or recent myocardial infarction.

Older subjects with a HONK coma may need very small doses of insulin to reduce plasma glucose levels; however, if the patient is catabolic or has marked insulin resistance, larger doses of insulin may be required.

Thrombotic complications may occur, or may well have occurred before hospitalization, in subjects with a HONK coma. A prophylactic regimen should be considered.

Older People and Hypoglycemia

In older patients, susceptibility to hypoglycemia is pronounced, and this is exacerbated by old people having little knowledge about the symptoms and signs of hypoglycemia [61]. Indeed, health professionals may misdiagnose hypoglycemia as a stroke, transient ischemic attack, unexplained confusion, or epileptic fit.

Patients with cognitive impairment and those with loss of the warning symptoms of hypoglycemia are vulnerable, as they may not recognize impending hypoglycemia and/or fail to communicate their feelings to their carers. Multiple risk factors underlie the increased susceptibility to hypoglycemia in the elderly and these include recent discharge from hospital with a recent change in sulfonylurea, renal and hepatic impairment, excess alcohol, and insulin therapy [62]. In addition, older subjects mount a diminished counterregulatory response to hypoglycemia [63] and this may lead to a delay in recovery.

They are often incapable of treating hypoglycemia themselves [56]. The educational program should include advice and information relating to the detection and treatment of hypoglycemia, including the criteria for admission in cases of unresponsive hypoglycemia.

Hypoglycemia with Sulfonylureas

An important clinical problem for older subjects taking glibenclamide and chlorpropamide is prolonged hypoglycemia, especially when many older people have so little knowledge of the symptoms of hypoglycemia [64]. Glibenclamide-induced hypoglycemia may be more pronounced because the drug accumulates within β-cells and its metabolites retain some hypoglycemic activity. Because of the long elimination half-life (35 h) of chlorpropamide, continued dosing results in drug accumulation (steady state being achieved by 7–10 days). In the presence of impaired renal function, further prolongation of hypoglycemia occurs. Gliclazide and tolbutamide are less likely to cause hypoglycemia [65] and glipizide has been considered unsafe in the elderly by some [66].

It should be remembered that insulin therapy carries a greater risk of hypoglycemia than do sulfonylureas but the introduction of insulin analogues may decrease this risk. Newer oral agents such as the glitazones and the meglitinides may also lower the risk of hypoglycemia in the elderly.

In the elderly, serious hypoglycemia appears to have a worse prognosis with high mortality following hospital admission; some may have permanent neurological damage, presumably because of an already compromised cerebral circulation. Most sulfonylureas have caused fatal hypoglycemia, although this is often associated with chlorpropamide or glibenclamide [67]. Other factors apart from old age that predispose to fatal hypoglycemia are alcohol consumption, poor food intake, renal impairment, potentiation of hypoglycemia by other drugs, and prescription of sulfonylureas. Many, if not all, of these factors are directly relevant in the elderly patient with type 2 diabetes.

Cognitive Impairment, Dementia, and Diabetes

Impaired cognitive function has been demonstrated in elderly subjects with diabetes, but these studies were generally not population based, excluded subjects with dementia, and generally used a large battery of tests to show the deficit [68]. Community-based studies in Melton Mowbray [69], Nottingham [28], and South Wales [29] have shown worse cognitive function in elderly diabetic subjects, using simple tests such as the Folstein MMSE, Hodkinson AMT, and the Clock Test.

Impaired glucose tolerance has also been shown to be associated with cognitive dysfunction [70]. It has been suggested that that many of the deficits seen in the metabolic syndrome (hyperglycemia, dyslipidemia, hypertension) may each play a role in memory disturbance in type 2 diabetes [71], and increased serum insulin may be associated with decreased cognitive function and dementia in women [72]. The Rochester study [73] has demonstrated that the risk of dementia is significantly increased for both men and women with type 2 diabetes with the risk for Alzheimer's disease achieving significance in men only. Poor glucose control may be associated with cognitive impairment, which recovers following improvement in glycemic control [74].

Cognitive dysfunction in older diabetic subjects has considerable implications which include increased hospitalization, less ability for self-care, less likelihood of specialist follow-up, and increased risk of institutionalization [75]. Impaired cognitive function should be borne in mind when treating elderly diabetic subjects as it has implications for their safe treatment; it may cause difficulty with glycemic control due to erratic taking of diet and medication, and may present as hypoglycemia if the patient forgets that he or she has taken the hypoglycemic medication and repeats the dose.

Depression and Diabetes

Major depressive disorder increases significantly the risk of diabetes [76], and in another study diabetes was significantly associated with depression, independent of age, gender, or presence of chronic disease [77]. The presence of depression was the single most important indicator of subsequent death in a group of diabetic patients admitted into hospital [78]. Failure to recognize depression can be serious since it is a long-term, life-threatening, disabling illness that can have a significant impact on quality of life. Depression may be associated with worsening diabetic control [79] and decreased treatment compliance [80].

There is a relative lack of specific evidence linking neuroendocrine abnormalities with diabetes and the probable explanation at this stage is that depression is due to the effect of increased stress and strain of having a chronic medical condition in a susceptible individual. Diabetes and depression share similar symptomatology—for example, fatigue, irritability of sexual dysfunction—and this may delay or confuse the diagnosis. However, commonly used diagnostic assessment scales are unlikely to be greatly affected by these overlapping symptoms. In routine practice, enquire about well-being, sleep, appetite, and weight loss as part of the assessment of older patients with diabetes. If alerted, take a more comprehensive psychiatric evaluation and use a geriatric depression scale score (>5) as indicative of probable depression. Treatment with serotonin selective reuptake inhibitors (SSRIs) such as fluoxetine may improve symptomatology with a consequent improvement in metabolic control [81]. In a recent Dutch community-based study of diabetic subjects with depression [82], the presence of comorbid disease increased significantly the prevalence of depressive symptoms in type 2 diabetes, which provides further support for identifying high-risk groups with this possible condition.

Diabetic Mortality

Type 2 diabetes in any group is a cardiovascular risk factor and has varying effects on life-expectancy. Early reports indicated that the ratio of death rates in diabetic subjects to rates in the general population falls progressively with age, especially in those 65 years and older. This has been confirmed largely by the Verona Study where excess mortality related to diabetes measured by the standardized mortality ratio (SMR) declined from a range of 2–3.5 for middle-aged subjects to a level of 1.75 in subjects aged 65–74, but remaining above unity in patients older than 75 years [83]. The impact of diabetes on the SMR was more pronounced in women at all ages. A recent systematic review of studies examining the relationship between mortality and age suggested that the incidence of premature death in older diabetic subjects was in fact higher [84]. Cardiovascular mortality is the principal cause of this excess mortality and accounted for 42% of the overall mortality in the Verona Study. In the Melton study by Croxson et al. [85], a substantial increase in excess mortality was seen in subjects 65 years and older, and impaired glucose tolerance was found to be associated with a relative risk of death of 1.7 (95% CI 0.8–3.5).

Age remains the strongest predictor of mortality but the other classic risk factors are present in older subjects with diabetes. Their contribution to cardiovascular mortality is uncertain: in a Finnish study [86] smoking, hypertension, low high-density lipoprotein cholesterol, and high total cholesterol did not affect overall mortality. In the Verona Study, long-term glycemic control had a greater effect in predicting outcome and those subjects whose glucose control was more variable (measured by the coefficient of variation fasting plasma glucose) had lower survival rates, especially in subjects 75 years and older [87].

Methodological variations have prevented consistent comparisons being made across different diabetic populations. It is important to determine whether premature death due to diabetes is observable in elderly patients because this evidence would provide guidance to those responsible for providing health services on how best to focus their resources. An unequivocal finding of increased mortality would argue for a more sustained commitment to diabetic health care provision and increased evidence of research. Alternatively, in the presence of no excess mortality, future care strategies could become focused on reducing morbidity and disability only.

METABOLIC TARGETING, DISABILITY, AND FRAILTY

The evidence base for metabolic interventions in type 2 diabetes in older subjects is limited since there have been few published studies that have focused on the elderly and no large trial data for microvascular disease. However, it seems entirely appropriate and justified to extrapolate data from studies in younger subjects and while there may be limitations to this approach [88], it ensures we pass on the potential benefits to older subjects. The benefits associated with achieving good glycemic control in type 2 diabetes are potentially substantial and apart from symptom control, may also lead to reduced hospitalization due to metabolic decompensation. Acceptable glycemic targets may also help to maintain visual acuity and cognitive function and reduce the risk of depression and the need for caregiver support.

I have previously introduced the concept of a five-step approach to prioritizing diabetes care in the elderly and this approach is represented in Table 5 [49]. This takes into account that diabetes in older subjects is invariably a major cause of functional impairment, both physically and cognitively. The care package must include, therefore, interventions designed to limit this impairment in addition to elements of metabolic targeting (see below).

Table 5 A five-step approach to prioritizing diabetes care in older adults

(1) Functional assessment, including cognitive testing and screening for depression
(2) Vascular risk assessment, especially vascular prophylaxis and lifestyle modification
(3) Metabolic targeting ("single disease" or "frailty" models)
(4) Devise appropriate interventions for diabetes-related disabilities
(5) Assess suitability for self-care vs. carer assistance

Identifying the Proportion of Diabetic Elders Who Require Metabolic Targeting

One approach to enhancing the appropriateness of intensive diabetes care with metabolic targeting is to review the functional status of individuals based on measures of physical and cognitive performance. Functional status can generally be used as a proxy for the combination of comorbidities, multiple medications, and diabetes-related vascular complications. In the Welsh Community Diabetes Study [29], we noted that diabetic subjects older than 65 years were nearly twice as likely to require assistance with personal care, to require a mobility aid, and to be in receipt of social services input. In addition, diabetic subjects had significantly higher levels of physical and cognitive disability when measured with well-validated tools. Data from the NHANES III, which was a nationally representative cross-sectional study of noninstitutionalized US citizens, revealed that diabetes was a major cause of physical disability among subjects 60 years and older [89]. Disability in at least one of the physical tasks examined was reported in 63% of diabetic women (controls, 42%) and 39% of diabetic men (controls, 25%), with stronger associations between diabetes and more severe forms of disability. Diabetes was shown to have a two- to threefold increased likelihood of a mobility disorder, with coronary heart disease being a major contributor to this excess disability in both sexes, and stroke being an important contributor among men.

However, despite these functional deficits, and based on analysis of objective ADL (activities of daily living) scores (as a marker of disability) and cardiovascular risk in subjects older than 65 years with type 2 diabetes [29], the majority (at least 60–70%) of older people with diabetes should be considered suitable for strategies which involve either strict or optimum glycemic control. It is important to identify those patients where a label of frailty is appropriate since their aims of care are modified, e.g. those in institutional care. Frailty, in this context, represents a vulnerability to a wide range of adverse outcomes secondary to the effects of aging, long-term vascular complications of diabetes, physical and cognitive decline, and the presence of other medical comorbidities. In the *Frailty Model of Diabetes* [49], a framework can be developed that provides further assistance with clinical decision making. This allows health professionals to define a series of factors such as recurrent hypoglycemia, cardiac disease, and reduced recovery from metabolic decompensation, which have three characteristics in common:

(1) These may represent a precursor state to disability

Table 6 Treatment targets for elderly diabetic patients

Blood glucose levels	Blood pressure	Blood lipid levels	Aspirin use
No specific studies in older people with diabetes	Increasing evidence of benefit from BP lowering UKPDS: ≤140/80 mmHg (not based on older subjects)	Increasing evidence of benefit of lipid lowering	ATS Study: 75–325 mg/day reduced major cardiovascular events in high-risk patients by 25%
UKPDS: HbA_{1c} <7%; fasting blood glucose <7 mmol/l	HOT Study: diastolic lowering to ≤83 mmHg SHEP Study: systolic BP <150 mmHg Syst-Eur Study: systolic BP <160 mmHg LIFE Study: target BP <140/90 mmHg ALLHAT Study: target BP <140/90 mmHg	LIPID, CARE, 4S, VA-HIT studies: total cholesterol <5 mmol/l; high-density lipoprotein cholesterol >1.0 mmol/l; triglycerides <2.0 mmol/l PROSPER and Heart Protection Study: 1 mmol/l lowering of LDL-cholesterol associated with 15–25% reduction in major vascular events	HOT Study: 75 mg/day reduced major cardiovascular events by 15% and myocardial infarction by 36%

(2) They are often a direct threat to independence
(3) They may have preventable or reversible components

In clinical practice, the presence of a mobility disorder or severe restriction of ADL, or the presence of several comorbidities, and/or advanced age (80 years and older) should be recognized as poor predictors of functional status and increases the risk of becoming confined to a chair or bed two- to threefold over 2 years [90].

Metabolic Targets for Older People with Type 2 Diabetes

In Table 6, a series of metabolic targets have been stated which should form a framework for imposing strict and optimal therapy programs. The evidence is based on data derived from important large-scale clinical trials, which are referenced in full in reference 50. It is now expected by clinicians that in addition to glucose and blood pressure control, lipid-lowering should be considered for subjects up to the age of 80 years. Thromboembolic prophylaxis is another important issue. A dose of 75–300 mg/day of aspirin (or use clopidogrel when aspirin is not tolerated) is suitable prophylaxis in aging subjects with evidence of macrovascular disease or who have risk factors such as hypertension, obesity, albuminuria (macro/micro), and cigarette smoking. The increased risk of atrial fibrillation in older diabetic subjects also increases the risk of thromboembolism but we have no specific evidence of benefit of formal warfarin anticoagulation in this age group with diabetes.

Estimation of cardiovascular risk is an essential prerequisite to metabolic targeting as it provides information about prognosis and the need for specific treatments both in the primary and secondary prevention of coronary artery disease. Several methods are available which usually provide a risk definition of 10–20% over a 5- or 10-year period. These include the New Zealand tables [91], Framingham study [92], and the Seven European Countries Study [93]. One limitation of these approaches is a lack of data from subjects older than 74 years.

In a New Zealand study, subjects with type 2 diabetes (70 years and older) had an increased mortality if they were hyperlipidemic [94]. In the Veterans Affairs Intervention Study (VA-HIT Study), treatment with gemfibrozil resulted in a greater than 20% reduction in cardiovascular mortality. Three quarters of subjects were aged 60–74 years and 25% had diabetes [95]. This provides some evidence that triglyceride reduction in older subjects may also be of benefit in reducing overall cardiovascular risk.

In the MicroHOPE study, the effects of ramipril, an angiotensin-converting enzyme inhibitor, on cardiovascular and microvascular outcomes in people 55 years and older were investigated over a 4.5-year follow-up [96]. Each of the patients recruited were at high risk of a cardiovascular event because of previous cardiac disease (e.g., stroke, myocardial infarction, peripheral vascular disease) or the presence of diabetes plus an additional cardiovascular risk factor such as hypertension of dyslipidemia. Primary endpoints (stroke or myocardial infarction, fatal or nonfatal) were reduced from 20 to 15%, with a relative risk reduction on all-cause mortality of 24%.

ISSUES IN TREATMENT AND CARE

Making the Diagnosis

An early diagnosis may reduce morbidity (detection and prevention of vascular complications) and cardiovascular mortality, although evidence for this is lacking. The diagnostic criteria are identical in young and old subjects but some concern has been expressed about the applicability of a fasting glucose level for diagnosis in many older subjects and mortality may be higher in those subjects diagnosed as diabetic with the 2-h glucose value than the new fasting criteria alone [97]. In addition, isolated postload hyperglycemia with normal fasting glucose (<7.0 mmol/l) is associated with increased fatal cardiovascular disease and heart disease in elderly women [98].

Many patients may not be able to give an accurate history of symptoms; classic hyperosmolar symptoms of polyuria and polydipsia may be absent because of a combination of altered thirst sensation and a variable renal threshold for glycosuria. A true fasted sample may be difficult to obtain and may be normal in any case [97] and an oral glucose tolerance test (OGTT) may be thought of as time-consuming and inconvenient.

In some cases, elderly patients have elevated plasma glucose levels, which are secondary to acute illness, diabetogenic therapy, or other stress-inducing disorders. Most cases will be diagnosed without the need for an OGTT but this should be employed where doubt exists. The demonstration of an elevated HbA_{1c} in this situation is a pointer to the likely presence of diabetes. Retesting following an acute illness may sometimes prevent false diagnosis being made.

Initial Management

The principal aims of managing diabetes in older adults are listed in Table 7. The priority of each may be provisionally established at an early stage but may change with disease duration, development of complications, and need for external help. Self-monitoring by patients or carers should be encouraged as part of an empowerment and educational approach to improving self-care activities.

For those presenting with type 2 diabetes in a nonacute presentation, four important steps are needed: establish the diagnosis of diabetes; screen for vascular complications and assess cardiovascular risk; assess the ability of the patient for diabetes self-care; and initiate treatment. An important aspect of care relates to producing an initial diabetes care plan (Table 8). No specific stepwise algorithm has been adopted for treatment and the guidelines of the International Diabetes Federation [99] are equally applicable to older subjects. In this section we shall limit our discussion to additional relevant comments.

Table 7 Major aims in managing older people with diabetes

Medical	Patient-orientated
Freedom from hyperglycemic symptoms	Maintain general well-being and good quality of life
Prevent undesirable weight loss	Acquire skills and knowledge to adapt to lifestyle changes
Avoid hypoglycemia and other adverse drug reactions	Encourage diabetes self-care
Screen for and prevent vascular complications	
Detect cognitive impairment and depression at an early stage	
Achieve a normal life-expectancy for patients where possible	

Table 8 Care plan for initial management of diabetes in an elderly person

(1) Establish realistic glycemic and blood pressure targets
(2) Ensure consensus with patient, spouse or family, general practitioner, informal carter, community nurse or hospital specialist
(3) Define the frequency and nature of diabetes follow-up
(4) Organize glycemic monitoring by patient or carer
(5) Refer to social or community services as necessary
(6) Provide advice on stopping smoking, increasing exercise, and alcohol intake

Initial Treatment

Dietary measures and lifestyle advice is given as for middle-aged subjects, irrespective of the presentation. This represents a low risk but potentially high-benefit strategy. In some cases, a specified exercise program is instituted. These may be sufficient for those subjects whose initial random glucose levels are less than 15 mmol/l, and in whom symptoms are minimal. If metabolic targets are not reached by 6–8 weeks, oral therapy is usually required. Strict glycemic targeting approaches are possible for many older subjects. However, a reasonable view applicable to patients with single system involvement (free of other major comorbidities) is to aim for control as follows: a fasting glucose range of 5–7 mmol/l (depending on their ability to self-care) and a random level of 6–9 mmol/l. A glycosylated hemoglobin (HbA_{1c}) range of 6.5–7.5% is also recommended but increases the risk of hypoglycemia. For frail subjects (dependent, multisystem disease, care home residency including those with dementia), a fasting glucose of 7–9 mmol/l and a HbA_{1c} range of 7.5–8.5% should be aimed for. In general, both sets of targets should reduce the occurrence of hyperglycemic malaise and the stricter target should have some preventative benefits in terms of vascular complication rate. Attention to lipid and blood pressure targets is essential to complement these approaches.

A range of options are available for dietary failures and these have been discussed in specific guidelines published in 1996 [100]. These require updating with the emergence of the thiazolidinediones, meglitinides, and insulin analogues.

Glucose Regulation: Use of Oral Agents in Type 2 Diabetes in Old Age

Sulfonylureas

These are often felt to be the oral agent of choice for the elderly diabetic subject failing on diet because they are generally well tolerated (apart from their risk of hypoglycemia) without the risk of gastrointestinal upset associated with other oral agents. They can achieve a fall of HbA_{1c} of about 1.5%.

Glibenclamide appears particularly likely to cause hypoglycemia and its use has been associated with fatalities more than do other sulfonylureas including chlorpropamide; this drug should be strictly avoided. Use of glipizide has been linked to deaths in elderly Swedish subjects due to hypoglycemia [66]; some elderly subjects experience a prolonged hypoglycemic effect from it. Gliclazide has a relatively low risk of hypoglycemia and it may be less likely to cause weight gain, the other common problem with sulfonylureas, and undoubtedly safer than glibenclamide [65]. If hypoglycemia is a major worry, then tolbutamide has the lowest risk, and this may be used in those with renal impairment. If compliance is a problem, then glimepiride is useful since the tablet range means that the dose for all patients is one tablet before breakfast; however, there are no good comparisons between this and gliclazide; alternatively, a modified release preparation of gliclazide is now available.

Metformin

Metformin is predictable and safe if used correctly, but there are contraindications to its use: these include renal impairment (creatinine >120 μmol/l), hepatic or cardiac failure, critical limb ischemia, any acute illness, and use of intravenous radiological contrast media. As a result, often about 40–50% of older subjects may be ineligible for use of metformin. Particular advantages of metformin are that it does not cause hypoglycemia on its own, it does not cause weight gain, and it is inexpensive. Its therapeutic benefits are similar to those with sulfonylureas, and in the UKPDS, all-cause mortality and any diabetes-related endpoint were significantly lower on intensive treatment with metformin than with insulin or sulfonylurea in obese subjects [101]. It has been shown to be an effective treatment in the elderly, with results similar to those with tolbutamide. The usual daily dose required is approximately 1.7 g, and it is as effective in the lean as in the overweight, and lowers HbA_{1c} by 1.5%. An extended-release form has the advantage of once-daily dosing.

The FDA in the United States limits the use of metformin to patients aged less than 80 years (unless they have normal renal function), presumably because of the increased risk of lactic acidosis; other side effects include gastrointestinal disturbance, which is minimized by gentle introduction of the agent. Metformin may also cause vitamin B_{12} malabsorption; hence, it is wise to check B_{12} level every 5 years.

An insulin secretagogue should be used in combination with metformin in overweight patients (BMI > 25 kg/m^2) where glycemic targets have not been achieved or maintained.

Acarbose

Since only 1–2% of oral acarbose is absorbed, it is relatively free of major systemic side effects and its main contraindications are inflammatory bowel disease and subacute obstruction. Acarbose can be successfully combined with metformin, sulfonylureas, or insulin. It is not as effective as other oral agents in older subjects. In practice, we prescribe 25 mg t.d.s. with the first mouthful of the meal for 1 month, and then increase to 50 mg t.d.s., which is at variance with the Glucobay data sheet (Bayer), which recommend starting with 50 mg before the main meal of the day, and then adding an extra tablet before another meal every few weeks. Doses above 50 mg t.d.s. seem to confer marginal increases in hypoglycemic effect, but do run a greater likelihood of gastrointestinal side effects in our experience.

Thiazoledinediones

These reduce insulin resistance by activating the peroxisome proliferator activated receptor gamma (PPAR-γ). They do not cause hypoglycemia and the only problems seem to be weight gain, mild edema, and anemia (less than 5% of subjects); although clinical trials did include subjects with New York Heart Association heart failure grade 2 and no patient developed acute left ventricular failure, they are contraindicated in heart failure (and consequently are not to be used with insulin at the present time). They are safe in mild to moderate renal impairment. They have the potential to cause liver function abnormalities and frequent monitoring of liver function is required especially during the first 12 months of treatment; this is an important disadvantage for many older subjects.

They can be used as monotherapy (although not all countries have a monotherapy license) or combined with metformin or sulfonylurea, or combined with insulin (where license permits). There are very few differences between the two agents in common use, with little difference in hypoglycemic effect and a modest improvement in lipid profile with pioglitazone; up to 6–8 weeks may occur before beneficial actions are observed following the introduction of a glitazone. They can be used as once-daily medications, and an HbA_{1c} fall of about 0.6–1.2% can be expected in combination with either metformin or a sulfonylurea.

Non-sulfonylurea Insulin Secretagogues

Repaglinide is a benzoic acid derivative of the meglitinide class which targets postprandial hyperglycemia. It is predominantly metabolized in the liver to inactive metabolites and is safe in mild to moderate renal impairment. It has

Table 9 Practice-orientated guidelines for insulin treatment in older people

	Indications	Advantages	Disadvantages
Once-daily insulin	Frail subjects Very old (>80 years) Symptomatic control	Single injection Can be given by carer or district nurse	Control usually poor Hypoglycemia common
Twice-daily insulin	Preferred if good glycemic control Suitable for type 1 diabetes	Low risk of hypoglycemia Easily managed by most older diabetic people	Normoglycemia difficult to achieve Fixed meal times reduce flexibility Expensive
Basal/bolus insulin	Well-motivated individuals Can reduce microvascular complications	Enables tight control For acute illness in hospital Flexible meal times	Frequent monitoring required to avoid hypoglycemia
Insulin plus oral agents	If glycemic control is unsatisfactory with oral agents alone To limit weight gain in obese subject	Limits weight gain by reducing total daily insulin Increased flexibility	May delay conversion to insulin in thin or type 1 patients

a rapid onset of action and a relatively low risk of symptomatic hypoglycemia compared with sulfonylureas and has better postprandial glucose profiles. Tablets can be missed if meals are not taken, introducing a degree of "flexibility" to its use. It has been used effectively in combination with metformin and with glitazones (where license permits). I recommend to start with 0.5 mg at the start of each meal for subjects on diet, and 1.0 mg for subjects transferring from other oral agents; up to 4 mg for each meal can be used. Nateglinide is a recent meglitinide that has faster and shorter duration of insulin secretory activity than does rapaglinide. In the United Kingdom, rapaglinide cannot be prescribed to those 75 years and older.

Insulin

Insulin use in older people has an important increasing role in management [102]. Recent improvements in the organization of care between hospital and primary care, together with the developing educational and diabetes care roles of diabetes specialist nurses and general practice nurses, have increased the availability and safety of insulin for older people with diabetes. Its main indications are in the treatment of type 1 diabetes at diagnosis, and in type 2 diabetes where metabolic targets have not been achieved with diet, exercise, and oral agents; other indications include its use in acute myocardial infarction, acute stroke, hyperglycemic coma, and major surgery. Its main disadvantage is hypoglycemia, although in the UKPDS less than 2% subjects treated with insulin had a major episode of hypoglycemia. Low visual aids are available to assist those with poor vision to administer insulin although some insulin pens have audible clicks for counting. Benefits of insulin include improvements in well-being (and possibly quality of life) [103–105] and cognitive function [74] in part due to improvements in glycemic control. However, these are not universal findings and treatment satisfaction may be lower in insulin-treated patients [106], suggesting that there is often a 'trade-off' between intensified control and quality of life, two important diabetes outcomes.

An insulin treatment grid is provided in Table 9. Rapidly acting insulin analogues such as insulin lispro or aspart may cause less hypoglycemia and weight gain and can be given after a meal where patient compliance with meals may be unpredictable, e.g. those with memory disorder. In patients with type 1 diabetes, premixed insulins (e.g., Humulin M range or Mixtard) given twice daily are often satisfactory. In older patients with type 2 diabetes, a twice-daily regimen of human isophane insulin (e.g., Humulin I or Insulatard) can be used with soluble, short-acting insulin added in later. The introduction of intermediate-acting insulin analogues (e.g., insulin glargine) with their reproducible kinetics, and absence of an early peak, should provide safer insulin usage in older subjects. Once-daily insulin regimens alone are now infrequently used except where glycemic control is not a priority, or where community support to give insulin is lacking.

My common clinical practice in using insulin is to add it to those failing on diet and oral agents and usually stop one oral agent. This can be achieved by using a nighttime dose of intermediate-acting insulin or insulin glargine (for example) and giving either a sulfonylurea (less plausible option) or metformin, which in the latter case has been associated with less weight gain, a lower frequency of hypoglycemia, and better glycemic control than does twice-daily insulin or combinations of glibenclamide with insulin or metformin [107]. Before prescribing insulin, the physician should make an assessment of the risk of hypoglycemia, and agree treatment goals with the patient (and/or carer).

INSTITUTIONAL DIABETES CARE

Residents with diabetes in care homes should receive a level of comprehensive diabetes care commensurate with their health and social needs [108]. The two most important aims of care are as follows:

(1) To maintain the highest degree of quality of life and well-being without subjecting residents to unnecessary and inappropriate medical and therapeutic interventions

Table 10 Importance of early detection of diabetes mellitus in care homes

- Improved metabolic control may improve cognition, decrease the risk of hyperosmolar coma, and lesson osmotic symptoms
- Earlier treatment may delay vascular complications and reduce disability
- Knowledge of diagnosis of diabetes prompts physician to be be alert to diabetes-related complications, e.g. hyperosmolar coma
- Earlier dietary intervention may delay treatment (and therefore limit adverse drug reactions) with oral agents
- Treatment can reduce symptoms and may increase quality of life and functional well-being

(2) To provide support and opportunity to enable residents to manage their own diabetes condition where this is a feasible and worthwhile option
Other crucial objectives of care include:
(3) To achieve a satisfactory (but optimal) level of metabolic control, which reduces both hyperglycemic lethargy and hypoglycemia, and allows the greatest level of physical and cognitive function
(4) To optimize foot care and visual health, which promotes an increased level of mobility, reduced risk of falls, and prevents unnecessary hospital admissions
(5) To provide a well-balanced nutritional and dietetic plan, which prevents weight loss and maintains nutritional well-being
(6) To effectively screen for diabetic complications regularly especially eye disease, peripheral neuropathy, and peripheral vascular disease, which predispose to foot infection and ulceration.

With recent demographic changes in developed countries, the numbers of care home residents is likely to increase dramatically as the populations age, and as the provision of hospital-based long-term care facilities is likely to continue falling. Inevitably, this will be associated with an increase in the prevalence of diabetes within these settings. A number of prevalence surveys of diabetes within care homes provide estimates of between 7.2 and 14.5%, depending on the method used for identifying those with diabetes [109–111]. In a recent UK study of screening care home residents for diabetes using two-point (fasting and 2-h post-glucose challenge values) oral glucose tolerance tests, the overall prevalence rate (newly diagnosed + known diabetes) was calculated as 26.7%, with a rate of 30.2% for impaired glucose tolerance [20]. However, the majority of diagnoses were made according to the 2-h values rather than the fasting glucose levels, although it may be argued that these residents are at greater cardiovascular risk and may benefit from an intervention [97]. The importance of early detection of diabetes in care homes is outlined in Table 10.

Diabetic residents of care homes appear to be a highly vulnerable and neglected group, characterized by a high prevalence of macrovascular complications, marked

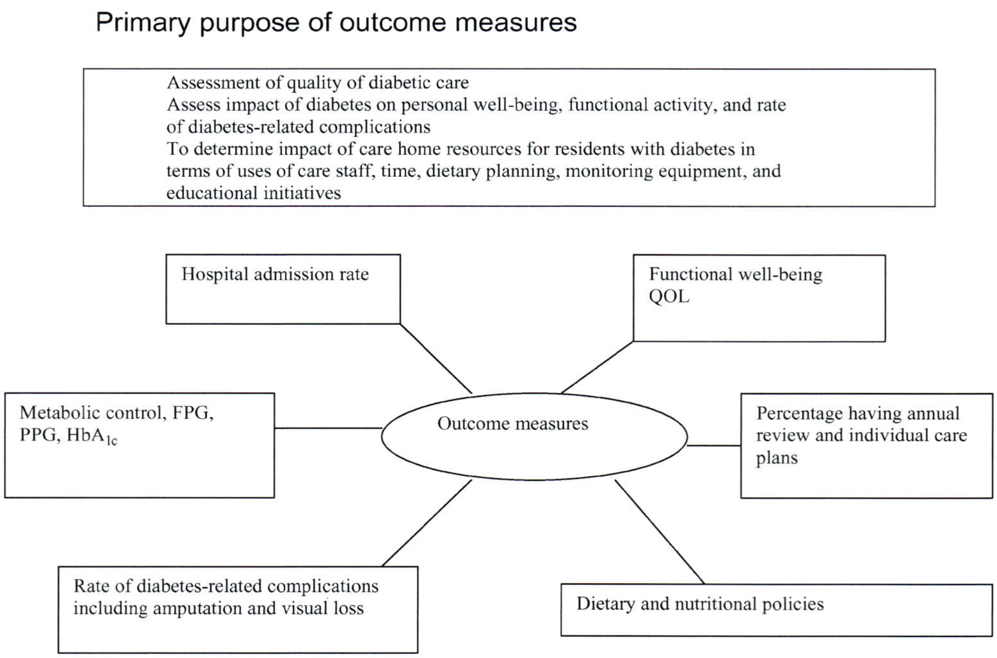

Figure 2 Development of robust outcome measures for diabetes care in long-term care settings QOL = quality of life; FPG = fasting plasma glucose; PPG = postprandial glucose [113]

Table 11 Strategies for improving diabetes care in care homes

- Establish National and International Standards of Quality Diabetes Care in Care Homes
- Establish National Diabetes Training and Educational Programmes for care home nursing and administrative staff
- Agreed Protocols of Diabetes Care within care homes covering medical, nursing, dietary, other health professional issues, and access to specialist care
- Involve care homes in an active Diabetes Audit Program

susceptibility to infections (especially skin and urinary tract), increased hospitalization rates, and high levels of physical and cognitive disability.

A number of deficiencies of diabetes care have been identified within these settings [110, 111] and include lack of individual care plans and case management approaches, inadequate dietary supervision, lack of specialist nursing and ophthalmology input, lack of knowledge and training for care staff, and inadequate medical review and follow-up practices.

Diabetes Care Home Provision—Modern Approaches

Several important strategies to improve the quality and outcomes of diabetes care within these settings have been proposed [110, 112, 113]. These have been summarized in Figure 2 and Table 11. Along with identifying suitable outcome measures, this includes choosing effective and appropriate outcome measures, providing educational and training programs for care staff, and ensuring that diabetes care is comprehensive, individualized, and cost-effective.

CONCLUSIONS

Structured diabetes care is particularly important for older people who are often missing out at present [114] and with the shift in health care from hospitals to the community and primary care setting, it is essential that general practitioners become well organized [115]. A detailed review of primary care diabetes and older people can be found elsewhere [116] but requires considerable motivation by the general practitioner, an effective screening for diabetes program, close liaison with diabetes specialist nurses whose many roles include teaching, advising counseling for older people (and carers/families), commencing insulin at home, and providing diabetic expertise within care homes, establishing an effective review and recall system, and ensuring that each patient with diabetes has an annual review. A shared-care approach (general practitioners working in partnership with hospital-based diabetic and surgical specialists) with agreed clinical protocols, including criteria for referral, is of particular value for older people.

The components of a modern day geriatric diabetes service is outlined in Figure 3. This uses a multidimensional intervention model [49] and emphasizes the importance of early intervention in vascular disease (retinal, microvascular, and macrovascular) and establishing rehabilitation programs for patients with a wide variety of disabling complications, e.g. amputation, peripheral neuropathy, immobility, falls, stroke, and cognitive change. Critical event monitoring is a system of monitoring those critical periods of ill health or social care need where patient vulnerability is high and opportunity for intervention is paramount, e.g. admission to hospital, amputation, or stroke illness.

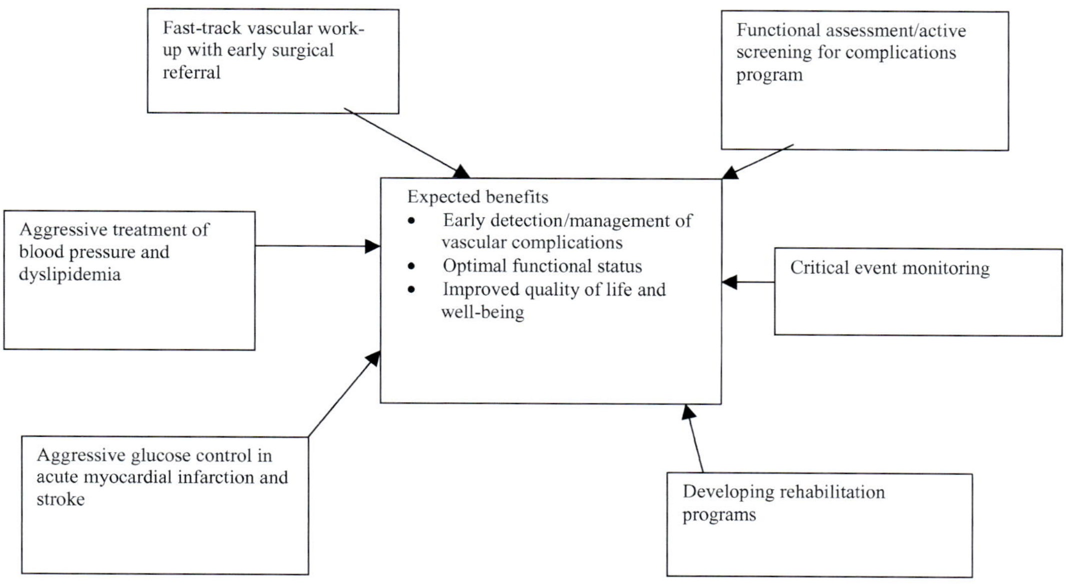

Figure 3 Components of a modern strategy for managing diabetes in the elderly

Ensuring cost-effective care becomes increasingly important *and is demanded* in our health care systems. Diabetes mellitus, in view of its high prevalence, long duration of impact, wide spectrum of complications, and multiple emotional and psychological sequelae provides a complex case for cost-effective studies. On older subjects, this is even more complex because of many other confounding factors. Two recent studies in this area [117, 118] suggest that aggressive treatment of diabetes in older individuals is not warranted because of reduced life-expectancy. However, implementing some of the strategies outlined above may lead to reduced acute hospitalization, lower outpatient costs, and less long-term disability. Only well-organized prospective clinical trials will be able to answer this important research question.

REFERENCES

1. Sinclair AJ. Issues in the initial management of type 2 diabetes. In Sinclair AJ, Finucane P (eds), *Diabetes in Old Age*, 2nd edn. Chichester: John Wiley & Sons Ltd, 2001; pp 155–64.
2. Finucane P, Popplewell P. Diabetes mellitus and impaired glucose regulation on old age: the scale of the problem. In Sinclair AJ, Finucane P (eds), *Diabetes in Old Age*, 2nd edn. Chichester: John Wiley & Sons Ltd, 2001; pp 3–16.
3. Krop JS, Shaffer TJ, Powe NR, Saudek CD, Anderson GF. Patterns of expenditures and use of services among older adults with diabetes. *Diabetes Care* 1998; 21: 747–51.
4. Hudson CN, Lazarus J, Peters J, Beck P, Sinclair AJ. An audit of diabetic care in three district general hospitals in Cardiff. *Pract Diab Intern* 1995; 13 (1): 29–32.
5. Damsgaard EM, Froland A, Green A. Use of hospital services by elderly diabetics: the Frederica Study of diabetic and fasting hyperglycaemic patients aged 60–74 years. *Diabet Med* 1987; 4: 317–22.
6. Beck-Nielsen H, and the European Group for the Study of Insulin Resistance (EGIR). General characteristics of the insulin resistance syndrome. *Drugs* 1999; 1: 7–10.
7. Haffner SM, Stem MP, Hazuda HP, Mitchell BD, Patterson JK. Cardiovascular risk factors in confirmed prediabetic individuals: does the clock of coronary heart disease start ticking before the onset of clinical diabetes? *JAMA* 1990; 263: 2893–8.
8. Kamel HK, Morley JE. Metabolic risk factors and their treatment. In Sinclair AJ, Finucane P (eds), *Diabetes in Old Age*, 2nd edn. Chichester: John Wiley & Sons Ltd, 2001; pp 187–98.
9. Sinclair AJ. Diabetes in the elderly: a perspective from the United Kingdom. *Clin Geriatr Med (USA)* 1999; 15: 225–37.
10. Hendra TJ, Sinclair AJ. Improving the care of elderly diabetic patients: the final report of the St Vincent Joint Task Force for Diabetes. *Age Ageing* 1997; 26: 3–6.
11. Spence JW. Some observations on sugar tolerance with special reference to variations found at different ages. *Q J Med* 1921; 14: 314–26.
12. Jackson RA. Mechanisms of age-related glucose intolerance. *Diabetes Care* 1990; 13 (suppl 2): 9–19.
13. Harris MI, Flegal KM, Cowie CC, Eberhardt MS, Goldstein DE, Little RR, Wiedmeyer H-M, Byrd-Holt DD. Prevalence of diabetes, impaired fasting glucose, and impaired glucose tolerance in US adults. The Third National and Nutrition Examination Survey, 1988–1994. *Diabetes Care* 1998; 21: 518–24.
14. Muller DC, Elahi D, Tobin JD, Andres R. The effect of age on insulin resistance and secretion: a review. *Semin Nephrol* 1996; 16: 289–98.
15. Meneilly GS, Hards L, Tessier D, Elliott T, Tildesley H. NIDDM in the elderly. *Diabetes Care* 1996; 19: 1320–75.
16. Meneilly GS, Elahi D, Minaker KL, Sclater AL, Rowe JW. Impairment of noninsulin-mediated glucose disposal in the elderly. *J Clin Endocrinol Metab* 1989; 63: 566–71.
17. Best JD, Kahn SE, Ader M, Watanabe RM, Ni TC, Bergman RN. Role of glucose effectiveness in the determination of glucose tolerance. *Diabetes Care* 1996; 19: 1018–30.
18. Croxson SCM, Burden AC, Bodington M, Botha JL. The prevalence of diabetes in elderly people. *Diabet Med* 1991; 8: 28–31.
19. Sinclair AJ, Croxson SCM. Diabetes Mellitus in the older adult. In Tallis R, Fillit H, Brocklehurst JC (eds), *Brocklehurst's Textbook of Geriatric Medicine and Gerontology*, 5th edn. Edinburgh: Churchill Livingstone, 1998; pp 1051–72.
20. Sinclair AJ, Gadsby R, Penfold S, Croxson SCM, Bayer AJ. Prevalence of diabetes in care home residents. *Diabetes Care* 2001; 24: 1066–8.
21. Levetan CS, Passaro M, Jablonski K, Kass M, Ratne RE. Unrecognised diabetes among hospital patients. *Diabetes Care* 1998; 21: 246–9.
22. Damsgaard EM, Froland A, Holm A. Ambulatory medical care for elderly diabetics: the Fredericia survey of diabetic and fasting hyperglycaemic subjects aged 60–74 years. *Diabet Med* 1987; 4: 534–8.
23. Wiliams DRR. Hospital admissions of diabetic patients: information from hospital activity analysis. *Diabet Med* 1985; 2: 2–32.
24. Harrower ADB. Prevalence of elderly patients in a hospital diabetic population. *Br J Clin Pract* 1980; 34: 131–3.
25. Cohen DL, Neil HAW, Thorogood M, Mann JI. A population based study of the incidence of complications associated with type 2 diabetes in the elderly. *Diabet Med* 1991; 8: 928–33.
26. Kannel WB, McGee DL. Diabetes and cardiovascular disease: the Framingham Study. *JAMA* 241: 2035–8.
27. Walters DP, Gatling W, Mullee MA, Hill RD. The prevalence of diabetic distal sensory neuropathy in an English Community. *Diabet Med* 1992; 9: 349–53.
28. Dornan TL, Peck GM, Dow JDC, Tattersal RB. A community survey of diabetes in the elderly. *Diabetic Med* 1992; 9: 860–5.
29. Sinclair AJ, Bayer AJ. All Wales Research in Elderly (AWARE). Diabetes Study. Department of Health Report 121/3040. London: UK Government, 1998.
30. Naliboff BD, Rosenthal M. Effects of age on complications in adult onset diabetes. *JAGS* 1989; 37: 838–42.
31. Ballard DJ, Humphrey LL, Melton LJ, et al. Epidemiology of persistent proteinuria in type II diabetes mellitus: population based study in Rochester, Minnesota. *Diabetes* 1988; 37: 405–12.
32. Knuiman MW, Welborn TA, McCann VJ, Stanton KG, Constable IJ. Prevalence of diabetic complications in relation to risk factors. *Diabetes* 1986; 35: 1332–9.

33. Grey RHB, Burns-Cox CJ, Hughes A. Blind and partial sight registration in Avon. *Br J Ophthalmol* 1989; 73: 88–94.
34. Butcher A, Dodson P. Visual loss. In Sinclair AJ, Finucane P (eds), *Diabetes in Old Age*, 2nd edn. Chichester: John Wiley & Sons Ltd, 2001; pp 119–32.
35. Sinclair AJ, Bayer AJ, Girling AJ, Woodhouse KW. Older adults, diabetes mellitus and visual acuity: a community-based case-control study. *Age Ageing* 2000; 29: 335–9.
36. The Diabetes Control and Complications Trial (DCCT) Research Group. The effect of intensive treatment of diabetes on the development and progression of long-term complications in insulin-dependent diabetes mellitus. *New Engl J Med* 1993; 329: 977–86.
37. The United Kingdom Prospective Diabetes Study (UKPDS) Group. Intensive blood-glucose control with sulphonylureas or insulin compared with conventional treatment and risk of complications in patients with type II diabetes, *Lancet* 1998; 352: 837–53.
38. The UKPDS Group. Tight blood pressure control and risk of macrovascular and microvascular complications in type II diabetes. *BMJ* 1998; 317: 703–13.
39. The Diabetic Retinopathy Research Group. Photocoagulation treatment of proliferative diabetic retinopathy: the second report of Diabetic Retinopathy Study findings. *Ophthalmology* 1978; 85: 82–106.
40. The Early Treatment Diabetic Retinopathy Study (ETDRS) Research Group. Treatment techniques and clinical guidelines for photocoagulation of diabetic macular oedema. *Ophthalmology* 1987; 94: 761–4.
41. The British Multicentre Study Group. Photocoagulation for diabetic maculopathy. *Diabetes* 1983; 32: 1010–6.
42. Young MJ, Boulton AJM. The diabetic foot. In Sinclair AJ, Finucane P (eds), *Diabetes in Old Age*, 2nd edn. Chichester: John Wiley & Sons Ltd, 2001; pp 67–88.
43. Van Houtum WH, Lavery LA, Harkless LB. The costs of diabetes-related lower extremity amputations in the Netherlands. *Diabet Med* 1995; 12: 777–81.
44. Palumbo PJ, Melton LJ. Peripheral vascular disease and diabetes. *Diabetes in America, Diabetes Data*, Vol 15. Washington, DC: US Government Printing Office, 1985; pp 1–21. NIH publication 85-1468.
45. Larsson J, Apelqvist J, Agardh DD, Stenstrom A. Decreasing incidence of major amputation in diabetic patients: a consequence of a multidisciplinary footcare team approach? *Diabet Med* 1995; 12: 770–6.
46. Cavanagh PR, Simoneau GG, Ulbrecht JS. Ulceration, unsteadiness and uncertainty: the biomechanical consequences of diabetes mellitus. *J Biomech* 1993; 26 (suppl 1): 23–40.
47. Backonja M, Glanzman RL. Gabapentin dosing for neuropathic pain: evidence from randomised, placebo-controlled clinical trials. *Clin Ther* January 2003; 25 (1): 81–104.
48. Flynn FD, Boolell M, Tooke J, Watkins PJ. The effect of insulin infusion on capillary blood flow in the diabetic neuropathic foot. *Diabet Med* 1992; 9: 630–4.
49. Sinclair AJ. Diabetes in old age—changing concepts in the secondary care arena. *J Roy Coll Phys (Lond)* 2000; 34: 240–4.
50. Sigurdsson HH, Macaulay EM, McHardy KC, Cooper GG. Long-term outcome of infra-inguinal bypass for limb salvage: are we giving diabetic patients a fair deal? *Pract Diab Intern* 1999; 16: 204–6.
51. Thomson FJ, Masson EA. Can elderly diabetic patients cooperate with routine foot care? *Age Ageing* 1992; 21: 333–7.
52. Vinik A, Richardson D. Erectile dysfunction. In Sinclair AJ, Finucane P (eds), *Diabetes in Old Age*, 2nd edn. Chichester: John Wiley & Sons Ltd, 2001; pp 89–102.
53. Feldman HA, Goldstein I, Hatzichristou DG, Krane RJ, McKinley JB. Impotence and its medical and psychosocial correlates: results of the Massachusett's Male Aging Study. *J Urol* 1994; 151: 54–61.
54. Braun M, Wassmer G, Klotz T, Reifenrath B, Mathers M, Engelmann U. Epidemiology of erectile dusfunction: results of the 'Cologne Male Survey'. *Int J Impot Res* 2000; 12 (6): 305–11.
55. Lakin MM, Montague DK, VanderBrug-Medendorp S, Tesar L, Schover LR. Intravenous Injection therapy: analysis of results and complications. *J Urol* 1990; 143: 1138–41.
56. Croxson SCM. Metabolic decompensation. In Sinclair AJ, Finucane P (eds), *Diabetes in Olde Age*, 2nd edn. Chichester: John Wiley & Sons Ltd, 2001; pp 53–66.
57. Basu A, Close CF, Jenkins D, et al. Persisting mortality in diabetic ketoacidosis. *Diabet Med* 1993; 10: 282–4.
58. Hamblin PS, Topliss DJ, Chosich N, et al. Deaths associated with diabetic ketoacidosis and hyperosmolar coma. *Med J Aust* 1989; 151: 439–44.
59. Small M, Alzaid A, MacCuish AC. Diabetic hyperosmolar non-ketotic decompensation. *Q J Med* 1988; 66: 251–7.
60. Wachtel TJ, Tetu-Mouradjian LM, Goldman DL, Ellis SE, O'Sullivan PS. Hyper-osmolarity and acidosis in diabetes mellitus: a three-year experience in Rhode Island. *J Gen Int Med* 1991; 6: 495–502.
61. Brierley EJ, Broughton DL, James OF, Alberti KG. Reduced awareness of hypoglycaemia in the elderly despite an intact counter-regulatory response. *QJM* 1995; 88 (6): 439–45.
62. Shorr RI, Ray WA, Daugherty JR, Griffin MR. Incidence and risk factors for serious hypoglycaemia in older persons using insulin or sulphonylureas. *Arch Intern Med* 1997; 157: 1681–6.
63. Meneilly GS, Cheung E, Tuokko H. Counter-regulatory hormone responses to hypoglycemia in the elderly patient with diabetes. *Diabetes* 1994; 43: 403–10.
64. Thomson FJ, Masson EA, Leeming JT, Boulton AJ. Lack of knowledge of symptoms of hypoglycaemia by elderly diabetic patients. *Age Ageing* 1991; 20: 404–6.
65. Tessier D, Dawson K, Tetrault JP, Bravo G, Meneilly GS. Glibenclamide vs gliclazide in Type 2 diabetes of the elderly. *Diabet Med* 1994; 11: 974–80.
66. Asplund K, Wiholm BE, Lundman B. Severe hypoglycaemia during treatment with glipizide. *Diabet Med* 1991; 8: 726–31.
67. Asplund K, Wiholm BE, Lundman B. Glibenclamide-associated hypoglycaemia: a report on 57 cases. *Diabetologia* 1983; 24: 412–7.
68. Strachan MWJ, Deary IJ, Ewing FME, Frier BM. Is type 2 (non-insulin-dependent) diabetes mellitus associated with an increased risk of cognitive dysfunction? *Diabetes Care* 1997; 20: 438–45.
69. Croxson S, Jagger C. Diabetes and cognitive impairment: a community based study of elderly subjects. *Age Ageing* 1995; 24: 421–4.
70. Vanhanen M, Koivisto K, Kuusisto J, Mykkanen L, Helkala EL, Hanninen T, Riekkinen P Sr, Soininen H, Laakso M. Cognitive function in an elderly population

with persistent impaired glucose tolerance. *Diabetes Care* 1998; 21: 398–402.
71. Kumari M, Brunner E, Fuhrer R. Minireview: mechanisms by which the metabolic syndrome and diabetes impair memory. *J Gerontol (Biol Sci)* 2000; 55A: B228–32.
72. Stolk RP, Breteler MM, Ott A, Pols HA, Lamberts SW, Grobbee DE, Hofman A. Insulin and cognitive function in an elderly population: the Rotterdam Study. *Diabetes Care* 1997; 20: 792–5.
73. Leibson CL, Rocca WA, Hanson VA, Cha R, Kokmen E, O'Brien PC, Palumbo PJ. Risk of dementia among persons with diabetes mellitus: a population-based cohort study. *Am J Epidem* 1997; 145 (4): 301–8.
74. Gradman TJ, Laws A, Thompson LW, Reaven GM. Verbal learning and/or memory improves with glycaemic control in older subjects with non-insulin-dependent diabetes mellitus. *JAGS* 1993; 41: 1305–12.
75. Sinclair AJ, Girling AJ, Bayer AJ. Cognitive dysfunction in older subjects with diabetes mellitus: impact on diabetes self-management and use of care services. *Diab Res Clin Pract* 2000; 50: 203–12.
76. Eaton WW, Armenian H, Gallo J, Pratt L, Ford DE. Depression and risk for onset of Type II diabetes: a prospective population based study. *Diabetes Care* 1996; 19: 1097–102.
77. Amato L, Padisso G, Cacciatore F, for The Observatorio Geriatrico of Campania Region Group. Non-insulin dependent diabetes mellitus is associated with a greater prevalence of depression in the elderly. *Diabetes Metab* 1996; 22 (5): 314–8.
78. Rosenthal MJ, Fajarde M, Gilmore S, Morley JE, Naliboff BD. Hospitalisation and mortality of diabetes in older adults. *Diabetes Care* 1998; 21: 231–5.
79. Robinson N, Fuller JH, Edmeades SP. Depression and diabetes. *Diabet Med* 1988; 5: 268–74.
80. Gavard JA, Lustman PJ, Clouse RE. Prevalence of depression in adults with diabetes mellitus. *Diabetes Care* 1993; 16: 1167–78.
81. Lustman PJ, Freedland KE, Griffith LS. Fluoxetine for depression in diabetes. *Diabetes Care* 2000; 23: 618–23.
82. Pouwer F, Beekman AT, Nijpels G, Dekker JM, Snoek FJ, Kostense PJ, Heine RJ, Deeg DJ. Rates and risks for comorbid depression in patients with Type 2 diabetes mellitus: results from a community-based study. *Diabetologia* July 2003; 46 (7): 892–8.
83. Muggeo M, Verlato G, Bonora E, Bressan F, Girotto S, Corbellini M, Gemma ML, Moghetti P, Zenere M, Cacciatori V. The Verona Diabetes Study: a population-based survey on known diabetes mellitus prevalence and 5-year all-cause mortality. *Diabetologia* 1995; 38: 318–25.
84. Sinclair AJ, Robert IE, Croxson SCM. Mortality in older people with with diabetes mellitus. *Diabet Med* 1997; 14: 639–47.
85. Croxson SCM, Price DE, Burden M, Jagger C, Burden AC. The mortality of elderly people with diabetes. *Diabet Med* 1994; 11: 250–2.
86. Kuusisto J, Mykkanen L, Pyorala K, Laasko M. NIDDM and its metabolic control predict coronary heart disease in elderly subjects. *Diabetes* 1994; 43: 960–7.
87. Muggeo M, Verlato G, Bonora E, Ciani F, Moghetti P, Eastman R, Crepaldi G, de Marco R. Long-term instability of fasting plasma glucose predicts mortality in elderly NIDDM patients: the Verona Diabetes Study. *Diabetologia* 1995; 38: 672–9.
88. Hendra TJ, Sinclair AJ. Improving the care of elderly diabetic patients: the final report of the St Vincent Joint Task Force for Diabetes. *Age Ageing* 1997; 26: 3–6.
89. Gregg EW, Beckles GL, Williamson DF, Leveille SG, Langlois JA, Engelgau MM, Narayan KM. Diabetes and physical disability among older U.S. adults. *Diabetes Care* 2000; 23: 1272–7.
90. Fried LP, Williamson JD, Kaspar J. The epidemiology of frailty: scope of the problem. In Perry HM, Morley JE, Coe RM (eds), *Aging and Musculoskeletal Disorders*. New York: Springer, 1993; pp 3–15.
91. Jackson R. Updated New Zealand cardiovascular disease risk-benefit prediction guide. *BMJ* 2000; 320: 709–10.
92. Wilson PWF, D'Agostino RB, Levy D, Belanger AM, Silbershatz H, Kannel WB. Prediction of coronary heart disease using risk factor categories. *Circulation* 1998; 97: 1837–47.
93. Menotti A, Lanti M, Puddu PE, Kromhout D. Coronary heart disease incidence in northern and southern European populations: a reanalysis of the Seven Countries Study for a European coronary risk chart. *Heart* 2000; 84: 238–44.
94. Florkowski CM, Scott RS, Moir CL, Graham PJ. Lipid but not glycaemic parameters predict total mortality from Type 2 diabetes mellitus in Canterbury, New Zealand. *Diabet Med* 1998; 15: 386–92.
95. Rubins HB, Robins SJ, Collins D, Fye CL, Anderson JW, Elam MB, Faas FH, Linares E, Schaefer EJ, Schectman G, Wilt TJ, Wittes J, for the Veterans Affairs High-Density Lipoprotein Cholesterol Intervention Trial Study Group. Gemfibrozil for the secondary prevention of coronary heart disease in men with low levels of high-density lipoprotein cholesterol. *New Eng J Med* 1999; 341: 410–8.
96. Heart Outcomes Prevention Evaluation Study Investigators. Effects of ramipril on cardiovascular and microvascular outcomes in people with diabetes mellitus: results of the HOPE and MICRO-HOPE substudy. *Lancet* 2000; 355: 253–9.
97. The DECODE Study Group on behalf of the European Diabetes Epidemiology Group. Consequences of the new diagnostic criteria for diabetes in older men and women. *Diabetes Care* 1999; 22 (10): 1667–71.
98. Barrett-Connor E, Ferrara A. Isolated postchallenge hyperglycaemia and the risk of fatal cardiovascular disease in older women and men. The Rancho Bernardo Study. *Diabetes Care* 1998; 21: 1236–9.
99. The European Diabetes Policy Group. *A Desktop Guide to Type 2 Diabetes Mellitus*. Brussels: International Diabetes Federation (European Region), 1999.
100. Sinclair AJ, Turnbull CJ, Croxson SCM. Document of care for older people with diabetes. *Postgrad Med J* 1996; 72: 334–8.
101. The UKPDS Group. Effect of intensive blood-glucose control with metformin on complications in overweight patients with Type 2 diabetes. *Lancet* 1998; 352: 854–65.
102. Hendra TJ. Insulin therapy. In Sinclair AJ, Finucane P (eds), *Diabetes in Old Age*, 2nd edn. Chichester: John Wiley & Sons Ltd, 2001; pp 165–76.
103. Berger W. Insulin therapy in the elderly Type 2 diabetic patient. *Diab Res Clin Pract* 1988; 4 (suppl 1): 24–8.
104. Yki-Jarvinen H, Kauppila M, Kujansuu E, et al. Comparison of insulin regimens in patients with non-insulin-dependent diabetes mellitus. *New Eng J Med* 1992; 327: 1426–33.

105. Goddijn PPM, Bilo HJG, Feskens EJM, Groenier KH, van der Zee KI, Meyboom-de Jong B. Longitudinal study on glycaemic control and quality of life in patients with Type 2 diabetes mellitus referred for intensified control. *Diabet Med* 1999; 16: 23–30.
106. Petterson T, Young B, Lee P, Newton P, Hollis S, Dornan T. Well-being and treatment satisfaction in older people with diabetes. *Diabetes Care* 1998; 21 (6): 930–5.
107. Yki-Jarvinen H, Ryysy L, Nikkila K, Tulokas T, Vanamo R, Heikkila M. Comparison of bedtime insulin regimens in patients with Type 2 diabetes mellitus. *Ann Intern Med* 1999; 130: 389–96.
108. Sinclair AJ, Gadsby R. Diabetes in Care Homes. In Sinclair AJ, Finucane P (eds), *Diabetes in Old Age*, 2nd edn. Chichester: John Wiley and Sons Ltd, 2001; pp 241–52.
109. National Center for Health Statistics. *The National Nursing Home Survey 1977. Summary for the United States*. Hyattsville, MD: US Government Printing Office, 1979.
110. Sinclair AJ, Allard I, Bayer AJ. Observations of diabetes care in long-term institutional settings with measures of cognitive function and dependency. *Diabetes Care* 1997; 20: 778–84.
111. Benbow SJ, Walsh A, Gill GV. Diabetes in institutionalised elderly people: a forgotten population? *BMJ* 1997; 314: 1868–9.
112. Sinclair AJ, Turnbull CJ, Croxson SCM. Document of diabetes care for residential and nursing homes. *Postgrad Med J* 1997; 73: 611–2.
113. British Diabetic Association. *Guidelines of Practice for Residents with Diabetes in Care Homes*. London: BDA, 1999.
114. Sinclair AJ, Barnett AH. Special needs of elderly diabetic patients. *BMJ* 1993; 306: 1142–3.
115. Goyder EC, McNally PG, Drucquer M, Spiers N, Botha JL. Shifting of care for diabetes from secondary to primary care, 1990–5: a review of general practices. *BMJ* 1998; 316: 1505–6.
116. Reenders K. Approaching primary care. In Sinclair AJ, Finucane P (eds), *Diabetes in Care Homes*, 2nd edn. Chichester: John Wiley and Sons Ltd, 2001; pp 229–40.
117. Eastman RC, Javitt JC, Herman WH, et al. Model of complications of NIDDM. *Diabetes Care* 1997; 20: (pt 1 and 2): 725–34 and 735–44.
118. Vijan S, Hofer TP, Hayward RA. Estimated benefits of glycaemic control in microvascular complications in type 2 diabetes. *Ann Intern Med* 1997; 127: 788–95.

90

Education of the Diabetic Patient[a]

J.L. Day

Ipswich Hospital, Ipswich, Suffolk, UK

If patients are not only to achieve glycemic targets, control of blood pressure and weight, and adopt other health-related measures to avoid long- and short-term complications, but also to live as nearly normal a lifestyle as possible, education must feature as a most important element of their care. This chapter reviews the historical literature, and provides an analysis of the reasons for success and failure, as well as recommendations for those planning or providing diabetes care and its educational component in particular.

HISTORICAL REVIEW

Recognition of the need for education and for self-management of subjects with diabetes is not new. In 1888, Bouchardat emphasized self-monitoring for those with diabetes. In the early 1900s the first patient education program was implemented in Portugal by Dr Roma. With the discovery of insulin and relatively crude insulin preparations, the effects of which were often unpredictable, the learning of injection skills, the ability to adjust dosage, and the timing and content of meals was paramount. The important role of education was enshrined in the doctrine of Joslin and his colleagues with the establishment of the classroom as a cornerstone of diabetes management in the Joslin clinic [1]. One of the earliest recipients of insulin, as well as the pioneer of British diabetes care, Dr R.D. Lawrence, continually stressed not only the information and skills needed but also the development of appropriate attitudes, if the goals of good diabetes control were to be accompanied by successful social adjustment [2]. However, in the years that followed the discovery of insulin, the emphasis on education waned with the search for new treatment regimens that might simplify self-management (for example, with long-acting insulins). More recently search for and application of potential pharmaco-technological solutions, despite their limited success, continue to overshadow the importance of patient education.

Close analysis of the educational processes necessary for subjects with diabetes to acquire the appropriate skills and attitudes remained in abeyance until the early 1980s. The pioneering work of Miller in 1972 demonstrated the dramatic effect of an educational program, combined with the development of nurse practitioners and a 24-h telephone service [3]. This study revealed that, over a 3-year period, admission rates per annum fell from 670 to 200 and episodes of ketoacidosis from 300 to less than 100 per annum. These results were achieved in a (perhaps atypical) group of low socioeconomic status with very high initial admission rates, but the major benefits were undeniable, not only in demonstrating improvement in patient outcome but also in reducing the cost of health care delivery. The stimulus that this gave to the development of the understanding and delivery of patient education was dramatic. Organizations such as the Diabetes Education Study Group (DESG) of the European Association for the Study of Diabetes (EASD) were established. Concurrently, the role of the diabetes nurse educator or specialist nurse [4, 5], was recognized, whose special educational skills have enabled enormous expansion of the scope of education and its skilled provision. In many countries national diabetes organizations created education sections, the most prominent of which must be that of Diabetes Educators in the United States. In addition dedicated centers were built for education provision [6]. These

International Textbook of Diabetes Mellitus, Third Edition. Edited by R. A. DeFronzo, E. Ferrannini, H. Keen, and P. Zimmet.
 ISBN: 0-471-48655-8.

[a] This article is based in part on a chapter of the same title that was published in an earlier edition of the *International Textbook of Diabetes Mellitus*, by J.L. Day and J.-P. Assal.

changes were accompanied by a major expansion of quality research into the theoretical aspects of patient learning and the efficacy of different methods.

Many educational programs have now been implemented and studied worldwide. Benefits are often highly significant and have been demonstrated in diabetes groups of all ages [7–9]. Reductions in admission rates are a common feature. In studies by Geller and Butler [10] in the United States, and by Scott and colleagues in New Zealand [11], educational failure was identified as the most common reason for admission to hospital. Analysis in the United Kingdom revealed unacceptably high admission rates for ketoacidosis, hypoglycemia, and diabetic foot ulcers, all of which should be preventable with appropriate education. That these ends can be achieved is demonstrated, not only by Miller's study [3], but also by a carefully designed educational foot-care program by Assal and colleagues [12], which resulted in significant reduction in amputation at any site, the proportion of above-knee to below-knee amputation rates, and duration of hospital stay. The Geneva–Düsseldorf group also reported a highly significant reduction in admission rates [13].

The goal of perfect glycemic control remains elusive, however. Despite greatly improved understanding of the pharmacokinetics of insulin, the development of genetically manufactured and modified insulins, and new delivery systems, standards of satisfactory diabetes control worldwide for type 1 diabetes remain disappointingly low [14–17], with as few as one quarter or one third of subjects attaining glycated hemoglobin results within the normal range. Results in persons with type 2 diabetes, for whom pharmacological advances have been extremely limited, are equally if not more disappointing.

It was predicted and has indeed now been demonstrated—in particular by the Geneva–Düsseldorf group, Mazucca et al. in the United States, and most recently by the Dose Adjustment for Normal Eating study (DAFNE)—that significantly better control can be achieved by better educational programs [13, 18–20]. The Diabetes Control and Complications Trial (DCCT), which demonstrated clear-cut relationships between glycemic control and complications, was heavily reliant on intensive education in the tightly controlled group [17]. Examination of the UK Prospective Diabetes Study (UKPDS) is salutary in that it revealed that the greatest fall in HbA_{1c} and weight occurred prior to randomization to different therapies [21]. This result could only be attributable to the education and change in eating behavior of the subjects. Furthermore, the degree of positive change could be related to the availability of dietetic advice.

It must be remembered that there is a wide range of important endpoints quite unrelated to glycemic control, which are essential components of diabetic self-care. Some of the most obvious include management and prevention of severe hypoglycemia, steps to be taken before driving or exercise, the carrying of identification cards, etc. Clinical attendance and foot self-care are vital if long-term complications are to be detected and prevented. Foot care has been exposed to considerable scrutiny. In addition to earlier studies of Miller [3] and Assal [12] referred to above, the most dramatic demonstration of efficacy of effective education is that provided be Malone et al. who achieved a 50% reduction in amputation rate, with a fairly short and simple intervention [22].

The breadth of educational studies over the last two decades is extensive and these range from observational, focus groups, longitudinal and cross-sectional analyses, to controlled trials (CTT) and randomized controlled trials (RCTT). Three meta-analyses have been performed with largely similar conclusions [23–25]. Despite a relatively small number of controlled trials the evidence strongly supports the efficacy of improved educational process. Unfortunately, the methodology in a large numbers of studies was inadequate; as a consequence, the authors were unable to provide firm guidance for best practice but did detect greater benefits from those using less didactic methods. Most recently the National Institute of Clinical Excellence (United Kingdom) undertook a study largely of CCTs and RCCTs and concluded that "All individuals with diabetes should be offered structured education at the time of diagnosis, and on-going education as required" [26].

Amidst the plethora of literature there are many negative studies. The reasons for their failure demand close scrutiny. Many of the earlier workers attempted to correlate knowledge acquisition with outcome. Not only were the scales of measurement insensitive but more importantly the weak relationship between knowledge acquisition and desired behavior went unrecognized. Many interventions were short, one-off courses and ignored the necessity of reinforcement and maintenance. Almost all educational studies are dependent on the "teachers" as the agents of change. Their skills are likely to be very variable and, with occasional exceptions, uncontrolled for [18]. Furthermore the theoretical basis for the interventions and their evaluation has often been limited.

In the last 10 years or so, those working in the field of psychology have given us much improved insights into factors governing behavior and their accurate assessment, with well-validated tools and innovative and more soundly based interventions. Important examples include the contributions from Dunn [27], Bradley [28], Cox [29], Snoek and Skinner [30], Anderson [31], Coles [32], Rollnick [33], and Day [34].

These and others have enabled us to develop, validate, and apply new models of behavior, and to recognize the importance of

- teacher training and a learner-centered approach,
- the context of learning,

- the influence of the attitudes, perceptions, and beliefs of the subject/patient and the professional/teacher,
- the role of health beliefs,
- concepts of self-efficacy/locus of control/self-empowerment,
- the lifelong necessity for continuing education, and
- the implications of patient satisfaction with treatment and quality of life.

Their insights have also provided a much greater understanding overall of the problems of compliance or self-adherence, and recognition that the principles applied to the care of those with diabetes are not disease-specific and should be applied generally to the management of all chronic diseases.

These aspects will be dealt with more fully in the following sections.

DETERMINANTS OF SUCCESS OR FAILURE OF EDUCATIONAL PROCESS

The Problem of Compliance/Self-adherence

It is well recognized in all spheres of medicine that patients' standards of adherence to the advice that is given often fall far short of those recommended by their physicians. Studies in tuberculosis, hypertension, antibiotic therapy, etc. all show that the medication swallowed maybe as little as 40–60% of that prescribed. Diabetes is no exception. A recent study of adolescents with type 1 diabetes in Scotland revealed that some individuals were injecting as little as 47% of the insulin dose recommended [35]. Failure of adherence to recommended eating patterns in type 2 diabetes is the commonest barrier to effective outcome. Standards of performance of other measures such as carrying identification, self-testing, recording results, and much other behavior required, frequently fall well short of the ideal. Even when there are statutory requirements, adherence may be low; for example, it was noted in one study that only a little over half of subjects reported the insulin control of their diabetes to the driving license authorities [36]. Despite the success of the DCCT study in improving glycemic control in the intensively treated group, only 8–9% of subjects in this group achieved the targets that were set for them [17]. Was this because the targets were inappropriate, unattainable, or perhaps unacceptable to the subjects due to the increased risk of severe hypoglycemia? We can only theorize, but it is certain that different factors were influencing different individuals. In view of the complexity of change needed in what is a mainly symptom free and lifelong disease, rather than be surprised and disappointed we should adopt the attitude expressed by Professor Dunn "Compliance is a very abnormal behavior pattern ... For one adult to do what another tells them on a continuous basis suggests that they are seriously disturbed!" [27].

Nonetheless, significant numbers of people do manage their diabetes extremely well and if complications are to be avoided we do need to find ways of persuasion—i.e. improved educational process—for the less successful majority of subjects who fall short of the targets we set. There are many reasons why patients may not comply with their treatment, and it is up to the doctor to discover them, just as it is up to the doctor to diagnose the organic lesions underlying patients' complaints.

To this end we need to examine the factors governing behavior and to compare the ways in which they operate to facilitate or hinder successful self-care.

Relationships Between Knowledge and Behavior

Disappointment was expressed in many early studies by those instigating new education programs designed to provide systematic and comprehensive information, in a number of innovative ways, who found no significant improvement in glycemic control or other outcomes such as foot self-care [37–40]. Some failures may have been related in part to inadequate scales for the measurement of knowledge. However, even though scales that are both validated and more sensitive are now available [41, 42], only weak relationships are demonstrable between knowledge acquisition and behavior [43]. The necessity to obtain new information is undeniable but its assimilation and application is frequently deficient. Expectations of health care providers are overoptimistic and overlook the long and complicated process between learning important information and the transformation of that knowledge into the development of skills. Most importantly, there is a necessity to maintain the desire not only to put the knowledge and skills into practice, but to continue to do so year in and year out. The "behavior gap," i.e. the difference between what people know and what they do, is continually evident in diabetic practice [37, 38].

The learning process may in part be at fault. Didactic, teacher-centered learning traditionally consists of what has been described as pot filling. Information is provided like pieces of a jigsaw that the patient must complete but without access to the picture. What the patient actually needs is a clear picture of the illness (overall aims and goals), a simple explanation of the shape of the pieces and their relationship to each other, and the provision of methods of assembly (assimilation and application). In this way, standards of learning will be far higher than those apparent in many programs that just provide factual information, and where rote learning is all that can be expected. Standards of achievement can be surprisingly high in those with apparently quite limited intellectual abilities, if the picture is made clear to them [32].

This is not to suggest that the provision of accurate, understandable, and appropriate information delivered at a time appropriate to the patients' needs is not an important first step in the education process. There is, however, still a long process of additional learning if the patient is going to use the information acquired in an appropriate and useful way.

Context of the Learning Process

There are three elements to the context that need consideration. Two are concrete or environmental—namely, the context in which the learning takes place, and the environment in which new learned behaviors are to be delivered—and the third is abstract, i.e. the patients' own perceptions of the illness itself, their life experience, and of what they have to learn.

First, the learning program should be delivered in an as near normal environment as possible and one in which the patient is comfortable. Hospital inpatient wards are quite unsuitable. All aspects of the teaching need to be related to the individual's daily life, using a problem-based learning approach.

Second, the context inevitably changes over time according to variations of lifestyle. This is one of the reasons for the inadequacy of one-off programs, such as single 5-day courses with no ongoing follow-up. The disappointments of those who found that improved control following the original intervention was not maintained 6–9 months or 2 years later were unrealistic [44–46]. The learning program must be adjusted over the years to deal with new life events including the (sadly still high) probability of complications and the necessity for new therapeutic interventions—especially in type 2 diabetes (see Diabetes Care Cycle, Figure 1), and provide reinforcement and encouragement to avoid "relapse" [47].

In addition, however, to the superimposition of diabetes on the lifestyle of the patient and vice versa it must be recognized that patients' perception of their disease, the efficacy of its treatment, and its likely course may be very different from those of their advisor, and hence there may be a significant mismatch between their expectations and those of the professionals.

Matching Agendas of Patient and Professional

Sources of information are extensive and because of the high prevalence of diabetes, the strong likelihood of other cases within the family, and information through the media, it is extremely unlikely that adults will know nothing of diabetes, despite their protestations of ignorance when asked. Their understanding, however, may well be hearsay-related and incorrect. Slama and his colleagues in France demonstrated that unaffected members of the public could have the most bizarre ideas of diabetes, for example that it is an infectious disorder and that sufferers demonstrate curious devious behavior, hiding forbidden sugar about their person and eating it in secret. Similar misconceptions and general ignorance have been demonstrated in the United Kingdom. In Jamaica there is a widespread belief that insulin treatment causes impotence—not entirely surprising since insulin is often only commenced when patients develop complications and these, including erectile dysfunction, get worse despite the therapy [48, 49].

One can assume therefore that everybody, regardless of class, educational status, or ethnic origin, knows something about the illness. Indeed one of the commonest mistakes is to overestimate the understanding of the illness by those of high intelligence or professional status. This

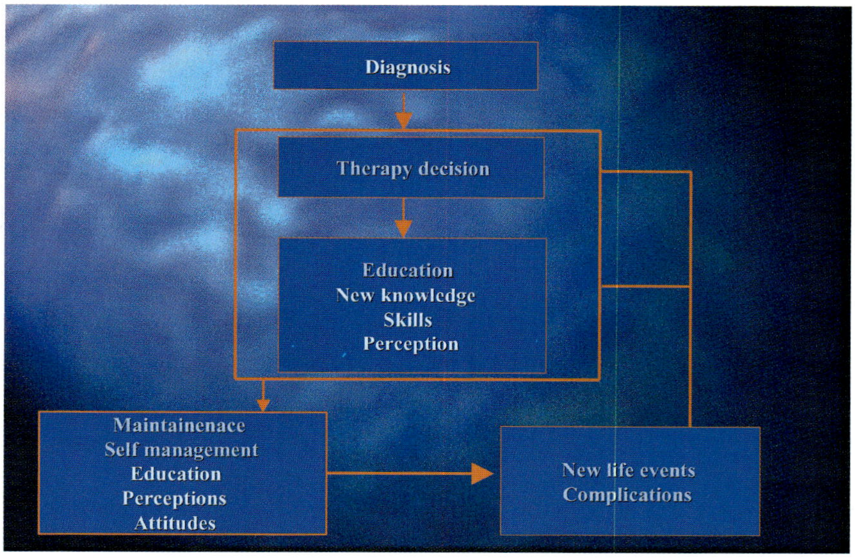

Figure 1 Diabetes Care Cycle

further emphasizes the need for the clinician to establish the patients' knowledge and vision of their illness, and modify it as necessary, prior to embarking on delivery of information of which the recipients perceive no relevance. The converse is also true. Patients with type 2 diabetes may expect information about hypoglycemia if all they know of diabetes comes from hypoglycemic episodes portrayed in the media. The physician, however, who is not planning to provide any hypoglycemic therapy, may fail to reassure the patient who is needlessly frightened at this prospect.

Patients' Perceptions of Their Disease and Its Treatment

Patients' willingness to comply with their treatment depends on their personal appreciation of the disease and its treatment. These correspond to patients' "health beliefs" [50, 51]. Agreement to comply with a treatment implies the tacit acceptance by the patient of four postulates concerning the disease, its consequences, its treatment, and the cost of the treatment to the patient. Patients will not be actively committed to their treatment unless they are convinced (1) that they have the disease, (2) that its consequences are serious, (3) that it can be treated, and (4) that the advantages of the treatment outweigh the disadvantages. Applied to diabetes this can be construed as follows:

(1) I am at risk of the complications of diabetes (e.g., acute complications such as hypoglycemic coma; long-term complications such as blindness, gangrene, etc.).
(2) These complications constitute a serious threat for me (in the widest sense; an emotional, professional and social threat, as well as a physical one).
(3) The treatment works.
(4) I accept the psychological, social, and financial cost involved (which must not outweigh the benefit that I can expect to derive).

These postulates must be accepted *en bloc* in order to ensure the patient's adherence to the different requirements of the treatment, from learning the requisite skills and complying with the daily obligation to take the medication to evaluating its effect on the blood sugar.

Nonacceptance of Disease

Illness weakens people's self-image and places them in a situation of inferiority in relation to others. When self-esteem is too severely threatened by disease, people use a series of defense mechanisms to protect themselves from the anxiety and depression engendered by their feelings of inferiority. This protection can take the form of delaying immediate "entry" into the state of disease by accomplishing a series of preliminary psychological steps known as the *work of acceptance of disease or mourning for health* [52, 53]. This psychological progression usually consists of five phases:

(1) Shock and denial of reality ("No it isn't true, I'm not sick . . . ").
(2) Revolt ("Why is this happening to me? It's unfair. It's all because of so-and-so . . . ").
(3) Bargaining ("Okay, I'll take your treatment, but just leave me alone for all the rest, I know perfectly well what to do . . . ").
(4) Hopeful depression ("I realize that I'm sick and that I've got to take my treatment, but shall I really be able to cope?").
(5) Acceptance ("I've come to terms with my disability and am learning to live with it, even if things aren't quite what they used to be . . . ").

The health care team must be capable of recognizing these stages, because patients' ability to listen and to learn varies greatly according to their stage of acceptance [50]. As patients who are going through the denial phase do not feel concerned by the illness, they are unlikely to derive benefit from any instruction. During the periods of revolt and bargaining they frequently distort and misinterpret the medical information that they receive. These are also difficult times for the health care team, who tend to be exasperated by the patients' inability to remember what they are told. The phase of emotional decompression is more propitious for learning. This is a time of sadness, also known as "hopeful depression," during which patients wonder how to cope with their illness. They express a great demand to learn at this time, but the health care team often remains impervious to it. This is a pity, but may be due to the recent difficulties that they have experienced with the same patients during the tumultuous phases of revolt and bargaining. It is when patients have finally come to terms with disease that they are most receptive: they listen attentively, take part in discussions, put their treatment into practice, and readily accept suggestions and corrections.

Who, or What, Ultimately Controls the Diabetes?

Even acceptance of the disease and the conviction that it can be treated do not necessarily guarantee patients' compliance. People's attitudes to treatment are also influenced by what is known as their "health locus of control." This concept corresponds to their perception of where the ultimate responsibility for their health is located.

Obviously, in the acute emergency setting this responsibility lies solely in the doctor's hands. However, the doctor is not always the unique repository of medical power, particularly where nonhospitalized patients with chronic disease are concerned. It has been shown that people vest power over health and sickness in three different sources [54–56]: (a) medical power in the widest sense, i.e. "official" and "alternative" medicine, locus of control:

external; (b) fate, locus of control: external; (c) themselves, locus of control: internal. The patients' "health locus of control" is external if they consider that the outcome of the disease depends on factors that are outside themselves, i.e. official or alternative medicine, and/or God; it is internal if patients consider that the outcome depends mainly on themselves. Patients often rely on more than one source of medical power, like the patient on the eve of an operation who said "I have faith in my doctor and if fate is kind ... all will be well, because I know that everybody's praying for me ... and anyway I'm going to do all I can to get well again as quickly as possible." Success in training patients to treat themselves, therefore, depends on their belief in the power of official medicine to treat the disease and in their own power to influence the outcome. Many examples of noncompliance may be due to the patient's adhesion to another system of medical reference (oriental medicine, fate, God, etc.). Acceptance of some responsibility, i.e. internal locus, is essential if the patient is to undertake the routine tasks necessary for them to remain healthy.

It is likely that the patients' perception of role is largely determined through public media channels, newspapers, magazines, popular drama, soaps, etc., which mainly focus on medical situations conforming to the "Acute Medical Model" roughly summarized as follows: doctor makes diagnosis, and medical team provides therapy and takes responsibility for outcome. In contrast in the "Chronic Disease model" doctor makes diagnosis, and medical team discuss, negotiate, and agree therapy with the patient who administers the therapy and shares responsibility for outcome. Often it is not only the patient whose role has to change. The traditional training of doctors and nurses, largely hospital-based, is often confined to the acute model [31]. Despite improvements in training in this regard, many remain unfamiliar with the different approach and reluctant to release control to the patient. These attitudes are also demonstrable in those managing other chronic diseases [57]. They are often predicated by their environment and the attitudes of their peers. Contrary to the stereotype of any professional group, i.e. doctors versus nurses, inappropriate attitudes can be observed in all.

Confirmation of the importance of feelings of internal control, self-efficacy, and hence empowerment are well demonstrated in diabetes by the study of type 1 subjects by Bradley et al. [55] who showed that strong feelings of internal control predicted better glycemic outcome; that of De Weerdt et al. who tested the model of Fishbein and Ajsen in a large population and demonstrated a negative correlation between self-testing behavior and the extent of external control (powerful others/professionals) [58]; and of Day et al. who demonstrated in both type 1 and 2 subjects significant correlations between feelings of self-efficacy and HbA_{1c} [59]. Bradley et al. also demonstrated the negative influence of strong feelings of medical control leading to the inappropriate search by the patient for an external technological solution to their problems, e.g. an infusion pump, which might control their diabetes without any self-intervention [55].

Fortunately, for both patients and professionals these attitudes, if inappropriate, are capable of change. In the first instance the professional carers must acquaint themselves with their patients' systems of medical reference before embarking on long-term treatment plans. This is no mean task, as patients frequently cannot define an explicit relationship between the treatment and their personal terms of reference. Moreover, it is not easy for doctors to take an impartial history of the patient's medical references, given that their own position in the medical power complex makes them both judge and jury. On the one hand they need to recognize actions they might take that could vitiate attempts to inculcate attitudes favoring self-efficacy (i.e., admission to hospital, dependence on permission from physician prior to dose adjustment) and on the other, to provide support and encouragement, especially for those who do not always succeed.

Perceived Benefits and Barriers

A key element of the impact of one's health beliefs on self-management are the judgments one makes about the potential benefits from the actions recommended versus the difficulty in applying them, and their impact on daily life. In the absence of symptoms the barriers provided by the arduous repetitive and often difficult actions demanded of them would at times seem insuperable. The benefits are largely those of maintenance of long-term good health though there are short-term gains that include avoidance of and ability to cope with both hypoglycemia and ketoacidosis, in type 1 diabetes. Other significant gains include those related to the ability to cope with normal daily life, e.g. driving, heavy exercise, etc. In the case of adolescents in whom immediate gratification is the norm, threat of long-term harm is ineffective. Furthermore, Bradley and colleagues, with well-validated scales of assessment of health beliefs, have demonstrated the important difference between knowing about late complications and believing that one is actually personally vulnerable to them, i.e. "It won't happen to me" [60]. Denial is a commonly used defense mechanism by up to 20% of the population. Once more the reference point of any one individual in this respect must be identified.

Those faced with a chronic disease diagnosis move from the "well" (no necessity to think about health on a daily basis) to the "sick" role (continual concern for their health). On the positive side, these feelings can be reversed if their perception of self-efficacy, and hence control over their illness and life and choices about their treatment, can be enhanced [61]. The provision of a care system that

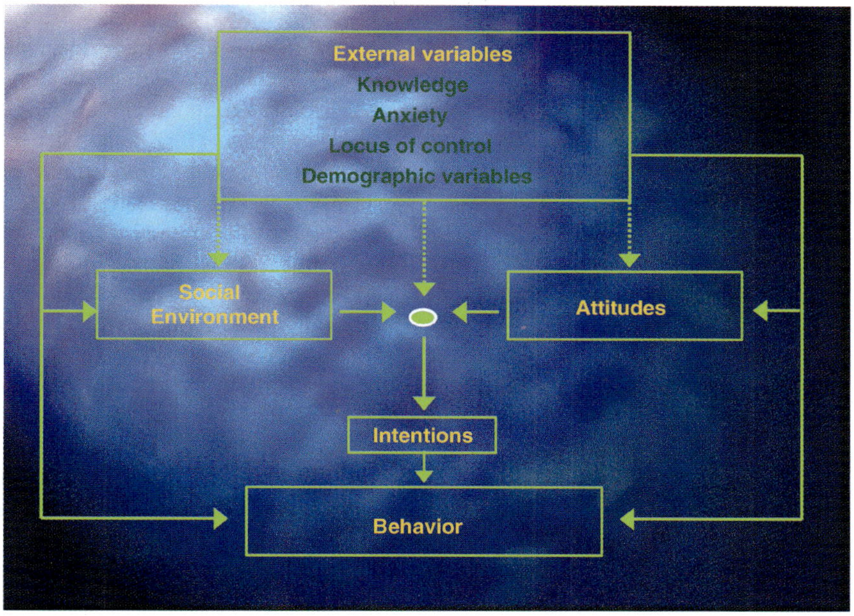

Figure 2 The behavioral model of Ajzen and Fishbein. (Reproduced with permission, from reference 63)

offers these opportunities to the patient is likely to lead to a much higher perception of benefits vs. barriers of therapy.

Patient Satisfaction and Quality of Life

It almost goes without saying that if the patient is not satisfied with his/her treatment, adherence is likely to be poor. The impact of the illness on the quality of life is also likely to be highly critical. Good scales of measurement of quality of life and satisfaction with treatment are now available [28]. However, high levels of satisfaction or quality-of-life ratings are not necessarily manifest in improved glycemic control or clinical outcomes. Patients may be more concerned about negative impact on lifestyle of self-care measures than long-term health benefits and hence more satisfied if they ignore desired care behaviors. However, Kinmouth and colleagues have shown that with careful training of carers in patient-centered interviewing, satisfaction rates could be considerably improved without detriment to glycemic control [62].

Needless to say, the emotional state of the patient also impacts on behavior. Excessive anxiety or depression may be crippling. Unfortunately, however, complete absence of anxiety, which may be manifest by a high satisfaction rating, can indicate neglect of any self-care behavior. A degree of "realistic anxiety" is a necessity.

The Behavioral Model of Education

Ultimately, education is designed to change behavior. As we have indicated, the factors that might determine this are basic knowledge, demographic characteristics of the person concerned (i.e. age, sex, etc.), perceptions about their disease, locus of control or the role of powerful others, perceived benefits and barriers to treatment, emotional state, general attitudes (i.e., anxiety, embarrassment, guilt, etc.), and the social environment/lifestyle of the person concerned. To these should be added the targets aimed for by the patients and their perceptions of whether they are achieving them. These have been combined neatly in the overall model of Ajzen and Fishbein (Figure 2), which relates demographic and attitudinal factors respectively to "intention" to change behavior on the one hand and actually making the changes on the other.

This model has been tested in a large number of subjects with diabetes and significant relationships demonstrated, especially the potentially powerful negative effect of powerful professional others on both knowledge and behavior [58, 63]. Clearly, different elements of this model will operate for different individuals, but Ajzen and Fishbein would stress the importance of establishing which elements are operative for each patient. This model is complemented by the change model/cycle of Prochaska et al. [47] through the different stages of intention to change broken down into

"Precontemplative" – "Contemplative" –
"Action" – "Maintenance" – "Relapse"

The latter is particularly relevant to diabetes care in that it includes the all-important maintenance and all too common relapse observed in practice, yet often not accommodated for in educational planning. Rollnick

Table 1 Steps in making decisions to change*

Importance (Why?)	Confidence (How? What?)	Readiness (When?)
Is it worthwhile?	Can I?	Should I do it now?
Why should I?	How will I do it?	What about other priorities?
How will I benefit?	How will I cope with x,y, and z	
What will change?		
At what cost?	Will I succeed if...	
Do I really want to?	What change....?	
Will it make a difference?		

*Reprinted from reference 64, Copyright (1999), with permission from Elsevier.

et al. working in a day-to-day clinical practice setting has simplified these models of the steps required to change as follows:

"Readiness to change" (Not ready – Unsure – Ready) together with "Decision to change" dependent on the "Importance of a change"/Why? and the "Confidence to change"/How?/What? and the "Degree of readiness to change"/When? (Table 1) [64]

Day et al. in studies designed to identify factors responsible for effective self-management in clinical practice designed a comprehensive questionnaire incorporating theoretical aspects of the health beliefs model and locus of control and the major domains of diabetes self-care. Satisfactory reliability and validity were established. Repeated factorizations were consistent in over 2000 insulin-treated subjects including adolescents (for whom the questionnaire required some modification). It should be noted that as well as confirming the factors described above a target factor ("ideal" and "aimed for"), a specific diet barrier factor and a separate weight concern factor were consistently and highly significantly identified. The factors correlating with HbA_{1c} were the target, self-efficacy, perception of control, emotional status, and self-management skills factors. These on multiple regression could explain 50% of variance of HbA_{1c}. Similar results have been achieved with a separate questionnaire for those treated with diet or tablets [59]. Evidence that these attitudes can be changed/improved was demonstrated using a brief educational intervention with a computer-based multimedia learning program [65]. The Fischbein–Ajzen model simplified in the light of these findings (Figure 3) confirms different factors contributing to two broad aims, namely factors related to living with diabetes and factors related to achieving health-related outcomes. The balance between the two will obviously vary from individual to individual. Identification of low-scoring factors predominant in any one individual will enable intervention to be more accurately focused.

The validity of these models is therefore sound, and a behavioral approach to their modification is recommended to all those involved in diabetes care. Their application is very well described in *Health Behavior Change—A Guide for Practitioners* by Rollnick et al. [33]. The steps required are summarized in Table 2.

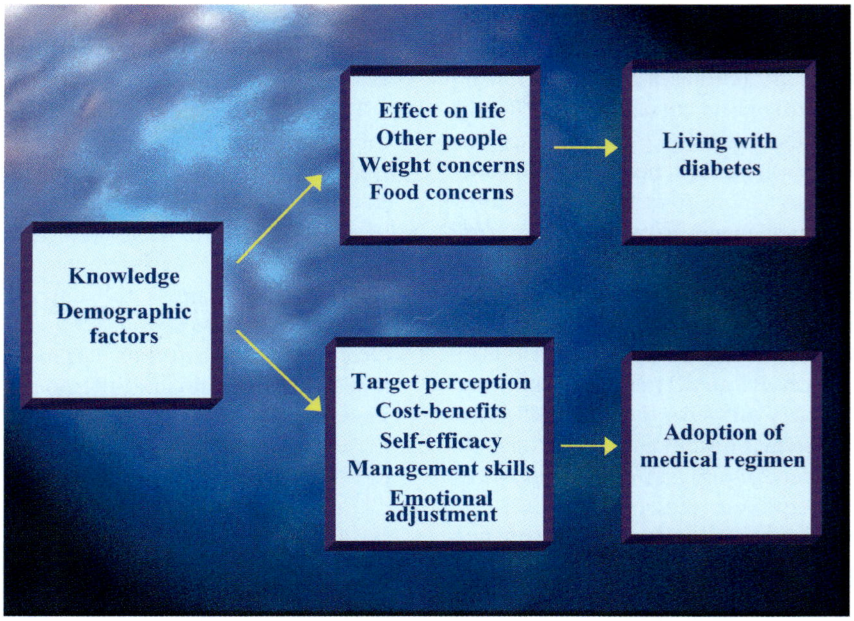

Figure 3 Simplified model of behavior

Table 2 Steps in Enabling Behavior Change

- Involving the patient
- Specify the problem
- Identify success and failures
- Negotiate a specific goal
- Identify ways to achieve the goal
- Contracting
- Tracking

The Teacher Effect

The skills of the teacher are obviously critical in learning process and far exceed the simple provision of information. Unfortunately, in most studies of new educational strategies the teacher variable is not taken into account.

It must be recognized that with any unit of average or moderate size, the number of staff is likely to be relatively small. In many studies where the same staff provide care for both treatment and control groups there is obvious potential for contamination. When different staff manage these separate groups, however, there is no guarantee that they all have equal teaching skills. The consideration, planning, and introduction of studies will also influence the behavior of all members of the health care group. Simply to allocate subjects to intervention and control (for example, one-to-one or group teaching) without eliminating such effects is likely to lead to a misleadingly negative result. For these reasons many authors have considered controlled studies to be inappropriate. The investigations of Mazucca and colleagues [18] are therefore particularly welcome. They had access to a very large number of physicians, significant numbers of whom had undergone training in the educational process. They were able, therefore, to conduct a study using a four-way design with patients allocated to (a) an educational program; (b) traditional management; (c) cared for by physicians with educational expertise; and (d) without educational expertise. Interestingly, the best glucose control was obtained in those undergoing an educational program and cared for by educationally trained physicians (a + c). Those whose physician was trained educationally, but who underwent no formal program (a + b), were nearly as successful. Elegant studies of the quality of doctor–patient interactions show that these are an important determinant of outcome. Despite the development of the diabetes educator the clinical consultation is still likely to be the most frequent contact between patient and professional, and therefore has a powerful educational impact, which may be positive or negative depending on the skills of the professional [61].

Further evidence of the critical importance of the teacher skill component is provided by the widely diverse results achieved by the same type of intervention in different hands, for example, in the numerous studies of changes in dietary therapy. Different dietary regimen may be equally successful in terms of weight loss and glycemic control. In contrast, similar diets applied by different groups may have quite different results. Hadden and colleagues [66], for example, obtained considerably more weight loss with apparently identical diets to those used by the UK Prospective Study Group [21]. Similarly, the implementation of home glucose monitoring techniques in some hands is associated with improved control while in others no such changes result [67–69]. It may not matter which method of testing (blood or urine) is used. One must conclude that the differences are due to the method of instruction and skills of persuasion, together with a wide range of beliefs or expectations of the individual to which the intervention may not be tailored. In the case of home glucose monitoring, success or failure depends on the subject's ability or willingness to respond to the results, rather than high standards of understanding or performance of tests *per se*. If the teacher remains in control the value of the tests is worthless.

These studies emphasize the need for training personnel in learning theory and practice, and for improving interactive skills.

Teacher Training—Who, What, How?

With the development of the diabetes specialist nurse/educator and diabetes centers devoted to education, the false and unreal assumption has arisen that this is the sole seat of learning to which all patients should have access. However, even in countries where these specialties and centers are most advanced, e.g. the United States, only a small percentage of patients have access to them. Secondly, even those that do still have regular contact with other professionals, especially in the primary care field. Even in the countries with the best-resourced health care systems it has been recognized that more than half the population of those with diabetes are, and probably should be, cared for in a primary care setting. It must be realized that every contact with any professional has a learning component. If unplanned, this may have a negative outcome rather than a positive one. All those involved in care do need training in the educational element. A good example of this is the cascade system of training of primary care physicians and practice nurses by Warwick Diabetes Care in the United Kingdom [70]. The content of this training has to take into account the need for some understanding of adult learning theory, improvement in communication skills and, as stressed above, ability to identify those critical factors governing behavior and delivery of behavioral modification techniques.

To achieve these ends a different style and content of the teaching programs are required. As a result of the pioneering work of Professor J.P. Assal working with the World Health Organization (WHO), a framework for such programs has been produced and is described in their recent publication *Therapeutic Patient Education* [71] and the pamphlet of the Diabetes Education Study group of the EASD, *Basic Curriculum for Health Professionals on Diabetes Education* [72]. Furthermore, Day et al. have reported the conclusions from a consensus workshop in the United Kingdom that there should be a national training program of similar style and content to that of the WHO group, and that it should be available to all care providers [73].

PLANNING AN EDUCATIONAL PROGRAM

As indicated above a structured education program is now recommended for all those with diabetes [26]. Contrasting types of educational programs include those described by groups in Geneva–Düsseldorf and Ipswich. The Geneva–Düsseldorf model has been well tested and is undoubtedly successful. The course is inpatient based, finite, and limited to 1 week (patients may be offered a second week). [74]. Both new and established cases are dealt with. It is effective in use of staff time and has the advantage that the participants are captive with a low dropout rate. Their program is well designed and encompasses the full range of domains of diabetes care. It allows effective use of group dynamics and, in their hands, uses modern interactive methods. Such limited-time courses may, however, be unsuitable for new cases who may not be receptive to courses of this intensity. And there is no facility for long-term maintenance and reinforcement, which is left to others in an unstructured way. The actual number of subjects that even sizeable units can deal with is small relative to the large population of those with diabetes for whom alternative strategies are required. They are however appropriate for small homogeneous groups of subjects such as those with type 2 diabetes, commencing insulin therapy. In contrast, the Ipswich program is delivered on an outpatient basis, most of the teaching being performed on a one-to-one basis and tailored to satisfy individual needs. Frequency of attendance is dependent on need. Although most concentrated in the first 2 weeks, the initial program is spread over 3 months. Follow-up is provided regularly during the first year with the diabetes educator, and telephone support is provided. The problem of reinforcement and long-term education is provided by scheduled sessions with the educator at a minimum frequency of once yearly. Weekly group sessions are scheduled for newly diagnosed subjects with type 2 diabetes. For certain categories of patient, interactive group sessions are provided, including type 2 subjects commencing insulin therapy or type 1 subjects commencing subcutaneous infusion therapy. Problems, however, are encountered in ensuring that all individuals attend the program. Subjects are less captive than those attending for a week's course, and greater difficulties are encountered in scheduling staff time. However, such programs are better suited to the long-term educational needs than the short one-off programs. Continuous and maintained improvements in HbA_1 concentrations have been demonstrated [75]. The DAFNE program, which is a recent extension of the Geneva–Düsseldorf model for training in intensive insulin therapy, does have the element of continuity and is provided on an outpatient basis but is expensive in staff time and limited to relatively small numbers of subjects.

It should be noted that these examples of well-designed programs are based on purpose-designed centers. The majority of patients, however, will be treated in a primary care setting now and for the foreseeable future. The educational principles and structure of the Ipswich program can be delivered largely on a one-to-one basis in primary care settings, given adequate level of skilled staff. Warwick Diabetes has led the way in development of a cascade training program in the technological and educational aspects of diabetes, which offers a population solution for those with diabetes treated in the community [70].

Choice of Program

For those responsible for planning a program for a population of subjects, therefore, choice of curricula and teaching methods will depend on the size and geography of the population, system of health care, case mix, definition of objectives, and identification of all those involved in care delivery.

Steps in Program Development

Traditionally, the development process consists of definition of objectives, planning a curriculum, selection of teaching methods, and evaluation. In the past this process has been predominantly teacher-centered or, in the case of medical/patient education, physician-driven. However, with the general acceptance of the need for the learner to be actively involved, combined with greater understanding of the principles governing patient behavior, the necessity for a learner-centered model is paramount [32]. In this way the patients' learning wants and needs are acknowledged, objectives and targets negotiated and agreed, and choice and ownership of the learning process invested in the learner/patient.

Planning Instructional Objectives

Mager's well-known aphorism, "If you don't know where you're going, you may very well end somewhere else and not even know it," beautifully summarizes the essential need for clear-cut objectives in the educational process [76]. This has traditionally been the prerogative of the teacher, but although the overall objectives have to be specified in the first instance by the professionals, who have the responsibility for improving health care outcomes, without the active participation of the patient in the choice of objectives specific to them the process is fruitless.

Since Mager, others have also stressed the necessity not only of listing aims, but of defining these in behavioral terms. The great advantage of doing so is that the endpoint is described in terms of what the learner can be expected ultimately to do, thus providing clear statements of these activities, whether intellectual (e.g. say, repeat, describe, etc.) or manual (draw up, inject, test, etc.) or attitudinal (demonstrates belief in treatment, etc). This done, these objectives can be shared and agreed, and there is a reasonable chance that different members of the team will all work toward commonly agreed goals. Contradictory messages and omissions are likely to be avoided. The simpler alternative of checklists fails in these respects. Given for example the heading "hypoglycemia," "diet," or "exercise," the specific outcomes desired may well vary from one teacher to another and important areas may be overlooked. Further, there is no implicit method of checking that the targets have been achieved. In contrast the description of "behavior" provides an obvious indication of how the objectives can be evaluated (e.g., patient carries a card, sugar, performs blood, or urine tests) [77]. A useful example of curriculum objectives for type 1 and 2 diabetes are provide in the list of competencies in *Therapeutic Patient Education* [78].

The desired attitudes are more difficult to describe but the profile provided in the same publication is helpful in this regard.

Profile of Attitudes

The patient [79]

- shows surprise and pays little attention when told of the diagnosis
- speaks of the disease in a detached manner
- is hostile but wishes to know more about the illness and complies more or less with the treatment
- asks for the least inconvenient type of treatment
- is sad but talks of the future though not yet aware of how to cope
- indicates willingness to cooperate and asks for help in coping
- makes specific and appropriate requests to the health care provider or the family
- takes some liberties with the treatment without much concern but also without being careless
- acknowledges his/her present state of health
- recognizes that the illness may have very serious consequences
- adheres confidently to treatment
- expresses the belief that the benefits of following treatment far outweigh its constraints
- changes lifestyle in accordance with the illness
- talks openly and without embarrassment of the illness
- adheres to treatment as a daily routine
- adjusts the treatment in case of a crisis

Furthermore, the discipline of the definition of objectives enables teams to identify differences between team members.

Translating Objectives into Specific Patient Targets

Different sets of objectives are required for different groups, most obviously for type 1 and 2 subjects.

This truth, apparently self-evident, is clearly ignored by many who provide the same teaching methods (lectures, groups, etc.) for both at the same time. Secondly, the objectives are spread over the lifetime of the subject. It is important, therefore, to categorize those objectives to be achieved immediately (e.g., first aid—injection techniques, recognition, and self-treatment of hypoglycemia), those desired over the next weeks or months (e.g., adjustment of dose of insulin), and lifelong objectives (continued self-monitoring and self-adjustment of regimen). By identifying an appropriate time scale the early stages of a program can be simplified. Timing is important not only to avoid information overload but also those objectives that are inappropriate in the presence of the severe emotional disturbance that the individuals may undergo at diagnosis. These may be profound, with a change from "not ill" to "ill," and similar to those associated with the grieving responses, e.g. shock, anger, guilt, and depression, before acceptance is achieved [80]. Overload may create depression and hopelessness, and delay the shift of the locus of control from the medical team to the individual, and the necessary experimentation of self-learning that is necessary for effective self-control. Careful documentation of objectives that are omitted will ensure coverage at a later date. The need to fulfill the intermediate and lifelong objectives at different stages of an individual's development emphasize the necessity for a lifelong program. Failure to consider this may account for the disappointment of those studying the long-term benefit of short self-contained programs.

Changes in behavior are only likely if the person concerned perceives the targets as achievable. The primary list of objectives has to be tailored to the patient's real and perceived needs, lifestyle, and current state of mind. It is well recognized in weight control that quite unattainable targets are often set and failure of weight reduction is usually the outcome. In contrast, if more limited weight loss is agreed, success is more likely [81]. It is now strongly recommended, therefore, that the final definition of objectives should be individualized to each patient, with objectives and targets agreed between the educator and the patient.

To achieve this, following steps are required:

- Identify patients existing knowledge, beliefs, perception, and expectations
- Dispel misconceptions
- Discuss with them what their immediate priorities are

Introduce to them those objectives you feel are appropriate in the context of

- the state of their illness
- their existing knowledge, skill, perceptions and beliefs,
- degree of acceptance of illness
- general emotional state
- Indicate those that are absolutely essential for their immediate health
- Select those considered feasible by the patient
- Record shared objectives and those deferred . . .

Who are the Teachers?

When planning education, care must be taken to include all those involved in care delivery. Failure to do so risks the danger of mixed messages for the patient and inadequate provision of the necessary training for all. All should be involved in the formulation of objectives and be familiar with the patient-centered approach to learning. Often overlooked are pharmacy staff and those providing care for the treatment of complications.

In pregnancy there need to be common attitudes, objectives, and therapeutic targets between diabetologists, diabetes nurses and the obstetric team. For those attending specialist centers, the primary team in frequent contact with the patient must be involved. Despite the requirement to involve everybody, an attempt should be made to keep the total numbers as small as possible in order to minimize misinformation, maintain consistency, and improve confidence. The core members of the diabetes team mainly responsible for care of any one patient should not exceed three or four people.

Where Does Education Take Place?

It has long been recognized that hospital wards and many outpatient departments are not good learning environments. In recent years, considerable efforts have been made to develop education units, separate from the clinical areas and staffed by trained diabetes educators. These enable curricula to be planned and tailored to the learners' needs and certainly are much better suited for the planning of 5-day courses, group programs, etc. Their development has enabled us to identify more clearly, and hence analyze, the educational component of care. However, there are disadvantages and impracticalities in such separation.

First, the majority of patients, and especially those with type 2 diabetes, are predominantly looked after in a primary care setting. The numbers are very large and increasing and greatly exceed the capacity of the centers.

Secondly, there is a problem in the selection of patients. Whether in specialist diabetes clinics or in primary care, assumptions are made that some are more "suitable" for education than others. Patients are often chosen as requiring education because of poor compliance or control. The large majority of more stable patients may not be so selected and therefore miss the benefits that they might acquire from a more intensified educational approach. Yet, it is these subjects who have been shown to gain the most benefit from further educational advice. It must be emphasized that during a lifetime of diabetes the majority of contacts with professionals will take place in a clinic/primary care environment. These provide opportunities for continuing education but also the threat of negative learning if the contacts are unsatisfactory. As already indicated, the consultation may have powerful positive or negative effects on patient behavior and outcome [61]. The educational philosophy must therefore be appropriate in all clinical situations, and it is strongly recommended that the delivery of care and education are integrated. This has been shown to be both feasible and successful [75].

Choice of Learning Methods

One-to-One Learning

For the majority, the most frequent contact and hence learning opportunity will be on a one-to-one basis with doctor, dietitian, or nurse educator. Even if group sessions are programmed they are of short duration relative to individual contacts, which are likely to predominate throughout the life of the patient. Studies of the process involved in adult learning suggest the need for considerable adjustment of the traditional consultative type of interview. Styles need changing if the knowledge and beliefs, misconceptions, and fears are to be successfully identified and dealt with. Formal attempts to make an active effort to use open-ended questions have been shown to be much more effective than reliance on standard medical interviewing skills [82]. Pauses and reiteration of questions are essential to check that messages have been understood. Interviews should be demand led, dealing with new symptoms or the immediate anxieties of the subject. Therefore the adjustment and timing of the carer's objectives becomes even more necessary. A problem-based style is most helpful ("What would you do if . . . .?) [83]. Kaplan et al. have demonstrated most skillfully that if the interview is adapted to allow the patient to feel some ownership and have some control over the content, he/she not only learnt more but also achieved better glycemic control [61].

The program must allow for the frequency of interviews to be adjusted to the learner's requirements and to ensure that all objectives are eventually dealt with. Care must be taken to recognize the blocking action of anxiety, with postponement of provision of important knowledge and skills until this is allayed. In the absence of absolutely overriding social reasons, sequential interviews on the same day, with different staff members should be avoided. The programming of sessions (for example on dietary advice) on subsequent days not only has enormous learning advantages, but also makes better use of nurse educators' and dietitians' time by enabling them to schedule their appointments more efficiently.

The requirement for maintenance and reinforcement should not be overlooked. The tendency for behavior to wane has already been described. Often, patients are returned to routine follow-up in an environment quite unsuited to ongoing learning and in which only the apparent clinical needs are dealt with [6]. A program of routine visits that ensures at least a minimum of one session per year with a nurse educator would seem ideal, and in view of the skills of many nurse educators, such educational appointments may, without harm, be substituted for some routine medical appointments [84]. Attention to detail may facilitate the learning approach—siting of chairs, avoiding the wearing of white coats, etc.

Many practitioners may need to develop new skills to achieve a high standard of one-to-one interaction. Whatever their professional background it is likely that they will have learnt a more traditional style of interviewer-led process. It should be emphasized that these methods are different from those used in counseling. Not only is training in these skills needed but also the opportunity to practice and reflect/review competency. To this end, self-recordings from time to time (audio or video) are invaluable.

Group Learning

This can be divided into three quite different styles:

(1) Traditional classroom-type learning.
(2) Interactive, task-orientated group learning.
(3) Therapeutic groups.

The lecture style of the traditional classroom setting is of relatively little value. It is teacher-centered with little facility for ascertainment of individual needs. Without interaction between the learners, the expression of attitudes and beliefs is negligible, and actual acquisition of new information also limited.

Although they would appear to offer solutions for dealing with large numbers, their low yield of effective learning suggests these methods are best avoided. However, using interactive educational groups, as pioneered by Groen and Pelser [85], has enormous advantages in that they facilitate the way in which individuals learn from one another.

Task-oriented groups need to be clearly distinguished from therapeutic ones. The latter have psychotherapeutic aims, for those with significant psychiatric disturbance, and are beyond the scope of this chapter. Educational groups use standard interactive group processes. The teacher acts as facilitator, only providing resource when necessary. This is the style that is fundamental to problem-based learning [83]. Participants much more easily express their concepts, beliefs, and concerns [86]. To the observer, a clear picture is provided of what individuals do and do not do, and why. The peer effect is often much more successful in enabling subjects to adopt difficult new behaviors, for example, altering insulin dosages for the first time, coping with illness, or dietary adherence. The studies of McCulloch and colleagues [87] and Aveline et al. [88] are good examples. The reasons for the behavior gap, which have remained quite covert in prolonged one-to-one consultation, may become obvious. Subjects may feel safer within a group and therefore declare their failures and the reasons for them, especially when such failures are found to be common to others.

For effective interaction, groups need to consist of no less than 5 and no more than 15 participants. The number of sessions will depend on the objectives of the group but can usually be limited to six or seven. Although groups may set their own objectives in any one session, the educator's objectives can be checked off as they are covered. Those that are omitted can be introduced at the leader's discretion. On occasions, however, the group process may need to be more open-ended and the number of sessions extended. Attempts to explore the use of lay facilitators, however, have been only partly successful in that most participants preferred the presence of a professional [85]. Professionally led interactive group processes are integral components of the Geneva–Düsseldorf, DAFNE, and Ipswich programs described above. They are particularly valuable for subjects with relatively homogeneous objectives, e.g. newly diagnosed type 2 patients, those starting insulin for the first time, embarking on intensified regimens including subcutaneous insulin infusion, or the prevention or management of complications.

A clear-cut timetable, i.e. number of sessions and duration, will help to encourage a good attendance rate. Many groups are scheduled outside office hours for the convenience of those in work, or parents of children. Experience suggests that this may encourage the view that group activity is an optional extra, having more of a social function than a direct learning effect. For type 2 patients where the incidence of the disorder is high, groups of sufficient size can be easily collected, and sessions can be scheduled in the working day and attendance rates improved. These may still not exceed 70% or 80%. Alternative strategies need, therefore, to be built in for the nonattenders. This is not, of course, a problem for the more captive participants of the residential or self-limited course of 1 or

2 weeks' duration, such as in the Düsseldorf or Geneva programs.

Adolescents are often selected as a target for group education. Attracting them to sessions is difficult. Camps for children and adolescents, which enable group activity, have been a feature of diabetes education for many years and are attractive. In the United Kingdom some 800 children attend such camps every year and similar activities take place in the United States and across Europe [89–92]. The Firbush scheme, [92], in which a number of teenagers were collected together for a week in a camp, was highly successful.

Finally as in the Nottingham study [93] it is notable that the beneficial effects of group learning often wane with the passage of time. This emphasizes yet again the need for a maintenance program; reconvening groups on an occasional basis is valuable in this respect.

Use of Audiovisual Aids

A wide range of audiovisual aids is now available to supplement teaching programs. These include the simplest, such as diet sheets, handbooks, and pamphlets, as well as the more complex, such as videotapes and packages combining workbooks, visual display material, self-evaluation check lists, and most recently, computer programs, especially new multimedia programs. Good examples include the handbooks [94, 95], lists of proprietary foods and their contents [96], and videotapes produced by *Diabetes UK* (British Diabetic Association), and the teaching packages of several pharmaceutical industries. However, very often such materials are used as a substitute for more appropriate tutor-led learning, in a haphazard way, regardless of the learner's needs. It is necessary to observe certain rules: the aids must be selected to satisfy individual learning objectives, the content must be appropriate, and the objectives and target audience of the aids or programs obvious; presentation and level should be correct and match the learner's abilities; materials are often prepared in which reading ages are ignored, and representational methods, e.g. graphs, or concepts are so complex or so specialized as to be beyond the abilities of the recipient. For average readership the content should be appropriate for a young teenager. This readership age can be increased if motivation is high. (The recent *Diabetes UK* handbooks have been estimated to have a reading age suitable for the average 17-year-old, but below that of a potential college graduate). In contrast, many leaflets may be far too complex [97]. Video programs should be short and their content limited. The number of new concepts should be restricted to two or three. Because videotapes are expensive to produce, many are far too long (up to 30 min), and misguided attempts are made to satisfy a variety of different audiences. Tapes embodying one or two concepts and lasting 7–10 min are much more suitable. The benefits of such materials when used to complement existing programs can be clear-cut [98]. Great care is necessary to avoid confusion. A recent examination of the advice in a number of commonly used leaflets on foot care, examples of which are given in Table 3, demonstrates contradictory information, both between leaflets and within them. Examples include demands for patients to "avoid wet feet" and yet to prevent their feet from becoming "dry" [99]. Advice must not only be correct but feasible. As recommended in the DESG of the EASD teaching letter, *Use, Misuse and Abuse of Audiovisual Aids* [100], audiovisual aids should not be a substitute for interaction with the learner, or place the patient in a passive role. Leaving videotapes to run in waiting rooms is a fruitless exercise because the recipients' minds are usually elsewhere. Aids that are mismatched to the learner group, i.e. designed for those with type 1 and shown to those with type 2 diabetes, or those that contain frightening or intellectually inappropriate material, must be avoided. Furthermore, it is essential that attempts are made to provide material in the native language of the subjects concerned. When translating material it should be back-translated to ensure that the original sense has not been lost.

Computer-based Learning Materials

A variety of computer programs are now available, from simple concept games to more sophisticated question-and-answer programs. It has been demonstrated that a well-organized quiz can have a significant learning benefit in its own right [42]. In addition, there are now a number of commercially available computer-based programs for establishing the correct dosage of insulin in relation to food and exercise, using a variety of different algorithms. These may have considerable learning effect but, ideally, should have immediate feedback, which they mainly lack [101, 102].

Table 3 Examples of contrasting advice from different leaflets on foot care

Never walk barefoot ...	Look after your feet	Rest if >50 years old
Do not cut with knives or razor blades yourself	Wear good shoes	Do not treat corns or sores
Avoid tight shoes	Must get infection treated	Do not walk barefoot
Wash feet alternate days	Have careful chiropody	Perform footbaths frequently
Never treat infection yourself	Do not smoke	Exercises
Avoid wet feet	Look after blood sugar	

Recent technical advances now allow the exploitation of all audiovisual materials to be combined using multimedia and CD-driven programs, which enable much more interactive use of audiovisual material. The most advanced such program, which combines the use of patient-generated material presented in a large number of short video clips, interactive exercises, strategy selection exercises, and presentation of factual information, has been produced for both type 1 and 2 diabetes (*Learning Diabetes*) [103]. This has been fully evaluated in a study designed to determine (a) the ease of access, difficulties encountered, and potential demographic factors (e.g., age, sex, educational or social status, and lack of computer expertise), which might create barriers to use and (b) to what extent the programs met patients perceived needs. Data were obtained from observation, focused interviews, and detailed analysis of the programs' use derived from the embedded tracking database. Analysis was also performed to determine whether changes in basic knowledge or attitudes and perceptions to diabetes self-care were achieved, using well-validated questionnaires pre- and postprogram use [103].

It was demonstrated that fears that older patients and those of lower educational or social status or with limited computer expertise would prohibit effective use of these programs were unfounded. Learner satisfaction was high with regard both to the ease of use and their value. Improvement in assessment of knowledge acquisition and attitudes to self-care were highly significant. Individual learners did use the programs differently, suggesting that they made choices of material to match their individual needs. It may be possible to apply these advances in distance learning materials, not only for those with diabetes but also for their carers and professional advisers (see also Chapter 68).

SPECIFIC PROBLEMS

Many of these have been subjects of a number of workshops of the DESG, the results of which have been published in a series of teaching letters [72, 104]. Certain learning requirements are so common as to deserve special mention and updating in the light of new technologies.

Initiation of Insulin Therapy

The initiation of insulin therapy is likely to be associated with considerable anxiety and possible depression in the patient. The objectives must be limited to those that are absolutely essential, hence the designation of specific "first-aid objectives" to tide patients over the first few days. To avoid prolonged anxiety, the first step must be to ensure that the patient gives himself or herself an injection at the time the decision is made to start insulin therapy. If the patient has driven to the clinic, or immediate therapeutic dosage is not clinically mandatory, a minimal dose can be given. It is not necessary to admit the patient to hospital and, indeed, this may be actually harmful in indicating an unnecessary reliance on a medical team to work out dosages, etc. thereby inhibiting the necessary transfer of the "locus of control" to the subject. If availability of personnel will allow, stabilization at home with home visits may be even more appropriate in removing much of the anxiety, especially with children [105]. Certainly, at some point during the early stages of the therapy, a home visit may be most useful in identifying the social context and any particular difficulties unique to the individual concerned. The use of relatively small dosages of insulin, initially combined with frequent blood tests, allows patients themselves to determine the relationships between food, exercise, insulin dosage, and blood glucose levels, with the self-achievement of the administration of more effective dosage within a couple of weeks. This self-learning element needs to be established as soon as possible. One-to-one sessions on three successive days should allow the achievement of all the other important early objectives. Significant hypoglycemia is unlikely to occur in the early stages, and it must be remembered that preventative or corrective techniques may be understood in theory but not put into practice.

Close contact must be maintained between the patient and educational team, with telephone consultation on subsequent nonvisit days for the first week or two. In the emotional turmoil, so much may be forgotten that simple written lists of advice given to the patient for subsequent reference may be most helpful. As in all areas of education, and of critical importance in the highly charged atmosphere of early treatment, the need to ensure uniformity of advice is paramount. Such clinical discrepancies as use or not of alcohol swabs, or choice of injection site, which may seem quite minor to the clinical team, may sow doubts in the patient's mind, which gravely threaten subsequent self-reliance.

Injection phobia is an uncommon but important barrier to insulin initiation. It demands early recognition and, once detected, must be treated seriously. Mollema and colleagues have identified that this is more commonly due to fear of the injected substance rather than of the needle itself. Specialist help is essential [106].

Learning About Hypoglycemia

For patients treated with insulin their attitude to hypoglycemic reactions and methods of dealing with them may well determine much of the day-to-day approach to their handling of their diabetes and, indeed, the standards of glycemic control that are achieved. The particular features of such reactions, their symptoms, methods for their prevention, related measures such as carrying identification and a source of glucose, and their treatment are among the most important in the list of learning objectives, and must be included in the first few days of a learning program. Whether or not hypoglycemia should be induced at this stage is usually hotly disputed. The proponents argue that, without this procedure, subjects are left wondering and anxious at the prospect of this "event," which they are encouraged to take pains to prevent and treat. However, it is frequently quite difficult to achieve on an outpatient or domiciliary basis. A failed attempt may provoke even greater anxiety. Certainly, it does tend to distract the individual from self-management and reinforce ideas of dependence on others. The most important elements of learning about hypoglycemia must be not merely the necessary precautions and avoidance of dangerous situations, but also the development of a tolerant and optimistic view of the occurrence and treatment of hypoglycemia. Studies have shown that feelings of vulnerability to hypoglycemia are very strong and may well outstrip concern about hyperglycemia and longer term complications [89, 90]. Day-to-day behavior is much more likely to be governed by short-term risk or gain than by long-term complications. The tendency to avoid hypoglycemia by maintaining high blood glucose levels is powerful and, indeed, it has been demonstrated that glycated hemoglobin may be as strongly related to this as to any other factor [107]. It is notable that in group discussions, without exception, a major amount of time is spent by participants spontaneously volunteering their fears or seeking reassurances about reactions.

Undoubtedly, severe hypoglycemia (that which requires help from others) can be socially disabling. However, the most powerful negative motivation must be the fear of death or brain damage with which the concept of coma is usually associated. The learning program must ensure that the usually very good prognosis of even severe hypoglycemia is fully explained and appreciated. These explanations are unlikely to be believed, however, without the reassurance of those who have experienced the condition.

Particular difficulty may be experienced after severe reactions, which are unperceived, and lead to emergency therapy with glucose or glucagon. Feelings of self-control/self-efficacy are severely threatened, and acquired high levels of feelings of internal control reversed. Undoubtedly, more frequent use of glucose self-testing may go some way to restoring confidence, but at such times careful and frequent counseling is also required. Particular care has to be paid by members of the medical team to their own attitudes and approaches. Watching the excited and dramatic behavior of many medical staff to a severe reaction on a ward will do little to allay an observer's fears of the "emergency" nature of the condition. It is of interest to note that among those using intensified insulin regimens, especially of the most rigorous kind aiming at normoglycemia, hypoglycemia does occur probably with greater frequency than during conventional therapy.

However, it has been shown that hypoglycemia can not only be tolerated, but even welcomed as demonstrating effective overall control, by subjects taught the advantages of self-control and the immediacy of self-treatment, within small groups [102]. Cox and others have developed methods for the early identification of impending hypoglycemia and specific intensive patient training programs for their application. These programs have been reproduced by others and show considerable promise [108].

Teaching of glucagon injection is included in most lists of learning objectives. However, its inclusion in the early stages of learning is usually unnecessary. When it is taught, it is common to overlook the fact that the procedure may not be required for 1–2 years or longer and then under circumstances of extreme anxiety (i.e. early in the morning with a convulsing child). Hence the need for repetition of instruction, say on a two-yearly basis.

In all respects the problems of learning to cope with hypoglycemia and avoid overdefensive attitudes and behavior cannot be achieved in one short-term education program. Plans must be made to check subjects' attitudes and behavior. A flexible education program needs to be developed to allow reinforcement and the support of peer groups to be provided when necessary throughout the life of the individual. The educator must also remain aware of the small proportion of subjects who actually feel better when hypoglycemic. This may be potentially dangerous and early identification of the problem is essential.

Finally, the particular problem of hypoglycemia emphasizes the need for public health education about diabetes. Observation or hearsay about insulin reactions largely determines lay attitudes and has an important influence on legislation in relation to driving, employment, insurance, etc. It is necessary to ensure intelligent understanding of the problem on a local and national basis.

Self-monitoring of Glucose

The introduction of self-monitoring of glucose was an important milestone in the self-management of diabetes [109] and provided a major instrument for changing the understanding, attitudes, and behavior of insulin-dependent subjects especially. Undoubtedly, early instruction in blood glucose estimation allows subjects to achieve a comprehension of the relationship between insulin, glucose, food, and exercise—concepts that are often surprisingly poorly understood by many with diabetes of quite long standing. Frequent testing in the first few weeks should be advised. The frequency can subsequently be adjusted to a subject's individual requirements. Originally, blood glucose testing was considered mandatory only for those treated with insulin. Those with diet or diet and tablets do not suffer the same wide range of glucose excursions, and (given a normal threshold) urine tests may provide a reasonable guide to overall control. However, many patients do not recognize fully the relationship between food and blood glucose, and this may not be easily understood without blood glucose testing. Furthermore, the gains from dietary adherence may be reinforced by the growth in self-satisfaction if individuals can attain normal blood glucose values, rather than the more easily achieved negative urine tests.

Learning blood glucose testing is not simple. It requires time, with careful demonstration and observation of individuals' standards of skill, not just initially but on repeated occasions. With the passage of time, techniques may become very poor and virtually worthless. In particular, when using meters, subjects may tend to regard the digital output as invariably correct, despite inadequate coverage of strip with blood or occlusion of the light beam aperture with dirt, due to poor machine maintenance.

Despite the obvious advantages of glucose control, the literature surrounding the subject indicates a degree of naivety. Studies have already been referred to that demonstrate no improvement in glycemic control with the introduction of home glucose monitoring [37, 45, 69]. Most, however, fail to distinguish between the learning of a skill and the use to which it might be put. For example, patients may only test to reassure themselves about hypoglycemia, hence the majority of tests recorded are likely to be done at times when they are at most risk. Hyperglycemia is overlooked; as a consequence, results will bear no relationship to glycated hemoglobin, nor will the latter value improve. There are those with persistent strong feelings of external control who will test frequently, regularly, and accurately but will take no action themselves in response to the results. The tests are being done for the doctor rather than for themselves. Some—especially those using meters—may regard the latter as a "black box," with the feeling that technique performance is in some covert way satisfying the requirements of control, without the need for any further action by themselves.

Glucose self-monitoring is only likely to achieve better control if accompanied by learning and application by the patient of dosage adjustment. The value of this is highlighted by intensified insulin regimens, especially those advocating not only variation in frequency of injections but also in timing and/or the use of intramuscular injections, on occasions, for rapid effect [96]. The principle that a high or abnormal level of glucose can be moderated by an immediate response does seem likely to augment feelings of "internal control" and to enhance the feeling that the technique is providing a benefit rather than a barrier. A number of monitoring systems have been developed, which record and relay results electronically to a professional advisor. Unfortunately, these promote dependence and predicate against self-adjustment and reinforce potential negative attitudes of "external control."

Attitudes of "learned hopelessness" must be detected. Clinical observation reveals this to be a common problem in diabetes clinics, in which patients not infrequently present sets of results for which they (and possibly their doctors) have no explanation or solution. If repeated, this can lead only to a response of despair and may well be one of the reasons for omission or fabrication of test results. Much has been made of the discovery of so-called "cheating" behavior, using memory meters [110–112]. That this should excite surprise suggests misunderstanding of the nature of the complicated requirements of compliance with diabetes regimens. Certainly, it is unproductive if recorded values are not valid. Open discussion of acceptability of self-testing, its value to the patient, targets aimed for, and the extent to which the patient's and physician's standards can be agreed will help resolve these problems. This maybe further helped by potential techniques of continuous monitoring systems. However, the solutions are still likely to depend on careful advice, support, and reassurance from a skilled practitioner.

Intensified Insulin Treatment

Introduction of intensified insulin treatment for those with insulin-treated diabetes is now recommended for most patients treated with insulin [17]. Originally, this was mostly achieved with multiple subcutaneous injection dose regimens. More recently, many patients are using subcutaneous infusion pumps. However, it has been well demonstrated that frequency of injections and/or testing *per se* have little relationship to outcome. Indeed, in the DCCT study those using pumps fared no better than those using multiple injections. The reasons for these surprising observations lie in the observations of Bradley et al. [55], who demonstrated with a study of users of the first generation of pumps that many subjects selected pump therapy as a solution to their diabetes, which did not require *their* active intervention. These intensive therapies only work if the patients have the knowledge, skills, and desire to drive the treatment themselves. This involves patients adapting their insulin, meals, etc. to their own day-to-day routines and test results to achieve optimum control. With regard to choice of insulin delivery system, reference to the theory of locus of control reminds us that quite large numbers of subjects may still be of the view that insulin dosage change is a matter for professional prescription, i.e. they rely on external control or, even worse, believe that what may happen to them is a matter of pure chance. The black box (i.e., the pump) will be worthless.

Furthermore, many clinicians working with these patients have noted that although appearing knowledgeable and willing, often with a long experience of insulin therapy, they still did not fully understand the relationship between food and insulin and had limited awareness of the relative carbohydrate content of their meals. Hence, dose adjustment was haphazard. This, at least in part, is due to the discarding of accurate carbohydrate counting with the introduction of the high versus low carbohydrate diet several years ago. This has led to the DAFNE regimen referred to above. Patients are trained to learn the glycemic effects of different foods and carbohydrates in particular, and to fine-tune their insulin doses accordingly. Programs of training are of 5 days duration, using interactive group methods. Significant improvements in glycemic control have been achieved in a randomized controlled trial, without increased rates of hypoglycemia or weight increase. Patient well-being and satisfaction were also improved [20]. The programs delivered to date are expensive in staff time and deal with relatively small numbers but there is no reason why the lessons learnt from them cannot be incorporated into more flexible outpatient systems similar to those described for the initiation of insulin therapy described above.

Learning Dietary Therapy

Studies of adherence to dietary treatment in the predominantly obese subjects with type 2 diabetes reveal repeated failure. Success is often only transitory [21, 66, 93]. This highlights the difficulty of achieving a major behavioral change in (very often) asymptomatic subjects. Unfortunately, most workers address themselves to the outcome rather than to the process, so that many of the causes of failure remain speculative. From an educational point of view, certain features stand out as important contributors. First, the goals may not be perceived as necessary or achievable. Once symptoms, if present, are rapidly relieved by avoiding sucrose, as is customary, the major objective is prevention of long-term complications. The risk of these may not be believed, i.e. subjects do not feel a threat. Subjects may desire weight reduction for cosmetic reasons, but this motive may well have been operative, unsuccessfully, for many years preceding the diagnosis of diabetes. Loss of glycosuria may be relatively easily achieved and further continuation of the struggle may be felt to be unwarranted. The goals that are set may be unacceptable—setting ideal body weight as a target may be hopelessly unattainable. Use of a stepwise approach with small but regular and achievable gains are more successful [81]. Some indication of a critical determinant is suggested by the analysis of factors responsible, by Day et al. [59]. Two factors, weight concerns and diet barriers, consistently separated from one another and in observations of several large groups of subjects there was only a weak relationship between the two. This would suggest that many people still perceive little relationship with what they eat and their weight. Dietary prescription may be far too complex. With the current emphasis upon restriction of fat and energy intake as well as of carbohydrate, and an increased fiber intake, the actual prescription may be too difficult to follow. It is common to find long lists of various foods categorized according to high or low carbohydrate, protein, and fat content. Patients are required to select appropriate foods with complex permutations from such lists. Ability to determine the exact constitution of different foods may be lacking. Alternatively, instruction may be too vague, with advice to develop a prudent diet or "cut calories," etc., with inadequate suggestions as to possible substitutes or alternatives.

Whatever the causes, certain strategies appear to be more successful than others. The setting of achievable goals has been alluded to and the use of an agreed (if not necessarily binding) contract works with some. The most striking benefits appear to be achieved when peer influence is supplied with group support [86, 87]. Unfortunately, it would appear that such effects also wane and for sustained effect the group process has to be maintained [93]. It would seem necessary to continue the process at least on an intermittent basis, albeit less frequently than the sessions every 2 or 4 weeks that seem to work in the first instance. Dietary advice is unlikely to be successful unless it is tailored to the individual's own goals, beliefs about outcome are fully explored, and adequate time is devoted to appropriate instruction about the actual content of different foods.

With regard to the management of type 1 diabetes the content and timing of meals are critical determinants of glycemic control and avoidance of severe hypoglycemia. The DAFNE study described above clearly indicate the need for more intensive training in the glycemic effects of what they eat. To this end recent determination of the glycemic index, which is not solely related to carbohydrate content, and compilation of this information in data banks of food are helpful [113].

Foot Care

The preventive value of education is undoubted. Many studies have been performed, examining the impact of educational interventions on acquisition of information, behavior change manifested by improved self foot-care, and clinical outcome (amputations, etc.). As with other aspects of education, knowledge acquisition *per se* has little influence on care behavior and outcome. But major reductions in hospitalization and amputation rates, and the ratio of above-knee to below-knee amputations have been achieved by behavioral change. The degree of success has been quite variable, however, and the study of Malone et al. is illustrative in this respect. They achieved a remarkable success in amputation rate reduction, using a really quite short and simple intervention. It was notable, however, that all their subjects already had significant foot problems and were therefore at high risk. Their success almost certainly related to the fact that the patients all recognized the risks themselves in contrast to asymptomatic subjects in other studies [22].

Examination of educational methods reveal a number of pitfalls. The confusing conflicts both between and within foot-care leaflets have been described in the section on audiovisual aids. In addition, however, the list of potential preventive measures that are commonly proposed is extensive (see Table 3). It would appear that although many items (e.g. appropriate shoe fitting) have a sound basis, there are others for which there is no substantive evidence of value (e.g., foot exercises). Indeed, it is probable that they are based on beliefs rather than on true knowledge. This is bound to lead to the discrepancies between and within different professionals within the team already described [99], and emphasizes the need for all to agree on the objectives. Furthermore, this list contains objectives that may be absolutely essential for certain individuals but are quite unnecessary for others. Thus advice for the young adolescent "not to walk barefoot" or "avoid high heels completely" may be ignored, and other more important objectives discarded. For those with no evidence of pathology of the feet, their actual foot care need be no different from that advised for healthy subjects. For this reason, Ward and colleagues have recommended a grading of risk for educational purposes [114]. Careful audit should detect early changes and more stringent educational programs can be instituted when and if required. This is particularly relevant in the light of the Malone study referred to above.

It should be remembered that each yearly examination provides an educational opportunity to reinforce the message of the importance of the steps necessary to continue glucose regulation to prevent foot (and of course, other) complications. Other general principles of education are equally appropriate. The need to target the appropriate advice is demonstrated by the overrepresentation of foot problems among the lower social classes and the behavior gap demonstrated by failure of individuals to purchase shoes for comfort [99] rather than for reasons of appearance and cost. This, too, may well have social causes.

"Sick Day" Rules

Failure of education is demonstrated more drastically by imperfect learning of "sick day" rules than in any other context. Numerous studies have demonstrated that the major contribution to admission for (and death from) ketoacidosis is inadequate instruction, and that this can be rectified by improved educational programs. For success, individuals do have to make major changes at a time when they are least capable of doing so, i.e. when feeling ill. Furthermore, if instruction is inadequate the changes may appear paradoxical, e.g. increasing insulin when eating less. Episodes of illness are usually quite infrequent, with a potentially long time between instruction and the need to put that advice into practice. These factors emphasize the need for ensuring that initial instructions are fully understood. Most importantly, the actions required (especially insulin dose adjustment) must be rehearsed in *detail*, not just in general terms. Many leaflets are too imprecise, but good examples are available [115]. One needs to also ensure that information has been retained even if not yet used, and that on the first occasion of significant illness (e.g. gastroenteritis or other cause of vomiting or severe anorexia) the patient or carer can with confidence contact their diabetes care team to talk through the necessary steps.

Children and Adolescents

The educational problems in childhood and adolescence are immense and mainly beyond the scope of this chapter. Certain recent developments, however, do require comment. It is notable that the domiciliary initiation of therapy was found many years ago to be of considerable value in diminishing anxiety and improving the early confidence in insulin dose adjustment, coping with hypoglycemia, etc., by the parents [105]. Education is, of course, a continuous process throughout childhood and adolescence to adult life, and therefore no single program can be appropriate. The conflicts between the needs of diabetic patients and the identity crises of adolescents require quite different strategies. Studies of individual programs often reveal a great deal of investment of time with the parents, and the assumption that their learning will be transferred to the child. Even allowing for the rejection that teenagers may exhibit, evaluation suggests that many failures may be due to omission of instruction to the youngsters themselves, and separate programs of reinstruction are necessary at the age of 13 or 14 years. Many countries have developed a system of camps that not only fulfil this function but also provide peer support, enabling youngsters to come to terms with their diabetes. However, despite the extensive organization in many countries (e.g., provision for 800 children in camps in the United Kingdom), this only provides facilities for a proportion of the individuals concerned (32 000 in the United Kingdom). Such camps do not suit all children. Steps are required in most areas, therefore, to develop peer support systems on a local basis.

Oral Agents

There is a wealth of evidence for failure of compliance with regard to tablet medication in asymptomatic diseases, such as hypertension and tuberculosis. Diabetes is no exception. Many of the reasons for this have already been discussed. However, there are certain factors specific to diabetes worthy of mention. Overreliance on urine testing may persuade people that all is well despite omission of therapy, or the learned hopelessness described above may be responsible. Beliefs by professionals of possible inefficacy of prevention of complications in type 2 diabetes will also contribute to patients' *laissez-faire* attitudes. George and colleagues have shown that subjects rarely know the names of or reasons for therapy [97]. Under these circumstances long-term maintenance in the face of continued well-being may falter. Dose adjustment is often not encouraged.

Pregnancy

The improved outcome of pregnancy in women with diabetes provides an excellent example not only of the beneficial effects of good glycemic control but also of how this can be achieved when motivation is high. The outcomes of pregnancy for those with diabetes have improved enormously over the last 30 years. In the main this has been due to greatly improved glycemic control resulting from much more effective self-care. Experience of the author in countries with less developed health delivery has shown that the principles of patient empowerment and achievement of successful outcomes in pregnancy, previously seen as inconceivable, is testament to the power of selfefficacy.

Improvements in obstetric practice have also contributed but to a lesser extent. One of the most critical improvements in this respect is the acceptance that the diabetes and obstetric teams should work as one. Combined antenatal clinics are strongly recommended to deliver common educational and clinical objectives. There is no dispute of the need for careful instruction about all aspects of pregnancy and now, in view of evidence of the importance of glycemic control at the time of conception, of the necessity for prepregnancy counseling. Many clinics now organize special sessions for the latter.

The postnatal period is sometimes neglected, however. During the pregnancy a great deal of time and attention is bestowed on the individual but often, as soon as successful delivery has taken place, the level of attention is (not unnaturally) greatly reduced. Withdrawal coincides with an extremely difficult time with the new baby for the woman concerned, and may increase her level of emotional disturbance. It is suggested that mothers should be "weaned," and that the level of support should be gradually tapered off, rather than terminated abruptly.

Counseling About Complications

Despite the critical importance of counseling about complications, there is surprisingly little data on the most appropriate educational approaches. Studies have been referred to [38, 40, 41] that demonstrate the variation of general knowledge among subjects, even those with quite long-standing diabetes. However, the individual's beliefs and expectations of the likelihood of complications, rather than knowledge *per se* [107], are much more likely to determine preventive action. Presence or absence of denial is likely to be a major factor determining not only behavior but also the response to educational input. This may indeed be an important defense mechanism in teenagers. Choice of timing of the introduction of a discussion about complications may be difficult. Delay, for fear of provocation of anxiety, would appear to be misguided. The vast majority of adults, despite explicit denials, will usually have some knowledge of diabetes and lay gossip is most likely to concern complications, i.e. knowledge of friends and relatives with eye or foot problems, etc. It is essential, therefore, at the diagnostic interview to establish the nature of the subject's knowledge and beliefs, and (in particular) any misconceptions about complications, if only to dispel unnecessary fears and refute mythology.

For younger subjects it seems unreasonable, once symptoms are relieved, to expect maintenance of high standards of glucose control, without clear statements of the reasons for imposition of the discipline that is required. Implicit in this discussion is the assumption that the professional staff not only agrees about the need for such education, but also recognizes that their own feelings will markedly affect those of their patients. Uncertainty about the effectiveness of the treatment will be transmitted to the patient. Variation of messages from different members of the team will be easily discerned and may well lead to confusion, if not rejection, of significant objectives by the patients.

The important educational component of the yearly clinic recommended for the screening for complications cannot be overemphasized. It may be the only point of contact with the patient for those whose attendance for educational sessions is haphazard, and special efforts should be made to encourage attendance at these clinics at the very least. It must not be assumed that the functions of these yearly clinic audits are solely technical. Those responsible need to understand the importance of the learning elements and have some skills to deliver them. It must be remembered that those who fail to attend carry the heaviest risks of complications. Skills in persuasion to achieve maximum attendance are vital.

Leaving aside preventive aspects, if regular attendance for medical audit is to be ensured together with immediate reporting of important physical symptoms (e.g., loss of vision, foot ulcers), a significant part of any program must be directed to full and frank discussion of complications.

The problem of counseling those with established complications is even more difficult. Each complication opens a new area of education in its own right. In this respect, diabetes probably differs little from other major chronic debilitating conditions. However, recent evidence suggests that intensified glycemic control, possibly demanding demand reeducation, may at least prevent further deterioration [17].

EVALUATION

Comprehensive and continuous evaluation must be a *sine qua non* of all effective educational programs to determine whether the stated objectives have been met. Despite this, assessment tends to be the Cinderella of the learning process. However, failure to meet the self-management targets massively increases the risk of the development of complications.

Four elements of evaluation require consideration:

(a) formative evaluation, i.e. assessment of progress of the individual
(b) certifying evaluation, i.e. placing students in order of merit or determining a pass or fail. The latter has little relevance to diabetes education, but might be appropriate for courses certifying nurses, for example. This section confines itself to formative evaluation
(c) assessment of *outcome*, i.e. whether the individual has or has not achieved the targets that have been set;
(d) evaluation of the *process* by which the outcomes have or have not been reached. This is mandatory for modification and redesign of the educational program or provision of reassurance that it can be continued in its present form. Techniques for individual vs. process assessment are different.

Assessment in Practice

Certain principles must be adhered to. First, attempts should be made to assess all the objectives/targets that have been set. If these are considered appropriate it is equally necessary to ensure that they have been achieved. Second, the lifelong nature of the process is critical. New objectives will be developed as the life of the individual matures and changes, with a need for checking these objectives periodically. The program itself and the need to adapt it to the individual may involve different timings for different objectives, with initial programs spread over weeks, months, or even years, thus allowing the subjects to achieve their objectives at their own rate and according to their own needs. The checking process needs to allow for this flexibility, yet ensure that objectives that have been postponed have not been omitted altogether.

What Has to Be Evaluated?

Perhaps the most common error in the educational literature is to consider glycemic control as the only measure of educational success or failure. Many educational objectives will in fact have little relationship to glycemic control and those that do are part of a long learning process, largely attitude dependent, and ultimately terminating in a level of glycated hemoglobin. Outcome measures need to be designed for all these factors, if sensible decisions are to be made either about the progress of the individual or about the success of the educational program. If however, as previously, suggested, objectives are expressed in behavioral terms, the whole process is much easier.

It is helpful to divide the objectives into different domains:

(1) the learning of new or basic knowledge;
(2) change in attitudes;
(3) performance, including basic skills, e.g., insulin injection, self-testing, and the recording of tests;
(4) decision making (adjustment of dose, variation in meal quantities and times).

Knowledge Assessment

There are well-known, reliable procedures for evaluation of knowledge. Questions and answers, whether on a one-to-one basis, using multiple choice questionnaires or computer interactive systems are all appropriate, and a number of different systems have been developed [41, 116, 117]. For day-to-day individual use, question-and-answer at interview with checklists on a repeated and regular basis may be quite satisfactory [104]. Knowledge is probably the easiest component of the educational status of the patient to evaluate, but is only the first step on the long road to effective self-care.

Attitudes

In contrast to the very weak relationship between basic knowledge and behavioral change, attitudes are much more powerfully correlated with behavioral outcomes. The verification of patients' attitudes poses considerable problems. Because of awareness of patients' reluctance to express their feelings freely in the clinical situation, much thought has been applied to the development of questionnaires to allow anonymous and therefore (it is hoped) more honest and accurate responses. However, relationships between attitudes, beliefs, health, and self-control are complex. Well-validated specific questionnaires are now available for measurement of diabetes-specific health beliefs, perceived control [28, 60, 118], locus of control [43, 119], quality of life, and patient satisfaction [120]. In contrast there are the more general, single questionnaires covering a broader range of outcomes, such as that of Dunn [19], and the diabetes profile of Davies et al. [121]. The former are better targeted to single areas with, for example, assessment of dependence on medical treatment, perceived benefits and barriers of treatment, beliefs about vulnerability and complications, or satisfaction outcomes. These questionnaires are cumbersome and tedious for patients to complete and staff to analyze. The unified questionnaires may be less specific and therefore require complex factorization to provide meaningful information, but are simpler to administer. A composite questionnaire for practical clinic use has recently been published and shown to be capable of distinguishing attitudes contributing to better glycemic control (medical outcomes) and those related to successful "living" with diabetes (social outcomes) [59]. Questionnaires are therefore mainly appropriate for *process* evaluation of samples or small groups of subjects than for individual evaluation. Individual *formative* assessment is almost entirely dependent on interview techniques during regular consultations. Although theoretically less objective this need not necessarily be so. It will depend on the skills of the professional, clear definition of objectives in behavioral terms, and accurate documentation of agreed targets at each clinic visit. Observation of standard interviews between professional—whether doctor, nurse, or dietitian—and patient still show that their content is predominantly related to clinical elements rather than attitudinal ones and still tend to be professional rather than patient-centered. More time than may be available in traditional clinics is needed for this process. Where group interactive learning is part of the program careful observation may supplement the one-to-one process, since important feelings previously withheld maybe revealed.

Performance

The skills required for diabetes self-management do need, if possible, to be observed rather than just reported. Systems must allow for this. As with any other type of learning, standards may wane, and in particular accuracy of self-testing or even insulin dose adjustment may fall well below the required standards. Time may well be saved by collecting subjects in groups to reassess many of these skills, and such sessions can also allow relearning or updating on new techniques. Home visits may be needed to assess performance in real life. One of the most difficult areas is that of blood testing, where false results may be reported, tests either not having been performed or results overoptimistically read [110, 111]. Memory meters, and levels of glycated hemoglobin, may suggest and identify discrepancies, but such failures are better handled in an interview or group situation, and only in extreme and perhaps pathological situations (i.e. brittle diabetes with gross self-manipulation) should secret surveillance procedures be employed.

Decision Making

Structured analysis of problems, with an interview at which hypothetical questions regarding possible problems are posed—"What would you do if . . . ?"—are probably the most helpful. Similar questions put to groups may be equally revealing, but if these groups are truly interactive it can be difficult to ensure that all the necessary areas are covered. New technology with multimedia-interactive programs involving the user in making choices, based as they are on CD-ROM, offer the possibility of a built-in process of intrinsic evaluation [103].

Self-management behavior in all patients will be the major determinant of glycemic control and hence prevention of complications as well as adjustment to day-to-day life. Identification of failure of patients to achieve the targets that have been set (and hopefully agreed!) is essential in clinical practice. An educational audit of each patient is as important as the yearly clinical examination. It is recommended, therefore, that all contributing factors (summarized in Table 4) should be evaluated on a yearly basis.

Table 4 Factors responsible for diabetes self-management

Knowledge
Self-management skills
Perception of desired goals
Perception of standards achieved
Perceived benefits
Perceived severity
Perceived vulnerability
Locus of control
Role of important others
General emotional adjustment

Methods of Process Evaluation

Different systems are needed for process evaluation. For accurate "diagnosis" of critical elements in the educational program in determining individual outcomes, it is necessary to take samples of the population at various stages of the process. The instruments must be designed for the purpose, and "before and after" comparisons are necessary. Questionnaires may well be most appropriate, in particular for sampling satisfaction, attitudes, or knowledge under these circumstances. However, if individual assessment programs are adequately structured and results recorded systematically, then these too can be sampled. It must be emphasized that in assessment of programs the instruments must be appropriate and valid. In addition, standard data collection of attendance rates are required. Biochemical outcomes, though desirable, are quite inadequate on their own. Health performance indicators (e.g., admission because of ketoacidosis, hypoglycemia, etc.) should also be included as important measures of educational quality.

It must be recognized that success or failure of education most probably depends on the interaction between learner and professional. The style and skills of the professional are major determinants of this. A mentoring of staff and performance evaluation are also essential. Self-development, however, is basically internally motivated. Opportunities need to be provided, therefore, for those delivering clinical care to reflect on their own practice. Audio and/or video recordings from time to time may well assist this process.

In conclusion, a systematic approach is essential for the development of effective evaluation of the individual and of the educational process. No one technique is going to achieve all objectives, and a number of different systems including interviews, questionnaires, and group observation are necessary. The individual skills of the educator will be critical in determining outcome.

CONCLUSIONS

- If complications are to be prevented and patients to minimize the impact on their daily life, high-quality structured education is essential.
- There is sound evidence that improved educational process contributes to more successful outcomes.
- Effective learning requires behavioral change
- It is a lifelong process with adaptation to lifestyle and concurrent health problems. All programs should recognize and plan for this.
- Factors governing behavior are complex and mainly dependent on attitudes, beliefs, and perceptions.
- These factors are however capable of identification and change, using learner-centered and behavioral modification methods.
- All professional carers require training in the educational aspects of care and skills to facilitate patient self-efficacy/empowerment.
- Continuous evaluation of patients' knowledge, skills, and attitudes is essential.
- These assessments are as important as clinical examinations.

REFERENCES

1. Joslin EP, Gray H, Root HF. Insulin in hospital and home. *J Metab Res* 1922; 2: 651–99.
2. Lawrence RD. *The Diabetic Life*. London: Churchill, 1925.
3. Miller LV, Goldstein G. More efficient care of diabetic patients in a county-hospital setting. *N Engl J Med* 1972; 286: 1388–91.
4. The place of nurses in management of diabetes [Editorial]. *Lancet* 1982; i: 145–8.
5. Dudley JD. The diabetes educator's role in teaching the diabetic patient. *Diabetes Care* 1980; 3: 127–33.
6. Day JL, Spathis M. District diabetes centres in the United Kingdom. *Diabet Med* 1988; 5: 372–80.
7. Davidson JK, Alogna M, Goldsmith M, Borden J. Assessment of program effectiveness at Grady Memorial Hospital. In Steiner G, Lawrence PA (eds), *Educating Diabetic Patients*. New York: Springer, 1981; pp 239–48.
8. Runyan JW. The Memphis chronic disease program. *JAMA* 1975; 231: 264–7.
9. Nersesian W, Zaremba M. Impact of diabetes outpatient education program—Maine. MMWR *Morb Mortal Wkly Rep* 1982; 31: 307–414.
10. Geller J, Butler K. Study of educational deficits as the cause of hospital admissions for diabetes mellitus in a community hospital. *Diabetes Care* 1981; 4: 487–9.
11. Scott RS, Brown LJ, Clifford P. Use of health services by diabetic persons, II: Hospital admissions. *Diabetes Care* 1985; 8: 43–7.
12. Assal J-P, Ekoé J-M, Lacroix A. L'enseignement au malade sur sa maladie et son traitement. Un succès thérapeutique; un échec du corps médical. *Journ A Diabétol Hôtel-Dieu (Paris)* 1984; 193–207.
13. Mühlhauser I, Jorgens V, Graninger W, Horke L, Kunz A, Shernthaner G, Scholz V, Voss HE. Bicentric evaluation of a teaching and treatment programme for type 1 (insulin dependent) diabetic patients: improvement of metabolic control and other measures of diabetes care for up to 22 months. *Diabetologia* 1983; 25: 470–6.
14. Mann NP, Johnston DI. Total glycosylated haemoglobin levels in diabetic children. *Arch Dis Child* 1982; 57: 434–7.
15. Gonen B, Rubenstein AH, Rochman H, Tenega S, Horwitz DL. Haemoglobin A_1: an indicator of the metabolic control of diabetic patients. *Lancet* 1977; ii: 734–7.
16. Tattersall RB, McCulloch DK. Modern aspects of conventional insulin therapy. *Ann Clin Res* 1984; 16: 107–17.
17. DCCT Research Group. The effect of intensive treatment of diabetes on development and progression of long term complications in insulin dependent diabetes. *N Engl J Med* 1993; 329: 977–86.
18. Mazucca SA, Morrman NH, Wheeler ML. The diabetes education study: a controlled trial of the effects of diabetes patient education. *Diabetes Care* 1986; 9: 1–10.
19. Dunn SM. Reaction to educational techniques: coping strategies for diabetics and learning. *Diabet Med* 1986; 3: 419–26.
20. DAFNE Study Group. Training in flexible, intensive insulin management in people with type 1 diabetes: dose adjustment for normal eating (DAFNE) randomised controlled trial. *BMJ* 2002; 325: 746–9.
21. UK Prospective Study of Therapies of Maturity-onset Diabetes, I: Effect of diet, sulphonylurea, insulin or biguanide therapy on fasting plasma glucose and body weight over one year. *Diabetologia* 1983; 24: 404–11.
22. Malone JM, Snyde M, Anderson G. Prevention of amputation by diabetic education. *Am J Surg* 1989; 158: 520–3.
23. Padgett D, Mumford E, Hynes M, Carter R. Meta-analysis of the effects of educational and psychosocial interventions on management of diabetes mellitus. *J Clin Epidemiol* 1988; 41 (10): 1007–30.
24. Brown SA. Studies of educational intervention and outcomes in diabetic adults: a meta-analysis revisited. *Patient Educ Couns* 1990; 16 (3): 189–215.
25. Griffin S, Kinmouth AL, Skinner C, et al. *Educational and Psychosocial Interventions, the Extent to Which They Have Been Evaluated in Controlled Trials and a Description of Their Relative Effectiveness as Reported in Existing Reviews*. A British Diabetic Association Report. London: British Diabetic Association, 1998.
26. National Institute for Clinical Excellence (UK) *Guidance on the Use of Educational Models for Diabetes* (Technology Appraisal 60). London: National Institute for Clinical Excellence, 2003.
27. Dunn SM. *Barriers and Challenges in Training Health Care Providers for Patient Education*. Amsterdam: Excerpta Medica, 1995.
28. Bradley C. *Handbook of Psychology and Diabetes: A Guide to Psychological Measurement in Diabetes Research and Practice*. Chur, Switzerland: Harwood Academic Publishers, 1994.
29. Cox D, Gonder-Frederick L, Lee J, Julian D, Carter W, Clarke W. Blood glucose awareness training among patients with IDDM: effects and correlates. *Diabetes Care* 1989; 12: 313–8.
30. Snoek FJ, Skinner TC (eds). *Psychology in Diabetes Care*. Chichester, UK: Wiley, 2000.
31. Anderson RM. Patient empowerment and the traditional medical model; a case of irreconcilable differences. *Diabetes Care* 1995; 18: 412–5.

32. Coles C. Adult learning. In Jolly B, Reef L (eds), *Medical Education in the Millenium—Taking Stock*. Oxford: Oxford University Press, 1998; pp 63–81.
33. Rollnick S, Mason P, Butler CC. *Health Behaviour Change—A Guide for Practitioners*. Edinburgh: Churchill Livingstone, 1999.
34. Day JL. Diabetic patient education: determinants of success. *Diabetes Metab Res Rev* 2000; 16 (suppl 1): S70–4.
35. Morris AD, Boyle DI, McMahon AD, Greene SA, MacDonald TM, Newton RW, for the DARTS/MEMO Collaboration. Adherence to treatment, glycaemic control, and keto-acidosis in insulin-depen-dent diabetes mellitus. *Lancet* 1998; 22 (350): 1505–10.
36. Frier BM, Steel JM, Mathews DM, Duncan LJP. Driving and insulin dependent diabetes. *Lancet* 1980; i: 1232–4.
37. Terént A, Hagfall O, Cederholm V. The effect of education and self-monitoring of blood glucose on glycosylated haemoglobin in type I diabetes. *Acta Med Scand* 1985; 217: 47–53.
38. Graber AL, Christman BG, Alogna MT, Davidson JK. Evaluation of diabetes patient education programmes. *Diabetes* 1977; 26: 61–4.
39. Beggan MP, Cregan D, Drury MI. Assessment of the outcome of an educational programme of diabetes self care. *Diabetologia* 1982; 23: 246–51.
40. Germer S, Campbell IW, Smith AWM, Sutherland JD, Jones IG. Do diabetics remember all they have been taught? A survey of knowledge of insulin-dependent diabetics. *Diabet Med* 1986; 3: 343–5.
41. Dunn SM, Bryson JM, Hoskins PL, Alford JB, Handelsman DJ, Turtle JR. The development of diabetes knowledge (DKN) scales: forms DKNA, DKNB and DKNC. *Diabetes Care* 1984; 7: 36–41.
42. Farrant S, Dowlatshahi D, Ellwood-Russell M, Wise PH. Computer based learning and assessment for diabetic patients. *Diabet Med* 1984; 1: 309–15.
43. Lockington TJ, Meadows KA, Wise PH. Compliant behaviour: relationships to attitudes and control in diabetic patients. *Diabet Med* 1987; 4: 56–61.
44. Lawrence PA, Cheely J. Deterioration of diabetic patients' knowledge and management skills as determined during outpatient visits. *Diabetes Care* 1980; 3: 214–18.
45. Worth R, Home PD, Johnston DG, et al. Intensive attention improves glycaemic control in insulin-dependent diabetes without further advantage from home blood glucose monitoring: results of a controlled trial. *Br Med J* 1982; 285: 1233–9.
46. Korhonen T, Huttenen JK, Aro A, Hentinen M, Ihalainen O, Majander H, Siitonen O, Uusitupa M, Pyorala K. A controlled trial on the effects of patient education in the treatment of insulin-dependent diabetes. *Diabetes Care* 1983; 6: 256–60.
47. Prochaska JO, DiClemente CC. *Toward a Comprehensive Model of Change. Treating Addictive Behaviours*. New York: Plenum Press, 1986.
48. Slama G. Sugar for diabetics? That's not the root of the problem. *Ann Med Interne (Paris)* 1987; 138 (7): 486–8.
49. Hoghton MR, Philipp R, Harvey K, Hughes AO, Fletcher GM, Burns Cox CJ. Understanding of diabetes mellitus in non-diabetic adults. *Pract Diabetes* 1987; 4: 60–2.
50. Rosenstock IM, Strecher VJ, Becker MH. Social learning theory and the health belief model. *Health Educ Q* 1988; 15: 175–83.
51. Rosenstock IM. Understanding and enhancing patient compliance with diabetic regimens. *Diabetes Care* 1985; 8: 610–16.
52. Gfeller R, Assal J-P. Le véce du malade diabétique avec sa maladie et avec son entourage. In Catelier C, Tchobroutsky E (eds), *Le diabète sucré*. Paris: Maloine, 1984: pp 222–31.
53. Assal J-P, Gfeller R, Kreinhofer M. Stades de l'acceptation du diabète, leur interférence avec le traitement, leur influence sur l'attitude de l'équipe soignante. *Journ Diabétol Hôtel-Dieu (Paris)* 1984; 223–35.
54. Wallston B, Wallston K. Locus of control and health. A review of the literature. *Health Educ Monogr* 1978; 6: 107–17.
55. Bradley C, Gamsu DS, Moses JL, Knight G, Boulton AJM, Drury J, Ward JD. The use of diabetes-specific perceived control and health belief measures to predict treatment choice and efficacy in a feasibility study of continuous subcutaneous insulin infusion pumps. *Psychol Health* 1987; 1: 133–46.
56. Sjöberg S, Carlson A, Rosenqvist U, Östman J. Health attitudes, self-monitoring of blood glucose, metabolic control and residual insulin secretion in type 1 diabetic patients. *Diabet Med* 1988; 5: 449–53.
57. Jones A, Pill R, Adams S. Qualitative study of views of health professionals and patients on guided self-management plans for asthma. *BMJ* 2000; 321: 1507–10.
58. De Weerdt I, Visser AP, Kok G, Van Der Veen EA. Determinants of active self-care behaviour of insulin treated patients with diabetes: implications for diabetes education. *Soc Sci Med* 1990; 30: 605–15.
59. Day JL, Bodmer CW, Dunn OM. Development of a questionnaire identifying factors responsible for successful self-management of insulin-treated diabetes. *Diabet Med* 1996; 13: 564–73.
60. Bradley C, Brewin CR, Gamsu DS, Moses JL. Development of scales to measure perceived control of diabetes mellitus and diabetes-related health beliefs. *Diabet Med* 1984; 1: 213–18.
61. Kaplan RM, Chadwick MW, Schimmel LE. Social learning intervention to promote metabolic control in type 1 diabetes mellitus: pilot experiment results. *Diabetes Care* 1985; 8: 152–5.
62. Kinmouth AL, Woodcock A, Griffin S, Spiegel N, Campbell MJ. Randomised controlled trial of patient centred care of diabetes in general practice: impact on current well-being and future risk. *BMJ* 1998; 317: 1202–8.
63. Ajzen I, Fishbein M. Understanding attitudes and predicting social behaviour. Englewood Cliffs, NJ: Prentice-Hall, 1980.
64. Rollnick S, Mason P, Butler CC. *Health Behaviour Change—A Guide for Practitioners*. Edinburgh: Churchill Livingstone, 1999; pp 17–39.
65. Graham AJ, Rayman G, Day JL. The evaluation study of "Learning Diabetes": a multi-media computer programme. *Diabet Med* 1999; 16 (suppl 1): A56.
66. Hadden DR, Blair ALT, Wilson EA, Boyle DM, Atkinson AB, Kennedy AL, Buchanan KD, Merrett JD, Montgomery DA, Weaver JA. Natural history of diabetes presenting age 40–69 years: a prospective study of the influence of intensive dietary therapy. *Q J Med* 1986; 59: 579–98.

67. Sönksen PH, Judd SL, Lowy C. Home monitoring of blood glucose. *Lancet* 1988; i: 729–31.
68. Clarson C, Daneman D, Frank M, Link J, Perlman K, Ehrlich R. Self monitoring of blood glucose: how accurate are children with diabetes at reading Chemstrip bG? *Diabetes Care* 1985; 8: 354–8.
69. Mazze RS, Pasmantier R, Murphy JA, Shamoon H. Self-monitoring of capillary blood glucose: changing the performance of individuals with diabetes. *Diabetes Care* 1985; 8: 207–13.
70. Warwick Diabetes Care 2000. Available at: www.diabetescare.warwick.ac.uk.
71. WHO Working Group. *Therapeutic Patient Education*. Copenhagen: WHO Regional office for Europe, 1998.
72. Diabetes Education Study Group of EASD. Basic curriculum for health professionals on diabetes therapeutic education. 2001. Available at: www.desg.org.
73. Day JL, Coles C, Walford S. Self-management in diabetes: training implications for professional carers. *Clin Med* 2003; 3: 1–5.
74. Mühlhauser I, Bruckner I, Berger M, Cheta D, Jorgens V, Ionescu-Tirgoviste C, Scholz V, Mincu I. Evaluation of an intensified insulin treatment and teaching programme as routine management of type I (insulin-dependent) diabetes. *Diabetologia* 1987; 30: 681–90.
75. Day JL, Metcalfe J, Johnson P. Benefits provided by an integrated education and clinical diabetes centre: a follow-up study. *Diabet Med* 1992; 9: 855–9.
76. Mager RF. *Preparing Instructional Objectives*. Palo Alto, CA: Fearon, 1967.
77. Guilbert JJ. *Educational Handbook for Health Personnel*. Geneva: WHO, 1987. WHO Offset Publication 35.
78. WHO Working Group. *Therapeutic Patient Education*. Copenhagen: WHO Regional office for Europe, 1998; pp 17–21.
79. WHO Working Group. *Therapeutic Patient Education*. Copenhagen: WHO Regional office for Europe, 1998; p 24.
80. Assal J-P, Berger M, Gay N, Canivet J (eds). *Diabetes Education: How to Improve Patient Education*. Amsterdam: Excerpta Medica, 1983.
81. Frost G. Comparison of two methods of energy prescription for obese non-insulin dependent diabetics. *Pract Diabetes* 1989; 6: 273–5.
82. Fox CJ, Gillespie CR, Kilvert A. Can the medical consultation be made more effective in diabetes care? *Diabetologia* 1986; 29: 538A.
83. Coles C. Differences between conventional and problem based curricula in their students approach to learning. *Med Educ* 1985; 19: 4–10.
84. Day JL, Johnson G, Rayman G, Walker R. The feasibility of a potentially 'ideal' system of integrated diabetes care and education based on a day centre. *Diabet Med* 1988; 5: 70–5.
85. Groen JJ, Pelser HE. Newer concepts of teaching, learning and education and their application to the patient–doctor cooperation in the treatment of diabetes mellitus. *Ped Adolesc Endocrinol* 1982; 10: 168–77.
86. Tattersall RB, McCulloch DK, Aveline M. Group therapy in the treatment of diabetes. *Diabetes Care* 1985; 8: 180–8.
87. McCulloch DK, Mitchell RD, Ambler J, Tattersall RB. Influence of imaginative teaching of diet on compliance and metabolic control in insulin dependent diabetes. *Br Med J* 1983; 287: 1858–61.
88. Aveline M, McCulloch DK, Tattersall RB. The practice of group psychotherapy with insulin-dependent diabetics. *Diabet Med* 1985; 2: 275–82.
89. Strickland AL, McFarland KF, Murtiashaw MH, Thorpe SR, Baynes JW. Changes in blood protein glycosylation during a diabetes summer camp. *Diabetes Care* 1984; 7: 183–5.
90. Walker R, Sharland V. Benefits of BDA educational holidays—chance or design? *Pract Diabetes* 1987; 4: 163–6.
91. Kerr D, Kerr S. Diabetic camps for children—effects on control and hypoglycaemia. *Pract Diabetes* 1988; 5: 74–6.
92. Newton RW, Isles T, Farquhar JW. The Firbush project—sharing a way of life. *Diabet Med* 1985; 2: 217–24.
93. Heller SR, Clarke P, Daly H, Davis I, McCulloch DK, Allison SP, Tattersall RB. Group education for obese patients with type 2 diabetes: greater success at less cost. *Diabet Med* 1988; 5: 552–6.
94. Day JL. *Living with Diabetes: The Diabetes UK Guide for Those Treated with Diet and Tablets*. Chichester, UK: Wiley, 2000.
95. Day JL. *Living with Diabetes: The Diabetes UK Guide for Those Treated with Insulin*. Chichester, UK: Wiley, 2002.
96. *Countdown*. London: British Diabetic Association, 1988.
97. George CF. Telling patients about their medicines. *Br Med J* 1987; 294: 1566–7.
98. Ward JD. Video cassette programmes in diabetes education. *Diabetes Educ/Spec* 1984; 48–50.
99. Day JL. Patient education—how may recurrence be prevented? In Connor H, Boulton AJM, Ward JD (eds), *The Foot in Diabetes*. Chichester, UK: Wiley, 1986; pp 135–43.
100. Alivisatos J, Halimi D (eds). *The Teaching letter. Use, Misuse and Abuse of Audiovisual Aids*. Paris: Diabetes Education Study Group, 1986.
101. Day JL, Metcalfe J, Alban-Davies H. Evaluation of new automatic recording system of diabetic patient information—Diadata. *Diabetologia* 1983; 25: 149.
102. Howorka K. *Funktionelle, nahenormoglykämische insulinsubstitution*. Berlin: Springer, 1987.
103. Day JL, Rayman G, Hall L, Davies P. Learning diabetes—a multi-media learning package for patients, carers and professionals to improve chronic disease management. *Med Inform* 1997; 22: 91–104.
104. Assal J, Alivisatos JG, Halimi D (eds). *The Teaching Letter, Evaluation*. Paris: Diabetes Education Study Group, 1986.
105. Walker J. The clinical management of the diabetic adolescent. *Postgrad Med J* 1970; 46: 625–9.
106. Mollema ED, Snoek FJ, Ader HJ, Heine RJ, van der Ploeg HM. Insulin treated diabetes patients with fear of self injecting or fear of self testing. *J Psychosom Res* 2001; 51: 665–772.
107. Burfield R, Walker R, Day JL. Good diabetes control. The role of patients' perceptions and beliefs. *Diabetologia* 1986; 29: 523A.
108. Gonder-Frederick L, Cox D, Clarke W, Julian D. Blood glucose awareness training. In Snoek FJ, Skinner C (eds), *Psychology in Diabetes Care*. Chichester, UK: Wiley, 2000; pp 169–206.
109. Tattersall R, Gale E. Patient self-monitoring of blood glucose and refinements of conventional insulin treatment. *Am J Med* 1981; 70: 177–82.

110. Smith MA, Greene SA, Kuykendall VG, Baum JD. Memory blood glucose reflectance meter and computer: a preliminary report of its use in recording and analysing blood glucose data measured at home by diabetic children. *Diabet Med* 1985; 2: 265–8.
111. Mazze RS, Shamoon H, Pasmantier R, Lucido D, Murphy J, Hartmann K, Kuykendall V, Lopatin W. Reliability of blood glucose monitoring by patients with diabetes mellitus. *Am J Med* 1984; 77: 211–17.
112. Wilson DP, Endres RK. Compliance with blood glucose monitoring in children with type 1 diabetes mellitus. *J Pediatr* June 1986; 108 (6): 1022–4.
113. Trichopoulou A. The DAFNE data bank as a simple tool for nutrition policy. *Public Health Nutr*. 2001; 4 (5B): 1187–98.
114. Assal J, Alivisatos JG, Halimi D (eds). *The Teaching Letter, Foot Care*. Paris: Diabetes Education Study Group, 1986.
115. *Catalogue of BDA Publications*. London: British Diabetic Association, 1988.
116. Hess GE, Davis WK. The validation of a diabetic patient knowledge test. *Diabetes Care* 1983; 6: 591–5.
117. McCowen C, Court S, Hackett AF, Parkin JM. An evaluation of multiple choice questionnaries for the assessment of knowledge in diabetic children and their families. *Diabet Med* 1988; 5: 474–88.
118. Given CW, Given BA, Gallin RS, Condon JW. Development of scales to measure beliefs of diabetic patients. *Res Nurs Health* 1983; 6: 127–41.
119. Lewis KSS, Bradley C, Knight G, Boulton AJM, Ward JD. A measure of treatment satisfaction designed specifically for people with insulin-dependent diabetes. *Diabet Med* 1988; 5: 235–42.
120. Ferraro LA, Price JH, Desmond SM, Roberts SM. Development of a diabetes locus of control scale. *Psychol Rep* 1987; 61: 763–70.
121. Davies WK, Hess GE, Harrison R Van, Hiss RG. Psychosocial adjustment to and control of diabetes mellitus: differences by disease type and treatment. *Health Psychol* 1987; 6: 1014.

91

Psychological Problems and Management of Patients with Diabetes Mellitus

Alan M. Jacobson

Joslin Diabetes Center, Harvard Medical School, Boston, MA, USA

In many ways, diabetes mellitus is the prototypical chronic illness. The patient enters a new world that involves increased visits to medical personnel, alterations in lifestyle, education in self-care activities, as well as the potential for painful, debilitating, and life-threatening complications. In addition to the medical assault of this chronic illness, patients may experience social and vocational dilemmas, such as rejection by friends, bias in hiring, and problems getting insurance. The treatment of diabetes depends on knowledgeable physicians, nurses, and other health care professionals working closely with the patient and his or her family. While type 1 diabetes always requires learning how to link insulin, diet, and exercise together to regulate glucose levels, patients with type 2 diabetes also must make significant changes in living style. These changes occur late in life, well after the time when health habits were formed. In addition, the patient with type 2 diabetes is often obese, so must address the very habits that are often most difficult to change—exercise and diet behaviors. Furthermore, later in the course of the disease process, this same patient may need to take insulin. This may require considerable social support by family and/or visiting health care personnel because of difficulties with vision and problems handling small objects [1–3].

The social, behavioral, and medical issues posed by diabetes often mean that the psychological management of the patient and the identification of emotional problems is an important aspect of successful treatment of diabetes mellitus. Moreover, achieving changes in behavior rests on the cornerstone of diabetes care: patient–health care professional interaction. This chapter examines an approach to the assessment and treatment of patients on the basis of considerations of the patient–health care professional relationship, a psychological understanding of the illness, as well as the comorbid psychiatric conditions that can influence the course of diabetes.

THE THERAPEUTIC RELATIONSHIP

The therapeutic relationship developed between the patient and his or her health care provider is at the center of any successful treatment of a chronic illness requiring the extent and type of behavioral changes demanded by either type 1 or type 2 diabetes. For linguistic simplicity we will generally use the physician as the prototypical health care provider during the course of this chapter—recognizing, however, that these comments are equally relevant as they pertain to the patient relationships with other clinicians, including dietitians, psychologists, and nurse educators.

Discussion of the therapeutic relationship can be fostered by consideration of a concept derived from psychotherapy: the *therapeutic alliance* [4, 5]. The therapeutic alliance refers to the extent to which there is underlying level of agreement about the goals of and approaches to treatment. When treatment is going well, i.e. physician and patient are working collaboratively toward agreed-upon goals, the nature of the alliance may not be recognized. In essence, the issue falls into the background as the physician–patient team works on the tasks of care. Ironically, the strength and/or weakness of the alliance usually becomes apparent at times of disagreement, i.e. when the patient is not following the physician's advice. Thus, therapeutic impasses manifest as failures in

International Textbook of Diabetes Mellitus, Third Edition. Edited by R. A. DeFronzo, E. Ferrannini, H. Keen, and P. Zimmet.
 ISBN: 0-471-48655-8.

adherence, missed appointments, and/or forgotten blood glucose testing records can reflect previously unrecognized problems with the therapeutic alliance. These problems, even when they are extremely problematic and frustrating, do not mean that the alliance is permanently impaired or that the patient should be characterized as noncompliant. Indeed, temporary breaks in the alliance may mask underlying strengths of the relationship that can be shored up over time. Moreover, the patient who is nonadherent in one aspect of care may follow through at other times around other treatment recommendations.

Example: A 45-year-old man with 10 years of type 1 diabetes had cared for his diabetes with one injection of insulin (using a split mix) per day over the course of his illness. He followed a prescribed diet, exercised regularly, and exhibited other healthy habits. He tested his blood glucose once or twice per week. He had no episodes of severe hypoglycemia or diabetic ketoacidosis requiring hospitalization. His HbA_{1c} was 10% (reference range 4–6%). The patient and physician had worked well together; the patient liked his physician, having recommended him to a cousin who had developed diabetes 3 years previously. Prior discussion about taking a second injection of insulin and testing more frequently had been brief and superficial. The patient agreed in principle that more frequent testing and injections would be helpful, but felt his life was too busy to allow him to manage the changes. Because of the results of the Diabetes Control and Complications Trial, his physician encouraged the patient to undertake a more intensive regimen. Reluctantly the patient agreed to this plan. After appropriate instruction by the physician and his nurse, the patient started the new therapeutic program. At the next visits the patient began complaining that he had trouble remembering to test and never felt right about the second injection of insulin. At these visits he was irritable and sometimes sullen. Although the physician had always looked forward to these visits he now felt uncomfortable with them. After several months the patient missed a planned visit and did not phone to reschedule. Since this was uncharacteristic, the physician phoned the patient, who seemed surprised to hear from the physician, but remained aloof until he blurted out that he had stopped the second injection because he just did not like how it made him feel. He had been hesitant to make another appointment because he was sure that the physician would be angry with him. The physician was able to allay this fear on the phone, thereby reestablishing their appointment schedule. At subsequent appointments they talked more openly of the problems the patient believed limited his ability to increase his involvement in the care of his diabetes.

The stress of the new therapeutic regimen posed a dilemma for the patient as to how he could discuss his differences openly with his physician. Since he had felt pressured to change, he was certain his physician would respond negatively. They had never faced this direct potential for confrontation and so the patient withdrew from treatment. This occurrence suggests an important principle of treatment: the therapeutic alliance must be addressed when problematic treatment issues present themselves. Since treatment of a chronic illness often shifts to more difficult problems, the therapeutic relationship will inevitably be challenged. For patients with type 2 diabetes, the common transitions from diet to oral agents, and from oral agents to insulin are likely to pose quality-of-life dilemmas that may lead patients to question their physicians and possibly default from regular follow-up. Starting an oral agent tells the patient he has a real illness; recommending insulin means it is serious and clearly threatening.

To help patients face these moments of challenge, it is important to understand the sources of strength and weakness in the therapeutic relationship, and how the therapeutic alliance can be strengthened as well as what may unwittingly weaken the alliance. As shown in Table 1, the therapeutic alliance rests on basic principles that can also inform many human relationships.

Table 1 Ways of improving therapeutic alliance

Striving for a collaborative relationship
Listening for and asking about hidden concerns and requests, and negotiating differences
Looking for differences in patient and physician models for treatment
Helping the patient to participate actively in setting the agenda

Striving for a Collaborative Relationship

The concept of the alliance directly leads to the first key issue: viewing the physician–patient relationship as collaborative. Being collaborative does not mean both members of the relationship have equal powers, knowledge, or choices of action. Since the patient is hiring the physician he/she can also fire the physician. However, the physician is endowed with technical expertise, power deriving from societal values, and information not directly accessible to the patient. Yet, collaboration can occur with the recognition that underlying the transactions in the dyad is a bargain that has been made. At times, as noted above, the deal may be unwittingly broken. Collaboration to achieve better understanding of differences between the parties is essential for restrengthening the working relationship. Indeed, technical and medical expertise leads the patient to the physician, yet it is transactional expertise that leads to an effective dialogue and ultimately to accomplishing the goals of the medical therapy [6, 7].

Identifying Hidden Concerns and Negotiating Differences

Lazare et al. [8] describe one method for dealing with important transactional aspects of the relationship. This approach revolves around eliciting unrecognized patient requests and concerns and negotiating between the patient and the physician to resolve differences. In this process the patient is explicitly viewed as a customer or consumer. Using this technique, the physician begins the interview by asking questions about specific patient requests or concerns, such as "Are there some specific things you would like me to address in our meeting today?" These types of queries give patients the opening to set their goals for the medical visit. Furthermore, this method may bring out new unexpected issues of concern for the patient that can be useful in planning treatment. Clinicians commonly think primarily in terms of their goals for treatment and education. The goal of the diabetes class is to teach home glucose monitoring; the goal of this medical appointment is to review blood glucose levels in order to revise the insulin schedule. These goals are often a function of our specialization. The role of the nurse educator may differ from that of the dietitian or the physician. Nonetheless the patient may come to any of these appointments with unrelated concerns and requests. While the patient may follow recommendations even when their own objectives for the appointment have not been addressed, follow through is far more likely if the interaction addresses the patient's requests.

Example: A woman came to a medical appointment knowing she wanted to get a different living situation where she did not have to climb as many stairs, and thinking that her physician might be helpful. Her husband did not wish to move; she thought her physician might convince the husband on medical grounds. She never raised the topic; rather the discussion focused on her high cholesterol and the need for a diet change. She was preoccupied, did not pay clear attention, and so did not follow through on the treatment recommendation.

The patient's concerns and requests in many instances may derive from and relate directly to the physician's recommendations for changes in medical therapy. In an earlier example, the physician recommended an increase in the intensity of therapy without first addressing carefully the patient's concerns. In essence, the physician pushed through the plan, anticipating that the weight of authority would lead the patient to follow through. When they met months later to discuss the negative outcome, the patient raised several concerns about the effects of evening insulin on nighttime blood glucose levels that had already been discussed, but the patient remained fixed in his worries and not fully satisfied with the physician's reassurance. When these were again discussed, the patient raised some specific requests for gradually trying out the second injection by using very low initial doses of insulin. While clearly below the required dose, these steps gave the patient confidence in the new regimen. The patient had never brought up the request because he thought it was childish and was certain the physician would react in the same manner. Now the physician sought out such hidden data and was able to negotiate a plan acceptable to both parties.

In some cases, the situation is emergent and so a negotiation of this type may be an inadequate solution. The patient in acute diabetic ketoacidosis (DKA) must be hospitalized. This cannot be avoided. If the physician–patient interactions have been characterized by a process of collaboration, facilitated by exploration for hidden requests and negotiation of differences, then it may be far easier to call on the patient to follow an order. The patient follows in part because of the implicit trust, i.e. on the basis of a solid therapeutic alliance [2, 3].

Example: One patient had a long history of suicidal thoughts and severe depression. This had led to recurrent psychiatric hospitalizations that were always voluntary. The patient had initially been extremely mistrustful of the psychiatrist treating her, but over the considerable period of treatment, had come to recognize that he had her best interests at heart, even though they had frequent disagreements about approaches to treatment. When she presented with an increase in depressive symptoms suggesting a high degree of suicidality, she refused voluntary admission because she did not recognize the seriousness of the problem and because she was terrified of losing control by returning to a locked inpatient unit. At this point, the psychiatrist expressed concern about the danger if she remained as an outpatient. During a similar, earlier crisis they had negotiated an initial settlement where she stayed with a close friend for 1 day to consider, in the safety of this environment, her status. She called within 12 h to inform the psychiatrist that she was ready for admission and was then admitted to the hospital on the exact unit that was originally recommended. This time, the psychiatrist recognized that the patient was at even greater risk, and so reflected on past decisions they had settled and insisted now on a more direct route to the hospital. Because of the trust built up through past interactions, the patient reluctantly agreed and was hospitalized.

While this is an example from a psychiatric treatment, there are parallel situations involving patients having severe psychological problems related to diabetes and its control. In some of these sticky situations, the physician may find it hard to maintain objectivity. Psychological consultation and ongoing collaboration with a mental health professional may be useful. The role of the mental health professional is to help the patient and the physician with a third party's perspective and alternative approaches to problem identification and dispute resolution.

Example: A 25-year-old man was hospitalized in DKA with previously undiagnosed type 1 diabetes mellitus. After initial stabilization in the intensive care unit, he was transferred to a medical floor where the first steps of teaching and diabetes treatment were instituted. The patient was terrified of taking insulin by injection, so refused all but two injections over the first few days on the unit. A psychiatric consultation was requested with the thought that the patient required immediate transfer to an inpatient psychiatric unit. The patient, according to the medical team, had had recognizable signs of diabetes for several months but had been avoiding contact with a physician. He had a history of psychiatric hospitalization for an apparent psychotic disorder and had remained marginally functional in the community. Although he had a supportive family, he was unable to maintain an independent living situation. The psychiatrist found the patient was guarded and frightened, but not overtly psychotic or clinically depressed. While he had been denying the possibility of diabetes until transfer to the medical unit, he was now making the first struggling attempts to accept the notion of taking insulin. During the consultation he started asking questions about the course of diabetes and its treatment and expressed some optimism because he had given himself one injection. The patient now wanted the staff to give him more time to get used to injections. The psychiatrist answered each question, suggested further discussions with the nursing staff, and indicated to the staff that the patient was now beginning to acknowledge his need for insulin. He indicated that transfer to a psychiatric unit was not needed and suggested the team give the patient another few days to grapple with the reality of his new diagnosis. During follow-up sessions he allowed the patient to vent feelings about having this new medical condition. Over the next few days the patient accepted twice daily injections and started learning self-injection and self-monitoring techniques. When the patient was discharged he was taking his own injections. The patient's own fears decreased as he came to experience the actuality of diabetes care. In turn he could gradually "accept" treatment without needing to be forced to change through confrontation. In essence, the illness did the confronting, and the staff, once comfortable with the patient's participation in control of decisions to start treatment in a less than optimal manner, provided expert support [3].

Agreeing on a Model for Therapeutic Intervention

Patient–physician disagreement and consequently a weakened therapeutic alliance may derive from differences in the implicit models of interaction. These implicit models are the products of cultural values and beliefs [9], and the differences often stand out in stark contrast when the patient and physician come from distinct cultures, religions, and countries of origin. However, key variations in culturally determined beliefs about medical care may occur within cultural groups from the same region or country [10]. For example, a 55-year-old with a 3-year history of type 2 diabetes was prescribed an oral agent. She resisted the recommendation because she believed that the diabetes was caused by a vitamin imbalance, for which she preferred to seek out help from a holistic health center. Attitudes derived from parental teachings and past illness experiences can also influence perspectives about the nature of the therapeutics.

Encouraging the Patient to Take an Active Role

Cultural factors as well as personality may influence the extent to which patients seek an active voice in the therapeutic dialogue. Variation may also occur over time, with patients preferring an active role in some but not other types of decisions. In acute medical situations, more patients may abdicate an active part in their care. Fear may drive the patient into extreme positions in either direction. In chronic conditions, such as diabetes, patients may also vary considerably in their desire to direct their own care. Interestingly, some research indicates that encouraging patients to take an active role in establishing the goals for medical appointments leads to higher levels of "adherence" to therapeutic recommendations made by the treating physician [11, 12]. In one controlled outcome study, diabetic patients were randomly assigned to one of two interventions: (a) interaction with a research assistant prior to the medical appointment for 20 min during which the patient was encouraged to take an active role in the upcoming medical visit; (b) similar time with a research assistant before a medical appointment, but without any specific focus on how the patient should behave during the meeting. The intervention designed to encourage the patient to take more responsibility for directing the medical interview led to better glycemic control and improved adherence [11]. Examination of the actual interactions within the interview showed that those patients who were most active had the best medical outcomes. This study was carried out in the United States. It remains to be seen if such patient activation is beneficial for medical outcomes in other countries and cultures. Furthermore, some physicians may welcome active patients while others may resist such activity as aggressiveness.

READINESS TO CHANGE

Recent studies have led to the conceptualization of a cross-theoretical model of behavior change that may be usefully applied to the treatment of diabetes [13–19]. This model draws together an evaluation of the patient's readiness to change a specific behavior with alternative intervention

Table 2 Readiness to change stages

Precontemplation—in denial
Contemplation—considering the possibility of change
Preparation—has made first attempts at change
Action—taking steps actively to change
Maintenance—keeping the process going

strategies that can be applied depending on the patient's readiness. Readiness to change can be divided into five levels or stages (see Table 2) [20].

- Precontemplation is the stage at which individuals exhibit no intention to change behavior in the foreseeable future. Although such individuals may express the desire to change, they are generally not concerned about their problems and may not recognize any faults or personal difficulties they may have. Thus, individuals in the precontemplation phase are in a sense denying their problems.
- Contemplation is the stage in which people are aware that a problem exists, and they are seriously thinking about overcoming it. However, they have not yet made a commitment to take action. This stage may last for long periods during which individuals recognize the problem, think they should try to work on it, but are not ready to take action.
- Preparation is a stage that combines intention as well as behavioral change. Individuals in this stage intend to take action in the near future, have unsuccessfully taken action in the recent past, and are likely to report small behavioral changes that represent preparation for the larger action.
- Action is the stage in which individuals modify their behavior, experiences, and/or environment to overcome their problems. This stage involves the most direct and clear behavioral changes and requires considerable commitment of time and energy.
- In the final stage, maintenance, people continue to work to prevent relapse and to consolidate gains. This stage is not described as a static period; rather it is a continual process of reworking previous changes in behavior.

Changes do not occur in a linear fashion but involve continual relapsing and reintroduction of changes. Strategies for change include consciousness-raising, self-reevaluation, stimulus control, reinforcement management, and use of helping relationships. Strategies vary in their value, depending on the stage of the individual. Thus, consciousness-raising may be an extremely useful tool in beginning the process of change in the precontemplation and contemplation stages; however, it may not be sufficient to induce action. Additional strategies, such as reinforcement management, are important in taking action on the basis of awareness of the nature of the problem. The most direct implication of this model of stages and processes of change is the need to evaluate the patient's stage of readiness to change and tailor interventions accordingly. Table 3 summarizes some linkages between stages and strategies for change [21].

While developed for use with addictive behaviors, this model of change provides a basis for evaluating and treating the adherence problems faced by patients with diabetes and clinicians who treat them [16–19]. Evaluating the patient's stage provides a method for discriminating between patients when devising effective treatment strategies. It is likely that some of the most difficult problems in clinical practice are posed by patients at the precontemplation phase. Making this explicit diagnosis may not lead to more rapid change, but it may allow the clinician to take a more thoughtful view of what interventions should be tried. The clinician should recognize that simply referring the patient for diet education or behavioral weight management will not be effective in a patient at the precontemplation stage. Repeated discussion of the nature of the problem is probably required to help the patient discard his denial of the problem.

According to Prochaska and associates, more than 80% of all smokers are in the precontemplation and contemplation stages [13, 15]. It would not be surprising if similar percentages were found among overweight patients with type 2 diabetes mellitus or those individuals with type 1 diabetes who purposely take too little insulin so as to lose or control weight. For these individuals, treatment must focus on consciousness-raising, family support to induce the individual to consider change, and if necessary, respect for the patient's initial unwillingness to consider change. Using the same diagnostic model may help the clinician recognize an individual at the preparation stage who would be more likely to respond positively to an action-oriented behavioral program. Patients in denial test the strength of the therapeutic alliance and often require repeated review of hidden requests, concerns, and goals. The physician must be prepared to discuss differences in goals and to find a balance between those of the patient and health-care team. Such struggles may recur over months to years with progress occurring only gradually.

Example: A patient with a 25-year history of type 1 diabetes, which had been poorly controlled, developed proliferative retinopathy leading to severe vision loss. He became increasingly depressed, and so agreed to psychiatric treatment. Treatment initially focused on the need for repeated ophthalmologic surgery and his alcohol abuse. Eventually the patient agreed to treatment of the alcohol abuse and successfully became abstinent. Over time he developed foot ulcers requiring medical hospitalization, repeated debridement, and other conservative management techniques. He persisted in smoking through the initial 16 months of these treatments until he gradually accepted the importance of cessation as part of his

Table 3 General guidelines for applying stages and processes of change to diabetes care*

Stage of readiness	Key factors associated with movement to next stage	Treatment do's at this stage	Treatment don'ts at this stage
Precontemplation	Increased information and awareness, emotional acceptance	Provide personalized information. Allow patient to express emotions about his or her disease. Raise consciousness about the problem	Do not assume patient has knowledge or expect that providing information will automatically lead to behavior change. Do not ignore patient's emotional adjustment to the disease, which could override ability to process relevant information
Contemplation	Increased confidence in ability to adopt recommended behaviors	Encourage support networks. Give positive feedback about a patient's abilities. Help to clarify ambivalence about adopting behavior, and emphasize expected benefits	Do not ignore the potential impact of family members, etc. on patient's ability to comply. Do not be alarmed or critical of a patient's ambivalence
Preparation	Resolution of ambivalence, firm commitment and specific action plan	Encourage patient to set specific, achievable goals (e.g. walk briskly for 15 min at least 3 times a week). Reinforce small changes that patient may have already achieved.	Do not recommend general behavioral changes (e.g. "Get more exercise"). Do not refer to small changes as "not good enough"
Action	Behavioral skill training and social support	Refer to education program for self-management skills. Provide self-help materials	Do not refer patients to "information-only" classes
Maintenance	Problem-solving skills, and social and environmental support	Encourage patient to anticipate and plan for potential difficulties (e.g. maintaining dietary changes on vacation). Collect information about local resources (e.g. support group shopping guides). Encourage patient to "recycle" if he or she has a lapse or relapse	Do not assume that initial action means permanent change. Do not be discouraged or judgmental about a lapse or relapse

* From reference 13, with permission.

treatment for peripheral vascular complications and then stopped smoking. However, he remained terrified of low blood glucose levels, so maintained a minimal glucose of 250 mg/dl (13.9 mmol/l). No amount of discussion could alter his intense preoccupation with hypoglycemia. In this instance the team wrestled with the differences in treatment goals between themselves and the patient. While they made progress in other areas of self-care, they came to recognize the immutability of his glycemic goals. Throughout this treatment, raising consciousness together with continual openness to the patient's own concerns and goals was the principal intervention.

Involvement of the family can be an important feature of this work. For example, it may be a spouse who contacts the physician about her husband who tests infrequently because he feels that he is OK, even though he has had periodic hypoglycemic episodes requiring assistance. The consciousness-raising process is entered jointly by the medical professional and appropriate loved ones. In all instances these confrontations must be carried out nonjudgmentally, with great care to avoid backlash that could lead to even greater problems with self-care. Group programs provide an additional nonmedical source of support for patients.

Example: A patient who consistently failed to follow recommendations about regular medical appointments and appropriate testing methods had complained to his physician that he wanted to enter a support group. Considerable effort was made to honor this request; the patient became an honored member of the group, respected by his co-attendees for his observations about his own diabetes. This became the first step in a process that led back to those very areas that he was not yet willing to face.

DEFAULTING FROM REGULAR CARE: A CRITICAL OUTCOME OF A FAILING ALLIANCE

There is some evidence that a substantial minority of patients may become so disinvested in treatment of their diabetes that they default from regular follow-up. One study found that 20% of an onset cohort of adolescents with type 1 diabetes were no longer coming in at least yearly within a few years after diagnosis [22]. Furthermore, other research suggests that such defaulters from regular care may default, at least in part, because they are not interested in discussing medical concerns with their physicians [23]. This is consistent with other studies in indicating that less actively involved patients are less adherent to physician recommendations [11]. Moreover, adolescent defaulters from regular care seem to come from disrupted family backgrounds with higher rates of divorce and less family warmth [22]. Finally, case-control studies indicate that defaulters have worse glycemic control [23] and, later in the course of illness, higher rates of diabetes complications than regular clinic attenders [24–26]. These findings highlight the critical importance of engaging patients by using methods to strengthen their therapeutic alliance. Successful implementation of treatment strategies designed to strengthen the therapeutic alliance and sensitively address psychological problems should lead to a more engaged and involved patient. One set of studies has suggested that use of paraprofessionals to provide basic support, education, and assistance in dealing with the logistics of appointment making and insurance can increase the regularity of appointments and decrease use of emergency rooms and improve other outcomes of care [27].

FAMILY AND PSYCHOPATHOLOGICAL EFFECTS OF DIABETES

The Family and Diabetes

A growing number of studies have examined the psychiatric and psychological impacts of diabetes mellitus. Because there are several useful reviews of this literature (e.g. [1, 28–30]) we will limit ourselves to a focused commentary about them. Most such studies have addressed the effects of type 1 diabetes on patients and their families and have specifically examined child and adolescent patients. These studies of children with type 1diabetes do not consistently demonstrate alterations in patient personality and maturation [30, 31]. There are suggestions that older adolescents and young adults experience problems in the development of close personal relationships, but the findings vary across the few studies examining the important transition of adolescence and young adulthood [32, 33]. Parents of children with diabetes, and young patients with diabetes experience considerable stress [34, 35]. However, families vary widely in their ability to adapt to the stresses of diabetes. Families who cope more successfully with diabetes tend to be more organized, more cohesive, and better able to maintain an affectively warm environment. Children with diabetes in these successful families appear to take better care of their diabetes [36–38]. This suggests that emphasis should be placed on making the family unit the focus of psychosocial intervention efforts. Strengthening the family could bolster the patient's adaptation to illness thereby influencing the course of illness.

Example: A 19-year-old with 5 years of diabetes was admitted for repeated episodes of DKA. On admission it became apparent that he would often stop his noon and evening insulin injections, because he hated any reminders that he was diabetic. He could tolerate the morning dose because he could do it while still feeling half asleep and then pretend he did not have diabetes. This had been occurring over the past 2 years, a period in which his parents were going through much marital conflict. He often felt that he had to side with one or another of the parents. Family therapy was undertaken and focused on the multiple family conflicts. The young man's wish to avoid insulin and develop DKA temporarily deflected the parents from their own struggles; this was his way of trying to get them back together. The family worked on ways of resolving conflict more effectively. The parents did divorce, but with less contentiousness and with the patient able to realize what he could and could not control.

Recent studies also now indicate that at least two forms of psychopathology, depressive and eating disorders, may be more common among patients with type 1 diabetes. In addition, these two forms of psychopathology are associated with glycemic control difficulties.

Depression

Several studies [28, 39–41; J. Samson, M. de Groot, and A.M. Jacobson, unpublished work, 2002] suggest that among patients with type 1 diabetes, there may be an increase in the frequency of depression. In particular it appears that major depression may be more common among adult patients with type 1 diabetes and at least in one study it would appear that this increase in prevalence is most clearly found among adult men with type 1 diabetes (J. Samson, M. de Groot, and A.M. Jacobson, unpublished work, 2002). It is also intriguing to note that the increased prevalence of depression among diabetic patients may be occurring well before the onset of chronic complications. The widely recognized increase in prevalence in other chronically ill patient groups is most likely because of the physical disability of medical illness. This does not appear to be necessarily the case among diabetic patients [42, 43]. While the advent of depression in patients with type 1 diabetes typically occurs after the onset of illness, the reverse is found among patients with type 2 diabetes. The timing of depression onset viz a viz diabetes may simply reflect the fact that depression is often an illness that manifests itself during young adulthood. However, some have suggested that depressive disorders may be a risk factor for type 2 diabetes; this intriguing suggestion [44] may reflect the neuroendocrine changes wrought by depression and the autonomic regulation of the endocrine pancreas.

In type 1 diabetes, it is not clear whether psychosocial or biological mechanisms mediate the relationship with depression [44].

A few studies of depression among patients with diabetes suggest that widely accepted forms of treatment, such as antidepressants and cognitive behavior therapy (CBT), are as effective in reducing psychiatric symptoms [45, 46] as would be expected in nondiabetic, depressed patients. Moreover, one study indicates that CBT for depression also led to substantial improvement in glycemic control [46]. These few studies suggest that we can alter the course of diabetes by treating depression aggressively. Since depressive symptoms include a bleak view of the future, loss of interest, and poor concentration, the symptoms of a particular depression might include pessimism about diabetes self-care, loss of interest in one's health, and/or trouble learning information about diabetes. Improving these symptoms could benefit the depressed patient in terms of their willingness and ability to care for diabetes. Because CBT addresses persistent and problematic attitudes, it can be modified to address diabetes-specific attitudes that interfere with learning and self-care techniques as part of the treatment of the depressed diabetic patient who is having diabetes self-care and/or glycemic control problems [47–49]. A similar approach, cognitive analytic therapy [47, 48] has now been used to treat diabetic patients with poor glycemic control and may also be useful. These are well-suited for short-term interventions, and so may be applicable to a wide array of patient situations at a time when there is increasing emphasis on cost-containment in health care.

Eating Disorders

One other area of considerable interest has been that of eating disorders in diabetes. Theoretically, the dietary requirements of diabetes mellitus may place the patient at greater risk for eating-related problems. Dietary expectations for the diabetic patient involve restricted food choices. Furthermore, treatment with insulin may be associated with weight gain. For example, intensive diabetes treatment in the DCCT experience led to increased weight when compared with patients undergoing conventional treatment. Type 2 diabetes typically has its onset well after the typical age of greatest risk for eating and body image related disturbances (ages 10–40). On the other hand, type 1 diabetes commonly occurs within the age of risk for eating disturbances. Thus, it is reasonable to assume that dietary restriction, weight gain from insulin treatment, the discovery that withdrawal of insulin leads to weight loss, and the age of onset can lead the female patient with type 1 diabetes to have a significantly increased risk for eating disorders. Available studies do not provide conclusive evidence for such assumptions, but do tend to support the contention that rates of anorexia nervosa and bulimia are increased in young women with type 1 diabetes [29].

Table 4 Percentage of type 1 diabetic women who omit insulin*

Ages (years)	Any omission (%)	Frequent omission (%)
All ages	30	9
≥15	8	0
15–30	40	16
31–45	30	4
46–60	20	6

* From reference 42, with permission.

Recent research underscores the dangers posed by eating disorders and weight-related concerns for the medical outcomes of diabetes. For example, it appears from one study [50] that 30% of adolescent and adult women with type 1 diabetes reported that they had omitted insulin. Moreover, 9% of these women reported frequent insulin omission (see Table 4). Women aged 15–30 reported the highest rates of omission. However, even in older women omission occurred. Insulin omission was associated with worse glycemic control. It is not uncommon for patients to feel awkward and embarrassed about attempts to regulate weight by underusing insulin, just as it may be for other forms of purging. Because of such experiences of shame, patients may not want to acknowledge their behaviors, thereby leading to underreporting in studies examining eating problems. In this study some patients reported that they underused insulin as a method to lose weight. Patients who acknowledged insulin omission to lose weight seemed to have the most psychological problems and also had the worst glycemic control. Those who omitted insulin, but did not report that they did it to lose weight, appear to have fewer psychological problems [50]. Preliminary data from a long-term follow-up of this cohort suggests those with history of eating disorders may experience earlier than expected deaths. In another study, a history of eating disorder was related, at follow-up, with an early development of retinopathy [51]. Taken together, these findings point to the important medical effects of eating problems in patients with diabetes. From a clinical perspective, the patients who do not have full-blown anorexia or bulimia may be the most difficult to identify, because they may not have acute problems with serious ketoacidosis or severe hypoglycemic events. Yet these underusers of insulin may have persistently high blood glucose levels that are apparently difficult to explain.

PRACTICAL PROBLEMS IN TREATING DIABETIC PATIENTS WITH PSYCHIATRIC PROBLEMS

Diagnosing and Treating Depression

As noted in the previous section, depressive disorders are common among patients with diabetes. While the general principles of evaluation and treatment are not altered, the presence of diabetes adds complexity to clinical decision making. Depressions may occur as primary disorders or secondary to the direct effects of medical conditions on aspects of brain physiology and anatomy. There is no clear, dependable symptomatic difference between primary and secondary depressions, and so certain medical illnesses need to be ruled out before limiting the treatment solely to use of antidepressants and psychotherapy. While diabetes, especially type 1 diabetes, appears to be a risk factor for depression, there is no clear evidence that the mechanism by which diabetes increases the risk for depression is biological rather than psychosocial. Thus, altering the treatment of diabetes, itself, will not typically improve a depression.

However, some symptoms of depression may occur in poorly controlled diabetes with ketonuria and hyperglycemia, and thus be confused with a depression. These include physical symptoms such as fatigue, excessive sleeping, nighttime awakening, and weight loss. Cognitive symptoms, such as decreased concentration and recent memory, may also occur in poorly controlled diabetes. Affective symptoms, such as depressed mood, loss of interest in activities, and increased guilt, shame, fear, or anxiety, and altered attitudes, such as pessimism about the future and a sense that actions cannot lead to positive consequences, are far less likely to be solely caused by poorly controlled diabetes. Patients usually come with some but not most of these symptoms. If physical and cognitive symptoms dominate the patient's report, then the situation is compatible with poorly controlled diabetes and a brief course of treatment focused on improving metabolic control may change the clinical picture. If 2 weeks of better metabolic control does not lead to a change in the physical and cognitive complaints, then treatment for depression should be implemented. If depressive attitudes and affective symptoms are present when the patient is first evaluated, then the clinician should assume that a depression has occurred and definitive therapy for the depression should begin at once [2, 3]. If suicidal ideation is reported, then depression is the most likely diagnosis, regardless of the mix of physical, cognitive, affective, and attitudinal symptoms.

Diabetes is often associated with other medical conditions that cause secondary depressions. These include, but are not limited to, hyperthyroidism, hypothyroidism, other endocrinopathies, and cerebrovascular events in older adults. Thus careful assessment of the patient should include evaluation of such conditions that may be causing the secondary depression.

Depressions are responsive to both antidepressant medication and forms of psychotherapy, such as CBT [49]. Antidepressants and CBT appear to be as effective in diabetic as nondiabetic patients [46, 52]. Some of the common side effects of antidepressants may be especially problematic in diabetic patients [53]. For example, antidepressants and lithium carbonate may influence glycemic regulation. Tricyclic antidepressants have been associated with increases in blood glucose levels and increased appetite; serotonin reuptake inhibitors may cause episodes of hypoglycemia. Lithium carbonate may also cause hypoglycemia. Thus, it is useful to explain this set of possibilities to patients beginning treatment for a depression. It is also useful to point out to the patient that depression often alters appetite and activity level so that successful treatment may require changes in dose of insulin or oral agents as the depression lifts [2, 3].

Antidepressants cause other side effects of special relevance to patients with diabetes. The tricyclic antidepressants are associated with orthostatic hypotension, constipation, and possibly slowed gastric emptying secondary to effects on the autonomic nervous system. In longer-term diabetes, frank gastroparesis and serious hypotension may be uncovered with the onset of therapy. If there are signs of cardiac disease, the risk of arrhythmias may be increased in patients on tricyclics. The serotonin reuptake inhibitors have fewer autonomic and cardiac side effects, rendering them generally safer in diabetic patients with complications. However, their gastric side effects may create problems in patients with gastroparesis. Furthermore, the serotonin reuptake inhibitors affect erectile functioning in men. While there is no clear evidence that this side effect is a greater problem in men with diabetes, it is reasonable to assume that minor erectile problems may be made worse by use of these agents. It is especially important to warn depressed men of this side effect because such a problem may heighten the problems of self-esteem that occur in depression. Lithium carbonate's side effects include renal toxicity and hypothyroidism; however, it can be used with the same regular reevaluation of kidney and thyroid function utilized in chronic treatment of nondiabetic patients.

The treatment of diabetic patients with painful neuropathy poses specific complexity as it appears that tricyclics, such as nortryptiline and desipramine, may decrease pain, while the serotonin reuptake inhibitors do not show this benefit. However, such patients may also have autonomic neuropathy, thereby limiting therapeutic choices.

Multiple trials of different antidepressants, as well as a very gradual increase in dose, are more likely to be necessary among patients with diabetes [2, 3]. Since the most frequent reasons for therapeutic failure with antidepressants are inadequate length of treatment and/or suboptimal dosing [54], special care is required to achieve an adequate therapeutic trial in patients with diabetes. The symptoms of depression, such as low self-esteem, poor concentration, psychomotor retardation, and pessimism, may themselves decrease the patient's capacity for learning and confidence in self-care. Thus patients recovering from depression may require additional diabetes education. Finally, depressions may improve but still leave the patient with diabetes care attitudes that are negative. Indeed, a sense of helplessness with diabetes care can be a precipitant for a clinical depression. Thus, after recovery from depression, careful reevaluation of such underlying negative beliefs is important for treatment planning and consideration of additional psychotherapy.

Anxiety Disorders

Some of the symptoms experienced by patients with anxiety syndromes may also occur in the course of diabetes [55]. While depressive disorder symptoms are most likely to be confused with those of hyperglycemia and ketonuria, symptomatic anxiety is more typically confused with acute hypoglycemic states. Panic states in particular present with adrenergic symptoms that include physical symptoms such as palpitations, sweats, headaches, as well as physical and emotional feelings of trembling, foreboding, and panic. The patient may need to evaluate the blood glucose repeatedly in order to compare the timing of symptoms with changes in glucose level. The occurrence of obsessive thoughts, compulsive acts, foreboding, or phobic avoidance usually suggests the presence of an anxiety disorder rather than hypoglycemia [2, 3]. Benzodiazepines, a class of drugs commonly used in the treatment of anxiety syndromes, may lead to lower blood glucose levels and might therefore increase the risk for hypoglycemia [56]. However, serious hypoglycemia is not a common outcome of such treatment.

Patients who report high levels of fear or worry about hypoglycemia may have underlying anxiety states. Thus patient complaints about fear of hypoglycemia should alert clinicians to the possibility of a co-occurring anxiety syndrome. Similarly, excessive home glucose monitoring beyond the recommendations of the clinician may also reflect an anxiety syndrome. In such patients psychotherapeutic interventions can help patients overcome such intense affective reactions to the sense of being out of control or severely endangered by excess insulin.

Example: A 33-year-old woman with 15 years of type 1 diabetes presented with complaints of frequent episodes of hypoglycemia over the prior 3-month period. She experienced palpitations, sweats, and headaches. The symptoms often occurred at night or just before bed. Occasional self-glucose monitoring did not reveal a clear pattern of hypoglycemia. Psychiatric evaluation revealed that the patient had become concerned about the diagnosis of early neuropathy 4 months previously. She had noted numbness and tingling in the toes of both feet. These symptoms meant to her that her diabetes was now going to wreak havoc on her life and that she could never lead a normal existence again. These thoughts often came up at quiet times when she had time to think over her day. In short-term therapy she came to see that these thoughts triggered considerable anxiety.

Eating Disorders

Eating disorders can be difficult to diagnose and treat. Cultural values regarding thinness so pervade many western societies in particular that weight becomes a critical method for self-evaluation. Failure to achieve the requisite thinness is the equivalent of failing to achieve a critical measure of value and therefore self-worth. These aspects of eating disorder are not particular to the patient with diabetes. The diabetic patient on insulin is differentiated because there is a ready method for weight regulation in which the patient is carefully trained: insulin use (or in this case underuse) [3]. This special method of purging, not available to the nondiabetic individual, also can interact with the patient's feelings about having diabetes. The patient who wishes she did not have diabetes can act on two wishes with a single act of missing an injection. It is possible that diabetic patients use insulin underdosing in preference to vomiting and laxatives [51]. Certainly, underdosing may be used alone and indeed may be found even when binge eating is not serious. The evaluation of a patient for eating problems should occur when there are repeated unexplained episodes of ketoacidosis or persistent hyperglycemia revealed through self-monitoring results or HbA_{1c} level. Evaluation requires repeated, careful, nonjudgmental questioning, for the sense of shame and embarrassment may lead such patients to hide their actions. If the patient feels she will be attacked for her behavior, she will not readily acknowledge it.

Reinsulinization may be quite difficult because insulin will cause water retention. The patient with distorted views of their body cannot readily distinguish weight changes by source. Indeed, weight loss due to dehydration may be seen as highly desirable. Thus restarting a regular insulin dose may require discussions related to rapid weight gain. Hospitalization is typically required during this phase of treatment. Indeed the hospitalization or other forms of supervision may be needed until weight is restabilized. Overt edema is especially frightening for the patient who is terrified by fat and weight gain [3].

SCHIZOPHRENIA: A POSSIBLE RISK FACTOR FOR DIABETES

There is a growing literature suggesting that patients with schizophrenia have a risk two to four times that of the general populations of developing type 2 diabetes [57]. The reasons for this added risk are unclear. It may reflect the generally poor lifestyle choices of these patients, i.e. they are quite sedentary, frequently smoke, and tend to overeat high carbohydrates/high fat foods. However, greater attention has recently been focused on the as yet poorly understood role played by treatment with antipsychotic medications. Many such medications lead to weight gain [57–65]. As yet no studies have identified other mechanisms of relevance to the added risk for diabetes. It appears that other metabolic changes associated with obesity also occur, e.g. elevated lipids. While newer antipsychotic medications (clozapine, olanzapine, and risperidone) have been implicated, the increased risk preceeds their use [57].

The most troubling aspect of this problem is reflected by occasional case reports suggesting that the onset of diabetes may occur suddenly and dramatically with emergent ketosis, hyperosmolar states, and extremely high blood glucose levels of diabetes among schizophrenic patients [57–65]. These typically recede once the antipsychotic medication is stopped. Patients on antipsychotic agents should therefore be assessed for their diabetes status when treatment is initiated and monitored for regularly to identify emerging glucose intolerance. In patients with known diabetes, antipsychotic medications can be used with appropriate attention to the care of the metabolic state. The clear clinical advantages of the newer antipsychotic may need to be balanced against these medical consequences.

PSYCHOSOCIAL MEASURES: ADJUNCTS TO THE INFORMATION GATHERING PROCESS

A broad array of measures have been developed that can be used to identify potential problem areas and to track outcomes of medical therapy. These can include assessment tools developed for the general population as well as those designed specifically with diabetic patients in mind [66]. There are now many generic measures in use to evaluate depressive and anxiety symptoms, eating attitudes and behaviors, functional health status, and quality of life. With the increasing pressure for physicians and other health care providers to use their time wisely, screening measures can guide the evaluation process. Most measures are now available in traditional paper formats, only, but computer-based and telephone-based inquiries are being developed. In the near future, it is likely that patients could answer questions, using an expert-system format that allows for skips in the protocol to areas of particular problems. Such inquiries will be available through phone contact and could generate patient-specific educational material and reports to the patient and provider prior to a scheduled appointment. A few potentially valuable measures are presented here as examples.

Table 5 Problem areas in diabetes scale (PAID)

Which of the following diabetic issues are currently aproblem for you (circle the number that best answers each question for you):

	Not a problem	Minor problem	Moderate problem	Somewhat serious problem	Serious problem
1. Not having clear and concrete goals for your diabetes care?	0	1	2	3	4
2. Feeling discouraged with your diabetes treatment plan?	0	1	2	3	4
3. Feeling scared when you think about living with diabetes?	0	1	2	3	4
4. Uncomfortable social situations related to your diabetes care (e.g., people telling you what to eat)?	0	1	2	3	4
5. Feelings of deprivation regarding food and meals?	0	1	2	3	4
6. Feeling depressed when you think about living with diabetes?	0	1	2	3	4
7. Not knowing if your mood or feelings are related to your diabetes?	0	1	2	3	4
8. Feeling overwhelmed by your diabetes?	0	1	2	3	4
9. Worrying about low blood sugar reactions?	0	1	2	3	4
10. Feeling angry when you think about living with diabetes?	0	1	2	3	4
11. Feeling constantly concerned about food and eating?	0	1	2	3	4
12. Worrying about the future and the possibility of serious complications?	0	1	2	3	4
13. Feelings of guilt or anxiety when you get off track with your diabetes management?	0	1	2	3	4
14. Not "accepting" your diabetes?	0	1	2	3	4
15. Feeling unsatisfied with your diabetes physician?	0	1	2	3	4
16. Feeling that diabetes is taking up too much of your mental and physical energy every day?	0	1	2	3	4
17. Feeling alone with your diabetes?	0	1	2	3	4
18. Feeling that your friends and family are not supportive of your diabetes management efforts?	0	1	2	3	4
19. Coping with complications of diabetes?	0	1	2	3	4
20. Feeling "burned out" by the constant effort needed to manage diabetes?	0	1	2	3	4

The Beck Depression Inventory [67] has been used extensively to evaluate symptoms of depression. It is a brief self-report that can be used to screen patients for depression, to identify issues for questioning during the medical visit, and to track the effects of treatment for depression. In using such measures in a medically ill population it is important to examine the responses to questions that address somatic symptoms, since, as noted above, these may elevate the depression scores, yet be caused by the presence of a concomitant medical problem.

Functional health and quality-of-life measures can characterize the influence of illness and treatment on patient views of their own well-being. These measures include both illness-specific and generic measures. Generic measures can be particularly helpful in characterizing the burden of illness on an entire population, and comparing the effectiveness of treatments across illness groups. Quality-of-life evaluation can also discriminate well between different areas, and so detect specific patient concerns. The Diabetes Quality of Life Measure developed for the DCCT [68–70] is one such diabetes-oriented measure. It has been found to have a high degree of reliability and can be used to detect differences between patients undergoing different therapies [68, 69]. It can be used with adult patients with type 1 and type 2 diabetes [71]. In addition to a core group of questions, there are questions of special relevance to adolescents and young adults. It has not been used extensively with older adults. In clinical practice, providers may find it useful to include questions of special interest to their own practices. The DQOL has been translated into multiple languages including Dutch, French, Chinese, and Malay. A copy of the measure can be found in C. Bradley [66].

Finally, Polonsky et al. [72, 73] have developed a screening measure designed to detect areas of distress related to diabetes. This measure, called the Problem Areas in Diabetes Scale (PAID), scrutinizes concerns about diabetes and the distress level associated with their presence. The measure is designed as a screen and covers multiple aspects of diabetes. Patient distress may be usefully evaluated periodically to see if the therapy is well-accepted or causing excess burden. Furthermore, the medical and psychosocial interventions can be targeted to specific domains of patient distress. Table 5 presents the PAID questions. The questionnaire has been widely used for clinical and research purposes and has been shown to be a sensitive indicator of change in distress related to diabetes. It can be used with type 1 and type 2 patients. The PAID has been translated into Japanese and Dutch [74] and has been found to be responsive to theoretically relevant changes in clinical states [75].

CONCLUSIONS

Diabetes demands of the patient considerable adaptive capacity in order to learn a new set of behaviors and to cope with the vagaries of the illness. This involves the development of a close working relationship with health care providers and with key family members. The patient's physician, as well as other health care team members, can enhance this collaborative relationship through attention to the elements of their transactions that are most likely to build trust, a therapeutic alliance, and mutually agreeable objectives for therapy. An understanding of the ways diabetes affects the patient and his or her family is an important condition for developing a successful working relationship. Indeed, such awareness may provide the patient with a sense of willingness to try increasingly more challenging aspects of the medical treatment. Even if the patient does not change behavior in the direction desired by the health care team, feeling understood can give the patient comfort and solace. The physician's office thereby becomes what Hemingway described as a "clean, well lighted, place" [76]: a setting that will be sought out when the demands and stresses of this illness are greatest.

Acknowledgment

Supported by NIH grants R01 DK 27845,42315, and 60754, and a donation from Herbert Graetz.

REFERENCES

1. Jacobson AM, Hauser S, Anderson B, Polonsky W. *Joslin's Diabetes Mellitus*. Philadelphia: Lea & Febiger, 1994.
2. Jacobson AM. Psychological care of patients with insulin-dependent diabetes mellitus. *N Engl J Med* 1996; 334: 1249–53.
3. Jacobson AM. *Psychiatric Secrets*. Philadelphia: Hanley and Belfus, 1996.
4. Greenson R. *The Technique and Practice of Psychoanalysis*. New York: International University Press, 1979.
5. Zetzel ER. Current concepts of transference. *Int J Psychoanal* 1956; 37: 369–76.
6. Wensing M, Elwyn G. Methods for incorporating patients' views in health care. *BMJ* 2003; 326: 877–9.
7. Elwyn G, Edwards A, Wensing M, Hood K, Atwell C, Grol R. Shared decision making: developing the OPTION scale for measuring patient involvement. *Qual Saf Health Care* 2003; 12: 93–9.
8. Lazare A, Cohen F, Jacobson AN, Williams MW, Mignone RJ, Zisook S. The walk-in patient as a 'customer': a key dimension in evaluation and treatment. *Am J Orthopsychiatry* 1972; 42: 872–83.
9. Kleinman A. Patients and healers in the context of culture. Berkeley, CA: University of California Press, 1980.
10. Arora NK, McHorney CA. Patient preferences for medical decision making: who really wants to participate? *Med Care* 2000; 38: 335–41.
11. Kaplan SH, Greenfield S, Ware JE Jr. Assessing the effects of physician–patient interactions on the outcomes of chronic disease. *Med Care* 1989; 27: S110–27.
12. Rost KM, Flavin KS, Cole K, McGill JB. Change in metabolic control and functional status after hospitalization. Impact of patient activation intervention in diabetic patients. *Diabetes Care* 1991; 14: 881–9.

13. Prochaska JO, DiClemente CC, Norcross JC. In search of how people change: applicaions to addictive behaviors. *Am Psychol* 1992; 47: 1102–14.
14. Prochaska JO, Norcross JC, Fowler JL, Follick MJ. Abrams DB. Attendance and outcome in a work site weight control program: processes and stages of change as process and predictor variables. *Addict Behav* 1992; 17: 35–5.
15. Prochaska JO, Diclemente CC, Velicer WF, Ginpil S. Norcross JC. Predicting change in smoking status for self-changers. *Addict Behav* 1985; 10: 395–406.
16. Peterson KA, Hughes M. Readiness to change and clinical success in a diabetes educational program. *J Am Board Fam Pract* 2002; 15: 266–71.
17. Boyle RG, O'Connor PJ, Pronk NP, Tan A. Stages of change for physical activity, diet, and smoking among HMO members with chronic conditions. *Am J Health Promot* 1998; 12: 170–5.
18. Parchman ML, Arambula-Solomon TG, Noel PH, Larme AC, Pugh JA. Stage of change advancement for diabetes self-management behaviors and glucose control. *Diabetes Educ* 2003; 29: 128–34.
19. Blanchard KA, Morgenstern J, Morgan TJ, Labouvie E, Bux DA. Motivational subtypes and continuous measures of readiness for change: concurrent and predictive validity. *Psychol Addict Behav* 2003; 17: 56–65.
20. Jacobson AM. Commentary: in search of how people change. *Diabetes Spectr* 1993; 6: 36–7.
21. Curry S. Commentary: in search of how people change. *Diabetes Spectr* 1993; 6: 34–5.
22. Jacobson AM, Hauser ST, Willett J, Wolfsdorf JI, Herman L. Consequences of irregular versus continuous medical follow-up in children and adolescents with insulin-dependent diabetes mellitus. *J Pediatr* 1997; 131: 727–33.
23. Jacobson AM, Adler A, Derby L, Anderson B, Wolfsdorf J. Clinic attendance and glycemic control: a study contrasting groups of patients with insulin-dependent diabetes mellitus [Abstract]. *Diabetes Care* 1991; 14: 599–601.
24. Krolewski AS, Warram JH, Christlieb AR, Busick EJ, Kahn CR. The changing natural history of nephropathy in type I diabetes. *Am J Med* 1985; 78: 785–794.
25. Hammersley MS, Holland MR, Walford S, Thorn PA. What happens to defaulters from a diabetic clinic? *Br Med J (Clin Res Ed)*, 1985; 291: 1330–2.
26. Deckert T, Pulsen JE, Larsen M. Prognosis of patients with diabetes onset before the age of thiry-one. *Diabetologia* 1978; 14: 371–7.
27. Laffel LM, Brackett J, Ho J, Anderson BJ. Changing the process of diabetes care improves metabolic outcomes and reduces hospitalizations. *Qual Manag Health Care* 1998; 6: 53–62.
28. Gavard JA, Lustman PJ. Clouse RE. Prevalence of depression in adults with diabetes. An epidemiological evaluation. *Diabetes Care* 1993; 16: 1167–78.
29. Rodin GM, Daneman D. Eating disorders and IDDM. A problematic association. *Diabetes Care* 1992; 15: 1402–12.
30. Dunn SM, Turtle JR. The myth of the diabetic personality. *Diabetes Care* 1981; 4: 640–6.
31. Jacobson AM, et al. Psychological adjustment of children with recently diagnosed diabetes mellitus. *Diabetes Care* 1986; 9: 323–9.
32. Lloyd CE, Robinson N, Andrews B, Elston MA, Fuller JH. Are the social relationships of young insulin-dependent diabetic patients affected by their condition? *Diabet Med* 1993; 10: 481–5.
33. Lloyd CE, Robinson N, Fuller JH. Education and employment experiences in young adults with type 1 diabetes mellitus. *Diabet Med* 1992; 9: 661–6.
34. Hauenstein EJ, Marvin RS, Snyder AL, Clarke WL. Stress in parents of children with diabetes mellitus. *Diabetes Care* 1989; 12: 18–23.
35. Wysocki T, Huxtable K, Linscheid TR, Wayne W. Adjustment to diabetes mellitus in preschoolers and their mothers. *Diabetes Care* 1989; 12: 524–9.
36. Wertlieb D, Hauser ST, Jacobson AM. Adaptation to diabetes: behavior symptoms and family context. *J Pediatr Psychol* 1986; 11: 463–79.
37. Hauser ST, et al. Interaction sequences in families of psychiatrically hospitalized and nonpatient adolescents. *Psychiatry* 1987; 50: 308–19.
38. Jacobson AM, et al. Family environment and glycemic control: a four-year prospective study of children and adolescents with insulin-dependent diabetes mellitus. *Psychosom Med* 1994; 56: 401–9.
39. Blanz BJ, Rensch-Riemann BS, Fritz-Sigmund DI, Schmidt MH. IDDM is a risk factor for adolescent psychiatric disorders. *Diabetes Care* 1993; 16: 1579–87.
40. Lustman PJ, Griffith LS, Clouse RE, Cryer PE. Psychiatric illness in diabetes mellitus. Relationship to symptoms and glucose control. *J Nerv Ment Dis* 1986; 174: 736–42.
41. Anderson R, Freedland KE, Clouse RE, Lustman PJ. The prevalence of comorbid depression in adults with diabetes. *Diabetes Care* 2001; 24: 1069–78.
42. Wells KB, Golding JM, Burnam MA. Psychiatric disorder in a sample of the general population with and without chronic medical conditions. *Am J Psychiatry* 1988; 145: 976–81.
43. Cohen T, Welch G, Jacobson A, de Groot M, Samson J. The association of psychiatric illness and increased prevalence of retinopathy in patients with type 1 diabetes mellitus. *Psychosomatics* 1997; 38: 998–1008.
44. Jacobson AM, Samson JA, Weinger K, Ryan CM. Diabetes, the brain, and behavior: is there a biological mechanism underlying the association between diabetes and depression? *Int Rev Neurobiol* 2002; 51: 455–79.
45. Cook RF, Katritsis D. Hypertensive crisis precipitated by a monoamine oxidase inhibitor in a patient with phaeochromocytoma. *BMJ* 1990; 300: 614.
46. Lustman PJ, Griffith LS, Freedland KE, Kissel SS, Clouse RE. Cognitive behavior therapy for depression in type 2 diabetes mellitus: a randomized, controlled trial. *Ann Intern Med* 1998; 129: 613–21.
47. Ryle A. Cognitive analytic therapy—active participation in change. Chichester, UK: J Wiley, 1990.
48. Fosbury JA, Bosley CM, Ryle A, Sonksen PH, Lowy C. Cognitive analytic therapy with poorly controlled type 1 diabetic patients [Abstract]. *Diabetologia* 1994; 37 (suppl 1): A175.
49. Beck AT. *Cognitive Therapy and the Emotional Disorders*. New York: International University Press, 1976.
50. Polonsky WH, et al. Insulin omission in women with IDDM. *Diabetes Care* 1994; 17: 1178–85.
51. Rodin G, Rydall A, Olmsted M, Daneman MB, Devenyi RG, A four year follow-up study of eating disorders and medical complication in young women with insulin-dependent diabetes mellitus. *Psychosom Med* 1994; 56: 179.
52. Lustman PJ, et al. Effects of nortriptyline on depression and glycemic control in diabetes: results of a double-blind, placebo-controlled trial. *Psychosom Med* 1997; 59: 241–50.

53. Goodnick PJ, Henry JH, Buki VM. Treatment of depression in patients with diabetes mellitus. *J Clin Psychiatry* 1995; 56: 128–36.
54. Weissman M, Klerman G. The chronic depressive inthe community: unrecognized and poorly treated. *Compr Psychiatry* 1977; 18: 523–32.
55. Grigsby AB, Anderson RJ, Freedland KE, Clouse RE, Lustman PJ. Prevalence of anxiety in adults with diabetes: a systematic review. *J Psychosom Res* 2002; 53: 1053–60.
56. Lustman PJ, et al. Effects of alprazolam on glucose regulation in diabetes. Results of double-blind, placebo-controlled trial. *Diabetes Care* 1995; 18: 1133–9.
57. Dixon L, et al. Prevalence and correlates of diabetes in national schizophrenia samples. *Schizophr Bull* 2000; 26: 903–12.
58. Buse JB. Metabolic side effects of antipsychotics: focus on hyperglycemia and diabetes. *J Clin Psychiatry* 2002; 63: (suppl 4): 37–41.
59. Ryan MC, Thakore JH. Physical consequences of schizophrenia and its treatment: the metabolic syndrome. *Life Sci* 2002; 71: 239–57.
60. Newcomer JW, et al. Abnormalities in glucose regulation during antipsychotic treatment of schizophrenia. *Arch Gen Psychiatry* 2002; 59: 337–45.
61. Koro CE, et al. Assessment of independent effect of olanzapine and risperidone on risk of diabetes among patients with schizophrenia: population based nested case-control study. *BMJ* 2002; 325: 243–5.
62. Henderson DC, Ettinger ER. Schizophrenia and diabetes. *Int Rev Neurobiol* 2002; 51: 481–501.
63. Henderson DC, Diabetes mellitus and other metabolic disturbances induced by atypical antipsychotic agents. *Curr Diabetes Rep* 2002; 2: 135–40.
64. Geller WK, MacFadden W. Diabetes and atypical neuroleptics. *Am J Psychiatry* 2003; 160: 388.
65. Lindenmayer JP, et al. Changes in glucose and cholesterol levels in patients with schizophrenia treated with typical or atypical antipsychotics. *Am J Psychiatry* 2003; 160: 290–6.
66. Bradley C. (ed). *Handbook of Psychology and Diabetes*. Chur, Switzerland: Harwood Academic Publishers, 1994.
67. Beck AT. *The Beck Depression Inventory*. New York: The Psychological Corporation, Harcourt Brace Jovanovich, 1978.
68. DCCT Research Group. Reliability and validity of a diabetes quality-of-life measure for the Diabetes Control and Complications Trial (DCCT). *Diabetes Care* 1988; 11: 725–32.
69. Jacobson AM, de Groot M, Samson JA. The evaluation of two measures of quality of life in patients with type I and type II diabetes. *Diabetes Care* 1994; 17: 267–74.
70. DCCT Research Group, Jacobson A, Cleary P, Baker L. The influence of intensive treatment on quality of life outcomes in the Diabetes Control and Complications Trial. *Diabetes Care* 1996; 19: 195–203.
71. Kotsanos JG, et al. Health-related quality-of-life results from multinational clinical trials of insulin lispro. Assessing benefits of a new diabetes therapy. *Diabetes Care* 1997; 20: 948–58.
72. Polonsky WH, et al. Assessment of diabetes-related distress. *Diabetes Care* 1995; 18: 754–60.
73. Welch GW, Jacobson AM, Polonsky WH. The Problem Areas in Diabetes Scale. An evaluation of its clinical utility. *Diabetes Care* 1997; 20: 760–6.
74. Snoek FJ, Pouwer F, Welch GW, Polonsky WH, Diabetes-related emotional distress in Dutch and U.S. diabetic patients: cross-cultural validity of the problem areas in diabetes scale. *Diabetes Care* 2000; 23: 1305–9.
75. Welch G, Weinger K, Anderson B, Polonsky WH. Responsiveness of the Problem Areas In Diabetes (PAID) questionnaire. *Diabet Med* 2003; 20: 69–72.
76. Hemingway E. *The Complete Short Stories*. New York: Scribners, 1987.

92

Computer-assisted Diabetes Education and Information Technology in Diabetes Care

Eldon D. Lehmann

St Bartholomew's Hospital, London, UK, and Imperial College, London, UK

INTRODUCTION

Much has been written about the Diabetes Control and Complications Trial (DCCT) and its implications for health care provision for patients with type 1 diabetes mellitus [1–4]. The long-term, randomized, prospective trial demonstrated conclusively that intensive insulin therapy (IIT) can delay the onset and slow the progression of retinopathy, nephropathy, and neuropathy in patients with type 1 diabetes.

However, achieving the benefits of IIT in the DCCT entailed substantial risks and costs [2]. The resources needed to achieve and maintain really tight diabetes control were enormous [5]. Specialist staff were recruited to maintain contact with patients who were often seen fortnightly in hospital, and contacted even more frequently by telephone during the day as well as at night. Efforts were redoubled at times of minor illness or emotional upset. Team meetings took place weekly to maintain these standards [3]. Over 560 health care professionals (HCPs) participated in the trial, looking after 1441 patients.

This level of expertise and HCP involvement has been hard to sustain in routine clinical practice. In particular, in the decade since the DCCT was published it has proven difficult to deliver the level of care offered in the trial, routinely, to a large number of diabetic patients in standard clinical practice.

A hypothesis will be developed in this chapter that one way of achieving the goals demonstrated by the DCCT in routine clinical care, while containing costs, may well be through the use of information technology (IT). As will be shown, there is still a great deal of work to be done. Current computer applications—including database systems, decision-support prototypes and educational tools—will be reviewed and some areas requiring further research and development will be discussed. A recurring theme of the need for rigorous validation and evaluation studies will be highlighted.

However, one thing that is important to stress from the outset is that any use of IT in clinical diabetes care is not envisaged to, in any way, replace diabetologists, endocrinologists, diabetes educators, or diabetes specialist nurses. Rather there is a growing realization that there are not enough HCPs available to deliver the type of care required by the large and growing number of patients with diabetes [6]. Therefore if IT can help to provide education and care to some of these patients, perhaps HCPs' time could be freed up to deal with some of the more complex cases, or simply to manage the expected larger number of people with diabetes.

In the words of the DCCT investigators "Because the resources needed are not widely available, new strategies are needed to adapt methods of intensive treatment for use in the general community at less cost and effort" [1]. The DCCT investigators were not specifically proposing the use of computers, but as will be highlighted here perhaps IT-based tools deserve closer attention.

Furthermore there have been other randomized controlled trials (RCTs) that have highlighted the potential benefits of a more flexible approach to diabetes care. The dose adjustment for normal eating (DAFNE) approach has been pioneered in Dusseldorf [7] and since trialled in Bucharest [8] and elsewhere [9], as well as more recently in the UK [10]. This has shown that a structured training

International Textbook of Diabetes Mellitus, Third Edition. Edited by R. A. DeFronzo, E. Ferrannini, H. Keen, and P. Zimmet.
 ISBN: 0-471-48655-8.

course designed to maintain blood glucose (BG) control while enabling dietary freedom—teaching diabetes self-management skills to patients with type 1 diabetes—can be effective in improving glycemic control [7–10]. The DAFNE educational model, which focuses on teaching patients the skills to self-adjust insulin dosages for carbohydrate, seems also to be associated with an improved sense of self-efficacy and treatment satisfaction [11].

There are clearly not enough diabetes educators to provide the sort of IIT offered in the DCCT, and even DAFNE-style structured teaching sessions can be workforce/HCP intensive and time-consuming. Therefore perhaps computer-assisted learning (CAL) tools may be able to help [12], particularly if there arises a need to offer repeat education to diabetic patients over a period of time.

COMPUTING BACKGROUND

Endeavors to apply IT routinely in diabetes care have been attempted for many years, but despite the novel work undertaken it is fair to say that the impact of computers in clinical diabetes practice thus far has been relatively limited.

Figure 1 summarizes the spectrum of IT applications relevant to clinical practice. The acceptance scale indicates how widely such applications have been adopted into routine clinical care. For example, BG meters (either with or without electronic memories) are well-accepted tools. By contrast at the other end of the spectrum computerized decision support is not at all widely used, at present [13].

It is clear that many of the earlier attempts at the "intelligent" application of computers in diabetes care were

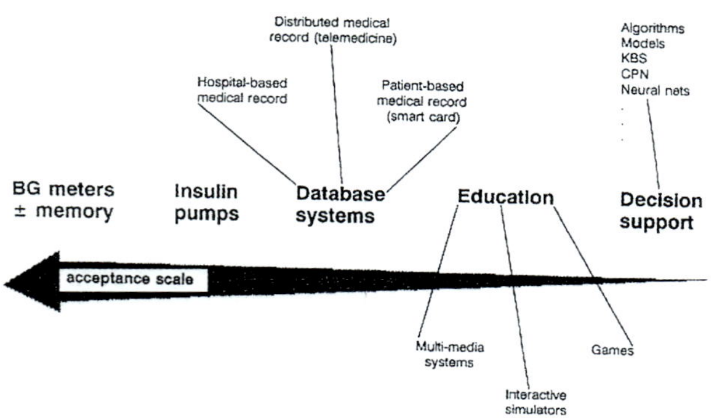

Figure 1 Spectrum of information technology applications in clinical diabetes care. The acceptance scale indicates how widely such applications have been adopted into routine clinical practice. Education and decision support could be for patients, relatives, students, or health care professionals. (BG = blood glucose, KBS = knowledge-based system, CPN = causal probabilistic network). All these different applications can equally be applied on standalone devices/computers, or via Internet-based programs, the exact implementation being less important than the functionality being provided (reproduced by permission from reference 13)

not sophisticated enough [14, 15]; user interfaces were primitive and prototypes difficult to use. However, further development and improvement of such systems was also limited by the fact that physicians with busy clinical practices did not see a need for, or have a desire to use, such software programs. In addition, system developers certainly can be faulted for not demonstrating, through rigorous retrospective and prospective clinical trials, the safety and efficacy of their applications.

Unfortunately, novel technologies can sometimes be introduced into medical practice with little by way of assessment or evaluation. This lack of validation is particularly marked with the application of computers in clinical diabetes care—where very few studies demonstrating the benefits of computer programs or IT systems have been reported [16]. In many cases system developers perceive the benefits as "self-evident," and therefore proponents consider it "intuitive" that a computer-based approach will have advantages over a conventional pen/paper-based predecessor. However in practice often these "advantages" are not quite so clear-cut. In addition the science of evaluating the utility of such programs and surveying users of such software is still very much in its infancy—particularly in diabetes care [17].

CURRENT COMPUTER APPLICATIONS

Many workers have suggested that IT may be able to assist in the transfer of knowledge and expertise from specialist diabetes centers to general practitioners (GPs) and practice nurses, as well as directly to patients [18–22]. The concept of providing a type 1 diabetic patient with a hand-held electronic log that could store BG readings and give the patient advice about the next meal or insulin injection may be seen as an exciting one [23]. However, the development of a hand-held log that could provide patient-specific advice and be able to justify its reasoning is a nontrivial problem that has not yet really been solved. Furthermore, such a system even if developed and validated would only really be of use in health care systems that could afford the costs of the relatively high technology involved.

A complimentary approach, however, might be to use similar IT techniques as a way of *teaching* patients about insulin dosage, dietary and exercise adjustments in diabetes. The idea being that once properly educated with a deeper understanding as to how changes in their therapeutic regimen could affect their BG control, motivated patients should be in a better position to optimize their own therapy with guidance from their HCPs. Such educational application of these techniques may be particularly pertinent because—rather than doing something for a patient all the time—teaching them how to do it for themselves may possibly lead to a much more lasting (and possibly better) result.

There has been in recent years a rapid growth in the development of prototype computer systems to assist in a number of different areas of clinical diabetes care: (a) as computerized outpatient clinic databases that store patients' clinical and biochemical data, in some cases also providing the HCP with management advice/access to electronic guidelines; (b) as statistical and graphical analysis programs that help the HCP and/or patient detect patterns and trends in the patient's home self-monitoring BG (SMBG) readings; (c) as dietary analysis programs that examine food composition and dietary exchanges and help devise meal plans; (d) as hand-held computers that store and graph BG data, and/or provide patients with insulin dosage adjustment advice either on a day-by-day or a meal-by-meal basis; (e) as interactive educational simulators that allow patients and students to practice and gain experience with insulin dosage and dietary/exercise adjustments, without actually exposing themselves to the risks of hypoglycemia; (f) as other computer-assisted teaching/learning tools; (g) as expert systems and question and answer programs for patient education; and (h) as educational games for diabetic children.

A selection of these computer applications will be reviewed in this chapter. However, it is important to stress that the software highlighted here represents just some of the hundreds of programs that have been developed and/or are available. Because of space limitations, computer prototypes solely offering dietary education and advice [24–30] will not be reviewed here.

DATABASE SYSTEMS

Personal Programs

A practical way by which people with type 1 and type 2 diabetes are already seeing benefits from IT applications is through the use of personal database programs. These generally can download data from BG meters to personal computers (PCs) and can graph and summarize the results (Figure 2). A wide range of these have been reviewed elsewhere [31]. However *BGTracker* is a good example of such a program. It works on IBM-compatible PCs running 32-bit Windows'95^{TM} (or later) operating systems. Available for free from www.bgtracker.com, the software allows SMBG data to be downloaded from a BG meter, or entered manually. A whole plethora of variables can be stored, summarized, and graphed. Reports can then be printed out for later discussion with a HCP.

Such programs allow motivated and interested patients to take these graphs to their clinic appointment. The rationale underlying the use of software like this is the recognition that in the limited time available for most routine clinical diabetes consultations there is simply no time for a physician to properly review all the BG data that a patient

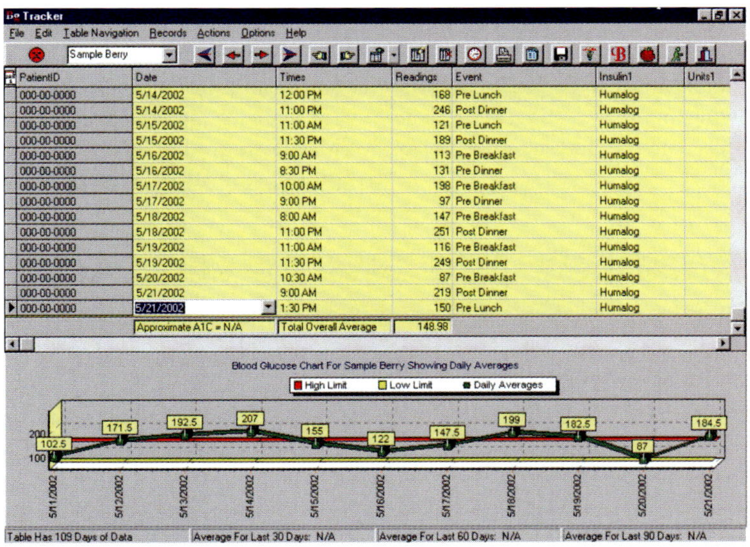

Figure 2 Screenshot from the free *BGTracker* software. This screen for insulin-dependent (type 1) diabetic patients provides the main entry point for recording data that is associated primarily with blood glucose (BG) meter testing. The data entry form records date, time, BG reading, event, time between events, and has a small notes field. Users can enter records either manually or with a wizard. Once collected the data can then be formatted into a comprehensive report for the doctor or personal use. There is a dynamic chart at the bottom that shows at a glance a week's worth of data averages, ensuring instant feedback regarding the user's BG levels. The form has a speed button tool bar for fast navigation of menu items. The status bar at the bottom is for showing users the average BG level for the previous 30, 60, and 90 days. The program, including all forms, allows for an unlimited number of users (e.g., for different members of a family) with separate data stored for each. The form can be customized for the users' individual needs. BG readings can be in either mg/dl or mmol/l (reproduced by permission of Mr. Jim Berry © www.bgtracker.com)

may have collected in a standard logbook. By contrast the hope is that perhaps by summarizing the data beforehand in graphical or tabular form the physician may be able to make better clinical use of the data [32].

While this approach is intuitively appealing—and offers dedicated patients some "rewards" for all the pain of collecting SMBG data—it needs to be recognized that there remains an absolute paucity of evaluation data in the literature showing a benefit from the use of such computer programs. Also it is still unclear what is the optimum way to present the data collected. For example, do physicians benefit most from graphs or tables of BG data? Or would it be better for the computer to simply highlight untoward or unexplained events such as hypo- and hyperglycemic episodes. Much further research is needed in this area [32].

GlucoControl is a free piece of software for handheld personal digital assistants (PDAs) running the Microsoft™ Pocket PC operating system. The program stores manually entered SMBG data and as such is intended to replace a standard paper-based diabetes notebook. Figure 3 shows some screenshots from this application. The program facilitates data entry and automatically calculates the average BG level for the last 7 and 30 days. It also can generate line graphs showing the BG level over a previous user-specified period. Furthermore, warning levels can be added for BG values over 200 mg/dl (11.1 mmol/l) and under 50 mg/dl (2.8 mmol/l), the aim being to facilitate increased understanding of the readings being collected. The data are stored in a Microsoft™ Access database, which allows the information to be exported to a conventional PC for further analyses. *GlucoControl*—available from www.glucocontrol.org/eng—is one of a growing number of programs that are being distributed widely on the Internet for PDA devices.

Hospital-based Systems

Although paper-based hospital medical records have served clinical medicine well for a long time, needs appear to be changing. In addition to being used for routine patient care there is a growing requirement to be able to regularly and rapidly access components of patient records for audit, research, and management purposes. Manually trawling through notes to retrieve such information is inefficient and prohibitively time-consuming. Furthermore if required on a frequent basis—for example to automatically identify patients who have missed an important test or follow-up appointment—paper-based audit becomes completely impracticable. Given this, in diabetes care where patient notes can grow to many volumes—and where the accuracy of the information recorded can become increasingly difficult to verify as time passes—increasing interest is focusing on the application of electronic patient records (EPRs).

This interest is being driven by the fact that the digital storage of data is becoming increasingly feasible and cheap. A megabyte of disc storage only costs a few cents and we now have the processing power to handle large quantities of data electronically. Therefore, at last there appear to be basic computer systems powerful enough to address some of the failings of paper-based clinical record systems, as well as potentially being able to assist doctors in the provision of high-quality medical care.

Computerized databases and clinical record systems offer the promise of much greater selective medical follow-up of patients, with opportunities for improved screening and health promotion/disease prevention. This is as true for diabetes mellitus as it is for other medical conditions. Monitoring outcomes in diabetes care, such as the degree or severity of retinopathy and microalbuminuria, also

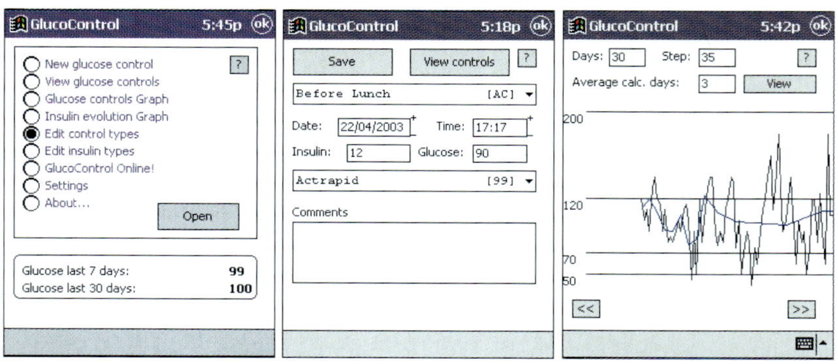

Figure 3 Shows some screenshots from the free *GlucoControl* diabetes personal digital assistant (PDA) software. Left: The main screen shows all available options. In the lower part of the screen the average glycemic control for the last 7 and 30 days are shown (in mg/dl). Middle: This is the data entry screen that aims to provide similar facilities to a standard diabetes logbook. Date and time data are completed automatically (but may be changed manually by the user). Right: This screen shows a graph with glucose values introduced during the previous *n* days. The rolling average glucose over that period is shown on screen in a different color. The graph aims to be an easier way to track the BG values over time, as compared with a more standard diabetes notebook, which only shows long lists of numbers (Reproduced by permission of Mr. Fernando Rafart © www.glucocontrol.org/eng)

potentially offers a valuable way of improving the provision and quality of such care. For this, computer-based records to keep track of clinical details and monitor when patients are due for their next appointment or specialist test could be invaluable. The incorporation of structured data entry screens into such systems could also provide a useful prompt to the user (clinician) when the time comes to recheck the patient's eyes, feet, renal function, etc. Prototype systems such as this have been described in the literature, and are being used in some dedicated centers for routine data storage [33].

However, various limiting factors to the widespread use of such applications exist. One issue remains the data itself. Unless a great deal of time and resource can be devoted to manual data entry of previous patient information (i.e., typing in whole clinic loads of data), paper-based and computerized medical record systems will need to be run in parallel for a considerable period of time. Furthermore the computerization of diabetes medical records needs to be managed in harmony with other medical record systems. While computer records will be of use in the diabetes clinic—unless the rest of the hospital records are computerized—paper-based diabetes records will need to be kept for some considerable time to maintain compatibility with the (old) pre-existing hospital-wide system of storing notes [34]. In addition, if for example the asthma clinic develops its own computer database system, and so does the hypertension clinic and the obstetric clinic, it is not difficult to envisage some of the logistical problems for storage of medical records that could ensue for a hypertensive, diabetic patient who became pregnant and developed some shortness of breath. To date, relatively few of these issues have been rigorously addressed. One solution might be to make patients responsible for holding their own medical records—for instance on a smart card [35–37], although issues of data security and backup still remain to be resolved. Another possibility is the use of distributed systems that could eventually see data reside on computers both at patients' homes and in hospitals, or even possibly both in primary and secondary care. However, as diabetic patients also have general medical and surgical problems—outside the specialist remit of diabetologists/endocrinologists—it seems highly probable that diabetes electronic medical records will need to fit in with computerization of the wider health care system [34]. Furthermore, the attempts to transfer diabetes care to primary care means that GPs also now need to access such databases, which must cater for a much wider variety of general medical data.

Electronic Patient Records

The St. Vincent Declaration [38] in part looked to use IT for quality assurance of diabetes health care provision and laboratory and technical procedures in diabetes diagnosis, treatment, and self-management. Now 14 years on, a multitude of database applications are available to monitor and document the level of care provided to patients with diabetes [39, 40]. Although it could be argued that too many different database programs are being developed—and therefore perhaps efforts are unnecessarily being duplicated—hopefully at least common datasets are starting to be being agreed upon [41] so that regardless of the application being used, data will eventually become compatible and therefore accessible locally, regionally, and nationally for research and audit. However, much work needs to be done to ensure data security and safeguard patient confidentiality, especially as data start to be transferred between primary and secondary care and between hospitals and regions, particularly with the use of the Internet.

Although databases may not be viewed as the most exciting area of medical informatics research, they are an area in which a clinical impact is being routinely made, now. Also perhaps one of the failings of earlier semi-intelligent decision-support prototypes (see below) rests with the lack of stable, computerized medical record systems that could "feed" the decision-support software with data. In this respect, as with EPRs, one of the major problems with decision-support systems has been their lack of integration into more standard hospital information systems [42]. The need for decision-support programmers to design and code their own individual small databases unnecessarily prolonged the development cycle, increased compatibility problems, and made the wider dissemination of the prototypes for evaluation by others all the more difficult.

It is expected that a proactive EPR, able to provide advice and access to guidelines and reminders, should be able to improve the quality of care [42, 43]; although, as with so many developments in the diabetes-computing field, formal evaluation studies will be required to confirm this.

However the jury is still out regarding whether such databases (EPRs) and registers, once evaluated, might offer an *affordable* method of improving care for patients with both type 1 and type 2 diabetes. The current trend seems to be to integrate guidelines and decision-support systems as reminders within EPRs, to support more complex primary care interventions. In this respect, to date in the diabetes field, researchers have at least shown that the use of computerized guidelines for diabetes management can improve *compliance* with accepted standards of care [42, 44].

DECISION SUPPORT

Algorithmic-based Systems

Clinical algorithms are general guidelines of empirical origin, most often encapsulated by a set of rules. Such rules of the form *if feature X is present then do action Y*

Table 1 Algorithms for adjusting insulin doses using an ultralente/3-dose regular insulin regimen, patient self-monitoring of blood glucose, and hyperglycemia not explained by unusual diet/exercise/insulin

If fasting BG on arising is greater than 7.2 mmol/l (130 mg/dl) for 2 days in a row, increase the ultralente insulin by 1–2 U.
If BG 2 h after breakfast is greater than 8.3 mmol/l (150 mg/dl), or if BG before lunch is greater than 7.2 mmol/l (130 mg/dl) for 2 days in a row, increase the morning regular insulin by 1–2 U.
If BG 2 h after breakfast is greater than 8.3 mmol/l (150 mg/dl), but less than 5.8 mmol/l (105 mg/dl) before lunch, consult HCP.
If BG 2 h after lunch is greater than 8.3 mmol/l (150 mg/dl), or if BG before supper is greater than 7.2 mmol/l (130 mg/dl) for 2 days in a row, increase the prelunch regular insulin by 1–2 U.
If BG 2 h after lunch is consistently greater than 8.3 mmol/l (150 mg/dl) and BG before supper is less than 5.8 mmol/l (105 mg/dl), consult HCP.
If BG 2 h after supper is greater than 8.3 mmol/l (150 mg/dl), or if BG at bedtime is greater than 7.2 mmol/l (130 mg/dl) for 2 days in a row, increase presupper regular insulin by 1–2 U.
If BG 2 h after supper is greater than 8.3 mmol/l (150 mg/dl), but less than 5.8 mmol/l (105 mg/dl) before bedtime snack, consult HCP.

Note: BG = blood glucose; HCP = health care professional.
Derived with permission from reference 45.

reflect the heuristics of the routine therapeutic strategy that attempts to lead the patient to progressively better control by suggesting stepwise changes to the dose or distribution of insulin in response to the observed patterns of BG control. Clinical algorithms may recommend changes to the basic insulin dosage regimen as well as to the anticipatory/supplementary insulin adjustments that may be required.

Advising on possible adjustments often is based on the assessment of time periods in which a particular insulin injection has a dominant role (for example, an injection of regular [short-acting] insulin will be active for approximately 6 h following the injection). One set of such production rules was published by Skyler and colleagues in 1981 [45] (Table 1). Similar algorithms have been implemented by other groups, and computer devices that work with BG measurements for split-mixed regimens, for continuous subcutaneous insulin infusions (pump therapy), and for various other insulin regimens have been developed [46].

Theoretically, hand-held computers incorporating clinical algorithms have the potential to bring the diabetologists' expert knowledge to the patient, at each injection. The algorithms built into such systems generally include formulae for suggesting supplementary insulin doses to cope with the anticipated and unwanted effects that unusual lifestyle events may produce in the future. Such changes can be made, if necessary, several times a day.

Most of these devices in the early days were based on commercial pocket calculators providing various degrees of data capture, therapeutic advice, and follow-up consultations. As an example, the hand-held Insulin Dosage Computer (IDC) was based on a HP-41CV programmable calculator [46]. This could be customized by the physician by setting its parameters, including the BG target, for each patient with certain safety limits and with a maximum permissible insulin dose [46–48]. At each injection, the device scanned its memory and analyzed the past as well as current BG data for features that determined the insulin dose to be administered. In addition to suggesting adjustments to the patient's basic insulin dosage, this device also allowed immediate therapeutic control adjustments to be made whenever a preprandial BG value was much higher or lower than the reference level set for that time period. Supplements could be calculated by means of simple formulae [46].

The patient only had to estimate the change from their usual carbohydrate intake, or the change in the intensity of anticipated physical activity (on a scale ranging between 1 and 5), and modify the timing and/or dose of the appropriate insulin injection accordingly. Thus an extra 4 units of regular (short-acting) insulin might be added if the patient ate an additional 60 g of carbohydrate. Use of such supplements coupled with appropriate changes in the insulin dosage regimen permitted some flexibility in the patient's lifestyle without apparently sacrificing BG control [48].

However, despite a number of interesting evaluation studies (although not all randomized) having been run with the IDC [23, 49, 50], with glycosylated hemoglobin (HbA_{1c}) levels as endpoints, and the item being sold commercially, the device does not seem to have achieved very widespread use in routine clinical practice. This may be because clinical algorithms do have some fundamental limitations. These include the fact that the rule-set needs to be very large to cover all anticipated situations in a consistent way. Incompleteness makes such systems inadequate when facing complex situations that either are not explicitly stated or in which more than one feature occurs that would require some response. Also algorithms cannot explain their reasoning.

Knowledge-based Systems

Knowledge-based systems (KBS) have been proposed as a possible alternative to algorithms. KBS with more comprehensive medical knowledge can be used in a variety of situations not anticipated in advance. Knowledge can be stored in various forms [51]. Some intelligent systems may use rule-based formalisms applied in context, explanations associated with each rule, and temporal reasoning. The knowledge bases of such systems consist of pathophysiological information, objects, actions, and diagnostic and therapeutic decisions. These qualitative reasoning techniques in general try to mimic the way in which HCPs select control actions (e.g., insulin-dosage adjustments) to correct the problems identified in SMBG data [52–54]. Introducing qualitative BG categories to replace continuous measurement data, time periods to replace the discrete time points at which BG data were sampled, and a description of problems in the glucose supply all help to formulate a technical description about what is observed, using a terminology that should be clear to fellow clinicians.

Problem-oriented reasoning may be a useful means of guiding decision making. However, coping with situations in which more than one problem exists becomes more complicated when the problems are of a different nature; for example, if data show hypoglycemia in one period of the day and severe hyperglycemia in another period—especially if these periods overlap or the events are causally interrelated (as is the case with rebound hyperglycemia). Moreover, therapeutic recommendations need to respond to a variety of patterns in longer-term BG data, and the temporal evolution of other markers such as HbA_{1c} or fructosamine equally need to be considered.

However, decision support is a complex area. The inability of current KBS prototypes to deal with complicated or conflicting situations severely limits the usefulness of current qualitative approaches, especially since it is in these difficult cases that the computer's assistance might be most useful. In this respect a detailed review of the use of computers in diabetes care some years back came to conclusion that none of the KBS-based approaches were sufficiently robust or safe to be used as insulin-dosage advisors [15]. Not much seems to have changed in the intervening period. Having reviewed the literature again and considered why KBS-based decision-support prototypes have not been more widely used, it has become apparent that algorithmic-based approaches do offer a computational robustness and practicality, difficult to provide at present by other means.

Algorithms Revisited: Telemedicine Advice

Algorithms by their very nature cannot cope with situations not explicitly stated. However they can cater for a large variety of situations—and if they can offer 90% coverage this could provide significant practical benefit to a considerable number of patients. Although intellectually it may not be so satisfying to use algorithms that are not comprehensive, they do seem to warrant closer attention.

An example of an algorithmic, telemedicine-based system is the *HumaLink* prototype [55]—formerly called *TeleDoc* [15]. Having measured their BG levels, patients can access the system remotely from any touch-tone telephone, whether at home or while travelling, 24 h a day. Patients are encouraged to call *HumaLink* at each BG measurement, if possible, and particularly when an insulin dosage is to be recommended. After identifying themselves with their own unique personal identification number, patients follow verbal instructions from the speech synthesizer in the computer, and key in their BG measurement(s) along with any other information about illness, hypoglycemia, changes in activity, unusual carbohydrate intake, and medication. The system verbally verifies each entry before accepting it into the patient's personal database.

The program is meant to then relay instructions in accordance with an individualized treatment plan programmed by the caller's physician. Following the computer's provision of verbal advice down the telephone line the system requires patient confirmation of the instructions given, by verbally requesting that patients key-in the new insulin dose(s).

The program can operate in manual or fully automated advisory mode. In manual recording/documenting mode the computer logs the patient's readings, and a physician reviews the data before leaving a verbal message for the patient on the system. The next time the patient telephones he/she will receive the physician's advice about what therapy adjustment(s) to make. All interactions by the HCP are documented and become part of the patient's legal medical record. A facility is also provided to forward courtesy reports automatically by fax from the *HumaLink* computer to the patient's referring physician [15].

The fully automated advisory mode applies algorithms to modify insulin dosages within predefined limits set by the physician. Using trigger levels, guidelines, and instructions that are meant to be individualized for each patient, the system can also automatically react on behalf of the physician immediately when a crisis (such as hypoglycemia) is reported or whenever BG control deviates from the targets set for that particular patient. Details of the advisory module that utilizes a pursuit algorithm have been reported elsewhere [46].

If the patient's BG profile does not respond in the manner expected, this is flagged by the computer for the physician's attention. The guidance provided and/or preset threshold levels are then reset in order to direct the pursuit algorithm in an alternative, more appropriate direction. These interactive capabilities, together with automatic safety limits built into the system, are intended to ensure patient safety. Although it is possible to construct rules and algorithms to be conservative and therefore that should *theoretically* be safe, apprehensions always exist about computers deciding on patient therapy, without human intervention. Clearly this is not a concern restricted to diabetes computing, but rather a much more general issue, with medicolegal implications [56] for the entire decision-support field of medical informatics [57]. With *HumaLink* such concerns are at least in part addressed by allowing periodic human clinical review of the data and possible human intervention, if required, via the central telemedicine computer. By contrast such supervisory input clearly could not be provided with earlier hand-held prototypes [46]. Preliminary safety and efficacy beta-testing experience with *HumaLink* has been described in three open case series [55, 58, 59]—although randomized validation studies in separate centers, and by independent workers, are still awaited.

Other Telemedicine-based Approaches

Although not focused on algorithms, an interesting piece of telemedicine-based work is currently receiving funding from the US Centers for Medicare and Medicaid Services. This organization is supporting a large-scale demonstration project evaluating the cost-effectiveness of telemedicine-based disease management in diabetes. A consortium led by Columbia University has been selected to carry out the project in the New York state area, and it has received a US$28 million grant [42, 60, 61]. The goal of this Informatics for Diabetes Education and Telemedicine (IDEATel) project is to establish a disease management program on the basis of telemedicine solutions for citizens in rural or urban underserved areas. Each patient has received a home telemedicine unit, a PC-based device that enables downloading of BG data, blood pressure readings, Internet access to educational material, and videoconferencing with a case manager. The case manager and GPs have access via the Internet to software that is linked to a clinical information system. Fifteen hundred patients will be randomized to a control and intervention group. The main outcomes of the study will be HbA_{1c} levels, blood pressure, and cost of care, but other outcomes will be considered, such as quality of life, patient compliance, and their use of clinical services [42]. It will be interesting to see what the effects of such a high profile, big budget IT project are on clinical diabetes care.

Descriptions of a range of other telemedicine-based prototypes can be found elsewhere in the literature [62–64]. It is also beyond the scope of this chapter to review all the hand-held devices—with or without telemedicine links—that have been developed to give patients therapeutic advice. However, descriptions of a number of these can be found elsewhere [65, 66].

EDUCATIONAL SYSTEMS

Collecting SMBG data is not sufficient to improve metabolic control [67, 68]. Although educational work may be considered less "glamorous" than the latest "artificial intelligence" decision-support endeavors, education is a key means of improving understanding in medicine. As CAL is changing the way that people are taught [69], so it is likely that CAL techniques applied to health care education may provide powerful tools for the teaching and motivation of both patients and health care students. Furthermore, with the massive expansion of the Internet over the past few years, there at last appears to be a stable common platform that will greatly increase accessibility to on-line teaching from (remote) centers of excellence.

Is diabetes education already not widely available? The simple answer is no. In a survey of over 2400 patients to determine the proportion of adults with diabetes in the United States who had received diabetes education, it was found that over 41% of type 1 diabetic patients had never attended a class or program about diabetes [70]. Furthermore, even when education is made available, there may be a tendency to explain the disease rather than ensure that patients acquire the reflexes and expertise that will genuinely enable them to manage their diabetes [71]. Therefore there is clearly room for improvement, and perhaps IT can help [72].

There are many different aspects to diabetes education, but learning facts is only one of these [73]. The ability to gain experience is also of great importance. In this respect, education is difficult if based only on verbal and written presentations of dry facts [74]. Teaching materials using multimedia presentations may provide a partial solution. However, the aim should also be to teach diabetes self-management to patients in an intuitive and enjoyable way, so that the knowledge can be enduring. Clearly it is not ideal to learn about diabetes control solely from real life experiences because of the long time frame involved, aside from the possible dangers to the patient of hypo- or hyperglycemia [75]. An interactive simulation of a diabetic patient might be one solution [76].

In the same way that aircraft pilots and air traffic controllers are trained for routine and emergency procedures on airplane and air traffic simulators, so it should be possible for diabetic patients and health care students to be trained to make appropriate responses to everyday situations using a diabetes simulator in absolute safety, and in a relatively short space of time [75]. In this respect, management of error is a key component of the learning process. Identifying the error, getting patients to discover it for themselves, and asking how they would correct it are essential steps in educating patients *how* to improve their BG control [71].

This point may be addressed by the use of diabetes simulators for the education of patients and their relatives, students, and even possibly some HCPs [76]. The purpose of such simulation tools is to create a learning environment for communicating and training intuitive thinking when dealing with insulin dosage, dietary, and lifestyle adjustments. As other researchers [77] have highlighted, such educational simulators are intended "neither to compete with normal diabetes education nor with dose adjustment algorithm programs, but rather to support these ... The increasing number of young persons with computer experience suggests an increasing acceptance of computer simulation and learning programs. This is particularly important where patient management of the disease is demanded" [77].

Use of Simulators for Education

One particular simulator, called *AIDA*, has been developed by this author in conjunction with colleagues [78] and seems to be one of the most widely distributed and currently used pieces of educational diabetes computer software. *AIDA* is a freeware program for IBM-compatible PCs, or Apple Macintosh computers running PC emulation software. It is not protected by any patents. The program permits the interactive simulation of plasma insulin and BG profiles for demonstration, teaching, self-learning, and research purposes. Since March 1996, it has been made available without charge on the World Wide Web as a noncommercial contribution to continuing diabetes education. In the 8 years since its original Internet launch, over 400 000 visits have been logged to the *AIDA* Web pages at www.2aida.org and over 80 000 copies of the program have been downloaded, free of charge. Further copies have been made available, in the past, on diskette by the system developers and from the former British Diabetic Association (now called Diabetes UK), London, UK [79].

The software has been described in detail elsewhere [73, 78, 80]. Briefly, it incorporates a compartmental physiological model that describes glucose–insulin interaction in patients completely lacking endogenous insulin secretion. It contains a single extracellular glucose compartment into which glucose enters via both intestinal absorption and hepatic glucose production. The *AIDA* model also contains separate compartments for plasma and active insulin [78, 81], the latter being responsible for glycemic control while insulin is removed from the former by hepatic degradation. The actual mathematics underlying the model have been documented elsewhere [78].

Numerous physiological (minimal) models of the human glucoregulatory system have been described [82–84]—but these are not really so useful to patients, their relatives, HCPs, or students without some sort of program to allow easy access to and interaction with the model. Also, although other interactive simulators of glucose–insulin interaction in diabetes have been described in the literature [76, 81, 85–89] to date these do not seem to have been distributed widely via the Internet, or been made particularly widely available. Furthermore for a number of these [85–88] it would seem that readers are wholly dependent on the authors' own descriptions of their prototypes in research articles, since no versions appear to be available for general use by others.

Figure 4 demonstrates a little of what *AIDA* can do. In the representation of an *AIDA* simulation shown, a baseline BG simulation is displayed by the grey line for a twice daily short and intermediate-acting (Actrapid and Lente) insulin injection regimen. Superimposed in black on the top graph, is a simulation for educational use demonstrating the hyperglycemia that would result from delaying the morning insulin injection until after breakfast [90]. The software comes with 40 such example case scenarios for simulation, and other cases can be added or created by users. Further examples of the sort of simulations that *AIDA* can provide, for free, can be found elsewhere in the literature [12, 17, 73, 75] or at www.2aida.org on the Internet.

Although *AIDA* represents one of an increasing number of diabetes-related programs that are becoming available, or being widely distributed, via the Internet, such diabetes

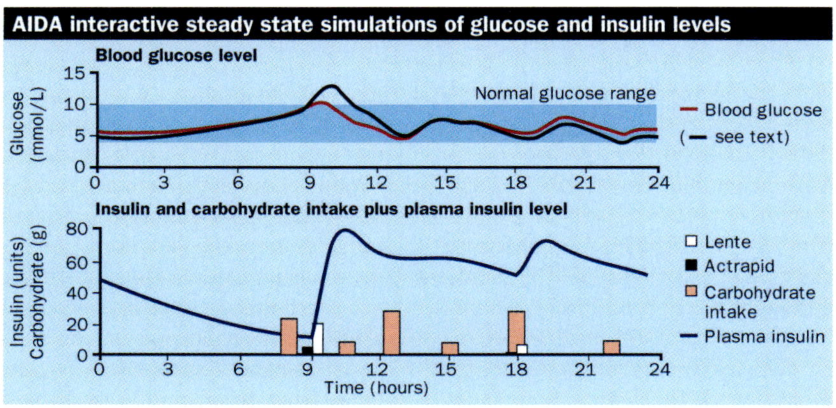

Figure 4 In the representation of an *AIDA* simulation shown, a baseline BG simulation is displayed by the grey line for a twice daily short- and intermediate-acting (actrapid and lente) insulin injection regimen. Superimposed in black on the top graph is a simulation for educational use demonstrating the hyperglycemia that would result from delaying the morning insulin injection until after breakfast (1 mmol/l = 18 mg/dl) (Reproduced by permission, from reference 90)

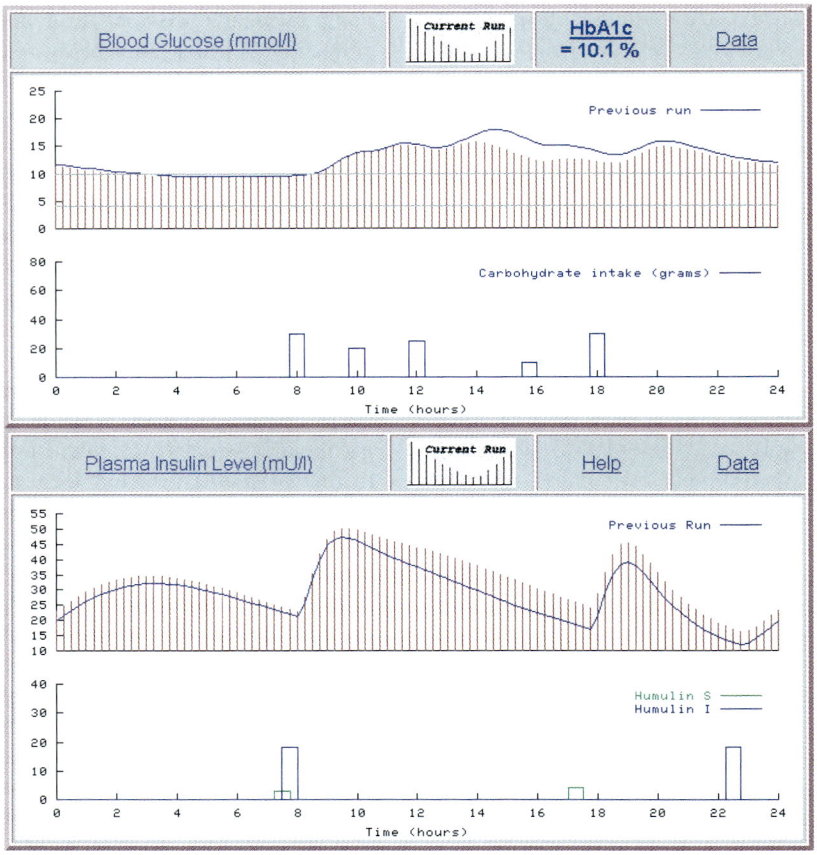

Figure 5 Simulation from *AIDA online* at www.2aida.net on the Web. The graphs show a BG simulation for an example case scenario from the *AIDA online* database. Further cases can be created by users. Upper panel: BG level and carbohydrate intake over a 24-h period. User definable normoglycemic ranges (4–10 mmol/l [72–180 mg/dl]) are shown superimposed. Lower panel: Plasma insulin level and injections of Humulin S (short-acting) and Humulin I (intermediate-acting) insulin. The baseline simulation is shown as the solid line (previous run), while the current simulation is shown by the vertical lines. For the current simulation run there has been an increase in the Humulin I insulin dose injected at 07:45 a.m., from 12 units to 18 units, and a decrease in the carbohydrate content of lunch, from 40 g to 25 g. As can be seen, injecting more insulin before breakfast and decreasing the size of lunch leads to a reduction in the BG profile predicted in the afternoon. If this change was effected long-term, this is also predicted to lead to an improvement in *AIDA*'s glycosylated hemoglobin (HbA_{1c}) level (10.6% at baseline [89] versus 10.1% after these adjustments). The HbA_{1c} value shown gives an indication—for educational purposes only—of the glycosylated hemoglobin level predicted by the *AIDA* model, if the current glycemic control were to be maintained in the medium- to long-term (reproduced by permission from reference 89)

simulations are not solely accessible as downloadable executables. A Web-based version of the same educational diabetes simulator—called *AIDA on-line* - is also accessible for free at www.2aida.net—no downloads or local installation being required. A prototype version of this was developed during 1996/1997 and the facility became available for widespread usage in August 1998 [91]. Since then, over 230 000 simulations have been run at *AIDA on-line*. Figure 5 shows a little of what *AIDA on-line* can do. A baseline Web-based diabetes simulation is shown by the solid line (previous run) while the vertical lines show the current simulation run, following an increase in the intermediate-acting Humulin I insulin dose injected before breakfast and a decrease in the carbohydrate content of lunch. Space precludes the inclusion here of further examples. However, direct usage of www.2aida.net will show how it is possible to experiment with adjusting sample diabetes regimens for educational, self-learning, demonstration or research purposes [92, 93], safe from the risks of hyper- or hypo-glycemia. For those Website visitors unfamiliar with the diabetes domain—or what to try simulating next—an interactive Diabetes/Insulin Tutorial can also be accessed directly at www.2aida.org/tutorial. This teaches a little about balancing insulin and diet in diabetes [94], and is integrated with *AIDA on-line* so that users can—at appropriate places in the tutorial—interactively simulate some of what they have learnt, using the *AIDA* model [89].

To date *AIDA* seems to have been one of the most extensively investigated and evaluated educational diabetes

Table 2 Levels of evidence for clinical/educational use of software

Level 1 –	Formal, open, clinical randomized-controlled trials (RCTs)
Level 2 –	Case controlled trials (comparisons made but not randomized)
Level 3 –	Observational studies (including surveys and questionnaires)
Level 4 –	Anecdotal evidence (including independent user comments and reviews)
Level 5 –	Methodological verification and validation studies

Derived with permission from reference 17.

simulators, so it may be useful to outline here how the program has been tested.

Prototype Evaluation—What is Required?

A key requirement for, and limitation to, the widespread use and acceptance of computer-based tools in diabetes care is the need for validation data to show that the applications really work as intended, and evaluation data to show that they can support clinical diabetes care, and actually do some good. There are many different ways that such evaluation studies may be done. These range from qualitative approaches to quantitative studies. Table 2 summarizes some of the different sorts of studies that can be undertaken, and the different levels of evidence that can be generated to support clinical use of a diabetes computer program. Level 1 studies (RCTs) are clearly the gold standard method for rigorously assessing educational/clinical utility. Nevertheless useful information can also be obtained from less formal studies, and in many cases these can be easier to undertake and involve more subjects than do RCTs. A range of these studies have been done with the *AIDA* software, and it may be helpful to overview these to demonstrate the sort of evaluation studies that really need to be undertaken for all diabetes computing prototypes.

In the case of *AIDA*, under level 5 (methodological verification and validation studies), a quantitative assessment has been reported to document the accuracy of the BG simulations in a cohort of 30 patients with type 1 diabetes [95]. While the simulations were shown to be unsuitable for individual patient glycemic prediction and therapy planning, they have nevertheless found widespread use for educational/demonstration/self-learning/research purposes where individual predictive accuracy is less critical [96, 97].

Under level 4 (anecdotal evidence—including independent user comments and reviews) various program users have written for the Website, and in print, their thoughts about the PC software [12, 98–100] and the Web-based simulator [101–103]. Some short comments/"sound bites" have also appeared elsewhere [104–106].

Under level 3 (observational studies—including the use of surveys and questionnaires [107]) several audits have been undertaken concerning the software. These have focused on finding out who has been downloading the program [17, 108] and why they have been turning to the Internet for such information [109, 110]. These surveys, which have so far yielded over 7660 responses, have provided an interesting insight into who the *AIDA* end users actually are—over two thirds of respondents being people with diabetes or their relatives. Furthermore, interesting information about why these people have been turning to the program for diabetes-related information has also been obtained [109, 110]. In addition, these surveys seem to confirm that there is considerable interest on the Internet amongst diabetic patients to learn more about balancing insulin and diet in diabetes, as well as possibly to get more involved in self-management of insulin dosages.

Level 2 case controlled trials have not been undertaken with *AIDA*, but a pilot level 1 prospective, clinical RCT has been done with lessons run from November 1999 to June 2000. For this, a detailed protocol was defined *a priori* [111]. The RCT randomized 24 patients with type 1 diabetes to one of two study groups, each receiving different teaching interventions. The *AIDA* group was exposed to the diabetes simulator, while the control group received conventional lessons with slides and transparencies. Six lessons were held for each group (one per week). At the end of the conventional lessons, after a "washout" period of 4 weeks, the control group entered a partial crossover phase with the simulator during a further 6-week block of lessons. Before and after the 6 weeks of lessons, all subjects had their HbA_{1c} measured. The subjects also carefully documented the incidence and severity of any symptomatic hypoglycemic episodes (hypos). HbA_{1c} levels dropped significantly from 7.2 to 6.4% after lessons with the diabetes simulator ($p = 0.01$) (Figure 6a). By contrast, no significant changes in HbA_{1c} were observed in the control group between baseline (7.1%) and the end of the control lessons (7.0%), or the end of the crossover phase lessons (6.8%). The number of hypos decreased significantly from 31 to 14 ($p = 0.03$) after *AIDA* lessons (Figure 6b), but did not change significantly in the control group from baseline ($n = 20$) to after the control lessons ($n = 22$). However, the number of hypos did decrease significantly (to $n = 10$) after exposure to the simulator during the crossover phase ($p = 0.03$, vs 6-week data) [112, 113]. Larger trials involving more patients in more centers are clearly needed, but this pilot study does demonstrate how such diabetes-computing tools need to be evaluated in RCTs to obtain evidence of utility or efficacy. In this respect, some recommended guidelines [114] and training requirements [115] have been drawn up for HCPs planning to give lessons with the software. Also the program has been tried out for teaching GPs [116] and student nurses [117].

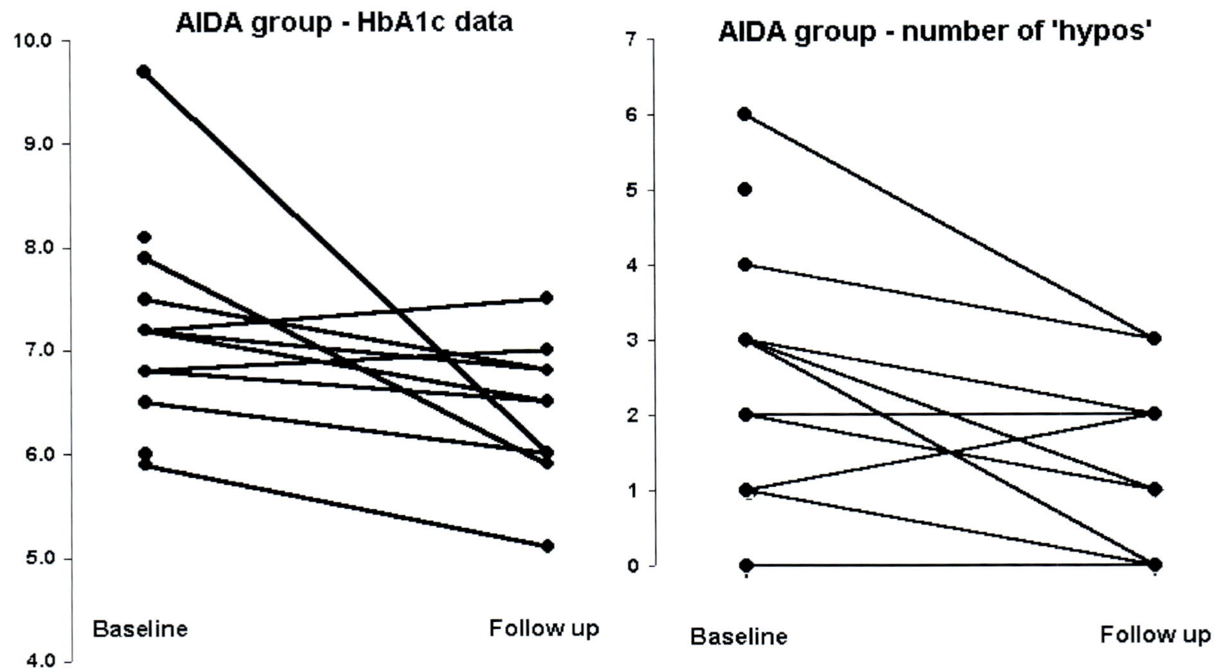

Figure 6 (a) Glycosylated hemoglobin (HbA_{1c}) data from a pilot randomized controlled trial testing out the *AIDA* diabetes simulator in small group teaching sessions. Baseline and follow-up HbA_{1c} data are shown in percent (%) for individuals in the *AIDA* simulator group. HbA_{1c} measured 4 weeks after end of cycle of 6 lessons. HbA_{1c} assay normal range = 4.5–5.5%; (b) Number of hypoglycemic episodes (hypos) in a pilot randomized controlled trial testing out the *AIDA* diabetes simulator in small group teaching sessions. Baseline and follow-up data for the number of symptomatic hypos for individuals in the *AIDA* simulator group (derived from reference 112 by permission of Editrice Kurtis s.r.l.)

An additional way of evaluating the use of such an educational diabetes simulator could test patients for proficiency in the management of a given simulated subject before and after some programmed instruction. The software could then evaluate the performance of the user by computing the number of hypos experienced by the simulated case, the average and standard deviations of the recorded BG levels, and the average and maximum amount of insulin administered during treatment, such quantitative analyses being used to (hopefully) demonstrate improvements in knowledge and ability following the simulator-based lessons. Comparisons of runs made before and after simulator-assisted instruction could also potentially be used to evaluate the effectiveness of this approach to education. Furthermore the use of a computer might remove some of the subjectiveness from the evaluation process and provide an impartial method of determining performance—i.e. using the computer to actually assist in the evaluation process. The Internet may also offer an ideal medium for running such studies, possibly via the use of Web-based tutorials [89] and on-line interactive simulations (Figure 5). Other issues for consideration about the use of RCTs for evaluation of educational diabetes simulators—including cost–benefit analyses—which are beyond the scope of this chapter have been discussed elsewhere [118, 119].

Educational Games for Children with Diabetes

When one considers that diabetes is for life, the importance of properly educating children with diabetes becomes apparent. One way of achieving this may be through the use of computers.

In this respect, a generation of patients with diabetes and relatives of patients are growing up for whom computers and the Internet are a completely natural and easy-to-use medium—people who are much more at ease with this technology than it is likely their parents will ever be.

Kids are at ease surfing the Internet and playing computer games. However, often when people think of games they do not consider serious applications. The dictionary definition of the word "game" includes amusement, diversion, entertainment, pastime, and recreation. However, none of these terms indicate that children learn a great deal about their environment simply by playing.

> It should be noted that children at play are not playing about; their games should be seen as their most serious-minded activity
> —Montaigne

Although traditional classroom lessons may provide more didactic content, a compelling video game can expose children to essential material repeatedly, as many children will typically play a game they like, for a considerable period of time. Games offer children opportunities to rehearse new skills and receive feedback on performance. Also playing video games with others can encourage children to talk about health topics and can serve as a springboard for discussion with friends, family, and HCPs about sensitive topics. There are good reasons to use the video game format to provide health education, since demand is high for both interactive games and for information about health [120]. In the United States more money is reported to be spent on video games than on films [121]. Along with interest in video games, interest is growing in health education and in health reference materials delivered on interactive media [122].

One of the first educational games for diabetic children was *BG Pilot* (Raya Systems, Inc., California, USA), which ran on most IBM PCs or compatibles. Underlying *BG Pilot* was a compartmental minimal model. In this program the user, typically a child with diabetes or a friend, was in control of a simple propeller-driven airplane. The purpose of the game was to pilot the airplane on a smooth course for a 3-day journey. Insulin, food, and exercise were provided as controls and the airplane's altitude represented BG. The user could administer shots of either short-acting or intermediate-acting insulin, take food, or exercise. As in any 36-h flight one had to sleep and therefore the user needed to ensure adequate glycemic control overnight. This might all sound simple enough, but if the airplane flew too high (hyperglycemia) it would hit the high-flying "dangerous ducks", while if it flew too low (hypoglycemia) it could hit the "treacherous trees" and crash (Figure 7a). Unlike other diabetes simulators

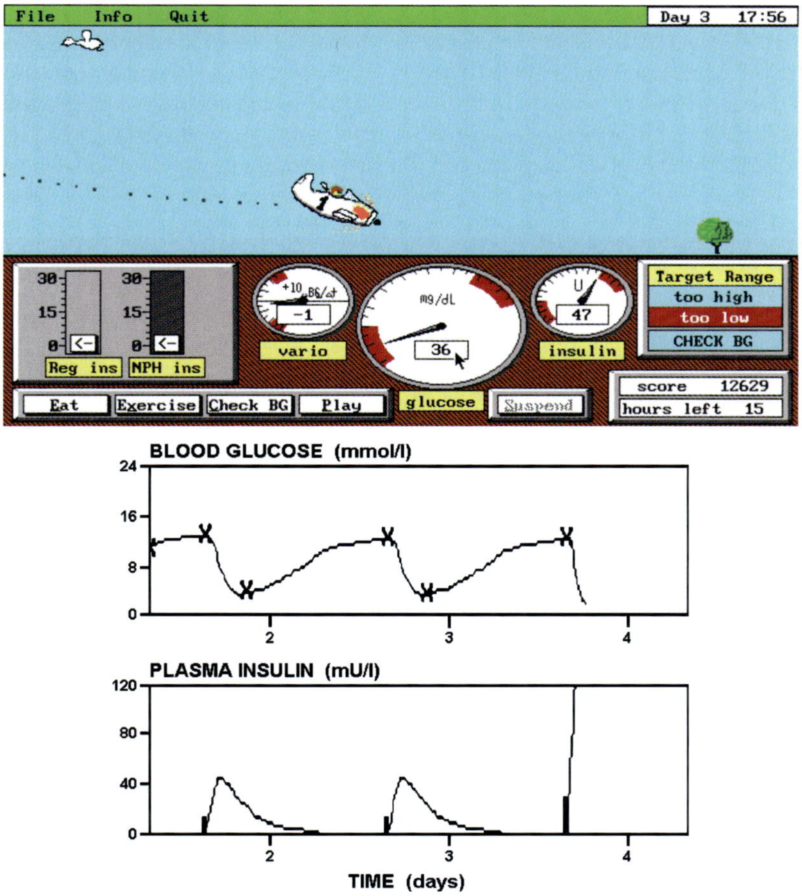

Figure 7 (a) Main interactive display of *BGPilot* showing the insulin, diet, and exercise controls for the airplane along with its flight path. The central large "speedometer" dial displays the BG reading in mg/dl (18 mg/dl = 1 mmol/l). The "vario" dial shows the change in BG with time while the insulin dial shows how much insulin is "on board". The user has to select the "Check BG" option to find out his/her actual BG level. As can be seen, the airplane is dropping rapidly following a large injection of insulin and is about to crash into one of the "treacherous trees"; (b) Summary graph of last flight of *BGPilot* shown in Figure 7a. In this example a child has been trying to control the airplane with just short-acting insulin. As a result the BG curve has been quite erratic. Eventually the child injected too much insulin and as a result the plasma insulin level sky-rockets and the BG level plummets. X = patient BG measurement (derived with permission from reference 76)

(Figures 4 and 5), with this game the user did not interact directly with the BG simulation, but rather the output from the model—the simulation—was used by the computer to fly the plane.

Controlling the airplane and adjusting the BG/altitude accordingly took skill, and it is expected that this would increase understanding of the underlying diabetes control processes involved. Furthermore, as the system was based on a compartmental model this methodology permitted the processes involved during a game to be studied in greater detail, which could be particularly of use for HCPs. Figure 7b shows one of the summary graphs that could be accessed either during or after a game. The ability to investigate the output from a compartmental model in more detail was one of the particular strengths of such approaches [123].

Captain Novocare (Raya Systems, Inc.) was the next game for diabetic children produced by this company on a PC platform, this time as an educational adventure. The game's super hero had diabetes and players had to manage his illness while fighting off sugary junk food aliens. The goal of the game was to rescue the mayor, who also had diabetes, before the supplies ran out. During the course of the game, information on managing diabetes was displayed on the screen. Using this information carefully gained additional points. The game occurred over two simulated days divided into stages that reflected a typical diabetes meal plan. Like *BG Pilot*, *Captain Novocare* was based on a compartmental model and was intended to provide diabetic children of school age with the opportunity to learn self-management skills in an interactive as well as fun and challenging way—something recognized to be very difficult to achieve using "traditional" educational techniques [76]. *Captain Novolin* (Raya Systems, Inc.) provided a re-engineering of the *Captain Novocare* approach on a Super Nintendo™ platform. Apart from the change in hardware, the big alteration involved the replacement of the compartmental modelling approach that had been used for both *BG Pilot* and *Captain Novocare* with a less physiological but simpler rule-based approach. The success of this Super Nintendo game (over 15 000 copies distributed in the first year alone) prompted the developers to introduce another game about diabetes called *Packy & Marlon* (Raya Systems, Inc.) for the Super Nintendo platform.

Packy & Marlon was designed to improve self-care, motivation, and behavior among children with diabetes. This was a role-playing game in which players managed the diet and insulin of two elephants who had diabetes (Figure 8).

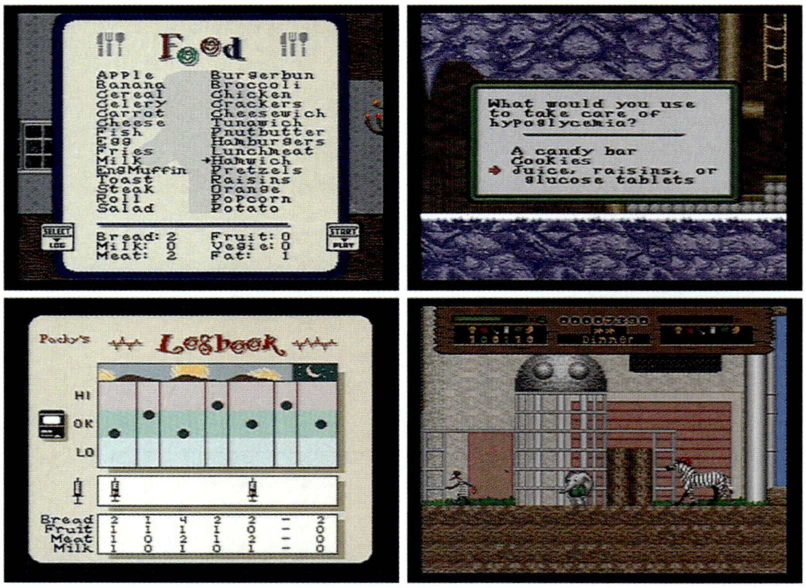

Figure 8 Screenshots from *Packy & Marlon* diabetes video/personal computer game. Packy and Marlon were two diabetic elephant pals who were involved in an action-adventure at a diabetes summer camp. Packy and Marlon followed a menu for 3 meals and 3 snacks each day. The game included 4 simulated days with 6 game levels per day, for a total of 24 game levels. To follow the menu, players could substitute one food for another as long as it was in the same food exchange group. Top left panel: Players could refer to a chart that showed the food exchanges of each food Packy and Marlon could find in the game. Then players decided whether the food fitted into the menu plan for the current meal or snack. Top right panel: Players of *Packy & Marlon* had to answer two multiple choice questions about diabetes in each of 24 levels of game play. Bottom left panel: The game recorded and displayed a cumulative logbook for each character. This logbook shows Packy's blood glucose levels, insulin doses, and food exchanges eaten during one simulated day. Bottom right panel: Packy visits the camp's playground in his search for missing food and diabetes supplies. The status bar shows the food exchanges of the foods he has eaten so far for dinner (reproduced by permission of Mr. Steve Brown © Health Hero Network, California, USA)

To optimize the educational benefits of this game, players could select insulin plans that matched their own. The scenario was a diabetes summer camp that had been raided by rats. The two elephants, Packy and Marlon, needed to defend themselves by blasting the attacking rodents with peanuts and water from their trunks. They also needed to find food and supplies, remembering to eat healthily, regularly check their BG levels, and take their insulin [124].

Not only did this game provide children with a fun way to learn about diabetes, but it was also intended to aid dialogue between children with diabetes and their non-diabetic friends.

Packy & Marlon was assessed in two US centers in a 6-month RCT, in a cohort of 59 type 1 diabetic children. Half the cohort received the diabetes game to use at home as much as they liked, while the other half (the control group) received a video game with no health care content. Although significant improvements in HbA_{1c} were not demonstrated, benefits were reported in diabetes self-efficacy, communication with parents about diabetes, and self-care behavior in the children who received *Packy & Marlon*. Also there was a decrease in unscheduled urgent doctor visits, a finding that if confirmed by larger studies would be most encouraging for children with diabetes [124].

CD-ROM based Diabetes Teaching

Another interesting diabetes educational program is a multimedia based self-learning package for patients, carers, and HCPs, called *Learning Diabetes* [125]. This comes in two forms, for type 1 and type 2 diabetes, and provides a whole host of practical information about diabetes and nutrition in an easy-to-access, interactive manner on CD-ROMs. As a valuable feature, rather than being "lectured" by HCPs, patients themselves have been filmed on video, recounting their own experiences with diabetes and these video clips—2 1/2 h in total—form one of the mainstays of the system. As an example of the sort of information stored, a patient recounting his own experiences of going hypoglycemic is provided. Intuitively this may well be more informative and a lot more interesting for other patients than being told by a doctor or nurse what it may feel like to have a hypo. An example display from the *Learning Diabetes* system is shown in Figure 9. This shows the main menu of the program, demonstrating the wide variety of topics that are covered.

Dr Day and colleagues from the Ipswich Diabetes Center (Ipswich, UK) have completed a study to look at the use of the program by a large heterogeneous group of people with diabetes. Data were obtained from observation, focused interviews, and detailed analysis of the programs' use as derived from the embedded tracking database.

Only 14% of the insulin-treated subjects required more than simple verbal instructions to use the program, with only 20% of older subjects needing more help. On average, subjects in the test evaluation spent 60 min actively working with the software.

Younger patients showed a greater preference for the interactive sections, while those with longer duration of diabetes showed a greater preference for learning from the experiences of others, using the video clips.

However, despite the relatively short exposure of the test evaluation, highly significant improvements were observed in basic knowledge scores and self-care scores—with programs for both insulin and non-insulin-treated

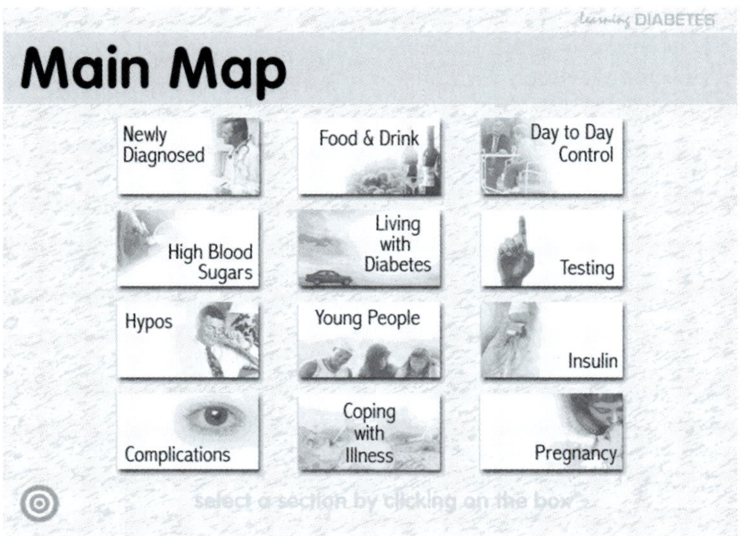

Figure 9 Main menu for *Learning Diabetes* CD-ROM educational diabetes software demonstrating the wide range of topics covered (reproduced by permission of www.interactiveeurohealth.com – Woodbridge, Suffolk, UK)

diabetes—as assessed using questionnaires. The researchers concluded that fears that older patients and those of lower educational or social status, or with limited computer expertise, would not be able to make effective use of these programs had proved unfounded (John Day, personal communication, 2003).

Such studies highlight some of the other novel ways by which educational diabetes software can be assessed. In particular the use of embedded tracking code to record which sections of the program have been accessed (and which sections have been bypassed) can offer an interesting insight in test circumstances into how the software is being used by people with diabetes.

The Way Forward for CAL?

So where do we go from here? That computers can "close the loop" for inpatient and perioperative BG control in diabetes mellitus has been well documented [126–129]. The problem is how to achieve similar ambulatory control through educational means. Providing diabetic patients with the knowledge and confidence to close the loop and act on their SMBG measurements is probably the single most important area in which computer-based simulation and education techniques can be applied with existing computer technology, today. The need for such systems is clear because even amongst interested and motivated patients, knowledge of the principles of insulin self-adjustment at present appears limited [130]. This is despite novel educational developments such as DAFNE [10] demonstrating the possible benefits of flexible therapy planning to diabetes care.

Prototype computer systems with the potential to improve patient education via the interactive simulation of various therapeutic options have been described. As outlined above, some have even been made available without charge [78, 81], in the words of Bergman and Buchanan [20], "to nascent diabetes hackers to try their own protocols and meal patterns." Time will tell whether such approaches provide a clinically useful method of teaching patients with diabetes to modify their therapy on the basis of their SMBG data.

OBSTACLES TO COMPUTERIZATION

Even though many of the prototypes developed up to now have had the *potential* to be useful tools in many aspects of clinical diabetes care, their use by the vast majority of the health care community has been extremely limited. It has been suggested that this may partly be due to the added cost, complexity, and difficulty in data acquisition imposed by the systems, as well as the absence of a smooth integration of these applications on the same computer platform [131]. Other researchers have suggested that the failure of computer programs to become incorporated into routine clinical practice may also, in part, be due to the fact that most of the software has been developed by specialists in information technology or computer scientists, i.e. by people who may be more interested in the functionality of computer-based systems rather than in the user interface or the impact on the health care environment [132]. Others have also felt that the failure of computer systems to attract the enthusiasm of people with diabetes, and their advisors, lay largely with the device–human interface and the lack of attention that was being paid to the very large and real problem of "packaging" [21].

The need for intuitive and easy-to-use graphical user interfaces for these applications is clear. Problems however run deeper than this. A survey of selected participants at a Computers and Quantitative Approaches to Diabetes workshop held in Sydney, Australia in 1988 summed it up by saying that "computers and related technology are unlikely to benefit diabetes management if they add more to the daily burdens of the patient and the supporting health authorities. In this day and age, the need is clearly for user-friendly and above all, simple systems so that patients will accept the tools for self-management" [133]. This analysis is as true now as it was 16 years ago.

Others have suggested that the lack of impact of some computing work on clinical diabetes care may relate to the paucity of serious efforts that have been devoted to validating them [20]. This is a very real issue, because without formal, well-conducted validation studies what confidence can physicians, nurses, dieticians, diabetes educators, pharmacists, or patients have in the safety of a computer program? Also, as in any systems science approach, it is vitally important not to just validate the "black box" but rather to systematically validate the individual components to verify their separate workings. While such validation studies are time-consuming to perform, and may be seen as tedious, they are a necessary part of any prototype's development, leading either to widespread acceptance of the work or to the identification of errors that would then be subject to improvement in an iterative feedback manner. Unfortunately very few of the applications developed to date have been validated in this way. Furthermore, any clinical evaluation work attempting to highlight a clinical benefit from the use of such systems is complicated by the very real difficulty of demonstrating that any one factor, such as patient education, has a significant impact on patient care—in view of the multiplicity of factors that are involved in the provision of such care.

Connected with this, decision support has been a "holy grail" for some researchers, aiming to produce a computer system that can give reliable, safe, and useful advice to people with diabetes. However, there is a slight conundrum here. Most diabetologists/endocrinologists do not need a computer to advise them what insulin dose to recommend for their patients. People with diabetes may wish to have such a system for themselves, but leaving aside the fact that no one so far has developed a decision-support system that has been demonstrated to be safe and efficacious in large-scale, independent RCTs, there are also substantial medicolegal issues surrounding what happens if a patient goes hypo as a result of advice from such a decision-support program. Who might be held medicolegally responsible? The programmer/software developer? A medical informatician? The diabetologist who recommended or prescribed use of the system? Will doctors' malpractice insurance cover HCPs against any such claims? At present this seems unlikely. There are, in fact, a whole "Pandora's box" of issues that need to be addressed regarding therapeutic decision-support tools in the broader field of medical informatics. For this reason, despite the understandable enthusiasm of some computer scientists, there is understandable scepticism on the part of many diabetes HCPs as to the possible uses for such decision-support programs in their diabetes practices.

Other issues to consider include the fact that most GPs do not have sufficient numbers of patients with diabetes in their practice to warrant the use of a dedicated or specialized program—just for this group of patients. Therefore, necessarily, diabetes information systems will need to fit into more general medical databases and programs, to be widely adopted.

Another issue is that of the actual software coding. Mission critical software, for instance in the nuclear industry or in weapons systems, are supposed to be tested in a rigorous manner—automated testing of each program procedure or function being undertaken to ensure that it responds as required. Such testing and coding is time-consuming and costly. However, it is not immediately apparent that such rigorous quality assurance processes are being applied in diabetes decision-support prototype development as would, for example, be expected in the nuclear or defence industries.

Declarations like the St. Vincent Declaration [38] try to encourage the use of audit, feedback, and quality circles to improve the process of delivery of diabetes care. Similar processes are needed to establish the safety of the actual coding used in diabetes decision-support developments.

However, another relative obstacle to the more widespread use of computer applications for diabetes is that of the "Not Invented Here" syndrome, where there may be difficulties in evaluating and applying programs in other independent diabetes centers, especially if those other centers have not been involved in some way in the program's initial development. Furthermore, sometimes even novel or good applications may not be properly tested because of a lack of clinical collaboration. Connected with this, many computer prototypes seem to flounder, after initially encouraging pilot validation studies, it would appear in part because of lack of clinical input. HCPs need to offer help to these developments by supporting the critical and independent evaluation of such computer prototypes. Without such clinical input, and grant support from funding bodies for evaluation studies, obstacles will remain to the wider use of computer-based tools in diabetes care.

Health Carer Perceptions

However, separate from all the above problems there may also be a "grass roots" resistance to the use of IT techniques to assist in the provision of therapy. Such resistance needs to be considered when trying to account for the lack of impact of computers in diabetes care—not least because it can also form a major hurdle to the formal validation of such IT systems. The problem, however, is not just restricted to the diabetes field. In the UK use of the Leeds Abdominal Pain System halved perforated appendix rates in a multicentre study, but its widespread application still proved problematic [134]. The resistance of some HCPs to accept the intelligent use of computers in health care may be a hurdle that will need to be generally overcome if IT techniques are to become more widely accepted in medicine. Part of the problem may lie in the fear that less-computer literate individuals may have about computers. However, gradually this seems to be changing with the more widespread use of the Internet and e-mail, even by quite computer-phobic individuals.

Unfortunately in the past some computer prototypes in the diabetes field have been viewed as an alternative to HCPs and therefore a threat to jobs. Clearly this is not the case. Some have feared that computers might detract from the autonomy of the clinician—possibly making the clinician's role superfluous. This will never happen. As highlighted above, the discussion is not about replacing HCPs, but rather supplementing their input, as resources and facilities are simply not in place at present to provide the benefits of studies like the DCCT [1] and DAFNE [10] to the majority of people with diabetes. Furthermore, the doctor and patient will always need to work together in partnership both with each other, as well as with dieticians, educators, nurses, and other HCPs. Any techniques that might be able to help clinicians and patients work together to *optimize* therapy, at a reasonable cost, are likely to have great clinical utility. In time, advanced IT techniques may well be able to fulfil this role and therefore—rather than being perceived as any sort of threat—should be clearly embraced as another useful tool to be applied to maintain and improve current standards of patient care.

DIABETES AND THE WORLD WIDE WEB

The Internet is increasingly becoming an alternative source of information for patients and their relatives, as well as students and some HCPs [135, 136]. A plethora of Websites and Internet-based applications related to

Table 3 A selection of diabetes Charity/Organization Website addresses

American Diabetes Association (ADA) – www.diabetes.org
Juvenile Diabetes Foundation – www.jdfcure.org
American Association of Diabetes Educators (AADE) – www.aadenet.org
American Association of Clinical Endocrinologists (AACE) – www.aace.com
World Health Organization (WHO) – www.who.int
International Diabetes Federation (IDF) – www.idf.org
International Diabetic Athletes Association – www.diabetes-exercise.org
National Institute of Diabetes and Digestive and Kidney Disease of the National Institutes of Health (NIH) Diabetes – www.niddk.nih.gov/health/diabetes/diabetes.htm
Centers for Disease Control (CDC) Diabetes – www.cdc.gov/health/diabetes.htm
Diabetes UK – www.diabetes.org.uk
Canadian Diabetes Association (CDA) – www.diabetes.ca
Diabetes New Zealand – www.diabetes.org.nz

Note: The World Wide Web is constantly changing, and being updated. Some sites cease to function, or change Web addresses. Therefore any printed list of Internet information will necessarily become out of date. A site with up-to-date information about the latest diabetes resources on the Web is Rick Mendosa's "On-line Diabetes Resources" at www.mendosa.com/diabetes.htm.

diabetes have appeared in recent years. Table 3 lists just a few of these. It is beyond the scope of this chapter to provide a review of all Websites about diabetes. A search on www.google.com for diabetes sites yields over 5 1/2 million Web addresses.

Intuitively the benefits of the Web as a method of disseminating knowledge are clear. By placing information on the Internet, the resource becomes very widely available to a vast potential audience, certainly in countries with ready Internet access. Much of this information is available without charge, which helps it reach an even wider audience. The resource becomes available 24 h a day, 7 days a week, 52 weeks a year. Although placing information on the Web is technically relatively straightforward, editing a large number of Web pages and keeping them up-to-date actually can be quite a time-consuming exercise. If subcontracted out, this can necessitate a considerable amount of resources or ongoing funding. Furthermore dealing with all the e-mail enquiries that can arise from a Website can also take time.

The number of diabetes Websites that were created in a "fit" of enthusiasm in the early days of the Internet, but which have not been updated since, is a testament to this. However, separating the "wheat from the chaff" and good Websites from the not so good is not so straightforward. Various vetting systems have been proposed (e.g. www.hon.ch/HONcode), but these have not yet been universally adopted and as with much of the Web it is a case of *caveat lector* (reader beware).

However, while there are a plethora of Websites devoted to diabetes care and diabetes education, there seems to have been relatively little evaluation of the true benefits of such sites. Intuitively it would seem self-evident that providing patients with accurate information about their condition can only be a "good thing." However, as with medical Internet sites generally there do not appear to have been many robust attempts to test out this hypothesis with RCTs comparing usage of diabetes Websites with other media. Furthermore while assessment of the perceived educational benefits of a standard informational diabetes resource such as, say, the American Diabetes Association Website at www.diabetes.org might be one thing, the need for evaluation becomes all the more relevant with less standard uses of the Web.

For instance there are Websites that offer people with diabetes facilities to upload their BG data onto the Internet and graph their results online. While such sites may offer patients and their HCPs greater *flexibility*, which of course is a good thing, the objective benefits of such tools—as with much of the use of Internet-based applications in clinical diabetes care—remains to be objectively proven and demonstrated in formal evaluation studies.

In addition to textual and graphical information on the Web, a fair amount of software that has been written for use by people with diabetes and/or their carers can also be found on the Internet. Some of this is even available without charge, for free, as so called "freeware" software. A good list of such programs, both freeware and commercial, can be found at www.mendosa.com/software.htm. Table 4 summarizes the categories and number of computer programs that can be found here. Further information about a wide range of other diabetes Websites can also be found at www.mendosa.com/diabetes.htm or in reference 137.

Additional uses of the Internet for sharing information about diabetes include e-mail and Web-based diabetes discussion forums and chat rooms. Table 5 lists a few of the larger of these. The views expressed in these are unedited, often unmoderated, and can sometimes be plainly wrong. Nevertheless, much of the information seems to be of interest to people with diabetes and their carers. Judging by the thousands of subscribers registered with some of these facilities and the countless e-mails that are exchanged, clearly people do find these services useful. Indeed there can be few GPs and hospital-based HCPs in industrialized

Table 4 Categories of diabetes computer software available on the Web

Web-based software – 20 programs
Commercial Windows Software – 26 programs
Shareware and Freeware Windows software – 24 programs
MS-DOS software – 10 programs
Software for Macintosh and other computers – 23 programs
Platform-independent software – 3 programs
Diet and Food Programs – 5 programs
Discontinued software – 19 programs

Note: Further details are available from the website address given below. Derived with permission from www.mendosa.com/software.htm © Rick Mendosa, Aptos, California, USA.

Table 5 Details of a selection of diabetes e-mail lists and discussion forums

Usenet newsgroups, many of which are now also accessible via the Web, for instance via http://groups.google.com
misc.health.diabetes – http://groups.google.com/groups?&group=misc.health.diabetes
alt.support.diabetes – http://groups.google.com/groups?&group=alt.support.diabetes
alt.support.diabetes.kids – accessible via same web address
alt.support.diabetes.uk – accessible via same web address

Yahoo! groups (http://dir.groups.yahoo.com) has a wide range of discussion groups freely available. A directory of all its diabetes-related groups can be found at
http://dir.groups.yahoo.com/dir/Health___Wellness/Support/Illnesses/Diabetes

Microsoft Network (MSN) Web Communities (http://communities.msn.com/home) all have message boards. The most active MSN message boards related to diabetes are
MSN Diabetes – http://communities.msn.com/Diabetes
MSN Diabetics Support Room – http://communities.msn.com/DiabeticsSupportRoom

The Lehigh "Diabetic" e-mail list is the oldest, and one of the largest and most active of all the on-line groups concerned with diabetes. To join the "Diabetic" list you need to send an e-mail to listproc@lehigh.edu containing the message: *subscribe diabetic firstname lastname*. Once subscribed you will receive instructions by e-mail about how to post messages

The Lehigh Diabetic Archives contains a repository of messages sent via the "Diabetic" mailing list. This archive can be viewed at http://listserv.lehigh.edu/lists/diabetic

Note: A Website with details of many more diabetes discussion forums and e-mail lists can be found at http://www.mendosa.com/diabetes.htm.

countries who have not had patients bring to them printouts from such diabetes discussion lists or the wider Internet.

Developing a Business Model

As illustrated by the dot com (.com) boom and crash, a number of Website owners have found that making money out of the Internet—despite the wide, potentially global, market—can be fraught with difficulties. In particular, a number of the .com software firms that developed and distributed diabetes-related programs in the early days of the Internet appear to no longer be trading now. Whether this is a result of the .com bubble bursting is not clear, but a number of commercially developed programs that were quite fun and/or medically/clinically useful are no longer around or easily available now because of commercial or other pressures. For instance Raya Systems, Inc., is no longer trading, and so *BG Pilot*, *Captain Novolin*, *Captain Novocare*, and *Packy & Marlon* referred to above are all no longer being sold. At www.mendosa.com/software.htm a list of over 18 other discontinued diabetes computer programs can be found.

Furthermore a number of software developers have reported commercial difficulties with actually selling their diabetes program(s) despite having novel, useful software—which in some cases has been encouragingly evaluated in RCTs. For instance the *Packy & Marlon* video game was unsustainable commercially, even though ported to a PC platform, and tens of thousands of copies were sold. This is despite being successful clinically, certainly in one RCT [124].

The interaction between software development and diabetes commerce is a complex area, beyond the scope of this chapter. Nevertheless, issues of business cases/financial overheads do become important in assessing the financial viability of the ongoing sale and distribution of diabetes software. Clearly, costs must be kept to a minimum if the commercial sale of some program is to succeed.

However, in addition to there being examples of diabetes software developers no longer trading, there are also cases of software no longer being supported, or not working with the latest operating systems, and so over time such programs may become out of date or unusable. Therefore ongoing simple maintenance of software, as well as updating programs, becomes an important issue for the widespread distribution of an application.

Basically it is not just enough to produce a useful program and validate it. In addition to clinically evaluating the program, unless it is going to be distributed for free, there also needs to be a well thought out business case. This is required to facilitate the long-term commercial distribution of the software. Without such a commercial case, fun products may be developed but they may not stay around long enough to really make an impact and benefit a large number of people with diabetes. What exactly that business model should be is unclear, but many commercial entrepreneurs seem to be moving toward subscription-based services where subscribers pay for ongoing use of a service, as opposed to paying just once to purchase the program. Such a subscription-based business model may possibly be one way to sustain ongoing development and distribution of IT-based applications in diabetes care.

However, if the motivation is not to make money, there are alternatives. A business model is by no means the sole approach to software development and distribution. Many useful diabetes-computing programs are distributed for free, and an open-access approach to software coding has been shown to have major benefits [138]—programs like Linux challenging even the domination of Microsoft™ Windows™ in the operating system market. There are also many computer software developments now that make use of a .GNU public licence (www.gnu.org), making the software source code accessible to all who wish to further develop such applications. Time will tell whether this approach catches on in the diabetes-computing field.

DISCUSSION

It is clearly not possible to cover in the limited space available for this chapter the entire diabetes-computing field. Extensive review articles [14, 15] and journal special issues [139–149] giving more detail are available elsewhere, and in the past 6 years a US journal, called *Diabetes Technology & Therapeutics*, dedicated to the application of technology (in its widest sense) in diabetes care has also been formed [150] (further information available at: www.liebertpub.com/dia/default.asp).

Rather, attention here has been focused on the more *clinically* relevant areas, especially those related to databases/EPRs, decision support—particularly using algorithms—education, and the clinical evaluation of such systems.

Regarding decision-support prototypes, the diversity of approaches described in the literature, effectively to solve a single problem—maintaining glycemic control—is intriguing [151]. Some researchers propose dose-by-dose adjustments, while others prefer longer-term visit-by-visit therapeutic interventions. Some prefer data-driven paradigms while others depend on model-based approaches. Some have tried to use qualitative advisors, others algorithms, and yet others causal probabilistic network-based approaches. Some rely on hand-held devices for the patient, whereas others make use of public telephone networks and the Internet.

Furthermore, as the trend for treatment, mainly driven by financial forces, is now towards self-administered management, education becomes an increasingly important component of the care offered to diabetic patients. Some clinicians who promote educational interventions have argued against a "crutch" for patients, which might increase reliance on a technological device while decreasing patients' ability to manage their own diabetes. However, it is self-evident that not all patients are the same. While some are motivated and interested and will take the time and trouble to learn more about their diabetes and truly understand how to adjust their insulin doses on the basis of SMBG data, and therefore could clearly benefit from further education, others appear to have no such interest and providing them with a solution whether it be in the form of a hand-held device, or telephone/Internet access to a central advisory service may be what they require.

Clearly there will always be patients who require greater freedom. However, such increased flexibility brings with it a requirement for increased complexity that may or may not be acceptable or usable by the vast majority of patients. For example, the *HumaLink* prototype [55] offers the possibility of patient flexibility but at the "price" of requiring frequent telephone calls. Not every patient will wish to have to telephone a central computer after each BG measurement or before each insulin injection, but some clearly could benefit from such support. Looking to the future, with the miniaturization of electronics and the extension of mobile telephone/WiFi wireless networks and internet access, it is not inconceivable to consider a day when a BG meter will incorporate a mobile telephone and be able to automatically dial a central computer, transmitting data after each BG measurement. The central computer's advice could be transmitted back and shown on the BG meter's display, *automatically*. By having the possibility of human review and intervention at the central computer, some of the concerns about patients acting solely on the basis of advice from a stand-alone machine may be mitigated.

However, one important question to be considered is whether current computational techniques are generally really sufficiently advanced to be used therapeutically to provide decision support for *individual* patients? The answer to this almost certainly is no—especially if explanations or the reasoning underlying the computer's decision-making process need to be accessible to HCPs and patients. As other researchers have pointed out, further work in this area is still very much required [131].

Related to this, obviously the field in which a program is to be applied needs to be clearly defined. Is the intended user a patient, a relative, a nurse practitioner, or a GP? Is the purpose of the application educational or therapeutic? The availability (and suitability) of current applications will very much depend on the answers to these questions.

A KBS written by hospital-based diabetes specialists, incorporating the sort of knowledge applied in the DCCT, and intended for use by GPs when treating their patients with type 1 diabetes in general practice, will use a different computer technology and a different sort of knowledge from that required by a hand-held log/advisor intended for use by patients themselves in-between clinic visits. Also concerns over evaluation methodologies will need to be addressed, before decision-support software will see widespread utilization and clinical acceptance. In this respect, systems intended for the generation of *individual* patient therapeutic advice will need to be much more rigorously tested and formally validated than systems utilizing similar technologies that are only intended for *educational* use.

However, when there are many ways of doing something in medicine, generally none of them manage the job very well. In diabetes computing, there have been a whole plethora of prototype decision-support systems—but few if any successful products. While things may be changing, as should be apparent from the diversity of approaches mentioned above, it would be oversimplistic to believe that a single computational technique will work for all patients. Different data requirements and demands on patients mean that different methodologies may be more or less suited to individual patients.

Of note, the spectrum of IT applications related to diabetes care illustration shown in Figure 1 was first produced in 1996. It is illuminating that while the technology/medium may have changed 8 years on, for example with Internet-based tools now being used more widely, the basic functions that people are trying to provide using IT have not actually changed that much. So while the technology may have moved on, the functionality still needing to be coded and the problems to be solved remain largely the same.

Patients' Needs

There may be a perception amongst some HCPs that certain computer programs, for instance diabetes simulators, may be too complex or complicated for people with diabetes to use. Also some HCPs may believe that patients are not really interested in getting so involved in their own diabetes care. However surveys, such as those that have been undertaken with freeware software [17, 108–110], repeatedly illustrate the large numbers of patients that seem to be actively seeking out more information about how to better manage their diabetes. Furthermore the use of some of these programs may actually increase patient empowerment [104]. Therefore the results of such surveys should encourage the refinement of diabetes software programs and the development of new applications.

Connected with this, the overall experience from a range of surveys seems to reinforce the view that patients are actually interested in getting more involved in managing their own insulin dosages. This may be of increasing importance as more DAFNE-style structured educational teaching sessions [7–11] are trialled and adopted.

It will be self-evident that much of the discussion in this chapter has focused on applications for people with type 1 diabetes, since these are the patients who might benefit most from IIT, especially because of their earlier age of onset. By contrast there are many more patients with type 2 diabetes. Nevertheless there are a whole range of database and graphing programs (Figures 2 and 3) that can be used equally well by patients with type 2 diabetes as by patients with type 1 diabetes. There are also educational programs available (Figure 9) that can benefit people with type 2 diabetes.

Evaluation Issues

All diabetes-computing prototypes need to be formally validated and clinically evaluated. Achieving this in practice is not without its difficulties. The testing of medical IT prototypes remains the subject of much debate, not just in the diabetes-computing field, but in medical informatics generally. In this respect it was commented 12 years ago that "The biggest challenge for each system and the unquestioned prerequisite is, however, its evaluation. In the field of evaluation more work needs to be done. This requires an agreed methodology for scientific evaluation of the impact of computer systems on health care" [152]. This seems to be as true now as it was when written. Unfortunately not much practical progress has been made in the past 12 years, and this appears to be one of the key factors holding back the development and more widespread usage of computer-based tools in diabetes care.

It has been suggested that what has happened with the application of electronic management systems in diabetes reflects what has also happened in many other fields of medical informatics [42]. A very high number of prototypes, pilot studies, and interesting solutions have been proposed, but a relatively low number of applications have been fully exploited to date in clinical practice. The reasons for this seem to be related to the fact that many of the prototypes have not been reliable or robust enough. However, the complexity of establishing and evaluating interventions that have a strong organizational impact on the process of care have also been problematical [42, 153, 154].

Connected with this it has been suggested that the maturity generally of IT and communications technology and the need for larger-scale organizational interventions are now providing the conditions for effective use of such technologies in the management of chronic diseases such as diabetes. Multifaceted interventions based on the integration of EPRs, electronic guidelines, and telemedicine solutions have been proposed as one of the directions in which technology and health care providers should be headed in order to try and improve patient outcomes in a cost-effective manner [42].

However, undoubtedly the greatest challenge facing those who seek to see IT and computer applications applied more widely in clinical diabetes care is that of evaluation. In this respect there is a well-recognized phenomenon in science that the effect of investigating or measuring something can lead to a change—especially if the scientific process affects the variable being measured. In diabetes clinical trials, this "Hawthorne" or placebo effect can be seen with the process of enrolling patients into a study, leading to improvements in their metabolic control (HbA_{1c}) separate from any effect of the intervention under investigation [112]. For this reason randomized trials with a control group are imperative to properly investigate the possible benefits of a computer-based intervention. While evaluation work is time-consuming (both for patients and HCPs) and can be expensive, such evaluations remain vital to the longer-term progress of this field.

As intimated above although a whole plethora of prototypes have been developed, very few have seen widespread clinical application, and even fewer have been properly evaluated in RCTs. In addition, of those that undergo some sort of preliminary evaluation study, this is rarely repeated or confirmed in a separate center with a different cohort of patients. Connected with this, commercially driven ventures often seem satisfied with a single evaluation study as "proof" of efficacy, which can then be used in marketing and press releases.

However this is not the way it should be. There is always much to learn not only in terms of "is a particular program efficacious?," but also with respect to the best way of applying a particular software program in the home or clinic setting. Furthermore as with pharmaceutical products and medical devices there should be some system of postrelease (postsales) monitoring of software and its users.

At one level it would just seem like good practice to obtain feedback from software users. But at another level this offers a method of ensuring some postdistribution surveillance of the program—to ensure that it functions as intended and that any "bugs" or problems can be identified and addressed in future versions or releases. Such surveying or auditing of the usage of diabetes software programs does not seem to happen often, compounding the problem of lack of data on which to base any conclusions about the widespread usage of such applications.

Looking to the Future

Looking to the future, what are the hopes for actually implementing the benefits of the DCCT in routine clinical practice using IT? Clearly, busy HCPs do not have time to access one program to provide a database, another piece of software for advice/guidance, and a third program to provide patients with education/simulations. Streamlined, integrated software with a consistent easy-to-use user interface is required. Similarly patients would benefit from access to one integrated program that would permit BG meter data download and graphing, database functionality, advice generation (if feasible)/highlighting of relevant features, education and simulations, with some method of communicating queries to a HCP, possibly via e-mail.

Telecommunications networks already exist for the transfer of data and expertise over telephone lines, and via the Internet. Such networks may offer a way of improving communication between patients and their physicians, as well as for also allowing patients access to on-line teaching by telephone and the Web. Such networks *per se* will never replace the doctor–patient consultation, but may provide patients who are less mobile or who live in rural areas with access to the advice, reassurance, and education that they need. Smart cards—credit cards with memories—that will permit the storage of large amounts of medical data are currently being evaluated as a way for patients to carry around their medical records. Technical and sociopolitical obstacles still need to be overcome before such cards become widely available, but they do offer a way of simplifying data collection and storage, especially in a data intensive field of medicine such as diabetes [35–37].

Undoubtedly the next advances in closing the loop will allow much greater feedback control of BG levels and will derive from noninvasive BG monitoring. Devices such as the *GlucoWatch*™ (www.glucowatch.com) are now available commercially. Such techniques in theory hold the promise of an end to finger-pricks, as well as much, much more. In time, continuous noninvasive glucose monitoring is likely to become widely available. In conjunction with either implantable or external insulin pumps—as well as possibly other novel methods of insulin delivery—noninvasive monitoring could make diabetes essentially forgettable with little or no attention being paid to diet, exercise, SMBG measurements, or insulin injections [155]. Unfortunately, we are not quite there yet.

However, one way that existing computational techniques may be able to help with continuous SMBG data is, once again, through education. In this respect, many diabetes HCPs have got used to handling sporadic data, such as BG values logged three or four times per day. But continuous BG data is actually quite different. Interpreting continuous 24-h BG profiles and knowing what actions to take based on them is not without its difficulties. For the most part HCPs and patients simply are not used to looking at such 24-h profiles. Therefore perhaps educational diabetes simulators that provide 24-h profiles (e.g. see Figures 4 and 5) might actually help, allowing the effects of changes in insulin and diet on these profiles to be simulated, 24-h patterns to be identified, and a better understanding of the data to be developed.

CONCLUSIONS

So what conclusions can be drawn about the application of IT in *clinical* diabetes care, as of 2004? As shown in Figure 1, BG meters and insulin pumps are well established tools. The use of database software is also widely accepted now (Figures 2 and 3). Furthermore, quite a wide variety of educational games and programs for patient use at home have started to become available (Figures 7–9). Some of these have started to be formally evaluated, but many have not. Decision-support research has not yet come to fruition although promising approaches are starting to be tested. In this respect, most of the papers in the literature do not propose, at present, to manage complicated patient cases, using computer-based decision-making tools—i.e. without human input. Rather the research consensus seems to be to focus on handling reasonably straightforward clinical cases with a computer—freeing up more of HCPs' limited time to devote to the more difficult cases [151].

Looking to the future, most current decision-support prototypes provide a feedback loop that is closed only at discrete times rather than continuously. Non-invasive glucose monitoring could help to change this, offering potentially much more frequent data sampling that could revolutionize the provision of modern-day diabetes care. However, what many diabetic patients, especially teenagers, fear most are not the later life complications of their diabetes, but rather quite understandably going hypo. Hypoglycemia alarms to alert patients to the possibility of nocturnal hypoglycemia could be another way in which computers may possibly be of direct benefit to patients.

How can further advances in diabetes-computing be ensured? There is a very real need for greater coordination of endeavors in this field. Clinically a multifactorial approach is required, combining concerted efforts at tightening BG control with improved patient education. Computers can help with both these processes. However, as should be self-evident from the foregoing, on its own measuring of BG levels will not achieve improved glycemic control; active interventions are required. HCPs can assist by being amenable to test out novel IT developments, and funding agencies can help move the field forward by providing grants to support such work.

In summary, computers and the application of IT techniques are going to play an increasingly important role in the provision of health care in the 21st century. This will be as true in the field of diabetes as in other branches of medicine. Major advances will come from the computerization of patient medical records with all the benefits that will so derive. In line with the provision of health care for other chronic diseases, such IT techniques should also permit much more selected medical follow-up, with greater opportunities for screening and health promotion/disease prevention.

Specific to diabetes care, IT techniques offer a great opportunity for improved collection, storage, display, and analysis of patient SMBG data. Clearly, further work is required to build systems that can reliably provide therapeutic advice for individual patients (a prerequisite being that such systems must be able to explain their reasoning, as the decision-making process should always be challengeable [156]). However, computing tools and techniques are *now* available for educating people with diabetes to close the loop and modify their therapeutic regimen—all that is required is a concerted effort to build an easy-to-use and widely acceptable system. Undoubtedly, stand-alone programs (that exist today) that can provide education only about, say, insulin-dosage adjustment—although useful—will not be as widely accepted as more comprehensive packages that can also teach patients about diet, exercise, and other important aspects of diabetes care. Building such integrated teaching tools is a realistic goal that the diabetes community should set itself, as through computer-assisted simulation and education it may well prove possible to provide the benefits of the DCCT and DAFNE trials to a much larger number of patients with diabetes.

However, in our possible enthusiasm for the widespread dissemination of such improvements in diabetes care we must always acknowledge that even motivated diabetic patients do not want to spend all their time worrying about their diabetes. They also want to get on with their lives. Given this, the application of technology in diabetes care needs to be managed sensitively, and progressively, in harmony with both patients and other HCPs.

REFERENCES

1. The Diabetes Control and Complications Trial Research Group. The effect of intensive treatment of diabetes on the development and progression of long-term complications in insulin-dependent diabetes mellitus. *N Eng J Med* 1993; 329: 977–86.
2. Lasker RD. The diabetes control and complications trial. Implications for policy and practice. *N Eng J Med* 1993; 329: 1035–6.
3. Watkins PJ. DCCT: the ecstasy and the agony. *Q J Med* 1994; 87: 315–6.
4. Hadden DR. The Diabetes Control and Complications Trial (DCCT): what every endocrinologist needs to know. *Clin Endocrinol* 1994; 40: 293–4.
5. The Diabetes Control and Complications Trial Research Group. Resource utilization and costs of care in the Diabetes Control and Complications Trial. *Diabetes Care* 1995; 18: 1468–78.
6. Siddons H. The cost of education. *Diabet Med* 1994; 11: 239–40.
7. Muhlhauser I, Jorgens V, Berger M, Graninger W, Gurtler W, Hornke L, Kunz A, Schernthaner G, Scholz V, Voss HE. Bicentric evaluation of a teaching and treatment programme for type 1 (insulin-dependent) diabetic patients: improvement of metabolic control and other measures of diabetes care for up to 22 months. *Diabetologia* 1983; 25: 470–6.
8. Muhlhauser I, Bruckner I, Berger M, Cheta D, Jorgens V, Ionescu-Tirgoviste C, Scholz V, Mincu I. Evaluation of an intensified insulin treatment and teaching programme as routine management of type 1 (insulin-dependent) diabetes: the Bucharest-Dusseldorf study. *Diabetologia* 1987; 30: 681–90.
9. Howorka K. *Functional Insulin Treatment*, 2nd edn Berlin [in English]. Springer Verlag, 1996.
10. DAFNE Study Group. Training in flexible, intensive insulin management to enable dietary freedom in people with type 1 diabetes: dose adjustment for normal eating (DAFNE) randomised controlled trial. *BMJ* 2002; 325: 746–9.
11. Howorka K, Pumpria J, Wagner-Nosiska D, Grillmayr H, Schlusche C, Schabmann A. Empowering diabetes outpatients with structured education: short-term and long-term effects of functional insulin treatment on perceived control over diabetes. *J Psychosom Res* 2000; 48: 37–44.
12. Lehmann ED. Preliminary experience with the Internet release of AIDA—an interactive educational diabetes simulator. *Comput Methods Programs Biomed* 1998; 56: 109–32.
13. Lehmann ED. Application of information technology in clinical diabetes care—A Special Issue. Part 1: databases,

algorithms and decision support. *Med Inform* 1996; 21: 255–8.

14. Lehmann ED, Deutsch T. Application of computers in diabetes care—a review, I: computers for data collection and interpretation. *Med Inform* 1995; 20: 281–302.
15. Lehmann ED, Deutsch T. Application of computers in diabetes care—a review, II: computers for decision support and education. *Med Inform* 1995; 20: 303–29.
16. Lehmann ED. Application of computers in clinical diabetes care. *Diabetes Nutr Metab* 1997; 10: 45–59.
17. Lehmann ED. The freeware AIDA interactive educational diabetes simulator—http://www.2aida.org—(1) A download survey for AIDA v4.0. *Med Sci Monitor* 2001; 7: 504–15.
18. Rodbard D. Potential role of computers in clinical investigation and management of diabetes mellitus. *Diabetes Care* 1988; 11 (suppl 1): 54–61.
19. Williams CD, Harvey FE, Sönksen PH. A role for computers in diabetes care. *Diabet Med* 1988; 5: 177–99.
20. Bergman RN, Buchanan TA. Impact of computer simulation on diabetes research and practice. *Diabetes Care* 1989; 12: 748–9.
21. Home PD. Diabetes and the number revolution. *Diabet Med* 1991; 8: 400–1.
22. Third Workshop of the EASD Study Group DO IT. Situation analysis: needs in diabetes care and existing IT solutions. *Diabetes Nutr Metab* 1993; 6: 173–82.
23. Schiffrin A, Mihic M, Leibel BS, Albisser AM. Computer-assisted insulin dosage adjustment. *Diabetes Care* 1985; 8: 545–52.
24. Turnin MC, Beddok RH, Clottes JP, Martini PF, Abadie RG, Buisson JC, Soule Dupuy C, Bonneu M, Camare R, Anton JP, Chrisment CY, Farreny H, Bayard F, Tauber J-PJ. Telematic expert system Diabeto. New tool for diet self monitoring for diabetic patients. *Diabetes Care* 1992; 15: 204–12.
25. Wheeler LA, Wheeler ML, Ours P. Computer selected exchange lists approximations for recipes. *J Am Diet Assoc* 1985; 85: 700–3.
26. Bassham S, Fletcher LR, Spanton RHJ. Dietary analysis with the aid of a microcomputer. *J Microcomput Appl* 1984; 7: 279–89.
27. Schrezenmeir J. Computer aids in dietetics. *Diabetes Nutr Metab* 1991; 4 (suppl 1): 175–9.
28. Lee RD, Nieman DC, Rainwater M. Comparison of eight microcomputer dietary analysis programs with the USDA Nutrient Data Base for Standard Reference. *J Am Diet Assoc* 1995; 95: 858–67.
29. Raidl MA, Bennett Wood O, Lehman JD, Evers WD. Computer-assisted instruction improves clinical reasoning skills of dietetics students. *J Am Diet Assoc* 1995; 95: 868–73.
30. Nebel IT, Bluher M, Starcke U, Muller UA, Haak T, Paschke R. Evaluation of a computer based interactive diabetes education program designed to train the estimation of the energy or carbohydrate contents of foods. *Patient Educ Counsel* 2002; 46: 55–9.
31. Lehmann ED. Database software for use with blood glucose meters. *Diabetes Technol Therapeut* 1999; 1: 229–32.
32. Lehmann ED. Database programs for use with blood glucose meters. *Diabetes Technol Therapeut* 1999; 1: 391–3.
33. Sönksen P, Williams C. Information technology in diabetes care 'Diabeta': 23 years of development and use of a computer-based record for diabetes care. *Int J Bio-Med Comput* 1996; 42: 67–77.
34. Lehmann ED. Electronic medical records in clinical diabetes care. *Diabetes Technol Therapeut* 1999; 1: 555–7.
35. Kuhnel E, Klepser G, Engelbrecht R. Smart cards and their opportunities for controlling health information systems. *Int J Bio-Med Comput* 1994; 35 (suppl): 153–7.
36. Engelbrecht R, Hildebrand C, Kuhnel E, Brenner G, Corcoy R, Eberhard G, Gapp C, Klepser G, De Leiva A, Massi-Benedetti M, Matthieb E, Mechtler R, Piwernetz K, Sembritzki J, Thiery J. A chip card for patients with diabetes. *Comput Methods Programs Biomed* 1994; 45: 33–5.
37. Gogou G, Mavromatis A, Maglaveras N, Engelbrecht R, Pappas C. DIABCARD CCMIS—a portable and scalable CPR for diabetes care. *IEEE Trans Biomed Eng* 2002; 49: 1412–9.
38. WHO/IDF Europe. Diabetes care and research in Europe. The Saint Vincent declaration. *Diabet Med* 1990; 7: 360.
39. Gorman C, Looker J, Fisk T, Oelke W, Erickson D, Smith S, Zimmerman B. A clinically useful diabetes electronic medical record: lessons from the past; pointers toward the future. *Eur J Endocrinol* 1996; 134: 31–42.
40. Flack JR. The impact of information technology on diabetes patient care. *Diabetes Nutr Metab* 1996; 9: 145–59.
41. Piwernetz K, Home PD, Snorgaard O, Antsiferov M, Staehr-Johansen K, Krans M, for the DIABCARE Monitoring Group of the St. Vincent Declaration Steering Committee. Monitoring the targets of the St. Vincent Declaration and the implementation of quality management in diabetes care: the DIABCARE initiative. *Diabet Med* 1993; 10: 371–7.
42. Bellazzi R. Electronic management systems in diabetes mellitus. Impact on patient outcomes. *Dis Manag Health Outcomes* 2003; 11: 159–71.
43. Zielstroff RD. On line practice guidelines: issues, obstacles and future prospects. *J Am Med Inform Assoc* 1998; 3: 227–36.
44. Lobach DF, Hammond WE. Computerized decision support based on a clinical practice guideline improves compliance with care standards. *Am J Med* 1997; 102: 89–98.
45. Skyler J, Skyler D, Seigler D, Sullivan MO. Algorithms for adjustment of insulin dosage by patients who monitor blood glucose. *Diabetes Care* 1981; 4: 311–8.
46. Albisser AM. Intelligent instrumentation in diabetic management. *CRC Crit Rev Biomed Eng* 1989; 17: 1–24.
47. Albisser AM, Schiffrin A, Schulz M, Tiran J, Leibel BS. Insulin dosage adjustment using manual methods and computer algorithms: a comparative study. *Med Biol Eng Comput* 1986; 24: 577–84.
48. Albisser AM. Six generations of the insulin dosage computer: a new clinical device for diabetes self management through specialized centres. *Horm Metab Res* 1990; 24 (suppl.): 140–4.
49. Mihic M, Pyper J, Albisser AM. Conventional insulin therapy in private practice: a one year controlled prospective study. *Diabetes Nutr Metab* 1988; 1: 125–31.
50. Chiarelli F, Tumini S, Morgese G, Albisser AM. Controlled study in diabetic children comparing insulin dosage adjustment by manual and computer algorithms. *Diabetes Care* 1990; 13: 1080–4.
51. Li LLX. Knowledge-based problem solving: an approach to health assessment. *Expert Syst Appl* 1999; 16: 33–42.
52. Carson ER, Carey S, Harvey FE, Sönksen PH, Till S, Williams CD. Information technology and computer

based decision support in diabetic management. *Comput Methods Programs Biomed* 1990; 32: 179–88.

53. Deutsch T, Boroujerdi MA, Carson ER, Harvey FE, Sönksen PH, Tamas G, Williams CD. Principles and prototyping of an AI-based diabetes management advisory system. *Comput Methods Programs Biomed* 1989; 29: 75–88.
54. Carson ER. Knowledge-based systems in diabetes care: an overview. *Diabetes Nutr Metab* 1991; 4 (suppl 1): 137–42.
55. Albisser AM, Harris RH, Sakkal S, Parson ID, Chao SCE. Diabetes intervention in the information age. *Med Inform* 1996; 21: 297–316.
56. Day JP. Some considerations of legal liability concerning the use and future development of knowledge based or expert systems in diabetes care. *Diabetes Nutr Metab* 1995; 8: 195–200.
57. Brahams D, Wyatt J. Decision-aids and the law. *Lancet* 1989; ii: 632–4.
58. Meneghini LF, Albisser AM, Goldberg RB, Mintz DH. An electronic case manager for diabetes control. *Diabetes Care* 1998; 21: 591–6.
59. Albisser AM, En Chao SC, Parson ID, Sperlich M. Information technology and home glucose clamping. *Diabetes Technol Therapeut* 2001; 3: 377–86.
60. Shea S, Starren J, Weinstock RS, Knudson PE, Teresi J, Holmes D, Palmas W, Field L, Goland R, Tuck C, Hripcsak G, Capps L, Liss D. Columbia University's Informatics for Diabetes Education and Telemedicine (IDEATel) Project: rationale and design. *J Am Med Inform Assoc* 2002; 9: 49–62.
61. Starren J, Hripcsak G, Sengupta S, Abbruscato CR, Knudson PE, Weinstock RS, Shea S. Columbia University's Informatics for Diabetes Education and Telemedicine (IDEATel) project: technical implementation. *J Am Med Inform Assoc* 2002; 9: 25–36.
62. Biermann E, Dietrich W, Rihl J, Standl E. Are there time and cost savings by using telemanagement for patients on intensified insulin therapy? A randomised, controlled trial. *Comput Methods Programs Biomed* 2002; 69: 137–46.
63. Bellazzi R, Larizza C, Montani S, Riva A, Stefanelli M, d'Annunzio G, Lorini R, Gomez EJ, Hernando E, Brugues E, Cermeno J, Corcoy R, de Leiva A, Cobelli C, Nucci G, Del Prato S, Maran A, Kilkki E, Tuominen J. A telemedicine support for diabetes management: the T-IDDM project. *Comput Methods Programs in Biomed* 2002; 69: 147–61.
64. Gomez EJ, Hernando E, Garcia A, Del Pozo F, Cermeno J, Corcoy R, Brugues E, de Leiva A. Telemedicine as a tool for intensive management of diabetes: the DIABTel experience. *Comput Methods Programs Biomed* 2002; 69: 163–77.
65. Holman RR, Smale AD, Pemberton E, Riefflin A, Nealon JL. Randomized controlled pilot trial of a hand-held patient-oriented, insulin regimen optimizer. *Med Inform* 1996; 21: 317–26.
66. Schrezenmeir J, Dirting K, Papazov P. Controlled multicenter study on the effect of computer assistance in intensive insulin therapy of type 1 diabetics. *Comput Methods Programs Biomed* 2002; 69: 97–114.
67. Worth R, Home PD, Johnston DG, Anderson J, Ashworth L, Burrin JM, Appleton D, Binder C, Alberti KGMM. Intensive attention improves glycaemic control in insulin-dependent diabetes without further advantage from home blood glucose monitoring: results of a controlled trial. *Br Med J* 1982; 285: 1233–40.
68. Daneman D, Siminerio L, Transue D, Betschart J, Drash A, Becker D. The role of self-monitoring of blood glucose in the routine management of children with insulin-dependent diabetes mellitus. *Diabetes Care* 1985; 8: 1–4.
69. McKimm J, Jollie C, Cantillon P. ABC of learning and teaching. Web based learning. *BMJ* 2003; 326: 870–3.
70. Coonrod BA, Betschart J, Harris MI. Frequency and determinants of diabetes patient education among adults in the US population. *Diabetes Care* 1994; 17: 852–8.
71. Assal JP. The Diabetes Education Study Group of the European Association for the Study of Diabetes. 15 years devoted to improving patient management. *Medicographia* 1995; 17: 15–20.
72. Lewis D. Computer-based approaches to patient education: a review of the literature. *J Am Med Inform Assoc* 1999; 6: 272–82.
73. Lehmann ED. Experience with the Internet release of AIDA v4 - an interactive educational diabetes simulator. *Diabetes Technol Therapeut* 1999; 1: 41–54.
74. Assal JP, Ekoe JM, Lacroix A, Liniger C. Teaching patients about their disease and its treatment: therapeutic success, professional failure. In Sakamoto N, Alberti KGMM, Hotta N (eds), *Recent Trends in Management of Diabetes Mellitus*. Amsterdam: Excerpta Medica, 1987; pp 63–74.
75. Lehmann ED. Interactive educational diabetes simulators: future possibilities. *Diabetes Nutr Metab* 1999; 12: 380–7.
76. Lehmann ED. Interactive educational simulators in diabetes care. *Med Inform* 1997; 22: 47–76.
77. Biermann E, Mehnert H. DIABLOG: a simulation program of insulin glucose dynamics for education of diabetics. *Comput Methods Programs Biomed* 1990; 32: 311–8.
78. Lehmann ED, Deutsch T. A physiological model of glucose–insulin interaction in type 1 diabetes mellitus. *J Biomed Eng* 1992; 14: 235–42.
79. Lehmann ED, Deutsch T, Broad D. *AIDA: An Educational Simulator for Insulin Dosage and Dietary Adjustment in Diabetes*. London: British Diabetic Association, 1997.
80. Lehmann ED, Deutsch T. A physiological model of glucose–insulin interaction. In *IEEE EMBS Proceedings, 13th Annual International Conference of the IEEE Engineering in Medicine and Biology Society, Vol 13, No 5.* 1991; pp 2274–5.
81. Berger M, Rodbard D. Computer simulation of plasma insulin and glucose dynamics after subcutaneous insulin injection. *Diabetes Care* 1989; 12: 725–36.
82. Cobelli C, Bergman RN (eds). *Carbohydrate Metabolism: Quantitative Physiology and Mathematical Modelling*. Chichester, Wiley, UK, 1981.
83. Albisser AM, Schulz M. Simulating human intermediary metabolism: OMNI et al. In Marks V, Alberti KGMM (eds), *Clinical Biochemistry Nearer the Patient II*. London: Bailliere Tindall, 1986; pp 59–67.
84. Bergman RN. Toward physiological understanding of glucose tolerance. Minimal-model approach. *Diabetes* 1989; 38: 1512–27.
85. Sivitz WI, Davidson PC, Steed D, Bode B, Richardson P. Computer-assisted instruction in intense insulin therapy using a mathematical model for clinical simulation with

a clinical algorithm and flow sheet. *Diabetes Educ* 1989; 15: 77–9.

86. Hedbrant J, Ludvigsson J, Nordenskjold K. Sarimner: a computer model of diabetes physiology for education of physicians and patients. *Diabetes Res Clin Pract* 1991; 14: 113–22.
87. Rutscher A, Salzsieder E, Fischer U. KADIS: model-aided education in type 1 diabetes. *Comput Methods Programs Biomed* 1994; 41: 205–15.
88. Plougmann S, Hejlesen OK, Cavan DA. DiasNet—a diabetes advisory system for communication and education via the internet. *Int J Med Inform* 2001; 64: 319–30.
89. Lehmann ED. Usage of a diabetes simulation system for education via the internet. *Int J Med Inform* 2003; 69: 63–9.
90. Lehmann ED. Diabetes moves onto the Internet. *Lancet* 1996; 347: 1542.
91. Lehmann ED, DeWolf DK, Novotny CA, Gotwals RR Jr, Rohrbach RP, Blanchard SM. Dynamic interactive educational diabetes simulations using the World Wide Web. *Diabetes Technol Therapeut* 2001; 3: A17–20.
92. Lehmann ED. Research use of the AIDA www.2aida.org diabetes software simulation program: a review. Part 1: Decision support testing and neural network training. *Diabetes Technol Therapeut* 2003; 5: 425–38.
93. Lehmann ED. Research use of the AIDA www.2aida.org diabetes software simulation program: a review. Part 2: Generating simulated blood glucose data for prototype validation. *Diabetes Technol Therapeut* 2003; 5: 641–51.
94. Hurter P, Travis LB. *Introductory Course for Insulin-Dependent Diabetics, 6th edn*. Frankfurt: Gerhards, 1991.
95. Lehmann ED, Hermanyi I, Deutsch T. Retrospective validation of a physiological model of glucose–insulin interaction in type 1 diabetes mellitus. *Med Eng Phys* 1994; 16 (3): 193–202. [Published erratum appears in *Med Eng Phys* 16 (4): 351–2].
96. Lehmann ED, Deutsch T. Computer assisted diabetes care: a 6 year retrospective. *Comput Methods Programs Biomed* 1996; 50: 209–30.
97. Lehmann ED, Deutsch T. Compartmental models for glycaemic prediction and decision-support in clinical diabetes care: promise and reality. *Comput Methods Programs Biomed* 1998; 56: 193–204.
98. Lehmann ED. User experience with the AIDA interactive educational virtual diabetes patient simulator. *Diabetes Technol Therapeut* 2000; 2: 165–71.
99. Wilson DM. Diabetes simulators: ready for prime time? *Diabetes Technol Therapeut* 1999; 1: 55–6.
100. Chausmer AB. Diabetes management tools for patients and physicians. *Med Software Rev CRI Health Care Publications* September/October 2002; 11 (5): 1–16.
101. Lehmann ED. User reviews of AIDA online: a web-based interactive educational diabetes simulator. *Diabetes Technol Therapeut* 2000; 2: 329–42.
102. The virtual diabetic patient: AIDA on-line. *Diabetes/Metab Res Rev* 1999; 15: 226.
103. Mendosa R. AIDA On-Line. [review]. Formerly available from the American Diabetes Association Website. Now accessible at: http://www.mendosa.com/aida.htm (Accessed 17th November 2003).
104. Lehmann ED. Spontaneous comments from users of the AIDA interactive educational diabetes simulator. *Diabetes Educ* 2000; 26: 633–43.
105. Lehmann ED. Short user comments ("sound bites") regarding usage of AIDA v4—http://www.2aida.org—an interactive educational diabetes simulator. *Diabetes Technol Therapeut* 2000; 2: 663–6.
106. Lehmann ED. Further user comments regarding usage of an interactive educational diabetes simulator (AIDA). *Diabetes Technol Therapeut* 2002; 4: 121–35.
107. Cleary PD. The increasing importance of patient surveys. *BMJ* 1999; 319: 720–1.
108. Lehmann ED. Who is downloading the freeware AIDA v4.3 interactive educational diabetes simulator? An audit of 2,437 downloads. *Diabetes Technol Therapeut* 2002; 4: 467–77.
109. Lehmann ED. Why are people downloading the freeware AIDA diabetes computing software program: a pilot study. *Diabetes Technol Therapeut* 2002; 4: 793–808.
110. Lehmann ED. Why people download the freeware AIDA v4.3a diabetes software program: a proof of concept semi-automated analysis. *Diabetes Technol Therapeut* 2003; 5: 477–90.
111. Tatti P, Lehmann ED. A randomised-controlled clinical trial methodology for evaluating the teaching utility of interactive educational diabetes simulators. *Diabetes Nutr Metab* 2001; 14: 1–17.
112. Tatti P, Lehmann ED. A prospective randomised-controlled pilot study for evaluating the teaching utility of interactive educational diabetes simulators. *Diabetes Nutr Metab* 2003; 16: 7–23.
113. Tatti P, Lehmann ED. Preliminary results from a randomised-controlled clinical trial for evaluating the teaching utility of an interactive educational diabetes simulator (AIDA). *Diabetes* 2001; 50 (suppl 2): A25.
114. Tatti P, Lehmann ED. Using the AIDA—www.2aida.org—diabetes simulator. Part 1: Recommended guidelines for health-carers planning to teach with the software. *Diabetes Technol Therapeut* 2002; 4: 401–14.
115. Lehmann ED, Tatti P. Using the AIDA—www.2aida.org—diabetes simulator. Part 2: Recommended training requirements for health-carers planning to teach with the software. *Diabetes Technol Therapeut* 2002; 4: 717–32.
116. Tatti P, Lehmann ED. Utility of the AIDA diabetes simulator as an interactive educational teaching tool for general practitioners (primary care physicians). *Diabetes Technol Therapeut* 2001; 3: 133–40.
117. Tatti P, Lehmann ED. Use of the AIDA diabetes simulation software—http://www.2aida.org—as an interactive educational tool for teaching student nurses. *Diabetes Technol Therapeut* 2001; 3: 655–64.
118. Biermann E. Comment on Lehmann and Tatti: proposed controlled trial on simulators in diabetes education. *Diabetes Technol Therapeut* 2002; 4: 255–7.
119. Lehmann ED, Tatti P. Randomised controlled trial design for simulator use in diabetes education: some issues for consideration. *Diabetes Technol Therapeut* 2002; 4: 258–69.
120. Lieberman DA, Brown SJ. Designing interactive video games for children's health education. In Morgan K, Satava RM, Sieburg HB, Mattheus R, Christensen JP (eds), *Interactive Technology and the New Paradigm for Healthcare*. Amsterdam: IOS Press and Ohmsha, 1995; pp 201–10.
121. Elmer-Dewitt P. The amazing video game boom. *Time Magazine*, September 27, 1993; 66–72.
122. Lieberman DA. The computer's potential role in health education. *Health Communi* 1992: 4: 211–25.
123. Lehmann ED, Deutsch T. An interactive, educational model for insulin dosage and dietary adjustment in type 1

diabetes mellitus. In Frisse ME (ed), *SCAMC Proceedings, 16th Annual Symposium on Computer Applications in Medical Care Vol. 16*. New York: IEEE Computer Society Press, 1992; pp 205–9.

124. Brown JS, Lieberman AD, Gemeny AB, Fan CY, Wilson MD, Pasta JD. Educational video game for juvenile diabetes: results of a controlled trial. *Med Inform* 1997; 22: 77–89.
125. Day JL, Rayman G, Hall L, Davies P. "Learning Diabetes"—a multi-media learning package for patients, carers and professionals to improve chronic disease management. *Med Inform* 1997; 22: 91–104.
126. Albisser AM, Leibel BS, Ewart TG, Davidovac Z, Botz CK, Zingg W. An artificial endocrine pancreas. *Diabetes* 1974; 23: 389–96.
127. Clemens AH. Feedback control dynamics for glucose controlled insulin infusion system. *Med Progress Technol* 1979; 6: 91–8.
128. Watson BG, Elliott MJ, Pay DA, Williamson M. Diabetes mellitus and open heart surgery. A simple, practical closed loop insulin infusion system for blood glucose control. *Anaesthesia* 1986; 41: 250–7.
129. Watson BG, Williamson M, Pay DA. A system for perioperative blood glucose control in diabetes mellitus. *Diabet Med* 1991; 8: 118–22.
130. Gill GV, Redmond S. Self-adjustment of insulin: an educational failure? *Pract Diabetes* 1991; 8: 142–3.
131. Berger M, Rodbard D. Towards the implementation of computers in diabetes practice. *Diabetes Nutr Metab* 1991; 4 (suppl 1): 77–86.
132. Piwernetz K, Fischer U. What are computers and models good for? Pros and cons. *Comput Methods Programs Biomed* 1990; 32: 171–5.
133. Opinion Leaders' Forum. The use of computers in the treatment of diabetes mellitus. *Diabetes Nutr Metab* 1989; 2: 319–21.
134. de Dombal FT, Dallos V, McAdam WAF. Can computer aided teaching packages improve clinical care in patients with acute abdominal pain? *BMJ* 1991; 302: 1495–7.
135. Lewis D. Computer-based patient education: use by diabetes educators. *Diabetes Educ* 1996; 22: 140–5.
136. Lewis D. The internet as a resource for healthcare information. *Diabetes Educ* 1998; 24: 627–32.
137. Lehmann ED. Diabetes information technology and WebWatch: general resources. *Diabetes Technol Therapeut* 1999; 1: 109–12.
138. Carnall D. Medical software's free future. *BMJ* 2000; 321: 976.
139. Beyer J, Albisser AM, Schrezenmeir J, Lehmann L (eds), *Proceedings, 1st International Symposium on Computer Systems for Insulin Adjustment in Diabetes Mellitus*, Mainz, Panscienta-Verlag, Hedingen, Switzerland, 1986; pp 1–183.
140. Schrezenmeir J, Kraegen EW, Beyer J (eds). Computers and quantitative approaches to diabetes. *Horm Metab Res* 1990; 24 (suppl.): 1–164.
141. Carson ER, Fischer U, Salzieder E (eds). Models and computers in diabetes research and diabetes care. *Computer Methods Programs Biomed* 1990; 32: 171–356.
142. Piwernetz K, Massi-Benedetti M, Bauersachs R, Sönksen PH (eds). Whither computers in diabetes care? *Diabetes Nutr Metab* 1991; 4 (suppl 1): 1–214.
143. Hovorka R, Carson ER (eds). Computers in diabetes 92. *Comput Methods Programs Biomed* 1994; 41: 151–303.
144. Carson E, Hovorka R, Andreassen S (eds). Computers in diabetes 94. *Comput Methods Programs Biomed* 1996; 50: 207–73.
145. Lehmann ED (ed). Application of information technology in clinical diabetes care. Part 1: databases, algorithms and decision support. *Med Inform* 1996; 21 (special issue): 255–378.
146. Lehmann ED (ed). Application of information technology in clinical diabetes care. Part 2: models and education. *Med Inform* 1997; 22 (special issue): 1–120.
147. Carson ER, Andreassen S, Hovorka R (eds). Computers in diabetes 96. *Comput Methods Programs Biomed* 1998; 56: 75–210.
148. Carson ER, Andreassen S, Cavan DA, Gomez EJ (eds). Computers in diabetes 98. *Comput Methods Programs Biomed* 2000; 62: 153–264.
149. Andreassen S, Gomez EJ, Carson ER (eds). Computers in diabetes 2000. *Comput Methods Programs Biomed* 2002; 69: 93–177.
150. Klonoff DC. Welcome to Diabetes Technology & Therapeutics. *Diabetes Technol Therapeut* 1999; 1: 1–2.
151. Lehmann ED. Application of information technology in clinical diabetes care—A Special Issue. Part 2: models and education. *Med Inform* 1997; 22: 1–3.
152. Piwernetz K, Massi Benedetti M, Bauersachs R, Sönksen PH. Forward. *Diabetes Nutr Metab* 1991; 4 (suppl 1): 1.
153. Friedman CP, Wyatt JC. *Evaluation Methods in Medical Informatics*. New York: Springer Verlag, 1997.
154. Wyatt JC. Clinical data systems. Part III: Developing and evaluating clinical data systems. *Lancet* 1994; 344: 1682–8.
155. Saudek CD. Future developments in insulin delivery systems. *Diabetes Care* 1993; 16 (suppl 3): 122–32.
156. Lehmann ED. Computer-based diagnostic systems. *N Eng J Med* 1994; 331: 1023.

93

Monitoring Diabetes with Urine Tests

A. Samad Shera

Diabetes Association of Pakistan and WHO Collaborating Centre, Karachi, Pakistan

It was not until 1674 that Willis rediscovered one of the most important indisputable symptoms of diabetes, the sweet flavor of urine, but it took sometime before "honey sweetness" of diabetic urine was identified as sugar and finally as glucose. Willis himself believed that the sweetness in the urine was due to a compound of salt and sulfur. It was not until 1776, a century later, that the Liverpool physician Dobson obtained a residue from the urine of several diabetic patients successfully, which was like sugar in flavor and appearance [1].

Dobson was also the first to observe hyperglycemia in diabetic patients and the presence of sugar in the blood of healthy individuals. He observed that the fermentation of diabetic urine could be used as a diagnostic test. Dobson's observations were taken up immediately by his Edinburgh compatriot Francis Home (1719–1813), who in 1780 developed the fermentation test, the first clinical method for detecting sugar in urine [2].

Glucose in urine has been used as a monitoring device for diabetes for long. Where facilities are limited, urine testing with reagent strips may be substituted for venous plasma testing. Urine glucose is used to monitor glycemic control for those who have a normal renal threshold and who cannot afford the cost of home blood glucose monitoring. Symptoms of diabetes alone are insufficient to replace biochemical testing. But if blood glucose testing facility is unavailable, the symptoms are helpful in creating an index of suspicion [3].

Urine tests are relatively cheap and easy to use, but their interpretation for patients with type 1 diabetes requiring tight control is difficult, because glucose can be found in the urine simultaneously as hypoglycemia. While urine testing can be helpful, patients need to be taught that it provides limited information. The results of urine tests can be used as a guideline for further treatment, dietary alterations, and activity schedules; however, major changes in insulin dose should not be made unless supported by blood sugar levels [4].

Self-monitoring of glycosuria in patients with type 2 diabetes is more effective because of the more stable and predictable changes in blood glucose levels. By aiming to maintain their blood glucose levels below the renal threshold, i.e. urine free of glucose, many of these patients can achieve fasting blood glucose concentrations of $<$10–12 mmol/l and freedom from hyperglycemic symptoms.

The attention of diabetes educators has mainly focused on home blood glucose monitoring, with little attention being given to the educational needs of patients who choose to perform home urine glucose monitoring [5]. To achieve the maximum benefit from self-monitoring of glucose, better education of people with diabetes and their health care providers is needed. Urine glucose test strips may sometimes be an adequate monitoring method if the aim is simply to detect the presence or absence of glycosuria [4]. Urine glucose testing may provide a reliable check for abnormally high blood glucose values and may prevent serious events as ketoacidosis requiring expensive hospitalization [6].

Urine glucose testing by patients in the home setting consists of semiquantitative measurements based on single voiding, or less often, by more quantitative "blocks" collected over 4–24 h. The rationale is that urinary glucose values reflect mean blood glucose during the period of urine collection. However, despite the relatively low cost and ease of specimen collection, the

International Textbook of Diabetes Mellitus, Third Edition. Edited by R. A. DeFronzo, E. Ferrannini, H. Keen, and P. Zimmet.
 ISBN: 0-471-48655-8.

well-described limitations of urine glucose testing make self-monitoring of blood glucose (SMBG) the preferred method of monitoring glycemic status on day-to-day basis.

If patients choose to perform urine glucose testing, they should fully understand the test limitations. Specifically, patients should be taught that although urine glucose measurements correlate with blood glucose measurements, urine glucose testing provides only a rough estimate of prevailing blood glucose levels. Patients should be taught that urine glucose testing provides no information about blood glucose levels below the renal threshold, which for most patients is 10 mmol/l (180 mg/dl) [7].

URINE GLUCOSE TESTING

The basis for using urine glucose tests is that the renal threshold for glucose is roughly correlated with hyperglycemia. Thus presence of glucose in urine, in people with a normal and stable renal threshold, may have an important role in monitoring glycemic control; however the following should be kept in mind:

(1) Some patients with raised blood glucose may show no glucose in the urine (high renal threshold), while others with normal blood glucose may show evidence of glucose in the urine (low renal threshold).
(2) In type 2 diabetic patients with a normal renal threshold, and being treated with diet alone, or diet and oral hypoglycemic agents (OHAs), it is desirable to get all the urine samples (pre- and postprandial) glucose free.
(3) In patients on insulin, one should try to get all the preprandial urine samples free of the presence of glucose.

Limitations of urine glucose tests are as follows:

(1) A negative test does not distinguish among hypoglycemia, euglycemia, and mild-to-moderate hyperglycemia.
(2) Urine glucose tests do not give warning of impending hypoglycemia.
(3) If urine glucose remains consistently very high, one should always check the blood glucose levels immediately.
(4) In the presence of very high blood glucose values, the urine should be checked for the presence of acetone [8].
(5) Urine dipsticks measure the urine glucose concentration, and therefore can be influenced by changes in urine volume. This concentration reflects the mean blood glucose level during the interval of the urine collection and not the value at the time of measurement. Urine glucose testing, given its limitations, should never be used alone to assess glycemic control or to make changes in the management. If used, it should always be supplemented by periodic blood glucose tests.

TESTING KETONES IN URINE

Ketones in urine indicate either an impending emergency or ketoacidosis requiring immediate treatment. Alternatively, it may reflect the fasting state.

Urine ketones should be tested in the following situations:

(1) During acute illness
(2) Consistently raised blood sugar >300 mg/dl
(3) Presence of symptoms of ketoacidosis as nausea, vomiting, abdominal pain, and drowsiness

False positive urine ketone results are found in the following situations:

(1) During fasting in normal subjects
(2) First urine specimen of pregnant women (30% cases)
(3) Methods using nitroprusside in the presence of sulfa group of drugs

False negative urine ketone results are found in the following situations:

(1) Use of test strips damaged by long exposure to air.
(2) Highly acidic urine due to intake of high doses of ascorbic acid

Blood ketone tests are more specific in diagnosing and monitoring ketoacidosis and are preferable to urine ketone test.

CONCLUSION

Although urine glucose testing is not an absolute method for monitoring glycemic control in diabetic patients, it is still an important tool for elderly people, who do not require a very tight control or in circumstances when socioeconomic conditions do not permit self blood glucose monitoring. If the limitations are kept in view, urine glucose estimations can be helpful by reducing the frequency of blood glucose estimations.

REFERENCES

1. Schadewaldt H. Die Geschichte des Diabetes. In *Allergie Immun Forsch*, Bd 2. Stuttgart, Germany: S 9–22, Schattuer, 1968.
2. Schadewaldt H. The history of diabetes mellitus. in Engelhardt D. (ed) *Diabetes: Its Medical and Cultural History*. Berlin: Springer-Verlag, 1989; p 64.
3. Rotchford AP, Rotchford KM, Machattie T, Gill GV. Assessing diabetic control—reliability of methods available

in resource poor settings. *Diabet Med* 2002; 19: 195–200.
4. Gallichan M. Self monitoring of glucose by people with diabetes [letter]. *Br Med J* 1997; 315: 184.
5. Smolowitz JL, Zaldivar A. Evaluation of diabetic patients, home urine glucose testing technique and ability to interpret results. *Diabetes Educ* 1992; 18: 207–10.
6. Kabadi UM. Urine glucose testing: reliable backup for whole blood glucose monitoring. *J Fam Pract* 1992; 34: 495–7.
7. American Diabetes Association. Tests of glycemia in diabetes. Position statement. *Diabetes Care* 2002; 25: S97–9.
8. Sadikot SM. *Monitoring Blood Glucose Control, The Indian Consensus 2002*, Diabetes India (www.diabetesindia.com).

94

Self-monitoring of Blood Glucose

Jay S. Skyler

University of Miami, FL, USA

In the twenty-first century, self-monitoring of blood glucose (SMBG) is an essential tool in the management of diabetes. The unfortunate exception to this is when SMBG is unaffordable or unavailable, which is tragically the case in many countries. In that situation, urine glucose monitoring provides an approximation of prevailing glucose and may be used. This chapter, however, will assume that SMBG is available and will discuss its use.

The first suggestion that patients should collect home blood samples for glucose determinations was made as early as 1961, but largely ignored [1]. The modern era of patient SMBG began in the late 1970s, when a number of groups proposed that SMBG was a useful tool to facilitate assessment of diabetes control on an ambulatory basis [2–9]. The development of SMBG was a revolutionary technological innovation. The evolution of use of SMBG has been chronicled in several review articles [10–24], punctuated in particular by two American Diabetes Association (ADA) Consensus Development Conferences on Self-monitoring of Blood Glucose, held in 1986 and in 1993 [25, 26]. As SMBG has evolved, it has become an important component of treatment, rather than an assessment tool [27–29]. This is a subtle but important distinction. SMBG values, monitored properly can be employed by the patient to make immediate treatment decisions. The decisions are based on a predetermined action plan, which consists of actions designed to achieve blood glucose values within a given target range.

The development of SMBG came at a time when there was mounting evidence of the relationship between prevailing glycemic control and diabetic complications [30–34]. SMBG became the linchpin in programs of "intensive therapy" aimed at meticulous glycemic control [27–29, 35–39]. The development of these strategies of intensive management of type 1 diabetes permitted the design of prospective randomized clinical trials to determine whether improved glycemic control decreases the incidence and slows the progression of chronic complications of diabetes. Now, the beneficial effects and impact of effective glycemic control on diabetic complications has been conclusively established in type 1 diabetes by the results reported from the Diabetes Control and Complications Trial (DCCT) [40] and the Stockholm Diabetes Intervention Study (SDIS) [41]. In type 2 diabetes, both the United Kingdom Prospective Diabetes Study (UKPDS) [42–44] and the Kumomoto Study [45] show risk reduction for microvascular complications. Collectively, these studies have ended the long-standing debate on whether or not glycemia is important in this regard, and refocused the debate on the best means of attaining effective glycemic control and on the therapeutic targets that should be sought [46]. Thus, "the quest for normoglycemia" [47], i.e. maintaining glycemic status as close to normal and as safely as possible, has become a realistic option, in large part because of the advent of SMBG.

The optimal treatment of diabetes is guided by the knowledge of prevailing blood glucose levels. Thus, a major advantage of SMBG is that it enables therapeutic goals to be clearly defined and permits assessment of glycemic control during ordinary life. In this regard, it complements glycated hemoglobin measurements. SMBG defines the extent of glycemic excursions while glycated hemoglobin documents average glycemic control. More importantly, SMBG determinations are used on an ongoing basis by patients, to aid in the adjustment of the therapeutic regimen. Thus, in the context of a comprehensive program of diabetes management, SMBG is an integral component of treatment, facilitating the attainment of improved glycemic control.

International Textbook of Diabetes Mellitus, Third Edition. Edited by R. A. DeFronzo, E. Ferrannini, H. Keen, and P. Zimmet.
 ISBN: 0-471-48655-8.

All contemporary diabetes treatment guidelines include SMBG as an integral part of their recommendations. These include those published by the American Diabetes Association [48], the American Association of Clinical Endocrinologists [49], the European Diabetes Policy Group [50, 51], and the International Society for Pediatric and Adolescent Diabetes [52], to cite just a few. These groups note that major clinical trials assessing the impact of glycemic control on diabetes complications invariably have included SMBG as part of multifactorial interventions, suggesting that SMBG is a component of effective therapy. Yet, a systematic health technology assessment review asserted that although SMBG is well established in clinical practice the optimal use of the technique has not been established [53, 54]. The authors argue that current evidence suggests that SMBG is not essential for all patients, and that randomized studies should be carried out to provide decisive evidence on the clinical and cost-effectiveness of SMBG in type 2 diabetes and gestational diabetes. Moreover, they seek a standard protocol for conducting and reporting evaluations of blood glucose monitoring devices. Other "systematic reviews" have drawn the same conclusions [55, 56]. These authors argue that SMBG should be compared to urine glucose monitoring or no monitoring, with all other components of treatment held constant. Quite frankly, this demonstrates the naéveti̇̈ of the reviewers and the danger of having nonclinically aware health assessors draw conclusions about clinical practice. To attempt to isolate SMBG from the other components of therapy is foolhardy. Without SMBG it would have been absolutely impossible to safely develop any of the treatment strategies that have resulted in improved glycemic control, or to conduct any of the major clinical trials that have demonstrated the importance of glucose control. It is ridiculous that such inane conclusions are allowed in print and, worse still, influence policymakers.

In fact, meta-analyses of the impact of comprehensive self-management education—which include SMBG as an integral component—have demonstrated both short-term and long-term beneficial effects [57, 58].

As noted in the ADA recommendations [48], it is important for health care providers to evaluate each patient's monitoring technique, both initially and at regular intervals thereafter, because the accuracy of SMBG is instrument- and user-dependent [59]. Optimal use of SMBG also requires proper interpretation of the data. Patients need to be taught how to use the data to adjust food intake, exercise, or pharmacological therapy to achieve specific glycemic goals. Health professionals should evaluate, at regular intervals, the patient's ability to use SMBG data to guide treatment.

Very recently, the Center for Devices and Radiologic Health of the United States Food and Drug Administration (FDA) has reported a strategy for evaluation of performance of blood glucose monitoring devices [60].

INDICATIONS AND USES FOR SMBG

To use SMBG properly, the goals of treatment must be clearly defined for each patient, thus providing the reason for performing SMBG. Ideally, patients or their designated care providers must be capable of learning the proper use of SMBG, must be motivated and willing to expend the effort necessary to ensure that SMBG measurements are accurate, and must be committed to modifying their treatment plans constructively in response to the feedback provided by SMBG.

Intensive Therapy

SMBG is an essential component of any intensive therapy program directed toward achieving meticulous glycemic control. Without SMBG, establishment of meticulous control may be neither feasible nor safe. SMBG provides the basis for the formulation and fine-tuning of insulin regimens and alerts patients on continuous subcutaneous insulin infusion (CSII) regarding possible pump failure [61–63].

A system of intensive therapy is appropriate for all patients with type 1 diabetes [29, 39, 48, 51, 52, 64–66]. The ideal candidate for meticulous control is the patient who is otherwise healthy and does not yet have signs of complications of diabetes. Patient motivation is crucial and perhaps the determining factor in treatment success or failure. Other criteria for assessing patients for implementation of a meticulous control program are

- Motivation to pursue meticulous glycemic control
- Suboptimal glycemic control with existing treatment plan
- Able and willing to perform frequent SMBG
- Sufficient education and technical ability to follow treatment program
- Psychological stability adequate to manage treatment program
- Trained and skilled medical staff to direct treatment program and provide necessary attention

A preliminary program of counseling, education, and training is desirable. Success in achieving meticulous glycemic control depends on daily SMBG and careful adherence to diet. It is desirable to have most patients demonstrate that they can do these things well. There should be ongoing surveillance to ensure that the patient is following the treatment plan, including being able to measure blood glucose levels accurately and adjust insulin doses reliably.

Hypoglycemia: Prevention, Detection, Avoidance

Hypoglycemia is a major complication in the management of diabetes [67]. The risk of hypoglycemia increases when meticulous glycemic control is sought. There was an overall threefold increased risk of severe hypoglycemia (including coma) in both the DCCT and the SDIS [40, 41]. In the DCCT, half of all severe hypoglycemic episodes occurred during sleep and one third of daytime episodes occurred without warning [40, 68]. Other studies have demonstrated an increased frequency of severe hypoglycemia in patients who are unable to recognize the early warning signs of hypoglycemia, so-called hypoglycemia unawareness [69–72]. Patients with type 2 diabetes, particularly elderly individuals, are also at risk for hypoglycemia if treated with either insulin or sulfonylureas [73]. SMBG is the only practical means of detecting asymptomatic hypoglycemia in the outpatient setting. SMBG may also be used to detect temporal glycemic patterns, so that therapy may be modified in an attempt to prevent hypoglycemia. This is especially important in individuals in whom hypoglycemia may have serious consequences, e.g., those with coexisting angina pectoris or cerebral vascular disease, or those on β-blockers (which both decrease recognition of hypoglycemia and impair glucose counterregulation).

Recent antecedent hypoglycemia is the major factor responsible for hypoglycemia unawareness [67, 73]. It has been shown that meticulous avoidance of hypoglycemia results in restoration of awareness of hypoglycemia in patients with hypoglycemia unawareness [74–76]. These crucial observations suggest that greater attention to avoidance of hypoglycemia, with slightly (but not substantially) raised glycemic targets, allows patients to avoid the more serious consequences of hypoglycemia and, in these series, without overall deterioration of glycemic control as measured by HbA_{1c}. There is greater reproducibility of insulin delivery with CSII, by virtue of using short-acting insulin only [77], and advantage may be taken of this to attain satisfactory glycemic control in patients with hypoglycemia unawareness, by combining use of CSII with raised blood glucose targets [78, 79]. Patients with hypoglycemia unawareness, and arguably all patients with type 1 diabetes, should determine their blood glucose level before performing critical tasks, such as operating a motor vehicle.

Avoidance of Severe Hyperglycemia

One of the great advantages of SMBG is its use in intercurrent illness or other emergency situations, which may increase the risk of severe hyperglycemia and/or ketoacidosis. In such circumstances, SMBG provides the ability to document objectively acute destabilization of diabetic control, and to prevent onset of ketoacidosis by quick implementation of appropriate therapy, thus often avoiding the need for hospitalization [80]. Therefore, patients should be instructed to initiate SMBG or increase the frequency of SMBG in these emergency situations. Patients may be provided with a home management plan, based on SMBG, to use during illness. Table 1 provides sample guidelines as to how to use SMBG data during illness.

Table 1 Sample action plan for illness

During illness

Check blood glucose every 3–4 h

- Check urine ketones at time of each blood glucose measurement
- If urine ketones are substantial *and* blood glucose is 16.7 mmol/l (300 mg/dl) or more, double the amount extra insulin taken

Drink plenty of fluids—more than you think you need

- If blood glucose is higher than 11.1 mmol/l (200 mg/dl), the fluids should be free of sugar
- If blood glucose is lower than 11.1 mmol/l (200 mg/dl), the fluids should contain sugar

Contact your physician or diabetes clinical specialist if

- You have taken 2–3 insulin supplements—to let them know you are having a problem
- You are unable to keep food down or are vomiting
- Your blood glucose does not seem to be responding to the supplements you have taken
- You have definite ketones two to three times in a row
- You are having to breathe fast or hard
- You have any question

These types of guidelines may be used both by patients with type 1 diabetes and by those with type 2 diabetes in whom diabetes decompensates with such intercurrent illness. It should be noted that patients with limited access to fluids or with increased fluid loss due to diarrhea, vomiting, or fever may be at increased risk. They should be in close contact with their physician if using guidelines such as those shown in Table 1.

Pregnancy

In women with diabetes, maintenance of blood glucose levels in the near-normoglycemic range before conception and during pregnancy has been shown to decrease rates of fetal malformation, morbidity, and mortality [81–88]. Normoglycemia should be striven for, not only throughout pregnancy, but also before conception, because congenital abnormalities, which are the main cause of perinatal mortality, are related to hyperglycemia during organogenesis. Strict glycemic control before conception and continued during the first weeks of pregnancy reduces the risk of malformations in infants of diabetic mothers [83, 86]. SMBG during pregnancy, together with intensive insulin treatment, has been shown to be effective in achieving euglycemia. Because insulin resistance occurs progressively during pregnancy, frequent SMBG is crucial in order to determine the need for progressively increased amounts of insulin in women with established diabetes. In addition, although it has been argued that SMBG is unnecessary in all women having gestational diabetes mellitus (GDM) [89–91], SMBG clearly is useful to determine the need for initiation of insulin therapy and to assure optimal pregnancy outcome.

Table 2 Representative target levels for self-monitoring of blood glucose suitable for a young otherwise healthy patient with type 1 diabetes in a program of intensive therapy

Time	Ideal	Acceptable
Fasting/preprandial	70–105 mg/dl (3.9–5.8 mmol/l)	70–130 mg/dl (3.9–7.2 mmol/l)
Postprandial (1 h)	100–160 mg/dl (5.6–8.9 mmol/l)	100–180 mg/dl (5.6–10.0 mmol/l)
Postprandial (2 h)	80–120 mg/dl (4.4–6.7 mmol/l)	80–150 mg/dl (4.4–8.3 mmol/l)
Bedtime	90–130 mg/dl (5.0–7.2 mmol/l)	100–140 mg/dl (5.6–7.8 mmol/l)
2:00–4:00 a.m.	70–105 mg/dl (3.9–5.8 mmol/l)	70–130 mg/dl (3.9–7.2 mmol/l)

Note: Ideal values approximate those seen in nondiabetic individuals; they are included for illustrative purposes. Acceptable values are attainable in a reasonable number of patients without creating an undue frequency of hypoglycemia; they are provided to appropriate patients.

A question that exists is whether it is best to monitor preprandial, 1-h postprandial, or 2-h postprandial glucose during pregnancy [89, 92–94]. The issue is complex, because the targets used in comparative studies have not been equivalent. However, postprandial monitoring is often required to achieve the stringent HbA_{1c} targets, i.e. normoglycemia, in pregnancy. The crucial issue is to be sure that monitoring is occurring and that appropriate care is provided.

Lifestyle Modifications

Changes in activity and diet have major effects on blood glucose levels. Regular exercise can increase insulin action, thereby decreasing the dose of either insulin or oral agents required to achieve a given level of glycemia [95]. Exercise can result in an increase, decrease, or no change in glucose levels (both during and after exercise), depending on the prevailing insulin concentration. Exercise can alter subcutaneous blood flow and therefore alter the rate of insulin absorption. SMBG can be useful in determining patterns of response to planned or unplanned exercise, permitting pharmacological therapy or diet to be appropriately modified. SMBG may be particularly important in children and adolescents who have wide day-to-day variations in activity. A reduction in caloric consumption can decrease insulin or oral agent needs. An increase in caloric consumption can have the opposite effect. Regular SMBG may be of assistance in modifying pharmacological therapy during periods of increased or decreased caloric consumption. It also provides the necessary information to determine whether pharmacological therapy should be modified when meal size is altered.

IMPLEMENTATION OF SMBG USE

Blood Glucose Targets

Instrumental to the use of SMBG as a component of diabetes management is the choice of blood glucose targets [30]. The selection of appropriate blood glucose targets is one of the most important aspects of management, and one that should be quite explicit. Each patient should have *defined* blood glucose targets. These must be *individualized* for the needs of each patient. The targets must be explicitly defined, in order to avoid confusion, and for the patient to understand his/her management goal.

Often the goal of therapy is meticulous glycemic control with near-normal glycemic targets. Table 2 shows an example of meticulous control targets for a young, otherwise healthy patient, who recognizes hypoglycemic symptoms and spontaneously recovers from hypoglycemia. In this example, the fasting blood glucose target is 3.9–7.2 mmol/l (70–130 mg/dl). These targets need to be lower during pregnancy. Table 3 shows an example of the even more stringent targets appropriate for a pregnant woman with diabetes. In this example, the fasting blood glucose targets is 3.3–5.0 mmol/l (60–90 mg/dl).

Yet such meticulous targets are inappropriate in patients who have difficulty perceiving hypoglycemic symptoms (hypoglycemic unawareness), patients who do not spontaneously recover from hypoglycemia (e.g., those with counterregulatory insufficiency or who are using β-blockers), patients in whom hypoglycemia might be particularly dangerous (e.g., patients with angina pectoris or transient ischemic attacks), or patients with other complicating features [73]. Such patients might require preprandial blood glucose targets of, for example, 6.7–11.1 mmol/l (120–200 mg/dl), or some other number.

Targets may also vary with age. A wider range may be desirable in toddlers or young children with diabetes, who may not readily recognize or report hypoglycemic symptoms, and who have active and varied lifestyles. Here, preprandial blood glucose targets might be 4.4–10.0 mmol/l (80–180 mg/dl). Similarly, in an elderly person, there may be a greater desire to avoid hypoglycemia,

Table 3 Representative target levels for self-monitoring of blood glucose suitable for a pregnant woman with type 1 diabetes

Time	Glucose
Fasting	60–90 mg/dl (3.3–5.0 mmol/l)
Preprandial	60–105 mg/dl (3.3–5.8 mmol/l)
Postprandial (1 h)	70–140 mg/dl (3.9–7.8 mmol/l)
Postprandial (2 h)	60–120 mg/dl (3.3–6.7 mmol/l)
Bedtime	60–120 mg/dl (3.3–6.7 mmol/l)
2:00–4:00 a.m.	60–100 mg/dl (3.3–5.5 mmol/l)

and greater tolerance of modest hyperglycemia. Here, for example, preprandial blood glucose targets might be 5.6–11.1 mmol/l (100–200 mg/dl).

Targets may also be changed with time. For example, when initiating flexible or intensive therapy, the initial targets might be preprandial blood glucose values of 5.6–11.1 mmol/l (100–200 mg/dl), even if the ultimate goal is meticulous glycemic control. Sequential changes might then be introduced, until the ultimate target is achieved.

It should be appreciated that the target range should be wide enough to be realistically achievable. A preprandial blood glucose target range of 5.0–6.1 mmol/l (90–110 mg/dl) is unrealistically narrow, and will lead to frustration, since it is not likely to be achieved on a regular basis. In motivated patients, realistic targets are achievable 70–80% of the time (it is unrealistic to expect targets to be achieved 100% of the time, and patients should appreciate this fact). If targets are not being regularly achieved, and the patient is adhering to his/her management program, then one should consider changing the targets to values that are achievable.

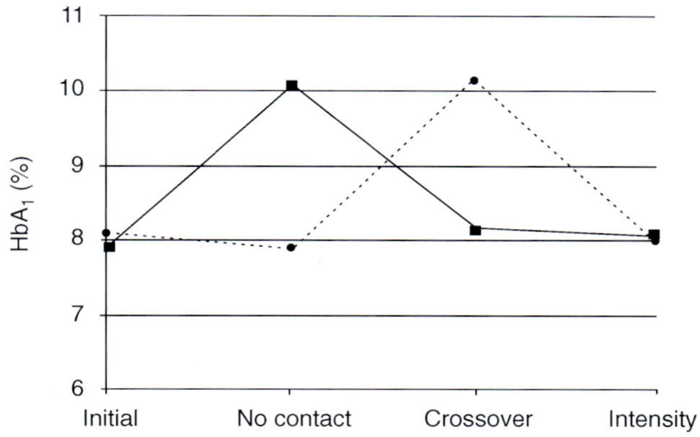

Figure 1 Glycemic control, assessed by glycated hemoglobin, in relation to number of daily blood glucose measurements. The "initial" HbA_1 was obtained after 1 year of "intensive therapy." After 6 months of "no contact," some subjects maintained near-normal HbA_1 values, and had continued to measure blood glucose four or more times daily, others had higher HbA_1 values and had measured blood glucose an average of two or less times daily. The next 3 months period ("crossover"), they changed the frequency of blood glucose monitoring, and the last 3 months period ("intensify"), they all resumed blood glucose measurement four or more times daily. (Adapted from reference 97)

Frequency of Monitoring

The frequency of monitoring depends on the treatment program of any individual patient and will vary considerably, depending on the clinical situation. As a general principle, insulin-treated diabetes requires more frequent monitoring than tablet-treated or diet-treated diabetes. As a second principle, unstable labile diabetes requires more frequent monitoring than does stable diabetes. As a third principle, fasting and preprandial glucose measurements alone underestimate the extent of postprandial glucose excursions and may be inadequate as the sole monitoring times if meticulous glycemic control is desired, especially during pregnancy.

A study from Montreal in patients with type 1 diabetes who had attained excellent control (near-normal glycated hemoglobin values) demonstrated that such control deteriorated if SMBG was reduced to less than four determinations per day [97] (Figure 1). Moreover, this prompted the investigators to institute a subsequent crossover study in which they demonstrated that better control was attained with four or more daily blood glucose determinations than with fewer measurements. This demonstrates the necessity of frequent daily SMBG, and taking action upon the information, if excellent control is desired.

These findings are congruent with other observations. For example, in a short-term study, one group of investigators have found that lower glycated hemoglobin values correlated with the number of blood glucose values charted per week [98]. In a long-term chart review, multiple linear regression analyses demonstrated that increased frequency of SMBG and of insulin injections were associated with lower glycated hemoglobin values in patients with type 1 diabetes [99].

The DCCT investigators noted the importance of frequent SMBG measurements as well [100]. For the intensive treatment group they recommended four or more daily determinations, with an overnight value at least once weekly. At least quarterly, profiles were obtained that included postprandial values as well. During the entire study, for which subjects were followed up for a mean of 6.5 years, on 86–92% of days there was compliance with at least three of the recommended four daily measurements. In addition, overnight values were obtained over 70% of the time. The DCCT Study Group noted the importance of frequent monitoring, careful record keeping, and actions taken upon the results, if meticulous control was to be achieved. Indeed, adjustment of insulin dosage, based on SMBG, was reported by 94–98% of intensive treatment patients throughout the DCCT. Other studies confirmed that good metabolic control is linked not only with the degree of knowledge but also with the application of this knowledge [101].

Knowledge of preprandial, bedtime, and nocturnal blood glucose concentrations is required to determine the appropriate basal and preprandial insulin doses. Therefore, in type 1 diabetes, in a program of intensive therapy, it would seem prudent to recommend that blood glucose be determined at least four times per day most days (before meals and at bedtime), with additional samples obtained in the middle of the night (2.00–4.00 a.m.) once every 1–2 weeks and any time that overnight insulin dosage is to be altered [29]. Additional samples are obtained any time hypoglycemia is suspected, and to measure the impact of alterations in food, activity, or insulin program. Periodically, postprandial samples are obtained as well. Certainly, there should be a minimum of one measurement per insulin component. Dosage decisions can then be based on a measured value rather than an unknown value.

During initiation of a program of intensive therapy aimed at meticulous control, and during pregnancy, more frequent sampling is recommended, i.e., 7–9 determinations daily: prebreakfast, postprandial breakfast, prelunch, postprandial lunch, presupper, postprandial supper, bedtime, midnight, and 2.00–4.00 a.m. When a relatively stable pattern is obtained, the frequency of monitoring is reduced to four daily samples as described above. If glycemic control deteriorates, it is necessary to increase the frequency of monitoring. Frequent sampling is also necessary during intercurrent illness and for problem assessment.

As noted earlier, there has been controversy over the utility of SMBG in type 2 diabetes. It should be noted, however, that these patients usually loathe urine testing and prefer SMBG. In type 2 diabetes a useful scheme for SMBG is to perform fasting measurements on a daily basis, since glycemia is generally stable from day to day [102]. The fasting measurement permits early detection of disruption of glycemic control as a consequence of intercurrent events (e.g., illness). Reasonable targets may be established, such as those shown in Table 4 [103]. In addition to fasting SMBG, insulin-treated type 2 patients should perform at least one additional daily test—either preprandial or bedtime. Once every 1–2 weeks, patients should perform a profile including fasting, preprandial, and bedtime measurements. Performing meal-related tests may also be desirable, as in one study, meal-related SMBG within a structured counseling program improved glycemic control in the majority of non-insulin-treated type 2 diabetic patients [104].

Table 4 Blood glucose targets for type 2 diabetes

Time	Target
Fasting/preprandial	80–120 mg/dl (4.4–6.7 mmol/l)
Postprandial	100–180 mg/dl (5.6–10.0 mmol/l)
Bedtime	100–140 mg/dl (5.6–7.8 mmol/l)

In the recent Treat to Target Trial a simple scheme of SMBG was incorporated, with a relatively simple algorithm based on a fasting blood glucose target of less than 5.6 mmol/l (100 mg/dl) [105]. In this study, patients with type 2 diabetes, inadequately controlled with oral agents, had bedtime insulin initiated at a low dose (10 units of insulin glargine or NPH insulin) and had the dose increased weekly, based on fasting SMBG values (Table 5).

Getting patients to believe in SMBG is important, since the best predictor of compliance with SMBG is the perception of improved control with such monitoring [96, 106]. In other words, patients who believed that SMBG improved glycemic control tended to monitor most frequently.

Records

Quite clearly, record keeping is essential to successful treatment, particularly if one is to consider the impact of previous responses. The patient should keep a diary

Table 5 Sample plan for bedtime basal insulin dosing in type 2 diabetes

Start with 10 units at bedtime of basal insulin (insulin glargine, insulin detemir, NPH insulin, or ultralente insulin). Adjust the dose weekly based on the following guidelines:

If mean fasting blood glucose during the previous 4 days is more than 10.0 mmol/l (180 mg/dl):

- Increase bedtime basal insulin dose by 8 units.

If mean fasting blood glucose during the previous 4 days is 7.8–10.0 mmol/l (140–180 mg/dl):

- Increase bedtime basal insulin dose by 6 units.

If mean fasting blood glucose during the previous 4 days is 6.7–7.8 mmol/l (120–140 mg/dl):

- Increase bedtime basal insulin dose by 4 units.

If mean fasting blood glucose during the previous 4 days is 5.6–6.7 mmol/l (100–120 mg/dl):

- Increase bedtime basal insulin dose by 2 units.

If mean fasting blood glucose during the previous 4 days is 3.9–5.6 mmol/l (70–100 mg/dl):

- Maintain current bedtime basal insulin dose.

If any fasting blood glucose during the previous week is less than 3.9 mmol/l (70 mg/dl):

- Return to previous bedtime basal insulin dose.

If any fasting blood glucose during the previous week is less than 3.1 mmol/l (56 mg/dl) or if there is any episode of severe hypoglycemia:

- Reduce the bedtime basal insulin dose by 2–4 units.

Note: This action plan assumes that the fasting blood glucose targets are 3.9–5.6 mmol/l. Plans should be individualized for each patient.

of daily blood glucose measurements, insulin doses, hypoglycemic episodes, and departures from daily routine (e.g., unusually large meals, increased physical activity, intercurrent illness). Careful recording, critical review by patient and health professional, and intelligent interpretation become an important element in successful management. The patient record becomes the focus of discussion at each follow-up visit. In particular, it is desirable to determine if the patient has followed the action plans and made appropriate changes in insulin dose or meals in response to prevailing blood glucose, meals, and activity. Explanation of hypoglycemic episodes and unusual hyperglycemia is sought. Blood glucose profiles and intervention measures undertaken by patients should be reviewed. The logic underlying clinical decisions based on SMBG data should, as far as possible, be explained to the patient, and the feasibility of their implementation discussed. Evaluation of the impact of any intervention steps adopted should be made. Glycated hemoglobin estimation should be performed as an independent complementary index of the patient's glycemic control. Explanations should be sought for any discrepancy between estimation of control by SMBG and by glycated hemoglobin [107]. It should be appreciated that records may be falsified [108], and that action based on recorded values may not be taken [109].

Unfortunately, some patients and physicians suffer from "data overload" when faced with blood glucose monitoring data. This can be crippling. A number of systems have been developed to handle the data and to provide graphic display and even advice according to customized action plans. Some use telecommunications to download the information. These various types of systems can greatly facilitate the management of both the data and the patient. On the other hand, the patient must have continual access to the data, in an appropriate format, if the data are to be useful in ongoing management. Data buried in the memory of a meter are useless for assessing glycemic patterns. For that purpose, the logbook (or an easily accessible electronic version) is essential.

Education and Action Plan

In response to blood glucose fluctuations, the patient must learn how to take appropriate action [27–29, 37–40]. To this end, the patient should learn a sequence of responses, predetermined by the physician. The system used for this purpose is that of *algorithms* for insulin dose alteration. These provide an action plan for the patient. The plan dictates that the patient intervene as necessary by altering the insulin dosage, changing the timing of insulin injections in relation to meals, or changing the size or content of food to be consumed.

Two general types of alterations in insulin dose may be defined: *supplements* and *adjustments*.

Table 6 Sample plan for premeal conventional regular (soluble) insulin dosing

Use the following scheme for premeal alteration of dosage of regular insulin:

If blood glucose is below 2.8 mmol/l (50 mg/dl):

- Reduce premeal regular insulin by 2–3 units
- Delay injection until immediately before eating
- Include at least 10 g of rapidly available carbohydrate in the meal.

If blood glucose is 2.8–3.9 mmol/l (50–70 mg/dl):

- Reduce premeal regular insulin by 1–2 units
- Delay injection until immediately before eating

If blood glucose is 3.9–7.2 mmol/l (70–130 mg/dl):

- Take prescribed premeal dose of regular insulin

If blood glucose is 7.2–8.3 mmol/l (130–150 mg/dl):

- Increase premeal dose of regular insulin by 1 unit

If blood glucose is 8.3–11.1 mmol/l (150–200 mg/dl):

- Increase premeal dose of regular insulin by 2 units

If blood glucose is 11.1–13.9 mmol/l (200–250 mg/dl):

- Increase premeal dose of regular insulin by 3 units
- Consider delaying meal an extra 15 min (to 45 min after injection)

If blood glucose is 13.9–16.7 mmol/l (250–300 mg/dl):

- Increase premeal dosage of regular insulin by 4 units
- Consider delaying meal an extra 20–30 min (to 40–60 min after injection)

If blood glucose is 16.7–19.4 mmol/l (300–350 mg/dl):

- Increase premeal dosage of regular insulin by 5 units
- Delay meal an extra 20–30 min (to 40–60 min after injection)
- Check urine ketones. If moderate to large, increase fluid intake, consider extra insulin (1–2 units). Recheck blood glucose and urine ketones in 2–3 h

If blood glucose is 19.4–22.2 mmol/l (350–400 mg/dl):

- Increase premeal dosage of regular insulin by 6 units
- Delay meal an extra 20–30 min (to 40–60 min after injection)
- Check urine ketones. If moderate to large, increase fluid intake, consider extra insulin (1–2 units). Recheck blood glucose and urine ketones in 2–3 h

If blood glucose is more than 22.2 mmol/l (400 mg/dl):

- Increase premeal dosage of regular insulin by 7 units
- Delay meal an extra 30 min (to 50–60 min after injection)
- Check urine ketones. If moderate to large, increase fluid intake, consider extra insulin (1–2 units). Recheck blood glucose and urine ketones in 2–3 h

If planned meal is larger than usual:

- Increase regular insulin by 1–2 units

If planned meal is smaller than usual:

- Decrease regular insulin by 1–2 units

If unusually increased activity is planned after eating:

- Eat extra carbohydrate and/or decrease regular insulin by 1–2 units

If unusually sedentary activity is planned after eating:

- Consider increasing regular insulin by 1–2 units

Note: This action plan assumes that the preprandial blood glucose targets are 3.9–7.2 mmol/l (70–130 mg/dl). It provides for changes to be made on the basis of prevailing blood glucose. Dose may also be altered on the basis of carbohydrate content of the meal. Plans should be individualized for each patient.

Table 7 Sample plan for premeal rapid-acting insulin dosing

Use the following scheme for premeal alteration of dosage of rapid-acting insulin (insulin lispro, insulin aspart, or insulin glulisine):

If blood glucose is below 2.8 mmol/l (50 mg/dl):

- Reduce premeal dose by 2–3 units.
- Delay injection until 10–15 min after starting to eat.
- Include at least 10 g of rapidly available carbohydrate in the meal.

If blood glucose is 2.8–3.9 mmol/l (50–70 mg/dl):

- Reduce premeal dose by 1–2 units.
- Delay injection until after starting to eat.

If blood glucose is 3.9–5.6 mmol/l (70–100 mg/dl):

- Take prescribed premeal dose.

If blood glucose is 5.6–8.3 mmol/l (100–150 mg/dl):

- Increase premeal dose by 1 unit.

If blood glucose is 8.3–11.1 mmol/l (150–200 mg/dl):

- Increase premeal dose by 2 units.

If blood glucose is 11.1–13.9 mmol/l (200–250 mg/dl):

- Increase premeal dose by 3 units.

If blood glucose is 13.9–16.7 mmol/l (250–300 mg/dl):

- Increase premeal dose by 4 units.
- Consider delaying meal to 10–20 min after injection.

If blood glucose is 16.7–19.4 mmol/l (300–350 mg/dl):

- Increase premeal dose by 5 units.
- Delay meal to 15–20 min after injection.
- Check urine ketones. If moderate to high, increase fluid intake, consider extra insulin (1–2 units). Recheck blood glucose and urine ketones in 2–3 h.

If blood glucose is 19.4–22.2 mmol/l (350–400 mg/dl):

- Increase premeal dose by 6 units.
- Delay meal to 20–30 min after injection.
- Check urine ketones. If moderate to high, increase fluid intake, consider extra insulin (1–2 units). Recheck blood glucose and urine ketones in 2–3 h.

If blood glucose is more than 22.2 mmol/l (400 mg/dl):

- Increase premeal dose by 7 units.
- Delay meal to ~30 min after injection.
- Check urine ketones. If moderate to high, increase fluid intake, consider extra insulin (1–2 units). Recheck blood glucose and urine ketones in 2–3 h.

If planned meal is larger than usual:

- Increase dose by 1–2 units.

If planned meal is smaller than usual

- Decrease dose by 1–2 units.

If unusually increased activity is planned after eating:

- Eat extra carbohydrate and/or decrease dose by 1–2 units.

If unusually activity is planned after eating:

- Consider increasing dose by 1–2 units.

Note: This action plan assumes that the preprandial blood glucose targets are 3.9–5.6 mmol/l (70–100 mg/dl). It provides for changes to be made on the basis of prevailing blood glucose. Dose also may be altered on the basis of carbohydrate content of the meal. Plans should be individualized for each patient.

Insulin *supplements* are dosage variations to prevent or correct momentary deviations of blood glucose outside the target range. They may be used when there is variation in the quantity or pattern of meals or activities, when there is intercurrent illness or other stress, or to correct variations in glycemia. Supplements, then, are temporary insulin doses. Conceptually, there are two types of supplements: (a) *anticipatory supplements*, given to limit expected hyperglycemia, e.g., before a large meal, and (b) *compensatory supplements*, given in response to glycemic levels outside the target range. Supplements may actually be decrements (negative supplements), for example a lowering of preprandial regular insulin in anticipation of an unusually small meal or in the face of prevailing

Table 8 Sample pattern adjustment action plan

Assumptions

- Basal insulin (bedtime insulin or basal rate of insulin pump) is the major insulin acting overnight. Its effect is reflected in the results of blood glucose tests during the middle of the night and on arising the next morning.
- Prebreakfast rapid-acting insulin has major action between breakfast and lunch. Its effect is primarily reflected in the results of blood glucose tests after breakfast and before lunch.
- Prelunch rapid-acting insulin has major action between lunch and supper. Its effect is primarily reflected in the results of blood glucose tests after lunch and before supper.
- Presupper rapid-acting insulin has major action between supper and bedtime. Its effect is primarily reflected in the results of blood glucose tests after supper and at bedtime.

Hyperglycemia not explained by unusual diet/exercise/insulin

- If prebreakfast blood glucose is greater than 5.6 mmol/l (100 mg/dl) for 3–5 days in a row, increase bedtime basal insulin by 1 or 2 units (0.05–0.1 units/h for CSII). Before making such changes, verify that the blood glucose nadir, usually around 3–4 a.m., is not below 3.9 mmol/l (70 mg/dl).
- If prelunch blood glucose is greater than 5.6 mmol/l (100 mg/dl) for 3–5 days in a row, increase prebreakfast rapid-acting insulin by 1 or 2 units.
- If presupper blood glucose is greater than 5.6 mmol/l (100 mg/dl) for 3–5 days in a row, increase prelunch rapid-acting insulin by 1 or 2 units.
- If bedtime blood glucose is greater than 5.6 mmol/l (100 mg/dl) for 3–5 days in a row, increase presupper rapid-acting insulin by 1 or 2 units.
- Only increase one insulin component at a time, starting with the one affecting the earliest blood glucose during the day.

Hypoglycemia not explained by unusual diet/exercise/insulin

- If prebreakfast blood glucose is less than 3.9 mmol/l (70 mg/dl), or if there is evidence of hypoglycemic reactions occurring during the night, reduce bedtime basal insulin by 1 or 2 units (0.05–0.1 units/h for CSII).
- If prelunch blood glucose is less than 3.9 mmol/l (70 mg/dl), or if you have a hypoglycemic reaction between breakfast and lunch, reduce prebreakfast rapid-acting insulin by 1 or 2 units.
- If presupper blood glucose is less than 3.9 mmol/l (70 mg/dl), or if you have a hypoglycemic reaction between lunch and supper, reduce prelunch rapid-acting insulin by 1 or 2 units.
- If bedtime blood glucose is less than 3.9 mmol/l (70 mg/dl), or if you have a hypoglycemic reaction between supper and bedtime, reduce presupper rapid-acting insulin by 1 or 2 units.
- Verify hypoglycemic symptoms with blood glucose measurements. Treat hypoglycemic reactions with 10–15 g of rapidly absorbed simple sugar.

Note: This action plan assumes that the preprandial blood glucose targets are 3.9–5.6 mmol/l (70–100 mg/dl). Plans should be individualized for each patient.

blood glucose levels lower than the preprandial target. It must be emphasized, too, that actions to be taken also include changes in food intake and in timing of insulin administration.

The intervention actions dictated by the plan include food intake (altering the size or content of food), activity, insulin dosage, and timing of injections in relation to meals. These actions are guided by self-monitored blood glucose determinations and daily records. The action taken may depend on the answers to four questions the patient needs to ask at the time of any premeal insulin injection. These include (1) What is my blood glucose now? (2) What do I plan to eat (i.e., usual size meal, large meal, or small meal; ideally based on carbohydrate content of the meal)? (3) What do I plan to do after eating (i.e., usual activity, increased activity, decreased activity)? (4) What has happened under these circumstances previously? With such questions, insulin supplements become sensible routine decisions. The answers dictate treatment response. Tables 6 and 7 provide sample supplement schedule that considers these questions.

The continuing need for compensatory insulin supplements to correct unexplained ambient glycemia outside the target range at a particular time of the day indicates that an adjustment should be made in the relevant insulin component. *Adjustments* are modifications in the basic insulin dose, made in response to a *pattern* of glycemia occurring over several days. Adjustments presuppose that the patient has a stable pattern of meals and activities, has no intercurrent illness, and is free from unusual stress. Table 8 provides a sample algorithm for insulin dose adjustments.

CONTINUOUS GLUCOSE MONITORING SYSTEMS

Two approaches to continuous glucose monitoring, both measuring interstitial fluid glucose, have made their appearance. These are the *continuous glucose monitoring system* (CGMS) [110, 111] and the *Glucowatch* [112, 113]. The former involves insertion of a small electrode sensor into the interstitial fluid, and records data obtained from a subcutaneous sensor over the course of 72 h and is designed to provide the clinician with a continuous profile of tissue glucose levels. The latter is transdermal and extracts interstitial fluid via iontophoresis and via a wristwatch-type device, provides readings for approximately 12 h, and can alert the patient for hypoglycemia or hyperglycemia outside a target level. Both have been evaluated by the NIH-sponsored Diabetes Research in Children Network (Direcnet) Study Group [114, 115]. Data from the CGMS have enabled clinicians to detect both frequency with which glucose levels change and trends of those changes—and thereby more precisely modify management and treatment measures used to make treatment recommendations, resulting in improved glycemic control [116].

As technology further evolves, development strategies for blood glucose monitoring include noninvasive glucose sensors and implantable glucose sensors [117–119]. One recent advance in this regard is a first-generation, long-term continuous glucose sensor that was implanted subcutaneously in 15 patients with type 1 diabetes, with data displayed to the patient for several months [120]. Another approach has used intravascularly implanted glucose sensors and has linked these to an implanted insulin pump, thus providing a key step toward the development of a closed-loop system [121].

CONCLUSION

The introduction of SMBG has been the single most important advance in the management of diabetes since the discovery of insulin. Yet, to some extent the need for potentially painful needle sticks several times daily has been a drawback in its acceptability and use. On the horizon are solutions to these obstacles, solutions that may further change the face of management of diabetes mellitus.

REFERENCES

1. Knight RK, Keen H. Blood sugar by post. *Br Med J* 1961; 1: 1168.
2. Danowski TS, Sunder JH. Jet injection of insulin during self-monitoring of blood glucose. *Diabetes Care* 1978; 1: 27–33.
3. Sonksen PH, Judd SL, Lowy C. Home monitoring of blood glucose. Method for improving diabetic control. *Lancet* 1978; i: 729–32.
4. Walford S, Gale EAM, Allison SP, Tattersall RB. Self-monitoring of blood glucose. Improvement of diabetic control. *Lancet* 1978; i: 732–5.
5. Skyler JS, Lasky IA, Skyler DL, Robertson EG, Mintz DH. Home blood glucose monitoring as an aid in diabetes management. *Diabetes Care* 1978; 1: 150–57.
6. Peterson CM, Jones RL, Dupuis A, Levine BS, Bernstein R, O'Shea M. Feasibility of improved blood glucose control in patients with insulin-dependent diabetes mellitus. *Diabetes Care* 1979; 2: 329–35.
7. Ikeda Y, Tajima N, Minami N, Ide Y, Yokoyama J, Abe M. Pilot study of self-measurement of blood glucose using the Dextrostix–Eyetone system for juvenile-onset diabetes. *Diabetologia* 1978; 15: 91–3.
8. Jovanovic L, Peterson CM, Saxena HB, Dawood MY, Saudek CD. Feasibility of maintaining normal glucose profiles in insulin-dependent pregnant diabetic women. *Am J Med* 1980; 68: 105–12.
9. Cohen M, Zimmet PZ. Home blood glucose monitoring. A new approach to the management of diabetes mellitus. *Med J Austr* 1980; 2: 713–6.
10. Tattersall RB. Home blood glucose monitoring. *Diabetologia* 1979; 16: 71–4.
11. Tattersall R, Gale E. Patient self-monitoring of blood glucose and refinements of conventional insulin treatment. *Am J Med* 1981; 70: 177–82.
12. Skyler JS. Self-monitoring of blood glucose. *Med Clin North Am* 1982; 66: 1227–49.
13. Bell PM, Walshe K. Benefits of self-monitoring of blood glucose. *Br Med J* 1983; 286: 1230–31.
14. Symposium on home blood glucose self-monitoring. *Diabetes Care* 1981; 4: 392–426.
15. Tattersall RB. Self-monitoring of blood glucose 1978–84. In Alberti KGMM, Krall LP (eds), *Diabetes Annual 1*. Amsterdam: Elsevier, 1985; pp 162–77.
16. Scott A, Tattersall R. Self-monitoring of diabetes. In Alberti KGMM, Krall LP (eds), *Diabetes Annual 2*. Amsterdam: Elsevier, 1986; pp 120–36.
17. Tattersall R, Peacock I. Assessment of diabetic control. In Alberti KGMM, Krall LP (eds), *Diabetes Annual 3*. Amsterdam: Elsevier, 1987; pp 143–58.
18. Singer DE, Coley CM, Samet JH, Nathan DM. Tests of glycemia in diabetes mellitus. Their use in establishing a diagnosis and in treatment. *Ann Intern Med* 1989; 110: 125–37.
19. Goldstein DE, Little RR, Lorenz RA, Malone JI, Nathan D, Peterson CM. Tests of glycemia in diabetes. *Diabetes Care* 1995; 18: 896–909.
20. Chmielewski SA. Advances and strategies for glucose monitoring. *Am J Clin Pathol* 1995; 104 (suppl 1): S59–71.
21. Chan JC, Wong RY, Cheung CK, Lam P, Chow CC, Yeung VT, Kan EC, Loo KM, Mong MY, Cockram CS. Accuracy, precision and user-acceptability of self blood glucose monitoring machines. *Diabetes Res Clin Pract* 1997; 36: 91–104.
22. Foster SA, Goode JV, Small RE. Home blood glucose monitoring. *Ann Pharmacother* 1999; 33: 355–63.
23. Yum SI, Roe J. Capillary blood sampling for self-monitoring of blood glucose. *Diabetes Technol Ther* 1999; 1: 29–37.
24. Reynolds LR, Karounos DG. Emerging technology in diabetes mellitus: glucose monitoring and new insulins. *South Med J* 2002; 95: 914–8.
25. American Diabetes Association Consensus Development Panel. Consensus statement on self-monitoring of blood glucose. *Diabetes Care* 1987; 10: 95–9.
26. American Diabetes Association Consensus Statement. Self-monitoring of blood glucose. *Diabetes Care* 1994; 17: 81–6.
27. Skyler JS, Skyler DL, Seigler DE, O'Sullivan MJ. Algorithms for adjustment of insulin dosage by patients who monitor blood glucose. *Diabetes Care* 1981; 4: 311–8.
28. Schade DS, Santiago JV, Skyler JS, Rizza R. *Intensive Insulin Therapy*. Princeton, NJ: Excerpta Medica, 1983.
29. Hirsch IB, Farkas-Hirsch R, Skyler JS. Intensive insulin therapy for treatment of type 1 diabetes. *Diabetes Care* 1990; 13: 1265–83.
30. Cahill GF, Etzwiler DD, Freinkel N. Blood glucose control in diabetes. *Diabetes* 1976; 25: 237–9.

31. Pirart J. Diabetes mellitus and its degenerative complications: a prospective study of 4400 patients observed between 1947 and 1973. *Diabetes Care* 1978; 1: 168–88, 252–63.
32. Tchobroutsky G. Relation of diabetic control to development of microvascular complications. *Diabetologia* 1978; 15: 143–52.
33. Skyler JS. Complications of diabetes mellitus: relationship to metabolic dysfunction. *Diabetes Care* 1979; 2: 499–509.
34. Brownlee M, Cahill GF. Diabetic control and vascular complications. *Arterioscler Rev* 1979; 4: 29–70.
35. Zinman B. The physiologic replacement of insulin. *N Engl J Med* 1989; 321: 363–70.
36. Howorka K. *Functional Insulin Treatment*. Berlin: Springer-Verlag, 1990.
37. Nathan DM. Modern management of insulin-dependent diabetes mellitus. *Med Clin North Am* 1988; 72: 1365–78.
38. Nolte MS. Insulin therapy in insulin-dependent (type I) diabetes mellitus. *Endocrinol Metab Clin N Am* 1992; 21: 281–312.
39. American Diabetes Association. *Intensive Diabetes Management*, 3rd ed. Alexandria, VA: American Diabetes Association, 2003.
40. The Diabetes Control and Complications Trial Research Group. The effect of intensive treatment of diabetes on the development and progression of long-term complications in insulin-dependent diabetes mellitus. *N Engl J Med* 1993; 329: 683–9.
41. Reichard P, Nilsson BY, Rosenqvist U. The effect of long-term intensified insulin treatment on the development of microvascular complications of diabetes mellitus. *N Engl J Med* 1993; 329: 304–9.
42. UK Prospective Diabetes Study Group. Intensive blood-glucose control with sulphonylureas or insulin compared with conventional treatment and risk of complications in patients with type 2 diabetes (UKPDS 33). *Lancet* 1998; 352: 837–53.
43. UK Prospective Diabetes Study Group. Effect of intensive blood-glucose control with metformin on complications in overweight patients with type 2 diabetes (UKPDS 34). *Lancet* 1998; 352: 854–65.
44. Stratton IM, Adler AI, Neil HAW, Matthews DR, Manley SE, Cull CA, Hadden D, Turner RC, Holman RR, on behalf of the UK Prospective Diabetes Study Group. Association of Glycaemia with Macrovascular and Microvascular Complications of Type 2 Diabetes (UKPDS 35): Prospective Observational Study. *BMJ* 2000; 321: 405–12.
45. Ohkubo Y, Kishikawa H, Araki E, Miyata T, Isami S, Motoyoshi S, Kojima Y, Furuyoshi N, Shichiri M. Intensive insulin therapy prevents the progression of diabetic microvascular complications in Japanese patients with non-insulin-dependent diabetes mellitus: a randomized prospective 6-year study. *Diabetes Res Clin Pract* 1995; 28: 103–17.
46. Skyler JS. Diabetic complications: glucose control is important. *Endocrinol Metab Clin N Am* 1996; 25: 243–54.
47. Tattersall RB. The quest for normoglycaemia: a historical perspective. *Diabet Med* 1994; 11: 618–35.
48. American Diabetes Association. Standards of medical care for patients with diabetes mellitus. *Diabetes Care* 2003; 26 (suppl 1): S33–60.
49. American Association of Clinical Endocrinologists. Medical guidelines for the management of diabetes mellitus. *Endocr Pract* 2002; 8 (suppl 1): 40–82.
50. European Diabetes Policy Group. A desktop guide to type 2 diabetes mellitus. *Diabet Med* 1999; 16: 716–30.
51. European Diabetes Policy Group. *A Guide to Type 1 (Insulin-Dependent) Diabetes Mellitus*. Brussels: International Diabetes Federation (European Region), 1998.
52. International Society for Pediatric and Adolescent Diabetes. *ISPAD Consensus Guidelines 2000*. Zeist, the Netherlands: International Society for Pediatric and Adolescent Diabetes, 2000.
53. Coster S, Gulliford MC, Seed PT, Powrie JK, Swamkinathan R. Monitoring blood glucose control in diabetes mellitus: a systematic review. *Health Technol Assess* 2000; 4: 1–93.
54. Coster S, Gulliford MC, Seed PT, Powrie JK, Swaminathan R. Self-monitoring in type 2 diabetes mellitus: a meta-analysis. *Diabet Med* 2000; 17: 755–61.
55. Faas A, Schellevis FG, Van Eijk JT. The efficacy of self-monitoring of blood glucose in NIDDM subjects: a criteria-based literature review. *Diabetes Care* 1997; 20: 1482–6.
56. Holmes V, Griffiths P. Self-monitoring of glucose levels for people with type 2 diabetes. *Br J Community Nurs* 2002; 7: 41–6.
57. Norris SL, Engelgau MM, Narayan KM. Effectiveness of self-management training in type 2 diabetes: a systematic review of randomized controlled trials. *Diabetes Care* 2001; 24: 561–87.
58. Norris SL, Lau J, Smith SJ, Schmid CH, Engelgau MM, Self-management education for adults with type 2 diabetes: a meta-analysis of the effect on glycemic control. *Diabetes Care* 2002; 25: 1159–71.
59. Sacks DB, Bruns DE, Goldstein DE, MacLaren NK, McDonald JM, Parrott M. Guidelines and recommendations for laboratory analysis in the diagnosis and management of diabetes mellitus. *Diabetes Care* 202; 25: 750–86.
60. Chen ET, Nichols JH, Duh SH, Hortin G. Performance evaluation of blood glucose monitoring devices. *Diabetes Technol Ther* 2003; 5: 749–68.
61. Lenhard MJ, Reeves GD. Continuous subcutaneous insulin infusion. A comprehensive review of insulin pump therapy. *Arch Intern Med* 2001; 161: 2293–300.
62. Bode BW, Tamborlane WV, Davidson PC. Insulin pump therapy in the 21st century. Strategies for successful use in adults, adolescents, and children with diabetes. *Postgrad Med* 2002; 111: 69–77.
63. Pickup J, Keen H. Continuous subcutaneous insulin infusion at 25 years. *Diabetes Care* 2002; 25: 593–8.
64. Ciofetta M, Lalli C, Del Sindaco P, Torlone E, Pampanelli S, Mauro L, Chiara DL, Brunetti P, Bolli GB. Contribution of postprandial versus interprandial blood glucose to HbA1c in type 1 diabetes on physiologic intensive therapy with lispro insulin at mealtime. *Diabetes Care* 1999; 22: 795–800.
65. Ludvigsson J, Bolli GB. Intensive insulin treatment in diabetic children. *Diabetes Nutr Metab* 2001; 14: 292–304.
66. Home PD. Therapeutic targets in the management of type 1 diabetes. *Diabetes Metab Res Rev* 2002; 18 (suppl 1): S7–13.
67. Cryer PE, Davis SN, Shamoon H. Hypoglycemia in diabetes. *Diabetes Care* 2003; 26: 1902–12.

68. Diabetes Control and Complications Trial Research Group. Hypoglycemia in the Diabetes Control and Complications Trial. *Diabetes* 1997; 46: 271–86.
69. Gold AE, MacLeod KM, Frier BM. Frequency of severe hypoglycemia in patients with type 1 diabetes with impaired awareness of hypoglycemia. *Diabetes Care* 1994; 17: 697–703.
70. Simonson DC, Tamborlane WV, DeFronzo RA, Sherwin RS. Intensive insulin therapy reduces counter-regulatory hormone responses to hypoglycemia in patients with type 1 diabetes. *Ann Intern Med* 1985; 103: 184–90.
71. Amiel SA, Tamborlane WV, Simonson DC, Sherwin RS. Defective glucose counter-regulation after strict glycemic control of insulin-dependent diabetes mellitus. *N Engl J Med* 1987; 316: 1376–83.
72. Lager I, Attvall S, Blohme G, Smith U. Altered recognition of hypoglycaemic symptoms in type 1 diabetes during intensified control with continuous subcutaneous insulin infusion. *Diabet Med* 1986; 3: 322–5.
73. Cryer PE. Hypoglycaemia: the limiting factor in the glycaemic management of type I and type II diabetes. *Diabetologia* 2002; 45: 937–48.
74. Fanelli CG, Epifano L, Rambotti AM, Pampanelli S, Di Vincenzo A, Modarelli F, Lepore M, Annibale B, Ciofetta M, Bottini P, Porcellati F, Scionti L, Santeusanio F, Brunetti P, Bolli GB. Meticulous prevention of hypoglycemia normalizes the glycemic thresholds and magnitude of most neuroendocrine responses to, symptoms of, and cognitive function during hypoglycemia in intensively treated patients with short-term IDDM. *Diabetes* 1993; 42: 1683–9.
75. Dagogo-Jack S, Rattarasarn C, Cryer PE. Reversal of hypoglycemia unawareness, but not defective glucose counter-regulation, in IDDM. *Diabetes* 1994; 43: 1426–34.
76. Cranston I, Lomas J, Maran A, Macdonald I, Amiel SA. Restoration of hypoglycemia awareness in patients with long duration insulin-dependent diabetes. *Lancet* 1994; 344: 283–7.
77. Binder C, Lauritzen T, Faber O, Pramming S. Insulin pharmacokinetics. *Diabetes Care* 1984; 7: 188–99.
78. Hirsch IB, Farkas-Hirsch R, Cryer PE. Continuous subcutaneous insulin infusion for the treatment of diabetic patients with hypoglycemia unawareness. *Diabetes Nutr Metab* 1991; 4: 41–3.
79. Kanc K, Janssen MM, Keulen ET, Jacobs MA, Popp-Snijders C, Snoek FJ, Heine RJ. Substitution of night-time continuous subcutaneous insulin infusion therapy for bedtime NPH insulin in a multiple injection regimen improves counterregulatory hormonal responses and warning symptoms of hypoglycaemia in IDDM. *Diabetologia* 1998; 41: 322–9.
80. Mann NP, Noronha JL, Johnston DJ. A prospective study to evaluate the benefits of long-term self-monitoring of blood glucose in diabetic children. *Diabetes Care* 1984; 7: 322–6.
81. Karlsson K, Kjellmer I. The outcome of diabetic pregnancies in relation to the mother's blood sugar level. *Am J Obstet Gynecol* 1972; 112: 213–20.
82. Landon MB, Gabbe SG, Piana R, Mennuti MT, Main EK. Neonatal morbidity in pregnancy complicated by diabetes mellitus: predictive value of maternal glycemic profiles. *Am J Obstet Gynecol* 1987; 156: 1089–95.
83. Fuhrmann K, Reiher H, Semmler K, Fischer F, Fischer M, Glockner E. Prevention of congenital malformations in infants of insulin-dependent diabetic mothers. *Diabetes Care* 1983; 6: 219–23.
84. Jovanovic L, Peterson CM. Optimal insulin delivery for the pregnant diabetic patient. *Diabetes Care* 1982; 5 (suppl 1): 24–37.
85. Langer O, Rodriguez DA, Xenakis EM, McFarland MB, Berkus MD, Arrendondo F. Intensified versus conventional management of gestational diabetes. *Am J Obstet Gynecol* 1994; 170: 1036–46.
86. Kitzmiller JL, Buchanan TA, Kjos SL, Combs CA. Preconception care of diabetes, congenital anomalies, and spontaneous abortions. *Diabetes Care* 1996; 19: 514–41.
87. Jovanovic L (ed). *Medical Management of Diabetes Mellitus During Pregnancy*, 3rd edn. Alexandria, VA: American Diabetes Association, 1999.
88. Mazze RS. Measuring and managing hyperglycemia in pregnancy: from glycosuria to continuous blood glucose monitoring. *Semin Perinatol* June 2002; 26 (3): 171–80.
89. Homko CJ, Reece EA. Self-monitoring of blood glucose in gestational diabetes. *J Matern Fetal Neonatal Med* 2002; 12: 389–95.
90. Jovanovic L. Point: yes, it is necessary to rely entirely on glycemic values for the insulin treatment of all gestational diabetic women. *Diabetes Care* 2003; 26: 946–7.
91. Buchanan TA, Kjos SL. Counterpoint: glucose monitoring in gestational diabetes: lots of heat, not much light. *Diabetes Care* 2003; 26: 948–9.
92. de Veciana M, Major CA, Morgan MA, Asrat T, Toohey JS, Lien JM, Evans AT. Postprandial versus pre-prandial blood glucose monitoring in women with gestational diabetes mellitus requiring insulin therapy. *N Engl J Med* 1995; 333: 1237–41.
93. Manderson JG, Patterson CC, Hadden DR, Traub AI, Ennis C, McCance DR. Preprandial versus postprandial blood glucose monitoring in type 1 diabetic pregnancy: a randomized controlled clinical trial. *Am J Obstet Gynecol* 2003; 189: 507–12.
94. Leguizamón G, Krupitzki H, Glujovsky D, Olivera Ravasi M, Reece EA. Blood glucose monitoring in gestational diabetes mellitus: 1- versus 2-h blood glucose determinations. *J Matern Fetal Neonatal Med* 2002; 12: 384–8.
95. Ruderman N, Devlin JT. *The Health Professional's Guide to Diabetes and Exercise*. Alexandria, VA: American Diabetes Association, 1995.
96. Wing RR, Koeske R, New A, Lamparski D, Becker D. Behavioral skills in self-monitoring of blood glucose: relationship to accuracy. *Diabetes Care* 1986; 9: 330–3.
97. Schiffrin A, Belmonte M. Multiple daily self-glucose monitoring; its essential role in long-term glucose control in insulin-dependent diabetic patients treated with pump and multiple subcutaneous injections. *Diabetes Care* 1982; 5: 479–84.
98. Peterson CM, Jovanovic L, Chanoch LH. Randomized trial of computer-assisted insulin delivery in patients with type 1 diabetes beginning pump therapy. *Am J Med* 1988; 81: 69–72.
99. Nathan DM, McKitrick C, Larkin M, Schaffran R, Singer DE. Glycemic control in diabetes mellitus: have changes in therapy made a difference? *Am J Med* 1996; 100: 157–63.
100. Diabetes Control and Complications Trial Research Group. Implementation of treatment protocols in the diabetes control and complications trial. *Diabetes Care* 1995; 18: 361–76.

101. Ziegher O, Kolopp M, Louis J, Musse JP, Patris A, Debry G, Drouin P. Self-monitoring of blood glucose and insulin dose alteration in type 1 diabetes mellitus. *Diabetes Res Clin Pract* 1993; 21: 51–9.
102. Holman RR, Turner RC. Maintenance of basal plasma glucose and insulin concentrations in maturity onset diabetes. *Diabetes* 1979; 28: 227–30.
103. Zimmerman B (ed). *Medical Management of Type 2 Diabetes*, 4th edn. Alexandria, VA: American Diabetes Association, 1998.
104. Schwedes U, Siebolds M, Mertes G, for the SMBG Study Group. Meal-related structured self-monitoring of blood glucose: effect on diabetes control in non-insulin-treated type 2 diabetic patients. *Diabetes Care* 2002; 25: 1928–32.
105. Riddle MC, Rosenstock J, Gerich J, on behalf of the Insulin Glargine 4002 Study Investigators. The Treat-to-Target Trial: Randomized addition of glargine or human NPH insulin to oral therapy of type 2 diabetic patients. *Diabetes Care* 2003; 26: 3080–6.
106. Wing RR, Lamparski DM, Zaslow S, Betschart J, Siminerio L, Becker D. Frequency and accuracy of self-monitoring of blood glucose in children: relationship to glycemic control. *Diabetes Care* 1985; 8: 214–8.
107. Citrin W, Ellis GJ, Skyler JS. Glycosylated hemoglobin: a tool in identifying psychological problems? *Diabetes Care* 1980; 3: 563–4.
108. Mazze RS, Shamoon H, Pasmantier R, Lucido D, Murphy J, Hartmann K, Kuykendall V, Lopatin W. Reliability of blood glucose monitoring by patients with diabetes mellitus. *Am J Med* 1984; 77: 211–7.
109. Mazze RS, Pasmantier R, Murphy JA, Shamoon H, Self-monitoring of capillary blood glucose: changing the performance of individuals with diabetes. *Diabetes Care* 1985; 8: 207–13.
110. Mastrototaro J. The MiniMed Continuous Glucose Monitoring System (CGMS). *J Pediatr Endocrinol Metab* 1999; 12 (suppl 3): 751–8.
111. Gross TM, Bode BW, Einhorn D, Kayne DM, Reed C, White NH, Mastrototaro JJ. Performance evaluation of the MiniMed® Continuous Glucose Monitoring System during patient home use. *Diabetes Technol Ther* 2000; 2: 49–56.
112. Tierney MJ, Tamada JA, Potts RO, Eastman RC, Pitzer K, Ackerman NR, Fermi SJ. The GlucoWatch biographer: a frequent automatic and noninvasive glucose monitor. *Ann Med* 2000; 32: 632–41.
113. Chase HP, Roberts MD, Wightman C, Klingensmith G, Garg SK, Van Wyhe M, Desai S, Harper W, Lopatin M, Bartkowiak M, Tamada J, Eastman RC. Use of the GlucoWatch biographer in children with type 1 diabetes. *Pediatrics* 2003; 111: 790–4.
114. The Diabetes Research in Children Network (Direcnet) Study Group. The accuracy of the CGMS in children with type 1 diabetes: results of the diabetes research in children network (DirecNet) accuracy study. *Diabetes Technol Ther* 2003; 5: 781–9.
115. The Diabetes Research in Children Network (Direcnet) Study Group. The accuracy of the GlucoWatch G2 Biographer in children with type 1 diabetes: results of the diabetes research in children network (DirecNet) accuracy study. *Diabetes Technol Ther* 2003; 5: 791–800.
116. Bode BW, Gross TM, Thornton KR, Mastrototaro JJ. Continuous glucose monitoring used to adjust diabetes therapy improves glycosylated hemoglobin: a pilot study. *Diabetes Res Clin Pract* 1999; 46: 183–90.
117. Gough DA, Armour JC. Development of the implantable glucose sensor. What are the prospects and why is it taking so long? *Diabetes* 1995; 44: 1005–9.
118. Koschinsky T, Heinemann L. Sensors for glucose monitoring: technical and clinical aspects. *Diabetes Metab Res Rev* 2001; 17: 113–23.
119. Robert JJ. Continuous monitoring of blood glucose. *Horm Res* 2002; 57 (suppl 1): 81–4.
120. Garg SK, Schwartz S, Edelman SV. Improved glucose excursions using an implantable real-time continuous glucose sensor in adults with type 1 diabetes. *Diabetes Care* 2004; 27.
121. Renard E. Implantable closed-loop glucose-sensing and insulin delivery: the future for insulin pump therapy. *Curr Opin Pharmacol* 2002; 2: 708–16.

This chapter is based in part on a chapter of the same title which was published in an earlier edition of the *International Textbook of Diabetes Mellitus*, by Jay S Skyler and Matthew Cohen.

95

Glucose Sensors: Present and Future

John C. Pickup

Guy's Hospital, London, UK

Glucose sensors are probe-type devices that measure glucose concentrations without added reagent. For a discussion of glucose sensors in the management of diabetes, it is useful to classify such devices on the basis of purpose, degree of invasiveness in the body, and the technology used (Table 1).

In vitro devices are used for intermittent measurements of blood glucose concentration, e.g. in self-monitored finger-prick capillary blood samples using a portable device, or in venous blood samples obtained in hospital and measured using a bench-top analyzer. The well-known dry-reagent strips that contain immobilized glucose oxidase and peroxidase were the original *in vitro* glucose sensors, in use since the 1960s, but many consider the MediSense Exactech glucose sensor (introduced in the 1980s), where there is electrochemical measurement of glucose, the first proper portable glucose sensor. The operation of this device was based on a mediated amperometric (current-measuring) enzyme electrode (see below) [1], the technology subsequently being developed along similar principles in currently available *in vitro* devices (Abbott MediSense Precision meters).

In vivo sensors monitor glucose levels in the body, usually continuously or semicontinuously. Invasive or minimally invasive sensors are implanted transcutaneously into the tissues such as the subcutaneum or a blood vessel for a short period, or totally implanted in the body. True non-invasive glucose sensors aim to detect glucose in the tissues from the body surface, without puncturing or damaging the skin; such devices have yet to enter routine clinical practice. This chapter focuses on *in vivo* glucose sensing [2–4] and its rapidly emerging impact in clinical diabetes.

MINIMALLY INVASIVE GLUCOSE SENSORS

Amperometric Enzyme Electrodes

By far the most experience with *in vivo* glucose sensing has been obtained with enzyme electrodes, one of which (the MiniMed-Medtronic Continuous Glucose Monitoring System, CGMS; see below) has now entered clinical practice. Enzyme electrodes are one type of "biosensor", i.e. a probe-type sensor where the analyte (glucose) is detected specifically by binding to a biological recognition molecule (the enzyme) which is in close contact with a transducer (e.g. an electrode), which then produces an analyte-dependent signal (e.g. current or voltage change) [5, 6]. Most enzyme electrodes for glucose detection are based on the immobilization of glucose oxidase at a platinum electrode. Glucose is oxidized to gluconic acid and hydrogen peroxide (H_2O_2), and at a positively charged electrode the H_2O_2 can be detected electrochemically as a current flow, which is proportional to glucose concentration (Figure 1). Sensors also have an inner membrane such as cellulose acetate which excludes electroactive interfering substances and an outer membrane such as polyurethane which controls biocompatibility, reduces oxygen dependence (since appropriate membranes are more permeable to oxygen than glucose), and reduces the diffusion of glucose to the enzyme, thereby increasing the linear range. Many sensors of this type have been described and tested *in vivo* in animals or humans [7–12].

Two variations in enzyme electrode design are noteworthy. Instead of measuring H_2O_2 production in the glucose oxidase reaction, the sensor can measure at a negatively charged electrode the oxygen consumption in

International Textbook of Diabetes Mellitus, Third Edition. Edited by R. A. DeFronzo, E. Ferrannini, H. Keen, and P. Zimmet.
 ISBN: 0-471-48655-8.

Table 1 A classification of glucose sensors

(1) *In vitro* (intermittent monitoring)
(2) *In vivo* (intermittent or continuous monitoring)
  (a) Minimally invasive
    (i) Amperometric enzyme electrodes
    (ii) Microdialysis
    (iii) Open-flow microperfusion
    (iv) Reverse iontophoresis (may also be considered noninvasive)
    (v) Other technologies under development (fiber-optic probes, etc.)
  (b) Noninvasive
    (i) Near-infrared spectroscopy
    (ii) Light scattering
    (iii) Fluorescence-based methods
    (iv) Other technologies under development (e.g. photoacoustic spectroscopy)

the reaction:

$$O_2 + 4e^- + 4H^+ \rightarrow 2H_2O$$

Sensors of this type have been used for long-term intravenous glucose monitoring in dogs [13], and for some experimental studies in humans [14], but have been less studied than the H_2O_2-based sensors. None are available for clinical use.

A second modification of the enzyme electrode concept is the "mediated sensor" (Figure 2) where small molecular weight redox mediators such as ferrocene transfers electrons directly from glucose oxidase to the underlying electrode, thereby bypassing oxygen and in theory making the sensor less dependent on changing oxygen tension in the tissues [1, 15, 16].

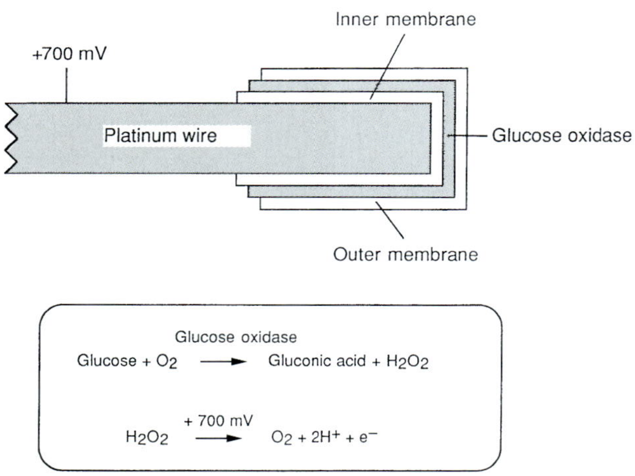

Figure 1 The principle of operation of the most commonly used amperometric enzyme electrode for glucose sensing. Glucose oxidase is immobilized at a platinum electrode. Hydrogen peroxide produced is detected electrochemically

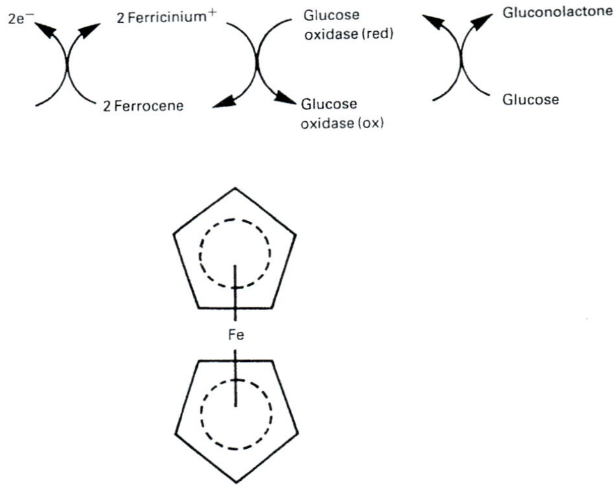

Figure 2 The molecular structure of ferrocene (lower) and the mechanism of action of mediated glucose sensors employing ferrocene. Electrons are shuttled directly from glucose to the electrode via the enzyme and ferrocene (not to oxygen as the final electron acceptor)

Enzyme Electrodes *In Vivo*

The most popular site for implantation of glucose sensors is the subcutaneous tissue, where the potential dangers of infection and thrombosis associated with bloodstream sensing are avoided. Most are of a needle-type design with the sensing element at the tip or side of the needle. Access to the subcutaneous site is simple and sensors can be inserted, removed, and replaced by the patient himself or herself. Moreover, there is now good evidence from wick experiments [17, 18] and from microdialysis [19, 20] (see below) that interstitial fluid glucose concentrations are similar to plasma glucose levels in the steady state. Many studies in animals and humans show that electrode responses measured by subcutaneously implanted sensors follow changes in blood glucose concentration [2, 7, 11, 12, 15, 16, 21], but with three important caveats: there are suppressed responses *in vivo*, indicating a lower than actual glucose level; there is unpredictable drift in the responses (usually a steady decline in sensitivity); and there are differing kinetics between changes in the blood glucose and the interstitial glucose concentrations.

When glucose sensors are calibrated *in vitro* in buffered glucose solutions of known concentration and then implanted subcutaneously, the apparent interstitial glucose level is up to one fifth of that in plasma [11, 15], though, as mentioned above, the true value is similar to that in plasma. Reponses usually decline unpredictably over the next day or so after implantation [21, 22], necessitating repeated calibration against the actual blood glucose concentration as measured by a reference method ("*in vivo* calibration") [11, 12, 23].

The explanation for these impaired responses is not certain, but possibilities include the effect of low oxygen tension in the tissue (unlikely, because sensors are usually unaffected at the Po_2 of about 7 kPa in the subcutaneum [24]); substances in the tissue that interact with the electrode, the enzyme, or its product (e.g., a catalase-like enzyme that would destroy H_2O_2); coating of the sensor with protein or cells; depletion layers caused by the slow and variable mass transport of glucose through the tissues; and a result of the wound response to sensor insertion (blood flow changes, inflammatory cells consuming glucose, etc.). The fact that the sensor sensitivity is similarly depressed after explantation compared to *in vivo* and recovers after repeated washing [11, 25] indicates a reversible accumulation of unknown substance on or in the sensor, rather than tissue-related phenomena such as depletion layers or wound responses. The reportedly better responses with a sensor incorporating microperfusion of the sensor tip *in vivo* with buffer or other fluid presumably works by the moving aqueous film preventing fouling [26]. There is some evidence that the interferrent is of small molecular weight [27] and can be excluded by a membrane placed between the electrode and the enzyme [28].

The dynamic relationships between interstitial glucose and plasma glucose concentrations are a subject of continuing controversy [29–31], the main issues being whether there is a time delay between the sensor reading and the plasma glucose value and whether this differs under different physiological circumstances. Unfortunately, the kinetics may well be influenced by the different species studied, the sensor type and size, the implantation site, the applied stimulus (test meal, oral glucose load, intravenous glucose load, intravenous insulin infusion, normal subcutaneous insulin regimen and meals), whether diabetic or nondiabetic subjects were investigated, and possibly their varying sensitivity to insulin. It is difficult to reach generalizable conclusions but many studies show that after an oral glucose load the sensor readings rise more slowly than the blood glucose levels and create a lag of about 5–15 min, though there is much variation between studies. Sensor readings then fall to baseline at a rate which can be slower, quicker, or the same as the blood glucose levels.

During insulin-induced hypoglycemia, some studies (including microdialysis experiments) have shown that sensor readings fall before the blood glucose levels decline, perhaps because insulin-stimulated glucose uptake by cells depletes the local interstitial fluid glucose before the blood [32, 33]. However, more recent work by some of the same authors [30] has found a slower decline in the sensor responses than in the blood glucose concentration. There is probably some agreement that after hypoglycemia, the interstitial glucose remains in the hypoglycemic range for some time, in spite of the return to normoglycemia. A recent study [31] where microdialysis sensors were inserted in either the subcutaneous fat or the loose subcutaneous tissue under the fat in nondiabetic humans suggests that the delay may be only associated with placement in fat: sensor and plasma glucose values were almost identical after an oral glucose load with the deeper insertion.

Clinical Studies with Enzyme Electrodes

The only commercially available enzyme electrode for glucose monitoring is currently the MiniMed-Medtronic CGMS [12, 34]. This has been in clinical use since about 1999. The system consists of a pager-sized monitor, usually worn around the waist, which logs current from the attached subcutaneously implanted sensor for later downloading to a portable computer and analysis (Figure 3). The intended wear period is up to 3 days. As yet, there is no real-time readout of blood glucose concentrations. Readings are taken every 10 s and averaged over 5 min.

The accuracy of the CGMS compared to conventional blood glucose self-monitoring is good when analyzed by error grids [34–36]—with about 95% of paired sensor and capillary blood glucose samples lying with zones A and B, i.e. either within 20% of the reference value and considered to be clinically correct or where errors would result in no treatment change or a benign one. However, when two sensors are implanted in the same individual, there may be substantial discrepancies in the readings [37]. Although CGMS readings closely parallel blood glucose levels during short-term insulin-induced hypoglycemia [38, 39], there is evidence that the CGMS reads significantly lower (average 38%) than the blood glucose levels during the night [40], perhaps because of drift uncorrected by calibration during the night. This indicates that the CGMS readings are best seen as a series that indicates trends in glycemia rather than an accurate reflection of blood glucose at one time, and therapeutic action should not be taken according to a single reading.

The two main clinical uses for the CGMS are detection of postprandial hyperglycemia (Figure 4) and hypoglycemia (Figure 5), which are not always recorded by frequent blood glucose self-monitoring [35–47]. In a recent study in type 1 diabetic subjects with poor control [35], we compared glycemic control as assessed by the CGMS, with blood glucose self-monitoring performed eight times daily. The duration of any hypoglycemia (nocturnal or daytime) and postprandial hyperglycemia were both significantly longer when assessed by CGMS, though the estimate of mean blood glucose concentration was the same by both methods. Continuous *in vivo* glucose sensing seems therefore to be more valuable as a measure of subtle moment-to-moment changes in blood glucose rather than average glycemia. It is increasingly being used to assess the quality of control in patients being considered for continuous subcutaneous insulin infusion (CSII) [35].

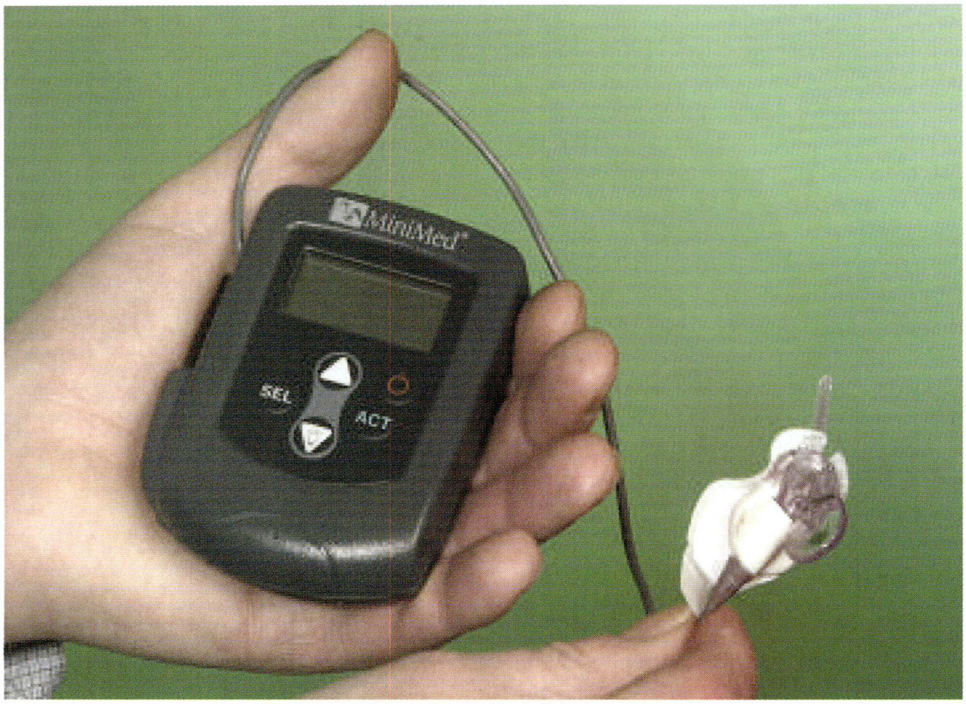

Figure 3 The Medtronic MiniMed CGMS

There is evidence that treatment adjustments made as the result of CGMS profiling can either improve overall glycemic control (HbA_{1c}) or reduce the frequency of hypoglycemia [41–43, 46], but most of these studies were uncontrolled.

The Future of Enzyme Electrodes: Total Implantation and Closing the Loop?

An alternative approach to subcutaneous glucose sensing is the total implantation of a glucose oxidase, H_2O_2-based

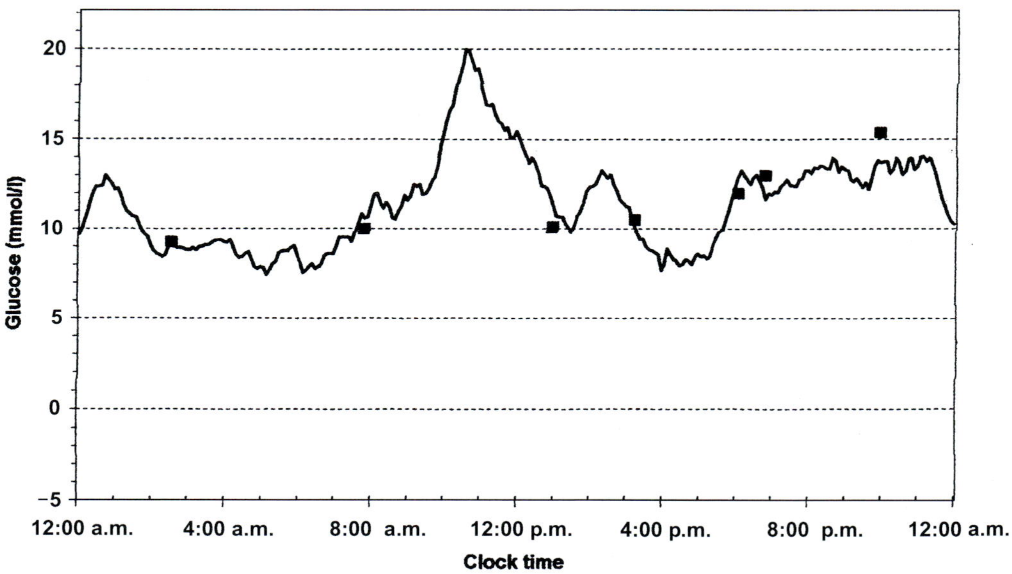

Figure 4 *In vivo* glucose monitoring in a type 1 diabetic patient using CGMS, compared with intermittent capillary blood glucose self-monitoring (squares). Note the marked postprandial hyperglycemia not detected by capillary sampling

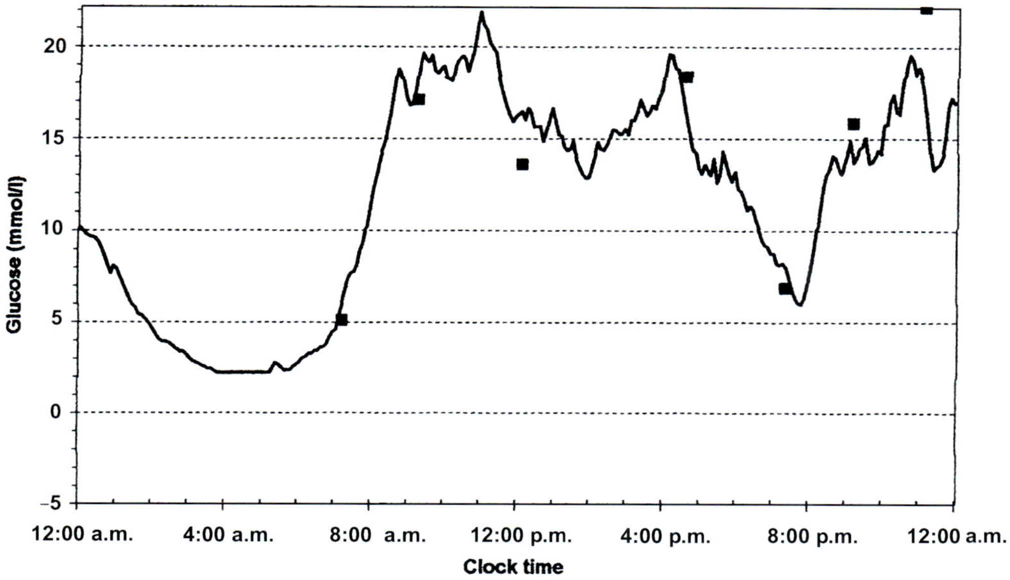

Figure 5 *In vivo* glucose monitoring in a type 1 diabetic patient using CGMS, compared with intermittent capillary blood glucose self-monitoring (squares). Note the period of nocturnal hypoglycemia detected by CGMS

glucose sensor. This allows a larger design, the ones described by Updike and colleagues for implantation in dogs are 7 cm in diameter and 14 cm thick, and data are communicated to outside the body via a radio transmitter and receiver [48, 49]. One design has an outer angiogenic membrane, with the aim of stimulating capillary formation around the sensor. After about 7 days, the sensors function well and some were reported to have a lifetime of >100 days.

Feedback-controlled, closed-loop systems have been described operating for a few days with a subcutaneous glucose sensor coupled to intravenous infusion of insulin in dogs [7, 50] and humans [51]. A glucose sensor totally implanted in the superior vena cava and based on immobilized glucose oxidase and detection of oxygen consumption has been tested experimentally in type 1 diabetic patients, with reportedly good correlation with capillary blood glucose after some months [14, 52]. Preliminary trials have been reported of this sensor used as a closed-loop system over 48 h [52].

Microdialysis and Open-Flow Microperfusion

In microdialysis, a fine hollow dialysis fiber is implanted in the subcutaneous tissue and perfused with isotonic fluid (Figure 6). Glucose diffuses into the fiber from the tissues and is pumped to the outside of the body for measurement by a biosensor, often a glucose oxidase enzyme electrode of the same design as described above, or some other analytical method [20, 53–56]. The potential advantages of microdialysis are that the sampled fluid is diluted and may cause less interference at the sensor, which is itself external and can be made larger and perhaps more stable than the miniature needle-type glucose sensor.

One system, the GlucoDay (Menarini Diagnostics), has recently been commercialized, shows promising stability, and uses a simple one-point calibration over one day [55]. Correcting for the 30-min delay caused by fluid transportation, there was a good correspondence between blood and sensor readings in first tests. An alternative microdialysis system under development by Roche Diagnostics shows good performance over 3 days [56].

An alternative, related technology for continuous *ex vivo* monitoring is open-flow microperfusion [57]. Here, a double-lumen catheter is inserted in the abdominal subcutaneous adipose tissue and isotonic, ion-free solution is slowly (2 μl/min) perfused through the inner lumen and diluted subcutaneous tissue fluid transported from the outer lumen to the sensor outside the body. The changing

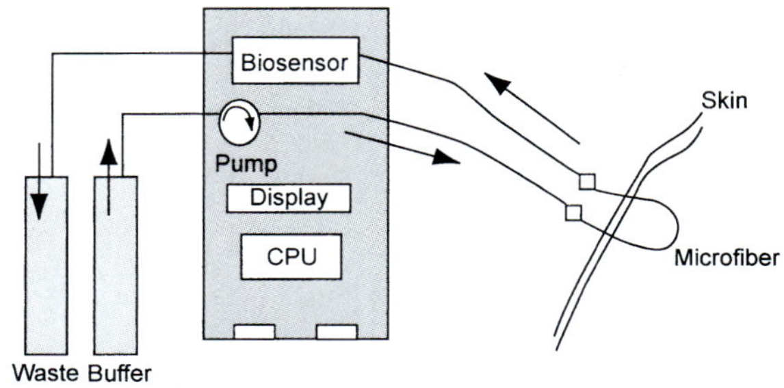

Figure 6 The principle of microdialysis. A fine dialysis fiber is implanted in the subcutaneous tissue, and isotonic fluid pumped through the fiber. An *ex vivo* biosensor measures glucose concentration (adapted from reference 56)

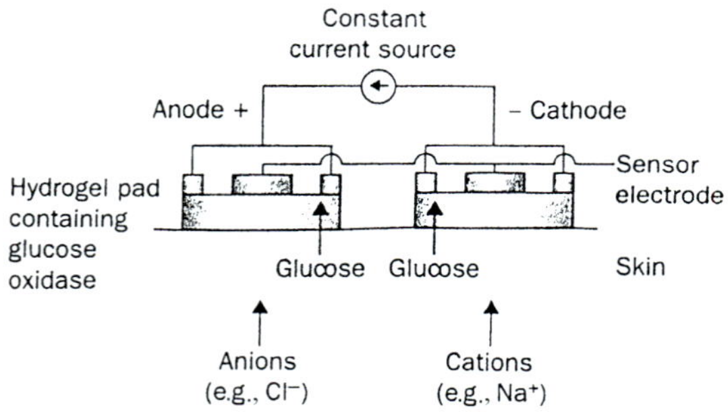

Figure 7 The principle of reverse iontophoresis. A current is passed between two electrodes on the skin surface. Ions are attracted to the surface and carry with them water and glucose. A pad absorbs glucose-containing fluid for measurement by a biosensor

recovery can be estimated by measuring the conductivity of the effluent (subcutaneous fluid conductivity is constant), and thus *in vivo* calibration is avoided. The system has not yet been tested extensively in diabetic subjects.

Reverse Iontophoresis

In reverse iontophoresis, a small current is passed between two electrodes on the skin surface and ions attracted to the anode and cathode carry water and glucose from the interstitial space to the surface by endosmosis (Figure 7). A hydrogel pad on the surface absorbs the glucose-containing fluid and the concentration is measured with a glucose oxidase based biosensor similar in principle to that of the CGMS [58, 60]. The technology has been commercialized as the Cygnus GlucoWatch, which is a watch-type device, usually worn on the arm (Figure 8). The operating and measuring cycle of the original GlucoWatch device consisted of two 10-min periods (3-min iontophoresis, 7-min sensing), and so three readings were made per hour. After a 3-h run in period, the sensor was calibrated against an initial capillary blood glucose sample and then run for up to 12 h before download to a portable computer. Unlike the CGMS, there is a real-time glucose readout on the face of the "watch." There are also low and high glucose concentrations and rapid decline alarms.

In initial clinical tests in type 1 diabetic subjects, a good correlation was reported between GlucoWatch sensor readings and capillary blood glucose concentrations [59, 60] and there was close tracking of blood glucose changes, the sensor lagging behind serial blood glucose values by a mean of 18 min [60]. The effectiveness of the device in detecting hypoglycemia has also been reported [61].

Several problems have been encountered with the original technology of reverse iontophoresis [62]. The GlucoWatch skips readings after excessive sweating, movement, and exposure to cold so it can prove unsuitable for those with an active lifestyle and during winter use. Nighttime use might also be a problem (because of sweating and movement) and in our series 10% of patients had automatic shutoff of the device during the night because of excessive skipped readings. A further problem is an itchy skin rash under the area of wear, which develops in many of the users and is sometimes severe enough to prevent multiple wear periods. Nevertheless, it is likely that alterations to current flow and other modifications to

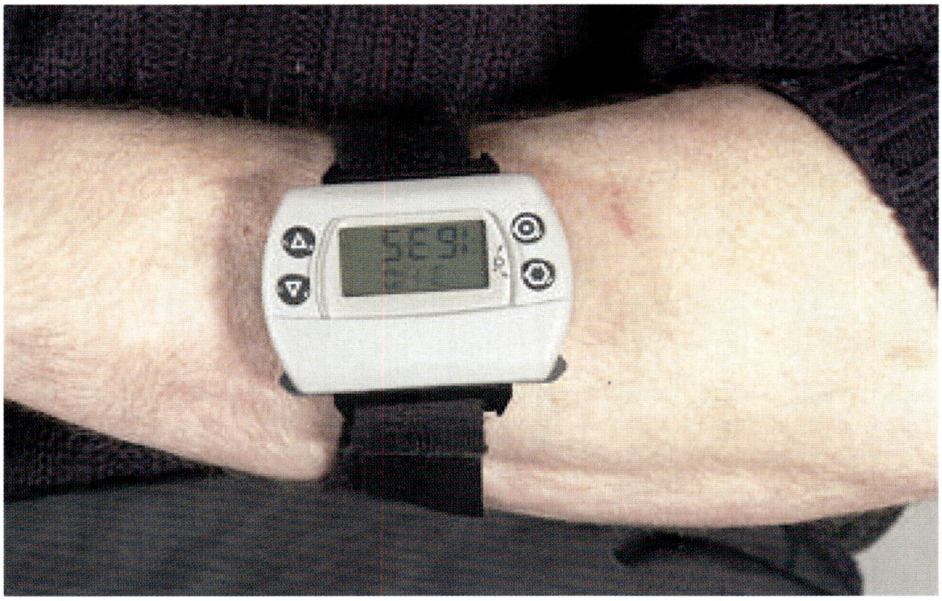

Figure 8 The GlucoWatch (Cygnus Inc.), a device operating by reverse iontophoresis

subsequent models can improve the performance of the technology. The latest model has a shorter warm-up period of 2 h, readings every 10 min, and a slightly longer 13-h intended wear period.

Other Minimally Invasive Technologies

A number of technologies have been described for probe-type glucose sensors that can be implanted in the subcutaneous tissue but have yet to be fully tested or developed for patient use. These include a "bioaffinity" fiber optic glucose sensor [63], where the glucose-binding lectin, concanavalin A, is attached to the inner wall of a hollow dialysis fiber. Fluoresceinated dextran of high molecular weight is confined inside the fiber and binds to the concanavalin A in competition with glucose. Increasing glucose displaces the dextran and increases fluorescence detected by the fiber optic. The slow reversibility of the system may be a problem for further development.

Another affinity-based sensing system detects glucose-dependent changes in the viscosity of a liquid containing dextran and concanavalin A, before and after perfusion through an implanted microdialysis probe [64]. We have described a concanavalin A based fluorescence assay for glucose which is particularly suitable for development as an implanted *in vivo* probe because it operates in the near-infrared NIR region and can thus be excited and interrogated from outside the body [64, 65]. In addition, glucose is detected by changes in fluorescence lifetime rather than intensity, and lifetimes are relatively independent of light scattering in the tissues. In this system, glucose induces a reduction in fluorescence resonance energy transfer between concanavalin A (labeled with the donor NIR fluorescent protein, allophycocyanin) and dextran (labeled with the dye acceptor, malachite green). A similar, but fluorescence intensity-based system uses fluorescein-labeled dextran and rhodamine-labeled concanavalin A, encapsulated in a polyethylene glycol hydrogel [66].

NONINVASIVE TECHNOLOGIES

NIR Spectroscopy

The most studied non-invasive method of measuring glucose is NIR spectroscopy [67, 70]. This technology is based on the fact that light in the NIR range of the spectrum travels through several centimeters of tissue, so that analyte-induced changes in the absorption or reflection spectrum can be sought from outside the body. Although there are only small glucose-related NIR changes *in vitro*, chemometric (i.e. multivariate statistical) techniques can be employed to relate *in vivo* NIR responses and blood glucose levels at several different wavelengths and thereby build models predicting glucose from body surface (e.g. finger, lip, tongue) NIR measurements [71–74]. However, precision so far has been too poor for routine clinical application, perhaps because of unpredictable variations in blood flow, tissue hydration, temperature, and interfering substances (especially water, fat, and hemoglobin) that also absorb NIR light [67, 70, 74]. Improved calibration procedures are said to give better results over longer periods in greater numbers of patients [75], but these procedures have not been extensively tested and validated.

Other Noninvasive Technologies

Although light scattering is a potential problem for NIR methods, it can also be used as a measuring technology [70, 76] since the amount of tissue light scattering is related to the ratio of the refractive indices of the plasma or interstitial fluid to the cell, fibril, and other particles. Increasing the glucose of the tissue fluid increases the refractive index and decreases the scattering coefficient by about 1% for each 5 mmol/l glucose change [76]. An acceptable correlation has been found between scattering and blood glucose in some (but not all) healthy subjects and type 2 diabetic patients [76]; and doubtless the same problems of varying tissue hydration and interfering non-glucose metabolites, etc. (which cause imprecision with *in vivo* NIR studies) are also operative here.

In photoacoustic spectroscopy, pulsed NIR light from a laser source at the body surface is absorbed by molecules such as glucose, causing thermal expansion and the generation of an ultrasound wave, which is detectable at the skin surface with a piezoelectric microphone [77, 78]. Studies in whole blood and tissue phantoms show encouraging relationships between glucose and the photoacoustic response, as do preliminary *in vivo* measurements during meal tests [79], but more development for clinical application is needed.

THE FUTURE

A possible non-invasive approach to metabolic monitoring is to measure changes in cellular autofluorescence, such as that due to NAD(P)H (the reduced form of nicotinamide adenine dinucleotide or its phosphate) [80]. Many glucose-dependent metabolic pathways increase NAD(P)H levels in the cell, including glycolysis, the sorbitol pathway, the tricarboxylic acid (Krebs) cycle, and the pentose phosphate pathway. NAD is nonfluorescent but since its reduced form, NAD(P)H, fluoresces at about 450 nm when excited at 370 nm, it is possible to relate glucose metabolism to NAD(P)H fluorescence [81]. We recently demonstrated a clear glucose-related increase in fluorescence in adipocyte and fibroblast cell lines in culture. As NADH fluorescence is known to be detectable at the skin surface [82], this might be translated into a system for non-invasive glucose monitoring. Since the fluorescence is related to cellular glucose metabolism, the relationship with blood glucose concentration will need to be established.

A major challenge for the future includes understanding more about the factors that create imprecision with non-invasive glucose sensors, whatever the technology. And though minimally invasive sensors have at last entered clinical practice, there is much to be learned about how to use the information from sensors so as to improve the metabolic control and the lifestyle of the diabetic patient.

REFERENCES

1. Cass AEG, Davis G, Francis CD, Hiu HAO, Aston WJ, Higgins IJ, Plotkin EV, Scott CO, Turner APF. Ferrocene-mediated enzyme electrode for amperometric determination of glucose. *Anal Chem* 1984; 56: 667–71.
2. Pickup J. Developing glucose sensors for *in vivo* use. *Trends Biotech* 1993; 11: 285–91.
3. Pickup J, McCartney L, Rolinski O, Birch D. *in vivo* glucose sensing for diabetes management: progress towards non-invasive monitoring. *BMJ* 1999; 319: 1289.
4. Koschinsky T, Heinemann L. Sensors for glucose monitoring: technical and clinical aspects. *Diab Metab Res Rev* 2001; 17: 113–23.
5. Turner APF, Karube I, Wilson GS (eds). *Biosensors: Fundamentals and Applications*. Oxford: Oxford University Press, 1987.
6. Thévenot DR, Toth K, Durst RA, Wilson GS. Electrochemical biosensors: recommended definitions and classification. *Pure Appl Chem* 1999; 71: 2333–48.
7. Shichiri M, Kawamori R, Yamasaki T, Hakui N, Abe H. Wearable-type artificial pancreas with needle-type glucose sensor. *Lancet* 1982; ii: 1129–31.
8. Rebrin K, Fischer U, Hahn von Dorsche H, von Woetke T, Abel P, Brunstein E. Subcutaneous glucose monitoring by means of electrochemical sensors: fiction or reality? *J Biomed Eng* 1992; 14: 33–40.
9. Bindra DS, Zhang Y, Wilson GS, Sternberg R, Thévenot DR, Moatti D, Reach G. Design and in vitro studies of a needle-type glucose sensor. *Anal Chem* 1991; 63: 1692–6.
10. Shaw GW, Claremont DJ, Pickup J. in vitro testing of a simply constructed, highly stable glucose sensor suitable for implantation in diabetic patients. *Biosens Bioelectron* 1991; 6: 401–6.
11. Pickup JC, Claremont DJ, Shaw GW. Responses and calibration of amperometric glucose sensors implanted in the subcutaneous tissue of man. *Acta Diabetol* 1993; 30: 143–8.
12. Mastrototaro JJ. The MiniMed Continuous Glucose Monitoring System. *Diabetes Technol Ther* 2000; 2 (suppl 1): 13–8.
13. Armour JC, Lucisano JY, McKean BD, Gough DA. Application of chronic intravascular blood glucose sensor in dogs. *Diabetes* 1990; 39: 1519–26.
14. Renard E, Shah R, Miller M, Stark-Weather T, Kolopp M, Costalat G, Bringer J. Accuracy of real-time blood glucose measurement by long-term sensor system allows automated insulin delivery in diabetic patients. *Diabetes* 2002; 51 (suppl 2): 126A.
15. Claremont DJ, Sambrook IE, Penton C, Pickup JC. Subcutaneous implantation of a ferrocene-mediated glucose sensor in pigs. *Diabetologia* 1986; 29: 817–21.
16. Pickup JC, Shaw GW, Claremont DJ. *in vivo* molecular sensing in diabetes mellitus: an implantable glucose sensor with direct electron transfer. *Diabetologia* 1989; 32: 213–7.
17. Fischer U, Ertle R, Abel P, Rebrin K, Brunstein E, Hahn von Dorsche H, Freyse EJ. Assessment of subcutaneous glucose concentration: validation of the wick technique as a reference for implanted electrochemical sensors. *Diabetologia* 1987; 30: 940–5.
18. Brückel J, Kerner W, Zier H, Steinbach G, Pfeiffer EF. *in vivo* measurement of subcutaneous glucose concentrations with an enzymatic glucose sensor and wick method. *Klin Wochr* 1989; 67: 491–5.
19. Jansson P-A, Fowelin J, Smith U, Lönroth P. Characterization by microdialysis of intercellular glucose level in subcutaneous tissue of humans. *Am J Physiol* 1988; 255: E218–20.
20. Bolinder J, Ungerstedt U, Arner P. Microdialysis measurement of the absolute glucose concentration in subcutaneous adipose tissue allowing glucose monitoring in diabetic patients. *Diabetologia* 1992; 35: 1177–80.
21. Moatti-Sirat D, Capron F, Poitout V, Reach G, Bindra DS, Zhang Y, Wilson GS. Towards continuous glucose monitoring: *in vivo* evaluation of a miniaturised glucose sensor implanted for several days in rat subcutaneous tissue. *Diabetologia* 1992; 35: 224–30.
22. Gerritsen M, Jansen JA, Lutterma JA. Performance of subcutaneously implanted sensors for continuous monitoring. *Neth J Med* 1999; 54: 167–79.
23. Velho G, Froguel P, Thévenot DR, Reach G. *in vivo* calibration of a subcutaneous glucose sensor for determination of subcutaneous glucose kinetics. *Diab Nutr Metab* 1988; 3: 227–33.
24. Fischer U, Hidde A, Herrmann S, von Woedtke T, Rebrin K, Abel P. Oxygen tension at the subcutaneous implantation site of glucose sensors. *Biomed Biochim Acta* 1989: 48: 965–71.
25. Thomé-Duret V, Gangnerau MN, Zhang Y, Wilson GS, Reach G. Modification of the sensitivity of glucose sensor implanted into subcutaneous tissue. *Diabetes Metab* 1996; 22: 174–8.
26. Rigby GP, Crump PW, Vadgama PV. Stabilised needle electrode system for *in vivo* glucose monitoring based on open flow microperfusion. *Analyst* 1996; 121: 871–5.
27. Kerner W, Keck FS, Zier H, Kiwit M, Linke B, Pfeiffer EF. The function of a hydrogen peroxide detecting electroenzymatic glucose electrode is markedly impaired in human subcutaneous tissue and plasma. *Biosens Bioelectron* 1993; 8: 473–82.
28. Linke B, Kiwit M, Thomas K, Krahwinkle M, Kerner W. Prevention of the decrease in sensitivity of an amperometric glucose sensor in undiluted human serum. *Clin Chem* 1999; 45: 283–5.
29. Rebrin K, Steil GM, van Antwerp WP, Mastrototaro JJ. Subcutaneous glucose predicts plasma glucose independent of insulin: implications for continuous monitoring. *Am J Physiol* 1999; 277: E561–71.
30. Aussedat B, Dupirie-Angel M, Gifford R, Klein JC, Wilson GS, Reach G. Interstitial glucose concentration and glycaemia: implications for continuous subcutaneous glucose monitoring. *Am J Physiol* 2000; 278: E716–28.
31. Tiessen RG, Rhemrev-Boom MM, Korf J. Glucose gradient differences in subcutaneous tissue of healthy volunteers assessed with ultraslow microdialysis and a nanolitre glucose sensor. *Life Sci* 2002; 70: 2457–66.

32. Thomé-Duret V, Reach G, Gangnerau MN, Lemmonier F, Klein JC, Zhang Y, Hu Y, Wilson GS. Use of a subcutaneous glucose sensor to detect decreases in glucose concentration prior to observation in blood. *Anal Chem* 1996; 68: 3822–6.
33. Sternberg F, Meyerhoff C, Mennel FJ, Bischof F, Pfeiffer EF. Does fall in tissue glucose precede fall in blood glucose? *Diabetologia* 1996; 39: 609–12.
34. Gross TM, Bode BW, Einhorn D, Kayne DM, Reed JH, White WH, Mastrotatare JJ. Performance evaluation of the MiniMed Continuous Glucose Monitoring System during patient home use. *Diabetes Technol Ther* 2000; 2: 49–56.
35. Sachedina N, Pickup JC. Performance assessment of the Medtronic-MiniMed Continuous Glucose Monitoring System and its use for measurement of glycemic control in type 1 diabetic subjects. *Diabet. Med* (in press).
36. Guerci B, Floriot M, Böhme P, Durain D, Benichou M, Jellimana S, Drouin P. Clinical performance of CGMS in type 1 diabetic patients treated by continuous subcutaneous insulin infusion using insulin analogs. *Diabetes Care* 2003; 26: 582–9.
37. Metzger M, Leibowitz G, Wainstein J, Glaser B, Raz I. Reproducibility of glucose measurements using the glucose sensor. *Diabetes Care* 2002; 25: 1185–91.
38. Monsod TP, Flanagan DE, Rife F, Saenz R, Caprio S, Sherwin RS, Tamborlane WV. Do sensor glucose levels accurately predict plasma glucose concentrations during hypoglycaemia and hyperinsulinemia? *Diabetes Care* 2002; 25: 889–93.
39. Caplin NJ, O'Leary P, Bulsara M, Davis EA, Jones TW. Subcutaneous glucose sensor values closely parallel blood glucose during insulin-induced hypoglycaemia. *Diabet Med* 2003; 20: 238–41.
40. McGowan K, Thomas W, Moran A. Spurious reporting of nocturnal hypoglycaemia by CGMS in patients with tightly controlled type 1 diabetes. *Diabetes Care* 2002; 25: 1499–503.
41. Bode BW, Gross TM, Thornton KR, Mastrototaro JJ. Continuous glucose monitoring used to adjust diabetes therapy improves glycosylated hemoglobin: a pilot study. *Diab Res Clin Pract* 1999; 46: 183–90.
42. Chase HP, Kim LM, Owen SL, MacKenzie TA, Klingensmith GJ, Murtfield R, Garg SK. Continuous subcutaneous glucose monitoring in children with type 1 diabetes. *Pediatrics* 2001; 107: 222–6.
43. Kaufman FR, Gibson LC, Halvorson M, carpenter S, Fisher LK, Pitukcheewanont P. A pilot study of the continuous glucose monitoring system. *Diabetes Care* 2001; 24: 2030–4.
44. Boland E, Monsod T, Delucia M, Brandt CA, Fernando S, Tamborlane WV. Limitations of conventional methods of self-monitoring of blood glucose. Lessons learned from 3 days of continuous glucose sensing in pediatric patients with type 1 diabetes. *Diabetes Care* 2001; 24: 1858–62.
45. Cheyne E, Kerr D. Making "sense" of diabetes: using a continuous glucose sensor in clinical practice. *Diabetes Metab Res Rev* 2002; 18 (suppl 1): 43–8.
46. Schiaffini R, Ciampalini P, Fierabracci A, Spera S, Borrelli P, Bottazzo GF, Crino A. The Continuous Glucose Monitoring System (CGMS) in type 1 diabetic children is the way to reduce hypoglycemic risk. *Diabetes Metab Res Rev* 2002; 18: 324–9.
47. Ludvigsson J, Isacson E. Clinical use of glucose sensors in children and adolescents. *Pract Diabetes Int* 2003; 20: 7–12.
48. Gilligan BJ, Shults MC, Rhodes RK, Updike SJ. Evaluation of a subcutaneous glucose sensor out to 3 months in a dog model. *Diabetes Care* 1984; 17: 882–7.
49. Updike SJ, Shults MC, Gilligan BJ, Rhodes RK. A subcutaneous glucose sensor with improved longevity, dynamic range, and stability of calibration. *Diabetes Care* 2000; 23: 208–14.
50. Rebrin K, Fischer U, von Woedtke T, Abel P, Brunstein E. Automated feedback control of subcutaneous glucose concentration in diabetic dogs. *Diabetologia* 1989; 32: 573–6.
51. Shichiri M, Kawamori R, Hakui N, Yamasaki Y, Abe H. Closed-loop glycemic control with a wearable artificial endocrine pancreas. *Diabetes* 1984; 33: 1200–2.
52. Renard E. Implantable closed-loop glucose-sensing and insulin delivery: the future for insulin pump therapy. *Curr Opin Pharmacol* 2002; 2: 708–16.
53. Meyerhof C, Bischof F, Sternberg F, Zier H, Pfeiffer EF. On line continuous monitoring of subcutaneous tissue glucose in men by combining portable glucosensor with microdialysis. *Diabetologia* 1992; 35: 1087–92.
54. Hashiguchi Y, Sakakida M, Nishida K, Uemura T, Kajiwara K-I, Shichiri M. Development of a miniaturised glucose monitoring system with microdialysis sampling method. *Diabetes Care* 1994; 17: 387–96.
55. Jungheim K, Wientjes K-J, Heinemann L, Lodwig V, Koschinsky T, Schoonen AJ. Subcutaneous continuous glucose monitoring. Feasibility of a new microdialysis based glucose sensor system. *Diabetes Care* 2001; 1696–7.
56. Maran A, Crepaldi C, Tiengo A, Grassi G, Vitali E, Pagano G, Bistoni S, Calabrese G, Santeusanio F, Leonetti F, Ribando M, Di Mario U, Annuzi G, Genovese S, Riccardi G, Previli M, Cucinotta D, Giorgino F, Bellomo A, Giorgino R, Poscia A, Varalli M. Continuous subcutaneous glucose monitoring in diabetic patients. A multicenter study. *Diabetes Care* 2002; 25: 347–52.
57. Trajanoski Z, Brunner GA, Schaupp L, et al. Open-flow microperfusion of subcutaneous adipose tissue for on-line continuous ex vivo measurements of glucose concentration. *Diabetes Care* 1997; 20: 1114–21.
58. Tamada JA, Bohannon NJV, Potts RO. Measurement of glucose in diabetic subjects using non-invasive glucose extraction. *Nat Med* 1995; 1: 1198–201.
59. Garg SK, Potts RO, Ackerman NR, Fermi SJ, Tamada JA, Chase HP. Correlation of fingerstick blood glucose measurements with GlucoWatch Biographer glucose results in young subjects with type 1 diabetes. *Diabetes Care* 1999; 22: 1708–14.
60. Tamada JA, Garg S, Jovanovic L, Pitzer KR, Fermi S, Potts RO. Non–invasive glucose monitoring. Comprehensive clinical results. *JAMA* 1999; 282: 1839–44.
61. Pitzer KR, Desai S, Dunn T, Edelman S, Jayalakshmi Y, Kennedy J, Tamada J, Potts RO. Detection of hypoglycaemia with the GlucoWatch Biographer. *Diabetes Care* 2001; 24: 881–5.
62. Pickup J. Technology advances in glucose monitoring. *Ped Diabetes* 2002; 3: 125–6.
63. Mansouri S, Schultz JS. A miniature optical glucose sensor based on affinity binding. *Biotechnology* 1984; 2: 885–90.
64. Rolinski OJ, Birch DJS, McCartney LJ, Pickup JC. A time-resolved near infrared fluorescence assay for glucose: opportunities for trans dermal sensing. *J Photochem Photobiol B* 2000; 54: 26–34.

65. McCartney LJ, Pickup JC, Rolinski OJ, Birch DJS. Near-infrared fluorescence lifetime assay for serum glucose based on allophycocyanin labelled concanavalin A. *Analyt Biochem* 2001; 292: 216–21.
66. Russel RJ, Pishko MV, Gefrides CC, McShane MJ, Coté GL. A fluorescence-based glucose biosensor using concanavalin A and dextran encapsulated in a poly(ethylene glycol) hydrogel. *Anal Chem* 1999; 71: 3126–32.
67. Khalil OS. Spectroscopic and clinical aspects of Non–invasive glucose measurements. *Clin Chem* 1999; 45: 165–77.
68. Arnold MA. Non-invasive glucose monitoring. *Curr Opin Biotechnol* 1996; 7: 46–9.
69. Klonoff DC. Non–invasive blood glucose monitoring. *Diabetes Care* 1997; 20: 206–11.
70. Heinemann L, Schmelzeise Redecker G. Non-invasive continuous glucose monitoring in type 1 diabetic patients with optical glucose sensors. *Diabetologia* 1998; 41: 848–54.
71. Robinson MR, Eaton RP, Haaland DM, Koepp GW, Thomas EV, Stallard BR, Robinson PL. Non-invasive glucose monitoring in diabetic patients: a preliminary evaluation. *Clin Chem* 1992; 38: 1618–22.
72. Marbach R, Koschinsky T, Gries FA, Heise HM. Non–invasive blood glucose assay by near-infrared diffuse reflectance spectroscopy of the human inner lip. *Appl Spectrosc* 1993; 47: 875–81.
73. Kajiwara K, Uemura T, Kishikawa H, Nishida K, Hashiguchi Y, Heharo M, Sakakida M, Ichinose K, Shichiri M. Non–invasive measurement of blood glucose concentrations by analysing Fourier transform infra-red absorbance spectra through oral mucosa. *Med Biol Eng Comput* 1993; 31: S17–22.
74. Burmeister JJ, Arnold MA, Small GW. Non–invasive blood glucose measurements by near-infrared transmission spectroscopy across human tongues. *Diabetes Technol Ther* 2000; 2: 5–16.
75. Garg SK, Fischer JS, Ruchti TL, Blank TB, Lorenz AD, Monfre SL. Calibration break-through for near-infrared, non-invasive blood glucose monitoring. *Diabetes* 2002; 51 (suppl 2): 122A.
76. Heinemann L, Krämer U, Klörster H-M, Hein M, Volz D, Hermann M, Heise T, Rave K. Non–invasive glucose measurement by monitoring of scattering coefficient during oral glucose tolerance tests. *Diabetes Technol Ther* 2000; 2: 211–20.
77. Christison GB, MacKennzie HA. Laser photoacoustic determination of physiological glucose concentrations in human blood. *Med Biol Eng Comput* 1993; 31: 284–90.
78. Quan KM, Christison GB, MacKenzie HA, Hodgson P. Glucose determination by a pulsed photoacoustic technique: an experimental study using a gelatin-based tissue phantom. *Phys Med Biol* 1993; 38: 1911–22.
79. MacKenzie HA, Aston HS, Spiers S, Shen Y, Freebern SS, Hannigan J, Lindberg J, Rae P. Advances in photoacoustic noninvasive glucose testing. *Chin Chem* 1999; 45: 1587–95.
80. Evans N, Gnudi L, Rolinski OJ, Birch DJS, Pickup JC. Non-invasive glucose monitoring in fibroblasts and adipocytes by measurements of intrinsic fluorescence. *Diabetes* 2003; 52 (suppl 1): 93A.
81. Piston DW, Knobel SM. Real-time analysis of glucose by microscopy. *Trans Endocr Metab* 1999; 10: 413–7.
82. Masters BR, So PTC, Gratton E. Multiphoton excitation fluorescence microscopy and spectroscopy of *in vivo* human skin. *Biophys J* 1997; 72: 2405–12.

96

Glycated Hemoglobin and Serum Proteins as Tools for Monitoring

Barry J. Goldstein, Serge Jabbour, and Intekhab Ahmed

Jefferson Medical College, Thomas Jefferson University, Philadelphia, PA, USA

INTRODUCTION

Technological advances have greatly improved our ability to monitor glycemic control in patients with diabetes. The wide availability of relatively inexpensive hand-held meters, for example, has facilitated the monitoring of spontaneous blood glucose levels at various times during the day. However, the notorious fluctuation of postprandial glucose values is a common source of frustration in patients with diabetes, as well as the physicians and nurses trying to determine the level of their glycemic control over a longer time frame. To this end, one of the most important clinical advances that has improved modern diabetes care is the recognition that glucose undergoes nonenzymatic chemical reactions with various proteins in the blood, including hemoglobin, in a manner that allows the estimation of an integrated value of the glucose excursions over a period of weeks to months, providing a useful window for glucose monitoring using the hemoglobin A_{1c} (HbA_{1c}) [1, 2]. The early 1980s also saw the emergence of a second group of tests, collectively called "fructosamine," that were based on a determination of glycated serum proteins, especially albumin, and found to be useful for similar clinical purposes over a shorter time period than that for the HbA_{1c} [3, 4]. There has also been growing interest in utilizing measurement of advanced glycosylation end products (AGEs) in serum and in tissues as laboratory correlates of some of the chronic tissue damage observed in patients with diabetes [5]. In the present chapter, starting from a chemical description of the glycation reactions, we will present the pathophysiological background necessary for an understanding of the variety of tests now used for glycated hemoglobin (GHb) and albumin determination and their interpretation in different clinical encounters. Finally, we will briefly describe AGEs and their potential relationship to the chronic complications of diabetes.

GLYCATION REACTIONS

During the early part of the twentieth century, Amadori, Maillard, and others characterized the fundamental chemical reactions that underlie the formation of HbA_{1c} and more advanced protein products associated with aging and tissue damage [6, 7]. Chemically, the basic reaction involves covalent attachment of the aldehyde group of an acyclic glucose molecule to protein amino groups (Figure 1). The first step of this reaction, resulting in the formation of a Schiff base, can be transient and reversible, while the second step yields a fixed ketoamine product. The potential clinical utility of these observation stems from the appreciation that these slow, nonenzymatic processes occur *in vivo*, and that the accumulation of protein glycation products is significantly increased in patients with hyperglycemia [8, 9]. The best known of these products is GHb and its related derivatives, including the hemoglobin HbA_{1c} subfraction, which has evolved over the past several decades from an intriguing finding in diabetic patients [10] to become a critically important clinical variable to evaluate the level of glycemic control in patients with diabetes over time [11–13]. In addition, protein glycation products undergo further rearrangements towards the development of AGEs, which have been associated with chronic complications of diabetes, including

International Textbook of Diabetes Mellitus, Third Edition. Edited by R. A. DeFronzo, E. Ferrannini, H. Keen, and P. Zimmet.
 ISBN: 0-471-48655-8.

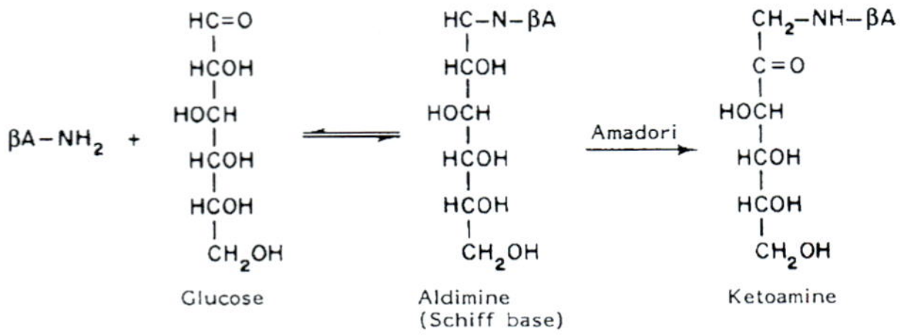

Figure 1 Reaction of glucose with the NH_2-terminal amino group of the β-chain of hemoglobin A (βA-NH_2) to form an aldimine linkage or Schiff base structure. This is an unstable structure (also called pre-A_{1c}) that can undergo rapid reversal to the two initial components. Alternatively, a slower reaction occurs involving an Amadori rearrangement to the more stable ketoamine linkage, forming HbA_{1c}

tissue damage and cardiovascular disease, as discussed below [4, 5].

In solution, the native glucose molecule exists primarily as an inert closed-ring structure. The open form, constituting 0.001% of the dissolved glucose, however, has a reactive aldehyde group with a unique capacity to bind covalently with proteins, generally to the free ε-amino group of lysine side chains [14]. In hemoglobin A, (HbA) the amino group of the β-chain N-terminal valine is also highly reactive with glucose [15, 16]. In both instances, the initial product is the unstable Schiff base or aldimine linkage, which may dissociate or spontaneously progress to a ketoamine or Amadori product, which is only partially reversible [17] (Figure 1). The rate of formation of the Schiff base depends predominantly on the ambient glucose concentration, while the formation of ketoamine is influenced by both the glucose concentration and the time of exposure of the protein to glucose [18–20].

GLYCATION OF HEMOGLOBIN

The glycation of HbA, leading to the formation of HbA_{1c} and other derivatives, the best characterized of the clinically important protein glycation reactions, is unique in several respects. One is the novel formation of a linkage between glucose and the amino group of the N-terminal valine of the hemoglobin β-chain, which serves as a unique recognition target for clinical biochemical assay methods, as described below [21]. Secondly, in contrast to the glycation of other serum proteins, it is crucial to recognize that the glycation of HbA is an *intracellular* process. Thus, determinants of the concentration of glucose within the red cells as well as factors that affect the turnover and life span of the erythrocytes will strongly influence the level of GHb.

Glucose first enters red blood cells by facilitated diffusion through membrane transport proteins with a Michaelis constant of about 0.5–2.0 mmol/l [22]. The intracellular glucose is phosphorylated by hexokinase and enters the three major pathways of erythrocyte glucose metabolism, including glycolysis to pyruvate/lactate, formation of 2,3-bisphosphoglycerate, and the pentose phosphate pathway. The activity of hexokinase and all three major metabolic pathways declines exponentially during the life of the red cell, with a major loss of the enzyme activities during the transition from reticulocyte to mature cell [23]. The loss in intracellular capacity to metabolize glucose causes a more rapid equilibration of extracellular glucose with the intracellular compartment and can lead to a subsequent rise in the glycation of hemoglobin in aging red cells. Further support for this hypothesis comes from the finding that HbA_{1c} concentrations are increased in nondiabetic patients with altered erythrocyte glucose metabolism such as those with glucose-6-phosphate dehydrogenase deficiency [24]. Interestingly, GHb is virtually undetectable in porcine red cells, since glucose transport across the pig erythrocyte membrane is very limited, and this minimizes the intracellular content of free glucose [25].

As pointed out above, glycation may also occur at other sites on hemoglobin, which may be detected or missed by some of the routinely used methods for GHb [14, 15]. Thus, ion-exchange chromatography, operating on the basis of a charge difference, separates hemoglobin modified at the N-terminal valine, while weak acid hydrolysis detects all the glycation sites of HbA that occur with varying degrees of reactivity (see below). Therefore, a physician using one of several available GHb assays for clinical patient management needs to be familiar with what form of the modified protein has actually been measured. These considerations will affect the clinical implications of the test results [2, 26].

Nomenclature

Glycosylation should be reserved to describe the enzymatic transfer of carbohydrates to proteins, such as during protein biosynthesis and posttranslational processing. In contrast, *glycation* is the term that best describes the process of nonenzymatic bonding of glucose to proteins, as in the formation of HbA_{1c}. The most commonly employed tests for GHb in current clinical practice involve the following glycated protein derivatives:

(1) *Hemoglobin A (HbA)* is "native" hemoglobin consisting of the unmodified globin tetramer formed from two α- and two β-chains.
(2) *Total glycated hemoglobin (GHb)* includes glycation at the N-terminal valine of β-globin in HbA (the actual HbA_{1c} component) as well as additional derivatives including glycation at other valines and lysines in the hemoglobin molecule. GHb also encompasses glycation of other hemoglobin types (HbS, HbC, HbF, etc.).
(3) *Hemoglobin A_1 (HbA_1)* refers to all the glycated species derived from adducts to the N-terminal valine

in the β-chain of HbA. It consists of several components classified according to the nature of the carbohydrate moiety. For example, fructose-1,6-diphosphate forms HbA_{1a1}, glucose-6-phosphate forms HbA_{1a2}, etc.

(4) *Hemoglobin A_{1c} (HbA_{1c})* is a component of HbA_1 formed by nonenzymatic addition of glucose to the N-terminal valine of the β-chain of HbA. As it is a subfraction of GHb and HbA_1, HbA_{1c} content is always a smaller percentage compared to the other two.

(5) *Hemoglobin A_0 (HbA_0)* is a major component of HbA that is posttranslationally modified, including addition of sugars but without an N-terminal valine adduct to the β-chain.

GLYCATION IN INDIVIDUALS WITH NORMAL GLUCOSE TOLERANCE

Kinetics of Glycation

Studies in normoglycemic individuals with radiolabeled iron documented that HbA_{1c} increases linearly during the life span of the erythrocyte [18], with the lowest HbA_{1c} content in the youngest population of erythrocytes and the highest content in the oldest cells [27]. In patients with diabetes, this relation is less clear, reflecting day-to-day changes in the serum glycemic profiles [27]. At any rate, there is no evidence that there is a certain period of the erythrocyte life-span when glycation occurs selectively. From these considerations it also follows that conditions causing a reduced life-span of the erythrocytes will cause a reduction in measured HbA_{1c} concentration [21]. In fact, it has been proposed that measurement of HbA_{1c} may serve as a measure of the erythrocyte life-span in individuals with normal glucose tolerance and without a hemoglobinopathy [28].

Glycated Hemoglobin in Nondiabetic Populations

The range of GHb values varies significantly in the normal population. Several groups of investigators have attempted to determine the factors associated with the distribution of GHb in nondiabetic individuals. From these studies it is clear that variation in the erythrocyte life-span does not seem to be the sole cause of variation in normal GHb values [29, 30]. In the large, cross-sectional "France Telecom" study, involving 3240 subjects without known diabetes, pregnancy, or hemoglobinopathies, HbA_{1c} rose with deterioration in glucose tolerance, age, body mass index, family history of diabetes, as well as in women with a history of delivering large babies, and after menopause [29]. No difference in the GHb (A_{1c}) was noted between males and females, and in both sexes HbA_{1c} was higher in smokers than in nonsmokers. Although some seasonal variation was observed, it did not assume a consistent pattern over a 2-year period of observation. In a stepwise multiple regression analysis, the most significant factors associated with HbA_{1c} level were age followed by fasting plasma glucose (FPG) [29]. Even so, the strongest correlation, i.e. between HbA_{1c} and FPG, was strikingly low ($r = 0.20$). Yudkin et al. [30] identified among nondiabetic individuals those who had relatively elevated or depressed GHb values, as confirmed by four different methods. The low and high glycators represented approximately 20% of the study population. The observed variation in GHb could not be explained on the basis of glucose level, age, gender, body mass index, hemoglobin levels, smoking, dietary habits, or vitamin intake.

Glycated Hemoglobin as a Screening Test for Diabetes

Since some of the variation in GHb levels in normal populations may be poorly explained by glycemia, and glycohemoglobin testing has been poorly standardized over the years, it has been difficult to recommend the use of these tests as a method of screening for diabetes mellitus in practice [31, 32]. However, the predictive value of a screening test also depends on the prevalence of the disease in the population under study. In populations known to have a high incidence of diabetes, the correlation between glycemia and GHb can be quite good [33, 34]. Glycated hemoglobin testing in these groups can have better sensitivity and specificity for detecting diabetes over random screening [35] but is generally not superior to fasting blood glucose measurements [36]. In a study of 381 Pima Native Americans with a high incidence of type 2 diabetes, an HbA_{1c} test was compared to formal oral glucose tolerance test criteria for the diagnosis of diabetes or impaired glucose tolerance (IGT). While an elevated HbA_{1c} usually indicates the presence of diabetes or IGT (sensitivities of 85 and 30%, respectively), a normal GHb was unable to *exclude* a diagnosis of diabetes or IGT [37] (Figure 2). Since a considerable number of individuals with IGT have HbA_{1c} values within the nondiabetic reference range, many experts, including the American Diabetes Association, do not currently support its use in diagnosis [2, 38, 39], although others support its diagnostic utility [40]. This issue may persist partly because of changing glycemic standards for diabetes diagnosis [39], as well as the challenges in developing national and international criteria for the performance and standardization of the HbA_{1c} assay [41].

GLYCATED HEMOGLOBIN IN PATIENTS WITH DIABETES MELLITUS

Kinetic Response of Glycated Hemoglobin to Alterations in Glycemic Control

A large body of data from early studies provided convincing evidence for the close correlation between GHb

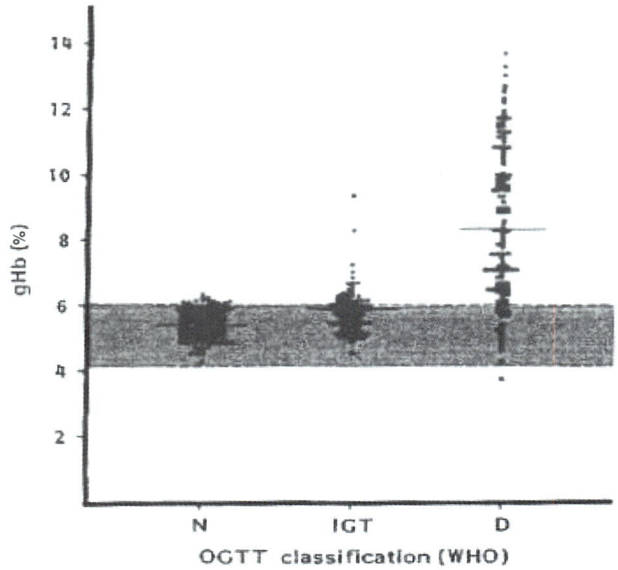

Figure 2 Glycated hemoglobin levels (GHb) in 159 subjects with normal glucose tolerance (N), 91 with impaired glucose tolerance (IGT), and 131 with diabetes (D), diagnosed by WHO criteria using an oral glucose tolerance test. Broken lines delimit the normal range of HbA_{1c} (from reference 37, reproduced by permission of the American Diabetes Association)

and glycemic control in patients with diabetes. In one well-characterized patient, the improvement in glycemic control, as estimated by glycosuria, was achieved over a 3-week period, while the reduction in HbA_{1c} lagged behind by 3–4 weeks and leveled off only after a period of 7–8 weeks had passed [11]. The rate of decline of HbA_{1c} in newly diagnosed diabetic patients generally begins only 2 weeks after the initiation of insulin therapy and tends to level off beyond the seventh week (Figure 3). A half-life of 28 days was shown for HbA_{1c} in patients with recently diagnosed type 1 diabetes who achieved a rapid normalization of glycemic control after initiation of insulin treatment [42].

The data on the kinetics of a rise in GHb values *in vivo* are limited. In non-insulin-dependent diabetic patients, HbA_1 rose from 12.6 to 14.1% after 1 week of deterioration in glycemic control induced by withdrawal of oral sulfonylureas [43]. Studies using partial pancreatectomy in dogs, allowing observation of a longer duration of hyperglycemia, revealed a curvilinear rise in the stable HbA_{1c} over a 12-week period [44].

Use of Glycated Hemoglobin to Quantify the Antecedent Glycemia

The quantitative nature of the relationship between glycemic control and HbA_{1c} was studied in a mixed group

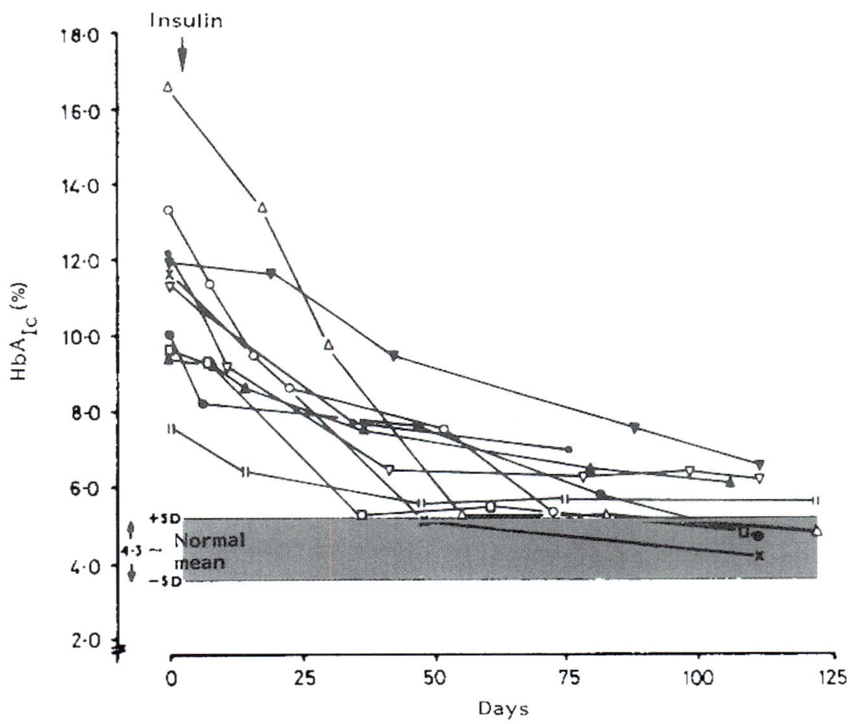

Figure 3 Time course of the decrease in HbA_{1c} concentrations during prolonged optimal regulation of blood glucose in 10 newly diagnosed diabetic patients (from reference 42, reproduced by permission of the British Medical Journal)

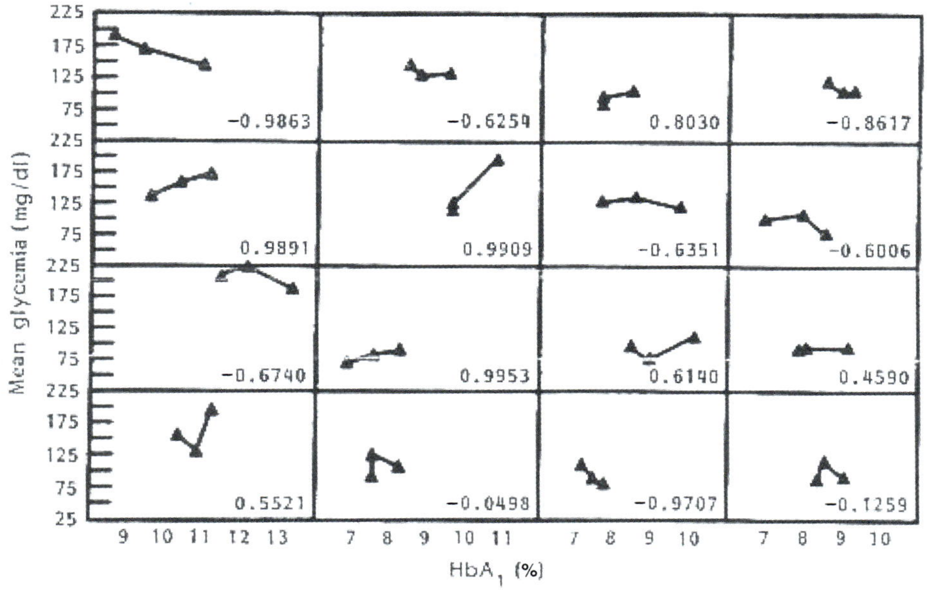

Figure 4 Mean glycemia determined by frequent glucose sampling at 1, 2, and 3 months; 3, 4, and 5 months; and 5, 6, and 7 months vs. HbA_1 level obtained at 4, 6, and 8 months, respectively, for 16 individual diabetic patients. In each box, the horizontal axis is the HbA_1 values and the vertical axis is the mean glycemia level. The individual correlation coefficients are shown (from reference 47, reproduced by permission of the American Diabetes Association)

of 40 type 1 and type 2 diabetic patients treated with insulin [45]. Each study participant performed a seven to eight sampling-point glycemic profile every 2 weeks for three consecutive months. A correlation of 0.93 was observed between mean glycemia from these data and the HbA_{1c} measured at the end of the study. Another study showed that glycemic profile collected over a 5-week period compared to HbA_{1c} measurements taken at the end of the study in 15 diabetic patients had a correlation coefficient of 0.98 [46]. While group correlations have generally demonstrated a close relationship between glycemic control and the GHb level, it is worth cautioning that these correlations can be poor in studies in individual patients, likely because of the inherent difficulties in the quantitation of the mean glycemia from glucose testing [47] (Figure 4).

Based on good group correlations (r values reaching 0.8–0.9), attempts have been made to estimate the mean blood glucose concentration in the preceding 1–3 months using various mathematical modeling equations [46, 48, 49]. As described above, although good correlations for the entire study group could be found, this may not necessarily hold true for correlations calculated on an individual basis [47, 50]. This individual variation might arise from the practical constraints of frequent blood glucose monitoring, consideration of the length of time required to reach a new steady state after an elevation of glycemia to a new constant level, and the slow dynamics of glycation, with reversibility of the Schiff base formation, which further confounds this issue [19, 46]. Nevertheless, the GHb test has proven to be a valuable measure of the adequacy of diabetic treatment and an index of the integrated changes in plasma glucose level over time in diabetic patients.

Glycated Hemoglobin as a Unique Index of Glycemic Control in Type 1 Diabetes

In diabetic patients, the level of GHb can provide the physician with a valuable monitor of the adequacy of control of hyperglycemia. Interestingly, early studies showed that physician judgment about the quality of the antecedent glycemic control based on historical and laboratory data (glycosuria and fasting and random glucose tests) was frequently discordant with the actual data provided by measuring the GHb [48]. Knowing the GHb has gradually become a fundamental feature of modern diabetes care. As a time-averaged monitor of blood glucose, it prompts the physician to work with the patient to intensify management when necessary in order to achieve treatment goals [51]. Measurement of GHb is especially valuable in type 1 diabetes when day-by-day oscillations in glycemia tend to be highly variable, making an accurate assessment of the adequacy of diabetic treatment based on home blood glucose measurement very difficult. In this respect, if there is frequently a discrepancy between glucose values and the GHb, with few rare exceptions (discussed in more detail below), the latter is usually more correct [52].

More detailed recent studies have tried to assess the relative contributions of fasting and postprandial glucose

Table 1 Correlation between hemoglobin A_{1c} level and mean plasma glucose in the DCCT cohort*

	Mean plasma glucose	
HbA_{1c} (%)	mg/dl	mmol/l
6	135	7.5
7	170	9.5
8	205	11.5
9	240	13.5
10	275	15.5
11	310	17.5
12	345	19.5

* From reference 1.

to the HbA_{1c} level. In general, pre- and postprandial glucoses as well as the mean plasma glucose concentrations (the average of multiple glucose measurements taken throughout the day) are highly correlated with HbA_{1c}. In contrast, postprandial glucose (PPG) excursions, the change in glucose concentration from before to after a meal, and the incremental glucose area, the area under the glucose curve that is above the premeal, are poorly correlated with HbA_{1c}. Interestingly, analysis of data from the Diabetes Control and Complications Trial (DCCT) in patients with type 1 diabetes showed bedtime and postlunch plasma glucose correlating most strongly with HbA_{1c}, and fasting and postbreakfast plasma glucose correlating less well. As expected, the mean plasma glucose was the best correlate of HbA_{1c} [1]. Differences in various study populations and methods have made it difficult to accurately determine the relative contribution of the FPG and PPG to HbA_{1c}.

The overall utility of the GHb in adjusting diabetes therapy is tempered by the fact that while it can help to identify patients with poorly controlled hyperglycemia, a high level by itself cannot guide the physician toward specific adjustments in the insulin regimen [49]. The GHb is thus an important ancillary test to be used in the ongoing assessment and treatment planning for the diabetic patient. Analysis of glucose data from the DCCT has provided some general correlations between the measured HbA_{1c} and the antecedent mean glycemia (Table 1) [1]. Comparison of the HbA_{1c} with the patient's own capillary glucose testing enables the physician to alter therapy, especially the timing and amount of multiple insulin injections, to improve the overall diurnal glycemic control.

Value of Glycated Hemoglobin Measurements in Type 2 Diabetes

As shown by a number of investigators [53, 54] the FPG in type 2 diabetes treated with diet or oral sulfonylureas does not vary markedly from day to day. Moreover, fasting hyperglycemia is a reasonably good correlate of preprandial and PPG levels in type 2 diabetes [53]. It thus follows that there is a good correlation between fasting blood glucose and the GHb level, leading several authors to initially suggest that the HbA_{1c} level may be a superfluous measurement in type 2 diabetes, especially in patients on diet or oral drug therapy [55]. In patients with type 2 diabetes requiring insulin treatment, the correlation between fasting glycemia and GHb is not as close as in type 2 patients not requiring insulin, but is still better than in type 1 diabetes. Thus, the periodic measurement of GHb as an assessment of the control of hyperglycemia in insulin-treated patients with either type 1 or type 2 diabetes is clearly justified [2]. A recent consensus conference concluded there are insufficient data to determine accurately the relative contribution of the FPG and PPG to HbA_{1c}, and that overall, the FPG is somewhat better than postprandial glucose in predicting HbA_{1c}, especially in type 2 diabetes [56]. In our opinion, if an elevated GHb level, in addition to an elevated fasting glucose, is required to prompt the care providers and their diabetic patients to adopt a more aggressive treatment strategy, then ordering the GHb assay may prove to be effective for the overall diabetes treatment program.

GLYCATED HEMOGLOBIN TESTING IN PREGNANCY

Maternal hyperglycemia in early pregnancy can lead to an increased incidence of fetal malformations and wastage, and poor glycemic control during later pregnancy is associated with perinatal morbidity [57]. The recognition that the risk of fetal malformations rises sharply with poor diabetic control prompted the use of GHb assays at the first prenatal visit to evaluate the patient's glycemic control over the initial few weeks of gestation [57]. Ideally, the diabetic patient should be managed aggressively prior to conception to achieve a normal or near-normal HbA_{1c} value and minimize the risk to the fetus early in gestation. This is often not possible, however, and the early GHb value may be used in counseling the patient with regard to possible effects on the fetus [58].

Frequent measurement of GHb is a useful adjunct to self-monitoring of blood glucose during a diabetic pregnancy. Since tight regulation of glycemic excursions is an important goal, HbA_{1c} measured at 6-week intervals can help in the overall assessment of the mean blood glucose as estimated from fasting and postprandial capillary values [59]. As in nonpregnant patients with diabetes, the GHb value should corroborate the glucose testing results and lead to a reassessment of the diabetic regimen if poor control is suggested [60]. It is important to note here that the average blood glucose concentration is about 20% lower in normal pregnant women than in nonpregnant women, leading to a small reduction in HbA_{1c} values; so the reference range for HbA_{1c} during pregnancy should be 20% lower than in normal people [59, 60].

GLYCATED HEMOGLOBIN AND CHRONIC COMPLICATIONS OF DIABETES

In long-lived proteins, once glycation has occurred, the protein modifications progress to more complex derivatives called AGEs. The involvement of AGEs in diabetic complications has been suggested by the observation that there is no significant correlation between the presence or severity of chronic complications of diabetes and the GHb level if the duration of observation is less than 2 years [61–64]. On the other hand, observations exceeding the threshold of 2 years have revealed an association of elevated GHb with the development or progression of diabetic retinopathy, nephropathy, and neuropathy.

Early studies demonstrated that A_{1c} was clearly predictive of the chronic complications of diabetes. In the seminal work by Klein and colleagues [65] on more than 1800 patients with diabetes, HbA_{1c} at the initial examination was predictive of the 4-year incidence and progression of diabetic retinopathy. In the group with onset of diabetes at less than 30 years of age, who were all treated with insulin, those with HbA_{1c} above the highest quintile compared with those below the lowest quintile had 1.9 times increased risk for developing any form of retinopathy; the relative risks for proliferative retinopathy and for the progression of retinopathy were 21.8 and 4.0, respectively. In older-onset patients not treated with insulin, the same comparison yielded a relative risk for any form of retinopathy of 4.0 and a relative risk for progression of 6.2. Further early studies confirmed that over a period of 3–9 years, microalbuminuria was 3.6 times and retinopathy 2.5 times more prevalent in patients with mean HbA_{1c} over 12.3% than in those with mean HbA_{1c} less than 10.9% [66]. This group also showed that none of the patients developed retinopathy and microalbuminuria if their GHb was consistently below 9.0% (using a normal range of 6.3–8.2%).

The strongest data supporting that long-term control of diabetes with monitoring of glycemia using the HbA_{1c} provides an index of the risk for development of microvascular diabetic complications comes from the DCCT [67]. This multicenter, 9-year study in a cohort of 1441 patients with type 1 diabetes compared conventional insulin therapy with diabetes management intensified by multiple daily insulin injections or use of an insulin infusion pump and rigorous attention to glycemic control. The intensive treatment resulted in significantly better glycemic control as estimated by HbA_{1c} measurements, reduced from ~9% in the conventionally treated group to ~7% in the intensively treated group (Figure 5). In the primary prevention group (no signs of retinopathy at the start of the study) intensive insulin therapy reduced the onset of retinopathy by ~34%, and reduced microalbuminuria and clinical neuropathy by 35 and 60%, respectively. In addition, there appeared to be a continuous relationship between the HbA_{1c} level and the risk of sustained progression of retinopathy in the entire study cohort (Figure 6). Consistent with these data is the notion that the higher incidence of chronic diabetic complications in the patients with elevated HbA_{1c} was somehow causally related, perhaps through a similar mechanism involving protein glycation in target tissues.

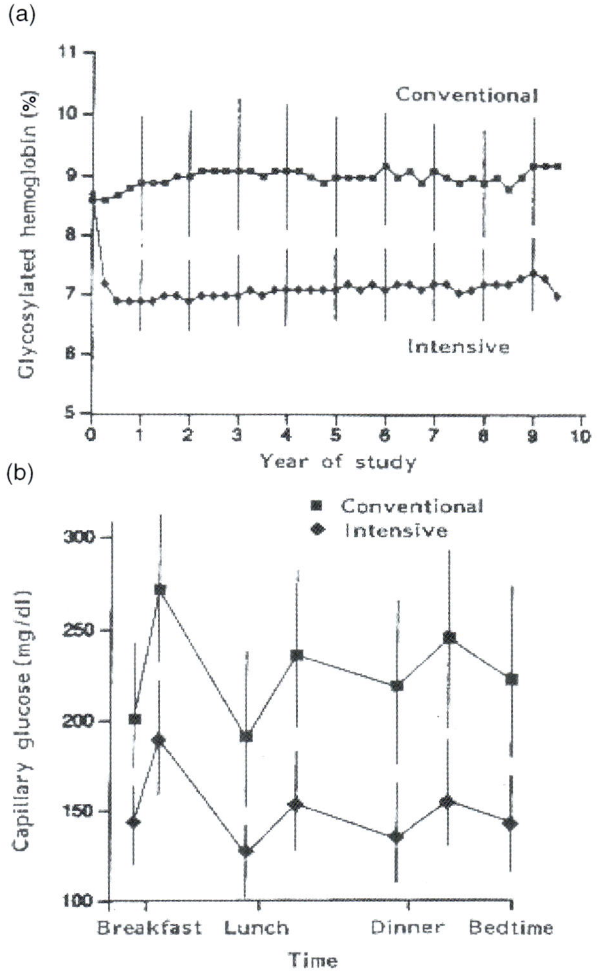

Figure 5 Measurements of glycated hemoglobin (HbA_{1c}) and blood glucose in patients with IDDM receiving intensive or conventional therapy in the DCCT study. (a) The upper panel shows the medians of all quarterly glycosylated hemoglobin values with the 25th and 75th percentiles of the yearly values shown by the vertical lines. (b) The lower panel shows the medians of the quarterly mean values of the seven capillary-blood glucose measurements over a 24-h period in each patient, with the 25th and 75th percentiles indicated by the vertical lines (from reference 67, reproduced by permission of the New England Journal of Medicine)

In a large cohort of more than 5000 patients with type 2 diabetes, the United Kingdom Prospective Diabetes Study (UKPDS) similarly reported that intensive treatment of glycemia using lifestyle modification in addition to oral agents and insulin, resulting in a lowering of the group mean HbA_{1c} from 7.9 to 7.1%, was associated with a

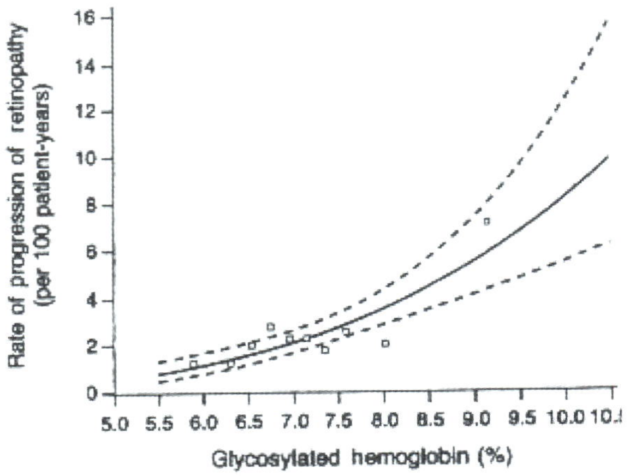

Figure 6 Risk of sustained progression of retinopathy in the patients receiving intensive therapy according to their mean glycosylated hemoglobin values during the DCCT study. Squares indicate the crude rates within deciles of the mean glycosylated hemoglobin (HbA_{1c}) values during the trial; each square corresponds to more than 400 patient-years. The solid line is a regression estimated as a function of the log of the mean glycosylated hemoglobin value; the dashed lines are 95% confidence intervals (from reference 67, reproduced by permission of the New England Journal of Medicine)

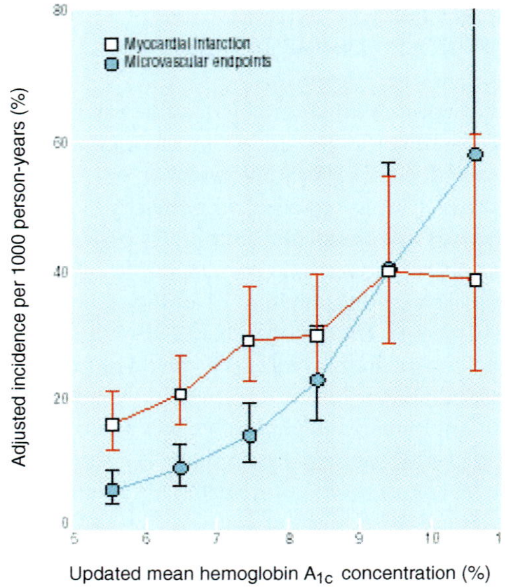

Figure 7 Incidence rates and 95% confidence intervals for myocardial infarction and microvascular complications by category of updated HbA_{1c} concentration, adjusted for age, sex, and ethnic group, expressed for White men aged 50–54 years at diagnosis and with mean duration of diabetes of 10 years (from reference 69, reproduced by permission of the British Medical Journal)

marked reduction in microvascular complications of diabetes [68]. In the updated epidemiological analysis of the UKPDS data, each 1% reduction in updated mean HbA_{1c} was associated with reductions in risk of 21% for any endpoint related to diabetes, 21% for deaths related to diabetes, 14% for myocardial infarction, and 37% for microvascular complications, with no threshold of risk observed for any endpoint [69]. Although not strictly proven in the intervention trial, these observational data suggest that in patients with type 2 diabetes, any reduction in HbA_{1c} is associated with reduced risk of complications, even with values extending into the normal range (<6%) (Figure 7).

Aggressive control of diabetes to improve outcomes with A_{1c} monitoring was also shown in the 8-year prospective Kumamoto Study of 110 Japanese patients with type 2 diabetes [70]. The initial data from this study in type 2 patients were remarkably similar to the DCCT results for patients with type 1 diabetes. Follow-up analyses have also demonstrated that within the intensively treated group, those individuals with a HbA_{1c} value of <6.5% had the lowest cumulative percentage of worsening retinopathy and nephropathy, suggesting that the upper limit of normal for HbA_{1c} may serve as a glycemic threshold for diabetic microvascular complications [71]. In the Norfolk cohort of the European Prospective Investigation of Cancer and Nutrition (EPIC-Norfolk), GHb was a predictor of death from cardiovascular and all causes in 4662 men aged 45–79 not known to be diabetic [72]. HbA_{1c} was continuously related to subsequent all cause, cardiovascular, and ischemic heart disease mortality through the whole population distribution, with lowest rates in those with HbA_{1c} concentration below 5%. An increase of 1% in HbA_{1c} was associated with a 28% increase in risk of death independent of age, blood pressure, serum cholesterol, body mass index, and cigarette-smoking habit. These provocative data suggest that the level of GHb even within the normal range may be closely associated with excess mortality in a population of men not known to be diabetic.

ASSAYS OF GLYCATED HEMOGLOBIN

Different analytical procedures measure one or more of the glycated species of HbA denoted as HbA_1, HbA_{1c}, or GHb (Table 2). Generally, the currently available technology

Table 2 Assay methods for glycated hemoglobin and serum proteins

- Methods based on charge difference
  - –Ion-exchange chromatography
  - –High performance liquid chromatography (HPLC)
  - –Isoelectric focusing
  - –Agar gel electrophoresis
- Methods measuring total GHb
  - –Weak-acid hydrolysis
  - –Affinity chromatography
- Immunoassay-based methods for HbA_{1c}
- Assays for glycated serum proteins
  - –Fructosamine assay
  - –Affinity chromatography

can be divided into two major groups. The first group consists of techniques where separation of glycated and nonglycated hemoglobin is based on the charge difference between HbA_1 and HbA_0, including ion-exchange chromatography, high performance liquid chromatography (HPLC), isoelectric focusing, and agar gel electrophoresis. The second group is based on the presence of glucose within the glycated species; thus, by definition, these techniques measure total GHb. Recently, a third group has emerged based on immunoassay techniques using new monoclonal antibodies with idiotypes that specifically recognize the glucose adduct of the N-terminal valine of HbA in the HbA_{1c} molecule.

Methods Based on Charge Difference

Ion-Exchange Chromatography and High Performance Liquid Chromatography

Ion-exchange chromatography, the most commonly used technique, is essentially based on the method of Trivelli [73]. The original method was laborious and time-consuming, and required the use of large columns and volumes of elution buffers containing cyanides, as well as very stringent control of pH and temperature [74]. The newer assays utilize microcolumns and temperature control column jackets and offer the advantage of speed and relative ease of handling [75]. Kits have been commercially available for some time that contain prepackaged columns with prepared buffers, standards, and additive to eliminate Schiff bases (labile component). Commercial minicolumns are capable of measuring either HbA_1 or HbA_{1c}.

HPLC also uses a principle of charge separation of HbA_1 or HbA_{1c} from HbA_0 but with much greater resolution and speed that lends the technique to automation. Some of the commercial HPLC systems have automatic samplers with a capacity to load up to 100 samples and an analysis time of only a few minutes per sample [76–78].

Isoelectric Focusing and Agar Gel Electrophoresis

Since the isoelectric difference between HbA_{1c} and HbA_0 is only 0.01–0.02 pH units, conventional electrophoresis is not capable of resolving HbA_0 and HbA_{1c} [79]. Isoelectric focusing using a thin-layer polyacrylamide gel containing ampholyte over a pH of 6–8 can resolve these species, but is prohibitively expensive for clinical use [80, 81]. Of this group of techniques, electroendosmosis is more commonly used. This method employs agar gel plates with a citrate buffer; the gels are analyzed by scanning densitometry and are capable of differentiating HbA_1 from HbA_0 in the clinical laboratory setting [82, 83].

Methods Measuring Total Glycated Hemoglobin

Weak-Acid Hydrolysis

This method relies on the ability of weak acids to release ketoamine from GHb and convert it to 5-hydroxymethyl furfural (5-HMF) [84]. The amount of 5-HMF can be determined colorimetrically after reaction with thiobarbituric acid. The initial methods had a number of disadvantages, including difficulty in achieving a complete hydrolysis, breakdown of 5-HMF, interference by glucose in the colorimetric assay, and other problems, but further technical modifications have been made to circumvent these shortcomings [85]. Although virtually every step in the method can be automated, the method is not widely used for clinical purposes.

Affinity Chromatography

The principle of this method lies in the affinity of boronic acids for the cis-diol groups of glucose and on the reversibility of the reaction in aqueous solutions [86]. The commercially available systems based on this principle employ prepacked affinity columns that contain *m*-aminophenylboronic acid immobilized on either cross-linked beaded agarose [87, 88] or Sepharose [89]. The GHb is retained on the columns, while the nonglycated hemoglobin passes through. In the next step the retained GHb is eluted from the column with a buffer containing a competing ligand such as sorbitol. Although it has been shown that a small proportion of GHb is not retained on the column [90] and the assay is sensitive to temperature change [91], the overall variation of replicate samples has been reported to be below 3%.

Method Based on Immunoassay

An immunoassay for HbA_{1c} has recently become available [92]. The method, which is based on microtiter plate technology, utilizes a mouse monoclonal antibody raised against an epitope that consists of the ketoamine linkage plus the first eight amino acids of the N-terminal end of the hemoglobin β-chain. The precision of this method is quite acceptable and the within-batch and between-batch coefficients of variation are equal to or less than 5%. One point to note is the low range of reference values (2.8–4.8%). The HbA_{1c} values determined by the new immunoassay correlates well with other standard methods of HbA_{1c} measurement, including HPLC. Since the antibodies used are specific for the underlying molecular structure of HbA_{1c}, the immunoassay does not detect glycation of other hemoglobin variants, although samples should be treated to remove the labile component (Schiff base), since this can cause falsely elevate the test results.

Which Assay Method to Choose?

The wide array of methods used by various clinical laboratories to measure GHb still causes significant confusion among physicians in spite of several excellent published guidelines. With some exemptions and precautions, in routine clinical or office practice each one of the commercially available methods is an acceptable tool for assessment of glycemic control in patients with diabetes. It is generally not recommended, however, to perform interconversion of results obtained by different methods, owing to lack of relevant standards. This precaution applies especially to attempts at estimating HbA_{1c} from HbA_1 or GHb. In his poignant analysis of the DCCT study, Santiago raised an appropriate note of caution in this regard, commenting that hospitals have often changed their method of analysis of GHbs over the years and that comparison of the results from one test to another can be fraught with difficulty [93]. This is particularly true since attempts at developing standard curves for the various tests demonstrate that they may follow different regression lines. As has been suggested in some published studies, it may be more useful to interpret a patient's HbA_{1c} result as a mean and standard deviation away from the normal value for that laboratory, in order to compare it to previous results using other methods to quantitate a GHb value. We would also advise practitioners not to use services of many laboratories but rather to choose one with an appropriate level of quality control to assure consistency and accuracy of the results. Most commercial methods employ steps to remove the "labile component" or Schiff bases from hemoglobin [19, 94] but it is a good practice to inquire whether the step is performed by an individual source laboratory to understand what has actually been measured. In general the HPLC method adopted for DCCT is probably the "gold standard" against which other methods may be standardized [67]. In the United States, a National Glycohemoglobin Standardization Program was initiated in 1996 to establish clinical laboratory standards and a certification program for HbA_{1c} analyses calibrated to the gold-standard HPLC method used in the DCCT study [41].

FREQUENCY OF GLYCATED HEMOGLOBIN TESTING

What is the appropriate frequency of clinical use of the GHb test? How often a clinician chooses to employ this test depends essentially on the nature of the information he/she wishes to receive. As mentioned above, fluctuations in the level of ambient hyperglycemia preclude the possibility that the glycation reaction ever reaches a true steady state. Therefore, a prerequisite for validation of conversion of GHb values to the level of antecedent hyperglycemia is not strictly met. In practice, the day-to-day oscillations in glycemia in the setting of an unchanged diabetic regimen (medication, diet, and lifestyle) do not prevent the GHb from ultimately stabilizing within a small range of values. Since the glycation reaction proceeds throughout the entire lifespan of the erythrocyte, however, it takes at least 4 months for the change from one relative steady state GHb value to a new "steady state" level to occur. Therefore, in an attempt to make a conversion of GHb to an actual level of antecedent glycemia, the physician must ascertain that no significant change in glycemic control has occurred in the last few months. On the other hand, if the purpose of employing the GHb test is to probe for trends in glycemic control, i.e., whether an improvement or worsening occurred compared to the previous relative steady state, the sampling of GHb is warranted more frequently, after at least 3–4 weeks have passed.

GLYCATED HEMOGLOBIN TESTING AFFECTED BY CO-MORBID ILLNESSES

Hemoglobinopathies

There are a number of potential pitfalls in the use of tests of GHb in the presence of a hemoglobinopathy or other complicating illnesses, affecting the erythrocyte life-span, such as hemolytic anemia (recently reviewed by [38, 95]. In some clinical situations, commonly used clinical assay methods may yield false values (Tables 3 and 4). Understanding the methodology currently used by the practitioner's clinical laboratory is essential to the proper interpretation of the test results. Over 700 hemoglobin variants are recognized worldwide, and some, like HbS, are common, affecting up to 9% of African Americans [96]. Since the presence of hemoglobinopathies can markedly affect HbA_{1c} test results, close attention should be paid to the interpretation of laboratory results in this setting. Bry et al. [95] have

Table 3 Conditions affecting measurement of GHb levels by chromatography*

- Increase measured levels
  - –Negatively charged hemoglobin variants
  - –Uremia (carbamylation of Hb)
  - –Alcoholism
  - –Lead poisoning
  - –Elevated triglycerides
  - –Iron-deficiency anemia
  - –Post-splenectomy
  - –Hyperbilirubinemia
  - –Opiate addiction
  - –Chronic aspirin therapy
- Decrease measured levels
  - –Positively charged hemoglobin variants
  - –Hemolytic anemias
  - –Acute or chronic blood loss
  - –Pregnancy

*Adapted from references 50, 96, and 97.

Table 4 Effects of frequently encountered hemoglobin variants on measurement of GHb*

	Method		
Variant or derivative	Cation exchange	Immunoassay	Boronate affinity
Carbamyl-Hb	Increase typical	NC†	NC
HbAS	NC or increased	NC or increased	NC
HbAC	NC	NC or increased	NC or reduced
HbAE	Falsely low or new reference range needed	NC	NC
HbSS	Unsuitable	May be OK with new reference range	NC or new reference range needed
HbCC	Unsuitable	May be OK with new reference range	NC or new reference range needed
HbSC	Falsely low or unsuitable	NC	NC
Increased HbF	Falsely low or unsuitable	NC or false readings	NC

* Modified from reference 95, where details on specific proprietary assay considerations can also be found.
† Unaffected.

recently reviewed the effect of hemoglobin variants on glycohemoglobin testing and provided practical guidelines for test applications and interpretation. If the HbA_{1c} testing does not roughly correlate with the patient's own monitoring of capillary blood glucose, the possibility of an underlying hemoglobin variant or disorder of erythrocyte stability should be explored. When dealing with populations in which HbSS, HbCC, or HbSC diseases are common and in which glycohemoglobin determinations have limited utility, laboratories should offer alternative forms of testing, such as glycated serum proteins or glycated serum albumin (as discussed below). Physicians taking care of patients with diabetes should especially be aware of hemoglobinopathies that may be prevalent in their patient populations.

HbF comprises 70% of the total hemoglobin at birth and falls to less than 1% in adults. In some individuals with hereditary persistence of HbF, its concentration can reach up to 30% of total hemoglobin, while in patients with β-thalassemia and sickle-cell anemia, HbF can comprise from 2 to 20% of the hemoglobin level [98]. Most boronate affinity column techniques separate HbF and GHb from HbA and HbA_{1c} and provide accurate measurements of GHb; the immunoassay method and cation exchange, may show erroneous values [95]. Similarly, with HbS disease and trait, the boronate affinity method is the best assay to use (Table 4). In patients homozygous for sickle-cell anemia, interpretation of GHb requires caution, given the pathological processes, including anemia, short red cell life span, and transfusion requirements. An alternative reference range may be used to correct for the shortened life span of red cells in HbS patients [99]. Additional measurements of glycemic control, such as glycated serum albumin should also be considered in these patients (see below).

HbC trait has a prevalence of 2.3% among African Americans and a false increase has been shown even with boronate affinity method [95]. The use of an altered protocol on certain analyzers may fully separate HbC from HbA for accurate reading [100]. Calculation of mean blood glucose and use of fructosamine assay (see below) may be an alternative in these conditions to assess long-term control.

HbE trait is most commonly encountered hemoglobin variant in Southeast Asia with a prevalence of up to 30% in the indigenous population [98]. Most of the cation-exchange chromatographic methods will report falsely decreased values whereas boronate affinity methods and immunoassays are free of error in such cases. Again, a reduced erythrocyte life span and increased turnover of red blood cells needs to be considered in affected cases, which will affect the time span of the GHb estimate of mean glycemia.

Uremia

HbA_{1c} levels have been found to be less reliable in renal failure because uremia *per se* has effects on HbA_{1c} level independent of a change in blood glucose level. Urea present at high levels in patients with renal failure may dissociate in the circulation to form cyanate. Protonation of cyanate leads to formation of isocyanic acid, which condenses with the N-terminal amino groups of hemoglobin in a process similar to glycation to form carbamylated hemoglobin [101]. Uremic patients may have carbamyl-Hb concentration as high as 3% of total Hb. Carbamylated hemoglobin tends to comigrate with HbA_{1c} in assays separating HbA_{1c} based on its electrical charge (cation-exchange chromatographic techniques) to give falsely high levels. This phenomenon only affects charge-dependent assays, such as column- and ion-exchange chromatography and agar gel electrophoresis, and the interference is only significant when serum urea levels are greater than 84 mg/dl (30 mmol/l) [102]. Immunoassay methods and boronate affinity columns to detect HbA_{1c} are more reliable in uremic patients [95].

HbA_{1c} levels also may be elevated in patients with renal failure because of an increase in rate of HbA_{1c} formation, possibly as a result of uremic acidosis. Some analyzers, e.g., the A_{1c} 2.2 HPLC analyzer, can apparently measure HbA_{1c} accurately in uremic patients [103]. While HbA_{1c} in the range of 6–7% may be estimated accurately in patients with severe renal impairment, values above 7.5% may overestimate the degree of hyperglycemia in patients with severe renal insufficiency [104]. These confounding factors arising from ion-exchange techniques can be avoided by use of boronate–agarose affinity chromatography or a thiobarbituric acid method, both of which can be used reliably in end-stage renal disease, but are time-consuming for routine determinations [103].

Overall, a boronate affinity chromatography method can be the method of choice in the setting of hemoglobin variants and end-state renal failure; however, affinity columns are unable to correct for the reduced life span of erythrocytes due to hemolysis or erythrocyte fragmentation. Clinicians also need to be aware of the changes in erythrocyte life span occurring during rapid blood loss or initial treatment with iron, folic acid, or vitamin B_{12} of the respective deficiency anemias [105].

Other Metabolic conditions

The presence of an elevated bilirubin or hyperlipidemia interferes with all available GHb assays, especially in situations when whole blood is used rather than an erythrocyte hemolysate [26]. Marked hypertriglyceridemia, hyperbilirubinemia, opiate addiction, lead poisoning, alcoholism, and long-term treatment with large doses of aspirin may spuriously elevate GHb measurements when determined by cation-exchange chromatography [50]. It has also been shown that vitamin C in doses of 1.0 gram daily for 3 months decreases GHb as measured by affinity chromatography by about 20%, while it increased HbA_1 determined by agar-gel electrophoresis by 16% [106, 107].

GLYCATION OF SERUM PROTEINS

The measurement of blood glucose is the *sine qua non* for the detection, treatment, and monitoring the progression of diabetes. The discovery of nonenzymatic glycation of hemoglobin, discussed above, paved the way for the possibility that other proteins could also be derivatized by glucose and serve a possible role as a measure of glycemia over time. Similar to hemoglobin, serum and intracellular protein molecules are subject to nonenzymatic glycation to form stable ketoamines, or fructosamines [108]. Fructosamine is the standard name for 1-amino-1-deoxy-fructose, also called isoglucosamine by Emil Fischer, who first synthesized the compound in 1886. The glycation of albumin accounts for approximately 90% of glycated serum proteins [109]. Glycation of serum proteins is similar to that of hemoglobin, except serum proteins do not contain β-amine terminals; therefore, attachment of glucose occurs at the ε-amino groups of lysine side chains [110]. Consequently, charge-dependent methods, like those used to separate HbA_{1c} from HbA cannot be used to measure fructosamine.

The rate of stable ketoamine formation is four to five times faster in glycated serum proteins than in hemoglobin [111]. Fructosamine reflects integrated glycemia during a period of 2–3 weeks, reflecting the half-lives of the derivatized serum proteins [112]. Use of the fructosamine assay has been well documented in clinical settings like hemolytic anemias and hemoglobinopathies where measurement of HbA_{1c} by conventional techniques may not provide a reliable index of glucose assessment (discussed above). In addition, fructosamine testing may be very helpful in patients with chronic renal failure who have increased levels of carbamylated hemoglobin, which can affect the clinical HbA_{1c} measurement assay [38]. However, falsely low fructosamine values in relation to mean blood glucose values will occur with rapid albumin turnover as occurs in patients with protein-losing enteropathy or the nephrotic syndrome [38]. For this reason, measurement of fructosamine has been on the rise especially in the developing world where significant numbers of patients have anemia and abnormal hemoglobin.

Assay Methods for Glycated Serum Proteins

In 1982, the fructosamine assay was developed and became commercially available [113]. To date, reduction of nitroblue tetrazolium dye (NBT) has been the most common method to estimate glycated serum proteins (fructosamine). It is a colorimetric test that is based on the ability of fructosamines to act as reducing agents in alkaline solution and convert NBT to a purple dye that can be monitored by absorbance at 530 nm. As with any other biochemical method, fructosamine assays have their limitations [114]. A number of problems have been found with this original automated fructosamine assay, such as standardization difficulties [115], lack of specificity [116], and interference by lipemia and urate [117, 118]. Of course, fructosamine values are affected by low serum albumin and plasma proteins, as in cases of protein-losing nephropathy or liver failure, and must be interpreted with caution under these circumstances.

A variety of biochemical methods have been developed for fructosamine [119, 120]. In the early 1990s, Boehringer–Mannheim and Roche Diagnostics developed an improved fructosamine assay [121], with reduced protein matrix effects and less interference by lipemia and urate. More recently, a nonseparation fluorescence quenching assay for the measurement of total glycated serum proteins has been introduced [122]. The principle of this method is that the fluorescence of a fluorophore, a boronic acid derivative, is quenched when it is bound to glycated proteins but not when it is unbound. The drop in fluorescence is proportional to the concentration of glycated protein.

Clinical Usefulness of Fructosamine Analysis in Diabetes Mellitus

Fructosamine assays may be used in clinical settings to detect short to medium-term changes in mean blood glucose. Fructosamine assays also assist in certain clinical conditions where measurement of HbA_{1c} is considered less reliable. The half-life of hemoglobin is approximately 60 days, of albumin 14–20 days, and that of various other proteins, 2.5–23 days. In a group of diabetic patients treated to achieve better glycemic control, the concentration of glycated albumin entered the normal range and plateaued, while the concentration of GHb continued to fall [123]. This study showed that the kinetics of the fructosamine test differs from those of the HbA_{1c}, and that is might serve as a more sensitive indicator of average blood glucose over a shorter time frame.

Austin et al. [124] showed that measurement of fructosamine could be a useful adjunctive test for management of outpatients with diabetes in situations where it is not practical to obtain same-day glycohemoglobin concentrations. This study also proved useful for patients less compliant with home glucose monitoring, or where recent changes in insulin dose or clinical presentation might not be reflected in the glycoHb levels. Weekly home testing of fructosamine, combined with therapeutic interventions based on the results, has also been found to lead to a more rapid and significant improvement in glycemic control than did a conventional regimen of testing based solely on capillary glucose testing [125].

The correlation between predicted HbA_{1c} and fructosamine was fair ($r = 0.88$) in diabetic patients but not in control subjects ($r = 0.01$) [126]. Other studies have questioned whether there is any additional benefit gained from measuring the fructosamine in the course of clinical monitoring of patients with diabetes that cannot be obtained from measuring capillary glucose or GHb [127]. A recent study has substantiated that HbA_{1c} measurement correlates better with home capillary blood glucose levels than with the fructosamine assay, even over the previous 2–3 weeks [128]. The most commonly cited problem confounding the interpretation and reliability of such data is related to short-term fluctuations in serum protein levels observed in diabetic patients [129, 130]. Thus, although tests such as the fructosamine assay are relatively inexpensive and simple to perform, they have been questioned as a reliable index of hyperglycemia. Accordingly, like HbA_{1c}, the fructosamine is not sufficiently sensitive or specific to be used as a screening tool for the diagnosis of diabetes.

Measurements of glycated serum proteins have also been employed for monitoring glycemic control in diabetic pregnancies. Although subject to the potential confounding influences of variations in serum protein concentration, glycated serum protein measurements may be conceptually more appropriate than HbA_{1c}, given the time constraints of normal gestation and the desire to maintain near-normal glycemia over short-term periods. Because of changes in the distribution of body water, a significant decrease in serum albumin and serum fructosamine concentration occurs during normal pregnancy [131]. In spite of this, the value of short-term monitoring of glycemic control has been substantiated in a few studies [132–134]. In general, the use of glycated serum protein assays in diabetic pregnancy cannot be used to replace the frequent monitoring of capillary glucose levels, but perhaps as a verification of the overall level of glycemic control that may lead to alterations in the treatment plan if the glycated proteins begin to increase with monitoring every 3–4 weeks [135].

ADVANCED GLYCOSYLATION END-PRODUCTS AND DIABETIC COMPLICATIONS

Multiple mechanisms have been described by which chronic hyperglycemia may contribute to the pathological end-organ complications that occur in diabetes mellitus. These include direct effects of elevated glucose on cells, hyperosmolality, oxidant stress, and nonenzymatic glycosylation. The irreversible ketoamine linkage that follows Schiff base formation of glycated proteins can undergo a series of multistep reactions potentially along several different pathways (Figure 8). Some of the formed products involve fragmentation to form deoxyglucosones, which may then lead to additional protein cross-links [137, 138]. The deoxyglucosones can form highly reactive dicarbonyl compounds that cyclize to form electrophilic pyrrole intermediates and more advanced cross-linked fluorescent derivatives [4, 38, 139]. The complex biochemistry of the AGEs and the implication of the formation of these

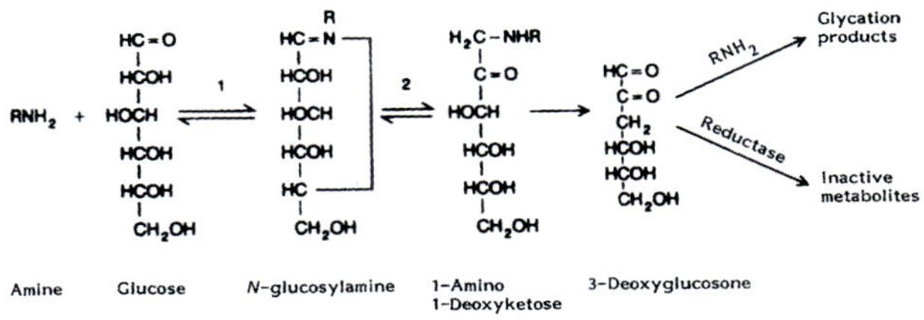

Figure 8 Formation of advanced glycosylation end-products from glucose. *N*-Glucosylamine is a reversible Schiff base product and the Amadori rearrangement leads to the formation of 1-amino-1-deoxyketose. The production of these reversible early products can give rise to irreversible advanced products through generation of highly reactive carbonyl compounds such as 3-deoxy-D-glucosone (from reference 136, reproduced by permission of the American Diabetes Association)

derivatives *in vivo* is incompletely understood, and remains an area of active research.

Once formed, AGE-protein adducts, such as carboxymethyllysine (CML) and pentosidine are biochemically irreversible and remain quite stable in the body. AGEs are a heterogeneous family of biochemical end products of nonenzymatic glycosylation. Circulating human AGE peptides are of variable size (molecular weight between 2000 and 6000) and characterized by intra- or intermolecular cross-linking products with cyclic aromatic rings that convey fluorescence [38]. In addition to their chemical reactivity, some AGE structures, for example *N*-carboxymethyllysine [140], lead to the formation of antibodies *in vivo* [141], which may portend an additional mechanism for tissue damage. AGE modification of proteins is potentially involved in the normal aging process as well as in the pathogenesis of diabetic nephropathy, atherosclerosis, diabetic retinopathy, and chronic renal failure [142–146].

An additional element of complexity in the effects of AGE products has been the discovery of a specific AGE receptor, called "RAGE" on a variety of cell types including macrophage/monocytes [147] and endothelial cells [148]. The AGE receptor may transmit effects of AGE products on signal transduction that may mediate its detrimental effects in tissues [148–150].

The discovery of RAGE has led to the development of a whole-cell radioreceptor assay for AGEs [151]. The principle of this assay rests on the assumption that the family of AGEs have similar affinity for the AGE receptor, and that those present in the sample will compete, in proportion to their concentration, with the binding of labeled AGE-modified albumin. The amount of AGEs in the sample is read from the standard curve showing competition binding of labeled and unlabeled AGE-modified albumin, and expressed in units defined as amount of the test protein required to inhibit the binding of 50% of the labeled AGE-modified albumin [151]. With this assay it is possible to detect AGEs in serum both in normal and diabetic patients. In the first report of this kind it has been documented that serum AGEs of molecular mass <10 kDa in nondiabetic patients with end-stage renal disease are increased 1.5-fold compared to those normal individuals, and increased 5-fold in patients with end-stage renal disease and diabetes [152]. This study raises two important questions, and the answers remain uncertain. First, the source of the circulating AGEs in serum is still unknown. Secondly, how do the AGEs themselves contribute to the development of chronic complications seen in diabetes? The authors of the cited report suggest that the AGEs in the serum (especially those of low molecular weight) are metabolites of AGE-modified proteins formed in the tissues. The major route of elimination of these metabolites, especially those of molecular weight of <10 kDa, is through the kidneys and the progression of renal failure leads to their retention in serum. The severalfold increased retention of low-molecular-weight AGEs in patients with end-stage renal disease and diabetes compared to the other study groups indicates that the turnover of AGEs in diabetes is greatly increased. Moreover as shown by the authors [152], the serum AGEs are poorly dialyzable and may contribute to the rapid progression of complications and mortality of patients with diabetes requiring dialysis.

At present, monitoring of serum AGEs remains a research tool that is not widely available. In the next few years, progress in this area of research may provide a new dimension in the clinical monitoring of diabetes and its complications that can extend the value of measurement of glycated proteins far beyond their present applications. A number of potentially therapeutic compounds are under extensive study in animals and humans for potential use in diabetics, in an effort to eliminate the accumulation of AGE products or minimize the deleterious effects of AGE [38].

Acknowledgment

The authors are grateful to Dr Jerzy Kolaczynski for his contributions to the writing of the previous version of this chapter.

REFERENCES

1. Rohlfing CL, Wiedmeyer HM, Little RR, England JD, Tennill A, Goldstein DE. Defining the relationship between plasma glucose and HbA(1c): analysis of glucose profiles and HbA(1c) in the Diabetes Control and Complications Trial. *Diabetes Care* 2002; 25: 275–8.
2. Sacks DB, Bruns DE, Goldstein DE, Maclaren NK, McDonald JM, Parrott M. Guidelines and recommendations for laboratory analysis in the diagnosis and management of diabetes mellitus. *Clin Chem* 2002; 48: 436–72.
3. Dolhofer R, Wieland OH. Increased glycosylation of serum albumin in diabetes mellitus. *Diabetes* 1980; 29: 417–22.
4. Wautier JL, Guillausseau PJ, Advanced glycation end products, their receptors and diabetic angiopathy. *Diabetes Metab* 2001; 27: 535–42.
5. Brownlee M. Negative consequences of glycation. *Metabolism* 2000; 49: 9–13.
6. Maillard LC. Action des acides amines sur les sucres; formation des melanoidines par voie methodique. *C R Hebd Seances Acad Sci* 1912; 154: 66–8.
7. Hodge JE. The Amadori rearrangement. *Adv Carbohydr Chem* 1955; 10: 169–205.
8. Monnier VM, Kohn RR, Cerami A. Accelerated age-related browning of human collagen in diabetes mellitus. *Proc Natl Acad Sci USA* 1984; 81: 583–7.
9. Monnier VM, Vishwanath V, Frank KE, Elmets CA, Dauchot P, Kohn RR. Relation between complications of type I diabetes mellitus and collagen-linked fluorescence. *N Engl J Med* 1986; 314: 403–8.
10. Rahbar S, Blumenfeld O, Ranney HM, Studies of an unusual hemoglobin in patients with diabetes mellitus. *Biochem Biophys Res Commun* 1969; 36: 838–43.

11. Koenig RJ, Peterson CM, Jones RL, Saudek C, Lehrman M, Cerami A. Correlation of glucose regulation and hemoglobin AIc in diabetes mellitus. *N Engl J Med* 1976; 295: 417–20.
12. Gabbay KH, Hasty K, Breslow JL, Ellison RC, Bunn HF, Gallop PM. Glycosylated hemoglobins and long-term blood glucose control in diabetes mellitus. *J Clin Endocrinol Metab* 1977; 44: 859–64.
13. Gonen B, Rubenstein A, Rochman H, Tanega SP, Horwitz DL. Haemoglobin A1: an indicator of the metabolic control of diabetic patients. *Lancet* 1977; 2: 734–7.
14. Bunn HF, Higgins PJ. Reaction of monosaccharides with proteins: possible evolutionary significance. *Science* 1981; 213: 222–4.
15. Bunn HF, Shapiro R, McManus M, Garrick L, McDonald MJ, Gallop PM, Gabbay KH. Structural heterogeneity of human hemoglobin A due to nonenzymatic glycosylation. *J Biol Chem* 1979; 254: 3892–8.
16. Garlick RL, Mazer JS, Higgins PJ, Bunn HF. Characterization of glycosylated hemoglobins. Relevance to monitoring of diabetic control and analysis of other proteins. *J Clin Invest* 1983; 71: 1062–72.
17. Koenig RJ, Blobstein SH, Cerami A. Structure of carbohydrate of hemoglobin AIc. *J Biol Chem* 1977; 252: 2992–7.
18. Bunn HF, Haney DN, Kamin S, Gabbay KH, Gallop PM. The biosynthesis of human hemoglobin A1c. Slow glycosylation of hemoglobin in vivo. *J Clin Invest* 1976; 57: 1652–9.
19. Goldstein DE, Peth SB, England JD, Hess RL, Da Costa J. Effects of acute changes in blood glucose on HbA1c. *Diabetes* 1980; 29: 623–8.
20. Mortensen HB, Christophersen C. Glucosylation of human haemoglobin a in red blood cells studied *in vitro*. Kinetics of the formation and dissociation of haemoglobin A1c. *Clin Chim Acta* 1983; 134: 317–26.
21. Bunn HF, Haney DN, Gabbay KH, Gallop PM. Further identification of the nature and linkage of the carbohydrate in hemoglobin A1c. *Biochem Biophys Res Commun* 1975; 67: 103–9.
22. Silverman M. Structure and function of hexose transporters. *Annu Rev Biochem* 1991; 60: 757–94.
23. Beutler E. How do red cell enzymes age? A new perspective. *Br J Haematol* 1985; 61: 377–84.
24. Donde UM, Baxi AJ, el Tawil H, Ghwarsha K. Glycosylated haemoglobin in glucose-6-phosphate dehydrogenase deficiency. *Lancet* 1985; 2: 47.
25. Higgins PJ, Garlick RL, Bunn HF. Glycosylated hemoglobin in human and animal red cells. Role of glucose permeability. *Diabetes* 1982; 31: 743–8.
26. John WG, Bullock DG, MacKenzie F. Methods for the analysis of glycated haemoglobins: what is being measured? *Diabet Med* 1992; 9: 15–9.
27. Fitzgibbons JF, Koler RD, Jones RT. Red cell age-related changes of hemoglobins AIa+b and AIc in normal and diabetic subjects. *J Clin Invest* 1976; 58: 820–4.
28. Panzer S, Kronik G, Lechner K, Bettelheim P, Neumann E, Dudczak R. Glycosylated hemoglobins (GHb): an index of red cell survival. *Blood* 1982; 59: 1348–50.
29. Simon D, Senan C, Garnier P, Saint-Paul M, Papoz L. Epidemiological features of glycated haemoglobin A1c-distribution in a healthy population. The Telecom Study. *Diabetologia* 1989; 32: 864–9.
30. Yudkin JS, Forrest RD, Jackson CA, Ryle AJ, Davie S, Gould BJ. Unexplained variability of glycated haemoglobin in non-diabetic subjects not related to glycaemia. *Diabetologia* 1990; 33: 208–15.
31. Verrillo A, de Teresa A, Golia R, Nunziata V. The relationship between glycosylated haemoglobin levels and various degrees of glucose intolerance. *Diabetologia* 1983; 24: 391–3.
32. Forrest RD, Jackson CA, Yudkin JS. The glycohaemoglobin assay as a screening test for diabetes mellitus: the Islington Diabetes Survey. *Diabet Med* 1987; 4: 254–9.
33. Flock EV, Bennett PH, Savage PJ, Webner CJ, Howard BV, Rushforth NB, Miller M. Bimodality of glycosylated hemoglobin distribution in Pima Indians: relationship to fasting hyperglycemia. *Diabetes* 1979; 28: 984–9.
34. Simon D, Coignet MC, Thibult N, Senan C, Eschwege E. Comparison of glycosylated hemoglobin and fasting plasma glucose with two-hour post-load plasma glucose in the detection of diabetes mellitus. *Am J Epidemiol* 1985; 122: 589–93.
35. Ferrell RE, Hanis CL, Aguilar L, Tulloch B, Garcia C, Schull WJ. Glycosylated hemoglobin determination from capillary blood samples. Utility in an epidemiologic survey of diabetes. *Am J Epidemiol* 1984; 119: 159–66.
36. Modan M, Halkin H, Karasik A, Lusky A. Effectiveness of glycosylated hemoglobin, fasting plasma glucose, and a single post load plasma glucose level in population screening for glucose intolerance. *Am J Epidemiol* 1984; 119: 431–44.
37. Little RR, England JD, Wiedmeyer HM, McKenzie EM, Pettitt DJ, Knowler WC, Goldstein DE. Relationship of glycosylated hemoglobin to oral glucose tolerance. Implications for diabetes screening. *Diabetes* 1988; 37: 60–4.
38. Beisswenger PJ, Szwergold BS, Yeo KT. Glycated proteins in diabetes. *Clin Lab Med* 2001; 21: 53–78, vi.
39. Report of the expert committee on the diagnosis and classification of diabetes mellitus. *Diabetes Care* 2003; 26 (suppl 1): S5–20.
40. Barr RG, Nathan DM, Meigs JB, Singer DE. Tests of glycemia for the diagnosis of type 2 diabetes mellitus. *Ann Intern Med* 2002; 137: 263–72.
41. Little RR, Rohlfing CL, Wiedmeyer HM, Myers GL, Sacks DB, Goldstein DE. The national glycohemoglobin standardization program: a five-year progress report. *Clin Chem* 2001; 47: 1985–92.
42. Ditzel J, Kjaergaard JJ. Haemoglobin AIc concentrations after initial insulin treatment for newly discovered diabetes. *Br Med J* 1978; 1: 741–2.
43. Boden G, Master RW, Gordon SS, Shuman CR, Owen OE. Monitoring metabolic control in diabetic outpatients with glycosylated hemoglobin. *Ann Intern Med* 1980; 92: 357–60.
44. Wood PA, Smith JE. Elevation rate of glycosylated hemoglobins in dogs after induction of experimental diabetes mellitus. *Metabolism* 1982; 31: 906–9.
45. Paisey RB, Macfarlane DG, Sherriff RJ, Hartog M, Slade RR, White DA. The relationship between blood glycosylated haemoglobin and home capillary blood glucose levels in diabetics. *Diabetologia* 1980; 19: 31–4.
46. Svendsen PA, Christiansen JS, Soegaard U, Nerup J. Synthesis of glycosylated haemoglobin in vivo. *Diabetologia* 1981; 21: 549–53.
47. Service FJ, O'Brien PC, Rizza RA. Measurements of glucose control. *Diabetes Care* 1987; 10: 225–37.
48. Nathan DM, Singer DE, Hurxthal K, Goodson JD. The clinical information value of the glycosylated hemoglobin assay. *N Engl J Med* 1984; 310: 341–6.

49. Nathan DM. Hemoglobin Alc–infatuation or the real thing? *N Engl J Med* 1990; 323: 1062–4.
50. Service FJ. Correlation between glycemia and glycated hemoglobin. *Compr Ther* 1990; 16: 33–40.
51. Larsen ML, Horder M, Mogensen EF. Effect of long-term monitoring of glycosylated hemoglobin levels in insulin-dependent diabetes mellitus. *N Engl J Med* 1990; 323: 1021–5.
52. Goldstein DE. Is glycosylated hemoglobin clinically useful? *N Engl J Med* 1984; 310: 384–5.
53. Holman RR, Turner RC. The basal plasma glucose: a simple relevant index of maturity-onset diabetes. *Clin Endocrinol (Oxf)* 1981; 14: 279–86.
54. Pecoraro RE, Koepsell TD, Chen MS, Lipsky BA, Belcher DW, Inui TS. Comparative clinical reliability of fasting plasma glucose and glycosylated hemoglobin in non-insulin-dependent diabetes mellitus. *Diabetes Care* 1986; 9: 370–5.
55. McCance DR, Ritchie CM, Kennedy L. Is HbA1 measurement superfluous in NIDDM? *Diabetes Care* 1988; 11: 512–4.
56. American Diabetes Association. Postprandial blood glucose [Consensus Statement]. *Diabetes Care* 2001; 24: 775–8.
57. Miller E, Hare JW, Cloherty JP, Dunn PJ, Gleason RE, Soeldner JS, Kitzmiller JL. Elevated maternal hemoglobin A1c in early pregnancy and major congenital anomalies in infants of diabetic mothers. *N Engl J Med* 1981; 304: 1331–4.
58. Greene MF, Hare JW, Cloherty JP, Benacerraf BR, Soeldner JS. First-trimester hemoglobin A1 and risk for major malformation and spontaneous abortion in diabetic pregnancy. *Teratology* 1989; 39: 225–31.
59. Singer DE, Coley CM, Samet JH, Nathan DM. Tests of glycemia in diabetes mellitus. Their use in establishing a diagnosis and in treatment. *Ann Intern Med* 1989; 110: 125–37.
60. de Veciana M, Major CA, Morgan MA, Asrat T, Toohey JS, Lien JM, Evans AT. Postprandial versus preprandial blood glucose monitoring in women with gestational diabetes mellitus requiring insulin therapy. *N Engl J Med* 1995; 333: 1237–41.
61. Lauritzen T, Frost-Larsen K, Larsen HW, Deckert T. Effect of 1 year of near-normal blood glucose levels on retinopathy in insulin-dependent diabetics. *Lancet* 1983; 1: 200–4.
62. Lauritzen T, Frost-Larsen K, Larsen HW, Deckert T. Two-year experience with continuous subcutaneous insulin infusion in relation to retinopathy and neuropathy. *Diabetes* 1985; 34 (suppl 3): 74–9.
63. Dahl-Jorgensen K, Brinchmann-Hansen O, Hanssen KF, Sandvik L, Aagenaes O. Rapid tightening of blood glucose control leads to transient deterioration of retinopathy in insulin dependent diabetes mellitus: the Oslo study. *Br Med J (Clin Res Ed)* 1985; 290: 811–5.
64. Beck-Nielsen H, Richelsen B, Mogensen CE, Olsen T, Ehlers N, Nielsen CB, Charles P. Effect of insulin pump treatment for one year on renal function and retinal morphology in patients with IDDM. *Diabetes Care* 1985; 8: 585–9.
65. Klein R, Klein BE, Moss SE, Davis MD, DeMets DL. Glycosylated hemoglobin predicts the incidence and progression of diabetic retinopathy. *JAMA* 1988; 260: 2864–71.
66. Chase HP, Jackson WE, Hoops SL, Cockerham RS, Archer PG, O'Brien D. Glucose control and the renal and retinal complications of insulin-dependent diabetes. *JAMA* 1989; 261: 1155–60.
67. The DCCT Study Group. The effect of intensive treatment of diabetes on the development and progression of long-term complications in insulin-dependent diabetes-mellitus. *N Engl J Med* 1993; 329: 977–86.
68. Turner RC, Holman RR, Cull CA, Stratton IM, Matthews DR, Frighi V, Manley SE, Neil A, Mcelroy K, Wright D, Kohner E, Fox C, Hadden D, Mehta Z, Smith A, Nugent Z, Peto R, Adlel AI, Mann JI, Bassett PA, Oakes SF, Dornan TL, Aldington S, Lipinski H, Collum R. Intensive blood-glucose control with sulphonylureas or insulin compared with conventional treatment and risk of complications in patients with type 2 diabetes (UKPDS 33). *Lancet* 1998; 352: 837–53.
69. Stratton IM, Adler AI, Neil HA, Matthews DR, Manley SE, Cull CA, Hadden D, Turner RC, Holman RR. Association of glycaemia with macrovascular and microvascular complications of type 2 diabetes (UKPDS 35): prospective observational study. *BMJ* 2000; 321: 405–12.
70. Ohkubo Y, Kishikawa H, Araki E, Miyata T, Isami S, Motoyoshi S, Kojima Y, Furuyoshi N, Shichiri M. Intensive insulin therapy prevents the progression of diabetic microvascular complications in Japanese patients with non-insulin-dependent diabetes mellitus: a randomized prospective 6-year study. *Diabetes Res Clin Pract* 1995; 28: 103–17.
71. Shichiri M, Kishikawa H, Ohkubo Y, Wake N. Long-term results of the Kumamoto Study on optimal diabetes control in type 2 diabetic patients. *Diabetes Care* 2000; 23 (suppl 2): B21–9.
72. Khaw KT, Wareham N, Luben R, Bingham S, Oakes S, Welch A, Day N. Glycated haemoglobin, diabetes, and mortality in men in Norfolk cohort of european prospective investigation of cancer and nutrition (EPIC-Norfolk). *BMJ* 2001; 322: 15–8.
73. Trivelli LA, Ranney HM, Lai HT. Hemoglobin components in patients with diabetes mellitus. *N Engl J Med* 1971; 284: 353–7.
74. Worth RC, Ashworth LA, Burrin JM, Johnston DG, Skillen AW, Anderson J, Alberti KG. Column assay of haemoglobin A1: critical effect of temperature. *Clin Chim Acta* 1980; 104: 401–4.
75. Welch SG, Boucher BJ. A rapid micro-scale method for the measurement of haemoglobin A1(a+b+c). *Diabetologia* 1978; 14: 209–11.
76. Davis JE, McDonald JM, Jarett L. A high-performance liquid chromatography method for hemoglobin A1c. *Diabetes* 1978; 27: 102–7.
77. Cole RA, Soeldner JS, Dunn PJ, Bunn HF. A rapid method for the determination of glycosylated hemoglobins using high pressure liquid chromatography. *Metabolism* 1978; 27: 289–301.
78. Schifreen RS, Hickingbotham JM, Bowers GN Jr. Accuracy, precision, and stability in measurement of hemoglobin A1c by "high-performance" cation-exchange chromatography. *Clin Chem* 1980; 26: 466–72.
79. Ryall RG, Graham JJ. Routine measurement of glycosylated haemoglobin. *Lancet* 1978; 2: 739–40.
80. Spicer KM, Allen RC, Buse MG. A simplified assay of hemoglobin AIc in diabetic patients by use of isoelectric focusing and quantitative microdensitometry. *Diabetes* 1978; 27: 384–8.
81. Simon M, Cuan J. Hemoglobin A1c by isoelectric focusing. *Clin Chem* 1982; 28: 9–12.

82. Menard L, Dempsey ME, Blankstein LA, Aleyassine H, Wacks M, Soeldner JS. Quantitiative determination of glycosylated hemoglobin A1 by agar gel electrophoresis. *Clin Chem* 1980; 26: 1598–602.
83. Thornton WE, Schellekens AP, Sanders GT. Assay of glycosylated haemoglobin using agar electrophoresis. *Ann Clin Biochem* 1981; 18: 182–4.
84. Fluckiger R, Winterhalter KH. In vitro synthesis of hemoglobin AIc. *FEBS Lett* 1976; 71: 356–60.
85. Parker KM, England JD, Da Costa J, Hess RL, Goldstein DE. Improved colorimetric assay for glycosylated hemoglobin. *Clin Chem* 1981; 27: 669–72.
86. Shapiro R, McManus MJ, Zalut C, Bunn HF. Sites of nonenzymatic glycosylation of human hemoglobin A. *J Biol Chem* 1980; 255: 3120–7.
87. Mallia AK, Hermansson G, Krohn RI, Fujimoto EK, Smith PK. Preparation and use of a boronic acid affinity support for separation and quantitation of glycosylated hemoglobins. *Anal Lett* 1981; 14: 649–61.
88. Bouriotis V, Scott J, Galloway A, Bellingham AJ, Dean PD. Measurement of glycosylated haemoglobins using affinity chromatography. *Diabetologia* 1981; 21: 579–80.
89. John WG, Albutt EC, Handley G, Richardson RW. Affinity chromatography method for the measurement of glycosylated haemoglobin: comparison with two methods in routine use. *Clin Chim Acta* 1984; 136: 257–62.
90. Fluckiger R, Woodtli T, Berger W. Quantitation of glycosylated hemoglobin by boronate affinity chromatography. *Diabetes* 1984; 33: 73–6.
91. Kortlandt W, van Rijn HJ, Hoeke JO, Thijssen JH. Comparison of three different assay procedures for the determination of HbA_1 with special attention to the influence of pre-HbA_{1c}, temperature and haemoglobin concentration. *Ann Clin Biochem* 1985; 22 (pt 3): 261–8.
92. John WG, Gray MR, Bates DL, Beacham JL. Enzyme immunoassay—a new technique for estimating hemoglobin A1c. *Clin Chem* 1993; 39: 663–6.
93. Santiago JV. Lessons from the Diabetes Control and Complications Trial. *Diabetes* 1993; 42: 1549–54.
94. Nathan DM, Avezzano E, Palmer JL. Rapid method for eliminating labile glycosylated hemoglobin from the assay for hemoglobin A1. *Clin Chem* 1982; 28: 512–5.
95. Bry L, Chen PC, Sacks DB. Effects of hemoglobin variants and chemically modified derivatives on assays for glycohemoglobin. *Clin Chem* 2001; 47: 153–63.
96. Schnedl WJ, Krause R, Halwachs-Baumann G, Trinker M, Lipp RW, Krejs GJ. Evaluation of HbA1c determination methods in patients with hemoglobinopathies. *Diabetes Care* 2000; 23: 339–44.
97. Eberentz-Lhomme C, Ducrocq R, Intrator S, Elion J, Nunez E, Assan R. Haemoglobinopathies: a pitfall in the assessment of glycosylated haemoglobin by ion-exchange chromatography. *Diabetologia* 1984; 27: 596–8.
98. Benz EJ. *Hemoglobinopathies, Vol 15*. New York: McGraw Hill, 2001; pp 666–73.
99. Weykamp CW, Penders TJ, Muskiet FA, van der Slik W. Influence of hemoglobin variants and derivatives on glycohemoglobin determinations, as investigated by 102 laboratories using 16 methods. *Clin Chem* 1993; 39: 1717–23.
100. Gibb I, Parnham A, Fonfrede M, Lecock F. Multicenter evaluation of Tosoh glycohemoglobin analyzer. *Clin Chem* 1999; 45: 1833–41.
101. Stim J, Shaykh M, Anwar F, Ansari A, Arruda JA, Dunea G. Factors determining hemoglobin carbamylation in renal failure. *Kidney Int* 1995; 48: 1605–10.
102. de Boer MJ, Miedema K, Casparie AF. Glycosylated haemoglobin in renal failure. *Diabetologia* 1980; 18: 437–40.
103. Scott MG, Hoffmann JW, Meltzer VN, Siegfried BA, Chan KM. Effects of azotemia on results of the boronate-agarose affinity and ion-exchange methods for glycated hemoglobin. *Clin Chem* 1984; 30: 896–8.
104. Chevenne D, Fonfrede M, Ducrocq R, Chauffert M, Trivin F. Uremia and HbA_{1c} measured by high-performance liquid chromatography. *Diabetes Care* 1998; 21: 463–4.
105. Gram-Hansen P, Eriksen J, Mourits-Andersen T, Olesen L. Glycosylated haemoglobin (HbA_{1c}) in iron- and vitamin B12 deficiency. *J Intern Med* 1990; 227: 133–6.
106. Weykamp CW, Penders TJ, Baadenhuijsen H, Muskiet FA, Martina W, van der Slik W. Vitamin C and glycohemoglobin. *Clin Chem* 1995; 41: 713–6.
107. Davie SJ, Gould BJ, Yudkin JS. Effect of vitamin C on glycosylation of proteins. *Diabetes* 1992; 41: 167–73.
108. Gottschalk A. Some biochemically relevant properties of N-substitued fructosamines derived from amino acids and N-arygucoslamines. *Biochem J* 1952; 52: 455–60.
109. Dolhofer R, Wieland OH. Improvement of the thiobarbituric acid assay for serum glycosylprotein determination. *Clin Chim Acta* 1981; 112: 197–204.
110. Dolhofer R, Wieland OH. Glycosylation of serum albumin: elevated glycosyl-albumin in diabetic patients. *FEBS Lett* 1979; 103: 282–6.
111. Schleicher E, Wieland OH. Specific quantitation by HPLC of protein (lysine) bound glucose in human serum albumin and other glycosylated proteins. *J Clin Chem Clin Biochem* 1981; 19: 81–7.
112. Olufemi S, Talwar D, Robb DA. The relative extent of glycation of haemoglobin and albumin. *Clin Chim Acta* 1987; 163: 125–36.
113. Johnson RN, Metcalf PA, Baker JR. Fructosamine: a new approach to the estimation of serum glycosylation. An index control of diabetic control. *Clin Chim Acta* 1982; 127: 87–95.
114. Baker JR, Metcalf PA, Johnson RN, Newman D, Rietz P. Use of protein-based standards in automated colorimetric determinations of fructosamine in serum. *Clin Chem* 1985; 31: 1550–4.
115. Schleicher ED, Vogt BW. Standardization of serum fructosamine assays. *Clin Chem* 1990; 36: 136–9.
116. Schleicher ED, Mayer R, Wagner EM, Gerbitz KD. Is serum fructosamine assay specific for determination of glycated serum protein? *Clin Chem* 1988; 34: 320–3.
117. Siedel J, Vogt B, Kerscher L, Ziegenhorn J. Serum frucostamine assay: two different color reagents compared with reference to a HPLC-procedure. *Clin Chem* 1988; 34: 1316.
118. Phillipou G, Seaborn CJ, Phillips PJ. Re-evaluation of the fructosamine reaction. *Clin Chem* 1988; 34: 1561–4.
119. Schleicher E, Prytulla S, Gerbitz KD. A new method for determination of glycated proteins using boronate ester. *Clin Chem* 1990; 36: 992–3.
120. Hayashi Y, Makino M. Fluorometric measurement of glycosylated albumin in human serum. *Clin Chim Acta* 1985; 149: 13–9.
121. Henrichs HR, Lehmann P, Vorberg E. An improved fructosamine assay for monitoring blood glucose control. *Diabet Med* 1991; 8: 580–4.
122. Blincko S, Colbert D, John WG, Edwards R. A reliable non-separation fluorescence quenching assay for total

glycated serum protein: a simple alternative to nitroblue tetrazolium reduction. *Ann Clin Biochem* 2000; 37 (pt 3): 372–9.

123. Rendell M, Kao G, Mecherikunnel P, Petersen B, Duhaney R, Nierenberg J, Rasbold K, Klenk D, Smith PK. Aminophenylboronic acid affinity chromatography and thiobarbituric acid colorimetry compared for measuring glycated albumin. *Clin Chem* 1985; 31: 229–34.
124. Austin GE, Wheaton R, Nanes MS, Rubin J, Mullins RE. Usefulness of fructosamine for monitoring outpatients with diabetes. *Am J Med Sci* 1999; 318: 316–23.
125. Edelman SV, Bell JM, Serrano RB, Kelemen D. Home testing of fructosamine improves glycemic control in patients with diabetes. *Endocr Pract* 2001; 7: 454–8.
126. Narbonne H, Renacco E, Pradel V, Portugal H, Vialettes B. Can fructosamine be a surrogate for HbA(1c) in evaluating the achievement of therapeutic goals in diabetes? *Diabetes Metab* 2001; 27: 598–603.
127. Ashby JP, Frier BM. Is fructosamine a clinically useful test? *Diabet Med* 1990; 5: 118–21.
128. Chen HS, Chen RL, Chang ZY, Li HD. A comparison of fructosamine and HbA_{1c} for home self-monitoring blood glucose levels in type 2 diabetes. *Zhonghua Yi Xue Za Zhi (Taipei)* 2002; 65: 151–5.
129. McCance DR, Coulter D, Smye M, Kennedy L. Effect of fluctuations in albumin on serum fructosamine assay. *Diabet Med* 1987; 4: 434–6.
130. Fluckiger R, Woodtli T, Berger W. Evaluation of the fructosamine test for the measurement of plasma protein glycation. *Diabetologia* 1987; 30: 648–52.
131. Dieijen-Visser MP, Salemans T, van Wersch JW, Schellekens LA, Brombacher PJ. Glycosylated serum proteins and glycosylated haemoglobin in normal pregnancy. *Ann Clin Biochem* 1986; 23 (pt 6): 661–6.
132. Nelson DM, Barrows HJ, Clapp DH, Ortman-Nabi J, Whitehurst RM. Glycosylated serum protein levels in diabetic and nondiabetic pregnant patients: an indicator of short-term glycemic control in the diabetic patient. *Am J Obstet Gynecol* 1985; 151: 1042–7.
133. Leiper JM, Talwar D, Robb DA, Lunan CB, MacCuish AC. Glycosylated albumin and glycosylated proteins: rapidly changing indices of glycaemia in diabetic pregnancy. *Q J Med* 1985; 55: 225–31.
134. Morris MA, Grandis AS, Litton JC. Longitudinal assessment of glycosylated blood protein concentrations in normal pregnancy and gestational diabetes. *Diabetes Care* 1986; 9: 107–10.
135. Parfitt VJ, Clark JD, Turner GM, Hartog M. Use of fructosamine and glycated haemoglobin to verify self blood glucose monitoring data in diabetic pregnancy. *Diabet Med* 1993; 10: 162–6.
136. Brownlee M. Glycation products and the pathogenesis of diabetic complications. *Diabetes Care* 1992; 15: 1835–43.
137. Kato H, Hayase F, Shin DB, Oimomi M, Baba S. 3-Deoxyglucosone, an intermediate product of the Maillard reaction. *Prog Clin Biol Res* 1989; 304: 69–84.
138. Njoroge FG, Monnier VM. The chemistry of the Maillard reaction under physiological conditions: a review. *Prog Clin Biol Res* 1989; 304: 85–107.
139. Cerami A, Vlassara H, Brownlee M. Role of advanced glycosylation products in complications of diabetes. *Diabetes Care* 1988; 11 (suppl 1): 73–9.
140. Ahmed MU, Thorpe SR, Baynes JW. Identification of N-epsilon-carboxymethyllysine as a degradation product of fructoselysine in glycated protein. *J Biol Chem* 1986; 261: 4889–94.
141. Ikeda K, Higashi T, Sano H, Jinnouchi Y, Yoshida M, Araki T, Ueda S, Horiuchi S. N-epsilon-carboxymethyllysine protein adduct is a major immunological epitope in proteins modified with advanced glycation end products of the Maillard reaction. *Biochemistry* 1996; 35: 8075–83.
142. Araki N, Ueno N, Chakrabarti B, Morino Y, Horiuchi S. Immunochemical evidence for the presence of advanced glycation end products in human lens proteins and its positive correlation with aging. *J Biol Chem* 1992; 267: 10211–4.
143. Imai N, Nishi S, Suzuki Y, Karasawa R, Ueno M, Shimada H, Kawashima S, Nakamaru T, Miyakawa Y, Araki N, Horiuchi S, Gejyo F, Arakawa M. Histological localization of advanced glycosylation end products in the progression of diabetic nephropathy. *Nephron* 1997; 76: 153–60.
144. Kume S, Takeya M, Mori T, Araki N, Suzuki H, Horiuchi S, Kodama T, Miyauchi Y, Takahashi K. Immunohistochemical and ultrastructural detection of advanced glycation end products in atherosclerotic lesions of human aorta with a novel specific monoclonal antibody. *Am J Pathol* 1995; 147: 654–67.
145. Hammes HP, Weiss A, Hess S, Araki N, Horiuchi S, Brownlee M, Preissner KT. Modification of vitronectin by advanced glycation alters functional properties in vitro and in the diabetic retina. *Lab Invest* 1996; 75: 325–38.
146. Yamada K, Miyahara Y, Hamaguchi K, Nakayama M, Nakano H, Nozaki O, Miura Y, Suzuki S, Tuchida H, Mimura N. Immunohistochemical study of human advanced glycosylation end-products (AGE) in chronic renal failure. *Clin Nephrol* 1994; 42: 354–61.
147. Vlassara H, Moldawer L, Chan B. Macrophage/monocyte receptor for nonenzymatically glycosylated protein is upregulated by cachectin/tumor necrosis factor. *J Clin Invest* 1989; 84: 1813–20.
148. Esposito C, Gerlach H, Brett J, Stern D, Vlassara H. Endothelial receptor-mediated binding of glucose-modified albumin is associated with increased monolayer permeability and modulation of cell surface coagulant properties. *J Exp Med* 1989; 170: 1387–407.
149. Kirstein M, Brett J, Radoff S, Ogawa S, Stern D, Vlassara H. Advanced protein glycosylation induces transendothelial human monocyte chemotaxis and secretion of platelet-derived growth factor: role in vascular disease of diabetes and aging. *Proc Natl Acad Sci USA* 1990; 87: 9010–4.
150. Oldfield MD, Bach LA, Forbes JM, Nikolic-Paterson D, McRobert A, Thallas V, Atkins RC, Osicka T, Jerums G, Cooper ME. Advanced glycation end products cause epithelial–myofibroblast transdifferentiation via the receptor for advanced glycation end products (RAGE). *J Clin Invest* 2001; 108: 1853–63.
151. Radoff S, Makita Z, Vlassara H. Radioreceptor assay for advanced glycosylation end products. *Diabetes* 1991; 40: 1731–8.
152. Makita Z, Radoff S, Rayfield EJ, Yang Z, Skolnik E, Delaney V, Friedman EA, Cerami A, Vlassara H. Advanced glycosylation end products in patients with diabetic nephropathy. *N Engl J Med* 1991; 325: 836–42.

This chapter is based in part on a chapter of the same title which was published in an earlier edition of the International Textbook of Diabetes Mellitus, by Jery W Kolaczynski and Barry J Goldstein.

97

Monitoring of Lipids in Diabetes

M.F. Laker and R.D.G. Neely

University of Newcastle upon Tyne, UK, and Newcastle upon Tyne Hospitals NHS Trust, UK

INTRODUCTION

Dyslipidemic diabetic patients may be investigated using a variety of techniques that vary in their complexity (Table 1) although most are managed by measuring total cholesterol, triglyceride, and high-density lipoprotein (HDL) cholesterol concentrations, this in turn being possible in clinical laboratories. For patients receiving pharmacological lipid-lowering therapy, the targets for optimal treatment remain a subject of considerable debate; however, there is increasing evidence to support the use of apolipoprotein B (apo B) and non-HDL-cholesterol in addition or as alternatives to low-density lipoprotein (LDL)-cholesterol, particularly in moderately hypertriglyceridemic diabetic patients. Other investigations are occasionally undertaken to establish the molecular basis of lipoprotein disorders, either at the protein level (enzymes or receptors) or at the DNA level (the genetic basis of disorders, genotyping). Such investigations are available in specialist and research laboratories, as are other complex laboratory procedures for investigating lipoprotein metabolism, including separation techniques to examine lipoprotein fraction and subfraction composition and investigations of the turnover and cellular metabolism of lipoproteins. Additional investigations for secondary hyperlipidemia due to causes other than diabetes mellitus will be important in some patients. The present chapter will consider the investigations that are used widely in clinical practice and sources of variation in these. Several reviews have been published in which more complex procedures are considered in depth [1–6].

ASSESSMENT OF LIPID STATUS

Screening

Cardiovascular morbidity and mortality is increased up to threefold in diabetic compared to nondiabetic populations [7, 8] and coronary artery disease is the major cause of mortality in patients with type 2 diabetes mellitus [9]. Some investigators have suggested that type 2 diabetes mellitus should be considered as a coronary heart disease (CHD) risk equivalent [10] and this has been recognized in recently published guidelines [11]. The cardiovascular risk factors that are found in the general population are important, particularly as the prevalence of some of these, including dyslipidemia, is increased in diabetes [12]. However, prospective data from the UKPDS study indicate that once diabetes has developed, increased concentrations of LDL-cholesterol, decreased concentrations of HDL-cholesterol, hypertension, hyperglycemia, and smoking appear to be the most important, potentially modifiable, risk factors for coronary artery disease [9]. The risk attributable to cholesterol increases more steeply with increasing cholesterol concentrations in diabetic compared with nondiabetic subjects [13] and atherogenic lipoprotein changes also occur in prediabetic patients [14]. In diabetes, the relative protection from the atherogenic effects of dyslipidemia seen in premenopausal nondiabetic females compared to males is lost [15] and serum total triglyceride concentrations are also predictors of cardiovascular events [16, 17]. Elevated serum triglycerides form part of the atherogenic lipoprotein phenotype in which a low HDL-cholesterol concentration is accompanied by increased numbers of small dense LDL particles [18], these abnormalities being common in type 2 diabetic patients without significant hypercholesterolemia [19]. Measurement of blood lipids, including total cholesterol, triglycerides, and HDL-cholesterol, is thus essential in the evaluation of both male and female diabetic patients.

Follow-Up

Following diagnosis the initial management will be aimed at improving glycemic control; when this has been

International Textbook of Diabetes Mellitus, Third Edition. Edited by R. A. DeFronzo, E. Ferrannini, H. Keen, and P. Zimmet.
 ISBN: 0-471-48655-8.

Table 1 Laboratory investigation of dyslipoproteinemia

Detection and management
Cholesterol, triglycerides, HDL-cholesterol, LDL-cholesterol, non-HDL-cholesterol
Apolipoproteins A1, B
Tests for other causes of secondary hyperlipidemia
Special investigations
Lipoprotein(a), apolipoprotein E phenotyping
Lipoprotein analysis
Fraction and subfraction analysis, LDL size
Lipoprotein composition
Lipoprotein metabolism (cell uptake, turnover)
Protein analysis (enzymes, receptors)
DNA analysis (genotyping, molecular defects)

achieved, blood lipid measurements should be repeated. However, normoglycemia is not required before dyslipidemia is addressed and no further improvements in blood lipids would be expected below an HbA_{1c} concentration of 8.5%. If levels are persistently high, which is often the case, other causes should be considered including a coexisting primary hyperlipoproteinemia or secondary hyperlipidemia due to causes other than diabetes mellitus (Table 2). The history should be checked for excessive alcohol consumption, medication reviewed, and screening investigations for hypothyroidism, renal disease, and liver disease performed. If a primary hyperlipidemia is suspected, this should be characterized, if necessary, with special investigations and family studies, where appropriate (Table 1). For persisting dyslipidemia, appropriate management should be introduced according to current guidelines, and patients monitored to ensure an adequate response has been achieved. The most appropriate choice of lipid parameter for monitoring drug therapy in diabetic dyslipidemia must take account of the pattern of lipid disturbance prior to treatment (see below).

For those in whom no dyslipidemia is apparent on initial evaluation, it has usually been recommended that lipids should be monitored merely on an annual basis. However, this advice may no longer be appropriate, as the Heart Protection Study showed uniform risk reduction with simvastatin treatment in high-risk patients, largely independent of baseline lipid status [20], suggesting that lipid-lowering treatment should be guided solely by assessment of absolute cardiovascular risk [21]. Inadequate cholesterol-lowering treatment may, however, result in failure to achieve the expected risk reductions, and it is therefore recommended that monitoring be undertaken to ensure that an adequate lipid-lowering response has been achieved [22].

Triglycerides are not usually considered a primary target of therapy, at least when only moderately elevated. However, elevated serum triglyceride concentrations may point to a constellation of metabolic abnormalities associated with insulin resistance and the metabolic syndrome. In particular, triglyceride >1.7 mmol/l is associated with the presence of reduced HDL-cholesterol and changes in the LDL subclass pattern to small dense LDL, which appears independently associated with progression of atherosclerosis in type 2 diabetes mellitus [23]. As triglycerides per se appear not to be inherently atherogenic, monitoring of fasting levels may be of lesser value after the initial evaluation. Although a recent meal elevates serum triglyceride levels (see below) it is inconvenient to insist that patients fast before routine lipid measurements and unnecessary in those without dyslipidemia or in those with severe hyperlipidemia. A reasonable compromise is to restrict the requirement for fasting to patients with borderline hypertriglyceridemia (1.7–10 mmol/l; 150–1000 mg/L). However, it should be remembered that calculation of LDL-cholesterol according to the widely used Friedewald equation is invalid in nonfasting samples or where triglyceride concentrations exceed 4.5 mmol/l (400 mg/dl) in a fasting sample.

Both apo B and non-HDL-cholesterol may be measured in nonfasting samples, and this provides an additional advantage over the calculated LDL-cholesterol method. As only a simple calculation is required to derive non-HDL-cholesterol, this parameter may be readily obtained from the majority of laboratories; however, as with the calculated LDL-cholesterol method, much depends on the choice of an HDL-cholesterol method that does not exhibit bias in dyslipidemic samples. Measurement of LDL-cholesterol in nonfasting samples, using homogeneous assays ("direct" LDL-cholesterol), has also been advocated. However, in dyslipidemic samples these may also underestimate LDL-cholesterol as measured by any of the reference methods.

Table 2 Major causes of dyslipidemia

Primary hyperlipoproteinemias	Common causes of secondary hyperlipoproteinemia
Familial hypercholesterolemia	Diabetes mellitus
Polygenic hypercholesterolemia	Obesity
Familial combined hyperlipidemia	Alcohol abuse
Familial dysbetalipoproteinemia (type III hyperlipoproteinemia)	Drug-related (see Table 5)
Familial hypertriglyceridemia	Hypothyroidism
Chylomicronemia syndrome	Renal disease
Hyperalphalipoproteinemia	Biliary obstruction

Target Values

Target values for serum lipids in type 2 diabetes mellitus have been proposed by the European Diabetes Policy Group [24], the National Service Framework (NSF) in the UK [25], and by the National Cholesterol Education Panel Adult Treatment Panel (NCEP ATP III) in the

Table 3 Target values for serum lipids in diabetes

	ATP III (2002)	NICE (2002)	IDF (1999)
Total cholesterol			
mmol/l	<5.2	<5.0	<4.8
mg/dl	<200	<190	<185
HDL-cholesterol			
mmol/l	>1.1	NS	>1.2
mg/dl	>40	NS	>45
Triglycerides			
mmol/l	<1.7	<2.3	<1.7
mg/dl	<150	<200	<150
LDL-cholesterol			
mmol/l	<2.6	<3.0	<3.0
mg/dl	<100	<115	<115
Non-HDL-cholesterol			
mmol/l	<3.4	NS	NS
mg/dl	<130	NS	NS
Apolipoprotein B			
g/l	<0.9	NS	NS
mg/dl	<90	NS	NS

Note: NS = Not specified.

United States [11] (Table 3). The values for total cholesterol are broadly consistent with those given in guidelines for CHD prevention in nondiabetic populations, which are supported by clinical trial data [11, 26]. The major national and international guidelines have emphasized the importance of LDL-cholesterol as the primary target for pharmacological lipid lowering therapy with HMG CoA reductase inhibitors (statins). Although treatment to reduce LDL-cholesterol has been successful in reducing cardiovascular events in diabetic subgroups in the major HMG CoA reductase inhibitor intervention trials, on-treatment LDL-cholesterol measurements appear to be a relatively poor predictor of outcomes, particularly in cases where pretreatment LDL-cholesterol is not particularly elevated [27]. This unexpected finding may be explained on the basis of the variability of LDL composition and the increasing significance of other atherogenic lipoprotein species at low LDL-cholesterol levels and in the presence of hypertriglyceridemia [28]. Indeed the validity of applying the Friedewald equation in diabetic dyslipidemia has been called into question [29]. Alternative lipid and lipoprotein markers, which reflect a broader range of atherogenic lipoproteins, may be better predictors of outcome. On-treatment concentrations of apo B, a measure of LDL, IDL (intermediate density lipoprotein), and VLDL (very low density lipoprotein) particle numbers independent of composition [30], appeared to be more consistent than concentrations of LDL-cholesterol as a predictor of outcome in several major prospective studies [31, 32]. A target of 0.90 g/l has been suggested for optimum risk reduction [33–35]. In the presence of moderate hypertriglyceridemia non-HDL-cholesterol is an alternative measure of atherogenic lipoprotein cholesterol content, including LDL, IDL, VLDL, and triglyceride-rich remnant lipoproteins (RLPs) [36]. At higher triglyceride concentrations, cholesterol in less atherogenic triglyceride-rich lipoprotein species may increasingly contribute to the non-HDL-cholesterol fraction, but despite this it also appears to be more strongly predictive of outcomes than is LDL-cholesterol in both diabetic and nondiabetic subjects [37, 38]. For this reason the recently published NCEP ATP III guidelines have recommended non-HDL-cholesterol as a secondary treatment target in patients with moderate hypertriglyceridemia once the LDL-cholesterol target has been achieved [35, 39].

Formal proof of benefit has not been demonstrated for the triglyceride and HDL-cholesterol targets, although patients with elevated triglyceride and low HDL-cholesterol concentrations benefited most from treatment with gemfibrozil in a primary CHD prevention study, the Helsinki Heart Study [40]. Others have argued that a more aggressive approach to lipid target values is warranted (total cholesterol <4.4 mmol/l, 170 mg/dl), since atherogenic compositional abnormalities of lipoproteins are found in diabetic patients with only modestly increased serum lipid concentrations [41].

Analytical Techniques

Total Cholesterol

Many different types of method have been described for the determination of cholesterol, although relatively few are used for clinical analysis [42]. Gas chromatography-mass spectrometry and colorimetric techniques are highly accurate procedures that are used for calibrating reference materials and for judging the performance of clinical methods. Enzymatic techniques have the advantage that preliminary extraction of serum is unnecessary and the reagents are not corrosive. They are rapid, sensitive, use small sample volumes, and can be readily adapted to modern clinical analyzers. Enzymatic techniques have also been adapted to dry reagent strips and used in portable desktop analyzers, which estimate cholesterol concentrations in small quantities of whole blood, the results being available within a short period [43]. However, each analysis takes several minutes and measuring a large batch of samples is time-consuming. If labor is included in a cost analysis, laboratory wet chemistry methods are more economic.

Triglycerides

Triglycerides may be quantified by a variety of methods, although enzymatic techniques are the most widely used [44]. Early enzymatic methods were applied to glycerol determination after initial saponification of triglycerides, but the introduction of lipases has allowed the development of wholly enzymatic procedures. Enzymatic techniques are direct, specific, and rapid. However, the quality of enzymes has been inconsistent, some lipases also requiring a protease to hydrolyze triglycerides completely. In addition, contaminating enzymes may cause interference and the shelf life of reagents is inconsistent. Despite these reservations, enzymatic techniques are used almost universally in clinical laboratories.

Blanking is required for the highest degrees of accuracy, since most methods measure free glycerol in serum in addition to glycerol derived from triglyceride. Free glycerol concentrations are sufficiently low in most subjects to be ignored (<0.15 mmol/l, 1.4 mg/dl) but can cause significant inaccuracies in patients receiving hyperalimentation fluids containing glycerol, or intravenous heparin, which induces increased lipase activity. In addition, high levels may occur in diabetes mellitus and in hemodialysis treatment [45, 46].

Triglycerides may also be measured using desktop analyzers, although these techniques have been investigated less for triglyceride than for cholesterol measurement. A pilot study has suggested that home monitoring of triglycerides by type 2 diabetic patients may be a useful adjunct to self-management, since improved lipid profiles were obtained [47].

High-Density Lipoprotein Cholesterol

Measurement of cholesterol in HDL requires either physical separation from other lipoprotein fractions or masking of these fractions prior to quantification. Ultracentrifugation, electrophoresis, high-performance liquid chromatography, or chemical precipitation based–methods can achieve physical separation of HDL from other fractions, the latter having been widely used in clinical laboratories. Masking of non-HDL fractions is achieved in homogenous methods by antibodies or other macromolecules that form complexes with chylomicrons, VLDL, and LDL. The cholesterol in these lipoprotein fractions is not accessible to enzymes used in quantification and therefore only HDL-cholesterol is quantified.

Homogenous assays do not use a physical separation stage and therefore have the distinct advantage that they can be automated. This results in improvements in precision, in addition to being more convenient. Thus, homogenous assays typically give within-run imprecision figures of ~1% and total imprecision figures of 2–3% compared to figures that are double of these for precipitation assays [48]).

The accuracy (or bias) of HDL methods is assessed by comparison to a Center for Disease Control and Prevention procedure that combines precipitation with ultracentrifugation in a three-stage procedure [49]. It can be difficult to make valid judgements of accuracy from published data because of factors such as differences in reagents. However, homogenous assays have been shown to have acceptable accuracy [50]. Studies of accuracy of homogenous assays in diabetes are lacking at present. Such studies would be important to enable conclusions to be reached as to the applicability of these procedures to the investigation of diabetic subjects. This is because RLPs have been shown to interfere with the homogenous measurement of HDL-cholesterol based on polyethylene glycol–modified enzymes in patients with dysbetalipoproteinemia [51] and such particles are elevated in the serum of diabetic patients [52].

Low-Density Lipoprotein Cholesterol

Guidelines for the detection and treatment of high blood cholesterol levels include action limits based on LDL-cholesterol levels in addition to total cholesterol values [11, 26]. Ultracentrifugation is used to measure LDL directly, either by separating lipoprotein fractions, or indirectly by combining ultracentrifugation—to separate VLDL—with precipitation to quantify HDL-cholesterol concentrations (beta quantification). Despite its recognised shortcomings, including the inclusion of lipoprotein(a) and IDL in the LDL fraction, the latter method has become the reference procedure for LDL- and HDL-cholesterol quantitation, as practiced by the Center for Disease Control and Prevention [49] and used in the major epidemiological studies used to develop the current guidelines for assessment of cardiovascular risk [53]. Ultracentrifugation is not available in most diagnostic laboratories and the traditional beta quantification technique is expensive and time-consuming, requires large sample volumes, and has limited analytical capacity. Although modified protocols have been proposed to address these shortcomings [54] the technique is unsuitable for processing workloads from busy clinics. The most widely used approach to LDL-cholesterol measurement is to estimate values indirectly using the Friedewald formula [55]. Total serum lipid and HDL-cholesterol concentrations are measured and VLDL-cholesterol concentrations calculated from serum triglycerides.

$$\text{LDL-cholesterol} = (\text{totalcholesterol}) - (\text{HDL-cholesterol}) - (\text{total triglycerides}/2.2)$$

where concentrations are expressed in mmol/l. (For LDL-cholesterol concentrations in mg/dl, triglycerides should be divided by 5.)

The Friedewald formula assumes that most circulating triglyceride is present in the VLDL fraction. Chylomicrons contain a lower proportion of cholesterol and the use of the Friedewald formula requires the subject to be fasting. In addition, the calculated LDL fraction includes IDL (density 1.006–1.019). The formula is thus inaccurate when increases in IDL occur, the percentage error increasing progressively with greater cholesterol/triglyceride ratios in IDL. Such changes occur in type III hyperlipoproteinemia (dysbetalipoproteinemia) and also in diabetes mellitus, chronic renal failure, and atherosclerotic vascular disease [56]. Inaccuracies also occur with precipitation techniques if serum triglyceride concentrations exceed 4.5 mmol/l (400 mg/dl), due to cholesterol enrichment of VLDL [57]. The use of LDL-cholesterol values calculated according to the Friedewald formula may therefore be less suitable for application in diabetic patients [29, 58] and alternative formulae [59] or direct measurements would seem preferable. Although commercial immunoseparation techniques for measuring LDL-cholesterol directly are now available [60], detailed evaluation of these has shown poor recovery of small dense LDL subfractions and variable, nonspecific reactions to VLDL particles [61, 62]. As equivalence to other LDL measurements in dyslipidemic sera cannot be assumed, these methods do not yet have an established place in monitoring dyslipidemic patients.

Several other techniques for quantifying LDL have been described, including chromatographic, electrophoretic, and precipitation procedures. Precipitation methods have the same difficulties as described for the calculated LDL method, while other techniques are time-consuming and require specialized instrumentation.

Apolipoproteins A1 and B

The advantages of apolipoprotein measurements over conventional and lipid and lipoprotein measurements in the assessment of cardiovascular risk [63, 64] and monitoring of lipid-lowering therapy [32, 65, 66] are now widely recognized [67]. These advantages indeed appear particularly relevant to the assessment and monitoring of dyslipidemic diabetic patients [28, 34, 68]. In recent years, the assays have become more widely available and with the advent of standardization [69–72], automated immunoassay methods, and the publication of reference intervals based on large populations [73–76] it has been suggested that these measurements should be preferred to lipid measurements [77, 78]. Although a wide variety of methods are available, including radioimmunoassay, enzyme-linked immunosorbent assays, and electroimmunoassay, the commercially available immunoturbidometric and immunonephelometric methods are most suited to automation and high throughput applications. Fasting samples are not required and calculation of the apo B/A1 ratio is considered highly predictive in the evaluation of cardiovascular risk [64].

Triglyceride-Rich Remnant Lipoproteins

Triglyceride-rich RLPs are considered to be a highly atherogenic lipoprotein fraction, increased concentrations of which are found in familial dysbetalipoproteinemia [79], visceral obesity [80], hypertriglyceridemia [81, 82], and diabetes [83] and are associated with progression of atherosclerosis [84]. The concentrations of triglyceride-rich RLPs are reduced by both statin [85] and fibrate therapies [86] and as they may contribute significantly to the risk reduction achieved by these classes of drugs they may be an important target for lipid-lowering therapy [87]. As they are variable in lipid and apolipoprotein composition, measurement of these lipoproteins is difficult [88] and despite the advent of more convenient methods [89, 90], these are not yet offered by many laboratories [87].

Table 4 Factors contributing to variation in lipid measurement

Analytical variation
Intraindividual variation
Biological variation
Physiological (e.g. temporal, seasonal, age, menstrual cycle)
Behavioral (e.g. diet, obesity, exercise, alcohol)
Clinical (e.g. drugs, myocardial infarction, infection, trauma)
Preanalytical variation
Patient preparation (fasting, posture)
Sample processing (e.g. venous occlusion, storage of samples)

SOURCES OF VARIATION IN LIPID MEASUREMENT

It is widely recognised that considerable variation is inherent in lipid measurement, independent of dyslipidemia or genetic variations in lipid metabolism. Several factors contribute to this variation (Table 4).

ANALYTICAL VARIATION

Cholesterol

The diagnosis and management of hypercholesterolemia is based on cardiovascular risk association rather than population-based reference intervals [11, 22, 24, 25]. Thus, great importance is attached to minimizing analytical bias (inaccuracy) and imprecision. Clinical laboratories should achieve an overall precision consistent with a coefficient of variation (CV) of 5% or less, with the goal of achieving a CV of 3% or less (Figure 1) [91]; many laboratories have already achieved the latter target. The accuracy of cholesterol assays may be improved by using calibrants in which values are assigned by reference methods [92, 93].

Portable dry chemistry analyzers have considerable potential for assessing serum lipids since results may be obtained rapidly, with immediate feedback to patients. The Reflotron[r] has been the most extensively investigated of these and an external quality assurance survey of the Reflotron in primary care has demonstrated that although many participants obtained satisfactory responses, 8.6% of results differed by 1.0 mmol/l or more from

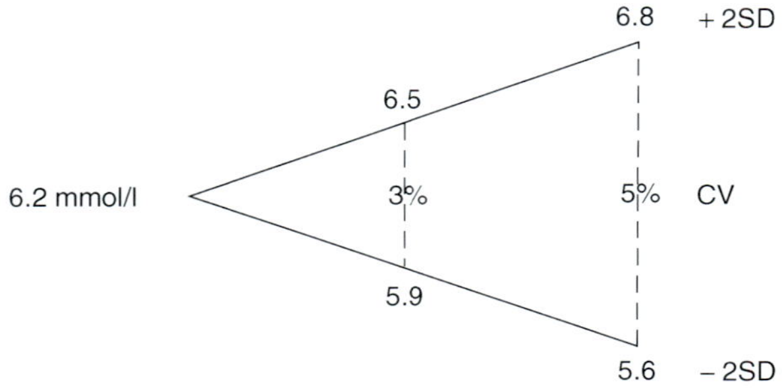

Figure 1 Effect of increasing imprecision on cholesterol measurement. The figure shows 95% confidence intervals for cholesterol values at the level of 6.2 mmol/l (240 mg/dl) when CVs are 3 and 5% (reprinted from reference 91, courtesy of the American Association for Clinical Chemistry, Inc.)

the target values, poor operator technique and outdated reagent strips being common sources of error [94]. Relatively wide limits of agreement between values obtained using the Reflotron and laboratory measurements (±0.9 mmol/l) have been demonstrated using bias plots [95]. Although desktop analyzers have much to offer, very careful attention to technique and participation in quality assurance schemes are mandatory for users.

Triglycerides

Consensus target values for serum triglycerides have received less attention than those for cholesterol because of uncertainty regarding their independent contribution to CHD risk. However, triglycerides are an independent risk factor in diabetes mellitus [16, 17] and modest increases occur in the atherogenic lipoprotein phenotype [18]. In addition, triglyceride measurement is required for calculated LDL values. Thus, the variation in triglyceride assays should be minimized. However, there is not yet a recognised hierarchy of reference assays against which clinical methods can be judged and by which reference values can be assigned to calibration material.

INTRAINDIVIDUAL VARIATION

In longitudinal studies, individuals not receiving lipid-lowering therapy show variations of up to 20% in cholesterol concentrations, with triglycerides showing variation of up to 23% [96–98]. These differences are greater than analytical variation and are large enough to affect the correct assignment of risk category. Thus, several determinations of lipid levels are required before advising major changes of lifestyle or drug therapy. Decisions concerning response to treatment should consider the effect of intraindividual as well as analytical variation, particularly when the mode of therapy might be expected to reduce lipid levels by only 5–10%. Intraindividual variation can be considered to result from factors that lead to biological changes in lipid concentrations and preanalytical factors.

Biological Variation

Physiological Variation

There is little diurnal variation in total or HDL-cholesterol levels although serum triglyceride concentrations rise during the day independent of meal patterns, within-day variation being over 30% [99, 100]. The increase in triglyceride levels is greater following breakfast than after meals later in the day, possibly due to a variable insulin response to meals [100]. The morning rise that occurs if breakfast is omitted may result from increased lipolysis, although plasma nonesterified fatty acid (NEFA) concentrations are not increased. Seasonal variations result in total cholesterol levels being 3–5% higher in winter than in summer, although trends in triglyceride and HDL-cholesterol levels are weaker [101, 102].

Total and LDL-cholesterol concentrations rise in early adult years in males to reach a plateau by the age of 45 years, with this increase occurring later in females; HDL-cholesterol levels are lower in all age groups in adult males compared to females [103, 104]. Total cholesterol levels are up to 9% higher in the follicular than the menstrual phase of the menstrual cycle, with no clear trends being seen in triglyceride concentrations [105, 106]. In pregnancy, total cholesterol levels fall slightly during the first 8–12 weeks and then rise progressively by 30% by term; triglyceride levels increase up to threefold by term [107, 108]. HDL-cholesterol concentrations rise until 24 weeks' gestation, after which they fall [107].

Behavioral Variation

Diet and fasting Serum cholesterol concentrations do not change significantly in the postprandial state [109], although triglyceride-rich chylomicrons may circulate for up to 12 h after a meal. Total serum cholesterol levels rise with increased dietary cholesterol and saturated fat intake, probably due to suppression of LDL receptor activity [110], although stearic acid (C18:0) appears to have no effect on serum cholesterol concentrations, possibly because it is converted to the mono-unsaturated oleic acid. The frequency of meals may also affect serum lipids. Subjects eating four or more meals per day have been found to have total cholesterol concentration 0.23 mmol/l (9 mg/dl) lower than for subjects eating 1–2 meals per day, due mainly to a lower LDL-cholesterol concentration. This occurred in spite of a higher total caloric and saturated fat intake [111], possibly because of reduced calorie density.

Following a fat-rich meal, triglyceride concentrations increase within 1 h, the peak concentration occurring at 4 h, with concentrations remaining elevated for up to 9 h

[112]. The extent of the increase after a fat-rich meal varies considerably between subjects but, on average, the peak concentration is more than double the fasting concentration. Postprandial lipemia tends to be greater in males than in females [112], and in older compared to younger subjects [112]. Mean total cholesterol concentrations do not change postprandially, although the response is variable in individual subjects [109, 112, 113]. Prolonged fasting for 6 days has been shown to increase both total cholesterol and triglyceride concentrations by 18% [114], with falls of 22% in HDL-cholesterol concentrations.

Coffee Serum total and LDL-cholesterol levels are 6–10% higher in boiled coffee drinkers than in nondrinkers [115, 116]. The hypercholesterolemic factor in boiled coffee is retained by a paper coffee filter, although its exact nature remains unknown [117–119]. Most studies have shown no effect of boiled coffee on triglycerides, although Zock et al. [120], using a lipid-rich fraction of boiled coffee, have reported triglycerides rising by 55%.

Alcohol Alcohol ingestion increases both triglycerides and HDL-cholesterol in the general population in addition to causing secondary hyperlipidemia in susceptible individuals. Modest consumption increases HDL-cholesterol concentrations by 10% [121, 122], with larger changes being seen with heavier intake. LDL-cholesterol levels show a negative correlation with alcohol consumption [121]. A moderate evening dose of alcohol has no effect on lipid concentrations the following morning in normotriglyceridemic individuals [123, 124]; in hypertriglyceridemic subjects, however, alcohol increases fasting triglyceride concentrations [125]. Hypertriglyceridemia appears to be due to both dietary factors and increased lipolysis in adipose tissue [126]. Alcohol taken with a meal increases and prolongs postprandial lipemia [123, 127], the degree of postprandial lipemia being greater in individuals with fasting hypertriglyceridemia [125]. Binge drinking (160 g alcohol/day over 3 days) results in a twofold increase in fasting triglycerides [128].

Exercise Moderate exercise has a variable effect on total cholesterol because of contrasting effects on lipoproteins, LDL-cholesterol falling, and HDL-cholesterol concentrations increasing [129]. The effects of exercise appear to be independent of dietary composition or caloric intake, much of the effect probably being due to decreased body fat content [130]. The rate of catabolism of triglyceride-rich lipoproteins is enhanced, lipoprotein lipase activity being increased in both adipose tissue and muscle of endurance runners, the effect of this being to increase the availability of NEFA for direct oxidation as an energy source in exercising muscles [129]. Total and HDL-cholesterol levels are increased by acute exertion (walking, vigorous cycling, and the standard Bruce protocol for exercise ECG testing), probably in part at least due to altered plasma volume [131, 132].

Table 5 *In vivo* effects of drugs on serum lipids and lipoproteins

Drug	TC	LDL-C	HDL-C	TG
Antihypertensive drugs				
Thiazide diuretics	↑	↑	→	↑
β-Blockers	→	→	↓	↑
α-Blockers	↓	↓	↑	↓
Calcium channel antagonists	→	→	→	→
ACE inhibitors	→	→	→	→
Gonadal steroids				
Estrogens	*a*	↓	↑	↑
Progestagens	*a*	→↑	↓	→↓

Note: *a* = Effects depend on the particular estrogen or progestagen used and the route of administration; see text for details. TC = total cholesterol; LDL-C = LDL-cholesterol; HDL-C = HDL-cholesterol; TG = triglycerides; ↑ = increased; ↓ = decreased; → = no significant effect.

Clinical Variation

Drugs The concomitant use of drugs for the management of diabetes and its complications may affect serum lipids (Table 5).

Antihypertensive drugs Antihypertensive drugs have various effects on lipoproteins, these being outlined in Table 5 (see also Chapter 97).

Estrogens and progestagens Oral estrogens increase concentrations of HDL-cholesterol, mainly HDL_2-cholesterol, through a suppression of hepatic lipase activity [133]. Triglyceride concentrations are also increased in a dose-dependent manner because of enhanced hepatic secretion of VLDL apo B. LDL composition is altered, with increased triglyceride content. The effects of progestagens depend to a large extent on their androgenicity, with the more androgenic progestagens causing a larger fall in HDL-cholesterol (mainly HDL_2-cholesterol) concentrations [134].

The net effect of combined therapy depends on the opposing effects of estrogens and progestagens. Older formulations of combined oral contraceptives increased LDL-cholesterol and lowered HDL-cholesterol [135]. Newer low-dose contraceptives are associated with more favorable lipid changes, although triglyceride levels are increased as a result of less androgenic progestagens being less able to oppose the estrogen-induced increase in VLDL synthesis [134]. After cessation of oral contraceptives, total cholesterol concentrations return to baseline within one cycle, whereas triglyceride concentrations remain elevated for longer [136].

In combined hormone replacement, the net effect depends on the balance between the opposing actions of estrogen and progestagen. Transdermally administered estrogens have less effect on lipids and, in contrast to oral estrogens, they lower serum triglyceride levels [137, 138]. This may be because serum estrogen concentrations are lower, or more constant, or due to the drug escaping first-pass clearance by the liver.

Other drugs Other drugs that affect lipoprotein metabolism include retinoids, which elevate serum triglyceride concentrations, and anticonvulsants, which raise HDL-cholesterol levels. A variety of metabolic complications result from antiretroviral therapy in patients with acquired immunodeficiency syndrome, including dyslipidemia, insulin resistance, and lipodystrophy. The lipid changes include increased LDL-cholesterol and reduced HDL-cholesterol concentrations, together with elevated triglycerides [139]. Hypercholesterolemia and hypertriglyceridemia, have been noted in patients with schizophrenia treated with clozapine or olanzapine [140, 141]. Hyperlipidemia, particularly hypertriglyceridemia, occurs in renal transplant recipients treated with the potent immunosuppressive agent Sirolimus [142].

Disease states Lipoprotein metabolism is affected by several diseases including myocardial infarction, infection, trauma, and malignancy.

Myocardial infarction Cholesterol concentrations measured 2 years prior to a myocardial infarction, within 24 h of admission, or 3 months 2 years following myocardial infarction do not differ [143, 144]. After 24-h postinfarction there is a fall in the concentrations of total, HDL-, and LDL-cholesterol, the extent of the decrease being related to the severity of the infarct [143, 145–147]. The maximum fall in cholesterol concentrations occurs 1 week following infarction. Triglyceride concentrations show no consistent changes, while falls in total and LDL-apo B, increases in VLDL-apo B, and decreases in apo A1 concentrations occur, these being maximal at 7 days [146].

Infection and inflammation Infection is an important cause of lipid, total, and HDL-cholesterol concentrations falling [148]. The lipid and lipoprotein changes seen during infection are consistent with falls in hepatic and lipoprotein lipase activities, possibly due to suppression by interleukin 1 [149], interferons, and tumor necrosis factor [150]. Recovery from sepsis is paralleled by a normalization of lipid values [151].

Trauma and surgery Major surgery is accompanied by a fall in both cholesterol (−31%) and triglyceride (−43%) concentrations [152]. VLDL-cholesterol and triglycerides both decrease by over 50% during the first week, while LDL-cholesterol also decreases but to a lesser extent. Concentrations return to normal within 1 month. HDL-cholesterol concentration falls following the operation (−35%) and remains low for longer than the other fractions. Following burns there are rises in total triglyceride, VLDL-, and LDL-triglyceride, concentrations peaking at 5–6 days [153], which are not explained by changes in free glycerol [154]. Total cholesterol concentrations fall, reaching a minimum 10–12 days postburn, with falls in both HDL- and LDL-cholesterol concentrations.

Malignancy Several longitudinal studies have shown falls in cholesterol concentrations of up to 0.6 mmol/l (23 mg/dl) 2 years prior to the diagnosis of cancer [155–157]. No consistent changes were seen in triglyceride or HDL-cholesterol concentrations, while LDL-cholesterol changes reflected those of total cholesterol [157]. For malignancy presenting more than 2 years after cholesterol measurement, or causing death after more than 5 years postmeasurement, initial cholesterol concentrations were lower than in patients without malignancy, although the difference was small [158]. The association seems to be limited to hematological malignancies, lung cancer, and other smoking-related tumors [158]. Because of the timescale it is unlikely that all these subjects had developed malignancy before the cholesterol measurement was undertaken and the association is, as yet, unexplained.

PREANALYTICAL VARIATION

Fasting

The effect of fasting is considered with diet (see above).

Posture

Serum cholesterol and triglyceride concentrations are higher on standing than on lying [158–162], with differences ranging between 9 and 19%. This is thought to be due to a fall in plasma volume on standing, with a resulting increase in the concentration of nondiffusible plasma components. Smaller changes are seen when changing from lying to sitting or sitting to standing [159, 160, 162, 163]. Howes et al. [161] showed that increases in cholesterol concentration on standing were correlated with increased noradrenaline levels but not with hematocrit changes. Lipid, lipoprotein, and apolipoprotein concentrations change within 5 min of altered posture [164].

Venous Occlusion

Occlusion of a vein for 0.5–1 min before venepuncture has no significant effect on serum lipid concentrations in normolipidemic subjects, although increases (of 20%) in serum cholesterol and triglyceride concentrations occur with prolonged venous occlusion [165, 166].

Type of Blood Sample

Lipid concentrations may differ between serum and plasma and are also affected by anticoagulants [167]. Low molecular weight anticoagulants such as citrate or oxalate cause large osmotic shifts of water from erythrocytes to plasma, reducing apparent lipoprotein concentrations [168, 169]. Heparin causes no detectable change in erythrocyte volume [170] and has negligible effects on cholesterol and triglyceride concentrations [171]. EDTA is often used as an anticoagulant for lipoprotein analysis. It causes decreases of 3% in cholesterol and triglyceride concentrations [172], and a correction factor of 1.03 has been suggested to convert EDTA plasma concentrations to the equivalent serum concentrations [173]. It is important that the collection tubes are filled to the volume mark, otherwise the osmotic effect of EDTA will lead to larger discrepancies between measurements in serum and plasma.

With increasing use of capillary samples obtained by finger-prick for cholesterol screening, comparability with venous cholesterol measurements is important. When the same analytical methods are used, capillary cholesterol concentrations vary between 4.4% higher and 8.7% lower than venous cholesterol concentrations with the same specimen type. Screening methods are now available for triglycerides and HDL-cholesterol, but for these analytes there is little information comparing capillary and venous blood.

Storage

Serum total cholesterol and triglyceride concentrations are stable for up to 5 years if stored at –20°C [174]. While total serum concentrations of lipids are relatively stable on storage, changes are seen in lipoprotein fractions. Much of the work in this field has been concerned with HDL-cholesterol concentrations determined after precipitation of apo-B-containing lipoproteins following storage of serum. Results of such studies are not consistent, some showing HDL-cholesterol to be stable at –20°C over several weeks [175, 176], while others report decreases in concentrations after 14 days at 4°C and over 6 months at –20°C [177], or increases in concentrations with storage for 6 months at –20°C [175]. These differences may be explained by high HDL-cholesterol levels falling and low levels rising on storage [178]. These changes are more marked in serum stored at 4°C than at –20°C, and while the changes are slowed they are not completely prevented by storage at –70°C [179]. HDL-cholesterol concentrations increase by 3% per day over 3 days in whole blood stored at room temperature [180].

Reports on the stability of lipoproteins in serum separated later by ultracentrifugation are contradictory, with reports that lipoproteins are stable if serum is stored at 0–5°C for 2 weeks, while showing changes after only a few days at –28°C [181]. Another investigation showed cholesterol concentrations in lipoprotein fractions to be stable for at least 27 weeks at –20°C, and triglyceride concentrations stable for at least 11 weeks [182], although the subjects studied had relatively normal lipid levels. Serum samples for lipoprotein electrophoresis are stable if stored at room temperature for 3 days, and are stable after one freeze–thaw cycle, but not after further freezing and thawing [183].

SUMMARY

Dyslipidemia should be monitored regularly in diabetes mellitus, and assessment should include the measurement of total cholesterol, HDL-cholesterol, and triglyceride concentrations. More detailed investigations may be required if a primary hyperlipoproteinemia is suspected and other causes of secondary hyperlipidemia should be considered. Several physiological factors cause variation in serum lipid concentrations, including age, sex, the menstrual cycle, and diet. Posture, venepuncture technique, concomitant medication, and clinical conditions other than diabetes mellitus also affect lipid levels.

REFERENCES

1. Laker MF, Game FL. Approaches to lipid and lipoprotein analysis. *Clin Endocrinol Metab* 1990; 4: 693–717.
2. Converse CA, Skinner ER (eds), *Lipoprotein Analysis. A Practical Approach*. Oxford: IRL Press, 1992.
3. Laker MF, Game FL. Laboratory investigations of dyslipoproteinaemias. In Betteridge DJ, Illingworth DR, Shepherd J (eds), *Lipoproteins in Health and Disease*. London: Edward Arnold, 1999; pp 381–98.
4. Stein E. Clinical chemistry annual review. *Curr Opin Lipidol* 1991; 2: 341–91.
5. Stein EA, Myers GL. Clinical chemistry—annual review. *Curr Opin Lipidol* 1992; 3: 359–98.
6. Assmann G, Hunt BJ. Clinical chemistry—annual review. *Curr Opin Lipidol* 1993; 4: 425–94.
7. Steiner C. Atherosclerosis, the major complication of diabetes. *Adv Exp Med Biol* 1985; 189: 277–97.
8. Panzram G. Mortality and survival in type 2 (noninsulin dependent) diabetes mellitus. *Diabetologia* 1987; 30: 123–31.
9. Turner RC, Millns H, Neil HA, Stratton IM, Manley SE, Matthews DR, Holman RR. Risk factors for coronary artery disease in non-insulin dependent diabetes mellitus: United Kingdom Prospective Diabetes Study (UKPDS 23). *Br Med J* 1998; 316: 823–8.
10. Haffner SM, Lehto S, Ronnemaa T, Pyorala K, Laakso M. Mortality from coronary heart disease in subjects with type 2 diabetes and in nondiabetic subjects with and without prior myocardial infarction. *N Engl J Med* 1998; 339: 229–34.
11. Expert Panel. Executive summary of the third report of the National Cholesterol Education Program (NCEP) Expert Panel on detection, evaluation, and treatment of high

blood cholesterol in adults (Adult Treatment Panel III). *J Am Med Assoc* 2001; 285: 2486–97.

12. Hanefield M, Schulze J, Fischer S, Julius U, Schmechel H, Haller H. The diabetes intervention study (DIS). A co-operative multi-intervention trial with newly manifest type 2 diabetes. *Monogr Atheroscler* 1985; 13: 98–103.
13. Kannel WB, McGee DL. Diabetes and cardiovascular disease. *J Am Med Assoc* 1979; 241: 2035–8.
14. Haffner SM, Stern MP, Hazuda HP, Mitchell BD, Patterson JK. Cardiovascular risk factors in confirmed prediabetic individuals. *J Am Med Assoc* 1990; 263: 2893–8.
15. Heyden S, Heiss G, Bartel AG, Hames CG. Sex differences in coronary mortality among diabetics in Evans County, Georgia. *J Chronic Dis* 1980; 33: 265–73.
16. West KM, Ahuja MMS, Bennett PA, Czyzyk A, De Acosta OM, Fuller JH, Grab B, Grabauskas V, Jarrett RK, Kosaka K. The role of circulating glucose and triglyceride concentrations and their interaction with other risk factors as determinants of arterial disease in nine diabetic populations from the WHO multinational study. *Diabetes Care* 1983; 6: 361–9.
17. Fontbonne A, Eschwège E, Cambien F, Richard J-L, Ducimetière P, Thibult N, et al. Hypertriglyceridemia as a risk factor of coronary heart disease mortality in subjects with impaired glucose tolerance or diabetes. *Diabetologia* 1989; 32: 300–4.
18. Austin MA, King MV, Vranizan KM, Krauss RM. Atherogenic lipoprotein phenotype. A proposed genetic marker for coronary heart disease. *Circulation* 1990; 82: 592–5.
19. Stewart MW, Laker MF, Dyer RG, Game FL, Mitcheson J, Winocour PH, Alberti KGMM. Lipoprotein compositional abnormalities and insulin resistance in type 2 diabetic patients with mild hyperlipidaemia. *Arterioscler Thromb* 1993; 13: 1046–52.
20. Heart Protection Study Collaborative Group. MRC/BHF Heart Protection Study of cholesterol lowering with simvastatin in 20,536 high risk individuals: a randomised placebo-controlled trial. *Lancet* 2002; 360: 7–22.
21. Inzucchi SE, Amatruda JM. Lipid management in patients with diabetes: translating guidelines into action. *Diabetes Care* 2003; 26: 1309–11.
22. Haffner SM. Management of dyslipidemia in adults with diabetes. *Diabetes Care* 2003; 26 (suppl 1): S83–6.
23. Vakkilainen J, Steiner G, Ansquer JC, Aubin F, Rattier S, Foucher C, Hamsten A, Taskinen MR; DAIS Group. Relationships between low-density lipoprotein particle size, plasma lipoproteins, and progression of coronary artery disease: the Diabetes Atherosclerosis Intervention Study (DAIS). *Circulation* 2003; 107: 1733–7.
24. European Diabetes Policy Group. A desktop guide to Type 2 diabetes mellitus. *Diabet Med* 1999; 16: 716–30.
25. Department of Health (UK). National service framework for coronary heart disease, 2001. Available at: http://www.doh.gov.uk/nsf/coronary.htm. Accessed September 15, 2003.
26. British Cardiac Society, British Hyperlipidaemia Association, British Hypertension Society. Joint British recommendations on prevention of coronary heart disease in clinical practice. *Heart* 1998; 80 (2S): 1S–29S.
27. Sacks FM, Pfeffer MA, Moye LA, Rouleau JL, Rutherford JD, Cole TG, Brown L, Warnica JW, Arnold JM, Wun CC, Davis BR, Braunwald E, for the Cholesterol and Recurrent Events Trial Investigators. The effect of pravastatin on coronary events after myocardial infarction in patients with average cholesterol levels. *N Engl J Med* 1996; 335: 1001–9.
28. Wagner AM, Perez A, Calvo F, Bonet R, Castellvi A, Ordonez J. Apolipoprotein(B) identifies dyslipidemic phenotypes associated with cardiovascular risk in normocholesterolemic type 2 diabetic patients. *Diabetes Care* 1999; 22: 812–7.
29. Rubies-Prat J, Reverter JL, Senti M, Pedro-Botet J, Salinas I, Lucas A, Nogues X, Sanmarti A. Calculated low-density lipoprotein cholesterol should not be used for management of lipoprotein abnormalities in patients with diabetes mellitus. *Diabetes Care* 1993; 16: 1081–6.
30. Durrington PN. Can measurement of apolipoprotein B replace the lipid profile in the follow-up of patients with lipoprotein disorders? *Clin Chem* 2002; 48: 401–2.
31. Pedersen TR, Olsson AG, Faergeman O, Kjekshus J, Wedel H, Berg K, Wilhelmsen L, Haghfelt T, Thorgeirsson G, Pyorala K, Miettinen T, Christophersen B, Tobert JA, Musliner TA, Cook TJ. Lipoprotein changes and reduction in the incidence of major coronary heart disease events in the Scandinavian Simvastatin Survival Study (4S). *Circulation* 1998; 97: 1453–60.
32. Gotto AM Jr, Whitney E, Stein EA, Shapiro DR, Clearfield M, Weis S, Jou JY, Langendorfer A, Beere PA, Watson DJ, Downs JR, de Cani JS. Relation between baseline and on-treatment lipid parameters and first acute major coronary events in the Air Force/Texas Coronary Atherosclerosis Prevention Study (AFCAPS/TexCAPS). *Circulation* 2000; 101: 477–84.
33. Alaupovic P, Fesmire JD, Hunnighake D, Domanski M, Forman S, Knatterud GL, Forrester J, Herd JA, Hoogwerf B, Campeau L, Gobel FL. The effect of aggressive and moderate lowering of LDL-cholesterol and low dose anticoagulation on plasma lipids, apolipoproteins and lipoprotein families in post coronary artery bypass graft trial. *Atherosclerosis* 1999; 146: 369–79.
34. Sniderman AD, Scantlebury T, Cianflone K. Hypertriglyceridemic hyperapob: the unappreciated atherogenic dyslipoproteinemia in type 2 diabetes mellitus. *Ann Intern Med* 2001; 135: 447–59.
35. Grundy SM. Low-density lipoprotein, non-high-density lipoprotein, and apolipoprotein B as targets of lipid-lowering therapy. *Circulation* 2002; 106: 2526–9.
36. Cui Y, Blumenthal RS, Flaws JA, Whiteman MK, Langenberg P, Bachorik PS, Bush TL. Non-high-density lipoprotein cholesterol level as a predictor of cardiovascular disease mortality. *Arch Intern Med* 2001; 161: 1413–9.
37. Bittner V, Hardison R, Kelsey SF, Weiner BH, Jacobs AK, Sopko G. Non-high-density lipoprotein cholesterol levels predict five-year outcome in the Bypass Angioplasty Revascularization Investigation (BARI). *Circulation* 2002; 106: 2537–42.
38. Lu W, Resnick HE, Jablonski KA, Jones KL, Jain AK, Howard WJ, Robbins DC, Howard BV. Non-HDL cholesterol as a predictor of cardiovascular disease in type 2 diabetes: the Strong Heart Study. *Diabetes Care* 2003; 26: 16–23.
39. Hsia SH. Non-HDL cholesterol: into the spotlight. *Diabetes Care* 2003; 26: 240–2.
40. Manninen V, Tenkanen L, Koskinen P, Huttunen JK, Mänttäri M, Heinonen OP, et al. Joint effects of serum triglyceride and LDL-cholesterol and HDL-cholesterol concentrations on coronary heart disease risk

in the Helsinki Heart Study. Implications for treatment. *Circulation* 1992; 85: 37–45.
41. Garg A, Grundy SM. Management of dyslipidemia in NIDDM. *Diabetes Care* 1990; 13: 153–69.
42. Richmond WR. Analytical reviews in clinical biochemistry: the quantitative analysis of cholesterol. *Ann Clin Biochem* 1992; 9: 577–97.
43. Warnick GR. Compact analysis systems. *Curr Opin Lipidol* 1991; 2: 343–8.
44. Klotzsch SG, McNamara JR. Triglyceride measurements: a review of methods and interferences. *Clin Chem* 1990; 36: 1605–13.
45. Jessen RH, Dass CJ, Eckfeldt JH. Do enzymatic analyses of serum triglycerides really need blanking for free glycerol? *Clin Chem* 1990; 36: 1372–5.
46. Naito HK, David JA. Laboratory considerations: determination of cholesterol, triglyceride, phospholipid, and other lipids in blood and tissues. In Storey JA (ed), *Lipid Research Methodology*. New York: Alan R Liss, 1984; pp 1–76.
47. Stewart MW, Laker MF, Alberti KGMM. Effects of self-monitoring of triglyceride concentrations in noninsulin dependent diabetes mellitus. *Br Med J* 1993; 306: 493.
48. Warnick GR, Nauck M, Rifai N. Evolution of methods for measurement of HDL-cholesterol: from ultracentrifugation to homogenous assays. *Clin Chem* 2001; 47: 1579–96.
49. Myers GL, Copper GR, Henderson LO, Hassemer DJ, Kimberley MM. Standardisation of lipid and lipoprotein measurement. In Rifai N, Warnick GR, Dominiczak MH (eds), *Handbook of Lipoprotein Testing*. Washington: AACC Press, 2000; pp 717–48.
50. Nauck M, März W, Jarausch J, Cobbaert C, Sägers A, Bernard D, Delanghe J, Honauer G, Lehmann P, Oestrich E, von Eckardstein A, Walch S, Wieland H, Assmann G. Multicenter evaluation of a homogenous assay for HDL-cholesterol without sample pretreatment. *Clin Chem* 1997; 43: 1622–9.
51. Lackner KJ, Schmitz G. β-VLDL of patients with Type III hyperlipoproteinemia interferes with homogenous determination of HDL-cholesterol based on polyethylene glycol-modified enzymes. *Clin Chem* 1998; 44: 2546–8.
52. Schaefer EJ, McNamara JR, Shah PK, Nakajima K, Cupples LA, Ordovas JM, Wilson PW. Elevated remnant-like particle cholesterol and triglyceride levels in diabetic men and women in the Framingham Offspring Study. *Diabetes Care* 2002; 25: 989–94.
53. The Lipid Research Clinics Coronary Primary Prevention Trial results, I: Reduction in incidence of coronary heart disease. *J Am Med Assoc* 1984; 251: 351–64.
54. Cole TG, Ferguson CA, Gibson DW, Nowatzke WL. Optimization of beta-quantification methods for high-throughput applications. *Clin Chem* 2001; 47: 712–21.
55. Friedewald WT, Levy RI, Fredrickson DS. Estimation of the concentration of low-density lipoprotein cholesterol in plasma without use of the preparative ultracentrifuge. *Clin Chem* 1972; 18: 499–502.
56. Senti M, Pedro-Botet J, Nogués X, Rubies-Prat J. Influence of intermediate-density lipoproteins on the accuracy of the Friedewald formula. *Clin Chem* 1991; 37: 1394–7.
57. Warnick GR, Knopp RH, Fitzpatrick V, Branson L. Estimating low-density lipoprotein cholesterol by the Friedewald equation is adequate for classifying patients on the basis of nationally recommended cutpoints. *Clin Chem* 1990; 36: 15–9.
58. Branchi A, Rovellini A, Torri A, Sommariva D. Accuracy of calculated serum low-density lipoprotein cholesterol for the assessment of coronary heart disease risk in NIDDM patients. *Diabetes Care* 1998; 21: 1397–402.
59. Planella T, Cortes M, Martinez-Bru C, Gonzalez-Sastre F, Ordonez-Llanos J. Calculation of LDL-cholesterol by using apolipoprotein B for classification of nonchylomicronemic dyslipemia. *Clin Chem* 1997; 43: 808–15.
60. Nauck M, Warnick GR, Rifai N. Methods for measurement of LDL-cholesterol: a critical assessment of direct measurement by homogeneous assays versus calculation. *Clin Chem* 2002; 48: 236–54.
61. Usui S, Kakuuchi H, Okamoto M, Mizukami Y, Okazaki M. Differential reactivity of two homogeneous LDL-cholesterol methods to LDL and VLDL subfractions, as demonstrated by ultracentrifugation and HPLC. *Clin Chem* 2002; 48: 1946–54.
62. Miller WG, Waymack PP, Anderson FP, Ethridge SF, Jayne EC. Performance of four homogeneous direct methods for LDL-cholesterol. *Clin Chem* 2002; 48: 489–98.
63. Lamarche B, Moorjani S, Lupien PJ, Cantin B, Bernard PM, Dagenais GR, Despres JP. Apolipoprotein A-I and B levels and the risk of ischemic heart disease during a five-year follow-up of men in the Quebec cardiovascular study. *Circulation* 1996; 94: 273–8.
64. Walldius G, Jungner I, Holme I, Aastveit AH, Kolar W, Steiner E. High apolipoprotein B, low apolipoprotein A-I, and improvement in the prediction of fatal myocardial infarction (AMORIS study): a prospective study. *Lancet* 2001; 358: 2026–33.
65. Moss AJ, Goldstein RE, Marder VJ, Sparks CE, Oakes D, Greenberg H, Weiss HJ, Zareba W, Brown MW, Liang CS, Lichstein E, Little WC, Gillespie JA, Van Voorhees L, Krone RJ, Bodenheimer MM, Hochman J, Dwyer EM Jr, Arora R, Marcus FI, Watelet LF, Case RB. Thrombogenic factors and recurrent coronary events. *Circulation* 1999; 99: 2517–22.
66. van Lennep JE, Westerveld HT, van Lennep HW, Zwinderman AH, Erkelens DW, van der Wall EE. Apolipoprotein concentrations during treatment and recurrent coronary artery disease events. *Arterioscler Thromb Vasc Biol* 2000; 20: 2408–13.
67. Grundy SM. Non-high-density lipoprotein cholesterol level as potential risk predictor and therapy target. *Arch Intern Med* 2001; 161: 1379–80.
68. Sniderman AD, Lamarche B, Tilley J, Seccombe D, Frohlich J. Hypertriglyceridemic hyperapoB in type 2 diabetes. *Diabetes Care* 2002; 25: 579–82.
69. Marcovina SM, Albers JJ, Dati F, Ledue TB, Ritchie RF. International Federation of Clinical Chemistry standardization project for measurements of apolipoproteins A-I and B. *Clin Chem* 1991; 37: 1676–82.
70. Marcovina SM, Albers JJ, Henderson LO, Hannon WH. International Federation of Clinical Chemistry standardization project for measurements of apolipoproteins A-I and B, III: Comparability of apolipoprotein A-I values by use of international reference material. *Clin Chem* 1993; 39: 773–81.
71. Marcovina SM, Albers JJ, Kennedy H, Mei JV, Henderson LO, Hannon WH. International Federation of Clinical Chemistry standardization project for measurements of apolipoproteins A-I and B. IV: Comparability of

apolipoprotein B values by use of international reference material. *Clin Chem* 1994; 40: 586–92.

72. Albers JJ, Marcovina SM, Kennedy H. International Federation of Clinical Chemistry standardization project for measurements of apolipoproteins A-I and B, II: Evaluation and selection of candidate reference materials. *Clin Chem* 1992; 38: 658–62.
73. Contois JH, McNamara JR, Lammi-Keefe CJ, Wilson PWF, Massov T, Schaefer EJ. Reference intervals for plasma apolipoprotein A-I determined with a standardized commercial immunoturbidimetric assay: results from the Framingham Offspring Study. *Clin Chem* 1996; 42: 507–14.
74. Contois JH, McNamara JR, Lammi-Keefe CJ, Wilson PWF, Massov T, Schaefer EJ. Reference intervals for plasma apolipoprotein B determined with a standardized commercial immunoturbidimetric assay: results from the Framingham Offspring Study. *Clin Chem* 1996; 42: 515–23.
75. Bachorik PS, Lovejoy KL, Carroll MD, Johnson CL. Apolipoprotein B and A-I distributions in the United States, 1988–1991: results of the National Health and Nutrition Examination Survey III (NHANES III). *Clin Chem* 1997; 43: 2364–78.
76. Jungner I, Marcovina SM, Walldius G, Holme I, Kolar W, Steiner E. Apolipoprotein B and A-I values in 147576 Swedish males and females, standardized according to the World Health Organization-International Federation of Clinical Chemistry First International Reference Materials. *Clin Chem* 1998; 44: 1641–9.
77. Miremadi S, Sniderman A, Frohlich J. Can measurement of serum apolipoprotein B replace the lipid profile monitoring of patients with lipoprotein disorders? *Clin Chem* 2002; 48: 484–8.
78. Sniderman AD, Furberg CD, Keech A, Roeters van Lennep JE, Frohlich J, Jungner I, Walldius G. Apolipoproteins versus lipids as indices of coronary risk and as targets for statin treatment. *Lancet* 2003; 361: 777–80.
79. Mahley RW, Rall SC Jr. Type III hyperlipoproteinemia (dysbetalipoproteinemia): the role of apolipoprotein E in normal and abnormal lipoprotein metabolism. In Scriver CR, Beaudet AL, Sly WS, Valle D (eds), *The Metabolic and Molecular Bases of Inherited Disease*, 7th edn. New York: McGraw-Hill, 1995; pp 1953–80.
80. Chan DC, Watts GF, Barrett PH, Mamo JC, Redgrave TG. Markers of triglyceride-rich lipoprotein remnant metabolism in visceral obesity. *Clin Chem* 2002; 48: 278–83.
81. Marcoux C, Tremblay M, Fredenrich A, Jacques H, Krimbou L, Nakajima K, Davignon J, Cohn JS. Plasma remnant-like particle lipid and apolipoprotein levels in normolipidemic and hyperlipidemic subjects. *Atherosclerosis* 1998; 139: 161–71.
82. Ooi TC, Cousins M, Ooi DS, Steiner G, Uffelman KD, Nakajima K, Simo IE. Postprandial remnant-like lipoproteins in hypertriglyceridemia. *J Clin Endocrinol Metab* 2001; 86: 3134–42.
83. Schaefer EJ, McNamara JR, Shah PK, Nakajima K, Cupples LA, Ordovas JM, Wilson PW, for the Framingham Offspring Study. Elevated remnant-like particle cholesterol and triglyceride levels in diabetic men and women in the Framingham Offspring Study. *Diabetes Care* 2002; 25: 989–94.
84. Hodis HN. Triglyceride-rich lipoprotein remnant particles and risk of atherosclerosis. *Circulation* 1999; 99: 2852–4.
85. Stein DT, Devaraj S, Balis D, Adams-Huet B, Jialal I. Effect of statin therapy on remnant lipoprotein cholesterol levels in patients with combined hyperlipidemia. *Arterioscler Thromb Vasc Biol* 2001; 21: 2026–31.
86. Karpe F, Taskinen MR, Nieminen MS, Frick MH, Kesaniemi YA, Pasternack A, Hamsten A, Syvanne M. Remnant-like lipoprotein particle cholesterol concentration and progression of coronary and vein-graft atherosclerosis in response to gemfibrozil treatment. *Atherosclerosis* 2001; 157: 181–7.
87. Jialal I, Devaraj S. Remnant lipoproteins: measurement and clinical significance. *Clin Chem* 2002; 48: 217–9.
88. Cohn JS, Marcoux C, Davignon J. Detection, quantification, and characterization of potentially atherogenic triglyceride-rich remnant lipoproteins. *Arterioscler Thromb Vasc Biol* 1999; 19: 2474–86.
89. Nakajima K, Saito T, Tamura A, Suzuki M, Nakano T, Adachi M, et al. Cholesterol in remnant-like lipoproteins in human serum using monoclonal anti apo B-100 and anti apo A-I immunoaffinity mixed gel. *Clin Chim Acta* 1993; 223: 53–71.
90. Leary ET, Wang T, Baker DJ, Cilla DD, Zhong J, Warnick GR, Nakajima K, Havel RJ. Evaluation of an immunoseparation method for quantitative measurement of remnant-like particle-cholesterol in serum and plasma. *Clin Chem* 1998; 44: 2490–8.
91. Laboratory Standardization Panel. Current status of blood cholesterol measurements in the United States: a report from the Laboratory Standardization Panel of the National Cholesterol Education Program. *Clin Chem* 1988; 34: 193–201.
92. Boerma GJM, Jansen AP, Jansen RTP, Leijnse B, van Strik R. Minimizing interlaboratory variation in routine assays of serum cholesterol through the use of serum calibrators. *Clin Chem* 1986; 32: 943–7.
93. Packard CJ, Bell MA, Eaton RH, Dagen MM, Cassidy M, Shepherd J. A pilot scheme for improving the accuracy of serum cholesterol measurement in Scotland and Northern Ireland. *Ann Clin Biochem* 1993; 30: 387–93.
94. Broughton PMG, Bullock DG, Cramb R. Quality of plasma cholesterol measurements in primary care. *Br Med J* 1989; 298: 297–8.
95. Neil HAW, Cassidy DM, Laker MF, Alberti KGMM. Within-clinic reagent strip measurement. *Diabet Med* 1989; 6: 824–8.
96. Friedlander Y, Kark JD, Stein Y. Biological and environmental sources of variation in plasma lipids and lipoproteins: the Jerusalem lipid research clinic. *Hum Hered* 1986; 36: 143–53.
97. Mogadam M, Ahmed SW, Mensch AH, Godwin ID. Within-person fluctuations of serum cholesterol and lipoproteins. *Arch Intern Med* 1990; 150: 1645–8.
98. Thompson SG, Pocock SJ. The variability of serum cholesterol measurements: implications for screening and monitoring. *J Clin Epidemiol* 1990; 43: 783–9.
99. Jones PJH, Schoeller DA. Evidence for diurnal periodicity in human cholesterol synthesis. *J Lipid Res* 1990; 31: 667–73.
100. Terpstra J, Hessel LW, Seepers J, van Gent CM. The influence of meal frequency on diurnal lipid, glucose and cortisol levels in normal subjects. *Eur J Clin Invest* 1978; 8: 61–6.

101. Robinson D, Bevan EA, Hinohara S, Takahashi T. Seasonal variation in serum cholesterol levels evidence from the UK and Japan. *Atherosclerosis* 1992; 95: 15–24.
102. Gordon DJ, Trost DC, Hyde J, Whaley FS, Hannan PJ, Jacobs DR Jr, et al. Seasonal cholesterol cycles: the Lipid Research Clinics Primary Coronary Prevention Trial Placebo Group. *Circulation* 1987; 76: 1224–31.
103. Lipid Research Clinics Program Epidemiology Committee. Plasma lipid distributions in selected North American populations: the Lipid Research Clinics Program Prevalence Study. *Circulation* 1979; 60: 427–39.
104. Heiss G, Tamir I, Davis CE, Tyroler HA, Rifkind BM, Schonfeld G, et al. Lipoprotein-cholesterol distributions in selected North American populations; the Lipid Research Clinics Program Prevalence Study. *Circulation* 1980; 61: 302–15.
105. Low-Beer TS, Wicks ACB, Heaton KW, Durrington P, Yeates J. Fluctuations of serum and bile lipid concentrations during the menstrual cycle. *Br Med J* 1977; 1: 1568–70.
106. Hemer HA, de Bourges VV, Ayala JJ, Brito G, Dýáz-Sánchez V, Garza-Flores J. Variations in serum lipids and lipoproteins throughout the menstrual cycle. *Fertil Steril* 1985; 44: 80–4.
107. Fåhraeus L, Larsson-Cohn U, Wallentin L. Plasma lipoproteins including high density lipoprotein subfractions during normal pregnancy. *Obstet Gynecol* 1985; 66: 468–72.
108. Rosing U, Samsioe G, Ölund A, Johansson B, Kallner A. Serum levels of apolipoprotein A-I, A-II and HDL-cholesterol in second half of normal pregnancy and in pregnancy complicated by pre-eclampsia. *Horm Metab Res* 1989; 21: 376–82.
109. Mann JI, Truswell AS. Effect of controlled breakfast on serum cholesterol and triglycerides. *Am J Clin Nutr* 1971; 24: 1300.
110. Grundy SM, Denke MA. Dietary influences on serum lipids and lipoproteins. *J Lipid Res* 1990; 31: 1149–72.
111. Edelstein SL, Barrett-Connor EL, Wingard DL, Cohn BA. Increased meal frequency associated with decreased cholesterol concentrations; Rancho Bernardo, CA, 1984–1987. *Am J Clin Nutr* 1992; 55: 664–9.
112. Cohn JS, McNamara JR, Cohn SD, Ordovas JM, Schaefer EJ. Postprandial plasma lipoprotein changes in human subjects of different ages. *J Lipid Res* 1988; 29: 469–79.
113. Rifai N, Merrill JR, Holly RG. Postprandial effect of a high fat meal on plasma lipid, lipoprotein cholesterol and apolipoprotein measurements. *Ann Clin Biochem* 1990; 27: 489–93.
114. Markel A, Brook JG, Aviram M. Increased plasma triglycerides, cholesterol and apolipoprotein E during prolonged fasting in normal subjects. *Postgrad Med J* 1985; 61: 395–400.
115. Pietinen P, Aro A, Tuomilehto J, Uusitalo U, Korhonen H. Consumption of boiled coffee is correlated with serum cholesterol in Finland. *Int J Epidemiol* 1990; 19: 586–90.
116. Stensvold I, Tverdal A, Foss OP. The effect of coffee on blood lipids and blood pressure. Results from a Norwegian cross-sectional study, men and women, 40–42 years. *J Clin Epidemiol* 1989; 42: 877–84.
117. Ahola I, Jauhiainen M, Aro A. The hypercholasterolaemic factor in boiled coffee is retained by a paper filter. *J Intern Med* 1991; 230: 293–7.
118. van Dusseldorp M, Katan MB, van Vliet T, Demacker PNM, Stalenhoef AFH. Cholesterol-raising factor from boiled coffee does not pass a paper filter. *Arterioscler Thromb* 1991; 11: 586–93.
119. Aro A, Teirilä J, Gref C-G. Dose-dependent effect on serum cholesterol and apoprotein B concentrations by consumption of boiled, non-filtered coffee. *Atherosclerosis* 1990; 83: 257–61.
120. Zock PL, Katan MB, Merkus MP, van Dusseldorp M, Harryvan JL. Effect of a lipid-rich fraction from boiled coffee on serum cholesterol. *Lancet* 1990; 335: 1235–7.
121. Castelli WP, Gordon T, Hjortland MC, Kagan A, Doyle JT, Hames CG, et al. Alcohol and blood lipids. *Lancet* 1977; 2: 153–5.
122. Gordon T, Ernst N, Fisher M, Rifkind BM. Alcohol and high-density lipoprotein cholesterol. *Circulation* 1981; 64 (suppl III): 63–7.
123. Veenstra J, Ockhuizen T, van de Pol H, Wedel M, Schaafsma G. Effects of a moderate dose of alcohol on blood lipids and lipoproteins postprandially and in the fasting state. *Alcohol* 1990; 25: 371–7.
124. Booth S, Clifton PM, Nestel PJ. Lack of effect of acute alcohol ingestion on plasma lipids. *Clin Chem* 1991; 37: 1649.
125. Ginsberg H, Olefsky J, Farquhar JW, Reaven GM. Moderate ethanol ingestion and plasma triglyceride levels. A study in normal and hypertriglyceridemic persons. *Ann Intern Med* 1974; 80: 143–9.
126. Wolfe BM, Havel RJ, Marliss EB, et al. Effects of a three-day fast and of ethanol on splanchnic metabolism of free fatty acids, amino acids and carbohydrates in healthy young men. *J Clin Invest* 1976; 57: 329–40.
127. Superko HR. Effects of acute and chronic alcohol consumption on postprandial lipemia in healthy normotriglyceridemic men. *Am J Cardiol* 1992; 69: 701–4.
128. Taskinen M-R, Nikkilä EA, Välimäki M, Sane T, Kuusi T, Kesäniemi YA, et al. Alcohol-induced changes in serum lipoproteins and their metabolism. *Am Heart J* 1987; 113: 458–64.
129. Wood PD, Haskell WL. The effect of exercise on plasma high density lipoproteins. *Lipids* 1979; 14: 417–27.
130. Marti B, Suter E, Riesen WF, Tschopp A, Wanner HU, Gutzwiller F. Effects of long-term, self-monitored exercise on the serum lipoprotein and apolipoprotein profile in middle-aged men. *Atherosclerosis* 1990; 81: 19–31.
131. Pay HE, Hardman AE, Jones GJ, Hudson A. The acute effects of low-intensity exercise on plasma lipids in endurance trained and untrained young adults. *Eur J Appl Physiol* 1992; 64: 182–6.
132. Krum H, Conway EL, Howes LG. Acute effects of exercise on plasma lipids, noradrenaline levels and plasma volume. *Clin Exp Pharmacol Physiol* 1991; 18: 697–701.
133. Burkman RT. Lipid and lipoprotein changes in relation to oral contraception and hormonal replacement therapy. *Fertil Steril* 1988; 49 (suppl): 39S–50S.
134. Crook D, Seed M. Endocrine control of plasma lipoprotein metabolism: effects of gonadal steroids. *Clin Endocrinol Metab* 1990; 4: 851–75.
135. Upton GV. Lipids, cardiovascular disease, and oral contraceptives: a practical perspective. *Fertil Steril* 1990; 53: 1–12.
136. Lussier-Cacan S, Xhignesse M, Desmarais J-L, Davignon J, Kafrissen ME, Chapdelaine A. Cyclic fluctuations in human serum lipid and apolipoprotein levels during the normal menstrual cycle: comparison with changes occurring during oral contraceptive therapy. *Metabolism* 1991; 40: 849–54.

137. Crook D, Cust MP, Gangar KF, Worthington M, Hillard TC, Stevenson JC, Whitehaed MI, Wynn V. Comparison of transdermal and oral estrogen–progestin replacement therapy: effects on serum lipids and lipoproteins. *Am J Obstet Gynecol* 1992; 166: 950–5.
138. Mattson LÅ, Samsioe G, von Schoultz B, Uverbrant M, Wilkund I. Transdermally administered oestradiol combined with oral medroxyprogesterone in postmenopausal women. *Br J Obstet Gynaecol* 1993; 100: 450–3.
139. Kuritzes DR, Currier J. Cardiovascular risk factors and antiretroviral therapy. *N Engl J Med* 2003; 348: 679–80.
140. Lindenmayer J-P, Czobor P, Volavka J, Citrome L, Sheitman B, McEvoy JP, Cooper TB, Chakos M, Lierberman JA. Changes in glucose and cholesterol levels in patients with schizophrenia treated with typical or atypical antipsychotics. *Am J Psychol* 2003; 160: 290–6.
141. Gaulin BD, Markowitz JS, Caley CF, Nesbitt LA, Dufresne RL. Clozapine-associated elevation in serum triglycerides. *Am J Psychol* 1999; 156: 1270–2.
142. Kahan BD, Podbielski J, Napoli, KL, Katz SM, Meier-Kriesche H-U, Van Buren CT. Immunosuppressive effects and safety of a sirolimus/cyclosporin combination regimen for renal transplantation. *Transplantation* 1998; 66: 1040–6.
143. Ahnve S, Angelin B, Edhag O, Berglund L. Early determination of serum lipids and apolipoproteins in acute myocardial infarction: possibility for immediate intervention. *J Intern Med* 1989; 226: 297–301.
144. Sewdarsen M, Vythilingum S, Jialal I, Nadar R. Plasma lipids can be reliably assessed within 24 hours after acute myocardial infarction. *Postgrad Med J* 1988; 64: 352–6.
145. Ryder REJ, Hayes TM, Mulligan IP, Kingswood JC, Williams S, Owens DR. How soon after myocardial infarction should plasma lipid values be assessed? *Br Med J* 1984; 289: 1651–3.
146. Avogaro P, Bittolo Bon G, Cazzolato G, Quinci GB, Sanson A, Sparla M, et al. Variations in apolipoproteins B and A1 during the course of myocardial infarction. *Eur J Clin Invest* 1978; 8: 121–9.
147. Fahie-Wilson M, Mills R, Wilson K. HDL cholesterol and the acute phase reaction following myocardial infarction and acute pancreatitis. *Clin Chim Acta* 1987; 167: 197–209.
148. Sammalkorpi K, Valtonen V, Kerttula Y, Nikkilä E, Taskinen M-R. Changes in serum lipoprotein pattern induced by acute infections. *Metabolism* 1988; 37: 859–65.
149. Beutler BA, Cerami A. Recombinant interleukin 1 suppresses lipoprotein lipase activity in 3T3-L1 cells. *J Immunol* 1985; 135: 3969–71.
150. Patton JS, Shepard HM, Wilking H, Lewis G, Aggarwal BB, Eessalu TE, et al. Interferons and tumor necrosis factors have similar catabolic effects on 3T3 L1 cells. *Proc Natl Acad Sci USA* 1986; 83: 8313–7.
151. Alvarez C, Ramos A. Lipids, lipoproteins and apoproteins in serum during infection. *Clin Chem* 1986; 32: 142–5.
152. Lindh A, Lindholm M, Holmquist L, Carlson LA. Time course for the changes of serum lipoproteins and apolipoprotein T concentrations after major surgical trauma in man. *J Parent Enter Nutr* 1986; 10: 265–73.
153. Coombes EJ, Shakespeare PG, Batstone GF. Lipoprotein changes after burn injury in man. *J Trauma* 1980; 20: 971–5.
154. Harris RL, Frenkel RA, Cottam GL, Baxter CR. Lipid mobilisation and metabolism after thermal trauma. *J Trauma* 1982; 22: 194–8.
155. Kritchevsky SB, Wilcosky TC, Morris DL, Truong KN, Tyroler HA. Changes in plasma lipid and lipoprotein cholesterol and weight prior to the diagnosis of cancer. *Cancer Res* 1991; 51: 3198–203.
156. Sherwin RW, Wentworth DN, Cutler JA, Hulley SB, Kuller LH, Stamler J. Serum cholesterol levels and cancer mortality in 361 662 men screened for the Multiple Risk Factor Intervention Trial. *J Am Med Assoc* 1987; 257: 943–8.
157. Gerhardsson M, Rosenqvist U, Ahlbom A, Carlson L. Serum cholesterol and cancer a retrospective casecontrol study. *Int J Epidemiol* 1986; 15: 155–9.
158. Law MR, Thompson SG. Low serum cholesterol and the risk of cancer: an analysis of the published prospective studies. *Cancer Causes Control* 1991; 2: 253–61.
159. Miller M, Bachorik PS, Cloey TA. Normal variation of plasma lipoproteins: postural effects on plasma concentrations of lipids, lipoproteins, and apolipoproteins. *Clin Chem* 1992; 38: 569–74.
160. Tan MH, Wilmshurst EG, Gleason RE, Soeldner JS. Effect of posture on serum lipids. *N Engl J Med* 1973; 289: 416–19.
161. Howes LG, Krum H, Louis WJ. Plasma cholesterol levels are dependent on sympathetic activity. *J Hypertens* 1987; 5 (suppl 5): S361–3.
162. Dixon M, Paterson CR. Posture and the composition of plasma. *Clin Chem* 1978; 24: 824–6.
163. Felding P, Tryding N, Hyltoft Petersen P, Horder M. Effects of posture on concentrations of blood constituents in healthy adults: practical application of blood specimen collection procedures recommended by the Scandinavian Committee on Reference Values. *Scand J Clin Lab Invest* 1980; 40: 615–21.
164. Eisenberg S. Postural changes in plasma volume in hypoalbuminemia. *Arch Intern Med* 1963; 112: 544–9.
165. Page IH, Moinuddin M. The effect of venous occlusion on serum cholesterol and total protein concentration a warning. *Circulation* 1962; 25: 651–2.
166. Koerselman HB, Lewis B, Pilkington TRE. The effect of venous occlusion on the level of serum cholesterol. *J Atheroscler Res* 1961; 1: 85–8.
167. Sperry WM, Schoenheimer R. A comparison of serum, heparinised plasma, and oxalated plasma in regard to cholesterol content. *J Biol Chem* 1935; 110: 655–8.
168. Grande F, Amatuzio DS, Wada S. Cholesterol measurement in serum and in plasma. *Clin Chem* 1964; 10: 619–26.
169. Alper C. Specimen collection and preservation. In Henry RJ, Cannon DC, Winkelman JW (eds), *Clinical Chemistry: Principles and Technics*. New York: Harper & Row, 1974; pp 373–88.
170. Cloey T, Bachorik PS, Becker D, Finney C, Lowry D, Sigmund W. Re-evaluation of serum–plasma differences in total cholesterol concentration. *J Am Med Assoc* 1990; 263: 2788–9.
171. Ladenson JH, Tsai L-MB, Michael JM, Kessler G, Joist JH. Serum versus heparinised plasma for eighteen common chemistry tests. Is serum the appropriate specimen? *Am J Clin Pathol* 1974; 62: 545–52.
172. Laboratory Methods Committee. Cholesterol and triglyceride concentrations in serum/plasma pairs. *Clin Chem* 1977; 23: 60–3.
173. National Cholesterol Education Program Expert Panel. Report of the National Cholesterol Education Program Expert Panel on detection, evaluation, and treatment of

high blood cholesterol in adults. *Arch Intern Med* 1988; 148: 36–69.

174. Kuchmak M, Taylor L, Olansky AS. Suitability of frozen and lyophilised reference sera for cholesterol and triglyceride determinations. *Clin Chim Acta* 1982; 120: 261–71.
175. Reckless JPD, Betteridge DJ, Wu P, Payne B, Galton DJ. Effect of storage on plasma-lipoproteins. *Lancet* 1977; 2: 350.
176. Stokes YM, Salmond CE, Carpenter LM, Welby TJ. Stability of total cholesterol, high-density-lipoprotein cholesterol, and triglycerides in frozen sera. *Clin Chem* 1986; 32: 995–9.
177. Warnick GR, Albers JJ. High-density-lipoprotein cholesterol quantitation: effect of plasma storage on heparin-Mn^{2+} supernanant cholesterol concentration. *Clin Chem* 1979; 25: 1098–9.
178. Bachorik PS, Walker R, Brownell KD, Stunkard AJ, Kwiterovich PO. Determination of high density lipoprotein-cholesterol in stored human plasma. *J Lipid Res* 1980; 21: 608–16.
179. Bachorik PS, Walker RE, Kwiterovich PO Jr. Determination of high density lipoprotein-cholesterol in human plasma stored at −70°C. *J Lipid Res* 1982; 23: 1236–42.
180. Hankinson SE, London SJ, Chute CG, Barbieri RL, Jones L, Kaplan LA, et al. Effect of transport conditions on the stability of biochemical markers in blood. *Clin Chem* 1989; 35: 2313–6.
181. del Gatto L, Nichols AV, Lindgren FT. Effects of freeze-thawing and storage on ultracentrifugal properties of human serum lipoproteins. *Proc Soc Exp Biol Med* 1959; 101: 59–61.
182. Tiedink HGM, Katan MB. Variability in lipoprotein concentrations in serum after prolonged storage at −20°C. *Clin Chim Acta* 1989; 180: 147–56.
183. Winkelman J, Wybenga DR, Ibbott FA. Phenotyping of hyperlipoproteinaemias. *Clin Chem* 1970; 16: 507–11.

This chapter is based in part on a chapter of the same title which was published in an earlier edition of the *International Textbook of Diabetes Mellitus*, by M F Laker and M W Stewart.

98

Infections, Immunity, and Diabetes

Paolo Pozzilli*† and R.D.G. Leslie†

**University Campus Bio Medico, Rome, Italy, and †St Bartholomew's Hospital, London, UK*

RATES OF INFECTION AND DIABETES

At the turn of the century many diabetic patients died of overwhelming infection. The introduction of insulin dramatically altered this situation and today noncommunicable diseases such as cardiovascular disease are the major cause of death in diabetic patients. However, infections in diabetic patients still represent an important issue.

A long-held and controversial clinical prejudice has been that infection tends to occur with greater frequency and severity in diabetic patients than in nondiabetic patients [1]. Two old studies have found that bacteriuria in adult women is more prevalent among diabetic patients [2, 3] and that this difference is associated with microangiopathic lesions including neuropathy. No similar observation has been reported in diabetic males, suggesting that the high level of infection in the urinary tract of diabetic women may be determined by microorganisms located in the vagina [3]. There is also evidence that a number of infections are uniquely associated with diabetes and that many infections are particularly life-threatening in diabetic patients [4–7] (Table 1). More recently a few studies have looked at the issue of infections and diabetes in an epidemiological fashion. Specific infections considered more prevalent in diabetic patients include both bacterial and fungal. Urinary tract infections (UTIs) are the most common bacterial infection accounting for nearly 7 million office visits and 1 million emergency department visits, resulting in 100,000 hospitalizations. The risk of UTI is increased in infants, pregnant women, the elderly, and patients with spinal cord injuries and/or catheters multiple sclerosis, HIV and also diabetes [8].

Of particular relevance is the occurrence of asymptomatic bacteriuria among diabetic women and treatment of such infections is recommended to prevent complications related to symptomatic UTIs [9].

Asymptomatic bacteriuria usually precedes overt UTIs in diabetic women. In a recent study asymptomatic bacteriuria defined by the occurrence of 100,000 or more colony forming units per milliliter was characterized by microbial growth in 40% of samples from diabetic women and 6% of samples from controls. *Eschericha coli* was the most frequently isolated strain in 55% of diabetic patients and 100% of controls. Duration of diabetes was longer among women with positive cultures than those with negative cultures; however glycosylated hemoglobin, fasting blood glucose, chronic complications of diabetes and treatment received appear not to affect microbiological results [10].

Data obtained *in vitro* (see section on Infection and Host Defense) indicate that immune function is compromised in diabetic patients. However, the risk of acquiring an infectious disease for a diabetic patient has never been quantified. Only very recently a cohort study using administrative data compared all patients with diabetes in Ontario, Canada, to matched nondiabetic subjects [11]. The risk ratio of suffering from an infectious disease or death caused by an infectious disease in diabetic and nondiabetic patients showed that risk ratio was up to 1.92 (1.79–2.05). Several infections occur more frequently in diabetes, especially severe bacterial infections. Diabetes therefore appears to increase the risk of developing an infectious disease and dying from an infectious disease, reinforcing both *in vitro* evidence and commonly held clinical belief.

An early study of 500 patients did suggest that there was an increased frequency in diabetes of skin infections, notably furunculosis, carbuncle, and erysipelas; however, the control group was inappropriate [12]. At the Dupont Company in the United States, of 622 diabetic employees followed for 1 year, 28% were absent from work for 10 days or more (because of infections and other illnesses), as

International Textbook of Diabetes Mellitus, Third Edition. Edited by R. A. DeFronzo, E. Ferrannini, H. Keen, and P. Zimmet.
 ISBN: 0-471-48655-8.

Table 1 Life-threatening infections in diabetic patients

Signs and symptoms	Causative organism	Diagnostic test	Treatment	% of diabetic patients	Mortality (%)
Otalgia Otorrhea Temporal headache	*Pseudomonas aeruginosa*	Cultures of drainage Cranial CT or MRI Bone scintigraphy WBC scintigraphy	Antipseudomonal antibiotics (carbenicillin + an aminoglycoside)	90	10–20
Lethargy Fever Headache Facial pain and swelling Nasal drainage Proptosis Black mucosal eschars	Fungi of the order Mucorales	Tissue biopsy Cranial CT or MRI	Control of hyperglycemia and acidosis Amphotericin B	75	34
Right upper quadrant colicky pain Nausea and vomiting Fever	*Clostridia* sp. or *Escherichia coli*	Culture of bile CT of abdomen US of abdomen WBC scintigraphy	Ampicillin, clindamycin, and an aminoglycoside Cholecystectomy	35	15
Fever Chills Nausea and vomiting Flank pain or tenderness	*Escherichia coli* and other Gram-negative rods	Cultures of urine and blood CT of abdomen Scintigraphy	Third-generation cephalosporin, imipenem or ciprofloxacin Nephrectomy or percutaneous drainage	90	10–37
Moderate pain Gas Seropurulent drainage Oedema Fever	Mixed aerobic–anaerobic flora	X-ray of involved area US scan WBC scintigraphy	Imipenem Extensive surgical debridement Amputation occasionally required Hyperbaric oxygen	75	20
Mild local pain Dark pus Foul odor Extensive gas	Mixed aerobic–anaerobic flora	X-ray of involved area US scan WBC scintigraphy	Imipenem Extensive surgical debridement Amputation occasionally required Hyperbaric oxygen	75	25–50
Rapid onset Severe pain Skin necrosis "Dishwater" pus No gas Mild muscle involvement	Mixed aerobic–anaerobic flora	X-ray of involved area US scan WBC scintigraphy	Imipenem Extensive surgical debridement Amputation occasionally required Hyperbaric oxygen	75	>60

compared with 15% of the control employees; this difference did not reach statistical significance [13]. An autopsy review of 307 diabetic patients aged more than 12 years and 2800 consecutive nondiabetic controls found a similar frequency of infections in both groups, with the exception of pyelonephritis and limb infections in the diabetic patients; some 2.4% of the diabetic patients had limb infections as compared with 0.5% of the controls [14].

As far as the severity of infections in the diabetic population is concerned, it is well known that chronic hyperglycemia impairs some host defense mechanisms and is associated with the increased mortality due to infection in diabetic patients (Table 1).

INFECTION AND HOST DEFENSE

Application of immunological techniques in the laboratory has facilitated early diagnosis of functional defects in the immune system. The World Health Organization (WHO) has included diabetes in its classification of secondary immunodeficiency diseases [15]. These secondary immunodeficiencies, unlike primary immunodeficiencies, can be resolved if their underlying cause (e.g. a tumor or steroid treatment) is eliminated.

The immune system is a system designed to fight infections while maintaining homeostasis, thus avoiding chronic inflammatory processes and autoimmune disease. It comprises two arms, one recognizing molecular patterns and the other recognizing variable molecular details. These two components of the immune system are called innate and adaptive, respectively [16, 17].

An immediate immune response is normally generated by the innate immune system in response to invading environmental signals. The less rapid adaptive immune response follows the innate response as it did in the evolutionary terms.

The innate and adaptive immune systems differ both in their mode of immune recognition of triggering factors and in their ability to respond to further signals. The adaptive response is generated in such a way as to retain memory, the basis for vaccine design. The innate response on the other hand does not have the ability to remember a previous challenge and therefore does not possess immune memory. The adaptive response employs T and B cells which, via their respective T- and B-cell receptors, recognize potentially dangerous molecules. The way these receptors are somatically generated provides each cell with a structurally unique receptor, thereby conferring the ability to memorize previous challenges. This system of receptor formation allows these cells to generate a very diverse response to different fragments of different pathogens, presented to T cells in the context of the HLA complex. By selecting the best response from the repertoire the system can adapt dynamically to the environmental signal. In this way the adaptive component of the immune system generates an efficient immune response after some 3–5 days, and more rapidly once immunological memory has been established. In contrast, the innate response is more rapid, even at the first challenge, but lacks flexibility and therefore the possibility to memorize antigenic challenge and also to adapt to new challenges. The innate response focuses on a few highly conserved structures normally shared with large groups of microorganisms [18]. (Since these structures are called pathogen-associated molecular patterns it follows that the receptors of the innate system are called pattern-recognition receptors.) There is a close relationship between innate and adaptive immunity, and changes in the former could provoke inappropriate responses in the latter. Since changes in innate immunity have been reported in type 1 diabetes, it is possible that these changes predispose not only to the disease but also to infections. For example, an innate effector, the CD1d-restricted NK-T cells, is present in reduced numbers and shows reduced production of IL-4 among other cytokines in type 1 diabetes in humans as well as in the nonobese diabetic (NOD) mouse [19]. In support of this hypothesis a stimulant of NKT cells decreases the incidence and rate of progression to diabetes in the NOD mouse [20].

Both BB rats and patients with type 1 diabetes may also have an innate abnormality of dendritic cells [21, 22]. There is no evidence that the immune response to infections is altered in subjects at risk of type 1 or type 2 diabetes. The evidence supports the concept that hyperglycemia *per se* or the metabolic abnormality of diabetes is sufficient to explain the impaired immune response in patients responding to infections [23].

Polymorphonuclear Cells

Polymorphonuclear (PMN) granulocytes represent the host's first defense barrier against bacterial agents. In diabetic patients these cells show functional alterations in chemotaxy and under some circumstances also in phagocytosis [23, 24]. A recent study showed that glycoxidation of two major extracellular-matrix collagens considerably altered their ability to modulate PMN migration and to produce reactive oxygen species. This imbalance in PMN metabolism may be a major event in the increased oxidative status that characterizes diabetes [25]. Moreover, accumulation of advanced glycation end products (AGEs) in the tissue and serum of subjects with diabetes could alter PMN function since AGE albumin enhances neutrophil phagocytosis of *Staphyloccal aureus* and inhibits bacterial killing [26].

Chemotaxy

This process involves the migration of white blood cells. PMN cells are attracted to the site of infection by various chemotactic substances secreted by microorganisms. In addition, complement activation and factors induced locally by PMN cells also play a role in this chemotactic process. The energy required for this process is supplied by anaerobic glycolysis and by the hexose monophosphate shunt.

Cells from diabetic patients have a reduced chemotaxy, especially when the diabetes is poorly controlled [23]. Monocytes in diabetic patients show a decreased cellular response to a chemokine, vascular endothelial growth factor α, because of a downstream signal transduction defect [27].

Phagocytosis

There are two phases of phagocytosis: (1) adhesion; (2) ingestion of foreign particles (e.g. microorganisms) into intracytoplasmic vacuoles. These processes are triggered by an intricate series of synergistic mechanisms involving the interaction of actin, myosin, and actin-linking proteins, expression of IgG Fc fragment receptor on cell membrane, and activation of a C3B complement component. Other mechanisms may also be involved (e.g. the link between lectin receptors and glycidic residues on target cell membranes). The energy required for this process is supplied by ATP produced during anaerobic glycolysis. Phagocytosis may be impaired in patients with long-standing diabetes [24, 28], and there is evidence for PMN functional impairment [29, 30]. This latter disturbance is correlated with an intrinsic defect in PMN rather than with a disturbance due to metabolic alterations. It has been suggested that an increase in sialidase enzyme secretion, together with a corresponding reduction in cell membrane sialic acid, may account for such a defect [31]. Other authors have suggested that defective lectin receptors, when saturated by high levels of glucose, lose their capacity to recognize the target and, as a result, fail to initiate phagocytosis [24]. In general terms, the metabolic disturbances associated with diabetes are probably important in impairing the function of immune effector cells.

Killing Activity

Once phagosome and lysosome fusion has taken place, killing is carried out by lysosomal enzymes. This process is dependent on integration of oxidative (primary phase) and nonoxidative metabolism. Killing activity is usually measured by two methods: (1) evaluating the capacity of phagocytes to interact with nitroblue tetrazolium dye, a yellow compound that turns blue during cytotoxic metabolic events; (2) measurement of PMN capacity to emit electromagnetic radiation following phagocytosis, a process known as chemiluminescence. Both tests show a decrease in the killing activity of PMN granulocytes associated with high blood glucose; its normalization following intensive insulin therapy augments killing activity within 48 h [32]. It has been suggested that the production of sorbitol in diabetes may also impair oxidative killing processes [33].

Lymphocyte Subpopulations and Their Function

Type 1 (insulin-dependent) diabetes is associated with alterations in some lymphocyte subpopulations. Several studies have reported a reduction in the total number of T lymphocytes, and more specifically in the number of CD4 phenotype ("helper") T lymphocytes, causing a subsequent reduction in the CD4/CD8 ratio [34–36]. This defect could be due to either decreased insulin levels or decreased insulin activity or both [37]. However, optimization of metabolic control is accompanied by normal lymphocyte transformation and normalization of the levels of T lymphocyte subpopulations [38]. In patients with good metabolic control, who have been exposed to different antigenic stimuli such as tuberculosis, tetanus, and diphtheria, and to species of *Trichophyton, Streptococcus, Proteus*, or *Candida*, there is a prompt secondary immune response, suggesting normal co-operational function between T memory cells and CD4-positive lymphocytes [39].

When diabetic patients are given an anti-influenza vaccine their antibody response is similar to that of normal subjects [40]. However, some components of the influenza vaccine may already have been processed by the host's immune system, and so the normal response is consistent with a normal secondary immune response. Hepatitis B vaccine, on the other hand, is only administered to subjects who have never encountered the viral antigen. In almost half of long-standing type 1 diabetic patients the antibody response to hepatitis B vaccine is poor, that is less than the titer proposed by WHO to ensure a sufficient level of protection [41]. Thus, reduced primary humoral and cellular immune responses (as for hepatitis B) can be attributed, in part, to defective antigen recognition. This defect may be due to insufficient macrophage recognition of antigen. On the other hand, changes in the secondary immune responses (such as activation of memory T cells following administration of the anti-influenza virus) probably depend on the metabolic state.

Immunoglobulins

Serum immunoglobulin levels (IgG and IgA) have been reported to be reduced in diabetic patients compared to normal subjects [42, 43]. However, the antibody response, in the diabetic population, for example to pneumococcal polysaccharide, is normal [44]. Appropriate controls have been a problem in these studies. Suitable matching was performed in one study in which a large number of nondiabetic individuals were also examined as part of a viral surveillance project during an outbreak of coxsackievirus infection (types B3, B4, and B5) [45]; antibody titers to coxsackie B3 and B4 were lower in diabetic than nondiabetic subjects and a low antibody titer was associated with an increased risk of diabetes.

Complement

It is only recently that attention has been paid to the possibility that a significant reduction in the quantity and functional activity of complement components may occur in diabetic patients. Low C4 levels, often associated with the possession of the C4A null gene, are present in approximately 25% of patients with type 1 diabetes [46] and abnormalities of other components, e.g. C1q and C3, have also been documented [47].

LOCAL FACTORS AND TARGET TISSUES

A number of factors make certain tissues in diabetic patients particularly prone to infections. The four most important elements are an underlying susceptibility to infection, vascular disease, nerve damage, and hyperglycemia. Hyperglycemia may predispose the diabetic patient to bacterial and fungal infections. Neuropathy can (1) alter pressure distributions contributing to ulceration and, as a result, infection of the feet [48]; and (2) lead to autonomic involvement of the bladder with urine retention, which predisposes to bacteriuria [48]. Vascular insufficiency and tissue hypoxia allow the growth of anaerobic organisms and limit host defense mechanisms.

The complex deterioration of both large and small blood vessels in diabetes can result in reduced peripheral circulation, relative hypoxia, and, as a result, a predisposition to proliferation of anaerobic bacteria [49]. Furthermore, hypoxia can modify the oxygen-dependent function of PMN granulocytes [33]. Finally, reduction in antibiotic absorption in diabetic patients with microangiopathy might lead to persistence of infections.

Peripheral and autonomic neuropathy are associated with infections of cutaneous tissues and ulcers [48]. Peripheral neuropathy reduces sensitivity to stimuli such as heat and pain, with loss of muscle tone. The resulting deformation of the foot with redistribution of normal pressure points predisposes to ulceration, and infection may then ensue [48].

Acute pyelonephritis may be more severe and more difficult to treat in diabetic patients, probably because of lesions in the microvascular system, which induce a reduction in renal blood flow. Such a reduction in blood flow and an increase in the frequency of bacterial infection are the principal causes of papillary necrosis. Fever, loin pain, hematuria, and deteriorating renal function characterize papillary necrosis. Sloughed papillary tissue can be found in the urine. The most frequent infective agent causing papillary necrosis is a Gram-negative bacillus. Cortical and perirenal cysts are more frequent in diabetic patients than in the normal population and 25% of all cases are caused by staphylococcal septicaemia [50].

Periodontal disease is related to diabetes. Patients with diabetes of long duration, with diabetic complications and with hyperglycemia, are particularly prone to this complication. Oral candidiasis is more prevalent in diabetic than nondiabetic patients, especially in those with dentures; diabetic patients who have dentures tend to grow a higher density of *Candida* than diabetic patients who do not have dentures [51].

Soft tissues and the skin are frequent targets of infection in patients with long-standing diabetes. Localized sepsis can arise from injections of insulin, although this is a surprisingly rare complication and the evidence is that routine hygiene without a local antiseptic is sufficient to limit its frequency. Abscess formation has also been reported at the infusion site for continuous subcutaneous insulin administration [52]. Even finger pricks to obtain blood for self-monitoring of blood glucose can be associated with soft tissue infections, sometimes complicated by underlying osteomyelitis [53].

Chronic foot ulcers result from a combination of peripheral and autonomic neuropathy and peripheral vascular disease. Bacteriological investigation is critical in the management of these patients if the ulcer becomes infected. Reliable bacteriological specimens without contamination are difficult to obtain and in one study at least 70% of the samples were deemed unreliable [49]. A striking observation is that those "reliable specimens" were significantly more likely to yield a single bacterial species. Mixed cultures containing five or more species are common in clinical practice. Corynebacteria and *Bacteroides* are particularly associated with necrotizing lesions. Prevention of problems by rigorous foot care is essential to limit the risk of ulceration [54]. When an ulcer has developed and become infected, then conservative management with antibiotics but without amputation is the initial target. Even in the presence of osteomyelitis, antibiotic therapy can be successful without the need for surgical intervention [55].

Soft tissue infections of an unusually aggressive nature can occur in patients with diabetes. Necrotizing fasciitis is a potentially lethal infection of superficial fascia [56] (Table 1). Minor surgical trauma, even an intramuscular injection, may precede the condition. The onset is rapid and the patient, often an elderly diabetic, develops toxic complications. The skin is smooth, red, and edematous. Subcutaneous gas may sometimes be detected. Multiple organisms appear to be responsible for the condition, although facultative streptococci are the prevalent organisms. The mortality rate in elderly diabetic patients has been reported to be as high as 80% [57]. Fournier's gangrene is also characterized by a subcutaneous infection although, in this case, of the penis, scrotum, and sometimes the abdominal wall [57]. It is also caused by a mixture of aerobic and anaerobic organisms. In both Fournier's gangrene and necrotizing fasciitis, treatment requires aggressive surgical debridement and antibiotic therapy. The potential for both aerobic and anaerobic organisms to be involved should direct the antibiotic policy.

RISK OF SPECIFIC INFECTIONS

Bacterial Infections

Staphylococcal Infections

There is not clear evidence that diabetic patients are more prone to staphylococcal infections than control subjects. In one study there was an increase in the nasal carriage of *Staphylococcus aureus* in diabetic children (76%) compared with controls (44%), and in insulin-treated adults (53%) compared with non-insulin-treated diabetic subjects (35%) and controls (34%) [58]. Other studies found no such association [59]. Patients with well-controlled diabetes do not have an increased risk of infection postoperatively. Of 8952 surgical procedures a postoperative staphylococcal infection was noted in only 143 (1.6%) and was not associated with diabetes or other chronic illnesses [60]. Older diabetic patients are at increased risk of significant bacteremia. There was an excess of diabetic patients aged 40 years or more in a study of 319 patients of whom

14 had staphylococcal bacteremia [61]. The mortality in patients with staphylococcal bacteremia and diabetes is higher than in those without this disease; the mortality rate in one study was 69% in the diabetic patients and 42% overall (diabetic and nondiabetic patients) [50].

Tuberculosis

While *Mycobacterium tuberculosis* used to be a major cause of mortality in diabetic patients, this is no longer the case in developed countries. There does not appear to be any increased prevalence of tuberculosis in diabetic patients in such countries. The rates of active disease have been found to be higher in those patients who take high insulin doses as compared with those who take less or no insulin. There is a suggestion that recrudescence of tuberculosis may account for the increased infection rate in diabetic patients in developing countries. There is, however, also evidence for an increased rate of both tuberculosis in diabetic patients and new diabetes in tuberculosis patients in Africa [62].

Erythrasma

This condition is due to a bacterial skin infection caused by *Corynebacterium minutissimum*. It appears in intertriginous areas, especially in obese patients [63]. It is therefore most prevalent in patients with type 2 diabetes. The bacteria produce a porphyrin that fluoresces red under a Wood's lamp. Those factors that enhance the growth of the organism include humidity, heat, obesity, poor hygiene, and debilitating illness such as alcoholism. The infection can spread to involve the trunk. It is responsive to erythromycin treatment and, if necessary, to imidazole derivatives [64].

Malignant External Otitis

The condition malignant external otitis (MEO) typically affects elderly diabetic patients and is caused by a chronic infection of the external auditory meatus due to *Pseudomonas aeruginosa*. The average age of patients is around 70 years, although any age may be affected; patients are usually insulin treated [65]. *Pseudomonas* is not normally found in the auditory meatus of normal subjects but is an invariant feature of MEO; bilateral disease is prevalent. The infection, left untreated, may extend to involve the temporal bone and, thereafter, the infection can spread to the base of the skull. A VIIth cranial nerve palsy is the most frequent herald of this malignant stage of the disease process. Some 50% of patients with MEO and cranial nerve pulsing die, and in those who survive permanent disability is common. The overall mortality of MEO is about 20%. The patient usually complains of pain and a purulent discharge, which has failed to respond to conventional treatment. Therapy consists of surgical debridement and a combination of carbenicillin with an aminoglycoside continued for up to 6 weeks and at least 1 week after negative cultures so as to ensure no recurrence.

Periodontal Disease

Periodontitis is twice as prevalent in diabetic individuals compared to nondiabetic individuals. In most industrialized countries approximately 15% of the population has enhanced risk for moderate to severe periodontitis. The disease is caused by infection by anaerobic Gram-negative bacteria, including *Porphyromonas gingivalis* and *Bacteroides forsythus*. There is evidence that *P. gingivalis* is a key pathogen. Once established in the diabetic host, this chronic infection complicates diabetes control and increases the occurrence and severity of microvascular and macrovascular complications. Mechanical removal of subgingival infection does not result in complete elimination of periodontal infection, though the evidence supports the notion that treatment of chronic periodontal infection in the diabetic patient is worthwhile [66]. Even though periodontitis in humans and in this animal model is a polymicrobial disease, immunization with a vaccine containing a single bacterial species, *P. gingivalis*, induced protection. Of all the *P. gingivalis* components that have been studied, the cysteine proteases have the greatest potential as vaccine antigens. In a pilot study using the same protocol, it has been shown that porphypain-2 purified from *P. gingivalis* is effective in inducing protection. In light of the increasing evidence that periodontitis significantly increases risk for potentially fatal diseases such as coronary heart disease, stroke, and complications from diabetes mellitus, a successful vaccine for periodontitis could have health benefits far exceeding the prevention of periodontitis [67].

Nonclostridial Gas Gangrene

This condition is the most common cause of gas gangrene in the diabetic patient. Of 49 cases of gas gangrene among 278 diabetic patients, only 1 had *Clostridium perfringens* infection and the remainder had a nonclostridial infection [68]. Usual organisms are a mixture of anaerobes including *Bacteroides* and anaerobic streptococci. The gas production is probably due to bacterial fermentation of high glucose levels in the tissues. Mortality is low with early diagnosis and aggressive antibiotic management, although most patients will lose part of a limb [68].

Fungal Infections

Candida *Infections*

Infection with *Candida albicans* is believed to be more prevalent in diabetic patients than in normal subjects. In one study of 100 diabetic and 100 control subjects, only

Candida was detected more frequently in diabetic patients (31% vs. 5%); other fungi including *Trichophyton* and *Epidermophyton* were not more prevalent in diabetic patients [69]. The infection can involve the vulva, penis, mouth, skin, and nails. Disseminated candidiasis is rare but occurs predominantly in patients with diabetes, liver, or renal disease. The explanation for this increased susceptibility to *Candida* remains unclear. A serum β-globulin anticandidal factor, detectable in most normal individuals, is decreased in patients with disseminated candidiasis. *C. albicans* is particularly prevalent in patients with high blood glucose levels. Glucose appears to promote the growth of this organism. In one study 77% of 160 diabetic girls had positive cultures for *C. albicans* from the vulva [70]. Chronic oral candidiasis was, however, only found in 3 of 350 diabetic patients [51]. It should be noted that up to 60% of normal healthy people may have oral *Candida* on culture; it is the density of the culture that is increased in diabetic patients and particularly in those who wear dentures. Chronic paronychia due to *Candida* has been detected in 10% of young diabetic girls as compared with just 3% of normal subjects [71]. Treatment of infection with *Candida* requires good control of blood glucose levels and then topical therapy with an imidazole. Therapy given at high blood glucose levels tends to be ineffective.

Rhinocerebral Mucormycosis

Mucormycosis relates to a group of fulminant infections caused by fungi of the class Phycomycetes. The four genera that affect humans are *Absidia*, *Mortierella*, *Mucor*, and *Rhizopus*. Infection with these organisms is rare as there is a strong natural immunity. The increased risk in diabetic patients is evident only in those patients who are debilitated, for example patients with ketoacidosis. About 75% of patients with mucormycosis have diabetes [72]. In such patients the natural inhibitory activity in serum against *Rhizopus*, and perhaps other Phycomycetes, is lost but can return following insulin treatment. The natural course of the condition can be chronic but is often rapid. The debilitated patient presents with fever, malaise, and headaches. The infection spreads from the nasal mucosa to involve the sinuses. Subsequently, the orbit and ocular nerves become infected. Invasion of arteries leads to thrombosis and if the internal carotid is infected, cerebral ischemia and death. Current survival rates are as low as 66%. Treatment involves control of the diabetes and aggressive surgery and antifungal therapy, often with systemic amphotericin B [73].

Onychomycosis

The prevalence of onychomycosis was assessed in India in 100 diabetic patients. Onychomycosis was more common in diabetic patients than in control groups (17% vs. 6.8%, respectively). Predisposing factors included increasing age, male gender, duration of diabetes, impaired peripheral circulation, peripheral neuropathy, and retinopathy [74].

PRINCIPLES OF TREATMENT AND PREVENTION

Prevention of infections in diabetic patients is directed toward predisposing factors, using a multidisciplinary approach [75]. First, there is the question of primary prevention, notably against influenza and pneumococcal infections. Second, the cause of diabetes may be relevant. Third, the degree of hyperglycemia influences disease outcome. Finally, infection in a diabetic patient may be complicated by a suboptimal immune response, by reduced vascular response, and by the presence of neurological and vascular disease.

Since influenza vaccines do not control epidemics they are only recommended for subjects at high risk should they develop severe influenza. Annual anti-influenza vaccination of diabetic patients has been recommended in Europe, particularly for those patients with long-standing diabetes. A polyvalent unconjugated pneumococcal polysaccharide vaccine is also used for the immunization of selected individuals over the age of 2 years. These subjects include patients with diabetes and are thought to be at high risk were they to develop pneumococcal pneumonia. The vaccine is effective in a single dose if the infection in the community is reflected in the polysaccharides contained in the vaccine. Revaccination is not recommended until after 5 years and then only in patients in whom the antibody response declines rapidly, such as those with aplenia [76].

The type of diabetes may influence the risk of infections. Alternatively, infections may influence the type of diabetes. It is important to establish the type of diabetes in order to assess the appropriate therapy. For example, transient diabetes can be found in infants with severe gastroenteritis. Another example is the development of diabetes secondary to therapy for HIV infection. Recently, combination therapy including HIV-1 protease inhibitors has dramatically improved the long-term survival of HIV-infected patients. However, such therapy is associated with a lipodystrophy syndrome characterized by selective loss of fat from the face and extremities and, in some patients, accumulation of fat around the neck, dorsocervical region, abdomen, and trunk. Lipodystrophy in HIV-infected patients (LDHIV) is associated with insulin resistance and its metabolic complications such as impaired glucose tolerance, diabetes, hypertriglyceridemia, and low serum high density lipoprotein cholesterol levels. The molecular basis of LDHIV remains unknown. There is no specific therapy for LDHIV. Avoiding weight gain by reducing energy intake and increasing physical activity may be beneficial in reducing fat accumulation as well as improving metabolic complications. Antihyperglycemic drugs may be used to treat diabetes. Substitution of protease inhibitors with other antiretroviral drugs can mitigate dyslipidemia and glucose intolerance [77].

Hyperglycemia should be corrected and metabolic control should be maintained as close to normal as possible. Diabetes Control and Complications Trial confirmed that maintaining near-normal blood glucose and glycosylated hemoglobin levels significantly reduces the risk of progression of diabetic complications [78]. These complications, including neuropathy and macrovascular disease, may predispose to infection as well as to the spread of infection. The maintenance of good metabolic control is of paramount importance for the limitation of established infections. This aspect has been discussed earlier and leads to more aggressive therapy both of the infections as well as of blood glucose control in infected diabetic subjects.

Having established the nature and severity of the infection, and performed investigations, a treatment plan should be drawn up. Early and aggressive treatment is important [79]. Surgical consultation should establish the degree of vascular impairment, if relevant, and the necessity for, and degree of, surgical intervention. If present, necrotic tissue will require surgical debridement. Deep space infection may require open drainage. In the case of limb infections, amputation may have to be considered. In order to promote skin healing after drainage, skin grafting and revascularization of a limb may be required. It is necessary, initially, to decide upon an empirical broad-spectrum antibiotic therapy, although laboratory results may subsequently necessitate revision. It is likely that antibiotic cover will be appropriate, even if laboratory samples are inadequate, albeit with the added possibility of unnecessary and potentially toxic therapy due to the presence of contaminating organisms, e.g. aminoglycoside therapy for aerobic Gram-negative bacteria.

In view of the preponderance of staphylococci and streptococci in infected foot ulcers, either a penicillin–cloxacillin combination or alternatively a cephalosporin (e.g. cefotaxime, cefuroxime) or a parenteral quinolone (e.g. ofloxacin) would be appropriate. Evidence suggesting an anaerobic infection would necessitate the use of metronidazole. Clindamycin might well be given as a suitable alternative, with the added benefit of activity against some aerobes. Aerobic Gram-negative bacteria, excluding *Pseudomonas aeruginosa*, are likely to be sensitive to cefotaxime and cefuroxime (or a similar cephalosporin) and/or to an aminoglycoside or a parenteral quinolone. Vancomycin may be necessary for penicillin-resistant streptococci, while fusidic acid would be suitable as additional antistaphylococcal therapy because of its particularly good tissue (including bone) penetration. Ciprofloxacin and oflaxacin have good activity against most aerobic pathogens but not against anaerobes, and imipenem has broad-spectrum activity but includes anaerobes. In more serious infections, and when surgery is necessary, inpatient management is obligatory, and antibiotics will be administered parenterally. However, in less severe cases, when there is no evidence of bone involvement and the patient is compliant, oral antibiotic therapy can be given on an outpatient basis with satisfactory results [80].

Conservative management without amputation is the cornerstone of management of infected foot ulcers. Distal lesions treated conservatively take about 10 weeks to heal, which contrasts with 13 weeks for more proximal lesions treated operatively [81]. However, some ulcers may fail to heal until many weeks later. Kaufman et al. [81] achieved limb salvage in 96% of distal lesions compared to only 48% in the proximal group; 12% required revascularization in order to achieve healing. Even in the presence of osteomyelitis, antibiotic therapy may be successful without surgical ablation [55].

Patients who develop foot ulcers are at risk of septic complications. Therefore, it is important to educate patients about the importance of rigorous foot care. In the experience of one large specialized foot clinic, preventive measures led to a significant improvement in wound healing and reduced the incidence of foot amputations [54]. Such an approach should improve the prognosis of this major complication.

The situation may be totally different in poor countries where access to care is limited. Foot and hand sepsis in adult diabetic patients in Africa is associated with significant morbidity and mortality. The pathogenesis of diabetic foot infections in these populations appears to be similar to that for patients in industrialized countries, ulcers and underlying peripheral neuropathy being the most important risk factors. Hence, preventive efforts for both foot and hand sepsis should include aggressive glucose control, and education regarding hand and foot care and the importance of seeking medical attention promptly at the earliest onset of symptoms [82].

Because of the high risk of infection in diabetic patients, it is recommended that special attention is paid to them especially for management of bacterial UTIs [83]. The need for treatment of asymptomatic bacteriuria remains controversial. No evidence is available on the optimal treatment of acute cystitis and pyelonephritis in patients with diabetes. Because of the frequent (asymptomatic) upper tract involvement and the possible serious complications, many experts recommend a 7- to 14-day oral antibacterial cystitis in these patients, with an antibacterial agent that achieves high concentrations both in the urine and in the urinary tract issues. The recommended treatment of acute pyelonphritis does not differ from that in patients without diabetes. Clinical trials specifically dealing with the treatment of UTIs in patients with diabetes comparing the optimal duration and choice of antibacterial agent are needed. In addition, new approaches to preventive strategies must prove their value in this specific patient group.

There is a greater likelihood UTIs affected by antimicrobial resistance or atypical uropathogens, and the risk of upper tract involvement is increased [84]. Pre- and posttherapy urine cultures are therefore indicated. The initial choice of empiric antimicrobial therapy should be based on Gram stain and urine culture. Choice of antibiotic therapy should integrate local sensitivity patterns of the infecting organism. Fluoroquinolones are a reasonable empiric choice for many patients with diabetes. For seriously ill patients, including patients infected with *Pseudomonas*, such agents as imipenem, ticarcillin-clavulanate, and piperacillin-tazobactam may also be considered. Treatment of asymptomatic bacteriuria in patients with diabetes is often recommended to prevent the risk of symptomatic UTIs.

HYPERBARIC OXYGEN

When the infection is severe, in particular when it affects the lower limb, additional therapies may be considered. Hyperbaric oxygen (HBO) treatment may have a role in selected cases. Several years ago, HBO therapy began to be used in the treatment of diabetic foot ulcers on the assumption that the force of oxygen diffusing through poorly perfused tissue would correct the hypoxia and acidosis.

The potential benefits of HBO therapy in diabetic patients with a foot ulcer is related to the role of oxygen in the physiology of wound healing. HBO can raise tissue oxygen tensions to levels where wound healing can be expected. HBO also increases the killing ability of leukocytes, is lethal for certain anaerobic bacteria, and inhibits toxin formation in other anaerobes [85]. Multiple anecdotal reports and retrospective studies in HBO therapy in diabetic patients suggest that HBO can be an effective adjunct in the management of diabetic wounds. Prospective studies also show the beneficial effects of HBO. However, in the only controlled trial of HBO no beneficial effects were observed [87]. Because most published studies suffer from methodological problems, there is an urgent need for a collaborative, international, randomized prospective clinical trial for the application of HBO in diabetic foot lesions, as part of a multidisciplinary treatment approach, before we can recommend HBO as standard therapy in patients with foot ulcers [86]. Access to HBO machines remains a major limitation.

CONCLUSION

Several points arise from the observations outlined in this review. It is now apparent that some clinical infections are indeed more prevalent in diabetic patients than in the general population. Recent studies have highlighted an underlying alteration in the innate immune system in patients with type 1 diabetes, which may predispose not only to diabetes but also to certain infections. Hyperglycemia, a characteristic of all types of diabetes, also impairs immune responses. In the event of an infection in a patient with diabetes the management policy differs from that for nondiabetic patients, in that there should be a high index of suspicion for certain types of infection, earlier introduction of antibiotic therapy, and a more aggressive and, in some cases, more prolonged use of antibiotics. Infections remain an important cause of morbidity in diabetes especially in developing countries. Awareness of those issues outlined here need to be considered both by doctors involved in caring for these patients and by the authorities responsible for calculating the costs of diabetes care.

REFERENCES

1. Smitherman KO, Peacock JE. Infectious emergencies in patients with diabetes mellitus. *Med Clin North Am* 1995; 79: 53–77.
2. Wheat LJ. Infection and diabetes mellitus. *Diabetes Care* 1980; 3: 187–97.
3. Vejilsgaard R. Studies on urinary infection in diabetes. Bacteria in patients with diabetes mellitus and in control subjects. *Acta Med Scand* 1966; 179: 173–8.
4. Bebrod L. Infections in the diabetic patients. *Clin Diabetes* 1985; 3: 98–105.
5. Berdade JD, Segreti J. The infectious emergencies of diabetes. *Endocrinologist* 1991; 1: 155–61.
6. Leslie CA, Sapico FL, Bessman AN. Infections in the diabetic host. *Compr Ther* 1989; 15: 23–32.
7. Sapico FL, Bessman AN. Infections in the diabetic patient. *Infect Dis Clin Pract* 1992; 1: 339–43.
8. Foxman B. Epidemiology of urinary tract infections: incidence, morbidity, and economic costs. *Dis Mon* 2003; 49: 53–70.
9. Harding GK, Zhanel GG, Nicolle LE, Cheang M. Antimicrobial treatment in diabetic women with asymptomatic bacteriuria. *N Engl J Med* 2002; 347: 1576–83.
10. Mendoza T, Garzia de los, Rios M, Lafourcade M, Soto C, Durruty P, Alvo M. Asymptomatic bacteriuria in type 2 diabetics women. *Rev Med Chil* 2002; 130: 1001–7.
11. Shah BR, Hux JE. Quantifying the risk of infectious diseases for people with diabetes. *Diabetes Care* 2003; 26: 510–3.
12. Greenwood AM. A study of the skin in five hundred cases of diabetes. *JAMA* 1927; 89: 774–80.
13. Pell S, D'Alonzo CA. Sickness absenteeism in employed diabetics. *Am J Public Health* 1967; 57: 253–8.
14. Robbins SL, Tucker AW Jr. The causes of death in diabetics. A report of 307 autopsied cases. *New Engl J Med* 1944; 231: 865–9.
15. World Health Organization. *Immunodeficiency: Report of a Scientific Group*. Technical Report Series 630. Geneva: World Health Organization, 1978.
16. Janeway CA. How the immune system works to protect the host from infection: a personal view. *PNAS* 2001; 98: 7461–8.
17. Shi FD, Wong HB, Li H, Hong S, Taniguchi M, Link H, Van Kaer L, Ljunggren HG. Natural killer cells determine the

outcome of B cell-mediated autoimmunity. *Nat Immunol* 2000; 1: 245–51.
18. Mackay I, Rosen FS. Innate immunity. *New Engl J Med* 2000; 343 (5): 338–43.
19. Wilson SB, Kent SC, Patton KT, et al. Extreme Th1 bias of invariant Valpha24JalphaQ T cells in type 1 diabetes. *Nature* 1998; 391: 177–81.
20. Sharif S, Arreaza GA, Zucker P, et al. Activation of natural killer cells by a-galactosylcermide treatment prevents the onset and recurrence of autoimmune type 1 diabetes. *Nat Med* 2001; 9: 1057–61.
21. Tafuri A, Bowers WE, Handler ES, et al. High stimulatory activity of dendritic cells from diabetes-prone BB/Worcester rats exposed to macrophage-derived factors. *J Clin Invest* 1993; 91: 2040–8.
22. Jansen A, Van Hagen M, Drehxhage HA, et al. Defective maturation and function of antigen-presenting cells in type 1 diabetes. *Lancet* 1995; 345: 491–2.
23. Moutschen MP, Scheen AJ, Lefebvre PJ. Impaired immune responses in diabetes mellitus: analysis of the factors involved. Relevance to the increased susceptibility of diabetic patients to specific infections. *Diabète Métab* 1992; 18: 187–201.
24. Wilson RM, Reeves WG. Neutrophil function in diabetes. In Nattrass M (ed). *Recent Advances in Type 2 Diabetes*. London: *Churchill Livingstone* 1986; pp 127–38.
25. Monboisse JC, Rittie L, Lamfarraj H, Garnotel R, Gillery P. *in vitro* glycoxidation alters the interactions between collagen and human polymorphonuclear leucocytes. *Biochem J* 2000; 3: 777–83.
26. Collison KS, Parhar RS, Saleh SS, Meyer BF, Kwaasi AA, Hammam MM, Schmidt AM, Stern DM, Al-Mohanna FA. RAGE-mediated neutrophil dysfunction is evoked by advanced glycation end products (AGEs). *J Leukoc Biol* March 2002; 71: 433–44.
27. Walenberger J, Lange J, Kranz A. Vascular endothelial growth factor-A-induced chemotaxis of monocytes is attenuated in patients with diabetes mellitus: a potential predictor for the individual capacity to develop collaterals. *Circulation* July 11, 2000; 102: 185–90.
28. Simmons D, Leong LNG, Bomford J. Abnormal myoinositol influx in human leukocytes in diabetes but not specifically in diabetic neuropathy. *Diabetes* 1992; 41: 760–65.
29. Wykretowicz A, Wierusz-Wysocka B. Infection and diabetes: role of polymorphonuclear neutrophils. In Pozzilli P, Signore A (eds). *Diabetes Prevention and Therapy, Vol. 6*. Chichester, UK: Wiley, 1992; p 27.
30. Sawant JM. Biochemical changes in polymorphonuclear leukocytes in diabetic patients. *J Postgrad Med* 1993; 39: 183–6.
31. Chiari SN, Nath N. Sialic acid content and sialidase activity of polymorphonuclear leukocytes in diabetes mellitus. *Am J Sci* 1984; 288: 1–5.
32. Gin H, Brottier E, Aubertin J. Influence of glycaemic normalization by an artifical pancreas on phagocytic and bacterial functions of granulocytes in insulin-dependent diabetic patients. *J Clin Pathol* 1984; 37: 1029–31.
33. Wilson RM, Tomlinson RA, Reeves WG. Neutrophil sorbitol production impairs oxidative killing in diabetes. *Diabet Med* 1987; 4: 37–40.
34. Horita M, Sunzuki H, Onodera T, Ginsberg-Fellner F, Fauci AS, Notkins AL. Abnormalities of immunoregulatory T-cell subsets in patients with insulin dependent diabetes mellitus. *J Immunol* 1982; 129: 1426–9.
35. Rodier M, Andary M, Richard JL, Mirouze J, Clot J. Peripheral blood T cell subsets studied by monoclonal antibodies in type 1 (insulin-dependent) diabetes: effect of blood glucose control. *Diabetologia* 1984; 27: 136–8.
36. Pozzilli P, Negri M, Visalli N, Pagani S, Beales P, Andreani D. Impaired CD4/CD8 lymphocyte ratio in patients with long-standing diabetes mellitus. *IRCS Med Sci* 1986; 14: 648–9.
37. Drell DW, Notkins AL. Multiple immunological abnormalities in patients with type 1 (insulin-dependent) diabetes mellitus. *Diabetologia* 1987; 30: 132–43.
38. Visalli N, Signore A, Pozzilli P. Immunodeficiency in long-standing diabetes: evidence and approaches to prevention. In Andreani D, Kolb H, Pozzilli P (eds). *Immunotherapy of Type 1 Diabetes*. Chichester, UK: Wiley, 1989; pp 185–92.
39. Pozzilli P, Pagani S, Arduini P, Visalli N, Cioccia GP, Negri D. *In vivo* determination of cell mediated immune response in diabetic patients using a multiple intradermal antigen dispenser. *Diabetes Res* 1987; 6: 5–8.
40. Pozzilli P, Gale EAM, Visalli N, Baroni MG, Crovari P, Frighi V, et al. The immune response to influenza vaccination in diabetic patients. *Diabetologia* 1986; 29: 850–5.
41. Pozzilli P, Arduini P, Visalli N, Sutherland J, Pezzella M, Galli C, et al. Reduced protection against hepatitis B virus following vaccination in patients with type 1 (insulin-dependent) diabetes. *Diabetologia* 1987; 30: 817–9.
42. Smith WI, Rabin BS, Huellmantel A, van Thiel DH, Drash A. Immunopathology of juvenile onset diabetes mellitus, I: IgA deficiency and juvenile diabetes. *Diabetes* 1978; 27: 1092–7.
43. Hoddinott S, Dornan J, Bear JC, Farid NR. Immunoglobulin levels, immunodeficiency and HLA in type 1 (insulin-dependent) diabetes mellitus. *Diabetologia* 1982; 23: 326–9.
44. Lederman MM, Rodman HM, Schaeter BZ, Jones PK, Schiffman G. Antibody response to pneumococcal polysaccharides in insulin-dependent diabetes mellitus. *Diabetes Care* 1982; 5: 36–9.
45. Palmer JP, Cooney MK, Ward RH, Hansen JA, Brodsky JB, Ray CG, et al. Reduced Coxsackie antibody titres in type 1 (insulin-dependent) diabetic patients presenting during an outbreak of Coxsackie B3 and B4 infection. *Diabetologia* 1982; 22: 426–9.
46. Vergani D, Johnston C, B-Abdullah N, Barnett AH. Low serum C4 concentrations: an inherited predisposition to insulin dependent diabetes? *Br Med J* 1983; 286: 943–8.
47. Charlesworth JA, Timmermans V, Golding J, Campbell LV, Peake PW, Pussell BA, et al. The complement system in type 1 (insulin-dependent) diabetes. *Diabetologia* 1987; 30: 372–9.
48. Boulton AJM. The importance of abnormal foot pressures and gait in the causation of foot ulcers. In Connor H, Boulton AJM, Ward JD (eds). *The Foot in Diabetes*. Chichester, UK: Wiley, 1987; pp 11–21.
49. Wheat LJ, Allen SD, Henry M, Kernek CB, Siders JA, Kuebler T, et al. Diabetic foot infections. *Arch Intern Med* 1986; 146: 1935–40.
50. Cluff LE, Reynolds RC, Page DL. Staphylococcal bacteremia: demographic, clinical and microbiological features of 185 cases. *Trans Am Clin Climatol Assoc* 1968; 79: 905–15.
51. Tapper-Jones LM, Aldred MJ, Walker DM, Hayes TM. Candidal infections and populations of *Candida albicans* in mouths of diabetics. *J Clin Pathol* 1981; 34: 706–11.

52. Pietri A, Raskin P. Cutaneous complications of chronic continuous subcutaneous insulin infusion therapy. *Diabetes Care* 1981; 4: 624–6.
53. Ryan EA, Miller J, Skyler JS. Finger sepsis. Possible complication of self-monitoring of blood glucose concentrations. *Br Med J* 1983; 286: 1614–5.
54. Edmonds ME, Blundell MP, Morris ME, Thomas EM, Cotton LT, Watkins PJ. Improved survival of the diabetic foot: the role of the specialised foot clinic. *Q J Med* 1986; 60: 763–71.
55. Bamberger DM, Daus GP, Gerding DN. Osteomyelitis in the feet of diabetic patients. Long-term results, prognostic factors and the role of antimicrobial surgical therapy. *Am J Med* 1987; 83: 653–60.
56. Giuliano A, Lewis F Jr, Hadley K, Blaisdell FW. Bacteriology of necrotizing fascitis. *Am J Surg* 1977; 134: 52–7.
57. Sen P, Louria DB. Infectious complications in the elderly diabetic patient. *Geriatrics* 1983; 38: 63–6.
58. Smith JA, O'Connor JJ, Welles AT. Nasal carriage of Staphylococcus aureus in diabetes mellitus. *Lancet* 1966; 2: 776–81.
59. Somerville DA, Lancaster-Smith M. The aerobic cutaneous microflora of diabetic subjects. *Br J Dermatol* 1973; 89: 395–401.
60. Minchew BH. Studies of the epidemiology of staphylococcal infections, VIII: infection in hospital personnel. *Bull Johns Hopkins Hosp* 1964; 114: 313–5.
61. Farrer SM, MacLeod CM. Staphylococcal infections in a general hospital. *Am J Hyg* 1960; 72: 38–58.
62. Mugusi F, Swai AB, Alberti KGMM, McLarty DG. Increased prevalence of diabetes mellitus in patients with pulmonary tuberculosis in Tanzania. *Tubercle* 1990; 71: 270–6.
63. Sarkany I, Taplin D, Blank H. Erythrasma—common bacterial infection of the skin. *JAMA* 1961; 177: 130–2.
64. Feingold DS, Wagner RF Jr. Antibacterial therapy. *J Am Acad Dermatol* 1986; 14: 535–48.
65. Chandler JR. Malignant external otitis: further considerations. *Ann Otol Rhinol Laryngol* 1977; 86: 417–28.
66. Grossi SG. Treatment of periodontal disease and control of diabetes: an assessment of the evidence and need for future research. *Ann Periodontol* 2001; 6: 138–45.
67. Page RC.Vaccination and periodontitis: myth or reality. *J Int Acad Periodontol* April 2000; 2 (2): 31–43.
68. Bessman AN, Wagner W. Nonclostridial gas gangrene. Report of 48 cases and review of the literature. *JAMA* 1975; 233: 958–63.
69. Alteras I, Saryt E. Prevalence of pathogenic fungi in the toe-webs and toe-nails of diabetic patients. *Mycopathologia* 1979; 67: 157–60.
70. Sonck CE, Somersalo O. The yeast flora of the anogenital region in diabetic girls. *Arch Dermatol* 1963; 88: 846–50.
71. Stone OJ, Mullins JF. Incidence of chronic paronychia. *JAMA* 1963; 186: 177–8.
72. Batra VK, Gaiha M, Gupta PS. Mucormycosis in a diabetic. *Postgrad Med J* 1982; 58: 781–2.
73. Hamill R, Oney LA, Crane LR. Successful therapy for rhinocerebral mucormycosis with associated bilateral brain abscesses. *Arch Intern Med* 1983; 143: 581–3.
74. Dogras S, Kumar B, Bhansali A, Chakrebarty A. Epidemiology of onycomycosis in patients with diabetes mellitus in India. *Int J Dermatol* 2002; 41: 647–51.
75. Caputo GM, Cavanagh PR, Ulbrecht JS, Gibbons GW, Karchmer AW. Assessment and management of foot disease in patients with diabetes. *New Engl J Med* 1994; 331: 854–60.
76. Zimmerman RK, Middleton DB, Smith NJ. Vaccines for persons at high risk due to medical conditions, occupation, environment, or lifestyle. *J Fam Pract* January 2003; 52 (1, suppl): S22–35.
77. Chen D, Misra A, Garg A. Clinical review 153: Lipodystrophy in human immunodeficiency virus-infected patients. *J Clin Endocrinol Metab* 2002; 87 (11): 4845–56.
78. The Diabetes Control and Complications Trial Research Group. The effect of intensive treatment of diabetes on the development and progression of long-term complications in insulin-dependent diabetes mellitus. *New Engl J Med* 1993; 329: 977–86.
79. Storm AJ, Bouter KP, Diepersloot RJ, Erkelens DW. Large variation in the treatment of foot infections in diabetic patients in The Netherlands. *Ned Tijdschr Geneeskd* 1994; 138: 569–73.
80. Lipsky BA, Pecoraro RE, Larson SA, Hanley ME, Ahroni JH. Out-patient management of uncomplicated lower-extremity infections in diabetic patients. *Arch Intern Med* 1990; 150: 790–7.
81. Kaufmann J, Breeding L, Rosenberg N. Anatomic location of acute diabetic foot infection. Its influence on the outcome of treatment. *Am Surg* 1987; 53: 109–12.
82. Abbas ZG, Gill GV, Archibald LK. The epidemiology of diabetic limb sepsis: an African perspective. *Diabet Med* 2002; 19: 895–9.
83. Meiland R, Geerlings SE, Hoepelman AI. Management of bacterial urinary tract infections in adult patients with diabetes mellitus. *Drugs* 2002; 62 (13): 1859–68.
84. Stapleton A. Urinary tract infections in patients with diabetes. *Am J Med* July 8, 2002; 113 (suppl 1A): 80S–84S.
85. Oriani G, Michael M, Meazza D, Sacchi C, Ronzio A, Montino O, et al. Diabetic foot and hyperbaric oxygen therapy: a ten-year experience. *J Hyperbaric Med* 1992; 7: 213–21.
86. Bakker DJ. Hyperbaric oxygen therapy and the diabetic foot. *Diabetes Metab Res Rev* 2000; 16 (suppl 1): S55–8.
87. Leslie CA, Sapico FL, Ginunas VJ, Adkins RH. Randomized controlled trial of topical hyperbaric oxygen for treatment of diabetic foot ulcers. *Diabetes Care* 1988; 11: 111–5.

This chapter is based in part on a chapter of the same title which was published in an earlier edition of the *International Textbook of Diabetes Mellitus*, by P Pozzilli, A Signore and R D G Leslie.

99

The Care of the Diabetic Patient During Surgery

G.V. Gill* and K.G.M.M. Alberti†

**University of Liverpool, Liverpool, UK, and †University of Newcastle upon Tyne, Newcastle upon Tyne, UK*

Most diabetic patients will require some sort of surgical procedure at some time in their lives [1, 2]. Indeed, the numbers undergoing major surgery such as cardiopulmonary bypass appear to be rising steadily [3]. Surgery seriously interferes with normal diabetic control, and a careful and logical method of planned management is therefore required.

There are many ways in which surgery interferes with carbohydrate metabolism and glucose homeostasis. These mechanisms are outlined in Table 1. They occur in nondiabetic patients, but are greatly exaggerated in states of partial or complete relative insulin deficiency, i.e. in type 2 and type 1 diabetes mellitus (DM) respectively.

The disease requiring surgical intervention may itself cause metabolic decompensation (e.g., abscesses, peritonitis, malignancy). Patient anxiety does not help, and anesthesia can also adversely affect carbohydrate metabolism [4]. Additionally, surgery is always associated with a period of starvation and some degree of infective risk. Finally, and perhaps most importantly, the trauma of surgical operation evokes a characteristic hormonal and metabolic response leading to catabolism, hyperglycemia, and ketogenic risks [5, 6].

METABOLIC RESPONSES TO SURGERY

In healthy subjects, the basic metabolic processes of anabolism and catabolism are finely and exactly balanced. The controlling influences on this system are essentially hormonal. Insulin is the only significant anabolic hormone, but several are associated with catabolism, notably cortisol, glucagon, and catecholamines. Thus, in very basic terms, insulin will promote tissue glucose uptake, and glycogen formation in liver and muscle, as well as promoting protein synthesis and lipogenesis. Conversely, the catabolic hormones (also known as "stress" or "counterregulatory" hormones) will oppose the actions of insulin by stimulating glycogen breakdown, gluconeogenesis, lipolysis, and inhibition of protein synthesis.

In the fed state, when insulin levels in the blood are high, anabolism predominates; on fasting, as insulin levels decline, metabolism swings toward catabolism. It should be noted, however, that even during fasting a small amount of insulin is secreted to prevent excessive and deleterious catabolism.

The key role of insulin can thus be readily seen, in containing the catabolic drive promoted by the "massed bands" of the counterregulatory ensemble. In the insulin-deficient state associated with, for example, untreated type 1 DM, restraints to excessive catabolism are limited or nonexistent. Even when a fixed amount of basal insulin is present, prolonged fasting, trauma, or infection may lead to dangerously excessive glucose production and lipid breakdown.

The hormonal and metabolic changes associated with surgical trauma are well described [7–10], and are outlined in Table 2. Generally, the degree of metabolic change is related to the severity of trauma, and responses are exaggerated and prolonged if complications, such as sepsis, occur [4]. The prime changes are hormonal, and secretory patterns seem to be altered mainly by neural mechanisms, although the release of stimulatory "wound hormones" is still postulated [5]. These may include tumor necrosis factor released in response to endotoxin [11] and interleukin 1

International Textbook of Diabetes Mellitus, Third Edition. Edited by R. A. DeFronzo, E. Ferrannini, H. Keen, and P. Zimmet.
 ISBN: 0-471-48655-8.

Table 1 Surgery and diabetes: factors adversely affecting diabetic control

1. Anxiety
2. Starvation
3. Anesthetic drugs
4. Infection
5. Metabolic response to trauma
6. Diseases underlying need for surgery
7. Other drugs, e.g. steroids

[12]. Almost immediately after the onset of trauma, the concentration of serum adrenocorticotropic hormone (ACTH) (and thereby of cortisol) rises, to be followed by catecholamines, glucagon, and growth hormone. More variable (and less important) are rises in levels of serum aldosterone, prolactin, vasopressin, and thyroid hormones. Insulin secretion is relatively reduced during trauma, and insulin resistance is commonly found [4, 13]. This insulin insensitivity occurs even after moderate uncomplicated surgery and is a postreceptor effect [14]. Brandi et al. [15] showed a dramatic eightfold increase in insulin requirements for parenteral feeding to maintain euglycemia in the 24 h after surgery. We found a 50% fall in insulin sensitivity 24 h after laparoscopic cholecystectomy compared with preoperative values [16]. A similar decrease following cholecystectomy was found by Thorell et al. [17], who also report a one-third decrease even after inguinal hernia repair. This resistance persists for at least 5 days following surgery [13] but does not appear to affect adipose tissue metabolism assessed by the microdialysis technique [18].

The metabolic results of these hormonal changes (Table 2) are glucose release into the circulation via glycogenolysis and gluconeogenesis, as well as fat and protein breakdown. Despite the insulin resistance there is sufficient insulin to suppress lipolysis and there is thus less nonesterified fatty acid available for ketogenesis [19]. The lack of ketone bodies is associated with increased proteolysis [20], the amino acids being used for gluconeogenesis. The overall scenario is one of intense catabolism, particularly in more traumatic surgical operations. Risks of metabolic decompensation are enhanced by the preoperative and postoperative starvation that accompanies operations. The key problem for the diabetic patient is the inability to increase insulin secretion to counteract the increases in the catabolic hormones.

Table 2 Summary of metabolic and hormonal responses to surgical trauma

Hormonal changes	Metabolic changes
"Stress hormone" secretion	Increased gluconeogenesis and glycogenolysis
Cortisol	Hyperglycemia
Catecholamines	Lipolysis
Glucagon	Protein breakdown
Growth hormone	
Cytokines	
Relative decrease in insulin secretion	
Peripheral insulin resistance	

Table 3 Principles of managing diabetes during surgery

Diabetic patients on insulin treatment	Assume to have no insulin reserves Provide continuous insulin and glucose for all grades of surgery
Diabetic patients not on insulin treatment	Assume to have limited insulin reserves Observe only (if reasonably controlled), unless surgery is major, when continuous insulin and glucose should be used as above

For more details of the metabolic and hormonal response to trauma in normal and diabetic humans, the reader is directed to other reviews on the subject [5, 6, 8, 12, 21–24].

PRINCIPLES OF MANAGING DIABETES DURING SURGERY

Principles of management depend mainly on whether the patient can secrete adequate amounts of insulin [25]. Thus, patients on insulin treatment should be considered to be insulin dependent, and assumed to have no effective insulin reserves. For these patients, a management protocol must include continuous provision of insulin and glucose if the intense catabolic drives of trauma and starvation are to be survived; this is true for all grades of surgery.

Patients *not* on insulin treatment (i.e., on dietary and/or drug treatment) may be considered to be non-insulin-dependent, and will have endogenous insulin reserves, albeit limited. Insulin therapy is less essential here for mild degrees of surgical trauma, although insulin supplementation will be needed for more severe operations. The patient's own insulin will inhibit lipolysis and ketosis, and usually prevent excessive hyperglycemia with minor stress, but will be inadequate for more severe grades of surgery. These principles are summarized in Table 3.

RISKS OF SURGERY ASSOCIATED WITH DIABETES

In the past, diabetes was considered to be a major cause of increased mortality during surgery. Precise and useful data from earlier years are hard to find. In the 1930s a mortality of 27% was reported, with more than 50% for those undergoing amputations [26]. In the United States in 1963 this had fallen to 4.9% (24 out of 487 patients) [27]. In the discussion of this latter paper the authors referred to considerably higher rates for other centers. The main causes of mortality were myocardial infarction, ketoacidosis, and infection. Important factors underlying these unacceptable risks probably included suboptimal glycemic control amongst the diabetic population in general at the time, and imperfect methods of operative and postoperative diabetic care.

Recent evidence, however, suggests that surgery is now safe for diabetic patients in terms of both mortality and morbidity. Thus, using treatment regimens based on the principles outlined above, Hjortrup and colleagues [28] reported a mortality of 5 out of 224 (2.2%) diabetic patients undergoing surgery, compared with 6 out of 224 (2.7%) nondiabetic controls. Postoperative complications occurred in 46 (20.5%) of each group, and in particular infections (wound, chest, and urinary) were not significantly different in either group. One curious feature of this study was that diabetic subjects who developed postoperative complications had slightly but significantly *lower* blood glucose values before, during, and after surgery, compared with those who had uncomplicated recoveries. This lack of an increase in morbidity and mortality was confirmed in another study by the same workers [29], as well as during biliary surgery [30, 31] and coronary artery bypass grafting (CABG) [32] and vascular surgery [33], although there was a tendency for there to be more postoperative sepsis in the biliary surgery patients. In the few studies showing increased surgical risk amongst diabetic patients, the excess has been small and almost certainly related to factors other than diabetes *per se* (for example, adverse associated preoperative factors such as coronary artery disease [34, 35]). In a very large series of patients [36] undergoing abdominal aortic surgery (153 diabetic, 970 nondiabetic), there was significantly increased morbidity only from myocardial infarction (5.2 vs. 2.1%) and infection, but even here numbers of cases were small. Similarly, infection rates in diabetic patients undergoing CABG may be increased when postoperative blood glucose control is poor [37]. Diabetic patients undergoing lower-limb revascularization procedures may have increased amputation and mortality compared with nondiabetic patients [38] (though it is known that diabetic patients with peripheral vascular disease are a poor prognostic group, generally). Overall, the literature suggests that surgical risk in diabetes is only significantly increased when glycemic control is particularly poor, or there are advanced large-vessel complications present.

AIMS OF TREATMENT

When preparing detailed protocols of care for diabetic patients during surgery, it is important to be clear about the exact aims of treatment. Ideal aims are outlined in Table 4, and it will be apparent from the discussion in the previous section that the first four aims, i.e. no excess in mortality and morbidity, should be achievable provided that a logical system of diabetic care is employed. The setting of metabolic targets is more difficult, however. Excessive hyperglycemia is to be avoided as it increases the risk of decompensation into ketoacidosis, and also promotes dehydration and electrolyte imbalance. Infection is also more likely because of impaired phagocytic function [39, 40], and wound healing is impaired, at least experimentally [41]. On the other hand, overdiligent attempts to induce normoglycemia may lead to hypoglycemia—a particular hazard for anesthetized or postoperative patients, who will have to rely on others for its detection. There is, indeed, no clear evidence that excellent glycemic control improves outcome; indeed, as mentioned previously, the study of Hjortrup et al. [28] suggested that particularly "good" control was associated with greater risks of postoperative morbidity. A reasonable practical compromise is to aim for operative and postoperative blood glucose levels in the region of 6–12 mmol/l [25].

Table 4 Management aims for diabetic patients undergoing surgery

1. No excess mortality
2. No increase in postoperative complications (especially infective)
3. Normal wound healing
4. No increase in the duration of hospitalization
5. No hypoglycemia
6. No ketoacidosis or severe hyperglycemia

PREOPERATIVE ASSESSMENT OF DIABETES

All diabetic patients requiring surgery will need assessment of their diabetes, and possibly some changes in management. Table 5 outlines the requirements of preoperative assessment. Admission a little earlier than usual may be needed, and blood glucose levels must be measured regularly. This is usually done by "bedside" monitoring with reagent test strips at least four times daily. Treatment

Table 5 Preoperative assessment and management of the diabetic patient undergoing surgery

1. Admit 2–3 days prior to surgery (ideally)*
2. Make general medical assessment (cardiac, renal, etc.)
3. Avoid long-acting blood glucose lowering agents (e.g., chlorpropamide, glibenclamide, ultralente insulins)
4. Avoid metformin
5. Closely monitor blood glucose levels
6. Optimize glycemic control—if necessary, use insulin
7. Arrange surgery in the morning
8. Cooperate closely with the anesthetist

* It is often not possible to admit patients more than 24 h preoperatively, and many may be dealt with as day cases. Improvement of glycemic control, adjustment of therapy, and full preoperative assessment should then be done on an outpatient basis.

may need to be rationalized, and in particular, excessively long-acting preparations such as the sulfonylureas, chlorpropamide and glibenclamide, and ultralente insulin, are best discontinued; their effect may last well into the operative and even postoperative period, and will complicate optimal management. It has been suggested that the new long-acting insulin, insulin glargine, can be continued but data are lacking [42]. The biguanide drug metformin is also best avoided, in case there is postoperative renal insufficiency, which is associated with lactic acidosis in metformin-treated patients.

If diabetic control needs to be improved, the treatments may include the addition of a short-acting sulfonylurea drug for those previously on diet alone, increase in drug doses for those already on sulfonylureas, or substitution with insulin if patients are on maximum doses of drugs or very poorly controlled. Metformin should be stopped 24–72 h before surgery and insulin used if control is suboptimal. The insulin system used in such patients should be as flexible as possible to allow rapid adjustments. Commonly, soluble (regular) insulin or short-acting insulin analogues are used three times daily before food, with a small amount of isophane or newer longer lasting insulins at night if morning hyperglycemia is a problem. These patients should be regarded as insulin dependent, and should be treated as such during and after surgery.

Patients with type 1 diabetes may need dose alterations to optimize control. Most patients will already be on twice-daily or multiple dose insulin injection regimens, so the basic form of treatment should not need changing. Once-daily regimens will usually require to be changed to two or three injections daily, except in insulin-treated type 2 patients who are not using ultralente insulins or glargine and who have adequate fasting blood glucose levels. This latter is an important requirement of any preoperative diabetic treatment. If the patient is hyperglycemic immediately preoperatively, blood glucose levels tend to remain high or may even escalate—despite reasonable protocols of operative management.

In addition to attending to diabetic control, general medical assessment is essential. Particular attention should be paid to those systems affected by diabetes: heart, peripheral circulation, peripheral and autonomic nervous systems, renal function, and blood pressure. These certainly contribute to postoperative complications, particularly heart failure [34]. Chest radiography and electrocardiography may well be needed, while renal function should be tested by measurement of serum creatinine and electrolyte levels. Urine culture should be routinely performed in older patients. Autonomic neuropathy is a particular risk because of its association with sudden death perioperatively [43] and the greater need for vasopressors intraoperatively [44]. Further emphasis on autonomic neuropathy comes from the report of Vohra et al. [45]. In 10 consecutive patients presenting for vitreous surgery all showed evidence of autonomic neuropathy. They showed no increase in heart rate when blood pressure fell after induction of anesthesia and also revealed a decreased cardiac index and stroke index. Finally, it is vital that full and complete liaison is made with the anesthetic staff involved, so that they are aware of the diabetic patient and any problems, as well as the operative management system planned.

Already 20 years ago, Podolsky [46] suggested that much of this preoperative assessment could be done on an outpatient basis. This is undoubtedly true, and it is regrettable that this system rarely operates. Excessive hospitalization of surgical diabetic patients almost always occurs in the preoperative phase. It is usually due to poor planning, and is very costly.

SURGICAL MANAGEMENT IN TYPE 2 DIABETES

Management of type 2 patients for minor surgery is outlined in Table 6. There is general agreement that a conservative approach is justifiable, provided that (a) blood glucose control is reasonable and (b) the planned surgery is not major. In the latter case, management should be as for insulin-treated patients (see next section). Otherwise, insulin is not required and only observation of blood glucose control is needed, together with omission of oral blood glucose lowering agents immediately before surgery, if the patient is on such treatment. Glucose and insulin delivery systems are unnecessarily complex, do not give any better glycemic control, and, indeed, may induce a rather distorted profile of blood metabolite levels [47, 48].

Morning surgery is not essential but it is helpful. If postoperative problems arise these are more easily dealt with in the afternoon or evening rather than the middle of the night. In fact, intervention is very rarely required for excessively high perioperative or postoperative blood glucose levels in response to regular monitoring. One important point is to ensure that the patient receives no glucose-containing intravenous (IV) fluids. Anesthetists

Table 6 Surgical management in type 2 diabetes

1. Ensure reasonable preoperative glycemic control
2. Operate in the morning, if possible
3. If the patient is taking oral blood glucose lowering agents, omit these on the morning of surgery
4. Avoid glucose-containing IV fluids
5. Restart oral blood glucose lowering agents with the first postoperative meal
6. Monitor glucose levels with test strips every 2 h initially, reducing frequency later as necessary

Note: If preoperative control is poor, or if the surgery is major, treat the patient as insulin dependent.

are particularly fond of 5% dextrose or dextrose–saline solutions. Similarly, lactate-containing infusion fluids (e.g. Hartmann's or Ringer–lactate solutions) should not be used as they can have hyperglycemic effects [49, 50]. Once again, this demonstrates the importance of liaison with anesthetic and surgical staff. The anesthetic management of patients with diabetes is well described by McAnulty et al. [51].

SURGICAL MANAGEMENT IN TYPE 1 DIABETES

Historical Aspects

Twenty-five years ago, recommendations for the management of type 1 patients undergoing surgery included the complete omission of insulin until after operation [52], a system not surprisingly associated with hyperglycemia and very significant ketotic risk (see reference 21 for review). Following this, there developed systems of continuing subcutaneous (SC) insulin and "covering" the period of fasting with IV glucose infusions. These systems were generally successful, but tended to be rather complex. They remained popular up to 10–15 years ago, and a great many were described and indeed are still used by some [52, 53]. Some recommended the usual morning SC insulin prior to operation [54], some isophane insulin only [55], and some a variety of fractions of morning doses [56, 57]. Regimens of IV glucose infusion usually involved fairly arbitrary amounts of 5 or 10% dextrose (glucose). Postoperative insulin delivery with all these methods was difficult and often haphazard until the patient was able to eat. Generally, intermittent boluses of soluble insulin were suggested, often by a *post hoc* "sliding scale" method. Review of the literature shows the rather poor glycemic control obtained with the SC regimens; postoperative mean glucose levels ranged from 11.3 mmol/l (203 mg/dl) [58] to 30.2 mmol/l (544 mg/dl) [59] with only one study showing values below 10 mmol/l (180 mg/dl) [60]; the latter was during minor surgery.

Dissatisfaction with these complicated and inflexible regimens led to the increased popularity of IV insulin systems over the last decade. The first major report [55] suggested the use of a low-dose insulin infusion with separate IV glucose delivery. This has evolved to a separate-line system still frequently used [61]. A constant glucose infusion (e.g. 100 ml 10% glucose/h) is given preferably by electronic drip counter, while "piggy-backed" to this (by Y-connector) is an IV insulin infusion given by syringe pump (usually 50 units short-acting insulin in 50 ml 0.9% saline, i.e. 1 unit/ml). The insulin infusion rate is altered according to regular bedside blood glucose monitoring, with the initial insulin dose usually 3 units/h. The system is flexible and physiological, but requires special apparatus and is labor intensive. It is best reserved for situations where close attention can be paid to the patient and the infusions—for example during labor in type 1 patients, and during serious intercurrent illness requiring care on intensive therapy or coronary care units.

A variety of complex algorithms have been developed using separate IV insulin and glucose infusions. The most complex is that of Meyers et al. [62]—the "two-step" protocol, which involves complex calculations and periodic IV insulin boluses. Such a system is ripe for catastrophe in the average surgical unit. Others are more simple, such as those of Woodruff et al. [63] and Watts et al. [64], although the latter, perhaps inadvisably, only starts postoperatively. There have been intermittent suggestions of giving insulin by hourly or 2-hourly boluses [65], but this is illogical and has been correctly criticized [3]. There has even recently been an unwelcome return to insulin-free treatment. A group of patients were given IV saline and insulin was added only if blood glucose levels exceeded 11.1 mmol/l (200 mg/dl) [66]. It was reported that only 40% of those previously on insulin needed this adjunctive insulin. However, no mention is made of other aspects of metabolism such as ketonemia and protein breakdown. More or less complex algorithms involving IV insulin are still in use particularly in the United States [42].

A particular worry of the separate-line glucose and insulin method is that if one line should block, fail or dislodge, then dangerous hypoglycemia or hyperglycemia will result, depending on which infusion stops. This problem, together with the need for a simpler system, has led to the widespread introduction of combined glucose and insulin infusions. Nonetheless many anesthetists still prefer to use separate lines for the glucose and insulin [67], and slightly better results were reported in one study than with a combined infusion [68].

Glucose, Potassium, and Insulin Infusion

Although there are many variations in use, the basic system of glucose, potassium, and insulin infusion remains essentially that described by Alberti and Thomas in 1979 [21]. Infusion of 500 ml 10% dextrose containing 10 U short-acting insulin and 10 mmol potassium chloride (KCl) was recommended to prevent hypokalemia. The infusion was given at a rate of 100 ml/h (i.e. 500 ml in 5 h), thus delivering 2 U insulin, 2 mmol KCl, and 10 g glucose each hour. The system has become known as GKI (glucose–KCl–insulin) or GIK.

It is interesting that the present GKI system was initially described in almost its exact present form by Galloway and Shuman in 1963 [27]. They recorded a method of management involving "regular insulin in IV glucose infusions, usually in doses ranging from 0.16 to 0.20 units/g of glucose," which equates with 10 U insulin in 500 ml 10% glucose.

Table 7 Algorithm for adjusting insulin content of GKI infusion

1. Measure blood glucose levels with test strips every 2 h*
2. Adjust infusion as follows:
   Blood glucose 6.5–11 mmol/l (117–200 mg/dl)—usual GKI (15 U/500 ml)
   Blood glucose over 11 mmol/l (200 mg/dl)—increase to 20 units
   Blood glucose under 6.5 mmol/l (117 mg/dl)—decrease to 10 units
3. Continue to adjust in 5-unit increments as necessary

* Frequency of monitoring is variable and depends on the individual clinical situation. Levels can usually be measured less frequently as time progresses.

As a result of the initial findings [21] the amount of insulin in GKI solutions was increased. Husband and colleagues in 1985 [69] increased the insulin to 16 U per 500 ml 10% glucose (0.32 U/g glucose). With this mixture, over 80% of their series of 128 patients achieved target blood glucose levels of 5–12 mmol/l (90–216 mg/dl) on the operative day, and most of the apparent failures were due to the system not being operated properly. Since the introduction of U100 insulin, the amount added to the glucose infusion has been adapted to the more metric 15 U of insulin (0.3 U/g). An alternative is to use 5% dextrose with 5–10 units/500 ml, again given at 100 ml/h [70]. We prefer the 10% glucose-based mixture as this gives more energy (5000 kJ rather than 2500 kJ/24 h).

GKI is started on the morning of surgery—the patient receiving no food or SC insulin—and is continued during and after surgery until diet and SC insulin can be safely restarted. Bedside blood glucose levels are measured regularly, and if too high, then a fresh GKI bag containing 20 U insulin is set up. Similarly, low levels will require a reduction of GKI to 10 U/bag. A suggested algorithm for GKI adjustment is shown in Table 7, although in fact such infusion changes are not often needed.

Continuous glucose and insulin infusions are simple and flexible, and give good glycemic results (Table 8). These results compare well with other reports of IV insulin regimens (reviewed in reference 23). Glucose and insulin infusion perioperatively has also been shown to maintain normal insulin sensitivity after surgery [71]. Because of the simultaneous mixed delivery of glucose and insulin, there is a much smaller risk of unexpected severe hypoglycemia or hyperglycemia compared with the separate-line system. The ratio of insulin to glucose remains constant whatever the infusion rate; the use of electronic dripcounters is, therefore, not essential.

Table 9 Conditions associated with increased insulin requirement during surgery in diabetic patients

	Insulin requirement (U/g glucose)
Uncomplicated	0.3–0.4
Liver disease	0.4–0.6
Severe obesity	0.4–0.6
Major infection/sepsis	0.6–0.8
Steroid therapy	0.5–0.8

In the elderly or those with heart failure, a standard GKI infusion may lead to fluid overload. Here, the infusion rate may be slowed (e.g. to 6–8 h/500 ml), or the concentration of glucose can be doubled to 20% (the rate of infusion is extended to 10-hourly or 50 ml/h, and the potassium and insulin content also doubled). In certain predictable conditions insulin requirement may be increased. These include severe obesity (body mass index greater than 30 kg/m^2), hepatic cirrhosis, sepsis, and steroid therapy (Table 9). In these situations the initial GKI mixture should contain an appropriately increased amount of insulin.

As with all patients on IV fluid therapy, plasma urea and electrolytes need to be measured daily. The KCl content of the infusion in particular may need altering, and for safety plasma potassium levels should be checked 4–6 h postoperatively. Others recommend giving the glucose in 0.45% saline [42]. With prolonged GKI, serious dilutional hyponatremia may occasionally occur. If plasma sodium levels begin to fall, and continued GKI is needed, then 0.9% (isotonic) saline infusion should be given at the same time. Absorption of insulin on to the plastic surfaces of infusion bags and giving sets is a theoretical rather than a practical problem [72]. The previously

Table 8 Results of a GKI-based system of surgical diabetes care*

Time	Blood glucose (mmol/l): Type 2 DM† – observation only	Type 2 DM‡ – GKI infusion	Type 1 DM‡ – GKI infusion
Preoperative	7.4 ± 2.0	7.9 ± 2.5	8.2 ± 3.0
Postoperative	8.5 ± 3.2	10.2 ± 3.9	9.6 ± 3.4
Mean operative day	8.2 ± 1.8	9.3 ± 2.2	8.9 ± 2.3
Mean first postoperative day	8.2 ± 1.9	8.7 ± 1.6	9.4 ± 1.9
Mean second postoperative day	8.4 ± 1.9	8.8 ± 1.8	10.2 ± 2.8

Note: Values represent mean ± SD.
* Adapted from reference 69.
† Minor surgery.
‡ Major and minor surgery.

suggested practices of adding blood or albumin to the infusion are unnecessary, although it is wise to discard the first 25–50 ml of GKI solution by running it through the infusion set, before connecting with the patient; this is said to saturate the "binding sites" of the plastic for insulin. Perhaps a more important problem concerns adding insulin to the drip bag via too short an insulin syringe, allowing "trapping" of the insulin near the entry port, and inadequate mixing [73].

ORGANIZATION OF CARE FOR THE SURGICAL DIABETIC PATIENT

Thai and colleagues [74] have advocated the formation of a "diabetic team" to supervize the care of diabetic patients undergoing surgery. The team consists of doctors belonging to the diabetic unit, who on a rotational basis act as the point of referral for diabetic surgical patients. The doctor visits appropriate surgical wards on a daily basis, making preoperative assessments, ordering operative protocols, consulting with ward and anesthetic staff, and adjusting postoperative treatment as necessary. Compared with care by surgical or anesthetic staff alone, better glycemic control and more consistent management systems amongst the team-cared patients were reported by Thai and coworkers [74]. Mortality and morbidity in both groups of patients were, however, similar.

Although attractive, the team approach is expensive in terms of physician time, and it is likely that only major teaching centers will have sufficient staff resources to mount such a scheme; most district hospitals will have to rely on surgical and anesthetic staff to operate diabetic care in surgical patients. Certain safeguards can be taken, however; there must be full agreement between medical, surgical, and anesthetic staff on the protocol to be used, and it is up to the diabetes specialist of the hospital to initiate and organize this dialogue. A simple, clear, and concise summary of the protocol must then be prepared (Table 10) and widely distributed among the medical and nursing staff involved. Use of a simple protocol has been shown to produce significantly better results than when the protocol was not adhered to [75]. Sufficient copies should be available so that it can be carried in any doctor's coat pocket and be seen on any notice board. The diabetes unit can then be used as a "troubleshooting" focus only, providing advice for particularly difficult problems.

In reality, it is unfortunately often difficult to ensure widespread adoption of such agreed protocols. Thus, Clark and colleagues have reported widespread variation in beliefs and practice in surgical diabetes care amongst anesthetists in three UK hospitals, despite the circulation of agreed protocols [67]. Both SC and IV insulin systems were in use, glycemic aims varied widely, and outmoded "sliding scales" were in use.

A final point of organization concerns the accuracy of bedside blood glucose monitoring. Serious errors in such extralaboratory tests can occur [76], which can seriously interfere with the smooth running and efficacy of a GKI infusion-based system. It is therefore wise to perform intermittent laboratory blood glucose level assessments on surgical diabetic patients, as a check on bedside testing. We routinely send the fasting blood glucose sample for laboratory measurement, as well as using the bedside test-strip method. Additionally, all hospitals should have some form of structured education program for test-strip blood glucose monitoring, as well as a quality control scheme to ensure its accuracy [77].

SPECIAL SURGICAL SITUATIONS

Open Heart Surgery

Although cardiac surgery is nowadays confined to specialist centers, within such centers diabetic patients represent a large proportion of the patients operated upon,

Table 10 Summarized protocol of diabetic care for surgical procedures

1. Ensure reasonable preoperative control. Operate in the morning, if possible
2. Cooperate closely with anesthetist
3. Omit patient's breakfast, and insulin or oral hypoglycemic drug, on morning of surgery
4. *Non-insulin treated diabetic patients* having nonmajor surgery need observation only. Chart 2-hourly test-strip glucose results on day of surgery. If patient on oral blood glucose lowering drugs, restart with next meal
5. *Glucose–potassium–insulin* (GKI) is used in all other cases, i.e. all insulin-treated diabetic patients and for major surgery in non-insulin-treated diabetic patients
   (i) At 8–9 a.m. on morning of surgery commence GKI infusion
   500 ml 10% dextrose
   +15 units soluble (regular) insulin
   +10 mmol KCl
   Infuse 5-hourly (100 ml/h)
   (ii) Check blood glucose levels 2-hourly initially with test strips: aim for 6.5–11 mmol/l (117–200 mg/dl). If glucose level above 11 mmol/l (200 mg/dl), change to GKI with 20 U soluble insulin; if glucose level below 6.5 mmol/l, change to GKI with 10 U soluble insulin. Continue to adjust in 5-unit steps as necessary. Check plasma potassium levels 4–6 h, postoperatively
   (iii) Continue GKI till patient eats, then revert to usual treatment. If GKI is prolonged (more than 24 h), check urea and electrolytes daily (and consider further nutritional support)

Table 11 Insulin requirements during cardiac surgery in diabetic patients controlled by Biostator*

Time	Insulin required (U/h)
Preoperatively	21.6 ± 0.2
Skin incision to onset of bypass	23.0 ± 1.0
Bypass	25.0 ± 1.2
Immediately after bypass	28.3 ± 0.9
Postoperatively	12.3 ± 2.6

Note: Values represent mean ± SEM.
*Adapted from reference 83.

because of the strong association between type 2 diabetes and coronary artery disease. It was reported in 1981 [78] that control of diabetic patients undergoing open heart surgery was difficult, and that insulin requirements during and immediately after surgery were variable and high (about three times that during "normal" types of operation). This has been confirmed by other workers [79] and implies severe insulin resistance [80]. This has been attributed to the severe degree of trauma, induced hypothermia, and inotropic cardiac drugs. The use of glucose-containing "priming" solutions at induction of cardiac bypass is also a major factor [78]. The hyperglycemic problems with such solutions are now well known [81, 82], and such fluids are best avoided. Lactate solutions are also inadvisable [50], and Elliott et al. [83, 84] have suggested plasmalyte as a much less metabolically hazardous priming solution.

Correction of the priming solution problem, however, is not the entire answer. Studies using the Biostator (or artificial pancreas) [83] have shown remarkable changes in insulin requirements throughout surgery to maintain acceptable degrees of glycemia (Table 11). Based on these observations, it has become accepted that the GKI infusion system is too inflexible, and separate-line control is needed [83, 85]. Frequent blood glucose testing must be done, and insulin infusion altered appropriately (large and frequent changes are needed). On the basis of their Biostator studies, Elliott and colleagues used such an open-loop system and achieved excellent control, comparable with or even better than in the Biostator-controlled patients [83]. This group also produced computer-based algorithms to aid such glycemic control during and after surgery. It should be noted that during bypass no glucose at all is given, just insulin.

Recent evidence demonstrates that careful use of GKI in diabetic patients undergoing CABG operations improves a number of outcome measures compared to those managed without GKI. These include length of hospital stay, risk of arrhythmias, and ventilation duration [86].

With systems for preoperative diabetic control as described above, as well as modern cardiac surgical and anesthetic techniques, CABG is highly successful in diabetic patients. Anginal relief and survival is equivalent to that in nondiabetic subjects [87, 88].

Cesarean Section

Delivery by cesarean section in diabetic patients is nowadays usually an elective procedure. The diabetic patient in labor who eventually needs an emergency section should already be on a glucose and insulin delivery system (often a separate-line type [89]), and this can simply be continued through surgery. For elective operations, however, a GKI system is simple and acceptable. The operation is brief, and food intake is usually rapidly resumed. It should be remembered, however, that diabetic patients in the later stages of pregnancy are insulin resistant, and are usually on insulin doses at least 50–100% greater than in their nonpregnant state [90]. It is thus sensible to start GKI with a solution containing 20 U insulin (0.4 U/g glucose), rather than the usual 15 U (0.3 U/g glucose). This insulin resistance of pregnancy rapidly disappears following delivery, in particular at delivery of the placenta, i.e. at completion of the third stage of labor. At this point, requirements drop to prepregnancy levels. A practical policy is to halve insulin delivery at this stage, whether it is being given separately or as GKI. Following this, insulin is adjusted as usual according to bedside blood glucose measurements, and SC insulin (in approximately prepregnancy amounts) is recommenced when normal diet is resumed.

Emergency Surgery

Fortunately, truly urgent surgery in diabetic patients is relatively rare. If the situation does arise, then immediate assessment of metabolic status must be made. In addition to a clinical history and examination, urine and plasma ketones, blood glucose, and plasma urea and electrolytes will need to be measured. Metabolic status should preferably be optimized before even emergency surgery, although the urgency of the surgical situation will also have to be considered. With regard to diabetic control, the GKI system is usually applicable. The time of the last SC injection of insulin is important. If the injection is recent (i.e. within the last 4 h for short-acting insulin analogues, 6 h for soluble insulin, or within the last 12 h for intermediate-acting insulins), then the system of IV insulin delivery may need to be altered to account for the continued absorption of the previously injected insulin. There will need to be particularly careful monitoring of blood glucose levels, especially by the anesthetist during the operation. In particularly unstable situations, a separate-line form of management may be advisable. In patients in whom glycemic control is severely disturbed or where ketosis or ketoacidosis are present, treatment should be initially without glucose and with GKI substituted for insulin alone when glucose levels reach 12–15 mmol/l. The possibility of an "acute abdomen" being purely due to ketoacidosis, particularly in younger patients, should also be remembered.

Other Surgical Situations

Minimal-access (or laparoscopic) surgery is increasingly popular. Though it would be expected that such operations are associated with less trauma, and perhaps an attenuated metabolic disturbance [16], this may not be the case. Thus, in one study comparing open and laparoscopic cholecystectomy, both procedures were associated with similar degrees of insulin resistance and metabolic disturbance [16].

With rising type 2 diabetes prevalence rates, and an aging population, surgery is increasingly being performed on elderly diabetic patients. Particular care is needed in this group of subjects—for example, many have macrovascular disease (which, as discussed earlier, puts them in a particularly high-risk group). They also tolerate hypoglycemia poorly, and have relatively inefficient systems for postoperative water homeostasis. Assessment and peri- and postoperative care of these patients must be especially meticulous [91].

CONCLUSIONS

The GKI system is widely accepted and used. Some authors have, however, questioned whether it is superior to traditional methods of administering SC insulin followed by IV glucose—particularly in terms of glycemic and metabolic control. Goldberg and colleagues in the United States [92] reported a study comparing the two methods in a small number of patients. No significant difference was found in blood glucose and hormonal responses between the two groups. As well as the small numbers, however, the treatment protocols were unusual in other respects; insulin was infused at only 0.5 U/h during surgery, and 0.5 U/h thereafter. Also, both in the IV and SC groups, dextrose was infused at arbitrary rates, and lactate-containing solutions were sometimes used. Glycemic control was often at levels in excess of 15 mmol/l.

In the United kingdom, Thomas and colleagues [58] compared the GKI system (10 U insulin/500 ml dextrose) with SC insulin and IV glucose (half to three quarters of the usual insulin dose, with 25 g IV glucose). As with the previous study, it can be seen that both regimens used here were suboptimal by modern standards. Eighteen patients were studied (12 GKI and 6 SC) and, again, no major differences were found in glucose and metabolic levels between the two groups, although blood glucose levels were lower ($p < 0.05$) at 4 h and 72 h postoperatively in the GKI group.

On the basis of results such as these, Hall [93] has criticized the overzealous acceptance of GKI, and has described it as a "promise unfulfilled." Review of the literature, however, shows the clear superiority of GKI regimens (see reference 23). GKI has, however, never promised or been promoted as having dramatic metabolic advantage, but it does offer simplicity and safety. Compared with SC-based regimens, it is easy to use and requires little in the way of staff or equipment resources. Insulin therapy is, moreover, only one part of the care of the diabetic patient during surgery. Management of diabetes during surgery is an exercise in logic, organization, cooperation, and communication. The diligent application of an accepted and efficacious system will result in reasonably good glycemic control, minimize avoidable disasters, and ensure patterns of mortality and morbidity that are equivalent to those of the nondiabetic population. [94].

REFERENCES

1. Root HF. Pre-operative care of the diabetic patient. *Postgrad Med* 1966; 40: 439–44.
2. Byyny RL. Management of diabetes during surgery. *Postgrad Med* 1980; 68: 191–201.
3. Milaskiewicz RM, Hall GM. Diabetes and anaesthesia: the past decade. *Br J Anaesth* 1992; 68: 198–206.
4. Allison SP, Tomlin PJ, Chamberlain MJ. Some effects of anaesthesia and surgery on carbohydrate and fat metabolism. *Br J Anaesth* 1979; 41: 588–93.
5. Elliott MJ, Alberti KGMM. Carbohydrate metabolism—effects of preoperative starvation and trauma. *Clin Anaesthiol* 1983; 1: 527–50.
6. McCowen KC, Malhotra A, Bistrian BR, Stress-induced hyperglycemia. *Crit Care Clin* 2001; 17: 107–24.
7. Hume DM, Egdahl RH. The importance of the brain in the endocrine response to injury. *Ann Surg* 1959; 150: 697–712.
8. Kehlet H. The stress response to anaesthesia and surgery: release mechanisms and modifying factors. *Clin Anaesthesiol* 1984; 2: 315–39.
9. Alberti KGMM, Marshall SM. Diabetes and surgery. In Alberti KGMM, Krall LP (eds), *The Diabetes Annual 4*. Amsterdam: Elsevier, 1988; pp 248–71.
10. Alberti KGMM. Diabetes and surgery. In Porte D, Sherwin R, Rifkin H (eds), *Ellenberg and Rifkin's Diabetes Mellitus*, 5th edn. Norwalk, CT: Appleton and Lange, 1997; pp 875–85.
11. Michie HR, Manogue KR, Spriggs DR, Revhaug A, O'Dwyer S, Dinarello CA, Cerami A, Wolff SM, Wilmore DW. Detection of circulating tumor necrosis factor after endotoxin administration. *N Engl J Med* 1988; 318: 1481–6.
12. Frayn KN. Hormonal control of metabolism in trauma and sepsis. *Clin Endocrinol* 1986; 24: 577–99.
13. Thorell A, Efendic S, Gutniak M, Haggmark T, Ljungqvist O. Insulin resistance after abdominal surgery. *Br J Surg* 1994; 81: 59–63.
14. Nordenstrom J, Sonnenfeld J, Arner P. Characterisation of insulin resistance after surgery. *Surgery* 1989; 105: 28–35.
15. Brandi LS, Frediani M, Oleggini M, Mosca F, Cerri M, Boni C, Pecori N, Buzzigoli G, Ferrannini E. Insulin resistance after surgery; normalization by insulin treatment. *Clin Sci* 1990; 79: 443–50.
16. Hawthorne GC, Ashworth L, Alberti KGMM. The effect of laparoscopic cholecystectomy on insulin sensitivity. *Horm Metab Res* 1994; 26: 474–7.
17. Thorell A, Efendic S, Gutniak M, Haggmark T, Ljungqvist O. Development of postoperative insulin resistance is associated with the magnitude of operation. *Eur J Surg* 1993; 159: 593–9.

18. Fellander G, Nordenstrom J, Ungerstedt U, Arner P, Bolinder J. Influence of operation on glucose metabolism and lipolysis in human adipose tissue: a microdialysis study. *Eur J Surg* 1994; 160: 87–95.
19. Foster KJ, Alberti KGMM, Binder C, Hinks L, Kassan S, Orskov H, Smythe P, Talbot S, Turnell D. Lipid metabolites and nitrogen balance after abdominal surgery in man. *Br J Surg* 1979; 66: 242–5
20. Smith R, Fuller DJ, Wedge JH, et al. Initial effect of injury on ketone bodies and other blood metabolites. *Lancet* 1975; i: 1–7.
21. Alberti KGMM, Thomas DJB. The management of diabetes during surgery. *Br J Anaesth* 1979; 51: 693–710.
22. Alberti KGMM, Gill GV, Elliott MJ. Insulin delivery during surgery in the diabetic patient. *Diabetes Care* 1982; 5: 65–77.
23. Alberti KGMM, Marshall SM. Diabetes and surgery. In Alberti KGMM, Krall LP (eds), *Diabetes Annual 4*. Amsterdam: Elsevier, 1988; pp 248–71.
24. Marshall SM, Alberti KGMM. Hyperglycaemic emergencies and surgery: an update. In Alberti KGMM, Krall LP (eds), *Diabetes Annual 5*. Amsterdam: Elsevier, 1990; pp 396–433.
25. Gill GV, Alberti KGMM. Surgery and diabetes. *Hosp Update* 1989; 15: 327–36.
26. Levin CM, Dealy FN. The surgical diabetic: a five-year survey. *Ann Surg* 1935; 102: 1029–39.
27. Galloway JA, Shuman CR. Diabetes and surgery. *Am J Med* 1963; 34: 177–91.
28. Hjortrup A, Sorensen C, Dyremose E, Hjortso N-C, Kehlet H. Influence of diabetes mellitus on operative risk. *Br J Surg* 1985; 72: 783–5.
29. Hjortrup A, Sorensen C, Dyrmose E, Kehlet H. Morbidity in diabetic and non-diabetic patients after abdominal surgery. *Acta Chir Scand* 1985; 151: 445–7.
30. Reiss R, Deutsch AA, Nudelmann J. Biliary surgery in diabetic patients: statistical analysis of 189 patients. *Dig Surg* 1987; 4: 37–40.
31. Walsh DB, Eckhauser FE, Ramsburgh SR, Burney RB. Risk associated with diabetes mellitus in patients undergoing gall bladder surgery. *Surgery* 1982; 91: 254–7.
32. Clement R, Rousou JA, Engelman RM, Breyer RH. Perioperative morbidity in diabetics requiring coronary artery bypass surgery. *Ann Thorac Surg* 1988; 46: 321–3.
33. Hamdan AD, Saltzberg SS, Sheahan M, Froelich J, Akbari CM, Campbell DR, LoGerfo FW, Pomposelli FB. Lack of association of diabetes with increased postoperative mortality and cardiac morbidity. *Arch Surg* 2002; 137: 417–21.
34. MacKenzie CR, Charlson ME. Assessment of perioperative risk in the patient with diabetes mellitus. *Surg Gynecol Obstet* 1988; 167: 293–9.
35. Sandler RS, Maule WF, Baltus ME. Factors associated with postoperative complications in diabetics after biliary tract surgery. *Gastroenterology* 1986; 91: 157–62.
36. Treiman GS, Treiman RL, Foran RF, Cossman DV, Cohen JL, Levin PM, Wagner WH, Davidson MB. The influence of diabetes mellitus on the risk of abdominal aortic surgery. *Am Surg* 1994; 60: 436–40.
37. Golden SH, Peart-Vigilance C, Kao WH, Brancati FL. Preoperative glycaemic control and the risk of infectious complications in a cohort of adults with diabetes. *Diabetes Care* 1999; 22: 1408–14.
38. Melliere D, Berrehal D, Desgranges P, Allaire E, Becquemin JP, Perlemuter L, Simon D. Influence of diabetes on revascularization procedures of the aorta and lower limb arteries: early results. *Eur J Vasc Endovasc Surg* 1999; 17: 438–41.
39. Wilson RM, Reeves WG. Neutrophil phagocytosis and killing in insulin-dependent diabetes. *Clin Exp Immunol* 1986; 63: 478–84.
40. McMahon MM, Bistrian BR. Host defences and susceptibility to infection in patients with diabetes mellitus. *Infect Dis Clin North Am* 1995; 9: 1–9.
41. McMurray JF. Wound healing with diabetes mellitus. *Surg Clin North Am* 1984; 64: 769–78.
42. Glister BC, Vigersky RA. Perioperative management of Type 1 diabetes mellitus. *Endocrinol Metab Clin N Am* 2003; 32: 411–36.
43. Page MMcB, Watkins PJ. Cardiorespiratory arrest with diabetic autonomic neuropathy. *Lancet* 1978; i: 14–6.
44. Burgos LG, Ebert TJ, Assiddao C, Turner LA, Pattison CZ, Wang-Cheng R, Kampine JP. Increased intraoperative cardiovascular morbidity in diabetics with autonomic neuropathy. *Anesthesiology* 1989; 70: 591–7.
45. Vohra A, Kumar S, Charlton AJ, Olukoga AO, Boulton AJM, McLeod D. Effect of diabetes mellitus on the cardiovascular response to induction of anaesthesia and tracheal intubation. *Br J Anaesth* 1993; 71: 258–61.
46. Podolsky S. Management of diabetes in the surgical patient. *Med Clin North Am* 1982; 66: 1361–72.
47. Thompson J, Husband DJ, Thai AC, Alberti KGMM. Metabolic changes in the non-insulin dependent diabetic undergoing minor surgery: effect of glucose–insulin–potassium infusion. *Br J Surg* 1986; 73: 301–4.
48. Malling B, Knudsen L, Christiansen CL, Schurizek BA, Alberti KGMM, Hermansen K. Insulin treatment in non-insulin dependent diabetic patients undergoing minor surgery. *Diabet Nutr Metab* 1989; 2: 125–31.
49. Thomas DJB, Alberti KGMM. The hyperglycaemic effects of Hartmann's solution in maturity-onset diabetics during surgery. *Br J Anaesth* 1978; 50: 185–8.
50. Fletcher J, Langman MJS, Kellock TD. Effects of surgery on blood glucose levels in diabetes mellitus. *Lancet* 1965; ii: 52–4.
51. McAnulty GR, Robertshaw HJ, Hall GM. Anaesthetic management of patients with diabetes mellitus, *Br J Anaesth* 2000; 85: 80–90.
52. Wheelock FC, Gibbons GW, Marble A. Surgery in diabetes. In Marble A, Krall LP, Bradley RF (eds), *Diabetes Mellitus*, 12th edn. Philadelphia: Lea and Febiger, 1985; pp 712–31.
53. Hughes TAT, Borsey DQ. The management of diabetic patients undergoing surgery. *Pract Diabetes* 1994; 11: 7–10.
54. Goldberg NJ, Wingert TD, Levin SR, Wilson SE, Viljoen JF. Insulin therapy in the diabetic surgical patient: metabolic and hormonal response to low dose insulin infusion. *Diabetes Care* 1981; 4: 279–84.
55. Taitelman U, Reece EA, Bessman AN. Insulin in the management of the diabetic surgical patient. Continuous intravenous administration versus subcutaneous administration. *JAMA* 1977; 237: 658–60.
56. Rossini AA, Hare JW. How to control the blood glucose level in the surgical diabetic patient. *Arch Surg* 1976; 3: 945–9.
57. Beaser SB. Surgical management. In Ellenberg M, Rifkin H (eds), *Diabetes Mellitus: Theory and Practice*. New York: McGraw-Hill, 1970; pp 746–59.
58. Thomas DJB, Platt HS, Alberti KGMM. Insulin-dependent diabetes during the peri-operative period. An

assessment of continuous glucose–insulin–potassium infusion, and traditional treatment. *Anaesthesia* 1984; 39: 629–37.

59. Meyer EJ, Lorenzi M, Bohannon NV, Amend W, Feduska NJ, Salvatierra O, Forsham PH. Diabetic management by insulin infusion during major surgery. *Am J Surg* 1979; 137: 323–7.
60. Christiansen CL, Schurizek BA, Malling B, Knudson L, Alberti KGMM, Hermansen K. Insulin treatment of the insulin-dependent diabetic patient undergoing minor surgery. Continuous intravenous infusion versus subcutaneous administration. *Anaesthesia* 1988; 43: 533–7.
61. Brogard JM, Diebunsch P, Guillausseau PJ, Grimaud D, Lambert H, Massable P, Scherpereel P. Diabète et anesthésie: prise en charge du diabétique en période opératoire. *Diabète Métab* 1995; 21: 197–206.
62. Meyers EF, Alberts D, Gordon MO. Perioperative control of blood glucose in diabetic patients: a two-step protocol. *Diabetes Care* 1986; 9: 40–5.
63. Woodruff RE, Lewis SB, McLeskey CH, Graney WF. Avoidance of surgical hyperglycemia in diabetic patients. *JAMA* 1980; 244: 166–8.
64. Watts NB, Gebhart SSP, Clark RV, Phillips LS. Postoperative management of diabetes mellitus: steady-state glucose control with bedside algorithm for insulin adjustment. *Diabetes Care* 1987; 10: 722–8.
65. Raucoules-Aime M, Ichai C, Roussel LJ, Romagnan MJ, Gastaud P, Dolisi C, Grimaud D. Comparison of two methods of i.v. insulin administration in the diabetic patient during the perioperative period. *Br J Anaesth* 1994; 72: 5–10.
66. Sato T, Hoshi H, Kumon T, Kitakaze Y, Watanabe R, Kobayashi T, Yoshinoga K. Managing diabetic surgical patients with glucose-free saline and insulin. *Diabetes Res Clin Pract* 1988; 5: 191–5.
67. Clark JDA, Currie J, Hartog M. Management of diabetes in surgery: a survey of current practice by anaesthetists. *Diabet Med* 1992; 9: 271–4.
68. Simmons D, Morton K, Laughton SJ, Scott DJ. A comparison of two intravenous regimens among surgical patients with insulin-dependent diabetes mellitus. *Diabetes Educ* 1994; 20: 422–7.
69. Husband DJ, Thai AC, Alberti KGMM. Management of diabetes during surgery with glucose–insulin–potassium infusion. *Diabet Med* 1986; 3: 69–74.
70. Shuman CR. Diabetes mellitus and surgery. In Galloway JA, Potvin JH, Shuman CR (eds), *Diabetes Mellitus*, 9th edn. Indianapolis: Eli Lilly, 1988; pp 242–51.
71. Nygren JO, Thorell A, Soop M, Efendic S, Brismar K, Karpe F, Nair KS, Ljungqvist O. Perioperative insulin and glucose infusion maintains normal insulin sensitivity after surgery. *Am J Physiol* 1998; 275; E410–8.
72. Petersen L, Caldwell J, Hoffman J. Insulin adsorption to polyvinylchloride surfaces with implications for constant infusion therapy. *Diabetes* 1976; 25: 72–4.
73. Talbot EM. Dangers of adding insulin to intravenous infusion bags with fixed needle syringes. *BMJ* 1984; 289: 678–80.
74. Thai AC, Husband DJ, Gill GV, Alberti KGMM. Management of diabetes during surgery. A retrospective study of 112 cases. *Diabète Métab* 1984; 10: 65–70.
75. Jaspers CAJJ, Elte JWF, Olthof G. Perioperative diabetes regulation with the help of a standard protocol. *Neth J Med* 1994; 44: 122–30.
76. Hutchinson AS, Shenkin A. BM strips: how accurate are they in general wards? *Diabet Med* 1984; 1: 225–6.
77. Price CP, Burrin JM, Nattrass M. Extralaboratory blood glucose measurement: a policy statement. *Diabet Med* 1988; 5: 705–9.
78. Gill GV, Sherif IH, Alberti KGMM. Management of diabetes during open heart surgery. *Br J Surg* 1981; 68: 171–2.
79. Thomas DJB, Hinds CJ, Rees GM. The management of insulin dependent diabetes during cardiopulmonary bypass and general surgery. *Anaesthesia* 1983; 38: 1047–52.
80. Ekroth R, Nilsson F, Berggren H, Feddersen K, Holm G, Holm J, Milocco I, Schersten T, William-Olsson G. Insulin sensitivity and glucose uptake in the course of surgical treatment for valvular aortic stenosis. *Scand J Thorac Cardiovasc Surg* 1982; 16: 137–40.
81. Stephens JW, Krause AH, Peterson CA, Bass JJ, Hartman JE, Solomon NW, Ward WK. The effect of glucose priming solutions in diabetic patients undergoing coronary artery bypass grafting. *Ann Thorac Surg* 1988; 45: 544–7.
82. Crock PA, Ley CJ, Martin IK, Alford FP, Best JD. Hormonal and metabolic changes during hypothermic coronary artery bypass surgery in diabetic and non-diabetic subjects. *Diabet Med* 1988; 5: 47–52.
83. Elliott MJ, Gill GV, Home PD, Noy GA, Holden MP, Alberti KGMM. A comparison of two regimens for the management of diabetes during open-heart surgery. *Anaesthesia* 1984; 60: 364–8.
84. McKnight CK, Elliott MJ, Pearson DT, Holden MP, Alberti KGMM. The effects of four different crystalloid bypass pump-priming fluids upon the metabolic response to cardiac operation. *J Thorac Cardiovasc Surg* 1985; 90: 97–111.
85. Watson BG, Elliott MJ, Pay DA, Williamson M. Diabetes mellitus and open heart surgery. A simple practical closed-loop infusion system for blood glucose control. *Anaesthesia* 1986; 41: 250–7.
86. Lazar HL, Chipkin S, Philippides G, Bao Y, Apstein C. Glucose–insulin–potassium solutions improve outcomes in diabetics who have coronary artery operations. *Ann Thorac Surg* 2000; 70: 145–50.
87. Devineni R, McKenzie FN. Surgery for coronary artery disease in patients with diabetes mellitus. *Can J Surg* 1985; 28: 367–70.
88. Lawire GM, Morris GC, Glaeser DH. Influence of diabetes mellitus on the results of coronary bypass surgery. *JAMA* 1986; 256: 1967–71.
89. Lean MEJ, Pearson DWM, Sutherland HW. Insulin management during labour and delivery in mothers with diabetes. *Diabet Med* 1990; 7: 162–4.
90. Leiper JM, Paterson KR, Lunan CB, MacCuish AC. A comparison of biosynthetic human insulin with porcine insulin in the blood glucose control of diabetic pregnancy. *Diabet Med* 1986; 3: 49–51.
91. Gill GV, Benbow S. Managing surgery in the elderly diabetic patients. In Sinclair AJ, Finucane P (eds), *Diabetes in Old Age*, 2nd edn. Chichester, UK: Wiley, 2000; pp 177–85.
92. Goldberg NJ, Wingert TD, Levin SR, Wilson SE, Viljoen JF. Insulin therapy in the diabetic surgical patient: metabolic and hormone response to low dose insulin infusion. *Diabetes Care* 1981; 4: 279–84.
93. Hall GM. Diabetes and anaesthesia—a promise unfulfilled? *Anaesthesia* 1984; 39: 627–8.
94. Hoogwerf BJ. Postoperative management of the diabetic patient. *Med Clin North Am* 2001; 85: 1213–28.

Diabetes and Public Health

100

Screening for Diabetes and Glucose Intolerance

Jonathan E. Shaw*, Gary Dowse†, Paul Zimmet*, and K.G.M.M. Alberti‡

**International Diabetes Institute, Melbourne, Australia, †Department of Health, Perth, Australia, and ‡University of Newcastle upon Tyne, Newcastle upon Tyne, UK*

Questions of "if," "when," and "how" to screen for diabetes, mellitus and related disorders of abnormal glucose tolerance have caused confusion, debate, and conflict for several decades. Contributing to this has been (1) the lack of standardized diagnostic criteria; (2) inadequate understanding of the natural history of glucose intolerance; (3) failure to include control populations in evaluation; (4) lack of appropriate cost–benefit analysis; and (5) naive enthusiasm for unsubstantiated therapeutic interventions.

Following the establishment of compatible and internationally accepted classifications and diagnostic criteria by the National Diabetes Data Group (NDDG) [1] and the World Health Organization (WHO) [2, 3], it was hoped that research workers might be able to answer many of the questions that remained concerning screening for diabetes. Unfortunately, to date some of these issues remain unresolved. However, enthusiasm for screening has increased in recent years for several reasons. There is now clear evidence that interventions in type 2 diabetes improve outcomes [4, 5]; that despite increasing awareness of diabetes, a substantial proportion of cases remain undiagnosed [6]; and that type 2 diabetes can be prevented or at least delayed [7–9].

This chapter focuses on screening directed toward detecting asymptomatic stages of diabetes [type 1, type 2, and gestational diabetes mellitus (GDM)], as well as screening for impaired glucose tolerance (IGT) and impaired fasting glycemia (IFG). Discussion of screening for specific complications can be found elsewhere in this book.

It is pertinent first to consider recognized definitions of screening; its potential scope within both the population and the health services; and those attributes of disease, screening test, and health system thought to be desirable for successful screening programs. Methods of evaluating screening services are discussed in general terms, before considering the historical development of screening as applied to diabetes detection, together with some reflections on limitations in our current knowledge of the relative prognostic value of glucose intolerance with normal basal glucose levels versus fasting hyperglycemias and raised glycated protein levels. Following this, various methods of screening are considered, and finally the potential application of screening to different categories of the diabetes syndrome is discussed.

DEFINITION AND RATIONALE FOR SCREENING

"Screening" was defined by the US Commission on Chronic Illness [10] as "the presumptive identification of unrecognized disease or defect by the application of tests, examinations or other procedures which can be applied rapidly. Screening tests sort out apparently well persons who probably have a disease from those who probably do not." The Commission further stated that "a screening test is not intended to be diagnostic," and specified that persons with conditions detected by screening exercises should be referred to their physician for definitive diagnosis and treatment if appropriate. This separation of screening and diagnostic tests, however, is not as clear for

International Textbook of Diabetes Mellitus, Third Edition. Edited by R. A. DeFronzo, E. Ferrannini, H. Keen, and P. Zimmet.
 ISBN: 0-471-48655-8.

diabetes as it is for many other diseases, since measurement of blood glucose is used for both.

Thus defined, screening is implicitly a tool for use in the prevention of onset of disease or complications of disease. Screening can be considered as a means of "primary" prevention of resultant diseases such as coronary heart disease and stroke through identifying individuals with modifiable risk factors such as cigarette smoking or hypercholesterolemia. By analogy, screening to detect IGT (considered here as a "risk factor" for onset of diabetes) and obesity could also be considered as primary preventive measures for type 2 diabetes.

More conventionally, however, screening fulfills a "secondary" preventive function through detection of presymptomatic disease, and intervention is directed toward preventing the development of complications. In some instances, treatment may lead to disease *cure* (e.g. tuberculosis discovered on screening radiograph), but in the context of chronic noncommunicable disease such as hypertension and diabetes, disease *control* is the aim, with a resultant reduction in associated morbidity and mortality.

SCOPE OF SCREENING

Screening may take place on a number of levels with varying implications for health sector costs. In the past, screening for diabetes has commonly taken place in tents or caravans situated in diverse locations such as municipal parks and suburban shopping centers. In such "mass" or "community" screening programs, whole populations are subjected to simple and quick tests. Mass screening exercises are often conducted by lay groups such as diabetes associations and, given their usual random occurrence, are "mass" only in a desultory fashion. This type of screening is probably more effective at fund-raising and creating community awareness than in positively influencing disease in screenees [11].

Alternatively, such programs may be sponsored by government health authorities. In these cases, coverage of the population is more complete, goals are more likely to have been clearly defined, and program planning more considered (although often not matched by results). At present, however, there are no noninfectious diseases for which mass indiscriminate screening of whole communities is likely to offer overall benefit.

For chronic diseases, "selective," "discriminate," or "high risk" screening offers the most attractive and cost-effective approach [12, 13]. This, too, can be considered on two levels. First, there are organized and usually government-sponsored programs where a serious attempt is made to cover all of the target group. These programs require a captive population, either through the responsible authorities visiting a common gathering point of the target screenees, or by requiring individuals to visit special facilities. In the first case, examples are routine screenings of school students carried out in some countries for conditions such as deafness or poor vision, and Mantoux or Heaf tuberculin testing to determine the requirement for BCG inoculation. In the latter case, immigrants are required to have a chest X-ray for tuberculosis detection before entrance to some countries. Similarly, although there is no obligation to attend, some countries have established organized breast cancer screening programs for middle-aged and elderly women, using mobile vans and/or central clinics.

Secondly, and more commonly, selective screening is conducted on an opportunistic "case-finding" basis by physicians or other health workers in subgroups of the population considered to be at high risk of the disease in question, at the time of a visit, usually for some unrelated matter. This is the situation in which most cervical cancer, diabetes, and cardiovascular disease (CVD) screening is undertaken in both developed and underdeveloped countries.

The extent to which such screening is institutionalized and standardized varies considerably both within and between countries. Factors determining the extent of screening activities in any particular country include the degree of economic development, the nature of the disease burden, the structure of—and resources available to—the primary health care network, and the extent of community, political, and physician interest in disease prevention activities.

"Multiphasic" screening, whereby a number of conditions may be screened for at one time, perhaps at regular intervals, has been considered a more cost-effective manner of screening [12, 13], and diabetes has been a component of such programs in the past [14]. Multiphasic screening is commonly performed in hospital practice, particularly in older patients, when a range of hematological, biochemical, and microbiological investigations are routinely and rather indiscriminately carried out at the time of admission. The extent of multiphasic screening within any community probably bears a positive relation to wealth, and an inverse relation to health status [13].

The diabetes screening literature is replete with epidemiological studies, the principal aims of which are to describe the prevalence and distribution of glucose intolerance, and to a greater or lesser extent, to investigate etiological factors and natural history. Although these studies often attempt to arrive at their prevalence estimate by application of "screening tests" [15, 16] or may compare the characteristics (in terms of sensitivity, specificity, and predictive value) of various procedures in relation to their "gold standard" definition [15, 17], they should be seen primarily as descriptive epidemiological studies. Their consideration as studies of screening, or even as "screening programs," [16, 18] may in part be responsible for

Table 1 Desirable characteristics for disease screening programs

Disease characteristics
(1) The disease should be an *important* health problem—this could be considered in terms of prevalence, severity (attributable morbidity and mortality), and economic and social cost to the community
(2) The natural history of the condition should be adequately understood, particularly the rate and determinants of progression from inapparent to symptomatic disease
(3) There should be a detectable preclinical phase to the condition
(4) A safe and accessible form of treatment must be available
(5) There should be clear indications of when, how, and in whom to use the treatment—it should necessarily improve the course and prognosis of the condition in detected presymptomatic individuals
Test characteristics
(6) The test should be safe and acceptable to screenees
(7) It should detect presymptomatic disease with appropriate validity (sensitivity and specificity) and repeatability, and the assessment of the usefulness of a screening test should include consideration of these indices
Program and health system characteristics
(8) Facilities and staff for follow-up of positive screenees for definitive diagnostic testing and subsequent treatment must be available
(9) Costs of screening, subsequent diagnostic testing, and resultant treatment should be acceptable in comparison with costs that would have been incurred in the absence of the program, and/or in the face of alternative uses
(10) Screening should be a continuing process, implying the need for at least some systematic integration into health care services and training of appropriate personnel. Moreover, the program must reach its target population

the lack of evaluated projects conceived and conducted as screening programs, and incorporating specific interventions.

Recommendations for screening for a range of conditions, such as diabetes, hypercholesterolemia, and breast and cervical cancer, have been made periodically by review bodies and as commentaries in leading medical journals, but considerable controversy surrounds many of the issues involved [19–32]. Even if recommendations were unanimous, there will always remain variation in the enthusiasm with which, firstly, doctors and other health workers offer the suggested screening service, and secondly, the target population takes advantage of services offered [33].

It has been a common observation in developed countries that those who tend to ask for and accept screening (the "worried well") are often those who least need it. Individuals from the lower socioeconomic groups, where rates of chronic diseases are higher, are less likely to be screened [13]. To counter this trend, awareness must be improved and resources made available in appropriate areas. A goal of complete uptake (even in clearly defined high-risk groups) seems unrealistically Utopian for most societies without some form of rigid institutionalism. Given the lack of convincing evidence for cost-effectiveness of most screening programs, it seems unlikely at this stage that governments will warmly embrace such major structural change to health services.

DESIRABLE CHARACTERISTICS FOR SCREENING PROGRAMS

Important principles that need to be considered before the establishment of screening programs were succinctly proposed by Wilson and Jungner [34] in 1968. Their points are presented in modified fashion under the three major headings of disease characteristics, test characteristics, and program and health system characteristics in Table 1.

ASSESSMENT OF SCREENING TESTS

The *repeatability* or *reliability* (the amount of agreement when a test is repeated or reassessed) of a screening test is not only an important determinant of its validity (the degree to which a test correctly classifies people with respect to the condition of interest), but it also influences the level at which referral for further testing is desirable. For tests with poor repeatability, thresholds lower than for tests with greater repeatability will be required to ensure that the same individuals are detected. A lack of repeatability is more important for screening tests (where subject misclassification has undesirable consequences) than for tests used in epidemiological surveys, where misclassification of individuals does not unduly influence estimates of disease frequency, on the assumption that the variation in measurements is random and will average out [35].

Although laboratory methods are available for measuring blood glucose accurately and precisely [36], there is still considerable random biological variation in any individual's blood glucose results, even under the standardized conditions of an oral glucose tolerance test (OGTT) [14, 37]; this has important implications for misclassification rates, particularly in subjects whose levels fall close to cutoff values. It should be noted, however, that a test can be highly repeatable but still have poor validity (as reflected by sensitivity and specificity).

The *sensitivity* of a screening test refers to its ability to identify correctly subjects with the disease or condition

Table 2 Method of determining screening test characteristics in relation to true disease status (all numbers are hypothetical)

	True disease status		
	Positive	Negative	Total
Screening test status			
Positive	a (40)	b (100)	$a+b$ (140)
Negative	c (10)	d (900)	$c+d$ (910)
Total	$a+c$ (50)	$b+d$ (1000)	$a+b+c+d$ (1050)

$$\text{Prevalence} = \frac{a+c}{a+b+c+d} = \frac{50}{1050} = 4.8\%$$

$$\text{Sensitivity} = \frac{a}{a+c} = \frac{40}{50} = 80.0\%$$

$$\text{Specificity} = \frac{d}{b+d} = \frac{900}{1000} = 90.0\%$$

$$\text{Predictive value (positive test)} = \frac{a}{a+b} = \frac{40}{140} = 28.6\%$$

$$\text{Predictive value (negative test)} = \frac{d}{c+d} = \frac{900}{910} = 98.9\%$$

of interest [12, 13]. A test with 80% sensitivity will correctly detect 8 out of 10 diseased individuals—those not identified are called "false negatives" (Table 2). These people gain little from a screening test and may be indirectly harmed if, for instance, they subsequently ignore the development of symptoms because of the false reassurance of a negative test. A lack of sensitivity may have disastrous consequences for conditions such as phenylketonuria, where a missed diagnosis may lead to irreparable brain damage. False-negative screenees in diabetes screening programs are less likely to come to great harm. In screening for GDM, however, it has been argued that tests with greater sensitivity are required than those employed in nonpregnant subjects—this implies a lowering of the values accepted as indicating a positive test [38–40].

Specificity is the ability of a screening test to identify correctly "normal" individuals [12, 13]. A test that misclassifies 1 out of 10 well persons as having the disease has a 90% specificity (Table 2). The misclassified subject is a "false positive" and suffers through the inconvenience, expense, and anxiety of undergoing unnecessary further diagnostic tests.

An ideal screening test should be both highly sensitive and specific, but unfortunately a compromise must usually be reached, as sensitivity and specificity have an inverse relationship–increasing specificity will result in more false-negative screenees and a lack of sensitivity (Figure 1). A lack of specificity (with corresponding increased sensitivity) will result in increased costs to a screening service, because of the need for false-positive screenees to undergo further diagnostic tests. Highly specific screening tests are desirable in situations where definitive diagnostic tests may be expensive, dangerous, or unpleasant, and when a lack of sensitivity is not critical (such as for diseases with long preclinical phases where the consequences of a false-negative screen for prognosis are unlikely to be grave).

Predictive value (PV) is a useful indicator in assessing the cost-effectiveness of a screening program [13]. The

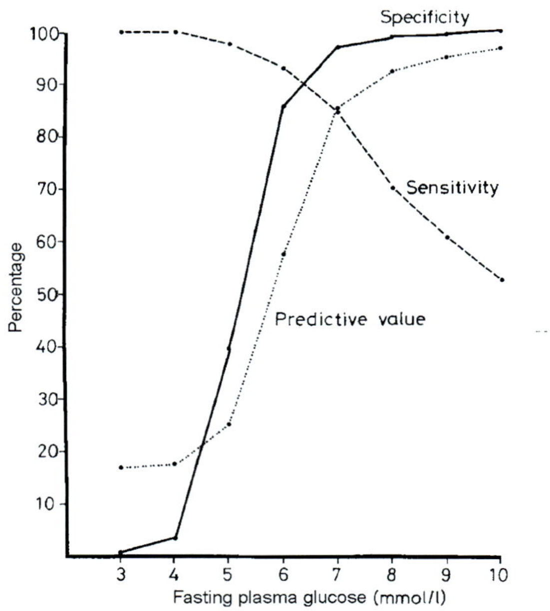

Figure 1 The relationship of sensitivity, specificity, and predictive value at different levels of fasting plasma glucose as a screening test for undetected or untreated type 2 diabetes in Micronesian Nauruans aged 20–74 years (type 2 diabetes defined as plasma glucose value 11.1 mmol/l or above, 2 h following a 75 g OGTT)

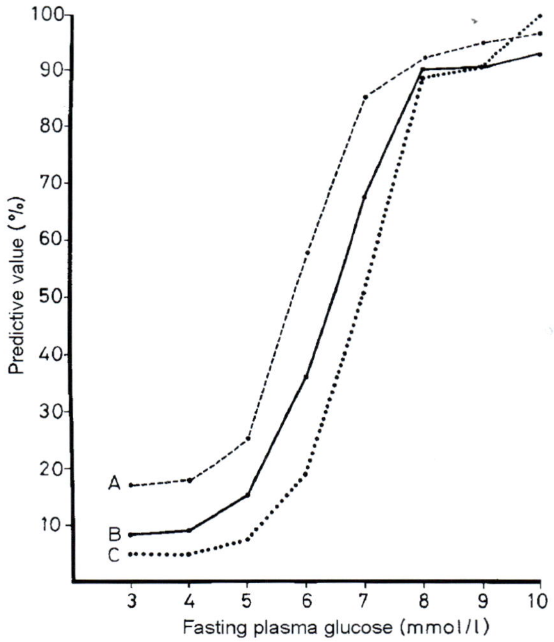

Figure 2 Predictive value of different levels of fasting plasma glucose as a screening test for undetected or untreated type 2 diabetes in adults aged 20–74 years in three populations with varying disease prevalence (type 2 diabetes defined as plasma glucose value 11.1 mmol/l or above 2 h following a 75 g OGTT). (A) Micronesian Nauruans (prevalence 17.1%); (B) Fijian Indians (prevalence 8.7%); (C) Fijian Melanesians (urban) (prevalence 5.1%)

PV of a positive test is the proportion of test positives who are proven to have the condition following definitive testing. For instance, if 100 of 1000 tested individuals have a positive screen, but only 25 are confirmed to have the condition, then the PV of the test is 25%. Conversely, the PV of a negative test is the proportion of those with a negative test who truly do not have the disease (Table 2). Predictive value is very prevalence-dependent; it can be improved by applying the test in subgroups with higher prevalence. This relationship is illustrated in Figure 2. It can be seen that, at any screening cutoff level, the PV of fasting plasma glucose testing for detection of type 2 diabetes (defined by the 2-h glucose value alone) is greater in the higher prevalence population.

High-risk screening takes advantage of the relationship between PV and prevalence: not only is expense spared by excluding the majority of the population from screening in the first place, but fewer unnecessary follow-up diagnostic tests are undertaken because of the higher PV of the screening test that arises implicitly through screening in higher prevalence subgroups. For abnormalities of glucose tolerance these include older age groups, the overweight, those with a family history, women with a history of GDM, and certain ethnic groups with high prevalence. The latter include Asian Indians in immigrant communities [41], Micronesian and Polynesian Pacific island populations [42], and aborigines of Australia [43] and the Americas [44].

A further point concerning screening for glucose intolerance in high-prevalence populations is that the sensitivity of screening tests is also improved [15, 45]. For categoric ("yes/no") conditions such as cancer, the sensitivity and specificity of screening tests are unrelated to disease prevalence. However, for a continuously distributed variable such as plasma glucose and where diagnostic thresholds are fixed, a screening test will have higher sensitivity in populations where the glucose distribution is shifted to the right, or where the distribution is bimodal [15]. This increased sensitivity has also been attributed to more severe hyperglycemia in diabetic patients of high-prevalence populations relative to those in low-prevalence populations [15]. The phenomenon can be appreciated from Figure 3 where the behavior of fasting plasma glucose levels as a screening test for type 2 diabetes in different populations is plotted. At any cutoff level the sensitivity of the test is greatest in the high-prevalence population. The relationship is somewhat more complicated, however, as indicated by the lower sensitivities in the intermediate-prevalence population.

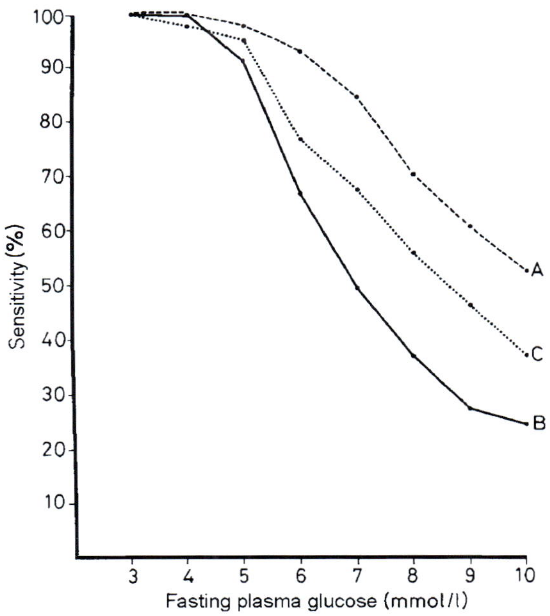

Figure 3 Sensitivity of different levels of fasting plasma glucose as a screening test for undetected or untreated type 2 diabetes in adults aged 20–74 years in three populations with varying disease prevalence (type 2 diabetes defined as plasma glucose value 11.1 mmol/l or above, 2 h following a 75 g OGTT). (A) Micronesian Nauruans (prevalence 17.1%); (B) Fijian Indians (prevalence 8.7%); (C) Fijian Melanesians (urban) (prevalence 5.1%)

EVALUATION OF SCREENING PROGRAMS

Many disease screening programs have been instituted in the past without proper evaluation either before their establishment or during their operation [46]. Both screening procedures and programs for diabetes have generally been poorly evaluated. Fortunately, there is now recognition of the need for proper evaluation [19, 27, 29, 47].

Costs and Benefits

Evaluation must rest finally with some form of cost–benefit analysis where an attempt is made to rationalize the costs and benefits that accrue to three diverse elements: screened individuals, the health services, and the community at large. The major points requiring consideration are summarized in Table 3. At the level of individuals, costs may include the following: financial loss due to travel, time off work, and further medical consultation and diagnostic testing; the pain and discomfort of procedures undergone; and the unnecessary anxiety caused to false-positive screenees. Benefits include the earlier diagnosis of disease with resulting improved health and longevity, and the reassurance of good health in correctly identified, disease-free individuals.

For health services, costs that need to be considered are the direct and indirect costs associated with staff and resources (test materials, facilities, etc.) involved in the screening program, and the ensuing costs of further consultations, diagnostic investigations, and treatment (which might in some cases be unwarranted). On the beneficial side, intervention in the early stages of disease might lead to monetary savings on more expensive treatment, hospitalization, and rehabilitation services. Although they carried out an incomplete cost–benefit analysis, Genuth et al. [48] calculated that expenses accrued over 6 years to a mass screening program in Cleveland in the United States could be offset if 4.2% of 8400 previously undetected diabetic patients were spared 1 week of hospitalization that they might have required if diagnosis was left until the appearance of symptoms. However, even if their figures for the direct and indirect costs of the program were correct, and although the possibility of such savings on hospitalization seems superficially to be eminently plausible, evaluation based on numerous assumptions is always questionable.

For the community, the costs of a screening program can be considered mainly in terms of the opportunity cost of scarce resources (money, personnel, and facilities) diverted from other potential uses, either within the health context (such as primary prevention) or outside it (social welfare, education, and so on). Benefits of the screening program to the community might conversely follow from overall savings on health expenditure, which can be put to other uses, and as described in the literature of diabetes screening, a much-vaunted role in increasing public awareness and education [14]. It is likely, however, that there are much more efficient methods of educating the public about diabetes than through screening programs.

Measures and Pitfalls

Important indices that need to be considered in evaluation of screening programs include the following *process* measures—the proportion of the target population who actually receive screening, the prevalence of disease detected in screenees, total expenditure on the program, the cost per screenee and case detected, and the PV of a positive test.

Additionally, important measures of *outcome* must be reckoned with. In the first instance, the frequency of complications such as proteinuria, retinopathy, hypertension, and ischemic heart disease, already present at the time of diagnosis, can be compared in screen-detected and symptom-detected cases. Subsequently, measures of morbidity (number of hospitalizations, days off work, frequency of development of particular complications, and mortality) can be determined and compared with a reference group.

It is important to consider, however, potential biases that act to exaggerate the efficacy of screening [13]. First, it is possible that those cases detected by screening represent the milder end of the disease spectrum with better prognoses (more severe cases present earlier in their course with symptoms) and might not normally have high

Table 3 Costs and benefits associated with disease screening programs

Level	Costs	Benefits
Individuals	Financial: travel, loss of earnings, medical consultation, diagnostic tests, treatment Other: pain and discomfort of procedures, anxiety	Improved health outcome Reassurance of health Potentially improved earning capacity
Health services	Direct and indirect costs of staff and resources allocated to screening Further diagnostic investigations and treatment	Potential savings on treatment costs if disease had not been detected early
Community	Opportunity cost of resources diverted from other potential uses to screening program	Potential benefit of savings on overall health expenditure diverted to other uses Public awareness and education

complication rates anyway. This is known as *length bias*. *Lead-time bias* operates where screen-detected cases appear to take longer to develop complications, and survive longer, than do symptom-detected cases; in reality this may be a false impression because of their diagnosis has effectively been brought forward in time.

Comparisons might also be biased by inclusion amongst screen-detected groups of a number of misclassified individuals, or those who may under normal circumstances (that is, without medical intervention) have reverted to normal glucose tolerance. This phenomenon is known as *pseudodisease* [13]. It is unclear how often this may occur amongst those whose glucose levels fall within the type 2 diabetes range, but the high frequency of "reversion" to normal tolerance in individuals originally classified as having IGT is well documented [49, 50].

A fourth factor that may bias evaluation of diabetes screening programs is *prognostic selection*, whereby those who are willing to attend screening services are likely to be more health conscious and amenable to undergoing treatment and changing lifestyle than are those not interested enough to undergo screening in the first place [13].

Methods of Evaluation

Comparison of clinical characteristics and outcome measures between screen-detected and symptom-detected cases is a common method of evaluation (often used for cancer screening programs), but is subject to the four sources of bias described above. The extent of such biases is difficult to determine, however, and little can be done to account for them beyond being aware of their potential influence, if this form of evaluation is undertaken.

Another less than satisfactory approach is to compare outcome measures before and after the start of screening activities. It may be difficult to discount the influence of temporal changes in disease patterns, although the incorporation of a control population into the "before and after" design may allow a reasonable assessment of the influence of secular trends. The use of a "before and after" comparison (with or without a control group) requires that appropriate measures of disease outcome have been collected in the past, and, in order to optimize the chance of drawing conclusions, that the newly introduced screening service is implemented widely [13, 51]. Case-control techniques have been utilized successfully in studies of cancer screening programs [13, 19], but are likely to be very difficult to apply to evaluation of diabetes screening.

Experimental methods will ultimately give the most objective answer to questions concerning the efficacy of screening services. Unfortunately, logistic and ethical considerations probably preclude the use of randomized controlled trials. It would be most difficult to randomize asymptomatic individuals to screening versus nonscreening groups, and it would be equally impractical and perhaps unethical to screen individuals for diabetes but act on the result in only half of the screenees. Thus, it would appear that the most satisfactory method of assessing diabetes screening programs will be by comparing outcome measures between control or reference communities and a demonstration "screening" community. The problems of ensuring comparability of such areas will need to be considered, but the method is the most likely to provide acceptable evidence for the impact of diabetes screening services.

The need for proper evaluation of diabetes screening programs has long been recognized. A meeting of experts held in Atlanta, USA, in 1979 [19] formally recommended that screening in nonpregnant populations should be conducted only in the context of well-designed research projects, some of which might specifically attempt to evaluate the effectiveness of screening. To date, apart from studies that have assessed the validity of alternative screening tests [15, 17], no properly controlled evaluated studies of diabetes screening programs have been reported. There is, therefore, no convincing evidence for the efficacy of screening asymptomatic nonpregnant persons for glucose intolerance.

HISTORY OF SCREENING FOR DIABETES

Early attempts to detect diabetes by screening were based on tests for glycosuria performed in World War I military recruits and life insurance applicants (see review by West [14]). After World War II, screening programs in the United States began to be instituted on a mass basis in a number of states, apparently following the lead of the American Diabetes Association (ADA), and often involving contributions from both government and lay groups [14, 48].

Screening for diabetes has not been so warmly embraced outside the United States. Surveys in places such as Birmingham, UK [52], Busselton, Australia [33], and Bergen, Norway [53], were primarily epidemiological studies, which also attempted to answer questions about community screening programs. A mass screening project in Ferrara, Italy, was reported to have favorably influenced the rate of progression of IGT to clinical diabetes, and to have led to a reduction in the incidence of type 2 diabetes in this community [54]; however, there are many potential biases in this study, and the optimistic conclusions of the authors seem unwarranted.

One of the better-documented and better-evaluated programs was that conducted during the 1960s and 1970s in Cleveland, USA, on over 600 000 persons, and based on a screening blood glucose test 2 h following a 75-g glucose load [47, 48, 55]. Eventually, this mass screening program was downgraded to a more discriminating program wherein community detection for GDM was initiated, and further screening was performed only on request, particularly in subjects over the age of 40 years [55]. The reasons for the change largely reflected the lack of specificity and poor PV of the screening test [48, 55], with consequent worries concerning incorrect disease labeling in false-positive screenees [47], and the recognition that not enough was known about either the natural history of lesser degrees of glucose intolerance or the effectiveness and safety of treatment in this group [47, 55].

A consensus conference in Atlanta, USA, in 1978 recommended that evidence available at that time did not support the need for either community *or* high-risk (except in pregnancy) screening programs for detection of states of asymptomatic glucose intolerance [19]. Their conclusions were drawn against the background of (1) availability of more objective assessment of diabetes screening programs [55]; (2) a growing interest by epidemiologists in the study of diabetes [14]; and (3) results of the University Group Diabetes Project (UGDP) which suggested that treatment of asymptomatic type 2 diabetes with oral hypoglycemic agents did not favorably influence disease end points [56].

In 1989 the ADA released a position statement [26] that appeared to legitimize community and physician screening programs for type 2 diabetes, although the statement did recommend that measurement of blood glucose should only be performed in subjects with demonstrated risk factors. As subsequently pointed out by Nathan and Singer [27], this liberalization of the "official" attitude to screening seemed unfounded, as there was little new evidence to challenge the previous consensus view that screening for type 2 diabetes is inappropriate [19, 20, 25, 57, 58].

Despite calls for more research into the effectiveness of diabetes screening programs [19, 29, 59], little new work has appeared recently. A report from New South Wales, Australia, looked at the results of mass detection exercises in that state on the basis of random blood glucose measurement ascertained with portable reflectance meters, and found the test to be insensitive and surprisingly nonspecific, and that a high proportion of positive screenees did not seek follow-up testing [11].

LIMITATIONS IN SCREENING FOR GLUCOSE INTOLERANCE—WHEN IS IT DIABETES?

There is no doubt that type 1 diabetes is a life-threatening disease, and that patients with clinically diagnosed type 2 diabetes require therapy. There remains some doubt, however, whether asymptomatic individuals (especially those with normal levels of fasting glucose, but who demonstrate abnormalities of glucose tolerance in response to glucose loads) who are identified by screening programs will benefit from detection and treatment [59, 60]. The current criteria for diagnosis of diabetes are largely based on longitudinal studies in two British cohorts [61, 62], and cross-sectional [63] and longitudinal [64] studies in Pima Indians, which demonstrated that "diabetes-specific" microvascular complications occurred only in subjects whose 2-h postload glucose concentrations exceeded 11.1 mmol/l. However, these studies did not adequately answer the question of whether the 2-h level was predictive of microvascular complications independently of the level of fasting glycemia [61–65].

In Pima Indians, retinopathy (but not nephropathy) did develop in 2 of 22 subjects with normal fasting plasma glucose (<7.8 mmol/l), but with 2-h levels ≥ 11.1 mmol/l [64]. Effectively, the legitimacy of the currently accepted 2-h diagnostic criterion as being sufficient for diagnosis of type 2 diabetes appears to rest on these two cases [65]. As they may well have had high fasting glucose levels in the past and/or soon after the single baseline OGTT, this seems rather insubstantial evidence on which to base disease definition.

Data from a longitudinal study conducted in the Micronesian Nauruan population, who have one of the highest incidence rates of type 2 diabetes yet recorded [49], support this view. Nauruans with high 2-h plasma glucose concentrations, but normal fasting glycemia, suffer microvascular complication rates (microalbuminuria and retinopathy) more compatible with rates seen in individuals with IGT than in diabetic patients who have fasting hyperglycemia [65].

Although the value of the 2-h glucose relative to fasting glycemia, as an independent predictor of microvascular disease, has not been established, evidence has emerged in the last few years of its importance in predicting CVD. Data from Mauritius, the Pacific, Japan, Europe, and the United States [66–69] have shown that 2-h glucose is a predictor of CVD and death. The effects appear to be independent of other traditional cardiovascular risk factors and of fasting glucose. The independence of the effect of 2-h over-fasting glucose is seen most markedly in those with nondiabetic fasting glucose levels. Limited data also suggest that the 2-h glucose is a better predictor of CVD than is glycated hemoglobin (HbA_{1c}) [70].

A major problem with these studies relates to the association of outcome events with unstable baseline information. The variability of the OGTT over both short and long time periods has been well documented [37, 49, 50, 71, 72] and initial misclassification of subjects in longitudinal studies may have a critical effect on outcome associations. It should be noted that the variability of the OGTT is mainly due to the 2-h value, rather than the more stable fasting value.

Thus, while some doubt and controversy remain, the balance of evidence is that there is merit in performing the OGTT, as the 2-h glucose value provides additional information about the disease status or risks of the individual.

METHODS AVAILABLE FOR DIABETES SCREENING FOR TYPE 2 DIABETES

The OGTT is the standard against which any screening test for type 2 diabetes must be compared. However, before fully accepting this, it is worth noting that each of HbA_{1c}, fasting, and 2-h glucose are similarly related to diabetic retinopathy [73]. Since this relationship with retinopathy is the primary means of setting diagnostic thresholds for diabetes, it might be reasonable to assign equal importance to each of the three tests, in terms of diagnosis and screening. Statements such as "fasting glucose is an insensitive test" for diabetes are therefore only true if it is accepted that the 2-h glucose is the "gold standard"—a belief that may have some supportive evidence, at least in terms of vascular disease [68], but is not proven. In reality, it is probably the case that abnormalities in any single glycaemic parameter are important, and that each parameter will detect many and miss some of the abnormalities identified by another.

Urine Glucose Testing

There is no place for urine testing as a screening tool where there is a means available (including reflectance meters) to measure blood glucose. Urine testing has neither acceptable sensitivity nor specificity [14, 71]. Its use can be advocated only where blood testing is either not available, or is particularly expensive. Even in the latter situation, however, costs involved in confirmatory testing in positive screenees (depending on the level accepted as positive) may eventually outweigh savings owing to initial use of urine tests. The renal threshold for glucose varies with age (higher), sex (lower in men), pregnancy (lower), and ethnic group, as well as demonstrating wide variability between individuals [14]. Hence the validity of urinary glucose as a standard screening test is highly questionable. Furthermore, sensitivity and specificity will vary depending on the level of glycosuria deemed significant, the state of hydration of subjects, and the type of test strips used.

Its sensitivity has been shown to rise from 16.7% for fasting values to 72.7% for 2-h postload values, with corresponding falls in specificity from 97.9% to 77.4% and PV (positive test) from 33.3% to 22.2%, using the previously promulgated diagnostic criteria in a British population [71]. In comparison with other potential screening tests such as fasting blood glucose, 2-h blood glucose, and glycohemoglobin, these figures are unappealing [14, 71].

Some research [61] and public-health-oriented [54] screening programs have in the past employed glycosuria as the initial screen in a multistage process. Such a method cannot be recommended, for a number of reasons. First, the prevalence of glucose intolerance will be underestimated because of the insensitivity of the first test. Second, if descriptive epidemiology and exploration of etiological hypotheses are to be pursued, then cases detected through such a multistage procedure are unlikely to be typical, leading to biased results. Third, if the principal aims relate to public health, and are presumably based on the belief that treating detected cases will improve their prognosis, then there seems little point in using an instrument acknowledged to be inferior.

The utility of testing urine with multitest strips as a screening tool during hospital admissions, primary health care contacts, and at general practitioner visits can also be questioned, unless there are specific indications for assessing other parameters such as hematuria and proteinuria. If one is really interested in screening for diabetes, then more sensitive and specific methods are indicated. However, where osmotic symptoms of diabetes are present, a positive urine test will be strongly supportive of the diagnosis.

Glycated Hemoglobin

Glycated hemoglobin is generally accepted as a useful guide to control blood glucose over the preceding 2–3 months. However, initial enthusiasm for its usefulness as a diagnostic and screening tool has waned in some [17, 74] but not all [29, 60, 71, 75–77] quarters.

Glycated hemoglobin has been shown to have superior sensitivity and specificity to casual blood glucose measurement in detecting type 2 diabetes [78], although these authors noted that glucose determination was cheaper, simpler, and quicker. However, depending on assay methods, studies have shown that glycated hemoglobin is either similar to [79, 80] or inferior to fasting blood glucose as a screening test for detecting type 2 diabetes or the combined group of IGT and type 2 diabetes [17, 78, 80].

Glycated hemoglobin measurement was also less effective when compared against 2-h postload glucose as a single screening test in a British population. With equivalent sensitivity of 90%, Forrest et al. [71] found that a screening 2-h postload glucose test had 93.3% specificity and 47.9% PV for type 2 diabetes confirmed in a second full OGTT (WHO criteria), as against 64.5 and 9.5%, respectively, for the screening glycohemoglobin. The latter's specificity was higher (85.3%), but still with a low PV of 14%, at the same level of sensitivity, when compared against "probable" diabetes as determined from the screening 2-h glucose value [71]. This difference apparently reflects the larger intraindividual coefficient of variation for the 2-h blood glucose level, compared with glycated hemoglobin.

Considerable but variable (perhaps related to methods) overlap has been observed in the glycated hemoglobin distributions of subjects with normal, impaired, and diabetic glucose tolerance, respectively [17, 71, 81, 82], which emphasizes the inadequacies of glycated hemoglobin measurement as a screening test, at least for IGT.

However, in the higher prevalence Pima Indian population, and using a superior liquid chromatography assay for HbA_{1c}, Little et al. [75] demonstrated a sensitivity of 85%, specificity of 91%, and positive PV of 73% for detecting diabetes defined by an OGTT. This suggests that with superior assays, and at least in high-prevalence groups, the performance characteristics of glycated hemoglobin as a screening test for diabetes (but not IGT) may be acceptable, particularly where it is logistically difficult to perform an OGTT, or for subjects to fast.

Serum fructosamine testing, largely because of its cheapness and ease of determination, was initially proposed as a potentially useful tool for diabetes screening [83], but this early enthusiasm was not vindicated in population screening exercises [84, 85]. The evidence suggests that the method has inappropriate sensitivity and PV for detection of glucose intolerance [74, 80, 82, 84, 85].

A recent study from Hong Kong [86] examined the utility of combining HbA_{1c} with fasting glucose, as an efficient means of screening for diabetes, and limiting the number of OGTTs that are required. Of all those subjects with FPG (fasting plasma glucose) $\geq$5.6 mmol/l, 19% had a "low risk" HbA_{1c} (below 5.5%); however, 14% of these in fact had undiagnosed diabetes (on the 2-h glucose). By comparison, 60% of those with the combination of FPG $\geq$5.6 mmol/l and HbA_{1c} $\geq$5.5%, and only 4% of those with FPG <5.6 mmol/l had undiagnosed diabetes. Thus, the addition of HbA_{1c} would have reduced the number of OGTTs required by 19%, would have labeled a small group of people as not needing further testing, even though 14% of this group had diabetes, and would have reduced the total number of people found to have diabetes by only 5%. Therefore, there may be some value in using HbA_{1c} as part of the screening process, although cost–benefit assessments would be needed.

The conclusion must be that with diabetes defined in terms of the glucose tolerance test, measurements of glycated proteins do not yet offer sufficient ability to discriminate between subjects with normal and abnormal glucose tolerance, although highly-specific assays for HbA_{1c} in high-prevalence populations may detect type 2 diabetes with acceptable sensitivity and specificity [75]. However, as has been discussed earlier, the validity of the OGTT for diagnosis of "real" diabetes [14, 60, 65, 81] has been questioned. Until further data on the relative prognostic value of glycated proteins and mild abnormalities of glucose tolerance are available, an open mind must be kept on the usefulness of glycated protein measurement as a screening and diagnostic test [29, 60, 76, 77, 81]. Furthermore, HbA_{1c} assays are still not fully standardized around the world. Thus, a cutoff value determined in any particular laboratory may not be directly applicable to all other laboratories, and so it is not possible, currently, to provide HbA_{1c} values that can be universally used in screening or diagnostic programs.

Blood Glucose and the OGTT

The various forms of abnormal glucose tolerance are defined in terms of raised blood glucose levels; with the diagnostic level depending on the nature of the specimen (venous or capillary; whole blood or plasma) and whether the blood is collected randomly (in relation to eating habit and time of day), in a fasting state, or at specified intervals following a standard glucose load [73, 87]. It is hardly surprising, therefore, that blood glucose levels are currently the best means of detecting states of glucose intolerance.

Fasting plasma glucose is often seen as the ideal first step in screening for glucose intolerance. It is simple and cheap, though requires overnight preparation (with the consequent cost and inconvenience implications of a further medical visit). Although used as a screening test, it may directly identify 60–70% of people with undiagnosed diabetes, without recourse to the OGTT [88, 89]. Furthermore, with the new category of impaired fasting glucose, it can also identify people with intermediate forms of glucose intolerance. Its limitations are that 30–40% of people with undiagnosed diabetes have a nondiabetic fasting glucose, and an even higher proportion of those with IGT have a completely normal fasting glucose. In one study, the median fasting plasma glucose of those with IGT was 5.4 mmol/l [90]. The properties of fasting plasma glucose (at a threshold of $\geq$6.1 mmol/l—i.e. the lower limit of IFG, rather than diabetes) as a screening tool for diabetes (diagnosed by the OGTT) have recently been reported in a number of studies using the new diagnostic thresholds for diabetes (Table 4). From these data, the median sensitivity for diabetes was 78%, and the median specificity was 91%. Thus, it is clear that using the FPG threshold of 6.1 mmol/l will result in approximately 20% of those with undiagnosed diabetes being missed. To improve this, a lower threshold (e.g., 5.5 mmol/l) could be used to select people who should be assessed further with an OGTT. This, of course, would necessarily lower the specificity of the test, and increase the number of individuals required to have the OGTT.

Random (or casual) blood glucose testing is the easiest and simplest form of blood glucose testing, since it requires no preparation of the patient. There are, however, only two studies [98, 99] that have examined the properties of random blood glucose testing (measured by reflectance meter in both studies) as a screening tool for diabetes (Table 5). Interestingly, in one of the studies [99], the performance of the test was related to postprandial time, and predicted diabetes better when measured in the earlier postprandial period (1–2 h). On the basis of the two studies, and by comparing Tables 4 and 5, it can be seen that in order to achieve a sensitivity of 80–90%, the specificity of a random glucose is likely to be considerably lower than that of a fasting glucose. There is, however, one caveat for this comparison. The design of the studies of

Table 4 Characteristics of fasting plasma glucose measurement as a screening test for type 2 diabetes in various populations*

Population	Number	Prevalence of undetected type 2 diabetes (%)	Sensitivity (%)	Specificity (%)	Predictive value (%)	
					Positive test	Negative test
United States (NHANES) [91, 92]	2 844	8.0	84	90	30	84
Holland [93]	2 540	6.9	88	88	30	91
United States (elderly) [94]	4 515	16.1	71	87	47	63
Hong Kong [95]	1 486	3.4	58	98	36	92
Australia [6]	11 247	3.6	72	91	17	89
Mauritius [96]	3 528	8.5	85	92	37	82
Japanese Brazilians [97]	647	21.9	92	92	72	83

* Fasting plasma glucose value of 6.1 mmol/l (110 mg/dl) or above constitutes a positive screening test. Type 2 diabetes is defined as a fasting plasma glucose value of 7.0 mmol/l (126 mg/dl) or over, or a plasma glucose value of 11.1 mmol/l (200 mg/dl) or over, 2 h following a 75 g OGTT.

random glucose measurements necessarily involved random testing and OGTTs to be performed on different days. However, the studies of fasting glucose involved only a single OGTT, in which classification by fasting glucose is compared to classification by the fasting and 2-h values combined. Given the day-to-day variation in blood glucose, these design differences would tend to favor the single-day studies of fasting glucose.

It has been suggested that a random plasma glucose of 5.6–11.0 mmol/l represents an uncertain range in which diabetes can be neither diagnosed nor confidently excluded [87, 100]. Such a result should be followed by an OGTT or fasting glucose, although it should be noted that the lower limit of 5.6 mmol/l has been selected rather arbitrarily. Overall, the limited data on random glucose testing would indicate that it is inferior to fasting glucose, and should only be used when there are difficulties in arranging a fasting test (e.g., work commitments or availability of glucose testing).

It should be noted that while a random glucose has significant limitations in screening asymptomatic individuals, it is generally unequivocal in individuals with clear symptoms of diabetes.

The 75 g OGTT has, in the last 20 years, become the gold standard for the diagnosis of diabetes. After several decades of varying practice, it has now been widely accepted, and the diagnostic thresholds recommended by the two most influential bodies (WHO and ADA) are identical [73, 87]. It should be noted that while many laboratories commonly measure and report 1-h glucose values, these cannot be used for diagnostic purposes, and indeed diagnostic thresholds for this time point are not available, although laboratories may quote "normal ranges." The recent revision of the fasting cut-point (from 7.8 mmol/l down to 7.0 mmol/l) [73, 87] has meant that the prevalence of diabetes by the fasting glucose is approximately the same as that according to the 2-h glucose (though this varies by age, obesity, and ethnicity), but the individuals identified as being diabetic by the two thresholds are not necessarily the same [89, 101]. At least in terms of CVD and mortality, those who are diabetic only on the 2-h value are at increased risk compared to normals [66].

Table 5 The performance of a random whole blood glucose as a screen for diabetes

Engelgau et al. (1995) [98]	
At sensitivity of 90%*	Median specificity 48–52% (according to age group)
At specificity of 90%	Median sensitivity 49–52%
Optimal	Median sensitivity 73–76%
	Median specificity 76–78%
Qiao et al. (1995) [99]	
Cutoff 5.8 mmol/l	Sensitivity 63%, specificity 85%†
Cutoff 5.2 mmol/l	Sensitivity 78%, specificity 62%†

* The cutoff value of random whole blood glucose for a sensitivity of 90% was 4.4–6.7, depending on age and postprandial period.
† Sensitivities and specificities were worse in women than men at all thresholds.

It should be emphasized again that, for clinical diagnosis, in those with symptoms, glucose tolerance tests are usually unnecessary [87]. For screening asymptomatic individuals to detect glucose intolerance, whether in the IGT or diabetes range, however, the inescapable conclusion is that casual and fasting blood specimens, and glycated proteins, are inadequate and that an OGTT is required.

Unfortunately, the OGTT has poor intraindividual repeatability, particularly in the IGT range and over short time periods [37, 50, 71, 72], and clinicians should therefore repeat tests from asymptomatic positive screenees before a final diagnosis is made. It also appears that there may be ethnic differences in the stability of an OGTT diagnosis of type 2 diabetes over time [72, 102]. Nevertheless, at least in Americans, the 2-h diagnostic level for type 2 diabetes seems to select individuals who, in the main, remain clearly diabetic when retested some years later [102]. It is standard practice that a diagnosis is only confirmed when both the first and repeat tests are above the diagnostic threshold, but it would probably be more logical to make a diagnosis in those whose *mean* value (from two tests) is over the diagnostic cut-point.

TO SCREEN OR NOT TO SCREEN?

Type 1 Diabetes

Unlike type 2 diabetes, type 1 diabetes does not have a prolonged asymptomatic period, and screening for unrecognized cases of the disease is not necessary. Therefore, for type 1 diabetes, screening might aim to identify those at risk of developing the disease in the future, and prevent it altogether. First-degree relatives of individuals with type 1 diabetes, particularly those who are either HLA identical or HLA haploidentical to a proband with type 1 diabetes, have an increased risk of developing the disease [103, 104]. Furthermore, a high proportion of those who ultimately develop diabetes carry islet cell antibodies (ICA), insulin autoantibodies (IAA), and antibodies to glutamic acid decarboxylase (GAD), for months to years before onset of disease, and overt decompensation may be heralded by a diminished acute insulin response during intravenous glucose tolerance tests [104–109]. On the basis of such evidence it is hoped that it might one day be possible to prevent progression to overt diabetes in individuals found to harbor these immunological, genetic, and biochemical markers [57, 104, 107, 110–112].

First-degree relatives are an easily identified "at-risk" group, and their numbers can be readily reduced to a "very high risk" group by ICA, IAA, and anti-GAD testing and glucose tolerance tests. If, however, onset of disease in this high-risk group cannot be prevented, then their identification through a series of increasingly invasive tests cannot be justified [113, 114]. Less intrusive education of family members in general concerning their increased risk, the identification of early symptoms, and the importance of not delaying medical attention in the event that such symptoms arise, is likely to be both considerably more cost-effective and humane than specific prediction of risk in individuals.

At present, it is generally accepted that screening of first-degree relatives of type 1 diabetes probands is justified only in the context of properly conducted intervention and other research studies [107, 110]. On the grounds that HLA haplotypes and alleles associated with type 1 diabetes are necessary, but not sufficient markers for disease, ICA and other autoantibody testing is recommended as the initial screening test in such studies, with combinations of immune and metabolic markers improving the PV for disease [104, 110].

To date, intervention trials of immunosuppressive and immunomodulatory agents in high-risk type 1 diabetes family members have had mixed success. While trials in recent onset type 1 diabetes with the immunosuppressive agents azothioprine or cyclosporine have demonstrated some short-term benefits in preserving islet B-cell function, long-term results have been disappointing [115–117], and the potential side effects of these therapies limit their use in prediabetic subjects [116–119]. Oral nicotinamide is another agent that had promising early results, but initial reports from the definitive trial have indicated that diabetes was not prevented (E. Gale, personal communication). Optimism about the potential of insulin to prevent type 1 diabetes has recently been dented by the Diabetes Prevention Trial, in which low-dose insulin neither delayed nor prevented the development of diabetes in children at high risk [109, 120]. More promisingly, a heat shock protein peptide [121], and an anti-CD3 monoclonal antibody [122] have been shown to preserve endogenous insulin production in recent onset type 1 diabetes, and long-term studies will now be required to determine if either of these drugs can prevent diabetes.

Notwithstanding the arguments above, the vast majority of cases of type 1 diabetes are sporadic in origin [123, 124], occurring in individuals with no family history of the disease. Hence even if primary prevention of onset were possible, screening would have to extend beyond families of known cases if any impact is to be made on the overall incidence of the disease. For this reason, there are high hopes that it may one day be feasible to screen all children for autoantibodies such as anti-GAD and for susceptibility genes [107, 117, 124]. However, the PV of particular immune or genetic markers in the general population is lower than in type 1 diabetes family members [104, 124], and hence population screening is not feasible unless a series of immune, genetic, and metabolic markers are used to improve PV [124].

Screening of the general population will only become efficacious if effective and safe interventions are first demonstrated in high-risk type 1 diabetes family members. Moreover, even assuming the latter is achieved, the presently available screening tests will need further refinement, as the cost of screening would otherwise be prohibitive for most countries.

The last decade has provided exciting insights into the etiopathogenesis and early natural history of type 1 diabetes, and the possibility of prevention. However, this remains only a possibility. Not until properly conducted experimental trials have demonstrated successfully that the incidence of type 1 diabetes can be significantly and safely reduced will it be reasonable to institute screening programs [107, 110, 118]. Once primary prevention in high-risk individuals does become tenable it may then be reasonable to extend screening to the general population, but only if the usual criteria for establishment of screening programs [12, 13] are satisfied. Nevertheless, hopes for prevention of the bulk of type 1 diabetes cases may well lie with environmental modification [123, 125].

Type 2 Diabetes

Ideally, any screening program should be assessed in controlled trials measuring health outcomes and costs in screened and unscreened populations. As yet, there have not been such studies for diabetes, and so screening should be considered in the light of whether or not type 2 diabetes satisfies all or most of the requirements listed in Table 1. Some of the relevant data for type 2 diabetes are outlined below.

(1) Type 2 diabetes affects up to 14% [126] of the adult population (aged 40–74) in the developed world, with higher rates seen in parts of the developing world. Approximately 50% of these individuals are undiagnosed.
(2) Diabetic complications are common at the time of clinical diagnosis, and less frequent among people diagnosed during screening surveys. It has been calculated that type 2 diabetes begins 4–7 years before the time of clinical diagnosis [127].
(3) The United Kingdom Prospective Diabetes Study (UKPDS) has shown that aggressive glucose and blood pressure lowering therapy in people with newly diagnosed (after clinical presentation) diabetes reduces the risk of long-term complications [5, 128].
(4) Hyperglycemia is an important CVD risk factor. The risk is apparent amongst people with diabetes, IGT, IFG [66, 68, 69, 129–132], and even high normal fasting glucose levels (FPG 4.7–6.0 mmol/l) [133, 134], and the absolute risk of CVD is significantly increased by the presence of diabetes. The recent HOPE study [135] demonstrated a significant reduction in CVD and mortality when ramipril was given to people with diabetes and one other cardiovascular risk factor. This indicates that knowledge of an individual's diabetes status is important in being able to institute treatment [with an angiotensin-converting-enzyme (ACE) inhibitor] that will prevent CVD.
(5) Computer modeling studies have indicated that a small improvement in overall health can be achieved by screening for diabetes, and that the cost per unit of health gained by screening high-risk populations (e.g. African Americans) is comparable to that for screening for other diseases, such as breast cancer [136].

There is mounting evidence to indicate that screening for diabetes would be beneficial to both individuals and communities. However, it should be noted that most of the relevant intervention data have been derived from people with clinically diagnosed diabetes (e.g. UKPDS and HOPE). As a group, such people have more advanced disease, and carry a greater risk of further complications than do people identified by screening. The risk reduction (especially the absolute risk reduction) may be considerably smaller in individuals identified by screening than has been shown in intervention trials in clinically diagnosed individuals. Conversely, one might argue that earlier intervention would ultimately have a greater potential to reduce risk, since it can be started before significant complications have developed. Additional concerns about screening relate to the nature of the relationship of hyperglycemia with CVD. It is unclear whether it is truly independent of other risk factors (such as dyslipidemia and hypertension). Some studies have indicated that it is an independent risk factor while others have not [137]. If hyperglycemia is not an independent CVD risk factor, screening for diabetes may not offer any advantages over screening for hypertension and dyslipidemia. In this scenario, diabetes screening could only be effective in reducing the risk of serious microvascular disease (e.g. blindness)—numerically a much smaller problem than CVD.

The question of the value of screening can only be answered by randomized trials comparing outcomes in screened and unscreened populations. Such studies would need to be very large, and carefully designed. The cost would necessarily be high, but the evidence is needed to support the adoption of screening programs. Similar studies have been performed in other areas such as breast and colorectal cancer, and should now be started in diabetes.

If it is accepted that screening for type 2 diabetes is worthwhile, the next question that arises is who should be screened. The prevalence of diabetes is not high enough in most countries to justify mass screening of the whole population. Moreover, most people with undiagnosed diabetes have easily identifiable risk factors [138], indicating that targeted screening of high-risk groups is likely to identify most cases of undiagnosed diabetes. Studies examining the utility of using such risk factors have found that the sensitivity for the detection of diabetes was 72–78%, the specificity was 55–56%, and the positive PV was 6–8% [139, 140]. The selection methods are shown in Table 6, and confirm that simple clinical parameters can be successfully used to select people for screening. Nevertheless, this still involved blood glucose testing of 40% of the population (over the age of 50), of whom only 8% had undiagnosed diabetes [139].

It is widely recognized that certain ethnic groups are at increased risk of type 2 diabetes. This was not analyzed in either of the two studies referred to in Table 6, since

Table 6 Results of two studies showing optimal combinations of risk factors for diabetes screening*

Any two of [140]:
Age 60+
Male
Obesity (BMI >29 kg/m^2 for women, >30 kg/m^2 for men)
Parent or sibling with diabetes
Chest pain or breathlessness on walking
Any two of [139]:
Age 60+
Male
Obesity (BMI >30 kg/m^2)
First-degree relative with diabetes
Treated hypertension

* The studies only included people over the age of 50.

Table 7 Suggested high-risk groups for targeting of screening for type 2 diabetes

Age ≥ 55 years
IGT or IFG (current or previous)
Previous GDM
All people with clinical CVD (myocardial infarction, angina, or stroke)
Any two of:
Age ≥ 45 years (35 in high-risk ethnic groups)
Obesity (BMI >30 kg/m^2)
First-degree relative with type 2 diabetes
Hypertension

they only included Caucasians. Interestingly, in a North American study, which included both Hispanics and Native Americans [138], ethnicity was not an independent risk factor for undiagnosed type 2 diabetes. The high risk of diabetes in these groups was also expressed through other factors, such as obesity and family history, suggesting that ethnicity itself may not need to be part of the algorithm for selecting people for diabetes screening. IGT, IFG, and previous GDM all carry a high risk of future diabetes, but were not selected as significant risk factors. The studies relied on clinically available information, and underdiagnosis of these three conditions (especially in the older adults included in these studies) probably accounts for their exclusion. Delivering a large baby also appears not to be an independent risk factor for diabetes [141]. Based on these findings on risk factors, as well as recent data that undiagnosed diabetes is present in more than 5% of those aged over 55 years in some Caucasian populations [6, 126], Table 7 shows suggested target groups for diabetes screening.

Virtually none of the data contributing to the above has been collected on people over the age of 75 years. However, the elderly are at high risk of diabetes and its complications. The UKPDS data showed that the benefits of intensive therapy for diabetes took approximately 10 years to become apparent [128]. These facts should be considered when deciding whether or not to screen an elderly person.

Symptoms of hyperglycemia (such as thirst and polyuria) have a poor sensitivity and specificity for diabetes [142]. Therefore, symptoms are unlikely to be a useful part of a formal screening program; however, it remains good clinical practice to look for diabetes in someone presenting with typical symptoms of hyperglycemia.

Impaired Glucose Tolerance

It is now clear from recent studies that progression from IGT to diabetes can be prevented or at least delayed by lifestyle measures [7, 9] and by drugs, such as metformin [7] and acarbose [8]. Over 3–5 years, these interventions reduced the incidence of diabetes by approximately 60, 35, and 25% respectively. The evidence on lifestyle is also consistent with earlier trials from Sweden [143] and China [144]. It has further been suggested that ACE inhibitors, thiazolidinediones, and statins may reduce the risk of progressing to diabetes. Successfully treating IGT therefore raises the possibility of preventing or at least delaying diabetes, and all its attendant problems and costs. However, while it is absolutely clear that the biochemical transition from IGT to diabetes can be influenced, there are no data yet on hard, clinical end points. In particular, we do not know if treating IGT will prevent CVD. Nevertheless, these new studies raise the question of screening for IGT. The issue is a difficult one, with major cost implications, since IGT is common (affecting approximately 10% of Caucasian adults [6]), can only be identified by performing an OGTT, and the best treatment (intensive lifestyle intervention) is beyond the capabilities of most health care systems. Until there is evidence that treating IGT prevents hard clinical end points, it is hard to recommend widespread screening for IGT. However, screening programs directed at type 2 diabetes are likely to identify significant numbers with IGT, and although using the fasting glucose as the first screen will miss many cases with IGT, those IGT individuals who are missed (i.e. have a normal fasting glucose) have a considerably lower risk of progressing to diabetes than do those with a fasting glucose above 6.0 mmol/l [7]. Depending on available resources, it can be useful to use a fasting plasma glucose threshold of 5.5 mmol/l, which will increase the number of people with IGT who are identified, but at the cost of performing more OGTTs. Once identified, people with IGT should, at the very least, be given the best available lifestyle advice, and if this does not achieve weight loss, drug therapy should be considered. Other cardiovascular risk factors should also be treated aggressively.

Gestational Diabetes Mellitus

Gestational diabetes mellitus (GDM) is important, because of the adverse consequences that it carries for both mother and child. However, little agreement exists worldwide on its definition or the most appropriate methods by which to screen for it. This confusion fuels the wide variations in practice, in which some centers employ universal screening, and others appear to have no formalized approach at all. However it is defined, its prevalence is only likely to increase in the future, as a consequence of the increasing age at which pregnancy occurs, and of the falling age at which type 2 diabetes now develops.

The broad basis for the concept of screening for GDM is sound, and relies on well-established data showing that hyperglycemia in pregnancy is associated with adverse outcomes (both fetal and maternal), and that intervention with glucose lowering in those with GDM improves fetal outcomes [145]. The difficulty arises in determining levels of hyperglycemia, that are associated with adverse outcomes, and above which interventions can be shown to be beneficial.

Despite the acceptance of standardized criteria for glucose intolerance outside pregnancy [73, 87], considerable confusion remains over standards for GDM [87, 146–149]. The WHO position is that pregnant women meeting standard WHO criteria for IGT or diabetes (using a 75 g OGTT) are classified as having GDM [87], whereas the ADA [149] continues to recommend a 1 h 50 g oral glucose screening test, followed by a 3 h 100 g diagnostic test, with diagnostic criteria that have their basis in those originally proposed by O'Sullivan and Mahan in 1964 [150]. The American criteria were developed statistically (mean glucose level plus two standard deviations) but were subsequently shown to be associated with maternal and perinatal outcomes [151], at a time when the general level of obstetric and perinatal care was inferior to current standards [57]. More recently, the ADA [149] has suggested an alternative of a 2 h 75 g OGTT, which uses the 0-, 1-, and 2-h cutoffs developed for the 3 h 100 g test. Thus, current diagnostic tests vary widely, with glucose loads of 50, 75, and 100 g being in use, fasting thresholds varying between 5.3 and 7.0 mmol/l, 2-h thresholds varying between 7.8 and 9.2 mmol/l, and values at 1 and 3 h being required in some but not other protocols.

West [59] considered that there was insufficient evidence that glucose intolerance in the absence of fasting hyperglycemia was an independent risk factor for complications in pregnancy. This view has been supported by studies using the relatively low fasting values of the O'Sullivan or similar criteria [152–154], and the higher fasting cutoff value of 7.8 mmol/l [155, 156].

Li et al. [155] compared the 1979 NDDG and 1985 WHO criteria [1, 3] in women at risk of developing GDM and found that 51% of women with GDM by NDDG standards had normal glucose tolerance according to WHO criteria. Moreover, in this group of Chinese women there were no major differences in perinatal outcome between treatment and control groups in women who were either normal or IGT by WHO standards.

Similarly, Roberts et al. [157] found no differences in fetal outcome, neonatal morbidity, or maternal antenatal complications in Irish women with normal vs. IGT (WHO), although the IGT group did have a higher rate of induced labor and cesarean section. In addition, a multicenter European study found that IGT in pregnancy was not associated with adverse obstetric outcomes (including macrosomia) [158]. The latter study even recommended raising the diagnostic threshold for diagnosis of IGT in pregnancy, although the necessity of recognizing IGT even at the higher levels is unclear, given the lack of outcome associations.

In contrast, Pettitt et al. [91] using WHO criteria but based only on the 2-h postload glucose level, concluded that screening for and recognition of IGT in pregnancy was worthwhile in the highly type 2 diabetes susceptible Pima Indian population. They found trends for increasing rates of perinatal mortality, macrosomia, and toxemia—but not for congenital malformations or prematurity—with increasing glucose intolerance. Examination of their data, however, shows that with the exception of macrosomia, the evidence for significantly higher rates in women with impaired glucose tolerance is not convincing. Indeed, the 2-h level of 11.1 mmol/l (200 mg/dl) seems to distinguish most clearly the group at risk of serious complications. A later paper from the same workers confirmed this [159]. There were no significant differences in rates for any perinatal or maternal complications between women with IGT in pregnancy and normal glucose tolerance (WHO criteria). A higher rate of cesarean sections in women with IGT may reflect obstetric practice more than necessity. Again, an obvious elevation in complication rates occurred only at 2-h glucose levels above 11.1 mmol/l. In a further study from the Pima population, the WHO single-step OGTT identified a greater percentage of women with adverse pregnancy outcomes (macrosomia or cesarean section), than did the two-step NDDG process [160].

Studies from other populations have presented findings supporting the hypothesis that milder degrees of glucose intolerance lead to adverse outcomes, and that these states may be better identified by WHO criteria. A Canadian study examining both the 1 h 50 g and the 3 h 100 g OGTTs in 3637 women showed that the risks of preeclampsia, macrosomia, and cesarean section increased in a continual fashion right across the maternal glucose range [161] for glucose measured at virtually every time point in both tests. For example, compared to those in the lowest quartile of 2-h glucose, those with a 2-h glucose of 6.5–7.3 mmol/l had a 97 and 59% increased risk of preeclampsia and macrosomia, respectively. A large study from Brazil reported data from almost 5000 women who had a 75 g OGTT between 20 and 28 weeks [162]. After excluding those with frank diabetes (fasting glucose >7.0 mmol/l or 2-h glucose >11.1 mmol/l), the data were interpreted separately according to WHO and ADA criteria. Those identified by either set of criteria were at significantly increased risk of adverse pregnancy outcomes (macrosomia, preeclampsia, and perinatal death) compared to women with normal glucose values, but there were approximately three times as many women identified by the WHO than by the ADA criteria. In a study of 700 women from Thailand [163], the WHO 75 g test identified 15.7% of women as having GDM, but the NDDG 100 g test only identified GDM in 1.4% (all of whom were picked up by the WHO test). There was a total of 15 macrosomic infants, of which 6 occurred in WHO GDM cases, and only 3 in ADA GDM pregnancies.

These studies provide important evidence that should lead to more widespread acceptance of the simpler WHO

Table 8 ADA and WHO criteria for GDM

	Glucose load	0 h	1 h	2 h	3 h	Criteria for GDM
ADA [149]	100 g	5.3	10.0	8.6	7.8	Two or more values at or above these levels
	75 g	5.3	10.0	8.6		Two or more values at or above these levels
WHO [168]	75 g	7.0		7.8		One or more values at or above these levels

Glucose values are in mmol/l.

criteria for GDM, but also indicate that doubt remains over the prognostic significance of IGT in pregnancy. The Hyperglycemia and Adverse Pregnancy Outcome Study [164] is an international epidemiological study involving 25 000 participants, which is due to be reported in 2004. It will attempt to definitively answer questions on the relationship between nondiabetic hyperglycemia and pregnancy outcomes and to shed light on screening and intervention. It should help determine if nondiabetic hyperglycemia (as defined by a 75 g test) is associated with adverse outcomes.

Glucose criteria may not be the only method of screening pregnant women to detect those who might benefit from insulin therapy. In a Hispanic population, a subgroup of those with mild GDM was identified on the basis of an ultrasound measurement of the fetal abdominal circumference above the 75th percentile. The mothers were randomized to diet or insulin plus diet, and fetal outcomes were better in the insulin group, despite the full criteria of GDM not being fulfilled [165].

The question of who should be screened is also a thorny one, with opinions divided between universal screening, and screening restricted to those with identifiable risk factors. Universal screening can be supported by data showing that adverse outcomes are just as likely in GDM pregnancies without maternal risk factors for GDM, as in those GDM pregnancies with risk factors, and that 40% of GDM pregnancies do not have risk factors [166]. Furthermore, in some ethnic groups, even teenage pregnancies have a prevalence of GDM of approximately 5% [167]. Nevertheless, the OGTT is often an unpleasant test and, like any screening program, expensive. Furthermore, with a degree of doubt remaining over the value of identifying lesser degrees of glucose intolerance, widespread screening has only been patchily adopted. The ADA recommends that screening is not necessary in low-risk women, as defined by having all of the following: being aged under 25 years, of normal prepregnancy weight, a member of a low-risk ethnic group, no family history of type 2 diabetes, and no personal history of abnormal glucose tolerance or obstetric problems [149]. In all other women, glucose tolerance testing is recommended at 24–28 weeks, and at presentation in women with multiple risk factors. The ADA recommends either a one-step approach, using either the 75 g or 100 g OGTT, or a two-step approach in which the glucose concentration 1 h after a 50-g oral glucose load is used as a screening test. The diagnostic 75 g or 100 g OGTT is reserved for those women with a 1-h value (in the 50 g test) above 7.2 or 7.8 mmol/l identifying approximately 80 and 90% respectively of women with GDM. The WHO recommends a simpler approach, only using the standard 75 g OGTT, and interpreting according to nonpregnant criteria (Table 8).

That the issue is a complex one is undoubted. However, unless screening and treatment regimens for GDM are established now on the basis of properly controlled and evaluated studies, physicians and pregnant women may bear the cost and discomfort of unnecessary procedures and treatment for many years to come. Until such definitive data become available, it seems sensible to recommend the WHO approach on the basis of simplicity, and the fact that the balance of evidence seems to favor it.

CONCLUSIONS

Many physicians nurture the hope that type 1 and type 2 diabetes may be preventable. There is evidence that primary prevention of many cases of type 2 diabetes is achievable through promoting a generally healthy lifestyle [7, 9] or with the use of pharmacological agents [7, 8]. Enthusiasts even foresee the day when primary prevention of type 1 diabetes might be possible through environmental modification [169] or screening all children in the general population [107, 117, 170], but in the meantime, hopes rest on preventing the small proportion of cases that occur in high-risk family members detected by immunogenetic screening [106, 107, 113, 171]. However, therapeutic intervention has not yet proved successful, and on humane grounds routine screening of first-degree relatives of type 1 diabetes probands cannot be advocated.

It is known that most communities harbor a considerable number of adults with asymptomatic glucose intolerance. The concept of "screening for diabetes" was born for the salvation of these individuals. With the establishment of the increased cardiovascular risk of these individuals, and increasing anxiety about the potential health care burden that they will bring if they remain unidentified and untreated (until they have a clinical event), the pendulum has, in recent years, swung in favor of advocating targeted screening. However, while this may turn out to be the correct approach, belief in it should not obscure the need for large-scale, properly controlled trials, which should determine whether or not detection and treatment of asymptomatic glucose intolerance results in improved longevity or quality of life. There are definite grounds for advocating some form of screening for diabetes in pregnancy, but the available evidence is inconclusive about the level of hyperglycemia that could benefit from intervention.

There is considerable need for well-planned and properly evaluated controlled trials of outcomes in screened and unscreened populations. Studies should continue to ask whether any form of screening for glucose intolerance or type 1 diabetes is appropriate in the general or high-risk population, and to clarify the nature of the screening test most appropriate to pregnancy. The questions are important and have long remained unanswered. The studies may be difficult, unglamorous, and time-consuming, but are essential if screening is to be based on sound scientific principles.

REFERENCES

1. The National Diabetes Data Group. Classification and diagnosis of diabetes mellitus and other categories of glucose intolerance. *Diabetes* 1979; 28: 1039–57.
2. World Health Organization. *Expert Committee on Diabetes Mellitus, Second Report*. Geneva: WHO, 1980.
3. Report of a World Health Organization Study Group. *Diabetes Mellitus*. Technical Report Series 727. Geneva: WHO, 1985.
4. The UK Prospective Diabetes Study (UKPDS) Group. Intensive blood glucose control with sulphonylureas or insulin compared with conventional treatment and risk of complications in patients with type 2 diabetes (UKPDS 33). *Lancet* 1998; 352: 837–53.
5. The UKPDS Group. Tight blood pressure control and risk of macrovascular and microvascular complications in type 2 diabetes: UKPDS 38. *BMJ* 1998; 317: 703–13.
6. Dunstan DW, Zimmet PZ, Welborn TA, De Courten MP, Cameron AJ, Sicree RA, Dwyer T, Colagiuri S, Jolley D, Knuiman M, Atkins R, Shaw JE. The rising prevalence of diabetes and impaired glucose tolerance: the Australian Diabetes, Obesity and Lifestyle Study. *Diabetes Care* 2002; 25 (5): 829–34.
7. Knowler WC, Barrett-Connor E, Fowler SE, Hamman RF, Lachin JM, Walker EA, Nathan DM. Reduction in the incidence of type 2 diabetes with lifestyle intervention or metformin. *N Engl J Med* 2002; 346 (6): 393–403.
8. Chiasson JL, Josse RG, Gomis R, Hanefeld M, Karasik A, Laakso M. Acarbose for prevention of type 2 diabetes mellitus: the STOP-NIDDM randomized trial. *Lancet* 2002; 359 (9323): 2072–7.
9. Tuomilehto J, Lindstrom J, Eriksson J, Valle T, Hamalainen H, Ilanne-Parikka P, Keinanen-Kiukaanniemi S, Laakso M, Louheranta A, Rastas M, Salminen V, Uusitupa M, for the Finnish Diabetes Prevention Study Group. Prevention of type 2 diabetes mellitus by changes in lifestyle among subjects with impaired glucose tolerance. *N Engl J Med* 2001; 344: 1343–50.
10. Commission on Chronic Illness. *Chronic Illness in the United States: Prevention of Chronic Illness, Vol 1*. Cambridge, MA: Harvard University Press, 1957.
11. Moses RG, Colaguiri S, Shannon AG. Effectiveness of mass screening for diabetes mellitus using random capillary blood glucose measurements. *Med J Aust* 1985; 143: 544–6.
12. Whitby L. Screening for disease: definitions and criteria. *Lancet* 1974; ii: 819–21.
13. Morrison A. *Screening in Chronic Disease. Monographs in Epidemiology and Biostatistics, Vol 7*. New York: Oxford University Press, 1985.
14. West K. *Epidemiology of Diabetes and Its Vascular Lesions*. New York: Elsevier, 1978.
15. Haffner S, Rosenthal M, Hazuda H, Stern M, Franco L. Evaluation of three potential screening tests for diabetes mellitus in a biethnic population. *Diabetes Care* 1984; 7: 347–53.
16. Hoskins P, Handelsman D, Hannelly T, Silink M, Yue D, Turtle J. Glycosylated hemoglobin as an index of the prevalence and severity of diabetes in biethnic Fiji. *Diabetes Res Clin Pract* 1987; 3: 257–67.
17. Modan M, Halkin H, Karasik A, Lusky A. Effectiveness of glycosylated hemoglobin, fasting plasma glucose, and a single post load plasma glucose level in population screening for glucose intolerance. *Am J Epidemiol* 1984; 119: 431–44.
18. Stern E, Blau J, Rusecki Y, Rafaelovsky M, Cohen M. Prevalence of diabetes in Israel: epidemiologic survey. *Diabetes* 1988; 37: 297–302.
19. Herron C. Screening in diabetes mellitus: report of the Atlanta Workshop. *Diabetes Care* 1979; 2: 357–62.
20. Screening for carbohydrate intolerance [editorial]. *Lancet* 1980; i: 1174–5.
21. McNeil JJ. Cholesterol: action or caution? *Med J Aust* 1988; 148: 1–3.
22. Screening for breast cancer [editorial]. *Lancet* 1985; i: 851–2.
23. Hakama M, Miller A, Day N. *Screening for Cancer of the Uterine Cervix*. Lyon: International Agency for Research on Cancer, 1986.
24. Canadian Task Force on the Periodic Health Examination. The periodic health examination. *Can Med Assoc* 1979; 121: 1193–254.
25. Frame P. A critical review of adult health maintenance: part 4. Prevention of metabolic, behavioral, and miscellaneous conditions. *J Fam Pract* 1986; 23: 29–39.
26. American Diabetes Association. Position statement: screening for diabetes. *Diabetes Care* 1989; 12: 588–90.
27. Nathan DM, Singer DE. Screening for diabetes [letter]. *Diabetes Care* 1990; 13: 542–3.
28. Harris M, Modan M. Screening for NIDDM: why is there no national program? *Diabetes Care* 1994; 17: 440–4.
29. Knowler W. Screening for NIDDM. Opportunities for detection, treatment, and prevention. *Diabetes Care* 1994; 17: 445–50.
30. Paterson KR. Population screening for diabetes mellitus. *Diabet Med* 1993; 10: 777–81.
31. Fletcher SW, Black W, Harris R, Rimer BK, Shapiro S. Report of the international workshop on screening for breast cancer. *J Natl Cancer Inst* 1993; 85: 1644–56.
32. Wright CJ, Mueller CB. Screening mammography and public health policy: the need for perspective. *Lancet* 1995; ii: 29–32.
33. Welborn TA, Cullen KJ, Balazs N. Diabetes detection in mass health examinations. Three-year experience from Busselton. *Med J Aust* 1972; 2: 133–7.
34. Wilson JMG, Jungner G. *Principles and Practice of Screening for Disease*. Geneva: WHO, 1968.

35. Rose G, Keen H, Jarrett AR. Epidemiologic methods in diabetic macrovascular disease. *Diabetes Care* 1979; 2: 91–7.
36. Burrin JM, Alberti KGMM. What is blood glucose: can it be measured? *Diabet Med* 1990; 7: 199–206.
37. Riccardi G, Vaccaro O, Rivellese A, Pignalosa S, Tutino L, Mancini M. Reproducibility of the new diagnostic criteria for impaired glucose tolerance. *Am J Epidemiol* 1985; 121: 422–9.
38. Merkatz IR, Duchon MA, Yamashita TS, Houser HB. A pilot community-based screening program for gestational diabetes. *Diabetes Care* 1980; 3: 453–7.
39. American Diabetes Association Workshop—Conference on Gestational Diabetes. Summary and recommendations. *Diabetes Care* 1980; 3: 499–501.
40. American Diabetes Association. Summary and recommendations of the 2nd International Workshop—Conference on Gestational Diabetes Mellitus. *Diabetes* 1985; 34 (suppl 2): 123–6.
41. Dowse G, Gareeboo H, Zimmet P, Alberti K, Tuomilehto J, Fareed D, Brissonnette L, Finch C. High prevalence of NIDDM and impaired glucose tolerance in Indian, Creole and Chinese Mauritians. *Diabetes* 1990; 39: 390–6.
42. Zimmet P, Dowse G, Finch C, Serjeantson S, King H. The epidemiology and natural history of NIDDM—lessons from the South Pacific. *Diabetes Metab Rev* 1990; 6: 91–124.
43. Guest CS, O'Dea K, Hopper JL, Nankervis AJ, Larkins RG. The prevalence of glucose intolerance in Aborigines and Europids of south-eastern Australia. *Diabetes Res Clin Pract* 1992; 15: 227–35.
44. Knowler W, Bennett P, Hamman R, Miller M. Diabetes incidence and prevalence in Pima Indians: A 19-fold greater incidence than in Rochester, Minnesota. *Am J Epidemiol* 1978; 108: 497–504.
45. Taylor R, Zimmet P. Limitation of fasting plasma glucose for the diagnosis of diabetes mellitus. *Diabetes Care* 1981; 4: 556–8.
46. Holland WW. Screening for disease. *Lancet* 1974; ii: 1494–7.
47. Houser HB, Mackay IR, Verma N, Genuth S. A three-year controlled follow-up study of persons identified in a mass screening program for diabetes. *Diabetes* 1977; 26: 619–27.
48. Genuth SM, Houser HB, Carter JR, Merkatz IR, Price JW, Schumacher OP, Wieland RG. Community screening for diabetes by blood glucose measurement. Results of a five-year experience. *Diabetes* 1976; 25: 1110–7.
49. King H, Zimmet P, Raper L, Balkau B. The natural history of impaired glucose tolerance in the Micronesian population of Nauru: a six-year follow-up study. *Diabetologia* 1984; 26: 39–43.
50. Yudkin J, Alberti K, McLarty D, Swai A. Impaired glucose tolerance. Is it a risk factor for diabetes or a diagnostic ratbag? *BMJ* 1990; 301: 397–402.
51. Barker DJP, Rose G. *Epidemiology in Medical Practice*, 3rd edn. Edinburgh: Churchill Livingstone, 1984.
52. Party BDSW. Five-year follow-up report on the Birmingham diabetes survey of 1962. *Br Med J* 1970; 3: 301–5.
53. Aspevik E, Jorde R, Raeder S. The diabetes survey in Bergen, Norway, 1956. *Acta Med Scand* 1974; 196: 161–9.
54. Morsiani M, Beretta P, Pareschi PL, Manservigi D, Bottoni L. Long-term results in preventive medicine for type II diabetes. *Acta Diabetol Lat* 1985; 22: 191–202.
55. Genuth S, Houser HB, Carter JR, Merkatz IR, Price JW, Schumacher OP, Wieland RG. Observations on the value of mass indiscriminate screening for diabetes mellitus based on a five-year follow-up. *Diabetes* 1978; 27: 377–83.
56. Program UGD. A study of the effects of hypoglycemic agents on vascular complications in patients with adult-onset diabetes, VI: supplementary report on non fatal events in patients treated with tolbutamide. *Diabetes* 1976; 25: 1129–53.
57. Bennett PH, Knowler WC. Early detection and intervention in diabetes mellitus: is it effective? *J Chron Dis* 1984; 37: 653–66.
58. Larkins R. To screen or not to screen—the diabetes dilemma. *Med J Aust* 1985; 143: 537.
59. West KM. Commentary. Community screening programs for diabetes? *Diabetes Care* 1979; 2: 381–4.
60. Duncan BB, Heiss G. Nonenzymatic glycosylation of proteins—a new tool for assessment of cumulative hyperglycemia in epidemiological studies, past and future. *Am J Epidemiol* 1984; 120: 169–89.
61. Jarrett R, Keen H. Hyperglycemia and diabetes mellitus. *Lancet* 1976; 2: 1009–12.
62. Al Sayegh H, Jarrett R. Oral glucose tolerance tests and the diagnosis of diabetes: results of a prospective study based on the Whitehall Survey. *Lancet* 1979; II: 431–3.
63. Rushforth NB, Miller M, Bennett PH. Fasting and two-hour post-load glucose levels for the diagnosis of diabetes. The relationship between glucose levels and complications of diabetes in Pima Indians. *Diabetologia* 1979; 16: 373–9.
64. Pettitt D, Knowler W, Lisse J, Bennett P. Development of retinopathy and proteinuria in relation to plasma glucose concentrations in Pima Indians. *Lancet* 1980; II: 1050–2.
65. Dowse G, Zimmet P. The prevalence and incidence of non-insulin-dependent diabetes mellitus. *Frontiers in Diabetes Research: Current Trends in Non-insulin-dependent Diabetes Mellitus*. Amsterdam: Elsevier, 1989.
66. Shaw J, Hodge A, de Courten M, Chitson P, Zimmet P. Isolated post-challenge hyperglycemia confirmed as a risk factor for mortality. *Diabetologia* 1999; 42: 1050–4.
67. Tominaga M, Eguchi H, Manaka H, Igarashi K, Kato T, Sekikawa A. Impaired glucose tolerance is a risk factor for CVD, but not impaired fasting glucose. The Funagata Diabetes Study. *Diabetes Care* 1999; 22 (6): 920–4.
68. DECODE Study Group. Glucose tolerance and mortality: comparison of WHO and American Diabetes Association diagnostic criteria. *Lancet* 1999; 354: 617–21.
69. Barzilay JI, Spiekerman CF, Wahl PW, Kuller LH, Cushman M, Furberg CD, Dobs A, Polak JF, Savage PJ. CVD in older adults with glucose disorders: comparison of American Diabetes Association criteria for diabetes mellitus with WHO criteria. *Lancet* 1999; 354 (9179): 622–5.
70. de Vegt F, Dekker JM, Ruhe HG, Stehouwer CD, Nijpels G, Bouter LM, Heine RJ. Hyperglycemia is associated with all-cause and cardiovascular mortality in the Hoorn population: the Hoorn Study. *Diabetologia* 1999; 42 (8): 926–31.
71. Forrest R, Jackson C, Yudkin J. The glycohemoglobin assay as a screening test for diabetes mellitus: the Islington diabetes survey. *Diabet Med* 1987; 4: 254–9.
72. Swai ABM, McLarty DG, Kitange HM, Kilima PM, Masuki G, Mtinangi BI, Chuwa L, Alberti KGMM. Study

in Tanzania of impaired glucose tolerance methodological myth? *Diabetes* 1991; 40: 516–20.

73. American Diabetes Association. Report of the Expert Committee on the diagnosis and classification of diabetes mellitus. *Diabetes Care* 1997; 20: 1183–97.
74. Ashby JP, Frier BM. Is serum fructosamine a clinically useful test? *Diabet Med* 1988; 5: 118–21.
75. Little RR, England JD, Wiedmeyer HM, McKenzie EM, Pettitt DJ, Knowler WC, Goldstein DE. Relationship of glycosylated hemoglobin to oral glucose tolerance Implications for diabetes screening. *Diabetes* 1988; 37: 60–4.
76. Liu QZ, Pettitt DJ, Hanson RL, Charles MA, Klein R, Bennett PH, Knowler WC. Glycated hemoglobin, plasma glucose and diabetic retinopathy: cross-sectional and prospective analyses. *Diabetologia* 1993; 36: 428–32.
77. McCance D, Hanson R, Charles M-A, Jacobsson L, Pettitt D, Bennett P, Knowler W. Comparison of tests for glycated hemoglobin and fasting and two-hour plasma glucose concentrations as diagnostic methods for diabetes. *BMJ* 1994; 308: 1323–8.
78. Ferrell RE, Harris CL, Aguilar L, Tulloch B, Garcia C, Schull WJ. Glycosylated hemoglobin determination from capillary blood samples. *Am J Epidemiol* 1984; 119: 159–66.
79. Forrest RD, Jackson CA, Gould BJ, Casburn-Budd M, Taylor JE, Yudkin JS. Four assay methods for glycated hemoglobin compared as screening tests for diabetes mellitus: the Islington diabetes survey. *Clin Chem* 1988; 34: 145–8.
80. Tsuji I, Nakamoto K, Hasegawa T, Hisashige A, Inawashiro H, Fukao A, Hisamichi S. Receiver operating characteristic analysis on fasting plasma glucose, HbA_{1c}, and fructosamine on diabetes screening. *Diabetes Care* 1991; 14: 1075–7.
81. Verrillo A, de Teresa A, Golia R, Nunziata V. The relationship between glycosylated hemoglobin levels and various degrees of glucose intolerance. *Diabetologia* 1983; 24: 291–393.
82. Guillausseau PJ, Charles MA, Paolaggi F, et al. Comparison of HbA_{1c} and fructosamine in diagnosis of glucose-tolerance abnormalities. *Diabetes Care* 1990; 13: 898–900.
83. Baker JR, O'Connor JP, Metcalf PA, Lawson MR, Johnson RN. Clinical usefulness of estimation of serum fructosamine concentration as a screening test for diabetes mellitus. *Br Med J* 1983; 287: 863–7.
84. Baker JR, Metcalf PA, Scragg R. Fructosamine concentrations in general population of Kawerau. *Diabetes Care* 1988; 11: 239–45.
85. Swai ABM, Harrison K, Chuwa LM, Makene W, McLarty DG, Alberti KGMM. Screening for diabetes: does measurement of serum fructosamine help? *Diabet Med* 1988; 5: 648–52.
86. Ko GT, Chan JC, Yeung VT, Chow CC, Tsang LW, Li JK, So WY, Wai HP, Cockram CS. Combined use of a fasting plasma glucose concentration and HbA_{1c} or fructosamine predicts the likelihood of having diabetes in high-risk subjects. *Diabetes Care* 1998; 21 (8): 1221–5.
87. Alberti K, Zimmet P. Definition, diagnosis and classification of diabetes mellitus and its complications, Part 1: diagnosis and classification of diabetes mellitus. Report of a WHO Consultation. *Diabet Med* 1998; 15 (7): 539–53.
88. Shaw JE, de Courten M, Boyko EJ, Zimmet PZ. Impact of new diagnostic criteria for diabetes on different populations. *Diabetes Care* 1999; 22 (5): 762–6.
89. DECODE Study Group. Will new diagnostic criteria for diabetes mellitus change phenotype of patients with diabetes? Reanalysis of European epidemiological data. *BMJ* 1998; 317: 371–5.
90. Shaw J, Zimmet P, Hodge A, de Courten M, Dowse G, Chitson G, Tuomilento J, Alberti K. Impaired fasting glucose: how low should it go? *Diabetes Care* 2000; 23: 34–9.
91. Pettitt D, Knowler W, Baird R, Bennett P. Gestational diabetes: infant and maternal complications of pregnancy in relation to third-trimester glucose tolerance in the Pima Indians. *Diabetes Care* 1980; 3: 458–64.
92. Harris M, Eastman R, Cowie C, Flegal K, Eberhardt M. Comparison of diabetes diagnostic categories in the US population according to 1997 American Diabetes Association and 1980–1985 World Health Organization diagnostic criteria. *Diabetes Care* 1997; 20: 1859–62.
93. de Vegt F, Dekker JM, Stehouwer CD, Nijpels G, Bouter LM, Heine RJ. The 1997 American Diabetes Association criteria versus the 1985 World Health Organization criteria for the diagnosis of abnormal glucose tolerance: poor agreement in the Hoorn Study. *Diabetes Care* 1998; 21 (10): 1686–90.
94. Wahl P, Savage P, Psaty B, Orchard T, Robbins J, Tracy R. Diabetes in older adults: comparison of diabetes mellitus with 1985 WHO classification. *Lancet* 1998; 352: 1012–5.
95. Ko G, Woo J, Chan JCN, Cockram CS. Use of the 1997 American Diabetes Association diagnostic criteria for diabetes in a Hong Kong Chinese population. *Diabetes Care* 1998; 21: 2094–7.
96. Shaw J, Zimmet P, de Courten M, Dowse G, Chitson P, Gareeboo H, Hemraj F, Fareed D, Tuomilehto J, Alberti K. Impaired fasting glucose or impaired glucose tolerance. What best predicts future diabetes in Mauritius? *Diabetes Care* 1999; 22: 399–402.
97. Gimeno S, Ferreira S, Franco L, Iunes M, The Japanese–Brazilian Diabetes Study Group. Comparison of glucose tolerance categories according to World Health Organization and American Diabetes Association diagnostic criteria in a population-based study in Brazil. *Diabetes Care* 1998; 21: 1889–92.
98. Engelgau MM, Thompson TJ, Smith PJ, Herman WH, Aubert RE, Gunter EW, Wetterhall SF, Sous ES, Ali MA. Screening for diabetes mellitus in adults. The utility of random capillary blood glucose measurements. *Diabetes Care* 1995; 18 (4): 463–6.
99. Qiao Q, Keinanen-Kiukaanniemi S, Rajala U, Uusimaki A, Kivela SL. Random capillary whole blood glucose test as a screening test for diabetes mellitus in a middle-aged population. *Scand J Clin Lab Invest* 1995; 55 (1): 3–8.
100. The European Diabetes Policy Group. A desktop guide to type 2 diabetes mellitus. *Diabet Med* 1999; 16 (9): 716–30.
101. Shaw J, de Courten M, Boyko E, Zimmet P. Impact of new diagnostic criteria for diabetes in different populations. *Diabetes Care* 1999; 22: 762–6.
102. Stern MP, Valdez RA, Haffner SM, Mitchell BD, Hazuda HP. Stability over time of modern diagnostic criteria for type 2 diabetes. *Diabetes Care* 1993; 16: 978–83.
103. Walker A, Cudworth AG. Type 1 (insulin-dependent) diabetic multiplex families. Mode of genetic transmission. *Diabetes* 1980; 29: 1036–9.

104. Ziegler A, Herskowitz R, Jackson R, Soeldner J, Eisenbarth G. Predicting type I diabetes. *Diabetes Care* 1990; 13: 762–75.
105. Srikanta S, Ganda O, Eisenbarth G, Soeldner J. Islet-cell antibodies and β-cell function in monozygotic triple and twins initially discordant for type 1 diabetes. *N Engl J Med* 1983; 308: 322–5.
106. Srikanta S, Ganda O, Rabizadeh D, et al. First degree relatives of patients with type I diabetes mellitus. *N Engl J Med* 1985; 313: 461–4, 300.
107. Palmer J, McCulloch D. Prediction and prevention of IDDM—1991. *Diabetes* 1991; 40: 943–47.
108. Atkinson M, Maclaren N, Scharp D, Lacy P, Riley W. 64000 M, autoantibodies as predictors of insulin-dependent diabetes. *Lancet* 1990; 335: 1357–60.
109. Eisenbarth GS. Molecular aspects of the etiology of type 1 diabetes mellitus. *J Diab Complications* 1993; 7: 142–50.
110. American Diabetes Association. Position Statement: prevention of type 1 diabetes mellitus. *Diabetes Care* 2002; 25 (suppl 1): S131.
111. Srikanta S, Ganda OP, Soeldner JS, Eisenbarth GS. First-degree relatives of patients with type I diabetes: islet cell anti-bodies and abnormal insulin secretion. *N Engl J Med* 1985; 313: 461–4.
112. Eisenbarth GS, Verge CF, Allen H, Rewers MJ. The design of trials for prevention of IDDM. *Diabetes* 1993; 42: 941–7.
113. Tuomilehto J, Wolf E. Primary prevention of diabetes mellitus. *Diabetes Care* 1987; 10: 238–48.
114. Bell DSH, Acton RT, Barger BO, Vanichanan C, Clements RS. Futility of predicting onset of type 1 diabetes mellitus. *Diabetes Care* 1987; 10: 788–9.
115. Bougneres PF, Landais P, Boisson C, Carel JC, Frament N, Boitard C, Chaussain JL, Bach JF. Limited duration of remission of insulin dependency in children with recent overt type 1 diabetes treated with low-dose cyclosporin. *Diabetes* 1990; 39: 1264–72.
116. Adreani D, DiMario U, Pozzilli P. Prediction, prevention and early intervention in insulin-dependent diabetes. *Diabetes Metab Rev* 1991; 7: 61–77.
117. Skyler J, Marks J. Immune intervention in type 1 diabetes mellitus. *Diabetes Rev* 1993; 1: 15–42.
118. Lipton R, LaPorte R, Becker D, Dorman J, Orchard T, Atchison J, Drash A. Cyclosporin therapy for prevention and cure of IDDM: epidemiological perspective of benefits and risks. *Diabetes Care* 1990; 13: 776–84.
119. Fathman C, Myers BD. Editorial. Cyclosporine therapy for autoimmune disease. *N Engl J Med* 1992; 326: 1693–5.
120. Diabetes Prevention Trial—Type 1 Diabetes Study Group. Effects of insulin in relatives of patients with type 1 diabetes mellitus. *N Engl J Med* 2002; 346 (22): 1685–91.
121. Raz I, Elias D, Avron A, Tamir M, Metzger M, Cohen IR. β-cell function in new-onset type 1 diabetes and immunomodulation with a heat-shock protein peptide (DiaPep277): a randomized, double-blind, phase II trial. *Lancet* 2001; 358 (9295): 1749–53.
122. Herold KC, Hagopian W, Auger JA, Poumian-Ruiz E, Taylor L, Donaldson D, Gitelman SE, Harlan DM, Xu D, Zivin RA, Bluestone JA. Anti-CD3 monoclonal antibody in new-onset type 1 diabetes mellitus. *N Engl J Med* 2002; 346 (22): 1692–8.
123. Bennett P. Changing concepts of the epidemiology of insulin-dependent diabetes. *Diabetes Care* 1985; 8 (suppl 1): 29–33.
124. Bingley P, Bonifacio E, Shattock M, Gillmor H, Sawtell P, Dunger D, et al. Can islet cell antibodies predict IDDM in the general population? *Diabetes Care* 1993; 16: 45–50.
125. Myers M, Mackay I, Rowley M, Zimmet P. Dietary microbial toxins and type 1 diabetes—a new meaning for seed and soil. *Diabetologia* 2001; 44 (9): 1199–200.
126. Harris M, Flegal K, Cowie C, Eberhardt M, Goldstein D, Little R, Wiedmeyer H, Byrd-Holt D. Prevalence of diabetes, impaired fasting glucose, and impaired glucose tolerance in U.S. adults. The Third National Health and Nutrition Examination 1988–1994. *Diabetes Care* 1998; 21: 518–24.
127. Harris MI, Klein R, Welborn TA, Knuiman MW. Onset of NIDDM occurs at least 4–7 yr before clinical diagnosis. *Diabetes Care* 1992; 15: 815–9.
128. The UKPDS Group. Intensive blood-glucose control with sulfonylureas or insulin compared with conventional treatment and risk of complications in patients with type 2 diabetes (UKPDS 33). *Lancet* 1998; 352: 837–53.
129. Fuller JH, Shipley MJ, Rose G, Jarrett RJ, Keen H. Mortality from coronary heart disease and stroke in relation to degree of glycemia: the Whitehall study. *Br Med J (Clin Res Ed)* 1983; 287 (6396): 867–70.
130. Charles M, Balkau B, Vauzelle-Kervroedan F, Thibult N, Eschwege E. Revision of diagnostic criteria for diabetes [letter]. *Lancet* 1996; 348: 1657–8.
131. Balkau B, Shipley M, Jarrett RJ, Pyorala K, Pyorala M, Forhan A, Eschwege E. High blood glucose concentration is a risk factor for mortality in middle-aged nondiabetic men. 20-year follow-up in the Whitehall Study, the Paris Prospective Study, and the Helsinki Policemen Study. *Diabetes Care* 1998; 21 (3): 360–7.
132. Barrett-Connor E, Ferrarra A. Isolated postchallenge hyperglycemia and the risk of fatal CVD in older women and men. *Diabetes Care* 1998; 21: 1236–9.
133. Balkau B, Bertrais S, Ducimetiere P, Eschwege E. Is there a glycemic threshold for mortality risk? *Diabetes Care* 1999; 22 (5): 696–9.
134. Bjornholt JV, Erikssen G, Aaser E, Sandvik L, Nitter-Hauge S, Jervell J, Erikssen J, Thaulow E. Fasting blood glucose: an underestimated risk factor for cardiovascular death. Results from a 22-year follow-up of healthy nondiabetic men. *Diabetes Care* 1999; 22 (1): 45–9.
135. Yusuf S, Sleight P, Pogue J, Bosch J, Davies R, Dagenais G, for the Heart Outcomes Prevention Evaluation Study Investigators. Effects of an angiotensin-converting-enzyme inhibitor, ramipril, on cardiovascular events in high-risk patients. *N Engl J Med* 2000; 342 (3): 145–53.
136. CDC Diabetes Cost-Effectiveness Study Group. The cost-effectiveness of screening for type 2 diabetes. *JAMA* 1998; 280 (20): 1757–63.
137. Coutinho M, Gerstein H, Wang Y, Yusuf S. The relationship between glucose and incident cardiovascular events: a metagression analysis of published data from 20 studies of 95,783 individuals followed for 12.4 years. *Diabetes Care* 1999; 22: 233–40.
138. Herman WH, Smith PJ, Thompson TJ, Engelgau MM, Aubert RE. A new and simple questionnaire to identify people at increased risk for undiagnosed diabetes. *Diabetes Care* 1995; 18 (3): 382–7.
139. Baan C, Ruige J, Stolk R, Witteman J, Dekker J, Heine R, Feskens E. Performance of a predictive model to identify

undiagnosed diabetes in a health care setting. *Diabetes Care* 1999; 22: 213–9.

140. Ruige JB, de Neeling JN, Kostense PJ, Bouter LM, Heine RJ. Performance of an NIDDM screening questionnaire based on symptoms and risk factors. *Diabetes Care* 1997; 20 (4): 491–6.
141. Larsson G, Spjuth J, Ranstam J, Vikbladh I, Saxtrup O, Astedt B. Prognostic significance of birth of large infant for subsequent development of maternal non-insulin-dependent diabetes mellitus: a prospective study over 20–27 years. *Diabetes Care* 1986; 9 (4): 359–64.
142. Welborn TA, Reid CM, Marriott G. Australian Diabetes Screening Study: impaired glucose tolerance and non-insulin-dependent diabetes mellitus. *Metabolism* 1997; 12 (suppl 1): 1–5.
143. Eriksson KF, Lindgarde F. Prevention of type 2 (non-insulin-dependent) diabetes mellitus by diet and physical exercise. The 6-year Malmö feasibility study. *Diabetologia* 1991; 34 (12): 891–8.
144. Pan X, Li G, Hu Y, Wang J, Yang W, An Z, Hu Z, Lin J, Xiao J, Cao H, Liu P, Jiang X, Wang J, Zheng H, Zhang H, Bennett P, Howard B. Effects of diet and exercise in preventing NIDDM in people with impaired glucose tolerance: the Da Qing IGT and Diabetes Study. *Diabetes Care* 1997; 20: 537–44.
145. Hadden DR. When and how to start insulin treatment in gestational diabetes: a UK perspective. *Diabet Med* 2001; 18 (12): 960–4.
146. Hunter A, Doery J, Miranda V. Diagnosis of gestational diabetes in Australia: a national survey of current practice. *Med J Aust* 1990; 153: 290–2.
147. Keen H. Gestational diabetes. Can epidemiology help? *Diabetes* 1991; 40 (suppl 2): 3–7.
148. Nelson-Piercy C, Gale E. Do we know how to screen for gestational diabetes? Current practice in one regional health authority. *Diabet Med* 1994; 11: 493–8.
149. American Diabetes Association. Gestational diabetes mellitus. *Diabetes Care* 2002; 25 (suppl 1): S94–6.
150. O'Sullivan JB, Mahan CM. Criteria for the oral glucose tolerance test in pregnancy. *Diabetes* 1964; 13: 278.
151. O'Sullivan JB. Establishing criteria for gestational diabetes. *Diabetes Care* 1980; 3: 437–9.
152. Little RR, McKenzie EM, Shyken JM, Winkelmann SE, Ramsey LM, Madsen RW, Goldstein DE. Lack of relationship between glucose tolerance and complications of pregnancy in nondiabetic women. *Diabetes Care* 1990; 13: 483–7.
153. Mestman J. Outcome of diabetes screening in pregnancy and perinatal morbidity in infants of mothers with mild impairment in glucose tolerance. *Diabetes Care* 1980; 3: 447–52.
154. Gabbe SG. Effects of identifying a high risk population. *Diabetes Care* 1980; 3: 486–8.
155. Li D, Wong V, O'Hoy K, Yeung C, Ma H. Is treatment needed for mild impairment of glucose tolerance in pregnancy? *Br J Obstet Gynaecol* 1987; 94: 851–4.
156. Pettitt DJ, Narayan KMV, Hanson RL, Nagi DK, McCance DR, Jacobsson LTH, Knowler WC. World Health Organization and National Diabetes Data Group criteria during pregnancy. *Diabetologia* 1993; 36 (suppl 1): A55.
157. Roberts R, Moohan J, Foo R, Harley J, Traub A, Hadden D. Fetal outcome in mothers with impaired glucose tolerance in pregnancy. *Diabet Med* 1993; 10: 438–43.
158. Lind T, Phillips P. Influence of pregnancy on the 75 g OGTT. A prospective multicentre study. *Diabetes* 1991; 40 (suppl 2): 8–13.
159. Pettitt DJ, Bennett P, Knowler WC, Baird HR, Aleck KA. Gestational diabetes mellitus and impaired glucose tolerance during pregnancy. Long term effects on obesity and glucose tolerance in the offspring. *Diabetes* 1985; 34 (suppl 2): 119–22.
160. Pettitt DJ, Bennett PH, Hanson RL, Venkat A, Narayan KM, Knowler WC. Comparison of World Health Organisation and National Diabetes Data Group procedures to detect abnormalities of glucose tolerance during pregnancy. *Diabetes Care* 1994; 17: 1264–8.
161. Sermer M, Naylor CD, Gare DJ, Kenshole AB, Ritchie JW, Farine D, Cohen HR, McArthur K, Holzapfel S, Biringer A, et al. Impact of increasing carbohydrate intolerance on maternal–fetal outcomes in 3637 women without gestational diabetes. The Toronto Tri-Hospital Gestational Diabetes Project. *Am J Obstet Gynecol* 1995; 173 (1): 146–56.
162. Schmidt MI, Duncan BB, Reichelt AJ, Branchtein L, Matos MC, Costa e Forti A, Spichler ER, Pousada JM, Teixeira MM, Yamashita T. Gestational diabetes mellitus diagnosed with a 2-h 75-g oral glucose tolerance test and adverse pregnancy outcomes. *Diabetes Care* 2001; 24 (7): 1151–5.
163. Deerochanawong C, Putiyanun C, Wongsuryrat M, Serirat S, Jinayon P. Comparison of National Diabetes Data Group and World Health Organization criteria for detecting gestational diabetes mellitus. *Diabetologia* 1996; 39: 1070–3.
164. Hanna FW, Peters JR. Screening for gestational diabetes; past, present and future. *Diabet Med* 2002; 19 (5): 351–8.
165. Buchanan TA, Kjos SL, Montoro MN, Wu PY, Madrilejo NG, Gonzalez M, Nunez V, Pantoja PM, Xiang A. Use of fetal ultrasound to select metabolic therapy for pregnancies complicated by mild gestational diabetes. *Diabetes Care* 1994; 17 (4): 275–83.
166. Weeks JW, Major CA, de Veciana M, Morgan MA. Gestational diabetes: does the presence of risk factors influence perinatal outcome? *Am J Obstet Gynecol* 1994; 171 (4): 1003–7.
167. Lao TT, Ho LF, Liu KL. Gestational diabetes mellitus in teenage pregnancy: a case-control study. *Diabet Med* 1998; 15 (12): 1036–8.
168. Alberti K, Zimmet P. New diagnostic criteria and classification of diabetes—again? *Diabet Med* 1998; 168: 593–4.
169. The Diabetes Epidemiology Research International Group. Preventing insulin dependent diabetes mellitus: the environmental challenge. *Br Med J* 1987; 295: 479–81.
170. Bingley P, Bonifacio E, Gale E. Can we really predict IDDM? *Diabetes* 1993; 42: 213–20.
171. Eisenbarth G, Verge C, Allen H, Rewers M. The design of trials for prevention of IDDM. *Diabetes* 1993; 42: 941–7.

101

Organization of Care: The "At Risk" Person in the Community

Karen S.L. Lam and Kathryn C.B. Tan

The University of Hong Kong, Queen Mary Hospital, Hong Kong, China

Diabetes is a global public health problem, because of its multiple acute and chronic complications and rising prevalence. In developed countries such as the United States of America, total medical expenditure incurred by people with diabetes amounts to nearly fourfold that for people without diabetes [1]. This economic burden is likely to be felt more keenly in the developing countries where an epidemic of type 2 diabetes is evident. In China, for instance, the prevalence of diabetes has more than tripled since the 1980s. In urban areas such as Hong Kong [2] and Shanghai, diabetes now affects 1 in 10 adults. Indeed, the World Health Organization (WHO) has forecasted that the prevalence of diabetes in the developing countries will increase by 170% between 1995 and 2025. A corresponding increase of about 40% is anticipated in the developed countries. This latter estimate may be too conservative, considering the findings of a recent population-based study in Australia [3], which revealed an over twofold increase in diabetes prevalence since 1981, with the overall prevalence in adults reaching 7.4%. As an additional 16.4% of the Australian adult population was found to have impaired glucose tolerance (IGT) or impaired fasting glycemia (IFG), the precursor of diabetes, it is anticipated that even in this developed nation with a predominantly Europid background, the health problems caused by diabetes will continue to grow, unless effective preventive measures are implemented without delay.

GENETIC AND ENVIRONMENTAL RISK FACTORS FOR TYPE 2 DIABETES

To be most cost-effective, measures to prevent the development of diabetes should be directed at individuals at increased risk of developing type 2 diabetes. Such at-risk individuals include those with genetic and/or environmental factors that predispose to insulin deficiency or insulin resistance. It has long been recognized that individuals with a family history of type 2 diabetes are more likely to become diabetic themselves. However, despite extensive research in the past decade, including genome-wide scanning, the major susceptibility genes for type 2 diabetes have remained elusive. On the other hand, various physical or environmental conditions associated with an increase in insulin resistance have been identified. These include the better known risk factors such as age, physical inactivity, high-calorie, high-fat diet, and obesity, especially central obesity. More recently, cigarette smoking and the presence of chronic systemic inflammation, as suggested by elevated levels of inflammatory markers such as C-reactive protein, have also been reported to be associated with an increased incidence of diabetes. Other individuals with an increased risk of diabetes on long-term follow-up include women with a past history of gestational diabetes and infants with low birth weight at full term. The presence of hypertension or dyslipidemia (low high-density lipoprotein cholesterol and/or hypertriglyceridemia) suggests an underlying insulin resistance. These conditions are also considered as risk factors for type 2 diabetes. Variable combinations of the above environmental factors, together with genetic predisposition, probably lead to the higher diabetes prevalence in some ethnic groups (Figure 1). In the United States, for instance, the American Diabetes Association has estimated that while the prevalence of diabetes is about 6.5% in Caucasians, higher prevalence rates of 13 and 10.2% respectively are found among Afro-Americans and Hispanics, while the Pima Indians in

International Textbook of Diabetes Mellitus, Third Edition. Edited by R. A. DeFronzo, E. Ferrannini, H. Keen, and P. Zimmet.
 ISBN: 0-471-48655-8.

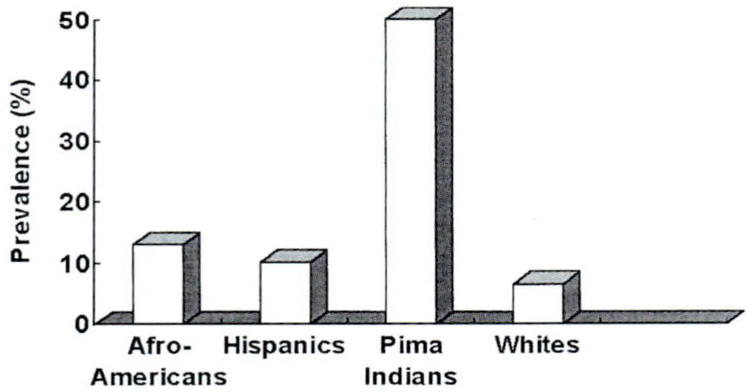

Figure 1 Ethnic differences in diabetes prevalence in the United States

Arizona has a prevalence of 50%, probably the highest in the world [4].

AGING

It has long been recognized that age is an important determinant for the development of type 2 diabetes in various population-based studies [5–8], as aging is accompanied by deterioration in both insulin secretion and insulin sensitivity. Lifestyle changes associated with advancing age, leading to a reduction in physical activity, may also contribute to a reduction in insulin sensitivity. Aging-related changes in the hormonal milieu, such as reductions in growth hormone and estrogen secretion, constitute another cause of insulin resistance in the elderly. In the age-stratified, population-based survey of cardiovascular risk factor prevalence study conducted in Hong Kong in 1995–1996 [2, 6], the prevalence of diabetes at the age of 25–34 years was somewhat higher for men, being 2% compared to 1.4% in women. In contrast, among those aged 65–74 years, a higher prevalence of diabetes was seen in the female sex, with the prevalence in men and women being 21.7 and 29.3% respectively. Estrogen deficiency, which accompanies menopause, probably accounts for the greater rise in diabetes prevalence with age in the female sex (Figure 2). The rapid increase in diabetes prevalence in the developing countries is at least in part attributed to an increasing longevity, consequent to the improvement in health care, control of infections, and increased food supply. The increased risk of diabetes with age has led the American Diabetes Association to recommend that all individuals 45 or older be screened for diabetes by testing the fasting plasma glucose at 3-yearly intervals [9].

OBESITY

Obesity is an established risk factor for type 2 diabetes, supported by the findings from long-term follow-up studies. Among women, the Nurses' Health Study [10] has demonstrated a definite quantitative relationship between body mass index (BMI) and the risk of diabetes. Even women who were considered to have normal weight, with a BMI of 23–24 kg/m^2, had a risk of diabetes 3.6 times that of those with a BMI $<$ 22 kg/m^2. A strong positive association between diabetes risk and overall obesity (and also the absolute weight gain throughout adulthood) was also found in men who participated in the Health Professionals' Follow-up Study. A multivariate relative risk of 42.1 was found for men with a BMI $\geq$ 35 kg/m^2, compared to those with a BMI $<$ 23 kg/m^2 [10]. BMI at the age of 21 was a significant independent risk factor [11], in accordance with the finding among women [10] that the amount of weight gain since early childhood significantly contributed to the risk of acquiring diabetes in later life. A cause–effect relationship is suggested by the benefit of weight reduction on glucose tolerance. In a 2-year randomized placebo-controlled study of 675 obese subjects [12], the group treated with orlistat, a gastrointestinal lipase inhibitor, lost a mean of 6.8% in weight, compared to 3.9% in the placebo group. This modest difference in weight loss was associated with significantly less deterioration in glucose tolerance, and more normalization of IGT, in the treatment group. More recent prospective studies suggest that central obesity, as represented by anthropometric measures such as waist/hip ratio (WHR) or waist circumference, is a better predictor of the development of diabetes than overall obesity as reflected by BMI measurements [13, 14]. Both WHR and waist circumference are indirect measures of visceral adiposity which, when measured directly as the intra-abdominal fat area using computerized tomography, has been demonstrated to be an independent predictor of diabetes in a 6-year prospective community-based follow-up study of 520 Japanese Americans [15]. There is also evidence to suggest that waist circumference, the simpler measurement, is in fact a better predictor than WHR [11, 13, 14]. In a prospective follow-up study of 644 nondiabetic southern Chinese [14], waist circumference was a stronger predictor of the development of diabetes, with those having a high baseline waist circumference (above the sex-specific median) showing an odds ratio of 3.81 relative to subjects with a waist circumference below the median (Table 1).

The increase in free fatty acids (FFAs) has been proposed to be an important link between obesity and type 2 diabetes. While their competitive inhibition of glucose oxidation may lead to a reduction in glucose transport, glucose oxidation, and glycogen synthesis, additional pathways for the adverse effects of FFAs have been suggested by more recent studies. The increased fat disposition in muscles and pancreatic β-cells may lead to insulin resistance [16] and reduced insulin secretion [17] respectively. The lipotoxicity of β-cells may also be mediated via the induction of uncoupling protein 2 by fatty acid oxidation [18], as uncoupling protein 2 has been shown to be a

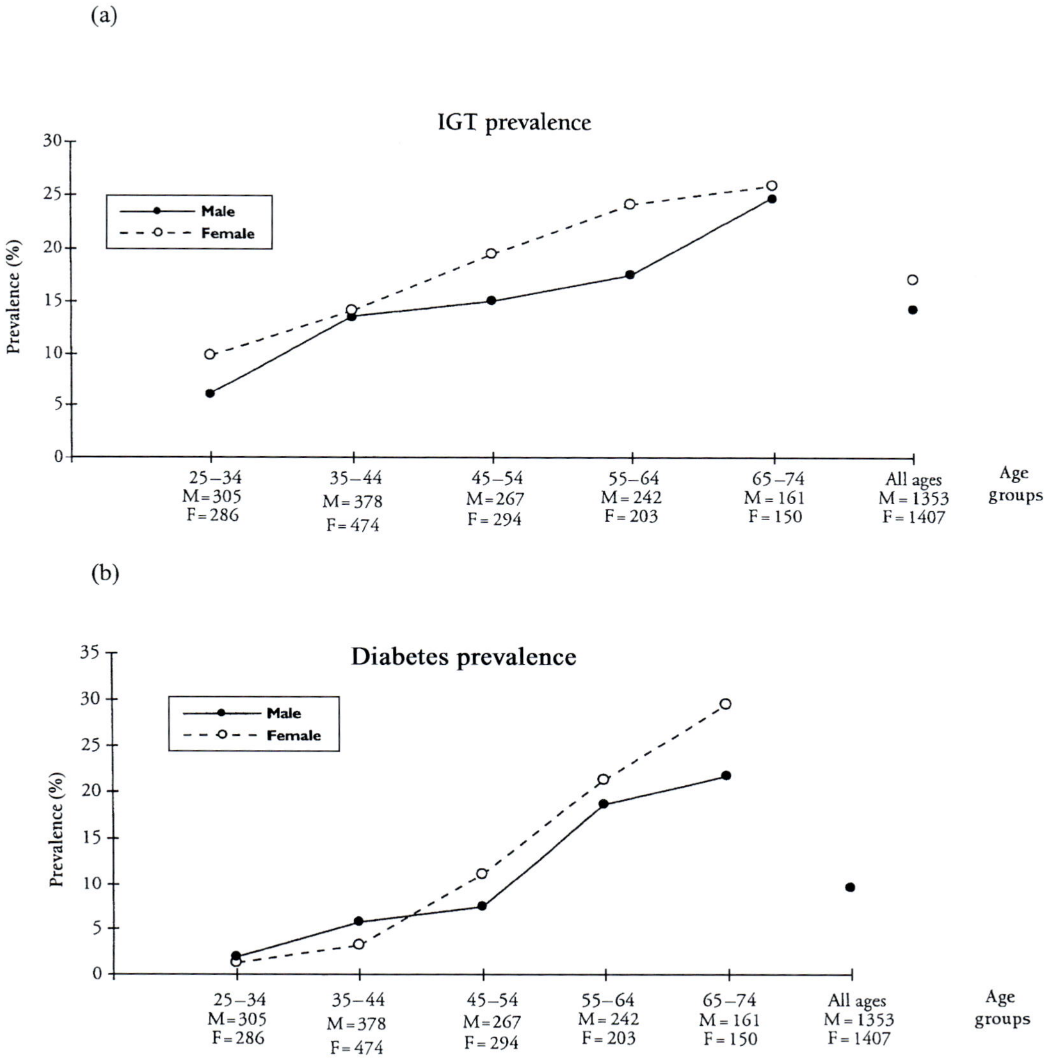

Figure 2 Increasing prevalence of (a) IGT and (b) diabetes with age in Hong Kong (reproduced with permission from reference 6)

key component of β-cell glucose sensing and a negative regulator of insulin secretion [19]. An increase in FFAs also stimulates gluconeogenesis and hence hepatic glucose production [20].

DIETARY AND LIFESTYLE RISK FACTORS

Several dietary and lifestyle factors have been shown to influence the risk of type 2 diabetes. In most previous

Table 1 Influence of baseline waist circumference and waist/hip ratio on outcome measures of glucose intolerance at 2 years*

Status at 2 years	Low	High	OR	*p*
Baseline waist circumference				
≥10% increase in fasting glucose	6.4%	11.7%	2.02	0.02
≥10% increase in 2-h plasma glucose	23.1%	29.8%	1.32	0.13
Development of diabetes mellitus	2.4%	8.6%	3.81	0.001
Baseline waist/hip ratio				
≥10% increase in fasting glucose	6.8%	10.4%	1.75	0.079
≥10% increase in 2-h plasma glucose	20.4%	30.2%	1.47	0.056
Development of diabetes mellitus	2.8%	7.4%	2.84	0.019

Note: OR = odds ratio adjusted for age and sex. Low = below; high = above or equal to gender-specific median.
*Reproduced with permission from reference 14.

studies, dietary and lifestyle factors have been considered individually even though behavioral factors are typically correlated with one another. The Nurses' Health Study has recently evaluated the impact of a set of dietary and lifestyle factors simultaneously and shown that overweight or obesity is the single most important predictor of diabetes [21]. However, lack of exercise, a poor diet, current smoking, and abstinence from alcohol use are all associated with a significantly increased risk of diabetes even after adjusting for BMI [21].

A recent epidemiological study has shown that even nonvigorous physical activity, carried out on a regular basis, is associated with higher insulin sensitivity [22]. In a large prospective study in British middle-aged men, those engaged in moderate levels of physical activity had a 60% reduction in the risk of diabetes relative to their physically inactive counterparts, independent of the effects of age and BMI [23]. On the other hand, a sedentary lifestyle, indicated by prolonged watching of television, was directly related to diabetes risk in a 10-year follow-up study [24]. Dietary habits like a Western dietary pattern (characterized by high contents of red meat and processed meat, high-fat dairy products and sugary food, and low fiber) or a low-fiber diet with high glycemic index have been reported to confer an adverse effect [25, 26]. During a 12-year follow-up of 42 504 US male health professionals, a Western dietary pattern was associated with an increased risk of diabetes relative to a prudent diet consisting mainly of fish, fruit, vegetables, and whole grains [25]. While the adverse effects of excessive total and saturated fat intake may be mediated through an increase in adiposity, the frequent consumption of processed meat has been found to be an independent risk factor for type 2 diabetes [27]. Whether this is mediated through the nitrosamines present in the processed meat, some of which are known to be toxic to β-cells, remains speculative. Smoking, a well-established causal factor for atherosclerosis, has recently been shown by prospective studies to be associated with the development of type 2 diabetes in men and women. Some, but not all, studies have shown a dose–response relationship with the number of cigarette smoked [28–31] and the benefit of giving up smoking is apparent only after 5 years of smoking cessation [31, 32]. The underlying mechanisms are not clear and it has been suggested that the effect of smoking may be mediated through alterations in fat distribution, insulin resistance, and/or chronic inflammation [32]. In recent reports, elevated levels of inflammatory markers appear to predict the development of type 2 diabetes [33, 34], possibly through the adverse effects of cytokines, such as interleukin 6 and tumor necrosis factor α, on insulin sensitivity. In contrast to smoking, the relationship between alcohol consumption and diabetes risk is nonlinear, with the risk being lowest in light and moderate drinkers, and highest in heavy drinkers [35]. The protective effect of moderate drinking may be mediated partly through an effect on insulin sensitivity [35] while the adverse effect of heavy drinking appears to act through the increase in body weight.

Table 2 Stepwise multiple linear regression models for insulin resistance measured as the homeostasis model assessment of insulin resistance index (HOMA-IR)*

	Estimate ± SE	p
$R^2 = 24.5\%$		
BMI (kg/m^2)	0.071 ± 0.010	<0.001
AHI (event/h)	0.005 ± 0.002	0.044
$R^2 = 24.5\%$		
BMI (kg/m^2)	0.070 ± 0.010	<0.001
Min. SaO_2	-0.008 ± 0.004	0.022

Note: AHI = apnea–hypopnea index; SaO_2 = arterial oxygen saturation. Other independent variables: AHI, time with oxygen saturation <90%, minimum oxygen saturation (Min. SaO_2), arousal index, age, gender, smoking.
*Modified with permission from reference 37.

OBSTRUCTIVE SLEEP APNEA

Obstructive sleep apnea (OSA) is another condition recently proposed to be a risk factor for type 2 diabetes. Data from the Nurses' Health Study suggested that women who regularly snored was associated with an over twofold increase in the risk of diabetes over 10 years, compared with nonsnoring women [36]. Snoring, which may suggest underlying OSA, remained an independent risk factor in analyses stratified by BMI, smoking history, and parental history of diabetes. Studies in men have shown that OSA is independently associated with insulin resistance [37, 38] and glucose intolerance [38]. Although patients with OSA tend to be overweight or obese, indices of sleep disturbance, including the apnea–hypopnea index and minimal oxygen saturation, are independently associated with insulin resistance (Table 2). Sympathetic activation or other effects of hypoxia may contribute to the increase in insulin resistance in these individuals.

GESTATIONAL DIABETES AND FETAL FACTORS

In women, gestational diabetes is another important risk factor for developing diabetes. Gestational diabetes affects up to 14% of pregnant women. It has been demonstrated that women with a history of gestational diabetes have chronic insulin resistance and impaired β-cell function [39] and they have a higher annual diabetes incidence rate than subjects with IGT from the general population [40]. In some ethnic groups like the Hispanic Americans, the cumulative incidence rate of type 2 diabetes 5 years after the index pregnancy is as high is 50% [41]. Hence, women with gestational diabetes are a high-risk group, which should be targeted for prevention. The infant of a woman with diabetes during pregnancy is also at an increased risk of developing obesity, IGT, or diabetes at an early age, even before entering adulthood [42, 43]. The infants of diabetic mothers tend to have a higher birth weight and their increased risk of future diabetes is thought to be the consequences of the hyperglycemic intrauterine environment superimposed on a genetic predisposition [42, 43]. The relationship between birth weight and obesity in adulthood is J-shaped [44] and an association between low birth weight at term and the incidence of obesity, IGT, type 2 diabetes mellitus, hypertension, and coronary heart disease has also been demonstrated in numerous, mainly cross-sectional, studies [44–46]. It has been postulated that these diseases may be the result of "fetal programming" whereby a stimulus or insult at a critical, sensitive period of early life has permanent effects on structure, physiology, and metabolism, with a resetting of major hormonal axes that control growth and metabolic processes [47, 48]. Irrespective of birth weight, adverse lifestyle changes with regard to physical activity and diet have led to an epidemic of childhood obesity and increasing prevalence of IGT in many countries, including the United States [49].

CONCLUSION

It is clear that active public education to promote a healthy lifestyle should be conducted at the community level, starting at the schools. More aggressive measures to prevent type 2 diabetes should be targeted at the "at risk" individuals. The effectiveness of diet and exercise in preventing type 2 diabetes in people with IGT was first reported in the Da Qing IGT and Diabetes Study [50]. In this 6-year intervention study, a reduction in the development of diabetes was achieved in 31, 46, and 42% of the participants in the centers randomized to diet, exercise, or diet plus exercise, respectively. These results have recently been confirmed by two large randomized-controlled studies conducted in Finland [51] and the United States [52] respectively. In both studies overweight individuals with IGT randomized to the intervention group underwent a vigorous lifestyle modification program with counseling and intensive reinforcement to achieve their goals for physical exercise and weight reduction, and the maintenance of a low-fat, low-calorie diet. A most impressive 58% reduction in diabetes incidence compared to the control group was achieved in both studies, after 3.2 and 2.8 years respectively [48, 49]. The effect of intensive lifestyle modification was even greater than that achieved with metformin, which resulted in a 31% reduction in diabetes incidence. These exciting results would suggest that, with appropriate public health measures, we could still hope to put a halt on the epidemic of type 2 diabetes.

REFERENCES

1. American Diabetes Association. Economic consequences of diabetes mellitus in the U.S. in 1997. *Diabetes Care* 1998; 21: 296–309.
2. Janus ED, Wat NMS, Lam KSL, Cockram CS, Siu STS, Liu LJ, Lam TH, on behalf of the Hong Kong Cardiovascular Risk factor Steering Committee. The prevalence of diabetes, association with cardiovascular risk factors and implications of diagnostic criteria (ADA 1997 and WHO 1998) in a 1996 community-based population study in Hong Kong Chinese. *Diabet Med* 2000; 17: 741–5.
3. Dunstan DW, Zimmet PZ, Welborn TA, De Courten MP, Cameron AJ, Sicree RA, Dwyer T, Colagiuri S, Jolley D, Knuiman M, Atkins R, Shaw JE. The rising prevalence of diabetes and impaired glucose tolerance: the Australian Diabetes, Obesity and Lifestyle Study. *Diabetes Care* 2002; 25: 829–34.
4. Marx J. Unraveling the causes of diabetes. *Science* 2002; 296: 686–9.
5. Pan XR, Yang WY, Li GW, Liu J, for the National Diabetes Prevention and Control Cooperative Group. Prevention of diabetes and its risk factors in China, 1994. *Diabetes Care* 1997; 20: 1664–9.
6. Janus ED, for the Cardiovascular Risk Factor Prevalence Study Group. Hong Kong Cardiovascular Risk Factor Prevalence Study (1995–1996) Monograph. Hong Kong, 1997.
7. Ramachandran A, Snehalatha C, Kapur A, Vijay V, Mohan V, Das AK, Rao PV, Yajnik CS, Prasanna Kumar KM, Nair JD, for the Diabetes Epidemiological Study Group in India (DESI). High prevalence of diabetes and impaired glucose tolerance in India: National Urban Diabetes Survey. *Diabetologia* 2001; 44: 1094–101.
8. Cuasay LC, Lee ES, Orlandeer PP, Steffin-Batey L, Hanis CL. Prevalence and determinants of type 2 diabetes among Filipino-Americans in the Houston, Texas metropolitan statistical area. *Diabetes Care* 2001; 24: 2054–8.
9. Report of the Expert Committee on the Diagnosis and Classification of Diabetes Mellitus. *Diabetes Care* 2002; 25 (suppl 1): S5–20.
10. Colditz GA, Willett WC, Rotnitzky A, Manson JE. Weight gain as a risk factor for clinical diabetes mellitus in women. *Ann Intern Med* 1995; 122: 481–6.
11. Chan JM, Rimm EB, Colditz GA, Stampfer MJ, Willett WC. Obesity, fat distribution, and weight gain as risk factors for clinical diabetes in men. *Diabetes Care* 1994; 17: 961–9.
12. Heymsfield SB, Segal KR, Hauptman J, Lucas CP, Boldrin MN, Rissanen A, Wilding JPH, Sjostrom L. Effects of weight loss with orlistat on glucose tolerance and progression to type 2 diabetes in obese adults. *Arch Intern Med* 2000; 160: 1321–6.
13. Wei M, Gaskill SP, Haffner SM, Stern MP. Waist circumference as the best predictor of non-insulin dependent diabetes mellitus (NIDDM) compared to body mass index, waist/hip ratio and other anthropometric measurements in Mexican Americans—a 7-year prospective study. *Obes Res* 1997; 5: 16–23.
14. Wat NMS, Lam TH, Janus ED, Lam KSL. Central obesity predicts the worsening of glycemia in southern Chinese. *Int J Obes* 2001; 25: 1789–93.
15. Boyko EJ, Fujimoto WY, Leonetti DL, Newell-Morris L. Visceral adiposity and risk of type 2 diabetes: a prospective study among Japanese Americans. *Diabetes Care* 2000; 223: 465–71.

16. Boden G, Lebed B, Schatz M, Homko C, Lemieux S. Effects of acute changes of plasma free fatty acids on intramyocellular fat content and insulin resistance in healthy subjects. *Diabetes* 2001; 50: 1612–7.
17. Unger RH, Zhou YT. Lipotoxicity of beta-cells in obesity and in other causes of fatty acid spillover. *Diabetes* 2001 (suppl 1): S118–21.
18. Li LX, Skorpen F, Egeeberg K, Jorgensen IH, Grill V. Induction of uncoupling protein 2 mRNA in beta-cells is stimulated by oxidation of fatty acids but not by nutrient oversupply. *Endocrinology* 2002; 143: 1371–7.
19. Zhang Cy, Baffy G, Perret P, Krauus S, Peroni O, Gujic D, Hagen T, Vidal-puig AJ, Boss O, Kim YB, Zheng XX, Wheeler MB, Shulman GI, Chan CB, Lowell BB. Uncoupling protein-2 negatively regulates insulin secretion and is a major link between obesity, beta cell dysfunction, and type 2 diabetes. *Cell* 2001; 105: 705–7.
20. Boden G, Chen X, Capulong E, Mozzoli M. Effects of free fatty acids on gluconeogenesis and autoregulation of glucose production in type 2 diabetes. *Diabetes* 2001; 50: 810–6.
21. Hu FB, Manson JE, Stampfer MJ, Colditz GC, Liu S, Solomon CG, Willett WC. Diet, lifestyle and the risk of type 2 diabetes mellitus in women. *N Engl J Med* 1997; 337: 1491–9.
22. Mayer-Davis E, D'Agnostino R, Karter AJ, Haffner SM, Rewers MJ, Sadd M, Bergman RN. Intensity of amount of physical activity in relation to insulin sensitivity: the Insulin Resistance Atherosclerosis Study. *JAMA* 1998; 279: 669–74.
23. Perry IJ, Wannamethee SG, Walker MK, Thomson AG, Whincup PH, Shaper AG. Prospective study of risk factors for development of non-insulin dependent diabetes in middle aged British men. *BMJ*. March 4 1995; 310: 560–4.
24. Hu FB, Leithzmann MF, Stampfer MJ, Colditz GA, Willett WC, Rimm EB. Physical activity and television watching in relation to risk for type 2 diabetes in men. *Arch Intern Med* 2001; 161: 1542–8.
25. van Dam RM, Rimm EB, Willett WC, Stampfer MJ, Hu FB. Dietary patterns and risk for type 2 diabetes mellitus in U.S. men. *Ann Intern Med* 2002; 136: 201–9.
26. Salmeron J, Manson JE, Stampfer MJ, Colditz GA, Wing AL, Willett WC. Dietary fiber, glycemic load, and risk of non-insulin-dependent diabetes mellitus in women. *JAMA* 1997; 277: 472–7.
27. van Dam RM, Willett WC, Rimm EB, Stampfer MJ, Hu FB. Dietary fats and meat intake in relation to risk of type 2 diabetes in man. *Diabetes Care* 2002; 25: 417–24.
28. Rimm EB, Manson JE, Stampfer MJ, Colditz GA, Willett WC, Rosner B, Hennekens CH, Speizer FE. Cigarette smoking and the risk of diabetes in women. *Am J Public Health* 1993; 83: 211–41.
29. Rimm EB, Chan J, Stampfer MJ, Colditz GA, Willet WC. Prospective study of cigarette smoking, alcohol use and the risk of diabetes in men. *BMJ* 1995; 310: 555–9.
30. Manson JA, Ajani UA, Liu S, Nathan DM, Hennekens CH. A prospective study of cigarette smoking and the incidence of diabetes mellitus among U.S. male physicians. *Am J Med* 2000; 109: 538–42.
31. Wannamethee SG, Shaper AG, Perry IJ, for the British Regional Heart Study Group. Smoking as modifiable risk factor for type 2 diabetes in middle-aged men. *Diabetes Care* 2001; 24: 1590–5.
32. Eliasson B, Attvall S, Taskinen MR, Smith U. Smoking cessation improves insulin sensitivity in healthy middle-aged men. *Eur J Clin Invest* 1997; 27: 450–6.
33. Pradhan AD, Manson JE, Rifai N, Buring JE, Ridker PM. C-reactive protein, interlukin-6 and risk of developing type 2 diabetes. *JAMA* 2001; 286: 327–34.
34. Festa A, D'Agostino R Jr, Tracy R, Haffner SM. Elevated levels of acute phase proteins and development of type 2 diabetes: the Insulin Resistance Atherosclerosis Study. *Diabetes* 2002; 51: 1131–7.
35. Wannanmethee SG, Shaper AG, Perry IJ, Alberti KG. Alcohol consumption and the incidence of type 2 diabetes. *J Epidemiol Community Health* 2002; 56: 542–8.
36. Al-Delaimy WK, Manson JE, Willett WC, Stampfer MJ, Hu FB. Snoring as a risk factor for type II diabetes mellitus: a prospective study. *Am J Epidemiol* 2002; 155: 387–93.
37. Ip MS, Lam B, Ng MM, Lam WK, Tsang KW, Lam KS. Obstructive sleep apnoea is independently associated with insulin resistance. *Am J Respir Crit Care Med* 2002; 165: 670–6.
38. Funjabi NM, Sorkin JD, Katzel LI, Goldberg AP, Schwartz AR, Smith PL. Sleep-disordered breathing and insulin resistance in middle-aged and overweight men. *Am J Respir Crit Care Med* 2002; 165: 677–82.
39. Buchanan TA. Pancreatic beta-cell defects in gestational diabetes: implications for the pathogenesis and prevention of type 2 diabetes. *J Clin Endocrinol Metab* 2001; 86: 989–93.
40. Maresh M. Diabetes in pregnancy. *Curr Opin Obstet Gynecol* 2001; 13: 103–7.
41. Kjos SL, Peters RK, Xiang A, Henry OA, Montoro MN, Buchanan TA. Predicting future diabetes in Latino women with gestational diabetes: utility of early postpartum glucose tolerance testing. *Diabetes* 1995; 44: 586–91.
42. Silverman BL, Metzger BE, Cho NH, Loeb CA. Impaired glucose tolerance in adolescent offspring of diabetic mothers. *Diabetes Care* 1995; 18: 611–7.
43. Dabelea D, Hanson RL, Lindsay RS, Pettitt DJ, Imperatore G, Gabir MM, Roumain J, Bennett PH, Knowler WC. Intrauterine exposure to diabetes conveys risks for type 2 diabetes and obesity: a study of discordant sibship. *Diabetes* 2000; 49: 2208–11.
44. Curhan GC, Chertow GM, Willett WC, Spiegelman D, Colditz GA, Manson JE, Speizer FE, Stampfer MJ. Birth weight and adult hypertension and obesity in women. *Circulation* 1996; 94: 1310–5.
45. Curhan GC, Willett WC, Rimm B, Spiegelman D, Ascheiro AL, Stampfer MJ. Birth weight and adult hypertension, diabetes mellitus, and obesity in U.S. men. *Circulation* 1996; 94: 3246–50.
46. Frankel S, Elowood P, Sweetnam P, Yarnell J, Davey Smith G. Birth weight, body mass index in middle age, and incident coronary heart disease. *Lancet* 1996; 348: 1478–80.
47. Godfrey KM, Barker DJ. Fetal nutrition and adult disease. *Am J Clin Nutr* 2000; 71 (suppl 1): 1344S–52.
48. Phenekos C. Influence of fetal body weight on metabolic complications in adult life: review of the evidence. *J Paediatr Endocrinol Metab* 2001; 14 (suppl 5): 1361–3.
49. Sinha R, Fisch G, Teague B, Tamborlane WV, Banyas B, Allen K, Savoye M, Rieger V, Takali S, Barbaretta G, Sherwin RS, Caprio S. Prevalence of impaired glucose tolerance among children and adolescence with marked obesity. *N Engl Med* 2002; 346: 802–10.
50. Pan XR, Li GW, Hu YH, Wang JX, Yang WY, An ZX, Lin J, Xiao JZ, Cao HB, Liu PA, Jiang XG, Jiang YY, Wang

JP, Zheng HM, Zhang H, Baenett PH, Howard BV. Effects of diet and exercise in preventing NIDDM in people with impaired glucose tolerance: the Da Qing IGT and Diabetes Study. *Diabetes Care* 1997; 20: 537–44.

51. Tuomilehto J, Eriksson JG, Hamalainen H, Hanne-Paarikka P, Keinanen-Kiukaanniemi S, Laakso M, Louheranta A, Rastas M, Salminen V, Uusitupa M, for the Finnish Diabetes Prevention Study Group. Prevention of type 2 diabetes mellitus by changes in lifestyle among subjects with impaired glucose tolerance. *N Engl J Med* 2001; 344: 343–50.

52. Diabetes Prevention Program Research Group. Reduction in the incidence of type 2 diabetes with lifestyle intervention of metformin. *N Engl Med* 2002; 346: 393–403.

102

Diabetes and Public Health in the United States

Frank Vinicor, Kathy Rufo, and Dara Murphy

Centers for Disease Control, Division of Diabetes, Atlanta, GA, USA

THE BURDEN OF DIABETES IN THE UNITED STATES

Diabetes mellitus (DM) in the United States is a chronic disease epidemic. The prevalence of those diagnosed with DM, especially type 2, has increased 61% since 1990 [1]. Further, (1) the *rate of increase* in the prevalence of diabetes, year to year, is increasing, with the most recent rate of 8.2% (2000 to 2001) [1], and (2) the onset of diabetes is at ever younger ages, with prevalence of type 2 diabetes now increasing at greatest rates among people in their 30s, and even in adolescent youth [2]. Should the epidemic of type 2 DM increase, even at its present rate, it is projected that there will be approximately 30 million persons with known DM in the United States by 2050 [3]. In essence, there will be more people with diabetes who have a longer duration of disease, with the devastating complications and associated morbidity, mortality, impaired quality of life, and costs; and this could increase substantially during the next two decades. The rise in prevalence observed in the United States is also happening throughout the world [4], and all countries can anticipate increasing challenges associated with DM.

WHY IS THE DIABETES BURDEN GROWING IN THE UNITED STATES?

There are three general reasons for the dramatic increase in the prevalence of DM: improved ascertainment, demographic changes, and increases in associated risk conditions and behaviors, such as obesity and physical inactivity. It is recognized in most countries that a substantial portion of DM is undiagnosed [5]. Thus, in terms of an increase in prevalence of diabetes and ascertainment, if *active and systematic* screening campaigns were to be implemented to find "missing diabetes," the prevalence of this disease would increase. (Likewise, if the mortality rate in persons with DM were to decrease, this also would result in an increased prevalence rate.) While the issue of screening for undiagnosed diabetes is controversial [6, 7] at present in the United States there is no coordinated and systematic "screening program" to identify persons with undiagnosed DM. Furthermore, other studies indicate an actual increase in the *incidence* of type 2 diabetes [8], and the increase in diabetes prevalence occurred prior to new glucose criteria for diabetes [9]. Hence, it is unlikely that "better ascertainment" contributes substantially to the increased prevalence. Demographic changes in the United States account for approximately two thirds of the increase in diabetes prevalence over the past two decades [3]. This is because of an increase in the number of elderly and specific minority communities who are already at great risk of DM. These two groups each account for one third of the diabetes epidemic. Furthermore, changes in associated risk conditions and behaviors, such as being overweight or obese, and physical inactivity, contribute to the final one third of the increasing prevalence of diabetes [3]. There is a close statistical correlation between overweight/obesity and diabetes rate increases over the past 10 years [1] . Further, the "epidemic" of overweight/obesity/physical inactivity has preceded the rapid rise in diabetes prevalence by about 5 years. This information in the aggregate, along with recent interventions studies regarding primary prevention of type 2 diabetes

International Textbook of Diabetes Mellitus, Third Edition. Edited by R. A. DeFronzo, E. Ferrannini, H. Keen, and P. Zimmet, 2004.
 ISBN: 0-471-48655-8.

in high-risk patients [10], indicates that improvement of nutritional and activity status of Americans would have a major beneficial impact on diabetes incidence [10, 11].

OPTIONS IN 2003

In the face of this epidemic of diabetes in the United States and throughout the world, we are not without options, today. Two basic approaches exist to reducing the overall diabetes burden, and these must be viewed as necessary and complementary: improved care (secondary and tertiary prevention) and decreased incidence (primary prevention.) It is likely that options for "cure" of diabetes, especially type 1, will be available to *some* individuals within 5 years [12]. The concept of "cure" for type 2 diabetes remains a future challenge at present [13].

Improved Care

Scientific and economic evidence provides the rationale for the expected benefits of secondary and tertiary diabetes prevention programs [14, 15]. In spite of the strength of extant efficacy science, there are however (1) many challenges in translating important efficacy studies into efficient and effective clinical and public health programs [16], and (2) "gaps" existing between what could be applied to persons with diabetes, and what is actually happening [17]. While many factors contribute to the genesis of this "gap" [16], evidence does indicate that in most health care systems in the United States, the differential between what should, and what is, happening to persons with diabetes, is diminishing [18]. However, challenges remain to ensure that *all* persons with diabetes—not just those with health insurance and reimbursed access—benefit from efficacious quality secondary and tertiary prevention programs [19].

Decreasing Diabetes Incidence

With the rapidly increasing prevalence of diabetes, there is serious concern that even "perfect care" will not be able control the burden of diabetes through complication prevention and control. That is, health systems may become "overwhelmed" with care demands of an increasing number of persons with diabetes [20]. Fortunately, several rigorous efficacy studies among those at high risk for subsequent type 2 diabetes—persons with impaired glucose tolerance, or "prediabetes" [5, 10, 11]—indicate that (1) modest behavioral improvements, such as weight loss and/or increased physical activity, can prevent or at least delay the onset of type 2 diabetes by over 50%, and (2) medication used presently in the treatment of DM also decreases the incidence of type 2 DM by about 30% [10, 11]. In the aggregate, these studies support the view that *if* modest improved nutrition, weight loss, and/or increased physical activity could be accomplished, the number of persons with diabetes would be reduced substantially, thus allowing health practitioners to focus on improved care for those who do develop DM. While many issues remain, for example identification of persons with prediabetes, development of feasible cost-effective primary prevention strategies, ensuring supportive implementation and reimbursement policies, and economic perspectives of primary prevention, the opportunity to implement targeted prevention strategies and programs that would decrease the incidence of type 2 diabetes provides a new option for reducing the individual and societal burden associated with DM.

THE ROLE OF PUBLIC HEALTH IN DIABETES PREVENTION AND CONTROL

Over the past century, remarkable improvements in the health of the United States have occurred [21], in large part due to investments in basic and clinical research, as well as *individual-targeted* clinical care systems located in the doctor's office or hospital setting. Persons with diabetes have also benefited from these strategies [18]. Still, excellent care for persons with diabetes remains an elusive goal, one that is perhaps magnified among those without adequate resources, insurance, and/or in various racial and ethnic communities [19]. Thus, serious questions about the basic design of US clinical care systems and its relevancy to chronic disease management are being asked [22–24]. Further, recognition that aspects of life *outside* the office or hospital setting dramatically influence processes of care and health outcomes [25] has led to the realization that the present US health care system [22–26], and dependency on the traditional *clinical* care mechanism alone, will not be able to control the emerging health and economic burden of diabetes, in particular the need to implement primary prevention programs for those at risk for type 2 DM. Does public health have a role in improving the health of persons at risk for and with DM [27]; what is public health; what are the relevant principles of public health; and what public health programs exist in the United States to address the challenges of DM?

PUBLIC HEALTH

An appropriate definition of public health (there are many) is "What we as a society do collectively to assure the conditions in which people can be healthy" [28]. Key words in this definition include "*society*": something beyond the one to one direct clinical process; "*collectively*": a decision among many people beyond the individual patient and health provider; "*conditions*": more than just biological phenomenon; "*people*": population health; and "*healthy*": greater than alive or dead, sick or well.

Several basic principles of public health define its role in diabetes prevention and control (Table 1):

1. *The Essential Place of Science*. The content, targets, and interventional methods of public health programs must have a solid scientific base—as much as any clinical treatment strategy for persons with DM. Thus, until clear efficacy evidence of glycemic control was established [29, 30], public health programs in the United States focused on tertiary prevention strategies: screening for, and prevention of, progression of diabetes complications. Similarly, the targets of public health programs—managed care organizations, cultural barriers, policies, laws, access and quality of care—must reflect valid surveillance and/or epidemiologic science. Further, both quantitative and qualitative science must be used to identify appropriate methodologies for public health interventions. Finally, the nature of the interventions, themselves, should reflect clear evidence of *effectiveness* of impact—whatever the nature of these interventions [31].
2. *Power of a Supportive Environment*. While both the individual health professional and patient must make personal decisions regarding preventive or management health strategies, the environments wherein these health practitioners provide care and where patients live, work, and play, dramatically influence the likelihood of these "correct decisions" being made [23, 32]. Thus, for example, the structure, design, and cultural relevancy of health care systems themselves, apart from what a health professional knows or would want to do, impacts greatly on whether appropriate recommendations are provided to patients [23–25, 33]. Similarly, efforts outside the doctor's office can significantly improve patient decision-making and indeed, outcomes [34]. Public health programs addressing diabetes do not provide direct care. Rather, the addressing and augmenting "environmental" factors is a corner stone of public health strategies.
3. *Need for Multiple and Coordinated Approaches*. Especially for chronic diseases like diabetes, an "if only" or single approach is unlikely to result in meaningful changes in long-standing societal and/or individual behaviors [35, 36]. It is the *coordination* of *several* strategies—individual, media, policy, laws, professional guidelines, community interventions, work site, reimbursement policies—all directed to a common purpose, that is likely to have a long-term impact on individuals at risk of, or with, chronic diseases like diabetes. It is the responsibility of the public health community to "see the forest," and to insure that *all* strategies are utilized and coordinated for the overall health of the population.
4. *A "System of Influence" Strategy*. Given that a relatively small percentage of the investment of the US society in health is directed to prevention and/or public health [37], and given that multiple approaches must be integrated in a coordinated fashion for maximum impact, the public health community often utilizes a "system of influence" in its implementation strategy [38]. Public health programs, especially those addressing chronic diseases, usually do not provide direct clinical care for individuals in need. Rather, public health focuses on "influencing the actions of others"—in the private, academic, community, state, federal, voluntary, and professional communities—to direct their expertise and resources to address problems such as diabetes. This philosophy of public health therefore requires that the public health community establish active, meaningful, and ongoing partnerships with all these other organizations if positive outcomes are to occur [39]. The process of partnership building is often slow and tedious at the beginning, but unless solidly established, will diminish how well public health can influence the action of others.
5. *Power of "Exposure*." Within the clinical system, doing the best for the individual patient is a highly laudable and ethically sound strategy [40, 41]. Consistent with this approach, the "impact" of a scientifically sound program has been primarily defined in terms of the efficacy of that program [42, 43]. However, a highly efficacious diabetes intervention available to only a few people would have minimal impact on the population or societal burden of diabetes [42]. "Exposure," or the number of people who can benefit from an efficacious program, is also an important consideration in determining the overall impact of scientifically validated diabetes program. Often, it is the public health community that is responsible for ensuring that as many people as possible are able to benefit from a diabetes strategy [44]. For example, while the clinical community would focus its efforts on who *does* come into the office or emergency room, public health strategies would also be concerned with those persons with diabetes who *do not* have access to appropriate diabetes management programs. Increasing access or exposure to even "good programs" would have a major impact on overall societal health around diabetes.
6. *Social Justice/Equity*. In the United States, highly efficacious care using advanced (and often expensive) technology is available, often in tertiary care centers and to some individuals. However, distribution of health care remains an essential element in defining a "good health care system" [45, 46]. While most health care professionals remain committed to preventing and managing chronic diseases like diabetes in all persons for whom they are responsible, a number of persons may not have equal access to even a basic level of

preventive and management services [19]. The challenges of equity in health services is an important dimension of the public health community, and a central tenet to a public health approach to diabetes. *All* persons at risk should benefit from the investments that society has made in basic, clinical, and health services research [47].

7. *Community Participation in Research/Programs.* If populations and/or communities are the targets of public health research and programs, the people who live, work, and play in these places must be involved actively, early, and continually in these efforts [48, 49]. The affected individuals are often not acutely ill, the programs often will last a lifetime, and will occur in places outside the doctor's office. They are not passive recipients of information and recommendations, but rather the major determiners of their fates. Thus, involved, active, and "empowered" people and communities must be a central part of public health programs for diabetes [50, 51] if these programs are to start, last, and have impact.
8. *Complementing the Clinical Care System.* In the later nineteenth and early twentieh centuries, clinical and public health professionals were often one in the same [52]. With the rapid growth of basic and clinical research and knowledge post-World War II, the two disciplines diverged, with separate schools, training programs, fundamental concepts, and organizations [53]. However, the emergence of chronic diseases as the major public health challenge in the United States, as well as a growing awareness of the important and powerful role of the larger environmental forces outside the doctor's office, means that a meaningful partnership between clinical and public health approaches to diabetes prevention and control is again essential in order to maximize what each community can provide for persons at risk of, or with, diabetes [53].
9. *Accountability.* As attention to chronic diseases and the role of public health increases, careful evaluation of program impact must occur. This "accountability" is both different from what might be expected in clinical medicine, and a challenge [31]. Given that (a) public health often does not directly deal with specific individuals, but large populations; (b) early preventive interventions for chronic diseases like diabetes may not have identifiable "hard outcome impact" for one to two decades; and (c) public health interventions often are not, and cannot, be applied in a randomized control format as in clinical efficacy studies [54, 55], other means of establishing accountability have to be implemented. Such paradigms have been proposed and used [54–56], but reliable evaluation systems must be further developed.

DIABETES PUBLIC HEALTH PROGRAMS IN THE UNITED STATES

Four elements characterize the dimensions of public health strategies for DM:

Surveillance/Epidemiology Science

Surveillance (the ongoing systematic collection, analyses, and interpretation of outcome-specific data for use in planning, implementation, and evaluation of public health practice) [57] and epidemiology (the design, implementation, and evaluation of specific and focused public health questions) [58] are examples of scientific studies supported by diabetes public health programs in the United States. Each type provides important information, for example, trend analyses of the burden of diabetes and associated complications [1], as well as its preventive treatment [17]. This defines the prevalence and incidence of diabetes among youth, including type 1 and 2 [59], identifying diabetes-related disparities in racial and ethnic populations [60]. These public health science programs provide essential information on the evolution of diabetes and its management in the United States—over time, in different geographical locations, with different populations, and in different clinical or community settings.

Translational/Health Services Research

This type of research represents (a) a complementary but different approach to public health science, whether surveillance, epidemiology, or the usual efficacy-focused clinical investigation [16] and (b) addresses issues of effectiveness, efficiency, availability, and distribution, as well as access to quality of care and disparities in health outcomes [43]. It includes both quantitative and qualitative behavioral science, particularly as pertains to population and community perspectives on diabetes prevention and control. Translational research addresses questions beyond "*what is going on*" and focuses on "*why is this happening*" and "*what changes should be implemented to address deficiencies*." Studies of the structure and design of health care systems [61], influence of economic forces in decision making [62, 63], and patient and community views of diabetes [64, 65] are examples of public health investigations that provide a greater understanding of *why* diabetes remains a major public health challenge in spite of remarkable basic and clinical knowledge. These types of translational research efforts should be closely linked to subsequent program design and implementation.

Public Health Programs

Consistent with the US Constitution, most public health program activity occurs at the state or local level. The major responsibilities of federal public health agencies are

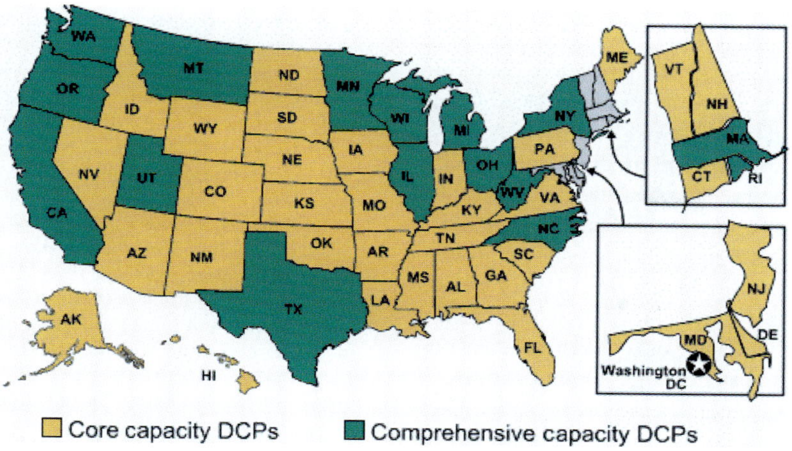

Figure 1 Distribution of state- and territorial-based public health programs in the United States: core and comprehensive

thus (a) to collect and analyze data relevant to the nation's health, (b) to develop broad strategies directed at national public health challenges like diabetes, and (c) to carefully evaluate program impact delivered at the state and local level. Consistent with these general principles, the Centers for Disease Control and Prevention (CDC) supports public health oriented Diabetes Prevention and Control Programs (DPCP) that are presently located in all states, territories, and the District of Columbia (66) (Figure 1). DPCPs, reflecting the principles of public health (Table 1), and incorporating the 10 Essential Public Health Strategies [67, 68] (Table 2), do not provide, or reimburse, for direct diabetes prevention and control activities for individual persons. Rather, these 59 DPCPs collect and analyze state and local diabetes data, establish active partnerships with various health organizations interested in or impacted by diabetes, develop state and territorial state diabetes plans for disease prevention and control, and assess program impact within each jurisdiction. At present, these DPCPs are incorporating the challenges of primary prevention programs for type 2 diabetes, establishing more formal and active interactions with other public health and clinical programs related to common diabetes complications, such as cardiovascular disease, targeting additional sites such as schools for program implementation, and addressing other high-risk populations, such as youth and elderly.

Table 1 Principles of public health

1. Role of science
2. Supportive environment
3. Multiple coordinated approaches
4. Systems of influence
5. "Good to many people"/power of exposure
6. Social justice
7. Participatory research/programs
8. Complementing the clinical care system
9. Accountability

In addition to governmental public health strategies, federal agencies such as CDC are also increasingly working in partnership with community entities and nongovernmental organizations (NGOs). Often, these NGOs fully reflect the culture and traditions of various community groups, have important insights into, and understanding about, basic determinants of the diabetes burden within communities and special populations, and use their own infrastructure and organizational system to disseminate information and implement programs. Faith, service, union, professional, economic, voluntary, and race- and ethnic-based organizations are some of the nongovernmental entities that are components of diabetes public health programs.

Finally, ensuring positive interactions between the governmental and nongovernmental organizations are important challenges to federal public health entities in efforts to ultimately reduce the burden of diabetes for all persons.

Table 2 Ten essential public health strategies

1. Monitor health status to identify community health problems
2. Diagnose and investigate health problems and health hazards in the community
3. Inform, educate, and empower people about health issues
4. Mobilize community partnerships to identify and solve health problems
5. Develop policies and plans that support individual and community health efforts
6. Enforce laws and regulations that protect health and ensure safety
7. Link people to needed personal health services and assure the provision of health care when otherwise unavailable
8. Assure a competent public health and personal health care workforce
9. Evaluate effectiveness, accessibility, and quality of personal and population-based health services
10. Research for new insights and innovative solutions to health problems

Communications

Information about diseases, including chronic conditions like diabetes, is increasingly being shared with large populations and the general public through media outlets—be they audio, television, or the print media [69]. Establishing active and multicomponent diabetes media activities is a major responsibility of a public health program in diabetes. Whether alerting the public about the growing challenges of diabetes [70], identifying greater general awareness of diabetes and its prevention and control [71], or implementing guidance and awareness of specific prevention strategies for potential complications in persons with diabetes [72], a broad-based and coordinated communications strategy is an essential part of a public health approach to diabetes prevention and control. Scientific approaches to these communications activities, e.g. social marketing concepts [73], and careful evaluation of program impact [55] are both important dimensions to a diabetes communications strategy.

SUMMARY

Much has been gained with improved clinical management of diabetes during the past few decades [14, 15]. With further improvements in chronic care health systems, additional benefits are to be expected as a result of a more effective individual clinical relationship between a health professional and patient [22–24]. However, given the reality of the size of the diabetes epidemic now and into the future, as well as the critical impact that the "environment" outside the doctor's office has on individual decisions, a complementary public health approach to diabetes is necessary to fully realize the benefits of traditional clinical science and care. Scientific and clinical knowledge, if not applied to all people, is knowledge wasted. Certainly, public health programs themselves need to improve, redesign, and show greater efficiency and accountability [28, 44, 45, 74] if they are to have maximum impact. These public health programs, however, do have the responsibility to ensure that *as a society*, we are aware of what is happening with chronic diseases like diabetes, and that all persons at risk of, or with, diabetes have access to quality prevention and control programs. The principles and activities of public health in the United States as described above delineate how public health and clinical medicine must work in concert to fully reduce the burden of diabetes. As it was during the early twentieth century, clinical and public health medicine is at present returning to coordinated and complimentary efforts to prevent and manage DM.

REFERENCES

1. Mokdad A, Ford E, Bowman B, Dietz W, Vinicor F, Bales V, Marks J. Prevalence of obesity, diabetes, and obesity-related health risk factors. *JAMA* 2003; 289: 76–9.
2. Fagot-Campagna A, Narayan V, Imperatore G. Type 2 diabetes in children: exemplifies the growing problem of chronic diseases. *BMJ* 2001; 322: 377–8.
3. Boyle J, Honeycutt A, Narayan V, et al. Projection of diabetes burden through 2050. *Diabetes Care* 2001; 24: 1936–40.
4. King H, Aubert R, Herman W. Global burden of diabetes, 1995–2025: prevalence, numerical estimates, and projections. *Diabetes Care* 1998; 21: 1414–31.
5. Unwin N, Shaw J, Zimmet P, et al. Impaired glucose tolerance and impaired fasting glycaemia: the current status on definition and intervention. *Diabetes Med* 2002; 19: 708–23.
6. Barrett-Conner E. The oral glucose tolerance test, revisited. *Eur Heart J* 2002; 23: 1229–31.
7. Engelgau M, Narayan V, Herman W. Screening for type 2 diabetes. *Diabetes Care* 2000; 23: 1563–80.
8. Burke J, Williams K, Gaskill S, et al. Rapid rise in the incidence of type 2 diabetes from 1987 to 1996: results from the San Antonio Heart Study. *Arch Intern Med* 1999; 159: 1450–6.
9. Expert Committee on the Diagnosis and Classification of Diabetes Mellitus. Report of the Expert Committee on the Diagnosis and Classification of Diabetes Mellitus. *Diabetes Care* 1997; 20: 1183–97.
10. Narayan V, Imperatore G, Benjamin S, et al. Targeting people with pre-diabetes. *BMJ* 2002; 325: 403–4.
11. Vinicor F, Bowman B, Engelgau M. Diabetes: prevention needed. *Lancet* 2003; 361: 544.
12. Ryan E, Lakey J, Paty B, et al. Successful islet transplantation: continued insulin reserve provides long-term glycemic control. *Diabetes* 2002; 51: 2148–57.
13. LeRoith D. Beta-cell dysfunction and insulin resistance in type 2 diabetes: role of metabolic and genetic abnormalities. *Am J Med* 2002; 113 (S6A): 3–11.
14. Keen H, Clark C, Laakso M. Reducing the burden of diabetes: managing cardiovascular disease. *Diabetes Metab Res Rev* 1999; 15: 186–96.
15. Peterson K, Vinicor F. Strategies to improve diabetes care delivery. *J Fam Pract* 1998; 47 (S1): 55–62.
16. Narayan V, Gregg E, Engelgau M, et al. Translation research for chronic disease: the case of diabetes. *Diabetes Care* 2000; 23: 1794–8.
17. Saaddine J, Engelgau M, Beckles G, et al. A diabetes report card for the United States: quality of care in the 1990s. *Ann Intern Med* 2002; 136: 565–74.
18. Vinicor F. Quality of care and diabetes mellitus. *Curr Opin Endocrinol Diabetes* 2001; 8: 58–66.
19. Schroeder S. Prospects for expanding health insurance coverage. *N Engl J Med* 2001; 344: 847–52.
20. Sandy L. Homeostasis without reserve—the risk of health systems collapse. *N Engl J Med* 2002; 347: 1971–5.
21. *Chronic Conditions: Making the Case for Ongoing Care*, Baltimore, MD: Johns Hopkins University, 2003.
22. Institute of Medicine. *Crossing the Quality Chasm: A New Health System for the 21st Century*. Washington, DC: National Academy Press, 2001.
23. Bodenheimer T, Wagner E, Grumbach K. Improving primary care for patients with chronic illness. *JAMA* 2002; 288: 1775–9, 1909–14.
24. Berwick D. *Escape Fire: Lessons For The Future of Health Care*. New York: The Commonwealth Fund, 2003.
25. McKinlay J, Marceau L. US public health and the 21st century: diabetes mellitus. *Lancet* 2000; 356: 757–61.

26. Kennedy E. Quality, affordable health care for all Americans. *Am J Pub Health* 2003; 93: 14.
27. Vinicor F. Is diabetes a public health disorder? *Diabetes Care* 1994; 17 (S1): 22–7.
28. Institute of Medicine. *The Future of Public Health*. Washington, DC: National Academy of Science Press, 1988.
29. The DCCT Study Group. The effect of intensive treatment of diabetes on the development and progression of long-term complications in insulin-dependent diabetes mellitus: the Diabetes Control and Complications Trial. *N Engl J Med* 1993; 329: 977–86.
30. The UK Prospective Diabetes Study Group. Intensive blood-glucose control with sulphonylureas or insulin compared with conventional treatment and risks of complications in patients with type 2 diabetes (UKPDS 33). *Lancet* 1998; 352: 837–53.
31. Centers for Disease Control and Prevention. Framework for program evaluation in public health. *MMWR Morb Mortal Wkly Rep* 1999; 48 (RR-11): 1–40.
32. Institute of Medicine. *Health and Behavior: The Interplay of Biological, Behavioral and Societal Influences*. Washington, DC: National Academy Press, 2001.
33. Cohen S. Potential barriers to diabetes care. *Diabetes Care* 1983; 6: 499–500.
34. Sadur C, Moline N, Costa M, et al. Diabetes management in a health maintenance organization: efficacy of care management using cluster visits. *Diabetes Care* 1999; 22: 2011–7.
35. Bodenheimer T, Lorig K, Holman H, et al. Patient self-management of chronic disease in primary care. *JAMA* 2002; 288: 2469–75.
36. Litzelman D, Slemenda C, Langefeld C, et al. Reduction of lower extremity clinical abnormalities in patients with non-insulin-dependent diabetes mellitus: a randomized, controlled trial. *Ann Intern Med* 1993; 119: 36–41.
37. McGinnis J, Williams-Russo P, Knickman J. The case for more active policy attention to health promotion. *Health Aff* 2002; 78–93.
38. Jack L, Liburd L, Vinicor F, et al. Influence of the environmental context on diabetes self- management: a rationale for developing a new research paradigm in diabetes education. *Diabetes Educ* 1999; 25: 775–90.
39. Weiss E, Anderson R, Lasker R. Making the most of collaboration: exploring the relationship between partnership synergy and partnership functioning. *Health Educ Behav* 2002; 29: 683–98.
40. Schwartz W. *Life Without Disease: The Pursuit of Medical Utopia*. Berkeley: University of California Press, 1998.
41. Tauber A. Medicine, public health, and the ethics of rationing. *Perspect Biol Med* 2002; 45: 16–30.
42. Vinicor F. The public health burden of diabetes and the reality of limits. *Diabetes Care* 1998; 21 (suppl 3): 15–8.
43. Detsky A, Naglie I. A clinician's guide to cost-effectiveness analysis. *Ann Intern Med* 190; 113: 147–54.
44. Vinicor F. New models of diabetes healthcare delivery. *Can J Diabetes Care* 2001; 25 (S2): 24–30.
45. Fuchs V. The best health care system in the world? *JAMA* 1992; 268: 916–7.
46. Report of the Scientific Peer Review Group on Health Systems Performance Assessment. Geneva: World Health Organization, 2001.
47. Starfield B. Equity in health. *J Epidemiol Community Health* 2002; 56: 483–4.
48. Cheadle A, Sullivan M, Krieger J, et al. Using a participatory approach to provide assistance to community-based organizations: the Seattle Partners community research center. *Health Educ Behav* 2002; 29: 383–94.
49. Naylor P, Wharf-Higgins J, Blair L, et al. Evaluating the participatory process in a community-based heart health project. *Soc Sci Med* 2002; 55: 1173–87.
50. Glasgow R, Fishe E, Anderson B, et al. Behavioral science in diabetes: contributions and opportunities. *Diabetes Care* 1999; 22: 832–43.
51. Tattersall R. The expert patient: a new approach to chronic disease management for the twenty- first century. *Clin Med* 2002; 2: 227–9.
52. Mullan F. Don Quixote, Machiavelli, and Robin Hood: public health practice, past and present. *Am J Public Health* 2000; 90: 702–6.
53. Lasker R. *Medicine and Public Health: The Power of Collaboration*. Chicago IL: Health Administration Press, New York Academy of Medicine, 1997.
54. Macintyre S. Evidence based policy making. *BMJ* 2003; 326: 5–6.
55. Glasgow R, Vogt T, Boles S. Evaluating the public health impact of health promotion interventions: the RE-AIM framework. *Am J Public Health* 1999; 89: 1322–7.
56. Safran M, Mukhtar Q, Murphy D. Implementing program evaluation and accountability for population health: progress of a national diabetes control effort. *J Public Health Manag Pract* 2003; 9: 58–65.
57. Teutsch S, Churchill R (eds). *Principles and Practice of Public Health Surveillance*. New York: Oxford University Press, 1994.
58. Brownson R, Remington P, Davis J (eds). *Chronic Disease Epidemiology and Control*. Washington, DC: American Public Health Association, 1998.
59. Imperatore G, Williams D, Vinicor F. Type 2 diabetes mellitus in childhood and adolescence in North America. In Silink, Rosenbloom, Kida (eds), *Type 2 Diabetes Mellitus in Childhood and Adolescence*. London: Martin Dunitz Publishers (in press).
60. Centers for Disease Control and Prevention. *National Diabetes Fact Sheet: General Information and National Estimates on Diabetes in the United States, 2000*. Atlanta, GA: US Department of Health and Human Services, Centers for Disease Control and Prevention, 2002.
61. The TRIAD Study Group. The Translating Research Into Action for Diabetes (TRIAD) Study: a multicenter study of diabetes in managed care. *Diabetes Care* 2002; 25: 386–9.
62. CDC Cost-Effectiveness Study Group. The cost effectiveness of screening for type 2 diabetes. *JAMA* 1998; 280: 1757–63.
63. CDC Diabetes Cost-Effectiveness Group. Cost-effectiveness of intensive glycemic control, intensified hypertension control, and serum cholesterol level reduction for type 2 diabetes. *JAMA* 2002; 287: 2542–51.
64. Brody G, Jack L, Murry V, et al. Heuristic model linking contextual processes to self- management in African-Americans adults with type 2 diabetes. *Diabetes Educ* 2001; 27: 685–93.
65. Goodman R, Liburd L, Green-Phillips A. The formation of a complex community program for diabetes control: lessons learned from a case study of Project DIRECT. *J Public Health Manag Pract* 2001; 7: 19–29.
66. Vinicor F, Engelgua M, Murphy D, Sniegowski R. A public health response to diabetes mellitus. In Davidson JK (ed), *Clinical Diabetes Mellitus: A Problem-Oriented Approach*, 3rd edn. New York: Thieme, 2000.

67. New tools can be used to gauge public health services. *The Nation's Health*, May 2002.
68. Roper W, Mays G. Performance measurements in public health: conceptual and methodological issues in building the science base. *J Public Health Manag Pract* 2000; 6: 66–77.
69. Johnson T. Medicine and media. *N Engl J Med* 1998; 339: 87–92.
70. The perfect diet. *Newsweek* January 20, 2003.
71. Clark C. Reducing the burden of diabetes. The National Diabetes Education Program. *Diabetes Care* 1998; 21 (S1): 1.
72. Vinicor F. Flu vaccination decreases relative morbidity risk for people with diabetes. *J Med Assoc Ga* 1998; 87: 330.
73. Andreasen A. Marketing social marketing in the social change marketplace. *J Public Policy Mark* 2002; 21: 3–13.
74. Hassmiller S. Turning Point: the Robert Wood Johnson Foundation's effort to revitalize public health at the state level. *J Public Health Manag Pract* 2002; 8: 1–5.

103

Organization of Care: Western Pacific Region (China and Hong Kong as Examples)

Juliana C.N. Chan and Clive S. Cockram

The Chinese University of Hong Kong, Shatin, Hong Kong, China

INTRODUCTION

In this chapter, the organization of diabetes care is examined in the setting of the Western Pacific Region. Since the Western Pacific Region is geographically huge, very diverse, and very complex, the discussion confines itself to organization of care in Hong Kong and China. This allows all of the major points to be made, including general points that will apply throughout the region, without overcomplicating the issues.

THE CONTEXT AND SIZE OF THE PROBLEM

The Western Pacific Region is at the forefront of the current diabetes epidemic. The epidemic is predominantly type 2 diabetes. As in other developing regions and areas, the emergence of the type 2 diabetes epidemic is closely associated with the epidemic of obesity and is increasingly having an impact in young individuals including children and adolescents as well as the older population [1]. This poses a particular threat to health care systems. Long-term diabetic complications and associated conditions are becoming a major threat in all parts of the region and the high costs associated with treating these diseases threaten to overwhelm the capacity of health care systems, even in richer or more developed countries and areas [2].

Apart from demonstrating the above points, Hong Kong and the remainder of China also highlight the degree of diversity and heterogeneity that can exist within health care systems. In Hong Kong (population approximately 6.5 million), it is estimated that about 600 000 adults have diabetes and 20% of them can expect to develop the disease before the age of 40. The burden of long-term complications is huge. Diabetes is the commonest cause of end-stage renal disease and of referral for renal replacement therapy. It is also a major contributor to cardiovascular morbidity and mortality and is present in 30–40% of people admitted to hospital with major cardiovascular events. Yet, estimates from epidemiological studies and health care utilization databases suggest that 50% of diabetic patients are undiagnosed. Among those who have been diagnosed, less than half are being managed in the public health care sector, while the remaining patients remain untreated, managed by private doctors or herbalists, or resort to self-medication. Among those managed in the public sector, probably less than half had optimal metabolic control [3, 4] (Figure 1).

Prevalence rates in China are generally lower than in Hong Kong but are rising at an alarming rate. Surveys conducted in Da Qing Province in 1986 and 1994 indicated a 3.4-fold rise in prevalence from 1.1 to 3.5% over a period of 8 years and similar rates of rise have been shown in national diabetes surveys. In the 1996 National Diabetes Survey, the overall prevalence of diabetes in China was reported to be 3.4% but with higher prevalence rates of 4.6% in provincial cities [5, 6]. Current estimates indicate more than 20 million people with diabetes in China, of whom, as in Hong Kong, less than half are diagnosed, this figure being even higher in some areas. In addition, prevalence rates of impaired glucose tolerance (IGT) exceed those

International Textbook of Diabetes Mellitus, Third Edition. Edited by R. A. DeFronzo, E. Ferrannini, H. Keen, and P. Zimmet.
 ISBN: 0-471-48655-8.

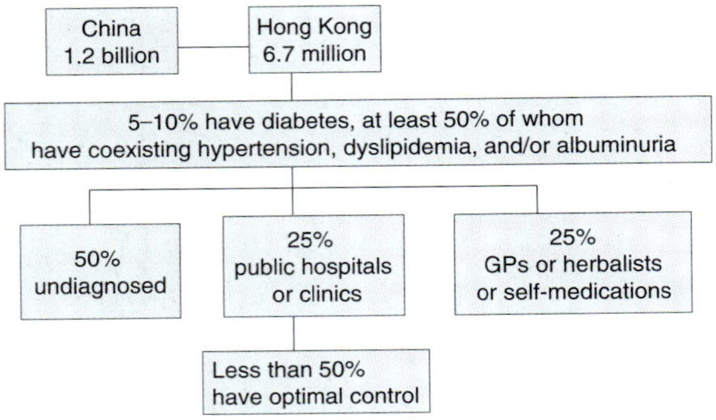

Figure 1 Challenges of chronic disease management using diabetes as a prototype

of diabetes in both China and Hong Kong. Given China's massive population (1.3 billion at the latest census), a 1% rise in adult prevalence corresponds to about 10 million people with diabetes. Conservative predictions indicate a doubling of prevalence in China over the next 20 years or so [7].

HEALTH CARE SYSTEMS—GENERAL CONSIDERATIONS

The health care system refers to the relationships that revolve around a caring individual or healer and a patient. All human societies create medical systems of one form or another. The carer may or may not be a conventionally trained physician and may be assisted by various categories of individuals. In the most complex settings, this evolves into the elaborate bureaucratic structures that provide the basis of modern health care systems—for example clinics, health maintenance organizations, and hospitals. Irrespective of complexity, all health care systems revolve around the core relationship between the healer and the patient. In all societies, the role of healer may be occupied by any one of a number of different categories of individuals. In simple preindustrial societies, the role of healer often overlaps with other roles, e.g. in relation to religion as in the case of Shaman. In certain parts of China, such systems continue to operate, and even in highly developed parts of the country, the naturalistic system that views disease as emanating from an imbalance in the male and female elements of yin and yang continues to be very important. In modern societies, family physicians may occupy this role as may herbalists, bonesetters, or western specialists such as cardiologists.

In Asia, there are three levels of medical systems designated as local, regional, and cosmopolitan systems. Local systems are folk systems of peasant communities and exist in remote parts of rural China. Regional systems, distributed over a relatively large area, include traditional Chinese medicine (TCM), which remains very important as a source of health care provision throughout China and among Chinese populations elsewhere. Many people will utilize TCM as a first resort and turn to "western medicine" only as a last resort. Similarly many individuals may return to TCM if they feel that western medicine has failed to fulfill their expectations, or may use both systems concurrently. Cosmopolitan systems refer to western medicine and its equivalents and will be the dominant system in some areas (e.g. Hong Kong) but not others [8, 9].

When considering health care systems in areas such as China, it is important to recognize the existence of these regional and local systems and to take steps where possible to utilize them in the overall strategy aimed at diabetes care. Unfortunately the practice of these forms of care is usually not based on evidence, which can be used in protocols or guidelines for care models.

COST-EFFECTIVENESS OF QUALITY DIABETES CARE

In most modern societies including Hong Kong, at least 12–15% of health care costs are spent on diabetes and its complications and this does not take into account indirect costs (sick days, loss of employment, disability allowances, hiring of additional carers) and intangible costs (poor quality of life and psychosocial stress). More than 80% of these health care costs are spent on treatment of complications rather than prevention [10].

Many important studies show that early detection and treatment of diabetes can substantially reduce the risk of complications and improve quality of life. In subjects with IGT, both nonpharmacological and pharmacological treatments can reduce the risk of progression from IGT to diabetes by 30–60% [11, 12]. In the Steno Type 2 Diabetes Study, optimization of metabolic control and use of appropriate treatment can lead to more than 70% risk reduction in the development of all microvascular complications [13].

The cost-effectiveness of control of diabetes can be reflected by the number-needed-to-treat. For example, using Hong Kong costs as an example, one only needs to treat 5 type 2 diabetic patients with insulin (HK$1–2/day; US$1 = HK$7.78) to prevent one event of retinopathy or nephropathy, 3 hypertensive diabetic patients with antihypertensive drugs (e.g. HK$1–2/day) to prevent one death or stroke or heart attack, 5 diabetic patients with a history of coronary heart disease with lipid-lowering drugs (HMG-CoA reductase) (e.g. HK$4–8/day) to prevent one cardiovascular event, 8 type 1 diabetic patients with an angiotensin-converting enzyme inhibitor (e.g. HK$1–2/day) or 16 type 2 diabetic patients with renal insufficiency with angiotensin II antagonist (HK$7–10/day) to prevent one case of end-stage renal disease. By contrast, screening 1075 healthy women is needed to prevent one

Table 1 The estimated treatment costs for each quality-adjusted-life-year (QALY) for different diseases

	Cost/QALY (HK$)* (August 1990)
Cholesterol testing and diet therapy (all adults aged 40–69)	2 640
Advice to stop smoking from family doctors	2 880
Antihypertensive treatment to prevent stroke (ages 45–64)	1 280
Coronary artery bypass graft for coronary heart disease	25 080–225 960
Kidney transplant	56 520
Continuous ambulatory peritoneal dialysis	238 440
Hospital haemodialysis	263 640
Erythropoietin treatment for anemia in dialysis patients	652 560–1 515 480

* US$1 = HK$7.78.

death from breast cancer. Table 1 shows some examples of how much it costs to gain one additional quality-adjusted-life-year for different diseases [14].

DIABETES CARE—A PROTOTYPE FOR CHRONIC DISEASE MANAGEMENT

Diabetes care is a classic model for chronic disease management, emphasizing the importance of pathophysiology, psychosocial, and behavioral sciences, evidence-based medicine, and consideration of patient preference. Complex diseases such as diabetes require a holistic and multidisciplinary approach using all available resources to cover a wide spectrum of need ranging from health promotion and disease prevention to treatment and eventually rehabilitation. Keys to success include *early diagnosis, risk stratification, individualized therapy, treatment to target values*, and *compliance reinforcement* [15].

Because of the complex and heterogeneous nature of diabetes management, there is a need for the diabetes specialist to adopt multiple roles as the leader of the multidisciplinary team. Apart from providing *comprehensive* care to high-risk individuals with complications, poor control, or multiple risk factors, the diabetes specialist team can provide *concurrent* care with other specialists such as ophthalmologists and cardiologists. At primary care level, the specialist team can provide *consultative* or *collaborative* assistance to primary care teams, together with provision of backup or ancillary services such as screening for complications and podiatry. The team also has important advocacy and leadership roles to lobby support from stakeholders. This includes the Government to set policy and create a conducive environment for healthy living and to reform the health care system so as to improve the provision of care for chronic diseases [16, 17].

A number of reports show that patients managed by a specialist multidisciplinary team have better metabolic control and lower complication rates compared to patients treated by primary care physicians [18]. For example in Hong Kong, the use of a structured protocol delivered by a diabetologist–nurse team, in the setting of a clinical trial, was associated with an annualized death rate of less than 1% (in 92 hypertensive, type 2 diabetic patients with no cardiovascular or renal complications followed up for 7 years) as compared to 4% amongst patients attending general medical clinics where quality of care processes were not monitored [19]. Similarly, after discontinuation of the 7-year Diabetes Control and Complication Trial (DCCT), there was progressive deterioration in glycemic control in those subjects who were assigned to intensified therapy, emphasizing the importance of protocol-driven care and continuous support [20].

The importance of protocol-driven care is also affirmed in a recent report issued by the National Institutes of Health (NIH) division, the National Institute of Diabetes, Digestive and Kidney Diseases (NIDDK) in the United States, which indicates that patients with type 2 diabetes are better treated by a team of health care professionals rather than a single primary-care provider. Type 2 diabetes can also greatly influence employment status, income, and family. Thus, another important component of the team approach is *family involvement*. The NIDDK also points to seven key domains of diabetic care for improving outcomes and minimizing costs [21] (Table 2).

BARRIERS TO QUALITY DIABETES CARE

Despite evidence, international recommendations, and increasing professional awareness, the prevalence of diabetes continues to rise and quality of diabetes care remains generally suboptimal in both community and hospital settings and in both developed and developing countries [22]. Challenges include the need for long-term care and medications, progressive deterioration of disease processes, and frequent admissions as complications develop. The

Table 2 Recommendations by the US National Institute of Diabetes and Diabetic Kidney Disease highlighting the seven key domains of diabetic care for improving patient functional outcomes and minimizing costs

- Diagnosing the type of diabetes
- Maintaining regular care for diabetes
- Teaching patients how to control their diabetes
- Appropriately treating high blood glucose levels and associated risk factors
- Continuously monitoring blood glucose levels
- Diagnosing and preventing diabetic complications (e.g. vascular disease)
- Regularly checking for onset of diabetic complications

need to empower patients to change their behavior and deal with social and emotional impacts of symptoms and disabilities adds further difficulty [23].

Reasons for failure to adhere to recommended standards of care include time pressure, lack of support staff and teamwork with other professionals, lack of formal training in diabetes management, poor financial incentives for implementation of preventive strategies, and overemphasis on treatment rather than prevention. The situation is worsened by low public awareness of diabetes and low motivation of at-risk subjects or patients to comply with healthy lifestyle or chronic medications because of the insidious nature of the disease and its complications [24].

PROVISION OF QUALITY DIABETES CARE—SPECIAL CHALLENGES IN ASIA

Asia is an economically, culturally, and socially diverse region. According to the World Bank data and statistics, in 2001, the gross domestic products (GDP) ranged from US$4 245 191 million in Japan to US$32 903 million in Vietnam and US$1684 million in Fiji. The public to private ratio of health care spending can vary from less than 1 in most Asian countries to approximately 1:1 in more affluent societies such as Hong Kong and Singapore and to more than 1 in highly developed countries such as Japan and Australia. In common with other countries [10], most diabetes-related health care spending is on treatment of complications rather than prevention. The situation is further exaggerated in Asia by a predominant focus on high technology, hospital-based care of complications, with lack of emphasis on coordinated, community-based prevention programs. This leads to injudicious use of finite resources and lack of balanced, formulated policy and is a problem throughout Asia, irrespective of relative wealth or poverty.

In Asia, management of chronic diseases such as diabetes by solo practice in the private sector, which usually adopts a "fee-for-service" approach (often putting it beyond the reach of the poor) also tends to discourage patients' commitment to continued care and increases treatment costs. This is compounded by the wide use of complementary and alternative medicine, either in replacement or conjunction with western medications. Because of lack of regulation and enforcement, pharmacological treatments for diabetes are also often available from community pharmacies without the need for prescription and are used by many patients with little, if any, monitoring by doctors.

In China, despite the socialist system, medical care is largely private with relatively little Government subsidy for the public sector. Nevertheless, China does have a strong, centrally reinforced policy emphasizing public health and prevention for chronic diseases and in this respect is more advanced than Hong Kong and other more developed countries and areas. One of the main challenges faced by many Asian countries including China and Hong Kong is the lack of comprehensive or compulsory national or private health care insurance schemes. As a result, the primary care systems are underdeveloped, often as solo practices, with little contact between community and hospital sectors or between private and public sectors. Despite rapid economic growth, the majority of people in China cannot afford the expensive western medications and periodic monitoring using even simple blood and urine tests. Besides, there is very little emphasis on the training of paramedics such as nurse educators and dietitians who play important roles in providing quality diabetes care [25–27]. Since many corporate or private insurance companies cover only hospital but not ambulatory care [28], many patients attending the outpatient clinics are not assessed or treated according to recommended guidelines. The lack of continuity of care, "doctor shopping," high usage of complementary or alternative medicine [29] as well as marked income differentials between the coastal cities and inland areas all contribute to a highly variable and generally substandard quality of diabetes care in China and Asia. This can be evidenced by an average HbA_{1c} of more than 9% in young diabetic patients according to the ASDIAB Study [30].

DIABETES CARE IN HONG KONG—PAST, PRESENT, AND FUTURE

Hong Kong with a predominantly Chinese population leading a westernized and affluent lifestyle represents an epitome of future China. Hong Kong has a heavily subsidized public health care system. With its low tax system (averaging 15–17%), approximately 6% of the GDP of Hong Kong is spent on health care. The Hospital Authority is a statutory and governing body for all public hospitals in Hong Kong and is largely funded by the Hong Kong Government. Historically, public hospitals in Hong Kong provide medical services to people from low socioeconomic classes and those with acute illnesses. These services are heavily subsidized and patients only need to pay a nominal fee that covers consultations, laboratory fees, medications, and all hospital charges.

On the other hand, the emphasis of the Department of Health is mainly on disease surveillance programs such as food hygiene and infection control, although it does also provide low cost primary health care as a safety net. As a result, over 70% of frontline community care is offered by the private sector, which charges a fee for service. Haphazard visits, doctor shopping, and self-medication are common, and single-handed medical practitioners often find it difficult to practice preventive medicine. This is largely due to the high costs and low profit margins

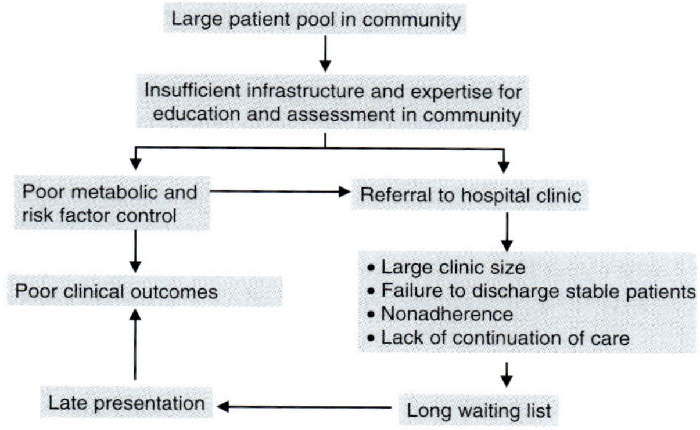

Figure 2 Overwhelming of hospital services owing to the lack of an effective interface between community and hospital settings

of providing education, performing laboratory tests, and supervising the administration of long-term medications. The incentive for medical practitioners to practice preventive medicine is further attenuated by the fact that less than 30% of people in Hong Kong have health care insurance and even when this is available, the scheme tends to provide cover for inpatient rather than ambulatory care. As a result, high-risk subjects are often not screened for risk factors, patients with risk factors are not fully assessed for complications, and treatment targets are not adequately attained in patients who are treated.

In 1989, the Hospital Authority was formed with a mandate to reorganize the health care system. This has led to dramatic improvement in the facilities and standards of medical care in public hospitals. However, this major hospital reform was not complemented by changes in the structure of primary health care or health financing policy. Although both the Hospital Authority and Department of Health are publicly funded, the two organizations have separate administrative bodies with different areas of priorities, leading to compartmentalization in service provision with both gaps and overlaps. Because of marked differentials in funding, drug formularies, and professional expertise, this lack of integration has led to many patients with chronic diseases such as diabetes seeking treatment in public hospitals and overloading the system beyond its capacity.

Figure 2 summarizes the consequences resulting from this lack of integration between community and hospital sectors. These include long clinic waiting times, overuse of emergency services, short consultation times, inability to discharge clinically stable patients, large clinic volumes, poor treatment compliance, suboptimal disease management, unnecessary advanced presentation of diseases, and overall, increased health care costs and poor quality of life. This situation in Hong Kong mirrors the situation in most parts of the Region.

DIABETES MODEL AT THE PRINCE OF WALES HOSPITAL

This section details attempts made at one hospital to overcome the barriers to diabetes care in Hong Kong, providing an example for the rest of the Region. Since this is a hospital-based model, it is still unable to address the needs of primary prevention. Large nongovernmental organizations and the Department of Health are increasingly engaged in many health promotion programs using mass media, publications, and exhibitions to highlight the importance of a healthy lifestyle. As in many countries, these health promotion programs tend to be conducted in isolation and may not be fully integrated into other disease detection and treatment programs (for example those targeting obesity, smoking, or vascular disease) that may have very similar agendas.

The Prince of Wales Hospital (PWH) is a 1700-bed regional hospital with a catchment population of 1 million. It is also the teaching hospital of the Chinese University of Hong Kong (CUHK). More than 40% of medical admissions and 15% of patients attending its medical clinics have diabetes. Since 1995, the CUHK/PWH Diabetes Group has introduced a series of diabetes-related quality improvement programs to enhance the cost-effective use of limited resources (Figure 3). These may be taken as examples applicable in the general setting to enhance quality of care by optimizing the use of existing resources.

The Importance of Diabetes Registries

Using a doctor–nurse–clerk team, 30–40 diabetic patients are assessed weekly using structured protocols and international guidelines. Documentation is made of demographic data, medical history, complications, metabolic profile, and cardiovascular risk profiles. These data are then computerized and reviewed by specialists who stratify patients into different risk groups and make treatment recommendations. Patients undergo structured assessments at referral and at 2–3 yearly intervals. Since

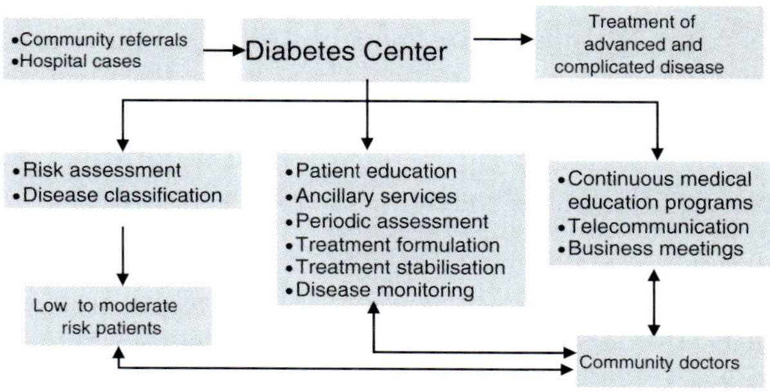

Figure 3 Reorganization of diabetes care at the Prince of Wales Hospital based on structured protocols to stratify risk and enhance multidisciplinary and intersectoral collaboration to promote more effective use of finite resources

1995, more than 5000 patients have been assessed. Many have undergone repeat assessments showing improvement in control of metabolic profile and cardiovascular risk factors. The Diabetes Registry has also provided a very useful tool for quality assurance and evaluation of care processes.

Diabetes Shared-Care Programs and Intersectoral Collaboration

After assessment, approximately 30% of patients with diabetes return to the community for shared care with the primary care sector while 30% stay at hospital medical clinics for secondary care and 30% remain in the diabetes specialist clinic for tertiary care. When clinically stable patients are discharged to community clinics, they receive education (knowledge and skills) on self-management, treatment goals, and modes of follow-up. The implementation of shared care was preceded by a series of workshops where community doctors were updated on diabetes management. These workshops have also established consensus on modes of follow-up and criteria to prioritize referral. This dialogue between community and hospital teams is reinforced by regular business meetings, telephones, and fax, and is coordinated by a specific shared-care nurse [31, 32].

Special Targeted Program: Young Diabetes Intensive Insulin Treatment

Over 30% of patients attending the PWH Diabetes Clinic have young onset of disease (<35 years). These patients pose particular therapeutic challenges due to the long future disease duration, increased risk of complications, busy lifestyles, and potentially low incentives to adhere to long-term therapy.

Since 1999, a Saturday clinic, coordinated by diabetes nurses, has managed young insulin-treated patients. At each visit, 15–20 patients attend a 4-h session with other patients, educators, and doctors. In addition to intensification of medical therapy, group dynamics are used to change behavior and attitudes. Among patients who have attended this clinic for at least 12 months, HbA_{1c} fell from 11 to 8% in a group with "poor control" (baseline HbA_{1c} $\geq$9.5%) and from 7.2 to 6.8% in a "fair control" group (HbA_{1c} between 8 and 9.5%) [31].

Special Targeted Program: Diabetic Nephropathy Clinic

In Hong Kong, diabetic nephropathy is a major problem. Over 40% of patients on dialysis have diabetes and the 5-year survival rate on dialysis is less than 50% [33]. Diabetic patients with renal impairment require intensified therapy for all risk factors and metabolic indices as well as careful dose titration of treatments and monitoring of adverse events. In the PWH Diabetes Clinic, 50% of patients have increased albuminuria, a powerful predictor for both cardiovascular events and end-stage renal disease [34]. Approximately 10–15% of patients have significant renal impairment (plasma creatinine $\geq$150 μmol/l). Many will develop end-stage renal disease within 24–30 months if not managed optimally [35].

In 55 type 2 diabetic patients with renal insufficiency (median plasma creatinine 200 μmol/l) who had been recruited into a clinical trial, delivery of protocol-driven care by a diabetologist–nurse team resulted in 50% or more reduction in the rate of decline of renal function. The stabilization of renal function implies that many of these patients will not need to enter dialysis, or at least that the process can be delayed by several years [36].

In June 2000, a dedicated Diabetic Nephropathy Clinic, coordinated by a research pharmacist and senior physicians, was set up from within existing resources to manage patients with moderate renal failure (plasma creatinine 150–350 μmol/l) using a protocol, treatment targets, and reinforcement of compliance, with similarly encouraging results [37]. Another study in Germany, involving 76 patients with type 2 diabetic nephropathy, has also shown that aggressive treatment and diabetes education following referral to a diabetes–nephrology combined clinic was associated with a reduction in the rate of decline in renal function in 39% of patients. This was attributed mainly to improvements in blood pressure, HbA_{1c}, and serum cholesterol [38].

THE PROBLEM OF CHRONIC DISEASES AND THE NEED FOR A NEW APPROACH

Although some of these translational research programs were not randomized in nature, the overall results support beneficial effects of various forms of structured care on clinical outcomes. Given the magnitude of the problem, the creation of a community-based system with appropriate financing should allow more cost-effective and rational use of fixed finite resources. This is especially important in developing countries, given that the main increase in diabetes prevalence will occur in young or middle-aged individuals.

In light of the finite nature of public funding, there is also a need to either increase or redistribute private expenditure to make quality diabetes care more readily available to all sectors of the society. There is now increasing consensus that no public-funded health care system in any country can provide care to 10% of the population on a long-term basis. In Hong Kong, in an attempt to do this, we have recently entered an academic–industrial venture to set up a Disease Management and Education Center funded by the business sector and managed by a university specialist team. Given the relatively high GDP and self-reliant nature of Hong Kong people, management of chronic diseases, especially at an early stage, is within the financial capacity of gainfully employed individuals. Admittedly, this will depend on the individual's values, perspectives, and priorities, the changes of which will need education and promotion [39]. In this regard, membership schemes or care plans in which patients can pay by installment rather than "fee for service" may be one alternative to increase the commitment of the individual and the affordability of these preventive programs through risk sharing.

CONCLUSIONS

Health care systems in Asia are in danger of being overwhelmed by the explosive rises in prevalence of diabetes and other chronic diseases. These problems can only be tackled effectively if new approaches and strategies are developed. To make the best use of limited resources, there is an urgent need for an increase in emphasis on prevention both of diabetes itself and of its complications. In Asia, this focus is now increasing although in a rather patchy manner. The more developed countries (such as Australia and Singapore) [40] and the socialist-based countries (particularly China and Vietnam) are leaders in this respect. Wherever possible, prevention programs should be integrated with programs targeting other chronic diseases and should involve as many sectors of society and areas of government as possible. This allows maximal utilization of available resources and economics of scale.

Health care systems for chronic disease care also need to be rethought. As discussed in this chapter, there is urgent need for review of traditional models of care that become both ineffective and inefficient when faced with the burden for complex, chronic, and complicated diseases such as diabetes. There is also need for integration of services and careful coordination between community and hospital-based sectors [41].

It seems unlikely that public-funded health care systems will be able to cope, even with optimal reallocation of resources, efficient use of those resources, and judicious use of funds. In many parts of Asia, such as Hong Kong and China, many patients turn to the private sector or alternative health care sectors such as TCM, and it is therefore very important to try to include these sectors in these health care reforms. In the case of the private sector, one of the most important issues relates to replacement of simple "fee-for-service" approaches by alternative schemes that allow for the long-term nature of the required care and that emphasize *maintenance of health* rather than *treatment of diseases*.

REFERENCES

1. King H, Aubert RE, Herman WH. Global burden of diabetes, 1995–2025: prevalence, numerical estimates and projections. *Diabetes Care* 1998; 21: 1414–31.
2. Zimmet P, Alberti KG, Shaw J. Global and societal implications of the diabetes epidemic. *Nature* 2001; 414: 782–7.
3. Chan JCN, Ng MCY, Critchley JAJH, Lee SC, Cockram CS. Diabetes mellitus—a special medical challenge from a Chinese perspective. *Diabetes Res Clin Pract* 2001; 54: S19–27.
4. Chan JCN, Cockram CS. Diabetes mellitus in Chinese and its implications on health care. *Diabetes Care* 1997; 20: 1785–90.
5. Pan XR, Yang WY, Li GW, Liu J, for the National Diabetes Prevention and Control Cooperative Group. Prevalence of diabetes and its risk factors in China, 1994. *Diabetes Care* 1997; 20: 1664–9.
6. Zhong XL. Diabetes mellitus survey in China. *Chin Med J* 1982; 95: 430–2.
7. Cockram CS, Chan JCN. Diabetes in China and Chinese populations. In Marshall SM, Home PD, Rizza RA (eds) *The Diabetes Annual 12*. The Netherlands: Elsevier, 1999; pp 87–110.
8. Baer HA, Singer M, Susser I. The pursuit of health as a human right: health praxis and the struggle for a healthy world. *Medical Anthropology and the World System*. Westport, CT: Bergin & Garvey, 1997; pp 232–44.
9. Dunn F. Traditional Asian medicine and cosmopolitan medicine as adaptive systems. In Leslie C (ed) *Asian Medical Systems. A Comparison Study*. Berkeley: University of California Press, 1976; pp 133–58.
10. Jonsson B. The economic impact of diabetes. *Diabetes Care* 1998; 21 (suppl 3): C7–10.
11. Tuomilehto J, Lindstrom J, Eriksson JG, Valle TT, Hamalainen H, Ilanne-Parikka P, Keinanen-Kiukaanniemi S, Laakso M, Louheranta A, Rastaas M, Salminen V, Uusitupa M, for the Finnish Diabetes Prevention Study Group. Prevention of type 2 diabetes mellitus by changes in lifestyle among subjects with impaired glucose tolerance. *N Engl J Med* 2001; 344: 1343–50.
12. Knowler WC, Barrett-Connor E, Fowler SE, Hamman RF, Lachin JM, Walker EA, Nathan DM. Reduction in the incidence of type 2 diabetes with lifestyle intervention or metformin. *N Engl J Med* 2002; 346: 393–403.
13. Gaede P, Vedel P, Parving H-H, Pedersen O. Intensified multifactorial intervention in patients with type 2 diabetes mellitus and microalbuminuria: the Steno type 2 randomised study. *Lancet* 1999; 353: 617–22.
14. Sackett DL, Sharon ES, Richardson WS, Rosenberg W, Haynes RB. *Evidence Based Medicine—How to Practice and Teach EBM*, 2nd edn. New York: Churchill Livingstone, 2000.
15. Ellrodt G, Cook DJ, Lee J, Cho M, Hunt D, Weingarten S. Evidence-based disease management. *JAMA* 1997; 258: 1687–92.
16. Quickel KE Jr. Diabetes in a managed care system. *Ann Intern Med* 1996; 124: 160–3.
17. Baer HA, Singer M, Susser I. Theoretical perspectives in medical anthropology. *Medical Anthropology and the World System*. Westport, CT: Bergin & Garvey, 1997; pp 20–36.
18. Zgibor JC, Drash AL, Songer TJ, Orchard TJ, Kelsey SF. Influence of health care providers on the development of diabetes complications. Long term follow up from the Pittburgh Epidemiology of Diabetes Complications Study. *Diabetes Care* 2002; 25: 1584–90.
19. So WY, Tong PCY, Ko GTC, Leung WYS, Chow CC, Yeung VTF, Chan WB, Cockram CS, Critchely Julian AJH, Chan JCN. The effects of protocol driven care

versus usual outpatient clinic care on survival rates in type 2 diabetic patients. *Am J Manag Care* 2003; 9: 41–51.

20. The Diabetes Control and Complications Trial/ Epidemiology of Diabetes Interventions and Research Group. Retinopathy and nephropathy in patients with Type 1 diabetes four years after a trial of intensive therapy. *N Engl J Med* 2000; 342: 381–9.
21. National Institute of Diabetes, Digestive and Kidney Disease. Team care: comprehensive lifetime management for diabetes. US National Institute of Health, 2001. Available at: http://ndep.nih.gov/materials/pubs/7-principles/7-english.htm.
22. Saaddine JB, Engelgau MM, Beckes GL, Gregg ED, Thompson TJ, Narayan KMV. A Diabetes report card for the United States: quality of care in the 1990s. *Ann Intern Med* 2002; 136: 565–74.
23. Wagner EH, Groves T. Care for chronic diseases. *BMJ* 2002; 325: 913–4.
24. Narayan KMV, Gregg EW, Engelgau MM, Moore B, Thompson TJ, Williamson DF, Vinicor F. Translation research for chronic diseases. The case for diabetes. *Diabetes Care* 2000; 23: 1794–8.
25. Assal J-Ph. Educating the diabetic patient: difficulties encountered by patients and health care providers who have to teach NIDDM and IDDM patients. In Mogensen C, Standl E (eds) *Concepts for the Ideal Diabetes Clinic*. Berlin: de Gruyter, Walter, 1992; pp 73–87.
26. Muhlhauser I, Berger M. Patient education—evaluation of a complex intervention. *Diabetologia* 2002; 45: 1723–33.
27. Sinnock P. Reduced hospital utilization and cost savings associated with diabetes patient education. *J Insur Med* 1986; 18: 24–30.
28. Sinnock P, Bauer DW. Reimbursement issues in diabetes. *Diabetes Care* 2984; 7: 291–6.
29. Egede LE, Ye X, Zheng D, Silverstein MD. The prevalence and pattern of complementary and alternative medicine use in individuals with diabetes. *Diabetes Care* 2002; 25: 324–9.
30. Thai AC, and the ASDIAB Study Group. Young Asian Chinese patients with newly diagnosed diabetes mellitus. *J Asean Fed Endocr Soc* (*JAFES*) 2000; 18 (suppl 1): 15.
31. Quality diabetes care—a model of disease management. In *32nd International Hospital Federation Congress*. Hong Kong Exhibition and Convention Centre, 2001. Available at: http://www.hospitalmanagement.net/informer/learning/learning6/index.html.
32. Chan JCN, Lau MSW, Wong YM, Chow CC, Yeung VTF, Loo KM, Mong M, Yeung T, Ko GTC, Li KY, So WY, Chan WB, et al. Delivery of diabetes care—the experience at the Prince of Wales Hospital. *Hosp Authority Qual Bull* 1997; 2: 3–21.
33. Lui SF, Ho YW, Chau KF, Leung CB, Choy BY. Hong Kong Renal Registry 1995–1999. *Hong Kong J Nephrol* 1999; 1: 53–60.
34. Chan JCN, Cheung CK, Cheung MYF, Swaminathan R, Critchley JAJH, Cockram CS. Abnormal albuminuria as a predictor of mortality and renal impairment in Chinese patients with NIDDM. *Diabetes Care* 1995; 18: 1013–4.
35. Brenner BM, Cooper ME, De Zeeuw D, Keane WF, Mitch WE, Parving HH, Remuizzi G, Snapinin SM, Zhang Z, Shahnifar S, for the RENAAL Study Investigators. Effects of Losartan on renal and cardiovascular outcomes in patients with type 2 diabetes and nephropathy. *N Engl J Med* 2001; 345: 861–9.
36. Leung WYS, So WY, Cockram CS, Critchley JAJH, Chan JCN. The renoprotective effects of intensive care in a clinical trial setting in Type 2 diabetic patients with nephropathy. *Diabetes* 2001; 50 (suppl 2): A465.
37. Leung WYS, So WY, Tong PCY, Ko GTC, Chan JCN. Implementation of a structured care system delayed renal disease progression in Type 2 diabetic patients with nephropathy. *Diabetes* 2002; 51 (suppl 2): A28.
38. Feest TG, Dunn EJ, Burton CJ. Can intensive treatment alter the progress of established diabetic nephropathy to end-stage renal failure? *Q J Med* 1999; 92: 275–82.
39. Schwarzer R. Social–cognitive factors in changing health-related behaviors. *Curr Dir Psychol Sci* 2001; 10: 47–51.
40. Cheah J. Chronic disease management: a Singapore perspective. *BMJ* 2001; 323: 990–3.
41. *Plan of Action for the Western Pacific Declaration on Diabetes 2000–2005*. Manila: World Health Organization Western Pacific Region, 2001.

104

Organization of Care: Problems in Developing Countries—The Asian Continent

A. Samad Shera

Diabetes Association of Pakistan and WHO Collaborating Centre, Karachi, Pakistan

INTRODUCTION

In 1988, I wrote in *Diabetes Digest* [1], the journal of the Diabetes Association of Pakistan,

> While the West is reaping the fruits of modern research, we are sadly decades behind. Particularly in the rural areas where the majority of our people live, a good number of young patients die undiagnosed because of a virtually non-existent health-care delivery system and very poor diagnostic facilities.

Those fortunate patients who survive, survive perilously due to lack of supply and proper storing facilities of life-saving drugs like insulin, high economic cost of diabetic care, low and poor living conditions with all their attendant miseries. Thus many of our diabetic children die prematurely due to acute complications to which they are particularly susceptible. Over longer periods of time (months and years), lack of control in children, coupled with inadequate diet, gives rise to the intermediate problems of growth failure and delayed development.

Since 1988, there has been progress in the management of type 2 diabetes, particularly with reference to awareness, early detection, treatment, and better compliance. The scenario with regards to type 1 diabetes, however, remains almost unchanged.

The last two decades have witnessed a revision of thinking in diabetes epidemiology, such that it is now recognized that it is the developing countries, and the migrant population from Indian subcontinent living in the developed countries, that presently face the greatest burden of diabetes.

Dr Hilary King of the World Health Organization (WHO) has compared the estimated diabetes prevalence in 1995 to that of 2025, highlighting that there will be a projected rise of 42% in the developed countries and a rise of 170% in the developing countries. By 2025 the number of people expected to have diabetes in India, Pakistan, and China will be more than 109 million. Of the expected 300 million diabetic patients in 2025, more than 75% will be from the developing countries [2, 3] (Table 1).

While the developed countries have almost eliminated communicable diseases from *their* countries, the developing countries are suffering from the dual burden of communicable and noncommunicable diseases, leading among them are diabetes, hypertension, and cardiovascular disorders [4] (Figure 1).

Asian countries need to develop a strategy to meet the requirements of better diabetes care delivery. It is neither sufficient nor practical to adopt the same strategies as in the industrialized societies. Our priorities and limiting factors are unique to our own setup. To be successful in the delivery of diabetes care, we in Asia must evolve our own strategies based on our technical knowledge, our limited resources, and on our own epidemiological studies. At the same time, interaction with experts from the developed world is necessary to keep in touch with the latest developments and technical progress in the field of diabetes.

National and international health authorities can no longer work alone. There is a need to form an alliance with nongovernmental agencies and private sectors with which they share aspirations for improvement in health care delivery.

International Textbook of Diabetes Mellitus, Third Edition. Edited by R. A. DeFronzo, E. Ferrannini, H. Keen, and P. Zimmet.
 ISBN: 0-471-48655-8.

Table 1 Top 10 countries for number of persons with diabetes (WHO estimates, 1995–2025)

	1995		2025	
	Country	Millions	Country	Millions
1.	India	19.4	India	57.2
2.	China	16.0	China	37.6
3.	United States	13.9	United States	21.9
4.	Russian Federation	8.9	Pakistan	14.5
5.	Japan	6.3	Indonesia	12.4
6.	Brazil	4.9	Russian Federation	12.2
7.	Indonesia	4.5	Mexico	11.7
8.	Pakistan	4.3	Brazil	11.6
9.	Mexico	3.8	Egypt	8.8
10.	Ukraine	3.6	Japan	8.5

In developing countries, especially in the Indian subcontinent, diabetes is a major cause of morbidity and mortality. According to recent surveys the prevalence of micro- and macrovascular complications in the people in India and Pakistan is also high. At the national level, medical facilities are too limited to combat the challenge of the rising prevalence of diabetes and its complications [5, 6].

Type 2 diabetes, in the Indian subcontinent, occurs at a relatively young age (15–18% people under 40 years) as compared to the Western world where type 2 diabetes usually occurs above the age of 40 among the Europeans. Nevertheless, the prevalence rates of type 2 diabetes and impaired glucose tolerance (IGT) increase with advancing age in both sexes, reaching a peak in the 55–64 age group in men, and in the 65–74 age group in women [7].

MAGNITUDE OF THE PROBLEM

Pakistan

In Pakistan, type 1 diabetes constitutes less than 2% of the total diabetic population. The other 98% is made up of people with type 2 diabetes.

Studies carried out within the last 30 years have produced some interesting results. In the 1970s and 1980s, for example, the prevalence of adult-onset diabetes (type 2) in Pakistan was estimated to be around 3%. Also, studies conducted during the 1980s and early 1990s indicate a higher prevalence of type 2 diabetes among the Asian-IndoPakistani migrant populations as compared to the indigenous population and other migrant groups.

Although a number of studies have been done on the indigenous population in the Indian subcontinent, they are not very reliable, as very few have used the WHO criteria for the diagnosis of diabetes mellitus. There also has been limited hospital data, and most of the surveys have been on small-scale and nonrepresentative.

As information on the true prevalence of the condition is considered essential for planning health care services, a national diabetes prevalence survey was initiated in 1994 and completed in 1998 by the Diabetes Association of Pakistan in collaboration with the WHO. This survey has clearly indicated that the prevalence of diabetes is very high among the indigenous population as well, which is comparable to that of the migrant population.

The prevalence of type 2 diabetes is about 12% and IGT is around 9% among the general population 25 years and above (Table 2). The prevalence of IGT was found to be higher than the prevalence of newly diagnosed type 2 diabetes [8–10].

Type 1 diabetes continues to be a rare disorder in Pakistan. In a recent study conducted in Karachi, the incidence of type 1 diabetes per 100 000 people per year was

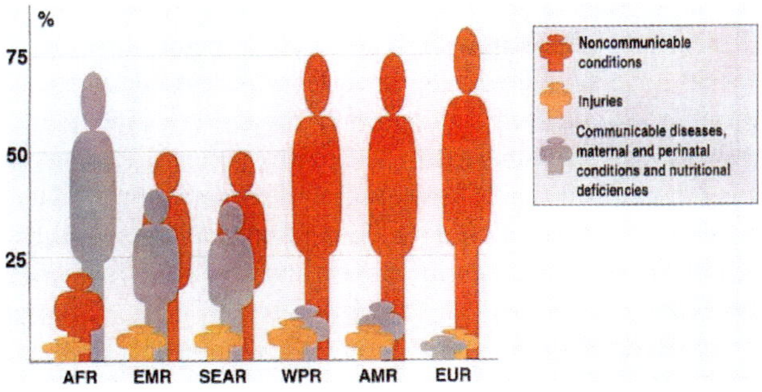

Figure 1 Deaths, by broad cause group and WHO region, 2000 (*Source*: Reference 4)

Table 2 Pakistan national diabetes survey

Province	Diabetes mellitus (%)	IGT (%)
Sindh (rural)	13.9	11.2
Sindh (urban)	16.5	10.4
Baluchistan (rural)	7.5	7.4
Baluchistan (urban)	10.8	10.4
NWFP (rural)	12.0	9.4
Punjab (rural)	6.39	5.39
Punjab (urban)	13.23	11.54
Overall total	*11.47*	*9.39*

1.01 for males and 1.04 for females. The peak incidence was between the ages of 10 and 12 in both genders, and the early peak was at the age of 1–2 years, rather than ages 5–7, as is usually the case in western Europe. The highest rate was for females aged 12 [11].

The survey of diabetes in pregnancy showed that of 12 877 females attending the antenatal clinic in a Karachi governmental teaching hospital (October 1986 to December 1993), 14.7% of women with risk factors for diabetes (e.g., family history, bad obstetric history, congenitally malformed babies, polyhydramnios, obesity, macrosomia) were found to have diabetes, whereas the corresponding figure for women with no risk factors was only 0.56%. The most cost-effective strategy, given the financial constraint in developing countries, is to screen at least those pregnant women who have risk factors [12].

India

A national urban diabetes survey was carried out in six major cities in India covering all the regions of the country. The study group of 11 216 subjects was representative of all socioeconomic strata. Age-standardized prevalence of diabetes and IGT were 12.1% and 14.0% respectively, and showed no gender difference. Newly diagnosed diabetic patients were 30%. Diabetes and IGT showed increasing trend with age. In subjects with <40 years of age, prevalence of IGT was higher than the prevalence of diabetes (13% vs. 5%). Prevalence of diabetes showed a positive and independent association with age, body mass index, waist-to-hip ratio, family history of diabetes, and monthly income. This national survey has shown that the prevalence of diabetes and IGT are high in the urban Indian population. The higher prevalence of IGT is probably an indicator of a further rise in the prevalence of diabetes in the years to come. Published data from Bangladesh has quoted the conversion rate as 2.36, 8.6, 19.83, 40.08, and 70.92% respectively in the first-, second-, third-, fourth-, and fifth-year follow-up [13].

In another study sponsored by the WHO in urban Chennai, the impact of poverty on the profile of diabetes and its complication was studied. The urban poor in the developing society has a lower prevalence of diabetes unlike the urban poor in developed societies. However, they have higher rates of complications of diabetes. Diabetic subjects in the lower income group had a higher prevalence of cardiac disease, neuropathy, and cataract and a lower prevalence of retinopathy than higher income group subjects. The prevalence of risk variables such as hyperglycemia, dyslipidemia, hypertension, smoking, and alcohol consumption were more in the low-income group. Low-income group was defined as the group having family income of less than Rs 30 000/annum (approx. £432) and high-income group was defined as the group having family income greater than or equal to Rs 60 000/annum (approx. £864) [14, 15].

Table 3 Prevalence of diabetes mellitus in Eastern Mediterranean and Middle East Region

County	Age in years	Prevalence of diabetes mellitus	Diagnostic methods
Jordan	25	13.4	75 g OGTT
Kuwait	20	14.8	75 g OGTT
Lebanon	30	13.2	75 g OGTT
Oman	20	10.0	75 g OGTT
Pakistan	25	11.47	75 g OGTT
Saudi Arabia	15	12.3	75 g OGTT
Syria	20	10.3	75 g OGTT
UAE	20	6.0	RCG

Note: OGTT: oral glucose tolerance test; RCG: random capillary glucose measurement.

Middle East

Several epidemiological surveys on diabetes have been conducted in the region over the past two decades. Many of these studies, however, are difficult to compare because of a lack of methodological standards. Various diagnostic criteria were used and sample selection varies from one study to another.

Nevertheless, those surveys that employed comparable methodologies and diagnostic criteria, based on WHO recommendations, indicate that diabetes in these populations is considerably more prevalent than in Europe and North America. Data on the epidemiological and clinical characteristics of type 2 diabetes have been reported from Jordan, Kuwait, Lebanon, Oman, Saudi Arabia, Syria, and United Arab Emirates (UAE). With the exception of UAE, the prevalence of diabetes in population samples aged 20 years and over has been reported to be high and is in most studies around 10%. There are also rural/urban differences in prevalence [16–22] (Table 3).

DIABETES CARE IN DEVELOPING COUNTRIES

Health Care Structure

Present health care delivery system in most developing countries is structured to deal with acute and episodic illnesses and not designed to provide the optimal array of services necessary to manage a complex, multisystem chronic illness like diabetes. Many healthcare providers are ill-equipped to manage chronic conditions effectively, and many governments cannot cope with the escalating disease burden and costs. As against this, the health care in developed countries is well organized and specialist-orientated with reliance on sophisticated technology and high cost [23].

Available Diabetes Care

There is limited availability of trained diabetes health care personnel. Even in areas with adequate health services, diabetes education and counseling is not readily available to patients. Western diabetes health care models are not replicable owing to problems of cost, organization, and accessibility.

Barriers and Suggested Solutions in the Organization of Diabetes Care

Despite the high prevalence of diabetes and its complications in developing countries, essential health care requirements and facilities for self-care and control of diabetes are often inadequate in many countries.

There is a wide disparity in the health care facilities available in the developed world and developing countries and again in the rural and urban areas in the Third World.

Many barriers stand in the way of adequate diabetes care in developing countries:

(1) Barriers affecting basic needs and rights: affordability and availability of insulin, syringes, needles, oral hypoglycemic agents (OHAs), and diagnostics; discrimination and lack of understanding about people with diabetes.
(2) Medical barriers: limited means of self-evaluation; high cost of self-monitoring; failure to gain all the information available about one's health status.
(3) Educational barriers: some health care programs are poorly conceived, delivered, and inadequately evaluated; failure to appreciate importance of education; high illiteracy rate; lack of awareness about diabetes and *importance of diet and exercise*.
(4) Emotional barriers: nonacceptance of diabetes; lack of contact with other people with diabetes and feeling of isolation; insufficient psychological support from relatives and friends.
(5) Lack of political will and commitment to diabetes control programs; lack of resources; parallel programs of diabetes and hypertension; nonintegration of diabetes care at the primary health care level.

Following measures are suggested to help combat these problems:

(1) Introduce measures to increase awareness of the problem of diabetes and its magnitude among policymakers, health care providers, the public, and health professionals.
(2) Reduce costs by removing import duty and taxes on insulin and other materials for diabetes health care.
(3) Encourage industry to manufacture insulin and OHA in developing countries to reduce costs.
(4) Encourage research in basic, clinical, and social aspects of diabetes.
(5) Encourage education through structured programs for people with diabetes, their friends and relatives, and for physicians, nurses, and paramedics.
(6) Use the press and electronic media to educate the public about diabetes. [24]

Actions That Improve Diabetes Care

Implementation planning, accelerating the implementation cycle, and good ongoing cooperative arrangements between the interested parties such as those in primary and secondary health care, local health authorities, and people with diabetes are the actions that improve diabetes care.

Actions That Do Not Improve Diabetes Care

Forming task forces, making reports, and governmental announcements without appropriate follow-up action are the actions that do not improve diabetes care.

Diabetes Care Planning

Diabetes care planning include the following: pick up resources when they become available; involve interested individuals; contract planning vs. consensus planning, discourage contract planning and encourage consensus planning; planning based on the available resources and not idealistic because idealistic planning soon runs into resource barriers; keep away nonoptimists from planning group as non-optimists become frustrated quickly. Do not think about implementing a diabetes programme until the government approves the programme plan, resources are available, infrastructure is established, and key persons are recruited.

The Challenge Ahead

The following actions are needed to introduce cost-effective care: invest in both primary and secondary prevention; structure health care services appropriately so that available resources can be used as wisely as possible; and provide diabetes education for people with diabetes and their families, health care providers, decision makers, and the general public.

REFERENCES

1. Samad Shera A. Editorial. *Diabetes Digest* August 1988; 1: 3.
2. King H, Rewers M. WHO Ad Hoc Diabetes Reporting Group: global estimates for prevalence of diabetes and impaired glucose tolerance in adults. *Diabetes Care* 1993; 16: 157–77.

3. King H, Aubert RE, Herman WH. Global burden of diabetes, 1995–2025, prevalence, numerical estimates and projection. *Diabetes Care* 1998; 21: 1414–31.
4. WHO. World Health Report, 2001.
5. Samad Shera A, Etu-Seppälä L. Increasing diabetes prevalence hits developing countries. *Diabetes Voice* September 1999; 44 (3): 6–9.
6. Ramachandran A, Snehalatha C, Satayavani K, Latha E, Sasikala R, Vijay V. Prevalence of vascular complications and their risk factors in type 2 diabetes. *J Assoc Physicians India* December 1999; 47 (12): 1152–6.
7. Samad Shera A. Diabetes in Pakistan. *IDF Bull* February 1998; 43: 14–6.
8. Shera AS, Rafique G, Khwaja IA, Ara J, Baqai S, King H. 'Pakistan National Diabetes Survey: prevalence of glucose intolerance and associated factors in Shikarpur, Sindh Province. *Diabet Med* 1995; 12: 1116–21.
9. Shera S, Rafique G, Khwaja IA, Baqai S, King H. Pakistan National Diabetes Survey: prevalence of glucose intolerance and associated factors in Baluchistan Province. *Diabetes Res Clin Pract* 1999; 44: 49–58.
10. Shera S, Rafique G, Ahmed KI, Baqai S, Khan IA, King H. Pakistan National Diabetes Survey: prevalence of glucose intolerance and associated factors in North West Frontier Province (NWFP) of Pakistan. *J Pakistan Med Assoc* September 1999; 49 (9): 206–11.
11. Staines A, Hanif S, Ahmed S, McKinney PA, Shera S, Bodansky HJ. 'Incidence of insulin dependent diabetes mellitus in Karachi, Pakistan'. *Arch Dis Childhood* 1997; 76: 121–3.
12. Samad N, Shera AS, Ara JH. 'Gestational diabetes mellitus—screening in a developing country'. *J Pakistan Med Assoc* 1996; 46 (11): 249–52.
13. Khan AR, Ahmed T, Mahtab H. Rate of conversion of IGT to diabetes mellitus: a retrospective study. *J Diab Assoc Bang* 1988; 17: 10–5.
14. Ramachandran A, Snehalatha C, Kapur A, Vijay V, Mohan V, Das AK, Rao PV, Yajnik CS, Prasanna Kumar KM, Nair JD. Diabetes Epidemiology Study Group in India (DESI). High prevalence of diabetes and impaired glucose tolerance in India: National Urban Diabetes Survey. *Diabetologia* September 2001; 44 (9): 1094–101.
15. Asha Bai PV, Murthy BN, Chellamariappan M, Gupte MD, Krishnaswami CV. Prevalence of known diabetes in Chennai City. *J Assoc Physicians India* October 2001; 49: 974–81.
16. Ala'Din Alwan. Type 2 diabetes in the Middle East/Eastern Mediterranean region. *IDF Bull* February 1998; 43: 8–13.
17. Ajlouni K, Jaddou H, Batieha A. Diabetes and impaired glucose tolerance in Jordan: prevalence and associated risk factors. *J Inter Med* 1998; 244: 317–23.
18. Aabdella N, Al Arouj M, Al Nakhi A, Al Assoussi A, Moussa M. Non-insulin dependent diabetes in Kuwait: prevalence rates and associated risk factors. *Diabetes Res Clin Pract* December 1998; 42 (3): 187–96.
19. Salti IS, Khogali M, Alam S, Abu Haider N, Masri A. Epidemiology of diabetes mellitus in relation to other cardiovascular risk factors in Lebanon. *Eastern Mediterranean Health J* 1997; 3 (3): 462–71.
20. Asfour MG, Lambourne A, Soliman A, Al-Behlani S, Al-Asfoor D, Bold A, Mahtab H, King H. High prevalence of diabetes mellitus and impaired glucose tolerance in the Sultanate of Oman: results of the 1991 national survey. *Diabet Med* December 1995; 12 (12): 1122–5.
21. Albach N. Epidemiological Studies Lay the Ground for Syrian Diabetes Campaign. *Diabetes Voice* October 2001; 46 (3): 18–21.
22. el Mugamer IT, Ali Zayat AS, Hossain MM, Pugh RN. Diabetes, obesity and hypertension in urban and rural people of Bedouin origin in the United Arab Emirates. *J Trop Med Hyg* December 1995; 98 (6): 407–15.
23. Epping-Jordan J, Bengoa R, Kawar R, Sabate E. The challenge of chronic conditions: WHO responds. *BMJ* 2001; 323: 947–8.
24. Ramachandran A, Shera S. *Indian Subcontinent, The Economics of Diabetes and Diabetes Care*. A Report of the Diabetes Health Economics Study Group. IDF-WHO, 1997; pp 75–81.

105

Organization of Care: Problems in Developing Countries—Sub-Saharan Africa

Jean Claude Mbanya

University of Yaoundé I, Yaoundé, Cameroon

INTRODUCTION

The global epidemic of diabetes has not spared sub-Saharan African countries. Diabetes mellitus is now a major health problem in Africa, and patient numbers will increase with the tremendous gain in life expectancy that has resulted from improvements in economic and educational standards. As life expectancy increases, more and more untreated diabetic patients with long-term complications will block hospital beds and put a vast strain on the limited resources. The problem in sub-Saharan Africa is whether proper diabetes care can be delivered in the present context of financial constraints, the lack of health infrastructure and trained staff, and the heavy health and social burden of the HIV/AIDS epidemic. The health care system of most countries in the region has to be amended to take on noncommunicable diseases including diabetes mellitus. This chapter discusses the present state of diabetes care in sub-Saharan Africa and highlights problems in the organization of diabetes care in the region.

IS DIABETES A PROBLEM IN SUB-SAHARAN AFRICA?

In 1901 Albert Cook, a medical missionary in Uganda, reported that "diabetes is rather uncommon and very fatal . . ." Over the next 50–60 years diabetes continued to be regarded as rare in sub-Saharan Africa. However, many countries in sub-Saharan Africa are at the early stage of modernization and are undergoing a demographic transition, with both the affluent and poor urban dwellers rapidly adopting western lifestyles, with an increase in the consumption of fat, sugar, and salt. These lifestyle changes have evolved along with increasing prevalence of diabetes mellitus, obesity, and hypertension in both rural and urban communities [1–4].

Type 1 Diabetes

The estimated incidence of type 1 diabetes in sub-Saharan Africa is 10/100 000 in children and adolescents and 15/100 000 in the adult population [5]. It is not known how many children die undiagnosed; nevertheless, type 1 diabetes may also account for the high infant mortality rate. Most often, traditional beliefs that the child is bewitched, especially if the presenting symptom is diabetic ketoacidosis, will lead the parents to consult firstly a "native doctor," or a traditional healer. They will seek medical attention only if there is no improvement in the child's condition. However, because of the poor prognosis of diabetic ketoacidosis in the region, the situation is usually fatal [6, 7].

Type 2 Diabetes

The prevalence of type 2 diabetes is low in both rural and urban Bantu communities, but it is 10 times higher in Indian migrants and Muslim and Hindu communities in Tanzania and South Africa, and in Chinese migrants in Mauritius. It is also higher in the urban than in the rural areas in view of the accelerated social change, with an increase in caloric intake, a decline in physical activity, and a marked increase in obesity taking place in the urban communities of Africa. Type 2 diabetes is already a major

International Textbook of Diabetes Mellitus, Third Edition. Edited by R. A. DeFronzo, E. Ferrannini, H. Keen, and P. Zimmet.
 ISBN: 0-471-48655-8.

public health problem in Africa and its impact is bound to continue if nothing is done to curb the rising prevalence of impaired glucose tolerance, which is between 2.2 and 32.2%. Moreover, from previous studies, the percentage of unknown diabetes varies from less than 50% in South Africa, to 57–67% in Cameroon, and up to 80% in Tanzania [8].

Africa had a population of nearly 600 million inhabitants in 1998, with an estimated diabetic population of 550 000 type 1 and 5 million type 2 diabetic patients. With the current trends, it is estimated that the African diabetic population would more than double by the year 2000 and quadruple by the year 2010 [1, 3].

ORGANIZATION OF DIABETES CARE IN SUB-SAHARAN AFRICA

In all sub-Saharan African countries, diabetes care is integrated in the overall national health care structures, with primary care bearing the main responsibility. The concept of a specialized diabetes care center is a novelty and where available it is limited only to those living in the cities and those of a certain socioeconomic group.

The organization of diabetes health care is based on three levels, with each of them having its own place and function. At the bottom of this chart, are the diabetic patients who, in the first instance, administer self-care or seek alternative care for their condition. Depending on the place where the patient lives, alternative care is sought at the primary, district, or tertiary health care systems. There is a great disparity in the care of diabetic patients between the rural and the urban areas of the region. Even within the same country, there are geographical disparities in the availability, organization, and quality of diabetes care.

Primary Health Care Centers

These range from dispensaries and satellite health centers to large clinics with a small number of beds for observation, delivery, etc. They are usually located in the rural areas and some suburban areas and they form the main focus of health care in the region. Primary health care centers are staffed by nurses and midwives who are often assisted by nursing aids and locally trained health workers. There are no specialized units for diabetes care in the primary care centers. At this level, diabetes care forms part of primary health care program. Where available, simple urine testing for glucose is carried out. Patients with glycosuria are usually referred to secondary health care centers. Diabetes health education is undertaken during general education sessions. However, a lot of emphasis is laid on nutrition, and diabetes and pregnancy. In most satellite health centers, which form the core of the primary health care delivery service, insulin and oral hypoglycemic agents are lacking. Diabetic patients, who cannot bear referral charges to hospitals, which are usually distant and inaccessible to the majority of the population, tend to seek alternative measures including consultation of witch doctors and other traditional healers. Primary health care services look after more than half the diabetic patients in the region.

District Health Care Centers

This level of health care is made of district hospitals with a bed capacity of 50–200 beds, and private clinics. These facilities are usually located in main towns and provincial headquarters. At this level, general health care physicians assisted by trained general nurses cater for the needs of diabetic patients. A minority of these centers has laboratory facilities for blood glucose measurements while a majority function like primary health care centers. Diabetic health education is imparted by the doctors at the outpatient consulting rooms.

Patients with diabetes are usually admitted to the hospital for insulin therapy for diabetes control. Ambulatory stabilization programs are rare at this level. Dietary counseling is undertaken by the nonspecialized nurses and the doctors. Hospital admission does not impose artificial regimes of meals because very few public hospitals in the region feed their inpatients. At this level, and in a minority of hospitals, insulin and oral hypoglycemic agents are sometimes available to those who can afford them.

Some problems are encountered at this level; the health professionals do not have sufficient management experience to keep up to date with diabetes care practices. The physicians have too high a general medicine patient load to allow them enough time to advise and assist patients with chronic diabetes-related problems. The infrastructure does not permit the health team to carry out diligently the routine screening procedures involved in monitoring control and determining the common diabetic complications. Even at this level, special health structures are not reserved for the care of diabetic patients. Patients' compliance with their treatment regimen is very poor, as most of the patients cannot afford the long and expensive prescriptions. Many patients are therefore lost to follow-up and are sometimes seen again with diabetic complications.

Tertiary Health Centers

These are large teaching, referral hospitals and specialized diabetes centers, which are mostly located in the capital city. In principle, tertiary health care services should receive patients from the secondary structures; however in a region where health services are paid for by the patients, this is not often the case. In the teaching hospitals, diabetes care centers are integrated into outpatients' clinics as independent units headed by the diabetes specialist. Members of the unit also include medical residents, nondiabetes specialist nurses, and dieticians. Diabetes specialist nurses and diabetes educators are most often absent. The outpatients' clinics serve as diabetic centers and incorporate services such as intervention for acute diabetes-related problems, stabilization and monitoring diabetes control, diabetes education, screening for diabetic complications, training of medical students and residents, as well as clinical research.

A wide range of laboratory tests for monitoring diabetes control and diabetic complications is carried out in these hospitals. Also, a variety of care can be offered to the diabetic patient, including proper diabetes care involving some form of self-monitoring by the patient and management of diabetic complications (cardiac surgery, renal dialysis, laser therapy, etc.). Follow-up visits are facilitated by a recall system. Home visits to diabetic patients are rare. The pitfall of the tertiary care system is that of cost. The system is very expensive and, since in most countries diabetic patients have to pay for the totality of their medical bills, only the privileged few can afford to be followed up in these health institutions.

PROBLEMS IN ORGANIZATION OF DIABETES CARE

The aims of any system of diabetes care are to facilitate diabetic self-management and control, thus enabling people with diabetes to make the necessary adjustments to remain well and have a good quality of life; to reduce morbidity, mortality, and hospitalization; and to allow for the early detection of complications by effective follow-up. It is impossible to meet these aims in sub-Saharan Africa because of the enormous problems encountered in the region, including organizational, socioeconomic, cultural, and geographic factors [9]. This section focuses on some of these problems.

Problems Related to the Health Service

The organization of the National Health Service in most sub-Saharan African countries is mostly oriented toward communicable diseases. The consequence is that little is known about the public health burden of diabetes and therefore awareness of diabetes both among health workers and among the general public is limited. Only the Republic of South Africa has developed a national diabetes program and in most countries there is no officer at the level of the ministry of health responsible for diabetes and other noncommunicable diseases. Diabetes therefore has a low health priority in most countries and diabetic patients are left to the vagaries of the disease or to die, as is the case with those suffering from type 1 diabetes.

Increased efforts must be made to integrate diabetes and other chronic diseases in the national network of care and these should involve primary, district, and tertiary levels of care. Primary health care is often falsely viewed in the region as an alternative to hospital-based care. It may exist autonomously in the delivery of immunization and maternal and child health care programs, but, in the care of chronic diseases, cooperation is essential between all levels of health care. In order to achieve this goal, there should be a rethink of the system of primary health care and a restructure of the existing health care system to integrate chronic diseases such as diabetes. A noncommunicable disease program with diabetes as an entry point should be developed with all stakeholders, with special emphasis on prevention, since many countries in the region have recorded marked increase in diabetes risk factors due to increasing life expectancy, changing lifestyles, urbanization, and smoking [4, 10, 11]. In this integrated management of diabetes, the provision of care should aim to be organized and individualized to the person concerned. Thus, during the lifetime of the patient with diabetes, care is provided by the primary care team or a specialist team, or both. The appropriate care provider will change according to the progress of the condition.

It is well recognized that a majority of diabetic patients in the region first seek alternative health care facilities before seeking Western-type health services. Indeed, because health beliefs are still deeply enshrined in the healing cultures of people in the region, most patients alternate between modern and traditional clinics. The alternating health seeking behavior is conditioned by the perceived causes of diabetes and the perceived benefits from the modern health unit when compared to the traditional. The modern clinics are believed to control the conditions and the traditional clinics to cure them. Attempts have therefore been made in some countries of the region to incorporate the contribution of traditional healers into the primary health care system; however, results have been variable, but generally the union has been fraught with difficulties.

Lack of Financial and Material Resources

There has been an improvement in the economic status in most sub-Saharan African countries over the past decade. Economic status should strongly affect outcomes by working through several proximal determinants including access to health services. However, this has not been the case with sub-Saharan Africa where there is still the unfinished agenda of communicable diseases, poverty, and a lack of proportional investments in health. The United Nations uses three criteria: low income based on the gross domestic product; human resource weakness involving a composite Augmented Physical Quality of Life Index based on indicators of (1) nutrition, (2) health, (3) education, and (4) adult literacy; and economic vulnerability to classify states as being "least developed countries" [12]. In 2000, 49 countries in the world were denominated under this category, of which 34 were from sub-Saharan Africa.

Table 1 The least developed sub-Saharan African countries in decreasing order of gross national product (GNP) per capita, 1998 (in dollars)

Country	GNP per capita
1. Cape Verde	1200
2. Equatorial Guinea	1110
3. Lesotho	570
4. Guinea	530
5. Senegal	520
6. Mauritania	410
7. Angola	380
8. Benin	380
9. Comoros	370
10. Gambia	340
11. Togo	330
12. Zambia	330
13. Uganda	310
14. Central African Republic	300
15. Sudan	290
16. Sao Tome and Principe	270
17. Madagascar	260
18. Mali	250
19. Burkina Faso	240
20. Chad	230
21. Rwanda	230
22. United Republic of Tanzania	220
23. Malawi	210
24. Mozambique	210
25. Eritrea	200
26. Niger	200
27. Guinea-Bissau	160
28. Burundi	140
29. Sierra Leone	140
30. Democratic Rep. of the Congo	110
31. Ethiopia	100
32. Djibouti	100
33. Liberia	100
34. Somalia	100

Source: Reference 12.

It is apparent that the gross domestic product of these countries, which varies between US$100 and US$1200, restrains improvement in provision of health care including diabetes (Table 1).

The major problems of the lack of investment in health care include (1) inadequate health infrastructure; (2) uneven distribution of health facilities and personnel; and (3) lack of government support or subsidy, with the result that costs of diabetes care have to be borne by the patients or their families. Moreover, very few countries in the region have an effective national health insurance policy; therefore the cost of health care is the responsibility of the patient, even for chronic diseases like diabetes. The consequence is that children with type 1 diabetes may die within 1 year of diagnosis because the desperately low incomes of individuals and families mean that insulin and supplies for diabetes management may consume as much as half or more of family income [13–16].

It is well known that money and time spent to provide quality diabetes care can prevent or minimize the long-term complications of diabetes, the major contributor to the overall cost of this chronic disease. The growing need to rationally allocate limited health care resources poses emotional, potentially divisive questions of science, politics, economics, and ethics that patients and physicians must each address. There is a need for better awareness and commitment at national, regional, and local government levels on the importance of integrating diabetes care in health care programs. Because diabetes is a chronic disease, certain aspects of diabetes cost should be subsidized by government agencies.

Problems Related to the Management of Diabetes

Lack of Knowledge on the Burden of Diabetes and Its Complications

The true burden of diabetes and its complications has not been well described in the region, therefore making health planning difficult. Community-based studies of diabetes prevalence using standard international protocols have been undertaken in Tanzania, South Africa, Cameroon, and Nigeria [4, 17–19]. It is based on these four studies that estimates of the burden of diabetes in the region has been made. Furthermore, awareness of diabetes both among health workers and among the general public is limited [20]. More studies, especially in specific occupational groups whose lifestyle has changed, are needed from the region.

Lack of Trained Personnel

There is a considerable variation in the standard of care provided to people with diabetes in sub-Saharan Africa. The majority of countries in the region do not have specialist diabetes clinics and therefore the patients are followed up in general medical clinics, health centers, and by staff not trained to administer diabetes care. Indeed, a majority of patients are either followed up by nonspecialist nurses or they receive no care at all. Diabetes care cannot be dependent on adequately trained physicians alone and here lies the major problem in the region. We need to have trained diabetes physicians/pediatricians, nurse specialists, dieticians, chiropodists, and podiatrists involved in diabetes care in the region. Unfortunately, very few trained personnel are available for training in these disciplines.

Lack of Drugs: Insulin and Oral Hypoglycemic Agents

Three quarters of a century after the discovery of insulin, access to insulin and equipment for sustaining life and health is still a major problem faced by patients with diabetes in sub-Saharan Africa. A recent questionnaire survey on insulin access conducted by the International Diabetes Federation's Insulin Task Force indicated that in 25 sub-Saharan African countries insulin was often unavailable in half the large city hospitals and only 5 countries reported regular insulin availability in rural areas. In consequence, the life expectancy of a child with newly diagnosed type 1 diabetes in much of sub-Saharan Africa may be as short as 1 year. In addition, restricted access to insulin will result in debilitating complications such as amputations and blindness and a much reduced life expectancy. The reasons for this poor insulin access included cost in 25 countries, distribution in 25 countries (roughly the same countries), difficulties in transport of the patients to sites of insulin distribution in 13 countries, and other reasons in 8 countries [21].

There have been concerns about the storage of insulin in the absence of refrigerators in the region; nevertheless, it is always possible to find suitable vessels including *clay pots* (a porous vessel filled with water or sand and water) and holes in the ground as long as the insulin is available [22, 23]. Although these systems are very popular, their efficiency is uncertain.

Oral hypoglycemic agents are still expensive in some countries in the region despite the introduction of generic forms. One of the commonest available sulfonylureas in the region is chlorpropamide, which has an extremely prolonged duration of action and causes severe hypoglycemia. In a region with mediocre health facilities coupled with poverty, the patients and staff should be well educated on the use of first and second generations of sulfonylureas.

Diabetic Control

The management of diabetes involves the self-monitoring of blood glucose by the patient and intermittent clinic measurements of glycosylated hemoglobin (HbA_{1C}). The majority of diabetic patients in the region do very little self-monitoring, except sometimes for urine glucose [24]. Home glucose testing has been successfully introduced in some countries of the region although it is generally far too expensive for the average patient. Testing of fasting blood glucose is offered by many clinics and hospitals to diabetic patients. It is still very difficult and expensive to measure HbA_{1C} although a few clinics in the region offer this facility to their patients.

As noted earlier, facilities are limited and resources short for the control of diabetes and its complications in the region. Standard systems for diabetic control are not usually possible in the region and laboratory support for the assessment and follow-up of acute diabetic complications notably diabetic ketoacidosis and hyperosmolar nonketotic coma is limited.

Patient Education

Diabetes affects all aspects of a person's life and functioning from the most particular (eating) to the most general (life expectancy). Diabetes is affected by other medical conditions and interventions, the progress and outcome of which may themselves be affected by the condition. Learning self-management is a life-long experience, requiring education, understanding, and appropriate support. Positive attitudes that are nonjudgemental are essential to the person with diabetes and the family who all require informed and appropriate medical care, friendship, and encouragement in order to live a healthy, happy, safe, and long life with diabetes. It is well recognized that knowledge about diabetes is integral to successful management, and indeed, diabetes education is the cornerstone of successful diabetes treatment. The challenge in sub-Saharan Africa is to disseminate this knowledge and to simultaneously provide optimal care for all people with diabetes. The major obstacle in the region is lack of trained diabetes specialist nurse educators. Although the Panafrican Diabetes Educators' Group has recently put in place a program of "educating the educators," nevertheless it will still take a long time to train enough diabetes educators who will deliver proper diabetes education in the primary health care centers in the region.

CONCLUSION

It is still a nightmare to deliver proper diabetes care in sub-Saharan Africa because of financial constraints, and lack of availability of health infrastructure and trained staff. Governments, diabetes associations, and other bodies comprising people affected with diabetes, physicians, nurses, nutritionists, and educators should cooperate with one another in improving diabetes care in the region. Governments and nongovernmental organizations should be urged to ensure consistent availability of insulin and other antidiabetic drugs and advocate for subsidy of certain aspects of diabetes care. Such bodies should also play a significant role in imparting education on various aspects of diabetes care to the patients, health care providers, and the community at primary, secondary, and tertiary health care levels.

REFERENCES

1. Amos AF, McCarty DJ, Zimmet P. The rising global burden of diabetes and its complications: estimates and projections to the year 2010. *Diabet Med* 1997; 14: S1–85.
2. King H, Rewers M. Diabetes in adults is now a Third World problem. World Health Organization Ad Hoc Diabetes Reporting Group. *Ethn Dis* 1993; 3: S67–74.
3. King H, Aubert RE, Herman WH. Global burden of diabetes, 1995–2025: prevalence, numerical estimates, and projections. *Diabetes Care* 1998; 21: 1414–31.
4. Mbanya JC, Ngogang J, Salah JN, Minkoulou E, Balkau B. Prevalence of NIDDM and impaired glucose tolerance in a rural and an urban population in Cameroon. *Diabetologia* 1997; 40: 824–9.

5. Swai AB, Lutale JL, McLarty DG. Prospective study of incidence of juvenile diabetes mellitus over 10 years in Dar es Salaam, Tanzania. *BMJ* 1993; 306: 1570–2.
6. Zouvanis M, Pieterse AC, Seftel HC, Joffe BI. Clinical characteristics and outcome of hyperglycaemic emergencies in Johannesburg Africans. *Diabet Med* 1997; 14: 603–6.
7. Rolfe M, Ephraim GG, Lincoln Dc, Huddle KRL. Hyperglycaemic nonketotic coma as a cause of emergency hyperglycaemic admission in Baragwanath Hospital. *S Afr Med J* 1995; 85: 173–6.
8. Levitt NS, Unwin NC, Bradshaw D, Kitange HM, Mbanya JC, Mollentze WF, Omar MA, Motala AA, Joubert G, Masuki G, Machibya H. Application of the new ADA criteria for the diagnosis of diabetes to population studies in sub-Saharan Africa. *Diabet Med* 2000; 17: 381–5.
9. Gill GV. Problems of diabetic care in tropical countries. *Practi Diabetes* 1988; 5: 156–8.
10. Cruickshank JK, Mbanya JC, Wilks R, Balkau B, Forrester T, Anderson SG, Mennen L, Forhan A, Riste L, McFarlane-Anderson N. Hypertension in four African-origin populations: current “Rule of Halves,” quality of blood pressure control and attributable risk of cardiovascular disease. *J Hypertens* 2001; 19: 41–6.
11. Cruickshank JK, Mbanya JC, Wilks R, Balkau B, McFarlane-Anderson N, Forrester T. Sick genes, sick individuals or sick populations with chronic disease? The emergence of diabetes and high blood pressure in African-origin populations. *Int J Epidemiol* 2001; 30: 111–7.
12. *UNDP Human Development Report 1997*. New York: Oxford University Press, 1997.
13. Castle W, Wicks A. A follow-up of 93 newly diagnosed African diabetics for 6 years. *Diabetologia 1980*; 18: 121–3.
14. Makame M for the Diabetes Epidemiology Research International Study Group. Childhood diabetes, insulin, and Africa. *Diabet Med* 1992; 9: 571–3.
15. Gill GV, Huddle KR, Rolfe M. Mortality and outcome of insulin-dependent diabetes in Soweto, South Africa. *Diabet Med* 1995; 12: 546–50.
16. Yudkin JS. Insulin for the world’s poorest countries. *Lancet* 2000; 355: 919–21.
17. McLarty D, Kitange H, Mtinangi B, Makene W, Swai A, Masuki G, Kilima P, Chuwa L. Prevalence of diabetes and impaired glucose tolerance in rural Tanzania. *Lancet* 1989; 871–4.
18. Levitt N, Katzenellenbogen J, Bradshaw D, Hoffman M, Bonnici F. The prevalence and identification of riak factors for NIDDM in urban Africans in Cape Town, South Africa. *Diabetes Care* 1993; 16: 601–7.
19. Olatunbosun ST, Ojo PO, Fineberg NS, Bella AF. Prevalence of diabetes mellitus and impaired glucose tolerance in a group of urban adults in Nigerian. *J Natl Med Assoc* 1998; 90: 293–301.
20. Riwa HT, Swai ABM, McLarty DG. Failure to diagnose diabetic ketoacidosis in Tanzania. *Diabet Med* 1986; 3: 181–3.
21. Access to Insulin: A Report on the IDF Insulin Task Force on Insulin 1994–1997. Brussels: International Diabetes Federation, 1998.
22. Harries AD, Maher D. Home insulin storage by patients with diabetes mellitus in Blantyre, Malawi. *Int Diabetes Digest* 1994; 5: 104.
23. Gill GV, Ngubane T. Insulin storage by diabetic patients in Soweto, South Africa. *Int Diabetes Digest* 1995; 6: 89.
24. Feleke Y, Abdulkadir J. Urine glucose testing: another look at its relevance when blood glucose monitoring is unaffordable. *Ethiop Med J* 1998; 36: 93–9.

106

Organization of Care: Problems in Developing Countries—South America

Pablo Arias*, Astrid M. Libman†, and Julio Libman†

**University of Buenos Aires Medical School, Buenos Aires, Argentina, and †University of Rosario Medical School, Rosario, Argentina*

THE GROUND: GEOGRAPHIC, DEMOGRAPHIC, AND EPIDEMIOLOGICAL FACTS

South America, stretching from Colombia to Tierra del Fuego (~18 000 000 km^2), includes 13 countries inhabited by approximately 340 million people. Its sanitary situation is imprinted by rapid demographic and epidemiologic changes, and by inequity in terms of morbidity and mortality profiles and in access to health care.

Health issues in South America need to be addressed with caution. There is limited information available and, in general, official epidemiological data are scarce. Considerable underreporting leads to underestimation of the total impact of many diseases. Diabetes is not listed on 30% or more of the death certificates of people with the disease, and there is a considerable variability across time and geographic areas concerning coding practices [1]. Thus, an accurate evaluation of the health problem posed by diabetes mellitus is still not possible.

Diabetes in Children

Regarding the epidemiology of type 1 diabetes, the situation has considerably improved in the past years because of the WHO Multinational Study on Childhood Diabetes [2]. Karvonen et al. [3] described the worldwide incidence of type 1 diabetes mellitus in children aged 0–14 years (Figure 1): in South America, the highest incidence rate (8.3/100 000) was found in Uruguay, while the lowest (0.1/100 000) was detected in Venezuela. Genetic and environmental causes may be responsible for this variation.

Diabetes in Adults

As reviewed by Barceló and Rajpathak [4], most South American studies report adult diabetes prevalence rates between 6 and 9%. However, these data have to be interpreted with caution. Different methodologies and cutoff values have been used for the diagnosis of diabetes mellitus in screening campaigns, and the representativity of the population sample is sometimes questionable.

The Pending Menace

Estimates by King et al. [5] suggest that the prevalence rates of diabetes will increase in the next 20 years (Figure 2). In some countries, such as Brazil and Colombia, the number of people with diabetes will double (Figure 3). The increase in the prevalence of diabetes is far more than would be expected from the population growth alone, and it may be related to the demographic, sociocultural, and epidemiologic changes taking place in the region.

AN EPIDEMIC EXPLAINED

Demographic and Epidemiologic Changes

A demographic transition is taking place in most regions of South America and can be characterized as follows (Table 1):

(1) The population is under continuous growth. Estimated to be of ~240 millions in 1980, it has reached

International Textbook of Diabetes Mellitus, Third Edition. Edited by R. A. DeFronzo, E. Ferrannini, H. Keen, and P. Zimmet.
 ISBN: 0-471-48655-8.

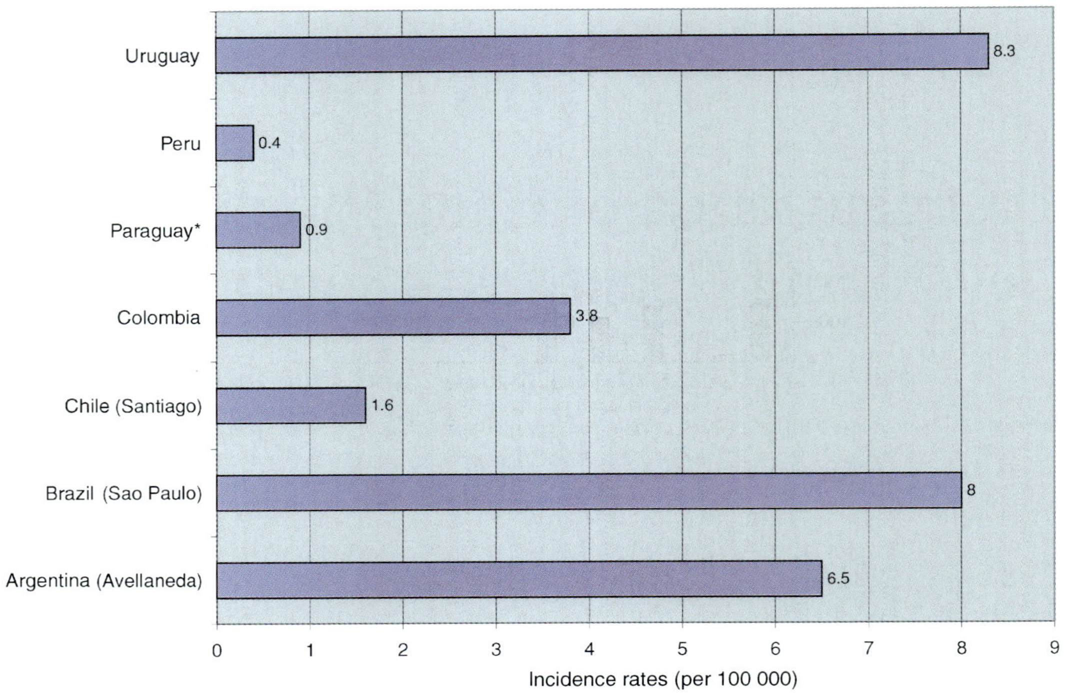

Figure 1 Incidence rates (per 100 000) of type 1 diabetes mellitus in children aged 0–14 years (adapted from reference 3)

~340 millions in the year 2000 (growth rate ≈42.1%).

(2) A considerable migration of inhabitants from rural areas into big cities is taking place: as of the year 2000, 88% of the population lived in urban areas.

(3) Birth rates have decreased and life expectancy has grown; the calculated growth rate of people aged 60 and older is 3–4% per year.

(4) Mortality from infectious diseases has fallen dramatically, while deaths from noncommunicable diseases and accidents are on the rise.

Nutritional Transition

Forced by economic and social changes, a considerable number of people living in rural areas (mostly from

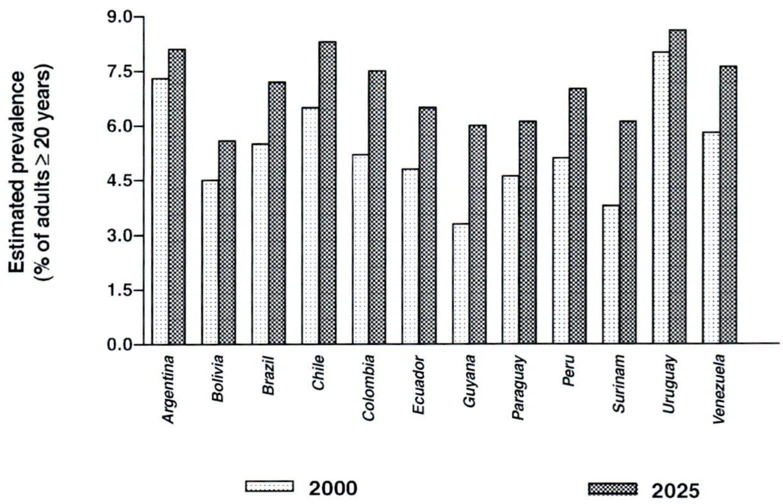

Figure 2 Estimated prevalence rate for diabetes in adults in several South American countries for the years 2000 and 2025 (adapted by permission of the American Diabetes Association [5])

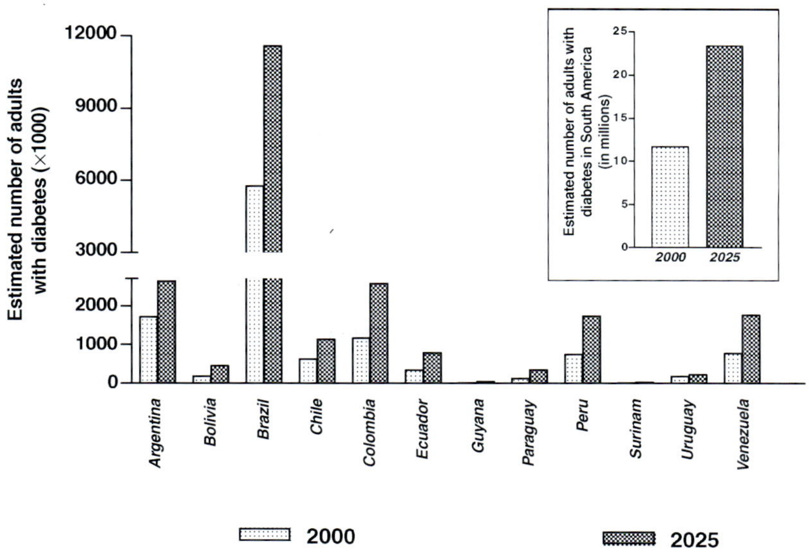

Figure 3 Number of adults with diabetes in several South American countries; estimation for 2000 and 2025 (adapted by permission of the American Diabetes Association [5])

aboriginal ascent) migrate to large urban centers. In order to fit the model set by the globalization process they have changed their dietary habits. The consumption of high-fat food has increased, and the intake of grains, vegetables, and fruits has diminished. These changes are frequently accompanied by a sedentary lifestyle. Under these circumstances, the protective effect of the rural way of life is lost: this combination triggers increasing adiposity, insulin resistance, and type 2 diabetes [7]. These changes affect a great part of the region, mostly the Andean countries and Brazil.

An example of the impact of environmental changes on the development of metabolic diseases in Chile is shown in Figure 4: the prevalence rates for diabetes and obesity in the rural Mapuche population of Chile, still preserving a physically active lifestyle and their traditional diet, are clearly lower than those detected in the Mapuche population living in Santiago, the capital. Moreover, this acculturation process with reduced physical activity and a hypercaloric diet seems to have stricken the native community even on its own ground: while the Mapuche Indians living in rural areas were practically free of diabetes in the mid-1980s, they show at present prevalence rates of 3.2% among males and 4.5% among females [9, 10].

Table 1 Demographic variables measured in South American countries and in the United States*

	South America		United States	
	1980	2000	1980	2000
Total population (millions)	239.2	339.9	255.1	308.6
Urban population (%)	70.0	88.3	73.9	77.2
Crude birth rate (×1000)†	28.5	21.8	15.6	13.6
Life expectancy at birth (years)†	66.0	70.0	74.7	76.9

* These variables show that a demographic transition is taking place in the former [6].
† Calculated for 1980–1985 and 1995–2000.

Poverty and Diabetes

A survey performed in Bolivia by Barceló et al. [11] shows that diabetes seems to be affecting people from the lower socioeconomic classes at an increased rate. As cited by the authors, "...the poorest people in one of the world's poorest countries are the most affected by the disease." Some of the reasons for this worrying affirmation have already been described. Moreover, hypothalamic arousal associated to psychosocial stress may also be a contributing factor, triggering endocrine abnormalities resulting in insulin resistance and type 2 diabetes [12].

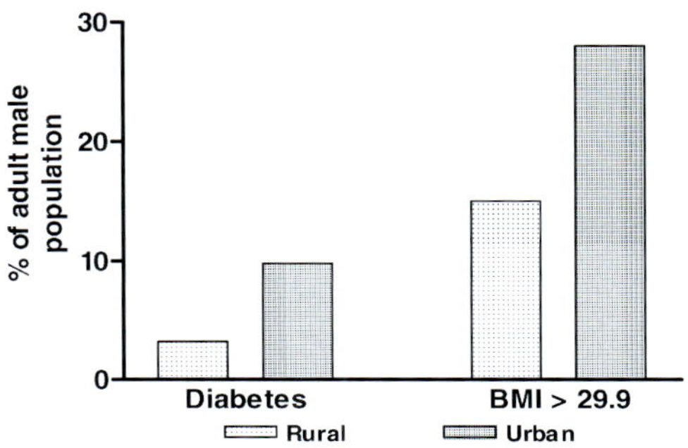

Figure 4 Prevalence of obesity (BMI > 29.9 kg/m^2) and diabetes in adult male members of the Mapuche population in Chile, according to rural/urban condition (modified from reference 8)

Last, but not least, poverty goes hand in hand with chronic malnutrition, and the disadvantaged aboriginal groups are the ones most likely to have endured severe nutritional stress in their recent histories. Hence, an elevated proportion of adults in these populations might have been exposed to fetal malnutrition, a known risk factor for type 2 diabetes and vascular disease [13, 14]. The vicious circle poverty–malnutrition–disease is far from being in the process of eradication in the region, since the number of people with unsatisfied basic needs seems to be rising steadily.

DIABETES CARE IN THE REGION: WHAT IS MISSING AND WHY

The Problem of Health Care Organization in South America

The organization of health care in the region is quite heterogeneous. Different social, political, and economic trends have led to dissimilar health care structures and social protection systems. Besides, in the context of repeated crises of authority and economic turmoil, many countries have begun to decentralize their health care systems, shifting more and more of the health care delivery to the private sector [15]. Public spending on health decreased [16], and these cutbacks in public-sector services are "favored" by international lending agencies [17, 18]. Thus, nonequity and absence of social solidarity have become a constant in most health care delivery systems of this region, restricting the accessibility of impoverished care seekers to health services. As stated by the authorities of the Pan American Health Organisation [19], a variable number of people (in some countries up to 66%) are effectively excluded from most health care services (Table 2). As a result of this lack of social coverage, one of the major factors associated with utilizing services or obtaining medical supplies is the ability to make out-of-pocket payments.

In most countries of the region three types of health care providers coexist:

(1) a public sector (run by national, state, provincial, or city governments);
(2) the social security system (funded in some countries by the state, and in others by contributions of the workers and employers);
(3) a private sector (managed care and health maintenance organizations).

Considering the region as a whole, approximately 56% of health expenditures are covered by the private sector, 20% by the public sector, and 24% by the social security system. There are important variations between countries, and there is no relationship between the percentage of individuals covered by each system and the country's income [19].

Economic resources assigned to health are limited. With the exception of Uruguay (13.4%), the percentage of the gross domestic product (GDP) allocated to health in all countries of the region is less than 10% (Table 2).

Diabetes Budgets: A Critical Issue

Diabetes and its complications are not considered as a health priority: of the total health care expenditure only 3–10% is invested in diabetes care [22]. It is known that the cost of caring for persons with diabetes is two to four times the amount spent on nondiabetic people in most health care systems [23]. These costs are mainly due to hospitalizations and secondary care needed for the treatment of chronic complications. In the United States, it was estimated to be 13% of the total health budget [23, 24]. According to Gagliardino and Olivera [25], the mean cost per

Table 2 Indicators reflecting health care situation in selected countries of South America, and health expenditure (in % of the GDP) in the same countries

Country	Infant mortality rate (per 1000 live births)*	Physicians per 10 000 inhabitants*	GDP (in billion US$)†	Health care expenditure (% of GDP)†	Accesibility to health services (% of total population)‡
Argentina	17.6	26.8	290	9.6	92
Bolivia	67.0	3.2	8.0	4.9	34
Brazil	33.1	14.4	760	7.3	72
Chile	10.1	13.0	74	3.9	93
Colombia	13.5	9.3	101	9.4	75
Ecuador	30.0	13.2	18.4	4.0*	61
Guyana	22.2	1.8	—	3.9*	—
Paraguay	19.4	4.9	9.2	9.8*	54
Peru	37.0	10.3	60.5	5.6	44
Uruguay	14.1	37	20	13.4	96
Venezuela	19.2	19.7	82.1	7.5	76

* Reference 20.
† Reference 21.
‡ Reference 19.

diabetic person per year in Latin America was US$352, far below the US$11 157 spent in the United States per diabetic person per year during 1996. Contrasting with the average calculated for the region, the annual cost per person with diabetes in Chile amounted US$1985 [26].

Problems with Insulin Supply

As an essential drug designated by the World Health Organization insulin should be available at all times. As stated by Alberti in 1994, "...ultimately, it is the duty of responsible governments to ensure the availability of insulin to those who need it, and it is the responsibility of people with diabetes and of the community as a whole to ensure that they do so" [27]. Almost all countries recognize the universal right to health. Nevertheless, sometimes they lack the appropriate resources and strategies to meet their needs. Even advocating a healthy lifestyle will not be successful unless there are means to obtain it.

Providing pharmaceuticals is one of the main pillars of western medicine, but in many low-income countries drugs make up half or more of health care costs. In some countries of South America, insulin and oral antidiabetic agents are not included on the list of essential medications, and the population faces many difficulties in obtaining them. Insulin shortages (acute or chronic) occur. Acute insulin shortage in the region can be the consequence of natural disasters or (more frequently) economic crises, while chronic insulin shortage can result from many causes: poverty, high cost, inadequate distribution system, and local policies resulting in high taxes. In some areas, some insulins are simply not available, and poor infrastructure (e.g., lack of refrigerators) combined with individual poverty can make insulin inaccessible to people who need it.

There are great differences in the utilization of insulin in the world: industrialized countries (900 million inhabitants) use 105 billions IU per year, while in developing countries (population ~4600 millions) 45 billions IU are utilized [28]. According to Gagliardino et al. [29], only 14% of type 2 diabetic patients in the region receive insulin treatment. In some countries, this percentage is as low as 6%. The low utilization of insulin in some areas of South America suggests that people with diabetes may suffer early complications or die from lack of insulin. The extent to which insulin treatment is administered to type 2 patients varies according to the degree of training of the treating physician, but also financial constraints, prejudice, or ignorance may play a role.

Taking into account that in most countries of the region a vial of insulin costs between US$12 and US$20, providing insulin to one family member can consume a substantial part of the total family income in countries where insulin is not free. On the other hand, the average cost arising from a year's insulin supply (approximately US$400) outgrows the mean cost per diabetic person per year in Latin America, US$352 [25]. In the face of other crucial health problems posed by malnutrition, infant mortality, and infectious diseases sometimes it is difficult, even for a well-intentioned government, to justify the assignment of scarce financial and health care resources. The issue in diabetes is further complicated by the lifetime need for medical support and education, dietary needs, eye care, foot care, and other medical supplies.

Quality of Diabetes Care: An Appraisal

There are limited data on the quality of diabetes care in South America, and, not surprisingly, most information arises from independent sources (e.g., nongovernmental organizations, scientific and patient associations). This fact, again, emphasizes most governments' low perception of diabetes as a priority and their reluctance to actively support and/or participate in related initiatives.

According to the existing data, diabetes care in the region can be considered suboptimal. A multicentric study (PEDNID-LA) assessed parameters of care in 446 patients with type 2 diabetes, showing that more than 70% of patients had HbA_{1c} levels > 6.5%, 45% had systolic hypertension, and 62% had elevated serum cholesterol levels [30]. QUALIDIAB, a multicenter study designed to assess the quality of care provided to more than 13 500 patients with diabetes in cities of Argentina, Brazil, Chile, Colombia, Paraguay and Venezuela, showed

(1) too infrequent assessment of relevant indicators, such as HbA_{1c}, proteinuria, and funduscopic examination;
(2) insufficient education, as showed by a high percentage of patients with type 1 (47%) and type 2 (80%) diabetes who do not check either blood or urine glucose levels. In some countries, the proportion of type 2 patients performing these measurements was as low as 1%;
(3) inadequate drug treatment for other cardiovascular risk factors, such as hypertension and/or dyslipidemia [29].

Moreover, specialized medical care is scarce and mostly found in some centers of important cities. Numerous patients who do attend health care facilities receive less than optimal medical care, limited to drug prescription to prevent decompensation. In general, complications are diagnosed at a stage when too little can be done. This reality shows the urgent need to improve the quality of care for patients with diabetes in the region.

Among other causes, these deficiencies could be related to the socioeconomic reality of the countries in the region, and to the characteristics of health care organization:

(1) absent public health tradition for chronic disease control;
(2) economic recession, resulting in restrictions on health care spending, or in redirection of resources;
(3) health care reforms including privatization and decentralization of health care;
(4) limited access to health care, medicaments, and medical supplies;
(5) insufficiently trained human resources;
(6) lack of awareness of the importance of education.

As stated by the PAHO, "...poverty adversely affects diabetes care. It influences the likelihood of being correctly diagnosed, the quality of education received, the adequacy of care, the affordability of treatment and the risk of developing serious complications" [31]. This suggests how beneficial it could be to introduce even limited improvements in care through national diabetes programs emphasizing screening, prevention, education of the population, and training of health care workers in diabetes care. Of course, it would be of paramount importance to bring about the necessary political and social processes that can lead to such improvements.

WHAT IS BEING DONE TO CLEAR THE HURDLES

Reducing costs by improving diabetes care seems achievable, especially for acute hospitalizations and amputations in the short term and for nephropathy in the long term [32, 33]. Education programs can improve the quality of care: a regional multinational diabetes intervention program (PEDNID-LA) demonstrated improved glycemic control as well as savings of 34% in the cost of medication following a diabetes education program [30]. But basically, the economic issue is not whether these interventions save money, but whether they will improve the health of the population at a reasonable cost, compared with other possible interventions.

According to a survey performed in 1997, and on the basis of a questionnaire sent to the Ministries of Health of the region, most South American countries reported having some type of national diabetes program [26]. However, only 5% of these programs were devoted exclusively to diabetes, while in most cases these were part of a general noncommunicable disease program. Accordingly, only one out of three countries assigns an exclusive part of its health budget to diabetes.

PAHO and its associates have been working to improve diabetes prevention and control in the Americas. As a result of their efforts, the Declaration of the Americas on Diabetes (DOTA) was implemented in 1996. One of the main goals of the DOTA is the development of national diabetes programs. Although these were already a priority in the region at the time DOTA was issued, very few have been implemented and have reached the evaluation phase. In 1994, Paraguay started its national program, covered mainly (95%) by the national health budget. At present, most of the regions in Paraguay have teams working in diabetes care education programs for people with diabetes; organized health promotion and prevention campaigns are running [22].

Some local nongovernmental organizations, supported by private funding (e.g., from pharmaceutical companies), have set up activities and programs to provide diabetes education and to improve diabetes care in the region. More than 20 years ago, the Argentine Diabetes Association (SAD) established a yearly program to train 12 physicians (from Argentina and Latin America) to become specialized in diabetes. Another program launched in 1998, PROCAMEG, has taught the fundamentals of diabetes care to more than 650 primary care physicians in different cities of Argentina. Since 1999, a 3-year program (CADIEQ) is being implemented to educate and train nonmedical health professionals [34].

It is very difficult to introduce control activities without knowing the magnitude of the problem. In the case of diabetes, programs must include an *a priori* epidemiological surveillance of diabetes, its complications, and the ensuing costs, as well as an evaluation of the impact of preventive strategies. In this sense the Ministry of Health of Brazil is implementing a National Plan for the Reorganization of Health Care for Hypertension and Diabetes Mellitus. The unavoidable initial stage of this plan was a national screening campaign, the first of its kind carried out by Public Health Services in Brazil and the largest epidemiologic evaluation in the region, studying more than 20 million people. This campaign represents a giant step for the restructuration of diabetes care in this country [35].

These as many other efforts are an example to be followed, always bearing in mind that success is mainly dependent on the commitment of those persons and institutions involved.

CONCLUSIONS

These are tough economic and sociopolitical times for the developing world, including South America. The menace placed on the health care resources by the diabetes epidemic underlines the urgent need for interventions aimed at prevention, but also at optimizing care, improving the quality of life of persons who suffer from diabetes, and diminishing the costs of the disease. Special emphasis is to be placed on access to primary care and basic treatment in the most economically disadvantaged areas. Patient education will surely contribute by giving information and methodological resources, but also by encouraging people (with diabetes) to actively demand services and manage their disease.

REFERENCES

1. Songer TJ, Deberry K, LaPorte R, Tuomilehto J. International comparisons of IDDM mortality. Clues to prevention and the role of diabetes care. *Diabetes Care* 1992; 15: 15–21.
2. WHO DiaMond Project Group. WHO Multinational Project for Childhood Diabetes. *Diabetes Care* 1990; 13: 1062–8.
3. Karvonen M, Viik-Kajander M, Moltchanova E, Libman I, LaPorte R, Tuomilehto J. For the Diabetes Mondiale (DiaMond) Project Group. Incidence of childhood type 1 diabetes worldwide. *Diabetes Care* 2000; 23: 1516–26.
4. Barceló A, Rajpathak S. Incidence and prevalence of diabetes mellitus in the Americas. *Pan Am J Public Health,* 2001; 10: 300–8.
5. King H, Aubert RE, Herman WH. Global burden of diabetes, 1995–2025. Prevalence, numerical estimates, and projections. *Diabetes Care* 1998; 21: 1414–31.
6. Pan American Health Organization (PAHO/OPS). *Selected Demographic Indicators by Subregion of the Americas, 1980 and 2000*. Available at: http://www.paho.org/English/SHA/subindb98dm.htm.
7. Zimmet PZ, Alberti KGMM. The changing face of macrovascular disease in non-insulin-dependent diabetes mellitus: an epidemic in progress. *Lancet* 1997; 350: 1–17.
8. Pérez-Bravo F, Carrasco E, Santos JL, Calvillén M, Larenas G, Albala C. Prevalence of type 2 diabetes and obesity in rural Mapuche population from Chile. *Nutrition* 2001; 17: 305–9.
9. Larenas G, Arias G, Espinosa O, Charles M, Lan-Daeta O, Villanueva S, Espinoza A. Prevalencia de diabetes mellitus en una comunidad mapuche de la IX Región, Chile. *Rev Méd Chile* 1985; 113: 1121–5.
10. Albala C, Vio F, Kain J, Uauy R. Nutrition transition in Latin America: the case of Chile. *Nutr Rev* 2001; 59: 170–6.
11. Barceló A, Daroca MC, Ribera R, Duarte E, Zapata A, Vohra M. Diabetes in Bolivia. *Pan Am J Public Health* 2001; 10: 318–23.
12. Björntorp P, Holm G, Rosmond R. Hypothalamic arousal, insulin resistance and type 2 diabetes mellitus. *Diabet Med* 1999; 16: 373–83.
13. Hales CN, Barker DJP. Type 2 (non-insulin-dependent) diabetes mellitus: the thrifty phenotype hypothesis. *Diabetologia* 1992; 35: 595–601.
14. Hattersley AT, Tooke JE. The fetal insulin hypothesis: an alternative explanation of the association of low birthweight with diabetes and vascular disease. *Lancet* 1999; 353: 1789–92.
15. Fleury S, Belmartino S, Baris E. *Reshaping Health Care in Latin America: A Comparative Analysis of Health Care Reform in Argentina, Brazil, and Mexico*. Ottawa: International Development Research Centre, 2000.
16. Musgrove P. The economic crisis and its impact on health and health care in Latin America and the Caribbean. *Int J Health Serv* 1987; 17: 411–41.
17. Stocker K, Waitzkin H, Iriart C. The exportation of managed care to Latin America. *N Engl J Med* 1999; 340: 1131–6.
18. *Investing in Health*. World Development Report 1993. World Bank: Washington, 1993.
19. PAHO/OPS. *Las condiciones de salud en las Américas*. Washington: PAHO/OPS, 1994.
20. PAHO/OPS, 1999.
21. *The Economist Pocket World in Figures*, 2001 edn. London: Profile Books Ltd., 2001.
22. Aschner P, Cañete F. Implementing National Diabetes Programmes in Latin America. *Diabetes Voice* 2001; 46: 6–10.
23. Rubin JR, Altman WM, Mendelson DN. Health care expenditures for people with diabetes mellitus. *J Clin Endocrinol Metab* 1994; 78: 809A–F.
24. Ray NE, Wills S, Thamer M, et al. *Direct and Indirect Costs of Diabetes in the United States in 1992*. Alexandria, VA: American Diabetes Association, 1993.
25. Gagliardino JJ, Olivera EM. Diabetes mellitus: Un problema de salud pública en América Latina. *Rev Asoc Lat Ame Diabetes* 1997; 5: 124–34.
26. White F, Vega J, Aedo C, Jadue L, Robles S, Salazar R. *Proyecto de demostración en educación en diabetes*. Informe final Washington: PAHO/OPS, 1998.
27. Alberti KGMM. Insulin-dependent diabetes mellitus: a lethal disease in the developing world. *BMJ* 1994; 309: 754–5.
28. Jervell J. Variations in utilization and cost of insulin. *IDF Bull* 1996; 41: 1–2.
29. Gagliardino JJ, de la Hera M, Siri F, and Grupo de Investigación de la red QUALIDIAB. Evaluación de la calidad de la asistencia al paciente diabético en América Latina. *Pan Am J Public Health* 2001; 10: 309–17.
30. Gagliardino JJ, Etchegoyen G, for the PEDNID-LA Research Group. A model educational program for people with type 2 diabetes. *Diabetes Care* 2001; 24: 1001–7.
31. PAHO/WHO. *Declaration of the Americas on Diabetes*. Washington: PAHO/WHO, 1996.
32. Assal JP, Muhlhauser I, Pernet A, Gfeller R, Jörgens V, Berger M. Patient education as the basis for diabetes care in clinical practice and research. *Diabetologia* 1985; 28: 602–13.
33. Borch-Johnsen K, Kreiner S, Deckert T. Diabetic nephropathy—susceptible to care? A cohort-study of 641 patients with type 1 (insulin-dependent) diabetes. *Diabetes Res* 1986; 3: 397–400.
34. Clark CM Jr. What we can learn from Argentina? [editorial]. *Diabetes Care* 2000; 23: 1721–2.
35. Barbosa RB, Barceló A, Machado CA. Campanha nacional de detecçao de casos suspeitos de diabetes mellitus no Brasil: relatório preliminar. *Pan Am J Public Health* 2001; 10: 324–7.

107

Organization of Care: Diabetes Community Programs

Warren Lee

KK Women's and Children's Hospital, Singapore

INTRODUCTION

Diabetes care must be available, affordable, and accessible, and must be the best we can provide. There is no one ideal model for the organization of care for people with diabetes mellitus. However, there is always room for improvement in the way we organize, supervise, and deliver this care, no matter how complex or rudimentary the existing health care services [1, 2]. Process and outcomes audits run at the local, regional, national, or international level can help benchmark care standards and identify problem areas [3, 4]. Stakeholder-led efforts to reorganize care and resource utilization, adoption of alternative care models such as rural health worker, nurse, or family practitoner led shared care, automatic patient recall systems and national diabetes associations with bulk buying will lead to measurable improvements in the way we provide care to people affected by diabetes.

The various models of health care delivery have developed in the context of local resource limitations and local needs. All too often, what has developed is only available to a few, especially in the more urbanized areas, or those who have health care insurance [5], leaving the poor and the ignorant and those living in remote communities less than ideally served. Political, societal, and commercial considerations also come into the equation. Governments prioritize and consider what they can afford in terms of health care. There is an ongoing debate about whether communicable diseases or noncommunicable diseases should receive priority. Sometimes the stark reality is that if all those with diabetes in a country were to be diagnosed and wish to have treatment, there would neither be the money nor the human resources available to treat them properly. People affected by diabetes are often from minority or disadvantaged groups and it may be a challenge to persuade them to come forward to receive care even when resources are available.

In view of the enormous economic burden of diabetes, preventive strategies for diabetes and other noncommunicable diseases must therefore be integral to any organized care for people with, or at risk of, diabetes.

WHAT IS REQUIRED?

Diabetes requires that the individual with diabetes first of all know that he or she is at risk, that he or she has the opportunity to be diagnosed, and if diagnosed, then has access to a recognized process of care, and then the ability and motivation to benefit from this process of care. Finally, the person with diabetes needs to know how, when, and why of the importance of good diabetes control and the prevention, early detection, and treatment of complications. The person with diabetes needs to know his or her options regarding aiming for intensity of care, drugs, and procedures. This includes the opportunity to learn about self-care, about diabetic complications and their prevention, and also to be screened for complications on a regular basis. The individual with diabetes should be encouraged and enabled to achieve the best HbA_{1c} possible through judicious use of drugs and lifestyle adjustments.

Despite the vast socioeconomic differences that exist in many societies, we must aim to organize the delivery of care, so that of those who are diagnosed, more might

International Textbook of Diabetes Mellitus, Third Edition. Edited by R. A. DeFronzo, E. Ferrannini, H. Keen, and P. Zimmet.
 ISBN: 0-471-48655-8.

receive the recognized process of care and actually attain their treatment goals.

There are several components of care:

(1) Community efforts to raise awareness of the disease and primary prevention efforts
(2) Opportunities to be screened, tested, and diagnosed
(3) Prescription of appropriate medication by a health care worker
(4) Education about the disease process and potential complications
(5) Teaching of self-care skills, including home blood glucose monitoring
(6) Education about lifestyle change, including dietary choices and exercise
(7) Complications screening
(8) Motivational support from caregivers, family, and friends

CONSIDERATIONS IN ORGANIZING CARE

In considering how we organize care, we need to consider the following:

(1) What is the size of the problem?
(2) Who is paying for the care?
(3) Who is available to deliver the care?
(4) What are critical issues impacting on our ability to deliver better care?
(5) How can we mobilize resources to address the critical issue?
(6) How can we sustain positive change?
(7) How can we emplace a self-sustaining cycle of continuous improvements in the way we organize the delivery of good diabetes care?

What Is the Size of the Problem?

Basic epidemiological knowledge about how many people are affected and the profile of those affected will help in planning prevention and screening programs, projecting needs and sourcing for resources. Audit studies will help demonstrate whether we are doing what we know we should be doing among those patients we already know and treat, and help the organization take corrective action [5]. Audit studies can target the process of care (i.e., did all patients get their HbA_{1c} at least once in a year?) or the outcomes of care (e.g., the mean HbA_{1c} levels in clinic patients). Audits can also give useful information about economics (e.g., lower limb amputation rates in clinic defaulters).

Audits can be done simply even by students or clinic assistants using paper forms or very sophisticated patient information management systems. The issue is that we should gather, review, and try to use this information to improve the way we organize and deliver care. Studies such as the DIABCARE Q-NET project [3] and the Diabcare Asia project have helped physicians and governments focus on identified needs with relevant data and helped to improve fundamental issues such as the recording of serial visits and medical notes in some countries [6]. How is care paid for?

Who Is Paying for the Care?

Where individuals pay for their own care, the limiting factor is often what the patient can afford [5]. Yet the problem may really be that the patient or his third-party payer is not prepared to pay because he does not see the need or the benefit of choosing to pay for needed interventions.

Who Is Available to Provide the Care?

It has often been emphasized that diabetes mellitus requires a team-based multidisciplinary approach. Yet often what is available to the patient is the lone medical practitioner and his practice nurse or auxillary health worker. Providing externally subsidized services may seem to address the immediate needs. It would be better for the care to be made more affordable, perhaps by using a cheaper but cost-effective alternative such as practice nurses health auxillaries, trained volunteers, patient support groups, or paramedical teams following established protocols and clear intervention plans.

PREVENTION STRATEGIES

Primary prevention for diabetes mellitus includes getting across concepts of healthy eating, sufficient exercise, and avoidance of smoking, stressful lifestyles, hypertension, and obesity [7, 8]. People must have knowledge, change their attitudes, and change their personal practices. Careful thought must be given to whether an upbeat, optimistic message or a dire warning type message will succeed in the local community. Demonstration projects involving local champions and community groups can lead the way, and may not cost much to implement. If they are successful, they may then be used to persuade government agencies to fund similar projects elsewhere. Public perceptions of diabetes may affect personal choices [9]. It is important to pitch public education programs with regard to local customs and sensitivities.

With tongue-in-cheek, I would offer the following analogy of diabetes care as a consumer item:

If too *expensive*, few will think they can afford it
If too *cheap*, no one wants it
If it is seen as a must have or a status symbol, people will find ways and means to get it
If it is seen as offering a competitive advantage to the buyer, likewise it will be more marketable

If it is seen as an area of meritorious public service, people will come forward to give of time and resource
Price it right to succeed
Pitch it right for people to buy

PRIMARY PREVENTION AND COMMUNITY EFFORTS

Increasing evidence points to exercise, lifestyle modification, and weight loss as effective measures to prevent the progression of impaired glucose tolerance to diabetes [7, 8]. National diabetes associations have traditionally been involved in screening for and helping people with diabetes, rather than in primary prevention. While national diabetes associations and professional bodies can lead efforts to educate the community about diabetes awareness, it often requires governments to lead by providing appropriate resources. Demonstration projects are useful in providing the evidence base for mass efforts, but nationwide campaigns bring together mass media, local government, health care providers, and patient support groups.

Preventive strategies are often decided at governmental level but implementation may be left to local authorities. In many countries, preventive strategies for diabetes mellitus are often linked to those of other noncommunicable diseases since they share the same risk factors such as obesity, inactivity, and smoking.

It is important to ensure that early detection strategies are included in such programs, especially to take into account new groups of at-risk individuals. Childhood obesity is increasingly linked to young-onset type 2 diabetes mellitus and early-onset impaired glucose tolerance [10, 11]. The schools are therefore a key organization for spreading the message about prevention of diabetes.

THE ROLE OF NATIONAL GUIDELINES AND BEST PRACTICE GUIDES

Numerous national guidelines and best practice models have been written and published. The most common criticism is that they often do little to change provider behavior. Reasons for this include a lack of resources to implement change, a resistance to change, or ignorance of the true state of affairs [5, 12].

National guidelines are useful however in the following circumstances:

(1) When isolated practitioners want and need a recognized standard of best practice, which they are willing to provide to the patients who can afford the best and are willing to pay;
(2) When guidelines include the recommendation of acceptable lower cost alternatives to best practice, in recognition of the fact that not everyone can afford the best;
(3) When guidelines are used as a benchmark for in-house or multicenter audit studies, so that the results of such studies can be used as a stimulus for change;
(4) When such guidelines are put in the hands of consumers, to inform them of the best practice available and to allow consumers themselves to press for the best possible care under the circumstances prevailing;
(5) When such guidelines are used by governments and health care provider organizations as benchmarks upon which to reorganize care and reprogram resources and as justification to fight for resources to provide recognized standards of care.

HOW MUCH INFORMATION SHOULD BE MADE AVAILABLE TO PEOPLE WITH DIABETES?

Well-informed consumer organizations can work with providers of care to provide low cost acceptable alternatives for the poorer segments of the population who might otherwise receive no care at all. Prevention strategies, whether primordial, primary, or secondary, also work better when the target population is well aware of health issues, and the concept of self-help and taking responsibility for one's own health prevails in the community [13].

It is important for the patient to have full access to reliable Web sites, and to be open in discussions about availability and feasibility of new interventions. It is also important to have frank discussions about the level of care that can be attained with the patient's level of commitment to self-management of his or her own condtion and to the economic realities at hand.

SCREENING FOR DIABETES AND IMPAIRED GLUCOSE TOLERANCE

Impaired glucose tolerance is now known to be independently associated with significant morbidity besides being a major risk factor for diabetes mellitus, thus posing a new challenge to health care systems already struggling to deal with large numbers of undiagnosed or undertreated people with diabetes. Many countries have opted for primary prevention strategies and healthy lifestyle campaigns to address this problem in the context of larger program for prevention of noncommunicable disease.

The new World Health Organization (WHO) and American Diabetes Association (ADA) criteria for diabetes, one being based on the results of the 75-g glucose tolerance test and the other on fasting blood sugars, will have major impact on the way we organize care. Subjects with impaired glucose tolerance but normal fasting plasma glucose are at greater risk of coronary heart disease. The new ADA definition fails to identify substantial numbers of such subjects, particularly among South Asians [14]. In countries where it is known that the 2-h postprandial glucose test will be needed to identify a large part of the population with diabetes and impaired glucose tolerance compared to just the fasting glucose criteria, decisions need to be made to either target all, or some of those at risk of postprandial hyperglycemia. Consideration will have to be made to organize oral glucose tolerance testing for high-risk individuals and their families.

BUSINESS MODELS IN PROVIDING CARE

Various evidence-based diabetes guidelines and best practice models abound, but it is often acknowledged that they do not always result in a change in behavior on the part of the doctor or caregiver. What are the reasons for this sorry situation? Leaving aside ignorance and resistance to change, there are good reasons why practitioners find the going difficult. Patients may forget because they do not realize the importance of the annual eye examination. A simple reminder letter may work well to improve compliance [13]. Diabetes education is also often left to the attending doctor. However, the doctor is often not remunerated according to the quality of the education given, but to episodes of care.

Some countries have adopted an annual diabetes check episode where the primary care practitioner is paid at a higher reimbursement rate than a normal general practitioner visit in order to partially redress the imbalance. Many countries have introduced practice nurses who take over the diabetes education and maintain a specialized register of diabetes patients, making it easier to keep track of and recall patients and also keep in touch with them regularly [15]. Some centers use internet-based interactive methodologies to keep in touch with their patients. Tertiary institutions have also used computerized medical records and staff with dedicated job descriptions to recall patients referred for diabetes complications. These interventions have generally proved successful [1, 16].

DIABETES OUTREACH CENTERS

The physician should ideally be part of a multidisciplinary team at a diabetes center that includes ophthalmic, podiatric, dietetic, and nursing expertise, with on-site measurement of glycosylated HbA_{1c}, fasting lipids, microalbuminuria and proteinuria, urine or serum ketones, and blood sugar levels, and a computerized database and recall system. However, this is not always possible.

One cost-effective solution to the problem of providing ophthalmic expertise is to use a fundal camera using ordinary film, polaroid process film, or digital photos that will be read by trained personnel at a remote site. This would reduce the cost and waiting time for a full ophthalmic examination, as ophthalmologists are often only available in urban centers.

Another solution adopted by countries like Singapore is to place trained diabetes nurse educators in government polyclinics. A nurse educator can be taught the basics of prescribing a healthy diet for people with diabetes, leaving specialized advice for people with diabetic nephropathy to trained dietitians, for example. Similarly, a nurse educator trained to examine a foot for signs of venous occlusion, arterial inadequacy, ulcers or ulcer-prone areas, nail hygeine, bunions or abnormal weight bearing patterns could triage patients for onward referral to the podiatrist or orthopedic surgeon. In some centers, the diabetes educator is the person who will actually do the on-site blood tests such as the HbA_{1c}. In addition, diabetes educators could help patients learn self-adjustment of insulin regimes, and also teach the use of insulin pumps.

The nurse educator or practice nurse could in addition help to run a database that will allow for timely reminders for annual complications reviews, identify defaulters, and track process and outcomes measures. These organizational processes will in turn impact greatly on the quality of care actually delivered.

Individuals with diabetes are encouraged to join support groups affiliated to these clinics. Low-cost blood glucose meters and blood glucose testing strips are made available, but costs have to be borne by the patient. Costs are kept low by generous government subsidies. Referral to dietitians, podiatrists, ophthalmologists, diabetologists, and other specialists in hospitals and tertiary centers are made by polyclinic doctors in conjunction with the nurse educators.

To address the issue of private practitioners not wanting to lose patients to the heavily subsidized government polyclinics, the local Diabetic Society of Singapore runs outreach clinics with similar facilities, but with one important difference. This is because the outreach clinic nurse acts as the agent of the patient's primary physician and results of tests and decisions for onward referral. The national association also runs support groups for individuals and families of those with diabetes. These outreach centers have the added advantage of allowing a hybrid cost structure, in that the private sector primary care practitioner is able to charge his commercial fee for service, but at the same time tap on the highly subsidized outreach center to provide the other components of care at a low cost to his patient.

REGISTRIES, DATABASES, AND CLINICAL INFORMATION SYSTEMS

Health care providers and diabetes care teams should ensure that there is comprehensive population-based diabetes register (either manual or computerized) that includes the names of all the target population (e.g. young or elderly people with diabetes) within a particular area or region. Regular register reviews and audits will assist in the evaluation of standards, assessment of outcome and to identify young people who default and thus help to ensure their consistent support and surveillance (ISPAD Guidelines on Paediatric Diabetes). In recent years there has been a move to put patient information on Web-based information systems. Different patterns of information security and privacy exist, including systems where the national health care authorities authorize physician access to a shared database of clinical data and other "double lock and key" commercial systems where the patient's information is posted on a secure website, and the patient agrees to allow the caregiver access to his information when both patient and physician supply the appropriate passwords. No matter whether the database is paper based or electronic, it is a powerful tool for better organisation of care and allocation of resources if properly managed.

Recently, there has been a proliferation of home blood glucose monitoring equipment and continuous glucose monitoring devices that can download data and allow computer-aided analysis of blood glucose data. Insulin pumps can also download data on dosages, times of administration, and total amount of insulin administered. Diabetes care teams need to know how to make use of this technology to work with patients as a team.

CARE OF CHILDREN AND ADOLESCENTS

Children and adolescents with diabetes should have access to age-appropriate support, care, and education in diabetes, with the aim of enhancing self-management as they grow up. Diabetes education will have to be repeated and reinforced as their capacity for understanding and acceptance increases. There should be provision for 24-h advice from a resource person (doctor, nurse, or educator) and written or electronic information and guidelines on the management of the different phases of diabetes in childhood and adolescence in the local language, and preferably multilingual staff and indigenous health workers.

Diabetes education is key to successful management of diabetes at all ages. It needs to be structured, patient-centered, and appropriate to the level of maturity and understanding of the patient and family (ISPAD guidelines, 2000). A written protocol detailing specific items to be covered before discharge from hospital is essential, as well as a check-off system to ensure that protocols are followed, especially when multiple staff share in the task of covering individual topics. In areas where diabetes occurs rarely, the numbers of children with diabetes will be small, a locally based pediatrician/physician who should have easy access to facilities, advice and the possibility of annual review by the diabetes care team based in the regional center of excellence.

CRISIS AND EMERGENCY MANAGEMENT

Centers that potentially will admit patients with diabetic ketoacidosis must have a written protocol for management of diabetic ketoacidosis and an admissions policy for diabetes patients. A resource person should be clearly identified, who can give regular updates for rotating staff, e.g. new residents, on management of diabetic ketoacidosis, and who can be contacted for advice whenever a child with diabetes is admitted. Ideally, diabetic ketoacidosis should be managed in a specialized children's inpatient facility, e.g. high dependency area or ICU where expertise can be concentrated, especially where diabetes is relatively rare.

REFERENCES

1. Renders CM, Valk GD, Griffin S, Wagner EH, Eijk JT, Assendelft WJ. Interventions to improve the management of diabetes mellitus in primary care, outpatient and community settings. *Cochrane Database Syst Rev* 2001; 1: CD001481.
2. Day JL, Humphreys H, Alban-Davies H. Problems of comprehensive shared diabetes care. *Br Med J (Clin Res Ed)* 1987; 294 (6587): 1590–2.
3. Piwernetz K. DIABCARE Quality Network in Europe—a model for quality management in chronic diseases. *Int Clin Psychopharmacol* 2001; 16 (suppl 3): S5–13.
4. Tabak AG, Tamas G, Zgibor J, Wilson R, Becker D, Kerenyi Z, Orchard TJ. Targets and reality: a comparison of health care indicators in the U.S. (Pittsburgh Epidemiology of Diabetes Complications Study) and Hungary (DiabCare Hungary). *Diabetes Care* 2000; 23 (9): 1284–9.
5. Saaddine JB, Engelgau MM, Beckles GL, Gregg EW, Thompson TJ, Narayan KM. A diabetes report card for the United States: quality of care in the 1990s. *Ann Intern Med* 2002; 136 (8): 565–74.
6. Lee WR, Lim HS, Thai AC, Chew WL, Emmanuel S, Goh LG, Lau HC, Lee CH, Soon PC, Tambyah JA, Tan YT, Jorgensen LN, Chua A, Yeo JP. A window on the current status of diabetes mellitus in Singapore—the Diabcare-Singapore 1998 study. *Singapore Med J* 2001; 42 (11): 501–7.
7. Tuomilehto J, Lindstrom J, Eriksson JG, Valle TT, Hamalainen H, Ilanne-Parikka P, Keinanen-Kiukaanniemi S, Laakso M, Louheranta A, Rastas M, Salminen V, Uusitupa M. Prevention of type 2 diabetes mellitus by changes in lifestyle among subjects with impaired glucose tolerance. *N Engl J Med* 2001; 344 (18): 1343–50.
8. Pan XR, Li GW, Hu YH, Wang JX, Yang WY, An ZX, Hu ZX, Lin J, Xiao JZ, Cao HB, Liu PA, Jiang XG, Jiang YY, Wang JP, Zheng H, Zhang H, Bennett PH, Howard BV. Effects of diet and exercise in preventing NIDDM in people with impaired glucose tolerance: the Da Qing IGT and Diabetes Study. *Diabetes Care* 1997; 20 (4): 537–44.
9. Muhlhauser I, Overmann H, Bender R, Bott U, Jorgens V, Trautner C, Siegrist J, Berger M. Social status and the

quality of care for adult people with type I (insulin-dependent) diabetes mellitus—a population-based study. *Diabetologia* 1998; 41 (10): 1139–50.
10. Sinha R, Fisch G, Teague B, Tamborlane WV, Banyas B, Allen K, Savoye M, Rieger V, Taksali S, Barbetta G, Sherwin RS, Caprio S. Prevalence of impaired glucose tolerance among children and adolescents with marked obesity. *N Engl J Med* 2002; 346 (11): 802–10.
11. Rosenbloom AL, Joe JR, Young RS, Winter WE. Emerging epidemic of type 2 diabetes in youth. *Diabetes Care* 1999; 22 (2): 345–54.
12. Delorme C, Boisjoly HM, Baillargeon L, Turcotte P, Bernard PM. Screening for diabetic retinopathy. Do family physicians know the Canadian guidelines? *Can Fam Phys* 1998; 44: 1473–9.
13. Legorreta AP, Hasan MM, Peters AL, Pelletier KR, Leung KM. An intervention for enhancing compliance with screening recommendations for diabetic retinopathy. A bicoastal experience. *Diabetes Care* 1997; 20 (4): 520–3.
14. Harris TJ, Cook DG, Wicks PD, Cappuccio FP. Impact of the new American Diabetes Association and World Health Organisation diagnostic criteria for diabetes on subjects from three ethnic groups living in the UK. *Nutr Metab Cardiovasc Dis* 2000; 10 (6): 305–9.
15. Pierce M, Agarwal G. Ridout D. A survey of diabetes care in general practice in England and Wales. *Br J Gen Pract* 2000; 50 (456): 542–5.
16. MacKinnon MM, Wilson RM, Hardisty CA, Ward JD. Novel role for specialist nurses in managing diabetes in the community. *BMJ* 1989; 299 (6698): 552–4.

108

Life with Diabetes Problems: Human and Social Rights

M. Massi Benedetti*, **G. Calabrese***, **M. Orsini Federici***, **J. Akwe***, **and A. Cesarini†**

**University of Perugia, Perugia, Italy, and †"Pretura Circondariale" of Perugia, Italy*

DEFINITION OF SOCIAL RIGHTS

Within the legal system of every country a cluster of rules exists to regulate issues of social importance. Considered as a whole, they define the social structure of a country which is codified by the lawmakers in order to fulfill the most widespread and prevalent expectations of that society with regard to both public and private activities. Such expectations are raised by individuals (either as single citizens or as groups or categories), and the scope of the related laws is to guarantee the utmost satisfaction of primary needs of people in the various phases of their life cycle and in different environments (family, education, free time, work activities, etc.).

In this context those conditions whose protection is to be considered a top priority are selected; this process identifies a series of rights, defined as "social rights," that have in common their social relevance and are legally homogeneous.

In modern societies, social rights are becoming an issue of increasing importance, and their systematic classification is being attempted in order to produce guidelines for those initiatives whose aim is a continuous improvement and widening of social equity.

IDENTIFICATION OF SOCIAL RIGHTS

To identify and categorize social rights, one must consider that the various situations that are regulated, and attain the ranking of rights (social rights), are characterized by an extremely wide variety of contents, as they reflect many aspects of individual and collective life. Moreover, their content may vary and be affected by the local environment, and by customs and traditions of the particular population and its current condition. Nevertheless, it is possible to identify aspects that are constant because of the universality of some fundamental social needs, and consequently an overall approach to this topic is feasible.

Without being exhaustive, the following major issues can be identified, bearing in mind that each of them could be further subdivided:

(1) Life expectations (birth, survival, physical autonomy, etc.)
(2) Expectations related to the family
(3) Expectations related to education and work
(4) Expectations related to leisure time
(5) Expectations related to the best exploitation of individual resources
(6) Expectations related to equal opportunities for everyone regarding all possible life events

It is the responsibility of the lawmaker to transform such expectations into rights using adequate technical instruments that transfer ethical concepts into the legal system and through it into daily life.

Several conditions related to health could lead to an impairment of social rights; illness that create disability expose individuals to a higher risk of having their rights reduced. The Disability Rights Task Force of the British Government reported in 1999 that disabled people had a double unemployment rate than nondisabled ones and were seven times more likely to be out of work and to claim benefits. Moreover, half of the disabled people had difficulties in accessing goods and services [1].

International Textbook of Diabetes Mellitus, Third Edition. Edited by R. A. DeFronzo, E. Ferrannini, H. Keen, and P. Zimmet.
 ISBN: 0-471-48655-8.

RELATIONSHIP BETWEEN DIABETES AND SOCIAL RIGHTS

Diabetes mellitus can be considered a paradigmatic social disease because of the large number of people affected, the chronic course, the highly disabling late complications, and the consequent high cost for the community [2–4]. For these reasons diabetes is a strong negative factor in regard to the individual social rights [1]. The 1973 Federal Rehabilitation Act of the US Government defined diabetes as a "handicap," resulting in the exclusion of qualified workers from a number of jobs [5]. However, the concept of diabetes as a disability is not widely accepted and is still an argument for strong debate. A recent statement of the Canadian Diabetes Association provides a balanced interpretation of the problem. It is stated that diabetes *per se* does not constitute a disability; the characterization of disability has to be done on an individual basis according to individual conditions with respect to a specific context. However, in the framework of the laws related to human rights, diabetes represents a disability and is protected against any kind of discrimination [6].

It is known that diabetes if not appropriately treated can interfere with life expectancy, with procreation, with the autonomy of the affected subjects, and, as a consequence, with family life. Furthermore, diabetes can largely condition the affected subject in various aspects of his/her life, often making it difficult to reach individual targets in the fields of education and work, where discrimination may produce irreversible effects, frustrating expectations of full development of personal resources [7–12].

In their daily life people with diabetes must cope with the difficulties of dealing with a society that is structured in principle and at every level to satisfy healthy subjects. Also, diabetes in the older generation is becoming increasingly burdensome and socially demanding: the health care system is asked to provide medical and psychological support to a category of patients which is continuously increasing because of the progressive aging of the general population [13, 14].

RELATIONSHIP BETWEEN ENVIRONMENT AND SOCIAL RIGHTS OF PEOPLE WITH DIABETES

When dealing with the relationship between diabetes and social rights it is necessary to consider carefully the impact of variable environmental conditions existing in different geographical areas and the characteristics of subpopulations in the same society [14–16]. Indeed, in many countries, knowledge, materials, tools, technologies, and support to treat diabetes and its complications are available, while in other countries these are not available or affordable [17, 18].

Let us consider the example of survival. Before the discovery of insulin, type 1 diabetes was characterized everywhere by early death. Subsequently, the availability of insulin demonstrated a clear-cut difference between richer and poorer countries. In the richer countries efforts in diabetes care are now focused on the achievement of near-normal metabolic control using sophisticated insulins, intensified insulin regimens, and adequate diets [19]. In the poorer countries shortage of therapeutic drugs and of food makes tight metabolic control an inappropriate and unattainable target, the real goal being the survival of the diabetic subject. In other regions, because of the shortage of resources, unfavorable environmental conditions, and characteristics of the population, the insulin era has not even started [17, 20]. So while ketoacidosis in industrialized countries rarely causes death in type 1 diabetes, the average survival after diagnosis, in some poor countries as in many African nations, is around 1 year. In the late 1990s the World Bank recognized 40 highly indebted underdeveloped countries that could not sustain the expenses for insulin therapy as the debt repayment overcame the available resources. Moreover, the cost for one year's insulin therapy for one patient corresponds to the cost of lifesaving chloroquine or antibiotic therapy for 75 individuals [21]. However, the problem of regular access to insulin and diabetes care in general is an issue not only in the poorest countries, but can also be present in more developed and industrialized ones. While in the developing countries the lack of insulin in general is the primary problem, differences of health care also exist in developing and industrialized countries. In these cases, differences are related to racial, ethnic, or socioeconomic disparities. A survey conducted in Egypt demonstrated that acute and chronic diabetic complications are more frequent among uninsured children than among the insured ones [22]. Musey et al. demonstrated that in urban African Americans living in Atlanta, USA, the commonest cause of ketoacidosis was the cessation of insulin therapy due to lack of money for insulin purchase or specialist care [23]. In 1999 the Third US National Health and Nutrition Examination Survey confirmed the racial and ethnic differences in quality of care received. In fact, it was demonstrated that among a multiethnic population with type 2 diabetes non-Hispanic Black women and Mexican American men constituted the majority of the group with poorest metabolic control, exposing them at a higher risk of complications [24]. The analysis of the London cohort of the World Health Organization (WHO) multinational study of vascular disease in diabetes showed a clear relationship between socioeconomic gradient and all causes of mortality according to the higher prevalence of common risk factors in the poorest classes [25]. A recent survey conducted in France in 1999 regarding the quality of care and the quality of metabolic control in children with type 1 diabetes evidenced a better control in those who were followed by university-affiliated hospitals or by centers following more than 50 children. In this case the disparity was created by the possibility to access to highly specialized structures [26].

In the case of procreation also, there are wide differences between populations relating to socioeconomic opportunities in different countries. In some countries the struggle for survival in the absence of insulin supply does not even allow young people with type 1 diabetes to reach the age of fertility, ruling out the most basic of rights. In other places the impossibility of achieving reasonable metabolic control, because of a large variety of environmental factors, produces infertility and severe disturbance of sexual life. In favorable environments diabetic individuals can experience a normal sexual life and near-normal procreation, but also in this case different groups of the same population can experience different levels of welfare [27–33].

Nutrition is a further field of difference: in some countries people with diabetes suffer relative or absolute shortage of food, while in others they have to cope with risks related to excessive food intake [34, 35]. The basic right of having regular access to food and to lifesaving drugs can also be denied in those countries in which it is usually guaranteed, in the event of natural calamities or conflicts, when the rights of the weakest sections of the population are likely to be given low priority [36]. On the other hand, it is true that some problems that are equally distributed among people with diabetes throughout the world, nevertheless, require different medical approaches in different environments and cultures [37–40].

It is evident, therefore, that although the ultimate aim worldwide is for all diabetic subjects to lead a near-normal life, it is necessary to set realistic targets for the care of people with diabetes, taking into account the socioeconomic and political situation of each country. Issues relevant in certain areas [41] are unrealistic in others. This concept cannot be disregarded by those who set the rules to guarantee social rights of a well-defined population [42].

At present lawmakers in various countries have mostly considered issues like employment, driving licence, and insurance, in order to protect the diabetic citizen, but even in these selected areas the approach has depended on the dominant culture in each environment and the local medical, social, and legal circumstances.

WORKING ACTIVITY—EMPLOYMENT

The possibility that people with diabetes have fewer opportunities than healthy people in finding their first employment has been documented [43–45]. This handicap may vary according to the level of education received, to the overall environmental economic conditions, and to other factors, but in fact it affects all people with diabetes.

It is also more difficult for diabetic employees to maintain their employment [46] than for nondiabetic employees, and discrimination can be more evident in periods of economic crisis inducing cuts in staffing [47]. Moreover, unduly negative evaluation of the diabetic employee, shared by employer and colleagues, is based on unscientific medical assumptions and on the erroneous opinion derived from widespread prejudice that employees with diabetes are unreliable and inefficient in their working performance [48].

Classifying the individual with diabetes as handicapped automatically results in discrimination and undervaluation of his working capacity. In 1984 the American Diabetes Association (ADA) stated that "any person with diabetes, whether insulin dependent or not, should be eligible for any employment for which he/she is otherwise qualified." Even if many actions were taken in that direction over the years, diabetes still represents a discriminatory factor for employment. The principal reason for this is justified by the fear that people with diabetes in working places could represent a safety risk [49], while an even stronger reason, although not clearly declared, is represented by the erroneous belief that a person with diabetes might have a reduced productivity.

This attitude can be reinforced by the fact that some activities should be avoided by people with diabetes [47, 50, 51]. The Disability Discrimination Act (DDA) in 1995 introduced new rules regarding the exclusion from specific jobs. Even though it was intended to avoid major limitations, a list of occupations that can refuse disabled people was identified. This list comprises the prison service, the armed forces, the fire service, the police service, work on board a ship, hovercraft, or aircraft [52]. The problem arising in such context is whether diabetes *per se* can be considered a disability or under which particular circumstances diabetes can be considered a disability. The ADA gives three criteria for disability: (1) an individual who has physical or mental impairment that substantially limits one or more major life activities, (2) someone who has a record of such an impairment, and (3) someone who is regarded as having such an impairment [53]. In that view the majority of people with diabetes cannot be considered as disabled and no discrimination should be applied to them. Problems could arise in case of poor metabolic control or in the presence of complications. The suggestion is that people with diabetes in these conditions should not attend work on dangerous areas but the relative decision should depend on the evaluation of the individual cases and should not be left to the employer's discretion [53]. People with diabetes when starting a new job can or cannot declare their diabetic conditions; in case they declare their condition they will be covered by the DDA, otherwise they will not necessarily be covered by this act. Declaring the diabetes status means that workers with diabetes could ask for specific advantages as extra rest times for glucose measurements or reasonable accommodation in order to permit them to work without undue hardship [53]. The DDA also defined a list of works that are not covered by the Act for people with diabetes. The following jobs are completely banned for people with diabetes treated with insulin: airline pilot, truck, or bus driver, working offshore regardless of the type of job, train driver. Other jobs permit people with diabetes to continue to work after the diagnosis of diabetes: armed forces, police and fire service, some airline crew. As a consequence it is relevant to define clearly the circumstances under which the worker with diabetes (or applicant) can experience equal opportunities with respect to workers nonaffected by diabetes. This possibility is obviously true for people with diabetes in good control; and this concept should be included in the legal system of each country as a general rule in the evaluation of a subject with diabetes, and not just in relation to one specific sector of activity [43]. The same general principle should be used by the law whenever it is considering the legitimacy of specific actions violating the right of the subject with diabetes in the field of working activity [47]. Furthermore, the right of the worker with diabetes to demonstrate his suitability for any type of employment, whether in the public or the private sector, in order to have equal chances of obtaining or maintaining a job, should be guaranteed [43].

Recently Chu et al. have published the results of an economic analysis of the data coming from the 1989 National Health Interview Survey highlighting the still existing discrimination for people with diabetes. The presence of diabetes *per se* was associated with 3.5% reduction of employment level, and the presence of complications with 12% if compared with the absence of complications. Moreover, while the presence of noncomplicated diabetes does not increase the number of working days lost in respect to subjects without diabetes, the presence of complications implies 3.2 working days lost every 2 weeks more than the others. The reduction of productivity related to diabetes was correlated with a one-third reduction of yearly earnings (ranging from $3700 to $8700 per annum) in respect to people without diabetes [54]. Similar results were found in a study conducted in Canada on a global population of around 25 000 persons, of whom 608 had diabetes. People with diabetes complications are likely to have a 50% lower rate of employment than people without diabetes. People with diabetes without complications had the same income as that of people without diabetes, while the presence of complications decreases the yearly earning by about 30% [55]. Different results were found in a survey in Australia where the presence of diabetes did not affect the employment rate. Nevertheless, when asked directly, people with diabetes felt a sense of discrimination and were negative in respect to a possibility for future employment [56].

DRIVING LICENCE

The analysis of laws that regulate the issue of driving licences to people with diabetes indicates a wide variety of approaches in different countries and also clear contradictions within the same legislation. In some countries diabetes is not taken into specific consideration and the citizen has only to pass a general medical examination. In others the medical evaluation is more complete and diabetes is specifically considered, but even here, the problem is dealt with differently depending on a more or less advanced medical evaluation and on variable relationships between lawmakers and the medical and scientific institutions.

A lack of standardization from international bodies (medical and nonmedical) is particularly evident in this field, and action would be highly desirable. In fact, a large variety of limits have been set, and in most cases these are rather questionable and relate to the type of therapy (insulin/non-insulin) or to the type of vehicle (under or over a certain weight) or to the type of activity (private or public transport) [57–62]. In most countries, only certain categories of driving licence are issued to people with diabetes. In case of diet treatment alone there is no need to notify the diabetic status. The presence of therapy with tablets usually only requires a notification to the Driver and Vehicle Licensing Authorities, while the insulin therapy other than the notification implies the exclusion of people from certain licences: insulin-treated people are not allowed to hold large goods vehicles or passenger carrying vehicles, D1 category licence, and C1 licences [63]. The Australian law foresees a notification for all cases of diabetes, also for those on diet alone. The hiding of the diabetic status, in case of car accident caused by a person with diabetes, could abolish insurance coverage [64]. A large variability of regulations exists in this field also in areas that should present a certain level of homogeneity, like the European Union, and in certain cases differences exist also within countries. However, new trends start to diffuse, as indicated, as an example, by the revision done in 2001 by the Irish government that allows people with diabetes treated with insulin to drive large vans or small lorries. It should be emphasized that a higher occurrence of accidents caused by diabetic drivers has never been documented, while a series of studies indicate that no difference exists between drivers with diabetes and the general population [65–70].

It must also be noted that the right to be allowed to drive is very important in developed countries where earning capacity and social life in general are highly dependent on individual mobility, while it might be a lower priority in some developing countries on account of the lack of resources and infrastructure and the different lifestyles.

INSURANCE

The right of people with diabetes to obtain insurance at equitable rates, or even to obtain insurance at all, is still unsatisfied in most countries because of strong resistance from the insurance companies [71]. In most cases only lay patients' associations have raised this topic. What is really needed is a complex approach able to guarantee both the rights of people with diabetes and the institutional economic interests of the insurance companies [72]. The balance between these two opposite interests needs to be clearly regulated by specific rules that are necessarily different from country to country, depending on their economic structure. The general target of the rules should aim at restoring the individual contractual strength of subjects with diabetes in negotiations with the insurance companies; a periodic updating of these rules is also relevant, taking into account progressive improvements in the care of the disease [73].

In a survey conducted in 1994 in the United States, Harris et al. showed that 13.5% of people with diabetes were not covered by insurance; even if the percentage is modest the number of people involved is quite relevant because of the diffusion of the disease, and the impact on the health status of the involved individuals is highly unfavorable. Moreover racial and ethnic disparities also exist in regard to the insurance coverage of people with diabetes. In fact only 66% of the Mexican Americans had insurance coverage with respect to 91% of the non-Hispanic ones. [74].

To reduce the burden for people with diabetes several institutions created specific programs. The North Dakota Department of Health in 1999 generated the health insurance coverage for diabetes in the North Dakota Plan that allowed the same opportunities for people with diabetes to have insurance coverage and almost at the same conditions than individuals without diabetes [75]. In the year 2000 the Canadian Diabetes Association introduced a Credit Life insurance Plan for Canadians living with diabetes in conjunction with the AIG Life Insurance Company of Canada to help people with diabetes to have their rights to be life-insured recognized [76]. Similar initiatives have been successfully undertaken also in other countries like France, the Netherlands, and Denmark.

EXISTING RULES FOR THE PROTECTION OF SOCIAL RIGHTS OF PEOPLE WITH DIABETES

In many countries regulations have been set specifically for diabetes in order to orientate existing governmental health care policy. Within this framework diabetes is classified as a social disease, thereby providing the diabetic citizen with an overall protection of his rights, as they are guaranteed to all people affected by any social disease. Nevertheless, it seems reasonable that, because of the peculiarity of the problems related to diabetes regarding individual rights, more emphasis needs to be given within the legal system to this topic.

In some countries specific laws for diabetes have been or are being adopted. Examples can be cited from three states of the United States: in Texas, the possibility of coordinating and optimizing the available resources at individual and family level is contemplated by law; in Connecticut, specific laws related to the care of children with diabetes are foreseen; in Montana, the law approaches the issue of education. In Italy, a national law [77] defines guidelines for primary, secondary, and tertiary prevention in diabetes and for safeguarding the rights of the citizen with diabetes.

These laws are quite innovative from the judicial point of view, addressing more the individual than the collective aspects, but, unfortunately, their content is not always transferred into practice owing to lack of resources or to lack of awareness of the relevance of the problem among those responsible for implementing the laws.

A NEW PROPOSAL FOR THE SAFEGUARD OF SOCIAL RIGHTS OF PEOPLE WITH DIABETES

In Europe a formal resolution [78] has been signed by the member of states of the WHO European Region to officially recognize and adopt the St Vincent Declaration [79] in which the protection of the social rights of people with diabetes is clearly stated.

The promotion of the role of Diabetes Associations as local ombudsman for problems specifically related to diabetes in order to assist those individuals with diabetes whose rights are violated, should be strongly pursued. This would have the advantage of providing a unique focal point for people with diabetes (or their families, or any other people caring for them) instead of having several organizations or institutions diluting the effectiveness of intervention in defence of violated rights.

In the last decades the Diabetes Associations have been playing a major role in the protection of human and social rights of the people with diabetes providing a reference point for assistance in case of abuses and violations, for the promotion of better legislation, and for the elimination of prevailing prejudices in the society. The most encouraging results have been obtained by initiatives whose aim was

(1) to make information regarding their rights available to people with diabetes;
(2) to legally represent people with diabetes when dealing with public and private institutions, thus promoting awareness of their rights;

(3) to promote investigation of potential violations of the social rights of people with diabetes in various environments (school, workplace, etc.);
(4) to provide guidance to people with diabetes in legal disputes;
(5) to solicit the formulation of proposals of laws and other local initiatives from public institutions able to safeguard the citizen with diabetes;
(6) to promote the activation of existing but rarely utilized specialized and nonspecialized health care resources at primary, secondary, and tertiary level; and
(7) to operate in general, in those fields where social and human rights of citizens with diabetes are neglected.

In the last years the development of information technologies and especially the Internet facilities has highly increased the possibility of associations to give support to people with diabetes. In fact all the major associations have developed their own Web sites that are available free of charge. Most of them have a specific area dedicated to the rights of people with diabetes, with general legal information covering the majority of the fields of social rights. Furthermore, usually they guarantee the possibility to formulate particular questions to specialized professionals and a list of supporting institutions in case of conflicts.

Of particular interest is the role that they played in correlating general national laws on disability with the practical application to diabetes. In this sense several experiences have been developed in recent years as for example the Diabetes UK initiatives for the application to diabetes of the DDA [80], the ADA program for the implementation of the Americans with Disabilities Act [81], and the Canadian Diabetes Association's Position on Disability that adjusted to diabetes the Canadian Human Rights Act [6].

Of particular interest is the example of the initiative dedicated by the ADA with a specific program for the protection of children with diabetes against discrimination in schooling activity based on the Individuals with Disabilities Education Act [82].

Other than the associations, several initiatives have been developed by governmental organizations.

In the United States the Minnesota Department of Health launched the Eliminating Health Disparities Diabetes program that comprised a series of initiatives to overcome the problem of discrimination: the Minnesota Diabetes Plan 2010 for the reduction of racial, ethnic, and socioeconomic disparities, the workout low-fat (WOLF) program to promote physical activity and low-fat diet in young people at school age, and the Diabetes Community Collaboration Project to target intervention to specific need locally identified [83].

The protection of the human and social rights of people with diabetes is characterized by a wide variability of needs and actions throughout the world because of socioeconomic and cultural gradients. However, a unifying platform can be represented by the systematic ethical approach to this issue that could provide the instrument for linking problems apparently distant and different but whose solution can only be obtained on a global perspective. In this direction is also moving the European Region of the International Diabetes Federation that has formally included the human and social rights of people with diabetes within the line of action on Ethics in Diabetes as first priority in its strategic plan (www.idf.org).

A further initiative of the International Diabetes Federation that could represent an extremely powerful instrument, although very simple and basic, for the reduction of discrimination is the policy on semantics of diabetes. It is suggested to consider politically noncorrect the terms *diabetic* and *patient* that convey a negative perception and deeply affect the dignity of the individual, to be replaced by "person with diabetes" or similar terms that put at the center of the attention the person and not the disease or the disability. It has been proven in other fields that apparently simple initiatives can produce extraordinary results when applied on a global scale.

REFERENCES

1. Department for Education and Employment, UK Government. Towards inclusion—civil rights for disable people. Government Response to the Disability Rights Task Force, 2001.
2. Krall LP, Entmacher PS, Drury TF. Life cycle in diabetes: socioeconomic aspects. In Marble A, Krall LP, Bradley RF, Chriestlieb AR, Soeldner JS (eds) *Joslin's Diabetes Mellitus*, 12th edn. Philadelphia: Lea and Febiger, 1985; pp 907–36.
3. Nenner RP, Imperato PJ, Will TO. Quality of care problems among Medicare patients in New York States. *NY State J Med* 1993; 93: 159–62.
4. Leese B. The costs of diabetes mellitus and his complications. *Soc Sci Med* 1992; 35: 1303–10.
5. Lundstrom RE, Rossini RN, Rossini MD. The healing handbook for person with diabetes—coping with diabetes, 1998. Available at: http://www.umassmed.edu/diabeteshandbook.
6. Canadian Diabetes Association. The Canadian Diabetes Association's position on disability. Available at: http://www.diabetes.ca/Section_Advocay/advHumanRightsCompliant.asp.
7. Hammonds GS, Aoki TT. Measurements of health status in diabetic patients. Diabetes impact measurement scales. *Diabetes Care* 1992; 15: 469–77.
8. The North Tyneside Diabetes Time. The diabetes annual review as an educational tool: assessment and learning integrated with care, screening and audit. *Diabet Med* 1992; 9: 389–94.
9. Lloyd CE, Robinson N, Fuller JH. Education and employment experience in young adults with type 1 diabetes mellitus. *Diabet Med* 1992; 9: 661–6.
10. Griffiths RD, Moses RG. Diabetes in the workplace. Employment experiences of young people with diabetes mellitus. *Med J Aust* 1993; 158: 169–71.

11. Padgett DK. Socio demographic and disease correlates of depressive morbidity among diabetic patient in Zagreb, Croatia. *J Nerv Ment Dis* 1993; 181: 123–9.
12. Rebelo L. Chronic disease, the chronic patient and his family. Psychosocial impact of diabetes mellitus. *Acta Med Port* 1992; 5: 383–7.
13. Funnel MM, Merritt JH. The challenges of diabetes and older adults. *Nurs Clin North Am* 1993; 28: 45–60.
14. Simons LA, McCallum J, Simons J, Friedlander Y. Health status and lifestyle in elderly Hawaii, Japanese and Australian men. Exploring known differences in longevity. *Med J Aust* 1992; 156: 188–90.
15. Douglas JG, Milligan SE. Race, ethnicity, and health: diabetes and hypertension. *Ethn Dis* 1991; 1: 151–3.
16. O'Dea K. Diabetes in Australian aborigines: impact of the western diet and life style. *J Intern Med* 1992; 232: 99–101.
17. King H, Rewers M. Diabetes in adults is now a Third World problem. *Bull WHO* 1991; 69: 643–8.
18. Khalid BAK. Status of diabetes in Malaysia. In Krall LP, Alberti KGMM, Turtle JR. (eds). *World Book of Diabetes in Practice*, Vol 3. Amsterdam: Elsevier, 1988; pp 341–2.
19. The Diabetes Control and Complications Trial Research Group. The effect of intensive treatment of diabetes on the development progression of long term complications in insulin dependent diabetes mellitus. *N Engl J Med* 1993; 329: 977–86.
20. Musaiger AO. Diabetes mellitus in Bahrain: an overview. *Diabet Med* 1992; 9: 574–8.
21. Yudkin JS. Insulin for the world's poorest counties. *Lancet* 2000; 335: 919–21.
22. Bassili A, Omar M, Tognoni G. The adequacy of diabetic care for children in a developing country. *Diabetes Res Clin Pract* 2001; Sep; 53: 187–99.
23. Musey VC, Lee JK, Crawford R, Klatka MA, McAdams D, Phillips LS. Diabetes in urban African-Americans, I: cessation of insulin therapy is the major precipitating cause of diabetic ketoacidosis. *Diabetes Care* April 1995; 18 (4): 483–9.
24. Harris MI, Eastman RC, Cowie CC, Flegal KN, Eberhardt MS. Racial and ethnic differencies in glycemic control of adults with type 2 diabetes. *Diabetes Care* 1999; 22: 403–8.
25. Chaturvedi N, Jarrett J, Shipley MJ, Fuller JH. Socioeconomic gradient in morbidity and mortality in people with diabetes: cohort study findings from the Whiteall study and the WHO multinational study of vascular disease in diabetes. *BMJ* 1998; 316:100–5.
26. Rosilio M, Cotton JB, Wieliczko MC, Gendrault B, et al. Factors associated with glycemic control. *Diabetes Care* 1998; 21: 1146–53.
27. Roger L, Nelson MD. Diabetes and pregnancy: control can make a difference. *Mayo Clin Proc* 1986; 61: 825–9.
28. Silverman B, Rizzo T, Green OC, Cho N, Winter RJ, Ogata ES, Richards GE, Metzger BE. Long-term prospective evaluation of offspring of diabetic mothers. *Diabetes* 1991; 40: 121–5.
29. Hadden DR. Geographic, ethnic, racial variations in the incidence of gestational diabetes mellitus. *Diabetes* 1985; 34: 8–12.
30. Kitzmiller JL, Gavin LA, Gin GD, Jovanovic-Peterson L, Main EK, Zigrang WD. Preconception care of diabetes, glycemic control prevents congenital anomalies. *JAMA* 1991; 265: 731–6.
31. Tardioli MC, Massi Benedetti M, Angeli G, Damiani F, Frascarelli A, Gigliarelli D, Masci D, Narducci P, Norgiolini R, Nicolucci A, Pastorelli G, Rossi AL, Settonce S, Toppetti ML, Brunetti PA. Pilot study for the screening of gestational diabetes mellitus. *Diabetes Nutr Metab* 1993; 6: 377–80.
32. Schiavi RC, Stimmel BB, Mandeli J, Rayfield J. Diabetes mellitus and male sexual function: a control study. *Diabetologia* 1993; 36: 745–51.
33. Watkins SE, Williams P, Ryder RE, Bowshier W. Psychometric assessment of diabetic impotence. *Br J Psychiatry* 1993; 162: 840–2.
34. Barnard RJ, Ugianskis EJ, Martin DA, Inkeles SB. Role of diet and exercise in the management of hyperinsulinemia and associated atherosclerotic risk factors. *Am J Cardiol* 69: 440–4.
35. Welch G, Smith RB. The evaluation of a behavioural food and weight control programme for obese patients with non-insulin dependent diabetes. *N Z Med J* January 22, 1992; 105 (926): 9–10.
36. Norkus A, Ostrauskas R, Zalinkevicius R. Prevalence of insulin-dependent diabetes mellitus and its complications in Lithuania. *Diabetes Nutr Metab* 1993; 6: 335–8.
37. AbuBakare A, Taylor R, Gill GV, Alberti KGMM. Tropical or malnutrition related diabetes: a real syndrome? *Lancet* 1986; i: 1135–8.
38. Bell JL, Bacchus RA, Madkour MM, Kilshaw BH. The prevalence of diabetes mellitus in male and female Saudi Arabs. In Bajaj JS (ed) *Diabetes Mellitus in Developing Countries.* New Delhi Interprint. 1984; pp 3–38.
39. Verma NPS, Mehta SP, Madhu S, Mather HM, Keen H. Prevalence of known diabetes in an urban Indian environment: the Dory and Ganj diabetes survey. *Br Med J* 1986; 293: 423.
40. Hinkle LE Jr, Wolff HG. Ecologic investigation of the realtionship between illness, life experience and the social environment. *Ann Intern Med* 1958; 49: 1373–88.
41. Alberti KGMM, Gries FA. Management of non-insulin dependent diabetes in Europe: a consensus view. *Diabet Med* 1988; 5: 251–75.
42. Azzopardi J, Barrett E, Gruber W, Home PD, Jervell J, Krans HMJ, de Leiva A, Massi Benedetti M, Piwernetz K, Staehr Johansen K. *Recommendations to Facilitate the Implementation of St Vincent Declaration Initiatives by National, Regional and Local Diabetes Task Forces.* Report on Consensus Workshop, Oslo, June 26–27, 1992. QCT Copenhagen: WHO Regional Office for Europe, 1992. EUR/ICP/CLR 055 0279g.
43. Robinson N, Yateman NA, Protopapa LE, Bush L. Employment problems and diabetes. *Diabet Med* 1990; 7: 16–22.
44. Zagoria RB. Employment rights: the tides are turning. *Diabetes Forecast* 1986; 38: 23–6.
45. Olivera EM, Pérez Duhalde E, Gagliardino JJ. Costs of temporary and permanent disability induced by diabetes. *Diabetes Care* 1991; 14: 593–6.
46. Songer TJ, et al. Employment spectrum of IDDM. *Diabetes Care* 1989; 12 (9): 615–23.
47. Baker J, Scragg R, Metcalf P, Dryson E. Diabetes mellitus and employment: is there discrimination in the workplace? *Diabet Med* 1993; 10: 362–5.
48. Robinson N, Stevens LK, Protopaper LE. Education and employment for young people with diabetes. *Diabet Med* 1993; 10: 983–9.
49. The American Diabetes Association. Hypoglycemia and employment/licensure. *Diabetes Care* 2002; 25 (suppl 1): S132.

50. Frier BM, Maher G. Diabetes and hypoglycemia: medico-legal aspects of criminal responsability. *Diabet Med* 1988; 5: 521–6.
51. Poole CJ, Wright AD, Nattrass M. Control of diabetes mellitus in shift workers. *Br J Ind Med* 1992; 7: 513–5.
52. National Health Service. The impact of social and environmental factors on diabetes, employment issues. The Disability Discrimination Act. Available at: http://cebmh.warne.ox.ac.uk/diabetes/patient/social/employment.
53. Dickson Mary B. Employment consideration for people who have diabetes. Program on employment and disability. New York State School of Industrial and Labour Relations, Cornell University, January 1994.
54. Chu YNG, Jacobs P, Johnson JA. Productivity losses associated with diabetes in the US. *Diabetes Care* 2001; 24: 257–61.
55. Kraut A, Wallis R, Tate R, Mustard C. Impact of diabetes on employment and income in manitoba, Canada. *Diabetes Care* 2001; 24: 64–8.
56. Griffits R, Moses R. Diabetes in the workplace: employment of young people with diabetes mellitus. *Med J Aust* 1993; 158:169–71.
57. Waller JA. Chronic medical conditions and traffic safety. Review of the California experience. *N Engl J Med* 1965; 273: 1413.
58. Ehrlich EN. Diabetes and the license to drive. *Wis Med J* 1991; 90: 115–8.
59. Gower IF, Songer TJ, Hylton H, Thomas NL, Ekoe JM, Lave LB, La Porte RE. Epidemiology of insulin-using commercial motor vehicle drivers. Major variability of state licensing requirements in the U.S. *Diabetes Care* 1992; 15: 1464–7.
60. Songer TJ, Love LB, La Porte RE. The risks of licensing persons with diabetes to drive trucks. *Risk Anal* 13, 1993; 3: 319–26.
61. Saunders CJ. Driving and diabetes mellitus. *BMJ* November 21, 1992; 305 (6864): 1265.
62. Frier BM. Driving and diabetes. *BMJ* 1992; 305: 1238–9.
63. National Health Service. The impact of social and environmental factors on diabetes, driving. The Legal Situation. Available at: http://cebmh.warne.ox.ac.uk/diabetes/patient/social/driving.
64. Diabetes Australia. Diabetes and driving. Available at: http://www.diabetesaustralia.com.au/multilingualdiabetes/HealthPros/Whatis/driving.htm.
65. Clarke B, Ward JB, Enoch BA. Hypoglycemia in insulin-dependent diabetic drivers. *Br Med J* August 30, 1980; 281 (6240): 586.
66. Cockram CS, Dutton T, Sönksen PH. Driving and diabetes: a summary of the current medical and legal postion based upon a recent heavy goods vehicle (HGV) case. *Diabet Med* 1986; 3: 137–40.
67. Songer TJ, LaPorte RE, Dorman JS, Orchard TJ, Cruickshanks KJ, Becker DJ, Drash AL. Motor vehicle accidents and IDDM. *Diabetes Care* 1988; 11: 701–7.
68. Ratner RE, Whitehouse FW. Motor vehicles, hypoglycemia and diabetic drivers. *Diabetes Care* 1989; 12: 217–22.
69. Hansotia P, Broste SK. The effect of epilepsy or diabetes mellitus on the risk of automobile accidents. *N Engl J Med* 1991; 324: 22–6.
70. Ekoe JM, Laberge-Nadeau C, Ghardirian P, Hamet P. Impact of diabetes mellitus on driving safety. *Diabete Metab* 1991; 17: 61–8.
71. Songer TJ, La Porte RE, Dorman JS, Orchard TJ, Becker DJ, Drash AL. Health, life and automobile insurnace characteristics in adults with IDDM. *Diabetes Care* 1991; 4: 318–24.
72. Wheeler ML, Warre-Boulton E. Diabetes patient education programs. Quality and reimbursegment. *Diabetes Care* 1992; 15 (suppl): 36–40.
73. Clark CM, Kinney ED. Standards for the care of diabetes. Origins, uses and implications for the third-party payment. *Diabetes Care* 1992; 15 (suppl): 10–4.
74. Harris M. Racial and ethnic differencies in health insurance coverage for adults with diabetes. *Diabetes Care* 1999; 22: 1679–82.
75. North Dakota Department of Health. Health insurance coverage for diabetes in North Dakota. Available at: http://diabetesnd.org/insurance.htm.
76. Canadian Diabetes Association. New credit life insurance plan launched for people with diabetes. Available at: http://diabetes.ca/Section_Main/NewsReleases.asp.
77. Disposizioni per la prevenzione e la cura del diabete mellito. Italian National Law No 115. *Gazz Ufficiale della Repubblica Ital* 1987; 128 (71): 6–8.
78. WHO Resolution on the Prevention and Control of Diabetes Mellitus. EUR/RC41/Conf. Doc./7 Rev. 1 4978B, adopted by the 41st Session of the Regional Committee for Europe, Lisbon, Europe: WHO/IDF, September, 10–14, 1991.
79. Diabetes care and research in Europe: the St Vincent declaration [appendix]. *G Ital Diabetol* 1990; 10 (suppl): 143–4.
80. Diabetes UK. Response towards equality and diversity. March 2002. Available at: www.diabetes.org.uk.
81. American Diabetes Association. Diabetes and employment discrimination. Available at: http://www.diabetes.org/main/application/commercew.
82. American Diabetes Association. Your school and your rights. Available at: http://www.diabetes.org/main/type1/parents_kids/away/scrights.jsp.
83. Minnesota Department of Health. Eliminating health disparities in diabetes. Available at: http://www.health.state.mn.us/divs/fh/chp/diabmiss.htm.

109

Economics of Care: Europe

Kamran Siddiqi and Rhys Williams

University of Leeds, Leeds, UK

INTRODUCTION

As this and the other chapters in this section show, there is a wide variation in the extent to which economic aspects of diabetes and diabetes care have been characterized worldwide. North America, particularly the United States, is well served with cost-of-illness studies relevant to diabetes and has taken a lead in many respects with regard to analytical studies of the cost-effectiveness of therapies and methods of delivering health care. The costs of diabetes in Latin American and Caribbean countries, while much less well studied in the past, have at least some new baseline data from which to draw comparisons both between countries of that region and with future costs.

Australia and New Zealand have their own accumulating literature on diabetes health economics, some of which is focused on indigenous groups—Aboriginal Australians and Maori communities—outlining the differences between these and other populations. These countries, too, have directed attention to the economics of diabetes health care delivery.

Middle Eastern countries differ considerably in their economic development and in their current prevalence of diabetes. The region contains countries with some of the highest per capita incomes in the world and, hardly surprisingly, some of the highest diabetes prevalences. Much of our information on the costs of care for people with diabetes in this continent is derived from studies of hospital clinics and inpatients. This information reveals the high personal costs of diabetes care. This theme is also illustrated by information from other parts of Asia and the Western Pacific—in many countries of the world diabetes care of any quality is not affordable by many of those who need and deserve it.

Africa is the continent least well served for economic information. Here the diabetes epidemic is still in its early stages. Nonetheless, national economies are already potentially threatened by it and much needs to be done to keep track of the economic impact of the disorder and to minimize it.

Europe, the subject of this chapter, in addition to its country-specific studies of the cost of diabetes care, now has one source of data—the CODE-2 Study—by means of which between-country comparisons can be made in the knowledge that the same method of study has been advocated throughout. The CODE-2 Study is the "Cost of Diabetes in Europe—Type 2" Study. The title is a registered trademark of GlaxoSmithKline plc. This information, however, is applicable only to the established market-economy countries that took part. The economic impact of diabetes and related conditions in eastern European and the former Soviet Union countries is virtually undocumented. While most studies of the indirect costs of diabetes (the "costs of lost production") have used the "human capital" approach to calculate them, researchers from one European country (the Netherlands) are developing an alternative approach—the "friction cost" method.

In all continents there is still a long way to go before we have reasonably robust, comparable data on these issues. However, it is clear from the data that we do have to hand that diabetes and, in particular, its complications have a large economic impact both directly and indirectly. This impact falls on individuals, families, the health care sector, and society in general. It is also clear that some methods for the delivery of diabetes health care are more cost-effective than others, but it is also likely (though as yet untested) that the most cost-effective approach of all is the primary prevention of the condition.

International Textbook of Diabetes Mellitus, Third Edition. Edited by R. A. DeFronzo, E. Ferrannini, H. Keen, and P. Zimmet.
 ISBN: 0-471-48655-8.

A considerable amount of data is now available on the incidence and prevalence of diabetes in European countries but there are still relatively few sources of cost data, particularly for direct nonmedical and indirect costs. The studies that are available have mainly focused on direct costs, for example, the costs of hospital care, consultations, insulin therapy, and drugs. Fewer studies have included indirect costs, such as the effect of time lost from work, early retirement, and premature death, mainly because of issues in assigning monetary values to these components [1].

DIRECT HEALTH CARE COSTS—THE GENERAL PICTURE

The CODE-2 Study, for the first time, has provided a comparison of the costs of care for people with type 2 diabetes in eight European countries [2]. The study used a "bottom-up" prevalence design to identify all health care episodes for a sample of 7000 people with type 2 diabetes. This study, therefore, differs from "top-down" studies, which estimate costs from aggregated, usually routinely collected, information for populations (usually national populations) of people with diabetes. A full account of the CODE-2 Study and the complementary T^2 ARDIS Study can be found in the monograph *The True Costs of Type 2 Diabetes in the UK—Findings from T^2 ARDIS and CODE-2 UK* available from GlaxoSmithKline UK, Uxbridge. By extrapolation from this sample, the cost of care for the more than 10 million patients with type 2 diabetes across Europe was estimated (1998 prices) to be 29 billion Euros (approx. US$26 billion) [2]. Table 1 compares the different costs estimated in CODE-2 for each country with costs estimated in previous studies.

Some care needs to be taken in interpreting these data since some of the comparison studies relate to type 1 and type 2 diabetes together or type 1 alone. (CODE-2 considered type 2 only.) Also, as in the literature from other continents, some studies estimate the *cost of care for people with diabetes* (as does CODE-2) whereas others estimate the *cost of diabetes care* (i.e. the incremental costs attributable to the condition). This is an important distinction not always made clear in published studies. The former term includes the costs of all episodes of care, irrespective of whether diabetes or diabetes-related conditions were the reasons for these episodes. The latter term includes only the costs of diabetes-related care. This is usually the main focus of attention. However, it is often necessary to estimate the overall costs of care for people with diabetes and then, by subtracting from this an estimate of the cost of care for people who do not have diabetes, arrive at an estimate for the incremental costs of diabetes. Proceeding by this method has the advantage of including the influence of diabetes on costs even when diabetes and diabetes-related conditions are not the main reason for any given episode. Also, it sidesteps the need to decide exactly what is and what is not "diabetes-related".

The general finding from CODE-2—that health care costs incurred by people with diabetes are more than double that of the average cost for the population, even taking age into account—is confirmed by Norlund et al. [8]. This is the result of higher levels of utilization in both primary and secondary care and in particular, more frequent and lengthier periods of hospitalization. According to a UK based economic model, the lifetime cost for an average male diagnosed with type 2 diabetes will be just under £33 000 as compared with £15 000 for a nondiabetic peer. For a woman with type 2 diabetes the estimated lifetime cost is £43 000 as compared with £22 000 for a non-diabetic peer [12].

A recent study from Finland compared the cost of medications used in both type 1 and 2 diabetic patients to that in matched non-diabetic controls. The costs for people with diabetes were 3.5 times greater than those for the control subjects. The higher cost amongst type 1 diabetic patients was mainly due to the use of insulin but the largest single component for type 2 diabetic patients was that for non-diabetes drugs (mainly drugs for cardiovascular diseases) [13].

Diabetes constitutes a major share in the health expenditure even prior to the onset of diabetic complications. In Sweden, 1 year after the diagnosis of diabetes, the annual excess costs of care were estimated as US$4743 for men and US$4976 for women (1997 prices). Fifty percent of this excess cost was due to hospital admissions. Another cohort in the same study 8 years after diagnosis still had annual excess costs of US$2010 for men and US$2734 for women [14].

The proportion of costs attributable to hospitalisation found in that Swedish study closely matches the 55% of the overall expenditure found in CODE-2 [2]. However within this overall total, there exists a fairly wide range. In Italy nearly 65% of direct medical expenditure is attributable to hospitalisation, while in the Netherlands the proportion is 30%. The United Kingdom spends 39% of type 2 diabetes costs on ambulatory (hospital outpatient) care, while in Germany this proportion is 11%.

CODE-2 also highlighted the fact that nearly two thirds of the total expenditure on drugs is on nondiabetes drugs [7]. Only 2–7% of the total direct costs overall across European countries is spent on oral hypoglycemic medication. In the Netherlands an estimated 39% of these direct costs are spent on nondiabetes drugs. In Italy the majority of health care expenditure in managing diabetic outpatients is spent on investigations in type 2 diabetic patients, and in those with type 1 diabetes, on medication directly related to diabetes [15].

Although most of the above studies concur with regard to the large economic impact of diabetes and, as mentioned

Table 1 A comparison of various cost-of-illness studies in each country

Country	Year	Diabetes	Cost type	Total cost of care per year in local currency	Total cost of care per year in US dollars*	Total cost as a proportion of health care expenditure (%)	Hospitalization cost (%)	Cost of care per person per year in local currency	Cost of care per person per year in US dollars*
Spain [2]	1998	Type 2	Direct medical	325 739 million pesetas	2.3 billion	4.4	32	217 158 pesetas	1 540
Spain [3]	1994	Type 2	Direct medical	90 000 million pesetas	684 million		58	63 000 pesetas	479
Spain [4]	1994	Type 1	Direct medical	9 134 million pesetas	70 million			12.7 million pesetas per life time	100 000 per life time
France [5]	1998	Type 2	Direct medical	25.8 billion francs	4.3 billion	3.2	50	20 100 francs	3 350
France [6]	1999	Type 1 & 2	Direct medical	31.9 billion francs	5.2 billion		45	25 700 francs	4 200
Germany [7]	1998	Type 2	Direct medical	31.4 billion deutsche marks	17.5 billion	6.3	50	7 012 deutsche marks	4 220
Sweden [8]	1992–1993	Type 2	Direct medical				65	17 276 SEK	2 450
			Direct nonmedical					19 127 SEK	2 710
			Indirect					25 297 SEK	3 590
Sweden [2]	1998	Type 2	Direct medical	6995 MSEK	868 million	4.5	42	24 983 SEK	3 103
Sweden [9, 10]	1994	Type 2	Direct medical	2455 MSEK	320 million		58		
			Indirect	3291 MSEK	425 million				
			Total	5746 MSEK	745 million				
Belgium [2]	1998	Type 2	Direct medical	44.1 billion Belgium francs	1.3 billion	6.7	55	133 000 Belgium francs	3 888
Italy [2]	1998	Type 2	Direct medical	11.2 trillion liras	6.8 billion	7.4	65	6.5 million liras	3 948
Netherlands [2]	1998	Type 2	Direct medical	976 million guilders	524 million	1.6	30	4,155 guilders	2 229
United Kingdom [11]	1992	Type 1	Direct	96 million pounds	175 million			1,021 pounds	1 840
			Indirect	113 million pounds	206 million				
United Kingdom [2]	1998	Type 2	Direct medical	1.8 billion pounds	3.1 billion	3.4	35	1,550 pounds	2 613

Note: * Local currencies are converted to US dollars (USD) at the mean conversion rate for the year of the study (1 Euro = 1.18 USD).
MSEK = one thousand Swedish Kronor; SEK = Swedish Kronor.

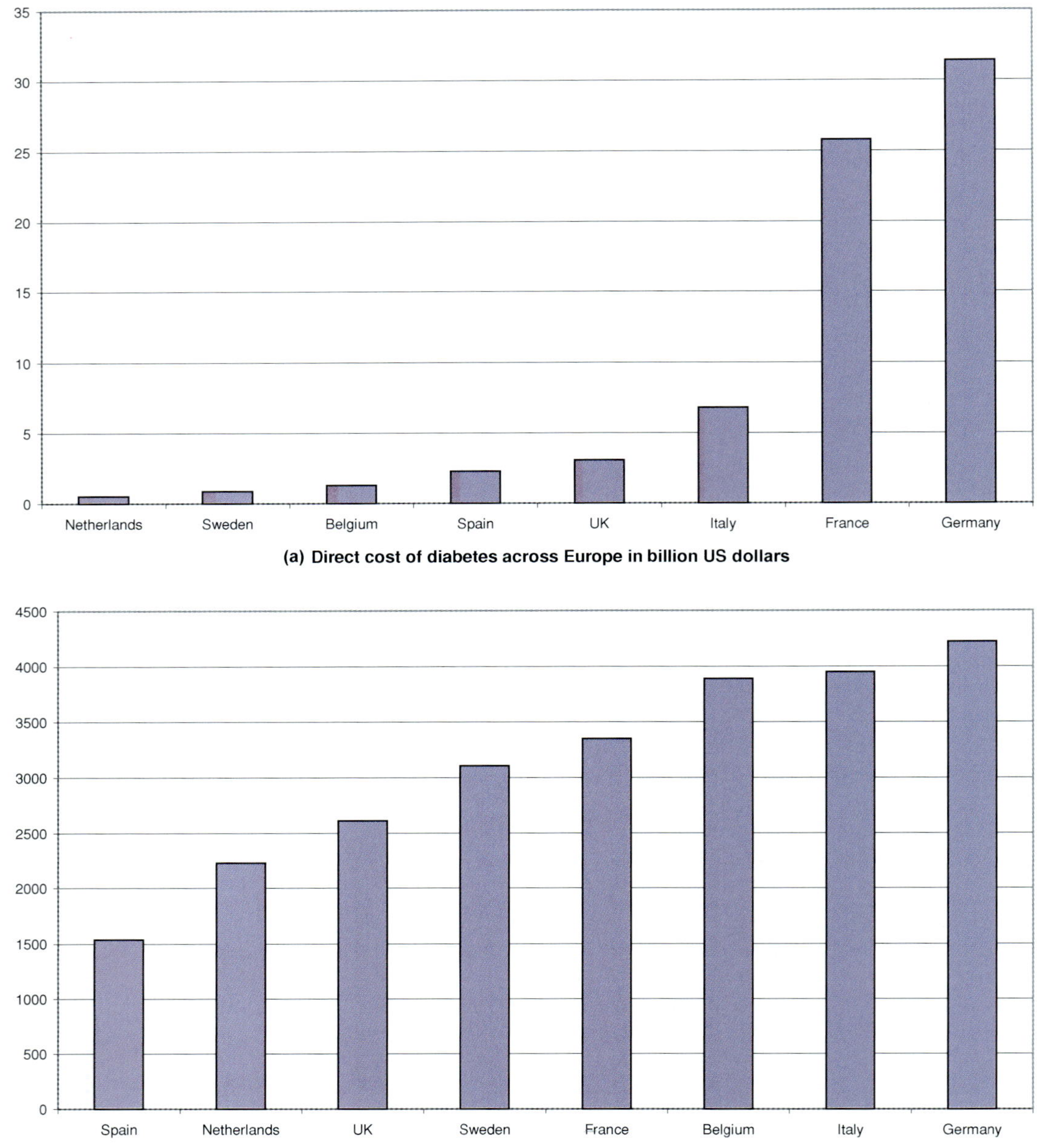

(a) Direct cost of diabetes across Europe in billion US dollars

(b) Cost per patient in US dollars

Figure 1 Cost comparisons in CODE-2 study

below, the importance, within the direct cost element, of the presence or absence of complications, they also show a range of health care costs between European countries (see Figure 1a and b). Within the CODE-2 Study, for example, the total direct costs per person with diabetes in the Netherlands were only marginally above the average per capita cost of care for the population as a whole. In contrast, in Italy, the costs for an individual with diabetes were 250% of these average per person costs. It remains uncertain whether this range is a result of the more efficient care of diabetes in the low-cost countries or of undertreatment in these countries. The question will remain unresolved until comparable data on outcomes are available.

DIRECT HEALTH CARE COSTS—THE IMPORTANCE OF COMPLICATIONS

The studies cited above and others agree that people with diabetes require disproportionately higher number of hospital admissions and stay for longer once admitted, as compared to non-diabetic patients. For a district hospital in UK this amounts to nearly 9% of the total expenditure on inpatient care [16]. The long-term complications of diabetes are major contributors to this effect.

The CODE-2 Study highlighted the difference between the cost of care for people with diabetes but with no complications, and the cost of care for people who had already developed the complications [2]. The presence of either macro- or microvascular complications is associated with nearly a doubling of costs compared with that for those without complications. The presence of both complications increases cost more than threefold. The T^{2}ARDIS Study (Type 2 Diabetes Accounting for a Major Resource Demand in Society; see under Direct Health Care Costs—The General Picture) confirms this relationship and that it is not the result of confounding with age or, by inference, with the duration of diabetes. Macrovascular complications contribute just as much to the overall cost of care of diabetes as the microvascular complications [7].

A similar study in Sweden found that costs as a result of diabetes become two to three times higher when diabetic complications are included in the cost estimation [8]. This highlights the need to intensify efforts to prevent or delay complications by means of better metabolic control and self-management. In Sweden in 1994, three times more resources were spent on treating complications compared to what was spent on the control of the disease [17].

Hypoglycaemia is an important complication in diabetes treatment. In some cases hospital admission is necessary and incurs further costs. With strategies to improve glycemic control, such episodes are likely to increase in frequency unless countered by appropriate educational and other preventive interventions. The probable annual cost of hospital care resulting from hypoglycaemia was estimated to be around 108–151 million francs (US$16–22 million) in 1995 in France [18].

There is a strong argument to invest in the prevention of diabetic complications as it is likely to curtail costs in terms of saving the long-term costs of treating these complications. In addition, and more importantly, the impact of such preventive strategies would be much wider in terms of improving the quality of life of people with diabetes and their families. Despite the long-term benefit of investing in preventive strategies, it still requires considerable investment in the short term [19].

INDIRECT COSTS ("COSTS OF LOST PRODUCTION")

Fewer attempts have been made to estimate the total cost of diabetes to the society, including not only direct health care costs but also indirect costs. These are the value of productivity lost as a result of "sickness absence," disability, early retirement, or premature death as a result of diabetes. Many studies that have attempted to measure these indirect costs have concluded that they are at least as great, sometimes greater, than direct costs. The methods used to value this lost production are controversial, however, and much needs to be done to standardize these and to reach agreement on their use.

A study in the Netherlands reported that diabetes along with its complications costs almost 1.67 milliard Dutch guilders (US$0.94 billion) to the society, out of which 0.2 milliard Dutch guilders (US$0.1 billion) are due to absenteeism [20]. In Sweden the excess indirect cost to the society in terms of early retirement and sickness absence was estimated to be approximately US$7000 per person with diabetes. Other studies have also estimated indirect cost of diabetes as presented in Table 1.

The Netherlands study cited above used the friction cost approach to estimate the cost of absenteeism due to diabetes. This estimates the cost to the industrial sector of bringing in other workers, either by recruitment or by retraining, to compensate for the fact that some of the workforce is "off sick" as a result of diabetes or its routine care. This method acknowledges the fact that sickness absence (and disability, premature retirement, and premature mortality) does not, inevitably, lead to work remaining undone but does convey a cost to society in order to minimize the consequences of that absence. This is in contrast to the human capital approach, which equates the value of lost productivity to the amount that would have been paid, in salaries and wages, for that work to be done. Most of the studies listed in Table 1 and in other chapters in this section have used the human capital approach. Neither method estimates the cost to society of time away from school nor of the loss of contributions from those not in paid employment (for example, those caring for children and the home).

ECONOMIC EVALUATION—THE COST-EFFECTIVENESS OF ACHIEVING BETTER GLYCEMIC CONTROL

Type 1 Diabetes

Evidence suggests that intensive therapy strategies in type 1 diabetes can achieve normal or near normal blood glucose levels and, as a result, reduce the risk of major complications. However, the cost of an intensive insulin-based strategy is approximately 50% more than that of conventional strategies. Cogent arguments can be made, however, that the extra costs of therapy are offset by savings made as a result of reductions in hospital care required for diabetic complications [21]. Evidence also exists to show that intensive therapy treatment is cost-effective in generating additional life years and quality-adjusted life years [22]. Although the most powerful evidence for this conclusion comes from the Diabetes Control and Complications Trial (DCCT) carried out in North America [23], the generally lower costs of care in European countries strengthen rather than weaken the argument.

Work from Moscow reveals that an intensive 5-day in-patient treatment supplemented by educational interventions can achieve better control in type 1 diabetes over a 2-year time period. This practice was shown to save resources due to less care required in patients with improved control. However this study was conducted with a small number of subjects followed up for only 2 years [24].

Type 2 Diabetes

The UK Prospective Diabetes Study (UKPDS) was a landmark study in highlighting the importance of intensive treatment in reducing mortality and morbidity secondary to type 2 diabetes. The data collected were analyzed to assess the cost-effectiveness of this intensive approach.

One analysis compared two groups of overweight subjects, one receiving metformin and the other on traditional therapy mainly consisting of dietary advice. The improved blood glucose control with metformin produced a net saving of GBP 258 per subject (1997 UK prices) over the trial period (median duration 10.7 years) as a result of the lower complication costs [25]. These results when applied, by means of computer modeling, to a Swiss third party payer system showed a net saving of CHF 927 [26].

UKPDS analysis including all subjects suggested that the incremental cost of intensive management is around GBP 478 (GBP 275 to GBP 1232) per subject. Subjects on intensive therapy gained 0.60 (0.12–1.10) years within trial event-free time and were estimated to achieve a lifetime gain of 1.14 (0.69–1.61) years. The incremental cost per event-free year gained was GBP 1166, and GBP 563 per year gained over a lifetime [27].

ECONOMIC EVALUATION—THE COST-EFFECTIVENESS OF OTHER SPECIFIC INTERVENTIONS

Obesity

Obesity is a common condition in type 2 diabetes. Treating obesity with Orlistat has been shown to be cost-effective, especially in the presence of hypertension and hypercholesterolemia. The cost-effectiveness varies between €3462 per year of life gained for obese patients with diabetes, hypertension, and hypercholesterolemia and €19986 per year of life gained for those with diabetes but without these other risk factors [28].

Treatment of Dyslipidemia

The Scandinavian Simvastatin Survival Study ("4S") provided an opportunity to analyze the cost-effectiveness of the use of one specific lipid lowering agent in a subanalysis of the group with diabetes. One economic analysis done in the context of Swedish costs published estimates of cost per life-year gained well within the range generally considered to be cost-effective (€1600–€3200) [29].

HYPERTENSION

Analyses from the UKPDS study showed that tight control of blood pressure in hypertensive patients with type 2 diabetes reduces the cost of care for diabetic complications by prolonging the interval between onset and survival. Treating hypertension with either β-blockers or ACE (angiotensin-converting enzyme) inhibitor to keep blood pressure control within the normal range has a cost-effectiveness ratio that compares favorably with many accepted health care programs. The incremental cost to gain 1 life year after discounting both cost and benefit at 6% is shown to be around GBP 720 [30].

Screening for Diabetic Retinopathy

A UK based study demonstrated that systematic retinopathy screening in people with diabetes is cost-effective in detecting vision threatening diabetic eye disease as compared to the less well-organized opportunistic screening currently practiced. The incremental cost of detecting one new case by the introduction of a systematic screening program is only GBP 34 [31].

A study from Italy concluded that screening for, assessing, and treating sight-threatening diabetic retinopathy may be a cost-effective procedure for society as a whole in Italy. This study compared different strategies for screening eye disease among people with diabetes and found that it would be more cost-effective to let clinicians do the screening as opposed to each person being referred to an ophthalmologist for initial tests. Early detection of sight-threatening eye disease in diabetes can also result in significant cost savings as demonstrated by a study conducted in Austria [32].

Diabetic Nephropathy

Evidence from the Netherlands suggests that strategies to screen and prevent diabetic renal complications are cost-effective [33]. Early treatment with ACE inhibitors in diabetic nephropathy is cost saving by reducing the incidence of end-stage renal failure and subsequent cost of renal care required [34]. Similar results have been found in Italy where a study demonstrated the economic benefits of treating patients with diabetes and with proteinuria with ACE inhibitors at an early stage [35].

Diabetic Foot

Diabetic foot ulcer and amputation are common and highly distressing complications of diabetes. The prevention of ulcers and amputation has shown to be cost-effective in patients with high risk of foot disease. Preventive interventions cost significantly less than the curative therapies in these foot complications [36]. Moreover, when estimating the costs for diabetic foot ulcers, it is necessary to include long-term costs, which can be high because of the need for increased home and social care and also because of the recurrence of the disease [37]. Interventions, including education directed at self-management, professional foot care, and footwear, can be very cost-effective if the risk of foot ulcers and amputations can be reduced to 25% [38].

ECONOMIC EVALUATION—THE COST-EFFECTIVENESS OF MULTIPLE INTERVENTIONS

Various simulation models have been used to estimate the cost savings and life years gained by introducing multiple interventions in type 2 diabetes. One such model was used to estimate the cost savings and life years gained by introducing multifactor interventions, including screening for nephropathy and retinopathy, educational programs, and control of cardiovascular risk profile in Swiss settings. The interventions led to a gain of 0.56 life years and a reduction of 10% in the total cost of care per patient compared to the current standard practice. Extrapolation to the whole Swiss type 2 diabetic population (285 000) suggested yearly cost savings of CHF 194 million as a result of the multifactor interventions [39].

The same research group studied the cost-benefit of multiple interventions in type 1 diabetes in Swiss settings and came up with similar conclusions. They concluded that optimal management of type 1 diabetic patients, including other preventive interventions, would lead to reduced costs and improved life expectancy [40].

Interventions using diet and physical activity programs are likely to be cost-beneficial in people with type 2 diabetes. A UK-based group estimated that such interventions can get an extra quality-adjusted life year for an incremental cost of US$9002 [41].

CONCLUSIONS

The evidence from European countries confirms that diabetes is a costly condition but that these costs can be contained and reduced by effective preventive interventions. There are many European countries and there are many interventions for which economic data on diabetes are lacking. The challenge of the next few years is to fill in the most important of these gaps so that more rational decisions may be made in health care planning. An additional challenge, however, is to explore what, if any, of the existing economic information can be translated from European studies (and from those based in other *developed* countries) to countries in the developing world. The goal should be to improve the delivery of care to people with diabetes worldwide, without the necessity to "reinvent the wheel" in every continent. Part of the answer to this will be the development of computer-based economic models of diabetes care constructed using the results of studies from Europe, North America, and Australasia but with data and assumptions relevant to health care delivery and the epidemiology of diabetes in the developing world.

REFERENCES

1. Leese B. The costs of diabetes and its complications. *Soc Sci Med* 1992; 35: 1303–10.
2. Baxter H, Bottomley J, Harvey J, Kernohan E, Lawlor D, Sheaves R, Sheldon P, Williams R, Young R. CODE-2 UK: the current costs of Type-2 diabetes in the UK. *Diabet Med* 2000; 17 (suppl 1): abstract.
3. Hart WM, Espinosa C, Rovira J. Costs of known diabetes mellitus in Spain. *Med Clin (Barc)* 1997; 109: 289–93.
4. Hart WM, Espinosa C, Rovira J. A simulation model of the cost of the incidence of IDDM in Spain. *Diabetologia* 1997; 40: 311–8.
5. Detournay B, Fagnani F, Pribil C, Eschwege E. Medical resources consumption of type 2 diabetics in France in 1998. *Diabetes Metab* 2000; 26: 225–31.
6. Ricordeau P, Weill A, Vallier N, Bourrel R, Fender P, Allemand H. The cost of diabetes in metropolitan France. *Diabetes Metab* 2000; 26 (suppl 6): 25–38.
7. Liebl A, Neiss A, Spannheimer A, Reitberger U, Wagner T, Gortz A. Costs of type 2 diabetes in Germany. Results of the CODE-2 study. *Dtsch Med Wochenschr* 2001; 126: 585–9.
8. Norlund A, Apelqvist J, Bitzen PO, Nyberg P, Schersten B. Cost of illness of adult diabetes mellitus underestimated if comorbidity is not considered. *J Intern Med* 2001; 250: 57–65.
9. Henriksson F, Agardh CD, Berne C, Bolinder J, Jonsson B. Health economics analysis of diabetes is necessary. It facilitates decision-making and international comparison. *Lakartidningen* 1999; 96: 3915–6, 3919.
10. Henriksson F, Jonsson B. Diabetes: the cost of illness in Sweden. *J Intern Med* 1998; 244: 461–8.
11. Gray A, Fenn P, McGuire A. The cost of insulin-dependent diabetes mellitus (IDDM) in England and Wales. *Diabet Med* 1995; 12: 1068–76.
12. Bagust A, Hopkinson PK, Maier W, Currie CJ. An economic model of the long-term health care burden of Type II diabetes. *Diabetologia* 2001; 44: 2140–55.
13. Reunanen A, Kangas T, Martikainen J, Klaukka T. Nationwide survey of comorbidity, use, and costs of all medications in Finnish diabetic individuals. *Diabetes Care* 2000; 23: 1265–71.
14. Jonsson PM, Marke LA, Nystrom L, Wall S, Ostman J. Excess costs of medical care 1 and 8 years after diagnosis of diabetes: estimates from young and middle-aged incidence cohorts in Sweden. *Diabetes Res Clin Pract* 2000; 50: 35–47.
15. Garattini L, Tediosi F, Chiaffarino F, Roggeri D, Parazzini F, Coscelli C. The outpatient cost of diabetes care in Italian diabetes centers. *Value Health* 2001; 4: 251–7.
16. Currie CJ, Kraus D, Morgan CL, Gill L, Stott NC, Peters JR. NHS acute sector expenditure for diabetes: the present,

future, and excess in-patient cost of care. *Diabet Med* 1997; 14: 686–92.

17. Bjork S. The cost of diabetes and diabetes care. *Diabetes Res Clin Pract* 2001; 54 (suppl 1): S13–8.
18. Allicar MP, Megas F, Houzard S, Baroux A, Le Thai F, Augendre-Ferrante B. Frequency and costs of hospital stays for hypoglycemia in France in 1995. *Presse Med* 2000; 29: 657–61.
19. Williams R. Applying recent findings to clinical care in type II diabetes. *Pharmacoeconomics* 1995; 8 (suppl 1): 80–4.
20. van Os N, Niessen LW, Koopmanschap MA, van der LJ. Detailed analysis of the societal costs of diabetes mellitus. *Ned Tijdschr Geneeskd* 2000; 144: 842–6.
21. Reichard P, Alm C, Andersson E, Warn I, Rosenqvist U. Intensified insulin treatment is cost-effective. *Lakartidningen* 1999; 96: 172–4.
22. Phillips CJ. The economic implications of implementing evidence-based diabetic treatment strategies. *Int J Clin Pract* 1998; 52: 181–7.
23. The Diabetes Control and Complications Trial (DCCT) Research Group. Lifetime benefits and costs of intensive therapy as practiced in the diabetes control and complications trial. *JAMA* 1996; 276: 1409–15.
24. Starostina EG, Antsiferov M, Galstyan GR, Trautner C, Jorgens V, Bott U, Muhlhauser I, Berger M, Dedov II. Effectiveness and cost-benefit analysis of intensive treatment and teaching programmes for type 1 (insulin-dependent) diabetes mellitus in Moscow—blood glucose versus urine glucose self-monitoring. *Diabetologia* 1994; 37: 170–6.
25. Clarke P, Gray A, Adler A, Stevens R, Raikou M, Cull C, Stratton I, Holman R. Cost-effectiveness analysis of intensive blood-glucose control with metformin in overweight patients with type II diabetes (UKPDS No. 51). *Diabetologia* 2001; 44: 298–304.
26. Palmer AJ, Sendi PP, Spinas GA. Applying some UK Prospective Diabetes Study results to Switzerland: the cost-effectiveness of intensive glycaemic control with metformin versus conventional control in overweight patients with type-2 diabetes. *Schweiz Med Wochenschr* 2000; 130: 1034–40.
27. Gray A, Raikou M, McGuire A, Fenn P, Stevens R, Cull C, Stratton I, Adler A, Holman R, Turner R. Cost effectiveness of an intensive blood glucose control policy in patients with type 2 diabetes: economic analysis alongside randomised controlled trial (UKPDS 41). United Kingdom Prospective Diabetes Study Group. *BMJ* 2000; 320: 1373–8.
28. Lamotte M, Annemans L, Lefever A, Nechelput M, Masure J. A health economic model to assess the long-term effects and cost-effectiveness of orlistat in obese type 2 diabetic patients. *Diabetes Care* 2002; 25: 303–8.
29. Jonsson B, Cook JR, Pedersen TR. The cost-effectiveness of lipid lowering in patients with diabetes: results from the 4S trial. *Diabetologia* 1999; 42: 1293–301.
30. UK Prospective Diabetes Study Group. Cost effectiveness analysis of improved blood pressure control in hypertensive patients with type 2 diabetes: UKPDS 40. *BMJ* 1998; 317: 720–6.
31. James M, Turner DA, Broadbent DM, Vora J, Harding SP. Cost effectiveness analysis of screening for sight threatening diabetic eye disease. *BMJ* 2000; 320: 1627–31.
32. Matz H, Falk M, Gottinger W, Kieselbach G. Cost–benefit analysis of diabetic eye disease. *Ophthalmologica* 1996; 210: 348–53.
33. van Os N, Niessen LW, Bilo HJ, Casparie AF, van Hout BA. Diabetes nephropathy in the Netherlands: a cost effectiveness analysis of national clinical guidelines. *Health Policy* 2000; 51: 135–47.
34. Hendry BM, Viberti GC, Hummel S, Bagust A, Piercy J. Modelling and costing the consequences of using an ACE inhibitor to slow the progression of renal failure in type I diabetic patients. *QJM: Int J Med* 1997; 90: 277–82.
35. Garattini L, Brunetti M, Salvioni F, Barosi M. Economic evaluation of ACE inhibitor treatment of nephropathy in patients with insulin-dependent diabetes mellitus in Italy. *Pharmacoeconomics* 1997; 12: 67–75.
36. Van Acker K, Oleen-Burkey M, De Decker L, Vanmaele R, Van Schil P, Matricali G, Dys H, De Leeuw I. Cost and resource utilization for prevention and treatment of foot lesions in a diabetic foot clinic in Belgium. *Diabetes Res Clin Pract* 2000; 50: 87–95.
37. Apelqvist J, Ragnarson-Tennvall G, Larsson J, Persson U. Long-term costs for foot ulcers in diabetic patients in a multidisciplinary setting. *Foot Ankle Int* 1995; 16: 388–94.
38. Ragnarson TG, Apelqvist J. Prevention of diabetes-related foot ulcers and amputations: a cost–utility analysis based on Markov model simulations. *Diabetologia* 2001; 44: 2077–87.
39. Gozzoli V, Palmer AJ, Brandt A, Spinas GA. Economic and clinical impact of alternative disease management strategies for secondary prevention in type 2 diabetes in the Swiss setting. *Swiss Med Wkly* 2001; 131: 303–10.
40. Palmer AJ, Weiss C, Sendi PP, Neeser K, Brandt A, Singh G, Wenzel H, Spinas GA. The cost-effectiveness of different management strategies for type I diabetes: a Swiss perspective. *Diabetologia* 2000; 43: 13–26.
41. Kaplan RM, Atkins CJ, Wilson DK. The cost–utility of diet and exercise interventions in non-insulin-dependent diabetes mellitus. *Health Promot* 1988; 2: 331–340.

110

Economics of Care: The Americas

Thomas J. Songer* **and Alberto Barcelo†**

**University of Pittsburgh, Pittsburgh, PA, USA, and †Pan American Health Organization, Washington, DC, USA*

INTRODUCTION

Economic issues in diabetes care are garnering great attention throughout the world today. This attention has been particularly pronounced in recent years. A look at the published literature in Medline concerning diabetes and economic issues shows that the number of published papers has increased dramatically since the early 1990s (Figure 1). Why is there such an interest right now in the costs of diabetes?

Cost issues in diabetes are of interest now because of three current and significant influences that have long-term implications. The first influence is the recognition that diabetes is a significant disease and one that is increasing. Research in the last 40 years has identified the global incidence of type 1 diabetes and the prevalence of type 2 diabetes. Cohort studies have noted a tremendous morbidity and mortality burden for both conditions. Recently, concern has been expressed about the rising frequency of diabetes [1, 2], and a continued increase projected in the future [3]. Diabetes imposes a particularly high burden on Latin America and the Caribbean where the prevalence of the disease will increase by 82% in the next 25 years [3]. The fact that several countries can now envision an epidemic of diabetes in the near future has led to questions about how they might be able to pay for it all.

The second influence affecting diabetes economics is the advent of several new treatments and intervention strategies in diabetes care. Both pharmaceutical manufacturers and researchers have recognized the emerging epidemic of diabetes as an opportunity for change. Tremendous advances in diabetes research and care have been the result. Starting first with the development of laser photocoagulation, and followed by the results of the Diabetes Control and Complications Trial (DCCT) and several angiotensin-converting enzyme (ACE) inhibitor studies, dramatic changes in the treatment of diabetes are now being recommended. Comprehensive care, which seeks to achieve tight metabolic control and regular screening for complications, is advised. This intensification of treatment translates into a greater use of health care resources by persons with diabetes.

The third influence is not specific to diabetes, but characteristic of the general prevailing winds affecting health care today. It is the worldwide push to implement health care reform. Over the last century, remarkable advances in life expectancy have been observed. As the priorities for health care have shifted from communicable diseases to noncommunicable diseases, expenditures for medical care have risen throughout the world. What is so frustrating to health care payers though, is the seeming inability to contain these rapidly rising health care costs. Health care reform initiatives seek cost containment as an underlying goal.

With rising health care costs and limited health care resources, there has been an expanding focus placed on the economic aspects of health care. Health economic data contribute to the decisions made by authorities and health providers regarding diabetes. In this light, there are a number of health economic approaches relevant to diabetes care [4]. These include (1) *descriptive* approaches, which provide information on the amount of resources that are used in diabetes; (2) *evaluative* approaches, which provide information for decisions regarding the appropriate use

International Textbook of Diabetes Mellitus, Third Edition. Edited by R. A. DeFronzo, E. Ferrannini, H. Keen, and P. Zimmet.
 ISBN: 0-471-48655-8.

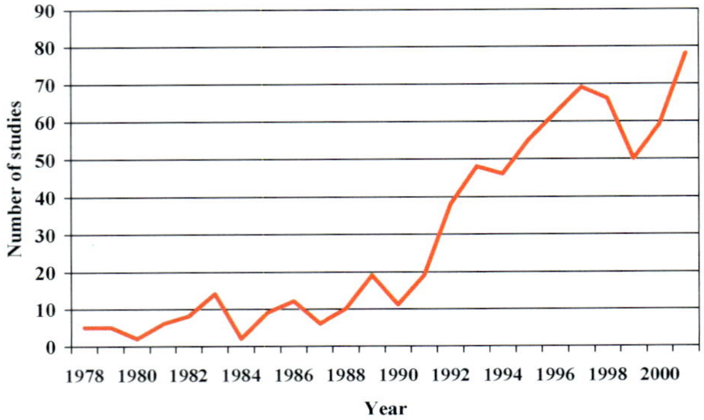

Figure 1 Studies in the published literature on diabetes and economic issues

of diabetes treatments; and (3) *explanatory* approaches, which provide information on the excesses and shortages in diabetes care and the conditions affecting diabetes care behaviors.

The most common exercises applied in the literature have been descriptive studies of the cost of diabetes and evaluative studies of the cost-effectiveness of diabetes interventions. This presentation addresses these two approaches as they have been applied in the Americas. Studies of both the economic costs of diabetes mellitus and the cost-effectiveness of diabetes interventions have been conducted for a number of years in this region. The lessons learned from this work may have extensions to other regions of the world.

THE COSTS OF DIABETES

In economic terms, the costs of diabetes are varied. They include items that one can easily recognize, such as the expenditures related to medical treatment for diabetes or the earnings lost to individuals prematurely disabled. Other less well-known costs exist as well. These include the opportunity costs to individuals with diabetes who forego other activities because they have to devote their financial or time resources to diabetes care. The psychosocial costs of diabetes, such as discrimination, are yet another dimension.

The cost-of-illness framework developed by Dorothy Rice is a common method used to quantify the economic costs of disease [5–8]. Cost-of-illness estimates integrate a variety of endpoints into one aggregate result (quantified in monetary terms), and thus, are often viewed as a comprehensive measure of the burden of a disease. With respect to diabetes, the cost-of-illness framework can describe the resources used in treating or coping with diabetes. These include resources related to hospital care, physician services, drugs, transportation to medical visits, and other items. These costs are often referred to as direct costs.

Indirect costs of diabetes can also be assessed in the cost-of-illness framework. These costs represent the present and future resources lost to individuals and families as a consequence of diabetes. Indirect costs are non-medical costs related to disability, morbidity, and premature mortality. Many debates surround the assessment and valuation of indirect costs [9–12]. The method of assessment of indirect costs, for example, can influence the overall results obtained. However, to date, all cost-of-diabetes studies have used the human capital approach. This method regards individuals as producing output in their lifetime that can be valued as equal to their earnings during that time.

Cost-of-Diabetes Estimates in the United States and Canada

Estimates of the overall economic costs of diabetes mellitus in the United States and Canada are listed in Table 1. The latest figures suggest that the burden of diabetes is quite substantial and growing. In the United States, total cost estimates appear to have risen from \$2.6 billion in 1969 to US\$98.2 billion in 1997 [13–27]. Additional information from Canada shows that the total cost of diabetes approaches US\$5 billion (28).

Several reasons have been cited for the increase noted in the economic costs of diabetes over time. They include the inflation of medical care prices, the increased prevalence of diabetes, the increased utilization of medical services among diabetic patients, and the development of new treatment technologies for diabetes. How much of a role do these factors play in the increases noted? The complete answer to this question is not entirely clear, but a partial answer is available when the estimates for changes in price inflation and the prevalence of diabetes are adjusted over time.

Adjusted estimates of the direct cost of diabetes in the United States (Table 2) show that inflation and the rising prevalence of diabetes contribute greatly to the increase in diabetes costs. In this assessment, direct costs rise from US\$12 billion to US\$44 billion; a more muted effect than seen in Table 1. Relatively small increases in the medical costs of diabetes are noted for the 1970s and 1980s. This observation differs in the estimates provided for the 1990s, where direct costs are markedly higher than previously thought. The jump in direct costs from the 1970s to the 1990s is not likely due to changes in diabetes treatment, but rather due to changes in the methods used to estimate the medical costs of diabetes.

A look at the methods and designs underlying the studies shows that approaches to estimating the cost of diabetes have changed over time [31]. The early studies, for instance, often followed the designs of Rice closely. This method considered diabetes costs as those related to health care visits where diabetes was the primary reason for the

Table 1 Estimates of the economic burden of diabetes in the United States and Canada

Study	Year	Design	Total costs (US$ billion)	Direct cost (%)	Indirect cost (%)
Statistical Bureau of the Metropolitan Life Insurance Company (SBMLIC) [13]	1969	Primary diagnosis data from federal surveys	2.6	38	62
SBMLIC [14]	1973	Primary diagnosis data	4.0	41	59
SBMLIC [14]	1975	Primary diagnosis data	5.3	47	53
SBMLIC [14]	1977	Primary diagnosis data	6.8	50	50
Policy Analysis, Inc. [15]	1977	Lifetime costs from diagnostic category data	10.8	34	66
Platt, Sudover [16]	1979	Cost projections	15.7	36	64
Miller [17]	1979	Diagnostic category data from federal surveys	12.4	60	40
SBMLIC [14]	1980	Primary diagnosis data	9.7	49	51
Smeeding, Booton [18]	1980	Diagnostic category data	18.9	30	53
SBMLIC [14]	1984	Cost projections	13.8	54	46
Huse [19]	1986	Diagnostic category data	19.8	59	41
Pracon, Inc. [20]	1987	Diagnostic category data	20.4	47	53
Roesler [21] (Minnesota)	1988	Estimates from national study applied to Minnesota	0.30	63	37
Kegler [22] (North Carolina)	1990	Diagnostic category data	1.24	46	54
Warner [23] (Texas)	1992	Principle diagnosis data and state survey data	4.0	40	60
American Diabetes Association (ADA) [24]	1992	Diagnostic category data	91.8	49	51
Thom [25]	1993	Primary diagnosis data	20	75	25
NIH/NIDDK [26]	1995	Cost projections	137.7	66	34
ADA [27]	1997	Diagnostic category data	98.2	45	55
Dawson [28]	1998	Diagnostic category data	4.76	73	27

visit. This assumption has been criticized as underestimating the impact of diabetes, particularly for individuals with complications. It is well known, for example, that diabetes is a leading cause of blindness, renal failure, and heart disease. Health events where diabetes is the underlying cause, but not the primary cause, are not included in estimates based upon this approach. Later studies in the 1990s diverged from this primary reason for a visit

Table 2 The direct costs of diabetes in the United States, 1969–1997, adjusted for inflation and diabetes prevalence

Study	Year	As reported (US$ billion)	Adjusted for inflation and diabetes prevalence (US$ billion – 1997)
SBMLIC	1969	1.00	12.04
SBMLIC	1973	1.65	13.28
SBMLIC	1975	2.52	15.04
SBMLIC	1977	3.40	16.53
Policy Analysis, Inc.	1977	10.80	52.52
Platt, Sudover	1979	5.64	22.01
Miller	1979	7.46	29.09
SBMLIC	1980	4.80	18.73
Smeeding, Booton	1980	5.66	20.28
SBMLIC	1984	7.43	18.81
Pracon, Inc.	1987	9.60	20.24
Rubin [29]	1992	85.71	134.19
ADA	1992	45.22	70.80
Thom	1993	15.10	23.04
Hodgson [30]	1995	47.87	56.93
ADA	1997	44.14	44.14

Note: US-based cost-of-illness estimates were adjusted to 1997 US dollars using the change in GDP deflator over time. Differences in prevalence were adjusted by considering the ratios of the prevalence of diabetes in 1997 to that in each study year.

Table 3 Studies showing the cost of diabetes in Latin America and the Caribbean

			Direct cost		Indirect cost	
Study, country	Year	Total cost	US$ million	%	US$ million	%
Phillips and Salmeron [32], Mexico	1992	US$429 936 000	330	77	99.936	23
White et al. [33], Chile	1998	US$1 000 000 000	319	29	792	71
Villareal-Ríos et al. [34], Mexico	2000	—	2 618 000	—	—	—
Barceló et al. [35], 23 countries	2000	US$65 216 500 000	10 720.1	16	54 495.9	84

standard. Researchers applied the epidemiologic concept of attributable risk to estimate costs related to diabetes complications. Attributable risk methods seek to identify the relative contribution that diabetes makes to the overall risk of the disorder. Studies using attributable risk methods have produced larger and more accurate estimates for the burden of diabetes.

Cost-of-Illness Studies in Latin America and the Caribbean

Information on the cost of diabetes in Latin America and the Caribbean is scarce. Few cost-of-illness studies exist in the region for diabetes, and all of them used the human capital approach in estimating cost. Table 3 provides information on the cost of diabetes in Latin America and the Caribbean. In 1992, Phillips and Salmerón reported on the cost of diabetes in Mexico [32]. The total cost of diabetes was estimated at US$430 million ($100 million in direct cost and US$330 million in indirect cost). They estimated that approximately three quarters of the government expenditures in health were dedicated to diabetes. Direct cost per person with known diabetes was US$450. This top–down study was based on a prevalence of diabetes of 1.2%, which was lower than the national estimate of 7.2% (5.2% diagnosed diabetes) [36].

In 1998, a cost-of-illness study conducted by the Pan American Health Organization estimated the total cost of diabetes in Chile at US$1000 million [33]. This exercise was done during an intervention program involving three clinics in Chile. A top-bottom approach was used to estimate cost. The contribution of indirect and direct costs was 71 and 29% respectively. This study considered only loss of work days due to temporary disability as indirect cost and did not include mortality and permanent disability.

In 2000, Villareal-Ríos et al. published a study estimating the total direct cost of diabetes mellitus in Mexico at US$2.6 billion [34]. This represented around 16% of the health budget and 0.8% of the gross domestic product (GDP) of Mexico. The cost per case was calculated at US$708. They also reported that among the services for people with diabetes, dialysis was the most expensive, which suggested that nephropathy may be one of the leading costly complications of diabetes.

A recent study analyzed the cost of diabetes in 23 countries of Latin America and the Caribbean in 2000 [35] (Table 4). The estimated prevalence of diabetes in included countries was 15.2 million people, of whom 726 575 were estimated to be permanently disabled. Mortality among those with diabetes was estimated at 330 035 (242 168 were estimated to be due to diabetes). The number of consultations and hospitalizations directly related to diabetes were estimated at 965 500 and 35 552 200 respectively. The study of the cost of diabetes in Latin America and the Caribbean included indirect cost caused by forgone earnings because of premature mortality and temporary and permanent disability (Figure 2). Even assuming a conservative 5% of permanently disabled people with diabetes the cost of lifetime forgone earnings was estimated at more than US$50 billion. Temporary disability and premature mortality contributed with US$3 billion and US$763 million respectively.

It has been estimated previously that the annual direct cost of diabetes in Latin America and the Caribbean would be around US$3 billion or US$353 per person [37]. This estimation assumed that 6% of the health budget of the region was allocated to diabetes. Estimations from Mexico placed the proportion of the health budget dedicated to diabetes at 16% [34]. More recent estimates placed the total cost of diabetes at US$65 billion. Only 16% of this was attributed to direct cost (Figure 3).

There is a contrast when comparing diabetes cost studies in the United States and in Latin America and the Caribbean. Direct cost represented only an estimated 16% of the total cost of diabetes in Latin America and the Caribbean, while it represented almost 45% of the total cost in the United States [27]. Direct cost in the United States accounted for a total of US$44.1 billion ($10 071 *per capita*), which is extremely high when compared with the one estimated for Latin America and the Caribbean at US$10.7 billion (only US$703 *per capita*, less than 1% of the cost in the United States) [35]. The major contributors to direct costs in Latin America and the Caribbean were oral medication with US$2.8 billion (27%), treatment of complications US$2.5 billion (23%), physician consultations US$2.5 billion (23%), insulin US$1.9 billion (18%), and hospitalizations US$1 billion (9%) (Figure 4).

Table 4 Estimated total indirect and direct cost (in US$ million) attributed to diabetes, per capita direct cost and per capita health expenditures by country in the Americas

Country	Total cost	Indirect cost	Direct cost	Per capita direct cost*	Per capita health expenditures*,†	Excess cost of diabetes (%)
North America						
Canada‡	4 756	1 277	3 478	1 745	2 185.4	80
United States of America	98 152	54 014	44 138	10 071	4 432.7	227
Mexico	15 118.3	13 144.1	1 974.2	528	221	239
Subtotal	118 026	68 435	49 590	4 115	2 280	180
Caribbean (Spanish)						
Cuba	1 346.6	624.4	722.2	1 219	139	877
Dominican Republic	625.1	399.4	225.7	888	112	793
Haiti	78.7	30.7	48.0	604	24	2 517
Subtotal	2 050.7	1 054.8	995.9	1 076	92	1 174
Caribbean (English)						
Bahamas	148.8	138.1	10.7	835	664	126
Barbados	151.2	138.4	12.8	551	506	109
Guyana	36.3	15.9	20.4	719	33	2 179
Jamaica	409.5	273.4	136.1	750	146	514
Trinidad/Tobago	284.5	246.5	38.0	533	162	329
Subtotal	1 030.5	812.4	218.1	687	302	227
Central America						
Costa Rica	473.2	376.6	96.6	624	285	219
El Salvador	499.5	362.1	137.4	626	161	389
Guatemala	840.8	549.6	291.2	790	94	840
Honduras	239.7	125.9	113.8	590	59	1 000
Nicaragua	128.8	43.8	85.0	624	41	1 522
Panama	434.7	330.3	104.4	866	354	245
Subtotal	2 616.4	1 788.1	828.3	695	166	420
South America						
Argentina	10 935.3	10 188.3	747.0	597	882	68
Bolivia	227.8	142.3	85.5	555	53	1 047
Brazil	22 603.8	18 651.5	3 952.3	872	270	323
Chile	2 417.9	2 122.9	295.0	594	449	132
Colombia	2 586.8	2 171.9	414.9	442	209	211
Ecuador	598.5	365.1	233.4	873	65	1 343
Paraguay	218.0	146.0	72.0	779	165	472
Peru	1 844.1	1 341.7	502.4	828	117	708
Uruguay	774.9	680.3	94.6	795	697	114
Venezuela	2 139.7	1 886.2	307.5	503	304	165
Subtotal	44 400.0	37 696.5	6 704.6	739	321	230
Total	168 071	109 787	58 337	1 448	632	633

* In US$.
† From reference 27 (United States), 28 (Canada), and 35 (Latin America and the Caribbean).
‡ Cost per case calculated with data from Dawson and an estimated prevalence of 3.4%.

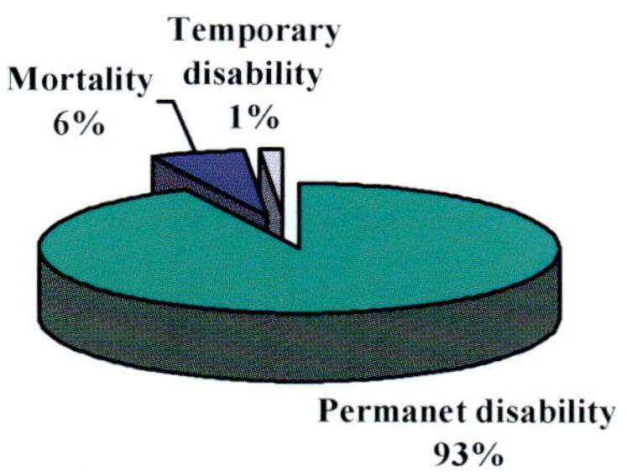

Figure 2 Indirect cost of diabetes in Latin America and the Caribbean in 2000

Indirect Costs in Diabetes

Several studies have included estimates of both direct and indirect costs in their cost-of-illness designs. In the United States (Table 1), there is a general trend for indirect costs to make up a slightly larger proportion of the total costs than direct costs. In Latin America and the Caribbean, the overall contribution of the indirect costs was 65% and 35% from direct cost [35]. The proportion of indirect and direct costs varied somewhat among countries in this region: the lowest proportion of direct cost was found in Argentina (7%) and the highest in Nicaragua (66%).

In general, a large impact for indirect costs is not unexpected. In Latin America and the Caribbean, it has been

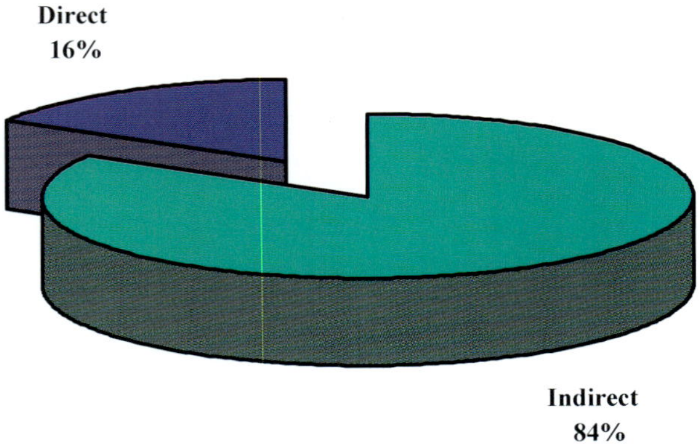

Figure 3 The cost of diabetes in Latin America and the Caribbean in 2000

demonstrated that the people with diabetes are 1.5 times less frequently employed (36% vs. 56%), 1.8 times less likely to achieve a technical or university degree (7.8% vs. 13.8%), and 2.6 times more frequently permanently disabled (8% vs. 3%) [38]. Recent reports for the United States show higher rates of disability and employment in the diabetes population [39–41], with markedly reduced earnings. The relationship of direct and indirect costs to total costs, however, is often influenced by the cost components included in the estimates. The recent estimates for Canada, for example, considered only the impact of premature mortality and did not include the effects of disability [28].

Estimates of the Cost of Diabetes Complications

As new treatment strategies and interventions are coming into place for the various complications of diabetes, there is now further interest in quantifying the costs related to specific complications. Our current understanding of the economic costs of diabetic complications, though, is incomplete. Despite a wide range of cost-of-diabetes studies, there have been relatively few reports on the burden of specific complications [42].

Three general trends emerge from the existing reports. First, data show that the late stage complications of diabetes are more costly than the early stage complications

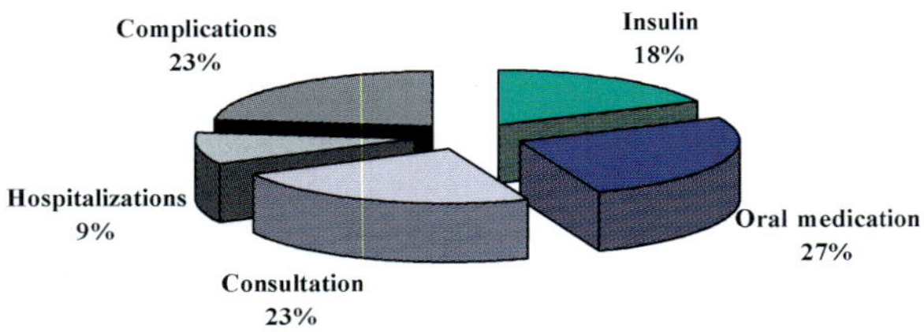

Figure 4 Direct cost of diabetes in Latin America and the Caribbean in 2000

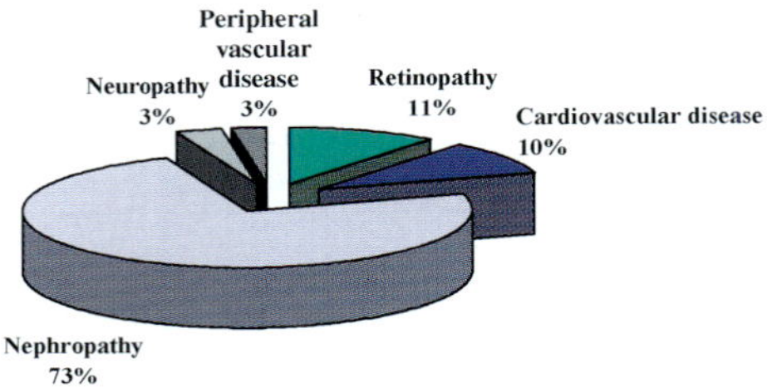

Figure 5 The cost of diabetes complications in Latin America and the Caribbean

[43]. Myocardial infarction ($27 630 per event) and end-stage renal disease ($53 659 per event), for example, are expensive conditions. In Argentina, research has shown that diabetes complications caused an excess loss of work days when comparing people with and without diabetes [44].

Second, the cost of care is generally higher in those with complications compared to those without complications. An interesting illustration is the work of Ramsey et al. [45], which compared subjects with and without diabetes over 3 years. In persons without complications, the annual cost of care for a person with diabetes was roughly 1.6 times greater than that in a person without diabetes. The ratio of the cost of care increased when complications were present (3–4 times higher for macrovascular disease, end-stage renal disease, and foot ulcer; 2–3 times higher for eye disease). Third, cardiovascular disease appears to account for the largest impact with respect to the burden of diabetes complications [45–49] in the United States and Canada. Both Jacobs [46] and Caro [47] noted that the costs of care for macrovascular disease account for more than one half of the cost of complications. Diabetic nephropathy accounts for the largest burden in Latin America and the Caribbean (Figure 5).

Estimates of the *Per Capita* Cost of Diabetes

A common question that arises in any discussion of the cost of diabetes relates to identifying the burden of diabetes on a patient basis. In Latin America and the Caribbean, Henry-Lee et al. estimated the individual cost of diabetes care in Jamaica at US$571 in 2000 [50]. In Argentina, Gagliardino et al. estimated the cost of diabetes care at US$1221 and US$330 for people with type 1 and type 2 diabetes, respectively in 1993 [37]. The Ministry of Health in Mexico estimated in 2002 that diabetes care would cost an average of between US$339 and US$1188 among those with diabetes without and with long-term complications respectively [36].

Assessments of the *per capita* (per person) medical costs of diabetes indicate that persons with diabetes account for more medical expenditures than do persons without diabetes. The most widely attributed figure for

Table 5 Annual medical costs for people with and without diabetes and excess cost of persons with diabetes, per person, in 1997 US dollars

Study	Year	Ratio of costs for diabetic to nondiabetic patients
Rubin [29]	1994	3.6
ADA [27]	1998	3.8
Selby [52]	1997	2.4
Brown [53]	1999	2.2
Jacob [54]	2000	2.1

this originates from Rubin et al. [29], who reported that health care expenditures among persons with diabetes account for one in seven of all the health care dollars spent in the United States. The cost of diabetes care in most countries of Latin America and the Caribbean is higher than the countries' investment in health.

In countries where services are not covered or are poorly covered by the national or government financed health services, people with diabetes face very high out of pocket expenses. Songer et al. [51] found higher out of pocket health care costs in families with type 1 diabetic children than in families having no diabetic children. In Jamaica, a study found that 57% of interviewed people with diabetes experienced financial difficulties because of the cost of health care and 50% of them reportedly avoided some medical treatment because of economic constraints [50].

Table 5 presents a summary of available studies [27, 29, 52–54] that outline the ratio of *per capita* expenses between persons with and without diabetes in the United States and Canada. Identified ratios vary from 2 to 5 times higher costs in persons with diabetes. Excess costs among persons with diabetes also differ by age, with higher excess costs more often identified in younger age groups.

In the Americas, *per capita* diabetes care cost was the highest in the United States ($10 071) and the lowest in Colombia ($442) [35]. The average *per capita* expenditure on health (latest available figures) in the region was US$604 while the average cost of care per person with diabetes was US$1482, and it was the lowest in Haiti ($24) and the highest in United States ($4432). In general, diabetes care cost was more than 400% higher than the average health expenditures in the Americas, and ranged from 68% in Argentina to 2517% in Haiti. The cost of medical diabetes care in the United States greatly influenced the average cost found in the region.

COST-EFFECTIVENESS ANALYSIS IN DIABETES CARE

A recent and rising practice in diabetes economics has been the use of cost-effectiveness studies to evaluate the economic efficiency of diabetes treatments and interventions. A cost-effectiveness analysis generally summarizes the impact of an intervention by characterizing the cost of the intervention relative to the health outcomes obtained (i.e. cost per number of lives saved) [55]. This evaluation assumes from the beginning that society has determined that doing something about treatment of diabetes is worth pursuing. The policy decision here is whether a new intervention is better able to meet a health care goal than the existing standard of care. The goal may be to maximize benefits for a given level of resources. Or, it may be to attain the greatest level of benefits for the least cost.

A current example of the role of cost-effectiveness analysis is the advocacy for intensive diabetes management regimens. This resource intensive practice raises several questions in light of the current emphasis on cost containment and the recognition that the number of people with diabetes will double in the next 25 years. Does the aggressive treatment of persons with diabetes represent value for money? We know that the aggressive management of diabetes likely will have several significant health benefits, but the underlying question is whether these benefits can be obtained at a reasonable cost.

Several cost-effectiveness studies have now been conducted to evaluate the economic efficiency of diabetes-related services and interventions [56–79]. Table 6 illustrates a sample of the studies undertaken in the United States and Canada. The first studies focused on the evaluation of strategies for identifying and treating diabetes complications. A large number of reports suggest that screening for and treating diabetes retinopathy and macular edema is extremely cost-effective, and in most situations it saves money [57–59, 63, 66, 77, 79]. A similar finding of cost savings is observed for interventions that reduce problems related to diabetes and pregnancy [60, 62]. Subsequent investigations focused on identifying the value of screening for microalbuminuria and the impact of treating diabetic nephropathy with ACE inhibitors [61, 64, 68, 69, 73, 74]. General indications here are that screening and treatment with ACE inhibitors would be beneficial and cost-efficient. That is, for a small amount of money, you will get a much improved health benefit. One report [68] even suggests cost savings for treatment with ACE inhibitors.

With the landmark results of two major clinical trials, the DCCT and the UKPDS (United Kingdom Prospective Diabetes Study), an additional economic question of interest is whether the intensive treatment of diabetes is cost-effective. Considering the costs and benefits that would be expected to occur over the lifetime of a cohort with type 1 diabetes, the DCCT investigators [65] found that the average costs associated with intensive treatment were considerably higher ($99 822 vs. US$66 076) than those for conventional treatment. However, the expected benefits were much greater with the intensive group. Overall, intensive therapy cost an additional US$19 987 per

Table 6 Cost-effectiveness ratios of diabetes care interventions in North America

Study	Year	Issue examined	Issue ratio
Kaplan [56]	1987	Diet and exercise intervention in type 2 diabetes	US$10 870 per well year gained
Javitt [57]	1989	Treatment and control of diabetic retinopathy in type 1 diabetes patients	US$966 per sight year saved
Javitt [58]	1990	Screening strategies for detecting retinopathy in type 1 diabetes patients	Cost savings
Dasbach [59]	1991	Screening and treatment strategies for retinopathy	Cost savings (type 1 diabetes)
Scheffler [60]	1992	Diabetes pregnancy intervention program	Cost savings
Siegel [61]	1992	Screening strategies for early renal disease and treatment with ACE inhibitors in type 1 diabetes	US$16 500 per life year saved
Elixhauser [62]	1993	Preconception care for diabetic women	Cost savings
Javitt [63]	1994	Screening and treatment for eye disease in type 2 diabetes	Cost savings
Kiberd [64]	1995	Screening and treatment for diabetic renal disease in type 1 diabetes	US$27 041 per QALY gained
DCCT [65]	1996	Intensive insulin treatment in type 1 diabetes	US$19 000 per QALY gained
Javitt [66]	1996	Screening and treatment for diabetic eye disease type 2 diabetes	US$3190 per QALY gained
Eastman [67]	1997	Intensive treatment in type 2 diabetes to attain normoglycemia	US$16 002 per QALY gained
Rodby [68]	1996	Treatment with ACE inhibitors to prevent nephropathy in type 1 diabetes	Cost savings
Douzdjian [70]	1998	Treatment strategies for diabetic subjects with end-stage renal disease	US$102 422–317 746 per QALY gained
CDC [72]	1998	Screening for type 2 diabetes	US$56 649 per QALY gained
Golan [73]	1999	Treating all type 2 diabetes patients with ACE inhibitors	US$7500 per QALY gained
Clark [74]	2000	ACE inhibitor treatment in type 1 diabetes	Cost savings
Vijan [75]	2000	Timing of screening interval for retinopathy in type 2 diabetes	US$49 760–US$107 510 per QALY gained
Elliott [76]	2000	Treatment to lower blood pressure to <130/85 mmHg	Cost savings
Sharma [77]	2000	Grid laser therapy for diabetic macular edema	US$3101 per QALY gained
CDC [78]	2002	Assessment of various treatment strategies in type 2 diabetes	
		• intensive glycemic control	US$41 384 per QALY gained
		• controlling blood pressure	Cost savings
		• reducing serum cholesterol	US$51 889 per QALY gained

Note: QALY = quality-adjusted life year.

quality-adjusted life year gained. The investigators concluded, and most agree, that intensive treatment in this situation is a cost-effective intervention. A second study by Eastman and colleagues [67] addressed the costs and benefits of intensive treatment in type 2 diabetes. In this work, it was estimated that an intervention that seeks to maintain normoglycemia (an HbA_{1c} of 7.2%) would cost an additional US$16 000 for each quality-adjusted life year gained.

Several treatment strategies in diabetes care have not yet received a full economic evaluation, and other areas, such as strategies to reduce lower extremity amputation, have conflicting results. Klonoff and Schwartz [79] reviews the literature and finds that many fundamental treatment strategies, including diabetes education, self-monitoring of blood glucose in type 2 diabetes, dietary counseling, and weight loss, among others, have an unclear economic benefit. Emerging work may, however, address the impact of weight loss and exercise as the results of the Diabetes Prevention Program study come to light.

Studies on the cost-effectiveness of diabetes care in Latin America and the Caribbean are scarce. A multicenter intervention in 10 countries demonstrated that an educational program can reduce the cost of drugs by 62% [33]. The program was implemented in centers of Argentina, Bolivia, Brazil, Chile, Colombia, Costa Rica, Cuba, Mexico, Paraguay, and Uruguay and coordinated by CENEXA (Centro de Endocrinologa Experimental y Aplicada), a WHO–PAHO collaborating center in Argentina. In another program also coordinated by CENEXA, results from 297 enrolled patients showed a reduction of 38% in diabetes-related cost.

FUTURE NEEDS

What are the future needs of economic research in diabetes care? As the field of diabetes economics is relatively new, there are several additional needs that can be identified. While it seems clear that the economic impact of diabetes in the Americas is quite extensive, it remains difficult to compare studies to establish accurate data on trends over time. There is a need to develop standard methods for addressing the cost of diabetes. Comparisons of costs or the distribution of costs between countries, for example, could provide clues about the possible advantages and disadvantages of alternative health care strategies. Further, the rationale behind economic reports and the methods applied therein should be clear and meaningful.

There is a need for incidence-based cost of diabetes and cost-of-complication estimates. Most of the existing work follows a prevalence-based model. However, incidence-based figures can give an indication of the costs that can be saved if the cases of diabetes or diabetes complications can be prevented. In addition, there remains a strong need to consider costs from the perspective of the individual and family. Many previous studies have considered costs and benefits from the standpoint of the country or a health care payer. Many organizations, though, may be more understanding, knowledgeable, and interested in diabetes care issues if they can see how diabetes directly affects the individual.

Examining the economic impact of diabetes and diabetes care can be a complex task, but does not have to be an educated guess. There are many possibilities in this sector that have been developed. These need to be further refined. There are other possibilities in this sector that should be developed. These need to be further explored.

REFERENCES

1. Harris MI, Eastman RC. Early detection of undiagnosed diabetes mellitus: a US perspective. *Diabetes Metab Res Rev* 2000; 16: 230–6.
2. Dokheel TM, for the Pittsburgh Diabetes Epidemiology Research Group. An epidemic of childhood diabetes in the United States? Evidence from Allegheny County, Pennsylvania. *Diabetes Care* 1993; 16 (12): 1606–11.
3. King H, Aubert RE, Herman WH. Global burden of diabetes, 1995–2025: prevalence, numerical estimates, and projections. *Diabetes Care* 1998; 21 (9): 1414–31.
4. Songer TJ. The economic costs of NIDDM. *Diabetes Metab Rev* 1992; 8 (4): 389–404.
5. Rice DP. *Estimating the Cost of Illness*. Washington, DC: US Government Printing Office, 1966. Health Economic Series No. 6, PHS publication No. 947-6.
6. Cooper BS, Rice DP. The economic cost of illness revisited. *Soc Secur Bull* 1976; 39 (2): 21–36.
7. Rice DP, Hodgson TA, Kopstein AN. The economic costs of illness: a replication and update. *Health Care Financ Rev Fall* 1985; 7: 61–80.
8. Hodgson TA, Meiners MR. Cost-of-Illness methodology: a guide to current practices and procedures. *Milbank Mem Fund Q* 1982; 60: 429–62.
9. Lubeck DP, Yelin EH. A question of value: measuring the impact of chronic disease. *Milbank Q* 1988; 66: 445–64.
10. Gold MR, Siegel JE, Russell LB, Weinstein MC. (eds) *Cost-Effectiveness in Health and Medicine*. New York: Oxford University Press, 1996.
11. Brouwer WB, Koopmanschap MA, Rutten FF. Productivity costs measurement through quality of life? A response to the recommendations of the Washington Panel. *Health Econ* 1997; 6: 253–59.
12. Weinstein MC, Siegel JE, Garber AM, Lipscomb J, Luce BR, Manning WG Jr, Torrance GW. Productivity costs, time costs and health-related quality of life: a response to the Erasmus Group. *Health Econ* 1997; 6: 505–10.
13. Entmacher PS. *Report of Economic Impact of Diabetes*. Washington, DC: US Government Printing Office, 1976. NIH publication no 76-1022, Vol 3, Part 2.
14. Entmacher PS, Sinnock P, Bostic E, Harris MI. The economic impact of diabetes. In Diabetes in America. National Diabetes Data Group, Diabetes Data Compiled 1984. Washington, DC: US Government Printing Office, 1985. NIH publication no 85-1468.
15. Policy Analysis, Inc. *Evaluation of Cost of Illness Ascertainment Methodology, Part II. Applications of Methodology to Ascertain Lifetime Economic Costs of Illness in an Incidence Cohort*. Final Report to the National Center for Health Statistics. DHHS Contract No. 233-79-2048. December 1981.
16. Platt WG, Sudover SG. *The Social and Economic Costs of Diabetes: An Estimate for 1979*. Elkhart, IN: Home Health Care Group, Ames Division, Miles Laboratories, Inc., 1983.
17. Miller LV. Socioeconomic impact of diabetes mellitus. In Brodoff BN, Bleicher SJ (eds) *Diabetes Mellitus and Obesity*. Baltimore: Williams & Wilkins, 1982; pp 799–803.
18. Smeeding TM, Booton LA. Measuring and valuing the economic benefits of diabetes control. In *Nineteenth National Public Health Conference on Records and Statistics*, August 1983. Hyattsville, MD: National Center for Health Statistics, 1983. DHHS publication no. (PHS) 81–1214.
19. Huse DM, Oster G, Killen AR, et al. The economic costs of non-insulin-dependent diabetes mellitus. *JAMA* 1989; 262: 2708–13.
20. Pracon, Inc. *Direct and Indirect Costs of Diabetes in the United States in 1987*. Alexandria, VA: American Diabetes Association, 1988.
21. Roesler J, Bishop D, Walseth J. Economic cost of diabetes mellitus Minnesota, 1988. *MMWR Morb Mortal Wkly Rep* 1991; 40: 229–31.
22. Kegler MC, Lengerich EJ, Norman M, et al. The burden of diabetes in North Carolina. *N C Med J* 1995; 56: 141–4.
23. Warner DC, McCandless RR, De Nino LA, et al. Cost of diabetes in Texas, 1992. *Diabetes Care* 1996; 19: 1416–9.
24. American Diabetes Association. *Direct and Indirect Costs of Diabetes in the United States in 1992*. Alexandria, VA: American Diabetes Association, 1993.
25. Thom TJ. Economic costs of neoplasms, arteriosclerosis, and diabetes in the United States. *In Vivo* 1996; 10: 255–60.
26. National Institutes of Health. *Disease-specific Estimates of Direct and Indirect Costs* of Illness and NIH support. Bethesda, MD: NIH, November 1995.
27. American Diabetes Association. Economic consequences of diabetes mellitus in the U.S. in 1997. *Diabetes Care* 1998; 21: 296–309.
28. Dawson KG, Gomes D, Gerstein H, Blanchard JF, Kahler KH. The economic costs of diabetes in Canada, 1998. *Diabetes Care* 2002; 25 (8): 1303–7.
29. Rubin RJ, Altman WM, Mendelson DN. Health care expenses for people with diabetes mellitus, 1992. *J Clin Endocrinol Metab* 1994; 78: 809A–F.
30. Hodgson TA, Cohen AJ. Medical care expenditures for diabetes, its chronic complications, and its comorbidities. *Prev Med* 1999; 29: 173–86.
31. Songer TJ, Ettaro L. *Studies on the Cost of Diabetes*. Atlanta, GA: Division of Diabetes Translation, Centers for Disease Control & Prevention, 1998. Available at: http://www.cdc.gov/diabetes/pubs/costs/. Accessed June 2003.
32. Phillips M, Salmerón J. Diabetes in Mexico— a serious and growing problem. *World Health Stat Q* 1992; 45 (4): 338–46.
33. White F, Vega J, Aedo C, Jadue L, Robles S, Salazar R, Delgado I. *Proyecto de demostración en educación en*

diabetes. Informe Final. Eli Lilly: Organización Pan Americana de la Salud, 1998.

34. Villareal-Ríos E, Salinas-Martinez AM, Medina-Jáuregui A, Garza-Elizondo ME, Nuñez-Rocha G and Chuy-Díaz ER. The cost of diabetes mellitus and its impact on the health spending in Mexico. *Arch Med Res* 2000; 31: 511–14.
35. Barceló A, Aedo C, Rajpathak S, Robles S. The cost of diabetes in Latin America and the Caribbean. *WHO Bull* 2003; 81 (1): 19–27.
36. Secretaria de Salud de México. Subsecretaria de Prevención y Protección de la Salud. Información Nacional sobre Diabetes. Ciudad Mexico, 2002.
37. Gagliardino J, Oliviera E. Latin America. In Gruber W, Lander T, Leese B, Songer T, Williams R (eds) *The Economics of Diabetes in Latin America. A Report of the Diabetes Health Economics Study Group*. Brussels, Belgium: International Diabetes Federation and World Health Organization.
38. Morice A et al. *Diabetes Mellitus en Costa Rica: Un análisis interdiciplinario*. Tres Rios: Costa Rica: Instituto de Investigación y Enseñanza en Nutrición y Salud, 1999.
39. Mayfield JA, Deb P, Whitecotton L. Work disability and diabetes. *Diabetes Care* 1999; 22 (7): 1105–9.
40. Ng YC, Jacobs P, Johnson JA. Productivity losses associated with diabetes in the US. *Diabetes Care* 2001; 24 (2): 257–61.
41. Valdmanis V, Smith DW, Page MR. Productivity and economic burden associated with diabetes. *Am J Public Health* 2001; 91: 129–30.
42. Summers K, Songer TJ. Cost of diabetes-related complications; current issues, future directions. *Expert Rev Pharmacoeconomics Outcomes Res* 2003; 3(1): 89–96.
43. O'Brien JA, Shomphe LA, Kavanagh PL, Raggio G, Caro JJ. Direct medical costs of complications resulting from type 2 diabetes in the US. *Diabetes Care* 1998; 21(7): 1122–8.
44. Olivera E, Duhalde E, Gagliardino JJ. Costs of temporary and permanent disability induced by diabetes. *Diabetes Care* 1991; 14 (7): 593–6.
45. Ramsey SD, Newton K, Blough D, McCullough DK, Sandhu N, Wagner EH. Patient-level estimates of the cost of complications in diabetes in a managed care population. *PharmacoEconomics* 1999; 16 (3): 285–95.
46. Jacobs J, Sena M, Fox N. The cost of hospitalization for the late complications of diabetes in the United States. *Diabet Med* 1991; 8 (suppl): S23–9.
47. Caro JJ, Ward AJ, O'Brien JA. Lifetime costs of complications resulting from type 2 diabetes in the US. *Diabetes Care* 2002; 25 (3): 476–81.
48. Brown JB, Nichols GA, Glauber HS, Bakst A. Ten-year follow-up of antidiabetic drug use, nonadherence, and mortality in a defined population with type 2 diabetes mellitus. *Clin Ther* 1999; 21: 1045–57.
49. Nichols GA, Brown JB. The impact of cardiovascular disease on medical care costs in subjects with and without type 2 diabetes. *Diabetes Care* 2002; 25: 482–6.
50. Henry-Lee A, Yearwood A. Protecting the poor and the medically indigent under health insurance: a case study in Jamaica. Small Applied Research No. 6. Partnership for Health Reform Project. Bethesda, MD: Abt Associate Inc, April 1999.
51. Songer TJ, LaPorte R, Lave JR, Dorman JS, Becker DJ. Health insurance and the financial impact of IDDM in families with a child with IDDM. *Diabetes Care* 1997; 20 (4): 577–84.
52. Selby JV, Ray GT, Zhang D, Colby CJ: Excess costs of medical care for patients with diabetes in a managed care population. *Diabetes Care* 1997; 20: 1396–402.
53. Brown, BJ, Glauber SH, Nichols AG, Bakst WA. Type 2 diabetes: incremental medical care costs during the first 8 years after diagnosis. *Diabetes Care* 1999; 22: 1116–24.
54. Jacobs, P, Blanchard JF, James RC, Depew N. Excess costs of diabetes in aboriginal population of Manitoba, Canada. *Can J Public Health* 2000; 91: 298–301.
55. Drummond MF, Stoddart GL. Principles of economic evaluation of health programs. *World Health Stat Q* 1985; 38: 355–76.
56. Kaplan RM, Hartwell SL, Wilson DK, Wallace JP. Effects of diet and exercise interventions on control and quality of life in non-insulin-dependent diabetes mellitus. *J Gen Intern Med* 1987; 2: 220–8.
57. Javitt JC, Canner JK, Sommer A. Cost-effectiveness of current approaches to the control of retinopathy in type I diabetics. *Ophthalmology* 1989; 96: 255–64.
58. Javitt JC, Canner JK, Frank RG, Steinwachs DM, Sommer A. Detecting and treating retinopathy in patients with type 1 diabetes mellitus; a health policy model. *Ophthalmology* 1990; 97: 483–95.
59. Dasbach EJ, Fryback DG, Newcomb PA, Klein R, Klein BEK. Cost-effectiveness of strategies for detecting diabetic retinopathy. *Med Care* 1991; 29: 20–39.
60. Scheffler RM, Feuchtbaum LB, Phibbs CS. Prevention: the cost-effectiveness of the California diabetes and pregnancy program. *Am J Public Health* 1992; 82: 168–75.
61. Siegel JE, Krolewski AS, Warram JH, Weinstein MC. Cost-effectiveness of screening and early treatment of nephropathy in patients with IDDM. *J Am Soc Nephrol* 1992; 3: S111–9.
62. Elixhauser A, Weschler JM, Kitzmiller JL, Marks JS, Bennert Jr, HW, Coustan DR, Gabbe SG, Herman WH, Kaufmann RC, Ogata ES, Sepe SJ. Cost–benefit analysis of preconception care for women with established diabetes mellitus. *Diabetes Care* 1993; 16 (8): 1146–57.
63. Javitt JC, Ferris FL, Aiello LP, Canner JK, Chiang YP, Greenfield S. Preventive eye care in people with diabetes is cost saving to the federal government: implications for health care reform. *Diabetes Care* 1994; 17 (8): 909–17.
64. Kiberd BA, Jindal KK. Screening to prevent renal failure in insulin dependent diabetic patients; an economic evaluation. *BMJ* 1995; 311: 1595–99.
65. The Diabetes Control and Complications Trial (DCCT) Research Group. Lifetime benefits and costs of intensive therapy as practiced in the DCCT. *JAMA* 1996; 276: 1409–15.
66. Javitt JC, Aiello LP. Cost-effectiveness of detecting and treating diabetic retinopathy. *Ann Intern Med* 1996; 124: 164–9.
67. Eastman RC, Javitt JC, Herman WH, et al. Model of complications of NIDDM. Analysis of health benefits and cost-effectiveness of treating NIDDM with the goal of normoglycemia. *Diabetes Care* 1997; 20: 735–44.
68. Rodby RA, Firth LM, Lewis EJ. An economic analysis of captopril in the treatment of diabetic nephropathy. *Diabetes Care* 1996; 19: 1051–61.
69. Kiberd BA, Jindal KK. Routine treatment of insulin-dependent diabetic patients with ACE inhibitors to

prevent renal failure: an economic evaluation. *Am J Kidney Dis* 1998; 31: 49–54.
70. Douzdjian V, Ferrara D, Silvestri G. Treatment strategies for insulin-dependent diabetics with ESRD: a cost-effectiveness decision analysis model. *Am J Kidney Dis* 1998; 31: 794–802.
71. Ollendorf DA, Kotsanos JG, Wishner WJ, Firedman M, Cooper T, Bittoni M, Oster G. Potential economic benefits of lower extremity amputation prevention strategies in diabetes. *Diabetes Care* 1998; 21: 1240–5.
72. CDC Diabetes Cost-Effectiveness Study Group. The cost-effectiveness of screening for type 2 diabetes. *JAMA* 1998; 280: 1757–63.
73. Golan L, Birkmeyer JD, Welch HG. The cost effectiveness of treating all patients with type 2 diabetes with angiotensin converting enzyme inhibitors. *Ann Intern Med* 1999; 131: 660–7.
74. Clark WF, Churchill DN, Forwell L, Macdonald G, Foster S. To pay or not to pay? A decision and cost–utility analysis of angiotensin converting enzyme inhibitor therapy for diabetic nephropathy. *CMAJ* 2000; 162: 195–8.
75. Vijan S, Hofer TP, Hayward RA. Cost–utility analysis of screening intervals for diabetic retinopathy in patients with type 2 diabetes mellitus. *JAMA* 2000; 283: 889–96.
76. Elliott WJ, Weir DR, Black HR. Cost effectiveness of the lower treatment goal (of JNC VI) for diabetic hypertensive patients. Joint National Committee on Prevention, Detection, Evaluation, and Treatment of High Blood Pressure. *Arch Intern Med* 2000; 160: 1277–83.
77. Sharma S, Brown GC, Brown MM, Hollands H, Shah GK. The cost-effectiveness of grid laser photocoagulation for the treatment of diabetic macular edema: results of a patient-based cost–utility analysis. *Curr Opin Ophthalmol* 2000; 11: 175–9.
78. CDC Diabetes Cost-Effectiveness Study Group. The cost-effectiveness of intensive glycemic control, intensified hypertension control, and serum cholesterol level reduction for type 2 diabetes. *JAMA* 2002; 287: 2542–51.
79. Klonoff DC, Schwartz DM. An economic analysis of interventions for diabetes [review]. *Diabetes Care* 2000; 23: 390–404.

111

Economics of Care: South and East Asia

P. Tong and Clive S. Cockram

The Chinese University of Hong Kong, Hong Kong, China

INTRODUCTION

Diabetes has now reached epidemic proportions with current estimates indicating that approximately 170 million individuals suffer from the disease, and has become one of the most important public health hazards on a global scale. It is associated with early death, disabling complications, reduced societal productivity, and poor quality of life. Rapidly developing countries are at the forefront of this epidemic, which is due mainly to rises in the prevalence of type 2 diabetes, but few societies or ethnic groups are spared. Current estimates, which are almost certainly conservative, indicate that of those who suffer from diabetes worldwide, two thirds live in developing countries [1]. It is also clear that the age at which diabetes presents is becoming lower and this is particularly true in developing countries where the peak age at diagnosis is now estimated to lie between 45 and 64 years (compared to 65 years and above in developed countries), and where alarming rises in prevalence are occurring in very young adults, adolescents, and children. This has direct economic consequences since economically productive members of the community are threatened, and occurrence of the disease in young people carries the potential need for very long periods of treatment together with risk of long-term complications while still young. Thus the public health and economic consequences of the diabetes epidemic threaten to hit hardest in developing countries, and these may be the very countries that are least well-equipped to deal with the problem.

Asia is at the forefront of the epidemic and is predicted to have the highest number of people with diabetes. By the year 2025 it is estimated that one third of the global population of people with diabetes will live in India and China alone. In India, there were 19.4 million persons with diabetes in 1995 and the projected number is expected to approach 60 million by 2025 [2]. In China current estimates indicate approximately 20 million people with diabetes with a conservatively predicted doubling to about 40 million by 2025 [2].

In addition to India and China, South and Eastern Asia includes a number of other countries that combine large populations with relatively high and increasing diabetes prevalence rates, relatively scarce health resources, and low levels of health care funding. Examples include Indonesia, the world's fourth largest nation with a population exceeding 200 million. Little is known about the current diabetes situation in Indonesia but extrapolation from a limited study in Jakarta in the early 1990s (which indicated a prevalence rate of 5.7%), together with the situation in nearby countries (such as Malaysia), suggests that a major problem may already exist. Other examples include Bangladesh, Vietnam, Philippines, and Sri Lanka.

In many countries in Asia there are also wide disparities between levels of health care available in different parts of the same country, for example between rural and urban areas. Inevitably this produces great variation in health care systems, costs, funding, and organization of care. As a result in many parts of the region there is a huge amount of unmet need. Although economic factors are very important contributors to this, a number of other factors are also important, for example geography, language, literacy and education, policy, and culture.

Despite the increase in the prevalence of diabetes in Asia, the health care systems in these countries are

International Textbook of Diabetes Mellitus, Third Edition. Edited by R. A. DeFronzo, E. Ferrannini, H. Keen, and P. Zimmet.
 ISBN: 0-471-48655-8.

Table 1 Estimated national health accounts indicators for 2000*

Countries	GNI per capita (US$)	Health expenditure per capita (US$)	Total expenditure on health as % of GDP	General government expenditure on health as % of total expenditure on health	Private expenditure on health as % of total expenditure on health
Bangladesh	370	12	3.8	36.4	63.6
Cambodia	260	17	8.1	24.5	75.5
China	840	40	5.3	36.6	63.4
India	450	20	4.9	17.8	82.2
Indonesia	570	8	2.7	23.7	76.3
Japan	35620	2243	7.8	76.7	23.3
Korea, Democratic People's Republic of	—	—	2.1	77.3	22.7
Korea, Republic of	8190	470	6	44.1	55.9
Laos	290	6	3.4	38.0	62.0
Malaysia	3380	81	2.5	58.8	41.2
Myanmar	—	97	2.2	17.1	82.9
Nepal	240	11	5.4	29.3	70.7
Pakistan	400	18	4.1	22.9	77.1
Philippines	1040	37	3.4	45.7	54.3
Singapore	24740	678	3.5	35.7	64.3
Sri Lanka	850	29	3.6	49	51
Thailand	2000	112	3.7	57.4	42.6
Viet Nam	390	17	5.2	25.8	74.2

Note: GNI per capita = gross national income divided by the midyear population; GDP = gross domestic product.
*Adapted from The World Health Report 2002, WHO and the Health, Nutrition and Population data from the World Bank.

ill-prepared to face the challenge. Access and provision of care are very variable and uneven, with needs remaining unmet in large sections of the population. To develop a cost-effective health care program in these countries, detailed information on the economics of diabetes care is required. Unfortunately, very limited published data are available from the Asia region. The following sections will consider such information as is available on the costs associated with diabetes in Asian countries. This information comes mainly from India, Taiwan, and Japan. Although limited in scope it does at least allow some comparison between high (Japan) and low (India) income countries in the Region. Table 1 provides some background information about economic indicators and health care expenditure in a few selected countries within the Region.

INDIA

In India, government health care expenditure accounts for just 2% of the monetary budget [3] and 0.8% of gross domestic product (GDP) (World Bank Development indicators). The per capita expenditure on health care is only 6.4% of the average global figure, while India accounts for 23.5% of the world's disability-adjusted life years lost due to diabetes [4]. Given the very limited resources available, the main thrust of health care provision is on eradication of communicable diseases. Most patients with diabetes can receive free health care from government-run institutions but access, quality, and availability of resources are limited. There are also services provided by private medical practitioners for those who can afford the cost. The difficulties with the public system place heavy reliance on the private system and many people may be driven to seek private care despite limited budget, leading to high out-of-pocket personal expenditure by individuals and families, especially when expressed as a percentage of household income. This scenario does not just apply in India but is very common throughout Asia, and in less developed countries elsewhere.

In the absence of a uniform health care system, it is difficult to estimate the cost of diabetes accurately. Nevertheless, there are recent studies on the economic cost of diabetes care in India, albeit in selected situations. The Bangalore Urban Diabetes Study estimated that the direct cost for diabetes ambulatory care in 1998 was about US$191 per person, and the mean direct cost per hospitalization was about US$208. The indirect cost was estimated to be US$451, giving a total annual economic burden of US$850 [5]. These figures may be compared to the estimated per capita gross national product (GNP) of India in the year 2000, which was US$500, and to the annual per capita health care spending by the Government, which is less than US$20.

Shobhana et al. studied the direct cost of diabetes in patients attending secondary care facilities in Chennai (Madras), in the private sector. The median direct cost for patients receiving diabetes care in the private sector was US$107. For those who required surgical care, the median expenditure was US$330. The proportion of annual family income spent on diabetes care depends on the duration of the disease. Those who had had diabetes for more than

5 years spent 11.5% of total family income compared to 7.8% among those with diabetes for less than 5 years [6].

In the Cost of Diabetes in India (CODI) study, more than 5500 subjects from all regions in India were studied. The direct cost, hospitalization cost, and indirect cost were estimated to be US$112, US$304, and US$410 respectively [7].

Despite the disparity in access to medical care, quality of care, education, employment, and earnings, results from these three studies were very similar. However, there are great differences between patients in the private sector and those who attended government institutions as well as those who were earners [7]. In a developing country such as India, patients with type 1 diabetes face additional financial burdens for insulin therapy. Shobhana et al. have reported that the median direct cost to the family of an individual with type 1 diabetes is US$310 (range US$45–1936). The percentages of the family income spent on diabetes care were 59%, 32%, 18%, and 12% in low, middle, upper-middle, and upper socioeconomic groups, respectively [8]. These percentages are higher than those seen in the United States, particularly in the lower socioeconomic groups.

JAPAN

The number of patients with diabetes has markedly increased over recent decades. In 1997, about 6.9 million subjects or 6% of the population suffered from diabetes [9]. The number of diabetes specialists is about 2500, and certified diabetes educators are about 4300 [10]. There are no available published data on the direct and indirect cost of diabetes. According to the Ministry of Health and Welfare, diabetes care accounts for about 4% of the total health care expenditure. According to World Bank figures, total health care expenditure in Japan is 7.6% of GDP of which 80% is accounted for by the public sector and only 20% by the private sector. All patients are covered by medical insurance schemes, either through their employers or through national health insurance. The cost of medical care to individuals is therefore heavily subsidized. The Social Welfare Programme provides free cover for those who cannot afford to pay. For people older than 65 years the cost for annual medical examination is covered by either local government budgets or health insurance policies.

Although basic health economic cost data are lacking in Japan, one earlier prospective study, the Kumamoto Study [11], which examines the effects of insulin therapy upon the development of long-term complications in type 2 diabetes, has allowed a cost-effectiveness analysis to be undertaken which examines this specific scenario.

Based on the Kumamoto Study, a cost-effectiveness analysis of intensive (versus conventional) insulin treatment for type 2 diabetes was carried out. With intensive insulin therapy, there were significant relative risk reductions in the progression of complications over a 10-year period (Figure 1).

At baseline, treatment costs were higher in the intensive therapy group (US$2807 vs. US$2272). The costs of treatment increased at the same rate in both groups during the 10-year follow-up period. Complication costs increased sharply from US$383 to US$3205 in the conventional treatment group. In contrast, the costs for treating complications rose steadily from US$453 to US$1314 in the intensive insulin therapy group. Hence, the cumulative total cost per patient in the conventional treatment group exceeded that in the intensive insulin group from the eighth year of the study. Wake et al. concluded that intensive insulin therapy could save money by prolonging the complication free period. In addition, the intensive insulin therapy improves quality of life. This study provides strong economic support for the use of intensive insulin therapy in patients with type 2 diabetes who require insulin [11]. It is also important as one of the very few analytical

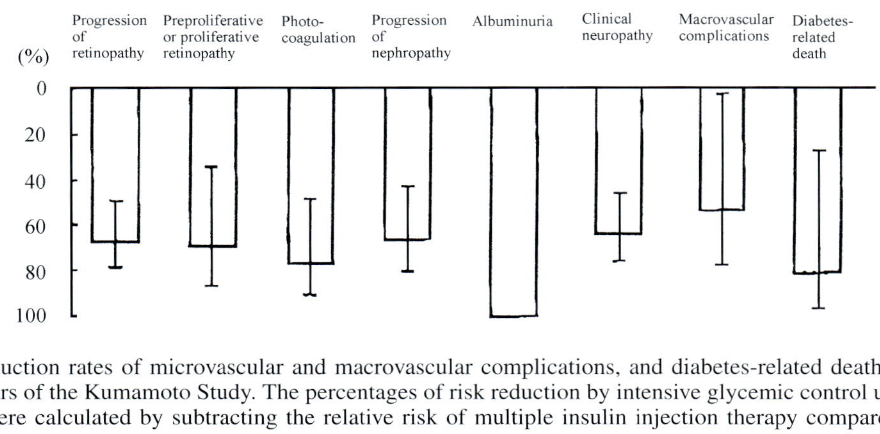

Figure 1 Risk reduction rates of microvascular and macrovascular complications, and diabetes-related death by intensive insulin therapy, over 10 years of the Kumamoto Study. The percentages of risk reduction by intensive glycemic control using multiple insulin injection therapy were calculated by subtracting the relative risk of multiple insulin injection therapy compared with conventional insulin injection therapy from one and multiplying by 100. Data represent the mean ± 95% CI. (reproduced from reference 11 by permission of Elsevier)

economic studies that examine issues relating to type 2 diabetes in non-Caucasian populations.

TAIWAN

During the period between 1985 and 1991, the prevalence of diabetes in Taiwan was estimated between 4.9 and 8.0% [12, 13]. More than 96% of inhabitants of the island were enrolled in the National Health Insurance scheme. The total cost of medical care represented 5.3% of the GNP in 1997 [14]. In a direct cost-of-illness study, the annual number of visits of patients with diabetes was 6.2% of total outpatient visits. Disproportionately, patients with diabetes represented 22.1% of total inpatient days. Diabetes and related diseases accounted for over 37% of all inpatient admissions. It is estimated that the direct cost for diabetes care was 11.5% of the total cost of health care in Taiwan. The average health care expenditure for patients with diabetes was 4.3 times higher compared to those without diabetes [15]. Most of the costs of diabetes care are related to treatment of complications, especially end-stage renal disease secondary to diabetes. In Taiwan, diabetes nephropathy is the second most common cause of underlying renal disease. The medical costs for dialysis in patients with diabetic nephropathy are 11.8% higher than in those without diabetes. The annualized medical costs per patient-year for patients with or without diabetes are US$26988 and US$24146 respectively. The higher costs in patients with diabetes are mainly due to more frequent hospitalization and longer hospital stay, resulting in a higher inpatient-to-annualized cost ratio [16].

Thus data from Taiwan, a developed area of Asia, show broadly similar themes to data from developed nations elsewhere, although only direct costs are available, with no estimates of either indirect or intangible costs. The common theme of high costs in relation to management of long-term complications and hospitalization is highlighted. The particularly high costs recorded in relation to renal disease also reflect the relatively high prevalence of end-stage renal disease due to diabetes, which has been recorded in Chinese populations [17].

CHINA

Despite the country's massive size and population (1.3 billion people), very little information with regard to the economics of diabetes is available from China. Several epidemiological studies have confirmed the rapid rise in the age-adjusted prevalence rates of diabetes during the last 15 years or so. For example a study in Beijing showed a prevalence of 3.63% for diabetes and 4.19% for impaired glucose tolerance in the early 1990s [18]. A National Diabetes Survey conducted in 1996 indicated an overall age-standardized prevalence of 3.6% for diabetes, and showed a clear prevalence gradient between provincial cities (approx. 4.6%) and other communities, with the lowest prevalence in poor rural areas (approx. 1.5%) [19].

Despite the reasonably reliable epidemiological information there are no current published data relating to the associated health costs. An approximate estimate of the direct costs incurred in the care of subjects diagnosed to have diabetes was made by the late Professor X.R. Pan in 1996 (X.R. Pan, 1996, personal communication to C.S.C.). He estimated the total direct cost of care for 5.25 million people with diabetes in China to be US$3.5 billion (29 billion Chinese yuen). This was based on a total diabetic population of 15 million with about one-third having been diagnosed. This estimated cost represents only a fraction of the total health care cost for diabetes if the indirect costs, intangible costs, and the costs incurred by undiagnosed subjects were also included. More recently the Health Minister, Zhang Wenkang, was quoted in the China Daily newspaper (8 May 2002) as giving an estimate for direct costs attributable to treatment of diabetes as approximately US$8 billion (in excess of 66 billion yuen), given a current prevalence rate of 3.6%.

CONCLUDING REMARKS

The Diabetes Control and Complications Trial (DCCT) and the UK Prospective Diabetes Study (UKPDS) have demonstrated clearly—in Caucasians—the benefits, in both human and economic terms, of improving glycemic control using intensive medical therapy for diabetes [20, 21]. This includes both type 1 and type 2 diabetes, and, particularly in the case of type 2 diabetes, associated conditions such as hypertension. There is a great need for information from cost–benefit analyses and cost-of-illness studies to quantify the situation in non-Caucasians, and nowhere is this need greater than in the countries of South and East Asia.

Given the rapid rise in the prevalence of both diabetes and impaired glucose tolerance, the development of programs aimed at preventing diabetes and its related complications should be a top priority in countries of East and South Asia, with very few, if any, exceptions. To help to allocate limited health care resources, properly conducted and thorough analysis of the economics of diabetes care is urgently needed. Without such information, it would be very difficult to assign priorities and establish cost-effective disease management programs.

REFERENCES

1. International Diabetes Federation. *Diabetes and Cardio-Vascular Disease: Time to Act.* International Diabetes Federation: Brussels, Belgium, 2001.

2. King H, Aubert RE, Herman WH. Global burden of diabetes, 1995–2025: prevalence, numerical estimates, and projections. *Diabetes Care* 1998; 21: 1414–31.
3. Ramachandran A. Health care system in India. In Gruber A, Leese B, Songer J, William R (eds) *The Economic of Diabetes and Diabetes Care.* A Report prepared by a Subgroup of the WHO/IDF Diabetes Health Care Economic Study Group. Geneva: WHO/IDF, 1988; pp 60–2.
4. Bank W. *World Development Report 1993: Investing in Health. World Development Indicators*. Oxford, World Bank, 1993; pp 213–4.
5. Rayappa PH, Raju KN, Kapur A, Bjork S, Sylvist C, DilipKumar KM. Economic cost of diabetes care—the Bangalore Urban District Diabetes Study. *Int J Diab Dev Countries* 1999; 19: 87–96.
6. Shobhana R, Rama Rao P, Lavanya A, Williams R, Vijay V, Ramachandran A. Expenditure on health care incurred by diabetic subjects in a developing country—a study from southern India. *Diabetes Res Clin Pract* 2000; 48: 37–42.
7. Kapur A. Influence of socio-economic factors on diabetes care. *Int J Diab Dev Countries* 2001; 21: 77–85.
8. Shobhana R, Rama Rao P, Lavanya A, Williams R, Padma C, Vijay V, Ramachandran A. Costs incurred by families having type 1 diabetes in a developing country—a study from Southern India. *Diabetes Res Clin Pract* 2002; 55: 45–8.
9. Ishii S, Kumasaka K. Choosing effective laboratory tests for diabetes care, and the reimbursement system. *Rinsho Byori* 2001; 49: 1218–23.
10. Matsuoka K. A diabetes care team—role of diabetes specialists and certified diabetes educator. *Rinsho Byori* 2001; 49: 1212–17.
11. Wake N, Hisashige A, Katayama T, Kishikawa H, Ohkubo Y, Sakai M, Araki E, Shichiri M. Cost-effectiveness of intensive insulin therapy for type 2 diabetes: a 10-year follow-up of the Kumamoto study. *Diabetes Res Clin Pract* 2000; 48: 201–10.
12. Chou P, Li CL, Kuo HS, Hsiao KJ, Tsai ST. Comparison of the prevalence in two diabetes surveys in Pu-Li, Taiwan, 1987–1988 and 1991–1992. *Diabetes Res Clin Pract* 1997; 38: 61–7.
13. Tai TY, Yang CL, Chang CJ, Chang SM, Chen YH, Lin BJ, Ko LS, Chen MS, Chen CJ. Epidemiology of diabetes mellitus among adults in Taiwan, R.O.C. *J Med Assoc Thai* 1987; 70: 42–8.
14. Department of Health, Health and Vital Statistics. *General Health Statistics 1997*. Republic of China: Department of Health, the Executive Yuan, 1998; p 24.
15. Lin T, Chou P, Lai MS, Tsai ST, Tai TY. Direct costs-of-illness of patients with diabetes mellitus in Taiwan. *Diabetes Res Clin Pract* 2001; 54: S43–6.
16. Yang WC, Hwang SJ, Chiang SS, Chen HF, Tsai ST. The impact of diabetes on economic costs in dialysis patients: experiences in Taiwan. *Diabetes Res Clin Pract* 2001; 54: S47–54.
17. Chi ZS, Lee ET, Lu M, Keen H, Bennett PH. Vascular disease prevalence in diabetic patients in China: standardised comparison with the 14 centres in the WHO Multinational Study of Vascular Disease in Diabetes. *Diabetologia* 2001; 44: S82–6.
18. Pan CY, Lu JM, Tian H, Kong XT, Lu XP, Yao C, Jiang CE, Deng XX, Wang SY, Zhang XL, Wang ZS, Cui L. Study of the prevalence of diabetes mellitus in adults in the Shougang Corporation in Beijing. *Diabet Med* 1996; 13: 663–8.
19. Wang K, Li T, Xiang H. Study on the epidemiological characteristics of diabetes mellitus and IGT in China. *Zhonghua Liu Xing Bing Xue Za Zhi* 1998; 19: 282–5.
20. Gray A, Raikou M, McGuire A, Fenn P, Stevens R, Cull C, Stratton I, Adler A, Holman R, Turner R, for the United Kingdom Prospective Diabetes Study Group. Cost effectiveness of an intensive blood glucose control policy in patients with type 2 diabetes: economic analysis alongside randomised controlled trial (UKPDS 41). *BMJ* 2000; 320: 1373–8.
21. The Diabetes Control and Complications Trial Research Group. The effect of intensive treatment of diabetes on the development and progression of long-term complications in insulin-dependent diabetes mellitus. *N Engl J Med* 1993; 329: 977–86.

112

Economics of Care: Australia and New Zealand

Jane Overland

Royal Prince Alfred Hospital, Camperdown, Australia, and The University of Sydney, Sydney, Australia

Diabetes will undoubtedly be one of the major health problems facing Australia and New Zealand in the twenty-first century. In the last two decades alone, the number of Australians with this disease has increased by more than 300%, from 250 000 in the early 1980s to a current level of 1 million [1, 2]. Moreover, the landmark Australian Diabetes, Obesity and Lifestyle Study has shown that one in four Australians either has diabetes or is at high risk of developing diabetes in the next 5–10 years [2]. Similar predictions have been made for New Zealand, with the total number of people diagnosed with diabetes expected to grow in the next 20 years by 20% in Europeans, 50% in the Maori population, and a staggering 130% for people of Pacific Islands descent [3].

Although Australia and New Zealand are nations that by world standards provide a high proportion of their population with opportunities for good health, health indices for its aboriginal populations are extremely poor. The prevalence of diabetes in Australian aborigines is the fourth highest in the world, with estimates reaching as high as 19.0% [4]. They also suffer exceptionally high rates of nerve damage, kidney disease, blindness, and infection. A diabetes epidemic is also apparent in New Zealand's Maori population, with the prevalence rising from 8 to 10% in middle age up to 18 to 20% among the older population [5, 6]. These figures are also mirrored in New Zealand's Pacific Islanders [5]. Whether this epidemic can be successfully halted is questionable. Although work by O'Dea and colleagues has shown that much of this diabetes can be reversed by returning to traditional lifestyles, there are complex social and economic barriers stopping these populations from doing so [7–9].

While this paints a bleak picture, research from the last decade offers hope. As discussed in other chapters, there is now convincing evidence from overseas studies that treatment to lower blood glucose as well as blood pressure and lipid levels can reduce the risk of death, disability, or morbidity due to diabetes. In many cases, these treatments are cost-effective. However, unless people have access to this care the personal and economic toll of diabetes will continue to rise.

THE CURRENT TOLL

There is no doubt that diabetes is expensive and already places a heavy burden on health care budgets. While exact figures vary, the cost of diabetes to Australia in the mid-1990s was estimated to be over A$550 million (Table 1), with inpatient costs accounting for nearly half of this total [4, 10, 11]. The largest contributor to inpatient costs was vascular disease. There are few figures available for New Zealand. However, Simmons estimated that diabetes cost New Zealand between NZ$250 million and NZ$600 million during a similar time period [3]. This compares with a more recent estimate that diabetes services will cost New Zealand NZ$247 million for the financial year 2001/2002 [12].

Diabetes also results in a substantial personal toll. The life expectancy for people with diabetes is, even in developed countries such as Australia and New Zealand, considerably lower than for people without diabetes. In Australia, for example, the life expectancy for people with diabetes is reduced by up to 15 years [13]. Moreover, the complications of diabetes can lead to permanent disability. In

International Textbook of Diabetes Mellitus, Third Edition. Edited by R. A. DeFronzo, E. Ferrannini, H. Keen, and P. Zimmet.
 ISBN: 0-471-48655-8.

Table 1 Estimates of the cost of diabetes health care in Australia, 1993–1994 and 1995

Study	Year	Health system costs (A$)	Cost per person (A$)
Mathers and Penm (1999) [10]	1993–1994	681 million	1919
McCarty et al. (1996) [4]	1995	561 million	2774
Dalton and Segal (1996) [11]	1995	553 million	2774

Australia this disability accounts for the loss of more than 53 000 years of equivalent "healthy" life [14]. Translation of this premature death and loss of quality of life into monetary units is difficult. Nevertheless, in the mid-1990s Segal and Carter estimated morbidity and premature mortality cost Australia a staggering A$418 million a year [15].

ACCESS TO CARE

As mentioned earlier, the potential to reduce this toll is dependent on ensuring that people with diabetes have access to appropriate health care. In Australia, the public hospital system together with the Medicare Program, a single government-controlled universal health insurance fund, provides "free" access to medical services for all residents. Under this program the majority of medical practitioner services are funded on a fee-for-service basis. While access to most specialist services is dependent on referral from a general practitioner, there are no other disincentives to the use of health care services. Services provided by allied health professionals are generally not covered by the Medicare system, thus supporting one-to-one medical service provision rather than multidisciplinary care. Multidisciplinary teams are offered by hospitals, which are funded by state (provincial) governments. Unfortunately, these services are vulnerable in times of restricted health budgets and in recent years there has been a decline in diabetes services available through the hospital system, regardless of the appropriateness or cost-effectiveness of multidisciplinary models of care.

In New Zealand the central government funds public hospital services as well as ambulatory care centers. Most patients see specialists at hospitals after referral from their general practitioner and so the cost of care is generally fully covered. However, for many years the country's health policy has relied on a rationing strategy as a way to manage within a limited budget, leading to shortages in many specialist and public hospital services. The central government also offers people with diabetes a free annual review with their general practitioner each year. Subsidy of most other nonhospital health services is skewed toward the very young or those at extreme socioeconomic risk, such as pensioners. Even these select patients may be faced with a copayment if their general practitioner charges above the subsidized fee. Moreover, the majority of diabetic patients are not provided subsidy and are therefore required to pay 100% of fees. These costs are a major barrier to many patients receiving the level and type of care they require [16]. New Zealanders who had private medical insurance cover prior to developing diabetes generally enjoy a more efficient level of services as needed. However, if diabetes is a previous condition it is commonly excluded from the insurance coverage or the cost of coverage is prohibitively high. It has therefore been argued that government health subsidies should be extended to all persons with diabetes.

On many levels this argument is a valid one. If the cost of diabetes is to be contained, it is important that health service utilization is commensurate with need rather than the ability to pay. It is clear that this is not the case in New Zealand. By contrast, the philosophy of health equity underpins Australia's Medicare system. Whether this has been successfully translated into practice was until recently unknown. However, a profile for people with diabetes living in the state of New South Wales (NSW) has recently been completed using Medicare occasions of service data. People with diabetes were identified using the Medicare item code for HbA_{1c}, a test where reimbursement is only paid if it is performed in a person with diagnosed diabetes. The profile showed that people with diabetes were more likely to be under the care of medical practitioners, with a heavy dependence on specialist services. In 1997, 41.8% of the diabetic population in NSW was under the care of consultant physician, a fourfold increase when compared with their nondiabetic counterparts. They also saw physicians more often (3.8 visits a year versus 2.7 visits a year) [17].

Obviously there are patients who, because of the severity of their disease, need specialist care. This is particularly so in diabetes where there is a high prevalence of vascular disease and other complications. Thus it would appear that health service utilization within Australia is driven by need. However, under the Medicare Program, reimbursement for specialist services is at least two to four times the rebate for services provided at the general practice level; thus the use of specialist services is placing extra strain on the health dollar. There is also a paradox in that people with diabetes who are socially disadvantaged or those living in rural areas are less likely to receive specialist care [18, 19]. In rural areas, the ratio of medical practitioners to population is low. In many of these areas patients also face a copayment (that is, the gap between the Medicare reimbursement amount and the amount charged by the medical practitioner), which is greater than in the case of their urban counterparts. In short, there are fewer services and those that are available are more expensive than those provided in metropolitan areas. Whether this difference in use of specialist services is reflected in better or worse health outcomes is not known. However, it is noteworthy that the proportion of people with diabetes undergoing laboratory investigations related to diabetes and its complications does not differ across NSW, despite some areas having fewer patients attending secondary care. This poses the question as to whether diabetes care would be better provided, at least in economic terms, at the primary care level.

REDUCING THE ECONOMIC BURDEN

There is no doubt that moving patients back to primary care has the potential to save millions of health dollars. However, there is also the potential to increase costs. In Australia, as part of the federal government's initiative to encourage chronic disease management at the primary care level, general practitioners are now financially rewarded for monitoring conditions such as diabetes and for seeking consultation with specialist diabetes services. As mentioned previously, over 40% of people with diabetes are currently using consultant physician services. The government's initiative is likely to see this number skyrocket with obvious effects on the health care dollar. It is also likely to place extra strain on allied health services that are already struggling because of other pressures on hospital and state budgets.

To try to reduce this strain, alternative models of care, aimed at facilitating improved integration of primary and secondary care to ensure efficient use of resources, will be crucial. There is already considerable interest in models of shared care. Most shared-care models rely on general practitioners being able to look after metabolic control in the majority of patients while making appropriate referrals for those patients that require specialist care. A randomized control trial conducted in Australia showed that diabetic control of uncomplicated patients was not compromised by the shared-care approach and that attendance rates were significantly improved. It was also shown to have a cost advantage when compared to a diabetic clinic or general practitioner care alone [20]. Experience also shows that general practitioners can distinguish between patients requiring different levels of care. An audit of over 400 patients showed that general practitioners differentiate between the "more complicated" patients, choosing to re-refer those with macrovascular disease, while maintaining the care of "less complicated" patients [21]. Although control of blood glucose levels can reduce microvascular complications, it is the aggressive treatment of macrovascular risk factors that significantly reduces the morbidity and mortality associated with diabetes [22, 23]. Referral of patients with macrovascular disease would therefore seem an appropriate use of specialist services.

THE COST AND EFFECTIVENESS OF AMBULATORY CARE

Other alternative approaches to diabetes care have received considerable attention in recent years. In Australia the traditional model of diabetes care is characterized by inpatient admission for acute episodes with long-term follow-up in an outpatient clinic. As the number of people with diabetes has risen, hospital clinics have found themselves facing increasing patient lists as well as a constantly changing array of doctors, many of whom are junior and unfamiliar with the nuances of caring for a person with chronic disease. Their inability to cope with this increased demand, together with declining hospital budgets, has led many of these clinics to downsize or close over recent years. There has also been a realization that the overall cost of treating diabetes could be lowered by adopting models of care that reduce hospital admission. This has led many institutions in Australia to shift from the traditional model of inpatient care to ambulatory care models.

There is no doubt that ambulatory care is "cheaper" than inpatient care. But rather than only seeking "cheaper" alternatives, it is important to look toward "effectiveness." There are few who would argue the feasibility and effectiveness of commencing insulin on an ambulatory basis even when a large number of patients need to be dealt with. For example, at the Diabetes Centre at Royal Prince Alfred Hospital in Sydney over 160 patients are commenced on insulin in this manner each year. The HbA_{1c} of these patients is significantly improved, falling from an average of 9.2% to 7.4% after 3 months of insulin therapy [24].

Initiation of insulin on an ambulatory basis is also clearly financially advantageous. An analysis in the mid-1990s showed that patients with type 2 diabetes commencing insulin used 0.7 h of medical and 9.6 h of nursing and allied health staff time (including case discussion and documentation) over a 3-month period. When infrastructure costs were included, the cost of initiation of insulin on an ambulatory basis came to A$979, which equated to 1.6 days of inpatient care (Table 2). Over the same period, the average length of stay for patients admitted to hospital for the same purpose was 4.3 days and cost A$2405 per patient [25]. Bruce et al. had similar results and concluded that an ambulatory approach was not only successful in achieving satisfactory diabetic control but also resulted in considerable savings in terms of hospital bed days [26]. A study by Flack et al. found that patients who were admitted to hospital for commencement of insulin therapy had significantly more clinical investigations than those who commenced insulin on an ambulatory basis [27]. Flack also found substantial savings in indirect costs through minimizing disruption to the patients' work and social life. Therefore, based on the average number of patients commencing insulin each year, total savings due to

Table 2 The cost of commencement of insulin and restabilization in an ambulatory care setting*

	Time (h)		Cost (A$)				
	Medical staff	Nonmedical staff	Direct salary	Administrative and clerical salary	Infrastructure	Total	Bed day equivalent
Commencement of insulin	0.7	9.6	279	395	305	979	1.6
Restabilization	0.2	5.9	144	201	177	522	0.9

* *Source*: Derived from reference 25.

initiation of insulin on an ambulatory basis is estimated to be in excess of A$0.25 million for the Diabetes Centre at Royal Prince Alfred Hospital alone.

While many clinicians and health care planners associate ambulatory care with ambulatory stabilization alone, if this approach is to have a major impact on the cost of diabetes care it needs to be viewed more broadly. It is well known that diabetes complications are the most important cost driver of diabetes care and that despite improvements in glycemic management in recent decades complications of diabetes remain highly prevalent [28] (Table 3). However, these can be delayed or minimized if effective treatment is implemented early. For this to happen it is essential that all patients with diabetes have access to regular and comprehensive complication assessment.

Traditionally, screening for complications has relied on the format of patients attending multiple appointments with specialists, allied health professionals, and laboratories. This can be inconvenient for the patient, expensive for the health care system, and in the end assessment may not be complete. A specific diabetes complications assessment service can address these issues. For example, at the Diabetes Centre at Royal Prince Alfred Hospital a complete complication assessment is performed during a 1-h appointment. Nursing staff perform most of the assessment, thus resulting in a considerable cost saving to the total health care budget. In addition, with less than 2.2% missing data for the status of individual complications the number of undiagnosed complications is low [29].

A single visit complications assessment service also decreases the overall cost of diabetes care by reducing

Table 3 The presence of complications among people with diabetes in Australia, 2000

Condition	Percent
Erectile dysfunction	28.1
Peripheral neuropathy	22.5
Peripheral vascular disease	11.7
Severe hypoglycemia*	3.3
Active foot lesion	3.2
Myocardial infarction*	2.0
Stroke*	1.6
New blindness*	1.3
Lower limb amputation*	0.7
End-stage renal disease*	0.08

* Denotes condition seen in last 12 months.

the number of appointments patients must attend. This is supported by a study by Sculpher et al. who showed that screening for complications such as retinopathy without the need for an additional appointment was a cost-effective approach in terms of appropriate referral for sight-threatening diabetic retinopathy [30]. Only 18% of patients attending the diabetes complications assessment service described above were found to have retinopathy requiring further ophthalmological assessment on their first presentation, thus preserving scarce specialist resources.

The area shown to produce the biggest cost saving is management of diabetic foot disease within a multidisciplinary ambulatory care setting. At present, diabetic foot disease leads to over 3000 amputations in Australia each year, which costs an estimated A$48 million per annum for health costs alone [31]. Obviously, if numbers of amputations increase, which has been the trend over recent years, the financial burden will rise further. The burden of diabetic foot disease is also increasing in New Zealand. An unpublished review reported by Simmons suggested that the number of hospital discharges due to diabetic foot disease had doubled over a decade [3]. This complication was also associated with long median lengths of hospital stay.

There is now convincing evidence that specialized ambulatory foot care services can both reduce the incidence of amputation and almost halve the average length of stay in those patients who cannot avoid hospitalization [32–34]. A review of patients with severe neuropathy or vascular disease who attended an ambulatory foot care service in Sydney showed that over 75% of neuropathic ulcers were healed within 1year. Moreover, 95% of the patients were treated without having to resort to hospitalisation. Treatment of a new ulcer used 2.8 h of staff time per month, falling to 1.5 h/month for prevention of ulcer recurrence. While this type of service may initially appear to be resource hungry the annual cost per patient represented only 15% of a medical and 10% of a surgical admission for diabetic foot disease [25] (Figure 1). Moreover, using these figures together with population studies of foot ulceration in diabetic patients, the authors of Australia's National Diabetes Strategy and Implementation Plan estimated that the cost of establishing specialist diabetic foot clinics in each health area throughout Australia would be recovered in

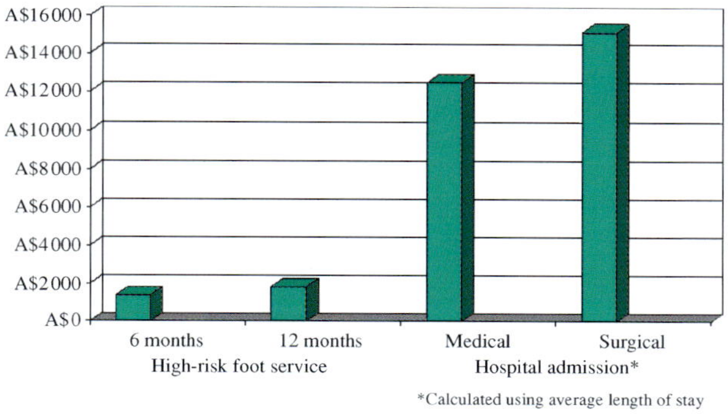

Figure 1 The cost of diabetic foot in an ambulatory care setting versus hospital inpatient care (derived from reference 25)

1–2 years, assuming these services reduced hospitalization for diabetic foot ulcers by a modest 2.5% [31]. Similar savings are likely to be realized in New Zealand.

THE FUTURE CHALLENGE

The challenge ahead is to continue to provide care to an increasing number of people with diabetes, taking into consideration available resources. To meet this goal the ongoing collection of relevant information to monitor future trends in diabetes service provision is of paramount importance. As shown earlier in this chapter, Australia's universal health insurance system, known as Medicare, offers a sustainable and reliable system that may play a vital role in this regard. Medicare occasions of service data have already provided unique information on health service utilization for people with diabetes living in the state of NSW. Its ability to provide an almost complete snap shot of the total picture means it has considerable potential in regard to ongoing monitoring of diabetes. In New Zealand, monitoring of health service utilization will be more difficult but it is a task that must be achieved.

REFERENCES

1. Glatthaar C, Welborn TA, Stenhouse NS, Garcia-Webb P. Diabetes and impaired glucose tolerance. A prevalence estimate based on the Busselton 1981 Survey. *Med J Aust* 1985; 143: 436–40.
2. Dunstan D, Zimmet P, Welborn T, Sicree R, Armstrong T, Atkins R, Cameron A, Shaw J, Chadban S. *Diabesity & Associated Disorders in Australia 2000. The Accelerating Epidemic. Australian Diabetes, Obesity and Lifestyle Report*. Melbourne: International Diabetes Institute, 2001.
3. Simmons D. Diabetes and its complications in New Zealand: an epidemiological perspective. *NZ Med J* 1996; 109 (1025): 245–7.
4. McCarty DJ, Zimmet P, Dalton A, Segal L, Welborn TA. *The Rise and Rise of Diabetes in Australia, 1996. A Review of Statistics, Trends and Costs*. Canberra: Diabetes National Action Plan, 1996.
5. Simmons D, Gatland BA, Leakehe L, Flemming C. Frequency of diabetes in family members of probands with non insulin dependent diabetes. *J Intern Med* 1995; 237: 315–21.
6. Baker J, Metcalf P, Scragg R. Fructosamine concentrations in the general population of Kawerau. *Diabetes Care* 1988; 11: 240–5.
7. McDermott R, O'Dea K, Rowley K, Knight S, Burgess P. Beneficial impact of the homelands movement on health outcomes in central Australian aborigines. *Aust NZ J Public Health* 1998; 22 (6): 653–8.
8. O'Dea K. Marked improvement in carbohydrate and lipid metabolism in diabetic Australian aborigines after temporary reversion to traditional lifestyle. *Diabetes* 1984; 33 (6): 596–603.
9. O'Dea K, Spargo RM, Akerman K. The effect of transition from traditional to urban life-style on the insulin secretory response in Australian Aborigines. *Diabetes Care* 1980; 3 (1): 31–7.
10. Mathers C, Penm R. *Health Systems Costs of Cardiovascular Disease and Diabetes in Australia 1993–94*. Canberra: Australian Institute of Health and Welfare, 1999. AIHW Cat. No. HWE11.
11. Segal L, Dalton A. *Cost Effectiveness of Strategies for the Prevention of NIDDM*. Fairfield, VIC: Monash University Centre for Health Program Evaluation, 1996.
12. New Zealand Inc. *Type 2 Diabetes: Managing for Better Health Outcomes*. New Zealand: New Zealand Inc., 2001.
13. Australian Bureau of Statistics (ABS). *Causes of death, Australia, 1998*. Canberra: ABS, 1999. ABS Cat. No. 3303.0.
14. Mathers C, Vos T, Stevenson C. *The Burden of Disease and Injury in Australia*. Canberra: Australian Institute of Health and Welfare, 1999. AIHW Cat. No. PHE 17.
15. Segal L, Carter R. The economics of diabetes care-Australia. In Alberti KGMM, DeFronzo R, Keen H, Zimmet P (eds) *International Textbook of Diabetes Mellitus*, 2nd edn. Chichester: Wiley, 1997; pp 1779–86.
16. Simmons D, Peng A, Cecil A, Gatland B. The personal costs of diabetes: a significant barrier to care in South Aukland. *NZ Med J* 2001; 112 (1097): 383–5.
17. Overland J, Yue DK, Mira M. The pattern of diabetes care in New South Wales: a five-year analysis using Medicare Occasions of Service Data. *Aust NZ J Public Health* 2000; 24 (4): 389–93.
18. Overland J, Yue DK, Mira M. The use of Medicare services related to diabetes: the impact of rural location. *Aust J Rural Health* 2001; 9: 311–6.
19. Overland J, Yue DK, Hayes L. Social disadvantage: its impact on the use of Medicare services related to diabetes in NSW. *Aust NZ J Public Health* 2002; 26 (3): 262–5.
20. Hoskins PL, Fowler PM, Constantino M, Forrest J, Yue DK, Turtle JR. Sharing the care of diabetic patients between hospital and general practitioners: does it work? *Diabet Med* 1993; 10 (1): 81–6.
21. Overland J, Mira M, Yue DK. Differential shared care for diabetes: does it provide the optimal partition between primary and specialist care. *Diabet Med* 2001; 18: 554–7.
22. Pyorala K, Pedersen TR, Kjekshus J, Faergeman O, Olsson AG, Thorgeirsson G. Cholesterol lowering with simvastatin improves prognosis of diabetic patients with coronary heart disease. A subgroup analysis of the Scandinavian Simvastatin Survival Study (4S). *Diabetes Care* 1997; 20 (4): 614–20.

23. The UK Prospective Diabetes Study (UKPDS) Group. Tight blood pressure control and risk of macrovascular and microvascular complications in type 2 diabetes: UKPDS 38. *BMJ* 1998; 317 (7160): 703–13.
24. Overland J, McGill M, Constantino M, Molyneaux L, Willey K, Hoskins P, Yue DK, Williamson M. *Diabetes Centre Based Ambulatory Care: Its Impact on Diabetes Health Outcomes*. Sydney: NSW Health Department, 1995.
25. Constantino M, Overland J, Hoskins P, Yue DK, Lagaida R. *Diabetes Ambulatory Care: Its Impact on the Approach and Cost of Treating People with Diabetes*. Sydney: NSW Health Department, 1994.
26. Bruce DG, Clark EM, Danesi GA, Campbell LV, Chisholm DJ. Outpatient stabilisation programme—an innovative approach in the management of diabetes. *Diabetes Res* 1985; 2: 85–8.
27. Flack JR, Strumfin G, Bauman A, Jan S. *An Assessment of Diabetes in South Western Sydney: Does Ambulatory Stabilisation Improve Health Outcomes*. Sydney: NSW Health Department, 1995.
28. National Association of Diabetes Centres. *Final Report ANDIAB 2000. Australian National Diabetes Information Audit and Benchmarking*. Canberra: National Association of Diabetes Centres, 2000.
29. Hoskins PL, Overland J, Constantino M, Molyneaux L, McGill M, Yue DK. *Demonstration Project for the Longitudinal Study of Diabetes Outcomes in the Community*. Sydney: NSW Health Department, 1995.
30. Sculpher MJ, Buxton BA, Ferguson BA, Humphreys JE, Altman JF, Spiegelhalter DJ, Kirby AJ, Jacob JS, Bacon H, Dudbridge SB. A relative cost-effectiveness analysis of different methods of screening for diabetic retinopathy. *Diabet Med* 1991; 8 (7): 644–50.
31. Colagiuri S, Colugiuri R, Ward J. *National Diabetes Strategy and Implementation Plan*. Canberra: Diabetes Australia, 1998.
32. McGill M, Collins P, Bolton T, Yue DK. Management of neuropathic ulceration. *J Wound Care* 1996; 5: 52–4.
33. Bakker K, Dooren J. A specialized outpatient foot clinic for diabetic patients decreases the number of amputations and is cost saving. *Ned Tijdschr Geneeskd* 1994; 138: 565–9.
34. Edmonds ME, Blundell MP, Morris ME, Thomas EM, Cotton LT, Watkins PJ. Improved survival of the diabetic foot: the role of a specialized foot clinic. *Q J Med* 1986; 60: 763–71.

113

Economics of Care: The Middle East

Morsi Arab

University of Alexandria, Alexandria, Egypt

GENERAL CONSIDERATIONS FROM THE REGIONAL AND WORLD ECONOMY

The economics of diabetes care cannot be separated from general health economics, and this in turn is not separable from the socioeconomic situation of a particular country or group of countries. Again, the economic aspects of a particular region of the world are part of the general world economy and development.

In the Middle East, with all of its countries belonging to the developing world, the limited economy in general may have a restrictive effect on the provision of health services and their standards, not excluding those for diabetes care.

Countries in the Middle East, however, may be classified into four categories:

(1) the high-income oil exporting group (above US$5000 per capita), such as Kuwait, Saudi Arabia, United Arab Emirates, Qatar, Bahrain, and Oman;
(2) the high middle-income group (above US$2000 per capita), such as Cyprus, Iraq, Lebanon, and Tunis;
(3) the low middle-income group (below US$2000 per capita), such as Egypt, Jordan, Algeria, Morocco, and Iran; and
(4) the very low-income group (less than US$1000), such as Yemen and Sudan [1–3].

However, apart from this single parameter of national income of a particular country, which certainly affects the economy, other additional factors may intervene. Poorer countries may not always have less access to proper health services, including those for diabetes.

For example, Egypt belongs to the lower middle-income group of the Middle East countries, but in certain aspects of health care Egypt rates quite high in the region. Examples include availability of physicians and other health care personnel, availability of hospital beds per head of population, adequacy of nutritional requirements (especially total caloric consumption per capita), and the very early establishment of diabetes care organizations in the country [4–7]. Table 1 gives some economic and health parameters for a range of Middle East countries.

STUDIES ON THE COST OF DIABETES IN MIDDLE EASTERN COUNTRIES

The Alexandria Hospitals Study 1986–1988

Certain studies on the cost of diabetes in Egypt were published in 1990. One of these studies was carried out on diabetic patients admitted to four groups of hospitals in the Governorate of Alexandria, with different administrative policies [8, 9]. The study included estimations of the direct cost of inhospital care at 10 hospitals with a total number of 3141 beds, including 800 for internal medicine. The total number of admissions during a 3-year period was 17 409, about 11% of which were cases of diabetes. Table 2 shows the results of that study, which included the basal cost of one day's stay in hospital, the additional cost of treatment to control noncomplicated cases of diabetes, and that for treatment of complicated cases, at the prevailing cost prices during this period (1986–1988).

It is to be noted that all the four groups of hospitals enlisted were in one way or the other supported by

International Textbook of Diabetes Mellitus, Third Edition. Edited by R. A. DeFronzo, E. Ferrannini, H. Keen, and P. Zimmet.
 ISBN: 0-471-48655-8.

Table 1 Economic and health parameters in Middle Eastern countries from World Data Bank (1990–2000) and WHO health parameters*

	Econmic parameters				Health parameters			
Country	Population (million)	GNI (US$ billion)	GNI per capita (US$)	Growth rate (annual) (%)	Life expectancy (years)	Infant mortality per 1000	Physicians per 100 000	Nurses per 100 000
Egypt	63.8	95.2	1490	5.1	66.6	37.0	202	233
Saudia Arabia	20.7	139.4	6900	0.4	72.2	18.8	166	330
Lebanon	4.3	16.2	3750	0.5	70.2	26.4	210	100
Oman	2.4	15.3			73.3	17.4	133	325
Qatar	0.585	9.1	13730		74.6	16.0		
Jordan	4.9	8.3	1680	3.9	71.3	26.2	166	296
Syria	16.1	16.5	990	1.4	69.5	24.0	144	189
Baharin	0.689	5.2	8640	3.1	73.0	7.7	100	283
Tunisia	9.6	20.1	2090	4.7	72.5	24.0	70	286
Algeria	30.4	48.3	1590	2.6	70.8	34.0	84	297
Iran	64.0	104.6	1630	5.2	71.1	36.0	85	259
Yemen	17.5	6.7	380	6.5	56.0	79.0	23	51
Morocco	28.7	33.8	1180	0.8	67.2	47.8	46	105
Palestine	2.9	4.7	1610	−6.2	71.8	22.8		
Iraq	23.3				69	32.0	55	236
Kuwait	2.0	32.3	19020	−3.3	76.6		189	475
Libya	5.5	35.5			71	22.0	128	360
Emirates	2.9	51.2	20830	10	75.2	7.6	181	341
Sudan	36.0	35.7	(1000)	7	56.9	68.6		
Pakistan	144.616					80.5	57	34

* From reference 1.

direct or indirect subsidization from the government, and it was therefore concluded that independent private hospital treatment could be appreciably more costly.

In that specific study it was observed that the period of stay in hospital and the basic costs per day were quite different at the different categories of hospitals because of their different policies governing the duration of stay, and because of the different standards of service facilities, such as running costs for salaries, equipments, water, electricity and fuel, laundry, maintenance, vehicles, and communications. On the other hand, the medical costs of treatment for diabetes control, such as insulin, oral agents, syringes, and fluids, plus the additional costs for treatment of complications such as infections, cardiovascular disease, and renal failure were dependent on market prices of medications and medical supplies. Therefore, the medical costs were more or less an equal burden added to the daily hospital expenses.

The average length of stay of a diabetic patient in those hospitals ranged between 12 and 22 days and was highest at the Health Insurance hospitals and lowest at the University hospitals. It may be quite understood that the period of stay in a University hospital may be affected by teaching requirements, while in private hospitals, where individual patients pay all the expenses, a shorter stay is always encouraged. At Health Insurance hospitals a more relaxed policy may encourage a longer stay.

Naturally, the period of stay and the cost of care per day, together constitute the final burden of hospital care for one individual. In the Alexandria Hospital Study 1986–1988 the cost of hospital care per patient per day ranged between E£5.27 and E£14.7 (Egyptian pounds). (In 1986, 1 US$ = E£1.37.)

The cost of hospital treatment for a diabetic patient in Egypt during one hospital admission was consequently estimated to be E£148.31/patient per one hospital admission, considering an average period of stay per one admission in all categories of hospitals.

The average outpatient care for the same group of patients in the above study was assessed from interviews with

Table 2 The hospital costs of diabetes—from the Alexandria Hospitals Study (1986–1988)

			Cost of treatment (E£/day)			
Hospital category	Diabetic admissions (% of total)	Average duration of stay (days)	Basal	Control of diabetes	Treatment of complications	Total cost
Ministry of Health	13.4	19.7	3.36	1.44	0.8	5.59
University	7.8	12.07	2.90	1.57	0.8	5.27
Semi-private	4.6	15.8	12.5	1.48	0.8	14.78
Health insurance	30.8	21.2	7.0	1.3	0.8	9.1

these patients, and it revealed an average expenditure of E£85.8/patient/year.

The total national direct cost of diabetes care (including inhospital and outpatient care) was estimated based on the following:

(1) The total population in Egypt 1990 was 55 million (10).
(2) The mean prevalence in the whole population (categories of all age groups and geographic sectors) was 4.3% [11–15]. About half were known diabetes cases and were receiving diabetes care (1 182 500 patients).
(3) All treated patients would require outpatient care, costing E£85.8/patient all through the year, at a total national cost of E£101.5 million.
(4) About one third of all diabetic patients would require an average of one hospital admission per year at a cost of E£148.31. Therefore the total national hospital cost would be E£58.5 million.
(5) The added costs of hospital and out-patient care for the diabetic population in Egypt in 1986 was therefore about E£160 million. This had to be corrected for the year 1990 according to the inflation rates of 1986–1990, which gave a figure of E£235.5 million.
(6) The huge burden of this cost (apart from the indirect cost) on the economy of the country is illustrated by comparing this figure to the available government expenditure on health during 1990 (i.e. E£351.8 million). Government expenditure on health at this time was just 2.8% of the total government expenditure, which in turn constituted about 40% of the national production during that year (E£31.3 billion).

This simply means that the direct cost of diabetes in 1990 would have required the consumption of about two thirds of the total national health budget in a country with per capita income of US$610 (6) (Table 3).

CHANGES FROM 1990 TO 2002

During 2001 another study was carried out in the same city of Alexandria. Three basic differences should be noted in analyzing the results compared with previous studies:

(1) An appreciable economical development in the country raised the per capita income from US$610 to US$1490 (apart from a higher purchasing power) [1–3].
(2) The 2001 study on hospital and out-patient costs of diabetes care was carried out on a middle-class diabetic population treated in a fully private hospital, but using the benefits of subsidized medication whenever compatible. This was thought to match better the expenditure capacity of individuals with the parameter of national per capita income, which represents the main bulk of the population, rather than the very rich or the very poor.
(3) The emergence during the past few years of several new forms of more expensive insulins, oral agents, and medical supplies put more stress on the capacity of individuals to balance their expenses with their incomes.

The 2001 study revealed that for a middle-class diabetic individual, the basic cost of treatment in hospital (that is, just for glycemic control and possibly minor pathologies) is approximately US$40/day (Table 4). More than half (55%) of this cost goes on medications and medical supplies. An extra burden is introduced when diabetes is complicated by one of the major pathologies such as cardiovascular disease, renal failure, or diabetic foot. In this case the cost of one day's hospital treatment is increased to 128, 354, or 346% respectively, compared to the non-complicated diabetes (Table 5).

As regards outpatient ambulatory treatment, an estimation was made for the cost of medication (insulin or

Table 3 The estimated impact of direct cost of diabetes on national economy in Egypt for the year 1990

1986	Population: 55 million
	Prevalence of diabetes mellitus: 4.3% (50% known diabetes)
	Treated patients: 1 182 500
	Presuming: All require outpatients care all through
	1 182 500 × 85.8 = E£101.5 million
	Require one hospital admission per year
	394.167 × 148.31 = E£58.5 million
	Total direct cost ∼E£160 million per year
1990	Total direct cost 1986: E£160 million
	Average inflation rate 1986–90: 11%
	Estimated total direct cost 1990: E£235.2 million
	National production 1990: E£31.3 billion
	Government expenditure 1990 (40%): E£12.6 billion
	2.8% Government expenditure on health: E£351.8 million
	Direct cost of DM/available government expenditure on health: 2/3

Table 4 Distribution of costs of hospital treatment of diabetic patients (E£/day) at a private hospital for middle-class Egyptian population at the city of Alexandria, Egypt, 2001

	E£	%
Cost of medications and medical supplies	99.00	55
Basic hospital expenses		
Food	9.00	5
Health care team	19.80	11
All other running expenses	52.20	29
Average total cost per day	E£180 (=US$40)	100

oral agents) plus the additional cost of laboratory and other follow-up procedures (ECG, radiology, etc.), and fees for physicians and other consultants at an average frequency per year. Apart from the cost of medications, the latter additional costs on average were estimated to be US$143/year (Table 6, part c).

Estimation of the cost of medication over 1 year for ambulatory care using one or other forms of insulin, oral agents, or both was based on market prices and the average daily doses. For insulins, the cost of one year's consumption varies widely according to whether animal or human insulin is used and whether it is U40 or U100. On one hand, this may drop steeply to US$3.6/year for a patient on animal U40 insulin heavily subsidized by the government, while on the other hand, it may rise to an extremely high cost of US$438/year for a patient on nonsubsidized human insulin U100 provided by a pen device (Table 6, part a).

Similarly, great variations exist in the cost of oral agents according to the form of tablet and the daily dose. This could range from US$10/year up to US$446/year (Table 6, part b).

It is worth noting that the newly introduced forms of oral insulin secretagogues and insulin sensitizers constituted the much higher cost (US$200–500/year) compared to the old classical sulfonylureas and metformin agents (US$10–162/year).

To assess the burden of the cost of diabetes ambulatory care on the individual economy, it was calculated that a patient who spends US$30/year on a cheap form

Table 5 The extra burden of cost of treatment of complicated diabetes at a private Alexandria Hospital, 2001 (average of 100 diabetic patients)

State of diabetes mellitus	Cost of 1 day in US$	Relative extra burden
Diabetes (uncomplicated); admitted for glycemic control	40.00	100%
Diabetes + cardiovascular disease	51.30	128%
DM + renal failure	141.70	354%
DM + diabetic foot	138.70	346%

Table 6 Estimated costs of ambulatory (outpatient) treatment of diabetes in Egypt at 2001 cost prices in US$/year

Type	Cost (US$/year)
(a) Insulin (dose 10–80 units/day)	
Animal insulin U40*	3.6–29.2
Human insulin U40†	14.6–116.8
Human insulin U100	32.8–262.8
Human insulin in pen device U100	54.7–438.0
(b) Oral antidiabetic agents‡	
Glibenclamide (5–20 mg)	14.0–56.0
Gliclazide (80–240 mg)	27.0–81.0
Glimepride (1–6 mg)	32.0–162.0
Metformin (500–1500 mg)	10.0–30.0
Rapiglinide (3 mg)	235
Nateglinide (360 mg)	405
Rosiglitazone (4 mg)	446
(c) Other costs at average frequencies per year	
Laboratory and other follow-up investigations (ECG, radiology, etc.)	76.4
Physician fees and other specialist consultations	66.6
Total	143

* Heavily subsidized.
† Moderately subsidized.
‡ Values in parentheses represent daily dose.

of animal insulin plus US$143/year for additional costs is able to tolerate well such expenditure, which constitutes about 11.6% of his average yearly income (US$1490). Similarly, a patient on oral medication of the older classical forms spending up to US$100/year, plus an additional cost of US$143/year, consumes 16.3% of his yearly income (US$1490) (Table 6).

On the other hand, a diabetic patient on expensive human insulin or on one of the new expensive forms of oral agents has to spend sometimes up to US$440/year, plus US$143/year for additional costs, which consumes about 40% of his annual income.

It was therefore concluded that treatment of simple diabetes (that is, just for glycemic control) by the new oral medications or by the expensive insulin devices is beyond the capacity of the middle-class population, unless subsidized by some form of health insurance. Furthermore, the possible requirement of hospital treatment for 10 days through a 1-year period in addition to the ambulatory treatment could add a burden of US$400–1410 (Table 5). It is quite evident that this huge cost is totally beyond the economical capacity of the middle class.

PROJECTING THE EGYPTIAN STUDIES ON OTHER MIDDLE EASTERN COUNTRIES—THE BALANCE OF COSTS AGAINST INCOMES

As previously indicated, Middle East countries have a very wide range of per capita income. Table 7 shows a list of

Table 7 The burden of the cost of ambulatory treatment of diabetes on individuals at low-income and high-income Middle East countries, based on the cost prices of insulins and oral antidiabetic agents (in US$/year)

	Egypt	Morocco	Qatar	Saudi Arabia
Percapita income in US$	1 490	1 180	13 730	6 900
Animal insulin U40 (40 units/day)	14.6*	134.3	NA	NA
Human insulin U40 (40 units/day)	55.5†	313.9	NA	NA
Human insulin U100 (40 units/day)	132.9	318.3	258.4	213.0
Human insulin in device U100 (40 units/day)	219.0	446.7	—	—
Glibenclamide (5–20 mg)	14–56	41–164	94–376	
Cliclazide (80–240 mg)	27–81	48–144	98–294	
Glimeperide (1–6 mg)	32–162	57–292	—	
Metformin (100–1500 mg)	20–30	24–36	44–66	
Rapiglinide (3 mg)	235	—	—	243
Nateglinide (360 mg)	405	—	—	—
Rosiglitazine (4 mg)	446	—	—	584

* Heavily subsidized.
† Moderately subsidized.

the market prices of some forms of insulin and oral agents in four Middle East countries: two of them at lower per capita incomes (Egypt US$1490 and Morocco US$1180) and two with appreciably higher incomes (Saudi Arabia US$6900 and Qatar US$13 700) [1–3]. From this table we may conclude the following:

(1) Government subsidization is essential and extremely effective in reducing the high cost burden on individual patients. This is quite evident in case of Egypt where animal insulin is highly subsidized and human insulin U40 is moderately subsidized. Without this subsidization, as in any other low-income country (like Morocco), the burden is less tolerated.
(2) Human insulin U100 is marketed in both lower and higher income Middle East countries without much difference in price. Therefore, human insulin, particularly when delivered by pen devices, is a relatively higher burden for patients with limited resources in the lower income group of countries.
(3) Oral agents also cost much more in higher income countries compared to the lower income group of countries (sometimes more than four- to sixfold). In Egypt, it may be lowered further because of a successful pharmaceutical industry existing there, even if it is only a partial process in some cases.
(4) The newly emerging oral medications, e.g., Rapiglinide, Nateglinide, and Rosiglitazone, are marketed at nearly the same prices in both categories of Middle Eastern countries.
(5) So, relating the costs of medications to individual incomes in Middle Eastern countries demonstrates a serious socio-economic contrast. To illustrate this, a new oral agent may require a consumption of 30–40% of the per capita income in Egypt or Morocco, while this constitutes a much more tolerable burden of 3–8% of the per capita income in Qatar or Saudi Arabia.

This must be seriously taken into consideration by physicians during socioeconomic planning of individual diabetes care, and by the decision makers and health authorities at national levels.

Unfortunately, we do not have further information on the cost of treatment of diabetic complications and hospital treatment in most of the Middle Eastern countries. However, guided by the data from the recent Alexandria study, the total direct cost of diabetes care must be an extremely high burden for all individual patients.

A LESSON FROM THE MIDDLE EASTERN MEDITERRANEAN COUNTRIES

A number of Middle Eastern countries belong to the Mediterranean group as well. It is of interest to refer to a study in 1990 in order to compare the cost of ambulatory outpatient diabetes care in some Mediterranean countries on both sides, that is, the European countries in the north and the North African Arab countries in the south (Table 8).

In that study, which included Egypt, Tunisia, and Algeria in comparison with Yugoslavia, Greece, and Italy, the total cost of ambulatory care was found to be the lowest in Egypt, probably as a result of a wide subsidization policy. This cost was also lower in the other southern Mediterranean countries compared to the northern European countries, possibly because of higher fees for physicians and other services, the wider use of self-monitoring, and possibly also because of several other factors [6, 16].

Table 8 Cost of ambulatory outpatient care in some Mediterranean countries in 1990, based on an average of 200 diabetic patients in each center (in US$/month/patient)

Centers	Cost of medicines		Self-monitoring	Total basic cost	Treatment of complications	Total cost of outpatient treatment
	Oral agents	Insulin				
Alexandria (Egypt)	1.12	2.44	2.49	6.06	2.28 (28.94*)	8.34 (35.0*)
Tunis (Tunisia)	2.85	12.24	3.23	6.69	4.17	10.86
Oran (Algeria)	9.87	23.41	15.45	27.54	71.08	98.62
Zagreb (Yugoslavia)	2.54	23.56	15.34	24.16	7.44	31.60
Athens (Greece)	7.53	38.48	15.35	39.15	71.45	110.60
Pavia (Italy)	3.33	27.38	5.52	12.65	25.10	37.75

* Including cost of dialysis for chronic renal failure.

REFERENCES

1. The World Bank Indicators Database, July 2001. Available at: http://devota.worldbank.org/external/CPProfile.asp/CCODE. Accessed January 15, 2003.
2. CIA. *The World Fact Book 2000*. Available at: www//ww.odci.gov/cia/publications/factbook/goes. Accessed January 15, 2003.
3. The World Bank Group. Available at: http://www.worldbank.org/data/. Accessed January 15, 2003.
4. WHO Estimates of Health Personnel (around 1998). Available at: http://www3 who.int/whosis/health_personnel/health_ personnel.cmf. Accessed January 15, 2003.
5. UNICEF Statistics. Available at: http://www.unicef.org.stat./country.html. Accessed January 15, 2003.
6. Arab M. The economics of diabetes care: the Middle East. In Alberti KGMM, Zimmet P, De Fronzo RA, Keen H (eds) *International Text Book of Diabetes Mellitus*, 2nd edn. New York: Wiley, 1997; pp 1793–7.
7. Arab MM. History of the diabetes care organizations in Egypt [in Arabic]. *Egypt Union Diabetes Assoc Bull* 1992; 1: 4.
8. Arab MM, A-Latif HM, Khalil SA, Hedayet N. *Cost of Diabetes Care for Hospital Patients in Alexandria* [MS thesis]. Egypt: University of Alexandria, 1989.
9. Gruber W, Lander T, Leese B, Songer T, Williams R (eds). *The Economics of Diabetes and Diabetes Care*. Report of Study Group of IDF and WHO. Geneva: WHO/IDF, 1997.
10. *The General Census Report*. Cairo: Department of Statistics and Census, 1987.
11. Arab M. Diabetes mellitus in Egypt. *World Health Stat* 1992; 45 (4): 334–7.
12. Arab M. Diabetes mellitus in Egypt. *Int Diabetes Dig* 1992; 3: 86–8.
13. Arab M. Epidemiology of diabetes mellitus in Egypt. In Proceedings first MGSD, Meeting Rome, 1986.
14. Arab M. The epidemiology of Diabetes mellitus in Egypt. *J Egypt Endoc Metab Diabetes* 1987; 19 (1): 5–23.
15. Arab M. Epidemiology of diabetes in Egypt. *Egypt J Diabetes* 1997; 2: 1–14.
16. Arab MM. The cost of outpatient care of diabetes in Alexandria compared to other Mediterranean Centers. In Proceedings of the third MGSD Meeting, Nice, November 1990.

114

Diabetes Cost: Sub-Saharan Africa Perspective

Jean Claude Mbanya

University of Yaoundé I, Yaoundé, Cameroon

INTRODUCTION

Diabetes mellitus is emerging as a major health problem in sub-Saharan Africa [1]. The economic burden of diabetes mellitus on the patient, family, community, and nation is enormous. However, medical innovations that can delay the onset and slow the progression of diabetes have tremendous potential to mitigate the associated clinical and cost repercussions. In sub-Saharan Africa, the HIV/AIDS pandemic is an unparallel catastrophe and coupled with the resurgence of tuberculosis and the unfinished agenda of communicable diseases, including malaria and childhood infectious diseases, most countries in the region have run a high health deficit. Health spending in these countries is insufficient to address the health challenges they face.

In contrast to developed countries where the majority of people with diabetes are over the age of 65 years, in sub-Saharan Africa by 2025 most people with diabetes will be in the economically productive age group of 20–25 years [1]. The consequence of developing diabetes in early age is that there is a greater potential for the development of its chronic complications, thus imposing additional financial costs. The emergence of diabetes and its consequent heavy burden of morbidity and premature mortality will result in extra high socioeconomic costs, in terms of both medical care and loss of human resources.

Health is defined in the countries of the region as a *social sector* and therefore politicians and finance ministers do not consider it as an *economic sector*. The importance of health investment has therefore been greatly underestimated by governments whereas increased investments in health would translate into hundreds of dollars per year of increased income in these countries. There is much to be achieved in the promotion of health and well being of individuals within these countries. In countries where the health needs are the greatest, the resources and means tend to be least available, and the relative poverty of these countries constrains their attempts to improve health care indicators. It is imperative that the available resources be used equitably and efficiently.

Table 1 shows the prevalence of diabetes and health expenditure and services in some sub-Saharan African countries [1–4]. The gross national product varied from US$483 in Tanzania to US$3040 in South Africa, with the percentage of gross domestic product spent on health care ranging from 0.7% in Nigeria to 7.15 in South Africa. The *per capita* expenditure is relatively low in international terms. It follows from these figures that the region has limited resources to invest in diabetes care. The late diagnosis of diabetes leads to early presentation of diabetic complications.

The burden of diabetic complications in some African countries is shown in Table 2. The prevalence of diabetic retinopathy varies from 16 to 77%, depending on the duration of diabetes and glycemic control, with severe retinopathy representing 15% of all cases. At diagnosis, 21–25% of type 2 patients and 9.5% of type 1 patients have retinopathy. The prevalence of nephropathy varies between 32 and 57% after a mean duration of diabetes of 5–10 years, and between 5 and 28% within the first year following the diagnosis of diabetes. The prevalence of neuropathy varies widely, depending on the methodology used. Macrovascular complications of diabetes are considered rare in Africa despite a high prevalence of hypertension. Coronary heart disease may affect 5–8% of type 2

International Textbook of Diabetes Mellitus, Third Edition. Edited by R. A. DeFronzo, E. Ferrannini, H. Keen, and P. Zimmet.
 ISBN: 0-471-48655-8.

Table 1 Prevalence estimates of diabetes and socioeconomic indicators for the year 2000 in some sub-Saharan African countries

Country	Total number of people with diabetes (000's)*		GNP per capita† (PPP $) (1998)	Health expenditure‡ as % of GDP from 1990 to 1998			Health expenditure‡ per capita (PPP $) (1990–1998)	Physicians‡ (1990–1998) Per 1000 people	Hospital beds‡ (1990–1998) Per 1000 people
	Type 1	Type 2 (20–79 age group)		Public	Private	Total			
Cameroon	2.14	61.1	1395	1.0	4.0	5.0	83	0.1	2.6
Congo, Democratic Republic of	4.80	252.6	733	1.2	1.3	2.5	—	0.1	1.4
Congo, Republic of	0.23	8.6	846	1.8	3.2	5.0	62	0.3	3.4
Côte d'Ivoire	1.27	42.7	1484	1.4	2.6	3.7	66	0.1	0.8
Ethiopia	4.95	268.1	566	1.7	2.4	4.1	42	0.0	0.2
Gabon	0.16	5.5	5615	0.6	—	—	—	0.2	3.2
Gambia	0.07	2.2	1428	1.4	1.7	3.1	46	0.0	0.6
Ghana	2.79	32.3	1735	1.8	2.9	4.7	82	—	1.5
Kenya	3.65	190.4	964	2.2	1.0	1.0	10	0.0	1.6
Madagascar	2.52	75.0	741	1.1	1.0	2.1	—	0.3	0.9
Mali	0.79	18.4	673	2.0	1.8	3.8	28	0.1	0.2
Mozambique	0.98	117.3	740	2.1	—	—	—	—	0.9
Nigeria	12.52	209.4	740	0.2	0.5	0.7	6	0.2	1.7
Senegal	0.82	33.5	1297	2.6	2.1	4.7	66	0.1	0.4
South Africa	57.56	886.4	8296	3.2	3.5	7.1	571	0.6	—
Tanzania	2.47	134.8	483	1.3	—	—	—	0.0	0.9
Togo	0.63	9.6	1352	1.1	2.1	3.2	46	0.1	1.5
Uganda	0.65	88.7	1072	1.8	2.9	4.7	50	0.0	0.9
Zambia	0.52	40.8	678	2.3	1.8	4.1	33	0.1	—
Zimbabwe	2.06	55.4	2489	3.1	3.3	6.4	191	0.1	0.5

Note. PPP = purchasing power parity (international dollars).
* From reference 2.
† Reference 3.
‡ Reference 4.

Table 2 Prevalence of diabetes complications in selected populations of Africa

Country	Author [reference]	Year	Type of diabetes	Sample size	Prevalence of diabetic complications
Sudan	Elbagir et al. [5]	1995	1	128	Nephropathy 22%; retinopathy 43%; neuropathy 37%; peripheral vascular disease 10%; cerebrovascular accidents 5.5%
Burkina Faso	Drabo et al. [6]	1996	1 and 2	400	Nephropathy 24.8%; retinopathy 15.8%; peripheral neuropathy 35.0%
Uganda	Nambuya et al. [7]	1996	1 and 2	252	Nephropathy 17.1%; peripheral neuropathy 46.4%; impotence 22.2% of the men; ischemic heart disease 4.8%; foot ulcers 4.0%
South Africa	Levitt et al. [8]	1997	1 and 2	300	Microalbuminuria 36.7%; retinopathy 55.4%; peripheral neuropathy 27.6%; absent foot pulses 8.2%; lower limb amputations 1.4%
Ethiopia	Rahlenbeck et al. [9]	1997	1 and 2		Microalbuminuria: type 1 33%; type 2 36%
Cameroon	Sobngwi et al. [10]	1999	1 and 2	64	Microalbuminuria 53.1%; retinopathy 37.5%
Lybia	Kadiki et al. [11]	1999	2	8922	Nephropathy 25.2%; retinopathy 30.5%; neuropathy 45.7%
Benin	Djrolo et al. [12]	2001	1 and 2	152	Nephropathy 28%

diabetic patients and cardiomyopathy up to 50% of all patients. Lower extremity amputation varies from 1.5 to 7%, and about 12% of all hospitalized diabetic patients have foot ulceration. Neuropathy underlies diabetic foot more often than peripheral vascular disease. While microvascular complications of diabetes are highly prevalent and occur early during the course of disease, macrovascular disease is rare [5–12].

WHO PAYS FOR DIABETES CARE IN THE REGION?

The lack of investment in the health care system described above, the limited availability of private medical insurance, and the absence of a free national health service in most countries of the region mean that the burden of diabetes care is on the patient or the family. For example, in Cameroon, diabetes care is paid for by patients (50%), family (44%), employer (2%), charities (2%), and others including government (2%) [13]. Persons living in this region, containing 33 of the 49 *least developed* countries according to the World Bank, have to pay for medication and or management tools to monitor diabetes [14]. This phenomenon leads to inequalities in accessing the main antidiabetes drugs including insulin, a drug declared by the WHO as an essential drug for the treatment of diabetes [15], and may account for the high prevalence of diabetes complications.

DIABETES HEALTH SERVICES DELIVERY COSTS

There is limited information on the economics of diabetes care in sub-Saharan Africa. Despite its limitations in developing countries [16], the human capital approach [17] (valuing human life according to the income stream produced by the employed individual during their lifetime) was used to estimate minimum cost of diabetes in Tanzania [17]. In the human capital approach, cost is divided into direct and indirect costs of the disease.

Direct Costs of Diabetes

Direct costs include the expenditure for medical care and treatment of diabetes. These costs are usually borne by the patient, family, and the health sector for the prevention, diagnosis, and treatment of diabetes. Chale et al. estimated that about US$4 million would have been required to take care of all patients with diabetes in Tanzania in the year 1989–1990, which translates to US$138 per patient per annum. This sum is equivalent to 8.1% of the total budgeted health expenditure for that financial year and well above the allocated per capita health expenditure in Tanzania of US$2 for the year 1989–1990 [18]. The total direct outpatient costs of diabetes care was estimated to be US$2.7 million, which was 68% of total direct costs of diabetes care whereas inpatient costs accounted for 32% of all direct costs. Approximately 50% of all outpatient expenditure was attributable to drugs while 40% of inpatient expenditure was attributable to investigations (Table 3).

In the same Tanzanian study, the annual direct outpatient cost per diabetic patient in 1989–1990 was US$229 for type 1 diabetic patients and US$69 for type 2 diabetic patients. Of these direct costs, 68.2% and 42.5% were used for the purchase of insulin and oral hypoglycemic agents. Treatment of infections and chronic complications accounted for 13.2% and 48.8% in type 1 and type 2 diabetic patients, respectively.

In Cameroon, the average direct medical cost of treating a patient with diabetes in 2001 was US$489, with 56% of this cost spent on hospital admissions, 33.5% on antidiabetic drugs, 5.5% on laboratory tests, and 4.5% on consultation fees. The direct medical costs for treating all diabetic patients in Cameroon represented about 3.5% of the national budget for the 2001–2002 financial year [13]. Diabetes care management estimates from Malawi based on international prices for essential drugs and Malawi hospital cost data suggest that a type 1 diabetic patient spends about US$100 per annum for the purchase of insulin while a type 2 patient spends US$25 annually on oral hypoglycemic agents [19].

Indirect Costs of Diabetes

These costs are difficult to determine in this region. A rough estimate of indirect cost of diabetes calculated as healthy life days (HLDs) lost by a diabetic patient because of premature death, disability before death, chronic disability, and acute illness due to diabetes has been published from Tanzania [18] (Table 4). The average age at onset of diabetes in Tanzania was 44 years and the average age at death was 46 years, with a general life expectancy of 53 years. Calculated HLDs lost because of diabetes was 4100 days per patient, of which 69% was due to premature mortality. This calculation was based on an average case-fatality rate after 5 years in Tanzania of 29%, with the rate of severe chronic disablement of 14%. The estimated HLDs lost per capita because of diabetes was 820 person-days per 1000 people per year (Table 4).

In Ghana [19], the average age at onset of diabetes was 40 years with 50% case-fatality rate after 15 years, and an average age at death of 55 years with 30% disablement before death. The total days lost were calculated as 217 per 1000 persons per year, of which 52% was due to premature death.

Table 3 Estimated 1-year costs (US$) of outpatient and inpatient care of all patients with diabetes in Tanzania (1989–1990)*

Cost category	Average costs (US$)	Proportion of total costs (%)
Outpatient costs		
Transport	32.4	1.2
Nursing	1.4	0.1
Physician	2.6	0.1
Blood/urine tests	51.2	1.9
Urine dipsticks	96.0	3.5
Spirit/cotton wool	119.3	4.4
Syringes and needles	42.2	1.5
Insulin	875.1	32.2
Oral hypoglycemic agents	661.6	24.3
Treatment of complications	839.4	30.8
Total outpatient costs	*2721.2*	*100.0*
Inpatient costs		
Investigations	507.4	40.4
Oral hypoglycemic agents	6.9	0.5
Insulin	74.3	5.9
Antibiotics	45.9	3.7
Antihypertensive drugs	18.0	1.4
Intravenous fluids	56.1	4.5
Syringes and needles	63.4	5.1
Other treatment	60.8	4.8
Food and accommodation	275.9	22.0
Nursing	114.8	9.1
Physician	31.8	2.5
Total inpatient costs	*1255.3*	*100.0*

*(Adapted with permission of Elsevier [9]).

Relevance of Economics of Diabetes Studies in Sub-Saharan Africa

The economics of diabetes studies undertaken in the region if anything are an underestimation of the burden of diabetes because of the completeness of the studies. The studies are all hospital-based and they therefore exclude outpatient services provided through community health centers and other community-based services including the use of allied health services and the private health service provision. These exclusions underestimate the true impact of diabetes on the use of health services. Indeed, in all of the studies, the average costs per patient were well above the allocated per capita health expenditure (Table 1). This may signify the inadequate provision of diabetes health services especially since in most countries of the region there are no specific health resources allocated to the management of diabetes and its complications. It therefore follows that there is a need for well-targeted studies on the economic burden of diabetes from sub-Saharan Africa.

In a region with limited resources and where every decision should be seen in terms of cost and outcomes, the use of cost-effectiveness and cost–benefit studies to evaluate the economic efficiency of diabetes treatment, interventions, and programs should be encouraged [20]. Cost-effectiveness studies usually summarize health outcomes in physical terms (such as the number of lives saved) while cost–benefit studies place monetary values

Table 4 Indirect costs of diabetes*

	Type 2 diabetes		Type 1 diabetes		Uncertain†		Overall	
	n	%	*n*	%	*n*	%	*n*	%
Premature death	1997	55.1	949	39.7	8885	96.8	2832	69
Disability before death	18	0.5	93	3.9	37	0.4	60	1
Chronic disability	1571	43.3	1332	55.7	219	2.4	1183	29
Acute illness	40	1.1	15	0.6	34	0.4	26	1
Total HLDs	*3626*	*100.0*	*2389*	*100.0*	*1975*	*100.0*	*4101*	*100.0*

* Calculated as future HLDs lost per patient in 8 years of diabetes because of premature death, disabilities, and acute illnesses associated with diabetes in Tanzania (18).
† Uncertain: patients not easily classified owing to death shortly after diagnosis, short follow-up period, or loss to follow-up.
(Reproduced by permission of Elsevier).

on the health outcomes of programs, for example, reducing the impact of diabetic foot amputations [21, 22]. There is an urgent need of both of these types of studies from Africa. Cost–benefit studies on one of the major diabetic complications in the region—diabetic foot and diabetic foot amputations—will sit very well with African health policymakers.

CONCLUSION

Diabetes health care costs consume a significant proportion of the annual health budgets of many sub-Saharan African countries and these costs will escalate with the increasing burden of diabetes and its complications in the region. The high cost of diabetes care hinders many people from getting proper care since most of these costs are met by the patient or the family. Cost–benefit studies are needed to assess health outcomes of diabetes programs, especially diabetic foot and diabetic foot amputations. We need studies to explore the feasibility, effectiveness, and cost-effectiveness of interventions, particularly brief interventions at primary care settings and of community-wide interventions using culturally appropriate methods to promote healthy diet, increased physical activity, and prevent obesity.

REFERENCES

1. King H, Aubert RE, Herman WH. Global burden of diabetes, 1995–2025: prevalence, numerical estimates, and projections. *Diabetes Care* 1998; 21: 1414–3.
2. International Diabetes Federation. *Diabetes Atlas 2000*. Brussels: International Diabetes Federation, 2000.
3. *World Bank Atlas – 2002*. The World Bank, 2002.
4. *World Bank Development Indicators – 2000*. The World Bank, 2000.
5. Elbagir MN, Eltom MA, Mahadi EO, Berne C. Pattern of long-term complications in Sudanese insulin-treated diabetic patients. *Diabetes Res Clin Pract* 1995; 30: 59–67.
6. Drabo PY, Kabore J, Lengani A. Complications of diabetes mellitus at the Hospital Center of Ouagadougou. *Bull Soc Pathol Exot* 1996; 89: 191–5.
7. Nambuya AP, Otim MA, Whitehead H, Mulvany D, Kennedy R, Hadden DR. The presentation of newly-diagnosed diabetic patients in Uganda. *Q J Med* 1996; 89: 705–11.
8. Levitt NS, Bradshaw D, Zwarenstein MF, Bawa AA, Maphumolo S. Audit of public sector primary diabetes care in Cape Town, South Africa: high prevalence of complications, uncontrolled hyperglycaemia, and hypertension. *Diabet Med* 1997; 14: 1073–7.
9. Rahlenbeck SI, Gebre-Yohannes A. Prevalence and epidemiology of micro- and macroalbuminuria in Ethiopian diabetic patients. *J Diabetes Complications* 1997; 11: 343–9.
10. Kadiki OA, Roaed RB. Epidemiological and clinical patterns of diabetes mellitus in Benghazi, Libyan Arab Jamahiriya. *East Mediterr Health J* 1999; 5: 6–13.
11. Sobngwi E, Mbanya JC, Moukouri EN, Ngu KB. Microalbuminuria and retinopathy in a diabetic population of Cameroon. *Diabetes Res Clin Pract* 1999; 44: 191–6.
12. Djrolo F, Attolou VG, Avode DG, Houngbe F, Akpona S, Addra B, Kodjoh N. Diabetic nephropathy: an epidemiological study based on proteinuria in a population of black African diabetics in Cotonou, Benin. *Sante* 2001; 11: 105–9.
13. Nkegoum AV. *Coût direct et indirect du diabéte en l'absence de complications chroniques a Yaoundé, Cameroon* [MD thesis]. Cameroon: University of Yaoundé I, 2002.
14. World Bank Report 2001. The World Bank, 2001.
15. Deeb LC, Tan MH, Alberti KG. Insulin availability among International Diabetes Federation member associations. Report of the Task Force on Insulin Distribution. *Diabetes Care* 1994; 17: 220–3.
16. Chale S. The economics of diabetes care in developing countries; focus on Tanzania. *Int Diabetes Dig* 1993; 4: 52–8.
17. Rice DP, Hodgson TA, Kopstein AN. The economic costs of illness: a replication and update. *Health Care Fin Rev Fall* 1985; 2: 61–80.
18. Chale S, Swai A, Mujinja P, McLarty D. Must diabetes be a fatal disease in Africa? Study of cost of treatment. *BMJ* 1992; 304: 1215–8.
19. Vaughan P, Gilson L, Mills A. Diabetes in developing countries: its importance for public health. *Health Policy Plan* 1989; 4: 97–109.
20. Drummond MF, Stoddart GI. Principles of economic evaluation of health programs. *World Health Stat Q* 1985; 355–76
21. Mills A, Drummond MF. Economic evaluation of health programmes: glossary of terms. *World Health Stat Q* 1985; 432–4
22. IDF Task Force on Diabetes Health Economics. *Diabetes Health Economics: Facts, Figures and Forecasts*. Brussels: International Diabetes Federation, 1999.

115

Prevention of Type 1 Diabetes Mellitus

Leonard C. Harrison, Spiros Fourlanos, Alison L. Every, Margo C. Honeyman, Raymond J. Steptoe, Nathan R. Martinez, Kent P. Jensen, David P. Funda, Stuart I. Mannering, Peter G. Colman, and Parth Narendran

The Walter and Eliza Hall Institute of Medical Research, Parkville, Australia

INTRODUCTION

Insulin-dependent or type 1 diabetes (T1D) results from the selective destruction of β cells in the islets of the pancreas, with consequent insulin deficiency and chronic hyperglycemia that may lead to complications involving primarily small blood vessels and nerves. T1D is considered to be an autoimmune disease triggered by environmental agents in genetically susceptible individuals, which in most cases begins months to years before loss of β-cell function heralds symptoms of hyperglycemia (Figure 1). The pathogenesis of T1D has been reviewed elsewhere [1–3] and will not be reiterated here except insofar as necessary to justify therapeutic approaches to the prevention of T1D. The ideal approach to T1D prevention would be primary prevention directed at the triggering events that initiate disease in genetically at-risk individuals. Secondary prevention, once the disease has been initiated, is directed at subverting pathogenic immunity and its effects on the β cell. Although the focus in T1D is on β-cell pathology and insulin deficiency, it is important to consider that blood glucose control reflects both insulin secretion and insulin action. T1D often presents clinically at times of "insulin resistance," e.g. puberty, and insulin resistance could accelerate the rate of progression to clinical disease. Therefore, agents that promote insulin action might also be considered for the secondary prevention of T1D.

The nonobese diabetic (NOD) mouse is a model of T1D that has contributed enormously to our understanding of the pathogenesis of the disease, and to our expectation that it is preventable. The NOD mouse develops spontaneous, autoimmune β-cell destruction that depends on activation of the innate immune cells followed by islet-reactive T cells [4]. The cellular immune infiltrate of the islets (insulitis) in NOD mice is more florid than that revealed from the limited number of autopsies performed on humans dying soon after diagnosis and diabetes occurs predominantly in females. Otherwise, the NOD mouse has features in common with human T1D, including polygenic inheritance dominated by specific genes within the major histocompatibility complex (MHC), autoimmunity to (pro)insulin, glutamic acid decarboxylase (GAD), and probably tyrosine phosphatase-like insulinoma antigen IA-2, transfer of disease by bone marrow, and a preclinical stage of disease prior to hyperglycemia (Table 1).

A variety of immune and other interventions substantially reduce the incidence of diabetes in NOD mice [5]. The question is whether any of these, if scientifically and ethically acceptable, are likely to be effective in humans. Knowledge of the immunopathogenesis of T1D over the last three decades has expanded to provide a rationale for the advent of controlled clinical trials to answer this question, but the answers have not yet been affirmative. Nevertheless, there are important lessons from the intervention/prevention trials conducted to date, and many improvements and refinements in trial design and translation from mice to humans remain to be implemented. Without knowing the environmental trigger agents or being able to modify genetic susceptibility, the prospect of primary prevention before the onset of disease is uncertain. It should not be forgotten, though, that primary prevention has already succeeded to a small extent through vaccination to prevent congenital rubella (German measles), the first-described and so far only known definite viral cause

International Textbook of Diabetes Mellitus, Third Edition. Edited by R. A. DeFronzo, E. Ferrannini, H. Keen, and P. Zimmet.
 ISBN: 0-471-48655-8.

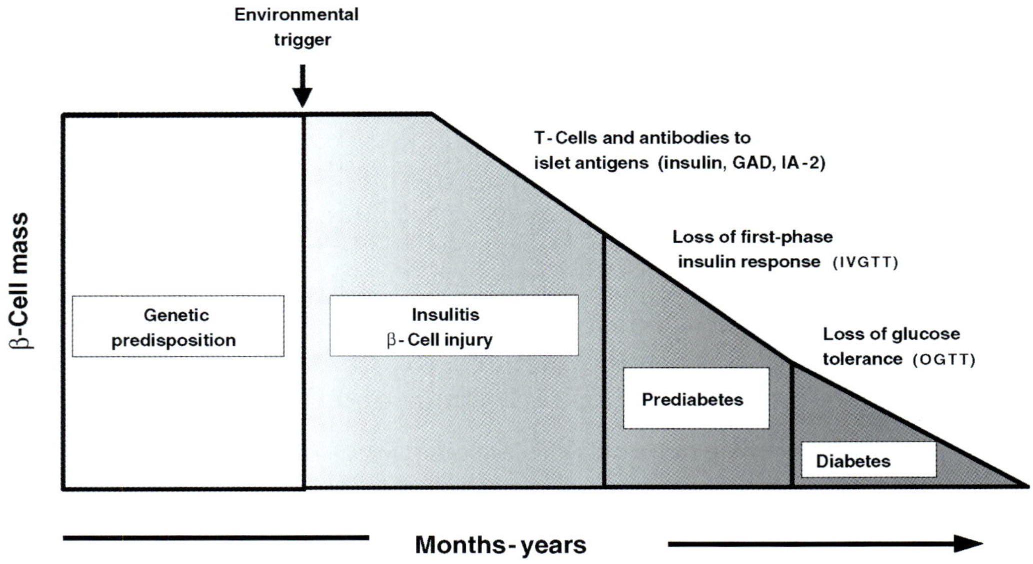

Figure 1 Natural history of preclinical T1D

of T1D (see below). Currently, most attention is focused on secondary prevention, to avert either progression to diabetes in people with autoantibody markers of islet autoimmunity or loss of residual β-cell function in those with recently diagnosed diabetes, by strategies aimed at suppressing pathogenic immune responses or promoting resistance of β cells to these responses.

The concept of T1D prevention is not irrelevant to people with established diabetes. T1D will not be cured, whether by transplantation of normal or engineered insulin-secreting cells or by stimulation of β-cell neogenesis, without preventing recurrent autoimmune disease. Here we examine the precepts and prospects for preventing T1D, with an emphasis on factors likely to be critical for successful clinical outcomes.

WHY?

Prevention is the ultimate treatment goal in T1D. The personal, social, and economic costs of T1D include those associated not only with day-to-day management but with longer term complications. Complications can be reduced but not prevented by intensive blood glucose control with injectable insulin. In the Diabetes Control and Complications Trial (DCCT), even intensively treated, motivated subjects in a study situation developed significant complications over the 10-year follow-up: 5% developed neuropathy, 10% retinopathy, and 15% nephropathy. Moreover, intensive treatment was accompanied by two- to threefold increase in severe, symptomatic hypoglycemic episodes [6]. Even retaining some β-cell function or

Table 1 The NOD mouse as a model of human T1D

Feature	NOD mouse	Human
Preclinical stage	Yes	Yes
Gender	F > M	M > F after puberty
Genetic susceptibility		
MHC class II β57 non-Asp	Yes (I-A^{g7})	Yes (DQ8)
Polygenic non-MHC	Yes	Yes
Environmental influence on gene penetrance	Yes	Yes
Disease transmission via bone marrow	Yes	Yes
Mononuclear cell infiltration of		
Islets (insulitis)	Marked	Moderate
Other organs	Yes	Sometimes
Impaired immune regulation	Yes	Yes
Autoantigens		
(Pro)insulin	Yes	Yes
GAD	Yes	Yes
IA-2	Yes	Yes
Response to autoantigen-specific therapy	Yes	?

Note: "?" indicates not yet known.

delaying the onset of clinical disease would reduce the burden of T1D. Patients who retain some β-cell function require lower doses of insulin and have better blood glucose control. In our experience of screening first-degree relatives, approximately 3% of whom will be confirmed positive for one or more islet autoantibodies, the cost of detecting one person with a 50% risk of diabetes within 5 years is approximately US$5500. As the annual cost of treating T1D in Australia is approximately US$2000, a relatively inexpensive means of prevention would only need to delay the onset of diabetes for 3 years for screening to be cost-effective in dollar terms. The Finnish IDDM Prediction and Prevention Project (DIPP) found that neonatal screening for HLA genetic risk was cost-effective as compared with autoantibody screening of the whole population [7]. Genetic risk-based screening alone may be economic in high incidence populations, provided of course that a safe and reasonably effective intervention is available.

WHO?

Target populations for prevention fall into two general categories: those with genetic and/or immune markers of risk who have not yet developed diabetes and those with recently diagnosed diabetes in whom residual β-cell function might be preserved or even regenerated. Most studies of at-risk individuals have followed first-degree relatives of a T1D proband who have circulating autoantibodies to one or more of the islet antigens (pro)insulin, GAD, and tyrosine phosphatase like insulinoma antigen IA-2 indicative of subclinical disease [8–11]. However, although islet autoantibodies have high (~90%) disease sensitivity and specificity in Caucasoid populations, about 10% of patients will have no detectable antibodies at diagnosis. First-degree relatives share susceptibility genes and possibly environmental risk factors and have at least a 10-fold higher prevalence of T1D than does the background population, but they represent only 10–15% of people diagnosed with T1D and whether their immunopathology is representative of T1D in the general population is uncertain. Studies in Finland, which has the highest incidence of T1D in the world, reveal that neonatal screening for high-risk HLA class II susceptibility genes can identify over half of those destined to develop T1D [12]. Neonatal screening to identify genetically at-risk populations is a basis for primary prevention but its predictive value, especially in populations with a lower incidence of T1D than Finland, would only be sufficient to justify intervention that was simple and safe, for example, diet modification.

An important prerequisite for intervention to prevent T1D in asymptomatic individuals is the ability to predict development of clinical disease. In first-degree relatives, autoantibodies to islet antigens are among several markers known to predict the rate of β-cell destruction and risk for diabetes development (Table 2). For example, the 5-year risk of diabetes in young, first-degree relatives is in the order <30%, 30–50%, and >50% for autoantibodies to one, two, and three islet antigens, respectively. In addition, impaired first-phase insulin response to intravenous glucose, at or below the first percentile, signifies end-stage disease and almost certain diabetes within 5 years. The risk associated with autoantibody markers cannot, however, be extrapolated from first-degree relatives to the general population, because the predictive value of a risk marker is proportional to the population prevalence of disease (Bayes' theorem). Autoantibody-positive first-degree relatives are therefore the main target population for primary or secondary prevention strategies in T1D.

Table 2 Factors that influence progression to diabetes in islet antibody-positive relatives

First-phase insulin response (FPIR) to IV glucose
Level of islet antibody
Number of antigen specificities of islet antibodies
Antigen specificity of islet antibody
Age at detection of islet antibody
HLA alleles for risk or protection
HLA haplotype sharing with proband
Relationship with proband

The pros and cons of trialling candidate prevention agents in asymptomatic, at-risk subjects versus symptomatic, recently diagnosed subjects is a topic of ongoing debate. The issue is not "either–or." Some agents, for example toxic immunosuppressive drugs, would not be justified in asymptomatic subjects, many of whom are children, whereas others, for example agents given to promote protective immune homeostasis, may be ineffective in end-stage disease. In at-risk individuals with subclinical disease, prediction of clinical disease is inexact but because their disease is less advanced intervention may be more effective. The majority of clinical trials for the prevention of T1D (Table 3) have been conducted with nonspecific, potentially toxic agents in subjects with recently diagnosed diabetes. The consideration of efficacy versus safety would appear to be less of a dilemma in these subjects, but this could be illusory. Irrespective of the mode of action of any candidate prevention agent, the major loss of β-cell function at the time of clinical diagnosis militates against therapeutic success. This is depicted in Figure 2 and is a theme that we will return to in the discussion of antigen-specific therapy below.

There are two possible exceptions to the idea that prevention should be directed to what is preventable, i.e. subclinical disease. First, treatment of NOD mice with anti-T-cell receptor (CD3) monoclonal antibody at the onset of diabetes surprisingly results in reversal of diabetes [57]. Removing the burden of pathogenic, effector T cells (T_{path}) at this stage is certainly an important principle (Figure 2) if we ever hope to see the emergence of

Table 3 Trials for prevention of T1D

	Subjects (n)	Follow-up (months)	Outcome	Chief investigator/ Reference
Primary prevention				
Non-antigen-specific immune modulation				
Cows' milk elimination (Trial to reduce IDDM in the genetically at-risk–TRIGR)	HLA at-risk infants (>2000)		Ongoing	Akerblom*
Gluten elimination	AR (7)	24	No effect on islet antibody levels	Hummel [13]
Secondary prevention				
Nonspecific immune suppression				
Azathioprine (2 mg/kg/day)	RD (24)	12	Higher basal and glucagon-stimulated C-peptide, and more remissions	Harrison [14]
Cyclosporine (7.5 mg/kg/day)	RD (122)	9	More remissions	Feutren [15]
Azathioprine (2 mg/kg/day) + prednisolone (reducing dose)	RD (46)	12	Higher meal-stimulated C-peptide and lower insulin dose	Silverstein [16]
Cyclosporin (20 mg/kg/day)	RD (188)	12	Higher glucagon C-peptide and more remissions. Greater benefit in most recently diagnosed	Canadian–European RCT Group [17]
Azathioprine (2 mg/kg/day)	RD (49)	12	Higher meal-stimulated C-peptide	Cook [18]
Azathioprine + thymostimulin	RD (45)	12	Higher glucagon-stimulated C-peptide and more remissions	Moncada [19]
Cyclosporine	RD (219)	24	Higher meal stimulated C-peptide and more remissions	Assan [20]
Cyclosporine (10 mg/kg/day, 4 months)	RD (43)	36	No difference in glucagon-stimulated C-peptide, HbA_{1c}, insulin dose	Chase [21]
Prednisolone (15 mg/day, 8 months); Indomethacin (100 mg/day, 8 months)	RD (25)	24	Lower insulin dose and higher urine C-peptide in prednisolone group	Secchi [22]
Cyclosporine (10 mg/kg/day)	RD (23)	12	Higher meal- but not glucagon- or glucose-stimulated C-peptide, no difference in insulin dose	Skyler [23]
Anti-CD5/ricin A chain (unblinded)	RD (15)	12	Higher meal-stimulated C-peptide	Skyler [24]
Glucocorticoid	RD (32)	12	Higher glucagon-stimulated C-peptide, but not remissions	Goday [25]
Anti-CD4 + glucocorticoid	RD (12)	12	No difference in insulin dose, or islet antibody titers	Kohnert [26]
Methotrexate (unblinded)	RD (10)	36	No effect on basal or meal-stimulated C-peptide. Insulin dose higher	Buckingham [27]
Anti-CD3 (hOKT3) (unblinded)	RD (18)	12	Increase in meal-stimulated C-peptide in first year. IL-10 detected in serum	Herold [28]
hCAMPATH 3 (6×8 mg IV)	RD (80)	?	Ongoing	Gorus*
Mycophenolate mofetil ± daclizumab	RD (90)	24	Ongoing	Gottlieb*
Daclizumab	RD (40)	24	Ongoing	Rodriguez*
Nonspecific immune stimulation				
BCG vaccine	RD (26)	18	No effect on glucagon-stimulated C-peptide, insulin dose or HbA_{1c}	Elliott [29]
BCG vaccine	RD (94)	24	No effect on mixed meal-stimulated C-peptide, insulin dose or HbA_{1c}	Allen [30]
Q fever vaccine	RD (39)	12	No effect on glucagon-stimulated C-peptide or insulin dose	Schmidli†
Oral IFN-α	RD (120)		Ongoing	Brod*
Nonspecific immune regulation				
Thymopoietin	RD (32)	6	Lower insulin antibodies and insulin dose. More remissions. No difference in C-peptide or HbA_{1c}	Giordano [31]
Gammaglobulin	RD (16)	6	Higher basal C-peptide Lower insulin dose, unchanged HbA_{1c}	Panto [32]
Linomide	RD (63)	12	Lower HbA_{1c}, insulin dose. No difference in glucagon-stimulated C-peptide	Coutant [33]
HSP60 p277 peptide (DiaPep)	RD (35)	10	Decrease in glucagon-stimulated C-peptide and insulin dose in placebo but not treated group	Raz [34]
1,25-Dihydroxy vitamin D_3	RD (40)	18	Ongoing	Ziegler*

Antigen-specific immune regulation				
Parenteral insulin (IV vs. SC 2 weeks)	RD (26)	12	Higher meal-stimulated C-peptide, lower HbA_{1c}	Shah [35]
Parenteral insulin	RD (49)	60	Higher glucagon-stimulated C-peptide and improved insulin sensitivity and glycemic control	Linn [36]
Parenteral insulin (IV vs. SC 2 weeks)	RD (19)	12	Higher meal and glucagon-stimulated C-peptide and lower HbA_{1c}	Schnell [37]
Parenteral insulin	RD (10)		Higher C-peptide response to oral glucose, HbA_{1c} unchanged	Kobayashi [38]
Parenteral insulin and sulfonylurea (Glipizide)	RD (27)	12	Higher basal and glucagon-stimulated C-peptide, more remissions	Selam [39]
Oral insulin	RD (80)	12	No effect on basal C-peptide, HbA_{1c}, insulin dose or insulin antibodies	Pozzilli*
Oral insulin	RD (131)	12	No effect on basal, glucagon- or meal-stimulated C-peptide, HbA_{1c}, insulin dose or islet antibody levels	Chaillous [40]
Parenteral insulin	AR (14)	84	Delay in onset of diabetes. No effect on islet antibody levels	Füchtenbusch [41]
Parenteral insulin (Diabetes Prevention Trial Type 1 – DPT-1)	AR (339)	44	No effect on diabetes development	DPT-1 Study Group [42] and Skyler*
Intranasal insulin (Melbourne Intranasal Trial – INIT I)	AR (38)	48	Increased antibody and decreased T-cell responses to insulin. Stable first-phase insulin response to IV glucose	Harrison [43]
Oral insulin (DPT-1)	AR (480)	To diabetes	Ongoing	Skyler*
Parenteral insulin B chain in incomplete Freund's adjuvant	RD (12)	24	Ongoing	Orban*
Parenteral insulin B chain 9–23 "altered peptide ligand" NBI-6024	RD (55)	28	Ongoing	"Neurocrine" Gottlieb*
Intranasal insulin (Diabetes Prediction and Prevention Project – DIPP)	AR (?)	?	Ongoing	Simell*
Parenteral GAD65	RD (?)	?	Ongoing	"Diamyd"
β-Cell protection				
Nicotinamide	RD (20)	12	Higher glucagon-stimulated C-peptide at 45 days, then decline. No difference in remissions	Mendola [44]
Nicotinamide	RD (23)	9	Higher basal and glucagon-stimulated C-peptide	Vague [45]
Nicotinamide	RD (35)	12	No difference in basal or glucagon-stimulated C-peptide	Chase [46]
Nicotinamide	RD (56)	12	Higher glucagon-stimulated C-peptide in subjects >15 years old	Pozzilli [47]
Nicotinamide ± cyclosporine	RD (90)	12	Lower insulin dose. No difference in remissions	Pozzilli [48]
Nicotinamide ± parenteral insulin	RD (34)	12	No difference in glucagon-stimulated C-peptide	Vidal [49]
Nicotinamide versus vitamin E (no control group)	RD (84)	12	No difference in basal or glucagon-stimulated C-peptide, HbA_{1c} or insulin dose	Pozzilli [50]
Nicotinamide (Deutsche Nicotinamide Intervention Study – DENIS)	AR (55)	36	No effect on diabetes development	Lampeter [51]
Nicotinamide (European Nicotinamide Diabetes Intervention Trial – ENDIT)	AR (552)		No effect on diabetes development	Philips [52]
Octreotide	RD (20)	12	Higher glucagon-stimulated C-peptide at 6 and 12 months; no difference in HbA_{1c} or insulin dose	Grunt [53]
Diazoxide	RD adults (40)	18	Higher basal C-peptide	Bjork [54]
Diazoxide	RD children (56)		Higher (?) stimulated C-peptide at 12, not 24, months	Bjork [55]
Antioxidants	RD (46)	30	No difference in meal-stimulated C-peptide, insulin dose or HbA_{1c}	Ludvigsson [56]

Note: "?" indicates not state, thus unknown.
* Trial is ongoing.
† Trial is finished, but in analysis.

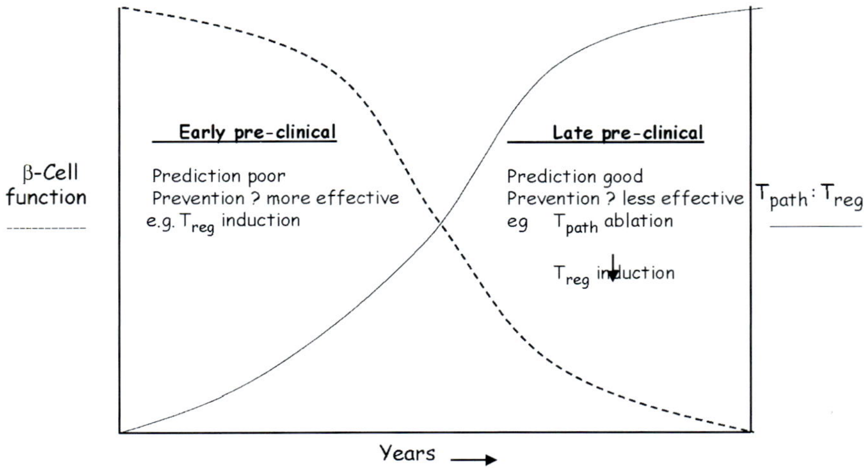

Figure 2 Type 1 diabetes: the prediction–prevention equation

protective, regulatory T cells (T_{reg}), as discussed below, or the potential for β-cell neogenesis. Anti-T cell agents such as anti-CD3 antibody not only are immunosuppressive but may also allow emergence of T_{reg} [57, 58]. To our knowledge, treatment with anti-CD3 antibody has not been shown to result in β-cell regeneration. The effect of anti-CD3 antibody to reverse diabetes suggests also, at least in the NOD mouse, that the onset of diabetes signifies a major degree of functional but not necessarily physical β-cell loss. This finding in the NOD mouse has been followed up by controlled trials of humanized anti-CD3 monoclonal antibody in humans with recently diagnosed diabetes (Table 3). Second, adults can present with a form of autoimmune diabetes, initially non-insulin-requiring, that accounts for approximately 10% of adult-onset diabetes [59–61]. Although they present with *type 2 diabetes*, these patients are seropositive for islet cell antibodies, specifically antibodies to GAD, and are therefore proposed to have a slowly progressive form of T1D. The small proportion of women with gestational diabetes who have antibodies to GAD and a high risk of insulin dependence also fall into this category of adult-onset, slowly progressive autoimmune diabetes. Adults with autoimmune diabetes have on average higher residual β-cell function at diagnosis compared to younger individuals with classical T1D [62]. This implies a potentially greater therapeutic window for secondary prevention, after the onset of symptoms.

HOW?

Starting with trials of glucocorticoids, azathioprine, and cyclosporine in the 1980s, a range of immunologic and nonimmunologic primary and secondary interventions have been or are being trialled in at-risk relatives and recently diagnosed patients [63, 64] (Table 3). No intervention, however, has yet demonstrated efficacy in the longer term. Trials in recently diagnosed subjects, for example the earlier trials of azathioprine and cyclosporine or the more recent trials of the HSP60 heat shock protein p277 ("DiaPep") and the humanised anti-CD3 monoclonal antibody (Table 3), demonstrated a beneficial effect on clinical remission and/or residual β-cell function (fasting or stimulated C-peptide secretion) in the first year after diagnosis. In the earlier trials, this "first-year effect" was not sustained and awaits evaluation in current trials. Greenbaum [64] has pointed out that the mean age of subjects in 9 such trials reporting such an initial positive outcome was higher than that in another 10 trials reporting a negative outcome (22 vs. 15 years, $p < 0.01$). She also observed that the proportion of trials reporting a positive outcome has decreased from the 1980s, along with a shift in the primary outcome measure away from clinical remission to the more rigorous measure of residual insulin (C-peptide) secretion. Trial design, including trial duration and the evaluation of primary and secondary outcomes, is critical, and standardization of design would facilitate comparative analysis of trials (Table 4). To this end, the Immunology of Diabetes Society (IDS) has published guidelines for trials of prevention agents in subjects with recently diagnosed T1D (http://www.idsoc.org/Guidelines.html) [65].

Not all trials have been based on preclinical data for efficacy or safety, or have incorporated surrogate disease markers. As emphasized, interventions particularly in asymptomatic, at-risk subjects must be deemed to be safe, and should ideally be based on proof-of-concept in animal studies. The primary outcome of trials should be to prevent diabetes. However, intermediate markers of disease, particularly measures of β-cell function, such as the oral glucose tolerance test (OGTT) or the mixed meal tolerance test (MMTT) in subjects with diabetes, or intravenous glucose for the measurement of first-phase insulin response

Table 4 Prevention trials in recently diagnosed T1D

Variables requiring standardisation
Criteria for diagnosis of diabetes
Documentation at diagnosis of clinical (symptoms, weight loss, insulin requirement, age, gender, pubertal status, family history), metabolic (blood glucose, HbA_{1c}, bicarbonate, ketones), genetic (HLA typing), and immune (islet autoantibodies) profile
Time from diagnosis
Measures of β-cell function, e.g. C-peptide fasting and after mixed meal stimulation
Subject number—sufficient for randomized controls and stratification
Trial duration—sufficient for efficacy and safety
Definition of primary and secondary outcome measures, e.g. "tight control" ($HbA_{1c} < 7\%$), β-cell function (area under curve of C-peptide response to mixed meal), and non-insulin-dependence (normal HbA_{1c} and OGTT off insulin)

(FPIR) in at-risk subjects, may provide critical interim information on efficacy. How immune markers—islet autoantibodies and T-cells reactive to islet antigens—reflect the nature and outcome of islet pathology is unknown, but these should be incorporated as surrogates into clinical trials in order to find out the same. Although humans at high risk for T1D have a relatively restricted set of HLA susceptibility genes, they are, in contrast to inbred NOD mice, likely to display significant heterogeneity in response to any therapeutic intervention. Clinical prevention trials in T1D provide an opportunity to gain insight into pharmacogenetics. For example, the immune response to proinsulin, which is likely to drive β-cell destruction [66, 67], could be determined by the length of the variable number of tandem repeats (VNTR) at the IDDM 2 susceptibility locus upstream of the proinsulin gene. The level of proinsulin gene transcription in the thymus, which may correlate with deletion ("negative selection") of proinsulin-specific T-cells during their intrathymic development, is proportional to the length of the VNTR [68, 69]: long (class III) and short (class I) VNTR alleles are associated, respectively, with low and high susceptibility to T1D.

The ideal strategy for T1D prevention would be to combine an inexpensive screening test that has a high positive predictive value with treatment that is safe and effective. The results of past and current trials (Table 3) show that this remains an ideal. Prevention of T1D falls under the headings of *primary* and *secondary*. Strategies for secondary prevention can be categorized as *nonspecific immune suppression*, *nonspecific immune stimulation*, *nonspecific immune regulation*, *antigen-specific immune regulation*, and *β-cell protection*. It is beyond the scope of this review to discuss each candidate agent in detail. As in cancer or HIV therapy, progress toward the prevention of T1D will be incremental, and is likely to involve a combination of agents—many yet to be developed—that act preferentially at different stages of disease development.

PRIMARY PREVENTION

Genetic manipulation of humans to avert risk is not feasible or ethical. Primary prevention therefore means targeting environmental factors that might trigger islet autoimmunity. The environment is implicated in T1D by several lines of evidence: in discordant identical twin pairs, the lifetime risk of diabetes for the nondiabetic twin is 50–70% [70, 71]; the incidence of T1D has increased over the last 15 years in many countries, particularly in the very young [72, 73]; in both hemispheres of the world a role for infectious agents is suggested by a spring–summer peak in births of children who develop T1D [74, 75] and a winter peak in diagnosis [72, 75, 76]; exposure to rubella virus *in utero* [77] and to the toxin Vacor [78] causes T1D.

Diet and the Role of the Mucosa

The hypothesis that early exposure of the infant to cows' milk and/or the lack of breastfeeding predisposes to T1D dates from the 1980s. It has important implications, but remains controversial because the evidence on which it is based is indirect and open to criticism [79]. Two meta-analyses of multiple studies in which diabetes prevalence was associated retrospectively with infant feeding revealed only a marginal increase in relative risk [80, 81]. In the Denver-based Diabetes Autoimmunity Study in the Young (DAISY), infant feeding patterns retrospectively analyzed up to 6 months of age were not found to be related to the development of islet autoantibodies up to 7 years of age [82]. In the Australian BabyDiab Study [83] and the German BabyDiab Study [84], there was no association between infant feeding patterns and the development of islet autoantibodies. To directly address the question whether cows' milk exposure is a risk, the Trial to Reduce IDDM in the Genetically At-Risk (TRIGR) has been initiated in Finland. Newborns with a T1D first-degree relative and with HLA risk alleles, initially exclusively breastfed, are being randomized to either a casein hydrolysate formula ("Neutramigen") or a conventional cow's milk-based formula until at least 6 months of age.

In the two rodent models of T1D, the NOD mouse and the biobreeding (BB) rat, recent reports indicate that in fact plant rather than milk proteins are associated with the development of islet autoimmunity [85]. Antibodies to wheat gluten proteins are found in a proportion of T1D patients at the time of diagnosis [86], but in a small unblinded pilot study 1 year of gluten-free diet had no effect on the natural history of islet autoimmunity [13]. Nevertheless, there is evidence that the prevalence of autoimmune diseases, including T1D, in individuals with celiac disease is related to the duration of exposure to gluten [87] and breastfeeding is reported to reduce the risk of celiac disease [88]. Further studies in this area are warranted.

Children with T1D have been reported to have an increased prevalence of immune responses to cows' milk proteins, but a review of published data suggests that this is not necessarily disease-specific, but reflects genetic predisposition to increased immunity to dietary proteins in general, associated with the HLA haplotype A1-B8-DR3-DQ2, which also predisposes to celiac disease and selective IgA deficiency. We have previously suggested that the cows' milk hypothesis could be productively reframed around mucosal immune function in T1D [79]. The essential role of a normal mucosal immune system in maintaining immune homeostasis is illustrated by the effect of germ-free versus "dirty" environments on diabetes incidence in NOD mice. The incidence of spontaneous diabetes in NOD mice differs greatly between colonies around the world and appears to be inversely correlated with exposure to microbial infection [89]. The high incidence of diabetes in NOD mice housed under pathogen-free conditions is reduced by conventional conditions of housing and feeding [90]. Under such conventional "dirty" conditions, bacterial colonization of the intestine is accompanied by an increase in the number of intraepithelial lymphocytes [91] and by maturation of mucosal immune function [92]. The recent increase in the prevalence of immunoallergic disorders in the first world has been attributed to "clean living" conditions—the "hygiene hypothesis" [93, 94]. If the NOD mouse is an example, then clean living comes at a cost. Apart from microbial stimuli, breast milk contains growth factors, cytokines, and other immunomodulatory agents that promote functional maturation of the intestinal mucosa and mucosal immune system. In addition, breast milk contains endogenous insulin that could induce "oral tolerance" to insulin and protect against the development of T1D, as described below. If correct, this implies that protection against T1D could be afforded by increasing exposure of the infant mucosa to (pro)insulin.

Viruses

Several viruses have been implicated as triggers of T1D. Viral mechanisms could include direct infection of β cells, infection of the exocrine pancreas with bystander death of β cells, molecular mimicry between T-cell epitopes in the virus and those in β-cell autoantigens, superantigenic stimulation of T cells, or any combination of these. If a virus was clearly implicated, vaccination of children early in life, if safe for the general population, would be protective (the caveat being molecular mimicry).

The first virus to be associated with T1D was rubella (German measles) [77]. Children with congenital rubella born to mothers who contracted rubella early in pregnancy had evidence of infection in the brain, pancreas, and other tissues and at least 20% developed insulin-dependent diabetes [95]. Subsequently, almost twice this proportion was reported to develop islet cell antibodies [96]. Children with congenital rubella and diabetes were noted to have a higher frequency of the T1D susceptibility haplotype HLA-A1-B8-(DR3-DQ2) [97]. More recently, molecular mimicry between rubella and GAD has been proposed [98]. Rubella vaccine has virtually eliminated congenital rubella and represents primary prevention of T1D. Clearly, many other environmental factors are involved, because the incidence of T1D has continued to increase in the first world. Despite the report of rubella–GAD mimicry, strengthened by the finding of islet cell antibodies in children infected with wild-type virus [99], there is little evidence from multiple studies [84, 100] that the rubella vaccine is harmful. Only 4% of girls receiving live attenuated vaccine developed islet cell antibodies, and these were transient and of low titer [101].

Mothers infected during pregnancy with some enteroviruses (including coxsackie and echoviruses) were found to be more likely to give birth to children developing T1D early in life [102, 103]. Recent studies, however, have not found an association between antenatal infection and T1D in offspring [104, 105]. Enterovirus RNA was isolated from peripheral blood mononuclear cells of 50% of recently diagnosed T1D cases in Scandinavia [106], 26% of siblings, and 0% of age- and sex-matched controls. In Germany and Australia, the BabyDiab studies show that coxsackie B virus infections are more common during the preclinical stage of T1D compared with controls but do not occur at the same time as islet autoantibodies are first detected [104] (J. Couper et al., submitted). This is consistent with infection of exocrine tissues rather than islets, as observed in rodent models [107, 108].

Enteroviruses may be involved indirectly in initiating β-cell autoimmunity. Evidence for mimicry, despite many studies, remains weak [109, 110], and the likely mechanism for any effect of enteroviruses is bystander inflammation [111]. The somewhat indirect nature of the enteroviral association with diabetes makes it less attractive as a vaccine target. Furthermore, there are 72 recognized serotypes and many thousands of strain variants within the enteroviruses, and no vaccines, except for polio virus, exist. However if diabetes-associated strains such as coxsackie B3, B4, echo 6 were clearly implicated, then vaccines for genetically at-risk children might be feasible.

Mumps virus epidemics have been associated with onset of T1D 2–4 years later [112, 113]. Intriguingly, the introduction of the mumps vaccine was associated with a plateau in the rising incidence of T1D in Finland [114], but as this was temporary, mumps vaccine is unlikely to be of much use for prevention of T1D.

Cytomegalovirus (CMV) can damage β cells [115] and contains a peptide sequence mimic of a T-cell epitope in GAD recognized by a T-cell clone from a subject with stiff man syndrome [110]. However, evidence for CMV in T1D is weak [116]. Furthermore, although CMV is now the major cause of congenital defects, development of a vaccine is problematic because of latency and possible carcinogenicity of an attenuated virus.

The discovery of strong sequence similarities between T-cell epitopes in IA-2 and GAD and the VP7 protein of rotavirus in islet antibody-positive relatives [117] suggested that molecular mimicry with rotavirus might initiate islet autoimmunity. Rotavirus epidemics occur each winter particularly in preschools and are the most common cause of gastroenteritis in children. They provide a profound inflammatory stimulus to the gut until sufficient IgA develops by about 5 years of age. In the Australian BabyDiab Study, rotavirus infections were temporally associated with the first appearance of or significant increases in islet antibodies in 24 children before they developed diabetes [118]. Rotavirus has now been shown to infect β cells specifically within islets from mice, pigs, and monkeys [119]. Vaccines under development for rotavirus contain the sequences that mimic both IA-2 and GAD. If molecular mimicry was proven to be a pathogenic mechanism, a vaccine may need to have the cross-reacting sequences deleted or modified to avoid the possibility of triggering islet autoimmunity.

Paradoxically, infection by rotavirus and other diabetogenic viruses in a noninflammatory context, such as during breastfeeding, could conceivably be protective against the later development of T1D. Enteroviruses and rotaviruses exemplify the concept that ubiquitous environmental agents might influence the development of T1D in genetically susceptible individuals. Understanding the role of environmental factors would be greatly advanced by large scale epidemiological studies, which are currently lacking.

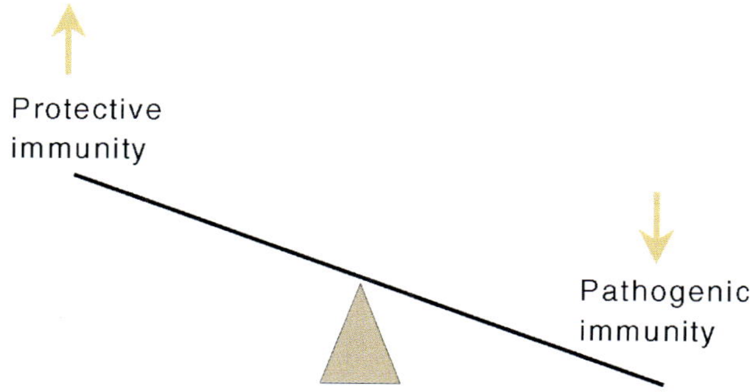

Figure 3 Prevention of autoimmune disease

SECONDARY PREVENTION

The one prevention approach that comes closest to the ideal for early subclinical disease, or even for primary prevention, is antigen-specific therapy [120]. This involves, paradoxically, the administration of an autoantigen as a therapeutic tool to induce protective immunity. This targeted approach avoids general immune suppression, is paraphysiological, and is aimed at restoring immune homeostasis. It is based on the precept that autoimmune diseases result from dysregulated immune responses to self-antigens. The presence of self-reactive lymphocytes in the blood of healthy individuals implies that self-antigen-specific immunoregulatory mechanisms are physiological and can be boosted or restored to prevent pathological autoimmunity (Figure 3). Antigen-specific strategies that induce "immune tolerance" (Table 5) have been shown to prevent or suppress experimental autoimmune diseases in rodents [120–122]. They operate either on pathogenic,

Table 5 Antigen-specific strategies that prevent experimental autoimmune disease

Strategy	Effect	Efficacy in animal models	Clinical trials in humans
Antigen administered via tolerizing route			
Mucosal	Induction of T_{reg};? deletion of antigen-specific T-cells (with high dose)	Yes	Yes
Dermal	Induction of T_{reg};? deletion of antigen-specific T-cells (with high dose)	Yes	No
Antigen administered in tolerogenic form			
As soluble high dose IV, IP, or SC	Deletion of antigen-specific T-cells;? induction of anergic T-cells	Yes	Yes
As soluble peptide – MHC IV	Deletion of antigen-specific T-cells;? induction of anergic T-cells	Yes	No
By "immature" dendritic cell	Induction of anergic T-cells/T_{reg}	Yes	No
During blockade of co-stimulation "second signal"	Induction of anergic T-cells/T_{reg}	Yes	Yes
As "altered peptide ligand"	Induction of anergic T-cells/T_{reg}	Yes	Yes
As aggregated Ig chimera	Induction of anergic T-cells/T_{reg}	Yes	No

effector T-cells to induce apoptosis-deletion or anergy, or by the induction of T_{reg} that secrete anti-inflammatory cytokines or compete with pathogenic effector T-cells at the level of the antigen-presenting cell (APC). How these mechanisms interrelate is not completely understood. T cells that are driven strongly by antigen may undergo apoptotic cell death and deletion, but those that respond "partially" may end up acquiring a state of anergy [13]. T_{reg} may in turn induce anergy directly or indirectly in pathogenic effector T-cells. The difference between anergic T cells and T_{reg} is becoming increasingly blurred, and may be more semantic than real. T_{reg} proliferate poorly to stimuli (which may explain their resistance to apoptosis-deletion) and anergic T cells, when tested in appropriate experimental systems, have the properties of T_{reg}. Of importance clinically is the ability of T_{reg} to exert what is called antigen-nonspecific "bystander suppression" in response to specific antigen recognized locally at the site of the lesion or in the draining lymph nodes [13, 120, 121]. For example, in response to antigen, T_{reg} secrete anti-inflammatory cytokines such as interleukin 10 (IL-10), transforming growth factor β (TGF-β), or interleukin 4, (IL-4), which have a local effect to downregulate the ability of dendritic APC to elicit T helper 1 (Th-1) T-cells that secrete gamma interferon (IFN-γ) and are characteristic of cell-mediated immune pathology as seen in T1D. Bystander suppression resolves the dilemma of multiple autoantigens in human autoimmune diseases by obviating the need to know if the autoantigen used to induce tolerance is the major or primary pathogenic autoantigen.

Mucosa-mediated Antigen-specific Therapy

Experimentally and clinically, antigen-specific therapy in autoimmune disease has been achieved primarily via the mucosal delivery of soluble protein or peptide antigen. This suppresses subsequent systemic priming by the antigen, a phenomenon originally called *oral tolerance*. While high-dose oral antigen has been associated with deletion of antigen-specific T cells, in most experimental animal models tolerance to oral or nasorespiratory antigen can be attributed to the induction of T_{reg}. Antigen-presenting dendritic cells with a functionally immature phenotype characterized by reduced expression of MHC class II molecules and essential co-stimulatory molecules exist naturally in the mucosal environment and other sites of "immune privilege," and can also be generated by exposure to anti-inflammatory cytokines such as IL-10 [123] or to other immune modulating agents such as vitamin D_3 [124]. These "tolerogenic" dendritic cells induce Th-2 or Th-3 rather than Th-1 T-cells, with the properties of T_{reg}. The context and state of the dendritic cell is therefore crucial and central to understanding the therapeutic manipulation of immune responses. Mucosa-mediated immunotherapy is an appealing strategy for autoimmune disease prevention that is supported by proof-of-concept in a range of experimental inbred rodent models (reviewed in references 120–122). The rationale for this approach is summarized in Table 6.

Table 6 Rationale for mucosa-mediated antigen-specific therapy in T1D

Prevention of diabetes in the NOD mouse	
Oral insulin	[125] [126]
Intranasal insulin B chain aa9–23	[127]
Aerosal insulin	[128]
Intranasal (pro)insulin peptide	[129]
Intranasal GAD peptides	[130]
Suppression of T-cell responses to the experimental neo- antigen, KLH, in human volunteers	
Oral KLH	[131]
Intranasal KLH	[132]

Numerous experiments have shown that it is possible to partially protect the NOD mouse from diabetes by the mucosal administration of islet autoantigen. Here we will use insulin as an example. Zhang et al. [125] initially reported protection after oral administration of porcine insulin. Bergerot et al. [126] showed that human insulin induced CD4 T_{reg} could transfer protection to naive mice. Protection following oral insulin was later found to be associated with decreased expression of IFN-γ-secreting Th-1 T-cells in the pancreas and pancreatic lymph nodes [133, 134]. Oral insulin-induced CD4 T_{reg} have also been shown to prevent immune-mediated diabetes induced by lymphocytic choriomeningitis virus (LCMV) infection of mice expressing the viral nucleoprotein of LCMV under control of the rat insulin promoter in their β cells [135]. Oral insulin decreased β-cell destruction, associated with downregulation of MHC class I and II and absence of antiviral cytotoxic T lymphocytes in the islets. The majority of T cells in the islets of oral-insulin-treated mice without diabetes secreted the Th-2 (IL-4, IL-10) and Th-3 (TGF-β) cytokines, in contrast to IFN-γ-secreting Th-1 cells in islets of mice developing diabetes. The protective effect of oral insulin was enhanced by simultaneous feeding with IL-10 [136], bacterial component OM-89 [137, 138], or Schistosome egg antigen [139], all of which promote Th-2 responses. Fusion of insulin to cholera toxin B (CTB) subunit significantly improved the ability of oral insulin to prevent diabetes [140]. Studies have since shown that oral CTB–insulin conjugates in NOD mice induce a shift from a Th-1 to a Th-2 immunity associated with the induction of regulatory CD4 T-cells [141]. NOD mice can be protected from diabetes by feeding potatoes that transgenically express CTB–insulin conjugates, demonstrating that food plants are feasible production and delivery systems for inducing oral tolerance [142]. Oral GAD has also been shown to suppress diabetes development in NOD mice [143]. It is generally believed that neonates are less susceptible to mucosal tolerance induction. However, oral administration of insulin, insulin B chain, or GAD peptide during the neonatal period still suppressed diabetes development in NOD mice [144]. This suggests that mucosal delivery of islet antigen, e.g. in milk, could be used to treat very young infants at risk of developing T1D.

Protection against diabetes in NOD mice can also be achieved by nasorespiratory administration of islet antigens. This route of delivery is direct to the mucosal surface and not associated with significant degradation of protein antigen. When insulin was administered as an aerosol to NOD mice at 8 weeks of age, after the onset of subclinical disease, pancreatic islet pathology and diabetes incidence were both significantly reduced [128]. Aerosol insulin induced novel antidiabetic CD8$\gamma\delta$ T cells that suppressed the adoptive transfer of diabetes to nondiabetic mice by T cells of diabetic mice. The type of T_{reg} induced by (pro)insulin delivered to the mucosa depends on the route and form of antigen. Naso-respiratory insulin, which is not degraded and remains conformationally intact, induces CD8$\gamma\delta$ T_{reg}, whereas oral insulin, which is degraded to peptides, or intranasal or oral (pro)insulin peptides induce CD4 T_{reg} [145]. Intranasal administration of a peptide comprising residues 9–23 of the insulin B chain, an epitope recognized by a majority of islet-infiltrating CD4 T-cell clones and capable of adoptively transferring diabetes to naive mice, induced CD4 T_{reg}, reduced the T-cell proliferative response to B9–23, and protected NOD mice from diabetes [127]. Not surprisingly, protection after intranasal insulin B chain was also associated with the induction of CD4 T-cells [146]. A peptide that spans the B–C chain junction in proinsulin also induces CD4 T_{reg} after intranasal administration [129]. This peptide, like insulin B9–23, binds to the NOD mouse class II MHC, I-A^{g7} [147], and is recognized by CD4 T-cells in NOD mice [148] and humans at risk for T1D [149]. T-cell epitope peptides from GAD administered intranasally were also protective, and associated with the induction of regulatory CD4 T_{reg} and with reduced IFN-γ responses to GAD [130]. All of these islet antigen peptides that induce T_{reg} are potential "vaccines" for intranasal delivery to prevent T1D in humans.

DNA-based Antigen-specific Therapy

DNA-based "gene therapy" offers particular advantages as a means of generating and delivering antigenic protein for induction of immunotherapy. Compared to protein, DNA is stable and easy to handle. DNA avoids the need to purify protein: after DNA delivery into mammalian cells the product is native protein—nature does the work. DNA can also be easily manipulated to modify the expressed product. DNA encoding genes for self-antigens or other genes, e.g. for cytokines, can be introduced into mammalian cells for immunotherapy by several routes and methods. Intramuscular injection of naked plasmid DNA containing the gene of interest and a strong promoter, e.g. from CMV, for mammalian expression is the most conventional approach. Delivery by the gene gun, which directly introduces DNA-coated gold particles under pressure into the skin or other tissues, greatly enhances cell uptake [150]. Viral vectors, particularly adenovirus, have also been used to deliver genes [151]. Just as for protein, the route of delivery may determine the nature of the immune response [152].

Several strategies have been employed to prevent T1D using gene therapy. Plasmids encoding islet antigens or peptides, cytokines, or co-stimulatory molecules have all been used with the aim of suppressing disease incidence. One of the advantages of gene therapy is that the DNA constructs can be tailored to contain elements that promote particular types of immune responses or direct expression in particular sites or cells. Thus, plasmid encoding a secreted form of GAD65 together with IL-4, when injected intramuscularly into NOD mice, suppressed β-cell-specific autoimmunity, as evidenced by a reduced incidence of insulitis and diabetes, thought to be mediated by antigen-specific Th-2 "regulatory" cells [153]. Suppression was not observed in mice given plasmid encoding GAD65 alone or an irrelevant antigen with IL-4. In contrast, a study that introduced IL-4 DNA by the gene gun showed a reduction in spontaneous diabetes incidence, possibly reflecting the increased efficiency of DNA uptake [154]. Intramuscular injection of a GAD65 plasmid was shown to reduce diabetes incidence in the cyclophosphamide-accelerated model of diabetes in NOD mice [155]. Intramuscular administration of plasmid encoding the anti-inflammatory cytokine, TGF-β1, was reported to reduce cyclophosphamide-accelerated diabetes in NOD mice [156]. Similarly, delivery of IL-10 DNA via an adenovirus vector was shown to reduce the incidence of disease in NOD mice and to induce regulatory T cells that suppressed the adoptive transfer of diabetes [151].

Intramuscular injection of plasmid encoding the insulin B chain reduced diabetes incidence in the RIP-LCMV model, postulated to be due to induction of CD4 T_{reg} [157]. However, this is inconsistent with other studies that showed plasmids encoding either the insulin B chain [158] or preproinsulin [159] injected intramuscularly did not reduce diabetes incidence in NOD mice. In the latter study, diabetes was reduced when CTLA-4 was targeted using a plasmid encoding a mutated gene for B7.1 (CD80), the ligand for CTLA-4. The incorporation of genes into the vector to target expressed protein or to direct its expression to a specific cell/site holds promise for refining gene therapy. We found that intranasal administration of a plasmid encoding mouse proinsulin II driven by the CMV promoter, while not suppressing diabetes, induced regulatory CD4 T-cells that could suppress the adoptive transfer of diabetes by "diabetogenic" T-cells. The lack of protection from diabetes in the treated mice suggested that pathogenic immunity was also stimulated, for example, by expression and presentation of MHC class I epitopes that induced diabetogenic cytotoxic CD8 T lymphocytes (CTL). The ability of mucosally administered antigen to induce both protective regulatory T cells and pathogenic CTL is well documented (CD154) [160]. However, induction of the latter can be prevented by concomitant blockade of co-stimulation with monoclonal antibody to CD40 ligand [161]. The same approach was also effective in allowing intranasal proinsulin DNA to reduce diabetes incidence in NOD mice (Every et al., submitted). Concomitant induction of protective and pathogenic immunity is a double-edged sword that cautions against implementing these strategies in humans without thorough preclinical testing.

Apart from specific encoded genes, DNA itself can modulate immune responses. Immunostimulatory (unmethylated) CpG motifs, 20 times more common in bacterial than in vertebrate DNA, are thought to stimulate Th-1 immunity [162], which could be considered problematic when trying to prevent a Th-1-mediated disease like T1D. However when injected intramuscularly as oligonucleotides (short DNA molecules), diabetes incidence was reduced [163]. Despite stimulating production of the Th-1 cytokine IFN-γ, CpG DNA treatment also stimulated production of the Th-2 cytokine IL-10, which may account for the observed reduction in disease incidence [163]. The effect of bacterial DNA to stimulate Th-1 immunity should not therefore preclude its use as an antigen delivery vehicle for preventing T1D. The relative ease with which DNA can be manipulated underscores the potential of DNA-based immunotherapy.

Hematopoietic Stem Cell-mediated Antigen-specific Therapy

Autoimmune diabetes in the NOD mouse can be transferred by bone marrow transplantation (BMT) [164–166]. This demonstrates that the mechanisms of disease development operate within the hematopoietic compartment and implies that autoimmune diabetes may be prevented by manipulating hematopoietic cells. Indeed, replacement of the NOD mouse hematopoietic compartment with that from diabetes-resistant mouse strains by BMT blocks development of diabetes [167, 168]. However, complete replacement of the hematopoietic compartment is not required as generation of mixed-allogeneic hematopoietic chimeras is equally effective [169–171]. The mechanism preventing autoimmune diabetes in mixed chimeras is most likely the introduction of thymic and/or peripheral tolerance-inducing antigen-presenting cells expressing diabetes-resistant MHC molecules. This would be analogous to the protection afforded by transgenic introduction of diabetes-resistant MHC molecules such as I-E and alternative I-A molecules [172–175], which may act by altering thymic selection of T cells [176, 177] or by inducing T_{reg} [174]. Induction of T_{reg}, however, does not appear to account for diabetes prevention in mixed chimeras [171]. Introduction of other non-MHC diabetes resistance genes into the hematopoietic compartment could also contribute.

Allogeneic- or mixed-allogeneic BMT strategies are being trialled in clinically severe autoimmune diseases [178]. However, this approach is unlikely to be suitable for T1D because of the requirement for cytotoxic conditioning of the host and the risk of graft rejection [179] or graft-versus-host disease [180]. A much safer approach would be the use of syngeneic or autologous, genetically engineered hematopoietic stem cells to introduce molecules into the hematopoietic compartment that could prevent autoimmune disease. In an autoantigen-specific approach, we found that transferring small numbers of syngeneic hematopoietic stem cells encoding proinsulin to young, irradiated NOD mice prevents diabetes [181]. It is plausible that this strategy could be adapted for application to humans.

Trials of Islet Antigen-specific Therapy in Humans

In the United States, the large multicenter Diabetes Prevention Trial 1 (DPT-1) was launched in 1994 to determine whether antigen-based therapy using systemic or oral insulin would delay or prevent the onset of diabetes in at-risk relatives. Previously, intensive systemic insulin therapy had been reported to prolong the "honeymoon phase" after diagnosis [35], and a pilot study of prophylactic systemic insulin in at-risk relatives had suggested that this approach might be of benefit [182]. In DPT-1, low-dose systemic insulin (annual intravenous insulin infusions and daily subcutaneous injections) was given to a high-risk group of relatives (>50% risk of diabetes over 5 years) who were matched with an untreated but closely monitored control group. However, as recently reported [42], this treatment had no effect on diabetes incidence. Currently, oral insulin is being compared to placebo in a double-blind study in relatives at intermediate risk (25–50% risk of diabetes over 5 years). No major safety concerns have been identified and outcome of the oral arm will be known after 2003. Pilot trials of nasal insulin have been conducted by ourselves (see below) and in Finland.

Two trials of oral insulin (up to 7.5 mg daily for 12 months) in recently diagnosed patients did not demonstrate a protective effect on residual β-cell function [40, 183]. Why have these trials failed? The reasons could include inadequate dose or bioavailability, the concomitant induction of pathogenic T cells [160, 161], and the selection of subjects with end-stage disease. Animal studies generally indicate that the induction of antigen-specific immunoregulation, without concomitant inactivation or deletion of pathogenic effector cells, is relatively ineffective in end-stage autoimmune disease. If a balance between pathogenic and protective T cells determines clinical outcome (Figure 2), then antigen-specific therapy should be more effective in early preclinical disease. Later, it might be applied most effectively after a limited course of treatment aimed at reducing the burden of pathogenic effector T cells. The route of administration may also be relevant. It is possible that the oral route may not be the most effective for induction of mucosa-mediated tolerance. Proteins are generally degraded after oral administration. Regulatory, antidiabetic CD8$\gamma\delta$ T cells, with the phenotype of intraepithelial lymphocytes, are induced only by conformationally intact insulin following nasal or aerosol, not oral, administration [128, 140]. Even in the case of a small peptide, however, therapeutic responses have been reported after nasorespiratory but not oral antigen delivery [184]. In the NOD mouse, nasal antigen elicited antigen-specific T-cell responses in cervical, mediastinal, and mesenteric mucosal lymph nodes, whereas oral insulin elicited responses only in the mesenteric nodes [160].

The Australian Intranasal Insulin Trial I (INIT I) [43] commenced in 1996. It was a randomized, controlled, crossover pilot trial of intranasal insulin, in young T1D relatives (median age 10.8 years) with islet antibodies, the majority with antibodies to at least two islet antigens and therefore at up to 50% risk of diabetes over 5 years. Two 400 μg doses of insulin per nostril were self-administered daily for 10 days, and then on two consecutive days each weekend, for 6 months. The aim was to determine if intranasal insulin was safe and would induce changes in surrogate immune and metabolic markers consistent with an immunoprotective effect. INIT I identified a dose of intranasal insulin that was safe and that induced the same changes in immunity to insulin as seen in NOD mice, namely an overall increase in serum IAb and a decrease in T-cell proliferation *ex vivo* to insulin (denatured). FPIR to IV glucose was measured at entry, 6, and 12 months and then at least yearly. After a median follow-up of 3.9 years, 13 subjects developed diabetes; all had FPIR $<$ 1st percentile at entry and their predicted time to diabetes based on FPIR was no different to historical controls. In the remaining 25 subjects with FPIR $>$ 1st percentile at entry, there has been no decrease in FPIR. Thus, intranasal insulin did not accelerate diabetes in subjects with measurable β-cell function at entry. In contrast, in similar subjects in the Melbourne Pre-Diabetes Family Study, initially with a normal FPIR, over half have had a roughly linear decrease in FPIR over time to diabetes [185]. However, because INIT I was a crossover trial in which all subjects received treatment with intranasal insulin for 6 months, it cannot determine if intranasal insulin prevents loss of β-cell function and diabetes. A follow-up trial to answer this is planned to begin in 2003.

In adults with autoimmune diabetes there has been only one published clinical trial of prophylactic insulin. This small study by Kobayashi et al. [38] demonstrated that low doses of subcutaneous insulin improved the C-peptide response to oral glucose and decreased HbA_{1c} at 6 and 12 months after diagnosis, compared to treatment with oral sulfonylurea drugs. Whether the beneficial effect of insulin treatment was due to metabolic or immunoregulatory mechanisms is not known.

Prevention of T1D in the Third Millennium

Most of what is known about the pathogenesis of T1D was learned at the very end of the second millennium. The rate of accumulation of knowledge has been remarkable and, on this basis, the prevention of T1D early in the third millennium can be confidently predicted. Increased funding for T1D research and the creation of the NIH-funded Immune Tolerance Network (ITN) and the NIH- and Juvenile Diabetes Research Foundation-funded TrialNet will facilitate the development and evaluation of candidate prevention agents and approaches based on an increasingly clearer knowledge of the cellular and molecular basis of β-cell destruction in T1D. This will be an incremental process and will involve a range of interventions depending on disease risk and stage, analogous to the treatment of cancer or HIV. Environmental agents involved in triggering or exacerbating islet autoimmunity are likely to be ubiquitous and interactive and therefore a single intervention, for example vaccination against a virus, is unlikely to be the total answer. Antigen-specific immunotherapy, which enhances natural mechanisms of immune homeostasis, promises to be a safe and widely applicable intervention at least in the early stages of disease. Later, combination treatment that not only enhances protective immunity but suppresses dominant pathogenic immunity is likely to be required. Rapid advances in identifying and manipulating stem cells may open new avenues for antigen-specific therapy, for example via hematopoietic stem cells. A major deficiency in all attempts to prevent T1D is the lack of surrogate markers that reliably reflect the nature of subclinical islet autoimmunity. In particular, there is a need for functional assays of T cells, both pathogenic T-cells as well as protective, regulatory T-cells that might be induced by intervention treatment. Preventing T1D will not only be a major achievement in its own right, but will enable the application of strategies to replace or regenerate β cells in people with established T1D.

Acknowledgments

The authors are supported by the National Health and Medical Research Council of Australia and by a Center Program Grant from the Juvenile Diabetes Research

Foundation. Catherine O'Shea provided excellent administrative assistance.

REFERENCES

1. Bach J-F. Insulin-dependent diabetes mellitus as an autoimmune disease. *Endocrinol Rev* 1994; 15: 516–42.
2. Harrison LC, Colman PG, Honeyman MC, Kay TWH. Type 1 diabetes—from pathogenesis to prevention. In Turtle JR, Kaneko T, Osata S. (eds) *Diabetes in the New Millennium*. Sydney: 1999; pp 85–100.
3. Adorini L, Gregori S, Harrison LC. Understanding autoimmune diabetes: insights from mouse models. *Trends Mol Med* 2002; 8: 31–8.
4. Leiter EH, Prochazka M, Coleman DL. The non-obese diabetic (NOD) mouse. *Am J Pathol* 1987; 128: 380–3.
5. Atkinson MA, Leiter EH. The NOD mouse model of type 1 diabetes: as good as it gets? *Nat Med* 1999; 5: 601–4.
6. The Diabetes Control and Complications Trial Research Group. The effect of intensive treatment of diabetes on the development and progression of long-term complications in insulin-dependent diabetes mellitus. *N Engl J Med* 1993; 329: 977–86.
7. Hahl J, Simell T, Ilonen J, Knip M, Simell O. Costs of predicting IDDM. *Diabetologia* 1998; 41: 79–85.
8. Verge CF, Gianani R, Kawasaki E, Yu L, Pietropaolo M, Jackson RA, Chase HP, Eisenbarth GS. Prediction of type I diabetes in first-degree relatives using a combination of insulin, GAD, and ICA512bdc/IA-2 autoantibodies. *Diabetes* 1996; 45: 926–33.
9. Bingley PJ, Williams AJ, Gale EA. Optimized autoantibody-based risk assessment in family members. Implications for future intervention trials. *Diabetes Care* 1999; 22: 1796–801.
10. Colman PG, Steele C, Couper JJ, Beresford SJ, Powell T, Kewming K, Pollard A, Gellert S, Tait B, Honeyman M, Harrison LC. Islet autoimmunity in infants with a Type I diabetic relative is common but is frequently restricted to one autoantibody. *Diabetologia* 2000; 43: 203–9.
11. Harrison LC. Risk assessment, prediction and prevention of type 1 diabetes. *Pediatr Diabetes* 2001; 2: 71–82.
12. Kimpimäki T, Kupila A, Hämäläinen A-M, Kukko M, Kulmala P, Savola K, Simell T, Keskinen P, Ilonen J, Simell O, Knip M. The first signs of β-cell autoimmunity appear in infancy in genetically susceptible children from the general population: The Finnish Type 1 Diabetes Prediction and Prevention Study. *J Clin Endocrinol Metab* 2001; 86: 4782–8.
13. Hummel M, Bonifacio E, Naserke HE, Ziegler AG. Elimination of dietary gluten does not reduce titers of type 1 diabetes-associated autoantibodies in high-risk subjects. *Diabetes Care* 2002; 25: 1111–6.
14. Harrison LC, Colman PG, Dean B, Baxter R, Martin FI. Increase in remission rate in newly diagnosed type I diabetic subjects treated with azathioprine. *Diabetes* 1985; 34: 1306–8.
15. Feutren G, Papoz L, Assan R, Vialettes B, Karsenty G, Vexiau P, Du Rostu H, Rodier M, Sirmai J, Lallemand A, et al. Cyclosporin increases the rate and length of remissions in insulin-dependent diabetes of recent onset. Results of a multicentre double-blind trial. *Lancet* 1986 19; 2: 119–24.
16. Silverstein J, Maclaren N, Riley W, Spillar R, Radjenovic D, Johnson S. Immunosuppression with azathioprine and prednisone in recent-onset insulin-dependent diabetes mellitus. *New Engl J Med* 1988; 319: 599–604.
17. The Canadian–European Randomized Control Trial Group. Cyclosporin-induced remission of IDDM after early intervention. Association of 1 yr of cyclosporin treatment with enhanced insulin secretion. *Diabetes* 1988; 37: 1574–82.
18. Cook JJ, Hudson I, Harrison LC, Dean B, Colman PG, Werther GA, Warne GL, Court JM. Double-blind controlled trial of azathioprine in children with newly diagnosed type I diabetes. *Diabetes* 1989; 38: 779–83.
19. Moncada E, Subira ML, Oleaga A, Goni F, Sanchez-Ibarrola A, Monreal M, Sevilla M, Goni MJ, Yoldi A, Teran D, et al. Insulin requirements and residual beta-cell function 12 months after concluding immunotherapy in type I diabetic patients treated with combined azathioprine and thymostimulin administration for one year. *J Autoimmun* 1990; 3: 625–38.
20. Assan R, Feutren G, Sirmai J, Laborie C, Boitard C, Vexiau P, Du Rostu H, Rodier M, Figoni M, Vague P, Hors J, Bach J-F. Plasma C-peptide levels and clinical remissions in recent-onset type I diabetic patients treated with cyclosporin A and insulin. *Diabetes* 1990; 39: 768–74.
21. Chase HP, Butler-Simon N, Garg SK, Hayward A, Klingensmith GJ, Hamman RF, O'Brien D. Cyclosporine A for the treatment of new-onset insulin-dependent diabetes mellitus. *Pediatrics* 1990; 85: 241–5.
22. Secchi A, Pastore MR, Sergi A, Pontiroli AE, Pozza G. Prednisone administration in recent onset type I diabetes. *J Autoimmun* 1990; 3: 593–600.
23. Skyler JS, Rabinovitch A, for the Miami Cyclosporine Diabetes Study Group. Cyclosporine in recent onset type I diabetes mellitus. Effects on islet beta cell function. *J Diabetes Complications* 1992; 6: 77–88.
24. Skyler JS, Lorenz TJ, Schwartz S, Eisenbarth GS, Einhorn D, Palmer JP, Marks JB, Greenbaum C, Saria EA, Byers V, for the The CD5 Diabetes Project Team. Effects of an anti-CD5 immunoconjugate (CD5-plus) in recent onset type I diabetes mellitus: a preliminary investigation. *J Diabetes Complications* 1993; 7: 224–32.
25. Goday A, Pujol-Borrell R, Fernandez J, Casamitjana R, Rios M, Vilardell E, Gomis R. Effects of a short prednisone regime at clinical onset of type 1 diabetes. *Diabetes Res Clin Pract* 1993; 20: 39–46.
26. Kohnert KD, Hehmke B, Keilacker H, Ziegler M, Emmrich F, Laube F, Michaelis D. Antibody response to islet antigens in anti-CD4/prednisolone immune intervention of type 1 diabetes. *Int J Clin Lab Res* 1996; 26:55–9.
27. Buckingham BA, Sandborg CI. A randomized trial of methotrexate in newly diagnosed patients with type 1 diabetes mellitus. *Clin Immunol* 2000; 96: 86–90.
28. Herold KC, Hagopian W, Auger JA, Poumian-Ruiz E, Taylor L, Donaldson D, Gitelman SE, Harlan DM, Xu D, Zivin RA, Bluestone JA. Anti-CD3 monoclonal antibody in new-onset type 1 diabetes mellitus. *N Engl J Med* 2002; 346: 1692–8.
29. Elliott JF, Marlin KL, Couch RM. Effect of bacille Calmette–Guerin vaccination on C-peptide secretion in children newly diagnosed with IDDM. *Diabetes Care* 1998; 21: 1691–3.
30. Allen HF, Klingensmith GJ, Jensen P, Simoes E, Hayward A, Chase HP. Effect of Bacillus Calmette-Guerin vaccination on new-onset type 1 diabetes. A randomized clinical study. *Diabetes Care* 1999; 22: 1703–7.

31. Giordano C, Panto F, Amato MP, Sapienza N, Pugliese A, Galluzzo A. Early administration of an immunomodulator and induction of remission in insulin-dependent diabetes mellitus. *J Autoimmun* 1990; 3: 611–7.
32. Panto F, Giordano C, Amato MP, Pugliese A, Donatelli M, D'Acquisto G, Galluzzo A. The influence of high dose intravenous immunoglobulins on immunological and metabolic pattern in newly diagnosed type I diabetic patients. *J Autoimmun* 1990; 3: 587–92.
33. Coutant R, Landais P, Rosilio M, Johnsen C, Lahlou N, Chatelain P, Carel JC, Ludvigsson J, Boitard C, Bougneres PF. Low dose linomide in Type I juvenile diabetes of recent onset: a randomised placebo-controlled double blind trial. *Diabetologia* 1998; 41: 1040–6.
34. Raz I, Elias D, Avron A, Tamir M, Metzger M, Cohen IR. Beta-cell function in new-onset type 1 diabetes and immunomodulation with a heat-shock protein peptide (DiaPep277): a randomised, double-blind, phase II trial. *Lancet* 2001; 358: 1749–53.
35. Shah SC, Malone JI, Simpson NE. A randomized trial of intensive insulin therapy in newly diagnosed insulin-dependent diabetes mellitus. *N Engl J Med* 1989; 320: 550–4.
36. Linn T, Ortac K, Laube H, Federlin K. Intensive therapy in adult insulin-dependent diabetes mellitus is associated with improved insulin sensitivity and reserve: a randomized, controlled, prospective study over 5 years in newly diagnosed patients. *Metabolism* 1996; 45: 1508–13.
37. Schnell O, Eisfelder B, Standl E, Ziegler AG. High-dose intravenous insulin infusion versus intensive insulin treatment in newly diagnosed IDDM. *Diabetes* 1997; 46: 1607–11.
38. Kobayashi T, Nakanishi K, Murase T, Kosaka K. Small doses of subcutaneous insulin as a strategy for preventing slowly progressive β-cell failure in islet cell antibody-positive patients with clinical features of NIDDM. *Diabetes* 1996; 45: 622–6.
39. Selam JL, Woertz L, Lozano J, Robinson M, Chan E, Charles MA. The use of glipizide combined with intensive insulin treatment for the induction of remissions in new onset adult type I diabetes. *Autoimmunity* 1993;16: 281–8.
40. Chaillous L, Lefevre H, Thivolet C, Boitard C, Lahlou N, Atlan-Gepner C, Bouhanick B, Mogenet A, Nicolino M, Carel JC, Lecomte P, Marechaud R, Bougneres P, Charbonnel B, Sai P, for the Diabete Insuline Orale Group. Oral insulin administration and residual β-cell function in recent-onset type 1 diabetes: a multicentre randomised controlled trial. *Lancet* 2000; 356: 545–9.
41. Füchtenbusch M, Rabl W, Grassl B, Bachmann W, Standl E, Ziegler AG. Delay of type I diabetes in high risk, first degree relatives by parenteral antigen administration: the Schwabing Insulin Prophylaxis Pilot Trial. *Diabetologia* 1998; 41: 536–41.
42. Diabetes Prevention Trial-Type 1 Diabetes Study Group. Effects of insulin in relatives of patients with type 1 diabetes mellitus. *N Engl J Med* 2002; 346: 1685–91.
43. Harrison LC, Honeyman MC, Steele C, Wright M, Gellert SA, Colman PG. Intranasal insulin trial (INIT) in preclinical type 1 diabetes. *Diabetes* 1999; 48 (suppl 1): A206.
44. Mendola G, Casamitjana R, Gomis R. Effect of nicotinamide therapy upon B-cell function in newly diagnosed type 1 (insulin-dependent) diabetic patients. *Diabetologia*. 1989; 32: 160–2.
45. Vague P, Picq R, Bernal M, Lassmann-Vague V, Vialettes B. Effect of nicotinamide treatment on the residual insulin secretion in type 1 (insulin-dependent) diabetic patients. *Diabetologia* 1989; 32: 316–21.
46. Chase HP, Butler-Simon N, Garg S, McDuffie M, Hoops SL, O'Brien D. A trial of nicotinamide in newly diagnosed patients with type 1 (insulin-dependent) diabetes mellitus. *Diabetologia* 1990b; 33: 444–6.
47. Pozzilli P, Visalli N, Signore A, Baroni MG, Buzzetti R, Cavallo MG, Boccuni ML, Fava D, Gragnoli C, Andreani D, Lucentini L, Matteoli MC, Crinò A, Cicconetti CA, Teodonio C, Paci F, Amoretti R, Pisano L, Pennafina MG, Santopadre G, Marozzi G, Multari G, Suppa MA, Campea L, De Mattia GC, Cassone Faldetta M, Marietti G, Perrone F, Greco AV, Ghirlanda G. Double blind trial of nicotinamide in recent-onset IDDM (the IMDIAB III study). *Diabetologia* 1995; 38: 848–52.
48. Pozzilli P, Visalli N, Boccuni ML, Baroni MG, Buzzetti R, Fioriti E, Signore A, Cavallo MG, Andreani D, Lucentini L, et al, for the The IMDIAB Study Group. Randomized trial comparing nicotinamide and nicotinamide plus cyclosporin in recent onset insulin-dependent diabetes (IMDIAB 1). *Diabet Med* 1994; 11: 98–104.
49. Vidal J, Fernandez-Balsells M, Sesmilo G, Aguilera E, Casamitjana R, Gomis R, Conget I. Effects of nicotinamide and intravenous insulin therapy in newly diagnosed type 1 diabetes. *Diabetes Care* 2000; 23: 360–4.
50. Pozzilli P, Visalli N, Cavallo MG, Signore A, Baroni MG, Buzzetti R, Fioriti E, Mesturino C, Fiori R, Romiti A, Giovannini C, Lucentini L, Matteoli MC, Crinò A, Teodonio C, Paci F, Amoretti R, Pisano L, Suraci C, Multari G, Suppa M, Sulli N, De Mattia G, Faldetta MR, Suraci MT. Vitamin E and nicotinamide have similar effects in maintaining residual beta cell function in recent onset insulin-dependent diabetes (the IMDIAB IV study). *Eur J Endocrinol* 1997; 137: 234–9.
51. Lampeter EF, Klinghammer A, Scherbaum WA, Heinze E, Haastert B, Giani G, Kolb H, for the DENIS Group. The Deutsche Nicotinamide Intervention Study: an attempt to prevent type 1 diabetes. *Diabetes* 1998; 47: 980–4.
52. Philips JC, Scheen AJ, Le Registre Belge du Diabete. Info-congress. Study of the prevention of type 1 diabetes with nicotinamide: positive lessons of a negative clinical trial ENDIT [in French]. *Rev Med Liege* 2002; 57: 672–5.
53. Grunt JA, al-Hakim H, Willoughby L, Howard CP. A randomized trial of a somatostatin analog for preserving beta cell function in children with insulin dependent diabetes mellitus. *J Pediatr Endocrinol* 1994; 7: 331–4.
54. Bjork E, Berne C, Kampe O, Wibell L, Oskarsson P, Karlsson FA. Diazoxide treatment at onset preserves residual insulin secretion in adults with autoimmune diabetes. *Diabetes* 1996; 45: 1427–30.
55. Bjork E, Ortquist E, Wallensteen M, Ludvigsson J, Aman J, Johansson C, Forsander G, Blom L, Berglund L, Persson B, Berne C, Karlsson AF. Diazoxide treatment at onset in childhood type 1 diabetes. *Diabetes* 2001; 50 (suppl 2): A90.
56. Ludvigsson J, Samuelsson U, Johansson C, Stenhammar L. Treatment with antioxidants at onset of type 1 diabetes in children: a randomized, double-blind placebo-controlled study. *Diabetes Metab Res Rev* 2001; 17: 131–6.
57. Chatenoud L. CD3-specific antibody-induced active tolerance: from bench to bedside. *Nat Rev Immunol* 2003; 3: 123–32.

58. von Herrath MG, Harrison LC. Antigen-specific regulatory T-cells [review]. *Nat Rev Immunol* 2003; 3: 223–32.
59. Hagopian WA, Karlsen AE, Gottsater A, Landin-Olsson M, Grubin CE, Sundkvist G, Petersen JS, Boel E, Dyrberg T, Lernmark A. Quantitative assay using recombinant human islet glutamic acid decarboxylase (GAD65) shows that 64K autoantibody positivity at onset predicts diabetes type. *J Clin Invest* 1993; 91: 368–74.
60. Gottsater A, Landin-Olsson M, Lernmark A, Fernlund P, Sundkvist G, Hagopian WA. Glutamic acid decarboxylase antibody levels predict role of β-cell decline in adult onset diabetes. *Diab Rev Clin Prac* 1995; 27: 133–40.
61. Turner R, Stratton I, Horton V, Manley S, Zimmet P, Mackay IR, Shattock M, Bottazzo GF, Holman R, for the UK Prospective Diabetes Study Group. UKPDS 25: autoantibodies to islet-cell cytoplasm and glutamic acid decarboxylase for prediction of insulin requirement in type 2 diabetes. *Lancet* 1997; 350: 1288–93.
62. Gottsater A, Landin-Olsson M, Fernlund P, Lernmark A, Sundkvist G. Beta-cell function in relation to islet cell antibodies during the first 3 yr after clinical diagnosis of diabetes in type II diabetic patients. *Diabetes Care* 1993; 16: 902–10.
63. Harrison LC, Kay TWH. Strategies for intervention therapy in type 1 diabetes. In Andreani D, Kolb H, Pozzilli P (eds) *Immunotherapy of Type 1 Diabetes*. Chichester: Wiley, 1989; pp 93–110.
64. Greenbaum C. Type 1 diabetes intervention trials: what have we learned? A critical review of selected intervention trials. *Clin Immunol* 2002; 104: 97–104.
65. Greenbaum C, Harrison LC. Guidelines for intervention trials in subjects with newly-diagnosed type 1 diabetes. *Diabetes* 2003; 52: 1059–65.
66. Eisenbarth GS, Moriyama H, Robles DT, Liu E, Yu L, Babu S, Redondo MJ, Gottlieb P, Wegmann D, Rewers M. Insulin autoimmunity: prediction/precipitation/prevention type 1A diabetes. *Autoimmun Rev* 2002; 1: 139–45.
67. Narendran P, Mannering SI, Harrison LC. Proinsulin—a pathogenic autoantigen in type 1 diabetes. *Autoimmun Rev* (in press).
68. Pugliese A, Zeller M, Fernandez A Jr, Zalcberg LJ, Bartlett RJ, Ricordi C, Pietropaolo M, Eisenbarth GS, Bennett ST, Patel DD. The insulin gene is transcribed in the human thymus and transcription levels correlated with allelic variation at the INS VNTR-IDDM2 susceptibility locus for type 1 diabetes. *Nat Genet* 1997; 15: 293–7.
69. Vafiadis P, Bennett ST, Todd JA, Nadeau J, Grabs R, Goodyer CG, Wickramasinghe S, Colle E, Polychronakos C. Insulin expression in human thymus is modulated by INS VNTR alleles at the IDDM2 locus. *Nat Genet* 1997; 15: 289–92.
70. Gale EA, Bingley PJ, Eisenbarth GS, Redondo MJ, Kyvik KO, Petersen JS. Reanalysis of twin studies suggests that diabetes is mainly genetic. *BMJ* 2001; 323: 997–8.
71. Redondo MJ, Yu L, Hawa M, Mackenzie T, Pyke DA, Eisenbarth GS, Leslie RD. Heterogeneity of type I diabetes: analysis of monozygotic twins in Great Britain and the United States. *Diabetologia* 2001; 44: 354–62.
72. Green A, Patterson CC. Trends in the incidence of childhood-onset diabetes in Europe 1989–1998. *Diabetologia* 2001; 44: B3–8.
73. Gale EA. The rise of childhood type 1 diabetes in the 20th century. *Diabetes* 2002; 51: 3353–61.
74. Laron Z. Seasonality of birth in children with diabetes. Maternally transmitted infection might increase risk of diabetes [letter]. *BMJ* 2000; 320: 716.
75. Willis JA, Scott RS, Darlow BA, Lewy H, Ashkenazi I, Laron Z. Seasonality of birth and onset of clinical disease in children and adolescents (0–19 years) with type 1 diabetes mellitus in Canterbury, New Zealand. *J Pediatr Endocrinol Metab* 2002; 15: 645–7.
76. Douglas S, McSporran B, Smail P, for the Scottish Study Group for the Care of Young Diabetics. Seasonality of presentation of type I diabetes mellitus in children. *Scott Med J* 1999; 44: 41–6.
77. Forrest JM, Menser MA, Burgess JA. High frequency of diabetes mellitus in young adults with congenital rubella. *Lancet* 1971; 2: 332–4.
78. Karam JH, Lewitt PA, Young CW, Nowlain RL, Frankel BJ, Fujiya H, Freedman ZR, Grodsky GM. Insulinopenic diabetes after rodenticide (Vacor) ingestion: a unique model of acquired diabetes in man. *Diabetes* 1980; 29: 971–8.
79. Harrison LC, Honeyman MC. Cows' milk and type 1 diabetes: the real debate is about mucosal immune function. *Diabetes* 1999; 48: 1501–7.
80. Gerstein H. Cows' milk exposure and type 1 diabetes mellitus. *Diabetes Care* 1994; 17: 13–9.
81. Norris JM, Scott FW. A meta analysis of infant diet and insulin-dependent diabetes mellitus: do biases play a role. *Epidemiology* 1996; 7: 87–92.
82. Norris JM, Beaty B, Klingensmith G, Yu L, Hoffman M, Chase HP, Erlich HA, Hamman RF, Eisenbarth GS, Rewers M. Lack of association between early exposure to cows' milk protein and β-cell autoimmunity: Diabetes Autoimmunity Study in the Young (DAISY). *JAMA* 1996; 276: 609–14.
83. Couper JJ, Steele C, Beresford S, Powell T, McCaul K, Pollard A, Gellert S, Tait B, Harrison LC, Colman PG. Lack of association between duration of breast-feeding or introduction of cows' milk and development of islet autoimmunity. *Diabetes* 1999; 48: 2145–9.
84. Hummel M, Fuchtenbusch M, Schenker M, Ziegler AG. No major association of breast-feeding, vaccinations, and childhood viral diseases with early islet autoimmunity in the German BABYDIAB Study. *Diabetes Care* 2000; 23: 969–74.
85. Beales PE, Elliott RB, Flohe S, Hill JP, Kolb H, Pozzilli P, Wang GS, Wasmuth H, Scott FW. A multi-centre, blinded international trial of the effect of A(1) and A(2) beta-casein variants on diabetes incidence in two rodent models of spontaneous Type I diabetes. *Diabetologia* 2002; 45: 1240–6.
86. MacFarlane AJ, Burghardt KM, Kelly J, Simell T, Simell O, Altosaar I, Scott FW. A type 1 diabetes-related protein from wheat (*Triticum aestivum*): cDNA clone of a wheat storage globulin, Glb1, linked to islet damage. *J Biol Chem* 2002; 278: 54–63.
87. Ventura A, Magazzu G, Greco L. Duration of exposure to gluten and risk for autoimmune disorders in patients with celiac disease (SIGEP study group for autoimmune disorders in celiac disease). *Gastroenterology* 1999; 117: 297–303.
88. Ivarsson A, Hernell O, Stenlund H, Persson LÅ. Breast-feeding protects against celiac disease. *Am J Clin Nutr* 2002; 75: 914–21.
89. Pozzilli P, Signore A, Williams AJ, Beales PE. NOD mouse colonies around the world—recent facts and figures. *Immunol Today* 1993; 14: 193–6.

90. Suzuki T. Diabetogenic effects of lymphocyte transfusion on the NOD or NOD nude mouse. In Rygaard J, Brunner N, Graem N, Spang-Thomson M (eds) *Immune Deficient Animals in Biomedical Research*. Basel: Karger, 1987; pp 112–6.
91. Imaoka A, Matsumoto S, Setoyama H, Okada Y, Umesaki Y. Proliferative recruitment of intestinal intraepithelial lymphocytes after microbial colonization of germ-free mice. *Eur J Immunol* 1996; 26: 945–8.
92. Kawaguchi-Miyashita M, Shimizu K, Nanno M, Shimada S, Watanabe T, Koga Y, Matsuoka Y, Ishikawa H, Hashimoto K, Ohwaki M. Development and cytolytic function of intestinal intraepithelial T lymphocytes in antigen-minimized mice. *Immunology* 1996; 89: 268–73.
93. Strachan DP. Hay fever, hygiene, and household size. *BMJ* 1989; 299: 1259–60.
94. Holt PG. A potential vaccine strategy for asthma and allied atopic disease during early childhood. *Lancet* 1994; 344: 456–8.
95. Menser MA, Forrest JM, Bransby RD. Rubella infection and diabetes mellitus. *Lancet* 1978; 1: 57–60.
96. Ginsberg-Fellner F, Witt ME, Fedun B, Taub F, Dobersen MJ, McEvoy RC, Cooper LZ, Notkins AL, Rubinstein P. Diabetes mellitus and autoimmunity in patients with the congenital rubella syndrome. *Rev Infect Dis* 1985; 7 (suppl 1): S170–6
97. Menser MA, Forrest JM, Honeyman MC, Burgess JA. Letter: Diabetes, HL-A antigens, and congenital rubella. *Lancet* 1974; 2: 1508–9.
98. Ou D, Mitchell LA, Metzger DL, Gillam S, Tingle AJ. Cross-reactive rubella virus and glutamic acid decarboxylase (65 and 67) protein determinants recognized by T-cells of patients with type I diabetes mellitus. *Diabetologia* 2000; 43: 750–62.
99. Lindberg B, Ahlfors K, Carlsson A, Ericsson UB, Landin-Olsson M, Lernmark A, Ludvigsson J, Sundkvist G, Ivarsson SA. Previous exposure to measles, mumps, and rubella—but not vaccination during adolescence—correlates to the prevalence of pancreatic and thyroid autoantibodies. *Pediatrics* 1999; 104: e12.
100. DeStefano F, Mullooly JP, Okoro CA, Chen RT, Marcy SM, Ward JI, Vadheim CM, Black SB, Shinefield HR, Davis RL, Bohlke K. Childhood vaccinations, vaccination timing, and risk of type 1 diabetes mellitus. *Pediatrics* 2001; 108: E112.
101. Bodansky HJ, Dean BM, Grant PJ, McNally J, Schweiger MS, Hambling MH, Bottazzo GF, Wales JK. Does exposure to rubella virus generate endocrine autoimmunity? *Diabet Med* 1990; 7: 611–4.
102. Dahlquist G, Frisk G, Ivarsson SA, Svanberg L, Forsgren M, Diderholm H. Indications that maternal coxsackie B virus infection during pregnancy is a risk factor for childhood-onset IDDM. *Diabetologia* 1995; 38: 1371–3.
103. Hyoty H, Hiltunen M, Knip M, Laakkonen M, Vahasalo P, Karjalainen J, Koskela P, Roivainen M, Leinikki P, Hovi T, et al., for the Childhood Diabetes in Finland (DiMe) Study Group. A prospective study of the role of coxsackie B and other enterovirus infections in the pathogenesis of IDDM. *Diabetes* 1995; 44: 652–7.
104. Füchtenbusch M, Irnstetter A, Jager G, Ziegler AG. No evidence for an association of coxsackie virus infections during pregnancy and early childhood with development of islet autoantibodies in offspring of mothers or fathers with type 1 diabetes. *J Autoimmun* 2001; 17: 333–40.
105. Viskari HR, Roivainen M, Reunanen A, Pitkaniemi J, Sadeharju K, Koskela P, Hovi T, Leinikki P, Vilja P, Tuomilehto J, Hyoty H. Maternal first-trimester enterovirus infection and future risk of type 1 diabetes in the exposed fetus. *Diabetes* 2002; 51: 2568–71.
106. Yin H, Berg AK, Tuvemo T, Frisk G. Enterovirus RNA is found in peripheral blood mononuclear cells in a majority of type 1 diabetic children at onset. *Diabetes* 2002; 51: 1964–71.
107. Horwitz MS, Bradley LM, Harbertson J, Krahl T, Lee J, Sarvetnick N. Diabetes induced by Coxsackie virus: initiation by bystander damage and not molecular mimicry. *Nat Med* 1998; 4: 781–5.
108. Mena I, Fischer C, Gebhard JR, Perry CM, Harkins S, Whitton JL. Coxsackievirus infection of the pancreas: evaluation of receptor expression, pathogenesis, and immunopathology. *Virology* 2000; 271: 276–88.
109. Marttila J, Juhela S, Vaarala O, Hyoty H, Roivainen M, Hinkkanen A, Vilja P, Simell O, Ilonen J. Responses of coxsackievirus B4-specific T-cell lines to 2C protein-characterization of epitopes with special reference to the GAD65 homology region. *Virology* 2001; 284: 131–41.
110. Roep BO, Hiemstra HS, Schloot NC, De Vries RR, Chaudhuri A, Behan PO, Drijfhout JW. Molecular mimicry in type 1 diabetes: immune cross-reactivity between islet autoantigen and human cytomegalovirus but not Coxsackie virus. *Ann N Y Acad Sci* 2002; 958: 163–5.
111. Horwitz MS, Ilic A, Fine C, Rodriguez E, Sarvetnick N. Presented antigen from damaged pancreatic beta cells activates autoreactive T-cells in virus-mediated autoimmune diabetes. *J Clin Invest* 2002; 109: 79–87.
112. Khakpour M, Nik-Akhtar B. Diabetes mellitus following a mumps epidemic. *J Trop Med Hyg* 1975; 78: 262–3.
113. Hyoty H, Leinikki P, Reunanen A, Ilonen J, Surcel HM, Rilva A, Kaar ML, Huupponen T, Hakulinen A, Makela AL, et al. Mumps infections in the etiology of type 1 (insulin-dependent) diabetes. *Diabetes Res* 1988; 9: 111–6.
114. Hyoty H, Hiltunen M, Reunanen A, Leinikki P, Vesikari T, Lounamaa R, Tuomilehto J, Akerblom HK, for the Childhood Diabetes in Finland Study Group. Decline of mumps antibodies in type 1 (insulin-dependent) diabetic children and a plateau in the rising incidence of type 1 diabetes after introduction of the mumps–measles–rubella vaccine in Finland. *Diabetologia* 1993; 36: 1303–8.
115. Jenson AB, Rosenberg HS, Notkins AL. Pancreatic islet-cell damage in children with fatal viral infections. *Lancet* 1980; 2: 354–8.
116. Hiltunen M, Hyoty H, Karjalainen J, Leinikki P, Knip M, Lounamaa R, Akerblom HK, for the The Childhood Diabetes in Finland Study Group. Serological evaluation of the role of cytomegalovirus in the pathogenesis of IDDM: a prospective study. *Diabetologia* 1995; 38: 705–10.
117. Honeyman MC, Stone NL, Harrison LC. T-cell epitopes in type 1 diabetes autoantigen tyrosine phosphatase IA-2: potential for mimicry with rotavirus and other environmental agents. *Mol Med* 1998; 4: 231–9.
118. Honeyman MC, Coulson BS, Stone NL, Gellert SA, Goldwater PN, Steele CE, Couper JJ, Tait BD, Colman PG, Harrison LC. Association between rotavirus infection and pancreatic islet autoimmunity in children at risk of developing type 1 diabetes. *Diabetes* 2000; 49: 1319–24.
119. Coulson BS, Witterick PD, Tan Y, Hewish MJ, Mountford JN, Harrison LC, Honeyman MC. Growth of rotaviruses in primary pancreatic cells. *J Virol* 2002; 76: 9537–44.

120. Harrison LC, Hafler DA. Antigen-specific therapy for autoimmune disease. *Curr Opin Immunol* 2000; 12: 704–11.
121. Faria AM, Weiner HL. Oral tolerance: mechanisms and therapeutic applications. *Adv Immunol* 1999; 73: 153–64.
122. Krause I, Blank M, Shoenfeld Y. Immunomodulation of experimental autoimmune diseases via oral tolerance. *Crit Rev Immunol* 2000; 20: 1–16.
123. Roncarolo M-G, Levings MK. The role of different subsets of T regulatory cells in controlling autoimmunity. *Curr Opin Immunol* 2000; 12: 676–83.
124. Penna G, Adorini L. 1α,25-Dihydroxyvitamin D_3 inhibits differentiation, maturation, activation and survival of dendritic cells leading to impaired alloreactive T cell activation. *J Immunol* 2000; 164: 2405–11.
125. Zhang ZH, Davidson L, Eisenbarth G, Weiner HL. Suppression of diabetes in nonobese diabetic mice by oral administration of porcine insulin. *Proc Natl Acad Sci USA* 1991; 88: 10252–6.
126. Bergerot I, Fabien N, Maguer V, Thivolet C. Oral administration of human insulin to NOD mice generates CD4+ T-cells that suppress adoptive transfer of diabetes. *J Autoimmunity* 1994; 7: 655–63.
127. Daniel D, Wegmann D. Protection of nonobese diabetic mice from diabetes by intranasal or subcutaneous administration of insulin peptide B-(9-23). *Proc Natl Acad Sci USA* 1996; 93: 956–60.
128. Harrison LC, Dempsey-Collier M, Kramer DR, Takahashi K. Aerosol insulin induces regulatory CD8 gamma delta T-cells that prevent murine insulin-dependent diabetes. *J Exp Med* 1996; 184: 2167–74.
129. Martinez NR, Augstein P, Moustakas AK, Papadopoulos GK, Gregori S, Adorini L, Jackson DC, Harrison LC. Disabling an integral CTL epitope allows suppression of autoimmune diabetes by intranasal proinsulin peptide. *J Clin Invest* 2003; 111: 1365–71.
130. Tian J, Atkinson MA, Clare-Salzler M, Herschenfeld A, Forsthuber T, Lehmann PV, Kaufman DL. Nasal administration of glutamate decarboxylase (GAD65) peptides induces Th-2 responses and prevents murine insulin-dependent diabetes. *J Exp Med* 1996; 183: 1561–7.
131. Husby S, Mestecky J, Moldoveanu Z, Holland S, Elson CO. Oral tolerance in humans. T cell but not B cell tolerance after antigen feeding. *J Immunol* 1994; 152: 4663–70.
132. Waldo FB, van den Wall Bake AW, Mestecky J, Husby S. Suppression of the immune response by nasal immunization. *Clin Immunol Immunopathol* 1994; 72: 30–4.
133. Hancock WW, Polanski M, Zhang J, Blogg N, Weiner HL. Suppression of insulitis in non-obese diabetic (NOD) mice by oral insulin administration is associated with selective expression of interleukin-4 and -10, transforming growth factor-beta and prostaglandin-E. *Am J Pathol* 1995; 147: 1193–9.
134. Ploix C, Bergerot I, Fabien N, Perche S, Moulin V, Thivolet C. Protection against autoimmune diabetes with oral insulin is associated with the presence of IL-4 type 2 T-cells in the pancreas and pancreatic lymph nodes. *Diabetes* 1998; 47: 39–44.
135. Homann D, Dyrberg T, Petersen J, Oldstone MB, von Herrath MG. Insulin in oral immune "tolerance": a one-amino acid change in the B chain makes the difference. *J Immunol* 1999; 163: 1833–8.
136. Slavin AJ, Maron R, Weiner HL. Mucosal administration of IL-10 enhances oral tolerance in autoimmune encephalomyelitis and diabetes. *Int Immunol* 2001; 13: 825–33.
137. Bellmann K, Kolb H, Hartmann B, Rothe H, Rowsell P, Rastegar S, Burghardt K, Scott FW. Intervention in autoimmune diabetes by targeting the gut immune system. *Int J Immunopharmacol* 1997; 19: 573–7.
138. Hartmann B, Bellmann K, Ghiea I, Kleemann R, Kolb H. Oral insulin for diabetes prevention in NOD mice: potentiation by enhancing Th-2 cytokine expression in the gut through bacterial adjuvant. *Diabetologia* 1997; 40: 902–9.
139. Maron R, Palanivel V, Weiner HL, Harn DA. Oral administration of schistosome egg antigens and insulin B-chain generates and enhances Th2-type responses in NOD mice. *Clin Immunol Immunopathol* 1998; 87: 85–92.
140. Bergerot I, Ploix C, Petersen J, Moulin V, Rask C, Fabien N, Lindblad M, Mayer A, Czerkinsky C, Holmgren J, Thivolet C. A cholera toxoid-insulin conjugate as an oral vaccine against spontaneous autoimmune diabetes. *Proc Natl Acad Sci USA* 1997; 94: 4610–4.
141. Ploix C, Bergerot I, Durand A, Czerkinsky C, Holmgren J, Thivolet C. Oral administration of cholera toxin B-insulin conjugates protects NOD mice from autoimmune diabetes by inducing CD4+ regulatory T-cells. *Diabetes* 1999; 48: 2150–6.
142. Arakawa T, Yu J, Chong DK, Hough J, Engen PC, Langridge WH. A plant-based cholera toxin B subunit-insulin fusion protein protects against the development of autoimmune diabetes. *Nat Biotechnol* 1998; 16: 934–8.
143. Ma SW, Zhao DL, Yin ZQ, Mukherjee R, Singh B, Qin HY, Stiller CR, Jevnikar AM. Transgenic plants expressing autoantigens fed to mice to induce oral immune tolerance. *Nat Med* 1997; 3: 793–6.
144. Maron R, Guerau-de-Arellano M, Zhang X, Weiner HL. Oral administration of insulin to neonates suppresses spontaneous and cyclophosphamide induced diabetes in the NOD mouse. *J Autoimmun* 2001; 16: 21–8.
145. Hänninen A, Harrison LC. Gamma delta T-cells as mediators of mucosal tolerance: the autoimmune diabetes model. *Immunol Rev* 2000; 173: 109–19.
146. Maron R, Melican NS, Weiner HL. Regulatory Th2-type T cell lines against insulin and GAD peptides derived from orally- and nasally-treated NOD mice suppress diabetes. *J Autoimmun* 1999; 12: 251–8.
147. Harrison LC, Honeyman MC, Trembleau S, Gregori S, Gallazzi F, Augstein P, Brusic V, Hammer J, Adorini L. A peptide-binding motif for I-A(g7), the class II major histocompatibility complex (MHC) molecule of NOD and Biozzi AB/H mice. *J Autoimmun* 1997; 10: 165–73.
148. Chen W, Bergerot I, Elliott JF, Harrison LC, Delovitch TL. Evidence that a peptide spanning the B–C junction of proinsulin is a primary autoantigen epitope in the pathogenesis of type 1 diabetes. *J Immunol* 2001; 167: 4926–35.
149. Rudy G, Stone N, Harrison LC, Colman PG, McNair P, Brusic V, French MB, Honeyman MC, Tait B, Lew AM. Similar peptides from two β-cell autoantigens, proinsulin and glutamic acid decarboxylase, stimulate T-cells of individuals at risk for insulin-dependent diabetes. *Mol Med* 1995; 1: 625–33.
150. Feltquate DM, Heaney S, Webster RG, Robinson HL. Different T helper cell types and antibody isotypes generated by saline and gene gun DNA immunization. *J Immunol* 1997; 158: 2278–84.

151. Yang Z, Chen M, Wu R, Fialkow LB, Bromberg JS, McDuffie M, Naji A, Nadler JL. Suppression of autoimmune diabetes by viral IL-10 gene transfer. *J Immunol* 2002; 168: 6479–85.
152. McCluskie MJ, Brazolot Millan CL, Gramzinski RA, Robinson HL, Santoro JC, Fuller JT, Widera G, Haynes JR, Purcell RH, Davis HL. Route and method of delivery of DNA vaccine influence immune responses in mice and non-human primates. *Mol Med* 1999; 5: 287–300.
153. Tisch R, Wang B, Weaver DJ, Liu B, Bui T, Arthos J, Serreze DV. Antigen-specific mediated suppression of beta cell autoimmunity by plasmid DNA vaccination. *J Immunol* 2001; 166: 2122–32.
154. Cameron MJ, Strathdee CA, Holmes KD, Arreaza GA, Dekaban GA, Delovitch TL. Biolistic-mediated interleukin 4 gene transfer prevents the onset of type 1 diabetes. *Hum Gene Ther* 2000; 11: 1647–56.
155. Filippova M, Liu J, Escher A. Effects of plasmid DNA injection on cyclophosphamide-accelerated diabetes in NOD mice. *DNA Cell Biol* 2001; 175–81.
156. Piccirillo CA, Chang Y, Prud'homme GJ. TGF-beta1 somatic gene therapy prevents autoimmune disease in nonobese diabetic mice. *J Immunol* 1998; 161: 3950–6.
157. Coon B, An LL, Whitton JL, von Herrath MG. DNA immunization to prevent autoimmune diabetes. *J Clin Invest* 1999; 104: 189–94.
158. Weaver DJ Jr, Liu B, Tisch R. Plasmid dnas encoding insulin and glutamic acid decarboxylase 65 have distinct effects on the progression of autoimmune diabetes in nonobese diabetic mice. *J Immunol* 2001; 167: 586–92.
159. Prud'homme GJ, Chang Y, Li X. Immunoinhibitory DNA vaccine protects against autoimmune diabetes through cDNA encoding a selective CTLA-4 (CD152) ligand. *Hum Gene Ther* 2002; 13: 395–406.
160. Hänninen A, Braakhuis A, Heath WR, Harrison LC. Mucosal antigen primes diabetogenic cytotoxic T-lymphocytes regardless of dose or delivery route. *Diabetes* 2001; 50: 771–5.
161. Hänninen A, Martinez NR, Davey GM, Heath WR, Harrison LC. Transient blockade of CD40 ligand dissociates pathogenic from protective mucosal immunity. *J Clin Invest* 2002; 109: 261–7.
162. Roman M, Martin-Orozco E, Goodman JS, Nguyen MD, Sato Y, Ronaghy A, Kornbluth RS, Richman DD, Carson DA, Raz E. Immunostimulatory DNA sequences function as T helper-1-promoting adjuvants. 1997; *Nat Med*: 849–54.
163. Quintana FJ, Rotem A, Carmi P, Cohen IR. Vaccination with empty plasmid DNA or CpG oligonucleotide inhibits diabetes in nonobese diabetic mice: modulation of spontaneous 60-kDa heat shock protein autoimmunity. *J Immunol* 2000; 165: 6148–55.
164. Serreze DV, Leiter EH, Worthen SM, Shultz LD. NOD marrow stem cells adoptively transfer diabetes to resistant (NOD × NON)F1 mice. *Diabetes* 1988; 37: 252–5.
165. Wicker LS, Miller BJ, Chai A, Terada M, Mullen Y. Expression of genetically determined diabetes and insulitis in the nonobese diabetic (NOD) mouse at the level of bone marrow-derived cells. Transfer of diabetes and insulitis to nondiabetic (NOD × B10) F1 mice with bone marrow cells from NOD mice. *J Exp Med* 1988; 167: 1801–10.
166. LaFace DM, Peck AB. Reciprocal allogeneic bone marrow transplantation between NOD mice and diabetes-nonsusceptible mice associated with transfer and prevention of autoimmune diabetes. *Diabetes* 1989; 38: 894–901.
167. Ikehara S, Ohtsuki H, Good RA, Asamoto H, Nakamura T, Sekita K, Muso E, Tochino Y, Ida T, Kuzuya H. Prevention of type I diabetes in nonobese diabetic mice by allogenic bone marrow transplantation. *Proc Natl Acad Sci USA* 1985; 82: 7743–7.
168. Beilhack GF, Scheffold YC, Weissman IL, Taylor C, Jerabek L, Burge MJ, Masek MA, Shizuru JA. Purified allogeneic hematopoietic stem cell transplantation blocks diabetes pathogenesis in NOD mice. *Diabetes* 2003; 52: 59–68.
169. Li H, Kaufman CL, Boggs SS, Johnson PC, Patrene KD, Ildstad ST. Mixed allogeneic chimerism induced by a sublethal approach prevents autoimmune diabetes and reverses insulitis in nonobese diabetic (NOD) mice. *J Immunol* 1996; 156: 380–8.
170. Kaufman CL, Li H, Ildstad ST. Patterns of hemopoietic reconstitution in nonobese diabetic mice: dichotomy of allogeneic resistance versus competitive advantage of disease-resistant marrow. *J Immunol* 1997; 158: 2435–42.
171. Mathieu C, Casteels K, Bouillon R, Waer M. Protection against autoimmune diabetes in mixed bone marrow chimeras: mechanisms involved. *J Immunol* 1997; 158: 1453–7.
172. Nishimoto H, Kikutani H, Yamamura K, Kishimoto T. Prevention of autoimmune insulitis by expression of I-E molecules in NOD mice. *Nature* 1987; 328: 432–4.
173. Lund T, O'Reilly L, Hutchings P, Kanagawa O, Simpson E, Gravely R, Chandler P, Dyson J, Picard JK, Edwards A. Prevention of insulin-dependent diabetes mellitus in non-obese diabetic mice by transgenes encoding modified I-A beta-chain or normal I-E alpha-chain. *Nature* 1990; 345: 727–9.
174. Singer SM, Tisch R, Yang XD, McDevitt HO. An Abd transgene prevents diabetes in nonobese diabetic mice by inducing regulatory T-cells. *Proc Natl Acad Sci USA* 1993; 90: 9566–70.
175. Singer SM, Tisch R, Yang XD, Sytwu HK, Liblau R, McDevitt HO. Prevention of diabetes in NOD mice by a mutated I-Ab transgene. *Diabetes* 1998; 47: 1570–7.
176. Schmidt D, Verdaguer J, Averill N, Santamaria P. A mechanism for the major histocompatibility complex-linked resistance to autoimmunity. *J Exp Med* 1997; 186: 1059–75.
177. Luhder F, Katz J, Benoist C, Mathis D. Major histocompatibility complex class II molecules can protect from diabetes by positively selecting T-cells with additional specificities. *J Exp Med* 1998; 187: 379–87.
178. Burt RK, Slavin S, Burns WH, Marmont AM. Induction of tolerance in autoimmune diseases by hematopoietic stem cell transplantation: getting closer to a cure? *Blood* 2002; 99: 768–84.
179. Castro-Malaspina H, Harris RE, Gajewski J, Ramsay N, Collins R, Dharan B, King R, Deeg HJ. Unrelated donor marrow transplantation for myelodysplastic syndromes: outcome analysis in 510 transplants facilitated by the National Marrow Donor Program. *Blood* 2002; 99: 1943–51.
180. Ratanatharathorn V, Ayash L, Lazarus HM, Fu J, Uberti JP. Chronic graft-versus-host disease: clinical manifestation and therapy. *Bone Marrow Transplant* 2001; 28: 121–9.
181. Steptoe RJ, Ritchie JM, Harrison LC. Transfer of hematopoietic stem cells encoding autoantigen prevents

autoimmune diabetes. *J Clin Invest* 2003; 111: 1357–63.

182. Keller RJ, Eisenbarth GS, Jackson RA. Insulin prophylaxis in individuals at high risk of type 1 diabetes. *Lancet* 1993; 341: 927–8.

183. Pozzilli P, Pitocco D, Visalli N, Cavallo MG, Buzzetti R, Crino A, Spera S, Suraci C, Multari G, Cervoni M, Manca Bitti ML, Matteoli MC, Marietti G, Ferrazzoli F, Cassone Faldetta MR, Giordano C, Sbriglia M, Sarugeri E, Ghirlanda G, for the, IMDIAB Group. No effect of oral insulin on residual β-cell function in recent-onset type I diabetes (the IMDIAB VII). *Diabetologia* 2000; 43: 1000–4.

184. Metzler B, Wraith DC. Inhibition of experimental autoimmune encephalomyelitis by inhalation but not oral administration of the encephalitogenic peptide: influence of MHC binding affinity. *Int Immunol* 1993; 5: 1159–65.

185. Colman PG, McNair P, Margetts H, Schmidli R, Werther G, Alford F, Ward G, Tait B, Honeyman MC, Harrison LC. The Melbourne Pre-Diabetes Study: screening for preclinical insulin-dependent diabetes in first-degree relatives of probands. *Med J Aust* 1998; 169: 81–4.

116

Prevention of Type 2 Diabetes Mellitus

Richard W. Simpson*, Jaakko Tuomilehto†, Jaana Lindstrom†, Jonathan E. Shaw‡, and Paul Zimmet‡

**Monash University, Box Hill Hospital, Victoria, Australia, †National Public Health Institute, Helsinki, Finland, and ‡International Diabetes Institute, Melbourne, Australia*

The rapid technological development that has characterized the automobile and computer era continues to reduce incidental physical activity. This, along with the aging of the population and the consumption of excess food energy (in relation to exercise), is driving the inexorable growth of an epidemic of type 2 diabetes in all countries. Rapid industrialization of the developing nations is spreading the epidemic globally [1, 2]. The global number of people with diabetes is expected to be at least 220 million by 2010, reaching 324 million by 2025 [3, 4] (Figure 1). The social and health care costs of the epidemic are now large and rising and are already beyond the economic capacity of most nations. In developed countries 10% or more of the total health budget is expended on people with diabetes [2]. In the United States [5] the most recent estimate of the total cost of managing diabetes is about US$132 billion per year, with over 10% of the health dollar spent on diabetes. Proportionately similar costs have now been reported from Australia [6]. A compelling case therefore exists for the prevention of this disease. Major advances in our understanding of the etiology and natural history of the disease and recent important published prevention studies show that type 2 diabetes can be prevented.

PREVENTION: DIFFERING LEVELS OF INTERVENTION

Type 2 diabetes is now recognized to be the end of a much bigger cardiovascular disease spectrum—the Metabolic Syndrome (MS), which itself is still an imprecisely defined entity. There have been a number of attempts to define criteria for the MS. The two most quoted are the World Health Organization (WHO) [7] and the NCEP ATP III [8], which published slightly differing sets of criteria. Both, however, recognize abnormalities in glucose metabolism, hypertension, obesity, and dyslipidemia as components of the syndrome. Effective prevention strategies for type 2 diabetes within the broader context of the MS could occur at a number of levels. In this larger medical paradigm these could be defined as primary interventions dealing with the whole population to prevent the early stages of the MS, secondary interventions identifying persons who are prediabetic [impaired glucose tolerance (IGT) and impaired fasting glucose (IFG)] [9], and tertiary interventions (beyond the scope of this review) implementing therapies to reduce the progression of hyperglycemia and development of complications of diabetes. However, these definitions are not in common usage and the currently accepted way of categorizing prevention strategies is in terms of population and targeted prevention approaches.

Population prevention deals with activities to change the lifestyle and thereby reduce environmental risk factors in the whole population or focused on particular at risk communities such as vulnerable ethnic subgroups. This population approach involves subjects with a wide range of susceptibility, differing levels of metabolic normality and abnormality, and all ages. It involves action from many levels or sectors of the community in addition to the health care sector. Health care personnel have the important role of influencing and providing leadership in national policymaking processes and where appropriate helping translate the measures at the patient level. Targeted prevention involves high intensity activities in those at particularly high risk with IFG and IGT. The health

International Textbook of Diabetes Mellitus, Third Edition. Edited by R. A. DeFronzo, E. Ferrannini, H. Keen, and P. Zimmet.

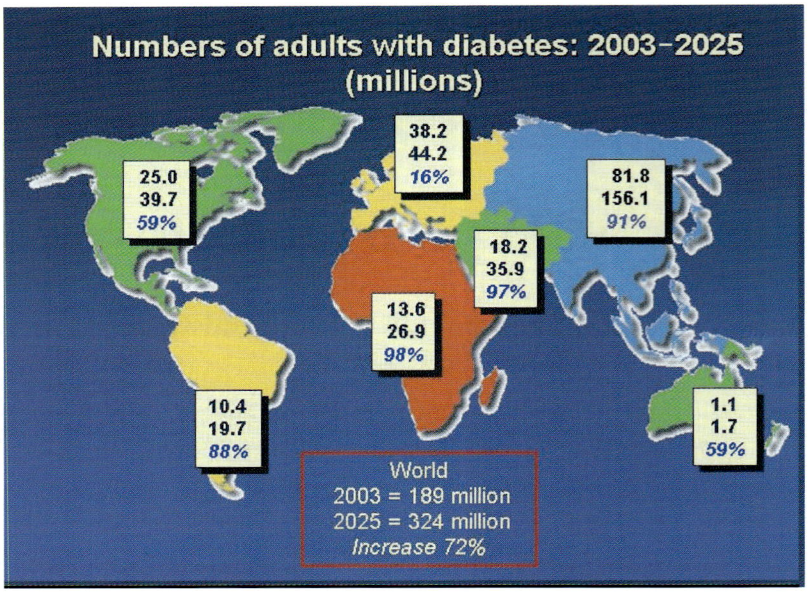

Figure 1 The predicted global distribution and increase of diabetes: 2003–2025. The estimate is based on expected growth and aging of the population. No account has been taken of the increasing incidence of obesity in many countries

care sector also has an important role here as many of these people are already known to and consumers of health care services. Again both levels of intervention are likely to be required for effective prevention of type 2 diabetes.

CLASSIFICATION OF DIABETES

The WHO [10] has recently reviewed the diagnostic criteria and classification of diabetes. These internationally accepted criteria facilitate a broad comparison of information on treatments of diabetes between countries. Of equal importance is the correct classification and phenotyping of subjects in prevention studies. Recent studies in type 2 diabetes have highlighted a high prevalence of subjects with antibodies to glutamic acid decarboxylase (anti-GAD) and other markers of autoimmunity [11, 12]. Thus, subjects who are probably developing type 1 diabetes may distort some studies aimed at type 2 diabetes. At the very least it would be wise to screen for anti-GAD antibodies in Caucasian subjects for type 2 diabetes prevention studies. It may also be important to consider that certain specific genetically determined forms of type 2 diabetes such as maturity-onset diabetes of the young (MODY) may also be unresponsive to preventative measures for the "common" form of the disease [13].

PATHOGENESIS OF TYPE 2 DIABETES

It is widely recognized that type 2 diabetes is a consequence of both increased insulin resistance and β-cell dysfunction and a result of an interaction between genetic and environmental factors. The relative contribution of insulin resistance and β-cell dysfunction to the disease evolution may vary between ethnically and perhaps nonethnically related individuals. In part, an individual's level of insulin resistance is inherited [14] but increases with age [15, 16] and levels of obesity [17] and inactivity [18]. Abnormal insulin resistance often predates prediabetes. The propensity for β-cell dysfunction also appears to have an inherited component. Studies in normoglycemic first-degree relatives of people with type 2 diabetes show that β-cell dysfunction also precedes the prediabetes state [19, 20]. By the time IGT has developed, clear evidence of a reduction in the first-phase insulin response to oral glucose is present [21]. As dysglycemia progresses to the early stages of diabetes and beyond, β-cell function continues to deteriorate.

A number of etiological and risk factors have been identified for type 2 diabetes (Table 1).

Genetic Susceptibility

There is strong familial aggregation of type 2 diabetes, with up to 40% of siblings of type 2 diabetic subjects developing the disease [22] and twin studies showing a higher concordance rate in monozygotic (between 60 and 90%) than dizygotic twins [23, 24]. Large numbers of studies examining different populations, including Native Americans and Canadians, Pacific Islanders, West Indian Blacks, Asian Indians, indigenous Australians, the Chinese, and Europeans, strongly point to a genetic predisposition in disturbance or adaptation of glucose metabolism to recent lifestyle changes [25]. A small percentage of cases (2–5% of all type 2 diabetes) can be explained by single gene

Table 1 Etiological determinants and risk factors of type 2 diabetes

A. Genetic factors
  Genetic markers, family history, "Thrifty gene(s)," etc.

B. Demographic characteristics
  Sex, age, ethnicity

C. Behavioral and lifestyle-related risk factors
  Obesity (including distribution of obesity and duration)
  Physical inactivity
  Diet
  Stress
  "Westernisation, Urbanization, Modernization"

D. Metabolic determinants and intermediate risk categories of type 2 diabetes
  Impaired glucose tolerance
  Impaired fasting glucose
  Insulin resistance
  Pregnancy-related determinants (parity, gestational diabetes, diabetes in offspring of women with diabetes during pregnancy, intrauterine mal- or overnutrition)

defects affecting key components of insulin secretion or action [26, 27]. These are usually associated with severe insulin resistance or with diabetes with a very early age of onset. It is highly likely that a number of genes other than these are involved in the pathogenesis of typical cases of type 2 diabetes. The complex or polygenetic mode of inheritance and the interaction with the environment have frustrated identification of the genes involved in the common forms of type 2 diabetes [2, 27].

The particularly high prevalence of type 2 diabetes in a range of ethnic communities led to the "thrifty" gene(s) hypothesis [28]. The current interpretation is that many of these different vulnerable groups carried one or more genes which were protective in a hunter-gatherer lifestyle but increase the risk of obesity and diabetes when there is a secure, nonseasonal (continual) food supply. However, diabetes is increasing globally and in all racial groups.

Environmental Factors

Many epidemiological studies have highlighted the significant role of the environmental factors, nutrition, physical exercise, and in turn, level of obesity, in the etiology of type 2 diabetes. Populations on all continents have shown an increasing prevalence of type 2 diabetes with increasing "westernization" or urbanization of their lifestyle. Many migrant groups have experienced dramatic increases in the incidence of type 2 diabetes within one generation in their new country [2, 25].

The association between obesity and diabetes has been well described in many cross-sectional and prospective studies in a range of Caucasian and non-Caucasian populations [29]. Risk ratios of between 2 and 60 have been reported [30–33], the highest risks in the very obese [30, 33]. Both duration [34] of obesity and particularly central, in addition to general, obesity are strongly associated with the risk of type 2 diabetes [17].

Overall physical activity levels have drastically decreased over recent decades in many populations and this has to be considered a major contributor to the current global rise of obesity [35]. Physical activity has been found in seven prospective or longitudinal studies to be independently associated with both prevalence and incidence of type 2 diabetes in men and women [25, 36, 37].

In epidemiological investigations it is difficult to separate out the components of the "westernized" diet: food types, calorie excess, increased dietary fat and refined carbohydrate, reduced complex carbohydrate and dietary fiber. The true risks associated with dietary components are still to be fully clarified. Table 2 summarizes the current state [13, 36].

A large but unrandomized prospective trial [38] of antihypertensive drugs found an increased risk (approximately 25%) of diabetes with β-blockers but not with diuretics. More recently the Antihypertensive and Lipid-Lowering Treatment to Prevent Heart Attack Trial (ALLHAT) [39], which was both randomized and prospective, reported an increased risk of diabetes with chlothalidone (a thiazide diuretic) compared with lisinopril [angiotensin-converting enzyme (ACE) inhibitor] and amlodipine (calcium-channel blocker). As neither trial was adequately designed to test the diabetogenic effects of these commonly used antihypertensive drugs, the issue remains unclear.

POPULATION PREVENTION APPROACHES

Until now there has been little evidence of truly population-based strategies being employed to reduce the environmental factors involved in the development of

Table 2 Proposed environmental risk factors of type 2 diabetes based on findings from cross-sectional and longitudinal studies

Risk Factors	Strength of association	Control for confounding factors
High BMI	High	Adequate
Increased central obesity	High	Adequate
Physical inactivity	High	Adequate
Excessive intake of		
Energy	Intermediate	Not satisfactory
Simple carbohydrates	Weak	Not satisfactory
Saturated fat	Weak	Not satisfactory
Trans fat	Intermediate	Not satisfactory
Glycemic load	Weak	Not satisfactory
Low intake of		
Dietary fiber	Intermediate	Not satisfactory
Certain trace elements	Weak	Not satisfactory
Antioxidants		
Smoking	Intermediate	Not satisfactory
Moderate alcohol*	Intermediate	Not satisfactory

* Inverse association.

the MS and therefore type 2 diabetes. Several studies have reported that a return to traditional lifestyle in aboriginal groups will improve various anthropometric and metabolic parameters [40, 41]. This is usually not an option for most ethnic communities and is likely to be less available with the global socioeconomic and technological changes underway. There have been few prevention programs targeting vulnerable communities (inevitably some of the subjects involved will be prediabetic or even have diabetes). These communities have been somewhat isolated aboriginal groups in Australia [42, 43] and North America [44]. The approach has been based on encouraging the communities to control food supply from the limited number of local commercial outlets in the communities and to develop self-help educational and activity groups. Again anthropometric and biochemical markers of glucose and lipid metabolism were improved. Neither studies examining return to traditional lifestyles nor the trials targeting the vulnerable communities have demonstrated a reduction in the incidence of diabetes, let alone cardiovascular disease morbidity and mortality. In 1992 the education ministry in Singapore commenced a "trim and fit" program for school children to reduce obesity and improve physical fitness [45]. Overweight students, parents, and teachers were targeted. Nutrition education was integrated into the curriculum; special exercise programs were established (for the overweight) and food and beverages available in the school environment were controlled. By 2000 the prevalence of obesity declined from 16.6 to 14.6% in 11–12-year-olds and 15.5–13.1% in 15–16-year-olds. This is an important program that could have wider international application.

PREVENTION TARGETED ON HIGH-RISK INDIVIDUALS

This level of intervention is dependent on being able to define a prediabetic stage. It is generally accepted that individuals proceed through IGT and/or IFG before progressing to type 2 diabetes [9, 10]. IGT and IFG thus identify individuals at high risk of developing type 2 diabetes and cardiovascular disease.

The Prediabetic State

The oral glucose tolerance test (OGTT) is the "gold standard" for categorizing patients with IGT but is poorly reproducible, cumbersome to administer for large studies, and unpleasant for the subjects [46]. In large studies examining the natural history of changes in glucose metabolism it has not been practical to repeat the test two or three times at each time point. This large physiological variation in postchallenge glucose levels may have resulted in some misclassification of individuals in studies based on a single OGTT and in turn clouded the interpretation of the natural history of subjects with IGT. Are subjects who apparently change from IGT to normal glucose tolerance (NGT) really reverting, were they normal all along (and thus misclassified) or were they at a much earlier stage of the disease? In Pima Indians it has been shown that if follow-up is extended from 5 to 10 years, the conversion level for individuals who demonstrate IGT increases from 25 to 61% [47]. Over 10 years 48% of subjects with "transient" IGT go on to develop diabetes [48]. Perhaps with time most survivors with IGT will ultimately progress to type 2 diabetes.

The risk experienced by patients with IGT for progression to type 2 diabetes is variable depending on obesity, fasting blood glucose, the 2-h post-glucose load level [49], and the number of other cardiovascular disease risk factors present [50, 51]. It is generally accepted that in comparison to those with NGT there is a 6–10-fold increase in risk overall, although one study [52] reported up to 23-fold increase in risk of developing type 2 diabetes from IGT. In particularly vulnerable groups of subjects, the evolution of type 2 diabetes appears to involve rapid transit through the stage of IGT [52, 53]. The annual conversion rate of subjects with IGT to type 2 diabetes varies but on average the rate of progression is 5% in middle-aged individuals; the reported range is 3.6% in Caucasians to 8.7% in Nauruans. IGT is also a significant risk factor for cardiovascular disease independent of other known risk factors [54, 55].

In recent years IFG has been defined as an additional risk factor for type 2 diabetes but not cardiovascular disease [56]. Just as IGT identifies individuals with elevated but nondiabetic postchallenge glucose values, IFG identifies those with elevated but nondiabetic fasting glucose values. The degree of overlap between the two conditions, however, is limited. Like IGT, IFG is associated with a higher risk of progression to type 2 diabetes than NGT. Within most populations IGT is much more common than is IFG [56].

Surgical or Drug-induced Weight Loss

As yet there are no randomized controlled trials of surgical treatment of obesity but in a group of severely overweight subjects with IGT undergoing gastric bypass surgery, the rate of conversion over 4–6 years to type 2 diabetes after an average weight loss of 22.5 kg was 0.15/100 persons/year. This was compared to a conversion rate of 4.72/100 persons/year in an unoperated group: a 30-fold reduction in risk with this intervention [57]. Likewise in the Swedish SOS Intervention Study [58] gastric surgery in very obese subjects reduced the 2-year incidence of diabetes 30-fold in grossly obese subjects (weight loss 28 kg) compared with control subjects who were receiving regular care (weight loss 0.5 kg). These results suggest that severe obesity can be treated surgically and lead to a marked reduction in the incidence of diabetes.

Recently, the results of Xendos [Xenical (orlistat) in the Prevention of Diabetes in Obese Subjects] [59], a placebo-controlled multicenter trial, were announced. This involved overweight (BMI $\geq$ 30 kg/m^2) subjects aged 30–60 years, of whom 21% had IGT at baseline. All subjects received lifestyle advice (calorie-reduced diet and exercise counselling) initially 2 weekly for 6 months and thereafter monthly. Over a period of 4 years the group receiving orlistat compared with the group on diet alone showed a reduced incidence [37% relative risk reduction (RRR) and 2.8% absolute risk reduction (ARR)] of type 2 diabetes. Weight reduction was 6.9 kg in the orlistat group and 4.1 kg in the placebo group. What are not yet known from the study are the relative prevention rates between the subjects with IGT and NGT. Also, it is unclear at present whether all the prevention of diabetes is solely attributable to weight loss. Unfortunately, there was a high dropout rate over the 4-year treatment phase in both groups: 52% in orlistat and 34% in placebo.

Both the surgical and the orlistat studies in obese subjects indicate that probably weight control alone is an efficient way to prevent the development of type 2 diabetes.

Lifestyle Intervention Studies

During the Franco-Prussian War (1870) and subsequently during the First and Second World Wars a decline in diabetes incidence, mortality, and/or morbidity was noted [60–62]. These periods were associated with food shortages, probably increased physical activity due to restricted transport facilities, and weight loss. A number of small, generally short-term studies involving subjects with various degrees of impaired glucose regulation have been reported over the last 20 years [63–68]. Most of them had problems with design. Generally however, these studies have shown a benefit of healthy (or traditional) lifestyle on improving or delaying deterioration of glucose tolerance.

There have now been four large controlled and longer term trials examining the effect of lifestyle changes on the progression from IGT to type 2 diabetes. The main lifestyle intervention targets were body weight, diet, and physical activity. The intervention methods used to modify lifestyle varied between the studies as sociocultural issues and the available facilities and personnel differed.

The Malmö Study

This feasibility study examined the benefits of diet and exercise in 217 middle-aged men in Malmö with IGT [69]. The subjects were "self" distributed into intervention and reference groups (in ratio 3:1). The subjects were therefore not randomly assigned to the study groups and this diminishes the ability to generalize the results. The treatment group received detailed dietary advice and support within an exercise program while the other received standard medical care according to requirements. Neither group received any form of antidiabetic drug. Over a period of 5 years the treated subjects significantly reduced and maintained weight loss (BMI reduced 2.5% in the intervention group, and increased 0.5% in the reference group). In addition the estimated maximal oxygen uptake increased by 10% in the intervention subjects while it decreased by 5% in control men. In the treated group 10.6% developed type 2 diabetes versus 28.6% of the reference subjects. The RRR in the intervention group was 59% and the ARR was 17%. Although the progression to diabetes in the reference group of Swedish men was lower than would be predicted from the observational studies, this study did demonstrate the feasibility of carrying out a diet–exercise program for 5 years among volunteers.

As will be apparent below, in a more recent intervention study, some subjects in the control group probably also made improvements in their lifestyle. The analysis of this study is based on intention-to-treat, and therefore probably underestimated the true effect of lifestyle changes.

The DaQing Study

The DaQing IGT and Diabetes Study, published in 1997, involved a large population-based screening program to identify people with IGT [70]. The effect of exercise and diet in preventing the development of type 2 diabetes in 577 subjects with IGT was examined over 6 years in 33 hospital clinics across China. There were four intervention groups: diet alone, exercise alone, diet–exercise combined, or no intervention. Randomization into these groups was undertaken on a clinic rather than an individual basis. For dietary intervention the participants were recommended a high-carbohydrate and low-fat diet and encouraged to reduce weight if BMI was $\geq$25 kg/m^2 aiming at 23 kg/m^2. A physician did counselling. Group sessions were organized weekly for the first month, monthly for 3 months, and then 3 monthly. For the clinics-assigned physical exercise, counselling sessions were arranged at a similar frequency. The participants were encouraged to increase their level of leisure-time physical activity by at least 1–2 "units" per day. One unit was defined as 30 min slow walking, 10 min slow running, or 5 min swimming.

The annual risk of progressing to type 2 diabetes from IGT in this population was reduced from 15.7% in the control group to 8% in the three intervention groups. The cumulative 6-year incidence of type 2 diabetes in the three intervention groups was 41–46% compared with 68% in the control group. The reported changes in risk factor patterns were modest. There was an approximate 1 kg/m^2 reduction of BMI in subjects with baseline BMI $\geq$ 25 kg/m^2, with no change in BMI for the lean subjects. The estimated changes in habitual dietary nutrient intakes were small and nonsignificant between groups. Thus, it appears that neither weight change nor even diet were the major determinates of the outcome. Physical activity and possibly subtle qualitative changes in diet played a key role.

There is a major methodological limitation in this study as allocation to intervention group was based on clinic (cluster) rather than the individual subject randomization. Individual data analysis must therefore be interpreted with caution. The study subjects were relatively lean (mean BMI 25.8 kg/m^2) compared to subjects with IGT from other ethnic groups, and the progression from IGT to diabetes was high (over 10% per year in the control group) compared to findings in observational studies. These issues make it difficult to generalize the conclusions for other ethnic groups.

The Finnish Diabetes Prevention Study

The Finnish Diabetes Prevention Study (FDPS) [71–73], the first properly controlled trial on prevention of type 2 diabetes with lifestyle modification (diet and exercise) alone, enrolled 523 subjects with IGT from five clinics in Finland between 1993 and 1998. Subjects (age 40–64 years, BMI over 25 kg/m^2) were individually randomly allocated into the intervention and control groups with stratification according to center, gender, and severity of IGT.

In the intervention group subjects received advice from a nutritionist seven times during the first year and then every 3 months. The intervention goals were as follows: reduction in weight of 5% or more, total fat intake to less than 30% of energy consumed, saturated fat intake to less than 10% of energy consumed, fiber intake of at least 15 g/1000 kcal, and moderate exercise of at least 30 min/day. The subjects were individually counselled to increase their level of endurance exercise (walking, jogging, swimming, aerobic ball games, skiing). Supervised and individually tailored resistance training sessions were also offered. The control group subjects were given general verbal and written advice about healthy lifestyle at the beginning of the study. An OGTT was performed annually but the study endpoint of type 2 diabetes was based on a confirmatory second OGTT.

By March 2000, after a median follow-up of 3 years, 86 cases of diabetes had developed, which was about half of the 160 cases predicted for the full period of the planned 6-year study. The cumulative incidence of diabetes after 4 years was 11% in the intervention group and 23% in the control group, a reduction of 58% ($p < 0.001$) in risk of diabetes in the intervention group. The reduction in the incidence of diabetes was directly associated with changes in lifestyle (Figure 2); none of the people (either in the intervention or control group) who had reached all five lifestyle targets by the 1-year visit developed diabetes.

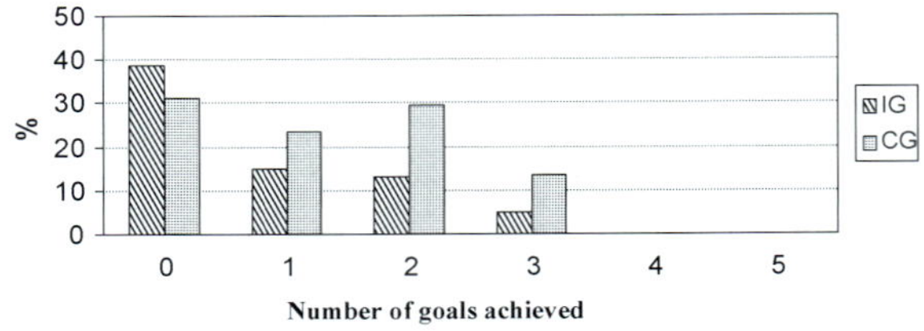

Figure 2 Occurrence of diabetes during the FDPS, according to number of intervention goals achieved. IG = intervention group; CG = control group

The Diabetes Prevention Program

The recently but prematurely completed Diabetes Prevention Program (DPP; the data safety and monitoring board advised closure) was a large multicenter, randomized, and placebo-controlled clinical trial carried out in the United States [74–76]. It involved an ethnically diverse population and was designed to investigate the effect of very aggressive lifestyle intervention (and metformin and troglitazone to be discussed below) in IGT patients. The study included 2161 (in lifestyle and placebo arms) high-risk individuals with IGT and a fasting plasma glucose over 5.5 mmol/l. Special educators ("case managers" who were not regular health personnel) primarily carried out the lifestyle intervention in the DPP. The lifestyle intervention involved a 16-session structured core curriculum within the first 24 weeks after Randomization. The focus of the dietary intervention was initially on reducing total fat intake but later calorie balance was introduced with a goal to achieve and maintain a weight loss of at least 7%. A physical activity target was set of approximately 700-kcal/week expenditure (this equaled approximately 150 min of moderate physical activity such as brisk walking every week). Clinical centers also offered voluntary supervised activity sessions.

In the DPP, of the participants assigned to intensive lifestyle intervention, 74% achieved the study goal of $\geq$150 min of activity per week at 24 weeks and at the 1-year visit the mean weight loss was 7 kg (about 7%). With intensive lifestyle intervention there was a 58% RRR in progression to type 2 diabetes compared with the placebo group. The lifestyle intervention was effective over a range of age, BMI, and racial or ethnic subgroups.

The lifestyle prevention trials have now provided unequivocal evidence that type 2 diabetes can be prevented (or at least delayed) in subjects with IGT. The major findings of the four studies are summarized and compared in Table 3.

The similarity of the RRR of the four studies is striking over a range of BMI values. The near identical RRR and ARR of Malmö, FDPS, and DPP are remarkable. The higher ARR in DaQing study was a result of the higher risk of diabetes in the Chinese participants. The effect of

Table 3 Summary of the findings of the four lifestyle intervention studies in IGT subjects

Study	Cohort size	Mean BMI (kg/m^2)	Duration (years)	RRR (%)	ARR (%)	NNT
Malmö	217	26.6	5	63	18	28
FDPS	523	31.0	3	58	12	22
DPP	2161*	34.0	3	58	15	21
DaQing	259*	25.8	6	46	27	25

Note: RRR = relative risk reduction; ARR = absolute risk reduction over 1 year; NNT = number needed to treat for 1 year to prevent one case of diabetes.
* Combined numbers for placebo and diet and exercise groups.

the intervention was rapid in the two well-designed studies (FDPS and DPP).

The Fasting Hyperglycemia Study II

The Fasting Hyperglycemia Study (FHS) [77, 78] in the United Kingdom and France is an ongoing study examining the potential of lifestyle changes (and sulfonylurea treatment) for preventing diabetes in 227 subjects with a fasting plasma glucose in the range of 5.5–7.0 mmol/l on two consecutive tests. These subjects were not identified by an OGTT. Participants were randomized to reinforced or basic healthy-living advice and/or a control group in a 2×2 factorial design. Basic advice encouraging dietary modification and increased exercise was given once at the initial visit and then reinforced every 3 months.

Preliminary data on 201 subjects who completed the first year have been disappointing, indicating no beneficial effect of diet and exercise in preventing type 2 diabetes. The treatment group achieved a significant mean reduction in body weight (1.5 kg) at 3 months but the weight subsequently returned to baseline. A small difference was achieved between treatment and control groups in measured physical fitness.

The FHS appears to be underpowered to detect a significant change with the "healthy-living advice" employed in a relatively small study in a predominantly Caucasian population with a low annual progression rate. Although IFG is a risk factor for type 2 diabetes, data are lacking on the prevention of diabetes in people screened for high fasting glucose. In addition, FHS has probably been weakened by the inclusion of subjects with asymptomatic diabetes.

Pharmacological Intervention Studies

Prior to the last couple of years, there were nine, generally small and poorly designed intervention studies using oral hypoglycemic agents, published that examined patients over 1–10 years. All were commenced prior to 1979 when there was no agreement on the definition of prediabetic states and the subjects on recent diagnostic criteria were probably a mixture of early type 2 diabetes and IGT. Seven studies investigated tolbutamide, and on an intention-to-treat analysis, four [79–82] reported improvement in glucose tolerance and/or reduced incidence of type 2 diabetes while three reported no benefit [63, 83, 84]. However, the Malmöhus Study [63] reported a large noncompliance rate in the tolbutamide group and found prevention of progression when analysis was based on treatment compliance. This is an intriguing observation in view of the four earlier positive studies and awaits further study. Two intervention studies with phenformin did not show benefit [85, 86]. Finally, two studies examined glibenclamide with mixed results [86, 87] and one study employing WHO criteria examined gliclazide and reported no benefit [88]. All these pharmacological studies, most containing fewer than 200 subjects in each of the intervention groups, would now be regarded as significantly underpowered.

The STOP-NIDDM Study

The STOP-NIDDM Study [89], a Canadian-European double-blind, placebo-controlled randomized trial, evaluated whether acarbose (an α-glucosidase inhibitor) could prevent the development of diabetes in 1429 high-risk subjects with IGT. After a mean of 3.3 years of follow-up, but including an approximate 25% discontinuation rate on acarbose, there was a 25% reduction in progression to diabetes (based on a single OGTT) attributable to acarbose. The main results were based on an intention-to-treat analysis. The drug was effective in the different subgroups of age, gender, and BMI. However, the benefit of treatment on prevention seemed to be reduced after only 3 months following cessation of active treatment.

The Diabetes Prevention Program

The DPP was initially set up to investigate individually the benefits of metformin, troglitazone [a peroxisome proliferator-activated receptor γ (PPAR-γ) agonist], and diet and exercise. As a result of the increased risk of severe liver damage and in some instances fatal hepatic toxicity caused by troglitazone, this arm was discontinued after 2 years. The DPP found that metformin reduced the risk of progression to type 2 diabetes from IGT by 31% while still taking the drug. The reduction in progression was less (24.9%) when metformin was ceased and allowing drug washout to occur before assessing glucose tolerance [90]. This benefit was not seen in subjects over the age of 60 years or with a BMI less than 30 kg/m^2 [74].

Troglitazone in the Prevention of Diabetes

Although the troglitazone arm of DPP was discontinued, a small 5-year double-blind study involving 250 Hispanic women living in Los Angeles with a history of gestational diabetes (approximately 70% with IGT) were randomized to either troglitazone or placebo [91]. Women with a history of gestational diabetes are at a high risk for developing type 2 diabetes. Over a median follow-up period of 31 months there was a 56% reduction in the conversion of these patients to type 2 diabetes. The average annual incidence of diabetes was 5.4% in women randomized to troglitazone and 12.1% in the placebo group ($p < 0.01$). The group of women most responsive to intervention with troglitazone was those who 3 months after Randomization showed the greatest reduction in insulin resistance and fall in insulin secretion to an intravenous glucose tolerance test. There was also evidence that the protection conferred by troglitazone against developing type 2 diabetes persisted for about 8 months after treatment ceased.

The Chinese Diabetes Prevention Study

In a small multicenter study [92] subjects ($n = 321$) with IGT were divided into four groups: control who received conventional education, diet and exercise, metformin, and acarbose. As in the DaQing Study, allocation into groups was not random, but took place by geographical location. Over a 3-year period 34.9%, 24.6%, 12.4%, and 6.0% of each group respectively progressed to diabetes. This represents an RRR of 76.8% for metformin and 87.8% for acarbose compared with the control group. The BMI for the three groups was approximately 25 kg/m^2, which in relation to metformin is inconsistent with the DPP findings.

Current Ongoing Pharmacological Diabetes Prevention Studies

There are at least four other placebo-controlled and blinded trials involving pharmacological therapy: three in patients with IGT and the other in subjects with fasting hyperglycemia. The Early Diabetes Intervention Trial (EDIT) [93] has a 2 × 2 factorial design to examine the effect of acarbose and metformin in 670 subjects. The Diabetes Reduction Assessment with Ramipril and Rosiglitazone Medication (DREAM) Trial is a multicenters, 2 × 2 factorially designed international study, which commenced in 2001 and will involve approximately 4000 subjects (H. Gerstein, personal communication, 2002). The Nateglinide (a fast-acting non-sulfonylurea insulin secretogogue) and Valsartan (an angiotensin II receptor blocker, ARB) in IGT Outcomes Research Trial (NAVIGATOR) commenced in 2002 and is also a multicenters, 2 × 2 factorially designed international study in approximately 7500 subjects [94]. Finally, the FHS, a small study also with a 2 × 2 factorial design, is examining the effect of gliclazide [95].

Another study ORIGIN (Outcomes Reduction with Initial Glargine Intervention) will commence in 2003 (H. Gerstein, personal communication, 2002) and will examine the use of insulin. Some of the subjects will have IGT but in this trial diabetes prevention is a secondary endpoint, with the main focus being on preventing cardiovascular outcomes.

Cardiovascular Intervention Studies with Diabetes Prevention as a Secondary Endpoint

In recent years there have been a number of completed trials where the development of type 2 diabetes has been a secondary endpoint. The characterization of the subjects' glycemic status was either inadequate or poorly defined at the entry and/or end of the study. None of the studies concentrated on IGT subjects and therefore the proportion of subjects with IGT at the beginning and end of the studies was unknown. Predictably, all the studies reported a low incidence of new diabetes in the control group, which makes it difficult to interpret the significance of the findings.

The Captopril Prevention Project (CAPPP) [96] was primarily a cardiovascular morbidity and mortality study in 10 413 hypertensive patients without biochemical evidence of diabetes. There was a 14% RRR for the development of diabetes over 6.1 years on captopril (angiotensin-converting enzyme inhibitor, ACEI) versus conventional therapy (β-blocker or thiazide diuretic). The study could not exclude the possibility that β-blockers and diuretics enhanced the risk of the development of diabetes, rather than captopril conferring protection.

In the Heart Outcome Prevention Evaluation (HOPE) [97] Study, 5720 individuals who were at high cardiovascular risk and reported no diabetes mellitus were either treated with placebo or ramipril. Over 4.5 years there was a significant reduction of 34% in the self-reported new diagnosis of type 2 diabetes mellitus (155 or 5.4% of the subjects on placebo versus 102 or 3.6% of the subjects assigned ramipril).

The Swedish Trial in Old Patients with Hypertension-2 Study (STOP Hypertension-2 Study) [98] involved 5893 hypertensive subjects without a history of diabetes at the baseline treated with a variety of antihypertensive agents including enalapril. No difference in the rate of diabetes was observed between the treatment groups. The design of the study involved significant numbers of subjects receiving both the ACEI and diuretics, which complicates the interpretation of the data.

The Losartan Intervention for Endpoint Reduction Study (LIFE) [99] was a large program designed to compare losartan (ARB) and atenolol in hypertensive subjects with left ventricular hypertrophy. Over a mean follow-up of 4.8 years significantly fewer subjects on losartan than on atenolol developed diabetes. Whether losartan is protective or atenolol is promoting diabetes cannot be determined.

In a *post hoc* analysis, the West of Scotland Coronary Prevention Study (WOSCOPS) [100], pravastatin appeared to significantly reduce (RRR 30%) the incidence of type 2 diabetes. Neither the Heart Protection Study (HPS) [101] with simvastatin nor a *post hoc* analysis of the Long-Term Intervention with Pravastatin in Ischemic Disease (LIPID) Study [102] with pravastatin confirmed a protective effect for a statin.

The Heart and Estrogen/Progestin Replacement Study (HERS) [103] investigated conjugated estrogen and medroxyprogesterone acetate as hormone replacement therapy (HRT) in postmenopausal women with coronary heart disease over 4.1 years. The incidence of diabetes based on self-report, a disease-related complication, or fasting blood glucose above 6.9 mmol/l was 6.2% in the HRT group and 9.5% in the placebo group ($p = 0.006$), a 35% reduction.

Potential Pharmacological Mechanisms of Diabetes Prevention

The possible mechanism(s) by which PPAR-γ agonists, metformin, acarbose, and more speculatively ACE blockade (ACEI, ARB), and statins could prevent diabetes are unknown. PPAR-γ agonists have been shown to preserve the cell mass [104, 105] and improve the insulin secretory function [106–108] of β–cells. These agents [109], as well as metformin [110], acarbose [111], and ACEI [112–114], increase insulin sensitivity, thereby decreasing the workload of the β-cell. There is also evidence that PPAR-γ agonists, metformin [115, 116], and ACEI [117] improve endothelial function, which may be of relevance to the microcirculation of the pancreatic islet. PPAR-γ agonists may temper a possible inflammatory response to islet amyloid, which is related to the level of insulin deficiency [118].

A single ("Grand") unified theory may be developed by extending the hypothesis of Yudkin [119, 120], whereby fat cell cytokines or high levels of free fatty acids (FFAs) have been implicated in endothelial dysfunction and therefore insulin resistance, hypertension, and dyslipidemia (Figure 3). The same fat cell "messengers" could be toxic to the β-cell. PPAR-γ agonists, ACEI, and metformin improve endothelial dysfunction and may also, through similar or other biochemical mechanisms, be β-cell protective. Acarbose and insulin secretogogues at an early stage of β-cell dysfunction may reduce postprandial glucose levels and in turn reduce levels of glucose-induced oxidative stress (glucose toxicity) [121] on the endothelial cell, thereby reducing endothelial dysfunction in the general vasculature and damage of the β-cell.

Cardiovascular Protection

Many studies have identified that glucose levels well within the impaired glycemic range (and perhaps below) exceed the threshold where blood glucose becomes a risk factor for atherosclerosis [54, 55, 122, 123]. The fasting blood glucose is less predictive of cardiovascular disease than is the 2-h glucose [54, 55]. The enhanced macrovascular risk associated with IGT is intermediate between normal and diabetes groups [54, 55], where the risk is further increased with poorer levels of diabetes control [124]. In the glycemic range below diabetes it remains to be defined whether the risk is directly related to glucose or to the associated components of the MS (hypertension, dyslipidemia, and visceral obesity).

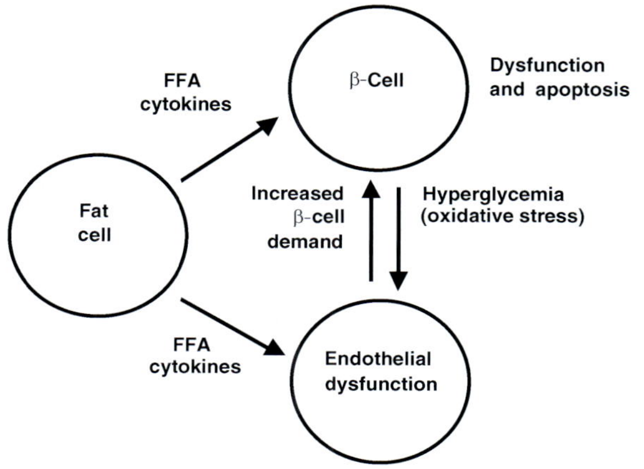

Figure 3 A "Grand" unified theory for the pathogenesis of type 2 diabetes and cardiovascular disease

The cost-effectiveness of diabetes prevention will be very dependent on demonstrating a reduction in risk of macrovascular disease.

The Malmöhus Study follow-up is continuing and increasing but so far statistically nonsignificant protection from macrovascular disease and total mortality has been reported in the compliant tolbutamide-treated group [125]. Most intriguingly, acarbose in STOP-NIDDM has been reported to both significantly reduce the development of hypertension and the number of total cardiovascular events [126]. The findings for cardiovascular disease, however, must be interpreted with caution owing to the very low event rate. There is also uncertainty as to whether the individuals in each part of the study received similar treatments with other vascular protective medications such as ACEI, statins, and aspirin. Currently, there is no published information on vascular event rates for FDPS and DPP although both reduced the frequency of vascular risk factors.

The major intervention studies [FDPS, DPP, STOP-NIDDM, CDPS (Chinese Diabetes Prevention Study)] have targeted patients with IGT and it is recognized that by preventing type 2 diabetes microvascular complications are prevented. If IGT reverts to NGT then the macrovascular burden would be expected to be reduced, although perhaps not normalized. Troglitazone appears to increase the reversion rate from IGT to NGT [127]. There is conflicting data for metformin [75, 92] whereas both STOP-NIDDM

[89] and the CDPS [92] reported increased reversion with acarbose. There is no information for ACEIs, ARBs, or fast-acting insulin secretagogues.

The major prevention trials now underway (DREAM, NAVIGATOR, ORIGIN) have cardiovascular events as endpoints.

Finally, it cannot be presumed that prevention of diabetes will always reduce the incidence of cardiovascular disease. While HERS reported that HRT in postmenopausal women prevented diabetes [103], in the main study HERS found no cardiovascular protection in women with coronary disease [128]. In the Women's Health Initiative Trial, HRT in healthy women was associated with an increased risk from cardiovascular disease [129]. ALLHAT [39] showed that ACEI and calcium-channel blockers reduced the incidence of diabetes (compared to chlorthalidone) but they were not associated with a reduced risk of death or cardiovascular outcomes in the general or diabetic populations.

THE PROBLEMS AND CHALLENGES AHEAD

The onset of type 2 diabetes is occurring at an increasingly younger age. Type 2 diabetes is increasingly seen in the third decade, and in some areas of the world is emerging in children [130–133]. The Singaporean [45] experience is relevant and important for this issue. The younger age of onset increases the potential vascular burden and makes even more urgent the need to prevent type 2 diabetes. The findings of the major prevention trials have now provided unequivocal evidence that diabetes can be prevented (or at least delayed) with reasonably modest lifestyle improvements. The increased risk of type 2 diabetes in certain ethnic and socioeconomic groups has caused concern that there might be differences in the levels of acceptance and compliance with lifestyle modification between the various communities. This highlights the need to ensure strategies developed to improve lifestyle are both culturally and socioeconomically relevant.

It is reassuring that in the DPP and FDPS, people older than 60 years at baseline benefited more from lifestyle intervention than did younger people. Thus age is not a barrier to preventing diabetes in people with IGT. Since type 2 diabetes has a greater deleterious impact on morbidity and mortality in younger subjects, better societal outcomes will result from treating the young.

The role of pharmacological therapy in prevention is unclear. Such therapy in the young, presumably for years or for life, raises major ethical and safety concerns. There are limited data about potential long-term side effects of powerful drugs taken for many decades by otherwise healthy adults and children. There is also the issue of the significant cohort of treated (or intolerant of the medication) subjects who will not derive benefit and will still develop type 2 diabetes. It is hoped that better targeting or selection of subjects for pharmacological treatment will be possible in the future. There is no information at this stage whether combination lifestyle and drug therapy will be an advantage over "monotherapy."

It has not been established whether the lifestyle or the pharmacological interventions will prevent or only delay the onset of type 2 diabetes. In FDPS it has been reported that the differences in incidence of diabetes between the two groups persist after 2 years from the study closure. The published data for HOPE (ramipril), DPP (metformin), and STOP-NIDDM (acarbose) appear to suggest delay rather than prevention. For troglitazone (troglitazone in the prevention of diabetes, TRIPOD) there may be an ongoing benefit as the prevalence curves appear to continue to diverge during the study and the protection seemed to continue for at least 8–12 months after treatment with troglitazone ceased. This may suggest true prevention but at this stage the data are very incomplete. It is of interest that in laboratory studies β-cell preservation with glitazones [104, 105] has been observed.

To date, there have been no published prevention studies with glucagon-like peptide 1 but this hormone has been reported to stimulate β-cell replication in laboratory studies [134–136].

If these drugs are successful in achieving a delay, it will be unclear whether treatment will be required lifelong or just for a finite period to enable other homeostatic or reparative mechanisms to come into play. In STOP-NIDDM, there appeared to be a "catch up" of the acarbose-treated subjects with many disease-free subjects developing diabetes when the drug was stopped. This suggests that at least for acarbose, treatment may need to be lifelong.

Since type 2 diabetes is a common disease the number of subjects at high risk of type 2 diabetes who would benefit from a lifestyle and/or pharmacological intervention program is very large. In the United States alone it is estimated that 11% of adults aged 40–74 years meet the strict DPP eligibility criteria [137]. Based on the findings of the DPP and with a range of reasonable assumptions it has been estimated that a prevention program in the United States [138], several European countries [139], and Australia [140] despite its costs would be cost-effective. The expense, especially if structured as in DPP, including the costs of a screening OGTT for such a nationally based lifestyle program would be daunting for any government. But with reasonable assumptions about mortality and morbidity rates, in Australia it is estimated that such a program will be generating overall health savings after 7–8 years [140]. Recently, a Diabetes Prediction Risk Score, based on the prospective study in Finland, has been developed which has the potential to replace the need for an OGTT to identify subjects at high risk for inclusion in a targeted prevention program [141]. Most of these high-risk subjects are already regular users of the primary health care system for various reasons.

For the successful prevention of type 2 diabetes in the community it will be necessary to combine population prevention measures directed at obesity with higher intensity programs directed at individuals identified as being at high risk. These are actions that will assure the shift of the risk factor distribution in the entire population to a lower level. The continuing growth in the level of obesity in all countries indicates that such an approach is urgently required. There is not much evidence that any country is making this a sufficiently high priority although perhaps it is belatedly about to happen. Effective prevention is a long-term program, which will include activities targeted to various age groups from fetal life to the elderly. They will need to be both culturally and socioeconomically appropriate. They will need implementation at an early age as programs in adults have often been unsuccessful and in many cases, too late. A formal and compulsory program on lifestyle (nutrition and exercise), including clear information about lifestyle-related ill health, should be an integral part of the school curriculum at all ages. Finally, governments have to take a more active role and should consider regulating dietary components in the food supply such as sugary drinks in schools and using the tax system to encourage healthy food choices.

Factors that currently limit a successful program are a sense of immortality in the young, apathy at all levels, vested commercial interests, adverse cultural beliefs, and socioeconomic factors. The long lead-in times before programs demonstrate benefits affect individual commitment to self-help. Furthermore, the short-term focus of successive governments impedes success. We have adequate knowledge to know that prevention of type 2 diabetes will work but the challenge will be the implementation of appropriate and practical programs.

REFERENCES

1. Zimmet P. Globalization, coca-colonization and the chronic disease epidemic: can the doomsday scenario be averted? *J Intern Med* 2002; 247: 301–10.
2. Zimmet P. Diabetes epidemiology as a trigger to diabetes research and care. *Diabetologia* 1999; 42: 499–518.
3. Amos AF, McCarty DJ, Zimmet P. The rising global burden of diabetes and its complications: estimates and projections to the year 2010. *Diabet Med* 1997; 14 (suppl 5): S1–87.
4. King H, Aubert RE, Herman WH. Global burden of diabetes, 1995–2025. Prevalence, numerical estimates and projections. *Diabetes Care* 1998; 21: 1414–31.
5. American Diabetes Association. Economic costs of diabetes in the U.S. in 2002. *Diabetes Care* 2003; 26: 917–32.
6. Colagiuri S, Colagiuri R, Grainger D, Graham-Clarke P, Davey P, Fitzgerald P, Conway B. DiabCost Australia—assessing the burden of type 2 diabetes in Australia. *Diabetologia* 2002; 45 (suppl 2): 931.
7. WHO Consultation. Definition, diagnosis and classification of diabetes mellitus and its complications, Part 1: Diagnosis and classification of diabetes mellitus. World Health Organization Non-communicable Disease Surveillance. Geneva: WHO, 1999.
8. National Institutes of Health. Third Report on the National Cholesterol Education Program Expert Panel on Detection, Evaluation and Treatment of High Blood Cholesterol in Adults (Adult Treatment Panel III). Executive Summary. Bethesda, MD: National Institutes of Health, National Heart, Lung and Blood Institute, 2001. NIH Publ. No. 01-3670.
9. World Health Organization (WHO). Diabetes Mellitus: Report of a WHO Study Group. Geneva: WHO, 1985.
10. World Health Organization Consultation. Definition, diagnosis and classification of diabetes and its complications, Part 1: diagnosis and classification of diabetes mellitus. *Diabet Med* 1998; 15: 539–53.
11. Turner RC, Stratton I, Horton V, Manleys, Zimmet P, Mackay IR, Shattock M, Bottazzo GF, Holman R, for the UK Prospective Diabetes Study Group. UKPDS 25: Autoantibodies to islet cell cytoplasm and glutamic acid decarboxylase for prediction of insulin requirement in type 2 diabetes. *Lancet* 1997; 350: 1288–93.
12. Zimmet P, Turner RC, McCarty DJ, Rowley MJ, MacKay IR. Crucial points at diagnosis. Type 2 diabetes or slow type 1 diabetes. *Diabetes Care* 1999; 22: (suppl 2) B59–64.
13. Simpson RW, Shaw JE, Zimmet PZ. The prevention of type 2 diabetes—lifestyle change or pharmacotherapy? A challenge for the 21st century. *Diabetes Res Clin Prac* 2003; 59: 165–80.
14. Eriksson J, Franssila-Kallunki A, Ekstrand A, Saloranta C, Widen E, Schalin C, Groop L. Early metabolic defects in persons at risk for non-insulin-dependent diabetes mellitus. *N Engl J Med* 1989; 321: 337–43.
15. DeFronzo RA. Glucose intolerance of aging. Evidence of tissue insensitivity to insulin. *Diabetes* 1979; 28: 1095–101.
16. Chen M, Bergman RN, Pacini G, Porte D Jr. Pathogenesis of age-related glucose intolerance in man: insulin resistance and decreased β-cell function. *J Clin Endocrinol Metab* 1985; 60: 13–20.
17. Bjorntorp P. Visceral obesity: a "civilization syndrome." *Obes Res* 1993; 1: 206–22.
18. Kahn SE, Larson VG, Beard JC, Cain KC, Fellingham GW, Schwartz RS, Veith RC, Stratton JR, Cerqueira MD, Abrass IB. Effect of exercise on insulin action, glucose tolerance and insulin secretion in aging. *Am J Physiol* 1990; 258: E937–43.
19. Ehrmann DA, Sturis J, Byrne MM, Karrison T, Rosenfield RL, Polonsky KS. Insulin secretory defects in polycystic ovary syndrome. Relationship to insulin sensitivity and family history of non-insulin-dependent diabetes mellitus. *J Clin Invest* 1995; 96: 520–7.
20. Elbein SC, Wegner K, Kahn SE. Reduced b-cell compensation to the insulin resistance associated with obesity in members of Caucasian familial type 2 diabetic kindreds. *Diabetes Care* 2000; 23: 221–7.
21. Kahn SE. The relative contributions of insulin resistance and beta-cell dysfunction to the pathophysiology of type 2 diabetes. *Diabetologia* 2003; 46: 3–19.
22. Kobberling J, Tillil H. Empirical risk factors for first degree relatives of non-insulin-dependent diabetics. In Kobberling J, Tattersall R (eds), *The Genetics of Diabetes Mellitus*. London: Academic Press, 1982; pp 201–10.
23. Kaprio J, Tuomilehto J, Koskenvuo M, Romanov VK, Reunanen A, Eriksson J, Stengard J, Kesaniemi YA.

Concordance for type 1 (insulin-dependent) and type 2 (non-insulin-dependent) diabetes mellitus in a population based cohort of twins in Finland. *Diabetologia* 1992; 35: 1060–7.
24. Pyke DA. Diabetes: The genetic connections. *Diabetologia* 1979; 17: 333–43.
25. De Courten M, Bennett PH, Tuomilehto J, Zimmett P. Epidemiology of NIDDM in non-Europids. In Alberti KGMM, Zimmett P, DeFronzo RA, Keen H (eds), *International Textbook of Diabetes Mellitus*, 2nd edn. Chichester, UK: Wiley, 1997; pp 143–70.
26. Hattersley AT. Maturity-onset diabetes of the young: clinical heterogeneity explained by genetic heterogeneity. *Diabet Med* 1998; 15: 15–24.
27. McIntyre EA, Walker M. Genetics of type 2 diabetes and insulin resistance: knowledge from human studies. *Clin Endocrinol* 2002; 57: 303–11.
28. Neel JV. Diabetes mellitus: a "thrifty" genotype rendered detrimental by progress? *Am J Hum Genet* 1962; 14: 353–62.
29. Hodge AM, de Courten MA, Zimmett P. Obesity and type 2 diabetes mellitus. In Bjorntorp P (ed), *International Textbook on Obesity*. Chichester, UK: Wiley, 2001; pp 351–64.
30. Westlund K, Nicolaysen R. Ten-year mortality and morbidity related to serum cholesterol. A follow-up of 3751 men aged 40–49. *Scand J Clin Invest* 1972; 30: (suppl 127) 1–24.
31. Medalie JH, Papier CM, Herman JB, Goldbourt U, Tamir S, Newfeld HN, Riss E. Diabetes mellitus among 10,000 adult men: five-year incidence and associated variables. *Isr J Med Sci* 1974; 10: 681–97.
32. Ohlson LO, Larsson B, Bjorntorp P, Eriksson H, Svardsudd K, Welin L, Tibblin G, Wilhelmsen L. The risk factors of type 2 (non-insulin-dependent) diabetes mellitus. Thirteen and one half years of follow up of the participants in the study of men born in 1913. *Diabetologia* 1988; 31: 798–805.
33. Colditz GA, Willett WC, Rotnitzky A, Manson JE. Weight gain as a risk factor for clinical diabetes mellitus in women. *Ann Intern Med* 1995; 122: 481–6.
34. Bennett PH, Bogardus C, Toumilehto J, Zimmett P. Epidemiology and natural history of NIDDM: non-obese and obese. In Alberti KGMM, DeFronzo RA, Keen H, Zimmett P (eds), *International Textbook of Diabetes*, 1st edn. Chichester, UK: Wiley, 1992; pp 147–76.
35. Prentice AM, Jebb SA. Obesity in Britain: gluttony or sloth? *Br Med J* 1995; 311: 427–9.
36. Toumilehto J, Toumilehto-Wolf E, Zimmett P, Alberti KGMM, Knowler WC. Primary prevention of diabetes mellitus. In Alberti KGMM, Zimmett P, DeFronzo RA, Keen H (eds), *International Textbook of Diabetes Mellitus*, 2nd edn. Chicester, UK: Wiley, 1997; pp 1799–827.
37. Kriska A, Bennett PH. An epidemiological perspective of the relationship between physical activity and NIDDM: from activity assessment to intervention. *Diabetes Metab Rev* 1992; 8: 355–72.
38. Gress TW, Nieto FJ, Sharhar E, Wofford MR, Brancati FL. Hypertension and anti-hypertensive therapy as risk factors for type 2 diabetes mellitus: Atherosclerosis Risk in Communities Study. *N Engl J Med* 2000; 342: 905–12.
39. The ALLHAT Officers and Coordinators for the ALLHAT Collaborative Research Group. Major outcomes in high-risk hypertensive patients randomized to angiotensin-converting enzyme inhibitor or calcium channel blocker vs diuretic: the Antihypertensive and Lipid-lowering Treatment to Prevent Heart Attack Trial. *J Am Med Assoc* 2002; 288: 2981–97.
40. O'Dea K, Spargo R. Metabolic adaptation to a low carbohydrate-high protein (traditional) diet in Australian aboriginals. *Diabetologia* 1982; 23: 494–98.
41. Shintani TT, Hughes CK, Beckham S, O'Connor HK. Obesity and cardiovascular intervention through the ad libitum feeding of traditional Hawaiian diet. *Am J Clin Nutr* 1991; 53 (suppl 6): 1647S–51S.
42. Lee AJ, Bailey AP, Yarmirr D, O'Dea K, Mathews J. Survival tucker: improved diet and health indicators in an aboriginal community. *Aust J Public Health* 1994; 18: 277–85.
43. Lee AJ, Bonson A, Yarmirr D, O'Dea K, Mathews J. Sustainability of a successful health and nutrition program in a remote aboriginal community. *Med J Aust* 1995; 162: 632–5.
44. Heath GW, Leonard BE, Wilson RH, Kendrick JS, Powell KE. Community-based exercise intervention: Zuni Diabetes Project. *Diabetes Care* 1987; 10: 579–83.
45. Cheong MT, Cutter J, Suok KC. School based intervention has reduced obesity in Singapore. *Br Med J* 2002; 324: 427.
46. Yudkin JS, Alberti KGMM, McLarty DG, Swai ABN. Impaired glucose tolerance. *Br Med J* 1990; 301: 397–401.
47. Saad MF, Knowler WC, Pettitt DJ, Nelson RG, Mott DM, Bennett PH. The natural history of impaired glucose tolerance in the Pima Indians. *N Engl J Med* 1988; 319: 1500–6.
48. Saad MF, Knowler WC, Pettitt DJ, Nelson RG, Bennett PH. Transient impaired glucose tolerance in Pima Indians: is it important? *Br Med J* 1988; 297: 1438–41.
49. Edelstein SL, Knowler WC, Bain RP, Andres R, Barrett-Connor EL, Dowse GK, Haffner SM, Pettitt DJ, Sorkin JD, Muller DC, Collins VR, Hamman RF. Predictors of progression from impaired glucose tolerance to NIDDM: an analysis of six prospective studies. *Diabetes* 1997; 46: 701–10.
50. Haffner SM, Stern MP, Hazuda HP, Mitchell BD, Patterson JK. Cardiovascular risk factors in confirmed prediabetic individuals. Does the clock for coronary heart disease start ticking before the onset of clinical diabetes? *J Am Med Assoc* 1990; 263: 2893–8.
51. McPhillips JB, Barrett-Connor E, Wingard DI. Cardiovascular disease risk factors prior to the diagnosis of impaired glucose tolerance and non-insulin dependant diabetes in a community of older adults. *Am J Epidemiol* 1990; 131: 443–53.
52. Saad MF, Knowler WC, Pettitt RG, Welson RG, Charles MA, Bennett PH. A two step model for development of non-insulin-dependent diabetes. *Am J Med* 1991; 90: 229–35.
53. Hamman RF. Genetics and environmental determinants of non-insulin-dependent-diabetes-mellitus (NIDDM). *Diabetes Metab Rev* 1992; 8: 287–338.
54. DECODE Study Group. Glucose tolerance and cardiovascular mortality: comparison of fasting and 2-hour diagnostic criteria. *Arch Intern Med* 2001; 161: 397–405.
55. DECODE Study Group. Is the current definition for diabetes relevant to mortality risk from all causes and cardiovascular and noncardiovascular disease? *Diabetes Care* 2003; 26: 688–96.
56. Unwin N, Shaw J, Zimmet P, Alberti KG. Impaired glucose tolerance and impaired fasting glycaemia: the

current status on definition and intervention. *Diabet Med* 2002; 19: 708–23.

57. Long SD, O'Brien K, McDonald KG Jr, Leggett-Frazier N, Swanson MS, Porries WJ, Caro JF. Weight loss in severely obese subjects prevents the progression of impaired glucose tolerance to type 2 diabetes: a longitudinal interventional study. *Diabetes Care* 1994; 17: 372–5.
58. Sjöström CD, Lissner L, Wedel H, Sjöström L. Reduction in incidence of diabetes, hypertension and lipid disturbances after intentional weight loss induced by bariatric surgery: the SOS Intervention Study. *Obes Res* 1999; 7: 477–84.
59. Sjöström L, Torgerson JS, Hauptman J, Boldrin M. XENDOS (Xenical in the Prevention of Diabetes in the Obese Subjects): a landmark study. In *9th International Congress on Obesity*, Sao Paulo, Brazil, 2002.
60. Himsworth HP. Diet and the incidence of diabetes mellitus, *Clin Sci* 1935; 2: 117–48.
61. Mann JI, Hueston A. A etiology of non insulin dependent diabetes. In: Mann JI, Pyorala K, Teuscher A (eds), *Diabetes in Epidemiological Perspective*, 1st edn. Edinburgh: Churchill Livingstone, 1983; pp 122–64.
62. Westlund K. Incidence of diabetes mellitus in Oslo, Norway 1925 to 1954. *Br J Prev Soc Med* 1966; 20: 105–16.
63. Sartor G, Schersten B, Carlström S, Melander A, Norden A, Persson G. Ten year follow up of subjects with impaired glucose tolerance. Prevention of diabetes by tolbutamide and diet regulation, *Diabetes* 1980; 29: 41–9.
64. Ramaiya KL, Swai ABM, Alberti KGMM, McLarty DG. Lifestyle changes, decreased rates of glucose intolerance and cardiovascular (CVD) risk factors. *Diabetologia* 1992; 35 (suppl 1): A60.
65. Bourn DM, Mann JI, McSkimming BJ, Waldron MA, Wishart JD. Impaired glucose tolerance and NIDDM: does a lifestyle intervention program have an effect? *Diabetes Care* 1994; 17: 1311–9.
66. Lynch J, Helmich SP, Lakka TA, Kaplan GA, Cohen RD, Salonen R, Salonen JT. Moderately intense physical activities and high levels of cardiorespiratory fitness reduce the risk of non-insulin-dependent diabetes mellitus in middle aged men. *Arch Intern Med* 1996; 156: 1307–14.
67. Torjesen PA, Birkeland KI, Anderssen SA, Hjermann I, Holme I, Urdal P, Lifestyle changes may reverse development of the insulin resistant syndrome. The Oslo Diet and Exercise Study: a randomized trial. *Diabetes Care* 1997; 20: 26–31.
68. O'Dea K, Marked improvement in carbohydrate and lipid metabolism in diabetic Australian aborigines after temporary reversion to traditional lifestyle. *Diabetes Care* 1984; 33: 596–603.
69. Eriksson KF, Lindgärde F. Prevention of type 2 (non-insulin-dependent) diabetes mellitus by diet and physical exercise: the 6-year Malmö feasibility study. *Diabetologia* 1991; 34: 891–8.
70. Pan XR, Li GW, Hu YH, Wang JX, Yang WY, An ZX, Hu ZX, Lin J, Xiao JZ, Cao HB, Liu PA, Jiang XG, Jiang YY, Wang JP, Zhang H, Bennett PH, Howard BV. Effects of diet and exercise in preventing NIDDM in people with impaired glucose tolerance: the Da Qing IGT and Diabetes Study. *Diabetes Care* 1997; 20: 537–44.
71. Eriksson J, Lindström J, Valle T, Aunola S, Hamalainen H, Ilanne-Parikka P, Keinanen-Kiukaanniemi S, Laakso M, Lauhkonen M, Lehto P, Lehtonen A, Louheranta A, Mannelin M, Martikkala V, Rastas M, Sundvall J, Turpeinen A, Viljanen T, Uusitupa M, Tuomilehto J. Prevention of Type II diabetes in subjects with impaired glucose tolerance: the Diabetes Prevention study (DPS) in Finland—study design and 1-year interim report on the feasibility of the lifestyle intervention programme. *Diabetologia* 1999; 42: 793–801.
72. Uusitupa M, Louheranta A, Lindström J, Valle T, Sundvall J, Eriksson J, Tuomilehto J. The Finnish Diabetes Prevention Study. *Br J Nutr* 2000; 83 (suppl 1): S137–42.
73. Tuomilehto J, Lindström J, Eriksson JG, Valle TT, Hamalainem H, Ilanne-Parikka P, Keinanen-Kiukaanniemi S, Laakso M, Lauhkonen M, Rastas M, Saminen V, Uusitupa M, for the Finnish Diabetes Prevention Study Group. Prevention of type 2 diabetes mellitus by changes in lifestyle among subjects with impaired glucose tolerance. *N Engl J Med* 2001; 344: 1343–50.
74. The Diabetes Prevention Program Research Group. The Diabetes Prevention Program: design and methods for a clinical trial in the prevention of type 2 diabetes. *Diabetes Care* 1999; 22: 623–34.
75. Knowler WC, Barrett-Connor E, Fowler SE, Hamman RF, Lachin JM, Walker EA, Nathan DM, for the Diabetes Prevention Programme Research Group. Reduction in the incidence of type 2 diabetes with lifestyle intervention or metformin. *N Engl J Med* 2002; 346: 393–403.
76. The Diabetes Prevention Program (DPP): description of lifestyle intervention. *Diabetes Care* 2002; 25: 2165–71.
77. Hammersley MS, Meyer LC, Morris RJ, Manley SE, Turner RC, Holman RR. The Fasting Hyperglycemia Study, I: Subjects, identification and recruitment for a non-insulin dependent diabetes prevention trial. *Metabolism* 1997; 46 (suppl 1): 44–9.
78. Dyson PA, Hammersley MS, Morris RJ, Holman RR, Turner RC. The Fasting hyperglycemia Study, II: randomized controlled trial of reinforced healthy-living advice in subjects with increased but not diabetic fasting plasma glucose. *Metabolism* 1997; 46 (suppl 1) 50–5.
79. Fajans SS, Cohn JW. Tolbutamide-induced improvement in carbohydrate tolerance in young people with mild diabetes mellitus. *Diabetes* 1960; 9: 83–8.
80. Engelhardt HT, Veccio TJ, The long term effect of tolbutamide on glucose tolerance in adults: asymptomatic latent diabetes. *Metabolism* 1965; 14: 885–90.
81. Belknap BH, Bagdade JD, Amaral JAP, Bierman EL. Plasma lipids and mild glucose intolerance, II: A double blind study of the effect of tolbutamide and placebo in mild adult diabetic outpatients. *Excepta Med Int Congr Ser* 1967; 149: 171–6.
82. Paasikivi J, Wahlberg F, Preventative tolbutamide treatment and arterial disease on mild hyperglycemia. *Diabetologia* 1971; 7: 323–7.
83. Camerini-Davalosra RA. Treatment of chemical diabetes. *Excepta Med Int Congr Ser* 1967; 149: 228–42.
84. Keen H, Jarrett RJ, McCartney P. The ten year follow up of the Bedford Survey (1962–1972): glucose tolerance and diabetes. *Diabetologia* 1982; 22: 73–8.
85. Jarrett RJ, Keen H, Fuller JH, McCartney M. Treatment of borderline diabetes: controlled trial using carbohydrate restriction and phenformin. *Br Med J* 1977; 2: 861–5.
86. Papoz L, Job D, Eschwege E, Aboulker JP, Cubeau J, Pequignot G, Rathery M, Rosselin G. The effect of oral hypoglycemic drugs on glucose tolerance and insulin

secretion in borderline diabetic patients. *Diabetologia* 1978; 15: 373–80.

87. Ratzmann KP, Witt S, Schulz B. The effect of long term glibenclamide treatment on glucose tolerance, insulin secretion and serum lipids in subjects with impaired glucose tolerance. *Diabet Metab* 1983; 9: 87–93.
88. Cederholm J. Short term treatment of glucose intolerance in middle-aged subjects by diet, exercise and sulphonylurea. *Ups J Med Sci* 1985; 90: 229–42.
89. Chiasson JL, Josse RG, Gomis R, Hanefeld M, Karasik A, Laakso M, for the STOP-NIDDM Trial Research Group. Acarbose for prevention of type 2 diabetes mellitus; the STOP-NIDDM randomized trial. *Lancet* 2002; 359: 2072–7.
90. The Diabetes Prevention Program Research Group. Effects of withdrawal from metformin on the development of diabetes in the Diabetes Prevention Program. *Diabetes Care* 2003; 26: 977–80.
91. Buchanann TA, Xiang AH, Peters RK, Kjos SL, Marroquin A, Goico J, Ochoa C, Tan S, Berkowitz K, Hodis HN, Azen SP. Preservation of pancreatic B-cell function and prevention of type 2 diabetes by pharmacological treatment of insulin resistance in high-risk Hispanic women. *Diabetes* 2002; 51: 2796–803.
92. Wenying Y, Lixiang L, Jinwu Q, Yang W, Pan X, Li G, Lin L, Qi J, Yu Z, Pei H, He G. The preventative effect of acarbose and metformin on the progression to diabetes mellitus in the IGT population: a 3-year multicenters prospective study. *Chin J Endocrinol Metab* 2001; 17: 131–5.
93. Holman RR, North BV, Tunbridge FK. Possible prevention of type 2 diabetes with acarbose or metformin. *Diabetes* 2000; 49 (suppl 1): 450P.
94. Haffner SM, Hotman R, Califf R, McMurray J, Pecher E. Targeting post-prandial hyperglycemia to prevent type 2 diabetes: rationale and design of the NAVIGATOR trial. *Diabetologia* 2002; 45 (suppl 2): A106.
95. Karunakaran S, Hammersley MS, Morris RJ, Turner RC, Holman RR. The Fasting hyperglycemia Study: III, Randomized controlled trial of sulphonylurea therapy in subjects with increased but not diabetic fasting plasma glucose. *Metabolism* 1997; 46 (suppl 1): 56–60.
96. Hansson L, Lindholm LH, Niskanen L, Lanke J, Hedner T, Niklason A, Luomanmaki K, Dahlof B, de Faire U, Morlin C, Karlberg BE, Wester PO, Bjorck JE. Effect of angiotensin-converting-enzyme inhibition compared with conventional therapy on cardiovascular morbidity and mortality in hypertension: the Captropril Prevention Project (CAPPP) Randomized Trial. *Lancet* 1999; 353: 611–6.
97. Yusuf S, Gerstein H, Hoogwerf B, Pogue J, Bosch J, Wolffenbuttel BH, Zinman B, for the HOPE Study Investigators. Ramipril and the development of diabetes. *J Am Med Assoc* 2001; 286: 1882–5.
98. Hansson L, Lindholm LH, Ekbom T, Dahlof B, Lanke J, Schersten B, Wester PO, Hedner T, de Faire U. Randomized trial of old and new antihypertensive drugs in elderly patients: cardiovascular mortality and morbidity in the Swedish Trial in Old Patients with Hypertension-2 study. *Lancet* 1999; 354: 1751–6.
99. Dahlof B, Devereux RB, Kjeldsen SE, Julius S, Beevers G, Faire U, Fyhrquist F, Ibsen H, Kristiansson K, Lederballe-Pedersen O, Lindholm LH, Nieminen MS, Omvik P, Oparil S, Wedel H, for the LIFE Study Group. Cardiovascular morbidity and mortality in the Losartan Intervention For Endpoint reduction in hypertension study (LIFE): a randomized trial against atenalol. *Lancet* 2002; 359: 995–1003.
100. Freeman DJ, Norrie J, Sattar N, Neely RD, Cobbe SM, Ford I, Isles C, Lorimer AR, Macfarlane PW, McKillop JH, Packard CJ, Shepherd J, Gaw A. Pravastatin and the development of diabetes mellitus; evidence for a protective treatment effect in the West of Scotland Coronary Prevention Study. *Circulation* 2001; 103: 357–62.
101. Heart Protection Collaborative Group. MRC/BHF Heart Protection Study of cholesterol lowering with simvastatin in 5963 people with diabetes: A randomized placebo controlled trial. *Lancet* 2003; 361: 2005–16.
102. Keech AC, Colquhoun D, Best J, Kirby A, Simes RJ, Hunt D, Hague W, Bellar B, Arulchelvam M, Baker B, Tonkin A, for the LIPID study group. Secondary prevension of cardiovascular events with long-term pravastatin in patients with diabetes or impaired fasting glucose: results from the LIPID trial. *Diabetes* (in press).
103. Kanaya AM, Herrington D, Vittinghoff E, Lin F, Grady D, Bittner V, Cauley JA, Barrett-Connor E, for the Heart and Estrogen/progestin Replacement Study. Glycemic effects of postmenopausal hormone therapy: the Heart and Estrogen/progestin Replacement Study. A randomized, double-blind, placebo-controlled trial. *Ann Intern Med* 2003; 138: 1–9.
104. Shimabukuro M, Zhou YT, Lee Y, Unger RH. Troglitazone lowers islet fat and restores beta cell function of Zucker diabetic fatty rats. *J Biol Chem* 1998; 273: 3547–50.
105. Finegood DT, McArthur MD, Kojwang D, Thomas MJ, Topp BG, Leonard T, Buckingham RE. Beta-cell mass dynamics in Zucker diabetic fatty rats. Rosiglitazone prevents the rise in net cell death. *Diabetes* 2001; 50: 1021–9.
106. Prigeon RL, Kahn SE, Porte D Jr. Effect of Troglitazone on B cell function, insulin sensitivity and glycemic control in subjects with type 2 diabetes mellitus. *J Clin Endocrinol Metab* 1998; 83: 819–23.
107. Porter LE, Freed MI, Jones NP, Biswas N. Rosiglitazone reduces proinsulin/insulin ratio and improves beta cell function in type 2 Diabetes. *Diabetologia* 2000; 43 (suppl 1): A192.
108. Cavaghan MK, Ehrmann DA, Byrne MM, Shneider DJ, Polansky KS. Treatment with the oral antidiabetic agent troglitazone improves beta cell responses to glucose in subjects with impaired glucose tolerance. *J Clin Invest* 1997; 100: 530–7.
109. Saltiel AR, Olefsky JM. Thiazolidinediones in the treatment of insulin resistance and type 2 diabetes. *Diabetes* 1996; 44: 1661–9.
110. Bell PM, Hadden D. Metformin. *Endocrinol Metab Clin North Am* 1997; 26: 523–37.
111. Chiasson J-L, Josse RG, Gomis R, Hanefeld M, Karasik A, Laakso M, for the STOP-NIDDM Trial Research Group. The effect of acarbose on insulin sensiti-vity in subjects with impaired glucose tolerance. *Diabetes Care* 1996; 19: 1191–4.
112. Pollare T, Lithell H, Berne CA. Comparison of the effects of hydrochlorothiazide and captopril on glucose and lipid metabolism in patients with hypertension. *N Engl J Med* 1989; 321: 868–73.
113. Berne C, Pollare T, Lithell H. Effects of anti-hypertensive treatment on insulin sensivity with special reference to ACE inhibitors. *Diabetes Care* 1991; 14 (suppl 4): 39–47.
114. Vuorinen-Markkola H, Yki-Jarvinen H. Antihypertensive therapy with enalapril improves glucose storage and

insulin sensitivity in hypertensive patients with non insulin dependent diabetes mellitus. *Metabolism* 1995; 44: 85–9.

115. Montanari G, Bondioli A, Rizzato G, Puttini M, Tremoli E, Mussoni L, Mannucci L, Pazzucconi F, Sirtori CR. Treatment with low dose metformin in patients with peripheral vascular disease. *Pharmacol Res* 1992; 25: 63–73.
116. Diamanti-Kandarakis E, Spina G, Kouli C, Migdalis I. Increased endothelin-1 levels in women with polycystic ovary syndrome and the beneficial effect of metformin therapy. *J Clin Endocrinol Metab* 2001; 84: 4666–73.
117. Mancini GB, Henry GC, Macaya C, O'Neill BJ, Pucillo AL, Carere RG, Wargovich TJ, Mudra H, Luscher TF, Klibaner MI, Haber HE, Uprichard AC, Pepine CJ, Pitt B. Angiotensin-converting enzyme inhibition with quinapril improves endothelial vasomotor dysfunction in patients with coronary artery disease: the TREND (Trial on Reversing Endothelial Dysfunction) Study. *Circulation* 1996; 94: 258–65.
118. Kahn SE, Andrikopoulos S, Verchere CB. Islet amyloid; a long-recognized but under appreciated pathological feature of type 2 diabetes. *Diabetes* 1999; 48: 241–53.
119. Pinkney JH, Stehouwer CD, Coppack SW, Yudkin JS. Endothelial dysfunction: cause of the insulin resistance syndrome. *Diabetes* 1997; 46 (suppl 2): S9–13.
120. Judkin JS, Stehouwer CDA, Emeis JJ, Coppack SW. C-reactive protein in healthy subjects: associations with obesity, insulin resistance and endothelial dysfunction. A potential role for cytokines originating from adipose tissue. *Arterioscler Thomb Vasc Biol* 1999; 19: 972–8.
121. Ceriello A, Taboga C, Tonutti L, Quagliaro L, Piconi L, Bais B, Da Ros R, Motz E. Evidence for an independent and cumulative effect of postprandial hypertriglyceridemia and hyperglycemia on endothelial dysfunction and oxidative stress. Effects of short-and long-term simvastatin therapy. *Circulation* 2002; 106: 1211–8.
122. Fuller JH, Shipley MJ, Rose G, Jarrett RJ, Keen H. Mortality from coronary heart disease and stroke in relation to degree of glycemia: the Whitehall Study. *Br Med J* 1983; 287: 867–70.
123. Khaw KT, Wareham N, Luben R, Bingham S, Oakes S, Welch A, Day N. Glycated haemoglobin, diabetes and mortality in men in Norfolk cohort of European prospective investigation of cancer and nutrition (EPIC-Norfolk). *Br Med J* 2001; 322: 15–8.
124. Stratton IM, Adler AL, Neil HA, Matthews DR, Manley SE, Cull CA, Hadden D, Turner RC, Holman RR. Association of glycaemia with macrovascular and microvascular complications of type 2 diabetes (UKPDS 35); Prospective observational study. *Br Med J* 2000; 321: 405–12.
125. Knowler WC, Sartor G, Melander A. Schersten B. Glucose tolerance and mortality, including a substudy of tolbutamide treatment. *Diabetologia* 1997; 40: 680–6.
126. Chiasson JL, Josse RG, Gomis R, Hanefeld M, Karasik A, Laakso M, for the STOP-NIDDM Trial Research Group. Acarbose treatment and the risk of cardiovascular disease and hypertension in patients with impaired glucose tolerance: the STOP-NIDDM trial. *J Am Med Assoc* 2003; 290: 486–94.
127. Antonucci T, Whitcomb R, McLain R, Lockwood D, Morris RM. Impaired glucose tolerance is normalised by treatment with the thiazolidiedione troglitazone. *Diabetes Care* 1997; 20: 188–93.
128. Grady D, Herrington D, Bittner V, Blumenthal R, Davidson M, Hlatky M, Hsia J, Hulley S, Herd A, Khan S, Newby LK, Waters D, Vittinghoff E, Wenger N, for the HERS Research Group. Cardiovascular disease outcomes during 6.8 years of hormone therapy: Heart and Estrogen/progestin Replacement Study follow-up (HERS 11). *J Am Med Assoc* 3002; 288: 49–57.
129. Rossouw JE, Anderson GL, Prentice RL, LaCroix AZ, Kooperberg C, Stefanick ML, Jackson RD, Beresford SA, Howard BV, Johnson KC, Kotchen JM, Ockene J, for the Writing Group for the Women's Health Initiative Investigators. Risks and benefits of estrogen plus progestin in healthy postmenopausal women: principal results from the Women's Health Initiative randomized controlled trial. *J Amer Med Assoc* 2002; 288: 321–33.
130. Dabelea D, Hanson RL, Bennett PH, Roumain J, Knowler WC, Pettitt DJ. Increasing prevalence of Type II diabetes in American Indian children. *Diabetologia* 1998; 41: 904–10.
131. Ehtisham S, Barrett TG, Shaw NJ. Type 2 diabetes mellitus in UK children: an emerging problem. *Diabet Med* 2000; 17: 867–71.
132. Sinha R, Fisch G, Teague B, Tamborlane WV, Banyas B, Allen K, Savoye M, Rieger V, Taksali S, Barbetta G, Sherwin RS, Caprio S. Prevalence of impaired glucose tolerance among children and adolescents with marked obesity. *N Engl J Med* 2002; 346: 802–10.
133. Invitti C, Guzzaloni G, Gilardini L, Morabito F, Viberti G. Prevalence and concomitants of glucose intolerance in European obese children and adolescents. *Diabetes Care* 2003; 26: 118–24.
134. Abraham EJ, Leech CA, Lin JC, Zulewski H, Habener JF. Insulinotrophic hormone glucagon-like peptide-1 differentiation of human pancreatic islet-derived progenitor cells into insulin-producing cells. *Endocrinology* 2002; 143: 152–61.
135. Xu G, Stoffers DA, Habener JF, Bonner-Weir S. Exendin-4 stimulates both beta-cell replication and neogenesis, resulting in increased beta-cell mass and improved glucose glucose tolerance in diabetic rats. *Diabetes* 1999; 48: 2270–6.
136. Tourrel C, Bailbe D, Meile MJ, Kergoat M, Portha B. Glucagon-like Peptide-1 (GLP-1) or exendin-4 treatment limited to the pre-diabetic period limits the progression to overt NIDDM in the adult GK rat. *Diabetes* 2001; 50 (suppl 2): A339.
137. Saydah SH, Byrd-Holt D, Harris MI. Projected impact of implementing the results of the Diabetes Prevention Program in the US population. *Diabetes Care* 2002; 25: 1940–45.
138. DPP Research Group. The cost-effectiveness of the DPP interventions to delay or prevent type 2 diabetes. *Diabetes* 2002; 51 (suppl 2): A74.
139. Palmer AJ, Roze S, Comte S, Cabrieres L. Cost-effectiveness of intense lifeste changes or metformin in overweight, glucose intolerant patients: modeling the long-term implications of the diabetes prevention program in the French, German and UK settings. *Diabetologia* 2002; 45 (suppl 2): A303.
140. Colagiuri S, Walker A. Type 2 diabetes screening and prevention—can we afford not to do? In *Proceedings of Australian Diabetes Society and Australian Diabetes Educators Association Annual Scientific Meeting*, Adelaide, 2002; p 179.
141. Lindstrom J, Tuomilehto J. The diabetes risk score: a practical tool to predict type 2 diabetes risk. *Diabetes Care* 2003; 26: 725–31.

Index